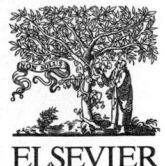
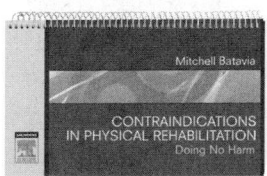
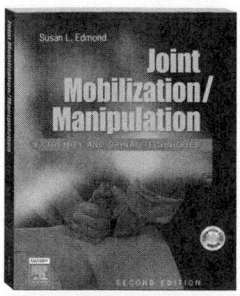
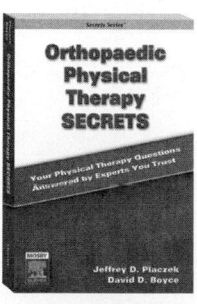
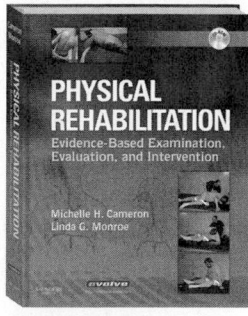

NEUROLOGICAL REHABILITATION

FIFTH EDITION

Darcy A. Umphred, PT, PhD, FAPTA
Professor Emeritus and Past Chair
Department of Physical Therapy
School of Pharmacy and Health Sciences
University of the Pacific
Stockton, California

WITH SECTION EDITORS:

Gordon U. Burton, PhD, OTR
Professor Emeritus
Department of Occupational Therapy
San Jose State University
San Jose, California

Rolando T. Lazaro, PT, DPT, MS, GCS
Assistant Professor
Department of Physical Therapy
Samuel Merritt College
Oakland, California

Margaret L. Roller, PT, MS, DPT
Associate Professor and Graduate Coordinator
Department of Physical Therapy
California State University, Northridge
Northridge, California
Clinical Instructor
NeuroCom International, Inc.
Clackamas, Oregon

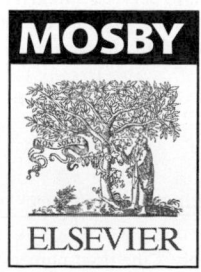

MOSBY

ELSEVIER

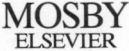

MOSBY
ELSEVIER

11830 Westline Industrial Drive
St. Louis, Missouri 63146

NEUROLOGICAL REHABILITATION,
FIFTH EDITION

ISBN-13: 978-0-323-03306-0
ISBN-10: 0-323-03306-7

Library of Congress Cataloging-in-Publication Data

Neurological rehabilitation / [edited by] Darcy Umphred ; with section editors, Gordon
   U. Burton, Rolando T. Lazaro, Margaret L. Roller.—5th ed.
       p. ; cm.
   Includes bibliographical references and index.
   ISBN-13: 978-0-323-03306-0 (hardback)
   ISBN-10: 0-323-03306-7 (hardback)
   1. Nervous system—Diseases—Physical therapy.   2. Nervous
system—Diseases—Patients—Rehabilitation.   I. Umphred, Darcy Ann.
   [DNLM: 1. Nervous System Diseases—rehabilitation. WL 140 N49265 2007]
   RC350.P48N487   2007
   616.8′0462—dc22
                                                                    2006050558

ISBN-13: 978-0-323-03306-0
ISBN-10: 0-323-03306-7

Publishing Director: Linda Duncan
Senior Editor: Kathy Falk
Senior Developmental Editor: Christie Hart
Publishing Services Manager: Patricia Tannian
Project Manager: Claire Kramer
Designer: Bill Drone

Printed in the United States of America

Last digit is the print number: 9   8   7   6   5   4

Dedicated: A sequential process of learning from the first to the fifth edition

to

Gordon, Jeb, Benjamin, and my mother, Janet, whose love, patience, and understanding constantly gave and have continued to give me strength.

to

All those special people whose insights, wisdom, guidance, and patience have helped to give the authors of these chapters their unique gifts and talents, as well as their willingness to share their thoughts with all of you.

to

Very dear friends, colleagues, and previous chapter authors who gave so much energy, dedication, and service, both as scholars and as practicing clinicians. Over the last 25 years, the book's family has changed, as has the evolution of the text. With great regret we have had to say good-bye to three authors, Mary Jane Bouska, Jane Schneider, and Laura Smith. The professions will miss all of you, but your gifts continue to make a difference.

to

Life, to each person's journey, and to all those who give opportunities for others' growth along that journey. Special thanks to my immediate family and all my friends and colleagues I hold so close to my heart. Because of all of you, my journey has been constantly renewed with love, warmth, and guidance. No one could feel wealthier than I.

to

Each day we are allowed to walk on this earth. Life is very precious, and how long we will be allowed to stay is an unknown. I have learned to appreciate this time and hope none of us become so busy that we forget its finiteness. Enjoy the journey and always find time to stop and appreciate who you are, what you are, and those gifts you have been given to share with the rest of us.

Contributors

Paula M. Ackerman, MS, OTR/L
Shepherd Center
SCI Day Program/OP Manager
Atlanta, Georgia

Janet Marie Adams, PT, MS, DPT
Professor
Department of Physical Therapy
California State University
Northridge, California
Licensed Kinesiological Electromyographer
Northridge, California

Leslie K. Allison, PhD, PT
Assistant Professor
East Carolina University
Greenville, North Carolina

Brent D. Anderson, PhD, PT, OCS
Adjunct Faculty
Department of Physical Therapy
University of Miami
Miami, Florida
Polestar Physical Therapy
Coral Gables, Florida

Joyce Ann, OTR/L, GCFP
Occupational Therapist, Guild Certified Feldenkrais
    Practitioner
Highland Park, Illinois

Myrtice B. Atrice, BS, PT
SCI Clinical Manager
Spinal Injury Program
Shepherd Center
Atlanta, Georgia

Sandra G. Bellamy, PT, DPT, PCS
Assistant Professor
Department of Physical Therapy
University of the Pacific
Stockton, California

Janet R. Bezner, PhD, PT
Senior Vice President
Division of Education
American Physical Therapy Association
Alexandria, Virginia

William G. Boissonnault, PT, DHSc, FAAOMPT
University of Wisconsin-Madison
Department of Orthopedics and Rehabilitation
Madison, Wisconsin

Jennifer M. Bottomley, PT, MS, PhD
Independent Geriatric Rehabilitation Consultant
Boston, Massachusetts

Annie Burke-Doe, PhD, MPT
Assistant Professor
California State University
Fresno, California

Gordon U. Burton, PhD, OTR
Professor Emeritus
Department of Occupational Therapy
San Jose State University
San Jose, California

Matthew N. Butler, DPT, CSCS
Physical Therapist and Fitness Trainer
Polestar Pilates Center
Coral Gables, Florida

Nancy N. Byl, PhD, PT, FAPTA
Professor and Chair, Department of Physical Therapy
    and Rehabilitation Science
School of Medicine
University of California
San Francisco, California

Beate Carrière, PT, CIFK
Certified Instructor Functional Kinetics
Private Practice
Hollywood, California

Laurie Ruth Chaikin, MS, OTR/L, OD
Wild Iris Optometric Group
Castro Valley, California
Guest Lecturer
Occupational Therapy Department
San Jose State University
San Jose, California

Carol M. Davis, PT, EdD, MS, FAPTA
Professor and Assistant Chair
Department of Physical Therapy
University of Miami Miller School of Medicine
Miami, Florida

Judith A. Dewane, MHS, PT, NCS
Faculty Associate
Physical Therapy Program
Department of Orthopedic Surgery
    and Rehabilitation Medicine
University of Wisconsin School of Medicine
    and Public Health
Madison, Wisconsin

Peter I. Edgelow, MA, PT
Assistant Clinical Professor
Graduate Program in Physical Therapy
University of California, San Francisco
San Francisco, California
Senior Physical Therapist
Physiotherapy Associates
Hayward, California

Barbara Edmison, PT
Center Coordinator of Clinical Education
Therapy Services Department
Santa Barbara Cottage Hospital
Santa Barbara, California

Donna El-Din, PT, PhD
Distinguished Professor Emerita
Eastern Washington University
Spokane, Washington

Robert A. Eskew, PT, MS, PCS
Pediatric Physical Therapist/ Pediatric Clinical Specialist
Mercy Health Center
Oklahoma City, Oklahoma
Vice Chair, Adolescents and Adults with Developmental
    Disabilities Special Interest Group Section on
    Pediatrics, American Physical Therapy Association

Teresa A. Foy, BS, OTR/L
Therapy Manager
SCI Program
Shepherd Center
Catastrophic Care Hospital
Atlanta, Georgia

Debra I. Frankel, MS, OTR
Senior Associate
Abt Associates Inc.
Cambridge, Massachusetts

Kenda Fuller, PT, NCS
Owner
South Valley Physical Therapy
Specialists in Neurologic Physical Therapy
Denver, Colorado

Mary Lou Galantino, PT, PhD, MSCE
Professor, Physical Therapy
Richard Stockton College of New Jersey
Pomona, New Jersey
Adjunct Research Scholar
University of Pennsylvania
Philadelphia, Pennsylvania

Rebecca M. Good, MA, RNC, ACRN, LPC, QTTT
Private Practice
Wholistic Counselor and Therapist
Therapeutic Touch Practitioner,
    Mentor, Teacher, Clinical Consultant, and Lecturer
Salt Lake City, Utah

Sharon L. Gorman, PT, MS, GCS
Assistant Professor
Samuel Merritt College
Oakland, California

Marcia Hall, PT, DPT, DSc-abd
Director of Clinical Education and Development
NeuroCom International, Inc.
Clackamas, Oregon

Ann Hallum, PhD
Dean of Graduate Studies
San Francisco State University
Professor
UCSF/SFSU Graduate Program in Physical Therapy
San Francisco, California

Osa Jackson Schulte, PhD, PT, GCFP/AT
Executive Director and Continuity Assistant Trainer
Feldenkrais Professional Training Program
Movement and Healing Center
Clarkson, Michigan
Contingent Physical Therapist
Community Care Services
Henry Ford Health System
Detroit, Michigan

Jeffery Kauffman, MD
Holistic Health Associate
Sacramento, California

Laurie Kenny, PT, OCS, FAAOMPT
Clinical Specialist
Occupational Health Department
Kaiser Permanente
Oakland, California

David M. Kietrys, PT, MS, OCS
Associate Professor
Developmental & Rehabilitative Sciences
University of Medicine and Dentistry of New
    Jersey–School of Health Related Professions
Stratford, New Jersey

Kristin J. Krosschell, PT, MA, PCS
Clinical Instructor
Department of Physical Therapy and
    Human Movement Sciences
Feinberg School of Medicine
Northwestern University
Chicago, Illinois

Rolando T. Lazaro, PT, DPT, MS, GCS
Assistant Professor
Department of Physical Therapy
Samuel Merritt College
Oakland, California

Rachel M. Lopez, MPT, NCS
Brain Injury Program Coordinator
Barrow Neurological Institute
St. Joseph's Hospital
Phoenix, Arizona

Marilyn MacKay-Lyons, PhD, PT
Associate Professor
School of Physiotherapy, Dalhousie University,
Halifax, Nova Scotia, Canada

Shari L. McDowell, PT
SCI Inpatient Program Manager
Shepherd Center
Atlanta, Georgia

Marsha E. Melnick, PT, PhD
Professor Emerita
San Francisco State University
Clinical Professor
University of California, San Francisco
UCSF/SFSU Graduate Program in Physical Therapy
San Francisco, California

Sarah A. Morrison, PT
Program Director of Spinal Cord Injury Services
Shepherd Center, Inc.
Atlanta, Georgia

Christine A. Nelson, PhD, OTR, FAOTA
Clinical Coordinator
Centro de Desarrollo
Cuernavaca, Morelos
Mexico

Mari Jo Pesavento, PT, PCS
Department of Pediatric Rehabilitation and Development
Advocate Christ Medical Center and
    Hope Children's Hospital
Oak Lawn, Illinois

Darbi Breath Philibert, MHS, LOTR
Assistant Professor
Clinic Coordinator of the Early Childhood Development
    Clinic
Early Intervention Institute of Louisiana State University
    Health Sciences Center
New Orleans, Louisiana

Rebecca E. Porter, PhD, PT
Executive Director of Enrollment Services &
Associate Vice Chancellor for Student Services
Indiana University Purdue University Indianapolis
Indianapolis, Indiana

Myla U. Quiben, DPT, PT, GCS, NCS
Faculty and Assistant Director of Clinical Education
Department of Physical Therapy
University of Central Arkansas
Conway, Arkansas

Walter Racette, CPO
Assistant Clinical Professor in Orthopedics;
Director
Orthotic and Prosthetic Centers at UCSF
San Francisco, California

Carol Ritberger, PhD
The Ritberger Institute for Esoteric Studies
Pollock Pines, California

Clinton Robinson, Jr.
8th Degree Tae Kwon Do Black Belt
Department of Physical Education
American River College
Sacramento, California

Margaret L. Roller, PT, MS, DPT
Associate Professor and Graduate Coordinator
Department of Physical Therapy
California State University, Northridge
Northridge, California
Clinical Instructor
NeuroCom International, Inc.
Clackamas, Oregon

Howell I. Runion, PA, MS, PhD
Emeritus Professor
Physiology & Pharmacology Dept.
T.J. Long School of Pharmacy
University of the Pacific
Stockton, California

Susan D. Ryerson, DSc, PT
Making Progress
Alexandria, Virginia
Research Scientist, Center for Applied Biomechanics and
    Rehabilitation Research
National Rehabilitation Hospital
Washington, District of Columbia

Dale L. Scalise-Smith, PhD, PT
Associate Professor and Director
Program in Physical Therapy
Utica College
Utica, New York

Claudia Senesac, PT, PhD, PCS
Lecturer
Department of Physical Therapy
University of Florida
Gainesville, Florida

Eunice Yu Chiu Shen, PT, DPT, MS, PCS
Regional Therapy Manager
California Children's Services
County of Los Angeles
Department of Health
El Monte, California

Timothy J. Smith, RPh, PhD
Department of Physiology and Pharmacology
Thomas J. Long School of Pharmacy and Health
    Sciences
University of the Pacific
Stockton, California

Corrie J. Stayner, MS, PT
Staff Physical Therapist
Barrow Neurological Institute
St. Joseph's Hospital
Phoenix, Arizona

James Stephens, PhD, PT, CFP
Physical Therapy Department
Temple University
Philadelphia, Pennsylvania

Bradley W. Stockert, PT, PhD
Professor
Department of Physical Therapy
California State University–Sacramento
Sacramento, California

Jane K. Sweeney, PhD, PT, PCS
Graduate Program Director
Doctoral Programs in Pediatrics
Rocky Mountain University of Health Professions
Provo, Utah

Stacey E. Szklut, MS, OTR/L
Executive Director South Shore Therapies, Inc.
National Lecturer
Weymouth, Massachusetts

Karla M. Tuzzolino, PT, NCS
Staff Physical Therapist
Barrow Neurological Institute
St. Joseph's Hospital
Phoenix, Arizona

Darcy A. Umphred, PT, PhD, FAPTA
Professor Emeritus and Past Chair
Department of Physical Therapy
School of Pharmacy and Health Sciences
University of the Pacific
Stockton, California

John Upledger, DO
Developer
Craniosacral Therapy
The Upledger Institute
Palm Beach Gardens, Florida

Richard Voss, DPC, MSW
Associate Professor
West Chester University
Department of Social Work
West Chester, Pennsylvania

John G. Wallace, Jr., PT, MS, OCS
President and CEO
BMS Reimbursement Management
Claremont, California

Therese Marie West, PhD, MT-BC, FAMI
Board-Certified Music Therapist & Fellow
    of the Association for Music and Imagery
Music Therapy Program Director
University of the Pacific
Stockton, California

Patricia A. Winkler, PT, DSc, NCS
Assistant Professor
Regis University
Private Practice
South Valley Physical Therapy
Denver, Colorado

Pat Winstead-Fry, RN, PhD
CAM Nursing Research
Pawlet, Vermont

George Wolfe, PT, PhD
Associate Professor
Department of Physical Therapy,
    California State University
Northridge, California

Preface

Each edition of this book brings new insights, new visions, and new avenues for therapists to advance their respective analytical and clinical skills when assisting individuals with neurological impairments to improve their quality of life. The explosion of new information within neuroscience and its effect on the evidence base of both evaluation and intervention strategies have modified and improved services to the many individuals seeking our expertise and will continue to do so. With this new knowledge, many individuals within the professions of physical and occupational therapy and other related health care disciplines will assist patients throughout the world to attain a level of life participation that they, as patients, define as quality of life. As the complex interactions of all systems slowly unravel their mysteries in front of the eyes and within the hands of practicing clinicians and researchers, the possibilities of new variables that affect outcomes will continue to arise and challenge the mind of the learner. Having a tether to basic neuroscience allows therapists of today and those of the future to stretch to limits and levels of understanding that boggle the rigid linear thinker of yesterday. With the explosion of new research over the last 5 years, this fifth edition has stretched our professions to the unknowns we might have considered the distant future a few years ago. These doors have led to integration of systems and help us discover what seem like unanswerable questions and continue to ground us to the evidence base of today's practice. This book mirrors a family dedicated to the advancement and quality of life of others. This book does not belong to the publisher, the editor, or even the chapter authors. We are just participants on life's journey and have come together to share what we have learned and to help future colleagues evolve further than we had at the same age. The book belongs to the learners, those students who are willing to question today's practice and look toward new and innovative ways to provide better and more effective patient care, to prevent loss of life participation, and to enhance the quality of life of all individuals who cross their paths.

Twenty-six years and four previous editions have passed since this book was conceived. In the evolution of a person, the attainment of 26 years usually signifies adulthood. Twenty-six years of evolution of this book has encompassed new visions; greater evidence base to practice within health care delivery; huge advancements in neuroscience and intervention strategies; and, without a doubt, many more questions. Mastery can never be obtained because new visions constantly suggest a new beginning, but mastery suggests knowledge and wisdom of the whole. The journey has led the reader from a book whose initial problem-solving focus was understanding medical diagnosis and science as it related to neurological problems to a book whose focus is placed on movement diagnosis and the ways to empower individuals in need of our services to the highest quality of life attainable. The evolution of the professions encompasses in-depth integration of movement science, a comprehension of disease/pathology, a high level of analysis and skill development in objective measurements of functional behavior, and intervention strategies based on best practice and evidence. During the last three decades, the therapeutic management of clients has undergone many stages of evolution. Evidence-based practice, which encompasses both effectiveness and efficacy through clinical studies and basic science research, should be guiding the choices of intervention procedures today. This shift in paradigm from specific treatment approaches to a problem-solving model that looks at the functional ability, activity limitations, and life participation of the client has led to a transformation of services throughout the world. As these problem-solving approaches become operational, more effective, reliable, and valid therapeutic examinations and management strategies are being presented in the literature. Yet, our understanding of how humans learn, relearn, or adapt is far from reaching closure. Neuroplasticity, once thought impossible, has become widely accepted as fact within the area of neurological rehabilitation. Given the many unknowns and the fact that what is "known" often changes daily, all learners are challenged to keep a mind open to change and to new learning while holding onto a flexible paradigm that allows for effective examination, evaluation, and treatment of clients within a dynamic, ever-changing environment. Client-centered care has shown that willing participation by the consumer of our services leads to the greatest potential outcomes and satisfaction of the client. No longer will therapy be done to the patient but instead will encompass and be enhanced by the family's and client's goals and expectations. Master clinicians of the past have always taken these patient goals into consideration, whether formally or informally. Thus their outcomes always exceeded others, and they never had problems with compliance.

Cost of services, managed care environments, limitations in visits, and practice patterns all create challenges to today's professionals. Young therapists are expected to graduate from school and immediately practice as experienced clinical problem solvers. Young colleagues think that they are expected to *know* the answers, not to discover them. Yet, within the clinical arena, problem-solving success is always dependent on one variable, and that variable is the patient. As long as the unique qualities of the patient are considered, a therapist will be able to select examination procedures and appropriate interventions using clinical reasoning. Graduates of today and tomorrow have the knowledge and skill and have practiced clinical problem-solving throughout their education. The only variables they will always need to add will be those unique characteristics of each patient.

This book is designed to provide the practitioner and advanced therapy student with a variety of problem-solving strategies that can be used to tailor treatment approaches to individual client needs and cognitive style. The treatment of persons with neurological disabilities requires an integrated approach involving therapies and treatment procedures used by physical, occupational, speech and language, music and recreational therapists; nurses; pharmacists; orthotists;

physicians; and a variety of other health care providers. Contributors to this book were selected for their expertise and integrated knowledge of various subject areas. The result is, I hope, a blend of state of the art information about the therapeutic management of persons with neurological disabilities.

This book is organized to provide the student with a comprehensive discussion of all aspects of neurological rehabilitation and to facilitate quick reference in a clinical situation. Section I, "Theoretical Foundations for Clinical Practice," constitutes an overview of foundational theories. This includes the entire diagnostic process used by movement specialists. The basis for this process ranges across many cognitive areas and theories, and thus concepts and integration are presented in a variety of chapters. Additional emphasis has been placed on both health and wellness, along with the visual analysis of functional movement development and change across the life span. To complete this foundational section, discussion ends with the need for reliable and valid documentation that should lead to reimbursement for services within various clinical environments. Section II, "Management of Clinical Problems," offers an in-depth discussion and analysis of the therapeutic management of the most common neurological disabilities encountered by physical and occupational therapists. A new chapter dealing with chronic movement problems over a lifetime incorporates the potential roles of therapists beyond acute or rehabilitation environments. Section III, "Neurological Disorders and Applications Issues," is devoted to recent advances in general approaches to intervention and rehabilitation that might affect any of the diagnostic categories discussed in Section II. The importance of other system problems, especially cardiopulmonary problems, has been emphasized to help the learner integrate the critical nature of an integrated systems model.

Special features within all three parts are examinations, evaluations, prognoses, and intervention strategies using sound clinical reasoning. Case studies are presented within each clinical-based chapter to help the reader with the problem-solving process.

During the conceptualization and preparation of all five editions, many individuals gave time, guidance, and emotional support. To all those individuals I extend my sincere appreciation. There are many people to thank in the preparation of this fifth edition: the authors, the researchers, the illustrators, each person assisting during the process of publication, and the patients. No person could have accomplished the end product alone. Yet, during the reediting process of this edition some specific individuals came to deserve special recognition and thanks:

The staff at Elsevier who worked on the publication of this edition: Christie M. Hart; Kathy Falk; Claire Kramer, most recently; and initially, Marion Waldman and Kathy Macciocca. Deep appreciation is given to all the teachers and healers who have crossed our paths in the last 35 years. They helped us to continually realize that before we can find answers, design research projects, and establish evidence-based practice, we must identify and acknowledge unknowns and formulate questions.

Each family member or significant other who encouraged and supported us from the moment we began the process to the day the book reached the learner.

My entire family, all of whom helped me make the time to complete this manuscript.

My two sons, Jeb and Ben, whose support I have had since the beginning of this book. Both are creative and brilliant young professionals in their own right yet have tirelessly helped me take very complex concepts and ideas and transformed them into illustrations that can be comprehended. As small children, during the book's conception, their tolerance far exceeded their age. As children, they allowed me to take pictures, many of which have been used to actualize the chapter on Movement Development across the Life Span. As young adults, their support and guidance always give me strength.

As a critical aspect of this edition, three section editors were asked to help guide and mold the book into what you have today. These three individuals will take the book into the future and help to establish its adulthood. Thus I extend a huge amount of gratitude, respect, and love to Gordon Burton, Rolando Lazaro, and Margaret Roller—three leaders, visionaries, and genuinely caring and loving individuals who have certainly made a significant impact on this edition and those to come.

Last, my husband, Gordon, who is the only one who truly knows what demands this book places on me and everyone around me. His support has never dwindled, nor his acceptance of my choices.

This book was conceived 26 years ago. It was presented in print to the world 21 years ago. Both dates signify young adulthood and the evolution from conception to a responsibility as an adult. We are all interconnected in a tapestry that has allowed this book to evolve into what it is today. For that, I give thanks as an author, as the editor, as a consumer, but most important as a learner. Our lives are finite, but the quality of those lives is extremely important to us and those around us. It is hoped that this book will guide colleagues to help consumers in attainment of that quality. It is hoped that with the eyes and minds of so many outstanding colleagues sharing their experiences and their desire to ground what they do into evidence-based practice, learners will embrace their adventure with the same vigor and enthusiasm that so many have in the past. For each of us the journey is today and the adventure tomorrow no matter how many tomorrows we may have. May all of you have the joy, the challenge, the excitement, and the learning adventure I have had throughout my professional career.

Darcy A. Umphred

Contents

CHAPTER 1

Theoretical Foundations for Clinical Practice

Darcy A. Umphred, PT, PhD, FAPTA
Donna El-Din, PT, PhD

KEY WORDS

clinical problem solving, diagnostic model:
    examination, evaluation, diagnosis, prognosis,
    intervention
disablement/enablement model
empowerment
holistic model for health care delivery
learning environment
systems model
visual-analytical problem solving (VAPS)

OBJECTIVES

After reading this chapter the student/therapist will be able to:
1. Comprehend the concepts of an interlocking systems model.
2. Analyze the diagnostic process using a disablement and an enablement model of bodily system problems/limitations in functional activities and disabilities or loss in the ability to participate in life.
3. Analyze the entire diagnostic process used by movement specialists including evaluation, diagnosis, prognosis, intervention, and documentation.
4. Relate each component of a systems model, including cognitive, affective, and motor subsections and how it influences function and dysfunction of the central nervous system.
5. Discuss the importance of the clinical triad and how each aspect of the triad affects the way the therapist interacts with the client and the environment.
6. Identify how the components of the clinical learning environment affect clinical practice.

Although a physical therapist (PT), occupational therapist (OT), or other health care professional may focus on a specific area of central nervous system (CNS) processing, a thorough understanding of the client as a total human being is critical for high-level professional performance. With the use of a problem-solving clinical diagnosis, prognosis approach, this book orients the student and clinician to the roles multiple systems within and outside the human body play in the causation, progression, and recovery process within a variety of common neurological problems. A secondary objective is the development of a theoretical framework that uses techniques for enhancing functional movement, enlarging the client's repertoire for movement alternatives and creating an environment for empowering the client to the highest level of functional activities and quality of life.

Evaluation, prognosis, and intervention methods incorporate all aspects of the client's nervous system and the influences of the external environment on those systems. The role of specific disciplines has not been defined. In the area of neurological disabilities, the overlap of basic knowledge and practical application of intervention techniques is so great that delineation of professional roles is often an administrative decision and billing practice. Selection of intervention strategies that have been demonstrated as evidence based is the focus of each chapter, yet approaches that have become or are in the process of becoming a common standard of intervention are included.

A clinical problem-solving approach is used because it is logical and adaptable, and it has been recommended by many professional during the past 30 years.[1-7] The concept of clinical decision making based in problem-solving theory has been stressed throughout the literature over the past decades and has guided the therapist toward an evidence-based approach. This approach clearly identifies the therapist's responsibility to examine, evaluate, analyze, draw conclusions, and make decisions regarding prognosis and treatment alternatives.[8-24]

Section I lays the foundation of knowledge necessary to understand and implement a problem-oriented approach to clinical care across the span of the human life. The basic knowledge of the human body is constantly expanding and often changing in content, theory, and clinical focus. Section I reflects that change in both philosophy and scientific research. The roles therapists are playing and will be asked to play in the future are changing.[25-27] Therapists have become experts in normal human movement across that life span (Chapter 2) and how that movement is changed after life events and disease or pathological conditions. Therapists have realized that health and wellness play a critical role in movement function as a client enters the health care system with neurological disease or condition (Chapter 6). Clients are now able to use direct access, which requires therapists to use differential diagnosis of disease and pathological conditions to make appropriate referrals (see Chapter 7) as well as make a differential diagnosis regarding movement dysfunctions within that therapist's respective scope of practice (see Chapter 8). Section I has been designed to weave together the issues of evaluation and treatment with other components of CNS function to consider the holistic approach to each client's needs (see Chapters 4, 5, and 9). This section delineates the conceptual areas that permit the reader to synthesize all aspects of the problem-solving process in the care of a client. Basic to the outcomes of care is accurate documentation of that process as well as the administration and reimbursement for that process (see Chapter 10).

Section II deals with specific clinical problems, beginning with pediatrics, progressing through adult problems and ending with aging with dignity and chronic impairments. In Section II each author follows the same problem-solving format to enable the reader either to focus more easily on one specific neurological problem or to address the problem from a larger perspective. Authors vary in their use of specific cognitive strategies or methods of addressing a specific neurological deficit. A variety of strategies for examining clinical problems are presented to facilitate the reader's ability to identify variations in problem-solving methods. Clinicians tend to adapt learning devices to solve specific problems, and many of the strategies used by one author may apply to situations presented by other authors. Readers are encouraged to use flexibility in selecting treatments with which they feel comfortable and to be creative when implementing any scheme.[16]

Changes in examination and evaluation methods are reflected in many of the clinical problem chapters. Identification of objective measurement tools, as well as a shift from a medical (disease/disorder) to an impairment/function/life participation with an empowerment focus as a critical aspect of the diagnostic process, is reflected in all clinical problem chapters. Change is inevitable and a problem-solving philosophy must reflect those changes.

Section III of the text focuses on clinical topics that might be appropriate for any one of the clinical problems discussed in Section II. Chapters have been added to reflect changes in the focus of therapy as it evolves as an emerging flexible paradigm with a multiple system approach. A specific system such as cardiopulmonary (see Chapter 35) or interactive responses of an intervention to multiply systems (see Chapter 37) are also presented as part of Section III. These changes incorporate not only the interactions of professional disciplines within the Western medical allopathic model of health care delivery but also additional delivery approaches including cultural and ethnic belief systems, family structure, and quality of life issues.

Evaluation tools presented throughout the text should help the reader identify many objective measurement scales. The reader is reminded that, although a tool may be discussed in one chapter, its use may have application to many other clinical problems. The same is true of treatment suggestions and problem-solving strategies used to analyze motor control problems.

CHANGING WORLD OF HEALTH CARE

For an understanding of how and why disablement and then enablement models have become the accepted models used by PTs and OTs when evaluating, diagnosing, deciding a prognosis, and treating clients with functional limitations resulting from neurological problems, it is important for the reader to review the evolution of health care within our culture. This review begins with the allopathic medical model because this model has been the dominant model of health care in Western society.[28] It forms the conceptual basis for health care in industrialized countries in the Western hemisphere. The model assumes that illness has an organic base that can be traced to discrete molecular elements. The origin of disease is found at the molecular level of the individual's tissue. The first step toward alleviating the disease is to identify the pathogen that has invaded the tissue and, after proper identification, apply appropriate treatment techniques.

It is implicit in the model that specialists who are professionally competent have the sole responsibility for the identification of the cause of the illness and for the judgment as to what constitutes appropriate treatment. The medical knowledge required for these judgments is thought to be the domain of the professional medical specialists and therefore inaccessible to the public. Yet PTs and OTs have never been responsible for the treatment of diseases or pathological conditions with which a specific client presents. Instead, we have always focused on the body system impairments resulting in activity limitations and inability to participate in life that have been caused by the specific disease or pathological condition. Simultaneously, we have also had to analyze the interactions of all other systems and how they compensated for or were affected by the original medical problem. As our roles within Western health care delivery have become clearer, so has the role of the consumer.

Levin[29] points out that there is a lot that consumers can do for themselves. Most people can assume responsibility to care for minor health problems. The use of nonpharmaceutical methods (e.g., hypnosis, biofeedback, meditation, and acupuncture) to control pain is becoming common. The recognition of the value of approaching illnesses with a holistic approach is receiving increasing attention in society. Treatment of emotional needs and physical needs during illness has been advocated as a way to help individuals regain some control over their lives (see Chapters 4 and 5).

A holistic model of health care seeks to involve the patient in the process and take the mystery out of health care for the consumer. Successful outcome measures are shifting from the traditional measure of whether the person lives or dies as the outcome indicator of success in health care to the quality of a person's life and his or her ability to participate in life. The use of the phrase "quality of life" or living implies more than physical health. It implies that the individual is mentally and emotionally healthy as well. It is a holistic (*holos,* from the Greek, meaning "whole") model of health care that takes the other dimensions of a person's being into consideration regarding health. Hippocrates emphasized treatment of the person as a whole. He also emphasized the influence of society and of the environment on health.

A holistic approach to health care acknowledges that multiple factors are operating in disease, trauma, and aging and that there are many interactions among the factors. Social, emotional, environmental, political, economic, psychological, and cultural factors are all acknowledged to influence health and the individual's potential to maintain health, to regain health after insult, or to maintain a quality of health in spite of existing disease or illness. An approach that takes this perspective centers its philosophy on the individual.[30] The individual with this orientation is less likely to have the physician look only for the chemical basis of his or her difficulty and ignore the psychological factors that may be present. Similarly, the importance of focusing on an individual's strengths while helping to eliminate system impairments and functional limitations in spite of existing disease or pathological conditions plays a critical role in this holistic model. Thus, the roles the PT and OT will play in the future of health care delivery will expand.

The health care delivery system in Western society has to serve all of the citizens. Given the variety of economic, political, cultural, and religious forces at work in American society, education of the people in regard to their health care is probably the only method that can work in the long run. With the limitations placed on delivery, the client's responsibility to health and healing is continuing to increase. The future task of PTs and OTs will be to cultivate people's sense of responsibility toward their own health and that of the community. The consumer has to be given and play a critical role in the decision-making process within the entire health care delivery model to more thoroughly guarantee compliance and optimal outcomes.[31-33] Education is an effective and vital approach to client management with perhaps the most potential to move us toward a concept of preventive care.

In-depth Analysis of the Holistic Model

Carlson[34] thinks that pressure to change to holistic thinking in medicine continues as a result of a societal change in its perspective of the rights of individuals. A concern to keep the individual central in the care process will continue to grow in response to continued technological growth that threatens to dehumanize care even more. The holistic model takes into account each person's unique psychosocial, political, economic, environmental, and spiritual needs as they affect the individual's health.

The nation faces significant social change in the area of health care. The coming years will change the access to health care for our citizens, the benefits, the reimbursement process for providers, and the delivery system. Health care providers have a major role in the success of the final product. The Pew Health Professions Commission[35] identified issues that must be addressed as any new system is developed, implemented, and addressed. Most, if not all, of the issues involve close interactions of the provider and client. These issues include (1) the need of the provider to stay in step with client needs; (2) the need for flexible educational structures to address a system that reassigns certain responsibilities to other personnel; (3) the need to redirect national funding priorities away from narrow, pure research access to include broader concepts of health care; (4) the licensing of health care providers; (5) the need to address the issues of minority groups; (6) the need to emphasize general care and at the same time educate specialists; (7) the issue of promoting teamwork; and (8) the need to emphasize the community as the focus of health care. There are other important issues, but the last to be included here is mentioned in more detail because of its relevance to the consumer.

The Pew Commission[35] concludes that the public has not been educated about the health care work force and the consumer's role in it. Without the consumer's understanding during development of a new system, the system could omit several opportunities for enrichment of design. Without the understanding of the consumer during implementation of a new system, the consumer might block delivery systems because of lack of knowledge. Thus, the delivery of service must be client centered and client/family driven and the focus of intervention needs to be in alignment with client objectives and desired outcomes.[30-33,36,37]

All the information about health care reform conveys with certainty the role of the client as the center of the focus of care. The client will assume greater involvement, greater responsibility, and greater control of the personal care process.

Providers will be more willing to include the client, will design care for the client, and will be better able to educate the client, address the issues of minority clients, and become proactive team caregivers. The influence of such methods will extend to the community and lead to greater patient/client satisfaction. Similarly, this direction will open to the consumer new direct access to providers within many health care delivery professions. The potential for occupational and physical therapy to become a primary provider of health care in the twenty-first century is becoming a reality within the military system as well as in some large health maintenance organizations. The role a therapist in the future will play as that primary provider will depend on that clinician's ability to screen for disease and pathological condition, examine and evaluate clinical signs that will lead to diagnoses and prognosis, and select appropriate interventions that will lead to the most efficacious, cost-effective treatment.

Client-centered care is a reality. As visionaries we will find new ways of sharing information with our client; computers will aid in this effort. The provider will set functional outcomes and work to accomplish performance goals. More people will be involved in the care process, and the process will extend on a continuum from acute care through the home setting. The provider must continue to enhance health care on a daily basis for each client. The case can be made that the most powerful tool for successful outcome is education.

Neurological rehabilitation is and will continue to take place in a changing environment and with a changing delivery system. The balance between visionary and pragmatist must be maintained. By the end of the twenty-first century, neurological rehabilitation will take place within a very different system and the client will be the center of the dynamic exchange of wellness, disease, function, and empowerment.

THERAPEUTIC MODEL OF HEALTH CARE DELIVERY

Traditional Therapeutic Models

Keen observers of human movement and how distortions or limitations of movement altered functional control developed models of therapeutic interventions. These models include Ayers, Bobath, Brunnstrom, Feldenkrais, Klein-Vogelback, Knott and Voss, and Rood approaches. These were the first behaviorally based models introduced within the health care delivery system, and they have been used by practitioners within the professions of physical and occupational therapy. These individuals, as master clinicians, tried to explain what they were doing and why their respective approaches worked using the science of the time. From their teachings, various philosophical models evolved. These models were isolated models of therapeutic intervention that were based on successful treatment procedures as identified through observation and described and demonstrated by the teachers of those approaches. The general model of health care under which these approaches were used was the allopathic model of Western medicine, which begins with disease and pathology. Today, our models must begin with health and wellness, with an understanding of variables that lead a client into the health care delivery system.

During the past decades, both short-term and full-semester courses, as well as literature related to treatment of clients with CNS dysfunction, have been divided into units labeled according to these techniques. Often, interrelation and integration among techniques were not explored. Clinicians bound to one specific treatment approach without the theoretical understanding of its step-by-step process may have lacked the base for a change of direction of intervention when a treatment was ineffective. It was difficult, therefore, to adapt alternative treatment techniques to meet the individual needs of clients. As a result, clinical problem solving was impeded, if not stopped, when one approach failed, because little integration of theories and methods of other approaches was ever stressed in the learning process. Similarly, because of a specific treatment having a potential effect on multiple systems and that treatment's specific interaction with the unique characteristics of the client's clinical problem, establishing efficacy using a Western research reductionistic model became extremely difficult. This does not negate the potential usefulness of any treatment intervention, but it does create a dilemma regarding efficacy of practice. Similarly, the rationale used to explain these therapeutic models was based on an understanding of the nervous system as described in the 1950s. That understanding has dramatically changed. With the basic neurophysiological rationale for explaining these approaches under fire for validity and the inability to demonstrate efficacy of these

approaches using traditional research methods, many of these treatment approaches are no longer introduced to the student during academic training. Yet, if these master clinicians were much more effective than their clinical counterparts, then the contrived therapeutic nature of their interventions may still be valid in certain clinical situations, but the neurophysiological explanation for the intervention may be very different. Similarly, to make statements today saying that these masters did not use theories of motor learning or motor control while motor learning was demonstrated by their clients seems contradictory. What can be said is that the practitioners, whether they were novices or masters, did not have knowledge of current theories. Although the verbal understanding of these behavior sequences to motor learning did not exist, they were often demonstrated by the client, thus directing the treatment and the successful intervention as described by masters.

Health Care Models

As clinicians, *especially PTs and OTs,* have moved toward establishment of models based on the functional needs of the client and the outcomes of the care process, more generic conceptualizations were created that were based on the interactions of multiple systems within the human body.

This systems model easily integrates into behavioral models for evaluation, diagnosis, prognosis, and intervention of physical disabilities. Today, the models are often considered *disablement models* as presented by Nagi[38,39] and the World Health Organization[40] (Table 1-1). As therapeutic emphasis has shifted away from a medical model to first a disablement[40] and then to an enablement model,[41] the primary focus of evaluation, prognosis, and intervention is on the impairment (systems interaction) and how those system interactions affect functional outcomes (Figure 1-1). Whether the functional limitations and strengths lead to a disability or to adaptation and adjustment will determine the eventual quality of life and empowerment that an individual will have over his or her life. Within each component of the disablement or enablement paradigm, risk factors occur that can be environmental,[42] psychosocial, or CNS related. These risk factors can positively or negatively affect the process and eventual outcome. Although therapists today are familiar with disablement models, other practitioners or providers of health services may not have the same depth of understanding. For that reason, PTs and OTs need to know how to communicate their models of practice to others who use

TABLE 1-1 ■ Disablement/Enablement Models Widely Accepted Throughout the World

IDENTIFIED MODEL	MEDICAL CONDITION	SUBSYSTEM CATEGORY	ACTIVITIES OF DAILY LIVING	SOCIAL LEVEL OF FUNCTION
World Health Organization (WHO) Disablement Model: *ICIDH* (1980)[40]	Disease/condition	Impairments	Disabilities	Handicaps
Nagi Disablement Model (1991)[39]	Disease/condition	Impairments	Functional limitations	Disabilities
World Health Organization Enablement Model: *ICF* (2001)[41]	Health condition	Body functions and structure	Activities	Participation or enablement

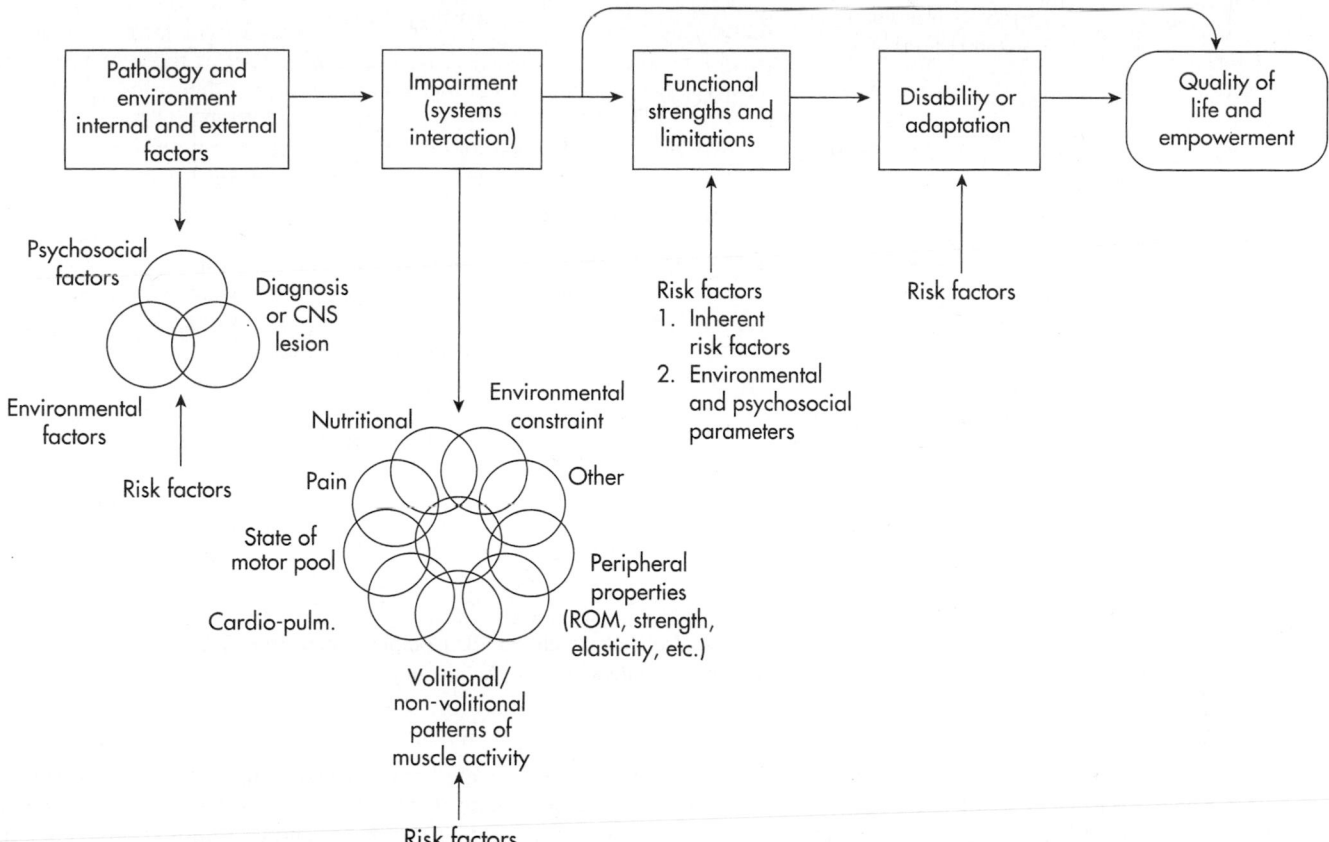

FIGURE 1-1 ■ Behavioral model for evaluation and treatment based on a disablement schema. *ROM,* Range of motion.

different frameworks when drawing conclusions regarding patient needs.

Within the current health care delivery system, three conceptual frameworks for client/provider interactions are commonly used. Each framework serves a different purpose and is used accordingly to the goals of the desired outcome and the group interpreting the results (Figure 1-2). The three primary models include (1) the statistical model, (2) the medical diagnostic model, and (3) the behavioral/disablement model. A fourth possibility may still be found using a philosophical or belief model such as those described by master clinicians from the past such as the Rood, Knott, Bobath, Ayers, or homeopathic models such as acupuncture or Chinese medicine. These philosophical models when applied to functional outcomes would be included with today's disablement model and incorporate a systems approach.

In today's health care arena, the PT and OT must make certain critical decisions before beginning service. With the limitations of visits and the extent of the clinical problems often contradictory, a therapist must determine how best to meet the needs of the patient given the environment of service. Similarly, the efficacy of any intervention may be questioned by anyone, including the client, the family, the physician, the third-party payer, or the lawyer. Thus, outcome tools that clearly measure the prognosis need to be carefully considered. Before selection of an appropriate evaluation tool, the specific purpose for the request for evaluation and the model by which to interpret the meaning of

the data must be identified. Regardless of the tool selected, third-party payers are concerned with the statistics obtained through the assessment. If the therapist scores a number 12 one week and a number 14 the next, and the payer knows a score of 16 means the individual's chance of falling is near normal, then the payer often permits additional visits. Those payers have little interest in the reasons why the client moved from a score of 12 to 14, only that the person is improving. This model is based on number crunching or gross quantitative measurements and relates closely to a statistical model. If today's clinicians do not provide these types of quantitative measurements, payment for services often is denied.

Physicians are educated to use a medical disease/pathological condition diagnostic model for setting expectations of improvement or lack thereof. In patients with neurological dysfunction, physicians generally formulate their medical diagnosis on the basis of complex, highly technical examinations such as magnetic resonance imaging, functional magnetic resonance imaging, computed tomography, positive emission transaxial tomography, evoked potentials, and laboratory studies. When abnormal results are correlated with gross clinical signs and patient history such as high blood pressure, diabetes, or head trauma, a medical diagnosis is made along with an anticipated course of recovery or disease progression. This medical diagnostic model is based on an anatomical and physiological belief of how the brain functions and may or may not correlate with the behavioral/disablement/enablement model used by therapists.

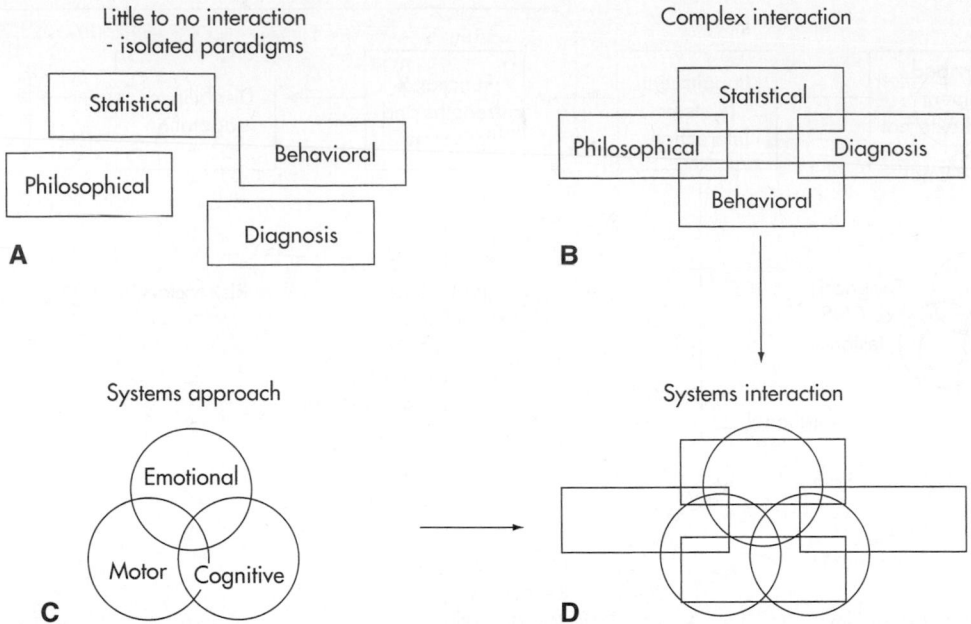

FIGURE 1-2 ■ Types of clinical models. **A,** Isolated paradigms. **B,** Complex interactive paradigms. **C,** Systems approach/paradigm. **D,** Systems interaction on traditional paradigms.

A behavioral/disablement/enablement model evaluates motor performance on the basis of two types of measurement scales. One type of scale measures functional activities, which range from simple movement patterns such as rolling to complex patterns such as dressing, playing tennis, or using a word processor. These tools would be considered disability/enablement measurements depending on the focus of the examination. Disablement focuses first on what the client cannot do, whereas enablement focuses first on those functional activities the patient can do. Both models stress the whole of the client's functional abilities in relation to his or her goals and environmental potential. Both use measurement tools that look at specific components of various systems and measures impairments within those respective areas or bodily systems. For example, if the system to be assessed was biomechanical, a simple tool such as a goniometer that measures joint range of motion might be used, whereas a complex motion analysis tool might be used to look at interactions of all joints during a specific movement. These types of measurements specifically look at impairments. Chapter 8 has been designed to help the reader clearly differentiate these measurement tools and how they might be used in the diagnosis, prognosis, and selection of intervention strategies.

All previously presented models can stand alone as acceptable models for health care delivery (see Figure 1-2, *A*) or can interact or interconnect (see Figure 1-2, *B*). These interconnections should validate the accuracy of the data derived from each model. The concept of an integrated problem-solving model using the systems within the CNS does not depend on any one of the previously mentioned models and does identify the components within the CNS (see Figure 1-2, *C*).

A model that identifies the three general neurological systems found within the human nervous system can be incorporated into each of the other models separately or when they are interconnected (see Figure 1-2, *D*). A systems/behavioral model that focuses on the neurological systems is much more than just motor and its motor components, or cognition with its multiple cortical facets, or the affective/emotion limbic system with all its aspects. The complexity of a neurological systems model (Figure 1-3), whether used for statistics, for medical diagnosis, for behavioral/functional diagnosis, or for documentation/billing, cannot be oversimplified. As the knowledge bank of central and peripheral system function increases, as well as knowledge about their interactions with other functions within and outside the body, the complexity of a systems model also enlarges. The reader must remember that each component within the nervous system has many interlocking subcomponents and that each of those components can be evaluated separately. Each component has many parts, and each of those parts could be assessed quantitatively. Those quantitative and qualitative measurements related to specific areas of function are the guidelines therapists use to establish problem lists and intervention sequences. Those small yet critical components, *considered impairments,* are of little concern within a general statistics model and may have little bearing on the medical diagnosis made by the physician.

In addition to the Western health care delivery paradigms are the interlocking roles identified within an evolving transdisciplinary model (Figure 1-4). Within this model, the environments experienced by the client both within the Western health care delivery system and those environments external to that system are interlocking and forming additional system components; they influence each other and affect the ultimate outcome demonstrated by the client. Because all these once-separate worlds encroach on or overlay each other and ultimately affect the client, practitioners are now operating in a holistic environment and must become open to alternative ways of practice. Some of those alternatives will fit neatly and comfortably with Western medical phi-

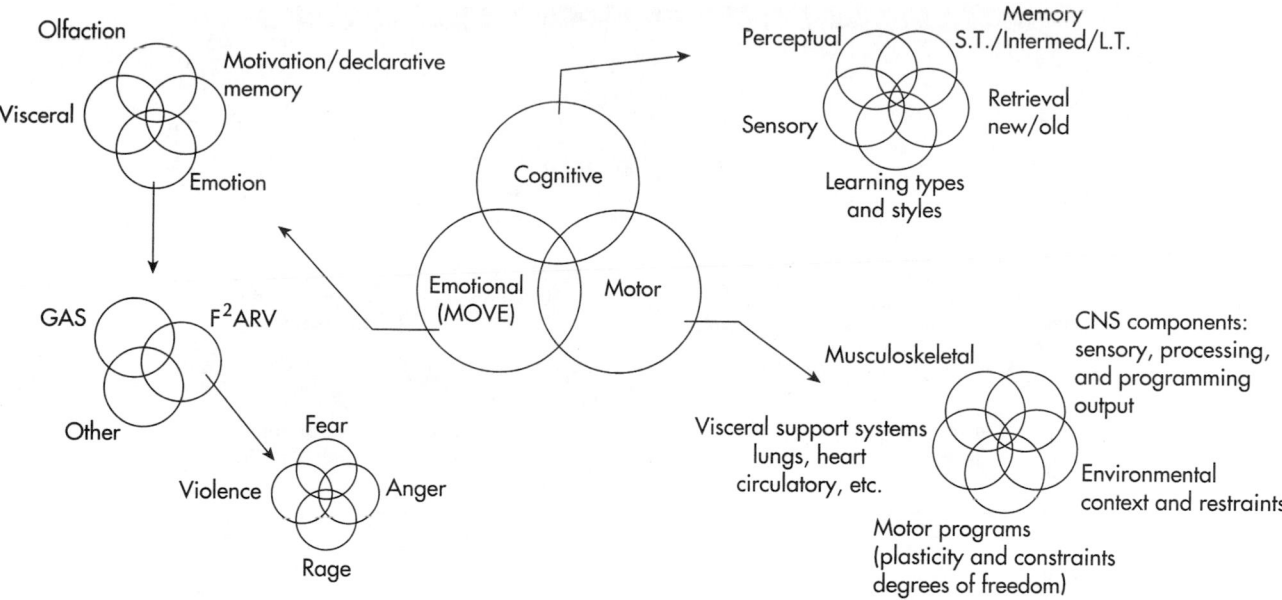

FIGURE 1-3 ■ Systems model: dynamic interactive subcomponents: whole to part to whole. *S.T.,* Short term; *L.T.,* long term; *GAS,* general adaptation syndrome; *F²ARV,* fear/frustration, anger, rage, violence.

EVOLVING TRANSDISCIPLINARY
Look at PT/OT/others

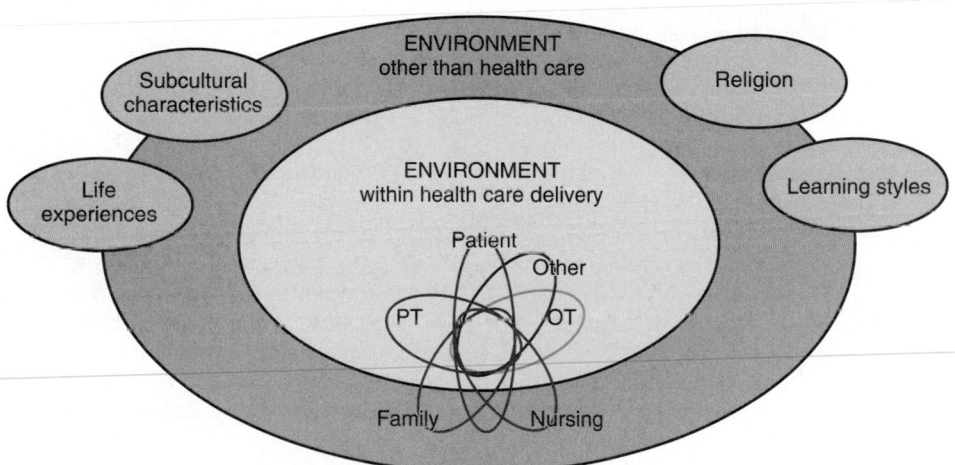

FIGURE 1-4 ■ Transdisciplinary model for delivery paradigms.

losophy and be seen as complementary. Others may be seen in sharp contrast, with conflicts seen as insurmountable. Until approaches have gone beyond belief of their effects, therapists will always need to expend additional focus measuring quantitative outcomes and analyzing accurately functional responses. Because the research is not available does not mean the approach has no efficacy. It may be that the complexity of the tools needed to measure the therapeutic interactions are not yet available. Thus, the clinician needs to learn to be totally honest with outcomes, and the importance of quality of care and quality of life remains the primary objective for patient management. Today, models that incorporate health and wellness have been added to these disablement/enablement models to delineate the complexity of the problem-solving process used by therapists.

This delineation should reflect accurate behavioral diagnoses based on functional limitations and strengths, preexisting system strengths and accommodations, and environmental-social-ethnic variables unique to the client. Similarly, it includes the family, caregiver, financial security, or health care delivery support systems. All these variables guide the direction of intervention[43] (Figure 1-5). These variables will affect behavioral outcomes and need to be identified through the examination/evaluation process. Many of these variables may not relate to the CNS disease/pathological condition medical diagnosis to which the patient has been assigned. The client brings to this environment life experiences. Many of these life events may have just been a life experience, others may have caused slight adjustments to behavior (e.g., running into a tree while

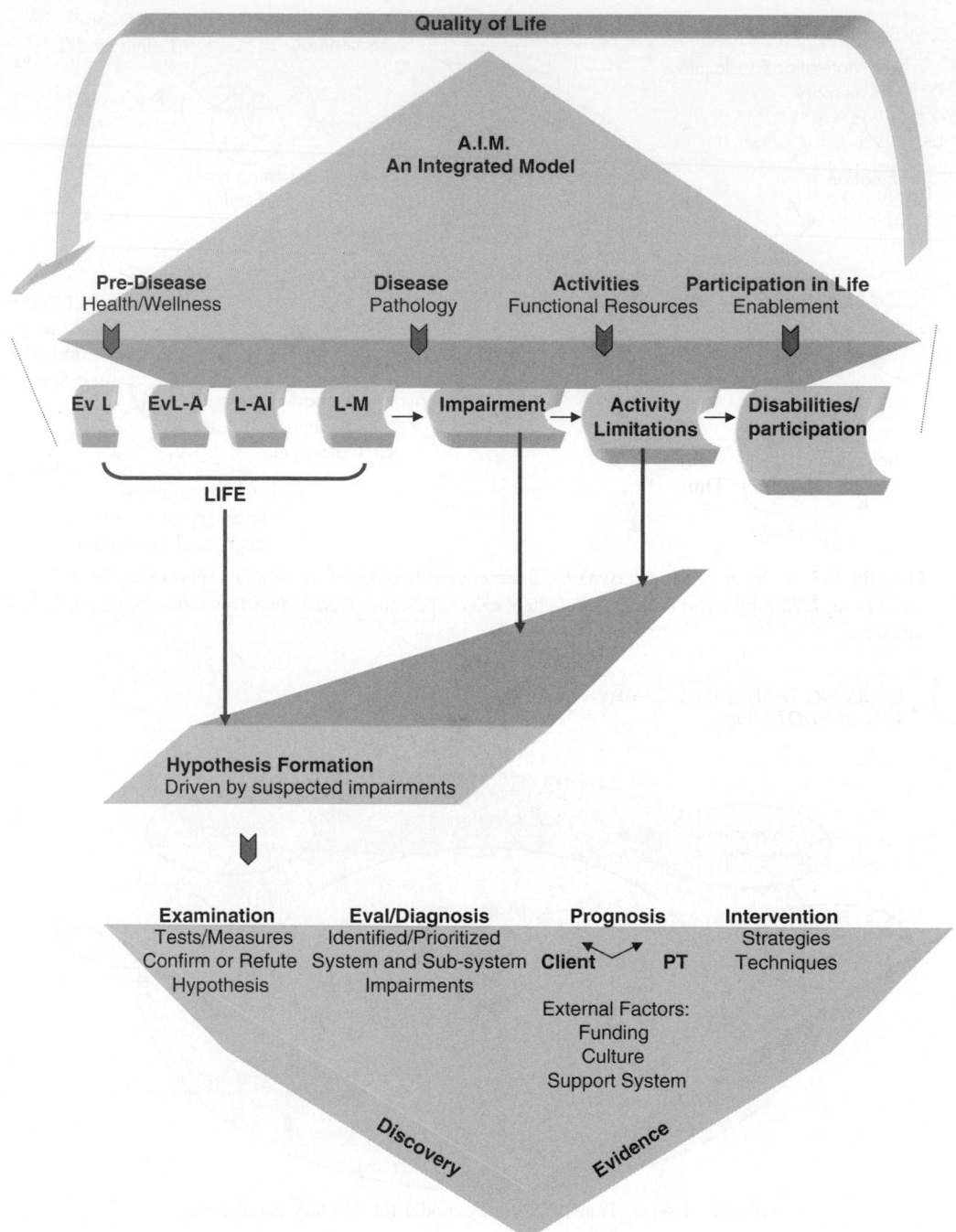

FIGURE 1-5 ■ Clinical problem-solving process incorporating life events, pathological condition, and postdisease state into a functional diagnosis. *L,* Life; *Ev,* event, disease; *L-A,* life with adaptation; *I,* identifiable impairment; *L-M,* life with modifications.

skiing out of patrolled downhill ski areas and then never doing it again), some may have caused limitations (e.g., after running into the tree, the left knee needed a brace to support the instability of that knee during any strenuous exercising), or caused adjustments in motor behavior and emotional safety before that individual enters into the heath care delivery system after CNS problems occur. The accommodations or adjustments can dramatically affect both positively and negatively the course of intervention. To quickly accumu-

late this type of information regarding a client, the therapist must become open to the needs of the client and family. This openness is not just sensory, using eyes and ears, but holistic and includes a bond that needs and should develop during therapy (see Chapter 4).

EFFICACY

When any model of health care delivery is considered, the question the therapist must ask is, which model will provide the most efficacious care? Therapists may not diagnose a pathological disease or its process, but they are in a position of responsibility to determine appropriate interventions for functional movement problems, including referral. Choosing interventions only because they are acceptable within a critical pathway of recovery after an identified neurological insult may not be questioned but also may not match the needs of the particular client.

Health care today demands that the therapeutic health care model be efficient and cost-effective and result in measurable outcomes. The message being given today might be considered to reflect the idea that the "end justifies the means." This hypothesis has come to fruition through the linear thought process of established scientific research. Yet, when a holistic model is accepted, it becomes apparent that the tools are not yet available to simultaneously measure the interactions of all systems and all models that purport to balance quality and cost of care. Thus, we must guard against the reductionistic research of today that has the potential to restrain our evolution and choice of therapeutic interventions. Therapeutic discovery usually precedes validation through scientific research and leads the way to, first, effective interventions, followed by efficacious care. If research and efficacious care always have to come before the application of therapeutic procedures, nothing new will evolve because discovery of care is most often, if not always, found in the clinic during interaction with a client. Thus the range of therapeutic applications will become severely limited and the evolution of neurological care stopped if that discovery is ignored because there is no efficacy as defined by today's research models.

Evidence-based practice is basic to the care process.[44-47] Clinicians need to identify which of their therapeutic interventions have demonstrated positive outcomes and which have not. Those that remain in question may still be judged as useful. The basis for that judgment may be a client satisfaction variable that is not measurable with today's research tools. For example, when a neurosurgeon recently asked the question of a therapist, "Do you know how to prove the theories of intervention you are teaching?" The answer was, "Yes, all I need is two dynamic positive-emission transaxial tomography units that can be worn on both the client's and the therapist's heads while performing therapeutic interventions. I also need a computer that will correlate simultaneously all synaptic interactions between the therapist and the client to prove the therapeutic effect." The physician said, "We don't have those tools!" The response was, "You did not ask me if the research tools were available, only if I know how to obtain an efficacious result." Thus, the creativity of the therapist will always bring the professions to new visions of reality. That reality, when proven to be efficacious, assists in validating the accepted interventions used by the professional. The therapist today has a responsibility to provide evidence-based practice to the scientific community . . . but more important, also to the client.

DIAGNOSIS: A PROCESS USED BY ALL PROFESSIONALS WHEN DRAWING CONCLUSIONS

Diagnosis is a conclusion drawn regarding specific diseases and pathological processes within the human body; when made by a physician it is considered a medical diagnosis.

Diagnosis made by a physical or occupational therapist is a conclusion drawn regarding functional movements and their interaction with life activities. Specific functional limitations and the bodily system impairments that affect the client's ability to control quiet or dynamic movement in any activity become a focus in the diagnostic process. The functional loss itself may or may not reflect specific diseases or pathological conditions within the CNS but does reflect specific impairments within that client's body. PTs and OTs, by use of functional behavioral models, are becoming comfortable with the term *functional diagnosis* and the conceptual understanding that the diagnosis made by a therapist is very different from that made by a physician. For the past 40 years, therapists have been receiving referrals from other health care practitioners stating "evaluate and treat." In the domain of neurological rehabilitation, similar referral patterns have been identified and physicians have made most of those referrals.[48] The process of evaluation includes both selection and administration of examination procedures, as well as interpreting those results. Once the interpretation has been made, a therapist must draw conclusions regarding those results and their interactions. That interpretation leads to the functional diagnosis. The interpretation of the evaluation results and their interaction with therapist's and client's desired outcomes, available resources, and client's potential lead to the prognosis. Selection of the best and most efficient resources or "road map" to the desired outcome will lead to treatment intervention.

The process used by therapists is complex and is clearly divided into two specific phases of differential diagnosis (Figure 1-6).

Phase 1: Differential Diagnosis: System Screening for Disease/Pathological Condition

With the increasing use of direct access and the length of time therapists spend with clients, clinicians have become acutely aware of the need to screen systems for disease and

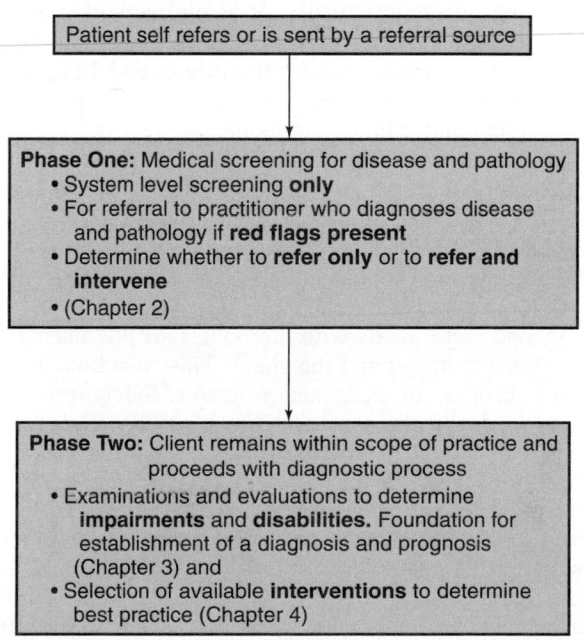

FIGURE 1-6 ■ The diagnostic process used for best practice by physical and occupational therapists.

pathological conditions. Accreditation standards for both PTs and OTs require the new learner to develop these skills before graduation. This screening process is used to determine whether the client should be referred to another practitioner, such as a physician, or can progress to diagnosis, prognosis, and intervention within the specific discipline. Thus, phase 1 of differential diagnosis separates a client's clinical problems into those that fall within a therapist's scope of practice and those that do not. If the phase 1 differential diagnosis shows signs and symptoms totally outside a therapist's scope of practice, then a referral to an appropriate practitioner must be made. If the signs and symptoms fall both within the clinician's scope of practice as well as overlap with other disciplines, the therapist must refer with adequate information and decide (1) to treat to prevent problems until the other practitioner's treatment can be performed, (2) to treat to eliminate functional disabilities in spite of the pathological process, or (3) to treat to eliminate functional loss and impairments and therefore correct the pathological cause. In some cases, the overlapping with other disciplines may not necessitate an immediate referral, but interactions must be made when needed to ensure the best outcome from intervention. Chapter 7 has been designed to help the reader grasp a better understanding of phase 1 of differential diagnosis. This form of system screening is part of history taking and may be redone periodically throughout treatment if the therapist has questions regarding changes in body systems. Once a clinician determines that the client's need for service falls within his or her respective scope of practice, then phase 2 differential diagnosis begins.

Phase 2: Differential Diagnosis within a Therapist's Scope of Practice

The client's signs and symptoms now fall clearly within an enablement/disablement model (see Figure 1-1), and the therapist needs to identify functional difficulties and limitations. Depending on the client's specific needs and expectations, these functional expectations may be activities of daily living, job requirements, or leisure activities. An indepth conceptual framework for selection of appropriate examination procedures needed to evaluate and draw appropriate diagnostic conclusion can be found in Chapter 8.

Two important clinical components affect the accuracy of the diagnostic conclusion drawn. First, the clinician must establish accurate, nonbiased results. This fact seems obvious, but with the pressures of third-party payers, family members, other providers of care, and the desire to have the client improve, it is not difficult to draw a conclusion regarding what is desired as outcomes versus what is truly present. The second factor deals with the honesty of the interaction between the therapist and the client. This "bonding" is critical for accuracy of examination results. Safety, trust, and acceptance of the client as a human being play a key role in outcome and thus in efficacy of practice. The reader is referred to Chapters 5 and 6 to get a greater understanding of the impact this bonding has on clinical outcomes.

The specific cognitive process used by therapists before formulation of a diagnosis might be conceptualized as a nine-step process. As the therapist enters into the clinical environment of the client, he or she starts collecting data that might be relevant to analysis of the clinical problem (step 1). The therapist must take that array of divergent information and incorporate his or her thought processes with relevant data while disregarding what may be nonrelevant information (step 2). This body of knowledge is then differentiated into various body systems that might be affected by identified problems. If a specific system does not seem to be affected, then it can be eliminated, at least temporarily, from the diagnostic process (step 3). Generally, a clinician performs functional activity testing at this time to obtain a general understanding of the functional strengths and limitations of the individual (step 4). After observing the patterns of movement and specific responses of the client to the evaluation procedures, the therapist once again diverges his or her thought processes back to separate large body systems to identify the system as having problems (step 5). The therapist further subdivides these systems into their components to assess specific subsystem deficits and strengths (step 6). This will give the therapist objective measurements of impairments that are recognized as deficits within any subsystem. This aspect of the problem-solving process will give clusters of specific signs and symptoms that will help direct the therapist to a clinical diagnosis. Once the therapist has obtained these clusters of symptoms within specific subsystems, two additional convergent steps need to be completed. First, subsystem identification of impairments and lack of impairments will help the clinician determine what aspect of each body system is affected by the impairments (step 7). Second, how those impairments affect the interaction of the major system with other major body systems is determined (step 8). The eight steps tell the therapist exactly why the client has difficulty with specific functional activities. The problem list that incorporates the severity of impairments that have interacted to cause loss of function gives the clinician a clinical diagnosis. The number and extent of impairments along with an understanding of the cause of loss of function will lead the therapist to establishment of various prognoses and identification of optimal intervention strategies. The last step (step 9) requires the therapist to diverge his or her thought processes back to the client's total environment to determine the accuracy of the diagnosis, prognosis, and selected treatment interventions as they interact with the client as a whole. Although some completion of this diagnostic process may occur within minutes after a client and therapist begin their interactions, the process is continual, and at any time a therapist may need to go back to previous steps to obtain and analyze new and relevant information.

PROGNOSIS: HOW LONG WILL IT TAKE TO GET FROM POINT A TO POINT B?

If a client has a variety of disabilities and impairments within a major system, then a variety of appropriate prognoses may be formulated. These prognoses could speculate regarding the time or number of treatments it will take to get from the existing functional limitations and identified disabilities (point A) to the desired outcomes (point B). The outcomes will state whether the intervention will eliminate functional limitations through (1) changes and learning within the client as an organism or (2) modification of the external environment. Once a diagnosis has been established, a therapist must consider many factors when making a prognosis. Some factors are related to the internal environment of the client, such as number and extent of impairments, physical conditioning or deconditioning of the client, the ability and motivation to learn, and the disease or condition that led to the existing neurological condition. The client's support systems have a dramatic impact on prognosis. Cultural and ethnic pressures, financial support to promote independence, availability of appropriate skilled professional services, prescribed medications, and the interaction of all of these factors need to be considered. Specific environmental factors such as belief in health care and agreement about who has the responsibility for healing can create tremendous conflict between current health care delivery systems; the client; the family; and you, the clinician. All of these variables affect prognosis. The last aspect of determining prognosis relates to empowerment of the client. Who sets the goals? Who determines function? Who identifies when a therapeutic intervention should be used versus a life activity? If consensus to these questions cannot be found by the therapist and the client, then conflict between anticipated and actual outcome will result and a definitive prognosis will not be achieved.

Once prognoses have been established, the therapist's next step is to identify the intervention strategies that will guide the client to the desired outcome within the time frame identified.

DOCUMENTATION

Documentation of the therapeutic intervention has always been integral to the process. However, there is added emphasis in today's health care environment, as well as a renewed respect for the importance of the issue.

Documentation communicates the process of care and the product or outcome of that process. The outcome is the realistic reflection of the effectiveness of care. Documentation must produce a clear framework from which to record and follow client progress. The goals should be stated in measurable functional terms throughout and developed in order

of importance to the client. The number of goals developed by the therapist takes into account the realistic probability of effectiveness of intervention, the environment in which the intervention will likely occur, and support systems available to the client. As the process goes forward, the therapist may add, delete, or change the functional goal, and so states that on the client's record. For further information about this process, refer to Chapter 10.

INTERVENTION

Clients with neurological diseases or conditions interact with the medical community for short or long periods. They present neurological problems of all types that are sudden or insidious. All aspects of human function are represented in the variety of problems. If individual beliefs and values energize and motivate physical behavior, think of the possibilities for stimulating wellness. Wellness might be considered return to previous function, maintenance of function, slowing progression of functional loss, habilitation of function never achieved, and striving for excellence in performance. Refer to Chapter 6 for additional discussion.

The therapist/client chooses nonrestrictive and restrictive treatment environments to best achieve the identified goal. It is the therapist's responsibility to guide the selection of appropriate intervention strategies that will allow the learner to achieve anticipated outcomes. Depending on the level of function of the client, some interventions will require the therapist to guide or limit the client's selection of CNS choices, whereas others will be directed toward the client's practicing functional control without clinician interference. The available choices will depend on the therapist's skill and available intervention strategies and on the client's ability to direct and control his or her CNS function. Yet, freedom within that established existing environment must exist if learning by the client is to occur. Another way to consider intervention is to refer to it as a clinical map (Figure 1-7).

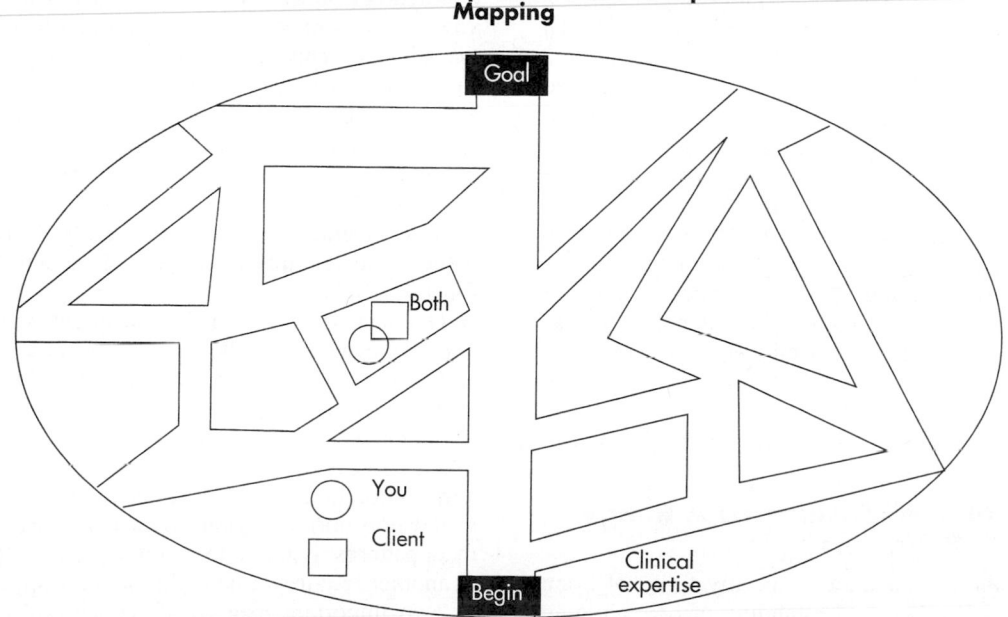

FIGURE 1-7 ■ Concept of clinical mapping.

Within the map, a therapist, through professional education, efficacy of preexisting clinical pathways, and clinical experience, can generally identify the most expedient way to guide a client toward the desired outcome. When the specific client enters into this interaction, slight variations off the existing pathway may lead to quicker outcomes. If the client diverges away from the desired end product, it is the therapist's responsibility to guide that individual back into the clinical map. For example, if a therapist and client are working on coming to standing patterns and the client begins to fall, the therapist would need to guide the client back into the desired movement patterns and not allow the fall. In that way the client is working on the identified outcome. Falling as a functional activity should be taught as a different intervention and would be considered part of a different clinical map. The degree to which the therapist needs to control the response of the client will determine the extent to which the intervention would be considered contrived. Contrived interventions can lead in time to functional independence of the client, but as long as the therapist needs to control the environment, functional independence has not been achieved. There are many ways to get to a desired outcome. Having the client be part of the goal setting and thus the intervention process will lead to the best result, but these interactions do require trust of the therapist as a guide or teacher. For a more thorough discussion of intervention strategies, the reader is referred to Chapter 9.

Most interventions used as treatment for clients with CNS pathological conditions incorporate principles of CNS function, neuroplasticity, and evaluation and treatment based on control over functional motor behaviors and adaptation to various environmental contexts. Thus, the consideration of the basic science of central and peripheral nervous system function (Chapter 3) and behavioral analysis of movement (Chapter 2) must be included in any conceptual model used as a foundation for the entire diagnostic process.

Of considerable significance also is the client-therapist interaction, which is labeled the *learning environment*. This may be the critical factor in clinical success or failure of therapeutic intervention. The interrelationships between understanding of neural function, variability in functional movement within the context of the environment, and the therapist-client learning environment can be considered a conceptual triad. All aspects occur simultaneously, yet each component has unique characteristics and influences the clinical performance. Although each component is explored separately in the following pages, the reader should retain the image of the entire model. This approach should help develop a gestalt, that is, a picture of the client as a total human being although a specific aspect of therapy may be the focus. When the client is not viewed as a whole being, the therapist often misses critical response patterns, such as movement in another body part, pain, or an autonomic nervous system response. These responses may be the key to successful goal attainment or client-therapist rapport.

Concept of Human Movement: A Range of Observable Behaviors

As researchers continue to unravel the mysteries of brain function and learning, their understanding of how children and adults learn initially or relearn after insult is often explained with new and possibly conflicting theories. Yet behavioral responses observed as functional patterns of movement, whether performed by a child, adolescent, young adult, or older person, are still visually identified by a therapist, family member, or innocent observer as either normal or abnormal.

Human beings exhibit certain movement patterns that may vary in tonal characteristics, aspects of the specific movement sequences, and even the sequential nature of development. Yet the range of acceptable behavior does have limitations, and variations beyond those boundaries are recognizable by most people. A 5-year-old child may ask why a little girl walks on her toes with her legs stuck together. If questioned, that same 5-year-old child may have the ability to break down the specific aspects of the movement that seem unacceptable even to that 5-year-old child. From birth a sighted individual observes normal human movement. Because the range of behaviors identified as normal within any functional activity does not vary from individual to individual, human movement patterns are predictable. This concept does provide flexibility in analysis of normal movement and its development. Some children choose creeping as a primary mode of horizontal movement, whereas others may scoot. Both forms of movement are normal for a young child. In both cases each child would have had to develop normal postural function in the head and trunk to carry out the activity in a normal fashion. Thus, for the child to develop the specific functional motor behavior, the various components or systems involved in the integrated execution of the act would require modulation in a plan of action. Because the action must be carried out in a variety of environmental contexts, the child would need the opportunity to practice those contexts, self-correct to regulate existing plans, identify error, and refine for skill development. Thus, each movement has a variety of complex systems interactions, which when summated are expressed by means of the motor pool to striated muscle function. The specifics of that function, whether fine or gross motor or total body or limb specific, still reflect the totality of the interaction of those systems. No matter the age of the individual, the motor response still reflects that interaction, and the behavior can be identified as normal and functional, functional but limited in adaptability, or dysfunctional and abnormal. Because of the simplicity or complexity of various movements and the components necessary for modulatory control over various movement, therapists can (1) look at any movement pattern, (2) evaluate its components, (3) identify what is missing, and (4) incorporate treatment strategies that help the client achieve the desired function outcome.

One can be confident that no infant will be born, jump out of the womb, walk over to the physician, and shake hands or say "hi" to mom and dad before learning rolling or postural control of the trunk and head. Instead, normal motor development requires motor programs that lead to the infant's ability to achieve functional movement. These plans will be modified and reintegrated along with other programs to develop normal motor control in more complex movement patterns. Each pattern and movement from one pattern to another requires time and repetition for mastery.

Two important aspects of the clinical problem-solving process emerge. First, the evaluation of motor function is based on the interaction of all the components of the motor system and the cognitive and affective influences over this motor system, as stated previously. Second, the therapist needs to recognize which aspects of the movement are deficient, absent, distorted, or inappropriate when cross-referenced with the desired outcome (the diagnostic/prognosis process). These behaviors, although dependent on many factors, are consistent regardless of age of the client. Some clients may not have had the opportunity to experience the desired skill, whereas others may have lost the skill as a result of changes within the CNS or disuse. In either case, the normal accepted patterns and range of behaviors remain the same. Refer to Chapter 2 for additional discussion of movement analysis across the life span.

Concept of CNS Control: a Multicomplex Control System

The concept of CNS control is based on a therapist's understanding of the CNS and motor performance patterns reflective of that system. This understanding, which requires in-depth background in neuroanatomy, neurophysiology, motor control, motor learning, and neuroplasticity, gives the therapist the basis for clinical application and treatment. Understanding the intricacies of neuromechanisms provides therapists with direction as to when, why, and in what order to use clinical treatment techniques. Behaviors are based on maturation, potential, and degeneration of the CNS. Each behavior observed, sequenced, and integrated as a treatment protocol should be interpreted according to neurophysiological and neuroanatomical principles as well as the principles of learning and neuroplasticity. As science moves toward a greater understanding of the neuromechanisms by which behaviors occur, the therapists will be in a better position to establish efficacy of intervention. Unfortunately, our knowledge of behavior is ahead of our understanding of the intricate mechanism of the CNS. Thus, the future will continue to expand the reliability and validity of the therapeutic environment. First, therapists need to determine what is effective within a clinical environment. Then, efficacy of specific variables can be studied and more clearly identified. The rationale for use of certain treatment techniques will change. At times the treatment will remain constant, and at other times the treatment will need to be changed. Within this practice environment the therapist must use evidence-based practice. Chapters 4 and 5 have additional information and references on CNS function. Chapter 9 has an in-depth discussion of intervention options.

Concept of the Learning Environment

The concept of the learning environment is the most abstract and complex of the three concepts in the clinical triad model. For that reason it is by far the hardest to present in concrete terms. Both simultaneous and sequential components formulate and maintain this environment. At any one moment multiple input events occur simultaneously and continuously. Thus, a temporal ordering of successive events plays a role in the CNS response to the environment. To comprehend the dynamics of this interaction and be able to function with optimal success, the clinician must do the following:

■ Comprehend the learning process to provide an environment that promotes learning

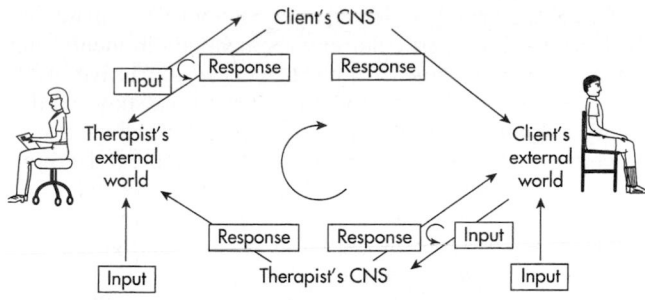

FIGURE 1-8 ■ Clinical learning environment.

■ Investigate the input, processing, feedforward, feedback, and output system as a vital servomechanism for higher-order learning.
■ Relate the concepts of learning to motor control and neuroplasticity principles to facilitate the carryover of treatment into other environments.
■ Compare the provider and client learning styles. If these learning styles are not compatible, then the clinician needs to teach through the client's preferential systems or learning styles.
■ Maintain an alertness to the motoric, affective, and cognitive aspects of the client, no matter what the clinical emphasis might be at any one time.

At all times there are four distinct components of the learning environment in operation: the internal and external environments of the client and the internal and external environment of the clinician (Figure 1-8). All four represent interactive components of the system.

A critical component of the client's learning is the internal environment. When a lesion occurs within the system, it affects both directly and indirectly the entire system. If the lesion occurs before initial learning, then habilitation must take place. Although a learning style might not have been established, the individual probably has a genetic predisposition. The therapist should test the inexperienced CNS by creating experiences in various contexts that require a variety of types of higher-order processing to discover optimal methods of learning that best suit the CNS of the client. Then the therapist can focus treatment on the most effective strategies. If previous learning has occurred and preferential systems have been established, then the therapist needs to know what those are and whether they have been affected by the insult so that proper rehabilitation can be instituted. The use of preferential modes such as visual compared with verbal or kinesthetic compared with verbal does not mean that other modes are ineffective, nor do all modes function optimally in any given situation.

One way to determine general preestablished preferential styles is by taking a thorough history. Leisure activities and job choice often give clues to learning styles. For example, a client who loved to take car engines apart or build model ships demonstrates a preference for the visual-spatial learning style, whereas another client, whose preference for pure enjoyment was sitting in a chair with a novel, demonstrates a probable preference toward verbal learning. Again, this does not mean that the clients in the examples mentioned could not selectively use both methods, but it does illustrate the issue of preference. Both the position of the lesion and preferential learning styles can play a key role in matching the learner with a particular environment and in identifying potential. For example, if a client has had a massive insult to the left temporal lobe and before the trauma showed poor ability in using the right parieto-occipital lobe, then spatial or verbal strategies may be ineffective in the relearning process. However, a client with the same lesion who had high-level right parieto-occipital function before the insult will probably learn at a much faster rate if visual-kinesthetic strategies are used to promote learning.

The client's external environment is the second critical component. All external stimuli, including noise, lighting, temperature, touch, humidity, and smell, modulate the client's internal responses. This external input can invoke either negative or positive influences on the internal mechanism and alter the client's ability to manipulate the world. A therapist should make every effort to be aware of what is happening to the client externally. It is important to know what is happening to the client both within and outside the hospital. Any behavioral change displayed by the client, such as mood, attitude, or muscle tone change, could serve as an indicator to the therapist that a change may have occurred. Following up that observation by determining what happened can help the therapist not only in understanding but also in assisting the client to deal with environmental change or in obtaining additional professional assistance.

The third critical component is the internal environment of the clinician. The clinician should be aware of personal internal factors that influence patient responses. Everyone has preferential styles of teaching and learning; yet many may be unaware of what they are and how they affect their outlooks on life and interactions with other people. A common example of a mismatch of styles is what happens when two people are arguing opposing sides of a political issue. Although both individuals may process the same data, they may also have different learning strategies and come up with very different conclusions.

The interplay of learning styles occurs continually in an academic setting. A student who is asked the question, "What do you want out of this course?" would probably say, "A good grade." Getting a good grade requires doing well on course requirements, including tests. High-grade test performance usually depends on not only a knowledgeable demonstration of a subject but also the way in which the teacher formulates the question and the teacher's expectation for a response. In a clinical setting, it is important that the clinician be aware of the client's response to the practitioner's request.

This external-internal interaction concept brings up another important clinical consideration. As students, most of us probably "clashed" with one or two teachers with whose learning styles we could never identify. As learners we cannot or will not adapt to all learning styles. For that reason there may be some clients who do not respond to our teaching. When that seems evident, a shift of therapists is appropriate for the rehabilitation process to succeed.

The fourth component of the learning environment is the clinician's external environment. It is generally expected that personal life should never affect professional work. To accept this assumption, however, may be to deny that emotions affect behavioral patterns (see Chapter 4). When an individual is emotionally upset or under stress, response patterns vary without cognitive awareness. For example, suppose that Mr. Smith, who has a hypertonic condition because of a cerebrovascular accident, comes down early for therapy each morning, has a cup of coffee, and chats while you write notes. If one day you are under extreme stress and do not feel like interacting as Mr. Smith rolls his wheelchair into your office, you might say, "Mr. Smith, I'll be with you in a few minutes. Go over to the mat, lock your brakes, pick up the pedals, and we'll transfer when I get there." Mr. Smith will quickly sense a change in your behavior. Society has taught him that you are a professional and that your personal life does not affect your job. Thus he may draw a logical conclusion—that he must have done something to change your behavior. When you go to transfer him, you notice he is more hypertonic than usual and ask, "Is something bothering you? You are tighter than usual," and so goes the interaction. Your external environment altered your internal state and, thus, normal response patterns. In turn, you altered Mr. Smith's external environment, changing his internal balance, and created a change of emotional tone that resulted in increased hypertonicity.[49,50] If, instead of interacting with Mr. Smith as if nothing were wrong, you informed him you were upset over something unrelated to him, you might have avoided creating a negative environment. Mr Smith's responses may have been different if you had shared with him the fact that there are days that you are upset and have mood changes. As he accepts your changes as normal, you may have created an opportunity for him to also exhibit a range of behavioral moods. You have also given him an opportunity to offer his assistance to comfort or help you if he so desires. Such behavior encourages interdependence and social interaction, long-term goals for all rehabilitation clients.

Although each client is unique and thus analysis of specifics related to the learning environment is difficult, certain basic learning principles can be formulated. Six clinically significant learning concepts have been selected from many that have been established.[51-53] Basic learning principles relevant to clinical performance may be summarized as follows:

1. Individuals need to be able to solve problems and practice those solutions as motor programs if independence in daily living is desired. They need to use intrinsic feedback systems to modulate feed-forward plans as well as correct existing plans.

2. Although assigned functional tasks must be challenging, there must be a possibility of success.

3. When tasks are difficult or unfamiliar (new problem), an individual will revert to safer or more familiar motor program or ways to solve the problem to succeed at the functional task.

4. When working on learning within one area of the CNS, learning also occurs simultaneously in many areas.

5. Motivation is necessary to drive the individual to try to experience what would be considered unknown. Simultaneously, success of the activity is critical to keep the individual motivated to continue to practice.

6. Clinicians need to be able to analyze an activity as a whole, determine its components, and use problem-solving strategies to design good individual programs. At the same time, if independence in living skills is an

objective, the therapist needs to teach the client those same problem-solving strategies rather than teaching the solution.

Although all six learning concepts seem simple, their application within the clinical setting is not always as obvious. Principles 1 and 2 are intricately linked with the appropriateness and difficulty of tasks presented to clients. If a client is asked to perform a task such as standing, rolling, relaxing, dressing, or maneuvering a wheelchair, a problem has been presented that requires a sequence of acts leading to a solution. To succeed, the client must be able to plan the entire task and modulate all motor control during the sequence of the entire activity. If steps are unmastered, if sequencing is inappropriate or absent, or if motor control systems are not modulated accurately, dependence on the clinician to solve the problem is reinforced. If the clinician can differentiate missing components (impairments) from functioning systems, creating an environment that encourages and allows the CNS to adapt and learn ways to regain that control, it will lead to optimal self-empowerment of the client and will help eliminate disabilities. Error in practice to intrinsically self-correct is critical for motor learning. Error that always leads to failure does not help the client learn avenues of adaptation. Linked intricately with success is the challenge of the task. The greater its difficulty or complexity, the greater the challenge and, consequently, the greater the satisfaction of success.

There is a subtle interplay in degree of difficulty, challenge, and success. Selecting tasks that are age appropriate, clinically relevant, and goal related is a challenge to the therapist. For the patient to be successful, the therapist must be a creative problem solver and knowledgeable about the client's needs, abilities, and goals. If the tasks are too simple or if the client considers them unimportant, boredom will ensue and progress may diminish. If the tasks are too difficult, the client may feel defeated and turn away from them. In such cases a child tends to withdraw physically, whereas an adult usually avoids the problem. Being late to therapy, having to leave early, needing to go to the bathroom, and scheduling conflicting sessions are all avoidance behaviors that may be linked to inappropriate tasks.

The third learning principle describes a behavior inherent in all people: reversal. When confronted by a problem, individuals revert to patterns that produce feelings of comfort and competence when solving the problem. In Figure 1-9, a 2-year-old child is confronted with just such a conflict. The bridge he wants to cross is unstable. The task goal is to cross the bridge; how that is accomplished is not as relevant as the task specificity. Therefore the child chooses a 6-month-old behavior and thus scoots. On gaining confidence, the child sequences from scooting to four-point bunny hopping, then crawling, on to cruising, and finally to reciprocal walking. The child's reversal lasted approximately 2 minutes. Although reverting to more familiar or comfortable ways of solving problems is normal, it creates constant frustration in the clinic if it is prolonged. For example, if a client with residual hemiplegia has spent a week modifying and controlling a hypertonic upper-extremity pattern during a simple task and is now confronted with a more difficult problem, the hypertonia within the limb will most likely return with the added complexity of the task. If another client has successfully worked to obtain the stand-

ing position and then is asked to walk, the strong synergistic patterns that had been controlled may return. The pattern or plan for standing is different than that of walking, and the emotional implications of walking are very high. The patient returning to a more stereotypical pattern should be anticipated by the clinician and the client should be prepared. Anticipating that less-efficient patterns will usually return as the tasks demanded increase in complexity, the clinician can attempt to modify the unwanted responses, let the patient know that the response is actually normal given the CNS, but the movement can be changed and normalized with practice. The key to comprehension of this concept is not the behavior itself; instead, it is the attitude of a therapist toward a new task presented to the client. If the clinician expects the client to be successful, the client will also expect success. If failure occurs, both parties will be disappointed and a potentially negative clinical situation will be created; however, if the client succeeds, both will have expected the result and their attitude will be neither excited nor depressed. On the other hand, a clinician that expects the client to revert to an old behavior can prepare the client. If the client reverts, neither party will be disappointed; but if no reversion occurs, both will be excited, pleased, and encouraged by the higher functional skill. By understanding the concept, the clinician can maintain a very positive clinical environment without the constant negative interference of perceived failure when a client does revert.

The fourth learning principle deals with the totality of the client. Whether the area of emphasis is motor performance, emotional balance, or perceptual integration, all areas are affected. Therefore understanding and respect for all areas are important if optimal client function is a primary objective. This does not suggest that therapists should address each aspect of personality; however, integration of the client's physical, mental, and spiritual areas should be a responsibility of the staff. Awareness of possible adverse effects of one learned behavior on other CNS functions can help avoid potential problems. For example, if working on lower extremity patterns creates extreme upper extremity hypertonicity through associated patterns, the clinician is not dealing with the client as a whole.

The unknown creates fear and curiosity for most individuals, and the fifth concept points out that for most clients the unknown is all encompassing whatever the degree of prior learning. For a client whose only difficulty is a flaccid upper extremity, functional activities such as toileting, dressing, or eating will be troublesome and unfamiliar. Motivation is a critical factor for success. Maintaining motivation to try while ensuring a high degree of success is an important teaching strategy that tends to encourage present and future learning.

An additional comment regarding clients who lack motivation should be made. If a client wants to be totally dependent and has no need to become independent, then a therapist will probably fail at whatever task is presented. For example, Mr. Brown, a 63-year-old bank president with a wife, 4 children, and 10 grandchildren, survives an operable brain tumor with residual right hemiparesis and minimal cognitive-affective deficits. The client's work history indicates that he was highly success oriented. Unknown to most persons is that for 63 years Mr. Brown desired to be a passive-dependent person, but circumstances never allowed

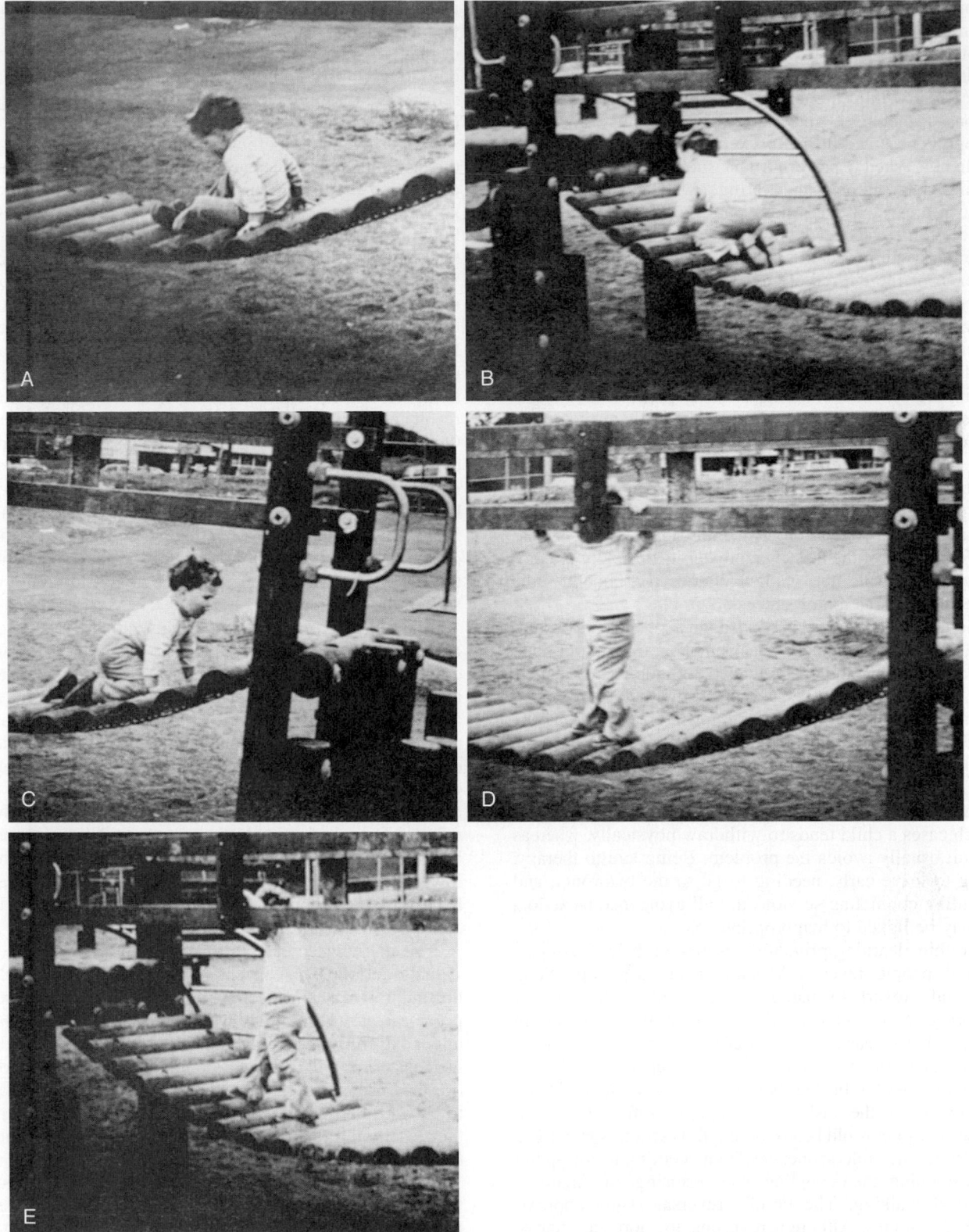

FIGURE 1-9 ■ Reverting to more comfortable behavior patterns when confronted with a problem. **A,** Scooting. **B,** Bunny hopping. **C,** Crawling. **D,** Cruising. **E,** Walking.

him to manifest those behaviors. With the neurological insult he is in a position to actualize his needs. Until the client desires to improve, therapy will probably be ineffective. Thus, motivating the client becomes critical and might be accomplished in a variety of ways. Knowing that Mr. Brown values privacy, especially with respect to hygiene, that he thoroughly enjoys dancing and bird watching in the forest, and that he ascribes importance to being accepted in social situations, such as cocktail parties, helps the therapist create a learning environment that motivates this client toward independence. Being independent in hygiene requires certain combinations of motor actions, including sitting, balance, and transfer skills. Being able to bird watch deep in an unpopulated forest requires ambulation skills, tolerance to the upright position for extended periods of time, and endurance. Being socially accepted depends to a large extent not only on grooming but on normal movement patterns, especially in the upper extremity and trunk. Creating a therapeutic environment that stresses independence in the three goals identified by the client will simultaneously create further independence in other areas. Whether the client decides to return to banking and other activities in conflict with his personality will need to be addressed later. Another way to motivate Mr. Brown is to place him in an environment in which he is not satisfied, such as a nursing home or his own home with an assistant rather than his wife to help him with his needs. Dissatisfaction with the current external environment will generally motivate an individual to change. Obviously, creating a positive environment for change versus a negative one would be the method of choice.

Many additional learning principles from the fields of education, development, and psychology can be used to explain the behavioral responses seen in our clients. It is not expected that all therapists will intuitively or automatically know how to create an environment conducive to help the patient achieve optimal potential. Yet all can become better at creating a maximal learning environment by understanding how people learn.

The principles presented in this chapter deliver a strong message: individuals need to solve problems and most want to solve the problem given a chance that the solutions will be successful. Unless the task fits the individual's current capability, adaptation using whatever is available will become the consensus that drives the motor performance. Learning is taking place in all aspects of life, and the client must ultimately take responsibility for the means to solve the problem.

THE CLIENT AND PROVIDER RELATIONSHIP

The Client's Role in the Relationship

Active participation in life and in relationships promotes learning. Rogers[54] defines significant learning as learning that makes a difference that affects all parts of a person. We have spoken of a relationship centered on an individual's health. One of the individuals involved in the relationship (the therapist) has knowledge that is to be imparted to or skills to be practiced by the other. The relationship "works" if the learning environment facilitates exchange between the participants. The concept of equal partners is crucial. The issue and practice of informed consent is not just political

or ethical; it is central to client care. Voluntarism has to be practiced by both practitioner and client alike. Each has a moral obligation to facilitate the process of health care within the moment. Although the Western world of medicine has steadily climbed a path toward excellence in medical technology, it has not as easily recognized the client's need to assume an equal role in the decision making or for the practitioner to seek the client's help. Consumers are now seeking to play a more active role in their health care.

Consumers of health care are becoming aware of the affect of medicine's control over their lives. This awareness has been fueled by the price they are paying for that health care. A recent Surgeon General's report confirms that expenditures for health are increasing. In addition, preventive care assumes major importance in view of the fact that 75% of all deaths today are the result of degenerative diseases, such as heart disease, cerebrovascular accidents, and cancer. Like other major causes of death, accidents (cited as the most frequent cause of death in persons younger than age 49 years) are increasingly linked to lifestyles.

Individuals in the health care professions during their training internalize values that reinforce the traditional professional attitude alluded to earlier. Many of these values do not support a partnership relationship with the client. Society is beginning to question the traditional role of the health care professional as the knowledge expert; however professional education and organizations resist the pressure to change the image. The professions still hold the image of great authority given to them by the public and fostered through increased political activity.

The major purpose of the patient's relationship with the health care professional is to exchange information useful to both in the health care of the client. McNerney[28] calls health education of the client the missing link in health care delivery. As the gap grows between technology and the users of that technology, client health education becomes more important than ever. McNerney[28] notes that although health care providers are now making efforts to educate their clients, they are doing so with little consistency, enthusiasm, theoretical base, or imagination and often with little coordination with other services. The health care professional continues to receive training and embrace professional organizational membership that places a premium on control of information and control of the decision making. There is and should be a special effort to introduce health education concepts into the basic educational programs of health care professionals. McNerney identified many of the problems three decades ago, and many still exist today.

When patients are given more information about their illnesses, and retain the information, they express more satisfaction with their caregivers. A study by Bertakis[55] tested the hypothesis that patients with greater understanding and retention of the information given by the physician would be more satisfied with the physician/patient relationship. The experimental group received feedback and retained 83.5% of the information given to them by the physician. The control group received no feedback and retained 60.5% of the information. Not surprisingly, the experimental group was more satisfied with the physician/patient relationship.

If the client is to be informed and included in the treatment process, client health education will have to go beyond the current styles of information giving. If the client is to assume some of the responsibility for his or her therapy, the therapist will have to facilitate that involvement. The attitude of the therapist toward educating clients about their health could affect his or her ability to facilitate client involvement in the care process.

The more the professional sees himself or herself as the expert, the less likely he or she will be to see the client as capable of responsibility or expertise in the care process. If communication skills and health education were an integral part of medical school and the health care professional school curricula, perhaps the health care professionals would temper their assumption of the "expert" professional role. Payton[56] points out that it is the client alone who can ultimately decide whether a goal is worth working for. Careful planning can be influential in helping all providers include the client in the process.

The health care delivery system in the United States has to serve all citizens. That is no easy task. The United States is a society of great pluralism. It is a free society. It is a society that is used to being governed by persuasion, not coercion. Given the variety of economic, political, cultural, and religious forces at work in American society, education of the people in regard to their health care is probably the only method that can work in the long run. The future task of health education will be to "cultivate people's sense of responsibility toward their own health and that of the community." Health education is an effective approach with perhaps the most potential to move us toward a concept of preventive care.

Becker and Maiman[57] discussed Rosenstock's Health Belief model as a framework to account for the individual's decision to use preventive services or engage in preventive health behavior. They cite noncompliance with a physician's recommendation in about one third of all patients. Action taken by the individual, according to the model, depends on the individual's perceived susceptibility to the illness, his or her perception of the severity of the illness, the benefits to be gained from taking action, and a "cue" of some sort that triggers action. The cue could be advice from a friend, reading an article about the illness, a television commercial, and so on. In some way, the person is motivated to do something.

Split-brain research, research in the functions of the left and right halves of the brain, seems to be a pertinent area of mind-body research. The left hemisphere of the brain processes experiences in a factual, logical, and analytical way, whereas the right half appears to process the same experiences in the form of images and impressions. The recognition that one half of the brain may be designed to record the impressionistic part of an experience gives further credibility to including the individual's accounts of his or her feelings and emotions as a part of the input for diagnosis of illness.

Freymann[58] ponders the strange logic of traditional medicine, which rewards the specialist who confines his or her practice to a very few and shows little concern for a public health physician whose field is broad and who treats so many. Dramatic traditional medicine does not result in many health benefits for large numbers of people.

McKay[59] asks to what extent health care providers are willing to commit themselves to explore and implement alternative forms of health care. The provider-client relationship becomes very important to a successful therapeutic outcome, as does health education and promotion of positive health behaviors. Health care providers seem to forget that well-being calls for wellness of the mind, body, and environment. Although they may talk about supporting a focus on health, they continue to focus on disease. The training that health care providers receive makes disease more interesting than wellness.

Saward and Sorenson[60] observe that the mass media has promoted the technology of health care. The consumer thus has a heightened expectation of the quality of care he or she will receive. However, we should avoid excesses in the other extreme. If society adheres to inappropriate lifestyles, the health care professional cannot blame the victim for bringing on the illness to absolve himself or herself from responsibility. Holistic health care carried to an extreme might result in "blaming the victim." Saward and Sorenson see that, in the extremes, the medical model and the holistic model of health care have different objectives; evolve from different historical, philosophical, and economic perspectives; and use practitioners with essentially different training and outlook on health care. Perhaps, they suggest, two health care systems should be available to people instead of one.

Szasz and Hollender[61] described five basic relationships between providers and clients on a continuum from a provider-dominated relationship, consistent with the medical model, through a mutual participation relationship, to a relationship where the client accepts the larger share of responsibility, which is consistent with the holistic model. Whether the client takes some responsibility for his or her care depends a great deal on whether the health care provider gives some to him or her.

Fink[62] also recognized the importance of the provider-patient relationship and made three points about it. The first is that a relationship between them is implicit. The second is that what the relationship becomes is mutually agreed on, consciously or not. Third, whatever the form of the relationship, it should meet the needs and health care requirements of the particular patient. The state of what we refer to as health varies for each client and includes both the simple and complex variables of that client's life, from the last nutritional meal to the totality of the client's life event history (see Figure 1-5).

The relationship of the therapist and client has also been called "the emotional bridge over which the more mechanical forms of treatment are conducted."[63] The psychological makeups of the therapist and of the client have an impact on the relationship that is established. The psychological development of both of them during their growth stages of dependence, aggressiveness, and ability to subordinate personal gratification must be acknowledged as having an effect on the relationship.

The illness or trauma of the client that represents a disintegrating force in his or her life may represent an opportunity for the therapist to grow professionally. The client and the therapist may have different psychological backgrounds, and, although the client's presence is usually related to a medical crisis, the therapist's presence may support the purposes of personal growth, financial gain, prestige, and unconscious gratification in influencing the lives of others through professional skill.

A large amount of time is spent by therapists in face-to-face patient contact.[64] In this respect, the therapist has an advantage over most other health care practitioners, who see the patient at infrequent intervals and who seldom touch the patient as a PT or OT does. The physical contact itself may provide psychological support and promote a close relationship between the therapist and the patient. It is important that the therapist be aware of the importance of the relationship itself. The therapist's attitudes and values can affect the expectations of patients regarding the outcome of treatment. The patient's expectations can be made realistic if he or she is an active participant in care from the start. Any process that involves personal commitment and purports to effect change should focus on the person seeking help. An attitude of acceptance of the patient as an equal in the process may be of healing value by itself and referred to as empowerment.

As the consumer becomes more involved, so should the family. The family is seldom brought into the practice. Sasano et al[65] described a patient program that includes the family. They made some comments relative to therapy's inclusion of the family in the care process. Patients were happier with the family involved; the family members felt less anxious and could be more supportive. All these factors facilitate the work of the therapist. The therapist, however, must be willing to facilitate the involvement of the family members and help them learn to take responsibility for some of the care and decision making. Most health care professionals are not conditioned to the patient's assuming greater authority and family members would not be given responsibility for care unless they are allowed to assume that role.

The therapist is caught up in the same problems of the health care system as are other health care professionals. Inflation has often caused profit to become a more important motive than human care considerations for setting priorities in our clinics. Research is heavily focused on technical procedures, yet the relationship with patients in the care process is vital. Singleton[66] labeled this phenomenon a paradox in therapy. Despite the commitment to humanistic service on which the profession was founded, the service rendered is mechanistic.

Is the patient approached as if he or she were a machine? Have scientific technology and evidence-based practice captured the therapist's attention to the extent that patient care procedures, which cannot or have not been scientifically analyzed, are ignored? Alexander[67] sees the necessity of reorganizing the education and work of the therapist to encourage a humanistic approach to care. To what degree, Alexander[67] asks, are we "masters or servants to our patients?" The educational programs should emphasize whole-patient treatment, increase communication skills, interdisciplinary awareness, and patient-centered care.[34-36]

If medicine succeeds in bringing humanistic medicine into focus and shifting some emphasis from a scientific technology approach, it is conceivable that some people currently suited to practicing therapy would find it intolerable to do so in the future.

The change in roles described previously requires a professional who demonstrates a potential for the assumption of many roles, responsibilities, and choices along the care pathway. The therapist working with the client with neuro-logical problems must always be ready to respond to triggers anywhere along the pathway from early intervention, midway during a crisis, or later during long-term care, because these triggers signal a need for change. Of equal importance, the path must be well documented to empower the therapist to reflect on current and prognosticated treatment intervention.

The Provider's Role in the Relationship

Gifted therapists are often thought to have intuition. Yet intuitive behavior is based on experience, a thorough knowledge of the area, sensitivity to the total environment, and ability to ask pertinent questions as the therapist evaluates, conceptualizes about, and treats clients. How these questions are formulated and the answers documented vary among therapists, but the result is the formulation of a profile for each client.

Cognitive-perceptual processing by the client will often determine the learning environment to be used, the sequences for treatment, and estimated time needed for therapeutic intervention. Thus, the client is in a position to play an important role with the therapist within the clinical problem-solving process. During that interactive environment, the therapist can ask questions regarding cognitive, affective, and motor domains that will help clarify, document, and guide future decisions regarding empowerment of the client. (See the client profile questions regarding cognitive, affective, and sensorimotor areas in Boxes 1-1, 1-2, and 1-3.) The motor output area is the main system the client uses to express thoughts and feelings and demonstrate independence to family, therapists, and community. This motor area cannot be evaluated effectively by itself while negating the cognitive-perceptual and the affective-emotional areas. If that rigidity becomes a standard of care, accurate prognosis and selection of appropriate interventions will continue to be inconsistent and lack effectiveness within the clinical environment.

Once the therapist has a clear understanding of the client's strengths and weaknesses, specific clinical problems can be identified and treatment procedures selected that allow flexibility in treatment sessions. Many treatment suggestions for various problems can be found in Chapter 9 and Chapters 11 through 37.

CONCLUSION

In this fifth edition of the textbook, the authors hope to bring the reader into the clinical practice of the twenty-first century. As the professions continue to evolve in depth and breadth, the future will encapsulate the knowledge, skill, and lessons of the past and the needs and problems of current and immediate health delivery systems while maintaining unique scopes and parameter of practice in an ever-changing environment. The professions must adapt and grow as they embrace change without losing the integrity and philosophical reasons they came into existence. The only concept that is guaranteed in the future is change. Both physical and occupational therapy are dynamic professions with the ability to adapt and evolve to provide the health care service expected and deserved by the consumer. The future is up to every practitioner. The consumer of our services is dependent on our willingness to learn, adapt, and provide quality of care at an appropriate cost for the best

BOX 1-1 ■ COGNITIVE AREA QUESTIONS FOR CLIENT PROFILE

A. Sensory input: awareness level
   1. What sensory systems are intact?
   2. Are any sensory systems in conflict with others?
   3. If conflict between systems is present, to which system does the client pay attention?
B. Perceptual awareness and development
   1. What specific perceptual processing deficits does the client have, and how would that affect motor performance?
   2. Do the perceptual problems relate to input distortion, processing deficits, or both? If input distortion is alleviated, is information processed appropriately?
C. Preferential higher-order cognitive system
   1. Was or is the individual's primary preferential system verbal or spatial?
   2. Is the client's preferential system different from yours? If so, can you work through the client's system?
   3. Is the client's preferential system affected by the clinical problems?
   4. Can the client adequately use nonpreferred systems?
D. Level of cognition
   1. Is the client functioning on a concrete, abstract, or fragmented level?
   2. Does the client's level of cognition change? If so, when and why?
   3. Is the client realistic? Does the client exercise judgment? If so, when? If not, when and why?
   4. Which systems or individuals are interfering with or distorting potential? (Systems within the individual and the environment around the client, such as the staff, the family, and the other patients, must be considered.)

BOX 1-2 ■ AFFECTIVE AREA QUESTIONS FOR CLIENT PROFILE

A. Level of adjustment or stage of adjustment to the disability
   1. At what level or stage of adjustment is the client with respect to the disability?
   2. At what level of adjustment is the family?
   3. Will the level of adjustment of the client or family affect treatment?
   4. If emotions are affecting treatment, what can be done to eliminate this problem?
B. Level of emotional control
   1. Can the client exercise impulse control?
   2. When does degree of emotional or impulse control vary?
   3. How did and does the client respond to stress?
   4. How did and does the client respond to perceived success and failure?
   5. What types of stresses outside of the specific physical disability are being placed on the client?
C. Attitude (attitude toward the disability is covered to some degree under level of acceptance, although additional information needs to be gathered)
   1. Before the onset of disability what was the client's attitude toward disabilities, and specifically, those related to his or her primary deficit?
   2. What is the client's attitude toward your professional domain?
   3. What is the family's attitude toward disabilities, especially those related to its family member?
   4. What is the family's attitude toward your professional domain?
D. Social adjustment
   1. At what social developmental stage is the client's performance?
   2. Is the social interaction in alignment with cognitive and sensorimotor stages of development?
   3. Are the family's social interactions and expectations at the level of the client's performance?
   4. Is the client's level of social adjustment the same as the rehabilitation team's level of expectation?
   5. Is the client aware of his, her, or others' socially appropriate behavior?

BOX 1-3 ■ SENSORIMOTOR AREA QUESTIONS FOR CLIENT PROFILE

A. Level of motor performance with respect to performance
   1. Is the client's level of motor performance or sensory and motor integration congruous with the staff's expected performance level?
   2. Is the client's level of motor control integration congruous with the family's expected performance level?
   3. Is the client's level of motor function congruous with his or her expected level of performance?
B. Functional skills
   1. What functional skills does the client perform in a normal fashion?
   2. What functional skills does the client perform in an abnormal manner?
   3. What functional skills has the client learned to perform that are reinforcing stereotypical patterns or hindering normal movement?
   4. What functional skills do the client and family consider of primary importance? Will splintering these skills hinder normal learning?

C. Abnormal patterns
   1. What patterns are present?
   2. When are these normal and abnormal patterns observed? Do they vary according to spatial positions?
   3. Is there ever a shifting or altering in degree of these abnormal patterns? If so, under what circumstances does this variance occur?
D. Degree of cortical override
   1. Does the client need to inhibit abnormal output by intentional thought, or does he or she use procedural adjustment through normal feedforward mechanisms?
   2. What amount of energy is being used to override abnormal output?
   3. Can the client use cognitive systems to control motor output?
   4. What amount of energy are you demanding the client to use when attending to the task? Are you asking the client to attend totally to the specific motoric task, or are you overloading the system to take away some cortical attending?

---

outcomes. We have done that in the past, are doing it in the present, and will continue doing it in the future.

REFERENCES

1. American Occupational Therapy Association: Standards of practice for occupational therapy in schools, *Am J Occup Ther* 34:900-903, 1980.
2. Barr J: Curriculum planning workshop, Midwinter Combined American Physical Therapy Association Sections Meeting, Washington, DC, 1976.
3. Edwards I, Jones M, Carr J et al: Clinical reasoning strategies in physical therapy, *Phys Ther* 84:984-987, 2004.
4. May BJ: An integrated problem-solving curriculum design for physical therapy education, *Phys Ther* 57:807-815, 1977.
5. Neistadt ME: Teaching clinical reasoning as a thinking frame, *Am J Occup Ther* 52:221-229, 1998.
6. Scaffa ME, Wooster DM: Effects of problem-based learning on clinical reasoning in occupational therapy, *Am J Occup Ther* 58:333-336, 2004.
7. Umphred D: Teaching, thinking and treatment planning. Unpublished master's thesis. Boston, 1971, Boston University.
8. Brookhart MA, Solomon DH, Wang P et al: Explained variation in a model of therapeutic decision making is partitioned across patient, physician, and clinic factors, *J Clin Epidemiol* 59:18-25, 2006.
9. Dennis JK: Problem-based learning in online vs face-to-face environments, *Educ Health (Abingdon)* 16:198-209, 2003.
10. Des Marchais JE, Dumais B, Pigeon G: From traditional to problem-based learning: a case report of complete curriculum reform, *Med Educ* 26:190-199, 1992.
11. Foster MA: Family systems theory as a framework for problem solving in pediatric physical therapy, *Pediatr Phys Ther* 3:70-73, 1992.
12. Gulpinar MA, Yegen BC: Interactive lecturing for meaningful learning in large groups, *Med Teach* 27:590-594, 2005.
13. Hayes KW: The effect of awareness of measurement error on physical therapists' confidence in their decisions, *Phys Ther* 72:515-525, 1992.
14. Hayes KW, Sullivan JE, Huber G: Computer-based patient management problems in an entry level physical therapy program, *J Phys Ther Educ* 1:65-71, 1991.
15. Jensen GM, Gwyer J, Shepard KF: Expert practice in physical therapy, *Phys Ther* 80:28-52, 2000.
16. Karasik RJ, Maddox M, Wallingford M: Intergenerational service-learning across levels and disciplines: "one size (does not) fit all," *Gerontol Geriatr Educ* 25:1-17, 2005.
17. Magistro C et al: Diagnosis in physical therapy: a roundtable discussion, *PT Magazine* 1:58-65, 1993.
18. Morris J: How strong is the case for the adoption of problem-based learning in physiotherapy education in the United Kingdom? *Med Teach* 25:24-31, 2003.
19. Norton BJ: Report on colloquium on teaching clinical decision making, *J Phys Ther Educ* 6:58-66, 1992.
20. Saarinen-Rahiika H, Binkley JM: Problem-based learning in physical therapy: a review of the literature and overview of the McMaster University experience, *Phys Ther* 78:195-211, 1998.
21. Schaber PL: Incorporating problem-based learning and video technology in teaching group process in an occupational therapy curriculum, *J Allied Health* 34:110-116, 2005.
22. Schmidt HG: The psychological basis of problem-based learning: a review of the evidence, *Acad Med* 67:557-565, 1992.
23. Stern P, D'Amico FJ: Problem effectiveness in an occupational therapy problem-based learning course, *Am J Occup Ther* 55:455-462, 2001.
24. Weinstein CJ: Movement science: its relevance to physical therapy, *Phys Ther* 70:759-762, 1990.
25. American Physical Therapy Association: Guide to physical therapy practice: second edition, *Phys Ther* 81:9-746, 2001.
26. Bennett S, Hoffmann T, McCluskey A et al: Introducing OTseeker (Occupational Therapy Systematic Evaluation of Evidence): a new evidence database for occupational therapists, *Am J Occup Ther* 57:635-638, 2003.
27. Moyers PA: The guide to occupational therapy practice, *Am J Occup Ther* 53:247-322, 1999.
28. McNerney WJ: The missing link in health services, *J Med Educ* 50:11-23, 1975.
29. Levin L: Forces and issues in the revival of interest in self-care impetus for redirection in health. *Health Educ Monogr* 5:115, 1977.
30. Duggan R: Reflection as a means to foster client-centred practice, *Can J Occup Ther* 72:103-112, 2005.

31. Harkness J: Patient involvement: a vital principle for patient-centered health care, *World Hosp Health Serv* 41:12-16, 40-43, 2005.

32. Law M, Darrah J, Rosenbaum P et al: Family-centred functional therapy for children with cerebral palsy: an emerging practice model, *Phys Occup Ther Pediatr* 18:83-102, 1998.

33. Palisano R: A model of physical therapist practice for children with cerebral palsy: integrating evidence, experience, and family centered services, III STEP 7-day Conference, Salt Lake City, Utah, July 16, 2005.

34. Carlson RJ: Holism and reductionism as perspectives in medicine and patient care, *West J Med* 131:466-470, 1979.

35. Pew Health Professions Commission: *Healthy America: Practitioners for 2005,* San Francisco, 1991, University of California.

36. Hale LA, Piggot J: Exploring the content of physiotherapeutic home-based stroke rehabilitation in New Zealand, *Arch Phys Med Rehabil* 86:1933-1940, 2005.

37. Mayo NE, Wood-Dauphinee S, Cote R et al: Activity, participation, and quality of life 6 months poststroke, *Arch Phys Med Rehabil* 83:1035-1042, 2002.

38. Nagi S: *Some conceptual issues in disability and rehabilitation,* Washington, DC, 1965, American Sociological Association.

39. Nagi S: *Disability concepts revisited: implication for prevention,* Washington, DC, National Academy Press, 1991.

40. Wood P: *International classification of impairments, disabilities and handicaps (ICIDH),* Geneva, Switzerland, 1980, World Health Organization.

41. World Health Organization: *The international classification of functioning, disability and health (ICF),* Geneva Switzerland, 2001, World Health Organization.

42. Schneidert M, Hurst R, Miller J et al: The role of environment in the international classification of functioning, disability and health (ICF), *Disabil Rehabil* 25:588-595, 2003.

43. Umphred D, Dewane J, Hall N, Roller M, Ryerson S, Winkler P: RMU model for neurological rehabilitation, Provo, Utah, 2001.

44. *Education standard for occupational therapy.* Bethesda, Maryland, Accreditation Council of Occupational Therapy Education 2006.

45. Commission on Accreditation in Physical Therapy Education: *Evaluative criteria for accreditation of education programs for the preparation of physical therapists,* Alexandria, Virginia, 2005, American Physical Therapy Association.

46. *A guide to physical therapist practice,* 2nd ed, Alexandria, VA, 2001, American Physical Therapy Association.

47. *Normative model of physical therapist professional education: version 2004,* Alexandria, VA, 2004, American Physical Therapy Association.

48. Byl NN, Duncan MS, Lewton DA et al: Characteristics of physician referrals to physical therapists, JSOPTA, unpublished.

49. Moore JC: The limbic system. Workshop presented in San Francisco, February 1980.

50. Moore JC: Neuroanatomical structures subserving learning and memory, San Diego, 1987, Fifteenth Annual Sensorimotor Integration Symposium.

51. Cronback LJ, Snow RE: *Aptitudes and instructional methods,* New York, 1977, Irvington.

52. Fauley JF, Bradley DF, Pauley JA et al: *Here's how to reach me: matching instruction to personality types in your classroom,* Baltimore, MD, 2002, Brookes Publishing Co. Inc.

53. Hunt DE: Matching models in education, Ontario Institute for Students in Education Monograph Series No. 10, Toronto, Ontario, 1974.

54. Rogers C: A humanistic concept of man. In Farsom R, editor: *Science and human affairs,* Palo Alto, CA, 1965, Science and Behavior Books.

55. Bertakis K: The communication of information from physician to patient: a method for increasing patient practice, *J Fam Pract* 5:217-222, 1977.

56. Payton OD: *Patient participation in program planning: a manual for therapists,* Philadelphia, 1990, FA Davis.

57. Becker M, Maiman L: Sociobehavioral determinants of compliance with health and medical care recommendation, *Med Care* 13:10-24, 1975.

58. Freymann JG: Medicine's great schism, prevention vs. cure: an historical interpretation, *Med Care* 13:525-536, 1975.

59. McKay S: Holistic health care: challenge to providers, *J Allied Health* 9:194-201, 1980.

60. Saward E, Sorenson A: The current emphasis on preventive medicine, *Science* 200:889-894, 1978.

61. Szasz TS, Hollender MH: A contribution to the philosophy of medicine, *Arch Intern Med* 97:585-592, 1956.

62. Fink D: Holistic health: The evolution of western medicine. In Flynn P, editor: *The healing continuum,* Bowie, MD, 1980, Robert J. Brady.

63. Leopold RL: Patient-therapist relationship: psychological considerations, *Phys Ther* 34:8-13, 1954.

64. Pratt JW: A psychological view of the physiotherapist's role, *Physiotherapy* 64:241-242, 1978.

65. Sasano E et al: The family in physical therapy, *JAPTA* 57:153-159, 1977.

66. Singleton M: Profession—a paradox? *JAPTA* 60:439, 1980.

67. Alexander DA: Yes, but what about the patient? *Physiotherapy* 59:391-394, 1973.

CHAPTER 2

Motor Development Across the Life Span

Dale L. Scalise-Smith, PhD, PT
Darcy A. Umphred, PT, PhD, FAPTA

KEY WORDS

abnormal movement strategies
developmental theory
normal movement strategies
stages of motor development
systems theory

OBJECTIVES

After reading this chapter the reader will be able to:
1. Analyze the complexity and interlocking nature of human development over a lifetime.
2. Differentiate traditional theories of development from a systems theory.
3. Analyze the differences between various subsystems within the human organism.
4. Identify elements of physiological changes over a lifetime.
5. Analyze normal movement strategies and identify subsystems responsibility for success of a motor task.
6. Identify normal changes in motor strategies over a lifetime and analyze differences between normal movement as one ages and pathological movement problems.

As physical and occupational therapists assume greater roles in primary care of patients/clients, they recognize the importance of approaching an individual using a multifactorial approach. To competently evaluate functional movement across the life span, clinicians must possess knowledge and skills in the development of skilled, refined movement across domains. Only then will therapists be prepared to perform the necessary evaluative and diagnostic testing and effectively develop and implement plans of care aimed at minimizing impairments, maintaining or regaining functional skills, and improving quality of life.

Throughout much of the twentieth century, developmental researchers were heavily focused on skill acquisition from infancy through early childhood.[1-3] In the 1970s, as research paradigms directed at motor development and motor learning evolved, it became evident that changes in motor skills were not limited to childhood but occurred throughout the life span. Consequently, the concept of life span development came to incorporate the prenatal period through older adulthood.

During infancy (birth to 1 year) and childhood (1 year to 10 years) acquisition of motor skills coupled with cognitive and perceptual development are the primary foci of developmental researchers and clinicians. As the young child transitions to adolescence (11-19 years) and has the opportunity to experience motor behaviors across different environmental contexts, more complex behaviors emerge. Adulthood (20-59 years) signals a period when skills are refined and motor behaviors mature. Only through practice and repetition are skills attained and retained. Individuals who continue to use motor learning strategies into late adulthood (60 years through death), often report more successful aging than those who do not engage in such motor skills.[4]

Identifying mechanisms that enable individuals to be successful in acquisition and retention of functional motor behaviors is critical to examining variables that alter or impair these same behaviors in other individuals. Kandel et al[5] suggested that "the task of neural science is to understand the mental processes by which we perceive, act, learn, and remember" (p. 3). This view supports the interactive and collaborative nature of intrinsic and extrinsic systems to accomplish motor learning tasks.

Given the interactive nature of different subsystems, it would seem most effective for clinicians to recognize the need for implementing a multidimensional approach when devising intervention programs. To discuss the interactive nature of these issues, this chapter will (1) briefly provide a historical perspective of theories of motor development, (2) discuss domains (cognition, memory, perception, etc.) associated with life span motor development from prenatal development through older adulthood, (3) discuss the impact of various body systems on motor skill acquisition, and (4) describe behavioral changes that may both positively or negatively influence motor performance across the life span.

With the focus of this book on neurological rehabilitation, it is imperative to incorporate the complex and interactive nature of the physiological, cognitive, and perceptual systems. Although readers can read about movement development across the life span, it will not integrate into clinical practice until the therapist understands the movements of the patients and how those movements reflect the summation of systems interacting to allow that individual to express movement, whether that be as a functional task, a written script, or the use of verbal language. Often without that link between identified movement and motor control expressing that movement, the therapist will miss critical clues to the analysis of the central nervous system (CNS) of the client and how best to provide an environment that provides the opportunity for that individual to improve functional skills and quality of life. For that reason, figures have been inserted to help the reader understand the differences between movement patterns across the life span.

THEORIES OF DEVELOPMENT

Development is often portrayed as a series of "stages" through which an infant progresses, with a fixed order to the sequence.[6] A developmental theory may be characterized as a systematic statement of principles and generalizations that provides a coherent framework for studying development. Historically, development was thought to be linear, occurring in an invariant sequence and resulting in behavioral changes that are direct reflections of the maturation of anatomical and physiological systems.[7,8] Development is generally examined in terms of quantitative and qualitative change. Although it is universally accepted that acquisition of developmental skills are not reversible, the underlying principles surrounding the emergence of these behaviors has evolved over the past 50 to 75 years.

Early developmental theorists used neuromaturational models of CNS organization as the framework for conceptualizing development.[1,2] These researchers provided elaborate descriptions of posture acquisition and a blueprint delineating skill development. Research focused on the emergence of cognitive and affective behaviors and ignored the processes and mechanisms involved in acquiring motor skills.[9] Several investigators attributed developmental changes to intrinsic variables such as maturation of the CNS, whereas others associated changes with extrinsic variables involving the environment.[1,2,10,11]

During the 1930s and 1940s, Arnold Gesell and Myrtle McGraw led a cadre of trailblazing researchers exploring the field of infant motor development. Gesell[1,12] described the normative time frame for when behaviors emerge and McGraw[2] examined the underlying mechanisms responsible for the emergence of these behaviors. The underlying premise, the foundation for their elaborate descriptions of motor development, was based on maturational processes in the CNS.

Gesell, a pioneer in developmental research, was a proponent of the theory that nature drives development.[13] He proposed that growth is a process so complicated and so sensitive that intrinsic factors are solely responsible for influencing development. He used the evolutional thinking of Darwin and Coghill to explain changes in motor behaviors. Coghill,[14] in his work with salamander embryos, reported that motor behaviors, like swimming, emerge in an orderly sequence as connections of specific neural structures appear. Coghill concluded from his observations of emergence of behaviors in the salamanders that human infant motor behaviors appear in a predictable sequence and at predictable chronological ages.

With Coghill's research as the foundation for his thinking, Gesell embraced the concept of a hierarchical organization of the CNS. He believed that the emergence of motor behaviors was contingent on maturation in the CNS and concluded that only after the emergence of higher level neural structures would complex motor behaviors appear. Within this constrained theoretical perspective, extrinsic or environmental stimuli, human or otherwise, were thought to have little impact on the appearance of motor behaviors. Gesell concluded that infant development is preprogrammed and appears at predetermined stages or periods in time.[13] Perhaps his greatest contribution to motor development was

the conceptualization of milestones as markers to evaluate infant behavior.

Although McGraw was a proponent of ontogenic development as one variable influencing motor development, she did not believe, as Gesell did, that it was the sole determinant.[15] Rather, McGraw attempted to explain the emergence of motor behaviors through environmental influences as well as CNS maturation.[2] She examined the temporal and qualitative aspects of motor skill acquisition through her study of Jimmy and Johnny,[16] a study of twin brothers in which one twin was provided an exercise program and no intervention was afforded to the other twin. She found temporal and qualitative differences in the boys' acquisition of motor skills and attributed differences in acquisition of these behaviors to disparities in practice opportunities.

McGraw believed that the acquisition of the movement (process) is as important as when the (chronological time frame) behavior is acquired (the outcome). She further elaborated that, within the constraints imposed by the developing CNS, a rich and challenging environment can and does facilitate temporal efficiency in acquisition of motor behaviors. And finally, she proposed that practicing motor skills influences emergence of the same behavior.

Sufficient evidence exists to support the idea that some predetermined processes occur at relatively similar points in development, but not all motor behaviors emerge at the same biological, chronological, or psychological age in every individual. Although motor milestones provide information regarding outcome, no information can be derived about the process of attaining motor skills from those specific milestones. Perhaps a more realistic explanation may be that emergence of new skills occurs out of a need to solve specific problems within the environment. Working within this context, it is evident that traditional theories of development and maturation fail to adequately encapsulate the innate variability in human development.[9,10]

More recently, researchers have used more current theories of development when designing studies involving infants and young children.[17-19] These investigators examined the process of skill acquisition rather than using traditional methods that assess outcome as a measure of motor development.[20]

Although early pioneers in developmental research described development as linear, uniform, and sequential, Thelan and Smith[21] depict development as "messy," "fluid," and context-sensitive. They also suggested that elements of a behavior may be evident before the task as a whole.

Thelan and Smith[21] suggested that, although traditional theories of development support the premise that behaviors emerge in accordance with a relatively fixed temporal sequence, an organism may exhibit presocial abilities when the context is altered and the demands of the system increased. These authors stated that immature systems exhibit behaviors that are variable and easily disrupted. Although development of some organisms in a controlled laboratory environment may reflect more traditional perceptions of development, outside, in a more naturalistic environment, development is more likely to be flexible, fluid, and tentative. Thelan and Smith also found that factors most likely to have an impact on performance are the "immediacy of the situation" and the "task at hand" rather than "rules" of the performance. Given this perspective, Thelan and Smith[21] identified six goals as essential to developmental theory. These goals are as follows:

1. "To understand the origins of novelty.
2. To reconcile global regularities with local variability, complexity, and context-specificity.
3. To integrate developmental data at many levels of explanation.
4. To improve a biologically plausible yet non-reductionist account of the development of behavior.
5. To understand how local processes lead to global outcomes.
6. To establish a theoretical basis for generating and interpreting empirical research"[21] (p. xviii).

Thelan and Smith urged developmental researchers to devise paradigms that attempt to explain development in terms of diversity, flexibility, asynchrony, and "the ability of even young organisms to reorganize their behavior around context and task" (p. 18).[21]

They suggested that behaviors are complex, interactive, cooperative, and capable of organizing and regrouping around task and context, rather than a rigid structure and rule-driven hierarchy, as many earlier cognitive researchers believed. These contemporary theorists inferred that developmental changes are nonlinear and emergent and may be the result of the interactive effects of intrinsic and extrinsic variables. This divergence from traditional thinking compelled avant-garde scholars to propose new theories.[21,22] One such theory of development, the systems theory, may more adequately account for changes in development than traditional theories identified previously described.

GENERAL SYSTEMS THEORY

Systems theory was first described by Bertalanffy in 1936 but not discussed in great detail until 1948. In 1954 Bertalanffy and colleagues from three other professions met to discuss systems movement.[23] Theorists then applied systems theory to a variety of human and nonhuman systems. As theorists became acquainted with systems theory, they became more receptive to alternate theoretical proposals of growth and development in living organisms.

Systems theory is defined as a transdisciplinary field examining relationships of structures as a whole.[24] "The notion of a system may be seen as simply a more self-conscious and generic term for the dynamic interrelatedness of components."[24] He proposed this theory to more adequately describe biological systems, investigate principles common to all complex organisms, and develop models that can be used to describe them.

Principles that embody general systems theory include nonsummative wholeness, self-regulation, equifinality, and self-organization.[24] Contrary to systems theory in disciplines such as physics where systems are said to be closed, Bertalanffy suggested that biological systems are open and modifiable and that changes in the system are the result of the dynamic interplay among elements of the system.

Embedded in the general systems theory is nonlinear dynamics, where behaviors are not described as the sum of their parts. Thus within a nonlinear dynamic systems theory, a mathematical description of a variety of systems evolves.[25] In this theory, systems may change in a sudden, discontinuous fashion. During development a small increase or decrease in a control parameter causes the system to change. This abrupt change, identified as a bifurcation, causes the system to move out of its previous state and toward a new state of being.

Scott[26] defined periods of rapid differentiation or change during development when an organism is most easily altered or modified as "critical periods." Physiological systems are most vulnerable during these periods and may be seriously affected by both intrinsic and extrinsic factors acting on the system. These periods occur at different times for different systems throughout the body. Understanding systems theory and the concept of critical periods is crucial to all aspects of motor development.

As scientists began to revisit theories of motor development, they discarded some of the traditional theories and embraced the concepts of general systems theory.[25] Proponents of systems theory contend that modifications in motor behaviors are the result of dynamic interactions among the musculoskeletal, peripheral and central neuromuscular, cardiovascular and pulmonary, and cognitive/emotional systems.[24] These interactive, multidimensional elements are vulnerable to changes in organizational and behavioral abilities (system) over time.[26,27] These theorists propose that, as skills are acquired and organizational or behavioral changes occur, the system is driven to identify the most efficient and effective strategy to produce motor behavior(s).

Implicit in systems theory is the concept of critical periods in development.[26-28] Critical periods are based on the premise that organisms are most easily altered or modified during period(s) of most rapid differentiation or change. Investigators suggested that interventions imposed during a critical period may more easily positively or negatively modify the behavior. Recognizing the crucial role systems theory and critical periods play in development is vital to comprehending how developmental skills emerge. The multifactorial nature of a systems theory illustrates the complexity of development and the difficulty in identifying the appropriate variables that influence motor skill development.

With use of concepts previously described, it is reasonable to expect that a small change in any subsystem may result in a large change in a motor behavior. This is evident in work by Thelan and colleagues examining stepping in infants eight weeks of age.[27-31] They reported that introducing a small change in one element of the system, identified as a small weight applied to an infant's leg, resulted in the infant being unable to step. The authors deduced that small changes in one subsystem, in this case the musculoskeletal system, may result in a change in the outcome. This lends support to the hypothesis that modifying one aspect of a multicomponent system, especially during a critical period, may evolve into an entirely new behavior.

Periods of rapid differentiation, although often observed during early life, have also been observed across the life span. Changes in anthropometric measures, such as weight gain during pregnancy, influence coordination between limbs and emergence as a different gait pattern. Changes in one system, in this case the endocrine system, result in increased ligamentous laxity at the pelvis and also contribute to gait alterations.

Menopause may for women be another critical period. During menopause, decreases in hormone production are thought to lead to osteoporosis and cardiac disease.[32] Examples described previously provide evidence across the lifespan that the dynamic interplay within a system and between systems may significantly influence emergence and disappearance of behaviors.

Although research in the beginning of the twentieth century was heavily focused on development of the very young, studies during the latter part of the century were directed toward research on aging. Technological advances in medicine have dramatically increased life expectancies. During the twentieth century, the number of individuals in the United States more than 65 years old grew from 3 million to 35 million.[33] Perhaps the most significant statistic is that the **oldest** grew from 100,000 in 1900 to 4.2 million in 2000.[33] By 2011, the Baby Boomer generation will begin turning 65 years old and the number of older individuals will increase sharply between 2010 and 2030.[33] By 2030, Americans over the age of 65 years will represent nearly 20% of the population and by 2050 the number of individuals over the age of 85 years could grow to 21 million.[33] Given this incredible demographic transformation and that current policymakers are, in large part, the generation directly affected by these statistics, a significant paradigm shift in funded research has evolved over the past quarter century. "As such, aging and death are inseparable partners to growth and development"[34] (p. 32). When it is recognized that a critical mass of Americans are entering older adulthood, it is imperative when referring to aging that terminology be applied consistently.

Biological and Chronological Age

Age can be referred to in terms of chronological age and biological age.[35] Chronological age is the period of time that a person has been alive, beginning at birth. In infants it is measured in days, weeks, or months, whereas in adults it is expressed in terms of years and at times decades.

Although chronological age is measured in terms of temporal sequencing, biological age is more related to function and physiological aging of organ systems.[36] For example, a triathlete may have biologically younger cardiovascular and pulmonary systems than same-age peers who do not perform high-level aerobic activities. Another example might be a child who underwent precocious puberty. Precocious puberty, identified as puberty earlier than 8 years of age in girls and 9.5 years in boys, results in acceleration in a biological system before same-chronological-age peers.[37] Physiological changes include elevated hormonal levels that would then stimulate development of breast tissue and early menstruation in girls. Changes in the musculoskeletal system include early closure of the epiphyseal plates, resulting in significantly smaller stature. Conversely, these young women's reproductive cycles are significantly skewed. Women would also have menopause and aging issues associated with hormonal changes earlier than other women of the same chronological age. Although no consistent method has been established for measuring biological age, there is general agreement that a wide variability of biological aging exists and that a number of factors contribute to accelerated or decelerated biological aging.

Aging

"Aging refers to the time-sequential deterioration that occurs in most animals including weakness, increased susceptibility to disease and adverse environmental conditions, loss of mobility and agility, and age-related physiological changes" (p. 9).[38] Although Goldsmith's description of aging is typically viewed as an inevitable fact of life, there is scientific evidence and theoretical support for the idea that age-related changes will eventually be more medically treatable than previously thought.[35,38,39]

Scientists are hesitant to attribute a decline in functional movement in older adults to a decline in physiological systems or to diminished opportunities for practice or conditioning.[4] Rowe and Kahn reported that "with advancing age the relative contribution of genetic factors decreases and the nongenetic factors increases" (p. 446).[4] Age-related factors that are modifiable may be used to identify individuals who may or may not age successfully. For instance, lifestyle choices, including diet, physical activity, and other health habits, and behavioral and social factors have a potent effect and accelerate or decelerate aging.

Factors associated with aging are generally identified as either age related or age dependent. Age-dependent changes within organ systems are observed in individuals at a similar age, whereas age-related changes may be accelerated or decelerated in same-age individuals on the basis of intrinsic or extrinsic factors related to lifestyle. Just as variables associated with lifestyle (extrinsic factors) influences aging, genetics (intrinsic factors) also play a significant role. From a genetic perspective, structural and functional changes are generally thought to be a consequence of aging and are, therefore, predictable and consistent across physiological systems. Variables thought to influence the genetic potential for longevity include environmental factors such as toxins, radiation, and oxygen free radicals. Free radicals are highly reactive molecules produced as cells turn food and oxygen into energy.[40] In summary, the use of biological age rather than chronological age may be a more accurate reflection of an individual's true age.

Theories of Aging

Throughout the twentieth century, the average life expectancy of individuals living in the United States increased. The second half of the twentieth century signaled a shift in the focus of human development research, from infant and child development to older adult development.

Scientists view aging as a progressive accumulation of changes over time that increases the probability of disease and death.[41] Given that portrayal of aging, researchers have proposed a myriad of hypotheses regarding aging. Aging theories evolved because there is no single factor or mechanism responsible for physiological aging.[35] Biological aging theories, similar to developmental theories, are attributed to complex, underlying mechanisms.[35,38,39,42] Although theorists attempt to classify aging theories, these theories are rarely mutually exclusive. Some theories were formulated around control of physiological functioning, others around cellular changes, and still others around genetic causes.

Neuroendocrine theory is based on the premise that hormones play a significant role in aging.[39,42] Hormones are vital to repairing and regulating bodily functions. Hormone production decreases significantly during aging and limits the body's ability to repair and regulate itself as effectively. Although hormonal decline is one plausible explanation for age-related changes, it does not account for all changes. Harman[43] proposed the free radical theory on the basis of his investigations that examined the effects of radioactive materials on human tissue.

Harman reported that when human tissue is exposed to radiation a byproduct is formed. He identified the byproduct, an unstable compound, as a free radical. Over time, human tissue with free radicals showed evidence of biological defects consistent with accelerated aging. Harman postulated that accumulation of free radicals in human tissue may also occur as a part of the normal aging process. This became known as the Free Radical Theory of Aging.[43-45]

Free radicals are highly reactive molecules that damage proteins, lipids, and deoxyribonucleic acid (DNA). In some instances the free radicals combine with enzymes and turn into water and a harmless form of oxygen that moves harmlessly through the cells.[44] In other instances the oxygen binds with intrinsic or extrinsic sources that influence the aging process.

Scientists have suggested several different ways that free radicals influence aging through intrinsic and extrinsic mechanisms.[44,45] An example of an intrinsic mechanism would be chronic infections that extend phagocytic activity and expose tissues to oxidants, creating cumulative oxidative changes in collagen and elastin. Extrinsic sources of free radicals include environmental toxins, for example, industrial waste and cigarette smoke.

Human exposure to intrinsic and extrinsic free radicals causes large numbers of reactive oxygen molecules to interact with DNA and lead to mutations thought to be the cause of a variety of diseases, including cancer, atherosclerosis, amyloidosis, age-related immune deficiency, senile dementia, and hypertension. Although some scientists suggest that aging has many factors that can accelerate or decelerate the process, other scientists suggest a much simpler, preprogrammed theory, known as the Hayflick limit.[35,44-46]

Hayflick and Moorehead[46,47] proposed that there is a finite number of times that a normal cell is capable of dividing. Current thinking is that cells are capable of dividing up to 50 times. Cell division is recognized as one way in which cells age and, after attaining the maximum number of divisions, finally die.

The factor thought to limit a cell's ability to divide infinitely is the presence of telomeres. Telomeres are minute units at the end of the DNA chain.[46] Each time a cell divides a small amount of the telomere is used in the process. Eventually, when cells have exhausted the supply of telomeres available, the cell is unable to divide and cell death ensues.

Telomerase, a substance that can lengthen telomeres, is available in human cells. Typically, telomerase is switched off in all cells except the reproductive cells. The availability of telomerase in reproductive cells allows for many more divisions than previously observed in the Hayflick limit. In addition to the presence of telomerase in reproductive cells, scientists have also discovered that telomerase remains active in cancer cells. Both reproductive and cancer cells divide well beyond the 50-division limit. Consequently, scientists are now working toward activating telomerase in all cells to slow or stop aging. If scientists are successful in activating telomerase in other cells, it may stimulate skin cell regrowth for burn patients and cure diseases that result from failure of aging cells to divide, as in macular degeneration or Hutchinson-Guilford progeria syndrome.[48,49] The downside of this is that scientists may have a difficult time controlling the telomerase and in fact may see more uncontrolled cell growth—cancer—one of the greatest threats to prolonged existence.

Although many of aging theories are directed at mechanisms that negatively influence aging, other theories are focused on factors that have a positive impact on aging processes. One such process is the caloric restriction theory.[43-46,50] Liang et al,[50] with use of several genetic mice models, investigated the impact of dietary control on the life span. The authors reported that the mice did, in fact, have their life spans extended when their dietary intake was controlled. Although these findings are potentially significant, given the small sample size and model examined, these data were not generalizable to all species. The researchers suggested that these preliminary data provide a foundation for scientists to examine whether dietary control will extend the life span in humans as it did in the mice models.

Although a large body of literature exists examining the underlying mechanisms associated with aging, it seems inconceivable that any one mechanism is responsible for age-related changes. More likely is that aging may be attributed to multiple factors, including lifestyle choices, in combination with the physiological and environmental factors.[51] Garilov and Gavrilova[51] conducted an exhaustive review of aging theories and concluded that additional research is necessary to further elaborate and validate existing aging theories and dispel unlikely theories.

In summary, scientists are unsure how much of the decline in motor behaviors, in older adults, is credited to true decline in physiological systems, how much is attributed to expected decline, and finally what percentage is due to decreased practice or conditioning.[52-54] This suggests that physical or occupational therapy intervention may provide older adults with strategies to positively influence successful aging, not only intervene after a negative outcome of aging is realized or a neurological insult has occurred.

The exogenous and endogenous variables of aging are thought to be interrelated and provide an expansive description of the deleterious changes at the cellular, organ, and systems level that accompany both aging and many age-associated diseases. The accumulation of damage is in DNA, proteins, membranes, and organelles, as well as the formation of insoluble protein aggregates. Many organ systems, such as the cardiovascular system, the brain, and the eye, are not programmed for indefinite survival. Consequently, the inability to maintain the integrity of tissues and organs is the end result of the multidimensional aspect of aging.

Physiological Changes in Body Systems Across the Life Span

Organ systems undergo critical physiological changes across the life span. These alterations are observed most often during periods of rapid differentiation. Applying concepts of dynamic systems theory to life span development may help to explain how small changes in biologic systems have a significant impact on the individual as a whole.

Examining interactions among variables within different body systems may provide insight into when one system may play a greater or lesser role in acquisition, retention, or deterioration of functional motor behaviors. The next section will examine how different systems develop and their contribution to functional movement.

Musculoskeletal System

Structural and functional adaptations in the musculoskeletal system are evident across the life span. The musculoskeletal system provides a structural framework for the body to move and serves as protection for the internal organs.

Skeletal muscle tissue first appears during the fifth week of embryonic development and continues into adulthood.[55,56] During this early period of embryonic development, the differentiation of musculoskeletal system is rapid: during the fifth week of embryonic life the limb buds appear, by the seventh week muscle tissue is present in the limbs, and limb movements emerge as early as the eighth week of prenatal life.[37,55,57]

Although many of the structural aspects of the musculoskeletal system are formed prenatally, muscle and bone continue to grow into adulthood. Although considerable variability exists among young children between the ages 5 months through 3 years, the rate of growth of muscle tissue is reportedly two times faster than that of bone.[58]

Structural and functional differences in the musculoskeletal system of a child compared with that of an adult are attributed to the presence and predominance of muscle fiber types. For example, infant muscles are composed predominantly of type I (slow-twitch) fibers, whereas adult muscles contain types I and II (fast-twitch) fibers. Behaviorally, infant movements are characterized predominantly by postural movements. The capacity to produce a greater repertoire of movements, including rapid or ballistic movements, emerges later in development.

Distinct differences also exist in temporal differentiation of the muscular systems of males and females of the same chronological age. Through adolescence, boys show evidence of a significantly greater increase in fiber size compared with girls.[59] Additionally, differences exist in the age at which the number of muscle fibers dramatically increases. Girls reportedly have a steady increase in the muscle fibers between 3.5 and 10 years of age. In contrast, boys have two periods of rapid differentiation in the number of muscle fibers. The first period occurs from birth until 2 years of age and the second between ages 10 and 16 years.[59] Although the pace slows considerably, muscle fiber development continues in men and women well into middle adulthood.

Age-related changes evident in the musculoskeletal system include decreased fiber size, loss of muscle mass, denervation of muscle fibers, decline of total muscle fiber number, and decreased quantity of fast-twitch fibers.[60-62] Muscle mass decreases beginning around age 50 years, and by age 80 years up to 40% of muscle mass is lost.[63] Muscle force production likewise decreases at a rate of about 30% between 60 and 90 years of age. Additional musculoskeletal changes documented in older adults include decreased tensile strength in bone, reduced joint flexibility, and limited speed of movement. Decreased muscle mass in a person more than 60 years old may be attributed to decreased size, fewer type II muscle fibers, and an increase in fat infiltration into the muscle tissue.[64,65] Clinically these factors present as reduced muscle force production during high-velocity movements.

Currently, scientists are examining the premise that, as an individual ages, muscular changes are more likely attributed to decreased motor activity levels and are age-related, rather than those changes being solely age dependent.[61,64] Acknowledging that investigators had previously found that muscle power deteriorates more quickly with age, scientists set out to measure training effects in older adults.[54,66] These investigators concluded that with training, older adults were capable of improving strength, power, and endurance.

The skeletal system develops similarly to the muscular system, exhibiting periods of growth, stability, and degeneration. The immature skeletal system is composed primarily of preosseous cartilage and physes (growth plates).[67] More simply, bone in infants and young children is flexible, porous (lower mineral count), and strong with a thick periosteum.[67,68] Given these properties of immature bone, a child is less likely to have a fracture because the periosteum is strong and, consequently, the bones absorb more energy before the break point is reached. Additionally, if a fracture does occur, healing is usually quicker because callous is formed faster and in greater amounts in children than in adults.

A primary difference between the child's and the adult's skeletal systems is the presence of the growth plate complex in children. Whereas primary ossification occurs prenatally, secondary ossification is not complete until the child reaches skeletal maturity, generally at 14 years in girls and 16 years in boys.[68,69]

Even after bones attain their full length, they continue to grow on the surface. This is termed appositional growth and continues throughout most of life. During childhood and adolescence, new bone growth exceeds bone resorption and bone density increases. Until age 30 years, bone density increases in most individuals and bone growth and reabsorption remain stable through middle adulthood. Later in adulthood, resorption exceeds new bone growth and bone density declines.[70]

Women exhibit more loss of bone mass than men do.[71] Decreased bone density in women is generally attributed to differences in the types and levels of hormones present. Although the difference is most significant during menopause, premenopausal women still lose bone density at a higher rate than their male peers do.

Osteopenia is the presence of a less-than-normal amount of bone and, if not treated, may result in osteoporosis. Progressive loss of bone density, observed into older adulthood, is commonly identified as osteoporosis. Osteoporosis is more common in women than in men and is a major cause of fractures and postural changes in both sexes.[72]

Overall, much of the growth in the musculoskeletal system is related to demands placed on the system. Intrinsic and extrinsic forces imposed on the musculoskeletal systems of typically and atypically developing children may lead to structural and functional differences in their respective skeletal structures. Consequently, temporal sequencing, acquisition, and characteristics of motor behaviors emerge differently in typically and atypically developing children. Similarly, age-related changes in older adulthood may be accelerated in direct proportion to decreased levels of activity.[73] Older adults who maintain more active lifestyles and place greater physical demands on their musculoskeletal systems are more likely to have an improved bone density and muscle mass than their peers who are not as active.[74]

Sarcopenia, the age-related loss of muscle mass, affects strength, power, and functional independence in older adults.[64,74] Although these changes are observed in many older adults, the degree of the muscular changes varies.[62] Researchers examining sarcopenia in older adults reported that men are affected more by sarcopenia than women are.[64,75] In fact, men with sarcopenia present four times the rate of activity limitations than do men with a normal muscle mass. Changes in the cross-sectional area of muscles directly affect the force production of a given muscle; consequently, as the cross-section of a muscle diminishes, its ability to produce force decreases. As an individual ages the number and size of the muscle fibers decrease, resulting in a reduction in strength.[72] Although this is true in all muscles, the impact is greater on muscles of the lower extremities than in those of the upper extremities.[64]

Although strength is critical to musculoskeletal function, flexibility is equally as important. Flexibility incorporates joint motion and the extensibility of the tissues that cross the joint. The degree of flexibility changes across the life span as a direct result of aging and activity level.[10] Changes in flexibility are evident throughout life: limited at birth, increasing until the individual approaches adolescence, and then gradually decreasing. Exceptions may be seen in athletes, dancers, and other individuals involved in activities that incorporate flexibility training. Loss of flexibility as a consequence of age may have a negative impact on functional independence in older adults. Flexibility is thought to be directly proportional to the amount, frequency, and variability of motor activities performed. As activity increases, so does flexibility. Conversely, as individuals exhibit decreased levels of motor activity, often associated with age, flexibility decreases.[70]

By age 70 years, flexibility is thought to decrease by 25% to 30%.[62] Although this appears to be age dependent, it may be more likely that it is age related.[61] Regularly performing exercise directed toward improving strength and flexibility can reverse the effects of inactivity for most individuals, even those older than 90 years of age.[61,73]

Although it may take longer for older individuals to regain strength or flexibility than a young adult or child, musculoskeletal tissue is modifiable throughout life. Modifying the strength and flexibility of an older adult requires that other bodily systems are capable of modifying performance levels to meet the increased needs of the musculoskeletal system.

As scientists continue to examine functional changes across different systems as a consequence of age, physical and occupational therapists must educate individuals regarding the importance of embracing a physically active lifestyle and methods to enhance quality of life at each stage in an individual's life. (See Chapter 6.) Although all systems contribute to an individual's health and wellness across the life span, the cardiovascular and pulmonary systems play a key role. (See Chapter 35.)

Cardiovascular and Pulmonary Systems

The cardiovascular system is composed of the heart, lungs, and associated vascular complex. It is responsible for pumping blood through the coronary, pulmonary, cerebral, and systemic circulations, with the goal of perfusing all bodily tissues for the delivery of oxygen and vital nutrients and picking up waste products for elimination. The pulmonary system is responsible for oxygen transport, gas exchange, and removal of airborne pollutants that may enter during respiration. (See Chapter 35.)

The interdependent nature of the cardiovascular and pulmonary systems is evident in the fact that, each minute, all of the body's blood travels through the lungs before being returned to the left side of the heart for ejection into the systemic circulation.[76] Because of this relationship, changes in heart function can dramatically affect lung function, and vice versa. In addition, these two systems are connected as part of a larger closed-pressure/volume loop through the peripheral circulatory structures. Likewise, any alteration in the function of the peripheral vessels will affect both the heart and lungs, and vice versa.

The function and homeostasis of the cardiovascular, pulmonary, and peripheral vascular systems are influenced by both internal and external forces.[76] Internal mechanisms of control are based on the autonomic nervous system, the relative health of the anatomic structures involved, the growth and development of the structures, and the behavioral/emotional adaptations of a particular individual. All those internal mechanisms are subject to changes with growth and development, aging, and the unique life experiences of an individual. Growth and development primarily affect the physics of the system by altering volumes, lengths, smooth and myocardial muscular tension, and physiological capacitance within the system to support the growing body. Numerous effects of aging have an impact on the adaptability of the system. Behavioral and emotional responses influence both autonomic and volitional cardiovascular and pulmonary reactions to stress. External forces include movement environment and activity level, which alter the gravitational forces on the closed pressure-volume system. An increased activity level causes exercise stress, which requires an altered demand for oxygen and nutrients to the structures providing the work. Finally, emotional stress needs to be considered as an external factor. Behavioral responses to stress can affect functional movement and cause maladaptive coping mechanisms on any or all systems. As with anything, the age, cognitive status, and relative health of an individual will dictate the potential success of these endeavors.

Because oxygen transport and exchange is the primary requirement for sustaining life, efforts toward maximizing the efficiency of the cardiovascular and pulmonary systems represent a fundamental component of therapeutic practice. It is critical that, no matter where a patient falls in the life span, strategies for screening, prevention, and rehabilitation of the cardiovascular and pulmonary systems are incorporated into a comprehensive plan to promote optimal mobility and independence.[77] It is essential for therapists to keep in mind that all interventions have a direct or indirect impact on these systems and that it is their responsibility to monitor and manage those responses to maintain safety.

A detailed understanding of the anatomy of the heart, lungs, and vessels, as well as the physiology and interrelationship of the organs involved, is essential to the practice of both physical and occupational therapy. For pediatric therapists, the added knowledge of normal growth and development of these structures is critical.

Between weeks 3 and 8 of fetal life, the cardiac structures are formed.[55,56,78] All other structures of the cardiovascular system are fully developed and functional shortly after birth. Although the left and right ventricles are of similar size at birth, by 2 months of age the muscle wall of the left ventricle is thicker than the right ventricle.[79] This is attributed to the fact that the left ventricle is responsible for pumping blood to the whole body, requiring a higher internal pressure and contractile force, whereas the right ventricle is responsible for pumping blood only to the lungs, a relatively low-pressure function in a healthy individual.

It bears mentioning that the heart's function begets structure. Therefore, if function becomes impaired, the structure is likely to adaptively change. For example, if the resistance in the vascular system from the right ventricle to the lungs becomes increased, the right ventricle must pump harder, with a greater volume of blood, to overcome the resistance.[80] Over time, this will increase the size of the ventricular walls because the myocardium is muscular tissue that is as equally capable of hypertrophy as skeletal muscle tissue.

Structurally, the heart doubles in size by year 1 and increases fourfold by year 5. Many of the changes associated with size are complete by the time the child has reached maturity. Recall that cardiac output is equal to stroke volume × heart rate. As the size of the heart increases (increasing the volume capacity for each stroke), the heart beat decreases and the blood pressure increases.[81] Heart rate in a newborn infant is generally 120 to 200 beats per minute (bpm), 80 bpm by 6 years of age, and 70 bpm by 10 years.[79,82] Systolic blood pressure (defined as maximal pressure on the artery during left ventricular contraction or systole) is 40 to 75 mm Hg at birth and increases to 95 mm Hg by 5 years of age.[79] Blood pressure continues to rise into adolescence. The capacity to maintain exercise for longer periods and greater intensities increases through early childhood. Although cardiovascular disease is generally associated with adults, children as young as 5 years of age may show signs of or be at risk for cardiovascular disease if they do not engage in regular aerobic activity.[79,83]

Development of the pulmonary system occurs late in prenatal and early postnatal life.[82] As the lungs increase in size, tripling in weight during year 1, the in capacity and efficiency increases while the respiratory rate decreases.[82] Although the vital capacity of a 5-year-old child is 20% of an adult's, this is not usually a limiting factor during exercise.[81] Overall, aerobic capacity increases during childhood and is slightly higher in boys than in girls. The overall work capacity of children increases most dramatically from 6 through 12 years of age.[81] Peak oxygen consumption is achieved early in adulthood and changes in direct relation to activity levels. Lungs of an average adult, at rest, take in about 250 ml of oxygen every minute and excrete about 200 ml of carbon dioxide.[84]

As activity decreases in older adulthood, so do the structural and functional capacities of the cardiovascular and pulmonary systems. Many of these changes are due to decreased elasticity of the tissues, decreased efficiency of the structures, and decreased ability to increase workload. Cardiac output (CO) decreases approximately 0.7% per year

after age 20 years so that by age 75 years the CO is 3.5 L/min, down from 5 L/min at age 20 years.[84] Functional changes include a decrease in the overall maximum heart rate from 200+ bpm through young adulthood to 170 bpm by age 65 years.[79] Older adults have less elastic vessels, and resistance to the blood volume increases. Consequently, older adults reach peak CO at lower levels than do younger individuals. These cardiovascular changes may be compounded by inactivity, resulting in decreased capacity to perform activities that raise metabolic demands and increase the requirement for oxygen transport.[85] The impact of these normal aging responses, however, can be reduced through structured aerobic and anaerobic activities. Conversely, physiological performance of the cardiovascular and pulmonary systems improves in response to growth and development.

Throughout life, performance of motor activities and activities of daily living (ADLs) is highly dependent on the integrity of an individual's cardiopulmonary and cardiovascular systems. Introduction of aerobic activities during early childhood has implications for improved health and wellness across the life span. Although aging has a negative impact on performance and efficiency of the cardiovascular and pulmonary systems, aerobic exercise has a positive impact on these systems. Changes in the cardiovascular and pulmonary systems have a significant impact on other systems and consequently on overall body function. Information from these systems, including blood pressure and oxygen saturation rates, is communicated through the nervous system. The nervous system, in turn, regulates responses of the cardiovascular and pulmonary systems through the autonomic nervous system.

Neurological System

The nervous system encompasses the CNS and the peripheral nervous systems (PNS). The CNS includes the brain and spinal cord, and it is responsible for all bodily functions. The PNS includes both the autonomic and somatic nerves and is responsible for transporting impulses to and from the CNS.[5] The capacity for humans to produce behaviors far beyond those of other animals is directly related to the complex abilities of the CNS and interneuronal communications.

Over the past two decades, technological advances have enabled neuroscientists to dramatically improve their understanding of the molecular changes in the nervous system over time. Development of the CNS is coordinated through intrinsic influences involving the temporal and spatial coordination of synaptic connections with genetic processes, along with extrinsic or environmental factors. Development of the CNS is dependent on precise connections formed between specific types of nerve cells and begins with the recruitment of cells that form the neural plate, which gives rise to the neural tube, and then differentiation of regions of the brain begins.[5] Changes in the nervous system are predicated on critical periods, or times when different regions of the brain are sensitive to change, and occur across the life span.[5,26]

Each region of the brain is thought to undergo critical or sensitive periods at different ages. One of the most critical periods in development of the CNS occurs from birth through 1 year of age. During this period, when the system is most vulnerable to change, intrinsic and extrinsic variables may influence the nervous system, structurally and functionally.

Differentiation of cells in the nervous system begins during the embryonic period and continues through adulthood.[5] Development of the nervous system during embryonic life involves the overproduction of glial cells and neurons that, after they are no longer useful, die. Additional developmental changes noted in the nervous system include increased myelination within the brain and an increase in neuronal size.[55] Much of the growth may be attributed to these changes in the nervous system and may account for the infant's brain development increasing to one half the size of the adult brain during the first year of life. Structural changes documented early in development may emerge out of a need to solve problems (tasks). Changes in neuronal structures continue to evolve as more complex problems are encountered.

Decline of the nervous system begins generally after age 30 years. Decline is noted in the death of thousands of neurons and in the decreased weight of the brain. Structural changes include a decrease in the number of corticospinal fibers, intracortical inhibition, and neuronal degradation in centers in the CNS, particularly the cerebellum and basal ganglia.[86] Loss of neurons in the centers controlling sensory information, long-term memory, abstract reasoning, and coordination of sensorimotor information negatively affect function. For some individuals this may not have significant implications. For others, CNS changes create serious functional losses. Alterations in the CNS, including altered neural control and decreased efficiency in temporal sequencing of muscle synergies, may play a role in postural instability and impaired sensation. Together these changes can result in falls.[60]

Although the CNS, similar to other bodily systems, may have the capacity to compensate for some age-related changes, the degree of compensation may be modulated by the complexity of the task. Investigators have reported that neuromuscular systems in older adults may not be as flexible as systems in younger adults. Neither are neuromuscular systems in older adults as capable of rapidly reorganizing muscle synergies to produce variable functional responses.[86] The researchers did say that this may not be solely related to the aging neurological system but to other factors including experience, cardiovascular and musculoskeletal fitness, and current level of functional independence. Other scientists suggested an alternative view that repetition of motor activities may stimulate new growth in dendrites located proximal to neurons previously lost.[60] The authors were quick to add that, although the pathways or connections may be activated, this may or may not result in improved functional ability. Implicit in performance of many functional activities is cognition. If changes in cognition coexist with changes in other systems, it may be difficult to accurately interpret the underlying causes.

Cognitive System

Cognition may be defined as awareness, perception, reasoning, and judgment.[87] Cognitive development involves processes of perception, action, attention, problem-solving, memory, and mental imagery. Action, from the perspective of physical or occupational therapy, may be referred to as functional movement(s) and incorporates all the processes described previously to successfully perform a specific task.

Jean Piaget, one of the most recognized scientists in developmental psychology of the twentieth century, was particularly intrigued with the how biological systems affect what individuals "know."[87,88] He observed interactions between children of different ages and hypothesized that younger children's thought processes were different from those of older children as evidenced through the differences in responses between them to the same questions.

Piaget proposed that cognitive development moved in a linear, stagelike progression, each stage of which involves radically different schemes.[88] He suggested four stages of cognitive development, identified as sensorimotor state (infancy), preoperational (toddler and early childhood), concrete operational (childhood and early adolescence), and formal operational (adolescence and adulthood).[87] He proposed that (1) sensorimotor behaviors stimulate cognitive development and (2) problem solving as a measure of cognition enables infants and young children to identify and modify motor behaviors.

Piaget's theory of cognitive development focused around how humans adapt within the environment and how these adaptations or behaviors are controlled.[88] He postulated that behavioral control is mediated through schemas or plans, generated centrally. These schemas provide a representation of the world in an effort to formulate an action plan. At birth, infants' earliest schemas were organized around reflexive behaviors that are modified as the infant adapts to the affordances and constraints of the environment.

Piaget suggested that adaptations occur through two processes: assimilation and accommodation.[88] He refers to assimilation as a process of altering the environment around cognitive structures. An example of assimilation is when an infant, initially breast-fed, is transitioned to bottle feeding. Accommodation refers to changes of the cognitive structures to meet changing demands of the environment. Accommodation may be involved when an infant transitions from nutritive (breast/bottle) to nonnutritive sucking (pacifier).

Much of Piaget's work was based on descriptive case studies. Although some aspects of his theory were supported by subsequent studies, other aspects of his work have not been shown to have empirical evidence. The inconsistencies of research findings examining Piaget's stages of development may be indicative of the dynamic and nonlinear nature of development and, more specifically, cognition.

Rather than postulating that infants are reflexive beings with little or no volitional movements early on, it may be more appropriate to view infants as competent beings with volitional and complex behaviors present at birth.[89] Brazelton[89] reported that newborn infants will turn toward their mother's voice rather than toward an unfamiliar voice. Additionally, research conducted by Meltzoff and Moore[90] provides evidence supporting the complex nature of infant behavior. They found that infants as young as 2 to 3 weeks of age can imitate facial gestures performed by adults. Their work was supported by subsequent studies performed by independent investigators using different procedures and in different environments.[91] These findings, contrary to Piaget's proposal that infants were not capable of imitative behaviors until 1 year of age, provided scientists with a new perspective on infant behavior.

Contemporary researchers approach developmental theory from a dynamic and nonlinear model.[21,92] Current thinking is that the cognitive system integrates multimodal input to process, interpret, store, and retrieve information as a mechanism for information processing and problem solving.[87] Changes in cognition, defined as relatively permanent changes in behavior, cannot be measured directly but rather must be inferred from changes observed across multiple systems.

As infants' ability to act on the environment develops, their ability to accurately detect and process relevant information becomes more efficient, lending support to the interdependence of the motor, cognitive, and perceptual systems.

Information processing, defined as the ability to understand human thinking, is a critical factor that must be examined within the cognitive system. Initially, infants and young children cannot recognize relevant cues or chunk information for storage. As children's developing systems become more adept at integrating information from multiple systems and more efficient in processing information, they begin to process relevant information more effectively. Consequently, infants and young children may not use or interpret information as efficiently as older children do.

The integrative nature of movement, cognition, and perception is evident in developmental psychology literature.[93] Given that these domains are interrelated, one area cannot be examined in isolation of other interrelated systems. Acquisition of motor skills is the primary mechanism for evaluating cognition and perception in prelinguistic children. Additionally, as individuals grow older, changes in any system may influence functional movement. Finally, when examining functional movements, therapists must always consider the individual's cognitive and perceptual abilities.

As higher level cognitive processing skills become apparent, the child can accurately identify relevant cues, filter irrelevant cues, and process information more efficiently. By young adulthood, as the individual approaches maturity, optimal cognitive processing becomes apparent.

Humans are continuously pelted with sensory information through some or all of the sensory modalities. At any one time much more sensory information is available than can possibly be processed. Consequently, the individual must learn to select information relevant to the task and chunk the information for processing.

Another example of the multidimensional processes involved in higher-order tasks such as functional movement is found in a study conducted by Hazlett and Woldorff.[94] They proposed that implicit in motor tasks are concepts of cognition including attention, perception, and information processes. This multimethodological approach examined (1) the influence of attention on sensory and perceptual processing, (2) the executive control of attention by higher centers of the brain, and (3) the processes underlying multisensory integration and the mechanisms by which attention interacts with such integration processes.[94]

Throughout the life span, physical growth and development of many systems have an impact on the acquisition and performance of motor skills. Changes in one system and the interactive effects on all other systems can lead to deleterious changes in motor performance as a whole.

A new paradigm that embraces the concept that memory and cognition do not deteriorate as part of normal aging is a topic of discussion in scientific literature.[95] This perspective was proposed after Gould et al[95] conducted a study that found that adult primates continue to develop new brain cells throughout life. The addition of new neocortical neurons throughout adulthood provides a continuum of neurons of different ages that may form a basis for marking the temporal dimension of memory. These late-generated neurons play an important role in learning and memory of older adults.

Changes in cognitive function are often revealed during tasks that require processing and retrieval of cognitive or motor memory. Consequences of aging include slowed information processing and increased time necessary to perform motor skills. Although learning may take more time in older adults, once a behavior is learned, retention is similar to that of younger individuals. Of significance for older adults is delayed performance of long-standing tasks such as driving a car, which may have serious consequences for the driver, passengers, or others in the immediate vicinity of the vehicle. Delays in processing and task execution pose risks to the older adult or individuals with CNS deficits and may affect the individual's level of independence and quality of life.[96]

Although older adults generally have a deterioration in the processing and retrieval of information, the degree of the decline is highly variable. Cognitive deficits most frequently observed in older adults include word retrieval, recall, dual-task execution, and activities involving rapid processing or working memory.

Memory

Memory can be broken down to three types: working, declarative, and procedural. Working memory, short-term memory, is the equivalent of the RAM of a computer.[87] This is the mechanism that enables a child, who does not appear to be attending to what the parent is saying, to repeat what the parent has just said. Given the temporary nature of this memory, no space in the hippocampus or amygdala is required. Working memory may in fact be more of a cortical phenomenon. Declarative memory is what is typically envisioned when we think of intermediate or long-term memory. Declarative memory is the area where long-term information about everything an individual has ever learned or information acquired is stored, including facts, figures, and names.[87] An example of declarative memory is a second-grade teacher recalling the name of a student that she had in her class 15 years previously. Declarative memory is analogous to the hard drive in the computer. The third type of memory is procedural memory. Procedural memory involves all motor activities, actions, habits, or skills that are learned through repetition in motor practice.[87] Examples of procedural memory include walking, playing an instrument, and driving a car.

Rovee-Collier et al[97-99] have conducted numerous studies related to memory retention in prelinguistic children. Evidence exists to support the premise that infants as young as 2 to 3 months of age are capable of identifying relevant cues and chunking this information for later retrieval. One caveat is that retrieval of such information is only possible when the specifics of the behavior are retained. Infant memories are tightly linked to the specific information related to the task, environment, and stimulus. Consequently, a slight change in any of these three components may result in an inability to retrieve information from infant memory. Retention of information is directly proportional to the infant's age. As an infant grows older, the period that information is retrained increases.

As children grow older, they develop more effective and efficient strategies to retain information. During adolescence the brain enters a plastic period, particularly in the frontal lobes. Neuronal connections that control sleeping and eating habits, regulate motor behavior, and modulate impulses, decision making, memory, and other high-level cognitive functions change significantly during adolescence. Given the plasticity of the adolescent's brain, it is highly probable that environmental stimuli influence intrinsic changes in the adolescent's CNS.

Across the life span, some aspects of cognition seem to be impaired or changed before others. One of the areas most susceptible to age-associated changes is the prefrontal cortex. This particular area of the brain is where information critical to executive function, attention, and working memory is stored.[100] Although memory is one component of cognition that is generally acknowledged to deteriorate as an individual moves toward older adulthood, not all aspects of memory are affected at the same time or in the same way.

Episodic memory is reportedly the first to be impaired, then working memory (short-term memory).[100] Implicit memory and semantic memory remain intact for a much longer period of time. Little information is available about procedural memory, memory of how to perform tasks. Researchers suggested that an older adult's declarative memory is also affected by normal and neuropathological aging.[39,100] These investigators suggested that, although older adults with deterioration in declarative memory are able to perform the task(s), the individual is unable to retain information and consequently unable to learn the task(s).[39] Many factors negatively or positively influence memory, including the nature of encoding or processing that information, such as the source of the material or time of day material is presented.[100]

Although evidence exists that many aspects of memory decline with age, recent evidence supports the premise that variables other than encoding and retrieving information may have a significant impact on memory and remembering in older adults.[101,102] Researchers at the University of Kuopio examined memory in older persons and focused on neuropsychological processes as a method for evaluating memory and other functions of the frontal lobe.[102] The investigators reported that elderly subjects with subsequent degradation of the frontal lobe had memory loss. These researchers suggested that some aspects of memory loss could be staved off through: memory sharpening activities/games, limiting alcohol consumption, and participating in activities designed to retain details of skills/tasks. Similar to these findings is work by May et al[101] examining the role of emotion in memory tasks for older adults. They reported that older adults seem to be motivated to remember information that is emotionally relevant and meaningful. These findings lend support to yet another system, the emotive system, which could add vital information to an older adult's memory and task performance. (See Chapter 4.)

Perceptual System

As researchers continue to examine the interactive and interdependent roles of body systems, the perceptual system must not be omitted. Perception, yet another process important to performance of functional movements, involves acquisition, interpretation, selection, and organization of sensory information. Perception is the very essence of the interaction between organism and environment. Every movement gives rise to perceptual information and in turn guides the organism to adapt movements accordingly.[10,103]

Initially perception revolves around the infant's visual exploration of people, objects, and environmental activities. Infants are capable, at birth, of visually exploring their environment, people, and objects.[89] Investigators have suggested that infants use information acquired through visual exploration to develop new methods of exploring and discovering cues about the environment such as depth, distance, surface definition, and dimensionality of objects.[104]

A second phase of perceptual exploration emerges as an infant's exploratory behaviors transition to functional movements such as reaching and kicking. Through these exploratory behaviors emerge additional mechanisms for acquiring information about the environment.[6,103] Throughout development, active exploration enhances perceptual information through each new encounter and enables the infant to recognize distinctive features and similar characteristics that allow the infant to differentiate between objects. The information generated from exploration provides new input to many subsystems, in particular the sensory, motor, and cognitive systems that enable the individual to gain new knowledge about the environment and the action.

Development of the infant's perceptual system is dependent on acquiring new information about the affordances of the task that may influence performance of the action. As the infant develops the capacity for independent mobility, the expanse of the environment increases, as do the opportunities to integrate prior knowledge with newly acquired information to discover unchartered surroundings. This again supports the interactive and interdependent nature of systems throughout development. As maturation progresses, infants develop the ability to evaluate information acquired from various systems and to make decisions about the optimal strategy for successfully navigating over or around a surface. With maturation, successful navigation of new environments depends on opportunities for exploration that may involve other processes in addition to motor. An example of this may be seen when trying to locate a building in an unfamiliar city. Adults typically use maps as a visual representation of the surroundings that allow them to find the location. Infants and young children are most accurate in locating desired targets through active exploration. This allows the child to acquire spatial information critical to locating the destination at a future time.

If perception is the process of integrating and organizing intrinsic and extrinsic input, then changes in sensory systems as a consequence of aging are certain to affect perception.[105] The visual perceptual processing system is most often identified as altered in older adults. Specifically, researchers have reported that, although older adults are capable of discriminating between variation in depth perception in a manner similar to that of younger adults, they were less able to discriminate between three-dimensional shapes of objects.[106] Clearly the perceptual system is closely associated with many other body systems and as such, age-related or age associated structural and functional changes in associated systems will impact the perceptual system.

Additionally, May et al[101] found that older adults placed less emphasis on perceptual aspects of an event than they did on the emotional components when encoding information. They suggested that older adults may find emotional information to be more meaningful than perceptual information and may retain more elaborate, detailed processing of emotional data than perceptual information.

Although there is no conclusive evidence regarding age-related changes of perception, evidence may be emerging that supports age-associated or individual differences.[107] Nonetheless, the role of perception in aging should continue to be investigated and not be underestimated or minimized until such time as adequate evidence exists.

Emotional System

Although current literature does examine the emotional development of children,[108-116] the normal emotional development of adults over a life span remains a mystery. Most people have accepted that emotional development occurs as a child and after that it no longer is considered development. A literature search of "normal emotional development across the life span" found one article.[117] This article stressed that emotional well-being of adults is based on parental care given during childhood. Problems in normal emotional development can be identified throughout medical literature, but again the emphasis is on children and adulthood emotional problems stemming from either pathological conditions or environmental childhood problems.[118-123] Within the literature, the reader can find discussions of emotional intelligence in adults and how those emotional skills such as empathy or cultural sensitivity might be taught.[124-130] But again, the reader will find it difficult to locate articles that emphasize changes within emotional intelligence across the life span and how that might alter cognition or motor system responses. Within the medical literature, a focus on pathological conditions and how they might change emotional health or development can be found, but again it is within a pediatric age span, not across a life span of healthy adult life. Specific aspects of an emotion or mood change and how that might assist or hinder an individual within a psychosocial environment can be located,[131-134] but the integration of the entire emotional system and its normal changes throughout life still alludes researchers. The link between intuition, emotional (development, sensitivity and intelligence), and cognitive abilities will also need to be delineated to more accurately create environments for learning within all domains. There are variables that seem to make a difference in social and professional success, but how they are measured or analyzed will be future scholars' dissertation studies.[135] (See Chapter 4 on the limbic system and its influence on motor control and Chapter 5 on psychosocial adaptation and adjustment for additional information.)

Motor Development

Movement is the primary mechanism by which prelinguistic children communicate with their environment. That said, it is no wonder that development of motor skills is greatest during the first 2 years of life. Motor development may be defined as the acquisition, refinement, and integration of biomechanical principles of movement in an effort to achieve a motor behavior that is proficient.[11]

Early developmental researchers referred to infants as reactive, inferring that, early on, infants are responsive to stimuli rather than capable of initiating functional movements. Young infants were characterized as "reflexive" beings producing stereotypic primitive and postural responses to stimuli. Emergence of these reflexive motor behaviors was based on traditional models of CNS organization and motor development theories. Traditional theories of human development emerged from animal models and studies involving spontaneously aborted fetuses.[14,136] Traditionally, sucking and stepping behaviors were examples of developmental reflexes. By definition, a reflex is a consistent response to a consistent stimulus. By use of traditional models of CNS organization, developmental reflexes, present at birth, become integrated as higher centers assume control over lower centers and then volitional movements begin to emerge.

Over the past two to three decades, advances in technology have enabled scientists to gain more insight into fetal and infant motor abilities. More recently, research has generated evidence that behaviors emerge out of a need to solve a problem in the environment rather than solely as a result of maturation in the CNS.[137] Given this evidence supporting the premise that newborn infants are capable of producing complex volitional movements, previous views of the infant as a passive "reflexive" is no longer accurate. In addition, continuing to refer to early infant motor behaviors as "reflexes" may also not accurately reflect the behavior. A reflex is defined as a consistent response given in response to a consistent stimulus. *Perhaps use of the term "innate motor behaviors" to reflect behaviors that are present at birth may be more appropriate.* See Figure 2-1, *A* to *C,* to visually understand how the complexity of the stepping reaction of a newborn infant and the learned programming for upright posture and balance, including biomechanical range and force production, will lead to the integration of stepping in standing. Similarly, as an individual ages, loss of some of the postural power, effectiveness of balance reactions, and fear can create a potentially dangerous environment for an elderly person (Figure 2-1, *D-E*). Similarly, an individual (Figure 2-1, *F*) with an abnormal or inefficient stepping pattern should automatically stand out to a therapist analyzing movement dysfunction. If a clinician does not have a clear picture in his or her mind of the movement pattern desired, then easily or quickly identifying the system or subsystem motor impairments seen in a client's movement dysfunction may be outside a therapist's analytical repertoire.

Contemporary research rebukes the assertion that infants are reactive organisms. In contrast, contemporary studies purport that infants are competent and capable of producing complex interactive behaviors at birth.[89,138] Additional support for the complex nature of a newborn infant is evident when the mother and another adult speak.

Evidence from studies examining motor development indicates that motor behaviors do not always emerge in a consistent sequence, nor do all individuals achieve the same

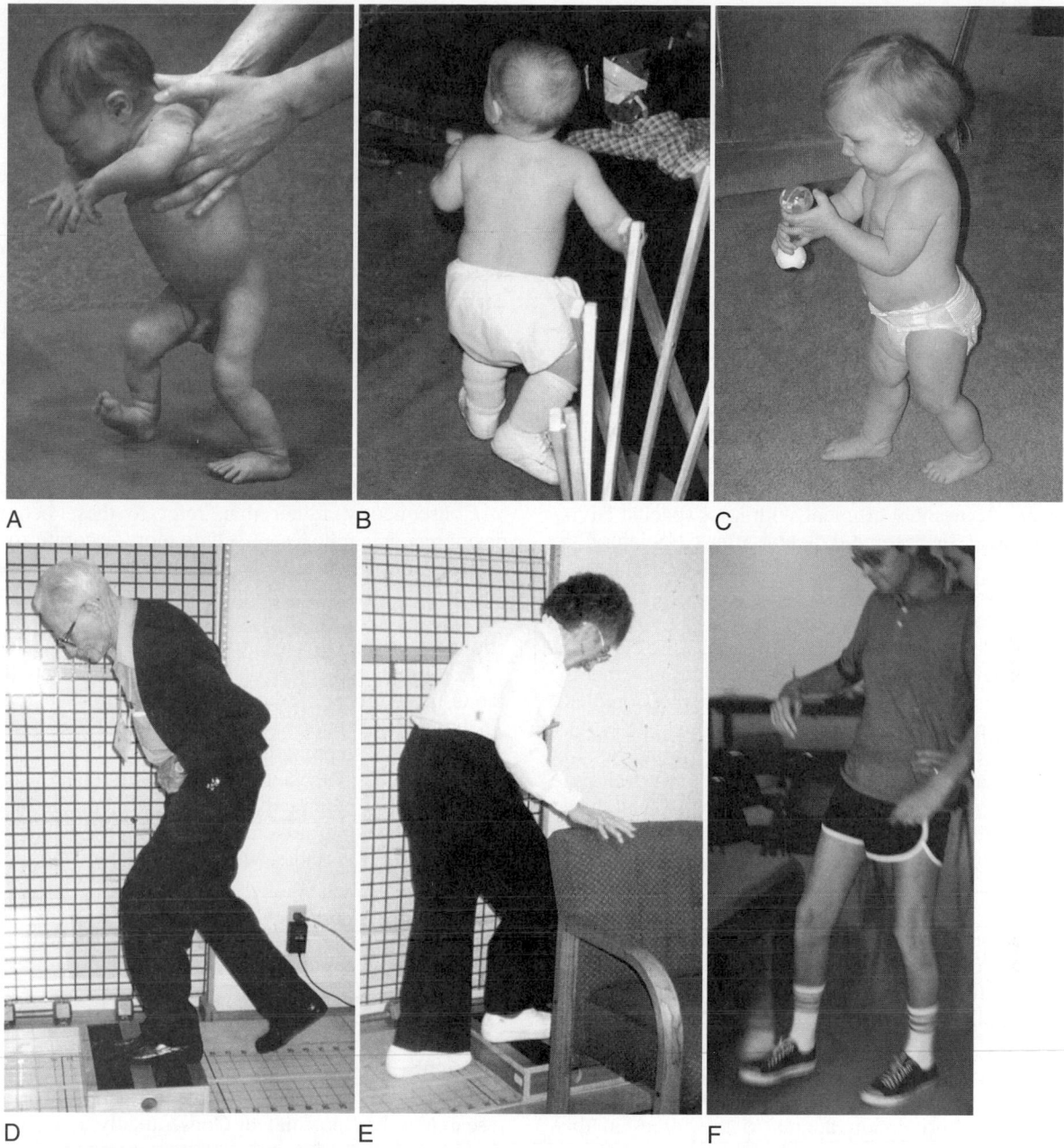

FIGURE 2-1 ■ Development and integration of stepping, upright vertical posture and vertical balance reaction: **(A)** automatic stepping in a newborn infant, **(B)** early cruising or side stepping using multiple points of support, **(C)** early bipedal independent stepping, **(D)** 90-year-old client stepping, **(E)** 78-year-old client with falling problems, **(F)** abnormal stepping after traumatic brain injury.

skills at the same chronological age.[8,138] Furthermore, emergence of motor behaviors in an alternate sequence is not indicative of later motor behaviors.

Motor performance, measured both qualitatively and quantitatively, is highly dependent on the task, the environment, and the individual. Changes in motor performance emerge in accordance with age-dependent changes, within different systems, and with respect to environmental affordances/constraints. As skills emerge in speech, language, and cognition, other previously achieved skills may "regress." In reality, acquisition of a new skill requires more attention than the previously attained skills; consequently, the infant or child's attention is divided between the tasks.

Lindenberger et al[139-141] conducted studies investigating life span changes in resource allocation during multitask activities. The researchers found that for young children certain tasks require more attention and attempting to perform such a task in conjunction with a task requiring less attention, causing deterioration in performance of both tasks. Hence, deterioration of a previously attained skill is more likely a result of attentional demands of young children performing high-attention tasks rather than a true "regression" of the skill. (See Chapter 1, Figure 1-9, p. 18.) This progression illustrates that a child confronted with a new environment will seem as if he regressed in motor performance as he confronted and solved the task-specific challenge of a moving compliant above ground bridge. Once the child began to succeed at the task, his attention was placed on retrieving a more efficient program to solve the problem. The child will progress to the most efficient learned motor program available if given the opportunity to explore and succeed at the desired task.

Relatively stable performance of motor behaviors and decreased intraindividual variability is generally achieved through practice and repetition. Conversely, decreased frequency in performing activities, as an effect of age, may be the factor that most contributes to a decline in motor skills. Motor skills emerge from a multifactorial interweaving of maturation and experience. Deterioration in motor performance may be attributable to alterations in various systems that occur as part of the aging process. Just as emergence of behaviors is never the same for any two individuals, neither does a decline in functional motor behaviors follow the same time line. Figure 2-2 illustrates how standing patterns will change with practice, be maintained as long as practice continues, become extremely efficient within an specific environmental context, or become deficient after CNS injury.

Prenatal (0 to 40 Weeks' Gestation) Development

Motor behaviors emerge early in embryonic life. By the tenth week of fetal life the variety of observed movements increases, as does the frequency of the movements. Complex movements are present by 12 weeks' gestational age (GA), and goal-directed movements may be seen as early as 13 weeks GA. Facial movements, including sucking, swallowing, and yawning, are evident between the second and third trimesters. The fetal activity level increases so that by week 14 GA, periods of quiet (no activity) are only 5 to 6 minutes in duration. Investigators have documented 15 fetal movements visible by 15 weeks of age.[142] After initial observation of a motor behavior, it remains part of the fetal repertoire. Pooh and Ogura's[142] research lends support to the premise that, before delivery, fetuses are in fact capable of producing complex motor behaviors.[142]

The dynamic nature of birth and the associated change from the intrauterine to the extrauterine environment alter the production of movements previously observed in fetal life.[57] As the newborn infant adapts to the forces in the extrauterine environment, motor behaviors emerge. These complex behaviors lend additional evidence to the premise that, at birth, infants are competent beings.

The extrauterine environment poses many challenges for the newborn infant. Consequently, fetal behaviors observed by ultrasonography may not be evident postnatally until the infant learns to adapt to the new environment by modifying movements to accommodate to the new forces imposed by gravity. Newborn infants must learn to use new strategies to generate functional motor behaviors, given the different environmental constraints.

Infancy (Birth to 12 Months)

As alluded to earlier, newborn infants possess a rich array of motor behaviors. During the first year of life, motor behaviors are the primary mechanism for learning. Every movement is a new and unique opportunity to gain knowledge about the environment. During each movement, new information is gathered in an effort to solve environmental

problems, and as a result this motor planning fosters cognitive development. Similarly, each movement provides feedback that intrinsically enables the infant to modify movements in accordance with changes in the environment, the skill, or growth parameters.[143] This interdependence between perception and motor behaviors allows one domain to facilitate acquisition of skills in the other domain in a reciprocal fashion.

Given the capabilities of a newborn infant, many behaviors previously identified as reflexes are in fact functional motor behaviors that the infant is capable of modifying. Evidence that one such behavior, sucking, is not a reflex was supported by studies examining sucking rates when stimuli were varied.[144,145] Researchers reported that the sucking response varied depending on the level of hunger or environmental stimuli. Additionally, when the stimulus was introduced after feeding, after the infant is satiated, the stimulus may produce no response or a diminished response, thus refuting the idea that sucking is reflexive.

Consequently, rather than refer to these behaviors as developmental reflexes, it seems more accurate to refer to such motor behaviors, evident at birth, as *innate motor behaviors*. Innate motor behaviors are, in essence, functional behaviors present at birth that are modifiable given alterations in feedback from intrinsic or extrinsic mechanisms.

Additional evidence exists to refute the concept that other motor behaviors are reflexes. Stepping is one such behavior. Thelan and Fisher[18,29,30] conducted a series of experiments examining the stepping reflex in young infants. Early developmentalists hypothesized that stepping reflexes, present at birth, became integrated and then later emerged as a volitionally controlled movement. Thelan and Fisher[18,30] found that when one variable, weight, was altered, infants mimicked "integration" or emergence of the behavior. Young infants who were stepping had weights added to their lower extremities, to simulate weight gain over the first few months. These infants stopped stepping. Similarly, infants who did not step were submersed in chest deep water, simulating less weight in the lower extremities, and stepping appeared. Obviously, the presence and absence of this behavior was mediated by weight gain in the lower extremities, and not by CNS control as early developmental researchers had postulated. Consequently, upright mobility emerges when the infant is able to garner the force production in the lower extremities to modulate stepping. This is just one example of the significance of one system on another and the interdependent nature of body systems. Recognizing the interdependence of systems may provide one explanation for the presence or absence of motor behaviors at any given time.

At birth, an infant is capable of turning toward the sound of her or his mother's voice and visually focusing on objects 8 to 12 inches from the face.[89] These behaviors are apparent when the infant's head is supported, given that at birth the newborn infant does not have the neck strength to maintain head control against gravity. Similarly, auditory and visual stimuli continue to bombard the infant and challenge the motor system, fostering the need to attain head control.

Infant motor behaviors during the first 3 months of life are focused on acquisition of head control in all planes of movement. Once the infant has achieved head control in the supine and prone positions, the complexity of the tasks

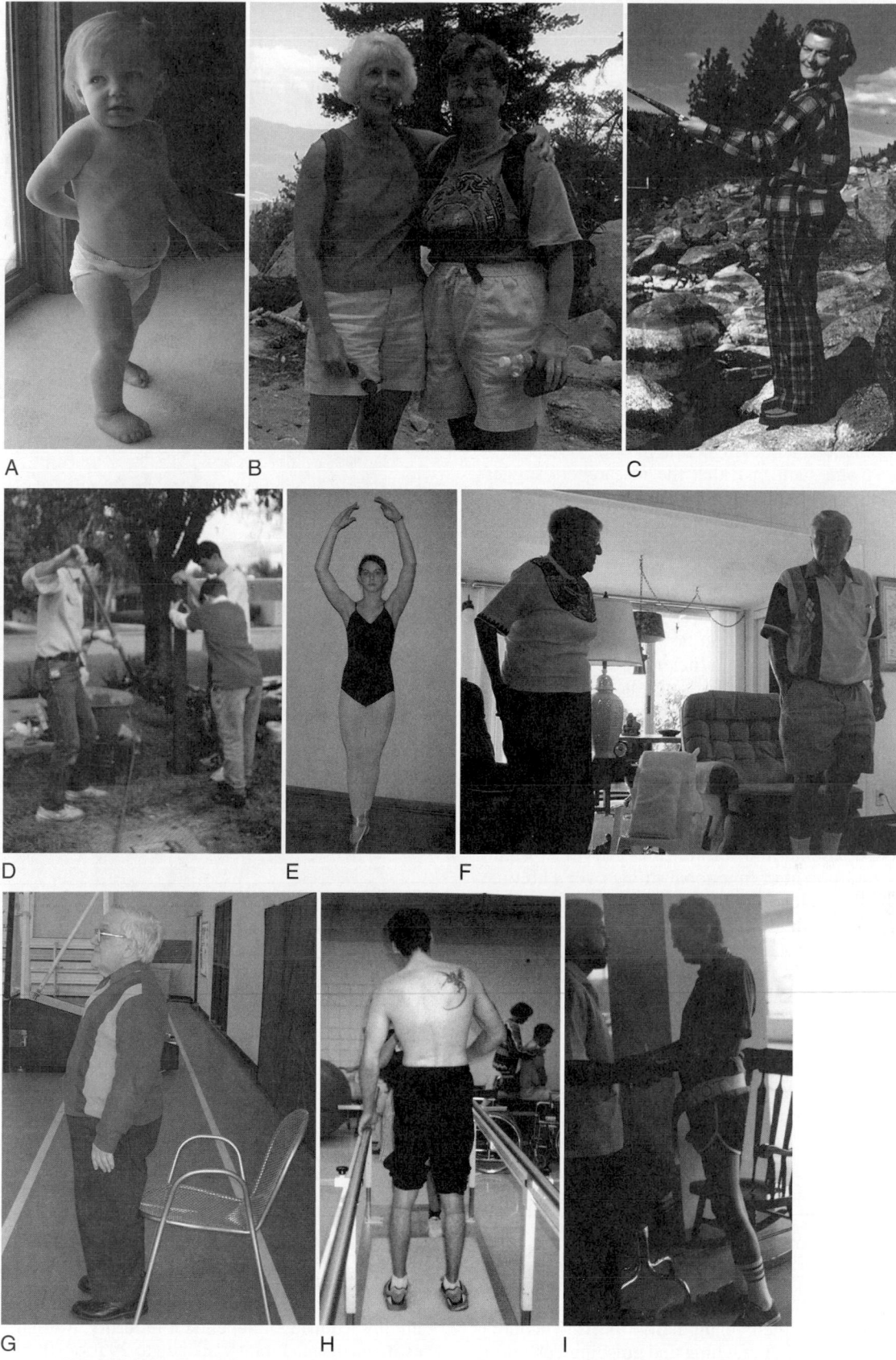

FIGURE 2-2 ■ Standing as a functional activity will become procedural with practice and be maintained over a lifetime as long as impairments do not preclude practice or injury to the CNS: **(A)** early standing, **(B)** relaxed standing as adults, **(C)** standing on uneven surfaces, **(D)** procedural standing during a functional activity, **(E)** advanced skill in standing as ballet dancer, **(F)** maintained functional standing in healthy 83-year-old elderly couple, **(G)** elderly man developing verticality impairment, **(H)** subtle abnormal standing after head injury, and **(I)** multiple subsystem problems in standing after CNS injury.

increases exponentially on the basis of the new challenges and stimuli presented to the infant. For example, while in the prone position, an infant may reach for an object out of reach and then roll to attain the desired object. Improvements in visual acuity enable infants to visually track people and objects at greater distances while challenging the infant to seek out the stimuli.

By age 3 to 4 months, as the infant is able to maintain head control in upright for longer periods, coordinated eye-hand activities begin to emerge. Acquisition of manipulative skills involves perception and lends support for the coupling of developing cognitive, sensory, and motor systems.[22,103] Bushnell and Boudreau[6] added that, if the infant is unable to achieve a motor skill and this skill is coupled with a sensory or cognitive task, that task may not be attained. Bushnell and Boudreau's[6] research focused on the role of motor development in achieving skills in other domains.

Reaching is one such task that the researchers suggest may serve to promote skills in cognitive and sensory domains. Initial reaching activities enable the infant to gain information relevant to depth perception and coupling this information then allows the infant to modulate parameters associated with reaching. For example, the infant must learn to vary the distance moved and force necessary to attain an object given a series of opportunities. Infant grasping and reaching may initially seem inefficient, but with practice under varying situations efficiency and accuracy improve across multiple domains with varying rates. Figure 2-3 illustrates both the error that provides feedback and the success during complex movement patterns after practice.

As infants develop an upright sitting posture, they use their upper extremities for support. Sitting, a functional motor behavior, is tightly linked to the performance of most ADLs and occupational and leisure-time activities. Figure 2-4 depicts development of functional sitting over a lifetime. Figure 2-4, A, illustrates the need for the upper extremities in supported sitting, whereas Figure 2-4, B to E, shows how independent sitting becomes procedural and linked with specific functional activities. Figure 2-4, F, shows how with age or disuse the postural component of sitting or hip range of motion may develop into an impairment that may not affect supported sitting but would certainly influence unsupported sitting. In Figure 2-4, G, multiple impairments are affected by functional sitting in an individual after a traumatic head injury. A delay in attaining independent sitting may directly affect upper extremity control, alter attainment of skills in other domains, and ultimately affect an individual's level of functional independence. Losing independent sitting after an insult to the CNS will have similar effects on that individual's ability to regain independence in any functional activity requiring interaction of those motor programs.

As upright trunk posture is attained and independent sitting emerges, usually by 6 months of age, and infants then begin to explore using their manipulative skills. Manipulative skills are composed of reaching and grasping behaviors. Upper extremity interlimb coordination bimanual and unimanual tasks include retrieving objects (placed within reach); holding two objects, one in each hand; using two hands to hold an object (bottle); and holding a toy in one hand while retrieving another object with the free hand.[146]

During the second half of year 1, the infant is focused on mobility, initially in prone (rolling, crawling), creeping on all

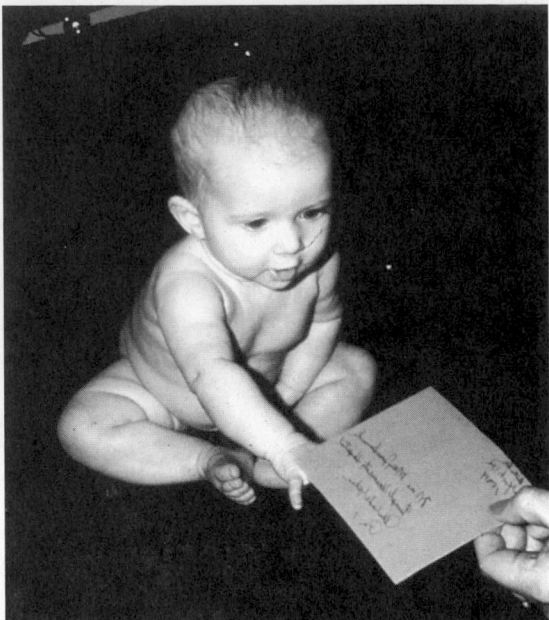

A

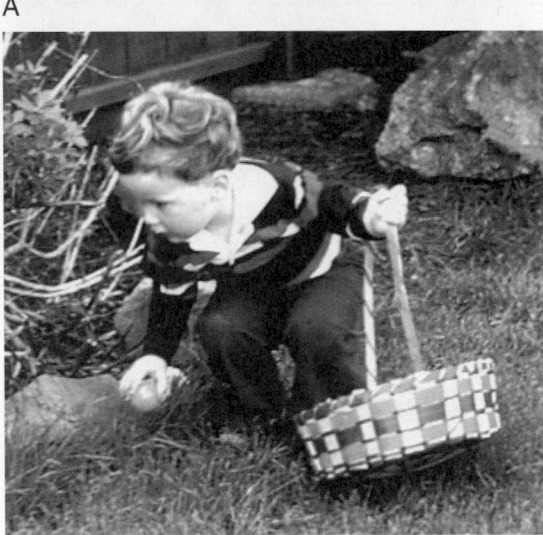

B

FIGURE 2-3 ■ Reaching activity: **(A)** error in reaching leads to learning and **(B)** reaching becomes accurate during a complex motor task.

fours, and then upright (cruising and ambulation). Adolph and Berger[22] reported that, as coordination of upper and lower extremity movements with trunk control emerges and infants begin upright mobility, they spend up to 50% of their day performing balance and mobility-based activities, varying the surface, distance, and other parameters each time task is performed. On the basis of research conducted with infants acquiring independent mobility, Adolph and Berger[22] estimate that an infant walks up to 29 football fields each day.

Acquisition of independent mobility is complicated by new manipulative skills, as discussed by Corbetta and Thelan.[146] They found that, while infants are achieving independent mobility, their manipulative skills are highly variable and vacillate between bimanual and unimanual tasks depending on the nature of other tasks with which the infant is simultaneously involved. Infants may revert to perform-

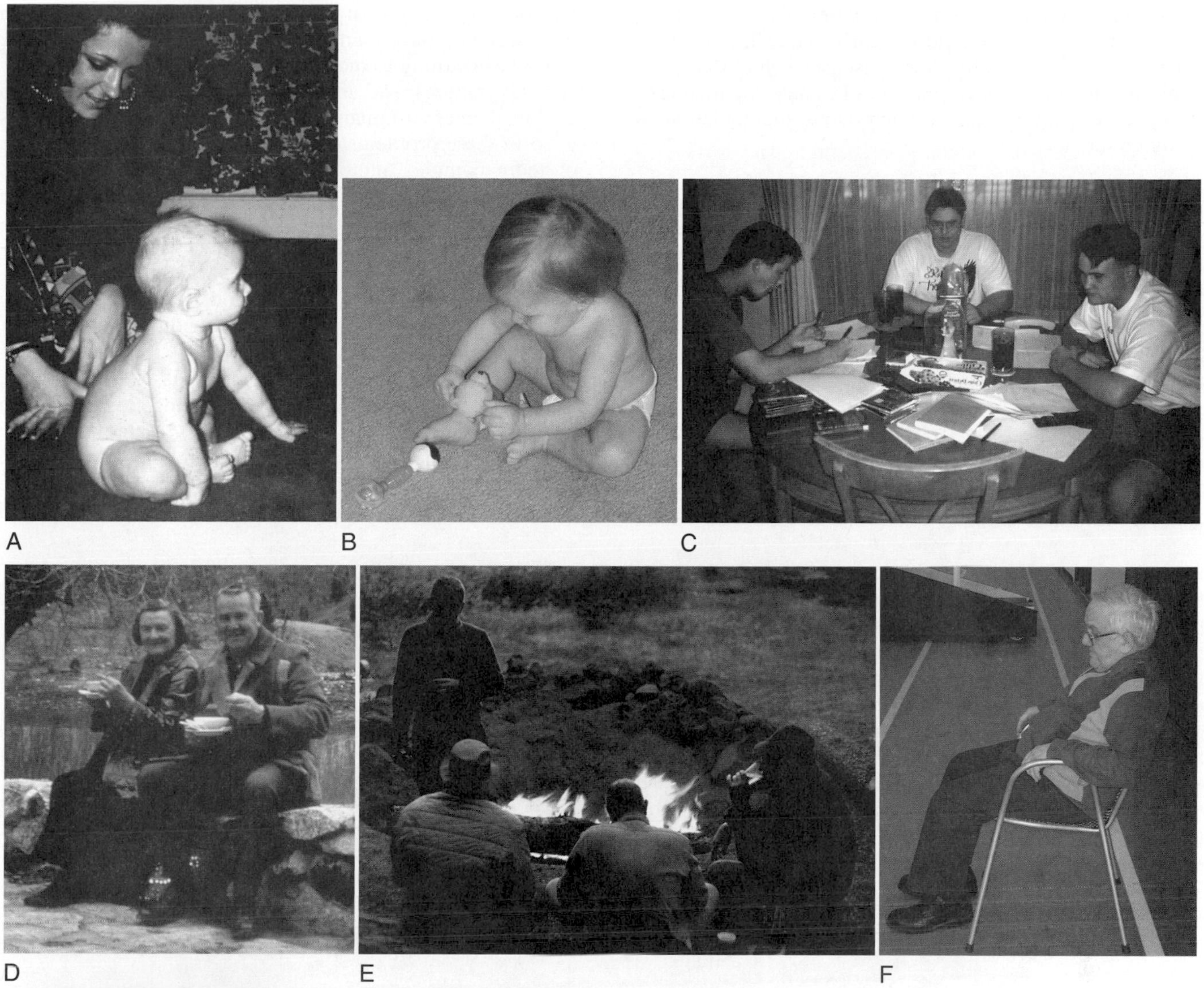

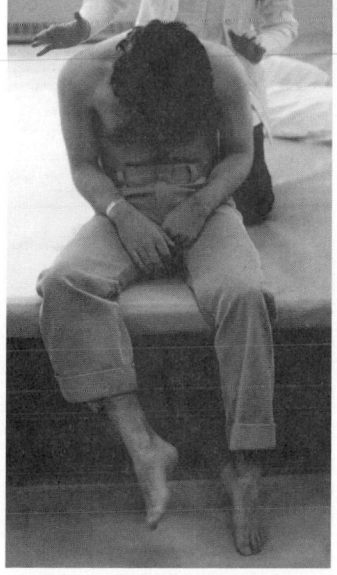

FIGURE 2-4 ■ Development and maintenance of functional sitting: **(A)** early support sitting during first year, **(B)** independent sitting during play, **(C)** functional sitting in adolescents while studying, **(D)** adults sitting without support while eating, **(E)** sitting as part of a social interaction of an adult group, **(F)** functional changes in sitting in the elderly, and **(G)** loss of adequate sitting programs after closed head injury.

ing bimanual activities, with upper extremities coupled and movements synchronized, during early acquisition of independent mobility, signaling the presence of multiple tasks requiring attention. Unimanual control signals uncoupling of the upper extremities and asynchronous manipulation in young children.

Early Childhood (1 Year to 5 Years)

Although the first year of life is characterized by periods of rapid physical growth and acquisition of motor skills, the second year signals a slower rate of growth, refinement of current skills, and acquisition of new motor skills.[147] Concurrently, the toddler experiences rapid differentiation in other areas of CNS function including cognition, speech, and social-emotional domains.

At the onset of the second year of life, independent ambulation becomes refined as other forms of mobility wane. Dynamic balance in an upright bipedal posture evolves as the infant develops more mature gait characteristics. Modification of parameters indicative of a more mature gait include

narrowing of the base of support, decreased cocontraction in the lower extremities, and improved intralimb coordination, as well as learning to modulate displacement and velocity.[22] As gait matures and toddlers have more opportunity to explore their environment, more challenges appear. Attempts to solve these problems/challenges result in the appearance of more complex motor behaviors that include running, climbing, and jumping. Toddlers find particular pleasure in throwing, kicking, and catching balls. Additionally, toddlers assert their independence through such activities as propelling themselves with riding toys.

Toddlers continue to explore and assert independence through activities involving bimanual and unimanual tasks. Challenges to fine motor skills of toddlers involve manipulating functional objects (large buttons, eating utensils, crayons, door knobs, blocks, and opening/closing jars to retrieve small objects [cereal, raisins]). Achieving these tasks enables the toddler to perform rudimentary aspects of ADLs such as eating and dressing and adds another degree of independence. Figure 2-5 illustrates development and

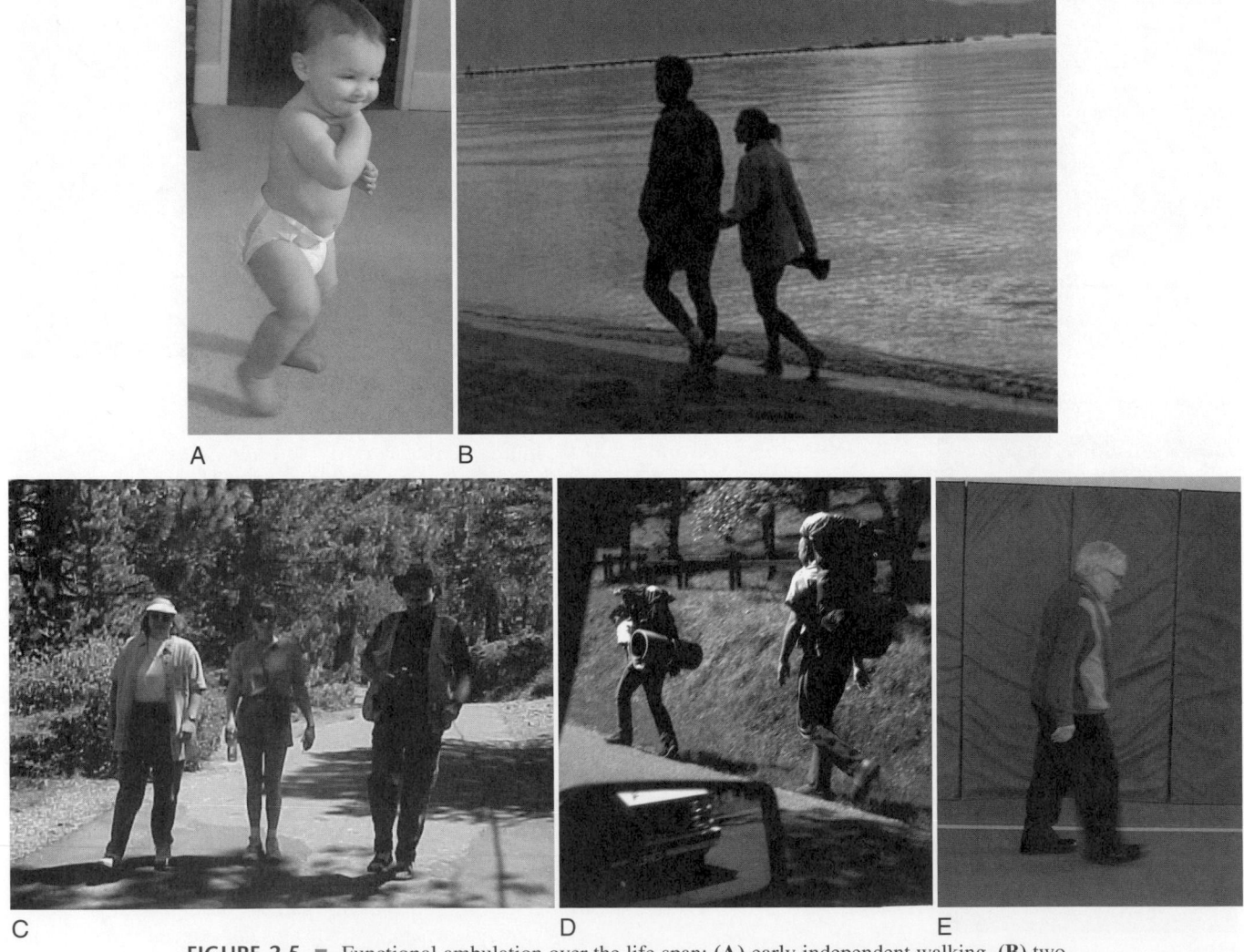

FIGURE 2-5 ■ Functional ambulation over the life span: **(A)** early independent walking, **(B)** two young adults walking on sand, **(C)** three different-sized adults show variation in ambulatory styles but all styles are considered normal, **(D)** adults hiking with backpacks requires motor adaptations, and **(E)** elderly man walking with visual guidance instead of visual anticipation creating potential functional impairments.

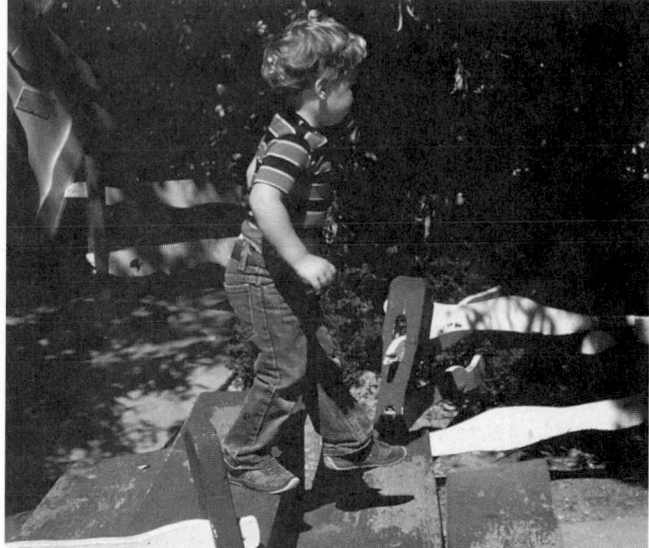

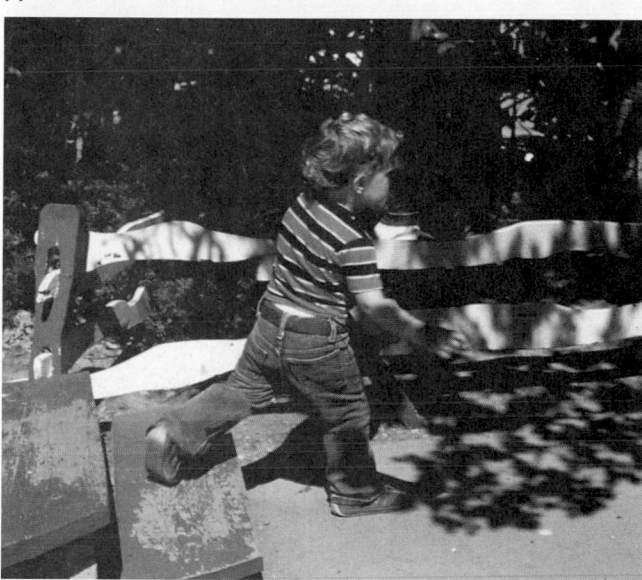

FIGURE 2-6 ■ Child descending stairs successfully: **(A)** attention on stepping down and **(B)** success at the task.

variance of ambulatory skill and task specificity over a lifetime. Figure 2-5, *E,* illustrates how someone may compensate for changes by using vision to guide the movement versus using vision to anticipate the environmental context two to three steps in the future.

The ambulatory pattern of a young child matures into reciprocal arm swing and a heel-to-toe gait pattern. Early in the preschool period, children mimic a "true" run and have difficulty efficiently controlling all aspects of the behavior. By age 3 years most children ascend stairs using alternating feet, and by 4 years most descend stairs alternately. Figure 2-6 shows a preschooler descending stairs. Initially the child will practice with intent (Figure 2-6, *A*). After successful practice the behavior becomes more relaxed and procedural (Figure 2-6, *B*). Preschool age children pedal a tricycle and use a narrow base of support to walk along a balance beam. Finally, receipt and propulsion of balls of all shapes and sizes improves qualitatively.

Fine motor skills expand significantly during the preschool period. The environmental demands of preschool and day care preparation for entering primary grades are the driving force behind acquisition of many manipulative behaviors. Most children begin to cut with scissors, copy circles or crosses, use crayons to color pictures, match colors, and often demonstrate hand preference. Although maturity certainly plays a role in skill performance, the efficiency in which skills are performed is also influenced by genetics, affordances/constraints of the environment, practice, and intrinsic motivation.

Childhood (5 to 10 Years)

Childhood is characterized as a period when children begin their formalized education, usually in a structured environment separate from their families. Consequently, a new set of dynamics comes into play. Children take on new roles with peers and adults outside of the family. During this period of social-emotional change, other systems also undergo changes.

Motor skills that children display during this period include galloping, hopping on one foot for up to 10 hops (hopscotch), jumping rope, kicking a ball with improved control (soccer), and bouncing a large ball (basketball). Often these skills emerge while playing with peers during directed (physical education or community-based team sports) and nondirected (recess) periods. Mobility, balance, and fine motor skills improve dramatically. Girls and boys exhibit similar abilities in speed up to age 7 years but by age 8 years boys begin to outperform girls.[147]

During early childhood, manipulative skills increase exponentially. Figure 2-7, *A* through *E,* shows the amazing skill developed between birth and age 4 years. Once the child begins school, manipulative skills assume a predominant role as part of the academic experience requiring high levels of practice and opportunities for refinement of the skills. Hand preference is confirmed by this age. As a component of independence, many of the manipulative skills achieved are directly related to self-care activities. Skills that improve dramatically include dressing, including fastening/unfastening clothing, tying shoes, and using an implement for writing (coloring and handwriting). As children approach preadolescence (9-12 years of age), manipulative skills again improve dramatically. Children produce cursive handwriting and complex drawings.

Perceptual development usually improves significantly, often in direct relationship to the demands of the tasks along with practice, feedback, and motivation.[147] Visual-perceptual systems are nearing maturity and allow children to participate in sophisticated activities such as archery, baseball, dance, and swimming. Figure 2-8 helps bring to light complex skill development during a lifetime. That skill development may begin with a fun team sport activity and lead to a lifetime of professional accomplishment.

The musculoskeletal system enters a period when muscle growth is rapidly increased, accounting for a large percentage of the weight gained during this period.[147] Constraints/affordances of the musculoskeletal system along with demands of the tasks and environment are highly interactive and influential in skilled activities. Children are generally flexible because muscle and ligamentous structures are not firmly attached to bones. Although this allows for flexibility, it also poses risks for musculoskeletal injury.

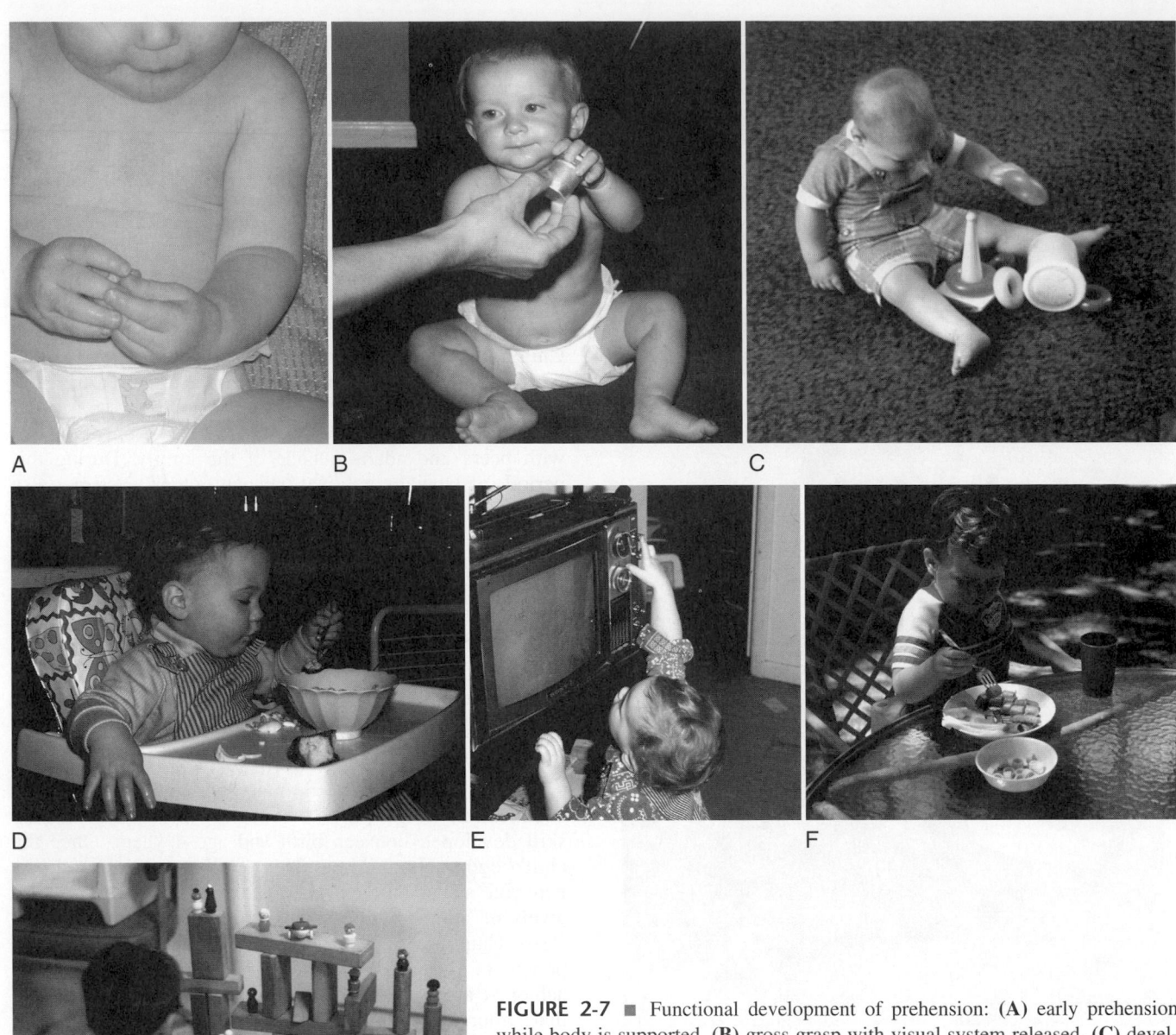

FIGURE 2-7 ■ Functional development of prehension: **(A)** early prehension while body is supported, **(B)** gross grasp with visual system released, **(C)** development and practice of eye-hand coordination during play, **(D)** early independent feeding with error, **(E)** functional use of individual digit, **(F)** eating with few errors while using utensils, and **(G)** fine motor prehension while simultaneously using force and direction of the upper extremity with little error during play.

Care should be taken when participation in high-level athletic activities is a consideration.

Qualitative changes in coordination, balance, speed, and strength improve while existing motor skills become more refined and controlled, more efficient, and more complex.[147] Qualitative improvements of motor skills may be attributed to an asynchronous growth in children's limbs in relation to the trunk. Consequently, better leverage is attained. Motor skills strongly influence social domains as boys and girls begin to perform in organized sports teams in school and the

community. Competition within sports becomes a powerful force in motivating children to practice motor skills or directing children away from organized sports. Children with poorly developed motor skills, as a result of either genetics or opportunity, may be excluded from team activities and experience social isolation.[147]

Adolescence (11 to 19 Years)
Early adolescence signifies a period characterized by improved quantitative performance and qualitative changes

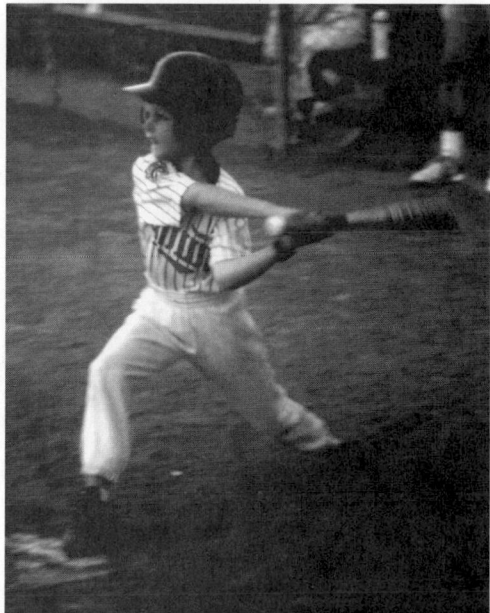

A

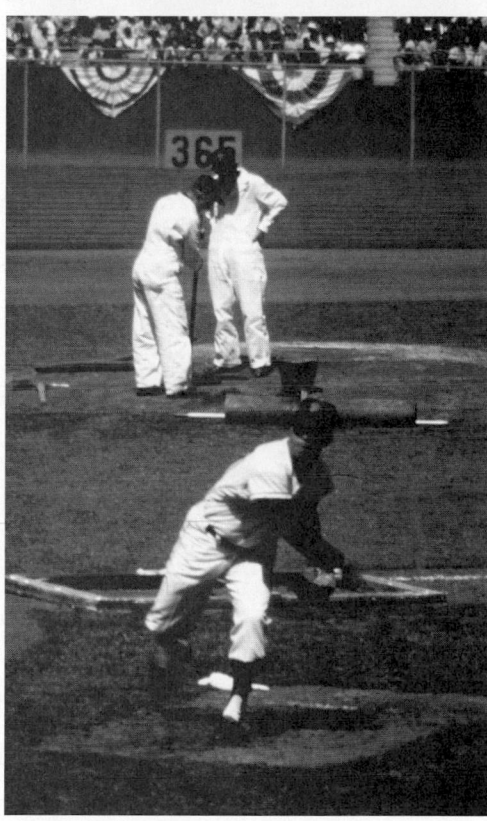

B

FIGURE 2-8 ■ Complex skill development: **(A)** child participating in a team sport and **(B)** adult demonstrating advanced skill development as a professional baseball player.

in skills along with physical growth (size and strength).[11] By age 12 years, reaction times closely resemble those of the mature adult. Although skills involving balance, coordination, and eye-hand coordination also continue to improve with respect to perceptual development and information processing, the rate is not as dramatic. Elite athletes, in

contrast, often continue to show steady improvement in qualitative and quantitative skill performance well into adulthood.

During later adolescence, when periods of physical growth have stabilized, motor skills acquired previously continue to develop and become more proficient in speed, distance, accuracy, and power. Many adolescents are involved in competitive sports. However, few exhibit performance levels identified with elite athletes. When analyzing individuals who attain a high level of athletic performance, other variables can usually be identified such as genetic predisposition, environmental affordances, adequate opportunities for high-level practice and performance, and strong motivation. More often, adolescents performing in competitive sports will find this is their avocation rather than serving as their vocation (see Figure 2-8).

Manipulative skills of adolescents resemble those of adults. Greater dexterity of the fingers for more complex tasks including art, sewing, crafts, knitting, and musical performance enables adolescents to perform these motor tasks with greater precision and proficiency.

Adulthood (20 to 39 Years)

Motor performance is relatively stable in adulthood, and consequently change is generally focused on leisure activities or elite athletic competition. Leisure activities of many adults involve exercise of some form. Maintaining a healthy lifestyle through exercise and fitness is one method for staving off effects of aging and degenerative diseases. Although many adults participate in exercise for health and wellness, others who do not routinely exercise are at risk for obesity and associated health problems. Often some of the physical activity expressed through the motor system is an example of parent-child bonds and creates a fun environment for play. When a task-specific activity is selected and challenged by family members, the motivation to perform becomes high. In Figure 2-9, *A,* the observer might think that all three individuals are performing with similar strategies and similar degrees of difficulty. In reality, single leg stance increases in difficulty as either the base of support decreases or the body size changes. Note that the smallest individual has the smallest foot and thus the largest base of support in proportion to his body size. The adolescent is not as tall as his dad but his foot size is significantly larger, which (1) decreases his base of support, (2) gives him less input proportional to his foot size or representation on the somatosensory cortex, and (3) gives him higher degrees of freedom when shifting his weight, which can either increase or decrease the task difficulty depending on practice. Figure 2-9, *B,* shows the way both the adolescent and the adult used strategies to initially assume the upright stance position while the smaller child stepped from a stump. Body height, weight, and amount of practice all are variables that will help determine outcome. All three individuals were successful, although the specific motor patterns and strategies used to succeed may have been different. In Figure 2-9, *C,* a child with severe sensory organization problems would not be able to solve the challenge in Figure 2-9, *A,* for he cannot even begin to stand independently on a large, stable surface. Again, therapists need to be able to match the motor program impairments causing the child with learning disabilities to fail at the task and identify what programs are

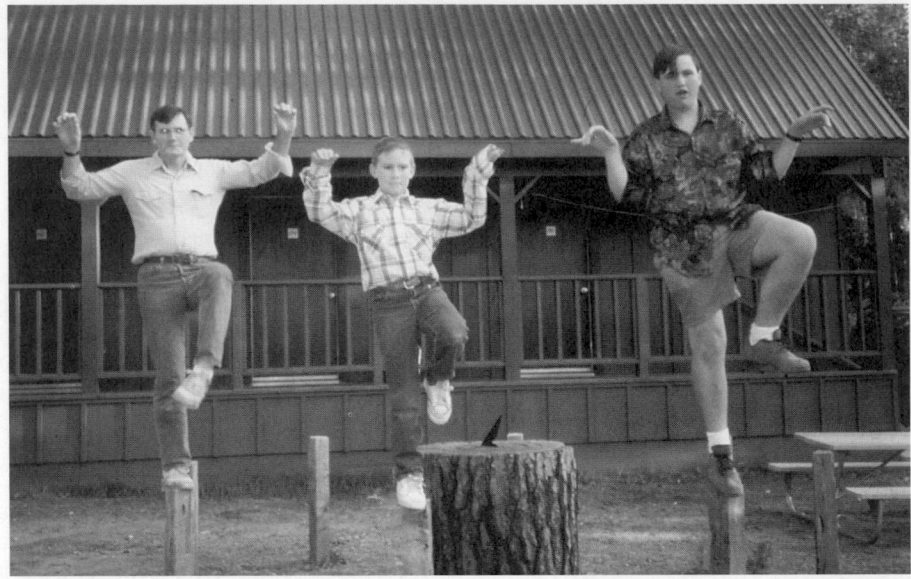

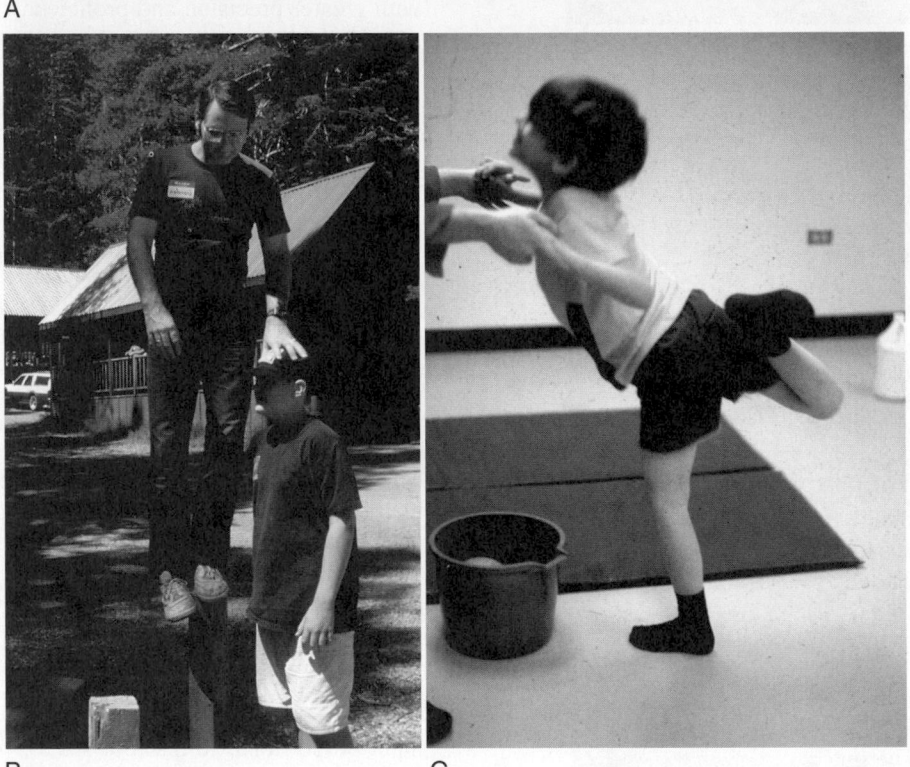

FIGURE 2-9 ■ A complex task performed by individuals with different foot size and body composition: **(A)** three individuals of differing age, body composition, and experience performing successfully the same task, **(B)** the strategy used by the adolescent and adult to find verticality, and **(C)** a child with learning difficulties and sensorimotor processing problems fails at independent one-legged stance.

needed or expressed in the success of all three individuals in Figure 2-9, *A*.

The peak of muscular strength occurs between 25 and 30 years of age in both men and women. After that period, muscle strength decreases as a result of a reduction in the number and size of the muscle fibers.[148] Loss is related to genetic factors, nutritional intake, exercise regimen, and daily activities.

Middle Adulthood (40 to 59 Years)

Changes associated with aging have been identified in the neuromuscular, musculoskeletal, and cardiovascular and pulmonary systems. These age-associated changes can greatly affect motor performance, although the degree is highly variable. Between 30 and 70 years of age, strength loss is moderate, with about 10% to 20% of total strength lost, for most activities insignificant and undetectable by the individual.[60,149] Participating in regularly scheduled exercise regimes that emphasize aerobic and strengthening activities may reduce effects associated with aging.

Older Adulthood (60+ Years)

Age-related changes may be attributed to alteration in perception, compensations in the neural mechanisms, and changes between and within the different systems involved in motor skill performance.[150] Integrated effects may include slowing in movement production and increased activation of agonist-antagonist muscle groups. An example of agonist-antagonist activation is during dynamic balance activities.[151] After age 70 years, most individuals incur losses in muscle strength of up to 30% over the next 10 years. Overall, the loss of muscle strength through adulthood may be as much as 40% to 50% by the time an individual reaches 80 years of age.[57] The percentage decline is inversely related to the demand by the individual for repetition of the movements. For example, repetitive movements, such as playing tennis daily, running, swimming, playing golf, downhill skiing, or working out regularly in a gym may significantly decrease the percentage of loss of strength compared with individuals who do not participate in such activities.

Although some effects are age associated and may be reduced with regular exercise and increased motor activity, not all are modifiable. Willardson[74] reported that older adults who maintain more active lifestyles are more likely to have a more favorable outcome than are peers who were not as active. As individuals age, they generally have a decreased ability to produce force, and they tend to coactivate agonist-antagonist muscles.[152] The researchers suggested that older adults may coactivate agonist-antagonist muscles as a strategy to (1) modulate movement variability and (2) maintain accuracy in movement. The investigators also reported that older adults' coactivation strategy compromised the subjects' ability to rapidly accelerate their limbs in exchange for improved accuracy of control.

In addition, information processing appears to be slowed in older adults.[150] Motor times were also found to be delayed in older adults, particularly when a higher-level force is required.

Temporal coupling also appears to be altered in older adults.[150] Perhaps as individuals age, they are less able to modulate timing of muscles during contraction and relaxation phases and are more likely to coactivate agonist-antagonist muscles. The outcome behaviors are typified by poorly coordinated motor activities and increased time to produce adequate muscle force to elicit the behavior.

In addition to being less efficient in movement production, variability in performance of motor skills also increases with age. Although small changes in individual systems may not have a significant effect on functional movements, the compounding effects of changes in several systems may have serious implications for older adults and place them at increased risk for falls and injuries.[60] Figure 2-10, A and B, are examples of movement dysfunctions seen within an elderly population. These alterations are limiting the individual's ability to response to a given motor task. As individuals age, there can be a large number of potential alterations in the body systems that limit CNS and musculoskeletal options when the individual tries to accomplish a motor activity. These limitations can place individuals at

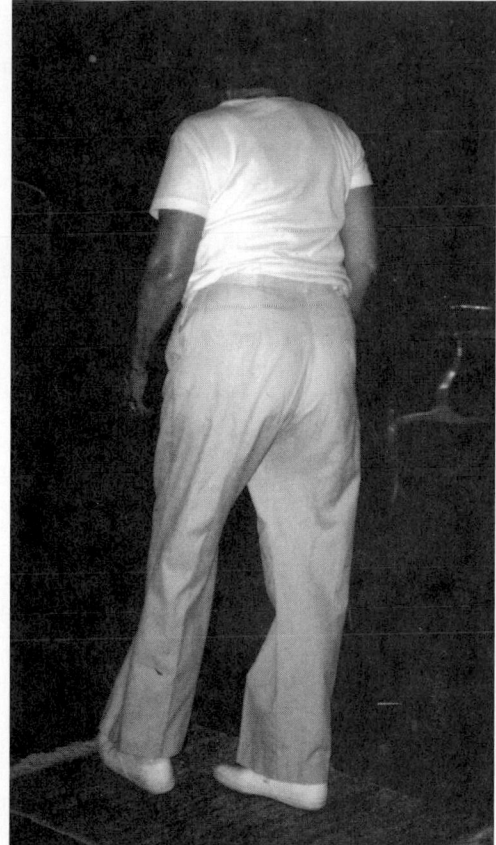

A

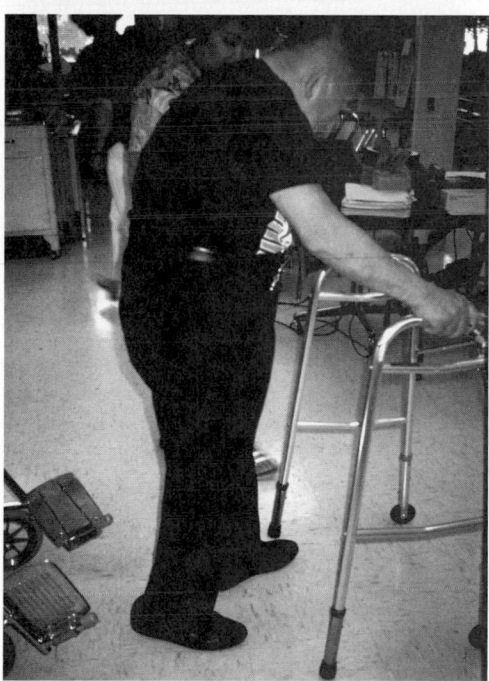

B

FIGURE 2-10 ■ As individuals age, more sedentary lifestyles, preexisting long-term health issues such as chronic obstructive pulmonary disease or chronic back pain and a decrease in environmental challenges can lead to a higher risk of falls: **(A)** woman with chronic back problems leading to a fixed trunk and little trunk rotation and **(B)** man with chronic obstructive pulmonary disease and a fixed flexed posture resulting from inactivity.

high risk of failure of any one motor task. The greatest fear within this group is not death; it is falling, and as a result losing independence. Prevention, as discussed in Chapter 6, will be more and more important as the world's population of elderly individuals enlarges on a yearly basis.

Thirty percent of all community-dwelling elderly persons fall at least once each year.[149] Factors contributing to falls include intrinsic and extrinsic variables.[153] Intrinsic alterations in the older adult have implications for performance of motor skills and potential for falls. Risks associated with falls increase with age and when functions of the neuromuscular, musculoskeletal, cardiovascular and pulmonary, and sensory systems deteriorate.

Researchers have examined manipulative skills in older adults and reported changes in muscle performance and flexibility.[49,154] These changes resulted in decreased hand function associated with impaired performance of ADLs.

STRATEGIES FOR FOSTERING ACQUISITION AND RETENTION OF MOTOR BEHAVIORS ACROSS THE LIFE SPAN

Movements occur out of a need to solve problems in the environment. Solving these problems is not dependent on any one system but rather in a collaborative effort of multiple systems. The clinician is responsible for examining the patient's performance by evaluating the underlying conditions and the strategies that the individual may use to modify a behavior. Figure 2-11, A to F, presents an example of individuals coming to stand from a chair. The first (Figure 2-11, a and b) shows a child whose feet are not on the surface because the child's legs are not long enough. No matter the variance of the task, the child was motivated to succeed. The second individual (Figure 2-11, C and D), an elderly gentleman, has lost the ability to shift his weight forward over his feet and thus is rising posterior on his heels, which will require anterior flexor power to prevent him from falling backward. The third individual (Figure 2-11, E and F) has residual motor problems after a stroke. She has been taught to come to stand over her less-involved leg versus centering her base of support between her two feet. The specific way an individual learns, maintains, and relearns a specific motor task as a functional activity will vary, but the important principle will be to empower the individual to success with fluid, dynamic motor pattern options. Therapists need to visualize movement and place the movement pattern or sequential patterns of the individual on top of that image(s). The specific motor impairments will then become obvious and treatment options will be generated. Examination is vital to this process, although it often occurs in an environment far removed from the client's natural surroundings.

Through acquisition of motor skills, individuals of all ages are afforded the opportunity to meet the environmental demands imposed by work, play, family, or personal activities. Refer to Figure 2-11 as an example of common motor activities used at work, play, and home. Motor skill acquisition, retention, and decline are influenced by constraints or affordances that affect opportunities for practice in an environment that challenges and drives the individual to perform optimally. The client's investment in achieving a successful outcome can help foster persistence in reaching the desired outcome.

Practice, the primary method for acquisition and retention of motor tasks, is exciting for very young children because each attempt is a new opportunity to achieve the outcome and reach a new level of independence. In contrast, practice in adolescent and adult populations may not be seen in the same light but rather referred to as tedious and boring. Instead, physical and occupational therapists have the capacity to challenge the cognitive, affective, motor, perceptual, sensory, and physiological systems in the same way through client-selected activities. Activities directed toward the age and needs of the individual, such as interactive dance mats for adolescent clients or ballroom dancing for the older adult, may provide the motivation necessary to practice the task a sufficient number of times and achieve the desired outcome. Figure 2-12, A to H, shows age-appropriate challenges to individuals. The activity used with a child may be inappropriate for use with an adult, although a similar motor program may be the desired outcome. If the individual identifies the activity, he will be more motivated and more likely to practice to maintain a desired skill. Carryover from a clinical setting to a home or environmental setting is critical when looking at movement function over a life span.

Strategies used to achieve desired motor outcomes may include a variety of feedback mechanisms to correct errors and identify more efficient strategies to attain the motor skill. Embracing the concept of an enablement rather than disablement may also serve to motivate the client because individual abilities are acknowledged and promoted while strategies are used for acquisition or relearning of motor skills. The needs of the adolescent and adult clients are unique and differ significantly from those of the young infant or child.

Opportunities for exploration that engage the infant or young child are the primary motivation for movement. Although motor activities serve as the primary focus, engaging the infant or child provides stimulation that promotes development across multiple domains (cognition, social, communication, etc.). Environmentally challenging activities place demands on the child that maintain a level of curiosity or motivation and encourage persistence in attaining a motor skill that is successful and efficient. As the child matures, play-based activities shift the focus, depending on the expected outcomes. Overall, play is the primary mechanism that children use to mimic adult-like behaviors. Finally, children and adults use play as a means of promoting skill acquisition and proficiency across all developmental domains.

SUMMARY

Scientists acknowledge that the development of motor skills in humans is nonlinear, emergent, and dynamic, rather than sequential, predictable, and stagelike. Despite certain limitations, dynamic systems theory appears to provide a better explanation for development than neuromaturational theories. This theory stresses that development is not emphasized in, nor the responsibility of, any one system, but varies across different systems as a consequence of age, genetics, or experience.[92] No system or skill develops in isolation; it is the complex interaction between multiple systems that results in the formulation of skills necessary to survive. Complex behaviors are evident beginning in utero and continuing throughout life. No one theory explains the devel-

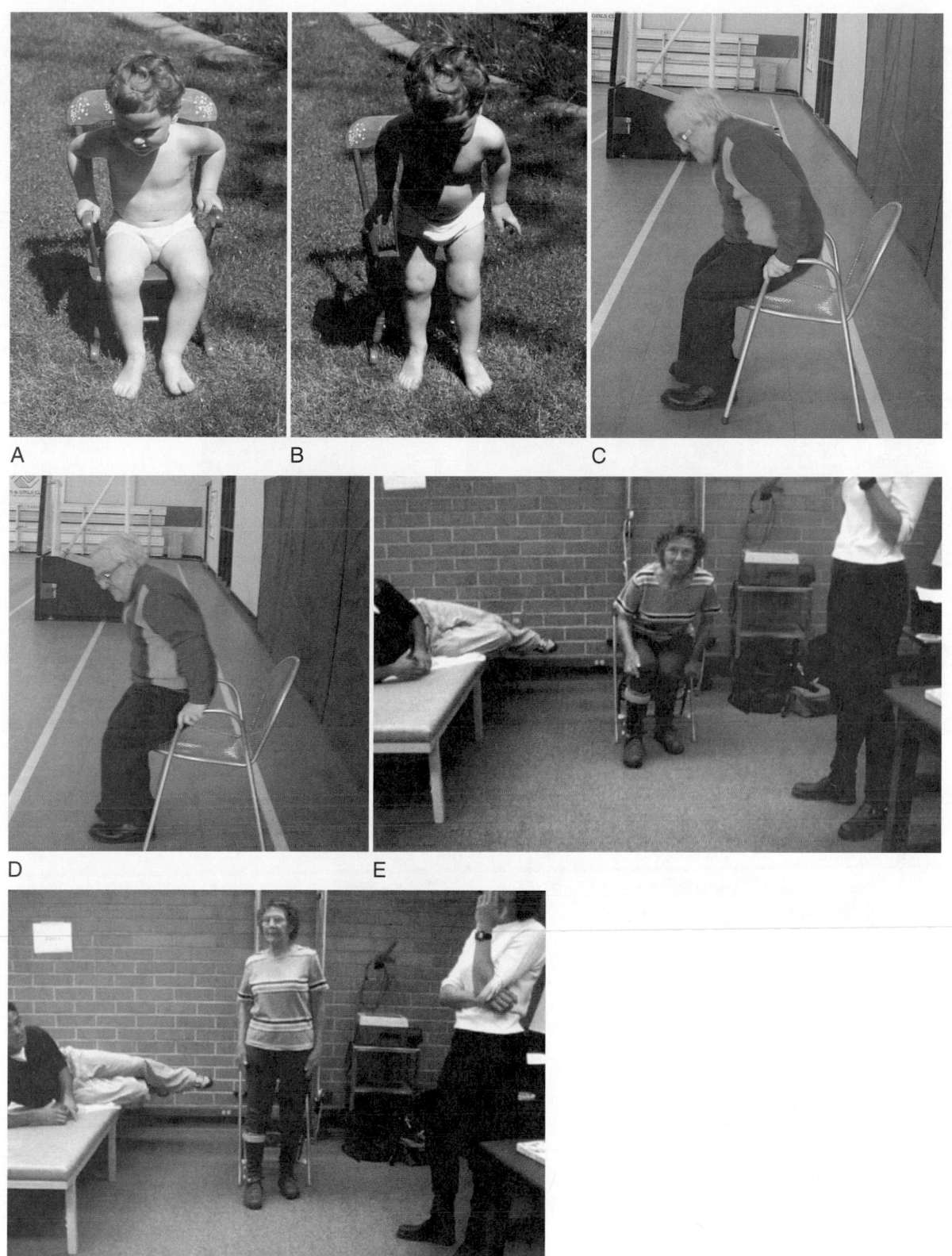

FIGURE 2-11 ■ Three individuals coming to stand using different motor patterns: (**A & B**) a child rising to stand from a chair by shifting his weight over his base of support and rising vertically, (**C & D**) an elderly man rising to stand without adequate weight shifting forward over his base of support requiring additional flexor power to prevent falling backward into the chair, and (**E & F**) a woman after stroke rising over her less involved leg thus decreasing her symmetrical weight distribution and ability to step in any direction with either foot as a response to center of gravity shifting outside her base of support.

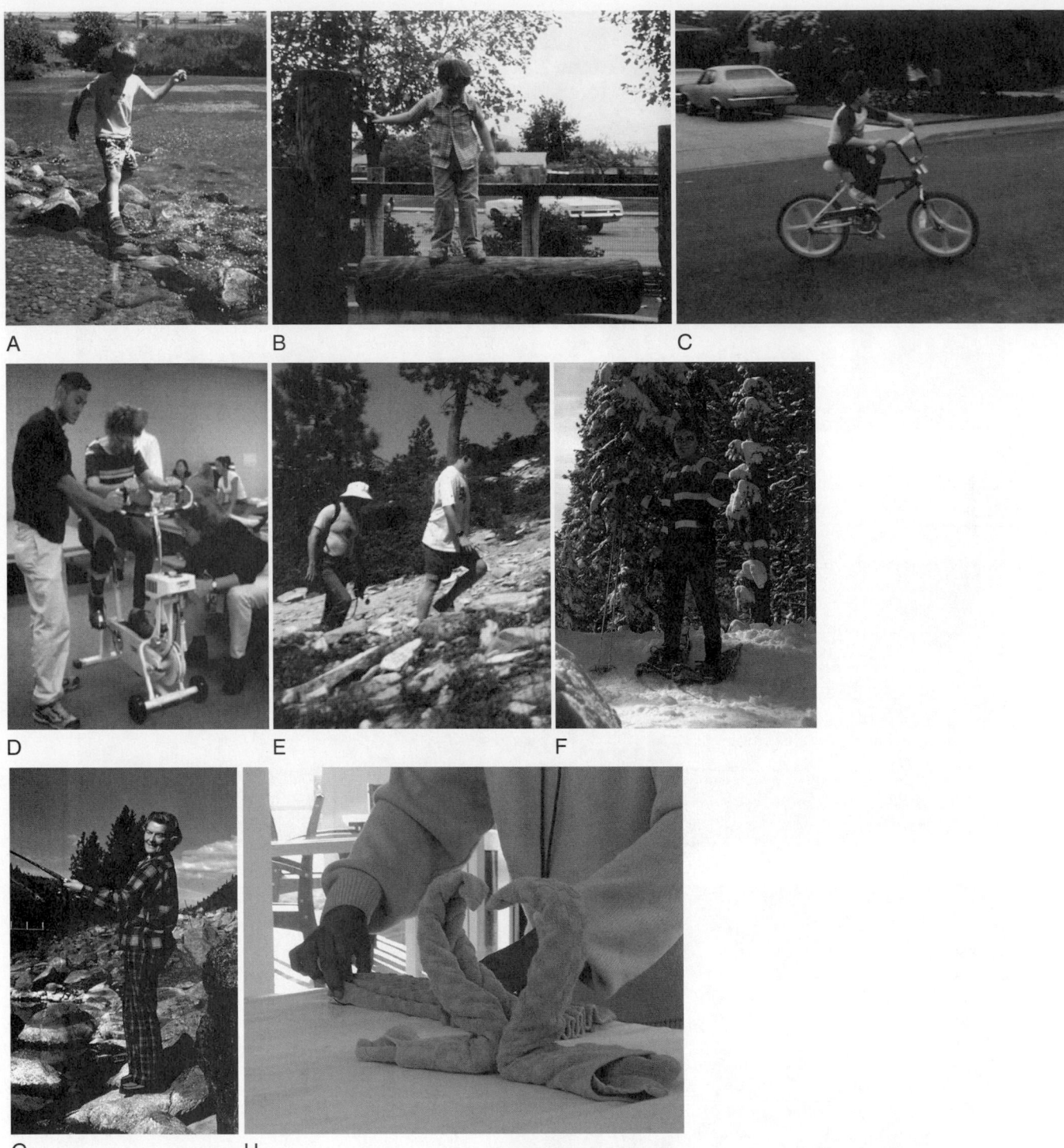

FIGURE 2-12 ■ Age appropriate self-select functional activities: **(A)** child walking across a creek, **(B)** child balancing on a moving surface for fun, **(C)** child riding a bike, **(D)** adult riding a bike, **(E)** adult walking up a hill, **(F)** adult using snow shoes, **(G)** adult fishing, and **(H)** adults folding towels into figures for fun.

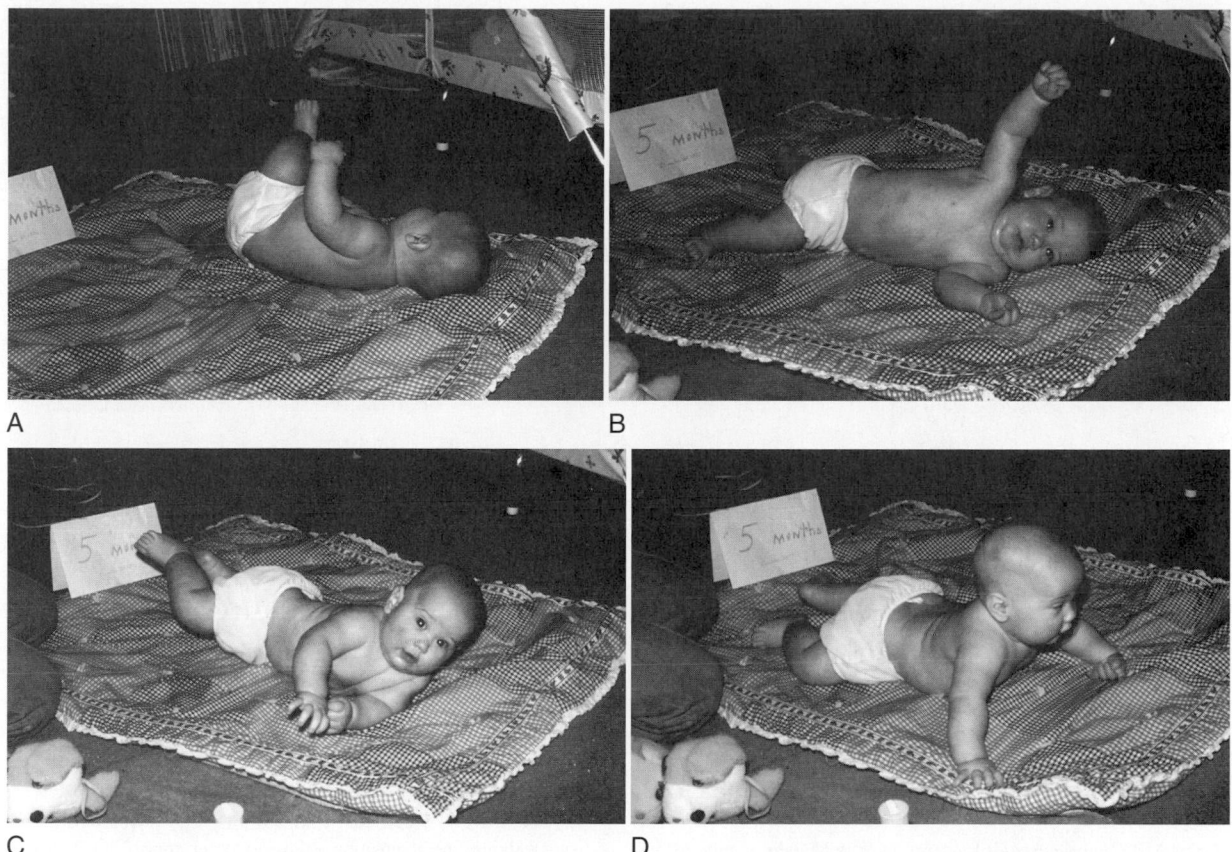

FIGURE 2-13 ■ Rolling—an activity attained within the first year: (**A**) child beginning rolling in supine, (**B**) child semiprone with trunk rotation, (**C**) child bring arm through to become symmetrical while proceeding toward prone, (**D**) child in prone with postural extension.

Continued

opment of complex motor behaviors, and none encompass the essence of interindividual and intraindividual variability in aging. Aspects of various theories provide evidence that an integrative perspective is a more accurate reflection of aging. As theorized earlier, lifestyle choices and other modifiable behaviors have potent effects on aging. Interventions designed to provide older adults with strategies to positively influence successful aging improve quality of life. Therapy should not only intervene after a negative problem of aging is realized. Optimal quality of life is what all individuals hope to obtain, whether learning to reach a toy, climbing the highest mountain, or playing a game of bridge. Maintaining that quality before the end of life, no matter the age, is often based on movement function. The identification of the necessary steps to get from existing skill to desired skill is the role of a movement specialist, whether dealing with preventive care or interventions after injury.

Clinicians must focus on best practice toward successful client management. This must include promotion of function and prevention of chronic illness or disability for the youngest of the young to the oldest of the old. Practitioners must embrace tenets central to the *Healthy People 2010* project, which aims to optimize health and well-being for all citizens. Physical and occupational therapists must educate individuals of all ages and backgrounds about the multifaceted, interactive systems involved in the acquisition, retention, and deterioration of motor behaviors. Recogniz-

ing internal and external constraints or affordances that influence motor behaviors enables the clinician to devise a plan of care and the scientist to design a study targeting the needs of the whole person. Analyzing, understanding, and visually recognizing normal movement patterns that are efficient, fluid, and goal oriented and that vary across the life span is the first step or prerequisite to evaluating abnormal movement patterns that do not fall within normal parameters. Rolling, which is a basic movement strategy controlled by the child midway through the first year of life (Figure 2-13, *A* to *D*) can become an extremely challenging activity after a CNS insult (see Figure 2-13, *E* to *G*). Differentiating between normal movement subsystem components from deviation that prohibit normal movement falls into the clinical skill of occupational and physical therapists treating individuals with CNS dysfunction. Without the knowledge of normal movement, analysis of the causation of abnormal movement would be difficult if not impossible. This chapter has been written to help the reader understand normal movement across the life span. It is the first step, and in sighted individuals this analysis is started as soon as visual images were recorded in the visual cortex. Memory of normal movement patterns has already been stored by students studying to become physical or occupational therapists. That memory just needs to be retrieved from general knowledge and renamed as a new file considered as vital images to be used throughout the therapist's clinical life when working with individuals with movement dysfunction.

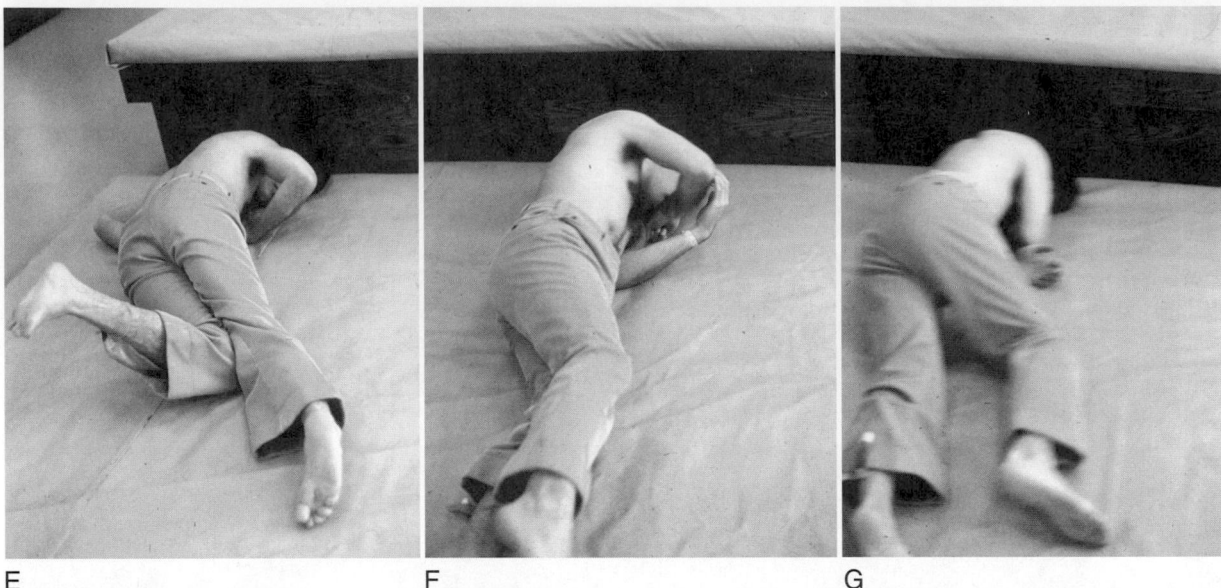

E   F   G

FIGURE 2-13, cont'd (**E**) Adult with traumatic brain injury, first try at rolling toward prone from supine, (**F**) adult's second try at rolling changing programming, and (**G**) once in prone he is stuck unable to extend.

REFERENCES

1. Gesell A: *The first five years of life,* New York, 1940, Harper and Brothers.
2. McGraw MB: *Neuromuscular maturation of the human infant,* ed 2, New York, 1945, Hafner. (Reprinted 1963, Columbia University Press).
3. Bayley N: *Bayley scales of infant development,* Berkeley, CA, 1969, Psychological Corporation.
4. Rowe JW, Kahn RL: Successful aging, *Gerontologist* 37:433-440, 1997.
5. Kandel ER, Schwartz JH, Jessel TM: *Principles of neural science,* ed 4, New York, 2000, McGraw-Hill.
6. Bushnell EW, Boudreau JP: Motor development and the mind: the potential role of motor abilities as a determinant of aspects of perceptual development, *Child Dev* 64:1005-1021, 1993.
7. Short-DeGraf M: *Human development,* New York, 1988, John Wiley.
8. Smith LB, Thelen E: *A dynamic systems approach to development,* Cambridge, 1993, MIT Press.
9. Singer RN: The readiness to learn skills necessary for participation in sport. In Magill RA, Ash MJ, Smoll FL, editors: *Children in sport: a contemporary anthology,* Champaign, 1978, Human Kinetics.
10. Gibson JJ: *The ecological approach to visual perception,* Boston, 1979, Houghton Mifflin.
11. Haywood KM: *Lifespan motor development,* Champaign, 1986, Human Kinetics.
12. Gesell A: The ontogenesis of infant behavior. In *Manual of child psychology,* pp. 295-331, New York, 1946, Wiley.
13. Thelen E, Adolph KE, Gesell AL: The paradox of nature and nurture, *Dev Psychol* 28:368-380, 1992.
14. Coghill GE: *Anatomy and the problem of behavior,* New York, 1969, MacMillan (original work published in 1929).
15. Oppenheim RW: Ontogenetic adaptations and retrogressive processes in the development of the nervous system and behaviour: the neuroembryological study of behavior—progress, problems, perspectives, *Stud Hist Philos Sci* 12:175-210, 1981.
16. McGraw MB: *Growth: a study of Johnny and Jimmy,* New York, 1935, Appleton-Century.
17. Heriza CB: Motor development: Traditional and contemporary theories. In Lister MJ, editor: *Contemporary management of motor control problems,* Alexandria, 1991, Foundation For Physical Therapy.
18. Thelan E: Developmental origins of motor coordination: Leg movements in human infants, *Dev Psychobiol* 18:1-22, 1985.
19. Zelazo PR, Weiss MJ, Leonard EL, The development of unaided walking: the acquisition of higher order control. In Zelazo PR, Barr R, editors: *Challenges to developmental paradigms: implications for theory assessment,* Hillsdale, 1976, Erlbaum Associates.
20. Thelan E: The role of motor development in developmental psychology: a view of the past and an agenda for the future. In Lockman J, Hazen N, editors: *Action in social context: perspectives in early development,* New York, 1990, Plenum.
21. Thelan E, Smith LB: *A dynamic systems approach to the development of cognition and action,* Cambridge, 1994, MIT Press.
22. Adolph KE, Berger SA: Motor development. In Damon W, Lerner R, series editors, Kuhn D, Siegler RS, volume editors: *handbook of child psychology,* vol 2: *Cognition, perception, and Language,* ed 6, New York, Wiley (in press).
23. Klir GJ: *Facets of systems science series: IFSR international series on systems science and engineering, vol 7,* New York, 1991, Plenum Press.
24. von Bertalanffy L: *General system theory,* New York, 1968, George Braziller.
25. Butterworth G: Dynamic approaches to infant perception and action: old and new theories about the origins of knowledge. In Smith LB, Thelen E, editors: *A dynamic systems approach to development,* pp. 171-187, Cambridge, 1993, MIT Press.
26. Scott JP: Critical periods in organizational processes. In Faulkner F, Tanner JM, editors: *Human growth,* pp. 181-186, New York, 1986, Plenum Press.
27. Thelan E: The (re) discovery of motor development: learning new things from an old field, *Dev Psych* 25:946-949, 1989.
28. Fischer KW: Relationship between brain and cognitive development, *Child Dev* 68:623-632, 1997.
29. Thelan E, Fisher DM: Newborn stepping: An explanation for a "disappearing reflex," *Dev Psychol* 8:447-453, 1982.
30. Thelan E, Fisher DM: From spontaneous to instrumental behavior: kinematic analysis of movement changes during very early learning, *Child Dev* 54:129-140, 1983.
31. Thelan E, Fisher DM, Ridley-Johnson R: The relationship between physical growth and a newborn reflex, *Infant Behav Dev* 7:479-493, 1984.

32. Bachman G: Menopause: E-Medicine (web site): August 10, 2005: http://www.emedicine.com/MED/topic3289.htm. Accessed Jan 20, 2006.

33. U.S. Census Bureau: United States census 2000: www.census.gov. Accessed Jan 20, 2006.

34. Carnes BA, Olshansky SJ, Grahn D: Biological evidence for limits to the duration of life, *Biogerentology* 4:31-45, 2003.

35. Chodzko-Zajko WJ: Biological theories of aging: implications for functional performance, In Bonder BR, Wagner MB, editors: *Functional performance in older adults,* ed 2, pp. 28-41, Philadelphia, 2001, FA Davis.

36. Karasik D, Hannan MT, Cupples AL et al: Genetic contributions to biological aging: the Framingham study, *J Gerontol* 59A:218-226, 2004.

37. DiGeorge AM, Parks JS: The endocrine system. In Behrman RE, Kliegman RM, Arvin AM: *Nelson's textbook of pediatrics,* ed 15, pp. 1580-1586, Philadelphia, 1996, WB Saunders.

38. Bengtson VL, Putney NM, Johnson ML: The problem of theory in gerontology today. In Johnson ML. editor: *Cambridge handbook of age and aging,* Cambridge, 2005, Cambridge University Press.

39. Goldsmith TC: *The evolution of aging,* Lincoln, NE, 2003, Iuniverse.

40. Goldstein S, Gallo JJ, Reichel W: Biologic theories of aging, *Am Fam Physician* 40:195-200, 1989.

41. Kelly KM, Nadon NL, Morrison JH et al: The neurobiology of aging, *Epilepsy Res* 68(suppl 1):S5-20, 2006.

42. Bengtson VL, Parrott TM, Burgess EO: Progress and pitfalls in gerontological theorizing, *Gerontology* 36:768-773, 1996.

43. Harman D: Aging: a theory based on free radical and radiation chemistry, *J Gerontol* 11:298-300, 1956.

44. Harman D: The aging process, *Proc Natl Acad Sci* 78:7124-7128, 1981.

45. Harman D: The aging process: major risk factor for disease and death, *Natl Acad Sci* 88:5360-5363, 1991.

46. Hayflick L, Moorhead PS: The serial cultivation of human diploid cell strains, *Exp Cell Res* 25:585-621, 1961.

47. Hayflick L: Theories of biological aging, *Exp Gerontol* 20:145-149, 1985.

48. de Magalhães JP: From cells to ageing: A review of models and mechanisms of cellular senescence and their impact on human ageing, *Exp Cell Res* 300:1-10, 2004.

49. Pesce K, Rothe J: The premature aging syndromes, *Clin Dermatol* 14:161-170, 1996.

50. Liang H, Masoro EJ, Nelson JF et al: Genetic mouse models of extended lifespan, *Exp Gerontol* 38:1353-1364, 2003.

51. Garilov LA, Gavrilova NS: Evolutionary theories of aging and longevity, *Sci World J* 2:339-358, 2002.

52. Jette AM, Branch LG, Berlin J: Musculoskeletal impairments and physical disablement among the aged, *J Gerontol* 45:M203-M208, 1990.

53. Binder EF, Yarasheski KE, Steger-May K et al: Effects of progressive resistance training on body composition in frail older adults: Results of a randomized controlled trial, *J Gerontol* 60A:1425-1431, 2005.

54. de Vos NJ, Singh NA, Ross DA et al: Optimal load for increasing muscle power during explosive resistance training in older adults, *J Gerontol* 60A:638-647, 2005.

55. Larsen WJ: *Human embryology,* Singapore, 1993, Churchill Livingstone.

56. Sadler TW: *Langeman's medical embryology,* Baltimore, 1984, Williams & Wilkins.

57. Kurjak A, Andopotono W, Stanojevic M et al: Longitudinal study of fetal behavior by four-dimensional sonography, *Ultrasound Rev Obstet Gynecol* 5:259-274, 2005.

58. Ashburn SS: Biophysical development during infancy. In Schuster CS, Ashburn SS, editors: *The process of human development: a holistic life-span approach,* pp. 118-140, Philadelphia, 1992, JB Lippincott.

59. Wilder PA: Muscle development and function. In Cech D, Martin S, editors: *Functional movement development across the lifespan,* pp. 137-157, Philadelphia, 1995, WB Saunders.

60. Wagner MB, Kaufman TL: Mobility. In Bonder BR, Wagner MB, editors: *Functional performance in older adults,* ed 2, pp. 61-85, Philadelphia, 2001, FA Davis.

61. Lieber RL: *Skeletal muscle structure, function, and plasticity: the physiological basis of rehabilitation,* Philadelphia, 2002, Lippincott Williams & Wilkins.

62. Bottomly JM: The geriatric population. In Boissonnault, editor: *Primary care for the physical therapist,* pp. 288-306, St. Louis, 2005, Elsevier.

63. Thompson LV: Physiological changes associated with aging, In Guccione AA, editor: *Geriatric physical therapy,* ed 2, pp. 28-55, St. Louis, 2000, Mosby.

64. Candow DG, Chilibeck PD: Differences in size, strength, and power of upper and lower body muscle groups in young and older men, *J Gerontol* 60A:148-156, 2005.

65. Visser M, Goodpaster BH, Kritchevsky SB et al: Muscle mass, muscle strength, and muscle fat infiltration as predictors of incident mobility limitations in well-functioning older persons, *J Gerontol* 60A:324-333, 2005.

66. Symons TB, Vandervoort AA, Rice CL et al: Effects of maximal isometric and isokinetic resistance training on strength and functional mobility in older adults, *J Gerontol* 60A: 777-781, 2005.

67. Staheli LT: Fundamentals of pediatric orthopedics, ed 2, Philadelphia, 1998, JB Lippincott.

68. Bowden VR, Dickey SB, Greenberg CS: *Children and their families: the continuum of care,* pp. 1217-1315, Philadelphia, 1998, WB Saunders.

69. Sullivan JA: Introduction to the musculoskeletal system. In Sullivan JA, Anderson SJ, editors: *Care of the young athlete,* pp. 242-258, 2000, American Academy of Orthopedic Surgeons and American Academy of Pediatrics.

70. Dutton M: *Orthopedic examination, evaluation and intervention,* New York, 2004, McGraw-Hill.

71. Moncur C: Posture in older adults. In Guccione AA, editor: *Geriatric physical therapy,* St. Louis, 2000, Mosby, pp. 265-279.

72. Lewis CB, Kellems S: Musculoskeletal changes with age: clinical implications. In Lewis CB, editor: *Aging the health-care challenge,* ed 4, pp. 104-126, Philadelphia, 2002, FA Davis.

73. Willardson JM, Tudor-Locke C: Survival of the strongest: A brief review examining the association between muscular fitness and mortality, *Strength Cond J* 27:80-85, 2005.

74. Willardson JM: Sarcopenia and exercise: mechanisms, interactions, and application of research findings, *Strength Cond J* 26:26-31, 2004.

75. Baumgartner RN, Koehler KM, Gallagher D et al: Epidemiology of sarcopenia among the elderly in New Mexico, *Am J Epidemiol* 147:755-763, 1998.

76. Morgan BJ, Dempsey JA: Physiology of the cardiovascular and pulmonary systems. In DeTurk WE, Cahalin LP, editors: *Cardiovascular and pulmonary physical therapy: an evidence-based approach,* pp. 95-122, New York, 2004, McGraw-Hill.

77. Brooks G: Physical therapy associated with prevention, risk reduction, and deconditioning. In DeTurk WE, Cahalin LP, editors: *Cardiovascular and pulmonary physical therapy: An evidence-based approach,* pp. 425-461, New York, 2004, McGraw-Hill.

78. Collins SM, ConCacour B: Anatomy of the cardiopulmonary system. In DeTurk WE, Cahalin LP, editors: *Cardiovascular and pulmonary physical therapy: an evidence-based approach,* pp. 73-94, New York, 2004, McGraw-Hill.

79. Jarvis C: *Physical examination and health assessment,* St. Louis, 2004, WB Saunders.

80. Cassady SL: Cardiovascular pathophysiology. In DeTurk WE, Cahalin LP, editors: *Cardiovascular and pulmonary physical therapy: an evidence-based approach,* pp. 123-150, New York, 2004, McGraw-Hill.

81. Stout J: Physical fitness during childhood and adolescence. In Campbell S, editor: *Physical therapy for children*, ed 2, pp. 141-169, Philadelphia, 2000, WB, Saunders.

82. Kelly MK: Physical therapy associated with respiratory failure in the neonate. In DeTurk WE, Cahalin LP, editors: *Cardiovascular and pulmonary physical therapy: an evidence-based approach*, pp. 647-663, New York, 2004, McGraw-Hill.

83. Overbay JD, Purath J: Self-concept and health status in elementary-school-aged children, *Iss Compr Nurs* 20:89-101, 1997.

84. DeTurk WE, Cassady SL: Essentials of exercise physiology. In DeTurk WE, Cahalin LP, editors: *Cardiovascular and pulmonary physical therapy: an evidence-based approach*, pp. 361-378, New York, 2004, McGraw-Hill.

85. Dean E: Cardiopulmonary development. In Bonder BR, Wagner MB, editors: *Functional performance in older adults*, ed 2, pp. 86-120, Philadelphia, 2001, FA Davis.

86. Barry BK, Riek S, Carson RG: Muscle coordination during rapid force production by young and older adults, *J Gerontol* 60A:232-240, 2005.

87. Papalia DE, Olds SW: *Human development*, ed 5, New York, 1992, McGraw-Hill.

88. Zuckerman BS, Frank DA: Infancy and toddler years. In Levine MD, Carey WB, Crocker AC, editors: *Developmental-behavioral pediatrics*, ed 2, pp. 27-38, Philadelphia, 1992, WB Saunders.

89. Brazelton TB: *Neonatal behavioral assessment scale*, London, 1984, Blackwell Scientific.

90. Meltzoff AN, Moore MK: Imitation of facial and manual gestures by human neonates, *Science* 198:75-78, 1977.

91. Field T, Goldstein S, Vega-Lahr N et al: Changes imitative behavior during early infancy, *Infant Behav Dev* 9:415-421, 1986.

92. Adolph KE: Babies' steps make giant strides toward a science of development, *J Infant Behav Dev* 25:86-90, 2002.

93. Sergiyenko Y: A revolution in developmental psychology, *Soc Sci* 36:91-102, 2005.

94. Hazlett CJ, Woldorff MG: Mechanisms of moving the mind's eye: planning and execution of spatial shifts of attention, *J Cognitive Neurosci* 16:742-750, 2004.

95. Gould E, Reeves AJ, Graziano MSA et al: Neurogenesis in the neocortex of adult primates, *Science* 286:548-552, 1999.

96. Ekelman BA, Mitchell S, O'Dell-Rossi P: Driving and older adults. In Bonder BR, Wagner MB, editors: *Functional performance in older adults*, ed 2, pp. 448-477, Philadelphia, 2001, FA Davis.

97. Rovee-Collier C: Memory systems of prelinguistic infants. In Diamond A, editor: *The development and neural bases of higher cognitive functions*, New York, 1990, New York Academy of Sciences, pp. 517-542.

98. Rovee-Collier C, Haynes H: Reactivation of infant memory: implications for cognitive development. In Reese HW, editor. *Advances in child development and behavior*, pp. 185-238, New York, 1987, Academic Press.

99. Greco C, Haynes H, Rovee-Collier C: The role of function, reminding, and variability in categorization by three-month-old infants, *J Exp Psychol* 16:617-633, 1990.

100. Riley KP: Cognitive development. In Bonder BR, Wagner MB, editors: *Functional performance in older adults*, ed 2, Philadelphia, 2001, FA Davis.

101. May CP, Rahhal T, Berry EM et al: Aging source memory and emotion, *Psychol Aging* 20:571-578, 2005.

102. Hänninen T, Hallikainen M, Koivisto K et al: A follow-up study of age-associated memory impairment: neuropsychological predictors of dementia, *J Am Geriatr Soc* 43:1007-1015, 1995.

103. Gibson EJL: Exploratory behavior in development of perceiving, acting, and the acquiring of knowledge, *Ann Rev Psychol* 39:1-41, 1988.

104. Kellman P, Short KR: Development of three-dimensional form perception, *J Exp Psychol Hum* 13:545-557, 1987.

105. Bohannon RW: Clinical implications of neurologic changes during the aging process. In Lewis CB, editor: *Aging the health-care challenge*, ed 4, pp. 127-142, Philadelphia, 2002, FA Davis.

106. Norman JF, Clayton AM, Shular CF et al: Aging and perception of depth and 3-D shape from motion parallax, *Psychol Aging* 19:506-514, 2004.

107. Hofer SM, Berg S, Era P: Evaluating the interdependence of aging-related changes in visual and auditory acuity, balance, and cognitive functioning, *Psychol Aging* 18:285-305, 2003.

108. Batty M, Taylor MJ: The development of emotional face processing during childhood, *Dev Sci* 9:207-220, 2006.

109. Dmitrieva ES, Gel'man VY, Zaitseva KA et al: Ontogenetic features of the psychophysiological mechanisms of perception of the emotional component of speech in musically gifted children, *Neurosci Behav Physiol* 36:53-62, 2006.

110. Edwards A, Shipman K, Brown A: The socialization of emotional understanding: a comparison of neglectful and nonneglectful mothers and their children, *Child Maltreat* 10:293-304, 2005.

111. Fries AB, Ziegler TE, Kurian JR et al: Early experience in humans is associated with changes in neuropeptides critical for regulating social behavior, *Proc Natl Acad Sci U S A* 102:17237-17240, 2005.

112. Katzman GH: Psychosocial development and school success: what more can be done? *J Dev Behav Pediatr* 27:42-43, 2006.

113. Lobaugh NJ, Gibson E, Taylor MJ: Children recruit distinct neural systems for implicit emotional face processing, *Neuroreport* 17:215-219, 2006.

114. Love JM, Kisker EE, Ross C et al: The effectiveness of early head start for 3-year-old children and their parents: lessons for policy and programs, *Dev Psychol* 41:885-901, 2005.

115. McCarty CA, Zimmerman FJ, Digiuseppe DL et al: Parental emotional support and subsequent internalizing and externalizing problems among children, *J Dev Behav Pediatr* 26:267-275, 2005.

116. Rose AJ, Rudolph KD: A review of sex differences in peer relationship processes: potential trade-offs for the emotional and behavioral development of girls and boys, *Psychol Bull* 132:98-131, 2006.

117. Fish EW, Shahrokh D, Bagot R et al: Epigenetic programming of stress responses through variations in maternal care, *Ann N Y Acad Sci* 1036:167-180, 2004.

118. Cocker C, Scott S: Improving the mental and emotional well-being of looked after children: Connecting research, policy and practice, *J R Soc Health* 126:18-23, 2006.

119. Egger HL, Angold A: Common emotional and behavioral disorders in preschool children: Presentation, nosology, and epidemiology, *J Child Psychol Psychiatry* 47:313-337, 2006.

120. Murray L, Halligan SL, Adams G et al: Socioemotional development in adolescents at risk for depression: The role of maternal depression and attachment style, *Dev Psychopathol* 18:489-516, 2006.

121. Nigg JT, Casey BJ: An integrative theory of attention-deficit/hyperactivity disorder based on the cognitive and affective neurosciences, *Dev Psychopathol* 17:785-806, 2005.

122. Porcerelli JH, West PA, Binienda J et al: Physical and psychological symptoms in emotionally abused and non-abused women, *J Am Board Fam Med* 19:201-204, 2006.

123. Sagvolden T, Johansen EB, Aase H et al: A dynamic developmental theory of attention-deficit/hyperactivity disorder (ADHD) predominantly hyperactive/impulsive and combined subtypes, *Behav Brain Sci* 28:397-419, 2005.

124. Barbuto JE Jr, Burbach ME: The emotional intelligence of transformational leaders: a field study of elected officials, *J Soc Psychol* 146:51-64, 2006.

125. Goldenberg I, Matheson K, Mantler J: The assessment of emotional intelligence: a comparison of performance-based and self-report methodologies, *J Pers Assess* 86:33-45, 2006.

126. Hopkins RO, Tate DF, Bigler ED: Anoxic versus traumatic brain injury: amount of tissue loss, not etiology, alters cognitive and emotional function, *Neuropsychology* 19:233-242, 2005.

127. Kemp AH, Hopkinson PJ, Stephan BC et al: Predicting severity of non-clinical depression: preliminary findings using an integrated approach, *J Integr Neurosci* 5:89-110, 2006.

128. Lewis NJ, Rees CE, Hudson JN et al: Emotional intelligence medical education: Measuring the unmeasurable? *Adv Health Sci Educ Theory Pract* 10:339-355, 2005.

129. Rao PR: Emotional intelligence: the sine qua non for a clinical leadership toolbox, *J Commun Disord* 39:310-319, 2006.

130. Taylor B: Emotional intelligence: a primer for practitioners in human communication disorders, *Semin Speech Lang* 26:138-148, 2005.

131. Elias MJ, Weissberg RP: Primary prevention: educational approaches to enhance social and emotional learning, *J Sch Health* 70:186-190, 2000.

132. Gohm CL: Mood regulation and emotional intelligence: individual differences, *J Pers Soc Psychol* 84:594-607, 2003.

133. Shammi P, Stuss DT: The effects of normal aging on humor appreciation, *J Int Neuropsychol Soc* 9:855-863, 2003.

134. Thomas KM: Assessing brain development using neurophysiologic and behavioral measures, *J Pediatr* 143(4 Suppl):S46-53, 2003.

135. Leonard D, Swap W: Deep smarts, *Harv Bus Rev* 82:88-97, 137, 2004.

136. Maret S: The evidence for a scientific "paradigm." In Stave U, editor: *Physiology of the perinatal period,* pp. 751-769, New York, 1978, Plenum.

137. Shumway-Cook A, Woollacott MH: *Motor control: theory and practical applications,* Philadelphia, 2001, Lippincott Williams & Wilkins.

138. VanSant AF: Motor control, motor learning and motor development. In Montgomery PC, Connolly BH, editors: *Clinical applications for motor control,* pp. 26-50, Thorofare, NJ, 2003, Slack.

139. Li KZH, Lindenberger U: Relations between aging sensory/sensorimotor and cognitive functions, *Neurosci Biobehav Res* 26:777-783, 2002.

140. Lindenberger U, Marsiske M, Baltes PB: Memorizing while walking: increase in dual task costs from young adulthood to old age, *Psychol Aging* 15:417-436, 2000.

141. Lovden M, Schellenbach M, Grossman-Hutter B et al: Environmental topography and postural control demands shape aging-associated decrements in spatial navgation performance, *Psychol Aging* 20:683-694, 2005.

142. Pooh RK, Ogura T: Normal and abnormal fetal hand positioning and movement in early pregnancy detected by three- and four-dimensional ultrasound, *Ultrasound Rev Obstet Gynecol* 1:46-51, 2004.

143. Bertenthal B: Origins and early development of perception, action and representation, *Annu Rev Psychol* 47:431-459, 1996.

144. DeCasper AJ, Fifer WP: Of human bonding: newborns prefer their mothers' voices, *Science* 208:174-176, 1980.

145. Chrisiensen S, Dubignon J, Campbell D: Variations in intra-oral stimulation and nutritive sucking, *Child Dev* 47:539-542, 1976.

146. Corbetta D, Thelan E: The developmental origins of bimanual coordination: a dynamic perspective, *J Exp Psychol Hum* 22:502-522, 1996.

147. Owens KB: *Child and adolescent development: an integrated approach,* Belmont, CA, 2002, Wadsworth.

148. Ashburn SS: Biophysical development during early adulthood. In Schuster CS, Ashburn SS, editors: *The process of human development: a holistic life-span approach,* pp. 556-577, Philadelphia, 1992, JB Lippincott.

149. Tinetti ME, Baker DI, McAvay G et al: A multifactorial intervention to reduce the risk of falling among elderly people living in the community, *N Engl J Med* 331:821-827, 1994.

150. Patten C, Craik RL: Sensorimotor changes and adaptation in the older adult. In Guiccone AA, editor: *Geriatric physical therapy,* ed 2, pp. 78-109, St. Louis, 2000, Mosby.

151. Benjuva N, Melzer I, Kaplanski J: Aging-induced shifts from a reliance on sensory input to muscle cocontraction during balanced standing. *J Gerontol A Biol Sci Med Sci* 59A:166-171, 2004.

152. Seidler-Dobrin RD, He J, Stelmach GE: Coactivation to reduce variability in the elderly, *J Mot Behav* 2:314-330, 1998.

153. Shumway-Cook A, Gruber W, Baldwin M et al: The effect of multidimensional exercises on balance, mobility and fall risk in community-dwelling older adults, *Phys Ther* 77:46-57, 1997.

154. Potvin AR, Syndulko K, Tourtellotte WW et al: Human neurological function and the aging process, *J Am Geriatr Soc* 28:1-9, 1980.

CHAPTER 3

Contemporary Issues and Theories of Motor Control, Motor Learning, and Neuroplasticity: Assessment of Movement and Posture

Sharon L. Gorman, PT, MS, GCS

KEY WORDS

motor and postural control theories
motor learning, motor control, and neuroplasticity
neurological assessment

OBJECTIVES

After reading this chapter the student/therapist will be able to:

1. Identify the difference between motor control–based theory from reflex or hierarchical-based theory.
2. Differentiate concepts of motor control from motor learning or neuroplasticity
3. Identify and analyze the parameters of motor control as an ability to maintain upright posture, movement within that posture, or change programming to allow movement away from that position.
4. Compare the various elements of motor control and identify how each factor might affect movement and the ability to maintain upright posture.
5. Recognize how motor and postural control theory can be applied to the examination and interventions of clients with neurological dysfunction.

Sciences fundamental to evaluation and selection of a treatment intervention in physical and occupational therapy are motor control, motor learning, and motor development. Therapists need an understanding of neural regulation of movements, how movement patterns or motor behavior are learned, and how motor behavior changes across the life span in healthy people, along with a current understanding of how neuroplasticity theories can affect changes after intervention. A framework for typical motor behavior is necessary to understand how motor behavior is altered in persons with neurological dysfunction and how the plastic properties of the nervous system interact to produce change. As new information about motor learning and neuroplasticity (Chapter 9), and life span development (Chapter 2) becomes available, principles that form the bases for examination and treatment are reassessed, modified, or replaced with newer principles of motor control.

Learning a behavioral sequence or motor program must occur before the individual's ability to control that motor pattern or behavior. Some motor learning occurs in utero, often called reflexive or pre-existing motor programs, and will be integrated and modified through life. Motor learning will continue throughout life as long as the environment asks for change and the central nervous system (CNS) has the pliability and desire to learn. Motor control is the study of how an individual controls movement already acquired.[1-5] Neuroplasticity is defined as the brain's ability to adapt or use cellular adaptations to learn or relearn functions previously lost as a result of cellular death by trauma or disease at any age. How much of this ability is created by internally driven mechanisms, such as disease or a change in height or weight compared with external environmental demands, such as

need to walk or eat, is yet to be identified. It has been found that, given the appropriate environment, the CNS can learn or relearn despite damage to the system.[6-8] Many of the in-depth concepts of motor learning and plasticity will be discussed throughout the book (especially Chapter 9). This chapter will focus on motor control and how the CNS during or after learning controls movements in relation to environmental demands or client choices. It is impossible to totally differentiate motor learning and plasticity from motor control because the CNS is responding, learning, adapting, and, in the most efficient way, directing motor action to meet life's demands. This chapter has three purposes: (1) to provide the reader with a review of current models used to represent neural regulation of motor control leading to posture and movement in all aspects of life activities, (2) to describe some deficits of motor control using these models and the ways in which therapists can use this schema to evaluate patients with neurological dysfunction, and (3) to describe neuroplasticity research in the context of physical and occupational therapy.

A model is a schematic representation of a theory, in this context, how the nervous system regulates motor behavior. Many motor and postural control models exist because researchers use different approaches to develop and test theories. All models have limitations and are constantly changing as researchers gain new information and as technological advances are made. A theory that is constantly tested and undergoing change is better than an outdated theory or no theoretical framework. Early researchers used visual observation and palpation to develop models of motor control. Today, researchers use a variety of techniques and tools reflective of their level of interest. These include, for example, electromyography, film analysis, force plates, electron microscopy, transcranial magnetic stimulation, and functional magnetic resonance. Finally, models may portray only a small part of the nervous system; for example, a model of the spinal cord control mechanisms examining regeneration of the lesioned spinal cord would not include higher-center control processes. Other models may be more holistic. For example, systems modeling may be used to investigate the interrelationships among various brain centers and spinal pattern generators to examine recovery of hand function in clients with hemiplegia resulting from a cerebrovascular accident.

Motor control theories serving as a basis for predicting motor responses during patient assessment and treatment and functional outcome should have a broad scope. A therapist using a spinal level reflex model, for example, may inaccurately predict motor behavior because this model does not consider regulation of motor behavior by higher brain centers. This model assumes the patient is a passive recipient rather than an active participant. Selecting and using a proper model is important for the analysis and treatment of posture and movement dysfunctions.

A CLASSIC MODEL OF MOTOR CONTROL

The hierarchy model is the base for traditional neurological therapy. A description of the hierarchy, its application to pathophysiological mechanisms and motor control, and its limitations are presented. The hierarchy model proposes that a higher-center commander select and delegate the motor program to subordinate centers for execution (Figure 3-1). The midbrain, brain stem, and spinal cord are considered subordinate centers. Motor programs are assumed to be stored at the highest level and not influenced by feedforward or feedback mechanisms during execution of the movement. Feedback loops are included in contemporary hierarchical models of motor control. Although information about the internal and external environment is available before and after the execution of the movement, the commander does not necessarily incorporate the information during subsequent movements.

When disease or injury damages the highest center, dissolution of the whole nervous system occurs.[9] The more stable lower and evolutionarily older nervous centers located in the midbrain and brain stem control movement. Movements represented at the lower levels of the nervous system are reflexive, that is, stereotypical and not capable of modification when the external or internal environmental conditions necessitate a change. Damage to the highest

centers also results in a poverty of motor responses (negative deficit) or an overreadiness of the nervous system to remain active (positive deficit).

The hierarchy model for motor control represents the state of science from the middle of the nineteenth century to the early twentieth century. Although this model has limitations, it was the basis for development of the disciplines of neurology and neurological physical and occupational therapy. Since the incorporation of the hierarchy model into therapeutic theory, researchers have developed other theories for the regulation of posture and movement. The hierarchical model is useful to examine motor activity that occurs without feedback and so is included here; however, this model is of limited use when trying to understand the interrelationships of brain centers for planning, initiating, or learning motor activities.

CONTEMPORARY MODELS OF MOTOR CONTROL

Researchers adopted the term *systems* from engineering to describe the relationship of various brain and spinal centers working together with the use of feedback (Figure 3-2). Sensation is the process whereby receptors receive information relative to the internal and external environment. The receptors encode the information for transmission to various regions of the nervous system. The CNS receives and interprets the sensations on the basis of present experiences, the present state of the internal and external environment, and memory of similar situations. This process is termed *perception*. Processing this information in the context of a goal, the motor activity to be achieved, leads to the development of movement and postural strategies. This operation is termed *response selection,* that is, choosing the most contextually appropriate movement strategy to meet the needs of the individual and the constraints of the environment. The strategy is executed (response execution) by the muscles and joints. The observable motor behavior is the result of perception and then the selection and execution of the appropriate motor and postural responses using both feed-forward and feedback mechanisms. This model differs significantly from the classical model in that both feed-forward and feedback are integral parts of the motor and postural responses. Additionally, this model includes the higher centers' active participation in the movement outcome through perception

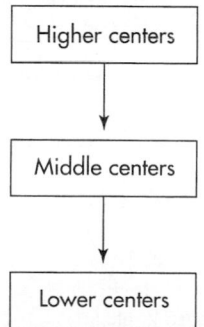

FIGURE 3-1 ■ Model of a hierarchy of motor control.

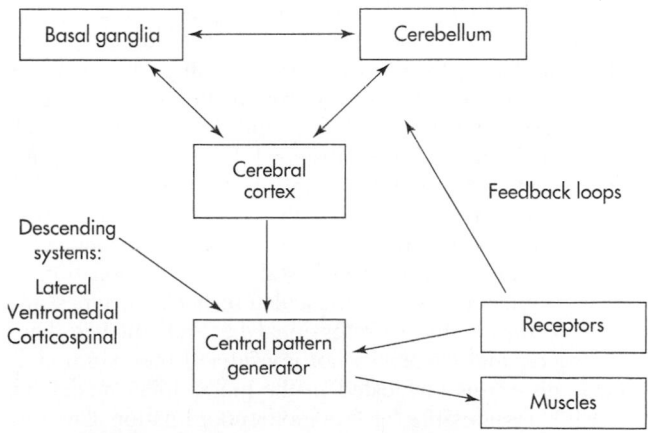

FIGURE 3-2 ■ Systems model of motor control.

of sensory input. Last, this model appreciates the subtle differences in motor output that can be driven by environmental context or situational needs of the individual relating the environment in which they are functioning as well as the emotional set (fear, relaxation, anger). This interplay between sensory input, motor output, and environmental concerns expands the function of persons from the classical model.

Researchers have garnered principles and concepts from different disciplines to develop the systems approach to motor control, for example, neuroscience theory, principles of nonlinear phenomena in physics, and Bernstein's[10] degrees of freedom. Some of the principles and concepts included in systems theory are described later. The concepts presented in this section are representative of systems theory and dynamic action theory and are by no means inclusive of all the concepts contained in these multifaceted and complex theories. Comprehensive discussions of these theories are found elsewhere.[10-17]

Principles and Concepts Related to Contemporary Motor Control Theories

As mentioned earlier, contemporary motor control models have a similar set of assumptions and concepts, yet each model contains additional discrete assumptions and concepts. Described in this section are elements from the various contemporary theories that are useful for the description of motor and postural control in clients with neurological dysfunction, as well as in healthy individuals. These elements can be components of a theory, or a single element can represent a theory. They do not stand alone to explain motor control in the healthy individual or the individual with neurological dysfunction. Rather, they are interrelated. The interaction of these various elements produces the emergent motor and postural behavior in response to the environmental and task demands of the situation.

Multiple Descending Pathways to Regulate Posture and Movement

A traditional hierarchical model assumes only one descending, voluntary pathway. Regulation of posture and movement is more complex, as demonstrated by a descending model proposed by Laurence and Kuypers.[18,19] The descending pathways are categorized into the medial descending system, the lateral descending system, and the cortical corticospinal system. The medial descending system, primarily represented by the vestibulospinal pathways, projects bilaterally to spinal level neuronal pools to provide antigravity regulation, that is, to control proximal limb girdle and trunk musculature to maintain the upright position so that the face is vertical and the mouth is horizontal. The lateral descending systems, primarily represented by the reticulospinal pathways, provide regulatory control over the axial and limb musculature. The third system, the corticospinal tract, provides regulation and control of fine motor control and regulation of movement, such as distal finger fractionation or intricate variance of axial musculature between types and speeds of throws by a professional baseball pitcher. Thus the corticospinal system is not considered the "volitional" control system as suggested in the hierarchical model but rather it is responsible for fine motor coordination. Creating lesions in the corticospinal system of monkeys did not result

in loss of volitional control. To expand their model, the cortical system, including the corticobulbar system, provides regulation and control over all synergies, both movement and balance movement patterns. The rubrospinal tract is smaller in humans than other primates, and its function in the regulation of upperextremity flexor activity is linked to the function of the lateral corticospinal tract.[8]

Central Pattern Generator or Reflex

Traditionally, in the hierarchical model the basic spinal level unit is the reflex. If a particular stimulus activates receptors, a single stereotypical motor response results. In systems theory developed from a neuroscience perspective, the basic spinal level unit is the central pattern generator (CPG).[20,21] Evidence for CPGs has been found in many vertebrates, including humans. CPGs are diagramed as oscillators to denote their rhythmical activity. One model postulates that one half of the oscillator controls flexor synergies and that the other half is responsible for extensor synergies, thereby controlling the muscles of an entire limb.[22] More discrete oscillators are postulated to regulate individual pairs of antagonistic muscles.[23] Coupling oscillators within a single limb permits multijoint intralimb coordination, and coupling oscillators between limbs produces interlimb coordination and allows for a variety of movement patterns. For example, a loose coupling of interlimb oscillators permits homolateral, homonymous, and cross-diagonal locomotor patterns.

If a single stimulus activates a CPG, a series of motor responses occurs. The rhythmical pattern (emergent property) produced by an oscillator can remain activated without additional sensory input. Rhythmical activity in a spinal level reflex occurs only by additional sensory stimuli (Figure 3-3).

Perturbations or disturbances during the rhythmical activity can affect the timing or amplitude of the response of the synergy. This is useful in the practical application of stimulating the CPG in humans. For example, a perturbation can occur during locomotion when an obstacle is placed in

A. A single response per stimulus

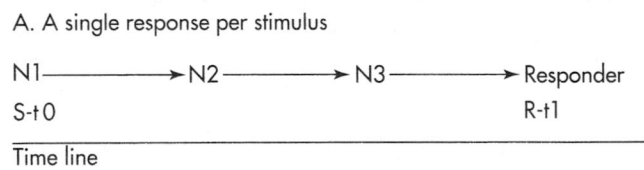

B. Emergent property: more than one response

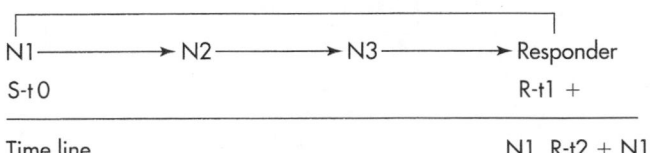

Key:
N = neuron
S-t0 = start time
R-t = response 1; response 2, etc.

FIGURE 3-3 ■ Emergent property.

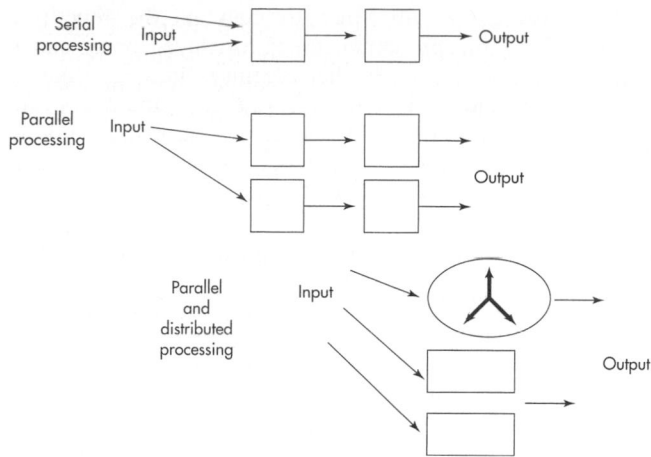

FIGURE 3-4 ■ Methods of information processing.

the path. Portions of the CPG can alter the timing or amplitude of the response without altering the rhythm. Spinal level neurons such as Renshaw cells or Ia inhibitory interneurons have been identified as potential contributors to this modulation.[24]

Information Processing

The configuration of the systems model lends itself to many modes to process information, primarily sensory information. Serial processing denotes a specific order of processing (Figure 3-4) of information by various centers. Information proceeds lockstep through each center. Parallel processing denotes processing of information by more than one center simultaneously or nearly simultaneously, and that information can be used for more than one activity. A third and more flexible type of processing of information is parallel-distributed processing.[25] This type of processing combines the best attributes of serial and parallel processing. That is, when the situation demands serial processing, this type of activity occurs. At other times, parallel processing is the mode of choice. For optimum processing of information from internal and external sensory information by various regions of the brain, a combination of both parallel and serial processing is the most efficient mode. The type of processing depends on the constraints of the situation. For example, maintaining balance after an unexpected external perturbation requires rapid processing, whereas learning to voluntarily shift the center of gravity to the limits of stability requires a different combination of processing modes.

In summary, processing reinforces and refines motor patterns. Processing permits the organism to initiate compensatory strategies if the wrong motor pattern is selected or if an unexpected perturbation occurs. Last, processing permits learning.

Movement Patterns Arising From Self-Organizing Subsystems

Coordinated movement patterns are developed from the dynamic interaction of subsystems in relation to internal and external constraints. Therefore, movement patterns used to accomplish a goal are contextually appropriate and arise as an emergent property of subsystem interaction. Several principles relate to self-organizing systems: reciprocity, distributed function, consensus, and emergent properties.[26]

Reciprocity implies information flow between two or more neural networks. These networks can represent specific brain centers, for example, the cerebellum and basal ganglia (see Figure 3-2). Alternatively, the neural networks can be interacting neuronal clusters located within a single center, for example, the basal ganglia. One model to demonstrate reciprocity is the basal ganglia regulation of motor behavior through direct and indirect pathways to cortical areas. One pathway, the more direct pathway from the putamen to the globus pallidus internal segment, provides net inhibitory effects. The more indirect pathway from the putamen through the globus pallidus external segment and subthalamic nucleus provides a net excitatory effect on the globus pallidus internal segment. Alteration of the balance between these pathways is postulated to produce motor dysfunction[27,28] (see Chapter 24). An abnormally decreased outflow from the basal ganglia is postulated to produce involuntary motor patterns, which produces excessive motion such as chorea, hemiballism, or tremor. Alternatively, an abnormally increased outflow from the basal ganglia is postulated to produce a paucity of motions, as seen in the rigidity observed in individuals with Parkinson's disease.

Distributed function presupposes that a single center or neural network has more than one function. The concept also implies that several centers share the same function. For example, a center may serve as the coordinating unit in one task and may serve as a pattern generator or oscillator to maintain the activity in another task. An advantage of distributing function among groups of neurons or centers is to provide centers with overlapping or redundant functions. Neuroscientists believe such redundancy is a safety feature. If a neuronal lesion occurs, other centers can assume critical functional roles, thereby producing recovery from CNS dysfunction.[5-8,15,29]

Consensus implies that motor behavior occurs when a majority of brain centers or regions reach a critical threshold to produce activation. Consensus also functions to filter extraneous information or information that does require immediate attention. If, however, a novel stimulus enters the system, it carries more weight and receives immediate attention. A novel stimulus may be new to the system, may reflect a potentially harmful situation, or may result from the conflict of multiple inputs.

Emergent properties may be understood by the adage "the whole is greater than the sum of its parts." This concept implies that brain centers, not a single brain center, work together to produce movement. An example of the emergent properties concept is continuous repetitive activity (oscillation). In Figure 3-3, A, a hierarchy is represented by three neurons arranged in tandem. The last neuron ends on a responder. If a single stimulus activates this network, a single response occurs. What is the response if the neurons are arranged so that the third neuron sends a collateral branch to the first neuron in addition to the ending on the responder? In this case (see Figure 3-3, B), a single stimulus activates neuron No. 1, which in turn activates neurons No. 2 and No. 3, causing a response as well as reactivating neuron No. 1. This neuronal arrangement produces a series of responses rather than a single response. This process is also termed *endogenous activity.*

Another example of an emergent property is the production of motor behavior. Rather than having every motor program stored in the brain, an abstract representation of the intended goal is stored. At the time of motor performance, various brain centers use the present sensory information, combined with past memory of the task, to develop the appropriate motor strategy. This concept negates a hard-wired motor program concept. If motor programs were hard-wired and if a motor program existed for every movement ever performed, the brain would need a huge storage capacity and would lack the adaptability necessary for complex function.

Controlling the Degrees of Freedom

Combinations of muscle and joint action permit a large number of degrees of freedom that contribute to movement. A system with a large number of degrees of freedom is called a *high-dimensional system.* For a contextually appropriate movement to occur, the number of degrees of freedom needs to be constrained. Bernstein[10] suggested that the number of degrees of freedom could be reduced by muscles working in synergies, that is, coupling muscles and joints of a limb to produce functional patterns of movement. Therefore the functional unit of motor behavior is a *synergy,* also called a coordinative structure. By reducing the degrees of freedom, a high-dimensional system becomes a low-dimensional system, that is, a system with fewer degrees of freedom. For example, a functional synergy pattern for the lower extremity can be a step. Locomotion occurs by linking together the functional synergies of other limbs (interlimb coordination).

Functional synergy implies that muscles are activated in an appropriate sequence and with appropriate force, timing, and directional components. These components can be represented as fixed or "relative" ratios, and the control comes from input given to the cerebellum from higher centers in the brain and the peripheral/spinal system and from prior learning[8,29,30] (see Chapter 26). The relative parameters are also termed *control parameters.* Scaling control parameters leads to a change in motor behavior to accomplish the task. For example, writing your name on the blackboard exemplifies scaling force and timing. Scaling is the proportional increase or decrease of the parameter to produce the intended motor activity.

Coordinated movement is defined as an orderly sequence of muscle activity in single functional synergy or the orderly sequence of functional synergies with appropriate scaling of activation parameters necessary to produce the intended motor behavior. Uncoordinated movement can occur at the level of the scaling of control parameters in one functional synergy or inappropriate coupling of functional synergies. The control parameter of duration will be used to illustrate scaling. If muscle A is active for 10% of the duration of the motor activity and muscle B is active 50% of the time, the fixed ratio of A/B is 1:5. If the movement is performed slowly, the relative time for the entire movement increases. Fixed ratios also increase proportionally. Writing your name on a blackboard very small or very large yields the same results—your name.

When a repetitive movement such as elbow flexion and extension is performed, the biceps and triceps muscles need to be active at certain times to maintain the repetitive motion. If the biceps demonstrates a delayed onset and a longer duration of activity that continues into the time of activation of the triceps muscle, the movement appears uncoordinated. If muscle A had a delayed onset and the same duration, the movement would not appear to be smooth. Patients with neurological dysfunction demonstrate alterations in the timing of muscle activity in a functional synergy or in coupling of functional synergies to produce movement.[31,32]

Fixed ratios such as amplitude and timing are incorporated into a synergy to decrease the degrees of freedom. The relative parameters of the synergy provide the flexibility or adaptability of the system for task accomplishment; however, the movement pattern may be self-limiting or limited by constraints imposed by the environment or the body. The amplitude of writing on a blackboard is limited by the height of the blackboard, the length of the arm, and the overall height of the person stretching to make the letter larger.

These functional synergies are not hardwired but represent emergent properties. They are flexible and adaptable to meet the needs of the task and the environmental constraints. They can be described in terms of timing, for example, timing of the flexion and extension phases, and in terms of phasing, that is, when the flexion and extension phases occur in relation to one another. The movement can also be described in terms of the positional relationship between joints. These descriptors of motor behavior have been termed *order parameters.* In summary, the nervous system is organized to limit the degrees of freedom to accomplish the task. Limiting the degrees of freedom implies that a finite number of strategies are available to accomplish the goal.

Finite Number of Movement Strategies

The concept of emergent properties could conceivably imply an unlimited number of movement strategies available to perform a particular task. As stated earlier, limiting the degrees of freedom decreases the number of strategies available for selection. In addition, constraints imposed by the internal environment (e.g., musculoskeletal system, cardiovascular system, metabolic activity, cognition) and external environment (e.g., support surface, obstacles, lighting) limit the number of movement strategies. Horak and Nashner[33] observed that a finite number of balance strategies were used by individuals in response to externally applied linear perturbations on a force plate system. With use of a life span approach, VanSant[34] identified a limited number of movement patterns for the upper limb, head-trunk, and lower limb for the task of rising from supine to standing.

The combination of these strategies produces the necessary variability in motor behavior. Although an individual has a preferred or modal profile, the healthy person with an intact neuromuscular system can combine the strategies in the various body regions to produce a different movement pattern to accomplish the task. Persons with neurological deficits may be unable to produce a successful efficient movement pattern because of their inability to combine strategies or adapt a strategy for a given environmental change (e.g., differing chair height for sit-to-stand transitions).

Variability of Movements Implies Normalcy

Age, activity level, the environment, constraints of a goal, and neuropathological conditions affect the selection of patterns available for use during movement tasks. When change occurs in one or more of the neural subsystems, a new movement pattern emerges. The element that causes change is called a control parameter. For example, an increase in the speed of walking occurs until a critical speed and degree of hip extension is reached, thereby switching the movement pattern to a run. When the speed of the run is decreased, there is a shift back to the preferred movement pattern, that is, walking. A control parameter then shifts the individual into a different pattern of motor behavior.

This concept underlies theories of development and learning. Development and learning can be viewed as moving the system from a stable state to a more unstable state. When the control variable is removed, the system moves back to the early, more stable state. As the control variable continues to push the system, the individual spends more time in the new state and less time in the earlier state until the individual spends most of the time in the new state. When this occurs, the new state becomes the preferred state. Moving or shifting to the new, preferred state does not obviate the ability of the individual to use the earlier state of motor behavior. Therefore new movement patterns take place when critical changes occur in the system because of a control parameter but do not eliminate older, less-preferred patterns of movement.

Motivation to accomplish a task in spite of functional limitations and neuropathological conditions can also shift the individual's CNS to select different patterns of motor behavior. The musculoskeletal system, by nature of the architecture of the joints and muscle attachments, can be a constraint on the movement pattern. An individual with a functional contracture may be limited in the ability to bend a joint only into a desired range, thereby decreasing the movement repertoire available to the individual. Such a constraint produces adaptive motor behavior. Dorsiflexion of the foot needs to meet a critical degree of toe clearance during gait. If there is a range of motion limitation in dorsiflexion, then biomechanical constraints imposed on the nervous system will produce adaptive motor behaviors (e.g., toe clearance during gait). Changes in motor patterns during the task of rising from supine to standing are observed when healthy individuals wear an orthosis to limit dorsiflexion.[9] The inability to easily open and close the hand with rotation may lead to adaptations that require the shoulder musculature to place the hand in a more functional position. This adaptation uses axial and trunk muscles and will limit the use of that limb in both fine and gross motor performance (see Chapter 27).

An individual uses preferred movement patterns that are stable yet flexible enough to meet the ever-changing environmental conditions. These preferred, not obligatory, movement patterns are considered *attractor* states. That is, the individual can choose to use another movement pattern to accomplish the task. Older adults may choose movement patterns that decrease the risk of falling. The choice may be in response to age-related declines in the sensory systems or a fear of falling. For example, when performing the Multi-directional Reach Test,[35] the older adult may choose to reach forward, backward (lean), or laterally without shifting the center of gravity toward the limits of stability. The older adult can perform a different reach if asked but prefers a more stable pattern.

An obligatory or stereotypical movement pattern suggests that the individual does not have the capability to adapt to a new situation or cannot use a different movement pattern to accomplish the task. This inability may be due to internal constraints that are functional or pathophysiological. The patient who had a cerebrovascular accident has CNS constraints that limit the number of different movement patterns that can emerge from the self-organizing system. With recovery, the patient may be able to select and use additional movement strategies. Cognition and the capability to learn may also limit the number of movement patterns available to the individual and the ability of the person to select and use new or different movement patterns.

Obligatory or stereotypical movement patterns also arise from external constraints imposed on the organism. Consider the external constraints placed on the concert violin player. These external constraints include, for example, the length of the bow and the position of the violin. Repetitive movement patterns leading to cumulative trauma disorder in healthy individuals can lead to muscular and neurological changes.[36-39] Over time, changes in dystonic posturing and changes in the somatosensory cortex have been observed. Although one hypothesis considers that the focal dystonia results from sensory integrative problems, the observable result is a stereotypical motor problem.

A key to the assessment and treatment of individuals with neurological dysfunction lies in variability of movement and in the notion that variability is a sign of normalcy and stereotypy is a sign of dysfunction.

To review, the nervous system responds to a variety of internal and external constraints to develop and execute motor behavior that is age appropriate and efficient to accomplish the task. Efficiency can be examined in terms of metabolic cost to the individual, type of movement pattern used, the preferred or habitual movement (habit) used by the individual, and time to complete the task. The term *attractor state* is used in dynamic systems theory to describe the preferred pattern or habitual movement.

The concepts of motor efficiency and preferred movement patterns are important for neurological rehabilitation. Because of the neurological insult, the patient with a neurological deficit may have a limited repertoire of movement strategies available. The patient experiments with different motor patterns to learn the most efficient and energy-conserving motor strategy to accomplish the task. Therapists can refine the task on the basis of safety issues and the patient's capability to accomplish the task by using a variety of movement strategies rather than using one stereotypical strategy, leading to an increase in function.

Role of Sensory Information

The CNS uses sensory information in a variety of ways to regulate posture and movement. Before movement is initiated, information about the position of the body in space and body parts to one another and environmental conditions is obtained from sensory receptors. This information is used in the selection and execution of the movement synergy. During movement, various neural centers (e.g., the cerebellum) use feedback to compare the actual motor behavior with the intended motor behavior. If the actual and intended motor behaviors do not match, an error signal is produced and alterations in the motor behavior are triggered. In some instances, the control system anticipates and makes corrective changes before the detection of the error signal. This anticipatory correction is termed *feed-forward* control. Changing one's gait path while walking in a busy shopping mall to avoid a collision is an example of how using visual information about the location of people and objects can be used in a feed-forward manner.

Another role of sensory information is to revise the reference of correctness (central representation) before the motor program is executed again. For example, a young child standing on a balance beam with the feet close together falls off the balance beam. An error signal occurs because of the mismatch between the intended motor behavior and the actual motor result. If the child knows that the feet were too close together when the fall occurred, then the child will space the feet farther apart on the next trial. The information about what happened, falling or not falling, is called knowledge of results. The CNS can store knowledge of results and use it when planning movement strategies for balancing on any narrow object, such as a balance beam, log, or wall, in the future. Therapists can use knowledge of results when formatting interventions with clients to improve motor control and motor learning by choosing appropriate activities and functional tasks for use when working with the client.[40] Ballistic movements do not rely on sensory feedback loops to modify the program as it is being executed because the execution phase occurs very quickly. In this instance, feedback is received in the form of knowledge of results after the execution of movement. Most naturally occurring movements are classified as nonballistic and therefore operate on both feed-forward and feedback mechanisms, allowing therapists to use knowledge of results to the client's benefit during treatment.

Several researchers investigated whether peripheral feedback is necessary during the execution phase of movement.[41-43] Rothwell et al[41,42] studied a patient with a unilateral deafferented upper extremity resulting from a peripheral sensory neuropathy. The man could write sentences with his eyes closed and drive a car with a manual transmission without watching the gearshift, but he had difficulty with fine motor tasks such as buttoning a shirt and using a knife and fork. He was unable to sustain a muscle contraction using a pincer grasp when asked to perform the task with eyes closed and he could not learn to drive a different car with a manual transmission. On the basis of these observations, continued peripheral feedback may not be necessary when executing a learned motor behavior in a stable context. However, peripheral feedback is necessary during the acquisition or learning of new motor behaviors that are not inherent in new, differing contexts or situations.

Sensory information must be weighed by the individual, unconsciously, in light of factors such as experience and other competing demands.[44] The importance may affect the timing of dual task activities. The amount of attention for maintaining postural control changes during increasing function, such as seen in sitting versus standing versus walking.[45-47] During dual task conditions, older people were found to respond to auditory tasks during the double-support, initial-contact phase of gait compared with younger participants who responded close to the time of stimulus regardless of the phase of gait.[46] Activities that require external timing, such as open tasks, will require more attention to the timing of the task, leaving less available attention for the actions required to maintain balance.[48] An example would be stepping onto an escalator. The balance control required for the stepping pattern is constant, but the individual must also time the stepping pattern precisely to coincide with the movement of the escalator for a successful action. Externally paced activities, dual task activities, and the complexity of the environment will provide a greater challenge to information processing.[44,49]

Neuroplasticity and Motor Rehabilitation

Neuroplasticity refers to the brain's ability to reorganize itself and form new neural connections. During early development, neuroplasticity is the norm in the nervous system, but it can occur in all humans after injury or insult to the CNS. Neuronal sprouting is thought to be the primary mechanism, allowing injured neurons to reconnect in new ways and allowing intact, undamaged neurons to form new connections to allow for increased function. In animal studies, intense exercise regimens when coupled with introduction to complex motor tasks have been shown to facilitate improvement in motor function and plastic neurological changes. Restoration of function by way of motor rehabilitation has been shown to call in mechanisms that repair, protect, rewire, or reactivate neurons. Rehabilitation techniques may prevent synaptic degeneration of neurons and may even help to reorganize or guide recovery to allow functional adaptations to occur. The timing of initiation of motor rehabilitation techniques has been shown in animals to be of the utmost importance; human studies will need to investigate the timing of rehabilitation to maximize the positive benefits provided by such programs and to limit any deleterious effects that timing may cause.

Research into neuroplasticity has shown the importance of attention to the somatosensory, proprioceptive, and kinesthetic aspects of the motoric task.[50] Plasticity outside infancy is strongly modulated by reward, judgment of error, punishment, and attention.[51] Determining the correct set of conditions for the task a patient is practicing will influence the difficulty of the task, which will in turn influence the brain's plasticity. Negative plasticity can occur when conditions for the motor tasks are not carefully considered or controlled (Table 3-1). The importance of using skilled motor behav-

TABLE 3-1 ■ Neuroprotective Motor Enrichment Factors Affecting Outcomes

	NEGATIVE PLASTICITY	POSITIVE PLASTICITY
Stimulation	Disuse, unskilled	Intensive, skilled
Quality of sensory input	Noisy, nonspecific	Appropriate, specific
Modulation	Not challenging	High stakes, novel, challenging
Outcome	Negative behaviors	Positive behaviors

iors in training to improve the plastic changes and the functional outcomes of clients/patients is just starting to be studied. The skill level required for task performance appears to influence plasticity changes. Exercise tasks in animal models, specifically skilled-type exercises, lead to increased angiogenesis in damaged cortical areas whereas unskilled activities did not show this positive change and additionally had no synaptogenesis in the damaged region.[51] It is believed that in humans focusing rehabilitation techniques on functional, meaningful, and skilled activities or tasks will enhance the neuroplastic changes and enhance recovery in the period immediately after the insult.[52-54]

Attention is one of the factors that can easily be monitored during therapeutic interactions with clients. Ensuring that the client is attentive to the task at hand during intervention will enhance the brain's ability to learn that task. This should sound familiar because you, as a student, have most likely noticed that attending a lecture will not ensure learning the material as well as attending the lecture and paying attention; being actively engaged in the content while it is being delivered helps learning and retention of the material.

Errors in Motor Control

When the actual motor behavior does not match the intended motor behavior, one or several errors may be postulated to produce this mismatch. This section describes these different types of errors. The following scenario can be used to illustrate various types of errors: A person is standing at a curb waiting for the light to change. The individual is unexpectedly pushed from behind and attempts to make a balance response, for example, a sway at the ankle to maintain the upright position, but ultimately falls. A loss of balance is indicative that one or several errors occurred. First, the individual selected the wrong movement strategy. Although sway about the ankle is a proper strategy to maintain balance, it was inadequate for this situation because the person fell. Second, the individual selected the appropriate motor program but used inappropriate scaling of relative parameters (in this instance an inappropriate scaling of amplitude of the response in relation to the perturbing force). Third, the individual may not have accurately accessed and perceived the initial sensory conditions (e.g., unable to ignore sensory conflicts). If a car were passing in front of the individual, the individual might perceive that he or she was moving sideways, thereby relying on altered or inaccurate information for selection of the motor program. Any one or any combination of these errors may have been the cause of the fall.

Errors also occur when unexpected factors disrupt the execution of the program. For example, an individual walks on a moving sidewalk. The more unpredictable moving surface has been called an "open environment" and will force the individual to adapt his or her responses more quickly. Other examples of open environments include catching a ball, because the ultimate trajectory of the ball on any given throw will vary and does not remain constant. Switching between open environments and more stable, or closed, environments will further challenge the individual to adapt motor responses. When the individual steps off the moving sidewalk, a disruption in walking occurs. The first few steps are not smooth because the person needs to switch movement strategies from one incorporating a moving support surface to one incorporating a stationary support surface.

Errors occur in the perception of sensory information, in selection of the appropriate motor program, in selection of the appropriate variable parameters, or in the response execution. Patients with a neurological deficit may demonstrate a combination of these errors. Therefore an assessment of motor deficits in clients includes analysis of these types of errors. If a therapist observes a motor control problem, there is no guarantee that the central problem arises from within the motor system. Somatosensory problems can drive motor dysfunction; cognitive and emotional problems express themselves through motor output. Thus it is up to the movement specialist to differentiate the cause of the problem through valid and reliable examination tools (see Chapter 8). Once the cause of the motor problem has been identified, selection of interventions should lead to more effective outcomes.

All individuals, both healthy individuals and those with CNS dysfunction, make errors in motor programming. These errors are assessed by the CNS and are stored in past memory of the experience. Errors in motor programming are extremely useful in learning. Learning can be viewed as decreasing the mismatch between the intended and actual motor behavior. This mismatch is a measure of the error; therefore, a decrease in the degree of the error is indicative of learning. Errors, then, are an important part of the rehabilitation process. However, this does not mean that the therapist allows the client to practice errors over and over. The ability of the patient to detect an error and correct it to produce appropriate and efficient motor behavior is one key to recovery and an important consideration when intervention strategies are developed.

Summary

The previous components of contemporary motor control theories are interrelated. Movement is an emergent property that arises from the cooperative working of neural centers that assess information from the internal and external environments, process the sensory information with past memories, and produce a movement strategy that is appropriate to the situation and accomplishes the task. The movement pattern has appropriate amplitude, duration, and sequencing of synergies. It is efficiently executed, both in terms of metabolic efficiency and movement efficiency. Movement efficiency in terms of energy expenditure relates to the appropriate controlling of the multiple of degrees of freedom at the various joints to accomplish the movement. The movement is accomplished with the flexibility and adaptability to be modified if new constraints are imposed during the execution of the movement. The movement pattern used is the preferred movement pattern selected by that individual to accomplish the task and not an obligatory pattern. Once the task is accomplished, elements of the task are stored in motor memory. The representation of the movement pattern that is stored may be modified as a result of learning and development. To enhance the neuroplastic changes that occur after CNS injury, the therapist must focus on engaging the client in a skilled motor task while attending to both the overall task and the sensory information produced during the task. The design of the intervention should consistently challenge the client to produce the most effective neuroplasticity possible. In the future, timing of the intervention may be found to heavily influence change and should be considered as evidence when rehabilitation interventions using timing as a variable are shown to be effective.

Regulation of Posture and Equilibrium

Postural and balance reactions are those automatic responses that maintain the organism in the erect position and maintain head orientation in space, primarily keeping the face vertical and the mouth horizontal. These responses are accomplished through the integration of sensory input from the vestibular, visual, and somatosensory systems. Stabilization of the head in space for gaze control will be described first, followed by a brief description of balance responses (see also Chapter 23).

Head Stabilization in Space

The phrase "stabilization of the head in space" refers to a dynamic equilibrium incorporating the alignment of the head on the trunk during movement to maintain gaze stability.[55] Vestibulocollic, vestibulospinal, tonic neck reflexes, and righting reactions assist with head stabilization in space by coordinating the neck, trunk, and limb musculature to maintain or regain a stable platform for the eyes. When the head or trunk is tilted or rotated in space or body parts are rotated in relation to one another (e.g., body on body righting reaction), automatic reactions are evoked. They oppose the motion resulting from the perturbing force to maintain or regain balance of the head and body in space. The motor control of the CNS to regulate and modify these simultaneous motor programs requires coordination of specific motor nuclei such as the cerebellum, the basal ganglia, the frontal lobes, the thalamus, and brain stem motor mechanisms.[8] Although many of these responses are seemingly automatic and are programmed early in life to respond, the control and sensitivity of the CNS allows these seemingly stereotypic reactions to vary depending on both the internal and external environmental demands.

Another function of the vestibular reflexes, particularly the vestibulocollic reflex, is to dampen the tendency for oscillatory motion of the head. On the basis of the biomechanics of the head/neck system, a resonant frequency of 2 to 3 Hz is likely to produce oscillation of the head. To maintain a stable gaze, this oscillation is regulated by a negative reflex loop associated with the vestibulocollic reflex system. The cervicocollic reflex also assists to stabilize the head.[56] Proprioceptors, primarily muscle spindles from muscles of the neck, provide sensory feedback for this reflex. Although this reflex has been demonstrated in decerebrate animals, it has been difficult to elicit in alert animals. The vestibular reflexes and this stretch reflex may be operating over the same circuitry, thereby making it more difficult to isolate and study. An investigation of these systems in a gravity environment and in a gravity-eliminated environment is in progress.[57,58]

The roles of the tonic neck reflexes and righting reactions are also important in the coordination of postural reactions. The tonic neck reflex can be considered to assist in the regulation of the neck-trunk-limb–coordinated linkage operated

through proprioceptors. Depending on the direction of the tilt, the tonic reflexes may oppose vestibular reflexes. For example, forward tilting of the head in a quadruped results in upper limb flexion by means of the tonic neck reflexes and upper limb extension by means of the vestibulospinal reflexes. When the reflexes are combined, tilting of the head maintains the neutral limb-trunk posture to support the animal.

Gaze stabilization is regulated by the vestibulo-ocular reflex and the optokinetic systems.[57] The function of these systems is to maintain a stable retinal image during head motion. Oscillopsia indicates that the retinal image is not stable during movement, that is, the stable world appears to move. The vestibulo-ocular system tends to operate during higher speeds of rotation so that the semicircular canals can monitor the precise velocity of head rotation. The optokinetic system tends to be most efficient at low speeds of rotation, so the photoreceptors detect both the speed and direction of the image passing across the retinal field. Both systems activate extraocular muscles to produce a counterrotation of the eyes, helping to keep an image stable on the retina. Failure to maintain gaze stabilization can result in the perception that the environment is blurry or in motion, thereby affecting the ability of an individual to stabilize himself or herself in relation to the world, resulting in motor limitations in balance. Functional deficits as a result of impaired balance include difficulty with ambulation and most instrumental activities of daily living, such as driving.[59]

The vestibulo-ocular reflex functions to produce counterrotation in the eyes in response to head rotation, thereby maintaining a stable gaze in the line of sight. Eye rotation is limited by the excursion in the eye socket; therefore, compensatory movements are necessary. Compensatory movement during maintained head rotation, which is termed *nystagmus,* consists of two phases, a slow phase that compensates for head rotation and a quick phase that returns the eye to the center of the orbit. If the counterrotation of the eyes matches the rotation of the head, then the strength of this linkage, or gain, is 1. If the gain is 0.5, it signifies a mismatch between the rotation of the head and counterrotation of the eyes so that the eye movement undercompensates head movement by one half. That is, the eyes rotate half as far as head rotation. Alternately, a gain of 2 indicates that the eyes are overcompensating and rotating twice as far as head rotation. The cerebellum assists in maintaining the gain of the vestibulo-ocular reflex.[60,61] Nystagmus can be seen with both central and peripheral vestibular disorders.

Other eye movements controlled by a complex neural system are saccades and smooth pursuit. Saccades are small gaze-shifting movements that operate quickly to keep the eyes in position. Input from visual, somatosensory, and auditory systems is used by the saccadic system to regulate eye movement to maintain the line of gaze.[24] Saccadic movements are necessary to scan the visual world, whereas smooth pursuit movements are used to maintain the eyes on target. The cerebellum is involved in the regulation of both these tasks. Eye movements are extremely important for aligning (righting) and maintaining (balancing) the body in space or within its limits of stability. Inability to control gaze stabilization or to shift gaze appropriately to scan the environment will severely limit the visual system's input into balance control, causing the increased potential for conflicting sensory input or inaccurate information, ultimately leading to poor balance control and often falling.[60]

Regulation of Balance

Balance reactions occur to maintain or regain the center of gravity (center of mass) over the base of support (see Chapter 23). Base of support is defined as the boundary where shifts of the center of gravity can occur by use of one movement strategy without losing balance or necessitating a change in the movement strategy. Alternately, posture defined from a biomechanical point of view is body segment orientation to one another and in space. These automatic reactions occur during static positions such as sitting and quiet standing, and they occur during transition phases, that is, from one position to another position (e.g., sit to stand, walk, and turn). Balance reactions operative over long ascending and descending pathways are sometimes termed *long-loop reflexes.*

Balance responses may be classified as *anticipatory* or *compensatory.* Anticipatory balance responses are those postural changes that occur before the perturbing force, whereas compensatory balance responses occur as a result of the perturbing force. A perturbing force may be voluntary, for example, reaching for an object moves the center of gravity close to the limits of the base of support. In anticipation of reaching, electromyographic activity occurs in lower-extremity musculature before the initiation of electromyographic activity in the upper extremity to counter the destabilizing effect that the reach will produce. Alternately, a compensatory balance response is activated by an external perturbing force such as responding from an unexpected bump from behind while standing in line at the market. The balance responses to maintain or regain the center of gravity over the base of support occur within 90 ms of the external perturbing force.

As discussed earlier, a finite number of movement strategies are available for response selection. This is true for all movements and combinations of programs.[5] With regard to balance, these strategies were observed during externally applied linear perturbations in the laboratory setting. The *ankle strategy* is a synergy where muscle activation occurs at the ankle and temporally spreads to more proximal musculature. A greater linear perturbation or unexpected rotation about the ankle results in the selection of a different movement strategy, *hip strategy.* If the perturbation is such that the hip and ankle strategies are not successful, then the individual takes a step to prevent falling, a *step strategy.* The time the individual has to react to maintain balance and prevent falling is extremely short, approximately 90 ms after the disturbance. Coupling muscles together into functional synergies and limiting the number of movement strategies available decreases the time for response. The specificity of these reactions, both with speed and accuracy, came through a huge amount of repetitive practice as the CNS was learning to control and adapt to whatever the external stimulus might be (flat, inclines, uneven surfaces, compliant surfaces). Every time the person challenges the nervous system with a new environment, such as walking on a sandy beach for the first time or walking in the ocean during an active tide shift, the nervous systems ability to learn and adapt

quickly will lead to controlled responses to these perturbations created by a new environment. Individuals with CNS problems may learn to walk and have adequate balance responses to a noncompliant surface but not be able to adapt when going to the beach. If the client's life included spending time at the beach and swimming in the ocean, then those environments need to be part of the balance and gait retraining intervention program.

Balance reactions occurring during routine activities of daily living incorporate a combination of these lower-extremity movement patterns along with trunk and upper limb patterns. Response selection is based on the conditions of the perturbation, the initial position of the individual, environmental conditions, past experiences, and the overall goal of the movement. These are the same conditions as those described earlier that pertain to the regulation of movement. Conditions of the perturbation include the amplitude, velocity, and direction of the perturbing force. The initial position of the individual incorporates the position of the individual in space and the relationship of the person's body parts to each other. Also included is the biomechanical, neurological, and general physiological status of the individual. Environmental conditions include the stability of the support surface, objects in the environment, and the condition of the lighting. If the goal of the individual is not to fall, then control in this particular scenario is to maintain or regain the center of mass over the base of support. Consequences of any loss of balance may also relate to the goal of movement. For example, the consequences of an improper response to an external perturbation while walking may change if the goal is carrying a hot cup of coffee rather than a book.

Errors in the selection and execution of balance responses occur in both healthy individuals and those with neurological disorders. Both groups of individuals may be unable to resolve conflicts that arise from the sensory processing of information from the visual, somatosensory, and vestibular systems. The result may be the selection and execution of an inappropriate or inadequate balance response. The appropriate balance response may be selected, but there may be an inappropriate scaling of control parameters. For example, an individual with cerebellar dysfunction may demonstrate an increased amplitude of the balance response in relation to an externally applied linear perturbation.[61] An individual with traumatic brain injury may select the appropriate movement strategy but with a delayed onset.[62] An individual with Parkinson's disease may have difficulty initiating a single movement strategy.[63] Selecting two movement strategies in response to externally applied linear perturbation results in decreasing all the degrees of freedom imposed by the selection of the two strategies. A more rigid posture ensues, with potential destabilization of the individual. Last, small deficits in any combination of systems required for balance regulation may have an additive effect, leading to postural instability or balance deficits. For example, normal age-related changes to both the visual system and the somatosensory system may not seem large when assessed individually, but when coupled together during a functional task, these deficits may cause an integrative balance disorder where the combination of these smaller deficits leads to inadequate or inappropriate balance responses in the elderly individual, causing a risk for falls. Once an individual begins to fall, the nervous system needs to select another program, such as falling. The autonomic reaction of fear can cause additional destabilization to the motor system and further increase an individual's risk or potential injury from the fall. Given these combinations of motor experiences, an individual who has a fear of falling will often become more sedentary, which decreases practice. As stated earlier, practice and motivation to practice is the key to maintaining or regaining motor control.[5,49]

ASSESSMENTS BASED ON CONTEMPORARY MOTOR AND BALANCE CONTROL THEORIES

Many evaluative methods are used to assess motor and postural control in clients with neurological dysfunction. How the therapist uses and interprets the data should be based on contemporary theories of motor and balance control and on considering the client as an active participant and not a passive recipient in the examination procedure.[49,64-66] Examination procedures are designed to determine how the individual's physical, mental, and cognitive status affects motor abilities. Furthermore, examination procedures must be valid and reliable tools to determine functional outcome.[67,68] A custom-designed evaluation approach is used because the mechanism of injury or disease, secondary brain damage, recovery rate, and functional outcome differ in every individual. One strategy to assess the client with neurological dysfunction is to assess the individual's previous and present activity levels.

Activity Level

Unobtrusive evaluation at the bedside or in the clinic provides an excellent opportunity to examine the functional activity level and observe compensatory or preferred movement strategies used by the individual. Another unobtrusive observation period can be "staged"; for example, the client is asked to assist the clinician to move objects off a low mat table, or the client is asked to remove his shoes and socks, any activity that is not explicitly stated to the client as a "test" but appears to be a normal, necessary function in the clinic. During these observation times, the patient does not perceive that he or she is "performing" a motor task but rather a daily function. The therapist can then observe a more natural pattern of motor behavior. A patient may sit on the floor to remove shoes and socks because the floor is more stable than sitting on a low mat table. In this instance, the therapist has the opportunity to observe the movements used by the patient to reach the floor, the mobility and stability patterns used while the shoes and socks are being removed, and the movement strategy used to get up from the floor. Stability, transition phases, and movements occurring with the various tasks are observed and documented. Obviously, this functional task for a senior citizen may be much more difficult than for a younger adult as a result of strength, range of motion, and so forth. Simultaneously, if the position is feasible, the patient is practicing coming upright from the floor, which is a motor program necessary to regain control after a fall.

Tasks or activities incorporated in an assessment of activity level vary depending on the age of the patient, the severity of the complaints, observational analysis before the examination, and the physical, cognitive, and behavioral status of the individual. For example, an elderly patient with CNS dysfunction may have preexisting movement and balance dysfunction owing to the aging process. Activity level, however, should not be assessed solely on the assumption that elderly persons are more inactive than younger adults. Inactive elderly and inactive college-aged individuals have lower functional patterns for righting reactions when coming to standing from supine than do their active cohorts.[34] Assessment of activity level involves employment status, including type of work (sedentary or active); participation in leisure activities, both organized and solo (sports, choir, bridge, walking, gardening); and the effect of preexisting and existing dysfunctions on current activity levels in terms of assistance with activities of daily living, work, and leisure activities. A thorough subjective examination or client history assessing prior level of function in a variety of contexts (work, home, community) can help determine the appropriate activity level for the client's examination.

Another important facet is to identify activities that the individual believes he or she can no longer perform because of the motor control problem or from loss of confidence. Tasks used in the examination should be similar to both those activities the patient can perform and those activities that are familiar to the individual. The inability to perform a new task may be due to CNS damage or the inability of the individual to understand and carry out an unfamiliar task. Tasks can incorporate transitional movements moving from supine to sit, sit to stand, bending down and reaching for something on the floor, walking and turning the head, and reaching in various directions. Functional activity permits analysis of motor and postural control, interplay between the individual and the environment, and the ability of the individual to function safely in the everyday home and work environment. Consideration of the task with regard to its predictability (or open tasks vs closed tasks) should also be considered.[48] If the client can successfully rise from the mat in the clinic, the therapist should consider assessment with a variety of other heights of surfaces and firmness of the surfaces to see if providing a more open environmental context (rising from a softer surface or a lower surface) will be difficult for the client. Recall that flexibility and adaptability of motor responses is normal and should be strived for in clients with neurological deficits.

Physical deconditioning decreases general flexibility, endurance, and strength and predisposes the individual to movement instability. Biomechanical factors such as the degree of motion between the head and neck, intersegmental rotation of the trunk, and degree of movement in the lower extremities are examined as the individual performs a functional activity. A decrease in range of motion may be due to a functional biomechanical loss or to a motor control problem that alters the timing of the movement. For example, a patient with a cerebrovascular accident may exhibit footdrop. Initially, the footdrop is due to alteration in the movement pattern resulting from the loss of CNS control for the timing and sequencing of interlimb muscle activity. If the footdrop persists, biomechanical changes contribute to the deficit in the lower-extremity movement pattern because of subsequent loss of range of motion or strength during recovery.

Another element to consider is metabolic change or reduced exercise capacity. Inactivity deconditions the cardiovascular and pulmonary systems, which results in a decreased ability to perform routine activities of daily living. The resulting decline increases stress on these physiological systems when the patient is asked to perform a task. A task as simple as walking up several steps can cause the individual to exceed his or her exercise capacity. When the decreased aerobic capacity is coupled with alterations in the CNS or biomechanical system, a cycle occurs in which a reduced exercise capacity leads to an increase in inactivity, which further reduces exercise capacity. This cycle can also cause a loss of self-confidence. The therapist always needs to be aware of the organ systems within the client because they will also affect fatigue and CNS's ability to learn. For example, someone with partial kidney failure may not be adequately filtering out waste products from muscles and other organs. With an increase in activity, there is an increase in waste products that would then be filtering through the CNS as a result of the kidney dysfunction. Confusion or a reduction in motor control can be the result. Last, the motor and postural control systems should be assessed according to the ability of the individual to perform the activity smoothly and efficiently, not just perform the activity.[69] A more detailed discussion follows.

USE OF MOTOR CONTROL PARAMETERS TO ASSESS POSTURE AND MOVEMENT DEFICITS IN CLIENTS WITH NEUROLOGICAL DISEASE OR TRAUMA

Patients with neurological disease are unable to generate "normal" motor behavior because the CNS deficit has altered the integrative capability of the brain. Biomechanical and metabolic factors are also altered whether from prior problems, primary insults from current trauma, or secondary problems associated with the disease or pathological condition. The movement pattern executed by the patient is considered a functional movement pattern used to accomplish the goal. Depending on the pathophysiological mechanisms of the trauma and secondary complications, the pattern may not be efficient in terms of neurological, biomechanical, or metabolic costs to the system. Nevertheless, the pattern is the preferred pattern (emergent property) arising from a self-organizing system that permits the individual to function. This preferred pattern is a result of the constraints imposed on the individual by the neurological condition, the constraints imposed by the environment, and the task. The use of assistive devices may further increase the costs to the system.[70] For example, a person using a walker will have an altered gait pattern, resulting in increased metabolic costs. Prolonged use of the walker alters the biomechanical and neurological relationship for postural alignment and the location of the center of mass, which can lead to long-term changes. Thus the client needs to

make decisions regarding the selection of assistive devices with regard to both their short- and long-term effects on motor performance and adaptability to various external environments.

Examination and intervention should focus on those movement parameters that have been altered and the way in which the individual can optimally function in a particular task. To guide the examination of posture and movement, several general questions can be addressed. For example, what is the activity level of the person? Is the person able to safely function in everyday environments of home and work? Does the person have the capability to generate movement strategies that achieve the task required, and is the person capable of learning new motor strategies? Is the patient motivated to regaining those movement strategies?

Another guiding factor is the life span developmental status of the person. A young child with cerebral palsy has a reference of correctness about movement that is based on the constraints imposed from the condition, never having experienced what would be considered normal.[69] An adult with an acute CNS deficit may have either a preinjury reference of correctness or a postinjury reference of correctness that may or may not be compatible with the new constraints imposed by the acute neurological condition.[69] For example, a client with a cerebrovascular accident may exhibit a list to the involved side while sitting but perceives that he or she is sitting upright.

Specific questions relative to motor control also guide the assessment. For example, is the individual appropriately processing sensory information? Is the person generating an appropriate motor response? Can the individual modify the motor response to accomplish the task, or does the person use limited or obligatory motor patterns? Is the person selecting the appropriate motor strategy, but parameters such as amplitude, timing, and phasing are not adequate to achieve the task? Clinicians identify inappropriate parameters of motor control. They then develop a hypothesis pertaining to alterations in the motor control system, in the physiological system, or in the biomechanical systems and use this hypothesis as a basis for treatment. Treating the patient and assessing the outcome are the means to test the hypothesis. Obviously, the patient needs to be the center of this discussion and decision making to achieve the best outcomes for the interventions.[71-74]

These examples are only a few of the guiding questions that can be asked relative to motor and postural control. Once the therapist observes the patient, he or she can formulate hypotheses on what factors are contributing to the deficits in motor behavior. Observational analysis can be used to focus the remainder of the examination in a more contextually appropriate manner. These more focused questions can be used to test the hypotheses. Often, a single factor does not produce the motor deficit but rather an interaction of present and past constraints. The satisfying part of an evaluation is to be able to test and rule out hypotheses. Theoretically, by ruling out hypotheses, the intervention can become more client focused and effective. A list of a large variety of assessment tools can be found at the end of Chapter 8.

CASE STUDY 3-1 ■ PERSON WITH PARKINSON'S DISEASE

When motor control deficits are evaluated in the client with Parkinson's disease, the severity of the disease, the activity level of the person, and the medication schedule are important considerations. Following are several motor control deficits that are evident in this disease. Figure 3-4 can be used to guide the evaluation.

Alterations in stride length, speed, and frequency produce changes in the gait pattern in the person with Parkinson's disease. The person may demonstrate a gait pattern with decreases in amplitude of leg movement, duration of the gait cycle, trunk rotation, and arm swing. Small, shuffling steps and a festinating gait pattern are also observed. The festinating gait occurs in an attempt to maintain the center of gravity over the base of support in the individual with a flexed posture. A decrease in righting and balance reactions also contributes to instability in gait. Whenever the preferred speed and frequency parameters are altered in any movement, they can increase metabolic costs and alter the ability of the individual to safely complete the functional movement with appropriate coordination of postural and motor control. In fact, any gait deficit increases metabolic costs. The Timed Up and Go Test (TUG) can be used to assess both gait and the transitional movements of standing up, walking, and turning.

The difficulty in initiating gait, or "freezing," is another observable motor control problem.[75] *Freezing* refers to a failure in gait initiation, which can be assessed at different times in the TUG. Freezing can occur when the person rises from the chair, turns at the end of 3 meters, turns, returns to the chair, and then sits down. Freezing also occurs when the target is approached (i.e., destination freezing), when an obstacle is encountered, or spontaneously. This deficit is attributed to the imbalance of the direct and indirect pathways from the basal ganglia.[76]

Overshooting or undershooting of the 3-meter line before turning may be demonstrated. Although clients with Parkinson's disease are able to prepare the motor strategy and use advance information, the primary problem is the slow onset of execution of movement; therefore changing motor patterns (e.g., switching from walking to turning) is most difficult.

To illustrate the multiple motor control deficits, imagine a patient performing the TUG.[77] The person is asked to stand up from a chair, walk a specified distance, turn around, walk back to the chair, and sit down. The person may have difficulty accelerating and decelerating to turn around and may have difficulty decelerating when approaching the chair and sitting down. These motor control deficits exhibited in the patient with Parkinson's disease are numerous and intertwined and their severity is influenced by the progression of the disease. As mentioned earlier, the client cannot appropriately control the increase and decrease in the rate of force production, which is evident in the acceleration and deceleration phases of the movement. If the rate of force production is altered; amplitude of force production may also be affected.

The person may have a decreased ability to predict and prepare the motor pattern for turning before the actual turn. There appears to be a slow initiation of the turning task. This phenomenon could be due to the inability to sequence the motor behavior as a whole. Several researchers have observed that the person completes one movement before starting the next movement in the sequence rather than executing a smooth, continuing movement pattern.[32] Another reason for the decrease in the ability to perform this task smoothly is the patient's dependence on visual feedback. Relying more heavily on visual feedback to accomplish a task slows the movement.

The movement deficits observed may also be due to the inability to effectively coordinate movements such as those observed between postural and motile components of the task. Postural strategies may be classified on a continuum that includes postural preparations, postural accompaniments, and postural reactions.[78] The person with Parkinson's disease may not predict and make appropriate postural adjustments before the movement and may have deficits in postural reactions (e.g., righting and equilibrium reactions). When patients are externally perturbed, some researchers[11,63] noted that simultaneous activation of two balance strategies occurs, whereas others[79,80] noted a decrease in functional activation of muscles, particularly around the ankle.

In the case of the TUG, movement and balance strategies are assessed when the client stands up and sits down. If the client does not use a controlled descent into the chair but rather flops, what are the possible causes for the sudden descent? The individual's preferred pattern may be to flop into the chair, the individual may not be able to predict the time and force needed to activate the muscles for a smooth descent, the individual may be deconditioned and does not have the strength or endurance to perform a smooth descent, or the individual may not have the balance strategies required to perform this maneuver.

In summary, to assess the patient with Parkinson's disease or any other neurological deficit, all aspects of motor control need to be examined as the individual executes a variety of functional tasks. The patient may have multiple gross and fine motor and postural control deficits; only a few were examined in the example. It is not within the scope of this section to present all the motor and postural control deficits but to highlight the complexity of patients with neurological pathophysiological conditions. Accurate identification of motor control problems in clients assists the therapist and client in the development of realistic functional goals and effective intervention programs (see Section II for recommendations regarding specific diseases or pathological conditions and their related functional movement limitations).

ACKNOWLEDGMENT

Roberta Newton, PT, PhD, laid the foundation both conceptually and structurally for the present chapter, and both the present author and the editor would like to thank her for her commitment to this text's evolution, as well as to the delivery of best practice to the elderly population.

REFERENCES

1. Alexandrov AV, Frolov AA, Horak FB et al: Feedback equilibrium control during human standing, *Biol Cybern* 93:309-322, 2005.
2. Buchanan JJ, Horak FB: Voluntary control of postural equilibrium patterns, *Behav Brain Res* 143:121-140, 2003.
3. Buchanan JJ, Horak FB: Transitions in a postural task: do the recruitment and suppression of degrees of freedom stabilize posture? *Exp Brain Res* 139:482-494, 2001.
4. Creath R, Kiemel T, Horak F et al: A unified view of quiet and perturbed stance: simultaneous co-existing excitable modes, *Neurosci Lett* 377:75-80, 2005.
5. Shumway-Cook A, Woolacott M: *Motor control: theory and practical applications,* ed 2, Philadelphia, 2000, Lippincott Williams & Wilkins.
6. Goldstein L, Kleim Merzenich M, Nudo RJ et al: Plenary session 3: neural plasticity: Basic mechanisms, III STEP Conference, Salt Lake City, Utah, July 17, 2005.
7. Nudo RJ: Functional and structural plasticity in motor cortex: implications for stroke recovery, *Phys Med Rehabil Clin North Am* 14:S57-S76, 2003.
8. Kandel ER, Schwartz JH, Jessel TM: *Principles of neural science,* ed 4, New York, 2000, McGraw-Hill.
9. King LA, VanSant AF: The effect of solid ankle foot orthoses on movement patterns used to rise from supine to stand, *Phys Ther* 75:952-964, 1995.
10. Bernstein N: *Coordination and regulation of movement,* New York, 1967, Pergamon Press.
11. Heriza C: Motor development: Traditional and contemporary theories. In *Contemporary management of motor control problems,* proceedings of the II STEP Conference, Fredericksburg, VA, 1991, Foundation for Physical Therapy.
12. Newell KM, Corcos DM (eds): *Variability and motor control,* Champaign, IL, 1993, Human Kinetics Publishers.
13. Schoner G, Kelso JAS: Dynamic pattern generation in behavioral and neural systems, *Science* 239:1513-1520, 1988.
14. Tuller B, Turvey MT, Fitch HL: The Bernstein perspective, II: the concept of muscle linkage or coordinative structure. In Kelso JAS, editor: *Human motor behavior: an introduction,* Hillsdale, NJ, 1982, Erlbaum.
15. Cheng S, Sabes PN: Modeling sensorimotor learning with linear dynamical systems, *Neural Comput* 18:760-793, 2006.
16. Fattore M, Arrigo P: Knowledge discovery and system biology in molecular medicine: an application on neurodegenerative diseases, *In Silico Biol* 5:199-208, 2005.
17. Pave A: By way of introduction: Modelling living systems, their diversity and their complexity: some methodological and theoretical problems, *C R Biol* 329:3-12, 2006.
18. Lawrence DG, Kuypers HGJM: The functional organization of the motor system in the monkey, I: the effects of bilateral pyramidal lesions, *Brain* 91:1-14, 1968.
19. Lawrence DG, Kuypers HGJM: The functional organization of the motor system in the monkey, II: the effects of lesions of the descending brainstem pathways, *Brain* 91:15-36, 1968.
20. Bussel B, Roby-Brami A, Yakovleff A et al: Late flexion reflex in paraplegic patients: evidence for a spinal stepping generator, *Brain Res Bull* 22:53-56, 1989.
21. Calancie B, Needham-Shropshire B, Jacobs P et al: Involuntary stepping after chronic spinal cord injury: evidence for a central rhythm generator for locomotion in man, *Brain* 117:1143-1159, 1994.
22. Gelfand IM, Orlovsky GN, Shik ML: Locomotion and scratching in tetrapods. In Cohen AH, Rossignol S, Grillner S (eds): *Neural control of rhythmic movements in vertebrates,* New York, 1988, Wiley.
23. Grillner S: Neurobiological bases of rhythmic motor acts in vertebrates, *Science* 228:143-149, 1989.
24. Glimcher PW: Eye movements. In Zigmond MJ, Bloom FE, Landis SC et al (eds): *Fundamental neuroscience,* pp 993-1010, San Diego, 1999, Academic Press.
25. Prihram KH: *Holonomic brain theory: Cooperation and reciprocity in processing the configural and cognitive aspects of perception,* Hillsdale, NJ, 1988, Erlbaum.
26. Davis WJ: Organizational concepts in the central motor networks of invertebrates. In Herman RM, Grillner S, Stein PSG, Stuart DG (eds): *Neural control of locomotion,* pp 265-291, New York, 1976, Plenum Press.
27. Alexander GE, DeLong MR, Crutcher MD: Do cortical and basal ganglionic motor areas use "motor programs" to control movement? In Cordo P, Harnad S (eds): *Movement control,* pp 54-63, New York, 1994, Cambridge University Press.
28. DeLong MR: Primate models of movement disorders of basal ganglia origin, *Trends Neurosci* 13:281-285, 1990.
29. Swinny JD, van der Want JJ, Gramsbergen A: Cerebellar development and plasticity: perspectives for motor coordination strategies, for motor skills, and for therapy, *Neural Plast* 12:153-160, 263-273, 2005.
30. Spencer RM, Ivry RB: Comparison of patients with Parkinson's disease or cerebellar lesions in the production of periodic movements involving event-based or emergent timing, *Brain Cogn* 58:84-93, 2005.
31. Nutt J, Marsden C, Thompson P: Human walking and higher-level gait disorders, particularly in the elderly, *Neurology* 43:268-279, 1993.
32. Sharmann S, Norton BJ: The relationship of voluntary movement to spasticity in the upper motor neuron syndrome, *Ann Neurol* 2:460-465, 1977.
33. Horak FB, Nashner LM: Central programming of postural movements: Adaptation to altered support surface configurations, *J Neurophysiol* 55:1369-1381, 1986.
34. VanSant AF: A lifespan perspective of age differences in righting movements, *Motor Dev Res Rev* 1:46-63, 1997.
35. Newton RA: Balance screening of an inner city older adult population, *Arch Phys Med Rehabil* 78:587-591, 1997.
36. Barr AF, Barbe MF, Vincent KK: Behavioral and histological changes in a rat model of an upper extremity cumulative trauma disorder, *Phys Ther* 79:S54, 1999.
37. Byl N, Merzenich MM, Cheung S et al: A primate model for studying focal dystonia and repetitive strain injury: effects on the primary somatosensory cortex, *Phys Ther* 77:269-284, 1997.
38. Hallett M: Is dystonia a sensory disorder? *Ann Neurol* 38:139-140, 1995.
39. Byl N, Roderick J, Mohamed O et al: Effectiveness of sensory and motor rehabilitation of the upper limb following the principles of neuroplasticity: patients stable poststroke, *Neurorehabil Neural Repair* 17:176-191, 2003.
40. Winstein: Knowledge of results, III STEP presentation, Salt Lake City, UT, 2005.
41. Marsden CD, Rothwell JC, Day BL: The use of peripheral feedback in the control of movement. In Evarts EV, Wise SP, Bousfield D, editors: *the motor system in neurobiology,* Amsterdam, 1985, Elsevier Biomedical.
42. Rothwell JC, Traub MM, Day BL et al: Manual motor performance in a deafferented man, *Brain* 105:515-542, 1982.
43. Taub E: Movements in nonhuman primates deprived of somatosensory feedback, *Exerc Sport Sci Rev* 4:335-374, 1976.
44. Huxham FE, Goldie PA, Patla AE: Theoretical considerations in balance assessment, *Aust J Physiother* 47:89-100, 2001.
45. Chen Y, Constantini S, Trembovler V et al: An experimental model of closed head injury in mice: pathophysiology, histopathology, and cognitive deficits, *J Neurotrauma* 13:557-568, 1996.

46. Lajoie Y, Teasdale N, Bard C et al: Upright standing and gait: Are there changes in attentional requirements related to normal aging? *Exp Aging Res* 22:185-198, 1996.

47. Teasdale N, Bard C, Fleury M et al: Determining movement onsets from temporal series, *J Mot Behav* 25:97-106, 1993.

48. Gentile AM, Beheshti Z, Held JM: Enrichment versus exercise effects on motor impairments following cortical removals in rats, *Behav Neural Biol* 47:321-332, 1987.

49. Adolph K: Learning, adaptation, recovery (neural systems level, perception-action considerations), III STEP Conference, Salt Lake City, Utah, July 18, 2005.

50. Shallert T: Neural plasticity: Basic mechanisms, III Step Plenary Session, Salt Lake City, Utah, July 17, 2005.

51. Nudo R III: Plasticity: Basic mechanisms, III Step Plenary Session, Salt Lake City, Utah, July 17, 2005.

52. Mattar AA, Gribble PL: Motor learning by observing, *Neuron* 46:153-160, 2005.

53. Meintzschel F, Ziemann U: Modification of practice-dependent plasticity in human motor cortex by neuromodulators, *Cereb Cortex,* published online October 12, 2005.

54. Sunderland A, Tuke A: Neuroplasticity, learning and recovery after stroke: a critical evaluation of constraint-induced therapy, *Neuropsychol Rehabil* 15:81-96, 2005.

55. Cromwell RL, Newton RA, Carlton LG: Horizontal plane head stabilization during locomotor tasks, *J Motor Behav* 2000, in press.

56. Peterson B, Goldberg J, Bilotto G et al: Cervicocollic reflex: its dynamic properties and interaction with vestibular reflexes, *J Neurophysiol* 54:90-109, 1985.

57. Herdman SJ: *Vestibular rehabilitation,* Philadelphia, 1994, FA Davis.

58. Peterson B, Richmond F (eds): *Control of head movement,* New York, 1988, Oxford University Press.

59. Shepard NT, Telian SA: *Practical management of the balance disorder patient,* 1996, Singular.

60. Lisberger SG: Properties of pathways subserving long-term adaptive plasticity in the vestibulo-ocular reflexes in monkeys. In Ruben RW et al, editors: *The biology of change in otolaryngology,* pp 171-183, Amsterdam, 1986, Elsevier.

61. Diener H-C, Dichgans J: Cerebellar and spinocerebellar gait disorders. In Bronstein AM, Brandt T, Woollacott M (eds): *Clinical disorders of balance, posture and gait,* pp 147-155, London, 1996, Arnold.

62. Newton RA: Balance abilities in individuals with moderate and severe traumatic brain injured patients, *Brain Injury* 9:445-451, 1995.

63. Horak FB, Nutt JG, Nashner LM: Postural inflexibility in parkinsonian patients, *J Neurol Sci* 111:46-58, 1992.

64. Dedding C, Cardol M, Eyssen IC et al: Validity of the Canadian Occupational Performance Measure: a client-centred outcome measurement, *Clin Rehabil* 18:660-667, 2004.

65. Litchfield R, MacDougall C: Professional issues for physiotherapists in family-centred and community-based settings, *Aust J Physiother* 48:105-112, 2002.

66. Schwartz JM, Begley S: *The mind and the brain: Neuroplasticity and the power of mental force,* New York, 2002, HarperCollins.

67. Whyte J: Interaction of science and practice in neurorehabilitation: What is a meaningful change? III STEP Plenary Session 7, Salt Lake City, Utah, July 19, 2005.

68. Wood-Dauphine S: Interaction of science and practice in neurorehabilitation: what is a meaningful change? III STEP Plenary Session 7, Salt Lake City, Utah, July 19, 2005.

69. Latash M, Anson G, Winstein C: Ecological validity related to practice outcomes: Promoting compensation or functional recovery: does the nervous system know best? III STEP Pleanary Session 9, July 20, 2005.

70. Holt KG: Toward general principles for research and rehabilitation of disabled populations, *Phys Ther Pract* 2:1-18, 1993.

71. Carswell A, McColl MA, Baptiste S et al: The Canadian Occupational Performance Measure: A research and clinical literature review, *Can J Occup Ther* 71:210-222, 2004.

72. Eng JJ, Chu KS, Kim CM, Dawson AS et al: A community-based group exercise program for persons with chronic stroke, *Med Sci Sports Exerc* 35:1271-1278, 2003.

73. Law M: Enhancing participation, *Phys Occup Ther Pediatr* 22:1-3, 2002.

74. McColl MA, Law M, Baptiste S et al: Targeted applications of the Canadian Occupational Performance Measure, *Can J Occup Ther* 72:298-300, 2005.

75. Brown P, Steiger MJ: Basal ganglia gait disorders. In Bronstein AM, Brandt T, Woollacott M, editors: *Clinical disorders of balance, posture and gait,* pp 156-167, London, 1996, Arnold.

76. Stelmach GE, Phillips IG: Movement disorders: Limb movement and the basal ganglia, *Phys Ther* 71:60-67, 1991.

77. Ng SS, Hui-Chan CW: The timed up & go test: Its reliability and association with lower-limb impairments and locomotor capacities in people with chronic stroke, *Arch Phys Med Rehabil* 86:1641-1647, 2005.

78. Frank JS, Earl M: Coordination of posture and movement, *Phys Ther* 70:855-863, 1990.

79. Lauk M, Chow CC, Lipsitz LA, Mitchell SL, Collins JJ: Assessing muscle stiffness from quiet stance in Parkinson's disease, *Muscle Nerve* 22:635-639, 1999.

80. Rogers MW: Motor control problems in Parkinson's disease. In *Contemporary management of motor control problems: Proceedings of the II STEP Conference,* Fredericksburg, VA, 1991, Foundation for Physical Therapy.

CHAPTER 4   The Limbic System: Influence over Motor Control and Learning

Darcy A. Umphred, PT, PHD, FAPTA
Marcia Hall, PT, DPT, DSc-abd
Therese Marie West, PhD, MT-BC, FAMI

KEY WORDS

amygdala
declarative memory
emotional behavior
F²ARV (Fear/Frustration, Anger, Rage, Violence)
    continuum
general adaptation syndrome (GAS)
hippocampus
intuition
limbic system
MOVE (*m*otivation/*m*emory, *o*lfaction, *v*isceral
    [ANS], *e*motional)
prefrontal lobe
reverberating loops or circuits
spirituality

OBJECTIVES

After reading this chapter the student/therapist will be able to:
1. Identify the complexity of the limbic complex and its influence over behavioral responses.
2. Analyze the interaction between the limbic, cognitive, and motor systems as expressed in behavior.
3. Differentiate between limbic motor control responses and cerebellar/basal ganglia motor regulation.
4. Identify different emotional or limbic responses and their influence on the spinal and brain stem motor generators.
5. Differentiate between declarative and procedural learning and the limbic system's role in cognition.
6. Analyze the client's functional responses to environmental demands and determine whether the limbic complex has negatively or positively influenced the observable behavior.
7. Analyze the influence intuition and spirituality may have on the therapist, the client, and the interactive behavior.

The understanding of the nervous system becomes more and more complex as scientists answer research questions and unravel new unknowns. Although neuroscience research has found answers to many questions, many additional questions about the limbic system still puzzle basic researchers. Neuroscience has helped to identify the critical nature of behaviors controlled or influenced by the limbic system. The motor system is just one of the many systems affected by the complex limbic network.[1-5] That research and knowledge is summating daily, and it forces today's therapist not only to recognize limbic behavior but also to develop an understanding of how that will positively and negatively affect each patient. As discussions in cell biology,[6-11] quantum physics,[12-17] and string theory[18-26] have merged into the arena of neuroscience, the complexity of the limbic system increases and the understanding of its influence over behavioral (motor) responses becomes more important. With areas of complementary or alternative medicine taking a huge chunk of health care dollars, new questions have and will develop regarding how emotions drive selection of health care delivery and how the limbic system influences outcomes of treatment such as compliance, belief in the outcomes, willingness to accept responsibility for home programs and maintenance of function, and empowerment over life activities.

Obviously, the complexity of the human organism is a totality made up of many interlocking parts. The medical system has traditionally divided the body into systems, and many specialists have forgotten that each specific system is codependent on many other systems for function. Specialists in movement function and dysfunction can fall into this same trap and look at movement from only a biomechanical, muscular, neurological, cardiopulmonary, or integumentary system and lose perspective of the movement as a whole. Subsystems within any one of the previous areas must also be acknowledged. For example, the motor system is a system in and of itself. But cognition and the limbic system can cause tremendous errors in motor responses even when the motor system is intact. Given many individuals with central nervous system (CNS) dysfunction, problems exist in motor, limbic and cognition, thus creating a complex set of behavioral responses resulting from both internal and external environmental influences. The totality of these problems is like interlocking pieces of a complicated puzzle. Considering the therapist as the learner that individual must always hold the visualization of the entire puzzle (the person or client and all his systems) while analyzing any one piece or component system. The learner must determine the number of pieces he or she can conceptually hold and analyze at any one time. The puzzle may initially consist of 2 pieces and progress to 5 or 10 pieces that can be analyzed as separate systems, units, or puzzle pieces but when rejoined give the learner a feeling of accomplishment and intellectual mastery of the causation of both normal movement and dysfunctional behavioral responses. The process of unlocking and reassembling the puzzle while either subdividing each original puzzle piece or adding new pieces is the journey a learner begins in school and can continue throughout life. The decision to continue on this journey is a LIMBIC function and is driven by desire to learn and answer questions regarding the unknown. The emotions felt by the learner and the ability to have the intellectual memory of the learning are also limbic functions. These behavioral responses play an important role in all our lives and cannot be set aside as insignificant.

In many curricula the limbic system is only discussed in a basic science course of neuroanatomy/neurophysiology. In others, the limbic role in declarative memory and emotional responses is presented as part of a discussion on memory or cognitive function within a psychology course. Few faculty members believe they have the opportunity or time to present the limbic system's role in observable motor behavior, whether that behavior is being expressed by the client or the therapist. This chapter has been written to provide the reader with the realization that, without an understanding of limbic interactions and modulations over motor expression, the reliability and validity of measurements of motor performance will always be in question and often inconsistent. Similarly, owing to the limitations of visits in today's health care delivery service models and the dependence on home programs, without a keen awareness of limbic responses to therapeutic interventions a therapist will have little guarantee of compliance by the patient or caregivers.

The limbic system drives behavior not through motor programming or comprehension of the task but rather through willingness to participate in the activity, engage in the learning, and believe that the outcome will lead to some quality of life that has never been achieved or had been lost as a result of a CNS dysfunction. Therapists today often say, "I have no time to talk to the patient." Given the limited time available, the response I give is, "I do not have enough time not to talk to the patient!" Bonding is even more important today because empowering the patient to self-learning through less-supervised or hands-on repetitive practice requires a patient who is willing and motivated to continue to learn and practice. Thus, the concept of patient (client)-centered therapy has evolved to become an important aspect of health care delivery.[27-37] Recognition of that possibility and desire to improve or regain function can be self-motivated, but very often it is instilled through the clinician to the patient that her or his best interests and unique primary goals are the focus of the health care team. This belief is based on trust, hope, and attainable steps toward desired goals. Through interactions, the patients know that their desires, interests, and needs as unique and valued members of society are considered. They first believe and then recognize that they are persons with specific problems and desired outcomes. Although they may have a specific medical diagnoses, placed on critical pathways, administered drugs, off to the next facility in a couple of days, patients need to feel that they, as individuals, have not lost all individuality and that someone cares. That need is a feeling of security and safety that bonds a patient to a therapist along the journey of learning.[38-40]

Before understanding and becoming compassionate to the needs of other people, such as patients with signs and symptoms of neurological problems, therapists need to understand their own limbic system fand how that affects others who might interact with them.[41-46] Because both occupational and physical therapy professions have evolved to using enablement models and systems interactions to explain movement responses of their respective client populations, the importance of separating limbic from true motor or cognitive impairments will help guide the clinician toward intervention strategies that will lead to the quickest and most effective outcomes.

The complexity of the anatomy, physiology, and neurochemistry of the limbic complex baffles the minds of basic science doctoral students. The changes in understanding of cellular metabolism, membrane potentials and the new mysteries of cell communication, and memory baffle the world of science and neuroscience.[6] How this microchasm relates to the macroworld and how the external environments influence not only consciousness but all levels of CNS function is still a mystery. Yet a therapist deals on a moment-to-moment functional level with the limbic system of clients throughout the day. Figure 4-1 illustrates the interlocking/codependency of all major CNS components with the environment. At no time does any system stand in isolation. Thus, from a clinical perspective the therapist should always maintain focus on the whole environment and all major interactive components within it, while directing attention to any specific component. How the feedback (internal and external) to the patient's CNS changes the neurochemistry and membrane potential, triggers memory, creates new pathways, or other potential responses is not the responsibility of the clinician/therapist. What is the responsibility of the clinician is accurate documentation of changes and consistency of those changes toward desired patient outcomes. The professions that focus on movement science are interacting more closely with neurosciences, other biological sciences and researchers within many related professions, to unravel many of these mysteries and create better assessment and intervention procedures for patients in the future.

The primary purpose of this chapter is to discuss the influence of the limbic system on motor learning, motor per-

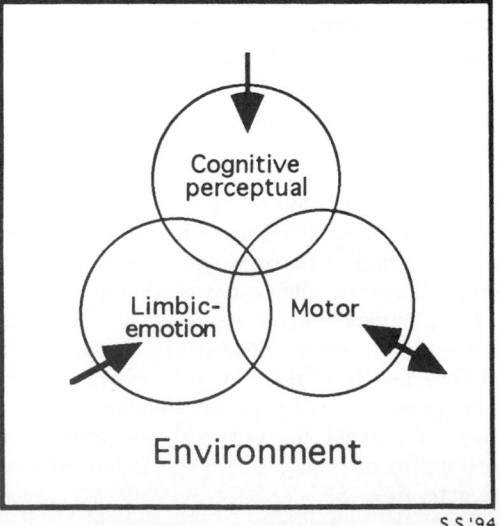

FIGURE 4-1 ■ Interlocking/codependence of all major CNS components.

formance, neuroplasticity, and functional independence in life activities. If a person is scared, fearful, or apprehensive, motor performance and ability to learn either a motor skill or intellectual information will be very different[47-53] from that of an individual who feels safe, is given respect, and becomes part of the decision-making process and thus functions inherently with control.[51,54-57]

After injury to any part of the body, but especially the CNS, an individual will naturally have feelings of loss and reservations or fears about the unknown future (see Chapter 5). Yet that individual needs to be willing to experience the unknown to learn and adapt. The willingness, drive, and adaptability of that individual will affect the optimal plasticity of the CNS.[58] The limbic system is a key player that drives and motivates that individual. The lack of awareness of that variable or its effect on patient performance will ultimately lead to questions and doubts about the effectiveness and efficacy of both assessment and intervention results. Similarly, if this system is overwhelmed either internally or externally, it will dramatically affect neuroplasticity and motor learning as well as cognitive, syntactical learning. At the conclusion of this chapter it is hoped that therapists will comprehend why there is a need to learn to modulate or neutralize the limbic system so that patients can functionally control movement and experience cognitive learning. Then therapists need to reintroduce emotions into the activity and allow the patient to once again experience movement and cognitive success during various levels of emotional demands and environments. Novelty of the task will help drive neuroplasticity and it is a critical motivator for learning.[59,60] For the new learner, the first section of the chapter is a discussion of limbic behavior and how to begin to differentiate true motor responses from those entangled in limbic interactions. For colleagues desiring more in-depth discussion of the basic neuroscience, the second section delves into the anatomy and physiology of the limbic system, the biology of learning and memory, neurochemistry, and neuroplasticity. The last section opens up paradigms and current research and possibilities for future research and presents questions that have not begun to be answered.

THE FUNCTIONAL RELATIONSHIP OF THE LIMBIC SYSTEM TO CLINICAL PERFORMANCE

The Limbic System's Role in Motor Control, Memory, and Learning

It is not easy to find a generally accepted definition of the "limbic system or complex," its boundaries, and the components that should be included. Mesulam[61] likens this to a fifth century BCE philosopher's quotation "the nature of God is like a circle of which the center is everywhere and the circumference is nowhere." Brodal[62] suggests that functional separation of brain regions becomes less clear as we discover the interrelatedness through continuing research. He sees the limbic system reaching out and encompassing the entire brain and all its functional components and sees no purpose in defining such subdivision. Although the anatomical descriptions of the limbic system may vary from author to author, the functional significance of this system is widely acknowledged in defining human behavior and behavioral

neurology. To go one step farther, the link between emotions, electrochemical energy, and healing has been researched for decades by a therapist who once practiced as a neuroscience therapist and worked with patients with CNS problems.[63] This system may be the link to establishing effectiveness and efficacy in alternative medical practices.[64,65]

Brooks[66] divides the brain into the limbic brain and the nonlimbic sensorimotor brain. The sensorimotor portion is involved in perception of nonlimbic sensations and motor performance. He defines a component of the limbic brain as primitive, essential for survival, sensing the "need" to act, and thereby initiating need-directed motor activity for survival. The limbic brain also has the capability for memory and can select what to learn from experience. Brooks also defines the two limbic and nonlimbic systems functionally and not anatomically because their anatomical separation according to function is almost impossible and changes with the task specificity (Figure 4-2).

Kandel et al[54] state that behavior requires three major systems: the sensory, the motor, and the motivational or limbic. When a seemingly simple action is analyzed, such as swinging a golf club, we recruit our sensory system for visual, tactile, and proprioceptive input to guide the motor systems for precise, coordinated muscle recruitment and postural control. The motivational (limbic) system does the following: (1) provides intentional drive for the initiation, (2) integrates the total input, and (3) plays a role in motor expression. The motivational system plays a role in control of both the autonomic and the somatic sensorimotor system. It thereby plays a role in controlling the skeletal muscles through input to the frontal lobe and brain stem and the smooth muscles and glands through the hypothalamus, which lies at the "heart" of the limbic system (Figure 4-3). Noback et al[67] state that "the limbic system is involved with many of the expressions that make us human; namely, emotions, behaviors, and feeling states." That humanness also has individuality. Our unique memory storage, our variable responses to different environmental contexts, and our control or lack thereof over our emotional sensitivity to environmental stimuli all play roles in molding each one of us. Because of this uniqueness, each therapist and each client need to be accepted for their own individuality.

Broca[68] first conceptualized the anatomical regions of the limbic lobe as forming a ring around the brain stem. Today, neuroanatomists do not differentiate an anatomical lobe as limbic but rather refer to a complex system that encompasses cortical, diencephalon, and brain stem structures.[54] This description is less precise and encompasses, but is not limited to, the orbitofrontal and prefrontal cortex, hippocampus, parahippocampal gyrus, cingulate gyrus, dentate gyrus, amygdaloid body, septal area, hypothalamus, and some nuclei of the thalamus.[54,69] Anatomists stress the importance of looking at interrelated segments or loops within the limbic region and include fiber bundles such as the fornix, mamillothalamic fasciculus, stria terminalis, medial forebrain bundle, and the stria medullaris as part of the system.[69-71] These multiple nuclei and interlinking circuits play crucial roles in behavioral and emotional changes,[72-77] declarative memory,[69-83] and motor expression.[84-93] The loss of any link can affect the outcome activity of the whole circuit. Thus, damage to any area of the brain can potentially cause

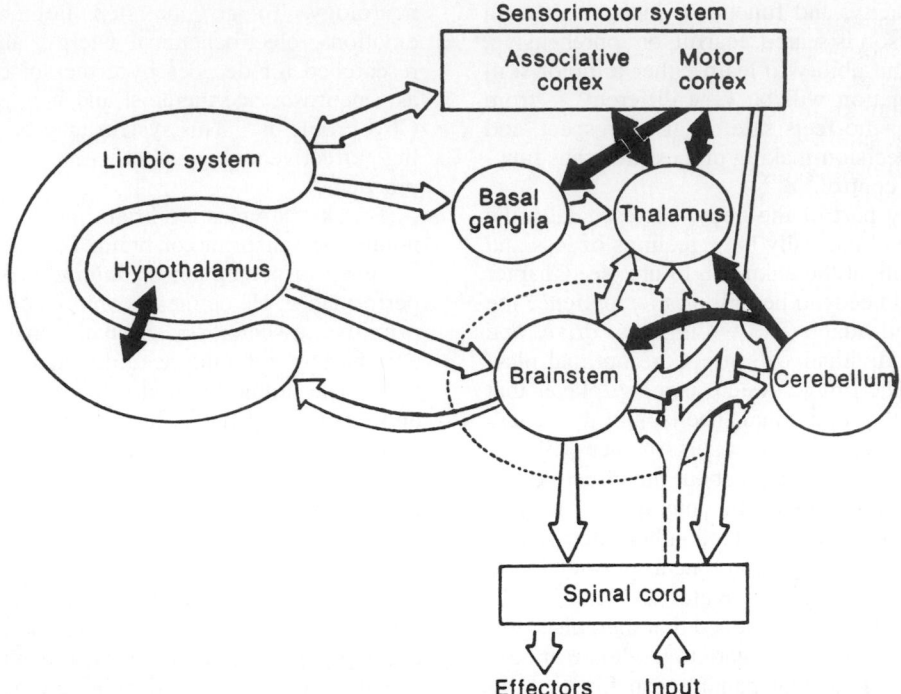

FIGURE 4-2 ■ Divisions and interconnections between the limbic and nonlimbic cortices (sensory and motor areas).

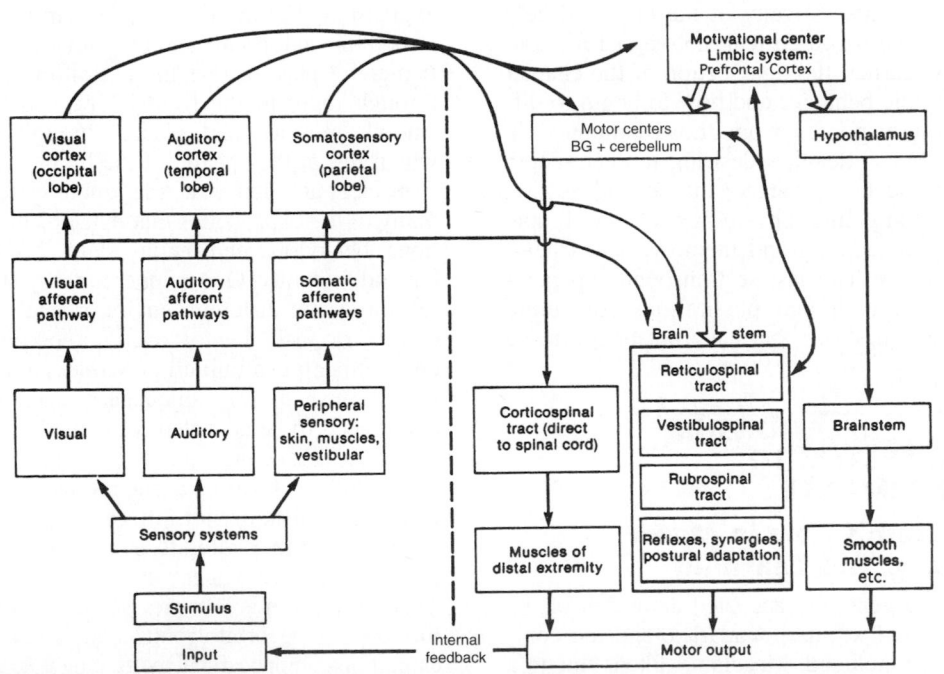

FIGURE 4-3 ■ Motivational system's influence over the sensorimotor and autonomic nervous systems. (Adapted from Kandel ER, Schwartz JH, Jessell TM: *Principles of neural science,* ed 4, New York, 2000, Elsevier Science.)

malfunctions in any or all other areas, and the entire circuit may need reorganization to restore function.

Researchers do not ascribe a specific single function to CNS formations but see each as part of a system participating to various degrees in the multitude of behavioral responses (see Chapters 2 and 3 for additional information).

Therefore, the loss of any part of higher centers or the limbic system may not be clearly definable functionally, and the return of function is not always easy to predict.

Recovery of function after injury may involve mechanisms that allow reorganizing of the structure and function of cortical, subcortical, and spinal circuits. In very young infants, areas within opposite hemispheres may "take over" function, whereas in more mature brains reorganization of existing systems seems to be the current accepted hypothesis within the expanding knowledge of neuroplasticity.[94-104] For complex behavior, such as in motor functioning requiring many steps, the limbic system, cortex, hypothalamus, basal ganglia, and brain stem work as an integrated unit, with any damaged area causing the whole system to initially malfunction. Without change or encouragement of appropriate external and internal environmental changes that will create neuroplasticity, the initial malfunction can become permanent. The timing for optimal neuroplasticity has not yet been established. The medical use of drugs to alter cellular activity and plasticity after CNS damage has become a huge pharmaceutics research area. (See Chapter 36.) Early as well as later drug therapy may encourage neuroplasticity.[105-108] The same questions must be asked about early instead of later rehabilitation intervention, as well as the limbic influence over motor responses. A loss of function or a change in behavior cannot necessarily be localized as to the underlying cause. A lesion in one area may cause secondary dysfunction of a different area that is not actually damaged.

The complexity of the limbic system and its associative influence over both the motor control system and cortical structures are enormous. A therapist dealing with a client with motor control or cognitive learning problems needs to understand how the limbic system affects behavioral responses. The knowledge base focuses not only on the client's deficits but also on the integrative function of the therapist. This understanding should lead to a greater awareness of the clinical environment and the factors within the environment that cause change. Without this knowledge of how to differentiate systems, objective measurements of motor performance or cognitive abilities may be inconsistent without any explanation. Similarly, with excessive limbic activity, clients' ability to store and retrieve either declarative or procedural learning may be negatively affected, thus limiting the patients' ability to benefit from traditional interventions and from potentially regaining their respective highest quality of life.

The Limbic System's Influence on Behavior: Its Relevance to the Therapeutic Environment

Levels of Behavioral Hierarchies: Where Does the Limbic System Belong?

Strub and Black[109] view behavior as occurring on distinct interrelated levels that represent behavioral hierarchies. Starting at level 1, a state of alertness to the internal and external environment must be maintained for motor or mental activity to occur. The brain stem reticular activating system brings about this state of general arousal by relaying in an ascending pathway to the thalamus, the limbic system, and the cerebral cortex. To proceed from a state of general arousal to one of "selective attention" requires the communication of information to and from the cortex, thalamus, and the limbic system and its modulation over the brain stem and spinal pattern generators.[54,86]

Level 2 of this hierarchy lies in the domain of the hypothalamus and its closely associated limbic structures. This level deals with subconscious drives and innate instincts. The survival-oriented drives of hunger, thirst, temperature regulation, and survival of the species (reproduction) and the steps necessary for drive reduction are processed here, as well as learning and memory. Most of these activities relate to limbic functioning. If an individual or patient is in a perceived survival mode, little long-term learning regarding either cognition or motor programming will occur. Thus, making the patient feel safe is initially a critical role for the therapist. This approach may require placing the therapist's hands on the patient initially to take away any possibility of falling. The therapist would first deal with the emotional aspect of the patient's environment and then shift to motor learning/control component where the patient is empowered to practice and self-correct within the program she or he can control.

On level 3 only cerebral cortical areas are activated. This level deals with abstract conceptualization of verbal or quantitative entities. It is at this level the somatosensory and frontal motor cortices work together to perceptually and procedurally develop motor programs. The prefrontal areas of the frontal lobe can influence the development of these motor programs, thus again illustrating the limbic influence over the motor system.[110]

Level 4 behavior is concerned with the expression of social aspects of behavior, personality, and lifestyle. Again, the limbic system and its relationship to the frontal lobe are vital. The shift to patient-centered therapy has actualized the critical importance of this level of human behavior.[27,31,34]

The interaction of all four levels leads to the integrative and adaptable behavior seen in the human. Our ability to become alert and protectively react is balanced by our previous learning, whether it is cognitive-perceptive, social, or affective. Adaptability to rapid changes in the physical environment, in lifestyles, and in personal relationships results from the interrelationships or complex neurocircuitry of the human brain. When insult occurs at any one level within these behavioral hierarchies, all levels may be affected.

As Western medicine is unraveling the mysteries behind the neurochemistry of the limbic system[56,111-121] and alternative medicine is establishing effectiveness and efficacy for various interventions philosophies (see Chapter 37), a fifth level of limbic function may become the link between the hard science of today and the unexplained mysteries. Those medical mysteries would be defined as unexplained, yet identified events that have either been forgotten or hidden from the world by those scientists. Mysteries such as why some people heal from terminal illnesses spontaneously, various others heal in ways not accepted by traditional medicine yet heal nonetheless,[121a] and still others just die without any known disease or pathological condition.[63,65,122] One critical component everyone identifies as part of that unexplained healing is a belief by the client that he or she will heal. That belief has a strong emotional component[65] and that may be the fifth level of limbic function. How conscious intent drives hypothalamic autoimmune function is being unraveled scientifically, and clinicians often observe these patient changes. Through observation it becomes apparent that clients who believe they will get better often do, and those who believe they will not often don't. Whether belief comes from a religious, spiritual, or hard science paradigm, that belief drives behavior and that drive has a large limbic component.

The Limbic System MOVEs Us

Moore[123] eloquently describes the limbic system as the area of the brain that moves us. The word "MOVE" can be used as a mnemonic for the functions of the limbic system.

Limbic System Function

Memory/motivation: drive
  Memory: attention and retrieval, declarative learning
  Motivation: desire to learn, try, or benefit from the external environment
Olfaction (especially in infants)
  Only sensory system that does not have to go through the thalamus as a second-order synapse in the sensory pathway before it gets to the cerebral cortex
Visceral (drives: thirst, hunger, and temperature regulation; endocrine functions)
  Sympathetic and parasympathetic reactions
  Hypothalamic regulation over autoimmune system
  Peripheral autonomic nervous system (ANS) responses that reflect limbic function
Emotion: feelings and attitude
  Self-concept and worth
  Emotional body image
  Tonal responses of motor system affected by limbic descending pathways
  Attitude, social skills, opinions

As seen in this outline, the "M" depicts the drive component of the limbic system. Before learning, an individual must be motivated to learn, to try to succeed at the task, to solve the problem, or to benefit from the environment. Without motivation the brain will not orient itself to the problem and learn. Motivation drives both our cortical structures to develop higher cognitive associations and the motor system to develop procedures or motor programs that will enable us to perform movement with the least energy expenditure and the most efficient patterns available. Once motivated, the individual must be able to pay attention and process the sequential and simultaneous nature of the component parts to be learned, as well as the whole. Thus there is an interlocking dependence between somatosensory mapping of the functional skills[124] (cognitive), attention (limbic) necessary for any type of learning, and the sequential, multiple, and simultaneous programming of functional movement (motor). The limbic amygdala and hippocampal structures and their intricate circuitries play a key role in the declarative aspect of memory.[125,126] Once this syntactical, intellectual memory is learned and taken out of short-term memory by passing through limbic nuclei, the information is stored in cortical areas and can be retrieved at a later time without limbic involvement.[127]

The "O" refers to olfaction, or the incoming sense of smell, which exerts a strong influence on alertness and drive. This is clearly illustrated by the billions of dollars spent annually on perfumes, deodorants, mouthwashes, and soap as well as scents used in stores to increase customers' desires to purchase. This input tract can be used effectively by therapists who have clients with CNS lesions such as internal capsule and thalamic involvement. The olfactory system synapses within the olfactory bulb and then with the limbic system structures and then may go directly to the cerebral cortex without synapsing in the thalamus. Although collaterals do project to the thalamus, unlike all other sensory information, olfaction does not need to use the thalamus as a necessary relay center to access the cortical structures, although many collaterals also project there.[54] Other senses may not be reaching the cortical levels, and the client may have a sensory-deprived environment. Olfactory sensations, which enter the limbic system, may be used to calm or arouse the client. The specific olfactory input may determine whether the person remains calm or emotionally aroused.[10] Pleasant odors would be preferable to most people. With the limbic system's influence on tone production through brain stem modulation, this is one reason aromatherapy causes relaxation and is used by many massage therapists.

A comatose, seemingly nonresponsive client may respond to or be highly sensitive to odor. The therapist needs to be acutely aware of the responses of these patients because these responses may be autonomic instead of somatomotor and may be reflected in a higher heart rate or an increase in blood pressure. Using noxious stimuli to try to "wake up" a patient in a vegetative state has the possibility of causing negative arousal, fear, withdrawal, or anxiety and an increase in base tone within the motor generators. Using this type of input places the patient at level 2 in a "protective state of survival." Using a pleasant and personal desirable smell will more likely place a client at level 2 "safety." The former can lead to strong emotions such as anger, whereas the latter often leads to bonding and motivation to learn. Research has shown that retrieval processing/retrieval of memory have a distinctive emotionality when they were linked to odor-evoked memories.[128,129]

The "V" represents visceral or autonomic drives. As noted earlier, the hypothalamus is nestled within the limbic system. Thus, regulation of sympathetic and parasympathetic reactions, both of the internal organ systems and the periphery, reflect continuing limbic activity. Obviously, drives such as thirst, hunger, temperature regulation, and sexuality are controlled by this system. Clients demonstrating total lack of inhibitory control over eating or drinking or manifesting very unstable body temperature regulation may be exhibiting signs of hypothalamic-pituitary involvement or direct pathways from hypothalamus to midbrain structures.[54]

Less obvious autonomic responses that may reflect limbic imbalances often go unnoticed by therapists. When the stress of an activity is becoming overwhelming to a client, she or he may react with severe sweating of the palms or an increase in dysreflexic activity in the mouth rather than with heightened motor activity. A therapist must continually monitor this aspect of the client's response behaviors to ascertain that the behaviors observed reflect motor control and not limbic influences over that motor system.

If the sensory input to the client is excessive whether through internal or external feedback, the limbic system may go into an alert, protective mode and will not function at the optimal level, and learning will diminish. The client may withdraw physically or mentally, lose focus or attention, decrease motivation, and become frustrated or even angry. The overload on the reticular system may be the reason for the shutdown of the limbic system and not the limbic system itself. Both are part of the same neuroloop circuitry. All these behaviors may be expressed within the hypothalamic-autonomic system as motor output, no matter where in the loop the dysfunction occurs. The evaluation of this system seems even more critical when a client's motor control system is locked, with no volitional movement present. Therapists often try to increase motor activity through sensory input; however, they must cautiously avoid indiscriminately bombarding the sensory systems. The limbic system may demonstrate overload, whereas the spinal motor generators reflect inadequate activation. Although the two systems are different, they are intricately connected, and the concept of massively bombarding one while ignoring the other does not make sense from any learning paradigm, especially from a systems model where consensus creates the observed behavior. To illustrate this concept, think of an orchestra leader conducting a symphony. It would make no sense to have the string section play louder if one half the brass section got sick. Instead, the conductor would need to quiet the string section to allow the brass component to be heard.

"E" relates to emotions, the feelings, attitudes, and beliefs that are unique to that individual. These beliefs include psychosocial attitudes and prejudices, ethnic upbringing, cultural experiences, religious convictions, and concepts of spirituality.[65] All these aspects of emotions link especially to the amygdaloid complex of the limbic system and orbitofrontal activity within the frontal lobe.[130-132] This is a primary emotional center, and it regulates not only our self-concept but our attitudes and opinions toward our external environment and the people within it.

To appreciate the sensory system's influential interaction with the limbic system directly, the reader needs only to look at the literature on music. Most people can give examples of instances where music has elicited immediate and compelling emotional responses of various types. Pleasant and unpleasant musical stimuli have been found to increase or decrease limbic activity and influence both cognitive and motor responses. Although the neurological mechanisms are not yet well understood, the limbic system seems to be implicated in both "positive" and "negative" emotions in response to musical stimuli.[132a-134] The clinical implications are huge. Excessive noise, loud speaker announcements, piped in music, and all the therapists' voices can affect the CNS of a client. Level of musical consonance or dissonance is just one element of the auditory stimulus that is subjectively experienced by the listener as pleasant or unpleasant. The implications that not only listening to music affects limbic emotional states but that the influence may direct the hypothalamus in regulation of blood flow within the CNS have also been shown.[134] With music or sound being just one input system, the therapist must realize that sensory influence from smell, taste, touch, proprioception, vestibular and organ system dysfunction can lead to potential limbic involvement in all aspects of CNS function.

Self-concept is the emotional aspect of body image. For example, assume that one morning I looked in the mirror and said, "The poor world, I will not subject it to me today." I then go back to bed and eat nothing for the rest of the day. The next day I get up and look in the same mirror and say, "What a change, I look trim and beautiful. Look out world, here I come!" In reality, my physical body has not been altered drastically, if at all, but my attitude toward that body has changed. That is, the emotional component of my body image has perceptually changed.

A second self-concept deals with my attitude about my worth or value to society and the world and my role within it. Again, this attitude can change with mood, but more often it seems to change with experience. This aspect of client-therapist interaction can be critical to the success of a therapeutic environment. The two following examples illustrate this point, with the focus of bringing perceived roles into the therapeutic setting:

Your client is Mrs. S., a 72-year-old woman with a left cerebrovascular accident (CVA). She comes from a low socioeconomic background and was a housekeeper for 40 years for a wealthy family of high social standing. When addressing you (the therapist) she always says "yes, ma'am" or "no, ma'am" and does just what was asked, no more and no less. It may be very hard to empower this client to assume responsibility for self-direction in the therapeutic setting. Her perceived role in life may not be to take responsibility or authority within a setting that may, from her perception, have high social status, such as a medical facility. She also may feel that she does not have the right or the power to assume such responsibilities. Success in the therapeutic setting may be based more on changing her attitudes than on her potential to relearn motor control. That is, the concept of empowerment may play a crucial role in regaining independent functional skill and control over her environment.[27,31,34,135]

Your client is a 24-year-old lumberjack who had a closed-head injury during a fall at work. It is now 1 month since his accident, and he is alert, verbal, and angry and has moderate to severe motor control problems. During your initial treatment you note that he responds very well to handling. He seems to flow with your movement, and with your assistance is able to practice much higher level motor control within a narrow biomechanical window; although at times he needs your assistance, you release that control whenever possible to empower him to control his body. At the end of therapy he sits back in his chair with much better residual motor function. Then he turns to you (the female therapist) and instead of saying, "That was great," he says, "You witch, I hate you." The inconsistency between how his body responded to your handling and his attitude toward you as a person may seem baffling, until you realize that he has always perceived himself as a dominant male. Similarly, he perceives women as weak, to be protected, and in need of control. If his attitude toward you cannot be changed to see you in a generic professional role, he will most likely not benefit as much from your clinical skills and guidance as a teacher. Before the accident the patient may have suppressed that verbal response but not tone and body language. After a traumatic brain injury affecting the orbitofrontal system, the inhibition of the behavioral response itself may be lost, further embarrassing the patient emotionally.

Preconceived attitudes, social behaviors, and opinions have been learned by filtering the input through the limbic system. If new attitudes and behaviors need to be learned after a neurological insult, the intactness, especially of the amygdaloid pathways, seems crucial. Damage to these limbic structures may prevent learning; thus, socially maladaptive behavior may persist, making the individual less likely to adapt to the social environment. It is often harder to change learned social behaviors than any other type of learning.[136-138] Because our feelings, attitudes, values, and beliefs drive our behaviors both through attention and motor responses, the emotional aspect of the limbic system has great impact on our learning and motor control. If a patient is not motivated and places little value on a motor output, then complacency results and little learning will occur. On the other hand, if a therapist places an extremely high value on a motor output as a pure expression of motor control without interlocking that control with the patient's limbic influence, the behavioral response may lead to inconsistency, lack of compliance, and thus lack of motor learning and carryover.

Motivation and Reward. Moore[123] considers motivation and memory as part of the MOVE system. Stellar and Stellar[139] link motivation with reward and help, illustrating how the limbic system learns through repetition and reward. They state that the concept of motivation includes drive and satiation, goal-directed behavior, and incentive. They recognize that these behaviors maintain homeostasis and ensure the survival of the individual and the species. Although the frontal lobe region appears to play an important role in self-control and execution activities, these functions seem to require a close interlocking neuronetwork between cognitive representation within the frontal regions and motivational control provided by limbic and subcortical structures.[130] An important aspect of motivated behavior is linked to patient- and family-centered therapy.[27,31,34,135] "The most powerful force in rehabilitation is motivation."[140] These words are strong and reflect the importance of the limbic system in rehabilitation.

Motivated behavior is geared to reinforcement and reward, which is based on both internal and external feedback systems. Repeated experience of reinforcement and reward leads to learning, changed expectancy, changed behavior, and maintained performance.[141] Emotional learning, which certainly involves the limbic system, is very hard to unlearn once the behavior has been reinforced over and over.[142] For that reason, motor behavior that is strongly linked to a negative emotional response might be a very difficult behavior to unlearn. For example, a patient that is willing to stand up and practice transfers just to get the therapist off his back is eliciting a movement sequence that is based on frustration or anger. When that same patient gets home and his spouse asks him to perform the same motor behavior, he may not be able to be successful. The spouse may say, "The therapist said you could." The patient may respond, "I never did like her/him!" Thus repetition of motor performance with either the feeling of emotional neutral or the feeling of success (positive reinforcement) is a critical element in the therapeutic setting. Consistently making the motor task more difficult just when the client feels ready to succeed will tend to decrease positive reinforcement/reward, lessen the client's motivation to try, and decrease the probability of true independence once the patient leaves the clinical setting. When pressure is placed on therapists to produce changes quickly, repetition and thus long-term learning are often jeopardized, which may have a dramatic effect on the quality of the client's life and the long-term treatment effects once he or she leaves the medical facility. Motor control theory (see Chapter 3) coincides with limbic research regarding reinforcement. Inherent feedback within a variety of environmental contexts allowing for error with correction leads to greater retention. Repetition or the opportunity to practice a task (motor or cognitive) in which the individual desires to succeed will lead to long-term learning. Without practice or motivation the chance of successful motor learning is minimal to nonexistent.

Positive emotional states may create a limbic environment where the therapist can link reward and pleasure associations to new motor sequences. Although it is well known that appropriate selections of music can stimulate states of highly pleasant positive affects and physical relaxation, the neurological mechanisms for these effects are not well understood. In an early study by Goldstein,[143] subjects reported pleasant physical sensations of tingling or "thrills" in response to music listening. After subjects were injected with naloxone, which blocks opiate receptors, thrill scores and tingling sensations were attenuated in some subjects. Although responses to music are highly individualized and this study has not been replicated, it suggests that endorphins may be released under certain music listening conditions that elicit pleasant physical sensations. Goldstein's study[143] does not allow us to determine which brain structures might be responsible for the apparent activation of endogenous opiate transmission in response to music, but one possible candidate could be the nucleus accumbens, a structure where opiate receptors have been found to be associated with behavioral reinforcement in a number of animal studies.[144]

In a positron emission tomography (PET) study of cerebral blood flow (CBF) changes measured during highly pleasurable "shivers or chills" in response to subject-selected music, Blood et al[133] found that, as the intensity of the chills increased, CBF increases occurred in the left ventral striatum, dorsomedial midbrain, bilateral insula, right orbitofrontal cortex, thalamus, anterior cingulate cortex, supplementary motor area, and bilateral cerebellum. As the intensity of chills increased, significant CBF decreases were also observed in the right amygdala, left hippocampus/amygdala, and ventral medial prefrontal cortex. The increases found in brain structures associated with reward or pleasant emotions and decreases in areas associated with negative emotional states suggest that music (1) reliably elicits such highly pleasurable experiences as "shivers down the spine" and (2) might be used therapeutically to positively affect limbic activity.

Other studies provide additional support for the notion that music may activate limbic and paralimbic areas associated with reward or pleasurable emotions Brown et al[132a] conducted a PET study of 10 nonmusicians who listened passively to unfamiliar music, which they later reported had elicited strongly pleasant feelings. Unlike previous studies of music, emotion, and limbic activity, this research design called for subjects to listen passively without engaging in any task such as evaluating affective components during the music. The authors noted that the music stimuli used was musically complex and strongly liked by the subjects. When the CBF during the music was compared with silent rest conditions in the same subjects, activations were seen, as expected, in areas presumed to represent perceptual and cognitive responses to music (primary auditory cortex, auditory association cortex, superior temporal sulcus bilaterally, temporal gyrus [BA 21] of the right hemisphere, in the right superior temporal pole [BA 38/22], and adjacent insula). In addition, responses were found in limbic and paralimbic areas, which included the left subcallosal cingulate (BA25/11), anterior cingulate (BA32), left retrosplenial cortex (BA 29/30), and right hippocampus and the left nucleus accumbens and cerebellum. The researchers compare these results with those from the earlier studies by members of the same team[133,134] and suggest that areas such as the subcallosal cingulate are related to the direct experience of occurrent emotions rather than discrimination processing for emotion and that different areas are specifically activated during the pleasant physical responses known as "chills." They go on to propose that the superior temporal pole (BA38/22) and adjacent insula may serve as a point of bifurcation in neural circuitry for processing music. They also suggest that neurons from that region project to limbic and paralimbic areas involved in emotional processing and to premotor areas possibly involved in discrimination and structural processing of music. Although research has increased our appreciation of the complexity of brain activation by music, much more study is needed to validate a model of limbic system activity in human emotional responses to musical stimuli. Clinically, music can be used to improve mood and increase patient motivation to participate in rehabilitation treatment. West has participated in rehabilitation settings as a music therapist in cotreatment with physical and occupational therapists. The music therapist provides music selected or composed to provide motivating energy, pleasant associations, and positive affective states to accompany the motor activity, modifying the musical elements as needed in the moment.

There are many types of emotions that create motivation, such as pleasure, reward processes, addiction, financial benefits, amusement, sadness, humor, happiness, and depression.[143-148] Some emotions tend to drive learning, whereas others may discourage learning, whether that learning be cognitive or motor.

Integration of the Limbic System as Part of a Whole Functioning Brain

Motivation, alertness, and concentration are critical in motor learning because they determine how well we pay attention to the learning and execution of any motor task. These processes of learning and doing are inevitably intertwined: "we learn as we do, and we do only as well as we have learned."[15]

Both motivation ("feeling the need to act") and concentration ("ability to focus on the task") are interlinked with the limbic system. The amygdaloid complex with its multitude of afferent and efferent interlinkages is specially adapted for recognizing the significance of a stimulus, and it assigns the emotional aspect of feeling the need to act. These neuroanatomical loops have tremendous connections with the reticular system. Hence, some authors call it the reticulolimbic system.[54,138] The interaction of the limbic system and the motor generators of the brain stem and ultimate direct and indirect modulation over the spinal system lead to need-directed and, therefore, goal-directed motor activity. It also filters out the significant from the nonsignificant information by selective processing and storing the significant for memory, learning, and recall. These interconnected neuroloop circuitries reinforce the concept that areas have both specialization and generalization and, thus, work closely together with other areas of the brain.[142]

Goal-directed or need-directed motor actions are the result of the nervous system structures acting as an interactive system. Within this system (Figure 4-4), all components share responsibilities. The limbic system and its cortical and subcortical components represent the most important level. In response to stimuli from the internal or external environment, the limbic system initiates motor activity out of the emotional aspect of feeling the need to act. This message is relayed to the sensory areas of the cerebral cortex, which could entail any one or all association areas for visual, auditory, olfactory, gustatory, tactile, or proprioceptive input. These areas are located in the prefrontal, occipital, parietal, and temporal lobes, where they analyze and integrate sensory input into an overall strategy of action or a general plan that meets the requirements of the task. Therefore these cortices recognize, select, and prepare to act as a response to relevant sensory cues when a state of arousal is provided by reticular input. The limbic cortex (uncus, parahippocampal gyrus/isthmus, cingulate gyrus, and septal nucleus) has even greater influence over the sensorimotor cortices through cingulate gyrus, both directly and indirectly through association areas. The thalamus, cerebellum, and basal ganglia contribute to the production of the specific motor plans. These messages of the general plan are relayed to the projection system. The limbic structures through the cingulate gyrus also have direct connections with the primary motor cortex. These circuits certainly have the potential to assist in driving fine motor activities through corticobulbar and corticospinal tracts interactions. The thalamus, cerebellum, basal ganglia, and motor cortices (premotor, supplementary motor, and primary motor) contribute to the production of the specific motor plans.[54] Messages regarding the sensory component of the general plan are relayed to the projection system, where they are transformed into refined motor programs. These plans are then projected throughout the motor system to modulate motor generators throughout the brain stem and spinal system.[54] Limbic connections with (1) cerebellum, basal ganglia, and frontal lobe[54,149-151] and (2) the motor generator within the brain stem[86] enable further control of limbic instructions over motor control or expression. If the limbic and the cognitive systems decide not to act, goal-driven motor behavior will cease. An individual's belief (emotional and spiritual) can inhibit even the most basic survival skills, as has been clearly shown throughout history when individuals' religious beliefs were pitted against vicious predators and those people chose not to defend themselves.

Within the projection system and motor planning complexes, the specifics are programmed and the tactics are given a strategy. In general, "what" is turned into "how" and "when." The necessary parameters for coordinated movement are programmed within the motor complex as to intensity, sequencing, and timing to carry out the motor task. These programs, which incorporate upper motor neurons and interneurons, are then sent to the brain stem and spinal motor generators, which in turn, through lower motor neurons, send orders regarding the specific motor tasks to the musculoskeletal system. (See Chapters 2, 3, and 9 for more specific in-depth discussion.) The actions performed by each subsystem within the entire limbic–motor control complex constantly loop back and communicate to all subsystems to allow for adjustments of intensity and duration and to determine whether the plan remains the best choice

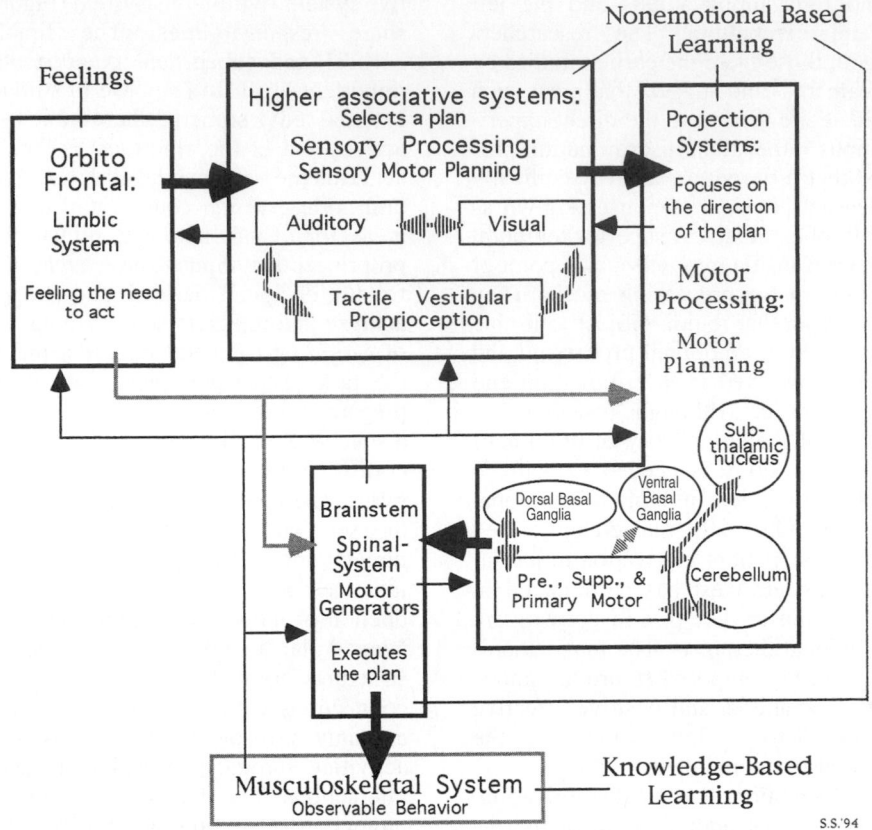

FIGURE 4-4 ■ Functional and dynamic hierarchy of systems based on both limbic and motor control interactions. (Adapted from Brooks VB: *The neural basis of motor control,* New York, 1986, Oxford University Press.)

of responses to an ever-changing three-dimensional world.[150,151]

The limbic system has one more opportunity to modify and control the central pattern generators and control the body and limbs through direct connections to the spinal neuronetwork.[86,152-154] That is, the limbic system can alter existing motor plans by modulating those generators up and down or altering specific nuclear clusters and varying the patterns themselves. Therapists as well as the general public see this in sports activities where emotions are high, no matter the emotion itself. Individuals who have excellent motor control over a specific sport may find high level performance difficult as the stress of competition increases. Having control over emotional variance as well as motor variance with a functional activity is an accurate example of empowerment. Thus, for a therapist to get a true picture of a patient's motor system's function, the limbic system should be flowing in neutral or balanced without strong emotions of any kind. Generally, that balance seems to reflect itself in a state of safety, trust, and compliance. Once the motor control has been achieved then the therapist must reintroduce various emotional environments during the motor activity to be able to state that the patient is independent.

In summary, the limbic complex generates need-directed motor activity and communicates that intent throughout the motor system[86,153] This step is vital to normal motor function

and thus client care. Clients need the opportunity to analyze correctly both their internal environment (their present and feedforward motor plans and their emotional state) and the external world around them requiring action on a task. The integration of all this information should produce the most appropriate strategy available to the patient for the current activity. These instructions must be correct and the system capable of carrying out the motor activity to observe effortless, coordinated movement expression. If the motor system is deficient, lack of adaptability will be observed in the client. If the limbic complex is faulty, the same motor deficits might present themselves. The therapist must differentiate what is truly a motor system problem versus a limbic influence over the motor system problem.

Schmidt[155] stresses the significance of "knowledge of results feedback" as being the information from the environment that provides the individual with insights into task requirements. This insight helps the motor system correctly select strategies that will successfully initiate and support the appropriate movement for accomplishing the task. This knowledge of results feedback is required for effective motor learning and for forming the correct motor programs for storage. The following example is presented to help the reader understand the limbic role in this motor programming.

You are sitting in your new car. The dealer has filled the tank with necessary fuel. The engine mechanism is totally functional with all its wires and interlocking components. The engine will not perform without a mechanism to initiate its strategies or turn on the system. The basal ganglia/frontal lobe motor mechanism plays this role in the brain. In a car you have a starter motor. Yet, the starter motor will not activate the motor system without your intent and motivation to turn the key and turn on the engine. The limbic complex serves this function in the brain. Once you have turned the key, the car is running and ready for your guidance. Whether you choose reverse or first gear usually depends on prior learning unless this is a totally new experience. Once the gear is selected, the motor system will program the car to run according to your desires. It can run fast or slow, but to change the plan both a purpose and a recognition that change is necessary are required. The car has the ability to adapt and self-regulate to many environmental variables, such as ruts or slick pavement, to continue running the feed-forward program, just as many motor systems within your CNS, especially the cerebellum, play that function. The limbic system may emotionally choose to drive fast, whereas your cognitive judgment may choose otherwise. The interactive result will drive your pedal and brake pressure and ultimately regulate the car. The components discussed play a critical role in the total function of the car, just as all the systems within your CNS play a vital role in regulating your behavioral responses to the environment.

Brooks[66] distinguishes insightful learning, which is programmed and leads to skills when the performer has gained insight into the requirements, from discontinuous movements, which need to be replaced by continuous ones. This process is hastened when clients understand and can demonstrate their understanding of what "they were expected to do." Improvement of motor skills is possible by using programmed movement in goal-directed behavior. The reader must be cautioned to make sure that the client's attention is on the goal of the task and not on the components of the movement itself. The motor plan needs programming and practice without constant cognitive overriding. The limbic/frontal system helps drive the motor toward the identified task or abstract representation of a match between the motor planning sequence and the desired outcome. The importance of the goal being self-driven by the patient cannot be overemphasized.[27,31,34,110]

Without knowledge of results, feedback, and insight into the requirements for goal-directed activity, the learning is performing by "rote," which merely uses repetition without analysis, and meaningful learning or building of effective motor memory in the form of motor holograms will be minimal. Children with cognitive and limbic deficits can learn basic motor skills through repetition of practice, but the insights and ability to transfer that motor learning into other contexts will not be high (see Chapters 12, 13, and 14).

Schmidt[155] suggests that, to elicit the highest level of function within the motor system and to enable insightful learning, therapy programs should be developed around goal-directed activities, which means a strong emotional context. These activities direct the client to analyze the environmental requirements (both internal and external) by placing the client in a situation that forces development of "appropriate strategies." Goal-directed activities should be functional and thus involve motivation, meaningfulness, and selective attention. Functional and somatosensory retraining

uses these concepts as part of the intervention (see Chapter 9). Specific techniques such as proprioceptive neuromuscular facilitation, neurodevelopmental therapy, the Rood method, and the Feldenkrais method can be incorporated into goal-directed activities in the therapy programs, as can any treatment approach so long as it identifies those aspects of motor control and learning that lead to retention and future performance and allows the patient to self-correct.[155] With insights into the learned skills, clients will be better able to adjust these to meet the specific requirements of different environments and needs, using knowledge of response feedback to guide them. The message then is to design exercise activities or programs that are meaningful and need directed, to motivate clients into insightful goal-directed learning. Thus, understanding the specific goals of the client is critical and will only be obtained by interaction with that client as a person with needs, desires, and anticipated outcomes. A therapist cannot assume that "someone wants to do something." The goal of running a bank may seem very different from that of bird watching in the mountains, yet both may require ambulatory skills. If a client does not wish to return to work, then a friendly smile and the statement, "Hi, I'm your therapist and I'm going to get you up and walking so you can get back to work," may lead to resistance and decreased motivation. In contrast, by knowing the goal of the client, a person highly motivated to ambulate may be present in the clinic every day to meet the goal of bird watching in the mountains although never wishing to walk back into the office again.

Clinical Perspectives

The Client's Internal System Influences Observable Behavior. At least once a year almost any local newspaper will carry a story that generally reads as follows:

Seventy-nine-year-old, 109-pound arthritic grandmother picks up car by bumper to free trapped 3-year-old grandson.

All of us read these articles and at first doubt their validity and then question the sensationalism used by the reporter. I would also question such news reporting if, at age 13 years, I had not seen three teenage boys pick up a 1956 Chevrolet and put it back in the garage in its correctly parked position. The boys had moved the car because they feared that if they did not put the car back into its original parked position, their parents would find out that they had driven the car without a license or permission. That elderly lady picked up the car out of fear of severe injury to her grandchild. Emotions can create tremendous high tonal responses, either in a postural pattern such as in a temper tantrum or during a movement strategy such as picking up a car. Similarly, fear can immobilize a person and make it impossible to create enough tone to run a motor program or actually move. Separating power or tone production because of strong emotions versus motor system control is an aspect of therapeutic evaluation often overlooked.

Limbic Continuums

All clinicians need to understand and recognize two powerful limbic motor response programs: the F^2ARV and the general adaptation syndrome (GAS). These continuums need to be monitored frequently with all patients with CNS injury and evaluated and recorded if response patterns exceed normal expectations.

F²ARV (Fear/Frustration, Anger, Rage, Violence) Continuum. One sequence of behaviors used to describe the emotional circuitry of the amygdala is called the F²ARV (Fear/Frustration, Anger, Rage, Violence or withdrawal) continuum[138,156] (Figure 4-5). This continuum begins with fear, often exhibited as frustration by children, teens, and young adults. If the event inducing the fear/frustration continues to heighten, anger will often develop. Anger is a neurochemical response perceived and defined by the cognitive aspect of our cortex as anger. If the neurochemical response continues to build, the anger of the person may go into rage (internal chaos) and, finally, violence (motor response). Women who attain the level of rage may become withdrawn and thus become victimized by a partner who is also in rage or inflicting physical/emotional violence.[157] How quickly any individual will progress from fear to violence depends on many factors. First, the initial wiring or genetic neurochemical predisposition will influence behavioral responses. Second, soft-wired or conditioned responses resulting from environmental influences and reinforcement patterns will determine output. For example, it is commonly known that abusive parents were usually abused children[156,158]; they learned that anger quickly leads to violence and that the behavior of violence was acceptable. Third, the quality and intensity of the stimulus initiating the continuum will influence the level of response.

The neurochemistry within the individual's CNS, whether inherently active or released into the system through drugs or injury, will have great influence on the plasticity of the existing wiring.[43,159] When the chemistry or wiring becomes imbalanced from damage, environmental stress, learning, or other potentially altering situations, then the control over this continuum may also change.[54,95]

Therapists need to be acutely aware of this continuum in clients who have diffuse axonal shearing within the limbic complex. Diffuse axonal shearing is most commonly seen and reported in research on individuals with head trauma. (See Chapter 17.) As a result, lesions within the limbic structures may result in an individual who progresses down this continuum at a rapid speed.[73] This point cannot be overemphasized. Patients who have difficulty in this area may physically strike out at a therapist out of frustration. The result may be a broken nose or blackened eye of the therapist. Once the patient strikes out, fear has been instilled in the therapist. Two continuums are interacting. By understanding "why the patient acted out," the therapist retains cognitive distance and potentially chemical control over her or his own limbic reactions. Knowing the social history of the client and the causation of the injury often can help the therapist gain insight into how an individual patient might progress down this continuum. Not all head-injured patients had prior difficulty with the F²ARV continuum, but, similarly, many individuals received their head injuries in violent confrontational situations.

General Adaptation Syndrome. The autonomic responses to stress have been identified as following a specific course of behavioral changes and are referred to as the general adaptation syndrome.[69,160-164] The sequential stages of this syndrome directly relate to limbic imbalance and can play a dramatic role in determining client progress. This stress can be caused by pain, the illness itself, ramification of the illness, confusion, sensory overload, and a large variety of other potential sources. Initial reaction to stress or neurochemical imbalance creates a state of alarm and triggers a strong sympathetic nervous system reaction. Heart rate, blood pressure, respiration, metabolism, and muscle tonus will increase. At this stage, the grandmother lifts the car off the child. If the overstimulation or stress does not diminish, the body will protect itself from self-destruction and trigger a parasympathetic response. At this time, all the symptoms reverse and the client exhibits a decrease in heart rate, blood pressure, and muscle tonus. The bronchi become constricted, and the patient may hyperventilate and become dizzy, confused, and less alert. As the blood flow returns to the periphery, the face may flush and the skin may become hot. The patient will have no energy to move, will withdraw, and again will exhibit signs of flexion, adduction, internal rotation, and lack of postural tone.

This stress or overstimulation syndrome is characterized by common symptoms.[130,165-170] If the acute symptoms are not eliminated, they will become chronic and the behavior patterns much more resistant to change.

General adaptation syndrome is often seen in the elderly, with various precipitating health crises,[163] and also in neonatal high-risk infants (see Chapter 11), victims of head trauma, and other clients with neurological conditions. What causes the initial alarm can range from moderate to maximal internal instability with less intensive external stress, to minimal internal instability, and severe external sensory bombardment. Medical conditions of head traumas (Chapter 17), inflammatory CNS problems (Chapter 20), and brain tumors (Chapter 25) often create hypersensitivity to external input such as noise, touch, or light. Normal clinical environments may create a sensory overload and trigger this general adaptation syndrome.

In the elderly, stresses such as change of environment, loss of loved ones, failing health, and fears of financial problems can each cause the client's system to react as if overloaded. Our elderly clients usually have two or more of these issues to deal with while trying to benefit from a therapeutic setting that demands their full attention for effective functioning. No wonder so many older clients shut down, withdraw from the therapeutic environment, and eventually withdraw from the entire world and become resistant and confused.

It is logical to assume that, because of the autonomic responses that this syndrome evokes, strong interactions exist with the hypothalamus and the limbic system. Stress, no matter what the specific precipitating incident (confusion,

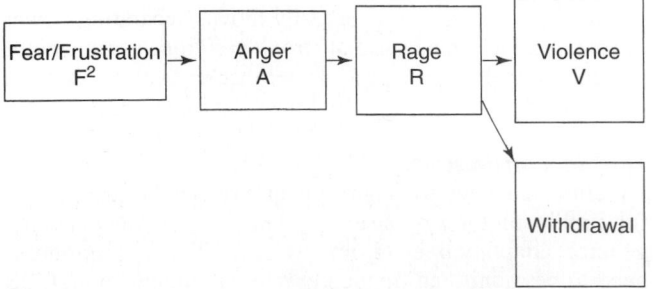

FIGURE 4-5 ■ Fear/Frustration, Anger, Rage, Violence: F²ARV continuum.

fear, anxiety, grief, and pain), has the potential to trigger the first steps in the sequence of this syndrome.[165-170] The clinician's sensitivity to the client's emotional system will be the therapeutic technique that best controls and reverses the acute condition.

These two continuums are interrelated in individuals who have direct or indirect limbic problems. If someone throughout life easily gets angry and may overreact with violence, then the F^2ARV continuum has always been on alert. After trauma, volitional control over this continuum may be diminished. The therapist needs to be aware that the patient may overrespond to frustration or fear of failure in both cognitive and motor activities. The initial response may be an escalation of the F^2ARV continuum with what then seems like a rapid withdrawal (general adaptation syndrome). There are many ways to help the patient balance these autonomic reactions and continue to learn within the therapeutic setting. The Bonny Method of Guided Imagery and Music is a music-centered psychotherapy method that has been used extensively with individuals recovering from various types of trauma.[171-174] In reviewing specific Bonny method treatment approaches used with trauma patients, Körlin[174] describes a cyclical process where an important initial treatment period emphasizes the mobilization of inner resources, alleviating vulnerability and increasing the patient's self-confidence. This phase uses carefully selected music that elicits positive limbic states and "bodily manifestations with qualities of warmth, energy, strength, movement, nourishing, and healing, all belonging to the implicit realm of positive vitality affects and mental models" (p. 398). The individual is then better equipped to face a period of confrontation with painful or traumatic material or the challenges faced within a therapeutic rehabilitation environment. Successful confrontation of difficult realities is then followed by a new phase of resource mobilization and consolidation of healthier behaviors that begin to replace dysfunctional defenses such as avoidance, behavioral extremes, or substance abuse.

This process continues in repeated cycles of rest/resourcing and working/confronting. The clinical success of this approach suggests that for some patients it may be advantageous to purposefully facilitate positive or pleasant physical and affective experiences before engaging in more challenging work. Although it may be impractical to provide appropriate music selections on the basis of individual assessment in a physical or occupational therapy setting (unless the therapist has access to consultation with a music therapist), other modalities such as heat, massage, or ultrasound treatment may also elicit relaxed, receptive physical states. The treating professional can also become aware during assessments or treatments of environmental auditory input that may trigger stress responses in patients who have limbic system involvement or who may have experienced traumatic physical or emotional injuries. These triggers can be something as simple as the therapist's tone of the voice in a sentence to the patient or as complex as the multiple-noise environment of a busy rehabilitation setting. Some patients may need to be scheduled for early morning, during lunchtime, or in the late afternoon to provide a decrease in the auditory environment.

Decreasing stimulation versus increasing facilitation may lead to attention, calmness, and receptiveness to therapy.

When the client feels that control over her or his life has been returned, or at least the individual is consulted regarding decisions, resistance to therapy or movement is often released and stress is reduced. Even clients in a semicomatose state can participate to some extent. As a clinician begins to move a client, resistance may be encountered. If slight changes are made in rotation or trajectory of the movement pattern, the resistance is often lessened. If the clinician initially feels the resistance and overpowers it, total control has been taken from the client. Instead, if the clinician moves the patient in ways her or his body is willing to be moved, respect has been shown and overstimulation potentially avoided. Most therapists are rushed by the full schedule of managed care, stressed by patients' early discharge, and by demands placed on the therapist for measurable outcomes of patient behaviors. As a result of these constraints, the clinician may physically move faster than the pace best tolerated by the patient, who needs more time to process stimuli and practice target skill. The challenge for both the therapist and the patient is to find harmony within the given environment to allow for optimal outcomes.

No single input causes these reactions, nor does one treatment counteract its progression. Being aware of clinical signs is critical. Another important therapeutic skill is not prejudging withdrawn clients by assuming that they need more stimulation to regain function. The specific techniques appropriate for treating this syndrome are tools all therapists possess. How each clinician uses those tools is a critical link to success or failure in clinical interaction.

Emotions Expressed Through Motor Programming. Throughout the existence of humankind, emotions have been identified in all cultures. A child knows when a parent is angry without the patient saying anything. A stranger can recognize someone who is sad or depressed. People walk to the other side of the road to avoid being close to someone who seems enraged. What is it that is recognized? Are emotions recognizable? Emotions are expressed through motor output and thus potentially have an impact on functional motor control. The extent and intensity are up to the therapist to evaluate.

Anger. Anger itself creates tone through the amygdaloid's influence over the basal ganglia and the sensory and motor cortices and their influence over the motor control system. This is clearly exhibited in a child throwing a temper tantrum (Figure 4-6) or an adult putting his fist through a wall. How far a client or a friend will progress through the F^2ARV continuum (discussed in the previous section) depends on a large number of variables. From observation, it is clear that clients do not want to lose control and progress to rage or violence, which often causes embarrassment. This fear, in and of itself, may be frustrating and trigger the continuum. When a client loses that control the therapist must first determine whether the therapist forced the client beyond her or his ability to control. If so, changes within the therapeutic environment need to be made to allow the client opportunities to develop control and modulation over that continuum.

For example, West was asked to consult with a rehabilitation team to devise a treatment program to address violent rage episodes in a 40-year-old man with moderate physical and severe cognitive functioning deficits resulting from a

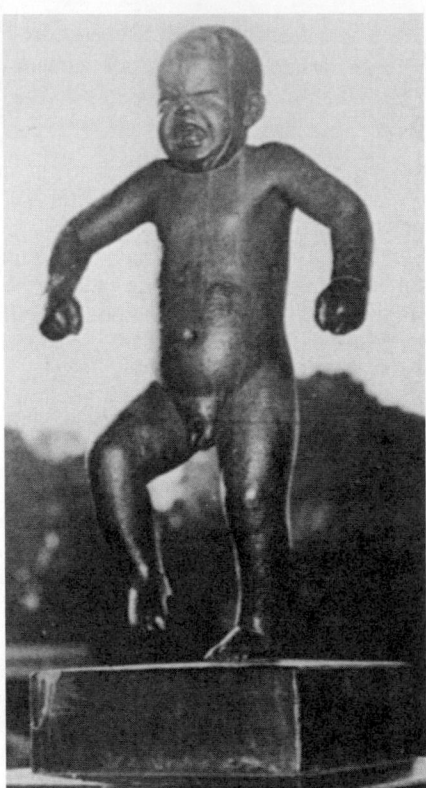

FIGURE 4-6 ■ Extensor behavior responses caused by anger. ("Angry Boy," Vigelund Sculpture Grounds in the Frogner Park, Oslo, Norway. Adapted from photo by Normann.)

brain aneurysm. He would escalate very rapidly along the F^2ARV continuum when presented with environmental challenges such as passing another patient with his wheelchair in the hallway. Although his physical rehabilitation had progressed well and he had regained much independence in mobility, because his assaultive outbursts posed risks to other patients as well as to caregivers, this patient appeared to be heading for placement in a locked facility, a more restrictive environment than he would need considering his level of physical limitation. Although this unfortunate man had no short-term memory function and no insight about his behaviors, West found during her assessment that he was highly responsive to calming music and was able to access some intact long-term memories that could be used to elicit a relaxation response. A highly positive limbic state of deep relaxation was thus elicited and simple verbal cues were then presented to develop a conditioned response that any staff member could then call forth with the verbal cue alone. The entire rehabilitation team was briefed on the use of this intervention and reported success using this approach in the milieu as well as during physical therapy and occupational therapy treatments, where the patient would become resistant and angry in response to therapist instructions. The patient was trained to self-regulate by giving himself the same verbal cue when confronted with challenging situations. This treatment supported the patient's ability to regain emotional controls and allowed him the opportunity to be placed in a less-restrictive community environment. The patient never recalled a previous music therapy treatment

session and asked each time to have the purpose of the treatment explained to him. But his body remembered the set of behavioral experiences, and he quickly complied with the relaxation procedure. The success of this approach demonstrates that, even in the absence of short-term memory and other cognitive functions usually considered essential for new learning, the skillful engagement of positive limbic states and intact areas of patient functioning (strengths) can support development of new adaptive skills.

Creating opportunities to confront frustration/fear or even anger in real situations while the client practices modulation will lead to independence or self-empowerment. The client simultaneously needs to practice self-directed motor programming without these emotional overlays. Thus, true motor learning can result. In time, practicing the same motor control over functional programs while confronted with a large variety of emotional situations should lead to independence in life activities and thus meet a therapeutic goal.

Similarly, being unaware of a client's anger may lead the therapist to the false assumption that that individual has adequate inherent postural tone to perform activities such as independent transfers. If the client is angry with the therapist and performs the transfer only to "get the therapist off her or his case," when the client is sent home she or he may be unable to create enough postural extension to perform the transfer. Thus, this transfer skill was never functionally independent because the test measurements were based on limbic/frontal influence over the extensor component of the motor system. The client needs to learn how to do the activity without the emotional overlay. When a therapist is unwilling, unaware, or unable to attend to these variables, the reliability or accuracy of functional test results becomes questionable.

Grief, Depression, or Pain. Emotions such as grief or depression can be expressed by the motor system.[54,121] The behavioral responses are usually withdrawal, decreased postural adaptation, and often a feeling of tiredness and exhaustion (Figure 4-7). Sensory overload, especially in the elderly, can create the same pattern of response of flexion, internal rotation, and adduction. Again, because of the strong emotional factor, these motor responses are considered to be the result of the limbic system's influence over motor control.[86] Learned helplessness is another problem that therapists need to avoid. When patients are encouraged to become dependent, their chances of benefiting from services and regaining motor function are drastically reduced.[175,176] The concept of pain and pain management is discussed in detail in both Chapters 15 and 32. Whether the pain is peripherally induced or centrally induced because of trauma or emotional overload, often the same motor responses will exist. That withdrawn flexor pattern makes postural activities exhausting because of the work it takes to override the existing central pattern generators. Thus, daily living activities, which constantly require postural extension against gravity, may be perceived as overwhelming and just not worth the effort. The therapist needs to learn to differentiate between peripheral physical pain and central or emotional pain and between mixed peripheral and central induced pain. To the patient, "pain is pain!"[177-181]

Bonding Projects Relaxation, Whereas Lack of Bonding Reflects Isolation. Because of the potency of the limbic system's connections into the motor system, a therapist's sensitivity to the client's emotional state would obviously be a key factor in understanding the motor responses observed during therapy. Before a therapist will be open and sensitive to a patient, he or she must first understand her or his own feelings, emotional responses, and communication styles that are being used within any given clinical or social environment.[182-186] In Figure 4-8 an entire spectrum of motor responses can be observed in the four statues. A client who feels safe can relax and participate in the learning without strong emotional reactions. The woman being held in Figure 4-8 is safe and relaxed. The man and woman are interacting through touch with warmth and compassion that is often observed when colleagues watch a "master clinician" treating a client. The client and clinician seem to flow together during the treatment as one motor system. When looking at the man and woman, it becomes obvious that the two figures could not be separated, for they are one piece of art. In today's health care environment and with the emphasis on the client running and self-correcting motor programming, many therapists assume that they need not or should not touch the patient. This conclusion may be accurate when considering the motor system in isolation and having concluded that the patient can self-correct error in motor programs. When correction by the therapist is through words rather than touch, it is external feedback where the auditory

system has replaced the somatosensory system. The voice, as well as touch, can be soothing and instill confidence. Yet language in and of itself will not replace the trust and safety felt both physically and emotionally through the deep pressure of touch. Bonding and trust occur much more often through touch than through conversation. Also, verbal instructions require intact auditory processing and translation from declarative to procedural information.

Referring again to Figure 4-8, the two men in the statue on the left could represent two unique pieces of art. Those two men demonstrate a lack of bonding. In fact, if the artist could have brought them closer together, they would just have rejected or repelled each other with greater intensity. If one of the men were the therapist and one the patient, little interaction would be occurring, and thus the assumption that learning is occurring is probably false. The therapist could not do anything to the other person (and vice versa) without that person perceiving the act as invasive, negative, or having little to do with what that individual values. The therapist's responsibility is to open the patient's receptiveness to learning, not to close it.

These pictures clearly illustrate two types of therapist/client interactions. If an artist can clearly depict the tonal characteristics of emotion, certainly the therapist should be able to recognize those behaviors in the client. If a client is

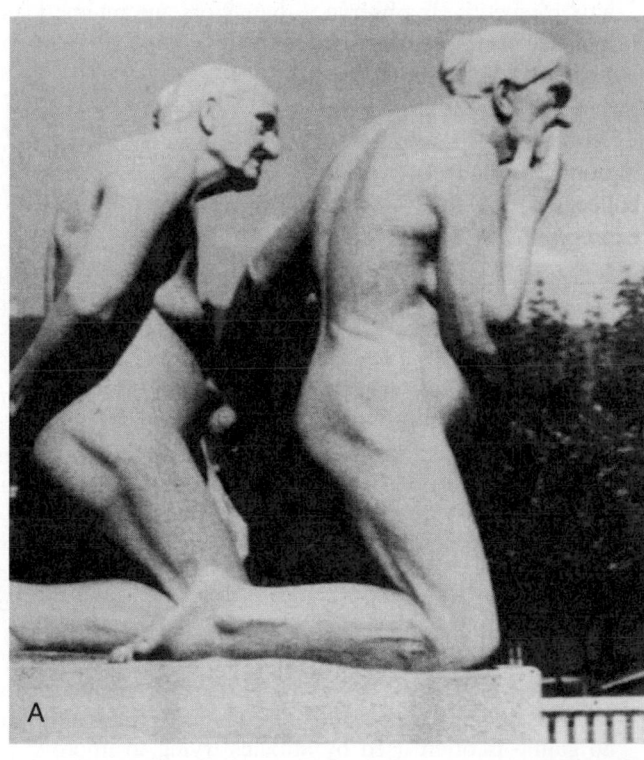

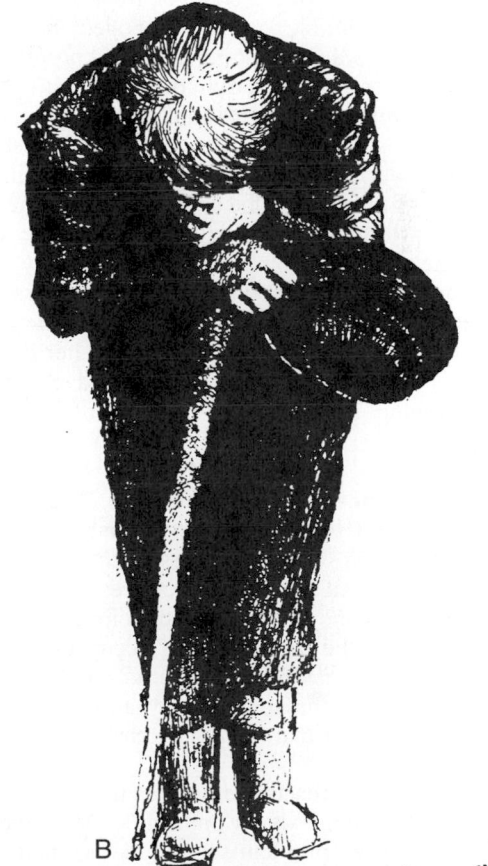

FIGURE 4-7 ■ **A,** Behavior responses elicited by concern, pain, and grief. **B,** Pain or grief elicits flexion and can modify postural extension. (**A,** Vigelund Sculpture Grounds in the Frogner Park, Oslo, Norway. Adapted from photo by Normann.)

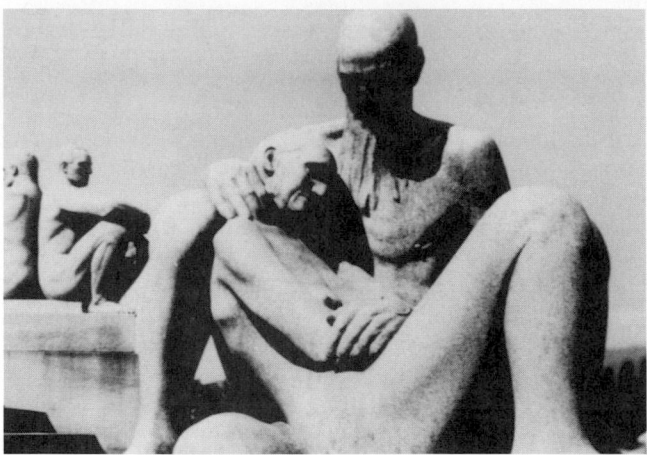

FIGURE 4-8 ■ Grief, depression, and compassion responses are seen in the center figures, and rigid, stoic, distancing behaviors are observed in the two left statues. (Vigelund Sculpture Grounds in the Frogner Park, Oslo, Norway. Adapted from photo by Normann.)

frustrated or angry and simultaneously has rigidity, spasticity, or general high tone, then a therapist might spend the entire session trying to decrease the motor response. If the client could be helped to deal with the anger or frustration during the therapy session and thus neutralize the emotion, then the specific problems could be treated effectively. Differentiating the limbic system component from the motor control system and establishing treatment protocols for each may not be within the spectrum of a therapist's skills. Thus, working simultaneously with another professional such as a psychologist, social worker, or neuropsychologist may be an acceptable alternative approach. This cotreatment will allow all aspects of the client to be addressed simultaneously. Carryover of procedural learning (motor learning; see discussion of neurobiology of learning and memory for details) into adaptive motor responses needs to be practiced with consistency.[54] The influence of the limbic system in a client with large mood swings may drastically alter the consistent responses of the motor systems and thus dampen the procedural learning and limit the success of the therapeutic setting.

Limbic Concepts that Influence Therapist/Client Interactions: Observations of Master Clinicians at Work. Although some colleagues might see this section as irrelevant to patient care, it has been presented for those who strive to understand and become the clinical masters of the future. Because the professions of occupational and physical therapy are considered both "arts" and "sciences," then linking the art to the science may allow new learners to obtain clinical skill and sensitivity earlier than "masters of the past."

How a clinician reacts at any given moment during a therapeutic session depends on both the client's and the clinician's declarative problem-solving skills, their procedural motor skills (see discussion of neurobiology of learning and memory and see Chapter 3), and their emotional drive to be part of the learning environment. Therefore, the sensitivity and specific level of attention of the therapist toward all responses of the client depend, to a large extent, on the clinician's limbic system and her or his interest and commitment to the patient and their mutual learning environment. Although therapists are trained to be skilled observers of patient behavior, the development of "master clinician" capabilities also requires self-awareness on the part of the helping professional. "Behavioral activity can tell us often about the inner state of another or ourselves"[187] (p. 19). The willingness to be aware of one's own internal state increases the therapist's ability to perceive subtleties in the patient's responses.

In an analysis of what differentiates a truly gifted or master clinician from a group of highly skilled and talented colleagues, the following philosophical verbal concepts are often expressed:

That person has a rare gift.

That person seems to intuitively know what to do or what the client needs.

When that clinician treats a client, the two seem to flow together in their movements.

The client seems to totally trust that clinician; I have never seen that before.

I cannot believe that the client accurately did that with that clinician; before, the client was too afraid.

Many factors in an interactive setting, such as therapy, cannot be identified, but certain limbic/emotional factors may play a role in that gifted clinician's skill. Some of those factors are discussed next. This discussion in no way encapsulates all limbic variables within an interaction, only those that Umphred believes safe to share and has had opportunity to repetitively observe as behaviors and interactions.

Trust/Responsibility. Trust is a critical component of a successful therapy session. The therapist gains the client's trust by his or her actions. Similarly, trust is gained by acknowledgment by the therapist that the patient has life-limiting functional problems and that those limitations have an emotional and motoric impact on life participation. Illustrating by the use of objective data where those functional limitations are and specifically how they may be treated creates a bond and trust between the patient and the therapist. In today's environment the use of reliable, valid objective tests and measures allows for this form of communication, which has not existed to the same extent in the past. Honesty and truth lead to trust.[63,188-192] Telling someone you will not hurt them is a contract between the therapist and the client. If the therapist continually ranges a joint beyond a pain-free range, that behavior is dishonest and untruthful and will not lead to trust. Trust can be earned by stopping as soon as the client verbalizes symptoms or shows pain with a body response such as a grimace. These symptoms can be overt or covert. In either case the therapist needs to be aware of both the physical and emotional responses of the patient. Some therapists say they feel the presence of pain. This concept of reducing or avoiding pain whenever possible cannot be overemphasized. The phrase "No pain, no gain!" is often used by athletes trying to improve performance, by athletic trainers, or by therapists and physicians trying to motivate their clients/patients. Why does something have to hurt to get better? Pain is present because of danger and potential harm, not for pleasure. Why can't the phrase "Gain without pain!" be just as appropriate? Symptoms are valuable to the therapist as well as the patient to create environments for change, but the intensity of those stimuli need close monitoring because they can dramatically affect motor responses and ultimately overwhelm the CNS and prevent learning. People often ask me, "How do I (Umphred) deal with pain?" I respond with, "I am not the colleague to ask because I first feel the pain, next I get rid of the pain, and then I treat the CNS problems!"

What does "feel the patient's pain" refer to? First, a therapist needs to assess the biomechanics of the joint(s) where pain is expressed. Second, the muscle fascial tightness needs to be examined. Third, the motor programming available to the patient during movement of the joint(s) during functional activities needs to be assessed. All three of these actions and their interactions do not necessarily explain the cause of the pain, but they do help a therapist draw conclusions about the pain. A fourth variable exists that is much harder to explain or validate scientifically. It seems as if "the therapist feels the patient's pain as well as its location." It is possible that a therapist might include all the above types of information from the examination and project that information onto her or his somatosensory cortex and into her or his body image, but as a result "the therapist feels the pain" and thus has limbic associations to that feeling. That information within the therapist would guide and direct intervention selection and be patient driven.

Second, the therapist should get rid of the pain, if possible. Using all the therapeutic techniques such as manual therapy for biomechanical alignment and joint mobility, fascial and muscle mobilization to get filament gliding, and rotation with elongation or compression to get changes in the motor programs helps. But, in addition, "a therapist feels the pain, bonds with it, and then, through visualization and touch, draws it away from the patient." While in Germany in 1996, Umphred asked Susanna Klein Vogelbach about this phenomenon. Susanna was a true master clinician. All the other early master clinicians in the area of neurorehabilitation whom Umphred had known were deceased. Susanna's responses to questions were preceded with long pauses because of the sensitivity and lack of scientific scrutiny that might accompany her responses. Yet she acknowledged she also felt the physical and emotional pain of her patients and that she too drew it out with her hands. She paused one moment, smiled, and then stated, "but sometimes they pull it back in!"

Pain is a complex phenomenon, and the more it is understood, the more complex it becomes[193-197] (see Chapter 32). Being sensitive to a patient's pain, no matter the cause, and working with the patient to eliminate that pain often lead to very strong bonding and trust that will lead to compliance and learning. Ignoring the pain may be perceived as insensitivity and lack of caring, which can lead to distrust and often resistance to learning or performance.

A personal limbic experience helped teach Umphred the previous lesson. It occurred while she was giving birth to her second son. The doctor finally said, "Push," and as she did her son's head compressed her left sciatic nerve and she stopped pushing. She said, "Please reposition my left leg (which was strapped into a stirrup) because the head of the baby is pushing on my sciatic nerve." Everyone ignored her, and as her pelvic muscles started to contract, the doctor again said, "Push." She refused and again stated the problem. The doctor then said, "Honey, you are having a baby and it is going to hurt!" She again stated her dilemma. The nurse finally said, "What did you say?" She repeated and the nurse said "Oh!" and adjusted her leg, and in one push her son was born. Compliance to participate is limbic, and limbic has tremendous control over intentional movement, no matter the context of the environment.[63] Patients with dizziness, particularly dizziness within visual environments, develop similar avoidance behaviors. These behaviors initially create feelings of panic and can develop into full panic attacks and agoraphobic responses.[198] These individuals avoid participating in activities that put them within visually overstimulating environments to be empowered to control the initial dizziness and prevent the autonomic reactions. Similar types of reactions have been documented, such as space-motion discomfort,[199] postural phobic vertigo,[198] visual vertigo,[200] and dizziness of "psychogenic" origin. Are these names and symptoms part of a spectrum of limbic responses to vestibular/cerebellar/brain stem interactions and thus create movement dysfunction that might lead to a referral to either a physical or occupational therapist? Of course, it may be referred to a psychologist or psychiatrist first.

Once a client gives her or his trust, a clinician can freely move with a client and little resistance caused by fear, reservations, or need to protect self will be felt or observed. What tightness or limitations in movement are present when the limbic system is emotionally neutral are problems with systems or subsystems that movement therapists specialize in. Examination and interventions at this time will more consistently reflect true motor limitations and impairments. It is recommended that, if after determining the pain is due to peripheral tightness or joint immobility and the limbic system has been neutralized, the therapist does not elicit pain during that session. Deal with those issues in the next session after gaining the trust of the client. Trust by the therapist or the client does not mean lack of awareness of potential danger. Trust means acceptance that, although the danger is present, the potential of harm, pain, or disaster is very slight and the expected gain is worth the risk. In Figure 4-9, the student's trust that the instructor will not hurt her can be seen by her lack of protective responses and by her calm, relaxed body posture. The student is aware of the potential of the kick but trusts her life to the skills, control, and personal integrity of the teacher. Those same qualities are easily observed in patient/therapist interactions when watching a gifted clinician treat clients. The motor activities in a therapeutic setting may be less complex than in Figure 4-9, but in no way are they less stressful, less potentially harmful, or less frightening from the client's point of view.

Therapists must first trust themselves enough to know that they can effect changes in their clients. Understanding one's own motor system, how it responds, and how to use ones hands, arms, or entire body to move someone else is based partly on procedural skills, partly on declarative learning, and partly on self-confidence or self-trust. Trusting that one, as a therapist, has the skill to implement the motor response within the patient has a limbic component. If a therapist has self-doubts about therapeutic skills, that doubt will change performance, which will alter input to the client. This altered input can potentially alter the client's output and vary the desired responses if the client's motor system cannot run independently.

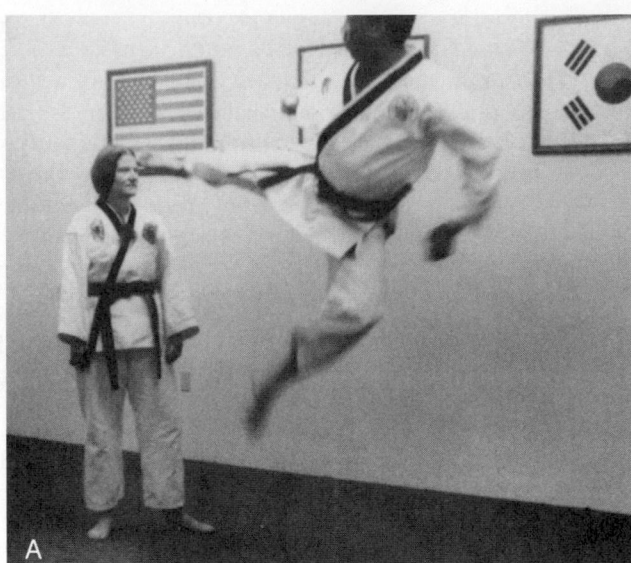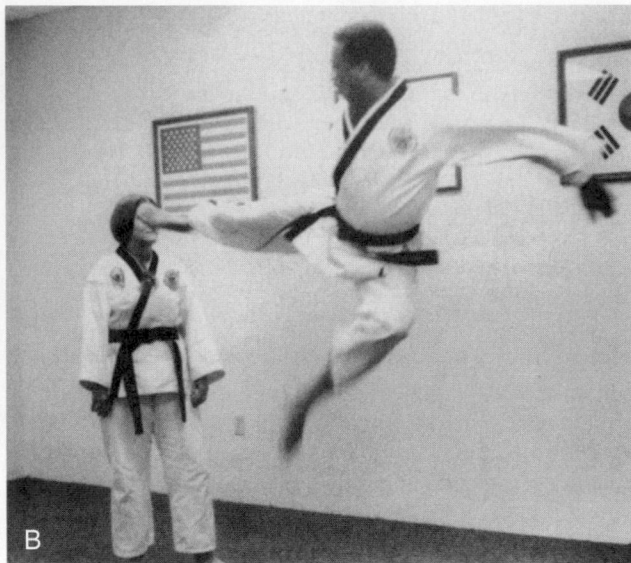

FIGURE 4-9 ■ Trust relaxes the limbic system's need to protect. **A,** The skill of the teacher is obvious. **B,** The student trusts that she is in no danger.

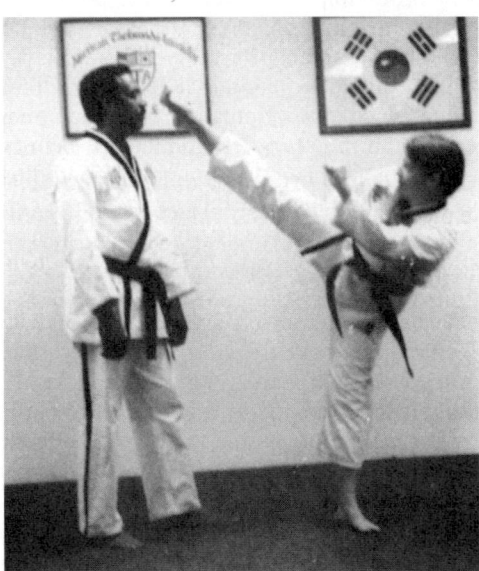

FIGURE 4-10 ■ The teacher relinquishes the task to the student, and the student trusts the teacher is right even if self-doubt exists.

Very close to the concept of trust is the idea of responsibility. Accepting responsibility for our own behavior seems obvious and is accepted as part of a professional role. Accepting and allowing the client the right to accept responsibility for her or his own motor environment are also key elements in creating a successful clinical environment and an independent person.* Figure 4-10 illustrates the concept through the following example:

The teacher (or therapist) asked the student (or client) to perform a motor act. In the figure, the act was to perform a kick to the teacher's head. The kick was to be very strong or forceful and completed. The student was told not to hold back or stop the kick in any way, yet the kick was to come within a few inches of the teacher's head. This placed tremendous responsibility on the student. One inch too far might dangerously hurt the instructor, yet one inch too short was not acceptable. The teacher knew the student had the skill, power, and control to perform the task and then passed the responsibility to the student. The student was hesitant to assume the responsibility, for the consequence of failure could have been very traumatic, but the student trusted that the teacher would not ask for the behavior unless success was fairly guaranteed. That trust reduced anxiety and helped neutralize emotions and thus the neurochemicial limbic response's effect on the motor system of the student/client, giving her optimal motor control over the act. Once the task was completed successfully, the student gained confidence and could repeat the task with less fear or emotional influence while gaining refinement over the motor skill.

Although the motor activities described in this example are complex and different from functional activities practiced within the clinic by therapists and clients, the dynamics of the environment relate consistently with client/therapist roles and expectations. A gifted clinician knows that the client has the potential to succeed. When asked to perform, the client trusts the therapist and assumes responsibility for the act. The therapist can facilitate the movement or postural pattern, thereby ensuring that the client succeeds. This feeling of success stimulates motivation for task repetition, which ultimately leads to learning. The incentive to repeat and learn becomes self-motivating and then becomes the responsibility of the client. As the therapist relinquishes control and empowers the client to more and more of the function, novelty to the learning is occurring. Current literature has shown that people are more motivated by novelty and change than by success at mastery or accomplishment of a goal.[203-205] The limbic complex and its interwoven network throughout the nervous system play a key role in this behavioral drive. The task itself can be

---

*References 27, 31, 34, 135, 201, 202.

simple, such as a weight shift or postural coactivating in a sitting pattern, or as complex as getting dressed or climbing onto and off of a bus. No matter what the activity, the client needs to accept responsibility for her or his own behavior before independence in motor functioning can be achieved. Although the motor function itself is not limbic, many variables that lead to success, self-motivation, and feelings of independence are directly related to limbic and prefrontal lobe circuitry. The variance and self-correction within the movement expression also creates novelty and motivation to continue to practice.[203-205]

As another clinical example of responsibility, in a patient with vestibular dysfunction and dizziness compounded by anxiety, symptoms of dizziness are necessary to drive CNS change. The therapist has a responsibility to prescribe the appropriate activities, dosing, and environment to retrain sensory organization and balance (motor output). The patient can be given the responsibility of monitoring and managing her or his own symptoms within these activities, for instance, by agreeing on the maximal level of dizziness the patient and therapist are willing to accept within the therapeutic activity. A tool as simple as a verbal or visual analog scale can empower the patient to manage symptoms, dampen the limbic system response, and improve motor output for balance control.

Dedication to Reality

Another component of a successful clinical environment deals with learning on the part of the therapist. A master clinician sees and feels what is happening within the motor control output system of the client. That therapist does not get stuck with what she or he has been taught but uses that as a foundation or tether for additional learning. Learning is constantly correlated to memories and new experiences. Each client presents to the therapist as a new map, sketchy at the beginning, that needs to be constantly revised as the terrain (client) changes. That initial map might be a critical care pathway for the client, given her or his neurological insult. That pathway is a map, but only a sketchy map, and may not be a map that a particular patient falls within. It is the therapist's responsibility to evaluate the patient and determine whether that pathway or map will work or is working and when changes in that map need to be altered. Similarly, the therapist needs to be able to transfer or change one motor activity into another spatial position. That is, the therapist can let go of an outdated map or treatment technique and create a new one as the environment and motor control system of the client changes. This transference or letting go of old maps or ideas is true for both the client and therapist. If a position, pattern, or technique is not working, then the clinician needs to change the map or directions of treatment and let the client teach the therapist what will work. The ability to change and select new or alternative treatment techniques is based on the attitude of the therapist toward selecting alternative approaches. Willingness to be flexible is based on confidences in oneself, a truly emotional strategy or limbic behavior. Master clinicians have learned that the answers to the patient's puzzle are within the patient, not the textbooks.

Figure 4-11 depicts two maps with a beginning point and a terminal outcome or goal in each. The parameters of the first map illustrate the boundaries of that therapist's experience and education. The clinician, through training, can

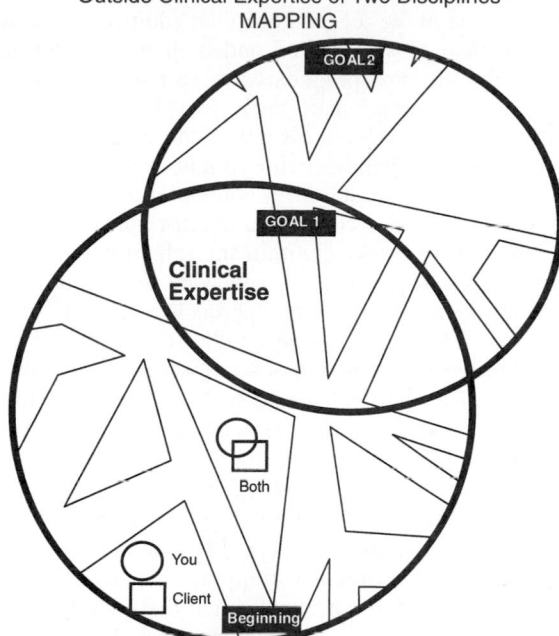

FIGURE 4-11 ■ Concept of clinical mapping including client and therapist and the interactions and importance of overlapping professional goals and staying within the professional expertise.

identify what would seem to be the most direct and efficient way or path toward the mutually identified goal of the therapist and client. When the client becomes a participant within the environment or map, what would seem like a direct path toward a goal might not be the easiest or most direct path for the client. If empowerment of the client leads to independence, then allowing and encouraging the client to direct therapy may provide greater variability, force the client to problem solve, and lead to greater learning. The therapist needs to recognize when the client is not going in the direction of the goal. For example, the client is trying to perform a stand-pivot transfer and instead is falling. If it is important to practice transfers, then practicing falling is inappropriate and the environment (either internal or external) needs modification. Falling can be learned and practiced at another time. Once both strategies are learned, the therapist must empower the patient to the ownership of the map. In the examples of transferring, if the therapist asks the client to practice transfers and if the client starts to fall, a change in required motor behavior must be made and the opportunity given to the client to self-correct. In that way the client is gaining independent control over a variety of environmental contexts and outcomes. Within the same figure (Figure 4-11) is a second map. That second map might represent another professional's interaction and goal with the same client. It is during these overlapping interactions that both professionals can empower the patient to practice and that practice will help lead to those functional goals established by both practitioners. In some situations one profession may guide a client toward obtaining the functional skill necessary for the second profession to begin guiding the client toward the expected outcomes of the second profession. These interlocking dependencies of the client and the professions are illustrated in Figure 4-11. If the client begins therapy striving for the first goal and ends at the functional outcome of the second goal, then additional functional outcomes have been achieved and both professions interacted for the ultimate prognosis for the patient. That interaction requires respect and openness of both professionals toward each other as well as toward the client. Those attitudes and ultimate behaviors are limbic driven.

Matching maps should be a collaborative effort instead of coincidence. These collaborative efforts include interactions with all professions within the rehabilitation setting. Occupational and physical therapists are very familiar with collaboration, and both often approach interventions as a team effort. There are a large number of additional therapists and individuals within that same setting who could also collaborate. Recreational therapists, psychologists, nurses, family members, and music therapists are but a few. Within a profession such as music therapy, the existence of two maps may overlap within a multidimensional environment. When a physical or occupational therapist needs to challenge a patient, the music therapist may be able to calm the system at the same time (overlapping maps). Research on affective responses to consonance and dissonance in music supports the creation of a map within a rehabilitation environment that could overlap with either physical, occupational, or speech therapy. Words such as "relaxed" or "calm" correlated positively with higher levels of consonance in the music, whereas adjectives associated with negative emotions (unpleasant, tense, irritable, annoying, dissonant, and angry) were found to correlate positively with higher levels of dissonance.[133] Creating a whole environment where potential frustrations within motor learning could be balanced with higher levels of consonance in the music would potentially balance the limbic system emotional response to the overlapping maps and bring balance or stability to the limbic system's influence on motor learning and control. A later study by Peretz et al[134] related the same variables to a happy-sad rating task. Given the research evidence for activity within the limbic system as it relates to music,[206] motor learning,[207] and cognitive enhancement, a natural multiple map system would be easy to incorporate within a therapeutic setting. The clinician needs to appreciate the uniqueness of each map while holding onto the concept of the interaction of the two maps.

Vulnerability. To receive input from a client that is multivariable and simultaneous, a therapist has to be open to that information. If a clinician believes that he or she knows what each client needs and how to get those behaviors before meeting the client, then the client falls into a category of a recipe for treating the problem. Using the recipe does not mean the client cannot learn or gain better perceptual/cognitive, affective, or motor control, but it does mean that the individuality of the person may be lost. A more individualized approach would allow the clinician to identify through behavioral responses the best way for the client to learn how to sequence the learning, when to make demands of the client, when to nurture, when to stop, when to continue, when to assist, when to have fun, when to laugh, or when to cry. An analogy might be going to a fast food restaurant versus a restaurant where each aspect of the meal is tailored to one's taste. It does not mean that both restaurants are not selling digestible foods. It does mean that at one eating place the food is mass produced with some choices,

but individuality, with respect to the consumer, is not an aspect of the service. Unfortunately, managed care, limited visits, reduced time for treatment, and therapists' level of frustrations all are pushing therapeutic interventions toward a "one size fits all" philosophy that may increase the time needed for learning, not reduce it.

To be open totally to processing the individual differences of the client, the clinician must be relaxed, nonthreatened, and feel no need to protect himself or herself from the external environment. The clinician is highly vulnerable because she or he is open to new and as-yet unanalyzed or unprocessed input. This vulnerability implies a role not of expert but of expert investigator. Being open must incorporate being sensitive to not only the variability of motor responses but also to the variability of emotional responses on the part of the client. This vulnerability leads to compassion, understanding, and acceptance of the client as a unique human being. It can also be exhausting. Therapists need to learn ways to allow openness without taking on the emotional responsibility of each patient.

Limbic Lesions and Their Influence on the Therapeutic Environment

Many lesions or neurochemical imbalances within the limbic system drastically affect the success or failure of physical, occupational, and other therapy programs. This chapter does not discuss in detail specific problems and their treatment but instead it is hoped that identification of limbic involvement may help the reader develop a better understanding of specific neurological conditions and carry that knowledge into Section II, where the specific clinical problems are discussed.

Substance Abuse (See Chapter 24). The anterior temporal lobe (especially the hippocampus and amygdala) has a lower threshold for epileptic seizures than do other cortical structures.[54] This type of epilepsy is produced by use of systemic drugs such as cocaine and alcohol. The seizure is often accompanied by sensory auras and alterations in behavior, with specific focus on mood shifts and cognitive dysfunction.[208] Obviously, the precise association between behavior and emotions or temporolimbic and frontolimbic activity is not understood, yet the associations and thus their impact on a therapeutic setting cannot be ignored.[69,209]

Whether street bought, medically administered, or ingested for private or social reasons (such as in alcohol consumption), drugs and alcohol can have dramatic effects on the CNS. Korsakoff's syndrome, caused by chronic alcoholism and its related nutritional deficiency, is identified by the structural involvement of the diencephalon with specific focus on the mamillary bodies, and the dorsal medial and anterior nucleus of the thalamus[54] usually shows involvement (see the anatomy section and Figure 4-12). This syndrome is not a dementia but rather a discrete, localized pathological state with specific clinical signs. The most dramatic sign observed in a client with Korsakoff's syndrome is severe memory deficits.[176,210-212] These deficits involve declarative memory and learning losses, but the most predominant problem is short-term memory loss. As the disease progresses, clients generally become totally unaware of their memory loss and are unconcerned. Initially, confabulation may be observed, but in time most clients with a chronic

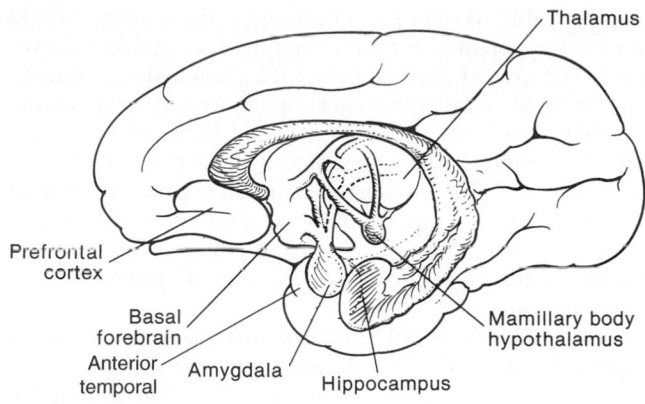

FIGURE 4-12 ■ Anatomy of the limbic system: schematic illustration.

condition become apathetic and somewhat withdrawn and are in a profound amnesic state. They are trapped in time, unable to learn from new experiences because they cannot retain memories for more than a few minutes and are unable to maintain their independence[176,210-212]; many may become social isolates and homeless.

The use of alcohol affects not only adults but also children and adolescents. Still another population of children suffering from alcohol abuse has surfaced as a specific clinical problem. These children are infants who have the effects of fetal alcohol syndrome. A variety of researchers have investigated the effects of alcohol and other toxic drugs on neuromotor and cognitive development.[213-219]

Alzheimer's Disease (see Chapter 28). In Alzheimer's disease, the hippocampus and nucleus basalis are the most severely involved structures, followed by neurofibrillar degeneration of the anterotemporal, parietal, and frontal lobes.[69,176,220,221]

Initially, the symptoms fall into several categories: emotional, social, and cognitive. Usually the symptoms have a gradual onset. Depression and anxiety often are seen during the early phases because of the neuronal degeneration within the prefrontal lobes and limbic system.[222-224] During the second stage, the emotional, social, and intellectual changes become more marked. Clients have difficulty with demands, business affairs, and personal management. Their memory and cognitive processing continue to deteriorate, whereas their awareness of the problem is often still insightful, causing additional anxiety and depression. During this phase clients may be unable to recognize familiar objects and become scared because they are losing control of the environment both internally and externally. Thus the client may become combative out of a defensive (fight/flight) autonomic response. For that reason, therapists need to make sure the client feels safe during therapy to optimize the learning and compliance. The third phase manifests itself with moderate to severe aphasic, apraxic, and agnostic problems. Object agnosia, the failure to recognize objects, is a typical sign of advancing Alzheimer's disease. Distractibility and nonattentiveness are also common signs of this third stage. The final stage is marked by an individual who is uncommunicative, with little meaningful social interaction, and who often takes on the features of the Klüver-Bucy syndrome. Thus, they exhibit emotional outbursts, inappropriate sexual behaviors, severe memory loss, constant mouth movements, and often a flexor-type postural pattern. In this latter phase, the client is virtually decorticate and clinically indistinguishable from persons with other dementias.

The continual degeneration of the limbic system is a key distinguishing factor in Alzheimer's disease.[109,225] Many clients are misdiagnosed as having other problems such as intracranial tumors, normal pressure hydrocephalus, multiinfarct dementia, or alcoholic/chronic drug intoxication.[226] Similarly, many clients with tumors, multifaceted dementias, alcoholism, or heart attacks resulting in hippocampal damage may be diagnosed with Alzheimer's disease. When the disease is correctly evaluated and diagnosed, however, it becomes obvious that the limbic-cortical area involved from phase 1 through the last phase is interacting with other areas of the brain and constantly affecting the behavioral patterns of the patient. Owing to the neurochemical sensitivity and production within the limbic system, drugs are often used to prevent or slow down the progression of Alzheimer's disease[227,228] (see Chapter 36). Similarly, a genetic predisposition has been found in some patients with Alzheimer's disease[54,229-231]; thus, gene therapy may prove to have great therapeutic value.

Head Injury (see Chapter 17)
Traumatic Injury. One potentially severe limbic problem that can be present after traumatic closed head injury is diffuse axonal injury.[232-236] The long associative bundles or fibers that transverse the cortex on a curved route can be sheared by an impact or a blow to the head. One of these long associative bundles is the cingulate fasciculus, which coordinates the amygdala and hippocampal projections to and from the prefrontal cortex. Many basic perceptual strategies, such as body schema, hearing, vision, and smell, are linked into the emotional and learning centers of the limbic system through the cingulate fasciculus.[237] Thus declarative learning through sensory/cognitive processing can become impossible. If the pathways to and from the hippocampus and amygdala are sheared bilaterally, total and permanent global anterograde amnesia will be present.[109,238] If destruction of both tracts on one side occurs, but the contralateral side is left intact, the individual can compensate, but learning will be slower or the rate of processing delayed.[138] If only one tract on one side is damaged, such as the tract to and from the hippocampus, the amygdaloid system on the same side will compensate but be slower than without the lesion.[138] Thus, the specific degree of involvement will vary and depend on the extent of shearing. Those with total shearing on both sides will usually be in a deep coma and will not survive the injury.[239] Those with less severe insult will show signs ranging from total amnesia to minor delays in declarative learning.[233,240]

When the interaction of the limbic system and higher control is considered, additional variables can be taken into consideration within the therapeutic environment. In treating more than 200 patients who had trauma, Körlin[174] found that certain kinds of musical elements often triggered intrusive and traumatic reexperiences of the event. These experiences may or may not be accessible to conscious memory and may include visual images, physical pain, pressure, nausea, and other sensory imagery. Körlin proposes that this triggering occurs through transmission of subcortical auditory input from the brain stem and thalamus to the amygdala. It is well known that music may elicit specific memories or associations related to the individual's personal and cultural history, and such memories and associations then stimulate various affective and cognitive responses. (For a theoretical discussion of this phenomenon, see Goldberg.[241]) What is of particular concern with trauma survivors is an auditory triggering process that does not necessarily activate specific memories or associations in relation to the music heard and that cannot be easily integrated psychologically. Rather, we observe an immediate and compelling alarm response that is triggered, according to Körlin,[174] by specific auditory properties such as dynamic changes (especially sudden, unexpected increases) or transients (onset or attack portions of sounds) and by high-volume levels of sound. High levels of distress, or numbing and dissociation, may accompany an overwhelming intrusion of sensory imagery and dramatically affect descending pathways to the spinal motor neuronetwork. This phenomenon has also been observed by West in several clinical populations, including children with developmental disabilities, adults with stroke or head injury, psychiatric patients, patients in the intensive care unit, and fragile medical-surgical patients. The phenomenon of auditory triggering also has implications for the rehabilitation setting, where patients may be recovering from traumas related to accident, injury, or difficult medical procedures. Both environmental noise and "background" music may present auditory triggers that elicit limbic system and ANS activity.

Negative or sympathetic limbic arousal may lead to increased levels of physical guarding, hypervigilance, and other behaviors that can limit successful engagement in the treatment process. Patients whose conscious memory of the traumatic events is limited or distorted may become confused or have difficulty understanding their physiological and sensory experiences in the context of the current therapy setting. Other patients who are more aware of the source of such posttraumatic experiences may not report odd sensations or intrusive trauma re-experiences to the clinician because of a need to deny or avoid the experience of continuing distress from the trauma or from fear of losing emotional control in an environment that does not support such vulnerability. Still others may lack cognitive or communication abilities to express their distress. Some individuals will silently struggle to regain control, suppressing the memories and sensations to avoid being evaluated as mentally unstable. But in spite of psychological or behavioral defensive maneuvers, the body continues to manifest responses to the limbic activation of alarm and defense systems. Individuals dealing with motor responses and motor behavior may have little awareness of these variables and thus no idea why the patient is behaving in the manner observed.

Cerebral contusions (bruises) have long been a primary sign of traumatic head injury.[242] Regardless of impact, the contusions are generally found in the frontal and temporal regions. There are long-term neuropsychological ramifications after mild traumatic brain injury even when there is no loss of consciousness.[243] The regions most frequently involved are orbitofrontal, frontopolar, anterotemporal, and lateral temporal surfaces.[233]

The limbic system's connection to these areas would suggest the potential for direct and indirect limbic involvement. The greater the contusion, the greater the likelihood that the limbic structures might simultaneously be involved. Impulsiveness, lack of inhibition, and hyperactivity are a few of the clinical signs associated with orbitofrontal/limbic involvement.[244] The dorsomedial frontal region, involved in the hippocampal-fornix circuit (once referred to as the Papez circuit,[245] when damaged, seems to induce a pseudodepressed state, including slowness, lack of initiation, and perseveration.

Nontraumatic Head Injuries: Anoxic/Hypoxic Brain Injury. Lack of oxygen to the brain, regardless of the cause, seems not only to have a dramatic effect throughout the cortex but also selectively damages the hippocampal regions.[233] The loss of hippocampal declarative memory systems bilaterally would certainly provide one reason for the slowness in processing so commonly observed in head injury.[246] A hypothesis could also be made regarding the limbic system's interrelation with other cortical and brain stem structures. In cases of hypoxia, many structures feeding into the limbic system are potentially affected, so information sent to the limbic system may be distorted. These distortions could cause tremendous imbalances within the limbic processing system, with not only attention and learning problems but also the hypothalamic irregularity often seen in head trauma. Individuals who demonstrate obstructive sleep apnea, another cause of hypoxia, have been shown to have an imbalance in the hippocampal area. This imbalance may lead to severe cognitive dysfunction.[247] This preexisting hypoxic environment certainly can have a long-term affect on any patient who has CNS damage at any age.

A therapist always needs to understand the environment within which the injury occurred as well as be aware of preexisting complications. If the injury was due to a violent confrontation, such as a fight or a frightful experience such as a near-drowning, the emotional system had to be at a high level of metabolic activity at the time of the insult. If the event was anoxic, then those areas with the highest oxygen need or at the highest metabolic state might be the most affected or damaged after the event. Knowing that information, a therapist's analytical problem-solving strategies should guide her or him toward limbic assessment.

Summary of Limbic Problems with Head-Injured Clients. The behavioral sequelae after any head injury reflect many signs of limbic involvement. In studies of both the pediatric and adult populations,[234-237,243,248] behaviors of impulsiveness, restlessness, overactivity, destructiveness, aggression, increased tantrums, and socially uninhibited behaviors (lack of social skills) are frequently reported. These behaviors all reflect a strong emotional or limbic component. After discussion of Moore's concept of a limbic system that MOVEs us and the F^2ARV continuum regarding emotional control over noxious or negative input, it is no wonder so many clients have difficulty with personal and emotional control over their reactions to the therapeutic world. If the imbalance were within the client, then the external environment would be one possible way to help center the client emotionally.[249,250] This centering requires that the therapist be sensitive to the emotional level of the client. As the client begins to regain control, an increase in external environmental demands would challenge the limbic system. If the demand is excessive, the client's emotional reaction as expressed by motor behavior should alert the therapist to downgrade the activity level.

Head injuries affect many areas of the CNS. A client with spasticity, rigidity, or ataxia may exhibit an increase in those motor responses when the limbic system becomes stressed. Learning to differentiate a motor control problem from a limbic problem that influences the motor control systems requires that the therapist be willing to address the cause of the problems and their respective treatments.[251] Each client is different, no matter commonalities of the site or extent of the lesions, because of prior learning and conditioning of the limbic system. Thus, the response of two clients to the same clinical learning environment may have great variance and should not surprise the clinician. Thus, the therapist needs to give undivided attention to the client at all times and be willing to make moment-to-moment adjustments within the external environment to help the client maintain focus on the desired learning.

Vestibular Disorders. The vestibular system has extensive neuronal connections and commissural influences on the limbic system and structures; the neuroanatomical basis is described later in this chapter. In general, vestibular dysfunction results in erroneous input to the central nervous system. This erroneous sensory information creates a mismatch between the external (afferent) cues and the internal conceptual model for movement contained by the cerebellum. This mismatch creates an imbalance in vestibular and cerebellar signals to the CNS, flooding the central limbic structures and resulting in symptoms such as vertigo, motion sickness, nausea, or decreased postural control. Detection of this mismatch results in an attempt by the cerebellum to compensate for the imbalance, which becomes a core tenet of recovery.[252] Thus vestibular dysfunction can influence the therapeutic environment both in the assessment and the treatment of this system.

Relative to assessment, vestibular system involvement is not a primary consideration by most physicians and therapists. On the basis of benchmarking data from within specialized balance centers, the average patient with a vestibular disorder (dizziness or imbalance) travels within the medical system an average of 52 months before finding a solution. During this time, he or she has seen on average four physicians. There is also at least one visit to the emergency department in crisis and one visit to a psychiatrist. Typically there has been no rehabilitation referral or intervention during this time.[253]

The patient with a chronic vestibular disorder can have a myriad of symptoms, including vegetative, motoric, psychological, and behavioral symptoms that are often misdiagnosed during this search for an outcome as other, more serious medical diagnoses. As an example, of those patients diagnosed with dizziness or imbalance of a psychologic origin, evidence has determined that more than 70% of these patients have underlying vestibular dysfunction on key vestibular function tests (electronystagmography/calorics, rotary chair, computerized dynamic posturography, auditory brain stem response, and acoustic reflexes).[198,200,254-256] Conversely, of those patients with chronic dizziness and imbalance, only 16% were found to have dizziness of a true

psychogenic origin.[257] As another example, military personnel with symptoms of motion sickness also have physiological changes identifiable by results of rotary chair (60% with abnormally long time constants) and computerized dynamic posturography (70% with abnormal sensory organization test [SOT] condition 5, and 6).[258]

Patients with mild head injury, postconcussive syndrome, and whiplash often have concomitant involvement of the vestibular apparatus or nuclei, which goes undetected within the initial medical workup and management plan.[258-262] When the disorder is undetected and left unchecked, the patients do not respond to standard treatment interventions. They also complain of atypical symptoms or responses to these typical treatments. When the patient does not respond in predictable ways to standard treatment, the label "aphysiological" is applied, particularly in situations where disability or secondary gain is a factor. Fortunately there are well-established performance criteria that can effectively differentiate true balance/vestibular impairment from embellishment for secondary gain.[263]

In treatment, given that recovery is based on long-term compensation mediated by the cerebellum, stimulation of the vestibular system must be controlled. Some patients have true vestibular dysfunction that affects only motor responses, whereas other patients have true limbic psychiatric problems that do not manifest themselves with vestibular symptoms. These two behaviors are located at the polar ends of the curve between limbic motor and vestibular motor dysfunction. Before a clinician can identify appropriate intervention strategies, the question "What are the best vestibular and limbic interactive environments that will challenge and drive neuroplastic change" must be answered. Although researchers[198,255] have identified tools that differentiate the two extremes, today researchers are trying to clarify the mid range of patients who clearly have symptoms on the basis of the interaction of both systems.[263] Development of tools that can further discriminate whether the behaviors are first driven by vestibular and followed by limbic responses, or vice versa, is a key to treatment planning.

Australian physiotherapists Murray et al[264] investigated the relationship between balance performance (SOT) and perceived handicap (Dizziness Handicap Inventory [DHI]) after a 4-week program of vestibular rehabilitation in patients with chronic vestibular dysfunction. A significant negative correlation was found between the variables, indicating that improved balance is related to decreased perception of handicap ($r = -0.6$). Important in their findings was that, when analyzed separately, the emotional component of the DHI showed no improvement over time with this program or correlation with balance performance. The authors concluded that vestibular rehabilitation alone was unable to address the broader *emotional* needs of patients with vestibular disorders.[264]

Cerebrovascular Accidents (See Chapter 27). The most common insult in CVA results in occlusions within tributaries of the middle cerebral artery.[54] When this occlusion is in the right hemisphere, studies have shown that clients are often confused and exhibit metabolic imbalance.[265] The primary problem of this confused state is inattention. After brain scans, it has been shown that focal lesions existed within both the reticulocortical and limbic cortical tracts, suggesting direct limbic involvement in many middle cerebral artery problems.[61]

Many clients with a CVA do not have direct limbic involvement, yet the stresses placed on the client, whether external or internal, are often reflected in the limbic system's influence over cognition and the motor control systems.[266] Everyday existence as well as performance of the motor task required during therapy is usually valued highly in the client's life. This value or stress placed on the limbic system overflows into the motor system and never allows it to relax, as observed by noting the increase of tonus in the unaffected leg. The client is usually unaware of this buildup of tonus but can release it once attention is drawn to it. If attention is never directed toward these tension buildups, a therapist trying to decrease tonus in the affected arm or leg will always be interacting with the associated patterns from the less-involved extremities.

Tumor (See Chapter 25). Any brain tumor, regardless of whether it directly affects the limbic structures, will certainly arouse the limbic system because of the stress, anxiety, and emotional overlays of the diagnosis. The degree of emotional involvement will obviously affect the declarative learning of the client as well as the limbic system's influence over motor response.

Tumors specifically arising within limbic structures[267] can cause dramatic changes in the client's emotional behavior and level of alertness, especially with hypothalamic tumors. The behaviors reported include aggressiveness, hyperphagia, paranoia, sloppiness, manic symptoms, and eventual confusion.[54] Tumors within the hypothalamus cause not only behavioral abnormalities but also autonomic endocrine imbalances, including body temperature changes, menstrual abnormalities, and diabetes insipidus.[109]

When the tumor is located within the frontal and temporal lobes associated with limbic structures, psychiatric problems may manifest, ranging from depression to anorexia to psychosis.[109,268] Obsessive-compulsive disorder resulting from limbic tumor has been used as a tumor marker for relapse.[269] Amnesia has been reported in patients with dorsomedial thalamus, fornix, midbrain, and reticulolimbic pathway lesions. This again reinforces the importance of the limbic system's role in storage.[109]

Ventricular Swelling after Spinal Defects in Utero, Central Nervous System Trauma, and Inflammation (See Chapters 17, 18, and 20). Although the effects of ventricular swelling after trauma, inflammation, and in utero cerebrospinal malformations are not discussed in great detail in the literature with respect to limbic involvement, the proximity of the lateral and third ventricle to limbic structures cannot be ignored. It is common knowledge that most people when exposed to hot, humid weather begin to swell; become more irritable, less tolerant, and moody; and may complain of headaches. Some people become aggressive, others lethargic. All these behaviors are linked to some extent with limbic function. Thus, ventricular swelling causing hydrocephalus, whether caused by trauma, inflammation, or obstruction, would potentially affect the limbic structures. Reported behavioral changes such as seizures, memory and learning problems, personality alternations, alertness,

dementia, and amnesia can be tied to direct or indirect limbic activity.[54]

Summary of Clinical Problems Affected by Limbic Involvement. It is easy to identify limbic problems when the behaviors deviate drastically from normal responses. It is much more difficult to determine subtle behavior shifts in clients. The therapist should be sensitive to these minor mood shifts because they may represent early signs of future problems. Similarly, noting that a particular client is always irritable and has difficulty learning on hot days should help direct the therapist toward establishing a treatment session that regulates humidity and temperature to optimize the learning environment. The limbic system is not just a neurochemical bundle of nuclei and axons found within the brain. It is a pulsating center that links perception of the world and the way an individual responds to that perception. Quality of life is a value and that value has a strong limbic component. If functional outcomes leading to maintaining or improving the quality of life of our clients is the goal of both physical and occupational therapy,[201,270,271] then the limbic system is no less important during examination, evaluation, prognosis, and intervention than the motor system itself.

THE NEUROSCIENCE OF THE LIMBIC SYSTEM

Basic Anatomy and Physiology

A brief overview of the anatomy and physiology of the limbic system is presented in the following sections. The reader is referred to a variety of textbooks for a more in-depth understanding of this system[54,63,65] and how higher thought might be much more complex than previously identified.[6,272-274]

Basic Structure and Function

The limbic system can best be visualized as consisting of cortical and subcortical structures with the hypothalamus located at the central position (Figures 4-12 and 4-13). The hypothalamus is surrounded by the circular alignment of the subcortical limbic structures vitally linked with each other and the hypothalamus. These structures are the amygdaloid complex, the hippocampal formation, the nucleus accumbens, the anterior nuclei of the thalamus, and the septal nuclei (see Figure 4-12). These structures are again surrounded by a ring of cortical structures collectively called the "limbic lobe," which includes the orbitofrontal cortex, the cingulate gyrus, the parahippocampal gyrus, and the uncus. Other neuroanatomists also include the olfactory system and the basal forebrain area (see Figure 4-13). Vitally linked and often included in the limbic system as the "mesolimbic" part is the excitatory component of the reticular activating system and other brain stem nuclei of the midbrain. Some consider components of the midbrain a very important region for emotional expression.[75] Derryberry and Tucker[75] found that attack behavior aroused by hypothalamic stimulation is blocked when the midbrain is damaged and that midbrain stimulation can be made to elicit "attack behavior" even when the hypothalamus has been surgically disconnected from other brain regions. Recent research has clearly identified the neurochemical precursors to this

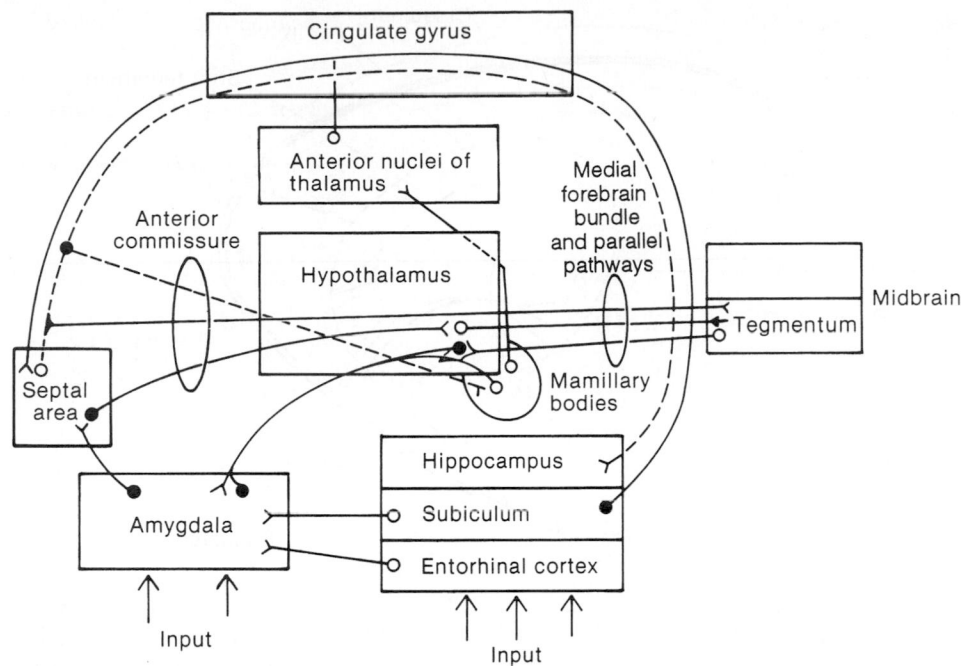

FIGURE 4-13 ■ Limbic system circuitry with parallel and reverberating connections and with medial forebrain bundle.

aggressive behavior.[52,54,275-277] This "septo-hypothalamic-mesencephalic" continuum, connected by the medial forebrain bundle, seems to be vital to the integration and expression of emotional behavior.[278] The linking of other brain structures to emotions came initially from the work of Papez,[245] who first identified the hippocampal-fornix circuit. He saw this as a way of combining the "subjective" cortical experiences with the emotional hypothalamic contribution. Earlier, Broca[68] labeled the cingulate gyrus and hippocampus "circle" as "the great limbic lobe." These concepts were combined by Maclean[279] into the construct of the limbic system.

Klüver and Bucy[280] linked the anterior half of the temporal lobes and the amygdaloid complex to the limbic system. They showed changes in behavior, with specific loss of the amygdaloid complex and anterior hippocampus input, resulting in (1) restless overresponsiveness, (2) hyperorality of examining objects by placing them in the mouth, (3) psychic blindness of seeing and not recognizing objects and the possible harm they may entail, (4) sexual hyperactivity, and (5) emotional changes characterized by loss of aggressiveness. These changes have been named the Klüver-Bucy syndrome.[69,70] A myriad of connections link the amygdala to the olfactory pathways, the frontal lobe and cingulate gyrus, the thalamus, the hypothalamus, the septum, and the midbrain structures of the substantial nigra, locus coeruleus, periaqueductal gray matter, and the reticular formation. The amygdala receives feedback from many of these structures it projects to by reciprocal pathways.

Music research has also shown clear activity within the limbic system. A novel melody with harmonization was used to control for possible effects of prior associations to a familiar piece of music.[134] Increasing levels of musical dissonance correlated with activity in right parahippocampal gyrus and precuneus regions. Inverse correlations were found between

these effects and responses to decreasing levels of dissonance (or increasing consonance), which correlated with activity in orbitofrontal, subcallosal cingulate, and frontal polar cortex areas. In addition, subjects' ratings of pleasantness correlated positively with activation in the left subcallosal cingulate gyrus and right orbitofronal cortex and negatively with activation in the right parahippocampal gyrus and precuneus.

At the heart of the limbic system is the hypothalamus. The hypothalamus, in close reciprocal interaction with most centers of the cerebral cortex, the amygdala, hippocampus, pituitary gland, brain stem, and spinal cord, is a primary regulator of autonomic and endocrine functions and controls and balances homeostatic mechanisms. Autonomic and somatomotor responses controlled by the hypothalamus are closely aligned with the expression of emotions.[276,281-283]

In the temporal lobe, anteromedially, are the amygdaloid complex of nuclei, with the hippocampal formation situated posterior to it. Located medial to the amygdala is the basal forebrain nuclei, which receive afferent neurons from the reticular formation, the hypothalamus, and the limbic cortex. From this basal forebrain, efferents project to all areas of the cerebral cortex, the hippocampus, and the amygdaloid body, providing an important connection between the neocortex and the limbic system. These nuclei represent the center of the cholinergic system, which supplies acetylcholine to limbic and cortical structures involved in memory formation. Depletion of acetylcholine in clients with Alzheimer's disease relates to their memory loss.[69,154,220,221]

Interlinking the Components of the System

The limbic system has many reciprocating interlinking circuits between its component structures, which provide for much functional interaction and also allow for continuing

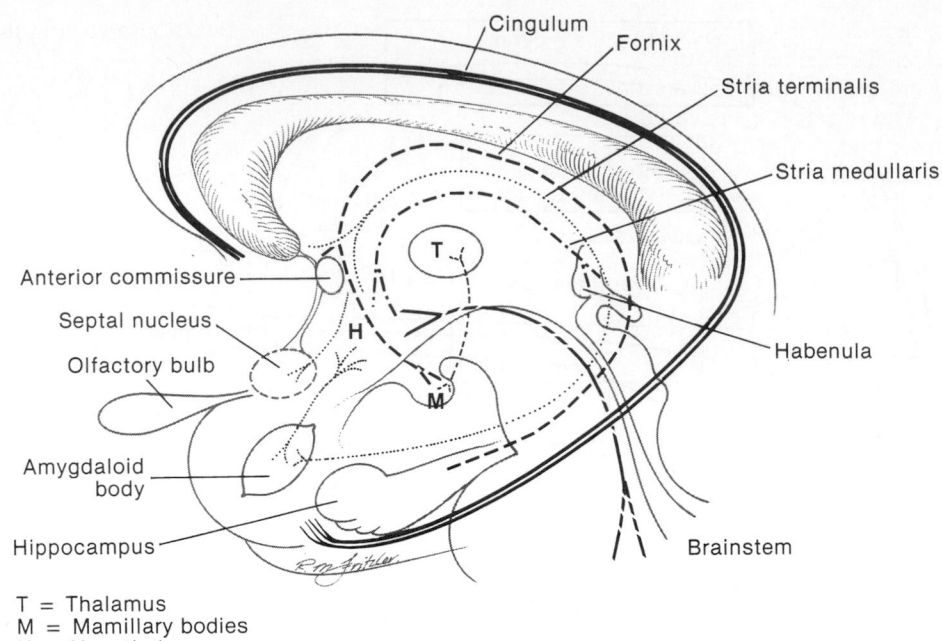

T = Thalamus
M = Mamillary bodies
H = Hypothalamus

FIGURE 4-14 ■ Interlinking neuron network within the limbic system. (Adapted from Kandel ER, Schwartz JH, Jessell TM: *Principles of neural science,* ed 5, New York, 2001, Elsevier Science.)

adjustments with continuous feedback (Figure 4-14).[54,276] The largest pathway is the fornix.[284]

Another limbic pathway is the stria terminalis, which originates in the amygdaloid complex and follows a course close to the fornix to end in the hypothalamus and septal regions. The amygdala and the septal region are also connected by a short direct pathway called the diagonal band of Broca. A third pathway, the uncinate fasciculus, runs between the amygdala and the orbitofrontal cortex.[54,285]

The medial forebrain bundle and other parallel circuits (see Figure 4-13) are vital connections of the limbic system.[286] These pathways course through the lateral hypothalamus to terminate in the cingulate gyrus in its ascending limb and in the reticular formation of the midbrain in its descending part; these pathways have strong interconnections and control over the periaqueductal gray area.[154] These links enable the limbic system itself and the non-limbic-associated structures to act as one neural task system. No portion of the brain, whether limbic or nonlimbic, has only one function.[54] Each area acts as an input-output station. At no time is it totally the center of a particular effect, and each site depends on the cooperation and interaction with other regions.

The parvicellular reticular formation (PCRF, or lateral medullary reticular formation), together with the nucleus tractus solitarius, receives both vestibular and nonvestibular input from the cortex, cerebellum, and limbic system and is considered functionally as the vomiting center. It also receives input from the area postrema (floor of the fourth ventricle), which contains the chemoreceptor region for the production of vomiting in response to noxious chemicals. Commissural fibers from the vestibular nuclei complexes run through the PCRF and connect the vestibular nucleus to the reticular formation through axon collaterals. The PCRF also projects fibers to the parabrachial nuclei that contain the

respiratory centers and to the hypoglossal nucleus.[252] Visceral autonomic input from multiple sources, including the vestibular nuclei, converge in the parabrachial nucleus. The locus ceruleus and autonomic brain stem nuclei also receive vestibular nuclear input.[287-291] Thus, cardiovascular activity and respiration (brain stem–mediated autonomic activity), as well as vomiting, are highly influenced by the status of the vestibular system. If we could understand how cold to the neck or forehead, pressure to the wrist, or taste/olfactory input of ginger interacts with known autonomic reactions and nausea in response to chronic vestibular or interneuronal connections problems, the synthesis of many aspects of health care delivery would no longer be a mystery. Obviously, these older treatment techniques are effective and have been for thousands of years, but to today's researchers the "why" drives the desire to better understand the neuromechanisms underlying the observable responses. There are three different types of drugs that neuroanatomically suppress or modulate vestibular input and thus have a dramatic effect on dizziness and nausea.[292]

Research involving functional magnetic resonance imaging supports the concept that there is an increased activity within the inferior frontal cortex when nausea is induced by either vestibular stimulation or ingestion of an emetic.[292a] This research verifies that there is a strong interconnection between vestibular input, limbic nuclei, and autonomic responses.[293]

There are also connections between the parabrachial nucleus and higher brain centers, including the amygdala, which is known to be critical in the development of conditioned avoidance, such as found in agoraphobia, as an example. Thus, vestibular input results in a sensory stimulus that may induce a state of general autonomic discomfort as a trigger of avoidance that precedes the onset of a panic attack.[252,287,293,294]

During the past decade anatomical pathways have been identified that are descending motor tracts that terminate in the caudal brain stem and spinal cord.[86] These pathways help modulate the activity level of somatic and autonomic motor neurons. Some of these tracts receive direct and indirect afferent information from the periphery and are part of the interneuronal projection system to motor neurons. They are found in the caudal brain stem, spinal cord, and between the two, and play a role in the generation of fixed action patterns such as biting and swallowing, which have a strong emotion context linked to the motor program.[295] Some of the pathways are linked with the ventromedial and lateral systems, identified for many years as part of both the proximal/axial and distal motor control system modulated by a variety of structures.[154] They connect the limbic system to the brain stem and spinal neuronal pools. These tracts do not seem to synapse on what would be considered true motor nuclei of the brain stem (e.g., red nucleus, vestibular nuclei, lateral reticular nuclei, interstitial nuclei of Cajal, or inferior olive). However, these pathways do connect with raphe nuclei, periaqueductal gray matter, and locus coeruleus. The medial components of these tracts originate within the medial portion of the hypothalamus, and the lateral portion originates in the limbic system (lateral hypothalamus, amygdala, and bed nucleus of the stria terminalis). The prefrontal area may be the master controller over this regulatory system.[296-299] The functional motor implication of these tracts is determined by whether the fibers project as part of a medial or lateral descending system. The medial system, through the locus coeruleus, periaqueductal gray matter, and raphe spinal pathways, plays a role in the general level of activity of both somatosensory and motor neurons. Thus, the emotional brain or limbic system has an effect on both somatosensory input and motor output. These fibers can alter the level of excitation to the first synapse of somatosensory information, thus altering the processing or importance of that information as it enters the nervous system. Similarly, it can alter the level of motor generators involved in motor expression, which may account for the extension with anger and flexion with depression. The lateral system seems to be involved in more specific motor output related to emotional behavior and may explain some of the loss of fine motor skill when placed in an emotional situation such as competition.[86] To differentiate whether the tonal conditions of a client are due to limbic imbalance or problems within the traditionally accepted motor system, the clinician would need to observe the emotional state and how it changes within the client. If the abnormal state consistently alters with mood shifts, then limbic involvement causing motor control disturbances would be identified.

Neurobiology of Learning and Memory
Functional Applications for an Intact System

"Ultimately, to be sure, memory is a series of molecular events. What we chart is the territory within which those events take place."[123] Although expressed more than two decades ago, these words are still accurate. They were expressed by a master clinician and researcher, a clinician who watched behavior, emphasized neuroscience, stressed accurate documentation, and always was respectful and aware of patient interaction and how that affected motor behavior.

The brain stores sensory and motor experiences as memory. In processing incoming information, most sensory pathways from receptors to cortical areas send vital information to the components of the limbic system. For example, extensions can be found from the visual pathways into the inferior temporal lobe (limbic system).[54,300] Visual information is "processed sequentially" at each synapse along its entire pathway, in response to size, shape, color, and texture of objects. In the inferior temporal cortex, the total image of the item viewed is projected. In this way the sensory inputs are converted to become "perceptual experiences." This also applies to other sensory stimuli, such as tactile, proprioceptive, and vestibular. The process of translating the integrated perceptions into memory occurs bilaterally in the limbic system structures of the amygdala and the hippocampus.[54,301-310]

Before the limbic system's impact on learning and memory can be delved into, a clear understanding of what is meant by these functions is needed. Current theories support a "dual memory system" that uses different pathways in the nervous system. Terms such as *verbal* and *nonverbal, habit* versus *recognition, intrinsic* and *extrinsic,* and *procedural* and *declarative* have been given to these two memory systems. These systems do not operate autonomously, and many therapeutic activities seem to combine these memory systems to achieve functional behavior.[54] In reality, the complexity of memory is not a two-category system. Verbal and nonverbal memory both interact with declarative function.[311] Even within spatial memory, additional areas of integration and parallel circuitry have been identified.[312]

For this discussion, two specific categories of learning—procedural and declarative—will be used, although in today's neuroscience environment implicit and explicit memory is used as frequently. Both categories of learning have been correlated to limbic function.[313,314] Declarative (explicit) memory entails the capability to recall and verbally report experiences. This recall requires deliberate conscious effect, whereas the procedural counterpart is the recall of "rules, skills, and procedures (implicit),"[54] which can be recalled unconsciously.

Procedural learning is vital to the development of motor control. A child first receives sensory input from the various modalities through the thalamus, terminating at the appropriate sensory cortex. That information is processed, a functional somatosensory map is formulated,[124,315] and the information is programmed and relayed to the motor cortex. From there, it is sent to both the basal ganglia and the cerebellum to establish plans for postural adaptations, refinement of motor programs, and coordination of direction, extent, timing, force, and tone necessary throughout the entire sequence of the motor act. Storage and thus retrieval of memory of these semiautomatic motor plans are thought to occur throughout the motor control system.[54] The complexity of this process has had an impact on the study of motor control and variables that might affect that control.[316]

The frontal lobe, basal ganglia, and cerebellum are critical nuclei for changing and modulating existing programs.[54] Many interlocking neuronetworks establish pathways allowing for the conceptualization of research on motor theory concepts of reciprocity, distributed function, consensus, and so on (see Chapters 3 and 9). Procedural learning and memory do not *necessitate* limbic system involvement so long as an emotional value is not placed on the task. This memory deals with skills, habits, and stereotyped behaviors. This motor system is involved in developing procedural plans used in moving us from place to place or holding us in a position when we need to stop.[54]

Unlike procedural learning and memory, declarative (explicit) learning and memory require the wiring of the limbic system. Recent literature has clearly identified that the basal ganglia and cerebellum both play roles in cognitive function, especially as it relates to category learning task.[317] This type of learning is closely associated with limbic function, further identifying the complexity of what was considered two entirely separate systems. Declarative thought deals with factual, material, semantic, and categorical aspects of higher cognitive and affective processing. A strong emotional and judgmental component is linked with declarative thought. Thus, as soon as a motor behavior has value placed on the act, it becomes declarative as well as procedural, and the limbic system may become a key element in the success or failure of that movement.[318,319] Most functional tasks or activities practiced in a clinical setting have value attached to them. That value can be clearly seen by observing the emotional intent placed on the activity by the client.[320]

The two reverberating or reciprocal pathways, or circuits, within the limbic system most intimately involved in declarative learning are (1) the amygdaloid, dorsomedial thalamic nucleus, and cortical pathways and (2) the hippocampal, fornix, anterior thalamic nucleus, and cortical pathways.

The hippocampus may be more concerned with sensory and motor signals relating to the external environment, whereas the amygdala is concerned with those of the internal environment. They both contribute in relation to the significance of external or internal environmental influences.[306,321-326] The hippocampus is rich in stem cells and may be a primary nuclear mass that directs the bodily systems to heal after injury. This is especially true when the

external environment is enriched and nurtures the emotional environment for that healing.[323]

The amygdaloid circuits seem to deal with strongly emotional and judgmental thoughts, whereas the hippocampal circuits are less emotional and more factual. The amygdala may be more involved in emotional arousal and attention, as well as motor regulation, whereas the hippocampus may deal with less emotionally charged learning. These limbic circuits seem crucial in the initial processing of material that leads to learning and memory. Once the thought has been laid down within the cortical structures, retrieval of that specific intermediate and long-term memory does not seem to require the limbic system, although new associations will need to be run through the system.[54,74,302,304,306]

A third component in the memory pathway involves the medial diencephalon, a structure that contains the thalamic nucleus. When this region is destroyed by neurotrauma such as strokes, neoplasms, infections, or chronic alcoholism, global amnesias result, owing to the destruction of the amygdala and hippocampus. The amygdala and hippocampus send fibers to specific target nuclei in the thalamus, and the destruction of these tracts also causes the same amnesic effect. It appears that the limbic system and the diencephalon cooperate in the memory circuits. The medial diencephalon seems to be another relay station along the pathway that leads from the specific sensory cortical region to the limbic structures in the temporal lobe to the medial diencephalic structures and ending in the ventromedial part of the prefrontal cortex (Figure 4-15).[54,327,328]

According to Figure 4-15, memories may be stored in the sensory cortex area, where the original sensory input was interpreted into "sensory impressions." Today, concepts regarding memory storage suggest that declarative memory is stored in categories similar to a filing system. Those categories or files seem to be stored in several cortical areas bilaterally depending on the context.[329,330] This system allows for easy retrieval from multiple areas. Memory has stages and is continually changing. Thus, to go from short-term to long-term memory, the brain must physically change

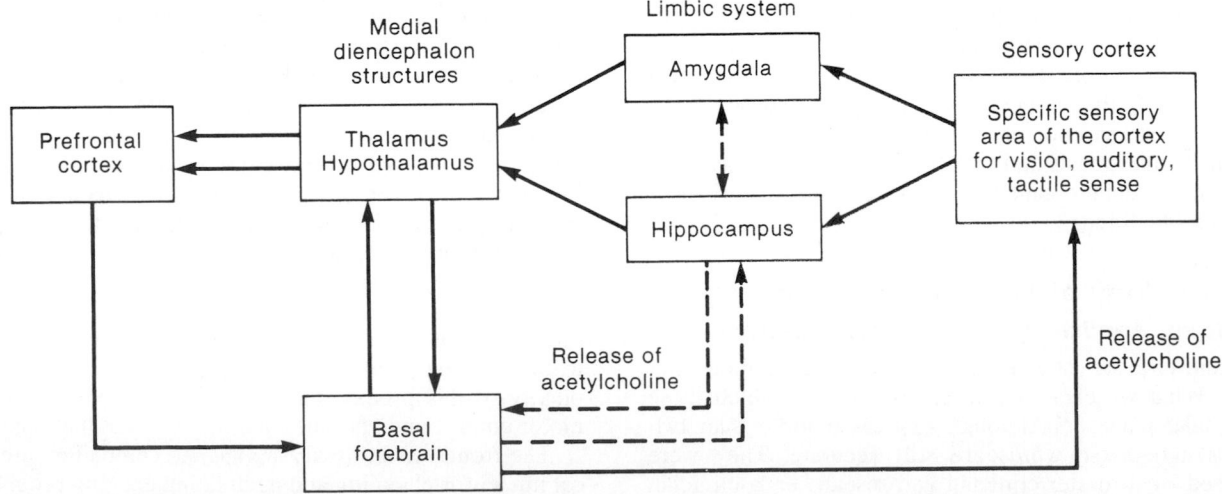

FIGURE 4-15 ■ The basal forebrain closes the circuit and causes changes in sensory area neurons, which could lead to correct perception and stored memory. This is neurochemical dependent.

its chemical structure (a plastic phenomenon). Memory first begins with a representation of information that has been transformed through processing of perceptual systems. The transferring of this new memory into a long-lasting chemical bond requires the neuronetwork of the limbic complex. Owing to the multiple tracts or parallel circuits in and out of the limbic system and throughout neocortical systems, clients, even with extensive lesions, can often learn and store new information.[54] This may also explain why damage to the limbic system structures does not destroy existing memory nor make it unavailable because it is actually stored in many places throughout the neocortex. The circular memory circuit illustrated in Figure 4-14 shows only one system. The reader must remember that many parallel circuits function simultaneously. The circular memory circuit shown reverts to the original sensory area after activation of the limbic structures to cause the necessary neuronal changes that would inscribe the event into retrievable stored memory. This information can be recognized and retrieved by activation of storage sites anywhere along the pathway.[54,331] This is why the power of music is so great, especially as observed in individuals with Alzheimer's disease (AD), who have lost declarative memory. In earlier phases of the disease, individuals who have lost words can recall words such as song lyrics through the linking with melody. When melody is lost, individuals still retain rhythmic responses. At the palliative stage of AD care, agitated patients are observed to calm to simple music such as familiar lullabies. Thus AD patients are able to continue to respond to music through the progression of the disease, and the response to rhythm may represent over learned motor responses that are tied to positive limbic states. For example, nonambulatory individuals, when presented with familiar and preferred music, may stand and move with the rhythm of the sound. Their bodies may remember how to dance with the spouse whose name they no longer know.

The last station or system to be added to the circuit is the "basal forebrain cholinergic system," which delivers the neurochemical acetylcholine to the cortical centers and to the limbic system, with which it is richly linked. The loss of this neurotransmitter is linked to memory malfunctioning in Alzheimer's disease. Performance of visual recognition memory can be augmented or impaired by administration of drugs that enhance or block the action of acetylcholine.[332-334]

It has also been shown that the amygdala and hippocampus are both interchangeably involved in recognition memory. The hippocampus is vital for memory of location of objects in space, whereas the amygdala is necessary for the association of memories derived through the various senses with a specific recognition recall. For example, a whiff of ether might bring to mind a painful surgical experience or the sight of some food may cause a recall of its pleasant smell. Removal of the amygdala brings out the behavior shown in Klüver-Bucy syndrome. For clients with this neurological problem, familiar objects do not bring forth the correct associations of memories experienced by sight, smell, taste, and touch and relate them to objects presented.[335] Association of previously presented stimuli and their responses appear to be lost. Animals without amygdaloid input had different response patterns that ignored previous fears and aversions. Thus, the amygdala adds the

"emotional weight" to sensory experience.[300] Loss of the amygdala takes away many positive associations and potential rewards, thereby altering the shaping of perceptions that lead to memory storage.

When stimuli are endowed with emotional value or significance, attention is drawn to those possessing emotional significance, selecting these for attention and learning. This would give the amygdala a "gatekeeping" function of selective filtering. The amygdala may enable emotions to influence what is perceived and learned by reciprocal connection with the cortex. Emotionally charged events will leave a more significant impression and subsequent recall. The amygdala alters perception of afferent sensory input and thereby affects subsequent actions.

In the human, memory functioning has been associated with the phenomenon of long-term potentiation observed in hippocampal pathways.[54] This potentiation of synaptic transmission, lasting for hours, days, and weeks, occurs after brief trains of high-frequency stimulation of hippocampal excitatory pathways.[69] Whether this phenomenon is caused by alteration at the presynaptic or postsynaptic terminals has not been established. The question remains whether there is an increased amount of neurotransmitter released presynaptically (glutamate) or whether the expected amount is producing a heightened postsynaptic response. Or, are both sites involved?[54] Even a third hypothesis regarding nonsynaptic neurotransmission or exocytoses with receptor sites on the surface of neuron beyond postsynaptic sites may help guide our understanding of memory and memory storage in the future.[54,154] Recent literature has linked a neurotropic factor usually considered for long-term potentiation within the hippocampus as a factor in amygdala-dependent learning, thus reiterating the interaction between these two nuclei and their role in memory and learning.[336]

Learning and memory evoke alterations in behavior that reflect neuroanatomical and neurophysiological changes.[54,115] These alterations include the phenomenon of long-term potentiation as an example of such changes. The hippocampus demonstrates the importance of input of long-term potentiation in associative learning. In this type of learning, two or more stimuli are combined. Tetanizing of more than one pathway needs to occur simultaneously. When only one pathway is tetanized, the effect is decreased synaptic transmission. Long-term potentiation, requiring the cooperative action of numbers of coactive fibers, is engendered and formed by the "associative" interaction of afferent inputs. Thus, long-term potentiation serves as one model for understanding the neural mechanism for associative learning. As the complexity of the limbic system evolves, questions regarding limbic responses to input stimuli need to be differentiated from limbic memory and initiation of a response without the stimuli. Recent research has shown that the amygdala is not only involved in learning related to emotional experiences but is also responsible for changing motor expression or conditioned response generated as part of an autonomic fear expression.[337]

Learning and Memory Problems after Limbic Involvement

For initial declarative learning and memory, the combination of hippocampus and amygdala of the limbic system is required.[54] For memory formation to occur, there must be a storing of the "neural representation" of the stimuli in the association and the processing areas of the cortex. This storage occurs when sensory stimuli activate a "cortico-limbo-thalamo-cortical" circuit.[54] Although there is not one single all-purpose memory storage system, this circuit serves as the "imprinting mechanism," reinforcing the pathway that activated it. On subsequent stimulation, a stimulus recognition or recall would be elicited. In associative recall, stored representations of any interconnected imprints could be evoked simultaneously.[54]

A vital processing area for all sensory modalities is located in the region of the anterior temporal lobe. This area is directly linked with the amygdala and indirectly with the hippocampus. The hippocampus and amygdala are also linked both structurally and functionally to each other and to specific thalamic nuclei. Clients, with temporal epileptic seizures and whose temporal lobes have been surgically removed, develop global anterograde amnesia; that is, amnesia developed for all senses and no new memories could be formed. Experimental removal of only the hippocampus does not bring about these changes, although processing is slowed down. When both the hippocampus and the amygdala are removed bilaterally, the amnesia is both retrograde and global. It is postulated that the amygdala is the area of the brain that adds a "positive association," the reward part to stimuli received and passed through processing. In this way, stimulus and reward are associated by the amygdala, and an emotional value is placed on it.[238,338]

It appears that limbic involvement in the declarative memory creates a chemical bond that allows cortical storage of "stimulus representation" necessary for subsequent recognition and recall of the information.[54,302,304,305,321]

When declarative and procedural learning from a clinical reference is analyzed, a separation of functional mediation can be observed. Clients with brain lesions localized in the limbic system components of the amygdala and hippocampus have the ability to acquire and function with "rule-based" games and skills but have lost the capacity to recall how, when, or where they gained this knowledge or to give a description of the games and skills learned. Relating this to clinical performance, clients may develop the skill in a functional activity but not the problem-solving strategies necessary to associate danger or other potentially harmful aspects of a situation that may develop once out of the purely clinical setting.[73,141,233,339,340] Similarly, if a client needs to learn a procedural task such as walking, transfers, eating, and so on, it may be extremely important to direct the attention off the task while the task is being practiced procedurally. As knowledge about the complexity of memory evolves, the clear dichotomy between explicit and implicit learning or declarative/procedural learning is being questioned by current research.[341] This study clearly demonstrates that anterograde amnesia affects learning that is dependent on combining a novel association with the development of memory compared with its accessibility to consciousness. As the specificity and generalizability of memory comes under scrutiny, a question arises regarding the differentiation of semantic memory from music perception, music production, and music memory.[342] If music memory is different than declarative memory and both are

different from procedural memory, then the use of music may become a link between declarative and procedural memory and learning.

Neurochemistry

Discussion of the limbic system's intricate regulation of many neurochemical substances is not within the scope of this chapter. Yet therapists need to appreciate how potent this system can be with respect to neurochemical reactions. The amount of research reflecting new understanding of the neurochemistry role on brain function is inundating the pharmacological research literature on a monthly basis.[310,343-348]

The hypothalamus, the physiological center of the limbic system (see Figures 4-2 and 4-13), is involved in neurochemical production and is geared for passage of information along specific neurochemical pathways.

Squire et al[349] consider it the major motor output pathway of the limbic system, which also communicates with every part of this system. Certain nuclei of the hypothalamus produce and release neuroactive peptides that have a long-acting effectiveness as neuromodulators. As such, they control the levels of neuronal excitation and effective functioning at the synapses. By their long-lasting effects, they regulate motivational levels, mood states, and learning. These peptide-producing neurons extend from the hypothalamic nuclei to the ANS components and to the nuclei of the limbic system, where they modulate neuroendocrine and autonomic activities.[349] The importance of these neuropeptides is being recognized as research begins to unravel the mysteries of the limbic system's role in the regulation of affective and motivated behaviors.[54,116,154,350-352] Lesions in the medial hypothalamus affect hormone production and thus alter regulation of many hormonal control systems.[54] For example, clients with medial hypothalamic lesions may have huge weight gain because of the increase of insulin in the blood, which increases feeding and converts nutrients into fat. Similarly, this weight gain may be caused by hyperphagic responses resulting from the loss of satiety. General hyperactivity and signs of hostility after minimal provocation can also be observed. These problems are often encountered in patients with head trauma.

Lesions in the lateral hypothalamus lead to damage of dopamine-carrying fibers that begin in the substantia nigra and filter through the hypothalamus to the striatum. Lesions, either along this tract or within the lateral hypothalamus, lead to aphagia and hypoarousal. Decreased sensory awareness contributing to sensory neglect is also present in lateral hypothalamic lesions. The decreased awareness may be caused by a decrease of orientation to the stimuli versus awareness of the stimuli once they are brought to conscious attention. These lesions cause the client to exhibit marked passivity with decreased functioning. Bilateral infarcts within the mammillothalamic tract create an acute Korsakoff's syndrome.[353]

As noted earlier, depression is clearly identified as a limbic function. A functional deficiency in monoamines, especially serotonin, is hypothesized to be a primary cause of depression.[354,355] The serotonin systems originate in the rostral and caudal raphe nuclei in the midbrain. Ascending serotonergic tracts start in the midbrain and ascend to the limbic forebrain and hypothalamus; they are concerned with mood and behavior regulation. Damage with direct or indirect limbic involvement results in the client exhibiting depression. Descending pathways to the substantia gelatinosa are involved in pain mechanisms and have also been linked through a complex sequence of biochemical steps to the increased sensitization of the presynaptic terminals of the cutaneous sensory neurons, leading to a hyperactive withdrawal reflex or hypersensitivity to cutaneous input.[54] This would account for the behavior patterns seen in clients with head trauma, when the therapist sees a flexed posture with a withdrawn or depressed affect yet with an extremely sensitive tactile system.

It is hypothesized that the underlying pathophysiological mechanism of one form of schizophrenia involves an excessive transmission of dopamine within the mesolimbic tract system.[54] The dopaminergic cell bodies are located in the ventral tegmental area and the substantia nigra. Some of these neurons project to the limbic system. These projections go to the nucleus accumbens, the stria terminalis nuclei, parts of the amygdala, and the frontal entorhinal and anterior cingulate cortex. It is the projection to the nucleus accumbens that seems critical because of its influence over the hippocampus, frontal lobe, and hypothalamus. This nucleus may act as a filtering system with respect to affect and certain types of memory, and the dopaminergic projections may modulate the flow of neural activity.[54] The masked facies due to the impaired motor activity seen in clients with Parkinson's disease and the paranoid/schizophrenic behaviors observed in some clients with CNS damage may directly reflect these mesolimbic dopaminergic systems.

The specific roles of the noradrenergic pathway are numerous and affect almost all parts of the CNS. The center for the noradrenergic pathways is located within the caudal midbrain and upper pons. Its nucleus is referred to as locus coeruleus. This nucleus sends at least five tracts rostrally to the diencephalon and telencephalon.[54] Of specific interest for this discussion are the projections to the hippocampus and amygdala. The axons of these neurons modulate an excitatory effect on the regions where they terminate.[54] Thus the activation of this system will heighten the excitation of the two nuclei within the limbic system intricately involved in declarative learning and memory. Hyperactivation may cause overload or the lack of focus of attention. Decreased activity may prevent the desired responses. Attention to task may depend on continuing noradrenergic stimulation. These tracts from the midbrain rostrally play a key role in alertness. The correlation of alertness and attention to performance of motor tasks as well as to learning can be demonstrated.[54] Again, these research findings reiterate previous statements regarding a therapist's role in balancing the neurochemistry within the client's limbic system. From a clinical perspective, a therapist will observe a relaxed, motivated, alert participant in the learning environment and will observe better carryover because the chemical interactions will only enhance the learning.

More than 200 neurotransmitters have been identified within the nervous system.[54] How each transmitter and the interaction of multiple transmitters on one synapse affect any portion of the CNS is still unclear. Certainly, some relationships have been identified. Novelty-seeking behavior of the limbic system seems to be dopamine dependent,[356] whereas melatonin receptors seem to coordinate circadian body rhythm.[357] Adrenal corticosteroids modulate hippocampal long-term potentiation.[340] The specifics of the total complexity are still beyond the grasp of human understanding.

In conclusion, the neurochemistry of the limbic system is intricately linked to the neurochemistry of the brain and the body organs regulated by the hypothalamus. All systems within the limbic circuitry seem to be interdependent, with the summation of all the neurochemistry being the determinants of the specific processing of information. Similarly, the interdependence of the limbic system to almost all other areas of the brain and the activities of those areas at any time reflect the complexity of this system.

THE LIMBIC CONNECTIONS TO THE "MIND, BODY, SPIRIT" PARADIGM

As neuroscientists, safe and deep within a Western allopathic model of linear research, establishing efficacy and evidence-based practice for what is taught to new learners is critically important[201,202,358] (see Chapter 37, section on music therapy). Yet there are too many unexplainable behavioral unknowns occurring daily in the clinical environment that cannot be researched using standard Western research tools common to physical or occupational therapists. Identifying with treatment approaches that base their philosophy on energy fields, flow patterns of those fields through the body, rhythms that do not seem to be proven as existing, or planes of consciousness and belief seems to contradict that comfortable groundedness of basic science. Thus, for many health care practitioners, denial of all those potential parameters that might affect evaluation and intervention outcomes is an easy way to feel safe and linked to what is believed to be efficacy or evidence-based practice within respective professions. Allopathic medical physicians within the clinical environment are often the first to reject what seem like irrational claims or ideas regarding philosophical approaches. Therapists are not far behind those physicians with their attitudes and verbal expressions toward both patients and colleagues that bring in ideas of potential approaches that seem to be outside of our reductionistic, linear research models used to establish efficacy. In the clinical arena, clinicians are realizing that effectiveness of practice with objective outcome measures is another way to establish evidence. Similarly, effectiveness can be subdivided into variables that pose questions. Researchers might be able to select variables that can be researched to establish efficacy of treatment approaches used within a clinical environment. Western medicine has taught both medical practitioners and therapists to strongly question anything that reflects concepts of energy, healing, or spiritual beliefs with regard to outcomes of therapy. Yet electromagnetic tools have been embraced by physicians and neuroscience researchers in the form of computed tomography, magnetic resonance imaging, positron emission tomography, or functional magnetic resonance imaging to diagnose and study neurodamage and neuroplasticity. These evaluation and research tools create their own electromagnetic field while the human body is placed within that field. Practitioners can still deny that there is a natural energy field and that this field has anything to do with health, but it is getting harder and harder to deny the presence of such a force. All of us have received an electric shock between our body and a metal surface. That shock is called an electromagnetic charge and the voltage depends on the inherent voltage of that individual. Where did this voltage come from? What is meant by inherent voltage of an individual? We all have learned that there is a static electromagnetic field around us, but it is very hard to identify how that charge might affect our body systems. As long as practitioners do not inquire about the physics of these energy fields and the bioelectric/biochemical reactions of our human cells to these fields, the idea that the electromagnetic and electrochemical fields have nothing to do with neuroplasticity and changes with patients after neurological insults can remain a myth.

Fortunately or unfortunately, there are enough scientists and therapists who are becoming "myth busters" and challenging the rigid paradigm of linear research, stating that there are many more variables and multiple systems involved in neurorecovery or neuroplasticity than have yet been identified. Physicians and neuroscientists studying the effects of disease and neuroplasticity after trauma or application of drugs[359-361] are trying to unravel a complex maze of chemical and electrical reactions at a level of the cell membrane.[6] Quantum physicists are studying the universe and the electromagnetic pull of suns on planets and solar systems on each other.

Science is a long way from unraveling the mysteries explored by cellular biologists and quantum physicists and how they might relate to each other. But many scientists trust that there is a relationship. As humans, we are made up of billions of these cells and each cell has a membrane potential and the ability to adapt and change, and they play an important role in the existence of our species. Similarly, the universe is made up of billions of masses; each has some relationship to energy pull, whether that be one solar system in relation to another, one planet in relationship to a sun, one moon in relationship to a planet's oceans, one person in relationship to the gravity on a planet, or one person in relationship to another person. If those cells are what makes a person human and what holds the person together is electromagnetic energy, then it is hard to ignore the possibility that one person might affect another person just by being present.[360]

Therapists want to study the interaction of brain responses between a practitioner and the client during a therapeutic treatment session. It is obvious that this interaction cannot be explained by one variable within linear space, nor that it is one variable alone that is causing all change over a linear set in time. Establishing efficacy on what seems to be a multidimensional construct using a basic science research model is not realistic. Thus efficacy research on the totality of the mind, the physical body, and the human spirit eludes basic scientist researchers in a similar way that understanding intuition eludes research in psychiatry.

As research practitioners we use various tools to manipulate both the internal and external environments within which our clients function to measure effectiveness of specific or generalized outcomes. Each person is so complex and unique, that finding the best combination of tools and environments has a very person-specific answer.[362] Thus what we as researchers are trying to do is find evidence that shows that one treatment paradigm has a better chance of creating change than another, without placing rigid restrictions that say all persons will optimally benefit from any one particular approach.[363-370] Magnetic resonance imaging, positron emission tomography, and functional magnetic resonance imaging tools are certainly capable of identifying changes in the CNS after interventions. Even when researchers or clinicians try to control as many variables as possible, many additional external and internal input possibilities exist.

This brings us full circle to the question regarding additional variables that might affect health, well-being, and recovery outcomes from therapeutic interventions.[371-375] After 30 years of clinical practice and hearing Western physicians saying "physical therapy and occupational therapy just make the patients FEEL BETTER," it is obvious that many physicians first do not understand the depth and breadth of our professions or what is provided to the clients. Second, those physicians do not understand the limbic interconnections to "feel better" and how that might drive the neuroplasticity of the CNS and the autoimmune system's response to disease or pathology.[376-379] Similarly, after many patients have been observed over the last 40 years regaining consciousness, whether the vegetative state lasted 6 months, 9 months, a year, or 4 years, the fact remains that each individual shifted from what might be considered a level 2, 3, or 4 on the Rancho Levels of Cognitive Functioning to a 6, 7, or 8 on the same scale after 5 to 20 minutes. This reality made Umphred ask the question from the beginning of her professional career, "What are the variables that cause changes in these clients?" The answers are still to be discovered, although the behavioral outcomes keep presenting themselves. Every time a patient comes out of this vegetative state this practitioner feels a wondrous, emotional, and humbling experience. Something happens that is far beyond our science understanding, simple but extremely complex, cellular and universal all at the same time. Similarly, the bond between that therapist and that client is very strong and deeply spiritual. The memory of those patients stay forever embedded in the mind of the therapist even if the clinical environment only lasted 30 minutes. All the words used to explain the above clinical experiences link closely to the limbic system and its role in creating change, both within the therapist and the patient, and certainly at this time fall outside the paradigm of Western medical science.

Medical schools and health science programs are becoming increasingly aware of the need to train the practitioners of the future to enter into a healing relationship with the whole patient, a relationship that empowers the patient to engage endogenous healing capacities, even while we work to better understand these mechanisms through both basic and applied research. Master clinicians have long appreciated this dynamic healing relationship that affects both the therapist and patient. Murray,[187] identified a need to train the clinician to appreciate the use of what he calls "limbic music" in the psychiatric assessment of affective components of patients with neurological issues. Here the word music does not refer concretely to auditory music, but rather may be perceived overtly by the clinician in response to various voice qualities, facial/gestural, and movement observations of the patient. Murray proposes that "limbic music" may differentiate cortical from limbic-controlled responses and assist in the clinician in assessment of which systems are impaired or intact. According to Murray, "limbic music is a term that denotes the existential, clinical, 'raw feel' emanating from the patient, and it is a more true rendering of the patient's clinical state than articulate speech," (p. 22).[187] Thus, even when our patients can verbally communicate with the therapist, it is still important to listen directly to the body, and on a deeper level, to more subtle input that we do not yet have the ability to describe and quantify with scientific method.

The success or failure of many forms of alternative medical practice, and for that matter Western allopathic medicine and therapeutic practices, may depend on the limbic system.[380] At times research can prove unequivocally that certain variables do not show a healing effect, after double blind studies.[381] If a patient "believes" an intervention will work, even if it is a placebo, the chances of success far exceed those when the patient does not think it will work.[382-385] If it is a placebo and the body heals, then logic dictates that the body and the mind did the healing. Similarly, when the drug itself aided in neuroplasticity and change, is it the drug itself or the individual's belief that the drug will work that creates the change or both? How these changes occurs is yet to be totally understood, but research substantiates that both neurochemical and neuroelectrical changes occur within an individual's physical body when the individual believes that change is possible.*

When Umphred was a novice therapist, a nurse once told her, "I am very glad you are not a nurse because you are so idealistic. You believe these patients in comas are going to wake up and walk out of here. And what is even worse is that most of them do!" That moment should have told Umphred that she was going to clash with allopathic doctrine throughout her professional career, but instead she was confused about the nurse's use of the term *idealistic*. For if the patients awoke and walked back into life with function and quality, then should not that be considered a realistic expectation? In that same job situation, her boss asked her to treat all the patients who were considered vegetative and, once they were awake, her colleagues would treat them from there. Umphred's response was, "Emotionally for both the patient and myself, I could not do that. Once I bonded with a person, gained his or her trust, and found the patient was willing and capable of regaining consciousness, I could not just abandon the patient and go on to another person." The significance of that statement took many years to understand, and it was not until Umphred began her study of the limbic system that she truly comprehended the accuracy of her once naïve perception.[373,378,380,386,387]

After 35 years of practice and often treating individuals in front of colleagues in workshop situations, Umphred cannot deny that something more than just "feeling good" occurs during physical or occupational therapy interventions. When working with clients, she finds herself feeling very open and bonding in some way that is neither "physical" nor "mental," and thus her only option left is a definition of "spiritual." If, when treating a patient in a vegetative state, that bond tells her the patient is lost within another plane of consciousness, wants to regain consciousness as defined by healthy people, and the physical body of the patient seems capable, then the treatment is goal directed, the direction of the intervention identified, and thus the outcome is selected by the patient. The map has been established, and together the patient and the therapist proceed. As with all therapists, the intervention will be guided by the motor responses and control of the patient and the window within which the patient can run those programs independently. At times, when treating clients in a vegetative state, Umphred is unable to locate the "spirit"; at other times it feels as if that person has not decided whether to venture to an awake state, but more often she senses a frightened, confused individual who just wants to find her or his way back to what we call "life or reality." Those patients often gain consciousness during therapy. It is not a miracle nor can Umphred even say, "I healed something." The term *healing* refers to a concept of "whole." The only person who can regain the structure of the whole is the patient.

As a therapist, Umphred is a teacher or a guide, helping others relearn and regain control over their respective lives. If after a 30-minute treatment session, a person regains feeling and control of an extremity after 18 years after a CVA or regains functional use of a hand 6 years after incomplete spinal cord injury, there is more to the intervention than merely following a clinical pathway or a treatment regimen geared to all individuals at a specific stage of a disease process.

One variable that always seems to be present when clients regain dramatic recovery is strong motivation by the patient to retain the control and an appreciation for the instruction on how to do that. A strong bond or compassionate appreciation for each other always seems to be present as another interlocking variable. Thus, the clinical question to this therapist arose more than 30 years ago, "What is spirituality?" It is a variable very difficult to define. That variable when researched has been shown to affect health and healing in individuals with health problems. The concept of "spirituality" and "healing" are both words that each individual defines according to her or his own beliefs, cultural experiences, and use of verbal language.[272,273,388-392] The literature is available for those who wish to pursue this topic.[239,335,393-400]

Over the last 5 years since the fourth edition was published, thousands of articles dealing with health, healing, spirituality, energy fields, quality of life, energy medicine, and emotional balance have been published in a large variety of types of journals.[401,402] Within this chapter, a system that affects all areas of the CNS and peripheral function has been discussed. How this system is affected by or affects one's spirituality is open for many lifetimes of future study. Yet, if spirituality affects healing and an individual believes that this potential is available, then this variable may play a critical role in patient compliance and the limbic interface with other treatment procedures. Ignoring this variable is no different from ignoring cognitive perceptual deficits when dealing with abnormal motor behavior.

Until we can measure simultaneous synaptic activity of all interactions within the therapist's and the client's CNS, we will not, from a grounded neuroscience efficacy base, be able to demonstrate exactly what occupational, speech, music, cognitive, or physical therapists do. Until then, outcomes need to be measured objectively. Even if interactions seem unmeasurable and subjective, clinicians still need to record the event change in the patient record and not bury that outcome deep somewhere in the subconscious level of the therapist's mind. The mind, the body, and the spirit are

---

*References 63, 65, 373, 376, 381, 384.

connected as a whole. If therapists treat only one part, it may help the whole, but if the whole is treated simultaneously, the outcome is more likely to change the whole. The concept is no different from focusing on strengthening an isolated muscle and hoping it will lead to functional use versus strengthening that muscle in functional patterns and in relation to other muscles that also work together within that movement sequence.

After years of clinical experience and thousands of patients responding positively to various interventions, the question arises regarding clinical decision making and choice of interventions. There is not a "variable" that has been identified that guides that decision. It has been shown that humans bring to consciousness about 10% of all incoming information. Yet the human brain is making decisions using 100% of the input information. Given that relationship, quite a bit of human decision making may be based on nonconscious information regarding the external and internal world.[63] Thus the word all neuroscientists shutter over, *intuition,* may, to a large extent, be the unraveling of that nonconsciously received data. Umphred has effectively taught colleagues how to feel blood pressure and heart beats of clinical partners by just barely touching the top of the hand, which might be explained by the high level of sensitivity of Meissner's corpuscles within our skin.[95] If a clinician can sense an autonomic response such as heart rate when touching a patient's skin, then knowing how the limbic system is interacting within a motor response can also be deduced. This would allow the clinician to modulate the rate used to move the patient during an activity such as bed mobility, while maintaining a consistent state of the motor generators. That steady state should decrease any need for limbic fear by the patient. In this case, it would look intuitive but it is not. When one clinician seems to know how fast to move the patient and another clinician has no idea how to determine that decision or control that variable, we say it is the art of therapy and not the science. Yet it is the science of therapy. Similarly, helping someone shift consciousness levels seems similar to hypnosis. The exact identification of these variables is very hard, let alone finding reliable and valid research tools. This may just be a case of one clinician being open to receiving information and processing it. The other therapist, for some reason, is either not receiving or not processing the available information. This is not an example of "intuition."

Intuition has been a source of fascination over centuries. Recently, with consumer dissatisfaction with health care and insurgence of alternative medical practices, intuition has again sparked the interest of scholars and the public. To many it reflects mystery, magic, and even voodoo. Those individuals with a strong ethnic, cultural, and even religious bias may find it hard to scientifically analyze this human strategy. For more than 30 years Umphred's husband has answered questions she had posed in her mind. It took at least the first decade for her left brain to actually accept that she was not subvocalizing the thought or that he could not have extrapolated the thought from an environmental stimuli. Yet he consistently has told her he hears her ask the question or state a fact. Obviously, her thoughts have traveled to his primary and associative receiving areas of his left temporal lobe and he "hears" the thought. The dilemma that confronted her as a scientist is, if the information did not

input through his eighth cranial nerve, how did it enter into his system? The answer would seem to be intuition. A definition might be knowing something without entering the data through traditional input systems. The next question is, what is intuition?

Unfortunately, after 30 years of study, Umphred cannot answer that question. She does acknowledge that it is something, it can be learned, and master clinicians use it as a part of their clinical decision making, even if they choose not to verbalize it to their colleagues or even acknowledge it within their conscious mind. There is much research and literature available regarding intuition.[63,403-422] Yet the answer to that simple question "what is intuition?" is unavailable and does not seem so simple. No answer exists that has shown to be definitively efficacious and reliable, although research over the last 5 years has begun to identify components of intuition.[403-422] It may be that intuition is more than one variable and can be accessed through more than one way. In fact, after studying various alternative medical practices, all using very different interventions based on different philosophies and belief systems, it seems as if all approaches may be tapping into the same human system, just opening to that system through different paradigms.

In the late 1960s, Umphred was beginning to present an integrated approach to neurological disabilities and integrating various treatment philosophies using the behavioral responses of patients and known science to guide intervention. She was told, at that time, that integrating approaches could not be done and that she would potentially injure patients by using approaches from different philosophical techniques. Today, of course, with our understanding of motor control, motor learning, and neuroplasticity, an integrated approach from the 1960s, based on a systems model, is what we now do. Umphred now presents the same model when looking at complementary approaches to intervention and the concept of intuition. There are a number of variables that seem to open one's intuition: bonding, dedication to the patient, openness to listening to the patient, letting preconceived knowledge be a tether from which to stretch that knowledge, not only a willingness to learn but an insatiable appetite to continue learning, and the ability to let go of one's importance and just be another person within the environment. These variables may be the best place for a learner to begin learning how to develop this skill. It would seem as if intuition is like an aptitude. Some individuals come into this life already with a high level of potential, others are nurtured to develop that potential, and still others never have an opportunity or have an environment in which to develop those strategies. Some individuals have had strong intuitive senses from childhood but share those experiences with few, if any, others.

Until 25 years ago, Umphred hid that aspect of her person because she was becoming a neuroscientist and wanted to be grounded in scientific efficacy like all her other colleagues. Unfortunately, her clinical experiences did not allow her to hide that intuitive aspect of her clinical decision making. Umphred treated a woman who had a severe head injury and who, after 6 months, was at a Rancho level 3. After 30 minutes of intervention the woman volitionally moved all of her limbs and trunk without cognitive confusion. Following the intervention, Umphred innocently stepped out of the safety of her science understanding. She shared with her colleagues this woman's medical and social history. That information was critical to their understanding the course of progression of this woman through the rehabilitation process. She discussed the patient's social background, her education, her family, her children, and her husband, who had shot her in the head. This all made perfect sense, until the head of the department asked her how she knew that information. Umphred said, "I read it in the chart." The director informed her that she had not seen the chart. Umphred said, "You told me?" The director responded with, "We did not discuss the case!" Umphred asked her if she was wrong and the director said "no." In fact, she was amazed at how accurate Umphred was and just wondered how she knew that about the patient.

At that moment, Darcy Umphred's life was changed. She could no longer hide whatever this "intuition" was, nor could she truthfully tell colleagues she was sharing what she did during interventions without bringing up this topic and saying she can only tell them ways to develop intuition but had no understanding of the basic neuroscience behind its function. She cannot tell anyone exactly what it was because she did not know. That unknown is still present. The future will unravel those answers. What she has found since that day is that "masters," whether they are physicians, therapists, or teachers, often use this additional source of information gathering to help them in their clinical reasoning. Umphred does not make this statement lightly nor without tremendous professional risk. Thus, she will leave you with an interaction that solidified her belief that this direction of scientific study needs to be pursued. A decade ago, she was a keynote speaker at an international neurosurgical conference on brain tumors. She was the token "other," and the only speaker who was not a neurosurgeon. She presented the topic "The Limbic System's Influence on Motor Output." With this audience of 500 neurosurgeons and 50 token others, she, of course, used charts and pictures and based every sentence on efficacy-based scientific research. At dinner that night when all the speakers were together, the master neurosurgeon whom everyone acknowledged asked if he could sit next to her. She was aghast, a little nervous but honored nonetheless. He opened by saying, "I think many physical and occupational therapists are intuitive." With that, she knew him, his life, his experiences, and so on. She let her left brain validate her intuition and said, "Yes, it is like walking into a room, looking at a patient, knowing where and what type of tumor he has, and using instruments such as PET studies to validate what you already know!" He responded with a smile and said, "Yes, it is exactly like that!" She does not need to continue to discuss the fascinating interactions of that night but leaves the reader with the thought that even the master of the masters in neurosurgery used intuition as a variable in clinical decision making. No physician or therapist uses intuition as the only variable; intuition just gives additional information that helps in the process of clinical reasoning. It would seem as though intuition has a strong limbic interaction.

Intuition is knowing something and as a result may bring on great emotion, such as "I know, thus I fear." If the sequence of events begins with an emotion or fear and leads to what is perceived as knowledge or truth, Umphred would question that intuition was a driving force behind the belief. When emotions become elevated an individual may progress with "I fear, thus I think I know." Fear is not what drives intuition; instead it is emotional balance. Emotional balance or centering is not a state of being without emotion but rather a heightened state of emotional awareness without emotion, all at the same time. To become truly intuitive, one needs to become emotionally centered. In our everyday world where each of us is overstimulated as a day-to-day experience, this emotional balance is extremely difficult to achieve. It is even harder to find that balance in a clinical arena where patients are arriving with more acute diseases along with chronic secondary problems, often patient's schedules overlap with other patients' time, and therapists not only are limited with time for intervention but also find that the number of allowed visits fall well short for optimal opportunity for learning by the patient. That reality does not mean that the therapists' responsibility has changed. It is always up to the therapist to find those avenues that provide better care within the existing environment. This reality just says the challenges and questions are enormous. Finding emotional balance with that environment is very hard. Yet intuition seems to be a variable that gives some colleagues additional information that is then used as part of the clinical reasoning process.

Intuition as a variable needs to be identified, studied, researched, and taught once it is clearly understood. It is up to all of us to find the answers to these questions and the solutions to today's clinical problems and develop evidence-based practice to progress into the twenty-first century.[423,424]

The concept of integration of mind, body, and spirit is not new to man as a critical element in maintaining or regaining quality of life between birth and death. Western society has tried to separate this concept into three distinct categories. The mind is made up of perception, cognition, and emotion. The body is made up of all systems external to the nervous system such as peripheral organs, muscles, bones, and skin. Both the peripheral and central motor systems that control the body are also included in the concept of body. The last component, the spirit, is a transcendental concept and is thought to depend on individuals' beliefs. Some individuals believe that spirit means belonging to a religious order. Others define spirit or spirituality as beyond religion and is the essence that links the person to a greater energy force. For decades this last category has been considered outside the domain of responsibilities of Western allopathy health care delivery and was comfortably relinquished to religious leaders or spiritual guides.

Today, everything is changing. Scientists refer to energy fields around cells while others talk about energy fields around solar systems. Complementary practitioners talk about energy fields around the living organisms. Physicians are being taught cultural sensitivity training while in medical school to be more empathetic to the populations of people they will service. Physical therapy curriculums are responsible for creating culturally sensitive professionals.[425] Occupational therapy programs are responsible for including spirituality as one of the competencies a graduate is to have met.[426] None of these professions has identified how these competencies relate to evaluation and intervention outcomes after treatment, but even the accrediting bodies believe they are important. Where does the interaction of the mind, body, and spirit play a critical role in quality-of-life issues and empowerment of the patient? The answers to that question cannot be found within this text or any other text in print today. Individuals with strong beliefs in a specific paradigm that includes spirituality can project the answer to this question, but finding efficacy is an entirely different issue. Our professions are tethered to research, science, behavioral observations, and current knowledge. That tether is a foundation from which we as clinicians can stretch. The unknowns are always present even as answers are discovered. Having those unknowns creates an exciting challenge and adventure for every clinician who has or will have the opportunity to interact with individuals who have been brought into the health care delivery system because of a CNS problem. Those individuals want to be considered as a whole human being even if part of their physical body is dysfunctional. A circle has been drawn and this chapter needs to end with a question. What is that whole? Refer to Case Study 4-1 as a clinical example.

SUMMARY

The complexity and interwoven neurological network of the limbic system may seem overwhelming. A reader who tries to grasp all parts on first study will feel lost and defeated,

which is a true limbic emotion. Thus this chapter was presented in three parts. The first part introduces the system and its potential clinical application. This section, in and of itself, has many interwoven components, for nothing in the limbic system functions in isolation. Yet the mysteries of this complex neurological network, when identified, may hold the answers to many clinical questions regarding the art and gift of a master clinician. The second part introduces in more detail the basic anatomy and physiology of the limbic system. It is hoped that once the student/clinician has been drawn to the conclusion that this system may be a key to clinical success, she or he might be willing to delve into the science of the system. This path of exploration is challenging, difficult, and frustrating at times but certainly worth the effort once understanding is achieved. The last section opens up the minds of the readers when and if they so choose to address these unknown variables. The limbic system is very complex, is very interactive with all parts of the human body, and may hold many answers about patients' responses and recovery. The reader's journey has just begun, and the future will open up many more avenues of research and clinical study as well as many more questions.

CASE STUDY 4-1

A 25-year-old first-grade teacher with whiplash is seen 5 months after a motor vehicle accident for severe dizziness and imbalance. She is unable to recall the accident; however, there was evidence to suggest that she struck her head on the steering wheel and briefly lost consciousness. Diagnostic testing is inconclusive (magnetic resonance imaging, electroencephalography). Medical management to date has been limited to central depressant medications (alprazolam [Xanax], diazepam [Valium]; see Chapter 36). She has received physical therapy since the accident for neck and back pain, which exacerbated her symptoms. She denies specific assessment or treatment of her dizziness or imbalance until this time. Her medical history is significant for hospitalization 3 months after the motor vehicle accident with "intractable migraine, postconcussive syndrome." Of note is a previous head injury 2 years before with moderate to severe postconcussive syndrome, including vertigo and migraines. She has been referred for psychological assessment and management and was recently diagnosed with obsessive-compulsive disorder. She is now referred to physical therapy by her neurologist for a full postural control and vestibular assessment. The differential medical diagnosis was postconcussive syndrome, rule out aphysiological performance (psychogenic, secondary gain). The physician believed that a large part of her problem was based with the medical psychiatric domain but was willing to widen his paradigm to include other possibilities. The patient's goal was to eliminate the dizziness and imbalance and return to normal activity and work.

PHASE I: EVALUATION

Unaware of being observed, the patient walks into physical therapy extremely slowly, holding the wall, watching the ground, and stopping periodically to close

her eyes. Her color is pale, her build small and thin, and her clothing loose. She is, however, well groomed. Her steps are shortened in length, widened in width, and limited in swing time. She demonstrates no segmental movement of the head or trunk, walking en bloc [rigid] without arm swing. As she sits down to begin our evaluation session, she smiles. She periodically closes her eyes as I or colleagues move around us. There are visible extraneous eye movements, though no immediate visualization of nystagmus [eyes opened or closed]. She is pleasant and cooperative with no overt signs of anxiety in quiet sitting.

Systems/Impairment:
- Dizziness with severe nausea and vomiting (at least once weekly)
- Dizziness Visual Analog Scale 7.5/10 and Dysequilibrium Visual Analog Scale 7.0/10 (with 10 representing the most severe symptoms imaginable)
- Decreased memory and forgetfulness
- Visual diploplia and blurriness with visual headaches
- Depression of central vestibular function (treated with medication)
- Her body mass was decreasing as observed by her loose clothing and severe nausea
- Her emotional stability was fight/flight: and went from calm/smile to fits of rage with family and other support systems
- She has photophobia but in reality she was hypersensitive to light and sound changes and again demonstrated fight/flight behavior with constant environmental searching for extraneous sensory data that might trigger anxiety.

Activity: Client Report
- Impaired balance for function, with near falls under dark/eyes closed environments. Patient reports one true fall in the shower with her eyes closed.

CASE STUDY 4-1—cont'd

- Impaired balance within visually challenging environments
- Sleep deprivation and fatigue
- Long-term stress and sensory intolerance/overstimulation

The long-term *stress* associated with a chronic disability of this nature can result in a decrease in serotonin, which influences the hypothalamus. Loss of sleep can alter levels of serotonin and other neurotransmitters. A decrease in serotonin results in further depression and *loss of sleep,* resulting in a physiological *fatigue*. It also can result in an increase in sensitization of presynaptic terminals of the cutaneous sensory nerves, contributing to the *sensory bombardment* and overstimulation.[427]

Participation in Life (Client Report)

- She attempted to return to work as a first-grade teacher but had a severe exacerbation of all symptoms in the classroom.
- She is unable to drive and requires assistance for shopping.
- She lives alone in an apartment and is independent in function modified by her symptoms.
- Disability Rating is 4/5 (recent severe disability/medical leave).[428]
- Dizziness Handicap Inventory (DHI) score was significant for physical and emotional impact of her dizziness, including depression. (Total disability score 78/100, functional subscore 28/32, emotional subscore 30/40, and physical subscore 20/28)[255]

From the signs and symptoms in the intake phase and subjective reporting, the preliminary physical therapy diagnosis would be that the patient has probable vestibular dysfunction, mixed with central and peripheral findings, sensory integration dysfunction, and anxiety overlay. The patient clearly has limbic system overload. It will be the therapist's responsibility to differentiate that from physical motor system problems with the assessment and treatment. The examination phase was designed to confirm or refute and redirect this hypothesis. (See Chapter 23 for clarification of these specific vestibular tests and measures.)

Oculomotor

Oculomotor examination was performed, with results supportive of the hypothesis of vestibular involvement, although inconclusive for peripheral versus central versus combination.

Gaze instability—clinical dynamic visual acuity test revealed a significant five- to six-line deterioration in dynamic visual acuity when head was moving with loss of postural control in posterior-left direction and symptom exacerbation during testing

Balance Stability

- Sensory Organization Test (SOT) of sensory balance function[429] showed an across-the-board dysfunction pattern,[1] although results were incomplete because the patient was not able to complete all 18 trials of the test protocol as a result of extreme symptoms (nausea, respiratory, and anxiety symptoms, particularly on conditions 2, 3, 5, and 6).

- Total dependence (overreliance) on visual information for balance stability
- Center of gravity position shift significantly leftward and anterior of midline
- Excessive use of a hip strategy for basic equilibrium (versus ankle), even with stable surfaces or the smallest perturbation
- Inability to effectively:
  - Use somatosensory or vestibular sensory cues on functional demand (reweight)
  - Organize the sensory inputs to the central nervous system to facilitate appropriate motor output
  - Dampen ANS/vegetative response, particularly in visual-vestibular mismatch conditions (SOT 3 and 6).
- Aphysiological criterion—Aphysiological responses on SOT raw data traces (exaggerated sway frequency and lateral sway responses). Motor Control Test (of automatic motor responses) results would have strengthened conclusions made regarding an aphysiological component but was unavailable to this clinician at the time of the examination.[429]

Function/Gait

Self-selected cadence of 1.82 ft/sec.[1] The patient watched the floor for the entire distance with no head or trunk or arm movement. Thus vision was clearly directing each step and to decrease extraneous visual flow/input. When she was encouraged to focus on a distant object, cadence decline to 1.34 ft/sec and the patient veered leftward 100% of the distance. She could be encouraged to walk at 2.86 ft/sec, with an increase in instability and a leftward loss of balance (regaining by self). With head turning, the patient became severely nauseous, cadence decreased to 2.0 ft/sec with loss of balance, bilaterally, requiring assistance. The interactions of the patient and therapist became a critical element in the examination. The patient had to trust the therapist that if she increased her speed or stopped looking down, she would not fall or incur additional emotional trauma. This trust is part of the limbic bonding referred to in previous sections within this chapter. The therapist, during the evaluation, empowered the patient to take responsibility for her functional movement while making sure the patient was successful if willing to take the risk. This aspect of the therapeutic interaction is limbic and will reflect success or failure through the motor responses of the patient.

Confirmatory Tests and Measures

- Intact sensation but extreme hypersensitivity to vibratory input (with ANS response).
- Normal strength and range of motion.

Multiple rests were required throughout the examination to decrease symptomatology (nausea, increased respiration, sweating) to patient tolerance. Testing reproduced all subjective dizziness and there was a resultant gross instability with loss of balance in the posterior direction, requiring assistance. Imbalance, nausea, and anxiety were residual for 10 minutes after testing.

Continued

CASE STUDY 4-1—cont'd

In the evaluative phase, the working hypothesis after the examination phase was as follows:

■ Diagnoses as identified by physical therapist: (Note that an occupational therapist could draw similar conclusions but would not draw conclusions based on the PT Practice Patterns. The occupational therapist would instead use OT Theory/Evidence-Based Research)

Medical—mixed central/peripheral vestibular presentation without confirmatory medical diagnostics/diagnosis. Further medical workup required.

PT Rehabilitation—Primary Problem–Practice Pattern 5D: Acquired impairment of the CNS and Secondary Problem Practice Pattern 5A: Primary prevention of falls

■ **Characterized** by (1) Vestibulo-ocular reflex impairment, probable high gain, with gaze instability, (2) central processing impairment with resultant, (3) postural control impairment with somatosensory dependence, and (4) heightened limbic responses with autonomic response to testing procedures and frequent rests required.

■ **Prognosis:** Fair for modified community level independence, physiologically complicated by history and chronicity. Improvement intratrial is a positive physiological sign. However, anxiety overlay and history may have psychogenic versus physiological impact on recovery.

■ **Red Flags:** Watch for (1) additional central signs, (2) signs of secondary gain, or (3) social service issues.

PHASE II: INTERVENTION

1. Assessment findings drive treatment decisions. There are three objectives of the treatment phase.
   a) Monitor and manage limbic symptoms through environment change of input systems (vision, auditory, kinesthetic) with the goal of the limbic system going neutral if possible.
   b) Maximize sensory integration, central processing, compensatory impairments of the vestibulospinal reflex (balance control) and vestibulo-ocular reflex (gaze control).
   c) Integrate gains in balance and gaze control into functional activity with and without emotional overlays.
2. Treatment approach
   a) Patient-oriented (limbic) approach
      Goal: Maximize internal locus of control and trust; quiet the limbic influence to set the tone for functional changes
      Techniques:
      ■ Awareness and validation of the problem. Provide the patient with objective findings of organic and functional involvement (sensory organization, dynamic visual acuity and other testing). Many of these patients have been told for years that it is "in their head." The statement is accurate but the intent condescending and implying some psychological dysfunction.
      ■ Awareness of and participation in the plan-approach. The treatment plan should have strong emotional meaning to the patient to turn the "limbic key" to maximize involvement and motivation. It should be goal directed intrasession and intersession. Achieving proper motivation and reward maximizes neuroplastic change.[430]
      ■ The correct patient-therapist pairing for effective execution of the plan. Safe clinician contact may actually be part of the rehabilitation plan with gradual reduction based on limbic and functional improvements.
      ■ The correct environment to effect change. Use appropriate voice (timber, pitch, volume), appropriate pacing (onset of sound or other stimuli), sound, light, consistency, and predictability.
   b) Balance retraining using sensory reorganization (reweighting)
      Gaze stability (vestibulo-ocular reflex) retraining
      Goal: Appropriate timing and predictability of sensory treatment: "dose" to achieve desired limbic and functional outcomes.
      ■ Expose the patient to the problem sensory conditions identified during the examination, presenting first the easier conditions and progressing the difficulty and complexity on the basis of patient response. Force the development of sensory integration, compensation or substitution, as well as the development of new and appropriate movement strategies.
      ■ Provide for selective attention through predictable, short segments of sensory integrative challenge.
      ■ Avoid sensory overload through proper "dosing" during sensory integrative treatment.
      ■ Provide for maximal motor learning environment by keeping the limbic system quiet while achieving the correct balance between error detection and correction versus demotivation through making mistakes.
      ■ Provide knowledge of performance and knowledge of results frequently. Computerized feedback provides direct one-on-one feedback of body position in space and motor performance.
      ■ This may be done using the following computerized or noncomputerized techniques. In this case, the treatment environment was controlled and progressed using SMART Balance Master custom sensory training. The visual stimuli was delivered in a predictable mode to the CNS (surround settings *responsive* in direction and amount to the patient's sway) at a level of difficulty no greater than the patient's balance ability (20%-40% of the patient's actual sway) and with minimal effect on symptoms by analog measures. With the

CASE STUDY 4-1—cont'd

goal of achieving a minor error message in postural control (sway) and in symptoms (mild dizziness), the task and environment were progressed on the basis of the patient's performance measures. Recognizing that neuroplasticity takes days, weeks, and years, and thus the patient and the therapist learn to recognize small changes in improvement that over a longer period of time will significantly alter quality of life.

c) Functional activity requires complex integration of balance and gaze control
   - Gait training at controlled pacing in stable environments, progressing changing pace within predictable visual environments, to unstable visual environments and variable surface environment.
   - Hippotherapy (the patient was positive regarding this element) at a controlled cadence provides predictable sensory input (somatosensory, vestibular, auditory, and olfactory), controlled rhythmic visual flow, neutral warmth in a meaningful, goal-directed activity (as identified by the patient).

d) If the patient does not progress in a physiologically normal manner or limbic signs remain unchanged (or increase) then psychological management may take precedent over (or be required before) recovery in rehabilitation (motor learning and neuroplasticity within the CNS) can be achieved.
   - Successful life outcome is affected by *early management*. The extent to which a mild dizziness problem becomes chronic is dependent mainly on the psychological reaction to the symptoms.[198]
   - There are specific management strategies associated with anxiety-type disorders within psychology, including use of medications. One theory of recovery from psychology problems is referred to as *exposure*. Although exposure is meant to cause habituation of the patient to the triggering events, in our case exposure actually will lead to forced use of the appropriate sensory system(s) as required in activities of daily living.

CONCLUSION

What makes this a clinical problem within the domain of the limbic system is that this woman's limbic system was overriding all other systems. At first glace this person was referred to therapy with typical vestibular/balance dysfunction. She was anything but typical and could not be approached in a "standard protocol," or failure for both the therapist and the patient was inevitable. The role of the patient within this setting is to gain an appreciation and integration of how her vestibular, motor, and limbic systems were interacting and when she went into system overload and why. The therapist's role was to (1) help the patient gain this body awareness, (2) empower the patient to her potential for recovery, (3) design interventions that nurture patient success, (4) collaborate with the patient on needed interventions regarding practice and novelty within the environment along with consistency of practice, and (5) allow the patient to improve at a pace her CNS can manage.

After 4 months of intervention the therapist moved and thus did not follow up on the long-term outcome of this case study. Although the therapist does not know whether the patient reached her ultimate goals, it was obvious after 4 months that the client was changing in the direction of functional control and participation in life.

The long-term permanent changes that may or may not have occurred with this patient's vestibular, motor, or limbic systems are not known. The essential role of complete history taking and dedication to reality by the therapist is obvious. The therapist's success within this case was dependent on her ability to listen and watch (visually, auditorily, and emotionally[limbic]) as the patient unfolded the mystery of her CNS problems. The patient was the key to successfully unlocking her complex subsystem problems. In the health care world of stress, limited visits, and expected outcomes after intervention, it is far too easy to blame the patient for our failure as clinicians. It is also easy to quickly identify that the patient has problems in other system areas outside our scope of practice and thus it is those areas that are limiting improvement. The difficulty is that all professions are doing the same thing and the patient is drowning in the repercussions of the waves. Partnering interventions both with other professionals and with the client should optimize an environment that nurtures long-term learning and plastic changes within the CNS. The limbic system drives our attention, our motivation, and our willingness to take risks into unknown environments. How you as a clinician accompany those patients throughout the learning experience will depend on your limbic system as much as theirs.

REFERENCES

1. Bababan CD: Projections from the parabrachial nucleus to the vestibular nuclei: potential substrates for autonomic and limbic influences on vestibular responses, *Brain Res* 996:126-137, 2004.
2. French SJ, Hailstone JC, Totterdell S: Basolateral anygdala efferents to the ventral subiculum preferentially innervate pyramidal cell dendritic spines, *Brain Res* 981:160-167, 2003.
3. Goto Y, O'Donnell P: Timing-dependent limbic-motor synaptic integration in the nucleus accumbens, *Proc Natl Acad Sci U S A* 99;13189-13193, 2002.
4. Harrison PJ: The hippocampus in schizophrenia: a review of the neuropathological evidence and its pathophysiological implications, *Psychopharmacology* 174:151-162, 2004.
5. Oliveri M, Babiloni C, Gilippi MM et al: Influence of the supplementary motor area on primary motor cortex excitability during

movements triggered by neutral or emotionally unpleasant visual cues, *Exp Brain Res* 149:214-221, 2003.

6. Lipton B: *The biology of belief: Unleashing the power of consciousness matter and miracles,* Santa Rosa, CA, 2005, Elite Books.

7. Ouyang M, Thomas SA: A requirement for memory retrieval during and after long-term extinction learning, *Proc Natl Acad Sci U S A* 102:9347-9352, 2005.

8. Rongo C: A fresh look at the role of CaMKII in hippocampal synaptic plasticity and memory, *Bioessays* 24:223-233, 2002.

9. Runyan JD, Dash PK: Distinct preforontal molecular mechanisms for information storage lasting seconds versus minutes, *Learn Mem* 12232-12238, 2005.

10. Wang R, Tang XC: Neuroprotective effects of huperzine A: A natural cholinesteraseinhibitor for the treatment of Alzheimer's disease, *Neurosignals,* 14:71-82, 2005.

11. Zhang WP, Guzowski JF, Thomas SA: Mapping neuronal activation and influence of adrenergic signaling during contextual memory retrieval, *Learn Mem* 12:239-247, 2005.

12. Bays H: Adiposopathy, metabolic syndrome, quantum physics, general relativity, chaos and the Theory of Everything, *Expert Rev Cardiovasc Ther,* 3:393-404, 2005.

13. Hyland ME: Does a form of "entanglement" between people explain healing? An examination of hypotheses and methodology, *Complement Ther Med Dec* 12:198-208, 2004.

14. Hyland ME: Extended Network Generalized Entanglement Theory: therapeutic mechanisms, empirical predictions, and investigations, *J Altern Complement Med,* 9:919-936, 2003.

15. Miller DW: Designing a bridge for consciousness: are criteria for a unification of approaches feasible? *Adv Mind Body Med,* 16:82-89, 2000.

16. Rein G: Bioinformation within the biofield: beyond bioelectromagnetics, *J Altern Complement Med,* 10:59-68, 2004.

17. Yamada S, Yamaguchi I: Magnetocardiograms in clinical medicine: unique information on cardiac ischemia, arrhythmias, and fetal diagnosis, *Intern Med* 44:1-19, 2005.

18. Buhrman H, Cleve R, Watrous J et al: Quantum fingerprinting, *Phys Rev Lett* 87:167902, 2001.

19. Greene BR, Morrison DR, Polchinski J: String theory, *Proc Natl Acad Sci U S A* 95:11039-11040, 1998.

20. Lewith GT, Brien S, Hyland ME: Presentiment or entanglement? An alternative explanation for apparent entanglement in provings, *Homeopathy* 94:92-95, 2005.

21. Milgrom LR: Patient-practitioner-remedy (PPR) entanglement, 5: Can homeopathic remedy reactions be coutcomes of PPR entanglement? *Homeopathy* 93:94-98, 2004.

22. Milgrom LR: Patient-practitioner-remedy (PPR) entanglement, 6: Miasms revisited: non-linear quantum theory as a model for the homeopathic process, *Homeopathy* 93:154-158, 2004.

23. Pauli HG, White KL, McWhinney IR: Medical education, research, and scientific thinking in the 21st century (part 3 of 3), *Educ Health* 13:173-186, 2000.

24. Polchinski J: *String theory,* Cambridge, UK, 1998, Cambridge University Press.

25. Saxena A, Jacobson J, Yamanashi W et al: A hypothetical mathematical construct explaining the mechanism of biological amplification in an experimental model utilizing pico Tesla (PT) electromagnetic fields, *Med Hypothesis* 60:821-839, 2003.

26. Smith CS: Quanta and coherence effects in water and living systems, *J Altern Complement Med* 10:69-78, 2004.

27. Duggan R: Reflection as a means to foster client-centred practice, *Can J Occup Ther* 72:103-112, 2005.

28. Dedding C, Cardol M, Eyssen IC et al: Validity of the Canadian Occupational Performance Measure: a client-centred outcome measurement, *Clin Rehabil* 18:660-667, 2004.

29. Epstein RM, Franks P, Fiscella K et al: Measuring patient-centered communication in patient-physician consultations: theoretical and practical issues, *Soc Sci Med* 61:1516-1528, 2005.

30. Harkness J: Patient involvement: a vital principle for patient-centred health care, *World Hosp Health Serv* 41:12-16, 2005.

31. Law M, Darrah J, Rosenbaum P et al: Family-centred functional therapy for children with cerebral palsy: an emerging practice model, *Phys Occup Ther Pediatr* 18:83-102, 1998.

32. Litchfield R, MacDougall C: Professional issues for physiotherapists in family-centred and community-based settings, *Aust J Physiother* 48:105-112, 2002.

33. Mossberg K, McFarland C: A patient-oriented health status measure in outpatient rehabilitation, *Am J Phys Med Rehabil* 80:896-902, 2001.

34. Palisano R: A model of physical therapist practice for children with cerebral palsy: integrating evidence, experience, and family centered services. III STEP 7-day Conference, Salt Lake City, Utah, July 16, 2005.

35. Palisano RJ, Snider LM, Orlin MN: Recent advances in physical and occupational therapy for children with cerebral palsy, *Semin Pediatr Neurol* 11910:66-77, 2004.

36. Schenkman M, Deutsch J, Gill-Body K: Models for rehabilitation applied to adults with neurological conditions. III STEP 7-day Conference, Salt Lake City, Utah, July 16, 2005.

37. Ward FR: Parents and professionals in the NICU: communication within the context of ethical decision making—an integrative review, *Neonatal Network* 24:25-33, 2005.

38. Graber DR, Mitcham MD: Compassionate clinicians: take patient care beyond the ordinary, *Holist Nurs Pract* 18:87-94, 2004.

39. Larson EB, Yao X: Clinical empathy as emotional labor in a patient-physician relationship, *JAMA* 293:1100-1106, 2005.

40. Schwerin JI: The timeless caring connection, *Nurs Adm Q* 28:265-270, 2004.

41. Autheir P: Being present—the choice that reinstills caring, *Nurs Adm Q* 28:276-279, 2004.

42. Black RM: Intersections of care: An analysis of culturally competent care, client centered care, and the feminist ethic of care, *Work* 24:409-422, 2005.

43. Cataldo KP, Peeden K, Geesey ME et al: Association between Balint training and physician empathy and work satisfaction, *Fam Med* 37:328-331, 2005.

44. Levy MM: Caring for the caregiver, *Crit Care Clin* 20:541-547, 2004.

45. Loewenstein G: Hot-cold empathy gaps and medical decision making, *Health Psychol* 24(4 suppl):S49-S56, 2005.

46. Tuckett AG: The care encounter: pondering caring, honest communication and control, *Int J Nurs Pract* 11:77-84, 2005.

47. Davis M: The role of the amygdala in fear and anxiety, *Annu Rev* 15:333-375, 1992.

48. Dougherty DD, Shin LM, Alpert NM et al: Anger in healthy men: a PET study using script-driven imagery, *Biol Psychiatry* 46:466-472, 1999.

49. Fendt M, Fanselow MS: The neuroanatomical and neurochemical basis of conditioned fear, *Neurosci Biobehav Rev* 23:743-760, 1999.

50. Gisquet-Verrier P, Dutrieuz G, Richer P et al: Effects of lesions to the hippocampus on contextual fear: evidence for a disruption of freezing and avoidance behavior but not context conditioning, *Behav Neurosci* 113:507-522, 1999.

51. Lachman ME, Howland J, Hennstedt S et al: Fear of falling and activity restriction: the survey of activities and fear of falling in the elderly (SAFE), *J Gerontol B Psychol Sci Soc Sci* 53:43-50, 1998.

52. LeDoux J: Fear and the brain: Where have we been, and where are we going? *Soc Biol Psychiatry* 44:1229-1238, 1998.

53. Liu CY, Wang SJ, Fun JL et al: The correlation of depression with functional activity in Parkinson's disease, *J Neurol* 244:493-498, 1997.

54. Kandel ER, Schwartz JH, Jessell TM: *Principles of neural science,* 5th ed, New York, 2000, Elsevier Science.

55. Melnyk BM, Alpert-Gillis L, Feinstein NF et al: Creating opportunities for parent empowerment: program effects on the mental health/coping outcomes of critically ill young children and their mothers, *Pediatrics* 11396:e597-607, 2004.

56. Ventegodt S, Gringols M, Merrick J: clinical holistic medicine: holistic rehabilitation, *Sci World J* 5:280-287, 2005.

57. Yorkston KM, Johnson KL, Klasner ER: Taking part in life: enhancing participation in multiple sclerosis, *Phys Med Rehabil Clin North Am* 16:583-594, 2005.

58. Khaslavskaia S, Sinkjaer T: Motor cortex excitability following repetitive electrical stimulation of the common peroneal nerve depends on the voluntary drive, *Exp Brain Res* 162:497-502, 2005.

59. Adolph KE: Flexibility and specificity in the development of action. III STEP 7-day Conference, Salt Lake City, Utah, July 18, 2005.

60. Sokolov EN, Nezlina NI: Long-term memory, neurogenesis, and signal novelty, *Neurosci Behav Physiol* 34:847-857, 2004.

61. Mesulam MM: *Principles of behavioral neurology,* Philadelphia, 1985, FA Davis.

62. Brodal A: *Neurological anatomy in relation to clinical medicine,* ed 5, New York, 1992, Oxford University Press.

63. Hunt VV: *Infinite mind: Science of the human vibrations of consciousness,* Malibu, CA, 1996, Malibu.

64. Esch T, Guarna M, Bianchi E et al: Commonalities in the central nervous system's involvement with complementary medical therapies: limbic morphinergic processes, *Med Sci Monit* 10:MS6-MS17, 2004.

65. Pert CB: *Molecules of emotion: the science behind mind-body medicine,* New York, 1997, Touchstone.

66. Brooks VB: *The neural basis of motor control,* New York, 1986, Oxford University Press.

67. Noback CR, Strominger NL, Demarest RJ: *The human nervous system: introduction and review,* ed 4, Philadelphia, 1991, Lea & Febiger.

68. Broca P: Anatomie compareáe des circonvolutions ceáreábrales: Le grand lobe limbique et la scissure limbique dans la seáries des mammifères, *Rhone Antropol* 1:385, 1878.

69. Barr ML, Kiernan JA, editors: *The human nervous system: an anatomical viewpoint,* 6th ed, Philadelphia, 1993, JB Lippincott.

70. Burt AM: *Textbook of neuroanatomy,* Philadelphia, 1993, WB Saunders.

71. Carpenter MB: *Core text of neuroanatomy,* ed 4, Baltimore, 1991, Williams & Wilkins.

72. Bielau H, Trubner K, Krell D et al: Volume deficits of subcortical nuclei in mood disorders: a postmortem study, *Eur Arch Psychiatry Clin Neurosci* 255:401-412, 2005.

73. Burns LH, Robbins TW, Everitt BJ: Differential effects of excitotoxic lesions of the basolateral amygdala, ventral subiculum and medial prefrontal cortex on responding with conditioned reinforcement and locomotor activity potentiated by intro-accumbens infusion of D-amphetamine, *Behav Brain Res* 55:167-183, 1993.

74. Decker MW, Curzon P, Brioni JD: Influence of separate and combined septal and amygdala lesions on memory, acoustic startle, anxiety, and locomotor activity in rats, *Neurobiol Learn Mem* 64:156-168, 1995.

75. Derryberry D, Tucker DM: Neural mechanism of emotion, *J Consult Clin Psychol* 60:329-338, 1992.

76. Sakata JT, Crews D, Gonzalez-Lima F: Behavioral correlates of differences in neural metabolic capacity, *Brain Res Rev* 48:1-15, 2005.

77. Winer JA: Decoding the auditory corticofugal systems, *Hear Res* 2005.

78. Aggleton JP, Keith AB, Rawlins JN et al: Removal of the hippocampus and transection of the fornix produce comparable deficits on delayed non-matching to position by rats, *Behav Brain Res* 52:61-71, 1992.

79. Gaskin DJ, Weinfurt KP, Castel LD et al: An exploration of relative health stock in advanced cancer patients, *Med Decis Making* 24:614-624, 2004.

80. Miyashita T, Williams CL: Peripheral arousal-related hormones modulate norepinephrine release in the hippocampus via influences on brainstem nuclei, *Behav Brain Res* 153:87-95, 2004.

81. Morgane PJ, Galler JR, Mokler DJ: A review of systems and networks of the limbic forebrain/limbic midbrain, *Prog Neurobiol* 75:143-160, 2005.

82. Zhang Y, Bailey KR, Toupin MM et al: Involvement of ventral pallidum in prefrontal cortex-dependent aspects of spatial working memory, *Behav Neurosci* 119:339-409, 2005.

83. Zola-Morgan S, Squire LR, Clower RP et al: Damage to the perirhinal cortex exacerbates memory impairment following lesions to the hippocampal formation, *J Neurosci* 13:251-265, 1993.

84. Cortese L, Caligiuri MP, Malla AK et al: Relationship of neuromotor disturbances to psychosis symptoms in first-episode neuroleptic-naïve schizophrenia patients, *Schizophr Res* 75:65-75, 2005.

85. Guigoni C, Li Q, Aubert I et al: Involvement of sensorimotor, limbic and associative basal ganglia domains in L-3,4-dihydroxyphenyl-alanine-induced dyskinesia, *J Neurosci* 25:2102-2107, 2005.

86. Holstege G, editor: *Descending motor pathways and the spinal motor system: limbic and non-limbic components,* New York, 1991, Elsevier Science.

87. Langenecker SA, Bieliauskas LA, Rapport LJ et al: Face emotion perception and executive functioning deficits in depression, *J Clin Exp Neuropsychol* 27:320-333, 2005.

88. Laurens KR, Kiehl KA, Liddle PF: A supramodal limbic-paralimbic-neocortical network supports goal-directed stimulus processing, *Hum Brain Mapp* 24:35-49, 2005.

89. Smith DM, Freeman JH, Nicholson D et al: Limbic thalamic lesions, appetitively motivated discrimination learning, and training-induced neuronal activity in rabbits, *J Neurosci* 22:8212-8221, 2002.

90. Spinella M: Prefrontal substrates of empathy: psychometric evidence in a community sample, *Biol Psychol* 70:175-181, 2005.

91. Tessitore A, Hariri AR, Fera F et al: Functional changes in the activity of brain regions underlying emotion processing in the elderly, *Psychiatry Res* 139:9-18, 2005.

92. Vinogradova OS: Hippocampus as comparator: role of the two input and two output systems of the hippocampus in selection and registration of information, *Hippocampus* 11:578-598, 2001.

93. Yamamoto Y, Struzik ZR, Soma R et al: Noisy vestibular stimulation improves autonomic and motor responsiveness in central neurodegenerative disorders, *Ann Neurol* 58:175-181, 2005.

94. Bergado JA, Almaguer W: Aging and synaptic plasticity: a review, *Neural Plast* 9:217-232, 2002.

95. Dobkin BH: Neuroplasticity: Key to recovery after central nervous system injury, *West J Med* 159:56-60, 1993.

96. Gomex-Pinilla F, So V, Kesslak JP: Spatial learning induces neurotrophin receptor and synapsin I in the hippocampus, *Brain Res* 904:13-19, 2001.

97. Goldstein LB: Pharmacotherapy for facilitating poststroke recovery: the challenge of translating preclinical studies to clinical trials. III STEP Conference, Salt Lake City, Utah, July 17, 2005.

98. Kleim JA: Neuroplasticity. III STEP Conference, Salt Lake City, Utah, July 17, 2005,

99. Kleim JA, Jones TA, Schallert T: Motor enrichment and the induction of plasticity before and after brain injury, *Neurochem Res* 28:1757-1769, 2003.

100. Liu L, Wong TP, Pozza MF et al: Role of NMDA receptor subtypes in governing the direction of hippocampal synaptic plasticity, *Science* 304:1021-1024, 2004.

101. Nudo RJ: Translating results between animal and human studies of brain plasticity after neuronal injury. III STEP Conference, Salt Lake City, Utah, July 17, 2005.

102. Merzenich M: Neuroplasticity. III STEP Conference, Salt Lake City, Utah, July 17, 2005.

103. Schallert T, Fleming SM, Leasure JL et al: CNS plasticity and assessment of forelimb sensorimotor outcome in unilateral models of stroke, cortical ablation, parkinsonism and spinal cord injury, *Neuropharmacology* 39:777-787, 2003.

104. Schallert T: Neuroplasticity. III STEP Conference, Salt Lake City, Utah, July 17, 2005.

105. Holmes GM, Van Meter MJ, Beattie MS et al: Serotonergic fiber sprouting to external anal sphincter motoneurons after spinal cord contusion, *Exp Neurol* 193:29-42, 2005.

106. Kemp A, Manahan-Vaughan D: Hippocampal long-term depression and long-term potentiation encode different aspects of novelty acquisition, *Proc Natl Acad Sci U S A* 101:8192-8197, 2004.

107. Majczynski H, Maleszak K, Cabaj A et al: Serotonin-related enhancement of recovery of hind limb motor functions in spinal rats after grafting of embryonic raphe nuclei, *J Neurotrauma* 22:590-604, 2005.

108. Thompson KR, Otis KO, Chen DY et al: Synapse to nucleus signaling during long-term synaptic plasticity: a role for the classical active nuclear import pathway, *Neuron* 44:997-1009, 2004.

109. Strub RL, Black FW: *Neurobehavioral disorders: a clinical approach,* Philadelphia, 1988, FA Davis.

110. Poldrack RA, Sabb FW, Foerde K et al: The neural correlates of motor skill automaticity, *J Neurosci* 25:5356-5364, 2005.

111. Arnsten AFT: The biology of being frazzled, *Science* 280:1711-1712, 1998.

112. Cahill L: Interactions between catecholamines and amygdala in emotional memory: subclinical and clinical evidence, *Adv Pharmacol* 42:964-967, 1998.

113. Carr DB, Sesack SR: Hippocampal afferents to the rat prefrontal cortex: Synaptic targets and reaction to dopamine terminals, *J Comp Neurol* 369:1-15, 1996.

114. Diano S, Naftolin F, Horvath TL: Gonadal steroids target AMPA glutamate receptor-containing neurons in the rat hypothalamus, septum and amygdala: a morphological and biochemical study, *Endocrinology* 138:778-789, 1997.

115. Izquierdo I, Medina JH: Memory formation: The sequence of biochemical events in the hippocampus and its connection to activity in other brain structures, *Neurobiol Learn Mem* 68:285-316, 1997.

116. Mitrovic I, Napier TC: Substance P attenuates and DAMGO potentiates amygdala glutamatergic neurotransmission within the ventral pallidum, *Brain Res* 792:193-206, 1998.

117. Saito H, Matsumoto M, Tagashi H et al: Functional interaction between serotonin and other neuronal systems: focus on in vivo microdialysis studies, *Jpn J Pharmacol* 70:203-225, 1996.

118. Sapolsky RM: Why stress is bad for your brain, *Science* 273:749-751, 1996.

119. Servan-Schreiber D, Perlstein WM, Cohen JD et al: Selective pharmacological activation of limbic structures in human volunteers: a positron emission tomography study, *J Neuropsychiatry Clin Neurosci* 10:148-159, 1998.

120. Smith BR, Dudek FE: Amino acid-mediated regulation of spontaneous synaptic activity patterns in the rat basolateral amygdala, *J Neurophysiol* 76:1958-1967, 1996.

121. Vizi ES, Kiss JP: Neurochemistry and pharmacology of the major hippocampal transmitter systems: Synaptic and nonsynaptic interaction, *Hippocampus* 8:566-607, 1998.

121a. Horii R, Akiyama F, Kasumi F et al: Spontaneous "healing" of breast cancer, *Breast Cancer* 12:140-144, 2005.

122. Segal B: *Love, medicine, and miracles: Lessons learned about self-healing from a surgeon's experience with exceptional patients,* New York, 1986, Harper Collins.

123. Moore JC: *Review of neurophysiology as it relates to treatment: personal notes,* San Francisco, 1980.

124. Rijntjes M, Dettmers C, Buchel C et al: A blueprint for movement: functional and anatomical representations in the human motor system, *J Neurosci* 19:8043-8048, 1999.

125. Moses SN, Cole C, Driscoll I et al: Differential contributions of hippocampus, amygdala and perirhinal cortex to recognition of novel objects, contextual stimuli and stimulus relationships, *Brain Res Bull* 67:62-76, 2005.

126. Rattiner LM, Davis M, Ressler KJ: Brain-derived neurotrophic factor in amygdala-dependent learning, *Neuroscientist* 11:323-333, 2005.

127. Bedwell JS, Horner MD, Yamanaka K et al: Functional neuroanatomy of subcomponent cognitive processes involved in verbal working memory, *Int J Neurosci* 115:1017-1032, 2005.

128. Herz RS: Are odors the best cues to memory? A cross-modal comparison of associative memory stimuli, *Ann N Y Acad Sci* 855:670-674, 1998.

129. Stevenson RJ, Boakes RA: A mnemonic theory of odor perception, *Psychol Rev* 110:340-364, 2003.

130. Burgdorf J, Panksepp J: The neurobiology of positive emotions, *Neurosci Biobehav Rev* 30:173-187, 2005.

131. Keele NB: The role of serotonin in impulsive and aggressive behaviors associated with epilepsy-like neuronal hyperexcitability in the amygdala, *Epilepsy Behav* 7:325-335, 2005.

132. Tucker DM, Derryberry D: Motivated attention: Anxiety and the frontal executive functions, *Neuropsychiatry Neuropsychol Behav Neurol* 5:233-252, 1992.

132a. Brown S, Martinez MJ, Parsons LM: Passive music listening spontaneously engages limbic and paralimbic systems, *NeuroRep* 15:2033-2037, 2004.

132b. Blood AJ, Zatorre RJ: Intensely pleasurable responses to music correlate with activity in brain regions implicated in reward and emotion, *Proc Natl Acad Sci U S A* 98:11818-11823, 2001.

133. Blood AJ, Zatorre RJ, Bermudez P et al: Emotional responses to pleasant and unpleasant music correlate with activity in paralimbic brain regions, *Nat Neurosci* 2:382-387, 1999.

134. Peretz I, Blood AJ, Penhune V et al: Cortical deafness to dissonance, *Brain* 124:928-940, 2001.

135. Townsend E, Wilcock AA: Occupational justice and client-centred practice: A dialogue in progress, *Can J Occup Ther* 71:75-87, 2004.

136. Lu L, Bao G, Chen H et al: Modification of hippocampal neurogenesis and neuroplasticity by social environments, *Exp Neurol* 183:600-609, 2003.

137. Meiser T, Hewstone M: Cognitive processes in stereotype formation: the role of correct contingency learning for biased group judgments, *J Pers Soc Psychol* 87:599-614, 2004.

138. Mosch SC, Max JE, Tranel D: A matched lesion analysis of childhood versus adult-onset brain injury due to unilateral stroke: another perspective on neural plasticity and recovery of social functioning, *Cogn Behav Neurol* 18:5-17, 2005.

139. Stellar JR, Stellar E: *The neurobiology of motivation and rewards,* New York, 1985, Springer-Verlag.

140. Gordon J: A top-down model for neurologic rehabilitation. III STEP 7-day Conference. Salt Lake City, Utah, July 16, 2005.

141. Kostandov EA: Organization of human higher cortical functions with different forms of reinforcement, *Neurosci Behav Physiol* 19:93-102, 1989.

142. Catani M, Ffytche DH: The rises and falls of disconnection syndromes, *Brain* 128 (pt 10):2224-2239, 2005.

143. Goldstein R: Thrills in response to music and other stimuli, *Physiol Psychol* 8:126-129, 1980.

144. Carlson NR. *Physiology of behavior,* ed 5, Boston, 1994, Allyn and Bacon.

143. Chesney MA, Darbes LA, Hoerster K et al: Positive emotions: Exploring the other hemisphere in behavioral medicine, *Int J Behav Med.* 12:50-58, 2005.

144. Esch T, Stefano GB: The neurobiology of pleasure, reward processes, addiction and their health implications, *Neuro Endocrinol Lett* 25:235-251, 2004.

145. Harvey PO, Possati P, Pochon JB et al: Cognitive control and brain resources in major depression: an fMRI study using the n-back task, *Neuroimage* 26:860-869, 2005.

146. Goldin PR, Hutcherson CA, Ochsner KN et al: The neural bases of amusement and sadness: a comparison of block contrast and subject-specific emotion intensity regression approaches, *Neuroimage* 27:26-36, 2005.

147. Mobbs D, Greicius MD, Abdel-Azim E et al: Humor modulates the mesolimbic reward centers, *Neuron* 40:1041-1048, 2003.

148. Small DM, Gitelman D, Simmons K et al: Monetary incentives enhance processing in brain regions mediating top-down control of attention, *Cereb Cortex* 15:1855-1865, 2005.

149. Hasselmo ME: A model of prefrontal cortical mechanisms for goal-directed behavior, *J Cogn Neurosci* 17:1115-1129, 2005.

150. Nakano K: Neural circuits and topographic organization of the basal ganglia and related regions, *Brain Dev* 22(1 suppl):S5-S16, 2000.

151. Sacchetti B, Scelfo B, Strata P: The cerebellum: synaptic changes and fear conditioning, *Neuroscientist* 11:217-227, 2005.

152. Groenewegen HJ, Wright CI, Beijer AVJ: The nucleus accumbens: Gateway for limbic structures to reach the motor system? *Prog Brain Res* 107:485-511, 1996.

153. Holstege G, Bandler R, Saper CB: The emotional motor system, *Prog Brain Res* 107:3-6, 1996.

154. Nieuwenhuys R: The greater limbic system, the emotional motor system and the brain, *Prog Brain Res* 107:510-580, 1996.

155. Schmidt RA: Motor learning principles for physical therapy. In Lister MJ, editor: *Contemporary management of motor control problems,* Norman, OK, 1991, Foundation for Physical Therapy.

156. Dawes J, Murphy P, Farber L et al: Work Group of the International Work Group on death, dying and bereavement: breaking the cycles of violence, *Death Stud* 29:585-600, 2005.

157. Feder L, Henning K: A comparison of male and female dually arrested domestic violence offenders, *Violence Vict* 20:153-171.

158. Molnar BE, Browne A, Cerda M et al: Violent behavior by girls reporting violent victimization: A prospective study, *Arch Pediatr Adolesc Med* 159:731-739, 2005.

159. Falls WA, Miserendino MJ, Davis M: Extinction of fear-potentiated startle: Blockage by infusion on an NMDA antagonist into the amygdala, *J Neurosci* 12:854-863, 1992.

160. Ancha L, Tucker P: A comprehensive approach to stress in primary care, *J Okla State Med Assoc* 94:451-454, 2001.

161. Cosen-Binker LI, Binker MG, Negri G et al: Influence of stress in acute pancreatitis and correlation with stress-induced gastric ulcer, *Pancreatology* 4:470-484, 2004.

162. Hamet P, Tremblay J: Genetic determinants of the stress response in cardiovascular disease, *Metabolism* 51(6 suppl):15-24, 2002.

163. Lewis CB: *Aging: The health care challenge,* Philadelphia, 1990, FA Davis.

164. Selye H: *The stress of life,* New York, 1959, McGraw Hill.

165. Corrigan FM: Psychotherapy as assisted homeostasis: activation of emotional processing mediated by the anterior cingulated cortex, *Med Hypoth* 63:968-973, 2004.

166. Godin I, Kittel F, Coppieters Y et al: A prospective study of cumulative job stress in relation to mental health, *BMC Public Health* 15:67, 2005.

167. Lacroix L, Spinelli S, Heidbreder CA et al: Differential role of the medial and lateral prefrontal cortices in fear and anxiety, *Behav Neurosci* 114:1119-1130, 2000.

168. Olff M, Langeland W, Gerson BP: Effects of appraisal and coping on the neuroendocrine response to extreme stress, *Neurosci Biobehav Rev* 29:457-467, 2005.

169. Sapolsky RM: Stress and plasticity in the limbic system, *Neurochem Res* 28:1735-1742, 2003.

170. Wolff B, Grabe HJ, Volzke H et al: Relation between psychological strain and carotid atherosclerosis in a general population, *Heart* 91:460-464, 2005.

171. Bishop S: *The use of guided imagery and music with adult female survivors of abuse in an inpatient psychiatric setting,* Salina, KS, 1994, Bonny Foundation.

172. Blake R: Vietnam veterans with posttraumatic stress disorders: findings from a music and imagery project, *J Assoc Music Imagery* 3:5-18, 1994.

173. Borling J: Perspectives of growth with a victim of abuse: a guided imagery and music (BMGIM) case study, *J Assoc Music Imagery* 1:85-98, 1992.

174. Körlin D: A neuropsychological theory of traumatic imagery in the Bonny method of guided imagery and music (BMGIM). In Bruscia KE, Grocke DE, editors: *Guided imagery and music: the Bonny method and beyond* (pp 379-415). Gilsum, NH, 2002, Barcelona.

175. Lachman HM: Alterations in glucocorticoid inducible RNAs in the limbic system of learned helpless rats, *Brain Res* 609:110-116, 1993.

176. Lewis CB, Bottomley JM: *Geriatric physical therapy: a clinical approach,* Norwalk, CT, 1994, Appleton & Lange.

177. Evans CJ: Secrets of the opium poppy revealed, *Neuropharmacology* 47(1 suppl):293-299, 2004.

178. Koyama T, McHaffie JG, Laurienti PJ et al: The subjective experience of pain: Where expectations become reality, *Proc Natl Acad Sci U S A* 102:12950-12955, 2005.

179. Kringelbach ML, Rolls ET: The functional neuroanatomy of the human orbitofrontal cortex: evidence from neuroimaging and neuropsychology, *Prog Neurobiol* 72:341-372, 2004.

180. Lenz FA, Bracely RH, Zirh AT et al: The sensory-limbic model of pain memory, *Pain Forum* 6:22-31, 1997.

181. Ramachandran VS: Plasticity and functional recovery in neurology, *Clin Med* 5:368-373, 2005.

182. Atac A, Guven T, Ucar M et al: A study of the opinions and behaviors of physicians with regard to informed consent and refusing treatment. *Mil Med* 17:566-571, 2005.

183. Kang SM, Shaver PR, Sue S et al: Culture-specific patterns in the prediction of life satisfaction: roles of emotion, relationship quality, and self-esteem, *Pers Soc Psychol Bull* 29:1596-1608, 2003.

184. Mills AE, Spencer EM: Values based decision making: A tool for achieving the goals of healthcare, *HEC Forum* 17:18-32, 2005.

185. Potter M, Gordon S, Hamer P: the physiotherapy experience in private practice: the patients' perspective, *Aust J Physiother* 49:195-202, 2003.

186. Schmidt S: Mindfulness and healing intention: concepts, practice, and research evaluation, *J Altern Complement Med* 10(1 Suppl):S7-S14, 2004.

187. Murray GB: Limbic music, *Psychosomatics* 33:16-23, 1992.

188. Beard EL Jr: Consumer trust in healthcare organizations is waning: how will 21st century learners bridge the gap? *Nurs Adm Q* 28:99-104, 2004.

189. Borbasi S, Gassner LA, Dunn S et al: Perceptions of the researcher: in-depth interviewing in the home, *Contemp Nurse* 14:24-37, 2002.

190. Leonard G: *The silent pulse,* New York, 1981, Bantam Books.

191. Raphael B, Wooding S: Debriefing: Its evolution and current status, *Psychiatr Clin North Am* 27:407-423, 2004.

192. Szawarski Z: Wisdom and the art of healing, *Med Health Care Philos* 7:185-193, 2004.

193. Walwyn W, Maidment NT, Sanders M et al: Induction of delta opioid receptor function by up-regulation of membrane receptors in mouse primary afferent neurons, *Mol Pharmacol* 68:1688-1698, 2005.

194. Koyama Y, Koyama T, Knocke AP et al: Effects of stimulus duration on heat induced pain: the relationship between real-time and post-stimulus pain ratings, *Pain* 107:256-266, 2004.

195. Rolls ET, O'Doherty J, Kringelbach ML et al: Representations of pleasant and painful touch in the human orbitofrontal and cingulate cortices, *Cereb Cortex* 13:308-317, 2003.

196. Mense SS: Functional neuroanatomy for pain stimuli: reception, transmission and processing. *Schemrz* 18:225-237, 2004.

197. Ramachandran VS: Plasticity and functional recovery in neurology, *Clin Med* 5:368-373, 2005.

198. Yardley L, Burgneay I, Nazareth I et al: Neuro-otologic and psychiatric abnormalities in a community sample of people with dizziness: a blind, controlled investigation, *J Neurol Neurosurg Psychiatry* 65:679-684, 1998.

199. Jacob RG, Furman JM, Durrant JD et al: Panic, agoraphobia, and vestibular dysfunction, *Am J Psychiatry* 153:503-512, 1996.

200. Bronstein AM: Visual vertigo syndrome: clinical and posturography findings, *J Neurol Neurosurg Psychiatry* 59:472-476, 1995.

201. *Guide to physical therapist practice,* ed 2, Alexandria, VA, 2001, American Physical Therapy Association.

202. American Occupational Therapy Association: Standards of practice for occupational therapy in schools, *Am J Occup Ther* 34:900-903, 1980.

203. Ito M, Fukuda M, Suto T et al: Increased and decreased cortical reactivation in novelty seeking and persistence: a multichannel near-infrared spectroscopy in health subjects, *Neuropsychobiology* 52:45-54, 2005.

204. Laurens KR, Kiehl KA, Liddle PF: A supramodal limbic-paralimbic-neocortical network supports goal-directed stimulus processing, *Hum Brain Mapp* 24:35-49, 2005.

205. Puttonen S, Ravaja N, Keltikangas-Jarvinen L: Cloninger's temperament dimensions and affective responses to different challenges, *Compr Psychiatry* 46:128-134, 2005.

206. Strange BA, Hurlemann R, Duggins A et al: Dissociating intentional learning from relative novelty responses in the medial temporal lobe, *Neuroimage* 25:51-62, 2005.

207. Thaut MH: The future of music in therapy and medicine, *Ann N Y Acad Sci,* 1060:303-308, 2005.

208. Spiers PA: Temporal limbic epilepsy and behavior. In Mesulum MM, editor: *Principles of behavioral neurology,* Philadelphia, 1985, FA Davis.

209. Adamec R: Kindling, anxiety, and limbic perspectives. In Wada JA, editor: *Advances in behavioral biology,* New York, 1990, Plenum Press.

210. Brand M, Fujiwara E, Borsutzky S et al: Decision-making deficits of Korsakoff patients in a new gambling task with explicit rules: associations with executive functions, *Neuropsychology* 19:267-277, 2005.

211. Caulo M, Van Hecke J, Toma L et al: Functional MRI study of diencephalic amnesia in Wernicke-Korsakoff syndrome, *Brain* 128:1584-1594, 2005.

212. van Asselen M, Kessels RP, Wester AJ et al: Spatial working memory and contextual cueing in patients with Korsakoff amnesia, *J Clin Exp Neuropsychol* 27:645-655, 2005.

213. Conry J: Neuropsychological deficits in fetal alcohol syndrome and fetal alcohol effects, *Alcohol Clin Exp Res* 14:650-655, 1990.

214. Gauthier TW, Drews-Botsch C, Falei A et al: Maternal alcohol abuse and neonatal infection, *Alcohol Clin Exp Res* 29:1035-1043, 2005.

215. Harris SR, Osborn JA, Weinberg J et al: Effects of prenatal alcohol exposure on neuromotor and cognitive development during early childhood: a series of case reports, *Phys Ther* 73:608-617, 1993.

216. Huizink AC, Mulder EJ: Maternal smoking, drinking or cannabis use during pregnancy and neurobehavioral and cognitive functioning in human offspring, *Neurosci Biobehav Rev* 30:24-41, 2006.

217. Osborn JA, Harris SR, Weinberg J: Fetal alcohol syndrome: Review of the literature with implication for physical therapists, *Phys Ther* 73:599-607, 1993.

218. Rosenthal M et al, editors: *Rehabilitation of the adult and child with traumatic brain injury,* Philadelphia, 1990, FA Davis.

219. Schneider JW, Chasnoff IJ: Motor assessment of cocanin/polydrug-exposed infants at age 4 months, *Neurotoxicol Teratol* 14:97-101, 1992.

220. Hone E, Martins IJ, Jeoung M et al: Alzheimer's disease amyloid-beta peptide modulates apolipoprotein E isoform specific receptor binding, *J Alzheimers Dis* 7:303-314, 2005.

221. Mungas D, Harvey D, Reed BR et al: Longitudinal volumetric MRI change and rate of cognitive decline, *Neurology* 65:565-571, 2005.

222. Gatz JL, Tyas SL, St John P et al: Do depressive symptoms predict Alzheimer's disease and dementia? *J Gerontol A Biol Sci Med Sci* 60:744-747, 2005.

223. Reding M, Haycox J, Blass J: Depression in patients referred to a dementia clinic: a three-year prospective study, *Arch Neurol* 42:894-896, 1985.

224. Takeuchi M, Kikuchi S, Sasaki N et al: Involvement of advanced glycation end-products (AGEs) in Alzheimer's disease, *Curr Alzheimer Res* 1:39-46, 2004.

225. Libon DJ, Boganoff B, Cloud BS et al: Declarative and procedural learning, quantitative measures of the hippocampus, and subcortical white alterations in Alzheimer's disease and ischaemic vascular dementia, *J Clin Exp Neuropsychol* 20:30-41, 1998.

226. Appel SH, editor: *Current neurology, vol 6,* Chicago, 1986, CV Mosby.

227. Alisky JM: Is the immobility of advanced dementia a form of lorazepam-responsive catatonia? *Am J Alzheimers Dis Other Demen* 19:213-214, 2004.

228. Voliver L: Management of severe Alzheimer's disease and end-of-life issues, *Clin Geriatr Med* 17:377-391, 2001.

229. Ehrenkrantz D, Silverman JM, Smith CJ et al: Genetic epidemiological study of maternal and paternal transmission of Alzheimer's disease, *Am J Med Genet* 88:378-382, 1999.

230. Levin JS, Larson DB, Puchalski CM: Religion and spirituality in medicine: research and education, *JAMA* 278:792-793, 1997.

231. Osterlund MK, Keller E, Hurd YL: The human forebrain has discrete estrogen receptor alpha messenger RNA expression: high levels in the amygdaloid complex, *Neuroscience* 95:333-342, 2000.

232. Adams JH, Graham DI, Murray LS et al: Diffuse axonal injury due to nonmissile head injury in humans: an analysis of 45 cases, *Ann Neurol* 12:557-563, 1982.

233. Auerbach SH: Neuroanatomical correlates of attention and memory disorders in traumatic brain injury: an application of neurobehavioral subtypes, *J Head Trauma Rehabil* 1:1-12, 1986.

234. Fork M, Bartels C, Ebert AD et al: Neuropsychological sequelae of diffuse traumatic brain injury, *Brain Inj* 19:1001-1008, 2005.

235. Goethals I, Audenaert K, Jacobs F et al: Cognitive neuroactivation using SPECT and the Stroop Colored Word Test in patients with diffuse brain injury, *J Neurotrauma* 21:1059-1069, 2004.

236. Levin HS, Hanten G: Executive functions after brain injury in children, *Pediatr Neurol* 33:79-93, 2005.

237. Soeda A, Nakashima T, Okumura A et al: Cognitive impairment after traumatic brain injury: a functional magnetic resonance imaging study using the Stroop task, *Neuroradiology* 47:501-506, 2005.

238. Haist F, Shimamura AP, Squire LR: On the relationship between recall and recognition memory, *J Exp Psychol Learn Mem Cogn* 18:691-702, 1992.

239. Anadaraijah G: Spirituality and medicine, *J Fam Pract* 48:389, 1999.

240. Witgen BM, Lifshitz J, Smith ML et al: Regional hippocampal alterations associated with cognitive deficit following experimental brain injury: a systems, network and cellular evaluation, *Neuroscience* 133:1-15, 2005.

241. Goldberg FS: A holographic field theory model of the Bonny method of guided imagery and music (BMGIM). In Bruscia KE, Grocke DE, editors: *Guided imagery and music: the Bonny method and beyond* (pp 359-378). Gilsum, NH, 2002, Barcelona.

242. Oehnichen M, Meissner C, Saternus KS: Fall or shaken: traumatic brain injury in children caused by falls or abuse at home—a review of biomechanics and diagnosis, *Neuropediatrics* 36:240-245, 2005.

243. Vanderploeg RD, Curtiss G, Berlanger HG: Long-term neuropsychological outcomes following mild traumatic brain injury, *J Int Neuropsychol Soc* 11:228-236, 2005.

244. Salmond CH, Menon DK, Chatfield DA et al: Deficits in decision-making in head injury survivors, *J Neurotrauma* 22:613-622, 2005.

245. Papez JW: A proposed mechanism of emotions, *Arch Neurol Psychiatry* 38:725, 1937.

246. Maguire EA, Frith CD, Rudge P et al: The effect of adult-acquired hippocampal damage on memory retrieval: an fMRI study, *Neuroimage* 27:146-152, 2005.

247. Bartlett DJ, Rae C, Thompson CH et al: Hippocampal area metabolites related to severity and cognitive function in obstructive sleep apnea, *Sleep Med* 5:593-596, 2004.

248. Starkstein SE, Robinson RG: Mechanism of disinhibition after brain lesions, *J Nerv Ment Dis* 185:108-114, 1997.

249. Fluharty G, Glassman N: Use of antecedent control to improve the outcome of rehabilitation for a client with frontal lobe injury and intolerance for auditory and tactile stimuli, *Brain Inj* 15:995-1002, 2001.

250. Gilmore R, Aram J, Powell J et al: Treatment of oro-facial hypersensitivity following brain injury, *Brain Inj* 17:347-354, 2003.

251. Ventegodt S, Morad M, Merrick J: Clinical holistic medicine: classic are of healing or the therapeutic touch, *Sci World J* 4:134-147, 2004.

252. Zajonc TP, Roland PS: Vertigo and motion sickness, 1: Vestibular anatomy and physiology, *Ear Nose Throat J* 84:581-584, 2005.

253. Executive summary. Clackamas, OR, 2004-2005, NeuroCom International.

254. Eagger S, Luxon LM, Davies RA et al: Psychiatric morbidity in patients with peripheral vestibular disorder: a clinical and neuro-otological study, *J Neurol Neurosurg Psychiatry* 55:383-387, 1992.

255. Jacob RG, Moller MB, Turner SM et al: Otoneurologic examination in panic disorder and agoraphobia with panic attacks: a pilot study, *Am J Psychiatry* 142:715-720, 1985.

256. Yardley L, Luxon LM, Haacke NP: A longitudinal study of symptoms, anxiety and subjective well-being in patients with vertigo, *Clin Otolaryngol Allied Sci* 19:109-116, 1994.

257. Kroenke K, Lucas C, Rosenberg M et al: Causes of persistent dizziness: a prospective study of 100 patients in ambulatory care, *Ann Intern Med* 177:899-904, 1992.

258. Hoffer ME, Gottshall KR, Kopke RD et al: Vestibular testing abnormalities in individuals with motion sickness, *Otol Neurotol* 24:633-636, 2003.

259. Longridge NS, Mallinson AI: Visual vestibular mismatch in work-related vestibular injury, *Otol Neurotol* 26:691-694, 2005.

260. Longridge NS, Mallinson AI: Across the board posturography abnormalities in vestibular injury, *Otol Neurotol* 26:695-698, 2005.

261. Mallinson AI, Longridge NS: Dizziness from whiplash and head injury: differences between whiplash and head injury, *Am J Otol* 19:814-818, 1998.

262. Mallinson AI, Longridge NS, Peacock C: Dizziness, imbalance, and whiplash, *J Musculoskel Pain* 4:105-112, 1996.

263. Furman JM, Jacob RG: Clinical taxonomy of dizziness and anxiety in the otoneurological setting [review], *J Anxiety Disord* 15:9-26, 2001.

264. Murray K, Carroll S, Hill K: Relationship between change in balance and self-reported handicap after vestibular rehabilitation, *Phys Res Int* 6: 251-263, 2001.

265. Schmidley JW, Messing RO: Agitated confusional states in patients with right hemisphere infarctions, *Stroke* 15:883, 1984.

266. Poulet R, Gentile MT, Vecchione C et al: Acute hypertension induces oxidative stress in brain tissues, *J Cereb Blood Flow Metab* (online): www.nature.com. Published 2005.

267. Ances BM, Vitaliani R, Taylor RA et al: Treatment-responsive limbic encephalitis identified by neuropil antibodies: MRI and PET correlates, *Brain* 128:1764-1777, 2005.

268. Trummer M, Eustacchio S, Unger F et al: Right hemispheric frontal lesions as a cause for anorexia nervosa report of three cases, *Acta Neurochir (Wien)* 144:797-801, 2002.

269. Gamazo-Garran P, Soutullo CA, Ortuno F: Obsessive-compulsive disorder secondary to brain dysgerminoma in an adolescent boy: a positron emission tomography case report, *J Child Adolesc Psychopharmacol* 12:259-263, 2002.

270. Commission on Accreditation in Physical Therapy Education: *Evaluative criteria for accreditation of education programs for the preparation of physical therapists,* Alexandria, VA, 2005, American Physical Therapy Association.

271. Accreditation Council of Occupational Therapy Education: *Education standard for occupational therapy,* Bethesda, MD, 2006, American Occupational Therapy Association.

272. Edelman GM: *Wider than the sky,* New Haven, CT, 2004, Yale University Press.

273. Restak R: *The new brain: how the modern age is rewiring your mind,* Emmaus, PA, 2003, Rodale.

274. Schwartz JM, Begley S: *The mind and the brain: Neuroplasticity and the power of mental force,* New York, 2002, HarperCollins.

275. Davis M: Are different parts of the extended amygdala involved in fear versus anxiety? *Soc Biol Pathways* 44:1239-1247, 1998.

276. Morris JS, Ohman A, Dolan RJ: Conscious and unconscious emotional learning in the human amygdala, *Nature* 393:467-474, 1998.

277. Pedersen CA: Biological aspects of social bonding and the roots of human violence, *Ann N Y Acad Sci* 1036:106-127, 2004.

278. LeDoux J: Emotional networks and motor control: A fearful view. In Holstege G, Bandler R, Saper, editors: *Progress in brain research, vol 107,* Amsterdam, 1996, Elsevier Science.

279. Maclean PD: Role of transhypothalamic pathways in social communication. In Morgane PJ, Panksapp J, editors: *Handbook of the hypothalamus,* vol 3, New York, 1981, Marcel Dekker.

280. Klüver H, Bucy PC: Preliminary analysis of functions of the temporal lobes in monkeys, *Arch Neural Psychiatry* 42:979, 1939.

281. Dalla C, Antoniou K, Drossopoulou G et al: Chronic mild stress impact: Are females more vulnerable? *Neuroscience* 135:703-714, 2005.

282. Harris GC, Wimmer M, Aston-Jones GA: A role for lateral hypothalamic orexin neurons in reward seeking, *Nature* 437:556-559, 2005.

283. Waxman SG: Clinical observations on the emotional motor system, *Prog Brain Res* 107:595-604, 1996.

284. Brasted PJ, Bussey TJ, Murray EA et al: Conditional motor learning in the nonspatial domain: effects of errorless learning and the contribution of the fornix to one-trial learning, *Behav Neurosci* 119:662-676, 2005.

285. Friedman DP, Aggleton JP, Saunders RC: Comparison of hippocampal, amygdala, and perirhinal projections to the nucleus accumbens: combined anterograde and retrograde tracing study in the Macaque brain, *J Comp Neurol* 450:345-365, 2002.

286. Dowd E, Dunnett SB: Comparison of 6-hydroxydopamine-induced medial forebrain bundle and nigrostriatal terminal lesions in a lateralised nose-poking task in rats, *Behav Brain Res* 159:153-161, 2005.

287. Balaban CD, Berkozkin G: Vestibular nucleus projections to nucleus tractus solitarius and the dorsal motor nucleus of the vagus nerve: potential substrates for vestibule-autonomic interactions, *Exp Brain Res* 98:200-212, 1994.

288. Jacob RG, Furman JM, Durrant JD et al: Panic, agoraphobia, and vestibular dysfunction, *Am J Psychiatry* 153:503-512, 1996.

289. Pompeiano O, Manzoni D, Barnes CD et al: Responses of locus ceruleus and subceruleus neurons to sinusoidal stimulation of labyrinthine receptors, *Neuroscience* 35:227-248, 1990.

290. Spiegel EA: Effect of labyrinthine reflexes on the vegetative nervous system, *Arch Otolaryngol* 44:61-72, 1946.

291. Yates BJ: Vestibular influences on the sympathetic nervous system, *Brain Res Rev* 27:51-59, 1992.

292. Zuccaro TA: Pharmacological management of vertigo, *J Neurol Phys Ther* 27:118-121, 2003.

292a. Dieterich M, Bense S, Stephan T et al: fMRI signal increases and decreases in cortical areas during small-field optokinetic stimulation and central fixation, *Exp Brain Res* 148:117-127, 2003.

293. Balaban CD, Thayer JF: Neurological bases for balance-anxiety links, *J Anxiety Disord* 15:53-79, 2001.

294. Balaban CD: Projections from the parabrachial nucleus to the vestibular nuclei: potential substrates for autonomic and limbic influences on vestibular responses, *Brain Res* 16:126-137, 2004.

295. Ledoux JE: Emotion, memory and the brain, *Sci Am* 270:50-57, 1994.

296. Bracha HS, Ralson RC, Williams AE et al: The clenching-grinding spectrum and fear circuitry disorders: clinical insights from the neuroscience/paleoanthropology interface, *CNS Spectr* 10:311-318, 2005.

297. Jones MW, Wilson MA: Phase precession of medial prefrontal cortical activity relative to the hippocampal theta rhythm, *Hippocampus* 15:867-873, 2005.

298. Seamans JK, Yang CR: The principal features and mechanisms of dopamine modulation in the prefrontal cortex, *Prog Neurobiol* 74:321, 2004.

299. Szameitat AJ, Lepsien J, Cramon DY et al: Task-order coordination in dual-task performance and the lateral prefrontal cortex: an event-related fMRI study, *Psychol Res* 2:1-12, 2005.

300. Mishkin M, Appenzeller T: The anatomy of memory, *Sci Am* 256:680, 1987.

301. Alkire MT, Haier RJ, Fallon JH et al: Hippocampal, but not amygdala, activity at encoding correlates with long-term, free recall of nonemotional information, *Proc Natl Acad Sci U S A* 95:14506-14510, 1998.

302. Bluck MA, Myers CE: Psychobiological models of hippocampal function in learning and memory, *Ann Rev Psychol* 48:481-512, 1997.

303. Bunsey M, Eichenbaum H: Conservation of hippocampal memory function in rats and humans, *Nature* 378:255-257, 1996.

304. Cohen NJ, Poldrack RA: Memory for items and memory for relations in the procedural/declarative memory framework, *Memory* 5:131-178, 1997.

305. Eichenbaum H: Declarative memory: Insights from cognitive neurobiology, *Annu Rev Psychol* 48:547-572, 1997.

306. Eichenbaum H: How does the brain organize memories? *Science* 277:330-335, 1998.

307. Helmstaedter C, Grunwalk T, Lehnertz K et al: Differential involvement of left temporolateral and temporomesial structures in verbal declarative learning and memory: evidence from temporal lobe epilepsy, *Brain Cogn* 35:110-131, 1997.

308. Gonsalves BD, Kahn I, Curran T et al: Memory strength and repetition suppression: multimodal imaging of medial temporal cortical contributions to recognition, *Neuron* 47:751-761, 2005.

309. Leutgeb S, Leutgeb JK, Barnes CA et al: Independent codes for spatial and episodic memory in hippocampal neuronal ensembles, *Science* 309:619-623, 2005.

310. Toni N, Buchs PA, Nikonenko I et al: LTP promotes formation of multiple spine synapses between axon terminal and a dendrite, *Nature* 402:421-425, 1999.

311. Postle BR, Desposito M, Corkin S: Effects of verbal and nonverbal interference on spatial and object visual working memory, *Mem Cognit* 33:203-212, 2005.

312. Mohr HM, Linden DE: Separation of the systems for color and spatial manipulation in working memory revealed by a dual-task procedure, *J Cogn Neurosci* 17:355-366, 2005.

313. Barry ES, Naus MJ, Rehm LP: Depression, implicit memory, and self: a revised memory model of emotion, *Clin Psychol Rev* Aug 16, 2005.

314. Forkstam C, Petersson KM: Towards an explicit account of implicit learning, *Curr Opin Neurol* 18:435-441, 2005.

315. Blais C: Concept mapping of movement: related knowledge, *Percept Mot Skills* 76:767-774, 1993.

316. Fang M, Li J, Lu G, Gong X et al: A fMRI study of age-related differential cortical patterns during cued motor movement, *Brain Topogr* 17:127-137, 2005.

317. Maddox WT, Aparicio P, Marchant NL et al: Rule-based category learning is impaired in patients with Parkinson's disease but not in patients with cerebellar disorders, *J Cogn Neurosci* 17:707-723, 2005.

318. Glisky EL: Acquisition and transfer of declarative and procedural knowledge by memory-impaired patients: a computer data-entry task, *Neuropsychologia* 30:899-910, 1992.

319. Tremblay L, Schultz W: Reward-related neuronal activity during go-nogo task performance in primate orbitofrontal cortex, *J Neurophysiol* 83:1864-1876, 2000.

320. Takakusaki K, Takahashi K, Saitoh K et al: Orexinergic projections to the midbrain mediate alternation of emotional behavioral states from locomotion to cataplexy, *J Physiol* 568(pt 3):1003-1020, 2005.

321. Poldrck RA, Gabrieli JDE: Functional anatomy of long-term memory. *J Clin Neurophysiol* 14:294-310, 1997.

322. Reber PJ, Knowlton BJ, Squire LR: Dissociable properties of memory systems: Differences in the flexibility of declarative and nondeclarative knowledge, *Behav Neurosci* 110:861-871, 1996.

323. Snyder E: Stem cells, Salt Lake City, UT, July 18, 2005, III STEP International Conference.

324. Squire LR: The medial temporal lobe memory system, *Science* 253:1380-1386, 1991.

325. Squire LR: Memory and the hippocampus: a synthesis from findings with rats, monkeys, and humans, *Psychol Rev* 99:195-231, 1992.

326. Squire LR, Zola SM: Structure and function of declarative and nondeclarative memory systems, *Proc Natl Acad Sci U S A* 93:13515-13522, 1996.

327. Ongur D, Zalesak M, Weiss AP et al: Hippocampal activation during processing of previously seen visual stimulus pairs, *Psychiatry Res* 139:191-198, 2005.

328. Simpson JR, Ongur D, Akbudak E et al: The emotional modulation of cognitive processing: an fMRI study, *J Cogn Neurosci* 12(2 Suppl):157-170, 2000.

329. Gabrieli JD: Disorders of memory in humans, *Curr Opin Neurol Neurosurg* 6:93-97, 1993.

330. McKee RD, Squire LR: On the development of declarative memory, *J Exp Psychol Learn Mem Cogn* 19:397-404, 1993.

331. Ros J, Pellerin L, Magara F et al: Metabolic activation pattern of distinct hippocampal subregions during spatial learning and memory retrieval, *J Cereb Blood Flow Metab* 26:468-477, 2006.

332. Knopman D: Long-term retention of implicitly acquired learning in patients with Alzheimer's disease, *J Clin Exp Neuropsychol* 13:880, 1991.

333. Lane RM, Potkin SG, Enz A: Targeting acetylcholinesterase and butyrylcholinesterase in dementia, *Int J Neuropsychopharmacol* 9:101-124, 2006.

334. Ge S, Dani JA: Nicotinic acetylcholine receptors at glutamate synapses facilitate long-term depression or potentiation, *J Neurosci* 25:6084-6091, 2005.

335. Muller JE, Koen L, Stein DJ: Anxiety and medical disorders, *Curr Psychiatry Rep* 7:245-251, 2005.

336. Rattiner LM, Davis M, Ressler KJ: Brain-derived neurotrophic factor in amygdala-dependent learning, *Neuroscientist* 11:323-333, 2005.

337. Knight DC, Nguyen HT, Bandettini PA: The role of the human amygdala in the production of conditioned fear responses, *Neuroimage* 26:1193-1200, 2005.

338. Turnbull OH, Evans CE: Preserved complex emotion-based learning in amnesia, *Neuropsychologia* 44:300-306, 2006.

339. Colon K: The healing power of spirituality, *Minn Med* 79:12-18, 1996.

340. Filipini D, Gijsbers K, Birmingham MK et al: Modulation by adrenal steroids in limbic function, *J Steroid Biochem Mol Biol* 39:245-252, 1991.

341. Park H, Quinlan J, Thornton E, Reder LM: The effect of midazolam on visual search: implications for understanding amnesia, *Proc Natl Acad Sci U S A* 101:17879-17883, 2004.

342. Sanchez V, Serrano C, Feldman M et al: Musical memory preserved in an amnesic syndrome [in Spanish]. *Rev Neurol* 39:41-47, 2004.

343. Coull JT, Buchel C, Friston KJ et al: Noradrenergically mediated plasticity in a human attentional neuronal network, *Neuroimage* 10:705-715, 1999.

344. Fetissov SO, Kopp J, Hokfelt T: Distribution of NPY receptors in the hypothalamus, *Neuropeptides* 38:175-188, 2004.

345. Gallinat J, Strohle A, Lang UE et al: Association of human hippocampal neurochemistry, serotonin transporter genetic variation, and anxiety, *Neuroimage* 26:123-131, 2005.

346. Gareri P, De Fazio P, De Sarro G: Neuropharmacology of depression in aging and age-related diseases, *Ageing Res Rev* 1:113-134, 2002.

347. Ogren SO, Schott PA, Kehr J et al: Modulation of acetylcholine and serotonin transmission by galanin: relationship to spatial and aversive learning, *Ann N Y Acad Sci* 863:342-363, 1999.

348. Phan KL, Fitzgerald DA, Cortese BM et al: Anterior cingulate neurochemistry in social anxiety disorder: 1H-MRS at 4 Tesla, *Neuroreport* 16:183-186, 2005.

349. Squire LR, Roberts JL, Spitzer NC et al, editors: *Fundamental neuroscience,* 2003, Elsevier Science.

350. Burgdorf J, Panksepp J: The neurobiology of positive emotions, *Neurosci Biobehav Rev* 30:173-187, 2006.

351. Genazzani AR, Bernardi F, Pluchino N et al: Endocrinology of menopausal transition and its brain implications, *CNS Spectr* 10:449-457, 2005.

352. Hellner K, Walther T, Schubert M et al: Angiotensin-(1-7) enhances LTP in the hippocampus through the G-protein-coupled receptor Mas, *Mol Cell Neurosci* 29:427-435, 2005.

353. Yoneoka Y, Takeda N, Inoue A et al: Acute Korsakoff syndrome following mammillothalamic tract infarction, *AJNR Am J Neuroradiol* 25:964-968, 2004.

354. Malhi GS, Parker GB, Greenwood J: Structural and functional models of depression: from sub-types to substrates, *Acta Psychiatr Scand* 111:94-105, 2005.

355. Ruat M, Traiffort E, Leurs R et al: Molecular cloning characterization and localization of a high-affinity serotonin receptor activating cAMP formation, *Proc Natl Acad Sci U S A* 90:8547-8551, 1993.

356. Menza MA, Golbe LI, Cody RA et al: Dopamine-related personality traits in Parkinson's disease, *Neurology* 43:505-508, 1993.

357. Lindross OF, Leinonen LM, Laakso ML: Melatonin binding to the anteroventral and anterodorsal thalamic nuclei in the rat, *Neurosci Lett* 143:219-222, 1992.

358. American Music Therapy Association/AMTA: *Standards of clinical practice committee news:* http://www.musictherapy.org/membersonly/official/com_standards.html. Accessed October 2, 2005.

359. Astrow AA, Sulmasy DP: Spirituality and the patient-physician relationship, *JAMA* 291:288, 2004.

360. Nelson LA, Schwartz GE: Human biofield and intention detection: individual differences, *J Altern Complement Med* 11:93-101, 2005.

361. Warder SL, Cornelio D, Straughn J et al: Biofield energy healing from the inside, *J Altern Complement Med* 10:1107-1113, 2004.

362. Egnew TR: The meaning of healing: transcending suffering, *Ann Fam Med* 3:255-262, 2005.

363. Barbeau H, Visintin M: Optimal outcomes obtained with body-weight support combined with treadmill training in stroke subjects, *Arch Phys Med Rehabil* 84:1458-1465, 2003.

364. Chen Y, Fetters L, Holt KG, Saltzman EL: Making the mobile move: constraining task and environment, *Infant Behav Dev* 146:1-26, 2002.

365. Duncan P, Studenski S, Richards L et al: Randomized clinical trial of therapeutic exercise in subacute stroke, *Stroke* 34:2173-2180, 2003.

366. Nilsson L, Carlsson J, Danielsson A et al: Walking training of patients with hemiparesis at an early stage after stroke: a comparison of walking training on a treadmill with body weight support and walking training on the ground, *Clin Rehabil* 15:515-527, 2001.

367. Page SJ, Levine P, Leonard AC: Modified constraint-induced therapy in acute stroke: a randomized controlled pilot study, *Neurorehabil Neural Repair* 19:27-32, 2005.

368. Page SJ, Sisto S, Levine P et al: Efficacy of modified constraint-induced movement therapy in chronic stroke: a single-blinded randomized controlled trial, *Arch Phys Med Rehabil* 85:14-18, 2004.

369. Sullivan KJ, Knowlton BJ, Dobkin BH: Step training with body weight support: effect of treadmill speed and practice paradigms on poststroke locomotor recovery, *Arch Phys Med Rehabil* 83:683-691, 2002.

370. Winstein CJ, Rose DK, Tan SM et al: A randomized controlled comparison of upper-extremity rehabilitation strategies in acute stroke: a pilot study of immediate and long-term outcomes, *Arch Phys Med Rehabil* 85:620-628, 2004.

371. Cook SJ: Use of traditional Mi'kmaq medicine among patients at the First Nations community health centre, *Can J Rural Med* 10:95-99, 2005.

372. Coyne C: Addressing spirituality issues in patient interventions, *PT Magazine* 13:38-44, 2005.

373. Daaleman TP, Perera S, Studenski SA: Religion, spirituality, and health status in geriatric outpatients, *Ann Fam Med* 2:49-53, 2004.

374. Harrison MO, Edwards CL: Religiousity/spirituality and pain in patients with sickle cell disease, *J Nerv Ment Dis* 193:250-257, 2005.

375. Weiner D, Burhansstipanov L, Krebs LU et al: From survivorship to thrivership: native peoples weaving a health life from cancer, *J Cancer Educ* 20(1 suppl):28-32, 2005.

376. Groopman J: The critical aspect of "hope" and thus empowerment. In *Anatomy of hope*, New York, 2004, Random House.

377. Lane MR: Spirit body healing-a hermeneurtic study examining the lived experience of art and healing, *Cancer Nurs* 28:285-291, 2005.

378. Perez JC: Healing presence, *Care Manag J* 5:41-46, 2004.

379. Sulmasy DP: A biopsychosocial-spiritual model for the care of patients at the end of life, *Gerontologist* 42:24-33, 2002.

380. Yentegrodt S, Merrick J: Clinical holistic medicine: the patient with multiple diseases, *Sci World J* 5:324-339, 2005.

381. Bishop JP: Retroactive prayer: lots of history, not much mystery, and no science, *BMJ* 329:1444-1446, 2004.

382. Connelly GE: The placebo effect and holistic intervention, *Holist Nurs Pract* 18:238-241, 2004.

383. Miller FG: William James, faith, and the placebo effect, *Perspect Biol Med* 48:273-281, 2005.

384. Rossi EL: Psychosocial genomics: gene expression, neurogenesis, and human experience in mind-body medicine, *Adv Mind Body Med* 18:22-30, 2002.

385. Walach H, Jonas WB: Placebo research: the evidence based for harnessing self-healing capacities, *J Altern Complement Med* 10(1 suppl):S103-S112, 2004.

386. MacPhee M: Medicine for the heart: The embodiment of faith in Morocco, *Med Anthropol* 22:53-83, 2003.

387. Yentegrodt S, Anderson NJ, Merrick J: Holistic medicine, III: the holistic process theory of healing. *Sci World J*3:1138-1146, 2003.

388. Boswell BB, Knight S, Hamer M: Disability and spirituality: a reciprocal relationship with implications for the rehabilitation process, *J Rehabil* 67:20-25, 2001.

389. Delgado C: A discussion of the concept of spirituality, *Nurs Sci Q* 18:157-162, 2005.

390. Faull K, Hills MD, Cochrane G, Gray J et al: Investigation of health perspectives of those with physical disabilities: the role of spirituality as a determinant of health, *Disabil Rehab* 26:129-144, 2004.

391. McColl MA, Bickenbach J, Johnston J et al: Spiritual issues associated with traumatic-onset disability, *Disabil Rehabil* 22:555-564, 2000.

392. Trieschmann RB: Spirituality and energy medicine, *J Rehabil* 67:26-32, 2001.

393. Fallot RD: Recommendations for integrating spirituality in mental health services, *New Dir Ment Health Serv* 80:97-100, 1998.

394. Goddard NC: Spirituality as integrative energy: a philosophical analysis as requisite precursor to holistic nursing practice, *J Adv Nurs* 22:805-815, 1995.

395. Hamilton J: Yes, religion and spirituality do matter in health, *Altern Ther Health Med* 5:18, 1999.

396. Hawks SR, Huyll ML, Thalman RL et al: Review of spiritual health: definition, role, and intervention strategies in health promotion, *Am J Health Promot* 9:371-378, 1995.

397. Karasu TB: Spiritual psychotherapy, *Am J Psychother* 53:143-162, 1999.

398. Kligman E: Alternative medicine, *Iowa Med* 87:232-234, 1997.

399. Koenig HG, Idler E, Kasl S et al: Religion, spirituality, and medicine: a rebuttal to skeptics, *Int J Psychiatr Med* 29:123-131, 1999.

400. Sulmasy DP: Is medicine a spiritual practice? *Acad Med* 74:1002-1005, 1999.

401. www.pubmed.gov.

402. www.pedro.fhs.usyd.edu.au.

403. Baumann N, Kuhl J: Intuition, affect, and personality: unconscious coherence judgments and self-regulation of negative affect, *J Pers Soc Psychol* 83:1213-1223, 2002.

404. Bolte A, Goschke T, Kuhl J: Emotion and intuition, *Psychol Sci* 14:416-421, 2003.

405. Cohen J, Steward I: That's amazing, isn't it? *New Sci* Jan 17, 1998.

406. Courchesme E: Neuroanatomic imaging in autism, *Pediatrics* 87:781-790, 1991.

407. Epstein S, Donovan S, Denes-Raj V: The missing link in the paradox of the Linda problem: beyond knowing and thinking of the conjunction rule, the intrinsic appeal of heuristic processing, *Personality Soc Psychol* 25:204-214, 1999.

408. Goodenough OR, Prehn K: A neuroscientific approach to normative judgment in law and justice, *Philos Trans R Soc Lond B Biol Sci* 359:1709-1726, 2004.

409. Greene JD, Nystrom LE, Engell AD et al: The neural bases of cognitive conflict and control in moral judgment, *Neuron* 44:389-400, 2004.
410. Grotstein JS: The seventh servant: the implications of a truth drive in Bion's theory of "O." *Int J Psychoanal* 85:1081-1101, 2004.
411. Hams SP: A gut feeling? Intuition and critical care nursing, *Intensive Crit Care Nurs* 16:310-318, 2000.
412. Johnson KE, Mervis CB: Impact of intuitive theories on feature recruitment throughout the continuum of expertise, *Memory Cogn* 26:382-401, 1998.
413. Mason A: Bion and binocular vision, *Int J Psychoanal* 81:983-989, 2000.
414. Piha H: Intuition: A bridge to the coenesthetic world of experience, *J Am Psychoanal Assoc* 53:23-49, 2005.
415. Radin DI, Schlitz MJ: Gut feelings, intuition, and emotions: an exploratory study, *J Altern Complement Med* 11:85-91, 2005.
416. Reiner A: Psychic phenomena and early emotional states, *J Anal Psychol* 49:313-336, 2004.
417. Rosanoff N: Intuition comes of age: workplace applications of intuitive skill for occupational and environmental health nurses, *AAOHN J* 47:156-162, 1999.
418. Shirley DA, Langan-Fox J: Intuition: a review of the literature, *Psychol Rep* 79:563-584, 1996.
419. Stitzman L: At-one-ment, intuition and "suchness," *Int J Psychoanal* 85:1137-1155, 2004.
420. Taggart WM, Valenzi E, Zalka L: Rational and intuitive styles: commensurability across respondents' characteristics, *Psychol Rep* 8:23-33, 1997.
421. Ventegodt S, Andersen NJ, Merrick J: Holistic medicine, IV: principles of existential holistic group therapy and the holistic process of healing in a group setting, *Sci World J*3:1388-1400, 2003.
422. Waldinger RJ, Hauser ST, Schulz MS et al: Reading others emotions: the role of intuitive judgments in predicting marital satisfaction, quality, and stability, *J Fam Psychol* 18:58-71, 2004.
423. Rosswurm MA, Larrabee JH: A model for change to evidence-based practice, *Image J Nurs Sch* 31:317-322, 1999.
424. Proceedings of the Symposium on Translating Evidence into Practice. III STEP, Salt Lake City, Utah,. Alexandria, VA, 2006, APTA.
425. Commission for Accreditation of Physical Therapy Education: www.apta.org.
426. Accreditation Commission of Occupational Therapy Education: www.aota.org.
427. Neeck G, Crofford LJ: Neuroendocrine perturbations in fibromyalgia and chronic fatigue syndrome, *Rheum Dis Clin North Am* 26:989-1002, 2000.
428. Shepard NT, Telian SA, Smith-Wheelock M: Habituation and balance retraining therapy: a retrospective review, *Neurologic Clinics.* 8:459-474, 1990.
429. Mallinson AI, Longridge NS: A new set of criteria for evaluating malingering in work-related vestibular injury, *Otol Neurotol* 26:686-690, 2005.
430. Mersenich M: *Neural plasticity: basic mechanisms.* III STEP: Symposium on Translating Evidence into Practice, University of Utah. Salt Lake City, July 17, 2005.

CHAPTER 5

Psychosocial Aspects of Adaptation and Adjustment during Various Phases of Neurological Disability

Gordon U. Burton, PhD, OTR

KEY WORDS

adaptation
adjustment
bonding
coping
family network
loss and grief
problem solving
sensuality
sexuality
support systems

OBJECTIVES

After reading this chapter the student/therapist will be able to:

1. Describe adaptation and adjustment as a flexible and flowing process, not as static stages.
2. Describe elements of the grief process that deal with age, cognition, and developmental level.
3. Respect aspects of sensuality and sexuality in treatment and consider them when treating the client.
4. Integrate the family of the client and the client's styles of coping into therapeutic treatment strategies to be used in the clinic.
5. Integrate the elements of problem solving, loss, cognitive functioning, coping, sensuality, as well as significant others' coping and learning styles into the treatment process to encourage adaptation.

This chapter explores the processes of adjustment and adaptation and the influences of culture and societal values as they affect the physically disabled person. The importance of loss as a psychological component will be examined as it relates to the body, sexuality, the personality, and the family. Age will also be discussed as a factor in adjustment to disability. The importance of focusing on the strengths of the client, the family, and the support system, rather than on the weaknesses of the disability, will also be explored.

This overview is designed to help therapists think of the client as a whole person, not as a diagnosis to be handled in some prescribed way. As fellow human beings, therapist and client are in the rehabilitation process together.

IMPAIRMENT, ACTIVITIES, AND PARTICIPATION

Every individual must adapt and adjust to changes in life on a daily basis. We hope to adjust to the everyday stresses, but there are situations that may overwhelm us. Work stress can create a situation that may stimulate a person who may not have "snapped" to break down and react in what appears to be inappropriate ways.[1] These are all examples of impairments that may result in functional problems in daily life as a result of stress. The advent of a physical limitation may provide the stress that will result in the failure of a person to adjust or adapt and lead to the ability to normally participate in life.

Why worry about adjustment or adaptation? If you have had a major stress in your life, such as the loss of a loved one or a divorce, you may have experienced a lack of concentration or an inability to function effectively. This is a natural experience and a part of life that all people have at some time, but it gives the therapist some minor insight into what a client goes through when confronted with the multiple major stresses that accompany a catastrophic physical disability.

The adjustment process is a dynamic state that is always in process.[2,3] We have some good days and some bad ones (feel good about ourselves or not). When we feel "in balance," we are more productive and are able to incorporate new strategies and concepts into our life. When we are out of balance, we find it hard to accept new concepts or incorporate new activities into our lives. Thus, the therapist must encourage growth and adaptation into the cognitive, emotional, and physical aspects of treatment of the client.[4-6] If these areas are not recognized or encouraged, the client may engage in maladaptive strategies.[7,8] Sometimes it is hard to distinguish between adaptive and maladaptive behaviors. The client may be angry, but this may be good if it stimulates positive strategies for change, or the anger can be used for negative self-defeating behaviors and strategies. Superficial observation may not be enough to distinguish between one and the other. The therapeutic session and the environment should be designed to stimulate positive adaptation for the client and help the client incorporate these strategies into everyday life for the growth of the client and the family.[5,8,9] If this is done, the chances for adherence, participation, and the incorporation of positive changes into the client's life will improve and so will the quality of that life.[2,5,10-13]

Impairments in relation to psychosocial adjustment relate to how the person is able to cope and adapt to the radical changes and demands of the situation.[14] The impairment may be new, such as in the case of brain damage or chemical imbalances, or it may have been premorbid in the case of a person who was just barely functioning before the stress and extra demands of a disability. The underlying problem will result in functional problems and resulting limitations and ability to participate in life. The psychosocial impairment or impairments are very often hard to tease out from the other impairments and activity restrictions in a traumatic event or even from a chronic problem. This, coupled with the fact that the person may have had several impairments or presently has several new impairments or a combination of these, complicates the problem for the therapist, the client, and the family. Think of yourself becoming physically disabled by a spinal cord injury at the C2-3 level. Might you have underlying psychological impairments that may never have been displayed or expressed if you had never been exposed to this stressful experience? The resulting functional disability may limit the person's ability to participate, enjoy, and be productive in life activities.[15] At times it may be hard or impossible to ascertain why specific behaviors are being displayed by the client.[16] Is anger the impairment that results in the disability, or is it the disability that results from another impairment? In some cases the physical disability may have been caused by the impairment, impulsiveness, or anger.

Just looking at a person's behavior will not necessarily tell you the motivation behind it. Some people use anger or religious activities to grow and adapt, and others use it to hide from adaptation. Compliance with therapy can also be a sign of future adaptation or of just going through the paces and not adapting. Unfortunately, if people go through therapy just doing what they have to do ("doing time"), when they get home or stop therapy they may not be able to adapt to the changes in the rest of their lives. Whenever possible, in therapy the functional activity should be presented and structured to promote empowerment, problem solving, and adjustment. Adjustment and adaptation to life is a dynamic process that allows for the person to interact with life in a meaningful and productive way that encourages the person to enjoy life (Figure 5-1).[5,16-20] We see the client at a very stressful time, and we need to make this time as productive for the client and the family as possible.

Psychological Adjustment

In clinical practice, theoretical foundations for adjustment to disability appear to be elusive because they represent a fluid process: all people are constantly changing. This is especially true for people who have recently become physically disabled. They do not reach a certain state of adjustment and stay there but progress through a series of adaptations. Therapists commonly see clients in a crisis state[21-23] and therefore identify their adjustment patterns from this frame of reference. How well the client adjusts to crisis, however, does not necessarily indicate how well the individual will adjust to all aspects of the disability or the rate of progress from one point adaptation to another.[24-31] Disabilities are a massive insult to a person's self-perception.[32,33] A month, or even a year, after the injury may not be long enough to put the disability into perspective.[27,32-35]

For most people, progressing from the shock of injury to the acceptance of, and later adaptation to, disability is a process fraught with psychological ups and downs. Several authors have discussed the possible stages of adjustment and

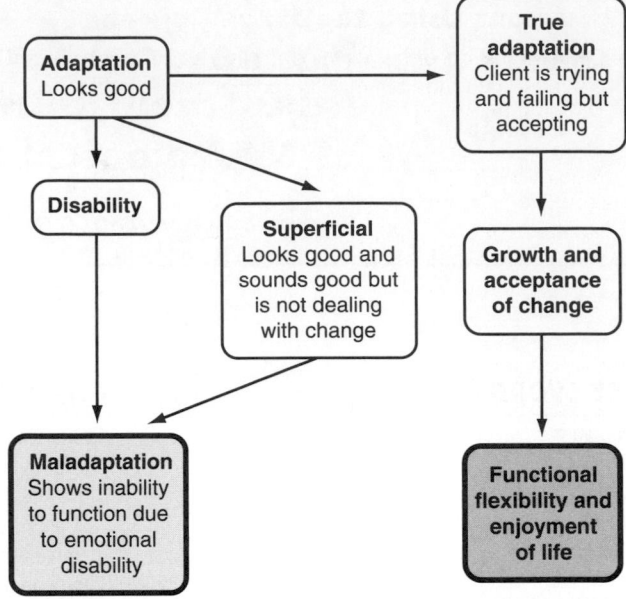

FIGURE 5-1 ■ Possible directions of the adaptive process.

grieving.[27,31] The research of Kubler-Ross[36] into death and dying also has application to this topic of adjustment to disability. She discussed the concept of loss and grief in relation to life; loss of function may result in just as profound a reaction. Peretz[37] and others[38,39] discuss the grieving process in relation to the loss of role function as well as loss of body function. These losses must be grieved for before the client can benefit from therapy or adjust to a changed body and lifestyle. Therapists must be aware that the client can and must deal with the death of certain functional abilities.

The concept of stages of adjustment has been questioned by some,[21,40] and a call for more empirical research into adaptation and adjustment has been made.[41] One alternative concept that has been developed is the cognitive adaptation theory.[42] This concept examines self-esteem, optimism, and control. In this theory, if the individual feels good about self and has an optimistic view of life and a sense of control over life, the individual will adapt to the functional limitations and will participate in life. Cognitive adaptation theory does not consider the organic changes that may take place when brain damage has occurred, but the basic goals are very much worth taking into consideration. These should be examined in relation to the limbic system (see Chapter 4) because limbic involvement is crucial to reaching all goals and plays the key role in establishment of motivation.

The components of successful psychological adjustment to a physical disability (activity limitations) are varied. To bring a client to a level of function that is of the highest quality possible for that individual, therapists must look holistically at the psychosocial aspects and at the adjustment processes involved, evaluate each component, and integrate the processes into the therapeutic milieu to promote growth in all areas. There is more to evaluation and treatment than just the physical component; the mind and body have interrelated influences, and both must be understood, evaluated, and treated individually and as a whole.

Adjustment Using the Stage Concept

Each person has his or her own coping style, and each should be allowed to be unique. Kerr[43] describes five possible stages of adjustment:

Shock: "This really isn't happening to me."

Expectancy for recovery: "I will be well soon."

Mourning: "There is no hope."

Defense: "I will live with this obstacle and beat it." (healthy attitude) "I am adjusted, but you fail to see it." (neurotic attitude)

Adjustment: "It is part of me now, but it is not necessarily a bad thing."

In light of current research, it is important for the therapist to realize that these are not lockstep stages and are to be thought of as concepts to help with the understanding of common reactions of all individuals.[44,45]

Shock

The client in shock does not recognize that anything is actually wrong. He or she may totally refuse to accept the diagnosis. The client may even laugh at the concern expressed by others. This stage is altered when the person has an opportunity to test reality and finds that the physical condition is actually limiting performance. If this stage continues, it may signify either a lack of mental health or an inability to cognitively realize the situation.

Expectancy for Recovery

The client in this stage is aware that he or she is "ill" but also believes that recovery will be quick and complete. The person may look for a "miracle cure" and may make future plans that require total return of function. Total recovery is the only goal, even if it takes a great deal of time and effort to achieve. Key signs of this stage are resentment of loss of function and the feeling that the whole body is necessary to do anything worthwhile. The staff can stimulate a change from this stage by giving clear statements to the client that the damage is permanent, by transferring the person home or to the rehabilitation unit, or by discontinuing therapy. Any one of these occurrences can help make the client realize the permanence of the disability.

Mourning

During the stage of mourning the individual feels all is lost, that he or she will never achieve anything in life. Suicide is often considered. The person may feel that characteristics of the personality (such as courage or fight) have also been lost and must be mourned as well. Thus, motivation to continue therapy, to work on improving, may be absent. The prospect of total recovery can no longer be held, but, at the same time, there appears to be no other acceptable alternative. This feeling of despair may be expressed as hostility, and, as a result, therapists may view the individual as a "problem patient." It is possible for a client to remain at this stage with feelings of inadequacy, dependence, and hostility. However, it is also possible for therapeutic intervention to facilitate movement to the next stage by creating situations in which the client may feel that "normal" aspirations and goals can be achieved. In this circumstance, "normal" would not include such low-level activities as dressing or walking; these are all activities that were taken for granted before the injury, but normal would include doing the work he or she

was trained to do. These activities would also include playing with or caring for a child or family. This would be seen as self-actualization by Maslow.[46]

Defense

The defense stage has two components. The first represents a healthy attitude in which the client actually starts coping with the disability. The client can take pride in his or her accomplishments, work to improve independence, and become as normal as possible. The person is still very much aware that barriers to normal functioning exist and is bothered by this fact but also realizes that some of the barriers can be circumvented. This healthy defensive stage can be undermined and possibly destroyed by well-meaning family, friends, and therapists who encourage the individual to see only the positive aspects and who do not allow the client to examine feelings about the restrictions and barriers of the condition. Conditions that lead to the final stage of adjustment may either be the client realizing that the whole body is not needed to actualize his or her life goals or that needs behind the goals can be actualized in other ways. A therapist should watch for opportunities to facilitate this transition. There is a fine line between hopelessness and hope of regaining function. Taking away any hope of regaining quality of life leads to helplessness and may take away the motivation for neuroplasticity within the patient's central nervous system. Thus, helping the patient be realistic and reality oriented while not taking away hope is a skill all therapists need to develop.

The negative alternative during the defensive stage is the neurotic defensive reaction. The client refusing to recognize that even a partial barrier exists to meeting normal goals typifies this. The client may try to convince everyone that he or she has adjusted.

Adjustment

In the final stage, adjustment, the person sees the disability as neither an asset nor a liability but as an aspect of the person, much like a large nose or big feet. Functional limitation or inability to participate in any life activity is not something to be overcome, apologized for, or defended. Kerr[43] refers to two aspects or goals of this stage. The first goal is for the person to feel at peace with his or her god: the client does not feel that he or she is being punished or tested. The second goal is for the client to feel that he or she is an adequate person, not a second-class citizen. Kerr[47] believes that, "It is essential that the paths to those more 'abstract goals' be structured if the person is to make a genuine adjustment." She also believes that it is the health care professional's job to offer that structure.

Acceptance or adjustment is at least as hard to achieve and maintain in life for the disabled person as happiness and harmony are for all people.[48] Adjustment connotes putting the disability into perspective, seeing it as one of the many characteristics of that person. It does not mean negating the existence of or focusing on the condition. Successful adjustment may be defined as a continuing process in which the person adapts to the environment in a satisfying and efficient manner. This is true for all human beings, able-bodied or disabled. There are always obstacles to overcome in attempting the goal of a happy and successful life.[32,48-50]

People and circumstances change. Maintaining a balanced state of adjustment is not easy, especially for the person with limitations. I recall a woman who had achieved a stable state of acceptance of her quadriplegic condition. One day she called in a panic because, as she saw it, she "wasn't adjusted anymore." She had moved into a college dormitory and wanted to go out for a friendly game of football with her new friends but suddenly saw how physically limited she was. She had grown up in a hospital and had never had to face this situation. After discussing this, she was able to put things into perspective and was able to talk over her feelings of isolation with her friends, who, without hesitation, altered the game to include her. Keeping a balanced perspective is hard in a world that changes constantly.

White[51] stated that without some participation, there can be no affecting the environment and, thus, no sense of self-satisfaction. Fine[52] and King[53] point out that, without satisfaction from affecting the environment, reinforcement is insufficient to carry on the behavior and the behavior will be extinguished. Thus, satisfaction and performance must be linked. If the patient has not adjusted to his or her new body, however, little satisfaction can be gained from such everyday activities as walking, eating, or rolling over in bed.[54] To define adjustment on a purely performance basis is to run the risk of creating a "mechanical person" who might be physically rehabilitated, but, once discharged, may find that he or she lacks satisfaction, incentive, and purpose. The psychological state of adjustment is what makes self-satisfaction possible.

King's Model of the Adaptive Process

The therapist can use the concept of the adaptive process to organize therapy sessions that promote the adjustment process as well as attain physical goals. In so doing, the therapist will be promoting and teaching performance and working toward the eventual achievement, client satisfaction.

King[53] described four characteristics of the adaptive process. They can be worked on singly or simultaneously, and they can be thought of as the means to reach the goal of Kerr's[47] final stage of adjustment. These characteristics are active response, incorporation of the environment, response organized unconsciously, and self-reinforcing adaptation.

Active Response

In general, therapy encourages an active response by the client toward the environment.[9] The client is expected to produce action to improve. Interaction with environmental factors can be seen even if there is little functional ability, as in the case of a client with high-level quadriplegia whose main avenue of interaction is verbal but whose influence can change the environment.

Incorporation of the Environment

Another characteristic of the adaptive process is use of the environment to stimulate adaptive responses.[9,18] An example of this would be setting up a graded walking program that takes the client from a smooth surface, to a rug, and eventually to grassy and rocky terrain. The adaptive process would be enhanced if at the time of discharge the client was not only able but also confident of his or her ability to walk over the lawn to reach the house from the surrounding perimeter.

Response Organized Unconsciously

King[53] believes that an unconsciously organized response is achieved most effectively by directing the client's conscious attention to a task or an object while allowing the subconscious centers to integrate the response. The example in the previous paragraph can be used to illustrate this characteristic. The client's objective (conscious mind) may be set on getting across a lawn to get into her or his house, but the therapist's goal would be to stimulate automatic balance reactions at a subconscious level. Unconscious adaptive responses generalize to other situations more easily than cognitively taught "splinter skill" reactions. As soon as the client cortically attends to balance, the automatic postural changes are, by definition, lost. That is, if the task is procedural, attention needs to be placed on something else while the client practices the activity.

Self-Reinforcing Adaptation

Each successful adaptation stimulates the next more complex step. It is essential for the client to succeed because this success stimulates progression to the next more complex "task." It should be remembered that the "task" is adjustment and that the activity only facilitates adaptation or adjustment. Thus, the therapist does not need to feel disheartened if the client learns to get into and out of his or her house but does not want to start mountain climbing: the goal of the adaptive process is adjustment in as near a normal pattern as possible for that client.

Summary of the Adjustment/Adaptive Process

Combining knowledge of Kerr's stages of adjustment, as outlined previously, with the adaptive process gives the therapist a reality-based, evaluative treatment framework. The stage of adjustment can be assessed, and the adaptive process characteristics can be drawn on in treatment to facilitate progression toward psychological acceptance of the activity limitations as well as to promote physical improvement.

For example, if a person is in the mourning stage of adjustment, the therapist, knowing that the defense stage usually follows, can encourage and support the client's entrance into this next stage by adapting a situation to one that meets the goal of the defense stage—beating the obstacles of physical limitations. The adaptive process may also be used to structure the therapeutic activities that facilitate an active response to overcome the functional physical problems, using the environment to organize the response subcortically in such a way that it is self-reinforcing. For example, the client might want to call his or her spouse, and the therapist may be working cortically on increasing upper extremity strength and wheelchair mobility. The client could be told that the only accessible phone is up a steep ramp and that the client must push the wheelchair up there to use the phone in privacy. The therapist might also add that it always seems that obstacles are in the way for the participation in life and that the client must explore methods to deal with these problems. As the client accomplishes the task, not only will the objectives of strength and wheelchair mobility be realized, the client may start thinking that he or she may be able to beat the effects of the disability, thus moving the client from the mourning stage to the defense stage. No single experience will cause this stage change to happen, but if therapy is designed to encourage adjustment and adaptation, the client will tend to progress faster and with less trauma.

AWARENESS OF PSYCHOLOGICAL ADJUSTMENT IN THE CLINIC, SOCIETY, AND CULTURE

The problem for the therapist in treating a person with a disability is to see the disability in perspective: to see the whole person in the client's own world and in the context of society and a given time. After this difficult task is achieved, the therapist must develop a program that will appropriately stimulate the client and all significant others around the client to pursue the highest-quality life possible. The successful and skilled therapist evaluates the client's physical capabilities but does not stop there. At some level, assessment of the more subtle psychological aspects of the client's ability to function is needed. This includes the client's family network (support system) and its ability to adjust to the imminent change in lifestyle.

Livneh and Antonak[55] have introduced a consolidated way to look at adaptation as a primer for counselors, which should be examined by therapists. They use some of the same basic concepts such as stress, crisis, loss and grief, body image, self-concept, stigma, uncertainty/unpredictability, and quality of life to frame their approach. They also use the concepts of shock, anxiety, denial, depression, anger/hostility, and adjustment in a format that is usable by the therapist.

Livneh and Antonak[55] mention that one of the aspects that the therapist must watch out for is a form of coping called *disengagement*. This style of coping may be demonstrated through denial or avoidance behavior that can take many forms. It can result in substance abuse, blame, or just refusal to interact. Research regarding people with head injuries has demonstrated that, if a premorbid coping style for a person was to use drinking or other drugs, the client may revert to these same styles of coping, which can result in poor physical and emotional rehabilitation.[56] It is important to help the client out of this quagmire. The skills of a therapist may not be enough to do this in the short time that the client is in treatment so a referral to social work, psychology, or psychiatry may be in order. It is still the therapists' job to help promote engagement activities. These activities are behaviors that are goal oriented (patient, family, and therapist driven), problem solving, information seeking, and doing things to positively "beat the condition" and demonstrate independence (promote function).

The rest of this section introduces the reader to some of the psychological change components that may be assessed. The last section will attempt to demonstrate possible ways that these components can be taken into account as an aspect of therapy.

Growth and Adaptation

The therapist must keep in mind the context from which the client is coming. Just days ago the person may have been walking around with no major problems and now is seeing you in your setting. The trauma may be multifaceted:

(1) there was the physical trauma that may have occurred to the client, (2), there was the emotional trauma occurring to the client and the clients' support system, and (3) there was the trauma of each of these systems interacting (the support system trying to protect the client and the client trying to protect the support system). The interaction of these multi-faceted components to one's life may lead to posttraumatic distress syndrome. This syndrome usually happens within the first 6 months after the injury. This syndrome may be observed more often in women[57] but because of cultural barriers it can be hidden in men. This happens more often when there has been a near death situation.[58,59] The client may blame others, try to protect others, or be so self-absorbed that little else in the world may be seen or heard. It may be helpful to get psychological help for the client early in therapy if this is preventing optimal outcomes or creating obstacles in therapy.[60-64]

It is the therapist's job to develop a trusting relationship with the client. Through this relationship the client can be helped to focus on the goals of therapy and work on a positive perspective about the future. One of the errors of the medical system is that of focusing on the disease outcomes and pathology and not on the person and the positive capabilities still within the client's grasp.[65] This focus on the negative or loss may cause the client to see only the injury, disease, or the pathological condition and nothing else. In a Veterans Administration hospital, spouses of people with spinal cord injuries formed a group in which the group's focus was on why the partners got married in the first place; the group never looked at the physical limitations as disabling. After a little while people came to the conclusion that they did not marry their spouses for their legs and the fact that the legs no longer worked was not a major issue after all. This started the decentering from the medical disability model and the focus started to be placed on the people and the families' future. If we can help clients focus on their functions and not their dysfunctions, the effect of therapy after treatment will be much better. More work needs to be done to help clients see the potential they will have in the future to live their lives with the highest quality possible.[66-68] Focusing on the how to participate, move, and function in the world is one of the keys to helping the client and the family work toward its future.[69,70]

The therapist needs to help the client focus on the direction of treatment objectives and to demonstrate how therapy translates into meeting the client's goals.[65] To discover the client's true goals, the therapist must gain the trust of the client and establish sound lines of communication. Distrust from health professionals may obstruct the adjustment process and lead to negative consequences.[71] Whenever possible, the client's support system should be enlisted to help establish realistic support for the client and the goals of both the client and the family. It has been found that if the client trusts the health professional that the client will be more adherent and will seek assistance when it is needed[72,73] (see Chapter 4 for additional information).

Societal and Cultural Influences

Culture, subcultures, and the culture and beliefs of the given family are all aspects of the client that the therapist must attend to.[4,70,74,75] This concept gets into the beliefs about the world and maybe a belief about the cause of the disability or at least how the client is viewing the disability. Asking "why do you think this happened to you?" can lead to an enlightening experience. "Causes" may range from "God is punishing me" to "I deserved it" to "life is against me."

From an early age, people in our society are exposed to misconceptions regarding the disabled person.[76-78] If in the therapeutic environment, however, the client and family have their misconceptions challenged constantly, they may start reformulating their concept of the role of the disabled person. As this process progresses, therapists and other staff can help make the expectations of the disabled person more realistic. Therapists can schedule their clients at times when they will be exposed to people making realistic adjustments to disabilities. Use of individuals who have attained successfully rehabilitated as staff members (role models) can help to dispel the misconception that people with disabilities are not employable.[79-81]

This process of adaptation to a new disability can be considered as a cultural change from a majority status (able bodied) to a minority status (disabled). Part of the adaptation process can be considered as an acculturation process, and the therapist can help facilitate this process.[32,78,82,83]

The cultural background of the individual also contributes to the perception of disability and to the acceptance of the disabled person. Trombly[84] states that perception and expression of pain, physical attractiveness, valuing of body parts, as well as acceptability of types of disabilities can be culturally influenced. One's ethnic background can also affect intensity of feelings toward specific handicaps, trust of staff,[84] and acceptance of therapeutic modalities.[16,85-87]

The successful therapist will be sensitive to the cultural values of the client and will attempt to present therapy to the client in the most acceptable way. For example, in the Mexican culture it is not polite to just start to work with a client; rapport must first be established. Sharing of food may provide the vehicle to accomplish rapport. Thus, the therapist might schedule the first visit with a Mexican client during a coffee break. The therapist must remember that the dysfunctional client may be the one who can least be expected to adjust to the therapist and that the therapist may need to adjust to the client, especially in the early stages of therapy.

Gaining trust is one of the crucial links in any meaningful therapeutic situation.[73,88] Trust will create an environment that facilitates communication, productive learning, and exchange of information.[80] Trust is important in all cultures and will be fostered by the therapist who is sensitive to the needs of the client. This sensitivity is necessary with every client but will be manifested in many different ways, depending on the background and needs of the individual in therapy. A client of one culture may feel that looking another person in the eyes is offensive, whereas in another culture refusal to look into someone's eyes is a sign of weakness or lack of honesty (shifty eyed).[89] Thus, although it is impossible to know every culture or subculture with which the therapist may come into contact, the therapist must attempt to be sensitive to the background of the client. Even if the therapist knows the cultural norms, not every person follows the cultural patterns, and thus every client needs to be treated as an individual in the therapeutic relationship. It should be the therapist's job to be sensitive to the subtle nonverbal and verbal cues that indicate the level of trust in the relationship. The therapist will obtain this information by being open to the client, not open to a textbook. The client is the owner of this information and will share it with everyone he or she trusts.

Trust is often established in the therapeutic relationship through physical activities. The act of asking a client to transfer from the chair to the bed can either build trust or destroy the potential relationship. If the client trusts the therapist just enough to follow instructions to transfer but then falls in the process, it may take quite some time to reestablish the same level of trust, assuming that it can ever be reestablished. This trusting relationship is so complex and involves such a variety of levels that the therapist should be as aware of attending to the client's security in the relationship as to the physical safety of the client in the clinic.[73,88] If the client believes that the therapist is not trustworthy in the relationship, then it may follow that the therapist is not to be trusted when it comes to physical manipulation of a disabled body. If the client does not know how to use the damaged physical body and thus cannot trust the body, then lacking trust in the therapist will only compound the stress of the situation.[73,88] Chapter 9 provides more information on the neurological components of this interaction during the interventions process.

The client's culture may be alien to the therapist, even though both the clinician and client may be from the same geographical region. A client's problems of poverty, unemployment, and a lack of educational opportunities[81,90] can all result in the therapist and client feeling that therapy will be unsuccessful, even before the first session has begun. Such preconceived concepts held by both parties may not be warranted and must be examined. These preconceived concepts can be more reflective of failure of rehabilitation than any physical limitation of the client.

Cultural and religious values may also result in the client feeling that he or she must pay for past sins by being disabled and that the disability will be overcome after atonement for these sins. Such a client may not be inclined to participate in or enjoy therapy. The successful therapist does not assault the client's basic cultural or religious values but may recognize them in the therapy sessions. If the therapist feels that the culturally defined problems are impeding the therapeutic process, the therapist may offer the client opportunities to reexamine these cultural "truths" and may help the client redefine the way the physical limitations and therapy is seen.[91] Religious counseling could be recommended by the therapist, and follow-up support in the clinic may be given to the client to view therapy not as undoing what "God has done" but as a way of proving religious strength. Reworking a person's cultural/religious (cognitive) structure is a sensitive area, and it should be handled with care and respect and with the use of other professionals (social workers and religious and psychological counselors) if needed.

The hospital staff can be encouraged to establish groups in which commonly held values of clients can be examined and possibly challenged.[32,50,91-96] Such groups can lead the client to a better understanding of priorities and may help the person see the relevance of therapy and the need to continue the adjustment process. This can also prepare the client to better accept the need for support groups after discharge. The therapist may be able to use information from such group sessions to adjust the way therapy sessions are presented and structured to make therapy more relevant to the client's values and needs. Value groups or exercises[97] can be another means used by the therapist for evaluation and understanding of the client.

Beliefs and values of cultures and families can play a profound role in the course of treatment. Such things as physical difficulties, which can be seen, are usually better accepted than problems that cannot be seen, such as brain damage that changed an individual's cognitive abilities or personality.[98] A person with a back injury may be seen as lazy where a person with a double amputation will be perceived as needing help. At the same time a person who has lost a body part, in some cultures, may be seen as "not all there" and should be avoided socially. Thus being attuned to the culture and beliefs of the client is imperative in therapy. The reader is encouraged to refer to texts on cultural issues in health care such as *Culture in Clinical Care* by Bonder, Martin, and Miracle[99]; *Cultural Competence in Health Care: A Practical Guide* by Rundle, Carvalho, and Robinson[100]; and *Caring for Patients from Different Cultures* by Galanti[101] for more detailed discussions on how culture and beliefs affect health care.

Body Image

Body image is an all-encompassing concept that looks at how the person and to some extent, the support systems view the person and roles that are expected to be assumed. Taleporos and McCabe[34] found that clients had negative feelings about their bodies and general negative psychological experiences after injury. Even when clients do not have disfigurements that are readily observable, they often still report changes in body image and negative feelings of self-worth.

One of the issues that may arise relating to body image is sexuality. This concept may take many behavioral forms: flirting, harassment, questions about fertility, or questions regarding whether the client is capable of performing the sex act at all. Flirting may be a sign that clients have had assaults on their femininity or masculinity. By flirting, clients are often trying to determine whether they still are seen as a sensual being. In this case a therapist may let the client down lightly by saying that he or she is not allowed to date or flirt with clients. This is to make sure that the client does not think that it is something about the disability that is the "turn off." Sensitivity should be used because the client could think that "if a medical person finds me repulsive then no one will ever see me as attractive." It is important for the therapist to try to ascertain the intent behind the behavior. Usually this can be accomplished by evaluating how he or she feels about the interaction. If the therapist feels unthreatened and does not feel demeaned when the client is flirting, he or she still needs to report this to the therapist of record. If the therapist feels defensive, demeaned, or very uncomfortable, then he or she may be experiencing harassment. The therapist should never be harassed on the job, and this client's behavior should be stopped immediately by telling the client that the behavior is making the therapist feel uncomfortable and that it should stop now. Again, the therapist should go to the supervisor or team to mention this behavior. If the behavior is considered a chronic problem by the staff, a treatment plan should be designed to stop the behavior. It is important to remember that sexual health should not be a neglected area of client treatment. It may take time for the appropriate questions to be asked by the client.[102,103]

Questions about any physical performance are within the domain of therapy. If the client is asking for information regarding positioning during sex it is an area that needs to be dealt with. If the questions are regarding fertility and the like, then these should be referred to an appropriate medical person. None of these questions should be discouraged or neglected because this area is important for your clients' motivation and sexual health.[104,105] It is important for the therapist to know that in spinal cord injury, fertility will generally not be impaired for the woman, but issues of lubrication before sex should be addressed by the appropriate person. Men may have erection problems and ejaculation issues, but this too can be addressed by the appropriate person. It is now thought that fertility in spinal cord–injured men may be dealt with and should not be ruled out.[106-108]

Establishment of Self-Worth and Accurate Body Image

Self-worth is composed of many aspects, such as body image, sexuality, and the ability to help others and to affect the environment. The body image of a client is a composite of past and present experiences and of the individual's perception of those experiences. Because body image is based on experience, it is a constantly changing concept. An adult's body image is substantially different from that which he or she held as a child and will no doubt change again as the aging process continues. A newly disabled person is suddenly exposed to a radically new body, and it is that individual's job to assess the body's sensations and capabilities and develop a new body image. Because the therapist is at least partially responsible for creating the environmental experiences from which the client learns about this new body, the therapist should be aware of the concept. In the case of an acute injury, the client has a new body from which to learn. The therapist can promote positive feelings as the therapist instructs the client how to use this new body and to accept its changes.*

Because in "normal" life we slowly observe changes in our bodies, such as finding one gray hair today and watching it take years for our hair to turn totally white, we have the luxury of slowly adapting to the "new me." This change usually does not happen quite so slowly and "naturally" when confronted with trauma or a disease that affects the central nervous system. This sudden loss of function creates a void that only new experiences and new role models can fill.

The loss of use of body parts can cause a person to perceive the body as an "enemy" that needs to be forced to work or to compensate for its disability. In all cases the body is the reason for the disability and the cause of all problems. The need for appliances can create a sense of alienation and lack of perceived "lovability" resulting from the "hardness of the hardware." People tend to avoid hugging someone who is in a wheelchair or who has braces around the body because of the physical barrier and because of the person's perceived fragility; a person with physical limitations is certainly not perceived as soft and cuddly.[34,39,70,101,109] Both the perception that these individuals are not lovable and their labored movements can sap the energy of the disabled and discourage social interaction or life participation. To accept the appliances and the dysfunctional body in a way that also

---

*References 21, 32, 34, 39, 109, 110.

allows the disabled person to feel sexy and sensual is surely a major challenge.

In the case of a person who will be disabled for the long term, such as the person with cerebral palsy or Parkinson's disease, the therapist is attempting to teach the client how to change the previously accepted body image to one that would allow and encourage more normal function. In short, the therapist has two roles. One role is to take away the disabled body image of such a disabled person. The second is the opposite sequence, that is, to teach a functional disabled body image to a newly disabled person. The techniques may be the same, but in both cases the client will have to undergo a great amount of change. The person with a chronic illness has based his or her life on the concept that the reason for not accomplishing many things was the disability. If the therapist can change the client's functional ability level, the individual must now change self-expectations. Similarly the newly disabled person must now also change expectations; however, he or she has little concept of what is realistic to expect of this new body. At this point, role models can be used to help shape the client's expectations. If the client does not adjust to this new body and change his or her body image and self-expectations, life will be impoverished for that individual. Pedretti[111] states that the client with low self-esteem often devalues his or her whole life in all respects, not just in the area of dysfunction.*

One way the client can start exploring this new body is by exploring it for sensation and performance. The client with a spinal cord injury may touch the whole body to see how it reacts.[114] For example, is there a way to get the legs to move using reflexes? What, if anything, stimulates an erection or lubrication? Can positioning the legs in a certain way aid in rolling the wheelchair or make spasms decrease? Such exploration will start the client on the road to an informed evaluation of his or her abilities.

The therapist's role is to promote expansion of the client's realistic perceptions of body functioning. Exercises can be developed that encourage exploration of the body by the individual and, if appropriate, the significant partner. Functioning and building an appropriate body image will be more difficult if intimate knowledge of the new body is not as complete as before injury.[26] The successes the client experiences in the clinical setting coupled with the client's familiarity with his or her new body will result in a more accurate body image and will contribute to the client's feelings of self-worth.

The last aspect of self-worth is often overlooked in the health fields. This aspect is the need that people have to help others.[13] People often discover that they are valuable through the act of giving. Seeing others enjoy and benefit from the individual's presence or offering increases self-worth. Situations in which others can appreciate the client's worth may be needed. Unless the client can contribute to others, the client is in a relatively dependent role, with everyone else giving to him or her without the opportunity of giving back. Achieving independence and then reaching out to others, with therapeutic assistance if necessary, facilitates the individual's more rapid reintegration into society. The therapist should take every opportunity to allow the client to express self-worth to others through helping.

---

*References 3, 28, 33, 34, 112, 113.

Hope and Spiritual Aspects

The process of hope can be a generalized and positive force to reduce depression, the sense of powerlessness, and grief.[115] Clients need a realistic sense of hope. The question of what is realistic is always open to interpretation. I had a client with tetraplegia who was a deer hunter. He swore he would go to the mountains in the fall and shoot a deer. All of the staff knew that he was not being realistic, but in the fall he came in with venison from the deer he shot. There was a client on the East Coast with tetraplegia who said when he left the hospital he would drive to the West Coast to live. The staff laughed about this, but sure enough, he was discharged and drove to the West Coast to live. It is hope that keeps most of us going in life. Hope is not always realistic. How many people really believe that they will win the lottery, if not this time, then maybe the next? Sometimes it is this hope that saves us from being overwhelmed by the other realities of life. Try not to take all of the client's hope away. They may win the lottery, shoot a deer, or drive to another part of the world.

Spirituality is something that provides hope, connection with others, and reason or meaning of existence for many (if not most) people. It is amazing that the medical community has been slow to accept the power of spirituality because this is an area that gives meaning to so many peoples' lives. Spirituality has been linked to health perception, a sense of connection with others, and well-being.[116-122] Anything that helps the client put the disability into perspective and helps the client move on with life in a healthy way is good. The Western medical system is based on pathology and focuses on that. Therapy focuses on functional activities, participation in life, and behavioral change, which is productive. One of the dangers of the medical system is the entrapment in pathology to the point that the client may not see anything but pathology. Spirituality may help the client and the family to see that there is more to life than pathology, stimulate interaction with others, put the functional limitations in perspective, give meaning to life (and the disability), and give the person hope and a since of well-being.[116,118,119] This is what we all want for the client and the family.

Awareness of Sexual Issues

Sexuality is usually one of the last areas to be assessed by clinical staff, but it is one area mentioned as having great importance to family members and the client.[3,110,113,123] Sexuality involves more than just the sex act; it incorporates characteristics such as sexual attraction, sexual identification, sexual confidence, and sexual validation.[3,110,113,123] It is a predictor of adjustment to disability, of success in vocational training, and of marital satisfaction when the woman is disabled.[113,123]

Sexuality (sensuality) is representative of how the person is dealing with his or her world. If the person feels inadequate as a sexual, sensual, and lovable human being, there is little chance that the person will also feel motivated to pursue other avenues of life.[113,123,124] This area of function must be assessed with great sensitivity to the individual's feelings.[54,124,125]

The framework for assessing sexuality differs with the therapist. Some therapists see sexuality as an activity of daily living and incorporate it into this evaluation. Others feel the client needs information about body mechanics to perform the sex act; thus, positioning and reflex inhibiting patterns are assessed. Still others have found it a motivating force when range of motion and muscle control are worked on. A further discussion of these concerns follows in the section on adult sexuality.

Development of Sensuality (Sexuality)

Even before birth, the sense of touch[126] and the ability to distinguish pleasurable and unpleasurable tactile sensations begin to develop. Pleasurable feelings are comforting, and attempts are made to prolong them; for example, a baby cries when nursing is stopped. If satisfaction is not derived from this interaction on a regular basis, a feeling of anxiety may develop and the child may withdraw from interaction with others and distrust may develop.[126] If pleasure in interaction with others is obtained in the first 3 years, the ability to maintain the warmth of being close and being nourished is translated into trust (that all needs will be satisfied by the caretaker) and lovability (bonding). It is here that a sense of intimacy is initiated.[114,127] Ego and sensuality are refined as the child develops the ability to stimulate and satisfy itself. By the age of 5 years, the ability to explore the world by using the hands and mouth, as well as other parts of the body, allows the person to develop communication, self-gratification, and a feeling of competence.[51,114,127]

This feeling of competence is derived from the effective use of the body to make itself feel good and to accomplish tasks. By the age of 8 years, body parts and body processes are usually named and the child perceives the body as good. At this time intimacy between the self and another person is further refined, as are roles. During puberty, body changes and sexual tension are heightened. Self-acceptance is based on the person's perception of how effectively he or she has accomplished the previous tasks.[114,127-129]

The preceding is an oversimplification of the first 20 years of life, but the role of sensuality and sensation cannot be overemphasized. This is especially true for those professionals who constantly interact with clients in a physical manner such as handling. The intervention the therapist provides when the client is, or feels he or she is, in a dependent state can have direct impact on how the client may perceive himself or herself in the future.

Pediatric Sensuality

The child needs to learn to enjoy the body. The therapist should help the client to distinguish between therapeutic touch and "fun" sensual touch, such as tickling or cuddling. It is important for clients to distinguish between the two so that they do not "turn their bodies off" to touch. For example, a woman with cerebral palsy stated during an interview that therapy was either painful or so clinical that she disassociated herself from sensations in her body during therapy. Later in life this became a problem when she was married. She stated that it took 7 years of marriage before she could enjoy the sensations of being touched by her husband. She also stated that it was a revolutionary concept for her that a vibrator could be used to give pleasure rather than just therapy.

The therapy session should also help the client develop a sense of personal ownership of the body.[3,85,130] This aspect is often neglected when working with children.[85,127] The therapist often does not ask permission to touch a client, thus suggesting that the client lacks the right to control being touched by others. The last thing the therapist would desire to communicate, especially to a child, is that any person has the right to handle and touch the client's body. Child molestation with a disabled population is just beginning to be recognized as a problem in this country, with possibly one third of the female and male population being victimized.[85] It is hard to think of a more likely victim than a person who has (unintentionally) been taught that he or she does not have the right to say "No" to being touched and who cannot physically resist unwanted advances and in some cases cannot even communicate that abuse has taken place. The effects of this can be seen in adults. When one client was asked why tone increased in her lower extremities when she was touched, her response was, "I was sexually abused by my father in the name of therapy, and therapy and sexual abuse are synonymous at this point." No wonder she had been resistant to reentering therapy!

One way of helping clients "own" their respective bodies (besides asking permission to touch) is by naming body parts and body processes using correct terminology (as opposed to baby talk), thus making it possible for the client to communicate and relate appropriately.[85,127,130,131] This can be accomplished as the need arises, or it can be encouraged through the use of anatomically correct puzzles or dolls during therapy sessions.

One goal of therapy may be to develop the concept that the body (in the case of persons with the congenital disabilities) or the "new body" (in the case of those with acquired disabilities) is acceptable and good,[127-131] thus giving the client a more positive attitude toward his or her body and toward therapy. Pointing out a particularly positive aspect of the client's body and mentioning this regularly can encourage this attitude. This feature could be the hair, eyes, or a smile, but it should be an aspect of the client that can be seen and commented on by others as well. Commenting on how well the body feels when it is relaxed or how good the sun feels on the body helps the client recognize that the body can be a positive source of pleasure.

Another message that can affect the client in later life is the concept that individuals with movement dysfunction are asexual and will never have sexual needs or partners.[129-133] Although it may not be appropriate to deal directly with the concept in therapy with a child, the therapist might mention that he or she knows of a person with a functional problem, such as the client's movement limitations, who is married or who has children. In this way the therapist communicates that there is a possibility that the "normal" sex roles of the child may be fulfilled in the future. Without this possibility being presented, the child may think that there is no chance that all the movies, books, and television programs that deal with normal adult interactions apply to individuals with functional limitations, a belief that leads to poor socialization and further alienation from participating in life.[114,130,131,133,134]

Adult Sexuality

Discussing positioning to reduce pain and spasticity or to enable the client to more comfortably engage in sexual relations will help the client deal with problems before they reveal themselves. Because sexual hygiene may be considered as an activity of daily living, it may fall within the domain of therapy.

The client may feel that his or her sexual identity is threatened by a newly acquired disability and may try to assert sexuality through jokes, flirting, or even passes toward the therapist. In these cases it is important for the therapist to realize that what is often being looked for is the confirmation that the client is still a sexual and sensual human being; thus, the therapist's response is very important.[114,130,131,133,134] If the therapist rejects or even ridicules the client, it may be a very long time before the client can even think of attempting such a confirmation of personal attractiveness. The client may feel that because the therapist rejects the client and the therapist is familiar with the disabled, there is little chance anyone who is not familiar with the disabled could accept the client as lovable.[135] The therapist should not be surprised by such advances and should deal with the situation in a professional manner. The therapist should also realize that approximately 10% of the population is homosexual and be prepared for advances from clients of the same sex. The therapist may need to remember that the therapist should not attempt to change the client's sexual orientation nor be offended but instead be as professional in dealing with this client as with any other. All of the therapist's interactions should be directed toward creating an environment that will promote a stronger and more well-adjusted client.[114,130,131,133]

The therapist's response to sexual advances must be tempered with an understanding of the possible cause for the behavior. The client may be cognitively impaired and may not even be aware of the inappropriateness of some forms of sexual behavior, or the client may be trying to control others through acting-out behaviors. The client may have been sexually aggressive even before the injury. At no time should the therapist allow himself or herself to be sexually harassed. If the therapist feels harassed, the therapist must take control of the situation and find a way to stop the client's behavior. This is usually achieved by confronting the issue. Not dealing with inappropriate behavior will allow it to continue and may be detrimental to the medical team and to the client's normal participation in life.[103,113,130,131]

The therapist can assist the client in moving through the stages of self-awareness to appreciate that the client is still sensual, sexual, and huggable. This process can be done through everyday interaction; it may entail encouraging the family to embrace the client and may even call for the therapist to role model these behaviors at times.[134] The therapist may provide reading materials to the client and family directly by reviewing and answering questions or indirectly by having such books as *Reproductive Issues for Persons with Physical Disabilities*,[135] *Sexuality and the Person with Traumatic Brain Injury: A Guide for Families*,[136] and *Sexual Function in People with Disability and Chronic Illness*,[137] available for their reading. In this way, the individual and significant others are made aware of possible options for the expression of intimacy and of the fact that this part of life is not over.

Because the therapist is in a situation of one-to-one treatment involving touching, moving, and handling the client's body, he or she may frequently be the natural person from whom the individual may seek information. If this natural curiosity does not appear to be forthcoming, however, the therapist can give the client an opening. For example, during an evaluation of motor skills, the person may be asked if there are any problems in such areas as sexual positioning. The topic need not be pursued any further by the therapist, but when the client is ready to deal with the subject area, he or she will probably remember that the therapist brought it up and may be a person to approach when dealing with these issues.[124,130,138]

Other ways of presenting sexual information are to have literature available on the client's ward so that those who are interested may pursue the topic in private, to have a group discussion (interested clients, clients and significant others, or whatever group the client and therapist might choose to assemble), or to have literature in the department waiting room.

It is important for the therapist to be aware of some of the aspects of sexuality that may or may not affect the client as a result of trauma or disease. Fertility is seldom affected in women.[10,139,140] Men, on the other hand, may experience dysfunction of the penis and testicles and/or fertility.[141-143] Devices may be used and adapted to allow for sexual gratification of the client (masturbation) or significant others. Stimulant drugs such as sildenafil citrate (Viagra) or other aids may be used to enhance a person's sex life. Safe sex is even more of a problem for clients who may be inclined to get infections,[135] especially in or around the genitals, because this may provide an avenue for transmission of disease. Sensation should be checked and sexual activities modified (or the client should be alerted to the problem) to avoid breakdowns or medical complications. Positioning modifications may be needed to allow for better energy conservation, joint protection, motor control, maintenance of muscle and skin integrity, and pleasure. Clients may have questions regarding modifications that may be needed for the use of birth control devices or contraindications regarding the use of such devices. Clients may also need equipment (e.g., vibrators) modified if hand function is involved. Complications that may affect function and mobility of the client may arise as a result of pregnancy. Delivery may present some unique situations that may also need to be dealt with. After delivery the disabled parent may require modifications to the wheelchair or consultations may be needed to achieve an optimal level of function in the parenting role. All of these possibilities point to the fact that sexual issues must be dealt with throughout the treatment of all individuals with disabilities whether the functional limitations are progressive, stable, or correctable.[10,135,144] The therapist may approach these needs or aspects of function while taking a client's sexual history. Clients have repeatedly called for more attention to be paid to sexual concerns. This is not sex counseling or therapy, and the therapist should not try to deal with deep psychosexual issues. The therapist should be informed and should provide information that relates to the therapist's areas of expertise, especially because other medical personnel may not have the knowledge to correctly analyze the components of some of these activities.[135,145,146]

Any of these issues may present themselves during the medical screening phase of evaluation while others become issues as the patient is adjusting to and questioning functional limitations caused by the disease or condition. Once the patient has identified need of this information, the therapist whether through referral, group work, or individual discussions needs to address the questions and should not deny the patient answers because the therapist is uncomfortable.

All the clinical problem areas that need assessment and evaluation and that have been mentioned previously are examined in relation to treatment planning in the clinical setting in the following sections.

Support System

Earlier literature hinted that partner relationships may be negatively affected by a member being disabled. Within the last 5 years this concept has been questioned in regard to some disabilities such as adult-onset spinal cord injuries,[146] whereas pediatric spinal cord injury and other disabilities may result in relationship problems.[147,148] It has been shown that adjustment and quality of life can be adversely affected by the physical environment being inadequate, thus making the person more dependent. The result of the dependence appears to be poor relationships.[149-151] This can also be seen with the families in which a member has had a brain injury.[152] In studies on muscular dystrophy it was found that physical dependence is not the only variable needing to be considered. Psychological issues need to be identified and considered as part of intervention.[153,154] Recent literature has identified a number of elements that the client and the family may need help to work on, such as "to assist them to develop new views of vulnerability and strength, make changes in relationships, and facilitate philosophical, physical and spiritual growth".[154] Turner and Cox[154] also felt that the medical staff could facilitate the following: "recognizing the worth of each individual, helping them to envision a future that is full of promise and potential, actively involving each person in their own care trajectory, and celebrating changes to each person's sense of self."[154] Man[155] observed that each family copes differently in relation to a brain-injured family member and that the family's structure should be explored to develop intervention guidelines. It has also been noted that health care professionals should view the situation from the family's perspective to approach and support the family's adaptation.[156] This should be done to help the client and the family accept the disability but at the same time to help them keep the negative views of society in perspective.[157] In general, it has also been found that family support is a significant factor in the client's subjective functioning[158,159] and that social engagement is productive.[90,160]

When dealing with children it is important to realize that they often feel responsible for almost anything that happens in life, such as divorce, siblings' getting hurt, or general arguments between parents. It is important that the therapist helps the client and the siblings realize that they are not responsible for the client's condition. Part of this magical thinking that often appears is the concept that "bad things happen to bad people." Thus, the child is bad because a bad thing has happened or the adult is bad just because the disease or trauma has occurred. It is important to be sensitive to this ideation and help dispel this maladaptive thought pattern because it is not true or productive for the client, the siblings, parents, or spouses within a family and may cause further adjustment problems later in treatment. Siblings of the client should be helped to see their roles as good siblings and should not be placed in the role of caretakers of a sibling

with special needs. In this way all children can grow naturally without any one of the children being overly focused on. At the same time, it is a fact of life that the disabled child will probably need physical assistance, therapy, increased medical care, and thus, more time devoted to him or her and this is just a fact of life.

It should always be noted by the medical establishment that having a disability is expensive in ways that we are often not aware of. There are the obvious medical costs of therapy, surgery, drugs, wheelchairs, or orthoses, but there are other costs such as the possibility of extra cost of transportation, catheters for urination, wheelchair maintenance, adaptive clothing, and the like that are continuing costs not covered by most insurance plans. These costs add up and contribute to the emotional costs and demands on the family. The significant others may feel the need to work more to have the money to cover such expenses, but then that person is not around to help out. This is but one of the many dilemmas that must be dealt with for the support system of the disabled person. The family may be encouraged to contact such groups as the Family Caregiver Support Network (www.caregiversupportnetwork.org) to get information and assistance with such diverse topics as being a caregiver, legal and financial aid, and communications (this group tends to focus on the adult but still may be a wonderful aid). Such groups will give information to all who need it and help to empower the family. This takes the focus off of the medical condition and may help the family to gain a better more balanced perspective on the condition.

Loss and the Family

In this chapter, the client's support system is referred to as the family. The family may be composed of spouses, parents, children, lovers (especially in gay and lesbian relationships), friends, employers, or interested others such as church groups, civic organizations, or individuals. The people in the support system may go through the same stages of reaction and adjustment to loss that the client does.[21,26,52,161-163]

Family Needs

The family will, at least temporarily, experience the loss of a loved member from the normal routine. During the acute stage the family may not have concrete answers to basic questions regarding the extent of injury, the length of time before the injured person will be back in the family unit, or possibly whether the person will live.

During this phase, the family network will be in a state of crisis.[26] New roles will have to be assumed by the family members, and the "experts" will not even tell them for how long these roles must be endured. If children are involved, they will probably demand more attention to reassure themselves that they will remain loved. Depending on the child's age, the child will have differing capabilities in understanding the loss (see the section on examination of loss). Each member of the family may react differently to bereavement, and each may be at a different stage of adjustment to the disability (see the section on adjustment). One member may be in shock and deny the disability, whereas another member is in mourning and verbalizes a lack of hope. The family crisis that is caused by a severe injury cannot be overstated.[97,162-165]

Role changes in the family may be dramatic.[50,74,79,166-168] Members who have never driven may need to learn that motor skill; one who has never balanced a checkbook may now be responsible for managing the family budget; and those who have never been assertive may have to deal forcefully with insurance companies and the medical establishment.[11,26,72,133,169]

The family may feel resentment toward the injured member. This attitude may seem justified to them because they see the person lying in bed all day while the family members must take over new responsibilities in addition to their old ones. The medical staff may not always understand the stress that family members are under and may react to the resentment expressed either verbally or nonverbally with a protective stance toward the client. Siding with the "hurt" client may alienate the family from the medical staff and may also drive a permanent wedge between family members. This long-term situation may undermine the compliance of family members' involvement in home programs and ultimately the successful outcome of long-term intervention.

Parental Bonding and the Disabled Child

The parent bonding process is complicated and is still being studied.[170] The process may start well before the child is even conceived. The parents often think about having a child and plan and fantasize about future interactions with the child; after conception the planning and fantasizing increase. During the pregnancy the mother and father accept the fetus as an individual, and after the birth of the child the attachment process is greatly intensified. The "sensitive period" is the first few minutes to hours after the birth. During this time the parents should have close physical contact with the child to strongly establish the attachment that will later grow deeper.[171,172] There is an almost symbiotic relationship between mother and child at this time: infant and mother behaviors complement each other (e.g., nursing stimulates uterine contraction). It is important at this point for the child to respond to the parents in some way so that there is an interaction. In the early stages of bonding, seeing, touching, caring for, and interacting with the child allow for the bonding process. When this process is disturbed for any reason, such as congenital malformations or hospital procedures for high-risk infants, problems may occur later.

When the parents are told that their child is going to be malformed or disabled, it is a massive shock. The parents must start a process of grieving. The dream of a "normal" child must be given up, and the parents must go through the loss or "death" of the child they expected before they can accept the new child. Parents often feel guilty. Shellabarger and Thompson[173] state that parents feel the deformed child was their failure.[21] Fathers are the most distressed about the child initially. The disabled child will always have a strong impact on the family, sometimes a catastrophic one.[21,25,26,173,174]

Parents must be encouraged to express their emotions, and they must be taught how to deal with the issues at hand. Techniques for accomplishing these goals are discussed in later sections.[68,172,174]

The Child Dealing with Loss

If a parent is injured, the young child may experience an overwhelming sense of loss. Child care may be a problem, especially if the primary caregiver is injured. The child will probably feel deserted by the injured parent and may demand the attention of the remaining parent. This will increase the strain on all family members.[74]

If the child is the client, his or her life will have undergone a radical change: every aspect of the child's world will have altered. Loved objects and people will help to restore the child's feeling of security. It is of major importance to explain to the child in very simple terms what is going on and to allow the child the opportunity to express feelings both verbally and nonverbally (perhaps by using play as the medium of communication).

The hospital setting is threatening to all people, but children are especially susceptible to loss of autonomy, feelings of isolation, and loss of independence. Senecac and Nelson (see Chapter 12) have stated that the severity of the disability is not as important a variable in the emotional development of the child as are the attitudes of parents and family.[22,25] Parents must attempt to be aware of the child's inability to understand the permanence (or transience) of the loss of function.[25] They will also need to help the child feel secure by bringing in familiar and cherished objects. A schedule should be established and kept to promote consistency. Play should be encouraged, especially that which allows the child to vent feelings and deal with the new environment. Any procedures or therapies should be presented in a relaxed way (fun, if possible), so that the child has time to think and to feel as comfortable as possible about the change. The parents may often need to be reminded to pay attention to the children in the family without disabilities during this acute stage.

The Adolescent Dealing with Loss

The adolescent is subject to all of the feelings and fears that other clients express. Adolescents are in a struggle to obtain autonomy and independence, and they often are ambivalent about these feelings. When an adolescent is suddenly injured and has to cope with being disabled, it can be a massive assault on the individual's development.[49,175]

The adolescent appears to react differently from other age groups to the knowledge of his or her own terminal illness. The adolescent often feels that he or she has gone through a very painful process (initiation) that will soon lead to the "joys and rights" of adulthood. Unlike persons in older age groups who might feel that they can look back and gain solace from the past, the adolescent feels that he or she will have what Brito et al[175] term "death before fulfillment" and thus may react by feeling cheated by life. This same pattern may occur with the disabled adolescent.[176] The therapist must be acutely aware of these feelings so that therapy may be presented in the most effective manner for the client to find challenge and fulfillment in life.[177]

Family Maturation

The family also has a maturational aspect. If the injured person is a child and if the family is young with dependent children at home, the adjustment may not be the problem that it would be for a family whose children are older. In the latter case, parents have begun to experience freedom and independence, and they may find adjusting to a return to a restricted lifestyle difficult or even intolerable. They may have the feeling that they have already "put in their time" and should now be free. If the disability interrupts the child's developmental process, future conflict may arise because the parents will eventually want retirement, relaxation, and freedom. Parents may feel guilty and try to repress this normal response.

The reverse may also be true. The parents may be feeling that the children have left them ("empty nest syndrome"), and they may be too willing to welcome a "dependent" family member back into the home. This may lead to excessive dependence or anger toward the parents on the part of the client. All these factors must be taken into consideration by the therapist when therapy is presented to the client and family.

The therapist can develop a greater understanding of the client and family by being aware of the normal human developmental patterns. These patterns identify some of the major hurdles that must be overcome in the client's life.

Coping with Transition

In the acute stage of a family member's injury, the family must be helped to deal with the crisis at hand. During this phase, the family must first be allowed to cope with the emotional impact of what is happening with a loved one. Second, the family should be helped to see the situation as a challenge that, if overcome, will facilitate growth. Third, adaptation within the family unit must occur to overcome the situation.

Brammer and Abrego[177] have developed a list of basic coping skills that they have broken into five levels. In the first level the person becomes aware of and mobilizes skills in perceiving and responding to transition and attempts to handle the situation. In the second level the person mobilizes the skills for assessing, developing, and using external support systems. In level three the person can possess, develop, and use internal support systems (develop positive self-regard and use the situation to grow). The person in level four must find ways to reduce emotional and physiological distress (relaxation, control stimulation, and verbal expression of feelings). In level five the person must plan and implement change (analyze discrepancies, plan new options, and successfully implement the plan). Using this model, the therapist and family can evaluate the coping skill level of the family. The therapist and staff can then help promote movement toward the next level of coping with the transition. These levels are also broken into specific skills and subskills so that the therapist can grade them further.

One of the more damaging aspects of hospitalization to all involved is that the hospital staff focuses on the disability rather than on the individual's strengths.[81,162,178] Centering on the disability can lead to a situation where client, family, and staff see only the functional limitations and not the potential ability of the client.

Decentering from the loss of function will be examined further in this chapter. If the family relationship was positive before the insult and if the client is cognitively intact, then the focus should be directed toward the relationship's strengths as well as toward the client's and family's individual cognitive and emotional strengths.[91] In the initial acute stage of adjustment, crisis intervention may help the family use its strengths and at the same time deal with the situation at hand.

To adequately deal with the crisis, the family should do the following:

1. Be helped to focus on the crisis caused by the disability; identify the situation to stimulate problem solving; identify and deal with doubts of adequacy, guilt, and self-blame; identify and deal with grief work; identify and deal with anticipatory worry; be offered basic information and education regarding the crisis situation; and be helped to create a bridge to resources in the hospital and in the community for support and to see their own family resources.[170,179-182]

2. Be helped to remember how they have dealt successfully with crises in the past and to implement some of the same strategies in the present situation.

3. Work with the family as a unit during crisis to help strengthen the family and facilitate more positive attitudes toward the client. These attitudes by the family will improve the client's attitudes or feelings toward the injury and hospitalization.[50,168,183-186] Encouraging family-unit functioning in this situation will decrease the amount of regression displayed by the client. If the family is encouraged to function without the client, however, more damage than good may be done.[21,49]

TREATMENT VARIABLES IN RELATION TO THERAPY

Livneh & Antonak[44] promote the following activities for the health professional:

1. *Assisting clients to explore the personal meaning of the disability.* "Training clients to attain a sense of mastery over their emotional experiences." A way of doing this would be to help the client not to demonstrate emotional outbursts or to help the client look at his or her emotions and to put them into perspective.

2. *Providing clients with relevant medical information.* "These strategies emphasize imparting accurate information to clients on their medical condition, including its present status, prognosis, anticipated future functional limitations, and when applicable, vocational implications." This may be done by helping the client and family access resources such as PubMed (pubmedcentral.nih.gov) online, or to find medical references in the library.

3. *Providing clients with supportive family and group experiences.* "These strategies permit clients (usually with similar disabilities or common life experiences) and, if applicable, their family members or significant others, to share common fears, concerns, needs, and wishes." This can be done in rather unobtrusive ways such as scheduling clients with the same disability at the same time so that they meet in the waiting room or while doing group mat activities. Another option is hiring individuals with limitations who are health care professionals and can discuss and role model positive behaviors and answer relevant questions from the client's perspective. Remember that clients are all potential teachers for you as well as other clients.

4. *Teaching clients adaptive coping skills for successful community functioning.* "These skills include assertiveness, interpersonal relations, decision making, problem solving, stigma management, and time management skills." This would entail role-playing situations that I have seen happen in the community such

as an able-bodied person asking why the client is in a wheelchair, preaching to the wheelchair user because he or she must have offended God in some way otherwise the person would not be in a wheelchair, or telling a woman that is such a shame that she is disabled because she is so good looking and could have found a man if it were not for the disability. Role playing can also be used to help a person deal with the possibly awkward experience of going to bed with a new partner and having to explain how to be undressed, or what those tubes coming out of the body are for, or what positions are best for someone with this condition.

ROLE OF THE THERAPEUTIC ENVIRONMENT

This section examines issues the therapist and staff should know to create a therapeutic environment that will facilitate psychological adjustment and independence of the client with activity limitations. The physical and the attitudinal environment of the treatment facility plays a major role in the way the client views the services that are rendered.

Recall a time before you became a member of the medical community. Think about how awe inspiring the people in white coats were, how strange the smells of the hospitals were, how busy it all seemed, and how puzzling the secret medical language was. It all seemed overwhelming then, and it still is to newcomers, especially newly admitted patients and their families. The hospital usually appears impersonal,[187] sterile, monotonous, and confusing, and all status accumulated outside the hospital means little inside.

The therapist needs to take the setting into account when dealing with the client. The environment can be altered in a variety of ways. Therapy staff could wear street clothes, decorate the department or hospital with posters and lively colors, and allow clients to bring some personal items into the hospital.

The nature of the therapy process can often lead the therapist to see only the disability and not the person, as occurs for example when a client is referred to by his or her disability rather than by name. This stereotyping of those with disabilities can lead the therapist to concentrate on the lack of abilities rather than on the strengths of the clients. The real danger is that the client and family will also start to focus on the functional limitations of the client and feel that their family relationship is now permanently altered. The accuracy of this perception may have to be evaluated as part of the adjustment process. The wife of a man with paraplegia said with a sudden burst of insight, "I didn't marry him for his legs—this doesn't change the relationship." Often so much attention is directed toward the disability that tunnel vision develops. One way to try to get a better perspective is to look at the bigger picture. A variety of questions can be asked that may help the therapist gain a greater insight into the client as a person (Box 5-1).

After the therapist is aware of the strengths of the client, these strengths may be capitalized on in therapy to help the client realize them and build confidence. Clients often reported that they were not complimented in therapy and especially that they never received feedback that their bodies were desirable[9] or that they were doing things correctly.[28,81,135,136,188] A logical thought by the client is "if the therapist cannot see anything desirable about me, and the

---

BOX 5-1 ■ QUESTIONS TO HELP GAIN INSIGHT INTO THE CLIENT AS A PERSON

What would this person be doing if he or she did not have this condition?
What is stopping the person from reaching these goals now?
Who will marry this person and why?
What are his or her good points?
What will this person do for a living?
What will this person do for enjoyment?
How will this person bring others enjoyment?
What would this person be doing if there was no disability?
How is the disability stopping the person from actualizing their goals? (these are the goals that need to be worked on)
Similar questions can be asked of the client to explore ways of helping the client have a meaningful life:
What do you look like and function like now?
What will you look like after therapy?
What important things would you be doing now if you were not in need of treatment?
What activities or forms of productivity were you involved in before and which were important to you?
Which of these things do you still do?
What if anything is preventing you from doing these things now?
How does this condition affect your being a lover of life, family, significant other, and so on?
How will this condition affect your important life goals, activities, and your ability to do meaningful activities?
How much different would your life look if it were not for this condition?
Will any of the above be stopped by your condition and if so how?

---

therapist deals with the individuals with similar problems all the time, then there must not be anything good about me." Positive, sincere comments to client and family can add a motivational factor to treatment that may have been missing.[81,185]

The last and possibly the most important aspect in creating an environment that will foster growth and adjustment in the client is a staff that is well adjusted and aware of their own personal needs. Just as coping skills are necessary for the client, the staff, too, must be capable of coping with the stresses of the emotional and physical pain of the client and the client's family. The therapist must also deal with his or her own personal reactions to the sometimes devastating situations others are in.[81,185,191] Exposure to such situations often elicits introspection on the part of the staff that can result in emotional turmoil for staff members and affect their own personal relationships. This emotional energy needs to be directed in a productive way so that the energy does not turn into chaos within the staff interaction or become a destructive force for the client.

To decrease the possibly distractive nature of this emotional energy, the staff should be made aware of their own coping styles, and they should be allowed to vent their reactions to particularly distressing client case loads in a positive, supportive group. Group meetings can be used to handle some of the inevitable tension, especially if there is a respected member who is skilled in group work. This is not a psychotherapy session but rather an opportunity to test reality and remove tension before it is incorrectly directed toward fellow staff members. These sessions can make use of the four elements of crisis intervention mentioned in the previous section, as well as information from others.[137,185] Other times that this stress reduction can be achieved are in supervision or during coffee breaks, as long as the sessions are productive.

The staff can use these sessions to better understand their reactions to stress and to explore their coping styles.[167,185,189,190] Ideally, this knowledge of coping styles and stress reduction will decrease staff burnout and aid the staff to help clients and their families deal with stress more successfully.[49,188-191]

The need to have a staff that is supportive is of paramount importance because the attitude of rehabilitation personnel has emerged as one of the chief motivating factors in rehabilitation.[21,47,50] Rogers and Figone[54] developed the following suggestions that the therapist could benefit from when trying to create a supportive environment:

1. It is helpful to use the same staff member to develop the relationship and to provide continuity of care.
2. Concerned silence is most appreciated, although pushing is sometimes necessary.
3. Staff members should anticipate the need to repeat information graciously.
4. Cumbersome, hard-to-repair adaptive equipment should not be used after discharge.
5. Give clients responsibility so that they feel they have some control over therapy.
   a. The client should be allowed to pick his or her own advocate from the team.
   b. The client should be given a choice of activities (e.g., which exercise comes first).
   c. Professionals should avoid placing the client in an inferior status. In time the client starts thinking this way (feeling like a "second-class citizen").
6. Psychological support was attributed to noncounseling personnel. Personal matters were better discussed with staff members with whom the client had developed a relationship.[22,133,180]
7. Willingness to allow the client to try and fail is more helpful than controlling the client.

CONCEPTUALIZATION OF ASSESSMENT AND TREATMENT

Assessment

The one component that weaves through all of Rogers and Figone's[54] seven points is the need for the therapist to be involved with the client in a therapeutic relationship, that is, to know where the client is "coming from." To know where the client is coming from is to be aware of and sensitive to the person's total psychosocial frame of reference.[22,180]

The therapist who knows his or her own beliefs, reference points, and prejudices can evaluate whether an assessment result or treatment sequence reflects the client's needs and values or those of the therapist. In the first half of this chapter, several assessments were discussed that could be summarized into the following three major components:

1. Preinjury
   a. Values and prejudices (value systems, culture, and prejudgments) of the client and family members before the injury
   b. Developmental stage of the client and family members
   c. Cognitive level of the client and family members
   d. Ability of the client and family members to handle crisis
2. Components to be evaluated leading to adjustment
   a. Loss and grief process for the client and family members
   b. Adjustment process for the client and family members
   c. Transitional stages for the client and family members
   d. Role changes for the client and family members
   e. Age or cognitive level of client and family members[26,49,180,192]
   f. Sexual adjustment for the client and spouse
3. Techniques used to elicit adjustment and independence
   a. Crisis intervention strategies
   b. Letting the client and family take control
   c. Expression of emotion—both verbally and nonverbally
   d. Problem solving
   e. Role playing
   f. Praise
   g. Education
   h. Support groups

Once an assessment has been made of the client and family members' stages of psychological adjustment, the client's occupational history and roles, and of their preinjury attitudes and beliefs, a treatment protocol can be established. This protocol will need to incorporate steps toward stage change and possibly attitudinal change. Because these changes require learning on the part of the client and family, an environment that optimally facilitates these changes must be established.*

Therapy can be seen as a form of education in which the client and the client's family are taught how the client should use his or her body. The education process is not limited to the physical aspects of therapy, however. The client is also taught how to look at and think about the body and the disability. If the staff is nonverbally telling the client and the family that the client is not capable of making decisions and of being independent, it follows that the client may indeed feel dependent and incapable of making decisions. Giles[167] and others[163,167,194-196] stated that there was an inverse relationship between independence and distress. Distress causes further anxiety and decreases the learning potential of the client. There are ways, however, for the therapist to encourage independence on the part of the client and his family.

Specific Therapeutic Interventions
Problem-Solving Process
The family unit, including the client, should be encouraged to take active control over as much of the client's care and decision making as possible.[70,164,167,194-200] This can be done

---

*References 8, 19, 32, 80, 82, 91, 159, 168, 180, 193.

in every phase of the rehabilitation process. A family conference with the rehabilitation staff should actively involve the client and family in all stages of planning and treatment, up to and including discharge. The family (including the client) should be briefed ahead of time to prepare questions that they want answered or problems that need to be addressed. Rogers and Figone[54] report that conferences with family members that excluded the client engendered suspicion[22,167]; therefore, if the client is capable, the client may educate the family in regard to what is happening in the hospital and in rehabilitation. Conversely, family involvement facilitates and shortens the rehabilitation process and reintegration into the community.[25,163,195,196] The family can also be educated regarding the side effects and interactions of medication with publications such as the *Physicians' Desk Reference*.[201] Later in the rehabilitation process the client and family can be encouraged to arrange transportation services, find and evaluate housing, and supervise attendant care. All these activities allow the client and the family to be more in control of the environment and, thus, to feel independent.

In the context of one-to-one therapy, giving choices can foster client responsibility and independence. Making a decision about the order of treatment activities (such as in which direction to roll one's wheelchair first) can give the individual a sense of self-worth that can continue to grow. This should lead the client and family toward believing that they are strong, with rights that need to be met. Moving out of the role of the victim, the client begins to exercise responsibility and to take action, such as applying for extended health benefits or getting a second consultation when an important medical decision needs to be made. If the client and family start to realize that they do not have to be a casualty of the medical establishment and if they find ways to control the medical establishment,[5,14,50] they are better able to discard the role of victim.

In some centers, such as the occupational therapy clinic at San Jose State University, the client is even taught the art of self-defense to make sure that the client never has to fall into the victim (dependent) role. It should be noted, however, that this knowledge on the part of the client and family can be used in ways that the therapist may not always agree with. At such times it may help to adopt a philosophical attitude toward the situation and to view it as a positive direction for the client in terms of moving from victim to advocate in the rehabilitation process.

The steps of crisis intervention, which were mentioned in the previous section, can be used to help the family understand and analyze their needs in the crisis situation. Once the family has discovered that they are in crisis, they will then be able to create strategies that they can use to overcome present and future problems.

Problem solving is another element the therapist may use to help the client and family gain independence and control.[70,163,167,194-200] Rather than having the client routinely learn how to accomplish a specific task, the client or family should be encouraged to think through the process, from the problem to the solution, and to accomplishment of the task. To achieve this activity analysis, the client would have to know the basic principles behind the activity[54] and may then be responsible for educating the family. An example of this would be a transfer from the wheelchair to the toilet. If the therapist simply has the client memorize the steps in the

task, the client or family members will not necessarily be able to generalize this procedure to a transfer to the car. If the client learns the principles of proper body mechanics, work simplification, and movement, the client or family member may be able to generalize this information to almost any situation and to solve problems later when the therapist is unavailable.[194] Rogers and Figone[54] have noted that, although the client and family may fail at times during these trials, the therapist should let them be as independent and responsible as possible: let them try it their way, even if they are not successful the first time.

Pictures or slides of a restaurant, movie theater, or public building can be used to facilitate discussion and problem solving by the family unit when analyzing potential architectural barriers in the environment. Thus, in the future, when the family is presented with a problem or a barrier, they will have the resources to overcome it rather than be devastated by it.

Role playing in combination with support groups can also be used to defuse potentially painful situations and operate independently. While still in the safe environment of the rehabilitation setting, simulations of incidents can be created for the family and client to practice problem solving with supervision. They can be asked what they would do when a stranger (possibly a child) approaches the client and asks why he or she is in a wheelchair or is disabled or what they would do when a waiter asks the family member to order for the disabled client. All of these situations are potentially devastating for all involved; however, if role playing and support groups are used in advance to help all members of the family (client included) to satisfactorily handle and feel in control of the situation, the family will not be as likely to be traumatized by a similar occurrence. The result is that the family will not be as inclined to be overwhelmed by social situations and will be able to socialize in a much freer, more gratifying way.[82,84,202]

Cognitive-behavioral therapy has been used for clients and spouses with success.[92-94] Psychosocial support groups have been called for throughout the literature.*

Throughout the therapeutic process, the client and the family need to be praised frequently, and credit needs to be given for the gains made by the client and family members. Granted, the therapist may have engineered the gains, but the family and client are the ones who need the reinforcement. Through gratifying experiences the family will unite to overcome the disability. They need to know that they can survive in the world without having the medical staff constantly there to solve the family's problems. In short, they need the strategies and resources that will allow them to be independent outside the medical model.

Yet another way to encourage independence can be applied to working with parents of disabled children.[30] The parents should be educated about normal and abnormal growth and development, including physical, cognitive, and emotional growth, so that the family can maintain some perspective and objectivity about their child's various levels.[18,25,50,127] The parents can then better understand the needs of those children with disabilities and those without in the family. Armed with this knowledge, the parents and children will not be frustrated with unreal expectations or

---

*References 11, 15, 18, 45, 134, 202-204.

unreal demands. Educations of the parents could take place at local colleges, the hospital, or even in a parent's group.

Support Systems

Groups are often used to increase motivation, provide support, increase social skills, instill hope, and help the client and family realize that they are not the only ones who have a disabled family member. This will help the client and family establish a more accurate set of perceptions about the disabled individual and allow for greater independence of the client and family.* Problem solving can be encouraged and value systems can be clarified. Client or family support groups can be used to relieve pressure that might otherwise be vented in therapy. Livneh and Antonak[44] found that in a chronic-care ward family involvement helped the client and the family improve their status. Schwartzberg[195] and Schulz[120] and others[†] have reported great success in the use of support groups with individuals who had brain damage. Support groups can also be used to educate the client about the client's disability to increase independence.[‡] Kreuter et al[207] and Taanila and colleagues[30,206] found that independent physical functioning and knowledge about one's condition were exceedingly important in moving through the phases of the rehabilitation process.[5,15,80,208] A guide to facilitating support groups has been published by Boreing and Adler,[207] and it has been found to be useful, especially by lay people establishing such groups.[§]

The Adult Client with Brain Damage

The adult client with brain damage and the needs of the family will be specifically, yet briefly, examined here because brain damage affects the cognitive and emotional system of the client. When a person receives a brain injury and is hospitalized, emotional support for the family (client included) is the primary need to be met initially. The therapist should attempt to convey warmth and a caring attitude, especially during the family's initial contacts.[211] Typical complaints about the acute period involve impersonal hospital routines and lack of definite information about the patient's status.[30,50,135,182,212] Unfortunately, definite information is usually not available at the earliest stages.

Later, the family must deal with the physical changes in the client's body; what may be even more injurious to the family is the psychological, cognitive, and social changes in the client.[21,25,26,32,213] People with cerebrovascular accidents have been found to be more clinically depressed than orthopedic patients are. The libido[214] and the emotional systems are also affected.[80,136-138,179] It has further been shown that persons who survive a cerebrovascular accident or other impairment and who have a full return of function do not return to normal life because of a lack of social and emotional skills.* Families of cerebrovascular accident victims have also reported that social reintegration is the most difficult phase of rehabilitation.[216] Lack of socially appropriate behaviors has been one of the most troublesome complaints of people who deal with the person with a chronic brain injury.[136] Therapists may be able to help alter this syndrome by encouraging appropriate behavior and by structuring therapy situations to reteach the client interaction skills. A technique called structured learning therapy[136,217] has been used with schizophrenics, and although this approach has not been used by enough clinics to judge its effectiveness completely, it appears to be a promising approach.

Better follow-up care needs to be implemented when dealing with the adult with brain damage.[†]

It may not be possible for the client and family to constantly come to the clinic for support and follow-up, but telephone conversations can be scheduled on a periodic basis, or the exchange of letters or audiotapes can also be used. With the increased availability of video recorders, the day may come when a follow-up may be performed on videotapes sent by clients living in rural areas. Support groups are being used increasingly to facilitate client and family adjustment and accommodation to disability, as well as reentry into the community.[‡]

CASE STUDY 5-1 ■ PUTTING EVALUATIONS AND TECHNIQUES INTO PRACTICE

Joan, a married 30-year-old woman, has had a T2 spinal cord injury. She has worked as a computer programmer for the past 8 years, except for a short maternity leave when she gave birth to her daughter, who is now 6 years old. Joan was always very active physically and often stated that she felt sorry for her physically disabled neighbor because the neighbor could not hike, be active, or enjoy the outdoors. Joan's husband, age 33 years, is attempting to visit Joan regularly and care for their daughter, a role that is new for him.

The therapist has assessed several things regarding Joan's developmental stage, adjustment stage, social/cultural influences, and family adjustment reactions. The two adult family members are probably in Sheehy's[219] "catch-30" stage, in which the person reevaluates his or her life and relationships. Joan already "knows" that the physically disabled cannot enjoy a physically active life and is also feeling that everything she has worked for in her career is lost. She appears to be in the mourning stage of adjustment. Her daughter and husband have to adjust to radical role changes. Cognitively, Joan's young daughter is not going to understand the permanence of the disability and may be inclined to act out as the result of the turmoil. The husband will have to be assessed to determine his stage of adjustment to her disability.

The therapist has determined that Joan's transfers need further work but would like to use the adaptive

Continued

---

*References 26, 50, 80, 97, 151, 166, 195, 198, 203.
†References 12, 13, 21, 97, 192, 193, 205.
‡References 21, 163, 192, 196, 206, 207.
§References 50, 80, 97, 163, 195, 206-210.

*References 18, 91, 179, 182, 195, 213-215.
†References 15, 21, 26, 45, 50, 202.
‡References 21, 32, 50, 185, 192, 205, 206, 218.

CASE STUDY 5-1 ■ PUTTING EVALUATIONS AND TECHNIQUES INTO PRACTICE— cont'd

process to stimulate adjustment. The therapist has devised a treatment session to meet the goals of promoting the defense stage of adjustment, decreasing her prejudice against the disabled, encouraging problem solving, increasing her feelings of self-worth, proving to her that she can take care of her daughter through interacting with children, and having her de-center her focus from her disability to her ability. The therapist has contacted the recreational therapist (who is a paraplegic) to plan a collaborative session at the park across the street from the hospital. Because the recreational therapist works in the pediatrics ward, it is determined that the children with spina bifida should come and play tag, transferring from log to log in the playground.

The stage is now set. Joan will be asked to help supervise the children. The adaptive process will be used to teach Joan how to transfer using the environment. The transfer will be organized subcortically because she will be attending cortically to the children's needs and to the game itself. Joan will be actively affecting her personal environment, and if everything goes well, the act of helping the children will increase her self-worth and will also be self-reinforcing. Within this treatment session, the therapist has used the recreational therapist as a role model to change Joan's prejudice against the disabled being active in the outdoors and to show Joan that she can still be a parent although she is disabled. The therapist may also increase Joan's knowledge of how to interact with children from a wheelchair by giving a few hints and then having Joan transfer up a set of stairs to reach one of the children.

If we want to carry this scenario further, the therapist could introduce Joan to a child who is interested in computers and who needs help with a programming problem (Joan's computer background will be used, which will increase Joan's feelings of self-worth and help her focus on her abilities rather than her disabilities). On the way back to the ward, the therapist and Joan may discuss how the family is dealing with the crisis they are in and help her realize how the family has made it through other crises in the past and how those previously successful strategies could be used in this situation. Support groups may be mentioned as resources. The session may end with Joan planning the next therapy session and thus starting to take control of her life.

REFERENCES

1. Gelenberg A: Depression is still unrecognized and undertreated, *Arch Intern Med* 159:1999.
2. Kibele A, Padilla R, Burton GU: The psychosocial issues of physical illness and disability. In Cara E, MacRae A (eds): *Psychosocial occupational therapy in clinical practice,* Albany, 1998, Delmar.
3. Mona LR, Krause JS, Norris FH et al: Sexual expression following spinal cord injury, *Neurorehabilitation* 15:121, 2000.
4. Salsgiver RO, Watson A, Cooke J et al: Spiritual/religious access for women with disabilities, *SCI Psychosoc Proc* 17:27-33, 2004.
5. Jonsson AL, Moller A, Grimby G: Managing occupations in everyday life to achieve adaptations, *Am J Occup Ther* 53:353-362, 1999.
6. Klausner EJ, Alexopoulos GS: The future of psychosocial treatments for elderly patients, *Psychiatr Serv* 50:1198-1204, 1999.
7. Weitzner MA, McMillan SC: Quality of life in cancer patients: use of a revised hospice index, *Cancer Pract* 6:282-288, 1998.
8. Martz E, Livneh H, Priebe M et al: Predictors of psyosocial adaptation among people with spinal cord injury or disorder, *Arch Phys Med Rehabil* 86:1182-1192, 2005.
9. Collins LF: Easing client transition from facility to community, *OT Pract* 1:36-39, 1996.
10. Verduyn WH: Spinal cord injured women, pregnancy, and delivery, *Sex Disabil* 1:29-143, 1993.
11. Vogel LC, Klaas SJ, Lubicky JP et al: Long-term outcomes and life satisfaction of adults who had pediatric spinal cord injuries, *Arch Phys Med Rehabil* 79:1496-1503, 1998.
12. Daniel A, Manigandan C: Efficacy of leisure intervention groups and their impact on quality of life among people with spinal cord injury, *Int J Rehabil Res* 28:43-48, 2005.
13. Yuen HK: Impact of an altruistic activity on life satisfaction in institutionalized elders: A pilot study, *Phys Occup Ther Geriatr* 20:125-135, 2002.
14. Moyers PA: The guide to occupational therapy practice. American Occupational Therapy Association. *J Occup Ther* 53:247-322, 1999.
15. Pain H: Coping with a child with disabilities from the parents' perspective: the function of information, *Child Care Health Dev* 25:299-312, 1999.
16. Mauras-Neslen E, Neslen SE: The therapeutic alliance: enhancing client-practitioner relationships, *OT Pract* 1:20-27, 1996.
17. Pentland W, Harvey AS, Walker J: The relationships between time use and health and well-being in men with spinal cord injury, *J Occup Sci* 5:14-25, 1998.
18. Viemero V, Krause C: Quality of life in individuals with physical disabilities, *Psychother Psychosom* 67:317-322, 1998.
19. Kennedy P, Duff J, Evans M et al: Coping effectiveness training reduces depression and anxiety following traumatic spinal cord injuries, *Br J Clin Psychol* 42:41-52, 2003.
20. Helgeson VS: Cognitive adaptation, psychological adjustment, and disease progression among angioplasty patients: 4 years later, *Health Psychol* 22:30-38, 2003.
21. Flagg-Williams JB: Perspectives on working with parents of handicapped children, *Psychol Schools* 28:238-246, 1991.
22. Moos R, Schaefer J: The crisis of physical illness: an overview and conceptual approach. In Moos R, editor: *Coping with physical illness: New perspectives,* New York, 1984, Plenum.
23. Moos R, Schaefer J: Life transitions and crises, a conceptual overview. In Moos R, editor: *Coping with life crises: an integrated approach,* New York 1986, Plenum.
24. Charlifue S, Gerhart K: Changing psychosocial morbidity in people aging with spinal cord injury, *Neurorehabilitation* 19:15-23, 2004.
25. Asarnow RF, Satz P, Light R: Behavior problems and adaptive functioning in children with mild and severe closed head injury, *J Pediatr Psychol* 16:543-555, 1991.
26. Brooks DN: The head-injured family, *J Clin Exp Neuropsychol* 13:155-188, 1991.

27. Garske GG, Turpin JO: Understanding psychosocial adjustment to disability: an American perspective, *Int J Rehabil Health* 4:29-37, 1998.
28. Gorman C, Kennedy P, Hamilton LR: Alterations in self-perceptions following childhood onset of spinal cord injury, *Spinal Cord* 36:181-185, 1998.
29. McCubbin MA, McCubbin HI: Family stress theory and assessment: the resiliency model of family stress, adjustment, and adaptation. In McCubbin HI, Thompson AI, editors: *family assessment inventories for research and practice,* Madison, WI, 1991, University of Wisconsin-Madison.
30. Taanila A, Jarvelin MR, Kokkonen J: Parental guidance and counselling by doctors and nursing staff: parents' views of initial information and advice for families with disabled children, *J Clin Nurs* 7:505-511, 1998.
31. Vander Kolk CJ: Client credibility and coping styles, *Rehabil Psychol* 36:51-62, 1991.
32. Braithwaite DO: From majority to minority: An analysis of cultural change from ablebodied to disabled, *Int J Intercultural Relations* 14:465-483, 1990.
33. Helgeson VS: Cognitive adaptation, psychological adjustment, and disease progression among angioplasty patients: 4 years later, *Health Psychol* 22:30-38, 2003.
34. Taleporos G, McCabe MP: Body image and physical disability-personal perspectives, *Soc Sci Med* 54:971-980, 2002.
35. Krause JS: Aging and life adjustment after spinal cord injury: Crawford Research Institute, Shepherd Center, Atlanta, Georgia, USA, *Spinal Cord* 36:320-328, 1998.
36. Kubler-Ross E: *On death and dying,* New York, 1969, Macmillan.
37. Peretz D: Reaction to loss. In Schoenberg B et al, editors: *Loss and grief,* New York, 1970, Columbia University Press.
38. Buscherhof JR: Diversity in adjustment to a leg amputation: case illustrations of common themes, *Top Stroke Rehabil* 5:19-29, 1998.
39. Rybarczyk B, Edwards R, Behel J: Diversity in adjustment to leg amputation: case illustrations of common themes, *Disabil Rehabil* 26:944-953, 2004.
40. Niemeier JP, Kennedy RE, McKinley WO et al: The Loss Inventory: preliminary reliability and validity data for a new measure of emotional and cognitive responses to disability, *Disabil Rehabil* 26:614-623, 2004.
41. Gerhart KA, Weitzenkamp DA, Kennedy P et al: Correlates of stress in long-term spinal cord injury, *Spinal Cord* 37:183-190, 1999.
42. Taylor SE: Adjustment to threatening events: a theory of cognitive adaptation, *Am Psychol* 38:1161-1173, 1983.
43. Kerr N: Understanding the process of adjustment to disability, *J Rehabil* 27:16, 1961.
44. Livneh H, Antonak RF: Reactions to disability: An empirical investigation of their nature and structure, *J Appl Rehabil Couns* 21:13-20, 1990.
45. Kemp BJ, Krause JS: Depression and life satisfaction among people aging with post-polio and spinal cord injury, *Disabil Rehabil* 21:241-249, 1999.
46. Maslow A: *Motivation and personality,* ed 2, New York, 1970, Harper & Row.
47. Kerr N: Understanding the process of adjustment to disability. In Stubbins J, editor: *Social and psychological aspects of disability,* Baltimore, 1977, University Park Press.
48. Riis J, Loewenstein G, Baron J et al: Ignorance of hedonic adaptation to hemodialysis: a study using ecological momentary assessment, *J Exp Psychol Gen* 134:3-9, 2005.
49. Cairns D, Baker J: Adjustment to spinal cord injury: a review of coping styles contributing to the process, *J Rehabil* 59:30-33, 1993.
50. Kasowski JC: Family recovery: an insider's view, *Am J Occup Ther* 48:257-258, 1994.
51. White W: The urge towards competence, *Am J Occup Ther* 26:271, 1971.
52. Fine SB: Resilience and human adaptability: who rises above adversity? 1990 Eleanor Clark Slagle Lecture, *Am J Occup Ther* 45:493-503, 1991.
53. King LJ: Toward a science of adaptive responses, *Am J Occup Ther* 32:429, 1978.
54. Rogers JD, Figone JJ: Psychosocial parameters in treating the person with quadriplegia, *Am J Occup Ther* 33:432, 1979.
55. Livneh H, Antonak RF: Psychosocial adaptation to chronic illness and disability: a primer for counselors, *J Couns Dev* 83:12-20, 2005.
56. MacMillan PJ, Hart RP, Martelli MF et al: Pre-injury status and adaptation following traumatic brain injury, *Brain Inj* 16:41-49, 2002.
57. Kennedy P, Evans MJ: Evaluation of post traumatic distress in the first 6 months following SCI, *Spinal Cord* 39:381-386, 2001.
58. Martz E: Death anxiety as a predictor of posttraumatic stress levels among individuals with spinal cord injuries, *Death Stud* 28:1-17, 2004.
59. Williams WH, Evans JJ, Wilson BA et al: Prevalence of *post-traumatic* stress disorder symptoms after severe *traumatic* brain injury in a representative community sample, *Brain Inj* 16:673-679, 2002.
60. Kennedy P, Rogers BA: Anxiety and depression after spinal cord injury: a longitudinal analysis, *Arch Phys Med Rehabil* 81:932-937, 2000.
61. Rybarczyk B, Edwards R, Behel J: Diversity in adjustment to a leg amputation: case illustrations of common themes, *Disabil Rehabil* 26:944-953, 2004.
62. Ownsworth T, Fleming J: The relative importance of metacognitive skills, emotional status, and executive function in psychosocial adjustment following acquired *brain injury, J Head Trauma Rehabil* 20:315-332, 2005.
63. McDermott S, Moran R, Platt T et al: Depression in adults with disabilities, in primary care, *Disabil Rehabil* 27:117-123, 2005.
64. Hughes RB, Robinson-Whelen S, Taylor HB et al: Characteristics of depressed and nondepressed women with physical disabilities, *Arch Phys Med Rehabil* 86: 473-479, 2005.
65. Mazaux JM, Croze P, Quintard B et al: Satisfaction of life and late psycho-social outcome after severe brain injury: a nine-year follow-up study in Aquitaine, *Acta Neurochir Suppl* 79:49-51, 2002.
66. Ayyangar R: Health maintenance and management in childhood disability, *Phys Med Rehabil Clin North Am* 13:793-821, 2002.
67. Kim SJ, Kang KA: Meaning of life for adolescents with a physical disability in Korea, *J Adv Nurs* 43:145-157, 2003.
68. Stewart DA, Law MC, Rosenbaum P et al: A qualitative study of the transition to adulthood for youth with physical disabilities, *Phys Occup Ther Pediatr* 21:3-21, 2001.
69. Putzke JD, Richards JS, Hicken BL et al: Predictors of life satisfaction: a spinal cord injury cohort study, *Arch Phys Med Rehabil* 83:555-561, 2002.
70. Stanley I, Innes I: Psychosocial factors and their role in chronic pain: A brief review of development and current status, *Chiropr Osteopat* 13:6, 2005. Published online April 27, 2005.
71. Gullacksen AC, Lidbeck J: The life adjustment process in chronic pain: Psychosocial assessment and clinical implications, *Pain Res Manag* 9:145-153, 2004.
72. Trachtenberg F, Dugan E, Hall MA: How patients' trust relates to their involvement in medical care, *J Fam Pract* 54:344-352, 2005.
73. McColl MA, Bickenbachoe J, Johnston J et al: Spiritual issues associated with traumatic-onset disability, *Disabil Rehabil* 22:555-564, 2000.
74. Fine S: Interaction between psychosocial variables and cognitive function. In Royeen CB, editor: *American Occupational Therapy Association self-study series on cognitive rehabilitation,* Rockville, MD, 1993, American Occupational Therapy Association.
75. Houston EM: What are the roles of spiritual and religious practices, attitudes, and beliefs in the lives of people with acquired *physical* disabilities? [doctoral dissertation], Madison, WI, 1999, University of Wisconsin-Madison.
76. de Klerk HM, Ampousah L: The physically disabled woman's experience of self, *Disabil Rehabil* 25:1132-1139, 2003.

77. Bogle JE, Shaul SL: Body image and the woman with a disability. In Bullard DG, Knight DE, editors: *Sexuality and physical disability*, St. Louis, 1981, CV Mosby.

78. Brown SE: Creating a disability mythology, *Int J Rehabil Res* 15:227-233, 1991.

79. Kim JJ: Spirituality and the disability experience: faith, subjective well being, and meaning and purpose in the lives of persons with disabilities [doctoral dissertation], Evanston, IN, 2002, Northwestern University.

80. Siosteen A, Kreuter M, Lampic C et al: Patient-staff agreement in the perception of spinal cord lesioned patients' problems, emotional well-being, and coping pattern, *Spinal Cord* 43:179-186, 2005.

81. Abresch RT, Seyden NK, Wineinger MA: Quality of life: issues for persons with neuromuscular diseases, *Phys Med Rehabil Clin North Am* 9:233-248, 1998.

82. Elfstrom ML, Kreuter M, Ryden A et al: Effects of coping on psychological outcome when controlling for background variables: a study of traumatically spinal cord lesioned persons, *Spinal Cord* 40:408-415, 2002.

83. Livneh H, Lott SM, Antonak RF: Patterns of psychosocial adaptation to chronic illness and disability: a cluster analytic approach, *Psychol Health Med* 9:411-430, 2004.

84. Trombly CA, Radomski MV: *Occupational therapy for physical dysfunction*, ed 2, Baltimore, 2002, Williams & Wilkins.

85. Andrews AB, Veronen LJ: Sexual assault and people with disabilities, *J Soc Work Hum Sexuality* 8:137-159, 1993.

86. Maze JR: The complementarity of object-relations and instinct theory, *Int J Psychoanal* 74:459-470, 1993.

87. Krause JS, Broderick LE, Broyles J: Subjective well-being among African-Americans with spinal cord injury: an exploratory study between men and women, *Neurorehabilitation* 19:81-89, 2004.

88. Guidetti S, Tham K: Therapeutic strategies used by occupational therapists in self-care training: a qualitative study, *Occup Ther Int* 9:257-276, 2002.

89. Hall ET: *The hidden dimension*, Garden City, NJ, 1966, Doubleday Anchor Books.

90. Holmbeck GN, Westhoven VC, Phillips WS et al: A multimethod, multi-informant, and multidimensional perspective on psychosocial adjustment in preadolescents with spina bifida, *Consult Clin Psychol* 71:782-796, 2003.

91. Elfström ML, Rydén A, Kreuter M et al: Relations between coping strategies and health-related quality of life in patients with spinal cord lesion, *J Rehabil Med* 37:9-16, 2005.

92. Craig AR, Hancock K, Chang E et al: Immunizing against depression and anxiety after spinal cord injury, *Arch Phys Med Rehabil* 79:375-377, 1998.

93. Craig AR, Hancock K, Dickson H et al: Long-term psychological outcomes in spinal cord injured persons: results of a controlled trial using cognitive behavior therapy, *Arch Phys Med Rehabil* 78:33-38, 1997.

94. Craig A, Hancock K, Chang E et al: The effectiveness of group psychological intervention in enhancing perceptions of control following spinal cord injury, *Aust N Z J Psychiatry* 32:112-118, 1998.

95. Craig A, Hancock K, Dickson H: Improving the long-term adjustment of spinal cord-injured persons, *Spinal Cord* 37:345-350, 1999.

96. Dunn KL: Sexuality education and the team approach. In Sipski ML, Alexander CJ, editors: *Sexual function in people with disability and chronic illness*, Rockville, MD, 1997, Aspen.

97. Barton J, Miller A, Chanter J: Emotional adjustment to stroke: a group therapeutic approach, *Nurs Times* 98:33-35, 2002.

98. Brown SA, McCauley SR, Levin HS et al: Perception of health and quality of life in minorities after mild-to-moderate traumatic brain injury, *Appl Neuropsychol* 11:54-64, 2004.

99. Bonder B, Martin L, Miracle A: *Culture in clinical care*, Thorofare, NJ, 2000, SLACK.

100. Rundle A, Carvalho M, Robinson M: *Cultural competence in health care: a practical guide*, Hoboken, NJ, 2002, Jossey-Bass.

101. Galanti G: *Caring for patients from different cultures*, ed 3, Philadelphia, 2003, University of Pennsylvania Press.

102. Fisher TL, Laud PW, Byfield MG et al: Sexual health after spinal cord injury: a longitudinal study, *Arch Phys Med Rehabil* 83:1043-1051, 2000.

103. Bezeau SC, Bogod NM, Mateer CA: Sexually intrusive behaviour following brain injury: approaches to assessment and rehabilitation, *Brain Inj* 18:299-313, 2004.

104. Phelps J, Albo M, Dunn K et al: Spinal cord injury and sexuality in married or partnered men: activities, function, needs, and predictors of sexual adjustment, *Arch Sex Behav* 30:591-602, 2001.

105. Nortvedt MW, Riise T, Myhr KM et al: Reduced quality of life among multiple sclerosis patients with sexual disturbance and bladder dysfunction, *Mult Scler* 7:231-235, 2001.

106. Brackett NL, Nash MS, Lynne CM et al: Male fertility following spinal cord injury: facts and fiction, *Phys Ther* 76:1221-1231, 1996.

107. Monga M, Dunn K, Rajasekaran M: Characterization of ultrastructural and metabolic abnormalities in semen from men with spinal cord injury, *J Spinal Cord Med* 24:41-46, 2001.

108. Sonksen J, Ohl DA: Penile vibratory stimulation and electroejaculation in the treatment of ejaculatory dysfunction, *Int J Androl* 25:324-332, 2002.

109. Cash TF, Santos MT, Williams EF: Coping with body-image threats and challenges: validation of the Body Image Coping Strategies Inventory, *J Psychosom Res* 58:190-199, 2005.

110. Reitz A, Tobe V, Knapp PA et al: Impact of spinal cord injury on sexual health and quality of life, *Int J Impot Res* 16:167-174, 2004.

111. Pedretti LW: *Occupational therapy: practice skills for physical dysfunction*, ed 5, St. Louis, 2000, Mosby.

112. Hartkopp A, Bronnum-Hansen H, Seidenschnur AM et al: Suicide in a spinal cord injured population: Its relation to functional status, *Arch Phys Med Rehabil* 79:1356-1361, 1998.

113. Taleporos G, McCabe MP: Relationships, sexuality and adjustment among people with physical disability, *Sex Relationship Ther* 18:25-43, 2003.

114. Cole SS, Cole TM: Sexuality, disability, and reproductive issues for persons with disabilities. In Haseltine FP, Cole SS, Gray DB (eds): *Reproductive issues for persons with physical disabilities*, Baltimore, 1993, Paul H Brookes.

115. Lohne V: Hope in patients with spinal cord injury: a literature review related to nursing, *J Neurosci Nurs* 33:317-325, 2001.

116. Delgado C: A discussion of the concept of spirituality, *Nurs Sci Q* 18:157-162, 2005.

117. Bartlett SJ, Piedmont R, Bilderberback A et al: Spirituality, well-being, and quality of life in people with rheumatoid arthritis. *Arthritis Rheum* 49:778-783, 2003.

118. Laubmeier KK, Zakowski SG, Bair JP: The role of spirituality in the psychological adjustment to cancer: a test of the transactional model of stress and coping, *Int J Behav Med* 11:48-55, 2004.

119. Faull K, Hills MD, Cochrane G et al: Investigation of health perspectives of those with physical disabilities: the role of spirituality as a determinant of health, *Disabil Rehabil* 26:129-144, 2004.

120. Schulz EK: Spirituality and disability: an analysis of select themes, *Occup TherHealth Care* 18:57-83, 2004.

121. Zauszniewski JA: Spirituality, resourcefulness, and arthritis impact on health perception of elders with rheumatoid arthritis. *J Holist Nurs* 18:311-336, 2000.

122. Treloar LL: Disability, spiritual beliefs and the church: the experiences of adults with disabilities and family members, *J Adv Nurs* 40:594-603, 2002.

123. Krause JS, Broderick LE, Broyles J: Subjective well-being among African-Americans with spinal cord injury: an exploratory study between men and women, *Neurorehabilitation* 19:81-89, 2004.

124. Sipski ML, Alexander CJ: Impact of disability or chronic illness on sexual function. In Sipski ML, Alexander CJ (eds): *Sexual function in people with disability and illness*, Rockville, MD, 1997, Aspen.

125. Lefebvre KA: Performing a sexual evaluation on the person with disability or illness. In Sipski ML, Alexander CJ (eds): *Sexual function in people with disability and chronic illness*, Rockville, MD, 1997, Aspen.

126. Kewman D, Warschausky LE, Warzak W: Sexual development of children and adolescents. In Sipski ML, Alexander CJ, editors: *Sexual function in people with disability and chronic illness,* Rockville, MD, 1997, Aspen.

127. Smith M: Pediatric sexuality: promoting normal sexual development in children, *Nurse Pract* 18:37-44, 1993.

128. Zani B: Male and female patterns in the discovery of sexuality during adolescence, *J Adolesc* 14:163-178, 1991.

129. Cole SS, Cole TM: Sexuality, disability, and reproductive issues through the life span, *Sexual Disabil* 11:189-205, 1993.

130. Burton GU: Sexuality and physical disability. In Pedretti LW, editor: *Occupational therapy: practice skills for physical dysfunction,* ed 6, St. Louis, 2006, Mosby.

131. Burton GU: Sexuality: an activity of daily living. In Early MB, editor: *Physical dysfunction practice skills for the occupational therapy assistant,* St. Louis, 2005, Mosby.

132. Kreuter M, Sullivan M, Dahllof AG et al: Partner relationships, functioning, mood and global quality of life in persons with spinal cord injury and traumatic brain injury, *Spinal Cord* 36:252-261, 1998.

133. Sandowski C: Responding to the sexual concerns of persons with disabilities, *J Soc Work Hum Sexual* 8:29-43, 1993.

134. Boyle PS: Training in sexuality and disability: preparing social workers to provide services to individuals with disabilities, *J Soc Work Hum Sexuality* 8:45-62, 1993.

135. Haseltine FP, Cole SS, Gray DB: *Reproductive issues for persons with physical disabilities,* Baltimore, 1993, Paul H. Brookes.

136. Griffith ER, Lemberg S: *Sexuality and the person with traumatic brain injury: a guide for families,* Philadelphia, 1993, FA Davis.

137. Sipski ML, Alexander CJ: *Sexual function in people with disability and chronic illness,* Rockville, MD, 1997, Aspen.

138. Lefebvre KA: Sexual assessment planning, *J Head Trauma Rehabil* 5:25-30, 1991.

139. Welner SL: Management of female infertility. In Sipski ML, Alexander CJ, editors: *Sexual function in people with disability and chronic illness,* Rockville, MD, 1997, Aspen.

140. Whipple B, McGreer KB: Management of female sexual dysfunction. In Sipski ML, Alexander CJ, editors: *Sexual function in people with disability and chronic illness,* Rockville, MD, 1997, Aspen.

141. Rivas DA, Cancellor MB: Management of erectile dysfunction. In Sipski ML, Alexander CJ, editors: *Sexual function in people with disability and chronic illness,* Rockville, MD, 1997, Aspen.

142. Linsenmeyer TA: Management of male infertility. In Sipski ML, Alexander CJ, editors: *Sexual function in people with disability and chronic illness,* Rockville, MD, 1997, Aspen.

143. Ducharme SH, Gill KM: Management of other male sexual dysfunction. In Sipski ML, Alexander CJ, editors: *Sexual function in people with disability and chronic illness,* Rockville, MD, 1997, Aspen.

144. Resources FRI: *Resources for people with disabilities and chronic conditions,* ed 2, Lexington, KY, 1993, Resources for Rehabilitation.

145. Zorzon M, Zivadinov R, Bosco A et al: Sexual dysfunction in multiple sclerosis: A case-control study, I: frequency and comparison of groups, *Mult Scler* 5:418-427, 1999.

146. Kreuter M: Spinal cord injury and partner relationships, *Spinal Cord* 38:2-6, 2000.

147. Vogel LC, Krajci KA, Anderson CJ: Adults with pediatric-onset spinal cord injuries, 3: impact of medical complications, *J Spinal Cord Med* 25:297-305, 2002.

148. Evans SA, Airey MC, Chell SM et al: Disability in young adults following major trauma: 5 year follow up of survivors, *BMC Public Health* 3:8, 2003.

149. Seki M, Takenaka A, Nakazawa M et al: Examination of living environment upon return to home for patients with cervical spinal cord injury—report of a case, *Gan To Kagaku Ryoho* 29(3 suppl):522-525, 2002.

150. Whiteneck G, Meade MA, Dijkers M et al: Environmental factors and their role in participation and life satisfaction after spinal cord injury, *Arch Phys Med Rehabil* 85:1793-1803, 2004.

151. Jaracz KL, Kozubski W: Quality of life in stroke patients, *Acta Neurol Scand* 107:324-329, 2003.

152. Kneafsey R, Gawthorpe D: Head injury: long-term consequences for patients and families and implications for nurses, *J Clin Nurs* 13:601-608, 2004.

153. Natterlund B, Ahlstrom G: Activities of daily living and quality of life in persons with muscular dystrophy, *J Rehabil Med* 33:206-211, 2001.

154. Turner DS, Cox H: Facilitating post traumatic growth, *Health Qual Life Outcomes* 2:34, 2004, doi: 10:1186/1477-7525-2-34: http://www.hqlo.com/content/2/1/34.

155. Man DW: Hong Kong family caregivers' stress and coping for people with brain injury, *Int J Rehabil Res* 25:287-295, 2002.

156. Taanila A, Syrjala L, Kokkonen J et al: Coping of parents with physically and/or intellectually disabled children, *Child Care Health Dev* 28:73-86, 2002.

157. de Klerk HM, Ampousah L: The physically disabled woman's experience of self, *Disabil Rehabil* 25:1132-1139, 2003.

158. Koukouli S, Vlachonikolis IG, Philalithis A: Socio-demographic factors and self-reported functional status: the significance of social support, *BMC Health Serv Res* 2:20, 2002.

159. Chan RC, Lee PW, Lieh-Mak F: Coping with spinal cord injury: personal and marital adjustment in the Hong Kong Chinese setting, *Spinal Cord* 38:687-696, 2000.

160. Mendes de Leon CF, Glass TA, Berkman LF: Social engagement and disability in a community population of older adults, *Am J Epidemiol* 157:633-642, 2003.

161. GAP, Group for the Advancement of Psychiatry: Caring for People with Physical Improvements: *The journey back,* Washington, DC, 1993, American Psychiatric Press.

162. Scholte OP, Reimer WJ, de Haan RJ et al: The burden of caregiving in partners of long-term stroke survivors, *Stroke* 29:1605-1611, 1998.

163. Schulz CH: Helping factors in a peer-developed support group for persons with a head injury, II: survivor interview perspective, *Am J Occup Ther* 48:305-309, 1994.

164. Neau JP, Ingrand P, Mouille-Brachet C et al: Functional recovery and social outcome after cerebral infarction in young adults, *Cerebrovasc Dis* 8:296-302, 1998.

165. Wineman NM, Schwetz KM, Zeller R et al: Longitudinal analysis of illness uncertainty, coping, hopefulness, and mood during participation in a clinical drug trial, *J Neurosci Nurs* 35:100-106, 2003.

166. Larner S: Common psychological challenges for patients with newly acquired disability, *Nurs Stand* 19:33-39, 2005.

167. Giles GM: Illness behavior after severe brain injury: Two case studies, *Am J Occup Ther* 48:247-255, 1994.

168. Hallett JD, Zasler ND, Maurer P et al: Role change after traumatic brain injury in adults, *Am J Occup Ther* 48:241-246, 1994.

169. Clarke PJ, Black SE, Badley EM et al: Handicap in stroke survivors, *Disabil Rehabil* 21:116-123, 1999.

170. Stewart DA, Law MC, Rosenbaum P et al: A qualitative study of the transition to adulthood for youth with physical disabilities, *Phys Occup Ther Pediatr* 21:3-21, 2001.

171. Coffman S: Parent and infant attachment: review of nursing research 1981-1990, *Pediatr Nurse* 18:421-425, 1992.

172. Yellott G: Promoting parent-infant bonding, *Prof Nurs* 6:519-520, 1991.

173. Shellabarger SG, Thompson TL: The clinical times: meeting parental communication needs throughout the NICU experience, *Neonat Network* 12:39-45, 1993.

174. Hooper SR, Alexander J, Moore D et al: Caregiver reports of common symptoms in children following a traumatic brain injury, *Neurorehabilitation* 19:175-189, 2004.

175. Britto MT, Solnit AJ, Green M: The pediatric management of the dying child. In Solnit A, Provence S, editors: *Modern perspectives in child development,* New York, 1963, International Universities Press.

176. Britto, MT, DeVellis RF, Hornung RW et al: Health care preferences and priorities of adolescents with chronic illnesses, *Pediatrics* 114:1272-1280, 2004.

177. Brammer LM, Abrego PJ: Intervention strategies for coping with transitions, *Counsel Psychol* 9:19, 1981.

178. Kettl P, Zarefoss S, Jacaby K et al: Female sexuality after spinal cord injury, *Sex Disabil* 9:287-295, 1991.

179. Kildal M, Willebrand M, Andersson G et al: Coping strategies, injury characteristics and long-term outcome after burn injury, *Injury* 36:511-518, 2005.

180. Song HY: Modeling social reintegration in persons with spinal cord injury, *Disabil Rehabil* 27:131-141, 2005.

181. Kalpakjian CZ, Lam CS, Toussaint LL et al: Describing quality of life and psychosocial outcomes after traumatic brain injury, *Am J Phys Med Rehabil* 83:255-265, 2004.

182. Boschen KA, Tonack M, Gargaro J: Long-term adjustment and community reintegration following spinal cord injury, *Int J Rehabil Res* 26:157-164, 2003.

183. Buscherhof JR: From abled to disabled: a life transition, *Top Stroke Rehabil* 5:19-29, 1998.

184. Charlifue SW, Gerhart KA, Menter RR et al: Sexual issues of women with spinal cord injuries, *Paraplegia* 30:192-199, 1992.

185. Koscuilek JF, McCublin MA, McCublin HI: A theoretical framework for family adaptation to head injury, *J Rehabil* 59:40-45, 1993.

186. McNeff EA: Issues for the partner of the person with a disability. In Sipski ML, Alexander CJ: *Sexual function in people with disability and chronic illness,* Rockville, MD, 1997, Aspen.

187. Heiskill LE, Pasnau RD: Psychological reaction to hospitalization and illness in the emergency dept, *Emerg Med Clin North Am* 9:207-218, 1991.

188. Romeo AJ, Wanlass R, Arenas S: A profile of psychosexual functioning in males following spinal cord injury, *Sex Disabil* 11:269-276, 1993.

189. Fisher M: Can grief be turned into growth? Staff grief in palliative care, *Prof Nurse* 7:178-182, 1991.

190. McLaughlin AM, Erdman J: Rehabilitation staff stress as it relates to patient acuity and diagnosis, *Brain Inj* 6:59-64, 1992.

191. Cohen MZ, Sarter B: Love and work: Oncology nurses' view of the meaning of their work, *Oncol Nurs Forum* 19:1481-1486, 1992.

192. Balcazar FE, Seekins T, Fawcett FB et al: Empowering people with physical disabilities through advocacy skills training, *Am J Commun Psychol* 18:281-296, 1990.

193. French S: Researching disability: the way forward, *Disabil Rehabil* 14:183-186, 1992.

194. Baker LL: Problem solving techniques in adjustment services, *Vocation Eval Work Adjust Bull* 25:75-76, 1992.

195. Schwartzberg SL: Helping factors in a peer-developed support group for persons with a head injury, I. Participant observer perspective, *Am J Occup Ther* 48:297-304, 1994.

196. Sigler G, Mackelprang RW: Cognitive impairments: Psychosocial and sexual implications and strategies for social work intervention, *J Soc Work Hum Sexual* 8:89-106, 1993.

197. McColl MA, Arnold R, Charlifue S et al: Aging, spinal cord injury, and quality of life: structural relationships, *Arch Phys Med Rehabil* 84:1137-1144, 2003.

198. Schandler SL, Cohen MJ, Vulpe M: Problem solving and coping strategies in persons with spinal cord injury who have and do not have a family history of alcoholism, *J Spinal Cord Med* 19:78-86, 1996.

199. Hammond FM, Hart T, Bushnik T et al: Change and predictors of change in communication, cognition, and social function between 1 and 5 years after traumatic brain injury, *J Head Trauma Rehabil* 19:314-328, 2004.

200. Kennedy P, Duff J, Evans M et al: Coping effectiveness training reduces depression and anxiety following traumatic spinal cord injuries, *Br J Clin Psychol* 42:41-52, 2003.

201. *Physicians' desk reference,* ed 60, Montvale, NJ, 2005, Medical Economics.

202. Keefe FJ, Caldwell DS, Baucom D et al: Spouse-assisted coping skills training in the management of knee pain in osteoarthritis: long-term followup results, *Arthritis Care Res* 12:101-111, 1999.

203. Martire LM, Lustig AP, Schulz R et al: Is it beneficial to involve a family member? A meta-analysis of psychosocial interventions for chronic illness, *Health Psychol* 23:599-611, 2004.

204. Schanke AK: Psychological distress, social support and coping behaviour among polio survivors: a 5-year perspective on 63 polio patients, *Disabil Rehabil* 19:108-116, 1997.

205. Fuhrer MJ, Rintala DH, Hart KA et al: Depressive symptomatology in persons with spinal cord injury who reside in the community, *Arch Phys Med* 74:255-260, 1993.

206. Miller L: When the best help is self-help, or everything you always wanted to know about brain injury support groups, *Cogn Rehabil* 10:14-17, 1992.

207. Kreuter M, Sullivan M, Dahllof AG et al: Partner relationships, functioning, mood and global quality of life in persons with spinal cord injury and traumatic brain injury, *Spinal Cord* 36:252-261, 1998.

208. Koplas PA, Gans HB, Wisely MP et al: Quality of life and Parkinson's disease, *J Gerontol A Biol Sci Med Sci* 54:M197-M202, 1999.

209. Richards JS, Bombardier CH, Tate D et al: Access to the environment and life satisfaction after spinal cord injury, *Arch Phys Med Rehabil* 80:1501-1506, 1999.

210. Boreing ML, Adler LM: Facilitating support groups: an instructional guide, Educational Monograph No. 3, San Francisco, 1982, Department of Psychiatry, Pacific Medical Center.

211. Sawchyn JM, Mateer CA, Suffield JB: Awareness, emotional adjustment, and injury severity in postacute brain injury, *J Head Trauma Rehabil* 20:301-314, 2005.

212. Neistadt ME, Freda M: *Choices: a guide to sex counseling with physically disabled adults,* Malabar, FL, 1987, Krieger.

213. Fleming JM, Mass F: Prognosis of rehabilitation outcome in head injury using the disability rating scale, *Arch Phys Med Rehabil* 75:159-162, 1994.

214. Kaitz S: Strategies to prevent caregiver fatigue, *Headlines* May/June:18-19, 1993.

215. Kemp BJ, Adams BM, Campbell ML: Depression and life satisfaction in aging polio survivors versus age-matched controls: relation to postpolio syndrome, family functioning, and attitude toward disability, *Arch Phys Med Rehabil* 78:187-192, 1997.

216. Kalpakjian CZ, Lam CS, Toussaint LL et al: Describing quality of life and psychosocial outcomes after traumatic brain injury, *Am J Phys Med Rehabil* 83:255-265, 2004.

217. Goldstein AP et al: *Skill training for community living,* New York, 1976, Pergamon Press.

218. Burton L, Volpe B: Sex differences in the emotional status of traumatically brain-injured patients, *J Neurol Rehabil* 2:151-157, 1993.

219. Sheehy G: *Passages,* New York, 1976, EP Dutton.

CHAPTER 6

Health and Wellness: The Beginning of the Paradigm

Janet R. Bezner, PhD, PT

KEY TERMS

paradigm
perceptions
well-being
wellness
whole person

OBJECTIVES

After reading this chapter the student/therapist will be able to:
1. Define and differentiate the terms health and wellness.
2. Describe the characteristics of wellness.
3. Compare and contrast illness, prevention, and wellness paradigms.
4. Identify and analyze a variety of wellness measures.
5. Synthesize a wellness approach into neurorehabilitation.

In learning to cope with the often chronic nature of their conditions, individuals with neurological disease, not unlike individuals with diseases of other systems, learn to rely on their abilities to adapt and compensate for their functional limitations to regain the ability to participate in life. Although not an uncommon approach to life for any human being, the achievement of health or wellness takes on an increased focus for individuals with chronic disease and it is strongly correlated to the quality of life they achieve. A casual consideration of the terms "health" and "wellness" indicates that they are similar, if not the same, in meaning, a commonly held belief among those without disease. This interpretation of the terms becomes problematic, however, in the presence of disease. Can an individual with a disease be well? Can a person without disease be ill? The concepts of health and wellness and their associated meanings and measures will be explored in this chapter to provide a perspective for movement specialists that will enhance their ability to promote health and well-being in clients with neurological disease.

DEFINITIONS AND RELATIONSHIPS AMONG TERMS

The classic understanding of the term "health" from a biomedical perspective is "absence of disease." The antonym of health, therefore, is disease. The World Health Organization contributed to the confusion between the terms health and wellness when, in 1948, it defined health as "a state of complete physical, mental and social well-being, and not merely the absence of disease or infirmity."[1] Indeed, there are numerous illustrations of the influence of the mind and spirit on the body and thus the importance, from a public health perspective, of considering more than the physical state of the body when formulating solutions to health problems. However, there is also value in differentiating health from more global concepts such as wellness and quality of life, if for no other reason than to explain the phenomenon that an individual can be diseased and well or can experi-

ence a high quality of life while simultaneously living with a chronic disease. Considering the catastrophic nature of many neurological diseases that compromise physical health, it is even more important to distinguish between health and wellness to recognize and pursue avenues to enhance overall quality of life and well-being.

H. L. Dunn first conceptualized the term wellness in 1961 and offered the first definition of the term: "an integrated method of functioning which is oriented toward maximizing the potential of which the individual is capable."[2] Since Dunn's introduction of the term, numerous researchers and educators have attempted to explain wellness by proposing various models and approaches.[3-11] Although the literature is full of references to and information about wellness, including numerous definitions of the term, a universally accepted definition has failed to emerge. Several conclusions can be drawn, however, from the abundance of literature regarding wellness.

For many people, including the public, health and wellness are synonymous with physical health or physical well-being, which commonly consists of physical activity, efforts to eat nutritiously, and adequate sleep. Research has indicated that when the public is asked to rate their general health, they narrowly focus on their physical health status, choosing not to consider their emotional, social, or spiritual health.[12] Referring to the definition of wellness from Dunn, and consistent with numerous other theorists, it is obvious that wellness, as it is defined, includes more than just physical parameters.

The common themes that emerge from the various models and definitions of wellness suggest that wellness is multidimensional,[2,4-13] salutogenic or health causing,[1,2,4,7,8,10,14] and consistent with a systems view of persons and their environments.[2,15-17] Each of these characteristics will be explored.

First as a multidimensional construct, wellness is more than simply physical health, as the more common understanding of the term might suggest. Among the dimensions

TABLE 6-1 ■ Definitions of the Dimensions of Wellness[18]

Physical	Positive perceptions and expectancies of physical health
Psychological	A general perception that one will experience positive outcomes to the events and circumstances of life
Social	The perception that family or friends are available in times of need, and the perception that one is a valued support provider
Emotional	The possession of a secure sense of self-identity and a positive sense of self-regard
Spiritual	A positive sense of meaning and purpose in life
Intellectual	The perception that one is internally energized by the appropriate amount of intellectually stimulating activity

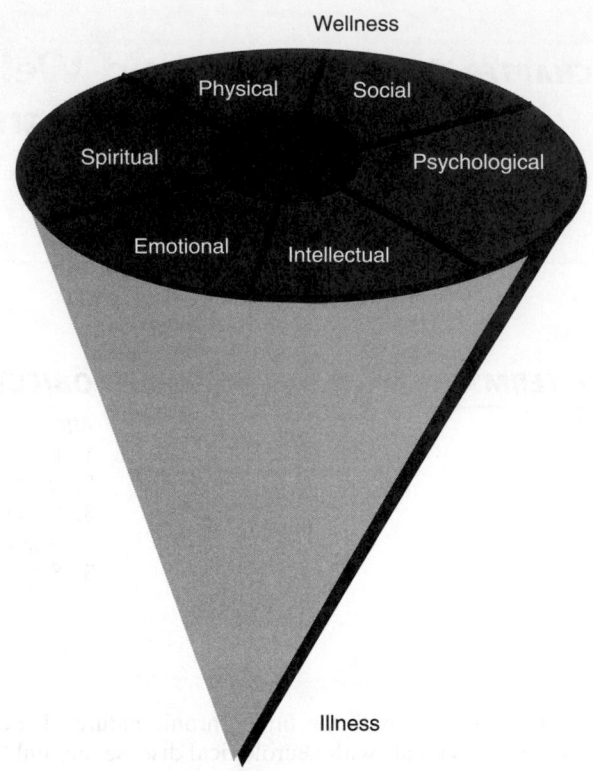

FIGURE 6-1 ■ The wellness model.

included in various wellness models are physical, spiritual, intellectual, psychological, social, emotional, occupational, and community or environmental.[18] Adams et al[18] in 1997, toward the aim of devising a wellness measurement tool, proposed six dimensions of wellness on the basis of the strength and quality of the theoretical support in the literature. The six dimensions and their corresponding definitions are shown in Table 6-1.

The second characteristic of wellness is that it has a salutogenic or health-causing focus,[14] in contrast to a pathogenic focus in an illness model. Emphasizing that which causes health (e.g., salutogenic) supports Dunn's[2] original definition that implied wellness involves "maximizing the potential of which the individual is capable." In other words, wellness isn't just preventing illness or injury or maintaining the status quo; rather, it involves choices and behaviors that emphasize optimal health and well-being beyond the status quo. Thus an individual may or may not be well before pathological conditions and diseases involve the body and similarly may be well during an acute episode or chronic pathology or disease whether that chronic problem results in static physical limitations or even progressive functional loss.

Third, wellness is consistent with a systems perspective. In systems theory each element of a system is independent and contains its own subelements, in addition to being a subelement of a larger system.[12,15,16] Further, the elements in a system are reciprocally interrelated, indicating that a disruption of homeostasis at any level of the system affects the entire system and all its subelements.[15,16] Therefore overall wellness is a reflection of the state of being within each dimension and a result of the interaction among and between the dimensions of wellness. Figure 6-1 illustrates a model of wellness reflecting this concept. Vertical movement in the model occurs between the wellness and illness poles as the magnitude of wellness in each dimension changes. The top of the model represents wellness because it is expanded maximally, whereas the bottom of the model represents illness. Bidirectional horizontal movement occurs within each dimension along the lines extending from the inner circle. As per systems theory, movement in every dimension

influences and is influenced by movement in the other dimensions.[18] As an example, an individual who has a knee injury and undergoes surgery to repair the anterior cruciate ligament will probably have at least a short-term decreased physical wellness. Applying systems theory and according to the model, this individual may also have a decrease in emotional or social wellness in the postoperative period. The overall effect of these changes in these dimensions will be a decrease in overall wellness, which anecdotally we know occurs when patients have an illness or injury.

A term related to wellness, quality of life, is also used to indicate the subjective experience of an individual in a larger context beyond just physical health. Quality of life has been defined as "an individual's perception of their position in life in the context of the culture and value systems in which they live and in relation to their goals, expectations, standards, and concerns. It is a broad ranging concept affected in a complex way by the person's physical health, psychological state, level of independence, social relationships, and their relationship to salient features of their environment."[19] Parallel to the issues related to the concept of wellness, there is lack of agreement in the literature on the definition of quality of life and its theoretical components,[20-23] as well as variation in the use of subjective or objective quality-of-life indicators.[21] Implied by the World Health Organization definition, and supported by several other authors, quality of life is best conceptualized as a subjective construct that is measured through an examination of a client's perceptions. In other words, quality of life, like wellness, is the subjective experience of health, illness, function, the environment, social support, and so forth, and it is best measured through an assessment of client perceptions.

A WELLNESS PARADIGM

The ultimate importance of gaining an understanding of health and wellness is to be able to apply it when interacting with patients/clients. In this sense, the goal would be to improve the health and well-being of the client, in addition to improving movement and function. A comparison of the traditional "illness" paradigm with both a "prevention" and "wellness" paradigm will serve to identify ways in which a physical or occupational therapist can incorporate a wellness paradigm into the treatment of a patient with a neurological disease in the context of rehabilitation. The three approaches or paradigms are contrasted in Table 6-2 on six parameters, including, the view of human systems, program orientation, dependent variables, client status, intervention focus, and intervention method.

As stated previously, in a wellness paradigm each dimension or part of the system affects and is affected by every other part, resulting in an integrative view of the human system. In contrast, in a traditional illness or medical model, the systems are independent. There are specialties in medicine by body system (e.g., neurology, orthopedics, gynecology), and in many physical and occupational therapy education programs, courses are arranged by body system (e.g., neurology, orthopedics, cardiopulmonary physical dysfunction, psychosocial), as indicators of the independence of the systems. In a prevention approach, there is recognition that the systems interact, or influence each other, but not in the reciprocal fashion characteristic of wellness.

The program orientation of an illness paradigm is the pathology or disease-causing issue, whereas the orientation of a prevention paradigm is normogenic, meaning efforts are aimed at maintaining a normal state or condition (e.g., normal muscle length, tone). Shifting to a wellness paradigm requires a salutogenic or health-causing approach,[14] with a focus on how to achieve greater well-being, health, or quality of life. This shift emphasizes the capabilities and abilities of the individual rather than the limitations and deficits.

The variables of interest in an illness paradigm are clinical variables, such as blood tests, VO_2 max (maximum volume of oxygen use), and tests of muscle strength. Changes in these variables result in labeling the patient more or less ill. In a prevention paradigm, the variables measured are behavioral, for example, whether the individual smokes, exercises, or wears a helmet. Positive improvement in a prevention approach typically results in a change in an individual's behavior. In contrast, the variables measured in a wellness paradigm are perceptual, indicating what the patient/client thinks and feels about herself or himself.

Although clinical, physiological, and behavioral variables are useful indicators of bodily wellness and are commonly used to plan individual and community interventions, their utility as wellness measures falls short.[24] Clinical and physiological measures assess the status of a single system, most commonly the systems within the physical domain of wellness. It can be argued that behavioral measures are a better reflection of multiple systems because of the importance and influence of motivation and self-efficacy on the adoption of behaviors, but they do not describe the wellness of the mind. On the other hand, perceptual measures, capable of assessing all systems and having been shown to predict effectively a variety of health outcomes,[18,25-28] can complement the information provided by body-centered measures insofar as they are valid, congruent with wellness conceptualizations, and empirically supportable.[24]

The influence of perceptions on health and wellness has been demonstrated repeatedly in the literature with a multiplicity of patient/client populations and in a variety of settings. Mossey and Shapiro[25] demonstrated more than 20 years ago that self-rated health was the second strongest predictor of mortality in the elderly, after age. Numerous other researchers have replicated these findings in other populations, lending support to the value of perceptions in understanding health and wellness and indicating that how well you *think* you are may be more important than how well you are as measured by clinical tests and measures or the judgment of a health professional. Wilson and Cleary[24] argued for the use of perceptions in understanding and explaining quality of life, proposing that health perceptions provide an important link between the biomedical model or clinical/illness paradigm with its focus on "etiological agents, pathological processes, and biological, physiological, and clinical outcomes" and the quality of life model or social science paradigm, with its focus on "dimensions of functioning and overall well-being"[24] (Figure 6-2). Citing studies that have used perceptual measures, including the Mossey and Shapiro[25] study, Wilson and Cleary[24] state that health perceptions "are among the best predictors of [outcomes from] general medical and mental health services as well as strong predictors of mortality, even after controlling for clinical factors."[24]

Shifting to client status in each of the three paradigms, the subject receiving treatment in an illness paradigm is called the patient, whereas in a prevention paradigm the subject is a person-at-risk because of the focus on risk factors and the maintenance of a state of normalcy. In a wellness paradigm, the client is considered a whole person, to emphasize the multiple systems interacting to produce a

TABLE 6-2 ■ The Wellness Matrix

	ILLNESS	PREVENTION	WELLNESS
View of human systems	Independent	Interactive	Integrative
Program orientation	Pathogenic	Normogenic	Salutogenic
Dependent variables	Clinical	Behavioral	Perceptual
Client status	Patient	Person at risk	Whole person
Intervention focus	Symptoms	Risk factors	Dispositions
Intervention method	Prescription	Lifestyle modification	Values clarification

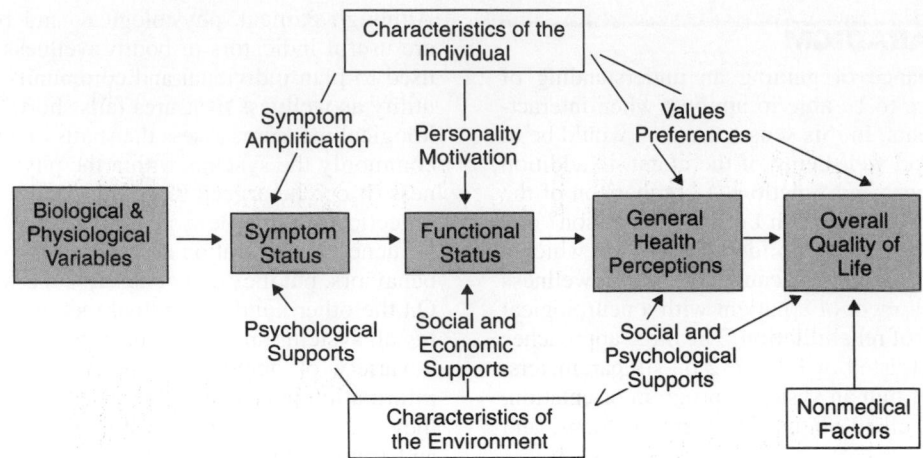

FIGURE 6-2 ■ Health-related quality-of-life conceptual model. (Modified from Wilson IB, Cleary PD: Linking clinical variables with health-related quality of life, *JAMA* 273:59-65, 1995.)

state of well-being, and, more important, that a high-functioning or intact physical dimension, although important, is not necessary to achieve a state of well-being or a high quality of life.

Consistent with the client status elements, the focus of intervention in an illness paradigm is on symptoms and in a prevention approach on risk factors. Consistent with a whole-person focus in a wellness approach, the intervention focuses on dispositions. Defined as a prevailing tendency, mood, or inclination or the tendency to act in a certain manner under given circumstances, dispositions produce perceptions, which can be measured to indicate a global or psychosocial assessment of the whole person, given input from all of the systems. Combined with symptom and risk factor assessment, perceptions of the individual provide valuable additional information about a client that can enhance the therapists' ability to intervene and the success of the interventions selected. Table 6-3 lists a few measurement tools that assess client perceptions.

The intervention method used in an illness paradigm is prescriptive. The prescriptive meaning is based on the system affected and symptoms reported. An intervention in an illness paradigm is prescribed to correct or improve the illness. Given that risk factors are the focus in a prevention paradigm and the aim is to maintain or return the person-at-risk to a normal state, the intervention method that is most appropriate is lifestyle modification in an attempt to change the behavior that is producing the identified risk. The intervention method in a wellness approach is called *values clarification*, and it is consistent with the focus on dispositions and measurement of perceptions. The aim of values clarification is to enhance self-understanding by surfacing the person's perceptions of the situation and its impact on his or her life. When values clarification can precede intervention prescription and lifestyle modification, wellness will be enhanced because the intervention will be more targeted and considerate of the person rather than the disease or condition.

MEASUREMENT OF WELLNESS

As a result of the varied way that wellness has been defined and understood, a variety of wellness measures exist. Con-

sistent with the characteristics of wellness described, a wellness measure should reflect the multidimensionality and systems orientation of the concept and have a salutogenic focus. In the literature, as well as in daily practice, clinical, physiological, behavioral, and perceptual indicators are all touted as wellness measures. Clinical measures include serum cholesterol level and blood pressure, physiological indicators include skinfold measurements and maximum oxygen uptake, behavioral measures include smoking status and physical activity frequency, and perceptual measures include patient/client self-assessment tools such as global indicators of health status (Compared with other people your age, would you say your health is excellent, good, fair, or poor?)[29] and the Short Form-36 Health Status Questionnaire[30] (see Table 6-3).

Although some perceptual measures assess only single system status (e.g., psychological well-being, mental well-being), numerous multidimensional perceptual measures exist that can serve as wellness measures. Perceptual constructs that have been used as wellness measures include general health status,[30] subjective well-being,[30,31] general well-being,[32,33] morale,[34,35] happiness,[36,37] life satisfaction,[38-40] hardiness,[41,42] and perceived wellness[18,43,44] (see Table 6-3). Refer to Figure 6-3 for the "Perceived Wellness Survey" used by many professions to help conceptualize the client's perception of her or his wellness. This survey was first published in the *American Journal of Health Promotion* in 1997.[18]

Physical therapists assess perceptions as a part of the patient/client history, as recommended in the "Guide to Physical Therapist Practice."[45] Occupational therapists assess perceptions as part of their focus on human performance and occupation. Some of the kinds of perceptions that can be assessed include perceptions of general health status, social support systems, role and social functioning, self-efficacy, and functional status in self-care and home management activities and work, community, and leisure activities. Although a few of these categories are included in overall wellness, such as general health status and social and role functioning, measuring wellness perceptions specifically can provide additional and more complete information about the patient that both the physical and occupational

TABLE 6-3 ■ Sample Items from Perceptual Measurement Tools

INSTRUMENT	PERCEPTUAL CONSTRUCT	SAMPLE ITEMS (RESPONSES)
Short Form-36[31]	General health perceptions	"In general, would you say your health is:" (excellent, very good, good, fair, or poor)
		"Compared with 1 year ago, how would you rate your health in general now?" (much better than one year ago, somewhat better, about the same, somewhat worse, much worse)
Satisfaction with Life Scale[44]	Life satisfaction	"In most ways my life is close to my ideal"
		"I am satisfied with my life" (7-point Likert scale from strongly disagree [1] to strongly agree [7])
Perceived Wellness Survey[28]	Perceived wellness	"I am always optimistic about my future"
		"I avoid activities that require me to concentrate" (6-point Likert scale from very strongly disagree [1] to very strongly agree [6])
NCHS General Well-Being Schedule[39]	General well-being	"How have you been feeling in general?" (In excellent spirits, In very good spirits, In good spirits mostly, I have been up and down in spirits a lot, In low spirits mostly, In very low spirits)
		"Has your daily life been full of things that were interesting to you?" (All the time, most of the time, A good bit of the time, Some of the time, A little of the time, None of the time)
Philadelphia Geriatric Center Morale Scale[40]	Morale	"Things keep getting worse as I get older"
		"I am as happy now as when I was younger" (yes, no)
Memorial University of Newfoundland Scale of Happiness[43]	Happiness	"In the past months have you been feeling on top of the world?"
		"As I look back on my life, I am fairly well satisfied" (yes, no, don't know)

therapist can use to formulate a plan that can be insightful to the patient/client. Therefore perceptual tools should be used when measuring wellness.

MERGING WELLNESS INTO REHABILITATION

Incorporating wellness into rehabilitation requires that the therapist or provider modify the traditional approach used to treat patients, which involves changing the focus from illness to wellness, being a role model of wellness, incorporating wellness measures into the examination, considering the client within his or her system, and offering services beyond the traditional patient-provider relationship. Establishing a wellness approach also requires that the provider assume the role of a facilitator or partner rather than that of an authority figure.[46]

When a patient is ill it is often appropriate for the health care provider to act as the expert because the patient has limited ability to provide self-care and is relying on the provider for information and skills to recover and improve. In a wellness paradigm the best approach is to believe that the client knows best in terms of maximizing her or his potential; therefore, assuming a partner or facilitator role is more appropriate and will create a relationship in which the client feels empowered to take control. Rather than "making" the client well, the provider can view the client as a whole person within a biopsychosocial context and partner with the client to discover the most appropriate path to achieve wellness. This approach is consistent with a client-centered perspective, in comparison to a biomedical

approach in which the emphasis is on impairment and physical function.[47-49] Recent discussion in the literature by a variety of health care providers suggest there is an important role for a client-centered approach within traditional medical settings.[47-51] Client-centered care requires the following:

- Assessment of and consideration for client thoughts, feelings, and expectations,
- Education about the client's condition to enhance the client's ability to take responsibility for her or his own well-being,
- A shift in professional identity from expert advisor to partner and facilitator,
- Excellent communication skills, including the use of language the client can understand and effective listening skills, and
- The provider to have a high level of confidence in his or her knowledge and skill to guide clients to optimize their potential (e.g., achieve greater wellness).[48,49]

Being a role model and fulfilling the role of facilitator will establish a relationship and environment in which clients can attain greater wellness.

It may be most instructive to consider first how a wellness approach could be adopted with clients who are seemingly healthy or without pathology. As experts in movement problems associated with the causes and consequences of pathological conditions, physical and occupational therapists should play a significant role in prevention. Indeed, intervention programs designed by therapists for patients/clients with pathology generally

Perceived Wellness Survey

The following statements are designed to provide information about your wellness perceptions. Please carefully and thoughtfully consider each statement, then select the <u>one</u> response option with which you <u>most</u> agree.

	Very Strongly Disagree				Very Strongly Agree	
1. I am always optimistic about my future.	1	2	3	4	5	6
2. There have been times when I felt inferior to most of the people I knew.	1	2	3	4	5	6
3. Members of my family come to me for support.	1	2	3	4	5	6
4. My physical health has restricted me in the past.	1	2	3	4	5	6
5. I believe there is a real purpose for my life.	1	2	3	4	5	6
6. I will always seek out activities that challenge me to think and reason.	1	2	3	4	5	6
7. I rarely count on good things happening to me.	1	2	3	4	5	6
8. In general, I feel confident about my abilities.	1	2	3	4	5	6
9. Sometimes I wonder if my family will really be there for me when I am in need.	1	2	3	4	5	6
10. My body seems to resist physical illness very well.	1	2	3	4	5	6
11. Life does not hold much future promise for me.	1	2	3	4	5	6
12. I avoid activities which require me to concentrate.	1	2	3	4	5	6
13. I always look on the bright side of things.	1	2	3	4	5	6
14. I sometimes think I am a worthless individual.	1	2	3	4	5	6
15. My friends know they can always confide in me and ask me for advice.	1	2	3	4	5	6
16. My physical health is excellent.	1	2	3	4	5	6
17. Sometimes I don't understand what life is all about.	1	2	3	4	5	6
18. Generally, I feel pleased with the amount of intellectual stimulation I receive in my daily life.	1	2	3	4	5	6
19. In the past, I have expected the best.	1	2	3	4	5	6
20. I am uncertain about my ability to do things well in the future.	1	2	3	4	5	6
21. My family has been available to support me in the past.	1	2	3	4	5	6
22. Compared to people I know, my past physical health has been excellent.	1	2	3	4	5	6
23. I feel a sense of mission about my future.	1	2	3	4	5	6
24. The amount of information that I process in a typical day is just about right for me (i.e., not too much and not too little).	1	2	3	4	5	6
25. In the past, I hardly ever expected things to go my way.	1	2	3	4	5	6
26. I will always be secure with who I am.	1	2	3	4	5	6
27. In the past, I have not always had friends with whom I could share my joys and sorrows.	1	2	3	4	5	6
28. I expect to always be physically healthy.	1	2	3	4	5	6
29. I have felt in the past that my life was meaningless.	1	2	3	4	5	6
30. In the past, I have generally found intellectual challenges to be vital to my overall well-being.	1	2	3	4	5	6
31. Things will not work out the way I want them to in the future.	1	2	3	4	5	6
32. In the past, I have felt sure of myself among strangers.	1	2	3	4	5	6
33. My friends will be there for me when I need help.	1	2	3	4	5	6
34. I expect my physical health to get worse.	1	2	3	4	5	6
35. It seems that my life has always had purpose.	1	2	3	4	5	6
36. My life has often seemed void of positive mental stimulation.	1	2	3	4	5	6

FIGURE 6-3 ■ The Perceived Wellness Survey.

include instruction in preventive behaviors and activities. Although appropriate and worthwhile, these efforts do not produce the significant outcomes that primary prevention programs might because they are applied after the onset of risk, illness, or injury. Contemporary practice includes a role for the physical and occupational therapist in primary prevention, that is, interacting with clients to promote health and improve wellness *before* they become patients.

Because individuals without overt disease are typically unmotivated to seek professional assistance, consideration must be given to how a provider recruits those without disease. A focus on wellness and health-causing activities is

a powerful solution to this dilemma. In a sports or athletic context, this approach would be considered "performance enhancing" and would be marketed to individuals who have goals and ambitions related to improving athletic performance in a specific context (e.g., improving 10K time, increasing cycling distance or speed). In a general wellness context, an appropriate marketing message might be to improve quality of life or productivity, or any subjective measure that a client deems important. The same knowledge and skills therapists use when intervening to prevent injury, delay or prevent the progression of disease, or enhance quality of movement are useful in a primary prevention context in which the goal is to improve quality of life, well-being, and productivity. The difference is the context in which the knowledge and skills are applied. Adopting a wellness paradigm and a client-centered perspective or focus creates an environment surrounding the client-provider relationship that both empowers the client to make meaningful changes and establishes a partnership that is most conducive to change and improvement. The improvement of quality of life or wellness requires a consideration of the client as a whole person, by definition, as discussed previously in this chapter. Using a client-centered, whole-person approach to the design of an intervention program requires a considerably different approach than the traditional, biomedical approach of measuring clinical and behavioral variables to identify impairments and functional loss and creating an intervention aimed at ameliorating the impairment.[48,49] Suddenly clients are more than their diseases, which sends a much different message and creates a much different relationship between the provider and the client.

Applying this same approach to individuals with chronic disease implies that the therapist must attend to more than just impairments and functional limitations and their causes when designing intervention programs and determining the best approach to adopt with an individual client. It requires consideration of issues such as social support given and received, intellectual curiosity, physical self-esteem, general self-esteem, optimism, and so forth. Recognition of these dimensions of the individual provides a unique opportunity to keep the client at the focus of the intervention and design interventions in partnership with the client that will stand a greater chance of producing positive, meaningful outcomes.[48] The following examples attempt to illustrate the adoption and application of a wellness paradigm within neurorehabilitation.

CASE STUDY ■ WELLNESS INTERVENTION CONCEPTS IN NEUROREHABILITATION

CASE STUDY 6-1

The client is a 56-year-old poststroke (CVA) man who expresses a desire to return to a pre-CVA hobby, fly fishing. In addition to the physical requirements necessary to fly fish, which the therapist would typically assess and then incorporate into the intervention plan for the goal of independence in fly fishing, a wellness approach requires additional considerations. Recognizing the client's desire to fly fish requires the therapist to have explored the client's goals and expectations and incorporate them into the intervention plan, as well as to appreciate the role of fly fishing in the achievement of well-being for this client. After the therapist provided education about living after a CVA, the client was aware that fly fishing was a realistic expectation. To understand the biomechanics and physical requirements of fly fishing, the therapist partners with the client to learn the process of fly fishing, thus gaining from the "expertise" of the client for the purpose of helping the client achieve his goal. The partnership relationship established in this case requires the therapist to be confident that she or he can identify the motor control, motor programming, and perceptual/cognitive aspects of movement program such as the strength, motion, postural requirements, and axial/distal motor relationships for fly fishing even though the therapist had never participated in or observed the activity. Throughout the process, excellent communication is required between the therapist and client to ensure that expectations are clear and that understanding is achieved to establish and meet goals. The task of learning how to fly fish may have also required the therapist to go beyond the typical boundaries of traditional care, including challenging reimbursement limitations, to assist the client in his quest for enhanced well-being.

CASE STUDY 6-2

The client is a 25-year-old man with a posttraumatic brain injury who would like to be able to spend more time with his friends. During the discussion about his desires, the therapist, learning that the group plays basketball one or two times per week, inquires about the client's interest in joining the group. The client indicates that he use to play basketball but is concerned about his ability to run and produce the movements necessary to play now. The therapist, in the role of facilitator and partner, assures the client that playing basketball is a realistic goal and expresses a willingness to assist the client in achieving his goal. To provide the interventions necessary, the therapist must understand the physical requirements of basketball, obtain access to a basket and ball, interact with the client's friends, be open to learning about basketball from the "expertise" of the client, and support and motivate the client. The therapist recognizes that playing basketball with his friends will contribute greatly to the client's overall well-being and is thus a worthwhile goal.

In both cases, the therapist functions as the movement specialist, also recognizing, however, the role of movement in the enhancement of emotional and social well-being within a paradigm of overall wellness. The potential contributions this approach can make to the overall quality of life of individuals living with neurological disease are immense and within the scope of practice and abilities of the physical and occupational therapist. Viewing the client within a larger context than the narrowly focused physical dimension provides increased opportunity to have an impact on well-being and quality of life.

REFERENCES

1. Preamble to the Constitution of the World Health Organization as adopted by the International Health Conference, New York, 19-22 June, 1946; signed on 22 July 1946 by the representatives of 61 States (Official Records of the World Health Organization, no. 2, p. 100) and entered into force on 7 April 1948.
2. Dunn HL: *High level wellness,* Washington, DC, 1961, Mt. Vernon.
3. Wu R: *Behavior and illness,* NJ, 1973, Prentice-Hall.
4. Lafferty J: A credo for wellness, *Health Educ* 10:10-11, 1979.
5. Hettler W: Wellness promotion on a university campus, *J Health Promotion Maintenance* 3:77-95, 1980.
6. Hinds WC: *Personal paradigm shift: A lifestyle intervention approach to health care management,* East Lansing, MI, 1983, Michigan State University.
7. Greenberg JS: Health and wellness: a conceptual differentiation, *J School Health* 55:403-406, 1985.
8. Ardell DB: *High level wellness,* Berkeley, CA, 1986, Ten Speed Press.
9. Travis JW, Ryan RS: *Wellness workbook,* ed 2, Berkeley, CA, 1988, Ten Speed Press.
10. Depken D: Wellness through the lens of gender: a paradigm shift. *Wellness Perspect* 10:54-69, 1994.
11. Ratner PA, Johnson JL, Jeffery B: Examining emotional, physical, social and spiritual health as determinants of self-rated health status, *Am J Health Promotion* 12:275-282, 1998.
12. Nicholas DR, Gobble DC, Crose RG, Frank B: A systems view of health, wellness and gender: implications for mental health counseling, *J Ment Health Couns* 14:8-19, 1992.
13. Whitmer JM, Sweeney TJ: A holistic model for wellness prevention over the life span, *J Couns Dev* 71:140-148, 1992.
14. Antonovsky A: *Unraveling the mystery of health: how people manage stress and stay well,* San Francisco, 1933, Josey-Bass.
15. Jasnoski ML, Schwartz GE: A synchronous systems model for health, *Am Behav Sci* 28:468-485, 1985.
16. Seeman J: Toward a model of positive health, *Am Psychol* 44:1099-1109, 1989.
17. Crose R, Nicholas DR, Gobble DC, Frank B: Gender and wellness: a multidimensional systems model for counseling, *J Couns Dev* 71:149-156, 1992.
18. Adams T, Bezner J, Steinhardt M: The conceptualization and measurement of perceived wellness: integrating balance across and within dimensions, *Am J Health Promotion* 11:208-218, 1997.
19. World Health Organization: *Measuring quality of life* (MNH/PSF/93.1), Geneva, 1993, World Health Organization.
20. Anderson KL, Burckhardt CS: Conceptualization and measurement of quality of life as an outcome variable for health care intervention and research, *J Adv Nurs* 29:298-306, 1999.
21. Gladdis MM, Gosch EA, Dishuk NM, Crits-Christoph P: Quality of life: expanding the scope of clinical significance, *J Consult Clin Psychol* 67:320-331, 1999.
22. Haas BK: Clarification and integration of similar quality of life concepts, *Image* 31:215-220, 1999.
23. Hendry F, McVittie C: Is quality of life a healthy concept? Measuring and understanding life experiences of older people, *Qual Health Res* 14:961-975, 2004.
24. Wilson IB, Cleary PD: Linking clinical variables with health-related quality of life, *JAMA* 273:59-65, 1995.
25. Mossey JM, Shapiro E: Self-rated health: a predictor of mortality among the elderly, *Am J Public Health* 72:800-808, 1983.
26. Idler E, Kasl S: Health perceptions and survival, do global evaluations of health status really predict mortality? *J Gerontol* 46:S55-S65, 1991.
27. Stewart A, Hays R, Ware J: Health perceptions, energy/fatigue, and health distress measures. In *Measuring functioning and well-being:* *the medical outcomes study approach,* Durham, NC, 1992, Duke University.
28. Eysenck H: Prediction of cancer and coronary heart disease mortality by means of a personality inventory: results of a 15-year follow-up study, *Psychol Rep* 72:499-516, 1993.
29. Ware JE, Sherbourne D: The MOS 36-item short-form health survey (SF-36), *Med Care* 30:473-483, 1992.
30. Andrews F, Robinson J: Measures of subjective well-being. In Robinson JP, Shaver PR, Wrightsman LS, editors. *Measures of personality and social psychological attitudes, vol 1,* pp 61-114, San Diego, 1991, Academic Press.
31. Diener E: Subjective well-being, *Psychol Bull* 95:542-575, 1984.
32. Campbell A, Converse P, Rodgers W: *The quality of American life,* New York, 1976, Russell Sage Foundation.
33. Fazio A: A concurrent validational study of the NCHS general well-being schedule, DHEW Publication No. (HRA) 2:78-1347, 1977.
34. Lawton M: The Philadelphia geriatric center morale scale: A revision, *J Gerontol* 30:85-89, 1975.
35. Morris J, Sherwood S: A retesting and modification of the PGC morale scale, *J Gerontol* 30:77-84, 1975.
36. Fordyce M: The PSYCHAP inventory: a multi-scale to measure happiness and its concomitants, *Soc Ind Res* 18:1-33, 1986.
37. Kozma A, Stones M: The measurement of happiness: Development of the Memorial University of Newfoundland scale of happiness (MUNSH), *J Gerontol* 35:906-912, 1980.
38. Diener E, Emmons R, Larsen R, Sandvik E: The satisfaction with life scale, *J Pers Assess* 49:71-75, 1984.
39. Neugarten B, Havighurst R, Tobin S: The measurement of life satisfaction, *J Gerontol* 16:134-143, 1961.
40. Wood V, Wylie M, Sheafor B: An analysis of a short self-report measure of life satisfaction: correlation with rater judgments, *J Gerontol* 24:465-469, 1969.
41. Kobasa S: Stressful life events, personality, and health: An inquiry into hardiness, *J Pers Soc Psychol* 37:1-11, 1979.
42. Williams P, Wiebe D, Smith T: Coping processes as mediators of the relationship between hardiness and health, *J Behav Med* 15:237-255, 1992.
43. Adams TB, Bezner JR, Drabbs ME et al: Conceptualization and measurement of the spiritual and psychological dimensions of wellness in a college population, *J Am Coll Health* 48:165-173, 2000.
44. Bezner JR, Hunter DL: Wellness perceptions in persons with traumatic brain injury and its relation to functional independence, *Arch Phys Med Rehabil* 82:787-792, 2001.
45. Guide to physical therapist practice, *Phys Ther* 81:471-593, 2001.
46. Ferguson T: Working with your doctor. In Coleman D, Gurin J, editors: *Mind body medicine,* New York, 1993, Consumer Reports Books, pp 429-450.
47. Litchfield R, MacDougall C: Professional issues for physiotherapists in family-centred and community-based settings, *Aust J Physiother* 48:105-112, 2002.
48. Black RM: Intersections of care: an analysis of culturally competent care, client centered care, and the feminist ethic of care, *Work* 24:409-422, 2005.
49. Duggan R: Reflection as a means to foster client-centred practice, *Can J Occup Ther* 72:103-112, 2005.
50. Mossberg K, McFarland C: A patient-oriented health status measure in outpatient rehabilitation, *Am J Phys Med Rehabil* 80:896-902, 2001.
51. Epstein RM, Franks P, Fiscella K et al: Measuring patient-centered communication in patient-physician consultations: theoretical and practical issues, *Soc Sci Med* 61:1516-1528, 2005.

Differential Diagnosis Phase 1: Medical Screening by the Therapist

William G. Boissonnault, PT, DHSc, FAAOMPT
Darcy A. Umphred, PT, PhD, FAPTA

KEY WORDS

Differential Diagnosis Phase 1
Differential Diagnosis Phase 2
medical screening
patient referral
review of systems screening

OBJECTIVES

After reading this chapter the student/therapist will be able to:

1. Identify the difference between Differential Diagnosis Phase 1, medical screening, and Phase 2, diagnosis of impairments, and functional limitations.
2. Analyze the concept for system and subsystem screening.
3. Develop a mechanism for body system screening to be used with clients with preexisting neurological dysfunction.
4. Analyze the significance and importance of performing a medical screening for all clients who interact in a therapeutic environment with occupational or physical therapists.

Traditionally, the term *differential diagnosis* has referred to a process used by physicians to diagnose disease. This process typically involves three distinct steps. Step 1 is taking a thorough history, including an investigation of the patient's medical history, presenting complaints, and a review of systems. Step 2 is the performance of the physical examination. This history and the findings of the physical examination will lead to a diagnosis or to step 3, the identification of necessary tests, including laboratory tests, diagnostic imaging modalities, and so on. The goal of the three steps is the formulation of a specific diagnosis that will lead to the implementation of the appropriate medical treatment and an accurate prognosis.

Although physical therapists (PTs) and occupational therapists (OTs) have long relied on examination findings to determine whether a patient should be referred to a physician or whether an appropriate treatment plan should be developed, the use of the term *differential diagnosis* is relatively new for both professions. For PTs, the differential diagnostic process fits within the Patient/Client Management Model described in *The Guide to Physical Therapist Practice*[1] (Figure 7-1). The therapist attempts to organize the history and physical examination (including tests and measures) findings into clusters, syndromes, or categories. There are certain clusters of findings that suggest the presence of disease or adverse drug event and warrant communication with a physician. There are other symptoms and signs that are consistent with conditions that fit the disablement framework. These conditions are inherent in the interrelationships between impairments, functional limitations or activities, and participation in life or disability and are appropriate for physical or occupational therapy interventions.[1-4] The process of differentiating the cluster of findings that warrant communication with a physician regarding con-

cerns about a patient's health status compared with those that do not will be called Differential Diagnosis Phase 1.[5] If the decision is reached that the symptoms and signs do fall within the scope of practice of PTs and OTs, a second level of differential diagnosis occurs. Now the therapist attempts to categorize the examination findings into the specific diagnostic categories that will specifically guide the choice of treatment interventions and the development of a prognosis. This second level of diagnosis is called Differential Diagnosis Phase 2[5] and is the focus of Chapters 8 and 9. Figure 7-2 illustrates where Differential Diagnosis Phase 1 and Phase 2 fit into the Patient/Client Management Model.

The purpose of this chapter is to discuss the medical screening components associated with Differential Diagnosis Phase 1, including identification of patient health risk factors, recognizing atypical symptoms and signs, review of systems, and within-systems review. Methods to collect this information during a patient examination are also presented. Patient case scenarios are used to illustrate the important medical screening principles.

DIFFERENTIAL DIAGNOSIS PHASE 1: MEDICAL SCREENING

The Guide to Physical Therapist Practice[1] and the Guide to Occupational Therapy Practice[2] clearly describe the therapists' responsibility to refer patients/clients with health concerns to other practitioners. The emphasis of the following discussion is detecting clinical manifestations that suggest the specific need for physician intervention. Typically, the initial warning signs associated with these scenarios include a recent onset or exacerbation of symptoms such as pain, weakness, numbness, dizziness, falls, confusion, etc., common complaints of patients with neurological disorders. Therapists may also detect symptoms or signs

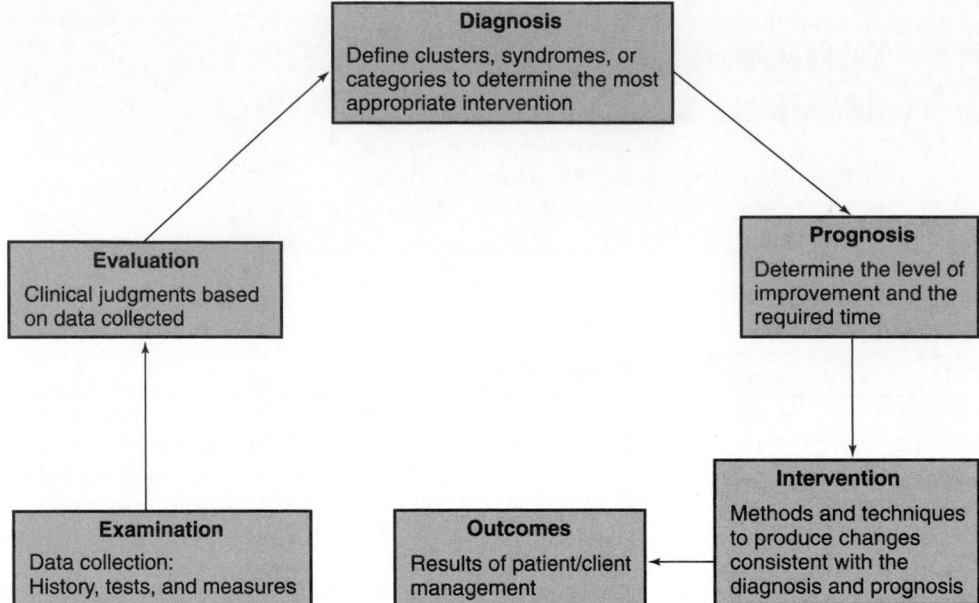

FIGURE 7-1 ■ Patient/client management model. (Adapted from American Physical Therapy Association: Guide to physical therapist practice, *Phys Ther* 81:43, 2001, with permission of the American Physical Therapy Association.)

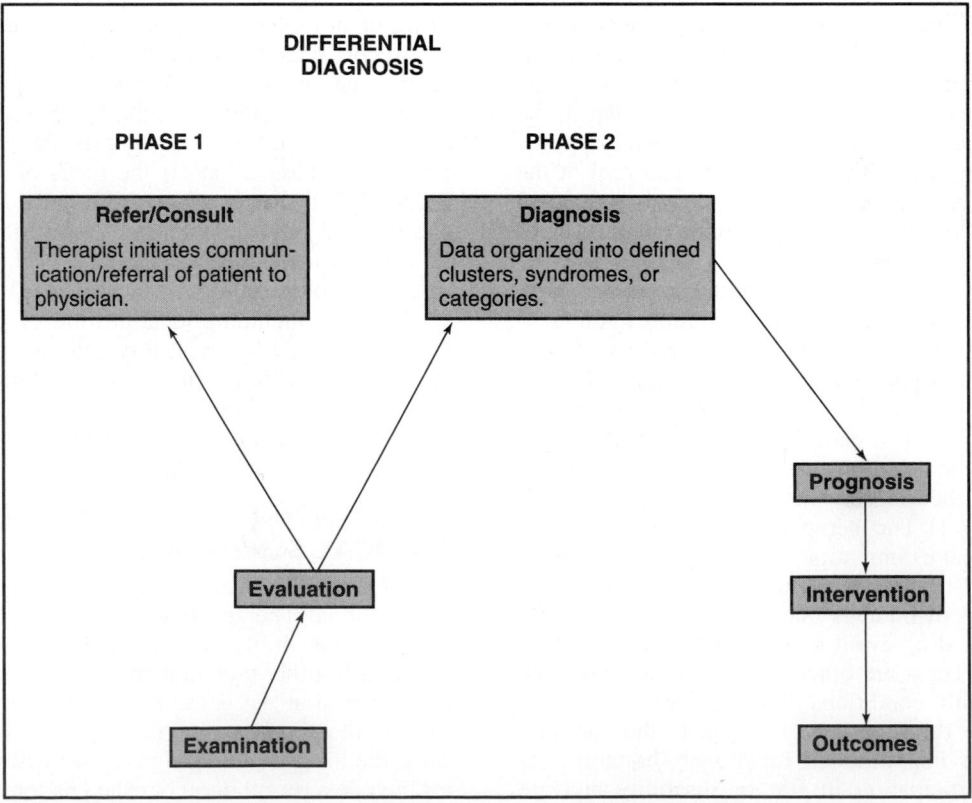

FIGURE 7-2 ■ Patient/client management model showing Differential Diagnosis Phase 1 and Phase 2. (Adapted from Umphred DA (Chair): Diagnostic Task Force, State of California, 1996-2000, California Chapter of American Physical Therapy Association.)

unrelated to the primary medical neurological condition. A general health and wellness screen may reveal a need for a psychological, dermatological, or other nonneurological medical consultation.

As opposed to Phase 2, the goal of Differential Diagnosis Phase 1 is NOT to formulate a specific diagnosis on the basis of these clinical manifestations. A therapist's Phase 2 diagnosis primarily deals with movement dysfunction and how it limits independence in life activities and an individual's ability to participate in life. Phase 1 deals with signs and symptoms that are health or disease/pathology driven and, when identified, directs a referral to a medical specialist. In fact, labeling a cluster of examination findings, when referring a patient to a physician because of health status concerns (e.g., peptic ulcer disease, endometriosis, new or progressive neurological problems), could place the therapist outside the scope of his or her practice. Having the ability to formulate such a specific disease/pathology diagnosis is not necessary to meet the responsibilities described in the Guides to practice and is outside the scope of practice for most health care practitioners other than physicians. Once the therapist's concerns have been communicated, it is then up to the physician to diagnose the presence of specific disease entities.

The purpose of the therapist's medical screening is to (1) identify existing medical conditions, (2) identify symptoms and signs suggesting that an existing medical condition may be worsening, (3) identify neurological manifestations that suggest an acute or life-threatening crisis, and (4) identify symptoms and signs suggestive of the presence of an occult disorder. This medical screening has always taken place informally within the clinical framework of physical and occupational therapists. As practitioners become more autonomous, this examination needs to become more formal requiring tools and documented evaluation results. Figure 7-3 is an example of an examination scheme leading to the decision of treating the patient, treating AND referring the patient, or referring the patient. The following material focuses on the components of this scheme most directly related to the medical screening process leading to a patient referral.

Identifying Patients' Health Risk Factors and Previous Conditions

An important aspect of the medical screening process is identifying existing health risk factors. There are numerous factors that increase the patient's risk for compromised health status, including age, sex, race, occupation, leisure activities, pre-existing medical conditions, medication usage (over-the-counter and prescription drugs), family medical history, tobacco use, and substance abuse or the interaction of some of these conditions.

Of these, a personal history of a current or recent medical condition, current medication use, and a positive family history (e.g., mother and aunt with a history of breast cancer, father diagnosed with prostate cancer at the age of 58 years) are the most relevant risk factors for the potential presence of an occult condition. For example, the history of a previous episode of depression significantly increases the risk of a second episode compared with the risk for someone who has never had an episode of depression having an initial episode.[6] The greater the number of existing risk factors, the

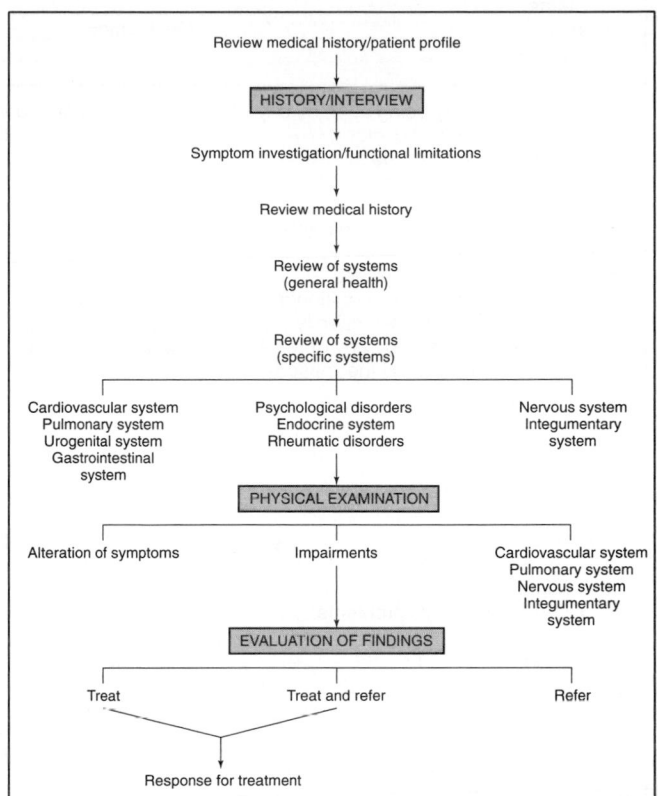

FIGURE 7-3 ■ Patient examination scheme. (Taken from notes from course by W. G. Boissonnault, 1998.)

more vigilant the therapist should be for the presence of warning signs suggestive of disease and the more extensive the other medical screening components will need to be.

There are different methods to collect this medical history/patient profile information, including a review of the medical record and use of a self-administered questionnaire. Figure 7-4 is an example of a self-administered questionnaire that could be completed by the adult patient, a family member, or a caregiver. As noted in Figure 7-3, a review of this information should occur, if possible, before the patient interview is begun. The therapist will have a head start in organizing the history and physical examination, knowing what to prioritize and at least initially what parts of the examination can be deemphasized. The utility and accuracy of using a self-administered questionnaire in patient populations germane to therapists' practice, similar to the one illustrated in Figure 7-4, has been described; with the conclusion that such a tool can be a valuable adjunct to the oral patient interview.[7]

Affirmative answers to previous or current illness questions should direct the therapist to consider what the potential impact may be on the patient's complaints, choice of examination and treatment techniques, rehabilitation potential, and risk for additional illness. For example, the presence of existing chronic kidney disease should alert the therapist to numerous potential complications. Chronic renal failure could result in fatigue, weakness, and impaired concentration, all of which could interfere with rehabilitation efforts. Chronic renal failure could also result in paresthesia and muscle weakness, which could mistakenly be associated with other neurological conditions. Osteoporosis can also

Medical History Questionnaire

Name:_____ Age _____

SS#: _____ Occupation: _____

Leisure activities: _____

I. Are you currently being seen by any of the following professionals:

A. General medical doctor (MD)	Yes	No
B. Medical specialist (MD)	Yes	No
If yes: please specify _____		
C. Osteopathic doctor	Yes	No
D. Physical/occupational therapist	Yes	No
E. Chiropractor	Yes	No
F. Psychiatrist/psychologist	Yes	No
G. Alternative medical practitioner	Yes	No
If yes: please specify _____		

If you have been seen by any of the above practitioners within the last year, please discuss the reasons:

_____

_____

_____

II. Have you EVER been diagnosed as having the following condition(s)?

A. Stroke	Yes	No
B. Seizure disorders	Yes	No
C. Migraines	Yes	No
D. Other neurologic problems:	Yes	No
Specify _____		
E. Depression	Yes	No
F. Cancer: Specify _____	Yes	No
G. High blood pressure	Yes	No
H. Heart condition	Yes	No
I. Emphysema	Yes	No
J. Asthma	Yes	No
K. Tuberculosis	Yes	No
L. Diabetes	Yes	No
M. Rheumatoid arthritis	Yes	No
N. Other arthritic disease	Yes	No
O. Kidney disease	Yes	No
P. Anemia	Yes	No
Q. Hepatitis	Yes	No
R. Circulatory problems	Yes	No
S. Thyroid problems	Yes	No
T. Skin problems	Yes	No
U. Digestive problems	Yes	No
V. Bowel or bladder problems	Yes	No
W. Chemical dependency (e.g., alcoholism)	Yes	No
X. Unexplained falls	Yes	No
Y. Cognitive dysfunction	Yes	No
Z. Genetic disorders	Yes	No
AA. Other _____	Yes	No

Please list all surgeries/hospitalizations including dates and reasons.

Date   Surgery/hospitalization/reason

_____ _____

_____ _____

Are you being or have you been treated for musculoskeletal injuries (fracture, dislocations, repetitive strains, joint instability)? If so, please state:

Date   Injury

_____ _____

_____ _____

Are you being or have you been treated for neuromuscular problems (weakness, pain, spasticity, incoordination, dizziness, tremor)? If so, please state:

Date   Injury

_____ _____

_____ _____

Has anyone in your immediate family (parents, sisters, brothers) ever been treated for any of the following:

A. Stroke	Yes	No
B. Seizure disorders	Yes	No
C. Parkinson's disease	Yes	No
D. Multiple sclerosis	Yes	No
E. Other neurologic problems _____	Yes	No
F. Mental illness	Yes	No
G. Cancer	Yes	No
H. High blood pressure	Yes	No
I. Heart condition	Yes	No
J. Breathing problems	Yes	No
K. Diabetes	Yes	No
L. Arthritic disease	Yes	No
M. Kidney disease	Yes	No
N. Anemia	Yes	No
O. Vascular problems	Yes	No
P. Thyroid problems	Yes	No
Q. Skin problems	Yes	No
R. Chemical dependency (e.g., alcoholism)	Yes	No
S. Learning disabilities	Yes	No
T. Cognitive dysfunction	Yes	No
U. Genetic disorders	Yes	No

Please list any PRESCRIPTION medications you are currently taking (include pills, injections, patches, etc.)

_____

_____

_____

Please list any OVER-THE-COUNTER MEDICATIONS you are taking:

_____

_____

_____

Please list any *prescriptions* or *over-the-counter* medications you were taking prior to your current problems

_____

_____

How much caffeinated coffee or other caffeinated beverages do you drink per day? (number of cups/cans/bottles) _____

Do you smoke?	Yes	No
If yes: How many packs per day?		_____

Do you drink alcohol?
  If yes: How many days per week
    do you drink? _____ days/week
  If yes: How many drinks per sitting? _____ drinks/sitting
    (Note: one beer or one glass of wine equals 1 drink)

If you use marijuana or other
  substances, how often? _____ days/week

FIGURE 7-4 ■ Self-administered questionnaire to collect medical history information. (Adapted from Boissonnault WG, Koopmeiners MB: Medical history profile: orthopaedic physical therapy outpatients, *J Orthop Sports Phys Ther* 20:2-10, 1994, with permission of the Orthopaedic and Sports Sections of the American Physical Therapy Association.)

be associated with chronic renal failure. This potential association should direct the therapist to use techniques that carry a reduced risk of skeletal injury. A series of follow-up questions for the affirmative answers will assist the therapist in determining the relevance (if any) of each item (see Figure 7-5 for examples of follow-up questions for some of the information categories).

Having the self-administered questionnaire completed before the scheduled time of the initial visit will improve the therapist's efficiency. Mailing the questionnaire to the patient before the visit or having the patient arrive 10 to 15 minutes before the appointment would allow for the form being completed without taking time away from the actual examination itself. Once completed, taking 1 to 2 minutes to scan the questionnaire before the interview should be all that is necessary for the therapist to begin formulating questions and organizing the physical examination. The inability of the patient to recall or complete the questionnaire may be another sign that medical clearance is necessary before progressing to Phase 2.

Chief Presenting Complaint or Functional Restriction

The chief complaint or the functional restriction typically provides the reason for therapy services being sought and can provide the initial warning sign(s) of potential issues needing to be addressed. Relatively mild pain is often the initial complaint associated with a serious pathological condition and it can be overlooked by therapists working with patients who are neurologically involved and presenting with symptoms (e.g., weakness, numbness) much more debilitating and causing more functional limitations than the pain complaints do. While investigating pain complaints may not be the initial priority for these therapists, at a later visit such questioning is very important, especially if it continues, increases in intensity, shifts, or enlarges its region with no causation. Effective medical screening involves the interpretation of a patient's description of symptoms, func-

tional limitations, and the corresponding physical examination findings. Descriptions of symptoms associated with neuromusculoskeletal impairments (loss or abnormality of physiological, psychological, or anatomical structure or function) generally reveal a fairly consistent and predictable pattern of onset and change over a defined period of time. In addition, the neurological and musculoskeletal impairments noted during the physical examination should match with the functional limitations described by the patient or the caregiver. If these expectations are not met, it does not necessarily mean the patient has cancer or infection, but doubt should be raised on the therapist's part whether therapy is indicated.

Patients many times are not aware that presenting symptoms or signs suggest a condition better addressed by a physician as opposed to a PT or OT. For example, Mr. S. had a cerebrovascular accident 6 months ago with resultant mild residual left hemiplegia. At the time of discharge from rehabilitation services he was independent in all activities of daily living, but residual left upper extremity weakness remained. When visiting his internist for a routine checkup, he complained that over the past 3 weeks he had lost some functional skills and was having difficulty with self-care. The physician then referred Mr. S. to the therapy clinic for evaluation and treatment. Mr. S. states he has been less active and just needs some help regaining his motor function. During the history taking he states he is experiencing a deep, dull, aching sensation in the lower lumbar spine and right buttock. He assumes it has developed as a result of his inactivity and thus saw no reason to bother the physician with this problem. As Mr. S. continues to describe his difficulties, he also notes a constant deep ache in the right shoulder that he relates to increased use of his right arm to compensate for the left arm weakness. The physical examination of the low back, pelvis, and right shoulder reveals that the existing symptoms do not vary with active or passive range of motion, resisted testing, or postural holding. In addition, quantity of motion is normal for these regions and motor programming appears intact. At this point the therapist cannot explain the symptoms from an impairment standpoint; therefore, depending on other examination findings, including the patient profile and medical history, communication with the internist may be warranted. The following information describes some of the subcategories associated with symptom investigation.

Location of Symptoms

A body diagram can be a valuable tool to document the location of symptoms expressed verbally or nonverbally by patients with identified neurological deficits. Besides pain and altered sensation, patterns of abnormal tone, asymmetrical posturing, and areas of weakness can also be noted on the body diagram (Figure 7-6). Numerous body structures are potential pain generators, including visceral structures. Figure 7-7 and Table 7-1 illustrate local and referred pain patterns from various visceral organs. Because there is so much overlap between pain locations associated with visceral disease and neuromusculoskeletal conditions, the results obtained in and of themselves have minimal use in differentiating musculoskeletal from nonmusculoskeletal conditions. Being familiar with the visceral pain patterns will be extremely important, however, when deciding which

---

Medical History Follow-up Form

1. Have you EVER been diagnosed as having the following condition(s)?

Heart condition   (Yes)   No

Follow-up questions:
- Describe your heart condition?/What is your heart condition?
- Current problem or previous problem and now fully resolved?
- If a current problem
  - Which doctor is following you for this condition?
  - When is your next follow-up visit?
  - What symptoms do you experience when your heart problem acts up?
  - How do you treat your problem if it's acting up?
  - How does your heart problem interfere with your daily activities/lifestyle?
  - Has the MD placed you on any restrictions owing to your heart problem?

2. Has anyone in your immediate family (parents, sister[s], brother[s]) ever been treated for any of the following:

Cancer   (Yes)   No

Follow-up questions:
- Who in your family has the history of cancer?
- What type of cancer?
- At what age were they diagnosed?
- What is their current health status?
- Does anyone else in your family have cancer?

FIGURE 7-5 ■ Potential follow-up questions for affirmative answers on the self-administered questionnaire. (From W. G. Boissonnault, course notes, 1998.)

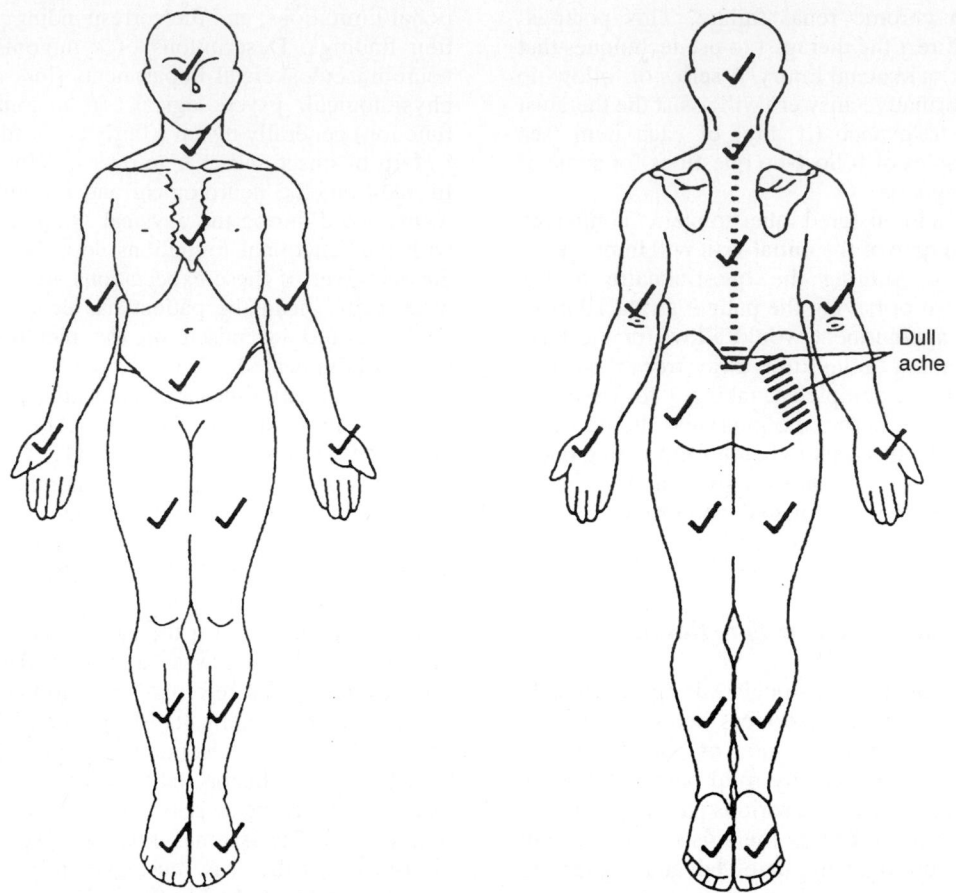

FIGURE 7-6 ■ Body diagram illustrating symptom location. Body areas with no known symptoms or abnormalities are marked with a "check" mark. (From Boissonnault WG, editor: *Examination in physical therapy practice—screening for medical disease,* ed 2, New York, 1995, Churchill Livingstone.)

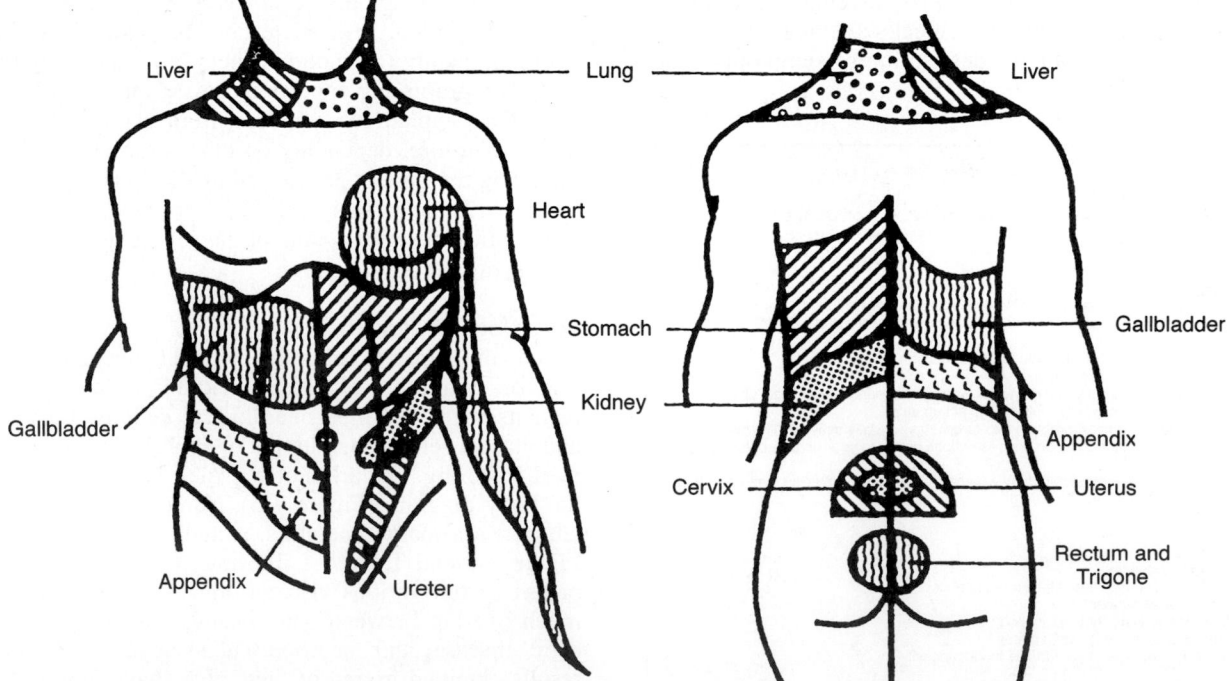

FIGURE 7-7 ■ Possible local and referred pain patterns of visceral structures. (From Boissonnault WG, editor: *Examination in physical therapy practice—screening for medical disease,* ed 2, New York, 1995, Churchill Livingstone.)

TABLE 7-1 ■ Visceral Pain Patterns

STRUCTURE	SEGMENTAL INNERVATION	POSSIBLE AREAS OF PAIN REFERRAL
PELVIC ORGANS		
Uterus including uterine ligaments	T10–L1, S2–4	Lumbosacral junction Sacral Thoracolumbar
Ovaries	T10–11	Lower abdominal Sacral
Testes	T10–11	Lower abdominal Sacral
RETROPERITONEAL REGION		
Kidney	T10–L1	Lumbar spine (ipsilateral) Lower abdominal Upper abdominal
Ureter	T11–L2, S2–4	Groin Upper abdominal Suprapubic Medial, proximal thigh Thoracolumbar
Urinary bladder	T11–L2, S2–4	Sacral apex Suprapubic Thoracolumbar
Prostate gland	T11–L1, S2–4	Sacral Testes Thoracolumbar
DIGESTIVE SYSTEM ORGANS		
Esophagus	T6–10	Substernal and upper abdominal
Stomach	T6–10	Upper abdominal Middle and lower thoracic spine
Small intestine	T7–10	Middle thoracic spine
Pancreas	T6–10	Upper abdominal Lower thoracic spine Upper lumbar spine
Gallbladder	T7–9	Right upper abdominal Right middle and lower thoracic spine, including caudal aspect scapula
Liver	T7–9	Right middle and lower thoracic spine
Common bile duct	T6–10	Upper abdominal Middle thoracic spine
Large intestine	T11–12	Lower abdominal Middle lumbar spine
Sigmoid colon	T11–12	Upper sacral Suprapubic Left lower quadrant of abdomen
CARDIOPULMONARY SYSTEM		
Heart	T1–5	Cervical anterior Upper thorax Left upper extremity
Lungs and bronchi	T5–6	Ipsilateral thoracic spine Cervical (diaphragm involved)
Diaphragm (central portion)	C3–5	Cervical spine

Adapted from Boissonnault WG, Bass C: Pathological origins of trunk and neck pain, I. Pelvic and abdominal visceral disorders, *J Orthop Sports Phys Ther* 12:192-207, 1990, with permission of the Orthopaedic and Sports Sections of the American Physical Therapy Association.

body systems to screen during the review of systems. Besides noting where symptoms are located, it is equally important to document areas of no complaints (Figure 7-6). Once the patient has reported symptoms (e.g., low back and right buttock aching, Figure 7-6), therapists should clarify. Screening to eliminate the possibility of symptoms being present down the back and up the front of the legs, pelvis, stomach, chest, neck and face areas, or between the shoulder blades and in the arms is critical. If there is one body area so involved that all the patient's and practitioner's attention is focused on it, that relatively mild, but potentially serious, symptoms may be overlooked elsewhere. Placing a check mark over each body region void of symptoms or other abnormal findings is one way to document such information and record change over time.

Symptom Pattern

Aspects of the patient's chief complaint other than symptom location are very relevant to the process of differential diagnosis, in particular a description of how and when the symptoms changed over a defined period of time. Complaints of pain, paresthesia, and numbness associated with primary musculoskeletal conditions typically change in a consistent manner over a 24-hour period. The patient will report that the symptom intensity increases with the assumption of specific postures such as left side lying or sitting or with specific activities such as walking, driving, or 2 hours of computer work. Conversely, patients typically can relate paresthesia or pain relief with avoiding certain postures or activities, the assumption of certain postures, wearing an arm sling, and so on. Night pain investigation also falls under this subcategory of patient data. If the pattern of symptom aggravation and alleviation is that there is no consistent pattern such as pain that comes and goes independent of the patient's posture, activities, or time of day, night pain is the patient's most intense pain, or paresthesia or pain that moves from one body region to another inconsistent with common pain referral patterns or identified medical conditions, the therapist should start thinking whether physical or occupational therapy is what the patient truly needs.[8]

In general, when symptoms such as weakness or numbness associated with primary neurological conditions are investigated, the 24-hour reference point to assess symptom change is not realistic. Except for an acute onset or exacerbation, these symptoms tend not to fluctuate that quickly with change in posture or position. Understanding the pathogenesis of primary neurological disorders will allow for detection of symptom change unusual for the patient. This will lead to follow-up questions to determine whether this change may represent a medically serious situation. Similarly, a change in the biomechanical alignment of a joint (e.g., the shoulder), may immediately alter the patient's pain response, indicating a direct relationship between musculoskeletal imbalance in joint stabilization and gravitational pull, for which therapy would be appropriate.

History of Symptoms

The therapist must also scrutinize the patient's report of the onset of the symptoms. Pain and paresthesia or numbness associated with neuromusculoskeletal impairments typically can be related to trauma, either on a macro or a micro level, or to a medical event such as a cerebrovascular accident.

More often than not it is repetitive overuse or cumulative trauma that leads to tissue breakdown and inflammation (see Chapter 15). Patients with neurological impairments resulting in postural abnormalities and abnormal movement patterns are at risk for such conditions. If a patient's symptoms are truly insidious, meaning not related to macro or micro trauma, or there has not been a significant change in activity level that reasonably accounts for the complaints, the therapist should again be concerned about the source of the symptoms. A worsening of symptoms (e.g., numbness, weakness, spasticity, swelling) associated with an existing medical condition should be investigated by the therapist with the same scrutiny. The therapist always needs to ask, "Is there a reasonable explanation for the worsening?" An increase in the intensity of the complaints or the involvement of additional body regions could signal a progression of the disease.

Review of Body Systems

By design, *review of systems* screening allows the therapist to detect symptoms secondary (and maybe unrelated) to the reason therapy has been initiated.[9] The review of systems allows for a general screening of body systems for symptoms suggesting the presence of an adverse drug reaction, occult disease, or worsening of an existing medical condition. Suspicions of any of these scenarios would warrant communication with a physician. Checklists of symptoms and signs for each body system can be used by the physical or occupational therapist during the patient interview (Box 7-1). To keep the checklists manageable in length, the therapist should investigate presenting complaints and symptoms and the patient's medical history before the review of systems, as noted in Figure 7-3. For example, on review of the cardiovascular/peripheral vascular system checklist items associated with heart conditions in Box 7-1, important items appear to be omitted, such as chest pain, claudication and a history of heart problems, hypertension, high cholesterol levels, and circulatory problems. If symptoms have already been investigated by use of a body diagram, the therapist would already know whether the patient has chest pain. If symptom change (aggravation or alleviation) over a 24-hour period has already been investigated, the therapist would know whether claudication was an issue. Finally, if the patient's medical history has already been discussed, the therapist would know whether heart problems, hypertension, or circulatory problems existed.

All of the checklists in Box 7-1 need not be used for every patient. The location of symptoms will direct the therapist in deciding which checklists should be included in the initial examination. Figure 7-7 and Table 7-1 can be used to link pain location with visceral systems that could be the source of the complaints. Table 7-2 provides a summary of potential pain locations and disease of the pulmonary, cardiovascular, gastrointestinal, and urogenital systems. Other symptom characteristics can also alert the therapist for the possible involvement of the endocrine, nervous, and psychological systems. Symptoms, including pain and paresthesias that come and go irrespective of posture, activity, or time of day and that appear to move among the various body regions can be associated with these systems as well as the visceral systems. In addition to the identification of the location and characteristics of symptoms, a patient's medical history will also help the therapist decide which systems to screen. A positive medical history, such as a heart problem, would direct the therapist to investigate the patient's condition, including possible use of the cardiovascular/peripheral vascular checklist as well as the questions listed in Figure 7-5. The therapist also needs to be aware of the medications taken by the patient to medically manage these pathological conditions. Similarly, therapists need to be able to analyze how the drugs potentially affect functional movements and functional loss. Often, that means a therapist must have a working professional relationship with a clinical pharmacist (see Chapter 36). Use of a general health checklist (Box 7-2) can assist the therapist in prioritizing the inclusion of the checklists in the review of systems checklists box during the initial visit. The symptoms noted in this checklist can be associated with disease of most of the body's systems, as well as with systemic disease and adverse drug events.

If the patient or caregiver (on the patient's behalf) replies yes to any *review of system* question, the therapist must determine whether there is a reasonable explanation for the complaint and whether the physician is aware of the complaint and, if so, has the complaint(s) worsened since the patient last saw the physician? When the given explanation is not satisfactory, the physician is unaware of the complaint, or the symptom is worsening, communication with the physician is warranted. All the checklists do not need to be covered during the initial visit. If the patient says "no" for each of the general health items, the patient's health history is uneventful and the therapist is comfortable with the description of the chief complaints (including pattern and onset), then the therapist can proceed with the evaluation of specific impairments and functional limitations with some confidence that Differential Diagnosis Phase 2 and therapy intervention is very likely appropriate. The review of systems then takes on a lower priority. The result is that the therapist could decide to delay the use of the appropriate review of systems checklists until the patient's second or third visit. If the patient answers "yes" to general health items and presents with an inconsistent pain pattern, the appropriate review of systems then takes on a higher priority and should be covered during the initial visit.

Musculoskeletal System

Box 7-3 provides the checklist for the musculoskeletal (MSK) system. In addition, as with all other body systems, the general health checklist also provides a level of screening for conditions of the MSK system such as infections, metastatic cancers, and rheumatic disorders (e.g., rheumatoid arthritis). Identifying patient risk factors for these conditions is a key for recognizing when to be suspicious. For example, those at highest risk for MSK cancers are those (1) over the age of 50 years and under 20 years, (2) a previous history of cancer (e.g., breast, lung, prostate, thyroid, and kidney—the most common cancers to metastasize to the axial skeleton), (3) a positive family history of cancer, and (4) exposure to environmental toxins. Those individuals at highest risk for MSK infections report or demonstrate (1) current or recent infection (e.g., urinary tract, tooth abscess, skin infection), (2) history of diabetes with use of large doses of steroids or immunosuppressive drugs, (3) elderly age, and (4) spinal cord injury with complete motor and sensory loss.[10] Last, the primary risk factors for

BOX 7-1 ■ REVIEW OF SYSTEMS CHECKLISTS

CARDIOVASCULAR/PERIPHERAL VASCULAR
dyspnea
orthopnea
palpitations
pain with sweating
syncope
peripheral edema
cold feet/hands
peripheral sensory loss
skin discoloration
open wounds/gangrene
cough

GASTROINTESTINAL
difficulty with swallowing
heartburn, indigestion
specific food intolerance
bowel dysfunction
   color
   frequency
   shape/caliber
   constipation/diarrhea
   incontinence

UROGENITAL
urinary
   frequency
   urgency
   incontinence
reduced force of stream
difficulty initiating/attention needed to urinate
dysuria
color

REPRODUCTIVE: MALE
urethral discharge
impotence
dyspareunia

REPRODUCTIVE: FEMALE
vaginal discharge
dyspareunia
change in menstruation
frequency and length of cycle
dysmenorrhea
blood flow
date of last period
number of pregnancies
number of deliveries
menopause

PSYCHOLOGICAL (DEPRESSION)
depressed/irritable mood
psychomotor agitation/retardation
apathy
sleep disturbance
weight gain/loss
fatigue
feelings of worthlessness
impaired concentration
suicide ideation (recurrent)
recent loss of family member

PULMONARY
dyspnea
onset of cough
change in cough
sputum
hemoptysis
clubbing of the nails
stridor
wheezing

SENSORY AND MOTOR NERVOUS SYSTEMS
sudden or slow onset of sensory loss
impaired balance
unexplainable frequent falls
impaired gross movement patterns
decrease/difficulty in fine motor skill
impaired mentation
tremors: intentional/nonintentional
muscle atrophy: symmetrical vs asymmetrical
asymmetrical facial features
asymmetrical tongue patterns
facial contour
ptosis
pupil abnormalities
strabismus

ENDOCRINE
arthralgias
myalgias
neuropathies
cold/heat intolerance
skin/hair changes
fatigue
weight gain/loss
polyuria
polydipsia

BOX 7-2 ■ GENERAL HEALTH CHECKLIST

Fatigue
Malaise
Fever/chills/sweating
Nausea
Unexplained weight change
Dizziness/light headedness
Unexplained paresthesia/numbness
Unexplained weakness
Unexplained cognitive and emotional changes

BOX 7-3 ■ MUSCULOSKELETAL SYSTEM SCREENING

Insidious onset of symptoms
Atypical pain pattern (aggravating/alleviating factors)
Night pain
Inadequate relief of symptoms with rest/rehabilitation
Inability to alter symptoms during the physical examination
Lack of impairments that match patients' functional limitations
Atypical physical examination findings (e.g., masses, unexplained atrophy, or weakness)

TABLE 7-2 ■ Linking Pain Patterns and Visceral Systems

PAIN LOCATION	VISCERAL SYSTEMS
Right shoulder (including shoulder girdle)	Pulmonary
	Cardiovascular
	Gastrointestinal
Left shoulder (including shoulder girdle)	Cardiovascular
	Pulmonary
Upper/midthoracic spine	Cardiovascular
	Pulmonary
	Gastrointestinal
Lower thoracic and upper/midlumbar spine	Peripheral vascular
	Pulmonary
	Gastrointestinal
	Urogenital
Lumbopelvic region	Gastrointestinal
	Urogenital
	Peripheral vascular

BOX 7-4 ■ SKIN LESION SCREENING— PATHOLOGICAL CHARACTERISTICS

Multivariant color
Black or blue-black color
Irregular borders
Nondistinct ("fuzzy") borders
Size: 6 mm or larger in diameter
Asymmetrical shape
Friable tissue
Ulcerations
Evolving (changing size, shape, color)

rheumatoid arthritis include (1) female sex, (2) age (peak) 30 to 40 years, and (3) positive family history.[11]

The other category of MSK conditions that therapists need to be vigilant for is fractures. The pain and deformity associated with most sudden-impact, traumatic fractures make for an obvious presentation. However, trauma sufficient to cause a fracture may not be so obvious in a patient with decreased bone density. Lifting a gallon of milk, a mild slip or bump, or trying to open a window that is stuck may be sufficient to cause a fracture in a patient with a history of chronic renal failure, multiple sclerosis, rheumatoid arthritis, hyperparathyroidism, gastrointestinal malabsorption syndrome, and long-term corticosteroid, heparin, anticonvulsant, and cytotoxic medication use. The most common locations for such fractures include vertebral bodies, neck of the femur, and radius. Observation of posture/body position may provide a clue that something may have changed structurally. For example, with vertebral compression fractures the thoracic kyphotic curve may be accentuated, accompanied by a very pronounced apex of the curve that was not present before. With femoral neck fracture the lower extremity is often positioned in external rotation and appears shortened compared with its counterpart.[12]

Causing potential confusion for the clinician is diseases of the MSK system, which may mimic mechanical MSK conditions. The patient may report a specific event or time of onset of symptoms, and a pain pattern of increased pain with weight bearing on the involved extremity and decreased pain with assumption of non-weight-bearing positions; all typical findings with impairment-driven symptoms. The therapist may also be able to provoke symptoms during the physical examination as the involved bony area is mechanically loaded. When the history and physical examination findings are evaluated, an unusual finding or pattern will emerge, making the therapist step back and consider alternative hypotheses regarding the origin of patient symptoms, especially if the risk factors listed above are present.

Integumentary System

Screening the integumentary system is not typically based on the presence or absence of pain, paresthesia, or numbness. As with the nervous system, some degree of screening of the integumentary system occurs with every patient regardless of the presenting diagnosis. Skin cancer has the highest incidence of all the cancers,[13] and therapists generally see a number of exposed body areas during the postural assessment and regional examination that make up the physical examination. In fact, as noted in Figure 7-3, screening the skin begins during the patient interview. During the interview the therapist can be looking at areas of exposed skin such as the face, neck, arms, and feet. As with screening the other body systems, the therapist's goal is not to identify a melanoma or differentiate squamous cell and basal cell carcinoma but simply to identify skin lesions with atypical presentations. Once the patient is referred to the physician, disease will be ruled out or diagnosed. Box 7-4 can be used to assess any mole or other skin marking. The items noted are atypical for a benign lesion, more suggestive of a pathological condition.[14] If the therapist notes any of these findings and the patient reports a recent change in the size, color, or shape of the lesion and that a physician has not looked at the lesion, a referral would be warranted.

Besides skin lesions, abnormal general skin color can be a manifestation of a number of conditions. Table 7-3 summarizes abnormal skin color changes. Occasionally, some of the most obvious abnormalities are the most difficult to note when one is so focused on items more directly related to therapeutic intervention.

Nervous System

As with the integumentary system, the nervous system is screened to a degree for all patients. The *review of systems* checklists in Box 7-1 includes items that provide a very gross, general screening of the nervous system. The therapist should be vigilant for the presence of any of these items in all patients during the initial and subsequent visits. For patients with pre-existing findings from this checklist, the therapist must be vigilant for a worsening of the observed abnormalities. Covering the items in the nervous system checklist should add little time to the therapist's initial examination. Assessing for facial asymmetries and tremors can take place during the interview. Observing balance, movement patterns, and muscle atrophy can occur while

TABLE 7-3 ■ Abnormal Color Changes of the Skin

COLOR CHANGE	PHYSIOLOGICAL CHANGE	COMMON CAUSES
White, pale (pallor)	Absence of pigment or pigment changes	Albinism, lack of sunlight
	Blood abnormality	Anemia, lead poisoning
	Temporary interruption or diversion of blood flow	Vasospasm, syncope, stress, internal bleeding
	Internal disease	Chronic gastrointestinal disease, cancer, parasitic disease, tuberculosis
Blue (cyanosis)	Decreased oxygen in blood (deoxyhemoglobin)	Methemoglobinemia (oxidation of hemoglobin), high blood iron level, cold exposure, vasomotor instability, cerebrospinal disease
Yellow	Jaundice, excess bilirubin in blood, excess bile pigment	Liver disease, gallstone blockage of bile duct, hepatitis (conjunctivae are also yellow)
	High levels of carotene in blood (carotenemia)	Ingestion of food high in carotene and vitamin A
Gray	High level of metals in body	Increased iron, bronze/gray; increased silver, blue/gray
Brown (hyperpigmentation)	Disturbances of adrenocortical hormones	Adrenal pituitary
		Addison's disease

From Shapiro C, Skopit S: Screening for skin disorders. In Boissonnault WG, editor: *Examination in physical therapy practice—screening for medical disease,* ed 2, New York, 1995, Churchill Livingstone.

watching the patient ambulate into the examination area, during the interview, and as the patient changes positions during the physical examination. Last, impaired mentation may become apparent during the interview or the physical examination as the patient struggles to appropriately answer questions or follow directions. Case Study 7-1 at the end of this chapter illustrates the importance of this general screening.

Depression

Depression is a commonly encountered psychological disorder that is associated with significant morbidity and mortality.[6,15-17] The *review of systems* checklists in Box 7-1 contains the checklist of items the therapist can use to help make the decision to refer a patient for consultation. If the patient has suicide ideation, the physician should be contacted before the patient leaves the clinic. For the first eight items on the depression checklist, concern should be raised when the therapist detects four to five of the items present daily for a minimum of 2 weeks and resulting in the patient having difficulty functioning at home, work, or school, socially, or in rehabilitation. Of the four to five items, one of them should be the depressed/irritable affect or apathy. An exception to the 2-week time frame is during periods of bereavement. When they are faced with a significant loss, it is not uncommon for people to experience a number of the checklist items as they work through the grieving process.[6] (Refer to Chapter 5.) It is reasonable for these people to experience these symptoms for up to 2 months. A neurological event such as a cerebrovascular accident could easily trigger a major clinical depressive disorder, and the depression could significantly impede rehabilitation progress. The therapist may be in the position to facilitate a psychological consultation.

Considering that approximately 15% of people with true major clinical depression commit suicide (Diagnostic and Statistical Manual, Fourth Edition, revised [DSM-IVR]), therapists need to be vigilant for warning signs that the patient may be considering this action. See the Suicide Screening shown in Box 7-5 for a list of warning signs. Once the patient acknowledges suicide ideation, follow-up ques-

BOX 7-5 ■ SUICIDE WARNING SIGNS

History of major clinical depression, chemical dependency, schizophrenia, and previous suicide attempt
Expressions of hopelessness
The sense the patient is "giving up"
An abrupt improvement in patient mood

tions would be appropriate to investigate the patient's plan and how readily available the resources are regarding the reported method of attempt. This is all-important information to be reported when the therapist contacts the physician. Therapists should be very familiar with their facility's "suicide protocol or procedure" in terms of what information should be collected from the patient and who should be contacted.

PHYSICAL EXAMINATION

Besides this discussion of observation screening for the integumentary and nervous systems, other screening principles are associated with the physical examination. The therapist should have expectations of physical examination findings based on the existing medical diagnosis and data from the history. There should be a correlation between the described functional limitations and the noted impairments. Using the clinical example previously described, the right shoulder pain Mr. S. was experiencing would be expected to increase or decrease in intensity with palpation, movement assessment, or special tests. Not only was the therapist unable to alter the ache, but the shoulder motion and motor control also appeared intact. Essentially there is nothing for the therapist to treat. The inability to alter a patient's complaints and the lack of neuromusculoskeletal impairments one would expect with the medical diagnosis and the reported functional limitations should again raise concern about the source of the symptoms. The physical examination also includes elements of the *systems review.*

The "Guide to Physical Therapist Practice" describes *systems review*, in part, as a brief or limited examination of the anatomical and physiological status of the cardiovascular/pulmonary, integumentary, musculoskeletal, and neuromuscular systems.[1] For the purposes of this chapter the discussion will focus on assessment of height and weight and assessing heart rate and blood pressure. Being overweight or obese can significantly increase the risk for development of a number of serious conditions (Table 7-4). Using patient height and weight to calculate body mass index (BMI) can be a valuable measure to identify patients who may need a dietary consultation to prevent disease states or minimize morbidity associated with current illnesses. BMI is calculated by dividing body weight (in kilograms) by height (in meters). Table 7-4 provides a summary of disease risk associated with BMI and waist circumference.

Resting blood pressure and pulse rate and rhythm are also important measures to be routinely collected. Table 7-5 pre-sents normal resting pulse rate parameters for therapists to consider when examining a patient. A 30-second monitoring period after a 2-5 minute rest period is recommended to obtain baseline rate values.[18] Resting blood pressure values can also provide important screening information. See Table 7-6 for a summary of blood pressure values for adults. As with assessing pulse rate, resting blood pressure should be assessed after a 5-minute rest period. Variations from the normative values may lead therapists to additional assessment of the vascular system and the central autonomic nervous system and then to a patient referral.

RESPONSE TO TREATMENT

Frequently during Differential Diagnosis Phase 1 the therapist will decide referral of the patient to a physician is not warranted and will proceed to Differential Diagnosis Phase 2. As treatment is initiated and progresses, the therapist must remain vigilant for the appearance of symptoms and signs

TABLE 7-4 ■ Disease Risk Relative to Normal Weight and Waist Circumference

	BMI (KG/M²)	OBESITY CLASS	MEN ≤102 CM (≤40 INCHES) WOMEN ≤88 CM (≤35 INCHES)	>102 CM(>40 INCHES) >88 CM (>35 INCHES)
Underweight	<18.5		—	—
Normal	18.5-24.9		—	—
Overweight	25.0-29.9		Increased	High
Obesity	30.0-34.9	I	High	Very high
	35.0-39.9	II	Very high	Very high
Extreme obesity	≥40	III	Extremely high	Extremely high

From the National Heart, Lung and Blood Institute: *Clinical guidelines on the identification, evaluation, and treatment of overweight and obesity in adults* (website): http://www.nhlbi.nih.gov/. Accessed August 28, 2006.
Classification by BMI, waist circumference, and associated disease risks.

TABLE 7-5 ■ Classification of Blood Pressure for Adults 18 Years or Older*†

CATEGORY	SYSTOLIC BLOOD PRESSURE (MM HG)		DIASTOLIC BLOOD PRESSURE (MM HG)
Optimal‡	<120	and	>80
Normal	120-129	and	80-84
High normal	130-139	or	85-89
Hypertension			
Stage 1	140-159	or	90-99
Stage 2	160-179	or	100-109
Stage 3	≥180	or	≥110

From The Sixth Report of the Joint National Committee on Prevention, Detection, Evaluation, and Treatment of High Blood Pressure, *Hypertension* 23:275-285, 1994, and The Sixth Report of the U.S. Department of Health and Human Services, Public Health Service, National Institutes of Health, National Heart, Lung and Blood Institute, Bethesda, MD, 1997.
*Not taking antihypertensive drugs and not acutely ill. When systolic and diastolic blood pressures fall into different categories, the high category should be selected to classify the individual's blood pressure status. In addition to classifying stages of hypertension on the basis of average blood pressure levels, clinicians should specify presence or absence of target organ disease and additional risk factors. This specificity is important for risk classification and treatment.
†Based on the average of two or more readings taken at each of two or more visits after an initial screening.
‡Optimal blood pressure regarding cardiovascular risk is less than 120/80 mm Hg. However, unusually low readings should be evaluated for clinical significance.

TABLE 7-6 ■ Resting Pulse Rate

	AVERAGE (BEATS/MIN)	LIMITS
Norms	120-160	—
Fetal	120	70-190
Newborn	120	80-160
1 year	110	80-130
2 years	100	80-120
4 years	100	75-115
6 years	99	70-110
8-10 years		
12 years		
Female	90	70-110
Male	85	65-105
14 years		
Female	85	65-105
Male	80	60-100
16 years		
Female	80	60-100
Male	75	55-95
18 years		
Female	75	55-95
Male	70	50-90
Well-conditioned athlete	50-60	50-100
Adult	—	60-100
Aging	—	60-100

Adapted from Jarvis C: *Physical examination and health assessment,* ed 4, Philadelphia, 1992, WB Saunders.

discussed throughout this chapter. In addition, correlating subjective and objective changes as treatment progresses will help the therapist decide whether further intervention is warranted or whether referral back to the physician is appropriate. For example, if a patient reports a significant improvement or worsening, one would expect the therapist to note a corresponding change in posture, movement ability, palpatory findings, or neurological status. If the expected correlation between patient report and physical examination findings is not found, the therapist should begin considering that therapy may not be warranted. A careful review of systems and symptom investigation would again be necessary as part of the return to Differential Diagnosis Phase 1.

CONCLUSION

If all diseases presented as a high fever, hemoptysis, and blood in the urine, the medical screening process would be a simple one. Unfortunately, many diseases are initially manifested by subtle complaints, intermittent symptoms or mild pain, stiffness, paresthesias, or acute dementia. If these complaints are brought to a physician's attention by the patient, they often are not severe enough to warrant extensive diagnostic testing. Many patients or family members simply ignore symptoms or physiological changes, rationalizing that everything is okay, the family member is just old, or it maybe he or she simply does not like to see physicians or is too busy. All of the scenarios can account for patients with occult disease seeing therapists. The fact that PTs and OTs tend to spend a moderate amount of time with patients over a period of weeks or months can facilitate the detection of subtle manifestations. In addition, as therapists develop rapport with patients, the patients may be willing to share information they were uncomfortable disclosing initially.

The responsibilities of the PT and OT related to screening for symptoms and signs that indicate the involvement of another health care practitioner are clearly stated in the "Guide to Physical Therapist Practice"[1] and "The Guide to Occupational Therapy Practice."[2] The process associated with Differential Diagnosis Phase 1 allows for the appropriate medical screening yet keeps therapists within their scope of practice. The therapist simply communicates to the physician the list of clinical findings. The physician will determine whether new or additional medical tests are needed to rule out or diagnose specific diseases. Facilitating the timely referral of patients to physicians is an important role for therapists working within a collaborative medical model. It is this model that best serves the needs of our patients. For additional information related to the medical screening process the readers are directed to three other textbooks.[19-21]

With changes in health care delivery and physicians also being asked to see more patients in less time, it is critical all health care practitioners include an adequate medical screening component to their examinations. If quality-of-life issues are truly an important component of health-care delivery, then Differential Diagnosis Phase 1, medical screening, has and will continue to be a professional expectation and responsibility placed on each PT and OT. Because consumers are accessing therapeutic services through more direct means, that responsibility will remain and grow in importance as part of both professions' education and practice.

In the future another choice will have to be considered as part of the role of a movement specialist. The results of Phase 1 and 2 assessments may determine that neither a medical referral nor therapeutic intervention itself is appropriate. In this situation, the patient might benefit from community activities but would not need a movement specialist, especially if the physician also determined that medical intervention was not necessary.

CASE STUDY

CASE STUDY 7-1

A 55-year-old elementary school teacher was referred with a diagnosis of cervical degenerative disk disease at C5-6 and C6-7. Her chief complaint was posterior cervical aching and a sense of neck weakness. Functionally, the patient's primary concern was her increasingly difficult time making it through her workday. She taught first-grade students, so much of her workday was spent with her neck and trunk in a forward flexed position. The patient stated this persistent flexion posturing is a significant factor for the worsening of her symptoms as her workday progresses. As the interview continued, a tremor of the patient's right hand and forearm was observed as the arm rested on her thigh. When questioned about the observed tremor she stated it started 4 or 5 months ago. She admitted the tremor appeared to be getting worse and that she did not mention it to her physician. No other positive neurological findings were noted. After the initial examination was completed, the concern about the tremor was discussed and the patient consented to allow her primary care physician (the referring physician) to be called to discuss the finding. The physician facilitated a referral of the patient to a neurologist. Approximately 1 month later, after the neurology consultation and tests, the patient was diagnosed with Parkinson's disease. During that month the patient continued to receive physical therapy care for her cervical complaints. In this example, performance of Differential Diagnosis Phase 1 showed the presence of a new symptom (tremor of the right hand) that is not consistent with the medical diagnosis of degenerative disk disease. This symptom triggered the decision by the therapist to refer the patient back to the physician for that specific clinical sign, which evidently led to the additional diagnosis of Parkinson's disease. While being referred to the physician, therapy was simultaneously initiated. Differential Diagnosis Phase 2 was performed, which resulted in the decision to treat the cervical complaints of the patient.

REFERENCES

1. American Physical Therapy Association: Guide to physical therapist practice, *Phys Ther* 81:9-744, 2001.
2. Moyers PA: The guide to occupational therapy practice, *Am J Occup Ther* 53:247-322, 1999.
3. Physical disability [special issue], *Phys Ther* 74:375-506, 1994.
4. Verbrugge L, Jette A: The disablement process, *Soc Sci Med* 38:1-14, 1994.
5. Umphred DA (Chair): Diagnostic Task Force and Special Project, California Physical Therapy Association, 1996-2000.
6. American Psychiatric Association: *Diagnostic and statistical manual of mental disorders-IV-TR,* Washington, DC, 2000, American Psychiatric Association.
7. Boissonnault W, Badke M: Collecting health history information: the accuracy of a patient self-administered questionnaire in an orthopedic outpatient population, *Phys Ther* 85:531-543, 2005.
8. Boissonnault W, DiFabio R: Pain profile of patients with low back pain referred to physical therapy, *J Orthop Sports Phys Ther* 24:80-191, 1996.
9. Bickley LS: *Bates' guide to physical examination and history taking,* ed 8, Philadelphia, 2003, Lippincott Williams & Wilkins.
10. Frisbie JH, Gore RL, Strymish JM et al: Vertebral osteomyelitis in paraplegia: Incidence, risk factors, clinical picture, *J Spinal Cord Med* 23:15-22, 2000.
11. Goodman CC, Snyder TE: *Differential diagnosis for the physical therapist,* ed 3, Philadelphia, 1999, WB Saunders.
12. Tronzo RG: Femoral neck fracture. In Steinburg ME, editor: *The hip and its disorders,* Philadelphia, 1991, WB Saunders.
13. Jemal A, Tiwari RC, Murray T et al: Cancer statistics, 2004, *CA Cancer J Clin* 54:8-29, 2004.
14. Sauer GC: *Manual of skin disease,* ed 6, Philadelphia, 1991, JB Lippincott.
15. Boissonnault WG: Prevalance of comorbid conditions, surgeries and medication use in physical therapy outpatient population: a multicentered study, *J Orthop Sports Phys Ther* 29:506-519, 1999.
16. Boissonnault WG, Koopmeiners MB: Medical history profile: orthopaedic physical therapy outpatients, *J Orthop Sports Phys Ther* 20:2-10, 1994.
17. Jette DU, Jette AM: Physical therapy and health outcomes in patients with spinal impairments, *Phys Ther* 76:930-941, 1996.
18. Tepper S, MeKeough M: Review of cardiovascular and pulmonary systems and vital signs. In Boissonnault WG, editor: *Primary care for the physical therapist—examination and triage,* Philadelphia, 2005, Elsevier/Saunders.
19. Boissonnault WG, editor: *Examination in physical therapy practice—screening for medical disease,* ed 2, New York, 1995, Churchill Livingstone.
20. Boissonnault WG: *Primary care for the physical therapist—examination and triage,* Philadelphia, 2005, Elsevier/Saunders.
21. Goodman C, Boissonnault W, Fuller K: *Pathology: implications for the physical therapist,* Philadelphia, 2002, WB Saunders.

CHAPTER 8

Differential Diagnosis Phase 2: Examination and Evaluation of Functional Movement Activities and System/Subsystem Impairments

Rolando T. Lazaro, PT, DPT, MS, GCS
Margaret L. Roller, PT, MS, DPT
Darcy A. Umphred, PT, PhD, FAPTA

KEY WORDS

delegation
diagnosis
differential diagnosis phase 2
evaluation
examination
functional limitations
impairments
prognosis

OBJECTIVES

After reading this chapter the student/therapist will be able to:

1. Differentiate diagnosis of impairments/bodily functions and functional limitations/activity limitations and disability/participation in life from medical diagnosis performed by the physician.
2. Identify the difference between a functional or activity limitation, a disability or participation in life activity, and impairments and their specific body systems function.
3. Analyze the scope of functional tools and impairment tools and analyze how the results of those tests accurately reflect the movement disorder causing functional loss.
4. Identify psychometric properties of measurement tools and discuss the efficacy of a chosen tool in relation to rehabilitation outcomes.
5. Identify available examination tools and locate them in the literature.
6. Discuss which examination tools would be appropriate to delegate to an assistant and under what conditions.
7. Discuss the process of establishment of a diagnosis on the basis of movement function and dysfunction and how that diagnosis interacts with prognosis and intervention outcomes.

From the beginning of the evolution of practice for movement specialists within the health care arena, clinicians have been expected to examine a client's functional performance and draw conclusions from the examination. The synthesis of information gathered has led to the establishment of short- and long-term goals and thus a prognosis concerning the likelihood of the goals being achieved, and the time it will take to achieve those goals. Similarly, the selection of the most effective and appropriate intervention strategies will guide the therapist and patient toward the desired outcomes. Today, clients are typically referred for physical and occupational therapy with "evaluate and treat" orders as the common referral pattern used by physicians or other health care providers. With direct access to physical and occupational therapy becoming a reality in many states across the United States and other countries, many patients are walking into clinics because they have decided that therapy is the best alternative to assist with their functional problems. Whether through self-referral or referral from another medical practitioner, once a client enters into a therapeutic environment, clinicians must first determine whether the individual is medically stable at a body system level (see Chapter 7) and an appropriate candidate for therapeutic intervention. Once medical screening has been completed and the therapist determines that there are no red flags to suggest that the client needs to be referred for additional disease/pathology examination or does not need therapeutic intervention, then the client enters into Phase 2 of the evaluation process (Figure 8-1). Critical to this phase is a solid understanding of empowerment and enablement/disablement models because these are the foundation of a strong diagnostic process (see Chapter 1). As stated in Chapter 1, both the International Classification of Functioning, Disability, and Health (ICF) model for enablement and the Nagi disablement models will be models used throughout this book. The reader must remember that other models exist and may use similar terminology to describe different aspects of enablement/disablement.

Numerous tools are used to examine clients with physical complaints and problems with functional movement. Many of these tools directly measure specific strengths and weaknesses within the body systems, helping the clinician to identify specific impairments of a client that are causes of functional loss. Each impairment tool is intended for a specific purpose and is designed to supply the user with a given outcome measure in a predetermined set of values.

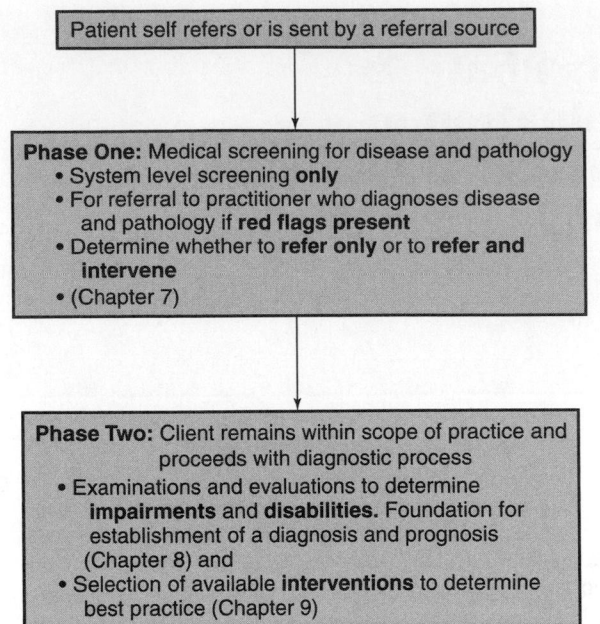

Patient self refers or is sent by a referral source

Phase One: Medical screening for disease and pathology
- System level screening **only**
- For referral to practitioner who diagnoses disease and pathology if **red flags present**
- Determine whether to **refer only** or to **refer and intervene**
- (Chapter 7)

Phase Two: Client remains within scope of practice and proceeds with diagnostic process
- Examinations and evaluations to determine **impairments** and **disabilities.** Foundation for establishment of a diagnosis and prognosis (Chapter 8) and
- Selection of available **interventions** to determine best practice (Chapter 9)

FIGURE 8-1 ■ The diagnostic process used for best practice by physical and occupational therapists.

Other tools measure a client's functional abilities or limitations. These tools are designed to examine the performance of a client during various functional skills and activities of daily living. Functional tools also supply the user with a predetermined set of values. These tools, however, do not directly supply information about the cause of the client's functional movement problems. The user must extrapolate information from the results of each functional test and then choose the appropriate impairment measurement tools to determine the combination of impairments that may be contributing to the limitations in the client's ability to perform daily living activities or participate in normal life interactions. The process of examination/evaluation is not a linear process. Thus, whenever the therapist is with the client, part of the therapist's focus needs to be on assessment. Initially, the therapist may miss something that does not become identified until more complex activities are introduced. Once the subtle impairments become obvious, the therapist may need to go back to identify more in-depth causes, to fine tune the intervention strategies. If the patient and therapist mutually agree that the goal should stress adaptation or compensation versus regaining motor learning, then the intervention strategy may proceed in different directions.

To be able to provide information that is meaningful in determining the best possible intervention for a particular patient, the examination tools selected by the clinician must be objective, reliable, valid, and appropriately matched with patient expectations. These tools should also communicate necessary information in a language that is understandable to all health care professionals and the payer responsible for funding the services (see Chapter 10). With the limitations on visits within the clinical setting and the critically important variable of motivation/compliance of the patient, the setting of goals and the selection of intervention strategies need to be established through patient-centered participation.[1-9]

This chapter has been developed to help the reader through the problem-solving and decision-making process for selecting appropriate tests. It is not within the scope of this chapter or text to explain each examination tool in detail. However, the reader is presented with an extensive list of impairment and functional tests with related references as a guide in determining the appropriate examination tools for a particular client (see Appendix 8-A at the end of this chapter).

THE DIAGNOSTIC PROCESS

The enablement/disablement models provide the clinician with a framework for understanding the relationships among the factors that affect the selection of appropriate examination and intervention strategies. The Nagi, ICF, and International Classification of Impairments, Disabilities, and Handicaps (ICIDH) models (Chapter 1), and the Top-Down Model (Chapter 4) are examples of models that are currently being used in occupational and physical therapy practice. As the clinician begins to sift through information obtained from the various examination procedures, it is appropriate to identify the impairments (body systems) that cause the particular activity limitation (disability or functional limitation). The clinician must consider all aspects of the client's multiple body and environmental systems during this process. The clinician should also be sensitive to the individual's perception of the effect these impairments have on the person and how they relate to participation in society, how they impose social limitations, or how they lead to a decrease in the quality of life.

In the clinical environment the clinician often identifies the client's presenting activity limitations through functional testing and then examines the subsystem impairments that directly cause or may have contributed to these limitations. Therefore, instead of approaching the examination process as "impairment leading to functional limitations," the clinician actually performs "functional limitations and then impairments causing the functional limitations" analysis. This process not only streamlines the examination but also assists the clinician in focusing on the problems and the interaction of the systems causing the various functional problems and thus helps to delineate how these will be affected by the resulting therapeutic intervention. Some impairments may be the result of the disease or pathological condition, reflecting a medical referral, and others may be reflective of life experiences and previous traumas.

Also in the clinical environment, the client's strengths are often emphasized as the foundation for intervention. In the enablement model, the clinician, whenever possible, asks what the client is able to do and then proceeds to work on those tasks that will provide the client with the most functionally oriented outcome. This approach is proactive and positive, truly capitalizing on the client's potential and goals, and it emphasizes the therapist-client partnership.

ACTIVITY LIMITATIONS

Activity limitations (ICF), functional limitations (Nagi), or disabilities (ICIDH) are defined as the restriction or lack there of in an individual's ability to perform—at the level of the whole person—a physical action, activity, or task in an efficient, typically expected, and competent manner.[10] It is important to observe the client during the performance of functional tasks and motor patterns to determine the functions that the client is unable to execute or has difficulty performing, to determine the cause of the dysfunctional movement patterns. Similarly, it is just as important to determine what functional motor behaviors the client can perform in daily life activities. Synthesizing both the enablement and disablement of the client in functional activities helps the therapist determine which specific subsystems are affecting those activities that the client is not able to perform. It is not uncommon for a client to have multiple system-related interactions causing activity limitations. In this case, the examiner must attempt to determine the primary functional loss or primary complaint. This will guide the process of choosing the appropriate functional tool(s) to use during the examination.

Functional tools are designed to measure and score a client during the performance of various functional tasks. Each functional tool is designed to measure a specific type of functional ability. Most tools test a range of skills from walking ability to balance ability during the performance of functional tasks, or a combination of the two. Some tests are quick and easy to set up and perform (e.g., Functional Reach Test, Tinetti Performance Oriented Mobility Assessment [POMA]), whereas others are lengthy and take longer to administer (e.g., Berg Balance Scale, Functional Independence Measure [FIM], Outcome and Assessment Information Set [OASIS], or Fugl-Meyer). There are advantages and disadvantages to both of these types of tests. Those that are the quickest to administer generally measure fewer functional skills and do not give information on the total functioning of a client. However, if the user properly identifies the client's problem and is able to focus on the most efficient way of measuring it, a quick functional test can be the most beneficial to use. Those tests that take a bit longer to administer and/or assess multiple skills typically supply the user with a more comprehensive picture of the client's functional abilities, generally in various domains such as gross mobility, self-care, cognitive ability, communication ability, and others.

Outcome scales for functional tests are generally in ordinal format (e.g., FIM, Barthel Index, Katz Index of Activities of Daily Living). Each has its own unique point value and range, varying from a two- to three-point scale (e.g., Tinetti POMA) to a seven-point scale (e.g., FIM). A few tools supply ratio scale data (e.g., the Timed Up and Go Test [TUG] and modified TUG, Functional Reach Test, and other measures of gait speed). Ratio scale data are easier to compare and to measure incremental changes in function.

Impairments

Impairment (ICF, Nagi, ICIDH) is defined as the loss or abnormality of physiological, psychological, or anatomical structure or function at the organ system level.[10] An efficient examination process first includes the use of activity-based measures and functional tools to identify the client's primary functional problems. From this information the clinician extrapolates the primary impairments that are suspected to be creating or contributing to the client's functional limitations. The clinician may then choose to proceed to examine these impaired systems directly by using tests and measures designed to supply objective information regarding the status of each involved body system. This entire process helps the clinician identify the most important problems affecting the client in the least amount of time. Knowledge

of the status of involved body systems helps guide choices for therapeutic intervention and goal setting. It also assists in predicting how the client's functional limitations may be affected by the resulting intervention.

Objective examination results are gained from both functional testing and impairment testing. These results supply the information base on which to set goals with the patient, determine intervention strategies, and measure progress. The clinician must also consider the nature of the neurological, neuromuscular, musculoskeletal, cardiopulmonary, or integumentary condition or medical diagnosis in the planning of treatment and goal setting. The potential impact of the intervention on the component problems in the disablement/enablement model for chronic, degenerative conditions is generally quite different from that of acute, nonprogressive, or acquired conditions. The projected length of time for intervention and to reach desired functional outcomes at the end of the intervention period will also differ greatly, depending on the nature of the disease or disorder.

After identifying the activity limitations (functional limitations/disabilities) and the impairments that may be causing them, the clinician may decide between three possible intervention scenarios: (1) the correction of impairments that may lead to the correction of functional problems, (2) the correction of the activity limitation itself through enhancement of existing strengths, or (3) compensation for uncorrectable limitations through alterations in the external environment.

The clinician needs to make the distinction between primary impairments, which are a direct consequence of the client's specific disease or pathological condition, and secondary impairments, which occur as sequelae to the disease or rehabilitation process or as the result of aging, disuse, repetitive strain, lifestyle, and so on. Moreover, the clinician must remember that, although functional limitations are usually caused by a combination of specific impairments, it is possible that impairments may not result in specific functional problems for a particular client. If this is the case, the clinician should make a determination regarding whether these impairments, if left uncorrected, will result in the development of activity limitations/functional limitations at a later time.

The ultimate goal of any therapeutic intervention program is to attain the highest level of health and wellness possible. Measurement tools that the clinician chooses to use also need to reflect this end result. For example, "traditional" impairment measurements may indicate that a client demonstrated increased shoulder range of motion (ROM) by 25 degrees. The more important question should be how this increase in ROM affects the client's ability to perform a functional task such as dressing or any other activity that the client sees as important. The clinician is therefore encouraged to consider the functional implications of these measurements to obtain results that are more meaningful for the client.

The clinician is always faced with the challenge of identifying and administering examination tools that will not only reflect the client's level of health and wellness but also reflect the client's functional improvement as a result of the intervention provided. Functional measurement tools can be used as a baseline measure for those functional skills. However, these tools typically require a large improvement

---

BOX 8-1 ■ IDENTIFICATION AND CLASSIFICATION OF IMPAIRMENTS

IMPAIRMENTS WITHIN THE CENTRAL NERVOUS SYSTEM

1. State of the motor pool
2. Synergies (volitional or reflexive)
3. Postural integration
4. Balance
5. Speed of movement
6. Timing
7. Reciprocal movements
8. Trajectory or pattern of movement
9. Accuracy
10. Task content
11. Emotional influences
12. Sensory organization: somatosensory mapping
13. Perception/cognition
14. Hormonal/nutritional
15. Levels of consciousness

IMPAIRMENTS WITHIN THE PERIPHERAL NERVOUS SYSTEM AND INTERACTION WITH THE ENVIRONMENT

1. Range of motion
2. Muscle strength or power
3. Cardiac function
4. Respiratory function
5. Circulatory function
6. Other organ and system interaction
7. Environmental task
8. Endurance
9. Psychosocial factors

---

in a client's functional performance for a corresponding change to be seen. Results obtained from impairment tests can fill in the large gaps between numerical scores on functional scales with objective measurements and trends in the direction toward improvement before any change is demonstrated on functional examination scales.

Box 8-1 illustrates impairments that are considered to be central neurological versus peripheral or environmental in origin. The column on the left illustrates the components of motor control within the systems that are traditionally considered central. These components are further discussed in detail in various sections of this book. Some qualitative and quantitative measures commonly used to assess these systems are referenced in Appendix 8-A.

The bottom column identifies impairments in systems traditionally considered peripheral and environmental. ROM is one example of a common musculoskeletal system examination procedure. Clinicians depend heavily on ROM measurements as an essential component of their examination and consequent evaluation process. It is imperative that the data obtained from this procedure be reliable. It has been suggested that the main source of variation in the performance of this procedure is method and that by standardizing the procedure reliability can be improved.[11]

An impairment of lack of ROM can be the result of other impairments. ROM measurements may be used to determine the effect of tone, balance, movement synergies, and so forth on the neuromuscular system and, ultimately, on behavior. Most important, the clinician needs to remember that the ROM needed to perform a functional activity is more critical than the "normal," anatomical, biomechanical ROM values and must be considered when labeling and measuring impairments. For example, full ROM in the shoulder is seldom needed unless activities of daily living require it, such as a tennis serve or placing objects overhead at work. When needed for specific tasks, goniometric measurements are appropriate, but at other times a functional range measurement may be just as reliable.

Muscle strength testing is another commonly used examination procedure. Clinicians use various methods of quantifying this measurement, including "traditional" manual muscle testing and the use of a dynamometer. As with ROM, strength should be correlated with the patient's functional performance. Again, the clinician may find a client to have 3/5 strength in the shoulder flexor muscle groups or find grip strength to be 50 kg, but the more important question should be "What does this mean in terms of the client's ability to perform activities of daily living"? The clinician is also advised to make the distinction among strength, power production, and muscular endurance as it relates to function. A client may have sufficient lower-extremity strength and power to get up from the seated position; however, this does not necessarily mean that the client has muscular endurance to perform the task repeatedly during the day as part of normal everyday activities.

The functioning of the cardiac, respiratory, and circulatory systems significantly affects a client's performance. Blood pressure, heart rate, and respiration give the clinician signs of the patient's medical stability and the ability to tolerate exercise. The clinician may also obtain pulmonary function tests for ventilation, pulmonary mechanics, lung diffusion capacity, or blood gas analysis after determining that the client's pulmonary system is a major factor affecting medical stability and functional progress. Various exercise tolerance tests also attempt to quantify functional work capacity and serve as a guide for the clinician performing cardiac and pulmonary rehabilitation.

A client who has difficulty performing activities of daily living and who has neurological impairments in the central motor, sensory, perceptual, or integrative systems needs to undergo examination procedures to establish the level of impairment of each involved system and to determine if and how that system is contributing to the deficit motor behaviors. Functional evaluation tools used may include the FIM, the Barthel Index, the Tinetti POMA, or the TUG test. The results of these tests will help to steer the clinician toward the most useful impairment tools to use to evaluate limitations in the various body systems. Impairment tools may include the modified Ashworth Scale for spasticity, the Upright Motor Control Test for lower-extremity motor control, the Clinical Test of Sensory Interaction on Balance or the Sensory Organization Test for balance and sensory integrative problems, or computerized tests of limits of stability on the NeuroCom Balance Master, among others (see Appendix 8-A).

The clinician is also advised to investigate the interaction of other organs and systems as they relate to the patient's functional limitations. For example, electrolyte imbalance, hormonal disorders, or adverse drug reactions (see Chapter 36) may explain impairments and activity limitations noted in the other interacting systems.

CHOOSING THE APPROPRIATE EXAMINATION TOOL

The ability to choose the appropriate examination tool(s) for a particular client will depend on several factors:

1. The client's current functional status (ambulatory vs. nonambulatory)
2. The client's current cognitive status (intact vs. confused/disoriented)
3. The clinical setting in which the person is being evaluated for treatment (acute hospital or rehabilitation or outpatient or skilled care or home care)
4. The client's primary complaints (pain vs. weakness vs. impaired balance)
5. The client's goals and realistic expectation of recovery, maintenance, or slowing down functional loss (acute injury or chronic problem or progressive disease process)
6. The type of information desired from the test (predictive or discriminative)

The evaluator should select examination tools that will measure the client's primary problems (impairments and activity limitations) and supply outcome measures that are needed to set realistic treatment goals and plan efficient and effective intervention strategies. To choose a functional tool, the clinician is advised to select one that contains component skills in which the particular client is having difficulty. Those component skills of the tool in which the client's performance is poor will disclose the client's activity limitations. Those skills in which the client performs well determine the client's strengths and abilities. The evaluator must then focus on the client's disablement measurements as determined by the results of functional test(s) to determine the impairment tests that will next be performed. For example, if the client demonstrates difficulty in rising from a chair during a functional test (e.g., FIM, Tinetti POMA) and scores low on this skill on the outcome measure, the clinician must then closely examine the skill of coming to stand to determine the cause of the mobility limitation. The problem may be that the client cannot generate adequate muscle power to push up from the chair or perhaps that the client does not have adequate ROM in the hip or the ankle joints to rise from the chair or the client no longer sees a reason to get out of the chair. It may be a problem with dynamic balance during the transitional movement or once standing. Any impairment that is identified during performance of the functional skill needs to be measured more specifically. It is up to the examiner to determine the next best steps to take to target the client's problems as efficiently as possible, to measure and record the needed outcomes as objectively as possible, and to then with the client set treatment goals and design the best intervention to remediate or manage the problems.

Many of the examination tools that measure a client's ability to perform functional activities have been accepted as valid, reliable, and useful for the justification of payment for services rendered. The number of activity limitations and the extent of the client's participation limitation is often a reason an individual either accessed therapy services directly or was referred by a medical practitioner. For this reason, the third-party payer expects to receive reports concerning positive changes in the client's functional status for therapeutic services to be justifiable. (See Chapter 10.) The initial list of functional/activity limitations or disabilities helps the therapist determine the extent, expectations, and direction of intervention, but it does not determine why those limitations exist. This is the question that is critical to answer as part of the evaluation process. Examination tests and procedures that identify specific system and subsystem impairments help the therapist determine causes for existing participation and activity limitations. These tools need to be objective, reliable, and sensitive enough to provide needed communication to third-party payers to explain the subsystem's baseline progress during and after the intervention. These tools should also supply explanations for residual difficulties in the event that the functional problems themselves do not demonstrate significant objective change or show progress within the time frame estimated.

USING THE EVALUATION PROCESS TO LINK IMPAIRMENTS AND ACTIVITY LIMITATIONS TO INTERVENTION

After objective measures for activity and participation limitations, as well as systems and subsystems impairments are obtained, clinicians must determine whether the impairments or the functional problems are changeable given the limitations in the number of treatment interventions. In certain situations a mobility limitation may be remediated and become more functional, although the component impairments contributing to it may remain unchanged. In other situations, impairment measures may significantly improve but the functional problem may remain unaltered. This is especially true when one impairment is significantly improved; however, functional progress is masked by the contribution of other impairments.

The examiner must be able to come to a conclusion regarding the relationship between the client's activity limitations/functional problems and the existing body systems impairments. Without an understanding of this relationship, it is difficult to assess the effect of the treatment intervention(s) on a particular patient.

The interactions and interrelationships of both the identified functional problems and impairments provide the clinician with an initial status or problem list specific to that individual. That list, or the interactions of the impairments and functional problems, helps to formulate a diagnosis for the movement dysfunction. Similarly, owing to the objective nature of the components within that diagnosis, a target status to be reached at the conclusion of therapeutic intervention can be estimated. That target status is both impairment and function driven and traditionally would be considered a list of outcome goals. The interactions between impairments and their related activity and participation limitations make up the unique problem map of that individual and direct the clinician toward selecting optimal interventions.

The difference between the initial and the target status and the time frame and estimated number of visits needed to reach the target outcome is the prognosis by the clinician. Once the clinician has measured and identified specific activity limitations and their respective impairments, he or she then has an excellent opportunity to conceptually understand how various impairments affect multiple functional problems and which impairments are activity specific.

The following case scenario clearly synthesizes the clinical examination and evaluation process used by physical and occupational therapists:

Assume that a clinician had been called in to examine a client who has had an anoxic event after heart surgery. The client's cognitive ability is within normal limits and he is highly motivated to get back to his normal activities. He is retired, loves to walk in the park with his wife, and go on bird watching experiences in the mountains with their group of friends. The clinician must select which functional tests to use to obtain an objective initial status and target the client's problems. Currently, the client requires assistance with all gross mobility skills and is demonstrating difficulty balancing in various postures and activities of daily living. After functional testing, the client demonstrates significant limitations in the activities of coming to sit, sitting, coming to stand, standing, walking, dressing, and grooming. If the client is moderately dependent in all seven activities and requires assistance to perform those functions, then, depending on the functional tests used, he will most likely be scored between "unable" and "independent" on a given scale. Assume that the client also displays impairment limitations in flexor range of motion at the hip joints because of both muscle/fascia tightness and hypertonicity within the extensor muscle groups, although he has compensated to some degree and is able to perform bed mobility independently. Upper extremity control is within normal limits, and thus the client is capable of performing many activities of daily living as long as his lower trunk and hips are placed in a supportive position and hip flexion is not required. The client has general weakness from inactivity and power production problems in his abdominals and hip flexor muscles owing to the dominance of extensor tonicity. Once he is assisted to stand, the extensor patterns of hip and knee extension, internal rotation, slight adduction, and plantarflexion are present. He can actively extend both legs after being placed in flexion, but he is limited in the production of specific fine and gross motor patterns. Thus, a resulting balance impairment is present owing to the inability to adequately access appropriate balance synergies caused by the presence of tone, limb synergy production, and weakness in the antagonists to the trunk and hip extensors. With the use of augmented intervention (see Chapter 9), the client is noted to possess intact postural and procedural balance programming; however, both functions are being masked by existing impairments. The decision is made to perform impairment measures, including range of motion at the hip, knee, and ankle joints; power production within both the abdominal and hip flexor muscle groups; volitional and non-volitional synergic programming; balance; posture; and volitional control over muscle tone. The amount of range and power production needed and the specific synergic programming required will vary according to the requirements of the functional activities performed.

Using a clinical decision-making process, the clinician will conclude that the impairments that are being targeted to measure will vary from one functional activity to the next. For instance, if this client is demonstrating difficulty rising from a chair, the target impairment may be an ROM measurement. This same ROM impairment may also contribute to problems with moving about the base of support in functional sitting. The clinician makes the determination as to the extent the impairment interferes with each functional problem for that particular client.

These objective measurements help the clinician explain which outcomes would be expected to be achieved first and why. These measurements are recorded as part of intervention charting and help to objectively demonstrate that the client is improving toward functional independence. They also give an indication of what the client still needs to reach the desired outcome, the rate of learning that is taking place, and an estimation of recovery time that is still required. These objective measurements give to the clinician and the client a better avenue to discuss expectations with family members, other medical practitioners, and third-party payers. In the previous example, assume that, after intervention, functional ROM in the hip was achieved. However, this improvement did not result in an improvement in the activity problems because synergic programming prevented adequate hip flexion during one or more functional activities. Understanding and measuring the difference between lack of range as a result of muscle/fascia tightness versus lack of range from synergic patterning helps clinicians communicate why a client is successful in one activity and still needing assistance in another.

Impairment and disability scores supply statistically important measurements that can then be used to discuss the limitations placed on the therapeutic environment by fiscal intermediaries. Therapists must be clear when documenting (see Chapter 10) the initial status and the target status for clients so that the recommended intervention and length of stay may be justified.

When making a determination of the potential impact of an intervention on improving a client's problems, clinicians must remember that a key factor in this process of examination and evaluation is the acceptance of the movement dysfunction or impairment by the client. A mobility problem or impairment may be clearly identified by a functional test or impairment test; however, the client may deny that the problem even exists. Acceptance of the problems by the client and a willingness to change are critical to the client's compliance with the intervention strategy.

As mentioned earlier, the identification of potential impairments was done after functional testing to streamline the examination process. After performing the functional examination, the therapist postulated that the client might have motor weakness, sensory deficits, pain, and a decrease in endurance that may have been causing the functional limitations. Manual muscle testing revealed lower-extremity strength of 1/5 in both ankle motions, 2/5 in both knees, and 3–/5 in both hips. Upper extremities tested as 1/5 finger flexors (incomplete grip), 2/5 wrist motions, and 3+/5 in both elbow motions. Shoulder and trunk strength were within functional limits for all motions. Sensory testing indicated absent touch and proprioceptive sensations from the foot to the knee of both lower extremities, with impaired sensation from the thigh to the hips. Both hands and wrists tested absent to touch and proprioception, with the elbows and shoulders testing intact. The client's endurance was limited to short bouts of activity (3 to 5 minutes), with rapid muscular and cardiovascular fatigue. The presence of these impairments helped to explain the resultant functional limitations tested earlier.

In terms of standardized functional tests, the multidisciplinary FIM could give insight into this patient's ability to function in multiple domains and categories. A baseline score on the Tinetti POMA and the Berg Balance Scale could be collected because this client is expected to regain further function in balance and postural control as recovery from the disease occurs. As the client regains strength and peripheral sensory ability, she may be able to perform the modified TUG Test and the Functional Reach Test. These functional assessments paint a better picture of what the

client can and cannot do, as well as provide a way to measure functional progress in various activities throughout rehabilitation.

When determining an appropriate tool to examine a client's functional status, the clinician must also consider the "ceiling and floor effect" of the functional tools. In this particular case, the patient is probably unable to perform the Functional Reach Test but may be appropriate for beginning the balance portion of the POMA. As the patient progresses, the predictive and discriminative properties of some of these tests could provide information regarding the patient's likelihood of falling, or ability to safely perform selected functional tasks.

CASE STUDY ■ C. B.

C. B. is a 27-year-old woman who was admitted to the hospital 3 days ago with acute onset and rapidly progressing distal to proximal weakness and sensory loss, greater in the lower extremities than in the upper extremities. The client reports right great toe numbness and weakness and tripping on the carpet at home the night before admission. She went to bed with increased weakness and numbness in both legs and with difficulty walking. At admission through the emergency department she also reported numbness in both hands.

Her medical diagnosis was Guillain-Barré syndrome. Her prior level of function indicates that the client was an active, independent woman who worked full time performing computer data entry. She lived at home with her husband and two children. There are four steps with a rail to enter the house and a flight of stairs to access the bedrooms.

The client was transferred to the neurology unit of the acute hospital. She was started on intravenous immunoglobulin treatment and pain medication every 4 hours. A Foley catheter was inserted for bladder control, and the client was supplied with thromboembolic disease hose and intermittent compression pumps on both legs for deep venous thrombosis prophylaxis.

Phase 1 screening indicates that the client's medical history is noncontributory. There are no acute or active diseases or pathological conditions that may contraindicate physical or occupational therapy

intervention. There is a precaution against overfatiguing the client; otherwise, the physician assessed the client's medical condition to be stable. At this point physical and occupational therapy examination and evaluation may be indicated to provide further insight into the necessity of therapeutic intervention. An order was received for "physical/occupational therapy evaluation and treatment as indicated." The patient's goal is to be able to walk, return home to the family, and return to work full time.

Phase 2 examination identified functional limitations and participation limitations and helped obtain an understanding of the potential systems interactions that may influence progress. In this particular case, a decision was made to perform functional testing first to identify the specific activity limitations of the patient and then to selectively identify possible systems impairments that may be causing the functional problems. The functional assessment indicated that the patient required moderate assistance to roll to the left/right side and to scoot. She also required moderate assistance to move from supine to sit and to transfer from sit to stand. Her blood pressure, heart rate, respiration, and oxygen saturation remained within safe limits throughout these changes in body position. She demonstrated fair sitting balance and poor standing balance. She was able to ambulate with a platform walker approximately 10 feet with moderate assistance of one person.

REFERENCES

1. Duggan R: Reflection as a means to foster client-centred practice, *Can J Occup Ther* 72:103-112, 2005.
2. Dedding C, Cardol M, Eyssen IC et al: Validity of the Canadian Occupational Performance Measure: a client-centred outcome measurement, *Clin Rehabil* 18:660-667, 2004.
3. Epstein RM, Franks P, Fiscella K et al: Measuring patient-centered communication in patient-physician consultations: theoretical and practical issues, *Soc Sci Med* 61:1516-1528, 2005.
4. Harkness J: Patient involvement: a vital principle for patient-centred health care, *World Hosp Health Serv* 41:12-16, 40-43, 2005.
5. Law M, Darrah J, Rosenbaum P et al: Family-centered functional therapy for children with cerebral palsy: an emerging practice model, *Phys Occup Ther Pediatr* 18:83-102, 1998.
6. Litchfield R, MacDougall C: Professional issues for physiotherapists in family-centred and community based settings, *Aust J Physiother* 48:105-112, 2002.
7. Mossberg K, McFarland C: A patient-oriented health status measure in outpatient rehabilitation, *Am J Phys Med Rehabil* 80:896-902, 2001.
8. Palisano R: A model of physical therapist practice for children with cerebral palsy: integrating evidence, experience, and family-centered services, III Step 7-day Conference. Salt Lake City, UT, 2005.

9. Palisano RJ, Snider LM, Orlin MN: Recent advances in physical and occupational therapy for children with cerebral palsy, *Semin Pediatr Neurol* 11:66-77, 2004.

10. American Physical Therapy Association: Guide to physical therapist practice. Second edition. American Physical Therapy Association, *Phys Ther* 81:9-746, 2001.

11. Gillian J, Barstow M: Range of motion. In Van Deusen J, Brunt D, Kaszczuk S, editors: *Assessment in occupational therapy and physical therapy,* Philadelphia, 1997, WB Saunders, pp. 50-51.

12. Karnath HO, Ferber S, Dichgans J: The origin of contraversive pushing: evidence for a second graviceptive system in humans, *Neurology* 55:1298-1304, 2000.

13. Roller ML: The pusher syndrome, *J Neurol Phys Ther* 28:29-34, 2004.

14. Bernhardt J, Ellis P, Denisenko S, Hill K: Changes in balance and locomotion measures during rehabilitation following stroke, *Physiother Res Int* 3:109-122, 1998.

15. Whitney SL, Poole JL, Cass SP: A review of balance instruments for older adults, *Am J Occup Ther* 52:666-671, 1998.

16. Wrisley DM, Whitney SL: The effect of foot position on the modified clinical test of sensory interaction and balance, *Arch Phys Med Rehabil* 85:335-338, 2004.

17. Richardson PK, Atwater SW, Crowe TK et al: Performance of preschoolers on the Pediatric Clinical Test of Sensory Interaction for Balance, *Am J Occup Ther* 46:793-800, 1992.

18. Cohen H, Blatchly CA, Gombash LL: A study of the clinical test of sensory interaction and balance, *Phys Ther* 73:346-354, 1993.

19. Shumway-Cook A, Horak FB: Assessing the influence of sensory interaction of balance: suggestion from the field, *Phys Ther* 66:1548-1550, 1986.

20. Shumway-Cook A, Woollacott M: *motor control: theory and practical application,* Philadelphia, 2001, Lippincott Williams & Wilkins.

21. Black FO: What can posturography tell us about vestibular function? *Ann N Y Acad Sci* 942:446-464, 2001.

22. Cevette MJ, Puetz B, Marion MS et al: Aphysiologic performance on dynamic posturography, *Otolaryngol Head Neck Surg* 112:676-688, 1995.

23. Furman JM: Posturography: uses and limitations, *Baillieres Clin Neurol* 3:501-513, 1994.

24. Krempl GA, Dobie RA: Evaluation of posturography in the detection of malingering subjects, *Am J Otol* 19:619-627, 1998.

25. Monsell EM, Furman JM, Herdman SJ et al: Computerized dynamic platform posturography, *Otolaryngol Head Neck Surg* 117:394-398, 1997.

26. Robertson DD, Ireland DJ: Dizziness Handicap Inventory correlates of computerized dynamic posturography, *J Otolaryngol* 24:118-124, 1995.

27. Sataloff RT, Hawkshaw MJ, Mandel H et al: Abnormal computerized dynamic posturography findings in dizzy patients with normal ENG results, *Ear Nose Throat J* 84:212-214, 2005.

28. Voorhees RL: The role of dynamic posturography in neurotologic diagnosis, *Laryngoscope* 99:995-1001, 1989.

29. Whitney SL, Marchetti GF, Schade AI: The relationship between falls history and computerized dynamic posturography in persons with balance and vestibular disorders, *Arch Phys Med Rehabil* 87:402-407, 2006.

30. Ekdahl C, Jarnlo GB, Andersson SI: Standing balance in healthy subjects: evaluation of a quantitative test battery on a force platform, *Scand J Rehabil Med* 21:187-195, 1989.

31. Di Fabio RP: Sensitivity and specificity of platform posturography for identifying patients with vestibular dysfunction, *Phys Ther* 75:290-305, 1995.

32. Cohen HS: Side-lying as an alternative to the Dix-Hallpike test of the posterior canal, *Otol Neurotol* 25:130-134, 2004.

33. Dix MR, Hallpike CS: The pathology symptomatology and diagnosis of certain common disorders of the vestibular system, *Proc R Soc Med* 45:341-354, 1952.

34. Kramer PD, Kleiman DA: Dix-Hallpike maneuver results are not influenced by the time of day of the test, *Acta Otolaryngol* 125:145-147, 2005.

35. Viirre E, Purcell I, Baloh RW: The Dix-Hallpike test and the canalith repositioning maneuver, *Laryngoscope* 115:184-187, 2005.

36. Goebel JA: The ten-minute examination of the dizzy patient, *Semin Neurol* 21:391-398, 2001.

37. Herdman SJ, Tusa RJ, Blatt P et al: Computerized dynamic visual acuity test in the assessment of vestibular deficits, *Am J Otol* 19:790-796, 1998.

38. Rine RM, Braswell J: A clinical test of dynamic visual acuity for children, *Int J Pediatr Otorhinolaryngol* 67:1195-1201, 2003.

39. Herdman SJ: *Vestibular rehabilitation,* Philadelphia, 2000, FA Davis.

40. Bonanni M, Newton R: Test-retest reliability of the Fukuda Stepping Test, *Physiother Res Int* 3:58-68, 1998.

41. Fukuda T: The stepping test: two phases of the labyrinthine reflex, *Acta Otolaryngol* 50:95-108, 1959.

42. Jordan P: Fukuda's stepping test: a preliminary report on reliability, *Arch Otolaryngol* 77:243-245, 1963.

43. Takahashi T, Ishida K, Yamamoto H et al: Modification of the functional reach test: analysis of lateral and anterior functional reach in community-dwelling older people, *Arch Gerontol Geriatr* 42:167-173, 2006.

44. Behrman AL, Light KE, Flynn SM et al: Is the functional reach test useful for identifying falls risk among individuals with Parkinson's disease? *Arch Phys Med Rehabil* 83:538-542, 2002.

45. Duncan PW, Studenski S, Chandler J et al: Functional reach: predictive validity in a sample of elderly male veterans, *J Gerontol* 47:M93-M98, 1992.

46. Duncan PW, Weiner DK, Chandler J et al: Functional reach: a new clinical measure of balance. *J Gerontol* 45:M192-197, 1990.

47. Jonsson E, Henriksson M, Hirschfeld H: Does the functional reach test reflect stability limits in elderly people? *J Rehabil Med* 35:26-30, 2003.

48. Lynch SM, Leahy P, Barker SP: Reliability of measurements obtained with a modified functional reach test in subjects with spinal cord injury, *Phys Ther* 78:128-133, 1998.

49. Smith PS, Hembree JA, Thompson ME: Berg Balance Scale and Functional Reach: determining the best clinical tool for individuals post acute stroke, *Clin Rehabil* 18:811-818, 2004.

50. Thapa PB, Gideon P, Brockman KG et al: Clinical and biomechanical measures of balance as fall predictors in ambulatory nursing home residents, *J Gerontol A Biol Sci Med Sci* 51:M239-M246, 1996.

51. Wallmann HW: Comparison of elderly nonfallers and fallers on performance measures of functional reach, sensory organization, and limits of stability, *J Gerontol A Biol Sci Med Sci* 56:M580-M583, 2001.

52. Weiner DK, Bongiorni DR, Studenski SA et al: Does functional reach improve with rehabilitation? *Arch Phys Med Rehabil* 74:796-800, 1993.

53. Weiner DK, Duncan PW, Chandler J et al: Functional reach: a marker of physical frailty, *J Am Geriatr Soc* 40:203-207, 1992.

54. Roma AA: Use of the head shake-sensory organization test as an outcome measure in the rehabilitation of an individual with head movement provoked symptoms of imbalance, *J Geriatr Phys Ther* 28:58-63, 2005.

55. D'Aquila MA, Smith T, Organ D et al: Validation of a lateropulsion scale for patients recovering from stroke, *Clin Rehabil* 18:102-109, 2004.

56. Clark S, Iltis PW, Anthony CJ et al: Comparison of older adult performance during the functional-reach and limits-of-stability tests, *J Aging Phys Act* 13:266-275, 2005.

57. NeuroCom International: *I: Operator's manual,* Clacamas, OR, 2003, NeuroCom International.

58. Holbein-Jenny MA, Billek-Sawhney B, Beckman E et al: Balance in personal care home residents: a comparison of the Berg Balance Scale, the Multi-Directional Reach Test, and the Activities-Specific Balance Confidence Scale, *J Geriatr Phys Ther* 28:48-53, 2005.

59. Newton RA: Validity of the multi-directional reach test: a practical measure for limits of stability in older adults, *J Gerontol A Biol Sci Med Sci* 56:M248-M252, 2001.

60. Leary P: Motor control assessment. In Montgomery P, Connoly B, editors: *Motor control and physical therapy: theoretical framework and practical applicaitons,* Chattanooga, 1991, Chattanooga Group.

61. O'Sullivan SB, Schmitz TJ: *Physical rehabilitation: assessment and treatment,* Philadelphia, 2001, FA Davis.

62. Vellas BJ, Rubenstein LZ, Ousset PJ et al: One-leg standing balance and functional status in a population of 512 community-living elderly persons, *Aging (Milano)* 9:95-98, 1997.

63. Vellas BJ, Wayne SJ, Romero L et al: One-leg balance is an important predictor of injurious falls in older persons, *J Am Geriatr Soc* 45:735-738, 1997.

64. Thomas JI, Lane JV: A pilot study to explore the predictive validity of 4 measures of falls risk in frail elderly patients, *Arch Phys Med Rehabil* 86:1636-1640, 2005.

65. Newton R: Review of tests of standing balance abilities, *Brain Inj* 3:335-343, 1989.

66. Bohannon RW, Larkin PA, Cook AC et al: Decrease in timed balance test scores with aging, *Phys Ther* 64:1067-1070, 1984.

67. Chandler JM, Duncan PW, Studenski SA: Balance performance on the postural stress test: comparison of young adults, healthy elderly, and fallers, *Phys Ther* 70:410-415, 1990.

68. Harburn KL, Hill KM, Kramer JF et al: Clinical applicability and test-retest reliability of an external perturbation test of balance in stroke subjects, *Arch Phys Med Rehabil* 76:317-323, 1995.

69. Jacobs JV, Horak FB, Tran VK et al: Multiple balance tests improve the assessment of postural stability in subjects with Parkinson's disease, *J Neurol Neurosurg Psychiatry* 77:322-326, 2006.

70. Wolfson LI, Whipple R, Amerman P et al: Stressing the postural response: a quantitative method for testing balance, *J Am Geriatr Soc* 34:845-850, 1986.

71. Black FO, Wall C III, Rockette HE Jr et al: Normal subject postural sway during the Romberg test, *Am J Otolaryngol* 3:309-318, 1982.

72. Ford-Smith CD, Wyman JF, Elswick RK Jr et al: Test-retest reliability of the sensory organization test in noninstitutionalized older adults, *Arch Phys Med Rehabil* 76:77-81, 1995.

73. Hu MH, Hung YC, Huang YL et al: Validity of force platform measures for stance stability under varying sensory conditions, *Proc Natl Sci Counc Repub China B* 20:78-86, 1996.

74. Nashner L: Evaluation of postural stability, movement, and control. In Hasson S, editor: *Clinical exercise physiology,* Philadelphia, 1994, Mosby.

75. Nashner L: Sensory, neuromuscular, and biomechanical contributions to human balance. In Duncan PW, editor: *Balance: Proceedings of the APTA forum,* Alexandria, 1990, American Physical Therapy Association.

76. Franchignoni F, Tesio L, Martino MT et al: Reliability of four simple, quantitative tests of balance and mobility in healthy elderly females, *Aging (Milano)* 10:26-31, 1998.

77. Berg K, Wood-Dauphinee S, Williams JI: The Balance Scale: reliability assessment with elderly residents and patients with an acute stroke, *Scand J Rehabil Med* 27:27-36, 1995.

78. Berg KO, Maki BE, Williams JI et al: Clinical and laboratory measures of postural balance in an elderly population, *Arch Phys Med Rehabil* 73:1073-1080, 1992.

79. Berg KO, Wood-Dauphinee SL, Williams JI et al: Measuring balance in the elderly: validation of an instrument, *Can J Public Health* 83:(2 Suppl):S7-S11, 1992.

80. Chiu AY, Au-Yeung SS, Lo SK: A comparison of four functional tests in discriminating fallers from non-fallers in older people, *Disabil Rehabil* 25:45-50, 2003.

81. Chou CY, Chien CW, Hsueh IP et al: Developing a short form of the Berg Balance Scale for people with stroke, *Phys Ther* 86:195-204, 2006.

82. Stevenson TJ: Detecting change in patients with stroke using the Berg Balance Scale, *Aust J Physiother* 47:29-38, 2001.

83. Kornetti DL, Fritz SL, Chiu YP et al: Rating scale analysis of the Berg Balance Scale, *Arch Phys Med Rehabil* 85:1128-1135, 2004.

84. Qutubuddin AA, Pegg PO, Cifu DX et al: validating the Berg Balance Scale for patients with Parkinson's disease: a key to rehabilitation evaluation, *Arch Phys Med Rehabil* 86:789-792, 2005.

85. Berg KO: Measuring balance in the elderly: preliminary development of an instrument, *Physiother Can* 41:304, 1989.

86. Berg K: Measuring balance in the elderly: validation on an instrument [dissertation], Montreal, 1993, McGill University.

87. Cress ME, Buchner DM, Questad KA et al: Continuous-scale physical functional performance in healthy older adults: a validation study, *Arch Phys Med Rehabil* 77:1243-1250, 1996.

88. McConvey J, Bennett SE: Reliability of the Dynamic Gait Index in individuals with multiple sclerosis, *Arch Phys Med Rehabil* 86:130-133, 2005.

89. Whitney S, Wrisley D, Furman J: Concurrent validity of the Berg Balance Scale and the Dynamic Gait Index in people with vestibular dysfunction, *Physiother Res Int* 8:178-186, 2003.

90. Wrisley DM, Marchetti GF, Kuharsky DK et al: Reliability, internal consistency, and validity of data obtained with the functional gait assessment, *Phys Ther* 84:906-918, 2004.

91. Di Fabio RP, Seay R: Use of the "fast evaluation of mobility, balance, and fear" in elderly community dwellers: validity and reliability, *Phys Ther* 77:904-917, 1997.

92. Dite W, Temple VA: A clinical test of stepping and change of direction to identify multiple falling older adults, *Arch Phys Med Rehabil* 83:1566-1571, 2002.

93. Thomas M, Jankovic J, Suteerawattananon M et al: Clinical gait and balance scale (GABS): validation and utilization, *J Neurol Sci* 217:89-99, 2004.

94. Deathe AB, Miller WC: The L test of functional mobility: measurement properties of a modified version of the timed "up & go" test designed for people with lower-limb amputations, *Phys Ther* 85:626-635, 2005.

95. Winograd CH, Lemsky CM, Nevitt MC et al: Development of a physical performance and mobility examination, *J Am Geriatr Soc* 42:743-749, 1994.

96. Binder EF, Storandt M, Birge SJ: The relation between psychometric test performance and physical performance in older adults, *J Gerontol A Biol Sci Med Sci* 54:M428-M432, 1999.

97. Brown M, Sinacore DR, Binder EF et al: Physical and performance measures for the identification of mild to moderate frailty, *J Gerontol A Biol Sci Med Sci* 55:M350-M355, 2000.

98. King MB, Judge JO, Whipple R et al: Reliability and responsiveness of two physical performance measures examined in the context of a functional training intervention, *Phys Ther* 80:8-16, 2000.

99. Reuben DB, Siu AL: An objective measure of physical function of elderly outpatients: the Physical Performance Test, *J Am Geriatr Soc* 38:1105-1112, 1990.

100. Sherman SE, Reuben D: Measures of functional status in community-dwelling elders, *J Gen Intern Med* 13:817-823, 1998.

101. VanSwearingen JM, Paschal KA, Bonino P et al: Assessing recurrent fall risk of community-dwelling, frail older veterans using specific tests of mobility and the physical performance test of function, *J Gerontol A Biol Sci Med Sci* 53:M457-M464, 1998.

102. Giorgetti MM, Harris BA, Jette A: Reliability of clinical balance outcome measures in the elderly, *Physiother Res Int* 3:274-283, 1998.

103. Cipriany-Dacko LM, Innerst D, Johannsen J et al: Interrater reliability of the Tinetti Balance Scores in novice and experienced physical therapy clinicians, *Arch Phys Med Rehabil* 78:1160-1164, 1997.

104. Lin MR, Hwang HF, Hu MH et al: Psychometric comparisons of the timed up and go, one-leg stand, functional reach, and Tinetti balance measures in community-dwelling older people, *J Am Geriatr Soc* 52:1343-1348, 2004.

105. Lombardi R, Buizza A, Gandolfi R et al: Measurement on Tinetti test: instrumentation and procedures, *Technol Health Care* 9:403-415, 2001.

106. Tinetti ME: Performance-oriented assessment of mobility problems in elderly patients, *J Am Geriatr Soc* 34:119-126, 1986.

107. Tinetti ME, Richman D, Powell L: Falls efficacy as a measure of fear of falling, *J Gerontol* 45:P239-243, 1990.

108. Mathias S, Nayak US, Isaacs B: Balance in elderly patients: the "get-up and go" test, *Arch Phys Med Rehabil* 67:387-389, 1986.

109. Podsiadlo D, Richardson S: The timed "Up & Go": a test of basic functional mobility for frail elderly persons, *J Am Geriatr Soc* 39:142-148, 1991.

110. Brooks D, Davis AM, Naglie G: Validity of 3 physical performance measures in inpatient geriatric rehabilitation, *Arch Phys Med Rehabil* 87:105-110, 2006.

111. Lundin-Olsson L, Nyberg L, Gustafson Y: Attention, frailty, and falls: the effect of a manual task on basic mobility, *J Am Geriatr Soc* 46:758-761, 1998.

112. Morris S, Morris ME, Iansek R: Reliability of measurements obtained with the Timed "Up & Go" test in people with Parkinson disease, *Phys Ther* 81:810-818, 2001.

113. Schoppen T, Boonstra A, Groothoff JW et al: The Timed "up and go" test: reliability and validity in persons with unilateral lower limb amputation, *Arch Phys Med Rehabil* 80:825-828, 1999.

114. Bischoff HA, Stahelin HB, Monsch AU et al: Identifying a cut-off point for normal mobility: a comparison of the timed "up and go" test in community-dwelling and institutionalised elderly women, *Age Ageing* 32:315-320, 2003.

115. Ng SS, Hui-Chan CW: The timed up & go test: Its reliability and association with lower-limb impairments and locomotor capacities in people with chronic stroke, *Arch Phys Med Rehabil* 86:1641-1647, 2005.

116. Shumway-Cook A, Brauer S, Woollacott M: Predicting the probability for falls in community-dwelling older adults using the Timed Up & Go Test, *Phys Ther* 80:896-903, 2000.

117. Wall JC, Bell C, Campbell S et al: The Timed Get-up-and-Go test revisited: measurement of the component tasks, *J Rehabil Res Dev* 37:109-113, 2000.

118. Williams EN, Carroll SG, Reddihough DS et al: Investigation of the timed 'up & go' test in children, *Dev Med Child Neurol* 47:518-524, 2005.

119. Eekhof JA, De Bock GH, Schaapveld K et al: Short report, functional mobility assessment at home: timed up and go test using three different chairs, *Can Fam Physician* 47:1205-1207, 2001.

120. Umphred DA: Reliability of the modified timed up and go test (mTUG), Unpublished research, 2000.

121. Umphred DA: Validity of the modified timed up and go test (mTUG), Unpublished research, 2000.

122. Creel GL, Light KE, Thigpen MT: Concurrent and construct validity of scores on the Timed Movement Battery, *Phys Ther* 81:789-798, 2001.

123. Whitney SL, Wrisley DM, Marchetti GF et al: Clinical measurement of sit-to-stand performance in people with balance disorders: validity of data for the Five-Times-Sit-to-Stand Test, *Phys Ther* 85:1034-1045, 2005.

124. Tran PV, Schwarz J, Gorman M et al: Validation of an automated up-timer for measurement of mobility in older adults, *Med J Aust* 167:434-436, 1997.

125. Holden MK, Gill KM, Magliozzi MR et al: Clinical gait assessment in the neurologically impaired: reliability and meaningfulness, *Phys Ther* 64:35-40, 1984.

126. Montero-Odasso M, Schapira M, Varela C et al: Gait velocity in senior people: An easy test for detecting mobility impairment in community elderly, *J Nutr Health Aging* 8:340-343, 2004.

127. Nelson AJ: Functional ambulation profile, *Phys Ther* 54:1059-1065, 1974.

128. Wolf SL, Catlin PA, Gage K et al: Establishing the reliability and validity of measurements of walking time using the Emory Functional Ambulation Profile, *Phys Ther* 79:1122-1133, 1999.

129. Baer HR, Wolf SL: Modified emory functional ambulation profile: an outcome measure for the rehabilitation of poststroke gait dysfunction, *Stroke* 32:973-979, 2001.

130. Bilney B, Morris M, Webster K: Concurrent related validity of the GAITRite walkway system for quantification of the spatial and temporal parameters of gait, *Gait Posture* 17:68-74, 2003.

131. Nelson AJ, Zwick D, Brody S et al: The validity of the GaitRite and the Functional Ambulation Performance scoring system in the analysis of Parkinson gait, *NeuroRehabilitation* 17:255-262, 2002.

132. Webster KE, Wittwer JE, Feller JA: Validity of the GAITRite walkway system for the measurement of averaged and individual step parameters of gait, *Gait Posture* 22:317-321, 2005.

133. McDonough AL, Batavia M, Chen FC et al: The validity and reliability of the GAITRite system's measurements: a preliminary evaluation, *Arch Phys Med Rehabil* 82:419-425, 2001.

134. VanSwearingen JM, Paschal KA, Bonino P et al: The modified Gait Abnormality Rating Scale for recognizing the risk of recurrent falls in community-dwelling elderly adults, *Phys Ther* 76:994-1002, 1996.

135. Whipple R, Wolfson LI: Abnormalities of balance, gait, and sensorimotor function in the elderly population. In Duncan PW, editor: Balance: *Proceedings of the APTA Forum,* Alexandria, VA, 1990, American Physical Therapy Association.

136. Professional Staff Association of Rancho Los Amigos Medical Center: *Observational gait analysis handbook,* Downey, CA, 1989, Rancho Los Amigos Hospital.

137. Salbach NM, Mayo NE, Higgins J et al: Responsiveness and predictability of gait speed and other disability measures in acute stroke, *Arch Phys Med Rehabil* 82:1204-1212, 2001.

138. Simonsick EM, Fan E, Fleg JL: Estimating cardiorespiratory fitness in well-functioning older adults: treadmill validation of the long distance corridor walk, *J Am Geriatr Soc* 54:127-132, 2006.

139. Rolland YM, Cesari M, Miller ME et al: Reliability of the 400-m usual-pace walk test as an assessment of mobility limitation in older adults, *J Am Geriatr Soc* 52:972-976, 2004.

140. Kosak M, Smith T: Comparison of the 2-, 6-, and 12-minute walk tests in patients with stroke, *J Rehabil Res Dev* 42:103-107, 2005.

141. Guyatt GH, Sullivan MJ, Thompson PJ et al: The 6-minute walk: a new measure of exercise capacity in patients with chronic heart failure, *Can Med Assoc J* 132:919-923, 1985.

142. Hamilton DM, Haennel RG: Validity and reliability of the 6-minute walk test in a cardiac rehabilitation population, *J Cardiopulm Rehabil* 20:156-164, 2000.

143. Pankoff BA, Overend TJ, Lucy SD et al: Reliability of the six-minute walk test in people with fibromyalgia, *Arthritis Care Res* 13:291-295, 2000.

144. Savci S, Inal-Ince D, Arikan H et al: Six-minute walk distance as a measure of functional exercise capacity in multiple sclerosis, *Disabil Rehabil* 27:1365-1371, 2005.

145. Moalla W, Gauthier R, Maingourd Y et al: Six-minute walking test to assess exercise tolerance and cardiorespiratory responses during training program in children with congenital heart disease, *Int J Sports Med* 26:756-762, 2005.

146. Kervio G, Carre F, Ville NS: Reliability and intensity of the six-minute walk test in healthy elderly subjects, *Med Sci Sports Exerc* 35:169-174, 2003.

147. King S, Wessel J, Bhambhani Y et al: Validity and reliability of the 6 minute walk in persons with fibromyalgia, *J Rheumatol* 26:2233-2237, 1999.

148. Larson JL, Covey MK, Vitalo CA et al: Reliability and validity of the 12-minute distance walk in patients with chronic obstructive pulmonary disease, *Nurs Res* 45:203-210, 1996.

149. McGavin CR, Gupta SP, McHardy GJ: Twelve-minute walking test for assessing disability in chronic bronchitis, *BMJ* 1:822-823, 1976.

150. Bernstein ML, Despars JA, Singh NP et al: Reanalysis of the 12-minute walk in patients with chronic obstructive pulmonary disease, *Chest* 105:163-167, 1994.

151. Botner EM, Miller WC, Eng JJ: Measurement properties of the Activities-specific Balance Confidence Scale among individuals with stroke, *Disabil Rehabil* 27:156-163, 2005.

152. Miller WC, Deathe AB, Speechley M: Psychometric properties of the Activities-specific Balance Confidence Scale among individuals with a lower-limb amputation, *Arch Phys Med Rehabil* 84:656-661, 2003.

153. Powell LE, Myers AM: The Activities-specific Balance Confidence (ABC) Scale, *J Gerontol A Biol Sci Med Sci* 50A:M28-M34, 1995.

154. Whitney SL, Hudak MT, Marchetti GF: The activities-specific balance confidence scale and the dizziness handicap inventory: a comparison, *J Vestib Res* 9:253-259, 1999.

155. Hotchkiss A, Fisher A, Robertson R et al: Convergent and predictive validity of three scales related to falls in the elderly, *Am J Occup Ther* 58:100-103, 2004.

156. Hellstrom K, Lindmark B: Fear of falling in patients with stroke: a reliability study, *Clin Rehabil* 13:509-517, 1999.

157. Yardley L, Beyer N, Hauer K et al: Development and initial validation of the Falls Efficacy Scale-International (FES-I), *Age Ageing* 34:614-619, 2005.

158. Southard V, Dave M, Davis MG et al: The Multiple Tasks Test as a predictor of falls in older adults, *Gait Posture* 22:351-355, 2005.

159. Hachisuka K, Okazaki T, Ogata H: Self-rating Barthel index compatible with the original Barthel index and the Functional Independence Measure motor score, *J Uoeh* 19:107-121, 1997.

160. Hsueh IP, Lee MM, Hsieh CL: Psychometric characteristics of the Barthel activities of daily living index in stroke patients, *J Formos Med Assoc* 100:526-532, 2001.

161. Neal LJ: Current functional assessment tools, *Home Healthc Nurse* 16:766-772, 1998.

162. Granger CV, Albrecht GL, Hamilton BB: Outcome of comprehensive medical rehabilitation: measurement by PULSES profile and the Barthel Index, *Arch Phys Med Rehabil* 60:145-154, 1979.

163. Green J, Forster A, Young J: A test-retest reliability study of the Barthel Index, the Rivermead Mobility Index, the Nottingham Extended Activities of Daily Living Scale and the Frenchay Activities Index in stroke patients, *Disabil Rehabil* 23:670-676, 2001.

164. Loewen SC, Anderson BA: Reliability of the Modified Motor Assessment Scale and the Barthel Index, *Phys Ther* 68:1077-1081, 1988.

165. Mahoney FI, Barthel DW: Functional evaluation: the Barthel Index, *Md State Med J* 14:61-65, 1965.

166. Nycin K, McMichael L, Turner-Stokes L: Can a Barthel score be derived from the FIM? *Clin Rehabil* 13:56-63, 1999.

167. van der Putten JJ, Hobart JC, Freeman JA, Thompson AJ: Measuring change in disability after inpatient rehabilitation: comparison of the responsiveness of the Barthel index and the Functional Independence Measure, *J Neurol Neurosurg Psychiatry* 66:480-484, 1999.

168. Bucks RS, Ashworth DL, Wilcock GK et al: Assessment of activities of daily living in dementia: Development of the Bristol Activities of Daily Living Scale, *Age Ageing* 25:113-120, 1996.

169. Byrne LM, Wilson PM, Bucks RS et al: The sensitivity to change over time of the Bristol Activities of Daily Living Scale in Alzheimer's disease, *Int J Geriatr Psychiatry* 15:656-661, 2000.

170. Brorsson B, Asberg KH: Katz index of independence in ADL: reliability and validity in short-term care, *Scand J Rehabil Med* 16:125-132, 1984.

171. Dowd S, Davidhizar R: Opening up to the Katz Index, *Elder Care* 11:9-12, 1999.

172. Hulter Asberg K: Disability as a predictor of outcome for the elderly in a department of internal medicine: a comparison of predictions based on index of ADL and physician predictions, *Scand J Soc Med* 15:261-265, 1987.

173. Katz S, Akpom CA: 12: Index of ADL, *Med Care* 14:116-118, 1976.

174. Katz S, Downs TD, Cash HR et al: Progress in development of the index of ADL, *Gerontologist* 10:20-30, 1970.

175. Katz S, Ford AB, Moskowitz RW et al: Studies of illness in the aged: The index of ADL: a standardized measure of biological and psychosocial function, *JAMA* 185:914-919, 1963.

176. Shelkey M, Wallace M: Katz Index of Independence in Activities of Daily Living, *J Gerontol Nurs* 25:8-9, 1999.

177. Schoening HA, Iversen IA: Numerical scoring of self-care status: a study of the Kenny self-care evaluation, *Arch Phys Med Rehabil* 49:221-229, 1968.

178. Klein RM, Bell B: Self-care skills: behavioral measurement with Klein-Bell ADL scale, *Arch Phys Med Rehabil* 63:335-338, 1982.

179. Nelson DL, Melville LL, Wilkerson JD et al: Interrater reliability, concurrent validity, responsiveness, and predictive validity of the Melville-Nelson Self-Care Assessment, *Am J Occup Ther* 56:51-99, 2002.

180. Marshall SC, Heisel B, Grinnell D: Validity of the PULSES profile compared with the Functional Independence Measure for measuring disability in a stroke rehabilitation setting, *Arch Phys Med Rehabil* 80:760-765, 1999.

181. Mahurin RK, DeBettignies BH, Pirozzolo FJ: Structured assessment of independent living skills: preliminary report of a performance measure of functional abilities in dementia, *J Gerontol* 46:P58-P66, 1991.

182. Oliver R, Blathwayt J, Brackley C et al: Development of the Safety Assessment of Function and the Environment for Rehabilitation (SAFER) tool, *Can J Occup Ther* 60:78-82, 1993.

183. Bohannon RW: Hand-grip dynamometry provides a valid indication of upper extremity strength impairment in home care patients, *J Hand Ther* 11:258-260, 1998.

184. Bohannon RW: Dynamometer measurements of hand-grip strength predict multiple outcomes, *Percept Mot Skills* 93:323-328, 2001.

185. Haward BM, Griffin MJ: Repeatability of grip strength and dexterity tests and the effects of age and gender, *Int Arch Occup Environ Health* 75:111-119, 2002.

186. Hillman TE, Nunes QM, Hornby ST et al: A practical posture for hand grip dynamometry in the clinical setting, *Clin Nutr* 24:224-228, 2005.

187. Mathiowetz V, Kashman N, Volland G et al: Grip and pinch strength: normative data for adults, *Arch Phys Med Rehabil* 66:69-74, 1985.

188. Schmidt RT, Toews JV: Grip strength as measured by the Jamar dynamometer, *Arch Phys Med Rehabil* 51:321-327, 1970.

189. Andrews AW, Thomas MW, Bohannon RW: Normative values for isometric muscle force measurements obtained with hand-held dynamometers, *Phys Ther* 76:248-259, 1996.

190. Bohannon RW: Intertester reliability of hand-held dynamometry: a concise summary of published research, *Percept Mot Skills* 88:899-902, 1999.

191. Bohannon RW: Reference values for extremity muscle strength obtained by hand-held dynamometry from adults aged 20 to 79 years, *Arch Phys Med Rehabil* 78:26-32, 1997.

192. Kellor M, Frost J, Silberberg N et al: Hand strength and dexterity, *Am J Occup Ther* 25:77-83, 1971.

193. Wadsworth CT, Krishnan R, Sear M et al: Intrarater reliability of manual muscle testing and hand-held dynametric muscle testing, *Phys Ther* 67:1342-1347, 1987.

194. Almekinders LC, Oman J: Isokinetic muscle testing: is it clinically useful? *J Am Acad Orthop Surg* 2:221-225, 1994.

195. Gaines JM, Talbot LA: Isokinetic strength testing in research and practice, *Biol Res Nurs* 1:57-64, 1999.

196. Kannus P: Isokinetic evaluation of muscular performance: implications for muscle testing and rehabilitation, *Int J Sports Med* 15(1 Suppl):S11-S18, 1994.

197. Brandsma JW, Schreuders TA: Sensible manual muscle strength testing to evaluate and monitor strength of the intrinsic muscles of the hand: a commentary, *J Hand Ther* 14:273-278, 2001.

198. Csuka M, McCarty DJ: Simple method for measurement of lower extremity muscle strength, *Am J Med* 78:77-81, 1985.

199. Kendall FP, McCreary EK, Provance P: Muscles, testing and function: With posture and pain, Baltimore, 1993, Williams & Wilkins.

200. Hislop HJ, Montgomery J: *Daniels and Worthingham's muscle testing: techniques of manual examination,* Philadelpia, 2002, WB Saunders.

201. Gajdosik RL, Bohannon RW: Clinical measurement of range of motion. Review of goniometry emphasizing reliability and validity, *Phys Ther* 67:1867-1872, 1987.

202. Goodwin J, Clark C, Deakes J et al: Clinical methods of goniometry: a comparative study, *Disabil Rehabil* 14:10-15, 1992.

203. Perret C, Poiraudeau S, Fermanian J et al: Validity, reliability, and responsiveness of the fingertip-to-floor test, *Arch Phys Med Rehabil* 82:1566-1570, 2001.

204. Tousignant M, Duclos E, Lafleche S et al: Validity study for the cervical range of motion device used for lateral flexion in patients with neck pain, *Spine* 27:812-817, 2002.

205. Breum J, Wiberg J, Bolton JE: Reliability and concurrent validity of the BROM II for measuring lumbar mobility, *J Manipulative Physiol Ther* 18:497-502, 1995.

206. Boone DC, Azen SP, Lin CM et al: Reliability of goniometric measurements, *Phys Ther* 58:1355-1390, 1978.

207. Norkin CC, White DJ: *Measurement of joint motion: a guide to goniometry,* Philadelphia, 2003, FA Davis.

208. Brashear A, Zafonte R, Corcoran M et al: Inter- and intrarater reliability of the Ashworth Scale and the Disability Assessment Scale in patients with upper-limb poststroke spasticity, *Arch Phys Med Rehabil* 83:1349-1354, 2002.

209. Pandyan AD, Johnson GR, Price CI et al: A review of the properties and limitations of the Ashworth and modified Ashworth Scales as measures of spasticity, *Clin Rehabil* 13:373-383, 1999.

210. Allison SC, Abraham LD, Petersen CL: Reliability of the Modified Ashworth Scale in the assessment of plantarflexor muscle spasticity in patients with traumatic brain injury, *Int J Rehabil Res* 19:67-78, 1996.

211. Gregson JM, Leathley M, Moore AP et al: Reliability of the Tone Assessment Scale and the modified Ashworth scale as clinical tools for assessing poststroke spasticity, *Arch Phys Med Rehabil* 80:1013-1016, 1999.

212. Haas BM, Bergstrom E, Jamous A et al: The inter rater reliability of the original and of the modified Ashworth scale for the assessment of spasticity in patients with spinal cord injury, *Spinal Cord* 34:560-564, 1996.

213. Mehrholz J, Major Y, Meissner D et al: The influence of contractures and variation in measurement stretching velocity on the reliability of the Modified Ashworth Scale in patients with severe brain injury, *Clin Rehabil* 19:63-72, 2005.

214. Sloan RL, Sinclair E, Thompson J et al: Inter-rater reliability of the modified Ashworth Scale for spasticity in hemiplegic patients, *Int J Rehabil Res* 15:158-161, 1992.

215. Clopton N, Dutton J, Featherston T et al: Interrater and intrarater reliability of the Modified Ashworth Scale in children with hypertonia, *Pediatr Phys Ther* 17:268-274, 2005.

216. Mackey AH, Walt SE, Lobb G et al: Intraobserver reliability of the modified Tardieu scale in the upper limb of children with hemiplegia, *Dev Med Child Neurol* 46:267-272, 2004.

217. Antonelli Incalzi R, Cesari M, Pedone C et al: Construct validity of the abbreviated mental test in older medical inpatients, *Dement Geriatr Cogn Disord* 15:199-206, 2003.

218. MacKenzie DM, Copp P, Shaw RJ et al: Brief cognitive screening of the elderly: a comparison of the Mini-Mental State Examination (MMSE), Abbreviated Mental Test (AMT) and Mental Status Questionnaire (MSQ), *Psychol Med* 26:427-430, 1996.

219. Swain DG, Nightingale PG: Evaluation of a shortened version of the Abbreviated Mental Test in a series of elderly patients, *Clin Rehabil* 11:243-248, 1997.

220. Jitapunkul S, Pillay I, Ebrahim S: The abbreviated mental test: its use and validity, *Age Ageing* 20:332-336, 1991.

221. Schramm U, Berger G, Muller R et al: Psychometric properties of Clock Drawing Test and MMSE or Short Performance Test (SKT) in dementia screening in a memory clinic population, *Int J Geriatr Psychiatry* 17:254-260, 2002.

222. Shulman KI: Clock-drawing: is it the ideal cognitive screening test? *Int J Geriatr Psychiatry* 15:548-561, 2000.

223. Sunderland T, Hill JL, Mellow AM et al: Clock drawing in Alzheimer's disease: a novel measure of dementia severity, *J Am Geriatr Soc* 37:725-729, 1989.

224. Watson YI, Arfken CL, Birge SJ: Clock completion: an objective screening test for dementia, *J Am Geriatr Soc* 41:1235-1240, 1993.

225. Wolf-Klein GP, Silverstone FA, Levy AP et al: Screening for Alzheimer's disease by clock drawing, *J Am Geriatr Soc* 37:730-734, 1989.

226. Hurley AC, Volicer BJ, Hanrahan PA et al: Assessment of discomfort in advanced Alzheimer patients, *Res Nurs Health* 15:369-377, 1992.

227. Chen-Sea MJ: Validating the Draw-A-Man Test as a personal neglect test, *Am J Occup Ther* 54:391-397, 2000.

228. Bassuk SS, Murphy JM: Characteristics of the Modified Mini-Mental State Exam among elderly persons, *J Clin Epidemiol* 56:622-628, 2003.

229. Bleecker ML, Bolla-Wilson K, Kawas C et al: Age-specific norms for the Mini-Mental State Exam, *Neurology* 38:1565-1568, 1988.

230. Braekhus A, Laake K, Engedal K: A low, "normal" score on the Mini-Mental State Examination predicts development of dementia after three years, *J Am Geriatr Soc* 43:656-661, 1995.

231. Crum RM, Anthony JC, Bassett SS et al: Population-based norms for the Mini-Mental State Examination by age and educational level, *JAMA* 269:2386-2391, 1993.

232. Grace J, Nadler JD, White DA et al: Folstein vs modified Mini-Mental State Examination in geriatric stroke: stability, validity, and screening utility, *Arch Neurol* 52:477-484, 1995.

233. Grigoletto F, Zappala G, Anderson DW et al: Norms for the Mini-Mental State Examination in a healthy population, *Neurology* 53:315-320, 1999.

234. Molloy DW, Standish TI: A guide to the standardized Mini-Mental State Examination, *Int Psychogeriatr* 9(1 Suppl):87-94, 143-150, 1997.

235. Folstein MF, Folstein SE, McHugh PR: "Mini-mental state": a practical method for grading the cognitive state of patients for the clinician, *J Psychiatr Res* 12:189-198, 1975.

236. Harrell LE, Marson D, Chatterjee A et al: The Severe Mini-Mental State Examination: a new neuropsychologic instrument for the bedside assessment of severely impaired patients with Alzheimer disease, *Alzheimer Dis Assoc Disord* 14:168-175, 2000.

237. Shyu YI, Yip PK: Factor structure and explanatory variables of the Mini-Mental State Examination (MMSE) for elderly persons in Taiwan, *J Formos Med Assoc* 100:676-683, 2001.

238. Tangalos EG, Smith GE, Ivnik RJ et al: The Mini-Mental State Examination in general medical practice: clinical utility and acceptance, *Mayo Clin Proc* 71:829-837, 1996.

239. Teng EL, Chui HC: The Modified Mini-Mental State (3MS) examination, *J Clin Psychiatry* 48:314-318, 1987.

240. Bravo G, Hebert R: Age- and education-specific reference values for the Mini-Mental and modified Mini-Mental State Examinations derived from a non-demented elderly population, *Int J Geriatr Psychiatry* 12:1008-1018, 1997.

241. Bravo G, Hebert R: Reliability of the Modified Mini-Mental State Examination in the context of a two-phase community prevalence study, *Neuroepidemiology* 16:141-148, 1997.

242. Helmes E: Multidimensional Observation Scale for Elderly Subjects (MOSES), *Psychopharmacol Bull* 24:733-745, 1988.

243. Helmes E, Csapo KG, Short JA: Standardization and validation of the Multidimensional Observation Scale for Elderly Subjects (MOSES), *J Gerontol* 42:395-405, 1987.

244. Pruchno RA, Kleban MH, Resch NL: Psychometric assessment of the Multidimensional Observation Scale for Elderly Subjects (MOSES), *J Gerontol* 43:P164-P169, 1988.

245. Novack TA, Dowler RN, Bush BA et al: Validity of the Orientation Log, relative to the Galveston Orientation and Amnesia Test, *J Head Trauma Rehabil* 15:957-961, 2000.

246. Flannery J: Using the levels of cognitive functioning assessment scale with patients with traumatic brain injury in an acute care setting, *Rehabil Nurs* 23:88-94, 1998.

247. Flannery J: Cognitive assessment in the acute care setting: reliability and validity of the Levels of Cognitive Functioning Assessment Scale (LOCFAS), *J Nurs Meas* 3:43-58, 1995.

248. Gouvier WD, Blanton PD, LaPorte KK et al: Reliability and validity of the Disability Rating Scale and the Levels of Cognitive Functioning Scale in monitoring recovery from severe head injury, *Arch Phys Med Rehabil* 68:94-97, 1987.
249. Kelly MP, Johnson CT, Govern JM: Recognition memory test: validity in diffuse traumatic brain injury, *Appl Neuropsychol* 3:147-154, 1996.
250. Roccaforte WH, Burke WJ, Bayer BL et al: Reliability and validity of the Short Portable Mental Status Questionnaire administered by telephone, *J Geriatr Psychiatry Neurol* 7:33-38, 1994.
251. Boake C: Supervision rating scale: a measure of functional outcome from brain injury, *Arch Phys Med Rehabil* 77:765-772, 1996.
252. Sherer M, Nick TG, Millis SR et al: Use of the WCST and the WCST-64 in the assessment of traumatic brain injury, *J Clin Exp Neuropsychol* 25:512-520, 2003.
253. Benaim C, Cailly B, Perennou D et al: Validation of the aphasic depression rating scale, *Stroke* 35:1692-1696.
254. Beck AT, Beamesderfer A: Assessment of depression: the depression inventory, *Mod Probl Pharmacopsychiatry* 7:151-169, 1974.
255. Beck AT, Rial WY, Rickels K: Short form of depression inventory: cross-validation, *Psychol Rep* 34:1184-1186, 1974.
256. Gallagher D, Nies G, Thompson LW: Reliability of the Beck Depression Inventory with older adults, *J Consult Clin Psychol* 50:152-153, 1982.
257. Green A, Felmingham K, Baguley IJ et al: The clinical utility of the Beck Depression Inventory after traumatic brain injury, *Brain Inj* 15:1021-1028, 2001.
258. Scogin F, Beutler L, Corbishley A et al: Reliability and validity of the short form Beck Depression Inventory with older adults, *J Clin Psychol* 44:853-857, 1988.
259. Visser M, Leentjens AF, Marinus J et al: Reliability and validity of the Beck depression inventory in patients with Parkinson's disease, *Mov Disord* 21:668-672, 2006.
260. Beck AT, Ward CH, Mendelson M et al: An inventory for measuring depression, *Arch Gen Psychiatry* 4:561-571, 1961.
261. Beck AT, Steer RA, Brown GK: *Beck Depression Inventory,* San Antonio, 1996, Harcourt Assessment.
262. Hoyl MT, Alessi CA, Harker JO et al: Development and testing of a five-item version of the Geriatric Depression Scale, *J Am Geriatr Soc* 47:873-878, 1999.
263. Rinaldi P, Mecocci P, Benedetti C et al: Validation of the five-item geriatric depression scale in elderly subjects in three different settings, *J Am Geriatr Soc* 51:694-698, 2003.
264. Arthur A, Jagger C, Lindesay J et al: Using an annual over-75 health check to screen for depression: validation of the short Geriatric Depression Scale (GDS15) within general practice, *Int J Geriatr Psychiatry* 14:431-439, 1999.
265. Burke WJ, Roccaforte WH, Wengel SP et al: The reliability and validity of the Geriatric Depression Rating Scale administered by telephone, *J Am Geriatr Soc* 43:674-679, 1995.
266. Ertan FS, Ertan T, Kiziltan G et al: Reliability and validity of the Geriatric Depression Scale in depression in Parkinson's disease, *J Neurol Neurosurg Psychiatry* 76:1445-1447, 2005.
267. Friedman B, Heisel MJ, Delavan RL: Psychometric properties of the 15-item geriatric depression scale in functionally impaired, cognitively intact, community-dwelling elderly primary care patients, *J Am Geriatr Soc* 53:1570-1576, 2005.
268. Yesavage JA, Brink TL, Rose TL et al: Development and validation of a geriatric depression screening scale: A preliminary report, *J Psychiatr Res* 17:37-49, 1982.
269. Hamilton M: A rating scale for depression, *J Neurol Neurosurg Psychiatry* 23:56-62, 1960.
270. Miller IW, Bishop S, Norman WH et al: The Modified Hamilton Rating Scale for Depression: Reliability and validity, *Psychiatry Res* 14:131-142, 1985.
271. Davidson J, Turnbull CD, Strickland R et al: The Montgomery-Asberg Depression Scale: reliability and validity, *Acta Psychiatr Scand* 73:544-548, 1986.
272. Biggs JT, Wylie LT, Ziegler VE: Validity of the Zung Self-rating Depression Scale, *Br J Psychiatry* 132:381-385, 1978.
273. Thurber S, Snow M, Honts CR: The Zung Self-Rating Depression Scale: convergent validity and diagnostic discrimination, *Assessment* 9:401-405, 2002.
274. Marder SR: Psychiatric rating scales. In Kaplan HJ, Saddock BJ, editors: *Comprehensive textbook of psychiatry,* Baltimore, 1995, Williams & Wilkins, pp. 619-635.
275. Rappaport M: The Disability Rating and Coma/Near-Coma scales in evaluating severe head injury, *Neuropsychol Rehabil* 15:442-453, 2005.
276. Rappaport M, Dougherty AM, Kelting DL: Evaluation of coma and vegetative states, *Arch Phys Med Rehabil* 73:628-634, 1992.
277. Giacino JT, Kalmar K, Whyte J: The JFK Coma Recovery Scale-Revised: measurement characteristics and diagnostic utility, *Arch Phys Med Rehabil* 85:2020-2029, 2004.
278. Giacino JT, Kezmarsky MA, DeLuca J et al: Monitoring rate of recovery to predict outcome in minimally responsive patients, *Arch Phys Med Rehabil* 72:897-901, 1991.
279. Kalmar K, Giacino JT: The JFK Coma Recovery Scale—revised, *Neuropsychol Rehabil* 15:454-460, 2005.
280. Gabbe BJ, Cameron PA, Finch CF: The status of the Glasgow Coma Scale, *Emerg Med (Fremantle)* 15:353-360, 2003.
281. Heron R, Davie A, Gillies R et al: Interrater reliability of the Glasgow Coma Scale scoring among nurses in sub-specialties of critical care, *Aust Crit Care* 14:100-105, 2001.
282. Juarez VJ, Lyons M: Interrater reliability of the Glasgow Coma Scale, *J Neurosci Nurs* 27:283-286, 1995.
283. Prasad K: The Glasgow Coma Scale: a critical appraisal of its clinimetric properties, *J Clin Epidemiol* 49:755-763, 1996.
284. Zafonte RD, Hammond FM, Mann NR et al: Relationship between Glasgow coma scale and functional outcome, *Am J Phys Med Rehabil* 75:364-369, 1996.
285. Jennett B, Bond M: Assessment of outcome after severe brain damage, *Lancet* 1:480-484, 1975.
286. Teasdale GM, Murray L: Revisiting the Glasgow Coma Scale and Coma Score, *Intensive Care Med* 26:153-154, 2000.
287. Teasdale G, Jennett B: Assessment of coma and impaired consciousness: A practical scale, *Lancet* 2:81-84, 1974.
288. Jennett B, Teasdale G: *Management of head injuries,* Philadelphia, 1981, FA Davis.
289. Espie CA, Watkins J, Duncan R et al: Development and validation of the Glasgow Epilepsy Outcome Scale (GEOS): a new instrument for measuring concerns about epilepsy in people with mental retardation, *Epilepsia* 42:1043-1051, 2001.
290. Anderson SI, Housley AM, Jones PA et al: Glasgow Outcome Scale: an inter-rater reliability study, *Brain Inj* 7:309-317, 1993.
291. Teasdale GM, Pettigrew LE, Wilson JT et al: Analyzing outcome of treatment of severe head injury: a review and update on advancing the use of the Glasgow Outcome Scale, *J Neurotrauma* 15:587-597, 1998.
292. Ansell BJ, Keenan JE: The Western Neuro Sensory Stimulation Profile: a tool for assessing slow-to-recover head-injured patients, *Arch Phys Med Rehabil* 70:104-108, 1989.
293. Ewing-Cobbs L, Levin HS, Fletcher JM et al: The Children's Orientation and Amnesia Test: relationship to severity of acute head injury and to recovery of memory, *Neurosurgery* 27:683-691, 1990.
294. Bode RK, Heinemann AW, Semik P: Measurement properties of the Galveston Orientation and Amnesia Test (GOAT) and improvement patterns during inpatient rehabilitation, *J Head Trauma Rehabil* 15:637-655, 2000.
295. Levin HS, O'Donnell VM, Grossman RG: The Galveston Orientation and Amnesia Test: a practical scale to assess cognition after head injury, *J Nerv Ment Dis* 167:675-684, 1979.
296. Davidoff G, Doljanac R, Berent S et al: Galveston Orientation and Amnesia Test: Its utility in the determination of closed head injury in acute spinal cord injury patients, *Arch Phys Med Rehabil* 69:432-434, 1988.

297. Shores EA: Further concurrent validity data on the Westmead PTA Scale, *Appl Neuropsychol* 2:167-169, 1995.

298. Tate RL, Perdices M, Pfaff A et al: Predicting duration of posttraumatic amnesia (PTA) from early PTA measurements, *J Head Trauma Rehabil* 16:525-542, 2001.

299. McDonald TW, Franzen MD: A validity study of the WAIT in closed head injury, *Brain Inj* 13:331-346, 1999.

300. Lai SM, Duncan PW: Evaluation of the American Heart Association Stroke Outcome Classification, *Stroke* 30:1840-1843, 1999.

301. Chae J, Labatia I, Yang G: Upper limb motor function in hemiparesis: concurrent validity of the Arm Motor Ability test, *Am J Phys Med Rehabil* 82:1-8, 2003.

302. Kopp B, Kunkel A, Flor H et al: The Arm Motor Ability Test: reliability, validity, and sensitivity to change of an instrument for assessing disabilities in activities of daily living, *Arch Phys Med Rehabil* 78:615-620, 1997.

303. Platz T, Pinkowski C, van Wijck F et al: Reliability and validity of arm function assessment with standardized guidelines for the Fugl-Meyer Test, Action Research Arm Test and Box and Block Test: a multicentre study, *Clin Rehabil* 19:404-411, 2005.

304. Desrosiers J, Bravo G, Hebert R, Dutil A, Mercier L: Validation of the Box and Block Test as a measure of dexterity of elderly people: reliability, validity, and norms studies, *Arch Phys Med Rehabil* 75:751-755, 1994.

305. Barreca SR, Stratford PW, Lambert CL et al: Test-retest reliability, validity, and sensitivity of the Chedoke arm and hand activity inventory: a new measure of upper-limb function for survivors of stroke, *Arch Phys Med Rehabil* 86:1616-1622, 2005.

306. Gowland C, Stratford P, Ward M et al: Measuring physical impairment and disability with the Chedoke-McMaster Stroke Assessment, *Stroke* 24:58-63, 1993.

307. Piercy M, Carter J, Mant J et al. Inter-rater reliability of the Frenchay activities index in patients with stroke and their careers, *Clin Rehabil* 14:433-440, 2000.

308. Post MW, de Witte LP: Good inter-rater reliability of the Frenchay Activities Index in stroke patients, *Clin Rehabil* 17:548-552, 2003.

309. Schuling J, de Haan R, Limburg M et al: The Frenchay Activities Index: assessment of functional status in stroke patients, *Stroke* 24:1173-1177, 1993.

310. Duncan PW, Propst M, Nelson SG: Reliability of the Fugl-Meyer assessment of sensorimotor recovery following cerebrovascular accident, *Phys Ther* 63:1606-1610, 1983.

311. Fugl-Meyer AR, Jaasko L, Leyman I et al: The post-stroke hemiplegic patient, 1: A method for evaluation of physical performance, *Scand J Rehabil Med* 7:13-31, 1975.

312. Gladstone DJ, Danells CJ, Black SE: The fugl-meyer assessment of motor recovery after stroke: a critical review of its measurement properties, *Neurorehabil Neural Repair* 16:232-240, 2002.

313. Lin JH, Hsueh IP, Sheu CF et al: Psychometric properties of the sensory scale of the Fugl-Meyer Assessment in stroke patients, *Clin Rehabil* 18:391-397, 2004.

314. Malouin F, Pichard L, Bonneau C et al: Evaluating motor recovery early after stroke: comparison of the Fugl-Meyer Assessment and the Motor Assessment Scale, *Arch Phys Med Rehabil* 75:1206-1212, 1994.

315. Sanford J, Moreland J, Swanson LR et al: Reliability of the Fugl-Meyer assessment for testing motor performance in patients following stroke, *Phys Ther* 73:447-454, 1993.

316. Mngoma NF, Culham EG, Bagg SD: Resistance to passive shoulder external rotation in persons with hemiplegia: evaluation of an assessment system, *Arch Phys Med Rehabil* 80:531-535, 1999.

317. Desrosiers J, Rochette A, Corriveau H: Validation of a new lower-extremity motor coordination test, *Arch Phys Med Rehabil* 86:993-998, 2005.

318. Wang CH, Hsueh IP, Sheu CF et al: Psychometric properties of 2 simplified 3-level balance scales used for patients with stroke, *Phys Ther* 84:430-438, 2004.

319. Carr JH, Shepherd RB, Nordholm L et al: Investigation of a new motor assessment scale for stroke patients, *Phys Ther* 65:175-180, 1985.

320. Poole JL, Whitney SL: Motor assessment scale for stroke patients: concurrent validity and interrater reliability, *Arch Phys Med Rehabil* 69:195-197, 1988.

321. Ferraro M, Demaio JH, Krol J et al: Assessing the motor status score: a scale for the evaluation of upper limb motor outcomes in patients after stroke, *Neurorehabil Neural Repair* 16:283-289, 2002.

322. Ahmed R, Zuberi BF, Afsar S: Stroke scale score and early prediction of outcome after stroke, *J Coll Physicians Surg Pak* 14:267-269, 2004.

323. Appelros P, Terent A: Characteristics of the National Institute of Health Stroke Scale: Results from a population-based stroke cohort at baseline and after one year, *Cerebrovasc Dis* 17:21-27, 2004.

324. Dewey HM, Donnan GA, Freeman EJ et al: Interrater reliability of the National Institutes of Health Stroke Scale: rating by neurologists and nurses in a community-based stroke incidence study, *Cerebrovasc Dis* 9:323-327, 1999.

325. Lyden P, Lu M, Jackson C et al: Underlying structure of the National Institutes of Health Stroke Scale: results of a factor analysis. NINDS tPA Stroke Trial Investigators, *Stroke* 30:2347-2354, 1999.

326. Lyden PD, Lu M, Levine SR et al: A modified National Institutes of Health Stroke Scale for use in stroke clinical trials: preliminary reliability and validity, *Stroke* 32:1310-1317, 2001.

327. Mao HF, Hsueh IP, Tang PF et al: Analysis and comparison of the psychometric properties of three balance measures for stroke patients, *Stroke* 33:1022-1027, 2002.

328. de Haan R, Limburg M, Bossuyt P et al: The clinical meaning of Rankin "handicap" grades after stroke, *Stroke* 26:2027-2030, 1995.

329. van Swieten JC, Koudstaal PJ, Visser MC et al: Interobserver agreement for the assessment of handicap in stroke patients, *Stroke* 19:604-607, 1988.

330. De Haan R, Horn J, Limburg M et al: A comparison of five stroke scales with measures of disability, handicap, and quality of life, *Stroke* 24:1178-1181, 1993.

331. Levin MF, Desrosiers J, Beauchemin D et al: Development and validation of a scale for rating motor compensations used for reaching in patients with hemiparesis: the reaching performance scale, *Phys Ther* 84:8-22, 2004.

332. Hsieh CL, Hsueh IP, Mao HF: Validity and responsiveness of the rivermead mobility index in stroke patients, *Scand J Rehabil Med* 32:140-142, 2000.

333. Hsueh IP, Wang CH, Sheu CF et al: Comparison of psychometric properties of three mobility measures for patients with stroke, *Stroke* 34:1741-1745, 2003.

334. Roden-Jullig A, Britton M, Gustafsson C et al: Validation of four scales for the acute stage of stroke, *J Intern Med* 236:125-136, 1994.

335. Wyller TB, Sodring KM, Sveen U et al: Predictive validity of the Sodring Motor Evaluation of Stroke Patients (SMES), *Scand J Rehabil Med* 28:211-216, 1996.

336. van Straten A, de Haan RJ, Limburg M et al: Clinical meaning of the Stroke-Adapted Sickness Impact Profile-30 and the Sickness Impact Profile-136, *Stroke* 31:2610-2615, 2000.

337. Ahmed S, Mayo NE, Higgins J et al: The Stroke Rehabilitation Assessment of Movement (STREAM): A comparison with other measures used to evaluate effects of stroke and rehabilitation, *Phys Ther* 83:617-630, 2003.

338. Daley K, Mayo N, Wood-Dauphinee S: Reliability of scores on the Stroke Rehabilitation Assessment of Movement (STREAM) measure, *Phys Ther* 79:8-23, 1999.

339. Wang CH, Hsieh CL, Dai MH et al: Inter-rater reliability and validity of the stroke rehabilitation assessment of movement (stream) instrument, *J Rehabil Med* 34:20-24, 2002.

340. Duarte E, Marco E, Muniesa JM et al: Trunk control test as a functional predictor in stroke patients, *J Rehabil Med* 34:267-272, 2002.

341. Franchignoni FP, Tesio L, Ricupero C et al: Trunk control test as an early predictor of stroke rehabilitation outcome, *Stroke* 28:1382-1385, 1997.

342. Fujiwara T, Liu M, Tsuji T et al: Development of a new measure to assess trunk impairment after stroke (trunk impairment scale): its psychometric properties, *Am J Phys Med Rehabil* 83:681-688, 2004.

343. Verheyden G, Nieuwboer A, Mertin J et al: The Trunk Impairment Scale: a new tool to measure motor impairment of the trunk after stroke, *Clin Rehabil* 18:326-334, 2004.

344. Edwards DF, Chen YW, Diringer MN: Unified Neurological Stroke Scale is valid in ischemic and hemorrhagic stroke, *Stroke* 26:1852-1858, 1995.

345. Treves TA, Karepov VG, Aronovich BD et al: Interrater agreement in evaluation of stroke patients with the unified neurological stroke scale, *Stroke* 25:1263-1264, 1994.

346. Morris DM, Uswatte G, Crago JE et al: The reliability of the wolf motor function test for assessing upper extremity function after stroke, *Arch Phys Med Rehabil* 82:750-755, 2001.

347. Wolf SL, Catlin PA, Ellis M et al: Assessing Wolf motor function test as outcome measure for research in patients after stroke, *Stroke* 32:1635-1639, 2001.

348. Wolf SL, Thompson PA, Morris DM et al: The EXCITE trial: Attributes of the Wolf Motor Function Test in patients with subacute stroke, *Neurorehabil Neural Repair* 19:194-205, 2005.

349. Goetz CG, Stebbins GT, Shale HM et al: Utility of an objective dyskinesia rating scale for Parkinson's disease: Inter- and intrarater reliability assessment, *Mov Disord* 9:390-394, 1994.

350. Hagell P, Widner H: Clinical rating of dyskinesias in Parkinson's disease: Use and reliability of a new rating scale, *Mov Disord* 14:448-455, 1999.

351. Smith RC, Allen R, Gordon J et al: A rating scale for tardive dyskinesia and Parkinsonian symptoms, *Psychopharmacol Bull* 19:266-276, 1983.

352. Jenkinson C, Fitzpatrick R, Peto V et al: The Parkinson's Disease Questionnaire (PDQ-39): development and validation of a Parkinson's disease summary index score, *Age Ageing* 26:353-357, 1997.

353. Peto V, Jenkinson C, Fitzpatrick R: Determining minimally important differences for the PDQ-39 Parkinson's disease questionnaire, *Age Ageing* 30:299-302, 2001.

354. Peto V, Jenkinson C, Fitzpatrick R: PDQ-39: a review of the development, validation and application of a Parkinson's disease quality of life questionnaire and its associated measures, *J Neurol* 245(1 Suppl):S10-S14, 1998.

355. Huntington Study Group: Unified Huntington's Disease Rating Scale: reliability and consistency, *Mov Disord* 11:136-142, 1996.

356. Siesling S, van Vugt JP, Zwinderman KA et al: Unified Huntington's disease rating scale: a follow up, *Mov Disord* 13:915-919, 1998.

357. Siesling S, Zwinderman AH, van Vugt JP et al: A shortened version of the motor section of the Unified Huntington's Disease Rating Scale, *Mov Disord* 12:229-234, 1997.

358. Goetz CG, Stebbins GT, Chmura TA et al: Teaching tape for the motor section of the unified Parkinson's disease rating scale, *Mov Disord* 10:263-266, 1995.

359. Richards M, Marder K, Cote L et al: Interrater reliability of the Unified Parkinson's Disease Rating Scale motor examination, *Mov Disord* 9:89-91, 1994.

360. Stebbins GT, Goetz CG: Factor structure of the Unified Parkinson's Disease Rating Scale: motor examination section, *Mov Disord* 13:633-636, 1998.

361. Stebbins GT, Goetz CG, Lang AE et al: Factor analysis of the motor section of the unified Parkinson's disease rating scale during the off-state, *Mov Disord* 14:585-589, 1999.

362. Mumford CJ, Compston A: Problems with rating scales for multiple sclerosis: a novel approach—the CAMBS score, *J Neurol* 240:209-215, 1993.

363. Sharrack B, Hughes RA, Soudain S et al: The psychometric properties of clinical rating scales used in multiple sclerosis, *Brain* 122:141-159, 1999.

364. Hohol MJ, Orav EJ, Weiner HL: Disease steps in multiple sclerosis: a longitudinal study comparing disease steps and EDSS to evaluate disease progression, *Mult Scler* 5:349-354, 1999.

365. Hohol MJ, Orav EJ, Weiner HL: Disease steps in multiple sclerosis: a simple approach to evaluate disease progression, *Neurology* 45:251-255, 1995.

366. Tesio L, Perucca L, Franchignoni FP et al: A short measure of balance in multiple sclerosis: Validation through Rasch analysis, *Funct Neurol* 12:255-265, 1997.

367. Hooper J, Taylor R, Pentland B et al: Rater reliability of Fahn's tremor rating scale in patients with multiple sclerosis, *Arch Phys Med Rehabil* 79:1076-1079, 1998.

368. Cella DF, Dineen K, Arnason B et al: Validation of the functional assessment of multiple sclerosis quality of life instrument, *Neurology* 47:129-139, 1996.

369. Hutchinson J, Hutchinson M: The Functional Limitations Profile may be a valid, reliable and sensitive measure of disability in multiple sclerosis, *J Neurol* 242:650-657, 1995.

370. Cohen RA, Kessler HR, Fischer M: The Extended Disability Status Scale (EDSS) as a predictor of impairments of functional activities of daily living in multiple sclerosis, *J Neurol Sci* 115:132-135, 1993.

371. Goodkin DE, Cookfair D, Wende K et al: Inter- and intrarater scoring agreement using grades 1.0 to 3.5 of the Kurtzke Expanded Disability Status Scale (EDSS): Multiple Sclerosis Collaborative Research Group, *Neurology* 42:859-863, 1992.

372. Hobart J, Freeman J, Thompson A: Kurtzke scales revisited: the application of psychometric methods to clinical intuition, *Brain* 123:1027-1040, 2000.

373. Kurtzke JF: Rating neurologic impairment in multiple sclerosis: an expanded disability status scale (EDSS), *Neurology* 33:1444-1452, 1983.

374. Kurtzke JF: Disability rating scales in multiple sclerosis, *Ann N Y Acad Sci* 436:347-360, 1984.

375. Kurtzke JF: A new scale for evaluating disability in multiple sclerosis, *Neurology* 5:580-583, 1955.

376. Amato MP, Fratiglioni L, Groppi C et al: Interrater reliability in assessing functional systems and disability on the Kurtzke scale in multiple sclerosis, *Arch Neurol* 45:746-748, 1988.

377. Fischer JS, Rudick RA, Cutter GR et al: The Multiple Sclerosis Functional Composite Measure (MSFC): an integrated approach to MS clinical outcome assessment: National MS Society Clinical Outcomes Assessment Task Force, *Mult Scler* 5:244-250, 1999.

378. Schwartz CE, Vollmer T, Lee H: Reliability and validity of two self-report measures of impairment and disability for MS: North American Research Consortium on Multiple Sclerosis Outcomes Study Group, *Neurology* 52:63-70, 1999.

379. Ravnborg M, Blinkenberg M, Sellebjerg F et al: Responsiveness of the Multiple Sclerosis Impairment Scale in comparison with the Expanded Disability Status Scale, *Mult Scler* 11:81-84, 2005.

380. Ravnborg M, Gronbech-Jensen M, Jonsson A: The MS Impairment Scale: a pragmatic approach to the assessment of impairment in patients with multiple sclerosis, *Mult Scler* 3:31-42, 1997.

381. Priebe MM, Waring WP: The interobserver reliability of the revised American Spinal Injury Association standards for neurological classification of spinal injury patients, *Am J Phys Med Rehabil* 70:268-270, 1991.

382. Waters RL, Adkins R, Yakura J et al: Prediction of ambulatory performance based on motor scores derived from standards of the American Spinal Injury Association, *Arch Phys Med Rehabil* 75:756-760, 1994.

383. Marino RJ, Shea JA, Stineman MG: The Capabilities of Upper Extremity instrument: reliability and validity of a measure of functional limitation in tetraplegia, *Arch Phys Med Rehabil* 79:1512-1521, 1998.

384. Middleton JW, Harvey LA, Batty J et al: Five additional mobility and locomotor items to improve responsiveness of the FIM in wheelchair-dependent individuals with spinal cord injury, *Spinal Cord* 44:495-504, 2006.

385. Marino RJ, Goin JE: Development of a short-form Quadriplegia Index of Function scale, *Spinal Cord* 37:289-296, 1999.

386. Yavuz N, Tezyurek M, Akyuz M: A comparison of two functional tests in quadriplegia: the quadriplegia index of function and the functional independence measure, *Spinal Cord* 36:832-837, 1998.

387. Boss BJ, Barlow D, McFarland SM et al: A self-care assessment tool (SCAT) for persons with a spinal cord injury: an expanded abstract, *Axone* 17:66-67, 1996.

388. McFarland SM, Sasser L, Boss BJ et al: Self-care assessment tool for spinal cord injured persons, *SCI Nurs* 9:111-116, 1992.

389. Ditunno JF, Jr., Ditunno PL, Graziani V et al: Walking index for spinal cord injury (WISCI): an international multicenter validity and reliability study, *Spinal Cord* 38:234-243, 2000.

390. Morganti B, Scivoletto G, Ditunno P et al: Walking index for spinal cord injury (WISCI): criterion validation, *Spinal Cord* 43:27-33, 2005.

391. van Hedel HJ, Wirz M, Dietz V: Assessing walking ability in subjects with spinal cord injury: validity and reliability of 3 walking tests, *Arch Phys Med Rehabil* 86:190-196, 2005.

392. Bennett R: The Fibromyalgia Impact Questionnaire (FIQ): a review of its development, current version, operating characteristics and uses, *Clin Exp Rheumatol* 23:S154-S162, 2005.

393. Burckhardt CS, Clark SR, Bennett RM: The fibromyalgia impact questionnaire: development and validation, *J Rheumatol* 18:728-733, 1991.

394. Wolfe F, Hawley DJ, Goldenberg DL et al: The assessment of functional impairment in fibromyalgia (FM): Rasch analyses of 5 functional scales and the development of the FM Health Assessment Questionnaire, *J Rheumatol* 27:1989-1999, 2000.

395. Zachrisson O, Regland B, Jahreskog M et al: A rating scale for fibromyalgia and chronic fatigue syndrome (the FibroFatigue scale), *J Psychosom Res* 52:501-509, 2002.

396. Chansirinukor W, Maher CG, Latimer J et al: Comparison of the functional rating index and the 18-item Roland-Morris Disability Questionnaire: responsiveness and reliability, *Spine* 30:141-145, 2005.

397. Childs JD, Piva SR: Psychometric properties of the functional rating index in patients with low back pain, *Eur Spine J* 14:1008-1012, 2005.

398. Feise RJ, Michael Menke J: Functional rating index: a new valid and reliable instrument to measure the magnitude of clinical change in spinal conditions, *Spine* 26:78-87, 2001.

399. Rocchi MB, Sisti D, Benedetti P et al: Critical comparison of nine different self-administered questionnaires for the evaluation of disability caused by low back pain, *Eura Medicophys* 41:275-281, 2005.

400. Grotle M, Brox JI, Vollestad NK: Concurrent comparison of responsiveness in pain and functional status measurements used for patients with low back pain, *Spine* 29:E492-E501, 2004.

401. Reneman MF, Jorritsma W, Schellekens JM et al: Concurrent validity of questionnaire and performance-based disability measurements in patients with chronic nonspecific low back pain, *J Occup Rehabil* 12:119-129, 2002.

402. Sigl T, Cieza A, Brockow T et al: Content comparison of low back pain-specific measures based on the International Classification of Functioning, Disability and Health (ICF), *Clin J Pain* 22:147-153, 2006.

403. Bombardier C, Hayden J, Beaton DE: Minimal clinically important difference: low back pain: Outcome measures, *J Rheumatol* 28:431-438, 2001.

404. Hart DL, Wright BD: Development of an index of physical functional health status in rehabilitation, *Arch Phys Med Rehabil* 83:655-665, 2002.

405. Paul A, Lewis M, Shadforth MF et al: A comparison of four shoulder-specific questionnaires in primary care, *Ann Rheum Dis* 63:1293-1299, 2004.

406. Beaton DE, Richards RR: Measuring function of the shoulder: a cross-sectional comparison of five questionnaires, *J Bone Joint Surg Am* 78:882-890, 1996.

407. Beaton D, Richards RR: Assessing the reliability and responsiveness of 5 shoulder questionnaires, *J Shoulder Elbow Surg* 7:565-572, 1998.

408. Shields RK, Enloe LJ, Evans RE et al: Reliability, validity, and responsiveness of functional tests in patients with total joint replacement, *Phys Ther* 75:169-179, 1995.

409. Kirkley A, Griffin S, McLintock H et al: the development and evaluation of a disease-specific quality of life measurement tool for shoulder instability: the Western Ontario Shoulder Instability Index (WOSI), *Am J Sports Med* 26:764-772, 1998.

410. Stratford PW, Binkley JM: A comparison study of the back pain functional scale and Roland Morris Questionnaire: North American Orthopaedic Rehabilitation Research Network, *J Rheumatol* 27:1928-1936, 2000.

411. Stratford PW, Binkley JM, Riddle DL: Development and initial validation of the back pain functional scale, *Spine* 25:2095-2102, 2000.

412. Magnussen L, Strand LI, Lygren H: Reliability and validity of the back performance scale: Observing activity limitation in patients with back pain, *Spine* 29:903-907, 2004.

413. Tan G, Jensen MP, Thornby JI et al: Validation of the Brief Pain Inventory for chronic nonmalignant pain, *J Pain* 5:133-137, 2004.

414. Corson JA, Schneider MJ: The Dartmouth Pain Questionnaire: an adjunct to the McGill Pain Questionnaire, *Pain* 19:59-69. 1984.

415. Gloth FM III, Scheve AA, Stober CV et al: The Functional Pain Scale: Reliability, validity, and responsiveness in an elderly population, *J Am Med Dir Assoc* 2:110-114, 2001.

416. Hagg O, Fritzell P, Romberg K et al: The General Function Score: a useful tool for measurement of physical disability: Validity and reliability, *Eur Spine J* 10:203-210, 2001.

417. Bird SB, Dickson EW: Clinically significant changes in pain along the visual analog scale, *Ann Emerg Med* 38:639-643, 2001.

418. Kane RL, Bershadsky B, Rockwood T et al: Visual analog scale pain reporting was standardized, *J Clin Epidemiol* 58:618-623, 2005.

419. Kelly AM: Does the clinically significant difference in visual analog scale pain scores vary with gender, age, or cause of pain? *Acad Emerg Med* 5:1086-1090, 1998.

420. Salo D, Eget D, Lavery RF et al: Can patients accurately read a visual analog pain scale? *Am J Emerg Med* 21:515-519, 2003.

421. Wheeler AH, Goolkasian P, Baird AC et al: Development of the Neck Pain and Disability Scale: Item analysis, face, and criterion-related validity, *Spine* 24:1290-1294, 1999.

422. Davidson M, Keating J: Oswestry Disability Questionnaire (ODQ), *Aust J Physiother* 51:270, 2005.

423. Fairbank JC, Couper J, Davies JB et al: The Oswestry low back pain disability questionnaire, *Physiotherapy* 66:271-273, 1980.

424. Gronblad M, Hupli M, Wennerstrand P et al: Intercorrelation and test-retest reliability of the Pain Disability Index (PDI) and the Oswestry Disability Questionnaire (ODQ) and their correlation with pain intensity in low back pain patients, *Clin J Pain* 9:189-195, 1993.

425. Fairbank JC, Pynsent PB: The Oswestry Disability Index, *Spine* 25:2940-2952, 2000.

426. Beurskens AJ, de Vet HC, Koke AJ et al: Measuring the functional status of patients with low back pain: assessment of the quality of four disease-specific questionnaires, *Spine* 20:1017-1028, 1995.

427. Chibnall JT, Tait RC: The Pain Disability Index: factor structure and normative data, *Arch Phys Med Rehabil* 75:1082-1086, 1994.

428. Jerome A, Gross RT: Pain disability index: Construct and discriminant validity, *Arch Phys Med Rehabil* 72:920-922, 1991.

429. Tait RC, Chibnall JT, Krause S: The Pain Disability Index: psychometric properties, *Pain* 40:171-182, 1990.

430. Tait RC, Pollard CA, Margolis RB et al: The Pain Disability Index: psychometric and validity data, *Arch Phys Med Rehabil* 68:438-441, 1987.

431. Gaston-Johansson F: Measurement of pain: The psychometric properties of the Pain-O-Meter, a simple, inexpensive pain assessment tool that could change health care practices, *J Pain Symptom Manage* 12:172-181, 1996.

432. Westaway MD, Stratford PW, Binkley JM: The patient-specific functional scale: Validation of its use in persons with neck dysfunction, *J Orthop Sports Phys Ther* 27:331-338, 1998.

433. Kopec JA, Esdaile JM, Abrahamowicz M et al: The Quebec Back Pain Disability Scale. Measurement properties, *Spine* 20:341-352, 1995.

434. Fritz JM, Irrgang JJ: A comparison of a modified Oswestry Low Back Pain Disability Questionnaire and the Quebec Back Pain Disability Scale, *Phys Ther* 81:776-788, 2001.

435. Jordan K, Dunn KM, Lewis M et al: A minimal clinically important difference was derived for the Roland-Morris Disability Questionnaire for low back pain, *J Clin Epidemiol* 59:45-52, 2006.

436. Kuijer W, Brouwer S, Dijkstra PU et al: Responsiveness of the Roland-Morris Disability Questionnaire: consequences of using different external criteria, *Clin Rehabil* 19:488-495, 2005.

437. Ostelo RW, de Vet HC, Knol DL et al: 24-item Roland-Morris Disability Questionnaire was preferred out of six functional status questionnaires for post-lumbar disc surgery, *J Clin Epidemiol* 57:268-276, 2004.

438. Riddle DL, Stratford PW, Binkley JM: Sensitivity to change of the Roland-Morris Back Pain Questionnaire: part 2, *Phys Ther* 78:1197-1207, 1998.

439. Stratford PW, Binkley J, Solomon P et al: Defining the minimum level of detectable change for the Roland-Morris questionnaire, *Phys Ther* 76:359-368, 1996.

440. Stratford PW, Binkley JM: Measurement properties of the RM-18: a modified version of the Roland-Morris Disability Scale, *Spine* 22:2416-2421, 1997.

441. Stratford PW, Binkley JM, Riddle DL et al: Sensitivity to change of the Roland-Morris Back Pain Questionnaire: part 1, *Phys Ther* 78:1186-1196, 1998.

442. Macdermid JC, Solomon P, Prkachin K: The Shoulder Pain and Disability Index demonstrates factor, construct and longitudinal validity, *BMC Musculoskelet Disord* 7:12, 2006.

443. Roach KE, Budiman-Mak E, Songsiridej N et al: Development of a shoulder pain and disability index, *Arthritis Care Res* 4:143-149, 1991.

444. Curtis KA, Roach KE, Applegate EB et al: Reliability and validity of the Wheelchair User's Shoulder Pain Index (WUSPI), *Paraplegia* 33:595-601, 1995.

445. Ren XS, Kazis L, Meenan RF: Short-form Arthritis Impact Measurement Scales 2: tests of reliability and validity among patients with osteoarthritis, *Arthritis Care Res* 12:163-171, 1999.

446. Taal E, Rasker JJ, Riemsma RP: Sensitivity to change of AIMS2 and AIMS2-SF components in comparison to M-HAQ and VAS-pain, *Ann Rheum Dis* 63:1655-1658, 2004.

447. Ditunno JF Jr: Functional assessment measures in CNS trauma, *J Neurotrauma* 9(1 Suppl):S301-S305, 1992.

448. Jacobson GP, Newman CW: The development of the Dizziness Handicap Inventory, *Arch Otolaryngol Head Neck Surg* 116:424-427, 1990.

449. Jacobson GP, Newman CW, Hunter L et al: Balance function test correlates of the Dizziness Handicap Inventory, *J Am Acad Audiol* 2:253-260, 1991.

450. Tesio L, Alpini D, Cesarani A et al: Short form of the Dizziness Handicap Inventory: construction and validation through Rasch analysis, *Am J Phys Med Rehabil* 78:233-241, 1999.

451. Perrot S, Dumont D, Guillemin F et al: Quality of life in women with fibromyalgia syndrome: validation of the QIF, the French version of the fibromyalgia impact questionnaire, *J Rheumatol* 30:1054-1059, 2003.

452. Gloth FM III, Scheve AA, Shah S et al: The Frail Elderly Functional Assessment questionnaire: its responsiveness and validity in alternative settings, *Arch Phys Med Rehabil* 80:1572-1576, 1999.

453. Gloth FM III, Walston J, Meyer J et al: Reliability and validity of the Frail Elderly Functional Assessment questionnaire, *Am J Phys Med Rehabil* 74:45-53, 1995.

454. Alcott D, Dixon K, Swann R: The reliability of the items of the Functional Assessment Measure (FAM): Differences in abstractness between FAM items, *Disabil Rehabil* 19:355-358, 1997.

455. Donaghy S, Wass PJ: Interrater reliability of the Functional Assessment Measure in a brain injury rehabilitation program, *Arch Phys Med Rehabil* 79:1231-1236, 1998.

456. McPherson KM, Pentland B, Cudmore SF et al: An inter-rater reliability study of the Functional Assessment Measure (FIM+FAM), *Disabil Rehabil* 18:341-347, 1996.

457. Turner-Stokes L, Nyein K, Turner-Stokes T et al: The UK FIM+FAM: Development and evaluation: Functional Assessment Measure, *Clin Rehabil* 13:277-287, 1999.

458. Bottemiller KL, Bieber PL, Basford JR et al: FIM score, FIM efficiency, and discharge disposition following inpatient stroke rehabilitation, *Rehabil Nurs* 31:22-25, 2006.

459. Hamilton BB, Laughlin JA, Fiedler RC et al: Interrater reliability of the 7-level functional independence measure (FIM), *Scand J Rehabil Med* 26:115-119, 1994.

460. Ottenbacher KJ, Mann WC, Granger CV et al: Inter-rater agreement and stability of functional assessment in the community-based elderly, *Arch Phys Med Rehabil* 75:1297-1301, 1994.

461. Pollak N, Rheault W, Stoecker JL: Reliability and validity of the FIM for persons aged 80 years and above from a multilevel continuing care retirement community, *Arch Phys Med Rehabil* 77:1056-1061, 1996.

462. Linacre JM, Heinemann AW, Wright BD et al: The structure and stability of the Functional Independence Measure, *Arch Phys Med Rehabil* 75:127-132, 1994.

463. Ravaud JF, Delcey M, Yelnik A: Construct validity of the functional independence measure (FIM): questioning the unidimensionality of the scale and the "value" of FIM scores, *Scand J Rehabil Med* 31:31-41, 1999.

464. Stineman MG, Shea JA, Jette A et al: The Functional Independence Measure: tests of scaling assumptions, structure, and reliability across 20 diverse impairment categories, *Arch Phys Med Rehabil* 77:1101-1108, 1996.

465. Keith RA, Granger CV, Hamilton BB et al: The functional independence measure: a new tool for rehabilitation, *Adv Clin Rehabil* 1:6-18, 1987.

466. *Guide for the uniform data set for rehabilitation (including the FIM [TM] instrument)*, version 5.1, Buffalo, NY, 1997, State University of New York at Buffalo.

467. Dikmen S, Machamer J, Miller B et al: Functional status examination: a new instrument for assessing outcome in traumatic brain injury, *J Neurotrauma* 18:127-140, 2001.

468. Sager MA, Rudberg MA, Jalaluddin M et al: Hospital admission risk profile (HARP): identifying older patients at risk for functional decline following acute medical illness and hospitalization, *J Am Geriatr Soc* 44:251-257, 1996.

469. Martin DP, Engelberg R, Agel J et al: Comparison of the Musculoskeletal Function Assessment questionnaire with the Short Form-36, the Western Ontario and McMaster Universities Osteoarthritis Index, and the Sickness Impact Profile health-status measures, *J Bone Joint Surg Am* 79:1323-1335, 1997.

470. Carr-Hill RA, Kind P: The Nottingham Health Profile, *Soc Sci Med* 28:885, 1989.

471. Hunt SM, McKenna SP, McEwen J et al: A quantitative approach to perceived health status: a validation study, *J Epidemiol Commun Health* 34:281-286, 1980.

472. Wiklund I: The Nottingham Health Profile—a measure of health-related quality of life, *Scand J Prim Health Care Suppl* 1:15-18, 1990.

473. Coons SJ, Rao S, Keininger DL et al: A comparative review of generic quality-of-life instruments, *Pharmacoeconomics* 17:13-35, 2000.

474. Hittle DF, Shaughnessy PW, Crisler KS et al: A study of reliability and burden of home health assessment using OASIS, *Home Health Care Serv Q* 22:43-63, 2003.

475. Kinatukara S, Rosati RJ, Huang L: Assessment of OASIS reliability and validity using several methodological approaches, *Home Health Care Serv Q* 24:23-38, 2005.

476. Neal LJ: OASIS inter-rater reliability, *Caring* 19:44-47, 2000.

477. Anagnostis C, Gatchel RJ, Mayer TG: The pain disability questionnaire: a new psychometrically sound measure for chronic musculoskeletal disorders, *Spine* 29:2290-2303, 2004.

478. Fann JR, Bombardier CH, Dikmen S et al: Validity of the Patient Health Questionnaire-9 in assessing depression following traumatic brain injury, *J Head Trauma Rehabil* 20:501-511, 2005.

479. McCarthy ML, MacKenzie EJ, Durbin DR et al: The Pediatric Quality of Life Inventory: an evaluation of its reliability and validity for children with traumatic brain injury, *Arch Phys Med Rehabil* 86:1901-1909, 2005.

480. Gerety MB, Mulrow CD, Tuley MR et al: Development and validation of a physical performance instrument for the functionally impaired elderly: the Physical Disability Index (PDI), *J Gerontol* 48:M33-M38, 1993.

481. Anderson C, Laubscher S, Burns R: Validation of the Short Form 36 (SF-36) health survey questionnaire among stroke patients, *Stroke* 27:1812-1816, 1996.

482. Brazier JE, Harper R, Jones NM et al: Validating the SF-36 health survey questionnaire: new outcome measure for primary care, *BMJ* 305:160-164, 1992.

483. Hagen S, Bugge C, Alexander H: Psychometric properties of the SF-36 in the early post-stroke phase, *J Adv Nurs* 44:461-468, 2003.

484. Jenkinson C, Wright L, Coulter A: Criterion validity and reliability of the SF-36 in a population sample, *Qual Life Res* 3:7-12, 1994.

485. Chrispin PS, Scotton H, Rogers J et al: Short Form 36 in the intensive care unit: assessment of acceptability, reliability and validity of the questionnaire, *Anaesthesia* 52:15-23, 1997.

486. Bergner M, Bobbitt RA, Carter WB et al: The Sickness Impact Profile: development and final revision of a health status measure, *Med Care* 19:787-805, 1981.

487. Bergner M, Bobbitt RA, Pollard WE et al: The sickness impact profile: validation of a health status measure, *Med Care* 14:57-67, 1976.

488. de Bruin AF, Buys M, de Witte LP, Diederiks JP: The sickness impact profile: SIP68, a short generic version: first evaluation of the reliability and reproducibility, *J Clin Epidemiol* 47:863-871, 1994.

489. Gerety MB, Cornell JE, Mulrow CD et al: The Sickness Impact Profile for nursing homes (SIP-NH), *J Gerontol* 49:M2-M8, 1994.

490. Gilson BS, Gilson JS, Bergner M et al: The sickness impact profile: development of an outcome measure of health care, *Am J Public Health* 65:1304-1310, 1975.

491. Pollard WE, Bobbitt RA, Bergner M et al: The Sickness Impact Profile: Reliability of a health status measure, *Med Care* 14:146-155, 1976.

492. Trigg R, Wood VA: The Subjective Index of Physical and Social Outcome (SIPSO): a new measure for use with stroke patients, *Clin Rehabil* 14:288-299, 2000.

493. Msall ME, DiGaudio K, Rogers BT et al: The Functional Independence Measure for Children (WeeFIM): conceptual basis and pilot use in children with developmental disabilities, *Clin Pediatr (Phila)* 33:421-430, 1994.

494. Piper MC, Pinnell LE, Darrah J et al: Construction and validation of the Alberta Infant Motor Scale (AIMS), *Can J Public Health* 83(2 Suppl):S46-S50, 1992.

495. Darrah J, Piper M, Watt MJ: Assessment of gross motor skills of at-risk infants: predictive validity of the Alberta Infant Motor Scale, *Dev Med Child Neurol* 40:485-491, 1998.

496. Jeng SF, Yau KI, Chen LC et al: Alberta infant motor scale: reliability and validity when used on preterm infants in Taiwan, *Phys Ther* 80:168-178, 2000.

497. Barbosa VM, Campbell SK, Sheftel D et al: Longitudinal performance of infants with cerebral palsy on the Test of Infant Motor Performance and on the Alberta Infant Motor Scale, *Phys Occup Ther Pediatr* 23:7-29, 2003.

498. Campbell SK, Kolobe TH, Wright BD et al: Validity of the Test of Infant Motor Performance for prediction of 6-, 9- and 12-month scores on the Alberta Infant Motor Scale, *Dev Med Child Neurol* 44:263-272, 2002.

499. Bartlett DJ, Fanning JE: Use of the Alberta Infant Motor Scale to characterize the motor development of infants born preterm at eight months corrected age, *Phys Occup Ther Pediatr* 23:31-45, 2003.

500. Isacsson A, Koutis AD, Cedervall M et al: Patient-number-based computerized medical records in Crete: a tool for planning and assessment of primary health care, *Comput Methods Programs Biomed* 37:41-49, 1992.

501. Squires J, Bricker D, Potter L: Revision of a parent-completed development screening tool: Ages and Stages Questionnaires, *J Pediatr Psychol* 22:313-328, 1997.

502. Klamer A, Lando A, Pinborg A et al: Ages and Stages Questionnaire used to measure cognitive deficit in children born extremely preterm, *Acta Paediatr* 94:1327-1329, 2005.

503. Glascoe FP, Byrne KE: The usefulness of the Battelle Developmental Inventory Screening Test, *Clin Pediatr (Phila)* 32:273-280, 1993.

504. Glascoe FP, Martin ED, Humphrey S: A comparative review of developmental screening tests, *Pediatrics* 86:547-554, 1990.

505. Berls AT, McEwen IR: Battelle developmental inventory, *Phys Ther* 79:776-783, 1999.

506. Hurt H, Malmud E, Betancourt LM et al: A prospective comparison of developmental outcome of children with in utero cocaine exposure and controls using the Battelle Developmental Inventory, *J Dev Behav Pediatr* 22:27-34, 2001.

507. Glascoe FP, Byrne KE: The usefulness of the Developmental Profile-II in developmental screening, *Clin Pediatr (Phila)* 32:203-208, 1993.

508. Aylward GP, Verhulst SJ: Predictive utility of the Bayley Infant Neurodevelopmental Screener (BINS) risk status classifications: clinical interpretation and application, *Dev Med Child Neurol* 42:25-31, 2000.

509. Gucuyener K, Ergenekon E, Soysal AS et al: Use of the bayley infant neurodevelopmental screener with premature infants, *Brain Dev* 28:104-108, 2006.

510. Hess CR, Papas MA, Black MM: Use of the Bayley Infant Neurodevelopmental Screener with an environmental risk group, *J Pediatr Psychol* 29:321-330, 2004.

511. Leonard CH, Piecuch RE, Cooper BA: Use of the Bayley Infant Neurodevelopmental Screener with low birth weight infants, *J Pediatr Psychol* 26:33-40, 2001.

512. Macias MM, Saylor CF, Greer MK et al: Infant screening: the usefulness of the Bayley Infant Neurodevelopmental Screener and the Clinical Adaptive Test/Clinical Linguistic Auditory Milestone Scale, *J Dev Behav Pediatr* 19:155-161, 1998.

513. Berk RA: The discriminative efficiency of the Bayley Scales of Infant Development, *J Abnorm Child Psychol* 7:113-119, 1979.

514. Chaudhari S, Shinde SV, Barve SS et al: A longitudinal follow up of neurodevelopment of high risk newborns—a comparison of Amiel-Tison's method with Bayley Scales of Infant Development, *Indian Pediatr* 27:799-802, 1990.

515. Crowe TK, Deitz JC, Bennett FC: The relationship between the Bayley Scales of Infant Development and preschool gross motor and cognitive performance, *Am J Occup Ther* 41:374-378, 1987.

516. Francis-Williams J, Yule W: The Bayley Infant Scales of Mental and Motor Development: an exploratory study with an English sample, *Dev Med Child Neurol* 9:391-401, 1967.

517. Gannon DR: Relationships between 8-mo. performance on the Bayley scales of infant development and 48-mo. intelligence and concept formation scores, *Psychol Rep* 23:1199-1205, 1968.

518. Horner TM: Test-retest and home-clinic characteristics of the Bayley Scales of Infant Development in nine- and fifteen-month-old infants, *Child Dev* 51:751-758, 1980.

519. Morgan LJ: Inappropriate interpretation of Bayley Scales of Infant Development, *J Pediatr* 100:173-174, 1982.

520. Naglieri JA: Extrapolated developmental indices for the Bayley Scales of infant development, *Am J Ment Defic* 85:548-550, 1981.

521. O'Connor MJ: A comparison of preterm and full-term infants on auditory discrimination at four months and on Bayley Scales of Infant Development at eighteen months, *Child Dev* 51:81-88, 1980.

522. Phatak P, Phatak AT: Application of Bayley scales of infant development (B.S.I.D.) to neurological cases, *Indian Pediatr* 10:147-154, 1973.

523. Frank DA, Jacobs RR, Beeghly M et al: Level of prenatal cocaine exposure and scores on the Bayley Scales of Infant Development: modifying effects of caregiver, early intervention, and birth weight, *Pediatrics* 110:1143-1152, 2002.

524. Gauthier SM, Bauer CR, Messinger DS et al: The Bayley Scales of Infant Development. II: Where to start? *J Dev Behav Pediatr* 20:75-79, 1999.

525. Glenn SM, Cunningham CC, Dayus B: Comparison of the 1969 and 1993 standardizations of the Bayley Mental Scales of Infant Development for infants with Down's syndrome, *J Intellect Disabil Res* 45:56-62, 2001.

526. Hack M, Taylor HG, Drotar D et al: Poor predictive validity of the Bayley Scales of Infant Development for cognitive function of extremely low birth weight children at school age, *Pediatrics* 116:333-341, 2005.

527. Harris SR, Megens AM, Backman CL et al: Stability of the Bayley II Scales of Infant Development in a sample of low-risk and high-risk infants, *Dev Med Child Neurol* 47:820-823, 2005.

528. Liao HF, Wang TM, Yao G et al: Concurrent validity of the Comprehensive Developmental Inventory for Infants and Toddlers with the Bayley Scales of Infant Development-II in preterm infants, *J Formos Med Assoc* 104:731-737, 2005.

529. Mcdoff-Cooper B, Gennaro S: The correlation of sucking behaviors and Bayley Scales of Infant Development at six months of age in VLBW infants, *Nurs Res* 45:291-296, 1996.

530. Provost B, Crowe TK, McClain C: Concurrent validity of the Bayley Scales of Infant Development II Motor Scale and the Peabody Developmental Motor Scales in two-year-old children, *Phys Occup Ther Pediatr* 20:5-18, 2000.

531. Raggio DJ, Massingale TW: Comparison of the Vineland Social Maturity Scale, the Vineland Adaptive Behavior Scales—survey form, and the Bayley Scales of Infant Development with infants evaluated for developmental delay, *Percept Mot Skills* 77:931-937, 1993.

532. Robinson BF, Mervis CB: Extrapolated raw scores for the second edition of the Bayley Scales of Infant Development, *Am J Ment Retard* 100:666-670, 1996.

533. Vincer MJ, Cake H, Graven M et al: A population-based study to determine the performance of the Cognitive Adaptive Test/Clinical Linguistic and Auditory Milestone Scale to Predict the Mental Developmental Index at 18 Months on the Bayley Scales of Infant Development-II in very preterm infants, *Pediatrics* 116:e864-e867, 2005.

534. Voigt RG, Brown FR 3rd, Fraley JK et al: Concurrent and predictive validity of the cognitive adaptive test/clinical linguistic and auditory milestone scale (CAT/CLAMS) and the Mental Developmental Index of the Bayley Scales of Infant Development, *Clin Pediatr (Phila)* 42:427-432, 2003.

535. Washington K: The Bayley Scales of Infant Development-II and children with developmental delays: a clinical perspective, *J Dev Behav Pediatr* 19:346-349, 1998.

536. Beer J, Fleming P: Relations of eye color to scores on Bruininks-Oseretsky Test of Motor Proficiency—Short Form. *Percept Mot Skills* 68:859-862, 1989.

537. Connolly BH, Michael BT: Performance of retarded children, with and without Down syndrome, on the Bruininks Oseretsky Test of Motor Proficiency, *Phys Ther* 66:344-348, 1986.

538. Duger T, Bumin G, Uyanik M et al: The assessment of Bruininks-Oseretsky test of motor proficiency in children, *Pediatr Rehabil* 3:125-131, 1999.

539. Flegel J, Kolobe TH: Predictive validity of the test of infant motor performance as measured by the Bruininks-Oseretsky test of motor proficiency at school age, *Phys Ther* 82:762-771, 2002.

540. Hassan MM: Validity and reliability for the Bruininks-Oseretsky Test of Motor Proficiency-Short Form as applied in the United Arab Emirates culture, *Percept Mot Skills* 92:157-166, 2001.

541. MacCobb S, Greene S, Nugent K et al: Measurement and prediction of motor proficiency in children using Bayley infant scales and the Bruininks-Oseretsky test. *Phys Occup Ther Pediatr.* 25:59-79, 2005.

542. Malloy-Miller T: Clinical interpretation of "use of the Bruininks-Oseretsky test of motor proficiency in occupational therapy," *Am J Occup Ther* 49:18, 1995.

543. Spiegel AN, Steffens KM, Rynders JE et al: The early motor profile: correlation with the Bruininks-Oseretsky Test of Motor Proficiency, *Percept Mot Skills* 71:645-646, 1990.

544. Wilson BN, Polatajko HJ, Kaplan BJ et al: Use of the Bruininks-Oseretsky test of motor proficiency in occupational therapy, *Am J Occup Ther* 49:8-17, 1995.

545. Ziviani J, Poulsen A, O'Brien A: Correlation of the Bruininks-Oseretsky Test of Motor Proficiency with the Southern California Sensory Integration Tests, *Am J Occup Ther* 36:519-523, 1982.

546. Carpenter L, Baker GA, Tyldesley B: The use of the Canadian occupational performance measure as an outcome of a pain management program, *Can J Occup Ther* 68:16-22, 2001.

547. Eyssen IC, Beelen A, Dedding C et al: The reproducibility of the Canadian Occupational Performance Measure, *Clin Rehabil* 19:888-894, 2005.

548. Kjeken I, Dagfinrud H, Uhlig T et al: Reliability of the Canadian Occupational Performance Measure in patients with ankylosing spondylitis, *J Rheumatol* 32:1503-1509, 2005.

549. Law M, Baptiste S, McColl M et al: The Canadian occupational performance measure: an outcome measure for occupational therapy, *Can J Occup Ther* 57:82-87, 1990.

550. Law M, Polatajko H, Pollock N et al: Pilot testing of the Canadian Occupational Performance Measure: clinical and measurement issues, *Can J Occup Ther* 61:191-197, 1994.

551. McColl MA, Paterson M, Davies D et al: Validity and community utility of the Canadian Occupational Performance Measure, *Can J Occup Ther* 67:22-30, 2000.

552. Petty LS, McArthur L, Treviranus J: Clinical report: Use of the Canadian Occupational Performance Measure in vision technology, *Can J Occup Ther* 72:309-312, 2005.

553. Ripat J, Etcheverry E, Cooper J et al: A comparison of the Canadian Occupational Performance Measure and the Health Assessment Questionnaire, *Can J Occup Ther* 68:247-253, 2001.

554. Toomey M, Nicholson D, Carswell A: The clinical utility of the Canadian Occupational Performance Measure, *Can J Occup Ther* 62:242-249, 1995.

555. Wressle E, Lindstrand J, Neher M et al: The Canadian Occupational Performance Measure as an outcome measure and team tool in a day treatment programme, *Disabil Rehabil* 25:497-506, 2003.

556. Wressle E, Marcusson J, Henriksson C: Clinical utility of the Canadian Occupational Performance Measure—Swedish version, *Can J Occup Ther* 69:40-48, 2002.

557. Carswell A, McColl MA, Baptiste S et al: The Canadian Occupational Performance Measure: a research and clinical literature review, *Can J Occup Ther* 71:210-222, 2004.

558. Cup EH, Scholte op Reimer WJ, Thijssen MC et al: Reliability and validity of the Canadian Occupational Performance Measure in stroke patients, *Clin Rehabil* 17:402-409, 2003.

559. McColl MA, Law M, Baptiste S et al: Targeted applications of the Canadian Occupational Performance Measure, *Can J Occup Ther* 72:298-300, 2005.

560. Pan AW, Chung L, Hsin-Hwei G: Reliability and validity of the Canadian Occupational Performance Measure for clients with psychiatric disorders in Taiwan, *Occup Ther Int* 10:269-277, 2003.

561. Georgalas C, Tolley N, Kanagalingam J: Measuring quality of life in children with adenotonsillar disease with the Child Health Questionnaire: a first U.K. study, *Laryngoscope* 114:1849-1855, 2004.

562. Gorelick MH, Scribano PV, Stevens MW et al: Construct validity and responsiveness of the Child Health Questionnaire in children with acute asthma, *Ann Allergy Asthma Immunol* 90:622-628, 2003.

563. Houghton FT: The Child Health Questionnaire (CHQ-PF50) studies: sincere congratulations and a sincere plea for terminological accuracy, *Clin Exp Rheumatol* 20:436-437, 2002.

564. Norrby U, Nordholm L, Fasth A: Reliability and validity of the swedish version of child health questionnaire, *Scand J Rheumatol* 32:101-107, 2003.

565. Panepinto JA, O'Mahar KM, DeBaun MR et al: Validity of the child health questionnaire for use in children with sickle cell disease, *J Pediatr Hematol Oncol* 26:574-578, 2004.

566. Raat H, Bonsel GJ, Essink-Bot ML et al: Reliability and validity of comprehensive health status measures in children: the Child Health Questionnaire in relation to the Health Utilities Index, *J Clin Epidemiol* 55:67-76, 2002.

567. Raat H, Botterweck AM, Landgraf JM et al: Reliability and validity of the short form of the child health questionnaire for parents (CHQ-PF28) in large random school based and general population samples, *J Epidemiol Community Health* 59:75-82, 2005.

568. Raat H, Landgraf JM, Bonsel GJ et al: Reliability and validity of the child health questionnaire-child form (CHQ-CF87) in a Dutch adolescent population, *Qual Life Res* 11:575-581, 2002.

569. Rentz AM, Matza LS, Secnik K et al: Psychometric validation of the child health questionnaire (CHQ) in a sample of children and adolescents with attention-deficit/hyperactivity disorder, *Qual Life Res* 14:719-734, 2005.

570. Sudan D, Iyer K, Horslen S et al: Assessment of quality of life after pediatric intestinal transplantation by parents and pediatric recipients using the child health questionnaire, *Transplant Proc* 34:963-964, 2002.

571. Sung L, Greenberg ML, Doyle JJ et al: Construct validation of the Health Utilities Index and the Child Health Questionnaire in children undergoing cancer chemotherapy, *Br J Cancer* 88:1185-1190, 2003.

572. Wake M, Hesketh K, Cameron F: The Child Health Questionnaire in children with diabetes: cross-sectional survey of parent and adolescent-reported functional health status, *Diabet Med* 17:700-707, 2000.

573. Waters E, Salmon L, Wake M et al: The Child Health Questionnaire in Australia: reliability, validity and population means, *Aust N Z J Public Health* 24:207-210, 2000.

574. Ruperto N, Ravelli A, Pistorio A et al: Cross-cultural adaptation and psychometric evaluation of the Childhood Health Assessment Questionnaire (CHAQ) and the Child Health Questionnaire (CHQ) in 32 countries: review of the general methodology, *Clin Exp Rheumatol* 19:S1-S9, 2001.

575. Wilson B, Pollock N, Kaplan BJ et al: Reliability and construct validity of the Clinical Observations of Motor and Postural Skills, *Am J Occup Ther* 46:775-783, 1992.

576. Johnson-Martin NM, Attermeier SM, Hacker BJ: *The Carolina curriculum for infants and toddlers with special needs,* Baltimore, MD, 2004, Brookes.

577. Johnson-Martin NM, Attermeier SM, Hacker BJ: *The Carolina curriculum for preschoolers with special needs,* Baltimore, MD, 2004, Brookes.

578. Adesman AR: Is the Denver II Developmental test worthwhile? *Pediatrics* 90:1009-1011, 1992.

579. Barratt MS, Moyer VA: Pediatric resident and faculty knowledge of the Denver II, *Arch Pediatr Adolesc Med* 154:411-413, 2000.

580. Brachlow A, Jordan AE, Tervo R: Developmental screenings in rural settings: a comparison of the child development review and the Denver II Developmental Screening Test, *J Rural Health* 17:156-159, 2001.

581. Frankenburg WK, Dodds J, Archer P et al: The Denver II: a major revision and restandardization of the Denver Developmental Screening Test, *Pediatrics* 89:91-97, 1992.

582. Glascoe FP, Byrne KE, Ashford LG et al: Accuracy of the Denver-II in developmental screening, *Pediatrics* 89:1221-1225, 1992.

583. Halioglu O, Topaloglu AK, Zenciroglu A et al: Denver developmental screening test II for early identification of the infants who will develop major neurological deficit as a sequalea of hypoxic-ischemic encephalopathy, *Pediatr Int* 43:400-404, 2001.

584. Johnson KL, Ashford LG, Byrne KE et al: Does Denver II produce meaningful results? *Pediatrics* 90:477-479, 1992.

585. Lim HC, Ho LY, Goh LH et al: The field testing of Denver Developmental Screening Test Singapore: a Singapore version of Denver II Developmental Screening Test, *Ann Acad Med Singapore* 25:200-209, 1996.

586. Pfannenstiel D, Lawhorn K: The Denver II replaces the Denver Developmental Screening Test, *Kans Nurse* 66:4-5, 1991.

587. Wade GH: Update on the Denver II, *Pediatr Nurs* 18:140-141, 1992.

588. Erhardt RP, Beatty PA, Hertsgaard DM: A developmental prehension assessment for handicapped children, *Am J Occup Ther* 35:237-242, 1981.

589. Ottenbacher KJ, Msall ME, Lyon NR et al: Interrater agreement and stability of the Functional Independence Measure for Children (WeeFIM): use in children with developmental disabilities, *Arch Phys Med Rehabil* 78:1309-1315, 1997.

590. Ottenbacher KJ, Taylor ET, Msall ME et al: The stability and equivalence reliability of the functional independence measure for children (WeeFIM), *Dev Med Child Neurol* 38:907-916, 1996.

591. Sperle PA, Ottenbacher KJ, Braun SL et al: Equivalence reliability of the functional independence measure for children (WeeFIM) administration methods, *Am J Occup Ther* 51:35-41, 1997.

592. Wong V, Au-Yeung YC, Law PK: Correlation of Functional Independence Measure for Children (WeeFIM) with developmental language tests in children with developmental delay, *J Child Neurol* 20:613-616, 2005.

593. Wong V, Chung B, Hui S et al: Cerebral palsy: Correlation of risk factors and functional performance using the Functional Independence Measure for Children (WeeFIM), *J Child Neurol* 19:887-893, 2004.

594. Yung A, Wong V, Yeung R et al: Outcome measure for paediatric rehabilitation: use of the Functional Independence Measure for children (WeeFIM): a pilot study in Chinese children with neurodevelopmental disabilities, *Pediatr Rehabil* 3:21-28, 1999.

595. Ziviani J, Ottenbacher KJ, Shephard K et al: Concurrent validity of the Functional Independence Measure for Children (WeeFIM) and the Pediatric Evaluation of Disabilities Inventory in children with developmental disabilities and acquired brain injuries, *Phys Occup Ther Pediatr* 21:91-101, 2001.

596. McCabe MA: Pediatric Functional Independence Measure: Clinical trials with disabled and nondisabled children, *Appl Nurs Res* 9:136-138, 1996.

597. Novacheck TF, Stout JL, Tervo R: Reliability and validity of the Gillette Functional Assessment Questionnaire as an outcome measure in children with walking disabilities, *J Pediatr Orthop* 20:75-81, 2000.

598. Avery LM, Russell DJ, Raina PS et al: Rasch analysis of the Gross Motor Function Measure: validating the assumptions of the Rasch model to create an interval-level measure, *Arch Phys Med Rehabil* 84:697-705, 2003.

599. Drouin LM, Malouin F, Richards CL et al: Correlation between the gross motor function measure scores and gait spatiotemporal measures in children with neurological impairments, *Dev Med Child Neurol* 38:1007-1019, 1996.

600. Gemus M, Palisano R, Russell D et al: Using the gross motor function measure to evaluate motor development in children with Down syndrome, *Phys Occup Ther Pediatr* 21:69-79, 2001.

601. Harries N, Kassirer M, Amichai T et al: Changes over years in gross motor function of 3-8 year old children with cerebral palsy: using the Gross Motor Function Measure (GMFM-88), *Isr Med Assoc J* 6:408-411, 2004.

602. Natroshvili I, Kakushadze Z, Gabunia M et al: Prognostic value of gross motor function measure to evaluate the severity of cerebral palsy, *Georgian Med News* Sep(126):45-48, 2005.

603. Nordmark E, Hagglund G, Jarnlo GB: Reliability of the gross motor function measure in cerebral palsy, *Scand J Rehabil Med* 29:25-28, 1997.

604. Nordmark E, Jarnlo GB, Hagglund G: Comparison of the Gross Motor Function Measure and Paediatric Evaluation of Disability

Inventory in assessing motor function in children undergoing selective dorsal rhizotomy, *Dev Med Child Neurol* 42:245-252, 2000.

605. Russell DJ, Avery LM, Rosenbaum PL et al: Improved scaling of the gross motor function measure for children with cerebral palsy: evidence of reliability and validity, *Phys Ther* 80:873-885, 2000.

606. Russell DJ, Rosenbaum PL, Lane M et al: Training users in the gross motor function measure: methodological and practical issues, *Phys Ther* 74:630-636, 1994.

607. Vos-Vromans DC, Ketelaar M, Gorter JW: Responsiveness of evaluative measures for children with cerebral palsy: the Gross Motor Function Measure and the Pediatric Evaluation of Disability Inventory, *Disabil Rehabil* 27:1245-1252, 2005.

608. Wang HY, Yang YH: Evaluating the responsiveness of 2 versions of the gross motor function measure for children with cerebral palsy, *Arch Phys Med Rehabil* 87:51-56, 2006.

609. Wong EC, Man DW: Gross motor function measure for children with cerebral palsy, *Int J Rehabil Res* 28:355-359, 2005.

610. Russell DJ, Rosenbaum PL, Cadman DT et al: The gross motor function measure: a means to evaluate the effects of physical therapy, *Dev Med Child Neurol* 31:341-352, 1989.

611. Nair MK, George B, Mathews S et al: Early intervention program for high risk babies—use of infant motor screen, *Indian J Pediatr* 59:687-690, 1992.

612. Nickel RE, Renken CA, Gallenstein JS: The infant motor screen, *Dev Med Child Neurol* 31:35-42, 1989.

613. Ellison PH: Scoring sheet for the Infant Neurological International Battery (INFANIB): suggestion from the field, *Phys Ther* 66:548-550, 1986.

614. Ellison PH: Infant Neurological International Battery has high predictive validity, and test author is a pediatric neurologist, *Am J Occup Ther* 46:855, 1992.

615. Ellison PH, Horn JL, Browning CA: Construction of an Infant Neurological International Battery (Infanib) for the assessment of neurological integrity in infancy, *Phys Ther* 65:1326-1331, 1985.

616. Stuberg WA, White PJ, Miedaner JA et al: Item reliability of the Milani-Comparetti Motor Development Screening Test, *Phys Ther* 69:328-335, 1989.

617. Cardoso AA, Magalhaes LC, Amorim RH et al: Predictive validity of the Movement Assessment of Infants (MAI) for Brazilian preterm children, *Arq Neuropsiquiatr* 62:1052-1057, 2004.

618. Harris SR: Identification of neurodevelopmental abnormality at four and eight months by the movement assessment of infants, *Dev Med Child Neurol* 34:1118-1119, 1992.

619. Harris SR, Haley SM, Tada WL et al: Reliability of observational measures of the Movement Assessment of Infants, *Phys Ther* 64:471-477, 1984.

620. Harris SR, Swanson MW, Andrews MS et al: Predictive validity of the "Movement Assessment of Infants," *J Dev Behav Pediatr* 5:336-342, 1984.

621. Schneider JW, Lee W, Chasnoff IJ: Field testing of the movement assessment of infants, *Phys Ther* 68:321-327, 1988.

622. Swanson MW, Bennett FC, Shy KK et al: Identification of neurodevelopmental abnormality at four and eight months by the movement assessment of infants, *Dev Med Child Neurol* 34:321-337, 1992.

623. Dubowitz LM, Dubowitz V, Palmer P et al: A new approach to the neurological assessment of the preterm and full-term newborn infant, *Brain Dev* 2:3-14, 1980.

624. Korner AF, Constantinou J, Dimiceli S et al: Establishing the reliability and developmental validity of a neurobehavioral assessment for preterm infants: a methodological process, *Child Dev* 62:1200-1208, 1991.

625. Als H, Tronick E, Lester BM et al: The Brazelton Neonatal Behavioral Assessment Scale (BNBAS), *J Abnorm Child Psychol* 5:215-231, 1977.

626. Anderson CJ: Integration of the Brazelton Neonatal Behavioral Assessment Scale into routine neonatal nursing care, *Issues Compr Pediatr Nurs* 9:341-351, 1986.

627. Beal JA: The Brazelton neonatal behavioral assessment scale: a tool to enhance parental attachment, *J Pediatr Nurs* 1:170-177, 1986.

628. Fowles ER: The Brazelton Neonatal Behavioral Assessment Scale and maternal identity, *MCN Am J Matern Child Nurs* 24:287-293, 1999.

629. Gibes RM: Clinical uses of the Brazelton Neonatal Behavioral Assessment Scale in nursing practice, *Pediatr Nurs* 7:23-26, 1981.

630. Kang R, Barnard K: Using the neonatal behavioral assessment scale to evaluate premature infants, *Birth Defects Orig Artic Ser* 15:119-144, 1979.

631. Lundqvist C, Sabel KG: Brief report: the Brazelton Neonatal Behavioral Assessment Scale detects differences among newborn infants of optimal health, *J Pediatr Psychol* 25:577-582, 2000.

632. Nugent JK: The Brazelton Neonatal Behavioral Assessment Scale: implications for intervention, *Pediatr Nurs* 7:18-21, 67, 1981.

633. Ohgi S, Arisawa K, Takahashi T et al: Neonatal behavioral assessment scale as a predictor of later developmental disabilities of low birth-weight and/or premature infants, *Brain Dev* 25:313-321, 2003.

634. Oyemade UJ, Cole OJ, Johnson AA et al: Prenatal predictors of performance on the Brazelton Neonatal Behavioral Assessment Scale, *J Nutr* 124:1000S-1005S, 1994.

635. Shin Y, Bozzette M, Kenner C et al: Evaluation of Korean newborns with the Brazelton Neonatal Behavioral Assessment Scale, *J Obstet Gynecol Neonatal Nurs* 33:589-596, 2004.

636. Stewart P, Reihman J, Lonky E et al: Prenatal PCB exposure and neonatal behavioral assessment scale (NBAS) performance, *Neurotoxicol Teratol* 22:21-29, 2000.

637. Tronick EZ: The neonatal behavioral assessment scale as a biomarker of the effects of environmental agents on the newborn, *Environ Health Perspect* 74:185-189, 1987.

638. Morgan AM, Koch V, Lee V et al: Neonatal neurobehavioral examination: a new instrument for quantitative analysis of neonatal neurological status, *Phys Ther* 68:1352-1358, 1988.

639. Palmer MM, Crawley K, Blanco IA: Neonatal Oral-Motor Assessment scale: a reliability study, *J Perinatol* 13:28-35, 1993.

640. Crowe TK, McClain C, Provost B: Motor development of Native American children on the Peabody Developmental Motor Scales, *Am J Occup Ther* 53:514-518, 1999.

641. Gebhard AR, Ottenbacher KJ, Lane SJ: Interrater reliability of the Peabody Developmental Motor Scales: fine motor scale, *Am J Occup Ther* 48:976-981, 1994.

642. Hinderer KA, Richardson PK, Atwater SW: Clinical implication of the peabody developmental motor scales: a constructive review, *Phys Occup Ther Pediatr* 9:81-106, 19889.

643. Palisano RJ: Concurrent and predictive validities of the Bayley Motor Scale and the Peabody Developmental Motor Scales, *Phys Ther* 66:1714-1719, 1986.

644. van Hartingsveldt MJ, Cup EH, Oostendorp RA: Reliability and validity of the fine motor scale of the Peabody Developmental Motor Scales-2, *Occup Ther Int* 12:1-13, 1005.

645. Berg M, Jahnsen R, Froslie KF et al: Reliability of the Pediatric Evaluation of Disability Inventory (PEDI), *Phys Occup Ther Pediatr* 24:61-77, 2004.

646. Dumas HM, Haley SM, Fragala MA et al: Self-care recovery of children with brain injury: descriptive analysis using the Pediatric Evaluation of Disability Inventory (PEDI) functional classification levels, *Phys Occup Ther Pediatr* 21:7-27, 2001.

647. Feldman AB, Haley SM, Coryell J: Concurrent and construct validity of the Pediatric Evaluation of Disability Inventory, *Phys Ther* 70:602-610, 1990.

648. Haley SM, Raczek AE, Coster WJ et al: Assessing mobility in children using a computer adaptive testing version of the pediatric evaluation of disability inventory, *Arch Phys Med Rehabil* 86:932-939, 2005.

649. Ho ES, Curtis CG, Clarke HM: Pediatric Evaluation of Disability Inventory: its application to children with obstetric brachial plexus palsy, *J Hand Surg [Am]* 31:197-202, 2006.

650. Iyer LV, Haley SM, Watkins MP et al: Establishing minimal clinically important differences for scores on the pediatric evaluation of

disability inventory for inpatient rehabilitation, *Phys Ther* 83:888-898, 2003.

651. Kothari DH, Haley SM, Gill-Body KM et al: Measuring functional change in children with acquired brain injury (ABI): Comparison of generic and ABI-specific scales using the Pediatric Evaluation of Disability Inventory (PEDI), *Phys Ther* 83:776-785, 2003.

652. Ostensjo S, Bjorbaekmo W, Carlberg EB et al: Assessment of everyday functioning in young children with disabilities: an ICF-based analysis of concepts and content of the Pediatric Evaluation of Disability Inventory (PEDI), *Disabil Rehabil* 28:489-504, 2006.

653. Tsai PY, Yang TF, Chan RC et al: Functional investigation in children with spina bifida—measured by the Pediatric Evaluation of Disability Inventory (PEDI), *Childs Nerv Syst* 18:48-53, 2002.

654. Dunn W: The sensations of everyday life: empirical, theoretical, and pragmatic considerations, *Am J Occup Ther* 55:608-620, 2001.

655. Dunn W: Performance of typical children on the Sensory Profile: an item analysis, *Am J Occup Ther* 48:967-974, 1994.

656. Dunn W, Brown C: Factor analysis on the Sensory Profile from a national sample of children without disabilities, *Am J Occup Ther* 51:490-499, 1997.

657. Dunn W, Westman K: The sensory profile: the performance of a national sample of children without disabilities, *Am J Occup Ther* 51:25-34, 1997.

658. Davies PL, Soon PL, Young M et al: Validity and reliability of the school function assessment in elementary school students with disabilities, *Phys Occup Ther Pediatr* 24:23-43, 2004.

659. Kimball JG: Using the Sensory Integration and Praxis Tests to measure change: a pilot study, *Am J Occup Ther* 44:603-608, 1990.

660. Mailloux Z: An overview of Sensory Integration and Praxis Tests, *Am J Occup Ther* 44:589-594, 1990.

661. Barbosa VM, Campbell SK, Smith E et al: Comparison of test of infant motor performance (TIMP) item responses among children with cerebral palsy, developmental delay, and typical development, *Am J Occup Ther* 59:446-456, 2005.

662. Campbell SK, Hedeker D: Validity of the Test of Infant Motor Performance for discriminating among infants with varying risk for poor motor outcome, *J Pediatr* 139:546-551, 2001.

663. Campbell SK, Kolobe TH, Osten ET et al: Construct validity of the test of infant motor performance, *Phys Ther* 75:585-596, 1995.

664. Einarsson-Backes LM, Stewart KB: Infant neuromotor assessments: a review and preview of selected instruments, *Am J Occup Ther* 46:224-232, 1992.

665. Miller LJ, Roid GH: Sequence comparison methodology for the analysis of movement patterns in infants and toddlers with and without motor delays, *Am J Occup Ther* 47:339-347, 1993.

APPENDIX 8-A ■ **Examination Tools**

Balance and Postural Control Tests
Clinical Scale of Contraversive Pushing[12,13]
Clinical Test of Sensory Interaction on Balance[14-20]
Computerized Dynamic Posturography[21-31]
Dix-Hallpike Test[32-35]
Dynamic Visual Acuity and Gaze Stabilization Tests[36-39]
Fukuda Stepping Test[40-42]
Functional Reach Lateral[43]
Functional Reach Test[15,44-53]
Head-shake Sensory Organization Test[54]
Lateropulsion Test[55]
Limits of Stability Test on NeuroCom System[51,56,57]
Modified Functional Reach Test[48]
Multidirectional Reach Test[58,59]
Nudge/Push Test[60,61]
One Leg Stand Test[62-66]
Postural Stress Test[67-70]
Postural Sway Tests[50,66,71]
Repetitive Reach Test[14]
Romberg Test[65,71]
Sensory Organization Test[29,51,72-75]
Sharpened Romberg Test[65,76]

Functional Tests of Balance and Mobility
Berg Balance Scale[15,49,77-86]
Continuous-Scale Physical Functional Performance[87]
Dynamic Gait Index[88-90]
Fast Evaluation of Mobility, Balance, and Fear[91]
Four Square Step Test[92]
Gait and Balance Scale[93]
L-Test[94]
Physical Performance and Mobility Examination[95]
Physical Performance Test[15,96-101]
Tandem Gait Test[102]
Tinetti Performance-Oriented Mobility Assessment[64,80,103-107]
Timed Up and Go Test[15,104,108-121]
Timed Movement Battery[122]
5 Time Sit to Stand Test[123]

Gait Tests
Automated Up-Timer[124]
Clinical Gait Assessments[125,126]
Functional Ambulation Profile[127-129]
Functional Gait Assessment[90]
GAITRite System[130-133]
Modified Gait Abnormality Rating Scale[101,134,135]
Observational Gait Analysis (Rancho)[136]
5-Meter Walk Test[137]
400 Meter Walk Test[138,139]
2-Minute Walk Test[110,140]
6-Minute Walk Test[98,140-147]
12-Minute Walk Test[140,148-150]

Falls Efficacy and Falls Prediction Scales
Activities-Specific Balance Confidence Scale[58,151-155]
Falls Efficacy Scale[107,155-157]
Multiple Tasks Test[158]
Survey of Activities and Fear of Falling in the Elderly[155]

Activities of Daily Living Scales
Barthel Index[159-167]
Bristol Activities of Daily Living Scale[168,169]
Katz Index of Activities of Daily Living[170-176]
Kenny Self-Care Evaluation[177]
Klein-Bell Activities of Daily Living Scale[178]
Melville-Nelson Self-Care Assessment[179]
PULSES Profile[161,162,180]
Structured Assessment of Independent Living Skills[181]
The Safety Assessment of Function and the Environment for Rehabilitation[182]

Nonequilibrium Coordination Tests
Coordination Tests[61]

Strength Tests
Grip Strength Dynamometry[183-193]
Isokinetic Testing[194-196]
Manual Muscle Test[193,197-200]

Range of Motion Tests
Objective Measurements of Joint Range of Motion[201-207]

Spasticity and Tone Tests
Ashworth Scale[208,209]
Modified Ashworth Scale[209-215]
Tardieu Scale[216]
Tone Assessment Scale[211]

Cognitive Function, Dementia, Alzheimer's Tests
Abbreviated Mental Test[217-220]
Clock Drawing Test for Dementia Severity in Alzheimer's[221-225]
Discomfort Assessment for Alzheimer's[226]
Draw a Man Test (neglect)[227]
Mental Status Questionnaire[218]

Mini-Mental State Examination[218,228-238]
Modified Mini-Mental State Examination[232,239-241]
Multidimensional Observation Scale for Elderly Subjects[242-244]
Orientation Log[245]
Rancho Los Amigos Levels of Cognitive Functioning Assessment Scale[246-248]
Recognition Memory Test[249]
Short Portable Mental Status Questionnaire[250]
Supervision Rating Scale[251]
Wisconsin Card Sorting Test[252]

Depression Scales
Aphasic Depression Scale[253]
Beck Depression Inventory[254-261]
Geriatric Depression Scale[262-268]
Hamilton Rating Scale for Depression[269,270]
Montgomery-Asberg Depression Scale[271]
Zung Depression Scale[272-274]

Coma Scales
Coma/Near Coma Scale[275,276]
Coma Recovery Scale[277-279]
Glasgow Coma Scale[280-288]
Glasgow Epilepsy Outcome Scale[289]
Glasgow Outcome Scale[285,288,290,291]
Western Neuro Sensory Stimulation Profile[292]

Amnesia Scales
Children's Orientation and Amnesia Test[293]
Galveston Orientation and Amnesia Test[245,294-296]
Post Traumatic Amnesia Scale[297,298]
Wolinsky Amnesia Information Test[299]

Stroke Tools
American Heart Association Stroke Outcome Classification Scale[300]
Arm Motor Ability Test[301-303]
Box and Block Test[303,304]
Chedoke Arm and Hand Inventory[305]
Chedoke-McMaster Stroke Assessment[306]
Frenchay Activities Index[307-309]
Fugl-Meyer[303,310-315]
Lateropulsion Scale for Stroke[55]
LIDO Active System: Resistance to Passive Shoulder ER[316]
Lower Extremity Motor Coordination Test[317]
Modified Berg Balance Scale for Stroke[81,318]
Modified Motor Assessment Scale[164]
Motor Assessment Scale[314,319,320]
Motor Status Score[321]
National Institutes of Health Stroke Scale[322-326]
Postural Assessment in Stroke Scale[318,327]
Rankin Scale[328-330]
Reaching Performance Scale[331]
Rivermead Mobility Index[163,332,333]
Scandinavian Stroke Supervision Scale[334]
Sodring Motor Evaluation of Stroke[335]
Stroke-Adapted 30-Item Sickness Impact Profile[336]
Stroke Rehabilitation Assessment of Movement[137,333,337-339]
Trunk Control Test[340,341]
Trunk Impairment Scale[342,343]
Unified Neurological Stroke Scale[344,345]
Upright Motor Control Test[200]
Wolf Motor Function Test[346-348]

Parkinson's and Huntington Disease Tools
Dyskinesia Rating Scales[349-351]
Parkinson's Disease Questionnaire[352-354]
Unified Huntington Disease Rating Scale[355-357]
Unified Parkinson's Disease Rating Scale[358-361]

Multiple Sclerosis Tools
Cambridge Multiple Sclerosis Basic Score[362,363]
Disease Steps[364,365]

EQUI-SCALE[366]
Fahn's Tremor Rating Scale[367]
Functional Assessment of Multiple Sclerosis[368]
Functional Limitations Profile[369]
Kurtzke Extended Disability Status Scale[370-376]
Multiple Sclerosis Functional Composite Measure[377]
Multiple Sclerosis Symptom Inventory[378]
Scripps Neurological Rating Scale[363]
The Multiple Sclerosis Impairment Scale[379,380]

Spinal Cord Injury Tools
American Spinal Injury Association Functional Classification of Spinal Cord Injury[381,382]
Capabilities of Upper Extremity Test[383]
Functional Independence Measure for Spinal Cord Injury with Five Additional Mobility and Locomotor Items[384]
Quadriplegia Index of Function[385,386]
Self-Care Assessment Tool[387,388]
Walking Index for Spinal Cord Injury[389-391]

Select Orthopedic Tools
Fibromyalgia Tools[143,147,392-395]
Functional Rating Index[396-398]
Low Back Pain Questionnaires and Functional Measures[399-403]
Physical Function Health Status[404]
Shoulder Questionnaires[405-407]
Total Joint Replacement Tests[408]
Western Ontario Shoulder Instability Index[409]

Pain Assessment Tools
Back Pain Functional Scale[410,411]
Back Performance Scale[412]
Brief Pain Inventory[413]
Dartmouth Pain Questionnaire[414]
Functional Pain Scale[415]
General Function Score[416]
Million Visual Analog Scale[417-420]
Neck Pain and Disability Scale[421]
Oswestry Low Back Pain Disability Questionnaire[422-426]
Pain Disability Index[421,427-430]
Pain-O-Meter[431]
Patient-Specific Functional Scale[432]
Quebec Back Pain Disability Questionnaire[433,434]
Roland-Morris Back Pain Disability Questionnaire[426,435-441]
Shoulder Pain and Disability Index[405,406,442,443]
Wheelchair Users Subjective Pain Index[444]

Health Status Tools: Disability, Handicap
Arthritis Impact Scale[445,446]
Disability Rating Scale[248,447]
Dizziness Handicap Inventory[26,448-450]
Fibromyalgia Health Assessment Questionnaire[394]
Fibromyalgia Impact Questionnaire[392,393,451]
Frail Elderly Functional Assessment Questionnaire[452,453]
Functional Assessment Measure (Functional Independence Measure + Functional Assessment Measure)[454-457]
Functional Independence Measure[161,166,386,458-466]
Functional Status Examination for Traumatic Brain Injury[467]
Hospital Admission Risk Profile[468]
McMaster University Osteoarthritis Index[469]
Musculoskeletal Function Assessment Questionnaire[469]
Nottingham Health Profile[163,470-473]
OASIS[161,474-476]
Pain Disability Questionnaire[477]
Patient Health Questionnaire-9 for Traumatic Brain Injury (PHQ-9)[478]
Pediatric Quality of Life Instrument[479]
Physical Disability Index[424,480]
Short-Form 36 Health Survey Questionnaire[469,473,481-485]
Sickness Impact Profile and Sickness Impact Profile 68[336,486-491]

Subjective Index and Physical and Social Outcome (for Stroke)[492]

Wee Functional Independence Measure[493]

Western Ontario Osteoarthritis Index[469]

Pediatric Tools

Alberta Infant Motor Scale[494-499]

Assessment, Evaluation, and Programming System for Infants and Children[500]

Ages and Stages Questionnaire[501,502]

Batelle Developmental Inventory[503-507]

Bayley Infant Neurodevelopmental Screener[508-512]

Bayley Scales of Infant Development[513-535]

Bruininks-Oseretsky Test of Motor Proficiency[536-545]

Canadian Occupational Performance Measure[2,546-560]

Child Health Questionnaire[561-573]

Child Health Assessment Questionnaire[574]

Children's Orientation and Amnesia Scale[293]

Clinical Observation of Motor and Postural Skills Test[575]

The Carolina Curriculum for Infants and Toddlers with Special Needs[576]

The Carolina Curriculum for Preschoolers with Special Needs[577]

DENVER II[578-587]

Erhardt Developmental Prehension Assessment[588]

Functional Independence Measure for Children (Wee Functional Indepence Measure)[493,589-596]

Gillette Functional Assessment Questionnaire[597]

Gross Motor Function Measure[598-610]

Infant Motor Screen[611,612]

Infant Neurological International Battery[613-615]

Milani-Comparetti Motor Development Screening Test[616]

Movement Assessment of Infants[617-622]

Neurological Assessment of the Preterm and Full-Term New Born Infant[623]

Neurobehavioral Assessment of Preterm Infant[624]

Neonatal Behavioral Assessment Scale[625-637]

Neonatal Neurobehavioral Examination[638]

Neonatal Oral Motor Assessment Scale[639]

Peabody Developmental Motor Scales[530,640-644]

Pediatric Clinical Test of Sensory Interaction on Balance[17]

Pediatric Evaluation of Disability Inventory[607,645-653]

Pediatric Quality of Life Instrument[479]

Infant/Toddler Sensory Profile[654-657]

School Function Assessment[658]

Sensory Integration and Praxis Test[659,660]

Test of Infant Motor Performance[497,498,661-663]

Toddler and Infant Motor Evaluation[664,665]

CHAPTER 9

Interventions for Clients with Movement Limitations

Darcy A. Umphred, PT, PhD, FAPTA
Nancy N. Byl, PhD, PT, FAPTA
Rolando T. Lazaro, PT, DPT, MS, GCS
Margaret L. Roller, PT, MS, DPT

KEY WORDS

augmented intervention
effectiveness in practice
functional training
impairment training
somatosensory retraining
therapeutic interventions
today/tomorrow's evidence-based practice

OBJECTIVES

After reading this chapter the student/therapist will be able to:

1. Appreciate the complexity of motor responses, the ways to influence those behaviors, and the theories that lay the foundation for intervention planning and design.
2. Identify variables that affect neuroplasticity and factors that create environments that optimize learning and motor performance.
3. Outline the differences in recovery related to healing, compensation, substitution, habituation, and adaptation.
4. Analyze the similarities and differences among functional training, impairment interventions, augmented therapeutic interventions, and somatosensory training.
5. Select appropriate intervention strategies to optimize desired outcomes.
6. Delineate variables that may both positively and negatively affect complex motor responses and a patient's ability to participate in functional activities.
7. Identify procedures and sequences required to attain the most successful therapeutic outcome that best meets the needs and goals of the client and the family.
8. Consider the contribution of the client, the client's support systems, research evidence, neurophysiology, and the best practice standards available to optimize outcomes after interventions.

Before discussing therapeutic intervention procedures, the therapist must identify the learning environment within which the client will perform. As discussed in Chapter 1, that environment is made up of the therapist and the client, all internal body control mechanisms of the client, and the external restraints and demands of the world. Although this text focuses on functional movement problems arising from internal peripheral and central nervous system (CNS) mechanism problems, the reader must always consider the client as a totality and include within the analysis how other organ or body systems will be affected by or will affect the outcome of therapeutic intervention both initially and in relation to long-term quality of life. An examination/evaluation (see Chapter 8) is performed before intervention to establish objective measurements, to help the clinician diagnose functional limitations or restrictions in activities and their causations (impairments), and to determine a prognosis of the outcomes on the basis of the patient's potential for functional improvement, taking into consideration factors such as motivation, family support, financial support, and cultural biases.[1] This process also guides the selection of intervention strategies. Although it could be assumed that some of these impairments would be directly correlated to the CNS trauma experienced by the client, it must also be determined whether some or most of these impairments have

developed over a lifetime as a result of small traumas and adjustments to life. This insidious cause of impairments needs to be differentiated from acute causation of activity limitations because goal setting and expectations related to prognosis and recovery can be different.

Through the use of current motor control, motor learning, and neuroplasticity theories and body systems models, the therapist must also determine the flexibility or inherent motor control the client demonstrates while executing functional activities and participating in life. During the evaluation phase, the therapist must break down the components of movement and determine which, if any, are causing distortions or inefficient execution of the overall motor plan. The therapist must examine, analyze, and diagnose the strengths and limitations of the client's motor subsystems, including but not limited to peripheral subsystems (joint range of motion [ROM], muscle strength, leg length), central subsystems (state of the motor pool or pattern generators, synergies [volitional and reflexive], postural integrity, balance, rate, timing, and trajectory of movement), and cardiopulmonary subsystems (circulation, heart rate, blood pressure, oxygen exchange). For example, if the clinician thinks there may be a potential problem in nutrition or internal organ subsystem function (e.g., physicians have stated the patient has some kidney function loss or has diverticulosis), then the therapist needs to understand how that will affect muscle physiological mechanisms and muscle/CNS fatigue. In addition, this motor analysis must occur within the larger context of the environment, ethnic and social diversity, sensory status, and learning capacity of the client. Functional goals must be established that lead to the client's ability to participate in life within his or her environment and whenever possible lead to or maintain the quality of life desired by the client. Similarly, the therapist must differentiate whether the observed motor problems are based on deficits within the motor, emotional, or cognitive systems. The conclusions drawn by the therapist from each one of these system/subsystem examinations will be critical variables for determining effective intervention strategies.

Before beginning any intervention, the therapist must determine the treatment strategies that will be used to help the client attain the desired outcomes. The categories for treatment strategies are defined in Box 9-1.

The specific environment used by the therapist to optimize patient performance will depend on the functional level and amount of motor control exhibited by the patient. The following classifications can be used to document the specific role of the therapist within the training session:

Functional training: Practice of a functional skill without the need of major program correction. Patient will experience error and self-correct as the program becomes more automatic and integrated. An example would be gait training with a cane to practice ambulation, needing stand by assistance only.

Impairment training: Treatment focus would be on correcting a subsystem impairment during an activity

---

BOX 9-1 ■ TREATMENT STRATEGY CATEGORIES

Compensation Training: Use of an assistive device or orthotic to compensate for a permanent impairment or lost body system function.

Substitution Training: Teaching the client to use a different sensory system or muscle(s) group to substitute for lost function of another system. An example of sensory substitution might be teaching the client to use vision to substitute for an impaired vestibular system or somatosensory system for balance function. Substitution within the motor system might be teaching hip hiking to substitute for lack of dorsiflexion of the ankle during swing phase of gait.

Habituation Training: Activity-based provocation of symptoms with the goal of symptom reduction with repetitive practice. An example would be teaching head movement in a patient who has a chronic labyrinthitis and severe nausea with any head movement.

Neural Adaptation: Driving changes in structure and function of the nervous system (CNS/PNS) with repetitive, attended practice. This category would be considered neural plasticity. This category of treatment strategy takes the greatest repetition of practice, a strong desire by the individual to gain the functional ability and the potential of the CNS to change.

(e.g., pure muscle strengthening, sensory training, endurance training).

Augmented feedback training: Patient needs external feedback (verbal, visual, kinesthetic moment to moment external feedback) and perimeter control over the motor program within the functional activity to express a portion of or a degree within an aspect of the total response necessary to perform the desired movement.

Somatosensory training: Treatment focus is placed on increasing sensory awareness as a result of somatosensory cortical involved from trauma or from overuse creating sensory dystonia. This is also referred to as learning-based sensory-motor training.

Clients with CNS damage often need interventions to encompass more than one of the preceding environments. An example of this might be the early phase of partial body weight treadmill training. Within the early phases, a therapist or assistant is guiding the client's leg during swing and stance phase (augmented feedback training) while the body harness supports a proportion of the client's total weight to assist the postural system in running appropriate programs and the decreasing the power needed to generate a normal gait pattern. The functional training is being done within an environment that perturbs the client's base of support under the normal center of gravity, thus moving the feet backward and the body forward, triggering a normal stepping reaction. In the case of an individual after a cardiovascular accident, one leg will still respond normally, thus helping to trigger a between-limb reciprocal stepping action of the involved leg. In the case of bilateral involvement, both legs may need placement, requiring two people to assist. The activity may be impairment training with the focus on appropriate power production, or cardiovascular fitness, leading to functional training to trigger normal motor programs necessary for gait. Simultaneously, augmented training done by a therapist includes manual assistance in the direction, rate, and placement of the involved leg throughout the gait cycle.

When selecting treatment interventions, the therapist must differentiate among somatosensory retraining, functional training, impairment training, and augmented feedback approaches. All four interventions include a variety of treatments, each based on different strategies and rationales that contribute to the expected outcome. All interventions should address the needs of the patient and must consider any emotional and cognitive restraints. Although these intervention methods can be used simultaneously or in various combinations, the clinician needs to consider which aspect of the intervention falls into which treatment classification. If not, although outcomes can be measured, the determination of how and why the outcomes were influenced by the intervention becomes confusing and hard to differentiate. Without understanding the interactions of intervention methods and the outcome, treatment effectiveness and future clinical decision making remains unpredictable, and unique practice patterns and pathways are hard to identify with consistency. A master clinician who is effective with all patients but does not know how and why the decisions are made along the intervention pathway cannot leave a legacy of effectiveness that will ever lead to efficacy. Although not all graduates or inexperienced clinicians may have the innate aptitude/potential to become or to be master clinicians, if professionals understand the verbal and spatial, cognitive, fine and gross motor, and emotional sensitivity variables that play a role in the evolution toward mastery, educational experiences might be able to nurture future colleagues along this pathway and help those with mastership potential reach that level of function earlier in their professional careers.

The reader must also remember that intervention encompasses multiple interactive environments where intervention decisions are often made moment by moment during any one treatment period. The challenge to the educated clinical professional is to determine what is being done, why it is working, how to continue its effectiveness, and how to determine the progress of the successful intervention. The clinician must also determine how to empower the client (emotionally, cognitively, and motorically) to take over the intervention with inherent, automatic mechanisms that lead to fluid, flexible, functional outcomes independent of both the therapist and the environment within which the activity is occurring. It is not until clinicians can determine effective treatment outcomes from various interventions that efficacy within a research laboratory can be studied without speculation and hypothesis formation based on speculation.[1] Effectiveness is the first way to determine evidence-based practice. Once effectiveness has been established through case studies and larger controlled studies within the clinical environment, researchers can begin to tease out separate variables and establish efficacy as part of evidence to justify clinical decision making.

OVERVIEW OF NEUROLOGICAL REHABILITATION AND MOTOR LEARNING THEORY

Therapeutic interventions that are focused on restoring functional skills to individuals with various forms of neurological problems have been part of the scope of practice of physical therapists (PTs) and occupational therapists (OTs) since the beginning of both professions. Similarly, nurses, speech pathologists, recreational therapists, orthotists, physical medicine and rehabilitation physicians, special educators, and dance and music therapists also focus on various aspects of regaining functional control. Each profession has a unique education, unique models for intervention, and often the belief that her or his respective professional training is the only and the best to guide the patient toward the desired outcome. In reality, no profession has the time or knowledge to develop a practitioner who can evaluate and treat all aspects of each client's mind, body, and spirit. Each professional has a unique skill to offer, and these skills need to be matched to the client, and the expertise needs to be available when needed. These professionals and their respective roles with patient interventions interact with both positive and negative effects on patient's spontaneous functional return, on learning, and on neuroplasticity. It is easy to blame the patient for lack of change or learning when in reality the poor outcomes are due to inconsistency and conflict between learning environments within the health care setting. Therapists have been aware for decades that often a patient does not improve until he or she goes home and has consistency and repetition of practice based on inherent motivation of the client to function independently within his natural environment.

When the educational training of PTs and OTs is considered, these two professions emerge with a complementary background to examine, evaluate, determine a prognosis, and implement interventions that empower clients to regain functional control of activities of daily living (ADLs) (e.g., getting out of bed, bathing, walking, and eating, as well as working, playing, and socially interacting) and resume active participation in life. Both professionals understand how all aspects of the nervous system and the organs that support that system express themselves through striated and smooth motor control and motor output. These two professionals are specialists in the analysis of movement with the scientific background to understand why the movement is occurring, what the strengths and limitations are within the system to support that movement, and how different types of intervention can facilitate functional movement strategies that ultimately carry over into functional life activities and social participation. PTs and OTs are also knowledgeable about neurological and organ system disease and how progression of these pathological states affects motor performance and quality of life as well as about assistance and support needed to help clients maintain functional skills during transitional disease states. Similarly, therapists are currently taught how to minimize impairments within the sensory and motor systems before functional loss. Individuals develop compensatory behaviors to adjust to impairments caused by life or acute pathological conditions. Difficulties in functional movements result, as well as a reduction in life participation. Appropriate intervention can help prevent dysfunction as well as save millions of health care dollars. (See Chapter 6, Health and Wellness.)

Effectiveness in Practice

All areas of practice within a Western medical model have been driven to establish efficacy for the interventions used by practitioners. Physicians take an oath stating "first do no harm." Their models for practice incorporate surgery and pharmacological interventions. The outcome of how either or both interface with the patient and his or her disease/pathological condition should drive the patient toward better health, slow down or stop a progressive disease process, and allow the patient to have a quality of life driven by pharmacological management. These types of interventions can easily be integrated into animal models and trial 1 and 2 human subject models because each specific variable can be controlled and studied. Clinical research in the area of functional movement control or motor learning after disease or trauma to the CNS cannot be as easily transferred into a single-subject (variable) design or linear research models (efficacy studies).[1] What is expressed through a functional or dysfunctional movement is consensus of many subsystems within the CNS and every bodily support system that interfaces with the CNS. Simultaneously the movement also represents that individual's CNS response to the external environment. The process of interpreting and responding to this environment requires sensory recognition, interneuronal communication between nuclei, neuroplasticity, and learning potential within the nervous system itself and the emotional drive of the individual to learn. Thus the movement itself may be measured as better, the same, or worse than previously measured, but understanding how and why that has occurred is complex. Thus therapists need to identify and document what treatment procedures are "effective" within patient populations. Once effectiveness has been established, researchers can begin to differentiate variables and establish efficacy within practice.[1] Both the professions of physical and occupational therapy have been and continue to stress the use of evidence to describe intervention. The American Physical Therapy Association (APTA) through the initiation of the California Physical Therapy Association has been collecting and classifying evidence-based articles through their "Hooked On Evidence" project.[2] Both the APTA and the American Occupational Therapy Association (AOTA) have created "Guides to Practice."[3,4] Yet neither guide can claim to be totally evidence based because the research is not available to substantiate claims.[5] Outcome measures that show change in the patient's quality and ease of movement during functional tasks need to be documented in such a way that the professions can establish effectiveness. That effectiveness will create a tether that will, in the future, allow clinical researchers to establish efficacy within the clinical environment. The therapist must always remember that effectiveness can be expressed in a functional movement, a verbal response by the patient, or an emotional expression. The clinician should never lose the ability to learn from evidence, from science, from patients, from families, and from life.[6]

History of Development of Interventions for Neurological Disabilities

In the mid 1900s, the interventions by PTs and OTs were separate. Generally, PTs worked on gross motor activities with specific emphasis on the lower extremities and the trunk, whereas OTs worked on the upper extremities and fine motor activities. Both professions focused on daily living skills, with those involving the arms falling within the domain of the OT and those involving the legs falling within the domain of the PT. Activities that required gross motor skills such as sitting, coming to stand, walking, walking with assistive devices, and running fell within the purview of the PT, whereas grooming, hygiene, and eating were the responsibility of the OT. Today, this approach is considered ridiculous owing to our understanding of motor learning, neuroplasticity, and motor programming/control. In the past, it was also accepted that the PT worked on specific impairment problems such as weakness, inflexibility, lack of coordination, and voluntary control, whereas the OT worked on functional activities integrated within the environment and the patient's emotional needs and desires. According to the terminology of the twenty-first century, PTs were trained to identify and correct impairments that could lead to functional limitations, whereas OTs were trained to identify and optimize the functional activities that resulted from the impairments. Few clinicians seem to focus on the sequential or interactive aspect of lack of function with specific impairments. Thus, after the onset of a stroke, the PT would strengthen and evaluate ROM of the leg, whereas the OT would encourage the patient to try to functionally use the arm. The PT would be preparing the patient to transfer out of bed and get into and out of a chair and then helping the patient walk, whereas the OT would be preparing the patient to use the arm in functional activities such as grooming or eating. Both therapists hoped the patient would accept life

with new challenges and embrace the attitude that it was up to the patient from there on. What both professions discovered was that the patient generally did not regain normal motor control. He or she might be able to walk and might be able to move the shoulder, but the movement strategies were generally stereotypical, abnormal in patterns, and took tremendous effort by the patient to perform. Over time, clients lost the motivation to even try, and thus what had been gained through therapy may have been lost from lack of practice. There was also minimal recovery of functional hand use, often because of the tremendous effort a patient had to use to move the shoulder to place the hand somewhere. Once that effort was used the tightness and increased tone in the hand prevented functional use. Although functionally independent skills as measured on the Functional Independence Measure were achieved, normal movement patterns and normal motor control were rarely restored, and quality of life was clearly affected for the patient and family.

During the decade or two before the 1960s, some talented and intelligent clinicians began to question the traditional intervention strategies used by the OT and PT. These pioneers[7-31] in neurological rehabilitation set the stage for the development of new concepts that infiltrated basic science into the clinical arena. Thus, the intervention strategies of Jean Ayers, Berta Bobath, Signe Brunnstrom, Margaret Johnstone, Susanne Klein-Vogelbach, Margaret Knott/ Dorothy Voss, Margaret Rood, and others became popular. Colleagues observed these master clinicians and could easily see that the "new" interventions were much more effective and provided better outcomes than previous interventions. Each approach focused on multisensory inputs introduced to the client in controlled and identified sequences. These sequences were based on the inherent nature of synergistic patterns[7,23,32,33] and motor patterns observed in humans[7,9,34] and lower-order animals[35] or a combination of the two.[21,23] Each method focused on the individual client, the specific clinical problems, and the availability of alternative treatment approaches within an established framework. Some of these approaches focused on specific neurological medical diagnoses. The treatment emphasis was then on specific patients and their related movement disorders. Children with cerebral palsy and head injuries[9,25,30] and adults with hemiplegia[10,11,23,34] were the two most frequently identified medical diagnostic categories. Since the 1970s, substantial clinical attention has also been paid to children with learning and language difficulties.[7,15,36] Now, these concepts and treatment procedures have been applied across the age spectrum for all types of medically diagnosed neurological problems seen in the clinical setting. This expansion of the use of any of the methods for any pathological condition seems to be a natural evolution given the structure and function of the CNS and commonalities in impairments and activity limitations manifested by insults from disease, injury, or degeneration of the brain.

Fortunately, most dogmatism no longer persists with respect to territorial boundaries identified by clinicians using some specific intervention methods. A conference in 1990 played a significant role in challenging the relevance of these territorial boundaries and stressed the adoption of a systems model when looking at impairments, activity limitations, and participation in life interactions.[37] As the boundaries for interventions began blurring, intervention approaches such as Proprioceptive Neuromuscular Facilitation (PNF) were then integrated into the care of clients with orthopedic problems and patients with neurological impairments. Today, few universities within the United States teach separate sections or units on specific approaches, but rather teach students to identify specific movement problems, when they are occurring, and what impairments might be the cause of those activity limitations.

For example, assume that a client with hemiplegia exhibited signs of a hypertonic upper-extremity pattern of shoulder adduction, internal rotation, elbow flexion, and forearm pronation with wrist and finger flexion. Brunnstrom[10] would have identified that pattern as the stronger of her two upper-extremity synergies. Michels,[23] although using an explanation similar to Brunnstrom's to describe the pattern, would have elaborated and described additional upper-extremity synergy patterns. Bobath would have asserted that the client was stuck in a mass-movement pattern resulting from abnormal postural reflex activity.[32] Although the conceptualization of the problem certainly determined treatment protocols, the pattern all three clinicians would have worked toward was shoulder abduction, external rotation, elbow extension, forearm supination, and wrist and finger extension. The rationale for the use of this pattern within an intervention period would vary according to the philosophical approach. One clinician might describe the pattern as a reflex-inhibiting position. Another would describe the pattern as the weakest component of the various synergies, whereas still another might identify the pattern as producing an extreme stretch and rotatory element that reciprocally inhibited the spastic pattern. How a clinician sequenced treatment from the original hypertonic pattern to the goal pattern correlated with functional movement would vary. Some would facilitate push-pull patterns in supine, side lying, and rolling. Others would look at propping patterns in sitting or at weight-bearing patterns in prone, over a ball or bolster, or in partial kneeling. All have the potential of eliciting the functional pattern and modifying the hypertonic pattern. One method may have been better than the others, but in truth improved performance may have stemmed not from the method itself but rather from the preferential CNS biases of the client and the variability of application skills among the clinicians themselves. That is, when augmented feedback is used to modulate the motor system's response to an environmental demand, without the understanding of all the additional augmented feedback applied simultaneously, the individual patient and the differences in outcome from patient to patient would vary, making the efficacy of intervention questionable, although the effectiveness of that therapist may be exceptionally high.

Because of the overlap of treatment methods and the infiltration of therapeutic management into all avenues of neurological dysfunction, various multisensory models were developed during the early 1980s,[15,38-41] and these have continued to evolve into acceptable methods in today's clinical arena. Although these models attempted to integrate existing techniques, in reality they have created a new set of holistic treatment approaches. The ultimate goal would be to develop one all-encompassing methodology that allows the clinician the freedom to use any method that is appropriate for the needs and individual learning styles of the client as well as to tap the unique individual differences of the clinician. Although intervention today is based on an integrated model, the influence of third-party payers, the need for efficacy of practice, and time limitations often factor in the therapist's choice of intervention. Visionary and entrepreneurial practice ideas that have the potential to be effective will always be a challenge to future therapists.

Today's therapists replaced many philosophical approaches with applications of motor control/motor learning, or dynamic systems theories. When confronted with a similar upper-extremity pattern described in the past, today's therapist may also work on the same pattern during a functional activity. Control of that combination of movement responses and modulation over those specific central pattern generators will allow the patient opportunities to experience functional movement that is task oriented and environmentally specific while allowing practice to enhance motor learning, neuroplasticity, and ultimate carryover.[42] With a better scientific basis for understanding the function of the human nervous system, how the motor system learns and is controlled and how other systems both internal and external to the CNS modulate response patterns, today's clinicians have many additional options for selection of intervention strategies.[43-52] Whether a patient would initially benefit best from somatosensory retraining, functional retraining, or a more traditional augmented/contrived treatment environment is up to the clinician and the specific needs identified during the examination and evaluation process.

No matter what treatment method is selected by a clinician, all intervention should focus on the active learning process of the client. The client should never be a passive participant, even if the level of consciousness is considered vegetative. With all interventions requiring an active motor response, whether to change an impairment such as increasing or reducing the rate of a motor response, or the tonal state of the combined central pattern generators or cause a functional response during an activity, the client's CNS is being asked to process and respond to the external world at multisegmental levels. That response needs to become procedural and run by the patient without any augmentation to be measured as functional independence. In time, the ultimate goal is for the client's internal drive system to self-regulate and orchestrate modulation over this adaptable and dynamic motor system in all functional activities and in all external environments.

A problem-oriented approach to treatment of any impairment or the residual disability implies that flexibility and neural adaptation are key elements in recovery. However, adaptation should not be random, disjointed, or non–goal oriented. It should be based on methods that provide the best combination of available treatment alternatives to meet individual needs. This adaptation achieved through development of a clinical knowledge bank enables the therapist to match treatment alternatives with the patient's impairments, activity limitations, desired quality of life, and objectives for improved function. A professionally educated therapist no longer bases treatment on identified recipes, although the ingredients for those recipes may be alternative treatment tools if, and only if, the client needs them. Treatment is based on an interaction among basic science, applied science, a therapist's skills, and client objectives.[47,50,53-63]

Motor Learning Concepts as a Basis for Intervention Design

Variables Controlled Outside the Motor System

When motor learning is considered, the therapist must first differentiate general factors affecting motor performance. Some factors are under the control of the cognitive and emotional systems, and others are controlled by the motor system itself. These various factors or concepts of motor learning are presented in Figure 9-1. There are many cognitive factors such as arousal, attention, and cortical pathways related to declarative or executive learning that have specific influences over observable disabilities after neurological insult. Other factors such as limbic connections to cortical pathways affected by motivation, fear and belief, and emotional stability/instability also dramatically affect motor performance and declarative learning. Some of these factors may also limit functional abilities. Therapists need to learn how to discriminate between motor, somatosensory, cortical, and limbic emotional problems. Similarly, clinicians need to identify how the latter two systems affect motor output. With that differentiation, PTs and OTs should be able to separate specific motor system deficits from motor control problems arising from dysfunction within other areas of the CNS. Similarly, motor learning concepts that relate specifically to the motor system need to be understood and incorporated into all interventions to achieve optimal outcomes in the least amount of time within the least restrictive environment.[62-68]

Another variable that is outside the motor system itself is consideration of the environmental context within which the client must perform functional activities. If motor programming and learning is limited, then practicing activities close to, if not specific to, the functional performance needed by the patient becomes critical. For example, assume that a client has limited visits and when returning home will spend most of the day on a boat in an armless chair while fishing. Independent sitting is the functional activity listed as the most important goal to the patient. The therapist has determined that the lack of adequate postural sitting balance as the impairment that limits the functional skill. Because the client will sit either in a lounge chair at home that requires no balance or in a chair on a boat while fishing that requires balance on a compliant surface, the environment in which the therapist needs to practice must incorporate either sitting on compliant surfaces or sitting on a hard-surfaced chair that has been placed on a compliant surface. In that way, the therapist is matching the therapeutic environment with the context of the life activity set as a goal by the patient. The closer the therapeutic environment matches the environmental context, the more likely the patient will learn the procedural program needed to gain functional independence within the established activity and again participate in a valued life activity.

Variables That Are Motor System Specific

If prior procedural learning has occurred, then creating an environment that allows the program to run in the least restrictive environment should lead to the most efficient outcome in the shortest time.[63,64] If a patient needs to learn a new program, such as walking with a stereotypic extension pattern, then goal-directed, attended practice with guided feedback is necessary. It may be easier to bring back an old ambulatory pattern by creating an environment to elicit that program than to teach a client to use a new inefficient movement program.[65,67,68]

Identifying what motor programs are available under what conditions allows the therapist to match existing programs with functional activities, to determine whether deficits are present, and to anticipate problems. Similarly, knowing available programs and the subcomponent necessary to run those programs aids the therapist in the selection of intervention procedures.

If the client has permanent damage to either the basal ganglia or the cerebellum, then retaining the memory of new motor programs may be difficult and substitution approaches may become necessary. Through evaluation the clinician needs to determine whether anatomical disease or a pathological condition is actually causing procedural learning problems. However, because of the plasticity of the CNS, significant recovery or adaptation may occur after attended goal-directed repetitive behavior.[69,70]

There are four traditional components of motor learning that must be considered during any intervention.[71,72] These four components include the type of movement required (Figure 9-2), the type of practice environment (Figure 9-2), the practice schedule itself (Figure 9-3), and the best reinforcement schedule to bring about the quickest, most efficient, and effective motor responses to environmental demands (Figure 9-4).

Timing of the intervention related to recovery of motor function is also important. There is evidence that aggressive therapy staged too close to the neural injury could increase the extent of damage to the brain and spinal cord. Thus, although goal-directed rehabilitation training has been shown to enhance recovery,[72-78] there is a window of healing that is needed. The time parameters of this window are not yet clearly defined, but they are particularly applicable in the acute inpatient setting.

Stages of Motor Learning

Motor learning is an intricate balance between the feedforward and feedback sensorimotor systems. When the sequential activities of the child walking off the park bench are observed, a clear (Figure 9-5, *A* through *C*) understanding of this relationship of height and falling is established. In frame *A*, the child is running a feed-forward program for

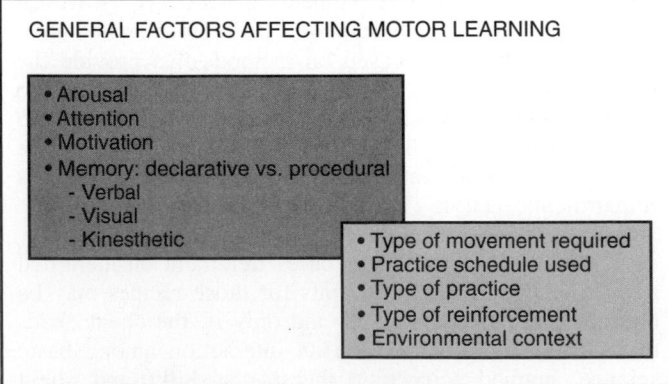

FIGURE 9-1 ▪ Concepts affecting motor learning.

walking. The cerebellum is procedurally responsible for modulating appropriate motor control over the activity and will correct or modify the walking when necessary to attain the directed goal. Unfortunately, a simple correction of walking is not adequate for the environment presented in frame *B*. The cerebellum has no prior knowledge of the feedback presented in this second frame and thus is still running a feed-forward program for stance on the left leg and swing on the right leg. The somatosensory cortices are processing a massive amount of mismatched information from the proprioceptive, vestibular, and visual receptors. In addition, the dopamine receptors are activated during the goal-driven behaviors, creating a balance of inhibition and excitation. Once the executive or higher cognitive system recognizes that the body is falling, a shift in motor control focus from walking to falling must take place. To prepare for falling, the somatosensory system must generate a sensory plan and then relay that plan to the motor system through the sensorimotor feedback loop. The frontal lobe will tell the basal ganglia and the cerebellum to brace and prepare for impact. The basal ganglia is responsible for initiating the new program, and the cerebellum carries out the procedure, as observed in Figure 9-5, *C*. The child succeeds at the task, which is innate and receives positive peripheral and central feedback. It is possible that this experience created a new procedural program that would be labeled jumping. The entire process of the initial motor learning took 1 to 2 seconds. Because of the child's motivation and interest, the program was mass practiced for the next 30 to 45 minutes. This would be the initial acquisition phase and will help the nervous system store the motor program to be used for the rest of his life. If this program is to become a procedural skill, practice must continue within similar environments and conditions. Ultimately, the errors will be reduced and the skill will be refined. Finally, with practice, the program will enter the retention phase as a high-level skill. The skill can still be modified in terms of force, timing, sequencing, and speed and be able to be transferred to different settings. This ongoing modification and improvement is the hallmark of true procedural learning. Modifications within the program will be a function of the plasticity within his CNS that occurs throughout life as the child ages and changes body size and distribution. Similar plasticity and the ability to change, modify, and reprogram will be demanded by individuals who age with chronic motor limitations. Unfortunately, in many of these individuals, the CNS is not capable of producing and accommodating change, which creates new challenges as they age with long-term movement dysfunction. (See Chapter 29.)

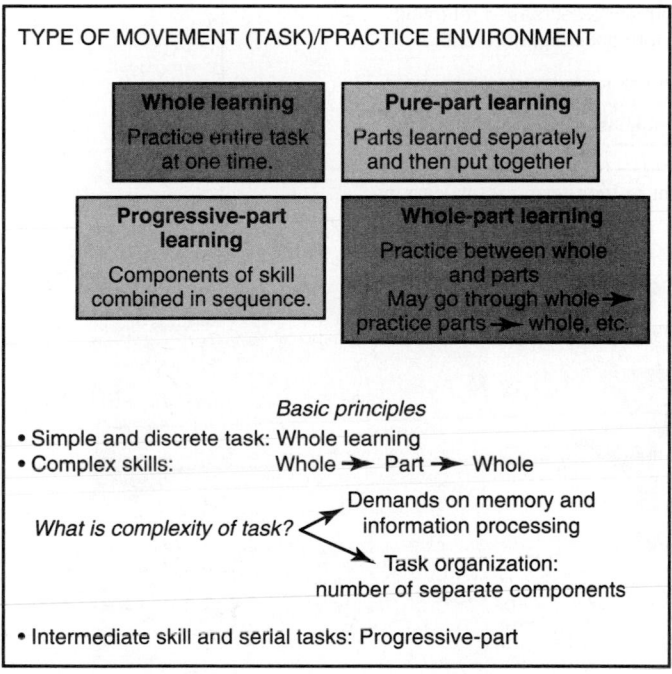

FIGURE 9-2 ■ Type of movement (task)/practice environment.

Systems Interactions: Motor Responses Represent Consensus of CNS Systems

Three Systems within the CNS

Motor behavior reflects not only motor programming but also the interaction of cognitive, affective, and somatosensory variables. Without a motor system, neither the cognitive nor the emotion systems have a way to express and communicate inner thoughts to the world. The cognitive and emotional systems can positively or negatively affect motor

PRACTICE SCHEDULE

Practice vs. rest periods (time between practice)

Mass practice
- Schedule: Daily consecutive session
- Similar to rehabilitation setting

Distributed practice
- Schedule
  - 3 × per week
  - 2 × per week
  - 1 × per week
- Similar to outpatient setting or fixed home program

Random practice
- No fixed schedule
- Empowered client to practice at own pace

General concepts
- Some activities mass practice leads to higher performance—others distributed or random.
- Novel skills probably require more intensive mass practice.
- Even if performance decreases during practice session, learning may increase.

FIGURE 9-3 ■ Practice schedule.

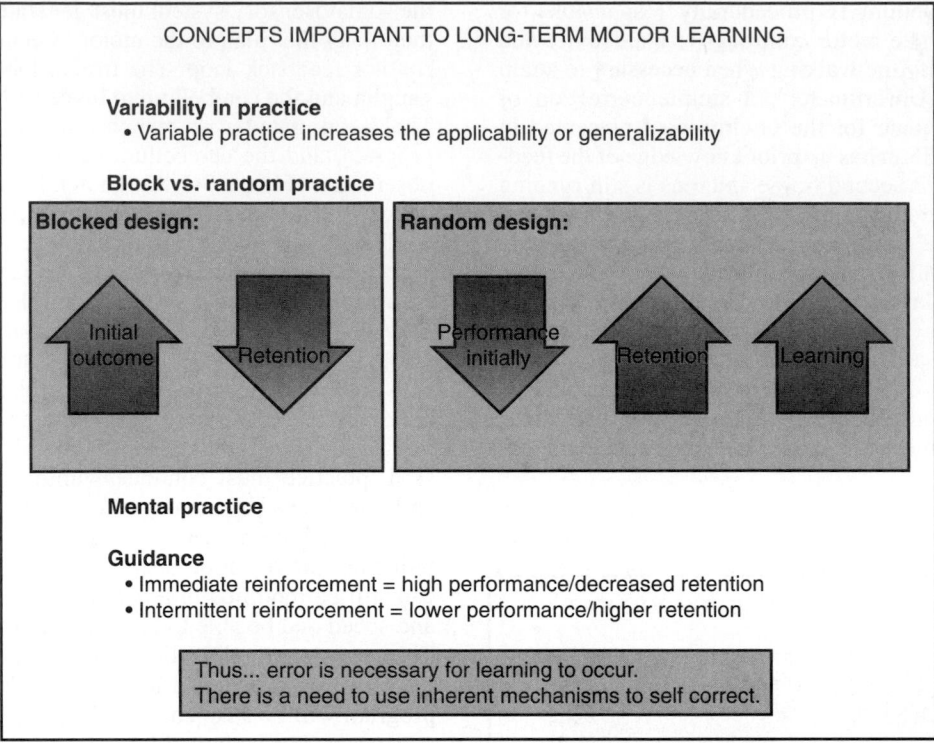

FIGURE 9-4 ■ Concepts important to long-term motor learning.

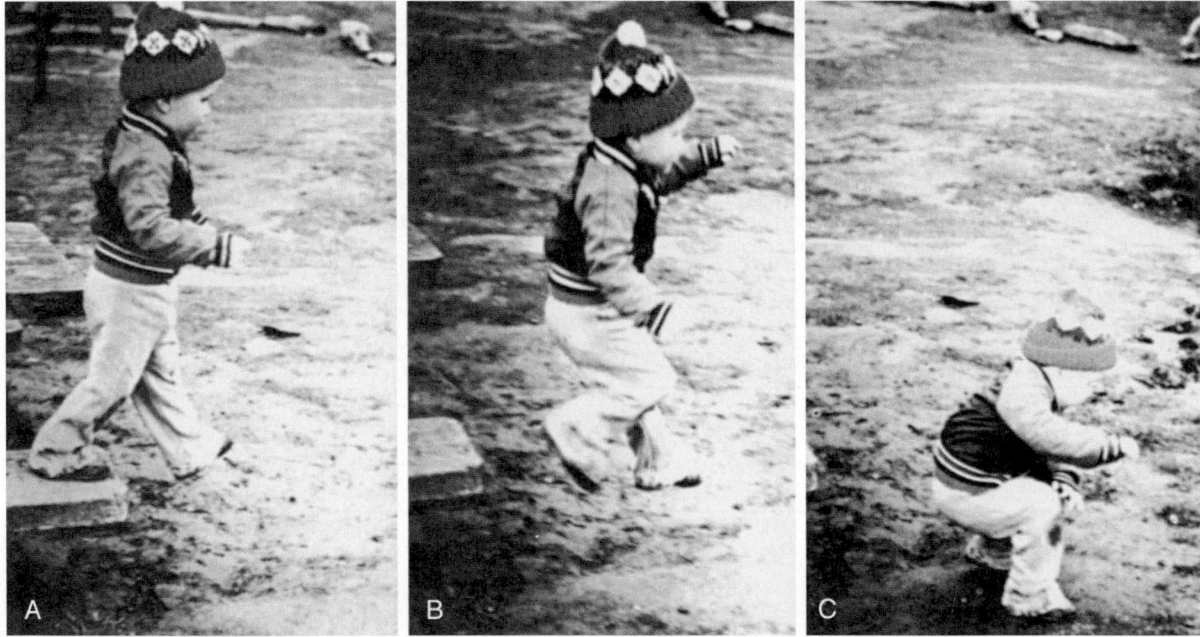

FIGURE 9-5 ■ **A,** Experiencing the unknown. **B,** Identifying the problem. **C,** Solving the problem.

responses. The significance of the somatosensory or perceptual/cognitive cortical system must be emphasized. The somatosensory association areas play a critical role in the ideational and constructional aspects of the motor program itself. When there are deficits within this system, clients will often demonstrate significant distortions in motor control even without a specific motor impairment. An example of this problem might be an individual who had a stroke and developed a "pusher syndrome." The motor behavior shown by this client would be pushing off vertical generally in a lateral or posterolateral direction.[79] Physically correcting the client's posture to vertical or asking the patient to self-correct will not eliminate the original behavior. Pusher syndrome does not stem from a motor problem but rather from a perceptual problem within the somatosensory cortices. Although a therapist might want to augment intervention by trying to push the patient to vertical, the patient will resist that movement pattern. Functional training becomes frustrating to both the patient and the therapist because the impairment does not fall within the motor system itself. Reliance on the use of vision and environmental cues might be the best intervention strategy for this type of problem because the impairment is within the sensory processing centers.[80] Asking the patient to find midline and reach across midline and then acknowledging success, and lack of falling, helps the somatosensory system to relearn and thus begin to inherently correct to vertical. By verbalizing to the patient that you (the therapist) acknowledge that she or he feels as if she or he is falling when placed in the vertical position demonstrates to the client that you have accepted her or him and his or her perceptions. Simultaneously maintaining tactile contact to prevent the patient from falling effectively lets the limbic system relax and reduces its need to trigger motor reactions. Taking all these variables into the treatment environment optimizes the potential that the patient will self-correct during a functional activity such as reaching with weight shift.

If a patient's insult falls within the limbic/emotional system, then motor behavior could also be affected. The motor dysfunction will be different from the dysfunction reflecting damage to the sensory cortices. For years it has been common knowledge that individuals who are depressed will demonstrate motor signs of withdrawal (e.g., flexion). If the posture of flexion was created by a chemical response related to depression, then somatosensory retraining would have a limited effect on behavior. Similarly, functional training may initially modify the impairments, but without changes within the limbic system itself no permanent change will be achieved. Instead, augmenting the input to alter the emotional system and then reinforcing self-control could create the best potential outcome.

For many clinical problems, functional retraining of the motor system through attended, sequenced, repetitive practice could lead to greater functional gains although the impairments may never be eliminated. That is, muscle strengthening and programming coactivation to enable joint stability could restore client independence. Given the complexity of impairments and function in a patient with a neurological insult, a therapist may need to use all three types of intervention procedures to affect all areas of the CNS simultaneously. The decision of which intervention is most appropriate or which should be emphasized falls within the professional judgment of the clinician.

In the clinical environment, the most effective and efficient treatment for the neural insult is the one that is matched to the client's expectations and motivation, the neural injury, the healing process, and the physiological potential for recovery. This requires a dynamic interaction between the client, the therapist, the family, science, and technology. The knowledge base of science includes an understanding of the disease process, all body system interactions both outside and within the nervous system, neuroanatomy and neurophysiological features, and the principles of neuroplasticity. Within the following section a more in-depth discussion of neuroplasticity has been presented to introduce or refamiliarize the reader with this rapidly enlarging and evolving component of neuroscience.

PRINCIPLES OF NEUROPLASTICITY: IMPLICATIONS FOR NEUROREHABILITATION

Research, Rehabilitation, and Practice

Rehabilitation is the process of maximizing learning. The integration of basic neuroscience into clinical practice is critical to guiding the questioning of the researcher and maximizing the recovery of the patient. The 1990s were referred to as the "Decade of the Brain." Over a 10-year period, researchers made striking discoveries that changed the perspective on the adaptability of the CNS. Neuroscientists and clinician researchers documented the adaptability of the CNS not only during development but throughout life. The CNS can recover from serious disease and injury through spontaneous adaptation and healing. However, we also know that the extent of the recovery can be enhanced with environmental enrichment and attended behavioral training. Even the physiological effects of aging can be slowed if neurons remain actively engaged and goal-oriented behavior is rewarded. This revolutionary growth of knowledge regarding the neural adaptation, the specific mechanisms, and the brain circuitry that facilitates neural adaptation are not as well understood. However, integration of the principles of neuroplasticity into clinical practice has become the focus of many colleagues.[81-83] The collaboration of basic scientists and clinicians can be attributed to the vision of researchers and clinicians who interact with patients, observe movement, are fascinated with the whys behind movement behavior, and whose appetite for learning is never satiated. Within the framework of basic science and clinical practice, the paradigm shift in intervention that is based on neuroplasticity has just begun.

It is not uncommon for researchers to become so involved in their experiments about neurological phenomenon that they forget about the impact of their findings on the larger learning environment and the clinical world. Other times, practicing neurorehabilitation clinicians are unaware of current research and apply basic science findings to change practice. Comfortable, familiar treatment approaches dominate practice even when there is little validation that they are the most effective intervention strategies. Other practitioners are familiar with recent basic research findings but do not know how to translate these findings into clinical practice. Still others are unwilling to accept animal-based neuroscience research findings as appropriate for human subjects. Unfortunately, failure to translate basic science findings into clinical practice significantly impairs the potential for recovery for patients with disabling neurological problems.

Three large conferences[84-86] have focused on these issues over a 40-year period. In 1966, the Northwestern University Special Therapeutic Exercise Project (NUSTEP) conference in Chicago, Illinois, brought researchers, basic scientists, educators, and master clinicians together for 6 weeks to identify commonalities in approaches to interventions and to integrate basic science into those commonalities. A huge shift from specific philosophies to a bodily systems model occurred in 1990 at Norman, Oklahoma, the site of the Second Special Therapeutic Exercise Project conference (II STEP). During this period, concepts of motor learning and motor control were beginning to affect the methodology and intervention philosophies of both occupational and physical therapy. The third STEP conference, Summer Institute on Translating Evidence into Practice (III STEP), occurred in July 2005 in Salt Lake City, Utah. At this time, unique clinical models for intervention were embraced that will direct professional education for decades. Changes in practice over the next 15 years will lead to embracing many older intervention techniques with current evidence-based practice. Simultaneously, newer approaches such as locomotion training with partial weight bearing on a treadmill,[67,87] task-specific training,[45,88] constraint-induced movement training,[77,89] neuroprotective effect of exercise,[56] mental and physical practice,[64,90] and patient-centered therapy[91-93] by 2005 was frequently seen in peer-reviewed literature. Four primary outcomes from the III STEP conference were (1) client-centered, empowerment models need to be the platform for all neurorehabilitation and postdisease models for all patients; (2) evidence-based practice needs to first start with clinical effectiveness based on reliable and valid measurement tools and then efficacy studies will follow; (3) there is a strong link between basic science, clinical science, and disease-specific motor dysfunction research and rejection of those integrative links does not provide the best patient management environments; and (4) movement science belongs to a world community that requires integration of many professions including but not limited to physical and occupational research practitioners, basic science researchers, educators, and the goals, cultural beliefs, and ethnic values of the clients and their families.

Patient-centered therapy has become one critical aspect affecting therapeutic outcomes after interventions. The patient could be the obstacle to successful recovery and neural adaptation[94,95] as well as a critical link to success.[96,97] To achieve optimum neuroplasticity, the patient must be engaged in attended, goal-directed behaviors. There is no measurable neural adaptation with passive movements or passive stimuli. To achieve a change in neural response, the stimulus needs to be novel and the patient has to attend to the stimulus and make a decision about it.[53] This has to be done repetitively. There are instances when patients are not convinced that their efforts will make a difference. In other cases, the patient is not motivated to be compliant. In still other situations, the neural insult itself alters patient motivation or cognition, creates emotional instability, or leads to neglect of one or more parts of the body. These latter conditions can interfere with the ability to participate in a meaningful way in goal-directed, even positively rewarded behaviors.

Another failure to bring scientific evidence into practice is the obstacle created by living in a society in which the economics of health care drive the system (see Chapter 10) rather than the science or the benefit to the patient. When a physician or a therapist recommends a new approach to intervention, the third-party payer may deny payment for service it considers "experimental." Further, third-party payers may disagree that findings from animal studies should be applied to human subjects. For example, studies show that the greatest spontaneous recovery after a cardiovascular accident occurs in the first 30 days. When the physician refers patients for continued therapy after 30 days, the third-party payer denies reimbursement for services despite the evidence that the CNS can be modified under conditions of goal-oriented, repetitive, task-relevant behaviors well after 30 days. It has also been shown that neural

adaptation is even greater when environmental conditions and sensory inputs are enriched.[51,52,75]

As the science of neuroplasticity continues to develop, it is critical that ways be found to improve the interface between the scientist, the practitioner, the patient, and the third-party payer. This partnership could be reinforced with increased collaborative research between basic scientists and clinician researchers. Clinicians need to become clinician researchers and accurately report effectiveness within a natural clinical environment. In addition, it is critical that third-party payers be regularly informed about current research findings both in the basic sciences and in the clinic.

To maximize neural adaptation, there are some basic principles to follow (see Appendix 9-A). Positive changes in neural structure can be measured by using a variety of imaging techniques (e.g., magnetic resonance imaging [MRI], functional MRI [fMRI], magnetoencephalography, magnetic source imaging [MSI]). The types of changes reported are summarized in Table 9-1. Positive neural adaptation can also be measured clinically in terms of improved performance. These changes are also summarized in Table 9-1. Although the specific type of intervention may vary, the principles of neuroplasticity must still be addressed.

Integration of Sensory Information and Motor Control

In virtually all higher-order perceptual processes, the brain must correlate sensory input with motor output to assess the body's interaction with the environment accurately. A problem in the somatic motor system affects the motor output system. Both systems are independently adaptive, but functional neural adaptation involves an interaction of adaptation in both systems. Although these two systems operate differently, they are hopelessly intertwined in the healthy nervous system.

The sensory system provides an internal representation of the outside world that guides the movements that make up our behavioral repertoire. These movements are controlled by the motor systems of the brain and the spinal cord. Our perceptual skills are a reflection of the capabilities of the sensory systems to detect, analyze, and estimate the significance of physical stimuli. (See the Augmented Therapeutic Intervention section within this chapter for a detailed discussion of each sensory system.) Our agility and dexterity represent a reflection of the capabilities of the motor systems to plan, coordinate, and execute movements. The task of the motor systems in controlling movement is the reverse of the task of sensory systems in generating an internal representation. Perception is the end product of sensory processing, whereas an internal representation (an image of the desired movement) is the beginning of motor processing.

Sensory psychophysics looks at the attributes of a stimulus: its quality, intensity, location, and duration. Motor psychophysics considers the organization of action, the intensity of the contraction, the recruitment of distinct populations of motor neurons, the accuracy of the movement, the coordination of the movements, and the speed of movement. In both the sensory and motor systems, the complexity of behaviors depends on the multiplicity of modalities available. In sensation, there are the distinct modalities of pain, temperature, light touch, deep touch, vibration, and

Text continued on page 201

TABLE 9-1 ■ Integrating the Principles of Neuroplasticity into Physical and Occupational Therapy Intervention

The scale of plasticity in progressive skill learning is massive. Although the greatest plasticity occurs during development, the potential for neural adaptation continues throughout life. Research suggests plasticity may even be excessive in some individuals (e.g., allowing an individual to drive aberrant changes). We know that learning is modulated as a function of behavioral state and although the nervous system can adapt with a powerful single behavioral event, enduring behavioral changes result from attended, repetitive, learning behaviors that modify the local neuroanatomy and neurophysiology within the CNS. This type of learning requires a commitment of the patient, insight of the therapist, support of the family, and integration of appropriate technology. Learning activities must be compelling and may include robotic devices, mental imagery and practice, computer gaming, and virtual reality experiences.

A. PRINCIPLES OF EXPERIENCE-DEPENDENT PLASTICITY[47,73,98-102]

1. Use it or lose it — *Stay active and keep challenging learning failure to regularly engage specific and general brain functions can lead to functional degradation.*
2. Use it and improve it — *Engaging in training behaviors that drive specific brain functions can lead to an enhancement of the function.*
3. Be specific — *The training experience must match the desired outcome; the nature of neural plasticity is dictated by the nature of the training.*
4. Repetition matters — *Learning requires repetition progressed in difficulty and spaced over time.*
5. Intensity matters — *Plasticity changes require a sufficient training intensity to ensure durability of pathways.*
6. Salience matters — *The training must be salient with the outcome behavior desired.*
7. Age matters — *Training induced plasticity occurs most readily in a young brain but neural adaptation continues across the life span with learning-based training.*
8. Transference — *Plasticity in response to one training experience can also enhance acquisition of similar behaviors and adaptation in other experiences and other parts of the body.*
9. Interference — *Plastic changes after one training experience may interfere with the acquisition of changes in similar systems.*
10. Patient expectation matters — *Patient expectation can facilitate the outcomes of training; patients who expect to get better can enhance their learning.*
11. Reward/feedback matters — *Feedback allows modification of training behaviors, correcting errors, and improving accuracy of learning.*

B. SPECIFIC SUGGESTIONS TO MAXIMIZE THE EFFECTIVENESS OF PHYSICAL THERAPY TRAINING

1. *Create activities that are attended-goal directed, repetitive, progressed in difficulty, increased in variety and depth, spaced over time, rewarded, and complemented with feedback on accuracy.*
2. *Link activities temporally and spatially but not simultaneously in time.*
3. *Make the stimulus strength adequate for detection and appropriate to avoid abnormal movement.*
4. *Integrate stimulus-induced behaviors into meaningful functional activities.*
5. *Be sure training activities are age appropriate.*
6. *Integrate training activities across multiple sensory modalities.*
7. *Perform training activities in different postural orientations.*
8. *Make sensory input relevant to desired outputs.*
9. *Match training behaviors with progression of healing and recovery as well as development.*
10. *Strengthen all positive responses with multisensory modalities.*
11. *Begin sensory training stimulation by using the most mature or accurate sensory receptors.*
12. *Create training situations where desired behaviors are performed in different environmental contexts.*
13. *Do the training in the gravitational positions that stimulate the best performance.*
14. *Create training activities that avoid abnormal movements.*

C. LEARNING-BASED NEUROPHYSIOLOGICAL AND NEUROANATOMICAL OUTCOMES

Neurophysiological and neuroanatomical changes can be measured in the CNS with learning. Measurements have been made with a variety of techniques (e.g., neurophysiological mapping after craniotomies, electroencephalography, MSI, fMRI, electromyography, cortical response mapping with positron emission tomography, and spectroscopy with the potential for neurochemical analysis of neurotransmitters, growth hormones, inhibitors, corticosteroids). With learning:

1. *Distributed cortical representations of inputs and brain actions "specialize" in their representations of behaviorally important inputs and actions for skill learning.*
2. *Important behavioral conditions are met in the learning phase of plasticity that enable growth in the number of neuron populations excited, progressively greater specificity in the neuronal representations, and progressively stronger temporal coordination.*
3. *Important behavioral inputs are selected as a product of strengthening input-coincidence–based connections (synapses).*
4. *Progressive, multiple-staged skill learning cortical plasticity processes are accelerated in child development.*
5. *Cortical field–specific differences in input sources, distributions, and time-structured inputs create different representational structures.*
6. *Temporal dimensions of behaviorally important inputs influence representational "specialization."*
7. *Integration time ("processing time") in cortical and noncortical areas is enhanced with training.*

Continued

TABLE 9-1 ■ Integrating the Principles of Neuroplasticity into Physical and Occupational Therapy Intervention—cont'd

8. *Topographical changes are measured by*
   a. Increased area of representation.
   b. Smaller receptive fields.
   c. Increased density of receptive fields.
   d. Improved organization and order of representation.
   e. Increased myelination.
   f. Increased complexity of dendrites and change in number and complexity of synapses.
   g. Increased strength (amplitude) of evoked responses.
   h. Decreased latency of response.
   i. Increased consistency of response (e.g., density of neuronal response).
   j. Improved selective excitation.
   k. Improved autogenic and surround inhibition.
   l. Improved neurochemical balance and transmission.
   m. Normalized location/translocation.
   n. Normalized pattern of response.
   o. Increased interconnectedness.
   p. Spread of healthy neurons to take over function in areas where damage occurred.
   q. Early achievement of developmental milestones.
   r. Increased specificity of neuronal firing.
   s. Improved synchrony of neuronal firing.
   t. Spatial representational mapping consistent with coincident temporal events.
   u. Increased salience of neuronal responses.
   v. Increased interrelatedness of temporally related neuronal firing.
   w. Improved resistance to representational degradation.
D. **CLINICAL DOCUMENTATION OF OUTCOMES AFTER LEARNING-BASED TRAINING FOR NEURAL ADAPTATION**
   Basic science and clinical research studies report positive correlations between functional outcomes and neural adaptation. With timely prevention, appropriate management of acute insults to the CNS, spontaneous recovery, and thoughtful attention to ADLs and task practice, disabling CNS problems can be minimized. Further, early treatment after CNS injury or onset of disease may prevent more extensive damage to the brain. Learning activities may not only be neuroprotective but also drive more complete recovery of function. Changes in neural adaptation can be measured clinically in terms of improvement in function including:
   1. *Fine and gross motor coordination.*
   2. *Sensory discrimination.*
   3. *Balance and postural control.*
   4. *Reaction time.*
   5. *Accuracy of movements.*
   6. *Rhythm and timing of movements.*
   7. *Memory storage, organization, and retrieval.*
   8. *Alertness and attention.*
   9. *Sequencing.*
   10. *Logic, complexity, and sophistication of problem solving.*
   11. *Language skills (verbal and nonverbal).*
   12. *Interpersonal communication.*
   13. *Positive self image, self-confidence, and sense of well-being.*
   14. *Insight.*
   15. *Self-confidence.*
   16. *Self-image.*
   17. *Signal/noise detection; able to make finer distinctions.*
   18. *Ability to "chunk" information for memory and use.*
   19. *Learning skills including faster learning.*
   20. *Achievement of developmental milestones.*
   21. *Appropriate sensitivity of the nervous system (e.g., reduction in hyperactivity and sensory defensiveness).*
   22. *Ability to perform a skill from memory.*
   23. *Flexible behaviors; variability in task performance.*
   24. *Flexibility for experience-based learning.*

TABLE 9-1 ■ Integrating the Principles of Neuroplasticity into Physical and Occupational Therapy Intervention—cont'd

E. INTERVENTION STRATEGIES TO FACILITATE NEUROPLASTICITY

There are many different intervention strategies to use when working with patients with neurological problems. These interventions need to be matched to the needs of the individual patient and be consistent with the patient's goals and objectives. All the intervention strategies should be goal directed and repeated with attention to both the input (motivation, sensory) and the output mechanisms (movement). The input and output mechanisms are multifactorial and they also involve all components of the sensory, sensorimotor, and motor systems. Although evidence is increasing about the benefit of learning-based activities, research is still needed to help define more precisely when intervention should occur, how intense the intervention should be, how much repetition is needed, how long the learning-based activities need to be continued and spaced, how specific the training needs to be, how quickly behaviors can be progressed and the magnitude of gradation needed, how to keep patients interested, motivated, and compliant in learning, and the magnitude of interference in learning relative to depression, stress, loss of self esteem. The intervention strategies can be broadly classified:

1. *General body responses leading to quieting of the nervous system*
   a. Slow rocking in a rocking chair or hammock.
   b. Slow anterior-posterior: horizontal or vertical movements (chair, hassock, mesh net, swing, ball bolster, carriage, glider chair).
   c. Rotating equipment such as a bed, chair, stool, or therapeutic or gymnastic ball (e.g., rhythmical bouncing).
   d. Slow linear, undulating movements, such as in a carriage, stroller, wheelchair, or wagon.
   e. Wrapping up tightly before rocking (e.g., roll self in sheet; put both arms inside tight tee shirt).
   f. Listening to quiet music or natural environmental sounds (e.g., waves).
   g. Repeating activities listed above first with eyes open and then closed.

2. *Techniques to heighten postural righting*
   a. Rapid or unexpected anterior-posterior or angular acceleration.
      1) Scooter board: pulled or projected down inclines.
      2) Prone over ball: rapid acceleration forward.
      3) Platform or mesh net: prone.
      4) Slides.
   b. Rapid anterior-posterior motion in prone, weight-bearing patterns such as on elbows or extended elbows while rocking and crawling.
   c. Weight-shifting in kneeling, half kneel, or standing.
   d. Do activities with eyes closed.
   e. Create dual-task activities such as walking and talking, stepping over obstacles while on unstable surfaces, reading while maintaining balance in a confusing environment.
   f. Challenge balance in distracting environments (e.g., moving surround, multisensory stimuli in visual surround).

3. *Facilitory techniques to influence whole-body responses*
   a. Movement patterns in specific sequences.
      1) Rolling patterns.
      2) Prop on elbows (prone and side lying) and extend and flex elbows as well as crawl (e.g., side by side, or linear and angular motion).
   b. Spinning.
      1) Mesh net.
      2) Sit and spin toy.
      3) Office chair on universal joint.
   c. Any activity that uses acceleration and deceleration of head.
      1) Sitting and reaching.
      2) Walking.
      3) Running.
      4) Moving from sit to stand.
      5) Do activities with eyes closed, head still and then eyes closed, head turning.
   d. Performing activities that require attention, memory, and cognitive processing at the same time.

4. *Combined facilitory and inhibitory technique: Inverted tonic labyrinthine*
   a. Inverted tonic labyrinthine activities:
      1) Semiinverted in-sitting (head between the legs).
      2) Squatting to stand (head below heart).
      3) Thirty degrees to total inverted vertical position beginning in supine.
   b. Somatosensory and sensorimotor stimulation.
      1) See learning-based sensorimotor training for tactile stimulation.
      2) Proprioceptive stimulation.
         a) Vibration over joints.
         b) Vibration in opposite direction of movement.

Continued

TABLE 9-1 ■ Integrating the Principles of Neuroplasticity into Physical and Occupational Therapy Intervention—cont'd

    c) Wear weights around ankles or on belt.

    d) Position the limbs and the trunk to match a position visually presented.

    e) Move slowly to the count of a metronome.

    f) Look at pictures and position the body to match the pictures.

  c. Auditory discrimination (localization).

5. *Techniques to facilitate specific task performance*

  a. Forced use.

    1) Create training activities where patients must use the affected extremity.

    2) Minimize the need to use the unaffected side.

  b. Constraint-induced movement therapy (forced use)[77,103-108] forced use emphasizes the repetitive use of an impaired limb in regular functional activities by restricting the movement of the less-affected or unaffected side.

    1) The patient is constrained from using the unimpaired limb on a concentrated basis.

    2) The impaired limb is used on a concentrated basis.

    3) The theory is to reduce motor deficits early in the recovery period.

    4) The assumption is the nervous system is adaptable and training for recovery should begin as soon as possible.

    5) If the good arm is constrained, the patient must use the affected limb.

    6) Set time limits to use the constraint; in one large randomized clinical trial the patients were asked to wear a protective safety mitt on the less affected upper limb for a goal of 90% of the waking hours for 14 consecutive days.

    7) During constraint, the individual works under supervision on designated functional tasks for 6 hours a day.

    8) The patient is encouraged to try to use the affected limb during waking hours.

    9) The constraint is paired with motor or behavioral objectives.

    10) Tasks are practiced and progressed in difficulty or speed.

    11) Functional activities are practiced for a set of 20 trials with explicit feedback provided.

    12) Tasks are practiced for 15 to 20 minutes.

    13) A bank of tasks is created.

    14) The therapist tries to match the tasks to the joint movements that have the greatest potential for recovery.

    15) The participant also has the opportunity to select a task of her or his preference.

    16) The minimal requirements for repetition, progression, intensity, and duration of training are under study.

  c. Body weight–supported treadmill training.[109-116]

    1) Use a harness system over a treadmill to safely unweight the full load of the body and stimulate stepping.

    2) Walk at different speeds on the treadmill.

    3) Select a speed where there is a natural rhythm and the pattern approaches normal.

    4) If the patient cannot step normally, the leg should be assisted by the therapist or by a mechanical device.

    5) Add learning activities while walking to facilitate learning and dual tasking.

    6) Integrate treadmill learning into over-ground walking (with or without unweighting or with or without a cane or walking stick depending on patient need for assistance).

  d. Mass practice.[117]

    1) Set aside a critical time period to practice a task repetitively.

    2) Practice the task until a target performance is achieved (accuracy, time, quality).

    3) Carefully progress the mass practice activities in small increments on the same task.

    4) Progress mass practice to increasingly difficult tasks.

    5) Research is needed to determine the number of repetitions and the duration of this type of training.

    6) Monitor blood pressure and heart rate regularly while on the treadmill.

    7) Begin with multiple short walking intervals (e.g., 2-5 minutes) followed by a break.

    8) Encourage walking for up to 30 minutes.

    9) Training parameters will vary by patient height, weight, and degree of impairment.

    10) Research is still needed to clarify the time needed for training, the frequency and duration of training needed, the ideal amount of unweighting and the most appropriate speed for speed, quality, and endurance of gait.

  e. Robotics.

    1) Incorporate the use of robotics in training.

    2) Robotic training may be passive or active.

    3) Facilitate general and task-specific movements with robotic assistance.

    4) Robotic instrumentation is designed to have "soft" guidance with patient participation.

    5) Robotic training may be combined with supervised, individual, or group physical therapy.

    6) Continued research is needed to lead to the most effective robots for training and the intensity and duration of the training needed with these devices.

stretch, whereas in the motor system can be found the modalities of reflex responses, rhythmic motor patterns within and between limbs, and voluntary fine and gross movements.[98-118] Although all motor movements require integration of sensory information for motor learning, once motor control is attained the system can run on very little feedback. The relationship of incoming sensory information is particularly complex in voluntary motor movements that constantly adapt to environmental variance. For voluntary motor movements, the motor system requires contraction and relaxation of muscles, recruitment of appropriate muscles and their synergies, appropriate timing and sequencing of muscle contraction and relaxation, the distribution of the body mass, and appropriate postural adjustments. As stated, once a motor program is learned, it does not take the same amount of sensory information to run the program feed-forward within the motor system as long as the information to the cerebellum is able to run and adjust all aspects of the program. (See Chapters 3 and 26.) To learn new programs, the CNS must go through the process of receiving sensory input, perceptual processing, communication with the frontal lobes, relays to basal ganglia and cerebellum, followed by intentional, goal-directed execution of the motor plan.

Within each movement, there must be adjustments to compensate for the inertia of the limbs and the mechanical arrangement of the muscles, bones, and joints both before and during movement to ensure and maintain accuracy. The control systems for voluntary movement include (1) the continuous flow of sensory information about the environment, position, and orientation of the body and limbs and the degree of contraction of the muscles; (2) the spinal cord; (3) the descending systems of the brain stem; and (4) the pathways of the motor areas of the cerebral cortex, cerebellum, and basal ganglia. Each level of control is based on the sensory information that is relevant for the functions it controls. This information is provided by feedback, feed-forward, and adaptive mechanisms. These control systems are organized both hierarchically and in parallel. The hierarchical organization permits lower levels to generate reflexes without involving higher centers, whereas the parallel system allows the brain to process the flow of discrete types of sensory information to produce discrete types of movements.[119,120]

Ultimately, the control of graded fine motor movements gets down to the sensory organ of the muscle spindle, which contains the specialized elements that sense muscle length and the velocity on changes in length. In conjunction with the Golgi tendon organ, which senses muscle tension, the muscle spindle provides the CNS with continuous information on the mechanical state of the muscle. Ultimately, the firing of the muscle spindles depends on both muscle length and the level of gamma motor activation of the intrafusal fibers on the basis of the interpretation by the CNS of the signals from the muscle spindles. Similarly, joint proprioceptors relay both closed and open chain input and mobility (range) within the joint structures to the CNS. This illustrates the close relationship between sensory and motor processing and the integral relationship between the two when neuroplasticity is discussed.[121]

Foundation for the Study of Neuroplasticity

The principal models for studying cortical plasticity have been based on the representations of hand skin and hand movements in the New World owl monkey *(Aotus)* and the squirrel monkey *(Saimire)*. These primate models have been chosen because their central sulci usually do not extend into the hand representational zone in the anterior parietal (S1) or posterior frontal (M1) cortical fields. In other primates the sulci are deep and interfere with accurate mapping. Albeit there are differences in hand use among primates, in all of the primates the hand has the largest topographical representation for the actual size of the extremity, the detail of this representation is distinct, and the hand has the greatest potential for skilled movements and sensory discrimination. However, the findings from studies of this cortical area are applicable across the cortex.[122,123] See Figure 9-6 to identify specific anatomical locations and their respective classifications.

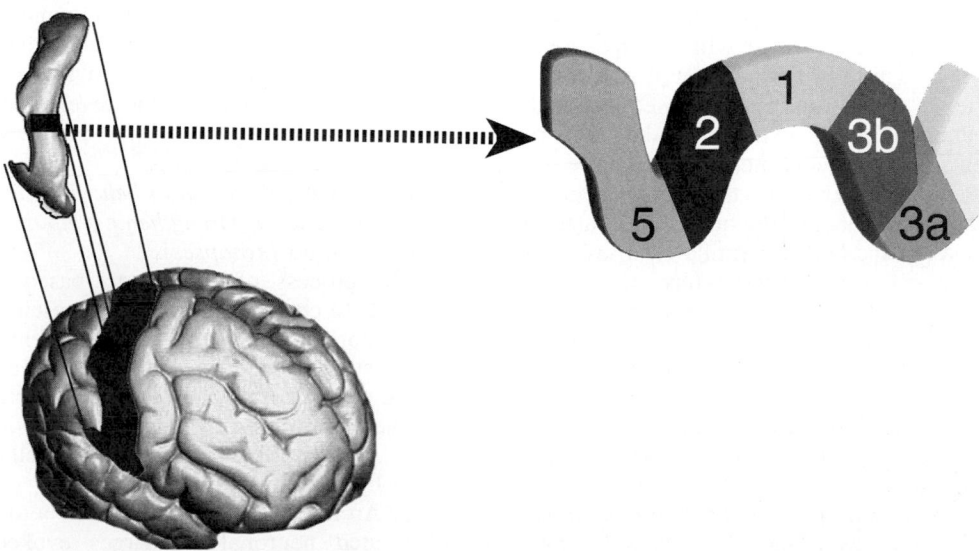

FIGURE 9-6 ■ Classification and anatomical locations of cortical map.

Neuroplasticity: Principles of Neural Adaptation

Learning drives neural adaptation. Plasticity is the mechanism for encoding and learning. During neural adaptation (neuroplasticity), the fundamental questions are as follows: As we learn, how does the brain change its representations of inputs and actions? What is the nature of the processes that control the progressive elaboration of performance abilities? In different individuals, what are the sources of variance for emergent performance abilities? What changes in cortical plasticity facilitate the development of "automatic" motor behaviors? Why are some behaviors hard to change? What limits the plasticity processes? What are the critical elements of brain circuitry, genes, synapses, neuronal networks, and neural connections that are needed to restore lost function? What guidelines need to be followed to drive the greatest change in brain structure and function? How do spontaneous compensatory behavioral strategies contribute to or interfere with restoring lost neuronal function? How does the unaffected side contribute or interfere with neuroplastic changes and restoration of function? Does damage to the brain alter the neuronal response to learning (e.g., cascade of cellular activity for healing altered circuitry, new neural connections)?

The most informative studies on neuroplasticity are those specifically directed towards defining changes induced by learning. One approach has been to document the patterns of distributed neural response representation of specific inputs before and after learning. In particular, neuronal responses have been measured in the primary auditory, somatosensory, and motor cortices in animals. These animal studies have been paired with behavioral studies in humans. Both the animal and human studies provide strong evidence documenting the ability of the brain to functionally self-organize. This capacity for change not only occurs during development but also in adulthood, specifically after learning-based activities. The basic cortical plasticity processes that contribute to learning are summarized in Table 9-1.

1. *Neural circuits must be actively engaged in learning-based activities to prevent degradation and atrophy.*
   We know that if infants are deprived of sensory and motor experiences during development, the brain does not develop normally. For example, without exposure to light, there is a reduction in the number of neurons in the visual cortex.[124] Similarly, if not exposed to sound, there is a reduction in the neurons in the auditory cortex.[125] Even in adults, when neural circuits are not used over an extended period of time, they begin to degrade and the unused area of the brain is allocated to serve another part of the body.[126] Similarly, if task performance is practiced, then the topography expands and becomes more detailed, as you might see in someone who is blind and reads Braille.[127] It is also interesting to note that, although a person is blind, the visual cortical areas may become active when the individual is reading Braille.[128] Similarly a person who is deaf may demonstrate activation of the auditory cortex when visual stimuli are presented.

2. *With learning, the distributed cortical representations of inputs and brain actions "specialize" in their representations of behaviorally important inputs and actions in skill learning.*

There seems to be a minimal level of repetitive practice needed to acquire a new skill that will be maintained over time. In fact, this may lead to specialization or change in the underlying neurophysiological processing.[129-131] This specialization develops in response to selective cortical neuron responses specialized to demands of sensory, perceptual, cognitive, and motor skill learning.[132-135] This adaptation has been clearly documented in animal studies. For example, if an animal is trained to make progressively finer distinctions about specific sensory stimuli, then cortical neurons come to represent those stimuli in a progressively more specific and progressively "amplified" manner.

3. *There are important behavioral conditions that must be met in the learning phase of plasticity.*
   a. If behaviorally important stimuli repeatedly excite cortical neuron populations, the neurons will progressively grow in number.
   b. Repetitive, behaviorally important stimuli processed in skill learning lead to progressively greater specificity in the spectral (spatial) and temporal dimensions.

4. *The growing numbers of selectively responding neurons discharge with progressively stronger temporal coordination (distributed synchronicity).*
   Through the course of progressive skill learning, a more refined basis for processing stimuli and generating actions critical to skilled tasks is enabled by the multidimensional changes in cortical responses. Consequently, specific aspects of these changes in distributed neuronal response are highly correlated with learning-based improvements in perception, motor control, and cognition.[74,78,136,137] In these processes, the brain is not simply changing to record and store content, but the cerebral cortex is also selectively refining its processing capacities to fit each task at hand by adjusting its spectral/spatial and temporal filters. Ultimately, it establishes its own general processing capabilities. This "learning to learn" determines the facility with which specific classes of information can be stored, associated, and manipulated. These powerful self-shaping processes of the forebrain machinery are operating not only on a large scale during development but also during experience-based management of externally and internally generated information in adults. This self-shaping with experience allows the development of hierarchical organization of perception, cognition, motor, and executive management skills.

5. *In learning, selection of behaviorally important inputs is a product of strengthening input coincidence-based connections (synapses).*
   The process of coincidence-based input coselection leads to changes in cortical representation. Coincident, temporally and spatially related events that fire together are strengthened together. In skill learning, this principle of concurrent input coselection results from repetitive practice that includes the following:
   a. A progressive amplification of cell numbers engaged by repetitive inputs.[136-138]
   b. An increase in the temporal coordination of distributed neuronal discharges evoked by successive events mark features of behaviorally important inputs is a consequence of a progressive increase in

positive coupling between nearly simultaneously engaged neurons within cortical networks.[136,139]

c. A progressively more specific "selection" of all of those input features that collectively represent behaviorally important inputs, expressed moment by moment in time.[138,139] Thus, skill learning results in mapping temporal neighbors in representational networks at adjacent spatial locations when they regularly occur successive in time.[70,140,141] Changes in activation patterns, dendritic growth, synapses, and neuronal activities may also be observed.

The basis of the functional creation of the detailed, representational cortical maps converting temporal to spatial representations is related to the Hebbian change principle.[142] The Hebbian plasticity principle applies to the development of interconnections between excitatory and inhibitory inputs within the cortical pyramidal neurons and their connections to extrinsic inputs and outputs. On the basis of the Hebbian principle, the operation of coincidence-based synaptic plasticity in cortical networks results in the formation, strengthening, and continuous recruitment of neurons within neuronal "assemblies" that "cooperatively" represent behaviorally important stimuli.

6. *Plasticity is constrained by anatomical sources and convergent-divergent spreads of inputs.* Every cortical field has the following:
   a. Specific extrinsic and intrinsic input sources.
   b. Dimensions of anatomical divergence and convergence of its inputs, limiting dynamic combination Hebbian input coselection capacities.[143,144]

Anatomical input sources and limited projection overlap both to enable change by establishing input-selection repertoires and to determine the limits for change. There are relatively strict anatomical constraints at the "lower" system levels, where only spatially (spectrally) limited input coincidence-based combined outcomes are possible. In the "higher" system hierarchies, anatomical projection topographies are more powerful with neurons and neuronal assemblies developing that respond to complex combinations of features of real-world objects, events, and actions.

7. *Plasticity is constrained by the time constants governing coincident input coselection and by the time structures and potentially achievable coherence of extrinsic and intrinsic cortical input sources.*

To effectively drive representational changes with coincident input-dependent Hebbian mechanisms, temporally coordinated inputs are prerequisite, given the short durations (milliseconds to tens of milliseconds) of the time constants that govern synaptic plasticity in the adaptive cortical machinery (see reference 145 for review). Consistently uncorrelated or low-discharge-rate inputs induce negative changes in synaptic effectiveness. In addition, stimuli occurring repetitively simultaneously in time can also degrade the representation. These negative effects also contribute importantly to the learning-driven "election" of behaviorally important inputs.

8. *Cortical field–specific differences in input sources, distributions, and time-structured inputs create different representational structures.*
   a. There are significant differences in the activity from afferent inputs from the retina, skin, or cochlea generated in a relatively strictly topographically wired V-1 (area 17), S-I proper (area 3b), or A-1 (area 43) compared with the inferotemporal visual, insular somatosensory, dorsotemporal auditory, or prefrontal cortical areas that receive highly diffuse inputs (see Figure 9-6). In the former cases, heavy schedules of repetitive, temporally coherent inputs are delivered from powerful, redundant projections from relatively strictly topographically organized thalamic nuclei and lower-level, associated cortical areas. Whereas neighboring neurons can share some response properties, neurons or clusters of neurons respond selectively to learned inputs. These neurons are distributed widely across cortical areas and share less information with neighboring neurons. In the "lower" levels, afferent input projections from any given source are greatly dispersed. Highly repetitive inputs are uncommon, inputs from multiple diffuse cortical sources are more common as well as more varied, and complex input combinations are in play. These differences in input schedules, spreads, and combinations presumably largely account for the dramatic differences in the patterns of representation of behaviorally important stimuli at "lower" and "higher" levels.[146]
   b. Despite these differences in representational organization across the cortex, the cortex does progressively differentiate cortical cells to accomplish specific operational tasks. There is a serial progression of differentiation to allow the development of functional organization that allows an individual to progressively master more and more elaborated and differentiated perceptual, cognitive, monitoring, and executive skills.
   c. The sources of inputs and their field-specific spreads and boundary limits, the distributions of modulatory inputs differentiated by cortical layers in different cortical regions, the basic elements and their basic interconnections in the cortical processing machine, and crucial aspects of input combination and processing at subcortical levels are inherited (see reference 147 for review). Although these inherited aspects of sensory, motor, and cortical processing circuit development constrain the potential learning-based modification of processing within each cortical area, representation changes can occur as a result of environmental interaction and purposeful behavioral practice.

9. *Temporal dimensions of behaviorally important inputs also influence representational "specialization."*
   In at least four ways, the cortex refines its representations of the temporal aspects of behaviorally important inputs during learning.
   a. First,
      1. The cortex generates more synchronous representations of sequenced and coincident associative input perturbations or events, not only recording their identities but also marking their occurrences (for examples, see references 134, 136, 139, and 148 to 151). These changes in representation appear to be primarily achieved through increases in positive coupling strengths between interconnected neurons participating in stimulus- or action-specific neuronal cell

assemblies.[134,150,152-171] The strength of the interconnectedness increases representational salience as a result of downstream neurons being excited as a direct function of the degree of temporal synchronization of their inputs.

2. Increasing the power of the outputs of a cortical area drives downstream plasticity. Hebbian plasticity mechanisms operating within downstream cortical (or other) targets also have relatively short time constants. The greater the synchronicity of inputs, the more powerfully those change mechanisms are engaged. The strength of the interconnections also helps protect against noise. For example, by simple information abstraction/coding, the distributed neuronal representation of the "signal" (a temporally coordinated, distributed neuronal response pattern representing the input or action) is converted at the entry levels in the cortex into a form that is not as easily degraded or altered by "noise." The strength of the interconnectedness also confers robustness of complex signal representation for spatially or spectrally incomplete or degraded inputs.

b. Second,
1. The cortex can select specific inputs through learning to exaggerate the representation of specific input time structures. Conditioning a monkey or a rat with stimuli that have a consistent, specific temporal modulation rate or interstimulus time, for example, results in a selective exaggeration of the responses of neurons at that rate or time separation. In effect, the cortex "specializes" for expected relatively higher-speed or relatively lower-speed signal event reception.
2. Both electrophysiological recording studies and theoretical studies suggest that cortical networks richly encode the temporal interval as a simple consequence of cortical network dynamics.[172,173] It is hypothesized that the cortex accomplishes time interval and duration selectivity in learning by positively changing synaptic connection strengths for input circuits that can respond with recovery times and circuit delays that match behaviorally important modulation frequency periods, intervals, or durations. However, studies on including excessive, rapid, repetitive fine motor movements can sometimes lead to serious degradation in representation if the adjacent digits are driven nearly simultaneous in time. This may be associated with negative learning and a loss of motor control.[174]

c. Third,
1. The cortex links representations of immediately successive inputs that are presented in a learning context.
2. As a result of Hebbian plasticity, it establishes overlapping and neighboring relationships between immediately successive parts of rapidly changing inputs yet retains its individualized, distinct cortical representation.[70,175]

d. Fourth,
1. The cortex generates stimulus sequence-specific ("combination-sensitive") responses, with neu-ronal responses selectively modulated by the prior application of stimuli in the learned sequence of temporally separated events.
2. These "associative" or "combination-sensitive" responses have been correlated with evidence of strengthened interconnections between cortical cell assemblies representing successive event elements separated by hundreds of milliseconds to seconds in time.[176,177] The mechanisms of origin of these effects have not yet been established.

10. *The integration time ("processing time") in the cortex is itself subject to powerful learning-based plasticity.*
   a. Cortical networks engage both excitatory and inhibitory neurons by strong input perturbations. Within a given processing "channel," cortical pyramidal cells cannot be effectively reexcited by a following perturbation for tens to hundreds of milliseconds. These integration "times" are primarily dictated by the time for recovery from inhibition, which ordinarily dominates poststimulus excitability. This "integration time," "processing time," or "recovery time" is commonly measured by deriving a "modulation transfer function," which defines the ability of cortical neurons to respond to identical successive stimuli within cortical "processing channels." For example, these "integration" times normally range from about 15 to about 200 ms in the primary auditory receiving areas.[178-180] Progressively longer processing times are recorded at higher system levels (e.g., in the auditory cortex, they are approximately a syllable in length, 200 to 500 ms in duration) in the "belt cortex" surrounding the primary auditory cortex.[181]
   b. These time constants govern—and limit—the cortex's ability to "chunk" (i.e., to separately represent by distributed, coordinated discharge) successive events within its processing channels. Both neurophysiological studies in animals and behavioral training studies in human adults and children have shown that the time constants governing event-by-event complex signal representation are highly plastic. With intensive training in the right form, cortical "processing times" reflected by the ability to accurately and separately process events occurring at different input rates can be dramatically shortened or lengthened.[182-185]

11. *Plasticity processes are competitive.*
   a. If two spatially or spectrally different inputs are consistently delivered nonsimultaneously to the cortex, cortical networks generate input-selective cell assemblies for each input and actively segregate them from one another.[139,184,186-188] Boundaries between such inputs grow to be sharp and are substantially intensity independent. Computational models of Hebbian network behaviors indicate this sharp segregation of nonidentical, temporally separated inputs is accomplished as a result of a wider distribution of inhibitory instead of excitatory responses in the emerging, competing cortical cell assemblies that represent them.
   b. This Hebbian network cell assembly formation and competition appears to account for how the cortex

creates sharply sorted representations of the fingers in the primary somatosensory cortex.[140,189] The Hebbian network probably accounts for how the cortex creates sharply sorted representations of native aural language-specific phonemes in lower-level auditory cortical areas in the auditory/speech processing system of humans. If inputs are delivered in a constant and stereotyped way from a limited region of the skin or cochlea in a learning context, that skin surface or cochlear sector is an evident competitive "winner."[136,190] By Hebbian plasticity, the cortical networks will coselect that specific combination of inputs and represent it within a competitively growing Hebbian cell assembly. The competitive strength of that cooperative cell assembly will grow progressively because more and more neurons are excited by behaviorally important stimuli with increasingly coordinated discharges. That means that neurons outside of this cooperative group have greater numbers of more coordinated outputs contributing to their later competitive recruitment. Through progressive functional remodeling, the cortex clusters and competitively sorts information across sharp boundaries dictated by the spectrotemporal statistics of its inputs. On the one hand, if it receives information on a heavy schedule that sets up competition for a limited input set, it will sort competitive inputs into a correspondingly small number of largely discontinuous response regions.[191,192]

c. Competitive outcomes are, again, cortical level dependent. The cortex links events that occur in different competitive groups if they are consistently excited synchronously in time. At the same time, competitively formed groups of neurons come to be synchronously linked in their representations of different parts of the complex stimulus and collectively represent successive complex features of the vocalization through the coordinated activities of many groups.

d. Neurons within the two levels of the cortex surrounding A-1 (see Figure 9-6) have greater spectral input convergence and longer integration times that enable their facile combination of information representing different spectrotemporal details. Their information extraction is greatly facilitated by the learning-based linkages of cooperative groups that deliver behaviorally important inputs in a highly salient, temporally coordinated form to these fields. With their progressively greater space and time constants, still higher-level areas organize competitive cell assemblies that represent still more complex spectral and serial-event combinations. Note that these organizational changes apply over a large cortical scale. In skill learning over a limited period of training, participating neuronal members of such assemblies can easily be increased by many hundredfold, even within a primary sensory area such as S-I area 3b or A-1.[136,139,174,184,193]

e. In extensive training in complex signal recognition, more than 10% of neurons within temporal cortical areas can come to respond highly selectively to a specific, normally rare, complex training stimulus. The distributed cell assemblies representing those specific complex inputs involve tens or hundreds of millions of neurons and are achieved by enduring effectiveness changes in many billions of synapses.

12. *Learning is modulated as a function of behavioral state.*
    a. At "lower" levels of the cortex, changes are generated only in attended behaviors.[137,138,146,193-195] Trial-by-trial change magnitudes are a function of the importance of the input to the animal as signaled by the level of attention, the cognitive values of behavioral rewards or punishments, and internal judgments of practice trial precision or error based on the relative success or failure of achieving a target goal or expectation. Little or no enduring change is induced when a well-learned "automatic" behavior is performed from memory without attention. It is also interesting to note that at some levels within the cortex, activity changes can be induced even in nonattending subjects under conditions in which "priming" effects of nonattended reception of information can be demonstrated.
    b. The modulation of progressive learning is also achieved by the activation of powerful reward systems releasing the neurotransmitters norepinephrine and dopamine (among others) through widespread projections to the cerebral cortex. Norepinephrine plays a particularly important role in modulating learning-induced changes in the cortex.[148,184,195]
    c. The cortex is a "learning machine." During the learning of a new skill, neurotransmitters are released trial by trial with application of behaviorally important stimulus or behavioral rewards. If the skill can be mastered and thereafter replayed from memory, its performance can be generated without attention (habituation). Habituation results in a profound attenuation of the modulation signals from these neurotransmitter sources; plasticity is no longer positively enabled in cortical networks.

13. *Top-down influences constrain cortical representational plasticity.*
    Attentional control flexibly defines an enabling "window" for change in learning.[182] Progressive learning generates progressively more strongly represented goals, expectations, and feedback[196,197] across all representational systems that are undergoing change and to modulatory control systems weighing performance success and error. Strong intermodal behavioral and representational effects have also been recorded in experiments that might be interpreted as shaping expectations.[198,199] These shaping expectations would be similar to those observed in a human subject using multisensory inputs such as auditory, visual, and somesthetic information to create integrated phonological representations, to create fine motor movement trajectory patterns that underlie precise hand control, or to make a vocal production.

14. *The scale of plasticity in progressive skill learning is massive.*
    a. Cortical representational plasticity must be viewed as arising from multiple-level systems that are broadly engaged in learning, perceiving, remembering,

thinking, and acting. Any behaviorally important input (or consistent internally generated activity) engages many cortical areas. Repetitive training drives all cortical areas to change.[133,144,200] Different aspects of any acquired skill are contributed from field-specific changes in the multiple cortical areas that are remodeled in its learning.

b. In this kind of continuously evolving representational machine, perceptual constancy cannot be accounted for by locationally constant brain representations; relational representational principles must be invoked to account for it.[133,201] Moreover, representational changes must obviously be coordinated level to level. It should also be understood that plastic changes are also induced extracortically. Although it is believed that learning at the cortical level is usually predominant, plasticity induced by learning within many extracortical structures significantly contributes to learning-induced changes that are expressed within the cortex.

15. *Enduring cortical plasticity changes appear to be accounted for by local changes in neural anatomy.*

Changes in synapse turnover, synapse number, synaptic active zones, dendritic spines, and the elaboration of terminal dendrites have been demonstrated to occur in a behaviorally engaged cortical zone.[144,202-207] Through many changes in local structural detail, the learning brain is continuously physically remodeling its processing machinery not only across the course of child development but also after behavioral training in an adult who has had a neural insult.

16. *Cortical plasticity processes in child development represent progressive, multiple-staged skill learning.*

a. There are two remarkable achievements of brain plasticity in child development. The first is the progressive shaping of the processing to handle the accurate, high-speed reception of the rapidly changing streams of information that flow into the brain. In the cerebral cortex, shaping appears to begin most powerfully within the primary receiving areas of the cortex. With early myelination, the main gateways for information into the cortex are receiving strongly coherent inputs from subcortical nuclei, and they can quickly organize their local networks on the basis of coincident input coselection (Hebbian) plasticity mechanisms. The self-organization of the cortical processing machinery spreads outward from these primary receiving areas over time to ultimately refine the basic processing machinery of all the cortex. The second great achievement, which is strongly dependent on the first, is the efficient storage of massive content compendia, in richly associated forms.

b. During development, the brain accomplishes its functional self-organization through a long parallel series of small steps. At each step, the brain masters a series of elementary processing skills and establishes reliable information repertoires that enable the accomplishment of subsequent skills. Second- and higher-order skills can be viewed as both elaborations of more basic mastered skills and the creation of new skills dependent on combined second- and

higher-order processing. That hierarchical processing is enabled by greater cortical anatomical spreads, by more complexly convergent anatomical sources of inputs, and by longer integration (processing, recovery) times at progressively higher cortical system levels. This hierarchical but integrating processing allows for progressively more complex combinations of information integrated over progressively longer time epochs as one ascends across cortical processing hierarchies.

c. As the cortical machinery functionally evolves and consequently physically "matures" through childhood developmental stages, information repertories are represented in progressively more salient forms (i.e., with more powerful distributed response coordination). Growing agreement directly controls the power of emerging information repertoires for driving the next level of elaborative and combinatorial changes. It is hypothesized that saliency enables the maturation of the myelination of projection tracts delivering outputs from functionally refined cortical areas. More mature myelination of output projections also contributes to the power of this newly organized activity to drive strong, downstream plastic change through the operation of Hebbian plasticity processes.

d. As each elaboration of skill is practiced, in a learning phase, neuromodulatory transmitters enable change in the cortical machinery. The cortex functionally and physically adapts to generate the neurological representations of the skill in progressively more selective, predictable, and statistically reliable forms. Ultimately, the performance of the skill concurs with the brain's own accumulated, learning-derived "expectations." The skill can now be performed from memory, without attention. With this consolidation of the remembered skill and information repertoire, the modulatory nuclei enable no further change in the cortical machinery. The learning machine, the cerebral cortex, moves on to the next elaboration. In this way the cortex constructs highly specialized processing machinery that can progressively produce great towers of automatically performable behaviors and great progressively maturing hierarchies of information-processing machinery that can achieve progressively more powerful complex signal representations, retrievals, and associations. With this machinery in a mature and thereby efficiently operating form, there is a remarkable capacity for reception, storage, and analysis of diverse and complexly associated information.

e. The flexible, self-adjusting capacity for refinement of the processing capabilities of the nervous system confers the ability of our species to represent complex language structures. This self-adjusting capacity also allows humans to develop high-speed reading abilities, and remarkably varied complex modern-era motor abilities, and abstract logic structures characteristic of a mathematician, software engineer, or philosopher. This nervous system refinement also creates elaborate, idiosyncratic, experience-based behavioral abilities in all of us.

How Are Learning Sequences Controlled? What Constrains Learning Progressions?

Perhaps the most important basis of control of learning progressions is representational consolidation. Through specialization, the trained cortex creates progressively more specific and more salient distributed representations of behaviorally important inputs. Growing representational salience increases the power of a cortical area to effectively drive change wherever outputs from this evolving cortical processing machinery are distributed (e.g., in "higher system levels distributed and coordinated [synchronized] responses" more powerfully drive downstream Hebbian-based plasticity changes).

A second powerful basis for sequenced learning is progressive myelination. At the time of birth, only the core "primary" extrinsic information entry zones (A-1, S-I, V-1) in the cortex are heavily myelinated.[208,209] Across childhood, connections to and interconnections between cortical areas are progressively myelinated, proceeding from these core areas out to progressively "higher" system levels. Myelination in the posterior parietal, anterior, and inferior temporal and prefrontal cortical areas is not "mature" in the human forebrain until 8 to 20 years of age. Even in the mature state, it is far less developed at the "highest" processing levels.

Myelination controls the conduction times and therefore the temporal dispersions of input sources to and within cortical areas. Poor myelination at "higher" levels in the young brain is associated with temporally diffuse inputs. They cannot generate reliable representational constructs of an adult quality because they do not as effectively engage input-coincidence–based Hebbian plasticity mechanisms. That ensures, in effect, that plasticity is not enabled for complex combinatorial processing until "lower" level input repertoires are consolidated (i.e., become stable, statistically reliable forms).

Although myelination is thought to be genetically programmed, some scientists hypothesize that myelination in the CNS is also controlled by emerging temporal response coherence and is achieved through temporally coordinated signaling from the multiple branches of oligodendrocytes that terminate on different projection axons in central tracts and networks. It has been argued that central myelination is positively and negatively activity dependent and that distributed synchronization may contribute to positive change.[210] If the hypothesis that coherent activity controls myelination proves to be true, then the emerging temporal correlation of distributed representations of behaviorally important stimuli is generated level by level. This is done by changes in coupling in local cortical networks in the developing cortex. It would also directly drive changes in myelination for the outputs of that cortical area. These two events in turn would enable the generation of reliable and salient representational constructs at that higher level. By this kind of progression, skill learning is hypothesized to directly control progressive functional and physical brain development through the course of child development. This is accomplished both by refining ("maturing") local interconnections through response dynamics of information processing machinery at successive cortical levels and by coordinated refinement ("maturing") of the critical information transmission pathways that interconnect different processing levels.

Another constraint in the development of neural adaptation may be the development of mature sleeping patterns, especially within the first year of life.[211] Sleep both enables the strengthening of learning-based plastic changes and resets the learning machinery by "erasing" temporary unreinforced and unrewarded input-generated changes produced over the preceding waking period.[212-214] The dramatic shift in the percentage of time spent in rapid-eye-movement sleep is consistent with a strong early bias toward noise removal in an immature and poorly functionally unorganized brain. Sleep patterns change dramatically in the older child, in parallel with a strong increase in its daily schedule of closely attended, rewarded, and goal-oriented behaviors. This research will need to be explored in greater detail when these data are related to patients with CNS damage. This population often has poor breathing habits and capabilities that lead to decreased oxygenation and often broken sleep cycles. How much either impairment breakdown or the interaction of the two diminishes neuroplasticity has yet to be determined.

Top-down modulation controlling attentional windows and learned predictions (expectations and behavioral goals) must all be constructed by learning. Delays in goal development could also create an important constraint for the progression of early learning. In the very young brain, prediction and error-estimation processes would be weakened because stored higher-level information repertoires are ill formed and statistically unreliable. As the brain matures, stored information progressively more strongly and reliably enables top-down attentional and predictive controls, progressively providing a stronger basis for success and error signaling for modulatory control nuclei and progressively enabling top-down syntactic feedback to increase representational reliability.

Attention, reward and punishment, accuracy of achievement of goals, and error feedback gate learning through a modulatory control system are critical for learning. The modulatory control systems that enable learning are also plastic, with their process of maturation providing constraint or facilitation for progressive learning. These subcortical nuclei are signaled by complex information feedback from the cortex itself. The salience and specificity of that feedback information grows over time. The ability to provide accurate error judging or goal-achievement signaling must grow progressively. The nucleus basalis, nucleus accumbens, ventral tegmentum, and locus coeruleus must undergo their own functional self-organization on the basis of Hebbian plasticity principles to achieve "mature" modulatory selectivity and power. The progressive maturation of the modulatory control system occurs naturally with development or training. This system can provide another important constraint on skill development progression and regulation of axial/trunk postural and balance control and fine-motor coordination.

What Facilitates the Development of Permanent "Automatic" Motor Behaviors?

The creation and maintenance of cortical representations are functions of the animal's or human's level of attention at a task. Cortical representational plasticity in skill acquisition is self-limiting. Because the behavior comes to be more "automatic," it is less closely attended and representational changes induced in the cortex fade and ultimately disappear or reverse (unlearning effects).[215,216] The element of behavioral performance that enables maintenance of the behavior with minimum involvement of the cortical learning machinery is probably stereotypical movement sequence repetition. As a movement behavior is practiced, an effective, highly statistically predictable movement sequence is adopted that enables the storage of the learned behavior in a permanent form that requires only minimal or no behavioral attention. If behavioral performance declines or behavioral or brain conditions change to render a task more difficult, attention to the behavior will again need to increase, producing an invigorated cortical response to the new learning challenge.

By this view, the cerebral cortex is clearly a learning machine. William James[217] was the first to point out that the great practical advantage for a self-organizing cortex was the development of what he called "habits." When a skill is overlearned, it will engage pathways that are so reliable that they can be followed without attention.

Why are some habits retained and others lost? Can sensorimotor learning be sustained when the adaptive representations of the learned behavior "fade" in the cerebral cortex? These areas have not been well researched. However, there are several possibilities. Habits could come to be represented in an enduring form extracortically. The cortex could modify processing in the spinal cord, the basal ganglia, red nucleus, or the cerebellum. For example, the learning of manual skills requires a motor cortex, but overlearned motor skills may not be significantly reduced by the induction of a wide area 4 lesion.

Another possibility is that behaviorally induced cortical changes endure in a highly efficient representational form that can sustain the representation of its key features on the cortex itself, engaging only limited distributed populations of cortical neurons to represent the behavior with high fidelity. Thus, recall of past learning may take less time to restructure than to reformat entirely new learning, whether it be a cognitive or motor task. The fact that a monkey improves discriminative abilities or movement performance after modifying the cortical neuron response with heavily practiced behaviors supports this alternative. However, many behaviors, such as musical performance, require constant, attended practice at a highly cognitive level to maintain both the representational changes and the performance. It also appears that continued learning with heavily practiced behaviors may be neuroprotective with aging, maintaining function despite loss of cortical neurons as a natural part of aging.

Summary

Over the years, learning has been tied to critical periods of development. Particularly in terms of language, it was assumed that if a particular skill or behavior was not accomplished during the critical period, the opportunity to acquire that skill had been lost. Although learning progression is heightened during certain periods, learning is not limited to that period alone.

Development actually refers to a process of neural and behavioral self-organization resulting from a physiological and developmental maturation of the nervous system. However, with increasing interaction with the environment, the brain changes its capacity from a simple to an incredibly specialized representational machine that is adapted to meet the specific inputs that engage it. Language is probably one of the most sophisticated examples of a specialized process at multiple levels. First, the brain has to learn to put meaning into words. Over time one is exposed to millions of English words although one may not consciously understand all of them. Yet, as an individual grows, attends school, and continues to interact in more sophisticated interactions, the brain adapts and develops massive, language-specific specialization.

The beauty of the brain is that as it self-organizes it also stores the contents of its learning, creating a foundation that increases in depth and breadth until it can begin to make predictions on even novel inputs to facilitate acute and efficient operations. The earlier the exposure occurs, the easier it is for the competitive neuronal processes to adapt and to make extensive connections. With growing neuronal specificity and salience, more powerful predictions are continued until there is greater learning and mastery.

Probably the most important thing that has been learned during the twentieth century is that the brain is a learning machine that operates throughout life. The aging process can take a toll on the ability to store information and may reduce both the complexity of the information that is processed and that individual's ability to remember. If an individual is conscious of good hydration and balanced nutrition and regularly engages in goal-directed activities that include intimate interactions with the environment and with people, then CNS pathways of representation and prediction can not only be preserved but also continue to adapt. Continuing to engage neuronal populations also has the potential to slow down the aging process. Thus, although the critical period can be viewed as developing more power specialization in the cortex, cortical plasticity does not shut down after the critical period. Instead, at times other than the critical period, therapists may well be driving improvements in individuals who have abnormalities in development or in whom abnormalities develop as a result of injury or disease.

It is now known that learning is not necessarily specifically staged. Rather, complex abilities develop more from systems interaction and integration. Therapists must develop the ability to determine what inputs are reliable and salient and which most effectively create functional and physical brain maturation, adaptation, and learning. As an individual continues to gather information, the nervous system adapts. In the face of different types of challenges (structural, emotional, pathological), clinicians must develop more effective strategies that can be used to facilitate neural adaptation, learning, substitution, and representational changes that will allow individuals to maintain meaningful function despite anatomical or physiological variances in structure.

To meet the conditions of neural adaptability, behaviors must be attended, repetitive, goal directed, integrated into functional activities, progressed in difficulty, and carried out over time with an increasing number of coincident events. Although strong behavioral events can be associated with measurable neural adaptability, new, more permanent neural connections and synapses must be strengthened with repetition and increased complexity. Clients with CNS disorders may have damaged certain areas of the brain, which may not recover; however, with learning-based activities it is possible to reorganize the brain, stimulate neurons from adjacent areas, establish new synapses and dendritic pathways,[218] and activate neurons in the contralateral, uninjured parts of the brain.[219-225] Creating the best environment to learn a skill may initially need to be contrived, with limitations controlled externally by the therapist's hands or clinical arena. In time, those limitations must be eliminated and variability within the natural environment reintroduced to obtain true learning and ultimate neuroplasticity.

The elements of neuroscience research on neural adaptation have been summarized into ten principles to guide rehabilitation programs designed to facilitate experience-dependent plasticity.[73,98,226] These principles, outlined in Table 9-1, are similar to those suggested by Nudo[131] as well as Byl et al.[227] Although these principles are particularly relevant to patients with a head injury, they are also relevant for aging adults[228-231] and those with neurodegenerative disease. These principles are not meant to be exhaustive or mutually exclusive but to highlight the principles of experience-dependent plasticity. However, they can serve as a reference for therapists who are designing creative intervention programs based on the translation of basic science to clinical practice and to help organize the extensive research neuroplasticity.

These principles can be applied across a broad range of exercises, not just "brain exercises" to improve cognition and intellect but also physical exercise. For example, we know that brain derivative neural factor (BDNF) is necessary for learning. BDNF decreases with aging, is severely reduced in animals with dementia, and can be increased with physical exercise.[232,233] Although learning-based exercises have the greatest effect during development, we know that physical and learning-based exercises can positively enhance brain plasticity in the elderly. Further, it is clear that timing of enrichment (e.g., mental stimulation, physical exercise, sensory and motor training) is important. Initiating an exercise program too early (e.g., acute post neural injury) may be associated with an exaggeration of cellular injury,[234] but waiting too long to intervene can limit the efficacy of the learning-based training experience.[235] It also appears that the efficacy of learning-based training may be enhanced with cortical stimulation[236] and repetitive transmagnetic stimulation (TMS).[237] Finally, it is critical to create a positive foundation to maximize learning (e.g., good hydration to maximize blood flow and oxygenation of tissues, adequate nutrition to energize the body, positive expectations). Rehabilitation specialists are in a great position to translate basic neuroscience into practice. However, to do this, it will be necessary for rehabilitation professionals to participate in clinical research, serve as advocates for patients and as access to appropriate rehabilitative services, and to be politically active to promote changes in health care policy to better care for patients with neural injury and those with neurodegenerative diseases.

To provide adequate repetition and learning, rehabilitation programs must include strong, carefully outlined home programs. Therapists need to invest significant time in educating patients and their families about the principles of neuroplasticity to empower them to continue to create progressive learning activities. Patients should come back periodically to see the therapist to discuss ways to continue to encourage learning. Patients must become their own best therapist. They must be motivated to continue to challenge themselves with progressive, attended behavioral activities that get integrated into functional activities. Individuals must work hard to avoid learning negative patterns of movement and behaviors that degrade the neuronal response as opposed to enriching it. It is also critical for learning to be engaging and fun. Learning should be an excuse to travel to new places and learn new skills. As we age, every day should include a new learning experience. Learning may not only be neuroprotective but could be critical for slowing down the natural neurodegenerative aspects of aging. Computer game–like activities may be an ideal mechanisms for reinforcing daily learning-based activities at home. Technology including robotics, electronic stimulations, auditory feedback systems, sensory devices, video displays, and virtual reality devices should be considered to facilitate repetition and correct patterns of movement.

The maximum attainment of skilled performance cannot necessarily be determined. The original injury can only be used as an estimate of the damage with some indicators for prognosis and recovery. The rest of the success of rehabilitation and restoration of function will reside with the motivation and commitment of the individual. See Box 9-2 for a summary of functional outcomes. How that motivation and commitment is initially established and continually reinforced is based on the patient, the therapist's interactive skills and emotional bond (see Chapter 4), and the family and support system surrounding the client (see Chapter 5).

INTERVENTION STRATEGIES

Functional Training

Functional training is a method of retraining the motor system using repetitive practice of functional tasks in an attempt to re-establish the client's ability to perform ADLs. This method of training is a common and popular intervention strategy used by clinicians owing to the fact that it is a relatively simple and straightforward approach to improving deficits in function. Because of its inherent simplicity, functional training is sometimes misused or abused by clinicians, often leading to additional problems for the client. The clinician is therefore advised to use a sound diagnostic process before making the decision to approach a specific clinical problem or condition through the use of functional training.

In Chapter 8 the steps involved in the examination process were explained in detail and the intricate relationship of impairments, functional activities and limitations, and participation in the rehabilitation process and life were discussed. Functional training can be implemented once the clinician has identified the client's functional limitations. The clinician must first answer the question "What can the client do?" followed by the question: "What limitations does the client have when engaging in functional activities?" Once these functional tasks have been identified, the clinician can proceed to guide the client in performing and practicing these difficult tasks.

The Effect of Functional Training on Task Performance and Participation

The main focus of functional training is the correction of functional limitations that prevent an individual from

BOX 9-2 ■ TREATMENT SUGGESTIONS*

GENERAL BODY RESPONSES LEADING TO RELAXATION

1. Slow rocking
2. Slow anterior-posterior: horizontal or vertical movement (chair, hassock, mesh net, swing, ball bolster, carriage)
3. Rocking bed or chair
4. Slow linear movements, such as in a carriage, stroller, wheelchair, or wagon
5. Therapeutic or gymnastic ball

TECHNIQUES TO HEIGHTEN POSTURAL EXTENSORS

1. Rapid anterior-posterior or angular acceleration
   a. Scooter board: pulled or projected down inclines
   b. Prone over ball: rapid acceleration forward
   c. Platform or mesh net: prone
   d. Slides
2. Rapid anterior-posterior motion in prone, weight-bearing patterns such as on elbows or extended elbows while rocking and crawling
3. Weight-shifting in kneeling, half kneel, or standing

FACILITORY TECHNIQUES INFLUENCING WHOLE-BODY RESPONSES

1. Movement patterns in specific sequences
   a. Rolling patterns
   b. On elbows, extended elbows, and crawling: side by side, linear and angular motion
2. Spinning
   a. Mesh net
   b. Sit and spin toy
   c. Office chair on universal joint
3. Any motor program that uses acceleration and deceleration of head
   a. Sitting and reaching
   b. Walking
   c. Running
   d. Moving from sit to stand

COMBINED FACILITORY AND INHIBITORY TECHNIQUE: INVERTED TONIC LABYRINTHINE

1. Semiinverted in-sitting
2. Squatting to stand
3. Total inverted vertical position

---

*Remember that all these treatment suggestions involve other input mechanisms and all aspects of the motor system and its components.

---

ion during transfer training will effectively place the ankles in functional positions. The act of standing also facilitates the trunk and neck extensors to affect postural control. Varying the speed of the activity during the treatment will stimulate cerebellar adaptation to the movement task. Moving from one position to another and with the head in a variety of positions stimulates the vestibular apparatus and may assist in habituating a hypersensitive vestibular system and allow the client to change body positions, resulting in a higher quality of life. Repetitive practice also affects the vasomotor system and may assist in habituating postural hypotensive responses.

If the presence of a particular functional problem can be explained as being caused by a specific impairment, then correcting the impairment may correct the problem. For example, if it was determined that a client's inability to stand up from the sitting position was caused by the presence of lower extremity weakness, then lower extremity strengthening exercises need to be targeted during therapeutic intervention. It is difficult to predict, however, whether lower extremity strengthening alone will create improved lower extremity function. The strengthening intervention selected should reflect the task and the environment within which the impairment was identified. Training within this context should facilitate the correction of the functional problem. The clinician should attempt to create a training situation so that the client may be able to run the necessary motor programs with all of the necessary subsystems in place. In this example, training the lower extremities using cuff weights is much less likely to automatically result in the improvement of sit-to-stand function than if the strength training was performed with repetition of practice in a functional activity of sit-to-stand. That is, it may be better to train the sit-to-stand pattern using various surface heights that closely resemble the same motor pattern to train the systems in the appropriate synergies, posture, and environment in which they are required to function than to perform strengthening exercises against resistant in an open-chain exercise program.

The decision to treat the impairments causing the activity/task limitations or to correct the functional problems themselves is influenced by a myriad of factors. It would appear that for certain tasks to be completed the client must possess a "threshold amount" of basic components to perform the task if movement is to be possible. These components include such factors as cognitive ability and motivation. Having the client control a pattern with use of a functional motor task within a narrow biomechanical window at first, then widening this window as motor learning improves, would be one way to use functional training and augmented impairment correction simultaneously. The therapist must accept that, when the biomechanical window is narrowed, the functional treatment intervention is controlled by the therapist and augmented to allow the client to succeed and correct errors within a limited environment. In this situation the patient is functionally training with environmental limitations. Without correcting these components, it would be impossible for the clinician to achieve any functional improvement. Moreover, if the clinician attempts to have the client run the entire motor program outside the available "normal" window by providing extrinsic assistance to enable the client to perform the task, the resulting movement is often minimally functional, if not unsafe for

participating in life. However, through repetitive practice of functional tasks and gross motor patterns, many of the client's impairments will also be affected. For example, if a therapist practices sit-to-stand transfers with a client in a variety of environments and performs multiple repetitions of each type of transfer, not only will learning be reinforced, but the client will also gain strength in the synergistic patterns of the lower extremities that work against gravity to concentrically lift the client off of the support surface and eccentrically lower him or her down. Weight bearing through the feet in a variety of degrees of ankle dorsiflex-

the client. Without analyzing impairments and their effect on function and only running functional training in distorted and abnormal patterns, this method of "intervention" may also have the potential of resulting in more impairments or functional problems in the future.

A good example of this is the "nag-and-drag" method of gait training in the parallel bars. This method finds the therapist literally dragging the client through the length of the parallel bars in an attempt to elicit some sort of movement response from the client. The therapist then labels this procedure "gait training." Clearly, this approach will result in the client eventually learning dysfunctional, inefficient motor programs. Before long, as the client learns to run these dysfunctional programs procedurally, the clinician will realize that he or she has created a bigger problem that may require a considerable amount of time and resources to undo the damage that was created by limiting the available movement strategies, limiting the variability within practice, and ultimately restricting the plasticity of the nervous system. Similarly, forcing the axial trunk musculature to compensate for lack of motor control within the elbow and wrist will result in dysfunctional upper extremity movement patterns.

Concept of Clinical Pathways

Another intervention approach that evolved as an offshoot of functional training is clinical pathways. These pathways have been established by health care institutions for many medical diagnoses to ensure consistency of practice between medical professionals, to ensure that all of a client's needs are met in a timely manner, and to facilitate discharge and maximize independence in the shortest amount of time possible. In the rehabilitation setting these pathways are time lines with corresponding "milestones" in the patient's functional progress. Figure 9-7 presents an example of one pathway.

These pathways assist the facility by reducing the amount of paperwork generated per client case. Charting is generally done by exception, rather than by narration. If the pathway is followed and the client stays on track with predetermined plans, then the component parts of the pathway are simply checked off. If the patient deviates from the primary pathway or has a complicating event that occurs during the duration of recovery, then the patient "falls off the pathway" and is handled according to a compilation of signs and symptoms that is generally customary for that clinical setting. The concept of clinical pathways works well for predictable diseases, diagnoses, and surgical procedures that follow a generally uncomplicated rehabilitation pathway, such as total joint arthroplasty, coronary angioplasty, and mild stroke. It becomes more difficult to predict the course of recovery and the functional outcomes when the disease or pathological condition is progressive, degenerative, or chronic, such as an exacerbation of multiple sclerosis or in the presence of neoplasms or after a severe insult to the CNS. Clinical pathways should never be used as a justification for denying care to a particular patient. When the patient is unable to follow a normal clinical pathway, the clinician should identify the unique factors in the patient's physical and medical functioning that prevent her or him from following a more "traditional" path of functional progress. As more and more institutions use the concept of clinical pathways as an essential and viable approach to the management

of the patient, there is a need to evaluate the outcomes after these pathways to ensure efficacy of the particular intervention strategy.

Selection of Functional Training Strategies

The question exists: what is the "ideal" procedure for effectively and efficiently using functional training as a treatment intervention? First, it is suggested that the clinician identify and select procedures that will use the client's strengths to regain lost function and correct impairments—"What can the client do?" The clinician is also advised to avoid activities that may be too difficult and elicit compensation strategies that may result in the development of abnormal, stereotypical movement and potentially create additional impairments. The therapist's decision regarding what functional patterns or activities to practice, and in what order, will depend on several factors. The therapist must choose functional activities that are necessary for the client to obtain independence before being discharged home or managed with less help. For PTs, safe transfers and ambulation are generally the functional activities that are focused on in this case. For OTs, independent bathing, dressing, and feeding are major foci. Yet both professionals also need to decide the activities that the patient or the patient's family wants to improve to enhance the quality of life for everyone involved in the person's case. The ability to get in and out of a car might be the most important activity for the client to learn because he or she needs to make frequent trips to the physician's office.

Last, it is suggested that the clinician modify or "shrink" the environment to allow normal motor programs to run. The environment can be progressively "enlarged" to allow the client to perform the activity in a functional context. Although this narrowing of the functional environment would be considered a contrived environment and must not be recorded as functional as defined in a functional/activities-based examination, it may allow the nervous system the opportunity to control and modify the motor programs within the limitations of its plasticity at the moment. As learning and repetition assist the CNS in widening the response pattern during a functional activity, the client's ability to respond to variance within the environment will enlarge and assist in gaining greater independence. An example of this application might be training a client to squat to pick up an object such as a shoe from the floor (stand-to-sit transfer). The client is first guided down to sitting onto a large ball or high-low table that only allows the client to sit one fourth to one half of the way down before returning to stand. As the client develops increased strength and balance and improved control over abnormal limb synergies and tone in this pattern, then a smaller ball or a lower point on a high-low table can be used. Finally, the client is asked to sit down on a ball that results in a 90-degree knee/hip angle or onto a chair. Once the client can sit down and regain a vertical position, the next task will be to sit down, relax, and then stand up. Once that activity is done easily, the client will be functional in sit-to-stand and reversing the movement pattern.

Although many clinicians understand the importance of running motor tasks within an appropriate biomechanical/musculoskeletal/sensorimotor window in which the client has the ability to perform procedures functionally, it may be argued that in many cases this particular type of treatment

UCLA MEDICAL CENTER
Name: Ischemic Stroke, Pathway 2, Severe Motor Deficit, Likely d/c to Rehab or Nursing Facility
Physician: ____
Case Manager/CNS: ____
Chief Resident: ____

ADDRESSOGRAPH

Indicators	Admit to: Neurology Service 0 to 12 Hours Post Onset	Day 1 12-72 Hours Post Onset	Day 2	Day 3	Day 4	Day 5	Day 6
MD Responsibilities	Immediately notify Stroke Team for hyperacute therapy evaluation; Notify Primary Care MD; Detailed physical/neurologic exam, history, review labs	Notify Primary Care MD*; Patient exam, review all labs; Discuss probable d/c date and needs with pt/family	Pt exam, review labs; Discuss Rehab/SNF placement with family	Pt exam, review labs; Arrange primary care, neuro f/up; Write d/c prescriptions	Pt exam, review labs; Arrange primary care, neuro f/up if d/c; Write prescriptions if d/c home or dictate d/c summary if d/c rehab/SNF	Patient exam, review all labs; Arrange primary care, neuro f/up if d/c; Write prescriptions if d/c home or dictate d/c summary if d/c rehab/SNF	Pt exam, review labs; Arrange primary care, neuro f/up; dictate d/c summary for rehab/SNF
Monitoring	VS/Neuro q 2 hours; Cardiac monitor; Strict I&Os	VS/Neuro q 2 hours; Daily weight; Cardiac monitor; Strict I&Os	VS/Neuro q 4 hours; Cardiac monitor, prn; Strict I&Os	VS/Neuro q 4 hours; Strict I&Os; Daily weight	VS/Neuro q 4 hours; Daily weight; Strict I&Os	VS/Neuro q 4 hours; Strict I&Os	VS/Neuro q 4 hours
Assessment	Nursing assess skin integrity, Assess for fall risk, aspiration risk, assess for usual bowel pattern	Assess for potential discharge needs	Assess for discharge options		Physicians assess need for daily weights	Physicians assess need for Strict I&Os	
Diagnostic/Lab	CXR, ECG, CBC, platelets, PT/PTT, lytes, BUN, creat, gluc, CPK, U/A; Additional Labs; Module #6: Neuroimaging	Module #6: Neuroimaging; Module #7: Carotid Duplex; Module #8: Cardiac ECHO; ECG, CXR, CBC, platelets, PT/PTT, lytes, BUN, creat, gluc, U/A; Module #1: Additional Labs	Fasting lipid panel; Module #6: Neuroimaging; Module #7: Carotid Duplex; Module #8: Cardiac ECHO				
Treatment/ Medications/IV	IV NS with 20meq KCl at 100 cc/hr; Thrombolysis protocol if qualifies; Module #2: Antithrombotics; Tylenol, prn, MOM, pm; Module #3: DVT prophylaxis; Pressure ulcer prevention protocol; Straight cath q 8 hr, pm; Seizure/aspiration/fall precautions	IV NS with 20meq KCl at 100 cc/hr, if indicated; Module #2: Antithrombotics; Tylenol, prn, MOM, pm; Module #3: DVT Prophylaxis; Straight cath q 8 hr, pm; Guaiac all stools; ROM q 8 hours	Module #2: Antithrombotics; Tylenol, prn, MOM, pm; Module #3: DVT Prophylaxis; Straight cath q 8 hr, pm; Guaiac all stools; ROM q 8 hours	Module #2: Antithrombotics; Tylenol, prn, MOM, pm; Module #3: DVT Prophylaxis; Straight cath q 8 hr, pm; Guaiac all stools; ROM q 8 hours	Module #2: Antithrombotics; Tylenol, prn, MOM, pm; Module #3: DVT Prophylaxis; Straight cath q 8 hr, pm; Guaiac all stools; ROM q 8 hours	Module #2: Antithrombotics; Tylenol, prn, MOM, pm; Module #3: DVT Prophylaxis; ROM q 8 hours	Module #2: Antithrombotics; Tylenol, prn, MOM, pm; Module #3: DVT Prophylaxis; ROM q 8 hours
Nutrition	NPO	Module #4: Dysphagia Assessment; Module #5: Diet Orders	Assess and advance as tolerated	Assess and advance as tolerated	Assess and advance as tolerated	Assess and advance as tolerated	Assess and advance as tolerated
Activity/Safety	Bedrest with head of bed ↑30°	Bedrest with head of bed ↑30°; Bathroom privileges after 24 hours, if patient safe to ambulate	OOB to chair, advance as tolerated	Advance as tolerated, advance as	Advance as tolerated	Advance as tolerated	Advance as tolerated
Education	Orient to 7West routine	Begin discharge teaching if appropriate: activity and meds; Begin stroke education program; Discharge planning	Discharge teaching activity and meds; Discharge options	Advance stroke education program; Discharge teaching	Advance stroke education program; Discharge teaching	Advance stroke education program; Discharge teaching	Advance stroke education program; Discharge teaching; Complete discharge teaching, provide appropriate hand-outs and follow-up appointments
Consults	PT, OT, Speech, pm; CNS Case Manager; Neurology if not neuro primary; Cardiology and Infect. Disease, pm	PT, OT, Speech, pm; CNS Case Manager; Discharge Planner; Social Worker, pm; Neuro Rehab Team; Neurology if not Neuro primary; Cardiology and Infect. Dis., pm	CNS Case Manager; Neurology if not Neuro primary; Cardiology and Infect. Dis., pm; Home Health Liaison, pm	CNS Case Manager; Neurology if not Neuro primary; Cardiology and Infect. Dis., pm; Home Health Liaison, pm	CNS Case Manager; Neurology if not Neuro primary; Cardiology and Infect. Dis., pm	CNS Case Manager; Neurology if not Neuro primary; Cardiology and Infect. Dis., pm	CNS Case Manager; Neurology if not Neuro primary; Cardiology and Infect. Dis., pm
Expected Outcomes	Initial assessment of stroke etiology concluded; Research protocol initiated; Adequate hydration maintained; Pt/family will verbalize usual hospital routine	Initial assessment of stroke etiology concluded; Adequate hydration maintained; No S&S of decreased bodily function; Pt/family will verbalize stroke definition, likely cause of own stroke; PTT in target range, if applicable; PT/OT/Speech Therapy evals initiated	Stroke etiology clarified; Adequate hydration maintained; No S&S of decreased bodily function; Pt/family will verbalize risk factors for stroke, s/s TIA and stroke; PTT in target range, if applicable; PT/OT/Speech Therapy evals complete, therapy initiated; Pt/family verbalize safe d/c plan	Long term stroke prevention strategy selected; Adequate hydration maintained; No S&S of decreased bodily function; Pt/family demonstrate progress in stroke education program; Pt/family verbalize safe d/c plan; PTT in target range, if applicable	Long term stroke prevention strategy selected; Adequate hydration maintained; No S&S of decreased bodily function; Pt/family demonstrate progress in stroke education program; PTT in target range, if applicable; Bowel and bladder program established; If discharged, all expected outcomes on Day 6 must be met	Pt/family demonstrate progress in stroke education program; Adequate hydration maintained; No S&S of decreased bodily function; PTT in target range, if applicable; If discharged, all expected outcomes on Day 6 must be met	Pt participates in ADLs with assistance; Pt can tolerate OOB and sit in chair 2 consecutive hours; Pt can tolerate 2-3 hours/day of acute rehab, if applicable; Pt/family understand and support rehab/SNF goals; Pt/family know facility to which patient will go, approx LOS, plan for Home Care upon d/c; Pt/family can state S&S of TIA/stroke, risk factors of stroke; Pt/family can state when to notify physician, activity restrictions, f/up appointments
Shift RN Signature	AM Admit; D.; N.	D.; N.	D.; N.	D.; N.	D.; N.	D.; N.	D.; N.
Initial/ Signature	___/___	___/___	___/___	___/___	___/___	___/___	___/___

FIGURE 9-7 ■ Example of critical pathway. (Copyright February 1996, Regents of the University of California [UCLA Clinical Effectiveness]. Adapted with permission.)

strategy is simply not possible in a real-world situation. For example, given the current health care environment, if the client is given a limited number of visits to achieve the desired outcome, the clinician may conclude that there is no choice but to "allow as many degrees of freedom as possible" or, in other words, to "force the window open" no matter the abnormal movement patterns used or the limitations in independent functional control that they may produce.

In summary, the clinician should first identify and emphasize the client's strengths ("What can the client do?") and use those strengths to efficiently and effectively achieve functional change. Next, the clinician must prioritize what systems or activities the client truly needs to change. The choice of what activities to emphasize during therapeutic training always poses a dilemma to therapists. Although it may be ideal for the client to eventually be able to ambulate independently on all surfaces without any assistance or reach for any object in and from any spatial position, it may be more important initially for the client to be able to safely transfer from the bed to the wheelchair, sit independently while someone assists with dressing, or walk and transfer onto and off of the commode independently at home. One should keep in mind that, although several skills may be learned by training them simultaneously, it may make more sense to concentrate on the safe performance of one or two necessary functional tasks rather than to end up being able to perform multiple tasks that require considerable outside assistance for safety. The need to work functionally on additional activities may also be an opportunity for the clinician to request additional therapy visits for the client, arguing that there is a reasonable expectation that more intervention would result in an increase in function and a decrease in the risk for potential injury than if the intervention were not continued. The use of valid and reliable functional outcome measures becomes critically important in case management. These tools objectively measure the effect of the intervention, help predict the potential risks if the therapy is not continued, and ultimately aid in the justification to continue therapeutic intervention.

CASE STUDY ■ BED MOBILITY

Teaching the client to roll in bed can be approached in a variety of ways to accomplish the goal. The entire rolling pattern may be practiced with enough assistance for the client to be able to accomplish the goal, but little enough such that the client must use the maximum amount of power and ROM available in key movement patterns.

ROLLING IN BED

The patient is a 73-year-old man, status post ischemic infarct in the frontoparietal cortex with resultant left hemiplegia, hemisensory deficit, and left homonymous hemianopia. The patient demonstrates visual-spatial inattention to the left environment. The client must learn to roll independently in bed for comfort and function. An example of a treatment session aimed at reaching the goal of independent rolling to the right and left may include the following sequence of activities: (1) begin in side lying on one side; (2) ask patient to tip back a few degrees and then return to the side-lying position; and (3) progressively increase the degree the patient must roll backward, assisting him as needed. By the end of several repetitions the patient may be rolling from supine to side lying.

Conclusion

Often, clients with neurological trauma or disease cannot begin therapy with functional training because of the degree and extent of both impairments and disabilities within the sensory cortices or the limbic or motor systems. Therapists must then choose augmented therapeutic interventions that externally guide the client's learning through hands-on and environmentally controlled treatment techniques. It is again cautioned that the therapist never consider these interventions as the client demonstrating functional independence because the individual's success is based on external control of the environment and not on internal self-regulation by the client. The clinician must continually strive to transfer that control to the client by widening the window of independence and limiting the hands-on or verbal guidance used during therapy.

One important variable that has clearly been identified with respect to functional training is "task specificity."[238-247] Although it is important that a patient be independent in as many ADLs as possible, often a therapist along with a patient and the family needs to prioritize which of these activities are most important to the quality of life of the patient. If walking into the mountains to do "bird watching" is one important goal to the patient, then creating an environment that would closely resemble the environment of that activity is crucial. Similarly, practice within that environment is a key to successful carryover. If the patient wants to walk into the mountains and the family expects him to walk into his old job, a therapist must accept that motivation will drive behavior and task specificity drive learning. Whether the patient ever goes back to work is not the variable that should be used as part of the motivational environment for task-specific training geared to walking in the mountains. Therapists need to allow the patient to tell them what will be the most important task and the specificity of that task to optimize motor learning and functional recovery.

Impairment Training

As mentioned in Chapter 8, examination results in the identification of functional limitations and possible system and subsystem impairments causing these functional movement disorders. Impairment training is another intervention strategy that involves the correction of impairments with the expectation that improving these impairments will result in a corresponding improvement in function. For example, in a client who has the inability to stand up without assistance (activity limitation) and the clinician determines that the cause of this is lower extremity weakness, an appropriate approach may be to strengthen the lower extremities (impairment training). Numerous studies have shown the effectiveness of impairment training in improving the functional performance of individuals with neurological conditions such as stroke,[248-254] multiple sclerosis,[255-257] Parkinson's disease,[258-260] and other neuromuscular diagnoses.[261-268]

The decision to provide this intervention must be predicated on a sound diagnostic process in which a reasonable expectation is made that impairment training will result in the improvement in function. Task specificity within this limited environment will result in more meaningful changes in function. Going back to the sit-to-stand example, if impairment training is the desired intervention pathway, the approach must focus on strengthening the specific muscles involved in sit-to-stand. It is important to remember, however, that the clinician must establish an environment which will still "put everything together"—that is, to go back and work with the patient on the actual sit-to-stand function. To enhance the response to impairment training, the therapist may also use augmented feedback, which will be presented in the next section. Use of hands-on facilitation or adaptive aids may improve the neuromuscular response, resulting in changes in the systems or subsystems that ultimately lead to improvement in function.

Augmented Therapeutic Intervention Classification

As discussed in the previous section, some treatment alternatives require little if any hands-on therapeutic manipulation of the client during the activity. For example, the patient practices transfers on and off many support surfaces with standby guarding only. Thus, the client self-corrects or uses inherent feedback mechanisms to self-correct error to refine the motor skill. This ultimate empowerment of the client allows each individual to adapt and succeed at self-motivated and identified objectives. Often, allowing the client to try to succeed independently enables the therapist to evaluate what components of the task the client can control and what components are not within the client's adaptable capabilities, especially if normal, fluid, efficient, and effortless movement is the desired outcome. In some cases the therapist may use hands-on skills or adaptive aids, which would augment the environment and allow the client to succeed at the task *but* would be considered contrived or noninherent feedback.

Such contrived techniques make up a large component of the therapist's specific intervention strategies. The difference between contrived and functional or intrinsic might be the need for the therapist to be part of the client's external environment for the client to succeed at the task. The therapist must recognize that as long as the therapist is part of that environment, the client is not functionally independent. Even if the client succeeds at the activity, the augmentation needed to succeed has changed the outcome, and without such intervention the patient would not have been successful. Thus, any contrived therapeutic technique or intervention must at some time be removed from the environment. The client must assume total ownership for the functional responses. Then and only then has independence been achieved. At that time, functional retraining can be used with

the intent of enlarging the environmental parameters to allow for maximal independence. Figure 9-8 illustrates this concept of functional versus contrived intervention, which must be constantly considered throughout any treatment session. At times, selecting functional activities without the use of contrived or augmented procedures may not help the patient achieve the desired outcome. Thus, contrived techniques are often the early choices for treatment. It cannot be emphasized enough that, once the client has the ability to perform without augmented methods and does so in functional, efficient ways, those techniques need to be selectively eliminated.

Although a clinician has chosen to augment the clinical environment, the client needs to learn efficient motor behaviors within the limitations of that environment. The client needs to direct the therapist's decision-making strategies by the plans selected as motor responses to a given task. If the response is effortless, efficient, and noninjurious to any part of the body and meets the client's expectations and goals, then the therapist knows the strategies selected were effective. If the response does not meet the desired goal for any reason, then the therapist must determine why. Many correct solutions may answer the question. Which solution is best may be more client than approach dependent. Yet, if flexibility means that the therapist selects any component of any method that helps the client reach an objective, then the therapist is confronted with hundreds—if not thousands—of various treatment procedures. If the treatment procedures used introduce information to the client through sensory systems, then, from a neurological perspective, a limited number of input systems or modalities are available. The myriad of treatment procedures are transduced into neurochemical and electrophysiological responses that must travel along a limited number of pathways. Thus, many different treatment procedures may produce similar types of neurotransmission. The temporal and spatial sequencing or timing of the input will vary according to the technique and the specific application. The clinician has little basis for decision making without a comprehensive understanding of the neurophysiological mechanisms of (1) the various techniques introduced to modify input, (2) the potential interactions that information will have with various connections within the CNS, (3) prior learning and ability for new learning, and (4) the client's willingness and motivation to adapt.

The number of available contrived or augmented feedback techniques is almost infinite. In this section an overview is presented of a classification system that can be used to help the reader develop a greater understanding of why certain responses occur and why the selection of certain techniques is appropriate, given the outcome expectations after intervention. This section focuses on intervention strategies accepted and used within the traditional Western health care model, whereas in Chapter 37 alternative approaches to intervention not necessarily classified as traditional within this chapter are introduced.

When considering the selection of a contrived intervention to augment sensory input, appropriate selection of specific techniques can be made by using a classification schema. The primary goal of this section is to help the reader develop such a classification system—a system based on the primary input modality used when introducing a stimulus or augmented treatment technique. The reader has been pro-

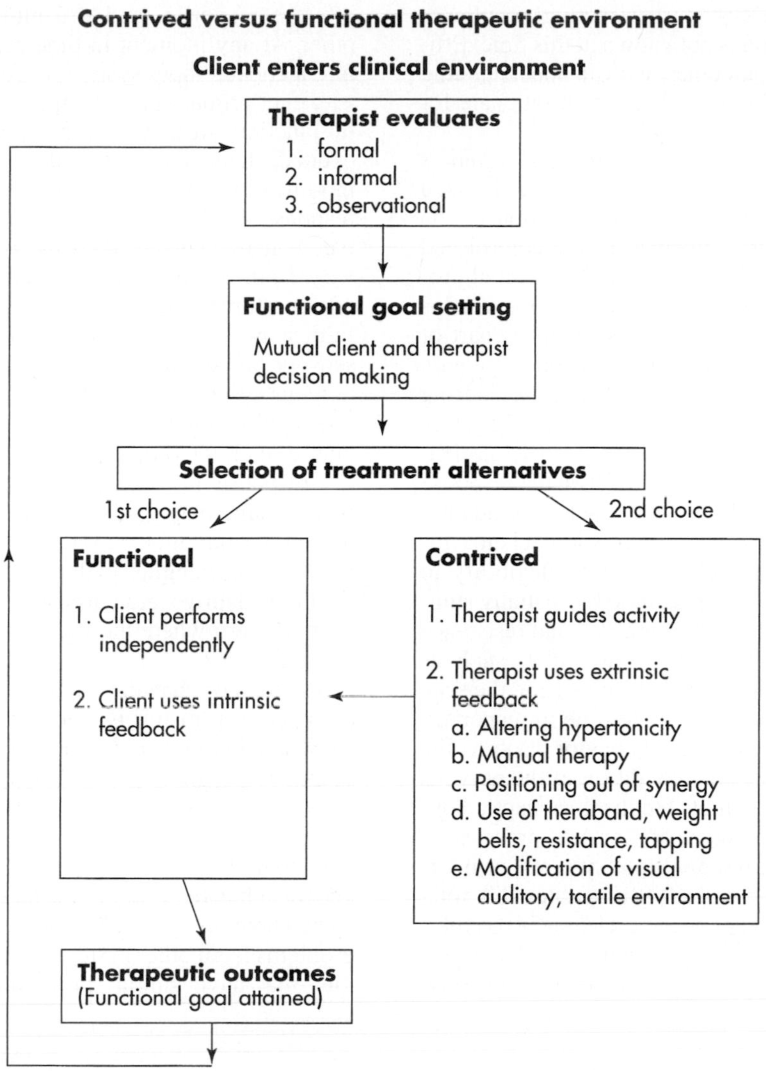

Contrived versus functional therapeutic environment

Client enters clinical environment

Therapist evaluates
1. formal
2. informal
3. observational

Functional goal setting

Mutual client and therapist
decision making

Selection of treatment alternatives

1st choice   2nd choice

Functional

1. Client performs
   independently

2. Client uses intrinsic
   feedback

Contrived

1. Therapist guides activity

2. Therapist uses extrinsic
   feedback
   a. Altering hypertonicity
   b. Manual therapy
   c. Positioning out of synergy
   d. Use of theraband, weight
      belts, resistance, tapping
   e. Modification of visual
      auditory, tactile environment

Therapeutic outcomes
(Functional goal attained)

FIGURE 9-8 ■ Contrived versus functional therapeutics. (Modified from the original work of Jan Davis, OTR, San Jose State University.)

vided with an in-depth reference to the specific neurophysiological basis behind each of these systems, and only a brief overview has been included. In-depth discussion of some basic treatment strategies, explanations of less-familiar techniques, and current approaches gaining popularity within the clinical area of movement analysis is found within the body of this section.

When the primary input system for a technique is identified, at no time do we suggest that it is the only input system affected. For example, when a proprioceptor is introduced, tactile cutaneous receptors are also simultaneously firing. If there is a "noise" component (such as with vibration), then auditory input has been triggered as well. There is evidence that a given sensory modality may "crossover" or fuse with a completely different modality, helping in the synthesis of motor responses. In addition, there is evidence that the principles of neuroplasticity are applicable across modalities (e.g., auditory, linguistic, visual, vestibular, somatosensory). Sometimes responses occur in a modality that does not appear to be related. For example, olfaction may improve tactile sensitivity of the hand. This concept is

called cross-modal training or stimulation.[269,270] Yet a classification schema based on a primary modality promotes logical problem solving because the therapist can select from available treatment procedures that theoretically provide similar information to the CNS and help in the organization of appropriate motor responses. The motor system and its various motor programmers adapt to the environment to achieve functional motor output toward a goal. Feedback is critical for adaptation and change. Feedback in this chapter is considered a mechanism to help the client's CNS optimally learn and adapt and not to facilitate a hard-wired reflexive response. Therapists must realize that even if the primary goal may be to facilitate or dampen a motor system response through multiple interlooping tracts, diverging pathways may also connect with endocrine, immune, and autonomic systems. At this time it is not known how much input leads to somatosensory remapping, which ultimately affects motor performance instead of directly affecting motor programming. According to motor control theory, the clinical picture is a consensus of all systems interacting (see Chapter 3). Research tools are not yet available to measure those systems interacting simultaneously; thus, isolated causation is not known at this time. Efficacy must then be based on outcomes, with an understanding of the best available scientific knowledge as a rationale for why the outcome is present.

Therefore, within this section, the classification system is based on identified input, observed responses, hypothesized neuromechanisms, current research on the function of the CNS, and the various systems involved in the control and modification of responses. An understanding of normal processing of input and its effect on the motor systems helps the clinician evaluate and use the intact systems as part of treatment. Research with fMRI is now helping to gain greater insight into specific brain regions being used during various cognitive and motor activities.[271-277] Yet, the specific interactive nature of multisensory input, memory, motivation and motor function is still unknown. When the response to certain stimuli does not help the client select or adapt a desired motor response, then the classification schema for augmented input provides the clinician with flexibility to select additional options. This can be done by spatially summating input, such as using stretch, vibration, and resistance simultaneously, or temporally summating input, such as increasing the rate of the quick stretch or increasing the time between inputs to give the system ample time to respond.

Many factors can influence motor behavior, such as the methods of instruction, the resting condition of the nervous system before introducing stimulus feedback, synaptic connections, cerebellar/basal ganglia or cortical processing, retrieval from past learning, motor output systems, or internal influences and balance. Figure 9-9 illustrates this total system. Its clinical implications become clearer if the therapist retains a visual image of the client's total nervous system, including afferent input, intersystem processing,

efferent response, and the multiple interactions on each other. At any moment in time multiple stimuli are admitted into a client's input system. Before that information reaches a level of primary processing, it will cross at least one synaptic junction. At that time the information may be inhibited, excited, changed or distorted, or allowed to continue without modification. If the information is inhibited, then no response will be observed, even if it were considered reflexive. If it is changed, then the processing of the input will vary from the one normally anticipated. The end product after multiple system interactions will either be close to or farther away from the desired motor pattern. Furthermore, sensory processing can take place at many segments of the nervous system. Although the CNS is not hierarchical, with one level in total control over another, certain systems are biased to affect various motor responses. At the spinal level the response may be phasic and synergistic. Brain stem mechanisms may evoke flexor or extensor biases, depending on various motor systems and their modulation. Cerebellar, basal ganglia, thalamic, and cortical responses may be more adaptive and purposeful.[278] Thus, the therapist must try to discern where the input or the feedback is being short circuited.

Remember that the same three alternatives—inhibiting (dampening), distorting, or normal processing—can occur anywhere in the system at a synaptic junction. Finally, motor output is programmed and a response is observed. If the response is considered normal, the clinician assumes that the system is intact with regard to the use and processing of the input. If the response is distorted or absent, little is known other than there is a lack of the normal processing somewhere in the CNS. One way to differentiate motor problems from other systems is to use other functional activities that have similar programs as the one identified as

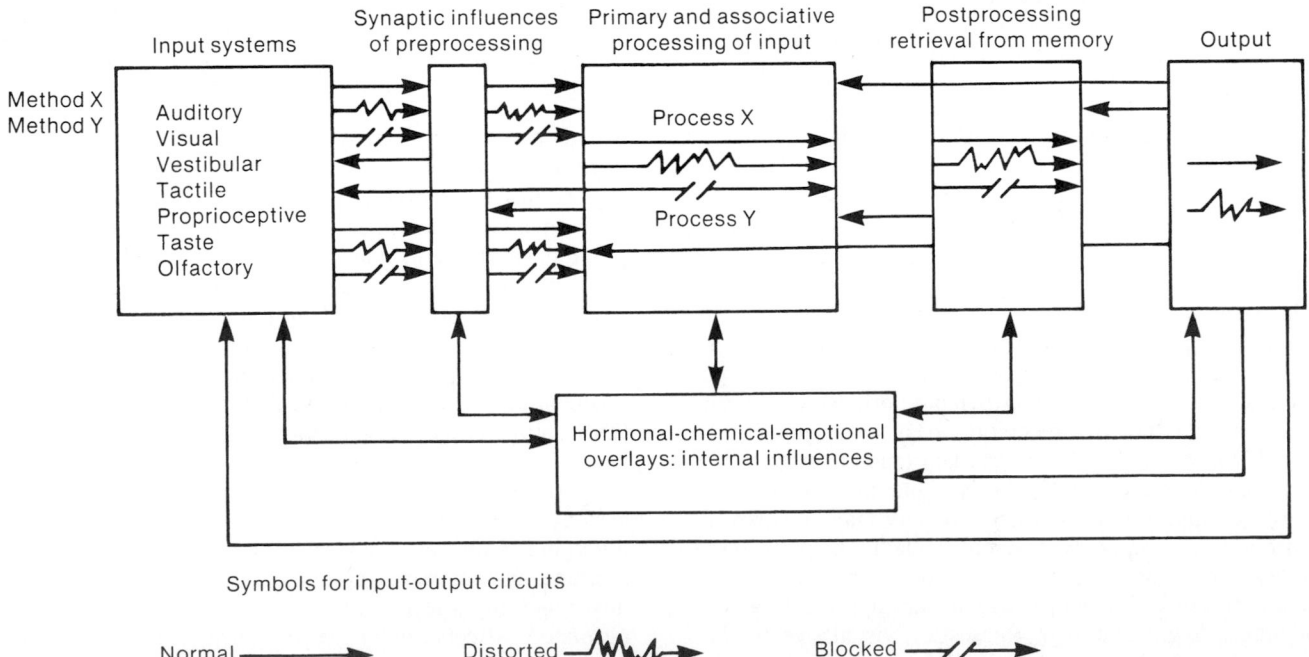

FIGURE 9-9 ■ Model of possible interactive effects among methods of treatment, input systems, processing and output systems, internal influences, and feedback systems.

impaired. If a program, such as posture, demonstrates deficiencies in other functional patterns, then it is likely that there is a motor problem. If, on the other hand, the program runs smoothly and effortlessly when certain demands are taken away, such as resistance from gravity, position in space, need for quick responses, and so forth, then it may be that the problem is within another subsystem such as perceptual/cognition, biomechanical, or cardiopulmonary. Differentially screening motor impairments as a pure CNS motor problem (strength, rate, balance) versus another system (perception of vertical) become critical in a managed-care system that only funds a certain number of treatment sessions. Internal influences also need to be considered because they affect each aspect of the system. Once normal processing is identified, understanding of deficit systems and potential problems can be analyzed more easily. To reiterate, this requires awareness of the totality of the individual, that is, the client's personal preference of stimuli and the uniqueness of processing and internal influences. A systems model requires simultaneous processing of multiple areas with interactions relaying in all directions. A client's CNS and peripheral nervous system (PNS) is doing just that, and the therapist must develop a sensitivity toward the client as a whole while interacting with specific components (see Chapters 4, 5, 6, and 37 for additional information). The classification system presented in this section will only help the reader organize one component affecting the entire clinical environment.

With input from the client and family, it is the therapist's responsibility to select methods most efficacious and effective for each client's needs. This viewpoint, based on a variety of questions, leads to a problem-oriented approach to intervention. Because the output or response pattern is based on alpha motor neuron discharge and thus extrafusal muscle contraction, the first question is posed: what can be done to alter the state of the alpha motor neuronal pool or motor generators? Second, what input systems are available, either directly or indirectly, that will alter the state of the motor pool? Third, which techniques use these various input systems as their primary modes of entry into the CNS? Fourth, what internal mechanisms need modification or adaptation to produce a desired behavior response from the client? Fifth, which input systems are available to alter the internal mechanism and what outcomes are expected? Sixth, what combination of input stimuli will provide the best internal homeostatic environment for the client to learn and rehearse a more optimal response pattern? For example, assume that a client with a residual hemiplegia resulting from a middle cerebral artery problem has a hypertonic lower extremity that produces the pattern of extension, adduction, internal rotation of the hip, extension of the knee, and plantarflexion inversion of the feet. The answers to the first two questions are based on the knowledge that the proprioceptive and exteroceptive systems can drastically affect spinal central pattern generators and that these input systems are intact at a spinal, brain stem, cerebellum, and thalamic levels and may even project to the cortex.

Appropriate selection of specific techniques—such as prolonged stretch using the tendon organ to modulate the hypertonic pattern, quick stretch or light touch to the antagonistic muscle, or any other treatment modality within the classification schema—provides viable treatment alternatives. Awareness that the client's response pattern is an inherent synergistic pattern and that it is further elicited by pressure to the ball of the foot leads to a better understanding of the clinical problem. Knowing that the client is unable to combine the alternative patterns, such as hip flexion and knee extension, needed for the latter aspects of swing through and early aspects of heel strike in gait, the therapist can use the other inherent processes to elicit these and other patterns. Body-supported treadmill training is an example of an augmented treatment intervention where the clinician assists the patient to place the leg and foot with each step to experience a normal gait pattern while needing only the strength to manage partial body weight.[279-284] Finally, techniques such as combining standing and walking with application of quick stretch, vibration, or rotation or having the client reach for a target or follow a visual stimulus while walking provide a variety of combinations of therapeutic procedures to help the client learn or relearn normal response patterns. Furthermore, this approach gives the clinician a choice of various procedures and promotes a learning environment that is flexible, changing, and interesting. The therapist must make the transition from applying contrived therapeutic procedures during functional tasks to allowing the client to practice the task without the therapist interceding with external feedback.[285] In that way the client uses inherent feedback to self-correct. This self-correction leads to independence and adaptability (see Figure 9-8).

A variety of sensory classification systems have been accepted by physiologists, neuroanatomists, and therapists. To avoid confusion about which nerve fiber is being discussed, the two primary methods of classification, along with a description of the functional component, have been included in Table 9-2 for easy referral. Each system will be presented separately to help the reader establish a classification scheme. The primary sensory input systems include proprioception, exteroception, vestibular, vision, auditory, taste, and smell. These inputs integrate pathways among the thalamus, the sensory and motor cortices, the cerebellum, the reticular formation, and the basal ganglia.

Proprioceptive System

Proprioception as an input system has a direct effect on program generators at the spinal level.[286] Because of its importance in motor learning and motor adaptation to new or changing environments, however, proprioception also has significant connections to the cortical and cerebellar neural networks. Its divergent pathways have synapses within the brain stem, diencephalon, and spinal system. It demonstrates how a systems model functions. Proprioceptive input can potentially influence multiple levels of CNS function, and all those levels can potentially modulate the intensity or importance of that information through many different mechanisms.[287,288] Proprioceptors are found in three peripheral anatomical locations: the muscle spindle, the tendon, and the joint. The afferent receptors responsible for relaying sensory information through those sites are discussed in the following subsections.

Muscle Spindle. Varied in function, the muscle spindle plays an important role in continuing modulation of the alpha motor neurons innervating the extrafusal muscle

TABLE 9-2 ■ Classifications of Peripheral Nerves According to Size

GASSER-ERLANGER	LLOYD	MOTOR (FUNCTIONAL COMPONENT)	SENSORY (FUNCTIONAL COMPONENT)
A Fibers: large myelinated fibers with a high conduction rate			
Aα	Ia	Large, fast fibers of alpha motor system (large cells of anterior horn to extrafusal motor fibers)	Muscle spindle: primary afferent endings (primary stretch or low threshold stretch: Ia tonic responds to length, Ia phasic responds to rate)
	Ib		Golgi tendon organ for contraction: responds to tendon stretch or tension
Aβ	II		Muscle spindle: secondary afferent endings: tonic receptors responding to length
			Exteroceptive afferent endings from skin and joints: respond to light or low threshold stretch
Aγ 1 and 2	II	Gamma motor system (small cells of anterior horn to intrafusal motor fibers)	Bare nerve endings: joint receptors, mechanoreception of soft tissues: exteroceptors for pain, touch, and cold (low threshold)
AΔ	III		
B Fibers: medium-sized myelinated fibers with a fairly rapid conduction rate			
Bβ		Preganglionic fibers of autonomic system (effective on glands and smooth muscle; motor branch of alpha): unknown function	
C fibers: small, poorly myelinated or unmyelinated fibers having slowest conduction rate; augmentation and recruiting occurs within the nervous system after stimulation of these fibers has ceased			
IV		Postganglionic fibers of sympathetic system	Exteroceptors: pain, temperature, touch

within which it is located. This is accomplished through simultaneous modulation of both the gamma and alpha motor neurons during functional activities. Spindle afferents also polysynaptically facilitate agonistic synergies while dampening antagonists and their synergies. Information is simultaneously sent through ascending pathways to the ipsilateral cerebellum and contralateral parietal lobe. Consequently, the spindle system seems to play an important role as an ongoing peripheral feedback mechanism to various centers within the CNS. These centers in turn regulate the continuous neuroexcitation at the brain stem and spinal cord level. Gamma innervation regulates the degree of internal stretch on the noncontractile portion of the spindle. Internal stretch, along with the external stretch of gravity, positioning, and therapeutic procedures, in turn helps modulate the efferent responses.[28]

Certain spindle afferents are length receptors and respond to length changes placed on the noncontractile portion of the spindle. This length change can result from a mechanical external force, such as positioning or stretch to the muscle, or from an internal mechanism caused by intrafusal muscle contraction. Spinal motor generators and supraspinal influences modulate both the alpha and gamma motor neuron activity to produce flexibility in regulation over patterns of striated muscle contraction. As long as the spindle has enough internal sensitivity, any therapeutic technique that creates a length change to the spindle has the potential of firing these length receptors. Other receptors respond to a rate of stretch versus length change. Techniques such as quick stretch, vibration, and tapping cause a rapid rate change within the spindle and thus potentially facilitate their receptors. The importance of muscle spindle afferent input as a treatment technique may lie in its ultimate influence over the cerebellum and basal ganglia to change existing programs permanently. Its direct influence over the spinal system is most likely short lived and has little long-term effect, although neuroplasticity within the spinal cord is possible. Cerebellar and basal ganglia/frontal lobe influence over brain stem motor nuclei and their modulation over interneurons within the spinal pattern generators should lead to change of existing output patterns (Figure 9-10).

Table 9-3 lists a variety of treatment procedures believed to use the proprioceptive muscle spindle system as a primary mode of sensory stimulation. The varying intensity, amount of tension, or rate of the stimuli, in addition to the original length of the muscle fiber before application of the stimulus, will determine which sensory receptor within the spindle is firing. Remember, afferent information is projecting to many areas above the spinal system, and the result will be regulation or modulation, ultimately affecting activity.[288]

Resistance. Resistance is often used to facilitate intrafusal and extrafusal muscle contraction. Resistance can be applied manually, mechanically, and by the use of gravity. Resistance recruits more motor units. Although muscles can contract both in an isometric and an isotonic fashion, most

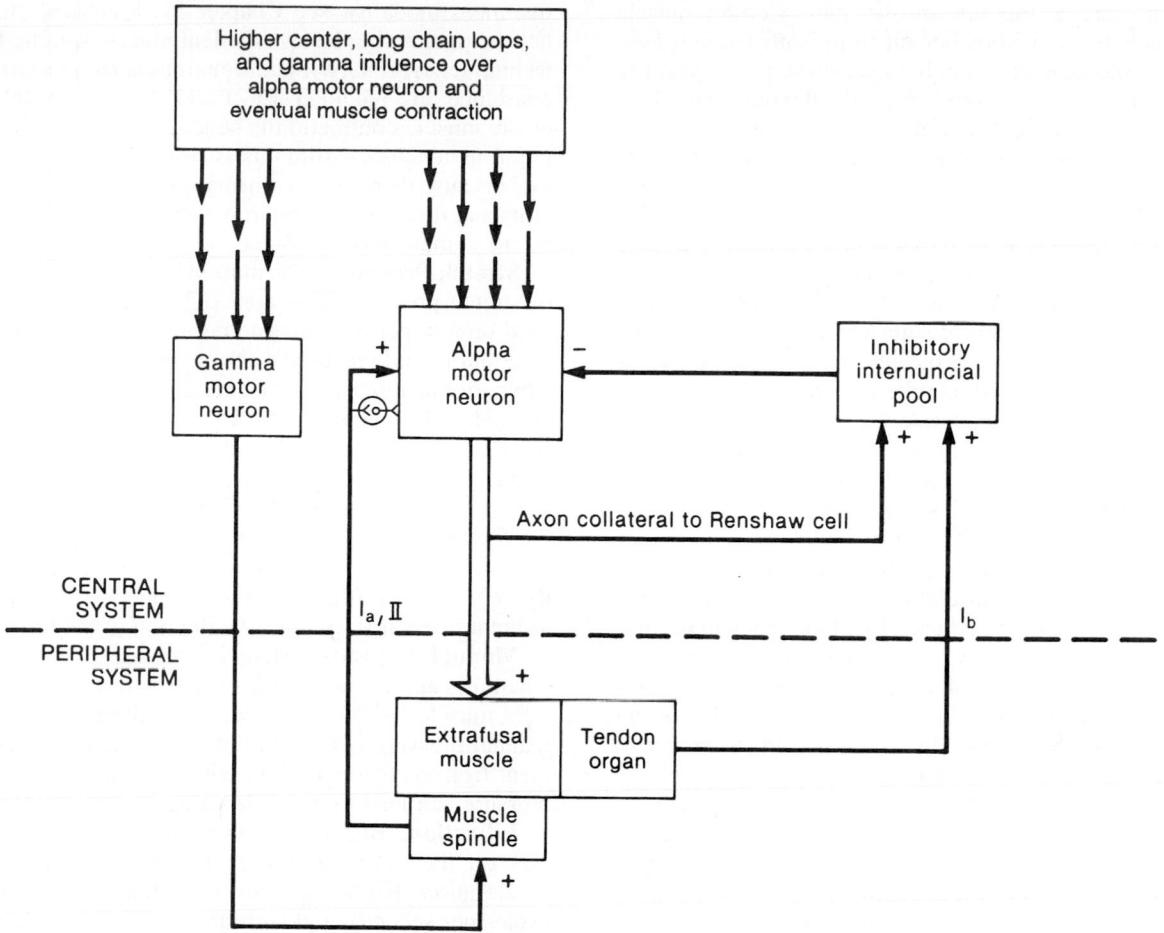

FIGURE 9-10 ■ Influences over the alpha motor neuron. The summation of all facilitory and inhibitory activity on the alpha motor neuron will determine the response of the muscle.

TABLE 9-3 ■ Proprioceptive Muscle Spindle System

RECEPTOR	STIMULUS	NATURE OF RESPONSE
Ia tonic	Length	Monosynaptic and polysynaptic facilitation of agonist
Ia phasic	Rate of change in length	Polysynaptic inhibition of antagonist and antagonistic synergy
		Polysynaptic facilitation of agonistic synergy
		Input to cerebellum
		Input to opposite parietal lobe
		Specific responses open for question:
II	Length	Monosynaptic facilitation of agonist
		Polysynaptic facilitation of specific muscle groups, depending on muscle function of tissue where II originates
		Transmittal of information to higher centers

POSSIBLE TREATMENT ALTERNATIVES

1. Resistance
2. Quick stretch to agonist
3. Tapping: tendon and muscle belly
4. Reverse tapping: gravity stretches; tapping agonist into shortened range
5. Positioning (range)
6. Electrical stimulation
7. Pressure or sustained stretch
8. Stretch pressure
9. Stretch release
10. Vibration within a facilitory frequency
11. Gravity as a prolonged stretch
12. Active motion

contractions are a mixture of the two. Certain muscle groups, such as the flexors, benefit from isometric exercise, as well as isotonic exercise in both eccentric and concentric modes. Under normal circumstances, the flexors are used for repetitive or rhythmical activities. The extensors, on the other hand, usually remain contracted in an effort to act against the forces of gravity. Therefore, the extensor groups benefit best from isometric and eccentric resistance.[289]

When resistance is applied to a voluntary muscle, spindle afferent fibers and tendon organs fire in proportion to the magnitude of the resistance. Resistance is more facilitative to an isometrically contracted muscle than to an isotonic contraction.[36] As isometric resistance is increased or continued, more motor units are recruited, thereby increasing the strength of extrafusal contraction.[28] Eccentric isotonic contraction refers to the lengthening of muscle fibers to resist force, as in lowering the arms while holding a heavy object. Eccentric contraction uses less metabolic output and promotes strength gains in less time.[28] However, all types of muscle contraction will promote increased strength. Resistance is an important clinical treatment and has been used and will continue to be used by clinicians within multiple treatment philosophies over the next millennium.*

Tapping. Three types of tapping techniques are commonly used by therapists. Tapping of the tendon is a fairly nondiscriminatory stimulus. Physicians use this technique to determine the degree of stretch sensitivity of a muscle. A normal response would be a brisk muscle contraction. Because of the magnitude of the stimulus and the direct effect on the alpha motor neuron, this technique is not highly effective in teaching a client to control or grade muscle contraction. Instead, tapping of the muscle belly, a lower-intensity stimulus, is more satisfactory. Reverse tapping is a less frequently described technique, but it can be used. The extremity is positioned so gravity promotes the stretch, instead of the therapist manually tapping or actively inducing muscle stretch. Once the muscle responds, the therapist taps or passively moves the extremity to help the muscle obtain a shortened range. An example of reverse tapping would be tapping the elbow when the client is bearing weight on the extended elbow and actively trying to achieve full elbow extension. Gravity quickly stretches the triceps. Timing of this technique is important. If the therapist taps the elbow toward extension when the flexors' motor neurons are sensitive, then those flexor muscles may respond to the stretch and contract. If the timing follows the quick stretch to the extensor, then the flexors will be dampened and active extension more likely a motor response.

Positioning (Range). The concept of submaximal and maximal range of muscles is highly significant to clinical application. Bessou et al[292] monitored the neuronal firing of muscle spindles at different ranges of motion. Upper motor neuron lesions can alter the sensitivity of the spindle afferent reflex arc fibers by not using presynaptic inhibition to normally dampen incoming afferent activity.[293] Therefore ROM should be carefully assessed on an individual basis, particularly in a patient with an upper motor neuron lesion, to determine the maximal or submaximal range for an individual.

Electrical Stimulation. For an in-depth discussion of the use of electrical stimulation both as an evaluation and a treatment modality, see Chapter 31. Electrical stimulation has the potential to be an excellent muscle spindle facilitory technique, especially if additional therapeutic tools, such as resistance, are included. Electrical stimulation delivered to create muscle contraction is beneficial, but electrical stimulation as a sensory stimulus is less effective as a learning tool because there are no sensory receptors for electrical currents and thus they are not represented as a unique stimulus on the somatosensory cortex.

Stretch Pressure. The muscle belly is the stimulus focus of stretch pressure. This approach would obviously not be used on a hypertonic muscle because it would increase the tone, but it could be used on the antagonist muscle to inhibit a hypertonic agonist.[269,294] Generally, this type of stimulus is applied and maintained for a period of time (e.g., 5 to 10 seconds). It is not a quick stimulus.

Stretch Release. This technique is performed by placing the fingertips over the belly of larger muscles and spreading the fingers in an effort to stretch the skin and the underlying muscle. The stretch is done firmly enough to temporarily deform the soft tissue so the cutaneous receptors and Ia afferent fibers may produce facilitation of the target muscle.

Manual Pressure. Manual pressure can be facilitory when it is applied as a brisk stretch or friction-like massage over muscle bellies. The speed and duration at which the manual pressure is applied determine the extent of recruitment from receptors. Paired with volitional efforts, manual pressure can lead to motor learning.

Vibration. Bishop[295,296] wrote an excellent series of articles on the neurophysiology and therapeutic application of vibration. High-frequency vibration (100 to 300 Hz or cycles per second) applied to the muscle or tendon elicits a reflex response referred to as the tonic vibratory response. Tension within the muscle will increase slowly and progressively for 30 to 60 seconds and then plateau for the duration of the stimulus.[297] Some researchers found that, at cessation of the input, the contractibility of the muscle was enhanced for approximately 3 minutes.[297,298] The discrepancy in the research may reflect the way the individual is using the input, both from a motor generator perspective and from supraspinal modulation over the importance of the input, which may affect the overall learning and plasticity of the CNS. To facilitate hypotonic muscle, the muscle belly is first put on stretch, and then vibratory stimuli are applied.[299] To inhibit a hypertonic muscle, the antagonistic muscle could be vibrated.[295,299] The use of vibration can be enhanced by combining it with additional modalities such as resistance, position, and visually directed movement. Vibration also stimulates cutaneous receptors, specifically the pacinian corpuscles, and thus can also be classified as an exteroceptive modality.[300] Because of its ability to decrease hypersensitive tactile receptors through supraspinal regulation, local vibration is considered an inhibitory technique (it is also discussed later in the section on exteroceptor-maintained stimulus). Therapists have reported that vibration over acupressure points can modulate localized pain syndromes. It seems to trigger A-delta exteroceptive fibers, which in turn dampen the effect of C fibers. (See Chapter 32 for more information on the treatment of pain.)

Farber[269] summarized the use of vibration and clearly identified precautions that must be taken. Frequencies greater than 200 Hz can be damaging to the skin. We have found frequencies greater than 150 Hz to cause discomfort

---

*References 10, 21, 27, 31, 290, 291.

and even pain. Thus, it is recommended that vibrators registering 100 to 125 Hz be used. Most battery-operated hand vibrators function at 50 to 90 Hz.[13] Frequencies less than 75 Hz are thought to have an inhibitory effect on normal muscle.[297] Cutaneous pressure is also known to cause inhibition, so if it is combined with a vibration technique that is being used to augment a muscle contraction, it can only serve to cancel the desired effects.

Amplitude or amount of displacement must also be considered when vibration is analyzed as a modality. It has been reported that high amplitude causes adverse effects, especially in clients with cerebellar dysfunction.[296] Vibration is not recommended for infants because the nervous system is not yet fully myelinated and it might cause too much stimulation. The reader is also cautioned about using vibration over areas that have been immobilized because of the underlying vascular tissue potential for clotting. Vibration on or near these blood vessels could dislodge a clot, causing an embolism. Vibration also needs to be used cautiously over skin that has lost its elasticity and is thin (e.g., that in older persons) because the friction itself from the vibration can cause tearing. The therapist must always keep in mind the environment and the functionality of an intervention procedure. The use of vibration may assist the client in contractions and somatosensory awareness, but it is an unnatural way to facilitate either system and thus needs to be removed as part of an intervention as soon as the patient demonstrates some sensory awareness and or volitional control over a movement component.

The Tendon Organ. The Golgi tendon organ is a specialized receptor located in both the proximal and the distal musculotendinous insertions. In conjunction with the muscle spindle, the tendon organ plays an important role in the mediation of proprioception.[286,301-304]

The principal role of the tendon organ is to monitor muscle tension exerted by the contraction of the extrafusal muscles. Research has demonstrated that the tendon organ is highly sensitive to tension and acts conjointly with the muscle spindle to inform higher centers of continuing environmental demands to modulate or change existing plans, which, in turn, regulate tonicity and compliance of extrafusal muscles.[42,288] The tendon organ (Ib) signals not only tension but also the rate of change of tension and provides the sensation of force as the muscle is working.[302,305] A fundamental difference between the Golgi tendon organ and the muscle spindle is that the muscle spindle detects length, whereas the tendon organ monitors tension and force. Motorically, the muscle spindle and the tendon organ spinal effect are exact opposites.[42,301,306] The muscle spindle regulates reciprocal inhibition, whereas the tendon organ modulates autogenic inhibition. In multiarthrodial muscles (superficial flexors and adductors), small-range repeated contractions will reduce hypertonicity in hypertonic muscles.[286,307] This is thought to occur as a result of flexor reflex afferent activity along with higher-center adaptation and modulation over those afferents.[308]

Clinically, this autogenic inhibition is seen in clients with upper motor neuron lesions. Usually, the patient has some degree of hypertonicity. As the hypertonic extremity is passively moved through range of motion, resistance is felt and then suddenly "melts away," allowing more freedom of movement. The exact mechanism that dampens the hyper-

tonicity is not known. It appears that other joint and cutaneous receptors could be sending signals to supraspinal centers, as well as the tendon organ, and it most likely is a cumulative effect.[288]

There appears to be a delicate balance between inputs that trigger inhibitory and excitatory loops within the central motor system. These peripheral input systems provide feedback control mechanisms to inform the CNS about the length, speed of movement, and contraction of a given muscle. Therefore, this balance among feedback mechanisms providing information to the CNS and the interpretation of that information is not only basic to the control of fine movements but also to decision making when feedforward plans need changing to adapt to the environmental demands. Table 9-4 lists a variety of known treatment approaches that use the tendon organ to inform higher centers regarding needed change and regulation over spinal generators.

Inhibitory Pressure. Pressure has been used therapeutically to alter motor responses. Mechanical pressure (force), such as cones, pads, or the orthokinetic cuff developed by Blashy and Fuchs,[309] provided continuously is inhibitory. That pressure seems most effective on tendinous insertions. It is hypothesized that this deep, maintained pressure activates pacinian corpuscles, which are rapidly adapting receptors. A variety of researchers have studied these receptors and their relationship to regulating vasomotor reflexes,[310] pain modulation,[311-313] and dampening other sensory system influence on the CNS.[298]

This inhibitory pressure technique also works when pressure is applied across the longitudinal axis of a tendon. The pressure is applied across the tendon with increasing pressure until the muscle relaxes. Constant pressure applied over the tendons of the wrist flexors may dampen flexor hypertonicity and elongate the tight fascia over the tendinous insertion (see Chapter 37 for additional information).

Pressure over bony prominences has modulatory effects. A common example is pressure on the medial aspect of the calcaneus, which dampens plantarflexors and allows contraction of the lateral dorsiflexor muscles. Pressure over the lateral aspect of the calcaneus also dampens calf muscles to allow for contraction of the medial dorsiflexor muscles.[27] Localized finger pressure applied bilaterally to acupuncture points has been shown to relieve pain and reduce muscle tone.[314-317] This technique has also been found to be particularly effective when used in a low-stimuli environment and when combined with deep breathing.

This combination of pressure (manually applied), environmental demands (low), and parasympathetic activity (slow, relaxed breathing) illustrates various systems interacting together to create the best motor response. The real world requires the client to respond to many environmental conditions while relaxed or under stress. Thus, once a client begins to demonstrate normal adaptable motor responses, the therapist needs to change the conditions and the stress level to allow the client to practice variability. That practice should incorporate motor error, especially error or distortions in the plan, yet still achieve the desired goal. As the client self-corrects, greater demand and variability should be introduced.[71]

The Joint. From a neurophysiological standpoint, joint movement provides the cerebellum and cortical sensory and

TABLE 9-4 ■ Proprioceptive Tendon Organs and Joints

RECEPTOR	STIMULUS	RESPONSE
TENDON ORGAN		
Tendon organ 1b	Tension on extrafusal muscle	Polysynaptic inhibition of agonist, facilitation of antagonist spinal level circuitry; supraspinal regulation

POSSIBLE TREATMENT SUGGESTIONS:
1. Extreme stretch
2. Deep pressure to tendon
3. Passive positioning in extreme lengthened range
4. Extreme resistance: more effective in lengthened and shortened range
5. Deep pressure to muscle belly to put stretch on tendon
6. Small repeated contractions with gravity eliminated

TYPE OF JOINT		
I (6-9 μ)	Static and dynamic joint tension: muscle pull	?: Facilitates postural holding: joint awareness
II (9-12 μ)	Dynamic: sudden change in joint tension	?: Facilitates agonist and awareness of joint motion: range
III (13-17 μ)	Dynamic: linked to Golgi tendon organ traction; activates in extreme range	?: Inhibits agonist
IV (2-5 μ $\leq$ 2 μ)	Pain	?: Inhibits agonist

POSSIBLE TREATMENT ALTERNATIVES:
1. Manual traction (distraction) to joint surfaces to facilitate joint motion
2. Manual approximation (compression) to joint surfaces to facilitate cocontraction or postural holding
3. Positioning: gravity used to approximate or apply traction
4. Weight belts, shoulder harnesses, and helmets to increase approximation
5. Wrist and ankle cuffs to increase traction
6. Wall pulleys, weights, manual resistance
7. Manual therapy[22]
8. Elastic tubing to provide compression during movement

motor nuclei with constant information about body position and movement.[318] It appears that the multiarthrodial joints contain the greatest number of receptors with the capacity to respond to the slightest change of angle between two bony articulations.

Four major types of joint receptors are described in the literature. Anatomically, these receptors are localized in the joint capsules and ligaments.[287,288] In general, joint receptors adapt slowly. Joint receptors have different thresholds for the rate of movement and the degree of angulation and thus play a key role in providing information about movement and position and also play a role in sensory mapping in area 3a.[174,319,320] These impulses project to many areas within the brain involved in both perception of the body in space and motor control over the body. Feedback to many areas is not crucial unless the existing environment does not match the predetermined feed-forward motor plan. If input matches the existing expectation, it is erased. When the input does not match what is expected from the predicted motor behavior, a change or modification in motor output or plan is needed to meet the desired goal. At this time feedback is critical, and without it the client will not have adequate adaptive mechanisms to rapidly change to environmental demands or demonstrate fine motor control. How the motor programmers adapt, learn, and change is discussed throughout this text both from a basic science and an outcome perspective.

Type III Golgi-type endings are slowly adapting joint receptors and seem to provide the brain with information about joint position.[12,287,296]

Type II Golgi-Mazzoni corpuscles are rapidly adapting. Higher concentrations of these receptors have been found in the connective tissues of the hands. These corpuscles function principally as detectors of rapid joint movements. They have also been found to discharge under deep pressure and vibration stimulus.[320]

Type I Ruffini's corpuscles respond vigorously with a volley of impulses at the beginning of joint movement and taper off to a steady state of firing at different angular positions. Ruffini's corpuscles monitor both the rate and direction of joint movement.[30,287]

Free nerve endings are contiguous with unmyelinated group IV or C fibers. It has been speculated that they provide a crude awareness of initial joint movement and the signaling of joint pain.[306,321,322] Although laboratory studies have analyzed these receptors in isolation, when they function together with all other input and regulatory systems it is thought that they operate more like an orchestra, where various rates of firing patterns are determined by both internal and external mechanisms. Thus, when treatment is considered, the therapist needs to consider the system as part of a whole, not as an isolated receptor whose rate of firing can be modified.

Studies reveal that an unidentified set of muscle afferent fibers and cutaneous receptors both contribute to the sense of movement and position.[306] Hence it may be safe to say that the somatosensory system works cooperatively as a unit in terms of both sensory processing and motor output.[323-327]

Because joint receptors are stretched and compressed during joint movement, they are in a good position to transmit signals regarding joint position, direction, and velocity of movement, but not force. Force sensations seem to be mediated by the receptors of the muscles and tendon organs. The joint receptors lend themselves well to treatment techniques. As already stated, the joint receptors are both slow and fast adapting. They exert strong influences on the motor system and ultimately on musculature. Joint receptors are sensitive to movement, position, traction, compression, and palpation. The specific role the joints play in somatosensory mapping is not known, but proprioception as a modality or sensory system is discussed further in this chapter on page 258. For clinical purposes, a variety of potential treatment approaches focus on the joint receptor (see Table 9-5).

Combined Proprioceptive Input Techniques. Many techniques succeed because of the combined effects of multiple input. Some of these combined techniques include jamming; ballistic movements; total-body positioning; PNF patterns; postexcitatory inhibition with stretch, range, rotation, and shaking; heavy work patterns; Feldenkrais (see Chapter 37)[328-330]; and manual therapy.[22,313,331]

Jamming. Jamming is usually applied to the ankle and knee with the intent of dampening plantarflexion while facilitating postural cocontraction around the ankle. The client can be placed in a side-lying position, can sit on a chair or mat, or can be positioned over a bolster with the hip and knee in some flexion. This flexion dampens the total extension pattern, including the plantarflexor muscles. With release of plantarflexion these muscles are placed on extreme stretch to maintain the modulation. In this position, intermittent joint approximation of considerable force is applied between the heel and knee. If the client is sitting, this approximation can easily be applied by pounding the heel on the floor and controlling a counterforce at the knee. Once cocontraction is minimally palpated, the clinician should initiate a movement pattern such as partial weight bearing to further encourage the CNS to readapt with postural control. This technique can also be used to dampen flexion of the wrist and fingers by focusing on appropriate upper-extremity patterns, modulating flexor reflex afferent activity, and applying a large amount of joint approximation between the heel of the hand and the elbow. To augment functional outcomes, the technique should be incorporated into functional training to get better somatosensory responses, improved representation of the involved body part, and greater functional carryover.

Ballistic Movement. Ballistic movements or pendular exercises are effective because of their combined proprioceptive interaction. The client is asked to initiate a movement, such as shoulder flexion while prone over a table with the arm hanging over the side. As the muscle approaches the shortened range, the amount of ongoing gamma afferent activity decreases. Thus both the agonist alpha motor neuron bias and the inhibition of Ia and II receptors of the antagonistic alpha motor neurons decrease. Simultaneously, the antagonistic muscle is being placed on more and more stretch. This stretch, as well as the lack of inhibition on the antagonistic alpha motor neurons, will encourage the antagonistic muscle to begin contraction and reverse the movement pattern. The tendon organs also play a key role in ongoing inhibition. As the muscle approaches the shortened range and tension on the tendon becomes intense, the tendon organ increases its firing, thus inhibiting the agonistic muscle in the shortened range while facilitating the antago-

nistic muscle. This technique is highly movement oriented, and the traction applied to the shoulder joint while swinging the arm further facilitates the movement. These ballistic movements are part of the program generators within the spinal system and are certainly more complex than a reflex response. The role of the Ib fibers during this open-chain or movement pattern is definitely different than its role in a closed-chair or weight-bearing environment.[303] Supraspinal influence over a preprogrammed activity also plays a role in the effectiveness of this treatment.[332] The specific rationale for why ballistic movements have functional carryover may be explained by recent research about cerebellar function and the importance of mechanical afferent input in regulation over movement (see Chapter 26).

The clinician using this technique must exercise caution. ROM can easily be obtained through pendular movement. Consequently, the clinician must always determine before therapy the reasons for specific clinical signs and whether the total problem will be corrected through an activity such as a ballistic movement. This is the diagnostic responsibility of the professional. If only one component of the problem is alleviated, such as limitation of range, while lack of postural tone or joint stability possibly increases in severity, then additional techniques must be combined with this treatment modality. For example, assume that the rotator cuff muscles are slightly torn and the movers of the shoulder are superficially splinting to prevent further tearing. Instructing the client to hold the humerus in the glenohumeral joint by active contraction of the rotator cuff muscles will facilitate postural holding and strengthen the torn muscles. Having the client simultaneously perform a ballistic movement with the arm will expedite shoulder movement, thus preventing unnecessary splinting and possible limitation of joint range.

Total-Body Positioning. Total-body positioning implies the use of positioning and gravity to dampen afferent activity on the alpha motor neurons and thus cause a decrease in tone, or relaxation.[333] Today, the rationale for why relaxation of striated muscle occurs after this treatment implies that the effect of the flexor reflex afferents is being dampened by a combination of input and interneuronal activity. These changes in the state of the muscle tone will not be permanent and will revert to the original posturing unless motor learning and adaptation within the central programmer occur simultaneously. Thus, for this treatment to effect permanent change, a large number of systems need modification. This modification can be augmented by techniques that facilitate autogenic inhibition, reciprocal innervation, labyrinthine and somatosensory influences, and cerebellar regulation over tone.[334] Changing the degree of flexion of the head also alters vestibular input and the state of the motor pool. But, again the CNS of the client needs to be an active participant and will ultimately determine whether permanent learning and change are programmed.

Proprioceptive Neuromuscular Facilitation Patterns. To analyze and learn the patterns and techniques that constitute PNF, a total approach to treatment, refer to the texts by Kottke[335] and Sullivan et al.[31] This approach is being used extensively for orthopedic and neuromuscular problems, and the research on this method has been studied more in lower motor neuron and musculoskeletal problems than in upper motor neuron lesions.[331,336-340]

Postexcitatory Inhibition with Stretch, Range, Rotation, and Shaking. The concept of postexcitatory inhibition (PEI) is based on the action potential or electrical response pattern of a neuron at the time of stimulation and on the entire phase response until the neuron returns to normal. At the time of stimulation, the action potential will build and go through an excitatory phase. The neuron then enters an inhibitory phase or refractory period during which further stimulation is not possible. This is referred to as the PEI phase or postsynaptic afferent depolarization.[269] These phase changes are extremely short and, in normal muscle, asynchronous with respect to multiple neuronal firing. In a hypertonic muscle more simultaneous firing occurs. When the muscle is lengthened, and thus tension is created, more fibers will be discharged. It is hypothesized that if the hypertonic muscle is placed at the end of its spastic range and a quick stretch is applied and held, then total facilitation followed by total inhibition will occur because of postexcitatory inhibition. As the inhibition phase is felt, the therapist can passively lengthen the spastic muscle until the facilitory phase sets in repolarization. At that time the clinician holds the lengthened position. Increased tone will ensue, followed by inhibition and continued lengthening. Holding the range (not allowing concentric contraction during the excitatory phase) is critical. If the muscle is held as the tone increases, the resistance and stretch are then maximal and probably further facilitate the inhibitory phase.

At a certain point in the range, if the muscle is not limited by fascial tightness, the hypertonic muscle will become dampened and tone will disappear. It is thought that at this time either the tendon organ activity takes over and maintains inhibition or flexor reflex afferents are modified, thus creating an inhibitory range where antagonistic muscles can be more easily initiated and controlled by the client. If this technique is performed in a pure plane of motion, the clinician will find it a time-consuming procedure. Range can be achieved quickly by integrating a few additional techniques, that is, incorporating rotatory patterns of movement. For example, if the spastic upper extremity is positioned in the pattern of shoulder adduction, internal rotation, elbow flexion, wrist pronation, and finger flexion, then a pattern in the opposite direction can be incorporated to include external rotation of the shoulder and supination of the wrist. Every time the clinician begins to lengthen the spastic extremity, those rotatory patterns should be used. This should be done both on initial stretch and hold and during the inhibitory phase. Rotation seems to lengthen the inhibitory phase and allows additional range. If the clinician adds a quick stretch to the antagonistic muscle during the inhibitory phase of the agonistic muscle, then further facilitation of the antagonistic muscle will occur. Because the agonistic muscle is in an inhibitory phase, movement in and out of its spastic range should not affect it. Yet the quick stretch facilitation of the antagonistic muscle inhibits the spastic agonistic muscle and again lengthens the inhibitory phase. This entire procedure occurs quite quickly. An observer might say that the clinician "shakes the hypertonicity out of the arm." The shaking action is thought to be the quick stretch as well as joint oscillations. The degree of success depends on the therapist's sensitivity to the tonal shifts or phase changes occurring in the client. These tonal shifts are automatic and not under the client's conscious control. The technique does not teach the client anything and

should only be used to maintain ROM and to create an optimal environment to encourage the client to initiate normal antagonistic control. This is also a good technique for a family to help with at home to set a better stage for exercises.

Rood's Heavy Work Patterns. Today, the concepts of motor learning more clearly explain why postural holding for periods of time and eccentric lengthening in and out of the shortened range are effective treatment techniques. If repetition within the environmental context leads to motor learning, then the postural systems need to learn coactivation within the shortened range of the postural pattern and need to practice directing the limbs during both closed-chain and open-chain activities.

Feldenkrais. Feldenkrais' concepts[328,329] of sensory awareness through movement place emphasis on relaxation of muscle on stretch and distracting and compressing joints for sensory awareness. Both techniques reflect combined proprioceptive techniques. Taking muscles off stretch slows general afferent firing and thus overload to the CNS. Compression and distraction of joints enhance specific input from a body part while simultaneously facilitating input of a lesser intensity from other body segments. This combined proprioceptive approach enhances body schema awareness in a relaxed environment. It also integrates empowerment of the client by use of visualization and asking for volitional control. (See Chapters 30 and 37 for additional information.)

Manual Therapy, Specifically Maitland's. "The peripheral and central nervous systems need to be considered as one since they form a continuous tissue tract."[313,328] Manual therapy or mobilization of joint or soft tissue structures is not specific to orthopedic conditions, nor are neurotreatment principles ineffective on orthopedic patients. Irrespective of the diagnostic reason, whether pathological condition or impairment leading to joint immobility, the functional consequences can be synonymous. With the immobility of joints, the peripheral nerve begins to lose its adaptability to change in the length of the nerve bed. This change in neural elasticity then creates additional problems in connective tissue function, which in turn may affect the function of the motor system's control over the musculoskeletal component.[331,341] For this reason alone, discussion of musculoskeletal mobilization needs to be included in this section as a component of classification.

"Pathological processes may interfere with both of these mechanisms: extraneural pathology will affect the nerve/interface relationship and intraneural pathology will affect the intrinsic elasticity of the nervous system."[341] Patient complaints of pain that limits functional movement constitute the primary reason clients are referred to a therapist for a musculoskeletal evaluation. Besides subjective and observational evaluation, the physical examination must include tension tests that are used to determine the degree of pain and joint limitation, to differentiate between somatic and radicular symptoms, and to identify adverse neurophysiological changes in the PNS.[341] "The increased muscle tone (in a peripheral injury) is considered to be a protective mechanism for the inflamed tissue."[342] This increase in tone may be due to a dampening of presynaptic activity of the flexor reflex afferent by supraspinal mechanisms. This same mechanism may be triggered by a CNS injury. The difference between the orthopedic patient and the neurological patient may be the trigger to the CNS. In a central lesion the motor generators are often not adequately maintained after injury, which results in hypotonicity. The hypotonicity causes peripheral instability, stretches peripheral tissue, and potentially causes peripheral damage. In both orthopedic and neurological cases, there is peripheral instability, the first the result of peripheral damage and the second the result of hypotonicity. The CNS response to the instability may be the same: an increase in muscle tone by dampening presynaptic inhibition. A result of a decrease in presynaptic inhibition on incoming afferents would cause an increase in spinal generator activity. With an isolated musculoskeletal problem and an intact CNS, the motor system would have the adaptability and control to modulate the spinal generators and isolate only those components in which an increase in tone might directly affect the problems. The client with CNS involvement may lose some of the flexibility of the motor system's control over the pattern generators, and thus high-tone synergistic patterns may develop.

In either case, the peripheral system needs to be evaluated and intervention provided when necessary. Tension tests look for adverse responses to physical examination of neural tissues. These adverse responses are muscle tone increases as a result of painful provocation of sensitized neural tissue nociceptors attempting to prevent further pain by limiting the movement of the neural tissue.[342] Pain increases tone and leads to limited range of passive movement.[342,343] Pain-free range suggests CNS sensitivity to the large, highly myelinated alpha fibers and functions in a discriminatory manner. Pain range encompasses the degree of joint motion where neural length, as well as nociceptors in the skin, fascia, muscles, and joints, plays a primary role in CNS attention and protection. Inflammation of neural tissue can also cause the nociceptors to become hypersensitized or more reactive to mechanical or chemical changes. This is particularly true in the joint when the nociceptors react significantly to movement at the end ranges.[341]

Treatment will be based on the degree of immobility, the pain range, the site of the irritability, and the degree of pain. Butler[331] not only looks at joint problems but also considers many joint problems as having adverse neural dynamics (tension on the PNS). Treatment still incorporates Maitland's grades of passive movement, listed in Figure 9-11, but with consideration across the length of the neural tissue across multiple joints.

Butler[341] divides treatment of the joint into three categories: limitations, pain, and adverse mechanical tension. When analyzing selective nervous system mobilization as identified by Butler, the therapist needs to mobilize the nervous system and its surrounding fascia rather than stretching it. These techniques may be either gentle (grade 1) or strong (grade IV), through the range (grades II and III), or at end range only (grade IV). Different disorders (irritable compared with nonirritable) will require different treatment approaches.

Treatment must interface with related tissues. When joint immobility is interfaced with muscle and fascia tightness, all components must be treated simultaneously. If the focus of treatment is the correction of joint and muscle signs, the constant reassessment of nervous system effect is crucial. This aspect would seem even more crucial in clients with CNS and PNS injuries. The treatment may be direct or indirect. Direct intervention refers to procedures aimed at rebalancing the neuromusculoskeletal system through strengthening and

Grades of Movement

Grade I   A small amplitude movement performed near the beginning of range.

Grade II   A large amplitude movement carried well into range. It's a movement that occupies any part of the range that is free of pain or resistance.

Grade III   A large amplitude movement that moves up to the limit of range or into resistance.

Grade IV   A small amplitude movement performed near the end of range or slightly into resistance.

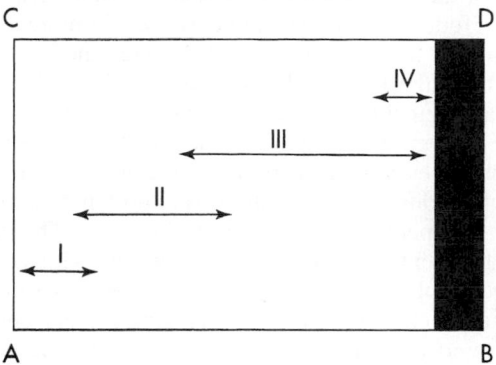

Maitland has also been using the pluses (1) and minuses (2) in his grades of movement for many years now. It enables the therapist to communicate better with other therapists as well as treat the patient with accuracy and skill.

Grade IV−−: just nicking resistance

Grade IV−: touching resistance

Grade IV: into resistance about 25%

Grade IV+: into resistance about 50%

Grade IV++: into resistance about 75%

FIGURE 9-11 ■ Grades of movement. (Adapted from Maitland's theory of joint and tissue mobilization by John Sievert, PT, GDMT. From Course notes, Graduate Diploma in Manipulative Therapy, Curtin University of Technology, Perth, WA, 1990; and from Maitland GD: Peripheral manipulation, ed 3, Boston, 1991, Butterworth Heinemann.)

increasing ROM to improve motor control. Indirect treatment includes the use of movement patterns, especially posture-based patterns. When individuals have nervous system changes, static and dynamic postural patterns often emerge as compensatory reactions to the problem state. Pain posturing, tension, or stiffness from prolonged positioning, and forced postures that are the result of synergy patterns, to name a few, all seem to respond well to indirect treatment with or without passive CNS mobilization. The use of posture-based movement patterns during functional activities also provides for variability and repetition and thus should lead to greater carryover in motor learning.

Many manual therapy approaches affect and use the proprioceptive system as a means to change motor responses. The reader is again reminded that the proprioceptive system affects all systems within the CNS and vice versa. The end effect of all systems interactions will be intrinsic reinforcement of existing behavior or will change and adapt behavior to meet intrinsic and extrinsic demands. The behavior observed by the therapist as the client initiates motor strategies in response to functional goals will be a consensus of all these interactions.

Exteroceptive/Cutaneous Sensory System

The somatosensory system is usually subdivided into two distinct systems. One system is phylogenetically older and nonspecific in nature. The other system is phylogenetically newer and specific in function. The concept of the dual quality of the somatosensory system was first suggested by Head.[344] Today, the systems are described in more anatomical terms as the spinothalamic (mediates more protective stimuli) and the lemniscal (mediates discriminative aspects of somatic sensibility) systems, which include both exteroceptive and proprioceptive information.[36,345]

A fundamental understanding of the anatomy and physiology of the dual sensory systems is important before undertaking therapeutic intervention techniques. The afferent information entering the lemniscal system originates from either a peripheral or cranial nerve. These interneurons are large and well myelinated. Therefore, signals are transmitted rapidly, with a minimum of three synaptic relays. A striking characteristic of this system is its somatotopic organization. There is an orderly spatial topographical representation of the surface of the skin in the fiber bundles of the dorsal columns and the synaptic organization of the thalamus. This highly developed organization of sensory relays allows discrimination among specific proprioceptive and tactile stimuli. This system transmits conscious proprioceptive and kinesthetic information such as touch, pressure, localization, contour, quality, and spatial details of mechanical stimuli.[287,345-348]

The spinothalamic system's ascending impulses either terminate in or send collateral connections to the reticular formation. These fibers continue upward to synapse with the nonspecific thalamic nuclei (medial) and then diverge to make connections with practically all regions of the cerebral cortex. Other collaterals of this system project to the regulators of the autonomic nervous system (ANS), limbic system, and brain stem nuclei.[287,288]

Because the spinothalamic system synapses with the reticular formation and the ANS, it serves more as an energizing or arousal mechanism to potentially harmful stimuli. Therefore this system is involved in perception of pain, light touch, pleasurable sexual sensations, and aversive stimuli and in the production of primitive orientations and preprogrammed and protective responses.[287,349,350]

This subdivision into spinothalamic and lemniscal systems can mislead one into thinking that they can be activated separately. Most sensory stimuli will activate both systems simultaneously, for example, light touch. The lemniscal system can carry both exteroceptive and proprioceptive stimuli. However, it is possible to "load" one system more than the other by using selective stimuli in a fast or slow manner.[36]

Poggio and Mountcastle[351] suggest that the lemniscal system can have an inhibiting influence on the spinothalamic system. Ayers[352] and Wilbarger[353] have proposed that "touch defensiveness" constitutes the predominance of the spinothalamic (protective) system over the lemniscal system. Many of the therapeutic techniques used in sensory integrative therapy are designed to activate the lemniscal system and establish a better balance between the two systems. In addition, the facial region receives its sensory innervation from the trigeminal nerve, which can be regarded as a third somatosensory system because it supplies a body surface that is outside the dermatomal segments supplied by the spinal cord.[145] A soft, low-intensity stimulation to the facial region can elicit a relaxation response because the soft tissues are also richly innervated by the parasympathetic nervous system.[354,355] Wilbarger[353] postulates that, if the protective system becomes hypersensitive, its generalized effect will lead to sympathetic overactivity, avoidance behaviors of all types, inability to handle or dampen extraneous input, and potential attention deficits. By desensitizing the touch system through maintained deep rubbing with a surgical-type scrub brush or other maintained stimuli, she states that the system will dampen its firing, and the discriminatory (lemniscal) system can begin to function. This discriminatory system will further override the older system and help to reestablish better homeostasis.

The exteroceptive system can be considered as a whole system or divided into sensory end organs located in the superficial layers of the skin, the subcutaneous layers, the dermis, and the external mucous membranes.[356] Some authors include the special sense organs or cranial nerves, such as gustatory, olfactory, visual, and auditory, as part of the exteroceptive system. This section describes only the nonencapsulated and encapsulated end organs found in the skin around hairs and does not include special senses.

The skin, being the organ of touch, is activated by stimuli from outside the body. Therefore, the exteroceptors inform the CNS about changes taking place in the external environment. These receptors tend to be especially sensitive to specific kinds of energy, such as pain, temperature, touch, and pressure. Before an exteroceptor will discharge, it must receive the appropriate amount of energy, which is called the adequate stimulus. Exteroceptors also have different thresholds. When the stimuli are adequate, the neuron reaches its action potential and discharges according to the intensity of the stimulus.[356,357] The duration of discharge depends on the receptor's ability to adapt. Some receptors adapt quickly, and others adapt slowly.

Exteroceptors innervate certain areas of the skin in a distinct fashion. The area of skin innervation is called a receptive field. There is a large variation in the number of receptors and the rate they transmit information from a given field of glabrous, nonhairy skin.[292,313] For example, the palmar surface of the hand contains a greater number of receptors than the dorsal surface does. There is a greater density of small receptor fields because the hands are used for fine motor skill, prehension, and touch and thus need to have greater representation within the cortical area.[288,358,359]

Differentiation of Receptor Site as Augmented Intervention. Humans have many different types of tactile receptors. Some are superficial, and others are deep. These receptors have been identified within the next subsection to discuss their use as augmented intervention strategies.

Free Nerve Endings. Free or bare nerve endings are phylogenetically the oldest unencapsulated receptors (see Table 9-2). Free nerve endings transmit pain, temperature, and light-touch sensations.[357] Sensitivity to cold stimuli is 10 times greater along the midline than in the extremities.[12,288] Free nerve endings seem to serve as primitive protective receptors because they are centrally located and alert the organism to potential dangers to vital organs.

Hair Receptors. In general, hair receptors cause an excitatory response because the reticular-activating system links to the ANS. Stimulation to hair follicles or skin located on a dermatome at the same segmental level can facilitate the underlying muscle.[142,360] However, this stimulus activates a cutaneous sensorimotor reflex. The reflex sends impulses along the alpha (group II) fibers to the interneurons and alpha motor neurons that terminate at the myoneural junction of the skeletal muscle.[142,360] This creates a dermatome-myotome relationship.

Merkel's Disks. Slowly adapting touch-pressure receptors, Merkel's disks (group II) are highly responsive to slow movements across the skin surface and to light pressures. These receptors have also been associated with the sense of tickly and pleasurable touch.[12,287]

Meissner's Corpuscles. Meissner's corpuscles as receptors are highly discriminative, providing an instantaneous sense of contact and flutter sensation. These receptors are used in two-point discrimination and stereognosis. There is some evidence that elderly individuals have a reduction of sensation resulting from a combination of skin inelasticity and loss of Meissner's corpuscles.[330,361]

Pacinian Corpuscles. Pacinian corpuscles are located deep in the dermis of the skin: in viscera, mesenteries, and ligaments, and near blood vessels. Interestingly, they are most plentiful in the soles of the feet, where they seem to exert some influence on posture, position, and ambulation.[362] The pacinian corpuscles adapt quickly, and they are activated by deep pressure and quick stretch of tissues.[360]

A list of treatment techniques using the tactile or exteroceptive system as their primary mode of entry can be found in Table 9-5.

Treatment Alternatives Using the Exteroceptive System. The function of the exteroceptive system is to inform the nervous system about the surrounding world. The CNS will adapt behavior to coexist and survive within this environment. Although many protective responses are patterned within the motor system, these patterned responses can be changed or modulated according to momentary inherent chemistry, attitude, motivation, alertness, and so on. Different from some of the other treatment approaches, the function of the exteroceptive input system is not reflexive but rather informative and adaptable.

Quick Phasic Withdrawal. The human organism reacts to painful or noxious stimuli at both conscious and unconscious levels. If the stimulus is brief and of noxious quality, it will elicit a protective reaction of short duration with use of the long-chain spinal reflex loops. Simultaneously, afferent impulses ascend to higher centers to evoke prolonged emotional-behavioral responses. Stimuli such as pain, extremes in temperature, rapid movement, light touch, and hair displacement are the most likely to cause this reaction by activating free nerve endings. These stimuli are perceived as potentially dangerous and communicate directly with the reticular-activating system and nonspecific thalamic nuclei. These structures have diffuse interconnections with all regions of the cerebral cortex, ANS, limbic system, cerebellum, and motor centers in the brain stem. Observing clients' behavior in chronic pain problems, these responses seem to become habitual and may lead to somatosensory remapping, making it hard to differentiate protective from discriminatory information.

There are some real therapeutic limitations to using stimuli that "load" the spinothalamic system. A painful stimulus will be excitatory to the nervous system and produce a prolonged reaction after discharge. According to Wall's "gate-control" theory,[321,363-366] all sensory afferent neurons converge and synapse in the dorsal horn in an area called the substantia gelatinosa. Curiously, the large, more discriminatory fibers do outnumber the small fibers.[353] Therefore, physical activity, frequent positioning, deep pressure, and proprioceptive and cutaneous stimulation should cause enough impulses to converge on cells within the substantia gelatinosa to close the gate and thus block transmission of pain messages to the brain. Studies have demonstrated that physical activity (types of physical stress) stimulates the production of endorphins, which in turn release opiate receptors and act as the body's own morphine for pain control[22,315,367-370] (see Chapters 32 and 36).

Because light touch has both a protective and discriminatory function, techniques such as brushing or stroking the skin with a soft brush have the potential of informing the CNS about (1) texture, object specificity, and error in fine motor responses or (2) danger (eliciting a protective response). If a protective response is triggered, the specific withdrawal pattern will depend on a variety of circumstances. If the stimulus is applied to an extensor surface, then a flexor withdrawal will be facilitated. If the stimulus is placed on a flexor surface, one of two responses occurs. First, the client might withdraw from the stimulus, thus going into an extensor pattern. Second, the stimulus may elicit a flexor withdrawal and cause the client to go into a flexor pattern. Which pattern occurs depends on preexisting motor programming bias as a result of positioning and the predisposition of the client's CNS. Both responses would be considered normal. The condition or emotional state of the nervous system and whether the stimulus is considered threatening also determine the sensitivity of the response, again reinforcing the systems' interdependence. These responses are protective and do not lead to repetition of movement or motor learning. For that reason, along with the emotional and autonomic reactions, a phasic withdrawal to facilitate flexion or extension is not recommended as a treatment approach unless all other possibilities have been eliminated.

Short Duration: High-Intensity Icing. Cold is another stimulus that the nervous system perceives as potentially dangerous. The use of ice as a stimulus to elicit desired motor patterns is an early technique developed by Rood. Her technique was referred to as repetitive icing. An ice cube is rubbed with pressure for 3 to 5 seconds or used in a quick-sweep motion over the muscle bellies to be facilitated. This method would activate both exteroceptors and proprioceptors and causes a brief arousal of the cortex. This method can produce unpredictable results. Although initially a phasic withdrawal

TABLE 9-5 ■ Exteroceptive Input Techniques

RECEPTORS	STIMULI	RESPONSE*
Free nerve endings: C + A fibers	Pain, temperature, touch	Seems to protect and alert, perception of temperatures, protective withdrawal
Hair follicles	Mechanical displacement of hair receptors	Increased tone of muscle below stimulus site
Merkel's disk	Touch: pressure receptors	Touch identification
Meissner's corpuscles	Discriminative touch	Postural tone; two-point discrimination
Pacinian corpuscles	Deep pressure and quick stretch to tissue, vibration	Position sense, postural tone and movement
Ruffini's corpuscles	Touch mechanoreceptor	Touch/spatial discrimination

SUGGESTED TREATMENT PROCEDURES USING CUTANEOUS STIMULI

Quick phasic withdrawal
1. Stimuli
   a. Pain
   b. Cold: one-sweep with ice cubes: Rood's quick ice
   c. Light touch: brush (quick stroking), finger, feather
2. Response
   a. Stimulus applied to an extensor surface: elicits a flexor withdrawal
   b. Stimulus applied to flexor surface: may elicit flexor withdrawal or withdrawal from stimulus into extension

Prolonged icing (repetitive icing should be used with caution because of rebound effect)
1. Stimulus
   a. Ice cube
   b. Ice chips and wet towel
   c. Bucket of ice water
   d. Ice pack
   e. Immersion of body part or total body
2. Response: inhibition of muscles below skin areas iced

Neutral warmth
1. Stimulus
   a. Air bag splints
   b. Wrapping entire body or individual body part with towel
   c. Tight clothing such as tights, fitted turtleneck jerseys
   d. Tepid water or shower
2. Response: inhibition of area under which neutral warmth was applied

Light touch/rapid stroking
1. Stimulus
   a. Light intermittent tactile stimulus to an identified dermatome/myotome interaction area
2. Response: facilitation of muscle(s) related to the stimulus area

Maintained pressure or slow, continuous stroking with pressure
1. Stimulus
   a. Slowly rubbing the target area with a towel
   b. Wearing Gore-Tex clothing
2. Response: sensory receptor adaptation and decrease in afferent firing

*Response: adaptation of many cutaneous receptors to stimulus, thus decreasing exteroceptive input, decreasing reticular activity, and decreasing facilitation of muscles underlying stimulated skin.

pattern generator response will be activated immediately after the reflex has taken place, the "rebound" phenomenon deactivates the muscle that has been stimulated and lowers the resting potential of the antagonistic muscle.[371] Therefore a second stimulus to the same dermatome/myotome neural network may not elicit a second response. But, because of reciprocal innervation, the antagonistic muscle may effect a rebound movement in the opposite direction. Icing may also cause prolonged reaction after discharge because of the connections to the reticular system, limbic system, and ANS. Thus, the ANS would be shifted toward the sympathetic end. Too much sympathetic tone causes a desynchronization of the cortex.[372] Although the resting state of the spinal generator may be altered briefly, if the heightened state persists it is most likely due to fear or sympathetic overflow (see Chapter 4). This state is destabilizing to the system and most likely will not lead to any motor learning. Because of unpredictable response patterns to Rood's repetitive icing, this technique is seldom used.

The therapist is cautioned not to use short-duration, high-intensity icing to the facial region above the level of the lips, to the forehead, or to the midline of the trunk. These areas have a high concentration of pain fibers and a strong connection to the reticular system.[12,373]

Ice should not be used behind the ear because it may produce a sudden lowering of blood pressure.[307] The therapist should also avoid using ice in the left shoulder region in patients with a history of heart disease because referred pain from angina pectoris manifests itself in the left shoulder area, indicating the cold stimulus might cause a reflexive constriction of the coronary arteries.[374] In addition, the primary rami located along the midline of the dorsum of the trunk have sympathetic connections to internal organs. The cold stimulus may alter organ activity and perhaps produce vasoconstriction, causing increased blood pressure and less blood supply to the viscera.[352,375]

Brief administration of ice can have beneficial effects if the nervous system's inhibitory mechanisms are in place. For instance, in children with learning disabilities or adults with sensorimotor delays, the application of ice to the palmar surface of the hands will cause arousal at the cortical level because of the increased activity of the reticular activating system. This arousal response presumably produces increased adrenal medullary secretions, resulting in various metabolic changes. Therefore, icing should be used selectively. If the patient has an unstable ANS, it should be eliminated as a potential sensory modality.[376]

Prolonged Use of Ice. A variety of approaches incorporate prolonged icing techniques. The proprioceptive neuromuscular facilitation approach may be the most common.[21] Inhibition of hypertonicity or pain is the goal for the use of any of these methods. With prolonged cold the neurotransmission of impulses, both afferent and efferent, is reduced. Simultaneously, the metabolic rate within the cooled tissue is reduced (see Chapter 32). Caution must be exercised with regard to the use of this modality. However, for effective treatment results, the client (1) should be receptive to the modality, (2) should be able to monitor the cold stimulus (sensory deficits should not be present), and (3) should have a stable autonomic system to prevent unnecessary adverse effects of hypothermia.

Ice massage is a form of prolonged icing and is often used to treat somatic pain problems. It is also used over high-toned muscles to dampen striated muscle contractions. Caution must be used when eliminating pain without correcting the problem causing pain. For example, if instability causes muscle tone and pain, then icing might decrease pain while causing additional joint instability and potential damage. The end result would be an increase, not a decrease, in pain and motor dysfunction.

Neutral Warmth. Like icing, neutral warmth alters the state of the motor generators, either directly or indirectly through afferent input. According to Farber,[14] the length of application depends on the client. A 3- to 4-minute tepid bath may create the same results as a 15-minute total body-wrapping procedure. As with any input procedure, the effects should be incorporated into the therapeutic session to maximize the results and promote client learning. Johnstone uses air splints effectively as a neutral warm treatment intervention in which she has clients work on functional activities.[19] If neutral warmth is applied as an isolated intervention, the client may feel relaxation or a decrease in discomfort, but neuroplastic CNS changes are unlikely, owing to the lack of repetition, attention, and error correction by the client during activities.

Maintained Stimulus or Pressure. Because of the rapid adaptation of many cutaneous receptors, a maintained stimulus will effectively cause inhibition by preventing further stimuli from entering the system. This technique is applied to hypersensitive areas to normalize skin responses. Vibration, used alternately with maintained pressure, can be highly effective. It should be remembered that these combined inputs use different neurophysiological mechanisms. It is often observed that low-frequency maintained vibration is especially effective with learning-disabled children who have hypersensitive tactile systems that prevent them from comfortable exploration of their environment. When children themselves use vibration on the extremities, their hypersensitive systems seem to normalize and they become receptive to exploring objects. If that exploration is accompanied by additional prolonged pressure, such as digging in a sandbox, the technique seems to be more effective because of the adaptive responses of the nervous system.

Maintained pressure approaches using elastic stockings, tight form-fitting clothing (e.g., wet suits, expanded polytetrafluoroethylene [Gore-tex] biking clothing), air splints, and other techniques can be incorporated into a client's daily activity without altering lifestyle. In this way clients can self-regulate their systems, allowing greater variability in adapting to the environment. Owing to the multisensory and multineuronal pathways used when peripheral input is augmented, traditional linear, allopathic research on human subjects is extremely difficult to design or measure with control. But outcome studies demonstrating efficacy are possible. Initially, efficacy was acceptable through observation. Now it is time to repeat studies by using objective measures to demonstrate the same outcome.

Vestibular System

The vestibular apparatus is a mechanoreceptor.[287] Peripheral proprioceptive receptors inform the CNS where the body is in space, and the vestibular system relays information about the head position and linear acceleration in space. Because the vestibular system is intimately connected to the auditory, visual, proprioceptive, and motor systems, it works interactively to modulate important functions.[318,377] The vestibular system has been credited with influencing muscle tone and maintaining visual gaze, spatial directionality, clarity of the image when the head is moving or the object is moving, and head and body orientation. It also influences learning and emotional development.[378,379]

The vestibular system has two distinct receptor areas. The vestibule (utricle and saccule) is located between the semicircular canals and the cochlea. It is often called the static labyrinth because it elicits tonic reflexes in postural muscles in response to changes in head and body positions and gravitational influences.[288] The anatomical arrangement of the hair cell receptors within the vestibule allows sensory receptors to be highly responsive to changes in head position. As the head is tilted to one side, the force of gravity displaces the otolithic membrane, which causes the cilia of the hair cell to bend. This bending or shearing action causes the hair cell to discharge and transmit afferent impulses to the CNS.[380]

The hair cells are tonic receptors and, even in the neutral position, are constantly discharging. The bending of the cilia in a single hair cell in one direction will cause an increase in firing, and bending in the opposite direction will cause a slowing of the rate of discharge.[287,288]

The saccule lies between the utricle and cochlear duct. Most of the cilia (hair cells) in the saccule are arranged in a side-lying fashion when the head is in the normal upright position. Therefore, if the head moves in a vertical plane (e.g., nodding), the cilia will discharge. Any up-and-down motion, including bouncing on a trampoline, is an adequate stimulus to the cilia in the saccule. In contrast, most of the cilia in the utricle are arranged vertically and the head is in the upright position. Thus linear acceleration and deceleration in the horizontal plane are adequate stimuli for the cilia in the utricle. One may think of a child in a prone position propelling down an incline on a scooter board. As the child hits the horizontal plane, the head is upright, causing the cilia to deflect and discharge. Quick deceleration, caused by running into a mat on the floor, causes the hair cells to whip forward, deflecting the cilia once again. In most instances, the cilia in both the sacculus and utriculus are sensitive to a variety of stimuli. For example, forward and backward movements will activate cilia in both chambers. In summary, the adequate stimuli for the cilia of the utricle and saccule (vestibule) are the static position of the head in space and linear acceleration and deceleration in horizontal and vertical planes. The greatest tonal changes occur in extensor groups of the postural muscles. In addition, the vestibule (saccule and utricle) contributes to the maintenance of righting reactions, especially head position in space.

Rood[27] suggested that the side-lying position of the head is useful to diminish unwanted extensor tone caused by poorly integrated labyrinthine information. In this position the symmetrical input of the vestibular receptors on the vestibular nuclei is eliminated, modifying the outflow of the vestibulospinal tract and thus its influence over postural extensors.

The semicircular canals are referred to as the kinetic labyrinth because they respond to movements of the head. The semicircular canals also exert influences on the limbs and the extraocular muscles of the eyes and assist in equilibrium responses and orientation in space. The semicircular canals are arranged approximately at right angles to one another, one for each axis of rotation. The anterior and posterior canals are sensitive to movement in the sagittal plane. The horizontal canal reacts to rotation around the central body axis.[184,381] Any angular (rotatory) acceleration or deceleration of the head will displace and causes the semicircular canal receptors to fire.[288,379,380]

The semicircular receptors are not responsive to prolonged spinning at constant velocity. Numerous physiological studies[354,382] have demonstrated that during the beginning of rotation the receptors fire at a greater rate. If the rotation is continued, the receptors gradually reassume their resting position in about 20 seconds. When rotation is stopped, deflection again occurs but in the opposite direction because the endolymph fluid continues to circulate through the canals. After 10 to 30 seconds, the endolymph stops circulating and the receptors return to their resting positions and resume a tonic level of discharge. During this time, a normal nystagmus can be observed.

On the basis of this information, prolonged spinning is physiologically unproductive. It should be remembered that the initial acceleration is the force that causes firing at a greater rate. Also, the semicircular canals are most responsive to short rotational movements as opposed to prolonged rotation.[318] A good formula for semicircular canal stimulation is to spin the subject approximately 10 times in 20 seconds, stop abruptly, wait about 20 seconds, and spin again at the same rate in the opposite direction. Spinning that includes alternation of direction (e.g., right then left) maintains adaptive firing. It is also beneficial to consider the position of the head during spinning. For example, if the subject is side lying on a large spinning apparatus, the endolymph fluid in both the anterior and posterior canals will circulate, causing a more powerful response. If functional movement is not incorporated along with attention (e.g., spelling words or counting), learning will not occur as motor programs.

Spinning is not to be used without proper precautions. In infants and disinhibited patients it may induce seizures or depress respiration. It is best to allow patients to control the initial rate of spinning or vestibular stimulation so they can accommodate to the stimulus.

To review, the receptors of the vestibule (macula) seem to be concerned with static orientation of the head in space and "directionality." In this context, directionality refers to the ability to move from a beginning point A to a designated point B without becoming disoriented or veering off in the wrong direction. For example, we rely on the macula for orientation when we are swimming underwater. Because the feet are not in contact with the ground and gravitational forces are altered, the proprioceptors in joints and muscles provide little information about position in space. Thus, the brain is not receiving its normal proprioceptive input from the legs and postural muscles. In addition, vision is of little assistance because to work properly the cornea must have air in front of it. Water causes a refractive error and vision becomes distorted.[383] Consequently, if the vestibular mechanism was not receiving gravitational feedback, the underwater swimmer would become disoriented and unable to determine the direction of the surface.

The semicircular canals detect movements of the head in all planes and are involved in the maintenance of the upright posture. The pathways of the semicircular canals are extremely important for visual gaze, ocular movements, and alignment of head and body. The connections of the semicircular canals and the otoliths work cooperatively with the joint receptors of the neck to accomplish head and neck-righting reactions.[7,15,381]

Vestibular Treatment Alternatives. Because the vestibular system is a unique sensory system, critical for multisensory functioning, it is a viable and powerful input modality for therapeutic intervention (see Chapter 23). Because any static position and any movement pattern will facilitate the labyrinthine system, vestibular function and dysfunction play a role in all therapeutic activities. To conceptualize vestibular stimulation as spinning or angular acceleration minimizes its therapeutic potential and also negates an entire progression of vestibular treatment techniques.[14,41,384-386] Horizontal, vertical, and forward-backward movements occur early in development and should be considered one viable treatment modality. These movements seem to precede side-to-side and diagonal movements, which are followed by linear acceleration and end with rotatory movements. All these movements can be done with assistance or by the client independently in all functional activities. It is important to remember that the rate of vestibular stimulation determines the effects. A constant, slow, repetitive rocking pattern, irrespective of plan or direction, generally causes inhibition of total-body responses, whereas a fast spin or fast linear movement tends to heighten both alertness and the motor responses. Again, the vestibular mechanism is only one of many that influence the motor system. Thus, the system interaction must be constantly reassessed.

General Vestibular Treatment Technique with Sensory Systems Intact. As already indicated, constant, slow, repetitive rocking patterns, irrespective of plane or direction, generally cause inhibition of the total-body responses. Yet any stimulus has the potential of causing undesired responses, such as increased or decreased tone. When this occurs, the procedure should be stopped and reanalyzed to determine the reason for the observed or palpated response. For example, assume that a client, whether a child with cerebral palsy, an adolescent with head trauma, or an adult with anoxia, exhibits signs of severe generalized extensor hypertonicity in the supine position. To dampen the general motor response, the therapist decides to use a slow, gentle rocking procedure in supine position and discovers that the hypertonicity has increased. Obviously, the procedure did not elicit the desired response and alternative treatment is selected, but the reason for increased hypertonicity needs to be addressed.

It is possible that the static positioning of the vestibular system is causing the release of the original tone and that by increasing vestibular input the tone also increases. It may also be that the facilitory input did indeed cause inhibition, but the movement itself caused fear and anxiety, thus increasing preexisting tone and overriding the inhibitory technique. Instead of selecting an entirely new treatment approach, a therapist could use the same procedure in a different spatial plane, such as side lying, prone, or sitting. Each position affects the static position of the vestibular system differently and may differentially affect the excessive extensor tone observed in the client. The vertical sitting position adds flexion to the system, which has the potential of further dampening extensor tone. This additional inhibition may be necessary to determine whether the slow rocking pattern will be effective with this client. It would seem obvious that if a vestibular procedure were ineffective in modifying the preexisting extensor tone, then use of a powerful procedure, such as spinning, is inappropriate. Selection of treatment techniques should be determined according to client needs and disability. Clients with either an acoustic tumor that perforates into the brain stem or with generalized inflammatory disorders may be hypersensitive to vestibular stimulation, whereas other clients, such as a child with a learning disability, may be in need of massive input through this system. Heiniger and Randolph[41] and Farber[14,269] present an in-depth analysis of various specific vestibular treatment procedures commonly used in the clinic. A general summary of the treatment suggestions is summarized in Table 9-1 on page 197.

General Body Responses Leading to Relaxation. Any technique performed in a slow, continuous, even pattern will cause a generalized dampening of the motor output.[387] During handling techniques, these procedures can be performed with the client in bed, on a mat while horizontal, sitting at bedside or in a chair, or standing. The movement can be done passively by the therapist or actively by the client. Carryover into motor learning will best be accomplished when the client performs the movement actively, without therapeutic assistance. In a clinical or school setting, a client who is extremely anxious, hyperactive, and hypertonic may initiate slow rocking to decrease tone or feel less anxious or hyperactive. The reduction of clinical signs allows the client to sit with less effort and to be more attentive to the environment, thus promoting the ability to learn and adapt.

It is the type of movement, not the technique, that is critical. The concept of slow, continuous patterns is used in Brunnstrom's rocking patterns[10] in early sitting, in proprioceptive neuromuscular facilitation mat programs, and in gymnastic ball exercise programs; the use of these patterns can be observed in every clinic. Although the therapist may be unaware of why Mr. Smith gets so relaxed when slowly rocked from side to side in sitting, this procedure elicits an appropriate response. The nurse taking Mr. Smith for a slow wheelchair ride around the hospital grounds may do the same thing. Once the relaxation or inhibition has occurred, the groundwork for a therapeutic environment has been created to promote further learning, such as ADL skills. The technique in and of itself will relax the individual but not create change or learning.

Pelvic mobilization techniques in sitting use relaxation from slow rocking to release the fixed pelvis. This release allows for joint mobility and thus creates the potential for pelvic movement performed passively by the therapist, with the assistance of the therapist, or actively by the client. This technique often combines vestibular with proprioceptive techniques, such as rotation and elongation of muscle groups, which physiologically modify existing fixed tonal response through motor mechanisms or systems interactions. Simultaneously, slow, rhythmic rocking, especially on diagonals, is used to incorporate all planes of motion and thus all vestibular receptor sites to get maximal dampening effect, whether directly through the vestibulospinal system or indirectly through the cerebellum or another motor system. The same pelvic mobility can be achieved by placing the patient (child or adult) over a large ball. The ball must be large enough for the patient to be semiprone while arms are abducted and externally rotated and legs relaxed (either draped over the ball or in the therapist's arms). Again, this position allows for maintained or prolonged stretch to tight muscles both in the extremities and trunk while doing slow, rhythmical rocking over the ball. The pelvis often releases, and the patient can be rolled off the large ball to stand on a relaxed pelvis preliminary to gait activities.

Techniques to Heighten Postural Extensors. Any technique that uses rapid anteroposterior or angular acceleration of the head and body while the client is prone will facilitate a postural extensor response. Scooter boards down inclines, rapid acceleration forward over a ball or bolster, going down slides prone, or using a platform or mesh net to propel someone will all facilitate a similar vestibular response of righting of the head with postural overflow down into the shoulder girdle, trunk, hips, and lower extremities. Rapid movements while on elbows, on extended elbows, and in a crawling position can also facilitate a similar response. Depending on the intensity of the stimulus, the response will vary. In addition, the client's emotional level during introduction to various types of stimuli may cause differences in tonal patterns. Clinical experience has shown that facilitory vestibular stimulation promotes verbal responses and affects oral motor mechanisms. Children with speech delays will speak out spontaneously and respond verbally.

Because facilitory vestibular stimulation biases the sympathetic branch of the ANS, drooling diminishes and a generalized arousal response occurs at the cortical level. Therefore the appropriate time to teach adaptive rehabilitative techniques is after vestibular stimulation.[288]

Facilitory Techniques Influencing Whole-Body Responses. Tactile, vestibular, and proprioceptive inputs also assist in the regulation of the body's responses to movement.[36,269] As stated previously, the vestibular system, when facilitated with fast, irregular, or angular movement, such as spinning, not only induces tonal responses but also causes massive reticular activity and overflow into higher centers. Thus increased attention and alertness are often the outcome. The tracts going from the spinal cord, brain stem, and higher subcortical structures must be sufficiently intact to permit the desired responses from this type of input. If a lesion in the brain stem blocks higher-center communication with the vestibular apparatus, then massive input may cause a large increase in abnormal tone. The therapist needs to closely monitor any distress or ANS anomalies.

Total-Body Relaxation Followed by Selective Postural Facilitation. The use of the inverted position in therapy has become increasingly more popular in recent years. Early research on the labyrinth's influence on posture and the influence of the inverted position showed that total inversion (angle of 0 degrees) produced maximal postural extensor tone, and the normal upright position elicited maximal flexor tonicity.[333] There seems to be much confusion in the literature about the clinical effects of inversion. The initial research was performed on anesthetized animals and may not be representative of how the human CNS responds to inversion as a system. Kottke[335] reports that the static labyrinthine reflex is maximal when the head is tilted back in the semireclining position at an angle of 60 degrees above the horizontal. Conversely, minimal stimulation occurs when the head is prone and down 60 degrees below the horizontal position. Stejskal[388] studied the effects of the tonic labyrinthine position in hypertonic patients. This study failed to show labyrinthine reflexes in subjects with hypertonia.

The explanation for this incongruity seems to be one of interpretation. Any time a subject is put on a tilt table or even a scooter board, the weight bearing of the body on the surface must cause firing of the underlying exteroceptors while gravity pulls on the proprioceptors. This position also has the potential of creating fear.[389] As the body shifts and presses onto the underlying surface, stretch reflexes associated with posture and movement must contribute some bias to muscle tone.[347] In addition, if the subject is flexing or extending the head, the proprioceptors of the neck could also alter the muscle tone of the limbs.[350]

Another factor that contributes to tonal changes in the extremities is the cervicoocular reflex.[382,390] Reflex eye movements to center the eyes as the body or neck rotates also exert influences on the muscles of the limbs. Because all the influences brought about by gravity and postural mechanisms in a clinical situation cannot be controlled, the inverted position appears to be an interplay of cutaneous receptors, proprioceptors, and tonal changes in the labyrinthine system.[391]

Several highly recognized therapists have reported using the inverted position as a therapeutic modality.[14,30,41] Generally, the inverted position produces three major changes. First, because of the gravitational forces on circulation, the carotid sinus sends messages to the medulla and cardiac centers that ultimately lower heart rate, respiration, and resting blood pressure through peripheral dilation, creating a parasympathetic response pattern. This position may be contraindicated for certain patients with a history of cardiovascular disease, glaucoma, or completed stroke. Clients with unstable intercranial pressure, for example, those with traumatic head injuries, coma, tumor, or postinflammatory disorders, and many children with congenital spinal cord lesions would also be at high risk for further injury if the inverted position were used. However, this position has been used with some success for adult patients with hypertension. In any case, scrupulous recording of blood pressure and other ANS effects should be taken before, during, and after positioning.

Another benefit of the inverted position is generalized relaxation. Farber[14] recommends its use as an inhibitory technique. Because the carotid sinus stimulates the parasympathetic system, the trophotropic system is influenced and muscle tonicity is reduced. This has been found to be beneficial to patients with upper motor neuron lesions and also to children who exhibit hyperkinetic behavior. Heiniger and Randolph[41] report that severe hypertonicity in the upper extremities is noticeably reduced.

The third benefit of the inverted position is an increased tonicity of certain extensor muscles. This phenomenon is not purely a function of the labyrinth; it is also a result of activation of the exteroceptors being stimulated by the body's contact with the positioning apparatus.[391] Therapists have capitalized on this reaction to activate specific extensor muscles of the neck, trunk, and limb girdles.[27,335,388]

Because the inverted position decreases hypertonicity and hyperactivity and facilitates normal postural extensor patterns, the responses to the technique should be incorporated into activities. For example, if the position of total inversion over a ball is used, then postural extension of the head, trunk, and shoulder girdles and hips should be facilitated next. Additional facilitation techniques, such as vibration or tapping, could help summate the response. Resistance to the pattern in a functional or play activity would be the ultimate goal. If the inverted position is used in a squat pattern, then squatting to standing against resistance would probably be a primary goal. This can be accomplished by the therapist positioning his or her body behind and over the child, not only to direct the child initially into the inverted position but also to resist the child coming to stand. If the inverted position is used in sitting, activities of the neck, trunk, and upper extremities would be the major focus after the initial responses.

Because the inverted position elicits both labyrinthine and ANS responses, this technique needs to be cross-referenced within the classification schema. Because of its ANS influence, close monitoring is important for all clients placed in an inverted position. As with all labyrinthine treatment techniques, this approach, considered a normal, inherent human response, is used outside the therapeutic setting. For example, standing on one's head in a yoga exercise causes the same physiological state as that observed in the clinic. In many respects the yoga stance is done for the same reasons: decreasing hypertonicity (generally caused by tension), relaxation, and increasing postural tone and altered states of consciousness. Clients can certainly be taught to control their own ANS activity and hypertonicity by placing their hands between their legs when they need a generalized dampening effect on motor generators. Thus, when accessing and incorporating other approaches, the therapist analyzes each specific technique with use of a critical neuroscience frame of reference.

This section has described procedures that use the vestibular system as a primary input modality to alter the client's CNS. If the client's vestibular system itself is dysfunctional, it has the potential of altering the functional state of the motor system. See Chapter 23 for additional information.

Peripheral and Central Vestibular Processing Deficits. A variety of clinical symptoms are associated with unilateral and bilateral vestibular dysfunction. Unilateral problems include vertigo, nausea, dizziness, and postural instability, whereas bilateral problems include those mentioned earlier along with blurred vision, oscillopsia, and gait ataxia.[392-394] When clinical symptoms persist, vestibular therapy seems to be an effective treatment approach but must be patient specific and based on whether the function of the vestibular system is reduced or absent.[393,395,396] In cases of total vestibular loss, treatment approaches will either teach the client a substitution approach using proprioception and vision or a combination approach using both substitution and adaptation in clients with reduced vestibular function. A number of researchers[384,385,392,393,397-401] have shown therapeutic intervention to be the most effective treatment for most clients. (See Chapter 23 for an in-depth discussion of vestibular deficits.)

Shumway-Cook and Horak[397,401,402] found that, with testing, some children and adults who demonstrated clinical vestibular impairment did not have true vestibular deficits but demonstrated impaired postural reactions under all conditions of sensory conflict among visual, vestibular, and somatosensory systems. They concluded that these patients had an integrative central processing disorder and recommended treatment that dealt with the total sensorimotor system. Approaches such as sensory integrative therapy,[403] Feldenkrais,[404] or neurodevelopmental treatment (NDT)[403] might be possible options. The critical link or recommendation would be to integrate all treatment activities into normal activities that the client is self-motivated to practice under conditions of specific attention in a variety of ways (e.g., walking on an unstable surface, on support surfaces with eyes closed while head turning, and while counting backward).

Autonomic Nervous System

The ANS has become a focus of clinical interest.[41] Traditionally, the ANS regulates, adjusts, and coordinates visceral activities. Many aspects of emotional behavior and primitive drives are controlled by the ANS.[32,375,405] The intricate interconnections between the ANS and CNS have led clinicians to discover viable treatment approaches that depend on both systems.[41,269] The importance of these interconnec-

tions seems obvious. If the external world is threatening the system, then both somatic and visceral systems need to modify responses to optimally protect the organism. For example, if your visual system identifies an angry bear ready to attack you as you walk through the forest, both autonomic and somatic responses are needed. Your somatic system needs to ready your neuromuscular system for immediate action. Your autonomic system needs to ready your heart and respiration for increased rate to provide oxygen and nourishment to muscles for increased metabolism. Your emotional system needs arousal to attend to and deal efficiently with the crisis. All systems must react simultaneously and at appropriate intensities to protect the organism from imminent danger. If any system malfunctions and creates too little or too much output, imbalance and inefficiency result. This decreases your flexibility and ability to solve the problem and remove yourself from the dangerous environment[374] (see Chapter 4).

The input and processing systems, as well as the ANS itself, are often impaired in clients with brain damage. This can create ANS responses that are not always appropriate to the situation and limbic responses that affect motor performance (see Chapter 4). Understanding the intricate balance of sympathetic and parasympathetic responses of the ANS and how these behaviors affect functional output is important to conceptualizing the client's total needs. All systems within the CNS will change if the person perceives imminent danger, whether real or imaginary. The clinician will observe these altered responses to the environment, for example, in a gait session or an ADL task. Anxiety level, emotional responses, increased blood pressure, heart rate, and respiration, hypertonicity, and hyperactivity are but a few of the signs a therapist might use to identify an ANS response. These signs should alert and orient the clinician to the causes of the change. Slight alterations in the external environment are often sufficient to produce homeostasis. For example, if when standing a client feels he is falling forward, it is important to check the patient's perception, even if the therapist believes it to be inaccurate. If the perception is wrong, then the clinician needs to help the client relearn perception of vertical. If the perception is correct, the client's response is appropriate and provides important internal feedback. Even more important, the therapist has respected and responded to the opinion and judgment of the client. This helps begin and kindle trust and mutual respect, important clinical tools for modifying the client's ANS responses to new situations.[376,406]

The ability to differentiate tone created by emotional responses compared with tone resulting from CNS damage is a critical aspect of the evaluation process. Emotional tone can be reduced when stress, anxiety, and fear of the unknown have been reduced. This is true for all individuals. The client with brain damage is no exception. Seven treatment modalities that normally produce a parasympathetic or decreased sympathetic (flight/fight) response are listed below[407]:

1. Slow, continuous stroking for 3 to 5 minutes over the paravertebral area of the spine
2. Inversion, eliciting carotid sinus reflex and tonic labyrinthine response (refer to vestibular section)
3. Slow, smooth, passive and active assistive movement within a pain-free range (Maitland's grade II movements)[22]

4. Maintained, deep pressure on the abdomen, palms, soles of the feet, peroneal area, and skin rostral to the top lip
5. Deep breathing exercises (see Chapter 15)
6. Progressive muscle relaxation
7. Cranial sacral manipulation (see Chapter 37)

When pressure is applied to both the anterior and posterior surfaces of the body, measurable reductions may be recorded in pulse rate, metabolic activity, oxygen consumption, and muscle tone.[307,308]

These pressure techniques are identified as an intricate part of the many intervention approaches such as therapeutic touch,[147,374] Feldenkrais,[328-330,404] Maitland,[22] massage,[408,409] and myofacial release.[8,315,410-412] Although not verbally identified, other techniques (e.g., NDT,[33,34] Rood,[31,41,269] Brunnstrom,[10] and PNF[31] also place an important emphasis on the response of the patient to the therapist's touch.

Treatment Alternatives by Use of the Autonomic Nervous System

Slow Stroking. Slow stroking over the paravertebral areas along the spine from the cervical through lumbar components will cause inhibition or a dampening of the sympathetic nervous system. The technique is performed while the client is in the prone position. The therapist begins by stroking the cervical paravertebral region in the direction of the thoracic area, using a slow, continuous motion with one hand. Usually a lubricant is applied to the skin, and the index and middle fingers are used to stroke both sides of the spinal column simultaneously. Once the first hand is approaching the end of the lumbar section, the second hand should begin a downward stroking at the cervical region. This maintains at least one point of contact with the client's skin at all times during the procedure. The technique is applied for 3 to 5 minutes—and no longer—because of the potential for massive inhibition or rebound of the autonomic responses.[36,387] It is also recommended that at the end of the range of the last stroking pattern, the therapist maintain pressure for a few seconds to alert both the somatic and visceral systems that the procedure has concluded. Eastern medicine recognizes the importance of the ANS in total-body regulation to a greater extent than Western medicine does. The concepts of meridians and acupressure/acupuncture points are all intricately intertwined with the ANS (see Chapter 37). For that reason, a technique such as slow stroking would potentially interact with meridians and does extend over the row of acupuncture points referred to as "shu points" and relates to visceral reflexes connecting smooth muscle and specific organ systems. It is believed that this continuous, slow, downward pressure modulates the sympathetic outflow, causing a shift to a parasympathetic reaction or relaxation. Whether the result of the pressure on the sympathetic chain, some energy pressure over meridian points, a pleasant sensation, or something unknown, slow stroking does elicit relaxation and calming.[41,269] Clients with large amounts of body hair or hair whorls are poor candidates for this procedure because of the irritating effect of stroking against the growth patterns and the sensitivity of hair follicles.

Slow, Smooth, Passive Movement within Pain-Free Range. Increasing ROM in painful joints is a dilemma frequently encountered by therapists caring for clients with neurological damage. Having the client communicate the first perception of pain and then moving the limb in a slow, smooth motion toward the pain range elicit a variety of behaviors. First, the client generally gestures or verbalizes that pain is present 10 to 15 degrees before it may, in reality, exist. This behavior may occur because the patient during previous treatment interventions learned that therapists often responded to the client's statement of pain by saying, "Let's just go a little farther." That additional range is usually 10 to 15 degrees. By stopping at the stated point of pain, retreating back into a pain-free area, and approaching again, possibly with a slight variation in the rotatory direction, the client will often relinquish the safety range and a true picture of the pain range is obtained. The second finding is that if the motion toward the pain range is slow, smooth, and continuous, then frequently much of the range that was initially painful becomes pain free. The hypothesis is that slow, continuous motion is critical feedback for the ANS to handle imminent discomfort. The slow pattern provides the ANS time to release endorphins, thus modifying the perception of pain and allowing for increased motion. If the therapist stabilizes the painful joint and prevents the possibility of that joint going into the pain range, rapid, oscillating movements can often be obtained within the pain-free range. This maintains joint mobility and often, as an end result, increases the pain-free range. This technique is not unique to the treatment of clients with neurological problems; it is often used as a manual therapy procedure.[315,321,413] Furthermore, one can move slowly into a range that actually shortens muscles. If held for 30 seconds, the muscle that is too short can relax, promoting greater motion in the opposite direction. This can be called strain/counterstrain, inhibiting firing by maintaining a position of active insufficiency, making the muscle too short.

Manual therapy[22,291,414-416] can be used to describe the pain and joint changes occurring at the joint level. As the fields of orthopedics and neurology merge into one system,[331] with the brain acting as an organ controlling the entire system and its components, the question of whether the pain reduction is centrally or peripherally triggered may be an important one. It is probably both. For example, thumb pain can increase the sensation of the nervous system to the point that even cutaneous and proprioceptive receptors act as nociceptors.

Maintained Pressure. Farber[14] discusses a variety of techniques that facilitate a reduction of tone or hyperactivity. Pressure to the palm of the hand or sole of the foot, to the tip of the upper lip, and to the abdomen all seem to produce this effect. The pressure need not be forceful, but it should be firm and maintained.[417] This same technique is defined as inhibitory casting when applied through the use of an orthosis (see Chapter 34).

Progressive Muscle Relaxation. Progressive muscle relaxation is practiced during both meditation and treatment approaches such as Feldenkrais.[404,417,418] These methods of relaxation tend to trigger parasympathetic reactions, which in turn slow down heart rate and blood pressure and trigger slow, deep breathing (see Chapters 15 and 37).

Cranial Sacral Manipulation. Summarizing the complexity of cranial sacral theory is not within the scope of this book. The reader is referred to references to gain a global understanding of the treatment interactions and the ANS response to cranial therapy as well as a brief discussion in

Chapter 37.[407,410] This treatment approach needs to be more intensively researched in terms of physiological effects and clinical effectiveness.

Olfactory System: Smell

The sense of smell is the least understood of all the senses. Because of the inaccessibility of the olfactory receptors, to date little research has been conducted. Unfortunately, there are more theories than facts about how odors are sensed.[355]

Although the olfactory epithelium occupies an area only about the size of a dime, it is estimated to contain 100 million receptor cells.[309] These have an equal number of fibers but converge on principal neurons at a ratio of 1000:1.[301] How the receptor cells transduce odors into meaningful perception of smell is not well understood. One theory suggests that different odors do selectively activate some receptors and not others.[12,419] Other theories suggest that odorous molecules simply alter the sodium permeability of the receptor membrane and cause an inactivation of enzymes, thus changing its chemical reactions and electrical states.[361]

Findings indicate that humans can distinguish between 2000 and 4000 different odors. What is more confusing is that individual perception of the same odor will vary considerably; what is nauseating to one may be fragrant to another.[14,420-422] Receptors for smell adapt rather quickly to a constant stimulus. Physiological studies indicate that olfactory receptors adapt as much as 50% during the first few seconds of stimulation.[423,424] The strength of the odor has to change by approximately 30% before the receptors are reactivated. There is also some evidence that part of the adaptation takes place in the CNS.

One of the most remarkable characteristics of the olfactory system is that some impulses travel from the receptors through alternative routes and synapses to the temporal and frontal lobes without passing through the thalamus. All other major sensory systems must pass through a relay in the thalamus en route to the cortex.

Smell evokes different responses by means of the limbic system's control over behavior. Pleasant odors, such as vanilla or perfume, can evoke strong moods. Unpleasant odors can facilitate primitive protective reflexes, such as sneezing and choking. Sharp-smelling substances such as ammonia can elicit a reflex interruption of breathing.[378,425]

As a result of arousal, protective reflexes, and mood changes caused by odors, the use of smell as a treatment modality has been implemented, especially during feeding procedures. Odors such as vanilla and banana have been used to facilitate sucking and licking motions.[405,426] Ammonia and vinegar have been used clinically to elicit withdrawal patterns and increase arousal in semicomatose patients.[427] When odors are used as a stimulant, the therapist must be aware of all behavior changes occurring within the client. Arousal, level of consciousness, tonal patterns, reflex behavior, and emotional levels all can be affected by odor. Because of limited research in this area, caution must be exercised to avoid indiscriminate use of the olfactory system. Odors such as body odor, perfumes, hair spray, and urine can affect the client's behavior although the smell was not intended as a therapeutic procedure. Some clients, especially those with head traumas and inflammatory disorders of the CNS, often seem to be hypersensitive to smell. In these cases the therapist needs to be aware of the external olfactory environment surrounding the client and to make sure those odors that are present facilitate or at least do not hinder desired response patterns.[428]

Many clinical questions arise regarding smell as a therapeutic modality. If the choice of odors is between pleasant and noxious, a pleasant odor will theoretically be perceived in a way that should be enjoyable, relaxing, and thus potentially tone reducing. On the other hand, noxious odors should have a sympathetic reaction and, although causing one to become alert, may also create a fight/flight internal reaction that, if repeated frequently, could cause an adverse response to the client's perception of the world. This has the potential of having a profound effect on her or his feelings toward the therapist and the therapeutic environment. The effect may not be observable until the client reaches a level of consciousness or motor skill in which there is some ability to react.

Individuals' perception of smell is not correlated to their actual olfactory ability.[429] Because of the complex neuronetwork of the olfactory system, the specifics between emotional responses and olfactory environment cannot be established, and determining which olfactory input will drive a pleasant, unpleasant, or neutral response is variable. There may be a culture sensitivity to various smells that would suggest a cultural learning linked with emotional responses to smell.[430] Yet, without a sense of smell an individual may not be able to respond appropriately to various olfactory environments, which may increase a client's feeling of isolation and lack of social interactive skills.[431,432] Smell is intricately linked to the sense of taste. Without these sensory systems, individuals tend to stop eating, thus creating an entirely different health care issue.[433,434]

Gustatory Sense: Taste

The sense of taste is a chemical sense, involving not only the receptors of the tongue but also olfaction and tactile receptors. Therefore, the term *taste* encompasses not only gustatory sensations derived from food but also the smell, temperature, and texture of the material to be ingested.[435,436]

Four primary taste sensations have been identified: salty, sour, bitter, and sweet. These primary tastes are believed to blend together in various combinations to form additional tastes, similar to the way mixing the colors yellow and blue produces green. Histologically, the taste buds appear to be the same, yet they tend to be selective to specific stimuli. Action-potential studies have shown that any one taste bud will respond to all four primary tastes.[288,437] However, the quantitative responses differ considerably, allowing some buds to respond more vigorously to bitter and some to sour, sweet, or salty stimuli. It is also commonly known that regions of the human tongue vary in sensitivity to the four primary tastes. The base of the tongue best detects bitter, the sides detect sour, and the tip is sensitive to sweet substances. The ability of taste buds to discriminate changes in concentration of a substance is relatively crude; a 30% change in concentration is needed before a difference in taste intensity is detected.[269,438,439]

Afferent transmission of impulses from taste receptors may travel to the CNS by three cranial nerves. Taste sensations from the base of the tongue are served by the glossopharyngeal nerve (cranial nerve IX); the sides and the tip are served by the vagus nerve (cranial nerve X) and the facial nerve (cranial nerve VII). The pharyngeal surface of the tongue is innervated by the laryngeal branch of the vagal nerve (cranial nerve X). Taste buds begin to degenerate during the fifth decade of life, contributing to diminished taste sensation in the elderly.[12,301]

Taste sensation adapts rapidly. Action-potential studies have shown that when first stimulated, taste buds fire a burst of impulses and only partially adapt. As with the olfactory system, the additional adaptation is suspected to come from the CNS.[288,440] As the neurons terminate on the somatesthetic region of the temporal lobe, adaptation may be occurring there.[287,288]

Gustatory input is generally used as part of feeding and prefeeding activities. As already mentioned, the oral region is sensitive not only to taste but also to pressure, texture, and temperature. For that reason feeding would be classified as a multisensory technique that uses gustatory input as one of its entry modalities. Specific input modalities are based on the combined taste, texture, temperature, and affective response pattern. That is, both a banana and an apple may be sweet, yet the textures vary greatly. When mashed, both fruits may have a pudding-like texture, yet the client's emotional response may differ. Disliking the taste of banana but enjoying apple may cause startling differences in the client's response to various sensations. Thus the importance of the clinician's sensitivity to the client's response patterns within each sensory modality cannot be overemphasized.[269] Similarly, a therapist needs to take into consideration normal changes with taste and smell that occur as a result of aging and adjust the input threshold appropriately.[441,442]

Auditory System

The auditory system is fundamental to survival and also to human communication. Together with vision, the auditory system enables human beings to perceive events in the external world that take place at a distance from the body and to localize in space the exact position of a sound.[284]

The auditory nerve shares a common cranial nerve (VIII) with the vestibular system, thus creating a close anatomical and physiological relationship between these two senses.[24,288,443] Thus, individuals with hearing loss may show simultaneous vestibular imbalances. Approximately 10% of adults have hearing loss to some extent, with hearing loss even greater in the elderly.[442,444] Therapists need to discuss with clients whether they have difficulty hearing specific tones or frequencies. Similarly, clients with auditory figure-ground problems will have difficulty hearing in noisy environments, and compensatory types of communication may need to be used.

The auditory pathway to the CNS is diffuse and complex. Information about sound is sent ipsilaterally and contralaterally to the auditory cortex at the superior temporal gyrus or Brodmann's area 41. As information ascends toward the cortex, synapsing within a variety of nuclear masses, all information will synapse in the inferior colliculus within the midbrain as well as the medial geniculate nucleus of the thalamus. Other collaterals pass directly to the reticular-activating system. There are also important connections to the cerebellum, particularly in the event of a sudden noise.[287,288] Once sound reaches the superior temporal, a sound is "heard," but more specific recognition requires connections with additional auditory associative centers.[288,300,445,446]

Descending fibers from the cortex and efferent pathways within the brain stem auditory complex project ipsilaterally through the cochlear nerve back to both the inner and outer hair cells of the cochlea. The efferents are important to auditory sensitivity and selective tuning of the cochlea. With this efferent control over the auditory afferents, the cortex has a way of focusing in on certain sounds while ignoring others.[288] This may be the mechanism for auditory figure-ground or selective hearing. Similarly, fibers leaving the inferior colliculi project into the tectum of the midbrain and help modify the effects of the tectospinal tract and automatic turning of the head in response to sound.[288]

Treatment Alternatives with Use of the Auditory System. Because of the complexity of the auditory system, a potentially large number of input modalities exists. Although some of them might not be considered traditional therapeutic tools, they are nonetheless techniques that affect the CNS. Some treatment alternatives focus on the following:

- Quality of voice (pitch and tone)
- Quantity of voice (level and intensity)
- Affect of voice (emotional overtones)
- Extraneous noise (sound)
- Auditory biofeedback
- Language
- Levels, volume, and affect of voice

The therapist's voice can be considered one of the most powerful therapeutic tools. Even constant sound has the ability to cause adaptation of the auditory system and thus inhibition of auditory sensitivity.[288] Similarly, intermittent, changing, or random auditory input can cause an increase in auditory sensitivity.[447] Because of auditory system connections, an increase or decrease in initial input or auditory sensitivity has the potential of drastically affecting many other areas of the CNS.[448] The connections to the cerebellum could affect the regulation of muscle tone. The collaterals projecting into the reticular formation could affect arousal, alertness, and attention, in addition to muscular tone. The importance of voice level has been acknowledged by colleagues for decades with respect to encouraging clients to achieve optimal output or maximal effort. The use of voice levels is a critical aspect of the entire PNF approach.[31] Yet the volume or intensity of a therapist's voice is only one aspect of this important clinical tool. Through clinical observation, it has been observed that clients respond differently to various pitches. The response patterns and specific range of comfortable pitch seem to be client dependent. The concept that each individual may have a range within the musical scale or even a specific note that is optimal for biorhythm function has been posed by one composer-musician.[449] This concept needs research verification but may prove to relate to one of those innate talents some therapists have that distinguish them as gifted therapists.

The emotional inflections used by the clinician certainly have the potential of altering client response. For example, assume the therapist asks Tim, a child with cerebral palsy, to walk. The specific response from the child may vary if the clinician's voice expresses anger, frustration, encouragement, disgust, understanding, or empathy. Knowing which emotional tone best coincides with a client's need at a particular moment may come with experience or sensitivity to others' unique needs.

Extraneous Noise. The varying level of sound or extraneous noise in a clinical setting can at times be overwhelming. Dropping of foot pedals, messages over loudspeakers, conversations, computers, printers, telephones, moans, a jackhammer outside the clinic, water filling in a tank, a drip in a faucet, whirlpool agitators, a burn patient screaming, and a child crying all are encountered in the clinical environment, and all could be occurring simultaneously. A therapist whose CNS is intact usually can inhibit or screen out most of the irrelevant sound. Clients with CNS damage may not have the ability to filter sensitivity to all these intermittent noise sensations. The protective arousal responses these sounds might produce in a client could certainly elevate tone, block attention to the task, heighten irritability, and generally destroy client progress during a therapy session. Awareness of the noisy environment and the client's response to it not only is important for treatment modalities but also is critical to the problem-solving process.

Decreasing auditory distracters or sudden noises can drastically improve the client's ability to attend to a task or to succeed at the desired movement.[442,450] The therapist is reminded that if the environment has been externally adapted for a client to procedurally and successfully practice the goal, then independence in that functional skill has not been achieved. Reintroduction of the noises of the external world must be incorporated into the client's repertoire of responses so that the individual can feel competent in dealing with any auditory environment the world might present.

Music as an adjunct to therapy has been suggested as a viable way to help clients develop timing and rhythm to a movement sequence (see Chapter 24 for a discussion of basal ganglia disorders and Chapter 37 for a discussion of music therapy). Consistent sound waves and tempos, such as soft music, allow the patient to develop a neuronal model or an engram for the stimulus. The use of background music during therapy sessions enables the patient to make an association to the sounds, producing an autonomically induced relaxation response to a particular musical composition.[451-453]

Music is used for encouraging not only motor function but also memory[454,455] and socialization.[456-458] Rhythmic sound perceived as an enjoyable sensation certainly has the effect of creating motor patterns in response to that rhythm. Individuals, young and old, will tap their fingers or feet to a beat. If the beat has words, people will often sing along, recalling from memory the appropriate words. The movement, memory, and willingness to interact are all critical aspects of the therapeutic environment. Having clients dance with a significant other twice a day to music they have enjoyed in the past encourages both the physical function and the social bonding so important for quality of life.[194] Music affects heart rate, blood pressure, and respiration.[459,460] It has even been suggested that easy listening music may bolster the immune system.[161,406,461-463]

Auditory Biofeedback. Biofeedback as a total therapeutic modality is discussed under the treatment sections in Chapters 31 and 37. Auditory biofeedback is generally thought of as a procedure in which sound is used to inform the client of specific muscle activity. The level or pitch may change in relation to strength of muscle contraction or specific muscle group activity. Yet auditory biofeedback also encompasses feedback as simple as a foot slap that communicates that a client's foot is on the floor or verbal praise after a successful therapeutic session. The importance of the auditory feedback system as a regulatory mechanism between internal and external homeostasis cannot be overlooked. However, the clinician should not assume that this system is intact and can automatically be used as a normal feedback mechanism for clients with CNS damage.[270,464]

Language. Although most therapists thoroughly appreciate the complexity of the language system as a whole, they have little if any in-depth background to help them understand the components or the sequences leading to the development of language.[465,466] Thus many therapists are extremely frustrated when confronted with clients who show perceptual or cognitive deficits involving the auditory processing system.

Therapists easily identify language comprehension difficulties with adults who have first language differences and with young children because of their age and lack of language experience. Nevertheless, many clients have a language processing dysfunction that leads to communication difficulties, both in reception and appropriate expression. The elderly often can understand a conversation in a quiet room but have difficulty in rooms that are noisy.[448,467,468] The environment within which communication occurs can drastically affect both reception and the ability to express to the world inner feelings and thoughts.[406] Creating an environment conducive to that exchange will dramatically affect the motivation and drive of a patient within the therapeutic setting.[469]

Visual System

Vision is considered the most important and dominant sensory modality. The eye is the most complex of all the sense organs in our body. Its uniqueness is attributed to the biochemical or biophysical mechanism used to transduce a light stimulus to a neurological action potential. The retina, which makes up a major portion of the inside of the eye, is where light energy is transformed into neuronal-electrical impulses. Once transformed, the information must reach one of two sensory photoreceptors: the rods and cones. The rods are reactive to light intensity, that is, shades of gray. Unable to distinguish different colors, rods are said to provide "night vision." The cones (about 6 million) are responsible for color vision and require more light energy to become activated. A central part of the retina, called the fovea, is in direct line with the lens and cornea. Therefore, when we fixate on an object, the image of that object is projected upside down and backward on the fovea.[288,470] Once information reaches these sensory receptors, a complex interaction among chemical reactions, cell membrane ion transport, action potential generation, and synaptic activity takes place that will terminate with axons of neurons leaving the eye and projecting down the optic nerve.[288,437]

Each optic nerve consists of about 1 million nerve fibers. The combined 2 million nerve fibers of both optic nerves make up about 38% of all sensory and motor fibers entering and leaving the CNS.[288] The optic nerve contains two types of fibers: large, fast-conducting fibers concerned with visual perception and small, slower-conducting fibers concerned with reflexive activity. Fibers originating in the nasal halves of each retina cross in what is referred to as the optic chiasm. Conversely, the fibers originating in the temporal portion of the retina pass through the chiasm without crossing. The fibers from the temporal side also carry the fibers from the fovea (macula), where visual acuity is sharpest.[288,470]

Once the optic nerve passes through the optic chiasm, it is referred to as the optic tract. These anatomical relationships of visual fields and distribution of axonal tracking help therapists understand why clients have specific field loss and the functional extent of the impairment. Once the optic tract reaches the thalamus, synapses, and proceeds as the geniculolocalcarine tract, it again divides and radiates onto the top and bottom of the calcarine fissure. If lesions occur along either portion of these radiations, variance in field deficits result and thus affect a client's functional sight.[470] Once primary sight has reached the occipital lobe, an individual sees, but for those images to have meaning additional associative aspects of this cortical lobe must be activated. Once that occurs, an individual will display visual perception[470] (see Chapter 30). The visual system is extremely helpful to medical personnel for diagnosing disorders of the CNS. The eye provides a window through which a physician can examine the integrity of blood vessels and neurological tissue. Because the system extends through so much of the subcortical and cortical regions of the brain, many disorders manifest themselves in the visual system. Aside from the more obvious visual field problems, nervous system disorders can interrupt visual reflexes and impede eye movements.

Eye movements are subserved at the cortical and subcortical levels. Brodmann's areas 18 and 19 of the occipital lobe produce a reflexive visual pursuit in response to visual stimuli. Voluntary eye movements elicited on command derive from neurons in the frontal lobe of the cortex (area 8). Protective reflexes, such as blinking and quick localization of eyes, head, and neck toward a startling stimulus, are mediated by the retinotectal system (superior colliculus). Reflex eye movements activated by rotation of the head are mediated at the brain stem level by the vestibular system. The sizes of the pupil and lens are reflexively controlled by light stimulus. Pretectal areas, such as the Edinger-Westphal nucleus of cranial nerve III, act on the sphincter muscle of the iris and the ciliary muscle. Psychosocial research has demonstrated that pupils dilate and constrict in response to emotional feelings elicited by a visual stimulus.[12] Objects that are pleasing to the eye cause the pupil to dilate, whereas repugnant visual stimuli constrict the pupil. The higher-level cortical association pathways are complex, and our understanding of them continues to grow.[288]

Child development studies suggest that the efficiency with which an infant uses its eyes is a strong indicator of verbal ability and performance on intelligence tests.[471] The therapist should reinforce eye pursuits by pointing out objects in the environment and by encouraging the hand to follow the eye toward the object. According to Stejskal,[388] the eyes turn toward an object, the head has a natural tendency to turn, and when the neck rotates, a volley of neuromuscular events take place that better enable the upper extremities to perform a task such as reaching. Program generators are much more than a pure reflex action and thus manifest motor response with great adaptability and variability within the environment.

Because of the complexity of the visual system, treatment procedures can vary from simple to extremely complex. Simple treatment alternatives, such as hues or types of lighting, are often overlooked by therapists; yet they have the potential of altering patient response. Complex treatment procedures, such as those discussed in Chapter 30, are also often ignored by therapists because of a lack of understanding of and frustration with the visual system. Although we are not suggesting that all therapists become experts in visual processing and training, clinicians should become more aware of this input system, its potency as a treatment modality, and, when damaged, its devastating effect on normal response patterns.

Treatment Alternatives with Use of the Visual System. Because light is an adequate stimulus for vision, any light, no matter the degree of complexity, has the potential to affect a client's CNS. That input not only reaches the optic cortex for sight recognition and processing but also projects to the brain stem and to the cerebellum through the tectocerebellar tract. Simultaneously, these afferents activate the reticular-activating and limbic systems through the interneuronal pathway.[288] It even has influence over cervical spinal generators through the tectospinal tract.[387,472] Thus, as long as light is entering a client's CNS, it has the potential of altering response patterns either directly—through the tectospinal system or the corticospinal system through occipitofrontal radiations—or indirectly through the influence of the ANS and limbic system on muscle tone resulting from emotional responses to light.[473]

The five categories of visual-system treatment alternatives should not be considered fixed, all-inclusive, or without overlap. The first three categories (color, lighting, and visual complexity) are common everyday visual stimuli. Combined, they make up the visual world.

Colors. By varying the colors or by changing hues, tones, or the type of lighting and degree of complexity of the combined visual stimuli, the treatment modality and the way the CNS processes it change.[474-476] Because the visual system tends to adapt to sustained, repetitive, even patterns, any input falling under those parameters should elicit visual adaptation.[288,324,424] This adaptation response will lead to decreased firing of sensory afferent fibers and have an overall effect of decreasing CNS excitation. A clinician would expect to see or palpate a decrease in muscle tone, a calming of the client's affective mood, and a generalized inhibitory response. Cool colors, a darkened room, and monotone color schemes all seem to have an inhibitory effect.

In contrast, intermittent visual stimuli, bright colors, bright lights, and a random color scheme seem to alert the CNS and have a generalized facilitory effect.[477-479] Research in the 1980s in the area of criminology has produced evidence to suggest that specific shades of colors can produce either a sedating response (such as certain pinks) or general arousal (certain blues).[480] Although a tremendous amount of research is required to substantiate these results if the clinician is to apply them with confidence, research is beginning to show that specific shades of colors and hues may drastically affect a client's general response to the world and specific response to a therapy session.[481] Within the next few years, many facts regarding the reaction of the CNS to specific visual stimuli may be uncovered, and the clinician will be responsible for integrating this new information into the present categorization scheme.[482] In the Netherlands at the

Institute de Hartenbuer, playrooms have been designed in different colors.[16] Except for color, all rooms are exactly the same and originate from a central hub or core.[16] Children are allowed to select which room they wish to play or be treated in. Children seem to pick the color room that most suits their moods and alertness and creates an environment in which they can learn.[16]

Lighting. Two types of lighting are found in a clinical environment. Fluorescent or luminescent lighting comes by definition from a nonthermal cold source. This type of lighting is generally emitted by a high-frequency pulse. Umphred (clinical observations, 1967 to 2005) has found that many individuals within a normal population complain that this high-frequency flutter is irritating and causes distraction. For this reason, it is recommended that each clinician observe clients' responses to various types of lighting to determine whether fluorescent visual stimuli cause undesirable output. This is especially true with clients who already have an irritated CNS, such as those with inflammatory disorders, head trauma, or seizure disorders.[483,484] The clinician should also remember that clients frequently lie supine and look directly at overhead lighting, whereas the therapist looking at the client is unaware of that particular visual stimulus.

Incandescent lights by definition come from hot sources and emit a constant light without a frequency. The brightness of this type of lighting has the potential of altering CNS response. The visual system quickly responds to bright lights with pupil constriction. After prolonged exposure to a bright environment, the visual system adapts and becomes progressively less sensitive to it.[288,324] Similarly, when exposed to darkness, the retina becomes more sensitive to small amounts of light. Because of the response of the visual system to incandescent lighting, it is recommended that a therapist monitor the brightness of the lighting, especially preceding any type of visual-perceptual training or visually directed movement.

Although the sun is a natural source of light, it is not generally the primary source in a clinical setting. The sun can effectively be used as indirect lighting, thus eliminating the problems produced by artificial lighting. Sunlight is also more acceptable psychologically. Some clinics have designed the buildings to allow for maximum use of natural light.[15]

Visual Complexity. The visual system is the primary spatial sense for monitoring moving and stationary objects in space.[485] An infant continually refines the ability to discriminate objects in external space until capable of identifying specific objects amid a complex visual array.[424] When brain damage occurs, the ability to identify objects, localize them in space, pick them out from other things, and adapt to their presence may be drastically diminished.[352] Because of the distractibility of many clients, reducing the visual stimuli within their external space can help them cope with the stimuli to which they are trying to pay attention. Using rooms that have been stripped of such stimuli as furniture and pictures can reduce not only distractibility but also hyperactivity and emotional tone. If this method of reduction of stimuli is used, the clinician must remember that this procedure has a sequential component. The client must once again adapt to extraneous visual stimuli. Thus, as the client's coping mechanisms improve, the therapist needs to monitor and change the visual environment. The therapist can monitor the amount of input according to the response patterns of the client but in time needs to have the client function in everyday environments and practice adaptation.

Cognitive-Perceptual Sequencing with the Visual System. In sighted individuals the visual system is important in integrating many areas of perceptual development, such as body schemes, body image, position in space, and spatial relationships.[352] Vision as a processing system is so highly developed and interrelated with other sensory systems that, when intact, it can be used to help integrate other systems.[486] Conversely, if the visual system is neurologically damaged, it can cause problems in the processing of other systems.

For example, assume that a child is asked to walk a balance beam while fixating on a target. The child is observed falling off the beam. On initial assessment vestibular-proprioceptive involvement would be primarily suspected. On further testing the therapist might discover that the child, while looking at the target, switches the lead eye in conjunction with the ipsilateral leg. As the child switches from right to left eye, the target will seem to move. Knowing the wall is stationary, the child will assume the movement is caused by body sway, will counter the force, and will fall off the beam. The problem is a lack of bilateral integration of the visual system in contrast to other sensory modalities. The visual system deficit is overriding normal proprioceptive-vestibular input to avoid CNS confusion. Unfortunately, the client is attending to a deficit system and negating intact ones. This visual conflict would be overriding the normal processing of intact systems.

This same problem of the visual system overriding other inputs is often seen when clients are trying to relearn the concept of verticality. Clients with hemiplegia who demonstrate a "pusher" syndrome illustrate this conflict. Because the intact visual system can often be used to help reintegrate other sensory systems, the reverse should also occur. Teaching clients to attend to vestibular-proprioceptive cues while vision is occluded or visual stimuli tremendously reduced will help them orient to intact systems. Once the orientation is re-established, visual input will often be perceived in a more normal fashion. This syndrome has been linked to the posterior thalamus as well as other integrative cortical areas within the brain.[79,487-489]

Familiarity with the visual-perceptual system and its interrelationships with all aspects of the therapeutic environment is crucial if the clinician is to have a thorough concept of the client's problem. (See Chapter 30 for specific information regarding visual deficits and treatment alternatives.)

Mental Imagery. As was mentioned under neuroplasticity and as is discussed further within the section on somatosensory retraining, having patients visualize the sensory awareness of input from the environment has a positive effect on treatment outcomes. Similar positive effects have been shown to be effective when having patients practice motor imagery as part of the treatment protocol.[490-494] Having the patient practice mental imagery of the functional activity practiced during a therapeutic session can be an excellent way to empower patients to practice when they cannot perform the activity itself independently, without extreme effort, or with ineffective movement strategies. A therapist will know whether the patient has mentally practiced the movement strategies by the carryover within the next session. Although imagery usually insinuates visualization, there are also other forms of imagery that can be used as part of intervention.[495,496] Refer to the music therapy section in Chapter 37 regarding mental imagery.

One extension of mental imagery that became a common word in the 1990s as a result of video game popularity was "virtual reality." Over the last decade the interface between virtual reality and the medical education was the use of a virtual environment to teach surgeon's fine motor skill without practicing on a live subject.[497] An inevitable link has currently been identified between virtual reality and motor rehabilitation.[498-501] Today, literature certainly reflects the potential advantage virtual reality may have with regard to not only motor learning but the use of these environments as an adjunct to therapy in individuals with CNS damage.[502-505] The future potential of this type of augmented intervention will be up to visionary thinkers who stretch the envelope of traditional therapeutic interventions.

Compensatory Treatment Alternatives with Use of the Visual System.

The visual system can be used effectively as a compensatory input system if the sensory component of the tactile, proprioceptive, or vestibular system has been lost or severely damaged. The procedure of using vision in a compensatory manner should not be attempted until the clinician is convinced the primary systems will not regain needed input for normal processing. Although vision can direct and control many aspects of a movement, it is not extremely efficient and seems to take a tremendous amount of cortical concentration and effort.[483,506] Vision was meant to lead and direct movement sequences.[388,485] If it is used to modify each aspect of a movement, it cannot warn or inform the CNS about what to expect when advancing to the next movement sequence. Thus, using vision to compensate eliminates one problem but also takes the visual system away from its normal function. For example, assume that a hemiplegic man is taught to use vision to tell him the placement of his cane and feet, thus decreasing his need to attend to proprioceptive cues. When advancing to ambulatory skills such as crossing the street, the client may be caught in a dilemma. As he is crossing the street, if he attends to the truck coming rapidly down the road, he will not know where his cane or foot are and thus become anxious and possibly fall. If, on the other hand, he attends to his foot and cane, he will not know if the truck is going to hit him. That may increase emotional tone and make it difficult to move. If normal sensory mechanisms could be reintegrated, this client would have freedom to respond flexibly to the situation. Thus, caution should be exercised to avoid automatic use of this high-level system to compensate for what seem to be depressed or deficit systems.

Visual input should be used to check or correct errors if other systems are not available. Movement should be programmed on a feed-forward mode unless change is indicated. Vision often recognizes the need for that change. If a client is taught a motor strategy in which vision is used as feedback to direct each component of the pattern, the pattern itself will generally be inefficient and disorganized and will lack the automatic nature of feed-forward procedural motor plans. If the client is too anxious to practice the procedure physically without overusing vision, then visual mental practice can be introduced.

Internal Visual Processing: "Visualization Techniques" or "Mental Imagery".

The use of visualization of some aspect of bodily function has been and continues to be used in many forms of therapy.[349] It has been shown that individuals can modulate their immune responses through visualization.[507] Smith et al[507] showed that individuals could dictate through their thoughts and visualization various control over what was thought to be mindless internal processes. These concepts have been used therapeutically but usually when the client is resting or totally relaxed.[328,329,404]

More recently, technology in neuroscience has allowed for the measure of blood flow (positive emitting transaxial tomography) and MRI while engaging the brain in functional mental tasks. All areas of the brain except the cerebellum appear to be activated during intense goal-directed mental imagery. Given that the task is not motorically executed, errors in rhythm and accuracy are not made, and thus the cerebellum is not recruited for correction. This suggests that mental imagery can be used to restore a function that might have been lost as the result of a stroke or other type of injury. Visual imagination has the benefit of allowing correct task performance when physical limitations may prevent normal task completion. This could prevent abnormal learning (e.g., like that developing from abnormal posturing in gait in a stroke patient who lacks the voluntary control to ambulate and integrate a primitive synergy). For additional information, see the section on somatosensory discrimination.

Today these concepts can be integrated during active treatment in a variety of ways. Before a client begins to initiate a plan of movement, the therapist could ask the client to close the eyes and imagine the movement and what it felt like in that functional activity before the CNS injury. In this way, the patient is using prior memory and visualization to access the motor systems and hopefully initiate better motor plans. Similarly, if during a movement plan the state of the motor generators builds to such a level that the client is becoming dysfunctional, the therapist can stop the movement; ask the client to visualize a calm, quiet place, and then continue with the movement pattern when the tone is reduced or extraneous patterns cease. The client can be asked to practice mental imagery of the task until she or he can accomplish it normally and then finally carry it over to the real environment.[508,509] For example, a client may have practiced transferring during an intervention session in which the therapist, using augmented treatment, kept the patient within a biomechanical window. During the interval between sessions, the patient is asked to visualize at least a couple of times an hour, performing transfers initially from the same surface practiced and later to other surfaces. At the follow-up session, the therapist will often be able to tell if the patient has done the visualization. If the patient did practice, there is often carryover into the skill performance. If the patient forgot to practice, often the skill has reverted back to the initial level of learning, with little carryover from the last intervention.

Another way to use the visual system to access the processing strategies of the client is to observe eye gaze. Neurolinguistic theory postulates that the eyes gaze in the direction of brain processing.[372,508] Figure 9-12 illustrates the eye gaze direction along with the suggested processing activity. For example, a client who needs to access and

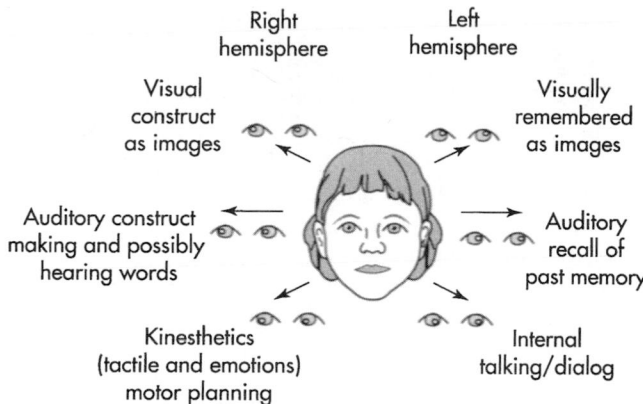

Right hemisphere

Left hemisphere

Visual construct as images

Visually remembered as images

Auditory construct making and possibly hearing words

Auditory recall of past memory

Kinesthetics (tactile and emotions) motor planning

Internal talking/dialog

FIGURE 9-12 ■ Eye gaze: correlation with lobe and hemispheric processing based on right-handed individuals. (Adapted from a handout from New Learning Pathways, Denver, 1988. Illustrations by Ben Burton.)

process motor plans through the frontal lobe will look down. A client who needs to visually construct an idea of something new will look up and to the right. Various cortical lobes and hemispheres serve specific global processing functions. There are many ways to apply and interpret this theory. By observing the patient's eye gaze, the therapist can determine whether processing is conducted in what would be believed to be the appropriate areas. Even more clinically relevant is observing where the eyes are gazing before and during successful functional activities. It may be that the area once used in processing is no longer available to do the function. If gazing to the right and down always leads to motor success, then the therapist can empower the patient to look down and right before dressing or transferring. Similarly, if a patient always looks down at the feet during ambulation, the reason may not be "to look at the feet" but instead may be accessing the motor cortex to gain better motor function. By asking the client to visualize the movement before and during the activity, the head often comes to a posturally correct position as the eyes gaze upward toward the occipital lobe. If the client is asked to walk while visualizing the movement, again the therapist may find a more upright, posturally efficient pattern. Once the program is set and practice scheduling begun, the patient may no longer need to look down and into the frontal lobe. Thus, in this case, the client not only learned the procedure but also avoided practicing and learning a posturally incorrect ambulation strategy.

Combined Multisensory Approaches

Although all techniques have the potential of being multisensory, the specific mode of entry may focus on one sensory system, as already described, or it may target two or more input modalities along with automatic motor programming. Table 9-6 categorizes a variety of treatment techniques that are clearly multisensory. The therapist, analyzing how the summated effect of the combined input and automatic responses influences client performance, gains direction in anticipating treatment outcomes in terms of the problem-solving process. Because the potential combinations of multisensory input classification are enormous, only a few examples of combinations are included in the text to illustrate the process a clinician might use when classifying

a new technique or a new approach to intervention. When clinicians select augmented treatment interventions to help a client as part of somatosensory retraining or functional retraining or to establish a procedural program, the basic science understanding behind the clinical decision helps develop questions for future research, determine a prognosis regarding outcomes, and rationally explain why or why not an intervention was effective. Clinical decisions must ultimately be made regarding which techniques or component of an approach should be eliminated first as the patient progresses. These decisions must be based on understanding and integration of neurophysiological mechanisms, learning environments, concepts of motor learning and control, and on client's needs, motivations, and goals. A simple rule a therapist might follow would be to take away the least natural technique first. That technique would be the most artificial or contrived. For example, a therapist might teach a client to assist with elbow flexion during a feeding pattern by (1) vibrating the biceps, (2) quick tapping the biceps, or (3) quick stretching the biceps a little beyond midrange by using gravity. The first option would be the least natural and obviously the least socially acceptable at a dinner party. The third option is the most natural and closest to the real environment the client will need to function within. Remember, these contrived techniques are used to assist clients who cannot control or perform the motor programs or functional activities without assistance or who need assistance in learning to modulate motor control for greater functional adaptability and independence.

Within the following section are examples of combined multisensory approaches that might be used to augment sensory feedback to obtain a better environment for regaining functional control.

Sweep Tapping. Many isolated techniques, such as sweep tapping[269] or rolling,[10] would be considered primarily proprioceptive-tactile in sensory origin. During sweep tapping the clinician first uses a light-touch sweep pattern over the back of the fingers of one of the hands. This stimulus is applied quickly over the dermatome area that relates to muscles the client is to contract. Second, the therapist applies some quick tapping over the muscle belly of the hypotonic muscle. The first technique is tactile and believed to stimulate the reflex mechanism within the cord to heighten motor generators and increase the potential for muscle contraction. The second aspect, tapping, is a proprioceptive stimulus used to facilitate afferent activity within the muscle spindle, thus further enhancing the client's potential for muscle contraction. At the same time the client will be asked to voluntarily activate the motor system, which then automatically augments tactile, proprioceptive, and auditory input with functional control.

Rolling of the Hand. Before Brunnstrom's rolling pattern is implemented, the client's upper extremity is placed above 90 degrees to elicit a Souques sign. This decreases abnormal, excessive tone in the arm, wrist, and hand.[10] This phenomenon may well be a proprioceptive reaction of joints and muscle. The rolling technique consists of two alternating stimulus patterns. The wrist and fingers are placed on extensor stretch. The ulnar side of the volar component of the hand is the stimulus target. A light-touch sweeping pattern is applied to the hypothenar aspect, which has the potential of eliciting an automatic opening of the hand beginning with the fifth digit.[10] Immediately after the

TABLE 9-6 ■ Combined Input Sensory Systems: Treatment Modalities

TECHNIQUE	PROPRIOCEPTIVE: JOINT, TENDON SPINDLE	EXTEROCEPTIVE	VESTIBULAR	GUSTATORY	OLFACTORY	AUDITORY	VISUAL	ANS	INHERENT RESPONSE LABELED	INHERENT RESPONSE NOT LABELED
Sweep tapping[94]	X	X							Automatic extension of hand	
Brumnstrom's rolling (hand)[40]	X	X								?
Raimiste's sign[40]	X	X								
Stretch pressure[94]	X	X								
Digging in sand, etc.	X	X					?			
Gentle shaking[94]	X	X	X							
Prone activities over ball[50,94]	X	X	X				X		Automatic righting of head (tectospinal/vestibulospinal)	
Sitting activities on ball[50]	X	?	X				X	X	OLR and balance (all systems)	
Mat activities	X	X	X			?	?			
Resistive exercises										
1. Resistive rolling	X	X	X			If verbal command	If visual leads			Rotatory integration
2. Resistive patterns: PNF[196,327]	X	X	Depends on pattern			X	X			
3. Resistive gait	X	?	Depends on pattern			If verbal command	X			
4. Isokinetics	X	Some					X			
5. Wall pulleys	X		X (if done in body rotation)				X (if guided toward target)			
6. Rowing[40]	X	?	X			If verbal command	X			Body rotation
Feeding[50,94,261]										
1. Maintained pressure: walking to back of tongue	X	X		?	?					
2. Resistive sucking										
a. Straw	X	X		?	?				X	
b. Popsicle	X	X		X	X				X	
3. Use of textures										
a. Peanut butter	X	X		X	X					
b. Apple sauce										

	Automatic closing of mouth	Decreased hypersensitive tactile system and thus withdrawal pattern: stereognosis	? (withdrawal to light touch)	Result of light touch	Labyrithine righting and equilibrium; possible OLR	OLR and equilibrium
4. Maintained pressure to top lip	X					
Inverted TLR[94,160]	X		?			
Touch bombardment[34]	X		X			
1. Tactile discrimination in sand, etc.		Decreased hypersensitive tactile system and thus withdrawal pattern: stereognosis				
2. Pool therapy						
Joint compression more than body weight[209,326]			X			
Throwing and catching						
1. Balloon			?	? (withdrawal to light touch)		
2. Heavy ball			Result of light touch	Result of light touch		
Variance in movement						
1. Quick action directed by vision			X			
2. Postural activities in front of mirror			X			
3. Therapist using voice command to assist client with movement			X			
High-level movement						
1. Walking balance beam			X	If visually corrected	Labyrithine righting and equilibrium; possible OLR	
2. Trampoline activities			X	If visually corrected		OLR and equilibrium
3. Running, jumping, skipping			X			

light touch, a quick stretch is applied to the wrist and finger extensors. These two techniques are applied quickly and repeatedly, thus giving the visual impression that the therapist is rolling his or her hand over the ulnar aspect of the dorsum of the client's hand. In reality, tactile and proprioceptive stimuli are being effectively combined to facilitate the central pattern generators responsible for the extensor motor neurons controlling the wrist and finger musculature. Because the tone is felt in the client's extensors and thus induces relaxation of the hypertonic flexors, the therapist can more easily open the client's hand. As the client obtains volitional control, some resistance can be added by the therapist to further facilitate wrist and finger extension. A hemiplegic client can also be taught to use this combined approach to open the affected hand and give it increased range. This technique is a noninvasive, relaxing approach to opening the hand stuck in wrist and finger flexion hypertonicity. The technique itself also seems to trigger spinal generator patterns that dampen the existing neuron network. It does not teach the patient anything unless that individual begins to assist or take over control of the extensor pattern. This usually occurs first by the therapist feeling the flexors relax when the patient is trying to extend the wrist and fingers even if no active extension is palpated. Encouraging the patient at this time to think correctly is important motivation for continued practice.

Withdrawal with Resistance. A therapist could combine the technique of eliciting a withdrawal with resistance to the withdrawal pattern. This can be an effective way to release hypertonicity, especially in the lower extremities. The withdrawal can be elicited by a thumbnail, a sharp instrument, a piece of ice, or any adequate light-touch stimulus to the sole of the foot. As soon as the flexor withdrawal is initiated, the therapist must resist the entire pattern. Once the resistance is applied, the input neuron network changes and the flexor pattern is maintained through the proprioceptive input caused by resistance to the movement pattern. The one difficulty with this technique is the application of resistance. The withdrawal pattern directly affects alpha motor neurons innervating those muscles responding in the flexor pattern and simultaneously suppresses alpha motor neurons going to the antagonistic muscles. If the antagonistic muscles are hypertonic, then initially the hypertonicity is dampened within the alpha motor neurons' neuronal pool. Because of the pattern itself, as soon as the flexor response begins, a high-intensity quick stretch is applied to the extensor muscles. If resistance is not applied to the flexors to maintain inhibition over the antagonistic muscles, the extensors will respond to the stretch. The client will quickly return to the predisposed hypertonic pattern and may even exhibit an increase of abnormal tone. This extensor response is a complex reaction within the spinal generators. The therapist should instruct the patient to assist with the flexor pattern to recruit other components of the motor system to enhance the system's modulation over the spinal generators.

Touch Bombardment. Another example of a proprioceptive-tactile treatment technique is modification of a hypersensitive touch system through a touch-bombardment approach. The goal of this approach is to bombard the tactile system with continuous input to elicit light-touch sensory adaptation or desensitization. Deep pressure is applied simultaneously to facilitate proprioceptive input and conscious awareness. Proprioceptive discrimination and tactile-pressure sensitivity are thought to be critical for high-level tactile discrimination and stereognosis. A hypersensitive light-touch system elicits a protective, altering, withdrawal pattern that prevents development of this discriminatory system and the integrated use of these systems in higher thought. This method of treatment can be implemented by having an individual dig in sand or rice. The continuous pressure forces adaptation of the touch system, and the resistance and deep pressure enhance the proprioceptive-discriminatory touch system by a complex adaptation process that most likely affects all areas involved in light and discriminatory touch, as well as the complex interaction of all motor system components.

Pool therapy can be used effectively for the same purpose, with the added advantage of neutral warmth. Any client perceiving touch as noxious, dangerous, and even life threatening will not greatly benefit from any therapeutic session in which touch is a component part. Touch includes contacts such as touching the floor with a foot, reaching out and touching the parallel bar railings, and touching the mat. The client may not respond with verbal clues such as "Don't touch me" or "When I touch the floor it hurts" but will often respond with increased tone, emotional or attitude changes, and avoidance responses. Nevertheless, this treatment approach has application in many areas of intervention with clients having neurological deficits. As an adjunct to this method, a clinician should cautiously apply light touch when in contact with the client. Deep pressure or a firm hold should elicit a more desirable response for the client even if the light-touch system is functional.[315,417] The use of Goretex material for clothing can greatly enhance the client's ability to tolerate the external world, where light-touch encounters cannot be avoided.

The therapist may also consider systematic desensitization as a strategy to integrate the touch system. By allowing patients to apply the stimuli to themselves, they can grade the amount that they can tolerate. In this respect they are empowered to control their own environment. They can practice adaptation in many situations. When the environment seems overwhelming, they have learned techniques to dampen the input both from within their own systems and by controlling the external world. For example, the therapist may place a box containing objects of different textures before the patient and encourage exploration and active participation to learn which textures are acceptable or offensive. A gradual exposure to the offensive stimuli will raise the threshold of the mechanoreceptors in the skin. There are also the benefits to the patient of being in control of the stimulus and having awareness of the treatment objective. In addition, vibratory stimuli through a folded towel provide proprioceptive input to desensitize the touch system.[298,352,417] Desensitizing the touch system from a need to protectively withdraw is an important process within the CNS if normal stereognosis is to develop.

Taping. Taping procedures used in peripheral orthopedic muscle imbalances and pain have the same potential for patients with neurological problems. This adaptation would be a modification of both splinting and slings. Although no research has been done to demonstrate efficacy for taping peripheral instability from CNS dysfunction, the concepts and ideas remain the same. Taping hypotonic muscle groups into a shortened range should effectively reduce the mechanical pull on both the muscle groups and joints and prevent the CNS from developing the need for compensatory stabilization. If hypertonicity is the result of peripheral instability, then taping a hypertonic muscle into its shortened range should stabilize the peripheral system and eliminate the need for the CNS to create the hypertonic pattern. On the other hand, taping can also be used to heighten information about proprioception and joint position, providing feedback to avoid hyperextension or hypermobility of a joint. This is especially true when there is an imbalance of intrinsics and extrinsics in the hand.

Oral-Motor Interventions. The complexity of combined proprioceptive-tactile input becomes enhanced by adding another sensory input, such as taste. Implementations of one of a variety of feeding techniques clearly identify the complexity of the total input system. When taste is used, smell cannot be eliminated as a potential input, nor can vision if the client visually addresses the food. The following explanation of feeding techniques is included to encourage the reader to analyze the sensory input, processing, and motor response patterns necessary to accomplish this ADL task. The complexity of the interaction of all the various systems within the CNS is mind boggling, but if the motor response is functional, effortless, and acceptable to the client and the environment, then the adaptation should be facilitated after attended repetitive behaviors.

Several feeding techniques have been developed in the past by master clinicians such as Mueller,[347] Farber,[269] Rood,[27] and Huss.[387] These techniques were not easily mastered or understood through reading alone. Competence in feeding techniques is best achieved from empirical experience under the guidance of a skilled instructor. Today, evidence base for implementation of feeding techniques can be found in the literature.[510]

The facial and oral region plays an important role in survival. Facial stimulation can elicit the rooting reaction. Oral stimulation facilitates reflexive behaviors, such as sucking and swallowing. Deeper stimulation to the midline of the tongue causes a gag reflex. These reactions and reflexes are normal patterns for the neonate. When these reactions/reflexes are depressed or hyperactive, therapeutic intervention is a necessity. Oral facilitation is an important treatment modality for infants and children with CNS dysfunction. Therapeutic intervention during the early stages of myelination can be crucial to the development of more normalized feeding and speech patterns.

Similarly, adults with neurological impairment often have difficulty with oral motor integration. Problems with swallowing, tongue control, and hypersensitive and desensitive areas within the oral cavity and also with mouth closure and chewing are frequently observed in adults with CNS damage.

Before basic feeding techniques are implemented, clinicians need to understand how the CNS and peripheral nervous system work collaboratively with the musculoskeletal system to control and perform these complex oral-motor functional movements.[287,288]

Feeding therapy is preceded by observation and examination. With a pediatric client, the therapist should observe breathing patterns while the client is feeding to determine whether the child can breathe through the nose while sucking on a nipple. In addition, the child's lips should form a tight seal around the nipple. Formal assessments should include functional assessments, developmental milestones, and behavioral manifestations. Medical charts and results from neurological examinations should be consulted for baseline data.

Postural mechanisms can influence feeding and speech patterns in clients with neurological dysfunction.[30,136] A client with a strong extensor pattern may have to be placed in the side-lying, flexed position to inhibit the forces of the extensor pattern. The ideal pattern for feeding is the flexed position, which promotes sucking and oral activity. Basic reflexes such as rooting, sucking, swallowing, and bite and gag reactions should be elicited and graded in children and evaluated in adults. The head needs to be in slight ventroflexion to pull in the postural stabilization of the neck and tongue. This is necessary to effectively facilitate programs that provide functional swallowing and control of foods by the tongue.

The facial region and the mouth have an extraordinary arrangement of sensory innervation. Therefore oral techniques must be used with utmost care. Anyone who has visited the dentist can attest to the feeling of invasiveness when foreign objects are placed in the mouth. With this in mind, the therapist should begin each treatment session by moving the autonomic continuum toward the parasympathetic end. Activation of the parasympathetic system should lower blood pressure, decrease heart rate, and, more important, increase the activity of the gastrointestinal system. Neutral warmth, the inverted position, and slow vestibular stimulation should help to promote parasympathetic "loading." Another approach that is applicable to feeding techniques is the application of sustained and firm pressure to the upper lip. An effective inhibitory device is a pacifier with a plastic shield that applies firm pressure on the lips. Perhaps this is why a pacifier is a "pacifier." Adults can acquire resistive sucking patterns with a straw and plastic shield and achieve the same results.

Sometimes children or adults are not cooperative and will not open their mouths. Rather than pry the mouth open, the jaw is pushed closed and held firmly for a few seconds. On releasing the pressure, the jaw reflexively relaxes. The receptors in the temporomandibular joint and tooth sockets may be involved in the production of this response.

A common problem seen in neurologically impaired infants and adults with head trauma is the "hyperactive tongue," which is often accompanied by a hyperactive gag reflex. To alleviate this problem, the receptors have to be systematically desensitized. The technique called tongue walking has met with clinical success.[14,41] It entails using an instrument such as a swizzle stick or tongue depressor to apply firm pressure to the midline of the tongue. The pressure is first applied near the tip of the tongue and progressively "walked back" in small steps. As the instrument reaches the back of the tongue, the stimulus sets off an automatic swallow response. The instrument is withdrawn the instant the swallow is triggered. This technique is repeated anywhere from 5 to 30 times a session, depending on individual responses.

Another technique, which might be called deep stroking, is used to either elicit or desensitize the gag reflex. Again, an instrument such as a swizzle stick is used to apply a light stroking stimulus to the posterior arc of the mouth. The instrument should lightly stretch the lateral walls of the palatoglossal arch of the uvula. Normally, the palatoglossal muscle elevates the tongue and narrows the fauces (the opening between the mouth and the oropharynx). Just behind the palatoglossal arch lies another called the palatopharyngeal arch. Normally, this structure elevates the pharynx, closes off the nasopharynx, and aids in swallowing. Touch pressure to either arc incites the gag reflex. This touch pressure should be carefully calibrated. A hyperactive gag reflex may be best diminished by prolonged pressure to the arcs, whereas light, continuous stroking may be more facilitory in activating a hypoactive gag reflex. A child or adult who has been fed by tube for extended periods of time will often have both hypersensitive reactions in various parts of the oral cavity and hyposensitive areas in other locations. This needs to be assessed to formulate a complete picture of the client's difficulties.

The use of vibration over the muscles of mastication appears to be physiologically valid. Muscle spindles have been identified in the temporal and masseter muscles.[39] Selected use of vibration on the muscles of mastication enhances jaw stability and retraction. For protraction to be facilitated, the mandible is manually pushed in.[269]

To promote swallowing, some therapists use manual finger oscillations in downward strokes along the laryngopharyngeal muscles and follow up with stretch pressure. Ice is beneficial as a quick stimulus to the ventral portion of the neck or the sternal notch. In addition, chewing ice chips provides a thermal stimulus to the oral cavity and a proprioceptive stimulus to the jaw and teeth; it also increases salivation for swallowing.

It is recommended that a therapist work closely with a colleague who has experience working with functional feeding before independently beginning to work with clients. The possible complications that might develop with individuals aspirating food cannot be overemphasized.

The therapist can quickly realize that feeding as a proprioceptive, tactile, and gustatory input modality is extremely complex and often incorporates other sensory systems. Breaking down the specific approaches into finite techniques helps the clinician categorize each component and then reassemble them into a whole. The job of dividing and reassembling the parts becomes more and more difficult as the number of input systems enlarges.[374]

Head and Body Movements in Space. Proprioceptive and vestibular input is one of the most frequently combined techniques used by therapists. In fact, client success in almost all therapeutic tasks depends on the coordinated input of these two sensory modalities.

If the head is moving in space and gravity has not been eliminated from the environment, vestibular and proprioceptive receptors will be firing to inform the CNS whether it should continue its feed-forward pattern or adapt the plan because the environment no longer matches the programmed movement. Depending on the direction of the head motion and the way gravity is affecting joints, tendons, and muscle, the specific body response will vary according to the degree of flexibility within the motor system. Bed mobility, transfers, mat activities, and gait all incorporate these two modalities. Although all these functional movements can be performed without these feedback mechanisms, the CNS cannot adapt effectively to changing environments without input from these systems. For that reason alone, a thorough examination of the integrity of both systems and the effect of their combined input seems critical if any ADL activity is to be used as a treatment goal.

The use of a large ball or a gymnastic exercise ball can be classified under the category of proprioceptive-vestibular input. Many activities can be initiated over a ball. When a child or adult is prone on a ball, righting of the head can often be elicited by quickly projecting the child forward while the therapist exerts control through the feet, knees, or hips. If the weight of the head is greater than the available power, then a more vertical and less gravitationally demanding position can be used. As the head begins to come up, approximation of the neck can be added. Vibration of the paravertebral muscles might also assist. Rocking forward or bouncing the client who is weight bearing on elbows or extended elbows would facilitate postural weight-bearing patterns through the two identified sensory input systems. Having a client sitting on a gymnastic ball doing almost any exercise will require vestibular and proprioceptive feedback to make appropriate adaptive responses. The combination seems to play a delicate role in the maintenance of normal righting and the equilibrium response so important in functional independence.

A trampoline, balance board, or a similar apparatus has the potential of channeling a large amount of vestibular-proprioceptive input into the client's CNS. In fact, a trampoline is so powerful it can often overstimulate the client and cause excitation or arousal in the CNS.

The trampoline and balance board are generally used to increase balance reactions, orient the client to position in space and to verticality, and increase postural tone. A client with poor balance, poor postural tone, or inadequate position in space and verticality perception may be justifiably fearful of these two apparatuses because of the rate, intensity, and skill necessary to accomplish the task. Because fear creates tone and that tone may be in conflict with the motor response from the client, caution must be exercised with either modality. (See Chapter 23 for further discussion of the interactions of sensory systems and balance.)

Gentle Shaking. A specific technique of gentle shaking can be listed under a combined vestibular, muscle spindle, and tendon category. This technique is performed while the client is in a supine position and the head ventroflexed in midline. The head is flexed 35 to 40 degrees to reduce the influence of the otoliths and unnecessary extensor tone through the lateral vestibulospinal tract. This flexed position should be maintained throughout the procedure. The therapist places one hand under the client's occiput and the other on the forehead. Light compression is applied to the cervical vertebrae. This technique activates the deep-joint receptors (C1 to C3) and muscle spindles in the neck along with the vestibular mechanism, which in turn connects with the cerebellum and motor nuclei with the brain stem. If the technique is performed slowly and continuously in a rhythmical motion, total-body inhibition will occur. If the pattern is irregular and fast, facilitation of the spinal motor generators will be observed.

Any one of these techniques can be implemented as a viable treatment approach in considering vestibular-proprioceptive stimuli. The selection of an approach or a method will depend on client preference, client response, the clinician's application skills, and the need for therapeutic assistance.

Summary of Techniques Incorporating Auditory, Visual, Vestibular, Tactile, and Proprioceptive Senses

Most therapeutic activities activate five sensory modalities: auditory, visual, vestibular, tactile, and proprioceptive. Auditory and visual inputs are used as the therapist talks to the client and demonstrates the various movement or response patterns to be accomplished during an activity. As the client moves, vestibular, tactile, and proprioceptive receptors are firing as inherent feedback systems. Thus, the complexity of any activity with respect to analysis of primary input systems is enormous. Even a sedentary activity such as card playing requires a certain amount of proprioception for postural background adaptations, tactile input from supporting body parts and limbs, and visual input for perception and cognition.

Thus, when the categorization of techniques—such as a PNF slow reversal,[21] a Brunnstrom marking time,[10] marking time with music,[511] Feldenkrais' sensory awareness through movement,[328,329] NDT,[33,512] Rood's mobility on stability,[27,30] or any mat or ADL activity is considered—the therapist must observe the sensory systems being bombarded during the activity. At the same time, if the therapist has determined which sensory systems are intact, which are suppressed or dysfunctional, and which seem to be registering faulty data; then altering duration and intensity of the input environment through any one system and the combined input through multiple systems creates tremendous flexibility in the clinical learning environment. Understanding this diagnostic process leads to more accurate prognosis and selection of appropriate interventions. Highly gifted therapists seem to instinctively go through this diagnostic process. One skill that seems consistent among master clinicians is a highly developed sensitivity to the client's responses, which represents a summation of expression of all systems within the CNS. Simultaneously, they adjust the quantity and duration of combined input to best meet the needs of the client. These masters release external control and encourage the client to use normal, inherent monitoring systems to adapt to changing environments as soon as the client is able to function independently no matter if that is only 5 degrees of motion or an entire functional pattern made up of many motor programs. Thus, that control may begin with a part of the range of a functional skill and not necessarily the entire functional activity itself. The key to carryover will be the client's empowerment over the motor control system and the degree of practice, self-monitoring, and adaptation available to the client. By analyzing and categorizing input and patient responses, many therapists may develop skills that were initially considered out of reach.

Innate CNS Programming

The responses of the PNS and CNS to various external stimuli determine the individuality of an organism and its survival potential within the environment. As organisms become more and more complex, the types of external stimuli and the internal mechanisms designed to deal with that input also increase in complexity. As the CNS develops structurally and functionally, inherent control over responses to certain common environmental stimuli seems to be manifested. Different areas of the motor system play different roles in the regulation of motor output. No area is dominant over another. Each area is interdependent on both the input from the environment and the intrinsic mechanisms and function of the nervous system.

As mentioned earlier, the PNS is intricately linked to the CNS and vice versa. Damage to one could potentially alter the neuropathways, their function, and ultimately behavior anywhere along the dynamic loops. Nevertheless, although researchers today emphasize the dynamic interactions of all components, clinicians have observed for decades different motor problems when different areas of the brain are damaged. Thus, when clients with neurological damage are discussed, it seems paramount to identify inherent synergy patterns available to humans, especially if those patterns become stereotypical and limit the client's ability to adapt to a changing environment.

The authors do not recommend or discredit the use of any stereotypical or patterned response as a treatment procedure. Acknowledging the presence and stressing the importance of knowing how these motor programs affect clients' functional skills are important. Without this knowledge, therapists working with either children or adults with CNS dysfunction limit their understanding of the normal CNS, normal motor control mechanism and its components, and the interactive effect of all systems on the end product: a motor response to a behavioral goal.

To conceptualize a systems model, the reader must replace the hypothesis of a stimulus response–based concept of reflexes[308] with a theory of neuronetworks that may be more or less receptive to environmental influences. That sensitivity is modulated by a large number of interconnecting systems throughout the CNS and by the internal molecular sensitivity of the neurons themselves. Specific patterns seem to be organized or programmed at various levels or areas within the CNS. These synergies or patterned responses are thought to limit the degrees of freedom available to programming centers such as the basal ganglia and cerebellum[13,334] and to enable more control over the entire body. Having soft-wired, preprogrammed, patterned responses allows organizing systems to activate entire sequences of plans and modify any components within the total plan. Modification and adaptation then become the goal or function of the motor system in response to both internal and external goal-directed activities. The specific location of soft-wired programs is open to controversy, as is the complexity of programming at any level within the CNS. Recognizing that these neuronetworks exist with or without external environmental influences would suggest that patterns can and will present themselves without an identified stimulus. In the past, when an external influence was not correlated with an identifiable stereotypical motor pattern, it was referred to as a synergy. When a stimulus was identifiable, the entire loop was called a reflex. Reflexes and preprogrammed, soft-wired neuronetworks such as walking are interactive or superimposed on one another to form the background combinations for more complex program interactions. This superimposed network may encompass spinal and supraspinal coactivity, which makes it difficult to specify a level of processing. The exact control mechanisms that regulate the specific pattern may again be a shared responsibility throughout the nervous system, thus providing the plasticity observed when disease, trauma, or environmental circumstances force adaptation of existing plans, as discussed in the neuroplasticity section.

One way to conceptualize this complex neuronetwork is to picture a telephone system linking your home to any other home in any city in any country on earth. If the relay between a friend in New York and you in California develops static, the system may self-correct, relay through another area, or even traject through a nonwired mechanism such as a satellite. The options are infinite, but priorities for efficiency and adaptability exist both within the telephone network and the brain. If the wires to your home are cut, the phone will not ring. If your peripheral nerve is cut or the alpha motor neuron damaged, the muscle will not contract. If the relay centers at one end of your block are short circuited and not working properly, then your phone and those of your neighbors may still function, but not in a fluid or specific manner. That is, someone may be calling your neighbor but both your phone and your neighbor's phone might ring. Spinal involvement can create a similar problem. The muscles are innervated and the input from the environment is accurate, but the neuronetwork is faulty. Regulation or modulation may be less efficient or controlled, but the system will use all available resources to try to respond to internal and external environmental requirements. This rule seems consistent throughout the nervous system, and the degree of plasticity is tremendous.[513]

When specific patterned responses are observed, the reader must always hold simultaneously the interaction of all other motor programming options. In this way the therapist can easily conceptualize the variations within one response and the reason why, under different environmental and internal constraints, the motor response pattern may show great variations within the same general plan. Similarly, the expected motor response may not be observable although it would seem appropriate and anticipated. The clinician must remember that the more complex the action (e.g., rolling compared with dressing compared with playing hockey), the greater the need for integration and coordination over pattern generators. Similarly, the more complex the desired action (especially in new learning), the greater the potential for needed perceptual/cognitive and affective interactions and the greater the potential for gratification and also for failure.

Certain patterned responses or neuronetworks might be considered more simplistic or protective in function. These patterns were once thought to be hard-wired spinal reflexes. It is now known that these reflexes, as well as complex pattern generators, exist at the spinal level and that their responses affect brain stem, cerebellar, and cortical actions. These centers simultaneously affect the specifics of the spinal neuronetwork responses. With clients who have low functional control over the spinal or brain stem motor networks, identification of existing patterns, optional patterns as a response to environmental demands, and obligatory patterns not within the control of the client's intentional repertoire of patterns becomes a critical evaluative component before prognosing or identifying the most appropriate interventions.

Recognizing specific patterns and how those patterns and others might affect functional movement or positional patterns has clinical significance. A child with spastic cerebral palsy, for instance, shows extension and "scissoring" when the pads of the feet are stimulated. Sometimes the extension pattern is so strong that the child will arch backward. Sustained positions that oppose pathological patterns are believed to elicit autogenic inhibition. Contraction-relaxation techniques also work on the autogenic inhibition principle.[21]

Just as afferent input can be used to alter tone and elicit movement, it can also become an obstacle when the therapist tries to coordinate complex movement patterns. A persistent grasp pattern is a common occurrence in children and adults with a CNS insult. This dominant grasp is often reinforced by the client's own fingers and frequently prevents functional use of the hand. If a withdrawal pattern is elicited every time a client is touched, the client not only will be unable to explore the environment through the tactile-proprioceptive systems but also will experience arousal by the influence of the cutaneous system over the reticular activating system. Severe agitation could likely be a behavioral outcome from such a persistent reflex.

As with any treatment procedure, a clinician should determine whether the technique will help the client obtain a higher level of function. The clinician must learn to recognize not only specific patterns but also what combinations of responses of pattern generators would look like. If the reader overlaid the map of the pattern generators for any combination of programs, a complex neuronetwork would result. To some it would verify chaos theory, and to others it would verify the end result of multiple systems interacting. The neuronetwork complexity of multiple input can be overwhelming. Thus, a therapist must always be observant of the specific behavioral response and the moment-to-moment changes in behavior during a treatment session, even if the specific neuronetwork is not understood.

The clinician needs to observe whether the specific patterned response is (1) triggered by afferent input, (2) triggered by volitional intent, or (3) activated without environmental input or cortical intent. In the third case, the entire motor system needs to be evaluated to determine which portion might be modulating the observable behavior. Differentiating these motor components will help in prognosing and selecting interventions.

Holistic Treatment Techniques Based on Multisensory Input

As already mentioned, a variety of accepted treatment methods exist. Each approach focuses on multisensory input introduced to the client in controlled and identified sequences. These sequences are based on the inherent nature of synergistic patterns,[7,32] the patterns observed in humans[7,9,343] and lower-order animals,[35] or a combination of the two.[21,30] Each method focuses on the total client, the specific clinical problems, and alternative treatment approaches available within each established framework. Certain methods have traditionally emphasized specific neurological disabilities. Cerebral palsy in children[9,25,30,178] and hemiplegia in adults[10,11,23,33] are the two most frequently identified. In the past two decades substantial clinical attention has been paid to children with learning difficulties.[14,36]

Yet the concepts and treatment procedures specific to all the techniques have been applied to almost every neurological disability seen in the clinical setting. This expansion of the use of each method seems to be a natural evolution because of the structure and function of the CNS and commonalities in clinical signs manifested by brain insult.

Two augmented therapeutic intervention approaches that have become accepted over the last decade have been *body-weight supported treadmill training* (BWSTT) and *constraint-induced movement therapy* (CIMT). Each is discussed as a separate intervention philosophy, but the reader must remember that these are augmented intervention programs. Before an individual would be considered functionally independent, the patient must be able to perform the functional activity in a natural environment such as ambulation within a home setting or eating using the more involved extremity without having the unaffected extremity restrained. A third augmented intervention approach, robotics, will also be presented to illustrate how therapists and patients have the capabilities to interface with new and sophisticated technology. More recently, another augmented approach, called the Accelerated Skill Acquisition Program, has been described. This approach is currently under testing. This approach is impairment oriented, emphasizes bimanual activities, and focuses on active, patient-centered collaboration reinforced with self management and self-efficacy.[514-516] This approach emphasizes attended, repetitive task practice progressing in difficulty and meets the principles for neuroplasticity.

Body-Weight Supported Treadmill Training
Over the last decade BWSTT has been accepted within the therapeutic community as an alternative approach to teaching gait to individuals after CNS damage. Students are introduced to the treatment procedures and potential sequences from total dependence to independence of the patient. Colleagues take continuing education courses to teach them how to position and drive the various motor components of the gait program while using BWSTT. With both a vertical support for the body weight and a treadmill that perturbs the feet backward or shifts the center of gravity forward, the environment unloads the CNS's need to (1) trigger and control an effective and efficient postural system, (2) drive the power necessary to perform upright ambulation, (3) control the balance strategy of stepping to prevent falling, and (4) have a cognitive interface with the various motor programs necessary to run this functional activity. The perturbation of the feet backward optimizes the stepping reaction forward, although this component can be controlled by one or two therapists at the patient's feet if the patient does not step, has a delayed stepping response, or only steps effectively with one foot. The rate of movement of the treadmill can also be controlled by the therapist to facilitate a patient's response even if it is slow or inadequate for normal over-ground ambulation. The question remains whether this type of augmented therapeutic intervention does create the best environment to empower the patient to learn or relearn normal locomotion after a neurological insult.

The literature is mixed with regard to the above question. Literature supports BWSTT for individuals with incomplete spinal injury,[517] the elderly with Parkinson's disease,[518] and some individuals after a stroke.[519,520] Other literature suggests that it is less effective than over-ground gait training,[521] whereas still others report that there is no difference among different forms of ambulation training.[522] With the literature so inconsistent, the clinician could be confused as to the effectiveness of BWSTT and whether this type of augmented intervention should even be considered. One primary problem with the literature is the great variance in identified variables selected by researchers within their respective studies, such as walking speeds, endurance, type and severity of neurological dysfunction, age of patients, and dependence on assistance.[519,523-525] There have been some excellent systematic reviews of the literature that help identify many of the reasons the literature seems so inconsistent.[525,526] The two populations of individuals most often studied by use of BWSTT are people with incomplete spinal cord injuries and individuals after stroke.* As stated, the number is huge when possible variables and functional ways to measure outcomes are considered when studying BWSTT or other types of training or studying other types of training along with BWSTT.[519,522,528-530] Even with all the confusion within the literature regarding these variables, this form of augmented intervention seems to show promise as a protocol for gait training. Future research studies will need to determine which patients, the degree of motor involvement, the optimal dosage, the time after insult, the best combination of other interactions (e.g., pharmacological, robotic), and the specific impairments within the gait cycle would most benefit from this type of intervention. As has been shown in the past, new treatment ideas gain popularity and become standards of practice without the rigor of establishing an evidence-based practice.[84-86,531] Physical and occupational therapy need to establish the evidence as a continuing evolution of the effectiveness of practice.

Constraint-Induced Movement Therapy
CIMT (or CI therapy) refers to the treatment of clients with motor system limitations that combines constraint or immobilization of the unaffected arm with use of a hand mitt or sling with forced-use type mass practice of meaningful motor tasks with the affected arm. The treatment focus of CIMT is on shaping behavior to improve functional use of the impaired upper limb.[532,533] CIMT is based on the theory that impairment in hand and arm function in clients after a stroke is compounded by learned nonuse of the upper extremity, which leads to a physical change in the cortical representation of the upper limb in the primary sensory cortex.[534] Learned nonuse develops in the early stages after a stroke in humans as the patient compensates for difficulty using the impaired limb by increasing reliance on the intact limb. This compensation has been shown to hinder recovery of function in the impaired limb.[535]

CIMT and the learned nonuse theory are based on deafferentation experiments in monkeys, many done by Dr. Edward Taub.[536,537] Early primate studies demonstrated that, if the upper limb was surgically impaired by dorsal rhizotomy to disrupt afferent input to the sensory cortex, the animal stopped using the limb for function. Active mobility was restored by immobilizing the intact upper limb for several days while training the animal to use the affected limb.[535] The first report of CIMT for hemiparesis

---

*References 282, 517, 519, 524, 525, 527.

in humans was by Ostendorf and Wolf in 1981.[538] Since then, investigations have demonstrated the effectiveness of CIMT with individuals who have residual upper-extremity weakness as the result of an upper motor neuron lesion.[104,106,107,538-545]

CIMT has been shown to be an effective therapy in persons with chronic stroke who have sufficient residual motor control to benefit from the exercises,[107,539,540,543,546-551] in brain-injured patients,[556,557] in children with hemiplegic cerebral palsy,[532,558-563] and in patients with Parkinson's disease.[564] The CI therapy approach has also been used successfully for the lower limb rehabilitation of patients with stroke hemiparesis, incomplete spinal cord injury, and fractured hip.[539] Other diverse chronic disabling conditions, including nonmotor disorders such as phantom limb pain and aphasia, may also benefit from CIMT.[539]

The criteria for the inclusion of subjects in most CIMT research studies have focused on voluntary movement ability in the involved upper extremity.[538-546,551] These criteria included the ability to start from a resting position of forearm pronation and wrist flexion and actively extend each metacarpophalangeal and interphalangeal joint at least 10 degrees and extend the wrist at least 20 degrees through a range of motion.[547] It is estimated that approximately 20% to 25% of the population of patients with chronic stroke with residual motor deficit meet this motor criterion.[565] Not all patients with hemiparesis have been found to benefit from CIMT. It has not been shown to be beneficial for clients with severe chronic upper extremity hemiplegia after a stroke.[566] Attempts to include individuals who did not meet the minimal motor criteria (at least 10 degrees finger extension and 20 degrees of wrist extension) have failed to demonstrate significant or lasting functional improvements in the involved upper extremity after CIMT.[539,566]

The successful therapeutic components of CIMT involve restraint of the unaffected arm with a mitt, sling, or glove for 90% of waking hours for a 2- to 3-week period combined with concentrated, repetitive task training of the more affected upper extremity with physical and occupational therapy.* Clients typically participate in 6 to 7 hours of therapy a day plus home activities and ADLs.[535,550,562,565] The ratio of therapist-to-client is typically 1:1, with the therapist present to give tactile and verbal feedback and instruction, along with assistance for the desired skill training. Clients also typically keep a daily treatment diary to document the amount and intensity of therapeutic intervention and the amount of time spent wearing the mitt or sling each day for the duration of the intervention.[562]

Subjects with chronic stroke hemiparesis who have participated in CIMT rehabilitation programs have demonstrated significant gains in functional use of the stroke-affected upper extremity with use of the Motor Activity Log,[565] and significant reductions in motor impairment on the upper extremity motor component of the Fugl-Meyer Test[566] and the Wolf Motor Function Test.[108,567-570] Fine motor improvements have been measured with use of the Grooved Pegboard Test and other dexterity tests.[534,535] These improvements in impairment and function have been shown to persist at follow-up evaluations up to 2 years after train-

ing.[534,545,563,569] Individuals participating in CIMT studies have demonstrated improvements in the amount of use and quality of movement in the more involved upper extremity and carryover of skills from the clinic to real-world activities.[104,106,538,562] This functional improvement may be significant even if the patient has previously participated in a conventional rehabilitation program.[571]

The question of when to begin CIMT after a stroke has not yet been definitively answered. Recently, CIMT has been applied to clients with subacute stroke with the hypothesis that earlier intervention may prevent learned nonuse from developing in the first place and may have a greater impact on overall function. Investigators found no adverse effects of CIMT in the subacute phase and only slightly greater improvement in motor function of the affected upper extremity.[572] There is some evidence to suggest that early application of CIMT may be detrimental to humans and may cause an increase in the size of the cortical lesion. This is based on studies of "forced overuse" in animal studies.[573-576] Kozlowski et al[576] found that early forced overuse of the affected limb within the first 7 days after a sensory motor cortex lesion impeded motor recovery of the affected limb and enlarged lesion volume. Bland et al[573] also forced overuse of the affected forelimb immediately after a focal cortical middle cerebral artery stroke, which increased the lesion size and impaired motor recovery. The relative risks and benefits of "acute" CIMT, and its optimal timing, remain to be determined.[535]

The neurophysiologic mechanisms that are believed to underlie the treatment benefit of CIMT include overcoming learned nonuse and plastic brain reorganization.[571,577] Studies have confirmed that CIMT produces use-dependent cortical reorganization in humans with stroke-related paresis of an upper limb.[106,545,577,578] There is some question, however, as to whether the improvements in upper extremity motor function after CIMT are due to the reduction of learned nonuse or to overcoming a sense of increased effort during movement.[534] Neuroimaging studies such as TMS, fMRI, and electroencephalogram[478,534] have been used to provide cortical change evidence of neuroplasticity after CIMT.[540,545,562,582] These studies have shown that massed practice of CIMT produces a massive use-dependent cortical reorganization that increases the area of cortex involved in voluntary movement of an affected limb, even in patients with chronic stroke.[105,535]

The application of CIMT to real-life clinical environments presents some challenges, including the time and physical demands on therapists and the resources of a rehabilitation unit, limiting its cost-effectiveness and overall effect.[535] Most patients in the acute rehabilitation setting do not qualify for CIMT on the basis of limited motor function.[535] CIMT, by its nature, can prove to be difficult and frustrating, intense, and slow, and it will only create beneficial effects if all participants put in the time and effort to make it successful.[562] Many subjects who have been presented with the opportunity to participate in CIMT programs and studies have refused because of the intense practice schedule and the necessity of the restrictive device.[580] Therapists have also voiced concerns about patient adherence and safety.[580] Although it has been shown to be effective in laboratory research, CIMT may have limited practicality in some clinical environments.[580]

---

*References 104, 106, 540, 541, 543, 544, 546, 551, 563, 564.

The future success of CIMT will depend on its ability to be modified according to disease factors, economic considerations, limitations of the practice setting, and the cognitive and physical status of the patient. Less intense practice schedule models[581-583] and combining CIMT with pharmacological interventions or robotic assistance will help to increase its cost benefit.[535,584] Patient satisfaction, overall cost, and the impact on quality of life are other areas that require further evaluation.[585]

Robotics

The third and probably the most recently augmented intervention procedure becoming popular in today's clinical environment is the use of robotics to assist the patient to regain control over functional movement. Robotics is being used to enhance motor function both in upper extremity and lower extremity movement patterns. The lower extremity treatment focus has been on functional ambulation,[530,586] whereas the upper extremity focus has been on shoulder, elbow, and wrist function during reach.[242,583,587,588] Individuals with spinal cord injuries are the most frequently studied group when robotics effect on retraining functional ambulation is analyzed,[530,586] whereas individuals after stroke are the most frequently studied population when robotics interface with upper extremity functional movement problems is analyzed.[242,587-592] The research is certainly looking encouraging when the interface between robotics and functional training is analyzed. The clinical reasoning needed to determine how and to what extent a patient would benefit from the combination of robotic assistance and functional movement training takes away any worry regarding robotics replacing the need for occupational or physical therapy. Robotics is just another therapeutic tool or orthosis that can assist in a task-specific training program that should lead to functional improvement and motor control outcomes for individuals who have had neurological trauma.[108] What research has not determined is what population of patients, time of onset compared with robotic intervention, dosage of intervention (both short and long term), or specific impairments within a functional pattern would best benefit from this type of intervention. With the interest shown both by the professionals and the robotic industry, these questions must be answered as clinician research unravels the effectiveness of inter-facing human movement control after a CNS insult with technology.

Summary of Augmented Intervention Strategies

As with many interventions, the therapist may need to start with augmented approaches and control the environment to allow the patient to practice effortlessly as an aspect of a functional activity training. At the same time, specific components of the intervention may be focusing on impairment training. Given the interactions between the patient, the therapist, and the environment during any one treatment session within a neurological rehabilitation setting all these strategies may be used.

Clinical Examples: How to Use a Classification Scheme When Selecting an Augmented Intervention Program

Clinical Problem 1: Client with Lack of Head Control. There is a potential for lack of head control

among young, developmentally delayed children or in individuals after a severe injury to the CNS. For that reason it is a common clinical problem. Furthermore, because of the importance of head and neck control, virtually all functional activities are affected by its absence.

Before a classification schema is discussed, the clinical problem must be analyzed and identification made of those sensory and inherent input systems to be facilitated. In considering the specific problem of lack of head control, let us assume that Timothy, a 16-year-old client with a closed-head injury, had a lesion within his CNS 3 months ago. He has the following signs regarding head control:

■ Mild extensor hypertonicity is present in the supine position, and Timothy is unable to flex and rotate his head off the mat.

■ In prone position, extensor hypertonicity is absent, and hypotonicity prevails. The client is able to briefly bob his head off the mat in a hyperextension pattern. Mild tonal shifts occur to either side when the head is turned and when it is symmetrically flexed or extended.

■ Timothy is unable to roll or perform any functional activity in the horizontal plane.

■ When placed in long sitting position, he is unable to hold the position or sit with flexed hips and extended knees. His head remains in total flexion with his chin on his chest.

■ When placed in a short sitting position on a mat table, he is unable to hold the position. General hypotonicity prevails, although slightly more flexion is palpable. His head remains flexed. When asked to pick up his head, he extends into a hyperextension pattern followed by extensor relaxation into flexion.

■ He is unable to hold the head in a postural coactivation pattern in a vertical position.

■ Timothy does not mind being touched and responds well to handling techniques.

From the analysis of these clinical signs, the following clinical interpretations are presented.

1. In the horizontal position, Timothy has persistence of a motor program that is enhanced by the spatial position and its influence on the vestibular system. The result might be considered persistence of a tonic labyrinthine reflex. In this client the dominant synergic pattern is extension. While he is supine, extension prevails. While he is prone, extension is inhibited, although flexion tone is not dominant. Because of the persistence of hyperactivity among the extensor motor generators, the ability to initiate rolling using a neck-righting pattern is prevented. The presence of a mild, asymmetrical tonic neck reflex to both sides and a symmetrical tonic neck reflex has been noted. Because of his instability and low tone, Timothy seems to be using these stereotypical patterns volitionally to assist in gaining some control over his motor patterns. In prone position, Timothy has the ability to move into a neck extension or optic and labyrinthine righting (OLR) pattern but is unable to hold it. Thus, movement and range are present but postural holding is missing.

2. As a result of ventroflexion of the head in sitting, the vestibular apparatus is placed in a position similar to that when prone. In a like manner, the total patterns

remain fairly consistent. The increase in flexor tone may result from the positioning of hip and knee flexion and kyphosis of the back. The inability to flex the hips with knee extension suggests that total tonal patterns or synergies are dominant. The client is unable to break out of those dominant patterns. Dominant OLR is not present.

3. When asked, Timothy carries out the command to the best of his motor ability. This suggests the presence of some intact verbal processing, which is translated into appropriate motor acts. Similarly, when asked to pick up his head, he does just that, suggesting some perceptual integrity of body image, body schema, and position in space. Knowing where his head is in space and where to reposition it also suggests that some proprioceptive-vestibular input and processing are occurring.

4. Timothy's enjoyment of being moved in space as related to handling techniques suggests proprioceptive-vestibular integrity. Similarly, his tactile systems seem to be functioning in a discriminatory manner and modifying negative responses of withdrawal and arousal. However, specific tactile perception would need a great deal of further testing. Thus, he demonstrates functional strengths in cognition and perception, in limbic motivation, in some areas of sensory integrity, and in control over available but limited motor programming. Yet, performance on any functional test would result in identification of an individual whose functional limitations prevent him from independence in any activity. Prognosis would need to be guarded until the therapist had an opportunity to augment the environment to determine how quickly he regained control and retained the learning. The initial prognosis is assumed to focus on development of head control as a preliminary and necessary motor program for all functional daily living activity. The estimated time it will take to regain this function would not be identified until after the first intervention session.

Behavioral Diagnosis. The client is unable to functionally control his head in any position in space, which limits independence in all functional activities. Lack of postural coactivation and adequate control over the motor generators has led to imbalances in the tonal characteristics of flexor and extensor patterns with the compensatory development of stereotypical patterns of movement.

Goal of Intervention Program. The goal is development of independent head control initially, in a narrow vertical window with the intent of enlarging that window to include all positions in space.

Now that the clinical problem has been analyzed and the goal of development of head control set, an intervention sequence or protocol must be established. Timothy lacks head control in all planes and in all patterns of movement. Thus, flexors and extensors must be facilitated to develop a dynamic coactivation or postural holding pattern of the neck. The categorization scheme can now be of some assistance. The therapist can ask, "Are there any inherent mechanisms that enhance flexors or extensors in a holding pattern?" OLR should elicit the desired response. Similarly, the clinician can ask, "Are there any inherent motor programs that would prevent righting of the head to face vertical OLR?" The tonic labyrinthine reflex (TLR) would block or modify the facilitation of OLR. Knowing that the TLR is most dominant in horizontal and least dominant (if at all affected) in vertical is of clinical significance. It is also important to know that the OLR is most frequently tested in a vertical position and seems most active in that position. Awareness that the client is sensitive to total patterns (e.g., flexion facilitates flexion or extension facilitates extension) gives additional treatment clues.

After all this information is assimilated, the following treatment protocol could be established.

To enhance neck flexors, the client will be placed in a totally flexed position in vertical, with the head positioned in neutral. The client will be rocked backward toward supine, allowing gravity to quick stretch the flexors (Figure 9-13, *A*). As soon as the neck flexors are stretched, the head should be tapped forward and then back to vertical but not

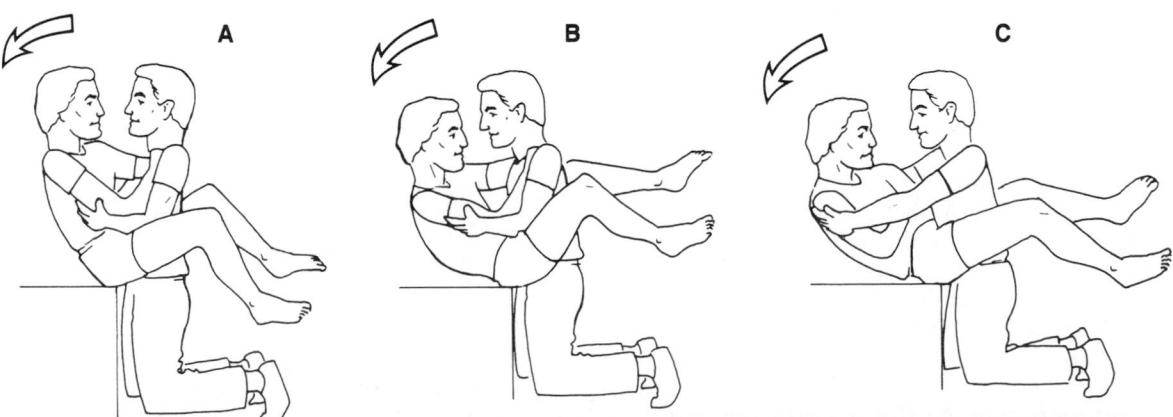

FIGURE 9-13 ■ Development of flexor aspect of head control. **A,** Vertical position: head at midline and midrange (total body flexion) to optimally facilitate neck flexors. **B,** Facilitating symmetrical neck flexion, using position, gravity, and flexor positions. **C,** Facilitating flexion and rotation to develop pattern necessary for neck-righting pattern.

beyond. This avoids hyperextension, extreme stretch to the proprioceptors, and the horizontal supine position of the labyrinths, all of which dampen the flexors and facilitate the extensors. The quick stretch and position should optimally facilitate OLR, which should activate the neck flexors. The total flexion of the body similarly facilitates the neck flexors. Once the neck flexors respond, Timothy can be rocked farther and farther backward while maintaining the head in vertical or ventroflexion (see Figure 9-13, B). Once Timothy can be rocked from vertical to horizontal and back to vertical while maintaining good flexor neck control, his CNS has demonstrated inherent control and modification over the stereotypical patterns, such as the TLR in supine with respect to its influence over the neck musculature. This rocking maneuver can be done on diagonals to practice flexion and rotation (see Figure 9-13, C), the key to eliciting a neck-righting, rolling pattern from supine to prone. The total flexed pattern can also be altered by adding more and more extension of the extremities. This decreases the external facilitation to the flexors and demands that Timothy's CNS take more and more control (internal regulation). Additional treatment procedures can be extracted from a variety of sensory categories. To add additional proprioceptive input, any one of those listed techniques might be used. The rotation and speed of the rocking pattern affect the vestibular mechanism. Auditory and visual stimuli can be used effectively. If the therapist takes a position slightly below the client's horizontal eye level, the client (to look at the therapist) will need to look down and flex his head, thus encouraging the desired pattern. Any type of visual or auditory stimulus that directs the client into the desired pattern would be appropriate. The therapist must remember that neck flexion is one of the identified goals. Rotation was added to incorporate and set the stage for inherent programming that will lead to rolling, coming to sit, and reaching while sitting. Because the postural extensor component still needs integration, total head control has not been attained. To facilitate neck extension, a procedure similar to the one for flexion can be established. A vertical position, thus eliminating the influence of the TLR, would again be the starting position of choice.

With extension facilitating extension, the client should be placed in as much extension as possible without eliciting excessive extensor tone. An inverted labyrinthine position, a kneeling position, or a standing position would be viable spatial patterns to facilitate OLR of the head and coactivation of postural extensors. The vestibular system sensory category can be checked to identify the treatment procedure for use with an inverted labyrinthine position. The kneeling or standing position places the client in a vertical position with hip and trunk extension. Kneeling rather than standing is used first because of the influence of the positive supporting reaction in standing and the massive facilitation of total extension. Kneeling avoids total extension while maintaining a predominant extensor pattern. As a result of the gravitational pull of body weight through the joints, approximation to facilitate postural extension is constantly maintained. The upper extremities can be placed in shoulder abduction and external rotation, which tends to inhibit abnormal upper extremity flexor tone and facilitate postural tone into the shoulder. This extensor tone has the potential through associated spinal reactions to facilitate neck and trunk extension. The arms can be placed in this position over a bolster or ball or by the therapist handling the client from the rear (Figure 9-14, A). The head should begin again in a neutral position. The client is rocked forward (see Figure 9-14, B) to facilitate optic and labyrinthine righting of the head and to elicit a quick stretch to the postural extensors. If the head begins to fall forward, the therapist can tap the client's forehead immediately after the quick stretch. This tapping action is the reverse tap procedure described under the muscle spindle proprioceptive category. The tapping is done to passively move the head back to vertical.

A variety of additional procedures can easily be combined to summate facilitation to the postural extensors. Tapping, vibration, and approximation through the head to the shoulders are only a few of the proprioceptive modalities. All would be facilitory. A variety of auditory and visual stimuli could be used to orient the client to a position in space and thus righting of the head. Techniques listed under the exteroceptive and vestibular systems could also be part of the treatment protocol. The therapist would want to sequence the client toward prone while the head remained in a vertical postural holding pattern. As the therapist rocks the client toward prone again, a rotatory component should be added (see Figure 9-14, C). The client will extend and

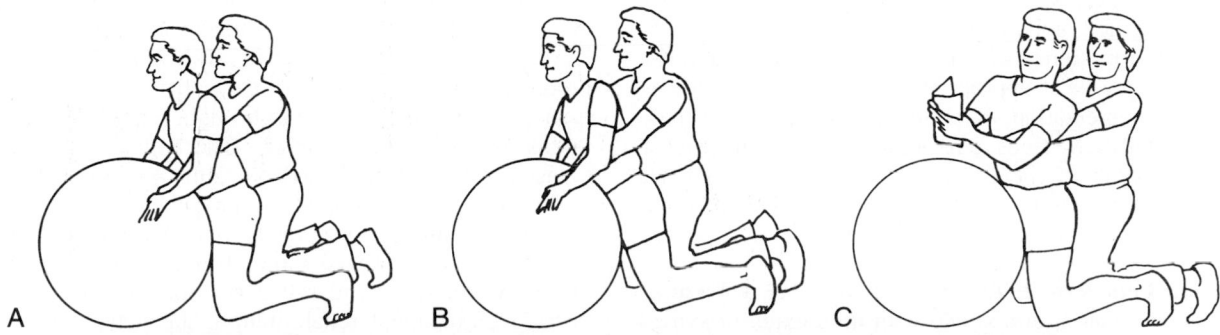

FIGURE 9-14 ■ Development of extensor aspect of head control. **A,** Vertical position: head midline with long extensor in midrange and postural extensors in shortened range; body in postural weight-bearing pattern. **B,** Facilitating symmetrical extension of head, trunk, and hips while inhibiting abnormal upper extremity tone. **C,** Facilitating head and trunk extension and rotation to encourage neck righting pattern; client reaches for an object, which is then placed on the opposite side.

rotate to counterbalance the movement, thus incorporating the neck-righting pattern of extension and rotation necessary when rolling from prone to supine. Resistance to neck extension with or without rotation is an important element in regaining normal functional control. The client is alert and has some functional use of the arms and legs. This rocking pattern in kneeling can be done as a functional activity. The therapist asks the client to assist in reaching toward an object with one upper extremity. The therapist can guide the client in the reaching pattern in a forward, sideward, or cross-midline direction. While reaching, the client can be rocked forward to elicit right and equilibrium reactions. By incorporating an activity into the treatment of head control, the client not only is entertained but also attends to the task rather than cognitively trying to keep his head up. In this way automatic head control is facilitated, and often postural patterns follow. In a partial kneeling pattern the client can be sequenced to on-elbow over a bolster or ball or on a chair. These activities should be sequenced from vertical to prone to ensure both total postural programming in prone and optimal integration of OLR, as well as letting the client experience control of various motor strategies in many different environmental contexts.

Once the client can maintain good flexor, extensor, and rotational components of head control, the activity should, if possible, be practiced with the client's eyes closed. If the client can still maintain head control, labyrinthine righting would be adequate for any functional activity. If the client loses head control, then additional labyrinthine facilitation would be indicated. If a client uses only vision to right the head, then any time vision is needed to lead or direct another activity, head control might be lost. Because symmetrical vestibular simulation plays a key role in activating the neck muscles to hold the head in vertical, it also is a key element leading to the perception of vertical and all the directional activities sequencing out of the concept of verticality. The postural extensor programming for head control needs to be practiced in a standing position and a sitting position. The client needs to be able to stand quietly without excessive extension to run both postural and balance programs. Similarly, he needs to be able to sit with hip flexion while coactivating postural extension in the trunk and neck.

Head control is a complex motor response. A therapist can facilitate inherent mechanisms to assist a client in regaining function. Simultaneously, multitudinous external input techniques classified under the various sensory modalities and combined modalities can be used to give the client additional information. Awareness of one technique and the ability to categorize it appropriately allow easy identification and implementation of many additional approaches. The therapist always needs to remember that the client must practice the behavior (head control) in a variety of spatial positions during various functional activities. This practice must be functional and no longer contrived.

Clinical Problem 2: An Individual after a Stroke.
A 66-year-old man after a stroke with mild extensor synergic hypertonicity within the right lower extremity and hypotonicity within the right upper extremity except within the shoulder girdle that has weak but functional movement patterns. His stroke was medically considered mild and his prognosis good in relation to the potential CNS regarding function.

Family, Patient, and Thus Long-Term Therapeutic Goals. Goals are to ambulate independently and use the right upper extremity to fly fish, an activity that he loves and does daily since he retired.

Occupational and Physical Therapy Management Decision. The patient would be taught to regain independent functional skills in dressing, feeding, hygiene, transfers, and other ADLs. To facilitate the patient's goal of fly fishing, his family was asked to bring in the rod and reel to augment a real situation with the functional skill he possessed within his right shoulder girdle.

Specific Physical Therapy Intervention with Regard to Fly Fishing. Besides ADLs, it was decided to use the BWST as a training tool for his right lower extremity. Manual assistance was used to guide the placement of the right foot at heel strike into dorsiflexion. The training began with a 30% weight reduction and the patient relaxed into the gait pattern. His right arm was suspended with the use of a shoulder harness and a robotic aid that swung through the arm in a reciprocal pattern to the left leg. This intervention was done twice daily for 3 weeks. During weeks 2 and 3, the patient's body weight support was reduced to 15%. By the end of the second week the patient was actively assisting the therapist with the entire gait cycle of both legs. By the end of week 3, the patient was able to walk on the treadmill independently. During the second week, over-ground ambulation was begun to transfer the treadmill learning into a functional activity. By the end of the fourth week, patient was independent on noncompliant surfaces. Over the next month the patient was in an outpatient environment with the primary goal of independent ambulation on compliant surfaces such as sand, dirt hills, and gravel environments.

Specific Occupational Therapy Intervention with Regard to Fly Fishing It was determined that the OT would work on postural endurance of the trunk and lower extremities while facilitating the right upper extremity to practice fly fishing. Initially, the training was done in sitting to create a stable environment for the right upper extremity. The arm was placed over a ball that the patient could roll back and forth as he visualized fly fishing. His right hand was placed in a glove that had a wrist support and was fastened to the rod with Velcro. The rod was placed in a bucket with a hinge joint that allowed for anterior and posterior movement of the rod attached to its base of support. Using this adaptation of the ball, rod brace and wrist support and glove, the patient was able to mimic one half of the range needed to fly fish. He so enjoyed the activity that his family would take it up to the room to allow him to practice in between therapy visits. After a week, the patient was brought to stand and the apparatus was adjusted for height. The ball was still used but placed on an adjustable bedside table. As normal motor programs began to be generated within the right upper extremity, modifications in size of the ball, angle of the wrist and hand, and range allowed within the hinge joint were changed to allow for error and self-correction. Within the 3-week period of inpatient rehabilitation, the patient was able to perform the activity normally with only the use of the ball for postural support within the shoulder girdle. The apparatus was taken home and the patient adjusted all components depending on his fatigue level. Within a 2-month period of the patient working at home, he went from a totally augmented intervention program to functionally being able to stand by a river or lake and fly fish independently. His endurance for this activity improved as he continued to practice.

Somatosensory and Sensorimotor Dysfunction and Interventions

When intervention options are considered, a fourth category of treatment must also be considered. Given that there is strong evidence that the nervous system is adaptable, when there are signs of neural dysfunction, planned, attended, repetitive behaviors can be designed to restore normal neural function. In this chapter on interventions, we have concentrated primarily on using the sensory input system as a way to facilitate motor output. However, there are times when the somatosensory system is dysfunctional as a result of developmental delay, injury, or high levels of repetitive fine-motor use of the hand, chronic pain, or learned dysfunction. Although the patient may not be complaining of sensory dysesthesia, numbness, or tingling, the therapist should determine the accuracy of sensory discriminative processing and the accuracy of performance of fine-motor skills such as writing, using a computer keyboard, or playing an instrument to be certain there are no underlying sensory problems, even though the patient may be complaining of pain or problems of motor control.

Brief Review of Somatosensory Neuroanatomy

The somatosensory system is complex.[288] It includes the primary sensory cortex in the parietal lobe and all of the pathways between the somatosensory cortex, the thalamus, the motor cortex, the basal ganglia, the cerebellum, and the spinal cord. The primary sensory cortex is an afferent input system, receiving information from the environment through the receptors in the skin and from the body through the muscle afferents, the Golgi tendon organs, and the joint proprioceptors. Information is carried from the receptors up the spinal cord to the medial lemniscus and the thalamus to the somatosensory cortex.

The somatosensory system includes four major modalities: discriminative touch, proprioception, nociception, and temperature. Discriminative touch helps us recognize the size, shape, and texture of objects and their movement across the skin. Proprioception is concerned with the sense of static position and movement of limbs and the body. Nociception is the signaling of tissue damage referred to as pain. Temperature sense includes warmth and coldness. The peripheral anatomy of the somatosensory system includes the sensory receptors, the peripheral nerve (carrying information to the spinal cord), the interneurons (excitatory and inhibitory), the dorsal column pathway in the spinal cord (carrying information to the medial lemniscus), the axons from the medial lemniscus projecting to the thalamus in the ventral posterior medial and ventral poster lateral nuclei, and then finally the projections to the primary somatosensory cortex in the postcentral gyrus of the parietal lobe. Sensations of pain and temperature are carried by the anterolateral system in the spinal cord to the thalamus. A discussion of these same receptors and their importance as feedback during hands-on augmented therapeutic interventions can be found in the section under "Intervention: Augmented Treatment Techniques" in this chapter. The sensations of pain and temperature are not addressed in this section but can be found in Chapters 15 and 32.

The somatosensory cortex has three major divisions: the primary (S-I) and the secondary (S-II) somatosensory cortices and the posterior parietal. See Figure 9-6 for orientation of cortical structures and their traditional classification. The primary S-I is divided into four areas: Brodmann's areas 1, 2, 3a, and 3b. Most of the thalamic fibers terminate in areas 3a and 3b. The cells in areas 3a and 3b then project to Brodmann's areas 1 and 2. Some of the thalamic neurons project directly to Brodmann's areas 1 and 2 and to the adjacent secondary somatosensory cortex (S-II). S-II is also innervated by neurons from each of the four areas of S-I. The projections from S-I are required for the perceptual function of S-II. If S-I connections are removed, it prevents stimuli applied to the skin of the hand from activating neurons in S-II. This outcome is most apparent when you obliterate area 3a. But removal of S-II has no effect on the response of neurons in S-I. Some thalamic neurons project to the posterior parietal cortex. The projections from the ventral posterolateral thalamus project to 3a and 3b and area 1. These pathways are most sensitive to cutaneous touch. Projections from the ventral posterolateral thalamus and the ventrolateral thalamus project to area 3a. Other neurons from the ventrolateral thalamus project to areas 1 and 2.

The sensory and motor hand regions in S-I and M-1 have been referenced most extensively in the study of neuroplasticity. In S-I, the area 3b has an unusually large topographical representation of the skin compared with the proportional size of the hand relative to the rest of the body. There is less precise representation in area 3a and areas 1 and 2. In area 3b, it is also most precisely and distinctly represented. The orderly representation of the digits makes it particularly sensitive to the measurement of change. However, these studies focusing on defining the characteristics of neuroplasticity are applicable to other somatotopic areas of the CNS. The hand representations in the cortical areas of 3b have a roughly mirror image topographical relationship to duplicative palmar representations between areas 3a, 3b, and 1.[122,593,594] These cortical representations have been described in S-I in humans,[585] macaque monkeys,[593] New World owl monkeys,[122,123] squirrel monkeys,[123,594,595] spider monkeys,[596] cebus monkeys, and marmosets.

Some New World monkeys have exaggerated representations of their fingernails that are used on a heavy behavioral schedule in grasping. The representation of the thumbs of humans and apes is proportionally large. In general, all primates have a similar general layout for the representation of the hand. The radial margin is lateralward and discontinuously related to the face. The digits and palmar pads are represented in order proceeding medialward in the cortex, in a radial to ulnar sequence across the hand. The wrist and forearm are represented medial to the hand representation. However, the representation of 3b is fairly consistent across species, with more variations by species and within species for 3a, 1, 2, and 5.[123]

Sensory information in all primates, including humans, is serially processed through relay regions. The relay nuclei are composed of projection neurons that send axons to the next relay nucleus in the ascending pathways. Each projection neuron receives synaptic input from many afferent axons. Most commonly, the sensory inputs to relay cells follow a pattern of extensive convergence and divergence. In addition to activating relay cells, afferent fibers also activate interneurons, both excitatory and inhibitory. These interneurons contribute to the processing of incoming sensory information by modulating the firing of the projection neurons. The firing pattern of the projection neurons reflects transformation of the signal by the cells of the nucleus.

There are three types of inhibitory pathways: feed-forward, feedback, and distal inhibition. These are local inhibitory mechanisms operating within a relay nucleus. Feed-forward (or reciprocal) inhibition allows activity in one group of neurons to inhibit a different group of neurons. Feed-forward inhibition permits a singleness of action (winner takes all). This ensures that only one of two or more competing responses is expressed. Feedback (recurrent inhibition) allows the most active neurons to limit the activity of all adjacent elements are less active. This enhances the contrast in firing patterns between the actively firing cells and the surrounding, less active neurons. These types of inhibition create a central zone of active neurons surrounded by a ring of less active neurons. By enhancing or amplifying the contrast between the highly active cells and their neighbors, the cellular interactions contribute to selective perception (attend to one stimulus and not another).

There is no inhibition in the peripheral receptor in the somatosensory system. Inhibitory actions are common in all relay nuclei (e.g., both feed-forward and feedback inhibitions are present in the dorsal column nuclei). The afferent fibers inhibit the activity of cells in the dorsal column nuclei that surround the cells they excite (feed-forward inhibition). Active cells in a nucleus inhibit the less active cells by recurrent collateral fibers (feedback inhibition), sharpening the contrast between the active cells and their neighbors. Neurons from more distant sites such as the motor cortex and the brain stem can also inhibit and control the flow of information from the relay nuclei (called distal inhibition), operating mostly on presynaptic terminals. Thus, higher areas of the brain are able to control the sensory inflow from the peripheral receptors.

Total removal of S-I (areas 3b, 3a, 1, and 2) produces deficits in position sense and the ability to discriminate size, texture, and shape. Thermal and pain sensibilities are altered but not abolished. Lesions in area 3b produce deficits in discrimination of the texture, size, and shape of objects. Lesions in area 2 alter only the ability to differentiate the size and shape of objects. Area 3b is the principal target for the afferent projections from the ventral posterolateral nucleus of the thalamus. The projections to area 1 are concerned primarily with texture, whereas the projections to area 2 are concerned with size and shape.

S-II receives inputs from all areas of S-I. Thus, a lesion of S-II causes severe impairment in the discrimination of both shape and texture and prevents animals from learning new tactile discrimination tasks on the basis of the shape of an object. Thus, damage to the posterior parietal cortex creates complex abnormalities in attending to sensations from the contralateral half of the body.

Sensory information is topographically organized in the primary somatic cortex. The body surface and deep tissues are also represented in a topographical order in the thalamus and the dorsal column nuclei. Each part of the body is represented in the brain in proportion to its relative importance in sensory perception. The face is large compared with the back of the head. The index finger is large compared with the big toe. This distortion reflects differences in innervation density in different areas of the body. Each of the four areas in Brodmann's classification has its own map (3a, 3b, 1, 2). In addition, area S-II has its own map. Each area has its own somatosensory inputs. Each central neuron has its own receptive field on the skin. The cortical neurons in the somatosensory system respond only to stimulation of a specific area of the skin. Any point on the skin is represented in the cortex by a population of cells connected to the afferent fibers that innervate that point on the skin. Stimulation of the skin excites specific cortical neurons.

The receptive fields have four important features: their size, distribution, modifiability, and fine structure. Where there is unusual sensitivity to touch in the body (e.g., lips and fingers), there are a large number of receptors per unit area and the receptive fields are small. The fingertips have the highest density of receptors (about $2500/cm^2$). Three fifths of these receptors are Meissner corpuscles, one third are Merkel cells, and the remainder are pacinian and Ruffini corpuscles. They are innervated by myelinated axons. Each afferent fiber connects to about 20 Meissner corpuscles, and each corpuscle receives two to five afferent fibers. As you move up the arm, the receptive fields become larger and decreased in density and there is a reduction in fineness of sensory discrimination.

The receptor cell has its greatest discharge at the center of the receptive field and its weakest around the perimeter. There is a gradient of excitatory activity within the receptive field and a gradient of inhibition. The inhibition is also greatest at the center of the field and decreases with distance from the center. Inhibition is delayed. Inhibition occurs after excitation. At each relay station in the somatic afferent system, a stimulus in the excitatory center of the receptive field produces a peak of excitation that is surrounded by a population of inactive (inhibited) cells. This spatial distribution sharpens the peak activity within the brain.

Spatial discrimination is the ability to distinguish two closely placed point stimuli as two rather than one. Two stimuli applied to different positions on the skin set up excitatory gradients of activity in two cell populations at every relay point in the somatosensory system. The activity in each population of cells has its own maximal region of activity or peak, and the perception of two points rather than one occurs because two distinct populations are active. Each neuron population has a central excitatory zone surrounded by a weaker excitatory zone. It is further depressed by the inhibitory surround, which sharpens each peak and further enhances the distinction between the two peaks.

When the two stimuli are brought closer together, the activity of the two populations tends to overlap so that the section between the two peaks can become blurred. As they get closer and closer, the inhibition produced by each summates. This allows the peaks of activity to be sharpened. When two stimuli keep getting closer and occur within a single large receptive field, the separation of the two stimuli becomes encoded as a single population of receptors. When two stimuli are widely separated they elicit separate, distinguishable, high-frequency responses. When these are coincident in time, it allows two different behaviors to be programmed and mapped together. This is a type of learning that facilitates improved skill, even automation of learning. As the separation narrows, the frequency decreases and the duration of neuronal firing decreases.

Somatosensory Discrimination Deficits: Degradation

Although rapidly adapting receptors can distinguish spacing between stimuli as small as 1 mm, ultimately the spacing is further reduced until no difference between stimuli can be distinguished. This can be a form of neuroplasticity that represents negative learning or degradation. Now two sensory stimuli come in to adjacent digits, for example, and no longer are interpreted as separate stimuli but the same stimulus. Thus, the stimulus is interpreted as the same one across the adjacent digits, which may interfere with individualized, coordinated, rapid fine-motor movement. This is hypothesized to be the underlying cause of occupational hand cramps that can develop in people who perform high levels of repetition as part of their jobs. The representation of the involved hand on the primary sensory cortex may become smaller than normal, with larger than normal receptive fields. In addition, the location of the hand area differs from normal and the order of the digits may not be sequential.[174,410,597,598] This same change in location and area of representation has also been observed in patients with chronic pain.[599,600]

This type of degradation might be more likely to occur when the stimuli are both cutaneous and deep, particularly when stretch stimuli affect fast-twitch, fatigable fibers. The fast-twitch fatigable fibers have a large cell body. The slow-fatigue resistance cells have a small cell body. The intermediate fibers, which are fast-twitch, fatigue-resistant fibers, have an intermediate-sized cell body. With stimulation or activation, the small cell bodies are activated first. With an increase in strength of contraction, the larger cell bodies are recruited. The slow fatigue-resistant fibers can fire with a consistent amplitude over 60 minutes; the fast-twitch, fatigue-resistant fibers can fire consistently up to 50 minutes, whereas the fast-twitch fatigable fibers lose their force at 4 minutes.[601-603]

In a muscle, when the firing rate gets to 80 Hz, there is an unfused tetanus. At 100 Hz, there is a fused tetanus and no muscle twitches are definable. The muscle stays in a fixed contraction. Interestingly, when an individual contracts a muscle voluntarily, even against resistance, the contraction rarely exceeds 25 Hz.[601]

Another possible learned degradation would be having the agonists and the antagonists always contract simultaneously instead of reciprocally. If this was repeated during all voluntary motor contraction, they could become learned. It is then possible that a stretch of the spindle would lead to an exaggerated muscle contraction of both the agonist and the antagonist rather than a reciprocal response. This simultaneous contraction of agonists and antagonists interferes with graded muscle contractions, again interfering with normal, coordinated voluntary muscle movements.[602-608]

Specific Afferent Sensitivity and Cortical Representation

Each nerve cell is responsive to one modality: touch, pressure, temperature, or pain. Neurons mediating touch are responsive to superficial tactile stimuli but not deep stimuli. Neurons responsive to superficial stimuli are more specialized. Some are responsive to movement of hairs, whereas others respond to a steady indentation of skin. One modality tends to dominate in each of Brodmann's areas. Muscle stretch is dominant in 3a, and information from cutaneous receptors is dominant in 3b. Deep-pressure receptors are dominant in area 2; and in area 1, rapidly adapting cutaneous receptors are dominant. Furthermore, there is a column for rapidly adapting and one for slowly adapting receptors in S-I, area 3b. Each relay nucleus has some level of adaptation similar to the receptors. The signal received by the input to the cortex reproduces the stimulus features encoded by the receptors in the skin.

The somatosensory cortex is arranged in six cellular layers, and there is no correlation between layers and neuron type. In all six layers, neurons within a column or slab of cortex running from the cortical structure to the white matter respond as one class of receptors. Some columns are activated by rapidly adapting cutaneous receptors of the Meissner type, some by slowly adapting cutaneous receptors of the Merkel type, and others by movement of the hair cells or the subcutaneous, rapidly adapting pacinian receptors.

Although each of the four areas of the primary somatosensory cortex (3a, 3b, 1, 2) receives input from all areas of the body surface, one modality tends to dominate in each area: area 3a = muscle stretch, area 3b = cutaneous, area 2 = deep pressure, and area 1 = rapidly adaptive cutaneous. Each layer also has connections with different parts of the brain. Layer 6 projects back to the thalamus, layer 5 projects to the subcortical structures, layer 4 receives information from the thalamus, and layers 1, 2, and 3 project to other cortical regions.

Tactile perception is determined by the response properties of the receptors that are matched with those of the CNS. Rapidly adaptive skin receptors connect to rapidly adapting neurons in the thalamus that connect to neurons in 3b and 3a. S-I slowly adapting receptors connect to neurons in the thalamus and areas 3b and 3a.

The neural representation of the surface texture of objects in areas 3b and 1 has been studied. Awake monkeys were stimulated with embossed letters. When the letter was moved across the skin, the response of a single neuron to a stimulus moved systematically across the receptive field could be assumed to represent the response of a pulsation of neurons with similar response properties of slowly and rapidly adapting receptors in the skin (e.g., Merkel cells, Meissner cells). In area 3b, the first stage of processing from the projections of the skin receptors gave rise to sharp images. In the later stages in area 1, the responses were more abstract.[606,607]

To sense the texture, form, and motion of an object, integration of information from many different mechanoreceptors sensitive to superficial tough, deep pressure and position of the finger and hand is required (stereognosis). Four factors are involved: (1) response properties of the neurons at successive levels of sensory processing become more complex, (2) submodalities converge on one common cell, (3) the size of the receptive field gets larger, and (4) profiles of responding populations of neurons change (e.g., cells in the hand region of the somatosensory cortex respond briskly to three-dimensional objects placed within the receptive fields, particularly movement of objects across the skin; the same cells do not respond to point stimuli like cells at earlier relays).

Neurons involved in inputs of 3b and 3a can respond to single and multiple static and dynamic point stimuli.

Neurons in areas 1 and 2 also respond to these types of stimuli. These neurons have complex response properties (e.g., responding to movement across the skin). This type of sensory analysis permits stereognosis (the perception of the three-dimensional shape of objects). The convergent projections for 3a and 3b into areas 1 and 2 permit neurons in areas 1 and 2 to respond to complex features such as edge orientation. Neurons in 3b and 1 respond only to touch. Neurons in 3a respond to position senses, and those in area 2 respond to both, particularly when an object is held in the hand.

Three types of neurons respond to movement. Motion-sensitive neurons respond to movement in all directions. Direction-sensitive neurons respond much better to movement in one direction. Orientation-sensitive neurons respond best to movement along a specific axis of the receptive field. Feature-detecting neurons are sensitive to stimulus direction and orientation and are found in area 1 and more extensively in area 2. These areas are more concerned with stereognosis and with discriminating the direction of movement of objects on the skin. These complex stimulus properties arise not from the thalamic input but from cortical projections from area 3a. The convergent projections from areas 3a and 3b into areas 1 and 2 also permit neurons in areas 1 and 2 to respond to other complex features. Neurons in areas 3b and 1 respond only to touch. Neurons in areas 3a respond only to position sense, and certain neurons in area 2 have both inputs.

Receptive fields are small in areas 3a and 3b (sites of initial inputs of S-I). Neurons in areas 1 and 2 receive inputs from 3a and 3b and also have their own neurons projecting on the fingers. Inputs for the finger areas are commonly adjacent to one another, and cells respond most effectively when adjacent fingers are stimulated, as when the hand is used to hold and manipulate an object. These complex cells in areas 1 and 2 become active during movements of the hand around an object. These complex cells also seem to have a role in stereognosis.

Inputs for finger areas are usually adjacent to one another, and cells respond most effectively when adjacent fingers are stimulated, as when the hand is used to hold and manipulate objects. Areas 1 and 2 are activated when the hand is actually moving objects.

Increase in complexity is important in perception and skilled movements. Area 2 sends somatosensory inputs from the entire body surface to the primary motor cortex. There is also some inhibition produced by neurotransmitters (e.g., gamma-aminobutyric acid [GABA]) that inhibit cortical cells. Reversible inhibition of neural activity in area 2 can be produced pharmacologically (GABA agonist). This leads to an inability to assume functional postures of the hand and coordinate the fingers. The somatosensory area protects the motor cortex and Brodmann's areas 5 and 7. Cells detecting complex information receive inputs from several modalities and are often related to movement. Cutaneous information is integrated into visual information and with other system activities in the brain stem, thalamus, and temporal lobe concerned with attention.

Tactile information from the periphery reaches the cortex by several pathways, all carrying redundant as well as unique information. Also, many pathways project to more than one cortical area. This parallel processing is designed to allow different neuronal pathways and brain relays to deal with the same sensory information in slightly different ways. Neurons in areas 2 and 1 are involved in the later stages of somatosensory processing and have more complex feature-detecting properties receiving convergent input from a number of other modalities. More complicated processing is carried out with object manipulation. In addition, the somatosensory cortex sends outputs to the posterior parietal cortex, where further integration takes place and an overall picture of the body is formed.

The convergent projections from 3a and 3b into areas 1 and 2 permit neurons in areas 1 and 2 to respond to complex features such as edge orientation. Neurons in areas 3b and 2 respond only to touch, and neurons in area 3a respond only to position sense. Area 2 neurons have both; thus, neurons respond best when an object is held in the hand and manipulated. Areas 1 and 2 also are activated when the hand is actually moving around objects.

The somatosensory areas also project to the posterior parietal cortex (Brodmann's areas 5 and 7). The cells that have complex projections receive inputs from several modalities that are often related to movement. Thus, information from tactile discrimination and position sense is integrated with visual information and neural information from the brain stem, thalamus, and temporal lobe.[428]

Sensory Receptor Interactions with Sensory Discrimination

Although each sensory receptor is described in detail under the augmented therapeutic intervention section of this chapter, these receptors are discussed within this section to help the reader develop an understanding of how these receptors work to aid somatosensory discrimination. These receptors are classified as proprioceptors or exteroceptors and make up the somatosensory system. Proprioceptors provide information about position sense and movement (kinesthesia). Exteroceptors provide information about the environment primarily through the superficial skin and some of the deep skin receptors.

Proprioception: Sensory Receptors in the Muscle and the Tendon. The proprioceptors include the muscle spindle, the Golgi tendon organ, and the joint receptors (free nerve endings, Ruffini corpuscles, and pacinian corpuscles). The proprioceptive system modulates the alpha motor neurons. Muscle spindle afferents also facilitate polysynaptically agonistic synergies while dampening antagonists. Information from the muscle spindle is simultaneously sent through ascending pathways to the ipsilateral cerebellum and contralateral parietal lobe.

The muscle spindle plays an important role in ongoing peripheral feedback mechanisms within the CNS, regulating continuous neuroexcitation at the level of the spinal cord and brain stem. These fibers do not contribute to muscle force but rather to length.

The Golgi tendon organ and the muscle spindles together provide complementary information about the mechanical state of muscle, length, and degree of tension. Information on length is used by the brain to determine the position of the limb segment. The length of the muscle varies with the angle of the joint. The information from the Golgi tendon organ is useful for maintaining a steady grip on objects and compensatory for fatigue (e.g., steady neural drive). Muscle stretch fires the spindle afferent, whereas, the Golgi tendon organ only shows light, inconsistent increases. When the muscle contracts after motor nerve stimulation, the firing rate of the Golgi tendon organ increases where the spindle decreases.

Exteroception: Sensory Receptors in the Skin. In the exteroceptor system, there are sensory end organs located primarily in the superficial and subcutaneous layers of the skin. The receptors are densest in the fingertips, the lips, and the tip of the tongue and have the greatest capacity for fine discrimination of touch stimuli. The sense of touch is most discriminative in the fingertips. Humans can feel the shape and texture of objects from information transmitted to the brain from mechanoreceptors in the fingers. The somatic modalities are segregated functionally in the CNS, and they are combined for coherent perception. These areas also contain more encapsulated receptors and more afferent neurons, also transmitting along thicker fibers. They also have the greatest representation on the cortical gyri.

There are four types of receptors in the skin. The rapidly adapting Meissner corpuscles are in the superficial skin (providing an instantaneous sense of contact and flutter).[606] The slowly adapting Merkel cells are also in the superficial skin. These group II receptors respond to slow movements across the skin and light pressure, which is associated with pleasure.[607] Meissner's corpuscles are used in two-point discrimination and stereognosis. The deeper subcutaneous tissue contains the rapidly adapting pacinian corpuscles, which respond to vibration (and provide information on posture, position, and ambulation).[608] These adapt quickly and are activated by deep pressure and quick stretch, which also stimulate the muscle spindle.[428,486,609] The slowly adapting Ruffini corpuscles are also deep.[606] They respond to rapid indentation of the skin.

Tactile information from the periphery reaches the cortex by several pathways, carrying unique and redundant information. Also, parallel ascending pathways project to multicortical areas. So there are five representations of the body surface in the parietal cortex: one in S-II and four in S-I. This allows parallel processing to enable neural pathways to send the brain relays to deal with the same information in different ways. Information from S-I (area 2) sends information from the entire body surface to the primary motor cortex.

Assessment of Somatosensory Function

When the somatosensory system is evaluated, it is important to provide multiple trials of stimuli to measure localization of light touch, kinesthesia, two-point discrimination, stereognosis, graphesthesia (interpretation of passive stimuli delivered to the skin), proprioception, and perception of sharpness and dullness. Two-point discrimination and detection of sharp and dull are traditionally included in the neurological examination. A discriminator can be used for easy testing of two-point discrimination.[610] Tests of localization, kinesthesia, stereognosis, and graphesthesia can be found in the Jean Ayres Sensory Integration and Praxis Test.[611] This test has normative values established for children; therefore tests of stereognosis may need to be elaborated, such as with the key test (matching a key by tactile exploration to a photocopy of the key).[612] There are other tests that contribute

information about somatosensory function. It is also important to measure the strength of grip,[613] pinch, and strength of intrinsics to make sure there is no weakness associated with the sensory dysfunction.[614] The patient should complete several standardized fine motor tasks, such as the Purdue Pegboard Test,[182] tapping speed,[615] and motor reaction time.[616] For measuring subtle changes over time, it can be helpful to videotape the patient doing several fine motor tasks, such as using the computer, playing an instrument, or writing. An ordinal scale can be created to grade the quality of movement to standardize the measurement and quantify change. Furthermore, the patient should complete some type of functional independence measure to document how much an upper extremity problem interferes with the ability to care for oneself and to work.

Intervention: Sensory Discriminative Retraining

The intervention strategies for retraining sensory discrimination are based on the principles of neuroplasticity (see Table 9-1). It should be remembered, however, that the sensory and motor systems are intimately linked. Thus, although the focus is on improving the responsiveness and the accuracy of the somatosensory system, the ultimate goal is usually to improve fine motor voluntary control.

To set the stage for the patient to benefit from sensory retraining of the hands in particular, the patient must become more aware of how she or he uses the involved extremity, particularly the hand. Appendix 9-A describes recommended strategies for how to use the hands in a stress-reduced way. If one works on sensory retraining and the individual continues to overuse unnecessary forces for self-care, then even effective retraining will not have the maximum benefit on restoration of function.

Appendix 9-B summarizes some activities recommended for sensory discriminative retraining. All activities must be attended, and all sensory modalities should be included. For the most part, the eyes must be closed because patients will depend on vision when the eyes are open, especially when somatosensory feedback is decreased. The sensory stimulation tasks must progress in difficulty. The emphasis initially should be on the cutaneous receptors (light touch). The performance accuracy should be close to 80%. All trials should involve feedback to determine whether performance was correct. The tasks should be performed in different contexts and with the patient in different positions to maximize information processing from all possible sensory areas. When a sensory stimulus is delivered to the fingers, the most involved digits should be targeted. Stimulation should be on the distal pads and the side of the fingers to help restore the individual nature of the digits. The stimulation should involve active and passive stimulation with static and moving stimuli. It is critical to have someone assist by providing these passive stimulation challenges. Furthermore, it is important to move from meaningful letters and numbers to designs to increase the challenge of the sensory task. The sensory task ultimately needs to be incorporated into functional tasks, particularly those that are difficult for the patient. There must be significant repetition in the performance of these tasks. The patient probably needs to spend at least 1 to 1.5 hours a day doing specific sensory discrimination tasks. Ultimately, computer-based sensory games may help drive faster change in the nervous system.

Some people with somatosensory degradation also have problems with movement control (e.g., focal hand dystonia).[174,410] There is an intimate close relationship between all higher-order perceptual and movement processes. The brain must correlate sensory inputs with motor outputs to accurately assess the body's interaction with the environment. Thus, dysfunction in sensory processing can lead to serious problems in motor control.[288] For effective sensory discriminative retraining to be carried out, it is important not to elicit abnormal movements and tension. When abnormal patterns of movement are repeated, they, too, can be learned; however, this would be considered negative learning. Movement problems have also been noticed in patients with chronic pain. Coincidentally, cortical differences have also been reported in the primary sensory cortex for patients with chronic pain, similar to those reported in patients with hand dystonia.[599,600]

The deep receptors should also be included in retraining. Appendix 9-B summarizes some activities that can be used to facilitate the sensitivity and accuracy of these deep receptors. Although the deep receptors are in area 3a, they provide information on proprioception and kinesthesia through deep pressure, tapping, weight bearing, and muscle stretch. These receptors also contribute information to the sensorimotor feedback loop that guides graded contractions and coordinated movements. Deep pressure can also contribute toward object recognition (size, shape, and attributes). Static and dynamic joint position and location sense should also be addressed to help improve motor control and control joint movement. These stimulation activities should be distinguished from discriminative touch. By having subjects practice lifting items of the same and different weights with rough surfaces, such as Velcro hook and loop fasteners applied, it is possible to begin to enhance gradations of force. Subjects will squeeze objects with a smooth surface harder than the same objects with a rough surface. Practicing controlled grasp and release strategies in functional tasks also contributes toward the development of proprioception and kinesthesia. Giving the extremity some resistance is another method of enhancing proprioception. Each of the behaviors must require a decision and be rewarded with feedback.

Sometimes it is difficult to perform sensory retraining activities without causing abnormal motor movements. This may be an indication to use imagery instead of physical practice. Imagery involves creating an internal representation of an object or a task without physical operation on the object or the task. Thus, in sensory discriminative programs, visual imagery, motor imagery, or mental rehearsal of a sequential task such as playing an instrument may assist the patient in restoring a sense of "normality." It has been well established that mental practice is successful in improving performance in sports.[617] It has also been used extensively in trying to control physiological states such as blood pressure[319,618-620] and to increase immunity to fight cancer.[210]

Current technology has allowed us to measure the blood flow in the brain while individuals are imaging. The hypothesis is that direct matching predicts the areas that contain the neurons that discharge during action execution regardless of how action is elicited. At least a subset of the neurons should encode the action as carried out as well as imagined. Thus, the cortical areas should have motor properties that become more active when the action to be executed is elicited by observation or imaging of the task. Recent research suggests that visual imagery is associated with increased activity in the somatosensory cortex, whereas motor imagery is associated with increased activity in the motor cortex.[621] In both types of imagery and in actual motor performance, the same cortical area is recruited.[619] However, during imaged performance, the cortical activity level is approximately 30% of that measured during actual task performance.[622] Abbruzzese et al[509] note that the excitability of the human cortex increases both during execution and mental imagination of a sequential finger task but not a repetitive finger movement. This suggests that retraining must be goal oriented, attended, and variable, not simple, simultaneous, or repetitious without attention.

Appendix 9-C outlines some of the functions that patients who have somatosensory problems associated with chronic pain or movement dysfunction are encouraged to visually image. Some patients can perform mental imagery more easily than others. Patients have to be able to isolate themselves, focus intensively on the task at hand, and be uninterrupted in this process. During a session, an individual should focus on this aspect of retraining for approximately 45 minutes to an hour. Patients may find it helpful to purchase a book on how to do imagery, take a course on mental imagery, or work with an individual counselor who can help them with this process.

In summary, sensory discriminative retraining as discussed within this section includes a complex process of retraining that adapts the principles of neuroplasticity to restore normal sensory and motor function. The retraining program is comprehensive, addressing first prevention and stress-free use of the arms. This specific sensory retraining includes both concerns about superficial somatosensory receptors and proprioceptive or deep receptors. The specific sensory discriminative activities are supplemented with visual imagery, motor imagery, and mental practice to facilitate maximum restoration of function.

CONCLUSION

There are treatment techniques that are universally applied to the very young and the very old. As discussed under the neuroplasticity section, the CNS is in a constant state of change throughout life. The brain is unique to each individual. Each brain has idiosyncrasies but also has an enormous number of predictable responses. These factors affect the success or failure of a client/therapist interaction. After thorough evaluation, the therapist must decide which treatment is appropriate and the most efficient course of intervention on the basis of the goals of the patient/family, the prognosis of the client, the resources available, and the skills of the therapist. Once a decision is made regarding whether the interventions should be based on compensation, substitution, habituation, neural adaptation, or a combination of the four, the team must select the best options available given all the resources. The options include functional retraining, impairment training, augmented and contrived intervention using a classification scheme, or somatosensory reintegration. No matter the specifics of the intervention selection, the therapist must cognitively organize intervention options in a sequential process, be willing to change direction or options as the patient changes, and develop a greater clinical repertoire of intervention strategies.

When specific augmented interventions are needed, the therapist must select specific treatments according to the needs of the client, the time available for therapy, the level and extent of the functional involvement, the motivation of the client and family, the creativity of the therapist, the pathological condition, and the course of a disease process. A therapist must choose whether somatosensory retraining, functional training, impairment training, augmented treatment interventions, or any combination of these four will provide the client with the most environmentally effective, cost-effective, and quickest map to functional independence or maximal quality of life. How each therapist combines the interventions with the client's specific needs will vary according to education, belief, skill, and openness to learning from the total environment itself. Learning should lead to further learning. Answers to unknowns will be found with new unknowns coming to consciousness. The brain is still more mystery than not, so for most of us the adventure has just begun.

REFERENCES

1. Portney LG, Watkins MP: *Foundations to clinical research: Applications to practice,* ed 2, Upper Saddle River, NJ, 2000, Prentice Hall Health.
2. APTA: Hooked on evidence project, 2006 (website): www.apta.org. Accessed July 14, 2005.
3. AOTA: Standards of practice for occupational therapy in schools, *Am J Occup Ther* 34:900-903, 1980.
4. APTA: Guide to physical therapist practice, *Phys Ther* 81:9-744, 2001.
5. Discussion Plenary Speakers: III STEP Conference: Summer institute on translating evidence into practice, Salt Lake City, UT, July 15-21, 2005.
6. Umphred D: Opening ceremony: Setting the stage—the history of the STEP conferences and today, Salt Lake City, UT, July 15, 2005.
7. Ayers AJ: *Sensory integration and learning disabilities,* Los Angeles, 1972, Western Psychological Services.
8. Bertoti DB: Effect of therapeutic horseback riding on posture in children with cerebral palsy, *Phys Ther Forum* 68:1505-1512, 1988.
9. Bobath K, Bobath B: Cerebral palsy. In Pearson PH, Williams CE, editors: *Physical therapy services in developmental disabilities,* Springfield, IL, 1972, Charles C Thomas.
10. Brunnstrom S: *Movement therapy in hemiplegia,* ed 2, Philadelphia, 1992, JB Lippincott.
11. Carr JH, Sheperd RB: *A motor relearning for stroke,* Frederick, MD, 1987, Aspen Publishers.
12. Colavita F: *Sensory changes in the elderly,* Springfield, IL, 1978, Charles C Thomas.
13. Crutchfield CA, Barnes MR, editors: *Motor control and motor learning in rehabilitation,* ed 2, Atlanta, 1993, Stokesville Publications.
14. Farber S: A multisensory approach to neurorehabilitation. In Farber S, editor: *Neurorehabilitation: a multisensory approach,* Philadelphia, 1982, WB Saunders.
15. Fisher AG, Murray EA, Bundy AC: *Sensory integration: theory and practice,* Philadelphia, 1991, FA Davis.
16. Flynn J: *Snoezelen,* Ede, the Netherlands, 1986, Hartenberg.
17. Freeman G: Hippotherapy/therapeutic horseback riding, *Clin Man Phys Ther* 4:20-25, 1984.
18. Gelb M: *Body learning—an introduction to the Alexander technique,* London, 1981, Auburn Press.
19. Johnstone M: *Restoration of normal movement after stroke,* New York, 1995, Churchill Livingstone.
20. Klein-Vogelbach S: *Functional kinetics,* New York, 1995, Springer-Verlag.
21. Knott M, Voss DE: *Proprioceptive neuromuscular facilitation,* New York, 1968, Harper & Row.
22. Maitland GD: *Peripheral manipulation,* ed 3, Boston, 1992, Butterworths.
23. Michels E: Motor behavior in hemiplegia, *Phys Ther* 45:759-767, 1965.
24. Moore JC: Cranial nerves and their importance in current rehabilitation techniques. In Henderson A, Coryell J, editors: *The body senses and perceptual deficit,* Boston, 1973, Boston University Press.
25. Page D: Neuromuscular reflex therapy as an approach to patient care, *Am J Phys Med* 46:816-837, 1967.
26. Quinn JF: Building a body of knowledge-research on therapeutic touch, 1974-1986, *J Holistic Nurs* 6:37-45, 1988.
27. Rood M: The use of sensory receptors to activate, facilitate and inhibit motor response, autonomic and somatic in developmental sequence. In Scattely C, editor: *Approaches to treatment of patients with neuromuscular dysfunction, Third International Congress, World Federation of Occupational Therapists,* Dubuque, IA, 1962, William Brown Group.
28. Seivert J: *Manual therapy: Maitland's concepts.* Unpublished handout from lecture, Department of Physical Therapy, University of Pacific, Stockton, CA, Oct. 15, 1993.
29. Seufert-Jeffer U, Jeffer EK: An introduction to the VOJTA Method, *Clin Man Phys Ther* 2:26-29, 1982.
30. Stockmeyer SA: An interpretation of the approach of Rood to the treatment of neuromuscular dysfunction, *Am J Phys Med* 46:900-961, 1967.
31. Sullivan PE, Markos PD, Minor MA: *An integrated approach to therapeutic exercise,* Reston, VA, 1982, Reston Publishing.
32. Bobath B: *Abnormal postural reflex activity caused by brain lesions,* ed 3, Frederick, MD, 1985, Aspen Publications.
33. Bobath B: *Adult hemiplegia: evaluation and treatment,* ed 2, London, 1978, William Heinemann Medical Books.
34. Noback CR, Strominger NL, Demarest RJ: *The human nervous system: introduction and review,* ed 4, Philadelphia, 1991, Lea & Febiger.
35. Fay T: The neurophysical aspects of therapy in cerebral palsy. In Payton OP, Hirt S, Newton RA, editors: *Neurophysiologic approach to therapeutic exercise,* Philadelphia, 1978, FA Davis.
36. Ayers AJ: *The development of sensory integrative theory and practice,* Dubuque, IA, 1974, Kendall/Hunt.
37. Lister M, editor: Contemporary management of motor control problems. Proceedings from II STEP Conference, Norman, OK, July 6-13, 1990, Alexandria, VA, 1991, Foundation for Physical Therapy.
38. Carr JH, Sheperd RB: *Movement science: Foundations for physical therapy in rehabilitation,* Frederick, MD, 1987, Aspen Publishers.
39. Cooper S: Muscle spindles in the intrinsic muscles of the human tongue, *J Physiol* 122:193, 1953.
40. Gilfoyle EM, Grady AP, Moore JC: *Children adapt,* Thorofare, NJ, 1981, Charles B Slack.
41. Heiniger MC, Randolph SL: *Neurophysiological concepts in human behavior,* St. Louis, 1981, CV Mosby.
42. Craik R: Abnormalities of motor behavior. In Lister MJ, editor: *Contemporary management of motor control problems,* Norman, OK, 1991, Foundation for Physical Therapy.
43. Byl N, Roderick J, Mohamed O et al: Effectiveness of sensory and motor rehabilitation of the upper limb following the principles of neuroplasticity: patients stable poststroke, *Neurorehabil Neural Repair* 17:176-191, 2003.
44. Chen R, Cohen LG, Hallett M: Nervous system reorganization following injury, *Neuroscience* 111:761-773, 2002.
45. Fisher BE, Sullivan KJ: Activity-dependent factors affecting poststroke functional outcomes, *Top Stroke Rehabil* 8:31-44, 2001.
46. Fraser C, Power M, Hamdy S et al: Driving plasticity in human adult motor cortex is associated with improved motor function after brain injury, *Neuron* 34:831-840, 2002.

47. Kleim JA, Jones TA, Schallert T: Motor enrichment and the induction of plasticity before and after brain injury, *Neurochem Res* 28:1757-1769, 2003.

48. Kleim JA: Neural mechanisms of motor recovery after stroke: plasticity within residual cortical tissue, III STEP Conference, Salt Lake City, UT, July 17, 2005.

49. Nudo RJ: Functional and structural plasticity in motor cortex: implications for stroke recovery, *Phys Med Rehabil Clin North Am* 14(1 Suppl):s57-76, 2003.

50. Nudo RJ: Translating results between animal and human studies of brain plasticity after neuronal injury. III STEP Conference, July 2005, Salt Lake City, UT. Available on CD from American Physical Therapy Association.

51. Nudo RJ, Plautz EJ, Frost SB: Role of adaptive plasticity in recovery of function after damage to motor cortex, *Muscle Nerve* 24:1000-1019, 2001.

52. Ward NS, Cohen LG: Mechanism underlying recovery of motor function after stroke, *Arch Neurol* 61:1844-1848, 2004.

53. Adolph KI: Flexibility and specificity in the development of action. III STEP Conference, July 2005, Salt Lake City, UT. Available on CD from American Physical Therapy Association.

54. Latash ML, Anson JG: Synergies in health and disease: relations to adaptive changes in motor coordination, *Phys Ther* 86:1151-1160, 2006.

55. Morris ME, Perry A, Bilney B et al: Outcomes of physical therapy, speech pathology, and occupational therapy for people with motor neuron disease: a systematic review, *Neruorehabil Neural Repair* 20:424-434, 2006.

56. Schallert T, Woodlee MT: Brain-dependent movements and cerebral-spinal connections: key targets of cellular and behavioral enrichment in CNS injury models, *J Rehabil Res Dev* 40:9-18, 2003.

57. Shim JK, Lay B, Zatsiorsky VM et al: Age-related changes in finger coordination in static prehension tasks, *J Appl Physiol* 97:213-224, 2004.

58. Law M, Darrah J, Rosenbaum P et al: Family-centred functional therapy for children with cerebral palsy: an emerging practice model, *Phys Occup Ther Pediatr* 18:83-102, 1998.

59. Remple MS, Bruneau RM, VandenBerg PM et al: Sensitivity of cortical movement representations to motor experience: evidence that skill learning but not strength training induces cortical reorganization, *Behav Brain Res* 123:133-141, 2001.

60. Tieman BL, Palisano RJ, Gracely EJ et al: Gross motor capability and performance of mobility in children with cerebral palsy: a comparison across home, school, and outdoors/community settings, *Phys Ther* 84:419-429, 2004.

61. Boyd LA, Winstein CJ: Providing explicit information disrupts implicit motor learning after basal ganglia stroke, *Learning Memory* 11:388-396, 2004.

62. Campbell SK, Vander Linden DW, Palisano RJ, editors: *Physical therapy for children,* ed 3, Philadelphia, 2006, Elsevier.

63. Winstein CJ: Designing practice for motor learning: Clinical implications. In Lister MJ, editor: *Contemporary management of motor control problem,* Norman, OK, 1991, American Physical Therapy Association.

64. Malouin R, Richards CL, Belleville S et al: Training mobility tasks after stroke with combined mental and physical practice: a feasibility study, *Neurorehabil Neural Repair* 18:66-75, 2004.

65. Shkuratova N, Morris ME, Huxham F: Effects of age on balance control during walking, *Arch Phys Med Rehabil* 85:582-588, 2004.

66. Shumway-Cook A, Wolllacott MH: *Motor control: theory and practical applications,* ed 2, Philadelphia, 2001, Lippincott Williams & Wilkins.

67. Sullivan K, Knowlton B, Dobkin B: Step training with body weight support: effect of treadmill speed and practice paradigms on poststroke locomotor recovery, *Arch Phys Med Rehabil* 83:683-691, 2002.

68. Van Sant AF: Life-span development in functional tasks, *Phys Ther* 70:788-798, 1990.

69. Merzenich MM: Neural plasticity: Basic mechanisms. III STEP: Symposium on Translating Evidence into Practice, Salt Lake City, UT, July 17, 2005.

70. Merzenich MM, Recanzone GH, Jenkins WM: How the brain functionally rewires itself. In Arbib M, Robinson JA, editors: *Natural and artificial parallel computations,* New York, 1991, MIT Press.

71. Schmidt RA: Motor learning principles for physical therapy. In Lister MJ, editor: *Contemporary management of motor control problems,* Norman, OK, 1990, Foundation for Physical Therapy.

72. Schmidt RA: Motor schema theory after 27 years: reflections and implications for a new theory, *Res Q Exerc Sport* 74:366-375, 2003.

73. Kleim JA, Hogg TM, VandenBerg PM et al: Cortical synaptogenesis and motor map reorganization occur during late, but not early, phase of motor skill learning, *J Neurosci* 24:628-633, 2004.

74. Nudo RJ, Milliken GW, Jenkins WM et al: Use-dependent alterations of movement representations in primary motor cortex of adult squirrel monkeys, *J Neurosci* 16:785-807, 1995.

75. Shepherd RB: Exercise and training to optimize functional motor performance in stroke: driving neural reorganization, *Neural Plast* 8:121-129, 2001.

76. Ward NS, Brown MM, Thompson AJ et al: Neural correlates of motor recovery after stroke: a longitudinal fMRI study, *Brain* 126:2476-2496, 2003.

77. Winstein CJ, Wing AM, Whitall J: Motor control and learning principles for rehabilitation of upper limb movements after brain injury. In Grafman J, Robertson IH, editors: *Handbook of neuropsychology,* ed 2, vol 9, Philadelphia, 2003, Elsevier.

78. Xerri C, Stern J, Merzenich MM: Alterations of the cortical representation of the rat ventrum induced by nursing behavior, *J Neurosci* 14:1710-1721, 1994.

79. Karnath HO, Ferber S, Dichgans J: The origin of contraversive pushing: evidence for a second graviceptive system in humans, *Neurology* 55:1298-1304, 2000.

80. Bohannon RW: Ipsilateral pushing in stroke, *Arch Phys Med Rehabil* 77:524-525, 1996.

81. Shumway-Cook A (moderator): Gordon panel discussion, July 18, 2005, Proceedings from the III STEP Conference, Salt Lake City, UT, 2006, American Physical Therapy Association. Available on DVD from American Physical Therapy Association Section on Pediatrics or Neurology.

82. Ochsner KN, Lieberman MD: The emergence of social cognitive neuroscience, *Am Psychol* 56:717-734, 2001.

83. Winstein CJ: Motor learning: from behavior to social cognitive neuroscience perspective. III STEP Conference, July 2005, Salt Lake City, UT. Available on CD from American Physical Therapy Association.

84. NUSTEP Conference: Northwestern University, Chicago, July 25–August 20, 1967.

85. II STEP Conference: University of Oklahoma, Norman, OK, July 6-13, 2000.

86. III STEP Conference: University of Utah, Salt Lake City, UT, July 15-21, 2005.

87. Barbeau H, Visintin M: Optimal outcomes obtained with body-weight support combined with treadmill training in stroke subjects, *Arch Phys Med Rehabil* 84:1458-1465, 2003.

88. Blennerhassett J, Dite W: Additional task-related practice improves mobility and upper limb function early after stroke: a randomized controlled trial, *Aust J Physiother* 50:219-224, 2004.

89. Page SJ, Levine P, Leonard AC: Modified constraint-induced therapy in acute stroke: a randomized controlled pilot study, *Neurorehabil Neural Repair* 19:273-289, 2005.

90. Michelon P, Vettel JM, Zacks JM: Lateral somatotopic organization during imagined and prepared movements, *J Neurophysiol* 95:811-822, 2006.

91. Dedding C, Cardol M, Eyssen IC et al: Validity of the Canadian Occupational Performance Measure: a client-centred outcome measurement, *Clin Rehabil* 18:660-667, 2004.

92. Law M, Darrah J, Rosenbaum P et al: Family-centred functional therapy for children with cerebral palsy: an emerging practice model, *Phys Occup Ther Pediatr* 18:83-102, 1998.

93. Palisano R: A model of physical therapist practice for children with cerebral palsy: Integrating evidence, experience, and family centered services, III STEP 7-day Conference, Salt Lake City, UT, July 16, 2005.

94. Langenecker SA, Bieliauskas LA, Rapport LJ et al: Face emotion perception and executive functioning deficits in depression, *J Clin Exp Neuropsychol* 27:320-333, 2005.

95. Sapolsky RM: Stress and plasticity in the limbic system, *Neurochem. Res* 28:1735-1742, 2003.

96. Mills AE, Spencer EM: Values based decision making: a tool for achieving the goals of healthcare, *HEC Forum* 17:18-32, 2005.

97. Yorkston KM, Johnson KL, Klasner ER: Taking part in life: enhancing participation in multiple sclerosis, *Phys Med Rehabil Clin North Am* 16:583-594, 2005.

98. Kleim JA, Barbay S, Cooper NR et al: Motor learning-dependent synaptogenesis is localized to functionally reorganized motor cortex, *Neurobiol Learn Mem* 77:63-77, 2002.

99. Kleim JA, Barbay S, Nudo RJ: Functional reorganization of the rat motor cortex following motor skill learning, *J Neurophysiol* 80:3321-3325, 1998.

100. Kleim JA, Bruneau R, VandenBerg P et al: Motor cortex stimulation enhances motor recovery and reduces peri-infarct dysfunction following ischemic insult, *Neurol Res* 25:789-793, 2003.

101. Kleim JA, Cooper NR, VandenBerg PM: Exercise induces angiogenesis but does not alter movement representations within rat motor cortex, *Brain Res* 934:1-6, 2002.

102. Kleim JA, Lussnig E, Schwarz ER et al: Synaptogenesis and Fos expression in the motor cortex of the adult rat after motor skill learning, *J Neurosci* 16:4529-4535, 1996.

103. Taub E, Crago JE, Burgio LD et al: An operant approach to rehabilitation medicine: Overcoming learned nonuse by shaping, *J Exp Anal Behav* 61:281-293, 1994.

104. Taub E, Miller NE, Novack TA et al: Technique to improve chronic motor deficit after stroke, *Arch Phys Med Rehabil* 74:347-354, 1993.

105. Taub E, Uswatte G, Morris DM: Improved motor recovery after stroke and massive cortical reorganization following constraint-induced movement therapy, *Phys Med Rehabil Clin North Am* 14:S77-S91, ix, 2003.

106. Taub E, Uswatte G, Pidikiti R: Constraint-induced movement therapy: a new family of techniques with broad application to physical rehabilitation—a clinical review, *J Rehabil Res Dev* 36:237-251, 1999.

107. van der Lee JH, Wagenaar RC, Lankhorst GJ et al: Forced use of the upper extremity in chronic stroke patients: results from a single-blind randomized clinical trial, *Stroke* 30:2369-2375, 1999.

108. Wolf SL, Lecraw DE, Barton LA et al: Forced use of hemiplegic upper extremities to reverse the effect of learned nonuse among chronic stroke and head-injured patients, *Exp Neurol* 104:125-132, 1989.

109. Barbeau H: Locomotor training in neurorehabilitation: emerging rehabilitation concepts, *Neurorehabil Neural Repair* 17:3-11, 2003.

110. Crompton S, Khemlani M, Batty J et al: Practical issues in retraining walking in severely disabled patients using treadmill and harness support systems, *Aust J Physiother* 47:211-213, 2001.

111. Dietz V: Neurophysiology of gait disorders: present and future applications, *Electroencephalogr Clin Neurophysiol* 103:333-355, 1997.

112. Dobkin BH, Harkema S, Requejo P et al: Modulation of locomotor-like EMG activity in subjects with complete and incomplete spinal cord injury, *J Neurol Rehabil* 9:183-190, 1995.

113. Hesse S, Konrad M, Uhlenbrock D: Treadmill walking with partial body weight support versus floor walking in hemiparetic subjects, *Arch Phys Med Rehabil* 80:421-427, 1999.

114. Werner C, Von Frankenberg S, Treig T et al: Treadmill training with partial body weight support and an electromechanical gait trainer for restoration of gait in subacute stroke patients: a randomized crossover study, *Stroke* 33:2895-2901, 2002.

115. Visintin M, Barbeau H, Korner-Bitensky N et al: A new approach to retrain gait in stroke patients through body weight support and treadmill stimulation, *Stroke* 29:1122-1128, 1998.

116. Wilson DJ, Swaboda JL: Partial weight-bearing gait retraining for persons following traumatic brain injury: preliminary report and proposed assessment scale, *Brain Inj* 16:259-268, 2002.

117. Wolf SL, Blanton S, Baer H et al: Repetitive task practice: a critical review of constraint-induced movement therapy in stroke, *Neurologist* 8:325-338, 2002.

118. Prochazka A, Hulliger M: Muscle afferent function and its significance for motor control mechanisms during voluntary movements in cat, monkey and man. In Desmedt JE, editor: *Advances in neurology: motor control mechanisms in health and disease, vol 39,* pp. 93-132, New York, 1983, Raven Press.

119. Bizzi E, Abend W: Posture control and trajectory formation in single and multi-finger movements. In Desmedt JE, editor: *Advances in neurology: motor control mechanisms in health and disease,* vol 39, pp. 31-45, New York, 1983, Raven Press.

120. Desmedt JE: Patterns of motor command during various types of voluntary movement in man. In Evarts EV, Wise SP, Bousfield D, editors: *The motor system in neurobiology,* pp. 133-139, New York, 1995, Elsevier.

121. Houk JD, Rymer WA: Neural control of muscle length and tension. In Brooks VB, editor: *Handbook of physiology, section 1: the nervous system, motor control part 1, vol 2,* pp. 257-323, Bethesda, 1981, American Physiological Society.

122. Merzenich MM, Kaas JH, Sur M et al: Double representation of the body surface within cytoarchitectonic areas 3b and 1 in "S1" in the owl monkey *(Aotus trivirgatus), J Comp Neurol* 181:41-73, 1978.

123. Merzenich MM, Nelson RJ, Kaas JH et al: Variability in hand surface representations in areas 3b and 1 in adult owl and squirrel monkeys, *J Comp Neurol* 258:281-296, 1987.

124. Hubel DH, Wiesel TN: Binocular interaction in striate cortex of kittens reared with artificial squint, *J Neurophysiol* 28:1041-1059, 1965.

125. Reale RA, Brugge JF, Chan JC: Maps of auditory cortex in cats reared after unilateral cochlear ablation in the neonatal period, *Brain Res* 431:281-290, 1987.

126. Merzenich MM, Nelson RJ, Stryker MP et al: Somatosensory cortical map changes following digit amputation in adult monkeys, *J Comp Neurol* 224:591-605, 1984.

127. Sterr A, Elbert T, Berthold I et al: Longer versus shorter daily constraint-induced movement therapy of chronic hemiparesis: an exploratory study, *Arch Phys Med Rehabil* 83:1374-1377, 2002.

128. Sadato N, Pascual-Leone A, Grafman J et al: Activation of the primary visual cortex by Braille reading in blind subjects, *Nature* 380:526-528, 1996.

129. Black JE, Isaacs KR, Anderson BJ et al: Learning causes synaptogenesis, whereas motor activity causes angiogenesis, in cerebellar cortex of adult rats, *Proc Natl Acad Sci U S A* 87:5568-5572, 1990.

130. Kleim J, Jones TA: Principles of experience–dependent neural plasticity: implications for rehabilitation after brain damage, *J Speech Lang Hear Res* (in press.)

131. Nudo RJ: Adaptive plasticity in motor cortex: Implications for rehabilitation after brain injury, *J Rehabil Med* (41 suppl):7-10, 2003.

132. Merzenich MM, Allard T, Jenkins WM: Neural ontogeny of higher brain function: implications of some recent neurophysiological findings. In FranzÈn O, Westman P, editors: *Information processing in the somatosensory system,* pp. 293-311, London, 1991, Macmillan.

133. Merzenich MM, deCharms RC: Neural representations, experience and change. In Llinas R, Churchland P, editors: *The mind-brain continuum,* pp. 61-81, Boston, 1996, MIT Press.

134. Merzenich MM, Jenkins WM: Cortical plasticity, learning and learning dysfunction. In Julesz B, Kovacs I, editors: *Maturational windows and adult cortical plasticity,* pp. 247-272, New York, 1995, Addison-Wesley.

135. Merzenich MM, Tallal P, Peterson B et al: Some neurological principles relevant to the origins of—and the cortical plasticity based remediation of—language learning impairments. In Grafman J, Cristen Y,

editors: *Neuroplasticity: building a bridge from the laboratory to the clinic,* pp. 169-187, New York, 1998, Springer-Verlag.

136. Recanzone GH, Merzenich MM, Schreiner CS: Changes in the distributed temporal response properties of SI cortical neurons reflect improvements in performance on a temporally-based tactile discrimination task, *J Neurophysiol* 67:1071-1091, 1992.

137. Recanzone GH, Schreiner CE, Merzenich MM: Plasticity in the frequency representation of primary auditory cortex following discrimination training in adult owl monkeys, *J Neurosci* 13:87-103, 1993.

138. Jenkins WM, Merzenich MM, Ochs M et al: Functional reorganization of primary somatosensory cortex in adult owl monkeys after behaviorally controlled tactile stimulation, *J Neurophysiol* 63:82-104, 1990.

139. Wang X, Merzenich MM, Sameshima K et al: Remodelling of hand representation in adult cortex determined by timing of tactile stimulation, *Nature* 378:71-75, 1995.

140. Allard TA, Clark SA, Jenkins WM et al: Reorganization of somatosensory area 3b representation in adult owl monkeys following digital syndactyly, *J Neurophysiol* 66:1048-1058, 1991.

141. Clark SA, Allard T, Jenkins WM et al: Receptive fields in the body-surface map in adult cortex defined by temporally correlated inputs, Nature 332:444-445, 1988.

142. Hebb DO: *The organization of behavior,* New York, 1949, Wiley.

143. Merzenich MM: Development and maintenance of cortical somatosensory representations: Functional "maps" and neuroanatomical repertoires. In Barnard KE, Brazelton TB, editors: *Touch: the foundation of experience,* pp. 47-71, Madison, WI, 1990, International Universities Press.

144. Merzenich MM, Sameshima K: Cortical plasticity and memory, *Curr Opin Neurobiol* 3:187-196, 1993.

145. Buomomano DV, Merzenich MM: Cortical plasticity: from synapses to maps, *Annu Rev Neurosci* 21:149-186, 1998.

146. Recanzone GH, Merzenich MM, Jenkins WM: Frequency discrimination training engaging a restricted skin surface results in an emergence of a cutaneous response zone in cortical area 3a, *J Neurophysiol* 67:1057-1070, 1992.

147. Quinn JF: Building a body of knowledge-research on therapeutic touch, 1974-1986, *J Holistic Nurs* 6:37-45, 1988.

148. Kilgard MP, Merzenich MM: Plasticity of temporal information processing in the primary auditory cortex, *Nature Neurosci* 1:727-731, 1999.

149. McAnally KE, Stein JF: Auditory temporal coding in dyslexia, *Proc Biol Sci* 263:961-965, 1996.

150. Wang X, Merzenich MM, Beitel R et al: Representation of species-specific vocalizations in the primary auditory cortex of the marmoset monkey: spectral and temporal features, *J Neurophysiol* 74:1685-1706, 1995.

151. Wright B, Lombardino LJ, King WM et al: Deficits in auditory temporal and spectral resolution in language-impaired children, *Nature* 387:176-177, 1997.

152. Baddeley A, Wilson BA: A developmental deficit in short-term phonological memory: implications for language and reading, *Memory* 1:65-78, 1993.

153. Benasich AA, Tallal P: Auditory temporal processing thresholds, habituation, and recognition memory over the first year, *Infant Behav Dev* 19:339-356, 1996.

154. Bishop DV: The underlying nature of specific language impairment, *J Child Psychol Psychiatry Allied Discipl* 33:3-66, 1992.

155. DeWierdt J: Spectral processing deficit in dyslexic children, *Appl Psychol* 9:163-174, 1989.

156. Eden GG, Stein JF, Wood HM et al: Temporal and spatial processing in reading disabled and normal children, *Cortex* 31:451-468, 1995.

157. Farmer ME, Klein R: The evidence for a temporal processing deficit linked to dyslexia: a review, *Psychonom Bull Rev* 2:460-493, 1995.

158. Giliam RB, Cowan N, Day LS: Sequential memory in children with and without language impairment, *J Speech Hear Res* 38:393-402, 1995.

159. Harel S, Nachson I: Dichotic listening to temporal tonal stimuli by good and poor readers, *Percept Motor Skills* 84:467-473, 1997.

160. Harl R, Kiesila P: Deficit of temporal auditory processing in dyslexic adults, *Neurosci Lett* 205:138-140, 1990.

161. Leonard LB: *Children with language impairment,* Cambridge, MA, 1998, MIT Press.

162. Leonard LB, Bortoline U: Grammatical morphology and the role of weak syllables in the speech of Italian-speaking children with specific language impairment, *J Speech Hear Res* 41:1363-1374, 1998.

163. Lundberg I: Why is learning to read a hard task for some children, *Scand J Psychol* 39:155-167, 1998.

164. Merzenich MM, Miller S, Jenkins WM et al: Amelioration of the acoustic reception and speech reception deficits underlying language-based learning impairments. In Euler CV, editor: *Basic neural mechanisms in cognition and language,* pp. 143-172, Amsterdam, 1998, Elsevier.

165. Mills M, Cohen BB: *Developmental movement therapy,* Amherst, MA, 1979, School for Body/Mind Centering.

166. Nagarajan S, Mahncke H, Salz T et al: Cortical auditory signal processing in poor readers, *Proc Natl Acad Sci U S A* 96:6483-6488, 1999.

167. Plaut DC, McClelland JL, Seidenberg MS, Patterson K: Understanding normal and impaired word reading: computational principles in quasi-regular domains, *Psychol Rev* 103:56-115, 1996.

168. Spitz RV, Tallal P, Flax J et al: Look who's talking: a prospective study of familial transmission of language impairments, *J Speech Lang Hear Res* 40:990-1001, 1997.

169. Tallal P, Miller SL, Bedi G et al: Acoustically modified speech improves language comprehension in language-learning impaired children, *Science* 271:81-84, 1996.

170. Tallal P, Piercy M: Defects of non-verbal auditory perception in children with developmental aphasia, *Nature* 241:468-469, 1973.

171. Tallal P, Piercy M: Developmental aphasia: Rate of auditory processing and selective impairment of consonant perception, *Neuropsychologia* 13:69-74, 1974.

172. Buonomano DV, Hickmott PW, Merzenich MM: Context-sensitive synaptic plasticity and temporal-to-spatial transformations in hippocampal slices, *Proc Natl Acad Sci U S A* 94:10403-10408, 1997.

173. Buonomano DV, Merzenich MM: Temporal information transformed into a spatial code by a network with realistic properties, *Science* 267:1028-1030, 1995.

174. Byl H, Merzenich MM, Jenkins WM: A primate genesis model of focal hand dystonia and repetitive strain injury, I: learning-induced dedifferentiation of the representation of the hand in the primary somatosensory cortex in adult monkeys, *Neurology* 47:508-520, 1996.

175. Merzenich MM, Grajski KA, Jenkins WM et al: Functional cortical plasticity: cortical network origins of representational changes, *Cold Spring Harbor Symp Quant Biol* 55:873-887, 1991.

176. Naya Y, Sakai K, Miyashita Y: Activity of primate inferotemporal neurons related to a sought target in pair-association task, *Proc Natl Acad Sci U S A* 93:2664-2669, 1996.

177. Sakai K, Miyashita Y: Neural organization for the long-term memory of paired associates, *Nature* 354:152-155, 1991.

178. Bieser A, Moller-Preuss P: Auditory responsive cortex in the squirrel monkey: neural responses to amplitude-modulated sounds, *Exp Brain Res* 108:273-284, 1996

179. Eggermont JJ: Temporal modulation transfer functions for AM and FM stimuli in cat auditory cortex: effects of carrier type, modulating waveform and intensity, *Hear Res* 74:51-66, 1994.

180. Schreiner CE, Urbas JV: Representation of amplitude modulation in the auditory cortex of the cat, II: comparison between cortical fields, *Hear Res* 32:49-63, 1988.

181. Kaas JH, Hacket TA, Tamo MJ: Auditory processing in primate cerebral cortex, *Curr Opin Neurobiol* 9:164-170, 1999.

182. Ahissar M, Hochstein S: Attentional control of early perceptual learning, *Proc Natl Acad Sci U S A* 90:5718-5422, 1993.

183. Karni A, Sagi D: Where practice makes perfect in texture discrimination: evidence for primary visual cortex plasticity, *Proc Natl Acad Sci U S A* 88:4966-4970, 1991.

184. Kilgard MP, Mezenich MM: Cortical map reorganization enabled by nucleus basalis activity, *Science* 279:1714-1718, 1998.

185. Merzenich MM, Jenkins WM, Johnson P et al: Temporal processing deficits of language-learning impaired children ameliorated by training, *Science* 271:77-81, 1996.

186. Grajski KA, Merzenich MM: Hebb-type dynamics is sufficient to account for the inverse magnification rule in cortical somatotopy, *Neural Computation* 2:74-81, 1990.

187. Grajski KS, Merzenich MM: Neuronal network simulation of somatosensory representational plasticity. In Touretzky DL, editor: *Neural information processing systems, vol 2,* San Mateo, CA, 1990, Morgan Kaufman.

188. Somers DC, Todorov EV, Siapas AG et al: A local circuit approach to understanding integration of long-range inputs in primary visual cortex, *Cerebral Cortex* 8:204-217, 1998.

189. Merzenich MM, Jenkins WM: Cortical representation of learned behaviors. In Anderson P, editor: *Memory concepts,* pp. 437-453, Amsterdam, 1993, Elsevier.

190. Recanzone GH, Merzenich MM, Dinse HR: Expansion of the cortical representation of a specific skin field in primary somatosensory cortex by intracortical microstimulation, *Cerebral Cortex* 2:181-196, 1992.

191. Kuhl PK: Human adults and human infants show a "perceptual magnet effect" for the prototypes of speech categories, monkeys do not, *Percept Psychol* 50:93-107, 1991.

192. Kuhl PK: Learning and representation in speech and language, *Curr Opin Neurobiol* 4:812-822, 1994.

193. Recanzone GH, Merzenich M, Jenkins WM et al: Topographic reorganization of the hand representational zone in cortical area 3b paralleling improvements in frequency discrimination performance, *J Neurophysiol* 67:1031-1056, 1992.

194. Ahissar E, Vaadia E, Ahissar M et al: Dependence of cortical plasticity on corelated activity of single neurons and on behavioral context, *Science* 257:1412-1415, 1992.

195. Weinberger NM: Learning-induced changes of auditory receptive fields, *Curr Opin Neurobiol* 3:570-577, 1993.

196. Chelazzi L, Duncan J, Miller EK et al: Responses of neurons in inferior temporal cortex during memory-guided visual search, *J Neurophysiol* 80:2918-2940, 1998.

197. Kaster S, Pinsk MA, deWeerd P et al: Increased activity in human visual cortex during directed attention in the absence of visual stimulation, *Neuron* 22:751-761, 1999.

198. Haenny PE, Maunsell JH, Schiller PH: State dependent activity in monkey cortex, II: Retinal and extraretinal factors in V4, *Exp Brain Res* 69:245-259, 1988.

199. Hsiao SS, O'Shaugnessy DM, Johnson KO: Effects of selective attention on spatial form processing in monkey primary and secondary somatosensory cortex, *J Neurophysiol* 70:444-457, 1993.

200. Merzenich MM, Jenkins WM: Reorganization of cortical representations of the hand following alterations of skin inputs induced by nerve injury, skin island transfers, and experience, *J Hand Ther* 6:89-104, 1993.

201. Phillips WA, Singer W: In search of common foundation for cortical computation, *Behav Brain Sci* 20:657-722, 1997.

202. Buonomano DV, Merzenich MM: Net interaction between different forms of short-term synaptic plasticity and slow-IPSPs in the hippocampus and auditory cortex, *J Neurophysiol* 80:1765-1774, 1998.

203. Engert F, Bonhoeffer T: Dendritic spine changes associated with hippocampal long-term synaptic plasticity, *Nature* 399:66-70, 1999.

204. Geinisman Y, deToledo-Morrell L, Morrell F et al: Structural synaptic correlate of long-term potentiation: formation of axospinous synapses with multiple, completely partitioned transmission zones, *Hippocampus* 3:435-445, 1993.

205. Greenough WT, Chang FF: In Peters A, Jones EG, editors: *Cerebral cortex,* vol 7, pp. 335-392, New York, 1988, Plenum.

206. Keller A, Arissian K, Asanuma H: Synaptic proliferation in the motor cortex of adult cats after long-term thalamic stimulation, *J Neurophysiol* 68:295-308, 1992.

207. Kleim JA, Swain RA, Czerlanis CM et al: Learning-dependent dendritic hypertrophy of cerebellar stellate cells: plasticity of local circuit neurons, *Neurobiol Learn Memory* 67:29-33, 1997.

208. Fleschig P: *Anatomie des menschlichen Gehirns und Ruckenmarks auf myelogenetischen Grundlage,* Liepzig, 1920, Georg Thieme.

209. Yakolev PI, Lecours AR: The myelogenetic cycles of regional maturation of the brain. In Minkowski A, editor: *Regional development of the brain in early life,* pp. 3-70, Oxford, 1967, Blackwell Scientific.

210. Derogatis R, Abeloff MD, Melisaratos N: Psychological coping mechanisms and survival time in metastatic breast cancer, *JAMA* 242:1504-1508, 1979.

211. Hopson JA: *The dreaming brain,* New York, 1989, Basic Books.

212. Buzski G: Memory consolidation during sleep: a neurophysiological perspective, *J Sleep Res* 1:17-23, 1998.

213. Karni A: When practice makes perfect, *Lancet* 345:395, 1995.

214. Qin YL, McNaughton BL, Skaggs WE et al: Memory reprocessing in corticocortical and hippocampocortical neuroral ensembles, *Phil Trans R Soc Lond* 352:1525-1533, 1997.

215. Haier RJ, Siegel BV, MacLachlan E et al: Regional glucose metabolic changes after learning a complex visuospatial/motor task: a positron emission tomographic study, *Brain Res* 570:134-143, 1992.

216. Nudo R, Jenkins W, Merzenich M: Unpublished observations, 1998.

217. James W: *The principles of psychology, vol 1,* New York, 1890, Dover.

218. Biernaskie J, Corbett D: Enriched rehabilitative training promotes improved forelimb motor function and enhanced dendritic growth after focal ischemic injury, *J Neurosci* 21:5272-5280, 2001.

219. Allred RP, Jones TA: Unilateral ischemic sensorimotor cortical damage in female rats: forelimb behavioral effects and dendritic structural plasticity in the contralateral homotopic cortex, *Exp Neurol* 190:433-445, 2004.

220. Allred RP, Maldonado MA, Hsu JE et al: Training the "less-affected" forelimb after unilateral cortical infarcts interferes with functional recovery of the impaired forelimb in rats, *Restorative Neurol Neurosci* 23(5-6):297-302, 2005.

221. Bury SD, Jones TA: Unilateral sensorimotor cortex lesions in adult rats facilitate motor skill learning with the "unaffected"forelimb and training-induced dendritic structural plasticity in the motor cortex, *J Neurosci* 22:8597-8606, 2002.

222. Bury SD, Jones TA: Facilitation of motor skill learning by callosal denervationn or foced forelimb use in adult rats, *Behav Brain Res* 150:43-53, 2004.

223. Hsu JE, Jones TA: Time-sensitive enhancement of motor learning with the less-affected forelimb after unilateral sensotimotor cortex lesions in rats, *Eur J Neurosci* 22:2069-2080, 2005.

224. Luke LM, Allred RP, Jones TA: Unilateral ischemic sensoimotor cortical damage induces contralesional synaptogenesis and enhances skilled reaching with the ipsilateral forelimb in adult male rats, *Synapse* 54:187-199, 2004.

225. Murase N, Duque J, Mazzocchio R et al: Influence of interhemispheric interactions on motor function in chronic stroke, *Ann Neurol* 55:400-409, 2004.

226. Kleim JA: III STEP: a basic scientist's perspective, *Phys Ther* 86:614-617, 2006.

227. Byl NN, Nagarajan SS, Merzenich MM et al: Correlation of clinical neuromusculoskeletal and central somatosensory performance: variability in controls and patients with severe and mild focal hand dystonia, *Neural Plast* 9:177-203, 2002.

228. Churchill JD, Galvez R, Colcombe S et al: Exercise, experience and the aging brain, *Neurobiol Aging* 23:941-955, 2002.

229. Cotman CW, Berchtold NC: Exercise: A behavioral intervention to enhance brain health and plasticity, *Trends Neurosci* 25:295-301, 2002.

230. Jin K, Minami M, Xie L Sun Y et al: Ischemia-induced neurogenesis is preserved but reduced in the aged rodent brain, *Aging Cell* 3:373-377, 2004.

231. Shapira S, Sapir M, Wengier A et al: Aging has a complex effect on a rat model of ischemic stroke, *Brain Res* 925;148-158, 2002.

232. Adlard PA, Perreau VM, Cotman CW: The exercise-induced expression of BDNF within the hippocampus varies across life-span, *Neurobiol Aging* 26:511-520, 2005.

233. Griesbach GS, Hovda DA, Molteni R et al: Voluntary exercise following traumatic brain injury: Brain-derived neurotophic factor upregulation and recovery of function, *Neuroscience* 125:129-139, 2004.

234. Griesbach GS, Gomez-Pinilla F, Hovda DA: The upregulation of plasticity-related proteins following TBI is disrupted with acute voluntary exercise, *Brain Res* 1016:154-162, 2004.

235. Biernaskie J, Chernenko G, Corbett D: Efficacy of rehabilitative experience declines with time after focal ischemic brain injury, *J Neurosci* 24:1245-1254, 2004.

236. Adkins-Muir DL, Jones TA: Cortical electrical stimulation combined with rehabilitative training: enhanced functional recovery and dendritic plasticity following focal cortical ischemia in rats, *Neurol Res* 25:780-788, 2003.

237. Kobayashi M, Hutchinson S, Theoret H et al: Repetitive TMS of the motor cortex improves ipsilateral sequential simple finger movements, *Neurology* 62:91-98, 2004.

238. Alexander NB, Galecki AT, Grenier ML et al: Task-specific resistance training to improve the ability of activities of daily living-impaired older adults to rise from a bed and from a chair, *J Am Geriatr Soc* 49:1418-1427, 2001.

239. Bayona NA, Bitensky J, Salter K et al: The role of task-specific training in rehabilitation therapies, *Top Stroke Rehabil* 12:58-65, 2005.

240. Canning CG, Shepherd RB, Carr JH et al: A randomized controlled trial of the effects of intensive sit-to-stand training after recent traumatic brain injury on sit-to-stand performance, *Clin Rehabil* 17:355-362, 2003.

241. Dobkin BH. Strategies for stroke rehabilitation, *Lancet Neurol* 3:528-536, 2004.

242. Ferraro M, Palazzolo JJ, Krol J et al: Robot-aided sensorimotor arm training improves outcome in patients with chronic stroke, *Neurology* 61:1604-1607, 2003.

243. Fisher BE, Sullivan KJ: Activity-dependent factors affecting post-stroke functional outcomes, *Top Stroke Rehabil* 8:31-44, 2001.

244. Jensen JL, Marstrand PC, Nielsen JB: Motor skill training and strength training are associated with different plastic changes in the central nervous system, *J Appl Physiol* 99:1558-1568, 2005.

245. Judkins TN, Oleynikov D, Narazaki K et al: Robotic surgery and training: electromyographic correlates of robotic laparoscopic training, *Surg Endosc* 20:824-829, 2006.

246. Michaelsen SM, Dannenbaum R, Levin M: Task-specific training with trunk restraint on arm recovery in stroke: randomized control trial, *Stroke* 37:186-192, 2006.

247. Volpe BT, Ferraro M, Krebs HI et al: Robotics in the rehabilitation treatment of patients with stroke, *Curr Atheroscler Rep* 4:270-276, 2002.

248. Marigold DS, Eng JJ, Dawson AS et al: Exercise leads to faster postural reflexes, improved balance and mobility, and fewer falls in older persons with chronic stroke, *J Am Geriatr Soc* 53:416-423, 2005.

249. Studenski S, Duncan PW, Perera S et al: Daily functioning and quality of life in a randomized controlled trial of therapeutic exercise for subacute stroke survivors, *Stroke* 36:1764-1770, 2005.

250. Olney SJ, Nymark J, Brouwer B et al: A randomized controlled trial of supervised versus unsupervised exercise programs for ambulatory stroke survivors, *Stroke* 37:476-481, 2006.

251. Teixeira-Salmela LF, Nadeau S, McBride I et al: Effects of muscle strengthening and physical conditioning training on temporal, kinematic and kinetic variables during gait in chronic stroke survivors, *J Rehabil Med* 33:53-60, 2001.

252. Teixeira-Salmela LF, Olney SJ, Nadeau S et al: Muscle strengthening and physical conditioning to reduce impairment and disability in chronic stroke survivors, *Arch Phys Med Rehabil* 80:1211-1218, 1999.

253. Pang MY, Eng JJ, Dawson AS et al: A community-based fitness and mobility exercise program for older adults with chronic stroke: a randomized, controlled trial, *J Am Geriatr Soc* 53:1667-1674, 2005.

254. Macko RF, Ivey FM, Forrester LW et al: Treadmill exercise rehabilitation improves ambulatory function and cardiovascular fitness in patients with chronic stroke: a randomized, controlled trial, *Stroke* 36:2206-2211, 2005.

255. Romberg A, Virtanen A, Ruutiainen J: Long-term exercise improves functional impairment but not quality of life in multiple sclerosis, *J Neurol* 252:839-845, 2005.

256. Romberg A, Virtanen A, Ruutiainen J et al: Effects of a 6-month exercise program on patients with multiple sclerosis: a randomized study, *Neurology* 63:2034-2038, 2004.

257. Brown TR, Kraft GH: Exercise and rehabilitation for individuals with multiple sclerosis, *Phys Med Rehabil Clin North Am* 16:513-555, 2005.

258. Hirsch MA, Toole T, Maitland CG et al: The effects of balance training and high-intensity resistance training on persons with idiopathic Parkinson's disease, *Arch Phys Med Rehabil* 84:1109-1117, 2003.

259. Inzelberg R, Peleg N, Misipeanu P et al: Inspiratory muscle training and the perception of dyspnea in Parkinson's disease, *Can J Neurol Sci* 32:213-217, 2005.

260. Scandalis RA, Bosak A, Berliner JC et al: Resistance training and gait function in patients with Parkinson's disease, *Am J Phys Med Rehabil* 80:38-43, 2001.

261. Bateman A, Culpan FJ, Pickering AD et al: The effect of aerobic training on rehabilitation outcomes after recent severe brain injury: a randomized controlled evaluation, *Arch Phys Med Rehabil* 82:174-182, 2001.

262. Lewis CL, Fragala-Pinkham MA: Effects of aerobic conditioning and strength training on a child with Down syndrome: a case study, *Pediatr Phys Ther* 17:30-36, 2005.

263. Miszko TA, Cress ME, Slade JM et al: Effect of strength and power training on physical function in community-dwelling older adults, *J Gerontol A Biol Sci Med Sci* 58:171-175, 2003.

264. Morton JF, Brownlee M, McFadyen AK: The effects of progressive resistance training for children with cerebral palsy, *Clin Rehabil* 19:283-289, 2005.

265. Polh M, Mehrholz J, Ruckriem S: The influence of illness duration and level of consciousness on the treatment effect and complication rate of serial casting in patients with severe cerebral spasticity, *Clin Rehabil* 17:373-379, 2003.

266. Taylor NF, Dodd KJ, Larkin J: Adults with cerebral palsy benefit from participating in a strength training programme at a community gymnasium, *Disabil Rehabil* 26:1128-1134, 2004.

267. Tsimaras VK, Fotiadou EG: Effect of training on the muscle strength and dynamic balance ability of adults with down syndrome, *J Strength Cond Res* 18:343-347, 2004.

268. Wilson DJ, Swaboda JL: Partial weight-bearing gait retraining for persons following traumatic brain injury: preliminary report and proposed assessment scale, *Brain Inj* 16:259-268, 2002.

269. Farber S: Sensorimotor evaluation and treatment procedures, ed 22, Indianapolis, 1974, Indiana University-Purdue University at Indianapolis Medical Center.

270. Greenberg JH, Reivich M, Alavi A et al: Metabolic mapping of functional activity in human subjects with the fluorodeoxyglucose technique, *Science* 212:678-680, 1981.

271. Busse L, Roberts KC, Crist RE et al: The spread of attention across modalities and space in a multisensory object, *Proc Natl Acad Sci U S A* 20:102, 2005.

272. Drobyshevsky A, Baumann SB, Schneider W: Neuroimage. a rapid fMRI task battery for mapping of visual, motor, cognitive, and emotional function, *Neuroimage* 16:18751-18756, 2006.

273. Kayser C, Petkov CI, Augath M et al: Integration of touch and sound in auditory cortex, *Neuron* 48:373-384, 2005.

274. Nakai T, Kato C, Matsuo K: An FMRI study to investigate auditory attention: A model of the cocktail party phenomenon, *Magn Reson Med Sci* 4:75-82, 2005.

275. Puttemans V, Wenderoth N, Swinnen SP: Changes in brain activation during the acquisition of a multifrequency bimanual coordination task: From the cognitive stage to advanced levels of automaticity, *J Neurosci* 25:4270-4278, 2005.

276. Ricciardi E, Bonino D, Gentili C et al: Neural correlates of spatial working memory in humans: a functional magnetic resonance imaging study comparing visual and tactile processes, *Neuroscience* 139:339-349, 2006.

277. Wenderoth N, Toni I, Bedeleem S et al: Information processing in human parieto-frontal circuits during goal-directed bimanual movements, *Neuroimage* 31:264-278, 2006.

278. Luft AR, Manto MU, Ben Taib NO: Modulation of motor cortex excitability by sustained peripheral stimulation: The interaction between the motor cortex and the cerebellum, *Cerebellum* 4:90-96, 2005.

279. Hesse S, Werner C, von Frankenberg S et al: Treadmill training with partial body weight support after stroke, *Phys Med Rehabil Clin North Am* 14(1 suppl):S111-S123, 2003.

280. Miyai I, Suzuki M, Hatakenaka M et al: Effect of body weight support on cortical activation during gait in patients with stroke, *Exp Brain Res* 169:85-91, 2006.

281. Moseley AM, Stark A, Cameron ID et al: Treadmill training and body weight support for walking after stroke, *Cochrane Database Syst Rev* CD002840, 2005.

282. Hornby TG, Zemon DH, Campbell D: Robotic-assisted, body-weight-supported treadmill training in individuals following motor incomplete spinal cord injury, *Phys. Ther* 85:52-66, 2005.

283. Sullivan KJ, Knowlton BJ, Dobkin BH: Step training with body weight support: Effect of treadmill speed and practice paradigms on poststroke locomotor recovery, *Arch Phys Med Rehabil* 83:683-691, 2002.

284. Van Peppen RP, Kwakkel G, Wood-Dauphinee S et al: The impact of physical therapy on functional outcomes after stroke: what's the evidence? *Clin Rehabil* 18:833-362, 2004.

285. Luft AR, Buitrago MM: Stages of motor skill learning, *Mol Neurobiol* 32:205-216, 2005.

286. Houk J, Hennemou E: Responses of Golgi tendon organs, *J Neurophysiol* 30:466-489, 1967.

287. Gilman S, Manter JT, Gatz AJ et al: *Manter and Gatz's essentials of clinical neuroanatomy and neurophysiology,* Philadelphia, 2002, FA Davis.

288. Kandel ER, Schwartz JH, Jessel TM: *Principles of neural science,* ed 4, New York, 2000, McGraw-Hill.

289. Gould JA: *Orthopedic and sports physical therapy,* St. Louis, 1990, CV Mosby.

290. Morris SL, Dodd KJ, Morris ME: Outcomes of progressive resistance strength training following stroke: a systematic review, *Clin Rehabil* 18:27-39, 2004.

291. Twomey LT, Taylor JR: *Physical therapy of the low back,* ed 2, New York, 1994, Churchill Livingstone.

292. Bessou P, Burgess PR, Perl ER et al: Dynamic properties of mechanoreceptors with unmyelinated (C) fibers, *J Neurophysiol* 34:116-131, 1971.

293. Butler RA: The cumulative effects of differential stimulus repetition rates on the auditory evoked response in man, *Electroencephalogr Clin Neurophysiol* 35:337-345, 1973.

294. Garliner D: *Myofunctional therapy,* Philadelphia, 1976, WB Saunders.

295. Bishop B: Vibration stimulation, I: Neurophysiology of motor responses evoked by vibratory stimulation, *Phys Ther* 54:1273-1281, 1974.

296. Bishop B: Vibratory stimulation, II: vibratory stimulation as an evaluation tool, *Phys Ther* 55:29-33, 1975.

297. Maisden DC, Meadows JC, Hodgson HJ: Observations on the reflex response to muscle vibration in man and its voluntary control, *Brain* 42:829-846, 1969.

298. Verrillo R: Change in vibrotactile thresholds as a function of age, *Sens Processes* 3:49-59, 1979.

299. Hagbarth KE, Eklund G: Tonic vibration reflexes in spasticity, *Brain Res* 2:201-203, 1966.

300. Purdue pegboard, model 32020, instructions and normative data, Lafayette, IN, Lafayette Instrument Company.

301. Cohen H, editor: *Neuroscience rehabilitation,* Philadelphia, 1993, JB Lippincott.

302. de Vlugt E, Schouten AC, van der Helm FC: Quantification of intrinsic and reflexive properties during multijoint arm posture, *J Neurosci Methods* Feb 25, 2006 (E pub).

303. Faist M, Hoefer C, Hodapp M et al: In humans Ib facilitation depends on locomotion while suppression of Ib inhibition requires loading, *Brain Res* 1076:87-92, 2006.

304. Moore JC: The Golgi tendon organ and the muscle spindle, *Am J Occup Ther* 28:415-420, 1974.

305. Guyton A: *Basic neuroscience: anatomy and physiology,* Philadelphia, 1991, WB Saunders.

306. McCloskey DI: Kinesthetic sensibility, *Physiol Rev* 58:763-813, 1978.

307. Downie RA: *Cash's textbook of neurology for physiotherapists,* Philadelphia, 1986, JB Lippincott.

308. Craik R: Spasticity revisited. In American Physical Therapy Association Combined Section Meetings, New Orleans, LA, 1996.

309. Blashy MR, Fuchs R: Orthokinetics: a new receptor facilitation method, *Am J Occup Ther* 8:226-234, 1959.

310. Tuttle R, McClearly J: Mesenteric baroreceptors, *Am J Physiol* 229:1514-1519, 1975.

311. Ge HY, Madeleine P, Arendt-Nielsen L: Sex differences in temporal characteristics of descending inhibitory control: an evaluation using repeated bilateral experimental induction of muscle pain, *Pain* 110:72-78, 2004.

312. Pertovaara A: Modification of human pain threshold by specific tactile receptors, *Acta Physiol Scand* 107:339-341, 1979.

313. Pickar JG: Neurophysiological effects of spinal manipulation, *Spine J* 2:357-371, 2002.

314. Melzack R: Myofascial trigger points: Relations to acupuncture and mechanisms of pain, *Arch Phys Med Rehabil* 62:47-50, 1981.

315. Melzack R, Konard KW, Dubrobsky B: Prolonged changes in the nervous system activity produced by somatic and reticular stimulation, *Exp Neurol* 25:416-428, 1969.

316. Melzack R, Stillwell DM, Fox EJ: Trigger points and acupuncture points for pain: Correlations and implication, *Pain* 1:3-23, 1977.

317. Merzenich MM: Development and maintenance of cortical somatosensory representations: functional "maps" and neuroanatomical repertoires. In Barnard KE, Brazelton TB, editors: *Touch: the foundation of experience,* pp. 47-71, Madison, WI, 1990, International Universities Press.

318. de Groot J: *Correlative neuroanatomy,* ed 21, San Mateo, CA, 1991, Lange Medical Publications.

319. Andrew BL, Dodt E: The deployment of sensory nerve endings at the knee joint in a cat, *Acta Physiol Scand* 28:287-296, 1953.

320. Talbot WH, Darian-Smith I, Kornhuber HH et al: The sense of flutter-vibration: companion of the human capacity with response patterns of mechanoreceptive afferents, *J Neurophysiol* 31:301-334, 1968.

321. Fields HL: *Pain,* New York, 1987, McGraw-Hill.

322. Vallbo AB, Hagbarth KE, Torebjork HE et al: Somatosensory, proprioceptive, and sympathetic activity in human peripheral nerves, *Physiol Rev* 59:919-957, 1979.

323. Gardner EP, Ro JY, Debowy D et al: Facilitation of neuronal activity in somatosensory and posterior parietal cortex during prehension, *Exp Brain Res* 127:329-354, 1999.

324. Geldard FA: *The human senses,* ed 2, New York, 1972, John Wiley.

325. Luft AR, Smith GV, Forrester L et al: Comparing brain activation associated with isolated upper and lower limb movement across corresponding joints, *Hum Brain Mapp* 17:131-140, 2002.

326. Matsuhashi M, Ikeda A, Ohara S et al: Multisensory convergence at human temporo-parietal junction—epicortical recording of evoked responses, *Clin Neurophysiol* 115:1145-1160, 2004.

327. Park HB, Koh M, Cho SH et al: Mapping the rat somatosensory pathway from the anterior cruciate ligament nerve endings to the cerebrum, *J Orthop Res* 23:1419-1424, 2005.

328. Feldenkrais M: *Awareness through movement,* New York, 1977, Harper & Row.

329. Feldenkrais M: *The elusive obvious,* Cupertino, CA, 1981, Meta Publication.

330. Jackson O: *Clinics in physical therapy, Therapeutic considerations for the elderly,* vol 14, New York, 1987, Churchill Livingstone.

331. Butler DS: *Mobilization of the nervous system,* New York, 1991, Churchill Livingstone.

332. Crown ED, Grau JW: Evidence that descending serotonergic systems protect spinal cord plasticity against the disruptive effect of uncontrollable stimulation, *Exp Neurol* 196:164-176, 2005.

333. Payton OP, Hirt S, Newton RA: *Scientific bases for neurophysiologic approaches to therapeutic exercise: An anthology,* Philadelphia, 1978, FA Davis.

334. Keshner EA: How theoretical framework biases evaluation and treatment. In Lister MJ, editor: *Contemporary management of motor problems,* Norman, OK, 1991, Foundation for Physical Therapy.

335. Kottke F: The neurophysiology of motor function. In Kottke F, Stillwell K, Lehmann J, editors: *Handbook of physical medicine and rehabilitation,* ed 3, Philadelphia, 1982, WB Saunders.

336. Chalmers G: Re-examination of the possible role of Golgi tendon organ and muscle spindle reflexes in proprioceptive neuromuscular facilitation muscle stretching, *Sports Biomech* 3:159-183, 2004.

337. Decicco PV, Fisher MM: The effects of proprioceptive neuromuscular facilitation stretching on shoulder range of motion in overhand athletes, *J Sports Med Phys Fitness* 45:183-187, 2005.

338. Gabriel DA, Kamen G, Frost G: Neural adaptations to resistive exercise: Mechanisms and recommendations for training practices, *Sports Med* 36:133-149, 2006.

339. Kofotolis N, Vrabas IS, Vamvakoudis E et al: Proprioceptive neuromuscular facilitation training induced alterations in muscle fibre type and cross sectional area, *Br J Sports Med* 39:e11, 2005.

340. Marek SM, Cramer JT, Fincher AL et al: Acute effects of static and proprioceptive neuromuscular facilitation stretching on muscle strength and power output, *J Athl Train* 40:94-103, 2005.

341. Butler DS: Adverse mechanical tension in the nervous system: a model for assessment and treatment, *Aust J Physiother* 35:227-238, 1989.

342. Elvey RL: Physical evaluation and treatment of neural tissues in disorders of the neuromusculoskeletal system: neural and brachial plexus tension. Course handout, San Jose, CA, Northeast Seminars.

343. Kornberg C, McCarthy T: The effect of neural stretching techniques on sympathetic outflow to the lower limbs, *J Orthop Sports Phys Ther* 16:269-274, 1992.

344. Head H: *Studies in neurology,* vol 2, Oxford, 1920, Oxford University Press.

345. Ciccarelli O, Toosy AT, Marsden JF et al: Identifying brain regions for integrative sensorimotor processing with ankle movements, *Exp Brain Res* 166:31-42, 2005.

346. Feldman DE, Brecht M: Map plasticity in somatosensory cortex, *Science* 310:810-815, 2005.

347. Mueller HA: Facilitating feeding and prespeech. In Pearson PH, Williams CE, editors: *Physical therapy services in the developmental disabilities,* Springfield, IL, 1972, Charles C Thomas, 1972.

348. Pleger B, Foerster AF, Ragert P et al: Functional imaging of perceptual learning in human primary and secondary somatosensory cortex, *Neuron* 40:643-653, 2003.

349. Brecker LR: Imagery and ROM combine to create, *Adv Phys Ther* 5:18-19, 1994.

350. Roberts TDM: *Neurophysiology of postural mechanisms,* New York, 1967, Plenum.

351. Poggio GF, Mountcastle VB: A study of the functional contributions of the lemniscal and spinothalamic systems to somatic sensibility, *Bull Johns Hopkins Hosp* 106:266-316, 1960.

352. Ayers AJ: *Sensory integration and the child,* Los Angeles, 1979, Western Psychological Services.

353. Wilbarger P: Advanced course for treatment of sensory defensiveness. In Symposium on intervention for persons with mild to severe dysfunction, Minneapolis, 1994.

354. Groen JJ: Vestibular stimulation and its effects from the point of view of theoretical physics, *Confin Neurol* 21:380-389, 1961.

355. Jacob S, Francone C: *Structure and function in man,* ed 3, Philadelphia, 1974, WB Saunders.

356. Sinclair D: *Cutaneous sensation,* London, 1967, Oxford University Press.

357. Granit R: *Receptors and sensory perception,* New Haven, CT, 1967, Yale University Press.

358. Iggo A: *A single unit analysis of cutaneous receptor with C afferent fibers: CIBA foundation groups,* Springfield, IL, 1967, Charles C Thomas.

359. Zotterman Y: *Sensory functions of the skin in primates,* Oxford, 1976, Pergamon Press.

360. Eldred E: Peripheral receptors: their excitation and relation to reflex patterns, *Am J Phys Med* 46:69-72, 1967.

361. Jackson O: The Feldenkrais method: a personalized learning model. In Lister MJ, editor: *Contemporary management of motor control problems,* Norman, OK, 1991, Foundation for Physical Therapy.

362. Quillian TA: Neuro-cutaneous relationships in fingerprint skin. In Kornhuber H, editor: *The somatosensory system,* Sachs, Germany, 1975, Thieme.

363. Godfrey H: Understanding pain, 1: physiology of pain, *Br J Nurs* 14:846-852, 2005.

364. Krames E: Spinal cord stimulation: Indications, mechanism of action, and efficacy, *Curr Rev Pain* 3:419-426, 1999.

365. Lim RK: Pain, *Annu Rev Physiol* 32:269-288, 1970.

366. Wall P: The gate control theory of pain mechanisms, *Brain* 101:1-18, 1978.

367. Booker J: Pain: It's all in your patient's head (or is it)? *Nursing* 82:47-51, 1982.

368. Gabis L, Shklar B, Geva D: Immediate influence of transcranial electrostimulation on pain and beta-endorphin blood levels: an active placebo-controlled study, *Am J Phys Med Rehabil* 82:81-85, 2003.

369. LaGraize SC, Borzan J, Peng YB et al: Selective regulation of pain affect following activation of the opioid anterior cingulate cortex system, *Exp Neurol* 197:22-30, 2006.

370. Marx J: Analgesia: How the body inhibits pain perception, *Science* 195:471-473, 1977.

371. Selbach H: The principle of relaxation oscillation as a special instance of the law of initial value in cybernetic functions, *Ann N Y Acad Sci* 98:1221-1228, 1962.

372. Bandler R, Grindler J: *The structure of magic,* Palo Alto, CA, 1975, Science and Behavior Books.

373. Reith E, Breidenback B: *Textbook of anatomy and physiology,* ed 2, New York, 1978, McGraw-Hill.

374. Weiss SJ: Psychophysiologic effects of caregiver touch on incidence of cardiac dysrhythmia, *Heart Lung* 15:495-502, 1986.

375. Normell LA: The cutaneous thermoregulatory vasomotor response in healthy subjects and paraplegic men, *Scand J Clin Invest* 4:133-138, 1974.

376. Gandhavadi B: Autonomic pain: features and methods of assessment, *Pain* 71:85-90, 1982.

377. Duncan PW, editor: *Balance proceedings of the APTA Forum,* Alexandria, VA, 1989, American Physical Therapy Association.

378. Moore JC: The limbic system. Class notes from Bay Area Sensory Symposium, San Francisco, CA, February 1980.

379. Wilson V, Peterson B: The role of the vestibular system in posture and movement. In Mountcastle VB, editor: *Medical physiology,* ed 14, vol 2, St. Louis, 1989, CV Mosby.

380. Barr ML, Kiernan JA, editors: *The human nervous system: an anatomical viewpoint,* ed 6, Philadelphia, 1990, JB Lippincott.

381. Moore JC, Umphred DA: *The vestibular-visual-cervical triad: Foundations for balance, posture, position sense and movement and treatment implications,* San Francisco, 1993, Pacific Coast Seminars.

382. Barnes GR: Head-eye coordination in normals and in patients with vestibular disorders: Proceedings of the Barany Society, Uppsala, Sweden, *Adv Otorhinolaryngol* 25:197-201, 1979.

383. Green JH: *Basic clinical physiology,* Oxford, 1973, Oxford University Press.

384. Herdman SJ: Assessment and treatment of balance disorders in the vestibular-deficient patient. In Duncan PW, editor: *Balance,* Alexandria, VA, 1990, American Physical Therapy Association.

385. Herdman SJ: Exercise strategies in vestibular disorders, *Ear Nose Throat* 68:961-964, 1990.

386. Herdman SJ, Schubert MC, Tusa RJ: Role of central preprogramming in dynamic visual acuity with vestibular loss, *Arch Otolaryngol Head Neck Surg* 127:1205-1210, 2001.

387. Huss J: *Sensorimotor treatment approaches in occupational therapy,* Philadelphia, 1971, JB Lippincott.

388. Stejskal L: Postural reflexes in man, *Am J Phys Med* 58:1-24, 1979.

389. Duensing F, Schaefer KP: The activity of various neurons of the reticular formation of the unfettered rabbit during head turning and vestibular stimulation [in German], *Arch Psychiatr Nervenkr* 201:97-122, 1960.

390. Barnes GR, Forbat LN: Cervical and vestibular afferent control of oculomotor response in man, *Acta Otolaryngol (Stockh)* 88:79-87, 1979.

391. Parker DE: The vestibular apparatus, *Sci Am* 243:118-130, 1980.

392. Horak FB, Shumway-Cook A, Crowe TK et al: Vestibular function and motor proficiency in children with impaired hearing, or with learning disability and motor impairment, *Dev Med Child Neurol* 30:64-79, 1988.

393. Horak FB, Jones-Rycewicz C, Black FO et al: Effects of vestibular rehabilitation on dizziness and imbalance, *Otolaryngol Head Neck Surg* 106:175-180, 1992.

394. Schubert MC, Herdman SJ, Tusa RJ: Vertical dynamic visual acuity in normal subjects and patients with vestibular hypofunction, *Otol Neuroltol* 23:372-377, 2002.

395. Gill-Body KM, Krebs DE, Parker SW et al: Physical therapy management of peripheral vestibular dysfunction: two clinical case reports, *Phys Ther* 74:130-142, 1994.

396. Rocchi L, Chiari L, Cappello A et al: Identification of distinct characteristics of postural away in Parkinson's disease: a feature selection procedure based on principal component analysis, *Neurosci Lett* 394:140-145, 2006.

397. Shumway-Cook A, Horak FB: Rehabilitation strategies for patients with vestibular deficits, *Neurol Clin* 8:441-457, 1990.

398. Shumway-Cook A, Hutchinson S, Kartin D et al: Effect of balance training on recovery of stability in children with cerebral palsy, *Dev Med Child Neurol* 45:591-602, 2003.

399. Silsupasol P, Siu KC, Shumway-Cook A et al: Training of balance under single- and dual-task conditions in older adults with balance impairment, *Phys Ther* 86:269-281, 2006.

400. Vearrier LA, Langan J, Shumway-Cook A et al: An intensive massed practice approach to retraining balance post-stroke, *Gait Posture* 22:154-163, 2005.

401. Horak FB, Henry SM, Shumway-Cook A: Postural perturbations: new insights for treatment of balance disorders, *Phys Ther* 77:517-533, 1997.

402. Shumway-Cook A: Equilibrium deficits in children. In Woolcott MH, Shumway-Cook A, editors: *Development of posture and gait across the lifespan,* Columbia, SC, 1989, University of South Carolina.

403. Montgomery PC: Neurodevelopmental treatment and sensory integrative theory. In Lister MJ, editor: *Contemporary management of motor control problems,* Norman, OK, 1991, Foundation for Physical Therapy.

404. Zemack-Bersin D, Zemach-Bersin K, Resse M: *Relaxercise: The easy new way to health and fitness,* New York, 1990, Harper & Row.

405. Steiner JE: Innate discriminative human facial expressions to taste and smell stimulations, *Ann N Y Acad Sci* 237:229-233, 1974.

406. Cherney L: Aging and communication. In Lewis C, editor: *Aging: the health care challenge,* Philadelphia, 1989, FA Davis.

407. Upledger J: *Craniosacral therapy,* ed 5, Seattle, 1986, Eastman Press.

408. Takagi K, Kobayahsi S: Skin pressure reflex, *Acta Med Biol* 4:31-37, 1956.

409. Tappan FM: *Healing massage techniques: Holistic, classic and emerging methods,* ed 2, Norwalk CT, 1988, Appleton & Lange.

410. Barnes JF: *Myofascial release,* ed 3, Paoli, PA, 1990, Rehabilitation Service.

411. Taylor TC: Myofascial release techniques, *Phys Ther Forum* 5:2-4, 1986.

412. Travell J: *Myofascial pain and dysfunction,* Baltimore, 1983, Williams & Wilkins.

413. McCormack GL: Pain management by occupational therapists, *Am J Occup Ther* 42:9:582-590, 1988.

414. Cleland JA, Fritz JM, Childs JD et al: Comparison of the effectiveness of three manual physical therapy techniques in a subgroup of patients with low back pain who satisfy a clinical prediction rule: study protocol of a randomized clinical trial (NCT00257998), *BMC Musculoskelet Disord* 7:11, 2006.

415. Bronfort G, Hass M, Evans RL et al: Efficacy of spinal manipulation and mobilization for low back pain and neck pain: a systematic review and the best evidence synthesis, *Spine J* 4:335-356, 2004.

416. Whitman JM, Fritz JM, Childs JD: The influence of experience and specialty certifications on clinical outcomes for patients with low back pain treated within a standardized physical therapy management program, *J Orthop Sports Phys Ther* 34:662-672, 2004.

417. Gerhart KD, Yezierski RP, Giesler GJ Jr et al: Inhibitory receptive fields of primitive spinothalamic tract cells, *J Neurophysiol* 46:1309-1325, 1981.

418. Mehling WE, DiBlasi Z, Hecht F: Bias control in trials of bodywork: a review of methodological issues, *J Altern Complement Med* 11:333-342, 2005.

419. Jain S, Janseen K, DeCelle S: Alexander technique and Feldenkrais method: a critical overview, *Phys Med Rehabil Clin North Am* 15:811-825, 2004.

420. Shepard GM: Synaptic organization of the mammalian olfactory bulb, *Physiol Rev* 52:864-917, 1972.

420a. Ottoson D: Experiments and concepts in olfactory physiology, *Progr Brain Res* 23:83-138, 1967.

421. Zwaardemaker H: *Physiology of smell,* London, 1895, Collier Macmillan.

422. Setlow B, Schoenbaum G, Gallagher M: Neural encoding in ventral striatum during olfactory discrimination learning, *Neuron* 38:518-519, 2003.

423. Cain WS: Scope and evaluation of odor counteraction and masking, *Ann N Y Acad Sci* 237:427-439, 1974.

424. Pribram KH: *Languages of the brain: experimental paradoxes and principles in neuropsychology,* Englewood Cliffs, NJ, 1971, Prentice-Hall.

425. Dringenberg HC, Saber AJ, Cahill L: Enhanced frontal cortex activation in rats by convergent amygdaloid and noxious sensory signals, *Neuroreport* 12:2395-2398, 2001.

426. Perl E, Shufman E, Vas A et al: Taste- and odor-reactivity in heroin addicts, *Isr J Psychiatry Relat Sci* 34:290-299, 1997.

427. Huss J: Neurophysiological approaches to treatment, Class notes, workshop, San Jose State University, 1980.

428. Eckert E: Muscle and movement. In *Animal physiology: mechanisms and adaptations,* ed 3, New York, 1988, Freeman.

429. Philpott CM, Wolstenholme CR, Goodenough PC et al: Comparison of subjective perception with objective measurement of olfaction, *Otolaryngol Head Neck Surg* 134:488-490, 2006.

430. Kobayashi M, Saito S, Kobayakawa T et al: Cross-cultural comparison of data using the odor stick identification test for Japanese (OSIT-J), *Chem Senses* 31:335-342, 2006.

431. Reiter ER, DiNardo LJ, Costanzo RM: Effects of head injury on olfaction and taste, *Otolaryngol Clin North Am* 37:1167-1184, 2004.

432. Soussignan R, Ehrle N, Henry A et al: Dissociation of emotional processes in response to visual and olfactory stimuli following frontotemporal damage, *Neurocase* 11:114-128, 2005.

433. Llorens J: The physiology of taste and smell: how and why we sense flavors, *Water Sci Technol* 49:1-10, 2004.

434. Small DM, Voss J, Mak YE et al: Experience-dependent neural integration of taste and smell in the human brain, *J Neurophysiol* 92:1892-1903, 2004.

435. Case J: *Sensory mechanisms: Current concepts in biology,* New York, 1966, Macmillan.

436. Spector AC, Travers SP: The representation of taste quality in the mammalian nervous system, *Behav Cogn Neurosci Rev* 4:143-191, 2005.

437. Groer MW, Shekleton ME: *Basic pathophysiology,* ed 2, St. Louis, 1983, CV Mosby.

438. Oakley B, Benjamin RM: Neurological mechanisms of taste, *Physiol Rev* 46:173-211, 1966.

439. Pfaffman C: Taste, its sensory and motivating properties, *Am Sci* 52:187-206, 1964.

440. Moulton DG, Turk A, Johnston JW, editors: *Methods in olfactory research,* London, 1975, Academic Press.

441. Fukunaga A, Uematsu H, Sugimoto K: Influences of aging on taste perception and oral somatic sensation, *J Gerontol A Biol Sci Med Sci* 60:109-113, 2005.

442. Souza PE, Boike KT: Combining temporal-envelope cues across channels: effect of age and hearing loss, *J Speech Lang Hear Res* 49:138-149, 2006.

443. Rauch SD, Zhou G, Kujawa SG et al: Vestibular evoked myogenic potentials show altered turing in patients with Meniere's disease, *Otol Neurotol* 25:333-338, 2004.

444. Howarth A, Shone GR: Ageing and the auditory system, *Postgrad Med J* 82:166-171, 2006.

445. Kacelnik O, Nodal FR, Parsons CH et al: Training-induced plasticity of auditory localization in adult mammals, *PLoS Biol* 4:e71, 2006.

446. Simon HJ: Bilateral amplification and sound localization: then and now, *J Rehabil Res Dev* 42(2 suppl):117-132, 2005.

447. Rabe K, Michael N, Kugel H et al: fMRI studies of sensitivity and habituation effects with the auditory cortex at 1.5 T and 3 T, *J Magn Reson Imaging* 23:454-458, 2006.

448. Martin JS, Jerger JF: Some effects of aging on central auditory processing, *J Rehabil Res Dev* 42(2 Suppl);25-44, 2005.

449. Brewer S: Personal correspondence with composer, pianist, and theoritician in use of sound in harmony with body rhythms, August 1983.

450. Howarth A, Shone GR: Ageing and the auditory system, *Postgrad Med J* 82:166-171, 2006.

451. De Sousa A: The role of music therapy in psychiatry, *Altern Ther Health Med* 11:52-53, 2005.

452. Hilliard RE: Music therapy in hospice and palliative care: a review of the empirical data, *Evid Based Complement Alternat Med* 2:173-178, 2005.

453. Jackendoff R, Lerdahl F: The capacity for music: what is it, and what's special about it? *Cognition* 100:33-72, 2006.

454. Koelsch S, Siebel WA: Towards a neural basis of music perception, *Trends Cogn Sci* 9:578-584, 2005.

455. Prickett CA, Moore RS: The use of music to aid in the memory of Alzheimer's patients, *J Music Ther* 28:101-110, 1991.

456. Koelsch S, Fritz T, V Cramon DY et al: Investigating emotion with music: an fMRI study, *Hum Brain Mapp* 27:239-250, 2006.

457. Olderog Millard KA, Smith JM: The influence of group singing on the behavior of Alzheimer's disease patients, *J Music Ther* 26:58-70, 1989.

458. Pollack NJ, Namazi KH: The effect of music participation on the social behavior of Alzheimer's disease patients, *J Music Ther* 29:54-67, 1992.

459. Bernardi L, Porta C, Sleight P: Cardiovascular, cerebrovascular and respiratory changes induced by different types of music in musicians and non-musicians: the importance of silence, *Heart* 92:445-452, 2006.

460. Etzel JA, Johnsen EL, Dickerson J et al: Cardiovascular and respiratory responses during musical mood induction, *Int J Psychophysiol* 61:57-69, 2006.

461. Frank A, Maurer P, Shepherd J: Light and sound environment: a survey of neonatal intensive care units, *Phys Occup Ther Pediatr* 11:27-45, 1991.

462. Hirokawa E, Ohira H: The effects of music listening after a stressful task on immune functions, neuroendocrine responses, and emotional states in college students, *J Music Ther* 40:189-211, 2003.

463. Nunez MJ, Mana P, Linares D et al: Music, immunity and cancer, *Life Sci* 71:1047-1057, 2002.

464. Aitkin LM: The auditory system. In Bjorklund A, Hokfeld T, Swanson LW, editors: *Handbook of chemical neuroanatomy: integrated systems of the CNS, Part II,* vol 7, New York, 1989, Elsevier.

465. Nelson HD, Nygren P, Walker M et al: Screening for speech and language delay in preschool children: systematic evidence review for the US Preventive Services Task Force, *Pediatrics* 117:298-319, 2006.

466. Szaflarski JP, Schmithorst VJ, Altaye M et al: A longitudinal functional magnetic resonance imaging study of language development of children 5 to 11 years old, *Ann Neurol* 59:796-807, 2006.

467. Bertoli S, Smurzynski J, Probst R: Effects of age, age-related hearing loss, and contralateral cafeteria noise on the discrimination of small frequency changes: psychoacoustic and electrophysiological measures, *J Assoc Res Otolaryngol* 6:207-222, 2005.

468. Caspary DM, Schatteman TA, Hughes LF: Age-related changes in the inhibitory response properties of dorsal cochlear nucleus output neurons: role of inhibitory inputs, *J Neurosci* 25:10952-10959, 2005.

469. Frank A, Maurer P, Shepherd J: Light and sound environment: a survey of neonatal intensive care units, *Phys Occup Ther Pediatr* 11:27-45, 1991.

470. Richter HO, Costello P, Sponheim SR et al: Functional neuroanatomy of the human near/far response to blur cues: eye-lens accommodation/vergence to point targets varying in depth, *Eur J Neurosci* 20:2722-2732, 2004.

471. Borenstein M, Sigman M: Infant intelligence quotient predictable by gaze, *Child Dev* 57:251-274, 1987.

472. Felton DL, Felton SY: A regional and systemic overview of functional neuroanatomy. In Farber SA, editor: *Neurorehabilitation: a multisensory approach,* Philadelphia, 1982, WB Saunders.

473. Gianakos D: Apathy, empathy, physicians, and Chekhov, *Pharos Alpha Omega Alpha Hone Med Soc* 60:10-11, 1997.

474. Gimbel T: *Healing through colour,* Suffron Halden, UK, 1980, CW Daniel.

475. Van Houten R, Rolider A: The use of color mediation techniques to teach number identification and single digit multiplication problems to children with learning disability, *Educ Treat Child* 13:216-221, 1990.

476. Zhai J, Barreto AB, Chin C et al: User stress detection in human-computer interactions, *Biomed Sci Instrum* 41:277-282, 2005.

477. Burgess HJ, Sharkey KM, Eastman CI: Bright light, dark and melatonin can promote circadian adaptation in night shift workers, *Sleep Med Rev* 6:407-420, 2002.

478. Cooper BA: Long-term care design: current research on the use of color, *J Healthc Des* 6:61-67, 1994.

479. Hill J, Baron JA: Psychology: red enhances human performance in contests, *Nature* 435:293-299, 2005.

480. Ninth National Conference on Juvenile Justice: Open forum discussion, Atlanta, GA, March 1982.

481. Valdez P: Emotion responses to color [dissertation], University of California at Los Angeles, 1993.

482. Roitman DM: Age-associated perceptual changes and the physical environment: Perspectives on environmental adaptation, *Isr J Occup Ther* 2:14-27, 1993.

483. Fisher RS, Harding G, Erba G et al: Epilepsy Foundation of America Working Group, *Epilepsia* 46:1426-1441, 2005.

484. Parra J, Kalitzin SN, Stroink H et al: Removal of epileptogenic sequences from video material: the role of color, *Neurology* 64:787-791, 2005.

485. Henderson A: Body schema and the visual guidance of movement. In Henderson A, Coryell J, editors: *The body senses and perceptual deficit,* Boston, 1973, Boston University Press.

486. Heinsen A: *Visual motor development,* Palo Alto, CA, 1973, Learning Opportunities: Stanford Professional Center.

487. Johannsen L, Broetz D, Naegele T et al: "Pusher syndrome" following cortical lesions that spare the thalamus, *J Neurol* 253:455-463, 2006.

488. Karnath HO, Johannsen L, Broetz D et al: Posterior thalamic hemorrhage induces "pusher syndrome," *Neurology* 64:1014-1019, 2005.

489. Malhotra P, Coulthard E, Husain M: Hemispatial neglect, balance and eye-movement control, *Curr Opin Neurol* 19:14-20, 2006.

490. Gentili R, Papaxanthis C, Pozzo T: Improvement and generalization of arm motor performance through motor imagery practice, *Neuroscience* 137:761-772, 2006.

491. Hamel MF, Lajoie Y: Mental imagery: Effects on static balance and attentional demands of the elderly, *Aging Clin Exp Res* 17:223-228, 2005.

492. Hornby TG, Zemon DH, Campbell D: Robotic-assisted, body-weight-supported treadmill training in individuals following motor incomplete spinal cord injury, *Phys Ther* 85:52-66, 2005.

493. Jackson PL, Lafleur MF, Malouin F et al: Functional cerebral reorganization following motor sequence learning through mental practice with motor imagery, *Neuroimage* 20:1171-1180, 2003.

494. Nyberg L, Eriksson J, Larsson A et al: Learning by doing versus learning by thinking: an fMRI study of motor and mental training, *Neuropsychologia* 44:711-717, 2006.

495. Stevenson RJ, Case TI: Olfactory imagery: a review, *Psychon Bull Rev* 12:244-264, 2005.

496. Zatorre RJ, Halpern AR: Mental concerts: musical imagery and auditory cortex, *Neuron* 47:9-12, 2005.

497. Aschwanden C, Sherstyuk A, Burgess L et al: A surgical and fine-motor skills trainer for everyone? Touch and force-feedback in a virtual reality environment for surgical training, *Stud Health Technol Inform* 119:19-21, 2005.

498. Holden MK: Virtual environments for motor rehabilitation: review, *Cyberpsychol Behav* 8:187-211, 2005.

499. Rizzo AA, Bowerly T, Buckwalter JG et al: A virtual reality scenario for all seasons: The virtual classroom, *CNS Spectr* 11:35-44, 2006.

500. Stansfield S, Dennis C, Suma E: Emotional and performance attributes of a VR game: a study of children, *Stud Health Technol Inform* 111:515-518, 2005.

501. Todorov E, Shadmehr R, Bizzi E: Augmented feedback presented in a virtual environment accelerates learning of a difficult motor task, *J Mot Behav* 29:147-158, 1997.

502. Albani G, Pignatti R, Bertella L et al: Common daily activities in the virtual environment: a preliminary study in parkinsonian patients, *Neurol Sci* 23(2 suppl):S49-S50, 2002.

503. Krebs HI, Hogan N, Hening W et al: Procedural motor learning in Parkinson's disease, *Exp Brain Res* 141:425-437, 2001.

504. Deutsch JE, Merians AS, Adamovich S et al: Development and application of virtual reality technology to improve hand use and gait of individuals post-stroke, *Restor Neurol Neurosci* 22:371-386, 2004.

505. Rose FD, Attree EA, Brooks BM et al: Virtual environments in brain damage rehabilitation: a rationale from basic neuroscience, *Stud Health Technol Inform* 58:233-242, 1998.

506. Umphred DA: Integrated approach to treatment of the pediatric neurologic patient. In Campbell SK, editor: *Clinics in physical therapy: pediatric neurologic disorders,* New York, 1984, Churchill Livingstone.

507. Smith GR Jr, McKenzie JM, Marmer DJ et al: Psychological modulation of the human immune response to varicela zoster, *Arch Intern Med* 145:2110-2112, 1985.

508. Knowles R: Through neurolinguistic programming, *Am J Nurs* 83:1010, 1983.

509. Abbruzzese G, Trompetto C, Schieppati M: The excitability of the human motor cortex increases during execution and mental imagination of sequential but not repetitive finger movements, *Exp Brain Res* 111:465-472, 1996.

510. Clark GF, Avery-Smith W, Wolf LS et al: Specialized knowledge and skills in eating and feeding for occupational therapy practice, *Am J Occup Ther* 57:660-678, 2003.

511. Allensworth A: A practical guide to the use of music with geriatrics, *Aging Perfections* 16:9, 1993.

512. Campbell S: *Clinics in physical therapy,* ed 2, *vol 5,* New York, 1992, Churchill-Livingstone.

513. Dobkin B: Neuroplasticity: Key to recovery after CNS injury, *West J Med* 159:56-60, 1993.

514. Platz T, Winter T, Muller N et al: Arm ability training for stroke and traumatic brain injury patients with mild arm paresis: a single-blind, randomized, controlled trial, *Arch Phys Med Rehabil* 82:961-968, 2001.

515. Carey LM, Abbott DF, Egan GF et al: Motor impairment and recovery in the upper limb after stroke: Behavioral and neuroanatomial correlates, *Stroke* 15:229-237, 2005.

516. Platz T, vanKaick S, Moller L et al: Impairment-oriented training and adaptive motor cortex reorganization after stroke: a fTMS study, *J Neurol* 252:1363-1371, 2005.

517. Behrman AK, Lawless-Dixon AR, Davis SB et al: Locomotor training progression and outcomes after incomplete spinal cord injury, *Phys Ther* 85:1356-1371, 2005.

518. Toole T, Maitland CG, Warren E et al: The effects of loading and unloading treadmill walking on balance, gait, fall risk, and daily function in Parkinsonism, *Neurorehabilitation* 20:307-322, 2005.

519. Barbeau H, Visintin M: Optimal outcomes obtained with body-weight support combined with treadmill training in stroke subjects, *Arch Phys Med Rehabil* 84:1458-1465, 2003.

520. Sullivan KJ, Knowlton BJ, Dobkin BH: Step training with body weight support: effect of treadmill speed and practice paradigms on poststroke locomotor recovery, *Arch Phys Med Rehabil* 83:683-691, 2002.

521. Brown TH, Mount J, Rouland BL et al: Body weight-supported treadmill training versus conventional gait training for people with chronic traumatic brain injury, *J Head Trauma Rehabil* 20:402-415, 2005.

522. Dobkin B, Apple D, Barbeau H et al; Spinal Cord Injury Locomotor Trial Group: Weight-supported treadmill vs over-ground training for walking after acute incomplete SCI, *Neurology* 66:484-493, 2006.

523. Chen G, Patten C, Kothari DH et al: Gait deviations associated with post-stroke hemiparesis: improvement during treadmill walking using weight support, speed, support stiffness, and handrail hold, *Gait Posture* 22:57-62, 2005.

524. Field-Fote EC, Lindley SD et al: Locomotor training approaches for individuals with spinal cord injury: a preliminary report of walking-related outcomes, *J Neurol Phys Ther* 29:127-137, 2005.

525. Moseley AM, Stark A, Cameron ID et al: Treadmill training and body weight support for walking after stroke, *Cochrane Database Syst Rev* CD002840, 2005.

526. Moseley AM, Stark A, Cameron ID et al: Treadmill training and body weight support for walking after stroke, *Stroke* 34:3006, 2003.

527. Hesse S, Werner C: Partial body weight supported treadmill training for gait recovery following stroke, *Adv Neurol* 92:423-428, 2003.

528. Hesse S, Uhlenbrock D, Sarkodie-Gyan T: Gait pattern of severely disabled hemiparetic subjects on a new controlled gait trainer as compared to assisted treadmill walking with partial body weight support, *Clin Rehabil* 13:401-410, 1999.

529. Pohl M, Rockstroh G, Ruckriem S et al: Immediate effects of speed dependent treadmill training on gait parameters in early Parkinson's disease, *Arch Phys Med Rehabil* 84:1760-1766, 2003.

530. Schindl MR, Forstner C, Kern H et al: Treadmill training with partial body weight support in nonambulatory patients with cerebral palsy, *Arch Phys Med Rehabil* 81:301-306, 2000.

531. Landsman GH: What evidence, whose evidence? Physical therapy in New York State's clinical practice guideline and in the lives of mothers of disabled children, *Soc Sci Med* 62:2670-2680, 2006.

532. Taub E, Ramey SL, DeLuca S et al: Efficacy of constraint-induced movement therapy for children with cerebral palsy with asymmetric motor impairment, *Pediatrics* 113:305-312, 2004.

533. van der Lee JH: Constraint-induced movement therapy: Some thoughts about theories and evidence, *J Rehabil Med* (41 suppl):41-45, 2003.

534. Sunderland A, Tuke A: Neuroplasticity, learning and recovery after stroke: a critical evaluation of constraint-induced therapy, *Neuropsychol Rehabil* 15:81-96, 2005.

535. Grotta JC, Noser EA, Ro T et al: Constraint-induced movement therapy, *Stroke* 35:2699-2701, 2004.

536. Taub E, Harger M, Grier HC et al: Some anatomical observations following chronic dorsal rhizotomy in monkeys, *Neuroscience* 5:389-401, 1980.

537. Taub E, Heitmann RD, Barro G: Alertness, level of activity, and purposive movement following somatosensory deafferentation in monkeys, *Ann N Y Acad Sci* 290:348-365, 1977.

538. Ostendorf CG, Wolf SL: Effect of forced use of the upper extremity of a hemiplegic patient on changes in function: a single-case design, *Phys Ther* 61:1022-1028, 1981.

539. Miltner WH, Bauder H, Sommer M et al: Effects of constraint-induced movement therapy on patients with chronic motor deficits after stroke: a replication, *Stroke* 30:586-592, 1999.

540. Liepert J, Bauder H, Wolfgang HR et al: Treatment-induced cortical reorganization after stroke in humans, *Stroke* 31:1210-1216, 2000.

541. Liepert J, Miltner WH, Bauder H et al: Motor cortex plasticity during constraint-induced movement therapy in stroke patients, *Neurosci Lett* 250:5-8, 1998.

542. Blanton S, Wolf SL: An application of upper-extremity constraint-induced movement therapy in a patient with subacute stroke, *Phys Ther* 79:847-853, 1999.

543. Kunkel A, Kopp B, Muller G et al: Constraint-induced movement therapy for motor recovery in chronic stroke patients, *Arch Phys Med Rehabil* 80:624-628, 1999.

544. Morris DM, Taub E: Constraint-induced therapy approach to restoring function after neurological injury, *Top Stroke Rehabil* 8:16-30, 2001.

545. Taub E, Uswatte G, King DK et al: A placebo-controlled trial of constraint-induced movement therapy for upper extremity after stroke, *Stroke* 37:1045-1049, 2006.

546. Alberts JL, Butler AJ, Wolf SL: The effects of constraint-induced therapy on precision grip: A preliminary study, *Neurorehabil Neural Repair* 18:250-258, 2004.

547. Dettmers C, Teske U, Hamzei F et al: Distributed form of constraint-induced movement therapy improves functional outcome and quality of life after stroke, *Arch Phys Med Rehabil* 86:204-209, 2005.

548. Fritz SL, Light KE, Patterson TS et al: Active finger extension predicts outcomes after constraint-induced movement therapy for individuals with hemiparesis after stroke, *Stroke* 36:1172-1177, 2005.

549. Page SJ, Sisto S, Levine P et al: Efficacy of modified constraint-induced movement therapy in chronic stroke: a single-blinded randomized controlled trial, *Arch Phys Med Rehabil* 85:14-18, 2004.

550. Rijntjes M, Hobbeling V, Hamzei F et al: Individual factors in constraint-induced movement therapy after stroke, *Neurorehabil Neural Repair* 19:238-249, 2005.

551. Suputtitada A, Suwanwela NC, Tumvitee S: Effectiveness of constraint-induced movement therapy in chronic stroke patients, *J Med Assoc Thai* 87:1482-1490, 2004.

552. Cho YW, Jang SH, Lee ZI et al: Effect and appropriate restriction period of constraint-induced movement therapy in hemiparetic patients with brain injury: A brief report, *Neurorehabilitation* 20:71-74, 2005.

553. Page S, Levine P: Forced use after TBI: Promoting plasticity and function through practice, *Brain Inj* 17:675-684, 2003.

554. Charles J, Gordon AM: A critical review of constraint-induced movement therapy and forced use in children with hemiplegia, *Neural Plast* 12:245-261, 263-272, 2005.

555. Gordon AM, Charles J, Wolf SL: Methods of constraint-induced movement therapy for children with hemiplegic cerebral palsy: development of a child-friendly intervention for improving upper-extremity function, *Arch Phys Med Rehabil* 86:837-844, 2005.

556. Taub E, Lum PS, Hardin P et al: AutoCITE: automated delivery of CI therapy with reduced effort by therapists, *Stroke* 36:1301-1304, 2005.

557. Willis JK, Morello A, Davie A et al: Forced use treatment of childhood hemiparesis, *Pediatrics* 110:94-96, 2002.

558. Eliasson AC, Krumlinde-Sundholm L, Shaw K et al: Effects of constraint-induced movement therapy in young children with hemiplegic cerebral palsy: an adapted model, *Dev Med Child Neurol* 47:266-275, 2005.

559. Gordon AM, Charles J, Wolf SL: Efficacy of constraint-induced movement therapy on involved upper-extremity use in children with hemiplegic cerebral palsy is not age-dependent, *Pediatrics* 117:e363-e373, 2006.

560. Tuite P, Anderson N, Konczak J: Constraint-induced movement therapy in Parkinson's disease, *Mov Disord* 20:910-911, 2005.

561. Bonnier B, Eliasson AC, Krumlinde-Sundholm L: Effects of constraint-induced movement therapy in adolescents with hemiplegic cerebral palsy: a day camp model, *Scand J Occup Ther* 13:13-22, 2006.

562. Bonifer N, Anderson KM: Application of constraint-induced movement therapy for an individual with severe chronic upper-extremity hemiplegia, *Phys Ther* 83:384-398, 2003.

563. Tarkka IM, Pitkanen K, Sivenius J: Paretic hand rehabilitation with constraint-induced movement therapy after stroke, *Am J Phys Med Rehabil* 84:501-505, 2005.

564. Bonifer NM, Anderson KM, Arciniegas DB: Constraint-induced therapy for moderate chronic upper extremity impairment after stroke, *Brain Inj* 19:323-330, 2005.

565. Uswatte G, Taub E, Morris D et al: Reliability and validity of the upper-extremity Motor Activity Log-14 for measuring real-world arm use, *Stroke* 36:2493-2496, 2005.

566. Duncan PW, Propst M, Nelson SG: Reliability of the Fugl-Meyer assessment of sensorimotor recovery following cerebrovascular accident, *Phys Ther* 63:1606-1610, 1983.

567. Morris DM, Uswatte G, Crago JE et al: The reliability of the wolf motor function test for assessing upper extremity function after stroke, *Arch Phys Med Rehabil* 82:750-755, 2001.

568. Wolf SL, Catlin PA, Ellis M et al: Assessing Wolf Motor Function Test as outcome measure for research in patients after stroke, *Stroke* 32:1635-1639, 2001.

569. Schaechter JD, Kraft E, Hilliard TS et al: Motor recovery and cortical reorganization after constraint-induced movement therapy in stroke patients: a preliminary study, *Neurorehabil Neural Repair* 16:326-338, 2002.

570. Wolf SL, Thompson PA, Morris DM et al: The EXCITE trial: attributes of the Wolf Motor Function Test in patients with subacute stroke, *Neurorehabil Neural Repair* 19:194-205, 2005.

571. Mark VW, Taub E: Constraint-induced movement therapy for chronic stroke hemiparesis and other disabilities, *Restor Neurol Neurosci* 22:317-336, 2004.

572. Dromerick AW, Edwards DF, Hahn M: Does the application of constraint-induced movement therapy during acute rehabilitation reduce arm impairment after ischemic stroke? *Stroke* 31:2984-2988, 2000.

573. Bland ST, Schallert T, Strong R et al: Early exclusive use of the affected forelimb after moderate transient focal ischemia in rats: functional and anatomic outcome, *Stroke* 31:1144-1152, 2000.

574. DeBow SB, McKenna JE, Kolb B et al: Immediate constraint-induced movement therapy causes local hyperthermia that exacerbates cerebral cortical injury in rats, *Can J Physiol Pharmacol* 82:231-237, 2004.

575. Humm JL, Kozlowski DA, James DC et al: Use-dependent exacerbation of brain damage occurs during an early post-lesion vulnerable period, *Brain Res* 783:286-292, 1998.

576. Kozlowski DA, James DC, Schallert T: Use-dependent exaggeration of neuronal injury after unilateral sensorimotor cortex lesions, *J Neurosci* 16:4776-4786, 1996.

577. Nudo RJ, Wise BM, SiFuentes F et al: Neural substrates for the effects of rehabilitative training on motor recovery after ischemic infarct, *Science* 272:1791-1794, 1996.

578. Kopp B, Kunkel A, Muhlnickel W et al: Plasticity in the motor system related to therapy-induced improvement of movement after stroke, *Neuroreport* 10:807-810, 1999.

579. Ro T, Noser E, Boake C et al: Functional reorganization and recovery after constraint-induced movement therapy in subacute stroke: case reports, *Neurocase* 12:50-60, 2006.

580. Page SJ, Levine P, Sisto S et al: Stroke patients' and therapists' opinions of constraint-induced movement therapy, *Clin Rehabil* 16:55-60, 2002.

581. Pang MY, Harris JE, Eng JJ: A community-based upper-extremity group exercise program improves motor function and performance of functional activities in chronic stroke: a randomized controlled trial, *Arch Phys Med Rehabil* 87:1-9, 2006.

582. Sterr A, Elbert T, Berthold I et al: Longer versus shorter daily constraint-induced movement therapy of chronic hemiparesis: an exploratory study, *Arch Phys Med Rehabil* 83:1374-1377, 2002.

583. Stein J, Krebs HI, Frontera WR et al: Comparison of two techniques of robot-aided upper limb exercise training after stroke, *Am J Phys Med Rehabil* 83:720-728, 2004.

584. Lum PS, Taub E, Schwandt D et al: Automated Constraint-Induced Therapy Extension (AutoCITE) for movement deficits after stroke, *J Rehabil Res Dev* 41:249-258, 2004.

585. Hakkennes S, Keating JL: Constraint-induced movement therapy following stroke: a systematic review of randomised controlled trials, *Aust J Physiother* 51:221-231, 2005.

586. Winchester P, McColl R, Querry R et al: Changes in supraspinal activation patterns following robotic locomotor therapy in motor-incomplete spinal cord injury, *Neurorehabil Neural Repair* 19:313-324, 2005.

587. Krebs HI, Ferraro M, Buerger SP et al: Rehabilitation robotics: pilot trial of a spatial extension for MIT-Manus, *J Neuroengineering Rehabil* 1:5, 2004.

588. Fasoli SE, Krebs HI, Hogan N: Robotic technology and stroke rehabilitation: translating research into practice, *Top Stroke Rehabil* 11:11-19, 2004.

589. Fasoli SE, Krebs HI, Stein J et al: Robotic therapy for chronic motor impairments after stroke: follow-up results, *Arch Phys Med Rehabil* 85:1106-1111, 2004.

590. Fasoli SE, Trombly CA, Tickle-Degnen L et al: Effect of instructions on functional reach in persons with and without cerebrovascular accident, *Am J Occup Ther* 56:380-390, 2002.

591. Stein J, Krebs HI, Frontera WR et al: Comparison of two techniques of robot-aided upper limb exercise training after stroke, *Am J Phys Med Rehabil* 83:720-728, 2004.

592. Hesse S, Schmidt H, Werner C et al: Upper and lower extremity robotic devices for rehabilitation and for studying motor control, *Curr Opin Neurol* 16:705-710, 2003.

593. Nelson RJ, Smith BN, Douglas VD: Relationship between sensory responsiveness and premovement activity of quickly adapting neurons in area 3b and 1 of monkey primary somatosensory cortex, *Exp Brain Res* 84:75-90, 1991.

594. Sur M, Nelson RHJ, Kaas JH: The representation of the body surface in somatic koniocortex in the Prosimian *(Galago senegalensis)*, *J Comp Neurol* 180:381-402, 1980.

595. Penfield W, Boldrey E: Somatic motor and sensory representations in the cerebral cortex of man as studied by electrical stimulation, *Brain* 60:389-443, 1937.

596. Pubois BH, Pubols LM: Somatotopic organization of spider monkey somatic sensory cerebral cortex, *J Comp Neurol* 141:63-76, 1971.

597. Chen R, Hallett M: Focal dystonia and repetitive motion disorders, *Clin Orthop Rel Res* 351:102-106, 1998.

598. Elbert T, Candia V, Altenmuller E et al: Alteration of digital representations in somatosensory cortex in focal hand dystonia, *Neuroreport* 9:3571-3575, 1998.

599. Flor H, Braun C, Elbert T et al: Extensive reorganization of primary somatosensory cortex in chronic back pain patients, *Neurosci Lett* 224:5-8, 1997.

600. Tinazzi M, Zanette G, Volpato D et al: Neurophysiological evidence of neuroplasticity at multiple levels of the somatosensory system in patients with carpal tunnel syndrome, *Brain* 121:1785-1794, 1998.

601. Burke RE, Rudomin P, Zajac FE: Catch property in single mammalian motor units, *Science* 168:122-124, 1974.

602. Desmedt JE, Godaux E: Fast motor units are not preferentially activated in rapid voluntary contractions in man, *Nature* 267:717-719, 1977.

603. Odergren T, Iwassaki N, Borg J et al: Impaired sensory-motor integration during grasping in writer's cramp, *Brain* 119:569-583, 1996.

604. Panizza M, Hallett M, Nilsson J: Reciprocal inhibition in patients with hand cramps, *Neurology* 39:85-89, 1989.

605. Ridding MC, Sheehan G, Rothwell JC et al: Changes in the balance between motor cortical excitation and inhibition in focal, task-specific dystonia, *J Neurol Neurosurg Psychiatry* 59:493-498, 1995.

606. Blake DT, Hsiao SS, Johnson K: Neural coding mechanisms in tactile pattern recognition: The relative contributions of slowly and rapidly adapting mechanoreceptors to perceived roughness, *J Neurosci* 17:7480-7489, 1997.

607. Blake DT, Johnson KO, Hsiao SS: Monkey cutaneous SAI and RA responses to raised and depressed scanned patterns: Effects of width, height, orientation, and a raised surround, *J Neurophysiol* 78:2503-2517, 1997.

608. Kaas JH: Evolution of somatosensory and motor cortex in primates, *Anat Rec A Discov Mol Cell Evol Biol* 281:1148-1156, 2004.

609. Mathews PBC: Proprioceptors and their contribution to somatosensory mapping: Complex messages required complex processing, *Can J Physiol Pharmacol* 66:430-438, 1988.

610. Louis S, Greene TL, Jacobson KE et al: Evaluation of normal values for stationary and moving two point discrimination in the hand, *Hand Ther* 9A:552-555, 1984.

611. Ayers A: *Sensory Integration and Praxis Test (SIPT) manual,* Los Angeles, 1989, Western Psychological Association.

612. McKenzie A: A new test to measure stereognosis: Key Test abstract. Presented at the annual meeting of the California Chapter of the American Physical Therapy Association, Sacramento, October 1997.

613. Schmidt RT, Tows JV: Grip strength as measured by the Jamar dynamometer, *Arch Phys Med Rehabil* 52:321-327, 1970.

614. Kellor M, Frost J, Silverberg N et al: Norms for clinical use, hand strength and dexterity, *Am J Occup Ther* 25:77-83, 1971.

615. *PAR finger tapper user's guide,* Odessa, FL, 1992, Psychological Assessment Resources.

616. Bohannon RW: Stopwatch for measuring thumb movement time, *Percept Mot Skills* 81:122-126, 1995.

617. Porter K, Foster J: *The mental athlete,* New York, 1986, Ballantine Books.

618. Achterberg J: *Imagery in healing: Shamanism and modern medicine,* Boston, 1985, Shambhala.

619. Decety J: Do imagined and executed actions share the same neural substrate? *Brain Res Cogn Brain Res* 3:87-93, 1996.

620. Rizzolatti G, Fadiga L, Gallese V et al: Premotor cortex and the recognition of motor actions, *Brain Res Cong Brain Res* 3:131-141, 1996.

621. Decety J, Perani D, Jeannerod M et al: The neurophysiological basis of motor imagery, *Behav Brain Res* 77:45-52, 1996.

622. Porro Ca, Francescato MP, Cettolo V et al: Primary motor and sensory cortex activation during motor performance and motor imagery: a functional magnetic resonance imaging study. *J Neurosci* 16:7688-7698, 1996.

623. Moseley GL: Is successful rehabilitation of complex regional pain syndrome due to sustained attention to the affected limb? A randomized clinical trial, *Pain* 114:54-61, 2005.

624. Byl NN, McKenzie AL: Treatment effectiveness of patients with a history of repetitive hand use and focal hand dystonia: a planned prospective follow up study, *J Hand Therapy* 13:289-301, 2000.

625. Byl NN, Nagarajan SS, McKenzie AL: Effective of sensory discrimination training on structure and function in patients with focal hand dystonia: a case series, *Arch Phys Med Rehabil* 84:1505-1514, 2003.

626. Candia V, Wienbruch C, Elbert T et al: Effective behavioral treatment of focal hand dystonia in musicians alters somatosensory cortical organization, *Proc Natl Acad Sci U S A* 100:7942-7946, 2003.

APPENDIX 9-A ■ Stress-Free Biomechanics of the Hand: Principles for Retraining Problems of Hand Control

Nancy N. Byl, PhD, PT, FAPTA Professor and Chair, Department of Physical Therapy and Rehabilitation Science, School of Medicine, University of California, San Francisco

A. GENERAL PRINCIPLES OF RETRAINING STRESS-FREE FUNCTIONAL USE OF THE HAND

1. *Create learning strategies that emphasize sensory input and feedback. This can be emphasized by placing sticky, coarse or rough surfaces on tools that are used in functional activities (e.g., pen, keyboard, glass, hammer, utensils).*

2. *Break down each task into manageable components that can be performed normally.*

3. *Perform each component of functional tasks without abnormal movements (e.g., pathological synergies, extraneous movements, excessive muscle firing, involuntary movements, strain, pain).*

4. *Be sure each activity is designed to require attention, repetition, progression of difficulty, feedback regarding accuracy of performance and positive reinforcement (reward).*

B. PREPARATION FOR TRAINING: STRESS-FREE HAND USE STRATEGIES

1. *Strengthen the small muscles inside the hand (intrinsic muscles) to facilitate stability of functional hand use.*
   a. Give resistance to spreading fingers apart (try not to use muscles that straighten the fingers).
   b. Try to hold the fingers together while you use your other hand to try and spread them apart.
   c. Bend the fingers at the large knuckle (metacarpophalangeal joint) to 90 degrees by placing the back of the hand against the edge of a table. Now, one finger at a time, try to keep the fingers straight as you use the other hand to try and bend the finger, giving resistance at the distal segment of the finger.

2. *Concentrate on using the small muscles of the hands in all functional activities.*
   a. Initiate bending the fingers from the base joint (the large metacarpophalangeal joint that joins the finger to the palm); try to do this without bending the fingers at the other joints, especially without using the muscles that bend the distal finger joints.
   b. Avoid heavy gripping; squeeze the fingers in a power grip only when necessary. For example, do not (1) squeeze the steering wheel, (2) exercise while holding on to free weights, or (3) squeeze a ball or strengthen the grip in other ways.
   c. Practice reaching for common objects with the eyes closed and the hand relaxed. When you contact the object, let the sensation of the surface of the object open the hand. For example, when you reach for your cup, let the cup open the hand (e.g., do not actively spread the fingers first). Do not use the handle of the cup.

3. *When practicing tool use, let the sensation of the object teach your hand how hard to squeeze.*
   a. Modify the sensation of the object (e.g., very rough, slightly rough, coarse, smooth, silky).
   b. Take practice lifts of the object to determine how heavy it is.
   c. Manipulate the object in your hands without visual monitoring before beginning functional use of the tool.

4. *Avoid aggressive, precise, rapid, alternating, forceful finger flexion and extension movements of the hand.*
   a. Transfer some of the work of the hand from the fingers to the forearm. For example,
      1) Lift the fingers by rotating the forearm into supination (e.g., turn palm up). If forearm rotation is limited, let the shoulder externally rotate if necessary.
      2) When the hand needs to be palm down (pronated), let the elbow swing away from the trunk if necessary to keep the hand relaxed (e.g., internal rotation of the shoulder can take the stress off the forearm).
   b. Use the hand in a natural functional position (e.g., rounded palm from the base of the thumb to the base of the fifth finger and rounded from the tips of the fingers to the wrist). Thus, all the finger joints are slightly bent, the palm is round, and the wrist is extended about 15 degrees. When your arms are at your side, this will usually be the position of the hand.
   c. Do not let the joints of the fingers collapse or hyperextend when they are down on a surface. This can be difficult if the joints are hypermobile or the intrinsic muscles (muscles inside the hand) are weak.
      1) Practice dropping the hand onto a surface and maintaining the roundness of the hand (a small soft ball under the palm may be used for assistance).
      2) Lean lightly onto the hand while it is on a flat pranated and keep the round shape of the hand (e.g., may need to initially keep small round ball under palm).
      3) Thread the fingers of one hand through the fingers of the other hand to help stabilize the hand when placing weight onto the hand, as in 2.
      4) Put a soft, rubber ball about 2 inches in diameter on the table; roll the palm of the hand over the ball while letting the finger pads (not the tips) drop onto the surface.

C. USING THE COMPUTER KEYBOARD SAFELY

1. *Position yourself comfortably to use the computer,*
   a. Sit with feet flat on the floor. Sit tall with hips about 90 degrees (vary this posture throughout the day).
   b. Place the computer screen at or slightly below eye level.
   c. Keyboard height should be adjusted to maintain elbow flexion at about 80 degrees (positioned in approximately 100 degrees of extension).
   d. Forearms should be angled toward the floor and not resting on the table. If it is difficult to let your hands rest lightly on the keyboard with the wrist floating, it may be helpful to have a pillow on your lap (or a lumbar roll around the waist), where the forearms receive positive sensory information to help them relax.
   e. Place the screen about 2 feet away from the eyes for most work; pull the screen closer as necessary for close work.
   f. Consider getting special antiglare glasses for computer terminal display work or use a screen glare protector.

2. *Keep your hands in a functional (e.g., round, not flat or angular) position on the keyboard.*
   a. Look at the contour of the hand when it is at your side; maintain that position as the finger pads (not the tips) are dropped on the keyboard

b. Place a rough surface on the keys (e.g., Velcro) to make it easier to feel the pads on the keys.

c. Avoid placing the tips of the fingers on the keys. This creates an obligatory cocontraction of the finger flexors and extensors.

3. *Keep the wrist in neutral (0-10 degrees' extension) while working on the keyboard (e.g., a floating wrist).*

a. Do not rest the wrist on a "wrist rest." Resting the wrist and forearm on the work surface will increase the pressure in the carpal tunnel and force all the work to be done with the fingers.

b. If there is a wrist pad on the computer keyboard tray, think of the pad as a "sensory tickle" to let you know that your wrists should be floating above the rest.

4. *Have all the fingers resting on the keyboard.*

a. Do not let any of the fingers fly up.

b. Continue to keep the fingers resting down even when one finger is engaged in depressing a key.

c. Avoid allowing the adjacent fingers to extend to get them away from the finger actively pressing down.

5. *It is not necessary to actively lift the fingers after pressing down. Usually it is sufficient to release the pressure without actively lifting up the digits.*

6. *Avoid resting the fingers on the keyboard with the finger tips. This leads to a contraction of the fingers and the wrist.*

a. Do not keep your fingers excessively curled. Then it is impossible to keep on the finger pads.

b. Initiate the movement down from the base joint of the fingers.

c. Imagine that you are using the muscles inside your hand and not the long muscles that bend the fingers.

d. Avoid reaching one finger out in isolation from the others.

7. *In general, change the primary fulcrum of movement from the fingers of the hand to the elbow and shoulder.*

a. Allow the elbow to move freely in flexion, extension, and rotation.

b. Use the trunk with a little shoulder movement when reaching for an object or a paper or to move closer to or away from the computer keyboard or screen.

8. *Use the mouse by using forearm rotation rather than individual finger movements.*

a. Do not squeeze the mouse; drape your hand on the mouse.

b. Keep your wrist in neutral.

c. Avoid clicking the button by lifting and bending the index finger.

d. Use rotation of the forearm to activate the button on the mouse.

e. Make sure the mouse is close to you and that the arm is not extended to the side. Place a cover for the mouse over the number keys, if necessary, to keep the arm closer to your trunk.

f. Consider interfaces other than a mouse (e.g., roller ball, a movement-sensitive pad, pen).

g. If it is not possible to use the hand in a stress-free way when on the computer, then consider voice-activated software to use your computer.
   1) Use your voice carefully and without excessive force or strain (e.g., loudness).
   2) Be careful to prevent cocontractions and stressful use of the vocal chords.

9. *Take regular breaks (e.g., every 15 minutes).*

a. Consider obtaining the software that forces a computer breakthrough screen reminder.

b. Do diaphragmatic breathing continually while working on your computer to minimize tension and facilitate good oxygen exchange.

c. When taking a break and staying at the desk, get your hands off the computer and change your sitting posture while doing gentle range of motion exercises. Occasionally, place the arms on the desk and bend the trunk over the arms.

10. *At least every 20 minutes, stand up for a few minutes and stretch.*

D. WRITING

1. *The fulcrum for the movement of writing should be the shoulder and elbow, not the fingers.*

2. *The hand should be round and relaxed.*

3. *Try putting a sticky or a rough surface on the pen/pencil before you begin to practice.*

a. A sticky surface (e.g., putting tape on with the sticky side facing out) can be strong enough to hold the pen in place without any squeezing.

b. A fatter pen is not as helpful as a sticky or a rough surface. It is possible to excessively grip a large pen.

4. *Practice writing when you are not at work or at a store when you have to write your name.*

5. *Practice writing non–work-related words and sentences and then progress to meaningful writing.*

6. *Try holding the pen by different fingers or using different movements.*

a. Try to hold the pen between the second (index) and third (middle) finger rather than the thumb (D1), index finger (D2), and middle finger (D3). The hand should be open, thumb resting down.

b. If you must hold the pen in the traditional way, try to hold the pen lightly between D1, D2, and D3 with D1 and D2 moving toward the thumb from the base joint with all joints of the digits extended.

c. With a sticky surface on the pen, it is possible to control the pen with minimal squeezing.

7. *Practice picking up the pen and putting it down without feeling any tension in your hand.*

8. *Control the movement of the pen primarily from the elbow and shoulder; keep wrist and fingers quietly positioned on the pen.*

a. Let the arm rest lightly on the table and comfortably on the ulnar (fifth finger) side of your hand. Avoid resting the elbow on the surface. If there is inadequate pronation (e.g., it is uncomfortable to have the hand be palm side down), allow the shoulder to move out away from the trunk (e.g., shoulder abduction /rotation).

b. Let all fingers rest down on the pen or the support surface. Do not hold any fingers up off the pen or the support surface.

c. Mentally review relaxed writing before beginning to write with a new technique.

d. Practice making circles, loops, large numbers, and letters. Consider practicing by writing in shaving cream, finger paints, or water.

e. If you see your fingers moving and your knuckles turning white, you are squeezing too hard and you are only using your fingers.

9. *Use a mirror to get some feedback to retrain your style of writing.*

a. Place a mirror in front of your affected hand as you write and notice whether it appears relaxed.

b. Place the unaffected hand in front of the mirror and the affected hand behind the mirror. Look at the image of the unaffected hand (e.g., looks like the affected side) and then have the affected hand behind the mirror copy the mirror image.

10. *Put the pen down if any signs of stress develop.*

E. DAILY ACTIVITIES IN THE KITCHEN

1. *Use two hands to hold a pot or a frying pan.*

2. *Use an electronic can opener and jar opener.*

3. *Use an electronic blender rather than hand stirring.*
4. *Use a chopper so you avoid heavy cutting.*
5. *Stand close to the sink and the work surface so you do not have to have your arms out too far in front of you.*
6. *Get close to the table for setting the table; avoid having to lean over; bend at the knees.*
7. *If you are short, stand on a stool to work at the sink.*
8. *If you are tall, consider raising the refrigerator up higher so you do not have to lean over.*
9. *Concentrate on eating and using utensils without stress in your hands.*
   a. Consider putting a sticky or a rough surface on the utensils (e.g., Velcro or flooring with a sticky back).
   b. When eating, hold the utensils lightly, even when trying to cut.
   c. When cutting, move the whole arm from the shoulder; use the weight of the trunk to assist putting force down on the knife.

F. DRIVING

1. *Use a lumbar roll in the back of your seat to support your lower back. Also consider placing a wedge in your seat (varying the placement of the wedge with the high side in front and then toward the back).*
2. *Pull the seat close to the steering wheel so that you do not have to reach out so far for the gas pedal.*
3. *Sit tall to ensure good visibility and try to drive without stress.*
4. *Consider putting a rough surface on the wheel so you do not want to squeeze it (you can buy ergonomic steering wheel covers).*
5. *When you need to look behind you, shift your weight in the opposite direction that you want to look. This will allow you to turn your whole trunk in the desired direction and avoid the isolated neck strain that occurs when you only turn your head.*
6. *Mentally rehearse and review calm, alert driving.*
7. *Do not squeeze the wheel in a death grip. Hold the steering wheel by gently pushing your arms together. You only need to hold the wheel with a palmar squeeze when turning.*
8. *Keep your arms comfortably at your sides.*
9. *Do not grip the shift knob; press the palm of your hand down on the shift bar to change gears. You may even want to allow your trunk to move with your arm while shifting.*
10. *If you continue to experience stress with driving, practice braking and turning the wheel in your garage and imagine different scenarios.*
11. *Also, if you need a diversion to avoid emotional confrontation with rude drivers, bring a plastic bag of buttons that you can manipulate and match to decrease your stress.*

G. OTHER HOUSEHOLD ACTIVITIES

1. *As before, do not grip objects too firmly; keep hands open and work with your arms close to the trunk.*
2. *Always bend your knees to pick up objects from the floor.*
3. *Be careful to avoid leaning over and straightening the bedding (e.g., when making the bed, ask someone to do it with you; otherwise, make one side of the bed at a time).*
4. *Put items at eye level; avoid putting things over your head for which you have to reach out and up.*
5. *Walk close to the vacuum cleaner; try to hold it where you do not have to reach your arms out (e.g., step forward and backward with the movement of the vacuum cleaner).*
6. *Do not lean over from the waist for dusting; if necessary, dust while kneeling or wipe the floor while you are on your knees; hold the dust cloth lightly.*

APPENDIX 9-B ■ Specific Learning-Based Sensorimotor Training

A. INSTRUCTIONS
Patients

We use our hands for many skilled fine motor and functional tasks. It is important for these movements to be smooth, efficient, and accurate. When there is dysfunction in the central or peripheral nervous system from congenital anomalies, injury, disease, overuse, degeneration, or chronic pain, skilled and functional movements can be impaired. Although it is still important to strengthen the muscles, increase flexibility, and restore normal motor control, it is critical to improve sensory processing. The purpose of learning-based sensorimotor activities is to place demands on the sensory receptors of the skin, the muscle, and the joints to restore normal sensitivity and accuracy of sensory input and feedback. Your brain can change with training. By improving the accuracy of sensory discrimination under conditions of high levels of attention, repetitive activities progressed in difficulty, reinforced with feedback and reward, should improve how the hand is mapped on your brain (e.g., primary sensory cortex). When specific tasks involve motor practice, topographical changes will also occur in other parts of the brain (e.g., thalamus, motor cortex, limbic system, basal ganglia, prefrontal cortex, supplementary motor cortex, brain stem). Although most think about the motor requirements for performing a task, it is essential to have accurate sensory information and feedback, which comes from accurate sensory differentiation of the hand. Dynamic sensory topography and function is a requisite for the restoration of fine motor control.

Research also suggests that positive expectations can facilitate recovery and maximize performance.[626] Physical impairments can lead to significant handicaps and disability. In these cases, it is challenging to maintain a positive attitude and be motivated for recovery and rehabilitation. Depression, anxiety, loss of self-worth, and compromised self-esteem can significantly impair the recovery process, especially when training activities are demanding, intensive, and possibly associated with discomfort or frustration. It is essential to progress activities without causing unnecessary anxiety, apprehension, or pain. Thus, with these issues in mind, the initial steps in the sensorimotor training may seem unusually simple and involve imagery in lieu of motor practice. Also, although the suggestions here focus on the hand, the principles apply to sensorimotor retraining for other parts of the body as well.

Specific randomized clinical trials have not been carried out on this series of training activities. However, Mosley[623] carried out several studies establishing the procedures to do recognition training of hand laterality, imagined hand movements, and mirror movements. He also carried out a randomized clinical trial for patients with Complex Regional Pain Syndrome using these training techniques. He randomly assigned 20 subjects to one of three different groups: hand laterality recognition, imagined movements, mirror training, or imagined movements; hand laterality recognition, imagined movements, or hand lateral recognition; mirror movements or hand recognition laterality. At 6 and 18 weeks after training for 2 weeks on these behaviors, subjects in all groups had a significant reduction in pain and disability ($p < 0.05$) with the group doing hand laterality recognition, imagined movements, and mirror training making significantly greater gains than the other two groups. Byl et al[624,625] also reported significant gains in patients with focal hand dystonia after 6 weeks of learning-based training. Candia et al[626] also reported significant gains in performance for musicians with focal hand dystonia after 1 year of training focusing on task practice while controlling the fingers with a splint to improve isolated control of the dystonic fingers. For patients who are stable after a stroke, Byl et al[43] also reported significant gains in fine motor performance after a sensory retraining program similar to the activities described here.

Therapists and Family Members

When giving these instructions to patients, it is important to supplement the written instructions with pictures or even videotapes. For patients with significant cognitive impairments, these instructions are almost more important for the family members who are helping reinforce the supervised therapy program.

B. PRINCIPLES OF LEARNING-BASED SENSORIMOTOR TRAINING

1. *Learning strategies focus on improving the discrimination of the somatosensory system in a range of tasks that focus primarily on sensory processing during sensory discrimination tasks and fine motor tasks.*
2. *Successful recovery is contingent on being able to imagine using the hands normally again without abnormal movements, apprehension, or pain.*
3. *The injured hand (affected limb) needs to recover laterality (right/left).*
4. *The patient needs to be able to look at a hand and imagine integrating the image of the hand into the movement or positioning of his or her own hand.*
5. *The hand must be able to interface with the target surface without creating tension, pain, or abnormal movement.*
6. *It is essential to be able to mentally imagine performing related and target tasks without abnormal movements or pain.*
7. *Sensory processing must achieve a minimum level of accuracy before functional fine motor movements are integrated.*
8. *Functional fine motor tasks need to be mentally practiced before they are physically practiced.*
9. *Tasks must be divided into the smallest components that can be normally executed (e.g., partial task performance), which will serve as the foundation for building skill-based learning on the whole task.*
10. *Learning requires attention and repetition of behaviors progressed over time.*
11. *Feedback and reward must be integrated into all learning activities, either by mental imagery, mirror imagery, visual reinforcement, auditory feedback or objective, accurate task performance.*
12. *Feedback from error correction may be critical for enhancing learning.*
13. *Each component of a functional task must be performed as normally as possible before progressing to a more difficult task (e.g., without pathological synergies, extraneous movements, excessive muscle firing, involuntary movements, strain, pain).*
14. *Repetitive activities must avoid stereotypical movements that occur nearly simultaneously in time.*
15. *Sensory discriminative retraining should eliminate visual cues to facilitate somatosensory learning (e.g., eyes closed, blindfolded, distorting lenses).*
16. *Begin sensory training on nontarget surfaces or with easy tasks that do not trigger abnormal responses (e.g., nontarget tasks).*
    a. Practice on nontarget tasks until sensory processing is improved and the task can be performed without any abnormal movement.
    b. Integrate sensory retraining in tasks that historically have been associated with abnormal movement (e.g., writers cramp, keyboarders cramp, hand functions associated with abnormal synergies related to hypertonicity, tremors, dystonia).

C. PRELIMINARY ACTIVITIES TO IMPROVE READINESS FOR LEARNING-BASED SENSORIMOTOR DISCRIMINATION TRAINING

1. *Restore hand laterality recognition.*
   a. Follow the guidelines developed by Moseley[623] to be able to quickly see the hand in different positions and identify whether the hand is right or left.
   b. Present pictures of the hand in different orientations and different positions of the wrist and fingers and identify whether right or left.
   c. Present the pictures in random order, faster and faster, and be able to accurately determine the side.[623]
2. *Restore ability to mentally imagine putting the affected hand into different positions.[623]*
   a. Show pictures of the appropriate hand (affected) in different positions.
   b. When picture is shown, mentally put your hand into the same position as the one in the picture.
   c. Practice doing this while changing the order of the positions and the time the position is visualized.
3. *Restore the ability to imagine performing normal movements while observing a videotape of the hands of someone else performing target and nontarget tasks.*
   a. Videotape different people performing target and nontarget tasks.
   b. Watch the videotapes and imagine that the hands being observed are your hands performing the tasks without pain or abnormal movements.
4. *Restore the ability to copy a mirror image of the affected side.[624]*
   a. Place the unaffected hand in front of a vertical mirror and the affected hand behind the mirror (out of sight).
   b. Look in the mirror and note that the mirror image of the unaffected hand looks like the affected hand.
   c. Do simple tasks using the mirror image to guide the movement of the affected side.
      1) Take the pictures from the visualization training and assume the position of the hand wrist.[624]
      2) Put different sensory objects within the reach of both hands and pick up the object and make the object feel the same on both sides.[624]
      3) Do simple functional tasks with both hands simultaneously (e.g., turn hand up/down, tap a finger, bring thumb to each finger, pick up a pen, circle the pen, pick up objects of different size or same size but different surfaces).[624]

D. INITIATE SPECIFIC LEARNING-BASED SENSORIMOTOR TRAINING

1. *Retrain cutaneous, muscle, and joint receptors at nontarget tasks.*
   a. Develop a variety of active sensory discrimination activities that you can do by yourself (e.g., actively exploring to interpret different object surfaces—stereognosis).
      1) Take the opportunity to feel objects in your environment and identify the objects without looking at the object.
      2) Put small objects in bowls of rice or beans and reach in and try to find and match the objects.
      3) Hang different objects from a string on a door jamb; start the objects swinging and allow them to stimulate your hand. See whether you can differentiate the different objects as they move across your hand.
   b. Modify the difficulty of the sensory task.
      1) Change the intensity of the sensory stimuli (e.g., make the surfaces less distinct).
      2) Increase the challenge or the complexity of the stimuli you are trying to identify.
      3) Change the environment in which you are exploring the sensory stimuli (e.g., hand in water, still or agitated, in shaving soap, in whipping cream as discriminate an object or manipulate a pen).

4) Change the position you assume when discriminating the stimulus (e.g., lie down on your back or your stomach, stand instead of sitting).
c. Palpate objects in water or other media for identification; have the water be still and then agitate the water.
d. Put pairs of coins and objects in your pocket (or a plastic bag) and try to match them or discriminate between them.
e. Purchase clay that can be molded and shaped and then heated until firm.
　1) Place or draw different shapes on the clay.
　2) Always include a pair of designs that can be matched.
f. Paste matched pairs of items on a card and try to find the matched pairs.
　1) Paste stickers with shapes on cards and try to find matched pairs.
　2) Paste matched pairs of buttons on a card.
　3) Paste alphabet soup letters on a card and match letters or spell words.
　4) Put magnetic letters and other shapes on a card or a refrigerator and move them to spell words.
g. Take construction paper and create pairs of letters, shapes, or other designs by pressing heavily with the pen; this will create a raised surface on the other side.
　1) With eyes closed, palpate and try to find matching pairs.
　2) Turn the paper in different directions to make the exploration different.
h. Make a grab bag of items and reach into the bag and identify the objects by gentle touch.
i. Obtain Braille workbooks and learn to read Braille.
　1) If you have trouble learning Braille with the affected side, try with the unaffected side.
　2) Do not tense your hand as you feel the letters and do not extend the adjacent digits away.
　3) Work your hands smoothly over the dots. You can improve your skill, getting other workbooks for the blind and ultimately purchasing books in Braille.
　4) Obtain "Braille object cards" where the object is described in Braille. Palpate the letters and sentences.
j. Place raised numbers and designs on the computer keyboard and try to determine what the number/shape is before striking the key; make some labeled letter match or mismatch the key itself.

2. *Practice activities requiring the interpretation of sensory information delivered to the skin (interpretation of sensory inputs without active exploration of the stimulus, graphesthesia).*
a. Ask a friend to stimulate your skin with different stimuli (e.g., hot, cold, sharp, dull, rough) and try to identify the stimuli.
b. Ask this friend to draw numbers, letters, words (upper and lower case or cursive) and designs on your forearm, hands, and fingers when you are not looking.
　1) Identify the letters/numbers/words/shapes verbally (e.g., start with capital letters).
　2) When it is easy to be correct on capital letters, have your friend draw lower case letters including words.
　3) Progress to having designs drawn on your skin; replicate the design by drawing it on a piece of paper or on your own skin.
　　a) Ask your friend to give you feedback about the drawing to make sure the drawing matches the stimulus.
　　b) Check the angles where the lines meet.
　　c) Note accuracy of detection of curves.
　　d) Note whether all parts of the design are placed in the right relationship and orientation (spatial accuracy).
　　e) Note whether the design is the correct size.
　　f) Check whether the drawing has some elaborate components that were not actually drawn on the surface of the skin.
　　g) Your friend should make the drawings smaller and smaller to increase the challenge of detection (e.g., 2-3 mm).
　　h) The drawing or the stimuli should be delivered two to three times. If the design is still missed, have the subject look at the design. Then repeat the design at the next trial (or the alternate trial) and before progressing determine whether the subject can recognize the drawing).

3. *Use other stimuli to reinforce somatosensory learning.*
a. Develop tasks to improve sound discrimination (either location or determination whether the subject heard one or two sounds delivered).
b. Provide a visual stimulus at the same time an object is touched to the skin (on the affected and unaffected side); the goal is for the subject to accurately describe the cutaneous stimulus (e.g., sharp, dull, smooth, rough, silky, hard, soft).

4. *Develop activities to emphasize proprioceptive/kinesthetic learning.*
a. Where necessary, use tape on the skin, use electrical or auditory biofeedback, or put weights around the wrist and ankle to increase feedback from joint, tendon, and muscle receptors.
b. Create games in which a part of an object has to be accurately placed on a topographical picture.
c. Create games in which objects have to be moved accurately across specific distances on a variable surface.
d. Create objects of the same weight and place different types of surfaces on the object (e.g., Velcro, sandpaper, flooring). Then practice picking up, moving, and putting down the object with minimal effort.
e. Assemble puzzles by feeling the matching pieces rather than looking with the eyes.
f. Work with a friend and practice copying movements together (first by looking and then by feeling).
　1) Tap one finger while the other fingers are resting down.
　2) Bring arms up over head and tap one finger at a time.
　3) Bend wrist with one arm and bend elbow with other arm.
　4) Circle wrist to the right (right hand) and circle to the left with left hand.
g. Have a friend give you some resistance as you move one finger, the wrist, or the forearm up and down.
h. On a piece of paper, draw hand diagrams with different angles of each finger and different angles of the wrist. Then put up a vertical screen where you cannot see your hand. Look at each picture and try to copy the pictures with your own hand. Look behind the screen to check to see how accurate you are.
i. See if you can rent a continuous passive motion machine.
　1) Set the machine at different speeds.
　2) Try to follow the movements of the machine.
　3) Vibrate on the skin over the joint in the direction opposite to the movement.
　4) Carefully time the movements to enable success.
j. Practice grasping objects with a light grip on the object. Use a spherical group (thumb pad to the pads of other

fingers). Practice this with objects of different size with minimum graded force.

   k. Practice bending and straightening the elbow, wrist, or fingers while vibrating at the appropriate joint.

      1) When bending (flexing) the joint, vibrate on the extensor surface.

      2) When straightening the joint, vibrate on the flexor surface.

E. SENSORY AND FINE MOTOR ACTIVITIES AT NON-TARGET TASKS

   1. Move in normal patterns in desired directions without excessive firing of the muscles.

     a. Consider a number of strategies to allow you to move the most difficult finger most easily (e.g., stabilize adjacent digits).

       1) Use a soft splint to stabilize the fingers adjacent to the finger you want to move.

       2) Mold a piece of clay and keep an area clear under the finger you want to move and place a hole in the clay for the other fingers to rest in.

       3) Put a buddy strap on fingers adjacent to most dystonic or painful finger.

       4) Use a finger interphalangeal splint on fingers adjacent to dystonic fingers.

     b. Increase sensory feedback on the finger you are trying to move (e.g., use tape on the finger).

   2. With the eyes closed, play games that require discrimination of sensory information through the skin of the fingers.

     a. Play dominoes.

     b. Play pick-up sticks.

     c. Play shape games (e.g., match a shape to an opening, such as Perfection).

     d. Put together puzzles that have a raised surface.

     e. Play Scrabble with raised or indented letters.

     f. Play games that require orientation in place without the benefit of vision.

       1) Play pin the tail on the donkey.

       2) Walk through the house with your eyes closed and hands out to feel objects in your way and to catch yourself if needed.

     g. Get a Braille deck of cards and play cards (e.g., Solitaire can be played alone or play hearts, bridge, pinnacle, or poker with others).

     h. Create other sensory games that require planning and control and that can be done without vision.

F. LEARNING BASED SENSORY MOTOR RETRAINING (PRAXIS)

   1. Feel objects and then define and demonstrate what to do with the objects.

   2. Have a friend provide a sensory stimulus and ask you to do something that indicates you felt the stimulus (e.g., "when I tap with this sharp object, I want you to tap once, but when I touch you with this dull object, I want you to tap twice").

   3. Feel a number of items in a bag that are related to performing a task and put the items together to do the task.

   4. Feel a number of objects put together in a specific design; give the patient a second set of the objects to replicate the or match the design.

   5. Practice throwing objects of different size; practice throwing them to a particular spot.

   6. Get accustomed to grading movements without uncontrollable contractions.

     a. Place the hand on a moving target and do not stop the movement.

     b. Manipulate objects without excessive force.

     c. Put your hand on a record player and do not stop the record movement (e.g., do not change the sound).

     d. Put your hand on the moving belt of a treadmill and feel the moving belt.

       1) Feel the belt moving under the hand.

       2) Hold objects under the fingers.

       3) Pass objects back and forth between the fingers and make the objects feel the same.

   7. When it is possible to perform the sensory activities in non-target tasks, begin the placing the hand on the target instrument without abnormal movements.

     a. With the hand on the target instrument, mentally rehearse the movements and the tasks you should perform.

     b. Add rough surfaces to the target instrument if necessary to change the interface with the hand.

G. SENSORY MOTOR AND FINE MOTOR TRAINING AT TARGET TASK

   1. Emphasize the sensory aspects of the task even when beginning to perform the target task.

   2. Perform a selected component of the task (e.g., drop one finger down on the keyboard).

   3. Progress the ability to complete more and more of a target task emphasizing sensory exploration as long as the tasks can be done normally.

   4. Be sure to get reinforcement for performing all tasks normally (e.g., use a mirror, use biofeedback, get verbal feedback).

   5. Have someone make a video performing the target task that you are having trouble with. Then try to copy the movements. Watch the movements carefully and imagine that the movements are your hands moving.

   6. Perform the target task in different, nontraditional positions (e.g., practice in nontraditional positions such as lying on the back, lying on the stomach, reaching hand behind you or over your head).

   7. Do the target task in different media (e.g., if having a problem with writing, draw shapes and letters in shaving soap; draw big letters and then small letters and then words).

   8. Provide external support of the affected hand to appropriately position the digits (e.g., a splint if necessary to prevent movement of adjacent digits) while doing sensory and sensory motor tasks on the target instrument.

     a. Begin with a single digit adjacent to the most involved digit, but not the most involved digit.

     b. When can do complex sensory exploration with a single finger without abnormal movement, combine sensory exploration with more complete target movements.

     c. Add multiple digits to the sensory motor tasks.

   9. Without externally supporting the position of the digits (e.g., all digits free) perform one simple movement on the target task.

     a. Integrate sensory exploration with the simple movements and do the movements slowly to a metronome.

     b. Increase the complexity of the sensory driven motor tasks (e.g., tapping single note to playing scales and chords to playing new music or new keyboard tasks).

     c. Increase the speed of the movements on the target task, keeping up with the metronome.

     d. Perform target task normally for brief periods and progress the practice time slowly with frequent breaks.

H. REINFORCING SENSORIMOTOR LEARNING WITH FEEDBACK

   1. Biofeedback can include visual, cutaneous, muscle, vibration, auditory, or stretch stimuli.

   2. Biofeedback can be supervised by another person, facilitated with robotic movements, controlled by electronic contraction (activation of muscles), controlled by a physical constraint of a limb, guided repetitive passive movements supplemented with active movements to control motor output.

    a. Put tape on the top of the skin over the extensor surface of the digits to limit motion or emphasize somatosensory input and feedback.

    b. Use multichannel biofeedback to learn how to avoid abnormal movement strategies.

       1) Practice isolated movements and stop practice of unnecessary cocontractions of agonists and antagonists.

       2) Use the small muscles inside the hand (intrinsic muscles) to move the digits instead of the extrinsic muscles.

I. FEEDBACK: USE OF IMAGERY (MENTAL REHEARSAL AND MENTAL PRACTICE) TO RESTORE NORMAL HAND REPRESENTATION AND NORMAL MOTOR CONTROL

If it is still difficult to perform tasks without abnormal movements, then retraining should focus on mental imagery and mental practice (see Appendix 9-C).

APPENDIX 9-C ■ Enhancing Learning-Based Sensorimotor Training: Use of Imagery, Mental Rehearsal, and Mental Practice

A. GENERAL COMMENTS ABOUT IMAGERY

It is critical to restore confidence, a sense of wellness, and normal control of the movements of the extremities and trunk. Initially, this may be difficult because of pain, lack of accurate sensory information, difficulty with the control of movement, or imagining that the hand/arm could be normal again. One way to begin to restore the accuracy of information processing system so you can use your hand normally is to begin by changing how the hand and the functional task you are trying to perform are represented on your brain (the internal representation of that injured part).

It is important to be able to restore the normal image of the involved limb, that is, how it used to be and how it will be normal again. In the process of restoring normal control, it is also important to begin to use the hand normally and not increase the pain or repeat the abnormal movements. Thus, visually imagine your hand and how it looks. Making your hand look like the other hand is a good beginning. Then begin to create an image of the hand and the task you want to perform. Imagine using the hand normally to perform all the usual and target tasks. You can start by imaging small parts of a larger task and then finally the whole task and then related skills and activities that would be associated with performing the task.

With advances in MRI, we can more readily confirm the recruitment of brain processes with imagery. It is possible to activate functional, motor, and sensory representations of the hand with mental imagery. The area of the brain recruited is dependent on the activities imagined by the individual. For example, you have many different maps of your body. Some of the topographical maps may be redundant across different parts of the central nervous system (e.g., motor cortex, sensory cortex, prefrontal cortex, thalamus, basal ganglia). Well-learned functions are also mapped separate from sensory and motor topography. When you visualize a body part, you will activate the somatosensory cortex. When you imagine doing the task (motor imagery), you will also activate the motor cortex. When you can visually and motorically imagine completing the task in your mind, you will activate the cortical areas representing the part of your body that is moving and the part of the brain that is devoted to completing that task (e.g., walking, writing, playing an instrument). The intensity with which the neurons fire when you are imaging is less than the intensity of firing when you are actually performing the task. Try to imagine performing your tasks without mistakes. This will reinforce the positive aspects of the sensorimotor feedback. You must imagine without interruption (e.g., attention) and you must repeat the imaging process with a high level of concentration to help the nervous system learn. If you are imaging and you run into difficulty completing a task normally, try to focus on the source of the difficulty, including asking your inner self what barriers are getting in the way. Once you can get insight into these barriers, you should be able to break them down.

During imaging or mental practice, approximately 30% of the neurons are recruited as would be recruited when the task is physically executed. Further, when learning a new task, more neurons are recruited than when the task is learned. An impairment of structure (e.g., neurological or musculoskeletal) could modify the ability to image performing a task normally. On the other hand, imaging normal function and task performance could be easier than actually executing normal performance. In addition, repetitive imaging could begin to drive neural adaptation and recovery.

When there are conditions of chronic pain, there are changes in the organization and representation of the painful part in the central nervous system (e.g., cortex, thalamus, prefrontal cortex, supplemental motor cortex). Similarly, repetitive, abnormal patterns of movement also can dedifferentiate the representation of the body part. Thus, intervention must focus on restoring the normal representation of the brain. Sometimes it is easier to imagine normal movement or pain reduction than it is to actually change the pattern of movement or turn off the "on cells" for pain.

B. SUGGESTIONS FOR GOAL-DIRECTED IMAGING

1. Set goals for yourself to specifically improve the function of your hand.

2. Follow a sequence for learning.

    a. Imagine that you are healthy and fit and have full normal control of all of your extremities.

    b. Focus on healing the involved tissues, particularly if you have signs of inflammation and pain.

       1) Focus on diaphragmatic breathing and bringing blood to the tissues.

       2) Imagine the blood carrying important elements to the area of injury (e.g., the growth factors and oxygen that are requisites for healing tissues).

       3) Imagine that an injury causes inflammation that triggers the healing response (e.g., laying down collagen [scar]). Also imagine that the body modifies the scar tissue and tries to keep it mobile.

    c. Visualize the anatomy, physiology, and kinesiology of the hand.

       1) Imagine the bones gliding smoothly on each other.

       2) Imagine the muscles being strong, with a balance between the intrinsic and extrinsic muscles that serve the hand.

       3) Imagine normal movement patterns.

       4) Imagine normal sensation in the hand.

    d. Imagine pain-free movement.

    e. Imagine the hand being quiet and relaxed.

    f. Imagine smooth control of the hand without involuntary extraneous movements.

    g. Imagine that the affected hand is working just like the unaffected hand.

    h. Imagine using the hand as you used to use it. Go back in time to when your hand felt good and you did not have any problems.

i. When mentally practicing and imaging, there should be no distractions. Spend at least 30 to 60 minutes a day normalizing the hand and imagining how good it feels.

j. Mentally practice and perform the target task without any signs of strain or pain.

k. Concentrate and mentally review each of the components of the hand working normally.

l. Concentrate on the free flow of rhythmic movements of the hand/arm as you walk.

m. Recapture the excitement of using your hand while playing your instrument or working at your job without pain or strain.

n. Reinforce the image of a normal hand by continuing to progress learning including more complex tasks and public performances

CHAPTER 10

Payment Systems for Services: Documentation through the Care Continuum

Barbara Edmison, PT,
John G. Wallace, Jr., PT, MS, OCS

KEY WORDS

capitation
CMS
CPT
HIPAA
ICD-9-CM
Medicaid
Medicare
prospective payment system
reasonable and necessary
skilled services
third-party payer

OBJECTIVES

After reading this chapter the student/therapist will be able to:

1. Value the importance of documentation and its relationship to payment for services.
2. Synthesize different inpatient and outpatient payment systems.
3. Differentiate the continuum of care and documentation needed in different treatment settings.
4. Appropriately assign an ICD-9-CM code to medical and functional diagnoses.
5. Identify and select the CPT codes that best describe therapeutic interventions used in treating patients.
6. Analyze how payment policy can affect patient outcomes.

IMPORTANCE OF DOCUMENTATION

Physical therapists (PTs) and occupational therapists (OTs) are in the *business* of providing a health care *service* to improve quality of life. Because of a myriad of insurance options available from both private and government-run programs, people rarely pay cash *(self-pay)* for physical and occupational therapy. Therapists want to be paid a "fair" amount for their skills and knowledge, but they generally rely on a third party to provide this payment. Clinicians must convince the *third-party payer,* an entity that was not present and did not receive the therapeutic interventions, that the patient received valuable, unique, and worthwhile services. This process is called *Documentation and Payment for Services.*

Documentation is a skill a therapist must acquire. Its importance is equivalent to other forms of therapy skills. Just as fellow practitioners and staff are witness to the therapeutic services provided by the therapist, physicians and insurance companies are witness to the documentation that a therapist leaves behind. Documentation creates a lasting impression of the practitioners who represent the profession. Occupational therapy and physical therapy are an imperative and integral part of patient care; the documentation must reflect that.

Accurate documentation affirms that services were delivered. Therapists then depend on other people to *interpret* their documentation, and, on the basis of contracted rates, determine how much each service should be paid. Third-party payers often submit documentation to peer reviewers to ascertain excessive, useless, or fraudulent treatments. In addition, PTs and OTs are legally responsible for interventions provided by personnel under their supervision.

Securing payment for services rendered is, and will continue to be, a crucial element for the therapist as a professional as well as for the therapist's livelihood. Documentation, which is a legal and professional responsibility, is the basis for billing and is the proof that treatment was provided. Documentation is critical for success in the payment appeals process. For these reasons, documentation and payment for services are tightly linked together. This chapter will look at the payer sources at the national level and their required documentation components for payment.

It is important to remember that all the federal programs mentioned in this chapter are constantly changing. The process of legislating health care is dynamic and will be significantly modified in the next several years because there are too many people who are entitled to, and who are requiring, health care under these programs. There are not enough dollars available to cover the total costs. As the "Baby Boomers" age and their chronic medical problems increase, the supply of funds is in direct conflict with both the increased numbers of patients and their need for services. Major changes must occur in the future to enable health care, as expected by the public, to survive. One of the keys to these changes lies in *documentation.*

Why document? Documentation provides baseline status, records pertinent information, measures progress and success, fulfills predictions, and declares the final outcomes. It creates a record of the appointments the patient or client had. It provides data for concurrent or retrospective audits as well as evidence for research. It serves as an itemized bill for services rendered. The medical record may also become evidence in legal proceedings, which can either defend or incriminate the clinician. Documentation provides a snapshot of a period of time that gives the reviewer a full and practical description of the status of patients and the impact care has made on their quality of life.

Who reads the medical record? Although many therapists seem to believe that documenting is a necessary evil with no particular purpose, the information that therapists provide is vitally important. Physical and occupational therapy documentation is read by colleagues in the same or related disciplines to affect or continue the plan of care. It is also read by physicians and discharge planners to assist in determining additional treatment/surgical options or placement opportunities. Insurance case managers rely on documentation for the assessment of proper utilization of services. OT and PT documentation is read by employees of third-party payers who may be screening for proper dates and codes or for predicted outcomes in a reasonable time frame. Therapists do not want to have payment denied for any reason; therefore, it is extremely important that the documentation clearly present all the pertinent information in a manner that is easily understood by all parties.

DEFINITION OF TERMS

There is an entire language of terms regarding payment issues. Please refer to the Quick Reference Guide to Acronyms (Appendix 10-A) to unscramble all the acronyms. When therapy services are received, either the person pays the therapist directly or someone else pays the bill. In the first instance, there is a *fee for service,* which is agreed on by the two parties. Generally, a patient will pay directly for therapy in three circumstances: (1) having a need for skilled services and not having insurance; (2) having had therapy interventions, understanding their value, and wishing to continue beyond what insurance is willing to cover; or (3) having a preference for a specific therapist who only accepts cash-based patients or who is not a preferred provider of the insurance company. When someone else pays the bill, it is the *third-party payer* that is billed for the services. Third-party payers are usually insurance carriers who, by contract or written agreement, may determine the maximum amount of money paid and under what circumstances.

Private health insurance is either purchased by a consumer or provided to people as a benefit of employment. People may have additional coverage as a result of being a dependent on an insurance plan sponsored by someone else or by purchasing additional coverage. This *secondary insurance* may pay for the portion of the bill that is unpaid by the patient's *primary insurance.* In the case of Medicare coverage, Medicare beneficiaries can purchase *supplemental insurance* that will pay some or all of the charges that are not part of their Medicare benefit.

Health care services, for purposes of payment, are generally divided into three groups: inpatient, outpatient, and home health services. *Inpatient services* are delivered to patients staying in a hospital or health care facility. *Outpatient services* are delivered to patients who receive service by going to a health care provider. *Home health agencies* deliver services to patients in their own homes. A *fiscal intermediary* (FI) is a company privately contracted with Medicare that is responsible for paying bills generated by Part A (inpatient) and some Part B (outpatient) services. A *Medicare carrier* is a private company contracted with Medicare that is responsible for paying bills generated for Part B services. Both the FI and the Medicare carrier have the ability to accept or deny claims made to them for payment on the basis of their interpretations of the *Centers for Medicare and Medicaid Services* (CMS) guidelines.

Medicare Parts A and B will be discussed in more detail in this chapter.

COBRA (from the Consolidated Omnibus Budget Reconciliation Act of 1985) refers to short-term interim insurance coverage. It allows people whose employment benefits have been terminated to have continuing protection until new coverage is acquired.

Workers' compensation is coverage for people who were injured on the job. These regulations are determined at both national and state levels. Workers' compensation is discussed in greater detail later in this chapter.

Coding systems: Correct billing and claims processing is also dependent on accurately communicating treatment diagnoses and interventions to third-party payers. Three primary coding systems are used to communicate diagnoses and interventions in health care. The *International Classification of Diseases, Ninth Revision, Clinical Modification* (ICD-9-CM) is a tabular list of medical diagnoses approved for use by CMS based on the World Health Organization's ICD-9 originally published in 1977. The *Current Procedural Terminology* (CPT) (a registered trademark of the American Medical Association [AMA]) is a coding system that describes health care interventions. CMS has developed its own coding system to meet the specific requirements of the Medicare and Medicaid programs. The *Healthcare Common Procedure Coding System* uses CPT and alphanumeric codes developed by CMS in conjunction with the AMA to describe interventions, procedures, and supplies for the Medicare and Medicaid programs.[1] Use of these coding systems will be discussed in greater detail later in this chapter.

FEDERAL PROGRAMS

Medicare

"Medicare is the national health insurance program for people age 65 or older, some people under age 65 with disabilities, and people with end-stage renal disease, which is permanent kidney failure requiring dialysis or a kidney transplant."[1] "Medicaid is a program that pays for medical assistance for certain individuals and families with low incomes and resources. Medicaid is the largest source of funding for medical and health-related services for people with limited income."[1] Medicaid is administered at the state level, allowing each state to define its own criteria and guidelines for coverage.

In 1945, President Truman "proposed a comprehensive, prepaid medical insurance plan for all people through the Social Security system."[2] Congressional debate about federal health care coverage continued for 20 years. In 1965, HR 6675, the "Mills Bill," was introduced. "Congressman Wilbur Mills, Chairman of the House Ways and Means Committee, created what was called the 'three-layer cake' by starting with President Johnson's Medicare proposal (Part A), adding to it physician and other outpatient services (Part B), and creating Medicaid which significantly expanded federal support for health care services for poor elderly, disabled, and families with dependent children. Medicare became Title 18 of the Social Security Act and Medicaid became Title 19."[3] Although HR 6675 passed the House without a single amendment, the Senate version required much more discussion and many amendments. Finally, Medicare Part A, which involves basic hospital benefits and other institutional services for the elderly; Medicare Part B, a *voluntary* program; and Medicaid were approved by both the House and Senate.

Medicare and Medicaid implementation did not begin until 1966. Initially, "Medicare was the responsibility of the *Social Security Administration* (SSA), while Federal assistance to the State Medicaid programs was administered by the *Social and Rehabilitation Service* (SRS). SSA and SRS were agencies in the *Department of Health, Education, and Welfare* (HEW). In 1977, the *Health Care Financing Administration* (HCFA) was created under HEW to effectively coordinate Medicare and Medicaid. In 1980, HEW was divided into the Department of Education and the *Department of Health and Human Services* (HHS). In 2001, HCFA was renamed the *Centers for Medicare and Medicaid Services* (CMS)."[1]

"Medicare beneficiaries who have low incomes and limited resources may also receive help from the Medicaid program. For such persons who are eligible for *full* Medicaid coverage, the Medicare health care coverage is supplemented by services that are available under their State's Medicaid program, according to eligibility category. These additional services may include, for example, nursing facility care beyond the 100-day limit covered by Medicare, prescription drugs, eyeglasses, and hearing aids. For persons enrolled in both programs, any services that are covered by Medicare are paid for by the Medicare program before any payments are made by the Medicaid program, since Medicaid is always the 'payer of last resort.' "[4]

The *Balanced Budget Act of 1997* (BBA) made the most significant changes to the Medicare and Medicaid programs since their implementation. One goal was to shift some of the financial stress to the private sector, which was accomplished by allowing Medicare beneficiaries options for additional types of health plans. The BBA also reduced hospital payments, which had considerable consequences in the health care industry. This was one reason that the Balanced Budget Refinement Act of 1999 was introduced. The BBA of 1997 was also designed to address fraud, abuse, and waste in the federal health care programs. Additionally, this legislation "created a new children's health insurance program called the *State Children's Health Insurance Program* (SCHIP). This program gave each state permission to offer health insurance for children, up to age 19, who are not already insured. SCHIP is a state administered program and each state sets its own guidelines regarding eligibility and services."[5]

SCHIP, known as Title XXI of the Social Security Act, still leaves some children without health care coverage. This may be related to fewer children being covered by employer-sponsored insurance or it may be related to the specific eligibility requirements of each state. Children may be able to access health care benefits associated with school programs or federal government legislation. The *Individuals with Disabilities Education Act* and *No Child Left Behind* are two examples of federal programs to assist children with special needs.

Health Insurance Portability and Accountability Act of 1996

The *Health Insurance Portability and Accountability Act (HIPAA) of 1996* is a legislative effort to improve insurance coverage of the work force and also to improve the continuum of care by switching health care records away from paper and into the computer age.

Title I of HIPAA refers to *health insurance reform.* This reform increases the opportunities for workers to maintain or acquire insurance coverage when they lose or change jobs.

Title II of HIPAA relates to *administrative simplification.* These provisions are more closely associated with documentation and payment for services. The purpose of *administrative simplification* is to create a national database for medical records to ease communication between health care agencies.

Communication between health care agencies led to concerns about privacy and security of information because once medical records are online, vital information is easily accessible. This prompted HIPAA to also include a *privacy rule* and a *security rule.* The privacy rule "mandates the adoption of Federal privacy protections for individually identifiable health information. It sets a Federal floor of safeguards to protect the confidentiality of information. The Rule does not replace Federal, State, or other law that provides individuals even greater privacy protections. In developing the Privacy Rule, *Health & Human Services* (HHS) worked to create a balance that would provide strong privacy protections, while not interfering with patient access to, or the quality of health care services."[6]

"While the Privacy Rule mandates policies and procedures to protect patient information in all forms, the purpose of the Security Rule is to adopt national standards to protect the confidentiality, integrity, and availability of *electronic* protected health information. This Rule is directed at the Covered Entities, which are health care providers, health care clearinghouses, and/or health plans, that transmit or maintain protected health information electronically, are required to implement reasonable and appropriate administrative, physical, and technical safeguards. The Security standards require that steps be taken to protect this information from reasonably anticipated threats or hazards."[7]

The federal government is helping businesses to achieve the HIPAA-mandated goals of improved and efficient health care while protecting the privacy of the recipients and the security of their information. The well-being of a person is reflected not only by her or his treatment but also by the integrity of the system to keep personal information confidential. HIPAA and its consequences directly relate to documentation standards and handling of protected health information.

Prospective Payment Systems

Years ago, people received therapy in hospitals, Medicare was billed, and the hospital was paid. Physical and occupational therapy departments were among the highest moneymakers in the hospital. This, unfortunately, led to excessive billing and resulted in the need for improved accounting. More recently, CMS has established stricter requirements in an effort to control spending and to have money available for future generations. These requirements also benefit the patients today by accelerating the establishment of a medical diagnosis, allowing for faster implementation of therapeutic interventions and preventing billing or payment for unskilled services. Currently, under the *prospective payment system* (PPS) hospitals are paid a set amount per patient. The amount depends on the medical diagnosis and related morbidities. Payments are no longer related to the length of stay or procedures ordered. It is the hospital's responsibility to maximize its income by minimizing the patient's stay.

The Social Security Amendments of 1983 were responsible for the plan to save taxpayers money by creating incentives to improve efficiency in acute care hospitals. This system applied to Part A Medicare beneficiaries and was designed to give the hospitals a lump sum for patients who fit into certain categories.

Section 1886(d) of the Social Security Act (the Act) sets forth a system of payment for the operating costs of acute care hospital inpatient stays under Medicare Part A (Hospital Insurance) based on prospectively set rates. This payment system is referred to as the *inpatient prospective payment system* (IPPS). Under the IPPS, each case is categorized into a *Diagnosis-Related Group* (DRG). Each DRG has a payment weight assigned to it, based on the average resources used to treat Medicare patients in that DRG.[8]

Use of the PPS and DRGs, where Medicare payments are established in advance and determined by the medical diagnosis at discharge, created the opportunity for the hospital to have money left over if the patient was discharged earlier than the system predicted. The hospital would lose money if the patient needed to stay longer than the agreement coverage. For this reason, it became essential to accurately determine the discharge diagnosis of patients in the hospital. Appropriate "coding" of patients developed in the Health Information Management Departments of hospitals to determine the correct DRG and corresponding payment.

Adjustments to the basic rate are made under certain other conditions. There is a *wage index* associated with labor costs related to the geographic location of the hospital. If the hospital receives a large number of low-income patients, the *disproportionate share hospital* adjustment is made. If it is a training hospital for medical residents, the *indirect medical education* adjustment is made. An *outlier* occurs when a patient's stay becomes unusually expensive because of a long and complicated medical course. The final Medicare payment to the hospital reflects the DRG base rate plus the adjustments made for each of the above applicable conditions.

With the success of the PPS in acute care hospitals, additional legislation mandated extension into other settings with Medicare Part A beneficiaries. The Balanced Budget Act of 1997, the *Balanced Budget Refinement Act* of 1999, and the *Benefits Improvement Act of 2000* moved the IPPS into skilled nursing and inpatient rehabilitation facilities, home health agencies, and long-term care hospitals. Payments for therapy services are now included in the lump sum.

The initial PPS has encouraged the use of modified versions of this payment system by nongovernment third-party payers. Today, most inpatient services are covered by prospectively paid contracts with hospitals and health care facilities. Services not covered by prospective payment arrangements are often covered by *per diem* contract arrangements that pay a flat rate per day for inpatient services.

Outcome Measures

Medicare has developed different methods of determining payment in the PPS on the basis of various settings. In almost every case, the initial status of the patient determines the amount of money the facility will receive. Generally, the more complicated the patient's condition, the higher the reimbursement rate. The facility must then have a system to create a preliminary comprehensive "snapshot" of patients within days of their arrival at that particular setting. To ensure that patients receive the same standard of care and are treated equally, all patients are assessed by use of the Medicare preferred tools, even if they do not have Medicare coverage.

In the inpatient acute rehabilitation facility, the preferred tool is the *Inpatient Rehabilitation Facility—Patient Assessment Instrument* (IRF-PAI) to assist in determining the payment amount. The *MDS (Minimum Data Set)* is the primary tool for reimbursement in subacute and skilled nursing facilities, whereas *OASIS (Outcome and Assessment Information Set)* is used in home health agencies. These tools are discussed in more detail later in this chapter.

With each of these outcome measurement tools and in each setting, therapy documentation in the medical record must validate the tool's ratings. Both the IRF-PAI and OASIS are completed when the patient is admitted to the program and also at the time of discharge. As the patient progresses, it is very important for the medical and functional record documentation to reflect improvement and goal achievement. Because of the relative insensitivity and ordinal scales of these comprehensive instruments, a significant amount of functional change is often required to document change from one level to the next. In reality, this degree of functional change might not occur over the available treatment period. Nevertheless, an optimist would expect considerable improvement from the initial to the discharge scores on each of the comprehensive tools.

It is certainly possible that third-party payers will begin to use the outcome measurement tools as a way of assessing the performance of different facilities. Evidence could demonstrate that an admission score on a particular measurement tool followed by appropriate therapeutic interventions may result in a consistent discharge score in a specific number of days. With this information available for comparison, physicians and payers may choose to admit patients to those facilities that provide the best outcomes in the fewest number of days.

The IRF-PAI, MDS, and OASIS were developed with essentially the same goals in mind: (1) to measure patient outcomes and (2) to improve quality of care. These tools are each used in conjunction with the Medicare PPS to determine reimbursement costs. However, the functional tools themselves are not related and therefore there is no one system available in the United States to provide "standardized, patient-centered outcome data that can provide policy officials and managers with outcome data across different diagnostic categories, over time, and across different settings where post-acute services are provided (p. 13)."[9] In the future, it is hopeful that "functional outcome data that is applicable to patients treated across different clinical settings and applications, more efficient and less costly to administer, and, sufficiently precise to detect clinically meaningful changes in functional outcomes (p. 23)"[9] will be developed.

Inpatient Rehabilitation Facility–Patient Assessment Instrument

The IRF-PAI is used for determining outcomes in the acute rehabilitation setting. It is best known for having incorporated the *Functional Independence Measure (FIM*)*[10] *Instrument* along with *function modifiers, quality indicators,* and additional patient information. "The FIM instrument is a basic indicator of severity of disability.... The need for assistance (burden of care) translates to the time/energy that another person must expend to serve the dependent needs of the disabled individual so that the individual can achieve and maintain a certain quality of life. The FIM instrument is a measure of disability, not impairment. The FIM instrument is intended to measure what the person with the disability actually does, whatever the diagnosis or impairment, not what (s)he ought to be able to do, or might be able to do under different circumstances (p. III-1)."*[10]

Demographic, payer, medical, admission, and discharge information are included in the IRF-PAI. *Quality indicators* include respiratory status, pain, pressure ulcers, and safety (balance and falls). The FIM Instrument addresses the amount of assistance required for the functional activities of self-care, sphincter control, transfers, locomotion, communication, and social cognition. The *Function modifiers*[11] apply to bowel and bladder control, tub and shower transfers, and distances covered by walking or in a wheelchair.

There are seven levels in the FIM Instrument associated with function that are then divided into three categories: (1) *No Helper,* (2) *Helper-Modified Dependence,* and (3) *Helper-Complete Dependence.* The highest score of "7" indicates the patient completes the task safely, in a timely manner, and without any assistive devices. A score of "6" indicates the patient requires a device, takes extra time, or safety is an issue. The Helper-Modified Dependence category refers to the amount of supervision ("5"), minimal assistance ("4"), or moderate assistance ("3") required. Finally, maximal assistance ("2") and total assistance ("1") conclude the Helper-Complete Dependence category. There is a training manual available to assist the clinician in completing this form.[10]

A similar data or documentation form is used in pediatrics. It is referred to as the WeeFIM II System[11] and can be used for children and adolescents up to age 21 years. This tool uses the same 1 to 7 ordinal scale, although some of the functional activities are different.

Minimum Data Set

In *skilled nursing facilities* (SNF) and *long-term care* (LTC) facilities, the prospective payment system is designed to cover the costs of providing care. This includes payment for ancillary services. The Balanced Budget Act of 1997 required that the payments be adjusted for *case mix.* Case mix refers to the diversity of patients/residents on the basis of their complexity of medical problems or need for resources. This accounts for the increase in costs of complicated or involved cases. It ensures that facilities accept a variety of patients, rather than only those who require the

least amount of services. A method of classifying residents was developed to adjust the payments relative to the staff resources required to care for the residents. All this information is determined by the MDS, which then forms the basis for *resource utilization groups, version III.*

In an SNF or LTC facility, a *Resident Assessment Instrument* is created for each resident. It is composed of three parts: the MDS, the *Resident Assessment Protocols* (RAPs), and the *Utilization Guidelines.* The Resident Assessment Instrument provides a structured method for the facility to create individualized care plans, communicate on an internal and external basis, and to monitor quality performance.

The MDS is completed on a set schedule. After the initial 5-day, then 14-, 30-, 60-, and 90-day reports, the MDS is filed on a quarterly and annual basis. The MDS requires input from residents, their families, physicians, therapists, and dieticians. Facility staff from direct care, social services, activities, billing, and admissions is also consulted. The resident's performance over the entire 24-hour day is reviewed and recorded to create an individual picture of strengths and needs. The MDS includes a complete review of the resident's health, sensory systems, activity levels, behaviors, continence, activities of daily living (ADLs), physical and functional status, medications, procedures, and discharge plans.

The RAPs are then used to organize the information from the MDS. The MDS is a screening tool from which the 18 areas in the RAPs are used to identify problems and to create individualized care plans. Certain responses from the RAPs initiate *triggers,* which identify potential or actual problems. From the triggers, areas of concern are further researched to determine complications and risk factors in addition to noting the need for referrals to appropriate health professionals. Utilization Guidelines are necessary to analyze the information gathered from the RAPs.

Resource Utilization Groups, version III, form the basis by which CMS has classified groups for various levels of payment. Theoretically, there is a higher cost associated with residents who require more resources or one-to-one care by staff. The facility should be reimbursed at a higher rate for these residents than for those who are more independent. Facilities are also reimbursed at a higher rate for residents who are receiving skilled services. The *number of minutes of therapy received* affects the reimbursement rate. This is why it is very important to correctly document the time spent treating the resident and the resident's functional status. The MDS has a training manual available to assist with completing the instrument.[12]

Outline and Assessment Information Set

"The *Outcome and Assessment Information Set (OASIS)* is a group of data elements that represent core items of a comprehensive assessment for an adult home care patient and form the basis for measuring patient outcomes for purposes of *outcome-based quality improvement.* The OASIS is a key component of Medicare's partnership with the home care industry to foster and monitor improved home health care outcomes."[13] It is also useful for care planning and performance improvement in *home health agencies,* similar to the MDS in SNFs and LTC facilities.

OASIS is not a sensitive assessment tool, particularly when it relates to transfers, ADLs, or gait. Although pro-

---

gression within a category is easily documented, it is much more difficult to demonstrate changes from one category to the next, such as minimal assistance to independence. Proper documentation in the OASIS tool will indicate a problem on admission to home health. Therapy documentation in the medical record should indicate therapeutic interventions to address the problem and enable a higher score at discharge. It may be challenging to have sufficient time to actually improve the OASIS scores from beginning to end of care. This is due to the large differences from one category on this ordinal scale to another category. The therapist's documentation will demonstrate the process and progress made. For example, a patient is discharged from the acute rehabilitation setting using a walker on noncompliant surfaces. After therapeutic interventions in the home health setting, the patient uses a cane for transfers and ambulation. There is obviously marked functional improvement but the OASIS category of "needs assistance" would not change.

DOCUMENTATION REQUIREMENTS

Documentation is used as a means of communication at many levels. The product of documentation should be the communication of the process of professional judgment that is used to establish a patient's plan of care. Documentation should also demonstrate the integration of the elements of patient management that will determine the services that, in the professional opinion of the therapist, will provide the best possible outcome for the patient. This process leads to a logical plan of care and requires skillful judgment and analysis.

Medicare guidelines provide the minimum context standards required for adequate documentation. Satisfying minimum guidelines is not sufficient for the therapist who is thinking critically. This therapist should always be asking determinative questions (Box 10-1).

When the answer to the first question is **NO,** document why services will not be rendered. This enables the rest of the team, or other involved parties, to quickly ascertain this perspective.

When the answer is **YES,** the therapist must be able to answer the additional questions above. These are important questions to answer. The patient may have insurance or may be receiving federal, state, or county aid. Either way the therapist must not forget that *someone* is paying the bill, and as a payer within the health care system, part of your taxes may going to pay for these services.

The American Physical Therapy Association (APTA) has published *Guidelines for Physical Therapy Documentation of Patient/Client Management.*[14] This can be found on the APTA Web site (www.apta.org) under Communities–Governance–Board of Directors Policies–Section I–Practice. The section "General Guidelines" is included in Box 10-2 for instruction in proper documentation.

Although these general guidelines were written as part of an APTA document, they should be pertinent to all health care professions. These guidelines set a standard for licensed professionals in the health care industry.

BOX 10-2 ■ GENERAL GUIDELINES

- Documentation is required for every visit/encounter.
- All documentation must comply with the applicable jurisdictional/regulatory requirements.
- All handwritten entries shall be made in ink and will include original signatures. Electronic entries are made with appropriate security and confidentiality provisions.
- Charting errors should be corrected by drawing a single line through the error and initialing and dating the chart or through the appropriate mechanism for electronic documentation that clearly indicates that a change was made without deletion of the original record.
- All documentation must include adequate identification of the patient/client and the physical therapist or physical therapist assistant (or occupational therapist or occupational therapist assistant):

 The patient's/client's full name and identification number, if applicable, must be included on all official documents.

 All entries must be dated and authenticated with the provider's full name and appropriate designation*:

- Documentation of examination, evaluation, diagnosis, prognosis, POC, and discharge summary must be authenticated by the PT who provided the service.
- Documentation of intervention in visit/encounter notes must be authenticated by the PT or PT assistant who provided the service.
- Documentation by PT or PTA graduates or other PT and PTAs pending receipt of an unrestricted license shall be authenticated by a licensed PT, or, when permissible by law, documentation by PT assistant graduates may be authenticated by a PTA.
- Documentation by students in PT or PTA programs must be additionally authenticated by the PT or, when permissible by law, documentation by PTA students may be authenticated by a PTA.
- Documentation should include the referral mechanism by which physical therapy services are initiated. Examples include:

 Self-referral/direct access

 Request for consultation from another practitioner
- Documentation should include indication of no shows and cancellations.[15]

---

*Occupational therapist or occupational therapist assistant should use the same documentation system and protocol. Space prohibited using all professionals' initials.

BOX 10-1 ■ DETERMINATIVE QUESTIONS

Is there any therapy-related skilled service that this patient requires?

If yes, what is the unique professional contribution to this person's rehabilitation?

Are therapy services medically reasonable and necessary and able to be correctly administered in a timely and beneficial way?

What are the therapy services and on what schedule will they be administered?

In addition to the APTA's *Guidelines for Physical Therapy Documentation of Patient/Client Management,* the medical record must follow requirements set forth by other agencies and regulating bodies. The CMS sets the minimum standards for documentation that are implemented on the local level by fiscal intermediaries or Medicare carriers, as appropriate. Fiscal intermediaries and Medicare carriers are responsible for acceptance or denial of claims made to them by the acknowledged provider of services. The standards pertaining to "reasonable and necessary" are available from individual fiscal intermediaries and Medicare carriers as *local coverage determinations* (LCD).

The LCD standards and other helpful information are available through specific Web sites or through the *Coverage* page of the CMS web site (www.cms.hhs.gov). Nongovernment third-party payers can follow guidelines of their own design. These may or may not be similar to Medicare guidelines. In general, when a therapist's documentation meets Medicare requirements, it satisfies the expectations of other third-party payers as well.

There are other regulating bodies, such as the Joint Commission on Accreditation of Healthcare Organizations or state Departments of Health Services, that set documentation standards to protect consumers and payers of health care services. It is important that therapists be aware of all documentation requirements that may apply to payers associated with their patients. The therapist may choose to communicate with the accounting department before seeing a patient with new or unusual policy requirements. All of these requirements must be kept in mind when it is time to document in the medical record. Because of the unique requirements of payers at the various state, county, and local levels, this chapter will primarily address CMS guidelines.

Medicare requires specific information with bills that are submitted for payment. Following these rules will facilitate reimbursement for services because any deviation may be used as a reason for *denial* of payment. Proper documentation is always necessary for the *appeals* process when a claim has been denied. Medicare billing must include the following, which are appropriate for both inpatient and outpatient settings.

First and foremost, the patient must be eligible for therapy services on the basis of an active written *plan of care* (POC). The plan of care must be certified by a physician or by another *licensed independent practitioner.* Time periods for certification and requirements for return physician visits may vary.

Second, therapy is a reasonable and necessary treatment for the particular illness or injury. *Reasonable and necessary* creates room for a broad interpretation, which is why documentation becomes so important. The following are components that establish medical necessity:

1. Intervention, as related to the specific profession, is an accepted standard of care for this diagnosis. There are specific and effective interventions (evidence-based practice) successfully used to treat the condition.
2. The treatments require the *skilled* services of a professional. Knowledge and judgment are required because of the complexity of the problem and sophistication of the therapist's unique body of knowledge.
3. Therapeutic intervention creates *significant improvement,* demonstrated by measurable gains in range of motion, strength, function, level of assistance, etc.
4. The *amount, frequency, and duration* of treatment are reasonable. This is clarified by a POC with short and long term goals, predicted end of treatment, and reasonable potential to achieve the stated goals. Weekly reassessments or changes in the patient's condition will require the plan to be modified as necessary.

Reasonable and necessary are key words for therapists to synthesize as part of the critical thinking process. Two examples are given to assist the reader to further analyze the meaning of these words.

CASE STUDY 10-1

A 60-year-old active, independent woman who falls and fractures her humerus may be, understandably, a little wobbly from the trauma, but she probably will not need therapy to achieve independent mobility. However, the situation changes completely when the same woman has an existing right hemiparesis, requires the use of a cane for balance, and then fractures her left humerus. Now therapy would be appropriate to address ADLs, safety, and gait to assist her in regaining her independence. Both physical and occupational therapy may be treating this woman, and both professions need to be following similar processes for thorough documentation.

CASE STUDY 10-2

A patient who lives independently and is admitted to the hospital with a ruptured appendix would not usually require therapy services. The patient would need to spend time out of bed and to ambulate in the hallways to regain endurance, but this may be done with nursing staff or family. If this same patient had comorbidities such as multiple sclerosis or Parkinson's disease that were exacerbated by the hospitalization, then therapy would be warranted. Therapy would establish a plan of care to address the issues that prevent a return to the prior level of function.

Independent of the medical diagnosis and the patient's functional limitations, each case must be examined individually. No two cases should be assumed to have the same problems and the same plans for resolution. What appears to be a routine assessment may present subtle and intricate challenges to both the patient and the therapist.

Skilled Services

People who experience trauma or a disease process that affect their ability to move or function would be readily labeled candidates for therapy services. Therapy intervention should be easy to justify. The challenge is twofold. The therapist must (1) be able to identify and then substantiate the need for skilled services and (2) be sure that the documentation allows other parties to follow and understand what has been written. The following example of documentation compares two sentences that a reviewer might read: "Gait training to facilitate weight shifting onto the affected extremity with minimal assistance required" versus "The patient ambulated down the hall." The first sentence conveys the need for the unique and necessary skills of a physical therapist. The second fails to even suggest the presence of a therapist. Avoid referring to *skilled* physical or occupational therapy, which then assumes *unskilled* therapy. Unskilled therapy, for which a reviewer should deny payment for services, could easily be represented by "The patient ambulated down the hall." *Skilled services,* on the other hand, reflect the therapy provided in the first example.

Duplication of services is also a concern when there is collaboration across the disciplines. Many patients will benefit from treatments where both OTs and PTs are present. However, if both therapists document, "Sat patient at edge of bed to work on balance," reviewers could easily question whether both therapists did the same thing at the same time. The reviewers might then have a problem approving payment for the care provided, with a possibility that both services would be denied payment. There are no questions of duplication when the medical record states that the PT treatment session included "instruction and demonstration of strategies for dynamic postural adjustments" and the OT treatment session was directed toward "ADL training with emphasis on dressing." The same is true for speech pathologists and PTs or OTs in a multidisciplinary approach. A treatment session may have one therapy facilitating head control and midline orientation, while another is addressing upper extremity function, coordination, cognition, and the third discipline focuses on the ability to swallow. Be sure the documentation reflects the specific skills and knowledge related to each therapy.

DOCUMENTATION RECOMMENDATIONS

The medical record is a legal document that is read by many people who are not therapists. Patients have much greater access to and interest in their medical records today than ever before. The medical record is available to insurance case managers and medical reviewers who are outside the medical facility. Patients may share their records with their families, new physicians and therapists, or even attorneys. Because of the various interests and needs of these diverse groups, it is necessary to be concise, legible, objective, and professional when documenting. It may be necessary to remind the reader at this time that no documentation can be released to others without a patient's

signed release of information form on file in the patient's medical record.

Therapists should realize that it is very possible that their notes may be subpoenaed in the future as part of a lawsuit. The lawsuit could reveal the quality of records to be either supporting the patient's injuries and case or confounding the facts. The lawsuit might determine that the therapist or the record keeper of the facility would be the key expert witness in the case. The person who is the keeper of the records at the time of the case may have to go to court and explain what was done for this patient by another therapist. Documentation can make or break a case for that patient and for the therapist's liability. It is even possible that a therapist may find himself or herself referring to his or her own notes several years later while sitting in a witness box. The therapist could be the defendant whose reputation is on the line while the verdict is balanced by the quality of documentation done by that professional.

When documenting, be aware of the following important and sensitive areas. Remember that therapists receive a long and expensive education to enable them to write in the official legal record. Reviewers are basing their decision to pay for therapy on what has been recorded; be mindful of the need to meet criteria for skilled services. Patients and their entire medical team appreciate professional interventions *and* professional documentation.

Patient Advocacy

The therapist is the patient's advocate. It is the clinician's responsibility to ensure that the record reflects the patient's best interests. Do not let therapy notes hinder the patient's forward progress in any way. Patients with neurological conditions may have deficits that affect their orientation, judgment, initiation, ability to respond or comprehend, or insight. They may have visual-perceptual or other sensory problems that affect their ability to participate in therapy. Their ability to process information may be delayed. None of these components are reasons to withhold treatment, but they may alter the goal expectations and the time needed for learning of functional movement. These patients can and will progress with a creative, patient, and knowledgeable therapist.

Timeliness

Whenever possible, document immediately after seeing the patient. This ensures that the session is recorded accurately. After others related to the case are contacted, be sure to include the relevant findings in the medical record.

Motivation

The patient is almost always motivated to improve functionally. Sometimes there is damage to the brain that affects initiation, insight, or judgment; sometimes there is depression, pain, or another medical reason. It is the therapist's responsibility to find the key to unlock the patient's ability to participate. Do not record that the patient is unmotivated. The lack of motivation usually belongs to the therapist. (See Chapter 6, *The Limbic System: Influence over Motor Control and Learning* for additional information.)

Personal Opinion

The therapist's documentation must be *absolutely* objective. The PT or OT may provide direct quotations or accurately record an event that happened during a therapy session to allow the reader to make his own judgment. It is very important to never let personal feelings about the patient enter the medical record. Bias and antagonism on the part of the therapist may leave the medical record open to speculation and become a problem regarding litigation. If the reader of the documentation senses animosity, the validity of the comments and thus the therapy provided becomes questionable. Thus, always keep personal opinions out of official documentation. (See Chapter 5, *Psychosocial Aspects of Adaptation and Adjustment during Various Phases of Neurological Disability* for additional information.)

Abbreviations

Be careful when abbreviating; the individual documenting may be the only one who knows what is being stated. Most facilities have an approved abbreviations list. This list should always be incorporated into the documentation process. The meaning of what has been written will change according to the reader's interpretation of the abbreviations used. It is possible that a reviewer will read the medical record and either find it incomprehensible or completely misunderstand the original intent. The purpose of documentation is to provide information. Claims may be denied because the claims reviewer does not understand the abbreviations used. It cannot be overemphasized that abbreviations used in school or in other facilities may not be understood by the reviewer within the current facility or service provider.

Pain

The Joint Commission on Accreditation of Healthcare Organizations has brought the patient's pain level to the forefront, making a patient's pain level the "fifth vital sign." It is required that a comprehensive pain assessment appropriate for the patient's age and condition be recorded at regular intervals. The most common pain scale is 0 to 10, with 0 being *no pain* and 10 being *the worst pain* the patient can imagine. To further explain the scale to the patient, the numbers 1 to 3 correspond to minimal pain, 4 to 7 to moderate pain, and 8 to 10 to severe pain. It is important to explain to the patient that his pain scale is accepted at face value and belongs only to him; his numbers are not compared with those of anyone else. For children, the FACES[16] pain rating scale may be easier to understand. The purpose of a pain scale is to ascertain the effectiveness of pain medication or pain-reducing modalities. It is important to document the pain number, whether pain interferes or prohibits participation in therapy, and what the therapist has done to remedy the painful situation. (See Chapters 8 and 32 for additional information.)

Reassessments

The plan and goals for care must include the patient's interests. Reassessments are done on a weekly basis at the minimum and also when short-term goals have been met or there has been a change in status. The reassessment should clarify the patient's situation and address the short-term goals, either explaining why the goals have not been met or setting new goals when the previous ones have been achieved. Objective documentation of impairment changes should accurately reflect when anticipated functional changes will occur in the future.

Patient, Family, and Caregiver Training

The education provided must be appropriate to the patient's abilities. It is important to assess the learning style and barriers to learning, then adjust the teaching accordingly. The patient or caregivers must be able to understand the information. For example, documenting that the patient is blind and that he was given written handouts would be inappropriate, unless it was also documented that the family was trained with the materials provided. With any teaching, it is important to record what was taught, the response, and how well the new information was comprehended, either by return demonstration or by knowledgeable questions. Record whether the patient will be safe after the training. With use of this format, it is documented that the patient is able to progress to the next level of care.

Patient Rights

Patients have many rights, including the right to be treated with respect and dignity. Use terms that focus on the patient as a person; avoid labeling patients by their diagnosis. Informed consent and confidentiality are extremely important, both ethically and legally. Patients always have the right to refuse treatment. Therapy cannot be forced on individuals against their will. Therapists offer a service that medical and health care professionals know will be beneficial, but patients are responsible for paying for their health care and they must be given a choice.

Interdisciplinary

Whenever possible, include references to the other health care team members to demonstrate an interdisciplinary approach to patient care. Perform a thorough review of the medical record. Information from other team members can aid therapists in their understanding of the patient's situation. Be sure to take a critical look at what has already been entered into the medical record. *Question* any findings that do not make sense, especially if previous documentation does not correspond to all the information and clinical symptoms present at the time of intervention. Take the initiative to solve problems and investigate inconsistencies. Patients depend on the skills and knowledge of their therapists. Therapists must be accountable for their own documentation.

CONTINUUM OF CARE

Acute Care

Different settings require a change in the focus of documentation. It is important for the therapist to understand this concept and to modify it as necessary. In the acute care setting, discharge planning begins as soon as the patient is admitted. The primary role of the therapist is to assess the patient to determine the next level of care and to introduce therapeutic interventions to expedite that process. Time is of the essence; the therapist may have only one or two visits to make a discharge recommendation and fewer than five visits to achieve initial short-term goals.

Depending on various circumstances, patients may transfer from the acute-care hospital to home either directly or indirectly by way of acute inpatient rehabilitation or a skilled nursing facility. Although the goal is to return the patient home and continue therapy at home or in an outpatient setting, some patients may never leave the skilled nursing facility. The emphasis is on safety. The patient must be safe in her or his own environment. Caregivers, if necessary, must be capable of safely assisting the patient. It is important to realize that patients may not access every level of care or they may require a combination of settings. In each location, the treatment techniques may vary and the short-term goals will be different, but the same documentation guidelines apply. The following section assumes the patient is initially admitted to an acute-care hospital and then describes the possible discharge options.

Subacute

A patient who is admitted to the hospital and then requires the use of both a ventilator and a feeding tube may benefit from a subacute setting before moving on to acute inpatient rehabilitation. In the subacute setting, respiratory therapists and the nursing staff have key roles. Patients who have had respiratory failure in addition to their neurological deficits require a much slower pace to achieve their rehabilitation goals (see Chapter 35). These patients, with extremely impaired endurance and low functional levels, may stay in subacute settings for several months before they develop sufficient strength to progress to acute inpatient rehabilitation or return home. Short-term goals are set month to month, in contrast to acute-care hospitals, where short-term goals may be met in a matter of visits or days.

Acute Inpatient Rehabilitation

The *Commission on Accreditation of Rehabilitation Facilities* monitors quality standards for acute inpatient rehabilitation care and is respected at an international level. Patients admitted to rehabilitation facilities accredited by this commission must meet several requirements. First, the patient must be medically stable and able to participate in at least 3 hours of therapy throughout the day. The overall medical stability must still require 24-hour nursing care and physician monitoring for medical diagnoses such as hypertension or diabetes. Second, the physical disability is such that the patient must need at least two of the three rehabilitation disciplines of speech, occupational, and physical therapy. Finally, the patient must have a community discharge plan. The discharge plan is imperative because acute inpatient rehabilitation is a dynamic process and patients *will* be discharged from this setting. A patient who was living alone before hospitalization but whose long-term goals do not include independence may not be eligible for acute inpatient rehabilitation care.

Skilled Nursing Facility

If the patient does not meet the requirements for acute inpatient rehabilitation or if the patient does not have financial, family, or other resources to enable him or her to live at home with assistance, then a SNF may be a better option. The SNF is able to provide the rehabilitation services. In this case, the patient benefits by receiving rehabilitation and having a place to live. The facility is able to bill the third-party payer at a higher rate than for someone who is not receiving therapy services. The patient is allowed to receive therapy at a slower pace for a longer period of time. As the patient improves, acute inpatient rehabilitation may then be considered.

Home Health

Patients who are discharged from hospitals and facilities may still require additional therapy. They may not have the ability or the endurance to travel to an outpatient setting and then also participate in the various therapies. In these cases, home health therapists provide the solution. To receive home therapy, a patient must be homebound. According to Medicare, the definition for *homebound* is "Normally unable to leave home unassisted. To be homebound means that leaving home takes considerable and taxing effort. A person may leave home for medical treatment or short, infrequent absences for non-medical reasons, such as a trip to the barber or to attend religious service. A need for adult day care doesn't keep you from getting home health care."[17] Documentation must include how and why the patient is homebound. As the patient improves, this becomes more difficult and facilitates a decision for outpatient therapy or discontinuing therapy services altogether.

Transitional Living Centers

Some communities are fortunate to have a *transitional living center* (TLC) available for additional therapy. TLCs move beyond inpatient facilities and into "real-world" situations. These are community-based neurocognitive rehabilitation programs where the standard of care includes occupational, physical, and speech therapy; case management; and neuropsychology services. This treatment team pulls their weekly documentation into a combined, goal-oriented individualized rehabilitation plan with monthly summaries prepared for the payer source, physicians, family, and team. TLCs provide "custom-designed" life plans to facilitate re-entry into home, school, or vocational settings. TLCs have been extremely successful as a way for older adolescents and young adults with neurological problems to progress from a rehabilitation center back into society.

Outpatient Therapy

Patients who have progressed to a level where they can easily leave home prefer to travel to therapy departments or offices for treatment. *Once in outpatient therapy, patients receive the fine-tuning necessary to maximize their potential function.* Usually these patients benefit from a gradually decreasing frequency with an increasing emphasis on independent home programs. The guidelines for documentation in outpatient therapy are the same as for inpatient therapy. The payment system for outpatient services is quite different from inpatient settings and will be covered in detail later in this chapter.

Therapy and Discharge Planning

Therapists in hospitals have the tremendous responsibility of seeing patients just a few times and making recommendations that may affect those patients for the rest of their lives. Those decisions are not made in a vacuum; other members of the health care team are involved and initial plans may be amended. Often, however, the team looks to the therapists to determine the best discharge plan.

When discharge options are considered, there are questions a therapist should ask as part of the critical thinking process (Box 10-3).

There are no simple answers to any of these questions, but the questions need to be asked to arrive at the best

BOX 10-3 ■ CONSIDERING DISCHARGE OPTIONS

The questions a therapist should consider before making a discharge recommendation may include the following:

Is the patient capable of being successful alone or with selective assistance to send the patient directly home?

If selective assistance is still needed, is outpatient therapy appropriate or would home health be a better choice?

Is the patient medically and physically stable enough to proceed to an acute inpatient rehabilitation facility?

Is the patient's medical condition at a level that warrants an SNF?

BOX 10-4 ■ POINTS TO PONDER ABOUT DISCHARGING A PATIENT

TO HOME

Was the home environment safe before the patient entered the hospital?

Does the patient have a history of falls? (Some patients know the paramedics by name.)

Are there stairs with rails or elevators available?

Are the rooms and halls wheelchair or walker accessible?

What kind of assistive equipment will need to be in the home?

Are there healthy and available family members willing to assist on a continuing basis?

Does the patient rely heavily on family, friends, or neighbors for assistance?

Is there any money available to hire caregivers in the home and will the patient consent to this?

Are there cultural aspects in the family unit that may affect caregiving?

Does the patient need dialysis and how will this be accomplished?

How compliant will the patient be with an independent exercise program?

Will it be possible and easy for the patient to travel to an outpatient program?

TO A RETIREMENT COMMUNITY

How far must the patient walk to reach the dining area or can meals be delivered to the room?

Are assistive devices allowed in public areas of this community?

If not, what options have been provided or recommended by this community?

discharge plan for the patient. When trying to ascertain the best solution, the therapist should remember that cognition is a major concern, as is the length of time expected for the patient to meet the long-term goals. The wishes of the patient *and* the family must always be involved in the decision-making process because sometimes they do not agree with each other or with the therapist's recommendations.

There are many aspects to consider. The patient's prior level of function is essential information, followed closely by the situation at home. The medical and surgical histories are also pertinent factors. Contemplate the questions listed in Box 10-4.

The therapist should consider the level of responsiveness, the ability to follow commands, the prior level of function, and the patient's support system before making a recommendation. To further challenge the therapist, insurance coverage may affect the discharge plans. There will be cases where particular insurance carriers will contractually mandate the patient's discharge disposition. In rare instances, patients must wait in an acute-care hospital until they become eligible for state or federal funding before moving on to the next level of care.

In situations such as multiple fractures with non-weight bearing on bilateral lower extremities, the patient only needs time to heal before being able to participate in a rehabilitation setting. Although the best-case scenario is for the patient to return home while recuperating, this is not always possible. The patient transfers to a LTC facility for *custodial care.*

Another possible discharge option is that of a retirement housing community. This plan usually includes three levels of care: the independent living setting, assisted living, and a health center/skilled nursing facility. People purchase a contract for a secure and predetermined health care future in the retirement community. The contract specifies receiving care at any and all of these levels. The members stay in independent living until they require medical intervention. They may slowly decline and move into assisted living for a few years before finally settling into the skilled nursing level of care.

Members of these three-tiered housing situations may have a medical emergency and be admitted to acute care. The hospital will then transfer them back to the community's health center for rehabilitation. These patients may stay in the assisted living facility temporarily before returning to their independent living setting.

In these cases, documentation for home health therapy, private attendants, or family members should also be provided to make the transition and continuity of care as seamless as possible.

Be careful! The therapist may adversely affect a patient's disposition on the basis of the plan of care. For example, a therapist in an acute-care hospital might routinely treat postoperative patients with orthopedic problems who elected to have surgery. These patients are expected to make major functional changes in just a few days. If a patient arrives with a new subarachnoid hemorrhage and a moderate-assist functional level, that same therapist may underestimate the amount of assistance and the duration of care that will be needed for this severely involved patient. The therapist's short-term goals might inappropriately project independent mobility within a 2-week time frame. If the therapist does not amend the plan of care, then the discharge planner, insurance case manager, and physicians may decide that the patient is not making any progress at all. The patient is determined to have little to no rehabilitation potential, when, in reality, the therapist's time line was too short. This kind of error could essentially end the patient's chances for acute inpatient rehabilitation and affect the patient's ultimate recovery level.

Less dramatic and possibly more common is the case of a patient who receives a total hip arthroplasty for a hip fracture after an unwitnessed fall. The patient does not progress as quickly as the therapist would expect. The therapist must consider the possibility that this patient had a mild stroke and *then* fell and fractured the hip. The patient underwent workup for the obvious fracture, but the neurological symptoms went undetected by the orthopedic surgeon. Sometimes the patient's subtle medical problems are only realized during evaluations that identify mismatches between the medical diagnosis and the anticipated functional skills and limitations. Open and clear lines of communication must be established between individuals working within the medical disease/pathology model and therapists working on impair-

ments, functional limitations, and quality of life issues. The therapists have the opportunity to assist the patient and influence the discharge plan by advocating for a facility that offers both orthopedic and neurological rehabilitation.

The third-party payer also has a say in the disposition of the case. Occasionally the discharge choice of the insurer, on the basis of the case manager's review of the medical records and the patient's coverage, is not the therapist's first choice for the patient. It may only be possible to affect the decision regarding the patient's future if the therapist has been a strong patient advocate and has consistently documented appropriately and thoroughly.

CASE STUDY 10-3

The following case illustrates the interaction of therapy on the continuum of care and the various assessment instruments used in different settings.

Ysabella D. is a 66-year-old woman, independent and healthy, who is diagnosed with atypical Guillain-Barré syndrome. She is admitted to the acute-care hospital, and subsequently respiratory failure, flaccid quadriplegia, and cardiac arrhythmias develop.

Over the course of 5 months in the acute-care hospital, with more than one visit to intensive care, Ysabella receives a tracheostomy, a gastrostomy tube, and a pacemaker. In the meantime, she also acquires pneumonia, dysphagia, and a decubitus ulcer. Although Ysabella receives occupational, physical, and speech therapy while in the acute-care hospital, she remains dependent in all areas. Because of the presence of the tracheostomy and percutaneous endoscopic gastrostomy tubes, Ysabella is transferred to a subacute setting, where she stays for another 8 months. Here she gradually improves in strength, endurance, and function.

After her tracheostomy and feeding tubes are removed, her skin has healed, and she has progressed to a regular diet, Ysabella is strong enough to meet the criteria for an acute inpatient rehabilitation facility and she is transferred there. She stays in the short-term rehabilitation facility for another 6 weeks before she reaches a minimal-assist level of care. At this point, she

and her very supportive family have been trained and she is able to be discharged home. Because she lives in a second-story apartment, is still using a wheelchair, and continues to require occupational and physical therapy, Ysabella is eligible for home health therapy.

Ysabella has Medicare Part A and B insurance coverage. This enables the acute-care hospital to be reimbursed on the basis of her DRG. In this case, her long and complicated stay would qualify her for the outlier adjustment, allowing the hospital to receive more money than it would have received for a patient with a typical or uncomplicated Guillain-Barré diagnosis. At the subacute facility, the initial PPS MDS would be completed after 5 days. The PPS MDS would again be completed after 14 days, 30 days, 60 days, 90 days, and then quarterly until her transfer to the short-term inpatient rehabilitation setting. Here the IRF-PAI, with the FIM score, would be completed after 3 days and at the time of discharge. When Ysabella finally returned home, the home health therapist opened the case by use of OASIS. Each facility would be reimbursed after the submission of the appropriate assessment and outcome instruments, assuming these tools were completed correctly and there was no reason for payment to be denied. Proper documentation by the therapists would justify all her therapy if there were to be an appeals process.

MEDICAL AND FUNCTIONAL DIAGNOSIS AND INTERVENTION CODING: DIAGNOSIS CODING

Payment for rehabilitation services is not only dependent on the quality of the medical record produced during the course of care but also on the accuracy of the codes used to describe medical and functional diagnoses and therapeutic and interventions used in treatment. Third-party payers and other health care system stakeholders rely on the accuracy of coding so that the appropriate payment policy can be applied during the claims adjudication process. This section will introduce the reader to the basics of diagnosis coding using ICD-9 codes and intervention coding using CPT codes.

The ICD-9-CM, or ICD-9 for short, is based on the official version of the World Health Organization's Ninth Revision of the International Classification of Diseases. ICD-9 classifies diagnosis, morbidity, and mortality information to allow systematic codification and standardized naming of diseases and injuries and allows indexing of data for outcome studies and for use in various payment, billing, and electronic information formats. Health care insurance companies and government agencies require the use of ICD-9 for billing/payment processes and for medical records as a result of HIPAA. To track outcomes, especially functional outcomes, standardized diagnosis nomenclature is absolutely essential. In rehabilitation settings the treating therapist is responsible for accurate identification of the physical therapy (treating) diagnosis and any comorbidities that could be factors during the course of care. Accurately identifying these diagnostic codes is an essential part of the advocacy role of the treating therapist because these coding decisions can have significant effects on third-party payer decisions for paying claims for patients and clients with potentially life-altering diseases and injuries.

Organization and Characteristics of ICD-9-CM

ICD-9-CM is organized into two volumes. Volume 1 is the tabular list of ICD-9 codes and five appendices. Codes from Volume 1 are not usually used for medical and functional diagnoses involved with rehabilitation. Volume 2 is an alphabetical list of ICD-9 codes. This listing contains a large number of medical and functional diagnoses that incorporate most of the diagnostic terms currently in use. A group comprised of the American Hospital Association, CMS, National Center for Health Statistics, and the American Health Information Management Association regularly update ICD-9 codes, resulting in annual editions that are updated throughout each calendar year. When ICD-9 resources are consulted, it is important to always be sure that the most current edition is used.

ICD-9 codes can be up to five digits long: at least three digits are to the left of the decimal and up to two digits to the right of the decimal. The three digits to the left of the decimal define the diagnosis category and the two available digits to the right of the decimal define more specific characteristics of the diagnosis by further defining site and location. We will look at several examples to illustrate the coding process (see Box 10-5).

Two terms need to be kept in mind when using ICD-9 codes. The first is *Not Elsewhere Classified*. This term is used when the ICD-9-CM does not provide a code that may be as specific as the diagnosis the therapist is trying to code, or when the clinician may not have enough information to code to a more specific diagnosis requiring the fourth-digit subcategory. The second term is *Not Otherwise Specified*. This term is used when the diagnosis is unspecified. Again, the reader will have an opportunity to look at examples of both abbreviations for illustration purposes.

Assigning ICD-9-CM Codes

In most cases the therapist will start with the name of a medical or functional diagnosis and will have to convert that name to the numeric ICD-9 code. In rare cases the opposite occurs; a diagnostic code is provided and the code will need to be converted to a name. For the purposes of this discussion it is assumed that a codebook is being used; however, readers will find that many software and Internet applications embed ICD-9 information within the application. When using embedded resources, it is important that the reader refer to the text included in the codebook because most of these applications use the "short language" form of the code and do not tell you whether fourth- or fifth-digit modification is required.

ICD-9 Coding Is a Five-Step Process

The following five-step process will guide the reader through the ICD-9 coding process:

Step 1: Start by consulting the alphabetical index (Volume 2) to identify the diagnostic category before using the tabular index (Volume 1). By identifying the correct name of the diagnostic category in the alphabetical index, therapists will avoid coding errors that will result in denied services.

Step 2: Identify the main medical or functional diagnostic term or category. The alphabetical index is arranged by condition. Conditions can be expressed as nouns, adjectives, and eponyms. Some conditions have multiple entries under their synonyms. Be sure to read any notes listed with the main term or category because these categories will help the reader identify the specific diagnostic code he or she is trying to identify.

Step 3: Interpret abbreviations, cross-references, and brackets. Cross-references used are "see," "see category," or "see also." The abbreviations NEC or NOS follow main terms or subterms. Identify a tentative code and locate it in the tabular index.

Step 4: By reading the entry in the tabular list, clinicians will be able to determine whether the code is at its highest level of specificity. Assign three-digit codes (category code) if there are no four-digit codes within the code category. Assign four-digit codes (subcategory codes) if there are no five-digit codes for that category. Assign five-digit codes (fifth-digit subclassification codes) for these categories where they are available.

Step 5: Assign the code.[15]

Box 10-5 provides two ICD-9 coding examples.

Depending on the treatment setting, patients/clients may come to the therapist with diagnoses that are already coded. In other situations, such as in acute-care and inpatient rehabilitation facilities, ICD-9 codes will be assigned by certified ICD-9 coders in the medical records department. In many outpatient settings the therapist will be required to "match" ICD-9 codes for their Medicare patients with specific CPT codes to establish medical necessity for the rehabilitation interventions according to the Fiscal Intermediary or Carrier Local Coverage Decisions. In any case, the treating therapist should be absolutely clear in the medical record about the treating diagnoses and comorbidities that define the treatment program and plan of care of the patient or client.

INTERVENTION CODING

Just as ICD-9 codes allow therapists to communicate to payers and other health care stakeholders the conditions and injuries being treated, CPT codes allow therapists to identify and communicate the interventions being used in the course of patient care. In a world where most billing information is transmitted electronically, it is essential for therapists to use the most appropriate CPT codes to communicate the breadth, depth, and complexity of the treatment plans required in the care of patients/clients. Appropriate intervention coding is also essential to the billing and claims adjudication process and to maximize the health care benefits available to the patient with complex neurological conditions and injuries.

Current Procedural Terminology

Current Procedural Terminology,[18] Fourth Edition, is maintained, updated, and published by the AMA and is a registered trademark of the AMA. It is a code set designed to

BOX 10-5 ■ ICD-9 CODING EXAMPLES

Following are two examples of common neurological conditions. You will need an ICD-9-CM book to do this exercise.

The name of the condition is the best place to begin. For example, code the diagnosis *complete paraplegia*.

- Go to Volume 2 (alphabetical index) and look up "Paraplegia, complete"
- Review the listings under 344 of Volume 2 under "Paraplegia." There is no listing that matches the term "complete."
- Go to "344.1 Paraplegia" in Volume 1 (tabular index). The main entry is "344 Quadriplegia and Paraplegia."
- Read the entries under 344 and find "344.1 Paraplegia." Notice what conditions are included and excluded by the listed codes. Read the note under "344.1 Paraplegia" that says "paralysis of both limbs." This represents the closest match to "complete paraplegia."
- "344.1 Paraplegia" is your diagnostic code.

Coding *nonspecific encephalopathy:*
- Go to Volume 2 (alphabetical index) and look up "Encephalopathy."
- Review the listings under "Encephalopathy." There is no listing that matches the term "nonspecific."
- Go to Volume 1 (tabular index) and look up "348.30 Encephalopathy."
- Read the notes and descriptions under "348.3 Encephalopathy." Notice what conditions are included and excluded by the listed codes.
- "348.30 Encephalopathy, unspecified" matches nonspecific Encephalopathy most closely.
- "348.30 Encephalopathy, unspecified" is your diagnostic code.

---

identify the interventions and other services performed by health care providers. Each intervention or service is described by a five-digit code. CPT is mandated by HIPAA as the appropriate code set for use in health care transactions in the United States.

CPT is used to report health care provider services to public and private/commercial insurance companies and payers. In addition, CPT codes are also used to report treatment encounter information to government agencies and private companies for the purposes of research, outcomes tracking, and education.

The AMA first published the CPT, Fourth Edition, in 1977. CPT is continually updated to keep the code current with the community standard of practice by a process led by the AMA CPT Editorial Panel.[19] For the rehabilitation disciplines, the Health Care Professional Advisory Committee develops CPT coding changes and updates. The Committee consists of representatives from 16 nonphysician provider groups, including physical therapy, occupational therapy, and speech and language pathology.

The CPT code set is organized into six major sections: Evaluation and Management, Anesthesiology, Surgery, Radiology, Pathology/Laboratory, and Medicine. Each section is divided into subsections based on anatomical, procedural, condition, and descriptor headings as appropriate to that specialty section. The AMA, in publishing the CPT code, recognizes that there may be significant overlap in the interventions, procedures, and services performed by health care providers and makes the following statement in the introduction:

It is important to recognize that the listing of a service or procedure and its code number in a specific of this book does not restrict its use to a specific specialty group. Any procedure or service in any section of this book may be used to designate the services rendered by any qualified physician or other qualified health care professional.[18]

Typically, most codes used by rehabilitation professionals to describe treatment of neurological conditions are in the 97000 series of the CPT; however, any code that adequately represents the interventions or services performed by a provider with the appropriate qualifications may be used.

Using the CPT Code

Selecting the correct CPT code that most adequately describes the intervention performed is often very challenging because most therapists have not had formal CPT training. Although in-depth coding training is beyond the scope of this text, this section will help the reader develop some basic skills in applying sound coding techniques to practice.

Most of the codes used to describe therapy interventions are found in the Physical Medicine Section of the CPT code. Although therapists use these codes, so do a large number of other health care professionals and providers. For this reason it is important for therapists to be able to adequately describe their use of interventions using the correct CPT code so the codes reflect the complex nature of the treatment plans implemented with their patients.

Physical Medicine CPT Codes

The Physical Medicine codes are located as a subsection of the Medicine section of the CPT code set. Some CPT codes in the Physical Medicine section represent interventions that occur in specified time intervals (e.g., 15 minutes) and are considered "timed" codes. Timed codes generally require constant attendance or direct (one-on-one) patient contact. Other codes are considered "occurrence" codes and do not have a time period associated with them. Some occurrence codes require direct contact, whereas others do not. Occurrence codes are only billed one time during a visit or treatment, but timed codes can be billed in multiple units as justified by the time it takes to provide the intervention. Consult a current CPT codebook for specific details because these codes and their associated descriptions can change each year.

The Physical Medicine codes are organized into six groups of codes. The codes in these subsections have specific attributes[18]:

Evaluation/Reevaluation

These codes are the evaluation and reevaluation codes for physical therapy, occupational therapy, and athletic training. These codes are occurrence codes requiring direct contact between the therapist and the patient.

Modalities

These codes are further divided into two groups: "Supervised" modalities (occurrence codes that do not require direct contact), and "Constant Attendance" modalities (timed codes that require direct contact).

Therapeutic Procedures

These codes require direct patient contact by the therapist. All but one of these codes are timed, so, if the time required for the intervention warrants, multiple units of a code can be charged.

Active Wound Care Management

These codes are occurrence codes that require direct contact.

Test and Measures

These codes represent specific assessment and testing interventions that are separate and distinct from evaluations and reevaluations. These interventions require separate written reports.

Other Procedures

This section consists of a single code used to describe any "unlisted" physical medicine service or intervention.

Each year therapists should review the codes and sections commonly use for changes and additions that will better describe the interventions performed with their patients. All therapists should consult the CPT code directly and avail themselves of training specifically designed to help them accurately describe their interventions. CPT coding resources are available from a number of sources, including the AMA and professional associations such as APTA.[20]

OUTPATIENT PAYMENT POLICY

The processes involved with billing, payment, and payment policy for outpatient services remains distinctly different compared with inpatient services. Although inpatient rehabilitation services are primarily paid on a *prospective* basis, outpatient rehabilitation services continue to be paid primarily on a *retrospective* basis. This means that, although services may have been authorized before delivery of care, the decision to pay for the services is made after care has been delivered and subject to reviews of medical necessity, appropriateness, and other policies. Financial class largely determines the types of policies and regulations that apply to any particular payer. There are four primary financial classes: Medicare/Medicaid/government programs, commercial insurance/private coverage, automobile/accident insurance companies, and workers' compensation. To be effective advocates for patient care, therapists must be vigilant to be aware of regulations and payment policies that determine how care is approved, billed, and paid.

Medicare/Medicaid

Both the Medicare and Medicaid programs are overseen and regulated by the CMS. Medicare, as a federal program, is heavily regulated. These regulations are readily available to providers through a number of resources, but the primary access to information is through the Internet at http://cms.gov. As previously discussed, Medicare pays for outpatient services through private contractors as FIs and carriers. Each of these entities must maintain a Web site for beneficiaries and providers to allow for ready dissemination of pertinent information. Carriers and FIs use Medicare's national policies to process and adjudicate claims. Although Medicare has national policies, carriers and FIs have some discretion in how these policies are implemented locally. Any carrier or FI regulations or policies specific to particular services, interventions, or provider types are contained in LCDs that must go through a lengthy draft and approval process before they are made available to providers and implemented. Most carriers and FIs have LCDs specific to physical rehabilitation providers (physical therapy, occupational therapy, and speech and language pathology) as well as specific services or interventions such as wound care, biofeedback for incontinence, vestibular problems, and cardiac rehabilitation. Because carriers and FIs have defined geographic coverage areas, it is advisable for therapists to be sure they are familiar with Medicare's payment policies in the areas where they practice.

Medicaid, as discussed earlier, is a health program for the economically disadvantaged. Although it is partially funded with federal dollars, it is also funded at the state level. Because Medicaid is implemented at the state level, states have significant leeway in how their programs operate, approve care, and pay for services. Consequently, there are large variations in the Medicaid program from state to state. Therapists should be aware within their individual work settings of the regulations and policies that may apply to them as a result of their employer's possible participation in the Medicaid program.

Medicare and other payers often attempt to mitigate their financial risk for costly episodes of rehabilitation by imposing arbitrary limits on care. These limits are often referred to as "caps." One example of such a limit is Medicare yearly cap on rehabilitation services. This cap was created as part of the Balanced Budget Act of 1997 and went into effect in 1999. The cap was $1500 in payments per year for physical therapy/speech therapy and a separate $1500 cap occupational therapy services. The cap applies in all outpatient settings except outpatient hospital rehabilitation units.

Another way Medicare and Medicaid attempt to mitigate their financial risk is to use outpatient service programs that are prospectively paid. These programs operate by use of *capitation,* a system by which health care providers are paid in advance of rendering care to a defined group of beneficiaries. In this payment system the capitated health care providers provide care out of the prepaid pool of funds. These programs use contracted insurance companies, using large groups of health care providers representing a wide array of specialties, to provide the anticipated health care needs of the covered patients. Capitation agreements must be carefully negotiated. If the negotiated prospective payment is too low, or, if the therapist overtreats, the payment for services rendered will be inadequate to cover the cost of providing care to the covered patient population.

There are a number of smaller government programs that also may have specific regulations and policies similar to those of Medicare. An example of such a program is CHAMPUS/TRICARE. This program provides for health care insurance coverage for the military and their dependents and for military retirees. Other federal health care programs, such as the Veterans Administration, may vary significantly from Medicare and Medicaid in their policies.

Coverage programs for children with congenital or acquired conditions requiring extensive rehabilitation are covered through a number of federal, state, and local programs. Because of the huge diversity in the payment policies related to these programs, therapists should be aware of the particular program covering the care and work closely with parents and agencies involved to ensure that proper coverage for services is achieved.

Commercial Insurance and Private Coverage

This financial class represents traditional health insurance companies, self-insured employers, and self-paying consumers. Commercial insurance companies are regulated at the state level and self-insured companies are regulated at the federal level. Cash-paying consumers must rely on their own understanding and self-education to make their purchasing decisions regarding therapeutic care.

Commercial insurance companies operate by charging premiums to the beneficiaries (employers or individual consumers) and then paying for services delivered to their insureds. Because these payers bear the risks associated with the health of their beneficiaries, they use a number of strategies to mitigate their risks in this delivery model. Many use preferred panels of health care providers to deliver services. These preferred providers agree to particular business processes, rates of payment, and utilization review/restrictions to have access to the beneficiaries of these payers. Some require the provider to obtain authorization before treatment is provided, whereas others provide strict review of care after delivery to decide whether payment is warranted. These companies also have a number of mechanisms to shift their financial risk to the patient and to the provider, including capitation and case-rate reimbursement. *Case-rate* reimbursement pays a flat rate for the entire course of care for a patient with a particular medical diagnosis.

Insurance companies often require the patient to pay different amounts toward their care on the basis of whether the patient sees a network provider (preferred provider) or an out-of-network provider (a provider who is not a contracted provider). These amounts can be based on a percentage of the charges, on a flat amount for each treatment (co-pay), or both. The required patient payment can have a significant effect on patients' and clients' financial abilities to participate in their respective treatments. By increasing co-pay amounts, payers know patients will have to make "harder" decisions regarding how much care they can afford. This can play an important factor when a therapist and his or her patient agree on a plan of care, how much therapy the patient can afford, and when the patient is discharged to a home program. For patients who pay cash for services, these decisions can be even more difficult and come far sooner in the plan of care. In other situations, especially in long-term management of an individual after central nervous system injury, the therapist's role may become consultative. When the patient or family identifies functional changes, the therapist may be asked to establish new goal interventions as a home program to be carried out by the patient's support system.

Payers can also place limitations on the amount of services a patient can receive each year by limiting the number of visits, days, and dollars spent on therapy services. Therapists must be aware of these limitations and how these limitations may affect the potential interactions between long-term care and patient potential. With this understanding, a therapist can help identify the best use of patients' resources and facilitate those individuals' abilities to participate in their own care. The nearly infinite number of ways payers can shift risk and financial responsibility to patients and providers makes it imperative that systems be in place in each clinical setting to check for limitations and alert the patient and therapist to potential financial challenges that can have chilling effects on treatment and the potential for recovery.

Automobile and Accident Coverage and Third-Party Liability

When individuals are injured in automobile and other accidents, financial liability for care may become the responsibility of others who were involved in or responsible for the accidents. In the case of automobile accidents, people are generally required by state law to carry some minimum amount of public liability insurance to cover such costs. Health insurance companies usually have stipulations in their policies that allow them to recover any costs they incur as the result of the liability of others.

To further complicate matters related to accidents, many of these cases end up in lawsuits and litigation. This represents several challenges for the treating therapist. In terms of payment for services, it is not always entirely clear who will be paying for services and when they will pay. Many patients injured from the actions of others may feel that they are not responsible for paying for the care they receive and they can be unaware of the cost of treatment as it mounts. This can be problematic if the party the patient believed was liable is exonerated or unable to pay.

Nearly all health care facilities have a policy that states that the patient, or their parent or guardian, is financially responsible for the treatment received although the facility may be willing to bill other parties for those services. Therapists should always be aware of the various possibilities that can occur during the course of care that can affect the ability of the patient to continue therapy. Therapists should also be aware that the medical records could end up being examined by a number of attorneys and end up in open court.

Workers' Compensation

Of all the insurance classes reviewed, workers' compensation has the highest degree of variability in regulation and payment policy. Each state legislates and regulates its treatment of injured workers independently of other states and federal involvement. This variability requires every facility treating workers' compensation patients to maintain a knowledge base of the laws and regulations governing the care of these patients as well as establishing procedures to ensure that they are followed. Many states use fee schedules that are based on CPT codes but are highly modified and have significant variations from "normal" coding. These types of fee schedules may require specific instruction to use so that the therapist can accurately describe the interventions used with patients covered by these fee schedules. In addition, the nature of work-related injuries produces other potential challenges for therapists.

Workers' compensation coverage is provided through purchased insurance or through self-insurance programs set up by employers. Workers' compensation cases are *concurrently* managed by insurance companies or by third-party administrators who manage self-insured employer programs. *Concurrently* managed care means that the payer requires the health care provider to preauthorize all proposed care and reviews documentation to ensure compliance with state-mandated fee schedules and use guidelines. Because of the assumed employer liability of work-related injuries, some of these cases progress to lawsuits and litigation as in the case of accidents. Therapists should remain aware, also, of the potential involvement of their patients' medical records in these legal proceedings. In the area of neurological rehabilitation, a workers' compensation package may become very complex. If the injury results in permanent CNS limitations, therapists are often asked to estimate the long-term needs of the patient to establish potential costs of long-term therapeutic management over the lifetime of the patient.

SUMMARY

Payment for rehabilitation services is a complex topic that involves many legal, regulatory, and contractual details. To completely explain the complexities involved in documentation of patient care, medical billing, and claims adjudication would fill a volume similar to the size of this text. The authors have attempted to provide the treating therapist with a basic understanding of the payment systems involved in inpatient and outpatient services, the importance of documentation to the billing and payment process, provided basic steps for inclusion of diagnosis and intervention coding, and provided an overview of payment policy for outpatient services. Therapists must keep in mind that the regulatory and legislative world of health care is in a continual state of flux and that there are a number of critical areas that affect payment for services that were not touched on in this chapter. These would include the areas of Medicare and corporate compliance, the HIPAA privacy and security rules, currently evolving issues related to the Medicare caps on therapy services, and individual state practice acts for various health care providers. The reader would be well served to get specific questions and concerns addressed by knowledgeable individuals or to consult source documents on these important areas.

ACKNOWLEDGMENT

With sincere appreciation for editorial contributions by Bob Niklewicz, PT, DHSc.

REFERENCES

1. Centers for Medicare and Medicaid Services. *Medical home page:* http://www.cms.hhs.gov/medicare. Accessed July 2005.
2. Centers for Medicare and Medicaid Services. *History of medical page:* http://www.cms.hhs.gov/about/history/ssachr.asp Accessed July 2005.
3. Centers for Medicare and Medicaid Services. History quiz page: http://www.cms.hhs.gov/about/history/quiz/answers.asp#10. Accessed July 2005.
4. Centers for Medicare and Medicaid Services. *A brief history page:* http://www.cms.hhs.gov/publications/overview-medicare-medicaid/default4.asp. Accessed July 2005.
5. Centers for Medicare and Medicaid Services. *State Children's Health Insurance Program page:* http://www.cms.hhs.gov/schip/consumers_default.asp. Accessed July 2005.
6. American Physical Therapy Association. *HIPAA page:* http://www.apta.org/Govt_Affairs/regulatory/fraud_abuse/hipaa/Privacy/HIPAA_Summary2. Accessed July 2005.
7. American Physical Therapy Association *HIPAA security summary page:* http://www.apta.org/Govt_Affairs/regulatory/fraud_abuss/hipaa.security/aptasummaryofsecurityrul. Accessed July 2005.
8. Centers for Medicare and Medicaid Services. *Acute inpatient prospective payment system page:* http://www.cms.hhs.gov/providers/hipps/background.asp. Accessed July 2005.
9. Jette AM, Haley SM, Ni P: Comparison of functional status tools used in post-acute care, *Health Care Financ Rev* 24:3, 13-24, 2003.
10. Inpatient Rehabilitation Facility—Patient Assessment Instrument: Training manual, 2002.
11. UDSMR. *WeeIMF information page:* http://www.udsmr.org/wee_subinfo.php. Accessed July 2005.
12. Heaton WH, editor: *Revised long term care resident assessment instrument user's manual,* version 2.0, Miamisburg, OH, 2003, MED-PASS.
13. Centers for Medicare and Medicaid Services. *Home health services information page:* http://www.cms.hhs.gov/oasis/hhoview.asp. Accessed July, 2005.
14. American Physical Therapy Association: *Guidelines for physical therapy documentation of patient/client management.* Accessed September 1, 2006.
15. Hart AC, Hopkins CA, editors: *ICD-9-CM expert for physicians,* ed 6, volumes 1 & 2, Eden Prairie, MN, 2004, Ingenix/Medicode/St. Anthony Pub.
16. Wong DL, Hockenberry-Eaton M, Wilson D et al: *Whaley and Wong's nursing care of infants and children,* ed. 6, St. Louis, 1999, Mosby-Year Book, Inc.
17. Centers for Medicare and Medicaid Services. *Home health definition page:* http://www.cms.hhs.gov/glossary/search.asp?Term=homebound&Language=English&SubmitTermSrch=Search. Accessed July 2005.
18. Beebe M, Dalton JA, Duffy C et al: *Current procedural, terminology, standard edition,* Chicago, 2005, American Medical Association.
19. American Medical Association: *CPT general information page:* http://www.amaassn.org/ama/pub/category/3113.html. Accessed July 30, 2005.

APPENDIX 10-A ■ Quick Reference Guide to Acronyms

ADLs = Activities of Daily Living
AMA = American Medical Association
BBA = Balanced Budget Act of 1997
BBRA = Balanced Budget Refinement Act of 1999
BIPA = Benefits Improvement Act of 2000
CARF = Commission on Accreditation of Rehabilitation Facilities
CMS = Centers for Medicare and Medicaid Services
COBRA = Consolidated Omnibus Budget Reconciliation Act of 1985
CPT = Current Procedural Terminology
DRG = Diagnosis-Related Group
DSH = Disproportionate Share Hospital
EPHI = Electronic Protected Health Information
FI = Fiscal Intermediary
FIM = Functional Independence Measure
HCFA = Health Care Financing Administration
HCPAC = Health Care Professional Advisory Committee
HCPCS = Healthcare Common Procedure Coding System
HEW = Department of Health, Education, and Welfare

HHA = Home Health Agency
HHS = Department of Health and Human Services
HIPAA = Health Insurance Portability and Accountability Act
HMO = Health Maintenance Organization
ICD-9-CM = International Classification of Diseases, Ninth Revision, Clinical Modification
IME = Indirect Medical Education
IPPS = Inpatient Prospective Payment System
IRF-PAI = Inpatient Rehabilitation Facility—Patient Assessment Instrument
JCAHO = Joint Commission on Accreditation of Healthcare Organizations
LCD = Local Coverage Decisions
LTC = Long Term Care
MDS = Minimum Data Set

NEC = Not Elsewhere Classified
NOS = Not Otherwise Specified
OASIS = Outcome and Assessment Information Set
OBQI = Outcome-based Quality Improvement
POC = Plan of Care
PPS = Prospective Payment System
RAI = Resident Assessment Instrument = MDS + RAPs + Utilization Guidelines
RAP = Resident Assessment Protocols
RUGs-III = Resource Utilization Groups, Version III
SCHIP = State Children's Health Insurance Plan
SNF = Skilled Nursing Facility
SSA = Social Security Administration
TLC = Transitional Living Center
WHO = World Health Organization

HHA = Home Health Agency
DHHS = Department of Health and Human Services
HIPAA = Health Insurance Portability and Accountability Act
HMO = Health Maintenance Organization
ICD = International Classification of Diseases, Ninth Revision
IME = Indirect Cost of Education
IPS = Inpatient Prospective Payment System
LTCH-PAI = Long-Term Care Hospital — Patient Assessment Instrument
OASIS = Based Coordination of Care Research in Healthcare Outcomes
LCD = Local Coverage Decision
LOS = Length of stay
MDS = Minimum Data Set

NEC = Not Elsewhere Classified
NOS = Not otherwise specified
OASIS = Outcome and Assessment Information Set
OMC = Outcome-based Quality Improvement
POC = Plan of Care
PPS = Prospective Payment System
RAP = Resident Assessment Instrument; MDS = RAP Utilization
RAI = Resident Assessment Instrument
RUG-III = Resource Utilization Group, Version III
SCHIP = State Children's Health Insurance Program
SNF = Skilled nursing facility
SSA = Social Security Administration
TPL = Third-party liability
RHC = Rural Health Clinic

CHAPTER 11

Neonates and Infants at Neurodevelopmental Risk

Jane K. Sweeney, PhD, PT, PCS

KEY WORDS

high-risk clinical signs
neonatal neuropathology
neuromotor assessment
neuromotor intervention
neonatal intensive care unit environment
parent instruction
physiological and musculoskeletal risks
subspecialty training

OBJECTIVES

After reading this chapter the student/therapist will be able to:

1. Discuss three theoretical frameworks guiding neonatal therapy services in the neonatal intensive care unit.
2. Identify the physiological and structural vulnerabilities of preterm infants that predispose them to stress during neonatal therapy procedures.
3. Outline supervised clinical practicum components and pediatric clinical experiences to prepare for entry into neonatal intensive care unit practice.
4. Describe how the grief process may affect behavior and caregiving performance of parents of low-birth-weight neonates.
5. Differentiate the developmental course and neuromotor risk signs in infants with emerging neuromotor impairment from the clinical characteristics of infants with transient movement dysfunction.
6. Identify instruments for neuromotor examination of high-risk infants in neonatal intensive care units and in follow-up clinics and compare psychometric features of the tests.
7. Describe program plans for low-birth-weight infants in neonatal intensive care unit and home settings.

In the past 4 decades, specialized neonatal intensive care units (NICUs) and technological advances have contributed to a dramatic decline in neonatal mortality rates, particularly among low-birth-weight (LBW) infants (defined as weighing less than 2500 g). Between 1960 and 1983 the rate of survival for infants of birth weights between 500 and 1000 g increased from 1% to 45%, and from 42% to 85% for neonates weighing between 1000 and 1500 g.[1-3] Within the past 10 years further gains have been achieved for the smallest group, extremely LBW (ELBW) infants (defined as weighing less than 1000 g). For neonates weighing between 500 and 800 g at birth, the survival rate increased from 40% in the 1980s to 60% in the 1990s.[3,4] Because premature birth is associated with an increased risk of neurological injury, the improved survival rates of very small infants are associated with an increased prevalence of major and minor neurodevelopmental disabilities. Over the past 20 years the prevalence of children with cerebral palsy has increased an estimated 20%, with the rise primarily occurring among very LBW (VLBW) infants (defined as weighing less than 1500 g), in whom the incidence of cerebral palsy has increased threefold.[1,2,4-6]

Although new diagnostic techniques such as cranial ultrasonography can document brain injury during the neonatal period, prediction of subsequent neurodevelopmental outcome is still unreliable and imprecise. Careful developmental assessment continues to be required during the outpatient phase of care for NICU graduates. Pediatric therapists serve the increasing numbers of surviving neonates at neurodevelopmental risk by (1) providing valuable diagnostic data through neurological and developmental examination, (2) facilitating and coordinating interdisciplinary case management for infants and parents, and (3) reinforcing the preventive aspects of health care through early intervention and long-term developmental monitoring.

Clinical management of preterm infants and their parents during the NICU and outpatient follow-up phases is the focus of this chapter. A theoretical framework for neonatal practice and an overview of neonatal neuropathology related to movement disorders are presented. In-depth discussion in the neonatal section includes indications for referral based on risk, neurodevelopmental examination instruments, high-risk profiles in the neonatal period, treatment planning, and therapy strategies in the NICU. The section on outpatient follow-up focuses on a service delivery model for a high-risk infant clinic and includes neuromotor examination and evaluation, clinical decision making, and selected intervention strategies.

THEORETICAL FRAMEWORK

Concepts of dynamic systems, neonatal behavioral organization, and parental hope and empowerment provide a theoretical framework for neonatal therapy practice. In this section are three models that provide a theoretical structure for practitioners designing and implementing neuromotor and neurobehavioral programs for preterm infants and their parents.

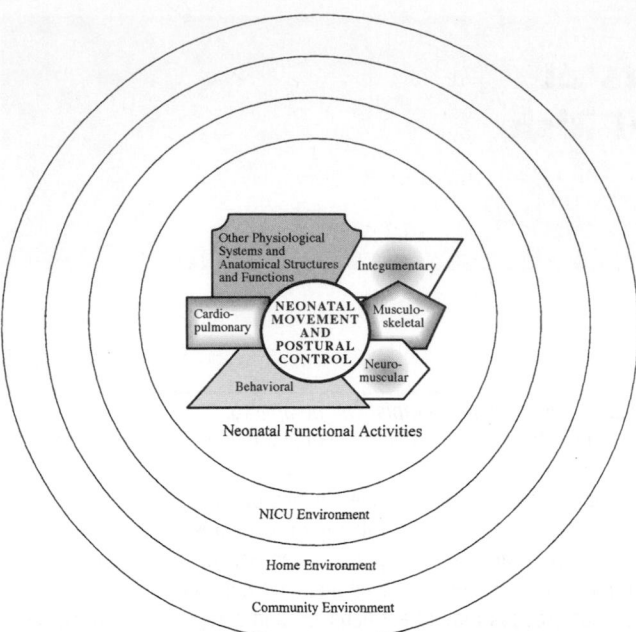

FIGURE 11-1 ■ Dynamic systems within neonates and interacting external environments influencing functional performance. (Reprinted from Sweeney JK, Heriza CB, Reilly MA, et al: Practice guidelines for the physical therapist in the neonatal intensive care unit [NICU], *Pediatr Phys Ther* 11:119, 1999.)

Dynamic Systems

Dynamic systems theory applied to infants in the NICU refers, first, to the presence of multiple interacting structural and physiological systems within the infant to produce functional behaviors and, second, to the dynamic interactions between the infant and the environment. In Figure 11-1, neonatal movement and postural control are targeted as a core focus in neonatal therapy, with overlapping and interacting influences from the cardiopulmonary, behavioral, neuromuscular, musculoskeletal, and integumentary systems. A change or intervention affecting one system may diminish or enhance stability in the other dynamic systems within the infant. Similarly, a change in the infant's environment may impair or improve the infant's functional performance.

This theory guides the neonatal practitioner to consider the many potential physiological and anatomical influences (dynamic systems within the infant) that make preterm infants vulnerable to stress during caregiving procedures, including neonatal therapy. In dynamic systems theory emphasis is placed on the contributions of the interacting environments of the NICU, home, and community in constraining or facilitating the functional performance of LBW infants.[7]

Synactive Model of Infant Behavior

The synactive model of infant behavioral organization is a specific neonatal dynamic systems model for establishing physiological stability as the foundation for organization of motor, behavioral state, and attention/interactive behaviors in infants. Als et al[8-10] described a "synactive" process of four subsystems interacting as the neonate responds to the stresses of the extrauterine environment. They theorized that

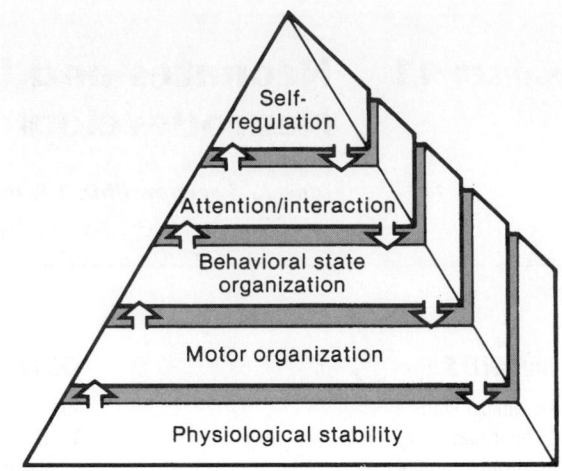

FIGURE 11-2 ■ Pyramid of synactive theory of infant behavioral organization with physiological stability at the foundation.

the basic subsystem of physiological organization must first be stabilized for the other subsystems to emerge and allow the infant to maintain behavioral state control and then interact positively with the environment (Figure 11-2).

To evaluate infant behavior within the subsystems of function addressed in the synactive model, Als et al[9,10] developed the Assessment of Preterm Infant Behavior. With the development of this assessment instrument, a fifth subsystem of behavioral organization, self-regulation, was added to the synactive model. The self-regulation subsystem consists of physiological, motor, and behavioral state strategies used by the neonate to maintain balance within and between the subsystems. For example, many preterm infants appear to regulate overstimulating environmental conditions with a behavioral state strategy of withdrawing into a drowsy or light sleep state, thereby shutting out sensory input. The withdrawal strategy is used more frequently than crying because it requires less energy and less physiological drain to immature, inefficient organ systems.

Fetters[11] placed the synactive model within a dynamic systems framework to demonstrate the effect of a therapeutic intervention on an infant's multiple subsystems (Figure 11-3). She explained that although a neonatal therapy intervention is offered to the infant at the level of the person, outcome is measured at the systems level, where many subsystems may be affected. For example, the motor outcome from neonatal therapy procedures is frequently influenced by "synaction," or simultaneous effects, of an infant's physiological stability and behavioral state. Physiological state and behavioral state are therefore probable confounding variables during research on motor behavior in neonatal subjects. Neonatal therapists may find this combined dynamic systems and synactive framework helpful in conceptualizing and assessing changes in infants' multiple subsystems during and after therapy procedures.

Hope-Empowerment Model

A major component of the intervention process in neonatal therapy is the interpersonal helping relationship with the family. A hope-empowerment framework (Figure 11-4) may guide neonatal practitioners in building the therapeutic partnership with parents; facilitating adaptive coping; and

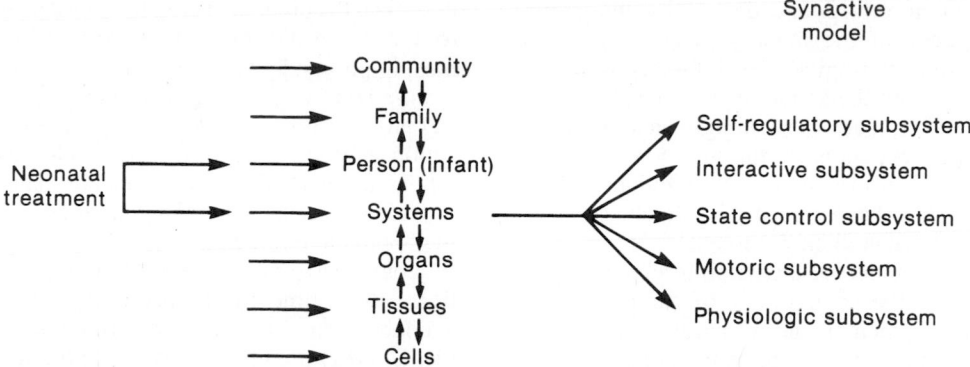

FIGURE 11-3 ■ Combined dynamic systems and synactive models. (Adapted from Fetters L: Sensorimotor management of the high-risk neonate. *Phys Occup Ther Pediatr* 6:217, 1986.)

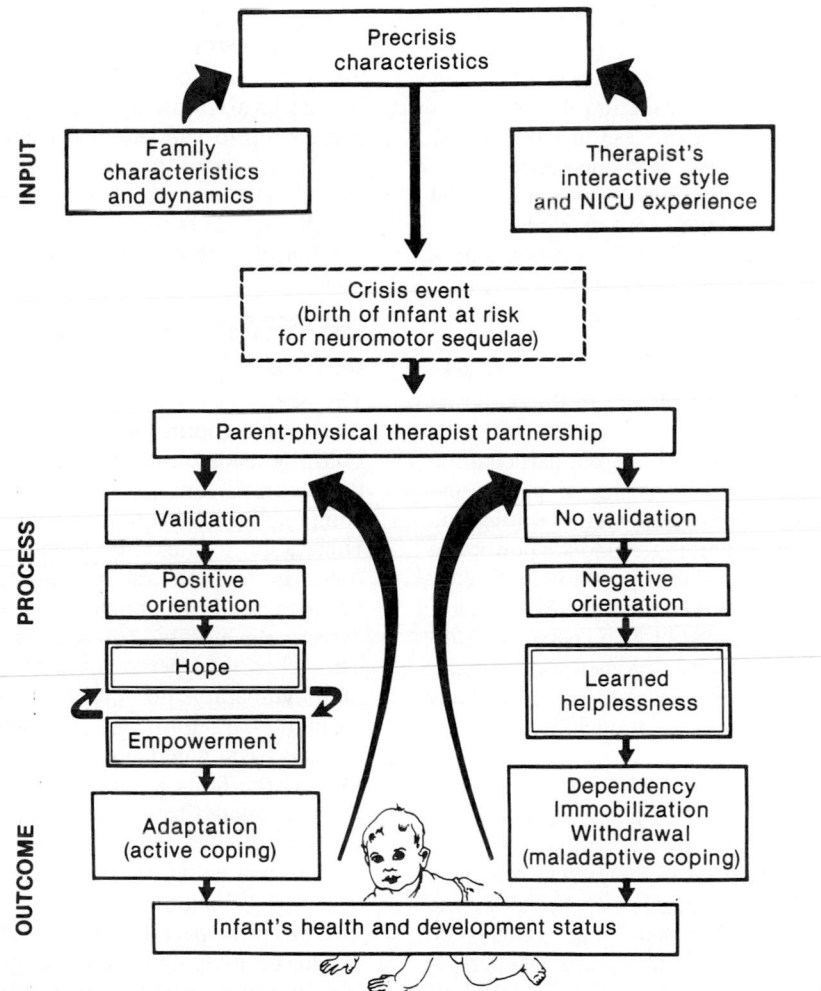

FIGURE 11-4 ■ Hope-empowerment *(left)* versus learned helplessness *(right)* processes of the therapeutic partnership between parents and the neonatal therapist.

empowering them to participate in caregiving, problem solving, and advocacy. The birth of an infant at risk for a disability, or the diagnosis of such a disability, may create both developmental and situational crises for the parents and the family system. The developmental crisis involves adapting to changing roles in the transition to parenthood and in expanding the family system. Although not occurring unex-

pectedly, this developmental transition for the parents brings lifestyle changes that may be stressful and cause conflict.[12]

A situational crisis occurs from unexpected external events presenting a sudden, overwhelming threat or loss for which previous coping strategies either are not applicable or are immobilized.[13] The unfamiliar, high-technology, often chaotic NICU environment creates many situational stresses that challenge parenting efforts and destabilize the family system.[14] The language of the nursery is unfamiliar and intimidating. The sight of fragile, sick infants surrounded by medical equipment and the sound of monitor alarms are frightening. The high frequency of seemingly uncomfortable but required medical procedures for the infant are of financial and humanistic concern to parents. No previous experiences in everyday life have prepared parents for this unnatural, emergency-oriented environment.

The quality and orientation of the helping relationship in neonatal therapy affect the coping style of parents as they try to adapt to developmental and situational crises (see Figure 11-4). Although parents and neonatal therapists come in to the partnership with established interactive styles and varying life and professional experiences, the initial contacts during assessment and program planning set the stage for either a positive or a negative orientation to the relationship.

Despite many uncertainties about the clinical course, prognosis, and quality of social support, a positive orientation is activated by validation or acknowledgment of parents' feelings and experiences. Validation then becomes a catalyst to a hope-empowerment process in which many crisis events, negative feelings, and insecurities are acknowledged in a positive, supportive, nonjudgmental context in which decision-making power is shared (S. O'Neil, personal communication, 1986). In contrast, a negative orientation may be inadvertently facilitated by information overloading without exploration and validation of parents' feelings, experiences, and learning styles. This may lead to magnified uncertainty, fear, and powerlessness with the misperception of excessive complexity in the proposed neuromotor intervention activities.

In a hope-empowerment framework, parent participation in neuromotor intervention allows sharing of power and responsibility and promotes continuous, mutual setting and revision of goals with reality grounding. Adaptive power can be generated by helping parents stabilize and focus energy and plans and by encouraging active participation in intervention and advocacy activities (S. O'Neil, personal communication, 1986). Exploring external power sources (e.g., Parents of Prematures or other parent-to-parent support groups) early in the therapeutic relationship may help parents focus and mobilize.[15]

Hope and empowerment are interactive processes. They are influenced by existential philosophy: the hope to adapt to what is and the hope to later find peace of mind and meaning for the situation, regardless of the infant's outcome. In describing the effect of a prematurely born infant on the parenting process, Mercer[16] related that "hope seems to be a motivational, emotional component that gives parents energy to cope, to continue to work, and to strive for the best outcome for a child." She viewed the destruction of hope as contributing to the physical and emotional withdrawal frequently observed in parents who attempt to protect themselves from additional pain and disappointment and then have difficulty reattaching to the infant.

Hope contributes to the resilience parents need to get through the arduous 1- to 4-month NICU hospitalization period and then begin to face the future in their home and community with an infant at neurodevelopmental risk. Groopman[17] proposed that hope provides the courage to confront obstacles and the capacity to surmount them. He described the process of creating a *middle ground* where truth (of the circumstances) and hope reside together as one of the most important and complex aspects in the art of caregiving.

In a hope-empowerment context, parent teaching activities are carefully selected to contribute to pleasurable interaction between infant and parent. Gradual participation in infant care activities and therapeutic handling in the NICU provide experience and build confidence for continuation in the home environment.

Conversely, if the parents' learning styles, goals, priorities, values, time constraints, energy levels, and emotional availability are not considered in the design of the developmental program, the parents may experience failure, loss of self-esteem, powerlessness, immobilization, or dependency. The neonatal therapist may recognize signs of learned helplessness in parents when they show nonattendance, noncompliance, negative interactions with infant and staff, or a hopeless outlook during bedside teaching sessions.

New events in the infant's health or developmental status may create new crises and destabilize the coping processes.[1] In long-term follow-up many opportunities occur within the partnership to validate new fears and chronic uncertainties within a hopeful, positively oriented, helping relationship. The alleviation of hopelessness is a critical helping task in health care. This model provides a conceptual framework for sharing with parents and caregivers the gifts of hope and power.

NEUROPATHOLOGICAL MOVEMENT DISORDERS

The neurodevelopmental outcome for infants born prematurely, or for term infants with prenatal or birth complications, depends on the *timing* of the brain injury as well as the *nature* of the insult to the developing brain. Different components of the fetal central nervous system are more vulnerable to noxious events or exposures at specific times in the maturational process. For example, insults occurring early in pregnancy typically result in neural tube defects, dysmorphic features, or congenital malformations. The subcortical periventricular region of the fetal brain is more vulnerable to injury during the gestational period, spanning the late second trimester and early third trimester, and the basal ganglia and cerebral cortex are more susceptible as the fetus approaches term. This selective vulnerability is related to the temporal sequence of maturation of specific structures and systems within the fetal brain, including vascular networks, metabolic processes, and myelination of the neural axons.

During the past decade improved technology and higher-resolution imaging equipment have provided more detailed insight into neurological structures and physiology, and previously held views regarding the development and pathological conditions of the fetal brain have been revised. The neuropathological conditions most directly related to movement disorders in preterm infants are now generally recognized to involve areas of the brain composed primarily of white matter as opposed to the gray matter areas such as the cerebral cortex, striatum, and cerebellum.[18] As stated by Paneth et al,[19] "The cardinal feature of brain damage in the preterm infant is injury to the hemispheric white matter."

The white matter is composed of axons and axon tracts that transmit nervous system impulses from one area of the

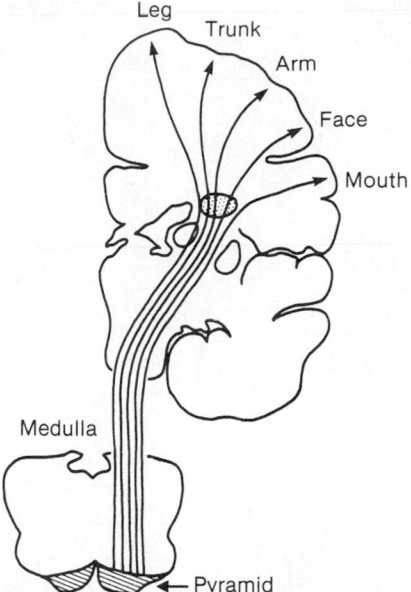

FIGURE 11-5 ■ Schematic diagram of corticospinal tract fibers that extend from the motor cortex through the periventricular region into the pyramid of the medulla.

brain to other areas of the central and peripheral nervous systems. The characteristic white color is derived from the myelin sheath of fatty acid that surrounds the axons. Because white matter regions include a predominance of motor projection fiber bundles, impairment of motor function is a logical consequence of injury in this location. In Figure 11-5 the vulnerability to injury is illustrated in the location of the medial corticospinal tract fibers that extend from the motor cortex through the periventricular region. In the next section two primary lesions of white matter, *periventricular leukomalacia* (PVL) and *periventricular hemorrhagic infarction* are described, as are other selected neuropathological conditions frequently found in preterm and term infants.

Germinal Matrix/Intraventricular Hemorrhage

The most common type of brain lesion occurring in the premature infant is hemorrhage, which typically originates in the subependymal layer of the germinal matrix (GM) and extends into the intraventricular space of the lateral ventricles (IVH). GM/IVH occurs in 20% to 30% of LBW infants, which represents a decline from a level of 40% to 50% more than a decade ago.[20-23] Reduction in the incidence of IVH is caused by improved neonatal management, including administration of indomethacin to high-risk neonates.

The GM is the source of the neuroblasts, or germinal cells of the cerebrum, and the glioblasts, which subsequently differentiate into astrocytes and oligodendrocytes. Toward the end of the second trimester of gestation, the GM is a region of high metabolic activity, and the endothelial walls of the vasculature in this area are immature and fragile. This anatomical vulnerability, coupled with the immaturity of vascular autoregulation at this time, contributes to the susceptibility to GM hemorrhage in response to fluctuations in cardiovascular pressure. In the majority of cases of GM

TABLE 11-1 ■ Grades of GM/IVH

GRADE	DESCRIPTION OF HEMORRHAGE
I	GM hemorrhage (no intraventricular hemorrhage)
II	Intraventricular hemorrhage into lateral ventricle(s) (no ventricular distention)
III	Intraventricular hemorrhage with distension of lateral ventricle(s)

hemorrhage blood extends into the lateral ventricles, and GM/IVH may or may not be accompanied by distention or dilatation of the ventricles.

Severity of GM/IVH is typically graded according to the location of the blood and the presence of ventricular dilatation. The criteria for grades I through III IVH are presented in Table 11-1. Older descriptions of IVH often included grade IV, described as an extension of the IVH into the brain parenchyma. However, this lesion is no longer recognized as a progression of IVH and is currently referred to as PHI.[21,23] Hydrocephalus, or progressive dilation of the ventricles, is a major complication of GM/IVH. A distinction is made by some neuropathologists between *hydrocephalus,* a ventricular enlargement resulting from disruption of cerebrospinal fluid absorption by a blood clot or other condition, and *posthemorrhagic ventriculomegaly,* which occurs subsequent to PVL or PHI.[23] In the posthemorrhagic type, ventricular enlargement is believed to result from passive expansion of the ventricles into adjoining periventricular areas of damaged white matter tissue, not because of increased intracranial pressure.[18,21]

The relation between GM/IVH and neurodevelopmental outcome has been investigated extensively since cranial ultrasonography became a routine NICU procedure for VLBW infants in the 1980s. However, reliable and consistent prediction is complicated by variations in the grading criteria used to describe the severity of IVH and in the outcome measures used in follow-up. Longitudinal studies that relate neonatal brain abnormalities to long-term outcome are often based on cranial ultrasound examinations performed with less-sophisticated technology as well as on less knowledge about neonatal pathological conditions than what is currently available. Consequently, earlier studies are more likely to associate adverse neurodevelopmental outcomes with GM/IVH, whereas more recent investigations evaluate outcome in relation to concurrent abnormalities, such as PHI and PVL, in addition to GM/IVH.[24] Because specific neonatal brain lesions usually do not occur in isolation but exist with other pathological features, attribution of a neurodevelopmental disability to a specific type of lesion can be misleading.

The neurodevelopmental outcome of infants with grade I or II hemorrhage is generally recognized to be favorable, with the majority of infants showing no adverse sequelae (Table 11-2).[25-27] Paneth et al[19] support this finding: "Since the germinal matrix is destined to involute,... and bleeding into the ventricles likewise in itself does not interfere with the function of any part of the brain: it is reassuring to discover that GM/IVH—the most common neurologic lesion in preterm infants, ... is not associated with a substantial risk of later disability." On the other hand, grade III IVH

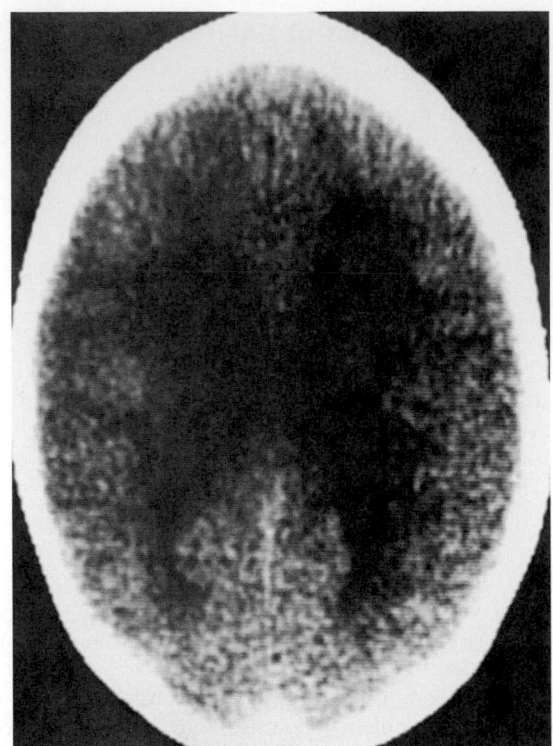

FIGURE 11-6 ■ Computed tomographic findings of dilated ventricles from a child with the spastic diplegia category of cerebral palsy.

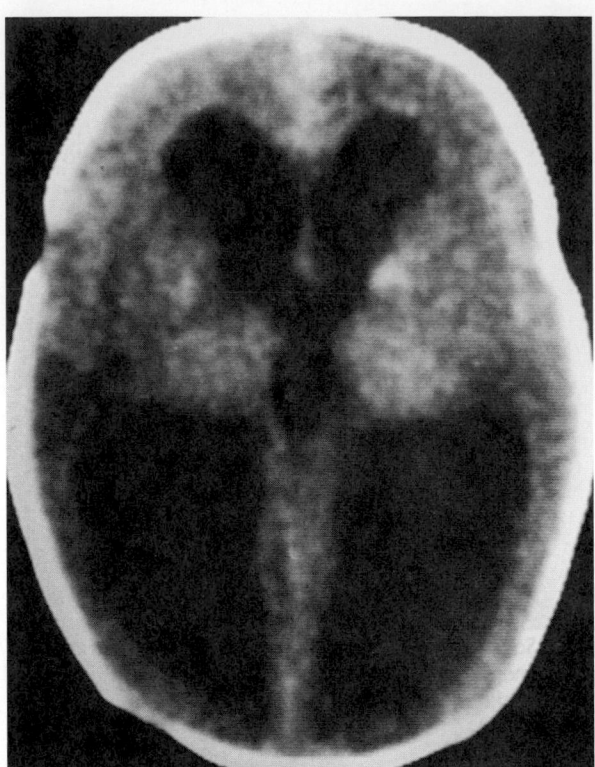

FIGURE 11-7 ■ Computed tomographic findings of ventriculomegaly and hydrocephalus in an infant with periventricular hemorrhagic infarction.

TABLE 11-2 ■ Neurodevelopmental Outcome of LBW and VLBW Infants Relative to Presence of GM/IVH

GRADE OF HEMORRHAGE	OUTCOME	
	MAJOR DISABILITY	CEREBRAL PALSY
I	5%	0%
II	15%	0%-5%
II	25%-60%	25%-50%

Data from references 19, 22, 24, 25, 27, 28, 29.

TABLE 11-3 ■ Neurodevelopmental Outcome of LBW and VLBW Infants Relative to PHI

SEVERITY OF PHI	OUTCOME	
	CEREBRAL PALSY	CONGENITAL DISABILITY
Localized	60%-80%	30%-50%
Extensive	80%-100%	40%-50%

Data from references 19, 23, 25, 32, and 37.

(i.e., IVH with ventriculomegaly) is associated with an increased risk of major neurological impairment.[25,26,28,29] Cerebral palsy has been reported to occur in 30% to 70% of neonates with persistent ventricular enlargement, and even transient ventriculomegaly appears to be associated with a greater incidence of neurodevelopmental disability (Figure 11-6).[18,25,28,30]

Periventricular Hemorrhagic Infarction

PHI refers to a relatively large region of hemorrhagic necrosis in the periventricular white matter. PHI occurs in approximately 15% of infants with GM/IVH, primarily those with grade III IVH.[23] Most PHI lesions occur in conjunction with a GM hemorrhage or IVH on the same side of the brain (Figure 11-7). PHI has a characteristic fan-shaped distribution that corresponds to the distribution of the medullary veins in the periventricular white matter.[19,23] These observations, as well as other characteristics of this lesion, con-

tribute to the current hypothesis that PHI is caused by venous infarction resulting from compression or obstruction of the medullary veins by a GM/IVH blood clot.[22] The concept of grade IV IVH that was described in earlier literature has generally been replaced by the current view of PHI as a lesion that is independent from IVH but may result as a complication of GM/IVH.[19] PHI in the LBW infant is associated with significantly increased risk for adverse neurological sequelae. Cerebral palsy, predominantly of the spastic quadriplegic or hemiplegic type, reportedly occurs in 60% to 80% of infants with this type of lesion (Table 11-3).[23,25,30,31]

Periventricular Leukomalacia

PVL refers to areas of cellular necrosis of the white matter in a specific location in the fetal brain adjacent to the external angles of the lateral ventricles. The terminology of PVL, which was derived from neuropathological studies conducted before the availability of routine ultrasonography, does not accurately describe the appearance of this lesion on cranial ultrasonograms of surviving preterm infants. Although some researchers recommend alternate designations, such as *white matter damage*, PVL remains the most widely used term. PVL occurs primarily in preterm infants, particularly those born between 28 and 32 weeks' gestation. Ultrasound studies with serial scans of VLBW infants indicated that 15% to 30% of surviving neonates demonstrate areas of periventricular echogenicity. For the majority of infants PVL is apparently transient; cystic PVL reportedly occurs in 5% to 11% of VLBW infants.[19,24,32,33]

The primary pathological manifestation of PVL consists of focal, or localized, areas of cellular necrosis believed to represent axonal degeneration. These areas are seen as echodensities on cranial ultrasonograms. Sequential cranial ultrasonograms of surviving neonates reveal a typical evolutionary course beginning with areas of increased echogenicity in the periventricular region. Over a period of days, cavitation occurs in the echodense areas, which then evolve into either small localized cysts, usually in the frontoparietal area, or extensive cystic lesions in the occipital and frontoparietal white matter.[19,26] This process of cyst formation occurs over a course of weeks so identification and classification of PVL depends on the timing and number of cranial ultrasound studies performed on the infant. Further investigation of these lesions with magnetic resonance imaging (MRI) revealed that the areas of localized brain injury are usually accompanied by broader, more diffuse regions of white matter damage extending beyond the periventricular area and often not detectable by routine cranial ultrasonography.[32,34] In contrast to the process of cyst formation, some echodense areas in the periventricular region resolve without evidence of residual abnormality and are referred to as transient periventricular echodensities (TPE), or *flares*.[33,35,36]

The pathogenesis of PVL is believed to involve ischemia coupled with unique aspects of the fetal brain. The characteristic location of PVL in the periventricular region appears to be related to the vascular distribution in this area. Earlier theories were based on the concept of "watershed" areas, described as boundary zones between arterial sources that might be inadequately perfused and therefore susceptible to ischemic injury.[23] Although this watershed view has not been upheld by recent neuropathological and ultrasonographic investigation, researchers continue to suspect that the localized distribution of PVL is related to a susceptibility to ischemia that is related to critical stages of vascular development in this region.[19]

A second key feature in the pathogenesis of PVL is the vulnerability of the cellular tissue at the time of injury. During the period between 28 and 34 weeks of gestation, myelin, which facilitates the transmission of nerve impulses, is deposited around the axons projecting through the periventricular region. Myelin is produced by glial cells, the oligodendrocytes, in a predictable sequence of time and location within the fetal brain during the latter half of gestation and the first year of life. Myelination appears to occur earlier in the deep white matter areas of the frontal, occipital, and parietal regions and later progresses to the temporal lobe and cortical areas.[2,18,37] Histological studies of areas of PVL reveal specific damage to the myelin-producing glial cells and infiltration by hypertrophic astrocytes, the progenitors of glial cells. The process of myelination, in which

TABLE 11-4 ■ Neurodevelopmental Outcome of LBW and VLBW Infants Relative to PVL

	OUTCOME	
SEVERITY OF PVL	MILD MOTOR DEFICITS	CEREBRAL PALSY
Transient echodensities (flares)	0%-30%	4%-10%
Persistent echodensities without cyst formation	0%-30%	7%-15%
Periventricular leukomalacia		
Localized cysts		25%-67%*
Extensive cysts		70%-100%*

*Bilateral cysts are associated with increased likelihood of poor outcome. Data from references 19, 25, 32, 33, and 41.

oligodendrocytes differentiate to produce the myelin sheaths, requires high levels of energy and glucose to synthesize the lipids and cholesterol necessary for myelin composition. During critical periods of gestation when the oligodendrocytes are differentiating within the fetal brain, these cells are hypothesized to be more susceptible to toxic influences, such as increased concentrations of glutamate and nitrous oxide.[18]

The relation between PVL observed on neonatal cranial ultrasonography and neurodevelopmental outcome depends primarily on the location, extent, and duration of periventricular echodensity and on the degree of cavitation or cyst formation (Table 11-4). Transient echodensities that resolve within 2 to 4 weeks appear to be of little prognostic significance relative to major disability. In contrast, infants with large cystic lesions, usually seen in the frontoparietal or frontoparietooccipital areas of the brain, are at high risk for major neurodevelopmental disability.[19,30,32,38,39] Bilateral cystic PVL is associated with spastic quadriparesis, whereas asymmetrical cysts are typically associated with spastic diplegia or hemiplegia.[40] Smaller areas of localized cystic PVL have been associated with less-severe cerebral palsy in 50% to 60% of cases.[32] Echodense areas that persist but without apparent cyst formation, observed in 10% to 20% of VLBW infants, are associated with a more variable outcome.[41]

The relation between neonatal PVL and subsequent motor disability is further supported by MRI studies of older children. MR images of children with spastic cerebral palsy have consistently revealed atrophy of white matter and high-intensity areas adjacent to the lateral ventricles.[32,34,35,42] In one study of *nondisabled* VLBW children at 6 years of age, periventricular gliosis observed in the white matter was associated with fine and gross motor deficits and inferior performance on tests of visual-perceptual function.[43]

Selective Neuronal Necrosis

Selective neuronal necrosis (SNN) refers to a type of brain injury that usually results from a neonatal hypoxic-ischemic event.[23] As the name indicates, it is characterized by necrosis of neurons, with a characteristic distribution in multiple areas of the brain. The primary regions of injury are the cerebral cortex, hippocampus, and cerebellum in the term infant; components of the brain stem (pons and inferior nuclei) in the LBW infant; and the basal ganglia and thalamus for both term and preterm infants. Severe oxygen deprivation appears to be a major factor in the pathogenesis of SNN, and it is frequently associated with intrapartum asphyxia in the term infant.[23] Although the hypoxic-ischemic event, such as total or near-total asphyxia, may be a global insult to the central nervous system, the selective vulnerability of specific areas of the brain is believed to reflect varying levels of metabolic activity in different regions at the time of injury. The neurological sequelae associated with SNN are related to the specific sites of necrosis. Injury in the cerebral cortex is associated with mental retardation and a high incidence of seizures. Neuromotor consequences, including hypotonia, spastic quadriplegia, and ataxia, result from damage in the cerebellum, basal ganglia, and regions of the motor cortex.

Parasagittal Cerebral Injury and Focal/Multifocal Ischemic Brain Necrosis

Two lesions primarily seen in term infants are parasagittal cerebral injury and focal/multifocal ischemic brain necrosis. Parasagittal cerebral injury, characterized by diffuse cortical atrophy and cystic lesions in the subadjacent white matter, occurs predominantly in the parietooccipital region. This type of injury, associated with perinatal asphyxia in term infants, is usually bilateral with fairly symmetrical distribution between the two hemispheres.[23] The most frequent long-term neurodevelopmental consequence of parasagittal cerebral injury is spastic quadriparesis. Focal ischemic brain necrosis refers to injury caused by infarction that leads to necrotic areas within a particular vascular distribution. The middle cerebral artery is the most common vascular site of injury in the term infant, occurring more frequently on the left side of the brain.[44] The neurodevelopmental consequences of this type of injury are determined by the location and extent of the lesion. Spastic hemiparesis, especially right hemiplegia, is the most common outcome, followed by spastic quadriparesis and seizures.

CLINICAL MANAGEMENT: NEONATAL PERIOD

Pediatric therapists with precepted, subspecialty training in neonatology and infant therapy can expand neonatal medicine efforts by creating clinical protocols and pathways designed to optimize the development and interaction of neonates and parents. The therapeutic partnership between parents and neonatal therapists during developmental intervention in the NICU sets the stage for competency in caregiving and compliance with follow-up in the outpatient period. General aims of NICU clinical management of infants at risk for neurological dysfunction, developmental delay, or musculoskeletal complications are to (1) promote posture and movement appropriate to gestational age and medical stability; (2) support symmetry and biomechanical alignment of extremities, neck, and trunk while multiple infusion lines and respiratory equipment are required; (3) decrease potential skull and extremity musculoskeletal deformities and acquired joint-muscle contractures; (4) foster infant-parent attachment and interaction; (5) modulate sensory stimulation in the infant's NICU environment to promote behavioral organization and physiological sta-

bility; (6) provide consultation or direct intervention for neonatal feeding dysfunction and oral-motor deficits; (7) enhance parents' caregiving skills (feeding, dressing, bathing, positioning of infant for sleep, interaction/play, and transportation); and (8) prepare for hospital discharge and integration into home and community environments.

Educational Requirements for Therapists

The examination and treatment of neonates are advanced-level, not entry-level, clinical competencies. Neonatology is a subspecialty within the specialty areas of pediatric physical therapy and pediatric occupational therapy. No amount of literature review, self-study, or experience with other pediatric populations can substitute for clinical training with a preceptor in a NICU. The potential for causing harm to medically fragile infants during well-intentioned intervention is enormous.[45-47] The ongoing clinical decisions made by neonatal therapists in evaluating and managing physiological and musculoskeletal risks while handling small (2 or 3 lb), potentially unstable infants in the NICU should not be a trial-and-error experience at the infant's expense. Therapists with adult-oriented training and even those with general pediatric clinical training (excluding neonatal) are not qualified for neonatal practice without a supervised clinical practicum (a minimum of 2 to 3 months). The NICU is not an appropriate practice area for physical therapy assistants, occupational therapy assistants, or student therapists on affiliations for reasons outlined by Sweeney et al[7]: "handling of vulnerable infants in the NICU requires ongoing examination, interpretation, and multiple adjustments of procedures, interventions, and sequences to minimize risk for infants who are physiologically, behaviorally, and motorically unstable or potentially unstable." The physical or occupational therapy assistant and student therapist are not prepared, even with supervision, to "provide moment-to-moment examination and evaluation of the infant and have the ability or modify or stop preplanned interventions when the infant's behavior, motor, or physiological organization begins to move outside the limits of stability with handling or feeding."[7]

Delineation of advanced-level roles, competencies, and knowledge for the physical therapist[7] and the occupational therapist[48] in the NICU setting have been described separately by national task forces from the American Physical Therapy Association and the American Occupational Therapy Association. These practice guidelines provide a structure for assessing competence of individual therapists working in NICU settings and offer a framework for designing clinical paths for specific neonatal therapy services.

A gradual, sequential entry to neonatal practice is advised by building clinical experience with infants born at term gestation as well as with physiologically fragile older infants and children and their parents. The experience may include managing caseloads of hospitalized children on physiological monitoring equipment, external feeding lines, and supplemental oxygen or ventilators. Participating in discharge planning and in outpatient follow-up of high-risk neonates are other options for providing exposure to examination, intervention, and family issues when the infants and parents are more stable. This clinical experience and a precepted practicum in the special care nursery offer the best preparation for appropriate, accountable, and ethical practice in neonatal therapy.[7,49]

Indications for Referral

Research efforts in recent years have been directed toward determining which neonates will have adverse neurodevelopmental outcomes. Specific prenatal, perinatal, and neonatal conditions associated with an increased likelihood of long-term neuromotor disability have been identified as risk factors. However, the predictive value of these risk factors is compromised by the absence of uniform or consistent definitions, differences in the study samples and follow-up procedures, and lack of standard measures of neurodevelopmental outcome. In addition, ongoing changes in obstetrical and neonatal procedures limit the applicability of findings from longitudinal studies of infants born in earlier eras of NICU care.

Tjossem's[50] categories of biological, established, and social risk provide a framework for categorizing indicators for neonatal therapy referral. An overview of developmental risk categories and risk factors for neonatal therapy referral is listed in Box 11-1 to assist clinicians in developing a referral mechanism for a clinical protocol based on risk categories.

Biological Risk

Biological risk refers to neurodevelopmental risk attributable to medical or physiological conditions in the prenatal, perinatal, or neonatal period.[50,51] Biological risks include placental abnormalities, labor and delivery complications, prenatal infection, and teratogenic factors. Examples of biological risk factors include asphyxia, neonatal seizures, prenatal exposure to cocaine or alcohol, and the cranial ultrasound abnormalities previously described. Birth weight is a strong predictor of outcome; in general, lower birth weight is associated with greater risk for adverse developmental outcomes.[1,3]

Respiratory disease is generally considered an important risk factor for motor and cognitive disability in LBW infants.[52] Although the presence of respiratory disease alone does not appear to be predictive of neurodevelopmental outcome, severity of disease does appear to be related to long-term outcome.[53] Infants with chronic lung disease or bronchopulmonary dysplasia have been found to be at increased risk for cerebral palsy and other neurodevelopmental abnormalities compared with preterm infants without bronchopulmonary dysplasia.[30,54] Prolonged mechanical ventilation and duration of supplemental oxygen were associated with increased risk of neurodevelopmental disability.[55] Administration of surfactant in the neonatal period has reduced the incidence and severity of respiratory disease in VLBW infants but has not been associated with a decline in neurodevelopmental disability in these children.[30]

Established Risk

Established risk is the risk for neurodevelopmental deficits associated with a diagnosis that is clearly established in the neonatal period. Included in this category are congenital malformations, chromosomal abnormalities, central nervous system disorders, and metabolic diseases with known developmental sequelae.

Environmental/Social Risk

Environmental/social risk involves developmental risk related to competency in parenting roles and factors in family dynamics. Such risk may be heightened by prolonged

---

BOX 11-1 ■ DEVELOPMENTAL RISK INDICATORS FOR NEONATAL THERAPY REFERRAL

BIOLOGICAL RISK

Birth weight of 1500 g or less
Gestational age of 32 weeks or less
Small for gestational age (less than 10th percentile for weight)
Prenatal exposure to drugs or alcohol
Ventilator requirement for 36 hours or more
Intracranial hemorrhage: grade III
Periventricular leukomalacia
Muscle tone abnormalities (hypotonia, hypertonia, asymmetry of tone/movement)
Recurrent neonatal seizures (three or more)
Feeding dysfunction
Symptomatic TORCH infections (*t*oxoplasmosis, *r*ubella, *c*ytomegalovirus infection, *h*erpesvirus type 2 infection)
Meningitis
Asphyxia with Apgar score less than 4 at 5 minutes
Multiple birth

ESTABLISHED RISK

Hydrocephalus
Microcephaly
Chromosomal abnormalities
Musculoskeletal abnormalities (congenitally dislocated hips, limb deficiencies, arthrogryposis, joint contractures, congenital torticollis)
Brachial plexus injuries (Erb's palsy, Klumpke's paralysis)
Myelodysplasia
Congenital myopathies and myotonic dystrophy
Inborn errors of metabolism
Human immunodeficiency virus infection
Down syndrome

ENVIRONMENTAL/SOCIAL RISK

High social risk (single parent, parental age younger than 17 years, poor-quality infant-parent attachment)
Maternal drug or alcohol abuse
Behavioral state abnormalities (lethargy, excessive irritability, behavioral state lability)

---

hospitalization of infants with the following characteristics: (1) suboptimal levels of stimulation and interaction (overstimulation or deprivation) in the NICU environment, (2) inadequate infant-parent attachment, (3) insufficient educational preparation of parents for caregiving roles, (4) meager financial resources of parents, and (5) limited or absent family support to assist in taking care of and nurturing the infant in the home environment.

It is common for LBW neonates to have a combination of risk factors from more than one major category. For example, an infant born prematurely to a single mother in a drug treatment program for heroin use during pregnancy is considered to be at both biological and environmental risk. In-depth study of perinatal and neonatal medicine and related obstetrical, neonatal nursing, and neonatal therapy literature is recommended before beginning to participate on the special care nursery team.

Neonatal Neurological and Pain Assessment

Multiple neonatal neurological and neurobehavioral examinations have been developed to calculate gestational age,[56,57] assess the integrity of the nervous system,[58,59] and describe newborn behavior.[8,59] Nine instruments with a range of neurological and behavioral tools used in current practice for management of both preterm and term infants are described. Most of these instruments offer quality data on motor performance and interactional behavior essential for developing individualized treatment plans. In addition, three pain assessment instruments for neonates are briefly reviewed.

Clinical Assessment of Gestational Age in the Newborn Infant

The Clinical Assessment of Gestational Age in the Newborn Infant was developed by Dubowitz et al[56] from data derived from a total of 167 preterm and term infants (28 to 42 weeks' gestation) tested within 5 days of birth. The tool focuses on criteria for calculation of gestational age from a composite of 10 neurological and 11 external (physical) characteristics.

This test rates criteria on a four-point scale; it is commonly administered by nurses or physicians in the newborn nursery. The accuracy (95% confidence limit) of the gestational age score is determined within a variation of ± 2 weeks on any single examination. This measurement error can be decreased to approximately ± 1.4 weeks when two separate examinations are performed. From the analyses of multiple tests on 70 of the 167 infants, the age score was equally reliable in the first 24 hours of age as during the next 4 days of life. The behavioral state of the infant during the examination is not considered a significant variable in testing.

Calculation of gestational age is an important adjunct to all other neonatal assessment tools. It guides practitioners in interpreting neurological and behavioral findings relative to the expected performance of neonates at various gestational ages. Additional guidelines on gestational differences in neurological, physical, and neuromuscular maturation can be found in the work of French pediatric neurologist Amiel-Tison.[57-59]

Newborn Maturity Rating

Ballard et al[60,61] designed a simplified modification of the Dubowitz gestational age tool. It has been widely adopted because of the time efficiency (3 to 4 minutes versus 10 to 15 minutes) and the elimination of active tone items, which are difficult to evaluate reliably in physiologically unstable newborns. The Ballard instrument involves only six physical and six neurological criteria, with a 0 to 5 scale and a maturity rating beginning at 20 weeks. It is designed to be used for neonates from birth through 5 days of age and has demonstrated concurrent validity with the Dubowitz gestational age calculation tool.

Neurological Examination of the Full-Term Infant

The Neurological Examination of the Full-Term Infant was designed by Prechtl[62] to identify abnormal neurological signs in the newborn period. The examination was developed from an investigation of more than 1350 newborns and was standardized on infants born at the gestational age of 38 to 42 weeks. If the test is used in premature infants who have reached an age of 38 to 42 weeks of gestation, lower resistance to passive movements (lower tone) may be expected. Delay of testing until a minimum of 3 days of age is advised to maximize the stability of behavioral states and neuromotor responses for improved reliability and validity of results.

The pattern of examination includes periods of both observation and examination. A 10-minute screening test is offered to determine if the full 30-minute examination of posture, tone, reflexes, and spontaneous movement is required. Although specific requirements for examiner training are not addressed, Prechtl offers a flow diagram (Figure 11-8) to assist clinicians with organizing the neurological examination process. Significant findings from the examination are summarized in the following categories: (1) quality of posture, spontaneous movement, and muscle tone (consistency and resistance to passive movement); (2) presence of involuntary or pathological movements (clonus, tremor, athetoid postures or movements); (3) behavioral state changes and quality of cry; and (4) threshold or intensity of responses to stimulation. Because of the transient pattern of neurological signs and rapid changes in the developing nervous system, Prechtl advised repeated examinations to monitor neurological status.

Neonatal Behavioral Assessment Scale

To document individual behavioral and motor differences in term infants, Brazelton and Nugent[63] developed a neonatal behavior scale to assess neuromotor responses within a behavioral state context. The 30- to 45-minute examination consists of observing, eliciting, and scoring 28 biobehavioral items on a 9-point scale and 18 reflex items on a 4-point scale. The reflex items are derived from the neurological examination protocol of Prechtl and Beintema.[64]

The scale was designed to assess newborn behavior in healthy 3-day-old term (40 weeks' gestation) white infants whose mothers had minimal sedative medication during an uncomplicated labor and delivery. Use of this examination with preterm infants requires modification of the examination procedure to the environmental constraints of an intensive care nursery and interpretation of findings relative to the gestational age and medical condition of the infant. For preterm infants approaching term (minimum of 36 weeks of gestation), nine supplementary behavioral items are offered. Many of these items were developed by Als[8] for use with preterm and physiologically stressed infants. In the manual,[63] methods of adapting the Neonatal Behavioral Assessment Scale (NBAS) for preterm neonates with accompanying case scenarios are described to illustrate use of the findings to enhance parent-infant interaction and guide developmental interventions.

Although the mean scores are related to the expected behavior of 3-day-old term infants, the NBAS is considered an appropriate assessment tool from 37 weeks of gestation until 44 weeks of gestation. Extended use of this scale for older infants was reported by Provost,[65,66] who described the methods for and results from administering the scale with the Kansas Supplements (five additional items on a 9-point scale) to 11 healthy, term infants during the first 4 months of life.

Six behavioral state categories are outlined in the NBAS: deep sleep, light sleep, drowsiness/semidozing, quiet alert,

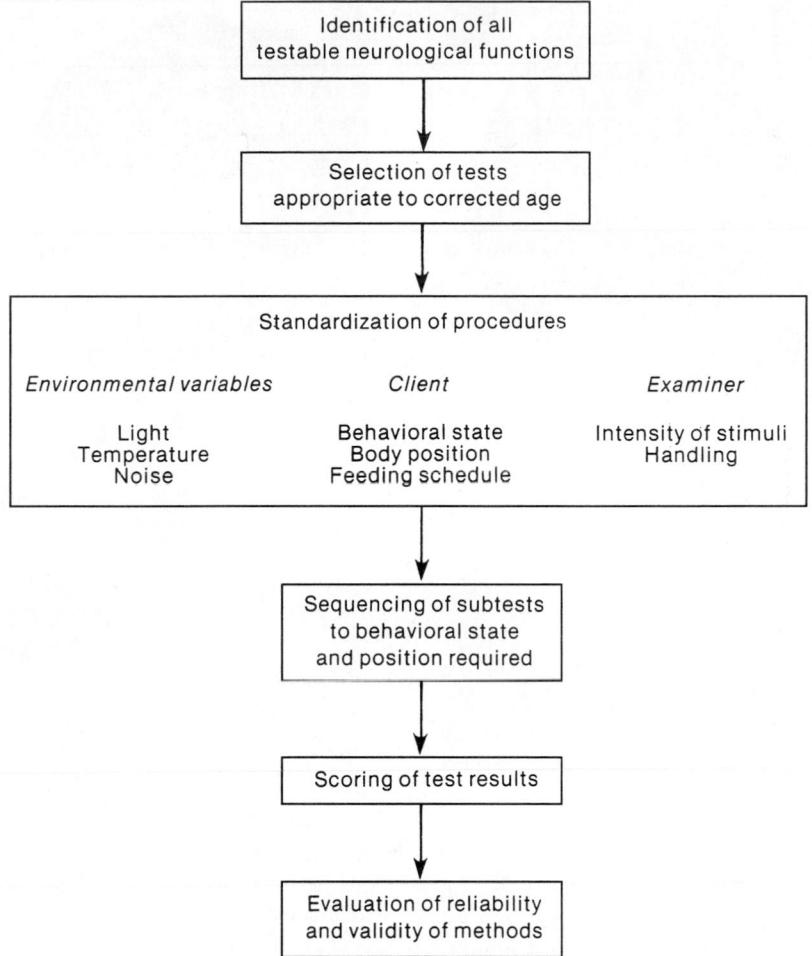

FIGURE 11-8 ■ Flow diagram illustrating decision steps in the neurological examination process.

active alert, and crying. Behavioral state prerequisites are provided for each biobehavioral and reflex item to reduce the state-related variables in testing. During the assessment the examiner systematically maneuvers the infant from the sleep states to crying and back to the alert states to evaluate physiological, organizational, motor, and interactive capabilities during stimulation and physical handling. The scoring is based on the infant's best performance, with flexibility allowed in the order of testing, repetition of items encouraged, and scheduling of the assessment midway between feedings to give the infant every advantage to demonstrate the best possible responses.

Four dimensions of newborn behavior are analyzed in Brazelton's NBAS: interactive ability, motor behavior, behavioral state organization, and physiological organization. Interactive ability describes the infant's response to visual and auditory stimuli (Figure 11-9), consolability from the crying state with intervention by the examiner, and ability to maintain alertness and respond to social or environmental stimuli.

Motor behavior refers to the ability to modulate muscle tone and motor control for the performance of integrated motor skills, such as the hand-to-mouth maneuver, pull-to-sit maneuver, and defensive reaction (e.g., removal of cloth from face). In the assessment of behavioral state organization, the infant's ability to organize behavioral

states when stimulated and the ability to shut out irritating environmental stimuli when sleeping are analyzed. Physiological organization is evaluated by observing the infant's ability to manage physiological stress (changes of skin color, frequency of tremulous movement in the chin and extremities, number of startle reactions during the assessment).

Performance profiles of worrisome or deficient interactive-motor and organizational behavior are identified by clusters of behavior associated with potential developmental risk. The cluster systems are highly useful for clinical interpretation and for data analysis in clinical research.[67]

Definite strengths of the NBAS are the well-defined indicators of autonomic stress, analysis of coping abilities of high-risk infants to external stimuli and handling, and quality of infant-examiner interaction. These features generate specific findings to assist therapists in grading the intensity of assessment and treatment within each infant's physiological and behavioral tolerance and in guiding the development of parent teaching strategies to address the individual behavioral styles of infants. The NBAS has proved to be more sensitive to the detection of mild neurological dysfunction in the newborn period than have classic neurological examinations that omit the behavioral dimensions.

Participation of the parent in the newborn assessment may yield long-term positive effects on infant-parent inter-

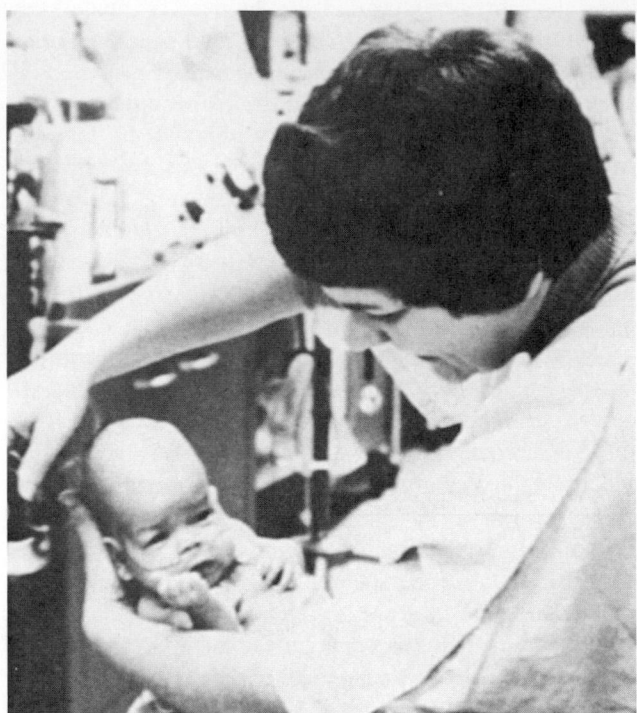

FIGURE 11-9 ■ Assessment of auditory orientation to the bell during neonatal assessment using the Brazelton Neonatal Behavioral Assessment Scale.

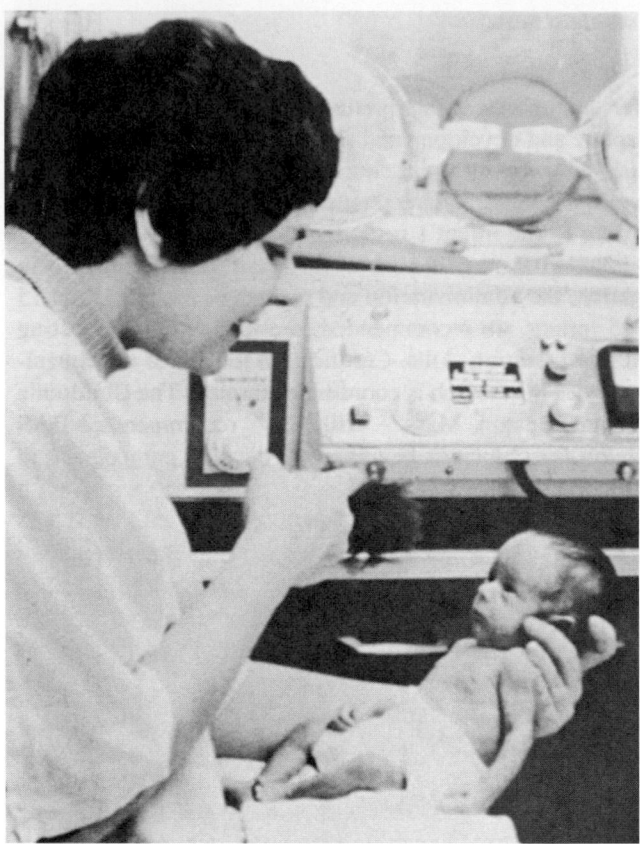

FIGURE 11-10 ■ Evaluation of visual orientation responses (i.e., visual fixation and horizontal tracking) during the Dubowitz Neurological Assessment.

action and later on cognitive and fine motor development. Widmayer and Field[68] reported significantly better face-to-face interaction and fine motor/adaptive skills at 4 months of age and higher mental development scores at 12 months of age when teenage mothers of preterm infants (mean gestational age at birth, 35.1 weeks) were given demonstrations of the NBAS. These demonstrations were scheduled when the premature infants had reached an age equivalence of 37 weeks of gestation.

Nugent[69,70] developed parent teaching guidelines for using the NBAS as an intervention for infants and their families. Published by the March of Dimes Birth Defects Foundation, the guidelines offer strategies for interpreting each item according to its adaptive and developmental significance, descriptions of the expected developmental course of the behavior (item) over several months, and recommendations for caregiving according to the infant's response to the item.

Four films are available for examiner training.[71] In addition, administration and scoring of the NBAS in 15 to 25 infants are recommended to establish reliable testing and interpretation skills. Certification for use of the NBAS in research is coordinated through The Brazelton Center for Infants and Parents, Children's Hospital, Boston, Mass.[72] Wilhelm[67] recommended NBAS training for clinicians beginning to develop competence in examining at-risk infants. She explained that it provides a system for developing basic handling skills with healthy, term infants without concerns of stressing medically fragile preterm infants during the training period. Learning the NBAS before the Assessment of Preterm Infant Behavior provides familiarity with similar testing and scoring procedures for preterm infants.[67]

Neurological Assessment of the Preterm and Full-Term Newborn Infant

The Neurological Assessment of the Preterm and Full-Term Newborn Infant is a streamlined neurological and neurobehavioral assessment designed by Dubowitz et al[73] to provide both a systematic, quickly administered newborn examination applicable to infants born preterm or at term gestation and a longer infant examination for children to 24 months of age. A distinct advantage of this tool is the minimal training or experience required by the examiner and the ease of adapting it to the infant and the environment. The adaptability of the test and use of the scoring form with stick figure diagrams have made it useful for implementation in developing countries where English is not widely spoken.

The test includes the six behavioral state categories of the NBAS and seven orientation and behavior items scored on a 5-point grading scale and sequenced according to the intensity of response. The orientation and behavior items consist of the following categories: (1) auditory and visual orientation responses (Figure 11-10); (2) quality and duration of alertness; (3) irritability: the frequency of crying to aversive stimuli during reflex testing and handling throughout the examination; (4) consolability: the ability after crying to reach a calm state independently or with intervention by the examiner; (5) cry: quality and pitch variations; and (6) eye appearance: absent, transient, or persistent appearance of sunset sign, strabismus, nystagmus, or roving eye movements.

The 15 items that assess movement and tone and the six reflex items evolved from clinical trials on 50 term infants using the Clinical Assessment of Gestational Age by Dubowitz et al,[56] the Neurological Examination of the Newborn by Parmelee and Michaelis,[74] and the Neurological Examination of the Full-Term Newborn Infant by Prechtl.[62] The examination format was then used during a 2-year period on more than 500 infants of varying gestational ages. After 15 years the authors revised the assessment in the second edition by eliminating seven items, expanding the tone pattern section, and developing an optimality score. Reliability data are not reported, but modification of examination procedures occurred during the pilot phase that promoted objectivity in scoring and a high interrater reliability among examiners, regardless of experience level.

The examination protocol is available in two formats: (1) Hammersmith Short Neonatal Neurological Examination and (2) Hammersmith Infant Neurological Examination (age range, 2 to 24 months). The examination forms are illustrated with stick figures and can accommodate both baseline and repeat assessments. For neonatal therapy examinations the forms can be effectively combined with a narrative impression, treatment goals, and plan of care. A numerical score for each item and a summary score are provided in the revised edition of the test. The authors advised that the scoring system was primarily intended for the purpose of research and for numerical charting of progress with sequential examinations. Because of the continued clinical emphasis on patterns of responses, selected parts of the protocol (without summary scoring) are appropriate for examining premature or acutely ill infants on ventilators, in incubators, or attached to monitoring or infusion equipment. Scheduling of examinations is recommended two thirds of the way between infant feeding sessions.

Evolution of neurological patterns in infants with IVH, PVL, and hypoxic-ischemic encephalopathy are described in the test manual and correlated with brain imaging. Abnormal neonatal clinical signs associated with long-term neurological sequelae were persistent asymmetry, decreased lower extremity movement, and increased tone. Infants with IVH had significantly higher incidence of abnormally tight popliteal angles, reduced mobility, decreased visual fixing and following, and roving eye movements. The authors cautioned that early signs of motor asymmetry in neonates with cerebral infarction may be associated with normal outcome, but normal neonatal neurological examinations after cerebral infarction do not exclude the possibility of later hemiplegia.[75]

Long-term follow-up data beyond 1 year have not been reported with this examination. Dubowitz et al[76] reassessed 116 infants (27 to 34 weeks of gestation) at 1 year of age. Of 62 infants assessed as neurologically normal in the newborn period, 91% were also normal at 1 year of age. Of 39 infants assessed as neurologically abnormal in the newborn period, 35% were found to be normal at 1 year of age. According to Wilhelm,[67] the predictive value of a negative test with this instrument was 92%, but the predictive value of a positive test was only 64%.

Interpretations of evaluative findings from the Neurological Assessment for Preterm and Full-Term Newborn Infants for neonatal therapy practice are comprehensively described in a case study format by Heriza[77] and Campbell.[78] Dubowitz[79] discussed the clinical significance of neurologi-

cal variations in infants and offered decision guidelines to clinicians on when to worry, reassure, or intervene with developmental referrals.

Assessment of Preterm Infant Behavior

Als[8] designed the Assessment of Preterm Infant Behavior (APIB) to structure a comprehensive observation of a preterm infant's autonomic, adaptive, and interactive responses to graded handling and environmental stimuli. As previously described in the theoretical framework section of this chapter, this assessment is derived from synactive theory and is focused on assessing the organization and balance of the infant's physiological, motor, behavioral state, attention/interaction, and self-regulation subsystems. The APIB has similar testing sequences and scoring format used in Brazelton's NBAS, with increased complexity and expansion for premature infants.

Administration and scoring of the APIB may require 2 to 3 hours per infant and often two or more sessions with the infant depending on examiner experience and infant stability. Although the APIB may be an instrument of choice for the clinical researcher, it is not practical (time efficient) for many neonatal clinicians with heavy caseloads in managed care environments. Extensive training and reliability certification are required to safely administer and accurately score and interpret the test for clinical practice or research.

Neonatal Individualized Developmental Care and Assessment Program

Als[10] and Als et al[10,80] developed the Neonatal Individualized Developmental Care and Assessment Program (NIDCAP) to document the effects of the caregiving environment on the neurobehavioral stability of neonates. This naturalistic observation protocol includes continuous observation and documentation at 2-minute intervals of an infant's behavioral state and autonomic, motor, and attention signals, with simultaneous recording of vital signs and oxygen saturation. Documentation occurs before, during, and after routine caregiving procedures. A narrative description of the infant's responses to the stress of handling by the primary nurse and to auditory and visual stimuli in the NICU environment is provided for developing bedside care plans. Options are described in the care plans for reducing aversive environmental stimuli and modifying physical handling procedures. This clinical tool allows neonatal therapists to determine the infant's readiness for assessment and intervention by observing the baseline tolerance of the infant to routine nursing care before superimposing neonatal therapy procedures.[81] Examiner training in the NIDCAP may be coordinated through the National Training Center at the Children's Hospital, Boston, Mass.[9]

NICU Network Neurobehavioral Scale

Lester and Tronick[82] developed a tool for preterm and drug-exposed infants from 30 weeks of gestation to 6 weeks postterm. The test consists of 115 items in general categories of neurological and neuromotor integrity, behavioral state and interaction, and physiological stress abstinence signs (drug-exposed infants). More than half (70) of the test items are infant observations, and 45 items require physical handling of the infant. Test-retest reliability of preterm infants indicated correlations of 0.30 to 0.44 at 34, 40, and 44 weeks of gestation. In the manual, normative neurobehavioral performance on the NICU Network Neurobehavioral Scale (NNNS) was reported for infants with prenatal polydrug exposure and for healthy, term infants. Training and certification on administration and scoring of the test are coordinated through Brookes Publishing Company and available in the United States and international sites with use of video-conferencing for lectures and demonstrations.

Test of Infant Motor Performance

Developed by Campbell et al,[83] the 42-item Test of Infant Motor Performance (TIMP) is focused on evaluating postural control, spontaneous movement, and head control for neonates at 32 weeks of gestation to 16 weeks postterm. Functional motor performance is assessed through observation of infant movement and through responses to various body positions and to visual or auditory stimuli. Psychometric qualities of the test include (1) construct validity[84] and ecological validity,[85] (2) concurrent validity at 3 months of age with the Alberta Infant Motor Scale,[86] and (3) predictive validity at 5 to 6 years of age with the Bruininks Oseretsky Test of Motor Proficiency[87] and at 4 to 5 years of age with the Peabody Developmental Motor Scales and Early Childhood Home Observation for Measurement of the Environment.[88] Training on test procedures is available through 2-day workshops or through a self-guided training method with a CD-ROM from the test developer.

Pain Assessment

Unlike early assumptions that immature myelinization prevented reception of pain or that memories of painful experiences were not retained in neonates, the current view is that infants *definitely* perceive pain. In fact, density of pain receptors in the skin of neonates at 28 weeks of gestation is considered similar to adult density and even exceeds adult density during maturation from birth to 2 years of age.[89-91] Blackburn[92] explained that although pain transmission in neonates occurs mainly through the slower, unmyelinated C fibers, the shorter distance in neonates that impulses travel to reach the brain compensates for the slower rate of transmission and creates substantial pain reception. Early pain experiences may create later increased sensitivity to pain and vulnerability to stress disorders.[93-95] If neonatal therapy procedures immediately follow a noxious medical procedure, precautions are needed in observing behavioral stress and motor responses and in modifying handling techniques or rescheduling the therapy session to avoid contributing to a cascade of aversive experiences for the infant.

In addition to practice guidelines on pain assessment and management developed primarily by neonatal nurses, numerous instruments are now available to assess pain in infants. Three multidimensional instruments used to assess pain in infants include (1) the Premature Infant Pain Profile (PIPP),[96] (2) CRIES: Neonatal Postoperative Pain Assessment Score,[97] and (3) Neonatal Infant Pain Scale (NIPS).[98] Psychometric data and clinical use of the pain tools are described for infants as early as 28 weeks of gestation. Indicators of pain summarized across the instruments include the following categories: (1) physiological (heart rate, oxygen saturation, breathing pattern), (2) behavioral (eye squeeze, brow bulge, facial grimace, behavioral state including crying, sleeplessness), or (3) motor (tone and movement in extremities).

Summary

Practitioners must be aware of the normative and validation data and of the predictive characteristics of the test(s) administered to allow appropriate interpretation of the results. Specific clinical training with a preceptor is essential to administer, score, and interpret neonatal assessment instruments accurately; to establish interrater reliability; and to plan treatment based on the evaluative findings. Even low-risk, healthy preterm infants are vulnerable to becoming physiologically and behaviorally destabilized during neurological assessment procedures.[99-101] This risk is reduced with precepted clinical training in the NICU.

Testing Variables

Neuromuscular and behavioral findings in the newborn period may be influenced by several variables. Increased reliability in examination results and in clinical impressions may occur when these variables are recognized. Medication may produce side effects of low muscle tone, drowsiness, and lethargy. Such medications include anticonvulsants, sedatives for diagnostic procedures (CT scan, electroencephalography, electromyography), and medication for postsurgical pain management. Intermittent subtle seizures may produce changes in muscle tension and in the level of responsiveness. Mild, ongoing seizures may present in the neonate as lip smacking or sucking, staring or horizontal gaze, apnea, and bradycardia. Stiffening of the extremities occurs in neonatal seizures more frequently than clonic movement. Fatigue from medical and nursing procedures can result in decreased tolerance to handling, decreased interaction, and magnified muscle tone abnormalities. Fatigue may also result when neurodevelopmental assessment is scheduled immediately after laboratory (hematologic) procedures, suctioning, ultrasonography, or respiratory (chest percussion) therapy. Tremulous movement in the extremities may be linked to conditions of metabolic imbalance (hypomagnesemia, hypocalcemia, hypoglycemia), and low muscle tone may be associated with hyperbilirubinemia, hypoglycemia, hypoxemia, and hypothermia.[102,103]

Treatment Planning

Level of Stimulation

The issue of safe and therapeutic levels of sensory and neuromotor intervention is a high priority in the design of developmental intervention programs for infants who have been medically unstable. The concept of "infant stimulation," introduced by early childhood educators in the 1980s to describe general developmental stimulation programs for healthy infants, is highly inappropriate in an approach based on concepts of dynamic systems, infant behavioral organization, and individualized developmental care.

For intervention to be therapeutic in a special care nursery setting, the amount and type of touch and kinesthetic stimulation must be customized to each infant's physiological tolerance, movement patterns, unique temperament, and level of responsiveness. Rather than needing more stimulation, many infants, especially those with hypertonus or those with tremulous, disorganized movement, have difficulty adapting to the routine levels of noise, light, position changes, and handling in the nursery environment. General, nonindividualized stimulation can quickly magnify abnormal postural tone and movement, increase behavioral state lability and irritability, and stress fragile physiological homeostasis in preterm or chronically ill infants. Implementation of careful physiological monitoring and graded handling techniques are essential to prevent compromise in patient safety and to facilitate development. Infant modulation, rather than stimulation, is the aim of intervention. Techniques of sensory and neuromotor facilitation and inhibition developed for caseloads of healthy infants and children are usually inappropriate for the developmental needs and expectations of an infant with physiological fragility or premature status (less than 37 weeks of gestation).

Physiological and Musculoskeletal Risk Management

Many maturation-related anatomical and physiological factors predispose preterm infants to respiratory dysfunction (Table 11-5). For this reason many LBW neonates require the use of a wide range of respiratory equipment and physiological monitors (Table 11-6). Pediatric therapists preparing to work in the NICU and those involved with designing risk management plans are referred to Crane's[104-106] overview of neonatal cardiopulmonary management for therapists and Peters'[5] analysis of physiological stress in preterm neonates during routine nursing procedures.

TABLE 11-5 ■ Factors Contributing to Pulmonary Dysfunction in Preterm Neonates

ANATOMICAL	PHYSIOLOGICAL
Capillary beds not well developed before 26 weeks of gestation	Increased pulmonary vascular resistance leading to right-to-left shunting
Type II alveolar cells and surfactant production not mature until 35 weeks of gestation	Decreased lung compliance
	Diaphragmatic fatigue; respiratory failure
Elastic properties of lung not well developed	Decreased or absent cough and gag reflexes; apnea
Lung space decreased by relative size of the heart and abdominal distention	Hypothermia and increased oxygen consumption
Type I, high-oxidative fibers compose only 10% to 20% of diaphragm muscle	
Highly vascular subependymal GM not resorbed until 35 weeks of gestation, increasing infant's vulnerability for hemorrhage	
Lack of fatty insulation and high surface area/body weight ratio	

Reprinted from Crane L: Physical therapy for the neonate with respiratory disease. In Irwin S, Tecklin JS, editors: *Cardiopulmonary physical therapy*, ed 2, St. Louis, 1990, Mosby.

In this subspecialty area of pediatric practice, neonatal therapists are responsible for the prevention of physiological jeopardy in LBW infants during developmental intervention in special care units. Before examination, discussion with the supervising neonatologist is advised regarding specific precautions and the safe range of vital signs for each infant. Medical update and identification of new precautions by the nursing staff before each intervention session are recommended because new events in the last few hours may not be recorded or fully analyzed at the time therapy is scheduled. The nurse should be invited to maintain ongoing surveillance of the infant's medical stability during neonatal therapy activities in case physiological complications occur. If medical complications develop during or after therapy, immediate, comprehensive co-documentation of the incident with the supervising nurse and discussion with the neonatology staff are essential to analyze the events, outline related clinical teaching issues, and minimize legal jeopardy.

Areas of particular concern during neonatal therapy activities include potential incidence of fracture, dislocation, or joint effusion during the management of limited joint motion; skin breakdown or vascular compromise during splinting or taping to reduce deformity; apnea or bradycardia during therapeutic neuromotor handling with potential deterioration to respiratory arrest; oxygen desaturation or regurgitation and aspiration during feeding assessment or oral-motor therapy; hypothermia from prolonged handling of the infant away from the neutral thermal environment of the incubator or overhead radiant warmer; and propagation of infection from inadequate compliance with infection control procedures in the nursery. Signs of overstimulation may include labored breathing with chest retractions, grunting, nostril flaring, color changes (skin mottling, paleness, gray-blue cyanotic appearance), frequent startles, irritability or drowsiness, sneezing, gaze aversion, bowel movement, and hiccups. Signals of overstimulation expressed through infants' motor systems are finger splay (extension and abduction posturing), arm salute (shoulder flexion with elbow extension), and trunk arching away from stimulation.[10]

Even a baseline neurological examination, usually presumed to be a benign clinical procedure, may be destabilizing to the newborn's cardiovascular and behavioral organization systems. The physiological and behavioral tolerance of low-risk preterm and term neonates to evaluative handling by a neonatal physical therapist was studied in 72 newborn subjects.[100] During and after administration of the Neurological Assessment of the Preterm and Full-Term Newborn Infant, preterm subjects (30 to 35 weeks of gestation) had significantly higher heart rates; greater increases in blood pressure; decreased peripheral oxygenation inferred from mottled skin color; and higher frequencies of finger splay, arm salute, hiccups, and yawns than in term subjects. Neonatal practitioners must examine the safety of even a neurological examination and weigh the risks and anticipated benefit of the procedure given the expected physiological and behavioral changes in low-risk, medically stable neonates.[99,100]

High-Risk Profiles

Three general high-risk profiles are observed from a dynamic systems perspective. These profiles identify movement abnormalities, related temperament or behavioral

TABLE 11-6 ■ Equipment Commonly Encountered in the NICU

EQUIPMENT	DESCRIPTION
Radiant warmer	Unit composed of mattress on an adjustable table top covered by a radiant heat source controlled manually and by servocontrol mode. Unit has adjustable side panels. Advantage: provides open space for tubes and equipment and easier access to the infant. Disadvantage: open bed may lead to convective heat loss and insensible fluid loss.
Self-contained incubator (isolette)	Enclosed unit of transparent material providing a heated and humidified environment with a servocontrol system of temperature monitoring. Access to infant through side portholes or opening side of unit. Advantage: less convective heat and insensible water loss. Disadvantage: infection control; more difficult to get to infant; not practical for an acutely ill neonate.
Thermal shield	Clear acrylic plastic dome placed over the trunk and legs of an infant in an isolette to reduce radiant heat loss.
Oxygen hood	Clear acrylic plastic hood that fits over the infant's head; provides environment for controlled oxygen and humidification delivery.
Mechanical ventilator	
Pressure ventilator	Delivers positive-pressure ventilation; pressure limited, with volume delivered dependent on the stiffness of the lung.
Volume ventilator	Delivers positive-pressure ventilation; volume limited, delivering same tidal volume with each breath.
Jet ventilator	Ventilator that delivers short bursts of air at high rates of flow; provides high-frequency jet ventilation.
Nasal and nasopharyngeal prongs	Simple system for providing continuous positive airway pressure; consists of nasal prongs of varying lengths and adaptor to pressure-source tubing.
Resuscitation bag	Usually a self-inflating bag with a reservoir (so high concentrations of oxygen can be delivered at a rapid rate) attached to an oxygen flowmeter and a pressure manometer.
Electrocardiogram; heart rate, respiratory rate, and blood pressure monitor (cardiorespirograph)	Usually one unit will display one or more vital signs on oscilloscope and digital display. High and low limits may be set, and alarm sounds when limits exceeded.
Transcutaneous oxygen ($TcPO_2$) monitor	Noninvasive method of monitoring partial pressure of oxygen from arterialized capillaries through the skin. The electrode is heated and placed on an area of thin epidermis (usually abdomen or thorax). The monitor has capability of providing both a digital display and a continuous recording of $TcPO_2$ values.
Intravenous infusion pump	Used to pump intravenous fluids, intralipids, and transpyloric feedings at a specific rate. Pump has alarm system and capacity to monitor volume delivered, obstruction of flow, and other parameters.
Neonatal vital signs monitor	Measures mean blood pressure and mean heart rate from plastic blood pressure cuff; values are digitally displayed on monitor.
Pulse oximeter	Measures peripheral oxygen saturation and pulse from a light sensor secured to the infant's skin; values are digitally displayed on the monitor; some models have continuous recording of values on strip charts.

Modified from Crane L: Physical therapy for the neonate with respiratory disease. In Irwin S, Tecklin JS, editors: *Cardiopulmonary physical therapy,* ed 2, St. Louis, 1990, Mosby.

characteristics, and interactional styles associated with motor status.

The first high-risk profile involves the irritable, hypertonic infant. These infants classically have a low tolerance level to handling and may frequently reach a state of overstimulation from routine nursing care, laboratory procedures, and the presence of respiratory and infusion equipment. They express discomfort when given quick changes in body position by caregivers and when placed in any position for a prolonged time. Predominant extension patterns of posture and movement are associated with this category of infants. Quality of movement may appear tremulous or disorganized with poor midline orientation and limited antigravity movement into flexion as a result of the imbalance of increased proximal extensor tone. Visual tracking and feeding may be difficult because of extension posturing or the presence of distracting, disorganized upper-extremity movement. In addition, increased tone with

related decreased mobility in oral musculature may complicate feeding behavior. Hypertonic infants frequently demonstrate poor self-quieting abilities and may require consistent intervention by caregivers to tolerate movement and position changes. These temperament characteristics and the signs of neurological impairment previously discussed may place infants at considerable risk for child abuse or neglect as the stress and fatigue levels of parents rise and as coping strategies wear thin during the demanding care required by irritable, hypertonic infants.[107,108]

Conversely, the lethargic, hypotonic infant excessively accommodates to the stimulation of the nursery environment and can be difficult to arouse to the awake states, even for feeding. The crying state is reached infrequently, even with vigorous stimulation. The cry is characteristically weak, with low volume and short duration, and related to hypotonic trunk, intercostal, and neck accessory musculature and decreased respiratory capacity. These infants are exceedingly comfortable in any position, and when held they easily mold themselves to the arms of the caregiver. Depression of normal neonatal movement patterns is common. To compensate for low muscle tone when in the supine position, some preterm infants appear to push into extension against the surface of the mattress in search of stability. Although potentially successful in generating a temporary increase in neck and trunk tone, the extension posturing from stabilizing against a surface in supine lying interferes with midline and antigravity movement of the extremities. Such infants dramatically respond to containment positioning in sidelying and prone. Drowsy behavior limits these infants' spontaneous approach to the environment and decreases their accessibility to selected interaction by caregivers. Feeding behavior is commonly marked by fatigue, difficulty remaining awake, weak sucking, and incoordination or inadequate rhythm in the suck-swallow process, with the need for supplementation of caloric intake by gavage (oral or nasogastric tube) feeding. The risk for sensory deprivation and failure to thrive is high for hypotonic infants because they infrequently seek interaction, place few if any demands on caregivers, and remain somnolent.

The third high-risk profile is the disorganized infant with fluctuating tone and movement who is easily overstimulated with routine handling but remains relatively passive when left alone. Disorganized infants usually respond well to swaddling or containment when handled. When calm, these infants frequently demonstrate high-quality social interaction and efficient feeding with coordinated suck-swallow sequence. When distracted and overstimulated, however, these infants appear hypertonic and irritable. Caregiving for intermittently hypertonic, disorganized, irritable infants can be frustrating for parents unskilled in reading the infant's cues, in implementing consolation and containment strategies, and in using pacing techniques during feeding.

Although these profiles address the extremes in motor and behavioral interaction, they suggest a need for identifying different tolerance levels of handling for neonates with abnormal tone and movement even though long-term developmental goals may be similar. Few neonates will demonstrate all behaviors described in the high-risk profile, but outpatient surveillance of neonates with worrisome or mildly abnormal motor and interactive behavior is advised to monitor the course of those behaviors and the developing styles of parenting.

Timing

The timing of neurodevelopmental examination and treatment for infants with high-risk histories or diagnoses is based on the medical stability of the infant and, in some centers, gestational age. All therapy activities need to be synchronized with the intensive care nursery schedule so that nursing care and medical procedures are not interrupted.

Neonatal therapists should not interrupt infants in a quiet, deep sleep state but instead wait approximately 15 minutes until the infant cycles into a light, active sleep or semiawake state. Higher peripheral oxygen saturation has been correlated with quiet rather than with active sleep in neonates. Preterm infants reportedly have a higher percentage of active sleep periods in contrast to the higher percentage of quiet sleep observed in term infants.[109] Allowing the preterm infant to maintain a deep, quiet sleep by not

interrupting is a therapeutic strategy for enhancing physiological stability.

Timing of parent teaching sessions is most effective when readiness to participate in the care of the infant is expressed. Some parents need time and support to work through the acute grief process related to the birth of an imperfect child before participation in developmental activities is accepted. Other parents find the neonatal therapy program to be a way of contributing to the care of their infant that also helps them cope with overwhelming fears, stresses, and grief.

Treatment Strategies

In this section, components of treatment are addressed for enhancing movement, minimizing contractures and deformity, promoting feeding behaviors appropriate to corrected age, developing social interaction behaviors, and fostering attachment to primary caregivers. The areas of developmental intervention presented are management approaches to body positioning, extremity taping, graded sensory and neuromotor intervention, neonatal hydrotherapy, and oral-motor/feeding therapy; parent teaching is discussed here and on page 329. In managing an intensive care unit caseload, the constant physiological monitoring; modification of techniques to adapt to the constraints of varying amounts of medical equipment; scheduling of intervention to coincide with visits of the parents and peak responsiveness of the infants; and ongoing coordination and reevaluation of goals, plans, and follow-up recommendations with the nursery staff create many interesting challenges and demand a high degree of adaptability and creativity from the clinician. Willingness to change an established assessment plan, treatment strategy, or therapy schedule to meet the immediate needs of the infant, parents, or nursery staff is paramount. For some infants with prolonged periods of only borderline stability with handling, a discharge examination with recommendations for follow-up care may be the best practice. Productivity standards of billable hours used for other caseloads of stable pediatric or adult clients in the hospital are not appropriate for the NICU setting and require negotiation and reinterpretation with rehabilitation or therapy department managers to protect both the infant and the neonatal therapist.

Positioning

A diligently administered positioning program can greatly assist infants on mechanical ventilators, under hood oxygen, or in incubators to simulate the flexed, midline postures of the neurologically intact term newborn swaddled in a bassinet. Preterm infants characteristically demonstrate low postural tone, with the amount of hypotonia varying with gestational age. Infants born prematurely do not have the neurological maturity or the prolonged positional advantage of the intrauterine environment to assist in the development of flexion. They are instead placed unexpectedly against gravity and presented with a dual challenge of compensating for maturation-related hypotonia and adapting to ventilatory and infusion equipment that frequently reinforce extension of the neck, trunk, and extremities.

Imbalance of excessive extension may occur in preterm infants with prolonged mechanical ventilation who appear to gain postural stability in the nonfluid extrauterine environment by leaning in to or stabilizing against a firm mattress while in the supine position. De Groot[110] explained the postural behavior of preterm infants as an imbalance between low passive muscle tone and active muscle power. She theorized that because preterm neonates have prolonged periods of immobility (often in the supine position), exaggerated active muscle power may be observed in the extensor musculature, particularly in the trunk and hips. This imbalance of extension is viewed as nonoptimal muscle power regulation that may negatively influence postural stability, coordinated movement, and later hand and perceptual skills.[110]

Some neonates, especially those born at less than 30 weeks of gestation, may attempt to posturally stabilize by hyperextending the neck in supine or side-lying positions to compensate for maturation-related hypotonia.[111] According to Bly,[112] neck hyperextension posturing, without a balance of movement into flexion, may trigger later development of a host of related abnormal postural and mobility patterns to compensate for inadequate proximal stability. In some high-risk infants, excessive postural stabilizing into neck hyperextension may contribute to sequential blocking of mobility in the shoulder, pelvis, and hip regions. The potential components of this high-risk, hypertonic postural profile appear in Box 11-2.

Shaping of the musculoskeletal system occurs during each body position experienced by neonates in the NICU. A variety of positional deformities in the extremities and skull can result from inattention to alignment. In Table 11-7, common neonatal positional deformities, musculoskeletal consequences, and functional limitations are outlined. Supporting the skeletal integrity of LBW infants is challenging in the midst of numerous equipment obstacles, restricted physical handling because of physiological instability, and limited spontaneous movement. Infants with gastroesophageal reflux are frequently positioned on wedges that make symmetrical, midline postures difficult to maintain. Skull flattening may continue to evolve after NICU discharge from overuse of infant seats and limited prone play experiences. Plagiocephaly (asymmetrical occipital flattening) and a secondary torticollis may emerge when a strong head turn preference remains and parents do not vary the direction of head turn for sleeping and infant seat use.

Retracted shoulder posture (scapular adduction with shoulder elevation and external rotation) may accompany excessive neck and trunk extension posture in preterm infants. This abnormal posture can interfere with later reaching, shoulder stability in the prone position, and rolling during the first 18 months of life.[113,114] Excessive tibial torsion and out-toeing gait were reported in preterm infants at 3 to 8 years of age and traced to prolonged "frog leg" (excessive abduction and external rotation with foot eversion) in the NICU.[115,116]

Goals of neonatal positioning procedures include the following:

■ Optimize alignment toward neutral neck-trunk position, semiflexed, midline extremity posture, and neutral foot position
■ Support posture and alignment within "containment boundaries" of rolls, swaddling blanket, or other positioning aids; avoid creating a barrier to spontaneous movement and allow space for controlled extremity movement
■ Create positions that promote alert states for enhanced short-duration interaction and sleep states that promote comfort and physiological stability

---

BOX 11-2 ■ POTENTIAL COMPONENTS OF HYPERTONIC POSTURAL PROFILE

Hyperextended neck
Elevated shoulders with adducted scapulae
Decreased midline arm movement (hand-to-mouth)
Excessively extended trunk
Immobile pelvis (anterior tilt)
Infrequent antigravity movement of legs
Weight bearing on toes, insupported standing

TABLE 11-7 ■ Musculoskeletal Malalignment and Functional Limitations in Neonates

POSITIONAL DEFORMITY	CONSEQUENCES	FUNCTIONAL LIMITATIONS
Plagiocephaly	Unilateral, flat, occipital region; head turn preference; high risk for torticollis	Limited visual orientation from asymmetrical head position; delayed midline head control
Scaphocephaly	Bilateral, flat, parietal, and temporal regions	Difficulty developing active midline head control in supine from narrowing of occipital region
Hyperextended neck and retracted shoulders	Shortened neck extensor muscles; overstretched neck flexor muscles; excessive cervical lordosis; shortened scapular adductor muscles	Interferes with head centering and midline arm movement in supine; interferes with head control in prone and sitting; limits downward visual gaze
"Frog" legs	Shortened hip abductor muscles and iliotibial bands; increased external tibial torsion	Interferes with movement transitions in and out of sitting and prone positions; interferes with hip stability in four-point crawling; prolonged wide-based gait with excessive out-toeing
Everted feet	Overstretched ankle invertor muscles; altered foot alignment from muscle imbalance	Pronated foot position on standing; retained, immature foot flat gait with potential delay in development of heel-to-toe gait pattern from excessive pronation

From Sweeney JK, Gutierrez T: Motor development chronology: a dynamic process. In Kenner C, McGrath JM, editors: *Developmental care of newborns & infants*, St. Louis, 2004, Mosby.

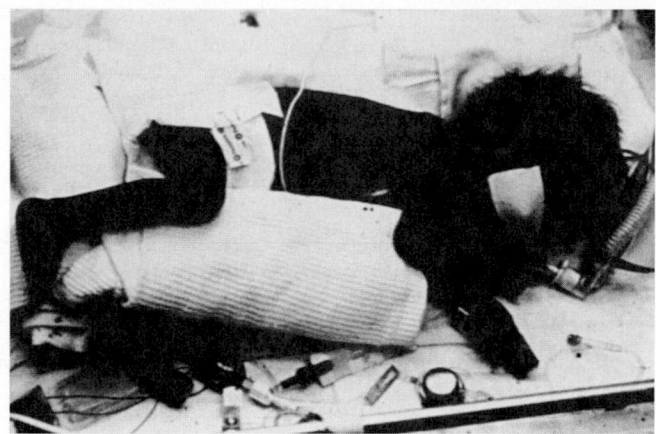

FIGURE 11-11 ■ Positioning with diaper rolls to reduce extension posturing.

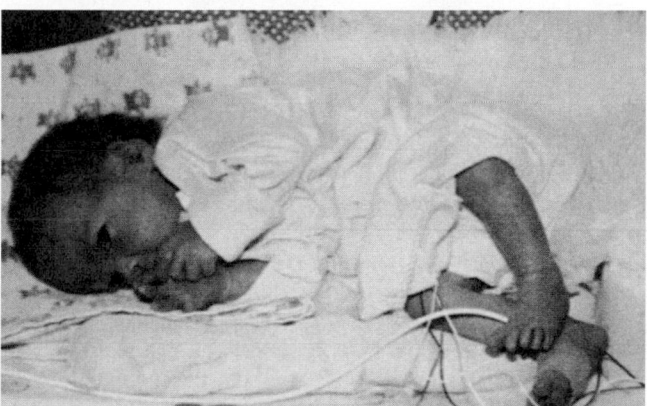

FIGURE 11-12 ■ Pacifier promotes flexion and long roll allows anterior and posterior containment of flexed side-lying position.

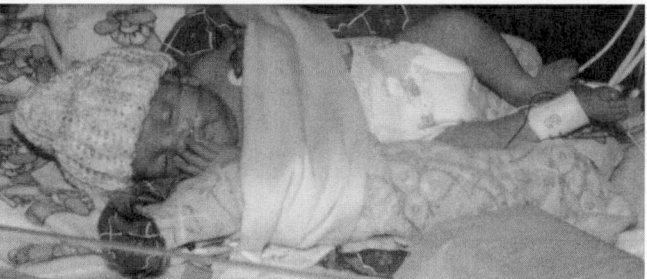

FIGURE 11-13 ■ A 6-inch-wide cotton stockinette is used to stabilize anterior and posterior rolls around the infant's body.

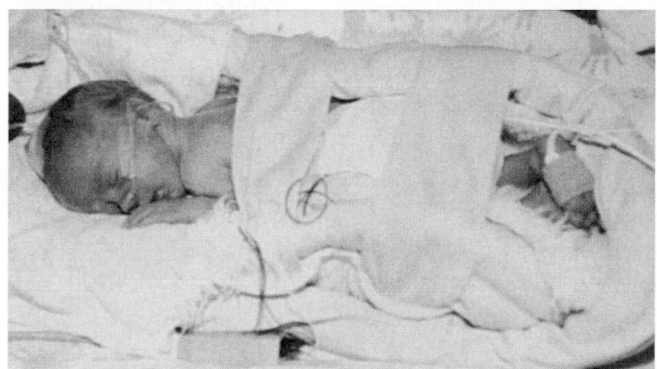

FIGURE 11-14 ■ Use of cloth bunting with circumferential straps, interior foot roll, lateral rolls, and sheepskin to promote body containment in prone flexion.

■ Offer positions that allow controlled, individualized exposure to proprioceptive, tactile, visual, or auditory stimuli while monitoring signs of behavioral and physiological stress from potential overstimulation

The use of blanket or cloth diaper rolls or customized foam inserts in a neonatal positioning program may modify increasing imbalance of extension in selected preterm or chronically ill infants and promote movement and postural stability from positions of flexion. After the infant is facilitated into a flexed posture in the side-lying position, posterior rolls behind the head, trunk, and thighs provide a surface against which the infant can posturally stabilize while a flexed midline posture is maintained (Figure 11-11). An additional anterior roll between the extremities and the use of a pacifier may promote further midline stabilization in flexion (Figure 11-12). Small neonates can be maintained in a flexed, symmetrical posture in a circular nest formed from a long blanket roll. Larger neonates may need additional stabilization from a folded blanket or stockinette band tucked over the nest of blanket rolls (Figure 11-13). Cloth buntings with circumferential body straps and a foot roll (Figure 11-14) provide positioning support and containment of extremity movement.

Endotracheal tube placement frequently contributes to the neck hyperextension posture in infants who require

mechanical ventilation (Figure 11-15). This iatrogenic component can be avoided by repositioning the ventilator hoses to allow enough mobility for slightly tucked chin and partially flexed trunk posture. For neurologically impaired infants with severe pulmonary disease necessitating prolonged ventilatory support, inattention to the alignment of the neck and shoulders may lead to the development of a contracture in the neck extensor muscles (Figure 11-16).

During the hospital stay, infants on ventilators (Figure 11-17) are now routinely positioned prone to enhance extremity and trunk flexion in the prone position, improve oxygenation, and decrease irritability.[117,118] Although placing infants on a sheepskin surface (see Figure 11-14) offers increased tactile input and has been correlated with increased weight gain in LBW infants compared with a matched group of infants on standard cotton sheets,[119] concern regarding the inhalation of microfibers from sheepskin has limited widespread use unless the sheepskin is covered by a thin blanket and used only to mid-chest level.[120]

Gel-filled, disc-shaped plastic head pillows of varying depths are options for distributing pressure on the side of the infant's head to reduce lateral head flattening in ELBW infants. In addition, water- or gel-filled mattresses may contribute to a nursery positioning program by providing a soft surface that is not conducive to postural stabilizing in extension. Other recognized advantages of waterbeds include increased vestibular and proprioceptive stimulation, decreased apnea, reduced head flattening, and improved skin condition.[121,122] After the infant is moved from intensive care to intermediate care, transition from a gel mattress or

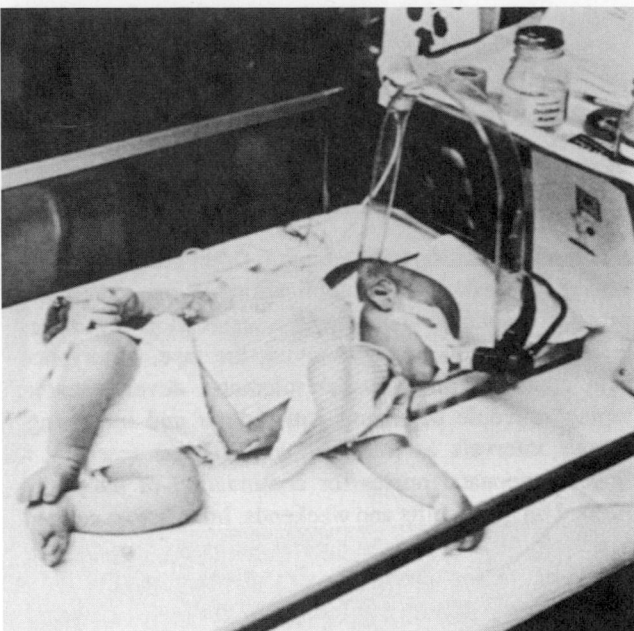

FIGURE 11-15 ■ Neck hyperextension posture magnified by the position of the endotracheal tube.

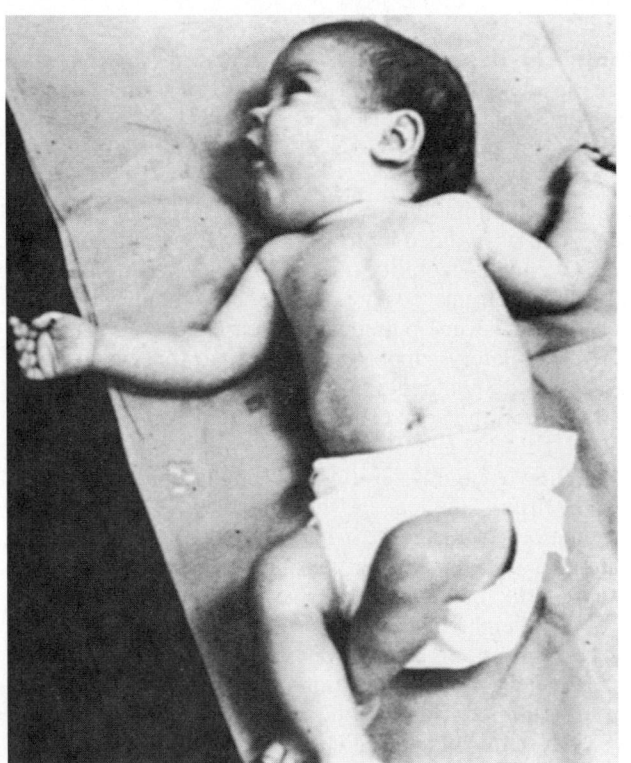

FIGURE 11-16 ■ Clinical presentation of contracture in neck extensor muscles related to hyperextension posture during prolonged mechanical ventilation.

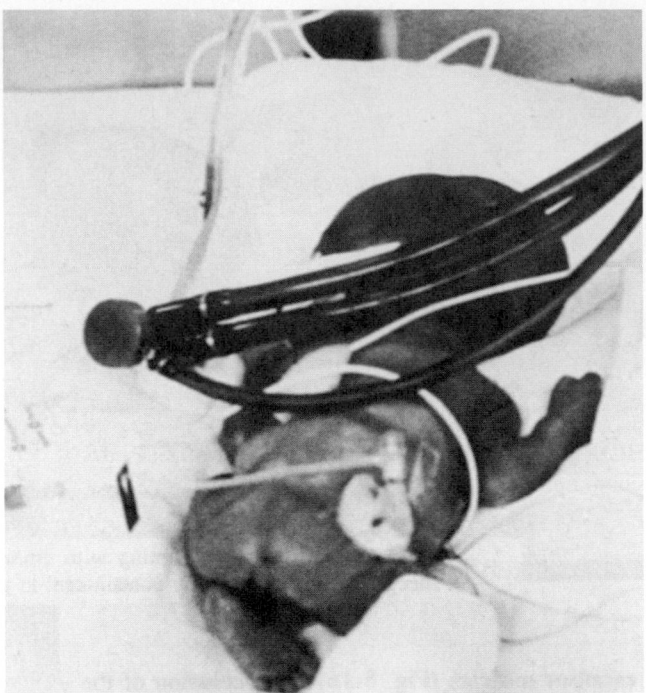

FIGURE 11-17 ■ Flexion posture enhanced in the prone position by the influence of the tonic labyrinthine reflex.

The neonatal therapist provides consultation on body alignment of infants in car seats when the LBW infant has not passed the peripheral oxygen saturation test in the car seat, which is usually conducted by the neonatal nurse before discharge. Some infants require the use of a car bed with body harness when they are unable to tolerate the semi-upright position of a car seat without oxygen desaturation.

Multiple studies of the effects of body positioning of neonates in NICU settings were reviewed and analyzed by Long and Soderstrom.[123] Continued research efforts are needed to measure effects of positioning and the risk-benefit effects of other neonatal therapy interventions to guide future directions of neonatal practice.

Extremity Taping

The presence of perinatal elasticity encourages early management of congenital musculoskeletal deformities in the neonatal period (birth to 28 days of age). A temporary ligamentous laxity is presumed to be present in the neonate because of transplacental transfer of relaxin and estrogen from the mother. In addition to the influence of maternal hormones, the rapid growth of the neonate can foster correction of malalignment if the deforming forces are expediently managed. This peak period of hyperelasticity offers pediatric therapists with advanced orthopedic expertise many opportunities to manage congenital joint deformities.[124]

Intermittent taping of foot deformities (Figure 11-18) has been more adaptable to the nursery setting than either casts or splints and is more effective in gaining mobility than range of motion exercises. Access to the heel for drawing blood, inspection of skin and determination of vascular status, and placement of intravenous lines can be accomplished with the tape in place or by temporary removal of the tape as needed. Therapists without a sound knowledge of arthrokinematic

waterbed to a standard mattress is recommended to allow time for adaptation to the type of mattress likely to be used at home. Infants are also transitioned to the supine sleeping position during the week before hospital discharge to reduce the risk of sudden infant death associated with the prone sleeping position and other factors.[120]

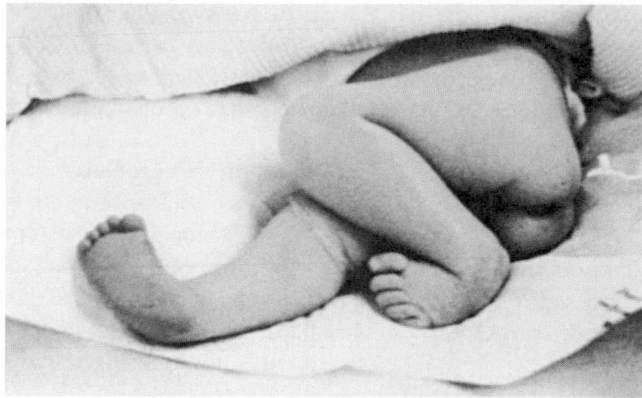

FIGURE 11-18 ■ Infant with lumbar meningomyelocele demonstrating marked varus foot deformities before taping.

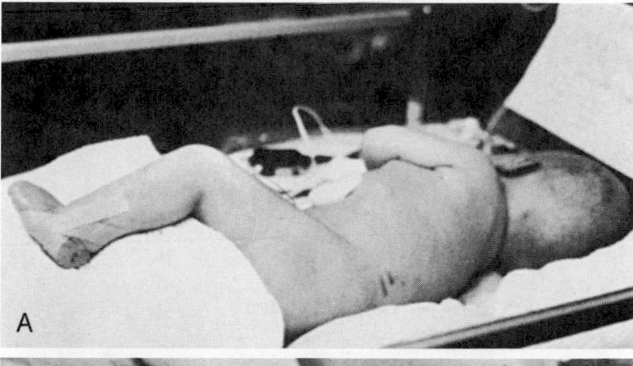

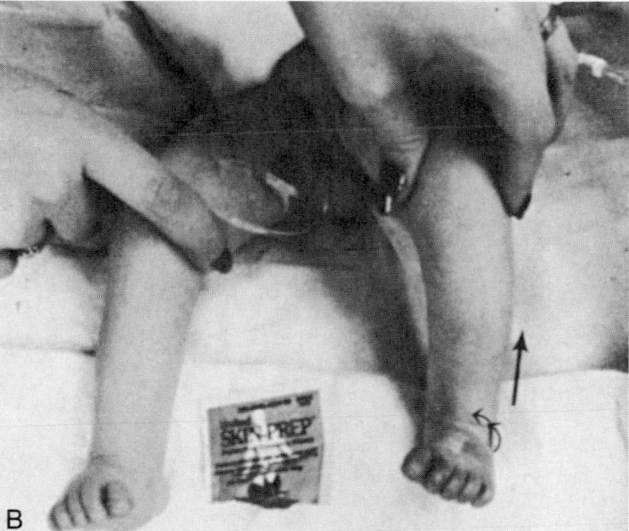

FIGURE 11-19 ■ Significant correction in alignment of varus foot deformities in neonate with a lumbar meningomyelocele. **A,** Lateral stirrup with open heel taping procedure. **B,** Moderate correction.

principles and techniques should not attempt the taping procedure, which involves articulation of the joint(s) into a corrected position before taping. Other components of the taping process include application of an external skin protection solution under the tape, application of an adhesive removal solution when removing the tape, observance of skin condition and vascular tolerance, development of a taping schedule beginning with 1 hour and increasing by 1-hour intervals as tolerated, and clinical teaching with selected neonatal nurses for continuation of the taping if needed on night shifts and weekends. Infants with congenital foot deformities required shorter periods of casting in the outpatient period after taping of the extremity (Figure 11-19) was implemented during the inpatient phase. Neither skin nor vascular complications have occurred during my 30 years of using silk tape to reduce deformity in neonates, even in infants with absent lower-extremity sensation resulting from meningomyelocele. Taping is not appropriate for medically fragile infants on minimal handling protocols or for infants younger than 30 to 32 weeks of gestation because of potential epidermal stripping from tape removal or vascular compromise from inadvertent, excessive compression by either the tape or the underwrap layer.

The availability of thin, self-adherent foam material now allows taping on an underwrap (bandage) layer rather than on the infant's skin (Figure 11-20). Although this method creates a definite advantage in skin protection, it may cover the calcaneal region for blood drawing. Compromise in alignment may occur if the underwrap layer is applied loosely; conversely, restriction in circulation may be observed by edema or purple-blue color changes in the toes if the underwrap is excessively tight around the foot or ankle.

Infants with wrist drop from radial nerve compression related to intravenous line infiltration also benefit from the use of taping (Figure 11-21). The wrist is supported in a functional position of slight extension. As muscle function returns, the taping is used intermittently to reduce fatigue and overstretching of the emerging, but still weak, wrist extensor musculature.

Therapeutic Handling

Use of tactile, vestibular, proprioceptive, visual, and auditory stimuli to facilitate infant development has been reported and reviewed by many authors.[125-133] Selection and application of the sensory or neuromotor treatment options in neonatal therapy must occur with judicious attention to the prevention of sensory overload and related physiological consequences. Decision making on the type, intensity, duration, frequency, and sequencing of intervention within the context of infant physiological and behavioral stability can be learned only in a mentored clinical practicum in the NICU setting. The current general guidance on intervention is more observation, less handling, protection from bright lights and loud conversation, and readiness for handling determined on the basis of behavioral and physiological cues of the infant.[10,126,132,133]

Primary aims of therapeutic handling include assisting the newborn to achieve maximal interaction with parents and caregivers and facilitating the experience of postural and movement patterns appropriate to the infant's adjusted gestational age. Helping infants reach and maintain the quiet, alert behavioral state and age-appropriate postural tone appears to enhance opportunities for visual and auditory interaction and for antigravity movement experiences. The typical early movement experiences include hand-to-mouth movement, scapular abduction and adduction, anterior and posterior pelvic tilt, free movement of the extremities

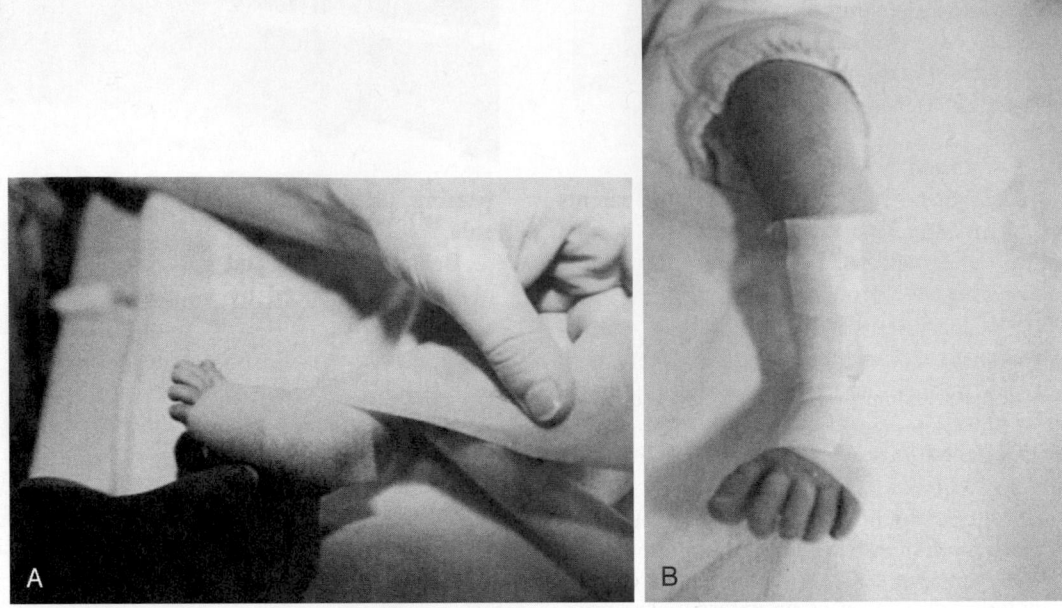

FIGURE 11-20 ■ Taping of varus foot deformity. **A,** Thin foam layer. **B,** Silk tape in lateral stirrup over foam layer.

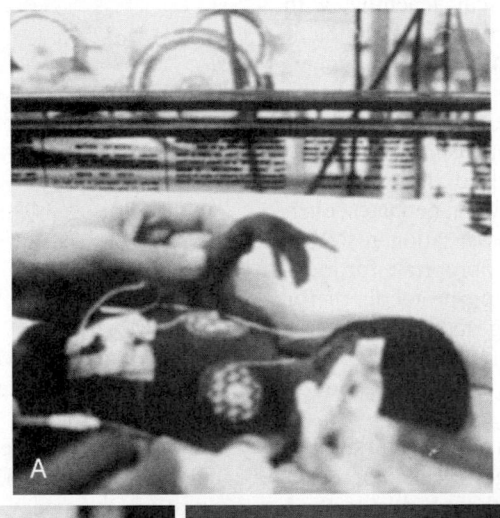

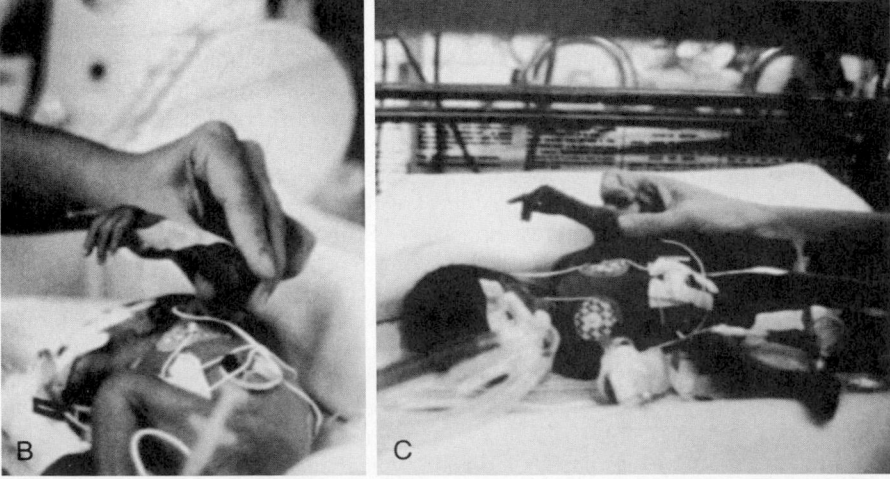

FIGURE 11-21 ■ Management of wrist drop in medically fragile neonate. **A,** Wrist drop before taping. **B,** Taping procedure. **C,** One week after taping.

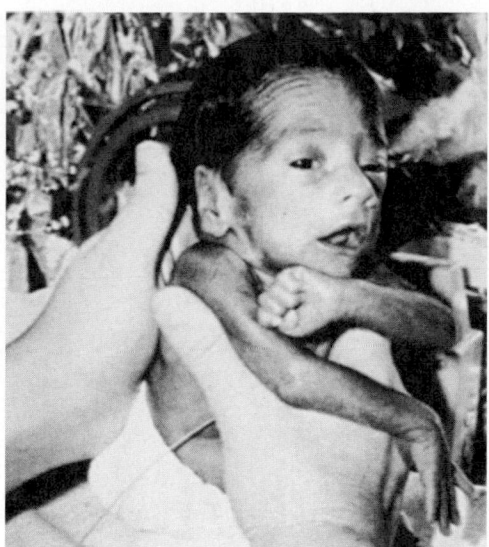

FIGURE 11-22 ■ Facilitation of head lifting by a neonatal nurse while burping the infant after feeding.

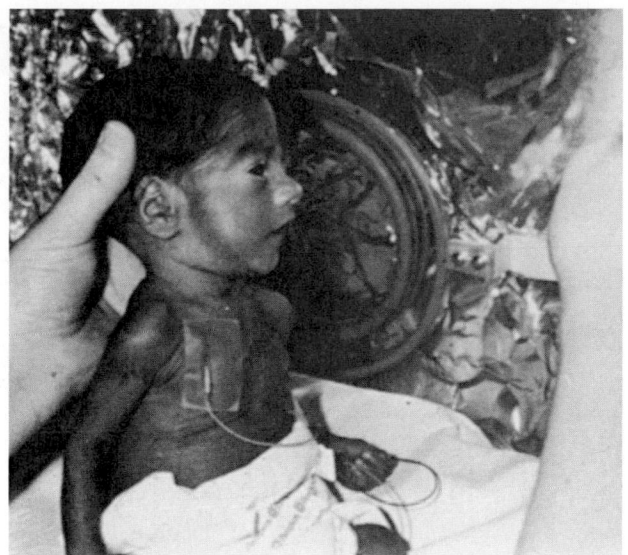

FIGURE 11-23 ■ Facilitation of visual following by a neonatal nurse during a change of the infant's position in the isolette.

against gravity, and momentary holding of the head in midline.[78,112]

Behavioral state and some movement abnormalities can be modified by creative swaddling and gentle weight shifts and nesting in the caregiver's lap. Swaddling the infant in a blanket with flexed, midline extremity position appears to promote flexor tone, increase hand-to-mouth awareness, inhibit jittery or disorganized movement, and elicit quiet, alert behavior. These effects can also be accomplished in skin-to-skin holding of infants against the parent's chest, a procedure now commonly adopted in NICUs in North America.[134,135] Application of neonatal therapy techniques must be contingent on both the infant's readiness for interaction and the need for a recovery break in interaction because of sensory overload. Teaching parents and caregivers to read and respond to the infant's motor cues for interaction, feeding, change of body position, and rest breaks is a critical quality-of-life component in the infant's NICU therapy program.

Incorporation of selected sensory and neuromotor activities into routine nursing care in the NICU increases developmental opportunities for the neonate during prolonged hospitalization. While feeding the infant in an incubator, the nurse may facilitate head lifting and momentary maintenance of the head in midline during the burping process in supported sitting (Figure 11-22). Techniques for inhibiting trunk and lower extremity hypertonus may be added during diaper changes. Modulated visual and auditory interaction may be integrated into nearly all parts of infant care (Figure 11-23), or they may be specifically reinforced as appropriate (e.g., visual orientation to human face, color photograph of family members' faces, or brightly colored animal toy; auditory orientation to human voice, taped soft conversation by parent reading a story, or taped sounds of nature).

A semi-inverted supine flexion position (Figure 11-24) with preterm neonates should be used with caution to facilitate elongation of neck extensor muscles and decrease the neck hyperextension posture. This position may compromise breathing from positional compression of the chest and

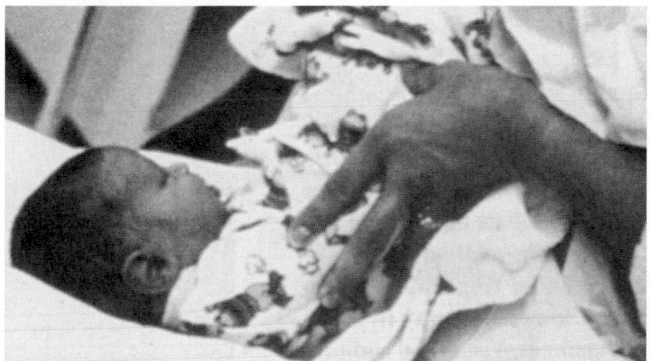

FIGURE 11-24 ■ Potential respiratory compromise to the infant from neck extensor muscle elongation in excessively flexed position while in supine position.

from potential airway occlusion associated with maximal flexion of the neck. The use of cardiorespiratory and oxygen saturation monitors during therapeutic handling activities is recommended for objective measurement of physiological tolerance. Although the peripheral oxygen saturation values from monitors may be intermittently unreliable because of motion artifacts from either the infant's spontaneous movement or the therapist's handling of the infant, reliable readings of oxygen saturation may be taken approximately 1 minute after the infant's body is not moved.

Easily overstimulated preterm infants may not tolerate multimodal sensory stimulation but may instead respond to a single sensory stimulus.[50,130] Implementation of a positioning program, oral-motor therapy, environmental modifications, and reinforcement of developmental activities with parents can be instituted only in collaboration with the shifts of bedside nurses who are in charge of the infant's 24-hour day in the NICU. Collaboration with nurses is a major component of precepted neonatal therapy training and requires integration into and valuing of the unique culture of the NICU.[81] Part of NICU culture is the unique ecology

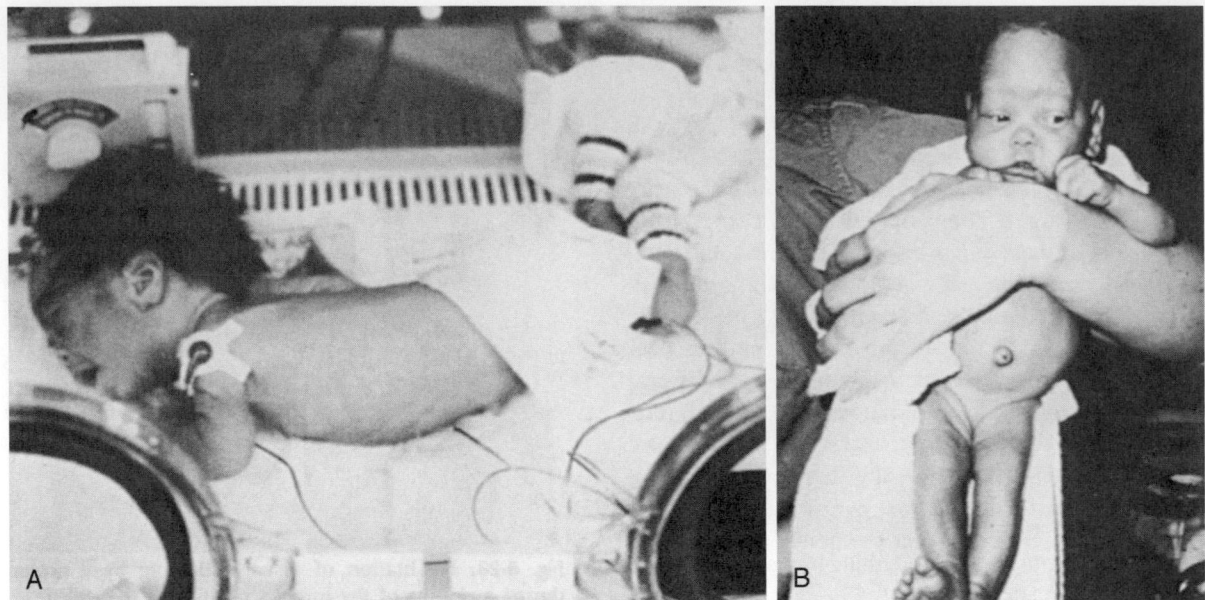

FIGURE 11-25 ■ Neonates demonstrating opisthotonic trunk posture (**A**) and marked lower-extremity hypertonus (**B**) before hydrotherapy.

of environmental light and sound modifications, medical procedures, equipment, and caregiving patterns. Observing and analyzing the effects of the environment on an infant's behavior, physiological stability, postural control, and feeding function are critical elements to establish a prehandling baseline status before each neonatal therapy contact.[81]

Neonatal Hydrotherapy

Modified for use in an intensive care nursery setting, the traditional physical therapy modality of hydrotherapy has been adapted and implemented into neonatal therapy programs. Neonatal hydrotherapy was conceptualized in 1980 at Madigan Army Medical Center in Tacoma, Wash., and results of a pilot study of physiological effects were reported in 1983.[136]

Indications for referral of medically stable infants to the hydrotherapy component of the neonatal therapy program include (1) muscle tone abnormalities (hypertonus or hypotonus) affecting the quality and quantity of spontaneous movement and contributing to the imbalance of extension in posture and movement (Figure 11-25); (2) limitation of motion in the extremities related to muscular or connective tissue factors; and (3) behavioral state abnormalities of marked irritability during graded neuromotor handling or, conversely, excessive drowsiness during handling that limits social interaction with caregivers and lethargy that contributes to feeding dysfunction.

Infants are considered medically stable for aquatic intervention when ventilatory equipment and intravenous lines are discontinued and when temperature instability and apnea or bradycardia are resolved. A standard plastic bassinet serves as the hydrotherapy tub, and the water temperature is prepared at 37.8° C to 38.3° C (100° F to 101° F). An overhead radiant heater is used to decrease temperature loss and enhance thermoregulation in the undressed infant. Agitation of the water is not included in the hydrotherapy protocol in the NICU.

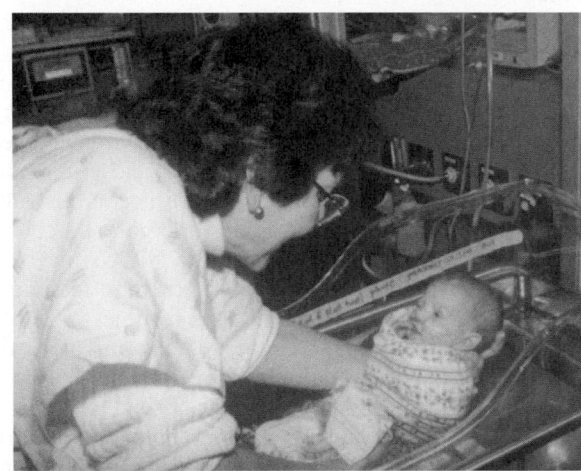

FIGURE 11-26 ■ Adjustment to water immersion before introducing guided movement during neonatal hydrotherapy.

After receiving medical clearance and individualized criteria for the maximum acceptable limits of heart rate, blood pressure, and color changes during hydrotherapy from the neonatal staff, the baseline heart rate and blood pressure values are recorded and pretreatment posture and behavioral states are observed. The undressed infant is swaddled and moved into a semiflexed, supine position. The blood pressure cuff is placed around the distal tibial region to continuously measure heart rate and blood pressure at 2-minute intervals during the 10-minute water immersion period. After being lifted into the water, the swaddled infant is given a short period of quiet holding in the water without body movement or auditory stimulation to allow behavioral adaptation to the fluid environment (Figure 11-26). A second caregiver (e.g., nurse or parent) is recruited to stabilize the infant's head and shoulder girdle region while the neonatal therapist provides support at the pelvis (Figure 11-27).

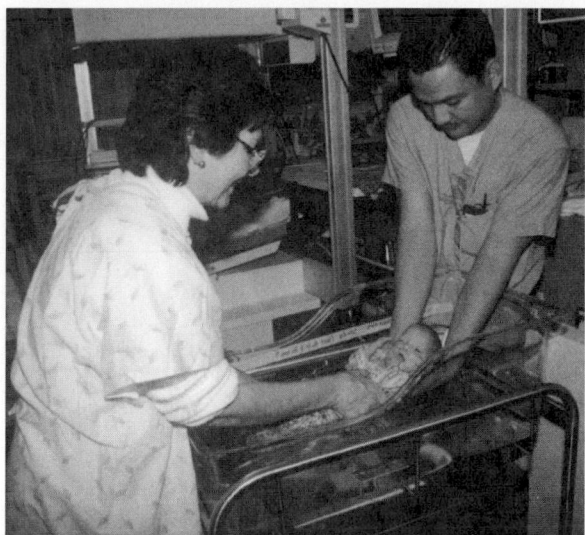

FIGURE 11-27 ■ Swaddled infant is supported in neonatal hydrotherapy tub by neonatal physical therapist and neonatal nurse. The blanket is gradually loosened to encourage spontaneous, midrange movement of the extremities.

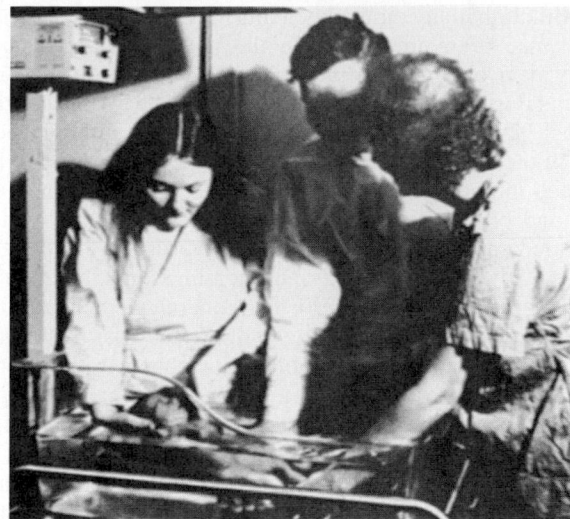

FIGURE 11-28 ■ Parents being trained in hydrotherapy techniques for later therapeutic bathing at home.

Within the loosened boundaries of the swaddling blanket, the movement techniques involve midline positioning of the head and slow, graded movement incorporating slight flexion and rotation of the trunk, followed (if tolerated) by progression distally to the pelvic girdle region and, finally, to the shoulder girdle region. After guided trunk extensor flexion with partially dissociated movement at the shoulder or pelvic girdle, most infants will demonstrate active extremity movement in the water and the swaddling blanket is adjusted (or removed) to allow more movement or more stability depending on the response of the infant. The improved range and smoothness of spontaneous extremity movement is facilitated by the buoyancy and surface tension of the water. Movement experiences in the supine, side-lying, and prone positions are offered as tolerated. If the movement therapy becomes stressful, with agitation or crying by the infant, body movement is stopped immediately, and the infant is either consoled or removed from the water and held with warmed towels. Compromise in hemodynamic stability (increased heart rate, increased blood pressure, decreased respiratory rate) and decrease in arterial oxygen tension during crying have been well documented in neonates.[137] Careful monitoring of behavioral tolerance to hydrotherapy (with avoidance of crying) is considered critical for reducing physiological risk with hydrotherapy.

Multiple therapeutic benefits have been observed from the selective use of 10-minute aquatic intervention sessions. Improved postural tone with semiflexed posture is obtained with less time and effort by the therapist and with higher behavioral tolerance by the infant than when a similar therapeutic handling approach is used without the medium of water. Postural tone changes are frequently maintained for 2 to 3 hours when aquatic intervention is followed by flexed, midline body positioning in the side-lying or prone position on a water mattress or supported against rolls. Mild flexion contractures of knees and elbows and dynamic hip adduction contractures can be safely and quickly reduced by

gentle muscle elongation techniques in warm water. Enhancement of visual and auditory orientation responses (e.g., visual fixing and tracking, auditory alerting, and localization to human voices), prolonged high-quality alertness, and longer periods of social interaction with caregivers are demonstrated during and after hydrotherapy sessions. Significant improvement in feeding performance may occur when hydrotherapy is scheduled 30 minutes before feeding to prepare the infant for arousal to the quiet, alert state and for flexed, midline postural changes for optimal feeding. As with all neonatal therapy interventions, possible adverse effects of fatigue and temperature loss during hydrotherapy must be carefully monitored so that exhaustion of the infant with a deterioration in feeding abilities does not establish a need for gavage feeding.

Therapeutic bathing techniques are incorporated into the parent teaching program to foster early parent participation in child care and in specific neonatal therapy activities during the inpatient period to prepare for carryover into the home environment. This early pleasurable involvement of parent and child in hydrotherapy and therapeutic bathing may provide a strong base for future participation in aquatics as a family leisure sports activity and, if needed, as an adjunct to an outpatient therapy program.

When oriented to treatment goals and trained in specific hydrotherapy techniques for individual infants, the nursing staff can effectively carry on the hydrotherapy program established by the neonatal therapist. This release of the neonatal therapist's role to nurses allows additional use of hydrotherapy on evening and night shifts and continued teaching and supervision of parents during evening and weekend visits (Figure 11-28).

An additional advantage of neonatal hydrotherapy is cost effectiveness with the use of equipment readily available in the newborn nursery and the short time (10 minutes) required for therapeutic bathing. Hydrotherapy becomes labor efficient for the neonatal therapist when it is incorporated into nursing care plans and conducted by nurses and parents, with the therapist assuming a supervisory role.

Although many clinical benefits may be obtained by judicious use of hydrotherapy in the newborn nursery, pilot study data obtained on physiological changes in high-risk infants during hydrotherapy clearly indicate a physiological risk.[136] This risk (7% increase in blood pressure and heart rate in the pilot sample) must be carefully evaluated relative to each infant's general medical stability and baseline heart rate and blood pressure status before hydrotherapy can be included safely in a neonatal therapy program. In collaboration with the neonatology and nursing staff, the therapist must use established criteria for general medical stability and the maximal limits during hydrotherapy for blood pressure, heart rate, and acceptable color changes; this step is essential for risk management. Physiological monitoring of mean blood pressure and heart rate by a neonatal vital signs monitor during aquatic intervention is recommended. The blood pressure cuff is a pneumatically driven device that is not electronically connected to the infant and can be safely immersed in water. Because hypothermia is a recognized risk with hydrotherapy, body temperature should be routinely measured before and after the hydrotherapy session by using a thermometer with a digital display. A risk-benefit analysis of the potential physiological risk to each infant and the expected therapeutic benefits is strongly advised before incorporating hydrotherapy techniques into a neonatal therapy program.

Oral-Motor Therapy

In LBW infants, feeding difficulties may be related to neurological immaturity, depressed oral reflexes, prolonged use of an endotracheal tube for mechanical ventilation and subsequent oral tactile hypersensitivity, or insufficient postural tone. Because behavioral state affects the quality of feeding behavior, feeding performance may be significantly improved by specific arousal or calming procedures before feeding. Other variables influencing feeding may include decreased tongue mobility, presence of tongue thrusting, decreased lip seal on nipple, nasal regurgitation, tactile hypersensitivity in the mouth, inefficient and uncoordinated respiratory patterns, insufficient proximal stability from hypotonic neck and trunk musculature, and hypertonic posturing of the neck and trunk in extension.[138,139]

Three instruments for assessing oral-motor and feeding behaviors in the nursery are the Neonatal Oral-Motor Assessment Scale (NOMAS),[140] the Nursing Child Assessment Feeding (NCAF) Scale,[141] and the Early Feeding Skills (EFS) Assessment for preterm infants.[142] The NOMAS is used to evaluate the following oral-motor components during sucking: rate, rhythmicity, jaw excursion, tongue configuration, and tongue movement (timing, direction, and range). Tongue and jaw components are analyzed during nutritive and nonnutritive sucking activity. Cut-off scores were derived from a pilot study with the instrument: a combined score of 43 to 47 indicated "some oral-motor disorganization"; a score of 42 or less indicated oral-motor dysfunction.[140] The absence of a category to evaluate breathing pattern, work of breathing/respiratory exertion, and physiological variables during feeding limits the use of this instrument to low-risk, healthy neonates.

The NCAF Scale is used to analyze parent-infant interaction during feeding. It provides a method for evaluating the responsiveness of parents to infant cues, signs of dis-

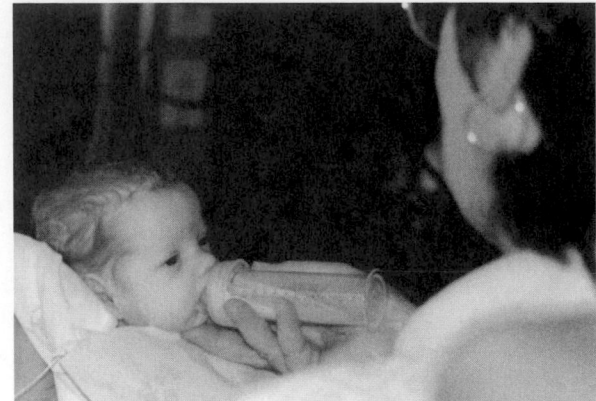

FIGURE 11-29 ■ Swaddled preterm infant fed in semiupright position with light support under chin.

tress, and social interaction opportunities during the feeding process. In concurrent validity studies, NCAF Scale scores were positively correlated with the Home Observation for Measurement of the Environment Inventory at 8 months (r = 0.72) and at 12 months (r = 0.79).[141]

The Early Feeding Skills Assessment is a 36-item observational measure of oral feeding readiness, feeding skill, and feeding recovery. The assessment tool includes examination of physiological and behavioral stability, behavioral feeding readiness cues, oral-motor coordination and endurance, coordination of breathing and swallowing, and postfeeding alertness, energy level, and physiological state. Preliminary content validity and intrarater and interrater reliability procedures were described as "stable and acceptable"(correlation data not reported) with predictive, concurrent, and construct validity testing in process.[142] This tool is specifically designed for feeding examinations in the NICU environment and with expanded psychometric testing will be a relevant instrument in managing neonates with feeding impairment.

General strategies during feeding may include semiflexed, upright positioning with light support under the chin (Figure 11-29). Techniques such as tactile facilitation of the facial muscles, judicious tactile stimulation of specific intraoral structures, use of a pacifier during gavage feedings, light manual support to the jaw or lip, and thickening of formula are frequent components of oral-motor therapy programs.[139]

For some infants, oral intake by bottle may be improved by selecting a nipple with a flatter shape, larger hole, and softer, lower resistance to compression than those for standard newborn nipples. Wolf and Glass[139,143] advised evaluation of the flow rate of liquid from various types of nipples and analysis of the effects of nipple size, shape, and consistency on an infant's sucking proficiency. Feeding infants in the side-lying position may improve tongue position, particularly if marked tongue retraction is present (Figure 11-30). The timing of movement therapy or neonatal hydrotherapy 30 minutes before feeding may significantly improve performance by preparation of postural tone, facilitation of oral musculature, and enhancement of alertness.

Infants with orofacial anomalies (e.g., cleft lip and palate, hypoplastic mandible) often respond to bottle feeding with a Haberman feeding system (Medela Inc., McHenry, Ill.),

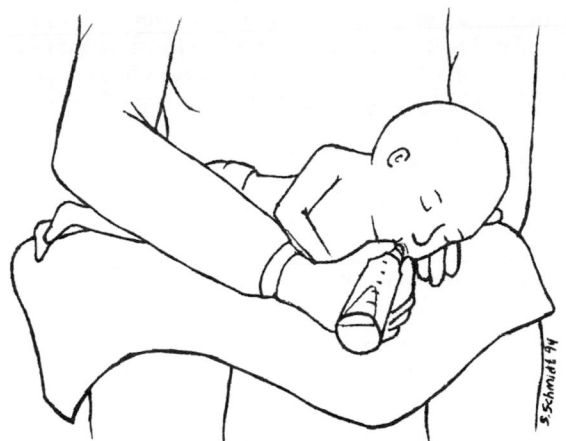

FIGURE 11-30 ■ Feeding in side-lying position for infants with marked tongue retraction.

which allows control of the flow rate through a valve in the bottle and manual compression of the nipple. The Haberman feeder is an ideal option for infants with large bilateral cleft lip and palate because of the long, flexible nipple, which allows formula to be released from manual compression of the nipple by caregivers instead of requiring negative pressure for suction by the baby. The feeding performance of infants with severe cleft palate deformities may be improved by a dental obturator. This custom-fabricated prosthesis is inserted before feeding to cover the defect in the palate. The increasing popularity of breastfeeding has encouraged the development of breastfeeding aids (e.g., Lact-Aid, J.J. Avery, Inc., Denver, Colo.). These devices allow supplementation of oral intake during breastfeeding through a small tube that goes to the mouth from a sterilized bag containing infant formula.

Expected outcomes of oral-motor treatment supported by clinical research include (1) increased number of nutritive sucks after perioral stimulation,[144,145] (2) increased volume of fluid ingested during nipple feedings,[146] (3) decreased number of gavage feedings and earlier bottle feeding,[145,147] (4) accelerated weight gain,[147] and (5) earlier hospital discharge.[147] Measel[147] found that use of a pacifier during tube feedings allowed hospital discharge 4 days earlier for experimental subjects (n = 29) than for control subjects (n = 30). With the cost of NICU care at approximately $5000 per day, a discharge 4 days earlier for infants with resolved feeding impairments may represent a saving of $20,000 per infant.

Monitoring the infant's physiological tolerance, breathing pattern, and work of breathing is critical during oral-motor examination, intervention, and feeding trials.[139] Heart rate values may be monitored from either the cardiorespirograph or with peripheral oxygen saturation from a pulse oximeter. Color changes, diminished tone in facial muscles, and behavioral stress cues (e.g., restlessness, trunk arching) must be carefully monitored to allow appropriate response to early signs of fatigue, overexertion, and potential airway management difficulty. Regurgitation with aspiration of milk or formula into the lungs may occur during feeding trials with complications of pneumonia, cardiopulmonary arrest, and associated asphyxia. Because of these risks, feeding trials should not be attempted by neonatal therapists

untrained in managing the respiratory and general physiological monitoring components of neonatal feeding.[143]

Success during feeding activities enhances parent-infant interaction and perceived competency in parenting. Parents of infants with feeding dysfunction describe higher stress than that reported by parents of infants who are gaining weight and feeding satisfactorily. Because oral-motor dysfunction has been reported as an early functional deficit in infants at high risk for later neuromotor sequelae,[148] early support to parents coping with a challenging feeding situation builds competence in caregiving and also commitment to continuity in outpatient developmental monitoring.

Parent Support

Grief Process

Strong, continuous support is essential to help parents through perhaps the most frightening crisis in their adult lives—the potential death or disability of their infant.[149,150] Parents sometimes initially establish emotional and physical distance from the infant as they cope with the knowledge that the infant may die. During this time of anticipatory grief, peer group support by other parents of prematurely born children can be of immeasurable value. Actively listening to the parents' feelings and concerns and providing support, without judgment, are critical through their episodes of detachment and anger. Although long-range plans include parent participation in all aspects of the developmental program, the timing and amount of initial teaching must be individualized to the levels of stress and acute grief present.

When an infant dies, the neonatal therapist begins the important work of closure. This work includes attending memorial or funeral services to support the family, writing a note expressing sympathy to the family, and initiating a personal closure process. Neonatal therapists are advised to find a senior nurse mentor to guide them through the closure process of identifying and dealing with feelings of loss regarding the infant and family. Finding meaning and value in the process of caregiving rather than solely in functional outcomes is an important task in the work of closure and in preventing professional burnout.

Parent Teaching

Components of the parent teaching process may include (1) discussion of the program goals and services in the NICU; (2) orientation to the interdisciplinary follow-up plan after discharge; (3) guidelines for recognizing and understanding the infant's temperament, stress and stability cues, and ability to interact with the environment; and (4) specific instructions on selected developmental activities and therapeutic handling techniques. When used in conjunction with verbal instructions and demonstrations, a packet of written guidelines and pictures that are individualized to the infant's needs may improve parents' overall skills and understanding of the program.

Occasionally, when geographical distance prevents participation by parents in the neonatal therapy program, the infant's individualized developmental plan may be mailed and later reviewed at discharge or during outpatient follow-up. During times of separation, telephone contact with parents helps foster attachment to the infant and explain the purpose and content of the home developmental intervention program as well as provide opportunity to discuss the critical need for follow-up. Parents need this ongoing dialogue to make the infant seem real to them and to allow communication of their fears and concerns during the separation.

Teaching strategies are most effective when they are adapted to the learning style of the parents. This adaptation may involve more demonstrations and an increased opportunity for supervised practice for some parents, particularly those with reading or language difficulties that limit use of a written instructional packet. Cultural caregiving practices of the family may require elimination of common procedures such as use of pacifiers for nonnutritive sucking or hand-to-mouth engagement.

With consultation from and collaboration with the neonatal therapist, neonatal nurses can incorporate recommendations to support skeletal and motor development into their routine discharge teaching activities. General considerations for discharge teaching by nurses may include the following[151]:

- Varying the direction of head turn for sleeping in the supine position to prevent plagiocephaly
- Placing the head in midline with lateral rolls extending along the side of the head and trunk for car seats and swings
- Limiting the use of infant seats and encouraging the use of prone play on the floor with a roll under the arms and upper chest to assist in head lifting and weight bearing on the arms
- Highlighting the importance of the prone play position for strengthening the neck, trunk, and arm musculature to prepare for sitting and rolling
- Reinforcing the value of interdisciplinary follow-up for musculoskeletal and neurodevelopmental monitoring
- Recommending expedient follow-up if parents notice signs of head flattening, persistent lateral head tilt, strong asymmetrical head turn preference, or asymmetrical arm use

In the neonatal period, the quality of infant-parent attachment and the comfort level and proficiency in routine caregiving and therapeutic handling set the stage for later parenting styles. Helping parents find and appreciate a positive aspect of the neonate's motor or other developmental behaviors gives them a spark of hope from which emotional energy can be generated to help them through the marathon of the NICU experience. Empowering parents early in their parenting experience with the infant is crucial. In the life of the child, the effects of parent empowerment will last far longer than neonatal movement therapy and positioning strategies.

CLINICAL MANAGEMENT: OUTPATIENT FOLLOW-UP PERIOD

Purpose of Outpatient Follow-Up for the At-Risk Infant

Systematic follow-up of the at-risk infant after discharge from the NICU is an essential component of the clinical management of high-risk infants. The purpose of this follow-up is threefold: (1) to monitor and manage ongoing medical issues, such as respiratory problems and feeding difficulties; (2) to provide support and guidance to parents and caregivers in care and nurturing of at-risk infants; and (3) to assess the developmental progress of infants to ensure that neuromotor impairments and delays in motor development can be identified and intervention initiated as early as possible. Issues of assessment, intervention, and developmental profiles of the high-risk infant after discharge from the NICU are discussed in this section.

Medical Management

The routine medical care of preterm infants after discharge may be provided by a pediatrician, family practitioner, or health professional. Infants at neurodevelopmental risk are frequently followed by a number of additional professionals, including neurologists, ophthalmologists, cardiac or pulmonary specialists, nutritionists, public health nurses, physical and occupational therapists, and infant educators. Communication among these specialists is often minimal, especially when they are located at different facilities, and access to providers may be restricted by policies of managed care systems. The parent or caregiver is often confronted with conflicting opinions, demands, and expectations of the family and the infant. The follow-up clinic can play a valuable role in this situation by providing case management to assist caregivers in coordinating necessary services, verify that all needs of the infant are being met, and help parents set realistic goals and priorities for themselves and their child.

Family Support

The stress that a vulnerable, premature, or at-risk infant brings to a family is well documented. Grief, anger, and depression are common reactions to the trauma and anxiety of an unanticipated premature birth.[149] The caregivers of high-risk infants are required to become knowledgeable about complex medical terminology and equipment. At discharge, they often become responsible for the administration of multiple medications of varying dosages, cardiopulmonary resuscitation procedures and equipment, and complicated feeding schedules requiring daily measurement and recording of nutritional intake and output. In addition, families are often faced with an unexpected, large financial obligation to the hospital and confusion of dealing with different billing agencies and funding sources.

These stresses and demands are even more overwhelming for parents who are young, are single, or do not speak English. In contrast to the 1980s, a greater proportion of at-risk infants now seen in follow-up clinics are living with caregivers other than their biological mothers. These caregivers may include other relatives, such as single fathers, grandparents, aunts and uncles, foster care providers, or preadoptive parents. At the same time the changing demographics of American society are reflected in the increasing ethnic diversity of LBW infants. Whether they are recent immigrants to the United States, seasonal workers, or residents of an ethnic neighborhood, parents from minority ethnic groups are frequently overwhelmed by the complexities and procedures of a large medical institution. To serve this population adequately, a follow-up clinic team should have access to interpreters and include social workers who are knowledgeable about community resources outside the predominant culture. Cultural competence, defined as performing "one's professional work in a way that is congru-

TABLE 11-8 ■ Incidence of Cerebral Palsy Relative to Birth Weight

BIRTH WEIGHT (G)	INCIDENCE
>2500	<1%
1500-2500	5%-8%
1000-1500	10%-17%
<1000	20%-30%

Data from references 1, 25, 29, 37, 41, and 161.

TABLE 11-9 ■ Incidence of Major Neurodevelopmental Disability among Preterm Infants Relative to Birth Weight

BIRTH WEIGHT (G)	DISABILITY*
>2500	4%-5%
1500-2500	5%-20%
1000-1500	15%-25%
<1000	20%-40%

*Cerebral palsy, mental retardation, blindness, seizures, sensorineural hearing loss, hydrocephalus.
Data from references 25, 26, 161, 162, and 165.

ent with the behavior and expectations that members of a distinctive culture recognize as appropriate among themselves," is an essential prerequisite for professionals working in a high-risk infant follow-up clinic.[152] For the physical therapist conducting an evaluation, cultural competence includes familiarity with differing cultural norms regarding personal interaction, child-rearing practices, and family dynamics.

The LBW or at-risk infant may be irritable, hypersensitive to stimulation, less responsive to the affective interactions of adults, and more irregular in sleeping and feeding schedules compared with the term infant.[153] The demands that such an infant places on caregivers can be extremely stressful, especially when other siblings in the home, financial concerns, and sleep deprivation are present. Although these stresses may resolve as the infant's schedule and temperament become more stable, some studies raise concerns about their long-term impact on the parent-infant relationship and the infant's social and affective development.[154,155]

The pediatric therapist in the follow-up clinic must be sensitive to these parent or caregiver stresses and concerns. Because social work and nursing services may not be routinely available, the therapist, within the context of the examination, needs to be alert to cues in the behavior of the infant or caregiver that may indicate problems in the home. Thoughtful questions regarding daily routines, feeding patterns, the sleep schedule of the caregiver as well as the infant, the caregiver's impression of the infant's temperament, and the availability of supportive resources can prompt a discussion of concerns that may not be readily communicated to a pediatrician or other professionals involved in the child's care.

Examination of Neurodevelopmental Status
Because LBW infants are at increased risk for neurodevelopmental disabilities, close follow-up is necessary during the first 6 to 8 years of life. Compared with term infants, the incidence of cerebral palsy is greater for LBW infants, and the rate of cerebral palsy increases with decreasing birth weight levels (Table 11-8).[1,156-159] Cerebral palsy is one of several major neurological conditions that are sequelae of prematurity; others include mental retardation, hydrocephalus, sensorineural hearing loss, visual impairment, and seizure disorder. When examined as a group, these major disabling conditions occur more frequently in LBW infants, and the incidence increases as the birth weight and gestational age of the infant decrease (Table 11-9).[156,160-162]

Preterm LBW infants are also at increased risk for more subtle neurodevelopmental disabilities, including visual-motor dysfunction, speech and language deficits, reading and math problems, balance and coordination impairment, and behavioral disorders such as attention deficit and hyperactivity.[3,6,162-165] Longitudinal studies indicate that by school age approximately half of all LBW infants will have educational and learning deficits compared with a reported rate of 24% in the general population.[161,162] Overall 10% to 30% of LBW infants are estimated to eventually have "major" disabilities and another 40% to have "minor" disabilities.[161,162]

A primary objective of developmental follow-up in at-risk infants is the early identification of neurodevelopmental disabilities and the expedient referral to therapeutic intervention services. LBW infants who participate in a follow-up clinic program have been shown to have advanced performance on cognitive measures and to receive more intervention services compared with unmonitored infants.[166,167] Motor benefits of early intervention for high-risk infants have not been clearly demonstrated by research findings.[168-175] The lack of substantiating evidence is caused in part by the methodological challenges presented by research in this area. The variability of LBW infants and the difficulty of early diagnosis, the heterogeneity of neurodevelopmental outcomes such as cerebral palsy, and the limitations of existing assessment instruments are some of the obstacles in the efforts to conduct efficacy studies of early intervention for this population.

Early identification of a developmental disability remains an important goal. A confirmed or tentative diagnosis can direct the family toward intervention services, financial resources, and social supports. Systematic follow-up and recognition of developmental problems in a high-risk infant provide a major role in supporting the relationship between an infant and the caregiver. The behavioral interaction of an infant with a developmental disability is often different than a typically developing infant, evoking negative maternal responses of anxiety, frustration, or withdrawal.[16,176] Diagnosis of a neurodevelopmental disability often facilitates dialogue about parental concerns and can assist caregivers in their process of accepting the disability and adjusting their expectations for the infant.

High-Risk Infant Follow-up Clinic: A Model
The developmental progress of an at-risk infant requires careful monitoring and regular evaluation at designated intervals in the first years of life. An organizational model of a high-risk infant follow-up clinic is shown in Figure 11-31.

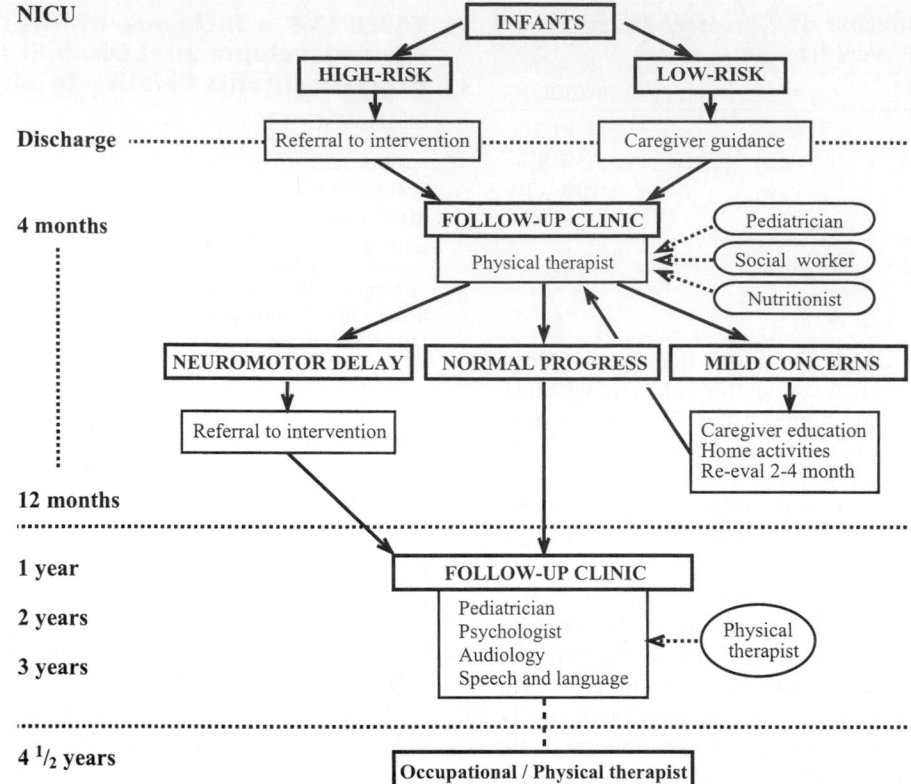

FIGURE 11-31 ■ Organizational model of a follow-up clinic for infants at risk for neurodevelopmental disabilities. Infants are evaluated through the interdisciplinary clinic from the time of discharge from the neonatal intensive care unit. When problems are identified, referrals are made to appropriate specialists.

It is based on the protocol of the High Risk Infant Follow-up Clinic (HRIF Clinic) of the Center on Human Development and Disability (CHDD) at the University of Washington in Seattle.

Before discharge from the NICU, infants who are considered to be at very high risk (infants with seizures, cystic PVL, chronic lung disease, feeding problems, or obvious neurological abnormalities) are identified. The high-risk infant receives therapeutic intervention as described in the section of this chapter on management in the neonatal period. Infants who do not exhibit specific signs of abnormality are closely monitored but do not receive individual intervention. For the LBW infant who is growing appropriately, the roles of the physical and occupational therapists are primarily to instruct nurses and caregivers in positioning and handling techniques that will support and promote normal development.

At discharge, infants who demonstrate atypical development or signs of abnormal neuromotor function are directly referred to therapy programs within the local community. Intervention is recommended to be provided in the home, if possible, to minimize the stress for the infant and family and to reduce exposure to infection. Infants who do not require therapy services at the time of discharge from the NICU are scheduled for an evaluation in the follow-up clinic and referred to a community pediatrician for medical management.

Age Correction

Premature infants are scheduled for evaluations in the follow-up clinic according to their corrected age (age adjusted for weeks of prematurity). The issue of whether to adjust for prematurity when assessing cognitive or motor development is an ongoing question. Several researchers have demonstrated that if chronological or unadjusted age is used for standardized testing, the premature infant who is developing appropriately will have a low developmental quotient and test scores indicative of motor delay.[177-181] If age is adjusted for prematurity, the performance of the premature infants is comparable to that of term infants at 1 year. Although some investigators caution that adjustment for prematurity tends to result in overcorrection, particularly for infants born at less than 33 weeks' gestation,[182] the general consensus is that infants born prematurely should be evaluated according to their corrected age.[182,183]

The decision regarding correction for gestational age in a follow-up clinic should be based on the objectives and testing protocol for that clinic. Consideration should be given to the following factors: (1) the testing instruments used, with attention to the competencies evaluated by the tool and the number of preterm infants in the normative sample, and (2) the overall purpose of the evaluation and whether the emphasis is on screening or diagnosis. In the HRIF Clinic premature infants born at 37 weeks' gestational age or younger are assessed according to their corrected age

TABLE 11-10 ■ High-Risk Infant Clinic: Scheduled Evaluations

CORRECTED AGE OF CHILD	EXAMINER(S)*	STANDARD TESTS ADMINISTERED
4 months	Physical therapist Pediatrician*	Movement Assessment of Infants (MAI), Bayley Scales of Infant Development (BSID)
1 year	Pediatrician Psychologist Audiologist Physical therapist*	Denver Developmental Screening Test (DDST), neurological examination BSID
2 years	Pediatrician Psychologist Physical therapist*	Neurological examination, DDST BSID
3 years	Pediatrician Psychologist Physical therapist* Speech/audiologist*	DDST, neurological examination Stanford-Binet, Peabody Picture Vocabulary Test
4.5 years	Pediatrician Psychologist Occupational therapist Physical therapist* Speech/audiologist*	DDST, neurological examination Wechsler Preschool and Primary Scale of Intelligence (WPPSI) Peabody Developmental Motor Scales (PDMS), Miller Assessment of Pre-Schoolers
6 years	Pediatrician	DDST, neurological examination
8 years	Psychologist Physical therapist* Speech/audiologist*	Wechsler Intelligence Scale for Children Revised (WISC-R) or WPPSI, Peabody Individual Achievement Test (PIAT)

*Consultant examiner.

until they are 8 years old. However, developmental quotients in the normal range do not preclude concerns or referral to intervention services when neuromotor or behavioral abnormalities are observed.

Follow-up Clinic Evaluation Schedule

The basic schedule of evaluations for infants and children in the follow-up clinic is shown in Table 11-10. Although the first routine appointment is at 4 months (corrected age), infants may be seen earlier at the recommendation of the hospital discharge team, physical therapist, community pediatrician, public health nurse, or caregiver. The examinations and test instruments typically administered by each specialist are also listed in Table 11-10.

Four-Month Evaluation

Four months of age is an optimal time for the initial follow-up evaluation for the following reasons:
1. Infant examinations are better predictors than neonatal examinations. The neonatal period and the first 2 to 3 months of life are characterized by variability in infant behavior and motor skills as well as instability of muscle tone and reflex activity.[8,9] Longitudinal studies with sequential examinations indicate that neonatal examinations are less accurate in long-term prediction of neurodevelopmental outcome than examinations administered to older infants.[184-186]
2. Four months is a critical time in the developmental maturation of infants. In the typically developing infant muscle tone tends to be stable,[187] the influence of primitive reflexes is minimal,[188] balance reactions are emerg-

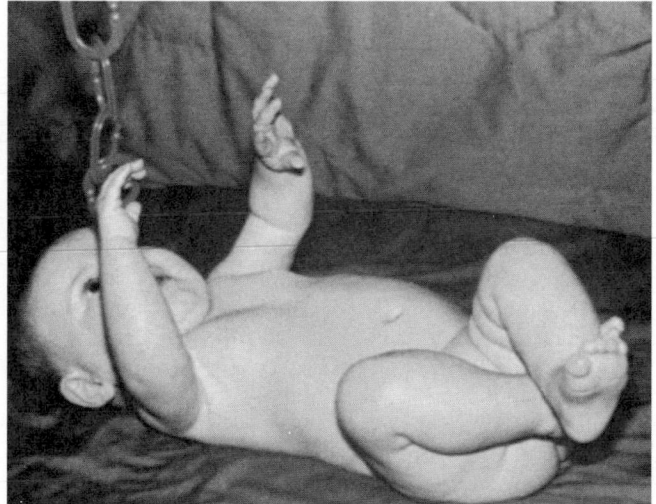

FIGURE 11-32 ■ Normal full-term infant at 4 months of age demonstrating symmetrical alignment of trunk and extremities, functional movement against gravity, and no influence of the tonic labyrinthine reflex.

ing, and functional skills are present with orientation around the midline (Figure 11-32). For most LBW infants, medical concerns have resolved at this age and caregivers are raising questions about developmental expectations. Although definitive predictions about long-term prognosis are not possible for a preterm infant at this age, the predictive accuracy of evaluation at 4 months has been shown to be comparable to that of evaluations at later ages.[189] A comprehensive developmental assessment at 4 months' adjusted age can document an infant's current level of performance and provide a baseline for subsequent evaluations.

In the HRIF Clinic the physical therapist assumes the role of case manager for the 4-month evaluation and for other scheduled evaluations up to 12 months of age. During the first year of life infants express their capabilities and neurological integrity primarily through movement, so the physical therapist, as a specialist in movement, is the most appropriate professional to observe and coordinate the examinations. By using the Movement Assessment of Infants (MAI)[190] and the Bayley Scales of Infant Assessment (BSID-II),[191] the therapist examines both the neuromotor and developmental status of the infant. (The infant examination and clinical decision-making processes of the physical therapist are described in greater detail later in this chapter.)

At the 4-month evaluation the developmental pediatrician provides medical consultation at the request of the therapist when health, neurological, or medical concerns are observed. A nutritionist is available to address feeding issues, growth concerns, and nutritional problems, which are common among preterm infants. Because of the increasing number of infants born to single women, mothers of minority ethnic groups, and women using illicit substances during pregnancy, a social worker is an important member of the follow-up clinic team. The social worker evaluates the family's home and living situation, identifies indicators of environmental risk, and assists the caregiver in accessing necessary financial and personal resources.

One-, Two-, and Three-Year Evaluations

Beginning at 1 year of age, the HRIF Clinic evaluations become increasingly multidisciplinary as the infant becomes a more complex individual. The clinic schedule is designed to allow for assessing many areas of developmental competency without exhausting the infant and family. Because the infant was evaluated by the physical therapist during the first year of life, a neuromotor evaluation is not routinely scheduled. Instead, motor skills are assessed by the psychologist and pediatrician with the BSID and the Denver Developmental Screening Test (DDST), respectively. The physical therapist is available for consultation if motor delay or neuromotor concerns are noted.

Evaluation at Four and One Half Years

A routine evaluation scheduled at 4.5 years of age enables the follow-up team to inform and assist families as they are making decisions regarding school entry. In addition to evaluation by the psychologist, speech pathologist, and pediatrician, the occupational or physical therapist examines the child's motor development. Particular attention is given to balance and coordination and to fine motor and perceptual-motor skills. Depending on the needs of the individual child, the concerns of the caregivers, and the time available for the evaluation, the therapist may use the Peabody Developmental Motor Scales (PDMS), the Beery Test of Visual-Motor Integration (VMI), the Miller Assessment of Pre-Schoolers, or other standard assessments. At this age, a major goal of the follow-up evaluation is to identify prob-

lems that might compromise learning and to assist the family in obtaining appropriate services to minimize the effect of any deficits on the child's school performance.

Neuromotor Assessment of the At-Risk Infant

Neuromotor Assessment Tools: Purpose and Clinical Use

Evaluation of the at-risk infant with a quantitative, standard assessment tool serves two major purposes in a follow-up clinic:

1. Documentation of the infant's motor status relative to developmental norms or relative to the infant's performance on previous examinations. The information is used to determine the child's developmental progress, rate of change, or extent of motor delay. Achievement of this objective is determined by the scope and focus of the assessment tools used in the evaluation.

2. Identification of a neuromotor impairment to initiate appropriate intervention services. Early identification is not simply a task of detecting signs of neuromotor deviation. The challenge is to identify those infants who are most likely to have an abnormal neurodevelopmental outcome. Achievement of this objective is determined by the predictive validity of the assessment tools that are used.

Evaluation of Predictive Validity of Infant Assessment Tools

A primary goal of the neuromotor evaluation is prediction of the long-term developmental outcome of the child on the basis of a clinical examination of the infant. The ability to achieve this goal accurately depends on the clinical experience and expertise of the therapist as well as the predictive accuracy or validity of the assessment tool used. The predictive validity of a test is defined by *sensitivity* and *specificity* and *positive* and *negative predictive values* (Table 11-11).[192]

The **sensitivity** of a test evaluates how *sensitive* the test is in its ability to identify a defined developmental problem, such as cerebral palsy. In the testing situation described here, sensitivity is calculated as the proportion of children with abnormal neurodevelopmental outcome who were correctly identified as "abnormal" when examined as infants. Specificity refers to how *specific* the test is in identifying *only* the defined developmental problem and not overdiagnosing by identifying children who do not have the problem. Specificity is calculated as the proportion of children with normal developmental outcome who were correctly identified as "normal" when examined as infants. The children with normal developmental outcome who were inaccurately classified as "abnormal" by the infant test are referred to as *false-positives;* that is, they were falsely determined by the test to be positive for the developmental problem. On the other hand, children who were classified as "normal" when tested as infants but subsequently are diagnosed with cerebral palsy are described as *false-negatives* because the test falsely indicated that they were negative for the developmental problem.

The **positive predictive value** of a test refers to the accuracy of the infant test in its classification of infants as "abnormal." For example, of the infants who were identified

TABLE 11-11 ■ Predictive Validity of an Infant Assessment Tool

INFANT TEST	OUTCOME (AT SPECIFIED AGE IN CHILDHOOD)		
	NORMAL	ABNORMAL	
No risk	a Correct nonreferrals	b Incorrect nonreferrals (false-negatives)	a + b = Total nonreferrals
Risk	c Incorrect referrals (false-positives)	d Correct referrals	c + d = Total referrals
	a + c = Total normal at outcome	b + d = Total abnormal at outcome	

Sensitivity = d/b, d × 100 = percentage of abnormal children who were correctly identified as "no-risk" by the infant test.
Specificity = a/a, c × 100 = percentage of normal children who were correctly identified as "risk" by the infant test.
Positive predictive value* = d/c, d × 100 = percentage of infants identified as "risk" by the infant test who had abnormal outcome.
Negative predictive value* = a/a, b × 100 = percentage of infants identified as "no risk" by the infant test who had normal outcome.

*Positive and negative predictive values will vary according to the prevalence of the abnormal outcome within the study population.

as "abnormal" or "suspect" by the infant test the proportion of infants who are actually diagnosed with cerebral palsy represents the *positive predictive value*. The *negative predictive value* refers to the accuracy of the infant test in its classification of infants as "normal." It is calculated as the proportion of infants categorized as "normal" who actually have normal developmental outcome. To the therapist in a follow-up clinic, it may appear that the positive and negative predictive values of a given test would be most useful because they indicate the probability of a given outcome for an infant being tested. However, predictive value is not a stable measure of the predictive validity of a test because the predictive values vary according to the prevalence of the developmental problem within a group or population of infants. When a condition is common, the positive predictive value will be relatively high. When the outcome of interest is rare, the positive predictive value will be relatively low. Further discussion about test evaluation and measurement can be found in a number of excellent resources available to pediatric therapists.[192,193]

Examples of Infant Assessment Tools

In addition to the tools previously described for the assessment of the neonate, a number of testing instruments have been designed for evaluation of the infant. On the basis of their content, infant assessment instruments can be viewed within two broad categories: comprehensive/developmental and neuromotor/motor. The BSID-II[191] and the DDST are comprehensive tests that assess the developmental status of infants across several domains of function. On the other hand, neuromotor assessment of gross motor skills such as the MAI[190] and the Neurological Evaluation of the Infant and Newborn[13] or the Alberta Infant Motor Scale (AIMS)[194] focus primarily on one functional area.

The choice of instrument for a particular clinical situation depends on the emphasis and purpose of the clinic as well as on the professional disciplines that are represented in the follow-up team. Neurological findings may be the most useful indicator of impairment in the neonate or young infant because this is a time when behavioral responses are influenced by the infant's affective state and motor skills are rudimentary. As the infant matures, neuromotor integrity is manifested by the acquisition of motor skills. For infants older than 3 months, longitudinal researchers indicated that

observed neuromotor abnormalities were predictive of later cerebral palsy only when accompanied by delay in one or more developmental milestones.[184,189] A brief review of the infant assessment tools commonly used in follow-up clinics is presented below.

Bayley Scales of Infant Development. The BSID-II[191] is a standardized assessment of the cognitive and motor abilities of infants and children between the ages of 2 months and 3 years. The test is divided into two primary areas. The Mental Scale is composed of items rating performance in the areas of problem solving, memory, visual perception, learning, and verbal communication. Gross and fine motor skills are evaluated in the Motor Scale. For infants younger than 12 months, successful performance on the Mental Scale requires competency in visual following and fine motor manipulation; the scale becomes more heavily weighted toward language items at the older age levels. The Motor Scale is predominantly an assessment of gross and fine motor milestones, with visual-perceptual skills included in the recent edition. The BSID-II also provides a Behavior Rating Scale that evaluates the child's behavior during the testing session.

The BSID was first published in 1969 in a format that has been used extensively in clinical and research settings throughout the United States. The BSID-II, a revised version of the BSID, was published in 1993. The goals of the revision process included updating the normative data, extending the upper age level of the test from 30 to 42 months, and adding more relevant test items and materials. The revised test was standardized on 1700 young children representing a distribution of race, gender, geographical region, and level of parent education as an indicator of socioeconomic status. In addition, approximately 370 children with various clinical diagnoses, including autism, Down syndrome, developmental delay, preterm birth, and prenatal exposure to drugs, were tested with the BSID-II. Test scores from these children were not included in the normative data and are intended to provide a baseline of performance for children with these diagnostic conditions.[191]

Administration procedures and grading criteria are clearly described in the manual. Items are scored on the basis of presence or absence of response. The raw scores are converted to standard scores, the Mental Developmental

Index (MDI) and the Psychomotor Developmental Index (PDI), both of which have a mean of 100 and a standard deviation variation of ±15. The authors note that scores on the BSID-II are lower than the scores derived from the original BSID, with the Mental Scale 12 points lower on average and the Motor Scale 10 points lower.[191] A "moderate" level of correlation was demonstrated between the original BSID and the BSID-II: r = 0.62 for the Mental Scale and r = 0.63 for the Motor Scale.

Test-retest reliability was evaluated for the BSID-II with a sample of 175 children aged 1, 12, 24, and 36 months.[191] The "stability coefficients" for ages 1 and 12 months were r = 0.83 for the Mental Scale and r = 0.77 for the Motor Scale. Interrater reliability, determined with a sample of 51 children, was 0.96 for the Mental Scale and 0.75 for the Motor Scale. Concurrent validity of the BSID-II was evaluated by comparing the BSID-II scores with those obtained for a variety of assessment tools, including tests of language, cognitive, and intellectual function. The correlations between the Mental Scale and subscales of language and cognitive tests ranged from 0.57 to 0.99, indicating positive correlations in the moderate to high range. The strongest correlation for the BSID Motor Scale was obtained with the motor subscale of the McCarthy Scales of Children's Abilities (r = 0.59).[191] The predictive validity of 4-month scores on the Motor Scale of the original BSID for identifying subsequent cerebral palsy was low but more accurate for older infants.[185,195] No predictive validity was reported in the revised manual for the BSID-II.

The expanded age range and updated normative data offered by the BSID-II enhanced its overall use as an assessment tool. However, several areas of weakness have been identified in using the BSID-II, particularly with preterm infants.[195-197] Unlike the protocol of the original test, the administration of items and the scoring procedures for the BSID-II are based on item sets. The appropriate item set for an individual child is usually determined according to the child's chronological age, but the examiner is told to "select the item set that you feel is closest to the child's current level of functioning based on other information you might have."[191] The option to begin testing at different item sets, which can yield different raw scores for the same infant, introduces a level of variability in administration procedures and test results that is inconsistent with the purpose of a standardized test.[197] This problem is magnified for preterm infants because it places even greater importance on the decision of whether to test the infant according to chronological or corrected age.[191]

In spite of these limitations the BSID-II is widely used throughout the United States. Until the administration and scoring issues are addressed by the test developers, and the testing procedures are clarified and universally followed, therapists using this tool should define and clearly state the protocol adopted by their clinical or research setting, particularly regarding item sets. Interpretation of test results, especially for high-risk or premature infants, should be done with caution, and the potential for variation in test results should be acknowledged.

Movement Assessment of Infants. The MAI[190] was originally developed by physical therapists specifically for use in a high-risk infant follow-up clinic. The MAI provides a systematic examination of muscle tone, primitive reflexes, automatic reactions of balance and equilibrium, and gross and fine motor skills.

In the MAI manual, the authors outlined the following clinical uses: (1) to identify motor dysfunction in infants up to 12 months of age, (2) to establish the basis for an early intervention program, (3) to monitor the effects of physical therapy on infants or children whose motor behavior is at or below the level for 1 year of age, (4) to assist in data collection and clinical research on motor development through the use of a standard system of movement assessment, and (5) to teach skilled observation of movement and motor development through evaluation of children with typical development or with neuromotor impairment.[190] The MAI has been used in clinical, research, and intervention settings with infants with a broad range of conditions and diagnoses, including Down syndrome,[198-200] prenatal exposure to alcohol and drugs,[201-203] human immunodeficiency virus (HIV)–positive status,[204] and premature birth.[189,199,205-208]

The MAI can be administered in 20 to 30 minutes, with additional time required for scoring, parent counseling, and rest or feeding breaks for the infant. A flexible order of testing is allowed, but grouping of items by the position of the infant (supine, prone, sitting, vertical suspension, standing, prone suspension) is advised to minimize fatigue and stress. The items in the categories of primitive reflexes, automatic reactions, and volitional movement are graded on a 4-point ordinal scale; muscle tone items are scored on a 6-point scale. The MAI manual includes a full description of the examination and administration procedures with detailed scoring criteria for each item.

The MAI provides a scoring profile based on the neuromotor performance expected for 4- and 8-month-old infants. A comprehensive full-scale score, the "total risk score," is derived, with higher scores indicating greater deviation from the norm. For a sample of typically developing term 4-month-olds, reported MAI total risk scores ranged from 0 to 13, with a mean of 5.9 and standard deviation of ±3.2; at 8 months the mean total risk score was 5.9 (range, 0 to 10) and standard deviation was ±2.4.[208] The MAI provides subscale scores for each of the four categories of the test as well as individual item scores.

Early studies of interrater reliability on the percent of agreement between the MAI scores given to term infants by different examiners indicated 90% reliability[190] compared with 72% interrater reliability and 76% test-retest reliability reported in a later study.[209] In a subsequent investigation of high risk-infants, interrater and test-retest reliability calculations with the MAI resulted in intraclass correlation coefficients of 0.91 and 0.79, respectively.[210] Concurrent validity between the MAI and the BSID Motor Scale was reported as –0.63.[211]

Preliminary findings originally reported in the MAI manual suggested that total risk scores greater than 7 indicated neuromotor delay or abnormality.[190] However, later studies with term and preterm infants showed that a score of 10 was a more useful cut-point for prediction of neuromotor disability (S. Hardy, personal communication, 1988).[189,212] Predictive validity of the MAI related to developmental outcome on the BSID and to pediatricians' assessments of childhood neurological status showed highly significant correlations between MAI scores at 4 and 8

TABLE 11-12 ■ Predictive Validity of Infant Assessment Tools

ASSESSMENT	SENSITIVITY (%)	SPECIFICITY (%)	POSITIVE PV (%)	NEGATIVE PV (%)
4-MONTH EXAMINATION				
BSID, Motor Scale	17	97	57	70
MAI	83	78	59	85
MAI	73	93	58	96
AIMS	77	82	39	96
8-MONTH EXAMINATION				
BSID, Motor Scale	77	88	63	82
MAI	96	65	52	91
MAI	96	80	43	99
AIMS	91	86	50	98

PV, Predictive value; *BSID,* Bayler Scales of Infant Development; *MAI,* Movement Assessment of Infants; *AIMS,* Alberta Infant Motor Scale.
Data from references 189, 205, 216.

months and MDI and PDI scores at age 1 and 2 years.[189,211] In a follow-up study of LBW infants weighing 1750 g or less, MAI total risk scores at 4 and 8 months of 10 or more were highly predictive of cerebral palsy at 18 months (Table 11-12).[189] The predictive validity of the MAI has also been demonstrated for preterm infants with bronchopulmonary dysplasia[213] and for predicting neurodevelopmental outcome in term infants at 2 years of age.[214]

Chandler Movement Assessment of Infants Screening Test. The Chandler Movement Assessment of Infants Screening Test (CMAI-ST) is a 10- to 15-minute screening tool for health care professionals in primary care (pediatricians, family practice physicians, and nurse practitioners) designed to identify infants needing referral for definitive neurological and developmental assessment.[215] The test retains the basic categories of the MAI but is limited to selected items considered to be most predictive of movement disorders. All items on the CMAI-ST are scored on a 3-point scale. Reported interrater and test-retest reliability ranges from 87% to 97% and from 81% to 92%, respectively.[215] Normative data have been collected on term infants from 1.5 to 12.5 months of age. Publication of the CMAI-ST will occur after the collection of normative data has been completed.

Alberta Infant Motor Scale. The AIMS[194] was designed to evaluate gross motor function in infants from birth to independent walking, or birth through 18 months. The stated purposes of the AIMS are (1) to identify infants who are delayed or deviant in motor development and (2) to evaluate motor maturation over time. The AIMS is described as an "observational assessment" that requires minimal handling of the infant by the examiner. The test includes 58 items, organized by the infant's position, designed to evaluate three aspects of motor performance: weight bearing, posture, and antigravity movements. The normative sample consisted of 2200 infants born in Alberta, Canada.

Raw scores obtained on the AIMS can be converted to percentile ranks for comparison with motor performance of the normative sample. Test-retest and interrater reliabilities, established on normally developing infants, ranged from 0.95 to 0.98 depending on the age of the child. The AIMS

reportedly had high agreement with the Motor Scale of the BSID and the Gross Motor Scale of the Peabody Developmental Motor Scales (PDGMS) (r = 0.93 and r = 0.98, respectively).[186] An evaluation of concurrent validity between the AIMS and the MAI at 4 and 8 months demonstrated acceptable agreement (r = 0.70 and r = 0.84, respectively)[205]

Predictive Validity of Infant Assessment Tools

In Table 11-12 the sensitivity and specificity of several infant assessment tools are described. The more comprehensive instruments, such as the Neurological Examination of the Newborn and Infant[58] and the MAI,[190] have a high sensitivity but a relatively low specificity. Instruments that are less detailed, such as the AIMS,[194] tend to have higher specificity but lower sensitivity. High sensitivity indicates that infants with a neuromotor impairment are unlikely to be "missed," or falsely identified as "normal," in a follow-up assessment; but low specificity suggests that infants who do not have a neuromotor impairment are more likely to be inappropriately identified as "abnormal." The balance between specificity and sensitivity can be altered by changing the cutoff score: a higher score will reduce the sensitivity of the test but increase the specificity.

In a sample of 164 high-risk infants the predictive ability of the AIMS, the MAI, and the PDGMS administered at 4 and 8 months of age was linked to motor outcome at 18 months.[216] At 4 months the MAI with a cut-point of 10 or higher provided the best combination of specificity and sensitivity values, as well as the highest positive predictive value, compared with the other assessments. For the AIMS, the 10th percentile rank was determined to provide the optimal predictive accuracy at this age. At 8 months, the MAI and the AIMS were comparable in their combined sensitivity and specificity, with a 5th or 10th percentile rank cut-point recommended for the AIMS. The positive predictive value of the AIMS was higher than that of the MAI at this age.

The positive predictive values for the MAI at 4 and 8 months were 58.3% and 42.9%, respectively, and 39.5% and 50.0%, respectively, for the AIMS (based on a cut-point of 10%).[216] These figures indicated that approximately half of the infants identified as "at risk" by the MAI or the AIMS had an abnormal outcome. On the other hand, negative predictive values for both the AIMS and the MAI were consistently greater than 90% at both the 4- and 8-month examinations. These results demonstrated that a negative, or "normal," rating for an infant was a more stable prediction of outcome than a positive, or "abnormal," rating.

The choice of assessment instrument and cutoff score should be determined according to the purpose and objectives of the follow-up clinic and the population of infants for evaluation. If the primary goal is to detect possible signs of early neuromotor abnormality so that infants at increased risk for disability can be monitored more closely, a test with a high sensitivity is desirable and an important consideration for a regional clinic or a clinic in a high-risk social environment where regular follow-up visits and ongoing medical supervision are not routine. When a high-risk infant will probably not be seen for 8 to 12 months, or the family may be lost to regular medical follow-up, even *potential* problems need to be identified and addressed. On the other hand, in a clinical situation where a high-risk infant is monitored regularly or where a test result of "abnormal" dictates referral to intervention services, high specificity in the assessment tool would be a greater priority to prevent unnecessary stress to the family or inappropriate use of limited therapy resources.

High-Risk Clinical Signs

Longitudinal studies of LBW infants have been used to identify specific clinical signs or conditions that are most predictive of abnormal neurodevelopmental outcome, such as cerebral palsy. The conclusions among studies are inconsistent because of the lack of standard criteria for the risk variables, demographic and clinical variation in the study samples, and use of different outcome measures. Results from these studies are summarized in Table 11-13.

Neonatal Period

During the neonatal period through 1 to 2 months after term (40 weeks of gestation), clinical signs suggestive of neuromotor abnormality include stiff, jerky movements or a paucity of movement. Prechtl et al[62] developed an assessment technique based on the recognition of "general movements" that occur at specific times during maturation. Abnormal general movements are characterized as movements with "reduced complexity and a reduced variation. They lack fluency and frequently have an abrupt onset with all parts of the body moving synchronously."[64] Persistence of these movements is considered to be predictive of cerebral palsy or cognitive impairment.[187]

Infancy

At 4 months of age, hypertonicity of the trunk or extremities is recognized as a high-risk clinical sign.[59,189,217,218] Neck extensor hypertonicity has been reported to be highly predictive of cerebral palsy.[184] This finding correlates with neck hyperextension and shoulder retraction associated with the tonic labyrinthine reflex in supine, which has been identified in other studies as a high-risk sign.[199] Although neck hypertonicity was the single item most predictive of cerebral palsy in one study, the majority of infants (60%) who exhibited this clinical sign did not subsequently develop cerebral palsy.[184] Hypotonicity of the trunk at 3 months of age has also been associated with abnormal developmental outcome (Figure 11-33).[218]

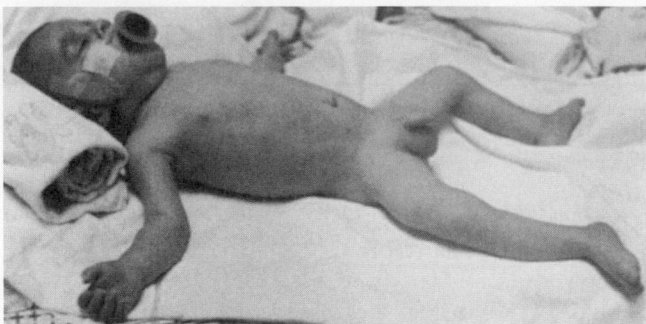

FIGURE 11-33 ■ Posture characteristic of hypotonia with minimal movement against gravity in unswaddled 4-month-old preterm infant with bronchopulmonary dysplasia.

TABLE 11-13 ■ Clinical Signs Indicative of Possible Neuromotor Impairment in LBW and VLBW Infants

NEONATAL PERIOD
Abnormal muscle tone
Jerky, stiff movements
Tremulousness
Abnormal or absent cry; abnormal eye movements

FOUR MONTHS OF AGE
Hypertonicity: limited passive mobility in hips, ankles, or shoulders; neck extensor hypertonicity
Truncal hypotonicity
Abnormal kicking with simultaneous bilateral leg movements of flexion and extension
Persistent, dominant reflexes: asymmetrical tonic neck reflex; tonic labyrinthine in supine
Motor delay in head control, hands to midline, support in prone position
Fisted hands

SIX TO EIGHT MONTHS OF AGE
Hypertonicity of extremities
Persistent, dominant reflexes: asymmetrical tonic neck reflex, tonic labyrinthine in supine, positive support
Delayed postural reactions: head righting, equilibrium reactions
Delayed motor skills: rolling, sitting, support in prone position, reach and grasp
Persistent asymmetry with differences in muscle tone and functional skill

The predictive value of primitive reflexes has been extensively debated. Reflexes and neurological signs, such as the asymmetrical tonic neck reflex (ATNR) and tremulousness, have been correlated with cerebral palsy in some studies[184,219] but not in others.[199] Of the four sections in the MAI, primitive reflexes were found to be the least predictive of later outcome.[189,211] The positive support reflex, characterized by stiff extension of the lower extremities when the infant is held in supported standing, is frequently cited as a high-risk sign, but this posture is seen in both term and LBW infants and has not been consistently associated with adverse sequelae.[181,189,199] Persistent primitive reflex activity and asymmetry have been identified as early signs of

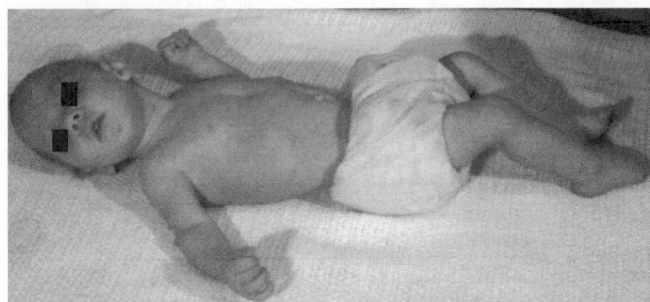

FIGURE 11-34 ■ Dominant asymmetrical tonic neck reflex in 4-month-old infant with athetoid cerebral palsy.

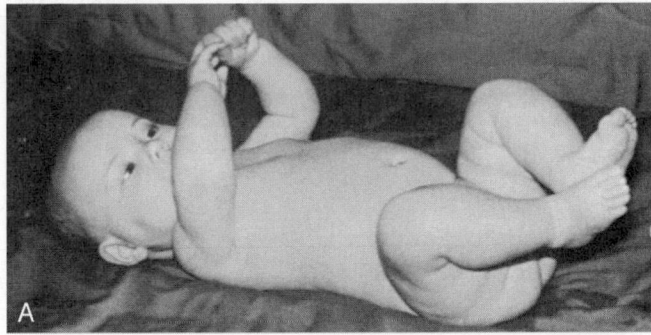

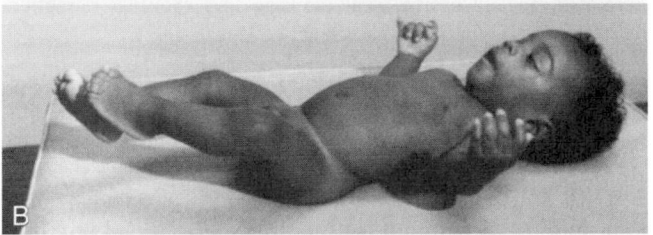

FIGURE 11-35 ■ **A,** Typically developing term infant at 4 months of age demonstrating ability to bring hands to midline and elevate legs with flexion and abduction of hips and dorsiflexion of ankles. **B,** Infant diagnosed with cerebral palsy at 5 months of age; note inability to bring hands to midline because of shoulder retraction, extension and adduction of hips with limited movement into flexion, and plantar flexion of ankles.

athetoid cerebral palsy, more common in infants born at term.[220] In Figure 11-34 a dominant ATNR posture is demonstrated by a 4-month-old infant with athetoid cerebral palsy. Immature automatic reactions of balance and equilibrium at 4 months, including head righting and the Landau reaction, have been found to be a significant predictor of abnormal neurological outcome.[199]

Comparing an infant's spontaneous, active movements with reflex or passive responses is important in determining risk for neurodevelopmental disability. Systematic observation of kicking activity in LBW infants indicated that infants with neurological impairment demonstrated less alternate kicking movement compared with typically developing LBW infants.[221] Abnormal patterns of kicking, including simultaneous flexion and extension of the hips and knees, were associated with subsequent cerebral palsy.[222] Abnormalities of kicking described by Prechtl as "cramped-synchronized," that is, limited in variety and characterized by "rigid movement with all limbs and the trunk contracting and relaxing almost simultaneously," were observed in 3-month-old infants who were subsequently diagnosed with cerebral palsy.[223]

In addition to qualitative differences in motor function, delayed acquisition of motor milestones is an important indicator of neuromotor impairment. Several investigations of the predictive validity of the MAI found volitional movement (gross and fine motor skills) to be the most predictive MAI category at 4 and 8 months.[189,211] This finding is supported by other studies in which delayed developmental milestones were significant predictors of later cerebral palsy (Figure 11-35).[184,224] In particular, delay in achieving upright, gross motor milestones, such as sitting without support, creeping on hands to knees, and pulling to stand, was found to be useful in identifying infants with neuromotor impairment.[224]

Challenges to Prediction of Neurodevelopmental Outcome

Accurate prediction of neurodevelopmental outcome of LBW infants on the basis of standard neuromotor tests is particularly challenging because of several complicating factors.

Impact of Medical Status on Test Performance

LBW infants often exhibit motor delay or neuromotor deviations because of their health or medical status, not because of neurological impairment. Two primary examples are

residual influences from habitual positioning in the NICU and chronic medical conditions.

Variations in Posture and Movement Caused by Residual Influences from Time in the NICU

Although current NICU positioning and handling procedures are increasingly sensitive to the developmental needs of the neonate, the application of life-sustaining interventions (e.g., mechanical ventilation) assumes priority in clinical management. Infants who have spent prolonged periods of time in the supine position, with minimal support to their shoulders or hips, are likely to maintain a posture of shoulder retraction and diminished flexion activity (see Fig. 11-33). On follow-up evaluation, these infants are typically delayed in reaching skills and in achieving antigravity postures.

LBW infants frequently exhibit asymmetry that may be related to intrauterine position or prolonged positioning in the NICU necessitated by surgical or medical intervention. On outpatient follow-up examinations, this asymmetry may appear as visual orientation to one side of the body, more mature upper extremity skill on the same side, and asymmetry of primitive reflex activity. Physical deviations, such as tightness of neck musculature on the preferred side and relative weakness of the opposing muscles, or skull deformities (plagiocephaly) may also be present.[178,208] Asymmetrical motor function resulting from intrauterine or NICU positioning can usually be distinguished from early spastic hemiplegia or other hemisyndromes by clinical examination and by review of the infant's medical history.[178,189] Positional asymmetry is generally not associated with differences in muscle tone between the two sides of the body or with neuromotor abnormalities, such as fisting of the hand on the

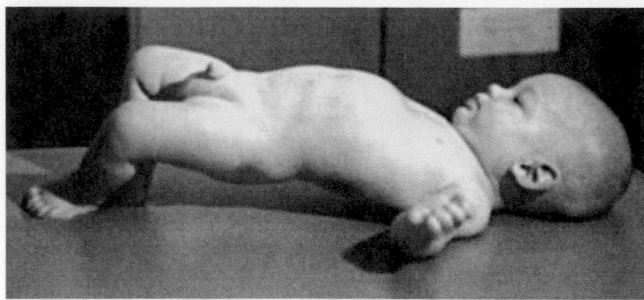

FIGURE 11-36 ■ Preterm infant at 4 months of corrected age demonstrating excessive trunk arching and shoulder retraction; developmental outcome was normal at 1 year.

TABLE 11-14 ■ Clinical Characteristics of Transient Dystonia

NEONATAL PERIOD
Neck extensor hypertonia
Hypotonia
Irritability; lethargy
FOUR MONTHS OF AGE
Increased muscle tone in extremities
Truncal hypotonia
Scapular adduction/shoulder retraction
Persistent reflexes: asymmetrical tonic neck reflex; positive
  support reflex
Asymmetry
SIX TO EIGHT MONTHS OF AGE
Increased muscle tone in lower extremities
Truncal hypotonia; minimal trunk rotation
Immature postural reactions
Immaturity of fine motor skills

less-active side. Caregivers are advised to promote symmetrical posture through their physical handling of the infant, placement of the infant in relation to toys, social activity in the room, and use of cushions or rolls to maintain midline positioning for the infant's head and proximal musculature.

Prolonged Retardation of Motor Development from Chronic Medical Conditions

Infants with chronic lung disease typically exhibit low muscle tone, delayed gross motor function, and immature balance reactions. Motor skills are often delayed as long as the infant's pulmonary capacity is compromised, but the rate of developmental progress typically accelerates when the respiratory condition resolves.[166,213] Intervention for infants with persistent respiratory disease includes providing reassurance and support to the caregivers who are dealing with the demands and stresses of parenting a medically fragile child. Caregivers are advised to avoid aggressive physical activity and excessive sensory stimulation that could cause fatigue or tax the infant's limited respiratory capacity. At the same time, the child should be given opportunities to develop skills in nonmotor tasks. Adaptive positioning techniques reduce energy expenditure and fatigue while enabling the infant to be supported in age-appropriate postures (e.g., prone or upright sitting) for developing hand function, vestibular responses, and social skills.

Transient Dystonia

During the first year of life up to 60% of all LBW infants, as well as a number of term infants, exhibit abnormal neurological signs that subsequently resolve without evidence of major neurodevelopmental sequelae.[207,225-229] This phenomenon is referred to as "transient dystonia." The abnormalities are initially observed in the first 4 months of life, are most prominent between 4 and 8 months, and usually resolve by 1 year of age (Figure 11-36). The clinical characteristics of transient dystonia described most frequently are summarized in Table 11-14.

The presence of these findings on clinical examination poses a challenge to the physical therapist because they are often undistinguishable from clinical signs considered to represent early cerebral palsy (see Table 11-13). From longitudinal studies researchers suggested that infants with transient neuromotor abnormalities may be at increased risk for long-term neurodevelopmental problems. Infants who demonstrated abnormal neurological findings during the first 12

months, although considered to be developmentally normal at 1 year of age, reportedly had a higher incidence of mental, motor, and behavioral deficits in preschool and at school age.[58,226-228] However, a definite relationship between transient abnormalities in infancy and long-term developmental outcome has not been confirmed in other studies.[226,229,230]

Abnormal neuromotor signs, even if they appear to be transient, should not be considered as clinically insignificant. These signs may indicate a child who is at risk for subtle neuromotor problems that will not be functionally evident until school age. Furthermore, neuromotor deviations, although transient, may interfere with the infant's ability to form attachments with caregivers. The infant who arches back into extension instead of cuddling, has poor head control and difficulty establishing eye contact, or stiffens when held may contribute to feelings of frustration, inadequacy, or resentment in caregivers. Instructing in handling techniques to minimize these postures, as well as informing caregivers that these behaviors reflect neurological instability commonly seen in LBW infants, are often valuable interventions during this transient period.

Differences between Preterm and Term Infant Neuromotor Function

Even when not compromised by chronic illness or neurological impairment, the motor development of preterm LBW infants differs from typical term infants. Compared with term infants, healthy preterm infants demonstrate variations in passive and active muscle tone and initially have greater joint mobility, such as an increased popliteal angles and low muscle tone in the trunk.[208,231] In the older infant, increased extremity tone is often present, particularly in the hips and ankles.[180,208] Comparison studies have frequently noted that preterm infants tend to exhibit more neck hyperextension and scapular adduction and fewer antigravity movements in supine (Figure 11-37).*

Primitive reflexes such as the ATNR, Moro reflex, and positive support reflex persist longer in LBW infants, even

---

*References 181, 208, 218, 228, 232, 233.

when assessed at corrected age.[110,181,234] Balance responses, such as protective extension reactions of the arms, are generally less mature in healthy premature infants compared with term infants of comparable age (Figure 11-38). Gross and fine motor skills are frequently delayed in preterm infants, especially activities requiring active flexion, such as (1) bringing hands to midline and feet to hands, (2) trunk stability required for head control and upright sitting, and (3) trunk rotation for rolling and transitional movements.[208,233]

LBW infants exhibit more asymmetry in active movement compared with term infants, but asymmetry is usually not observed in passive tone or reflex activity.[178,208] One group of investigators concluded that "these findings convey an important clinical message: if motor asymmetries are only restricted to the facet of active muscle power, then they are unlikely to be of central origin and as such should not be seen as a sign of neurological impairment. In short, they constitute a typical feature of the post-term development of relatively healthy preterm infants."[178] For most premature infants, these early variations in movement and posture eventually resolve. However, in the first months of life neuromotor deviations may influence the infant's performance on a standard assessment of motor function or neurological status.

Prenatal Exposure to Drugs and Other Substances

Infants with a history of intrauterine exposure to illicit drugs, such as marijuana, cocaine, or methadone, may exhibit deviations in neuromotor behavior. Neonatal abstinence syndrome, predominantly observed in infants exposed to heroin or methadone, is characterized by irritability, tremulousness, and inconsolability. Treatment of neonatal abstinence syndrome with morphine or other medications during the neonatal period usually leads to resolution of the symptoms within 2 to 4 weeks.

Since 1985, when crack cocaine became widely available to women of child-bearing age, many term gestation and LBW infants have been prenatally exposed to cocaine. Reliable documentation on intrauterine effects of cocaine exposure on the neurobehavioral outcome of the neonate and infant is limited. Results vary, and reported findings are frequently compromised by methodological limitations of the research.[203] Researchers suggest that prenatal cocaine exposure is associated with tremulousness, irritability, hypertonia, abnormal reflexes, and motor impairment in the neonatal period.[235-238] These findings are not consistently observed and, when present, do not usually persist beyond 2 to 4 months of age.

Longitudinal research specifically addressing motor outcomes in infants beyond the neonatal period has yielded inconsistent results. In follow-up studies using the BSID no statistically significant differences have been observed in the Motor Scale scores of exposed and nonexposed infants when examined at 6, 12, 24, or 30 months of age.[236,239-241] Cocaine exposure also was not associated with significant differences

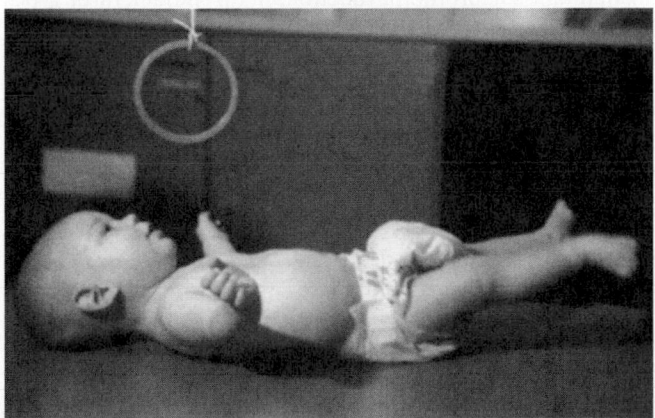

FIGURE 11-37 ■ Healthy preterm infant at 4 months of corrected age demonstrating neck hyperextension, scapular adduction/shoulder retraction, and limited antigravity movement into flexion.

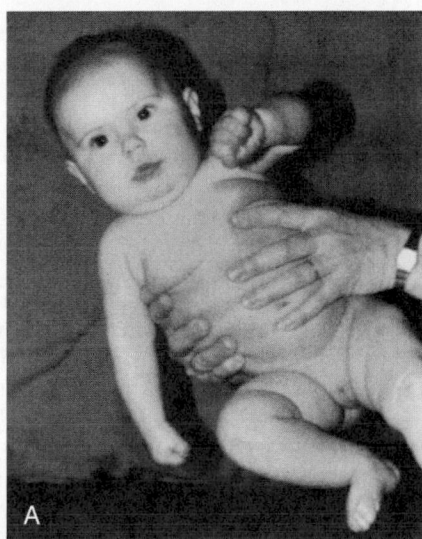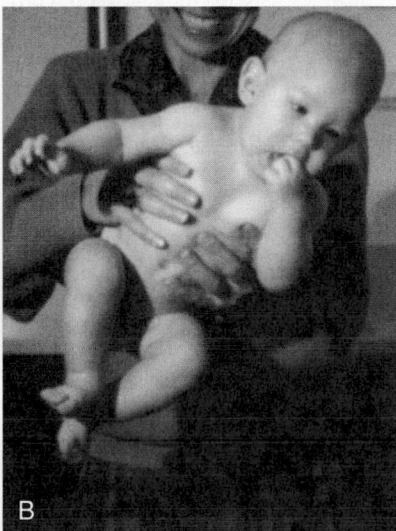

FIGURE 11-38 ■ **A,** Normal term infant at 4 months of age demonstrating lateral head righting. When tipped to the side she is able to maintain her head in midline. **B,** Healthy preterm infant at 4 months of age demonstrating immature lateral head righting. When the body is tipped to one side, the head also leans toward that side.

in scores on the PDMS at 6 or 15 months.[201] However, a preliminary report from one study indicated inferior fine motor performance on the PDMS at 24 months of age in a group of infants prenatally exposed to cocaine.[242]

Researchers using the MAI as an outcome measure have detected subtle, but statistically significant, differences in the neuromotor function of cocaine-exposed infants.[201-203] Prenatal cocaine exposure was associated with higher total risk scores at 4 and 8 months, with significant differences in muscle tone, primitive reflexes, and volitional movement. Individual clinical findings included tremulousness, extension posturing with shoulder retraction, fisted hands, inability to bring hands to midline, and less mature head balance in the infants prenatally exposed to cocaine.[202,243] Further evidence suggests that infants exposed through the third trimester of pregnancy may be at increased risk for adverse neuromotor outcomes.[243]

The long-term implications of cocaine-related neuromotor or behavioral deviations observed in exposed infants are not known. Follow-up studies have generally found no significant differences on standardized test performance between children with prenatal cocaine exposure and a control group. However, in some recent longitudinal studies of children at school age, prenatal cocaine exposure was associated with increased risk for deficits in visual-motor skills, language, and attentional behavior.[244-246] Further research is required to determine if neuromotor abnormalities detected in infancy are related to adverse long-term developmental outcome.

Clinical Decision Making in the High-Risk Infant Follow-up Clinic

During the past 10 to 20 years, advances in multiple areas have dramatically increased the amount of information and knowledge available to the therapist working in a high-risk infant follow-up clinic. Evidence-based medical practice requires the therapist to access objective, scientifically based evidence and to incorporate this knowledge into the formation of diagnostic and therapeutic decisions. More sophisticated imaging techniques, assessment tools with improved predictive accuracy, and high-risk factors identified by longitudinal research provide the substance for evidence-based decisions. Yet, as is indicated by the material presented earlier, no single source of information currently offers a means of establishing a definitive and reliable prognosis for the neurodevelopmental outcome of the preterm infant.

During the follow-up clinic evaluation, the therapist administers the standardized assessment procedures, obtains information from the caregivers, and observes the movements and behavioral responses of the infant. The information and impressions gained are evaluated within the context of the infant's medical, social, and environmental history to form a hypothesis regarding the infant's neuromotor status and prognosis. Although this process is individualized because it is influenced by the therapist's own clinical experience and by the characteristics of the infant, an informed clinical judgment should be reached in an organized, systematic way. Clinical decisions should be made on the basis of the integration of knowledge derived from valid research with the therapist's clinical experience and expertise and with the values and priorities of the family.

General Guidelines

The clinical decision-making process for at-risk infants occurs within a framework of general guidelines regarding the neurodevelopmental outcome of LBW infants. These guidelines are based on the clinical and research evidence previously presented.

1. Risk for adverse neurodevelopmental outcome is increased by the presence of specific abnormal neurological signs, but the majority of infants with any abnormal sign develop normally.
2. A normal neonatal or infant assessment is more predictive than an abnormal examination.
3. Multiple factors are more predictive of neurodevelopmental outcome than single factors, emphasizing the need for a comprehensive evaluation.
4. Periodic, sequential examinations over time are the most useful method of determining the developmental outcome of an individual infant.

A conceptual model provided by Aylward[247] is used to understand and categorize the variations that are observed in an infant's neuromotor function. In this model, three types of developmental abnormality are described: (1) *delay,* which occurs when a child does not achieve an expected developmental milestone; (2) *dissociation,* a difference in the developmental rate of two different aspects of development (e.g., cognitive and motor); and (3) *deviation,* "an atypical developmental indicator."[247]

Clinical Decision-Making Pathway

A model of the clinical decision-making process for the pediatric therapist in a follow-up clinic is shown in Figure 11-39. It is based on a model of clinical decision making that was developed for pediatric physical therapists working within an interdisciplinary assessment team.[248] The model is composed of a series of alternating "action steps" of data collection and assessment procedures and "decision steps" of analysis, interpretation, and planning. The sequential order of the steps is intended to reflect the thought process and is not necessarily a linear progression of events.

Action Step 1: Obtain Relevant History

The therapist reviews the infant's medical history with particular attention to events or conditions known to be associated with neurological risk or adverse outcomes. For the infant born prematurely, key risk factors should be noted, including ELBW (less than 1000 g), abnormal cranial ultrasonographs, neonatal seizures, or infectious conditions. Indicators of birth asphyxia or trauma, infection, and genetic or metabolic disorders are highlighted for infants born at term. Evidence should also be documented of prenatal exposure to illicit drugs or alcohol and the timing and extent of such exposures during pregnancy. Attention is given to the source and reason for the referral: is this a routinely scheduled examination for a graduate of the NICU, or is this an infant who has raised specific concerns for caregivers or medical professionals? Specific concerns of caregivers are an important consideration, although parents' overall perceptions of the developmental status of their high-risk infant do not correlate well with clinical assessment.[249] Background information about the social environment is also reviewed to identify risk factors and ascertain available resources and level of support for the caregivers.

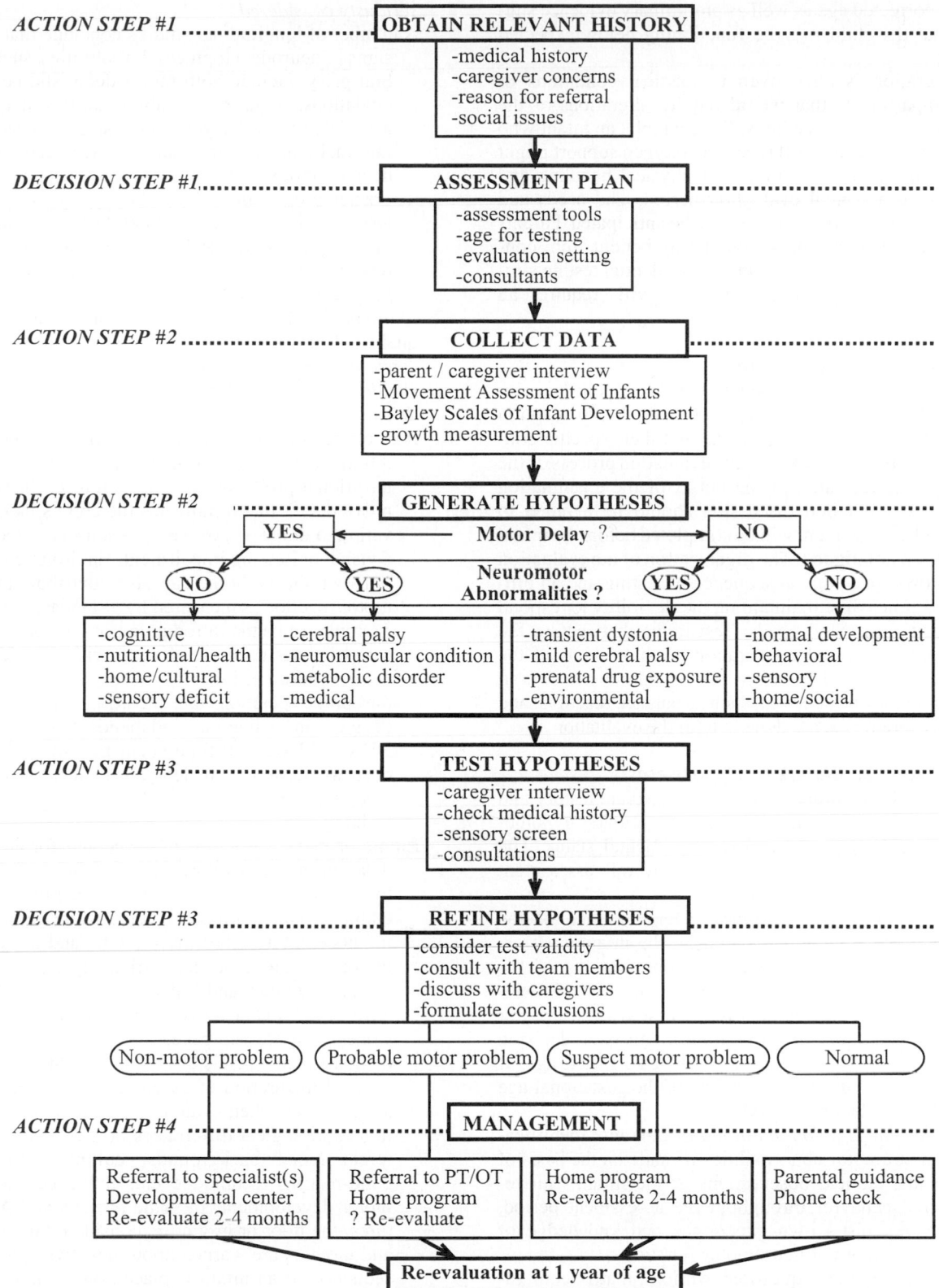

ACTION STEP #1 .... **OBTAIN RELEVANT HISTORY** ....

-medical history
-caregiver concerns
-reason for referral
-social issues

DECISION STEP #1 .... **ASSESSMENT PLAN** ....

-assessment tools
-age for testing
-evaluation setting
-consultants

ACTION STEP #2 .... **COLLECT DATA** ....

-parent / caregiver interview
-Movement Assessment of Infants
-Bayley Scales of Infant Development
-growth measurement

DECISION STEP #2 .... **GENERATE HYPOTHESES** ....

| YES | ← **Motor Delay** ? → | NO |

Neuromotor Abnormalities ?

NO   YES   YES   NO

-cognitive	-cerebral palsy	-transient dystonia	-normal development
-nutritional/health	-neuromuscular condition	-mild cerebral palsy	-behavioral
-home/cultural	-metabolic disorder	-prenatal drug exposure	-sensory
-sensory deficit	-medical	-environmental	-home/social

ACTION STEP #3 .... **TEST HYPOTHESES** ....

-caregiver interview
-check medical history
-sensory screen
-consultations

DECISION STEP #3 .... **REFINE HYPOTHESES** ....

-consider test validity
-consult with team members
-discuss with caregivers
-formulate conclusions

(Non-motor problem) (Probable motor problem) (Suspect motor problem) (Normal)

ACTION STEP #4 .... **MANAGEMENT** ....

Referral to specialist(s)	Referral to PT/OT	Home program	Parental guidance
Developmental center	Home program	Re-evaluate 2-4 months	Phone check
Re-evaluate 2-4 months	? Re-evaluate		

Re-evaluation at 1 year of age

FIGURE 11-39 ■ Decision-making pathway in the high-risk infant follow-up clinic.

Decision Step 1: Assessment Plan

On the basis of the information gained, the therapist antici-pates the central questions and issues that need to be addressed in the evaluation and decides on an appropriate assessment plan. This includes consideration of the testing instruments to be used, the evaluation setting and format, and the interdisciplinary team members to be included. For standardized tests to be administered, the therapist must determine the appropriate age level for initiation of testing. The age level will be determined by the choice of chronological or corrected age as well as preliminary evidence suggesting that the child may be functioning below expected age level.

Consideration is also given to medical conditions or sensory impairments that would require alterations of the standardized testing procedures. For example, an infant who is medically fragile and still receiving oxygen support might be unable to tolerate the amount of physical handling and stimulation in a typical evaluation period. The needs and concerns of the caregivers should also be anticipated. Parents from a high-risk social background may benefit from consultation with a social worker and a confidential testing situation; non–English-speaking parents will require an interpreter.

Action Step 2: Collect Data
The initial interview enables the therapist to establish a relationship with the parents or caregivers, elicit their perception of the infant's developmental status and their specific concerns and questions, and explain the evaluation process. If the infant is awake and alert at the outset of the examination period, lengthy detailed discussion should be avoided to ensure that the assessment will be completed before the infant becomes tired or fatigued. The organization of the evaluation session allows for a logical sequence of testing and an efficient use of time while maintaining the flexibility to respond to the infant's cues and needs. Test items that require the infant's compliance and cooperation, such as items of the Mental Scale of the BSID, are ideally administered first; activities that may be stressful, such as balance reactions and growth measurements, are done later in the evaluation.

Decision Step 2: Generate Hypotheses
Beginning with the initial review of the medical history and throughout the evaluation, the therapist formulates hypotheses regarding the infant's neurodevelopmental status. The following two questions underlie the overall assessment process:
1. *Is motor development delayed?* Determination of the level of motor function is based on the infant's performance on the standardized tests, observations of the child's movement activities, and the therapist's knowledge of normal development in the first year of life. For the preterm infant this question involves a decision regarding the use of chronological or corrected age; if corrected age is used, the accuracy of the gestational age estimate must be considered.
2. *Is neuromotor function abnormal or deviant?* Identification of neuromotor abnormalities is made on the basis of test results, clinical observations of the infant's movements and behavior throughout the assessment period, and the therapist's own experience and knowledge of atypical or abnormal neuromotor function.

By considering these questions within a matrix configuration, four potential hypothetical situations can be derived. Although such a matrix is a simplistic representation, it accurately presents the major issues to be addressed in the evaluation of a high-risk infant.
1. If motor development is delayed relative to the infant's age (corrected or adjusted age for the preterm infant) and the quality of movement is abnormal, *the possibility of cerebral palsy or other neuromuscular condition must be seriously considered.*

A number of longitudinal studies conclude that the early signs of neurodevelopmental disabilities, such as cerebral palsy, include both motor delay and neuromotor deviations. Neuromotor abnormalities that are not associated with delayed motor skills appear to be of minimal clinical significance. When accompanied by delayed motor function, neuromotor deviations have greater prognostic value. The age of the infant and testing conditions are critical factors because, at a given age, absent skills may be just emerging and deviant responses may be exaggerated by stress, fatigue, or illness.
2. If motor development is delayed or immature, but the quality of movement appears to be normal with no evidence of neuromotor abnormalities, *nonmotor problems should be considered as potential causes of the motor delay.*

Possible reasons for a motor delay include medical conditions such as bronchopulmonary dysplasia; health or nutritional problems such as failure to thrive; a cognitive deficit that diminishes the child's lack of motivation to move or explore; or a sensory defect such as a vision or hearing impairment. Environmental conditions within the home can also contribute to delayed motor function as measured by a standardized test. For example, since the introduction of the "back to sleep" campaign designed to reduce the risk of sudden infant death syndrome, infants typically spend less time in the prone position and healthy, term infants are delayed in achieving independent rolling on the DDST.[250] Extended time spent in a baby walker has been associated with delayed acquisition of sitting, creeping on hands and knees, and independent walking.[169,251]

Ethnic or racial variations may account for an apparent delay in motor development if an infant is evaluated by a test that has been normed on infants of other ethnic groups. Compared with white infants, black infants exhibit higher muscle tone and achieve gross motor milestone at an earlier age.[224,252-254] Asian, Asian-American, and Native American infants born at term reportedly achieve gross and fine motor milestones at a slower pace.[253] Asian-American infants demonstrated persistence of primitive reflexes, delayed maturation of automatic reactions, and more asymmetries when evaluated by the MAI.[255] In addition to biological differences between infants of different racial backgrounds, cultural variations in child-rearing techniques can influence the rate of motor development. In some African and Asian cultures, the floor or ground is considered to be unclean and mothers are warned about negative spiritual consequences if an infant is placed on the floor before 6 months of age.
3. If neuromotor abnormalities are observed but motor development is not delayed, early signs of mild cerebral palsy should be considered as one of several possible conditions.

Between 4 and 8 months of age mild diplegia or hemiplegia may first appear as subtle asymmetries or muscle tone variations that are not likely to compromise motor function until the infant begins to crawl on hands and knees, pulls to stand, or performs skilled bimanual activities. However, in the preterm infant neuromotor variations without motor delay are more likely to be manifestations of transient dystonia. If the infant has a history of prenatal exposure to cocaine or other substances such as methamphetamines or heroin, characteristic neuromotor deviations may be observed but are usually not associated with permanent delay in motor skills. Environmental influences may also account for deviations in the quality of movement. For example, infants who spend extended time in baby walkers, jumpers, or nonmobile standing devices may exhibit excessive toe-standing and limited mobility in ankle dorsiflexion.

4. If the examination reveals no delay in motor function and no abnormalities in the quality of the infant's movement, *the therapist may assume normal neurodevelopmental status but also needs to explore alternative conditions.*

Consideration should be given to other possible reasons for the caregiver's or referring professional's concerns. A problem that is perceived as a neuromuscular impairment, such as paucity of active movement, minimal exploration of the environment, or failure to manipulate toys, may in fact be the consequence of a cognitive or sensory impairment. Parents may be concerned by differences observed between the motor development of their child and that of other infants of comparable age or between siblings, especially among nonidentical multiple birth siblings. For parents or caregivers of a preterm infant, the therapist should emphasize the importance of using the infant's corrected age to determine developmental expectations, especially during the first 1 to 2 years of life. Furthermore, an infant's individual personality or body type can be a major factor in rate and style of development. Active infants with firm, strong neuromuscular structures typically achieve gross motor milestones earlier than infants with calm, placid personalities or overweight infants. A therapist in a follow-up clinic must be aware of the broad range of variability in the pace and age of acquisition of gross motor milestones in the typically developing infant.[205]

Action Step 3: Test Hypotheses

Initial hypotheses and assumptions can be verified or substantiated by additional testing and probing into the infant's medical or environmental history. Further discussion with the infant's caregivers may reveal health or nutritional conditions that could compromise physical growth or indicate other developmental influences within the infant's home. In general, open-ended questions elicit more relevant and informative responses and may be less threatening and intrusive than inquiries directed toward a specific answer. For example, a request to "Tell me what your baby's typical day is like" or "Where does your baby like to spend her time?" will provide a more complete view of the home environment and appear less challenging than "Do you put your baby in a baby walker?"

A review of the infant's birth and neonatal history may validate examination findings or cast doubts on a hypothesis under consideration. For example, cranial ultrasound documentation of PVL on the right side of the brain would provide support for suspicion of a neuromotor impairment on the left side of the body. On the other hand, a benign birth history for a term infant with a tendency for toe-standing posture and immature motor development would argue against a hypothesis of early cerebral palsy and in support of environmental influences.

Consultation with or examination by other specialists may be warranted. For an infant with motor delay who exhibits no neuromotor abnormalities but shows inadequate physical growth, examination by the pediatrician or nutritionist may reveal health conditions that account for the motor delay. Immaturity in fine motor skills or asymmetrical development with persistent orientation to one side (i.e., preferred arm use or persistent head turn) may be evidence of a visual impairment.

Decision Step 3: Refine Hypothesis

In formulating a final hypothesis, validity of the test results must be considered. Performance on a standardized test in the follow-up clinic may be compromised if the infant is fatigued, ill, exhibiting stranger anxiety, or unable to cope with the demands and stimulation of a testing situation. If this is a concern the therapist can verify with the caregiver whether the observed responses and behaviors represent the infant's abilities and temperament typically observed at home.

Discussion with other members of the interdisciplinary follow-up clinic team is often helpful, especially when ambiguities or inconsistencies are present in the overall clinical picture. Although other team members may not have examined or observed the infant, they may be able to offer insights on the basis of their own clinical experience when presented with a given constellation of factors. For example, a psychologist may recognize early signs of autistic behavior or a pediatrician may suspect a particular genetic disorder in an infant whose developmental profile is inconsistent with the therapist's expectations.

Finally, but most importantly in the clinical decision-making process, the therapist reviews the test results, clinical observations, and tentative conclusions with the infant's caregivers. A diagnosis is made on the basis of expertise of the interdisciplinary professionals and the clinical, medical, and technological resources available to the follow-up clinic. However, the individuality of the developmental course and outcome of each high-risk infant, the broad range of factors that influence an infant's development, and the limitations of a single assessment in an unfamiliar environment should all be acknowledged. A summary discussion with the parents or caregivers allows the therapist to present the clinical impressions of the follow-up team as well as the limitations of long-term prognosis for LBW infants and to assess the compatibility between the diagnostic hypotheses and the caregivers' perception of their infant.

Action Step 4: Management

In the HRIF Clinic protocol, infants who demonstrate normal neuromotor and developmental progress at the 4-month evaluation are scheduled for follow-up evaluations at 1 year of corrected age. Parents or caregivers are informed of their infant's performance on the standard tests as well as the therapist's overall impressions and conclusions. In addition to reviewing the infant's abilities in various domains of

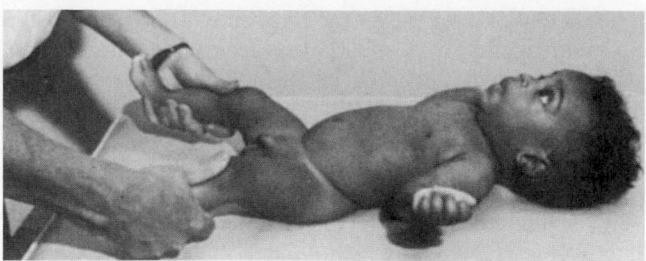

FIGURE 11-40 ■ Infant diagnosed with cerebral palsy at 5 months of corrected age; limited hip abduction is demonstrated with passive mobility.

competency (e.g., gross motor, fine motor, language), the child's personal strengths, such as sociability, alertness, inquisitiveness, or persistence, are emphasized. Recommendations for developmental activities and handling skills are given when appropriate, and caregivers are advised regarding expectations for their child's developmental activities in the next months. They are encouraged to call the therapist if questions arise about their child's developmental progress. If the therapist has noted a minor concern such as a subtle asymmetry, an interim telephone call can verify that motor development is proceeding appropriately.

If the infant demonstrates definite neuromotor abnormality with motor delay (Figure 11-40) or shows strong evidence of a neurodevelopmental disability, the child is referred to an appropriate therapeutic intervention program. An infant who has only motor disability without evidence of deficits in other areas is usually referred to a pediatric therapist in the local community. The infant with delays in multiple areas of development are commonly referred to a developmental program with comprehensive, interdisciplinary services including pediatric physical and occupational therapy.

At 4 months of age, many LBW infants demonstrate immaturity or mild neuromotor abnormality. In this situation, the therapist gives parents or caregivers recommendations for methods of handling and positioning as well as activities to facilitate normal developmental progress. Reevaluation is scheduled at an interval of 2 to 4 months depending on the therapist's level of concern; the caregivers' preferences and concerns; and geographical, financial, and transportation considerations. At the follow-up examination the infant's neurodevelopmental status is reassessed. If neuromotor abnormalities are still present, or if the infant's progress in acquisition of motor skills is below the expected rate, the infant is referred for intervention. If previous neuromotor concerns have resolved and motor development is progressing appropriately, the infant is scheduled to return for the 1-year evaluation.

At all follow-up visits caregivers are advised about appropriate expectations for development in the subsequent months as well as hazards and risks. Particular emphasis is given to issues of safety, which often include injuries associated with infant walkers and the need for a safe place where an infant who has learned to crawl or walk can be confined. Caregivers are advised to introduce their infants to a playpen or other restrictive area before the time of independent mobility and to place the infant in this safe place whenever they are unable to provide constant supervision for their child.

NEUROMOTOR INTERVENTION
Levels of Intervention

Therapeutic intervention for the high-risk infant in the outpatient phase after discharge from the NICU occurs at multiple levels. Type and intensity of intervention depend on (1) the needs of the infant and family, (2) the structure and organization of the follow-up clinic, and (3) the availability of resources in a particular clinical and geographical setting.

Assessment as Intervention

The clinical assessment of an infant is a unique opportunity for intervention on behalf of the infant and family. For the full potential of this interaction to be realized, parents or caregivers must be informed and involved participants in the assessment process, not passive observers. The focus of intervention in this context is on parent or caregiver support with two primary components: *education* and *positive reinforcement for parenting skills.*

Education

The educational component of intervention includes enabling the parents of an at-risk infant to recognize their child's unique capabilities and strengths as well as his or her ability to respond to and influence the surrounding environment. Caregivers learn about their infant's individual responses to stimuli: for example, what causes their child to attend to a stimulus and what elicits stress reactions. Parent education includes describing typical characteristics and common developmental patterns of the LBW or medically fragile infant that may differ from expectations that are based on observations or published descriptions of healthy, full-term infants. Parents of at-risk infants are informed about the appropriate sequence and pace of development for their child so they will be realistic in their expectations and interpretation of the child's progress. This anticipatory guidance enables parents to prepare for and maximize learning opportunities.

Reinforcement for Parenting Skills

During the follow-up examination, opportunities to provide positive reinforcement to caregivers need to be emphasized. Parents of a high-risk infant who responds inconsistently to affective cues should particularly be given positive feedback and affirmation for their investment of emotion and energy.[256] They should be reassured that they are providing appropriate and beneficial parenting and reminded that the infant's behavioral responses reflect neurobehavioral immaturity or instability rather than an unpleasant personality or negative affective feelings toward the caregiver.

Instruction in Home Management

A critical component of intervention is instruction in specific activities and handling techniques for home management. The recommendations are made on the basis of the therapist's knowledge of the infant's medical and neurological history, current health status, and findings from the neurodevelopmental assessment. The overall purpose may be to maximize a healthy child's growth potential or to promote developmental progress in an infant who demonstrates delay or neuromotor abnormality. In either case, the parent or caregiver must have a clear understanding of the purpose of the activity, what motor behavior it is intended to facilitate or counteract, the underlying neurodevelopmental process that the activity will support, and the desired response on the part of the infant. This enables the parent to participate more creatively in the process of intervention by adapting and modifying the recommendations according to the infant's responses and progress of the infant at home.

Although neuromotor handling recommendations are specific to the individual child, some intervention activities are applicable to many preterm infants.

Activities to Counteract Shoulder Retraction

Up to 50% of LBW infants reportedly demonstrate shoulder retraction.[232] This posture inhibits the infant's ability to bring hands to midline and often results in delayed achievement of upper-extremity skills and rolling. To overcome shoulder retraction, play activities and carrying techniques that bring shoulders forward and hands to midline are encouraged.

Reaching

Most premature infants are immature in reaching skills, reducing their ability to interact with the environment. Activities to counteract shoulder retraction will promote reaching, but LBW infants should also be provided with other opportunities to practice this skill. Infants who are ready to initiate reaching at 3 to 4 months of age often have only a visually stimulating mobile suspended beyond their reach in the crib. Caregivers are advised to hang toys *within the child's reach* in the crib, playpen, infant seat, or other suitable places. Objects that are suspended, rather than handed to or placed in front of the infant, are preferred to promote the development of directed reach and grasp as well as shoulder stability (Figure 11-41). Commercially available, relatively inexpensive activity gyms that stand upright on the floor are highly recommended for infants at neurodevelopmental risk.

Centering and Symmetrical Orientation

Midline positioning of the head with symmetrical alignment of the trunk and extremities is encouraged to counteract the residual effects of asymmetrical positioning in utero or during hospitalization. Midline orientation will reduce the

influence of the ATNR and promote symmetrical function of the right and left sides of the body. Asymmetry that is not caused by neurological dysfunction tends to resolve when positioning and environmental influences are modified.

Prone Positioning

Active play time in the prone position with weight bearing on the arms is beneficial for the development of neck and trunk postural and shoulder girdle stability. The prone position also counteracts extension posturing tendencies because the influence of the tonic labyrinthine reflex in prone contributes to extremity flexion. However, parents of vulnerable premature infants are often hesitant to place their infants in the prone position for play. Many LBW infants demonstrate a low tolerance for prone positioning, particularly if they have relatively large heads and are visually attentive. Gradually increased duration of the prone play position with visually stimulating objects, including mirrors, musical toys, and the faces of siblings or caregivers, can be placed on the floor in front of the infant to encourage acceptance of the prone position. A roll or wedge positioned under the infant's axillae and upper chest will facilitate the ability to push up in prone, particularly for the infant with low muscle tone. An infant who is apprehensive or stressed when placed on the stomach may tolerate prone lying on the caregiver's chest, where reassuring eye contact can be maintained.

Head Balance

Balance activities to develop active head control are frequently recommended for LBW infants. Tilting responses are usually achieved most effectively with the infant in the parent's lap. Instruction to the caregivers often includes demonstration and practice using a doll before attempts with the infant. Emphasis is placed on the importance of (1) adequate trunk support; (2) movement through small ranges; (3) slow, graded motion; (4) desired head-righting response; and (5) sensitivity to indications of stress or fatigue.

Limited Use of Infant Jumper or Baby Walker

For infants with increased lower-extremity tone or a tendency for toe-standing, the use of baby walkers and jumpers is discouraged because they may increase stiffness and extension posturing of the legs.[257] Moreover, mobile baby walkers are associated with a high risk of injury, including serious trauma such as burns, drowning, and severe head injuries resulting from falls down stairs.[251,258-260] However, baby walkers are usually enjoyable for infants and may provide caregivers with some needed moments of respite in a stressed household. When recommending that time in a baby walker or jumper be restricted, the therapist should help the caregivers find alternative methods of positioning and amusement for the infant. Parents are often reluctant to discard a baby walker, believing that it promotes early ambulation and is beneficial for infants. Informing caregivers of the hazards of infant walkers and of research findings that indicate walker use may delay the acquisition of gross and fine motor skills enhances the likelihood of their cooperation.[169,251,258,261]

Ongoing Therapy

Referral to a regular program of therapeutic intervention is usually made after at least two assessments and a simulta-

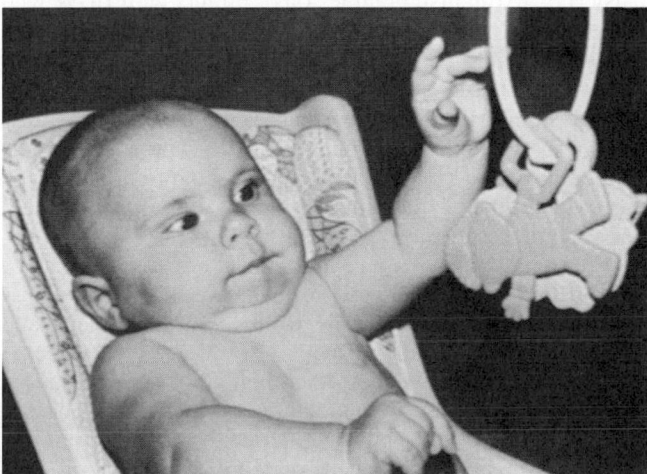

FIGURE 11-41 ■ Toys suspended directly in front of infant to encourage symmetrical reaching and midline orientation of head.

neous, short-term trial of interim home activities from the follow-up clinic. Criteria for pediatric therapy referrals include the following:

1. Persistent or progressive indications of abnormal tone
2. Developmental delay in motor skills or postural reactions
3. Increasing asymmetry or disparity between right and left sides of the body, especially if accompanied by tone differences
4. Loss of joint mobility
5. Feeding difficulties

As described in the clinical decision-making pathway previously described, a referral for intervention is determined after considering several key factors, including the following:

1. Infant's medical status
2. Concerns and priorities of parents or caregivers
3. Home environment
4. Availability of therapy services relative to geographical, financial, and personnel factors

Effectiveness of Early Therapy for Infants

Critical Analysis of Evidence

The effectiveness of pediatric therapy for high-risk or neurologically abnormal infants has been addressed by numerous studies and reviews with inconclusive and, at times, conflicting results.[168,170-174,206,262,263] The therapist whose clinical responsibilities include referring high-risk infants to intervention programs or providing intervention to high-risk infants must critically analyze these studies regarding the validity of the research methods and clinical relevance. Specific questions for consideration include the following:

1. Is the sample of infants or subjects receiving intervention at risk or neurologically abnormal? Are these infants similar to the infants seen in the therapist's clinic situation?
2. Are the comparison groups of subjects similar in all relevant factors other than the intervention being studied?
3. Are the intervention techniques used clearly described, and are they consistent with conventional therapy practice?
4. Is the frequency of therapy an accurate and realistic representation of the standard of practice?
5. Is the duration and timing of intervention appropriate and relevant to what is known about change in motor function and critical periods of development?
6. Is the quality and amount of parent or caregiver participation documented, evaluated, and realistic?
7. Are the outcome measures of the study appropriate relative to the subjects included in the study sample and to the methods and objectives of the intervention?

Characteristics of Positive Intervention for the At-Risk Infant

A review of early intervention programs that demonstrated measurable positive change highlights several characteristics of effective intervention.*

High Degree of Parent Involvement

The parents or caregivers must be active participants in the therapy session as well as in the therapy program at home.

---

*References 170, 172, 173, 175, 263, 264.

Activities and techniques for home therapy programs must be meaningful and manageable. Because infants often spend much of their time in the care of adults other than parents (e.g., relatives, day care providers), verbal and written instructions given in therapy sessions must be communicated to all caregivers.

Comprehensive Program of Developmental Intervention

Motor skills cannot be addressed in isolation from other aspects of an infant's development. To improve quality of life, not just quality of movement, pediatric therapists must include the broad perspective of infant learning and development.

Well-Defined Curriculum of Sequential Activities

Physical and occupational therapy for infants has traditionally been implemented through a flexible and variable selection of therapy activities rather than a structured curriculum. However, a defined program of learning objectives and activities enables the therapist and caregivers to have a clear and consistent understanding of the current therapeutic activities, the goals of the program, and the steps involved in achieving those goals.

Individualized, Goal-Oriented Infant Intervention

Infant therapy programs ideally incorporate the preceding recommendations into a treatment plan individualized for the infant and the home environment. Progress is monitored by systematic, quantified evaluation performed at regular intervals. Effectiveness of therapy is determined relative to the rate of progress and the specified goals for each infant.

The long-range goals of an intervention program for an infant with a neurodevelopmental disability must be realistic and stated in terms of clear, measurable objectives. When defining goals, therapists should make distinctions among (1) objectives that are generally accepted as achievable by therapy, (2) objectives that are presumed to be achievable through therapy but objective evidence is not available, and (3) changes that are not within the domain or capability of physical or occupational therapy. Examples of objectives in these categories are provided in Table 11-15.

For example, physical therapy cannot "cure" cerebral palsy (i.e., extinguish brain lesions). Infants with LBW who demonstrate neurological abnormalities, receive therapy, and subsequently show no residual signs of neuromotor abnormality demonstrate a clinical course typical of transient dystonia, in which neuromotor abnormalities largely resolve. Nevertheless, the benefit of the support and intervention provided by therapists to infants and families during this critical time of transient neuromotor impairment should not be underestimated.

Therapists and other professionals are encouraged to support and conduct research to evaluate the effectiveness of interventions that purport to modify movement and posture or improve motor function in infants with neurodevelopmental impairments. Other benefits of intervention, including prevention of contractures or deformities, design and modification of adaptive equipment, functional training, assistance in home management, parent satisfaction, and quality of life also need to be assessed and documented. Further research on the efficacy of physical and occupational

TABLE 11-15 ■ Efficacy and Feasibility of Physical Therapy Intervention for At-Risk Infants

REALISTIC GOALS OF PHYSICAL THERAPY	POTENTIAL GOALS OF PHYSICAL THERAPY NOT YET DOCUMENTED	GOALS NOT IN DOMAIN OF PHYSICAL THERAPY
Home management of disability (feeding, handling)	Change abnormal motor patterns	Cure cerebral palsy
Evaluation and construction of orthoses and splints for extremity alignment and function	Prevent physical deformities	Release contractures
Equipment selection for position and function	Minimize long-term neurodevelopmental abnormalities by early therapy	
Parent support and guidance		
Documentation of motor development in at-risk infants		

therapy is required, especially by therapists working with this population who can address the clinical questions that are most important to the quality of life for the LBW infant and family.

SUMMARY

This chapter on the NICU management and follow-up of at-risk neonates and infants presented three theoretical models for NICU practice, reviewed neonatal neuropathological conditions related to movement disorders, and described expanded professional services for at-risk neonates and infants in a relatively new subspecialty within pediatric practice. Pediatric therapists participating in intensive care nursery and follow-up teams in the care of high-risk neonates and their parents are involved in an advanced-level practice area that requires heightened responsibility for accountability and for precepted clinical training (beyond general pediatric specialization) in neonatology and infant therapy techniques. Practice guidelines for the NICU from national task forces representing the American Physical Therapy Association and American Occupational Therapy Association indicate roles, proficiencies, and knowledge for neonatal therapy and designate the NICU as a restricted area of practice to therapy assistants, aides, and entry-level students on affiliation.

Inherent in this subspecialty practice is the challenge to design comprehensive neonatal therapy protocols and clinical paths that include standardized examination instruments, comprehensive risk-management plans, long-term follow-up strategies, and systematic documentation of outcome. Ongoing analyses of the physiological risk-therapeutic benefit relationship of neuromotor and neurobehavioral treatment for chronically ill and LBW infants must guide the NICU intervention process. The quality of collaboration

between therapists and neonatal nurses largely determines the success of neonatal therapy implementation during the 24-hour care environment of the nursery.

Pediatric therapists working in neonatal units are encouraged to participate in follow-up clinics for NICU graduates to identify and analyze the development of movement dysfunction and behavioral sequelae that may, in the future, be minimized or prevented with creative neonatal treatment approaches. The important preventive aspect of neonatal treatment must be guided by careful analyses of neurodevelopmental and functional outcomes in the first year of life.

The LBW or medically fragile infant is at increased risk for major and minor neurodevelopmental problems that may be manifested in infancy or not became evident until childhood. Prenatal and perinatal risk factors may identify infants who have a greater likelihood of neurological complications, but the relation between single factors and outcome is neither direct nor consistent. Abnormal neurological signs in the first year are also not reliably predictive of abnormal outcome. Attempts to identify factors that definitively indicate significant brain injury are complicated by changing NICU technology, management procedures, environmental variables, and variability among and within individual infants.

In deciding whether and when an infant requires regular intervention, consideration must be given both to the potential for abnormalities to resolve during the first year and to the time span that may elapse before definitive evidence of cerebral palsy. The pediatric therapist's long-term clinical management of the at-risk infant is guided by the developmental course of the individual infant over time, including behavioral and cognitive growth as well as neuromotor progress, considered within the context of the priorities and values of the family.

CASE STUDY 11-1 ■ HIGH-RISK INFANT A

The infant was born prematurely at 29 weeks of gestation with a birth weight of 940 g. Her neonatal course was complicated by idiopathic respiratory distress syndrome, which was treated with surfactant.

She was first evaluated in the high-risk infant follow-up clinic at 4 months' corrected age (6 months' chronological age). Her mother stated that the infant had several respiratory illnesses after discharge from the

NICU. She reported that her infant felt "tense" compared with her older child born at term and seemed to be "a little behind" in overall development. Performance on the BSID-II generated an MDI of 94 and PDI of 82. On the MAI, this infant had a total risk score of 7. She had mildly increased lower extremity muscle tone evident in mild resistance to passive range of motion of her hips and ankles. She demonstrated

Continued

CASE STUDY 11-1 ■ HIGH-RISK INFANT A—cont'd

persistent primitive reflexes, including the asymmetrical tonic neck reflex, Moro reflex, and tonic labyrinthine reflex influence in supine. Head balance was immature, but emerging righting reactions were noted. When the infant was observed in the supine position her posture was extended, but she was beginning to bring her hands to midline. In prone, she had started to push up on elbows but posture was immature and unstable. Her parents were given recommendations for handling to include holding and carrying positions with shoulders forward to inhibit retraction, frequent play in the prone position, and increased opportunities for reaching in supine.

When the infant returned at 8 months' corrected age, her mother reported that progress had been made in the areas of rolling, talking, and sitting. She indicated that the body "stiffness" was less evident, but the infant still did not like to play on her "tummy" and instead preferred to use the baby walker. BSID-II scores at this time were MDI of 101 and PDI of 81. The MAI total risk score was 9. Increased muscle tone observed previously was less evident and she had full hip mobility but some resistance to passive ankle movement. Muscle tone of the trunk was mildly hypotonic but age-appropriate antigravity movements were demonstrated in all positions. Primitive reflexes were no longer evident except for the positive support reflex, characterized by toe-standing tendency during weight bearing. Balance reactions were present but immature in some areas, including head righting into flexion and protective extension reactions. In volitional skills, the infant was now sitting independently for up to 30 seconds, could roll from supine to prone, and could pivot sideways in the prone position. She could pick up a block with either hand and transfer objects. Immaturity was observed in sitting balance, inability to move out of

sitting, and failure to move forward on the floor (i.e., low two-point crawl). She attempted to pick up a pellet but was unable to do so. Her parents were advised to discontinue using the baby walker and to maximize play time on the floor. Because the infant reportedly enjoyed watching her 4-year-old sibling the therapist recommended that he play on the floor beside her. Her mother was also advised to provide the infant with tiny bits of food (e.g., Cheerios) to practice fine motor dexterity.

When seen at 12 months' corrected age, the infant had an MDI of 108 and a PDI of 88. Although not yet walking independently, she was cruising with good weight shift and balance. She was able to creep reciprocally on hands and knees and pulled to stand. She picked up a pellet with an inferior pincer grasp. No deviations of muscle tone or reflex development were observed during examination by the developmental pediatrician. The infant was developing normally and will return for follow-up at 2 years of age. Her parents were advised to call if she was not walking within 2 months or if they had any concerns regarding her pattern of independent walking.

In the management of this child who demonstrated abnormal signs, the primary responsibilities of the pediatric therapist were ongoing assessment and parental guidance and teaching. Although initial concerns about this infant's muscle tone and reflex deviations were present, diagnosing her with a particular condition would have been inappropriate. When followed up over time, the abnormalities resolved and proved to be transient. This child should continue to be followed up in the high-risk infant clinic because she remains at risk for other neurodevelopmental problems that may not become evident until school age.

CASE STUDY 11-2 ■ HIGH-RISK INFANT B

The infant was born prematurely at 29 weeks of gestation with a birth weight of 1200 g. The neonatal course was complicated by idiopathic respiratory distress syndrome and persistent apnea and bradycardia. Cranial ultrasonography revealed a left subependymal hemorrhage with ventriculomegaly and left-sided periventricular leukomalacia.

She was first seen in the high-risk infant follow-up clinic at 4 months' corrected age (6 months and 17 days' chronological age). The parents stated that they had no specific concerns regarding their daughter's development. On the BSID-II the infant received an MDI of 96 and a PDI of 87. On the MAI she received a total risk score of 14. Muscle tone was normal at rest but increased when she was active or agitated. Tone in the lower extremities was mildly increased with restricted passive movement in the hip adductor and gastrosoleus muscles bilaterally. In supine she was frequently in an extended posture and brought her hands to midline

only once during the examination. In prone she was able to push up and elevate her head while kicking actively. In the prone suspended position, she showed good postural elevation but movements were stiff. Persistent primitive reflexes included the tonic labyrinthine reflex in supine, asymmetrical tonic neck reflex, neonatal positive support reflex, and bilateral ankle clonus. Plantar grasp with toe curling was observed on the right. Righting and equilibrium reactions were emerging. She showed a mature Landau with full extension in prone suspension, which is atypical for her age. In volitional movement, mild asymmetry was evident because she had difficulty bringing her right arm forward in prone and brought her left arm to midline more frequently. Her kicking pattern in supine was low (close to the surface), and she did not elevate her hips. On the right side, hip extension was accompanied by knee extension and plantar flexion of the ankle. She was not yet reaching

CASE STUDY 11-2 ■ HIGH-RISK INFANT B—cont'd

for objects, and her hands were frequently fisted, particularly on the right. Her parents were assisted with handling skills to reduce shoulder retraction and extension posturing and to facilitate symmetry in movements and posture.

When the family returned for a follow-up visit at 6 months they reported that their daughter was making good progress, but she continued to prefer use of her left hand in spite of their efforts to encourage use of the right hand. At this evaluation, Bayley Scale scores were an MDI of 94 and a PDI of 83; the MAI total risk score was 13. The infant had made the following developmental progress: (1) rolling from supine to prone (over the right side only), (2) beginning sitting balance, and (3) reaching out and grasping objects. She showed a preference for and greater skill and dexterity with her left hand. Occasional fisting was still observed on the right hand. She transferred objects only from right to left. Muscle tone continued to be increased in the lower extremities with restricted passive mobility of the gastrosoleus muscles bilaterally. Toe clawing was observed on the right with minimal spontaneous dorsiflexion observed on this side. Primitive reflexes were integrated except for persistent neonatal positive support and asymmetrical tonic neck reflex to the right. Automatic reactions were improved, but balance responses were asymmetrical with equilibrium reactions and protective extension reactions delayed on the right. Although the developmental progress was encouraging, the persistent asymmetry remained a major concern. The infant was referred to a developmental intervention program with the recommendation that she receive consistent pediatric therapy in her home at least once a week.

The infant was seen in the follow-up clinic at 12 months' corrected age (14 months' chronological age).

On the BSID the MDI was 95 and the PDI was 82. She now was creeping reciprocally on hands and knees. When she pulled to stand she consistently brought the left foot up first. She cruised holding on to furniture with a tendency to stand on her toes on the right. She picked up cubes with either hand but showed partial palmar grasp on the right. She picked up a pellet with an inferior pincer grasp on the left but scooped it into the palm of the right hand. Muscle tone continued to be mildly increased in the lower extremities with Achilles tendon tightness, particularly on the right. She sat independently with a mildly flexed thoracic spine. When moving into and out of sitting, she lacked full trunk rotation and weight was predominately over the left hip. Language development was considered appropriate for her age. The infant was diagnosed with mild right hemiplegic cerebral palsy. It was recommended that she continue in the intervention therapy program and return for reevaluation at 2 years of age.

In the management of this child, the role of the pediatric therapist was assessment of neurodevelopmental status and referral to therapy when it became evident that the abnormalities of muscle tone were persisting and interfering with developmental progress. Of note, this child's MDI scores were in the normal range at both the 4- and 8-month examinations. Because the BSID-II does not require infants to perform tasks with both hands, a normal score can be obtained by using just one side of the body. This child should continue to be followed up in the high-risk infant clinic after 2 years of age to provide periodic reassessment and guidance to the family as they confront questions of school placement and program planning for their child.

ACKNOWLEDGMENT

I thank Marcia Swanson, PT, MPH, PhD, for significant contributions to the sections on neuropathology, NICU follow-up, and case studies.

REFERENCES

1. Bhushan V, Paneth N, Keily JL: Impact of improved survival of very low birth weight infants on recent secular trends in the prevalence of cerebral palsy, *Pediatrics* 91:1094-1100, 1993.
2. Brothwood M, Wolke D, Gamsu H et al: Mortality, morbidity, growth and development of babies weighing 501-1000 grams and 1001-1500 grams at birth, *Acta Paediatr Scand* 77:10-18, 1988.
3. Hack M, Friedman H, Fanaroff AA: Outcomes of extremely low birth weight infants, *Pediatrics* 98:931-937, 1996.
4. O'Shea TM, Klinepeter KL, Goldstein DJ, et al: Survival and developmental disability in infants with birth weights of 501 to 800 grams, born between 1979 and 1994, *Pediatrics* 100:982-986, 1997.
5. Peters K: Does routine nursing care complicate the physiologic status of the premature neonate with respiratory distress syndrome? *J Perinat Neonatal Nurs* 6:67-84, 1992.
6. Sommerfelt K, Markestad T, Ellertson B: Neuropsychological performance in low birth weight preschoolers: a population-based, controlled study, *Eur J Pediatr* 157:53-58, 1998.
7. Sweeney JK, Heriza CB, Reilly MA et al: Practice guidelines for the physical therapist in the neonatal intensive care unit (NICU), *Pediatr Phys Ther* 11:119, 1999.
8. Als H, Butler S, Kosta S et al: The Assessment of Preterm Infant Behavior (APIB): furthering the understanding and measurement of neurodevelopmental competence in preterm and full-term infants, *MRDD Research Rev* 11:94-102, 2005.
9. Als H: A synactive model of neonatal behavioral organization: framework for the assessment of neurobehavioral development in the premature infant and for support of infants and parents in the neonatal intensive care environment, *Phys Occup Ther Pediatr* 6:3, 1986.
10. Als H, Lawhorn G, Brown E et al: Individualized behavioral and environmental care for the VLBW preterm infant at high risk for bronchopulmonary dysplasia: NICU and developmental outcome, *Pediatrics* 78:1123-1132, 1986.
11. Fetters L: Sensorimotor management of the high-risk neonate, *Phys Occup Ther Pediatr* 6:217, 1986.
12. Affleck G, Tennen H, Rowe J: Mothers, fathers, and the crises of newborn intensive care, *Inf Mental Health J* 11:12, 1990.
13. Kenner C: Caring for the NICU parent, *J Perinat Neonatal Nurs* 4:78-87, 1990.
14. Pohlman S: Father's role in NICU care: evidence-based practice. In Kenner K, McGrath JM, editors: *Developmental care of newborns & infants,* St. Louis, 2004, Mosby.

15. Mitchell JS: *Taking on the world: empowering strategies for parents of children with disabilities,* New York, 1982, Harcourt Brace Jovanovich.

16. Mercer RT: *Nursing care for parents at risk,* Thorofare, NJ, 1977, Slack.

17. Groopman J: *The anatomy of hope,* New York, 2004, Random House.

18. Leviton A, Gilles F: Ventriculomegaly, delayed myelination, white matter hypoplasia, and "periventricular" leukomalacia: How are they related? *Pediatr Neurol* 15:127-136, 1996.

19. Paneth N, Rudelli R, Kazam E et al: *Brain damage in the preterm infant,* London, 1994, MacKeith Press.

20. Ment LR, Vohr B, Oh W et al: Neurodevelopmental outcome at 36 months' corrected age of preterm infants in the multicenter indomethacin intraventricular hemorrhage prevention trial, *Pediatrics* 98:714-718, 1996.

21. Parer JT: Evaluation of the fetus during labor, *Curr Probl Pediatr* 12:1-58, 1982.

22. Perlman JM, Rollins N, Burns D, et al: Relationship between periventricular intraparenchymal echodensities and germinal matrix–intraventricular hemorrhage in the very low birth weight neonate, *Pediatrics* 91:474-480, 1993.

23. Volpe JJ: *Neurology of the newborn,* ed 4, Philadelphia, 2001, WB Saunders.

24. Whitaker AH, Feldman JF, Van Rossem R et al: Neonatal cranial ultrasound abnormalities in low birth weight infants: relation to cognitive outcomes at six years of age, *Pediatrics* 98:719-729, 1996.

25. Aziz K, Vickar DB, Sauve RS et al: Province-based study of neurologic disability of children weighing 500 through 1249 grams at birth in relation to neonatal cerebral ultrasound findings, *Pediatrics* 95:837-844, 1995.

26. Fawer CL, Diebold P, Calame A: Periventricular leucomalacia and neurodevelopmental outcome in preterm infants, *Arch Dis Child* 62:30, 1987.

27. Piecuch RE, Leonard CH, Cooper BA et al: Outcome of extremely low birth weight infants (500 to 999 grams) over a 12-year period, *Pediatrics* 100:633-639, 1997.

28. Krishnamoorthy KS, Kuban KC, Leviton A et al: Periventricular-intraventricular hemorrhage, sonographic localization, phenobarbital, and motor abnormalities in low birth weight infants, *Pediatrics* 85:1027-1033, 1990.

29. Pinto-Martin JA, Riolo S, Cnaan A et al: Cranial ultrasound prediction of disabling and nondisabling cerebral palsy at age two in a low birth weight population, *Pediatrics* 95:249-254, 1995.

30. Allan WC, Vohr B, Makuch RW et al: Antecedents of cerebral palsy in a multicenter trial of indomethacin for intraventricular hemorrhage, *Arch Pediatr Adolesc Med* 151:580-585, 1997.

31. Cooke RW: Cerebral palsy in low birthweight infants, *Arch Dis Child* 65:201-206, 1990.

32. de Vries LS, Eken P, Groenendaal F et al: Correlation between the degree of periventricular leukomalacia diagnosed using cranial ultrasound and MRI later in infancy in children with cerebral palsy, *Neuropediatrics* 24:263-268, 1993.

33. Ringelberg J, van de Bor M: Outcome of transient periventricular echodensities in preterm infants, *Neuropediatrics* 24:269-273, 1993.

34. Koeda T, Suganuma I, Kohno Y et al: MR imaging of spastic diplegia: comparative study between preterm and term infants, *Neuroradiology* 32:187-190, 1990.

35. Cioni G, DiPaco MC, Bertuccelli B et al: MRI findings and sensorimotor development in infants with bilateral spastic cerebral palsy, *Brain Dev* 19:245-253, 1997.

36. Dammann O, Leviton A: Duration of transient hyperechoic images of white matter in very-low-birthweight infants: a proposed classification, *Dev Med Child Neurol* 39:2-5, 1997.

37. Weisglas-Kuperus N, Baerts W, Fetter WP, et al: Minor neurological dysfunction and quality of movement in relation to neonatal cerebral damage and subsequent development, *Dev Med Child Neurol* 36:727-735, 1994.

38. Murphy DJ, Hope PL, Johnson A: Ultrasound findings and clinical antecedents of cerebral palsy in very preterm infants, *Arch Dis Child* 74:F105-109, 1996.

39. Roth SC, Baudin J, McCormick DC et al: Relationship between ultrasound appearance of the brain of very preterm infants and neurodevelopmental impairment at eight years, *Dev Med Child Neurol* 35:755-768, 1993.

40. Murphy DJ, Hope PL, Johnson A: Neonatal risk factors for cerebral palsy in very preterm infants: case-control study, *BMJ* 314:404-408, 1997.

41. Jongmans M, Mercuri E, De Vries L et al: Minor neurological signs and perceptual-motor difficulties in prematurely born children, *Arch Dis Child Fetal Neonatal Ed* 76:F9-14, 1997.

42. Olsen P, Paakko E, Vainionpaa L et al: Magnetic resonance imaging of periventricular leukomalacia and its clinical correlation in children. *Ann Neurol* 41:754-761, 1997.

43. van der Bor M, den Ouden L, Guit GL: Value of cranial ultrasound and magnetic resonance imaging in predicting neurodevelopmental outcome in preterm infants, *Pediatrics* 90:196, 1992.

44. Kuban KCK, Leviton A: Cerebral palsy, *N Engl J Med* 330:188-195, 1994.

45. Blackburn S: Environmental impact of the NICU on developmental outcomes, *J Pediatr Nurs* 13:279-289, 1998.

46. Perlman JM: Neurobehavioral deficits in premature graduates of intensive care: potential medical and neonatal environmental risk factors, *Pediatrics* 108:1339-1348, 2001.

47. Graven SN, Bowen FW, Brooten D et al: The high-risk infant environment. Part 1: the role of the neonatal intensive care unit in the outcome of high-risk infants, *J Perinatol* 12:164-172, 1992.

48. American Occupational Therapy Association, Neonatal Intensive Care Unit Task Force: Knowledge and skills for occupational therapy practice in the neonatal intensive care unit, *Am J Occup Ther* 47:1100, 1993.

49. Sweeney JK, Chandler LS: Neonatal physical therapy: medical risks and professional education, *Inf Young Child* 2:59, 1990.

50. Tjossem TD: Early intervention: Issues and approaches. In Tjossem TD, editor: *Intervention strategies for high risk infants and young children,* Baltimore, 1976, University Park Press.

51. Blackburn ST: Assessment of risk: perinatal, family, and environmental perspectives, *Phys Occup Ther Pediatr* 6:105, 1986.

52. Bhushan V, Paneth N, Kiely JL: Hyaline membrane disease, birth weight, and gestational age, *Am J Dis Child* 136:888, 1982.

53. Bhushan V, Paneth N, Keily JL: Impact of improved survival of very low birth weight infants on recent secular trends in the prevalence of cerebral palsy, *Pediatrics* 91:1094-1100, 1993.

54. Vohr BR, Coll CG, Lobato D et al: Neurodevelopmental and medical status of low-birthweight survivors of bronchopulmonary dysplasia at 10 to 12 years of age, *Dev Med Child Neurol* 33:690-607, 1991.

55. Skidmore MD, Rivers A, Hack M: Increased risk of cerebral palsy among very low-birthweight infants with chronic lung disease, *Dev Med Child Neurol* 32:325-332, 1990.

56. Dubowitz LM, Dubowitz V, Goldberg C: Clinical assessment of gestational age in the newborn infant, *J Pediatr* 77:1-10, 1970.

57. Amiel-Tison C: Neurological evaluation of the maturity of newborn infants, *Arch Dis Child* 43:89-93, 1968.

58. Amiel-Tison C, Grenier A: *Neurological assessment during the first year of life,* New York, 1986, Oxford University Press.

59. Amiel-Tison C: Does neurological assessment still have a place in the NICU? *Acta Paediatr* 416(suppl):31-38, 1996.

60. Ballard JL, Novak KK, Driver M: A simplified score for assessment of fetal maturation of newly born infants, *J Pediatr* 95:769-774, 1979.

61. Ballard JL, Khoury JC, Wedig K, et al: New Ballard score, expanded to include extremely premature infants, *J Pediatr* 119:417-423, 1991.

62. Prechtl H: The neurological examination of the full-term newborn infant. In *Clinics in developmental medicine, no. 63,* Philadelphia, 1977, JB Lippincott.

63. Brazelton TB, Nugent JK: Neonatal behavioral assessment scale. In *Clinics in developmental medicine, No. 137,* London, 1995, Mac Keith Press.

64. Prechtl H, Beintema D: The neurological examination of the newborn infant. In *Clinics in developmental medicine, No. 12,* London, 1964, Heinemann Educational Books.

65. Provost B: Normal development from birth to 4 months: extended use of the NBAS-K: part I, *Phys Occup Ther Pediatr* 2:39, 1980.

66. Provost B: Normal development from birth to 4 months: extended use of the NBAS-K: part II, *Phys Occup Ther Pediatr* 1:19, 1981.

67. Wilhelm IJ: The neurobehavioral assessment of the high-risk neonate. In Wilhelm IJ, editor: *Physical therapy assessment in early infancy,* New York, 1993, Churchill Livingstone.

68. Widmayer SM, Field TM: Effects of Brazelton demonstrations for mothers on the development of preterm infants, *Pediatrics* 67:711-714, 1981.

69. Nugent JK: The Brazelton Neonatal Behavioral Assessment Scale: implications for intervention, *Pediatr Nurs* 42:18-21,67, 1981.

70. Nugent JK: *Using the NBAS with infants and their families: guidelines for intervention,* White Plains, NY, 1985, March of Dimes Birth Defects Foundation.

71. *Brazelton neonatal behavioral assessment scale training films,* Cambridge, MA, Educational Development Corporation, www.brazelton-institute.com/. Accessed September 2006.

72. Brazelton Center for Infants and Parents: *Brazelton neonatal behavioral assessment scale certification program,* Boston, MA. The Brazelton Institute. www.brazelton-institute.com/. Accessed September 4, 2006.

73. Dubowitz L, Dubowitz V, Mercuri E: The neurological assessment of the preterm and full-term newborn infant. In *Clinics in developmental medicine, No. 148,* London, 1999, Mac Keith Press.

74. Parmelee AH, Michaelis MD: Neurological examination of the newborn. In Hellmuth J, editor: *Exceptional infant, vol 2,* New York, 1971, Brunner/Mazel.

75. Mercuri E, Dubowitz L, Rutherford M, et al: Early prognostic indicators of outcome of infants with neonatal cerebral infarction: a clinical, EEG, and MRI study, *Pediatrics* 103:39-46, 1999.

76. Dubowitz LM, Dubowitz V, Palmer PG, et al: Correlation of neurologic assessment in the preterm newborn infant with outcome at 1 year, *J Pediatr* 105:452-456, 1984.

77. Heriza C: The neonate with cerebral palsy. In Scully R, Barnes ML, editors: *Physical therapy,* Philadelphia, 1989, Lippincott.

78. Campbell SK: The infant at risk for developmental disability. In Campbell SK, editor: *Decision making in pediatric neurologic physical therapy,* Philadelphia, 1999, Churchill Livingstone.

79. Dubowitz L: Neurologic assessment. In Ballard R, editor: *Pediatric care of the ICN graduate,* Philadelphia, 1988, Saunders.

80. Als H, Lawhon G, Duffy FH et al: Individualized developmental care for the very low-birth-weight preterm infant: medical and neurofunctional effects, *JAMA* 272:853-858, 1994.

81. Sweeney JK: Assessment of the special care nursery environment: effects on the high risk infant. In Wilhelm IJ, editor: *Physical therapy assessment in early infancy,* New York, 1993, Churchill Livingstone.

82. Lester BM, Tronik EZ: *NICU network neurobehavioral scale manual,* Baltimore, 2005, Brookes.

83. Campbell SK, Osten ET, Kolobe TH, et al: Development of the test of infant motor performance, *Phys Med Rehabil Clin North Am* 4:541, 1993.

84. Campbell SK, Kolobe TH, Osten ET et al: Construct validity of the Test of Infant Motor Performance, *Phys Ther* 75:585-597, 1995.

85. Murney ME, Campbell SK: The ecological relevance of the Tests of Infant Motor Performance elicited scale items, *Phys Ther* 78:479-489, 1998.

86. Campbell SK, Kolobe TH: Concurrent validity of the Test of Infant Motor Performance with the Alberta Infant Motor Scale, *Pediatr Phys Ther* 12:1, 2000.

87. Flegel J, Kolobe TH: Predictive validity of the Test of Infant Motor Performance as measured by the Bruiniks-Oseretsky Test of Motor Proficiency at school age, *Phys Ther* 82:762-771, 2002.

88. Kolobe TH, Bulanda M, Susman L: Predicting motor outcome at preschool age for infants tested at 7, 30, 60, and 90 days after term age

using the Test of Infant Motor Performance, *Phys Ther* 84:1144-1156, 2004.

89. Fitzgerald M, Anand KJS: Developmental neuroanatomy and neurophysiology of pain. In Schnechter NL, Berde CB, Yaster M, editors: *Pain: infants, children, adolescents,* Baltimore, 1993, William & Wilkins.

90. Vanhatalo S, van Nieuwenhuizen O: Fetal pain? *Brain Dev* 22:145-150, 2000.

91. Anand KJS: Effects of perinatal pain and stress, *Prog Brain Res* 122:117-129, 2000.

92. Blackburn ST: *Maternal, fetal & neonatal physiology: a clinical perspective,* ed 2, St. Louis, 2003, Saunders.

93. Grunau RV, Whitfield MF, Petrie JH: Pain sensitivity and temperament in extremely low-birth-weight premature toddlers and preterm and full-term controls, *Pain* 58:341-346, 1994.

94. Porter FL, Grunau RE, Anand KJ: Long-term effects of pain in infants, *J Dev Behav Pediatr* 20:253-261, 1999.

95. Smythe JW, McCormick CM, Meaney MJ: Median eminence corticotropin-releasing hormone content following prenatal stress and neonatal handling, *Brain Res Bull* 40:195-199, 1996.

96. Stevens B, Johnston C, Petryshen P et al: Premature infant pain profile: development and initial validation, *Clin J Pain* 12:13-22, 1996.

97. Bildner J, Krechel S: Increasing staff nurse awareness of postoperative pain management in the NICU, *Neonatal Network* 15: 11-16, 1996.

98. Lawrence J, Alcock D, McGrath P, et al: The development of a tool to assess neonatal pain, *Neonatal Network* 12: 59-66, 1993.

99. Sweeney JK: Physiological adaptation of neonates to neurological assessment, *Phys Occup Ther Pediatr* 6:155, 1986.

100. Sweeney JK: Physiological and behavioral effects of neurological assessment in preterm and full-term neonates [abstract], *Phys Occup Ther Pediatr* 9:144, 1989.

101. Wilhelm IJ: The neurologically suspect neonate. In Campbell SK, editor: *Pediatric neurologic physical therapy,* New York, 1985, Churchill Livingstone.

102. Avery GB: *Neonatology: pathophysiology and management of the newborn,* ed 5, Philadelphia, 2005, Lippincott, Williams & Wilkins.

103. Blackburn ST, VandenBerg KA: Assessment and management of neonatal neurobehavioral development. In Kenner C, Lott JW, editors: *Comprehensive neonatal nursing care,* ed 3, Philadelphia, 2003, Saunders.

104. Crane L: Physical therapy for the neonate with respiratory disease. In Irwin S, Tecklin JS, editors: *Cardiopulmonary physical therapy,* ed 2, St. Louis, 1990, Mosby.

105. Crane L: Cardiorespiratory management of the high-risk neonate: implications for developmental therapists, *Phys Occup Ther Pediatr* 6:255, 1986.

106. Crane L: The neonate and child. In Frownfelter DL, editor: *Chest physical therapy and pulmonary rehabilitation: an interdisciplinary approach,* ed 3, Chicago, 1983, Year Book.

107. Miles MS: Parents of critically ill premature infants: sources of stress, *Crit Care Nurs Q* 12:69-74, 1989.

108. Lawton G: Facilitation of parenting the premature infant within the newborn intensive care unit, *J Perinat Neonat Nurs* 16:71-82, 2002.

109. Hansen N, Okken A: Transcutaneous oxygen tension of newborn infants in different behavioral states, *Pediatr Res* 14:911, 1980.

110. de Groot L: Posture and motility in preterm infants [annotation], *Dev Med Child Neurol* 42:65-68, 2000.

111. Dusing S, Mercer V, Yu B et al: Trunk position in supine of infants born preterm and at term: an assessment using a computerized pressure mat, *Pediatr Phys Ther* 17:2, 2005.

112. Bly L: *Motor skills acquisition in the first year of life,* Tucson, AZ, 1994, Therapy Skill Builders.

113. Gorga D, Stern FM, Ross G, et al: Neuromotor development of preterm and full-term infants, *Early Hum Dev* 18:137-149, 1988.

114. Georgieff MK, Bernbaum JC: Abnormal shoulder muscle tone in premature infants during their first 18 months of life, *Pediatrics* 77:664-669 1986.

115. Davis PM, Robinson R, Harris L et al: Persistent mild hip deformation in preterm infants. *Arch Dis Child* 69:597-598, 1993.

116. Katz K, Krikler R, Wielunsky E, et al: Effect of neonatal posture on later lower limb rotation and gait in premature infants, *J Pediatr Orthop* 11:520-522, 1991.

117. Martin RJ, Herrell N, Rubin D et al: Effect of supine and prone positions on arterial oxygen tension in the preterm infant, *Pediatrics* 63:528-531, 1979.

118. Wagaman MJ, Shutack JG, Moomjian AS, et al: Improved oxygenation and lung compliance with prone positioning of neonates, *J Pediatr* 94:787-791, 1979.

119. Scott S, Lucas P, Cole T, et al: Weight gain and movement patterns of very low birthweight babies nursed on lambs wool, *Lancet* 2:1014-1016, 1983.

120. Lockridge T, Taquino L, Knight A: Back to sleep: is there room in that crib for both AAP recommendations and developmentally supportive care? *Neonatal Network* 18:29-33, 1999.

121. Korner AF, Kraemer HC, Haffner ME et al: Effects of waterbed flotation on premature infants: a pilot study, *Pediatrics* 56:361-367, 1975.

122. Marsden DJ: Reduction of head flattening in preterm infants, *Dev Med Child Neurol* 22:507-509, 1980.

123. Long T, Soderstrom E: A critical appraisal of positioning infants in the neonatal intensive care unit, *Phys Occup Ther Pediatr* 15:17, 1995.

124. Hensinger RN, Jones ET: *Neonatal orthopedics,* New York, 1981, Grune & Stratton.

125. Field T: Supplemental stimulation of preterm neonates, *Early Hum Dev* 4:301-314, 1980.

126. Kahn-D'Angelo L: The special care nursery. In Campbell SK, Vander Linden D, Palisano RJ, editors: *Physical therapy for children,* ed 2, Philadelphia, 2000, Saunders.

127. Korner AF, Thoman EB: The relative efficacy of contact and vestibular-proprioceptive stimulation in soothing neonates, *Child Dev* 43:443-453, 1972.

128. Rice RD: Neurophysiological development in premature infants following stimulation, *Dev Psychol* 13:69, 1977.

129. Scafidi FA: Effects of tactile/kinesthetic stimulation on the clinical course and sleep/wake behavior of preterm neonates. *Infant Behav Dev* 9:91, 1986.

130. White-Traut R, Nelson MN, Silvestri JM et al: Responses of preterm infants to unimodal and multimodal sensory intervention, *Pediatr Nurs* 23:169-175, 1997.

131. Creger PJ: *Developmental interventions for preterm and high-risk infants: self-study modules for professionals,* Tucson, 1989, Therapy Skill Builders.

132. Vergara ER, Bigsby R: *Developmental & therapeutic interventions in the NICU,* Baltimore, 2004, Brookes.

133. Hunter JG: The neonatal intensive care unit. In Case-Smith J, Allen AS, Pratt PN, editors: *Occupational therapy for children,* ed 4, St Louis, 2001, Mosby.

134. McGrath JM, Brock N: Efficacy and utilization of skin-to-skin care in the NICU, *Newborn Nurs Rev* 2:17, 2002.

135. Ludington-Hoe SM, Nguyen N, Swinth JY, et al: Kangaroo care: research results and practice implications and guidelines, *Neonatal Network* 13:19, 1994.

136. Sweeney JK: Neonatal hydrotherapy: an adjunct to developmental intervention in an intensive care nursery setting, *Phys Occup Ther Pediatr* 3:20, 1983.

137. Ludington-Hoe SM, Cong X, Hashemi F: Infant crying: nature, physiologic consequences and select interventions, *Neonoatal Network* 21:29-36, 2002.

138. Palmer MP: Identification and management of the transitional suck pattern in premature infants, *J Perinat Neonatal Nurs* 7:66, 1993.

139. Wolf LS, Glass RP: *Feeding and swallowing disorders in infancy: assessment and management,* Tucson, AZ, 1992, Therapy Skill Builders.

140. Braun MA, Palmer MM: A pilot study of oral-motor dysfunction in "at-risk" infants, *Phys Occup Ther Pediatr* 5:13, 1985.

141. Barnard KE, Eyres SJ: Feeding scale. In *Child health assessment,* Hyattsville, MD, 1978, U.S. Department of Health, Education, and Welfare.

142. Thoyre SM, Shaker CS, Pridham KF: The early feeding skills assessment for preterm infants, *Neonatal Network* 24:7-16, 2005.

143. Glass RP, Wolf LS: Feeding and oral-motor skills. In Case-Smith J, editor: *Pediatric occupational therapy in early intervention,* ed 2, Boston, 1998, Butterworth-Heinemann.

144. Leonard E, Trykowski LE, Kirkpatrick BV: Nutritive sucking in high risk neonates after perioral stimulation, *Phys Ther* 60:299-302, 1980.

145. Fucile S, Gisel E, Lau C: Oral stimulation accelerates the transition from tube to oral feeding in preterm infants, *J Pediatr* 141:230-236, 2002.

146. Trykowski LE, Kirkpatrick BV, Leonard EL: Enhancement of nutritive sucking in premature infants, *Phys Occup Ther Pediatr* 1:27, 1982.

147. Measel CP: Non-nutritive sucking during tube feedings: effect on clinical course in premature infants, *Obstet Gynecol Neonat Nurs* 8:265-274, 1979.

148. Rogers B, Arvedson J: Assessment of infant oral sensorimotor and swallowing function, *Ment Retard Dev Disabil Res Rev* 11:74-82, 2005.

149. Leander D, Pettett G: Parental response to the birth of a high-risk neonate: dynamics and management, *Phys Occup Ther Pediatr* 6:205, 1986.

150. Affleck G, Tennen H, Rowe J: *Infants in crisis: how parents cope with newborn intensive care and its aftermath,* New York, 1991, Springer-Verlag.

151. Sweeney JK, Gutierrez T: Musculoskeletal implications of preterm infant positioning in the NICU, *J Perinat Neonatal Nurs* 16:58-70, 2002.

152. Lynch EW, Hanson MJ, editors: *Developing cross-cultural competence: a guide for working with young children and their families,* Baltimore, 1992, Brookes.

153. Davis DH, Thoman EB: Behavioral states of premature infants: implications for neural and behavioral development, *Dev Psychobiol* 20:25-38, 1987.

154. Barnard KE, Bee HL, Hammond MA: Developmental changes in maternal interactions with term and preterm infants, *Infant Behav Dev* 7:101, 1984.

155. Crnic KA, Rogozin AS, Greenburg MT, et al: Social interaction and developmental competence of preterm and full-term infants during the first year of life, *Child Dev* 54:1199-1210, 1983.

156. Escobar GJ, Littenberg B, Petitti DB: Outcome among surviving very low birthweight infants: a meta-analysis, *Arch Dis Child* 66:204-211, 1991.

157. Hagberg B, Hagberg G: The changing panorama of cerebral palsy—bilateral spastic forms in particular, *Acta Paediatr* 416(suppl):48, 1996.

158. Pharoah PO, Platt MJ, Cooke T: The changing epidemiology of cerebral palsy, *Arch Dis Child Fetal Neonatal Ed* 75:F169-173, 1996.

159. Stanley FJ: Survival and cerebral palsy in low birthweight infants: implications for perinatal care, *Paediatr Perinat Epidemiol* 6:298-310, 1992.

160. Blitz RK, Wachtel RC, Blackmon L et al: Neurodevelopmental outcome of extremely low birth weight infants in Maryland, *Maryland Med J* 46:18-24, 1997.

161. Hack M, Klein NK, Taylor HG: Long-term developmental outcome of low birth weight infants, *The Future of Children* 5:176-196, 1995.

162. Whitfield MF, Eckstein RV, Holsti L: Extremely premature (<800 g) schoolchildren: multiple areas of disability, *Arch Dis Child* 77:F85, 1997.

163. Saigal S, Szatmari P, Rosenbaum P et al: Cognitive abilities and school performance of extremely low birth weight children and matched term control children at 8 years: a regional study, *J Pediatr* 118:751-760, 1991.

164. Teplin SW, Burchinal M, Johnson-Martin N et al: Neurodevelopmental, health, and growth status at age 6 years of children with birth weights less than 1001 grams, *J Pediatr* 118:768-777, 1991.

165. Msall ME, Buck GM, Rogers BT et al: Multivariate risks among extremely premature infants, *J Perinatol* 14:41-47, 1994.

166. Luchi JM, Bennett FC, Jackson JC: Predictors of neurodevelopmental outcome following bronchopulmonary dysplasia, *Am J Dis Child* 145:813-817, 1991.

167. Slater MA, Naqvi M, Haynes K: Neurodevelopment of monitored versus nonmonitored very low birth weight infants: the importance of family influences, *J Dev Behav Pediatr* 8:278-285, 1987.

168. Goodman M, Rothberg AD, Houston-McMillan JE et al: Effect of early neurodevelopmental therapy in normal and at-risk survivors of neonatal intensive care, *Lancet* 2:1327-1330, 1985.

169. Kauffman IB, Ridenour M: Influence of an infant walker on onset and quality of walking pattern of locomotion: an electromyographic investigation, *Percept Mot Skills* 45:1323-1329, 1977.

170. Mayo NE: The effect of physical therapy for children with motor delay and cerebral palsy, *Am J Phys Med Rehabil* 70:258-267, 1991.

171. Rothberg AD: Six-year follow-up of early physiotherapy intervention in very low birth weight infants, *Pediatrics* 88:547-552, 1991.

172. Shonkoff JP, Hauser-Cram P: Early intervention for disabled infants and their families: a quantitative analysis, *Pediatrics* 80:650-658, 1987.

173. Turnbull JD: Early intervention for children with or at risk of cerebral palsy, *Am J Dis Child* 147:54-59, 1993.

174. Weindling AM, Hallam P, Gregg J et al: A randomized controlled trial of early physiotherapy for high-risk infants, *Acta Paediatr* 85:1107-1111, 1996.

175. Resnick MB, Eyler FD, Nelson RM et al: Developmental intervention for low birth weight infants: improved early developmental outcome, *Pediatrics* 80:68-74, 1987.

176. Yoder PJ, Farran DC: Mother-infant engagements in dyads with handicapped and nonhandicapped infants: a pilot study, *Appl Res Ment Retard* 7:51-58, 1986.

177. Allen MC, Alexander GR: Gross motor milestones in preterm infants: correction for degree of prematurity, *J Pediatr* 116:955-959, 1990.

178. de Groot L, Hopkins B, Touwen B: Motor asymmetries in preterm infants at 18 weeks corrected age and outcomes at 1 year, *Early Hum Dev* 48:35-46, 1997.

179. Palisano RJ: Use of chronological and adjusted ages to compare motor development of healthy preterm and fullterm infants, *Dev Med Child Neurol* 28:180-187, 1986.

180. Piper MC, Darrah J, Byrne P: Impact of gestational age on preterm motor development at 4 months chronological and adjusted ages, *Child Care Health Dev* 15:105-115, 1989.

181. Valvano J, DeGangi GA: Atypical posture and movement findings in high risk pre-term infants, *Phys Occup Ther Pediatr* 6:71, 1986.

182. Lems W, Hopkins B, Samson JF: Mental and motor development in preterm infants: the issue of corrected age, *Early Hum Dev* 34:113-123, 1993.

183. Aylward GP: Conceptual issues in developmental screening and assessment, *J Dev Behav Pediatr* 18:340-349, 1997.

184. Ellenberg JH, Nelson KB: Early recognition of infants at high risk for cerebral palsy: examination at age four months, *Dev Med Child Neurol* 23:705-716, 1981.

185. Paban M, Piper MC: Early predictors of one year neurodevelopmental outcome for "at risk" infants, *Phys Occup Ther Pediatr* 7:17, 1987.

186. Piper MC, Darrah J, Pinnell L et al: The consistency of sequential examinations in the early detection of neurological dysfunction, *Phys Occup Ther Pediatr* 11:27, 1991.

187. Hadders-Algra M: The assessment of general movements is a valuable technique for the detection of brain dysfunction in young infants, *Acta Paediatr* 416(suppl):39-43, 1996.

188. Bartlett D: Primitive reflexes and early motor development, *J Dev Behav Pediatr* 18:151-157, 1997.

189. Swanson MW, Bennett FC, Shy KK, et al: Identification of neurodevelopmental abnormality at four and eight months by the movement assessment of infants, *Dev Med Child Neurol* 34:321-337, 1992.

190. Chandler LS, Andrews MS, Swanson MW: *Movement assessment of infants: a manual*, Rolling Bay, WA, 1980, Authors.

191. Bayley N: *Manual for the Bayley Scales of Infant Development*, ed 2, New York, 1993, Psychological Corp.

192. Rothstein JM, Echternach JL: *Primer on measurement: an introductory guide to measurement issues*, Alexandria, VA, 1993, American Physical Therapy Association.

193. Portney LG, Watkins MP: *Foundations of clinical research: applications to practice*, ed 2 Upper Saddle River, NJ, 2000, Prentice Hall.

194. Piper MC, Darrah J: *Motor assessment of the developing infant*, Philadelphia, 1994, Saunders.

195. Ross G, Lawson K: Using the Bayley II: unresolved issues in assessing the development of prematurely born children, *J Dev Behav Pediatr* 18:109-111, 1997.

196. Nellis L, Gridley BE: Review of the Bayley scales of infant development, ed 2, *J Sch Psychol* 32:201, 1994.

197. Gauthier SM, Bauer CR, Messinger DS et al: The Bayley scales of infant development II: where to start? *J Dev Behav Pediatr* 20:75-79, 1999.

198. Haley SM: Sequence of development of postural reactions by infants with Down syndrome, *Dev Med Child Neurol* 29:674-679, 1987.

199. Harris SR: Early neuromotor predictors of cerebral palsy in low-birthweight infants, *Dev Med Child Neurol* 29:508-519, 1987.

200. Rast MM, Harris SR: Motor control in infants with Down syndrome, *Dev Med Child Neurol* 27:682-685, 1985.

201. Fetters L, Tronick EZ: Neuromotor development of cocaine-exposed and control infants from birth through 15 months: poor and poorer performance, *Pediatrics* 98:938-943, 1996.

202. Schneider JW, Chasnoff IJ: Motor assessment of cocaine/polydrug exposed infants at age 4 months, *Neurotoxicol Teratol* 14:97-101, 1992.

203. Swanson MW: Neuromotor outcomes of infants exposed prenatally to cocaine: issues of assessment and interpretation, *Phys Occup Ther Pediatr* 16:35, 1996.

204. Harris-Copp M: The HIV-infected child: a critical need for physical therapy, *Clin Management* 8:16, 1988.

205. Danesak M: Concurrent validity of two infant motor scales: the Alberta Infant Motor Scale (AIMS) and the Movement Assessment of Infants (MAI), *Dev Med Child Neurol* 35(suppl)69:4, 1993.

206. Piper MC, Kunos VI, Willis DM, et al: Early physical therapy effects on the high-risk infant: a randomized controlled trial, *Pediatrics* 78:216-224, 1986.

207. Piper MC, Mazer B, Silver KM et al: Resolution of neurological symptoms in high-risk infants during the first two years of life, *Dev Med Child Neurol* 30:26-35, 1988.

208. Swanson MW: Neuromotor assessment of low-birthweight infants with normal developmental outcome, *Dev Med Child Neurol* 31(suppl 59):27, 1989.

209. Harris SR, Haley SM, Tada WL et al: Reliability of observational measures of the Movement Assessment of Infants, *Phys Ther* 64:471-477, 1984.

210. Brander R, Kramer J, Dancsak M et al: Inter-rater and test-retest reliabilities of the Movement Assessment of Infants, *Pediatr Phys Ther* 5:9, 1993.

211. Harris SR, Swanson MW, Andrews MS et al: Predictive validity of the Movement Assessment of Infants, *Dev Behav Pediatr* 5:336-342, 1984.

212. Schneider JW, Lee W, Chasnoff IJ: Field testing of the Movement Assessment of Infants, *Phys Ther* 68:321-327, 1988.

213. Luther M, Ornstein M, Asztalos E: Predictive value of the Movement Assessment of Infants (MAI) and bronchopulmonary dysplasia as a confounding variable, *Pediatr Res* 31:254A, 1992.

214. Rose-Jacobs R, Cabral H, Beeghly M et al: The Movement Assessment of Infants (MAI) as a predictor of two-year neurodevelopmental outcome for infants born at term who are at social risk, *Pediatr Phys Ther* 16:212, 2004.

215. Chandler LC: Neuromotor assessment. In Gibbs ED, Teti DM, editors: *Interdisciplinary assessment of infants: a guide for early intervention professionals*, Baltimore, 1990, Brookes.

216. Darrah J, Piper M, Watt MJ: Assessment of gross motor skills of at-risk infants: predictive validity of the Alberta Infant Motor Scale, *Dev Med Child Neurol* 40:485-491, 1998.

217. Amiel-Tison C: Does neurological assessment still have a place in the NICU? *Acta Paediatr* 416(suppl):31-38, 1996.

218. Georgieff MK, Bernbaum JC, Hoffman-Williamson M et al: Abnormal truncal muscle tone as a useful early marker for developmental delay in low birth weight infants, *Pediatrics* 77:659, 1986.

219. Zafeiriou DI, Tsikoulas IG, Kremenopoulos GM: Prospective follow-up of primitive reflex profiles in high-risk infants: clues to an early diagnosis of cerebral palsy, *Pediatr Neurol* 13:148-152, 1995.

220. Yokochi K, Shimabukuro S, Kodama K et al: Motor function of infants with athetoid cerebral palsy, *Dev Med Child Neurol* 35:909-916, 1993.

221. Droit S, Boldrini A, Cioni G: Rhythmical leg movements in low-risk and brain-damaged preterm infants, *Early Hum Dev* 44:201-213, 1996.

222. Yokochi K, Inukai K, Hosoe A et al: Leg movements in the supine position of infants with spastic diplegia, *Dev Med Child Neurol* 33:903-907, 1991.

223. Van Der Heide J, Paolicelli PB, Boldrini A et al: Kinematic and qualitative analysis of lower-extremity movements in preterm infants with brain lesions, *Phys Ther* 79:546-557, 1999.

224. Allen MC, Alexander GR: Using gross motor milestones to identify very preterm infants at risk for cerebral palsy, *Dev Med Child Neurol* 34:226-232, 1992.

225. Coolman RB, Bennett FC, Sells CJ et al: Neuromotor development of graduates of the neonatal intensive care unit: patterns encountered in the first two years of life, *J Dev Behav Pediatr* 6:327-333, 1985.

226. D'Eugenio DB, Slagle TA, Mettelman BB et al: Developmental outcome of preterm infants with transient neuromotor abnormalities, *Am J Dis Child* 147:570-574, 1993.

227. Drillien CM: Abnormal neurologic signs in the first year of life in low-birthweight infants: possible prognostic significance *Dev Med Child Neurol* 14:575-584, 1972.

228. Gorga D, Stern FM, Ross G et al: The neuromotor behavior of preterm and full-term children by three years of age: quality of movement and variability, *J Dev Behav Pediatr* 12:102-107, 1991.

229. Michaelis R, Asenbauer C, Buchwald-Saal M et al: Transitory neurological findings in a population of at risk infants, *Early Hum Dev* 34:143-153, 1993.

230. Stewart KB, Deitz JC, Crowe TK et al: Transient neurologic signs in infancy and motor outcomes at 4 1/2 years in children born biologically at risk, *Topics in Early Childhood Education* 7:71, 1988.

231. Majnemer A, Brownstein A, Kadanoff R et al: A comparison of neurobehavioral performance of healthy term and low-risk preterm infants at term, *Dev Med Child Neurol* 34:417-424, 1992.

232. Georgieff MK, Bernbaum JC: Abnormal shoulder girdle muscle tone in premature infants during their first 18 months of life, *Pediatrics* 77:664-669, 1986.

233. Gorga D, Stern FM, Ross G: Trends in neuromotor behavior of preterm and full-term infants in the first year of life: a preliminary report, *Dev Med Child Neurol* 27:756-766, 1985.

234. Marquis PJ, Ruiz NA, Lundy MS et al: Retention of primitive reflexes and delayed motor development in very low birth weight infants, *J Dev Behav Pediatr* 5:124-126, 1984.

235. Beltran RS, Coker SB: Transient dystonia of infancy: a result of intrauterine cocaine exposure? *Pediatr Neurol* 12:354-356, 1995.

236. Chiriboga CA, Vibbert M, Malouf R et al: Neurological correlates of fetal cocaine exposure: transient hypertonia of infancy and early childhood, *Pediatrics* 96:1070-1077, 1996.

237. Napiorkowski B, Lester BM, Freier MC et al: Effects of in utero substance exposure on infant neurobehavior, *Pediatrics* 98:71-75, 1995.

238. Neuspiel DR, Hamel SC, Hochberg E et al: Maternal cocaine use and infant behavior, *Neurotoxicol Teratol* 13:229-233, 1991.

239. Alessandri SM, Bendersky M, Lewis M: Cognitive functioning in 8- to 18-month-old drug-exposed infants, *Dev Psych* 34:565-573, 1998.

240. Hurt H, Brodsky NL, Betancourt L et al: Cocaine-exposed children: follow-up through 30 months, *Dev Med Child Neurol* 16:29-35, 1995.

241. Jacobson SW, Jacobson JL, Sokol RJ et al: New evidence for neurobehavioral effects of in utero cocaine exposure, *J Pediatr* 129:581-590, 1996.

242. Fewell R, Rine RM, Landau D et al: Motor ability of children prenatally exposed to cocaine: the effect of age on motor test results [abstract], *Pediatr Phys Ther* 9:194, 1997.

243. Swanson MW, Streissguth AP, Sampson PD et al: Prenatal cocaine and neuromotor outcome at four months: effect of duration of exposure, *J Dev Behav Pediatr* 20:325-334, 1999.

244. Bender SL, Word CO, DiClemente RJ et al: The developmental implications of prenatal and/or postnatal crack cocaine exposure in preschool children: a preliminary report, *J Dev Behav Pediatr* 16:418-424, 1995.

245. Heffelfinger A, Craft S, Shyken J: Visual attention in children with prenatal cocaine exposure, *J Int Neuropsychol Soc* 3:237-245, 1997.

246. Richardson GA, Conroy ML, Day NL: Prenatal cocaine exposure: effects on the development of school-age children, *Neurotoxicol Teratol* 18:627-634, 1996.

247. Aylward GP: Conceptual issues in developmental screening and assessment, *J Dev Behav Pediatr* 18:340-349, 1997.

248. Hay A, Breiger AG: The role of pediatric physical therapy in the interdisciplinary assessment process. In Guralnick MJ, editor: *Interdisciplinary clinical assessment for young children with developmental disabilities*, Baltimore, 2000, Brookes.

249. Kim MM, O'Conner KS, McLean J et al: Do parents and professionals agree on the developmental status of high-risk infants? *Pediatrics* 97:676-681, 1996.

250. Jantz JW, Blosser CD, Fruechting LA: A motor milestone change noted with a change in sleep position, *Arch Pediatr Adolesc Med* 151:565-568, 1997.

251. Thein MM, Lee J, Tay V et al: Infant walker use, injuries, and motor development, *Inj Prev* 3:63-66, 1997.

252. Capute AJ, Shapiro BK, Palmer FB et al: Normal gross motor development: the influence of race, sex, and socioeconomic status, *Dev Med Child Neurol* 27:635-643, 1985.

253. Cintas HM: Cross-cultural variation in infant motor development, *Phys Occup Ther Pediatr* 8:1, 1988.

254. Cohen E, Boettcher K, Maher T et al: Evaluation of the Peabody Developmental Gross Motor Scales for children of African American and Hispanic ethnic backgrounds, *Pediatr Phys Ther* 11:191, 1999.

255. Toy CC: *Performance of 6-month-old Asian American infants on the Movement Assessment of Infants: a descriptive study* [thesis], Seattle, 1997, University of Washington.

256. Yoder PJ: Relationship between degree of infant handicap and clarity of infant cues, *Am J Mental Defic* 91:639-641, 1987.

257. Holm VA, Harthun-Smith L, Tada WL: Infant walkers and cerebral palsy, *Am J Dis Child* 137:1189-1190, 1983.

258. Johnson CF, Ericson AK, Caniano D: Walker-related burns in infants and toddlers, *Pediatr Emerg Care* 6:58-61, 1991.

259. Partington MD, Swanson JA, Meyer FB: Head injury and the use of baby walkers: a continuing problem, *Ann Emerg Med* 20:652-654, 1991.

260. Garrett M, McElroy AM, Staines A: Locomotor milestones and baby-walkers: cross sectional study, *BMJ* 324:1494, 2002.

261. Siegel AC, Burton RV: Effects of baby walkers on motor and mental development in human infants, *J Dev Behav Pediatr* 20:355-361, 1999.

262. Barrera ME, Rosenbaum PL, Cunningham CE: Early home intervention with low-birth-weight infants and their parents, *Child Dev* 57:20-33, 1986.

263. Palmer FB, Shapiro BK, Wachtel RC et al: The effects of physical therapy on cerebral palsy, *N Engl J Med* 318:803-808, 1988.

264. McCormick MC, McCarton C, Brooks-Gunn J: The Infant Health and Development Program: interim summary, *J Dev Behav Pediatr* 19:359-370, 1998.

CHAPTER 12

Management of Clinical Problems of Children with Cerebral Palsy

Christine A. Nelson, PhD, OTR, FAOTA
Claudia Senesac, PT, PhD, PCS

KEY WORDS

cerebral palsy
direct intervention
family
indirect intervention
postural and movement compensation
research
spasticity
treatment strategies

OBJECTIVES

After reading this chapter the student/therapist will be able to:

1. Identify the parameters of the diagnosis of cerebral palsy including motor, family, and psychosocial components.
2. Analyze the multifaceted aspects of the clinical problem and appreciate a multifaceted approach to evaluation and treatment.
3. Analyze treatment strategies and their application to clinical problems.
4. Identify and critique current research for the pediatric client with cerebral palsy.
5. Identify the therapist role in the treatment of the child with cerebral palsy, with family involvement, in different settings, and with other health professionals.

OVERVIEW

Historical Perspective

Cerebral palsy is a misnomer at best. Little[1] suggested the name in the mid 1800s, but there is still no established direct relationship between the identifiable state of the brain and the distortions in posture and movement control that we are able to observe in the individual.[2,3] The condition is not always evident at birth, although the work of Prechtl[4] statistically supports the possibility of a link between the quality of spontaneous movements in the first months of life and later difficulties in coordinated movement expression. In only a minor number of children has a specific lesion been identified that corresponds to the observed motor responses of the child, and this elite group includes children with porencephaly and other early developmental malformations of the brain. Whether there is a biochemical element in the brain of a child that distorts the actual motor learning process is not established. There is a shocking variability in the age at which intervention is initiated for individual children and a wide variety of programs that do not necessarily take into account the current information available from clinical studies on efficient motor development and brain function. This confusion has led us astray in understanding the process of movement and postural distortion that characterizes children who carry the label of "cerebral palsy."

Historically, the evolution of diagnosis and treatment intervention or management is clear and relates to the recognition of the special needs of this minority of society. The British physician Little identified the condition on the basis of observable characteristics of movement and posture, or—in other words—the external features of the condition, so the initial efforts at remediation fell to orthopedists such as Deaver and Phelps.[3,5,6] Deaver placed importance on external bracing that was periodically reduced in the hope that the child would take over control of increasing parts of his own body.[5] Phelps used bracing and surgery and was a sig-

nificant force in obtaining schooling for these children in the United States.[6] He pointed out that they did not belong in academic classes with children diagnosed as retarded or mentally handicapped, and children with cerebral palsy should be exposed to a traditional academic curriculum. In his Children's Rehabilitation Institute in Reisterstown, Maryland, he also advocated restriction of a more functional limb to encourage use of the one less used, particularly in work with the upper extremities.

In the 1950s and 1960s there emerged simultaneously new theories of neuromotor behavior that redefined the clinical characteristics of cerebral palsy and permitted clinicians to orient their intervention strategies to the principles of motor development and motor learning. Kabat in conjunction with Knott introduced proprioceptive neuromuscular facilitation, known as PNF, which was applied to children with movement disorders and to adults with a history of trauma.[7] The use of diagonal patterns of movement in this approach changed the customary postures of the child and introduced more functional movement patterns in logical learning sequences. Physical therapist Rood added the more specific sensory components of ice and light quick brushing of the skin surface to guide the desired motor response.[8] She spoke of the need to focus our attention on both "heavy work" and "light work" during the early development of movement skills. These terms referred to the central body moving over limb support and limb movement with central stability. Bobath was working in London at this same time and observed the need to have a dynamic interaction between stability and mobility, after finding the inhibition of the reflexive movements was not sufficient to change the functional outcome of the child with cerebral palsy.[9] They pointed out that the areas of the child's body that appeared to be spastic changed when the body was placed in a different relationship to gravity. This observation held up for reexamination the prevailing view of the time, namely, that spasticity existed in a tendon or muscle, a specific structure.

Cerebral palsy was identified in the mid 1900s as an incident that occurred shortly before, during, or shortly after the birth of the infant. Early intervention was recommended. This time line was extended to cover the first 2 years of life, which included early cases of meningitis, encephalitis, near-drowning accidents, and so forth. although the clinicians mentioned tried to define cerebral palsy as a "disorder of posture and movement control," many of the children also presented learning problems and inadequate general brain development. There was a general agreement on categories according to movement characteristics that included spasticity, athetosis, flaccidity, ataxia, and rigidity. Categorization according to the part of the body affected was added to identify hemiplegia, quadriplegia, diplegia, and even monoplegia, affecting one limb, and triplegia, affecting three limbs. It was noted that some children moved from one category to another as they matured and therapists began to be aware that a child with high tone could have some low tone underneath when spasticity was inhibited. Fluctuating tone could be confused with ataxia and the precise intervention strategy might be elusive.

The birth process is complex at many different levels. Sequential hormonal changes alert both the fetus and the mother that it is time for a separation. The infant moves into position for exiting the uterus through the birth canal while the mother's body prepares to participate in the work/labor of the expulsion. When all goes smoothly, the head of the infant is molded by the passage through the birth canal and the membranous-like cranial plates return to their balanced alignment and functional motion.

When the birth process is prolonged for any of many reasons, the physiological timing of these changes is interrupted. Unique combinations of pressure may make it difficult for the membranous structures to maintain their structural alignment. That lack of structural alignment may persist long after birth and affect future movement and development. Rapid changes of pressure, with minor misalignments of the head and body during the birth process, result in sufficient trauma to affect the nervous system and the delicate fascia and in a small percentage of infants to affect the expression of spontaneous movements. In the majority of healthy infants born at term the spontaneous movements seem to assist in the activation of the central body and the limbs so that physiological changes in the fascia are sufficient to permit a normal expression of developmental movement responses after birth. Body movement and respiration are coordinated with the infant's physiological rhythms in this initial adaptation to the world of gravity. With complications of the pregnancy or the birth process, these spontaneous movements that are so easily made by the healthy infant become laborious and sometimes impossible, affecting motor actions, postural mechanisms, and the basic physiological rhythms. Cerebral palsy is a heterogeneous collection of clinical syndromes, not a disease or pathological or etiological entity.[10] Little described cerebral palsy as "a persistent disorder of movement and posture appearing early in life and due to a developmental nonprogressive disorder of the brain."[3] Current definitions have reiterated that abnormal execution of movement and interference with postural mechanisms are the key characteristics of this nonprogressive disorder affecting the developing brain.[10]

Diagnostic Categorization of the Characteristics of Cerebral Palsy

In general, a diagnosis of cerebral palsy suggests that the individual has a lesion within the motor control system with a residual disorder of posture and movement control. In addition, the labeling process often identifies the parts of the body that are primarily involved. Diplegia, hemiplegia, and quadriplegia, respectively, indicate that the lower extremities, one side of the body, or all four extremities are affected. This can be misleading to the therapist who is working with infants because these children often change their clinical signs and symptoms and their respective disabilities. The disorder is not progressive, but the presentation of involvement of body segments may manifest itself differently as the child grows and his or her structure changes against gravity.

The clinician must be aware that the categorization of cerebral palsy is based on descriptions of observable characteristics; thus, it is a symptomatic description. The hypertonus of spasticity prevents a smooth exchange between mobility and stability of the body. Constriction of respiratory adaptability occurs with poor trunk control. Incrementation of postural tone occurs with an increase in the speed of even passive movement, and clonus may occur in response to sudden passive movement. Although diagnostic terms reflect the distribution of excessive postural tone, the entire body must be considered to be involved. Spasticity, by nature, involves reduced quantity of movement, which makes its distribution easier to identify. Recruitment of the corticomotor neuron pool is affected in the presence of spasticity, and therefore timing issues result in the poor grading of agonists and antagonists.[11,12] There is also a risk of reduction in the range of limb movements over time when therapy does not include active adaptation in end ranges and organization of postural transitions.[13] There are several spastic types of cerebral palsy that require clarification. Spastic diplegia implies that the lower extremities are more involved than the upper extremities but could present with varying degrees of hand function, and often the involvement is asymmetrical.[12] Hemiplegia displays involvement of one side of the body and can manifest itself with the arm involved more than the leg or the leg involved as much or more than the arm.[10] Quadriplegia, as the term implies, involves the entire body.[10]

Dyskinetic syndromes, which include athetosis and dystonic types of cerebral palsy, are characterized by involuntary movements. The term *dyskinetic* is commonly used with children who lack posture and axial/trunk coactivation. The excessive peripheral movement of the limbs occurs without central coactivation. Dystonic types of cerebral palsy are dominated by tension, and athetosis usually has a hypotonic base or underlying tone. Dyskinetic syndromes may occur with greater involvement in particular extremities, although it most often interferes with postural stability as a whole. When pathological/primitive reflexes are used to accomplish movement, there is a difficulty with midline orientation. Dyskinetic distribution of postural tone is changeable in force and velocity, particularly during attempted movement by the individual. Midrange control is limited if present at all, and frequently end ranges of motion are used to accomplish a motor task.[10] For these reasons, these children have a reduced risk for contractures over time.

Hypotonicity is another category of cerebral palsy, but it may also mask undiagnosed degenerative conditions (see Chapter 13). Hypotonia in a young infant may also be a precursor of a dyskinetic syndrome. Often, athetoid movements or spasticity are not noticed until the infant is attempting antigravity postures, although there may be some disorganization apparent to the careful observer. Generalized hypotonia often masks some specific areas of deep muscle tension with accompanying local immobility.

True ataxia is a cerebellar disorder that is seen more frequently as a sequela of tumor removal (see Chapters 24 and 25) than as a problem occurring from birth. Ataxic syndromes are more commonly found in term infants. This type of cerebral palsy is a diagnosis of exclusion. In a small number of patients there is congenital hypoplasia of the cerebellum. Most of these children are hypotonic at birth and display delays in motor acquisition and language skills.[10] Recruitment and timing issues remain problems in this population. Midline is often achieved but control of midrange movements of the extremities and control of trunk postural reactions is affected.

These classifications, even when accurately applied, give the therapist only a general idea of the treatment problem and must be supplemented by a specific analysis of posture and movement control during task performance, an interview for home care information, and assessment of treatment responses (see Chapters 8 and 9). The therapist is then ready to establish treatment priorities for the individual child.

Many of the characteristics described in the preceding paragraphs also apply to children who have had closed head traumas or brain infections. Further information can be obtained in Chapters 17 and 20. Some of the treatment suggestions that follow may also be applied in such cases. As with cerebral palsy, early positioning and handling after trauma may deter later problems.

EVALUATIVE ANALYSIS OF THE INDIVIDUAL CHILD

Initial Observations and Assessment

Examination of the individual child begins with careful observation of the interaction between parents and the child, including parental handling of the child that occurs spontaneously. Some additional insight can be gained about the relationship between parent and child by observing how the child is handled both physically and emotionally. Does the child receive and respond to verbal reassurance from the parent in the therapy situation? Are immediate bribes offered to the child? Does parent eye contact increase the child's confidence in responding? Does family communication convey the idea of negativity in the therapy situation or a difficult experience that will soon come to an end? The family orientation will affect the response of the child while working with the therapist.

The therapist working as part of a team may have the advantage of a social worker or psychologist who will relate to the problems and motivations of the parents. Parental responses toward the disabled child arise from their uncertainty, fear, concern for the future, disappointment, distress, and other normal reactions to this unforeseeable life experience. The therapist will observe positive changes in parent

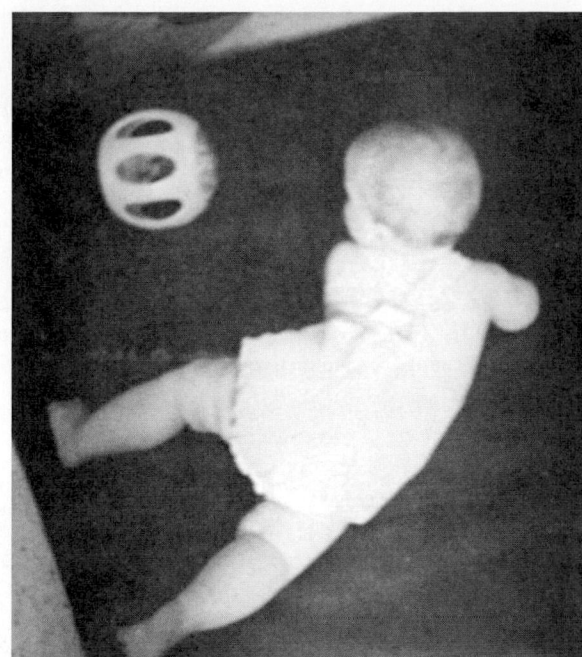

FIGURE 12-1 ■ Normal infants accumulate a multitude of experiences as they move smoothly in their environments.

orientation to the child as the parents are educated as to what can be done to help the child move forward. They may be further assisted by opportunities to interact with well-adjusted parents of older children.

While observing the child, the experienced therapist will want to periodically elicit from the parents their view of the problem. By listening carefully, the therapist will also be able to discern the emotional impressions that have surrounded previous experiences with professionals. Sometimes what is not said is more important than what is verbally offered immediately. Listening carefully and clarifying facts are more important than overwhelming the parents with excessive information and suppositions during early contacts. Observation of the family response to information will keep the therapist on track in developing a positive relationship with parents that deepens over time.

The next general step is to observe, in as much detail as possible, the spontaneous movement of the child when separated from the parent (Figure 12-1). Is the child very passive? Does he or she react to the supporting surface (Figure 12-2)? Are there abnormal patterns of movement to reach a toy? Are clearly normal responses occurring with specific interference by reflexive synergies or total patterns of movement? Does the child rely heavily on visual communication? Do the eyes focus on a presented object or does the postural abnormality increase with an effort to focus the eyes? Do they lead or follow hand activity? Does an effort to move result only in an increase of postural tone with abnormal distribution? Does respiration adapt to new postural adaptations (Figure 12-3)? Is the child able to speak as well while standing as while sitting?

This type of observation is valuable because movement patterns directly reflect the state of the central nervous system and can generally be seen while the parent is still handling the child.[14] Once the child is on the mat or

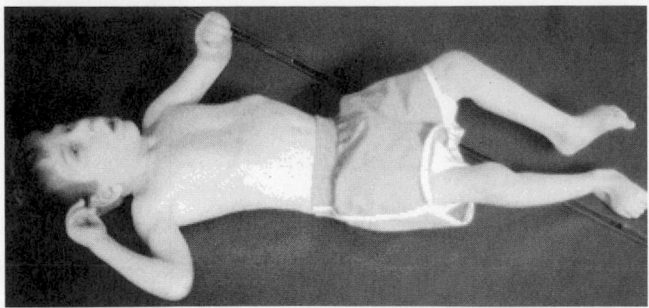

FIGURE 12-2 ■ Lack of support surface contact demonstrates difficulty conforming to and activating off of the supporting surface.

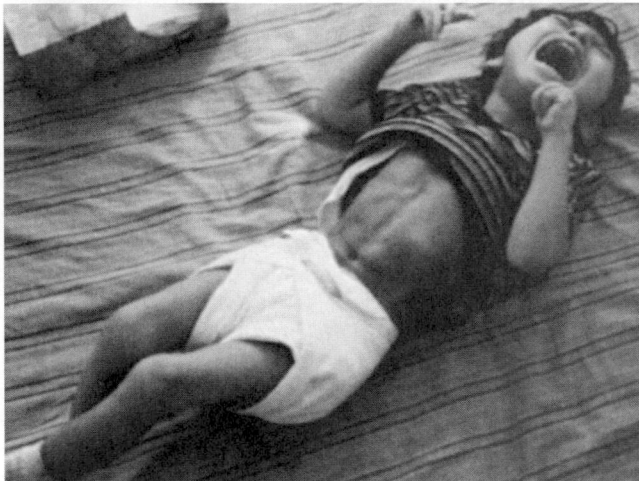

FIGURE 12-3 ■ Emotional reactions are also translated into stronger spastic reactions influencing respiratory adaptation (see Chapter 4 on the limbic system).

treatment table, outer clothing can be removed to observe interactions of limbs and trunk. Movement responses of the child can gradually be influenced directly by the therapist. Many disabled children associate immediate undressing in a new environment with a doctor's office, and the chance to establish rapport is lost. In some instances it is preferable to have the parent gently remove some of the child's clothing or even to leave the child dressed during the first therapy session.

Examination of the child's status is more likely to be adequate if the therapist follows the child's lead when possible. Notes can be organized later to conform to a specific format. It is often possible to jot down essential information while observing the child moving spontaneously or while the parent is holding the child. Reactions to the supporting surface will differ in these circumstances. After the session, the therapist may dictate the salient information into a tape recorder, or a videotape or digital tape can be made to capture the interactions and movement patterns. Attention should be given to the normal movements of the child and to those postures that the child spontaneously attempts to control. Eye alignment is important; the correspondence between visual and postural activity relates directly to quality movement control. It is important to notice the inter-

action between the two sides of the body. In noting abnormal reactions and compensatory movement patterns, the therapist must also indicate the position of the body with respect to the supporting surface. There is a tendency to compile more pertinent data by learning to cluster observations and relating one to the other. Children are vibrant beings. Their choices of position tell us something about their habits and how comfortable they are in this situation. To be the slave of a preformulated sequence destroys the decision-making initiative appropriate to the situation at hand. This is true for the therapist as well as for the child.

Standardized assessments are often used by facilities to document the developmental level of the functioning of a child with disability and to justify treatment. The Gross Motor Function Measure (GMFM) was developed to assess children with cerebral palsy with good reliability and validity for children aged 5 months to 16 years.[15,16] The Pediatric Evaluation and Disability Inventory assess children aged 6 months to 7.5 years in three domains: social, self-care, and mobility.[17] The Functional Independence Measure for Children was developed as a test of disability in children aged 6 months to 12 years. This assessment covers self-care, sphincter control, mobility, locomotion, communication, and social cognition.[18-20] This tool has been used to track outcomes over time. Although several instruments have been developed that meet psychometric criteria to document function in children with disabilities, the GMFM and the Pediatric Evaluation and Disability Inventory are thought to be the most responsive to change in this population of children because of their good reliability and validity.[21] Often the decision to use an instrument to assess development will be left up to the clinician. To date, there is no one tool that will cover all the categories necessary to document change in a child with cerebral palsy, so the clinician will need to rely on observational skills to describe quality of movement and response to changes in position in space and handling.

Each child will differ in the ability to separate from her or his parents. Spontaneity of movement, interest in toys, general activity level, and communication skills will also vary from child to child.[22] Responding to the specific needs of the child enables the therapist to set priorities more effectively. If fatigue is likely to be a factor, it is important to evaluate first those reactions that present themselves spontaneously, followed by direct handling to determine near-normal potential for movement. Those movements or abilities for which there is a major interference by spasticity, reflexive responses, or poor balance may be better checked at the termination of the assessment so that the child remains in a cooperative mood as long as possible. Information regarding favorite sleeping positions, self-care independence, and chair supports used at home can be requested as the session comes to a close.

Reactions to Placement in a Position

If the child totally avoids certain postures during spontaneous activity, these are likely to be the more important positions for the therapist to evaluate. Placement of the child in the previously avoided position will permit the therapist to feel the resistance that prevents successful control by the child.[22] The parent should play an active role in the assessment whenever possible. Continued dialog with the parents reveals factors such as the frequency of a poor sitting align-

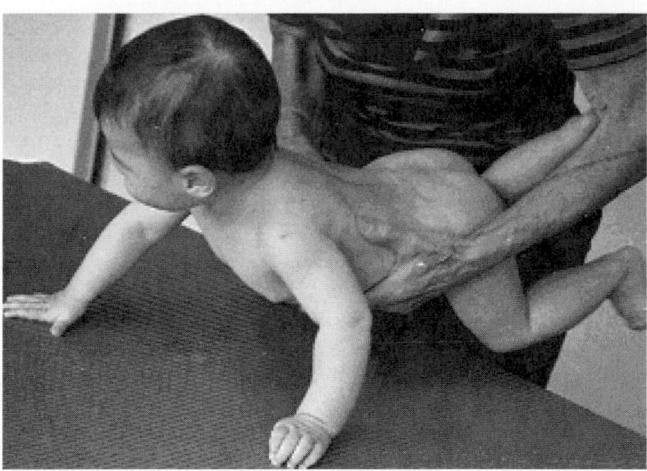

FIGURE 12-4 ■ Baby treatment must be dynamic and precisely oriented to individual needs.

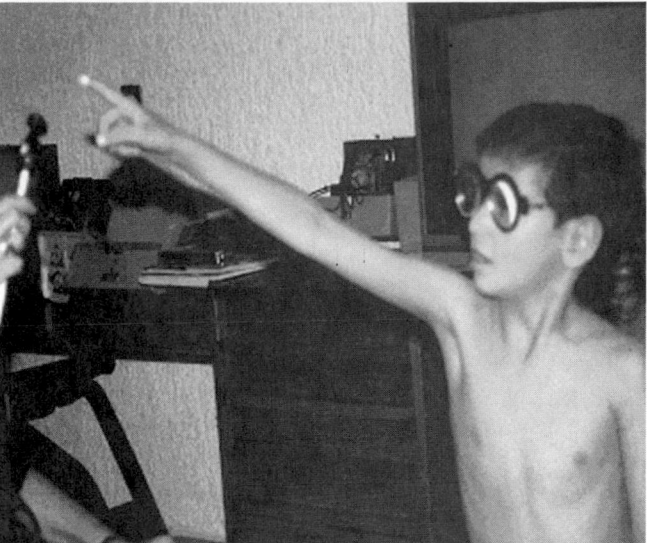

FIGURE 12-5 ■ Touching the target integrates the new visual perception with the motor response.

ment at home or a habitual aversion to the prone position. Sitting close to the television set or tilting the head when looking at books should also be noted so that functional vision skills can be related to other therapy interventions.[23] These contributions by the parents establish the importance of good observation and the need for parents and the therapist to work cooperatively. Therapists of different specialties need to initiate continuing communication to coordinate therapy objectives.

According to the guide for normal development, infants should be able to maintain the posture in which they are placed before they acquire the ability to move into that position alone.[24,25] The problems presented by cerebral palsy occur to some extent as a reaction to the field of gravity in which the child moves.[24] Visual perceptions of spatial relationships motivate and determine movement patterns while the child must react at a somatic level to the support surface. It is helpful, therefore, to attempt placement of the infant or child into developmentally or functionally appropriate postures that are not assumed spontaneously (Figure 12-4). Resistance to placement indicates an increase in tone, a structural problem, or an inability to adapt to the constellation of sensory inputs for that alignment. *A movement that resists control by the therapist will be even less possible for the child.* What appears to be a passive posture may hide rapid increases in hypertonicity when movement is initiated or instability of a proximal joint when weight bearing is initiated. A child may have learned to avoid excitation of the unwanted reactions and may fix the body position to avoid the alignment that cannot be controlled. Another child may enjoy the sensory experience of accelerated changes in postural tone and deliberately set them off as a means of receiving the resulting stimulation to his or her system.

VISUAL-MOTOR ASSESSMENT

It is the visual-motor aspect of performance function that is a primary concern to the therapist because spatial judgments are needed to control movement of the body in an upright alignment. The infant who is able to stand and walk along a support and then seems unable to let go of the support is often found to have functional vision interferences. The child with cerebral palsy most often demonstrates significant

neuromotor delay in the developmental process, which often results in the inadequate establishment of matching of inputs from the postural and visual systems (Figure 12-5). Visual-motor learning experiences are filled with compensatory responses from both systems.

The visual system in its development has many parallels with the postural system.[26] Binocular control and freedom of movement are necessary for the system to function properly. Ambient visual processing must be integrated with central visual processing to take in information that relates to position in space and to focus on a particular target. A simple screening examination may check acuity at 20 feet on the E chart and declare vision to be normal. An ophthalmological examination is needed to determine the health of the eye structures, particularly in the case of infants born preterm. Equally important is a functional vision examination given by a behavioral or developmental optometrist to reveal the level of efficiency that the two eyes have achieved in working together and whether the ability to focus in far and near ranges is smoothly established. Strabismus dysfunctions commonly coexist with cerebral palsy and may cause the child to receive a double image of environmental objects. Judgments about space are related to a three-dimensional perception of the surrounding environment, which requires coordinated use of the two eyes. Conservative management of eye alignment problems is done with the use of lenses and prisms by the experienced optometrist, which permits the therapist to work for basic head control by the child before any irreversible changes are made to the eye muscles. Eye movement differentiates from head movement in much the same way that the hand differentiates from general arm movement, corresponding to general maturation of the central system.

Because the visual system is first a motor system, children with cerebral palsy most often have difficulty separating eye movement from head movement and controlled convergence for focal changes. When their posture is supported, eye movement can proceed to evolve in accuracy and complexity. With inadequate alignment of the head in relation to the

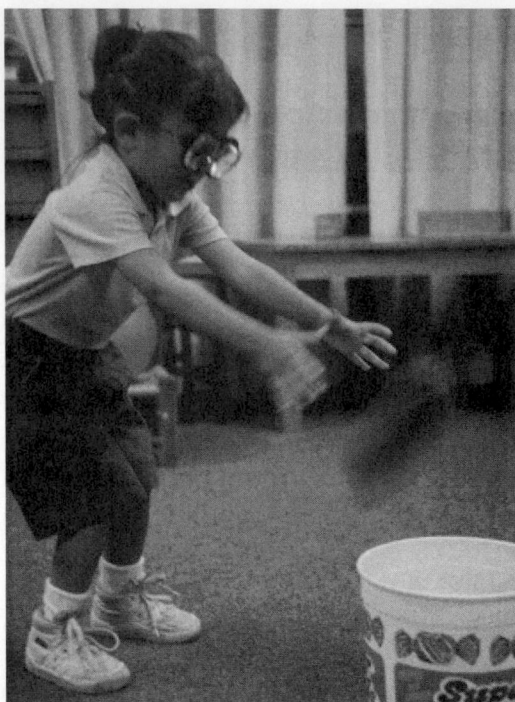

FIGURE 12-6 ■ This 3-year-old girl with diplegia takes her weight evenly over two feet with the help of prism lenses to shift her perception of space while engaged in a motor task.

base of support, the visual system accumulates distortions and inconsistent input, which leads to the formation of an inadequate perceptual base for later motor learning (see Chapter 30). Even after improvement in the control of posture and movement, the visual system continues to adapt to the previous faulty visual-motor learning, resulting in perceptual confusion and inefficient organization of body movement in space. The therapist who is working for improved motor control may notice that such a child reacts with adequate postural adaptations when facing the therapist or a support and that the movement quality seems to disintegrate when the child faces an open space. This immediately jeopardizes the ability of the child to use her or his new responses after leaving the therapy environment.

Padula, a behavioral optometrist specializing in neuro-optometric rehabilitation, has described a posttrauma vision syndrome in adults with acquired central dysfunction and has applied this information to children with cerebral palsy.[27] A perceptual distortion in the perceived midline of the body, known as visual midline shift syndrome, is corrected with the use of prescribed prism lenses, which then permits the child to step into the perceived space with more confidence (Figure 12-6). The observant therapist will begin to notice that the sudden increase in neuromuscular tension in a child taking steps in a walker is often accompanied by closing of the eyes. This seems to be a momentary inability of the central processing system to integrate the information arriving from different sources. With the use of prism correction, the child experiences the body as more coherent with visual-spatial perceptions. By incorporating an understanding of visual observations into intervention strategies, physical and occupational therapists are able to note compensatory adaptations by the complementary systems and use that to their advantage in effective treatment intervention.

Some children who walk on their forefeet or even on their toes and who have made little if any permanent gait change after the use of inhibitory casting or orthotics also fall into the population described above. With prisms that correct the perception of forward space, the child places the entire foot in contact with the support. Such prism lenses are used during therapy handling as a perceptual learning experience for the child, with the optometrist and the therapist coordinating their efforts. Hand coordination activities also require timing of reach and grasp that is based on feedforward by the visual system. In some cases the therapist observes the visual system to over-focus in the moment that the child loses control of his or her postural stability. This suggests that the visual system may be attempting to compensate for the inadequacy of the postural control, much in the same way that we all adjust our head position to see better. Understanding the nature of the continuing dynamic interaction between these two functional subsystems of the central nervous system and attending to the needs of a visual-postural orientation will increase the successful evolution of clients with cerebral palsy.

POSTURE AND MOVEMENT COMPENSATIONS

Compensatory patterns of movement arise from the motivation of the child to move in spite of various restrictions on the expression of that movement. Visual impressions of the environment motivate movement, and the infant attempts to influence nearby objects or confirm visual impressions by touching. As visual awareness enlarges to include more distant targets, the infant is motivated to move toward the object or person seen. When the child's body does not respond in a smooth way, the child begins to learn and perfect the uncoordinated reaction. Repetition of inadequate ranges of movement and limited variability of movement patterns begin to establish the abnormal appearance of posture in the child with cerebral palsy.

The quality of a body posture or position in space determines the quality of the movement that is expressed. From a distorted starting position the movement initiated is one that is restricted (Figure 12-7). The lack of central stability in the body restricts the full mobility of a limb. This limitation is increased by fascial restrictions on smooth coordinated muscle action. The child continues to learn the abnormal responses because the movement patterns tend to be reinforced by either accomplishment or reinforcement of some kind from the environment. Compensatory movement patterns evolve because of necessity rather than any feedback as to efficiency or functional smoothness.

Habitual movement patterns are established on the basis of frequency of use, so the child with cerebral palsy tends to repeat the abnormal responses that have been learned. In the therapy situation the child has the opportunity to learn new combinations of input to create the basis for a more stable postural control. Careful analysis of the postural adjustments and movement patterns of the child with cerebral palsy is crucial to initiate effective intervention strategies. There are many factors to be considered in the context of the continuing developmental changes in the child, which makes a simple solution impossible.

Active therapy intervention allows the sensorimotor learning of the child to be modified so that some part of the compensatory response becomes unnecessary and the move-

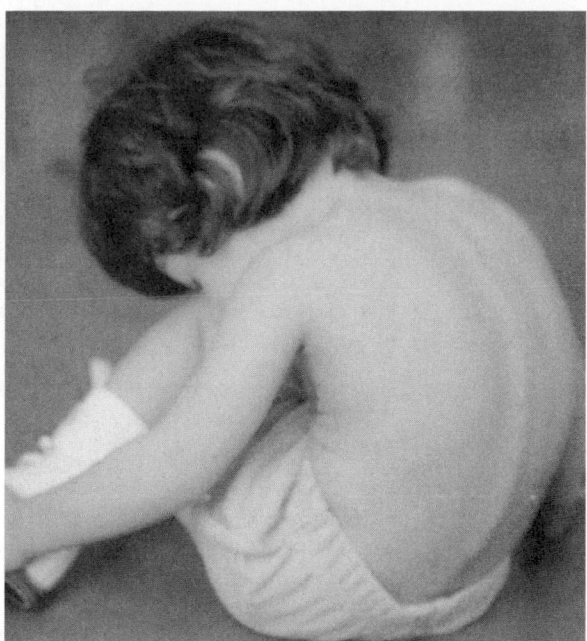

FIGURE 12-7 ■ Compensatory postures restrict movement initiation.

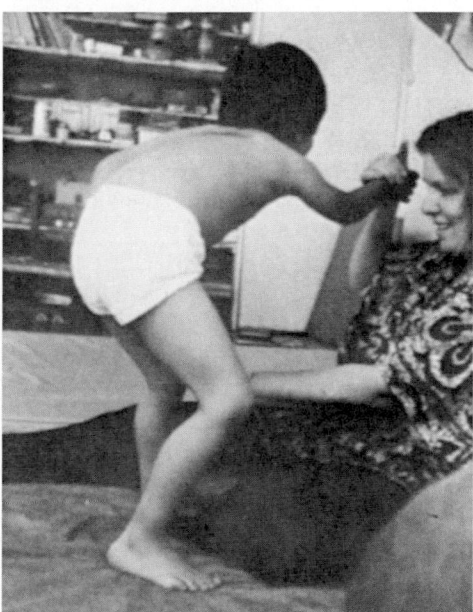

FIGURE 12-8 ■ The experience of coming to stand over the more affected side activates diagonal patterns of postural adjustment.

ment becomes more normal (Figure 12-8). This relative approximation to what is expected in a normal response may occur in the area of initiation, timing, strength, or ability to sustain an antigravity alignment. As movement expression and postural stability are better established, the compensatory patterns are used less often and new motor learning occurs on a base of closer-to-normal experience.

Compensatory processes have their positive aspects.[28] The independence finally achieved by the older child reflects her or his intelligence and motivation and the family's attitude toward the child and the disability. The most debilitat-

ing handicap of cerebral palsy in an intelligent child may be social or psychological when the child is not accepted by the family and therefore cannot develop a positive self-image. Compensatory movement patterns may permit greater independence, if and when they do not limit or block the active learning of new motor strategies.

OTHER ASSESSMENT CONSIDERATIONS

Nutritional Aspects of Neuromotor Function

Nutrition is viewed as providing an important biochemical base for enhanced human performance. Williams,[29] author of the classic reference *Biochemical Individuality,* was one of the first to point out the existence of significant variability in the need for specific individualized nutrients because of differences in assimilation and other factors. Physicians Crook and Stevens,[30] Smith,[31] Pfeiffer,[32] and Cott[33] are a few of the leaders who have analyzed the link between nutrient intake and behavioral differences in children and adults. Many of these references address issues of attention and learning. To have efficient function of the transmitters at the myoneural junction and good health for the myelinated neurons of the nervous system, a variety of trace elements must be present.[32] Lack of dendritic proliferation is associated with malnutrition regardless of the cause.[34] The ambulatory child with cerebral palsy will need to be considered for a new level of energy expenditure to avoid short stature and poor nutritional status.[35]

Another body of work explains more about the direct link between food intake and muscle efficiency for high performance and normal function. The need for water is paramount for healthy fascia. In children with cerebral palsy and related disorders there is often from the beginning a difficulty in the smooth automatic sucking needed for nutritive intake. Uncoordinated patterns of mandibular and tongue motion persist when not addressed in early and precise intervention strategies. Even the digestive process is affected negatively by inadequate chewing, a higher than typical percentage of food allergies, and less than efficient physiological functions.[36]

It is likely that brain dysfunction in some of these children extends to the hypothalamus, thus influencing the entire digestive process. Duncan et al[37] have documented the risk of osteopenia in nonambulatory children with cerebral palsy. This retrospective study showed that fewer than 75% of the calories needed were administered to 95% of the children with gastrostomy tubes. Nutrients were also deficient. This may explain part of the poor physical response level of such children. Sonis et al[38] looked specifically at energy expenditure in children and adolescents with spastic quadriplegia in relation to food intake. They found dietary intake to be markedly overreported for this population and determined that nutrition-related growth failure was likely related to inadequate energy intake. Reflux is also common in infants with developmental problems. In some infants reflux subsides as the physical stress is reduced in the tissues bordering the upper thoracic and cervical spine, but it can be related to milk sensitivity or even susceptibility to environmental contaminants.

To supplement nutritional intake in the child with cerebral palsy, the individual child must be considered with regard to age, size, activity level, and growth factors.[39]

Ideally, blood, urine, or hair analyses would be done to determine nutrient imbalances, and supplementation with specific nutrients would be guided by a specialist. Environmental medicine has taken the lead in this type of work. In the absence of other resources, the therapist can always encourage parents to follow their intuition and use a balanced vitamin-mineral supplement appropriate for the age of the child.

Consideration of Supplemental Oxygen

Oxygenation of muscle tissue is considered essential for smooth movement control, and it is generally accepted that respiratory support increases automatically to permit faster or stronger movement patterns in a normal subject. Therapists often note that children with cerebral palsy resist moving into new ranges of movement and that respiratory adaptation does not occur automatically. Supporting the child in the novel posture until a respiratory adaptation is noted results in acceptance of the new experience. Oxygen needs increase in children during growth spurts or when mastering more vertical postural alignments. There is also increased oxygen required for sustained activity such as continuous walking.

Shintani et al[40] have done a careful study of 233 children with cerebral palsy to determine the presence of obstructive sleep apnea. In 10 children with cerebral palsy who were received at the hospital for treatment of severe obstructive sleep apnea, these authors determined that adenoidal or tonsillar hypertrophy were noted in only four children and that the main cause of sleep apnea in the other six children was pharyngeal collapse at the lingual base. Fukumizu and Kohyama[41] looked at central respiratory pauses, sighs, and gross body movement during sleep in 19 healthy children, ages 3 months to 7 years. Central pauses occurred more often during non-rapid-eye-movement sleep and increased with age. Developmental differences need further study.

In the presence of inadequate peripheral oxygen saturation, low levels of oxygen can be administered during the night. This practice has been used with selected low-tone and athetoid children for improved energy during the day during growth changes, but formal study is needed on a larger group of children with cerebral palsy. Better oxygenation of the tissues can also result in increased food intake and consequently improved energy levels.

ROLES OF THE THERAPIST

Role of the Therapist in Direct Intervention

The primary role of the therapist is in direct treatment or physical handling of the child in situations that offer opportunities for new motor learning. This should precede and accompany the making of recommendations to parents, teachers, and others handling the child. Positioning for home and home handling recommendations should always be tried first by the therapist during a treatment session. As noted with the initial assessment, many interventions will cause a reaction unique to the particular youngster.[22,42] It is the role of the therapist to analyze the nature of the response that is accompanied by adaptation inadequacies, to analyze the movement problems, and to choose the most effective intervention (Figure 12-9). It will then be possible for other persons to manage play activities and supervise independent functioning that reinforce treatment goals.[43]

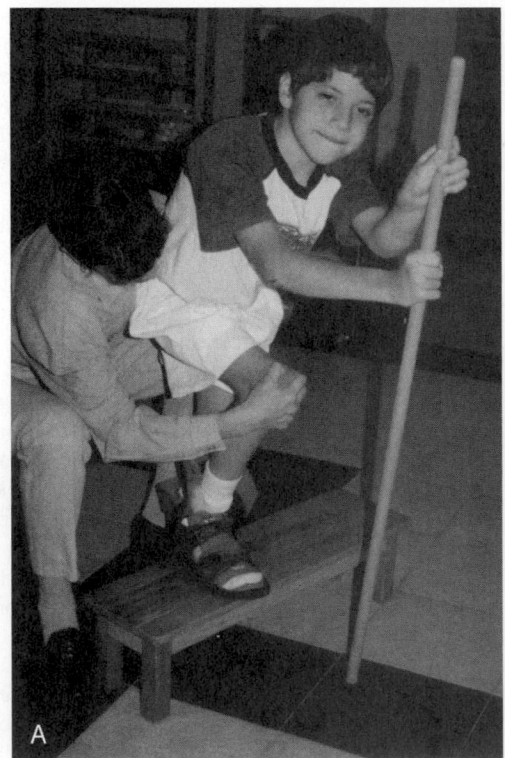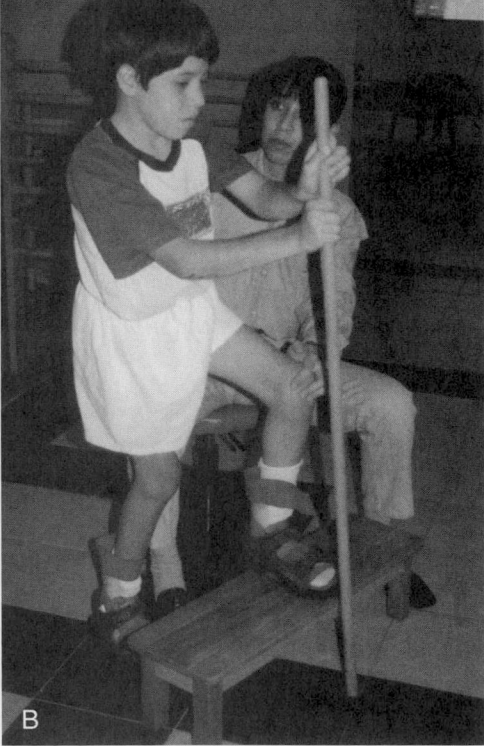

FIGURE 12-9 ■ The two sides of the body (**A** and **B**) often respond very differently to the same task, and therapy must be adapted accordingly.

The therapist working with these children becomes an important and trusted resource to the family. At times the therapist who has had the more consistent contact with the child becomes the facilitator of better communication between the parents and medical or health care professionals. The child who starts early and continues with the same therapist may make of this person a confidant and share concerns that are difficult or uncomfortable for the child to explain to parents. It is a challenge for the therapist who follows the same child for an extended time to come up with appropriate goals and new activities to continue positive change. Part of direct intervention is to recognize when the amount of therapy can be reduced and replaced with recreational activities with peers.

Case Management/Direct Intervention

Simple documentation of observed changes in a child over a series of regular clinic visits is still too common for many children with cerebral palsy. Regular appointments, with periodic assignment of a new piece of apparatus, do not constitute active treatment. Although physical intervention in the form of direct handling of the child is considered a conservative treatment by most physicians, there are relatively few children who receive sufficient physical treatment at an early age.[44,45] Therapists need to demonstrate their unique preparation and describe their interventions in ordinary language so that families as well as other health care professionals understand the importance of specific treatment versus general programs of early stimulation that are designed for neurologically normal infants.

The prognosis for change in cerebral palsy is too often based on records of case management rather than on the effect of direct and dynamic treatment by a well-prepared therapist. Bobath[24,46] documented accurately the developmental sequence expected in the presence of spasticity or athetosis. Her book consolidates some observations of older clients that help professionals understand the uninterrupted effects of the cerebral palsy condition. In any institution one can observe the tightly adducted and internally rotated legs, the shoulder retraction with flexion of the arms, and the chronic shortening of the neck so common as the long-term effects of cerebral palsy. The long-term influence of athetosis results in compensatory stiffness or limited movement patterns to create a semblance of the missing postural stability while a limited number of movement patterns with limited degrees of freedom are used to function (Figure 12-10).

Within the clinical community there is increasing evidence that soft tissue restrictions further limit spontaneous movement in children with cerebral palsy. The fact that these fascial restrictions are often found in infants suggests that they originate early rather than as a gradual result of limited ranges in movement. Because of the tendency of fascial tissue to change in response to any physical trauma or strong biochemical change, some of these characteristics might be originating with traumatic birth experiences, and they would be continued by daily use of limited patterns of movement. Tissue restrictions can also occur with immobilization or general infectious processes.[47-49] Soft tissue begins to change its physiological structure with the application of gentle sustained pressure, so it serves as documentation that there are changes caused by the therapist's simple hand contact. Some

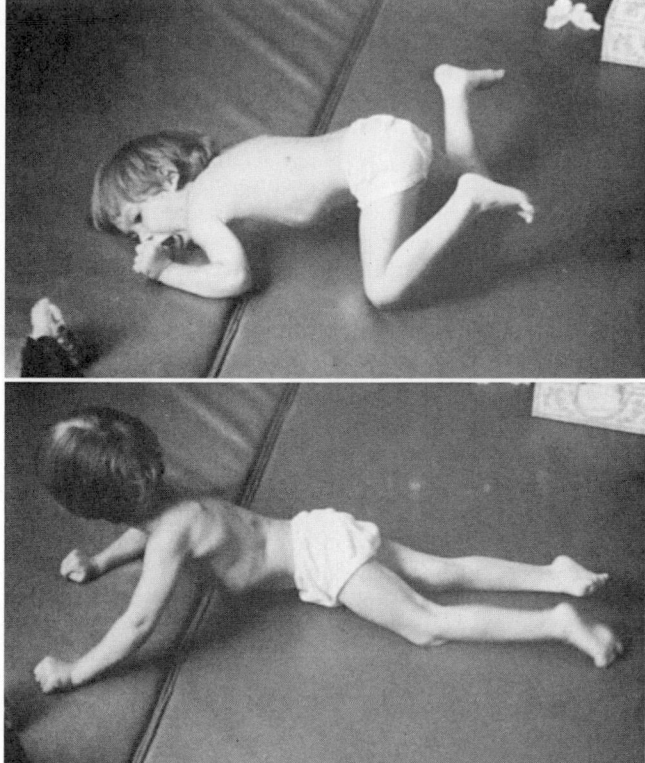

FIGURE 12-10 ■ Attempted movement activates abnormal patterns and restrictions; restrictions are revealed with limited degrees of freedom available for function.

of the sensory information in the form of tapping or holding or application of pressure affects fascial meridians and muscle alignments.[50]

Applying specific soft tissue treatment techniques to any person with a neuromotor disorder creates the need for immediate follow-up with practice of new skills using this improved range of motion. Creating excessive tissue mobility in a given area of the body can destroy the delicate patterns of coordination that permit synergic function in the person with cerebral palsy, so functional activation of the body after each specific mobilization is strongly recommended to integrate the tissue change. Well documented in the literature on current motor control and motor learning is the need to practice, practice, practice.[51] Practice time is related to skill performance; the amount and type of practice is determined by the stage of learning that an individual is in and the type of task to be learned[51-53] (see Chapter 3 on motor control/learning). Interestingly, most of what we know about motor control/motor learning is based on normals, and it is yet to be determined whether the same principles that are considered important in healthy individuals apply to people with disability. However, it makes sense that practice would be a part of any new or relearned skill.

An occupational therapist, Josephine Moore, stressed Bach-Y-Rita's[54] works to emphasize some important points for therapists regarding concept of increasing functional demands on the central system and the importance of the neck structures in developmental movement sequences. Children with spasticity often have a lack of developmental elongation of the neck, whereas children with athetoid or dystonic movement lack neck stability and consistent postural activation. Tone changes often originate with changes in the delicate postural interrelationship between head and body or with ambient visual processing.

By appreciating the abundance of polysynaptic neurons and parallel processing in the central nervous system, the therapist will become more optimistic regarding his or her role as facilitator and feedback organizer to guide new movement. Restak,[55] in his book *The New Brain*, has confirmed the continual reorganization of the brain in response to new input. Several animal and human studies on neuroplasticity have confirmed that the brain reorganizes after an injury and that this reorganization is shaped by rehabilitation and motor skill learning.[56-59] In the child with cerebral palsy, the therapist looks for subtle changes in the child's response to determine newly integrated sensorimotor learning. For example, excessive emphasis on extensor responses in the prone posture for the older child can jeopardize the quality of neck elongation in sitting, so it is essential to work on the components necessary for control of the new posture desired.

Therapy intervention is far from innocuous when it is responsibly applied. A truly eclectic treatment approach comes with clinical experience and personal consideration of observations of the functional problems presented by the complex issue of cerebral palsy at different ages. Priorities in intervention strategies have a practical aspect, while new developments in our knowledge lead us forward in clinical applications. The intricacies of normal development offer many new clues for new effective interventions. With quality treatment intervention the need for direct therapy service as a crucial aspect of case management for these children is confirmed. Clinical findings in individual case studies need to become part of the professional literature to strengthen the efficacy of intervention in this population.

Special Needs of Infants

The direct treatment of infants deserves special mention because there are significant differences in intervention strategies for the infant and the older child. Aside from the delicate situation of the new parents, the infant is less likely to have a diagnosis and presents a mixture of normal and abnormal characteristics. It is essential that the clinician have a strong foundation in the nuances of normal developmental movement and early postural control.[4,60] Soft tissue issues must be addressed in detail. Direct intervention can be offered as a means of enhancing development and overcoming the effects of a difficult or preterm birth. It will be important, however, to pursue a diagnosis for the infant who reaches 8 or 9 months of age and continues to need therapy because third-party payers often require a diagnosis beyond developmental delay or prematurity.

Infants with early restrictions in motor control should be followed until they are walking independently, even if they no longer need weekly therapy. Infant responses can change rapidly as the therapist organizes the components of movement control. Soft tissue restrictions should be treated initially to have more success with facilitated movement responses. Careful observation is essential because all but the severely involved infant will change considerably between visits. The therapist should invest some time in

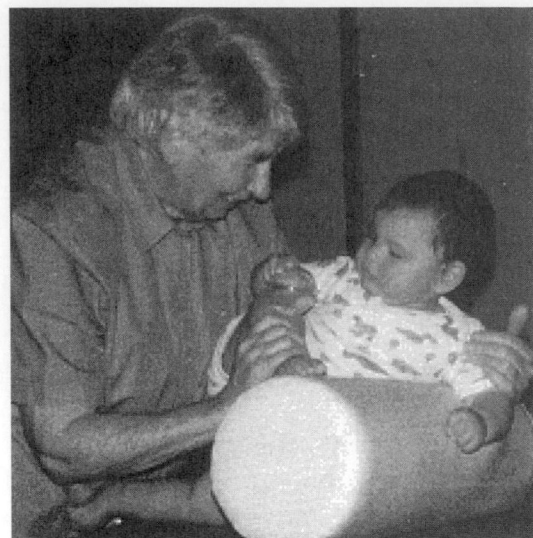

FIGURE 12-11 ■ Mary Quinton, British physiotherapist, is widely recognized as the originator of effective infant intervention.

training the parents to become skilled observers while appreciating the small gains made by their infant. Physiotherapist Mary Quinton[61] has written down specific intervention strategies for babies (Figure 12-11). Infant massage is important to improve the bonding of mother and child and to improve physiological measures.[62,63]

Referral to other health care professionals is essential in the presence of possible allergies, new neurological signs, visual or auditory alterations, and persistent reflux or nutritional issues. There is always the possibility of convulsions when some brain dysfunction is present, and neurological evaluation should be recommended if this is a concern.

ORIENTATION TO TREATMENT STRATEGIES

The child whose movement is bound within the limitations of hypertonicity suffers first of all from a paucity of movement experience. Because early attempts to move have resulted in the expression of limited synergistic postural patterns, the child often experiences the body as heavy or awkward and loses incentive to attempt movement. The therapist will want to focus on the child's ability to sustain postural control in the trunk. Central stability to support directed arm movement or weight shifts for stepping have not developed, so they need to be addressed during therapy intervention. Improved upper extremity control opens the possibility for new learning of more coordinated tasks. Specific work on hand preparation for reach and grasp follows use of the arm for directed movement and often results in improved balance in standing. Any freedom gained in upper body control results in more efficient balance in the upright posture.

Inhibition or stopping the movement of one part of a movement range or even one limb must be done in a way that permits the child to activate the body in a functional way. The child who lies in the supine position with extreme pushing back against the surface is rarely seen when therapy intervention has started early. The therapist initially eliminates the supine position entirely but would incorporate into the treatment plan the activation of normal flexor in sitting

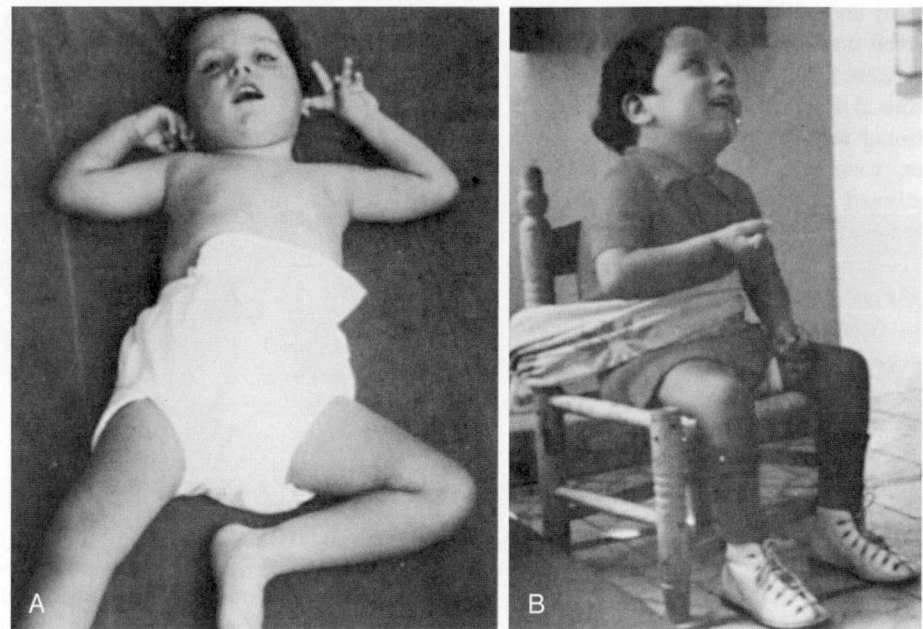

FIGURE 12-12. ■ **A,** Strong asymmetry and abnormal tone in the supine position. **B,** Simple seating can inhibit strong asymmetry and make function a possibility.

with variations of pelvic tilt (Figure 12-12). The child might later be reintroduced to a supine position with postural transitions that support balanced control of the body with more differentiated movement.

One of the primary considerations for the child with spasticity is adequate respiratory support for movement. Mobility of the thoracic cage and the midtrunk must be combined with trunk rotation during basic postural transitions (Figure 12-13). Consideration of age-appropriate movement velocity will guide the therapist in choosing activities that challenge better respiratory adaptability and prepare for speech breathing to support vocalization. The therapist will find it helpful to hum or sing or even make silly sounds that encourage sound production by the child during therapy. Movement of the child's body changes respiratory demands and frequently spontaneous sound production during therapy.

In some children respiratory patterns remain immature and superficial, which may be related to the causative factors of the impairment. A lack of postural control limits even the physiological shaping of the rib cage itself because the ribs do not have an opportunity to change their angle at the spine. The therapist must give careful support to sustain the transitional posture of the older child during transient respiratory change. An active respiratory adaptation will increase the variability of postural adaptation. Improved respiratory adaptation will improve trunk tone, just as dynamic trunk alignment facilitates better respiration.

Weight bearing changes postural tone. The trunk can be helped to experience weight bearing in a variety of alignments by using inflated balls or rolls that offer a contoured surface. The threshold of the original response is gradually altered so that the child begins to learn the new sensations and can follow guided postural transitions. When there are distinct differences between the two sides of the body, attention must be given to lateral weight shifts in sitting and

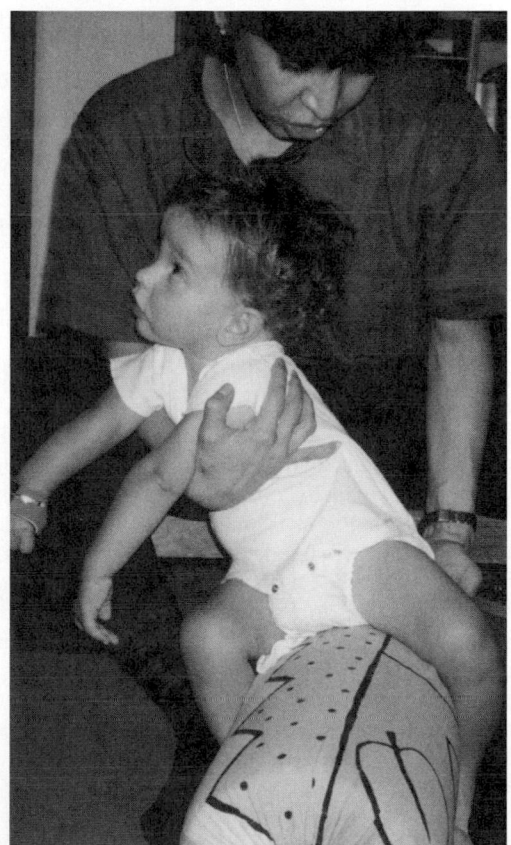

FIGURE 12-13 ■ Rotational patterns combined with transitional movements can be used to mobilize the thoracic cage.

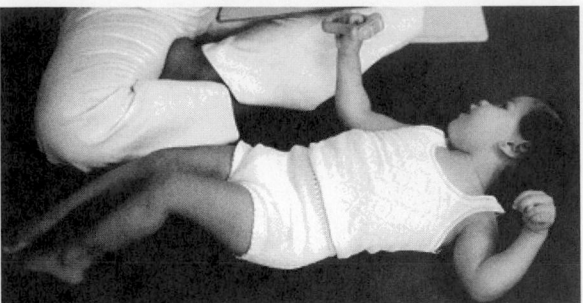

FIGURE 12-14 ■ This child has little contact with the supporting surface, resulting in poor movement initiation.

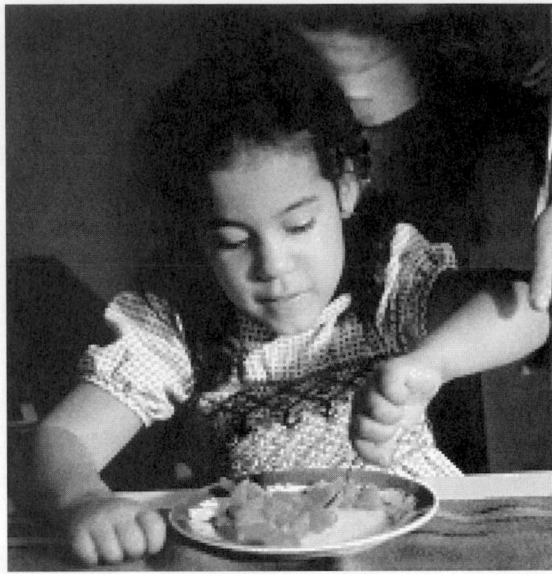

FIGURE 12-15 ■ Maintaining the child's elbow in this high position initially permits forearm pronation and activates the shoulder in the normal developmental pattern for improved motor learning.

standing. Changes near the vertical midline of the body seem to represent the more difficult input for the compromised system to integrate. It may be necessary to assist sustained weight over one side and then the other to initiate the change. It is important to assist the shoulders to align with the hips and that the visual orientation of the individual brings the head to a correct alignment. Young children need special help with segmental rotation of the trunk in the vertical alignment so that the weight-bearing side is relatively forward with dynamic balance of flexion and extension influences.

Children and adolescents with cerebral palsy often require a more intense or prolonged sensory cue to obtain a desired movement response. Weight bearing against the surface may need to be sustained for a prolonged period of time and a range of movement prepared beyond the essential range for the functional goal. The therapist is addressing a system that is deficient in its ability to receive, perceive, and use the available input. This makes careful analysis and functional orientation of the sensory input essential. If the microcosm of experience given the child during a therapy session is no more intense than an equal amount of time in her or his living environment, the therapist has failed to use this unique opportunity to deliver a meaningful message to encourage the learning of new motor behavior.

The therapist working with the child with cerebral palsy constantly monitors the quality of the child's motor response. These continuing observations guide the manipulation of the environment and the assistance given the child to move toward a functional goal. Is the body tolerating the position? Does the child adapt to the supporting surface and use the support surface contact for movement initiation (Figure 12-14)? Is the movement of a limb graded and without unwanted associated reactions in other parts of the body? By analyzing the answers to such questions, the therapist is guided to an appropriate sequence of the therapy session and is enabled to set functional treatment goals and realistically change prognoses.

The therapist makes constant judgments as to the child's responses during therapy, challenging the child's system while ensuring success and moving toward improved control. By using specific intervention strategies, the therapist works to introduce new somatosensory and motor learning. The therapist may introduce a slight modification of the child's response, such as an elongation of a limb as it is being moved. At other times the therapist augments sensory

information that helps direct a movement. Weight bearing over the feet may be simulated with the young child's foot against the therapist's hand and pressure given through the knee. Visual-motor experiences can be altered with the child's use of prism lenses prescribed by an optometrist for use during therapy.

To be meaningful, sensory input must be contextual and meaningful to the individual who is receiving it. Multiple sensory systems are simultaneously activated by most therapeutic input, whereas a variety of sights and sounds may be available in the immediate environment. Memory, previous learning, and cognition are activated during the therapy interaction. The therapist makes a continuous reassessment of the child's experiential needs compared with the current input provided. When the therapist works with the child in a more upright alignment during at least part of the session, the central nervous system is alert and more receptive to the incoming information.

The developmental meaning attached to the sensation of normal movement is complex and starts with the ability to process contrasting stimuli. While several parts of the body are stable, another is moving. Stability of the proximal body permits a limb to extend forcefully or to be maintained in space. Each new level of developmental dissociation of movement increases the complexity of central nervous system processing. The process of self-feeding illustrates how internal and external stimuli impinge simultaneously on the central nervous system. The process of guiding a full spoon toward the mouth initially engages the child's attention. The arm is lifted at the shoulder to bring the fragrant food odor to the level of the mouth before elbow flexion takes the spoon to the face (Figure 12-15). Between 2 and 6 years of age the self-feeding pattern is modified and the elbow moves down beside the body. Now the motor aspect of the task has become procedural and more efficient, permitting the child to participate in social exchanges with the family at the same time that she or he manages independent self-feeding. The complexity of the task increases with the secondary task of social exchange.

A solid understanding of normal developmental sequences is essential for the clinician providing direct treatment intervention.[14,64] Early responses of the normal infant change from a self-orientation to an environmental orientation as new developmental competence emerges. More sophisticated balance in independent sitting occurs as the ability to pull to standing at a support begins to develop. Such knowledge of developmental details supports the therapist in introducing postural activities at a higher developmental level to integrate more basic abilities. The assisted self-dressing process is an effective way to introduce and integrate new movement and sensorimotor learning while using established movement skills. To sit well, the child needs practice moving over the base of support, coming in and out of sitting, and control of coming to stand from sitting. To walk well, the child may need to practice running to allow practice in changing rate, direction, range, and balance. Sitting is made more dynamic by using a gymnastic ball as a seat. Transitional adaptations of posture may be elaborated during therapy sessions to include more complex alignments. Specific techniques are reviewed in Chapter 9.

With the child dominated by athetoid movement, the therapist's role relates primarily to organization and grading of seemingly erratic movement responses. These children have the ability to balance, but their balance reactions are often extreme in range and velocity. By working to improve central control, the therapist gradually introduces taking of body weight over the limbs, with assistance to grade the postural control of the central body. By working closely with a behavioral optometrist the therapists can use visual input to improve the child's balance reactions. In these children the therapist may note that disruption of eye alignment or focusing results in a momentary disorganization of postural control.

Movement control must become procedural so that it is not interrupted by every environmental distraction. This is more likely to happen when balanced activity of the visual, vestibular, and proprioceptive systems has been achieved. Independent ambulation becomes practical when the individual is able to think of something else at the same time. The therapist begins this process by carrying on a conversation with the child to engage the cognitive attention so that the motor act becomes more automatic. The concept of graded stress is discussed in Chapters 4 and 5.

Direct intervention for the hemiplegic child takes into account the obvious difference in postural tone between one side of the body and the other. Treatment for children that addresses itself only to the more affected side of the body will not prove to be effective. The critical therapeutic experience seems to be that of integration of the two sides of the body (Figure 12-16). This begins early for the normal infant, with lateral weight shifts in a variety of developmental patterns, and leads to postural organization that permits later reaching for a toy while the body weight is supported with the opposite side of the body. The child with a contrast in the sensorimotor function of the two sides of the body needs to experience developmental patterns that include rotation within the longitudinal body axis and lateral flexion of the trunk, the more affected side forward. The more affected

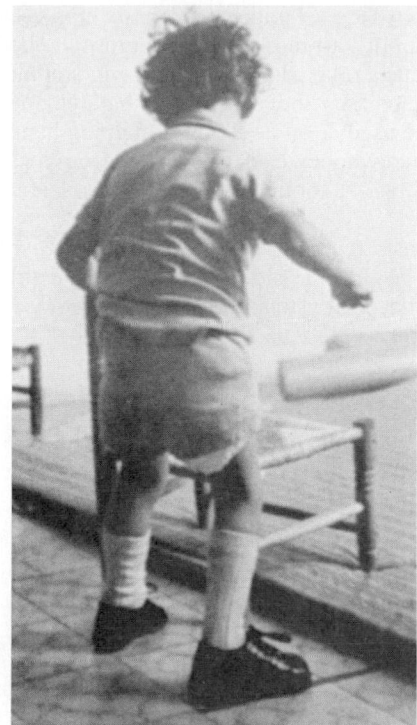

FIGURE 12-16 ■ This boy with hemiplegia tries to move a chair by orienting only his more active side to the task and bearing weight only briefly on the more affected side.

side needs the experience of supporting the body and the experience of initiating movement.

Development of hand use first focuses on bilateral arm activity while keeping the affected hand well within the functional visual field (Figure 12-17). The infant or young child works primarily in sitting until dynamic trunk flexion is activated. Pelvic mobility is essential to activate the necessary trunk responses. The therapist may find that true lateral flexion of the more-affected side of the body is fully as difficult for some children as the initial active elongation of that side. There tends to be a high incidence of soft tissue restrictions in the shoulder and neck of the affected side. Children with hemiplegia have difficulty in sustaining a balanced posture against the influence of gravity, and some begin to struggle to do everything with the less-affected side. This characteristic contrast in function may contribute to the development of seemingly hyperactive behavior that is related to the inability of the central nervous system to resolve contrasting incoming information. Hyperkinetic responses in one side of the body may compensate for relative inactivity in the opposite side. Leg length discrepancy, scoliosis, pelvic obliquity, and shortening between the ribs and pelvis may develop. One goal of treatment is to bring these divergent response levels closer together so that the child can experience more comfortable postural change and adapt to later school demands.

The limbs of the hemiplegic child will change in postural tone as the trunk reactions are brought under active control and lateral weight shifts more clearly to the more-affected side. The two hands need the experience of sustaining the body weight simultaneously, as do the two feet. Although the more-affected hand may not develop sensation adequate for skilled activity, an important treatment goal is sufficient shoulder mobility to move the arm across the body midline and to assume a relaxed alignment during ambulation. Early treatment increases the possibility that the more-affected hand will be used as an assisting or helping hand. There are some children who have such severe sensory loss that active use is minimal, although considerable relaxation can be achieved.

The greater the discrepancy between the sensorimotor experience of the one side of the body and the other, the more tendency the system seems to have to reject one of the

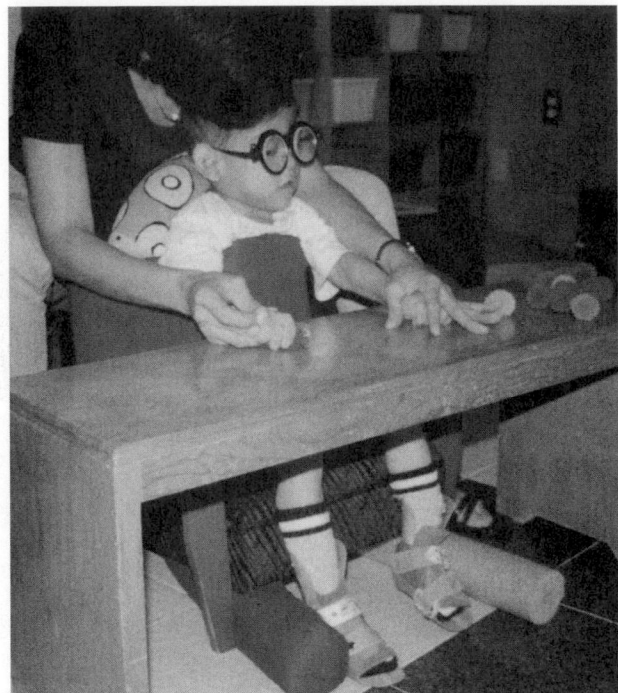

FIGURE 12-17 ■ Bilateral arm activity with visual regard that corresponds to hand motion incorporated into therapy.

messages. This can lead to distortions in verticality and is a major interference in bilateral integration. Functional vision evaluation is important to avoid the midline shift problem that will distort postural control. As body weight is shifted to the more-normal side, flexor withdrawal patterns of the limbs increase in frequency and strength in some children. These postural reactions are often associated with lack of full weight bearing on the more affected side. The presence of a lateral visual midline shift or some visual field loss may increase the avoidance of weight on the more-affected side.[60] One important therapy goal is the achievement of graded weight shift through the pelvis during ambulation (Figure 12-18).

Treatment strategies must incorporate a wide variety of more basic developmental alignments in which pelvic weight shift is a factor. The choice of prone, moving from sitting to four-point support, or a simple weight shift while sitting on a bench will depend on the movement characteristics observed by the therapist during the evaluative session. Diagonal adaptations are useful in normalizing the distribution of tone for upright function. Careful attention must be given to pelvic alignment and mobility because the pelvis has a tendency to be rotated posteriorly on the more-affected side in children who have not had good early therapy. This can cause increased hip flexion and incomplete hip extension at terminal stance later if the child begins to walk with the more-affected side held posteriorly, a characteristic that may be observed during analysis of leg position in gait. Dynamic foot supports will facilitate a more functional weight shift when the child is not in the treatment session. The goal of functional movement is best reached through a wide variety of weight-bearing postures, from the obvious developmental alignments to horizontal protective responses or reaching above the shoulders in sitting and standing to incorporate practical and commonly used adaptations.

The child with low muscle tone is perhaps the greatest challenge for both therapist and parent. Adequate developmental stimulation is difficult unless positioning can be

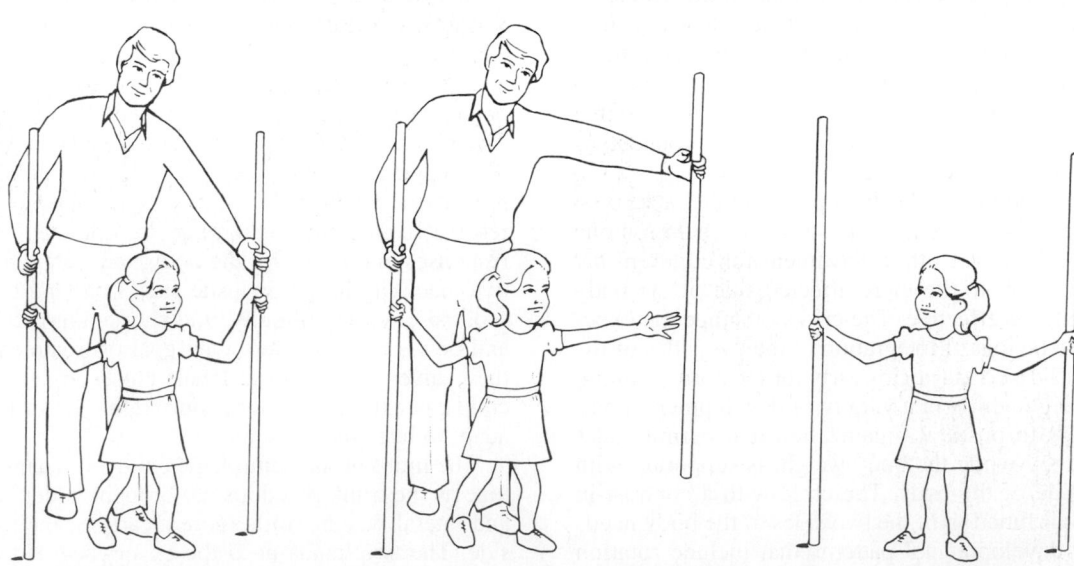

FIGURE 12-18 ■ The use of poles was introduced by the Bobaths as a way to achieve graded weight shift for increasingly complex postural adjustments in standing and walking.

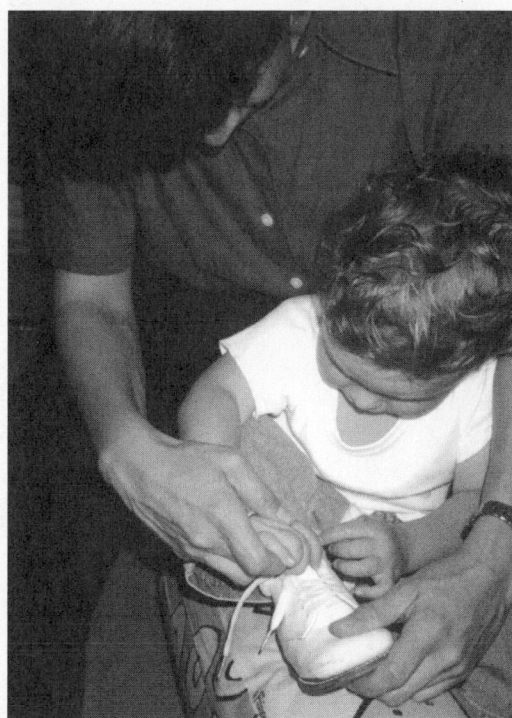

FIGURE 12-19 ■ With assistance, this boy with right hemiplegia is helped to improve his self-esteem by exploring dressing.

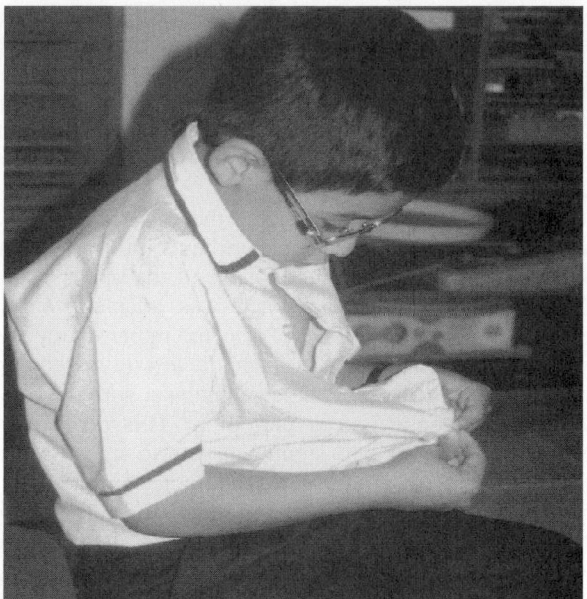

FIGURE 12-20 ■ Straddle-sitting on a bench gives this diplegic boy postural stability while he concentrates on the buttoning process.

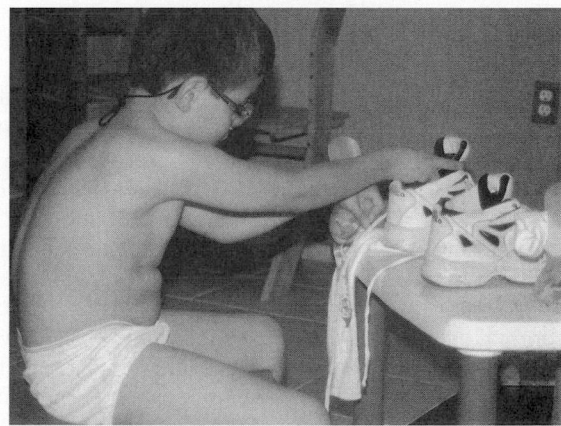

FIGURE 12-21 ■ Organization of clothing within reach is essential for success in independent dressing.

varied. Placing the child in a more upright alignment, although it is achieved with complete support initially, seems to aid the incrementation of postural control. To prepare the low-tone body for function, it is helpful to review the articulations for possible soft tissue restrictions. The neck and shoulder girdle are particularly vulnerable. Strong proprioceptive input while accurate postural alignment is ensured is an important part of the treatment session. A direct push-pull motion of the limbs, which is gentle traction alternated with approximation as described by the Bobaths,[65] also assists in maintaining antigravity positions and creates postural variance in the practice of antigravity postural reactions. Positioning at home may include a high table that supports the arms, allows for increased trunk extension in good alignment, and permits voluntary horizontal arm motion. The therapist must be cautious of the tendency to fixate in response to trunk instability and initial hypotonicity. This seemingly hypertonic response, which can be distributed in the deeper musculature, contributes to limited adaptability rather than differentiated postural control. It is difficult to ramp up the corticomotor neuron pool even though the child's motor output may remain limited; changes in positioning and opportunities for the child to have visual and other sensory experiences will aid learning. Home handling needs to include a variety of positions during each day for seating and play. Consistency in these practices is essential for the child with low tone to progress.

The process of undressing and dressing can be a dynamic part of the treatment program for any child (Figure 12-19). Diagonal patterns of movement that are incorporated into the removal of socks and shoes assist in the organization of midline orientation. Weight shifts and changes in stability-mobility distribution occur throughout the dressing process.

Concepts of direction and spatial orientation are applied to the relationship of body parts and clothing. Directional vocabulary terms and names of clothing and body parts are learned with this experience. A bench is useful because it permits the adult to sit behind the child who is just beginning to participate actively. The older child with difficult balance reactions can use the bench in a straddle-sit alignment (Figure 12-20). Aside from the physical and perceptual benefits, this achievement of dressing independently is one that offers the child a feeling of pride and independence. It is also a very practical preparation for the future when it is introduced in keeping with individual developmental and emotional needs (Figure 12-21).

RESEARCH

Pediatric clinicians are faced with selecting treatments that are efficacious for children with cerebral palsy. Increasing pressure on clinicians to establish that treatments are effective in improving functional abilities is often dictated by third-party payers. In the past there was little research on pediatric treatment approaches and protocols that withstood the rigors of scientific investigation. Today, several methods that warrant mentioning are beginning to undergo systematic investigation.

Constraint-induced movement therapy (CIMT) was developed from basic science experiments on deafferentated monkeys to overcome learned nonuse of the upper extremity.[66,67] This forced use approach was adapted to adult patients after a stroke where the affected upper extremity is forced to participate in activities and the less-involved upper extremity is constrained. Practice is intense, with 6 hours of mass practice for a 2-week period.[68-70] This protocol has been quite successful, with significant improvement in upper extremity movement and use of the affected limb. CIMT is very popular and is now beginning to appear in the clinical setting. The pediatric client has also demonstrated a favorable response to this treatment protocol in several single case studies.[71-75] In a recent clinical randomized trial by Taub et al,[76] children with hemiplegia or brain injury receiving CIMT for 21 consecutive days, 6 hours a day, demonstrated significant improvement in the amount of use, quality of movement, and spontaneous use of the affected upper extremity. These results were sustained at 6-month follow up. Clinicians are beginning to adapt these studies to their therapeutic settings and modify the protocols for clinical use and reimbursement potential.

Treadmill training has also been used in children with cerebral palsy.[77-81] The treadmill has been instrumental in rehabilitation for many years with a variety of purposes. This treatment began with animal studies on spinalized cats and rats and their responses to training on a treadmill in the recovery of a walking pattern.[82-85] Today, this treatment is used in many populations, including those with spinal cord injury, traumatic brain injury, Parkinson's disease, stroke, and cerebral palsy.[86] The use of the treadmill in children with cerebral palsy has shown promising results: improvement in gait pattern, decreased coactivation in lower extremity musculature, and improved and stabilized energy expenditure (Figure 12-22).[77-81] Commercial equipment is now available to assist with supporting the body weight of those individuals who otherwise would not be candidates for such a treatment. Clinical adaptations have also been incorporated to accommodate smaller bodies on a treadmill, which allows the therapist to assist from behind or from the side. Setting goals for this treatment must be precise, with an understanding of the purpose intended for its use: improving endurance, changing the parameters of the gait pattern, strengthening, and gait training. Each goal must be based on a sound theoretical foundation, which is now available from the literature.

Strength training was never thought possible in the presence of spasticity in children with cerebral palsy. Several studies have now shown that strength can improve in children with spastic cerebral palsy.[87-90] Circuit training was used in an afterschool training program for 4 weeks, two times a week for 1 hour of intense group training, resulting in improved strength and functional performance.[87] Strength was maintained in this group of individuals at an 8-week follow-up posttest. Dodd et al[88] set up a home-based lower

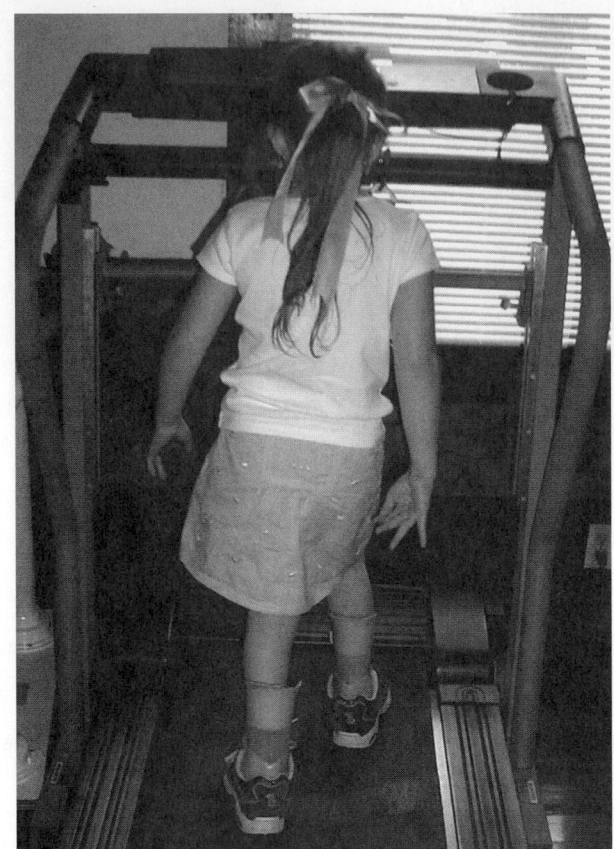

FIGURE 12-22 ■ This young girl is practicing walking on the treadmill without holding on and incorporating arm swing to improve her stride length.

extremity strengthening program in a randomized clinical trial with 21 individuals with cerebral palsy. All subjects in the treatment group had improved lower extremity strength that was maintained at follow-up periods of 6 and 12 weeks. In a study focused on biofeedback and strength training to improve dorsiflexion and range of motion, Toner et al[90] demonstrated significant changes in active range of motion and dorsiflexion strength.[90] Strength training in the presence of spasticity is also documented in adults as beneficial not only for conditioning, improving range of motion and psychological well being, but in some cases reducing spasticity.[91-94] A variety of methods for strength training can be incorporated into a clinical treatment setting or home exercise program with anticipated improvement in muscle strength, which may also result in improved functional status for children with cerebral palsy. Strength training encompasses free weights, aerobic workouts, stretch bands/tubing, and machines that address resistive exercise (Figure 12-23).

Many adjuvant therapies that are popular in combination with other treatments are available to individuals with cerebral palsy. Electric stimulation (ES) has been used in a variety of ways with children with cerebral palsy. In several case reports by Carmick,[95-97] neuromuscular electrical stimulation used in conjunction with task-oriented practice was found to improve sensory awareness, strength, gait parameters, and passive/active range of motion. Neuromuscular electrical stimulation was used as an adjunct therapy with

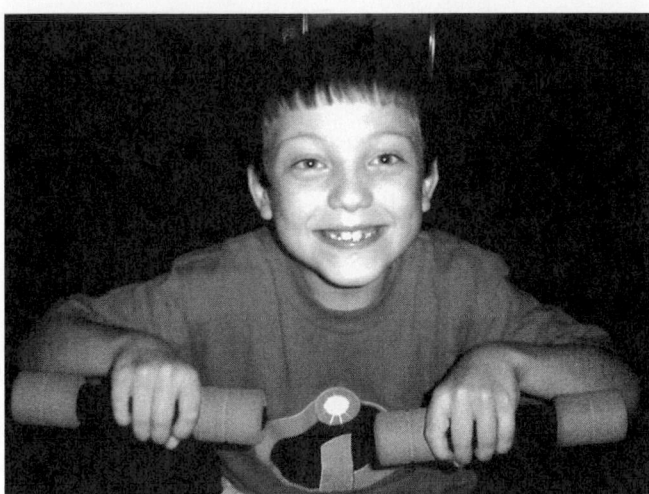

FIGURE 12-23 ■ Using free weights to strengthen the upper extremities while stabilizing the trunk seated on an incline bolster.

upper and lower extremity practice protocols.[95-98] ES has been used in conjunction with 6 weeks of intensive therapy to improve sitting posture and trunk control for children with spastic cerebral palsy. Radiographic studies confirmed the statistical significance in decreasing the kyphotic angle of the spine and sitting score on the GMFM.[99] ES has been in the therapy arena for many years, and its selective use with children who have cerebral palsy may supplement regular therapy sessions with enhanced results. (Therapeutic subthreshold electric stimulation at meridian points is discussed in the Electroacupuncture Treatments section and in Chapter 37.)

Botulinum toxin A (BtxA) has been used to assist in decreasing spasticity because it provides a permissive condition that improves and increases range of motion and practice of new motor patterns without the interference of increased muscle tone. Gait velocity, stride length, range of motion, and decreased spasticity were noted to be significant in 33 subjects with cerebral palsy after local injections of BtxA.[100] Several studies have shown a decrease in spasticity, successful treatment of foot deformities, and improved gait parameters with BtxA.[101-104] In a study by Galli et al,[105] dynamic dorsiflexion improved during stance and swing phases of gait with significant improvement in foot placement at initial contact. BtxA has been used with varying results as an adjunct treatment for the management of upper extremity spasticity.[106] It allows for the reduction of muscle tone and opens a window of practice opportunity, in combination with other treatments, to learn new movement possibilities. BtxA has a temporary effect, so therefore the critical element is its combination with other treatment modalities. It has also been used as an alternative to control the progression of hip dislocation and hip pain in children with cerebral palsy.[107]

Joint and trunk taping and strapping have been used to provide sensory input and alignment for posture, balance, and strengthening. To date, there is no evidence that these adjunctive treatments actually provide these benefits, but there is also no evidence that they do not. Further objective investigation will be necessary to address the issues presented by these additives to therapy. Both are considered noninvasive with few side effects other than adhesive allergy to tape and autonomic nervous system responses such as sweating and overheating. Several different types of tape (athletic, Leuko P Patellatape [Notoden, The Netherlands], and Kinesio Tape [Kinesio USA Corp., LTD.]) and strapping devices are available commercially.

Soft tissue mobilization is a method of stretching tight structures that have become restricted from overuse, spasticity, deformities, muscle shortening, surgeries, trauma, and poor nutrition. This type of stretching has strong roots in osteopathic medicine but is not limited to that area of expertise. Over the years, research investigating the cellular and tissue changes that occur with immobilization have revealed some interesting and shocking alterations in the muscle and collagen fibers. With immobilization, slow muscle fibers show greater atrophy than fast fibers do.[47] There is atrophy, a decrease in peak torque, an increase in fatigue resistance, loss of strength, and reduced central activation when the plantar flexors of the ankle are immobilized.[108,109] In a recent study of children with severe spasticity, muscle biopsies were performed on the vastus lateralis to determine collagen accumulation in the spastic muscle. An increased accumulation of collagen I fibers in the endomysium of the muscle was noted, with thickening and decreased muscle fiber content in the more severe cases.[110] This study, in combination with what we understand about healthy muscle, reinforces the need to keep the muscles flexible and active to help prevent this accumulation of collagen. Soft tissue mobilization and deep tissue stretching are methods that can improve the ability of the tissue to lengthen and fold, allowing for a more efficient activation of the muscle fibers, thus optimizing the formation of normal synergies during practice of motor skills.

As mentioned earlier, children with cerebral palsy often have visual difficulties that are not acuity problems and that are not correctable with a standard lens. Vision therapy has demonstrated good results when emphasis is placed on ocular motility and accommodation.[111] When children were given intense visuo-oculomotor training, improvement was noted in visuo-oculomotor control.[112] Changes in the child's ability to execute smooth pursuit precision and maximum velocity, an improvement of saccadic movement precision and stability, and a shortening of the saccadic reaction time were significantly improved after training.[112] Although many clinicians are not experts in the area of vision, vision is an important part of every therapy session. Incorporating vision as an integral part of a therapy session will not only improve the child's orientation in space but will address their ability to scan the environment as they learn to move through space.

Many therapies become popular by purporting a "fix" for a particular problem associated with cerebral palsy. The clinician accepts responsibility in making sound judgments concerning treatment and outcomes for children with cerebral palsy. Not all the treatments used in therapy will be investigated rigorously in a scientific manner. However, when a treatment approach is presented as advantageous for many diagnoses and conditions, with claims of success beyond what is reasonable for those conditions, it is your duty to proceed with caution. Always stop and think what theory and frame of reference the approach will fit best. Does this "new" therapy make sense with the knowledge you have of anatomy, physiology, neurology, and motor learning? As clinicians we will always be tempted to try new approaches before the scientific community has investigated them thoroughly. Clinicians, because they are creative and innovative, have advanced our professions. It is essential to advance patient care with treatments that are safe and do no harm. Every environment affords itself to research opportunities that contribute to the treatment of children with cerebral palsy. Single case reports and single case studies are the beginning of this process and, although descriptive in nature and with limited generalization, provide evidence for new therapeutic approaches and further systematic investigation.

MEDICAL INFLUENCES ON TREATMENT

Because the problems of cerebral palsy are so varied, the condition lends itself to diverse interventions, some of which have a longer life than others. Management of spasticity has always been an area of great concern and interest, and over the years several treatments have been offered to control this positive sign. Various medications have been used to control spasticity; baclofen, diazepam, and dantrolene remain the three most commonly used pharmacological agents in the treatment of spastic hypertonia. (See Chapter 36 for additional information.)[113] The baclofen pump has been used in children with excessive spasticity. This pump is implanted in the lower abdomen with a catheter leading to the intrathecal space for the administration of the drug. This treatment for spasticity has been effective for some types of cerebral palsy but led to complications in some patients with mixed cerebral palsy, low body weight, younger age, gastrostomy tubes, and nonambulatory status.[114-116]

The cerebellar implant so popular in the late 1970s offered the possibility of regulating tone by supplementing cerebellar inhibition.[117-120] As time passed, the procedure was used less often, and patients had difficulty getting repairs or replacement parts for the implant. The procedure that largely replaced the cerebellar implant was the placement of four electrodes in the cervical area to offer more control over postural tone.[121] These had the advantage of being adjustable so that the individual or a family member could make daily choices as to the optimal tone distribution. In some cases early success gave way to disappointment as the system adapted to the inputs. In some cases the child or adolescent had to make a decision whether movement or speech was more important on a given day. Therapy was always recommended after the procedure, although the nature of the specific program was left to the family to decide. The success of the cerebellar stimulator is considered moderate when used on a select group of individuals with cerebral palsy.[117-120] Other more recent spasticity management programs are less invasive and are often considered before use of this invasive procedure.

In 1968 a posterior rhizotomy surgical intervention was developed with some success reported in reducing spasticity.[122,123] It remained for Peacock and Arens[124] to apply the procedure more selectively and functionally and to bring it to the United States from South Africa. On the basis of their experience, Peacock and colleagues insisted on daily neurodevelopmental (Bobath) treatment for at least 1 year after the surgical intervention. Electromyographic testing before and during the surgery is used to determine which posterior

nerve rootlets are creating the spasticity in the lower extremities.[125] The foundation for success is accurate selection of the child, an experienced surgeon, and careful analysis of therapy goals.

A more recent improvement in the rhizotomy procedure was developed by Lazareff et al,[126] who enter a limited number of levels rather than five levels of the spinal column and prefer to work close to the cauda equina, according to the technique of Fasano.[127] Several recent studies have documented improvement in function, strength, and reduction of spasticity outcomes as far out as 3 to 5 years.[122,128] Careful selection of the appropriate candidate for this surgery followed by intense therapy intervention is essential for the success of the procedure and for optimizing motor outcomes.

Alcohol (phenol) blocks and the use of botoxin (BtxA) have been used locally to affect a change in the individual muscle or motor point injected.[113,129-135] Both orthopedists and neurologists have taken an interest in the use of botulism toxin to block selected muscle responses for a temporary period. BtxA has been reported to have fewer side effects than the phenol blocks and is now considered the drug of choice for this type of procedure.[103] These conservative interventions serve to delay surgery until the child is more capable of responding to postsurgical therapy programs.

Orthopedic surgical intervention continues to be effective in cerebral palsy when there are tendon contractures or specific structural limitations that are not accompanied by excessive levels of spasticity.[136,137] In any surgery the outcome is much improved by close coordination between therapist and surgeon, with a functional orientation toward goal setting for the child. Early standing after surgery and use of dynamic footplates inside the casts and orthotics after cast removal will generally improve functional outcomes. Bony surgeries that offer better joint stability are usually planned for the termination of growth. The orthopedist is also able to guide conservative positioning measures to prevent hip problems resulting from spasticity while direct treatment intervention continues. Bracing of the trunk, which is sometimes warranted for scoliosis or kyphosis, is prescribed by the orthopedist. Surgical intervention for spinal deformities is determined by the physician, with consideration of the child's age, condition and health, and the degree of curvature.

Children with cerebral palsy differ in their ability to relax completely during sleep, and a small number of these children can benefit from inhibitive casting or splints to be used at night. More often this type of positioning is used during therapy sessions and independent ambulation to combine control with weight bearing.[138] The orthopedist should participate in any plan for prolonged immobilization or temporary casting that will be used on a 24-hour schedule, such as serial casting to improve range of motion.[139,140] A variety of lower extremity bracing is available and its selection is dependent on the segment to control and the outcomes sought in positioning or dynamic action, as in ambulation (Figure 12-24).

EQUIPMENT

Equipment recommendations must take into account the physical space in the home and the amount of direct treat-

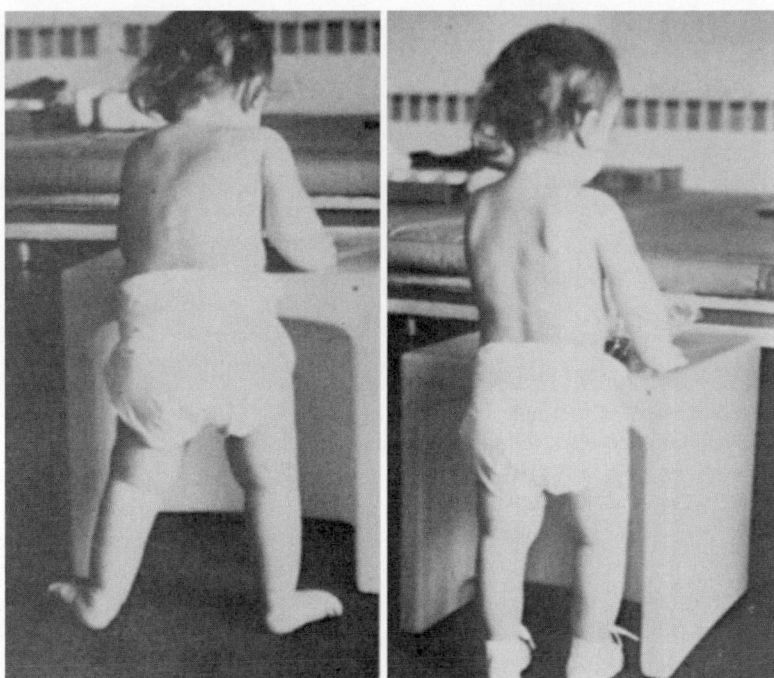

FIGURE 12-24 ■ A supportive shoe with footplates inside for this low-tone child facilitates more normal trunk reactions and permits use of the hands for play.

ment available to the child (Figure 12-25). Young children in particular can often use normal seating with slight adaptations. This is not only more socially and financially acceptable but also permits changes as required by the child's developmental progress. The portability of supportive seats or standers encourages the family to take the apparatus along for weekend outings or visits to relatives. Chair designs should place children at an age-appropriate level in their environments. This permits a better quality of visual exploration and facilitates social exchange with siblings and visiting peers. When planning the amount of physical support needed by the child, the therapist considers varying the structural control in relation to activity (Figure 12-26). The child who is merely watching the play of others or a television presentation may successfully control trunk and head balance independently with minimal support. However, concentration on hand skills or self-feeding may necessitate trunk control assistance by a chair insert to avoid the child's use of abnormal reactions. As postural reactions become more integrated and hence more automatic, support should be diminished.

For the more severely disabled child, equipment should be easily and completely washable. Mothers should be able to place special seating inserts into wheelchairs or travel chairs with one hand while holding the child. Wheelchairs should be ordered with consideration for family needs and the child's environment. The most costly does not always offer the best solution. Control straps and seating should be adaptable and allow for future change on the basis of growth and improved function. The severely limited child needs seating changes at least once every hour during the day to prevent pressure and provide environment changes as in normal development. Pleasing color, good-quality upholstery, and professional finishing are important not only for

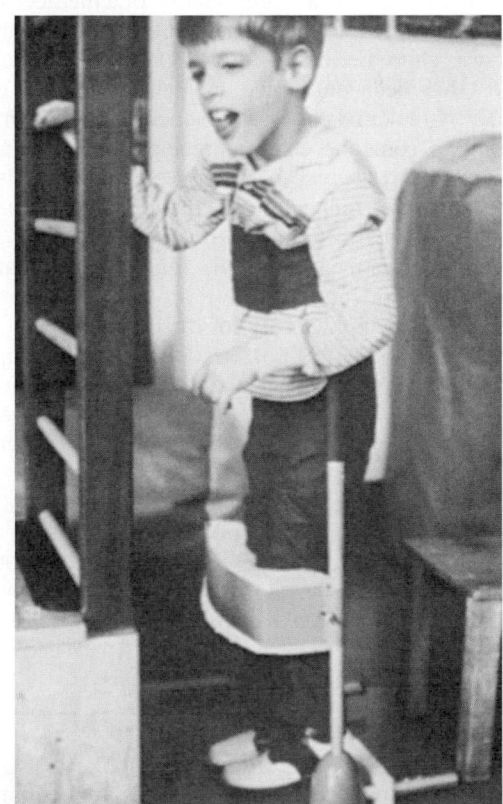

FIGURE 12-25 ■ An upright stander is easily incorporated into the home environment, providing the child with an upright position, stimulation, and an opportunity to participate in activities.

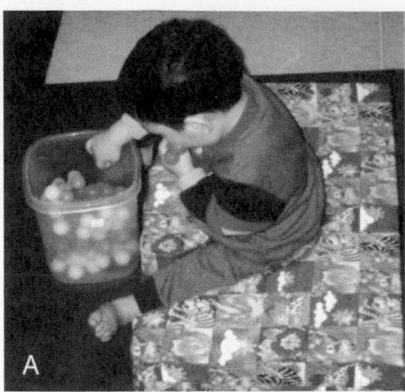
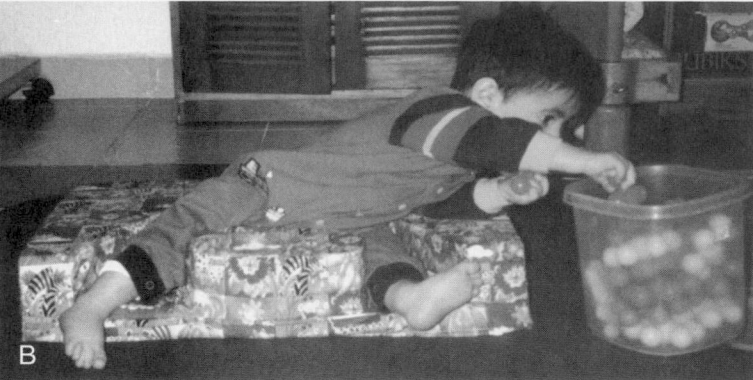

FIGURE 12-26 ■ Use of a simple cut-out space in 3-inch foam gives this 1-year-old child security while requiring more active trunk adaptation during play.

the child but also for family members, who are accepting the equipment as part of their personal living environment.

As prices rise and the applicability of insurance changes, the therapist must consider cost-effectiveness more carefully. Parents are often desperate to do everything possible for the child and tend to be very susceptible to high-powered advertising and reassuring sales personnel. By providing a list of essential equipment features, the therapist will aid the parents in becoming informed consumers. Perusal of several catalogs permits some comparison of quality and prices. Adaptive equipment fairs are often open to parents and therapists and are great opportunities to actually try the equipment without the burden of the cost. Therapists can forge a relationship with a representative of a medical supply company and then access equipment on loan to try with their patients for short periods of time. Once the appropriate equipment has been purchased, periodic review of equipment used by the child can serve to encourage the family to pass along to someone else equipment items that are no longer needed. Investment in expensive equipment also has the hidden effect of influencing both parent and therapist to continue its use well beyond its effectiveness as a dynamic supplement to treatment. For this reason more than any other, large investments must be thoroughly researched as to their long-term applicability for the child.

Adaptive equipment is not the only type of equipment that the therapist must consider for clients. Conditioning and strengthening, now recognized as beneficial to children and adults with cerebral palsy, opens the door for equipment that lends itself to these parameters.[87-94] Exercise bikes, treadmills (see Figure 12-22, p. 372), light weights (see Figure 12-23, p. 373), and balance equipment (Figure 12-27) are all valuable adjuncts to a home exercise program and should be considered, when appropriate, for a particular individual. Many of the commercially available items found at a sporting goods store can be well adapted to fit the needs of the higher functioning person with cerebral palsy.

ALTERNATIVE THERAPIES

Hyperbaric oxygen treatment is gaining popularity as a treatment for cerebral palsy in children. Clinics are beginning to spring up worldwide for this type of therapy. Research on this treatment has been inconclusive, and scientific evidence for its efficacy is lacking.[141,142] Clinicians should keep

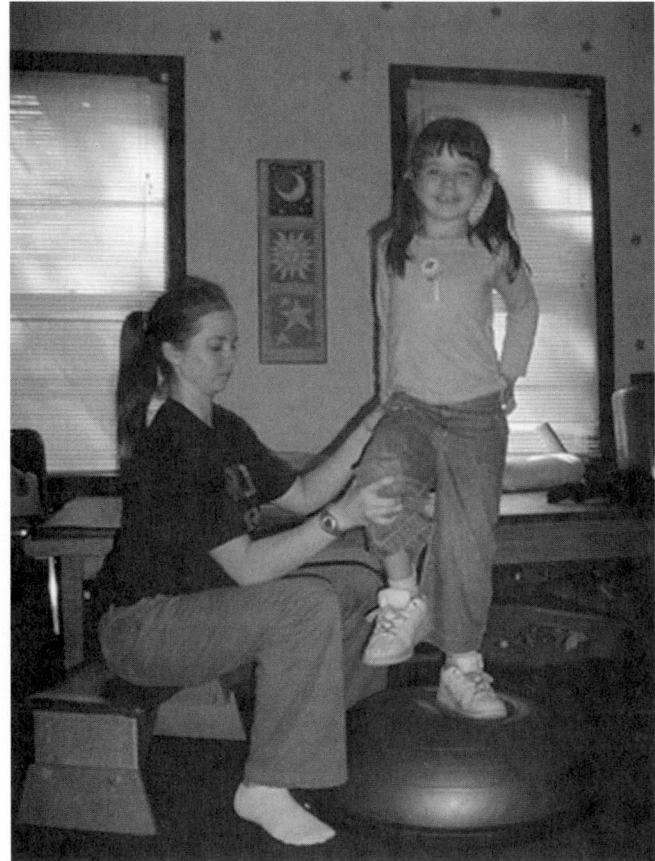

FIGURE 12-27 ■ Balance equipment allows for increased complexity in the therapy program with the refinement of balance reactions.

abreast of the latest developments in the treatment of cerebral palsy and inform families about the pros and cons of designer treatments. Currently the Undersea and Hyperbaric Medicine Society states that there is not enough evidence to recommend the use of hyperbaric oxygen therapy for cerebral palsy.[143,144]

The Adeli suit is a compression garment with bungee cord–like elastic cords attached to the suit along the trunk and extremities. This suit, once referred to as the therapeutic space suit or treatment-loading suit (space-designated PINGUIN), was developed for Russian cosmonauts to counteract the adverse effect of long-term zero gravity on the skeletal muscles.[145] There are a few studies that suggest that there are benefits for children with cerebral palsy when they receive therapy in the suit.[143,145-148] The suit allows for controlled practice of activities with resistance, and assistance when necessary; the cords are attached in a variety of ways to give different types of practice repetitions. As is prescribed by the proponents of this approach, intense practice is warranted to reap the benefits. This therapy is expensive and the suit, if bought to use at home, is also very expensive. Rosenbaum[143] has suggested that the benefits of this therapy vary with the type and severity of the involvement, the child's ability to participate in controlled movement, and the tolerance to wearing the suit for extended periods of time. In Australia the Upsuit described in the article as made of a stretchy material has been investigated for use with children with cerebral palsy and similar results have been noted: the type of cerebral palsy and the person's ability to participate in movement forecast the potential outcomes.[149,150] The Upsuit was also noted to compromise lung capacity, which interfered with the child's ability to participate.[149] As clinicians, it is important for us to stay abreast of the latest developments and to provide families with reasonable alternatives. Although intense practice is well known in the literature as being beneficial for motor learning, the addition of the suit brings in a component that "appears" to provide stability and graded control during practice. Caution when describing this approach to families is warranted because some evidence suggests that it may not be for every child with cerebral palsy. The long-term effects and measurable outcomes after the use of the Adeli suit and the Upsuit are not documented in the literature. The following questions must be asked: what happens to the motor abilities of the child when the suit is removed, and has the suit actually prevented the development of postural antigravity coactivation of the trunk and proximal axial joints?

In the mid-1980s Pape[151] published a case series involving five children with cerebral palsy receiving therapeutic (subthreshold) electrical stimulation. Reported in this case series was that overnight use of low-intensity ES in combination with standard therapy demonstrated significant improvement in gross motor, balance, and locomotor skills as measured by the Peabody Developmental Motor Scales in children with mild cerebral palsy.[151] Results reported were based on observations by individuals who were not blinded to the purpose of the study, and therefore the research design was biased. In a follow-up study Steinbok et al[152] followed children who had undergone selected dorsal rhizotomy and received therapeutic ES for 1 year. Although this study reported improvement in gross motor function, no other measures were changed: range of motion, spasticity, or strength. Two well-controlled clinical trials investigated this method of TES delivery and concluded that no objective effects on motor, ambulatory function, or clinical benefit for children and youths with cerebral palsy were detected.[153,154] Parents often report changes with this therapy, but the objective measures do not demonstrate significant results. Clinicians in the field have reported that overnight use of TES builds muscle bulk but, unless combined with active participation of the musculature, stimulated overall improvement

in movement may not be seen. This therapy, for children with cerebral palsy, requires a special simulation unit that is subthreshold and capable of being used at night with a shutoff setting if the electrodes become disconnected from the child. The unit is costly and further requires a clinician that is specially trained in its use to evaluate and periodically update the treatment protocol. Significant benefits for this type of electric stimulation have not been documented.

The Peto method or "conductive education" (CE) developed by Andres Peto in Budapest after World War II has been used in children with disabilities.[155] This approach is an educational versus medical model, as the name implies, and the focus is on the many aspects of child development.[156] It is based on practice and repetition combined with verbal guidance of a trainer (conductor) and self-verbalization by the child as he or she performs the task or activity.[143] Most of the claims that promote its value have come from the Peto Institute in Budapest, Hungary. The institute has been very selective in choosing candidates for this approach on the basis of the child's potential for independent mobility and function with a good overall prognosis.[143,155,157] Research into this method of delivery of services to children with cerebral palsy has been sparse outside the Peto institute's studies. In two studies in Australia conductive education was found to have encouraging results in developmental changes.[158,159] In a randomized controlled study with children assigned to a CE group or a neurodevelopmental intervention group, no significant differences were noted in the two groups.[160] This approach advocates intense practice of all skills, motor and educational, with emphasis on self-doing regardless of whether a compensatory pattern is used. Various pieces of equipment are used to facilitate independent skills: wooden slatted beds to allow the child to pull and maneuver, wooden ladders mounted on the wall to assist with dressing and transitions. The literature on CE does stress the concept of intense practice for motor learning. Similarly, promoting practice in the CE environment must transfer to home and community for carryover to everyday life situations.[161] To fully optimize the outcomes of CE, a commitment from the family is essential, as is the case in most therapeutic approaches. Further investigation into this approach is warranted before this philosophy is fully supported. For a selected group of individuals, CE research results seem hopeful, although transfer to unpracticed tasks and different environments may be minimal.

The Feldenkrais method was developed by an Israeli engineer Moshe Feldenkrais while looking for a solution to his own knee problem. He started analyzing body alignment for more efficient movement.[162,163] This form of body work has been used to help dancers, gymnasts, and other skilled persons improve their performance. Some therapists have undertaken the long training necessary to understand normal movement in more detail and to improve the movement coordination for their clients with neuromotor challenges. There is no published research on this method, but several books and training courses exist that promote its use.

Ida Rolf, trained in physics, had a son with some postural disorganization.[164] She developed a structural approach, called the Rolfing technique, to improve body alignment that uses specific release of deep soft tissue to restore effortless postural control against gravity.[165] She was able to make positive changes in the movement patterns of many children with cerebral palsy, but she never claimed to treat the disorder itself. This approach requires special training in the Rolfing technique, which is a type of deep tissue massage.

Dr. William Sutherland,[166] an osteopathic physician, developed direct treatment of the cranium, which is referred to commercially as cranial therapy, or cranial sacral treatment. This type of therapy is believed to have wide application to many disabilities and conditions.[167] Today there are persons trained at many different levels, so the family of a child with cerebral palsy seeking this treatment will need to be certain that the practitioner is a professional and that she or he has experience with small children.[168] Cranial treatment is purported to restore the physiological motion of the craniosacral system, improving circulation of fluids to the brain as well as respiratory function, to which it is believed to be closely linked. Research has been encouraged in this area to substantiate the claims of this approach.

DEVELOPING A PERSONAL PHILOSOPHY OF TREATMENT

The practicing therapist continues to learn much about the nuances of normal human development (see Chapter 2).[169] The dynamic interaction of developmental movement components becomes more significant as the therapist acquires greater clinical experience and recognizes developmental change as a reflection of central nervous system maturation. Increasing knowledge of the functional nature of sensory systems and central nervous system processing will influence the choice of treatment techniques. Direct intervention will have more depth and specificity that improve the child's control of posture and movement while the therapist appreciates the complex interaction of developmental factors in cerebral palsy. On the basis of individual experience, each therapist develops a personal philosophy of treatment that incorporates new research findings and evolving perceptions of the problem of central nervous system dysfunction. Without a philosophical/theoretical orientation for decision making the therapist may succumb to following each promising treatment idea that is learned without having a clear image of the potential benefits for the specific client. "Commercial" programs may benefit the child whose needs match the program objectives. An "individualized" program adapts to the needs of the particular child and is shaped by the response of that child during therapy. Without an internalized treatment goal toward which independent techniques are applied, the result may remain ineffective and unconvincing. The therapist in a direct treatment situation must develop a concise visualization of what is to be achieved in each session with the individual child. Repetition and practice that is so critical for learning must often be carried out at home, and the therapist becomes responsible for family instruction. Home exercise programs must be tailored for both the child and family situation and must be in alignment with the goals and expectations of the family. These programs need to be practical, fun ideas for practice that can be incorporated into the child's home life with reasonable assurance that the activities can and will be carried out regularly. Creative therapeutic ideas for playtime, dressing, grooming, mealtime, and relaxation time are best addressed in the home exercise program because these are everyday tasks that every family encounters and the family is likely to be compliant.[170]

Specialized therapy, like normal development, is potentially a preparation for functional performance. Training in specific coordination skills may be necessary for the older child or adolescent and must begin with a thorough analysis of the whole person who happens to demonstrate the effects of cerebral palsy. Some children have learned self-care along with brothers and sisters. Others have needed therapy guidance for each achievement. Intelligent children with strong motivation may only need some assistance in avoiding use of abnormal reactions, whereas others have poor spatial orientation and minimal motivation to achieve independence. The therapist most often needs to create a dialog with the individual who has the problem because parents are often fatigued and without energy to solve the issue of adolescent life skills.

INVOLVING THE FAMILY

To be successful, therapy for the child with cerebral palsy includes active family participation. Variability of practice in different environments tends to promote more effective motor learning and parents who learn to help their child early begin to understand the importance of their participation as well as the nature of their child's disability. Parents are in the process of healing their own self-image that was so injured when they learned of their child's disability. They should not be expected to become therapists per se but learn to observe small gains in treatment sessions that offer insight into the child's current strengths and weaknesses.

Parents need to adapt their expectations in keeping with the child's continuing change and emotional maturity. Parenting a child with cerebral palsy is no easy task, and the therapist will do well to develop respect for this demanding role. No one provides more for the child with cerebral palsy than the nurturing parent who guides the child to self-acceptance of limitations without destroying personal initiative. This is the child who most often becomes an independent working adult (Figure 12-28).

The therapist must give serious thought to priorities in home recommendations. Therapists must consider the size of the family, outside employment of the mother and father, physical capabilities of the child, general health status of the child, and psychological acceptance of the problem within

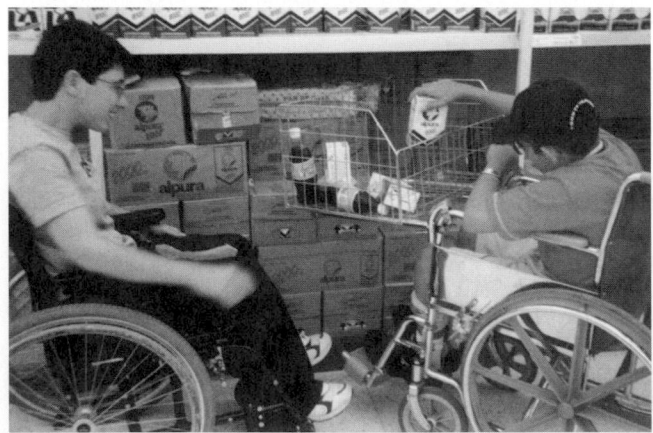

FIGURE 12-28 ■ Therapy goals must incorporate functional activities that lead to personal independence if they are to be pertinent for the older child and adolescent.

the family. The emotional needs of some parents demand a period of less, rather than more, direct involvement with the child. Other parents must be cautioned that repetition of an activity more times than recommended will not result in faster improvement. This impression is sometimes gained from wide advertising of commercial programs that offer the same activity sequence for every child and demand a large number of daily repetitions. Both parent and therapist must appreciate the need for the central nervous system to have some time to integrate new sensorimotor experiences and to perfect emerging control of postural adjustments. Excessive control of movement patterns and overprotection by an adult tends to reduce the child's initiation of postural change and decrease active sensorimotor learning. Health needs for good nutrition and adequate rest must also be considered by parents and professionals. The attitude of teachers in the first years is extremely important for the child with cerebral palsy.

ROLE OF THE THERAPIST IN INDIRECT INTERVENTION

For many children with cerebral palsy, active treatment is not available. Geographical isolation, socioeconomic factors, and lack of qualified therapists may interfere with the delivery of direct service. The therapist must then assume the role of teacher, counselor, or consultant. More often the new role emerges as one in which the therapist tries to meet a combination of needs and is frequently frustrated by lack of time, energy, and community resources. The therapist may be a member of a community team that includes a psychologist, a social worker, and a public health nurse. This sometimes creates more of a behavioral than a traditional medical orientation. Therapists can also be primarily responsible to the public school systems, introducing therapeutic positioning to classroom teachers. For these types of situations the clinician will find videotape a valuable adjunct to direct instruction. The individual child may be filmed with equipment, adequate positions, or therapeutic procedures. Useful topic-oriented videotapes are also available for professionals and families.

When children have no access to direct treatment, positioning is of paramount importance. The selected support is used to avoid contractures, scoliosis, and permanent limitations in range of movement. Even the most severely limited child should have a minimum of three positions that can be alternated during the day. In addition, the position selected should be as functional as possible for the individual child to allow access to the child's environment. In some cases this may mean encouraging eye contact. For another child, hand use becomes a possibility with proper trunk support.

Communication for the nonverbal client with cerebral palsy must be an integral part of the therapy or school program.[171] A simple start may be made with pictures to permit choices in food, clothing, and therapy activities. The parents need encouragement to begin the process of letting the child make some simple choices in food, clothing, or preferred activities. Although computers have their place, the child should have the communication device with him or her at all times. Language development in the young child is enhanced by having this type of alternative while articulation is still difficult. Use of head movement is a powerful influence on muscle tone changes that may cause negative

regression in postural or visual control. Postural and visual control is essential toward the goal of better function and communication. A solution that was successful with one 9-year-old athetoid girl was moving the elbow back to a switch mounted on the vertical bar of the wheelchair backrest to access her communication device. Any activity that is repeated on a daily basis should be examined in light of possible interference by abnormal patterns.

Affordable electronic systems with voice recording, portability, and growth features are available. Communication, which can be achieved by coordinating efforts with the speech pathologist, can make the difference between passivity and active participation in the environment.[171] Play can be encouraged with the use of switch toys and touch-screen computers. Many new programs are being developed for computers and electronic interactive books.

THERAPY IN THE COMMUNITY

Children with mild dysfunction as a result of cerebral palsy may be successfully incorporated into physical education classes if the teacher is prepared to make some small adaptations. Teachers generally appreciate the opportunity to discuss with the therapist specific limitations of the child and those movements that should be encouraged. For better success the child with functional limitations can be incorporated into a class that follows the British form of movement education, which places much less emphasis on intragroup competition and encourages each child to progress at her or his own rate.

Classroom teachers who lack experience with children who have special needs are understandably reluctant to incorporate a child with movement limitations into the classroom until they know the child. A meeting with the therapist might be used to help the child demonstrate his or her strengths, physical independence, and ability to participate in classroom activities. The child may often play an active role in the problem-solving process necessary for a successful classroom experience. Children often have developed their own ways of managing the water fountain, the locker door, or personal care needs. Demonstrating these abilities reinforces strengths rather than limitations and empowers the child to some positive responses for curious peers.

As programs that hire therapists move into the fields of prevention and early intervention, the therapist is dealing directly with a population that is not familiar with therapy per se nor aware of the need for this intervention. The therapist may discover a need to reorient previously accepted concepts of general rehabilitation. Clarification of one's own ideas is essential to establish effective communication with others. In some instances, active intervention to help the child will precede the labeling or diagnostic process, and referral to other specialists becomes part of the therapist's responsibility. Philosophically, early therapy becomes an enhancement of normal development rather than a remedial process, and it is advocated in the natural environment by federal funding agencies for children 0 to 3 years of age. This implies introducing new concepts of quality in early child development to the public. Day care programs are an example of new early childhood settings that incorporate children with impairments.

It is important to keep direct, active treatment available for older children, adolescents, and adults who are motivated to change. Now that more effective procedures are available for changing some of the basic neurophysiological movement characteristics observed in children with cerebral palsy, it is possible to obtain change with direct treatment of the older client. The adolescent often responds best to short-term, goal-oriented therapy programs that are patient centered. Motor learning concepts are better understood by both the therapist and the client (see Chapters 3 and 9) and can be incorporated in activities after mobilizing tissues that have been unused for so many years. With current program directions many older clients may not have had the opportunity for direct treatment over time by a qualified therapist. For the minimally involved teenager, young adult, and adult with cerebral palsy the local gym offers an alternative to direct therapy. A therapist can be consulted to establish an appropriate program for the individual who wants to work out at the gym on equipment, attend special classes that are offered, or work out in the pool. When asked, it is the therapist's area of expertise to help identify and make recommendations regarding functional movement and activity participation for adults with developmental disabilities such as cerebral palsy. (See the section in Chapter 29 on Adults with Developmental Disabilities.)

The movement toward a health orientation as opposed to crisis intervention for illness will also affect services for children and adults with cerebral palsy. This population does not have an illness or an active disease process, and they strive to lead as normal a life as possible. Many adults with neuromotor disabilities express their preference to participate in the decisions that are made for them regarding their ultimate lifestyle in the community. Optimal health for the adult with cerebral palsy has yet to be described, and much more data must be collected (see Chapter 29).

PSYCHOSOCIAL FACTORS IN CEREBRAL PALSY

We have defined cerebral palsy as a condition existing from the time of birth or infancy. The developing child has no memory of life in a different body. Movement limitations circumscribe the horizon of the child's world unless the family is able to provide enriching experiences. The development of both intelligence and personality relies heavily on developmental experiences and the opportunity for self-expression.

The child with spastic diplegia or spastic quadriplegia may be hesitant in making decisions or reaching out for a new opportunity because the world may seem overwhelming and threatening. The child may find it easier to withdraw toward social isolation. Parents and professionals can help children, adolescents and adults with cerebral palsy avoid these reactions by encouraging independence in thought and in physical tasks. Early choices can be made by the child regarding which clothes to wear or which task to do first. Understanding the child's limitations helps build successes rather than failures. To function in spite of the constraints of spasticity or other movement problems demands considerable effort on the part of the child.

Athetoid children, in contrast, have adapted to failures as a transient part of life. However disorganized their movements, they repeatedly attempt tasks and eventually succeed. Their social interactions reflect this life experience. Most people will sooner or later succumb to the positive smiling approach without analyzing the deeper communication offered by the child. These children are difficult for parents to discipline and structure during their early years. Early treatment with concomitant guidance for young parents ameliorates some of the problems by making the developmental expectations for the child more appropriate. The words of professionals who are in contact with the parents at the time of the diagnosis echo through time to influence future decision making for the child.

Intelligent children with low tone demand that the world be brought to them. Mentally limited children may fail to receive sufficient stimulation for optimal development at their functional levels. Many of these children need visual or auditory evaluations and intervention, and some of them need a special educational approach. Whatever the learning potential of the child with cerebral palsy, it is not always evident early in the child's life. Parents find it difficult to know how to guide a child when they are not certain that an assigned task or calm explanation is understood by the child.

Parental guidance of the child with functional limitations is also influenced by the adults' adaptation to their offspring's problem. Parents need to resolve in their own way the emotional impact of the child's disability. Most parents feel inadequate, ignorant, and relatively helpless at being unable to remedy the situation for their child. They need help in feeling good about themselves before they can effectively guide the child toward self-acceptance as an adequate human being. Parents need guidance to provide themselves with opportunities to rest and renew their energies.

The therapist plays an important role in the psychosocial development of children who receive regular treatment. The child may perceive the therapist as a confidant, disciplinarian, counselor, or friend at various stages of development. Some children accept the therapist as a member of their extended family. This is natural considering the extent to which therapists influence clients' own self-awareness through changes in their physical bodies. However, it also places a personal responsibility on the therapist to be aware of the continuing interaction and its effect on the maturational process of the child. Long-term relationships with patients and their families must remain professional for the therapist to be effective.

Any evaluation of personality characteristics in a disabled child must take into account the unnatural lifestyle that is imposed by the need for therapy, medical appointments, and hospitalization. The child is expected to separate from parents earlier than the average child and usually confronts many more novel situations. There is little time or physical opportunity for free play. Continuous demands are placed on children to prove their intellectual potential in evaluations of various types. Adults most often monitor their social interaction while they assume a dependent role. Nonetheless, these children's social acceptance frequently rests on their skill in interacting with persons in their environments. It is not fair to the child to evaluate the evolution of personality without considering these experiential factors.

DOCUMENTATION

Data collection is an important task in the treatment of cerebral palsy. Change occurs at variable rates, but it is important to document the cause and effect of change whenever possible. Slides or videotapes are useful in recording functional comparisons over time. Digital video now allows a specific analysis of movement sequences. A motor drive unit or automatic advance on a 35-mm single-lens reflex camera can record a sample of movement five or more times per second. Placing the subject against a spaced grid in a specific alignment to perform a movement task allows for measurement of efficiency of movement. These ideas may be applied to documentation of treatment effectiveness or analyzed for an understanding of similar movement problems in other clients.

Methods of intervention or treatment are measurable for research and applicable to the functional problems presented by a diagnosis of cerebral palsy. Once a specific research question has been formulated, systematic recordings of appropriate data can be gathered over time to accumulate the number needed for a viable study. There is value in longitudinal reporting of a single case or a small group of individuals who have some characteristics in common because this aids our understanding of what we need to prevent in the young child to permit optimal function later. (See Chapters 8 and 10 regarding suggestions of impairment and disability measurements to be used as objective measures for functional outcome studies and record keeping.) Clinicians have a difficult time putting into words exactly what takes place during intervention, which further complicates research investigation into the efficacy of treatment. Descriptive analysis of treatment is essential to document and begin to understand what a therapist does during a therapy session. Understanding what takes place in therapy will help identify those questions that could be investigated more closely.

The way in which therapists learn to view a problem determines, to a large extent, the potential range of solutions available to them. Cerebral palsy is a complex of motor and movement inabilities that cluster about the inadequacy of central nervous system control, visual and soft tissue restrictions, and the amazing ability of the human body to compensate. Therapists need to look critically at developmental processes, qualities of movement, postural adjustments, timing and limitations of movements, and the range of dynamic functional movement. New areas of motor learning and systems and chaos theories offer the researcher novel approaches to the challenge of cerebral palsy and the resultant disorder of posture control and movement learning. Environmental factors may have as much influence as specific central nervous system limitations. Early intervention should be analytical and specific and based on a theoretical foundation. Posture and movement control begins to change with direct treatment. Analysis of the postural components and movement characteristics of children with cerebral palsy will lead to meaningful research more quickly than will professional reliance on the traditional definitions of the medical condition. Thorough documentation of therapy changes is critical to develop more effect intervention strategies in the future (see Chapter 10).

CASE STUDIES

To understand the problems of children with cerebral palsy, it is essential to follow some children over time to capture the evolution of family problems. Functional treatment must change according to the developmental level, chronological age, and neuromotor responses of the child. Intervention must be specific to the presenting problem of the moment while the missing aspects of complete motor development are considered. The case study comparison of two boys illustrates the typical lack of clinical correlation between history and manifest characteristics of cerebral palsy.

CASE STUDY ■ 12-1

A young woman was pregnant with her first child. She was middle class, well nourished, and had no identified risk factors. In the seventh month of pregnancy, her older sister died, causing considerable emotional upheaval. The much-anticipated infant was born, small for gestational age, at the correct date. It was theorized that there had been inadequate intrauterine nourishment during the first 6 to 7 months. The child, L. P., weighed 3.5 pounds (1587 g) and was fed initially by nasogastric tube. Her movements were quick and eye movement was very active for a newborn infant. She was seen for therapy at 17 days of age, immediately after hospital discharge.

The initial therapy focus was on the practical task of adequate nutritional intake so that the nasogastric tube could be removed before scarring occurred from repeated passage of the tube. Swaddling was suggested to calm the infant and assist her organization of body movement. Simple handling was oriented to moving the trunk over midline to let the head follow and assisting the infant to assume age-appropriate antigravity postures.

At 3 years of age L. P. continued to have difficulty with control of her head position in space and was unable to initiate postural changes with her head. The clinical picture was one of low tone with athetoid movement. She could not speak, communicated with looks and a few word approximations, and hitched along the floor in a seated position with one supporting hand.

By 5 years of age L. P. was still receiving therapy three times per week and could walk in a hesitating way with her hands held. At this stage she was evaluated by a behavioral optometrist and started vision therapy to prepare her to participate in preschool activities. As a secondary benefit her balance in walking improved markedly. L. P. began walking up and down 27 steps daily in her new home.

Now, at 7 years of age, L. P. can walk independently on level surfaces. She has physical therapy once a week and vision therapy once a week to maintain her control of posture and movement. Her school performance is adequate to keep her with her age peers and she attends a regular school.

CASE STUDY ■ 12-2

D. D. and E. D. were born within 6 months of each other at 6 months 1 week of gestation. Both were first-born infants for their respective mothers. D. D.'s mother was discovered to have a double uterus when she had a miscarriage early in the pregnancy. E. D. had malnutrition during his intrauterine development. D. D. started therapy just before he was 5 months old, and E. D. began therapy at almost 7 months old.

At 6 years of age D. D. walks alone with very mild athetotic "overflow." He wears corrective lenses that were fit at 2 years of age, and he returns for follow-up examinations with the behavioral optometrist once a year. Vision therapy was an important adjunct to physical handling because it introduced changes in spatial perception on the basis of specific sessions with prism lenses. At age 4 years D. D. was discovered to have a mild to moderate hearing loss; he still uses a hearing aid in one ear. He speaks English and Spanish, as do his parents, and he understands the French spoken to him by his grandparents. He functions in a regular school with his age peers and is a well-adapted, active child.

At 6 years of age E. D. is a moderately severe diplegic, with some immaturity of hand use and trunk control. He speaks English and Spanish well, although he demonstrates some emotional instability and difficulty in dealing with his disability. He is creative in storytelling and offers to tell original stories for other children in therapy. He is just beginning to walk with a walker within interior environments and with low resistance.

REFERENCES

1. Little WJ: On the influence of abnormal parturition, difficult labours, premature birth and asphyzia neonatorum on the mental and physical condition of the child, especially in relation to deformities, *Clin Orthop Relat Res* 46:7-22, 1966.
2. Accardo PJ: William John Little and cerebral palsy in the nineteenth century, *J Hist Med Allied Sci* 44:56-71, 1989.
3. MacKeith R: The Little Club memorandum on terminology and classification of cerebral palsy, *Cereb Palsy Bull* 1:34-37, 1959.
4. Prechtl HF: General movement assessment as a method of developmental neurology: New paradigms and their consequences, The 1999 Ronnie MacKeith lecture, *Dev Med Child Neurol* 43:836-842, 2001.
5. Kottke FJ, Knapp ME: The development of physiatry before 1950, *Arch Phys Med Rehabil* 69:4-14, 1988.
6. Crosland JH: Winthrop M. Phelps, *Cereb Palsy Bull* 3:205-206, 1961.
7. Knott M, Voss D: *Proprioceptive neuromuscular facilitation, patterns and techniques,* New York, 1968, Harper & Row.
8. Rood MS: Neurophysiological reactions as a basis for physical therapy, *Phys Ther Rev* 34:444-449, 1954.
9. Bobath K: *A neurophysiological basis for the treatment of cerebral palsy,* London, 1980, William Heinemann.
10. Miller G, Clark G: *The cerebral palsies: causes, consequences, and management,* Boston, 1998, Butterworth-Heinemann.
11. Kandel ER, Schwartz JH, Jessell TM: *Principles of neural science,* New York, 2000, McGraw-Hill, Health Professions Division.
12. Sussman M: *The diplegic child: evaluation and management,* Rosemont, IL, 1992, American Academy of Orthopaedic Surgeons.
13. Bryce J: The management of spasticity in children, *Physiotherapy* 62:353-357, 1976.
14. Brazelton T: *Infants and mothers: Differences in development,* New York, 1969, Dell.
15. Nordmark E, Hagglund G, Jarnlo GB: Reliability of the gross motor function measure in cerebral palsy, *Scand J Rehabil Med* 29:25-28, 1997.
16. Russell D, Rosenbaum P, Avery L et al: *Gross Motor Function Measure (GMFM-66 & GMFM-88) user's manual,* London, 2002, Mac Keith Press.
17. Berg M, Jahnsen R, Froslie KF et al: Reliability of the Pediatric Evaluation of Disability Inventory (PEDI), *Phys Occup Ther Pediatr* 24:61-77, 2004.
18. Ottenbacher KJ, Msall ME, Lyon NR et al: Interrater agreement and stability of the Functional Independence Measure for Children (WeeFIM): use in children with developmental disabilities, *Arch Phys Med Rehabil* 78:1309-1315, 1997.
19. Ottenbacher KJ, Msall ME, Lyon N et al: The WeeFIM instrument: its utility in detecting change in children with developmental disabilities, *Arch Phys Med Rehabil* 81:1317-1326, 2000.
20. Msall ME, DiGaudio K, Rogers BT et al: The Functional Independence Measure for Children (WeeFIM): Conceptual basis and pilot use in children with developmental disabilities, *Clin Pediatr (Phila)* 33:421-430, 1994.
21. Ketelaar M, Vermeer A, Helders PJ: Functional motor abilities of children with cerebral palsy: a systematic literature review of assessment measures, *Clin Rehabil* 12:369-380, 1998.
22. Montgomery P, Connolly B: Motor control and physical therapy: *Theoretical framework, practical application,* Hixson, TN, 1991, Chattanooga Group.
23. de Benabib RM, Nelson C: Efficiency in visual skills and postural control: a dynamic interaction, *J Occup Ther Pract* 3:57-68, 1991.
24. Bobath B: The very early treatment of cerebral palsy, *Dev Med Child Neurol* 9:373-390, 1967.
25. Kong E: Very early treatment of cerebral palsy, *Dev Med Child Neurol* 8:198-202, 1966.
26. Benabib R: *Goal-oriented curriculum to establish functional vision skills in the clinic and classroom,* Albuquerque, NM, 1997, Clinician's View.
27. Padula WV, Argyris S, Ray J: Visual evoked potentials (VEP) evaluating treatment for post-trauma vision syndrome (PTVS) in patients with traumatic brain injuries (TBI), *Brain Inj* 8:125-133, 1994.
28. Horak F: Assumptions underlying motor control for neurologic rehabilitation: contemporary management of motor control problems. In Lister MJ, editor: Proceedings of the II STEP Conference, Fredericksburg, VA, 1991, Bookcrafters.
29. Williams R: *Biochemical individuality: the basis for the genetotrophic concept,* New Canaan, CT, 1998, Keats Publishing.
30. Crook W, Stevens L: *Solving the puzzle of your hard-to-raise child,* New York, 1987, Random House.
31. Smith L: *Feed your body right: Understanding your individual body chemistry for proper nutrition without guesswork,* New York, 1994, M Evans.
32. Pfeiffer C: *Dr. Carl C. Pfeiffer's updated fact/book on zinc and other micro-nutrients,* New Canaan, CT, 1978, Keats Publishing.
33. Cott A: *Help for your learning disabled child: the orthomolecular treatment,* New York, 1985, Times Books.
34. Diamond M, Hopson J: *Magic trees of the mind,* New York, 1998, Dutton.

35. Bell KK, Davies PS: Body composition of ambulatory children with mild cerebral palsy, *Asia Pac J Clin Nutr* 12:S57, 2003.

36. Mandell M, Scanlon L: *Dr. Mandell's 5-day allergy relief system,* New York, 1988, Harpercollins.

37. Duncan B, Barton LL, Lloyd J et al: Dietary considerations in osteopenia in tube-fed nonambulatory children with cerebral palsy, *Clin Pediatr (Phila)* 38:133-137, 1999.

38. Sonis A, Castle J, Duggan C: Infant nutrition: implication for somatic growth, adult onset diseases, and oral health, *Curr Opin Pediatr* 9:289-297, 1997.

39. Hogan SE: Energy requirements of children with cerebral palsy, *Can J Diet Pract Res* 65:124-130, 2004.

40. Shintani T, Asakura K, Ishi K et al: [Obstructive sleep apnea in children with cerebral palsy], *Nippon Jibiinkoka Gakkai Kaiho* 101:266-271, 1998.

41. Fukumizu M, Kohyama J: Central respiratory pauses, sighs, and gross body movements during sleep in children, *Physiol Behav* 82:721-726, 2004.

42. Tecklin J: *Pediatric physical therapy,* Philadelphia, 1999, Lippincott Williams & Wilkins.

43. Gilfoyle E, Moore J, Grady A: *Children adapt,* Thorofare, NJ, 1990, Slack.

44. Palmer FB, Shapiro BK, Capute AJ: Physical therapy for infants with spastic diplegia, *Dev Med Child Neurol* 31:128-129, 1989.

45. Parkes J, Hill N, Dolk H et al: What influences physiotherapy use by children with cerebral palsy? *Child Care Health Dev* 30:151-160, 2004.

46. Bobath B: *Abnormal postural reflex activity caused by brain lesions,* London, 1983, William Heinemann.

47. Appell HJ: Muscular atrophy following immobilisation: a review, *Sports Med* 10:42-58, 1990.

48. Stevens JE, Walter GA, Okereke E et al: Muscle adaptations with immobilization and rehabilitation after ankle fracture, *Med Sci Sports Exerc* 36:1695-1701, 2004.

49. Hendricks T: The effects of immobilization on connective tissue, *J Man Manip Ther* 3:98-103, 1995.

50. Myers T: *Anatomy trains: myofascial meridians for manual and movement therapists,* New York, 2001, Churchill Livingstone.

51. Schimidt R, Lee TD: *Motor control and learning: a behavioral emphasis,* Champaign, IL, 2005, Human Kinetics.

52. Shumway-Cook A, Woollacott MH, editors: *Motor control: theory and practical applications,* Philadelphia, 2001, Lippincott Williams & Wilkins.

53. Cech D, Martin S, editors: *Functional movement development across the life span,* Philadelphia, 2002, WB Saunders.

54. Bach-y-Rita P: *Recovery of function: theoretical considerations for brain injury rehabilitation,* Berne, Switzerland, 1980, Hans Huber.

55. Restak R: *The new brain: how the modern age is rewiring your mind,* New York, 2003, Rodale Press.

56. Hallett M: The plastic brain, *Ann Neurol* 38:4-5, 1995.

57. Karni A, Meyer G, Jezzard P et al: Functional MRI evidence for adult motor cortex plasticity during motor skill learning, *Nature* 377:155-158, 1995.

58. Kleim JA, Barbay S, Nudo RJ: Functional reorganization of the rat motor cortex following motor skill learning, *J Neurophysiol* 80:3321-3325, 1998.

59. Hallett M: Functional reorganization after lesions of the human brain: Studies with transcranial magnetic stimulation, *Rev Neurol (Paris)* 157:822-826, 2001.

60. Leach P: *Babyhood,* New York, 1983, Knopf.

61. Quinton M: *Concepts and guidelines for baby treatment,* Albuquerque, NM, 2002, Clinicians View.

62. Weissenbock M: [Baby massage—a chance for a careful encounter between parents and child], *Osterr Krankenpflegez* 47:20-21, 1994.

63. McClure V: Infant massage, *MCN Am J Matern Child Nurs* 25:276, 2000.

64. Bly L: *Motor skills acquisition in the first year: an illustrated guide to normal development,* San Antonio, TX, 1994, Therapy Skill Builders.

65. Bobath B: *Motor develpment in the different types of cerebral palsy,* New York, 1975, William Heinemann Medical Books.

66. Taub E, Ellman SJ, Berman AJ: Deafferentation in monkeys: effect on conditioned grasp response, *Science* 151:593-594, 1966.

67. Taub E, Perrella P, Barro G: Behavioral development after forelimb deafferentation on day of birth in monkeys with and without blinding, *Science* 181:959-960, 1973.

68. Taub E, Crago J, Uswatte G: Constraint-induced movement therapy: a new approach to treatment in physical rehabilitation, *Rehabil Psychol* 43:152-170, 1998.

69. Wolf SL, Blanton S, Baer H et al: Repetitive task practice: a critical review of constraint-induced movement therapy in stroke, *Neurologia* 8:325-338, 2002.

70. Taub E, Morris DM: Constraint-induced movement therapy to enhance recovery after stroke, *Curr Atheroscler Rep* 3:279-286, 2001.

71. Yasukawa A: Upper extremity casting: adjunct treatment for a child with cerebral palsy hemiplegia, *Am J Occup Ther* 44:840-846, 1990.

72. Crocker MD, MacKay-Lyons M, McDonnell E: Forced use of the upper extremity in cerebral palsy: a single-case design, *Am J Occup Ther* 51:824-833, 1997.

73. Charles J, Lavinder G, Gordon A: Effects of constraint-induced therapy on hand function in children with hemplegia cerebral palsy, *J Pediatr Phys Ther* 13:68-76, 2001.

74. Karman N, Maryles J, Baker RW et al: Constraint-induced movement therapy for hemiplegic children with acquired brain injuries, *J Head Trauma Rehabil* 18:259-267, 2003.

75. Pierce SR, Daly K, Gallagher KG et al: Constraint-induced therapy for a child with hemiplegic cerebral palsy: a case report, *Arch Phys Med Rehabil* 83:1462-1463, 2002.

76. Taub E, Ramey SL, DeLuca S et al: Efficacy of constraint-induced movement therapy for children with cerebral palsy with asymmetric motor impairment, *Pediatrics* 113:305-312, 2004.

77. Keefer DJ, Tseh W, Caputo JL et al: Within- and between-day stability of treadmill walking VO2 in children with hemiplegic cerebral palsy, stability of walking VO2 in children with CP, *Gait Posture* 21:80-84, 2005.

78. Maltais DB, Pierrynowski MR, Galea VA et al: Minute-by-minute differences in co-activation during treadmill walking in cerebral palsy, *Electromyogr Clin Neurophysiol* 44:477-487, 2004.

79. Maltais D, Wilk B, Unnithan V et al: Responses of children with cerebral palsy to treadmill walking exercise in the heat, *Med Sci Sports Exerc* 36:1674-1681, 2004.

80. Bodkin AW, Baxter RS, Heriza CB: Treadmill training for an infant born preterm with a grade III intraventricular hemorrhage, *Phys Ther* 83:1107-1118, 2003.

81. Schindl MR, Forstner C, Kern H et al: Treadmill training with partial body weight support in nonambulatory patients with cerebral palsy, *Arch Phys Med Rehabil* 81:301-306, 2000.

82. Smith JL, Edgerton VR, Eldred E et al: The chronic spinalized cat: a model for neuromuscular plasticity, *Birth Defects Orig Artic Ser* 19:357-373, 1983.

83. Lovely RG, Gregor RJ, Roy RR et al: Effects of training on the recovery of full-weight-bearing stepping in the adult spinal cat, *Exp Neurol* 92:421-435, 1986.

84. Roy RR, Hutchison DL, Pierotti DJ et al: EMG patterns of rat ankle extensors and flexors during treadmill locomotion and swimming, *J Appl Physiol* 70:2522-2529, 1991.

85. Hodgson JA, Roy RR, de Leon R et al: Can the mammalian lumbar spinal cord learn a motor task? *Med Sci Sports Exerc* 26:1491-1497, 1994.

86. Hesse S: Locomotor therapy in neurorehabilitation, *Neurorehabilitation* 16:133-139, 2001.

87. Blundell SW, Shepherd RB, Dean CM et al: Functional strength training in cerebral palsy: a pilot study of a group circuit training class for children aged 4-8 years, *Clin Rehabil* 17:48-57, 2003.

88. Dodd KJ, Taylor NF, Graham HK: A randomized clinical trial of strength training in young people with cerebral palsy, *Dev Med Child Neurol* 45:652-657, 2003.

89. McBurney H, Taylor NF, Dodd KJ et al: A qualitative analysis of the benefits of strength training for young people with cerebral palsy, *Dev Med Child Neurol* 45:658-663, 2003.

90. Toner LV, Cook K, Elder GC: Improved ankle function in children with cerebral palsy after computer-assisted motor learning, *Dev Med Child Neurol* 40:829-835, 1998.

91. Garbe G: [Critical observation of selected exercises of power training in relation to prevention of postural damage and physical handicaps], *Rehabilitation (Stuttg)* 28:123-128, 1989.

92. Sharp SA, Brouwer BJ: Isokinetic strength training of the hemiparetic knee: effects on function and spasticity, *Arch Phys Med Rehabil* 78:1231-1236, 1997.

93. Teixeira-Salmela LF, Olney SJ, Nadeau S et al: Muscle strengthening and physical conditioning to reduce impairment and disability in chronic stroke survivors, *Arch Phys Med Rehabil* 80:1211-1218, 1999.

94. Rochester L, Vujnovich A, Newstead D et al: The influence of eccentric contractions and stretch on alpha motoneuron excitability in normal subjects and subjects with spasticity, *Electromyogr Clin Neurophysiol* 41:171-177, 2001.

95. Carmick J: Clinical use of neuromuscular electrical stimulation for children with cerebral palsy, 2: upper extremity, *Phys Ther* 73:514-522, 1993.

96. Carmick J: Managing equinus in children with cerebral palsy: electrical stimulation to strengthen the triceps surae muscle, *Dev Med Child Neurol* 37:965-975, 1995.

97. Carmick J: Use of neuromuscular electrical stimulation and [corrected] dorsal wrist splint to improve the hand function of a child with spastic hemiparesis, *Phys Ther* 77:661-671, 1997.

98. Maenpaa H, Jaakkola R, Sandstrom M et al: Electrostimulation at sensory level improves function of the upper extremities in children with cerebral palsy: a pilot study, *Dev Med Child Neurol* 46:84-90, 2004.

99. Park ES, Park CI, Lee HJ et al: The effect of electrical stimulation on the trunk control in young children with spastic diplegic cerebral palsy, *J Korean Med Sci* 16:347-350, 2001.

100. Wissel J, Heinen F, Schenkel A et al: Botulinum toxin A in the management of spastic gait disorders in children and young adults with cerebral palsy: a randomized, double-blind study of "high-dose" versus "low-dose" treatment, *Neuropediatrics* 30:120-124, 1999.

101. Kalinina LV, Sologubov EG, Luzinovich VM et al: [Botox in combined treatment of cerebral palsy in children], *Zh Nevrol Psikhiatr Im S S Korsakova* 100:60-63, 2000.

102. Wong V: Evidence-based approach of the use of Botulinum toxin type A (BTX) in cerebral palsy, *Pediatr Rehabil* 6:85-96, 2003.

103. Boyd RN, Hays RM: Current evidence for the use of botulinum toxin type A in the management of children with cerebral palsy: a systematic review, *Eur J Neurol* 8(5 Suppl):1-20, 2001.

104. Garcia Ruiz PJ, Pascual Pascual I, Sanchez Bernardos V: Progressive response to botulinum A toxin in cerebral palsy, *Eur J Neurol* 7:191-193, 2000.

105. Galli M, Crivellini M, Santambrogio GC et al: Short-term effects of "botulinum toxin a" as treatment for children with cerebral palsy: kinematic and kinetic aspects at the ankle joint, *Funct Neurol* 16:317-323, 2001.

106. Wasiak J, Hoare B, Wallen M: Botulinum toxin A as an adjunct to treatment in the management of the upper limb in children with spastic cerebral palsy, *Cochrane Database Syst Rev* CD003469, 2004.

107. Pascual-Pascual SI: [Use of botulinum toxin in the preventive and palliative treatment of the hips in children with infantile cerebral palsy], *Rev Neurol* 37:80-82, 2003.

108. Vandenborne K, Elliott MA, Walter GA et al: Longitudinal study of skeletal muscle adaptations during immobilization and rehabilitation, *Muscle Nerve* 21:1006-1012, 1998.

109. Shaffer MA, Okereke E, Esterhai JL Jr et al: Effects of immobilization on plantar-flexion torque, fatigue resistance, and functional ability following an ankle fracture, *Phys Ther* 80:769-780, 2000.

110. Booth CM, Cortina-Borja MJ, Theologis TN: Collagen accumulation in muscles of children with cerebral palsy and correlation with severity of spasticity, *Dev Med Child Neurol* 43:314-320, 2001.

111. Duckman RH: Vision therapy for the child with cerebral palsy, *J Am Optom Assoc* 58:28-35, 1987.

112. Gauthier GM, Hofferer JM: Visual motor rehabilitation in children with cerebral palsy, *Int Rehabil Med* 5:118-127, 1983.

113. Katz RT: Management of spasticity, *Am J Phys Med Rehabil* 67:108-116, 1988.

114. Albright AL, Barry MJ, Painter MJ et al: Infusion of intrathecal baclofen for generalized dystonia in cerebral palsy, *J Neurosurg* 88:73-76, 1998.

115. Meythaler JM, Guin-Renfroe S, Law C et al: Continuously infused intrathecal baclofen over 12 months for spastic hypertonia in adolescents and adults with cerebral palsy, *Arch Phys Med Rehabil* 82:155-161, 2001.

116. Murphy NA, Irwin MC, Hoff C: Intrathecal baclofen therapy in children with cerebral palsy: efficacy and complications, *Arch Phys Med Rehabil* 83:1721-1725, 2002.

117. Schulman JH, Davis R, Nanes M: Cerebellar stimulation for spastic cerebral palsy: preliminary report; on-going double blind study, *Pacing Clin Electrophysiol* 10:226-231, 1987.

118. Davis R, Schulman J, Nanes M, Delehanty A: Cerebellar stimulation for spastic cerebral palsy—double-blind quantitative study, *Appl Neurophysiol* 50:451-452, 1987.

119. Davis R, Schulman J, Delehanty A: Cerebellar stimulation for cerebral palsy—double blind study, *Acta Neurochir Suppl (Wien)* 39:126-128, 1987.

120. Davis R: Cerebellar stimulation for cerebral palsy spasticity, function, and seizures, *Arch Med Res* 31:290-299, 2000.

121. Hugenholtz H, Humphreys P, McIntyre WM et al: Cervical spinal cord stimulation for spasticity in cerebral palsy, *Neurosurgery* 22:707-714, 1988.

122. Mittal S, Farmer JP, Al-Atassi B et al: Long-term functional outcome after selective posterior rhizotomy, *J Neurosurg* 97:315-325, 2002.

123. Lazareff JA, Garcia MA: Selective dorsal rhizotomy, *J Neurosurg* 76:1047-1048, 1992.

124. Peacock W, Arens L: Selective posterior rhizotomy for the relief of spasticity in cerebral palsy, *S Afr Med J* 62:119-125, 1982.

125. Cahan LD, Kundi MS, McPherson D et al: Electrophysiologic studies in selective dorsal rhizotomy for spasticity in children with cerebral palsy, *Appl Neurophysiol* 50:459-462, 1987.

126. Lazareff JA, Garcia-Mendez MA, De Rosa R et al: Limited (L4-S1, L5-S1) selective dorsal rhizotomy for reducing spasticity in cerebral palsy, *Acta Neurochir (Wien)* 141:743-751, 1999.

127. Fasano V: Long-term results of posterior functional rhizotomy, *Acta Neurochir* 30(Suppl):435-439, 1980.

128. McLaughlin J, Bjornson K, Temkin N et al: Selective dorsal rhizotomy: meta-analysis of three randomized controlled trials, *Dev Med Child Neurol* 44:17-25, 2002.

129. Koman LA, Paterson Smith B, Balkrishnan R: Spasticity associated with cerebral palsy in children: guidelines for the use of botulinum A toxin, *Paediatr Drugs* 5:11-23, 2003.

130. Gooch JL, Patton CP: Combining botulinum toxin and phenol to manage spasticity in children, *Arch Phys Med Rehabil* 85:1121-1124, 2004.

131. Wallen MA, O'Flaherty S J, Waugh MC: Functional outcomes of intramuscular botulinum toxin type A in the upper limbs of children with cerebral palsy: a phase II trial, *Arch Phys Med Rehabil* 85:192-200, 2004.

132. Gracies JM, Elovic E, McGuire J et al: Traditional pharmacological treatments for spasticity, I: local treatments, *Muscle Nerve Suppl* 6:S61-91, 1997.

133. Karepov VG: [Selective pharmacological correction of muscle tonus during rehabilitation of stroke patients], *Vrach Delo* 6:56-57, 1984.

134. Morrison JE Jr, Hertzberg DL, Gourley SM et al: Motor point blocks in children: a technique to relieve spasticity using phenol injections, *AORN J* 49:1346-1347, 1349-1351, 1354, 1989.

135. Morrison JE Jr, Matthews D, Washington R et al: Phenol motor point blocks in children: plasma concentrations and cardiac dysrhythmias, *Anesthesiology* 75:359-362, 1991.

136. Bleck EE: *Orthopedic management in cerebral palsy,* Philadelphia, 1987, JB Lippincott.

137. Sprague JB: Surgical management of cerebral palsy, *Orthop Nurs* 11:11-19, 1992.

138. Watt J: A prospective study of inhibitive casting as an adjunct to physiotherapy for cerebral-palsied children, *Dev Med Child Neurol* 28:480-488, 1986.

139. Brouwer B, Wheeldon RK, Stradiotto-Parker N et al: Reflex excitability and isometric force production in cerebral palsy: the effect of serial casting, *Dev Med Child Neurol* 40:168-175, 1998.

140. Brouwer B, Davidson LK, Olney SJ: Serial casting in idiopathic toe-walkers and children with spastic cerebral palsy, *J Pediatr Orthop* 20:221-225, 2000.

141. Collet JP, Vanasse M, Marois P, Amar M et al: Hyperbaric oxygen for children with cerebral palsy: a randomised multicentre trial: HBO-CP Research Group, *Lancet* 357:582-586, 2001.

142. Papazian O, Alfonso I: [Hyperbaric oxygen treatment for children with cerebral palsy], *Rev Neurol* 37:359-364, 2003.

143. Rosenbaum P: Controversial treatment of spasticity: exploring alternative therapies for motor function in children with cerebral palsy, *J Child Neurol* 18(1 Suppl):S89-S94, 2003.

144. Undersea and Hyperbaric Medicine Society: Position statement, 2003, www.uhms.org.

145. Sologubov EG, Iavorskii AB, Kobrin VI et al: [Role of vestibular and visual analyzers in changes of postural activity of patients with childhood cerebral palsy in the process of treatment with space technology], *Aviakosm Ekolog Med* 29:30-34, 1995.

146. Semenova KA: Basis for a method of dynamic proprioceptive correction in the restorative treatment of patients with residual-stage infantile cerebral palsy, *Neurosci Behav Physiol* 27:639-643, 1997.

147. Semenova KA, Antonova LV: [The influence of the LK-92 "Adeli" treatment loading suit on electro-neuro-myographic characteristics in patients with infantile cerebral paralysis], *Zh Nevrol Psikhiatr Im S S Korsakova* 98:22-25, 1998.

148. Shvarkov SB, Davydov OS, Kuuz RA et al: New approaches to the rehabilitation of patients with neurological movement defects, *Neurosci Behav Physiol* 27:644-647, 1997.

149. Blair E, Ballantyne J, Horsman S et al: A study of a dynamic proximal stability splint in the management of children with cerebral palsy, *Dev Med Child Neurol* 37:544-554, 1995.

150. Chauvel PJ, Horsman S, Ballantyne J et al: Lycra splinting and the management of cerebral palsy, *Dev Med Child Neurol* 35:456-457, 1993.

151. Pape KE, Kirsch SE, Galil A et al: Neuromuscular approach to the motor deficits of cerebral palsy: a pilot study, *J Pediatr Orthop* 13:628-633, 1993.

152. Steinbok P, Reiner A, Kestle JR: Therapeutic electrical stimulation following selective posterior rhizotomy in children with spastic diplegic cerebral palsy: a randomized clinical trial, *Dev Med Child Neurol* 39:515-520, 1997.

153. Dali C, Hansen FJ, Pedersen SA et al: Threshold electrical stimulation (TES) in ambulant children with CP: A randomized double-blind placebo-controlled clinical trial, *Dev Med Child Neurol* 44:364-369, 2002.

154. Sommerfelt K, Markestad T, Berg K et al: Therapeutic electrical stimulation in cerebral palsy: A randomized, controlled, crossover trial, *Dev Med Child Neurol* 43:609-613, 2001.

155. Robinson RO, McCarthy GT, Little TM: Conductive education at the Peto Institute, Budapest, *BMJ* 299:1145-1149, 1989.

156. Sutton A: Conductive education, *Arch Dis Child* 63:214-217, 1988.

157. Bairstow P, Cochrane R, Rusk I: Selection of children with cerebral palsy for conductive education and the characteristics of children judged suitable and unsuitable, *Dev Med Child Neurol* 33:984-992, 1991.

158. Catanese AA, Coleman GJ, King JA et al: Evaluation of an early childhood programme based on principles of conductive education: the Yooralla project, *J Paediatr Child Health* 31:418-422, 1995.

159. Coleman GJ, King JA, Reddihough DS: A pilot evaluation of conductive education-based intervention for children with cerebral palsy: the Tongala project, *J Paediatr Child Health* 31:412-417, 1995.

160. Reddihough DS, King J, Coleman G et al: Efficacy of programmes based on Conductive Education for young children with cerebral palsy, *Dev Med Child Neurol* 40:763-770, 1998.

161. Schmidt RA, Lee TD, editors: *Motor control and learning: A behavioral emphasis,* Champaign, IL, 1999, Human Kinetics.

162. Feldenkrais M: *Awareness through movement,* San Francisco, 1972, Harper.

163. Rywerant Y, Feldenkrais M: *The Feldenkrais method,* North Bergen, NJ, 1983, Basic Health Publications.

164. Rolf I, Lodge J: Rolfing: *The integration of human structures,* New York, 1978, HarperCollins.

165. Rolf I, Thompson R: Rolfing: *Reestablishing the natural alignment and structural integration of the human body for vitality and well-being,* Rochester, VT, 1989, Healing Art Press.

166. Sutherland WG: The cranial bowl, 1944, *J Am Osteopath Assoc* 100:568-573, 2000.

167. Deoora T: *Healing through cranial osteopathy,* London, 2004, Frances Lincoln.

168. Carreiro J: *An osteopathic approach to children,* New York, 2003, Churchill Livingstone.

169. Finnie N, Bavin J, Bax M et al: *Handling the young cerebral-palsied child at home,* New York, 1997, Butterworth-Heinemann.

170. Geralis E: *Children with cerebral palsy: a parent's guide,* Bethesda, MD, 1998, Woodbine House.

171. Langley M, Lombardino L: *Neurodevelopmental strategies for managing communication disorders in children with severe motor dysfunction,* Austin, TX, 1991, Pro-Ed.

CHAPTER 13

Genetic Disorders: A Pediatric Perspective

Sandra G. Bellamy, PT, DPT, PCS
Eunice Yu Chiu Shen, PT, DPT, MS, PCS

KEY WORDS

evaluation
functional skills
genetic disorders
natural environments
occupational therapist
physical therapist

OBJECTIVES

After reading this chapter the student/therapist will be able to:

1. Describe the main types of genetic disorders and give examples of each type.
2. Describe the diagnostic approach for genetic disorders.
3. Describe three modes of inheritance for single-gene disorders.
4. Explain why it is important to include family members in the planning and development of therapy programs for children with genetic disorders.
5. Describe and give examples of three types of assessment tools and state the intended purpose of each.
6. Describe the importance of developing therapy programs for children that are outcome focused on functional skills in natural environments.
7. Identify three medical treatments that may be used for children with genetic disorders to ameliorate the effects of the disorder.
8. Explain why it is important for physical and occupational therapists to have knowledge of the services available through genetic counseling.
9. Describe strategies for accessing information and increasing knowledge about genetic disorders for use in clinical decision making.

Genetic disorders in children can result in wide variety of movement impairments and disabilities. The resultant impact of a genetic condition on the child may be evident before or immediately after birth, whereas other disorders are not diagnosed until later in life when problems are manifested. In this chapter we discuss disorders of known genetic origin that physical and occupational therapists are most likely to encounter in therapy programs for children.

An overview of the diagnostic process and the general categories and subtypes of genetic disorders are presented first. Specific examples of each type are given along with a brief description. A summary of typical clinical signs observed in genetic disorders is presented in the second section. The third section focuses on the physical or occupational therapist's role in the clinical management of children with genetic disorders. Evaluation procedures, treatment goals and objectives, and general treatment principles and strategies are discussed from a family-centered perspective. The final section includes a discussion of the medical management of genetic disorders and genetic counseling and the ethical implications of genetic screening and testing. Last, we discuss the need for therapists to develop competence in clinical practice when working with patients and families affected by a genetic disorder. A list of educational resources for clinicians and families is given.

AN OVERVIEW: CLINICAL DIAGNOSIS AND TYPES OF GENETIC DISORDERS WITH REPRESENTATIVE CLINICAL EXAMPLES

The Human Genome Project completed in 2003 expanded the knowledge about the genetic basis for disease and congenital malformations.[1] The impact of this project is not yet realized because new diagnostic techniques and treatment options for genetic disorders will surely follow. Pediatric health care professionals will be faced with questions from families who, in seeking diagnostic and prognostic information, will access this new information through the lay scientific press and the World Wide Web.[2]

An accurate diagnosis for a specific genetic disorder (syndrome or disease) is necessary to provide a prognosis, to determine eligibility for therapy and education services, and to provide the basis of genetic counseling for the child's family.[3] The diagnostic process for genetic disorders includes a combination of clinical assessment by the physician who collects the child's medical history and a clinical geneticist who may construct a family history or "pedigree" to recognize disorders with familiar inheritance patterns. Molecular studies can confirm a clinical diagnosis and identify the genetic cause of the disorder.[3] Some genetic disorders are not easily identified, and laboratory testing can be extensive, prolonged, and often inconclusive; therefore pediatricians may refer children to occupational and physical therapy before the nature of their condition is fully known.[4] Although sometimes far removed from the hospitals and specialized centers that perform genetic testing and diagnosis, the pediatric therapist is often able to contribute clinical evidence that will assist the diagnostic process.[5]

Genetic disorders are typically divided into four categories: chromosomal, single gene, multifactorial, and mitochondrial. Chromosomal disorders arise when there is an alteration in either the number or structure of chromosomes that exist in either autosomal or sex (X,Y) chromosomes.[6] Numerical or large structural chromosomal abnormalities can be seen through a microscope; therefore, a sample of the patient's peripheral blood can be used in detection of disorders such as Down syndrome. When there is a suspicion of a clinical spectrum associated with some of the known chromosomal microdeletions, translocations, or inversions, direct DNA analysis techniques such as fluorescence in situ hybridization (FISH) with use of specific sequence DNA probes, can confirm a specific suspected diagnosis. Indirect DNA analysis techniques such as linkage analysis can be performed to confirm single-gene disorders where the gene or genomic region associated with the disorder is unknown.[7]

Of our 20,000 to 25,000 protein-coding genes,[1] a single gene may be responsible for approximately 6000 known genetic traits. Approximately 4000 of these known traits are diseases or disorders.[8] Single-gene disorders may be transmitted through three different patterns: autosomal dominant, autosomal recessive, and sex linked. *Dominant* refers to the case where a mutated gene from one parent is sufficient to produce the disorder in offspring. *Recessive* refers to the case where the disorder will not be expressed unless offspring inherited a mutated copy of that gene from both parents. It is incorrect to say that a *gene* is recessive or dominant, rather the *trait,* or disorder, is dominant or recessive.[9]

Inheritance is usually a term reserved for the transmission of a previously recognized family *trait* to subsequent offspring. However, many genetic disorders are due to new, spontaneous mutations in a *gamete,* the single egg cell from the mother or a sperm cell from the father. The remainder of the gametes from either parent are most likely normal. In this case, their offspring will be the first in the family to display the *sporadic* disorder and now the faulty gene can be passed onto subsequent generations. A disorder that results from a single copy of a mutated gene is referred to as a dominant disorder, even if it is acquired by a spontaneous mutation. Not all literature sources will include spontaneous mutations in the description of *inherited* disorders.

It is important to understand how a disorder was acquired because the relative risks to other offspring for the disorder vary according to mode of transmission. For example, the risk of having another child with the same genetic disorder that occurred as a result of a spontaneous mutation is low. However, when one parent is affected by an inherited dominant mutation, the risk of passing that faulty gene onto each child is 50%.[6]

Most congenital malformations and many serious diseases that have an onset in childhood or adulthood are not caused by single genes or chromosome defects; these are called multifactorial disorders.[3,6,9]

Mitochondrial disorders are caused by alterations in the cytoplasmic mitochondrial chromosomes passed from the mother to her unborn child. The clinical manifestation of mitochondrial DNA-related disorders extremely variable[10]

and the occurrence is reportedly rare (5.0/100,000)[6,11]; however, collectively as a group of neuromuscular disorders, they account for substantial use of health care resources.[11]

Table 13-1 shows clinical examples of specific disorders, organized into categories by the most common mechanism by which they occur.

Specific DNA testing may soon be able to identify nearly all human genetic disorders. This not only allows for accurate and more complete diagnosis but should pave the way for the development of mechanisms for treatment, cure, and prevention of certain genetic conditions.[3-7]

Chromosome Disorders

Cytogenics is the study of chromosomal abnormalities. A karyotype is prepared that displays the 46 chromosomes; 22 pairs of autosomes arranged according to length, and then the two sex chromosomes that determine male or female sex. Modern methods of staining karyotypes enable analysis of the various numerical and structural abnormalities that can

TABLE 13-1 ■ Partial Listing of Typical Genetic Syndromes or Diseases

SYNDROME OR DISEASE	APPROXIMATE INCIDENCE
CHROMOSOMAL ABNORMALITIES	
Autosomal Trisomy	
Trisomy 21 (Down syndrome)	1:700-1:10,000
Trisomy 18	1:6000
Trisomy 13	1:15,000-2:20,000
Sex Chromosome Abnormality	
Turner's syndrome	1:2500-10,000 females
Klinefelter's syndrome	1:1000 males
Partial Deletion	
Prader-Willi syndrome	1:10,000
Cri-du-chat syndrome	1:20,000
SINGLE-GENE ABNORMALITIES	
Autosomal Dominant	
Osteogenesis imperfecta	1:20,000-30,000
Tuberous sclerosis	1:10,000
Neurofibromatosis	1:3500
Autosomal Recessive	
Cystic fibrosis	1:2500-4000 whites
Hurler syndrome	1:100,000
Phenylketonuria	1:10,000-15,000
Werdig-Hoffmann disease	1:20,000
Sex-Linked	
Fragile X syndrome	1:1500 males, 1:2500 females
Hemophilia A	1:10,000 males
Duchenne muscular dystrophy	1:3500
MULTIFACTORIAL	
Cleft lip with/without cleft palate	1:500-1000
Clubfoot (talipes equinovarus)	1:1000
Spina bifida	1:200-1000
MITOCHONDRIAL	
Mitochondrial myopathy	Rare
Kearns-Sayre disease	Rare
OTHER	
Rett syndrome	1:15,000

occur. Most chromosomal abnormalities appear as numerical abnormalities (aneuploidy) such as one missing chromosome (monosomy) or an additional chromosome, as appears in trisomy 21 (Down syndrome).[6] Structural abnormalities occur in many forms. They include a missing or "extra portion" of a chromosome or a translocation error, which is an interchange of genetic material between nonhomologous chromosomes. The incidence of chromosomal abnormalities among spontaneously aborted fetuses may be as high as 60%.[6,12] About 1 in 150 live-born infants has a detectable chromosomal abnormality; and in about half of these cases the chromosomal abnormality is accompanied by congenital anomalies, mental retardation, or phenotypic changes that are manifested later in life.[6] Of the fetuses with abnormal chromosomes that survive to term, about half have sex chromosome abnormalities and the other half have autosomal trisomies.[13]

The following section provides a brief overview on common genetic disorders seen by physical and occupational therapists working with children.

Autosomal Trisomies

Trisomy is the condition of a single extra nuclear chromosome. Trisomies occur frequently among live births, usually as a result of the failure of the parental chromosomes to disjoin normally during meiosis. Trisomy can occur in autosomal or sex cells. Trisomies 21, 18, and 13 are the most frequently occurring trisomies.

Trisomy 21 (Down Syndrome). Trisomy 21 occurs in 1 in every 800 live births[14] and its incidence is distributed equally between the sexes.[8] Information compiled by the Centers for Disease Control and Prevention for years 1968 through 1997 indicates that the median survival age is 49 years, compared with 1 year in 1968. Improvements in the median survival age were less in races other than white, although the reasons for this are unclear.[14] The pathophysiological features of Down syndrome include the presence of an extra twenty-first chromosome, found in 95% of individuals with the diagnosis. The remaining 5% have the mosaic and translocation forms. The incidence of Down syndrome increases with advanced maternal, and possibly paternal, age.[15,16]

The impairments associated with Down syndrome are numerous. It is the most common chromosomal cause of moderate to severe mental retardation.[17,18] A list of 10 features characterizing newborn infants with Down syndrome was published by Hall in 1966.[19] These features included hypotonicity, a poor Moro reflex, joint hyperextensibility, excess skin on the back of the neck, a flat facial profile, slanted palpebral fissures, anomalous auricles, dysplasia of the pelvis, dysplasia of the midphalanx of the fifth finger, and simian creases. In his study of 48 neonates with Down syndrome, Hall[19] reported the frequency of these characteristics to vary from 45% to 90% (Figure 13-1).

In a longitudinal study of 79 infants with Down syndrome from birth to 10 months of age, Cowie[20] reported the universal finding of marked hypotonicity (which appeared to gradually diminish with age) and the persistence of several primitive reflexes, including the palmar and plantar grasp reflexes, the stepping reflex, and the Moro reflex. She also observed a delay in the development of normal postural

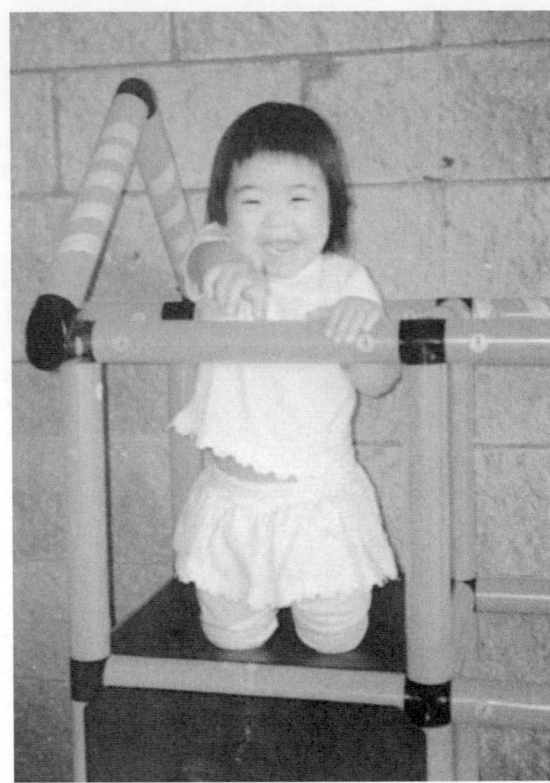

FIGURE 13-1 ■ Two-year-old girl with Down syndrome climbing up playground equipment.

tone, as indicated by the severe head lag evident during elicitation of the traction response and the lack of full antigravity extension noted when the Landau response was tested.

Craniofacial impairments, such as a shortened palate and midface hypoplasia, have been noted. These craniofacial differences, together with oral hypotonia, tongue thrusting, and poor lip closure, frequently result in feeding difficulties at birth.[21] The prevalence of obesity in adults with Down syndrome is estimated to be as high as 70% in male subjects and 95% in female subjects.[22] Children with Down syndrome also appear to have a higher risk for being overweight or obese,[23-25] which may be, in part, due to the retarded growth and endocrine and metabolic disorders associated with trisomy 21.[25] In a small population study of children with Down syndrome, Dyken et al[26] reported that there was a high prevalence of obstructive sleep apnea and that it was associated with a higher body mass index.[26]

Impairments of visual and sensory systems are also common in individuals with Down syndrome. As many as 77% of children with Down syndrome have a refractive error (myopia, hyperopia) or astigmatism. Convergent strabismus and nystagmus are also reported.[27] Hearing losses that interfere with language development are reportedly present in 80% of children with Down syndrome. In most cases the hearing loss is conductive; in up to 20% of cases the loss is sensorineural or mixed.[21] Additional impairments observed in individuals with Down syndrome include congenital heart disease (occurring in 40% of children) and musculoskeletal anomalies such as metatarsus primus varus, pes planus, thoracolumbar scoliosis, patellar instability, and an increased risk for atlantoaxial dislocation.[15]

It is particularly important for persons working with infants and children with Down syndrome to be aware of this propensity for atlantoaxial dislocation, which has been observed through radiography in up to 10% to 30% of individuals with this syndrome.[28,29] There is some controversy in the medical community as to the necessity and efficacy of radiographic screening for the instability.[29,30] Proponents of radiographic screening argue that neurological symptoms of atlantoaxial instability may often go undetected in this population because symptoms are often masked by the wide-based gait and motor dysfunction already associated with the disorder. If the child is unable to verbalize complaints, or the child is uncooperative with physical and neurological examinations, symptoms may be missed. There is particular concern about cervical instability if these children undergo surgical procedures requiring general anesthesia[30] and in participation in recreational sports such as the Special Olympics.[29] Symptomatic instability can result in spinal cord compression leading to myelopathy with leg weakness, decreased walking ability,[31] and increased spasticity or incontinence.[21] Although reportedly rare, there have been cases where atlantoaxial dislocation has resulted in quadriplegia.[28]

Several researchers have explored the neuropathology associated with Down syndrome. The relatively small size of the cerebellum and brain stem has been reported.[17,32] Marin-Padilla[33] studied the neuronal organization of the motor cortex of a 19-month-old child with Down syndrome and found various structural abnormalities in the dendritic spines of the pyramidal neurons of the motor cortex. He suggested that these structural differences may underlie the motor incoordination and mental retardation characteristic of individuals with Down syndrome. Loesch-Mdzewska[34] also found neurological abnormalities of the corticospinal system (in addition to reduced brain weight) in his neuropathological study of 123 individuals with Down syndrome aged 3 to 62 years. Crome[35] reported lesser brain weight in comparison with normal persons. Finally, Benda[36] noted a lack of myelinization of the nerve fibers in the precentral area, frontal lobe, and cerebellum of infants with Down syndrome. As McGraw[37] has pointed out, the amount of myelin in the brain reflects the stage of developmental maturation. The delayed myelinization characteristic of neonates and infants with Down syndrome is thought to be a contributing factor to the generalized hypotonicity and persistence of primitive reflexes characteristic of this syndrome.[38]

Trisomy 18. Trisomy 18, or Edwards' syndrome, is the second most common of the trisomic syndromes to occur in term deliveries, although it is far less prevalent than Down syndrome (Figure 13-2). The birth prevalence (live and still births) is reported as 1 in 8000 live births,[8] with females affected more often than males (3 : 1).[8,12] As with Down syndrome, advanced maternal age is positively correlated with trisomy 18.[27] Most cases of Edwards' syndrome occur as random events during the formation of reproductive cells, fewer cases occur as errors in cell division during early fetal development, and inherited, translocation forms rarely occur.[39] Only 10% of infants born with trisomy 18 survive past the first year of life; female and non-Caucasian children survive longest.[40] The survival of girls averages 7 months; the survival of boys averages 2 months.[40]

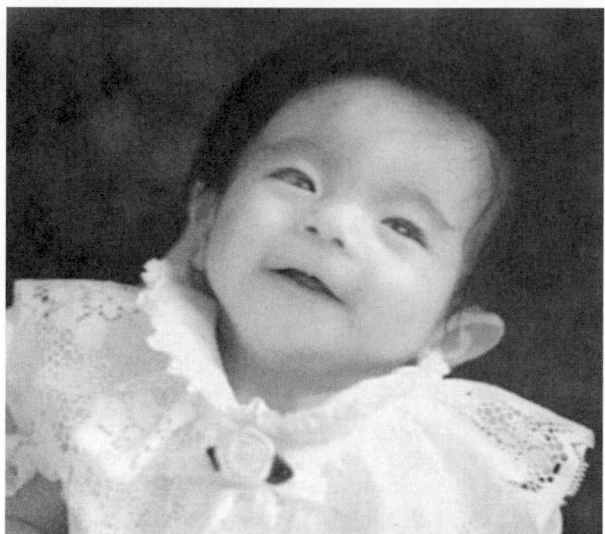

FIGURE 13-2 ■ One-year-old girl with trisomy 18.

Individuals with trisomy 18 generally have far more serious organic malformations than seen in those with Down syndrome.[41] Typical malformations affect the cardiovascular, gastrointestinal, urogenital, and skeletal systems. Infants with trisomy 18 have low birth weight and small stature, with a long narrow skull, low-set ears, flexion deformities of the fingers, and rocker-bottom feet. Muscle tone is initially hypotonic, but it becomes hypertonic.[41] The period of hypertonicity in the early years may change to low tone and joint hyperextensibility by preschool and school age. Microcephaly, abnormal gyri, cerebellar anomalies, myelomeningocele, hydrocephaly, and corpus callosum defects have been reported in individuals with trisomy 18.[42]

Common skeletal malformations that may warrant attention from the developmental physical or occupational therapist include scoliosis,[42] limited hip abduction, flexion contractures of the fingers, rocker-bottom feet, and talipes equinovarus.[41] Infants with trisomy 18 may also have feeding difficulties as a result of a poor suck.[31] Profound mental retardation is another clinical factor that will affect the developmental therapy programs for children with trisomy 18.[42]

Trisomy 13. Trisomy 13, also commonly called Patau's syndrome, is the least common of the three major autosomal trisomies, with an incidence of 1 in 10,000 to 20,000 live births.[6] As in the other trisomic syndromes, advanced maternal age is correlated with the incidence of trisomy 13.[43] Fewer than 10% of individuals with trisomy 13 survive past the first year of life[43]; girls and non-Caucasian infants appear to survive longer.[43] As with Edwards' syndrome, most cases of Patau syndrome occur as random events during the formation of eggs and sperm, such as nondisjunction errors during cell division.[44]

Trisomy 13 is characterized by microcephaly, deafness, anophthalmia or microphthalmia, coloboma, and cleft lip and palate.[32,44] As in trisomy 18, infants with trisomy 13 frequently have serious cardiovascular and urogenital malformations and typically have severe to profound mental retardation. Skeletal deformities and anomalies include flexion contractures of the fingers and polydactyly of the hands and feet.[8] Rocker-bottom feet also have been reported, although less frequently than in individuals with trisomy 18. Reported central nervous system (CNS) malformations include arhinencephalia, cerebellar anomalies, defects of the corpus callosum, and hydrocephaly.[45]

Sex Chromosome Disorders

The human X chromosome is large, containing approximately 5% of a human's nuclear DNA. The Y chromosome, much smaller, contains few known genes.[6] Females, with genotype XX are mosaic for the X chromosome, meaning that one copy of their X chromosome is inactive in a given cell; some cell types will have a paternally derived active chromosome, and others a maternally derived X chromosome. Males, genotype XY, have only one copy of the X chromosome; therefore diseases caused by genes on the X chromosome, called X-linked diseases, can be devastating to males, and less severe in females.[6] In the presence of abnormal numbers of sex chromosomes, neither male nor female will be phenotypically normal.[6] Two of the most prevalent sex chromosome anomalies are Turner's syndrome and Klinefelter's syndrome.

Turner's Syndrome. Turner's syndrome affects females with monosomy of the X chromosome. The syndrome, also known as gonadal dysgenesis, occurs in 1 in 2,500 births.[46,47] Turner's syndrome is the most common chromosomal anomaly among spontaneous abortions.[48,49] Most infants who survive to term have the mosaic form of this syndrome, with a mix of cell karyotypes, 45,X and 46,XX. The SHOX gene, found on both the X and Y chromosomes, codes for proteins essential to skeletal development. Deficiency of the SHOX gene in females accounts for most of the characteristic abnormalities of this disorder.[47] Three characteristic impairments of the syndrome are sexual infantilism, a congenital webbed neck, and cubitus valgus.[50] Other clinical characteristics noted at birth include dorsal edema of hands and feet, hypertelorism, epicanthal folds, ptosis of the upper eyelids, elongated ears, and shortening of all the hand bones.[13,46] Growth retardation is particularly noticeable after the age of 5 or 6 years, and sexual infantilism, characterized by primary amenorrhea, lack of breast development, and scanty pubic and axillary hair, is apparent during the pubertal years. Ovarian development is severely deficient, as is estrogen production.[8] Congenital heart disease is present in 20% of individuals with Turner's syndrome[51]; 33% to 60% of individuals with Turner syndrome have kidney malformations.[46]

There are numerous incidences of skeletal anomalies, some of which may be significant enough to require the attention of a pediatric therapist. Included among these are hip dislocation, pes planus and pes equinovarus, dislocated patella,[46] deformity of the medial tibial condyles, and deformities resulting from osteoporosis.[8,52] Decreased lumbar lordosis[53] and idiopathic scoliosis are also common.[42]

Sensory impairments include decrease in gustatory and olfactory sensitivity, deficits in spatial perception and orientation,[54] and moderate hearing loss. Although the average intellect of individuals with Turner's syndrome is within normal limits, the incidence of mental retardation is higher than in the general population.[41] Noonan's syndrome, once thought to be a variant of Turner's syndrome, has several common clinical characteristics; however, advancements in genetics research have shown that the they have different genetic causes.[55]

Klinefelter's Syndrome. Klinefelter's syndrome is an example of aneuploidy with an excessive number of chromosomes. The most common type, 47,XXY, is usually not clinically apparent until puberty when the testes fail to enlarge and gynecomastia occurs.[27] Eighty percent of males with Klinefelter's syndrome possess a karyotype of XXY, and the other 10% of cases are variants.[27] The incidence of Klinefelter's syndrome (XXY) is about 1 in 1000 males and an estimated half of 47,XXY conceptions are spontaneously aborted.[6,31] The extra X chromosome(s) can be derived from either the mother or father; 50% of cases are maternally derived and incidence increases with advanced maternal age.[6] Parental age does not appear to be a factor in the incidence of the more severe types of Klinefelter's syndrome.[27]

Most individuals with karyotype XXY have normal intelligence, a somewhat passive personality, and a reduced libido. Eighty-five percent of individuals having the nonmosaic karyotype are sterile. Individuals with the karyotypes 48,XXXY and 49,XXXXY tend to display a more severe clinical picture. Individuals with 48,XXXY usually have severe mental retardation, with multiple congenital anomalies, including microcephaly, hypertelorism, strabismus, and cleft palate.[8] Skeletal anomalies include radioulnar synostosis, genu valgum, malformed cervical vertebrae, and pes planus.[8]

Partial Deletion Disorders

Deletions are one example of mutations that cause changes in the sequence of DNA in human cells. A sequence change that affects a gene's function can cause the final protein product to be altered or not produced at all.

Cri-du-Chat Syndrome. Cri-du-chat syndrome, also referred to as cat-cry syndrome, results from a partial deletion of the short arm of chromosome 5. Example nomenclature for a female with this syndrome is (46,XX,del[5p]). The incidence of the syndrome is estimated to be 1 case per 20,000 to 50,000 live births.[8] Although approximately 70% of individuals with cri-du-chat syndrome are female, there is an unexplained higher prevalence of older males with this disorder[56] (Figure 13-3). Advanced parental age is not a

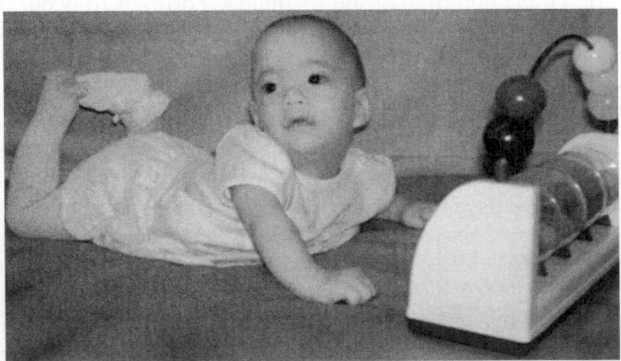

FIGURE 13-3 ■ Nine-month-old girl with cri-du-chat syndrome.

causal factor. A study completed in 1978 indicated that life expectancy was 1 year for 90% of infants born with this disorder,[57] but now life expectancy is nearly normal with routine medical care.[58]

Primary identifying characteristics at birth include a definitive high-pitched catlike cry, microcephaly, and evidence of intrauterine growth retardation.[8] The characteristic cry, which results from abnormal laryngeal development, disappears in the first few years of life.[31] It is not present in all individuals. Other features of individuals with this syndrome include hypertelorism, strabismus, "moon face," and low-set ears.[8] Associated musculoskeletal deformities include scoliosis, hip dislocations, clubfeet, and hyperextensibility of fingers and toes. Muscular hypotonicity is associated with this syndrome, although cases with hypertonicity have also been noted.[59] Severe respiratory and feeding problems have also been reported.[31] Postnatal growth retardation has been documented with the median near the 5th percentile of the normal growth curve.[60]

Although mental retardation and physical deformities are more severe with larger deletions,[61] there is evidence that with early developmental intervention these children can develop language, functional ambulation, and self-care skills.[62,63]

Prader-Willi Syndrome and Angelman's Syndrome. Prader-Willi syndrome (PWS) and Angelman's syndrome (AS) are discussed together because they result from a loss of the PWS/AS region of chromosome 15, which can occur by one of several genetic mechanisms.[64,65] Each syndrome has an incidence of 1 in 15,000 live births.[64,65] These two syndromes illustrate the effect of *genomic imprinting,* which is the differential activation of genes of the same chromosome and location, depending on the sex of the parent of origin[6] (Figure 13-4).

PWS results when a segment of paternal chromosome 15 is deleted or entirely absent.[66] Conversely, AS results when the maternal copy of chromosome 15 is incomplete or absent.[6] *OCA2* is a gene located within the PWS/AS region of chromosome 15 that codes for the protein involved in melanin production. With loss of one copy of this gene, individuals with PWS or AS will have light hair and fair skin. In the rare case that both copies of the gene are lost, these individuals may have a condition called oculocutaneous albinism, type 2, which causes severe vision problems.[65]

Characteristics of PWS include hypogonadism, short stature, hypotonia, dysmorphic facial features, dysfunctional CNS performance,[67] and obesity associated with a compulsive preoccupation with food.[64,68] Diagnosis is confirmed by chromosome studies and molecular studies showing a loss of the *OCA2* gene.[64] Most cases of PWS are due to random mutations in parental reproductive cells.[64] Other cases may result from translocation errors.[69] Parental studies are important in translocation cases because 20% of cases cited in the literature involved familial rearrangements, which may significantly increase the risk for recurrence.[70]

Infants with PWS have a 300% increased incidence of breech and cesarean deliveries,[71] suggesting that hypotonia is present even in this fetal stage.[68] Generalized hypotonia persists at birth and is severe in most cases.[72] Most infants have an expressionless face, flaccid muscles, a weak cry, and little spontaneous movement. Muscle tone generally

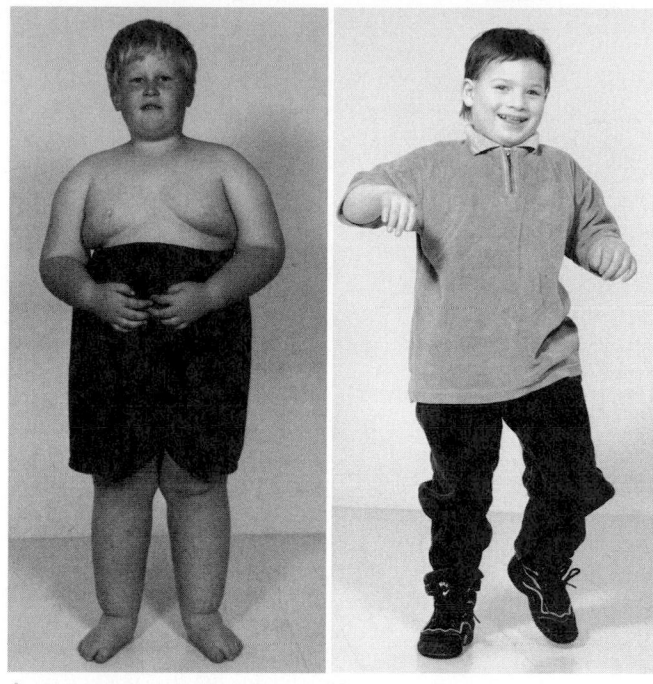

A   B

FIGURE 13-4 ■ Illustration of the effect of imprinting on chromosome 15 deletions. **A,** Inheritance of the deletion from the father produces PWS. **B,** Inheritance of the deletion from the mother produces AS. (From Jorde L, Carey J, Bamshad M, White R: *Medical genetics,* ed 3, St. Louis, 2005, Mosby.)

improves after the first few months of life; however, poor coordination and motor delays persist. Hypotonia often results in a poor suck, with early feeding difficulties and slow initial weight gain.[72] At an average age of 2 years, children develop a persistent appetite and the focus shifts from initial concerns about weight gain to preventing obesity.[73]

Most individuals with PWS have mild to moderate mental retardation, although some individuals have intelligence quotient (IQ) scores within normal limits.[73] Maladaptive behaviors such as temper tantrums, aggression, self-abuse, and emotional lability have been reported.[74] As a result of extreme obesity, many individuals with PWS have impaired breathing that can produce sleepiness, cyanosis, cor pulmonale, and heart failure.[74] Scoliosis is common but does not appear to be related to obesity.[75]

AS is characterized by developmental delay or mental retardation, seizures, ataxia, progressive microcephaly, and severe speech impairments. Tongue thrusting, drooling, and sucking and swallowing disorders occur in 20% to 80% of children. Individuals often display spontaneous bouts of laughter accompanied by hand-flapping movements and a characteristic walking posture of arms overhead and flexed elbows.[6] Infants appear normal at birth but severe developmental delay becomes apparent by 6 to 12 months of age; more unique features of the disorder do not appear until after 1 year of age, so molecular studies can confirm the disorder before all of the clinical criteria for this diagnosis are met.[65]

Most cases of AS occur as a result of mutations involving deletion or deficient function of the maternally inherited *UBE3A* gene. This gene codes for an enzyme, ubiquitin protein ligase UBE3A, involved in the normal process of removing damaged or unnecessary proteins in healthy cells. In most of the body's tissues except the brain, both copies (maternal and paternal) of the *UBE3A* gene are active. Only the maternal copy of the gene is normally active in the brain, so if this copy is absent of deficient, the normal cellular housekeeping process breaks down.[65] The risk of having another child with AS can vary from 1% to 50%, depending on which of the six known genetic mechanisms is responsible for the disorder. Molecular studies can identify the genetic cause in children with suspected AS before a clinical diagnosis can be made.[76]

Translocation Disorders

Translocation errors have been identified in many childhood hematologic cancers and sarcomas.[77,78] Translocation errors are also commonly seen in couples with infertility.[79] Translocation abnormalities occur when genetic material is exchanged and rearranged between two nonhomologous chromosomes (those not in the same numbered pair). The structural abnormality can result in the loss or gain of chromosomal material (an unbalanced arrangement) or no loss or gain of material (a balanced arrangement). Unbalanced arrangements can produce serious disease or deformity in individuals or their offspring. Carriers of balanced arrangements, estimated to occur in 1 in 500 individuals, often have a normal phenotype, but their offspring may have an abnormal phenotype.[6] There are two basic types of translocations, a reciprocal translocation or a Robertsonian translocation. Reciprocal translocations occur when two different chromosomes break and the genetic material is mutually exchanged. A Robertsonian translocation occurs when there is a break in a portion of two different chromosomes, the longest remaining portions of both chromosomes forming a single chromosome. The shorter portions that broke away usually do not contain vital genetic information; therefore the individual may be phenotypically normal.[6] An example notation of a reciprocal translocation is 46,XY,t(7;9)(q36;q34). This individual is female with a normal number of chromosomes but with a translocation of genetic material on chromosomes 7 and 9; "q" refers to the short arm of these chromosomes and the numbers "36" and "34" refer to the location.

Translocations occur in children seen in therapy settings, including about 3% to 5% of children with Down syndrome,[8] and translocations are found in 40% of all cases of acute lymphoblastic leukemia.[80]

Acute Lymphoblastic Leukemia. Acute lymphoblastic leukemia (ALL) accounts for one fourth of all childhood cancers, and it is the most common type of childhood leukemia.[81,82] ALL reportedly occurs more frequently in white males in developed countries.[81-84] Sixty percent of cases of ALL occur in children, with the peak incidence in the first 5 years of life. A rise in the incidence of ALL has been reported during major periods of industrialization worldwide,[83,85] and it is probably associated with exposure to radiation and other environmental teratogens.[82,85]

There are numerous forms of translocation mutations associated with ALL; an example is the Philadelphia chromosome, which takes place between chromosomes 9 and 22.[82] There are some translocation forms of ALL that do not respond well to combination chemotherapy treatment, but 70% to 80% of all pediatric patients with ALL will have long-term remission of the disease.[82]

Frequently, diagnosis is made when a physician relates the child's history of a persistent viral respiratory infection with other characteristic clinical signs and symptoms. Signs and symptoms of ALL include those consistent with hematopoietic leukemia: pallor, poor appetite, lethargy, easy fatigue and bruising, fever, and mucosal bleeding. Bone pain occurs in 40% to 50% of children with ALL.[82] A complete blood count will show a shortage of all types of blood cells, including red, white, and platelets. Diagnosis is confirmed by the presence of lymphoblasts in bone marrow. Radiographs may be necessary to determine metastases, and cerebrospinal fluid will be examined because early involvement of the CNS has important prognostic implications.[85]

Single-Gene Disorders

Other genetic disorders commonly seen among children in a therapy setting include those that result from specific gene defects. The inheritance patterns of single-gene traits were described by Gregor Mendel in the nineteenth century. These patterns, autosomal dominant, autosomal recessive, and sex linked, are discussed separately and specific examples of syndromes or disorders associated with each type are presented.

Autosomal Dominant Disorders

Mutations on one of the 22 numbered pairs of autosomes may result in isolated anomalies that occur in otherwise normal individuals, such as extra digits or short fingers. Each child of a parent with an autosomal dominant trait has a 50:50 chance of inheriting that trait.[6] Other autosomal dominant disorders include syndromes characterized by profound musculoskeletal and neurological impairments that may require intervention from a physical or an occupational therapist. Three examples of autosomal dominant disorders are osteogenesis imperfecta, tuberous sclerosis, and neurofibromatosis.

Osteogenesis Imperfecta. Osteogenesis imperfecta (OI) is a spectrum of diseases that results from deficits in collagen synthesis[31] associated with single-gene defects of *COL1A1* and *COL1A2* located on chromosomes 17 and 7, respectively.[8] OI is characterized by brittle bones, hyperextensible ligaments, blue sclerae, cardiopulmonary abnormalities, discolored and fragile teeth,[86] and hypotonia.[87] Deafness, resulting from otosclerosis, appears in adulthood and is found in 35% of individuals by the third decade of life.[41] New knowledge about this disease from molecular genetic studies and bone histomorphometry has expanded the classification subtypes of OI into types I through VII.[88] These classifications are helpful in determining prognosis and management, although there is a continuum of severity of clinical features and much overlap in the features among the different classifications.[88] OI types V and VI account for only 5% of cases and type VII has been found to date only in a Native Canadian population.[88] This section will focus on discussion of types I through IV.

The overall incidence of OI is 1 in 20,000 to 30,000, with types I and IV being the most common. Types II and III have an incidence of 1 in 62,000 and 1 in 68,000, respectively.[8]

Type I is the least severe form, followed by types IV and III, with type II being the most severe.

Types I and IV follow the autosomal dominant pattern of inheritance.[88] Type I is characterized by blue sclera, mild-to-moderate bone fragility, and joint hyperextensibility. There are no significant deformities, and individuals with this type are usually ambulatory. Type IV OI is characterized by more severe bone fragility and joint hyperextensibility than is type I. Bowing of long bones, scoliosis, and short stature are common.[86,88] Children with type IV OI are often ambulatory but may require splinting or crutches.[86]

Children with type III OI have severe bone fragility and osteoporosis; often there are fractures in utero. Type III occurs primarily in autosomal dominant inheritance in North Americans and Europeans.[88] The less-frequent, autosomal recessive form of OI, type III is characterized by progressive skeletal deformity, scoliosis, triangular facies, large skull, normal cognitive ability, short stature, and limited ambulatory ability.[86,88,89] The long bones of the lower extremities are most susceptible to fractures, particularly between the ages of 2 to 3 years and 10 to 15 years,[41] with the frequency of fractures diminishing with age.[31] Intramedullary rods inserted in the tibia or femur may minimize recurrent fractures.[33]

Type II, the most severe form, is most often lethal before or shortly after birth although there are a few cases of children living to 3 years.[88,89] Infants with type II OI have multiple fractures, often in utero, and underdeveloped lungs and thorax, and many die from respiratory complications after birth. Most type II cases are the result of spontaneous mutations; because only one copy of the gene is sufficient to cause the disorder, it is still commonly classified as an autosomal dominant condition. There are fewer cases of autosomal recessive inheritance.[6]

Prevention of fractures through careful handling and positioning is the most important goal in working with individuals with OI. Mobility aids and splinting also can be helpful in preventing fractures.[31,90] Aquatic therapy can be a valuable treatment strategy for children with OI.[90]

Tuberous Sclerosis Complex. Tuberous sclerosis complex is characterized by a triad of impairments: seizures, mental retardation, and sebaceous adenomas[32]; however, there is wide variability in expression, with some individuals displaying skin lesions only.[41] Although tuberous sclerosis is inherited as an autosomal dominant trait, 86% of cases occur as spontaneous mutations, with older paternal age a contributing factor. Tuberous sclerosis complex is a relatively rare condition, affecting both sexes equally, with a frequency of 1 in 10,000 births.[3] Infants are frequently normal in appearance at birth, but 70% of those who go on to show the complete triad of symptoms display seizures during the first year of life. Mutations in the *TSC1* and *TSC2* genes are known to cause tuberous sclerosis.[8] The normal function of these genes is to regulate cell growth; if these genes are defective, cellular overgrowth and noncancerous tumor formation can occur.[91] Tumor formation in the CNS is responsible for most of the morbidity and mortality with TSC.[91]

Hypopigmented macules are often the initial finding. These lesions vary in number and are small and ovoid. Larger lesions, known as leaf spots, may have jagged edges.[31] Sebaceous adenomas first appear between the ages of 4 and 5 years, with early individual brown, yellow, or red lesions of firm consistency in the nose and upper lips. These isolated lesions may later coalesce to form a characteristic butterfly pattern on the cheeks. Known also as hamartomas (tumor-like nodules of superfluous tissue), the skin lesions are present in 83% of individuals with tuberous sclerosis.[41]

Delayed development is another characteristic during infancy,[92] particularly in the achievement of motor and speech milestones. Mental retardation occurs in 62% of individuals with tuberous sclerosis.[41] Because of the retardation in motor development and the associated rigidity or hemiplegia seen in some cases, children with this disorder may be referred to a developmental physical or occupational therapist.

Ultimately, 93% of individuals who are severely affected will have seizures, usually of the myoclonic type, in early life, progressing in later life to grand mal seizures. Seizure development is the result of formation of nodular lesions in the cerebral cortex and white matter.[41] Tumors are also found in the walls of the ventricles. Neurocytological examination reveals a decreased number of neurons and an increased number of glial cells and enlarged nerve cells with abnormally shaped cell bodies.[8] Surgical excision of seizure-producing tumors has been successful in some cases.[32]

Other associated impairments include retinal tumors and hemorrhages, glaucoma, and corneal opacities.[32] Cyst formation in the long bones and in the bones of the fingers and toes contributes to osteoporosis. Cardiac and kidney involvement[31] and catatonic schizophrenia have also been reported.[32]

Neurofibromatosis. There are two recognized forms of this disease, neurofibromatosis I and neurofibromatosis II.[93] Commonalities in the two forms are the presence of flat, light brown skin patches, known as café-au-lait spots, and neurofibromas, or connective tissue tumors of the nerve fiber fasciculus.[93,94] Tumors typically increase in number with increasing age. About half of all cases of neurofibromatosis are due to sporadic mutation in parental germ cells or during fetal development.[93]

Neurofibromatosis type 1 is also known as von Recklinghausen's disease, or peripheral neurofibromatosis. Compared with type II, type I is more common (1:3000 births)[8] and usually identified in younger children. It is associated with mutations in the *NF1* gene, which produces a protein that is a tumor suppressor. Café-au-lait spots and skin tumors are reported to be the only consistent clinical feature of type I neurofibromatosis.[8] Other clinical features include scoliosis, pseudarthrosis of the tibia, pheochromocytoma, meningioma, glioma, acoustic neuroma, optic neuroma, mental retardation, hypertension, and hypoglycemia. Fewer than 10% of individuals are mentally retarded, but about 30% to 50% of affected children have learning disabilities.[51,95]

Infants usually appear normal at birth, with the initial café-au-lait spots first appearing in early childhood[41] (Figure 13-5).

Neurofibromatosis type II, also called central neurofibromatosis, is caused by a mutation in the gene encoding neurofibromin-2, also called *Merlin*.[8] Merlin is produced in the nervous system, particularly in Schwann cells that surround and insulate the nerve cells of the brain and spinal cord. Although type II shares characteristics with neurofi-

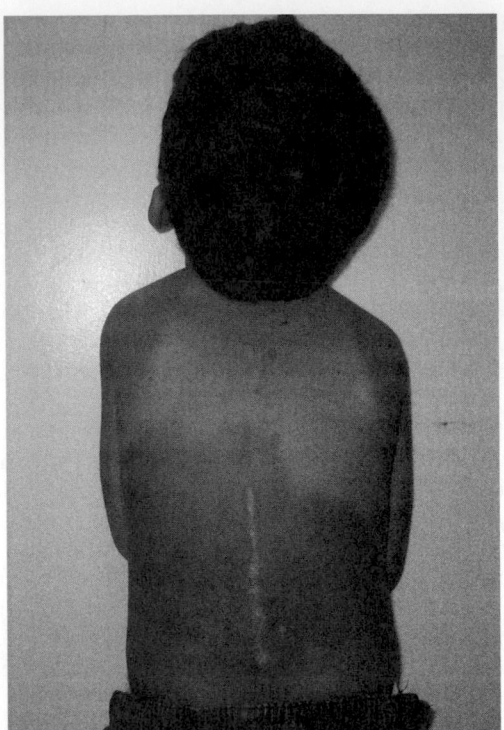

FIGURE 13-5 ■ Four-year-old boy with neurofibromatosis and characteristic café-au-lait spots on trunk.

bromatosis type I, it is commonly characterized by tumors of the eighth cranial nerve (usually bilateral), meningiomas of the brain, and schwannomas of the dorsal roots of the spinal cord.[8] Signs and symptoms usually appear during adolescence or in the person's early 20s[93] and it occurs less frequently than type I does (1:40,000 births).[8]

In summary, neurofibromas may be found in either the peripheral nervous system or the CNS[13] and can lead to secondary impairments such as optic and acoustic nerve damage, paraplegia, quadriplegia,[32] or hemiparesis.[96] Muscle weakness or incoordination, rather than complete paralysis, may be evident.[31] Neurofibromas may also develop in the kidneys, stomach, or heart.[41] Puberty and pregnancy may exacerbate dermatological symptoms of this disorder.[94] Ultimately, 47% of individuals with neurofibromatosis will have some type of neurological impairment.[41]

Cervical paraspinal neurofibromas may develop in late childhood or early adulthood and are a major cause of long-term disability.[97] Scoliosis occurs in up to 10% to 20% of individuals with neurofibromatosis.[51] Severe kyphoscoliotic deformities may lead to spinal cord compression or impaired cardiopulmonary function. Kyphosis usually becomes apparent between ages 6 and 10 years. Other skeletal deformities include pseudarthrosis of the tibia and fibula, tibial bowing, craniofacial and vertebral dysplasia,[31,51] rib fusion, and dislocation of the radius and ulna. Differences in leg length also have been noted and may contribute to scoliosis.[51]

Autosomal Recessive Disorders

An unaffected carrier of a disease-causing trait is *heterozygous* for the abnormal gene (possessing one normal and one mutated copy of the gene). If both parents are unaffected carriers of the gene, each of their offspring faces a 25% risk of exhibiting the disorder.[6] Consanguinity involving close relatives increases the chance of passing on autosomal recessive traits.[6] Certain types of limb defects, familial microcephaly, and a variety of syndromes such as Hurler's syndrome are passed on through autosomal recessive genes. Four examples of autosomal recessive disorders that may be of interest to physical or occupational therapists are presented in this section: cystic fibrosis, Hurler's syndrome, phenylketonuria, and spinal muscle atrophy.

Cystic Fibrosis. Cystic fibrosis (CF) is one of the most common autosomal recessive disorders affecting whites, with an incidence of 1 in 2000 to 4000.[8] The incidence in nonwhites is much less and has been reported at 1 in 17,000 among African Americans. The CF gene has been mapped to chromosome 7, and the protein CF transmembrane regulator (CFTR), which is the product of the gene, has been cloned.[6] CFTR is involved in the regulation of chloride channels of the bowel and lung, which is dysfunctional in patients with CF.

The primary impairments include fibrotic lesions of the pancreas, and up to 85% of patients have been reported to have pancreatic insufficiency. The inability of the pancreas to secrete digestive enzymes can result in chronic malnutrition. Ten percent to 20% of newborn infants with CF also have intestinal tract involvement with a meconium ileus. The sweat glands are commonly affected, with high levels of chloride found in the sweat, which is the basis for the sweat chloride test used in diagnosis. The most serious impairment in CF is the obstruction of the lungs by thick mucus, which leads to chronic pulmonary obstruction, infection that destroys lung tissue, and eventual death from pulmonary disease in 90% of individuals.[6]

Although CF has markedly variable expression, the overall median survival time has improved from about 6 years of age in the 1940s to 30 years of age in the 1990s.[6] This improved survival rate is a result of improved antibiotic management, aggressive chest physical therapy, and pancreatic replacement therapy. Postural drainage, percussion, vibration, and breathing exercises are key components of the management program provided by the therapist. Attention to diet is important, and every attempt should be made to maintain a routine exercise program with a goal of helping the children be more active to improve their respiratory status. Overexertion and fatigue are to be avoided in prescribing an exercise program.

Hurler's Syndrome (Mucopolysaccharidosis I). Hurler's syndrome, or gargoylism, are common names for mucopolysaccharidosis I, an inborn error of metabolism that results in abnormal storage of mucopolysaccharides in many different tissues of the body.[87] The incidence is estimated to be 1 in 100,000 live births for the severe forms[8] and 1 in 500,000 for milder forms.[98] *IDUA* is the only gene currently known to be associated with this multisystem disorder.[98]

Infants born with Hurler's syndrome are usually normal in appearance at birth[32] and may be larger in birth weight than their siblings. Symptoms of this progressively deteriorating disease usually appear during the latter half of the first year of life,[13] with the full disease picture apparent by 2 to 3 years of age.[8]

Characteristic physical features include a large skull with frontal bossing, heavy eyebrows, edematous eyelids, corneal clouding, a small upturned nose with flat nasal bridge, thick lips, low-set ears, hirsutism, and gargoyle-like facial features. Growth retardation results in characteristic dwarfism.[87] Some individuals with the physical characteristics of Hurler's syndrome have normal intelligence, but most have mental retardation.[8]

Spastic paraparesis or paraplegia and ataxia[8] also have been observed in individuals with Hurler's syndrome. Commonly reported orthopedic deformities include flexion contractures of the extremities, thoracolumbar kyphosis, genu valgum, pes cavus,[87] hip dislocation, and claw hands as a result of joint deformities.[41] Restriction of neck flexion and extension also may result from hypoplasia of the odontoid process.[31] Atlanto-occipital instability occurs more commonly with the milder form of the disorder and may require surgical stabilization.[98]

Deafness is another frequently reported anomaly. Progressive mental and physical deterioration leads to early death, usually before adulthood. Death is usually due to the result of deposits of mucopolysaccharides in the cardiac valves, myocardium, or coronary arteries.[87]

Delayed motor milestones have been noted in later infancy and early childhood, with severe disabilities occurring with increasing age. Adaptive equipment often is needed, and most children with Hurler's syndrome become wheelchair users in their later years.[31]

Phenylketonuria. Phenylketonuria (PKU) is the result of one of the more common inborn errors of metabolism. Mutations of the *PAH* gene located on chromosome 12 cause a deficiency in the production of phenylalanine hydroxylase.[99] Without this enzyme, there is no conversion of phenylalanine to tyrosine, resulting in an abnormally excessive accumulation of phenylalanine in the blood and other body fluids.[99] If untreated, this metabolic error results in mental and growth retardation, seizures, and pigment deficiency of hair and skin.[100] PKU is most prevalent among individuals of northern European ancestry, with a frequency of 1 : 10,000 to 1 : 15,000 births.[13] It is estimated that 1 of every 50 individuals is heterozygous for PKU.[6]

Children born with PKU are usually normal in appearance, with delayed development becoming apparent toward the end of the first year. Parents usually become concerned with the child's slow development during the preschool years.[100] If PKU is untreated, the affected child may go on to develop hypertonicity (75%), hyperactive reflexes (66%), hyperkinesis (50%), or tremors (30%),[101] in addition to mental retardation. IQ levels generally fall between 10 and 50, although there have been reported rare cases of untreated individuals with normal intelligence.[100]

A simple blood plasma analysis, which is mandatory for newborn infants in many states in the United States, can detect the presence of elevated phenylalanine levels. This test is ideally performed when the infant is at least 72 hours old. If elevated phenylalanine levels are found, the test is repeated, and further diagnostic procedures are performed. Placing the infant on a low phenylalanine diet (low protein) can prevent the mental retardation and other neurological sequelae characteristic of this disorder.[100] Follow-up management by an interdisciplinary team consisting of a nutritionist, psychologist, and appropriate medical personnel is advised in addition to the special diet.

Spinal Muscle Atrophy. Spinal muscle atrophy (SMA) is characterized by progressive muscle weakness because of degeneration and loss of the anterior horn cells in the spinal cord and brain stem nuclei.[102] Mutations in the *SMN1* gene (named for survival of motor neuron 1), location 5q13, are associated with SMA. Another gene, *SMA2*, can modify the course of SMA. Individuals with multiple copies of *SMA2* can have less severe symptoms or symptoms that appear later in life as the number of copies of the *SMN2* gene increases.[103] The overall disease incidence of SMA is 5 in 100,000 live births.[103]

SMA has historically been classified by subtypes on the basis of age at symptom onset and expectations for maximum physical function. There are four commonly accepted subtypes of SMA (types I-IV) and one proposed form (SMO O) that is diagnosed prenatally.[102]

SMA I, otherwise known as Werdnig-Hoffmann disease or acute infantile SMA,[8] has an onset before 6 months of age.[102] Incidence is estimated to be 1 in 20,000 live births.[8] It is characterized clinically by severe hypotonicity, generalized symmetrical muscle weakness, absent deep tendon reflexes, and markedly delayed motor development. Intellect, sensation, and sphincter functioning, however, are normal.[104] In one third of individuals with this disorder, onset occurs in utero with a prenatal history of decreased fetal movements during the third trimester. Children usually sit with support but have poor head control.[105] They may develop mild joint contractures and have some facial and oral-motor weakness[102] and swallowing difficulties.[102,105] Intercostal muscle weakness leads to diaphragmatic breathing and contributes to the greatly increased susceptibility to pulmonary infection, which usually results in death before the age of 2 years.[8,103]

SMA II, otherwise known as intermediate, or chronic infantile, SMA has an onset at age 6 to 12 months. Finger trembling is almost always present.[102] Children with SMA II can usually sit independently if placed. Seventy percent of children diagnosed with SMA II are alive at 25 years of age.[102]

SMA III is characterized by onset of symptoms in childhood after 12 months.[102] It is also known as juvenile SMA or Kugelberg-Welander syndrome.[8] These individuals have a normal life span and usually attain independent ambulation and maintain it until the third or fourth decade of life.[102] Lower extremities are often more severely affected than the arms. Strength is often not sufficient for stair climbing and balance problems are common.[102]

SMA IV typically has an adult onset. It is also called distal spinal muscle atrophy, or spinal muscle atrophy, Charcot-Marie-Tooth type.[8]

For all types of SMA, a clinical diagnosis may be accomplished through electromyography and muscle biopsy, which reveal neurogenic atrophy.[105] There are multiple and complex mutations of the *SMN* gene, so molecular testing can be laborious and inconclusive with today's technology.[102] With the likelihood that methods will improve in the future, DNA banking (storing DNA samples of affected individuals or suspected carriers) is recommended so that DNA samples will be available to family members seeking future genetic counseling.[102]

Sex-Linked Disorders

The third mechanism for transmission of specific gene defects is through sex-linked inheritance. Two well-known sex-linked diseases are Duchenne muscular dystrophy (see Chapter 16, Neuromuscular Diseases) and hemophilia. In most sex-linked disorders, the abnormal gene is carried on the X chromosome. Female individuals carrying one abnormal gene usually do not display the trait because of the dominant normal gene on the other X chromosome. Each son born to a carrier mother, however, has a 50:50 chance of inheriting the abnormal gene and thus exhibiting the disorder. Each daughter of a carrier mother has a 50:50 chance of becoming a carrier of the trait.[6] Four syndromes that result in disability are discussed in this section: hemophilia A, fragile X syndrome, Lesch-Nyhan syndrome, and Rett syndrome.

Hemophilia. Hemophilia is a bleeding disorder caused by a deficient clotting process. Affected individuals will have hemorrhage into joints and muscles, easy bruising, and prolonged bleeding from wounds. The term *hemophilia* refers to hemophilia A (coagulation factor VIII deficiency), hemophilia B or Christmas disease (coagulation factor IX deficiency), and von Willebrand's disease (deficiency of factor VIII and von Willebrand factor).[8] All three forms of hemophilia can occur as X-linked recessive traits.[8]

Hemophilia A is reported to affect 1 in 5,000 to 10,000 males worldwide.[8] Hemophilia B is less common, affecting 1 in 20,000 to 35,000 males worldwide.[8] The severity and frequency of bleeding in hemophilia A are inversely related to the amount of residual factor VIII (<1%, severe; 2%-5%, moderate; and 5%-30%, mild). The proportions of cases that are severe, moderate, and mild are about 50%, 10%, and 40%, respectively.[106] The joints (ankles, knees, hips, and elbows) are frequently affected, causing swelling, pain, decreased function, and degenerative arthritis. Similarly, muscle hemorrhage can cause necrosis, contractures, and neuropathy by entrapment. Hematuria and intracranial hemorrhage, although uncommon, can occur after even mild trauma. Bleeding from tongue or lip lacerations is often persistent.[6]

Treatment includes guarding against trauma and replacement with factor VIII derived from human plasma or recombinant techniques.[6] In the late 1970s to mid 1980s it was estimated that half of the affected individuals in the United States contracted hepatitis B or C or human immunodeficiency virus infection when treated by donor-derived factor VIII. The initiation of donor blood screening and use of heat treatment of donor-derived factor VIII has almost completely eliminated the threat of infection.[6] Although replacement therapy is effective in most cases, 10% to 15% of treated individuals have neutralizing antibodies that decrease its effectiveness.[6]

Fragile X Syndrome. Fragile X syndrome is the most common sex-linked inherited cause of mental retardation, with a frequency of 1:1250 in males and of 1:2500 in females.[8] A fragile site on the long arm of an X chromosome is present, with breaks or gaps shown on chromosome analysis. A region of the X chromosome, named FMR1, normally codes for proteins that may play a role in the development of synapses in the brain. Mutations of this region are errors of trinucleotide repeats, where the number of CGG triplets at this region is expanded, thereby making the gene segment unable to produce the necessary protein.[107]

Eighty percent of males are reported to have mental retardation, with IQs of 30 to 50 being common but ranging up to the mildly retarded to borderline range.[107] *Penetrance* (the proportion of individuals with a mutation that actually exhibit clinical symptoms) in the female is reported at only 30%.[6] Other impairments include delayed acquisition of motor milestones, emotional lability, and autistic-like behaviors, such as hand biting, that have been reported to improve at puberty.[107] Life span is normal for individuals with this condition.[107]

Lesch-Nyhan Syndrome. Also known as hereditary choreoathetosis, Lesch-Nyhan syndrome, a sex-linked disorder, leads to profound neurological deterioration.[108] First described in 1964 by Lesch and Nyhan,[109] it is associated with a mutation in the *HPRT1* gene on the X chromosome. This gene codes for an enzyme, hypoxanthine guanine phosphoribosyltransferase, which allows cells to recycle purines, some of the building blocks of DNA and RNA.[110] Without this gene's normal function, there is an overproduction of uric acid (hyperuricemia),[108,110] which accumulates in the body. Individuals may have gouty arthritis and kidney and bladder stones. High uric acid levels are thought to cause neurological damage.[110]

The syndrome has an incidence of 1 in 10,000 in males.[51] Females born to carrier mothers have a 25% chance of inheriting the mutation. There are rare reports of females demonstrating this syndrome as a result of X chromosome inactivation. Most female carriers are considered to be asymptomatic, but some may have symptoms of hyperuricemia in adulthood.[110]

Lesch-Nyhan syndrome is detectable through amniocentesis, and genetic counseling is advisable for parents who have already given birth to an affected son.[111]

Infants appear normal at birth but begin to self-mutilate at 1 to 2 years of age by biting their lips. The disorder progresses to more severe forms of self-mutilation in which individuals have been known to bite off their fingertips.[108,110] Because of the extreme self-mutilation that characterizes this disorder, it has been questioned whether these children have normal pain perception.[112] One hypothesis is that these children have abnormal catecholamine metabolism that is seen in other patients with congenital pain insensitivity.[113] A single individual with Lesch-Nyhan syndrome ceased self-mutilating behavior after deep brain stimulation of the globus pallidus internus.[114]

A reported survey of parents of children with Lesch-Nyhan syndrome indicated that parents often find behavioral programming techniques helpful in modifying aggression toward self or others. In addition, parents report that they frequently elected tooth distraction and used physical restraints to prevent biting. It was interesting to note that the restrictive devices were often items such as a glove or band aid that would not actually prevent biting and that the patients frequently requested them.[115]

Motor development in these children is often normal during the first 6 to 8 months of life. Progressive spastic paresis and athetosis, however, become evident during the latter half of the first year of life. Other neuromotor symptoms include chorea, ballismus, tremor, hyperactive deep tendon reflexes, severe dysarthria, and dysphagia. Bilateral dislocation of hips may occur as a result of the spasticity.[108,110] An increased incidence of clubfoot deformity has been noted.[97] Growth retardation is also apparent, as well as moderate to severe mental retardation.[8]

Blood and urine levels of uric acid have been decreased successfully through the administration of allopurinol, with a resultant decrease in kidney damage.[97] With current management techniques, most individuals survive into their second or third decade of life.[110]

Rett Syndrome. Rett syndrome is an X-linked dominant condition affecting females almost exclusively, and it is most often lethal in males.[8] The inheritance pattern has yet to be fully delineated.[8] More recently, Rett syndrome has been reported in males with a extra X chromosome in many or all of the body's cells.[116-118] The estimated incidence is 1 in 15,000 to 20,000 females.[8,119] It has been reported that 99% of all cases of Rett syndrome are to the result of sporadic mutations.[120]

The syndrome is characterized by apparently normal development during the first 6 months of life, with deterioration occurring between 6 to 18 months of age.[121] Virtually all language ability is lost, although some children may produce echolalic sounds and learn simple manual signing. Evidence of minimal receptive language skills may be observed. Previously acquired purposeful hand skills are also lost and replaced by stereotypical hand movements. These nonspecific hand movements have been described as hand wringing, clapping, waving, or mouthing. Almost all individuals with Rett syndrome function in the range of severe to profound mental retardation. Although head circumference is normal at birth, deceleration of rate of head growth occurs between 5 months and 4 years of age.[122]

The onset of walking is usually delayed until about 19 months of age; almost one fourth of girls with Rett syndrome never develop independent ambulation skills.[122] Initially, hypotonia may be evident, but with advancing age, spasticity of the extremities develops.[123] Increased muscle tone is usually observed first in the lower extremities, with continued greater involvement than in the upper extremities. Peripheral vasomotor disturbances and muscle wasting have been noted as associated characteristics.[122]

In a report of 16 patients with Rett syndrome, Hennessey and Haas[124] described musculoskeletal deformities in nearly all patients. Fifteen patients showed clinical evidence of scoliosis, nine showed heelcord tightening, and hip instability was identified as an area of potential concern. Trevathan and Naidu[122] reported scoliosis in 50% of girls with Rett syndrome after the age of 10 years, many of whom required surgical correction.

Seventy percent to 80% of individuals with Rett syndrome have seizures in the first 5 years of life. Early electroencephalography results can be normal before 2 years of age. Cranial computed tomography results are normal or show mild generalized atrophy. Breathing dysfunction, including wake apnea and intermittent hyperventilation,[122] is also associated with Rett syndrome. Interventions reported in the literature have focused on splinting,[125] behavioral modification techniques to teach self-feeding skills,[126] music therapy, physical therapy, and occupational therapy.[127]

Mitochondrial DNA Disorders

In addition to the nuclear genome, humans have another set of genetic information within their mitochondria. Mitochondrial DNA (mtDNA) is small, circular, and double stranded. It is well studied and was mapped long before the human nuclear genome. mtDNA, inherited maternally, is highly susceptible to mutation and is responsible for a wide variety of disorders and syndromes.[10] These disorders affect the metabolic functions of the mitochondria, such as the generation of the body's energy currency, adenosine triphosphate.

Nuclear genes exist in pairs of one maternal and one paternal allele. In contrast, there are hundreds or thousands of copies of mtDNA in every cell. Normal and mutated versions of mtDNA can coexist within a patient's body; when a certain critical number of mutations exist, the body's tissues will show clinical signs of dysfunction. Tissues that have a high demand for oxidative energy metabolism, such as brain and muscle, are vulnerable to mtDNA mutations.[10]

Many patients with point mutations of mtDNA exhibit symptoms in early childhood; these mutations may be the most frequent cause of metabolic abnormality in children.[10] The minimum birth prevalence of childhood mitochondrial respiratory chain disorders is reported to be 6.2 per 100,000.[11,128-130] An example of a childhood disorder that can result from a mtDNA mutation is Leigh syndrome.

Leigh Syndrome

Leigh syndrome, or subacute necrotizing encephalomyopathy, may also be transmitted by X-linked recessive and autosomal recessive inheritance. Approximately 20% of all cases of Leigh syndrome are caused by mitochondrial mutations.[131] The discussion in this section will focus on characteristics of mtDNA-associated Leigh syndrome.

Leigh syndrome has an onset in infancy, typically at 3 to 12 months of age. Initial features may be nonspecific, such as a failure to thrive and persistent vomiting.[131,132] It is a progressive disorder caused by lesions that can occur in the brain stem, thalamus, basal ganglia, cerebellum, and spinal cord. Common clinical features include seizures, epilepsy, muscle weakness, peripheral neuropathy, speech and feeding difficulties, gastrointestinal and digestive problems, and heart problems. Most affected children have hypotonia, movement disorders such as chorea, and ataxia. Life expectancy is 2 to 3 years; death most often results from respiratory or cardiac failure.[131]

Multifactorial Disorders

Multifactorial disorders are believed to be a result of the combined effects of mutations in multiple genes combined with environmental factors.[6] Environmental factors may be those that have an impact on a developing fetus, such as prenatal diet or those that have an impact on humans as we age, such as cigarette smoking. Disorders in this category can result in congenital malformations such as spina bifida and clubfoot. An in-depth discussion of spina bifida can be found in Chapter 18. Management information on clubfoot can be found in pediatric textbooks that include orthopedic information.[133-136]

Many diseases such as cancer can result when the environment interacts with genetic variations that exists in all humans.[6] Scientists are exploring genetic contributions to premature births.[137-139] Premature birth is the leading cause of infant mortality and morbidity,[140] and its causes are most likely due to multiple genetic and environmental determinants that tend to run in families.[137-139] Premature infants are at higher risk of neurological, musculoskeletal, and respiratory problems than term infants are. Management of infants with low birth weight can be found in Chapter 11 of this text.

TYPICAL CLINICAL SYMPTOMS AND COMMON PROBLEMS

Specific examples of genetic disorders in children were presented in the foregoing section. Table 13-2 summarizes the impairments common to many genetic disorders that are most relevant for physical or occupational therapists.

Hypertonicity

Children with hypertonus generally display stiff or jerky movements that are limited in variety, speed, and coordination. Movements tend to be limited to the middle ranges. Total patterns of flexion or extension may dominate, with limited ability for selective joint movements. Motor development of children with hypertonicity may be further com-

plicated by the retention of primitive reflexes, which can result in stereotyped movements associated with sensory input.[141]

Children may learn to use stereotypical patterns of movement to achieve functional goals by activating the muscle synergies of a reflex without sensory feedback.[141] If a goal of therapy is to facilitate functional movement that is not dominated by persistent reflexes, it is critical to practice new motor patterns to accomplish the functional activity for which that reflex is being used. The focus of therapy activities needs to be on active movement of the child and not on passive inhibition techniques of abnormal reflexes for the sake of "normalization" of tone and movement.[142-145]

Differences and similarities observed in children with hypertonicity and hypotonicity are listed in Table 13-2. Although hypertonicity is often used interchangeably with the term *spasticity* (defined as increased resistance to passive stretch), there is growing recognition that muscles may be stiff but not spastic. One explanation for muscles that are stiff but not spastic is that such hypertonicity results from an attempt to control excessive movement at a joint.[141,146] This may be observed during the learning of a new skill in which there is a need to eliminate some of the excessive movement. Such "fixing" keeps the involved joints fairly rigid, thereby "freezing" nonessential movements and resulting in increased muscle tone or stiffness around that joint. As skill increases, a child learns to control the forces of movement and no longer needs to "fix," thereby allow-

TABLE 13-2 ■ Typical Impairments in Selected Genetic Disorders

GENETIC DISORDER	HYPO-TONICITY	HYPER-TONICITY	HIP DISLOCATION	SPINAL DEFORMITY	UPPER EXTREMITY DEFORMITY	OTHER DEFORMITY	MOTOR DELAYS	COGNI-TIVE DELAYS	CEREBELLAR DYSFUNCTION
Trisomy 21	X			X		X	X	X	X
Trisomy 18	X	X		X	X	X	X	X	
Trisomy 13	X	X			X	X	X	X	
Turner's syndrome			X	X	X	X			
Klinefelter's syndrome					X	X			
Cri-du-chat syndrome	X	X	X	X		X	X	X	
PWS	X			X		X	X	X	
OI				X	X	X	X		
Tuberous sclerosis		X					X	X	
Neurofibromatosis		X		X		X			
Untreated PKU				X					
Hurler's syndrome		X	X	X	X	X	X	X	X
Werdig-Hoffmann syndrome	X			X	X	X	X	X	X
Kugelberg-Welander syndrome	X			X			X	X	
Fragile X syndrome	X			X			X	X	
Lesch-Nyhan syndrome		X	X			X	X	X	X
Hemophilia A					X	X			
Rett syndrome					X	X	X	X	—

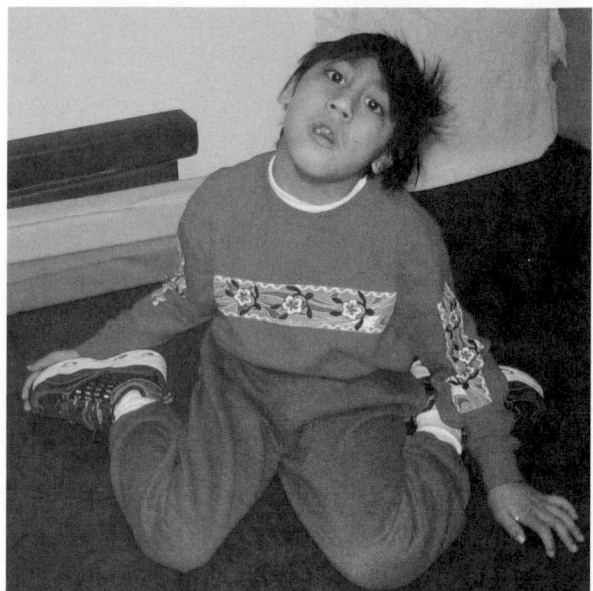

FIGURE 13-6 ■ Eight-year-old boy with hypotonia associated with a chromosomal translocation error. Note the broad base of support in this "W" sitting position.

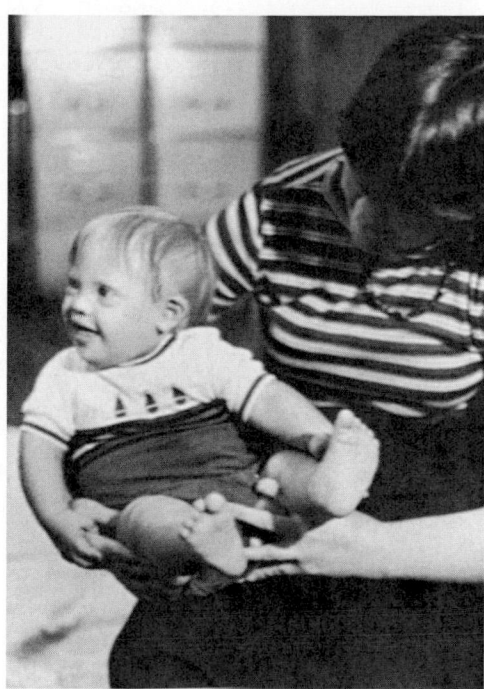

FIGURE 13-7 ■ Facilitation of equilibrium reactions in a 10-month-old child with Down syndrome.

ing a greater variety of movements to occur. If skill does not increase, however, a child may "fix" to compensate for his or her lack of active control, resulting in hypertonus. Another reason for stiffness without the evidence of spasticity may be an increase in connective tissue in the muscle, which has been shown to be a factor in children with cerebral palsy.[146,147]

Hypotonicity

Although movements of the child with high muscle tone are generally limited to the mid ranges, children with low muscle tone typically display movements in the extremes of the range. Children with hypotonicity tend to lock weight-bearing joints or assume positions that provide a broad base of support to maximize their stability (Figure 13-6). Although retention of primitive reflexes is less likely in children with hypotonia compared with those with hypertonia, delays in the development of postural reactions are a major concern (Figure 13-7). As a result of delays in postural development, children with hypotonicity often learn to rely on sources of external support to maintain upright positions. Limited strength and lack of endurance are often concerns with children who have hypotonicity. Hypotonicity and joint laxity are often associated with motor delay; however, therapists should not assume that hypotonia and joint laxity are absolutely predicative of persistent motor delay.[148] For example, many premature infants, with or without a genetic disorder, have global hypotonia at birth that resolves and does not cause long-term functional impairment.[148,149]

Hyperextensible Joints

Hyperextensible joints are commonly observed in children with hypotonicity and are noted in many children with genetic disorders. Activities should be modified to avoid undue stress to these joints and the surrounding ligaments, tendons, and fascia. For example, positions that allow the knee or elbow joints to lock into extension should be mod-

ified so that weight bearing occurs through more neutral alignment. Varying the placement of toys and support surfaces, providing physical assistance, and using adaptive equipment can help modify weight-bearing forces to achieve more neutral alignment.[150] For example, if hyperextensibility of ligaments leads to excessive pronation in stance (Figure 13-8), the use of ankle-foot orthoses may provide enough support to the structures to allow functional activities in standing (see Chapter 34, Orthotics). For a child who stands with knee hyperextension, a vertical stander may allow that child to stand and play at a water table with or her or his classmates for extended periods with the knees in a more neutral position. Rather than restricting a child's repertoire of upright positions, it is preferable to modify an activity or provide external support to enable a child to participate fully (Figure 13-9).[151]

Contractures and Deformities

Skeletal anomalies and deformities are associated with many genetic disorders. The physical or occupational therapist may work with orthopedists, prosthetists, and orthotists to detect and prevent the progression of a variety of conditions. The therapist should be aware of factors that can contribute to the development of deformities to prevent or minimize such problems.

Conditions that cause hypertonicity or spasticity are well known to place children at risk for joint contracture.[152] Children with hemophilia are at great risk of joint contractures associated with hemarthroses and intramuscular hemorrhages.[153] Therapists should consider the nature of the disorder that places the child at risk for contractures when choosing treatment techniques; disorder-specific techniques can be found in pediatric occupational and physical therapy textbooks.[133,154]

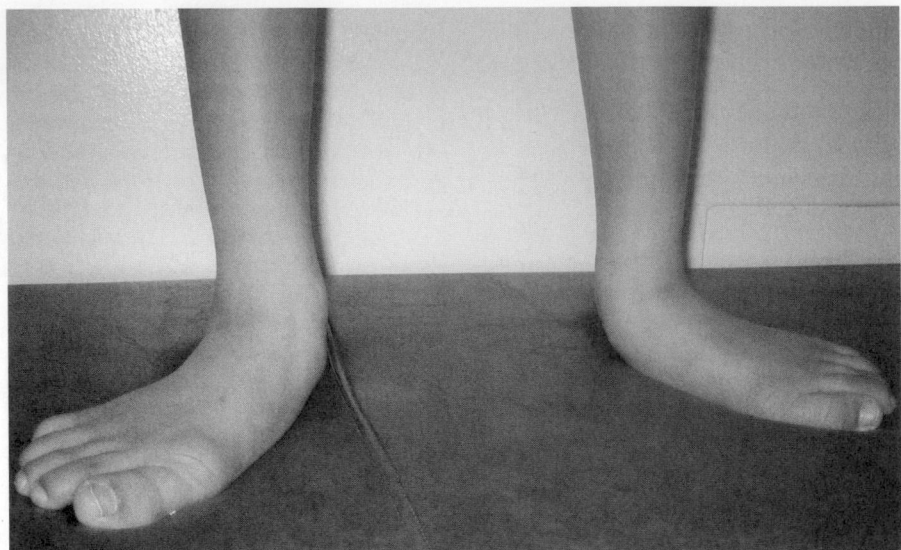

FIGURE 13-8 ■ Excessive bilateral pronation and flat feet associated with hyperextensibility in 8-year-old boy with global hypotonia.

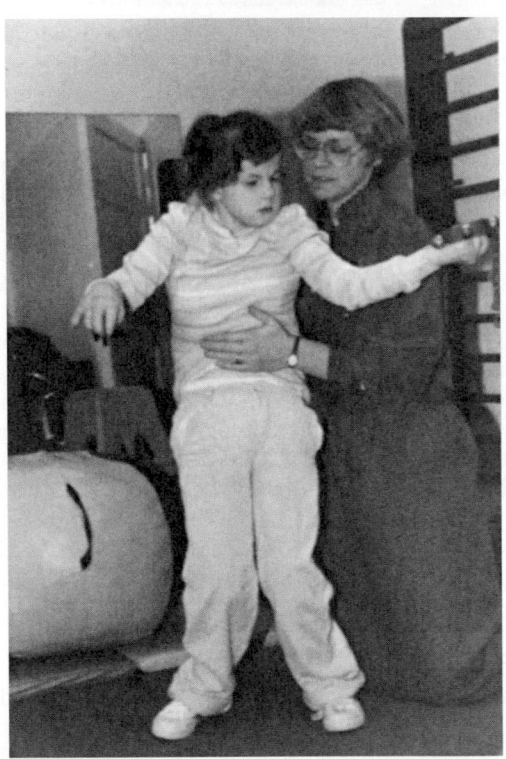

FIGURE 13-9 ■ Facilitation of standing in a girl with trisomy 18.

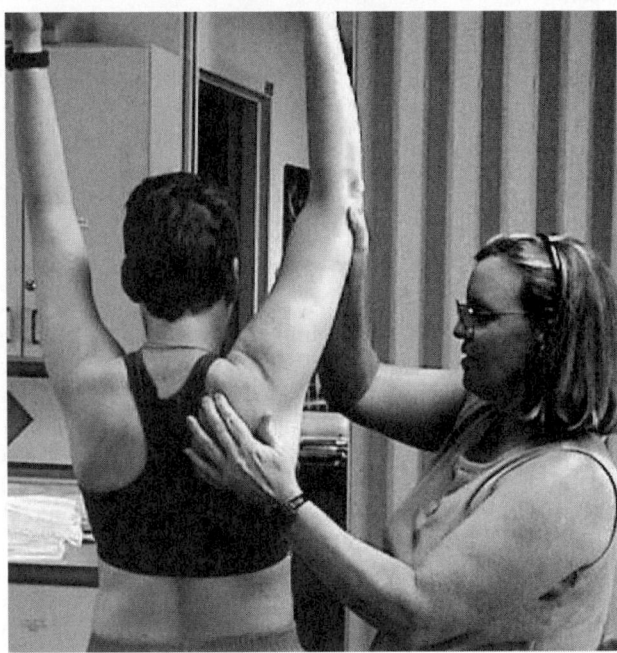

FIGURE 13-10 ■ Test of scapulothoracic mobility during assessment of normal chest wall mobility in an adult client.

Although joint contractures are less likely to occur in a child with hypotonicity, habitual positioning may lead to soft tissue restrictions. For example, children with hypotonia often adopt a constant position of wide abduction, external rotation, and flexion at the hips ("frog" or "reverse W" position)[137]; in these children, soft tissue contractures can develop at the hips and knees. Children whose hips are maintained in a position of adduction, flexion, and internal rotation are at risk for hip subluxation or dislocation.[137] Spinal deformities, such as lumbar lordosis and thoracic kyphosis and scoliosis, are also common concerns in children with abnormal muscle tone. An imbalance of muscle tone or strength or immobility may increase the risk of spinal deformity.

Chest wall deformity is common with hypotonicity because the anterior chest wall muscles tighten as a result of the long-term rounded, internally rotated shoulders and protracted scapulae. Therapists should assess scapulothoracic mobility[155-157] as a component of normal chest wall mobility; assessment techniques for children can be similar to those used in adults (Figure 13-10).

In general, contractures and deformities are a concern for most children who display a limited variety of postures and movements. Therapists should consider the nature of the disorder that places the child at risk for contractures when choosing treatment techniques. For example, premature infants are susceptible to chest wall deformity because of the imbalance of weak chest wall and respiratory musculature working against forces of gravity.[155-157] Premature infants can benefit from therapeutic positioning[158] to prevent contractures of the shoulder girdle[159] and to aid in proper respiratory function.

Respiratory Problems

A genetic risk for respiratory distress in infancy has been suggested by reports of family clusters.[160] Furthermore, comparison of short- and long-term respiratory function in infants with respiratory distress syndrome suggests that if all other factors of nutrition, previous mechanical ventilation, and gestational development are comparable, genetic risk may account for cases of chronic and potentially irreversible respiratory failure.[160]

Respiratory problems are often observed in children with limited mobility. If the mobility impairments are the result of hypotonicity or hypertonicity, impaired respiration may be due to chest and skeletal deformities.

Many infants with genetic disorders are born prematurely.[137-139] Premature infants who are on prolonged mechanical ventilation may spend much of their day in a supine position to facilitate observation. A long-term supine position for the infant with weak abdominal muscles increases the tendency for lateral flaring of the rib cage because it takes the path of least resistance in the gravity-eliminated plane.[155,161] Therefore, premature infants are more susceptible to respiratory problems associated with abnormal chest wall development as a result of the imbalance of a weak chest wall and respiratory muscles against forces of gravity.[155-157,161] Refer to Chapter 11 for additional information.

Some children may find it difficult to tolerate one position for an extended time owing to respiratory difficulties. For these children, frequent changes of position and use of adapted positioning devices may be necessary. Premature infants in the neonatal intensive care unit may benefit from regular prone positioning to facilitate restorative sleep,[162] improved arterial oxygen saturation,[163] and improved respiratory synchrony.[164] Children with respiratory problems may require mobilization techniques, deep breathing, chest expansion exercises, and postural drainage. In the case of children with CF, a comprehensive program of respiratory care is the primary therapy goal.[165]

Developmental Delay

Genetic disorders that affect neuromuscular, somatosensory, and cognitive function are frequently associated with developmental delays in children. The genetic basis for multisystem syndromes such as Down syndrome or Lesch-Nyhan syndrome can be identified by cytogenetic and molecular techniques. Congenital malformations, hearing impairment, and mental or growth retardation are examples of common components of developmental delay that often have a genetic basis.

Developmental delay is typified by the failure to meet expected age-related milestones in one or more of five areas: physical, social/emotional, intellectual, speech and language, and adaptive life skills. Developmental milestones that are typically assessed in the first 5 years of life can be found in Box 13-1.

Physical and occupational therapists can observe the interaction between each of the five areas of development in an infant or child. For example, a child with severe hypotonia who has limited movement experiences will not develop a well-adapted sensory system. Children with problems processing sensory information often withdraw from social interaction where they would otherwise find opportunities to develop speech, language, and social skills. Dynamic systems theory[166] explains this relationship between all of the developing components in a child; language does not develop independently of gross motor skills, and the ability to feed or dress oneself is as related to social, emotional, and intellectual development as it is to fine motor skills.

Suspicion of developmental delay often leads to physician referral. An accurate medical diagnosis is important in that it facilitates knowledgeable surveillance for potentially associated health problems. A delayed diagnosis can preclude timely implementation of beneficial medical, therapeutic, and educational services. Children who are identified to be at risk for developmental delay may be referred to early intervention programs. Examples of assessment techniques and interventions for children with developmental delay can be found in pediatric physical therapy textbooks.[167,168]

FAMILY-CENTERED INTERVENTION FOR CHILDREN WITH GENETIC DISORDERS

This section examines the role of the physical or occupational therapist in providing therapy services for children with genetic disorders. After a discussion of ways in which therapists can support families of children with genetic disorders, evaluation strategies, goals and objectives, and general treatment principles are presented. Throughout this section, emphasis is placed on supporting and including family members in all aspects of therapy and ensuring that therapy programs meet the priorities and needs of family members.[169]

Supporting Families

Therapists working with children with genetic disorders need to recognize and acknowledge the multitude of tasks that all families work to accomplish. In addition to tasks specifically related to caring for a child with a disability, families must perform functions to address the economic, daily care, recreational, social, and educational/vocational needs of both individual members and the family as a whole. As Turnbull and Turnbull[170] have cautioned, each time professionals intervene with families and children, they can potentially enhance or hinder the family's ability to meet important family functions. For example, intervention that promotes a child's social skills can be an important support to positive family functioning. On the other hand, intervention that focuses on a child's deficits can have a negative impact on how the family perceives that child and the place of the child in the family. For therapists to be supportive of families, they must (1) acknowledge the importance of family priorities, (2) respect the family's cultural values, (3) include families as integral team members, and

---

BOX 13-1 ■ SIGNS OF POSSIBLE DEVELOPMENTAL DELAY IN THE FIRST 5 YEARS OF LIFE[231]

BY 1 MONTH

Sucks poorly and feeds slowly

Lower jaw trembles constantly even when infant is not crying or excited

Does not respond to loud sounds or bright light

Does not focus on and follow a nearby object moving side to side

Rarely moves

Extremities seem loose and floppy or very stiff

BY END OF THIRD MONTH

No Moro reflex

Does not notice own hands by 2 months

Does not grasp and hold objects

Eyes cross most of the time or eyes do track well together

Does not coo or babble

BY END OF FOURTH MONTH

Head flops back when pulled up to sitting by his or her hands

Does not turn head to locate sounds

Does not bring object to mouth

Does not smile spontaneously

Inconsolable at night

BY END OF FIFTH MONTH

Persistent tonic neck reflexes

Cannot maintain head up when placed on stomach or in supported sitting position

Does not reach for objects

Does not roll in both directions

BY THE END OF SEVENTH MONTH

Reaches with one hand only

Cannot sit with help by 6 months

Does not follow objects at a distance

Does not bear some weight on legs

Does not laugh; does not try to attract attention through actions

Refuses to cuddle; shows no affection for caregiver

BY END OF TWELFTH MONTH

Does not creep on all fours

Cannot stand when supported

Does not search for toy hidden while he or she watches

Says no single words (e.g., "mama" or "dada")

Does not use gestures such as waving hand or shaking head; does not point to objects or pictures

BY END OF SECOND YEAR

Cannot walk by 18 months

Failure to develop heel-toe walking pattern after several months of walking

Does not speak at least 15 words by 18 months

Does not use two-word sentences by 2 years

Does not know the function of common objects (brush, telephone, spoon) by 15 months

Does not imitate actions or words; does not follow simple instructions

BY END OF THIRD YEAR

Frequent falling and difficulty with stairs

Persistent drooling or unclear speech

Inability to build a tower of more than four blocks

Difficulty manipulating small objects

Cannot copy a circle

Cannot communicate in short phrases

No pretend play

Little interest in other children

Extreme difficulty separating from caregiver

BY END OF FOURTH YEAR

Cannot throw a ball overhand

Cannot jump in place with both feet

Cannot ride a tricycle

Cannot grasp a crayon between thumb and fingers; cannot scribble

Resists dressing, sleeping, using the toilet

Does not use sentences of more than 3 words; does not use "me" and "you" appropriately

Ignores other children or people outside the family

Does not pretend in play; no interest in interactive games

Persistent poor self-control when angry or upset

BY END OF FIFTH YEAR

Does not engage in a variety of physical activities

Has trouble eating, sleeping, using the toilet

Cannot differentiate between fantasy and reality

Seems unusually passive or aloof with others

Cannot correctly give her or his first and last names

Does not use plurals or past tense when speaking

Does not talk about daily experiences

Does not understand two-part commands

Cannot brush teeth efficiently

Cannot take off clothing

Cannot wash and dry hands

Cannot build a tower of six to eight blocks

Does not express a wide range of emotions

Seems uncomfortable holding a crayon

---

(4) promote and deliver services that build on family and community resources.

Assisting the family in identification of a support group is often helpful for adjustment and continuing encouragement in coping with issues. A comprehensive Web site provided by the Alliance of Genetic Support Groups to locate support groups can be found at http://www. geneticalliance.org.

Assessment Strategies

Knowledge of a child's diagnosis can aid in the selection of appropriate assessment tools and can alert the therapist to any potential medical problems or contraindications associated with the specific syndrome that might affect the assessment procedures (tests and measures). Therapists must be careful, however, not to develop preconceived opinions about a child's capabilities on the basis of how other children with similar diagnoses have performed. It is critical to remember that there is wide behavioral and performance variability among children within each genetic disorder. For example, wide variability in the achievement of developmental milestones has been reported among children with Down syndrome.[171]

The assessment process includes many components that in certain areas are specific to the practice of either physical or occupational therapy. For the physical therapist, use of the *Guide to Physical Therapist Practice*[172] is recommended as a framework to identify appropriate tests and measures for impairments or disabilities. For the occupational therapist a useful reference is the assessment section of the textbook *Occupational Therapy for Children*.[154]

Typically, a therapist's assessment includes observation and testing of the neuromuscular status of the child, such as primitive reflexes, automatic reactions, and muscle tone. For children with orthopedic involvement, assessment of muscle strength, joint range of motion, joint play, and soft tissue mobility is also important. An assessment of the child's developmental level and functional ability should be completed. Such assessments can be used to discriminate between typical and delayed development, to identify the constraints interfering with the achievement of functional skills, and to guide the development of treatment goals and strategies. Most developmental assessment tools fall into one of the following categories: (1) discriminative, (2) predictive, and (3) evaluative measures.[173] Each of these three types of developmental assessment tools yields a different type of information. It is important to understand these differences and the intended purpose for each type of assessment to ensure that evaluation tools are used appropriately. A list of tests and measures commonly used by pediatric physical therapists is summarized in Table 13-3.

Discriminative Assessment

A discriminative assessment is used to compare the ability of an individual with the ability of members of a peer group or with a criterion selected by the test author.[173] Such instruments provide information necessary to document children's eligibility for special services but rarely provide information useful for planning or evaluating therapy programs.[105] Norm-referenced tests such as the Alberta Infant Motor Scale,[174] the Bayley Scales of Infant Development (motor and mental scales),[175] the Peabody Developmental Motor Scales,[176] and the Revised Gesell & Amatruda Developmental & Neurological Examination (adaptive, gross and fine motor, language, and personal/social development)[177] are examples of tests used with infants and young children to verify developmental delay or to assign age levels (Figure 13-11). The Test of Infant Motor Performance is used to identify the risk for developmental delay in infants from 32 weeks post concept to 16 weeks after term.[178] An example of a norm-referenced assessment tool for older children is the Bruininks-Oseretsky Test of Motor Proficiency.[179]

It may be possible to detect improved motor performance by administering a developmental test used to identify children who have motor delays. Such tests, however, usually cannot detect small increments of improvement because there are relatively few test items at each age level and developmental gaps between items are often large. In assessing whether intervention has been effective, the use of most discriminative tools does not examine a child's performance of functional activities in natural environments.[105]

Predictive Assessments

Predictive measures are used to classify individuals according to a set of established categories and to verify whether an individual has been classified correctly.[173] Measures designed to predict future performance are often used to detect early signs of motor impairment in infants who are at risk for neuromotor dysfunction.[105] The Movement Assessment of Infants was designed to assess muscle tone, reflex development, automatic reactions, and volitional movement of infants in the first year of life.[180] The ability of the Movement Assessment of Infants to predict later cerebral palsy has been examined.[181]

Evaluative Assessments

An evaluative measure is used to document change within an individual over time or change occurring as the result of intervention.[173] Helping Babies Learn[182] is a curriculum-referenced test that provides information about a child's developmental progress relative to a prespecified curriculum sequence.

To determine whether a child's ability to perform meaningful skills in everyday environments has improved, a functional assessment should be used. Functional assessments focus on the accomplishment of specific daily activities rather than on the achievement of developmental milestones. Emphasis is placed on the end result in terms of the achievement of a functional task, although the form or quality of the movement should never be ignored by the therapist. Assistance in the form of people or devices is incorporated into the assessment of progress, with the measurement of progress focusing on the achievement of independence.[53] Qualitative aspects of movement that have important functional implications, such as accuracy, speed, endurance, and adaptability, are also considered.

Functional assessments can be used to screen, diagnose, or describe functional deficits and to determine the resources needed to allow the child to function optimally in specific environments (e.g., school, home). Another use of functional assessments is to evaluate the nature of the problem and the specific task requirements limiting function to develop educational plans and teaching strategies.[53] A final use of functional assessments is to examine and monitor for changes in functional status. Such assessments can be used for program evaluation and for determining the cost-effectiveness of services or programs. (See Chapter 8 for additional information regarding evaluation tools.)

The Functional Independence Measure (FIM) is an example of a functional assessment. The FIM assesses the effectiveness of therapy on functional dependence in the areas of self-care, sphincter control, mobility, locomotion, communication, and social cognition.[183] Seven levels of functional dependence ranging from total assistance to complete independence are used to determine an individual's status. An adaptation of the FIM places greater emphasis on functional gains as opposed to the level of care. The WeeFIM[184] has been developed for use with children through the age of 6 years.

TABLE 13-3 ■ TESTS AND MEASURES COMMONLY USED IN PEDIATRIC PHYSICAL THERAPY

TESTS AND MEASURES	AGE RANGE	PURPOSE
Alberta Infant Motor Scale (AIMS)[174]	Birth to 18 months	Identifies motor delays and measures changes in motor performance over time
Batelle Developmental Inventory[232]	Birth to 8 years	Identifies developmental level and monitors changes over time
Canadian Occupational Performance Measure (COPM)[233]	Any age	Identifies changes in parent or child's self perception of performance over time
Bayley Scales of Infant Development, 2nd ed. (BSID-II)[175,231]	1 to 42 months	Identifies developmental delay in gross motor, fine motor, and cognitive domains; monitors progress over time
Berg Balance Scale[234]	5 years and older	Performance-based measure of balance during specific movement tasks
Bruininks-Oseretsky Test of Motor Proficiency (BOTMP)[179]	4.5 to 14.5 years	Identifies motor abilities and can be used for program planning; monitor change over longer periods of time for child with mild disabilities
Child Health Assessment Questionnaire (CHAQ)[235]	Any age	Measures quality of life from patient's or parents' perspective
Child Health Questionnaire[236]	2 months to 15 years	Measures quality of life from patient's or parents' perspective
Denver Developmental Screening Test II[237]	2 weeks to 6.5 years	Screening tool for developmental delay
Early Intervention Developmental Profile[238]	Birth to 3 years	Measures development of gross and fine motor, language, perception, social skills, and self-care skills
Energy Expenditure Index (EEI)[239]	3 years and older	Measures endurance level for activity; monitors changes over time
Functional Independence Measure (FIM)[183]	7 years and older	Measures changes in mobility and activities of daily living skills; used for program evaluation and rehabilitation outcomes assessment
Functional Independence Measure for Children (WeeFIM II)[184]	6 months to 7 years	Measures changes in mobility and activities of daily living skills; used for program evaluation and rehabilitation outcomes assessment
Functional Reach Test (FRT)[240]	4 years and older	Measures anticipatory standing balance during reach
Gross Motor Function Measure (GMFM)[241]	5 months to 16 years	Measures change in gross motor function over time
Harris Infant Neuromotor Test (HINT)[242]	Birth to 12 months	Screening tool to detect early signs of cognitive and neuromotor
Health Utilities Index Mark 3[243]	Any age	Measures child's functional health status; computes cardinal utility value that represents health-related quality of life
Modified Ashworth Scale (MAS)[244]	4 years and older	Qualitative measurement of spasticity through resistance to passive joint movement
Modified Tardieu Scale[245,246]	4 years and older	Qualitative measurement of spasticity through resistance to passive joint movement
Movement Assessment of Infants (MAI)[180]	Birth to 12 months	Identifies motor abilities or dysfunction
Peabody Developmental Motor Scales (PDMS-2)[176]	Birth to 5 years	Identifies gross and fine motor delays; used to monitor progress
Pediatric Clinical Test of Sensory Integration for Balance (P-CTSIB)[247]	4 to 10 years	Measures sensory system contributions to standing balance and postural control
Pediatric Evaluation of Disability Inventory (PEDI)[185]	6 months to 7.5 years	Measures self-care and mobility performance in the home and community Used to monitor progress over time
Revised Gesell and Amatruda Developmental and Neurologic Examination[177]	4 weeks to 36 months	Identify minor deviations in development of gross motor, fine motor, language, and personal/social adaptive domains
School Function Assessment (SFA)[186]	Kindergarten to 6th grade	Measures function in the school environment
Sensory Integration and Praxis Test[248]	4 to 9 years	Measures sensory systems contribution to balance and motor coordination
Sensory Profile[249]	3 to 10 years	Determines which sensory processes contribute to child's performance with activities of daily living
Six Minute Walk Test[250]	5 years and older	Measures walking endurance; monitors progress over time
Test of Infant Motor Performance (TIMP)[178]	32 weeks' gestation to 4 months	Provides early identification of motor delay; assesses postural control for early skills acquisition
Test of Sensory Function in Infants[251]	4 to 18 months	Identifies sensory processing dysfunction and those at risk for developmental delay or learning problems
Timed Up and Go (TUG)[252]	4 years and older	Performance based measure of anticipatory standing balance, gait and motor function
Toddler and Infant Motor Evaluation (TIME)[253]	4 months to 3.5 years	Identifies children with mild to severe motor problems; measures sensory development; monitors progress over time

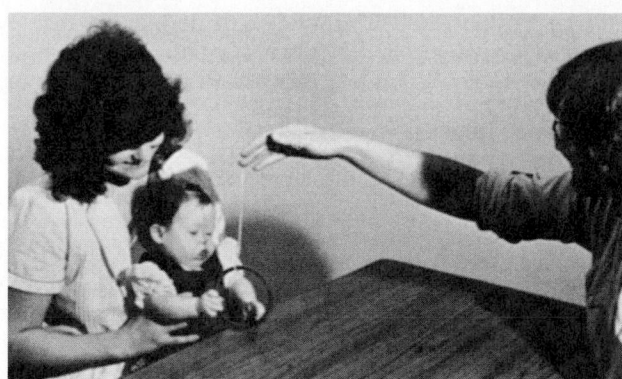

FIGURE 13-11 ■ Four-month-old infant with Down syndrome being assessed with the Bayley Scales of Infant Development.

The Pediatric Evaluation of Disability Inventory (PEDI) is a functional assessment that focuses on the domains of self-care, mobility, and social cognition.[185] The PEDI incorporates three measurement scales: (1) the capability to perform selected functional skills, (2) the level of caregiver assistance that is required, and (3) identification of environmental modifications or equipment needed to perform a particular activity. The PEDI has been standardized and normed and is intended for use with children whose abilities are in the range of a typical 6-month-old to 7-year-old child.

The final example of a functional assessment is the School Function Assessment (SFA).[186] The SFA is designed to measure a student's performance in accomplishing functional tasks in the school environment. It is composed of three sections that focus on (1) the student's participation in major school activities, (2) the task supports needed by the student for participation, and (3) the student's activity performance. The SFA is standardized and was conceptually developed to be reflective of the functional requirements of a student in elementary school.

Family-Driven Goals and Objectives

After a child's strengths and needs are evaluated and the family's objectives identified, therapy goals and objectives can be developed. In the past, establishment of these goals has primarily been the responsibility of professionals and often did not incorporate the needs and desires of the family. More recently, however, professionals have recognized the value of having families guide the process of establishing intervention goals and objectives.[187,188] This shift toward collaborative goal setting and family-centered care has occurred largely as a result of the belief that families should determine their vision of the future for their children and that professionals should act as consultants and resources to assist families in achieving that vision. The stress that caregivers experience with the everyday care of a child can reduce compliance with a home therapeutic program,[189] which further supports the notion that parents should be jointly involved with therapists to determine goals and the means by which to attain identified outcomes.[190] For children living in the United States, these goals are developed within the context of individualized service plans.

Individualized Service Plans

In the United States, children with disabilities are guaranteed the right to free and appropriate public education. Beginning with the enactment of United States Public Law 94-142 in 1975[191] and several important legislative revisions in 1990 (Individuals with Disabilities Education Act),[191-193] 1991 (PL 102-119), 1997 (PL 105-17), and 2004 (PL 108-446, Individuals with Disabilities Education Improvement Act of 2004),[194] physical and occupational therapists working in public school settings are required to establish long-term annual goals and short-term therapy objectives within the framework of each child's educational needs. The document that defines a child's educational needs, including therapy services, from preschool to twelfth grade is the individualized education program (IEP). The components of an IEP are as follows[192-194]:

1. A statement of the child's current levels of educational performance
2. A statement of measurable annual goals, including short-term instructional objectives
3. A statement of the specific special education and related services to be provided to the child and a statement of program modifications or supports for school personnel
4. The projected dates for initiation of services and the anticipated duration of the service
5. Appropriate objective criteria and evaluation procedures and schedules for determining, at least annually, whether short-term instructional objectives are being achieved
6. An explanation of the extent to which the child will not participate with nondisabled children in the regular class
7. A statement of transition services that will be provided for the child

Similar requirements are in effect for infants to preschool-age children, documented in the individualized family service plan (IFSP). An IFSP must be written after a multidisciplinary assessment of the strengths and needs of the child is completed. This assessment must include a family-directed assessment of the supports and services necessary to enhance the family's capacity to meet the needs of their child with a disability.[193,194] The IFSP must contain the following:

1. A statement of the child's current levels of development (cognitive, speech/language, psychosocial, motor, and self-help)
2. A statement of the family's resources, priorities, and concerns related to enhancing the child's development
3. A statement of major outcomes expected to be achieved for the child and family
4. The criteria, procedures, and time lines for determining progress
5. The specific early-intervention services necessary to meet the unique needs of the child and family, including the method, frequency, and intensity of service
6. The natural environments in which services shall be provided
7. The projected dates for the initiation of services and expected duration
8. The name of the service coordinator
9. The procedures for transition from early intervention to the preschool program

Functional Objectives

The development of behaviorally written, measurable therapy objectives is crucial for monitoring the effects of intervention in a child with a genetic disorder. Many of the clinical symptoms listed in the descriptions of genetic disorders described earlier in the chapter may be monitored through systematic, periodic, data-keeping procedures. One example is the monitoring of functional hand skills in girls with Rett syndrome. Periodic vital capacity measures for a child with OI or a child with Werdnig-Hoffmann disease can reflect progress toward a goal of maintaining respiratory function.

Typically, in the past, therapy objectives focus on a child's deficits. For example, delays in achieving motor milestones are often used to identify gaps in development, and therapy objectives are written and programs established to address these deficits. When the child meets an objective, new deficits are identified and new objectives are developed. A different model for goal development that is consistent with a family-centered intervention philosophy, is the "top-down" approach, described by Campbell[195] and later by McEwen[196] and Effgren.[135] In this model, the child and family identify a desired functional outcome that is the driving factor for the therapeutic intervention plan. An example of this approach is seen in Goal Attainment Scales. Goal attainment scaling is a variation of behavioral objectives that detects small, clinically important changes over time.[197] Similar to behavioral objectives, goal attainment scaling requires (1) identification of observable goals, (2) reproducibility of conditions under which performance is measured, (3) measurable criteria for success, and (4) a time frame for goal achievement. In contrast to behavioral objectives, however, goal attainment scaling identifies five possible outcomes with accompanying score values: two outcomes that surpass the expected level, the expected-level outcome, and two outcomes that fall below the expected level. By using five possible levels of attainment, it can be determined whether a child has made progress despite not achieving the expected outcome or whether progress has exceeded the expected outcome.

Following is an example of the use of goal attainment scaling to assess Maile's first functional objective:

−2 = With physical assistance, Maile will climb up the rungs of a 4-foot-high slide by (date)

−1 = With physical assistance, Maile will climb up the rungs of a 4-foot-high slide and seat herself at the top with feet pointed down the decline of the slide by (date).

  0 = With standby assistance, Maile will climb up the rungs of a 4-foot-high slide and seat herself at the top with feet pointed down the decline of the slide by (date).

+1 = Maile will climb up and seat herself at the top of a 4-foot-high slide independently, slide down, and stop at the bottom with assistance to prevent losing her balance by (date).

+2 = Maile will climb up and seat herself at the top of a 4-foot-high slide, slide down, and stop at the bottom independently by (date).

Rather than focusing on a child's deficits, such "outcome-focused" objectives provide a more positive and supportive context for therapy and at the same time address the family's needs and priorities. This approach to developing therapy goals and objectives in ways that support positive family functioning is also an important aspect of delivering therapy services to children and their families.

General Treatment Principles

Several general treatment principles guide the delivery of therapy services to children with genetic disorders. A description of each of these principles is followed by examples illustrating their applicability to particular children. A discussion of treatment techniques that target specific impairments is beyond the scope of this chapter and are included in pediatric textbooks of clinical practice. The reader is also referred to Chapter 9 on Interventions for Clients with Movement Dysfunction.

Focus on Functional Skills

Many of the classic therapeutic exercise approaches for individuals with neurological disorders are oriented toward making qualitative changes in motor tasks, such as normalizing muscle tone or improving gait symmetry. Often, there is little regard for the functional significance of those changes.[198] More recent therapeutic approaches place less emphasis on such qualitative changes and instead focus on the motor behaviors necessary to acquire functional skills. In this approach, environmental adaptations and assistive technology are used to attain functional outcomes such as independence in self-help skills, communication, and mobility[198] (Figure 13-12).

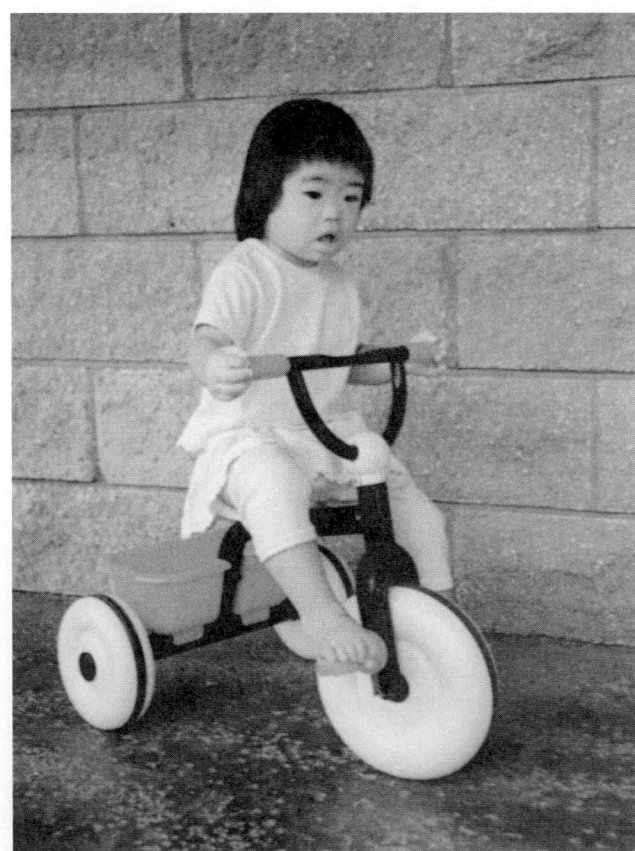

FIGURE 13-12 ■ Child with Down syndrome during practice of functional motor skills.

This shift to a focus on functional skills is consistent with recent task-oriented approaches to neurological rehabilitation. The task-oriented model assumes that control of movement is organized around goal-directed, functional behaviors rather than on muscle or movement patterns.[146,199] Intervention, therefore, is aimed at teaching motor problem solving (adaptability to varied contexts), developing effective compensations that are maximally efficient, and providing practice of new motor skills in functional situations. Rather than teaching individuals to perform movement patterns in a controlled therapy setting, this approach focuses on the learning that must take place for an individual to function independently of a therapist's guidance.[146,200]

Delivery of Services in Natural Environments

Functional skills are most meaningfully taught and practiced within the context in which they will be used.[201] The movement toward integrating therapy into classroom settings is one example of providing services in a natural environment.[202-204] In an integrated model of service delivery, therapists work in the classroom with teachers, rather than removing students to an isolated therapy room to provide services. Therapists work closely with the teacher to establish common goals for the student and to devise programs that will allow therapeutic activities to be interwoven into a variety of activities throughout the day in a natural manner.

Another example of providing therapy in a natural environment is providing home-based services for infants and young children. Home-based programs are "normal" options for young children because the natural environment for most infants and toddlers is the home—either their own or that of a day-care provider.[202-204] For children who are medically fragile, it is the preferred option for therapy.[205] For other families, transportation to a center-based program may be difficult because of the expense or length of travel required.

Incorporating Therapy Activities into Daily Routines

Therapists need to work collaboratively with families to develop activities that incorporate therapeutic activities into the family's daily routine (e.g., during play, dressing, bathing, meals). Rather than practicing narrowly defined tasks in a controlled clinic environment, therapy activities should be interwoven into a variety of activities throughout the day in a natural manner. Practicing skills in the context of daily routines allows the child to learn to adapt to the real-life contingencies that arise during a functional task.[200] In addition, activities become more meaningful to both the child and the family (Figure 13-13).

Use of Assistive Technology Devices

As noted previously, an important aspect of providing developmental therapy services is the use of assistive technology devices to maximize a child's functional abilities, level of independence, and inclusion in school and community activities with peers. Examples of assistive technology include mobility devices, augmentative communication devices, and adapted computer keyboards. Assistive technology also includes adaptive devices such as splints, bath chairs, prone standers, and other positioning equipment that can be used to provide optimal body alignment and minimize the risk for contractures or deformities while encouraging a greater

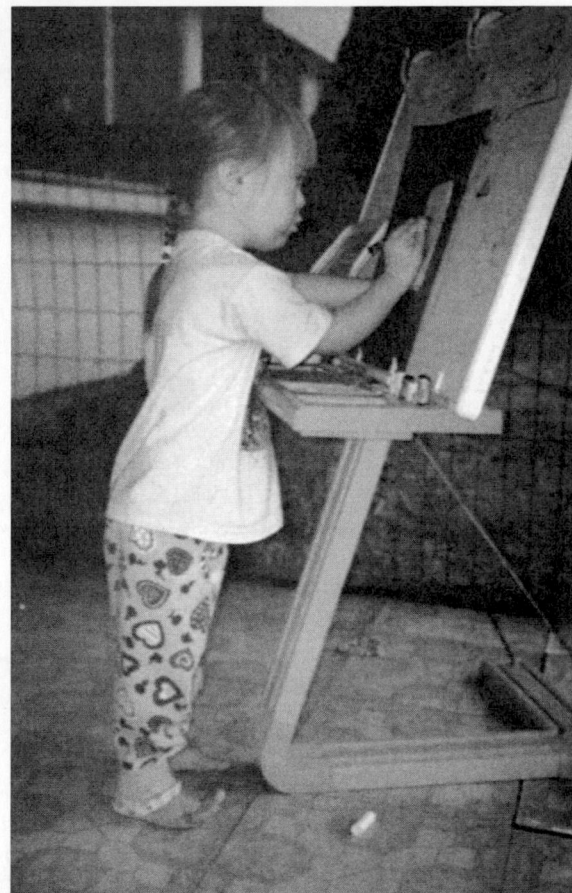

FIGURE 13-13 ■ Practice of developmental skills during daily routine at home.

variety of movement patterns. Such devices can be constructed from readily available materials or obtained commercially. The developmental physical or occupational therapist works with the family and other team members to select, construct, or order assistive devices and to assist caregivers in the use of the devices.

The case example demonstrates how these general treatment principles are applied to a particular child receiving therapy services. The case example also shows how the family's priorities and needs are considered and supported in the planning and delivery of services (see Case 13-1: Part 3, pg. 408).

MEDICAL MANAGEMENT AND GENETIC COUNSELING

The physical or occupational therapist should have general knowledge of both medical management of children with genetic disorders and genetic counseling for family members. This information allows the therapist to answer the family's general questions and to refer family members to the appropriate persons for more specific information.

Medical Management

Few medical therapies have been successful in treating genetic disorders in children, although a number of strategies for ameliorating isolated symptoms have been reported.[206] Of the genetic disorders discussed in this

CASE STUDY 13-1 ■ PART 1—USE OF THE WORLD WIDE WEB TO ACCESS INFORMATION ON PATHOPHYSIOLOGY AND IMPAIRMENTS

Maile is a 3-year-old girl with Down syndrome (trisomy 21) who was referred to you for development of a therapy program. You have not worked with children with Down syndrome, but having access to the WWW you decide to look up the syndrome on the electronic database called Online Mendelian Inheritance in Man (OMIM), which is maintained by the National Center for Biotechnology.[8] You activate your WWW browser (a program that runs on an Internet-connected computer and provides access to the WWW) and type in http//www.ncbi.nlm.nih.gov/omim, which is the Internet home page address for OMIM.* At the OMIM home page you select "Search the OMIM Database," which takes you to the area of OMIM where you can

search using key words. By typing in "Down syndrome" you are taken to information on trisomy 21, and additional information on Down syndrome can be found on the OMIM Web site or the suggested link sites on the WWW. The link sites from the OMIM site include direct access to PubMed, which is the National Library of Medicine search service for Medline and other related databases.[229] These reference tools are highly recommended to the clinician because the information on and number of new syndromes or diseases with genetic etiology are increasing each year. A concise synopsis of genetic syndromes can also be found in *Smith's Recognizable Patterns of Human Malformation* by Jones if WWW access is not available.[42]

*More detailed information on accessing the WWW for genetic information can be found in a review article by Phillips.[228] The article also includes an annotated bibliography of WWW sites related to genetics.

CASE STUDY 13-1 ■ PART 2—PROGRAM PLANNING

On developmental testing, Maile displays deficits in single-leg stance stability. A typical developmental therapy objective might be, "Maile will balance on one foot for at least 3 seconds, two out of three trials." In Maile's IFSP meeting, however, her parents expressed the hope that Maile would be able to play safely with her peers at a neighborhood playground—a more functionally relevant goal. The following therapy objectives were developed to address her need to

develop single-limb stance stability within the context of the family-identified goal:

1. With standby assistance, Maile will climb up the rungs of a 4-foot-high slide and seat herself at the top with feet pointed down the decline of the slide by June 1994.
2. Maile will be able to walk independently across a 25-foot stretch of uneven ground (sand or lawn) without falling by June 1994.

CASE STUDY 13-1 ■ PART 3—INTERVENTION

The primary concerns of the parents were Maile's motor skills involving her playground abilities. Therefore, the therapist scheduled Maile's weekly therapy session during the classroom playground time. In this way, the therapist would be able to help Maile improve her strength, endurance, and coordination in the context in which these skills need to be used. Therapy occurring on the playground will provide opportunities for Maile to learn how to assess the demands of the environment and to match them with her abilities. In this natural setting, she will also learn a

variety of strategies to adapt to changing conditions. For example, when faced with the task of negotiating the playground slide, Maile will have to learn how to compensate for her low muscle tone and joint laxity so that she can climb up the ladder to sit on the top of the slide. Working on postural stability, single-leg stance, and shoulder girdle stabilization in this context will be more motivating than practicing these same skills in an isolated therapy room and will likely be facilitated by Maile's classmates, who can serve as models.

chapter, the only one for which dramatic results have been achieved through early medical management is PKU. With early diagnosis and immediate implementation of a low-phenylalanine diet, the infant with PKU can be spared the severe mental retardation and other progressive neurological impairments that have resulted without treatment.[100]

Medical treatment for the other disorders is not curative but rather palliative or directed at specific associated anomalies. The congenital heart defects present in an estimated

40% to 60% of individuals with Down syndrome can, in most instances, be corrected by cardiac surgery.[21] Orthopedic surgery in the form of insertion of intramedullary rods in the tibia or femur may minimize the recurrence of repeated fractures associated with OI.[137]

Surgical correction of scoliosis may be warranted in individuals with neurofibromatosis, Rett syndrome,[122] or Werdnig-Hoffmann disease [207,208] if the deformity is severe and bracing is not successful. Radiographic screening for atlantoaxial instability in children with Down syndrome can be initiated beginning at age 2 years.[21] If atlantoaxial instability is excessive or results in a neurological deficit, a posterior fusion of the cervical vertebrae is recommended.[31] Surgical removal of obstructive or malignant tumors is advisable in certain cases of neurofibromatosis, as is removal of cerebral nodular growths for the control of seizures in individuals with tuberous sclerosis.

The use of appetite-regulating drugs for individuals with PWS has had equivocal results. Surgical interventions such as gastric bypass, small intestinal bypass, and jaw wiring have been attempted for weight control with these individuals but have met with limited success.[73]

Respiratory therapy is an important adjunctive treatment strategy for children with CF or Werdnig-Hoffmann disease[207] and should be implemented as part of the overall therapy program. Specific medical therapies include estrogen therapy to promote feminization in individuals with Turner's syndrome and testosterone therapy to enhance secondary sex characteristics in boys with Klinefelter's syndrome.[209] The use of anticonvulsants is an important part of seizure management for individuals with Rett syndrome[122] and tuberous sclerosis.[94] Allopurinol has been used for individuals with Lesch-Nyhan syndrome to prevent urological complications, although it has no effect on the progressive neurological symptoms.[97]

The use of large, potentially toxic amounts of vitamins and minerals (the orthomolecular hypothesis) has been proposed for children with many different types of developmental disabilities.[210] This approach has been rejected for children with Down syndrome on the basis of the results of several investigations. In addition, supplementation of individual metabolites such as 5-hydroxytryptophan or pyridoxine for children with Down syndrome is ineffective.[211]

Proponents of cell therapy, which involves intramuscular injection of fetal lamb brain tissue, claim that many of the morphological and developmental characteristics of Down syndrome can be altered. These claims have not been supported by clinical investigations, and opponents of cell therapy warn of the potential risk for serious allergic reactions.[212]

Gene therapy could potentially correct defective genes responsible for disease, but there has not yet been much success in clinical trials. Gene therapy is still only experimental and is moving along cautiously in the United States. In 1999, and again in 2003, individuals died while participating in gene therapy trials.[1] As of April 2006, the U.S. Food and Drug Administration has not approved any human gene therapy products for sale[213] but more than 600 gene therapy protocols have been developed.[1] In addition to Food and Drug Administration approval, trials that are funded by the National Institutes of Health (NIH) must be registered with the NIH Recombinant DNA Advisory Committee. The NIH, which includes more than 20 institutes and offices, is the federal focal point for biomedical research in the United States.

Gene therapy can take on many different forms, from altering human somatic cells to techniques that involve the replacement of a missing gene product by inserting a normal gene into a somatic cell. Because viruses have the ability to insert their genes into somatic cells, attention is being focused on using viruses that have been modified to include the desired genetic information. To date, a gene therapy protocol is under way for Duchenne muscular dystrophy but not for any of the disorders described in this chapter. The interested reader can obtain an up-to-date listing of current gene therapy protocols from the NIH's Office of Biotechnology on the World Wide Web (WWW) at http://www.nih.gov/od/oba/.

In light of the limited medical treatment strategies available for children with genetic disorders, the physical or occupational therapist must be concerned with maximizing the child's developmental or functional potential within the limitations imposed by the lack of possible cures and the prospect of the shortened life span that characterizes many of these disorders. When deterioration of skills is expected, therapy must be directed at maintaining current functioning levels, minimizing decline, and minimizing caregiver support as possible.

Genetic Counseling

Developmental physical or occupational therapists must have an understanding of the modes of inheritance of the various genetic disorders and information about the services that can be offered through genetic counseling. Although the physician has primary responsibility for informing the parents of a child with a genetic disorder about the availability of genetic counseling, the close professional and personal relationships that therapists often develop with families may prompt family members to seek this type of information from the therapist.

Although a physical or occupational therapist cannot substitute for the role of a qualified genetic counselor, it is important that therapists be aware of the availability and location of genetic counseling services so that they may be assured that parents of a child with a genetic disorder have this information. Most major university-affiliated medical centers provide genetic counseling.

Process of Genetic Counseling

Six steps or procedures in genetic counseling have been discussed by Novitski.[214] The first is to make an accurate medical diagnosis of the child's disorder. In the case of a suspected chromosome abnormality, this usually involves determining the karyotype of the child and possibly the karyotypes of the parents. Other diagnostic procedures may include a medical examination, FISH, DNA studies, biochemical studies, muscle biopsy, and other laboratory tests.

The next step in genetic counseling is to construct a pedigree or family tree of all known relatives and ancestors of both parents.[214] Pedigree information includes the age at death and cause of death of ancestors, a history of stillbirths and spontaneous abortions, and a history of appearance of any other genetic defects or unknown causes of mental retardation. The country of origin of ancestors is also important because certain genetic defects, such as PKU, are far more prevalent in families of a particular ethnic origin. Once the defect has been identified and a pedigree constructed, Novitski[214] advises that further information be obtained from one of the comprehensive resource texts on genetic disorders. Informing family members about the characteristics of the disorder and its natural history may diminish fears of the unknown.

The third procedure in genetic counseling is to estimate the risk of recurrence of the disorder.[213] In specific gene defects, the probability of recurrence is fairly straightforward, with a risk of 25% for autosomal recessive disorders and a 50% risk for each male child in sex-linked disorders. These percentages, however, do not hold true in cases of spontaneous mutations. In cases of chromosomal abnormalities, such as Down syndrome, karyotyping is mandated to determine whether the child has the translocation type of Down syndrome. In that case the risk of recurrence is much greater than with a history of standard trisomy 21 Down syndrome.

Informing parents of the probability of recurrence is the next procedure. Novitski[214] points out the common misunderstanding that if a risk is 1:4 for a child to be affected, as in an autosomal recessive disorder, many parents assume that if they have just given birth to a child with the disorder, the next three children should be normal. It is important to explain that each subsequent child faces a 1:4 risk of inheriting the disorder regardless of how many siblings with the disorder have already been born. Estimating the risk of multifactorial disorders is a complex process. Although these conditions tend to cluster in families, there is no clear-cut pedigree pattern. The risk for recurrence of a multifactorial disorder is typically low, but if a couple has had two children with the same condition, the recurrence risk is presumed higher with either a high genetic susceptibility or a chronic environmental insult suspected.

The fifth step in genetic counseling is for the parents to decide on the course of action they will take for future pregnancies once the counselor has presented all available facts to them.[213] Some parents may choose not to have any more children; others may elect to undergo prenatal diagnostic procedures for subsequent pregnancies. These decisions rest entirely with the parents and may be influenced by their individual religious or ethical preferences.

Follow-up counseling and review of the most recent advances in medical genetics are the final steps in the genetic counseling procedure.[214] Genetic counseling can play an important role in opening channels of communication between parents, other family members, and their friends; connecting parents and siblings to support groups; and helping families to address their grief, sadness, or anger.[17] The effect of a child's disability on the family may modify the parents' earlier decision to have or not to have more children. Recent medical advances may allow a more certain prenatal diagnosis of specific genetic disorders.

Early Detection of Genetic Conditions

Many genetic disorders are made clinically, as in observation of a congenital malformation; however, many serious conditions are not immediately apparent after birth. Detection of genetic conditions is performed through various screening procedures, followed by specific diagnostic testing to confirm a suspected disorder. With technological advancements in genetics, these procedures have been expanded for the unborn and the newborn. Couples planning to have children can be tested for specific genetic disorders before conception or embryonic implantation.[215] Health care professionals and parents should be informed about both the positive and negative aspects of exercising this new knowledge and technology.

Newborn Screening

Routine newborn screening is required practice in the United States. Screening is performed on whole populations for common disorders. The purpose of screening is the early identification of infants who are affected by a certain condition for which early treatment is warranted and available. Of the 4 million newborn infants screened each year, approximately 3000 have detectible disorders.[216] Currently, all 50 states require screening for three disorders: PKU, congenital hypothyroidism, and galactosemia (national newborn screening and genetic report). Some populations known to be at higher risk of certain disorders may be screened automatically, or individuals may elect screening, state specific.[216] Tandem mass spectrometry (MS/MS) is a laboratory technique that allows for the identification several metabolic disorders using a single analysis of a small blood sample drawn from the neonate. Many states use MS/MS for newborn screening for various disorders and have expanded their list of those that are mandated and those that are part of limited pilot programs.[217] Some genetic screening is performed primarily for research purposes when the disorder is not preventable, for example, type I diabetes. Screening for type I diabetes is available in some states and early reports are that 90% of parents consent to the test.[218]

Benefits of newborn screening are earlier definitive diagnosis and medical intervention for the affected child. Concerns about expanded newborn screening include hasty medical decisions before conclusive evidence is available, and parental stress because of a lag time in screening and definitive results. A study by Waisbren et al[219] conducted with parents of children screened for biochemical genetic disorders recognized that parents generally reported less stress the earlier a diagnosis could be made. However, in the same study, in cases where the test yielded a false-positive result, parents reported a higher stress index and their children were twice as likely to experience hospitalization (usually the emergency department) than in mothers of children with normal screening results.[219] In the case of a positive screening result, infants will typically undergo more definitive genetic testing.

Genetic Testing in Infants and Children

Many genetic disorders can be diagnosed by clinical criteria specific to that disorder. If a diagnosis cannot be made on the basis of the patient's clinical presentation, then genetic testing may be warranted. There are currently about 900 genetic tests that can be offered by diagnostic laboratories; specific information can be found at http://www.genetests.org. In the United States, the standards and methods of all laboratories performing clinical genetic tests are governed at the federal level.[215]

Prenatal Testing

Tests to diagnose a genetic disorder in a developing fetus can be placed into the two broad categories of invasive and noninvasive procedures. Currently, in contrast to the most common invasive procedures, noninvasive methods typically cannot give a definitive diagnosis, but they can be performed with less risk to the fetus. Invasive procedures are recommended in cases of high risk for a serious disorder, when definitive diagnosis could lead to treatment, and to allow parents to make decisions about the pregnancy.[220] The ethical implications for prenatal testing are many. Parents are often given information that requires a sophisticated understanding of biology and medicine to fully understand the implications and results of a diagnostic procedure. For example, amniocentesis can detect many chromosomal abnormalities, but the functional outcome of some disorders can have great variety.[221]

Invasive Procedures. The most common prenatal diagnostic procedure is amniocentesis, which is used to detect early genetic disorders in the fetus at 11 to 20 weeks' gestation.[220] This method involves inserting a long, slender needle through the mother's abdominal wall and into the placenta to extract a small amount of amniotic fluid.[222] Laboratory tests of amniotic fluid reveal all types of chromosome abnormalities and a number of specific gene defects, including Lesch-Nyhan syndrome, and some disorders of multifactorial inheritance, such as neural tube defects. This procedure carries a risk of miscarriage of about 0.5% to 1.7%,[223] and the risk increases the earlier that it is performed.[220]

Chorionic villus sampling involves extracting and examining a portion of the placental tissue. It has nearly a 99% detection rate for chromosome abnormalities[220] and it can be definitive earlier than amniocentesis; however, the risk of severe limb defects (amniotic band syndrome) increases the earlier that it is performed. The miscarriage rate with this procedure is estimated to be 0.5%.[220]

Noninvasive Procedures. Ultrasonographic examination of a fetus has been used to identify congenital malformations since 1956. It is currently offered to most women in the United States. It is currently believed that there is no inherent risk from this procedure. First-semester sonography is performed mainly to confirm the gestational age, to identify multiple pregnancy, and to measure nuchal thickness (NT). NT is a measure of the subcutaneous space between the skin and the cervical spin in the fetus; increased NT is often associated with trisomies. Second-trimester ultrasonography can detect problems in the quantity of amniotic fluid, large fetal structural defects, and certain smaller defects associated with a genetic disorder. A definitive diagnosis is not made on the basis of the presence of small defects alone, but the findings are considered along with the other risk factors present.[224] Again, there are ethical questions about the risk to the parents (emotional stress and uncertainty) versus the benefits of early detection.

Tests of maternal serum screening done about 15 to 20 weeks' gestation can detect chromosomal abnormalities, but the accuracy depends on many factors, such as gestational age, maternal weight, ethnicity, multiple pregnancy, maternal type I diabetes, and maternal smoking.[220] Finally, it is possible to perform cytogenic analysis of fetal blood cells that can be isolated from a sample of the mother's blood, but this requires expensive equipment and expertise.[220]

Assisted Reproduction and Preimplantation Genetic Diagnosis

Couples who want to conceive often seek genetic counseling if one or more parents is aware of a familial genetic condition, if they are having difficulty conceiving, and commonly in cases of advanced maternal or paternal age. More than 1000 babies have been born worldwide after as a result of in vitro fertilization.[225] In vitro fertilization has enabled couples with fertility problems to conceive and more recently is used to diagnose a genetic disease or condition in an embryo when it has differentiated into just eight cells.[225] Chromosomal abnormalities are the most common detected abnormality, and approximately 100 single-gene disorders have been diagnosed.[225] The ultimate purpose of preimplantation genetic diagnosis is to implant only mutation-free embryos into the mother's uterus.

Ethics in Genetics

Advancements in genetics have led to important ethical questions about testing and screening for genetic disorders during the course of a couple's family planning and after the birth of the child. Ethical debates about genetic testing are inevitable. Traditionally in pediatric medicine, parents are presumed to be best suited to make the decision whether to pursue genetic testing, but organizations such as the American Academy of Pediatrics have argued that parental autonomy should not be absolute.[2] Pediatricians and other health care professionals should be able to help families with the decision-making process about genetic testing. Ross and Moon[2] propose a decision algorithm that weighs the risks and benefits of genetic testing. A decision to pursue genetic testing would be advised if the child was symptomatic, had a suspected genetic condition or was from a high-risk family, if early diagnosis would decrease morbidity or mortality, and if the testing method was considered ethical and it would lead to a beneficial treatment.

INTEGRATING GENETICS INFORMATION FOR PRACTICAL USE IN PEDIATRIC CLINICAL SETTINGS

Therapists in all settings frequently find it challenging to keep up on practice issues and the growing body of knowledge and evidence in rehabilitative medicine. In clinical settings where most of a therapist's day is spent in actual hands-on treatment, the wealth of information that is available may seem burdensome and practically inaccessible. Patients and their families will present the therapist with many questions about medical interventions, diagnostic procedures, and research. Although therapists know that a working knowledge of all of these areas is important, often time constraints and access to resources are limited.

Pediatric therapists know the importance of a collaboration with other professionals, including a type of collective knowledge about the child and his or her diagnosis, impairments, functional limitations, and quality of life issues identified by the family. A 1998 survey of individuals from six different health professionals, including physical therapists, revealed that most professionals are not confident in their education and working knowledge in the field of genetics.[226] There are additional studies that have indicated that there are not enough genetic counselors[2,219] to meet the growing need of patients and families and that those patients often express the most stress and dissatisfaction because their primary care physician does not appear to be informed about their child's disorder.[219]

Basic Knowledge and Skills Competence

Most physical therapists responding to the survey reported by Long et al[226] reported that they received most of their information through nonscientific media and that they had limited or no education in genetics. Furthermore, it was expressed that physical therapists wanted continuing education in genetics to include topics such as the role of genetics in common disorders such as cancer and heart

---

BOX 13-2 ■ RESOURCES ON TOPICS IN GENETICS FOR CLINICIANS AND FAMILIES

TEXTBOOKS

1. Jorde LB, Carey JC, Bamshad MC et al: *Medical genetics,* ed 2. St. Louis, 2000, Mosby.
   Review for clinicians of basic genetic science, helpful illustrations.

JOURNAL ARTICLES

1. Therrell BL: Integrating genetic services into public health-guidance for state and territorial programs from the National Newborn Screening and Genetics Resource Center (Austin). *Commun Genet* 4:175-196, 2001.
   Useful reference for therapists working in early intervention services to aid in understanding a model of collaboration with other health care agencies.

WORLD WIDE WEB

1. Human Genome Projects Information (U.S. Department of Energy–funded site): http://www.ornl.gov/sci/techresources/Human_Genome/home.shtml.
   Research, updates on the Human Genome Project and current gene therapy:
2. Clinical Trials.gov (National Institutes of Health): http://www.clinicaltrials.gov/search.
   Current information on state of clinical trials for gene therapy.
3. Virtual Children's Hospital. Children's Hospital of Iowa:http://www.vh.org/pediatric/provider/pediatrics/ClinicalGenetics.
   Clinical genetics self-study courses (free) for health care providers.
4. American College of Medical Genetics: http://www.acmg.net/.
   Information about educational courses in genetics for health care professionals.
5. Genetics and Public Policy Center: http://www.dnapolicy.org/about/mission.jhtml.html.
   Information on current available genetics testing and family planning.
6. National newborn screening report. National Newborn Screening and Genetics Resource Center, Austin, TX: http://genes-r-us.uthscsa.edu/resources/newborn/oo/2000report.pdf.
   Lists what genetic screening tests are being performed in the 50 United States. Gives definitions of various genetic disorders.
7. Genetics and public health in the 21st century. Using genetic information to improve health and prevent disease: http://www.cdc.gov.genomics/info/books/21stcentury.htm.
   Describes how data are collected for public surveillance of genetic disorders. Guidelines for professional training and integration of genetics knowledge in practice.

---

disease, an overview of human genetics, what treatments were available, and how to direct clients to information resources. Although occupational therapists were not part of this study, it is felt colleagues would stress similar needs.

The National Coalition for Health Professional Education in Genetics is an organization of individuals from approximately 120 health profession. They have proposed basic competencies for all health care professionals.[9] With a working knowledge about genetics, therapists can develop competence in eliciting and accessing genetic information from subjective interviews with proper patient consent, can learn how to protect patient privacy while making appropriate recommendations to genetics professionals, and understand the social and psychological implications of genetic services.[226,227]

SUMMARY

In this chapter we have addressed several chromosomal abnormalities and specific gene defects that are most likely to be seen in children in a typical developmental therapy setting. The inclusion of family members in all aspects of therapy has been stressed, along with the need to consider family goals, priorities, and resources in the development and implementation of therapy services. The importance of developing functional goals and delivering services in natural environments has also been emphasized. Last, many diseases or conditions have a genetic component that must be considered in the course of medical management. Physical and occupational therapists should expand their working knowledge of genetics to appropriately refer patients for genetic services.[228-230] Readers are encouraged to consult Box 13-2 for a list of resources about genetic disorders, education, testing, and interventions not described in this chapter.

ACKNOWLEDGMENTS

We wish to acknowledge the contributions of Wayne A. Struberg, PhD, PT, PCS, and Warren G. Sanger, PhD, to the writing of the previous edition's version of this chapter.

REFERENCES

1. Wellcome Trust Sanger Institute, International Partners of Human Genome Project: http://www.sanger.ac.uk/HGP/draft2000/mainrelease.shtml. Accessed February 6, 2005.
2. Ross L, Moon M: Ethical issues in genetic testing of children, *Arch Pediatr Adolesc Med* 154:873-879, 2000.
3. Weatherall DJ: *The new genetics and clinical practice,* ed 3, New York, 1991, Oxford University Press.
4. Sanger WG, Bhavana D, Struberg W: Overview of genetics and role of the pediatric physical therapist in the diagnostic process, *Pediatr Phys Ther* 13:164-168, 2001.
5. Poirot L: Genetic disorders and engineering: Implications for physical therapists, *PT Magazine* 13:54-60, 2005.
6. Jorde LB, Carey JC, Bamshad MJ et al: *Medical genetics,* ed 2, St. Louis, 2000, Mosby.
7. Gene tests: Medical genetics information resource, University of Washington, Seattle, 1993-2005: http:///www.genetests.org. Accessed February 14-20, 2005.
8. Online Mendelian Inheritance in Man: Center for Medical Genetics, Johns Hopkins University (Baltimore, MD) and national center for biotechnology information. US National Library of Medicine (Bethesda, MD), 1998-2005: http//www.ncbi.nlm.nih.gov/omim. Accessed January 19-February 20, 2005.

9. McInerney JD: *Principles of genetics for health professionals.* National Coalition for Health Professional Education in Genetics (NCHPEG), 2004: http://www.nchpeg.org/eduresources/core/core/asp. Accessed February 19, 2005.

10. Shanske A, Shanske S, DiMauro S: The other human genome, *Arch Pediatr Adolesc Med* 155:1210-1216, 2001.

11. Skladal D, Halliday J, Thorburn D: Minimum birth prevalence of mitochondrial respiratory chain disorders in children, *Brain* 126:1905-1912, 2003.

12. Simpson JL, Golbus MS: *Genetics in obstetrics and gynecology,* Philadelphia, 1992, WB Saunders.

13. Smith DW: Clinical diagnosis and nature of chromosomal abnormalities. In Yunis J, editor: *New chromosomal syndromes,* New York, 1977, Academic Press.

14. Centers for Disease Control and Prevention: Racial disparities in median age at death of persons with Down syndrome—United States, 1968-1997, *Morb Mortal Wkly Rep* June 8, 2001, http://www.cdc.gov/mmwr. Accessed February 18, 2005.

15. Harris SR, Shea AM: Down syndrome. In Campbell SK, editor: *Pediatric neurologic physical therapy,* ed 2, New York, 1991, Churchill Livingstone.

16. Thacker P: Biological clock ticks for men, too: Genetic defects linked to sperm of older fathers, *JAMA* 291:1683-1685, 2004.

17. Crome L, Stern J: *Pathology of mental retardation,* ed 2, Edinburgh, 1972, Churchill Livingstone.

18. Robinson NM, Robinson HB, editors. *The mentally retarded child: a psychological approach,* New York, 1976, McGraw-Hill.

19. Hall D: Mongolism in newborn infants, *Clin Pediatr* 5:4-12, 1978.

20. Cowie VA: *A study of the early development of Mongols,* Oxford, 1970, Pergamon Press.

21. Msall ME, DiGaudio KM, Malone AF: Health, developmental and psychosocial aspects of Down syndrome, *Infants Young Child* 4:35-45, 1991.

22. Bell AJ, Bhate MS: Prevalence of overweight and obesity in Down's syndrome and other mentally handicapped adults living in the community, *J Intellect Disabil Res* 36:359-364, 1992.

23. Luke A, Roizen NJ, Sutton, M et al: Energy expenditure in children with Down syndrome: correcting metabolic rate for movement, *J Pediatr* 125:829-838 1994.

24. Cronke CE, Chumlea WC, Roche AF: Assessment of overweight children with trisomy 21, *Am J Ment Defic* 89:433-436, 1985.

25. Cronke CE, Chumlea WC: Is obesity a problem in trisomy 21? *Trisomy 21* 1:1, 1985.

26. Dyken ME, Lin-Dyken DC, Poulton S et al: Prospective polysomnographic analysis of obstructive sleep apnea in Down syndrome, *Arch Pediatr Adolesc Med* 157:655-660, 2003.

27. Gorlin RJ: Classical chromosome disorders. In Yunis J, editor: *New chromosomal syndromes,* New York, 1977, Academic Press.

28. Whaley WI, Gray WD: Atlanto-axial dislocation and Down's syndrome, *Can Med Assoc J* 123:35-37, 1980.

29. Pueschel SM: Should children with Down syndrome be screened for atlantoaxial instability? *Arch Pediatr Adolesc Med* 152:123-125, 1998.

30. Cohen WI: Atlantoaxial instability: what's next? *Arch Pediatr Adolesc Med* 152:119-121, 1998.

31. Oski FA, Feigin RD, Deangelis CD et al: *Principles and practice of pediatrics,* Philadelphia, 1990, Lippincott.

32. Rubinstein TH: Cranial abnormalities. In Carter CH, editor: *Medical aspects of mental retardation,* ed 2, Springfield, IL, 1978, Charles C Thomas.

33. Marin-Padilla M: Pyramidal cell abnormalities in the motor cortex of a child with Down's syndrome: A Golgi study, *J Comp Neurol* 167:63-81, 1976.

34. Loesch-Mdzewska D: Some aspects of neurology of Down's syndrome, *J Ment Defic Res* 12:237-246, 1968.

35. Crome L: The pathology of Down's disease. In Hilliard LT, Kirman BH, editors: *Mental deficiency,* ed 2, Boston, 1965, Little, Brown.

36. Benda CE: *The child with mongolism (congenital acromicria),* New York, 1960, Grune & Stratton.

37. McGraw MB: *The neuromuscular maturation of the human infant,* New York, 1966, Hafer.

38. Cowie VA: Neurological aspects of the early development of Mongols, *Clin Proc Child Hosp DC* 23:64-69, 1967.

39. Genetics Home Reference: Edwards syndrome, National Library of Medicine (Bethesda, MD, United States), 2003-2005: http://ghr.nlm.nih.gov/condition=edwardssyndrome. Accessed February 14, 2005.

40. Rasmussen SA, Wong LY, Yang Q et al: Population-based analysis of mortality in trisomy 13 and trisomy 18, *Pediatrics* 111:777-784, 2003.

41. Jones KL: *Smith's recognizable patterns of human malformation,* ed 5, Philadelphia, 1997, WB Saunders.

42. Goldberg MJ: *The dysmorphic child: An orthopedic perspective,* New York, 1987, Raven Press.

43. Genetics Home Reference: Patau syndrome, National Library of Medicine (Bethesda, MD, United States), 2003-2005: http://ghr.nlm.nih.gov/condition=patausyndrome. Accessed February 14, 2005.

44. Patau K, Smith DW, Therman E et al: Multiple congenital anomaly caused by an extra chromosome, *Lancet* 1:790-793, 1960.

45. Warkany J, Passarge E, Smith LB: Congenital malformations in autosomal trisomy syndromes, *Arch Pediatr Adolesc Med* 112:502-517, 1966.

46. Hall JG, Gilchrist DM: Turner syndrome and its variants, *Pediatr Clin North Am* 37:1421-1440, 1990.

47. Genetics Home Reference: Turner syndrome, National Library of Medicine (Bethesda, MD), 2003-2005: http://ghr.nlm.nih.gov/condition=turnersyndrome. Accessed February 14, 2005.

48. Carr DH: Chromosome anomalies as a cause of spontaneous abortion, *Am J Obstet Gynecol* 97:283-293, 1967.

49. Petrozza JC, O'Brien B: Early pregnancy loss, *eMedicine* [Internet]. [Updated October 5, 2004]: http://www.emedicine.com/med/topic3241.htm. Accessed February 20, 2005.

50. Turner HH: A syndrome of infantilism, congenital webbed neck, and cubitus valgus, *Endocrinology* 23:566-574, 1938.

51. Connor JM, Ferguson-Smith MA: *Essential medical genetics,* ed 4, Boston, 1993, Blackwell Scientific Publications.

52. Hoffenberg R, Jackson WPU: Gonadal dysgenesis: modern concepts, *BMJ* 2:1457-1462, 1957.

53. Haley SM, Hallenborg SC, Gans BM: Functional assessment in young children with neurological impairments, *Top Early Childh Special Educ* 9:106-126, 1989.

54. Milunsky A, editor: *Genetic disorders and the fetus,* ed 3, Baltimore, 1992, Johns Hopkins University Press.

55. Ibrahim J, McGovern M: Noonan syndrome, *eMedicine* [Internet]. [Updated October 30, 2002]: http://www.emedicine.com/PED/topic1616.htm. Accessed February 12, 2005.

56. Breg WR, Steele MW, Miller OJ et al: The cri du chat syndrome in adolescents and adults: clinical findings in 13 older patients with partial deletion of the short arms of chromosome no. 5 (5p–), *J Pediatr* 77:782-791, 1970.

57. Campbell DJ, Carlin ME, Justen JE et al: Cri-du-chat syndrome: a topical overview, *5p Minus Society Online Journal* [Internet] 2004-2005 (Arkansas State University): http://www.fivepminus.org. Accessed February 14, 2005.

58. Chen H: Cri-du-chat syndrome, *eMedicine* [Internet]. [Updated November 21, 2002]: http://www.emedicine.com/ped/topic504.htm. Accessed February 12, 2005.

59. Schneegans E, Rohmer A, Levy-Silagy J: Un cas de maladie du cri du chat: déaléation partielle du bras court du chromosome 5, *Pediatrie* 21:823-834, 1966.

60. Marinescu RC, Mainardi PC, Collins MR et al: Growth charts for cri-du-chat syndrome: an international collaborative study, *Am J Med Genet* 94:153-162, 2000.

61. Genetics Home Reference: Cri-du-chat syndrome, National Library of Medicine (Bethesda, MD), 2003-2005: http://ghr.nlm.nih.gov/condition=criduchatsyndrome. Accessed February 14, 2005.

62. Wilkins LE, Brown JA, Nance WE et al: Clinical heterogeneity in 80 home-reared children with cri-du-chat syndrome, *J Pediatr* 102:528-533, 1983.

63. Wilkins LE, Brown JA, Wolf B: Psychomotor development in 65 home-reared children with cri-du-chat syndrome, *J Pediatr* 97:401-405, 1980.

64. Cassidy SB, Schwartz S: Prader-Willi syndrome, *Genereviews at genetests: Medical genetics information resource* [Internet] [Updated April 8, 2004], University of Washington, Seattle, 1997-2005: http://www.genetests.org. Accessed February 17, 2005.

65. Williams CA, Dong, HJ, Driscoll DJ: Angleman syndrome, *Genereviews at genetests: Medical genetics information resource* [Internet] [Updated September 3, 2004], University of Washington, Seattle, 1997-2005: http://www.genetests.org. Accessed February 14, 2005.

66. Butler MG, Meaney FJ, Palmer CG: Clinical and cytogenetic survey of 39 individuals with Prader-Labhart-Willi syndrome, *Am J Med Genet* 23:793-809, 1986.

67. Holm VA: The diagnosis of Prader-Willi syndrome. In Holm VA, Sulzbacher S, Pipes PL, editors: *Prader-Willi syndrome*, Baltimore, 1981, University Park Press.

68. Ledbetter DH, Cassidy SB: The etiology of Prader-Willi syndrome: Clinical implications of the chromosome 15 abnormalities. In Caldwell ME, Taylor RL, editors: *Prader-Willi syndrome: selected research and management issues*, New York, 1988, Springer-Verlag.

69. Robinson WP, Bottani A, Xie YG et al: Molecular, cytogenetic, and clinical investigations of Prader-Willi syndrome patients, *Am J Hum Genet* 49:1219-1234, 1991.

70. Zellweger H, Spoer RT: The Prader-Willi syndrome, *Med Hyg* 37:3338-3345, 1979.

71. Lewis CL: Prader-Willi syndrome: a review for pediatric physical therapists, *Pediatr Phys Ther* 12:87-95, 2000.

72. Cassidy SB: Management of the problems in infancy: hypotonia, developmental delay, and feeding problems. In Caldwell ME, Taylor RL, editors: *Prader-Willi syndrome: selected research and management issues,* New York, 1988, Springer-Verlag.

73. Luiselli JK: Issues in Prader-Willi syndrome: diagnosis, characteristics and management. In Caldwell ME, Taylor RL, editors: *Prader-Willi syndrome: selected research and management issues*, New York, 1988, Springer-Verlag.

74. Taylor RL: Cognitive and behavioral characteristics. In Caldwell ME, Taylor RL, editors: *Prader-Willi syndrome: selected research and management issues*, New York, 1988, Springer-Verlag.

75. Wagner CW: Surgical considerations in Prader-Willi syndrome. In Caldwell ME, Taylor RL, editors: *Prader-Willi syndrome: selected research and management issues*, New York, 1988, Springer-Verlag.

76. Stalker HJ, Williams CA: Genetic counseling in Angelman syndrome: the challenges of multiple causes, *Am J Med Genet* 77:54-59, 1998.

77. Kupfer GM: Childhood cancer, epidemiology, *eMedicine* [Internet], [Updated October 15, 2003]: http://www.emedicine.com/ped/topic2585.htm. Accessed February 20, 2005.

78. Rubnitz JE: Acute lymphoblastic leukemia, *eMedicine* [Internet], [Updated January 17, 2005]: http://www.emedicine.com/ped/topic2587.htm. Accessed February 20, 2005.

79. Nussbaum RL, McInnes RP, Williard HF: *Thompson and Thompson genetics in medicine*, ed 6, Philadelphia, 2001, WB Saunders.

80. Margolin JF, Poplack DG: *Principles of pediatric oncology*, ed 3, Philadelphia, 1997, Raven Publishers.

81. O'Donnell MR: Acute leukemias. In *Cancer management: a multidisciplinary approach*, ed 8, Philadelphia, 2004, FA Davis.

82. Adde M: Case report: Childhood acute lymphoblastic leukemia, *International network for cancer treatment and research newsletter* [Internet]: http://www.inctr.org/publications/2001_v02_n03_n07.shtml. Accessed February 20, 2005.

83. Cancer Data Registry of Idaho Annual Report 1998 [Internet]: Leukemia: http://www.idcancer.org/report98/leukemia.html. Accessed February 20, 2005.

84. Hrusak O, Trka J, Zuna J et al: Acute lymphoblastic leukemia incidence during socioeconomic transition: selective increase in children from 1 to 4 years, *Leukemia* 16:720-725, 2002.

85. Crist WM, Pui CH: Acute lymphoblastic leukemia. In Nelson WE, Behrman RE, Kliegman RM et al, editors: *Nelson's textbook of pediatrics*, ed 15, Philadelphia, 1996, WB Saunders.

86. Marini JC: Osteogenesis imperfecta: Comprehensive management, *Adv Pediatr* 35:391-426, 1988.

87. Aita JA: *Congenital facial anomalies with neurologic defects*, Springfield, IL, 1969, Charles C Thomas.

88. Steiner RD, Pepin MG, Byers PH: Osteogenesis imperfecta, *Genereviews at genetests: medical genetics information resource* [Updated January 28, 2005], University of Washington, Seattle, 1997-2005: http://www.genetests.org. Accessed February 14, 2005.

89. Plumridge D, Bennett R, Dinno N et al, editors: *The student with a genetic disorder*, Springfield, 1993, Charles C Thomas.

90. Gerber LH, Binder H, Weintrob J et al: Rehabilitation of children and infants with osteogenesis imperfecta: a program for ambulation, *Clin Orthop* 251:254-262, 1990.

91. Northrup H, Au KS: Tuberous sclerosis complex, *Genereviews at genetests: medical genetics information resource* [Updated September 27, 2004], University of Washington, Seattle, 1997-2005: http://www.genetests.org. Accessed February 14, 2005.

92. Critchley M, Earl CJC: Tuberose sclerosis and allied conditions, *Brain* 55:311-346, 1932.

93. Genetics Home Reference: Neurofibromatosis, National Library of Medicine (Bethesda, MD, United States), 2003-2005: http://ghr.nlm.nih.gov/condition=neurofibromatosis. Accessed February 14, 2005.

94. Berg BO: Current concepts of neurocutaneous disorders, *Brain Dev* 13:9-20, 1991.

95. Crawford A: Neurofibromatosis, *eMedicine* [Internet], [Updated December 1, 2002]: http://www.emedicine.com/orthoped/topic525.htm. Accessed February 18, 2005.

96. Hornstein L, Borcher D: Stroke in an infant prior to the development of manifestations of neurofibromatosis, *Neurofibromatosis* 2:116-120, 1989.

97. Emery AEH, Rimoin DL: *Principles and practice of medical genetics*, ed 2, New York, 1990, Churchill Livingstone.

98. Clarke LA: Mucopolysaccharidosis type I, *Geneteviews at genetests: medical genetics information resource* [Internet] [Updated August 6, 2004], University of Washington, Seattle, 1997-2005: http://www.genetests.org. Accessed February 14, 2005.

99. Genetics Home Reference: Phenylketonuria, National Library of Medicine (Bethesda, MD, United States), 2003-2005: http://ghr.nlm.nih.gov/condition=phenylketonuria. Accessed February 14, 2005.

100. Scott CR: Inborn enzymatic errors. In Smith DW, editor: *Introduction to clinical pediatrics,* ed 2, Philadelphia, 1977, WB Saunders.

101. Know WE: Phenylketonuria. In Stanbury JB, Wyngaarden JB, Fredrickson DC, editors: *The metabolic basis of inherited disease*, ed 3, New York, 1972, McGraw-Hill.

102. Prior TW, Russman BS: Spinal muscle atrophy, *Gene reviews at gene tests: medical genetics information resource* [Updated September 3, 2004], University of Washington, Seattle, 1997-2005: http://www.genetests.org. Accessed February 14, 2005.

103. Genetics Home Reference: Spinal muscular atrophy, National Library of Medicine (Bethesda, MD, United States), 2003-2005: http://ghr.nlm.nih.gov/condition=spinalmuscularatrophy. Accessed February 14, 2005.

104. Haslam RHA: Neurological disorders. In Smith DW, editor: *Introduction to clinical pediatrics,* ed 2, Philadelphia, 1977, WB Saunders.

105. Harris SR, McEwen I: Assessing motor skills. In McLean M, Bailey D, Wolery M, editors: *Assessing infants and preschoolers with special needs*, ed 2, Englewood Cliffs, NJ, 1996, Prentice Hall.

106. Antonarakis SE, Waber PG, Kittur SD et al: Hemophilia A: detection of molecular defects and carriers by DNA analysis, *N Engl J Med* 313:842-848, 1985.

107. Saul RA, Tarleton JC: Fragile X syndrome, *Genereviews at genetests: medical genetics information resource* [Internet] [Updated September 13, 2004], University of Washington, Seattle, 1997-2005: http://www.genetests.org. Accessed February 18, 2005.

108. Holmes LB, Moser HW, Halldorson S et al: *Mental retardation: an atlas of diseases with associated physical abnormalities,* New York, 1972, Macmillan.

109. Lesch M, Nyhan WL: A familial disorder of uric acid metabolism and central nervous system function, *Am J Med* 36:561-570, 1964.

110. Nicklas JA, O'Neill JP, Jinnah HA et al: Lesch-Nyhan syndrome, *Gene reviews at gene tests: Medical genetics information resource* [Internet] [Updated February 8, 2005], University of Washington, Seattle, 1997-2005: http://www.genetests.org. Accessed February 18, 2005.

111. Boyle JA, Raivio KO, Astrin KH et al: Lesch-Nyhan syndrome: preventive control by prenatal diagnosis, *Science* 169:688-689, 1970.

112. Pellicer F, Buendia-Roldan I, Pallares-Trujillo VC: Self-mutilation in the Lesch-Nyhan syndrome: a corporal consciousness problem?—A new hypothesis, *Med Hypotheses* 50:43-47, 1998.

113. Raw I, Schmidt BJ, Merzel J: Catecholamines and congenital pain insensitivity, *Braz J Med Biol Res* 17:271-279,1984.

114. Taira T, Kobayashi T, Hori T: Disappearance of self-mutilating behavior in a patient with Lesch-Nyhan syndrome after bilateral chronic stimulation of the globus pallidus internus: case report, *J Neurosurg* 98:414-416, 2003.

115. Anderson LT, Ernst M: Self-injury in Lesch-Nyhan disease, *J Autism Dev Disord* 24:67-81, 1994.

116. Schwartzman JS, Bernadino A, Nishimura A et al: Rett syndrome in a boy with a 47,XXY karyotype confirmed by rare mutation in the MECP2 gene, *Neuropediatrics* 32:162-164, 2001.

117. Clayton-Smith J, Watson P, Ramsden S et al: Somatic mutation in *MECP2* as a non-fatal neurodevelopmental disorder in males, *Lancet* 356:830-832, 2000.

118. Meloni I, Bruttini M, Longo I et al: A mutation in the Rett syndrome gene, *MECP2*, causes X-linked mental retardation and progressive spasticity in males, *Am J Hum Genet* 67:982-985, 2000.

119. Hagberg B: Rett syndrome: Swedish approach to analysis of prevalence and cause, *Brain Dev* 7:276-280, 1985.

120. Schanen NC, Dahle EJ, Capozzoli F et al: A new Rett syndrome family consistent with X-link inheritance expands the X chromosome exclusion map, *Am J Hum Genet* 61:634-641, 1997.

121. Hagberg B, Goutieres F, Hanefeld F et al: Rett syndrome: criteria for inclusion and exclusion, *Brain Dev* 7:372-373, 1985.

122. Trevathan E, Naidu S: The clinical recognition and differential diagnosis of Rett syndrome. *J Child Neurol Suppl* 3:S6-16, 1988.

123. Hagberg B,Aicardi J, Dias K et al: A progressive syndrome of autism, dementia, ataxia and loss of purposeful hand use in girls: Rett syndrome, report of 35 cases, *Ann Neurol* 14:471-479, 1983.

124. Hennessey MJ, Haas RH: Orthopedic management of Rett syndrome. *J Child Neurol Suppl* 3:48-50, 1988.

125. Naganuma GM, Billingsley FF: Effects of handsplints on stereotypic behavior of three girls with Rett syndrome, *Phys Ther* 68:664-671, 1988.

126. Piazza CC, Anderson C, Fisher W: Teaching self-feeding skills to patients with Rett syndrome, *Dev Med Child Neurol* 35:991-996, 1993.

127. Stewart KB, Brady DK, Crowe TK et al: Rett syndrome: a literature review and survey of parents and therapists, *Phys Occup Ther Pediatr* 9:35-55, 1989.

128. Jaksch M, Kleinle S, Scharfe C et al: Frequency of mitochondrial transfer RNA mutations and deletions in 225 patients presenting with respiratory chain deficiencies, *J Med Genet* 38:665-673, 2001.

129. Blakely E, He L, Taylor R et al: Mitochondrial DNA deletion in "identical" twin brothers, *J Med Genet* 41:e19, 2004.

130. Hutchin, T, Thompson K, Parker M et al: Prevalence of mitochondrial DNA mutations in childhood/congenital onset non-syndromic sensorineural hearing impairment, *J Med Genet* 38:229-231, 2001.

131. Thorburn DR, Rahman S: Mitochondrial DNA-associated Leigh syndrome and NARP, *Gene reviews at gene tests: Medical genetics information resource* [Internet] [Updated October 30, 2003], University of Washington, Seattle, 1997-2005: http://www.genetests.org. Accessed February 18, 2005.

132. The Leigh's Center Newsletter [Internet], The Mitochondrial and Metabolic Disease Center, University of California San Diego: http://biochemgen.ucsd.edu/mmdc/index.htm. Accessed February 21, 2005.

133. Campbell SK, VanderLinden DW, Palisano RJ, editors: *Physical therapy for children*, ed 2, Philadelphia, 2000, WB Saunders.

134. Campbell SK, editor: *Decision making in pediatric neurologic physical therapy*, Philadelphia, 1999, Churchill Livingstone.

135. Effgren SK: *Meeting the physical therapy needs of children*, Philadelphia, 2005, FA Davis.

136. Ratliffe KT: *Clinical pediatric physical therapy*, St. Louis, 1998, Mosby.

137. Tachdjian MO: *Pediatric orthopedics*, ed 2, Philadelphia, 1990, WB Saunders.

138. Hao K, Wang X, Niu T et al: A candidate gene association study on preterm delivery: application of high-throughput genotyping technology and advanced statistical methods, *Hum Mol Genet* 13:683-691, 2004.

139. Ward K, Wang X: Overview of the genetics and mechanisms of preterm birth [abstract presented at workshop of National Institute of Child Health and Human Development May 4, 2001: The role of genetics in health disparity of premature birth and low birth weight infants] [Internet]: http://www.nichd.nih.gov/cdbpm/pp/geneticshealth_disparities.pdf. Accessed February 19, 2005.

140. Macones G: Genetic variation and its relationship to premature birth: bacterial vaginosis, tumor necrosis factor-alpha and spontaneous preterm delivery [abstract presented at workshop of National Institute of Child Health and Human Development, May 4, 2001: The role of genetics in health disparity of premature birth and low birth weight infants] [Internet]: http://www.nichd.nih.gov/cdbpm/pp/geneticshealth_disparities.pdf. Accessed February 19, 2005.

141. Infant mortality fact sheet: Centers for Disease Control and Prevention [Internet] [Updated February 8, 2005]: http://www.cdc.gov/omh/AMH/factsheets/infant.htm. Accessed February 21, 2005.

142. Bly L: A historical and current view of the basis of NDT, *Pediatr Phys Ther* 3:131-135, 1991.

143. Harris SR: Early intervention: does developmental therapy make a difference? *Top Early Childh Special Educ* 7:20-32, 1988.

144. Winstein CJ: Motor learning: from behavior to social cognitive neuroscience perspectives. Proceedings of III Step Conference, Salt Lake City, UT, 2005.

145. Shumway-Cook A, Woollacott MH: *Motor control: theory and practical applications*, ed 2, Philadelphia, 2001, Lippincott Williams & Wilkins.

146. Ketelarr M, Vermeer A, Hart H et al: Effects of a functional therapy program on motor abilities of children with cerebral palsy, *Phys Ther* 81:1534-1545, 2001.

147. Wilson Howle, JM: Cerebral palsy. In Campbell SK, editor: *Decision making in pediatric neurologic physical therapy*, Philadelphia, 1999, Churchill Livingstone.

148. Tardieu G, Tardieu C: Cerebral palsy: mechanical evaluation and conservative correction of limb joint contractures, *Clin Orthop Rel Res* 219:63-69, 1987.

149. Pilon JM, Sadler GT, Bartlett DJ: Relationship of hypotonia and joint laxity to motor development during infancy, *Pediatr Phys Ther* 12:10-15, 2000.

150. Sheahan MS, Brockway NF: The high-risk infant. In Tecklin JS, editor: *Pediatric physical therapy*, ed 3, Philadelphia, 1999, Lippincott Williams & Wilkins.

151. Lowes L, Orlin MN: Musculoskeletal system: Considerations for interventions for specific pediatric pathologies. In Effgren SK, editor: *Meeting the physical therapy needs of children*, Philadelphia, 2005, FA Davis.

152. Olney SJ, Wright MJ: Cerebral palsy. In Campbell SK, VanderLinden DW, Palisano RJ, editors: *Physical therapy for children*, ed 2, Philadelphia, 2000, WB Saunders.

153. McGee SM: Hemophilia. In Campbell SK, VanderLinden DW, Palisano RJ, editors: *Physical therapy for children*, ed 2, Philadelphia, 2000, WB Saunders.

154. Case-Smith J, Allen AS, Pratt PN: *Occupational therapy for children*, ed 4. Philadelphia, 2000, Mosby.

155. Massery MP: Chest development as a component of normal motor development: implications for pediatric physical therapists, *Pediatr Phys Ther* 3:3-8, 1991.

156. Massery MP: The patient with neuromuscular or musculoskeletal dysfunction. In Frownfelter DL, Dean E, editors: *Principles and practice of cardiopulmonary physical therapy*, ed 3, St. Louis, 1996, Elsevier Science

157. Massery MP, Frownfelter D: Facilitating ventilation patterns and breathing strategies. In Frownfelter DL, Dean E, editors: *Principles and practice of cardiopulmonary physical therapy*, ed 3, St. Louis, 1996, Elsevier Science.

158. Kahn-D'Angelo L, Unanue RA: The special care nursery. In Campbell SK, VanderLinden DW, Palisano RJ, editors: *Physical therapy for children*, ed 2, Philadelphia, 2000, WB Saunders.

159. Monfort K, Case-Smith J: The effects of a neonatal positioner on scapular rotation, *Am J Occup Ther* 51:378-384, 1997.

160. Cole FS, Hamvas A, Nogee LM: Genetic disorders of neonatal respiratory function, *Pediatr Res*, 50:157-162, 2001.

161. Wolfson MR, Greenspan JS, Deoras KS et al: Effect of position on the mechanical interaction between the rib cage and abdomen in preterm infants, *J Appl Physiol* 72:1032-1038, 1992.

162. Fox RE, Viscardi RM, Taciak VL et al: Effect of position on pulmonary mechanics in healthy preterm newborn infants, *J Perinatol* 13:205-211, 1993.

163. Mizuno K, Itabashi K, Okuyama K: Effect of body position on blood gases and ventilation volume of infants with chronic lung disease before and after feeding, *Am J Perinatol* 12:275-277, 1995.

164. Maynard V, Bignall S, Kitchen S: Effect of positioning on respiratory synchrony in non-ventilated pre-term infants, *Physiother Res Int* 5:96-110, 2000.

165. Tecklin JS: Pulmonary disorders in infants and children and their physical therapy management. In Tecklin JS, editor: *Pediatric physical therapy*, ed 3, Philadelphia, 1999, Lippincott Williams & Wilkins.

166. Thelen E, Smith LB: A dynamic systems approach to the development of cognition and action, Cambridge, 1994, MIT Press.

167. Campbell SK: The infant at risk for developmental disability. In Campbell SK, editor: *Decision making in pediatric physical therapy*, Philadelphia, 1999, Churchill Livingstone.

168. Connolly BH, Montgomery PC: The children: history and systems review. In Connolly BH, Montgomery PC, editors: *Therapeutic exercise in developmental disabilities*, ed 3, Thorofare, NJ, 2005, SLACK.

169. Dunst CJ: A family systems assessment and intervention model. In Hanft BE, editor: *Family centered care*, Rockville, 1989, American Occupational Therapy Association.

170. Turnbull AP, Turnbull HR: *Families, professionals and exceptionality: a special partnership*, ed 2, Columbus, OH, 1990, Merrill.

171. Melyn MA, White DT: Mental and developmental milestones of non-institutionalized Down's syndrome children, *Pediatrics* 52:542-545, 1973.

172. *Guide to physical therapist practice*, revised ed 2, Alexandria, VA, 2003, American Physical Therapy Association.

173. Kirshner B, Guyatt GH: A methodological framework for assessing health indices, *J Chron Dis* 38:27-36, 1985.

174. Piper MC, Darrah J: *Motor assessment of the developing infant*, Philadelphia, 1993, WB Saunders.

175. Bayley N: *Bayley scales of infant development*, ed 2. San Antonio, TX, 1993, Psychological Corporation.

176. Folio MR, Fewell RR: *Peabody developmental motor scales: examiner's manual*, ed 2, Austin, TX, 2000, Pro-Ed.

177. Knobloch H, Stevens F, Malone AF: *Manual of developmental diagnosis: The administration and interpretation of the revised Gesell & Amatruda developmental and neurological examination*, Houston, TX, 1987, Gesell Developmental Materials.

178. Campbell SK: *Test of infant motor performance*, Chicago, IL, 2001, Test of Infant Motor Performance.

179. Bruininks RH: *Bruininks-Oseretsky test of motor proficiency: examiner's manual*, Circle Pines, MN, 1978, American Guidance Service.

180. Chandler L, Andrews M, Swanson M: *The movement assessment of infants: a manual*, Rolling Bay, WA, 1980, Infant Movement Research.

181. Harris SR: Early diagnosis of spastic diplegia, spastic hemiplegia, and quadriplegia, *Arch Pediatr Adolesc Med* 143:1356-1360, 1989.

182. Furuno S: *Helping babies learn: Developmental profiles and activities for infants and toddlers*, San Antonio, TX, 2000, Communication Therapy Skill Builders.

183. Granger CV, Hamilton BB, Sherwin FS et al: *Guide for the use of the uniform data set for medical rehabilitation*, Buffalo, NY, 1987, Research Foundation, State University of New York.

184. Uniform Data System for Medical Rehabilitation: *WeeFIM II^{SM} System clinical guide*, Buffalo, NY, 2004, Uniform Data System for Medical Rehabilitation.

185. Haley SM, Coster WJ, Ludlow LH et al: *Pediatric evaluation of disability inventory (PEDI), version 1: development, standardization and administration manual*, Boston, MA, 1992, Infant Research Group, Department of Rehabilitation Medicine at New England Medical Center.

186. Coster W, Deeney T, Haltiwanger et al: *School function assessment*, San Antonio, TX, 1998, Therapy Skill Builders.

187. Stewart K: Collaborating with families: reflections on empowerment. In Hanft BE, editor: *Family centered care*, Rockville, MD, 1989, American Occupational Therapy Association.

188. Palisano RJ, Snider LM, Orlin MN: Recent advances in physical and occupational therapy for children with cerebral palsy, *Semin Pediatr Neurol* Mar 11:66-67, 2004.

189. Rone-Adams SA, Stern DF, Walker V: Stress and compliance with a home exercise program among caregivers of children with disabilities, *Ped Phys Ther* 16:140-148, 2004.

190. Bailey D: Collaborative goal setting with families: resolving differences in values and priorities for services, *Top Early Childhood Special Educ* 7:59-71, 1987.

191. Public Law 94-142. Education for all handicapped children act of 1975 (5.6), 94th Congress, 1st Session, 1975.

192. Federal Register, Part II, Department of Education, 34 CFR Parts 300 and 303, Vol 64, No 48, March 12, 1999.

193. McEwen I, editor: *Providing physical therapy services under Parts B & C of the Individuals with Disabilities Education Act (IDEA)*, Alexandria, VA, 2000, Section on Pediatrics, American Physical Therapy Association.

194. David K: IDEA 2004, PL108-446: Impact on physical therapy related services, Section on Pediatrics, Alexandria, VA, 2005: http://www.pediatricapta.org/members/peds-govt-affairs.cfm. Accessed September 6, 2005.

195. Campbell PH: Evaluation and assessment in early intervention for infants and toddlers, *J Early Intervent* 15:36-45, 1991.

196. McEwen IR: Children with cognitive impairments. In Campbell SK, VanderLinden DW, Palisano RJ, editors: *Physical therapy for children*, ed 2, Philadelphia, 2000, WB Saunders.

197. Palisano RJ: Validity of goal attainment scaling in infants with motor delays, *Phys Ther* 73:651-660, 1993.

198. Harris SR: Functional abilities in context. In Lister MJ, editor: *Contemporary management of motor control problems: proceedings of the II-Step Conference*, Alexandria, VA, 1991, Foundation for Physical Therapy.

199. Horak FB: Assumptions underlying motor control for neurologic rehabilitation. In Lister MJ, editor: *Contemporary management of motor control problems: proceedings of the II-Step Conference*, Alexandria, VA, 1991, Foundation for Physical Therapy.

200. Higgins S: Motor skill acquisition, *Phys Ther* 71:123-129, 1991.

201. Noonan MJ, McCormick L: *Early intervention in natural environments*, Pacific Grove, CA, 1993, Brooks/Cole.

202. Cole K, Harris SR, Eland SF et al: Comparison of two service delivery models: In class vs. out of class therapy approaches, *Pediatr Phys Ther* 1:49-54, 1989.

203. Sternat J, Messina R, Nietupski J et al: Occupational and physical therapy services for severely handicapped students: toward a natural-

ized public school service delivery model. In Sontag E, editor: *Educational programming for the severely and profoundly handicapped,* Reston, VA, 1977, Council for Exceptional Children.

204. Effgen SK: The educational environment. In Campbell SK, Vander-Linden DW, Palisano RJ, editors: *Physical therapy for children,* ed 2, Philadelphia, 2000, WB Saunders.

205. Sandall SR: Developmental interventions for biologically at-risk infants at home, *Top Early Childhood Special Educ* 10:1-13, 1990.

206. Nelson WE, Behrman RE, Kliegman RM et al, editors: *Nelson textbook of pediatrics,* ed 15, Philadelphia, 1996, WB Saunders.

207. Koehler J: Spinal muscular atrophy of childhood. In Bleck EE, Nagel DA, editors: *Physically handicapped children: a medical atlas for teachers,* New York, 1975, Grune & Stratton.

208. Osawa M, Shishikura K: Werdnig-Hoffmann disease and variants, *Handbook Clin Neurol* 15:51-80, 1991.

209. Myhre SA, Ruvalcaba RH, Johnson HR et al: The effects of testosterone treatment in Klinefelter's syndrome, *J Pediatr* 76:267-276, 1970.

210. Berg BO: Convulsive disorders. In Bleck EE, Nagel DA, editors: *Physically handicapped children: a medical atlas for teachers,* New York, 1975, Grune & Stratton.

211. Guralnick MJ, Bennett FC: Early intervention for at-risk and handicapped children: current and future perspectives. In Guralnick MJ, Bennett FC, editors: *Effectiveness of early intervention for at-risk and handicapped children,* Orlando, FL, 1987, Academic Press.

212. Pruess JB, Fewell RR: Cell therapy and the treatment of Down syndrome: a review of research, *Trisomy 21* 1:3-8, 1985.

213. U.S. Food and Drug Administration: http://www.fda.gov/Cber/gene.htm. Accessed June 3, 2006

214. Novitski E: *Human genetics,* New York, 1977, Macmillan.

215. Lea DH, Williams JK: Genetic testing and screening, *AJN* 102:36-43, 2002.

216. Botto LD, Mastroiacovo P: Surveillance for birth defects and genetic diseases. In Khoury MJ, Burke W, Thomson EJ, editors: *Genetics and public health in the 21st century: using genetic information to improve health and prevent disease,* Oxford University Press [Internet version] (2000): http://www.cdc.gov/genomics/info/books/21stcent2.htm. Accessed February 12, 2005.

217. Therrell BL: *National newborn screening report—2000,* Austin TX, National Newborn Screening and Genetics Resource Center: http:genes-r-us.uthscsa.edu/resources/newborn/00/200report.pdf. Accessed March 15, 2005.

218. Dorman JS: Need for genetic education for type I diabetes, *Arch Pediatr Adolesc Med* 57:935-936, 2003.

219. Waisbren SE, Albers S, Amato S et al: Effect of expanded newborn screening for biochemical genetic disorders on child outcomes and parental stress, *JAMA* 290:2564-2572, 2003.

220. Agarwal R: Prenatal diagnosis of chromosomal anomalies: pictorial essay, *Ind J Radiol Imag* 13:173-187, 2003.

221. Pine D: Ethics in medicine: fetal diagnosis and treatment, *P&S Journal of Columbia University Medical Center* 17(2), 1997: http://cumc.columbia.edu/news/journal/journal-o/archives/jour_v17n2_0021.html. Accessed June 3, 2006.

222. Werch A: Amniocentesis: indications, techniques, and complications, *South Med J* 69:824-827, 1976.

223. Sangalli M, Langdana F, Thurlow C: Pregnancy loss rate following routine genetic amniocentesis at Wellington Hospital, *N Z Med J* 117:818-823, 2004.

224. Anderson G: Routine prenatal ultrasound screening. In *Canadian Task Force on the Periodic Health Examination,* Ottawa, 1994, Health Canada.

225. Fasouliotis SJ, Schenker JG: Preimplantation genetic diagnosis principles and ethics, *Hum Reprod* 13:2238-2245, 1998.

226. Long TM, Brady R, Lapham EV: A survey of genetics knowledge of health professionals: implications for physical therapists, *Pediatr Phys Ther* 13:156-163, 2001.

227. Nora JJ, Fraser FL: *Medical genetics: principles and practice,* Philadelphia, 1989, Lea & Febiger.

228. Phillips JA: Surfing the net for information on genetic and hormone disorders, *Growth Genet Horm* 15:17-22, 1999.

229. PubMed: US National Library of Medicine, Bethesda, MD (United States): http://www.ncbi.nlm.nih.gov/PubMed. Accessed February 6, 2005, to June 3, 2006.

230. Hobbs C, Cleves M, Simmons C: Genetic epidemiology and congenital malformations: from the chromosome to the crib, *Arch Pediatr Adolesc Med,* 156:315-320, 2002.

231. Black MM, Matula K: *Essentials of Bayley Scales of Infant Development-II Assessment,* New York, 2000, John Wiley.

232. Newborg J, Stock JR, Wnek L et al: *Battelle Developmental Inventory,* Allen, TX, 1998, DLM.

233. Law M, Baptiste S, McColl M et al: The Canadian occupational performance measure: an outcome measure for occupational therapy, *Can J Occup Ther* 57:82-97, 1990.

234. Berg KO, Wood-Dauphinee S, Williams JI et al: Measuring balance in the elderly: preliminary development of an instrument, *Physiother Can* 41:304-311, 1989.

235. Len C, Goldenberg J, Ferraz MB et al: Crosscultural reliability of the childhood health assessment questionnaire, *J Rheumatol* 21:2349-2352, 1994.

236. Landgraf JL, Abetz L, Ware JE: *The CHQ user's manual,* Boston, 1996, Health Institute at New England Medical Center.

237. Frankenburg WK, Dodds J, Archer P et al: *Denver II technical manual,* Denver, 1990, Denver Developmental Materials.

238. Schafer DS, Moersch MS, editors: *Developmental programming for infants and young children,* Volumes I, II, III. Ann Arbor, 1981, University of Michigan Press.

239. Rose J, Gamble JG, Lee J et al: The energy expenditure index: a method to quantitate and compare wailing energy expenditure for children and adolescents, *J Pediatr Orthop* 11:571-578, 1991.

240. Duncan PW, Weiner DK, Chandler J et al: Functional reach: a new clinical measure of balance, *J Gerontol Med Sci* 45:M192-M197, 1990.

241. Russell D, Rosenbaum PL, Cadman DT et al: The gross motor function measure: a means to evaluate the effects of physical therapy, *Dev Med Child Neurol* 1:341-352, 1989.

242. Harris S, Daniels L: Reliability and validity of the Harris Infant Neuromotor Test, *J Pediatr* 139:249-253, 2001.

243. Feeney D, Furlong W, Boyle M et al: Multi-attribute health status classification systems: Health Utilities Index, *Pharmacoeconomics* 7:490-502, 1995.

244. Bohannon RW, Smith MB: Interrater reliability of modified Ashworth scale of muscle spasticity, *Phys Ther* 67:206-207, 1987.

245. Boyd RN, Graham HK: Objective measurement of clinical findings in the use of botulinum toxin type A for the management of children of cerebral palsy, *Eur J Neurol* 6(4 suppl):S23-S35, 1999.

246. Fosang AL, Galea MP, McCoy AT et al: Measures of muscle and joint performance in the lower limb of children with cerebral palsy, *Dev Med Child Neurol* 45:664-670, 2003.

247. Deitz JC, Richardson P, Crowe TK et al: Performance of children with learning disabilities and motor delays on the Pediatric Clinical Test of Sensory Interaction for Balance (P-CTSIB), *Phys Occup Ther Pediatr* 16:1-21, 1996.

248. Ayers AJ: *Sensory integration and praxis tests,* Los Angeles, 1989, Western Psychological Services.

249. Dunn W: *Sensory profile,* San Antonio, 1999, Psychological Corporation.

250. Lipkin DP, Scriven AJ, Crake T et al: Six minute walking test for assessing exercise capacity in chronic heart failure, *BMJ* 292:653-655, 1986.

251. DeGangi GA, Greenspan SI: *Test of sensory function in infants (TSFI),* Los Angeles, 1981, Western Psychological Services.

252. Podsiadlo D, Richardson S: The timed "up & go": a test of basic functional mobility for frail elderly persons, *J Am Geriatr Soc* 39:142-148, 1991.

253. Miller LJ, Roid GH: *Toddler and infant motor evaluation: a standardized assessment,* Tucson, 1994, Therapy Skill Builders.

CHAPTER 14 Learning Disabilities

Stacey E. Szklut, MS, OTR/L
Darbi Breath Philibert, MHS, LOTR

KEY WORDS

developmental coordination disorder
learning disabilities
life span disability
model of disablement
motor control
motor learning
neurodevelopmental treatment
nonverbal learning disabilities
praxis
sensory integration
verbal learning impairments

OBJECTIVES

After reading this chapter the student/therapist will be able to:

1. Be aware of characteristics that typically identify a child with learning disabilities.
2. Become familiar with accepted definitions and terminology used in the field of learning disabilities.
3. Develop a historical perspective of brain dysfunction theories in the field of learning disabilities.
4. Understand the clinical presentation of subgroups within the learning-disabled population.
5. Become familiar with members of the specialist team and service provision types for children with learning disabilities.
6. Recognize the characteristics of the child with developmental coordination disorder.
7. Identify areas of evaluation to assess motor deficits effectively in the child with a learning disability.
8. Become familiar with theoretical development and intervention techniques applicable to children with learning disabilities and motor deficits.
9. Understand the lifelong ramifications for the individual with learning disabilities.

AN OVERVIEW OF LEARNING DISABILITIES

Characteristics

Learning disabilities are not a singular disorder, but a term that refers to a group of varied and often multidimensional disorders.[1] Difficulties in learning may manifest themselves in various combinations of impairments in language, memory, visual-spatial organization, motor function, and the control of attention and impulses.[2,3] The characteristics of a child with a learning disability are often diverse and complex. Each child presents with a different composite of impairments, disabilities, functional deficits, and societal limitations. The most commonly recognized performance difficulties in learning are associated with academic success. In most instances, the focus has been on deficits in verbal learning, including difficulties with reading, the acquisition of spoken and written language, and arithmetic. Functional limitations in nonverbal learning are equally important and more recently recognized. The three primary impairment areas affected by nonverbal learning disorders include visual-spatial organization, social-emotional development, and sensorimotor performance.[4] In addition to verbal and nonverbal disabilities, specific motor impairments also can be present and affect academic achievement or daily life tasks.[5] Accompanying behavioral manifestations may include problems with self-regulatory behaviors, such as lack of attention, hyperactivity and poor impulse control, as well as difficulties in social perception and social interactions.[4,6,7] These learning and behavioral difficulties may be isolated (e.g., academic, motor, or behavioral), combined (e.g., academic and motor), or global (academic, motor, and behavioral).[8]

Definition

The heterogeneity of persons with learning disabilities has made consensus on a single definition difficult. Many disciplines describe learning disabilities according to their own frames of reference. Medical professionals have tended to relate the deficit to its cause, particularly to cerebral dysfunction. Terms historically used include *brain injured,*[9] *minimal brain dysfunction,*[2] and *psychoneurological disorder,*[10] all implying a neurological cause for the deviation in development. Educational professionals, however, prefer to describe the child's difficulties in behavioral or functional terms. Educators view children with learning disabilities as "children who fail to learn despite an apparently normal capacity for learning."[11] Preferred terminology within the academic environment includes *reading disorder, mathematics disorder,* and *disorder of written expression.*[12] Associated behaviors observed include poor impulse control, restlessness, and frustration. Functional difficulties often include ineffective participation in classroom activities, playground games, and peer interactions.

These differences in frame of reference have resulted in numerous definitions, labels, and inconsistencies in terminology for children having difficulties in learning.[3,13-17] Regardless of the inconsistencies, the salient features of learning disabilities are at least average intelligence and adequate hearing and vision coupled with a deficiency in acquiring basic academic skills.[1] Despite these common features and a variety of proposed guidelines, the issue of creating a single, standard definition has not been resolved.[18,19] The scientific community continues to attempt to predict and explain learning disabilities, whereas the political discipline's goal is advocacy and policies directed to create programs and services to meet the needs of students with learning difficulties.[20] The lack of consensus toward one accepted definition continues to affect consistency in diagnosis, research, and intervention of persons with learning disabilities.

After multiple revisions, the National Joint Committee on Learning Disabilities (NJCLD), which represents several professional organizations, proposed the following definition:

Learning disability is a general term that refers to a heterogeneous group of disorders manifested by significant difficulties in the acquisition and use of listening, speaking, reading, writing, reasoning, or mathematical abilities. These disorders are intrinsic to the individual and are presumed to be due to central nervous system dysfunction and may occur across the life span. Problems of self-regulatory behaviors, social perception, and social interaction may exist with learning disabilities but do not themselves constitute a learning disability. Although learning disabilities may occur concomitantly with other handicapping conditions (for example, sensory impairment, mental retardation, serious emotional disturbance) or with extrinsic influences (such as cultural differences, insufficient or inappropriate instruction), they are not the result of those conditions or influences.[6]

This definition identifies a proposed cause but does not provide a clear exclusion statement regarding what learning disabilities may not result from. The inclusion of mental retardation as a concomitant handicapping condition could further confuse classification and subgrouping because the widely accepted criterion of intelligence in learning disabilities is average or above average. A positive addition to this revision by the NJCLD is the lifelong nature of the condition, which had been stressed in an earlier definition from the Learning Disabilities Association of America. Also, by including the behavioral manifestations of regulatory and social difficulties, a more complete picture of functional problems for the individual with learning disabilities is presented. These additions could assist in the creation of more comprehensive and life-spanning programs of service and could therefore ultimately help in the recognition and remediation of functional and societal limitations.

The definition used in educational settings was initially passed in Public Law 94-142 and later incorporated into the Individuals with Disabilities Education Act (IDEA) (Section 602.26). These federal educational regulations specified seven potential areas of specific academic difficulties children with learning disabilities may exhibit: oral expression, listening comprehension, written expression, basic reading, reading comprehension, mathematics calculation, and mathematics reasoning.[11] The development of a uniform educational definition provided guidelines for setting policies and

securing funds.[18] On a foundational level it formed the basis for creating academic programs and delineating appropriate services for children with learning disabilities. Children with learning disabilities are defined by IDEA as[19]:

Those children who have a disorder in one or more of the basic psychological processes involved in understanding or in using language, spoken or written, which may manifest itself in imperfect ability to listen, think, speak, read, write, spell, or do mathematical calculations. The term includes conditions such as perceptual disabilities, brain injury, minimal brain dysfunction, dyslexia, and developmental aphasia. This term does not include a learning problem that is primarily the result of visual, hearing, or motor disabilities, of mental retardation, of emotional disturbance, or of environmental, cultural, or economic disadvantage.

The differences between these two definitions of learning disabilities are striking. This description does not specifically address etiology but does highlight psychological processes versus neurological impairments. It is clear in its exclusionary statement but does indicate that these disabilities may occur concomitantly. The primary disability focus is on language, which may exclude difficulties in learning that involve visual-spatial and perceptual reasoning. Further, by not mentioning regulatory, reasoning, and social perception within the definition those individuals who do not have a classic verbal learning disability may not be clearly represented. This could have a significant impact on families trying to secure accommodations and remedial services for children with nonverbal learning disabilities through the school. Interestingly, despite the numerous definitions proposed over the years and gains in understanding the subtleties and variations in learning disabilities, this educational model still includes all the basic components first proposed by Kirk as early as 1962 and continues to lack precision.[18,20]

IDEA mandates that all children will have free and appropriate education and authorizes aid for special education and related services for children with disabilities. IDEA influences how children with learning disabilities are identified and classified. The 1997 amendments of IDEA redirected the focus of special education services by adding provisions that would enable children with disabilities to make greater progress and achieve higher levels of functional performance by promoting the early identification and provision of services. The rationale for this was based on research and experience demonstrating that the practice of waiting to refer children with significant reading or behavior problems for special education services increased their problems.[21] The new regulations also permitted states and local education agencies to service children aged 3 to 9 years who have learning problems by using "developmental delay" eligibility criteria instead of specific disability categories, which are limited in scope.

On December 3, 2004, President George W. Bush signed into law a newly amended Individuals with Disabilities Education Improvement Act (P.L. 108-446), which included several significant revisions to IDEA 97. New provisions regarding how schools can determine whether a child has a specific learning disability eliminates the requirement that students must exhibit a severe discrepancy between intellectual ability and achievement for eligibility. This "severe discrepancy" policy often mandated that children would have to experience failure for several years to demonstrate the requisite degree of discrepancy.[22] Congress also sought to recognize current evidence that the "IQ achievement" approach to determining eligibility may not be valid because it does not predict a student's response to instruction.[22,23] IDEA 2004 limits the schools from finding a student eligible for special education services if the learning problems are determined to be caused by a lack of appropriate instruction. It gives the schools the option of using scientific, research-based interventions to attempt to maximize a student's opportunity to be successful within the general education before being placed in special education. The goal is to identify ways of serving students more quickly and efficiently once they begin to show signs of difficulty.[22] These law changes may encourage educators to revise their definition of learning disabilities to stress the importance of identifying individual differences and patterns of ability within each child struggling with learning as a means of creating the best instructional methods for greater success.

Classifications

Binet and Simon's[24] test of intelligence, which enabled an intelligence quotient (IQ) to be calculated, was a landmark in the history of learning disorders.[25] This test was accepted to provide an objective, scientific, and accurate measurement of a child's intellectual potential. Learning disabilities were diagnosed on the basis of a discrepancy model in which the child's intellectual ability was disparate with his or her current level of academic achievement. Within the educational model a 2-year discrepancy between the child's age and school achievement was historically the criterion used for the classification of a learning disability. Intellectual ability, as determined through testing, is influenced by the reliability of the test and examiner as well as the child's ability to pay attention and understand directions. Academic achievement relies heavily on the effectiveness of the teacher and the instructional techniques. In the discrepancy model of classification a child could possibly become labeled as learning disabled as a result of a testing or examiner bias or placement in an ineffective learning environment. Studies indicate that learning disabilities do not fall evenly across racial and ethnic groups, with a higher incidence of special education services needed for black, non-Hispanic children.[26] One could argue that teaching factors could be influencing these children's appearance of having learning disabilities because of poor educational quality. This forms the foundation of the recent No Child Left Behind Act, which challenges states and school districts to become more accountable for improving educational standards for all students through intensifying their efforts to close the achievement gap between underachieving students and their peers.

Fletcher et al[23] conclude that classification research over the last 15 years has provided little evidence to support IQ discrepancy as a clear categorization of learning disabilities as different from underachievement. They outline two models that have emerged for the classification of children with learning disabilities. The first model focuses on abilities and discrepancies within the child as a basis for classification (intraindividual differences). The second model is outcome oriented, reflecting an empirical approach toward identifying the most effective instructional techniques (problem solving). Both models are based on a notion of discrepancy, either internally or in the teaching environment, and have the ultimate goal of developing effective strategies for intervention. Yet neither model fully encompasses dual levels of classification. The intraindividual model centers on the identification of strengths and weaknesses, which does not necessarily identify effective treatment strategies, and the problem-solving model may not take into account the individual strengths and weakness of a child. Fletcher et al[23] suggest that neither of these single classification models is suitable for all purposes and emphasize the importance of a multivariate approach within an integrated model. They argue that for both identification and eligibility learning disabilities should be characterized as "unexpected" because the child is not learning up to expectations despite adequate instruction. If these models are used in conjunction, a child should not be placed in special education without evidence of failure to respond to quality instruction. These changes in classification have been reflected in the current IDEA 2004.

The two most widely used classification systems are those of the American Psychiatric Association (*Diagnostic and Statistical Manual of Mental Disorders* [DSM]) and the World Health Organization (WHO) (*International Classification of Diseases* [ICD]). Educational professionals prefer the DSM classification for its academic relevance. A variety of specific academically related disorders are outlined in the DSM. The latest edition, DSM-IV,[27] now classifies learning disabilities under developmental disorders as "disorders usually first diagnosed in infancy, childhood, or adolescence." It subclassifies disorders into the following categories:

Learning disorders:
- Reading disorder
- Mathematics disorder
- Disorder of written expression

Motor skills:
- Developmental coordination disorder

Communication disorders:
- Expressive language disorder
- Mixed receptive-expressive disorder
- Phonological disorder
- Stuttering

The classification system commonly used by therapists is the ICD. The ICD codes are state mandated and recognized diagnostic codes used for billing and information purposes. In the recent revision, ICD-10,[28] "specific delays in development," which included "other specific learning difficulties," was changed to "disorders of psychological development." The term "learning" is no longer part of this classification. This updated classification is as follows:

Disorders of psychological development
- Including specific developmental disorders (SDD) of speech and language (including acquired aphasia with epilepsy)
- SDD of scholastic skills
- SDD of motor function
- Pervasive developmental disorder

Model of Disablement

Beyond classifying learning disabilities as a diagnosis, the National Center for Medical Rehabilitation Research

(NCMRR)[29] and the WHO have integrated related approaches to classify functional performance. The conceptual approach, The Model of Disablement (see Chapter 1) describes the multiple dimensions of disability and identifies various internal and external factors that affect the way a disability manifests. The purpose of this model is to shift classification of a disability to include assessment of functional performance and societal participation as opposed to solely identifying component deficit areas.

Five dimensions are outlined in the model of disablement. They include pathophysiology, impairments, functional limitations, disabilities, and societal limitations. *Pathophysiology* refers to the underlying disease or injury processes at the tissue or cellular level. Proposed etiological factors related to learning disabilities at this level include brain damage, biochemical abnormalities, genetics, or metabolic disorders. The challenge for interventionists is to recognize the signs and symptoms that verify the diagnosis.[30]

The second dimension of *impairment* includes the organ and system dysfunction that potentially has a negative effect on functional performance. Children with learning disabilities may demonstrate impaired balance, endurance, and coordination of movements. Impairments that occur in one or more systems may lead to functional limitations, the third dimension. The challenge for the clinician is to treat impairments within the context of daily functional performance because impairments do not always result in functional limitation.

Functional limitations involve whole-body functions that are typically assessed, but may or may not receive remediation.[30] For a child with learning disabilities this may include poor hand function in the performance of manipulation activities involved in dressing and handwriting. When functional limitations persist, which are not remediable and cannot be adequately compensated for with assistive technology or other supports, *disabilities* in daily life occur. The child then fails to be an active participant in normal life roles, such as activities of daily living and school tasks. Emotional difficulties, such as depression and decreased self-esteem, which may result from learning difficulties, can ultimately impair social interactions.

Community and environmental barriers, called *societal limitations,* also can lead to restriction in social participation. An example of structural or attitudinal barriers that prevent optimal participation in society is a child who cannot use playground equipment because of lack of accessibility. The ultimate goal for the clinician is to facilitate functional abilities and performance as well as provide necessary supports so the child can become an active participant in society.

The Model of Disablement proposes that the environment, purpose, and level of participation should all be considered when evaluating performance. Determination of the presence, severity, or kind of disability should be made on the basis of a combination of these factors. Within this framework a clinician does not assume a handicap exists because of an impairment but rather considers levels of functional and societal abilities. This allows the therapist to determine intervention needs on the basis of functional performance in relevant environments rather than being driven purely by diagnosis. A 9-year-old child with learning disabilities, for example, might have impairments in motor components of muscle strength and balance. Although these impairments can be identified on assessment, the Model of Disablement suggests that a disability does not exist unless these deficits affect functional performance (e.g., ascending/descending stairs) that limit societal participation (e.g., child cannot leave house independently to go to school or play). If assessment occurs within an academic setting the identified impairments would have to affect successful participation within the educational environment to warrant intervention.

Incidence and Prevalence

According to a 2002 report to Congress on the implementation of IDEA, nearly 2.9 million students aged 6 to 21 years are currently receiving special education services for learning disabilities.[26] Children with specific learning disabilities represent the highest incidence (number of new cases identified in a given period) among 13 disability categories, representing 50% of the total population of children receiving special education. Overall, the estimated prevalence (total number of cases in a population at a given time) of learning disabilities is approximately 5% to 7% of children enrolled in public schools.[26,31] Yet a wide disproportion exists across states, with the latest data ranging from a low of 2.36% in Kentucky to a high of 7.1% in Massachusetts.[26] This disparity reflects the variations in identifying learning disabilities and defining eligibility criteria around the country.[22] Inconsistencies in the definition of learning disabilities continue to affect the ability to determine accurate numbers of incidence and prevalence, although both have continued to rise steadily, with an approximately 28% rise in incidence of identified cases since 1992.[26] Recently the growth trend has slowed and prevalence has varied only slightly since 1997.[31] Boys are more likely than girls to be identified as having a learning disability. According to Child Trends, 10% of boys and 6% of girls aged 3 to 17 years had a learning disability in 2002.[31]

Perspectives on the Causes of Learning Disabilities

Learning disability is a diverse diagnosis with varied manifestations. Searching for a single cause for this often multifaceted difficulty would therefore be inadequate. Historically researchers have studied etiological factors including (1) brain damage or dysfunction caused by birth injury, perinatal anoxia, head injury, fetal malnutrition, encephalitis, and lead poisoning; (2) allergies; (3) biochemical abnormalities or metabolic disorders; (4) genetics; (5) maturational lag; and (6) environmental factors, such as neglect and abuse, a disorganized home, and inadequate stimulation.[32-34] Hereditary links have been observed, with learning difficulties often seen across generations within families. The National Center for Learning Disabilities lists the possible causes of learning disabilities as heredity, problems with pregnancy and birth (e.g., drug and alcohol use, low birth weight, anoxia and premature or prolonged labor), and incidents after birth (e.g., head injuries, nutritional deprivation, and exposure to toxic substances such as lead).[35] Although researchers in the past have considered emotional and environmental issues as a possible cause of learning disabilities, current understanding is that learning disabilities have a biological basis.[18]

Children with learning disabilities frequently display a composite of neuropsychological symptoms that interfere with the ability to store, process, or produce information. These symptoms typically include disorders of speech, spatial orientation, perception, motor coordination, and activity level. Researchers have attempted to identify areas of the brain that may be responsible for these functional limitations. Recent research includes empirical measures of physiological function such as electroencephalograms (EEG), event-related potentials (ERP), brain electrical activity mapping (BEAM), regional cerebral blood flow (rCBF), positron emission tomography (PET), and functional magnetic resonance imaging (fMRI). These measures expand the understanding of brain functioning but are best used in conjunction with data on functional and behavioral manifestations coupled with effective teaching methods to help the individual with learning disabilities most efficiently.

Early attempts at classifying the causes of functional deficits of learning disabilities generated many theories. These theories were often based on experimental studies of animals, studies of adults with gunshot wounds or other forms of cerebral trauma, or studies of people with epilepsy who have had brain surgery. The three most accepted theories were delayed development of cerebral dominance, visual-perceptual deficits, and auditory-perceptual deficits with associated language inefficiencies.[36] Although each of these theories has been criticized for being too simplistic to cover the broad spectrum of learning disabilities, all of them have contributed greatly to research and subgrouping within the field of learning disabilities.

Orton's theory of delayed cerebral dominance, for example, was based on his clinical observation of higher incidence of reading problems in children with mixed handedness. He asserted that the left hemisphere did not develop dominance for preferred hand and language processes, which therefore led to deficiencies in organizing language information necessary for reading.[37] Although this theory of a dominant side of the brain was refuted by empirical data, several research models evolved, including left hemisphere maturational lag or damage, lack of hemispheric specialization, and inefficient interhemispheric integration.[36]

Left Hemisphere Maturational Lag
In the early 1970s researchers proposed that reading problems resulted from a lag in the development of left hemisphere lateralization.[38,39] These authors suggested a left hemisphere *maturational lag* affecting motor, somatosensory, and language functions in children with dyslexia. This resembled behavioral patterns of chronologically younger children as opposed to a unique syndrome of disturbance. The fact that these children did not catch up with their peers over time questioned the basic tenet of this theory.[40] Geschwind and Galaburda[41] proposed an elaborate model attributing the underdevelopment of the left hemisphere to testosterone, which selectively inhibits maturation of the left hemisphere. Other studies[42,43] have suggested hemispheric lateralization is present at birth, further questioning the tenability of the left hemisphere maturational lag theory. The progression of research has suggested the right hemisphere has a role in language development, which highlights this theory as too simplistic.[44,45]

Lack of Hemispheric Specialization
Research findings on brain structure have documented that certain functions are specialized within each hemisphere.[46,47] Semmes[47] first hypothesized that the left hemisphere has a more focal, precise organization, with functional units located near each other, facilitating the accurate coding needed for speech. The left hemisphere processes information in a sequential, linear fashion and is more proficient in analyzing details. Academically, this hemisphere is responsible for recognizing words and comprehending material read, performing mathematical calculations, and processing and producing language.

The right hemisphere is organized diffusely, allowing dissimilar information to be processed simultaneously. This type of organization is advantageous for spatial processing and visual perception. The right hemisphere processes input in a more holistic manner, grasping the overall organization or the "gestalt" of a pattern.[43,47a] Functionally, the right hemisphere synthesizes nonverbal stimuli, such as environmental sounds and voice intonation, recognizes and interprets facial expressions, and contributes to mathematical reasoning and judgment. Although the hemispheres vary in the method of organization of input, they both participate in specific academic outcomes such as reading and mathematical concepts. Over time these differences in left and right brain processing have become accepted and are commonly labels of cognitive style (i.e., left-brained versus right-brained learner).

Researchers over the years have suggested that specialization of cerebral hemisphere functioning is optimal for efficient learning. Ayres[47b] suggested that in some children with learning disabilities, the two hemispheres do not specialize in their functions, implying that neither hemisphere is as effective for specified tasks. Levy et al[46c] reviewed a number of studies that support the hypothesis that development of language function in both hemispheres is achieved at the expense of the development of visual-spatial skills. Witelson hypothesized that children with learning disabilities have bilateral representation for spatial function, leading to poor performance on linguistic tasks such as reading, which demands sequential analysis.

Measures of hemispheric specialization are largely inferential, and definitive statements of function are compounded by the complex organization of the brain and the heterogeneity of learning disabilities. Research suggests that children with learning disabilities show different patterns of cerebral organization than normal children.[36,43] A strict left-right dichotomy is oversimplified because it does not take into account many aspects of functional brain organization.[36,43] Recently, as physiological measures have improved, the emphasis of research has shifted to looking at differential patterns of cortical activation, emphasizing the highly complex nature of information processing within the brain.

Inadequate Hemispheric Communication
Adequate communication between the cerebral hemispheres is essential for many academic tasks. Reading, for example, is a process that requires the participation of both hemispheres and the transfer of information between them. Gazzaniga[48] first suggested that aspects of learning difficulties might reflect problems in the "shuttling of information

between various specialized processing centers in the brain." Myklebust[49] believed that the primary deficit in some children with learning disabilities was attributable to one hemisphere not communicating with the other. This lack of hemispheric communication could be reflected cognitively by the child's inability to convert verbal learning (left hemisphere) into nonverbal meanings (right hemisphere) and to convert nonverbal learning into verbal expression. Hardy et al[49a] reported that this auditory-to-visual processing is critical to academic achievement. Recent research on reading difficulties and dyslexia also points to an auditory-visual connection in reading. Miller et al[50] indicate that although the primary deficit in this disorder appears to be phonological processing, that visual processing is also implicated. They suggest that research should continue to examine the relationship between the prevalence of both auditory and visual processing difficulties in dyslexia.

The adequacy of hemispheric communication also has been assessed by using motor tasks; the left brain governs actions of the right and vice versa. Badian and Wolff[51] examined motor sequencing abilities in boys aged 8 to 15 years with reading disabilities by using both single-hand tapping and alternating-hand tapping. The boys with reading disabilities showed marked deterioration when performing alternating-hand tapping. The authors suggested that the motor sequencing deficit of children with reading disabilities was the result of inadequate interhemispheric communication. This communication is necessary to coordinate control over the motor actions in the left hand (right hemisphere), motor actions of the right hand (left hemisphere), and hemispheric specialization for temporal sequencing (left hemisphere). More recently, numerous studies have looked at brain activation patterns in bimanual tasks. Recent work by Gerloff and Andres[52] has illustrated dynamic changes in hemispheric interaction as a motor task is learned. Initially, hemispheric communication is heightened and believed to be especially important in acquiring the motor sequence, but as a task becomes mastered it becomes less so. Through this decrease in hemispheric interaction, the brain is hypothesized to better inhibit mirror movements and override previously learned but not applicable motor patterns. This study illustrates the dynamic nature of learning within the brain and illustrates that a simple, unchanging theory cannot explain the complexities of learning.

In addition to the communication that occurs between the hemispheres by the corpus callosum, essential communication within the hemispheres is also present. Intrahemispheric communication is critical for developing higher level cognitive functions such as memory, language, visual-spatial perception, and praxis.[53] Functional brain imaging techniques such as MRI, PET scans, and cerebral blood flow (rCBF) have given researchers a mechanism to view specific networks of brain activation. These scans have shown dynamic changes in the brain mapping when a task is novel versus well learned, as well as if a task is done successfully or unsuccessfully.[54] This indicates the dynamic process of learning, in which minor difficulties in shuttling information effectively could limit learning in some way. The complexity and changeability of the human brain create a significant challenge for researchers attempting to clearly understand interhemispheric and intrahemispheric communication involved in learning tasks. Yet for clinicians, brain plasticity

is the basis of designing and implementing a variety of intervention techniques aimed at improving processing.

Subgroups

As debate continues regarding definition and causes of learning disabilities, discrete subgroups identifying specific learning difficulties also are inconsistent. Although similarities can be found in grouping individuals with learning disabilities by patterns of academic achievement, the categorization appears to vary with the orientation of the researcher, the types of assessments and observations used, and the age and heterogeneity of the sample.[23,47a,55,56] This ongoing dilemma affects how a diagnosis is determined and who receives services and how research studies are interpreted.[19,56,57]

In early attempts to classify learning disabilities, Denckla and Rudel[58] determined that approximately 30% of the 190 children they assessed by neurological examination could be classified into three recognizable subgroups. The other 70% exhibited an unclassifiable mixture of signs. Of the 30%, the first subgroup was classified as children having a *specific language disability*. These children, who were failing reading and spelling, showed a pattern of inadequacy on repetition, sequencing, memory, language, motor, and other tasks, all of which require rote functioning. The second group had a specific *visual-spatial disability*. These children had average performance in reading and spelling with delayed arithmetic, writing, and copying skills. This subgroup all had social and/or emotional difficulties. The third group manifested as a *dyscontrol* syndrome. These children had decreased motor and impulse control, were behaviorally immature, and were average in language and perceptual functioning.

Rourke[55] first identified discrete patterns of performance and neuropsychological functioning with his research. He initially drew from research on adults with brain damage by using the Weschler Adult Intelligence Scale (WAIS) to yield a "verbal IQ" (based primarily on language tasks) and a "performance IQ" (based primarily on visual-perceptual and perceptual-motor tasks).[59] Research on adults with brain damage found that patients with left hemisphere dysfunction showed a low-verbal, high-performance WAIS profile with language deficits. Adults with right hemisphere dysfunction presented the opposite profile of high verbal, low performance on the WAIS and exhibited predominantly visual-constructive deficits. Based on patterns of scores on the Weschler Intelligence Scale for Children (WISC),[60] children aged 9 to 14 years were placed into similar subgroups.[61-64] The performance of the high-verbal, low-performance group was superior for tasks that primarily involved verbal skills, language, and auditory-perceptual skills. In contrast, the high-performance, low-verbal subgroup was superior on tasks that primarily involved visual-spatial skills.

In additional studies of children with learning disabilities, similar subgroups of children were identified.[65] The first group exhibited age-appropriate visual-spatial-organizational, tactile-perceptual, motor, and nonverbal problem-solving skills coupled with poor language skills, including reading and spelling. The second group exhibited strengths in language skills, spelling, and rote verbal memory with difficulties in visual-spatial-organizational, mathematics, balance and equilibrium, discerning social cues, and nonverbal problem solving. This group often had difficulties understanding nonverbal cues, with greater frequencies of emotional problems reported by their parents.[66]

Recent thoughts on subgroups with learning disabilities are far more complex and do not provide strong support of the validity of classification based on IQ discrepancy alone.[23] The authors suggest that strides towards subtyping children through patterns of academic strengths and weakness are as important as those based on neuropsychological or cognitive measures. Within an academic classification the heterogeneity of learning disabilities can be more clearly recognized and learning modalities can be adjusted to the individual child to facilitate academic performance. For example, a child with a specific reading difficulty could be differentiated by patterns of strength and weaknesses in the components of word recognition, fluency, or comprehension, and those deficit areas could be specifically addressed.[23] Most important in these decisions are the future implications for future research and intervention.

Trends based on a variety of studies have led to the following general subgroups: verbal learning impairments, nonverbal learning disorders, specific motor impairments, and behavior disorders.

Verbal Learning Impairments

Verbal learning impairments typically include dyslexia, dyscalculia, and dysgraphia. Harris[12] classifies these deficits in functional terms, with dyslexia including disorders of reading and spelling, dyscalculia labeling a mathematics disorder, and dysgraphia describing a disorder of written expression. These learning disorders may occur individually or concurrently. Each of these verbal learning impairments will significantly affect academic performance.

Dyslexia. Children with dyslexia demonstrate a specific learning disability characterized by reading problems and language disorder[8] and proposed to be neurologically based.[50,67] The International Dyslexia Association adopted the following definition in 2002: "Dyslexia is a specific learning disability that is neurological in origin. It is characterized by difficulties with accurate and/or fluent word recognition and by poor spelling and decoding abilities. These difficulties typically result from a deficit in the phonological component of language that is often unexpected in relation to other cognitive abilities and the provision of effective classroom instruction. Secondary consequences may include problems in reading comprehension and reduced reading experience that can impede the growth of vocabulary and background knowledge."[68] Dyslexia is the most common learning disorder, affecting as many as 80% of individuals identified as learning disabled.[69] Prevalence rates range from 5% to 17% of the school-aged population, with as many as 40% of the entire population reading below grade level.[69,70] Boys were previously believed to be affected by dyslexia at a higher rate than girls, but recent data indicate an equal distribution between the sexes.[70]

Neuroanatomical abnormalities, atypical brain symmetry in the temporal-parietal region, size differences in the corpus callosum, and anomalies in cerebral blood flow have been observed in children with reading disorders.[12,50,56] Investigations using functional brain imagining techniques (PET, fMRI, and the newer ultrafast echo planar imagining [EPI])

continue to provide information on brain functioning during cognitive tasks such as reading.[70] Converging evidence is present indicating that dyslexic readers exhibit deficits in left hemisphere posterior brain systems during reading tasks, creating a phonological deficit in understanding that spoken words can be pulled apart into phonemes and that written letters represent these sounds.[70] In addition, evidence of an associated increased reliance on ancillary systems during reading tasks exists, including the frontal lobe and right hemisphere posterior circuitry. This suggests that the child with dyslexia may be compensating for poor phonological skills with other perceptual processes, helping to explain why individuals with dyslexia can develop reading skills, although they often remain slow and nonautomatic.[70]

Various classifications and subtypes within dyslexia have been proposed, involving both language and visual spatial difficulties.[12,71,72] Reading skills consist of a combination of visually perceiving whole words and phonetically decoding letters, morphemes, and words.[71,72] Visually based disorders could account for the poor comprehension of "visual word form,"[72] with a tendency to reverse letters, read words backwards, and misread similar words (e.g., "when" and "which").[71] Auditory-language word analysis difficulties would cause difficulties in relating letter symbols to sounds and with poor word sounding and spelling.[70,71,73] By further examining the neural systems for reading, Shaywitz and Shaywitz[70] hope to develop specific interventions based on the neural circuitry in subtypes of poor readers.

Dyscalculia. Children with dyscalculia have specific difficulties in performing arithmetic functions. This heterogeneous disorder may involve both intrinsic and extrinsic factors.[74] Intrinsic factors are hypothesized to include deficits in visual-spatial skill, quantitative reasoning, sequencing, memory, or intelligence. Extrinsic factors can be a combination of poor instruction in the mastery of prerequisite skills as well as attitude, interest, and confidence in the subject. The neurological cause of dyscalculia was initially hypothesized to be right hemisphere dysfunction because of the strong relation of visual-spatial skills to numerical computation.[75] Additional research supports the involvement of both hemispheres because mathematics computation involves a complex relation of spatial problem solving, sequential analysis, language processing, and memory. Compared with reading disorders, limited research has been done on the neural mechanisms that contribute to arithmetic disorders. Part of the difficulty in research stems from limited knowledge of the normal development and associated competencies in mathematics.[76]

No universal definition of dyscalculia exists. The British Department of Education and Skills offers a comprehensive definition of dyscalculia as "a condition that affects the ability to acquire arithmetical skills. Dyscalculic learners have difficulty understanding simple number concepts, lack an intuitive grasp of numbers and have problems learning number facts and procedures. Even if they produce a correct answer or use a correct method, they may do so mechanically and without confidence."[77] Large-scale studies on the prevalence of arithmetic disorders have not been conducted. Smaller samples have demonstrated that dyscalculia occurs in approximately 5% to 8% of school-aged children.[76] Geary[76] concludes that arithmetic disabilities currently appear to constitute at least two subgroups: those with only arithmetic disorders and those with concomitant reading disorders and/or attention deficit disorder.

Various classifications of subtypes within dyscalculia have been proposed on the basis of the development and functional structure of mathematical skills. Geary[76] recently proposed a taxonomy of three general subtypes of mathematical disability, including procedural, semantic memory, and visuospatial. He identifies these subtypes through differences in cognitive and performance features as well as developmental manifestations. Specific skills that may be impaired in dyscalculia include linguistic skills for mathematical terms and concepts and decoding written problems; perceptual skills for recognition of number symbols; attentional ability to copy figures correctly and follow sequenced procedures; and development and retrieval of basic math facts.[77] Children with mathematics disorder may demonstrate a variety of these mathematical difficulties, including recognizing numbers and symbols, performing and applying basic mathematical functions (e.g., addition and subtraction), and maintaining proper order of numbers when performing mathematical calculations.[74,78] Some children have difficulty with written math problems but can learn practical concepts in functional applications (e.g., using money or measurement concepts in cooking).[78]

Dysgraphia. Children with dysgraphia have specific difficulties in written language production, which may include problems putting thoughts into words, using words inappropriately, or mastering the mechanics of writing. This heterogeneous disorder is frequently found in combination with other academic, learning, and attention disorders.[12,79] Dysgraphia has been suggested to be a neurological disorder that seldom occurs in isolation and can result from a number of other dysfunctions, including attention deficit, auditory or visual processing weakness, and sequencing problems.[80] The complex nature of written expression makes finding the cause difficult. Writing involves integration of spatial and linguistic functions, planning, memory, and motor output. This suggests involvement of both the left and right hemispheres for skill in decoding, spelling, formulating and sequencing ideas, and producing work in correct spatial orientation, all coupled with rules of punctuation and capitalization.

Diagnosis of "disorder of written expression" depends on recognition of "writing skills . . . substantially below those expected given the person's chronological age, measured intelligence, and age appropriate education," which "significantly interferes with academic achievement or activities of daily living that require composition of written texts."[27] Limited data are available on the prevalence of dysgraphia; it is often misdiagnosed and frequently occurs concomitantly with other learning difficulties. Difficulties in written expression are frequently underidentified and can be masked by reading disorders or considered to be attributable to poor motivation. Studies have suggested that it may be as common as reading disorders and may occur in 3% to 4% of the population.[12,81]

Classifications of dysgraphia can include penmanship-related aspects of writing (e.g., motor control and execution), linguistic aspects of writing (e.g., spelling and composing), or a combination.[81] The common difficulty is in the expression of thoughts through written language.[12] Sandler et al[82] proposed four subtypes within dysgraphia based on assessment of 190 children aged 9 to 15 years with average intelligence. These subgroups include writing disorder coupled with *fine motor and linguistic deficits, visual-spatial deficits, attention and memory deficits,* and *sequencing deficits.* The subgroup that exhibited fine motor and linguistic difficulties also demonstrated delays in decoding and comprehension during reading. Written output was slow, with spelling, punctuation, and capitalization errors. Soft neurological indicators of finger agnosia and mirror movements were present, influencing motor output. Children who exhibited visual-spatial deficits as the primary component of writing disorder had normal reading skills. Their difficulties were in written production with inconsistent letter formations and poor spatial organization, including sloping lines, inconsistent spacing, and undefined margins. Decoding difficulties were observed with attention and memory deficits. Spelling was poor and inconsistent. For these children written production and speed were within expected ranges. When sequencing deficits were present the children exhibited strong reading skills but delayed math computation. A variety of deficits also were noted in written production, including spelling, letter formation, and legibility.

Nonverbal Learning Disabilities

Nonverbal learning disorders affect children in both academic performance and social interactions. Three primary areas affected by nonverbal learning disabilities include visual-spatial organization, sensory-motor integration, and social-emotional development. These functions are all mediated by the right hemisphere. These deficit areas impede the child's performance in constructional tasks, handwriting, and fine and gross motor skills. The social and emotional difficulties for individuals with nonverbal learning disorders are paramount, leading some researchers to label this a *social-emotional learning disability.*[12,83] Deficits include the inability to read facial expressions and change performance in response to interactional cues. These children cannot appropriately interpret emotional responses made by others or make correct inferences regarding emotional behavior.[12] They are often intrusive and disruptive and are frequently labeled as behavior problems or emotionally disturbed.[4] Cues received through body language, facial expressions, and voice intonations are unnoticed or misinterpreted. Jokes, metaphors, and implied meanings are not understood, and figures of speech are interpreted on a concrete level.

Nonverbal learning disability is considered by some to be a neuropsychological disability. Although the condition has been identified for more than 30 years, it has not yet been included as a diagnostic category in the DSM.[55,61-63,66] It is generally defined by a distinct pattern of strengths and deficits, with early speech and vocabulary development, notable rote memory skills, early reading, and strong spelling abilities. Sensory-motor deficits in tactile discrimination, body awareness, balance, and graphomotor delays, executive functioning difficulties, and social ineptitude are salient weaknesses.[12,44,47a,84] Accurate diagnosis often involves identification of lowered performance IQ compared with verbal IQ on the WISC. Differential diagnosis is essential because nonverbal learning disabilities can occur in conjunction with dyscalculia, attention deficit, adjustment disorder, anxiety and depression, and obsessive-compulsive tendencies.

Nonverbal learning disabilities are frequently overlooked in the educational arena because children with this disorder are highly verbal and develop an extensive vocabulary at a young age. Well-developed memory for rote verbal information positively influences early academic learning of reading and spelling. Yet these students will have difficulty performing in situations where adaptability and speed are necessary, and their written output will be slow and laborious.[47a] Nonverbal learning disorders are therefore challenging to identify at younger ages but become progressively more apparent and debilitating by adolescence and adulthood. This disorder is considered a low-incidence disability and is thought to be less prevalent than language-based disorders. Although approximately 10% of the general population is suspected to have an identifiable learning disability, only 1% to 10% of that population is estimated to have a nonverbal learning disability (0.1% to 1% of the general population). This type of learning disability affects both sexes equally.[4]

Classification of nonverbal learning disorders is made on the basis of the domains for processing social signals and include *expressive, receptive,* and *mixed*.[12] Expressive deficits are observable in limited facial expression, flat affect, unchanging voice intonation, and robotic speech. Receptive difficulties result in impairments in social understanding with intact affective expression. Mixed disorders couple both expressive and receptive features. Children often lack social reciprocity and awareness of social space.

Specific Motor Impairments

Children with learning disabilities may or may not present with motor coordination problems. Conversely, some children have motor and coordination problems but do not experience learning difficulties. Children with motor impairments typically have difficulty acquiring age-appropriate motor skills and move in an awkward and clumsy manner. Difficulties in daily functional tasks and performance areas (e.g., school and leisure skills) are common. Motor deficits can result from a wide variety of neurological, physiological, developmental, and environmental factors. These impairments can manifest in diverse ways depending on the severity of the disorder and the areas of motor and social performance affected.

An International Consensus Meeting on Children and Clumsiness was held in 1994 with expert educators, kinesiologists, occupational therapists, physical therapists, psychologists, and parents. These experts discussed a common name to identify "clumsy" children with movement, coordination, and motor planning difficulties. The term *developmental coordination disorder* (DCD) was identified to distinguish these children from those with severe motor impairments (such as those with cerebral palsy or paraplegia) and children with normal motor movements.

Developmental coordination disorder is a childhood disorder characterized by poor coordination and clumsiness. As described in the DSM-IV as one of the motor skill disorders, DCD is a "marked impairment in the development of motor coordination that significantly interferes with academic achievement or activities of daily living that is not due to a general medical condition."[27] This condition is not considered benign and is distinct from normal developmental variance, maturational delays, and other medical conditions.[5] Difficulties in movement skills are not primarily caused by impairments in intellectual functioning, primary sensory, or neurological disorders.[85,86] An estimated 6% of children aged 5 to 11 years have DCD.[67] Boys diagnosed with DCD outnumber girls 2 : 1. This difference may reflect a higher referral rates for boys as a result of increased behavioral difficulties of boys with motor incoordination.[87]

Various approaches have been used to investigate subtypes of DCD, including classification by underlying causes, clinical and descriptive approaches, and statistical clustering.[86] Initial attempts at classifying subtypes within DCD support the heterogeneity of this group of children.[88] Henderson and Hall[89] first divided "clumsy" children into three groups on the basis of academic skill, motor ability, and behavior. Although a distinct motor impaired group was present, the other two groups involved combinations of motor, academic, and behavioral difficulties without distinct clarity. Dewey et al[90] took this classification further by teasing out distinctions in motor planning and motor execution deficits. The three motor deficit subgroups they identified included severe motor impairments (planning and execution), deficits in balance, coordination and gestural performance (motor execution), and motor sequencing (planning).[86] As in the Henderson study the composite of academic, language, and perceptual skills was varied. In a more recent classification attempt, five patterns of dysfunction were observed in a sample of 80 children identified as having DCD.[88] The two largest subgroups had average to above-average visual-perceptual and visual-motor performance, with mild to moderate delays in two of the three gross motor measures (i.e., kinesthetic acuity, static balance, and running). Difficulty with visual-perceptual and visual-motor tasks, as well as kinesthetic acuity and balance, delineated the third largest subgroup. The smallest two clusters had average kinesthetic acuity but had difficulty in either visual-perceptual or balance and running.

Behavior Disorders

Behavior disorders associated with learning disabilities include attention deficits, conduct problems, depression, and global behavior problems. Ames[91] stressed that no single behavior pattern is prevalent in children with learning disabilities. Issues in learning and related behaviors affect each other in a complex manner.

Attention problems can affect behavior, often relating to difficulties with impulse control, restlessness, and irritability, with the inability to sustain attention for learning and peer interactions. These issues frequently coincide with frustration, anger, and resentment, which may manifest as a conduct problem (e.g., verbal and nonverbal aggression, destructiveness, and significant difficulties interacting with peers). Children with learning disabilities often become discouraged and fearful, lose motivation, and develop negative and defensive attitudes. These patterns of behavior can worsen with age, contributing to juvenile deliquency.[3] Low self-esteem and depression are common during school years and escalate around age 10 years.[92]

Children with learning disabilities may initially be an integral part of the social and educational milieu. Poor academic progress, additional prompting needed from teachers, and negative attention for disruptive behaviors can cause children with learning disabilities to perceive themselves as being "different."[93] Lack of success in school experiences can influence the development of positive self-perception and have powerfully negative effects on self-esteem.[94] A self-defeating cycle may be established: the child experiences learning problems, school and home environments become increasingly tense, and disruptive behaviors become more pronounced. These responses, in turn, further affect the child's ability to learn. Lack of success generates more failure until the child anticipates defeat in almost every situation.

Assessment of and Intervention for the Child with Learning Disabilities

Specialists

Evaluation of and intervention for children with learning disabilities must involve interdisciplinary procedures because of the differing constellations of problems present. Remediation of foundational and skill-related deficits is beyond the competency of any one professional group. Most children with learning disabilities are seen by a group of professionals, the make-up of which depends on the purpose, location, philosophical orientation, or availability of resources of a particular program. Box 14-1 lists the different professionals and specialists who might participate in assessment or remediation of children with learning disabilities. The types of professionals are grouped into the four categories of education, medicine and nursing, psychology, and special services; they have been listed only once, although some professions could be categorized in more than one way.

Therapists should be familiar with the roles of the various medical specialists and of primary care physicians. School nursing is mentioned, however, because it is a specialty within nursing. The school nurse is usually the key health care professional in a school system and is responsible for maintaining information about the child's health history, current health status, medication, home environment, family cooperation, and family problems. The school nurse is the primary liaison between the child and the doctor or health clinic and relays information from the school to medical professionals.

Psychologists have two distinct and often separate roles in the care of children with learning disorders. The first role is in identification of learning strengths and weaknesses. Psychological testing is often essential in the recognition of specific learning problems and may be done by clinical psychologists, school psychologists, or clinical neuropsychologists, who specialize in diagnosis of learning disorders. The second role of psychologists is to provide mental health services and support systems. Children with learning disabilities often have problems with self-esteem and peer relationships, resulting from either primary behavior problems or reactions to failure.

A child with learning disabilities with a primary behavior problem, such as impulsiveness, disinhibited behavior, or hyperkinetic activity, may receive special treatment for the behavior disorder. A behavior modification specialist may be working with parents and teachers to help the child

---

BOX 14-1 ■ TYPES OF SPECIALISTS WORKING WITH CHILDREN WITH LEARNING DISABILITIES

EDUCATION
Classroom teacher
Special educator
Learning disability specialist
Psychoeducational diagnostician
Reading specialist
Early childhood education teacher
Physical educator
Adaptive physical educator

MEDICINE AND NURSING
Family physician
Pediatrician
Pediatric neurologist
Psychiatrist
School nurse
Biochemist
Geneticist
Endocrinologist
Nutritionist
Ophthalmologist
Otologist

PSYCHOLOGY
Clinical psychologist
Neuropsychologist
School psychologist
Child psychologist
Counseling psychologist
Guidance counselor

SPECIAL SERVICES
Occupational therapist
Physical therapist
Speech and language pathologist
Psycholinguist
Audiologist
Optometrist
Social worker
Recreational therapist
Motor therapist
Perceptual-motor trainer
Vocational education specialist

---

control behavior. The child may receive psychotherapy from a psychologist or psychiatrist, or family therapy may be provided by a social worker, psychologist, or psychiatrist. These latter interventions are usually provided by public or private mental health clinics. Children with learning disabilities with general adjustment problems in peer relationships are often treated within the school setting. School adjustment or guidance counselors offer support and advice on specific academic difficulties, social conflicts, and affective issues. The school psychologist, in addition to the diagnostic role, may offer psychological counseling to students and may help plan strategies for classroom management.

Physical educators, adaptive physical educators, physical therapists, occupational therapists, and developmental optometrists also may be involved in the evaluation. Overlap in the areas assessed may occur. The unique training of each professional influences both the selection of tests and the qualitative aspects of assessment on the basis of observations of a child's performance. Although the evaluations may appear similar, differences between professions are apparent in orientation and rationale when interpreting dysfunction.

Differences in professional orientation and emphasis in assessment contribute to a comprehensive overview of the child's abilities and relative concerns related to the impairments resulting from the learning disability. Physical educators and adaptive physical educators typically assess skilled tasks necessary for sports-related activities. These include abilities in ball throwing, kicking, catching, jumping, running, and climbing skills. The primary concern of these professionals is the child's physical fitness. Physical therapists' assessment of the child's gross motor development and physical fitness integrate neuromuscular and neurodevelopmental factors. The physical therapy assessment includes observations of muscle strength and tone, postural refinement, reflex integration including automatic reactions, and sensory-motor functions. Occupational therapists consider developmental motor skills and sensory integrative functions that underlie skill development and affect functional performance. Within the academic environment fine motor and visual-perceptual motor skills are emphasized with consideration of the impact on academic achievement. The developmental optometrist assesses bilateral eye movements as they relate to visual-perceptual motor skills, recognizing the relation between vision and movement in development and eye-hand coordination.

Planning an assessment protocol can prevent unnecessary duplication of testing and provide comprehensive information related to the referral concerns. The areas assessed and particular evaluations chosen dependent on the make-up of the professional team, the setting, and the service delivery model. The assessment is driven by the referral concerns and the functional difficulties the child is experiencing. Communication of information between professionals and the parents will generate a comprehensive picture of the child's areas of strength and weakness necessary for effective intervention planning.

Coordinating Multiple Interventions

As the number of therapeutic disciplines involved in the assessment and therapeutic management of children with learning disabilities has steadily increased, communication for effective programming has become more challenging. Despite the benefits of specific skills brought to the case by each professional, the huge variety of well-meaning recommendations can result in service delivery overkill. Case Study 14-1 provides an example of the negative impact of overabundant specialized intervention on the child and family.

Effective coordination of intervention services presents a dilemma because no single discipline has trained its students to handle that role.[95] Rather, the assumption is made that all professionals acquire the ability to coordinate services by virtue of learning their own special skills. Kenny and Burka[95] stress the need for a person to act as coordinator for the management and integration of the multiple interventions received by the child with learning disabilities. They suggest that the coordinator be the team member who could best service the needs of the child. This thought is similar to that of the philosophy of case management, an area of practice within a profession rather than a profession in itself. The case manager helps identify appropriate providers and options throughout the continuum of services while ensuring that available resources are being used to obtain outcomes. These services are best offered in a climate that promotes and practices direct communication among

---

CASE STUDY 14-1 ■ MATT

Matt is an 8-year-old boy referred for clinic-based physical therapy intervention 1 hour per week for remediation of severe motor coordination and planning problems that accompanied his learning disability. In addition to Matt's weekly treatment sessions, suggestions were made to his mother for a home program to be accomplished three times a week for 15 to 30 minutes each time. Meanwhile, Matt also received other services. Although he was mainstreamed into a regular classroom in accordance with the special education law, he was seen by the resource room teacher on a daily basis and by the adaptive physical education teacher twice a week to meet his specialized needs. The classroom teacher told Matt's mother that Matt must read at least one book a night because he needed additional reading practice. A reading tutor came to Matt's house Saturday morning. Ocular motor problems were identified, so he was evaluated by an optometrist, who recommended weekly visits plus ocular exercises for 30 minutes a day. Matt developed secondary emotional problems, partly because he was bright yet aware of his learning disability and frustrated by it. Thus Matt also saw a psychotherapist on a weekly basis. The psychotherapist recommended participation in weekly group sessions, in addition to Matt's individual sessions, to help improve peer relationships. Thus Matt's "therapists" had developed a 12-hour-a-day program for him and his family. It is no wonder that Matt had difficulty in developing peer relationships—he never had time. Matt's schedule also affected interaction in his own family. His mother believed that being a "therapist" to Matt interfered with her role as his mother. She felt unable to carry out the home program and felt guilty for not doing it.

What became apparent with Matt's case is that although each professional involved with him made an important contribution to evaluation and intervention, the massive input, to some extent, had a detrimental effect on Matt and his family. Coordinating interventions and providing additional support at home can create a drain on the family and limit time for family activities and extracurricular participation.

the case manager, the student, the family, and service personnel.[96]

Service Delivery Models

Cruickshank et al[97] indicated that one of the major problems confronting the child with learning disabilities is the lack of a true interdisciplinary approach. Each discipline has traditionally been concerned with its own viewpoint in the field of learning disabilities, resulting in research and remediation approaches that are limited in scope. Gaddes[3] reiterates that territoriality is not necessary because none of the procedures by itself is complete and adequate, and superiority of any one method has not been demonstrated over another for all children with learning disabilities. In creating a plan that truly encompasses and addresses the issues hindering the child's learning within the academic setting, the team must work together to fabricate relevant and inclusive goals and objectives that are functionally based.[98]

IDEA currently requires that all children in special education be educated in the least restrictive environment (LRE). This environment is often mistakenly interpreted as meaning a regular or general special education environment. The LRE should be determined after assessing the individual needs of the child. If services in a regular classroom with supplemental aids and services do not meet the needs of the child, an alternate environment should be considered.

In some educational settings, children with learning disabilities are given full-time instruction in a special classroom with a small group of other children with learning disabilities. A special education teacher or a learning disability teacher is in charge of the classroom. More commonly, the child is placed in a regular classroom and leaves class for special instruction for some part of the day. The child may go to a resource room, where a special education teacher provides regularly scheduled remedial education for children with a variety of educational delays, or the child may receive tutoring from a reading specialist or a private tutor.

Although the model of inclusion has much support, it requires members of the team to work closely together with the regular education teacher. This collaborative effort ensures an understanding of the child's special learning needs and incorporation of therapeutic procedures into the regular classroom to facilitate the best learning environment. Within the model of inclusion, a continuum of services exists to enable interventionists to be responsive to all children's needs. The continuum includes direct service, integrated or supervised therapy, and consultation.[99] Regardless of the choice of service provision, the therapist must, at the very least, observe the child within the classroom and other appropriate environments, ensuring that intervention addresses the functional issues of the child within the educational setting.

Direct therapy occurs when an interventionist designs individualized interventions and carries them out with the child individually or in a small group. Best practice dictates that direct therapy should always be provided with one of the other service models to ensure generalization of skills to natural settings.[99] Without the use of other models, therapists cannot be confident that changes observed in the isolated setting are affecting the child's overall performance.

Integrated or supervised therapy allows the therapists to support a child within the natural environment while working with other care providers, such as the teachers who are with the child every day. This allows for therapeutic consistency and repeated practice, thereby increasing the chances for skill acquisition with contextual supports. With this model, the therapist designs an intervention plan to meet individual needs of the child and remains responsible for the outcome of the plan. The therapist trains another person within the child's natural environment (e.g., classroom) to implement the plan. The therapist must remain in contact with the person carrying out the plan to make necessary modifications.[98] Therefore ongoing contact between the therapist and implementer is imperative to integrated therapy.[99]

The consultative model of service provision incorporates the use of another team member's expertise to be responsible for the outcome of the child.[98,99] The teacher, for example, may be responsible for carrying out the program and the outcome of the child and the therapist responsible for the collaborative efforts with the teacher. Dunn and Campbell[98] found that teachers who participated in a collaborative consultation model of services reported that the therapists contributed to EIP goal attainment in 24% more instances than teachers whose children participated in isolated direct services. This collaborative effort supports the shared responsibility for identifying the problem or weakness of the child, creating possible solutions, implementing the intervention as the solution, and altering the plan as necessary for increased effectiveness.[99]

Summary

Learning disabilities are heterogeneous and multidimensional in their presentation, making consensus on a definition and classifications extremely challenging. A great deal of attention has been focused on the definition of learning disabilities without much change from earlier versions. Various models of classification have evolved with continued revisions. Assessment and classification methods are being revamped to identify both underlying deficits and effective remediation strategies in an attempt to delineate more clearly a learning disability from underachievement as a result of inadequate instruction.

Research continues to work on identifying the causes and the associated functional deficits of learning disabilities as well as developing effective intervention techniques. The heterogeneity of the group suggests a spectrum of neurological processing difficulties. As physiological measures of brain function improve, our theoretical understanding increases. On the basis of research, subgrouping within learning disabilities has assisted in delineating functional areas of dysfunction and distinguishing associated deficits. The challenge for the clinician is to recognize the multitude of components that interact to impede functional abilities and social participation for the child with learning disabilities.

THE CHILD WITH LEARNING DISABILITIES AND MOTOR DEFICITS

Occurrence of Developmental Coordination Disorder

Motor deficits are often the most overt sign of difficulty for the child with learning disabilities. Yet they are only one of the multifaceted problems facing these children. As evidence mounts that children do not "outgrow" clumsiness, more efforts have been made to identify causes and interventions to enhance remedial strategies for these students. Occupational and physical therapists are frequently asked to provide intervention to enhance functional performance for children with a variety of motor coordination difficulties. The emphasis of this section relates to children with DCD.

Specific focus on motor performance does not imply that the motor deficits are the paramount problems of children with learning disabilities or that motor deficits should receive priority over other symptoms. The therapist providing intervention must be aware of the child's strengths and weaknesses and the characteristics of the child's educational program to plan and implement optimal intervention strategies effectively.

Historical Terminology of Developmental Coordination Disorders

Terms used to describe motor deficits have varied greatly in the literature, research, and clinical practice. Developmental clumsiness was documented as early as the 1900s, when Collier used the term *congenital maladroitness*.[100] Orton[37] first adopted the term *clumsy* or *developmentally clumsy* to refer to children with motor coordination difficulties. He recognized that disorders in praxis and gnosis resulted in clumsiness in physical performance, which he described as similar to a right-handed person trying to use the left hand, and said that the child seemed to have two left feet. Children with learning disabilities and motor incoordination were described in the literature most frequently as "clumsy."[86,89,101-104] Clinicians suggested that this term is pejorative and had unfavorable connotations.[105] Other terminology used to describe children with motor deficits have included motor delayed, physically awkward, perceptual motor deficient,[5] developmentally dyspraxic/apraxic,[104,106,107] or having sensory integration dysfunction or developmental output failure.[5]

The DSM-III introduced the diagnostic label of developmental coordination disorder.[108] This descriptive term was adopted in 1994 at the International Consensus Meeting on Children and Clumsiness to identify and describe the heterogeneous group of children with motor deficits and facilitate communication within the field.[5] In this chapter, the term DCD is used to describe a subgroup of children identified in the DSM-IV[27] who demonstrate marked impairment in the development of motor coordination that significantly interferes with academic achievement or activities of daily living. A child may exhibit difficulty with motoric academic tasks such as handwriting and gym class, self-care skills such as dressing and using utensils, and leisure activities including playground activities and social interactions.[109] *Motor coordination deficit, disorder,* or *disturbance* is used as a general term to identify disorders that have a motor component.

Motor coordination refers to functions that are more clearly and traditionally defined as motoric and includes gross motor, fine motor, and motor planning (praxis). Gross motor coordination includes motor behaviors concerned with posture and locomotion ranging from early developmental milestones to finely tuned balance.[110] Fine motor coordination involves motor behavior such as discrete finger movements, manipulation, and eye-hand coordination. Motor planning is used specifically to denote the ability to plan and execute skilled, nonhabitual motor tasks.[111] Visual-motor function can be considered an aspect of motor coordination and is predominantly used in the literature as a synonym for visual constructional abilities. Visual-motor tasks involve the ability to reproduce shapes, figures, or other visual stimuli in written form.

Prevalence

Motor difficulties manifest in multiple variations, which skews the ability to document the prevalence of motor deficits within learning disabilities accurately. The child's motor disturbances may be predominantly in gross or fine motor skills, but not necessarily both.[112] Other factors influencing prevalence rates include the criteria used to determine motor dysfunction, differences in terminology, types and methods of testing, reliability of the tests used, and heterogeneity of the test sample.[109,113,114] Within the general population the prevalence rates of motor dysfunction for school-aged children are estimated at 6%.[27] In 1996, Wright and Sugden[115] found in a random sample that 4% of children aged 6 to 9 years had motor coordination difficulties. In this study only children whose motor impairments interfered significantly in their functioning in everyday life were included.

The current rate of comorbidity between DCD and learning disabilities has been reported to be approximately 50%.[116] Over the years, studies attempting to identify the prevalence of motor problems in children with learning disabilities have yielded quite varied estimates. In 1997 Tarnopol and Tarnopol[117] reported that approximately 90% of the children with learning disabilities have motor coordination and visual-motor defects. Ten years later, Sugden and Wann[118] found that 29% to 33% of children with learning disabilities also had coordination problems. In other studies, the estimates of motor deficits range from 35% to 60%.[113,119] A recent study looked at incidence of primitive reflex patterns and motor coordination difficulties in children with reading difficulties.[120] The group with the lowest reading scores had a significantly higher rate of asymmetrical tonic neck reflex (ATNR) and motor impairments when compared with good readers. The study by Jongmans et al[116] indicates that children with concomitant perceptual-motor and learning problems are more severely affected in motor difficulties than those with only DCD or only learning disabled.

Causes of Developmental Coordination Disorders

Debate among researchers and clinicians exists regarding the causes of DCD. Prenatal or neonatal insult,[85] developmental delays, variance from normal development,[5] and neurological and physiological factors are the major theories proposed to explain the basis of DCD.[121] To explain the high co-occurrence of developmental and learning problems, Kaplan et al[122] have proposed that abnormal brain development (ABD) is the underlying impairment manifesting in variable symptoms. Recently, Hadders-Algra[123] has suggested that DCD is a result of damage at the cellular level in the neurotransmitter and receptor systems rather than a specific region of the brain. Resulting coordination difficulties can be from a combination of one or more impairments in proprioception, motor programming, timing, or sequencing of muscle activity.[85]

Possible physiological origins of motor coordination deficits have addressed unisensory and multisensory processing. The visual system, kinesthetic system, and vestibular system have been explored, individually and in combination. Depth perception and figure-ground perception have been hypothesized to provide a foundation for motor movements.[124] Kinesthetic awareness (i.e., awareness of body position in space) can be an important factor in coordination problems and motor skill learning for children with developmental coordination difficulties. The vestibular system mediates movement in space and postural control and stabilizes the eyes during head movements.[125,126] Fisher[126] suggests the visual and kinesthetic systems work in conjunction for accurate motor performance, hence the support of the multisensory processing theories. Ayres[107,111] developed the theory of sensory integration that suggests that the integration between sensory systems is imperative for motor performance in children. She suggested that normal development depends on intrasensory integration, particularly from the somatosensory and vestibular systems.[107] When examining vestibular functioning in children with learning disabilities and coordination problems, difficulty with the integration of vestibular, visual, and somatosensory inputs was exhibited, thereby affecting postural stability.[127]

The heterogeneity of DCD makes finding a unitary cause difficult. Children with DCD present wide variability in both locus of specific problems and functional disabilities.[87] Perspective on the cause of DCD then affects intervention. Barnhart[87] suggests an integrated approach to facilitating development in the child with DCD including both bottom-up, physiological interventions and top-down, cognitive strategies. Physiological theories support intervention that is specific to identified sensory deficits, encouraging bottom-up, multisensory activities to be done with the child at different developmental stages.[121] Top-down approaches are task-specific cognitive approaches or strategies that emphasize the context in which motor behavior occurs. The theoretical foundation for this type of intervention is based on functional results in which children have demonstrated gains in motor skills with this approach.[87]

Descriptions of Children with Coordination Deficits

The motor deficits of children with learning disabilities are variable, with different levels of severity and functional deficit. At times, extreme discrepancy in competence over a range of motor skills exists, with strengths in some motor areas and significant weaknesses in others.[128] If a diagnosis of DCD is made the essential component is a marked impairment in motor coordination that interferes with academic achievement or activities of daily living.[27] The salient features are coordination difficulties in gross and fine motor skills that include decreased anticipation, speed, reaction time and quality and grading of movement.[85,128] Secondary difficulties in psychosocial development can occur with associated behavioral and emotional difficulties caused by poor self-esteem. Presentation of difficulties may change over time depending on developmental maturation, environmental demands, and interventions received.

Two approaches are proposed to describe the characteristic motor deficits of the child with DCD. The first approach is based on observations and is *descriptive,* highlighting the general characteristics of the motor problems. These characteristics are frequently reported by parents and teachers. The second method, termed the *neurological approach,* is based on direct assessment of soft neurological signs. Evaluation of soft neurological signs is typically part of an examination by a pediatric neurologist, although therapists can assess these areas in conjunction with standardized testing. Soft signs may include minor neurological indicators, coordination difficulties, postural and motor impairments, and tactile discrimination deficits.[129] A number of soft sign batteries have been published that include tests of sensory function, coordination, motor speed, and abnormal or associated movements.[130]

Descriptive/Observational Approach

Children with DCD are generally described as awkward, with clumsy movements and poor coordination. They often fall, trip, and bump into things, acquiring more than the usual number of bruises. Motor movements are performed at a slower rate despite practice and repetition.[128] These motor problems can affect gross and fine motor skills with related functional limitations, such as running, ball skills, manipulating fasteners, tying shoelaces, and handling objects. Although motor milestones of rolling, sitting, standing, and walking may develop within normal or slow-normal limits, the child often has a history of relative slowness in self-care skills. Self-care tasks such as dressing, feeding, and use of tools (e.g., a toothbrush) also may be problematic and delayed.

In school, children with DCD may have lowered academic achievement, with any or all areas of learning affected (reading, spelling, writing).[5] When playing, these children may be sedentary and engage in solitary play because of their poor coordination and planning. They may have difficulty assembling puzzles, building models, and playing games.[27] Other play skills, such as riding a tricycle and bicycle, skipping rope, and catching a ball, are often achieved at a later age and seem to take extra effort for the child to perform. Children with DCD often experience secondary low self-esteem and emotional and behavioral problems because of their motor difficulties.[121] Anxiety may be more prevalent in adolescence, most notably in boys.[131] Feelings of incompetence, depression, or frustration are common and are lifelong problems.[5,132,133]

Fine motor coordination problems specifically related to academic and play skills also are evident. They may be manifested by reluctance to engage in, or incompetence in, small motor tasks such as coloring and cutting with scissors, or constructive manipulatory play such as block building, Tinker Toys, Legos, and puzzles. Inefficiencies of fine motor performance may manifest educationally in difficulties with drawing and writing. Impaired drawing ability is characterized by poor motor control, with wobbly lines, inaccurate junctures, and difficulty coloring within the lines. Handwriting is often labored, with spacing and sizing problems evident. Letters may be irregular, illegible, and poorly organized on the page. To compensate for inadequate pencil manipulation, the child may develop a maladaptive grasp and use excess pressure when writing, further contributing

CASE STUDY 14-2 ■ PAUL

The following is a mother's description of her child, Paul, who had motor coordination problems and learning disabilities: "I think when Paul was first born I tried to ignore the problem. Paul is a child who never climbed or ran or drew pictures the way other kids did. But until he went to nursery school, I didn't pay much attention to it. Maybe I didn't want to pay attention to it. Maybe I knew it was there and I didn't want to know about it. I'm not sure. But Paul was always a verbal child and a creative and imaginative child. He and I had something special because I used to enjoy that kind of creative imaginative play. We used to have our own world of various fantasies, heroes, and places."

"Paul sat up at about 7 months; he crawled and crept on time. He didn't learn to walk until he was about 15 months old. He walked cautiously, holding on and not letting go. He walked late, but he talked early. He said his first clear word, 'cat,' at 6 months. He knew what a cat was and could relate to it. My husband and I were so enthusiastic about his sounds. In those days they said that if you stimulated your child and talked to him and got him ready to talk, he could read early. I was concerned that Paul would be able to talk and have a marvelous vocabulary and read because I had a reading disability and a spelling disability."

"When Paul was 4 years old and in nursery school, at my first conference the teacher said, 'Look out the window, Mrs. B. See Paul sitting at the bottom. All the other kids are climbing on top of the jungle gym.' And then she showed me some art work. Paul couldn't cut, he couldn't paste, he couldn't do any of it. We could definitely, at the age of 3 or 4, see his problems. He was bright, but he couldn't cut, paste, or draw, he couldn't climb, and he really didn't know how to run. That was where his handicaps were first being noticed, more by other teachers and professionals than by my husband and myself."

"When we had to make the decision as to whether to put Paul into kindergarten or hold him back, we were frustrated because Paul was very bright and very alert. He has always known everything that was going on in the world."

"Now, the kids Paul knows and the kids who know Paul know that he can't do motor tasks and they'll come over and play rocket ships with him. But there will come a time, as the kids are getting older, that they won't want to do this."

Paul's mother, who also had learning and motor difficulties, described her own disability as follows:

"The hardest course for me was gym. I was unfortunate enough to have the same gym teacher throughout high school. The teacher always used to think I was a lazy kid, that I just never wanted to try to do the exercises. Although I tried, I couldn't do the stunts and tumbling for anything. The other girls would do a somersault and I would still do it like a 4 year old. I'd just about get over."

"I took dance a couple of times. I never could figure out as a kid why I couldn't point my toes. The teacher would say, 'Point your toes' and it never made any sense to me. I always curled my toes up. Only when somebody sat down with me and actually showed me did I know that that was how you were supposed to point your toes. With other kids, they just did what the teacher did. Nobody had to stop and tell them. I was the klutzy kid. I never could do the nice leaps across the floor. But I would try. After two or three sessions my mother stopped giving me lessons. She was probably embarrassed."

"As a girl, it wasn't as traumatic not being athletic. As I got older, the need for a woman to be athletic tended to decrease, whereas for a boy, the need to be athletic and competitive tends to increase. I foresee this as one of the major problems for Paul."

"Most of my life my friendships have always relied on other people. I met most of my friends through other friends because I've gone along to things. I think it goes back to being teased as a child about the things I couldn't do or the way I looked. If you looked at me, I probably looked like a lot of the learning-disabled kids that you see—my clothes were not put together properly, my shoelaces were untied, and my hair was never quite combed properly."

"It was very difficult for me to learn how to put on make-up and use a hairdryer. It would take many hours of trying to learn. For a long time, my fingernails were cut very short because I didn't know how to file them. It is still very hard for me to put on eye make-up and look in the mirror and try to figure it out. I still don't feel as though I am completely put together. And I put a lot of effort and energy into looking good."

---

to making writing prolonged and laborious. Associated articulatory deficits are often present, possibly because of the fine motor nature demanded for articulation.[107,111,134,135] Poor motor coordination may present as total-body balance difficulties. Ineptness is most apparent when complex motor activities are attempted. Physical education class often presents major problems. A 9-year-old boy described his motor problems as follows: "When the gym teacher tells us to do something, I understand exactly what he means. I even know how to do it, I think. But my body never seems to do the job."[136] Case Study 14-2 describes the motor difficulties frequently encountered in children with DCD.

Neurological Approach

Children with DCD do not exhibit obvious evidence of neuropathological disease (i.e., "hard" neurological signs such as a cerebral lesion). They therefore are often not referred for evaluation until they reach school age. Parents, however, report long-standing coordination problems and associated difficulties.[137] Classic neurological examinations may not identify motor deficits,[5,93] and neurological involvement is not a necessary concomitant of learning disabilities.[13,138] Subtle abnormalities of the central nervous system are frequently noted by the presence of "soft" neurological signs.[5,33,139,140] Deficits indicative of soft neurological signs include abnormal movements and reflexes, delayed motor milestones, and poor coordination.[141,142] Box 14-2 lists soft neurological signs frequently used to assess this population. Tupper,[143] Touwen and Prechtl,[144] and Levine et al[136] provide more information on the evaluation of soft neurological signs.

Researchers suggest that a high percentage of children with learning disabilities exhibit certain soft neurological signs. In a study of preschoolers,[145] children who exhibited a greater number of minor neurological indicators had a high likelihood of demonstrating difficulty with tasks of visual perception and gross and fine motor tasks on developmental scales. A National Collaborative Perinatal Project reported that 75% of the more than 2300 children with positive total "neurological soft sign" ratings had the symptom of poor coordination.[146] In a recent study, 169 children between the ages of 8 and 13 years were assessed for a relation between soft neurological signs and cognitive functioning, motor skills, and behavior.[130] Those children with a high index for soft neurological signs were found to have significantly worse scores in each domain. A soft neurological sign score above the 90th percentile had a sensitivity of 38% for detecting cognitive impairment, 42% for detecting motor problems, and 25% for possible attention disorders.[130]

In general, a composite of signs is more predictive of dysfunction than single signs. Children without notable motor difficulties can frequently exhibit one or more soft signs; therefore identification of a single sign must be interpreted cautiously. In a study of 80 children with learning disabilities, the total number of soft signs exhibited was not predictive of learning disabilities.[147] Neurological signs requiring complex processes were found to be the most predictive. Peters et al[148] compared boys with learning disabilities with a normative sample for the presence of 80 signs and found that 44 of the signs significantly discriminated between the groups. Research has suggested that soft neurological signs could be more predictive if they were subgrouped, but no one sign or discrete group of signs currently presents a consistent relation to learning disabilities.[114]

Kinsbourne[149,150] stressed the need to view soft signs from a developmental perspective and stated that "soft signs differed from hard signs in that the child's age is the factor that determines whether the sign represents an abnormality." Denckla[151] divided soft signs into two groups: developmental and neurological. Developmental signs imply a state of immature neurological function considered to be normal in a younger normal child. These signs include functional articulatory substitution or distortion, motor overflow, right-left confusion, and mild oculomotor difficulties. Neurological soft signs, such as reflex asymmetries, are subtle abnormalities that do not occur at any time during normal development and are possible evidence of brain damage. Tupper[152] has added a third category of signs that results from causes other than neurological damage.

BOX 14-2 ■ COMMON SOFT NEUROLOGICAL SIGNS USED IN ASSESSMENT OF CHILDREN WITH LEARNING DISABILITIES AND MOTOR DEFICITS

MINOR NEUROLOGICAL INDICATORS
  Left-right discrimination
  Finger agnosia
  Visual tracking
  Extinction of simultaneous stimuli
  Choreiform movement
  Tremor
  Exaggerated associated movements
  Reflex asymmetries

COORDINATION
  Finger-to-nose touching
  Sequential thumb-finger touching
  Diadochokinesia
  Heel to shin
  Slow controlled motions
  Postural/motor measures
  Muscle tone
  Schilder's arm extension posture
  Standing with eyes closed (Romberg test)
  Walking a line
  Tandem walking (forward and backward)
  Hopping, jumping, skipping
  Ball throw and catch
  Imitation of tongue movements
  Pencil and paper tasks
  Fine motor tasks (stringing beads, building block towers)

SENSORY
  Graphesthesia
  Stereognosis
  Localization of touch input

Assessment measures of soft neurological signs vary considerably for children with learning disabilities, both in what signs are included in assessment and how they are grouped. This list represents a compilation of possible soft neurological signs.

Social and Emotional Consequences of Motor Impairments

Poor motor coordination often results in significant social and emotional consequences. Play, which in the early years of life is in large part motoric, is essential to psychosocial aspects of development, including self-concept and ego development.[153] As early as 1912, Montessori[153a] believed that movement was the basis for personality. In addition, the stimulation stemming from socialization and play was essential to the development of motor behavior.[153a] The child with poor play skills and coordination is affected in both aspects.

Development of gross and fine motor skills, coupled with the child's ability to master body movements, enhances feelings of self-esteem and confidence. The challenges of motor exploration build self-reliance, whereas the frustrations and accomplishments enhance confidence and the ability to take risks. By engaging in group activities children develop essential social skills, including how to compromise, work as a team, and deal with conflicts and different personality styles.[154] Success in these areas further builds confidence and self-esteem. When a child is poorly coordinated she or he is often teased and shunned from group play. Their peers may ostracize them. Children with motor coordination difficulties often feel shame in their poor ability to perform motor tasks, especially those required for participation in sports and those required for school achievement (e.g., cutting with scissors, coloring, drawing, writing). Clumsy children tend to be more introverted and anxious, frequently judging themselves to be both physically and socially less competent.[155] In one recent study, boys with learning and motor coordination problems were found to demonstrate significantly less-effective coping strategies in all domains of functioning than the normative sample.[156] Boys with learning disabilities and poor motor coordination also were found to have lower ratings on measures of self-esteem, happiness, and the establishment of same-sex social relationships than a matched group of boys with learning disabilities and adequate motor coordination.[157] Shaw et al[157] called this phenomenon "double developmental jeopardy," which refers to the double risk factors of poor self-esteem coupled with learning disabilities and motor deficits.

Because they are unsuccessful in peer competition, have difficulty with the changing demands of cooperative play, or feel self-conscious because of a lack of coordination, children with learning disabilities often shy away from participation in games. Adolescents with motor deficits were found to have fewer social pastimes and hobbies than peers their age.[158] Failure at play and social interactions, coupled with the inability to succeed at school serve to compound the child's feelings of worthlessness, increasing inappropriate responses to the demands of society.[153] The impact of motor coordination difficulties on social behavior is exemplified by this statement from a child with learning disabilities and motor deficits.

They always pick me last. This morning they were all fighting over which team had to have me. One guy was shouting about it. He said it wasn't fair because his team had me twice last week. Another kid said they would only take me if his team could be spotted four runs. Later, on the bus, they were all making fun of me, calling me a "fag" and a "spaz." There are a few good kids, I mean kids who aren't mean, but they don't want to play with me. I guess it could hurt their reputation.[136]

Assessment of Motor Impairments

The use of standardized tests can help identify the overall developmental status of a child and examine patterns of impairments, thereby providing clues to underlying deficits and functional limitations.[159] Appendix 14-A provides an overview of standardized tests available for the assessment of motor dysfunction in children with learning disabilities. Uses and limitations of the individual tests and test batteries are listed. Knowledge and understanding of the rules for use and interpretation of standardized tests is a prerequisite. The use of any evaluation tool requires specific training or practice. A therapist should become familiar with all aspects of test administration and scoring procedures of an evalua-

tion and should comply with the training requirements described in the test manual. Administration and interpretation of some tests such as the Sensory Integration and Praxis Tests require special coursework and training.

The test descriptions in Appendix 14-A include data on test construction and reliability but not validity. Criteria for a satisfactory standardized test should include validation against external criteria. The fragmented knowledge regarding patterns of motor impairments and functional implications of coordination disorders make selecting appropriate external criteria difficult. Few of the tests for children with learning disabilities reach a desirable level of external validity.[160] The judicious use of the evaluations described in Appendix 14-A must rest on the content validity of the test items. Clinical judgment of the therapist is important in the selection of tests for an assessment protocol. The evaluations must be logical and accurate in assessing the concerns from the parents, teachers, and referral source.

Within the school system the child is assessed for deficits that are educationally relevant. The frame of reference is to evaluate functional skills needed for success in the school environment. Evaluation procedures noted in IDEA (Section 300.532) state that each child's evaluation must be comprehensive to identify all the child's special education and related service needs. When conducting the evaluation, the use of a variety of assessment tools and strategies to gather relevant functional and developmental information is mandated by IDEA (Section 614). Additional information should be collected from parents, existing data, classroom-based assessments, and observations and assessments made by the teacher and other related personnel. Eligibility for special education or related services is determined by a team of qualified personnel with a copy of the evaluation and eligibility report given to the parent or guardian of the child.[161]

Evaluation also may occur outside the context of the academic environment. Hospital- and clinic-based assessments focus on both medical (physical and psychological health) and educational issues. The frame of reference is diagnostic to determine the type and extent of difficulties in foundational development and skill performance. A variety of standardized and nonstandardized evaluation tools should be used to assess these areas extensively. Information is gathered from direct observations as well as reports from parents and input from other professionals interacting with the child. Performance should be assessed in a variety of environments and should include components of skill, functional performance areas, and social and societal participation. Recommendations may be made for further diagnostic assessment, direct remediation, and consultation. Specific recommendations should include activities to enhance performance in the environments and contexts the child functions in on a daily basis.

Qualitative Assessment of Motor Deficits

Identification of subtle motor difficulties is critical and challenging. These subtle motor difficulties initially can be undetected, leading to unrealistic expectations of age-level motor performance. The child's difficulty with skilled, purposeful manipulative tasks or with finely tuned balance activities may not be readily apparent in the classroom or may be perceived as lack of effort. Children with DCD may be able to perform certain motor tasks with a level of strength, flexibility, and coordination that is qualitatively average but must use increased effort and cognitive control for sustained success. Levels of performance in gross and fine motor composites may encompass borderline function. Careful observations are of paramount importance, because the child's deficits are often qualitative rather than quantitative. A child might have age-appropriate balance on testing but lack ability in weight shifting and making quick directional changes, which affects the ability to participate in extracurricular activities such as soccer or baseball. When assessing children with subtle motor deficits, realizing that evaluation tools, for the most part, have been developed for children with moderate-to-severe neurological impairments is important.

Compiling a complete picture of motor deficits in children with learning disabilities involves assessing the following complex skills: (1) postural control and gross motor performance, (2) fine motor and visual motor performance, (3) motor planning, (4) sensory integration, and (5) physical fitness. Each of these interrelated functions is described in this chapter as an area of clinical assessment. Greater reliance on tests with normative data may be necessary because children with learning disabilities often exhibit subtle motor dysfunction. Information on age-appropriate performance is not always available, but sources for provisional information are included when possible. Formal tests and test batteries are described in Appendix 14-A to provide sources of normative data that can be used as guides for clinical assessment.

Postural Control and Gross Motor Performance

Muscle Tone and Strength. Low muscle tone and poor joint stability have been identified as characteristic of some children with learning disabilities.[111,162] Increased tone is not common in children with learning disabilities and may be indicative of mild cerebral palsy. Children with low tone may develop patterns of compensation called *fixing patterns*. These patterns often include elevated and internally rotated shoulders, internally rotated hips, and pronated feet. The child compensates for low tone by using the stable joint positions and holding himself or herself stiffly for increased stability. These patterns may resemble those of children with slightly increased tone. Judgments of inadequate tone are primarily made through clinical observations and felt in a hands-on assessment.

On observation, the child with low tone may look "floppy," have an open-mouth posture, lordotic back, sagging belly, and knees positioned closely together. Muscles may be poorly defined and feel "mushy" or soft on palpation, and joints may be hyperextensible. A common method for assessing muscle tone and proximal joint stability involves placing the child in a quadruped position and observing the ability to maintain the position without locking elbows, winging of the scapula, or sagging (lordosis) of the trunk. The therapist can determine joint stability by asking the child to "freeze like a statue." The therapist then provides intermittent pushes to the trunk assessing the child's ability to remain in a static position.

Manual muscle testing can provide detailed information about impairment in strength of individual muscles but is not regularly used in assessing children with learning disabilities, unless concerns of a possible degenerative disease exist. More appropriately, strength should be assessed by the child's functional ability to move against gravity during activities. Within developmental assessments, the therapist is observing range of motion against gravity in skills such as reaching, climbing, throwing, and kicking. The therapist also can have the child hold positions against gravity to assess strength and endurance (e.g., prone extension and supine flexion).

Early Postural Reflexes. Early reflexes are essential for the development of normal patterns of motor development. These reflexes facilitate movement patterns that are later integrated into purposeful motions.[163] Stereotyped or obligatory responses only occur in pathology and are not expected in the child with a learning disability and motor dysfunction. The residual reactions (e.g., asymmetrical tonic neck [ATNR] and symmetrical tonic neck reflex [STNR]) that might be noted in this population are subtle and most often are seen in stressful, nonautomatic tasks. Full integration of these postural reflexes of children who are typically developing is not anticipated until they are 8 or 9 years old[143] or even later.[164,165] Assessment for persistence of primitive reflex patterns in children with learning disabilities should emphasize impact on functional aspects of performance.

The effect of lack of integration can be observed during tasks such as writing at a table or gross motor activities such as ball skills and rope jumping. Persistence of these primitive reflexes may be seen in the child's inability to sit straight forward at the table for fine motor or writing tasks. The ATNR influence might be observed by a sideways position at the table with the arm on the face side used in extension. During ball games the child may have diminished ability to throw with directional control because head movements will influence extension of the face-side arm. Another observation of residual ATNR can be seen when the child is asked to pull a rope at midline to propel a swing or scooter board. If the reflex is affecting function, the child may lose the bilateral hold on the rope with changes in head position. Although residual reflex involvement may affect performance on these tasks, many other components are involved that require consideration.

Righting, Equilibrium, and Balance. Righting and equilibrium are dynamic reactions essential for the development of upright posture and smooth transitional movements. Righting reactions help maintain the head in an upright alignment and are the background for movement between positions.[163,166] Equilibrium reactions occur in response to a change in body position or surface support to maintain body alignment.[166] In simpler terms, equilibrium reactions get us into a position and righting reactions keep us in that position. Together these reactions provide continuous automatic adjustments that maintain the center of gravity over the base of support and keep the head in an upright position.

Righting and equilibrium (balance) reactions are assessed on an unsteady surface such as a tilt board or large therapy ball. These reactions occur in all developmental and/or functional positions, and complete assessment will consider a range of positions during functional performance in gross and fine motor activities. When testing equilibrium, the child's center of gravity is quickly tipped off balance. The equilibrium response is one of phasic extension and abduction of the downhill limbs for protection and of flexion of the uphill body side for realignment. In daily actions, most of the balance reactions are subtle and occur continuously to relatively small changes in the center of gravity.[166] Subtle shifts of the support surface can be made to assess the child's ability to maintain the head and trunk in a continuous upright position.

The vestibular system plays a role in the mediation and facilitation of reactions for the development of balance.[167,168] Automatic righting and equilibrium reactions occur as a response to changes in the center of gravity that stimulate the utricles and semicircular canals of the vestibular system. This stimulation "acts on antigravity extensor muscles so as to elicit compensatory head, trunk, and limb movements, which serve to oppose head perturbations, postural sway, or tilt."[169] Sensory input of proprioception and vision plays an even more integral role in balance control than the vestibular system.[168] When assessing balance, it is important to always consider these combined sensory inputs. The therapist should test balance skills while child's eyes are open and again with their eyes closed. Assessment can include items that involve visual, proprioceptive, and vestibular dissociation, such as balancing on an unsteady surface (e.g., dense foam or a tilt board) with and without visual orientation.[168] DeQuiros and Schrager,[170] for example, changed consistency of the board to demonstrate vestibular proprioceptive dissociation. The board is a wide walking beam with irregular lengths of polyurethane foam alternating with wood for an inconsistent walking surface. Traditional tests of balance include (1) the Romberg position-standing with feet together and eyes closed, (2) Mann's position-standing with feet in tandem with eyes closed, and (3) standing on one leg with eyes open and eyes closed. The Sensory Integration and Praxis tests include a 16-item test of standing and walking balance (see Chapter 23).[171]

Posture. The quality of posture is affected by decreased strength and endurance of the trunk musculature and diminished automatic postural reactions required to maintain a dynamic upright position. The relation between posture and muscle tone is important to consider. A child has adequate trunk stability when control of the trunk is sufficient "to maintain an erect posture, shift weight in all directions, and use rotation within the body axis."[169] These areas are often deficient in children with learning disabilities and motor dysfunction, affecting both gross and fine motor performance.

The child may fatigue quickly and fall often during gross motor play. Other body parts may be used for additional support because of weak postural musculature, such as placing the head on the ground when crawling up an incline or sticking out the tongue when climbing or pumping a swing. In sitting, a child with diminished postural control will fatigue quickly, either leaning on his or her hands for additional support or moving frequently in and out of the chair. These compensations affect the child's ability to perform fine motor tasks or maintain attention for cognitive learning because so much effort is exerted on sitting up. Observing the effects of fatigue is important because both sitting and standing postures may deteriorate over the course of a day. Generally, the problem stems from motor programming problems versus muscle power.

Gross Motor Skills. Children with learning disabilities and DCD may attain reasonably high degrees of motor skill in specific activities. Motor accomplishments frequently remain highly specific to particular motor sequences or tasks and do not necessarily generalize to other activities, regardless of their similarities. When variation in the motor response is required, the response often becomes inaccurate and disorganized. Smyth[172] found that movement time for complex responses was longer for these children. Although children with DCD can sit, stand, and walk with apparent ease, they may be awkward or slow in rolling, coming to standing, running, hopping, and climbing. Skilled tasks such as skipping may be accomplished with increased effort, decreased sequencing and endurance, and associated movements. Gilfoyle and Grady[173] and others[174] have described qualitative differences in gross motor skills when observing twins, one demonstrating motor dysfunction and the other demonstrating age-appropriate skills.

Evaluation of motor skills should therefore include novel motor sequences and age-appropriate skills.[175] The child, for example, can be asked to imitate a hopping sequence or maneuver around a variety of obstacles. Skills that have been accomplished can be varied slightly (e.g., hopping over a small box). Age-appropriate social participation tasks, such as tag and dodge ball, can be observed for qualitative difficulties in timing and spatial body awareness. Developmentally earlier skills also should be observed to assess the quality of performance. The Bruininks-Oseretsky Test of Motor Proficiency[176] and the Peabody Developmental Motor Scales[177] are examples of standardized assessment of motor skills (see Appendix 14-A). Hughes and Riley[178] have described several other gross motor tasks useful in evaluating minor motor dysfunction.

Fine Motor Performance

Fine Motor Skill. A child with learning disabilities often demonstrates multiple fine motor concerns. Areas of difficulty typically include the grasp and manipulation of small objects and tools such as a pencil, spoon, or knife. Delays in activities of daily living requiring dexterous hand use such as buttoning, zippering, and shoe tying may be observed. Assessment should include both standardized assessments and structured observations of functional performance.

A complete fine motor evaluation should include assessment of proximal trunk control to distal finger movements. Upper-extremity reach and manipulation patterns are thought to be controlled by dual systems.[178] Proximal movements of the trunk and shoulders directly affect distal function.[179] Trunk control and shoulder stability affect the accuracy and control of reaching patterns and create a stable base from which both hands can be used to perform bilateral skills.

The assessment of distal control considers wrist stability, development of hand arches, and separation of the two sides of the hand, all providing a structural basis for the control of distal movement.[180] Qualitative observations of distal fingertip control are separated into manipulative motions labeled translation, shift, and rotation.[181] Translation involves finger motions to move objects into and out of the palm of the hand. Shift is an alternation pattern of the thumb and first finger generally used for the final adjustment of an object. Rotation involves turning an object within the hand. Exner[181] and Pehoski[181a] have studied these developmental trends.

Although standardized assessments such as The Test of Motor Proficiency by Bruininks[176] and the Peabody Developmental Motor Scales have fine motor sections, they do not adequately measure manipulative elements previously described.[177] Careful observations of movement components during a variety of fine motor tasks are necessary for qualitative analysis. The clinician must have a strong reference base in normal development for accurate assessment. Soft neurological signs, including diadochokinesia (rapid alternation of forearm supination and pronation), sequential thumb-to-finger touching, and stereognosis (identifying objects and shapes without visual input) can provide further qualitative information. Several excellent sources provide provisional information on age-appropriate performance.[33,136,144,152,182]

Eye-Hand Coordination and Handwriting. The evaluation of eye-hand coordination is best achieved by using standardized test measures. Examples include the Bruininks-Oseretsky Test of Motor Proficiency,[176] Movement-ABC,[183] the Motor Accuracy Test of the Sensory Integration and Praxis Tests,[171] and the Purdue Pegboard Test.[184] Supplemental clinical observations include the assessment of ball catching and throwing, fine motor tasks such as stringing beads and building block towers, and written accuracy tasks of drawing or coloring within a boundary.

Handwriting requires complex integration of fine motor control, motor planning, sensory feedback, and visual-motor integration.[184] Refinements of accuracy and control have been documented up to the age of 14 years.[185,186] Despite developmental trends in the child's finger and hand position during writing, the actual type of grasp on the pencil has not been proven to significantly affect the speed and legibility of written work.[186] More important to accuracy is grasp pressure (observationally measured by the angle of flexion in the index finger and the breaking of the pencil during writing) and forearm position.[185] Children who have difficulties with handwriting commonly produce sloppy work with incorrect letter formations or reversals, inconsistent size and height of letters, variable slant, and irregular spacing between words and letters.[187]

Visual motor integration is the ability to perceive a form and reproduce it with a written response. It can be assessed through standardized measures such as The Developmental Test of Visual Motor Integration[188] and the Test of Visual Motor Skills.[189] The production of handwritten work can be assessed by using the Evaluation Tool of Children's Handwriting (ETCH)[190] and the Test of Handwriting Skills.[191] Handwriting samples provide important information regarding functional abilities in written production.

Praxis and Motor Planning. Praxis involves the ability to plan and carry out a new or unusual action when adequate cognitive and motor skills are present. Derived from the Greek work for acting or doing, praxis means "action based on will."[192] The components of praxis include *ideation* or generating an idea of how one might act in the environment, *planning* or organizing a program of action, and *execution* of the action sequence.[193] Motor planning involves the same components relative to a motor task. Sensory information is considered essential for initiation, execution, and adaptation of motor actions.

Children with praxis difficulties, or dyspraxia, may exhibit a paucity of ideas. The child may enter a room filled with toys or equipment and have limited capacity to experiment and play. Other children with dyspraxia may move from one activity to the next without generating effective plans for participating in, or completing, tasks. Lack of variation and adaptation in play can be another indication of planning problems. At times, children with dyspraxia also may exhibit poor anticipation of their actions. They can quickly engage in play with the equipment but demonstrate little regard for safety (e.g., kicking a large ball across the room where other children are playing). Observations of typically developing children show continuous modifications in play, with spontaneous adaptations to motor sequences, making explorations varied and increasingly successful.

Kephart[194] describes trouble adapting to changes in external conditions as being a reflection of a child's inability to plan movements. Children with dyspraxia often have difficulties in situations characterized by changing demands, such as unstructured group play. Transitions also may be difficult because they involve the creation or adaptation of a plan. Frustration and difficulties with peer interactions frequently are part of the composite. Often children with planning problems can clearly see the differences between their performance and that of other children the same age, which significantly affects their self-esteem.

The child with motor planning deficits has difficulty performing in, and acting on, the environment.[193] Observations of motor planning deficits may include difficulties figuring out new motor activities, disorganized approaches, resistance or inability to vary performance when a task is not successful, and awkward motor execution. Movements are performed with an excessive expenditure of energy and with inaccurate judgment of the required force, tempo, and amplitude.[194a] They are unable to relate the sequence of motions to each other.

Manifestations of poor motor planning ability are apparent in many daily tasks. Dressing is often difficult. Children are not able to plan where or how to move their limbs to put on clothes. Problems are often demonstrated in constructive manipulatory play, such as building with toys, cutting, and pasting. Similarly, learning how to use utensils, such as a knife, fork, pencil, or scissors, is difficult. The child with dyspraxia often has problems with handwriting.

Standardized assessments of praxis include the tests of Postural Praxis, Sequencing Praxis, Praxis on Verbal Command, Oral Praxis, Constructional Praxis, and Design Copy of the Sensory Integration and Praxis Tests.[171] The FirstSTEP[195] is a preschool screening tool with a section assessing motor planning abilities. Clinical observations can add valuable information regarding the child's ability to see the potential for action, organize and sequence motor actions for success, and anticipate the outcome of an action.

Sensory Integration. Ayres[111] originally defined sensory integration as "the ability to organize sensory information for use." Information is received through the senses and simultaneously processed and organized throughout the nervous system to learn about and act on the environment. Integration of sensory input affects regulatory cycles, arousal state, planning, and skilled motor execution.

Information is registered by the sensory receptors, organized, and used in social, motor, and academic learning. The process of scanning incoming information for relevance is called *sensory modulation.* Sensory modulation is important in determining the appropriate action for a situation and regulating arousal. *Discrimination* of sensory input involves discerning subtle differences in sensation to learn about the qualities of objects and refine body movements within space. Both sensory modulation and discrimination are thought to play integral roles in organized motor behavior.[167]

Impairments in processing sensory input can result in motor dysfunction, including immature postural reactions, delayed eye-hand coordination, deficient safety awareness, and motor planning problems.[107,111,196] Deficits in registering and discriminating sensory input may be responsible for qualitative motor difficulties in children with developmental coordination disorder. Observations may include awkward timing and movement, poor grading of force, and difficulty performing in situations involving integration of multiple inputs (e.g., gym class).

Types of Sensory Integration Dysfunction. Ayres[47b,125,171,197] described certain characteristics that often co-occur in the child with learning disabilities and relate to deficits in the processing of specific sensory input. These types of sensory integration dysfunction often are associated with deficits in tactile or vestibular-proprioceptive processing. The patterns that emerged most consistently through factor and cluster analyses affecting motor performance include (1) disorders in vestibular-proprioceptive discrimination influencing postural-ocular movements, bilateral integration, and sequencing; and (2) deficits in somatosensory discrimination resulting in somatodyspraxia.

Certain indicators of inadequate vestibular functions have been noted in children with learning disabilities. One of the most frequently used measures is the postrotatory nystagmus response (i.e., the back-and-forth movements of the eyes following rotation of the head). This response is a manifestation of the vestibulo-ocular reflex and is a normal adaptive response designed to reestablish the original fixation on a visual field.[198] DeQuiros and Schrager[170] and Ayres[196,198] both found that more than 50% of the children with learning disabilities studied had shortened duration of nystagmus.

Nystagmus is only one manifestation of vestibular functioning. Other indicators, such as *postural and ocular problems,* have been associated with vestibular system dysfunction.[199] The vestibular system serves a primary role in the maintenance of tone, development of postural control, and equilibrium reactions. Inadequate muscle tone and proximal joint stability may be noted on assessment.[111,199-201] The child also may show an inability to assume and maintain the prone extension position (head, trunk, and leg extension against gravity). Many children with learning disabilities have immature or poorly developed equilibrium and delayed automatic postural reactions. Standing balance is often deficient, and standing with eyes closed is even more impaired because the child cannot use vision and must rely on vestibular and proprioceptive input.[198,202] The ability to use the eyes efficiently in space may be hindered because the vestibular system stabilizes the eyes during head and neck movements so that a fixed visual image may be perceived.[111]

Bilateral integration and sequencing deficits are represented by difficulties in coordination of the two body sides, avoidance of crossing the body midline, failure to develop a preferred hand for skill, and possible right-left confusion. Tasks demonstrating these difficulties include problems in jumping with both feet together, reciprocal stair climbing, or skipping. The child who tends to avoid crossing the midline may shift the entire body to avoid crossing the midline or tend to use the right hand on the right body side and the left hand on the left body side. This may interfere with the development of a preferred skilled hand. Difficulties sequencing and projecting body movements in space can be observed through deficits in timing, sequencing, and terminating a series of jumps and running to kick a moving ball.[126] *Somatodyspraxia* refers to the subgroup of children with motor planning delays that are hypothesized to result from deficits in tactile and proprioceptive discrimination.[192] Somatosensory input is important for developing awareness of where the body is in space and body scheme. "If the information that the body receives is not precise, the brain has a poor basis on which to build its body scheme."[203] During early development the child experiences much of the environment through the tactile system to gain awareness of the body and discover the nature of objects. Proprioceptive input from the muscles, tendons, joints, and vestibular input from the inner ear work in conjunction with the tactile system to establish body scheme. According to Ayres,[111] motor planning depends strongly on an adequate body scheme to understand one's relation to the environment.

Ayres has repeatedly linked poor tactile, proprioceptive, and kinesthetic perception with problems in motor planning.[47b,197,202] Kinesthesia, the conscious perception of the position of body parts and movement, is suggested to have a close association with motor performance and learning.[204] Laszlo and Bairstow[159] developed the Kinesthetic Sensitivity Test (KST), which measures acuity, perception, and memory. Initial results of a study of 40 children with motor impairments indicated that 73% had deficits in processing kinesthetic input.[205] Hoare and Larkin[206] tested 80 children with motor difficulties with the KST and found that three of the seven kinesthetic measures were deficient in these children. Johnston et al[114] found that 40% of a sample of 95 children had abnormal proprioception. Slower processing of proprioceptive information was identified in children with motor deficits.[207] Other researchers have emphasized the visual and kinesthetic contributions to movement.[89,124,159,208]

In a current view of sensory integration assessment, Bundy and Murray[209] outline four broad groupings of children identified through synthesizing the results of factor and cluster analysis. Dyspraxia now includes patterns earlier described as bilateral integration and sequencing deficits, as well as somatodyspraxia. The dyspraxic group had indications of central sensory processing deficits such as poor tactile discrimination and postural deficits.[209] A second group, sensory modulation dysfunction, is not easily identified with standardized measures such as the Sensory Integration and Praxis Tests[171] because these test measures do have the physiological basis for measuring deficits in sensory modulation. The modulation group often exhibits sensory defensiveness, gravitational insecurity, and aversive reactions to movement. Visual perception and visual-motor coordination deficits highlight the third group. Relating these deficits solely to a sensory integration deficit is not feasible because of the strong cognitive component of visual-perceptual development. This is also true of the last group, which reflects deficits in auditory-language measures.

Clinical observation of a child's responses to a variety of sensory inputs and the ability to organize multiple inputs provides essential information regarding the integration of sensory input. Gross and fine motor tasks that involve postural and ocular responses, bilateral motor coordination, planning, and sequencing are end products that reflect sensory integration. The Sensory Integration and Praxis Tests[171] and The Miller Assessment for Preschoolers[210] are used most commonly to assess various aspects of sensory integration function.

Physical Fitness. Children with DCD often have performance difficulties in games and athletic activities. As a result, the level of physical fitness, strength, muscular endurance, flexibility, and cardiorespiratory endurance may be poorly developed. Fitness testing of a group of "clumsy" children in a movement program in Australia indicated that the group performed well below average on a number of fitness tests of aerobic/anaerobic capacity, flexibility, strength, and muscular endurance, even when the tasks selected required minimal motor coordination.[211] Tests of flexibility indicated that children who were "clumsy" performed at both ends of the range. Seventy-two percent of the sample scored either below the 25th or above the 75th percentile. One task of the physical therapist is to differentiate between poor physical fitness as a result of low motor activity and problems of low muscle tone, joint limitations, decreased strength, and reduced endurance that reflect a developmental lag or deviation in motor function. Collaboration among the physical educator, the adaptive physical educator, and the physical therapist is critical in these areas. Arnheim and Sinclair[153] and Larkin and Hoare[211] further discuss a physical fitness developmental program for children with problems in motor coordination.

Linking Evaluation to Intervention

After evaluation the therapist must synthesize areas of strength and weakness to address the functional implications of identified deficits. If impairment areas are clearly affecting the child's functional performance within the environment, intervention may be warranted. The intervention process begins with identification of the child's specific concerns coupled with corresponding statements of the type and quality of behavior desired as a result of remediation. In other words, the therapist must set treatment goals to be achieved through intervention.

Interpreting test data, integrating findings, identifying functional limitations, and creating goals is a complex process. Initial impressions of the child's areas of difficulty may result in the recommendation for further examination before outlining refined goals relevant to functional performance. Collecting additional assessment information may involve observations in other environments or during functional daily tasks, and/or additional formal testing.

Setting goals for the child with learning disabilities with motor deficits must be made by considering a variety of factors:
1. Referral information and age of the child
2. Medical, developmental, and sensory processing history
3. Parents' and teachers' perception of the child's strengths and concerns of functional impairments
4. Educational information
   a. Major difficulties experienced in school
   b. How motor problems are interfering with the child's school performance
   c. Current services being received
5. Child's peer relationships, play and leisure activities, and self-esteem
6. Therapists' observations/assessment of the child through informal and formal evaluation, both standardized and nonstandardized
7. Functional expectations and abilities at home and school

Goals for the child with learning disabilities can be stated in terms of long-term or short-term objectives. According to Arnheim and Sinclair,[153] the major long-term objective in remediation of motor impairments for the child with DCD should be "effective total body management in a wide variety of activities requiring dynamic balance and agility; object management including manipulation, propulsion and reception; emotional control; ability to socialize effectively; a positive self-concept; and a sense of enjoyment in movement."

Short-term objectives should be written to reflect a specific behavior or set of behaviors that are attainable within a predetermined time frame of intervention, usually 6 months to 1 year. Bundy[212] indicates that "well written objectives are predictions about how a client will be different, in some meaningful way, as a result of intervention." Behavioral short-term objectives are composed of three parts: (1) the *behavioral statement* is what will be accomplished by the child; (2) the *condition statement* provides details regarding how the skill or behavior will be accomplished; and (3) the *performance statement* denotes how the skill or behavior will be measured for success. The most important consideration is ensuring that the goals and objectives chosen are relevant to the child's functional daily performance and are meaningful to the team, including the family, working with the child. Case Study 14-3 provides an example of functional objectives.

Intervention for the Child with Learning Disabilities and Motor Deficits

Roles of the Therapist

Historically, occupational and physical therapy was provided in special schools or classes for multiply handicapped children or in clinics that were completely separated from the educational environment. Integration of services into the public school arena occurred with the establishment of the Education for All Handicapped Act (PL 94-142) and IDEA. The provision of related services, including occupational and physical therapy, as well as special education, is now a mandated and typically well-integrated part of the educational process.

Kalish and Presseller[213] identified five areas of function for the physical or occupational therapist in the educational environment:
1. Screening and evaluating children with a wide variety of functional deficits
2. Program planning based on evaluating results and related to a child's ability to receive maximal benefit from educational experiences
3. Treatment activities designed to meet program goals
4. Consultation with teachers, other school personnel, and parents around carryover of services into the classroom and home programming

CASE STUDY 14-3 ■ JONATHAN

Jonathan was a 6 year old referred for an occupational therapy evaluation by his parents and teacher because of concerns regarding motor skill development. Assessment results revealed several areas of impairment, including poor discrimination of his body position and movement in space, diminished postural control and balance reactions, motor planning deficits, delayed eye-hand coordination, qualitative fine motor deficits, and delayed visual-motor integration affecting his handwriting. Jonathan's mother reported that he was clumsy and seemed to bump into things constantly. Of greater concern was that Jonathan seemed fearful of activities that his peers found pleasurable, such as climbing the jungle gym and coming down the slide at the neighborhood playground. Jonathan tended to play on the outskirts of groups. When he did attempt to interact he became angry because the children would not play the game by his rules. At home, Jonathan often was frustrated by tasks of daily living such as putting on his coat, snapping his pants, and tying his shoes. His mother reported that Jonathan frequently called himself "stupid" when he could not independently complete self-care skills.

When determining appropriate behavioral objectives for Jonathan, looking at the areas of functional relevance such as pleasure and safety in gross motor play, peer interactions, and independence in age-appropriate activities of daily living is critical. These areas of concern for Jonathan were consistent with those of his parents. His parents wanted him to feel more competent and less frustrated in play, at home, and at school. Jonathan's goal was to "not be so stupid that kids won't play with me." The occupational therapist believed that through remediation of sensory discrimination and motor deficits Jonathan could develop improved motor competence and planning abilities. This would lead to greater success in peer interactions and improved feelings of self-confidence. Based on these common desires the following goals and objectives were made. Among the many excellent references on writing goals and objectives and functional outcome measures are Arnheim and Sinclair,[153] Dunn and Campbell,[98] Fisher et al,[167] and LaVesser and Bloomer.[119]

One of the general/long-term goals became to *improve Jonathan's gross motor skill development.* Jonathan was interested in learning to ride a bicycle without training wheels and his parents were hopeful that he could become more confident at the neighborhood playground. These behavioral objectives would measure the development of improved

proficiency in discrimination of his body in space, postural control balance reactions, and motor planning. The following objectives were written:

1. Jonathan will independently climb the ladder and come down the slide without exhibiting fear, bumping into other children, or falling.
2. Jonathan will develop the ability to ride his bicycle without training wheels in straight lines and will learn to turn corners. (*Note:* Successfully riding the bicycle becomes the performance measure of behavior in this objective.)

To address improvement in independence for self-care:

1. Jonathan will put on his coat independently in correct orientation and successfully zip it four out of five times.
2. Jonathan will successfully tie his shoes without assistance in a timely manner.

To address greater success in peer interactions:

1. Jonathan will participate in a structured game, following the rules, for 10 minutes.
2. Jonathan will play outside with the children in the neighborhood without conflict for at least 1 hour.

Although impairment level objectives could have been written to address the same areas, they would have been of limited relevance to Jonathan and the team working with him. Balance and postural control also could be addressed by an objective stating that Jonathan would stand on one foot for 10 seconds. The functional implications of this objective would not have been clear, and Jonathan and his parents would be without an outcome measure that was measurable and meaningful to them. Thus it would have negated the effects of working as a cohesive team toward a common goal.

When working as a member of a team within the school, behavioral objectives will have implications for the child's performance in the school environment. Within the school system, statements of goals and specific objectives are included in the Individualized Educational Plan (IEP). In Jonathan's case, specific objectives that were meaningful to the classroom situation included the ability to sit in the chair to complete written assignments for 15 minutes and increase accuracy of letter formation, size, and spacing on written assignments. Other areas related to gross and fine motor skills and peer interactions also were influential to Jonathan's success at school. Specific objectives written pertaining to school would have functional outcome measures chosen from tasks within the school environment such as gym class, playground interactions, and classroom expectations.

5. In-service training for individuals or groups relative to the needs of disabled children

Because each of these functions is usually required of the public school therapist, the time available for providing direct services to children may be limited. Intervention services must be done, in part, through consultation to parents, classroom teachers, and physical educators. The child's motor development needs can sometimes be met, wholly or in part, within the physical education program. Through assessment and observation the therapist can identify deficit areas and suggest therapeutic activities that could be incorporated into an adaptive physical education program.

Kalish and Presseller[213] point out the necessity of integrating therapy into the educational process, first by adapting intervention to reinforce educational goals and then by incorporating therapy into routine classroom activities. The therapist must be flexible and discover alternate methods of reaching goals, such as positioning and using unobtrusive adaptive equipment. The teacher's responsibility for all the children in the classroom must always be kept in mind. Before proposing the incorporation of a therapeutic activity into a classroom, feasibility of the activities must be ensured. In some classrooms a teacher's aide might be available for individual attention, but in all instances both the child's time and the teacher's time must be considered in relation to the total program requirements.

Intervention Techniques

Models of intervention used in treating children with motor deficits include direct and indirect therapeutic techniques. Both approaches are necessary when addressing the variety of motor impairments in the child with learning disabilities. Indirect methods provide the foundation for the development of components for functional performance and the generalization of skills. Direct methods enhance a child's motor performance and social participation through skill training. Indirect methods involve "training the brain"[3] and direct methods teach the child by practice and repetition. Ottenbacher[214] proposed that the medical model of intervention resembles the indirect therapeutic approach and the educational model resembles the direct therapeutic approach. Intervention should be provided in an atmosphere in which these models are synergistic rather than antagonistic.[214] Proportions of direct and indirect therapy used are relevant to the child's age, developmental status, and the severity of the disability.[3]

Many of the treatment approaches later discussed integrate indirect and direct concepts of intervention. Sensory integration, for example, attempts to modify the neurological dysfunction interfering with motor performance while emphasizing functional adaptive performance and motor skill development. The neurodevelopmental treatment approach uses handling techniques to inhibit abnormal movement by facilitating normal movement patterns to encourage the acquisition of functional movement skills needed for learning and daily living skills.[215] Motor learning theories aim to adapt the neural structures required to control movement by task-related intervention. Successful intervention for children with learning disabilities should derive from all existing procedures for the management of impairments.

No delineated formulas exist for determining the best intervention approach for an individual child. Each child is unique and presents a new challenge to the therapist when fabricating a functional outcome plan. A chosen intervention approach typically reflects the setting the child is referred to, the therapist's experience and expertise, and the parents' beliefs and goals. Selection of intervention methods is integrally tied to the child's presenting problems and the goals and objectives established as part of the intervention plan.

The intervention methods presented in this chapter for remediation of motor deficits in the child with learning disabilities include sensory integration; neurodevelopmental; motor control, learning, and development; sensorimotor; motor skill training; and physical fitness. None is mutually exclusive, and each requires a level of training and practice for competence as well as experience in normal development. Most therapists synthesize information from different intervention techniques and use an eclectic approach, pulling relevant pieces from a variety of intervention modalities to best meet the needs of each child.

Sensory Integration. The sensory integration theory was developed and articulated by A. Jean Ayres,[111,171,203,216] with concepts drawn from neurophysiology, neuropsychology, and development. Her purpose in theoretical development was to explain the observed relation between difficulties organizing sensory input and deficits in academic and neuromotor "learning" observed in some children with learning disabilities and motor deficits.[217] The theory proposes that "learning is dependent on the ability of normal individuals to take in sensory information derived from the environment and from movement of their bodies, to process and integrate these sensory inputs within the central nervous system, and to use this sensory information to plan and organize behavior."[217] Ayres[171] used "learning" in a broad sense to include the development of concepts, adaptive motor responses, and behavioral change. The goal of sensory integration intervention is to elicit responses that result in better organization of sensory input and facilitate the generalization of functional skills.

Ayres[111] proposed that the integration of sensory inputs could be facilitated by providing opportunities for enhanced sensory intake in the context of meaningful activities, resulting in adaptive responses. During intervention, sensory input is provided in a planned and organized manner while eliciting progressively harder adaptive motor responses. The therapist strives to find activities that are motivating and tap the child's inner drive to encourage adaptation. "Evincing an adaptive behavior promotes sensory integration, and, in turn, the ability to produce an adaptive behavior reflects sensory integration."[111] Effective intervention requires melding the science of a neurophysiological theory with the art of "playing" with the child.

An example of sensory integration intervention for a child with postural difficulties might involve having the child riding a swing pretending to be a fisherman while keeping a lookout for whales that might bump his boat. This "pretend play" scenario taps the child's motivation and inner drive to be productive (fishing), while challenging himself in a dangerous situation (whales). The therapist will adapt this activity in a variety of ways to maintain an appropriate level of challenge and adaptation (adaptive response). The required type and amount of sensory input, postural demands, bilateral control, timing, and planning are all considered and can be adapted to an easier or harder level to maintain adaptation and learning. Sensory input can be controlled through the speed and direction the boat moves and the amount of work the child must do with his arms to propel the boat and catch fish. Additional sensory input can be provided through "rocky seas" and "whales crashing the side of the boat." The boat can facilitate more or less postural adaptation by the amount of support it provides and the speed of its movement. The child can pull a rope to propel the swing, or the therapist can provide the movement to decrease the bilateral coordination and postural demands. A more demanding bilateral response could include pulling a rope and catching a fish simultaneously. Unexpected movements of the boat, fish, and whales will require greater timing and planning for success.

For this intervention technique to be appropriate, the motor and planning difficulties observed in a child with learning disabilities need to be a result of deficits in processing sensory information. Each child's intervention plan should be individualized based on the results of a comprehensive evaluation and responses to sensory input within therapy. Aspects of modulation and discrimination of sensation will be considered for their impact on functional motor performance. Sensory modulation difficulties can result in heightened responsiveness to sensation, thereby increasing the child's arousal level, which can affect successful peer interactions and safety on the playground. Sensitivity to movement input can cause the child to avoid playground equipment or become nauseated during car rides. Discrimination difficulties can significantly affect the quality of motor performance and the acquisition of prepositional concepts (up, down, left, right, in front of, behind, next to). The child who has difficulty discriminating information from the body can exhibit deficits in body awareness, force grading, balance, timing movements in space, bilateral and eye-hand coordination, fine motor control, and handwriting.

Vestibular, proprioceptive, and tactile sensory inputs used in therapy are powerful and must be applied with caution. The autonomic and behavioral responses of the child must be monitored carefully. The therapist should be knowledgeable about sensory integration theory and intervention before using these procedures. Monitoring behavioral responses after the therapy session also is suggested through parent or teacher consultation. Intervention precautions are elaborated by Ayres,[111] Koomar and Bundy,[218] and Bundy.[219]

Research on the Effects of Sensory Integration Procedures. Within the field of occupational therapy, sensory integration is the most well-documented intervention procedure. According to Gaddes,[3] sensory integration is one of the most articulated and best-developed programs of sensorimotor training for children with learning disabilities. Despite this, disagreement persists on the value of this therapeutic modality.

When considering the multiple reviews of sensory intervention *effectiveness,* a lack of consistency and agreement exist.[139,220-230] In relation to children with learning disabilities, Hoehn and Baumeister[224] concluded that sensory integration therapy was both unproven and ineffective.

Henderson,[231] however, concluded that "the studies . . . [of sensory integration] provide preliminary evidence of the value of sensory integrative therapy for children with learning disabilities."[231] Clinicians using sensory integration procedures also are convinced of the effectiveness of this treatment approach in making important functional changes. Testimonials from parents of children who have received occupational therapy with sensory integration procedures are frequently heard. Perhaps the inconsistencies noted in research on sensory integration effectiveness are caused by the complex characteristics of children receiving intervention and to the challenge of creating a structured research model for an intervention that adapts frequently to the child's changing needs. The diagnostic and screening tools used in studies may not, however, be appropriate for assessing change over time.[229]

The empirical data continue to raise questions about *who, how,* and *what* sensory integration procedures affect.[232] Studies have not adequately controlled for the heterogeneity of children with sensory integration dysfunction. A study by Densem et al[233] included subjects who "exhibited a wide array of handicapping conditions, including mild mental retardation, behavioral disturbance, mild cerebral palsy, and epilepsy." The variation of this population confused the study results and encouraged the authors to consider not "How effective was the program?" but, rather, "How does it work and for whom?"[233]

Sensory integration effectiveness research also is confounded by variable treatment designs and outcome measures. Clark and Pierce[234] found 26 effectiveness studies that included four different independent variables, including sensory integration procedures, systematically applied vestibular stimulation, multisensory input, and perceptual-motor training. In reviewing effectiveness studies, Cermak and Henderson[221,222] identified at least six different outcome measures, including academic measures, language outcomes, motor skills, postrotatory nystagmus, self-stimulatory behaviors, and behavioral outcomes. In a recent meta-analysis Vargus and Camilli[235] noted that studies using fewer outcome measures (one to four) had a greater effect sizes, but that many studies use higher number of outcomes to increase the studies' reliability. As with many areas of research, the heterogeneity of the population and variation in approaches continue to confound any consensus on intervention effectiveness.

Several studies have demonstrated some improvements in sensory integrative measures.[225-227] In a 3-year follow-up study, Wilson and Kaplan[236] found that sensory integration intervention had a more sustained impact on gross motor performance. Humphries et al[227] found that subjects treated with a sensory integration approach showed an advantage in motor planning. Vargus and Camilli[235] found larger effect sizes in the motor and psychoeducational categories. A recent study of intensive short-term sensory integration intervention with children with special needs demonstrated a reduction in soft neurological signs, extremes of activity level, and increased predictability and adaptability compared with a matched group.[237] Self-esteem was shown to significantly increase in a sample of 67 children with learning disabilities randomly assigned to two groups after sensory integration intervention.[230] The results of these studies suggest that motor and behavior measures may be more effective outcome measures for sensory integration intervention.

Several studies[227,230,238] have suggested that sensory integration intervention is not more effective in motor skill development than more traditional skill-based therapies. Vargus and Camilli's[235] meta-analysis indicates that sensory integration treatment measures were at least as effective as various alternate methods. One recognized confounding variable is the heterogeneity of the study subjects.[239] Another difficulty is in determining the best outcome measures of improved sensory integration. Traditional motor tests may not best reflect the changes in organization, adaptability, and planning that children with sensory integration therapy consistently appear to make. Cermak and Henderson[221,222] suggest that "organization, learning rate, attention, affect, exploratory behavior, biological rhythm (sleep-wake cycle), sensory responsivity, play skills, self-esteem, peer interactions, and family adjustment" are domains that may change with sensory integration treatment. Cohn and Cermak's[240] research, which focused on the parent perspective of changes with sensory integration intervention, targeted these areas. Parents identified two important outcome measures for intervention. The first included change in the child, such as improved self-regulation, perceived competence, and social participation. The second was related to parents developing the ability to understand their child's behavior in a new way and having their experiences validated to better support and advocate for the child.

In her review of sensory integration research with children with learning disabilities, Henderson concluded that the studies "certainly . . . provide sufficient evidence to warrant further investigation of the effects of sensory integrative therapy."[231] In their recent review of sensory integration effectiveness, Miller and Kinnealey[228] suggest that future studies need better controls for homogeneous samples, treatment approach, and more clearly defined hypotheses. The complexity of sensory integration theory, the individualized approaches that treatment warrants, and the difficulty finding sensitive outcome measures create many challenges in designing appropriate and valid research studies.

Neurodevelopmental Theory. Neurodevelopmental treatment (NDT) is a technique formulated by Bobath and Bobath[241,242] to enhance the development of gross motor skills, balance, quality of movement, and hand skills in individuals with movement disorders.[243] The original framework was based on the hierarchical levels of reflex integration in the nervous system. Abnormal and normal postural reflexes were thought to be the basis of automatic changes in muscle activity.[163,244] Abnormal postural responses were lower-level hierarchical reactions that did not integrate into a typical time frame (e.g., ATNR, STNR), thereby inhibiting the development of automatic postural mechanisms. The normal postural reflex action used higher-level righting and equilibrium responses as a foundation for automatic postural reactions, balance, and transitional movement patterns. In this framework the nervous system was viewed as a passive system controlled by sensory feedback.[244] The NDT approach emphasized specific ways to inhibit abnormal reactions and facilitate more normal movement patterns.[245] Treatment techniques were originally designed for individuals with cerebral palsy.

More recently, the hierarchical model of reflex integration has been replaced by the distributed control model of the nervous system. In this model the nervous system is viewed as a dynamic system capable of initiating, anticipating, and controlling movements with ongoing sensory feedforward and feedback.[244] Many factors are recognized as contributing to abnormal movement patterns, including abnormal muscle tone, influence of primitive reflex patterns, delayed development of righting and equilibrium reactions, weakness of specific muscles, inability to counteract the forces of gravity, and deficits in sensory input. This framework of NDT works to facilitate normal movement patterns so that the individual does not develop abnormal or compensatory patterns, which lends its use to children with more minimal motor involvement. Of particular relevance to the child with learning disabilities with motor deficits is facilitation of improved righting and equilibrium responses, automatic postural adjustments, and balance reactions.

Neurodevelopmental treatment uses physical handling techniques directed toward developing the components of movement that underlie functional motor performance. Movement components of neuromotor maturation, postural alignment and stability, mobility skills, weight bearing, weight shifting, and balance are all foundations for smoothly executed movements in space.[243] This is accomplished through a combination of facilitation and inhibition techniques that use sensory input, particularly tactile-proprioceptive cues. Abnormal movement patterns are prevented, whereas normal postural adjustments are guided through key points of control on the body.[215] The ultimate goals of NDT are the normalization of abnormal tonus, facilitation of active adaptive posture and movement, and integration of postural reactions to encourage the acquisition of functional movement patterns needed for learning and daily living skills.[215]

As theory and intervention practices have evolved, the need to promote better movement within the context of functional task performance has been greatly emphasized. Activities incorporate targeted reactions into the specific functional skills the child is working on. The therapist's hands guide the reactions, with the child actively participating in problem solving and adapting performance. Practice of more effective postural reactions and reduction of abnormal movement patterns are embedded into meaningful activities. A skilled therapist balances the quality of movement patterns with the importance of active problem solving and participation in learning new motor tasks.[244] At times, participation and independent task completion are more important than qualitatively normal movement patterns. Knowledge of normal movement patterns, postural control, base of support, and weight shifting are important aspects of this intervention approach.[245]

Research on the Effects of Neurodevelopmental Therapy. NDT is based on principles derived from research in motor development and neurophysiology. The techniques, however, arise from careful and extensive clinical observations. Few studies have quantitatively assessed the effectiveness of this intervention technique. One difficulty with designing effectiveness studies to assess NDT is defining appropriate and measurable outcomes. Two studies[246,247] that used standardized developmental motor tests as a dependent variable did not find significant differences between children treated with NDT techniques and children who were not treated. In her study of infants and toddlers with Down syndrome, Harris[246,248] used individualized, specific, objective measures as a dependent variable. According to her findings, 80% of the treatment group reached individualized objectives compared with 57% of the control group. Harris, however, did not find any significant differences on the standardized motor measures. The appropriateness of these standardized tests in assessing the qualitative motor changes associated with the use of NDT is therefore questioned.

Of the 41 studies initially identified by Royeen and DeGangi[243] for a review of NDT effectiveness, only one quantitative study was performed.[139] They concluded that the effectiveness studies had methodological problems attributable to the lack of objective outcome measures, overreliance on subjective clinical observations, and small sample size. Of the 19 studies they reviewed, sample populations varied greatly, including adults and children with cerebral palsy and Down syndrome as well as high-risk infants.

In 1986, Ottenbacher et al[139] performed a meta-analysis on the use of NDT procedures in the pediatric population and found that the effect was small because of the small number of samples, difficulty in measuring the changes in the quality of movement and posture, and lack of rigorous control. The findings did suggest that individuals receiving NDT or some combination of NDT and other related therapy performed better than 62.2% of the subjects not receiving therapeutic services. A recent review of efficacy for the pediatric population diagnosed with neurological dysfunction indicated that the results supporting the benefits of NDT were inconclusive.[249] In their sample of 17 studies they found six published studies supporting the benefit of NDT intervention and nine that reported no benefit, with two being inconclusive. Specifically, they found that treatment for the child with cerebral palsy had inconsistent results, where as NDT treatment with the high-risk, low birth weight infants was not supported as useful.

No studies were found on the use of this technique for children with learning disabilities and motor deficits. Royeen and DeGangi[243] suggested that more studies are needed. They proposed that the benefits of NDT intervention over time should be investigated before comparison of NDT and other therapeutic approaches.

Motor Control, Motor Learning, and Motor Development Theories. *Motor control* is the study of the nature and cause of movement, encompassing the control of both posture and movement.[250] The organization and control of processes underlying motor behavior are considered.[194a] The mechanism responsible for the control of motor behavior is the primary focus.

The motor control model is developed on the assumption that the neural structures controlling movement must adapt to the constraints of the musculoskeletal system and the physical laws governing motion.[251] Bernstein[252] proposed that the brain has difficulty controlling the many different joints and muscles of the body. The body's biomechanical system has a large number of *degrees of freedom*. Degrees of freedom in the upper extremity, for example, occur within each joint that flexes, extends, or rotates. This creates an incredible complexity and variation of movement patterns that control for functional activities such as handwriting.[252]

Bernstein believed that synergy plays an important role in decreasing degrees of freedom. Synergy is achieved when muscles work together as a unit.

Another mechanism that decreases the degrees of freedom problem are *motor programs*. Motor programs are "command sets" characterized by specific motor patterns that activate in invariant order.[143] When throwing a baseball, for example, the motor program used (the order the muscles fire, the duration of the muscular contraction, and the force levels used) is fixed. A theory incorporating motor programs is the "open-loop theory," or feedforward system. With the feedforward system of control, the nervous system does not rely on peripheral feedback but uses previous motor learning to detect errors in a movement plan before it has been executed so that the individual can avoid errors in motor performance. The work of Nashner and McCollum[253] indicates that postural control works on a feedforward system. A person makes preparatory postural adjustments before he or she ever initiates a movement.

A feedback, or closed-loop system, depends on the recognition and correction of errors from peripheral feedback for performance. Feedback can be intrinsic or extrinsic. Intrinsic feedback is provided by sensory receptors (e.g., muscle spindles) before, during, and after movement. Extrinsic feedback is provided externally by visual or verbal information or cues.[254] If all movement depended on this type of error correction, human behavior would be extremely slow and inefficient.[255]

Feedforward and feedback work collaboratively during movement. Feedforward is used when initiating movement, and feedback assists in regulating and adapting movements. Both are learned experientially, by practice, and cannot be taught.[244]

Functional motor behaviors are critical regardless of the specific motor control theories adopted. These functional behaviors should occur in the context of a meaningful environment. The influences of environmental factors make task-related interventions essential to the development of motor control. For interventionists, the environments in which children are required to function is of paramount importance. The environment can be considered stable or variable.[143] Home and classrooms can be stable, in that many elements within these settings are fixed and do not change. The heights of the tables, sizes of chairs, and so forth are considered "variable features" within these stable environments. These variable features require a greater amount of motor control because the child must adjust movements and actions to the changing demands. Therapists generally practice in stable environments and therefore must ensure that the children are able to function under varied circumstances encountered in daily life situations. All environments must be critically assessed to determine the actions and adaptations needed to perform functional tasks relative to the child's abilities and demands.[194a]

Motor learning refers to the process of acquiring the ability to produce skilled movements[195] or the modifications of movements.[250] The acquisition of motor skills through practice and experience is emphasized.[194a] Acquiring skilled movements not only depends on integration within the nervous system but also is influenced by environmental factors and human biomechanics. Attainment of the motor behavior, whether through practice or experience, is the focus. Motor learning occurs when the skill becomes a permanent response, regardless of the environment.[254] Actual motor learning cannot be directly observed, only noted through the performance of a motor skill.[194a] Variables of motor learning applicable to intervention include feedback, practice, and motivation.[254]

During the process of learning, often called the skill acquisition phase, extrinsic feedback (often called knowledge of results) usually is given to the learner. "Feedback is essential for learning, but may not be necessary for the performance of a well learned task."[194a] Therapists tend to provide excessive feedback, especially when the performance is below what is expected. Low frequency and fading feedback, progressively decreasing the rate at which feedback is provided, appear to be most effective in facilitating learning.[194a] One proposed reason is that when feedback is less, the individual can more readily engage in the processes that enable learning versus focusing on the external support. During intervention, therapists should allow children the opportunity to self-evaluate and correct their own performance, with only accurate and necessary feedback given. Children should be provided with motor problems that require similar processing but varying outcomes.[254]

Regardless of the intervention approach used, repetition occurs. Practice, in general, is believed to increase learning of a skill or movement. Variations in practice can occur in the order tasks are performed and in the environment where the tasks are practiced and by changing the aspects of the task. Opportunity and variety in practice appear to improve motor learning, particularly when skills are practiced in a random manner. Practice should therefore be varied and occur in multiple environments (e.g., home and school) to maximize motor learning (see Chapters 3 and 9).

Motor development is the evolution of motor changes across the life span. This age-related process has been examined in specific age groups and the life span. Changes in motor behavior over time is the primary focus.

A life span approach to motor development has sparked research in the variety of movement patterns used to perform motor tasks from infancy throughout life. Variability in performance has been found to differ with age and activity levels. Two systems theories have explained the variety of motor development. The perceptual-action theory views motor development as functions of the perceptual system and motor system. The dynamic action theory promotes increasing the dimensions of variables until a new action is formed. A child's growth, for example, changes motor behavior. A child's motor behavior when grasping a baseball changes as the size of the hand increases. The emphasis in intervention should therefore be on age-appropriate skills and motor patterns during functional activities, regardless of the impairment.

Components of these theories of motor control appear particularly relevant to the treatment of children with learning disabilities and motor deficits. Progress is seen more rapidly when a task-related behavior that is meaningful to the child is used. Eye-hand coordination tasks, for example, become more meaningful within the context of a game of hot potato or baseball.

Motor learning and control problems typically seen in children with learning disabilities and motor difficulties include clumsiness, difficulty with judging force, timing and amplitude of motions, and deficits in anticipating the results of a motor action. These children often take longer to initiate a motor action and many move in a slow, plodding fashion. By using the concepts of the motor control theories presented here, these children can be hypothesized to be experiencing difficulties with feedforward and feedback systems. Feedforward would be essential to the development of timing body movements in space in relation to another object. Smyth[172] compared children with motor difficulties with a normal control group on a series of simple and complex movements and found that the group with motor difficulties had a longer reaction time and movement time for complex motions. He hypothesized that these children have a deficit in programming the movements; they need to rely more heavily on feedback for movement control.

Intervention using theories of motor control and learning considers how the child solves movement problems in the environment.[256] For completion of a successful task-oriented movement, the child must conform to the spatial and temporal demands of the environment. Visual and verbal cognitive strategies are used to assist the individual in performing the movement more appropriately. At times specific movement components of a task might be practiced, but they are combined in the context of the entire motor task, concentrating on the specific goal or end product of the task. The clinician should communicate the goal of the task to the child but encourage independent problem solving.

Critique of Motor Control Theories. Current motor control research involves a multidisciplinary effort, including neurophysiology, anatomy, muscle physiology, biomechanics, and behavioral sciences.[251,257] The great number and variation of theories presented on motor control, learning, and development limit consensus on terminology and definitions. These variations impede the ability to test and compare these theories adequately by using samples of children with mild motor difficulties. The variety of theories and terms used to describe motor functioning impede researchers from understanding and interpreting related research and limit the ability to search for underlying neural mechanisms of dysfunction.[258]

Sensorimotor Intervention. The premise of this type of intervention is that sensorimotor performance requires organizing sensory information from the environment for use in executing motor actions.[259] Evolution of sensorimotor intervention has not revolved around a single, unified theory but has incorporated a variety of theoretical foundations.[260,260a] Techniques developed for children with learning disabilities are a combination of perceptual-motor, neurodevelopmental, motor control, and sensory integration procedures.[174,259,261,262]

The goal of sensorimotor intervention is outcome based, with emphasis on the development of age-appropriate perceptual-motor and gross motor skills. The therapist chooses activities to meet the child's developmental levels, promote sensory and motor foundations, and encourage practice of appropriate motor skills. Gross motor outcomes of improved muscle strength, postural control, balance, equilibrium, and planning are promoted. For the child having difficulty keeping up with the skilled activities in gym class such as rope jumping, components of these activities will be encouraged, with emphasis on sequencing and timing. The therapist may use a heavier jump rope or wrist and ankle weights to provide more sensory information for improved task performance.

In sensorimotor intervention, tasks are chosen for their innate sensory and motor components. The child is directed to activities that encourage the use of the body in space to complete a structured motor sequence. Activities incorporate sensory components such as movement (vestibular), touch (tactile), and heavy work for the muscles and joints (proprioception). Environmental concepts such as spatial and temporal sequencing are included in the structure of a motor activity. Play interactions are considered important to encourage sensorimotor integration within the context of meaningful interactions with persons and objects.[259] Children may propel themselves prone on a scooter board through an "obstacle maze" while looking for matching shapes, for example. This activity provides tactile and proprioceptive and vestibular sensory input and encourages the development of postural strength and endurance while addressing perceptual skill development.

Gilfoyle and Grady,[173,174] Knickerbocker,[260a] Ayres,[111] and DeQuiros and Schrager[170] provide more information on sensorimotor therapy. These sources also describe many therapeutic activities for the development of postural functions in children with learning disabilities.

Research on Sensorimotor Intervention. DeGangi et al[263] identified a gap between theoretical reasoning and current research in sensorimotor intervention. Studies in this intervention technique are limited. In a comparison study, they found that children provided with structured sensorimotor therapy made greater gains in sensory integrative foundations, gross motor skills, and performance areas such as self-care than children who engaged in child-centered activity.

Motor Skill Training. Motor skill training involves learning skills and subskills functionally relevant to the child's daily performance. Tasks are taught in a sequenced manner by developmental ages or by steps from simple to complex. Evaluation identifies the point at which a child fails, and intervention involves a hierarchy of tasks from gross to fine.[101,102] Thus a graded system that includes ongoing evaluation of performance and task acquisition is developed.

Abbie[264] described the motor skills training approach: "One can . . . break down the skills into their simplest forms and give the child opportunities to practice each in as many varied ways as possible so that he does not learn one isolated splinter skill." As an example, Abbie suggested that a child with poor balance in standing practice balance in all positions—kneeling, all fours, sitting, and prone—and on both stable and mobile surfaces. Abbie used multiple approaches, including neurodevelopmental theory, modern dance, and gymnastics.

In general, motor skill training can involve both indirect and direct facilitation of specific motor tasks. Much of the treatment is directed toward the acquisition of basic skills as described by Abbie.[162,264] The goal is to provide a great variety of motor activities at the child's developmental motor level to promote motor generalizations. The activities recommended include balance, locomotion, body awareness, and hand-eye coordination. The functional relevance

of these skill areas includes being able to sit at a desk within the classroom and complete written work as well as having greater success in recess games such as basketball. Specific skills such as dribbling and foul shooting also may be taught and practiced to facilitate improved social participation.

A final area of skill that should be addressed is activities of daily living. Children with DCD are frequently delayed in the basic self-care skills of tying shoelaces, using a knife and fork, and blowing the nose as well as generally inefficient in dressing for school.[85,102] Inadequacy in self-care is a sensitive area for children whose peers have no such difficulty, and teachers and therapists should be aware of the child's need to learn these basic skills.

Monitoring Physical Fitness. Statistics for the United States indicate that since 1980 the number of children who are overweight has nearly doubled and the number of overweight adolescents has tripled. Approximately 15% of children are currently overweight.[265] For children with motor impairments the addition of deficits in sensory foundations and motor skill development contribute further to risk factors. A child with learning disabilities and motor deficits is at risk for poor posture, body mechanics, and physical fitness. Physical fitness, as defined in this chapter, includes strength, endurance, speed, agility, flexibility, and cardiorespiratory endurance. Arnheim and Sinclair[153] pointed out that the relation between motor ability and physical fitness forms a vicious cycle. The child with poor motor ability avoids physical activity, and the poor fitness that develops through lack of exercise lessens motor ability. A study of 24 7- to 9-year-old boys with DCD found significantly decreased anaerobic performance and peak power and speed, with increased fatigue.[266]

The physiologically based poor posture and inefficient body use can be exaggerated by a secondary disability. The child's poor self-concept may be reflected in a hunched, withdrawn posture and the avoidance of any physical activity beyond that needed in everyday activities. This latter pattern also can be found in children with learning disabilities without a primary motor disability.

The physical educator within the school system should monitor physical fitness in all children. For those children receiving supportive services for motor coordination delays the physical therapist should collaborate with the physical educator to ensure that a child receives sufficient exercise to maintain physical fitness. Arnheim and Sinclair[153] presented graded levels of activities for fitness in the four areas of strength and muscular endurance, flexibility, agility and large muscle coordination, and cardiorespiratory endurance. See Arnheim and Sinclair,[153] Larkin and Hoare,[211] and the Presidents Council for Physical Fitness[267] for further discussion of physical fitness and a developmental program for children with problems in motor coordination.

Summary

Children with learning disabilities frequently have motor coordination problems. The presenting motor deficits may be subtle and difficult to pick up by neurological evaluation or standardized testing. When undetected, motor difficulties may have a significant impact on the qualitative development of age-appropriate motor skills, limiting functional performance at home and school. The child's inability to master basic motor skills such as dressing and bicycle riding further affects self-esteem, peer relations, and societal participation.

Motor performance and movement are important aspects of a child's total development, including academic growth. Automatic postural control provides stability needed to sit upright in a chair for participation in academic tasks and freedom of movement for exploration within the environment. Movement through space and body awareness precedes prepositional concept development. Children first understand the words up, down, left, and right on their own body. A multitude of factors must be considered in the development of each individual's learning capacities. Lerner[268] stated that:

"We cannot conclude that motor development is unimportant or that this aspect of learning should be discarded. Rather, these studies suggest that plans are needed for building the bridge between motor training and academic learning. Efficient motor movement may be a prerequisite but alone it is insufficient."

Many theoretical models have been developed in an attempt to explain the qualitative motor deficits observed in children with learning disabilities as well as provide constructs to develop intervention programs. All have certain relevance to this population and perhaps to each individual child. Many of the approaches share common assumptions, although rationales and intervention strategies may vary markedly. Several theories and intervention approaches have been presented to give a spectrum of alternatives in working with children with DCD.

Each child presents a unique composite of clinical signs and functional deficits, and the therapist is challenged to assess the child appropriately, identify strengths and weaknesses, and formulate an intervention program that best addresses the underlying deficits in foundation skills and the functional weaknesses in daily life tasks. The experienced interventionist will combine knowledge from many areas of theoretical development and remediation to facilitate the best performance in each child.

LEARNING DISABILITIES ACROSS THE LIFE SPAN

Research with adolescents and adults with learning disabilities has indicated that, for the most part, children do not outgrow learning disabilities. Learning disabilities are lifelong challenges. Problems tend to persist in some or all of the following areas: attention and activity, cognitive and academic performance, motor skills, emotional adjustment, and social interactions.

Follow-up studies of children with high activity levels indicate that although hyperactivity may become less of a problem as children get older, many other problems exist. Routh and Mesibov[269] found that, of 83 teenagers who had been hyperactive as children, 58% had failed one or more grades in school, many had low self-esteem, and several had been involved in delinquent behavior. In a small longitudinal sample, Barkley et al[270] identified that after 8 years most children sampled continued to have attention issues, but 59% also had oppositional defiant disorder or conduct disorder. Other significant issues noted in adolescents and

adults with persistent attentional problems include increased incidence of antisocial behaviors and substance abuse.[271] Overall, studies indicate that childhood attention and activity difficulties are often predictive of continued academic failure, low self-esteem, and social and behavioral problems.

Helper[272] reviewed follow-up studies of children with learning disabilities and found that, both emotionally and behaviorally, boys continued to have a much higher frequency of problems than control subjects. In addition, persistent deficits in learning skills (e.g., reading achievement), along with deficits in attention and information processing, were noted. Research also has indicated that learning disabilities carry long-term academic effects during the school years. To ascertain whether children outgrow learning disabilities, Book[176a] tested 472 Utah kindergarten children on standardized tests and assigned each student to one of three categories of presumed risk. Students were retested on academic achievement tests in the first through fourth grades. Less than 11% of the students assigned to the high-risk group ever performed above the 50th percentile. Only 4% in the lowest risk group ever performed below the 25th percentile. Parham's[273] recent 4-year longitudinal study of elementary school children supported the belief that children with learning disabilities do not outgrow perceptual-motor problems related to academic achievement.

Within the motor domain, increasing evidence shows that children do not outgrow their deficits despite some arguments to the contrary.[274] Denckla[146] and Denckla et al[275] pointed out that although many children with motor difficulties do eventually master specific motor skills, they fail new age-appropriate ones. Longitudinal studies have found an association between childhood motor deficits and later learning difficulties and psychological problems.[133,276] Cantell et al[158] provided additional evidence in a longitudinal study that adolescents with DCD have lower academic achievement, fewer spare time activities, poor opinion of their competence, and lower aspirations.

Learning disabilities and motor impairments appear to have a persistent effect on self-concept. Of the adolescent populations with learning disabilities or hyperactivity studied, 40% to 60% have low self-esteem.[277] Depression, thoughts of suicide, and low expectations for the future also seemed to be more prevalent in the adolescent with a learning disability.[278]

In recent years, the relation between learning disabilities and juvenile delinquency has been explored.[279,280] A high rate of antisocial behavior in adolescence, "trouble with the law," or "police contact" are found frequently in follow-up studies of children with learning disabilities.[133,281] Several studies of delinquent adolescent boys have shown that 25% to 30% have learning disabilities,[282] and Mauser[283] reported that 50% to 70% of juvenile delinquents in his sample exhibited evidence of learning disabilities. Some clinicians believe that the educational and psychological trauma within the classroom may be expressed later as aberrant social functioning in the community.[280]

Less information is available on adults with learning disabilities, in part because learning disabilities were not diagnostic entities until the 1960s. Many of the reports on learning disabilities in adulthood are from persons who were diagnosed in their teenage or adult years. Thus they did not receive the early intervention services that children with learning disabilities currently receive. Therefore the effectiveness of treatment or its impact on long-term disabilities cannot be evaluated.

Much of our knowledge about the adult with a learning disability today is anecdotal and in the form of case histories. Few research studies have systematically explored the continued effects of a learning disability in adulthood. Review of the literature regarding adults with learning disabilities indicates that difficulties can be expressed throughout the total personality—cognitively, perceptually, and emotionally.[91] Functional difficulties also persist and are seen in vocational adjustment, work management, and social and family interactions.[284]

The same cycles of ineptitude, frustration, and anxiety experienced by the child with learning disabilities may be repeated as an adult. Mrs. B., Paul's mother in Case Study 14-2, articulates this. She was not diagnosed with learning disabilities until age 20 years. Nevertheless, she completed both bachelor's and master's degrees in counseling. Although the academic frustrations were no longer an issue, the learning disability interferes with her work and home performance. Mrs. B. describes her organizational difficulties and identifies a continuous need to make lists to function in her job. She concentrates on not looking "clumsy" and is fearful she will trip over things and look foolish. Learning and accomplishing things continue to require increased effort compared with her peers. Thus as an adult, the learning disability continues to present difficulty in functional performance.

A letter from a woman with learning disabilities, motor coordination impairments, and sensory integration problems is included in Box 14-3. She describes how her learning dis-

---

BOX 14-3 ■ A LETTER FROM AN ADULT WITH A LEARNING DISABILITY

I am 26 years old, a professional bassoonist with a master's degree in music performance. My name is Wendy. Through Jane, an occupational therapist, I discovered when I was 24 years old that I had learning problems and sensory integration problems.

I invert letters and especially numbers. When people speak English to me, I feel it's a foreign language. There's translation lag time. When learning new things, I either understand intuitively or never. I can't seem to go through step-by-step learning processes.

Physically, I'm extremely sensitive to motion. When I was little, we moved every year. I spent the first 5 years of my life feeling sick. It seems that I feel everything more strongly than most people. I have an extremely low threshold of pain and even pleasure tends to overload me. If I am touched unexpectedly it hurts, it's so jarring. This causes a lot of problems with interpersonal relationships. I can't stand to have people close to me; it produces an adrenalin reaction.

Motor activities are also a problem; my muscles don't seem to remember past motions. Despite the many times I've walked down steps and through doors, I still have to think about how high to lift my foot and about planning my movements. When eating, I have to think about chewing or I bite my tongue or mouth. I don't think other people think about these things. I'm physically inept; I can bump into the same table 10 times running. I'm always bruised, and as a child people constantly labeled me as clumsy. Physical education courses were hell as a child, especially gymnastics, where you are forced to leave the ground and swing or walk on balance beams or uneven bars. I cannot begin to explain the terror or disorientation.

Academically, I was labeled stupid or, more frequently, lazy. I was told that I was not trying. Actually, my IQ is high and my coping mechanisms are complex. If they only knew how hard I was trying. I was lucky because I taught myself to read at an early age. I would never have learned to read otherwise. Even so, my first grade teacher wouldn't believe that I could read so far past my age. She called me a liar when I said that I had finished each "Dick and Jane" book. I was forced to read each one 50 times before she would give me a new one.

Not all teachers were so insensitive. My fourth grade teacher made every effort to let me go at my own pace, letting me read on a college level and do 2 years of math on my own. Left to my own devices, I can learn and love to do so. My fifth grade teacher forced me to do math the long way with steps. I just know the answer by looking at multiplication or division problems, even algebra problems, but to this day I cannot understand how one does it in steps. If a teacher didn't accept this, I was in for a year of hell. I cried a lot in school, from frustration mostly, and I pretended to be sick a lot.

I never had friends until college. I guess I was too different to be acceptable. I grew up in a rigid, repressive, religious community, which made it especially difficult to be accepted. My differences were labeled evil or, at best, I was ignored. I left high school at age 16 for college, where at least I could structure what I wanted to learn. It's never been easy for me to make friends, although it's better now. Music circles tend to be a bit crazy so I fit in more easily.

My learning disabilities still are problems. My motor and learning problems get in the way of my music, but my coping mechanisms are strong. I deal better with my clumsiness now. Just being diagnosed by Jane has made a big difference. To have things labeled, to be told and realize that it's not my fault, has given me a sense of peace. It's also allowed me to turn from inward depression to outward anger at those who labeled me stupid and clumsy. Just being able to admit anger allows one to let it go.

Other than my testing and subsequent conversations with Jane, I have not received treatment for my problems. I believe that adults with my problems can be helped. I wish programs were available in all areas of the country. At age 26, I feel much better about myself than I did even at age 24. It's a matter of growth and coping with major differences.

The greatest advice I would give to educators and therapists working with problem children is to accept. Accept what they can do well; don't make an issue of what they can't do. We all have our strengths and weaknesses. If a child can't do math, so what! Buy the child a calculator and the child will do a lot better with it than with a label of stupidity following her through life.

ability affects her current functioning and how it affected her when she was a child.

SUMMARY

Meeting the needs of the child with learning disabilities offers new challenges in occupational and physical therapy. As a result of the passage of PL 94-142 and IDEA, intervention with children is moving from the clinical to academic arena. Providing comprehensive service requires variety in patterns of service delivery, with an increase in consultation and inservice education. When presented with the subtle motor deficits that are frequently part of DCD the therapist must develop and refine skills in assessment and intervention.

Occupational and physical therapists assume an important role in educating the team of professionals and parents to the importance of motor deficits regarding functional performance and societal participation. Within the school system motor deficits must have educational relevance to warrant remediation. Service provision within the LRE might begin with education of the teacher and accommodations to the classroom. If this approach does not facilitate adequate functional abilities, intervention in or out of the classroom may be warranted.

The child's motor needs must be assessed in the context of overall educational and emotional development. The question is not whether the child *would* benefit from therapy but *which types* of remediation are the most essential for the child at a given time in development. Some children with coordination difficulties cope quite well as long as their problem is recognized. Gubbay[102] says, "Bringing the child into focus by the recognition of his problem immediately reduces the pressures to conform." In an environment where parents, teachers, peers, and the child recognize the nature of the deficit and set reasonable expectations, some children accept their motor disability, and academic skills and alternative forms of recreation assume greater importance.

As this review has indicated, evidence supporting the effectiveness of intervention of motor deficits in children with learning disabilities is as yet fragmentary. Children with learning disabilities present highly variable patterns of disability that make predicting or measuring response to therapy difficult. Continued formal research and careful documentation of clinical outcomes are needed to explore and define the dimensions of motor disorders in children with learning disabilities that are relevant to therapy. Only then can we better categorize children, improve the precision of treatment, and validate theory.

REFERENCES

1. National Center for Learning Disabilities: *What is a learning disability?* (website): www.nichcy.org/pubs/factshe/fs7txt.htm. Accessed June 27, 2006.
2. Clements SD: *Minimal brain dysfunction in children: Terminology and identification,* Washington, DC, 1966, U.S. Department of Health, Education, and Welfare.
3. Gaddes WH: *Learning disabilities and brain function: a neuropsychological approach,* ed 2, New York, 1985, Springer-Verlag.
4. Thompson S: Nonverbal learning disorders, The LDA Gram, Fall 1996, Winter 1997, www.nldline.com.
5. Polatajko HJ: Developmental coordination disorder (DCD): Alias the clumsy child syndrome. In Whitmore K, Hart H, Willems G, editors: *A neurodevelopmental approach to specific learning disorders,* London, 1999, MacKeith Press.
6. National Joint Committee on Learning Disabilities: *Letter to NJCLD Member Organizations.* Washington, DC, 1988, National Joint Committee on Learning Disabilities.
7. Cutting LE, Denckla MB: Attention: Relationships between attention-deficit hyperactivity disorder and learning disabilities. In Swanson HL, Harris KR, Graham S, editors: *Handbook of learning disabilities,* New York, 2003, The Guilford Press.
8. Gallico R, Lewis MEB: Learning disabilities. In Batshaw ML, Perret YM, editors: *Children with disabilities: a medical primer,* ed 3, Baltimore, 1992, Paul H. Brookes.
9. Strauss AA, Lehtinen LE: *Psychopathology and education of the brain-injured child,* New York, 1947, Grune & Stratton.
10. Myklebust HR: Learning disabilities: Definition and overview. In Myklebust HR, editor: *Progress in learning disabilities, vol 1,* New York, 1968, Grune & Stratton.
11. Office of Education: Education of Individuals with Disabilities (IDEA), 1990, 20 U.S.C., §1401(1) (15) p. 4.
12. Harris JC: *Developmental neuropsychiatry: Assessment, diagnosis, and treatment of developmental disorders, vol II,* New York, 1998, Oxford University Press.
13. Adelman HS, Taylor L: *An introduction to learning disabilities,* Glenview, IL, 1986, Scott Foresman & Co.
14. Black PE: *Brain dysfunction in children: etiology, diagnosis and management,* New York, 1981, Raven Press.
15. Black PE: Introduction: changing concepts of "brain damage" and "brain dysfunction." In Black PE, editor: *Brain dysfunction in children: etiology, diagnosis and management,* New York, 1981, Raven Press.
16. MacKeith RM: Defining the concept of minimal brain damage. In Bax M, MacKeith RM, editors: *Minimal cerebral dysfunction,* London, 1963, William Heinemann Medical.
17. Rie HE: Definitional problems. In Rie HE, Rie ED, editors: *Handbook of minimal brain dysfunctions: a critical view,* New York, 1980, John Wiley & Sons.
18. Hallahan DP, Mock DR: *A brief history of the field of learning disabilities,* In Swanson HL, Harris KR. Graham S, editors: *Handbook of learning disabilities,* New York, 2003, The Guilford Press.
19. Kavanagh JF, Truss TJ, editors: *Learning disabilities, proceedings of the national conference,* New York, 1988, York Press.
20. Kavale KA, Forness SR: Learning disability as a discipline. In Swanson HL, Harris KR. Graham S, editors: *Handbook of learning disabilities,* New York, 2003, The Guilford Press.
21. Policymaker Partnership for Implementing IDEA: *IDEA 1997 and final part B regulations. Benefits to children with disabilities,* 1999, Policymaker Partnership. www.ideapractices.org/law_res/doc/resources/topic.php?subcatID=88. Accessed June 27, 2006.
22. National Center for Learning Disabilities: *IDEA 2004 brief summary of changes and new provisions* (website). www.nrcld.org/research/rti.shtml. Accessed June 26, 2006.
23. Fletcher JM, Morris RD, Lyon GR: Classification and definition of learning disabilities: An integrated perspective. In Swanson HL, Harris KR, Graham S, editors: *Handbook of learning disabilities,* New York, 2003, The Guilford Press.
24. Binet A, Simon T: Le dévelopment de l'intelligence chez l'enfant, *Année Psychol* 14:1, 1908.
25. Whitmore K, Bax M: What do we mean by SLD? A historical perspective. In Whitmore K, Hart H, Willems G, editors: *A neurodevelopmental approach to specific learning disorders,* London, 1999, MacKeith Press.
26. U.S. Department of Education: *Twenty-fourth annual report to Congress on the implementation of the Individuals with Disabilities Act* (website): www.ed.gov/about/reports/annual/osep/2002/index.html.
27. American Psychiatric Association: *Diagnostic and statistical manual of mental disorders,* ed 4, Washington, DC, 1994, American Psychiatric Association.

28. World Health Organization: *The ICD-10 classification of mental health and behavioral disorders: Clinical descriptions and diagnostic guidelines,* Geneva, 1992, World Health Organization.

29. National Institutes of Health: *Research plan for the National Center for Medical Rehabilitative Research,* Bethesda, MD, 1993, National Institutes of Health.

30. Palisano KJ, Campbell SK, Harris SR: Clinical decision-making in pediatric physical therapy. In Campbell SK, editor: *Physical therapy for children,* Philadelphia, 1995, W.B. Saunders.

31. Child Trends Data Bank: *Learning disabilities* (website). *www.childtrendsdatabank.org/indicators/65LearningDisabilities.cfm.*

32. Finucci MM: Genetic considerations in dyslexia. In Myklebust HR, editor: *Progress in learning disabilities, vol 4.* New York, 1978, Grune & Stratton.

33. Touwen BCL, Sporrel T: Soft signs and MBD, *Dev Med Child Neurol* 21:528, 1979.

34. Towbin A: Neuropathologic factors in minimal brain dysfunction. In Rie HE, Rie ED, editors: *Handbook of minimal brain dysfunctions: a critical view,* New York, 1980, John Wiley & Sons.

35. National Center for Learning Disabilities: *What are the causes of learning disabilities?* (website): www.nichcy.org/pubs/factshe/fs17txt.htm. Accessed June 27, 2006.

36. Willis AG, Hooper SR, Stone BH: Neuropsychological theories of learning disabilities. In Singh NN, Beale IL, editors: *Learning disabilities: nature, theory, and treatment,* New York, 1992, Springer-Verlag.

37. Orton ST: *Reading, writing, and speech problems in children,* New York, 1937, W.W. Norton.

38. Sparrow S: Dyslexia and laterality: Evidence for a developmental theory, *Semin Psychiatry* 1:270, 1969.

39. Sparrow S, Satz P: Dyslexia, laterality, and neuropsychological development. In Bakker BJ, Satz P, editors: *Specific reading disabilities: advances in theory and method,* Rotterdam, The Netherlands, 1970, University of Rotterdam.

40. Bishop DVM, Edmundson A: Language-impaired 4-year-olds: distinguishing transient from persistent impairment, *J Speech Hearing Disord* 52:156-173, 1987.

41. Geschwind N, Galaburda A: Cerebral lateralization: biological mechanisms, associations, and pathology: I, II, III. *Arch Neurol* 42:428-459, 521-552, 634-654, 1985.

42. Crowell DH, Jones RH, Kapuniai LE, et al: Unilateral cortical activity in newborn infants: An early index of cerebral dominance? *Science* 180:205-208, 1973.

43. Murray EA: Hemispheric specialization. In Fisher AG, Murray EA, Bundy AC, editors: *Sensory integration: theory and practice,* Philadelphia, 1991, FA Davis.

44. Locke JL: Towards a biological science of language development. In Barrett M, editor: *The development of language.* London, 1997, UCL Press.

44a. Thompson S: The source for nonverbal learning disorders, East Moline, IL, 1997, LinguiSystems.

45. Poremba A: Auditory processing and hemispheric specialization, *Psychological Science Agenda,* 28:10, 2004.

45a. Ayres AJ: Characteristics of types of sensory integrative dysfunction, *Am J Occup Ther* 25:329, 1971.

46. Brown JK, Minns RA: The neurological basis of learning disorders in children. In Whitmore K, Hart H, Willems G: *A neurodevelopmental approach to specific learning disorders,* London, 1999, MacKeith Press.

47. Semmes J: Hemispheric specialization: a possible clue to mechanism, *Neuropsychologia* 6:11, 1968.

47a. Thompson S: *The source for nonverbal learning disorders,* East Moline, IL, 1997, LinguiSystems.

47b. Ayres AJ: Characteristics of types of sensory integrative dysfunction, *Am J Occup Ther* 25:329, 1971.

47c. Levy J, Trevarthen C, Sperry RW: Perception of bilateral chimeric figures following hemispheric deconnexion, *Brain* 95:61, 1972.

47d. Witelson SF: Developmental dyslexia: two right hemispheres and none left, *Science* 195:309, 1977.

48. Gazzaniga MS: Brain theory and minimal brain dysfunction, *Acad Sci* 205:89, 1973.

49. Myklebust HR: Learning disabilities and minimal brain dysfunction in children. In Tower DB, editor: *The nervous system, vol 3, human communication and its disorders,* New York, 1975, Raven Press.

49a. Hardy M, Smythe PC, Stennett RG: Developmental patterns in elemental reading skills: phoneme-grapheme and grapheme-phoneme correspondences, *J Educ Psychol* 63:433, 1972.

50. Miller CJ, Sanchez J, Hynd GW: Neurological correlates of reading disabilities. In Swanson HL, Harris KR, Graham S, editors: *Handbook of learning disabilities,* New York, 2003, The Guilford Press.

51. Badian NA, Wolff PH: Manual asymmetries of motor sequencing in boys with reading disabilities, *Cortex* 13:343, 1977.

52. Gerloff, C, Andres FG: Bimanual coordination and interhemispheric interaction, *Acta Psychologica* 110:161-186, 2002.

53. Kitterle FL: *Hemispheric communication,* Hillsdale, NJ, 1995, Lawrence Erlbaum Associates.

54. Diamond SJ: *Processing speed and motor planning: the scientific background to the skills trained by Interactive Metronome® Technology* (website): peakpotental.net/pdf/diamond0/020-whitepages.pdf.

55. Rourke BP, editor: *Neuropsychology of learning disabilities: essentials of subtype analysis,* New York, 1985, The Guilford Press.

56. Singh NN, Beale IL: Learning disabilities: Nature, theory, and treatment, New York, 1992, Springer-Verlag.

57. Ingersoll BD, Goldstein S: *Attention deficit disorder and learning disabilities, realities, myths and controversial treatments,* New York, 1993, Doubleday.

58. Denckla MB, Rudel R: Rapid automatized naming (RAN): Dyslexia different from the other learning disabilities, *Neuropsychologia,* 14:976, 1976.

59. Kaufman AS, Lichtenberger EO: *Essentials of WAIS-III assessment,* New York, 1999, John Wiley & Sons, Psychological Corporation, San Antonio TX.

60. Flanagan DP, Kaufman AS: *Essentials of WISC-IV,* New York, 2004, John Wiley & Sons, Psychological Corporation, San Antonio TX.

61. Rourke BP: Brain-behavior relationships in children with learning disabilities: a research program, *Am Psychol* 30:911, 1975.

62. Rourke BP, Telegdy GA: Lateralizing significance of WISC verbal-performance discrepancies for older children with learning disabilities, *Percept Mot Skills* 33:875, 1975.

63. Rourke BP, Young GC, Flewelling RW: The relationship between WISC verbal-performance discrepancies and selected verbal, auditory-perceptual, visual-perceptual and problem solving abilities in children with learning disabilities, *J Clin Psychol* 27:475, 1971.

64. Siegel LS, Metsala J: Subtypes of learning disabilities. In Singh NN, Beale IL, editors: *Learning disabilities: nature, theory, and treatment,* New York, 1992, Springer-Verlag.

65. Harnadek MCS, Rourke BP: Principal identifying features of the syndrome of nonverbal learning disabilities in children, *J Learning Dis* 27:144-154, 1994.

66. Rourke BP: Socioemotional disturbances of learning disabled children, *J Consult Clin Psychol* 58:801-810, 1988.

67. Gordon N: Dyslexia—why can't I learn to read? In Whitmore K, Hart H, Willems G, editors: *A neurodevelopmental approach to specific learning disorders,* London, 1999, MacKeith Press.

68. International Dyslexia Association: *Definition of dyslexia* (website): www.interdys.org. Accessed June 27, 2006.

69. Shaywitz SE, Shaywitz BA: *The neurobiology of reading and dyslexia* (website): ncsall.gse.harvard.edu/fob/2001/shaywitz.html.

70. Shaywitz SE, Shaywitz BA: The neurobiological indices of dyslexia. In Swanson HL, Harris KR, Graham S, editors: *Handbook of learning disabilities,* New York, 2003, The Guilford Press.

71. Boder E: Developmental dyslexia: A diagnostic approach based on three typical reading-spelling patterns, *Dev Med Child Neurol* 15:663-687, 1973.

72. Bakker D: Neuropsychological classification and treatment of dyslexia, *J Learn Disabil* 25:102-109, 1992.

73. Logan G: Toward an instance theory of automatization, *Psychological Rev* 95:492-527, 1988.

74. Gordon N: Children with developmental dyscalculia [annotation], *Dev Med Child Neurol* 34:459-463, 1992.

75. Nixon Education Services: *Subtypes of dyslexia* (website). *www.alphabetmats.com/facts.html.*

76. Geary DC: Learning disabilities in arithmetic: Problem solving differences and cognitive deficits. In Swanson HL, Harris KR, Graham S, editors: *Handbook of learning disabilities,* New York, 2003, The Guilford Press.

77. Sharma M: What is dyscalculia? (website): www.dfes.gov.uk/readwriteplus/understandingdyslexia/introduction/whatdoweknowaboutdyslexia/. Accessed June, 27, 2006.

78. Schwartz SE, Budd D: Mathematics for handicapped learners: a functional approach for adolescents. In Meyer E, Vergason GA, Whelan BP, editors: *Promising practices for exceptional children—curriculum implications,* Denver, 1983, Love Publishing.

79. International Dyslexia Association: *About dysgraphia* (website). www.dyslexia-ca.org/dysgraphia.html.

80. Dysgraphia Low Incidence Project: *Causes and prevalence* (website): www.arachne.cofc.edu/classes/EDFS710/Student/Dysgraphia.html#Causes_and_Prevalence.

81. O'Hare A: Dysgraphia and dyscalculia. In Whitmore K, Hart H, Willems G: *A neurodevelopmental approach to specific learning disorders,* London, 1999, MacKeith Press.

82. Sandler AD, Watson TE, Footo M, Levine MD, Coleman WL, Hooper SR: Neurodevelopmental study of writing disorders in middle childhood, *J Dev Behav Pediatr* 13:17-22, 1992.

83. Denckla MB: The neuropsychology of social-emotional learning disability, *Arch Neurol* 40:461-462, 1983.

84. Nonverbal Learning Disorders Association: *What is NLD?* (website): www.nlda.org/index.php?submenu=Education&src=gendocs&link=WhatIsNLD/. Accessed June 27, 2006.

85. Gubbay SS: *The clumsy child,* New York, 1975, W.B. Saunders.

86. Cermak SA, Larkin D: *Developmental coordination disorder,* Albany, NY, 2002, Delmar.

87. Barnhart RC, Davenport MJ, Epps SB, Nordquist VM: Developmental coordination disorder, *Phys Ther* 83:722-732, 2003.

88. Hoare D: Subtypes of developmental coordination disorder, *Adapted Phys Activity Q* 11:158-169, 1994.

89. Henderson SE, Hall D: Concomitants of clumsiness in young school children, *Dev Med Child Neurol* 24:448, 1982.

90. Dewey D, Kaplan BJ, Crawford SG: Developmental coordination disorder: associated problems in attention, learning, and psychosocial adjustment, *Human Movement Sci* 21:905-918, 2002.

91. Ames TH: Post secondary problems: an optimistic approach. In Weber RE, editor: *Handbook on learning disabilities: a prognosis for the child, the adolescent, the adult,* Englewood Cliffs, NJ, 1974, Prentice-Hall.

92. Rasmussen P, Gillberg C: AD(H)D, hyperkinetic disorders, DAMP, and related behaviour disorders. In Whitmore K, Hart H, Willems G, editors: *A neurodevelopmental approach to specific learning disorders,* London, 1999, MacKeith Press.

93. Gottlieb MI: The learning-disabled child: Controversial issues revisited. In Gottlieb MI, Zinkus PW, Bradford LJ, editors: *Current issues in developmental pediatrics: the learning disabled child,* New York, 1979, Grune & Stratton.

94. Elbaum B, Vaughn S: *Can school-based interventions enhance self concept in students with learning disabilities* (website)? ld.org/research/ncld_self_concept.cfm.

95. Kenny TJ, Burka A: Coordinating multiple interventions. In Rie HE, Rie ED, editors: *Handbook of minimal brain dysfunctions: a critical view,* New York, 1980, John Wiley & Sons.

96. Case Management Society of America: *Definition of case management* (website): www.cmsa.org/ABOUTUS/DefinitionofCaseManagement/tabid/104/Default.aspx. Accessed March 13, 2005.

97. Cruickshank WM, Hallahan DP: *Learning disabilities, the struggle from adolescence toward adulthood,* Syracuse, NY, 1980, Syracuse University Press.

98. Dunn W, Campbell PH: Designing pediatric service provision. In Dunn W, editor: *Pediatric occupational therapy: facilitating effective service provision,* Thorofare, NJ, 1991, Slack.

99. Dunn W: Designing best practice services for children and families. In Dunn W, editor: *Best practice occupational therapy,* Thorofare, NJ, 2000, Slack.

100. Ford FR: *Diseases of the nervous system in infancy, childhood and adolescence,* ed 5, Springfield, IL, 1966, Charles C Thomas.

101. Gubbay SS: The management of developmental apraxia, *Dev Med Child Neurol* 20:643, 1978.

102. Gubbay SS: The clumsy child. In Rose FC, editor: *Pediatric neurology,* London, 1979, Blackwell Scientific, p 157.

103. Gubbay SS, Ellis E, Walton JN et al: Clumsy children: a study of apraxic and agnosic deficits in 21 children, *Brain* 85:295, 1963.

104. Walton JN, Ellis E, Court DM: Clumsy children: a study of developmental apraxia and agnosia, *Brain* 85:603, 1963.

105. Schaffer R, Law M, Polatajko H, Miller J: A study of children with learning disabilities and sensorimotor problems or let's not throw the baby out with the bathwater, *Phys Occup Ther Pediatr* 9:101-117, 1989.

106. Ayres AJ: Sensorimotor foundations of academic ability. In Cruickshank WM, Hallahan DP, editors: *Perceptual and learning disabilities in children vol 2, research and theory,* New York, 1975, Syracuse University Press.

107. Ayres AJ: *Sensory integration and the child,* Los Angeles, 1980, Western Psychological Services.

108. American Psychiatric Association: *Diagnostic and statistical manual of mental disorders,* ed 3, revised, Washington, DC, 1987, American Psychiatric Association.

109. Miller LT, Missiuna CA, Macnab JJ et al: Clinical description of children with developmental coordination disorder, *Can J Occup Ther* 68:5-15, 2001.

110. Hoskins T, Squires J: Developmental assessment: a test for gross motor and reflex development, *Phys Ther* 53:117, 1973.

111. Ayres AJ: *Sensory integration and learning disorders,* Los Angeles, 1972, Western Psychological Services, p 17.

112. Haley S, Coster W, Binda-Sundberg K: Measuring physical disablement: The contextual challenge, *Phys Ther* 74:74-82, 1994.

113. Deuel RK, Robinson DJ: Developmental motor signs. In Tupper DE, editor: *Soft neurological signs,* New York, 1987, Grune & Stratton.

114. Johnston O, Short H, Crawford J: Poorly coordinated children: a survey of 95 cases, *Child Care Health Dev* 13:361-376, 1987.

115. Wright HC, Sugden DA: A two-step procedure for the identification of children with developmental co-ordination disorder in Singapore, *Dev Med Child Neurol* 38:1099-1105, 1996.

116. Jongmans MJ, Smits-Engelsman BC, Schoemaker MM: Consequences of comorbidity of developmental coordination disorders and learning disabilities for severity and pattern of perceptual-motor dysfunction, *J Learn Disabil* 36:528-539, 2003.

117. Tarnopol L, Tarnopol M: *Brain function and reading disabilities,* Baltimore, 1977, University Park Press.

118. Sugden D, Wann C: The assessment of motor impairment in children with moderate learning difficulties, *Br J Educ Psychol* 57:225-236, 1987.

119. LaVesser P, Bloomer MA: Using functional performance outcomes in a school setting, *OT Week* 4(38):7, 1990.

120. McPhillips M, Sheehy N: Prevalence of persistent primary reflexes and motor problems in children with reading difficulties, *Dyslexia* 10:316-338, 2004.

121. Willoughby C, Polatajko HJ: Motor problems in children with developmental coordination disorder: Review of the literature, *Am J Occup Ther* 49:787-789, 1995.

122. Kaplan BJ, Wilson BN, Dewey DM, Crawford SG: DCD may not be a discrete disorder, *Hum Mov Sci* 17, 471-490, 1998.

123. Hadders-Algra M: The neuronal group selection theory: a framework to explain variation in normal motor development, *Dev Med Child Neurol* 42:566-572, 2000.

124. Hulme C, Biggerstaff A, Moran G, McKinley I: Visual, kinaesthetic and cross-modal judgements of length by normal and clumsy children, *Dev Med Child Neurol* 24:461, 1982.

125. Ayres AJ: Types of sensory integrative dysfunction among disabled learners, *Am J Occup Ther* 26:13, 1972.

126. Fisher AG: Vestibular-proprioceptive processing. In Fisher AG, Murray EA, Bundy AC, editors: *Sensory integration: theory and practice,* Philadelphia, 1991, F.A. Davis.

127. Horak F, Shumway-Cook A, Crowe TK, et al: Vestibular function and motor proficiency of children with impaired hearing, or with a learning disability and motor impairments, *Dev Med Child Neurol* 30:64-79, 1988.

128. Missiuna C: Motor skill acquisition in children with developmental coordination disorder, *Adapted Phys Activity Q* 11:214-235, 1994.

129. Galaburda AM: Neurology of developmental dyslexia, *Curr Opin Neurobiol* 3:237-242, 1993.

130. Fellick JM, Thomson APJ, Sills J, Hart CA: Neurological soft signs in mainstream pupils, *Arch Dis Child* 85:371-374, 2001.

131. Sigurdsson E, Fombonne E: Childhood motor impairment is associated with male anxiety at 11 and 16 years, *Evid Based Ment Health* 6:18-22, 2003.

132. Cermak SA, Trimble H, Lebby M, Kinsbourne M, Coryell J, Drake C: The persistence of motor deficits in older students with learning disabilities, *Jpn J Sensory Integration* 2:17-31, 1991.

133. Losse A, Henderson SE, Elliman D et al: Clumsiness in children: do they grow out of it? A 10-year follow-up study, *Dev Med Child Neurol* 33:55-68, 1991.

134. Cermak S, Ward E, Ward L: The relationship between articulation disorders and motor coordination in children, *Am J Occup Ther* 40:546, 1986.

135. Levine M: *Pediatric examination of educational readiness at middle childhood,* Cambridge, MA, 1985, Educators Publishing Service.

136. Levine MD, Brooks R, Shonkoff MD: *A pediatric approach to learning disorders,* New York, 1980, John Wiley & Sons, p 83.

137. Cermak S: Developmental dyspraxia. In Roy E, editor: *Neuropsychological studies of apraxia and related disorders,* New York, 1985, Elsevier Science.

138. Wolff PH, Gunnoe CE, Cohen C: Associated movement as a measure of developmental age, *Dev Med Child Neurol* 25:417, 1983.

139. Ottenbacher K, Biocca Z, DeCremer G, et al: Qualitative analysis of the effectiveness of pediatric therapy, *Phys Ther* 66:462-468, 1986.

140. Shafer S, Stokman CJ, Shaffer D et al: Ten-year consistency in neurological test performance of children without focal neurological deficit, *Dev Med Child Neurol* 28:417, 1986.

141. Cratty BJ: *Perceptual and motor development in infants and children,* Englewood Cliffs, NJ, 1986, Prentice-Hall.

142. Sugden D, Keogh J: *Problem and movement skill development,* Columbia, SC, 1990, University of South Carolina Press.

143. Tupper DE: *Soft neurological signs,* New York, 1987, Grune & Stratton.

144. Touwen BCL, Prechtl HFR: *The neurological examination of the child with minor nervous dysfunction,* Philadelphia, 1970, JB Lippincott.

145. Landman GB, Levine MD, Fenton T, Solomon B: Minor neurological indicators and developmental function in preschool children, *Dev Behav Pediatr* 7:97-101, 1986.

146. Denckla MB: Developmental dyspraxia: the clumsy child. In Levine MD, Satz P, editors: *Middle childhood development and dysfunction,* Baltimore, 1984, University Park Press.

147. Rie ED: Soft signs in learning disabilities. In Tupper DE: *Soft neurological signs,* New York, 1987, Grune & Stratton.

148. Peters JE, Romine RA, Dykman RA: A special neurological examination of children with learning disabilities, *Dev Med Child Neurol* 17:63-78, 1975.

149. Kinsbourne M: Minimal brain dysfunction as a neurodevelopmental lag, *Ann NY Acad Sci* 205:268, 1973.

150. Kinsbourne M: MBD—a fuzzy concept misdirects therapeutic efforts [editorial], *Postgrad Med* 58:211, 1975.

151. Denckla MB: MBD and dyslexia: Beyond diagnosis by exclusion, *Top Child Neurol* 19:253, 1977.

152. Tupper DE: The issues with "soft signs." In Tupper DE: *Soft neurological signs,* New York, 1987, Grune & Stratton.

153. Arnheim DD, Sinclair WA: *The clumsy child: a program of motor therapy,* St. Louis, 1979, C.V. Mosby.

153a. Montessori M: *The Montessori method: scientific pedagogy as applied to child education in the children's houses,* E. George (trans). New York, 1912, F.A. Stokes.

154. Today's child: *Gross motor* (website): www.angelfire.com/on3/todayschild/grossmotor.htm.

155. Schoemaker MM, Kalverboer AF: Social and affective problems of children who are clumsy: how early do they begin? *Adapted Phys Activity Q* 11:130-140, 1994.

156. Miller AE: *Differences in coping strategies between boys with motor incoordination and learning disabilities and normally developing peers* [thesis]. Boston, 1994, Boston University.

157. Shaw L, Levine M, Belfer M: Developmental double jeopardy: a study of clumsiness and self-esteem in children with learning problems, *J Dev Behav Pediatr* 3:191, 1982.

158. Cantell MH, Smyth MM, Ahonen TP: Clumsiness in adolescence: educational, motor, and social outcomes of motor delay detected at 5 years, *Adapted Phys Activity Q* 11:115-129, 1994.

159. Laszlo JI, Bairstow PJ: Kinaesthesis: its measurement, training, and relationship to motor control, *Q J Exp Psychol* 35A:411, 1983.

160. Goodwin WL, Driscoll LA: *Handbook for measurement and evaluation in early childhood education,* San Francisco, 1980, Jossey-Bass.

161. Individuals with Disabilities Education Act (IDEA): 1990 Public Law 101-476.

162. Abbie MH, Douglas HM, Ross KE: The clumsy child: observations in cases referred to the gymnasium of the Adelaide Children's Hospital over a three-year period, *Med J Aust* 1:65, 1978.

163. Bly L: *The components of normal movement during the first year of life and abnormal motor development,* Oak Park, IL, 1983, NDT.

164. Hanson C: *A study of the presence of the asymmetrical tonic neck reflex in fifth and seventh grade children* [thesis], Boston, 1976, Sargent College.

165. Rylander P: *The ATNR in eight and twelve year old LD and normal boys* [thesis], Boston, 1977, Sargent College.

166. Koomar JA, Bundy AC: The art and science of creating direct intervention for theory. In Fisher AG, Murray EA, Bundy AC, editors: *Sensory integration: theory and practice,* Philadelphia, 1991, F.A. Davis.

167. Fisher AG, Murray EA, Bundy AC, editors: *Sensory integration: theory and practice,* Philadelphia, 1991, FA Davis.

168. Shumway-Cook A, Horak F, Black FO: A critical examination of vestibular function in motor impaired learning disabled children, *Int J Pediatr Otorhinolaryngol* 14:21-30, 1987.

169. Fisher AG, Bundy AC: Vestibular stimulation in the treatment of postural and related disorders. In Payton OD, editor: *Manual of physical therapy techniques,* New York, 1989, Churchill Livingstone, pp 92, 240.

170. DeQuiros J, Schrager O: *Neuropsychological fundamentals in learning disabilities,* San Rafael, CA, 1979, Academic Therapy Publications.

171. Ayres AJ: *The sensory integration and praxis tests,* Los Angeles, 1988, Western Psychological Services.

172. Smyth TR: Abnormal clumsiness in children: a defect of motor programming? *Child Care Health Dev* 17:283-294, 1991.

173. Gilfoyle EM, Grady A: A developmental theory of somatosensory perception. In Henderson A, Coryell J, editors: *The body senses and perceptual deficit. Proceedings of the Occupational Therapy Symposium on somatosensory aspects of perceptual deficit,* Boston, 1972, Boston University.

174. Gilfoyle EM, Grady AP, Moore J: *Children adapt,* Thorofare, NJ, 1981, Charles B. Slack.

175. Miller LJ: *FirstSTEP (screening test for evaluating preschoolers),* San Antonio, TX, 1993, The Psychological Corporation.

176. Bruininks RH: Bruininks-Oseretsky test of motor proficiency, Minneapolis, MN, 1978, American Guidance Service.

176a. Book RM: Identification of educationally at risk children during the kindergarten year: A four-year follow-up study of group test performance. Psycho Schools 17:153, 1980.

177. Folio MR, Fewell RR: *Peabody developmental motor scales—second edition (PDMS-2),* Austin, TX, 2000, Pro-Ed.

178. Hughes JE, Riley A: Basic gross motor assessment, *Phys Ther* 61:503, 1981.

179. Danella E, Vogtle L: Neurodevelopmental treatment for the young child with cerebral palsy. In Case-Smith J, Pehoski C, editors: *Development of hand skills in the child,* Rockville, MD, 1992, American Occupational Therapy Association.

180. Benbow M: *A neurodevelopmental approach to teaching handwriting* [unpublished manuscript], 1990.

181. Exner CE: In-hand manipulation skills. In Case-Smith J, Pehoski C, editors: *Development of hand skills in the child,* Rockville, MD, 1992, American Occupational Therapy Association.

182. Pehoski C: Central nervous system control of precision movements of the hand. In Case-Smith J, Pehoski C, editors: *Development of hand skills in the child,* Rockville, MD, 1992, American Occupational Therapy Association.

183. Henderson SE, Sugden D: *Movement assessment battery for children (ABC),* Kent, England, 1992, Psychological Corporation.

184. Tseng MH, Cermak SA: The influence of ergonomic factors and perceptual-motor abilities on handwriting performance, *Am J Occup Ther* 47:919-926, 1993.

185. Ziviani J: Qualitative changes in dynamic tripod grip between seven and 14 years of age, *Dev Med Child Neurol* 25:778-782, 1983.

186. Ziviani J, Elkins J: Effect of pencil grip on handwriting speed and legibility, *Educ Rev* 38:247-257, 1986.

187. Tseng MH, Cermak SA: The evaluation of handwriting in children, *Sensory Integration Q* 19:1-6, 1991.

188. Berry KE: *Developmental test of visual-motor integration (VMI),* ed 4, Cleveland, 1997, Modern Curriculum Press.

189. Gardner MF: *Test of visual-motor skills (TVMS),* San Francisco, 1995 Psychological and Educational Publications.

190. Amundson SJ: *Evaluation of children's handwriting (ETCH),* Homer, AK, 1995, OT Kids.

191. Gardner MF: *Test of handwriting skills (THS),* San Francisco, 1998, Psychological and Educational Publications, Inc.

192. Cermak SA: Somatodyspraxia. In Fisher AG, Murray EA, Bundy AC, editors: *Sensory integration: theory and practice,* Philadelphia, 1991, F.A. Davis.

193. Ayres AJ: *Developmental dyspraxia and adult onset apraxia,* Torrance, CA, 1985, Sensory Integration International.

194. Kephart NC: Teaching the child with a perceptual-motor handicap. In Bortner M, editor: *Evaluation and education of children with brain damage,* Springfield, IL, 1968, Charles C. Thomas.

194a. VanSant A: Motor control, motor learning, and motor development. In Montgomery PC, Connolly BH: *Motor control and physical therapy: theoretical framework and practical application,* Hixton, TX, 1991, Chattanooga Group, p 121.

195. Miller LJ: FirstSTEP (Screening Test for Evaluation Preschoolers). San Antonio, TX, The Psychological Corporation, 1993.

196. Ayres AJ: Learning disabilities and the vestibular system, *J Learn Disabil* 11:18, 1978.

197. Ayres AJ: Cluster analyses of measures of sensory integration, *Am J Occup Ther* 31:362, 1997.

198. Ayres AJ: *Southern California postrotary nystagmus test,* Los Angeles, 1975, Western Psychological Services.

199. Montgomery P: Assessment of vestibular function in children, *Phys Occup Ther Pediatr* 5:33, 1985.

200. DeGangi GA, Berk RA, Larson LA: The measurement of vestibular based dysfunction in pre-school children, *Am J Occup Ther* 34:452, 1980.

201. Ottenbacher K: Identifying vestibular processing dysfunction in learning disabled children, *Am J Occup Ther* 33:317, 1979.

202. Ayres AJ: *Interpreting the Southern California sensory integration tests,* Los Angeles, 1976, Western Psychological Services.

203. Ayres AJ: *Southern California sensory integration tests manual, revised,* Los Angeles, 1980, Western Psychological Services, p 170.

204. Sage G: *Motor learning and control: A neurophysiological approach,* Dubuque, IA, 1984, W.C. Brown.

205. Laszlo JI: Child perceptuo-motor development: Normal and abnormal development of skilled behavior. In Hauert CA, editor: *Developmental psychology: cognitive, perceptuo-motor, and neuropsychological perspectives,* North Holland, Amsterdam, 1990, Elsevier Science.

206. Hoare D, Larkin D: Kinaesthetic abilities of clumsy children, *Dev Med Child Neurol* 33:671-678, 1991.

207. Smyth TR, Glencross DJ: Information processing deficits in clumsy children, *Aust J Psychol* 38:13-22, 1986.

208. O'Brien V, Cermak S, Murray E: The relationship between visual-perceptual motor abilities and clumsiness in children with and without learning disabilities, *Am J Occup Ther* 42:359, 1988.

209. Bundy AC, Murray EA: Sensory integration: A. Jean Ayres theory revisited. In Bundy AC, Lane SJ, Murray EA, editors: *Sensory integration theory and practice,* ed 2, Philadelphia, 2002, F.A. Davis.

210. Miller LJ: *Miller assessment for preschoolers, manual 1988 revision,* San Antonio, TX, 1988, The Psychological Corporation.

210a. Miller LJ: *The toddler and infant motor evaluation (TIME),* Littleton, CO, 1992, The KID Foundation.

211. Larkin D, Hoare D: *Out of step,* Nederlands, West Australia, 1991, The Active Life Foundation.

212. Bundy A: *A conceptual model of school system practice for occupational and physical therapists* [unpublished manuscript], 1991.

213. Kalish R, Presseller S: Physical and occupational therapy, *J Sch Health* 50:264, 1980.

214. Ottenbacher K: Occupational therapy and special education: some issues and concerns related to public law 94-142, *Am J Occup Ther* 36:81, 1982.

215. DeGangi GA: Perspectives on the integration of neurodevelopmental treatment and sensory integrative therapy, *NDTA Newsletter* 1(4), 1990.

216. Ayres AJ, Mailloux Z, Wendler C: Developmental dyspraxia: is it a unitary function? *Occup Ther J Res* 7:93, 1987.

217. Fisher AG, Murray EA: Introduction to sensory integration theory. In Fisher AG, Murray EA, Bundy AC, editors: *Sensory integration: theory and practice,* Philadelphia, 1991, FA Davis, p 4.

218. Koomar, JA, Bundy AC: Creating direct intervention from theory. In Bundy AC, Lane SJ, Murray EA, editors: *Sensory integration theory and practice,* ed 2, Philadelphia, 2002, FA Davis.

219. Bundy AC: The process of planning and implementing intervention. In Bundy AC, Lane SJ, Murray EA, editors: *Sensory integration theory and practice,* ed 2, Philadelphia, 2002, FA Davis.

220. Arendt RE, MacLean WE, Baumeister A: Critique of sensory integration theory and its application in mental retardation, *Am J Ment Defic* 92:401, 1988.

221. Cermak SA, Henderson A: The effectiveness of sensory integration procedures: I, *Sensory Integration Q* 17:1-5, 1989.

222. Cermak SA, Henderson A: The effectiveness of sensory integration procedures: II, *Sensory Integration Q* 18:1-17, 1990.

223. Clark FA, Pierce D: *Synopsis of pediatric occupational therapy effectiveness: studies on sensory integrative procedures, controlled vestibular stimulation, other sensory stimulation approaches, and perceptual-motor training,* Presented at the Occupational Therapy for Maternal and Child Health Conference, Santa Monica, CA, 1986.

224. Hoehn TP, Baumeister AA: A critique of the application of sensory integration therapy to children with learning disabilities *J Learn Disabil* 27:6, 1994.

225. Humphries TW, Snider L, McDougall B: Clinical evaluation of the effectiveness of sensory integrative and perceptual motor therapy in improving sensory integrative function in children with learning disabilities, *Occup Ther J Res* 13:3, 1993.

226. Humphries T, Wright M, McDougall B, Vertes J: The efficacy of sensory integration therapy for children with learning disabilities, *Phys Occup Ther Pediatr* 10:3, 1990.

227. Humphries T, Wright M, Snider L, McDogall B: A comparison of the effectiveness of sensory integrative therapy and perceptual-motor

training in treating children with learning disabilities, *Dev Behav Pediatr* 13:31-40, 1992.

228. Miller LJ, Kinnealey M: Researching the effectiveness of sensory integration, *Sensory Integration Q* 21, 1993.

229. Polatajko HJ, Kaplan BJ, Wilson BN: Sensory integration for children with learning disabilities: Its status 20 years later, *Occup Ther J Res* 12:6, 1992.

230. Polatajko HJ, Law M, Miller J et al: The effect of a sensory integration program on academic achievement, motor performance, and self-esteem in children identified as learning disabled: Results of a clinical trial, *Occup Ther J Res* 11:3, 1991.

231. Henderson A: Research in occupational therapy and physical therapy with children. In Camp BW, editor: *Advances in behavioral pediatrics,* Greenwich, CT, 1981, Jai Press, p 45.

232. Ottenbacher K: Sensory integration therapy: Affect or effect, *Am J Occup Ther* 36:9, 1982.

233. Densem JF, Nuthall JA, Bushnell J et al: Effectiveness of a sensory integrative therapy program for children with perceptual-motor deficits, *J Learn Disabil* 22:221-229, 1989, p 223, 228.

234. Clark F, Pierce D: Synopsis of pediatric occupational therapy effectiveness, *Sensory Integration Q* 16, 1988.

235. Vargus S, Camilli G: A meta-analysis of research on sensory integration treatment, *Am J Occup Ther* 53:189-198, 1999.

236. Wilson BN, Kaplan B: Follow-up assessment of children receiving sensory integration treatment, *Occup Ther J Res* 14:4, 1994.

237. Kinnealey M, Koenig K, Eichelberger-Huecker G: Changes in special needs children following intensive short term intervention, *J Dev Learn Disabil* 3:85-103, 1999.

238. Kaplan BJ, Polatajko HJ, Wilson BN et al: Reexamination of sensory integration treatment: A combination of two efficacy studies, *J Learning Dis* 26:342-347, 1993.

239. Law M, Polatajko HJ, Schaffer R, Miller J: The impact of heterogeneity in a clinical trial: motor outcomes after sensory integration therapy, *Occup Ther J Res* 11:3, 1991.

240. Cohn ES, Cermak SA: Including the family perspective in sensory integration outcomes research, *Am J Occup Ther* 52:540-546, 1998.

241. Bobath K: The motor deficits in patients with cerebral palsy. In *Clinics in developmental medicine, no. 23,* London, 1966, William Heinemann Medical.

242. Bobath K, Bobath B: Neuro-developmental treatment. In Scrutton D, editor: *Management of the motor disorders in children with cerebral palsy,* ed 2, Philadelphia, 1984, JB Lippincott.

243. Royeen CB, DeGangi GA: Use of neurodevelopmental treatment as an intervention: annotated listing of studies, 1980-1990, *Percept Mot Skills* 75:175-194, 1992.

244. Bly L: A historical and current view of the basis of NDT, *Pediatr Phys Ther* 3:131-135, 1991.

245. Rast M: NDT in continuum: micro to macro levels in therapy, *Dev Disabil Spec Interest Section Q* 22:1-4, 1999.

246. Harris SR: Effects of neurodevelopmental therapy on motor performance of infants with Down's syndrome, *Dev Med Child Neurol* 23:477-483, 1981.

247. Piper MC, Kunos VI, Willis DM, Mazer BL, Ramsay M, Silver KM: Early physical therapy effects on the high risk infant: A randomized control trial, *Pediatrics* 78:216-224, 1986.

248. Harris SR: Physical therapy and infants with Down's syndrome: the effects of early intervention, *Rehab Literature* 42:339, 1981.

249. Brown GT, Burns SA: The efficacy of neurodevelopmental treatment in paediatrics: a systematic review, *Br J Occup Ther* 64:235-244. 2001.

250. Shumway-Cook A, Woollacott M: *Motor control: theory and practical applications,* Baltimore, 1995, Williams & Wilkins.

251. Gordon J: Assumptions underlying physical therapy intervention: theoretical and historical perspectives. In Carr JH, Shepard RB: *Movement science: foundations for physical therapy in rehabilitation,* Rockville, MD, 1987, Aspen Publications.

252. Bernstein N: *The coordination and regulation of movements,* Elmsford, NY, 1967, Pergamon Press.

253. Nashner LM, McCollum G: The organization of human postural movements: a formal basis and experimental synthesis, *Behav Brain Sci* 8:135-172, 1985.

254. Baker B: Principles of motor learning for school-based occupational therapy practitioners, *School System Special Interest Section Q* 6:1-4, 1999.

255. Sabari JS: Motor learning concepts applied to activity-based intervention with adults with hemiplegia, *Am J Occup Ther* 45:523-529, 1990.

256. Ostronsky KM: Facilitation vs motor control: Clinical management, *Am PT Assoc* 10:34-40, 1990.

257. Bradley NS: Motor control: Developmental aspects of motor control in skill acquisition. In Campbell SK, editor: *Physical therapy for children,* Philadelphia, 1995, WB Saunders.

258. Horak FB: Assumptions underlying motor control for neurologic rehabilitation. In Lister MJ, editor: *Contemporary management of motor problems,* Alexandria, VA, 1991, Foundation for Physical Therapy.

259. Linquist JE, Mack W, Parham LD: A synthesis of occupational behavior and sensory integration concepts in theory and practice: I. theoretical foundations, *Am J Occup Ther* 36:365-374, 1982.

260. Goldman L: Sensory motor activity not necessarily SI, *OT Week* 2:8, 1988.

260a. Knickerbocker BM: *A holistic approach to the treatment of learning disorders,* Thorofare, NJ, 1980, Charles B. Slack.

261. Farber SD: *Neurorehabilitation: a multisensory approach,* Philadelphia, 1982, W.B. Saunders.

262. Miller TG, Goldberg MA: Sensorimotor integration, *Phys Ther* 55:501, 1975.

263. DeGangi GA, Wietlisbach S, Goodin M, Scheiner N: A comparison of structured sensorimotor therapy and child-centered activity in the treatment of preschool children with sensorimotor problems, *Am J Occup Ther* 47:777-786, 1993.

264. Abbie MH: Physical treatment for clumsy children—not enough? *Physiotherapy* 64:198, 1978.

265. Healthier USGov: *Physical fitness: Be physically active each day* (website): www.healthierus.gov/exercise.html.

266. O'Beirne C, Larkin D, Cable T: Coordination problems and anaerobic performance in children, *Adapted Phys Activity Q* 2:141-149, 1994.

267. Department of Health and Human Services: *The Presidents Council on Fitness and Sports* (website) www.fitness.gov.

268. Lerner J: *Children with learning disorders,* Boston, 1976, Houghton-Mifflin, p 155.

269. Routh DK, Mesibov GB: Psychological and environmental intervention: toward social competence. In Rie HE, Rie ED, editors: *Handbook of minimal brain dysfunctions: a critical view,* New York, 1980, John Wiley & Sons.

270. Barkley RA, Fischer M, Edelbrock CS, Smallish L: The adolescent outcomes of hyperactive children diagnosed by research criterion: an 8-year prospective follow-up study, *J Am Acad Child Adolesc Psychiatry* 29:546-557, 1990.

271. Biederman J: Attention deficit-hyperactivity disorder: a lifespan perspective, *J Clin Psychiatry* 59:4-16, 1998.

272. Helper MJ: Follow-up of children with minimal brain dysfunctions: outcomes and predictors. In Rie HE, Rie ED, editors: *Handbook of minimal brain dysfunctions: a critical view,* New York, 1980, John Wiley & Sons.

272a. Book RM: Identification of educationally at risk children during the kindergarten year: a four-year follow up study of group test performance, *Psychol Schools* 17:153-164, 1980.

273. Parham D: Is sensory integration related to achievement? A longitudinal study of elementary school children, *Sensory Integration Q* 18:9, 16, 17, 1990.

274. American Academy of Pediatrics: Committee on children with disabilities: school-age children with motor disabilities, *Pediatrics* 76:648-649, 1985.

275. Denckla MB, Rudel RG, Chapman C, Krieger J: Motor proficiency in dyslexic children with and without attentional disorders, *Arch Neurol* 42:228, 1985.

276. Cermak SA, Trimble H, Coryell J, Drake C: Bilateral motor coordination in adolescents with and without learning disabilities, *Phys Occup Ther Pediatr* 10:5-18, 1990.

277. Stewart MA, Mendelson WB, Johnson NE: Hyperactive children as adolescents: How they describe themselves, *Child Psychiatr Hum Dev* 4:3, 1973.

278. Mauser AJ: Learning disabilities and delinquent youth, *Acad Ther* 9:389, 1974.

279. Lane BA: The relationship of learning disabilities to juvenile delinquency: current status, *J Learning Dis* 13:20, 1980.

280. Zinkus PW: Behavior and emotional sequelae of learning disorders. In Gottlieb MI, Zinkus PW, Bradford LJ, editors: *Current issues in developmental pediatrics: the learning disabled child,* New York, 1979, Grune & Stratton.

281. Cannon IP, Compton CL: School dysfunction in the adolescent, *Pediatr Clin North Am* 27:79, 1980.

282. Faigel HC: The learning disabled adolescent, Practicioner 214 (1280): 181-191, 1975. In Gottlieb MI, Zinkus PW, Bradford LJ, editors: *Current issues in developmental pediatrics: the learning disabled child,* New York, 1979, Grune & Stratton.

283. Mauser AJ: Learning disabilities and delinquent youth, *Acad Ther* 9:389, 1974.

284. Cermak SA, Murrary E: The adult with learning disabilities: where do all the children go? *Work* 2:41-47, 1991.

285. Provost B, Heimerl S, McCain C, Kim NH, Lopez BR, Kodituwakku P: Concurrent validity of the Bayley scales of infant development II motor scales-2 in children with developmental delays, *Pediatr Phys Ther* 16:3, 2004.

286. Rosenthal A, Sterling HM, Spalding NV: An evaluation of the Quick Neurological Screening Test (QNST), *Int J Neurosci* 21:85-95, 1983.

287. Miller LJ: *Miller assessment for preschoolers (MAP),* Littleton, CO, 1982, The Foundation for Knowledge in Development.

288. Tiffin J: *Purdue pegboard test,* Lafayette, IN, 1968, Lafayette Instrument.

289. Gardner RA, Broman M: The Purdue pegboard: normative data on 1334 school children, *J Clin Child Psych* 1:156, 1979.

290. Mathiowetz V, Rogers SL, Dowe-Keval M, Donahoe L, Rennells C: The Purdue pegboard: norms for 14-19-year olds, *Am J Occup Ther* 40:174, 1986.

APPENDIX 14-A ■ A Summary of Standardized Motor Tests

Bruininks-Oseretsky Test of Motor Proficiency (1978)[176]

Author: Robert H. Bruininks, PhD

Source: American Guidance Service, Inc., Circle Pines, MN 55014

Ages: 4 to 14 years

Administration: Individual; 45 minutes to 1 hour

Equipment: Test kit needed

Description: The Bruininks-Oseretsky Test of Motor Proficiency is the most recent revision of the Oseretsky Tests of Motor Proficiency first published in Russia in 1923. The Oseretsky Tests were first adapted by Doll in 1946 and then by Sloan in 1955 as the Lincoln-Oseretsky Motor Development Scale. As with the earlier versions, the Bruininks-Oseretsky Test yields an age equivalency score, but standard scores and percentile ranks also are available. The test assesses motor functioning in eight areas, each with standard score information:

1. Running speed and agility: runs 15 yards, picks up blocks, and returns
2. Balance: eight items ranging in difficulty from standing on one leg to stepping over object on a balance beam
3. Bilateral coordination: seven items that require use of upper and lower extremities simultaneously or in sequential movement (e.g., tapping feet and fingers, and jumping and clapping); final item requires pencil use with both hands simultaneously
4. Strength: three items: standing broad jumps, sit-ups, and push-ups

5. Upper-limb coordination: five items that involve catching and throwing balls and an additional four items assessing precise finger movements
6. Response speed: requires a quick catch of falling stick
7. Visual motor control: eight pencil, paper, and scissor items
8. Upper-limb speed and dexterity: eight items that range from putting pennies in a box to making dots in circles

Construction and reliability: The Bruininks-Oseretsky Test has been carefully standardized on 765 subjects from differing geographical regions and community size. Test-retest reliability coefficients for the subtests ranged from 0.50 to 0.89, and that of the total battery was 0.87 for second graders and 0.86 for sixth graders. With the exception of "response speed," the subtests differentiated significantly between normal children and children with learning disabilities.

Comment: The Bruininks-Oseretsky Test of Motor Proficiency appears to be one of the better standardized tests of motor performance. A short form, taking 15 to 20 minutes, can be used for screening. In testing children with motor dysfunction, careful attention must be paid to performance on individual items. For example, a child who compensates for poor proprioceptive postural control with vision can score in the normal range on the balance subtest, even though he or she fails the single item of balance with eyes closed. A problem with finger sequencing in the upper limb coordination subtest could be masked by good ball skills. These kinds of problems could result in not identifying a child's deficit. Another problem with the subtests is that a single item has a disproportionate effect on a child's age equivalence. Nevertheless, this is an excellent test for monitoring the motor development of a dysfunctioning child.

Movement Assessment Battery for Children (Movement-ABC) (1992)[183]

Authors: S. E. Henderson and D. Sugden

Source: Psychological Corporation, 555 Academic Court, San Antonio, TX 78204-0952

Ages: 4 to 12 years

Administration: Individual; 20 to 30 minutes

Equipment: Test kit required

Description: The Movement-ABC is a revision and expansion of the Test of Motor Impairment (TOMI)-Henderson Revision. The Movement-ABC includes three aspects. *Screening and evaluation:* The Movement-ABC Checklist provides classroom assessment of movement difficulties, screening for at-risk children, and monitoring of treatment programs. *Assessment:* The Movement-ABC Test (similar to the TOMI) provides a more comprehensive assessment and includes both normative and qualitative measures of movement competence. The test is divided into four age brackets: for children aged 4 to 6 years; 7 to 8 years; 9 to 10 years; and 11 to 12 years. *Treatment:* The manual provides guidelines for organizing intervention programs. The Movement-ABC Test includes eight categories, with a single item for each age in each category:

1. Manual dexterity 1: speed and sureness of movement by each hand
2. Manual dexterity 2: coordination of two hands for a single task
3. Manual dexterity 3: hand-eye coordination using the preferred hand
4. Ball skills 1: ball task emphasizing aiming at a target
5. Ball skills 2: ball task emphasizing catching a ball
6. Static balance: balance task
7. Dynamic balance 1: balance task emphasizing spatial precision
8. Dynamic balance 2: balance task emphasizing control of momentum

Construction and reliability: Standardization of the test was done in the United States, whereas work on the checklist was based in the United Kingdom. Normative data on the test were gathered on 1234 children in the United States. The sample was approximately representative of the general population of children in the United States in terms of sex, region, and ethnic origin. Test-retest reliability for consistency of individual item scores with children ages 5, 7, and 9 years showed a median percentage of agreement between test and retest from 80% to 90%. Percent agreement for total impairment score ranged from 73% for age 9 years to 97% agreement for age 5 years.

Comment: This revision offers several advantages: (1) the checklist helps teachers identify children with movement problems; (2) information is provided for a cognitive-motor approach to intervention; and (3) the qualitative component of the test is more clearly defined and incorporated on the record form, and the scoring systems have been refined.

Peabody Developmental Motor Scales, Second Edition (PDMS-2) (2000)[177]

Authors: M. Rhonda Folio and Rebecca R. Fewell
Source: Pro-Ed, 8700 Shoal Creek Boulevard, Austin, TX 78757
Ages: Birth to 5 years
Administration: 40 to 60 minutes (test items may be scored by direct observation or by parent or teacher report)
Description: An early childhood motor development program that provides, in one package, both in-depth assessment and training or remediation of gross and fine motor skills. The assessment is composed of six subtests that measure interrelated motor abilities that develop early in life. The PDMS-2 can be used by occupational therapists, physical therapists, diagnosticians, early intervention specialists, adapted physical education teachers, psychologists, and others who are interested in examining the motor abilities of young children. The PDMS was designed for use with children who show delay or disability in fine and gross motor skills. Test items are similar to those on other developmental scales, but only motor items are included. Items are scored on a 3-point scale: 0 for unsuccessful, 1 for partial, and 2 for successful performance. Age-equivalent scores, motor quotients, percentile rankings, and standard scores are provided. Scoring software for the PDMS-2 is available to convert the PDMS-2 scores into standard scores, percentile ranks, and age equivalents and generate composite quotients. The software also can be used to compare PDMS-2 subtest performances and composite performances to identify intra-individual differences and provide a printed report of the student information, including treatment goals and objectives.

Subtests

1. Reflexes: This 8-item subtest measures a child's ability to automatically react to environmental events. Because reflexes typically become integrated by the time a child is 12 months old, this subtest is only given to children from birth through 11 months.
2. Stationary: This 30-item subtest measures a child's ability to sustain control of his or her body within its center of gravity and retain equilibrium.
3. Locomotion: This 89-item subtest measures a child's ability to move from one place to another. The actions measured include crawling, walking, running, hopping, and jumping forward.
4. Object Manipulation: This 24-item subtest measures a child's ability to manipulate balls. Examples of the actions measured include catching, throwing, and kicking. Because these skills are not apparent until a child has reached the age of 11 months, this subtest is only given to children aged 12 months and older.
5. Grasping: This 26-item subtest measures a child's ability to use his or her hands. It begins with the ability to hold an object with one hand and progresses up to actions involving the controlled use of the fingers of both hands.
6. Visual-Motor Integration: This 72-item subtest measures a child's ability to use his or her visual perceptual skills to perform complex eye-hand coordination tasks such as reaching and grasping for an object, building with blocks, and copying designs.

Composites

1. Gross motor quotient: This composite is a combination of the results of the subtests that measure the use of the large muscle systems:
   ■ Reflexes (birth to 11 months only)
   ■ Stationary (all ages)
   ■ Locomotion (all ages)
   ■ Object manipulation (12 months and older)
2. Fine motor quotient: This composite is a combination of the results of the subtests that measure the use of the small muscle systems:
   ■ Grasping (all ages)
   ■ Visual-motor integration (all ages)
3. Total motor quotient: This composite is formed by a combination of the results of the gross and fine motor subtests. Because of this, it is the best estimate of overall motor abilities.

Construction and reliability: Reliability coefficients were computed for subgroups of the normative sample (e.g., individuals with motor disabilities, African Americans, Hispanic Americans, girls, and boys) as well as for the entire normative sample. The normative sample consisted of 2003 persons residing in 46 states and was collected in the winter of 1997 and spring of 1998. Normative samples relative to geography, sex, race, and other critical variables are therefore representative of the current U.S. population.

A test-retest reliability of 0.84 for the Gross Motor Scale and of 0.73 for the Fine Motor Scale (0.89 Total Motor) was reported based on a sample of 30 children from Austin, Texas, in the age range of 2 to 11 months. A second group of 30 children from Nacogdoches, Texas, ages 12 to 17 months, were tested with a test-retest reliability of 0.93 for the Gross Motor Scale and 0.94 for the Fine Motor Scale (0.96 Total Motor). These values are of sufficient magnitude for a tester's confidence in the test scores' stability over a period of time. The correlation coefficients between the PDMS and the PDMS-2 for criterion-prediction validity in the Gross and Fine Motor Quotients exceed 0.80, which supports the equivalency of the tests.

The PDMS-2 scores were correlated with those of the Mullen Scales of Early Learning: AGS Edition (MSEL:A) when both tests were administered on the same day to 29 children, aged 2 months to 66 months, in Evansville, Ind. The relations of the PDMS-2 and MSEL:A gross and fine motor quotients exceed 0.80, high enough to support the equivalency of the tests. When the concurrent validity of the age equivalent and standard scores of the Bayley Scales of Infant Development II (BSID 11) Motor Scale and PDMS-2 were calculated, the standard scores show poor agreement and had low concurrent validity, particularly the BSID II Motor Scale and the PDMS-2 Locomotion Subscale.[285] The differences in the scores of these two tests warrant concern when using one test to make clinical decisions for service eligibility.

Comment: The PDMS-2 is primarily useful for children with mild to moderate motor deficits, such as a child with learning disabilities or a child with developmental delay. The test does not discriminate among children with moderate to severe motor disability because they fall far below the standard scores given. The skill categories are unevenly distributed and have too few items at some age levels to be meaningful. Despite their drawbacks, the PDMS-2 is probably the most valuable motor scale test currently available for preschool children.

Quick Neurological Screening Test (QNST) (1978)[286]

Authors: M. A. Mutti, H. M. Sterling, and N. V. Spalding
Source: Academic Therapy Publications, 20 Commercial Boulevard, Novato, CA 94947
Ages: 5 years and older
Administration: Individual; 20 minutes
Equipment: None

Description: The QNST was developed as a screening device to identify children who have possible learning disabilities. The tasks are adapted from pediatric neurological examinations and developmental assessments. The test is composed of the following 15 subtests:

1. Hand skill: writing his or her name and a sentence
2. Figure recognition and production: naming, then drawing, five geometric forms
3. Palm form recognition: recognizing numbers written on the palm by examiner with his or her finger
4. Eye tracking: following pencil back and forth and up and down
5. Sound patterns: with hands on knees and eyes closed, imitating patterns demonstrated by the examiner
6. Finger to nose test: includes observation
7. Thumb and finger circle: forming circle with thumb and each of the fingers; laterality also observed
8. Double simultaneous stimulation of hand and cheek with eyes closed: child must identify hands and cheeks touched by examiner in various combinations simultaneously
9. Rapid reversing, repetitive hand movements: observation of diadochokinesis
10. Arm and leg extension: with eyes closed, extending legs, arms, and tongue for 1 to 15 seconds
11. Tandem walk: walking straight line, heel to toe, forward and backward
12. Stand on one leg: balancing first on one leg, then on the other, 10 seconds each; eyes open, then closed; right-left differentiation observed
13. Skip: skipping across the room
14. Left-right discrimination: scored from subtests 6, 7, and 12
15. Behavior irregularities: general observation for behaviors such as distractibility, perseveration, defensiveness, and hyperactivity

The test is scored by careful observation and requires a subjective evaluation of performance. The manual provides ages at which 75% of neurologically intact children pass each test as well as total scores indicative of probable neurological dysfunction.

Construction and reliability: The QNST has been used in numerous research studies of normal children and children with suspected learning disabilities. Although the manual reported these studies, the test has not been formally standardized. Reliabilities on the whole test on children with learning disabilities of 0.81 and 0.71 are reported, but the data are incomplete. Ages at which 25%, 50%, and 75% of normal children pass each subtest are given on the basis of a compilation of subjects from many studies. Norms for the total test are not given.

Comment: The QNST is a screening device that identifies children with possible neurological dysfunction. It is not, and should not be, used as a standardized test but rather as an adjunct to clinical observation. The test is primarily of motor function. It does not include language tests and therefore will not identify all children with learning disabilities. The test does screen for possible minimal brain dysfunction or motor deficits.

Miller Assessment for Preschoolers (MAP) (1988)[210,287]

Author: Lucy Jane Miller, PhD
Source: Psychological Corporation, 555 Academic Court, San Antonio, TX 78204-0952
Ages: 2 years, 9 months to 5 years, 8 months
Administration: Individual; 20 to 30 minutes, including scoring
Equipment: The MAP Test Kit
Description: The MAP was designed to identify children who exhibit mild to moderate developmental delays. The MAP is a developmental assessment intended for use by educational and clinical personnel to identify those children in need of further evaluation and remediation. It can also be used to provide a comprehensive, clinical framework that would be helpful in defining a child's strengths and weaknesses and that would indicate possible avenues of remediation. The test is composed of 27 items and a series of structured observations. The test items are divided into five performance indexes:

1. Foundations: items generally found on standard neurological examinations and sensory integrative and neurodevelopmental tests
2. Coordination: gross, fine, and oral motor abilities and articulation
3. Verbal: cognitive language abilities, including memory, sequencing, comprehension, association, following directions, and expression
4. Nonverbal: cognitive abilities such as visual figure-ground, puzzles, memory, and sequencing
5. Complex tasks: tasks requiring an interaction of sensory, motor, and cognitive abilities

Construction and reliability: The MAP has been well standardized on a random sample of 1200 preschool children. The sample was stratified by age, race, sex, size of residence, community, and socioeconomic factors. Data were collected nationwide in each of nine U.S. Census Bureau regions. Reported reliabilities are good. In a test-retest on 90 children, 81% of the children's scores remained stable. The coefficient of internal consistency on the total sample was 0.798. Interrater reliability on 40 children was reported as 0.98.

Comment: The MAP was developed by an occupational therapist and provides information that is of particular relevance to therapists. It is carefully standardized and fills a need for early identification of learning and motor deficits in children. Several articles have now been published supporting the validity of this test as a screening instrument.[188-190,196] Reviews of the MAP in the *Ninth Mental Measurements Yearbook* have described it as "the best available screening test for identifying preschool children with moderate preacademic problems"[68] and "an extremely promising instrument which should find wide use among clinical psychologists, school psychologists, and occupational therapists in assessing mild to moderate learning disabilities in preschool children."[184] A more complete review of this test is provided by King-Thomas and Hacker.[156]

FirstSTEP (Screening Test for Evaluating Preschoolers) (1993)[287]

Author: Lucy J. Miller, PhD
Source: Psychological Corporation, 555 Academic Court, San Antonio, TX 78204-0952
Ages: 2 years, 9 months to 6 years, 2 months
Administration: Individual; 15 minutes
Equipment: Test kit
Description: The FirstSTEP is a quick screening test for identifying developmental delays in all five areas defined by IDEA and mandated by PL 99-457: cognition, communication, physical, social/emotional, and adaptive functioning. Twelve subtests assess cognitive, communication, and motor domains. An optional Social-Emotional Scale includes 25 items from five areas (task confidence, cooperative mood, temperament and emotionality, uncooperative antisocial behavior, and attention communication difficulties) that are scored on the basis of behaviors observed by the examiner during the test session. The Adaptive Behavior Checklist is an optional measure completed by parent interview to assess the child's self-help and adaptive living skills. The Parent/Teacher Scale provides additional information about the child's typical behavior.

Cognitive Domain

Money Game (quantitative reasoning)
Description: The child is asked a series of questions about coins regarding quantity, amount, comparisons, size, and numeration. This subtest requires cognitive understanding of simple arithmetic concepts.

What's Missing Game (picture completion)

Description: The child is asked to identify what is missing from the pictures of common objects or events by naming or pointing. This subtest measures visual figure-ground as well as gestalt closure abilities.

Which Way? Game (visual position in space)

Description: The child is asked to look at a stimulus figure that is turned in a specific direction. The child then selects the response figure that matches. This subtest measures visual discrimination and the ability to perceive directionality visually.

Put Together Game (problem solving)

Description: The child is asked to select the pieces that best fit a certain space. The subtest requires abstract thinking.

Language Domain

Listen Game (auditory discrimination)

Description: This two-part activity requires the child to listen as the examiner names and points to three similar-sounding pictures. Then the child chooses the pictures that represent the words. The second part requires the child to discriminate between words that are the same and words that are different. This task taps phoneme discrimination and requires good auditory processing skills.

How Many Can You Say? Game (word retrieval)

Description: The child's linguistic fluency and word-finding skills are measured by asking the child to count, recall animals, and recite rhyming words.

Finish Up Game (association)

Description: The child is asked to complete a phrase that is initiated by the examiner. The subtest requires the child to demonstrate an understanding of the association between concepts (e.g., big and little).

Copy Me Game (sentence and digit repetition)

Description: The child is asked to repeat a series of meaningful verbal stimuli and then a series of numbers. This subtest measures verbal memory, grammatical abilities, and verbal expression skills.

Motor Domain

Drawing Game (visual-motor integration)

Description: The child is presented with paper and pencil tasks. This subtest requires the integration of fine motor and visual-perceptual abilities.

Things with Strings Game (fine motor planning)

Description: The child is asked to perform a series of motor movements with the upper extremities with a wooden cube and a string. These items tap the ability to plan and execute a series of motor actions and measure fine motor planning or praxis.

Statue Game (balance)

Description: The child is asked to assume a series of increasingly more difficult positions that require the child to balance with eyes open and vision occluded. The subtest taps the abilities needed to maintain equilibrium and screens for proprioception, vestibular perception, and visual processing difficulties.

Jumping Game (gross motor planning)

Description: The child is asked to imitate the examiner through a series of increasingly more difficult tasks that involve jumping in specific patterns. Gross motor and motor planning abilities are measured.

Construction and reliability: The FirstSTEP is norm referenced and was standardized on 1433 children. Norms are provided in 6-month intervals for each of seven age groups. Standardization sample closely matches demographic characteristics provided by the U.S. Census Bureau. Scores are reported in standard scores as well as a three-category, color-coded risk status to indicate whether the child is functioning in the normal or delayed range. The FirstSTEP is a highly reliable instrument. Overall test reliability (split half) is 0.90, with individual domains ranging from 0.71 to 0.87. Test-retest reliability indicated a high degree of consistency in the classification of a child's performance across two test sessions (90% agreement for composite score; 85% to 93% for individual domain scores). Results also indicated a high level of interrater agreement ($r = 0.94$ on composite scores).

Comment: The FirstSTEP is a new test that shows exceptional promise as a screening instrument. A Spanish version, Primer Paso, will be published in the near future. The FirstSTEP was developed by the occupational therapist who also developed the MAP (The Miller Assessment for Preschoolers) and, like the MAP, the test provides information that is of particular relevance to therapists. Although individual items on the FirstSTEP differ from the MAP, many are derived from the MAP, and the test is based on the same theoretical framework as the MAP.

Initial validity studies of the FirstSTEP appear highly promising and indicate that FirstSTEP has good construct, content, and discriminant validity. The FirstSTEP can effectively identify children with developmental delays. A study of 900 children demonstrated that children with delays perform 1.5 to 2 standard deviations below the mean in all domains.

With regard to the motor domain of the FirstSTEP, which taps motor skills, the results of a concurrent validity study suggest that the motor domain measures constructs similar to those measured by the Bruininks-Oseretsky Test of Motor Proficiency and support the use of the motor domain of the FirstSTEP as an indicator of the child's motor functioning.

The Sensory Integration and Praxis Tests (SIPT) (1989)[171]

Author: A. Jean Ayres

Source: Western Psychological Services, 12031 Wilshire Boulevard, Los Angeles, CA 90025

Ages: 4 years to 8 years, 11 months

Administration: Individual; 2 hours; examiner certification required

Equipment: SIPT Test Kit

Description: The SIPT is a major revision and restandardization of the Southern California Sensory Integration Tests.[22] Four new tests of praxis were added, five tests underwent major revisions, eight tests underwent minor revisions, and four tests were deleted. The tests are designed to identify sensory integration and praxis deficits in children with learning disabilities. The 17 tests are described as follows:

1. Space visualization: Select from two blocks the one that will fit into a form board. Mentally manipulating the forms is required to arrive at the correct choice on the more difficult test items.
2. Figure-ground perception: The child selects from six pictures the three that are superimposed or embedded with other forms on the test plates.
3. Manual form perception: Part I: A geometric form is held in the hand and the counterpart is selected from a visual display. Part II: A geometric form is felt with one hand while its match is selected from several choices with the other hand.
4. Kinesthesia: With vision occluded, the child attempts to place his or her finger on a point at which this finger had been placed previously by the examiner; a separate recording sheet is provided for each child.
5. Finger identification: With hands screened from view, the examiner touches the child's finger, the shield is removed, and the child then points to the finger touched.
6. Graphesthesia: The examiner uses his or her finger to draw a design on the back of the child's hand without the child looking; the child then reproduces the design.
7. Localization of tactile stimuli: With vision occluded, the child touches the spot on his or her hand or arm that was touched by the examiner with a specially designed pen.
8. Praxis on verbal command: The examiner verbally describes a series of body movements and the child executes them.
9. Design copying: Part I: The child copies a design by connecting dots on a dot grid. Part II: The child copies a

design without the use of a dot grid; both process and product are scored.

10. Constructional praxis: Working with blocks, the child attempts to duplicate two different block structures. In the first structure, the child observes the examiner building the model; the second structure is preassembled.

11. Postural praxis: The child imitates unusual body positions demonstrated by the examiner.

12. Oral praxis: The child imitates movements of the tongue, lips, and jaw demonstrated by the examiner.

13. Sequencing praxis: The child imitates a series of simple arm and hand movements demonstrated by the examiner.

14. Bilateral motor coordination: The child imitates a series of bilateral arm and foot movements demonstrated by the examiner.

15. Standing and walking balance: This subtest consists of 15 items in which the child assumes various standing and walking postures.

16. Motor accuracy: The child traces a printed, curved black line with a red, nylon-tipped pen, first with the preferred hand and then with the nonpreferred hand.

17. Postrotatory nystagmus: The child is rotated first counterclockwise and then clockwise on a rotation board; the duration of postrotatory nystagmus, a vestibuloocular reflex, is observed.

In addition to these 17 tests, a series of clinical observations aids in interpreting the SIPT. These clinical observations include the following:

■ Eye dominance
■ Eye movements
■ Muscle tone
■ Co-contraction
■ Postural background movements
■ Postural security
■ Equilibrium reactions and protective extension
■ Schilder's arm extension posture
■ Supine flexion
■ Prone extension
■ Asymmetrical tonic neck reflex
■ Hyperactivity, distractibility
■ Tactile defensiveness
■ Ability to perform slow motions
■ Thumb-finger touching
■ Diadochokinesis
■ Tongue-to-lip movements
■ Hopping, jumping, skipping

Construction and reliability: The construction of the SIPT was based on a theoretical model developed from observation of children with learning disabilities and supported by factor analytical and cluster analysis studies. Interpretation follows a clinical model based on patterns of scores rather than a poor score on any one test.

The SIPT was nationally standardized on 1997 children from across the United States and Canada. Sex, geographical location, ethnicity, and type of community are represented in proportion to the 1980 U.S. Census.

Test-retest reliability was evaluated in a sample of 41 dysfunctional children and 10 normally function children and ranges from moderate to high. As a group, the praxis tests had the highest reliabilities. Interrater reliability is excellent, with most correlations between raters at 0.90 or higher.

Comment: The SIPT is computer scored and interpreted, and a full eight-color profile (WPS Chronograph) is provided that summarizes major SIPT testing and statistical results in a clear manner. Initial validity studies of the SIPT indicate a good ability to discriminate between normal and dysfunctional groups and across ages. The SIPT is the most comprehensive assessment of sensory integration and praxis; however,

it requires specialized training for administration and interpretation, and the test kit and scoring of protocols are expensive.

Developmental Test of Visual-Motor Integration (VMI), 4th Revision (4R) (1997)[188]

Author: K. Berry
Source: Modern Curriculum Press, 13900 Prospect Road, Cleveland, OH 44136
Ages: 3 years to adult (standard scores to 17 years, 11 months)
Administration: Individual or group; 10 to 15 minutes
Equipment: Protocol booklets (test forms)
Description: The VMI tests the ability to copy geometric forms. A booklet is provided with 24 designs in an age-graded sequence. A shorter format including the first 15 forms is available for children aged 3 to 7 years. The child copies each design in a space directly below it. The first three items are presented twice and may be demonstrated for imitation. Items are judged pass or fail on criteria given in the manual. One point is awarded for each passed item, with a total of 27 possible points.

Construction and reliability: Additional specificity was added for the scoring of some items in the 1989 revision. The VMI manual contains information relating to ages at which forms are passed based on Gesell and other researchers. Developmental drawing trends are illustrated. Age equivalences, standard scores, percentile equivalents, and T scores are based on a sample of more than 6000 children. This reflects normative samples from 1964, 1981, and 1989. Various studies of reliability and validity are reported in the manual. Studies of test-retest reliability were reported for groups of children of all ages and range from 0.63 (7-month interval) to 0.92 (2-week period), with a median of 0.81. There are no reports of reliability at individual ages. Split-half reliability was 0.88, and interscorer agreement was 0.94.

Comment: The VMI provides a quick and easy method to assess the development of a child's ability to copy geometric forms. It is useful as an adjunct to other assessments of the child with learning disabilities. When the test is presented to the child, he or she is told that the booklet must remain parallel to the edge of the table. This prevents some of the problems of other tests, such as the child turning the individual paper on which designs are reproduced. However, the structured format does not allow the assessment of overall organization of copying forms, as can be done when the child copies forms on a blank sheet of paper (e.g., Bender Gestalt Test). Therefore overall organization also should be tested.

Test of Visual-Motor Skills Revised (TVMS-R) (1995)[189]

Author: Morrison F. Gardner
Source: Children's Hospital of San Francisco, Publication Department OPR-110, P.O. Box 3805, San Francisco, CA 94119
Ages: 3 to 13 years
Administration: Individual or group; 3 to 6 patients
Equipment: Protocol booklet
Description: The TVMS-R consists of a series of 23 forms to be copied by the child. Each form is on a separate page of the booklet. The booklet contains some forms commonly used in visual-motor tests (e.g., lines and circles), but many forms are unique to this test. Care was taken to avoid forms that resemble language symbols. The revision of the TVMS has updated norms, standardization, and scoring criteria.

Two different scoring methods are now available. Modifications in scoring the TVMS-R include a classification system to characterize errors in one of eight categories. The eight classifications are closure, angles, intersecting and overlapping lines, size of design, rotation or reversals, line length, overpenetration or underpenetration, and modification of design. Scoring of each design is completed by following a definitive criterion with errors and strengths identified. The examiner can identify specific areas of strength and weakness in visual-motor integration on the basis of the number of errors and accuracies recorded. Standard scores, scaled scores, percentile ranks, and stanines are available for both weaknesses and strengths. An alternative scoring method (ASM) was also designed to allow a straight point system designation to each form. The forms are scored on a 0- to 3-point scale. A score of 0 indicates that the child is unable to copy the form with any degree of motor accuracy. Scores of 1 and 2 indicate various visual-motor errors for which criteria are both written and illustrated. A score of 3 demonstrates precision in execution. Age equivalents, standard scores, scaled scores, percentile ranks, and stanines are provided.

Construction and reliability: The TVMS-R was administered to 1484 children in the San Francisco Bay area aged 3 years to 13 years, 11 months. The overall sample was 51.9% male and 48.1% female. Cronbach's coefficient alpha was used to determine the internal consistency of the test. These reliability coefficients ranged from 0.72 to 0.84 over the age ranges, with a value of 0.90 for the sample as a whole. Test-retest reliability was not reported in the manual, but the author noted the need for research in that area.

Comment: The TVMS-R is a companion test to the Test of Visual-Perceptual Skills (TVPS), which is a motor-free test of form perception. Using the tests together can determine whether the child's form reproduction reflects incorrect visual perception or whether the problem is in motor execution. The TVMS-R places greater expectations on motor precision than do other visual-motor tests. For example, a line must touch an intersecting line without crossing over it. Therefore it should be used only when motor control and constructive abilities are important.

Evaluation Tool of Children's Handwriting (ETCH) (1995)[190]

Author: Susan J. Amundson
Source: O.T. Kids, P. O. Box 1118, Homer, AK 99603
Ages: First through sixth grades (6 to 11 years)
Administration: Individual
Equipment: Protocol booklet, task sheets and wall charts, stopwatch, #2 pencil
Description: The ETCH is designed to evaluate manuscript and cursive writing for components of legibility and speed. Specific components of the child's handwriting, including letter formation, spacing, size, and alignment, are included for assessment. The following tasks are presented in order:

1. Lower case alphabet letters (from memory)
2. Upper case alphabet letters (from memory)
3. Numeral writing (from memory)
4. Near point copying (visual model)
5. Far point copying (visual model)
6. Dictation (verbal)
7. Sentence composition (independent)

   A quick reference card is included with standardized directions and timing criterion. Written and illustrated scoring criteria have been designed to assist the evaluator in determining the legibility of letters and numbers. The primary focus of scoring is whether the written material is readable.
Construction and reliability: Pilots of the ETCH were designed by using adaptations of written tasks from existing tools. Three editions of the ETCH have been sampled by practitioners working in school systems with feedback on the examiner's manual, ease of administration and scoring, item selection, scoring procedures, and face validity of the instrument. Normative data have not yet been collected on the ETCH tasks, although the author suggests that occupational therapists and classroom educators might collaboratively collect data. Eight studies of handwriting speed have been included for reference

in the manual. No test-retest or internal reliability studies have been conducted. Interrater reliability ranged from 0.63 to 0.94 for individual manuscript items and 0.64 to 0.97 for cursive. Overall, the total word reliability is more stable than task scores, ranging from 0.90 to 0.98.

Comment: The ETCH assesses functional writing skills that are relevant to academic performance. The varied tasks allow the examiner to identify areas of strength and weakness in written performance, including legibility components, speed, and composition models (visual, verbal, and memory). Information received from the ETCH is qualitative at this point because of the lack of normative samples. The author suggests that the ETCH be used in conjunction with observations of the child's writing activity in natural environments, such as classroom and home, as a determination of difficulties in functional written performance.

Test of Handwriting Skills (THS) (1998)[191]

Author: Morrison F. Gardner
Source: Psychological and Educational Publications, Inc.
Ages: 5 through 11 years; manuscript norms 5 to 8 years, cursive norms 9 to 11 years
Administration: Individual or group administration; 15 to 20 minutes
Equipment: THS manual, manuscript or cursive test booklet, #2 pencil, and stopwatch
Description: The purpose of the THS is to assess a child's neurosensory integration ability in handwriting, with focus on upper and lower case letter formations as well as numbers. It is designed to assess strengths and weaknesses in the motoric aspects of handwriting, including legibility and speed. Varied aspects of written performance are assessed, including:

1. Spontaneously writing, from memory, upper and lower case letters of the alphabet in sequence
2. Writing, from dictation, upper and lower case letters of the alphabet out of alphabetical sequence
3. Writing, from dictation, numbers out of numerical order
4. Copying selected letters of the alphabet
5. Copying selected words
6. Copying selected sentences
7. Writing selected words from dictation

   Scoring criteria are outlined in the manual and sample visual representations are given to illustrate the quality needed to achieve each score. Possible errors include overextended or underextended lines, broken lines, overlapping or reworked lines, parts missing, distortion of shape, or omitted dots or line crossings. Additional scoring looks at the speed of performance as well as reversed letters, case substitutions, and touching letters.
Construction and reliability: The THS was standardized with children from various parts of the United States. Approximately equal numbers of boys and girls were tested, with representation for both right and left handedness. The manuscript version was administered to 494 children with a median age of 6 years, 11 months; 406 were right handed and 61 were left handed. The cursive version was administered to 345 children with a median age of 9 years, 8 months; 309 were righted handed and 36 were left handed. Norms were derived for each of the 10 subtests as well as the additional scores. Cronbach's alpha was used to calculate the internal consistency of the test at each age level. These reliability coefficients ranged from 0.51 to 0.78 for the manuscript version and 0.29 to 0.87 for the cursive version. Two items on each version had low reliabilities (writing eight numbers and copying 10 letters), probably a result of the small number of items in the subtest. Scores on the manuscript version correlated positively with scores on the TVMS-R, indicating that the handwriting skills being tested involve a visual-motor component.
Comment: This test was developed primarily as a means for various professionals to measure children's handwriting skills.

The THS can be administered by various professionals such as occupational therapists, teachers, psychologists, resource specialists, educational diagnosticians, learning specialists, and optometrists. While gathering pertinent information for test development, the author arranged two conferences with teachers from kindergarten to fifth grade and obtained information from various professionals throughout the United States. In designing this test he recognized that three main methods of handwriting are taught—D'Nealian, Palmer, and Zaner-Bloser—and that children, in general, have better accuracy for copied letters and words versus dictation that involves holding symbols in memory.

This test is functional and relevant to academic performance. The varied tasks and additional scoring allow the clinician to identify areas of strength and weakness in written performance. This can provide the foundation for recommendations within the classroom and/or guide intervention. Scoring criteria are well delineated and the visual samples provide information on typical developmental performance and error types.

Purdue Pegboard Test (1948, 1968)[288]

Author: Joseph Tiffin, PhD

Source: Lafayette Instrument Co., P.O. Box 5728, Lafayette, IN 47903

Ages: 5 years through adult

Administration: Individual; 10 to 15 minutes

Equipment: Pegboard with pins, collars, and washers required

Description: This test of manual dexterity consists of four parts, each described as follows:
1. Right hand: the subject inserts small pegs into holes in pegboard with right hand for a 30-second trial
2. Left hand: the subject inserts pegs into pegboard with left hand for a 30-second trial
3. Both hands: both hands pick up and insert pegs into board at same time for a 30-second trial
4. Assembly: using hands cooperatively, the subject assembles sequences of pins, collars, and washers for a 60-second trial

Construction and reliability: This test has recently been standardized with 1334 normal schoolchildren, aged 5 to 16 years, from New Jersey. Means, standard deviations, and percentile scores are presented as a function of age (6-month intervals) and sex. Reliability data on children are not presented in the test manual, although reliability with college students ranged from 0.60 to 0.71. A number of validity studies indicate that learning-disabled subjects perform more poorly than normal controls on this test. Additional normative data are presented in the manual for various age and diagnostic groups.

Comment: This test was originally designed for adults to assist in the selection of employees for manual industrial jobs. It has recently been standardized with school-aged children[289] and adolescents.[290]

CHAPTER 15   **Beyond the Central Nervous System: Neurovascular Entrapment Syndromes**

Bradley W. Stockert, PT, PhD
Laurie Kenny, PT, OCS, FAAOMPT
Peter I. Edgelow, MA, PT

KEY WORDS

neural mobility
neural sensitization
neural irritability
neurovascular entrapment
pain mechanisms
physical therapy

OBJECTIVES

After reading this chapter the reader should be able to:
1. Identify the anatomical and physiological mechanisms involved in the development of neurovascular entrapment syndromes.
2. Describe modifications to the physical examination on the basis of the presence of neural sensitization or neural irritability.
3. Identify six common signs of dysfunction in neurovascular entrapment.
4. Describe the importance of self-assessment techniques in giving patients control of their rehabilitation.

OVERVIEW

The purpose of this chapter is twofold. The first purpose is to develop the concept that the entire nervous system forms a continuous tissue tract. This concept is central to the idea that movements of the trunk or limbs can have a profound biomechanical and physiological impact on the peripheral and central nervous systems. Mobility of the nervous system and some of the responses of the system to movement in normal and sensitized states are discussed.

The second purpose of this chapter is to develop in the reader an understanding of neurovascular entrapment syndrome. This is an underrecognized impairment present in some patients with a wide variety of diagnoses (e.g., nonspecific arm pain, repetitive strain injury, and thoracic outlet syndrome). These patients frequently are failed by standard medical care. The theoretical mechanisms involved in the development and perpetuation of neurovascular entrapment syndrome are presented. Background information regarding the syndrome is provided and the appropriate screening tools for assessment of the impairment are discussed. Treatment suggestions and a case study are presented at the end of the chapter.

PERIPHERAL NEUROANATOMY

The peripheral nervous system (PNS) is generally regarded as that portion of the nervous system that lies outside the central nervous system (CNS) (i.e., the brain and spinal cord).[1,2] The major components of the PNS include motor, sensory, and autonomic neurons found in spinal, peripheral, and cranial nerves. Although this partitioning is valid from an anatomical perspective, it often leads to a lack of appreciation of the truly continuous nature and integrative function of the nervous system as a whole. The concept that the entire nervous system is a continuous tissue tract reinforces the idea that limb and trunk movements can have a

mechanical effect on the PNS and the CNS that is local and global.

The nervous system is composed of two functional tissue types. One type of tissue is concerned with impulse conduction. This functional category includes nerve cells and Schwann cells. The second functional tissue type provides support and protection of the conduction tissues (i.e., the connective tissues).

Three levels in the organization of a peripheral nerve have been described (Figure 15-1).[2,3] At the innermost level the nerve fiber is the conducting component of a neuron (nerve cell). A connective tissue layer called the endoneurium surrounds each nerve fiber. The endoneurium surrounds the basement membrane of the neuron and plays an important role in maintaining fluid pressure within the endoneurial space. The pressure within the endoneurium changes dramatically with compression.[4]

The second level of organization is a collection of many nerve fibers (a fascicle) surrounded by a layer of connective tissue called the perineurium.[2,3] The perineurium acts as a selective barrier to diffusion and as such exerts significant control over the local movement of fluid and ions. This connective tissue layer acts like a pressurized container (i.e., extrusion of the contents occurs if the membrane is cut). The compartment enclosed by the perineurium does not contain lymphatic channels.[4] This may be a problem during inflammatory states when edema is present deep to the perineurial layer. The perineurium is the last connective tissue layer to rupture in tensile testing of peripheral nerves.[5] The outermost connective tissue layer of a peripheral nerve is called the epineurium. The epineurium protects the fascicles as well as enhances gliding between them. Lymphatic channels are found within the epineurial compartment.

All three connective tissue layers are interconnected. They are not separate and distinct but continuous tissue layers.[2,3] Each of the connective tissue layers contains free

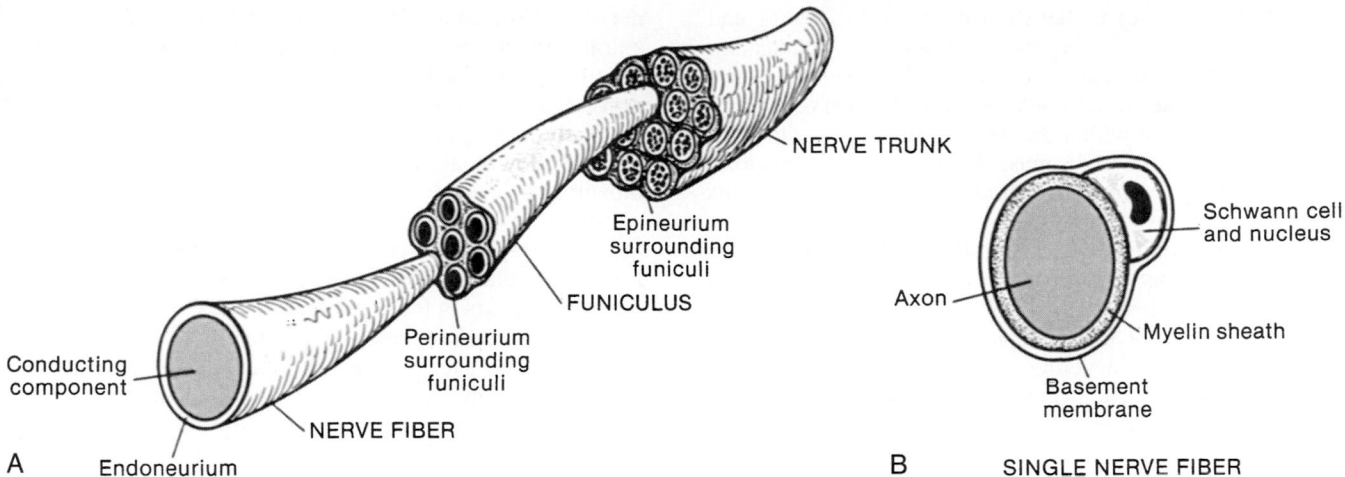

FIGURE 15-1 ■ Three levels of organization of a peripheral nerve or nerve trunk. **A,** Nerve trunk and components. **B,** Microscopic structure of nerve fiber.

nerve endings from the *nervi nervorum*. As a result, all three connective tissue layers are a potential source of pain. In addition, all three layers are continuous with the homologous dura mater and epineurium connective tissue layers of the CNS.

The vascular supply for peripheral nerves is designed to provide uninterrupted blood flow regardless of the position of the trunk and limbs. Extrinsic vessels provide blood flow to "feeder" vessels that in turn supply an extensive intrinsic (intraneural) vasculature within the nervous system. The feeder vessels branch off the extrinsic vessels and enter peripheral nerves in areas of low nerve mobility relative to the surrounding tissue. The intrinsic vasculature supplies all three connective tissue layers within the peripheral nervous system, but only capillaries cross the perineurium.[6]

Peripheral nerves are regularly subjected to elongation (stretching) and compression, which increases intraneural pressure. An increase in intraneural pressure can decrease the diameter of the intrinsic blood vessels and result in a reduction in blood flow within the nerve. A strain of 6% to 8% has been shown to decrease intraneural blood flow significantly and alter neuronal conduction.[4] Complete arrest of the blood flow has been shown to occur in the sciatic nerve of a rabbit at 8% elongation.[6] Complete arrest of blood flow has been shown to occur at about 15% elongation.[7] Changes in intraneural pressure and blood flow have the potential to interfere with neuronal conduction, metabolism, and axonal transport.

The cytoplasm moves in all cells. Cytoplasm has thixotropic properties (i.e., the viscosity of cytoplasm is lower when it is continuously moving).[4] In neurons the movement of the cytoplasm from the cell body through the axons (anterograde movement) occurs at two speeds. Fast axoplasmic flow, which occurs at a rate of about 100 to 400 mm per day, is used to carry ion channels and neurotransmitters to the nerve terminals, which are materials required for normal impulse conduction. Slow axoplasmic flow occurs at a rate of about 6 mm per day; it is used to transport cytoskeleton proteins, neurofilaments, and other materials used to maintain the physical health of the cell. A third flow occurs in the opposite direction (retrograde) at a

rate of about 200 mm per day. Retrograde transport carries unused anterograde material and exogenous materials taken up at the terminus (e.g., neurotrophic factors). The material carried back to the cell body has been shown to influence activity in the cell nucleus.[4]

Compression raises intraneural pressure and has a negative impact on the flow of cytoplasm.[4] The anterograde and retrograde flow of axoplasm is impaired with mild compression of the nerve (30 mm Hg) or hypoxia.[8,9] Prolonged or intense exposure to compression can result in conduction abnormalities, endoneurial edema, fibrin deposition, demyelination and axonal sprouting. Each of these events increases the likelihood for development of adhesions and abnormal impulse-generating sites (AIGS).[4] (The negative impact of AIGS is discussed in the section on adaptive responses to pain, p. 465.)

MOBILITY OF THE PERIPHERAL NERVOUS SYSTEM

Bone, fascia, and muscle surround peripheral nerves as they "travel" to target tissues. Peripheral nerves can be thought of as passing through a series of tissue tunnels composed of various biological materials. The composition of the tunnel changes during the passage of the nerve from the vertebral column (an osseous tunnel) to the target tissue, which might be soft tissue or a fibro-osseous tunnel. A "mechanical interface" exists at the junction between the nerve and the material adjacent to the nerve that forms the tissue tunnel. Movement of the trunk or limbs can cause three types of movement to occur in the peripheral nerves: unfolding, sliding, and elongation.[6]

When there is no tension on a peripheral nerve, the axon typically contains undulations (folds). As tension is applied, the axon will unfold, causing the undulations to disappear. Sliding can be defined as movement between the nerve and the surrounding tissues at the mechanical interface (extraneural movement). Sliding does not cause significant elongation or tension to develop within the nerve. Elongation of the nerve occurs when tension is applied to an unfolded nerve and there is little or no movement at the mechanical interface. Elongation causes sliding to occur between the fascicles or between the neural elements and connective tissue layers (intraneural movement). Elongation can result in a significant decrease in the diameter of the nerve, an increase in the tension within the nerve, and an increase in pressure within the nerve.[6] The increase in pressure has the potential to decrease the flow of blood and axoplasm resulting in altered neural function (see previous section).

Both extraneural and intraneural movements may occur simultaneously, but they may not be uniformly distributed within a nerve. When the body is moved, some parts of the nervous system will undergo primarily extraneural movement with little or no development of tension, whereas other areas undergo intraneural movement (elongation), resulting in an increase intraneural tension. As a consequence, some areas within a nerve develop little or no tension, and other areas of the same nerve develop a significant amount of intraneural tension, which often develops into a "tension point." In areas repeatedly exposed to high amounts of tension (e.g., the median nerve at the wrist), the nerves are found to contain a higher-than-average amount of connective tissue.[6]

If the entire nervous system is considered as a continuous tissue tract, then the idea that movement or tension developed in one region of the nervous system can be distributed and dissipated throughout the entire nervous system becomes apparent.[10,11] The inability of a component within the nervous system to dissipate or distribute movement and tension can lead to abnormal force development and lesions elsewhere in the continuous tissue tract.[12]

PERIPHERAL NERVE ENTRAPMENT

Seddon's classification of nerve injury is based on mechanical trauma.[13] Schaumberg[2] modified this paradigm into an anatomically based scheme containing three classes of injury (Table 15-1). Injuries in class II and III are due to macrotrauma that results in some disruption to the integrity of the nerve fiber. The following discussion of entrapment is focused on microtrauma in which there is no breach in the anatomical integrity of the nerve fiber (class I). Mechanical microtrauma resulting in nerve entrapment can occur with excessive or abnormal (1) friction, (2) compression, or (3) tension (elongation).[2]

Tissue tunnels, peripheral nerves, and the mechanical interfaces between them are all vulnerable to mechanical microtrauma (i.e., abnormal friction, compression, or tension).[2,6] Some peripheral nerves are exposed to bony hard interfaces (e.g., the lower cords of the brachial plexus at the first rib), which are potential sources of abnormal friction. Inflammation and swelling within a tissue tunnel can produce compression of a nerve, such as the median nerve within the carpal tunnel. Abnormal tension can develop in nerves where excessive intraneural movement occurs or extraneural movement is restricted. An example would be the tibial nerve in the popliteal fossa. The point at which a nerve branches limits the amount of gliding (extraneural movement) available at that location and increases the amount of local intraneural tension developed with movement.[2,6]

Microtrauma can produce an intraneural lesion.[2,6] Injuries to conducting tissues can result in a decrease in intraneural flow of axoplasm, demyelination, or conduction defects. If the lesion occurs in the connective tissues of the nerve, there may be pain, inflammation, proliferation of fibroblasts, and scar formation (fibrosis). An intraneural scar decreases the compliance of the nerve and increases the amount of tension and intraneural pressure generated with movement.[11] Intraneural changes can impair or completely block the ability of the nerve to conduct action potentials.[2,6,14] Partial or complete conduction blocks can result in positive or negative sensory phenomena, loss of motor function, autonomic dysfunction, and atrophy of muscle or skin tissue.

Microtrauma can produce an extraneural lesion.[2,6,11,14] The damage in an extraneural lesion can occur in the tissue surrounding the nerve or at the mechanical interface. Swelling within the tissue tunnel can produce compression of the nerve. Fibrosis can produce adhesions at the mechanical interface, leading to a decrease in sliding of the nerve. A decrease in the ability of a nerve to slide within a tissue tunnel will result in an abnormal increase in intraneural tension and pressure as movement is imposed on the nerve. The increase in local intraneural tension will be distributed in an aberrant pattern throughout the continuous tract of the nervous system, predisposing the system to abnormal tension and lesions at other sites.[6]

Friction, compression, and tension can produce microtrauma that results in intraneural and extraneural pathological conditions.[2,6] For example, fibrosis can produce a combined pathological state that results in a substantial reduction in the ability of a nerve to slide within the tissue tunnel and a substantial increase in tension within the nerve as the compliance of the nerve is decreased. These changes result in an abnormal distribution of sliding and tension throughout the nervous system with movement of the trunk or limbs. The abnormal distribution of tension within a nerve increases the probability of a second injury or abnormality developing within the nerve. This scenario has led to the use of the term "double crush injury" first used by Upton and McComas[15] in 1973. This term should be considered a misnomer because a "crush" does not necessarily occur. For example, entrapment of the median nerve at the carpal tunnel can cause the development of abnormal tension in cervical spinal nerves, resulting in an injury at that site. Upton and McComas[15] have shown that a lesion at the carpal

TABLE 15-1 ■ **Classification of Acute Traumatic Peripheral Nerve Injury**

ANATOMICAL CLASSIFICATION	CLASS I	CLASS II	CLASS III
Previous nomenclature	Neurapraxia	Axonotmesis	Neurotmesis
Lesion	Reversible conduction block resulting from ischemia or demyelination	Axonal interruption but basal lamina remains intact	Nerve fiber and basal lamina interruption (complete nerve severance)

Adapted from Schaumberg HH, Spencer PS, Thomas PK: *Disorders of peripheral nerves,* Philadelphia, 1983, FA Davis.

tunnel increases the risk of having a second neural lesion in the cervical region.

PATHOGENESIS OF NEUROVASCULAR ENTRAPMENT

Sunderland[16] has reasoned that a change in the normal pressure gradients within the carpal tunnel can lead to compression of the median nerve. For proper nutrition of the median nerve to occur, blood must flow into the carpal tunnel, then into the nerve and back out of the tunnel. For normal blood flow to occur in the median nerve, the blood pressure must be highest within the epineurial arterioles and becomes progressively less in the capillaries, fascicles of the nerve, epineurial venules, and least within the extraneural space of the carpal tunnel. Any increase in the pressure of a single compartment has the potential to disrupt the normal pressure gradients and impair the flow of blood within the compartments of the median nerve and the carpal tunnel. Impaired intraneural blood flow can lead to localized hypoxia, edema, and fibrosis.[16]

An increase in pressure within the carpal tunnel can occur for a variety of reasons (e.g., inflammation, thickening of tendons, synovial hyperplasia, venous congestion, or edema). Venous blood flow will be impaired or blocked, and venous stasis will develop if pressure within the carpal tunnel becomes greater than the pressure within the epineurial venules. This phenomena could occur with pressures as low as 20 to 30 mm Hg.[6,17] Motor and sensory abnormalities begin to present at about 40 mm Hg, and complete blockade of the median nerve has been shown to occur at 50 mm Hg.[18]

The pressure within the carpal tunnel is normally about 3 mm Hg with the wrist in a neutral position.[4] Studies have shown that the pressure within the carpal tunnel in someone with carpal tunnel syndrome can be 30 mm Hg, or more, with the wrist in neutral and increase to 100 mm Hg when the wrist is in flexion.[4,8,9] These abnormal pressures are clearly adequate to disrupt the normal flow of blood or axoplasm within the median nerve and cause severe consequences to normal nerve functions.

Sunderland[16] has proposed that venous congestion or stasis within the carpal tunnel will lead to hypoxia, edema, and fibrosis. Hypoxia can cause alterations in axoplasmic flow, abnormal impulse conduction, and a deterioration of the capillary endothelium. C fibers may also play a role in the degeneration of the capillary endothelium. C fibers contain vasoactive peptides (e.g., substance P and calcitonin gene-related peptide), which can be released onto the capillary endothelial cells.[4] These vasoactive substances cause the endothelial cells to become flatter, larger, and leakier, resulting in exudation and edema. In addition, substance P is known to promote mast cell degranulation that releases serotonin or histamine, which augments the inflammatory state.[19,20] A localized inflammatory state is known to decrease the threshold and increase the firing rate of nociceptors and increase their sensitivity to other modes of stimulation, such as mechanical.[4]

A breakdown of the capillary endothelium results in exudation and the formation of a protein-rich edema in the interstitial space. Protein-rich edema (1) stimulates proliferation of fibroblasts resulting in fibrosis and (2) intensifies the abnormal pressure gradients, resulting in more tissue hypoxia, which initiates a positive feedback or self-perpetuating cycle of pathological states. Intraneural fibrosis decreases compliance of the nerve and extraneural fibrosis results in the formation of adhesions at the mechanical interface between the nerve and tissue tunnel. Fibrosis causes a nerve to become stiffer and less mobile, resulting in an abnormal increase in tension when movement is imposed on the nerve.

The set of circumstances describe above may be referred to as a *neurovascular entrapment;* it has the potential to cause the development of problems elsewhere in the system, which is referred to as a "double crush injury" (see previous section). Upton and McComas[15] studied 115 subjects with carpal tunnel syndrome or ulnar impingement at the elbow. They found that 81 of the 115 subjects had evidence of a neural lesion at the neck. Because all nerves essentially travel within tissue tunnels, the potential exists for this scenario to occur elsewhere in the continuous tissue tract of the nervous system, such as the capsule of the dorsal root ganglion and the thoracic outlet.[5,6,21]

ADAPTIVE RESPONSES TO PAIN

A thorough discussion of the pain associated with neurovascular entrapment is beyond the scope and intent of this chapter. The topic of pain is discussed in Chapter 32 of this book. However, there are a couple of issues related to the pain associated with neurovascular entrapment that need to be discussed.

"Normal" or physiological pain occurs when peripheral nociceptors are subjected to a stimulus that is at or above threshold. "Abnormal" or pathological pain can occur when there is a change in the sensitivity (threshold) of the somatosensory system.[22] Devor[23] wrote that ". . . the crucial pathophysiological process triggered by nerve injury is an increase in neuronal excitability."

Axons that become inflamed, hypoxic, or demyelinated can enter a hyperexcitable state.[2,23,24] A nerve in a hyperexcitable state can begin to discharge spontaneously, become mechanosensitive, or develop a sustained rhythmic discharge after stimulation, all of which can result in the production of pathological pain.[23,25] These changes in the "behavior" of a nerve can occur in the absence of detectable degeneration in the nerve.[24]

Mechanosensitivity and spontaneous impulse generation are characteristics of an AIGS.[4] A hyperexcitable state and an AIGS can occur with the mechanical microtraumas such as compression, tension, friction, and inflammation normally associated with peripheral nerve pathology.[2,23,25,26]

The dorsal root ganglion appears to play a significant role in the pain associated with peripheral nerve pathological conditions.[22] Abnormal amounts of compression, tension, inflammation, or other injuries to peripheral nerves can cause the dorsal root ganglion to become hyperexcitable (sensitized). The change in sensitivity (threshold) allows what were weak, subthreshold stimuli to evoke pain and suprathreshold stimuli to evoke exaggerated pain. In addition, the dorsal root ganglion and peripheral nerves may become mechanosensitive. In this case they may generate pain signals in response to movement. This change in sensitivity reflects a change in the physiological features of the nerve and may be a component in the development of enhanced central sensitivity to pain and a chronic pain state.[22]

As stated previously, the PNS and CNS represent a continuous tissue tract. The pain and symptoms associated with musculoskeletal injury or peripheral nerve pathology can include changes that are the result of an alteration in the autonomic nervous system, which is considered part of the continuous tissue tract of the nervous system.[2,27] For example, catecholamines do not normally elicit pain. However, if a nerve is injured or if there is local inflammation, the catecholamines can induce pain and they can maintain or enhance pain in inflamed tissues.[4]

Wyke[28] demonstrated that stimulation of nocioceptors in spinal joints resulted in reflex changes in the cardiovascular, respiratory, and endocrine systems. Feinstein[29,30] has shown that injecting saline solution into the thoracic paraspinal muscles caused pallor, diaphoresis, bradycardia, and a drop in the blood pressure. These changes are often associated with an alteration in the output from the autonomic nervous system.[21,27,31]

Some patients who are treated for musculoskeletal injuries have signs that may be related to autonomic dysreflexia.[21] In patients with cumulative trauma disorder (CTD), signs of abnormal autonomic nervous system output can include (1) vasomotor reflexes leading to cool, pale skin,[32] (2) changes in the pattern of sweating (hypohidrosis or hyperhidrosis), (3) trophic changes in the skin, (4) hyperactive flexor withdrawal reflexes, or (5) paradoxical breathing patterns.[21] Edgelow[21] has described paradoxical breathing as the use of the scalene muscles for ventilation during quiet breathing instead of normal ventilation, which is predominantly a function of the diaphragm. Edgelow[21] found that paradoxical breathing is present in most patients with CTD of the upper extremity. A better appreciation of the contribution of the autonomic nervous system to the pathological conditions and symptoms present in some patients with neurovascular entrapment may enhance the effectiveness of their treatment.

CLINICAL EXAMINATION AND TREATMENT OF NEUROVASCULAR ENTRAPMENT

For an effective evaluation of a patient with a neurovascular entrapment problem, the whole person must be addressed and involved in the evaluation and treatment processes. This philosophy requires the therapist to become the evaluator, teacher, and guide for the patient. Wherever possible the testing procedures should be performed by the patients so that they can learn to self-assess their status before and after treatment procedures. This self-assessment gives the patient control, thus decreasing their fear of movement or reinjury. In some cases, if a therapist uses his hands it may be detrimental to the patient in a lifelong sense if it leads to dependence. The concept of the patient gaining control of the problem(s) is fundamental and must be integrated into the initial patient contact to develop an effective self-management approach. Without an effective self-management strategy, the patient is at risk for recurrent problems and development of a chronic condition.

The Edgelow protocol for examination and treatment of neurovascular entrapment challenges the traditional musculoskeletal paradigm by placing the primary emphasis on the response of the neurovascular and neuromotor systems to injury.[33-35] The standard musculoskeletal evaluation centered on a biomechanical model of the musculoskeletal and nervous systems is adequate for patients with straightforward symptoms that appear to be of biomechanical origin. However, a biomechanical approach is inappropriate for patients with severe or irritable signs and symptoms that may be neurological or vascular in origin. Patients with neurovascular entrapment often have severe, irritable symptoms. First, a subjective evaluation is conducted in a patient with a potential neurovascular entrapment problem to determine how the objective examination should proceed. The history of the condition is discussed with the patient. Key components that should be discussed include history of trauma, repetitive activities, sustained static or tension postures, such as computer keyboard work, or physical activities performed with a high level of cognitive demand, as seen in a pianist. The history should include a discussion of general health, including any potentially relevant medical conditions (e.g., asthma, diabetes, hypothyroidism). Phase I of differential diagnosis (medical screening) should be completed to ensure that the patient is appropriate for evaluation and intervention. (See Chapter 7, Differential Diagnosis Phase I.)

A discussion of the patient's symptoms and complaints should include questions that determine whether the neural or vascular systems are potential sources of the problem. Symptoms relevant to the potential problem of neurovascular entrapment include complaints of fullness in the upper extremity, a feeling of swelling, tingling, pain, coldness, numbness, or dropping things. In addition, the progression of the symptoms or complaints and the level of irritability should be determined. If pain is a major factor, then a functional pain questionnaire should be completed (see Chapter 32). Motor changes of relevance to the potential problem of neurovascular entrapment include complaints of dropping things, weakness, or an inability to perform motor tasks that were done previously without difficulty. The level of neural irritability and the presence of peripheral or central sensitization should be determined by asking the patient what activities aggravate and ease the symptoms. Irritability may be indicated when an extended period of time is required for symptoms to ease after provocation. Sensitization is indicated when minor mechanical or normally nonnoxious stimuli, such as clothing on the skin, provoke pain. Vascular complaints relevant to the potential problem of neurovascular entrapment include complaints of fullness, swelling, abnormal skin color, or cool skin temperatures. A change in the vascular symptoms with a change in limb position is particularly significant.

In a biomechanical evaluation model the therapist examines the quantity and quality of active movements and determines whether there is pain, spasm, or resistance at an end feel. In patients with neurovascular entrapment this procedure may evoke a significant flare and worsening of symptoms. In patients with neurovascular entrapment the "feel" of involuntary muscle tension can be the first sign of abnormality in assessing movement. This tension is often subtle and may occur earlier in the range of motion than where traditional biomechanical symptoms or the end feel normally occurs.[36] Moving into the range of motion to the initial onset of tension minimizes the risk of provoking adverse neurological or vascular consequences. In patients with suspected neurovascular entrapment who have symptoms suggestive of neural irritability and sensitization, the biomechanical

TABLE 15-2 ■ Suggested Modifications to a Standard Biomechanical Evaluation

OBSERVATION

Cervical/thoracic:	WNL	kyphosis	flat
Scapula:	equal	high R/L	low L/R
Lumbar:	WNL	lordosis	flat

Hands and feet: swelling, discoloration, other

ACTIVE RANGE OF MOTION
(FOR A PATIENT WITH UPPER QUADRANT SYMPTOMS)
Cervical:

Flexion: _____° causes/increases symptoms
Extension: _____° causes/increases symptoms
Rotation: (R): _____° causes/increases symptoms
Rotation: (L): _____° causes/increases symptoms
Lateral flexion (R): _____° causes/increases symptoms
Lateral flexion (L): _____° causes/increases symptoms

Shoulder Flexion

(R):(with elbow extension): ___° causes/increases symptoms
(L):(with elbow extension): ___° causes/increases symptoms
(R):(with elbow flexion): ___° causes/increases symptoms
(L):(with elbow flexion): ___° causes/increases symptoms

Shoulder Internal Rotation (reaching behind back)
(functional tension test with radial nerve bias)

(R): position   causes/increases symptoms
(L): position   causes/increases symptoms

NEURAL EXAMINATION
Passive Neck Flexion

no/yes _____° causes/increases symptoms

Upper Limb Neural Dynamic Test[4]

(R): position _____ causes/increases symptoms
(L): position _____ causes/increases symptoms

Straight Leg Raising Test or Lasegue's Test[37]

Right: _____° causes/increases symptoms
Left: _____° causes/increases symptoms

Tinel's sign[37]
(Normal = 0; Mild = 1+; Moderate = 2+; Severe = 3+)

Supraclavicular region:		Right	Left
Elbow:		Right	Left
Wrist:	Median	Right	Left
	Ulnar	Right	Left

KABAT TESTS[42]
Strength Tests[42]

Flexor carpi ulnaris: (R)/5 (L)/5
Adductor pollicis: (R)/5 (L)/5

Thinker Pose[42] (isometric contraction of longus colli)
(temporary strengthening of the flexor carpi ulnaris
and adductor pollicis)

no/yes—which muscles are effected and by what amount?

VASCULAR INTEGRITY
Temperature of hands (ambient room temperature)

Right: (index)   (digiti minimi)
Left: (index)   (digiti minimi)

Adson's Test[37] (change in pulse pressure)

Right after: 1 minute 2 minutes 3 minutes
Left after: 1 minute 2 minutes 3 minutes

EAST Test[37] (change in pulse pressure)

Right after: 1 minute 2 minutes 3 minutes
Left after: 1 minute 2 minutes 3 minutes

SENSATION[37] (LOCALIZATION, STEREOGNOSIS,
GRAPHAESTHESIA AND OTHERS)
BREATHING PATTERN (ABILITY TO RELAX THE SCALENE
MUSCLES WITH QUIET BREATHING)

Normal or dysfunctional pattern

PALPATION FINDINGS (TENDERNESS: NORMAL = 0;
MILD = 1+; MODERATE = 2+; SEVERE = 3+)

Scalene muscles:	Right:	Left:
Subclavius:	Right:	Left:
Pectoralis minor:	Right:	Left:

---

examination and treatment techniques should be modified or deferred until the sensitivity and irritability of the nervous system are improved. (See Table 15-2 for suggested modifications to a standard biomechanical evaluation.)

One component of the examination involves evaluating the integrity of the vascular system in the extremities. The hands or feet should be inspected for discoloration and the skin temperature should be determined in each of the peripheral nerve territories present in the affected limb. Cool, cyanotic skin can be an indication of arterial insufficiency or sympathetic dysreflexia in the area, whereas swelling can be an indication of inflammation and venous or lymphatic insufficiency. An Adson's test and the elevated arm stress test (EAST) can be used to evaluate vascular integrity by determining whether the pulse pressure decrease with a change in the position of the limb.[37] The Adson's test and the EAST test should be performed on both upper extremities and the pulse pressure evaluated at 1, 2, and 3 minutes. These tests may be modified or deferred depending on the level of neural irritability found.

Sensory changes may be subtle and are not always accompanied by obvious motor dysfunction. The most common complaint with neurovascular entrapment of the upper extremity is that "I drop things," yet standard tests of strength, light touch, and two-point discrimination may have normal results. Therapists often think of this problem as motor until our standard tests fail to demonstrate motor dysfunction. Subtle changes in the somatosensory cortex can occur as a consequence of repetitive motions, particularly when performed under conditions of intense concentration or in the presence of pain.[38-40] Byl[39] observed severe degradation in the representation of the hand in the somatosensory cortex of owl monkeys that were trained in a behavior of rapid, active opening/closing of the hand under conditions of high cognitive drive. In addition, Byl[38] found a significant difference in the response on some sensory integration and praxis tests in human subjects with diagnoses of tendonitis and focal dystonia. Byl has postulated that similar changes can be identified in humans with repetitive strain injuries with the use of Jean Ayers tests of sensory localization, stereognosis, and graphesthesia.[40]

An assessment of the patient's breathing pattern at rest and palpation of the subclavius, pectoralis minor, and scalene muscles should be performed. The normal breathing pattern at rest is primarily diaphragmatic (Figure 15-2). However, patients with neurovascular entrapment often

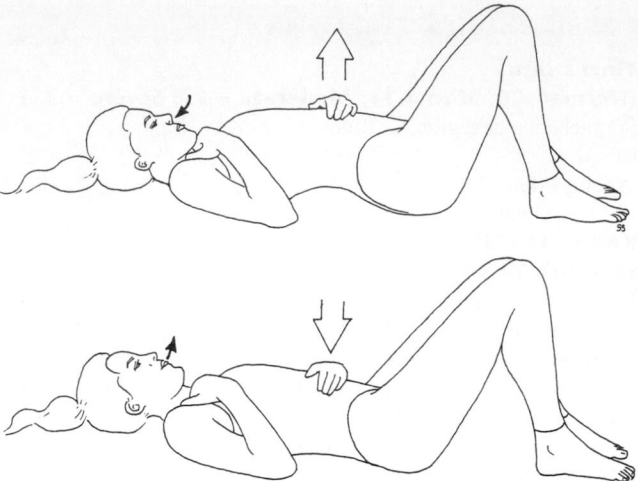

FIGURE 15-2 ■ Diaphragmatic breathing. As the client inhales, the stomach should rise and the lordosis in the low back should increase. During exhalation the stomach should fall and the back flatten against the floor.

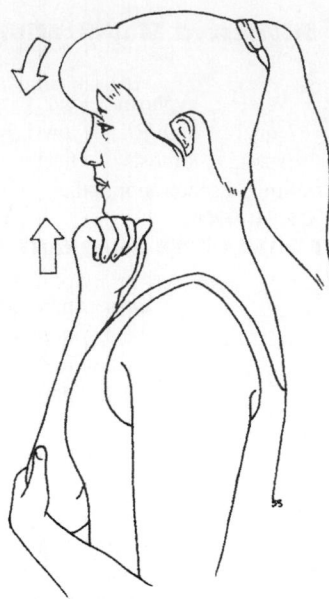

FIGURE 15-3 ■ The "thinker pose." Self-traction is applied by using gentle upward pressure from one upper extremity onto the chin.

demonstrate a breathing pattern at rest that relies predominantly on the scalene muscles. The scalene breathing pattern mechanically narrows the thoracic outlet area, thus potentially perpetuating a neurovascular entrapment syndrome in the area. The scalene breathing pattern may be a sign of protective posturing. Palpation is used to determine whether tenderness or tightness is present. Palpation of the subclavius, pectoralis minor, and scalene muscles is significant because of the relationship these muscles have with the subclavian vein, brachial plexus components, and subclavian artery, respectively. The results of the palpation should be correlated to the neurological and vascular changes found elsewhere in the extremity.

Neurovascular Entrapment Examination

There are some common symptom patterns characteristic of neurovascular entrapment that alert the practitioner to modify the physical examination. In addition to the symptoms mentioned previously, the following patterns help the practitioner recognize a patient with a potential sensitized nervous system.

Symptom Patterns Characteristic of Neurovascular Entrapment
1. Symptoms are severe and irritable.
2. Function is markedly reduced in the target task (injury producing activity) and activities of daily living.
3. The patient reports feeling that his or her emotions are in a state of "being out of control."

In a modified examination scheme designed to evaluate for the presence of a neurovascular entrapment syndrome, patients typically have six signs. These signs, in addition to the more traditional musculoskeletal signs, are used as guides in determining the effectiveness of treatment.

Six Common Signs of Neurovascular Entrapment
1. Abnormal hand temperature within the following parameters:

a. Cold hands defined as in the 70° F range at rest and during activity at the target task.
b. Asymmetry between the temperatures of the second digit and the fifth digit, with the fifth digit being colder.[41]
c. Asymmetry between hands in which there is an abnormal temperature cooling response to diaphragmatic breathing, aerobic walking, and repeated use of the upper extremities in an activity such as bouncing a gymnastic ball.
2. Abnormal breathing pattern: accessory, chest, or paradoxical rather than diaphragmatic.
3. Abnormal mobility and sensitivity of the nervous system: specifically the dura, the brachial plexus, or the sciatic nerve/sacral plexus.
4. Cardiovascular deconditioning: patient has a low level of endurance and is easily fatigued.
5. Sensory dysfunction of the hand at the cortical level: abnormal tactile localization, graphesthesia, and stereognosis.
6. A positive Kabat[42] sign: weakness of the flexor pollicis brevis in the shortened range of adduction that is unilateral and reversed with a gentle 30-second isometric contraction of the longus colli obtained with the "thinker pose" (Figure 15-3).

This combination of symptoms and signs identifies neurovascular consequences of the injury. Improvements in these signs and symptoms serve as markers that identify treatment effectiveness; namely, decrease in pain, improvement in function, and a feeling of being more in control.

Neurovascular Entrapment Examination Procedures

Hand temperature is assessed with an infrared hand-held thermometer. Measurements are made of the second digit (innervated by the upper roots of the brachial plexus) and fifth digit (innervated by the lower roots). Temperature is assessed during rest, diaphragmatic breathing, walking on a treadmill, and during repeated movements of the upper extremities while bouncing a gymnastic ball. A normal response is an increase in temperature in response to these activities. A cooling response is considered abnormal.

Breathing pattern is assessed by palpating the scalene muscles in the area between the inferior border of the sternocleidomastoid and superior to the clavicle. This procedure is best done while the patient performs relaxed inhalation. The scalene muscles are normally quiet during relaxed inhalation. Contraction of the scalene muscles and elevation of the sternum is considered to be abnormal during quiet inhalation. Patients are instructed to breathe with the "belly" only (diaphragmatic breathing). If they are unable to do this, breathing is considered to be paradoxical.

Neurodynamics is assessed with the use of upper limb neural dynamic tests (ULNT) for the upper extremity, as described by Butler.[4] Passive neck flexion is used as an assessment of dural sensitivity. Straight leg raise is tested to assess the sensitivity of the sciatic nerve/sacral plexus.

Cardiovascular fitness is assessed by treadmill walking. The patient is instructed to walk at a speed that does not cause an increase in symptoms for up to 20 minutes. Over time, patients are encouraged to increase their walking speed until they reach a level where they are aerobically fit on the basis of standard measures.

CNS sensory dysfunction of the hand (specifically tactile localization, graphesthesia, and stereognosis) is assessed by the methods of Byl.[40]

Hand strength is assessed by examining for the presence of a Kabat sign.[42] The patient is instructed to hold the arm at the side with the elbow flexed to 90 degrees and fully supinated. The wrist is positioned in neutral flexion/extension with the fingers fully extended and the thumb in the shortened range of adduction and flexion (thumb in the plane of the palm). The distal phalanx of the thumb is held in full extension. This starting position inhibits the median innervated muscles of the palm and finger flexors. A manual muscle test is done to test the strength of flexor pollicis brevis/adductor pollicis in the shortened range. If there is a "giving way" at the metacarpophalangeal joint, then this is quantified using a "thumbometer," an inexpensive device consisting of an eye drop bottle attached to a blood pressure cuff sphygmomanometer. Clinical experience demonstrates that after longus colli isometric contraction there is a strengthening of the affected muscles in the thumb. There will be a weakening effect on thumb strength if the patient has cervical instability during the performance of activities or exercises. This indicates the activity is too much for the patient at that time. If there is no effect on thumb strength then the patient is stable enough for the activity.

Neurovascular Entrapment Interventions

Treatment must follow the same principles that guide the examination. The patient is taught self-assessment techniques and strategies so that the patient has control of the progression of treatment and activities of daily living. The patient may use any of the following self-assessment techniques, as appropriate, to guide the course of treatment: a pain scale, a thermometer to test skin temperature, a neuro-

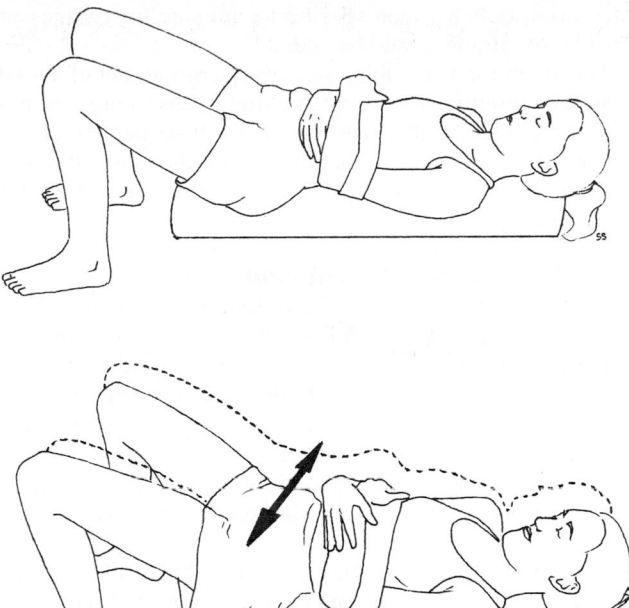

FIGURE 15-4 ■ Foam roller exercise for mobilization of the spine. The roller is placed underneath the spine with the client in the supine position. The client gently rolls from side to side to increase mobility of the spine.

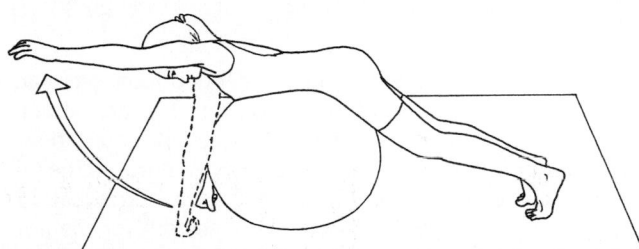

FIGURE 15-5 ■ Patient in a quadruped position on a therapy ball with the chin tucked and the neck straight. The patient can lift an upper or lower extremity to provide a challenge to the muscles that stabilize the spine.

dynamic test, or a Kabat strength test. Any treatment or activity that increases symptoms, protective posturing, or tension is modified or discontinued.

Treatment is begun using sensory motor integration with an emphasis on functional skills (e.g., breathing, balance, and hand function) in a manner that does not cause irritation of the patient's condition. The patient is guided through a series of breathing exercises designed to improve the circulation to the extremities, calm the nervous system, and retrain the scalene muscles, if appropriate. The breathing exercises are progressed through the use of foam rollers (Figure 15-4). These are used to increase the mobility of the spine and rib cage. The breathing exercises are combined with functional movements of the trunk and extremities in a manner that mobilizes the nervous system. Once the patient is able to manage the symptoms, the treatment can progress to stabilization exercises with a gym ball (Figure 15-5). If the patient has vestibular, balance, or sensory integration deficits, then specific techniques for balance or sensory retraining would be added.

Our intention is not to present every component of a total treatment program but rather highlight those core components that address the neurovascular consequences of the injury. Our experience is that modifying these neurovascular consequences is the first step and the foundation for recovery.

Core Components of Treatment

The reversible weakness of the thumb is addressed by strengthening the longus colli muscle. This is accomplished by a 30-second isometric contraction using the "thinker pose" (see Figure 15-3) and specific muscle reeducation for longus colli with Jull's protocol.[43] The expected effect of the thinker pose is to reverse the identified weakness of the thumb. The patient is taught to minimize mechanical stress to the cervical/thoracic spine through instruction in body mechanics. An important concept is to train the patient to identify the coactivation position for stability of the neck and to visualize that position before moving the body away from the center of gravity or moving the arm. This method has the patient assume the thinker pose to stimulate the deep neck flexors to contract before the movement is performed.

The temperature, neurodynamic, and breathing dysfunctions are addressed by training the patient to perform relaxed diaphragmatic breathing with spinal motion (see Figure 15-2). The expected outcomes are to normalize hand temperature and increase the range of motion while decreasing sensitivity to the neurodynamic tests. Low cardiovascular endurance is addressed by having the patient begin a progressive aerobic conditioning program of walking. Because the examination identifies six signs of dysfunction, the goals of treatment are to normalize these six signs. Clinical experience teaches that, as these signs improve, there is a reduction in pain and an increase in function.

Role of the Patient

Maximizing the treatment response requires a unique partnership between the physical therapist and the patient that facilitates the patient's "feeling of being in control." The "feeling of being in control" is thought to have a positive impact on the response to treatment. Patients are taught methods for self-assessment of the immediate effect of their treatment. They are taught to assess their responses to the core program on the basis of signs of hand strength and hand temperature and mobility and sensitivity of the nervous system. The patients are provided with self-assessment tools and treatment devices. The details of the exercise program are provided in a patient booklet, two audiotapes, and a videotape, which can be purchased at www.edgelow.com.

CASE STUDY

PATIENT DESCRIPTION

The patient is a 35-year-old right-handed legal secretary who has worked at her present job for 16 years. About 2 years ago her office switched to software applications requiring increased use of the computer mouse. She reports a 2-year history of right arm pain of gradual onset that worsened and has been constant for the last 4 months. She has been off work for 4 months because of the symptoms in her right arm. Her recreational activities include aerobics and softball, but she has done neither for several months as a result of her arm symptoms. She has experienced sensations of numbness and tingling on the dorsal surface of both hands and "tension" in her neck. She has had "four or five" cortisone injections in the elbow, participated in physical therapy for "stretching and strengthening," and switched to a trackball pointing device at her computer workstation without significant benefit. Ten days before the current physical therapy evaluation she had right elbow surgery (debridement). The sutures were removed 4 days ago. She reports her current symptoms as a constant "throb" at the elbow, 3/10 intensity at rest, on a 0-10 pain scale. The neck tension is still present, but the hand numbness has not been present since surgery. She states her arm pain increases with trying to take a shirt off over her head or if she does any task that involves gripping with the right hand. She is avoiding using her right arm.

Her significant history includes a meat cutter accident at age 5 years that resulted in the amputation of fingertips 2 and 3 on the right hand. She reports no residual limitation in function from that injury. Five years ago she fell injuring her right wrist and left ankle. The wrist symptoms resolved without intervention, and the ankle recovered after 1 month of physical therapy. One year ago she fell while playing softball, which resulted in a sore neck for 1 day.

She reports no general health problems. She denies use of anticoagulant and steroid medications. She reports normal sensation in both feet and denies any dizziness. She is currently able to sleep through the night. Her medications include hydrocodone with acetaminophen and acetaminophen with codeine.

CLINICAL REASONING

Diagnostic hypothesis based on the subjective examination:

1. *Potential soft tissue edema* in the forearm extensor muscles 10 days after surgery.
2. *Potential altered neural dynamics with sensitization* on the basis of:
   a. Duration of symptoms
   b. Pattern of symptoms that do not fit localized tendonitis or cervical radiculopathy
   c. Lack of response to multiple interventions

Physical Examination

In this patient the nervous system is considered a potential source of dysfunction. (See Table 15-2 for suggested modifications to a biomechanically based musculoskeletal examination.) The referring physician specified a precaution of "no resistive exercises right upper extremity until 6 weeks post operatively"; therefore, no strength tests or Kabat tests were done.

The incision at the right lateral epicondyle area was well healed with mild ecchymosis. The right upper extremity otherwise had normal skin color and temperature. Girth measurements at 2 inches below the olecranon were +1.9 cm and at the olecranon +1.3 cm on the right versus the left. The patient sat with a mild forward head posture and a flat upper thoracic kyphosis while she held the right arm at her side with her elbow flexed.

The patient was instructed to complete active movement testing just to the point of feeling tension or resistance to movement. This precaution is meant to minimize the potential for a significant flare of symptoms from provocation testing of potentially irritable neurovascular structures while still providing a repeatable measurement for reassessment. The patient moved through full cervical flexion and bilateral rotation without report of tension or symptoms. Cervical extension at 45 degrees produced a feeling of neck stiffness. On further investigation, left lateral flexion at 75% range produced vague soreness in her right arm that was similar, but less intense, than her present symptoms. Right lateral flexion was 100% and did not provoke symptoms. Isolated right upper extremity movements that were done without provocation of her symptoms included elbow flexion 120 degrees, extension –10 degrees, pronation 80 degrees, and supination 70 degrees. Passive neural provocation testing was performed to the onset of tension or a change in symptoms (Table 15-3). The ULNT was the only passive neural provocation test performed because of the patient's suspected nervous system irritability. (See the list of suggested readings at the end of this chapter for a more complete description of how to perform this and other ULNTs.) On palpation the scalene muscles were noted to be active during quiet breathing.

CLINICAL REASONING

Diagnostic hypothesis based on physical examination:
1. Postoperative edema in forearm extensor muscles (confirmed by circumferential measurements)
2. Altered neural dynamics based on the presence of:
   a. Reproduction of elbow pain with cervical movement in a direction that required elongation of the affected brachial plexus (indicator of neural sensitivity to mechanical elongation of the brachial plexus)
   b. Early onset of protective muscle tension and reproduction of symptoms with ULNT (indicator of possible neurovascular entrapment)
   c. Scalene breathing pattern (Indicator of possible adaptive response to chronic pain)

Intervention

The patient was instructed to perform active range of motion exercises for the upper extremity in "out of tension" positions (i.e., in positions that allowed for minimal tension on neural structures and did not provoke symptoms). For example, she was able to do relaxed right wrist flexion/extension as long as she was lying on her left side with her right arm supported on her body and the elbow flexed. This position did not result in abnormal tension-related symptoms and probably provided her with a minimal amount of tension on the brachial plexus. She was instructed in relaxed diaphragmatic breathing in the supine position. She was issued a foam roller and instructed in spine mobilization exercises (see Figure 15-4). She was instructed to walk daily, supporting her right arm as needed. Use of ice and edema reduction measures for the right upper extremity was reviewed. A trial of cervical traction with use of a towel was found to increase cervical range in left lateral flexion without producing forearm symptoms. The patient was instructed in the towel traction technique for symptom management (Figure 15-6).

At her second visit she was instructed in self-assessment techniques to evaluate her response to activity. If she had a negative response to an exercise or activities of daily living, as evidenced by an increase in symptoms or a decrease in the range of her upper limb neural dynamic self-test, she was instructed to modify or discontinue the activity and perform a self-treatment that restored her tension-free range. The techniques that she found successful in restoring her mobility were diaphragmatic breathing (see Figure 15-2) and supine cervical traction.

At 4 weeks after the operation the surgeon gave the approval to start light resistive exercises. At this stage the patient no longer demonstrated signs of neural irritability. Treatment was progressed with the addition of foam roller exercises to improve spinal mobility (see Figure 15-4). The patient was started on gentle strengthening for the wrist extensors. Neural mobilization exercises progressed from active exercise in tension-free range to active exercise into mild resistance (i.e., to a feeling of "stretch" in the upper limb neural dynamic test position). Once full mobility was gained in the standard ULNT, then the radial nerve biased test position was examined and determined to be restricted. The radial biased ULNT was taught to the patient as a treatment technique to restore mobility in the branches of the radial nerve that cross the extensor surface of the forearm. The patient was placed prone on fists and knees and prone on a therapy ball to perform exercises that promote scapular stabilization, postural strengthening, and progressive weight bearing through the wrist and elbow joints (see Figure 15-5).

Final treatment sessions focused on problem solving related to symptom management and postural training with simulated work tasks and recreational activities. Diaphragmatic breathing and cervical traction techniques were adapted to the upright position so that the patient could manage symptoms while performing work tasks. Emphasis was placed on continued self-assessment of the response of the nervous system to the progression of activity.

Continued

CASE STUDY—cont'd

Outcome

At the first follow-up visit 2 days after the initial evaluation, the patient reported a significant reduction in symptoms after walking for 1 hour. Her girth measurements at the right elbow were improved by 1 cm, indicating a reduction in edema. The right upper limb neural dynamic test was performed to the onset of tension: shoulder depression (neutral), abduction (90 degrees), external rotation (80 degrees), forearm supination (85 degrees), wrist extension (60 degrees), and elbow extension (−70 degrees), indicating a significant improvement in tension-free range (compare with Table 15-3). The patient was able to objectively see and experience the benefit of the activities that were prescribed. The intent of the treatment program was to improve function in the vascular, neural, and lymphatic systems without provoking a protective tension response. The early success with self-guided treatment set the stage for teaching the patient to evaluate the effect of any activity, manage symptoms with one or two easing techniques, and ultimately progress her own activity level. This approach gave the patient control of her problem.

The patient had received a total of nine treatments at the time of discharge (3 months postoperatively). Grip strength was equal bilaterally at 75 pounds. At this point she was working full-time, regular duty with ergonomic improvements to her workstation. She reported a residual symptom of spot pain at the elbow that she could control with exercise. Through trial and error and self-assessment, she determined that her aerobic exercise class was a consistent irritant so she switched her aerobic activity to walking.

Discussion

This case illustrates the importance of evaluating the role of the nervous system in patients with chronic or irritable symptoms. Sensitization[4] and possible processing changes in the central nervous system[38-40] necessitate evaluation of the nervous system as a potential source of symptoms in patients with chronic or irritable symptoms (e.g., cumulative trauma disorder). If the issues of nervous system irritability and sensitization are not addressed during evaluation and throughout treatment, then the risk for increasing the patient's symptoms and continuing the cycle of nervous system hypersensitivity is high.

TABLE 15-3 ■ Changes Observed in the Upper Limb Neurodynamic Test

SHOULDER

DEPRESSION	ABDUCTION	EXTERNAL ROTATION
Right neutral	80 degrees	neutral
Left neutral	Full	full

FOREARM

Supination
Right 70 degrees without symptoms
Left full without symptoms

WRIST

Extension
Right 40 degrees without symptoms
Left full without symptoms

ELBOW

Extension
Right deferred
Left 10 degrees

CERVICAL

Lateral flexion
Right increase in forearm symptoms
Left full with no symptoms

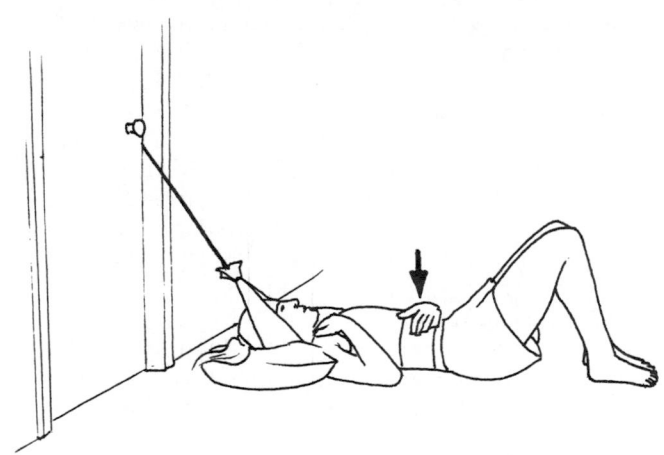

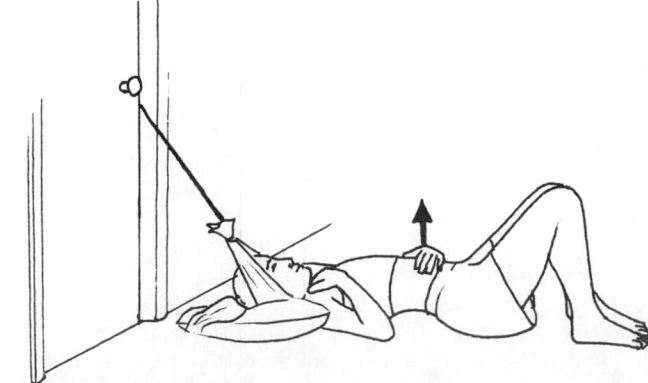

FIGURE 15-6 ■ Towel traction unit. By arching the low back the amount of traction is increased slightly. By flattening the low back the amount of traction is decreased slightly.

CASE STUDY—cont'd

The indicators that this patient may have had a nervous system dysfunction were her history of repetitive work, prior trauma, pattern of symptoms, and her lack of response to standard medical care. The indicators on physical examination were the restricted upper limb neural dynamic test, the reproduction of symptoms with selected neck movements, and the altered breathing pattern. Other objective indicators not assessed initially that may have further guided the

treatment would be Kabat testing, measuring the temperature of the hands and sensory testing of localization, graphesthesia, and stereognosis. A key concept to keep in mind is the role of education in treating patients with a long-term problem such as neurovascular entrapment. Teaching the patient a self-assessment tool restores the patient's control, allowing the patient to guide his or her own treatment and to be more responsible for his or her own well being.

REFERENCES

1. Mather LH: *The peripheral nervous system: Structure, function and clinical correlations,* Reading, 1985, Addison-Wesley.
2. Schaumberg HH: *Disorders of peripheral nerves,* Philadelphia, 1983, FA Davis.
3. Pratt NE: Neurovascular entrapment in the regions of the shoulder and posterior triangle of the neck, *Phys Ther* 66:1894-1900, 1986.
4. Butler DS: *The sensitive nervous system,* Adelaide, 2000, Noigroup Publications.
5. Sunderland S: *Nerves and nerve injuries,* ed 2, Baltimore, 1978, Williams & Wilkins.
6. Butler DS: *Mobilization of the nervous system,* Edinburgh, 1991, Churchill Livingstone.
7. Ogata K, Naito M: Blood of peripheral nerve: effects of dissection, stretching and compression, *J Hand Surg* 11B:10-14, 1986.
8. Gelberman RH, Hergenroeder PT, Hargens AR et al: The carpal tunnel syndrome: a study of canal pressures, *J Bone Joint Surg* 63:380-383, 1981.
9. Werner CO, Elmquist D, Ohlin T: Pressure and nerve lesions in the carpal tunnel, *Acta Orthop Scand* 54:312-316, 1983.
10. Elvey RL: The investigation of arm pain. In Grieve GP, editor: *Modern manual therapy of the vertebral column,* Edinburgh, 1986, Churchill Livingstone.
11. Grieve GP: *Common vertebral joint problems,* ed 2, Edinburgh, 1988, Churchill Livingstone.
12. Breig A: *Adverse mechanical tension in the central nervous system,* Stockholm, 1978, Almqvist & Wiksell International.
13. Seddon HJ: Three types of nerve injury, *Brain* 66:237-288, 1943.
14. Ochoa J, Fowler TJ, Gilliatt RW: Anatomical changes in peripheral nerves compressed by a pneumatic tourniquet, *J Anat* 113:433-455, 1972.
15. Upton ARM, McComas AJ: The double crush injury in nerve entrapment syndromes, *Lancet* 2:359-362, 1973.
16. Sunderland S: The nerve lesion in carpal tunnel syndrome, *J Neurol Neurosurg Psychiatry* 39:615-626, 1976.
17. Rydevik B, Lundborg G, Bagge U: Effects of graded compression on intraneural blood blow: an in-vivo study on rabbit tibial nerve, *J Hand Surg* 6:3-12, 1981.
18. Szabo RM, Bay BK, Sharkey NA et al: Median nerve displacement through the carpal canal, *J Hand Surg* 19A:901-906, 1994.
19. Hagermark O, Hokfelt T, Pernow B: Flare and itch induced by substance P in human skin, *J Invest Derm* 71:233-235, 1978.
20. Ebertz JM, Kettelkamp NS: Substance-P induced histamine release in human cutaneous mast cells, *J Invest Derm* 88:682-685, 1987.
21. Edgelow PI: Neurovascular consequences of cumulative trauma disorders affecting the thoracic outlet: a patient-centered treatment approach. In Donatelli RA, editor: *Physical therapy of the shoulder,* ed 3, New York, 1997, Churchill Livingstone.
22. Woolf CF: The dorsal horn: State-dependent sensory processing and the generation of pain. In Wall PD, Melzack R, editors: *Textbook of pain,* ed 3, Edinburgh, 1994, Churchill Livingstone.

23. Devor M: The pathophysiology of damaged peripheral nerves. In Wall PD, Melzack R, editors: *Textbook of pain,* ed 3, Edinburgh, 1994, Churchill Livingstone.
24. Eliav E, Herzberg U, Ruda MA: Neuropathic pain from an experimental neuritis of the rat sciatic nerve, *Pain* 83:169-182, 1999.
25. Gifford L: Fluid movement may partially account for the behavior of symptoms associated with nocioception in disc injury and disease. In Shadlock M, editor: *Moving in on pain,* Sydney, 1995, Butterworth-Heinemann.
26. Devor M, Seltzer Z: Pathophysiology of damaged nerves in relation to chronic pain. In Wall PD, Melzack R, editors: *Textbook of pain,* ed 4, Edinburgh, 1999, Churchill Livingstone.
27. Grieve GP: The autonomic nervous system in vertebral pain syndromes. In Grieve GP, editor: *Modern manual therapy of the vertebral column,* Edinburgh, 1986, Churchill Livingstone.
28. Wyke BD: The neurological basis of thoracic spinal pain, *Rheum Phys Med* 10:356-367, 1970.
29. Feinstein B, Langton JNK, Jameson RM et al: Experiments on pain referred from deep somatic tissues, *J Bone Joint Surg* 36A:981-997, 1954.
30. Feinstein B: Referred pain from paravertebral structures. In Buerger AA, Tobias JS, editors: *International conference on approaches to the validation of manipulative therapy,* Springfield, IL, 1981, Charles C Thomas.
31. Grieve GP: Referred pain and other clinical features. In Grieve GP, editor: *Modern manual therapy of the vertebral column,* Edinburgh, 1986, Churchill Livingstone.
32. Greening J, Lynn B, Leary R: Sensory and autonomic function in the hands of patients with non-specific arm pain (NSAP) and asymptomatic office workers, *Pain* 104:275-281, 2003.
33. Falla D, Jull G, Dall'Alba P et al: Electromyographic analysis of the deep neck flexors in performance of craniocervical flexion, *Phys Ther* 83:899-906, 2003.
34. Falla D: Unraveling the complexity of muscle impairment in chronic neck pain, *Man Ther* 9:125-133, 2004.
35. Falla D, Bilenkij G, Jull G: Patients with chronic neck pain demonstrated altered patterns of muscle activation during performance of a functional upper limb task, *Spine* 29:1436-1440, 2004.
36. Coppieters M, Stappaerts K: Aberrant protective force generation during neural provocation testing and the effect of treatment in patients with neurogenic cervicobrachial pain, *J Manip Physiol Ther* 26:99-106, 2003.
37. Magee D: *Orthopedic physical assessment,* ed 4, Philadelphia, 2002, WB Saunders.
38. Byl N: Sensory dysfunction associated with repetitive strain injuries of tendonitis and focal hand dystonia: a comparative study, *JOSPT* 23:234-244, 1996.
39. Byl N: A primate model for studying focal dystonia and repetitive strain injury: effects on the primary somatosensory cortex, *Phys Ther* 77:269-284, 1997.

40. Byl N, Melnick M: The neural consequences of repetition: clinical implications of a learning hypothesis, *J Hand Ther* 10:160-174, 1997.

41. Ellis W, Cheng S: Intraoperative thermographic monitoring during neurogenic thoracic outlet decompressive surgery, *Vasc Endovasc Surg* 37:253-257, 2003.

42. Kabat H: *Low back and leg pain from herniated cervical disc,* St. Louis, 1980, WH Green.

43. Jull G, Trott P, Potter H et al: A randomized controlled trial of exercise and manipulative therapy for cervicogenic headache, *Spine* 27:1835-1843, 2002.

CHAPTER 16

Neuromuscular Diseases

Ann Hallum, PhD

KEY WORDS

amyotrophic lateral sclerosis
disuse atrophy
Duchenne muscular dystrophy
Guillain-Barré syndrome
overwork damage
polyradiculoneuropathy

OBJECTIVES

After reviewing this chapter the student/therapist will be able to:
1. Describe the basic pathology and medical treatment of amyotrophic lateral sclerosis, Guillain Barré syndrome, and Duchenne muscular dystrophy.
2. Describe the current goals and treatment program for each condition.
3. Describe the "safe" exercise windows related to disuse atrophy and exercise (overwork) damage.
4. Be able to apply treatment concepts discussed in this chapter to other neuromuscular diseases.

This chapter traces the connections between the central nervous system (CNS) and musculoskeletal system by three disorders: amyotrophic lateral sclerosis (ALS), which damages upper and lower motor neurons; Guillain Barré syndrome (GBS), which affects the peripheral nervous system; and Duchenne muscular dystrophy (DMD), which impairs muscle function. The upper motor neurons that are affected in ALS originate in the motor cortex of the brain (Betz cells). These upper motor neuron axons descend by means of the corticobulbar and corticospinal tracts to synapse with lower motor neurons (primary motor cranial neurons) in the brain stem and spinal cord (anterior horn cells). Simultaneously, corticobulbar tract fibers innervate descending motor tracts originating within the brain stem. Initially the lateral descending system is more affected than the ventromedial system. But, with progress of the disease, all motor systems are affected. From the lower motor neurons within both the brain stem and spinal cord, the axons run within the peripheral nerves, which include motor and sensory fibers, to synapse with muscle fibers. Depending on the site of the pathological condition, neuromuscular diseases can be classified as neurogenic or myopathic. ALS and GBS are neurogenic disorders; DMD is a primary myopathy (Figure 16-1).

AMYOTROPHIC LATERAL SCLEROSIS
Pathology and Medical Diagnosis

ALS, commonly known in the United States as Lou Gehrig's disease, is a relentless, degenerative, terminal disease affecting both upper and lower motor neurons. Massive loss of anterior horn cells of the spinal cord and the motor cranial nerve nuclei in the lower brain stem results in muscle atrophy and weakness (amyotrophy). Demyelination and gliosis of the corticospinal tracts and corticobulbar tracts caused by degeneration of the Betz cells in the motor cortex result in upper motor neuron symptoms (lateral sclerosis).

Diagnosis of ALS depends primarily on the identification of a constellation of motor system changes. Little is known about the early changes occurring in the motor neurons; however, histologically, extensive neuronal loss with astrocytic gliosis occurs. Some neurons seem to remain intact, whereas others show nonspecific cytoplasmic and nuclear shrinkage associated with the accumulation of lipofuscin.[1-3] The differential diagnosis for ALS is extensive. The possibility of cervical or lumbar spondylosis, syringomyelia, multiple sclerosis, and diseases associated with lower motor neuron diseases, among other diagnoses, needs to be excluded.[4]

ALS is the most common form of motor neuron disease, with an incidence of approximately 3 to 5 cases per 100,000 persons. Mean age at onset is 57 years, with two thirds of patients aged 50 to 70 years old at time of onset.[5] Men are affected 1.5 to two times more frequently than are women.[1] Ninety percent to 95% of cases are classified as sporadic, with 5% to 10% of cases classified as a familial form of ALS.[6] The clinical presentation of the familial form is identical to that of the patients with a sporadic form of ALS.[7] ALS occurs approximately as often as muscular dystrophy and is three times more common than is myasthenia gravis.[8]

The cause of ALS is unknown; however, numerous theories have been proposed. Toxic theories related to increased lead and aluminum levels and abnormalities in calcium and magnesium levels have been suggested,[1] as have a deficiency of nerve growth factor, hypersensitivity or abnormal expression of glutamate transport in the CNS, and an autoimmune process.[9] A viral origin for ALS has been proposed by Berger et al,[5] who identified traces of a virus in the spinal cord tissue of 15 of 17 patients who died of ALS but in only one of 29 patients who died of other causes; however, no clear viral or bacterial source has been implicated. Mutations in the superoxide dismutase (SOD1) gene, located on chromosome 21, leading to a gain of toxic properties, have been identified as a cause of the motoneuron

Neuromuscular diseases

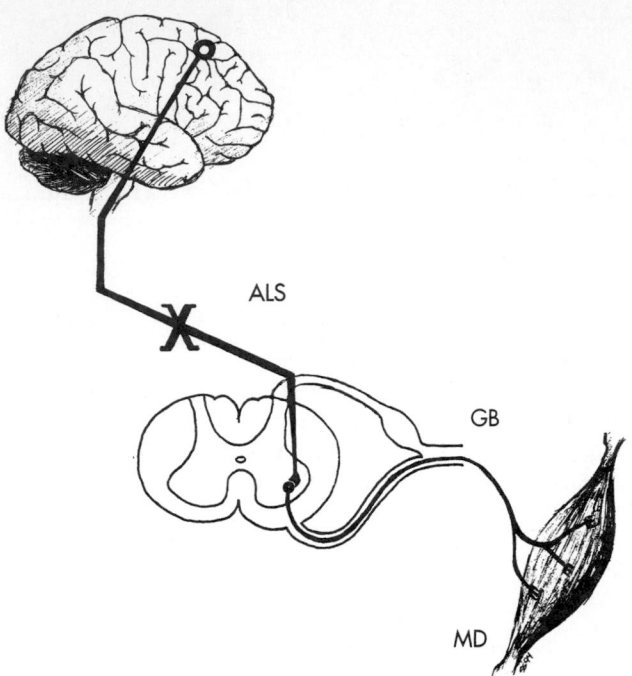

ALS

GB

MD

FIGURE 16-1 ■ Primary sites of pathological features of ALS, GBS *(GB)*, and DMD *(MD)*.

degeneration evident in 10% of patients with the familial form of ALS.[6] Current research supports the view that mitochondrial damage, which heralds the preclinical onset and early stages of ALS, and oxidative stress and aberrations in the excitotoxicity pathways may be implicated as components in the complex pathways leading to the programmed cell/neuronal death (apoptosis).[10-13] The apoptosis is triggered by the activity of the caspases, enzymes that cleave apart essential cell proteins.

No single laboratory test is currently available to confirm a diagnosis of ALS, although creatine phosphokinase levels are elevated in approximately 70% of patients.[2] Genetic testing to identify the mutation in the *Cu, Zn SOD1* gene is available when a family history of ALS is present. Other laboratory tests, such as identification of biochemical markers in the blood and cerebrospinal fluid, and neuroimaging techniques are used to exclude other neurological diseases. Electromyography (EMG) and nerve conduction studies can be helpful to confirm the presence of widespread lower motor neuron disease without peripheral neuropathy or polyradiculopathy. Nerve conduction velocities of patients with ALS are usually within normal limits. EMG studies typically show spontaneous fibrillations and fasciculations with giant or large unit spikes with voluntary activity.[1,14,15] Magnetic resonance imaging shows evidence of Wallerian degeneration of both the corticospinal and corticobulbar tracts.[10] Because of the absence of clear laboratory markers of ALS, the clinical diagnosis must be made on the basis of recognition of a pattern of observed and reported symptoms and persistent declines in physical functions supported by inclusionary and exclusionary diagnostic testing.

Clinical Presentation

The World Federation of Neurology (WFN) has developed suggested diagnostic criteria (suspected, possible, probable, and definite) for patients with ALS entering clinical research trials. Essentially, a patient with "definite" ALS must show concomitant upper motor neuron and lower motor neuron signs in three spinal regions or in two spinal regions with bulbar signs. Either upper or lower motor signs must also be evident in other regions of the body.[16,17] Exclusionary criteria are oculomotor nerve pathway abnormalities, significant movement disorder patterns, sphincter control problems, the presence of sensory and autonomic nervous system (ANS) dysfunction, and cognitive deterioration.[14,18] (Refer to the World Federation of Neurology Amyotrophic Lateral Sclerosis site, section on Guidelines and Rating Scales, www.wfnals.org/guidelines/index.html, for diagnostic criteria used for clinical studies.[19])

Although a consistent diagnostic criterion for ALS has been the absence of sensory involvement, several researchers have reported that a small percentage of patients have shown possible dysfunction in somatosensory evoked potentials transmitted in the posterior columns.[20,21] In addition to the possible sensory deficits, subclinical abnormalities of the ANS, both sympathetic and parasympathetic, have been identified in 34 of 74 patients with ALS. The authors suggested that the problems appear to be associated with atrophy and bulbar changes, and that this subgroup of patients may have a faster rate of progression.[22] (See Rowland[17] and Belsh[14] for succinct reviews of the differential diagnosis for ALS.)

Similarly, cognitive deficits are considered exclusionary criteria for an ALS diagnosis. However, a small subgroup of patients with both familial and sporadic forms of ALS has been identified as having evidence of frontotemporal dementia (FTD). A combination of ALS and FTD suggests a common cause may be possible.[23] Because of these findings, therapists should be aware of the possibility of cognitive deficits in their ALS patients associated with a decrement in executive skills, such as planning, organization, and language problems. This small subgroup of patients may have more difficulty following through on medication and therapeutic recommendations, and their families may need more support.

The earliest clinical markers heralding ALS are fasciculations (especially unequivocal fasciculation in the tongue), muscle cramps, fatigue, weakness, and atrophy.[17,24] During initial diagnostic visits, patients frequently report to their physicians a profound sense of fatigue or the loss of exercise tolerance.[24] Ninety percent of patients reported weakness occurring in a striated muscle or group of muscles. Because the onset of ALS is insidious, most patients are not aware of the strength changes, or they have adjusted to the changes until they have difficulty with a functional activity such as tying shoes or climbing stairs. Physical examination usually demonstrates more widespread weakness and atrophy than reported by the patient.[1,8,20] By the time most patients report weakness, they have lost approximately 80% of their motor neurons in the areas of weakness. This demonstrates the plasticity of the nervous system and its drive to adapt to meet functional goals. The weakness spreads over time to include musculature throughout the body. Succeeding symptoms of weakness in other muscles depend on the continued loss of motor neurons to the 20% threshold needed for perception of weakness.[25,26] A typical, but not absolute, pattern of motor progression is early distal involvement followed by proximal limb involvement. In some cases bulbar symptoms herald the onset of ALS, but bulbar symptoms more commonly occur later in the disease. Flexor muscles tend to be weaker than extensor muscles.[27]

Although the atrophy and weakness component of ALS is most obvious, 80% or more of patients show early clinical evidence of pyramidal tract dysfunction (e.g., hyperreflexia in the presence of weakness and atrophy, spasticity, and Babinski and Hoffman reflexes).[17,20] Although in some cases the upper motor neuron signs may be absent clinically, Chou[28] has shown on autopsy that significant involvement may be present despite the lack of clinical evidence.

The pattern of ALS onset is highly varied, with several patterns identified by primary area of onset. Lower-extremity onset is slightly more common than upper-extremity onset, which is more common than bulbar onset. Some patients show initial symptoms in distal musculature of upper and lower extremities. A significant diagnostic feature of the pattern of disease is the asymmetry of the weakness and the sparing of some muscle fibers even in highly atrophied muscles. For example, a patient may present with weakness of the right intrinsics and shoulder musculature or weakness of the left anterior tibial muscles. Bulbar symptoms are presaged by tongue fasciculations and weakness, facial and palatal weakness, and swallowing difficulties, which result in dysphagia and dysarthria. Oculomotor nuclei are almost always spared.[1] Despite the pattern of onset, however, the eventual course of the illness is similar in most patients, with an unremitting spread of weakness to other muscle groups leading to total paralysis of spinal musculature and muscles innervated by the cranial nerves. Death is usually related to respiratory failure.[29]

In a multisite study of 167 patients with ALS, subjects were followed up for 2 years on a monthly basis with 42 strength and functional assessments. Data confirmed findings of other studies that showed a more rapid loss of strength in the upper extremities than in the lower extremities. No difference was found between men or women in the rate of progression. In contrast to other studies, results indicated that older patients did not show a faster rate of deterioration, although they did enter the study in a weaker, more debilitated state, which may be related to their apparent shorter disease course.[29] In an ongoing study using monthly questionnaires, direct patient interviews, record reviews, physician interviews, and family member interviews, Brooks et al[25] followed 702 patients with ALS. Their findings suggest that spread of neuronal degeneration occurred more quickly to adjacent areas than to noncontiguous areas. The spread to adjacent areas was more rapid at the brain stem, cervical, and lumbar regions. Limb involvement after bulbar onset was more aggressive in men than in women.[25]

One study focused on developing methods to assess the natural history of the progression of ALS so that medical and supportive treatment planning and interventions can be instituted.[30] Hillel et al[31,32] have developed the ALS Severity Scale for rapid functional assessment of disease stage. Their 10-point ordinal scale allows clinicians and therapists to score patients in four categories of function: speech, swallowing, lower extremity, and upper extremity (Box 16-1).

A five-point scale of severity is currently being used in ALS clinical drug trials. Patients in stage 1 (mild disease) have a recent diagnosis and are functionally independent in ambulation, activities of daily living (ADLs), and speech. Stage 2 (moderate) identifies patients with mild deficits in function in three regions or a moderate to severe deficit in one region and mild or normal function in two other regions.

BOX 16-1 ■ AMYOTROPHIC LATERAL SCLEROSIS SEVERITY SCALE: LOWER EXTREMITY, UPPER EXTREMITY, SPEECH, SWALLOWING

LOWER EXTREMITIES (WALKING)

Normal

10	Normal ambulation	Patient denies any weakness or fatigue; examination detects no abnormality.
9	Fatigue suspected	Patient experiences sense of weakness or fatigue in lower extremities during exertion.

Early Ambulation Difficulties

8	Difficulty with uneven terrain	Difficulty and fatigue when walking long distances, climbing stairs, and walking over uneven ground (even thick carpet).
7	Observed changes in gait	Noticeable change in gait; pulls on railings when climbing stairs; may use leg brace.

Walks with Assistance

6	Walks with mechanical device	Needs or uses cane, walker, or assistant to walk; probably uses wheelchair away from home.
5	Walks with mechanical device and assistant	Does not attempt to walk without attendant; ambulation limited to less than 50 ft; avoids stairs.

Functional Movement Only

4	Able to support	At best, can shuffle a few steps with the help of an attendant for transfers.
3	Purposeful leg movements	Unable to take steps but can position legs to assist attendant in transfers; moves legs purposely to maintain mobility in bed.

No Purposeful Leg Movement

2	Minimal movement	Minimal movement of one or both legs; cannot reposition legs independently.
1	Paralysis	Flaccid paralysis; cannot move lower extremities (except, perhaps, to close inspection).

Continued

BOX 16-1 ■ AMYOTROPHIC LATERAL SCLEROSIS SEVERITY SCALE: LOWER EXTREMITY, UPPER EXTREMITY, SPEECH, SWALLOWING—cont'd

UPPER EXTREMITIES (DRESSING AND HYGIENE)

Normal Function

10 Normal function — Patient denies any weakness or unusual fatigue of upper extremities; examination demonstrates no abnormality.

9 Suspected fatigue — Patient experiences sense of fatigue in upper extremities during exertion; cannot sustain work for as long as normal; atrophy not evident on examination.

Independent and Complete Self-Care

8 Slow self-care — Dressing and hygiene performed more slowly than usual.

7 Effortful self-care performance — Requires significantly more time (usually double or more) and effort to accomplish self-care; weakness is apparent on examination.

Intermittent Assistance

6 Mostly independent — Handles most aspects of dressing and hygiene alone; adapts by resting, modifying (e.g., use of electric razor), or avoiding some tasks; requires assistance for fine motor tasks (e.g., buttons, ties).

5 Partial independence — Handles some aspects of dressing and hygiene alone; however, routinely requires assistance for many tasks such as applying makeup, combing, and shaving.

Needs Attendant for Self-Care

4 Attendant assists patient — Attendant must be present for dressing and hygiene; patient performs the majority of each task with the assistance of the attendant.

3 Patient assists attendant — The attendant directs the patient for almost all tasks; the patient moves in a purposeful manner to assist the attendant; does not initiate self-care.

Total Dependence

2 Minimal movement — Minimal movement of one or both arms; cannot reposition arms.

1 Paralysis — Flaccid paralysis; unable to move upper extremities (except, perhaps, to close inspection).

SPEECH

Normal Speech Processes

10 Normal speech — Patient denies any difficulty speaking; examination demonstrates no abnormality.

9 Nominal speech abnormalities — Only the patient or spouse notices speech has changed; maintains normal rate and volume.

Detectable Speech Disturbance

8 Perceived speech changes — Speech changes are noted by others, especially during fatigue or stress; rate of speech remains essentially normal.

7 Obvious speech abnormalities — Speech is consistently impaired; rate, articulation, and resonance are affected; remains easily understood.

Intelligible with Repeating

6 Repeats message on occasion — Rate is much slower, repeats specific words in adverse listening situation; does not limit complexity or length of messages.

5 Frequent repeating required — Speech is slow and labored; extensive repetition or a "translator" is commonly used; patient probably limits the complexity or length of messages.

Speech Combined with Nonvocal Communication

4 Speech plus nonverbal communication — Speech is used in response to questions; intelligibility problems need to be resolved by writing or a spokesman.

3 Limits speech to one-word responses — Vocalizes one-word responses beyond yes/no; otherwise writes or uses a spokesperson; initiates communication nonvocally.

Loss of Useful Speech

2 Vocalizes for emotional expression — Uses vocal inflection to express emotion, affirmation, and negation.

1 Nonvocal — Vocalization is effortful, limited in duration, and rarely attempted; may vocalize for crying or pain.

X Tracheostomy

SWALLOWING

Normal Eating Habits

10 Normal swallowing — Patient denies any difficulty chewing or swallowing; examination demonstrates no abnormality.

9 Nominal abnormality — Only patient notices slight indicators such as food lodging in the recesses of the mouth or sticking in the throat.

BOX 16-1 ■ AMYOTROPHIC LATERAL SCLEROSIS SEVERITY SCALE: LOWER EXTREMITY, UPPER EXTREMITY, SPEECH, SWALLOWING—cont'd

Early Eating Problems

8 Minor swallowing problems

Reports some swallowing difficulties; maintains essentially a regular diet; isolated choking episodes.

7 Prolonged times/smaller bite size

Meal time has significantly increased and smaller bite sizes are necessary; must concentrate on swallowing thin liquids.

Dietary Consistency Changes

6 Soft diet

Diet is limited primarily to soft foods; requires some special meal preparation.

5 Liquefied diet

Oral intake adequate; nutrition limited primarily to liquefied diet; adequate thin liquid intake usually a problem; may force self to eat.

Needs Tube Feeding

4 Supplemental tube feedings

Oral intake alone no longer adequate; patient uses or needs a tube to supplement intake; patient continues to take significant (greater than 50%) nutrition orally.

3 Tube feeding with occasional oral nutrition

Primary nutrition and hydration accomplished by tube; receives less than 50% of nutrition orally.

No Oral Feeding

2 Secretions managed with aspirator and/or medications

Cannot safely manage any oral intake; secretions managed with aspirator and/or medications; swallows reflexively.

1 Aspiration of secretions

Secretions cannot be managed noninvasively; rarely swallows.

Adapted with permission from Hillel AD, Miller RM, Yorkston K, et al: Amyotrophic lateral sclerosis severity scale, *Neuroepidemiology* 8:142, 1989.

Stage 3 (severe) defines patients who need assistance because of deficits in two or three regions; for example, the patient needs assistance to walk or transfer, needs help with upper-extremity activities, and/or is dysarthric/dysphasic. Stage 4 identifies patients with nonfunctional use of at least two regions and moderate or nonfunctional use of a third area. Stage 5 is death.[27] (See Brooks[16] and Pradas et al[33] for information on the natural history of ALS and its importance in the design of clinical treatment trials.)

Medical Prognosis

In almost all cases ALS progresses relentlessly and leads to death from respiratory failure. The rate of progression seems to be consistent for each patient but varies considerably among patients. Patients with an initial onset of bulbar (dysarthria, dysphagia) and respiratory weakness (dyspnea) tend to have a more rapid progression to death than patients whose weakness begins in the distal extremities.[29] Caroscio[1] reported that in a study of 397 patients with ALS, the median survival time was 4.08 years after onset of symptoms, with a shortening of median survival time with increasing age at onset. A small number of patients have lived for 15 to 20 years after onset. Although time of onset is determined primarily by the patient's recognition of the disease manifestations, autopsies of patients who have died of respiratory failure soon after diagnosis have shown evidence of more widespread disease in the skeletal musculature even though no clinical evidence was present of skeletal muscle involvement.[20] Years of survival after diagnosis may change as drug therapies are developed.[34] In addition, increasing numbers of patients are electing to prolong life with home-based mechanical ventilation as opposed to palliative or comfort care only.

Medical Management

ALS has no known cure and no known treatment. Drug therapies under investigation include gabapentin (to decrease the synthesis of glutamate); supplemental doses of tocopherol (vitamin E), an antioxidant and free-radical scavenger; and insulinlike growth factors (rhIGF-1).[34] The use of viral vectors to introduce gene products into the CNS is also under investigation. Recently, however, several multicenter drug treatment trials with riluzole have shown slight evidence of a positive effect on the length of survival (several months), although the effect is marginal.[35-37] Riluzole, a drug that inhibits the presynaptic release of glutamate, is the first drug approved by the U.S. Food and Drug Administration (FDA) for use with ALS. Strict monitoring of liver enzymes is necessary for patients on riluzole.[38] Most recently, investigators are identifying the relation between cell death pathways and novel drug treatments to inhibit apoptosis, such as antiinflammatory drugs, which have been shown to slow cell death in rat models of ALS. Double-blind studies of minocycline, an antiinflammatory drug, are currently underway.[39] On the basis of mouse model findings, a large multicenter trial of celecoxib (Celebrex) with 300 patients with ALS randomly assigned to three groups was undertaken. The study consortium released findings stating that celecoxib did not have a demonstrated beneficial effect on the disease process of patients with ALS at the dosages used.[40]

The popular press has reported on nutritional cures for ALS. Recently, Ascherio et al,[41] studying the relation between oxidative stress and ALS by using data from a large cancer study, found an association suggesting that regular use of vitamin E may have a role in ALS prevention. However, Graf et al[42] and Orrell et al,[43] in a literature review of studies related to use of vitamin E and ALS, found insufficient evidence to support clinical use of vitamin E supplements as an additive to riluzole treatment or as adjunctive therapy, although no apparent contraindication was found to taking the supplement.

Cannabis has been studied in its effect on spasticity in patients with multiple sclerosis and spinal cord injury. In a study of 131 people with ALS, 13 used cannabis. This small group showed evidence that spasticity and pain and depression were reduced.[44] A novel treatment intervention with repetitive transcranial magnetic stimulation (rTMS) of the brain was tested on transgenic rats and four patients with ALS.[45] The therapeutic effect of low-frequency rTMS was postulated to diminish glutamate-driven excitotoxicity, which may be related to apoptosis in ALS. In preliminary results, two patients with ALS treated with low-frequency rTMS of the brain may have had slower rates of progression after treatment than before treatment. The rTMS treatment had no effect on the transgenic rats. Controlled human trials will be essential.[46]

Because of the apparent hopelessness of the diagnosis, many physicians, especially those not associated with major medical centers having neuromuscular disease units, do not refer patients with ALS for services. In a survey of ALS patients, 90% stated that their referring neurologists made no referrals or follow-up appointments. Most patients had been told to expect death within 1 to 3 years, although evidence shows that the median life span is approximately 4 years. Some physicians are concerned that providing aggressive treatment will only increase or prolong the patient's distress.[47] Other physicians, however, believe that withholding care and symptom relief seriously impairs the patient's quality of life.[48] Supportive medical and therapy interventions are available.[49,50] Some evidence exists to suggest that treatment in a multidisciplinary center improves prognosis over patients monitored by a single practitioner.[51]

Muscle Spasms and Pain

Some patients experience muscle cramps and spasms related to the upper motor neuron changes. Although most spasms can be relieved with stretching or increased movement, some patients require medications such as quinine or baclofen to relieve symptoms (see Chapter 36 for information on drug therapies). In a review of studies on the treatment of spasticity in ALS, Ashworth et al[52] found one randomized study showing that an exercise regimen decreased spasticity at 3 months after initiation of the program. Kesiktas et al[53] reports that in a controlled study of spasticity in patients after spinal cord injury, adding hydrotherapy to a program of medication and exercise decreased severity of spasms and decreased the amount of medication required. A similar response could be hypothesized in patients with ALS. In addition to muscle spasms, patients report nonspecific aching and muscle soreness, probably related to immobility and trauma to paralyzed muscles during caregiving procedures. However, many patients do not receive adequate pain medication, or the pain is not controlled by the medication taken.[54] Because many patients have compromised respiratory function, the physician must take great care when prescribing pain medication, especially opiates. Patients should be instructed to keep a daily reporting log of the effectiveness of the medication so that the dosage can be adjusted if necessary.[55]

Dysphagia

Dysphagia, a difficulty swallowing liquids, foods, or saliva, accounts for considerable misery in the patient with advanced ALS, and it must be dealt with aggressively.[56,57] Patients with dysphagia present with both nutritional and swallowing problems associated with weakness of the lips, tongue, palate, and mastication muscles.[58] As the progressive loss of swallowing develops, patients are also at extreme risk for aspiration. Most patients with dysphagia also have severe problems with management of their saliva (sialorrhea). Normal average flow is approximately 1 ml/min from the parotid, submaxillary, sublingual, and minor salivary glands. With stimulation, this amount can increase to 8 ml/min. If a patient has difficulty transporting saliva back to the oropharynx for swallowing, choking and drooling are common.[57] This condition is disconcerting to the affected person, who must constantly wipe the mouth or have someone do it for him or her.

In addition, secretions are often thickened because of dehydration. With pooling of the thickened saliva, the possibility of aspiration is increased. Viscosity of saliva can best be treated by hydration and, in some cases, with tablets that contain papain and bromelain, the enzymes in papaya that are used in meat tenderizer. Drugs such as decongestants, antidepressant drugs with anticholinergic side effects, and atropine-type drugs have been used to help control the amount of saliva, provided the patient is well hydrated.[59] In extreme cases, various surgical procedures such as ligation of the salivary gland ducts, severing the parasympathetic supply to the salivary glands, and excision of the salivary glands have been used effectively.[60-62] Newer treatments to decrease excessive secretions are radiotherapy and botulin A toxin injections into salivary glands.[63]

Although dietary treatment is not known to be effective in changing the course of the disease, a nutritious diet to meet caloric, fluid, vitamin, and mineral needs must be maintained. Seventy-three percent of patients with ALS have difficulty bringing food to the mouth, making them dependent on others for their dietary needs. Because of the time it takes to be fed, many patients decrease their intake. All patients with dysphagia should be referred for a dietary consultation to determine the choice and progression of solid and liquid foods and supplements. Appel et al[64] describe nutritional plans to maintain nutrition and hydration in patients with motor neuron diseases. The ALS Association also publishes manuals on dealing with swallowing problems.[65] Patients with bulbar symptoms and severe dysphagia who are no longer able to consume nutrients orally because of motor control problems and recurrent aspiration may need placement of a percutaneous endoscopic gastrostomy (PEG), depending on the patient's wishes for long-term care.[66] Although placement of a PEG does not appreciably lengthen survival time,[67] patients may have less fear of choking or aspiration. The number of patients choosing to have a PEG has increased since 1989, with a decrease in 1-month mortality rates after PEG placement because of better patient selection. Placement of a PEG does not prevent the person from taking food orally if desired.

Aspiration can be the cause of sudden death in the patient with ALS, although it is not common. With mild aspiration problems in a patient who is still able and wants to eat, dietary changes and instruction in swallowing techniques by speech, occupational, or physical therapists can be helpful. Techniques as simple as changing the eating position, head position, or the temperature, texture, or viscosity of the food may lengthen the time that the patient can enjoy eating safely.[68]

Dysarthria

Dysarthria, impairment in speech production, is the result of abnormal function of the muscles and nerves associated with coordinated functions of the tongue and lips, larynx, soft palate, and respiratory system. Speech impairments are the initial symptom in most patients with bulbar involvement. Speech intelligibility is compromised by hypernasality, abnormalities of speed and cadence of speech, and reduced vocal volume. Speech is further compromised by inadequate breath volumes for normal phrasing. A possible option to help patients with severe hypernasality is a palatal lift prosthesis to augment velopharyngeal function.[69,70] Because little can be done medically to delay the loss of speech control, early referral to a speech therapist is essential. Numerous augmentative communication systems are now available, the simplest being voice amplification systems or homemade point boards. For some patients, computer-based communication devices adapted to the needs of the patient—single-finger pointing or eye-pointing systems that can translate typed words into voiced words—are useful.[71]

Respiratory Management

Progressive respiratory failure is the primary cause of death in ALS patients. Respiratory failure is related to primary diaphragmatic, intercostal, and accessory respiratory muscle weakness; decreased pulmonary compliance; a weak cough; and bulbar symptoms such as a decreased gag reflex with aspiration.[72] Physiological factors indicating respiratory failure are vital capacity and maximal voluntary inspiratory and expiratory ventilation of 30% of predicted or less, hypoxemia, mild hypercapnia, and acidosis. Clinical signs are dyspnea with exertion or lying supine; hypoventilation; weak or ineffective cough; increased use of auxiliary respiratory muscles; tachycardia (also a sign of pulmonary infection with fever and tachypnea); changes in sleep pattern; daytime sleepiness and concentration problems; mood changes; morning headaches; and diffuse pain in the head, neck, and extremities. Chronic respiratory insufficiency should be assessed with tests of standing and supine forced vital capacity, or transcutaneous nocturnal oximetry may be necessary to determine oxygen saturation levels. Scheduled, serial evaluations of respiratory status are essential so that the patient and the treatment team can make informed decisions about appropriate treatment relative to both acute illnesses and progressive respiratory difficulties.[72,73]

Approximately half the patients with ALS have dyspnea as a secondary symptom of an acute respiratory illness. Concurrent infection and disease that may respond to medication or short-term respiratory support measures must be ruled out and treatment or nontreatment, as desired by the patient, should be initiated. Early involvement of respiratory or pulmonary physical therapists is advantageous. Physical therapists may be involved in the treatment of gradual respiratory failure by providing postural drainage with cough facilitation (suctioning if necessary), especially during acute respiratory illnesses. The patient and care providers should also be taught breathing exercises, chest stretching, and incentive spirometry techniques.[72] An assessment of the home environment is imperative to identify sleeping positions and energy conservation techniques that can be incorporated into the patient's daily life.

As respiratory symptoms increase, oxygen at 2 L/min or less can be used intermittently at home. When hypoventilation with a decline in oxygen saturation becomes common during sleep, resulting in morning confusion and irritability, patients have the option to initiate noninvasive, positive-pressure ventilation such as bilevel positive airway pressure (BiPAP). BiPAP, which provides greater inspiratory pressure than expiratory pressure to decrease the effort of breathing, can be administered by either mask or contoured nasal delivery systems. Some evidence indicates that early use of noninvasive ventilation (NIV) can increase survival time by several months; however, some indication exists that the patient's functional vital capacity (FVC) decreases more rapidly after beginning BiPAP.[74,75] To determine the best time to initiate BiPAP, Pinto et al[76] suggest measurement of diurnal respiratory insufficiency with nocturnal pulse oximetry. Tracheostomy or death is likely once the baseline pulse oximetry saturation indicates frequent episodes of desaturation throughout the day and night.[77]

When a patient can no longer benefit from NIV, a decision must be made about initiating ventilation by tracheostomy or palliative care.[78] (See Miller et al[79] for an excellent discussion of practice parameters in the decision-making process related to ventilatory support.) Although in the initial stages of ALS most patients indicate they would not want prolonged respirator dependence at home, patients may change their minds as they adapt to the disease restrictions.[80] Oliver[73] states that when counseling patients about outcome and treatment options, the "aim should be to avoid inappropriate treatment, which could cause harm to the patient, may merely prolong a poor quality of life and could lead to further distress." In a study of 121 patients, Albert et al[81] determined that patients with slower disease progression tended to choose technological interventions less often than patients with more aggressively progressive disease. In their study, preferences stated early after diagnosis predicted later treatment decisions; however, only a few patients expressed a preference for any specific intervention.

Decisions about long-term respirator use should be made by the patient and involved family members or partners, with input from the interdisciplinary team caring for the patient. Discussions of preferred long-term care options should be revisited as the patient's condition changes. However, lurking in the decision-making process are ethical considerations, especially those related to the relation between patient autonomy or self-determination and justice as well as the secondary family and societal effects associated with any decision about long-term technological interventions. For example, Lechtzin et al[82] have shown that lower income patients are less likely to use supported ventilation, which brings into question possible disparities in health care. (See Russell[83] for references on studies of ethical issues in the treatment of ALS.)

If a patient decides that home ventilation is a reasonable option, those involved in the decision should visit another patient who is using in-home mechanical ventilation, if possible.[84] Because the decision for home mechanical ventilation (HMV) also affects the life of the patient's spouse, children, and extended family who may be responsible for some aspects of home care, or whose lives may be affected by the presence of in-home nurses or attendants, the decision for HMV should not be taken lightly. Extensive preparation, ongoing support, and respite options for caregivers are necessary if HMV is to be successful. Success of HMV also depends on such variables as third-party payment for home care equipment and nurse/attendant staffing, working status of the partner/spouse, age and physical fitness of spouse and children, pre-ALS family psychosocial interactions, and financial factors. HMV should be viewed as long term, often extending for more than 1 year. Initiation of HMV results in a reasonable perceived quality of life for the patient, yet caregivers report that their quality of life may be lower than the patient's because of the burden of care that must be provided.[85]

In a Kaiser Foundation Hospital program from 1987 to 1992, 34 patients with ALS were discharged to HMV. On average, the patients were on the ventilator 23 hours per day and needed 24-hour, 7-day-a-week care (at least three trained caregivers per week).[86] Eighty-seven percent of the patients were alive at the end of 1 year, 58% at the end of 3 years, and 33% at the end of 5 years. Less than 25% of the ALS patients in the Kaiser study had elected HMV in advance of the decision to begin ventilator assistance.[84]

With chronic respiratory insufficiency, the patient and family must be involved in the long-term care decisions related to instituting mechanical assistance under either emergency situations or in response to gradual deterioration. This discussion should occur before the patient develops respiratory failure (see Chapter 35). Acute respiratory failure can be so frightening, however, that few patients or family members are prepared to forego intubation and artificial ventilation during the emergency. Patients and caregivers should understand that *not* making a decision about mechanical ventilation, noninvasive or invasive, is a decision to support mechanical ventilation.[87] A patient who arrives at an emergency department in severe respiratory distress will be placed on ventilation unless documentation is provided to withhold treatment and provide comfort care only. If patients have stated that they do not want mechanical ventilation, appropriate use of medications such as morphine can markedly control the person's sense of air hunger during the dying process.[73]

Although NIV and HMV are known options for patients at end-stage ALS, a new pilot clinical trial is underway in a small group of patients with ALS.[88] The investigators hope to determine if a laparoscopically placed "diaphragm pacing system can provide stimulation to the diaphragm to maintain its strength and potentially help with the breathing problems associated with ALS." These patients, however, have atrophy of the diaphragm secondary to degeneration of phrenic nerves, so effectiveness of the treatment to support respiration is questionable. However, stimulation may delay the need to use positive pressure breathing systems.

Physicians and health care workers who work with the patient and family must be aware of their own feelings and beliefs about prolonging life. For example, a healthy physician or therapist who values control and an active lifestyle may envision a life on a ventilator as intolerable and pass that value on to the patient, who may or may not have the same needs. The patient's decision, or change in decision, must be respected by the medical team involved in care.[89] In medical centers that use a team approach, patients and families may find support by meeting with counselors or peers with ALS who are making or have made decisions about long-term ventilator care.

Therapeutic Management of Impairments and Activity Limitations

When determining therapeutic goals and treatment, the rate of the patient's disease progression, the extent and areas of involvement, and the stage of illness must be considered. This is particularly important today considering the increasing number of patients choosing NIV or tracheostomy ventilation, which may extend life span. Patients with severe respiratory and bulbar complications may not benefit as greatly from active exercise programs. The goal in the end stages, however, is to optimize health and increase the quality of life. With guidance and environmental adaptations, patients with slowly progressing weakness may be able to continue many of their ADLs for an extended number of years. In the final stages of the disease, when the patient is bedridden, physical or occupational therapy interventions such as stretching may not effectively control contractures. However, patients may benefit from range of motion (ROM) exercises to decrease muscle and joint pain related to immobility. The efficacy of therapeutic interventions is also related to the timing of interventions, the motivation and persistence of the patient in carrying out the program, and support from family members.[90]

Evaluation

The extent of the therapeutic evaluation of a patient with ALS may depend on whether the therapist is working as a member of a neuromuscular team or as an independent or clinic-based therapist receiving a referral to evaluate and treat. Physical and occupational therapists working as team members may have a more circumscribed role related to gross motor function and ADLs, with other consultants focusing on bulbar, respiratory, and environmental adjustments. The therapist working in a facility without a neuromuscular disease clinic or in a community or rural environment, however, should be aware of the need to carry out a broad-based assessment. In addition to the standard neuromuscular, musculoskeletal, and functional level examinations, the therapist should also evaluate the patient's stated or observed functional problems relative to bulbar and respiratory impairments, environmental blocks to independence, and caregiving demands. Evidence exists to suggest that patients treated by a multidisciplinary team fare better than do those treated by single-source providers.[91]

Before the patient's initial visit, the therapist should contact the patient and request that he or she keep an activity log for 5 days. If an early contact is not possible, the therapist can assign that task during the initial session. The log should include 15-minute time increments in which the patient or caregiver can record what she or he was doing during a specific period. Space also should be included to indicate whether the patient was experiencing fatigue or pain during the activity and how the patient perceived her or his respiratory status. An example of an activity log and how it is used is shown in Figure 16-2. The sense of fatigue with

Name: J. Costello

DATE: 5 - 10 - 00
DAY: Saturday

DAILY ACTIVITY LOG

Instructions: 1) In column I write in what you are doing during the 24 hour period. You may draw a line or an arrow to indicate when the activity occurs for more than one 15 minute time period.

2) In column II indicate whether you are lying down, sitting, standing, or moving actively (walking, etc.) during the activity.

3) In column III on a 10 point scale, indicate how fatigued you feel while performing the activity (No fatigue = 0, extreme fatigue = 10.)

4) In column IV indicate where you feel pain if any and score the intensity on a 10 point scale (No pain = 0, extreme pain = 10.)

Try to fill out your log three or four times a day so you don't forget what you have been doing. An example is shown below.

	I What are you doing? Type of activity	II What position are you in (lying, sitting, standing, moving)	III Fatigue level 0 – 10	IV Pain Location	IV Pain Intensity 0 – 10
5:30 AM	Sleep	lying	0		
45					
6:00					
15					
30	Bathroom	standing	2	neck	3
45	Shave, etc				
7:00					
15	Breakfast	sitting	3	neck	3
30					
45					
8:00	Reading	sitting	3	neck	3
15				shoulder	
30					
45	walk	standing, walking	4	neck	2
9:00					
15	nap				
30		lying	2	neck	4
45			1	hips	1
10:00	Reading/TV	sitting	4	neck	3
15				hips	
30					
45	walk	standing, walking	5	hips	3
11:00					

FIGURE 16-2 ■ Example of a log for monitoring activity level of patients with ALS.

repetitive muscle activity or functional activity should be specifically tracked by the patient. Later, the therapist who is assessing muscle strength should keep in mind that muscle weakness and the experience of fatigue may be independent measures of ALS pathology.[92]

The therapist's evaluation will vary depending on the patient's situation; however, a typical initial assessment may include the following:

■ Review of the patient's medical and activity record
■ Discussion of the patient's lifestyle, ADL tasks, hobbies or interests, work focus, respiratory status, fatigability, safety issues, psychosocial support issues (family and agencies), and patient concerns and goals
■ Baseline testing of muscle strength (manual muscle testing or electronic handheld dynamometer testing if standards are clear and can be replicated) and ROM assessment
■ Evaluation of functional activity level (a standardized test or assessment tool is preferable)
■ Examination of pain (type, site, and intensity; use body chart and subjective pain scale); identify what makes pain worse or better
■ Evaluation of bulbar and respiratory function (For an in-depth evaluation of bulbar function, the patient should be referred to an ear, nose, and throat clinic or communications disorders clinic unless full evaluation is available in a comprehensive ALS clinic. See Table 16-1 for bulbar and respiratory evaluation suggestions.)

Therapists who work in a clinic environment with a number of patients with ALS or other motor neuron disease should refer to the WFN's Research Group on Neuromuscular Diseases *Guidelines for the Use and Performance of Quantitative Outcome Measures in ALS Clinical Trials.* This excellent document, available at the WFN website,[93] identifies standards for assessment in clinical trials. However, the review of recommended tests and measurements is extremely valuable for any therapist assessing and treating patients with neuromuscular diseases.

Therapeutic Intervention Goals

Intervention goals and the recommended exercise/activity program designed by physical or occupational therapists must be based on the patient's personal goals. Goals are often a difficult area for therapists to discuss with the patient because both know that the disease is progressive despite interventions. Patients, therapists, and physicians commonly assume that because nothing can be done to "cure" the disease, not making additional demands on a patient who is already coping with daily loss is somehow kinder. Some believe that exercise programs may create false hopes that exercise will delay progression. The literature on rehabilitation in neuromuscular disorders, however, suggests that patients with ALS can benefit from carefully designed exercise and activity programs. Active participation in determining goals for therapy can provide the patient and the family with some sense of control over a difficult situation.[4]

The general, broad goals for both patient and therapist are related to maintaining maximal independence in daily living and a positive quality of life for as long as possible. More specific therapeutic goals are (1) maintenance of mobility and ADLs, to include safety issues for patient and caregiver; (2) maintenance of maximal muscle strength within limits imposed by ALS; (3) prevention and minimization of secondary consequences of the disease, such as contractures, thrombophlebitis, decubitus ulcers, and

TABLE 16-1 ■ Common Physical Findings in Bulbar Amyotrophic Lateral Sclerosis

ANATOMICAL SITE	INNERVATION	METHOD OF EVALUATION	PROGRESSION OF FINDINGS	PROGRESSION OF SYMPTOMS
GROUP I				
Tongue	XII	Inspect for fasciculations at rest	Fasciculations evident	Dysarthria (disturbance of lingual-alveolar consonants "t," "d," "l," etc.)
		Range of motion	Slow, incomplete lateral movements	Inability to clear buccal sulcus of food
			Loss of lateral force	Marked dysarthria (slow rate and slurring of consonants)
			Unable to reach palate with mouth open	
		Protrusion	Unable to protrude beyond lips	Oral transport difficulties
				Dietary changes
		Perform rapid lateral motion	Unable to protrude beyond incisors	Speech intelligibility problems
			Atrophy evident	
			Paralysis	
Lips	VII	Suck on gloved finger	Lack of suction	Inability to whistle
		Smile or curl lips over teeth	Inability to complete a seal	Inability to use a straw
				Dysarthria (loss of bilabial consonants "p" and "b")
		Hold seal and blow out cheeks	Inability to purse lips	Drooling

TABLE 16-1 ■ Common Physical Findings in Bulbar Amyotrophic Lateral Sclerosis—cont'd

ANATOMICAL SITE	INNERVATION	METHOD OF EVALUATION	PROGRESSION OF FINDINGS	PROGRESSION OF SYMPTOMS
GROUP 2				
Palate	V, X, XI	Visual examination during phonation and stimulation of gag. Puff out cheeks to check for nasal air leak (hold lips closed if necessary)	Unsustained or slow palatal elevation. Soft palate fails to reach Passavant's ridge. Absence of palatal movement	Dysarthria (hypernasal speech). Inability to use a straw. Nasal air emission during speech. Nasopharyngeal reflex on swallowing
Muscles of mastication Masseter/temporalis	V	Palpate during bite. Visual inspection for wasting	Noticeable wasting. Unable to palpate contraction	Chewing fatigue. Elimination of specific, tough foods from diet. Dietary changes (soft foods and liquids). Mouth breathing and drying of secretions
Pterygoids		Move jaw from side to side	No observable lateral jaw movement	Unable to use dentures
GROUP 3				
Neck and shoulder	XI			
Trapezius		Hold arm in coronal plane, hand externally rotated, as patient elevates arm against resistance while the trapezius is palpated	Progressive inability to raise the arm (often asymmetrical weakness)	Inability to comb hair. Inability to perform facial grooming
Sternocleidomastoid or mounted head support		Turn the head against resistance applied to opposite side of patient's chin	Progressive weakness in turning the head against resistance (often asymmetrical)	Inability to lift head when supine. Inability to support head while sitting; wears neck collar, has weakness
Vocal cords	X	Mirror or fiberoptic laryngoscopy	Progressive loss of abduction of vocal cords: mild abductor weakness, near-midline paralysis. Paradoxical vocal cord movement	Strained/strangled voice. Short of breath (stridor usually not present because of impaired respiratory function)
GROUP 4				
Extraocular muscles	III, IV, VI	Assessment of extraocular movements	Limitation of extraocular movement	Limitation of gaze
Respiratory group Diaphragm	$C_{3,4,5}$	Pulmonary function test or handheld respirometer for vital capacity	Diminishing vital capacity: 1.5-2.0 L	Shortness of breath during exertion if patient has remained active
Intercostal	C_7-L_3			
Accessory muscles of respiration	VII, XI, XII, C_{5-8}	Cough. Sustain a vowel. Blow against a tissue	1.0-1.5 L	Weak cough. Change in speech phrasing (5-10 syllables per breath)
			0.5-1.0 L	Speech produced in syllable-by-syllable fashion (if vocal). Shortness of breath on swallowing

Adapted with permission from Hillel AD, Miller RM: Bulbar amyotrophic lateral sclerosis: patterns of progression and clinical management, *Head Neck* 11:51-59, 1989. Copyright 1989. Reprinted by permission of John Wiley & Sons, Inc.

respiratory infections[4,90]; (4) management of energy conservation techniques and respiratory comfort; (5) determination of adaptive equipment needs to include mobility, self-help and feeding devices, augmentative communication units, and hygiene equipment that supports both patient and caregiver.[4]

Therapeutic Considerations

To prevent more rapid functional loss than expected by the natural history of the disease, both the patient and therapist must delicately balance the level of activity between the extremes of inadequate exercise and excessive exercise. Two major factors must be considered when planning and implementing an activity or exercise program for patients with ALS: prevention of disuse atrophy and prevention of overuse injury.

Disuse Atrophy. The first consideration for the therapist working with a patient with ALS is to prevent further deconditioning and disuse atrophy beyond the level caused specifically by the disease process. Although no studies have shown a relation between disability and disuse atrophy in persons with ALS, a number of reasons exist as to why it would be plausible. Because ALS is a disease of older adults, patients may not have maintained their aerobic fitness or muscle strength before the onset of their neuromuscular problem.[94] Newly diagnosed patients also commonly report that they had markedly decreased their activity level in the months before diagnosis because of a sense of fatigue or increasing clumsiness. If the patient had led a sedentary lifestyle before diagnosis, the additional decrease in activity level after the onset of ALS can lead quickly to marked cardiovascular deconditioning and disuse weakness.[95,96] The disuse weakness lowers muscle force production and reduces muscle endurance.[97] Disuse atrophy in combination with pathological weakness and spasticity of specific muscle groups contribute to poorly coordinated, less-efficient movements that require more energy expenditure. Disuse atrophy therefore contributes to the patient's level of functional loss and disability (see Chapter 29).

Exercise or Overwork Damage. The second, and perhaps more critical, consideration in designing an intervention program is to do no harm. Anecdotal evidence that muscle activity or overwork exercise can lead to a loss of muscle strength has been reported since the poliomyelitis epidemic of the 1940s and 1950s.[98] During that epidemic, physicians and therapists noted that patients with poor- and fair-grade muscles who exercised repeatedly or with heavy resistance after reinnervation often lost the ability to contract the muscle at all (see Chapter 29).[99]

Reitsma[100] noted that vigorous exercise damaged muscles if less than one third of motor units were functional. If more than one third of the motor units remained, exercise led to hypertrophy. Therefore the extent of strengthening attained seems to be proportional to the number of intact or undamaged motor units. Exercise at a level to elicit a training effect in normal muscle, however, may cause overwork damage in weakened, denervated muscle. Others have also expressed concern about the possible relation between high-resistance exercise and muscle fiber degeneration.[101] Because of the concerns about damage from stressing an abnormal neuromuscular system, Sinaki and Mulder[102] suggested that patients not engage in any vigorous exercise and focus instead on exercise associated with walking and daily activities. Later, several researchers demonstrated that repeated maximal eccentric contractions in normal muscle damaged muscle fibers, resulting in muscle weakness of several weeks' duration. Although normal muscle eventually adapts to repeated eccentric exercise, whether the reparative effect is possible in patients with neuromuscular diseases is uncertain.[103]

In contrast, Sanjak et al[104] suggested that muscle damage does not necessarily result from resistance exercise testing or training, although fatigue occurs more easily during both anaerobic and aerobic exercise. Exercise energy requirements during bicycle ergometry testing were greater than expected, possibly because of motor inefficiency caused by weakness. Work capacity and maximal oxygen consumption were decreased, but heart rate, respiratory responses, and blood pressure were within normal limits. In addition, patients in several case studies had lowered responses in force production and oxygen use related to their decreased muscle mass. Milner-Brown and Miller[105] found that mild progressive resistance exercise was helpful if the patient had muscle strength in the good (4/5) to normal (5/5) range. They determined that patients should begin their exercise program early because strength training of muscles with less than 10% of normal function was generally not effective. In more recent studies, Chan and Sinaki[106] have suggested that patients follow a program of six maximal isometric contractions held for 6 seconds and isotonic elastic band exercises at submaximal levels to maintain and improve muscle strength.

In general, impairments in muscle strength, the presence of spasticity, and decreases in ROM are clearly associated with decreases in functional abilities, hence the interest in correlating changes in level of impairment with level of functional loss. Although some research has shown improvements in muscle force production with strengthening and endurance training, functional improvements were not clear.[107] Jette et al[108] calculated the percentage of predicted normal maximal isometric force (%PMF) relative to four walking levels: unable to walk, walking within the home only, walking in the community with assistance, and independent walking in the community. Although they found great variation in muscle force production between and within the different levels of walking for each patient, they demonstrated that relatively small changes in force production were associated with losses of functional levels. For example, on average, when an independent ambulator began to need assistance in the community, the lower extremity %PMF dropped to less than 54%. When the patient became an in-home ambulator only, the average %PMF dropped to approximately 37%, and it was approximately 19% when the patient was no longer able to walk. Jette et al[108] acknowledge that many factors need to be considered when interpreting their work; however, their study is valuable to therapists because it relates functional skills to isometric muscle force production, which by itself is not sufficient evidence to predict functional status. Many studies focus on the impact of exercise on muscle strength; however, knowledge of impairments does not necessarily correlate directly with functional status. Factors such as spasticity, age at onset of ALS, prior levels of fitness and activity, and psychological factors, including past responses to extremely challenging situations and satisfaction with social support, must be considered.

Kilmer et al[109] and Wright et al[110] found positive physiological effects of directed exercise programs and aerobic walking programs, respectively. The positive effects of focused exercise programs can have a positive psychological effect on a patient's coping strategies.[111] Most recently, Drory et al[112] randomly assigned 25 patients with ALS to a group continuing their normal daily activities and a group participating in a moderate daily program of exercise individualized for each patient. The primary exercise focus was to have muscles of the trunk and limbs work against "modest" loads while undergoing significant changes in length (not lengthening or eccentric contractions). The program was completing twice daily for 15 minutes at home with phone contact by the treating therapist every 14 days. Data were evaluated for 3 and 6 months after initial assessment. All patients showed continued disease progression; however, in all cases, at the 6-month assessment patients who exercised showed positive effects in maintenance of muscle strength, less fatigue, less spasticity, less pain, and higher functional ratings. Although the investigators identified problems with the study related to adherence beyond the 3-month period, the findings show that nonstrenuous physical activity does have a positive effect on level of disability, fatigue, and quality of life, and they suggest that moderate physical activity should be encouraged. These findings are supported by studies of exercise in mouse models with SOD1 mice.[113] Ongoing, gentle exercise programs may also help decrease persistent pain and muscle stiffness that often accompany weakened, overtaxed muscle groups.[114] In addition to exercise programs, some preliminary evidence exists to suggest that creatine supplementation may increase isometric power in patients with ALS over the short term.[115]

Kilmer and Aitkens,[94] in an excellent review of the literature on exercise for patients with neuromuscular disorders, developed the following seven exercise prescription recommendations:

1. To improve compliance, consider both a formal exercise program and enjoyable physical activities.
2. Include activities with opportunities for social development and personal accomplishment.
3. Strengthening programs should emphasize concentric rather than eccentric muscle contractions.
4. High-resistance strengthening programs probably have no benefit over moderate-resistance programs.
5. Muscles with less than antigravity strength have little capacity to improve; the program should focus on stronger muscles.
6. Periodically monitor muscle strength to assess for possible overwork weakness, particularly in unsupervised programs.
7. Activity modifications should include periods of physical activity with rest.

Vignos[90] suggests that for a patient to make any gain in function, a therapist (or physician) should be prepared to

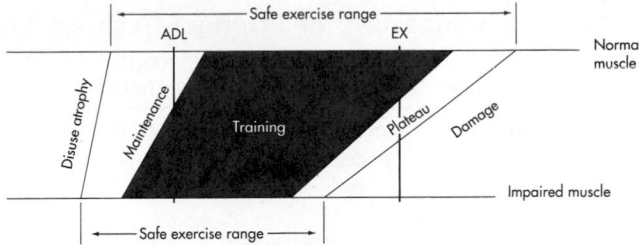

FIGURE 16-3 ■ Exercise window for normal and damaged or denervated muscles. (From Coble NO, Maloney FP: Effects of exercise on neuromuscular disease. In Maloney FP, Burks JS, Ringel SP, editors: *Interdisciplinary rehabilitation of multiple sclerosis and neuromuscular disorders,* New York, 1985, J.B. Lippincott.)

accept the possible consequences of overwork weakness when establishing an exercise program. The therapist should carefully monitor the patient's exercise or activity program to ensure that any decrement in strength is related to the progression of the disease rather than excessive overwork of weakened muscles. When determining the possible detrimental effects of exercise, a distinction must be made between the transient muscle fatigue from moderate heavy work and the prolonged, persistent decrease in muscle strength and endurance after excessive exercise of weakened muscles.[99] If a patient shows evidence of significant, persistent weakness after institution of an exercise program or persistent morning fatigue after exercise on the previous day, the therapist must carefully redesign the patient's exercise program and activity level and increase the frequency of monitoring the patient's home program. Because the possible positive and negative effects of resistive exercises are not clear, the therapist must take an assertive yet cautious approach to exercise. Although the therapist cannot determine the number of intact motor units available to a patient or whether the patient is evoking maximal motor unit recruitment during activities, the therapist must make decisions about underwork and overwork and adjust the patient's program on the basis of his or her response to exercise. The program must be adjusted as the disease progresses to prevent possible damage from excessive overwork and fatigue. Figure 16-3 is a diagram showing the appropriate exercise "window" for use in working with a patient with a neuromuscular disorder.

Therapeutic Interventions

Maintenance of strength and endurance requires daily activity and repetitive muscle contractions. In normal persons, absence of muscle contraction can result in 3% to 5% decreases in muscle strength per day. If the patient's exercise level requires less than 20% of the maximal voluntary contraction of the muscles, a decrease in strength will occur; yet overwork must be monitored.[96] A summary of the literature on strength training in neuromuscular disease is presented in Table 16-2.

When designing an intervention program, the therapist should know what the patient has been told about the disease process and the expected course of symptom development. If diagnostic and prognostic information is not explicit,

TABLE 16-2 ■ Summary of Strength Training Studies in Neuromuscular Disease

AUTHOR	STUDY POPULATION AND SAMPLE SIZE	DURATION OF TRAINING	TRAINING MODALITY	TRAINING PROTOCOL	RESPONSE(S)
Vignos and Watkins, 1966[295]	Various neuromuscular diseases (NMDs) (24)	12 months	Weight training (multiple muscle groups)	Unspecified, but based on 10-repetition maximum (RM)	Strength increased; percentage increase correlated with initial strength
Milner-Brown and Miller, 1988[105]	Various NMDs (12)	>12 months (variable)	Weight training (elbow flexion and knee extension)	Initially 1 set of 10 reps based on 15 RM performed on alternate days; gradually increased to a maximum of 5 sets 4 days/week; protocol individualized	Strength increased significantly when the initial degree of strength loss was not severe (<10%)
McCartney et al, 1988[294]	Various NMDs (12)	9 weeks	Weight training (arm curl and leg press)	3 days/week; initially 2 sets of 10-12 reps at 40% maximum; gradually progressed to 3 sets of 10-12 reps (1 set at 50%, 60%, and 70% maximum); contralateral arm control	Strength and muscular endurance increased; considerable intersubject variability
Aitkens et al, 1993*	Slowly progressive (12 weeks); NMD (27) and able-bodied controls (14)	12 weeks	Weight training (elbow flexion, knee extension, grip)	3 days/week; submaximal exercises	Significant improvement in most strength measures (not grip) in both groups; cross-training effect
Kilmer et al, 1994[109]	Slowly progressive NMD (10) and able-bodied controls (6)	12 weeks	Weight training (elbow flexion, knee extension)	3 days/week; high-resistance exercise	Results mixed; some increase in leg strength coupled with decrease in arm strength in NMD
Lindeman et al, 1995†	NMD (33) and HMSN (29); nonexercise control group	24 weeks	Weight training (knee extension and flexion, hip extension and flexion)	3 days/week; initially 3 sets of 25 reps at 60% of 1 RM; progressed to 3 sets of 10 reps at 80% of 1 RM	In NMD group, no change in strength In HMSN group, increased strength of knee extensors

*Aitkens SG, McCrory MA, Kilmer DD et al: Moderate resistance exercise program: its effect in slowly progressive neuromuscular disease, *Arch Phys Med Rehabil* 74:711-715, 1993.
†Lindeman E, Leffers P, Spaans F et al: Strength training in myotonic dystrophy and hereditary motor and sensory neuropathy: a randomized clinical trial, *Arch Phys Med Rehabil* 76:612-620, 1995.

neither therapist nor patient will be able to make appropriate goals and treatment plans. Before finalizing an intervention plan based on patient goals, the therapist must consider the following:

■ The typical rate of the patient's disease progression
■ Distribution of weakness and spasticity, respiratory factors leading to hypoxemia, and easy fatigability and bulbar involvement
■ Phase of the disease
■ Any preexisting impairments and/or activity limitations (see Chapter 7)

Sinaki[116] has described three phases and six substages of ALS with recommended exercise levels. Although therapists should not assume that all patients will fit precisely within the stages as described, the stages do provide suggestions for interventions on the basis of degree of impairment, functional limitations, and level of disability. Therefore, in the following section, staging patterns are used as the framework for therapy interventions. Staging information is particularly helpful to therapists who do not have the opportunity to work with large numbers of patients with ALS. Box 16-2 shows an adapted version of the Sinaki[116] phases and substages.

BOX 16-2 ■ **EXERCISE AND REHABILITATION PROGRAMS FOR PATIENTS WITH ALS ACCORDING TO STAGE OF DISEASE**

PHASE I (INDEPENDENT)
Stage 1
Patient Characteristics
- Mild weakness
- Clumsiness
- Ambulatory
- Independent in ADLs

Treatment
- Continue normal activities or increase activities if sedentary to prevent disuse atrophy
- Begin program of ROM exercises (stretching, yoga, tai chi)
- Add strengthening program of gentle resistance exercises to all musculature with caution not to cause overwork fatigue
- Provide psychological support as needed

Stage 2
Patient Characteristics
- Moderate, selective weakness
- Slightly decreased independence in ADLs, such as:
  - ■ difficulty climbing stairs
  - ■ difficulty raising arms
  - ■ difficulty buttoning clothing
- Ambulatory

Treatment
- Continue stretching to avoid contractures
- Continue cautious strengthening of muscles with MMT grades above F+ (3+); monitor for overwork fatigue
- Consider orthotic support (e.g., ankle-foot, wrist, thumb splints)
- Use adaptive equipment to facilitate ADLs

Stage 3
Patient Characteristics
- Severe selective weakness in ankles, wrists, and hands
- Moderately decreased independence in ADLs
- Easily fatigability with long-distance ambulation
- Ambulatory
- Slightly increased respiratory effort

Treatment
- Continue stage 2 program as tolerated; caution not to fatigue to point of decreasing patient's ADL independence
- Keep patient physically independent as long as possible through pleasurable activities such as walking
- Encourage deep breathing exercises, chest stretching, postural drainage if needed
- Prescribe wheelchair, standard or motorized, with modifications to allow eventual reclining back with head rest, elevating legs

PHASE II (PARTIALLY INDEPENDENT)
Stage 4
Patient Characteristics
- Hanging-arm syndrome with shoulder pain and sometimes edema in the hand

- Wheelchair dependent
- Severe lower-extremity weakness (with or without spasticity)
- Able to perform ADLs but fatigues easily

Treatment
- Heat, massage as indicated to control spasm
- Preventive antiedema measures
- Active assisted passive ROM exercises to the weakly supported joints; caution to support, rotate shoulder during abduction and joint accessory motions
- Encourage isometric contractions of all musculature to tolerance
- Try arm slings, overhead slings, or wheelchair arm supports
- Motorized chair if patient wants to be independently mobile; adapt controls as needed

Stage 5
Patient Characteristics
- Severe lower-extremity weakness
- Moderate to severe upper-extremity weakness
- Wheelchair dependent
- Increasingly dependent in ADLs
- Possible skin breakdown as a result of poor mobility

Treatment
- Encourage family to learn proper transfer, positioning principles, and turning techniques
- Encourage modifications at home to aid patient's mobility and independence
- Electric hospital bed with antipressure mattress
- If patient elects HMV, adapt chair to hold respirator unit

PHASE III (DEPENDENT)
Stage 6
Patient Characteristics
- Bedridden
- Completely dependent in ADLs

Treatment
- For dysphagia: soft diet, long spoons, tube feeding, percutaneous gastrostomy
- To decrease flow of accumulated saliva: medication, suction, surgery
- For dysarthria: palatal lifts, electronic speech amplification, eye-pointing electronics
- For breathing difficulty: clear airway, tracheostomy, respirator if patient elects HMV
- Medications to decrease impact of dyspnea

Adapted with permission from Sinaki M: Exercise and rehabilitation measures in amyotrophic lateral sclerosis. In Yase Y, Tsubaki T, editors: *Amyotrophic lateral sclerosis: recent advances in research and treatment,* Amsterdam, 1988, Elsevier Science.

Most patients need specific guidance about what type of activities and exercises they should do.[90] Although many physicians may suggest to patients that they increase their activity level, their suggestions are seldom specific. Examples of exercise advice that patients have recalled are "Try to move around as much as possible," "Walk some more," and "Be active, but don't overdo it." Because changing their typical exercise pattern is difficult for most patients, even when they know doing so is important, referral for a physical therapy consultation can be helpful.

Phase I: Stages 1 to 3. The first step in working with a patient in phase I, stages 1 to 3 (independent), of ALS is to determine the patient's current activity level. A program to increase activity must be specifically designed, with input from the patient about willingness to participate and knowledge of the patient's environmental situations and social support systems. In the early stages of the disease, patients should be encouraged to continue as many prediagnosis activities as tolerated. For example, a golfer should continue to golf as long as possible. Walking the course should be encouraged if it is not too fatiguing. When walking or balance becomes difficult on uneven terrain, the golfer can use a golf cart, decrease the number of holes played, move to a par 3 course, or hit balls at a driving range. If upper-extremity weakness is a major problem that interferes with swinging the club for distance shots, the player can continue playing the greens or on putting courses. Some golfers may need adaptations to club handles with nonskid material such as Dycem (Dycem Technologies: Non-skid solutions, http://www.dycem.com/) or Scoot Guard (often found at marine stores; manufacturer ID: V10975; see Appendix 16-A) to prevent the club from rotating on impact.

Older patients with newly diagnosed ALS who had a sedentary lifestyle before diagnosis should be encouraged to increase their activity level. This may include activities that require muscular effort within or around the home, such as sharing household and gardening tasks or beginning a walking program around the neighborhood. After diagnosis, some patients begin searching for in-home exercise devices such as bicycles and rowing machines. As with healthy persons who start an exercise program after the purchase of exercise equipment, patients with ALS are not likely to use the equipment consistently if they did not before a diagnosis. The search for a "perfect" exercise machine may reflect the patient's desperation to do something tangible. Without taking away the patient's motivation to exercise, therapists can encourage participation in exercise programs that do not require expensive equipment, such as walking or working out to specific exercise videos. A clever therapist can make a videotape for each patient that includes stretching and gentle exercise programs that elicit muscle contractions from all functional muscle groups (by using inexpensive elastic bands or small weights) with follow-up breathing, "warm down," and relaxation exercises. As mentioned earlier, Chan and Sinaki[106] have suggested that patients follow a program of six maximal isometric contractions held for 6 seconds and isotonic elastic band exercises at submaximal levels to maintain and improve muscle strength. Patients should exercise for short periods several times a day rather than attempt to exercise all muscle groups in one session.

For most patients in the early stages of ALS, pleasurable, natural activities such as swimming, bowling (can gradually decrease weight of ball if shoulder strength is a problem), walking, bicycling (three-wheeler may be needed or in-home stationary bicycle, either of which must be evaluated for easy mounting and dismounting), or tai chi should be recommended. Some patients prefer to exercise alone, whereas others will gain confidence and companionship by joining a group activity. Listening to the patient's desires related to group activities is important. The dropout rate is high among those who have been pressured to participate. Some spouses or family members are supportive of the patient's activity needs and will join the patient in his or her regimen. If possible, the spouse and family members should be engaged in the treatment planning process.[117]

The therapist must observe the patient completing her or his entire recommended activity program. The patient's response to the program must be monitored because fatigue from exercise sessions can interfere with the ability to carry out other normal daily activities. If the patient becomes too exhausted at the end of a session, he or she may learn to fear exercise and may become depressed about the decreased activity status. This depression may lead to decreased activity and further deconditioning (see Chapter 5).

Phase II: Partially Independent. During phase II (partially independent), the goal of physical and occupational therapy intervention should be to help the patient adapt to limitations imposed by weakness and spasticity, an increasingly compromised cardiorespiratory status, and possible pain from stress related to weakness or muscle imbalance. This transition stage is often frightening for patients because the decrease in function and independence becomes clear; therefore therapists should accentuate what the person can do and how accommodations can be made to help maintain independence. After a full physical assessment of the patient's motor status similar to the initial evaluation, the patient, family members, and the therapists (including PT, OT, and speech therapists if a team approach is possible) should discuss treatment options and adaptive devices that can help the patient remain as independent as possible.

During late phase I, stage 3, and during phase II, stages 4 and 5, many patients show significant weakness of both upper- and lower-extremity musculature, but each patient has his or her own pattern and rate of progression of weakness and onset of spasticity, bulbar, and respiratory symptoms. A typical patient at this time may have marked weakness of the intrinsic muscles, shoulder muscle weakness (in some cases "hanging arm" syndrome) with shoulder pain, and generalized lower-extremity weakness (in some cases more severe distally). Patients may be able to walk within the home environment, but many patients have precarious balance and fall easily because of muscle weakness. At this stage, most patients report fatigue with minimal work and have to rest frequently when carrying out ADLs.[118] Patients at this point, even if ambulatory, should use a wheelchair outside the home to conserve energy. Because a motorized chair will eventually be necessary, therapists should develop a plan to purchase this equipment. For example, the nonmotorized chair may not need the same level of adjustability as a motorized chair. However, for families whose finances are a major issue, or those that do not elect to purchase a van necessary to transport a motorized chair, the standard wheelchair should be purchased with the future required features, such as a reclining back and pressure-relieving seat systems. At this stage, patients with more advanced bulbar symptoms begin to experience dysarthria and may need guidance in dealing with communication issues. Murphy[119] indicated four major reasons for communication: to identify needs or request help, share information, respond politely in social situations, and maintain social closeness. The primary focus of communication for the study participants was to maintain social closeness. Although few patients had any instruction in ways to deal with communication problems, most patients and caregivers created ways to make themselves understood, such as giving cues about the topic and context, creating a "shorthand" language, and checking with the dysarthric speaker to ensure that the listener is understanding the patient correctly. A number of patients in the study who had significant dysarthria commented that attempting to communicate socially was extremely tiring. Therapists who are guiding patients with energy conservation techniques should be aware of the exhaustion that can be associated with communication. A number of strategies recommended by the American Speech-Language-Hearing Association[120] can be used by the person with ALS to deal with the effects of dysarthria, including the following:

■ Reduce background noise in the room.
■ Face the person being talked to.
■ Use short, simple phrases rather than long, complicated ones.
■ Take the time to say what needs to be said; do not allow people to rush conversation.
■ Make extra use of body language, such as gestures and facial expressions, and use writing to supplement speech, if possible.
■ Do not worry about saying things correctly; if the basic message being conveyed is understood, then that is enough.

In addition, some patients and families may need support to identify adapted feeding systems (special utensils, adapted plates, adjustable tables) and hygiene equipment if transfers within the family bathroom are problematic.[71] Because Mr. Turner in Case Study 16-1 was cared for in a neuromuscular disease clinic, he benefited from input from multiple specialists working as a team to help him maintain his independence. Unfortunately, many patients do not have the benefit of such a coordinated treatment environment. Therefore, when necessary, the therapist must be in a position to provide input on adaptive and safety devices and bulbar issues if other specialist input is not available. Therapists working in smaller communities and rural areas most likely need to be chameleon-like to play many therapeutic roles when working with the patient with ALS.

Phase III: Dependent. Physical and occupational therapists are usually less involved in the care of the patient in phase III, stage 6 (dependent), and nursing personnel become more active. During this phase, therapists make home visits to support caregivers and respond to questions about pain control, bed mobility, positioning, ROM, and equipment adaptations. Therapists should be sure to teach all caregivers some basic body mechanics to use during

lifting and patient care activities. If possible, caregivers should be taught how to safely move the person with ALS from the bed to a reclining wheelchair or neuro-chair during specific times of the day so that the person can continue to be part of the family activities. However, the ease of caregivers in transferring and caring for the person in the wheelchair must also be considered. Although some patients want to be in the midst of family activities even when dependent on HMV, other patients feel uncomfortable with their dependency and appearance and are reasonably content to stay in their room with television and visits from family members. This highly personal decision by patients must be respected. The therapist should review ROM procedures with family and professional caregivers and provide splinting or positioning devices if spasticity or paralysis leads to caregiving difficulties (e.g., excessive adductor tone and contractures interfering with hygiene and bowel care) or tissue damage and pain. If nursing care providers do not give advice on pressure relief beds or mattresses, therapists should be prepared to do so. Unfortunately, many insurance providers and Medicare may not fund special mattresses, and they can be costly. Therapists may also need to review postural drainage techniques with caregivers.

Of greatest importance in phase III, and sometimes in earlier stages, is the patient's ability to communicate. In the earliest manifestation of dysarthria, therapists train patients to slow the speech rate and cadence, exaggerate lip and tongue movements, and manage phrasing through breath control.[101] Although spouses and caregivers can often interpret their partner's or patient's severely dysarthric speech (see discussion of phase II above), most patients who use NIV or invasive ventilation for a prolonged periods need to find nonverbal methods to communicate. If severe bulbar impairments precede extremity paralysis, paper and pencil, alphabet/word boards, and adapted computer keyboards can be used with minimal upper-extremity or finger control for pointing. The American Speech-Language-Hearing Association provides suggestions for developing communication boards with the specific language most appropriate for the patient's situation.[120] For example, the board may be designed with commonly needed sentences, words used in the person's daily life, and the alphabet. As the person's ability to finger point or eye point decreases, the language board can be redesigned. When no extremity movement is possible, subtle neck movements or pressures, eye gaze, eye blink, upper facial movements, and electroencephalographic activity can be harnessed to operate communication devices.[121,122] Learning to use EEG interfaces, however, takes months of intense training that may not provide a reasonable system for communication for most patients with ALS.[123]

Some patients with hypernasality benefit from using an orthodontic palatal appliance. Patients with a tracheostomy may benefit from use of the Passy-Muir (Irvine, Calif.) speaking valve tracheostomy tube. These devices need to be recommended by communication specialists. As speech quality deteriorates and sound projection wanes, the spouse or caregiver can use an electronic speech amplifier to magnify the patient's speech. Speech pathologists and therapists have information on commercially available amplifying devices that are often used by persons with hearing problems but can be used by hearing people to amplify the speech of a person with severe weakness of phonation.

When selecting a communication device, therapists must work closely with the patient and family members to ensure that the system is compatible with patient skills and communication needs and preferences. Expensive systems commonly lie unused because of simple factors such as lack of proximity to the patient, interference of the unit with personal care, increased caregiver workload to manage the unit, and slowness of communication processing. The best systems are tailored to the precise needs of the patient; however, many patients do not have the financial or insurance support to purchase the device, and many patients in the end stages of ALS do not have the time to wait for systems designed for their specific needs. Therefore commercially manufactured systems may be most appropriate. (See Cook and Hussey[121] for a comprehensive list of communication devices and control interfaces.)

Some patients and caregivers learn to communicate effectively with simple eye gaze, eye blinking, and clicking techniques with Morse code or self-developed codes. At minimum, patients with no ability to communicate or move and their caregivers must have some system to communicate emergency needs; for example, looking to the right means "help" and looking to the left means "pain." Therapists should help patients develop alternative modes of communication before intelligible speech becomes impossible. (See also Cobble[124] for information on language impairments.) In addition to communication systems, environmental control systems can be programmed to turn on and off television, lights, and other electronic units with the same type of switching units used for communication (e.g., eye blink, infrared beam, head movement pressure). Unfortunately, these devices are often expensive and may not be available to all patients. (See Cook and Hussey[121] for a comprehensive review of environmental control systems.) Financial support is often not extended for high-tech equipment by third-party payers because of the patient's limited life expectancy. The ability to communicate and call for help, however, is of paramount importance with completely dependent patients.

By phase III most patients have significant problems eating and maintaining nutrition, although these problems may manifest in earlier stages. Patients often report choking or coughing after swallowing liquids or problems moving food around in the mouth or to the back of the throat for swallowing. These problems are best handled medically and can be assessed with videofluoroscopy or videoendoscopy. The aggressiveness of treatment intervention depends on the patient's preference and whether she or he still wants to attempt any oral feeding (e.g., syringe feeding, oral gastric tubes) or wishes to have a PEG or another alternative to oral feedings implemented. Therapists, however, can help patients and caregivers develop strategies that improve eating and nutrition, such adjusting eating position, head and neck alignments, adding thickeners to liquids, and adjusting portion sizes and texture of foods.[4]

Psychosocial Issues

Giving the bad news of a terminal diagnosis is difficult for even the most experienced clinician. In dealing with the diagnosis of ALS, most physicians now believe that the diagnosis, prognosis, and possible patterns of progression should be shared with the patient and family or partners and caregiving friends. Only by knowing the truth can patients and families deal openly with each other and make plans for the future.[125] McCluskey et al[126] suggest that those giving the medical or therapeutic diagnosis should attend to good practice parameters when giving bad news, such as creating the appropriate setting, identifying patient and caregiver needs, asking what patients and caregivers want to know, providing knowledge, exploring feelings of the patients and caregivers, and formulating a strategy for dealing with the situation. In addition, the presenter of bad news must be prepared to spend adequate time to give information—at least 45 minutes. Patients and family members, however, seldom remember what they are told when first given a terminal diagnosis. They do, however, remember how the information was given. Therefore information should be given honestly but with a sense of hope. When giving the diagnosis, the physician or team members must be careful to present a plan for treatment and support so that the patient and the family do not feel abandoned.[87] All information need not be given at the time of diagnosis. Rather, the patient and family can be exposed to more in-depth information over a number of sessions when they have the opportunity to ask questions that occur during the assimilation process. Therapists, especially those working in isolation from a comprehensive clinic, should also follow these guidelines by providing information, helping the patient and family identify goals, and establishing a plan for intervention. Patients should know that the goals will have to be adjusted and plans reset as the disease process continues. But if patients and families know that they can contact the therapist for support and advice, many of the negative aspects of the illness can be confronted in a positive manner. Preferably, an appointment for a follow-up visit will be set so patients and family members feel that contact with the care provider is expected.

Once the patient has adjusted to the diagnosis, information about transitions related to nutrition, communication, and respiratory functions should be delivered to patients and families in time to make thoughtful decisions rather than just before a time of crisis, such as after a choking episode or during a respiratory arrest. Care should also be taken to respect the cultural and spiritual views of the patient and family. Preferably, patients and family members will prepare an advanced medical directive that should be reviewed with the physician at least every 6 months.[79] If patients are referred to a specialty clinic from a rural area, contacting patients regularly at home by phone is imperative after the initial diagnosis to allow follow-up questions and make appropriate support referrals if needed. Local medical providers should also be contacted and provided information on the treatment goals and processes. Therapists treating patients who do not have access to a multidisciplinary ALS clinic should remember that they are often the person who works most closely with the patient and they should plan on spending enough time with the family to respond to concerns and help with problem solving.

Patients will progress through the diagnostic process with different responses and at different rates on a continuum from taking a cognitive approach by asking many questions and reviewing the most current research to the extreme of marked denial and disinterest in participating in any medical or therapeutic recommendations. Although some degree of denial can be a useful coping strategy, Oliver and Cardy[86] have found that most patients with motor neuron disease want to talk about their prognosis and future. The opportunity to express fears and concerns is essential. The overall goal of helping the patient and family members express themselves is to provide a forum for self-reflection and insight about the process of living while dying.[127] Nevertheless, the view by some health care workers that patients and families cannot deal with the disease effectively unless they express complete acceptance may be as faulty as hiding the diagnosis from the patient.

Purtilo and Haddad[127] identified four major fears of the patient who has a terminal condition: fear of isolation, fear of pain, fear of dependence, and fear of death itself. Patients with progressive diseases often see their social contacts decrease. Mr. Turner in Case Study 16-1 was concerned when he was no longer able to join his colleagues in the company cafeteria. After he received his motorized wheelchair he was able to continue his social contacts until his bulbar symptoms progressed to a point that he chose not to eat in public. When Mr. Turner lost the ability to speak and had to use his computerized speech system, he noticed that fewer colleagues stopped by his office to talk because of the slowness of the communication process. Although he understood the problem, Mr. Turner mourned the loss of friendship and his loss of standing as a competent computer expert. Because of his need for social contact, Mr. Turner continued to work until he could no longer tolerate the sitting position.[128] His fear of isolation increased when he became homebound. Although colleagues came for visits regularly at first, as Mr. Turner progressed to a near locked-in state only a few close friends came by for brief visits. Mr. Turner's greatest fear was being separated from his family and abandoned to hospital care with the usual inconsistent staffing patterns. Fortunately, in his community, Mrs. Turner was able to set up visitations from several church members, clerics, and hospice volunteers.

Fear of uncontrolled pain is common among people with terminal diseases. Patients need assurance that their pain will be controlled. Many patients can recall postsurgical horrors of being in severe pain but being told they had to wait another 2 hours for their next dose. Fortunately, today pain medications can be administered in many forms, dosages, and frequencies that can be tailored to the patient's specific needs. Because many patients are routinely undermedicated for pain, patients with ALS and their families need to be assertive about pain management.[54] In a study of the final month of life with ALS, caregivers reported that a major emphasis of care was to eliminate as much pain and discomfort as possible, even if it shortened the patient's life.[129] Keeping a pain log of intensity, type, location, and time of pain may provide the physician with information necessary to best prescribe dosages. Although sensory systems of patients with ALS are essentially normal and are not the cause of pain, many patients do experience significant pain from musculoskeletal sources, persistent spasms, or spasticity and pressure sores. Most of these problems can be handled with appropriate pain medications, muscle relaxants, careful positioning, frequent ROM, and tissue massage. Undertreated and uncontrolled pain is associated with a patient's seeking information on assisted suicide.[130] Some patients who expressed interest in assisted suicide

options did not follow up because of religious beliefs and concerns about possible loss of life insurance coverage for surviving family members.[131]

A major concern of patients with ALS is the dependence necessary for ADLs associated with late phase II and phase III of the disease. Because the process is gradual, most patients have the opportunity to make adjustments. The dependency issues and resulting privacy issues are more uncomfortable for some patients than for others, especially for the person who has always valued self-control and independence. Some patients are concerned about their increasing dependence because of the consequences or increasing burden of care on spouses or other caregivers.[132] That concern for others sometimes causes patients to choose hospital, nursing home, or in-patient hospice care over home care during the terminal stage of the disease. (See Damiano et al[133] for information on measurement of health-related quality of life.)

Not all patients with terminal illness react the same way during the dying process. Throughout the process, patients and family members may cycle and recycle through a range of different reactions, such as the stages described by Kübler-Ross: depression, anger, hostility, bargaining, and acceptance/adaptation (order is not implied).[127] How the patient coped with life's difficulties before the illness and her or his prior relationship patterns often direct how the patient will deal with the terminal illness. In one study, patients adjusted most successfully to the changes in their functional status if they did not look back to the past and compare their losses to their future.[134]

Health care providers and family members often have great difficulty coping with a patient who is depressed, and they make repeated efforts to "talk the person out of" the depression. Smith[135] stresses the importance of distinguishing between depression that can be destructive and the mourning or grieving that is a necessary and vital response to dealing with loss. In both states the person may feel a level of withdrawal, sadness, apathy, loss of interest in activities, and cognitive distortions. In a depressive state, however, the patient experiences an accompanying loss of self-esteem. A person in mourning rarely experiences that loss of self-esteem essential to a diagnosis of depression. The grieving person's feelings are congruent with the degree of loss experienced.[136] A person who grieves for what is lost but who has adapted to the prognosis may make plans for the impending death. Such behaviors are positive coping strategies. However, depressive symptoms related to hopelessness, uncontrolled suffering, and perceived burden on caregivers are more related to a choice for treatment discontinuance of feeding or ventilatory support.[131]

The issue of depression is complicated by the pseudobulbar effect of emotional lability (inappropriate laughing and crying), which is manifested by approximately 50% of patients with ALS. This emotional lability is not under complete control of the patient and is often misunderstood by family members and caregivers. Although current treatment is antidepressant medications, underlying clinical depression may or may not be present that would respond to higher doses of antidepressant medication and counseling.[79]

Because overt grieving or emotionality causes observers discomfort, some professional caregivers try to rush the patient and family into formal counseling as soon as mourning occurs. This option should be offered, but other recommendations such as guidance from a cleric, support groups, hospice volunteers, and informal support from friends are also invaluable resources for the person uncomfortable with formal counseling situations.

With today's pressure to express oneself and talk about one's feelings, patients are often pressed to "talk out" their problems and feelings. Although caregivers should give a patient the opportunity to talk about dying and to feel comfortable with the topic, each patient's personal style in talking about death must be respected. For example, some persons are not comfortable sharing feelings with a professional counselor or psychologist. This is especially true for older patients or those who were raised with the view that one should maintain the appearance of control or that seeking emotional help shows weakness or defect. Pressuring a patient to see a mental health clinician can lead to loss of trust. Therefore occupational and physical therapists and other persons involved in the care of a dying patient should feel comfortable talking with their patients about death and be prepared to suggest various options if the patient expresses the need for emotional support.

Caregiver Issues

Often in the concern for the patient's needs professionals pay little attention to the effect a person's degenerative illness has on other members of the family. ALS significantly affects the person's extended family because the patient gradually becomes increasingly dependent on family members, partners, or caregiving friends for physical care, social arrangements, cognitive stimulation, and emotional support. For some families, the spouse may have to take on additional work, return to work or, in the case of some older women, join the workforce for the first time to deal with the financial stresses that occur when chronic illness invades the family unit. Family members must absorb the former family duties of the dependent person. For example, a spouse or child may have to handle all the cooking, cleaning, or other household chores or work to help support the family. Once the patient becomes dependent, the caregiver may need to reduce or discontinue employment to take care of the patient. All family members may have to become involved in the physical care of the increasingly dependent person with ALS.

Families have differing levels of long-term care coverage. Some families are fortunate to have excellent coverage that provides extensive home nursing support, whereas other families are unable to cope with the financial stresses and must accept public assistance during the final stages of the person's disease. As opposed to Germany and Japan, which provide long-term nursing care insurance, financial stress on patients with ALS in the United States can reach more than $150,000 per year for ventilation support at home.[87] For example, the Springer family, consisting of the father with ALS (aged 61 years), mother (aged 59 years), and son (aged 25 years), was forced to live on a combination of Supplemental Security Income, general assistance, and food stamps after the father became ill. The family had little savings and catastrophic insurance coverage that did not cover any long-term care. Mrs. Springer returned to work full time and cared for her husband all evening. When he reached the point of needing full-time care, the wife had to quit work to care for her husband because she did not make an adequate salary to pay for nursing care and maintain the family finances. Because the son had to care for his own family of four, he was not able to help out the family financially, although both he and his wife provided several half-days of respite care for their mother so she could do shopping and spend some time out of the home. The process of "going on welfare" was upsetting to the family. After numerous discussions about options for home care, Mr. Springer decided that continuing his life was too great a burden on his family and he requested that his life be terminated. Because that was not considered an option, his family and primary physician worked out a plan to allow a peaceful death without placing Mr. Springer on any artificial feeding, respiration, or antibiotics. He died at home 3 months after the decision was made.

In another case, a young single woman who lived alone and had no family found that she could not rely on friends for her care even though they were supportive and visited her often. When she was no longer able to care for herself safely she was admitted to a nursing home, where she died 2 years later.

Children of patients with ALS also have to deal with major changes in their lifestyle. Although they may love their parent who is sick, at some level most are frustrated with factors such as the need to provide physical care to parents. This is a difficult problem for children who have not had a positive relationship with that parent. Children living in the home of a parent who is dying of ALS also express frustration about the lack of privacy in their home when nursing personnel and attendants are present, interruptions in family and personal life plans, embarrassment because of the parent's appearance and dependency, lack of attention from the caregiving/working parent, and fear of financial crises (e.g., possible loss of home, no financial support for college).

The entire family is affected by the sick person's increasing dependency and impending death.[137] The changes the family must make to anticipate and deal with the dependent person's needs have a significant emotional overlay. Anger, helplessness, frustration, sadness, or mourning for an impending loss; guilt; and remorse commonly occur and recur at different stages as the sick person and family try to adjust to the progression toward death. Weariness and exhaustion from day-to-day caregiving and frequent interactions with health and social agencies can try the soul of the most adaptable persons.[138] In a small study of 11 family caregivers, many caregivers felt frustrated and resentful because their lives were consumed with the caregiving responsibilities. Most caregivers had adjusted to some degree after 2 to 4 years. Caregivers who adjusted most successfully learned to take time for themselves without guilt and to tap their social support systems for help.[134] Similarly, investigators working with 40 caregivers of young adults with severe disabilities reported being overwhelmed by the physical requirements of daily care and felt a severe loss of spontaneity in their lives. They also reported a sense of isolation from everyday social interactions. Although they highly valued their social support systems, they expressed frustration that few people offered instrumental or direct service support, such as respite care or help with medical appointments, housekeeping, or shopping. Despite the stresses of caregiving, the caregivers felt positive about their roles in helping their dependent adult by finding meaning in their acts of caregiving.[139] Fortunately, most families manage to cope with the process—the major contributing factor being the coping ability of families before the illness. To be really effective, the therapist working with the patient with ALS must be prepared to help families and caregivers find appropriate ways of coping with the emotional, social, and physical stress of caregiving (Case Study 16-1).

CASE STUDY 16-1 ■ MR. TURNER

Mr. Turner is a 45-year-old man diagnosed 2 years ago with ALS. He lives at home with his wife, who works full time, and two teenaged children. Mr. Turner is a computer programmer for an engineering firm in the area. Since his diagnosis, Mr. Turner has been able to continue his full-time work schedule, although he states that he is no longer able to touch type and can type with the index fingers only. He has noticed that his shoulders and neck hurt after an hour at the computer. In the last 2 weeks he has found it fatiguing to walk to the cafeteria for lunch, and he fears that he will be knocked down when walking in crowds. He dropped his tray last week, which was embarrassing, so he decided to eat in his office even though he misses the socialization and opportunity to discuss work issues with his colleagues.

Mr. Turner has been able to continue most of his nonwork activities, although he is no longer able to operate his sailboat independently and is having trouble maintaining his balance when golfing. He states that his wife and children are supportive and that they have made some changes in the home environment to accommodate his increasing weakness. He also revealed, however, that his children seem frustrated with him because he is so much slower than he was before the illness.

On assessment, Mr. Turner showed marked wasting of hand intrinsics. He was unable to abduct or flex either shoulder past 90 degrees. His right shoulder showed considerable atrophy, especially of the deltoid and supraspinatus muscles. All other upper-extremity movements were weakened but in the G– (4–) range. His neck posture was forward: neck extension is F+ (3+), neck flexion is G– (4–). Scapular winging was noted bilaterally. No spasticity was evident in the upper extremities.

Lower-extremity musculature showed generalized weakness at about the F (3) to F+ (3+) range, with left musculature weaker than right, marked wasting of the foot intrinsics, and a cavus foot position bilaterally. Spasticity of the hip adductors and hamstrings was noted on passive motion. Most obvious during gait was inadequate dorsiflexion for heel strike and no propulsion during heel-off. He showed bilateral corrected gluteus medius pattern on weight bearing. He needed to pause to lock each knee during weight bearing and at times he pushed his knee into extension with his hand. He had great difficulty ascending and descending steps in his home. There were no stairs to negotiate at work.

Until this appointment, Mr. Turner had not been willing to discuss the use of adaptive equipment or a wheelchair. During prior clinic visits his decisions were supported and he was told that when he was ready, therapists would work with him and his family to help with equipment decisions. Therapists should present but not press adaptive equipment options to patients when they first start to show impairment in functional ability. If shown how the equipment will help them maintain independence, most patients are receptive to its use. Even when presented in a positive way, however, a wheelchair or adaptive devices may be resisted long after the adaptations would facilitate mobility and ADLs. Therapists must be attentive to patients' feelings and fears at this time because use of a wheelchair heralds to many patients the beginning of the end.

Mr. Turner also showed some early bulbar signs. He noted that he sometimes had to catch drool when working intensely, and that his pillow was moist in the morning. Food sometimes got stuck in his cheek area and he could not move it out with his tongue. Swallowing was still adequate for eating all foods; however, he had had a few coughing episodes when drinking coffee and wine. He showed increased use of accessory musculature when breathing but had no reports of respiratory distress. His cough was adequate to clear secretions.

With input from the therapist, Mr. Turner and his wife identified the following general goals:
1. Increase mobility
2. Control fatigue and pain of upper extremities and neck during computer work
3. Maintain maximal muscle strength and ROM (patient reported that he felt stiff)
4. Identify safety issues within the home and work environment and adjust household and work environment to prepare for the time when Mr. Turner could not ascend and descend stairs safely

A treatment plan was discussed to achieve the following:
1. **Increase mobility.** Because of his increased walking difficulties, Mr. Turner decided to use a front-wheeled walker with a seat attachment at home. Because of his hand grip weakness, he felt most stable using attached forearm troughs. For his worksite, he selected a motorized wheelchair so that he could maintain his independence at work. Although he found that he could push an ultralight manual chair, his upper-extremity strength was clearly decreasing. To prevent overworking and further damaging weakened musculature, he was discouraged from self-propelling a manual chair because of the repetitive pushing action and the

Continued

CASE STUDY 16-1 ■ MR. TURNER—cont'd

effort necessary to cope with inclines. Although most patients will need a motorized device such as a wheelchair or scooter to maintain independent mobility, some homes would need adaptations to allow electric wheelchair access. Some patients are initially horrified at the appearance of disability when using a motorized wheelchair and prefer the electric scooter, which is more socially accepted. The scooter, however, does not provide adequate support for the patient in the later stages of the disease. Therefore its purchase should be discouraged unless the patient has adequate financial resources to make the transition later to a motorized chair.

Factors to consider include extent of insurance coverage or financial assistance programs for purchase of wheelchair (some policies or programs may provide only one type of wheelchair or only one wheelchair, either motorized or manual); transportability of motorized chair from home to community and work (few motorized wheelchair brands fold for stowing in car trunk and few families can afford to purchase a van that will allow patient to drive or be driven while in motor chair); reclining potential of chair back and head rest (preferably electric) to allow the patient to shift weight and rest while in the chair during later stages of the disease; removable arm rests for ease of transfer; potential for head rest attachment or extension; potential mounting area for portable respirator equipment if needed; and ease with which caregiver can help patient with chair mobility transfers. Because Mr. Turner's insurance and Medicare would not fund an additional manual chair and because the family had no way to transport the electric wheelchair, the ALS Society loaned the family a manual wheelchair for home use. Although not ideal, it was functional. Mr. Turner's son made some inexpensive adjustments to adapt the chair for a head rest and his daughter and grandchildren repainted the chair to his specifications.

Because Mr. Turner wanted to keep as active as possible and use his walker within the home, he was fitted with bilateral ankle-foot orthoses (AFOs) with a flexible ankle joint and pretibial shell to facilitate knee extension. Straps were simple overlap style because Mr. Turner had poor thumb and grasp control.

2. **Decrease fatigue and pain of upper extremities.** Mr. Turner was taught some simple ROM exercises of the neck and arms to perform every half hour while working at the computer. In a simulated work environment the therapist noted that Mr. Turner had a forward head position when working at a computer similar to his workstation. The height of the computer was adjusted to decrease his neck strain, and the desk height was adjusted to allow his wheelchair to fit under the desk so that his arms could rest fully on the surface. He

felt immediate relief with the adaptations. He was also fitted for a soft neck collar to wear when he felt he needed more neck support. (As his condition worsened, he learned to rest his head on the headrest of his chair and recline slightly for a few minutes every 15 minutes.)

3. **Maintain maximal muscle strength and ROM.** Mr. Turner was taught as many self-ranging maneuvers as possible, which he was encouraged to do in small segments frequently throughout the day. For example, his series of motions included neck rotations, side bends, and flexion and extension within strength limits, upper-extremity motions with the exception of shoulder flexion and abduction past 90 degrees, hip flexion, abduction and rotations, full knee extension, and all ankle motions. When using the walker, Mr. Turner was encouraged to extend each hip fully and to stretch his heel cords. Mrs. Turner and their adult children were taught to administer full ROM exercises, including trunk rotations, with special attention to ranging of the shoulder to prevent impingement. Simple massage techniques were also taught to all family members who felt comfortable with the task.

Maintaining maximal muscle strength is difficult because any program must be designed to prevent disuse activity and prevent overwork damage. No exercise program should be recommended that would cause enough fatigue to require extensive periods of postexercise rest or interfere with participation in normal ADLs. Mr. Turner had been active before the onset of ALS and he liked to exercise. Therefore he rented a portable pedaling unit to attach to a chair at home. He pedaled two to four times a day, with no additional resistance, to the point at which he felt fatigue (usually 3 to 5 minutes at this stage). He carefully monitored his soreness and fatigue level after exercise and increased and decreased his pedaling depending on how he felt immediately and several days after exercise. Mr. Turner felt invigorated by this exercise, which he usually did while watching television. He was also taught a series of simple elastic band exercises, with tensile strength adjusted according to his ability to contract his muscles without fatigue. Mr. Turner was also shown a series of isometric exercises for all muscle groups to do throughout the work day. Because he had some foot and ankle edema, he was encouraged to wear lightweight pressure stockings while sitting. Mr. Turner also had access to a swimming pool, and he was encouraged to carry out walking and upper-extremity exercises as long as another adult was with him in the water at all times.

4. **Assess environment of home and work.** Occupational therapy input was requested to help with ADL aids such as reachers, utensil adaptors to facilitate grip, rubber pen grippers, key adaptors to permit turning, and thumb abduction

CASE STUDY 16-1 ■ MR. TURNER—cont'd

splints to assist in pincer grasp. Mr. Turner's occupational therapist made several visits to his worksite and home to identify adaptations of the environment for safety and independence. His wheelchair was eventually adapted with universal joint arm troughs to decrease his effort during self-feeding and basic upper-body hygiene. Ramps were recommended for home entry, and nonpermanent safety rails were placed in the bathroom. Mr. Turner was able to assist with transfer to a shower chair and the shower head was replaced with a handheld unit.

A speech pathology consultation was also requested. Using information from the physical therapist's MMT, the speech pathologist carried out a thorough bulbar evaluation and provided information about swallowing techniques. The speech therapist focused on ways to decrease drooling and ways to cope with food pocketing (tongue mobility was impaired) by using techniques such as hand pressure on the cheek to push food back to the center of the mouth. The therapist also instructed Mr. Turner and his wife how to prepare foods with textures that were easily swallowed and manipulated. Mr. Turner had lost 5 pounds during the last 6 months so he was also referred to the dietitian for information about how to maintain nutritious calorie intake.

Mr. Turner had great difficulty adjusting to his physical dependence. Because of his slow onset of dysphagia and his augmented communication system, he was able to continue control over his expressive, cognitive, and emotional life until the last 5 or 6 months of his life. Initially Mr. Turner angrily resisted his wife's attempts to help him with eating and dressing tasks. This began to alienate her and the children until a family meeting was held with their medical social worker and physical and occupational therapists. All family members had the opportunity to express their frustrations. A major irritation to the children was what they perceived to be their constant waiting for their father to complete a task. Mrs. Turner was most irritated when Mr. Turner yelled at her when she attempted to help even though he frequently expressed anger about his clumsiness. Mr. Turner sadly admitted that he was having increasing difficulty with his ADLs and was sometimes too tired after dressing to participate in family activities. At the end of the meeting, the family had worked out a compromise plan. Mr. Turner would continue to do as much as possible for himself. He would specifically ask for help from Mrs. Turner when he wanted it so she did not get caught in his anger about needing help. He preferred that the children not have to take any role in his care at this point but realized that he might need their help later. Visiting nurse support was requested twice a week to help with bathing, and the occupational therapist was requested to make another home visit to help with toileting needs. Mr. Turner felt comfortable with his wife and children carrying out ROM exercises. A therapy home visit was arranged to review the exercise/positioning program as well as respiratory exercises and postural drainage techniques.

As Mr. Turner became totally dependent, he needed 24-hour care. Professional nurses were provided through his insurance contract 14 hours a day from 6:30 AM to 8:30 PM. Family members provided care until midnight. Initially Mr. Turner was able to activate a bell at night to call for help. His wife and children followed a schedule to turn him every 3 hours throughout the night. When Mr. Turner became respirator dependent and was no longer able to call for help, it became clear that the nighttime responsibilities were taking a heavy toll on his wife, who worked full time, and the children, who were in high school and college. Fortunately the family was able to pay for a nurse assistant to remain at Mr. Turner's bedside throughout the night, although the family members all felt that they had no privacy. Although the family was committed to having Mr. Turner remain at home until his death, all agreed that they needed respite. Thus several week-long hospitalizations were made to give the family a break in the constant care needs.

Although Mr. Turner had elected HMV, he also had signed a durable power of attorney for health care, indicating that he did not want treatment for infections and that palliative care for comfort should direct his treatment. He had a strong lust for life, but he had come to accept his impending death. He did not have strong religious views, but he had talked with all his caregivers and therapists about his concerns related to death. He freely expressed his fear of "non-being." Because his caregivers and therapists were willing to talk about his and their own feelings, Mr. Turner came to believe that he would live on in the minds, hearts, and behaviors of those he had known. This idea seemed to give him great comfort. He particularly liked to talk to others about special times they had had together and how their interactions had affected each other. To help Mr. Turner process his death, his family, friends, and medical team put together an album of pictures and statements about their time together. Mr. Turner frequently liked to have his wife read through the book with him. His family continued to carry out his ROM exercises and massage because Mr. Turner had indicated that the treatments provided him physical comfort and the spiritual closeness he needed with his family. His primary treatment during the last few days consisted of morphine to decrease his respiratory discomfort. After 5 to 6 months of being totally dependent for all care and respiratory function, Mr. Turner died at home in his sleep after a respiratory illness.

DEMYELINATING INFLAMMATORY POLYRADICULONEUROPATHY

Pathology and Medical Diagnosis

In the past 15 years a broad spectrum of demyelinating inflammatory polyradiculoneuropathy has been identified. GBS, or acute inflammatory demyelinating polyradiculoneuropathy, is the most common form of the disease that affects nerve roots and peripheral nerves leading to motor neuropathy and flaccid paralysis.[140] The incidence of GBS is approximately one to four cases per 100,000 persons. A variant form is acute motor axonal neuropathy, which, like GBS, has a good prognosis. Less common forms are acute motor and sensory axonal neuropathy, which has a less positive prognosis (which some consider to be a distinct type of peripheral neuropathy); Miller-Fisher syndrome with primarily cranial nerve symptoms, ataxia, and areflexia[141]; and chronic inflammatory demyelinating polyradiculoneuropathy (CIDP), which causes progressive or relapsing and remitting numbness and weakness.[142] Epidemiological studies show that males are affected by GBS twice as often as are females.[143]

Approximately 27% of patients with GBS have no identified preceding illness; however, more than two thirds had symptoms of an infectious disease 2 weeks before the onset of GBS symptoms. Although no consistent predisposing factors are known, evidence exists to support connections with *Campylobacter jejuni,* mycoplasma pneumonia, cytomegalovirus, and Epstein-Barr virus. In GBS the spinal roots and peripheral nerves are infiltrated with macrophages and T-lymphocytes. Macrophages then attack and strip the myelin sheaths. In milder cases of GBS the axons are left intact and the nerves are remyelinated. However, in some cases, the axons also degenerate. In acute axonal motor neuropathy, macrophages invade the axon directly, leaving the myelin intact.[144] Some evidence exists in a substantial number of patients with GBS that axonal loss is related to long-lasting or permanent muscle weakness.[145]

Recent studies into the complex pathogenesis of the forms of demyelinating inflammatory polyradiculoneuropathy have demonstrated significant associations with autoimmune reactions, such as autoantibodies against myelin constituents, and against gangliosides and glycolipids of axonal and myelin membranes. (See Steck et al[146] for a comprehensive review of the pathogenesis of inflammatory demyelinating diseases.)

Because of damage to the myelin sheath, saltatory propagation of the action potential is disturbed, resulting in slowed conduction velocity, dyssynchrony of conduction, disturbed conduction of higher frequency impulses, or complete conduction block.[147] Partial conduction block (CB) is most often seen in the early stages of GBS, and the CB increases as the patient reaches a plateau. The most common CB findings were in the peroneal nerve followed by the tibial nerve. Proximal CB was evident more often than distal CB. In axonal neuropathy, CB is more severe and the number of functional motor units is decreased (Figure 16-4).[148] For a readable review of reactions of neurons and peripheral nerves to injury, see Kandel et al.[149] See Hartung et al[150] and Trojaborg[151] for reviews of GBS and other forms of inflammatory, immune-mediated neuropathy such as chronic inflammatory demyelinating polyradiculoneuropathy and

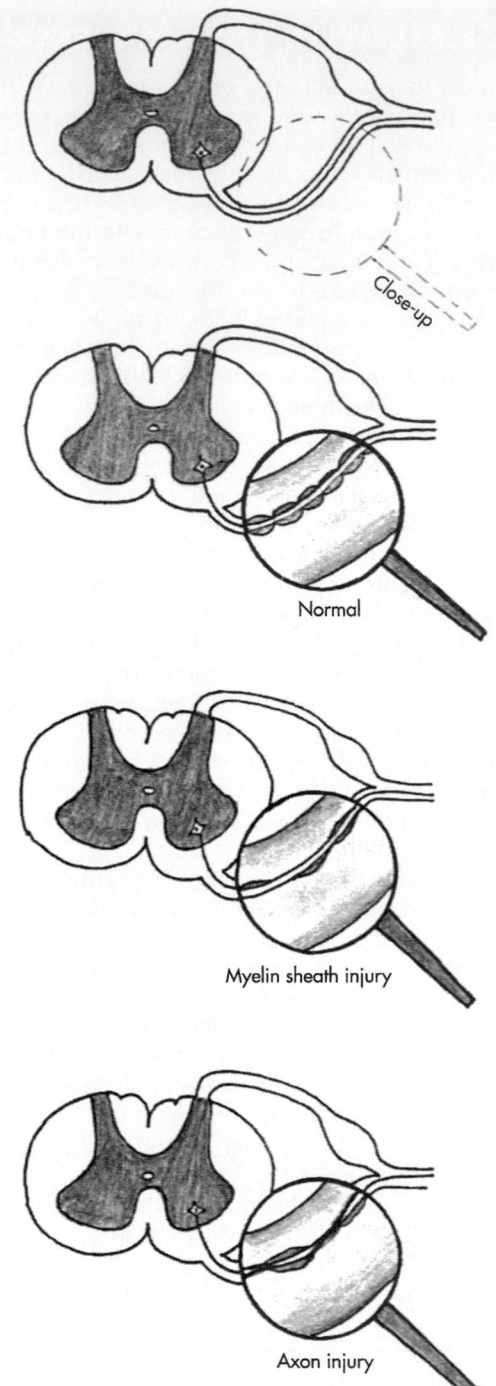

FIGURE 16-4 ■ Peripheral nerve showing axonal degeneration and demyelination.

acute motor axonal neuropathy. The diagnostic criteria for GBS are detailed in Box 16-3.

Clinical Presentation

GBS in both children and adults is characterized by a rapidly evolving, relatively symmetrical ascending weakness or flaccid paralysis. Motor impairment may vary from mild weakness of distal lower-extremity musculature to total paralysis of the peripheral, axial, facial, and extraocular musculature. Tendon reflexes are usually diminished or

BOX 16-3 ■ COMMON DIAGNOSTIC FEATURES OF GBS

A. Motor weakness
  1. Progressive symptoms and signs of motor weakness that develop rapidly
    a. Relative symmetry of motor involvement
    b. Usual progression of weakness from distal to proximal; self-limiting to distal limbs of upper and/or lower extremities or may extend to full quadriplegia with respiratory and cranial nerve involvement
  2. Areflexia of at least distal tendon responses
B. Mild sensory symptoms or signs, particularly paresthesias and hypesthesias
C. Autonomic dysfunction such as tachycardia and arrhythmias, vasomotor symptoms
D. Absence of fever at onset of symptoms; history of flulike illness common
E. Laboratory tests nonspecific but may have elevation of cerebrospinal fluid protein; cerebrospinal fluid cells at 10 or fewer mononuclear leukocytes per cubic millimeter of cerebrospinal fluid
F. Electrodiagnostic testing, nerve conduction velocities usually abnormal
G. Recovery usually begins 2 to 4 weeks after plateau of disease process

absent. Twenty to 30% of patients may require assisted ventilation because of paralysis or weakness of the intercostal and diaphragm musculature.[152] Impaired respiratory muscle strength may lead to an inability to cough or handle secretions and to decreased vital capacity, tidal volume, and oxygen saturation. Secondary complications such as infections or organ system failure lead to death in approximately 5% of patients with GBS.[153] Approximately 50% of patients develop some cranial nerve involvement, primarily facial muscle weakness, although patients may also develop oropharyngeal and oculomotor involvement.[154]

ANS symptoms are noted in approximately 50% of patients. Low cardiac output, cardiac dysrhythmias, and marked fluctuations in blood pressure may compromise management of respiratory function and can lead to sudden death. Other typical ANS symptoms may result in peripheral pooling of blood, poor venous return, ileus, and urinary retention.[155]

Sensory symptoms such as distal hyperesthesias, paresthesias (tingling, burning), numbness, and decreased vibratory or position sense are common. The sensory disturbances often have a stocking-and-glove pattern rather than the dermatomal distribution of loss. Although the sensory problems are seldom disabling, they can be disconcerting and upsetting to patients, especially during the acute stage.[156-158]

Pain was identified as a significant presenting symptom reported in the original articles describing GBS.[159] In 1949, 1963, and 1984 studies of 50, 35, and 29 patients with GBS, respectively, approximately 55% of patients reported pain preceding their illness or early during onset. Seventy-two percent reported pain at some time during the full course of the disease process. When pain was prominent, patients spontaneously revealed its presence during a medical

history. Therefore, therapists who may be working with patients who present with the onset of low back pain not associated with known injury or stress and reports of paresthesias and vibratory or decreased tendon reflexes should be evaluated or monitored for possible GBS.[160,161]

The most common description of presenting pain was of muscle aching typically associated with vigorous or excessive exercise. Pain was usually symmetrical and reported most frequently in the large-bulk muscles such as the gluteals, quadriceps, and hamstrings and less often in the lower leg and upper-extremity muscles. Some pain reported during late stages of the illness was described as "stiffness." Pain was consistently more disturbing at night.[161] As the disease progresses, some patients experience severe burning or hypersensitivity to touch or even air movement, which can interfere with nursing care and limit therapy interventions. The types of pain reported include paresthesias, dysesthesias, axial and radicular pain, joint pain, and myalgias.[162] A patient with GBS describing his pain while in an intensive care unit stated that he had "very severe pins and needles all over my body, especially in my hands and feet. My skin was so sensitive that the slightest touch felt like salt and vinegar was being rubbed into an open wound. My hips were also giving me a lot of pain, just a dull ache on both sides."[163] Pain may have neuropathic, musculoskeletal, or autonomic origins. Ropper[164] hypothesized that the paresthesias and pain experienced by patients are probably related to the spontaneous discharges of the demyelinated sensory nerves. In addition, the serum creatine kinase level was elevated in 10 of 13 patients with pain and in only one of eight patients without pain. This finding suggests that changes in muscle related to neurogenic origin may also be the cause of pain, especially pain described as a dull aching.[162]

Dysautonomia (orthostatic hypertension, blood pressure instability, cardiac arrhythmias) is most often related to patients with GBS requiring ventilatory support and can be life threatening.[143] In patients with paraplegia or quadriplegia, approximately one fourth had problems with urinary retention caused by detrusor areflexia or overactivity, overactive urethral sphincter, and disturbed bladder sensation.[143,162] The possibility of deep vein thrombosis and pulmonary embolus must also be monitored and prophylactic treatment used.[162]

Prognosis

Although some patients have a fulminating course of progress with maximal paralysis within 1 to 2 days of onset, 50% of patients reach the nadir (the point of greatest severity) of the disease within 1 week, 70% by 2 weeks, and 80% by 3 weeks.[154] In some cases, the process of increasing weakness continues for 1 to 2 months. Onset of recovery is varied, with most patients showing gradual recovery of muscle strength 2 to 4 weeks after progression has stopped or the condition has plateaued. Although 50% of the patients may show minor neurological deficits (e.g., diminished or absent tendon reflexes) and 15% may show persistent residual deficits in function, approximately 80% become ambulatory within 6 months of onset of symptoms. The most common long-term deficits are weakness of the anterior tibial musculature, and less often weakness of the foot and hand intrinsics, quadriceps, and gluteal musculature. Three percent to 5% of patients die of secondary cardiac, respiratory, or other systemic organ failure.[143,162,164] Fatigue or poor endurance was also noted as a long-term consequence of GBS, possibly attributable to deconditioning.[165] Vasjar et al[166] also report that fatigue and poor exercise tolerance were common persisting symptoms in children who appeared to have fully recovered from acute GBS.

Although often not the focus of most studies on the long-term impact of GBS, sensory deficits (impaired pinprick, light touch, vibration, and proprioception in combination with other sensory losses) are an ongoing problem for patients 3 to 6 years after recovery from acute GBS. In a study of 122 subjects, 38% showed sensory deficits in the upper extremities[167] and 66% had ongoing sensory deficits of the lower extremities.[162] The muscle aches and cramps experienced by some of these patients appeared to be related to sensory rather than persistent motor dysfunctions as usually thought.[162] Overall, factors associated with a poor prognosis are severity of muscle weakness (especially quadriplegia), the need for respiratory support, cranial nerve involvement associated with loss of eye movement and swallowing, rapid rate of progression from onset, length of time to nadir, older age at onset, history of gastrointestinal illness, and recent cytomegalovirus infections.[143,152]

Medical Intervention

Medical treatment depends on the rate and degree of ascending paralysis. Because most patients return to their prior functional status, excellent supportive care during the acute stage is imperative. Respiratory compromise should be expected and all patients, including those with limited paralysis and sensory dysfunction, must be closely monitored for the rapid onset of pulmonary and cardiac decompensation or cardiac arrhythmias caused by dysautonomia. Because of the possibility of sudden respiratory failure, patients with evidence of GBS must be hospitalized so that immediate cardiorespiratory support can be given if FVC falls below 20 ml/kg or oxygen saturation falls below 75%.[153] Patients who progress to respiratory paralysis must be treated in an intensive care environment where adequate respiratory function can be maintained, secondary infections can be prevented or limited, and metabolic functions can be carefully monitored. The patient should be intubated if the FVC falls below 12 ml/kg or if the patient is increasingly dyspneic even if FVC is above the cutoff level.[154,168] Twenty-five percent of patients who experience respiratory failure will develop pneumonia.[162] Older patients who may have comorbid conditions such as chronic obstructive pulmonary disease will be particularly susceptible to pneumonia and have difficulty with weaning from supported respiration. After extubation, aspiration can be a serious complication because of oral muscle weakness and dysphagia.

In addition to the intensive monitoring of progression and supportive care required for patients with GBS, two specific immunotherapy-based treatments, plasma exchange (PE) (removal of plasma from withdrawn blood with retransfusion of the formed elements back into the blood) and intravenous immunoglobulin (IVIg), have been under investigation for their ability to decrease the duration of respirator dependence and the time to onset of improvement. Two large clinical trials carried out in the United States and France have shown that patients undergoing plasmapheresis had shorter periods on mechanical ventilation and walked earlier than subjects who did not undergo exchange.[159,169]

PE, however, has some serious possible complications that relate to an increased incidence of hypotension and arrhythmias, which makes it unsuitable for GBS patients with autonomic instability. The need for multiple infusion lines increases the possibility of septicemia and thrombosis. The technique is also expensive and requires highly skilled personnel and equipment.[170]

More recently, a study comparing PE and IVIg demonstrated that the outcome measures did not differ between the two groups, although the incidence of complications was slightly higher in the PE group. The relapse rates were similar in the two groups.[171] Therefore evidence supports the use of either intervention provided that it is initiated within the first 1 or 2 weeks of treatment.[154] Although corticosteroids were used to decrease the inflammatory process in GBS beginning in the 1960s, a clinical study of corticosteroid effectiveness in 1993 suggested that corticosteroids were not useful in the treatment of GBS,[172] although they may have some place in the treatment of other chronic demyelinating polyneuropathies. On the basis of these large studies of PE and IVIg, practice parameters and guidelines for the treatment of GBS have been delineated. The evidence-based study led to the following recommendations: PE hastens recovery in patients with GBS and is recommended for nonambulatory patients within 4 weeks of onset and for ambulatory patients within 2 weeks of onset; IVIg is recommended for patients who require aid to walk within 2 to 4 weeks from onset of symptoms; the effects of PE and IVIg are equivalent; sequential treatment with PE followed by IVIg is not recommended; corticosteroids are not recommended for treatment of GBS; and treatment with PE and IVIg is an option for children although there have been no adequate randomized drug trials in this population. The report also states that further research must be done to determine whether patients with primary axonal forms and Miller Fisher syndrome have different responses to PE, IVIg, or corticosteroid medications.[173]

Therapeutic Evaluation

A comprehensive therapeutic evaluation of the patient with GBS includes factors shown in Box 16-4.

Motor System Examination

The extent of the evaluation depends on the patient's condition and ability to participate in the assessment. In many situations, therapists carry out manual muscle testing (MMT) procedures by testing functional muscle groups. In GBS, however, testing muscle strength and ROM as specifically as possible is important so the patient's course of progression or improvement can be tracked, possible patterns leading to contractures can be predicted and prevented, and the appropriate level of exercise can be implemented. Because full MMT cannot be completed every week with a debilitated patient, a few specific muscles are commonly selected (e.g., sternocleidomastoids, deltoids, triceps, flexor carpi ulnaris, lumbricals, iliopsoas, gluteus medius, anterior tibialis, flexor hallucis longus) to test weekly.

More complete testing should be performed once the acute stage is over or for specific evaluation end points only. Patients who report considerable pain during handling or active movement may not tolerate testing or may be unwilling or unable to cooperate with muscle testing. Therefore the therapist may wish to track the patient's level of pain on

BOX 16-4 ■ FACTORS TO CONSIDER IN EVALUATION OF PATIENTS WITH GBS

HISTORY

Patterns and sequence of symptom onset

Recent illness, injury, prior episodes of sensorimotor problems

MOTOR FUNCTION

Visual inspection to identify symmetry of muscle bulk and function

Myotatic reflexes, rule out tonic reflexes

MMT carefully identifying pattern of weakness (testing should be as muscle specific as possible rather than assessing muscle groups only; use form for serial recording)

Presence of muscle fasciculations

Cranial nerves

ROM (use form for serial recording)

Equilibrium reactions sitting and standing (if testable)

Current functional status (ADLs, including bowel and bladder function, ambulation)

SENSORY SYSTEM

Identify pattern of sensory loss or changes (use body chart)

Identify specific type of sensory change (e.g., paresthesias, anesthesia, hypesthesias); use body chart

Identify pain type and location (use body chart): what makes it better, what makes it worse?

Identify pressure points or areas that might lead to pressure sores

AUTONOMIC SYSTEM

Blood pressure resting and immediately after activity (prone, sitting, standing, if possible)

Heart rate resting and immediately after activity, dysrhythmias

Body temperature stability

Bowel and bladder control

PSYCHOSOCIAL SYSTEMS

Identify patient and family concerns in acute circumstances and concerns about long-term issues that may affect patient and family. Assessment need not be extensive if referral can be made for social service evaluation of patient and family financial concerns, day-to-day living problems (e.g., transportation, child care), support systems, and coping strategies.

ELECTRODIAGNOSTIC TESTING

Nerve conduction velocity. (Physician will order these studies to be performed by a clinician skilled in the procedures. This may be a physical therapist, physician, or technician depending on facility.)

---

a pain scale to help determine weakness related to pathological condition or apparent weakness caused by pain. Changes in the patient's condition should be monitored with serial MMT, ROM assessments, sensory testing, and functional status evaluations. Care should be taken not to fatigue the patient in any single evaluation session. (See Appendix 8-A for references on specific examination tools. Also see Karni et al[174] and Lewis and Bottomley[175] for suggestions on serial functional assessments.)

Respiratory and Dysphagia Evaluation

Therapists are usually involved early in the care of patients with GBS. For patients with respiratory or bulbar paralysis, the therapist's initial contact may be in the intensive care unit (ICU). Although most hospitals have fully equipped ICUs, a therapist working in rural or smaller community hospitals may be the first person to note a patient's changing respiratory status during an evaluation and treatment session for muscle weakness or back pain. Therefore the therapist must be prepared to advise nursing and medical staff about the need to test oxygen saturation levels and FVC. Therapist attention to respiratory complications is particularly important in the managed care environment, which discourages hospitalization if presenting symptoms are not life endangering.[154] A simple estimate of FVC can be done at bedside. If after taking a large breath the patient can count only to 10, the forced vital capacity is approximately 1 L and intubation should be considered. Complete information on the physical therapist's evaluation of patients in acute respiratory failure is provided by Irwin and Tecklin.[176] Patients who have been intubated or who have cranial nerve involvement with oral motor weakness commonly have a high incidence of aspiration. Patients with severe oral-motor

problems and dysphagia should be evaluated thoroughly and treated by a therapist skilled in oral-motor dysfunction and feeding. This may be a speech therapist, occupational therapist, or physical therapist depending on the facility. Patients with a feeding tube (PEG) should receive their feedings in a relatively upright position and should remain in that position for 30 to 60 minutes after feeding to decrease the chance of aspiration. According to Logemann,[177] approximately 40% of patients receiving bedside swallowing assessments have undetected aspiration. Therefore the bedside evaluation should be considered only a preliminary step in the diagnostic process. In addition to careful evaluation of oral-motor control, some clinicians recommend cervical auscultation to listen to swallowing sounds, particularly during the acute phase of the illness.

With evidence of swallowing difficulties and possible aspiration, the patient should be referred for comprehensive testing with videofluoroscopy. Swallowing also can be assessed by techniques such as fiberoptic endoscopy, ultrasound, electroglottography to determine laryngeal movement, and scintigraphy, which involves scanning a radioactive bolus during swallowing.[178] (Refer to section on Medical Management of ALS, for suggestions on dealing with dysphagia on page 480.)

Intervention Goals

Goals for the care of the patient with GBS include the following:

■ Facilitate resolution of respiratory problems and dysphagia

■ Minimize pain

■ Prevent contractures, decubitus ulcers, and injury to weakened or denervated muscles

■ Introduce a graduated program of active exercise while monitoring overuse and fatigue

Therapeutic Interventions

Ropper,[164] an expert in the treatment of GBS, states that no systematic studies of the effectiveness of physical therapy in the treatment of GBS have been undertaken. However, the treatment programs used for patients with poliomyelitis, ALS, and spinal cord injuries can be adapted for use with patients with GBS.

Respiratory and Cranial Nerve Dysfunction

Depending on the facility, physical therapists may be involved in the respiratory care of patients with GBS. Goals of treatment are related to increasing ventilation or oxygenation, decreasing oxygen consumption, controlling secretions, and improving exercise tolerance. See Irwin and Tecklin[176] for coverage of treatment programs and techniques appropriate for the GBS patient with acute or residual respiratory dysfunction. The text includes chapters dealing with practice standards for patients with airway clearance problems, respiratory failure, respirator dependence, and deconditioning as a result of prolonged immobilization.

In the more severe cases of GBS, cranial nerve involvement can lead to multiple complications such as dysphagia and vocal cord paralysis. In many facilities, speech pathologists or occupational therapists are responsible for establishing a dysphagia treatment program. Therapists responsible for treatment of patients with dysphagia and swallowing problems should refer to Logemann's classic text on the evaluation and treatment of swallowing disorders.[177] Basic treatment goals are the prevention of choking and aspiration and the stimulation of effective swallowing and eating. The act of chewing and swallowing is complex and requires coordinated reflexive and conscious action. Treatment is focused on positioning, head control, and oral-motor coordination (e.g., sucking an ice cube, stimulating the gag response, facilitating swallowing with pressure on neck and thyroid notch timed with intent to swallow). A conscious swallowing technique is introduced with thick liquids and progressed to thinner liquids after the patient's oral-motor coordination response is enough to control movement of fluids. Once the patient has good lip closure, fluids should be introduced one sip at a time from a straw cut to a short length to minimize effort. Semisoft, moist foods are gradually introduced (pasta, mashed potatoes, squash, gelatin). Any crumbly or stringy foods (coffee cakes, cookies, snack chips, celery, cheeses) should be avoided, and the patient should not attempt to talk or be interrupted during eating until choking does not occur and swallowing is comfortable and consistent.[179] Feeding training should occur during frequent, short sessions to prevent fatigue. Therapists should be prepared to use the Heimlich maneuver if choking occurs or have a suction machine available at bedside.

Pain

If pain seems to be a major factor in limiting the patient's passive or active motion, the treatment team should determine the best approach to alleviating pain. According to one study, patients with GBS did not seem to show a consistent response to any specific pain medication, although six of the 13 patients seemed to have a positive response to codeine, oxycodone, acetaminophen (Percocet), and oxycodone with aspirin (Percodan).[157] Some patients may find relief with medications used to treat neurogenic pain, such as the tricyclic antidepressants, carbamazepine, or gabapentin (anticonvulsants).[162] For patients who do not respond to conventional analgesics or tricyclic antidepressants, a short course of high-dose corticosteroids can lead to pain relief.[154]

Some patients with neuropathy have noted decreased pain after using transcutaneous electrical nerve stimulation (TENS)[180,181] Although no study has examined the effect of TENS specifically on pain associated with GBS, it might be a treatment option to help with desensitization in patients whose pain is not controlled with passive movement or pain medications (see Chapters 31, 32, 36, and 37). Another option suggested by Meythaler et al[162] is capsaicin, the active ingredient in chili peppers, which when applied topically interacts with the sensory neurons to relieve pain of peripheral neuropathies. Therapists, wearing gloves, apply a topical anesthetic until the area is numb. The capsaicin is then applied topically. The capsaicin remains on the skin until the patient starts to feel the heat, at which point it is promptly removed. Because the nerves are overstimulated by the burning sensation, the sensory gateway is unable to report pain for an extended period.[182] Some patients who experience extreme sensitivity to light touch, such as from movement of sheets, air flow, and intermittent touch contact, benefit from a "cradle," which holds sheets away from the body. Some find relief if the limbs are wrapped snuggly with elastic bandages, which provide continuous low pressure while warding off light and intermittent stimuli. Because persistent pain can seriously interfere with the rehabilitation process, physicians and therapists must be willing to try various medications and desensitization techniques until the patient can tolerate passive and active motion.

Contractures, Decubitus Ulcers, and Injury to Weakened or Denervated Muscles

Positioning. To prevent pressure sores, the therapist needs to be involved within the first few days of hospitalization, especially for the patient who has complete or nearly complete paralysis. A positioning program for the dependent patient is the first line of defense. The therapist should arrange for a special mattress or unit that constantly changes the pressure within the mattress to shift the patient's position or is designed to spread pressure over wide surfaces. For patients who are slender with prominent bony surfaces, the therapist may need to fashion foam "doughnuts" or pads or use sheepskin-type protection for pressure relief. Patients who have muscle pain may prefer to have their hips and knees flexed. In these cases the patient must be taken out of the flexed position for part of each hour.

As part of a complete positioning program, therapists should consider how to best maintain the physiological position of the hands and feet. Research has shown that mild continuous stretch maintained for at least 20 minutes is more beneficial than stronger, brief stretching exercises.[183] Therefore the use of splints for prolonged positioning is superior to the use of short bursts of intermittent, manually applied passive stretching for maintaining functional range. Although some facilities still use a footboard to control passive ankle dorsiflexion, most therapists now use moldable plastic splints that can be worn when the patient is in any position. Because ankle-foot splints often prevent visual inspection of the heel position, care must be taken to ensure that the heel is firmly down in the orthosis and that the strapping pattern is adequate to secure the foot. The strap system must be simple enough to be positioned properly by all staff and family members caring for the patient. The ankle-foot splint should extend slightly beyond the end of the toes to prevent toe flexion and skin breakdown from the toes rubbing on sheeting. Care should be taken not to compress the peroneal nerve with the splint as it crosses the fibula.[158] Wrist and hand splints may be prefabricated, resting-style splints or molded to meet the patient's specific needs. Because increased tone is not a problem in the patient with GBS, a simple cone or rolled cloth may be adequate to maintain good wrist, thumb, and finger alignment.

Another concern is regaining tolerance to the upright position. A review of the literature on dysautonomia found that between 15% and 50% of patients with GBS have problems with hypotension as a result of prolonged immobility in the supine position.[155] Most patients must be placed on a graduated program to regain tolerance to the upright position. A program to improve tolerance to upright position can be started in the ICU if the patient is on a circle electric or Nelson standing bed. If a standing bed is not available, a sitting program can be initiated as soon as it is tolerated. A progressive standing program can be instituted when the patient's respiratory system and ANS are no longer unstable and the patient can be moved to a tilt table. Caution should be taken to stabilize the patient fully to maintain alignment and to limit activity in muscles below the fair range. When beginning training, some patients benefit from using an abdominal binder or foot-to-thigh compression stockings if tolerated. Because of the relation between poor hydration and hypotension, therapists must ensure their patient is well hydrated before beginning upright or standing tolerance programs.[147]

Range of Motion. The onset of connective tissue shortening in response to immobilization caused by paralysis is rapid.[184] To be effective, the ROM program must include both accessory and physiological motions to increase circulation; provide lubrication of the joints; and maintain extensibility of capsular, muscle, and tendon tissue. ROM can usually be maintained with standard positioning and ROM programs. Nevertheless, some patients, especially those who have reported severe extremity and axial pain early during the disease process and those who have been quadriplegic and respirator dependent for prolonged periods, may develop significant joint contractures despite preventive interventions. As with patients with spinal cord or severe head injuries, heterotopic ossification has been reported in patients with GBS.[185] Meythaler et al[186] note that early mobilization was related to therapeutic decreases in serum calcium levels and suggest that aggressive range of motion may impede the effects of heterotopic bone overgrowth that can have a severe impact on range of motion.

Soryal et al[187] reported on three patients who had marked residual contractures that limited function after strength improved. None of the patients had radiological signs of erosive arthropathy or inflammatory joint disease. They hypothesized a number of possible mechanisms for the limitations in ROM: (1) therapists and nurses may have been reluctant to take patients who reported marked pain during passive movement through the full ROM; (2) the contractures may have been a result of pain or damage caused by inappropriate excessive passive movement of hypotonic and sensory-impaired joints and muscles (often caused by poor movement of the patient in bed or by poorly trained staff or family members moving limbs); (3) the paralysis may have resulted in lymphatic stasis with accumulation of fluid in tissue spaces and nutritional disturbances; and (4) vasomotor disturbances resulting from autonomic neuropathy may have led to adhesions and fibrosis. Although the authors found few reports describing contractures as a significant residual problem, they suggested that ROM programs must be defined precisely as to frequency and duration, particularly for patients reporting early joint pain.[187]

Some patients will continually position their limbs so muscle and tendons are in the shortened range in an attempt to decrease muscle pain. This may lead to capsular contractures. The therapist should be aware of changes in "end feel" over time when testing ROM of each joint to determine if capsular and ligamentous structures are also becoming more restricted as the muscle and tendon tissue shortens. Patients who have intact sensation of pain and temperature may respond positively to the use of heat to decrease muscle pain and to facilitate tissue elongation before stretching. Several basic studies of the relation between load and heat that used rat tail tendon have shown that attaining permanent length increases in collagenous tissue is possible with a combination of heat and stretch.[188-191] On the basis of these studies, Warren[192] suggests that stretch be combined with the highest tolerable therapeutic temperature (approximately 45° C or 113° F). He also recommends that the application of stretch should be of long duration, that moderate forces should be used, that tissue temperature should be elevated before stretching, and that elongation of tissue should be maintained for at least 8 to 10 minutes while the tissue is cooling. (*Caution:* Heat should not be used on a patient with a sensory deficit related to an inability to distinguish differences in temperature.) Because heating muscle and tendon tissue before sustained stretching was a mainstay in prevention of contractures caused by muscle spasms attributable to poliomyelitis, it may have a place in treatment of muscle spasm and contractions in GBS provided no sensory impairment is present.[193]

Denervated or weakened muscles can be injured easily; therefore the therapist is responsible for ensuring that joint structures are not damaged and that ROM is done with appropriate support of the limb to prevent sudden overstretching. This is particularly true at the shoulder because many caregivers, especially those with minimal or no training in ROM, do not know to carefully rotate the shoulder externally during abduction to prevent impingement and capsular damage.[194] Caution also should be taken when "ranging" or stretching the ankle into dorsiflexion to ensure that the subtalar joint is in neutral or locked position so that the Achilles tendon is effectively elongated and the midfoot structures are not overstretched. In hospitals where the patient is treated by a changing therapy or nursing staff or by family members, a positioning schedule with diagrams, a splinting plan, and ROM recommendations should be presented in poster format at the patient's bedside to provide consistent treatment.

ROM stretching of all involved joints should be performed at least twice a day and more frequently if the patient has no active movement. Patients should be encouraged to move actively when they can do so without causing pain or fatigue. They should be observed carrying out their active range to determine whether change has occurred in the quality of movement that may be related to decreasing strength. If the patient cannot complete ROM through full range independently, the therapist or nursing staff must carefully assist the patient in moving to the end range. This may not be easy if the patient has pain with motion. Knowing whether to "push through the pain" or stay within the limits of pain is often a great dilemma for the therapist. The therapist needs to find a balance between working for full joint range and reacting to the patient's reports of pain.

On the basis of evidence that continuous passive motion (CPM) is effective in maintaining joint range in both rabbits and human beings,[195] Mays[196] described a case study of a patient with GBS (quadriplegia with 7 days of mechanical ventilation) who had persistent pain and stiffness of the upper extremities and fingers approximately 3 months after the onset of GBS. Therefore CPM of the hands and fingers was added to a program of occupational therapy that included ROM, splinting, and ADLs. The author reported an increase in the rate of recovery of finger range and a decrease in pain after use of CPM. Numerous other studies have reported the value of CPM in maintaining or increasing ROM after hip and knee surgery. It may be a useful adjunct to traditional therapy for patients with GBS, especially those who continue to develop contractures with standard, intermittent ROM programs. Patients with severe paresthesias or dysesthesias may not be able to tolerate CPM equipment.

Massage also may play a positive role in maintaining muscle tissue mobility and tissue nutrition. In a study of crush injuries of muscle in rat tails, investigators reported that massage may lessen the amount of fibrosis that develops in immobilized, denervated, or injured muscle.[197] The use of massage in patients with GBS has not been reported; however, it makes intuitive sense that it may be a useful adjunct to ROM exercises in patients who do not have marked hypersensitivity to touch, significant muscle pain, or a history of deep vein thrombosis (DVT). For patients with or without a history of DVT who are immobile for long periods or who have concomitant cardiac illnesses may have marked swelling of the distal limbs. After medical clearance, edema-specific massage and limb-elevation techniques may be useful if tolerated by the patient. Even early active ROM creating "muscle pumping" contractions in muscles with at least fair strength can help prevent uncomfortable edema.

Progressive Program of Active Exercise While Monitoring for Overuse and Fatigue

Although most patients with GBS recover from the paralysis, the course and rate of recovery may vary significantly between patients. Strength usually returns in a descending pattern—opposite of the pattern noted during onset of the disease. *The most important concept to remember in designing an exercise program is that exercise will not hasten or improve nerve regeneration or influence the reinnervation rate during the rehabilitation process.*[198] The major goal of therapeutic management therefore must be to maintain the patient's musculoskeletal system in an optimal ready state, prevent overwork, and pace the recovery process to obtain maximal function as reinnervation occurs.

The rule in developing an exercise program for patients with GBS is that muscle fatigue must be avoided and rest periods must be frequent.[183,199] Bensman[200] reported on eight patients who had stabilized after acute polyradiculoneuritis (among them patients with GBS). All eight patients had a temporary loss of function after strenuous physical exercise. Three patients apparently had significant decreases in strength. All patients were then placed on a program of passive ROM and an increase in muscle strength was noted. Recurring episodes of a temporary loss of function appeared to be related to strenuous exercise and fatigue. Studying the effect of exercise on rat muscle after nerve injury, Herbison et al[199] identified a loss of contractile proteins during initial reinnervation. After reinnervation the same amount of exercise resulted in muscle hypertrophy. Reitsma[100] noted that vigorous exercise damaged muscles if fewer than one third of motor units were functional. If more than one third of the motor units remained, exercise led to hypertrophy. Therefore the amount of strengthening attained seems proportional to the number of intact or impaired motor units. Exercise at a level to elicit a training effect in normal muscle may cause overwork damage in damaged muscle. Because the therapist cannot determine the number of intact motor units available to a patient, the therapist must be cautious when initiating exercise with any patient who is undergoing reinnervation. The safe exercise range differs for normal and impaired muscle, with the therapeutic window being smaller for muscles undergoing reinnervation (see Figure 16-3).

Bensman[200] recommended that once the condition has stabilized, active exercise may begin as follows:

- Short periods of nonfatiguing exercise appropriate to the patient's strength
- An increase in activity or exercise level only if the patient improves or if no deterioration occurs after 1 week
- A return to bed rest if a decrease in function or strength occurs
- A program of exercise directed at strengthening for function rather than strength itself
- A limit of fatiguing exercise for 1 year with a gradual return to sport activities and more strenuous exercise

Steinberg[198] suggested that patients be allowed to exercise to the first point of fatigue or muscle ache. Abnormal sensations (tingling, paresthesias) that persist for prolonged periods after exercise may also indicate that the exercise or activity level was excessive.

When neural recovery begins, the initiation of active exercise must be implemented with a clear understanding that excessive exercise during early reinnervation when only a few functioning motor units are present can lead to further damage rather than to the expected exercise-induced hypertrophy of muscle.

On the basis of this information, a graduated exercise program can be viewed as a pyramid with passive ROM at the base; antigravity and specific, functionally focused, resistive exercises in the middle levels; and integrated, coordinated, and functional exercises and activities at the top.[201]

During the initial stages of exercise, the repetitions per exercise period should be low and the frequency of short periods of exercise should be high.[183] As reinnervation occurs and motor units become responsive, the early process of muscle reeducation exercise used by the therapist may be similar to that used during the polio era. To encourage active contraction of the muscle the therapist should carefully demonstrate to the patient the expected movement. The therapist then passively moves the patient's limb while the patient observes. After gaining a clear picture of what movement is expected, the patient is encouraged to contract muscles. Facilitatory techniques such as skin stroking, brushing, vibration, icing, and tapping may be used in conjunction with the muscle reeducation process. The patient is taught to reassess his or her movements and make corrective responses. As the patient gains strength, the movements are translated into functional activities.[199]

Functionally directed exercise should be initiated judiciously, and the activities should be appropriate for the muscle grade of that muscle or muscle group. For example, if the patient's deltoid muscle receives a poor (2/5) grade (full range of motion with gravity eliminated), the patient should be cautioned not to repeatedly attempt to elevate her or his arm against gravity (e.g., to shave or do one's hair). Exercises should be developed to allow the patient to exercise in the gravity-free position (overhead slings, powder boards, pool exercises) that allow the patient to move actively through a full range until he or she can take resistance in the gravity-eliminated position. Many younger patients have to be reminded to pace their activity so they do not overly fatigue and possibly injure their recovering muscles. Children, teenagers, or adults with impaired judgment often need a strict schedule of rest and activity. Patients and staff also need to be reminded that prolonged sitting in bed or in a wheelchair, even when supported, may tax the axial musculature. A program of gradual sitting should be instituted, with the final goal being independent, unsupported sitting with functional adaptive reactions. In busy hospitals a schedule of sitting and activity should be posted in clear view at the patient's bedside.

As reinnervation progresses and strength and exercise tolerance increases, the therapist may choose to use facilitative exercise techniques such as proprioceptive neuromuscular facilitation (PNF), which intentionally recruits maximal contraction of specific muscle groups. Although PNF techniques are excellent for eliciting maximal contraction, care must be taken not to overwork the weaker components of the movement pattern. A positive aspect of PNF techniques is that they can be tied in with functional patterns such as rolling, which is necessary for bed mobility, transitions to quadruped, kneeling, sitting, standing stability, and gait.[202-204]

Because patients with GBS are transferred from acute care facilities to rehabilitation, skilled nursing, or home environments more quickly than in the past, therapists must be careful to document any serial negative changes or plateaus in motor, sensory, or respiratory impairments or functional status that may herald a relapse.[147] Standard measures of impairment, including MMT, ROM, and sensory tests, should be completed before and after discharge from the acute setting, as should assessments of functional status or disability, such as the Functional Independence Measure (FIM) or Barthel Index (BI).[205,206] In addition, before discharge from the hospital or rehabilitation unit, therapists should complete an assessment of the patient's home environment so that appropriate safety and adaptive equipment can be in place in time for the patient's return home. Schmitz[207] has written a comprehensive review of home assessment protocols.

Although 65% to 75% or more of patients with GBS show a return to clinically normal motor function, between 2% and 5% of patients have a recurrence of symptoms similar in onset and pattern to the original illness. The recurrence differs from a chronic inflammatory demyelinating polyneuropathy.[208] In addition, anecdotal and empirical evidence shows that some patients continue to show deficits during strenuous exercises that require maximal endurance. Four soldiers who were considered clinically recovered from GBS (normal motor power with or without reappearance of reflexes and the absence of sensory impairment) were unable to pass the Army Physical Fitness Test (APFT), which is designed to measure a minimal acceptable age-related level of physical fitness (maximal effort to challenge respiratory and muscular endurance, strength, and flexibility). Before onset of GBS, the four patients had all exceeded the APFT standards. None was able to pass the APFT as long as 4 years after the illness, indicating that the sustained effort required in the fitness testing unmasked a significant, persistent deficit that interfered with their ability to continue their military careers.[209] Therefore the possibility of long-term endurance deficits should be considered when patients appear to have reached full recovery but report difficulty when returning to work or activities that require sustained maximal effort.[210]

Cardiovascular fitness may also be compromised after recovery from GBS. This may be caused by altered muscle function, but it is also related to deconditioning from an imposed sedentary lifestyle.[166] Several studies have attempted to determine the effect of endurance exercise training after GBS. In one case study a 23-year-old woman with a chronic-relapsing form of GBS (usually a slow-onset polyneuropathy with a remitting/relapsing course and persistent slowing of nerve conduction velocities) with onset at age 15 years was placed on a walking and cycling program at 45% or less of her predicted maximal heart rate reserve. The low-intensity exercise program was selected to prevent possible fatigue-related relapse. After the program, the subject had increased her walking time 37%, walking distance approximately 88%, and cycle ride time more than 100%. Although no standardized or formalized recording of functional level was recorded before and after the exercise program, the patient reported that her energy level for ADLs was a "little higher" and that stair walking was easier.[210] In another single-subject study of a 54-year-old man 3 years after onset of GBS with residual weakness, the authors demonstrated similar improvements in cardiopulmonary and work capacities as well as leg strength after a 16-week course of a thrice-weekly aerobic exercise program. The subject also reported expanded ADL capabilities. The authors suggested that their training regimen may disrupt the cycle of inactivity after recovery from GBS that leads to disuse atrophy and further deconditioning in patients with mild residual weakness.[211] Fehlings et al[212] tested the muscle strength and endurance in a group of children at least 2 years

TABLE 16-3 ■ Medical Status of Patients with GBS and Possible Treatment Outline

MEDICAL STATUS	TREATMENT*
Tracheostomy Respirator dependent Complete cranial nerve paralysis Quadriplegia	*Week 1:* Postural drainage every 3 hours around the clock Passive ROM to all joints Splinting (molded plastic) of hands and feet to maintain functional position Positioning, splinting, and ROM program schedule posted at bedside *Weeks 2-5:* Postural drainage decreased to two times each shift (every 8 hours) Passive ROM, physiological and accessory motions, gentle stretching of intercostal musculature, trunk rotations Continue splinting and positioning program Family education: family members taught gentle physiological ROM techniques, with attention to correct shoulder patterns and simple massage techniques
Respirator set on intermittent mandatory ventilation Weaning to respirator at night by end of week 7 No active muscle contractions except eye opening and lip movements Dysphagia	*Weeks 6-7:* Postural drainage two times each shift (every 8 hours) Continue ROM program, splinting, and positioning Begin to build tolerance of upright sitting with good trunk alignment Begin facilitation of active facial/tongue muscle activity in patterns necessary for swallowing, eating, and speaking; speech pathology, occupational therapy consultation for dysphagia training Family members active in care, helping with ROM, splinting, and positioning schedule as they choose
Palpable muscle activity in neck, trunk, proximal musculature of upper and lower extremities	*Weeks 8-12:* Postural drainage one time each shift Chest stretching, breathing exercises Dysphagia program in collaboration with speech consultant Muscle reeducation program with EMG biofeedback progressing to gravity-eliminated exercises using suspension slings attached to bed Tilt table standing program to increase tolerance to upright (wearing positioning splints if necessary) Collaborate with occupational therapy for treatment in wheelchair with suspension slings to facilitate active arm motion in gravity-limited position Exercise, rest, positioning schedule posted Family, patient educated about stimulating activity level to prevent fatigue, overuse of reinnervating muscles

*Treatment depends on rate of recovery.

after acute onset of GBS. Although the children appeared essentially recovered, endurance of the arm muscles was lower than that of the lower extremities. They hypothesize that the typical walking, running, and cycling activities that the children participating in were sufficient to improve strength and endurance of lower-extremity muscles and they recommended that children be encouraged to participate in activities such as swimming to improve upper-extremity endurance. Controlled tetherball and volleyball activities are also appropriate. Most recently, Tuckey and Greenwood[213] reported positive results of treatment with partial body weight support (PBWS) treadmill exercise for a patient with severe GBS. Prior studies of PBWS treatment of patients with total hip arthroplasty,[214] stroke,[215] and back pain[216] support the findings for the patient with GBS and may present a reasonable option for therapy in patients with prolonged weakness and deconditioning after acute GBS.

Although the traditional thought has been that little clinical improvement occurs after 2 to 3 years, Bernsen et al[217] found that 21% of the patients in a study of 150 patients after recovery from acute GBS reported improvement after 2.5 to 6.5 years, although the authors thought the perception of improvement was related to improved sensory function. Of future research and clinical interest are the long-term consequences of GBS and how the normal aging process will affect patients who have some mild residual, for example, whether some patients will develop increasing weakness over time similar to persons with postpolio syndrome.[147] For an example of treatment progression during the acute stage from week 1 through week 12, see Table 16-3.

Adaptive Equipment and Orthoses

Judicious use of orthotic devices and adaptive equipment should be considered an integral part of the rehabilitation process. The purpose of the orthotic and adaptive devices is twofold: (1) to protect weakened structures from overstretch and overuse and (2) to facilitate ADLs within the limits of the patient's current ability. Orthotic devices and adaptive equipment should be introduced and discontinued on the basis of serial evaluations of strength, ROM, and functional needs. For example, a hospitalized patient who has poor (2/5) middle deltoid strength may practice upper-extremity activities such as eating while using suspension slings. A thumb position splint may be used temporarily to aid thumb control in grasping tasks.

Most patients will need a wheelchair for several months until strength and endurance improve. As strength returns, patients recovering from severe paralysis may need to change from use of a wheelchair with a high, reclining back with a head rest to use of a lightweight, easily maneuverable chair. A quandary for the therapist is to predict how long a wheelchair will be necessary and whether it should be rented or purchased as the patient progresses through different stages of recovery. While moving from wheelchair mobility to independent ambulation, patients will usually progress from parallel bars to a walker with a seat to allow frequent resting, and then to crutches or a cane. Because wheelchairs, walkers, crutches, and canes, especially custom appliances, are expensive and not always covered by insurance, the therapist should carefully consider the cost to the patient during the recovery process.

Although most patients with GBS have a complete functional recovery, many show a more prolonged residual weakness of calf and, most commonly, anterior compartment musculature, requiring the use of an ankle-foot orthosis (AFO). The decision whether to use a prefabricated orthosis or custom appliance is not always simple. Several temporary orthotic measures can be considered. For example, if the patient shows good gastrocnemius-soleus strength with mild weakness of the dorsiflexors, a simple elastic strap attached to the shoelaces and a calf band may be sufficient to prevent overuse of the anterior compartment muscles. An old-fashioned, relatively inexpensive spring wire brace, which can be attached to the patient's shoes to facilitate dorsiflexion, is a good choice for patients who report sensory hypersensitivity when wearing a plastic orthosis.

Most therapy units today have access to varied sizes of plastic, fixed-ankle AFOs that can be used until a decision is made to have the patient fitted with custom AFOs. A newer system of prefabricated AFOs with adjustable ankle motion cams has been developed that allows the therapist to limit plantar flexion and dorsiflexion to the specific needs of the patient. For patients with reasonable control of plantar flexion and dorsiflexion, but with lateral instability because of peroneal weakness, a simple ankle stirrup device such as the Aircast Swivel-Strap stirrup splint (Aircast, Inc., Summit, N.J.) can be used temporarily to provide lateral ankle stability. Although few patients with GBS need knee-ankle-foot orthoses (KAFOs) on a long-term basis, inexpensive air splints or adjustable long-leg metal splints to control knee position are sometimes helpful when working on standing weight bearing and during initial gait training. See Chapter 34 for additional information on orthotics.

Psychosocial Issues

Although most patients with GBS have a good recovery over a period of 2 or more years, the acute stage of the disease can be frightening, especially to patients who progress to complete paralysis and respiratory failure. Nancy, in Case Study 16-2, reported that she was terrified during the time she was totally paralyzed (including eyelid movement) and on a respirator. She said that nurses, doctors, and hospital staff seemed to assume she could not hear because she was unable to respond in any manner. In her words,

"They acted like I was already dead, and I thought I would be from the way they were talking. The thing I hated the most was when the night nurses from the registry would come in and ask how to make the ventilator work! I felt panicked. Can you imagine having your life depend on a machine and knowing that the person who was supposed to make it work had no idea what to do if a tube came unconnected? They were always worried about my blood pressure. Who wouldn't have high blood pressure in that situation! The thing I liked about my therapists was that they told me what they were going to do even when I couldn't respond. They didn't just start doing things or pulling on me like other people did."

Skirrow et al[218] remind clinicians that the "intensive care patient is plunged into a world of machines that flash and beep; of tubes and wires that seem to spring from almost every orifice; and of mind-numbing sedative and analgesic medications." Needless to say, evidence is increasing that patients treated in acute trauma rooms or ICUs can have posttraumatic stress syndrome (PTSD). Particularly vulnerable are patients who have had previous traumatic experiences. PTSD places patients at marked risk for increased startle responses, extreme vigilance or anticipation of painful events, sleep disorders, terrifying dreams, and dissociative flashbacks after leaving the ICU and left untreated for years after the experience.[219] Patients discharged from prolonged ICU experiences, especially those who had respiratory failure, have an increased incidence of anxiety, depression, and panic disorders years after discharge.

In a nursing study of patient experiences in the ICU, researchers found that patients often felt anxious, apprehensive, and fearful. The patients expected ICU nurses to be experienced and technically adept, but those who felt most secure despite the traumatic ICU experiences felt that the nurses were vigilant to their needs and offered personalized care,[220] a point clearly made by Nancy. Although one might expect ICU staff to be carefully tuned in to patient needs, the highly technical nature of modern ICUs may attract personnel less focused on individual patient care or it may prevent caring staff from attending to the little kindnesses that are so comforting to critically ill patients. Baxter[219] suggests that caregivers in the ICU try to orient patients to what is being done, to approach the patients within their field of vision, and to minimize unexpected noises and sudden touching. To decrease the long-term consequences of PTSD, Skirrow et al[218] recommend that hospitals consider use of an ICU follow-up clinic to offer patients an opportunity to talk about their experiences in a group format and to get information about their recovery process.

Although most patients recover well from GBS, 3 to 6 years after onset of GBS 38% of patients in a Dutch study had to make a job change to accommodate their physical status, 44% had to alter their leisure activities, and nearly 50% described ongoing psychosocial changes.[217] Similar findings were reported in a study of Japanese patients recovering from GBS.[221]

In summary, the rehabilitation program for a person with GBS must be graded carefully according to the stage of illness. In the acute care environment when respiratory deficits are present, the initial emphasis is directed toward support of maximal respiratory status through postural drainage, chest stretching, and breathing exercises. Because of prolonged bed rest and immobility related to weakness, accessory and physiological ROM must be maintained with around-the-clock efforts. Splinting or positioning devices are recommended to maintain functional positions during prolonged periods of immobility. A gradual program to increase upright tolerance is begun when respiratory and autonomic functions have stabilized. Therapists must keep in mind the potential to damage denervated muscles with aggressive strengthening programs when developing a rehabilitation plan and a home-based conditioning program. Adaptive equipment and orthoses should be used as needed to protect weakened muscles, facilitate normal movement, and prevent fatigue during the reinnervation process. Although a rehabilitation program has been found to make a measurable difference in patient long-term recovery, many patients are being discharged without follow-up care.[222] Therefore therapists should be assertive in ensuring that their patients with GBS have ongoing contact with rehabilitation specialists who can guide the recovery process (Case Study 16-2).

MUSCULAR DYSTROPHY

Pathology and Medical Diagnosis

Muscular dystrophy refers to forms of hereditary myopathy characterized by progressive muscle weakness, deterioration, destruction, and regeneration of muscle fibers. During the process, muscle fibers are gradually replaced with fibrous and fatty tissue. Each of the inherited forms of myopathy (i.e., Becker's dystrophy, myotonic dystrophy, limb-girdle dystrophy, and facioscapulohumeral dystrophy) has its own unique genetic and phenotypic characteristics. (For comprehensive review of the forms of muscular dystrophy and myopathy, see Dubowitz.[223])

Because Duchenne (pseudohypertrophic) muscular dystrophy (DMD) is one of the most commonly known forms of muscular dystrophy, it is used as a model for discussion of treatment implications for therapists. DMD is a disease of progressive muscle weakness leading to total paralysis and early death in the late teens or young adulthood. It has an incidence of between 13 and 33 cases per 100,000 live births and a new mutation rate of approximately 1 in 10,000 (i.e., one third or more cases occur in families without a history of DMD). In the past few years the abnormal gene for DMD has been detected on the X chromosome at band Xp21, which encodes for dystrophin, a 427-kD cytoskeleton protein in the membrane. Because it has an X-linked, recessive pattern, the disease affects males almost exclusively.[224] However, in nearly one third of DMD cases, DNA analysis is normal and diagnosis must be confirmed by protein analysis or immunohistology tests.[225]

In almost 100% of patients with DMD, immunoblotting or immunostaining techniques show complete absence of dystrophin from muscle tissue. An early abnormality during the process of muscle fiber destruction is the breakdown of the muscle fiber plasma membrane. The membrane destruction results in an influx of calcium-rich extracellular fluid and complement components into the muscle fibers. In addition, activation of intracellular proteases and complement occurs, with the ultimate removal of necrotic fibers by macrophages.[226] This loss of dystrophin results in a weakened cell membrane that is easily damaged in muscle contraction.[224] However, loss of dystrophin alone is not considered the sole explanation of the severity and lethality of muscular dystrophy.[227]

Laboratory studies show serum creatine kinase (CK) elevated more than 100 times normal in early stages of the disease. These CK levels decrease over time with loss of muscle mass. Elevated CK level is evident at birth long before symptoms are evident. Muscle biopsy specimens show degeneration with gradual loss of fiber, variation in fiber size, and a proliferation of connective and adipose tissue. Histochemical studies indicate loss of subdivision into fiber types, with a tendency toward type I fiber pre-

---

CASE STUDY 16-2 ■ NANCY

Nancy, a 16-year-old girl with a history of repeated hospitalizations for asthma, was admitted to the hospital with tingling in the hands and feet and mild respiratory distress. Because staff thought her asthma attacks had a significant emotional component, her repeated complaints of paresthesias, muscle pain, and weakness were largely ignored or attributed to anxiety attacks. The day after admission, Nancy began staggering while walking and became extremely agitated and hysterical, screaming that she was dying and could not breathe. A medical assessment showed evidence of wheezing with a normal chest radiograph and decreased FVC. She was uncooperative during strength testing, although strength was estimated to be within normal limits except for approximately F+ (3+) strength of the dorsiflexors and everters and G (4) strength of the plantar flexors. She became extremely upset when her feet were touched.

Because of her psychological history, she was referred for psychiatric assessment and was placed on an anxiolytic medication. Two hours later she had a full respiratory arrest and was intubated and maintained on mechanical ventilation. Over the next 3 days she developed flaccid quadriplegia and within 5 days she had complete cranial nerve involvement. She was weaned from the respirator after 29 days after several episodes of pneumonia. After extubation, she had swallowing and speech problems that resolved by discharge at 3 months after onset. During the acute stage, she was catheterized because of urinary retention and was treated for a bowel obstruction. Sensation was normal for perception of temperature changes and deep pressure.

Proprioception was diminished at the ankle, knee, and fingers. Paresthesias and hypesthesias, aggravated by light touch, were present in a glovelike pattern of both hands and feet.

Nancy's physical therapy treatment began in the ICU. Although her postural drainage treatment was performed by using respiratory therapy techniques in conjunction with aerosol medication by iPPV, physical therapists began a course of chest stretching techniques in coordination with a fastidious ROM program performed twice a day by a therapist and on the evening and night shifts by a nurse. A pressure relief mattress was ordered for her bed. To prevent contracture development, an occupational therapist fabricated bilateral wrist and finger splints; a physical therapist molded ankle splints to maintain 90 degrees of dorsiflexion with neutral eversion-inversion. A positioning and ROM schedule in poster form with pictures of positions and ROM patterns was posted at Nancy's bedside.

Because Nancy reported severe hypersensitivity to light touch or to any passive movement of her limbs, a cradle was placed on the bed to prevent sheets from touching her and to prevent air flow changes from irritating her skin. She was fitted for above-knee light pressure stockings, which seemed to decrease her sensitivity to light touch.

Progression of the GBS process seemed to plateau at approximately 15 days after onset with a gradual return of respiratory function complicated by infections. Weaning from the respirator was difficult and the physical therapist played a major role in instructing Nancy, the staff, and her family in appropriate breathing exercises to be performed every 1 or 2 hours. Because her parents wanted to be involved with her care, they were taught ROM techniques with special attention to correct shoulder ROM techniques. The physical therapists continued to follow Nancy twice a day to ensure that accessory motions were completed with the physiological motions. Moist hot packs similar to those used during the polio era were used effectively before ROM for 1 week during which Nancy reported severe muscle pain.

As part of her positioning program, Nancy was placed in supported semisitting position while on the respirator. As muscle control returned, a muscle reeducation program was initiated that focused initially on the head and trunk and then on the upper and lower extremities. Exercise periods were limited to 15 minutes twice a day. Ideally, she would have benefited from more frequent short sessions; however, this was not possible. Therefore her parents were shown how to guide her active exercise program cautiously so that she was able to exercise more frequently at low repetitions. When each muscle group reached an MMT grade of F+ (3+) or greater, Nancy was allowed to use the muscles in functional activities with proscribed limitations in activity duration. When she was able to tolerate upright sitting and had some bed mobility, Nancy was transferred to a Nelson bed in which she could begin a gradual standing weight-bearing program.

A speech therapist worked with Nancy in the ICU to help her relearn safe swallowing patterns and to reintroduce her to different-textured foods. A dietitian had been working with Nancy throughout her hospitalization to ensure adequate nutrition while intubated, and she worked closely with the speech therapist to progress Nancy's diet as she became able to handle liquids and solids.

After being weaned from the respirator and transferred to the general floor, Nancy was brought to the physical therapy department for treatment, which was frequently done in conjunction with occupational therapy. As strength increased, she began a program of resisted exercise. Trunk and upper- and lower-extremity PNF patterns were used as the primary exercise technique; however, great caution was used to avoid overworking weak muscle groups evoked during use of the PNF pattern. A full mat program with rolling and coming to sitting was also instituted. Occupational therapists focused on graduated use of Nancy's upper extremities, first using overhead slings attached to a wheelchair and later using a lap board to support her weakened shoulder musculature while practicing hand activities.

After 2 months of hospitalization, Nancy was discharged home to return for daily outpatient rehabilitation. Because Nancy appeared to be regaining strength well, she was provided with an ultralight rental wheelchair through her insurance for use until a final determination was made for long-term need. Nancy was also fitted with prefabricated adjustable AFOs, which were purchased through the physical therapy department. After 4 to 6 months a determination would be made about expected return of her persistently weakened dorsiflexors. If Nancy appeared to need AFOs for a prolonged period, a set of specifically molded AFOs would be ordered. At discharge, both the physical and occupational therapists made a home visit with the hospital social worker and parents to determine what home adaptations and support services would be necessary.

Follow-up of Nancy's outpatient therapy showed that she continued to make gradual recovery over the next 1.5 years. She initially returned to school 3 months after discharge using a wheelchair. She graduated to a walker, then to forearm crutches, and finally to independent ambulation. She refused to be seen using a walker at school so she continued to use the wheelchair at school until she was independent on crutches. She continued to wear bilateral AFOs but was weaned from full-time use approximately 14 months after discharge. During the weaning process, Nancy wore her AFOs at school while walking and for any walking distance over four city blocks or if she heard her feet begin to slap from fatigued dorsiflexors. By 14 months, Nancy showed no evidence of overuse weakness after her regular activities, although she had difficulty with endurance activities in her physical education classes. When hiking, she carried her AFOs to use when she expected a long downhill trek to prevent overwork from eccentric muscle activity. By age 19 years, Nancy had returned fully to her normal activity level.

dominance. EMG studies show patterns of low-amplitude, short-duration, polyphasic motor unit action potentials.

Although the absence of dystrophin is usually discussed relative to skeletal muscle, dystrophin is also evident on the membrane surfaces of the cardiac Purkinje fibers and is thought to contribute to the cardiac conduction problems seen in DMD. Cardiac involvement is present in more than 60% of boys with DMD across all ages; however, the common electrocardiogram and electrocardiographic abnormalities are reflected in clinical complications in only 30% of boys until late stages of the disease, and death caused by cardiac dysfunction occurs in only approximately 10% of patients.[228] Weakness of the respiratory muscles (diaphragm, chest wall, and abdominal musculature) is usually evident by the tenth or twelfth year, although the diaphragm remains functional longer than do the intercostal and accessory muscles. A progressive, sometimes severe scoliosis may contribute to respiratory compromise. Pure respiratory failure, restrictive lung disease, or respiratory failure caused by infection is the usual cause of death, most commonly between the ages of 18 and 25 years.[229] Other less-common causes of death include gastric dilation and aspiration.

The average intelligence quotient (IQ) of boys with DMD is approximately 85, with one third of the boys testing below 75. A specific deficit of verbal intelligence and verbal memory has been identified.[230,231] Although the relation between lower IQ and DMD was initially thought to be related to limited life experience caused by the disease, recent studies have shown that dystrophin is also found in brain tissue. This suggests a possible relation between the gene defect, which may cause a decrease in dystrophin in brain tissue and impaired IQ. In contrast to the progressive pattern of muscle deterioration, intellectual impairment is not progressive.[231,232]

Clinical Presentation

Although histological studies have indicated that DMD may be identified in the fetus as early as the first trimester, symptoms are seldom noted until the child is between 2 and 5 years of age. When recalling the child's early development, parents often state that the affected child was more placid and less physically active than expected.[233] The earliest obvious manifestations of DMD, however, may be the delay of early developmental milestones, particularly crawling and walking. In many cases the onset is gradual. Parents or teachers may first identify a problem because the boy is noted to have difficulty keeping up with peers during normal play activities and to be somewhat clumsy, with frequent falling when attempting to run, jump, climb structures, or negotiate uneven terrain. By age 5 years, symmetrical muscle weakness can usually be clearly identified by MMT. Deep tendon reflexes may be absent by 8 to 10 years or earlier. Sensation is normal.[234]

The typical progression of weakness is symmetrical from proximal to distal, with marked weakness of the pelvic and shoulder girdle musculature preceding weakness of the trunk and more distal extremity muscles. Muscles innervated by cranial nerves (except the sternocleidomastoids) are not involved, and bowel and bladder function is usually spared. Progression of weakness is slow but persistent. Weakness of trunk and lower extremity musculature typically leads to changes in gait between 3 and 6 years of age.

Muscle mass continues to decline with increasing weakness of the trunk, anterior neck, and upper-extremity musculature, affecting functional activities. A typical child will continue walking until about age 12 years, at which time the process of transition to a wheelchair becomes imperative. A rapid decrease in strength may occur after prolonged periods of immobilization caused by illness, injury, or surgery.[235]

Progression of Lower-Extremity Weakness

Before age 5 years, hypertrophy of the calf muscles is frequently noted. Pseudohypertrophy is evident as the muscle tissue is replaced by fat and fibrous tissue. Even in the early stages of the disease, few boys with DMD walk with a normal gait pattern. Because of early pelvic girdle muscle weakness, most young boys retain a developmentally immature, wide-based gait pattern. An early distinctive feature of DMD is the Gowers maneuver, in which the child gets up from the floor by using his arms to crawl up his own legs (Figure 16-5).[233]

Muscle imbalance occurs in typical patterns as a result of weakness and contractures. As the posterior hip muscles weaken, the child must arch his back when standing and retract his shoulder girdle to maintain the center of gravity behind the hip joint. This creates a pattern of lumbar lordosis with protrusion of the abdomen. As the quadriceps weaken, the child must maintain his knees in hyperextension to place the axis of rotation posterior to the line of gravity. At this point, mild equinus contractures caused by a muscle imbalance between the plantar and dorsiflexors may help the child maintain knee control because the gastrocnemius-soleus group provides a torque opposing knee flexion. If plantar flexion contractures become severe, however, the child will not be able to maintain standing balance because his base of support is too small and his ankle adaptive strategies are nonfunctional.

Once the child stops weight bearing, development of severe equinovarus deformities is common. Figure 16-6 shows a pattern of progression of muscle imbalance affecting the trunk and lower extremities in stance. Note the increasing lordosis and plantar flexion as the boys attempt to maintain their center of gravity posterior to the hip joint and anterior to the knee joint.

Progression of Gait Pattern Changes

The typical changes in gait pattern over time are identified in Figure 16-7; however, age alone is not an adequate index of predicted gait pattern. Many factors influence how long a child will be able to ambulate. Contributing factors are rate of progression of weakness; severity of contractures (hip flexion, external rotation, abduction, knee flexion, and plantar flexion–inversion contractures occur as disease progresses); influence of body weight; degree of respiratory compromise; type of treatment interventions such as bracing, surgery, and exercise; extent of family support; and the child's personal motivation to ambulate. When the child can no longer ambulate functionally, a wheelchair must be ordered to fit the specific needs of that child within his home and community environment. (For an extensive analysis of changes in gait pattern see Sutherland et al.[236])

Progression of Upper-Extremity Weakness

The upper-extremity pattern of weakness is similar to that in the lower extremities, with proximal musculature being

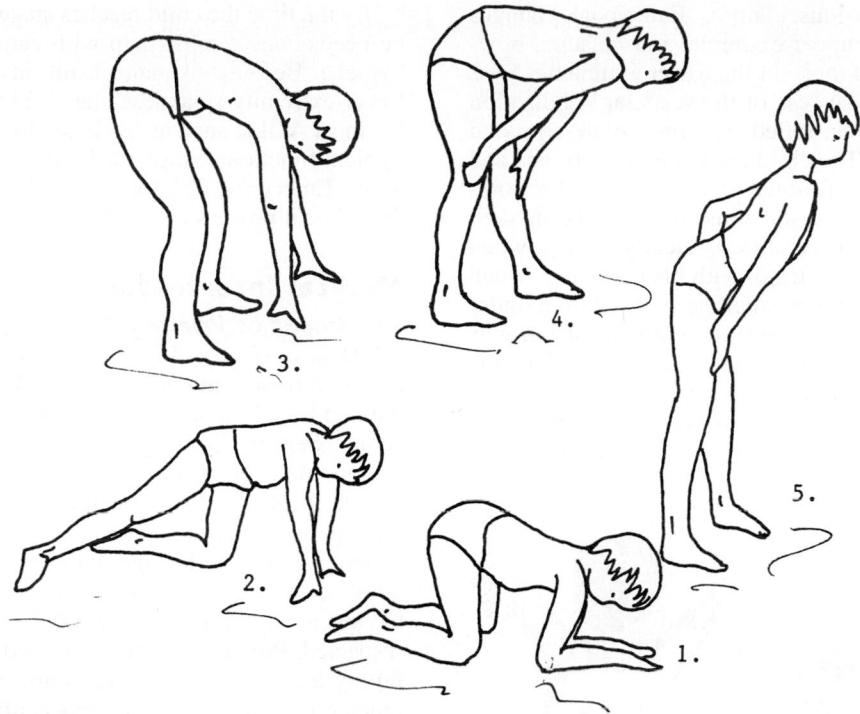

FIGURE 16-5 ■ Child demonstrating Gowers maneuver necessary to achieve upright posture because of pelvic and trunk weakness caused by DMD.

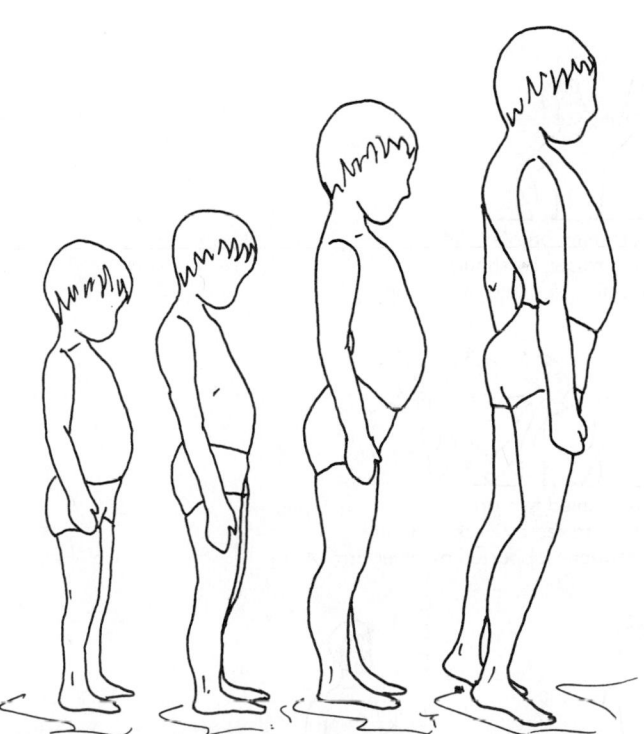

FIGURE 16-6 ■ Pattern of progression of muscle imbalance affecting trunk and lower extremities in DMD.

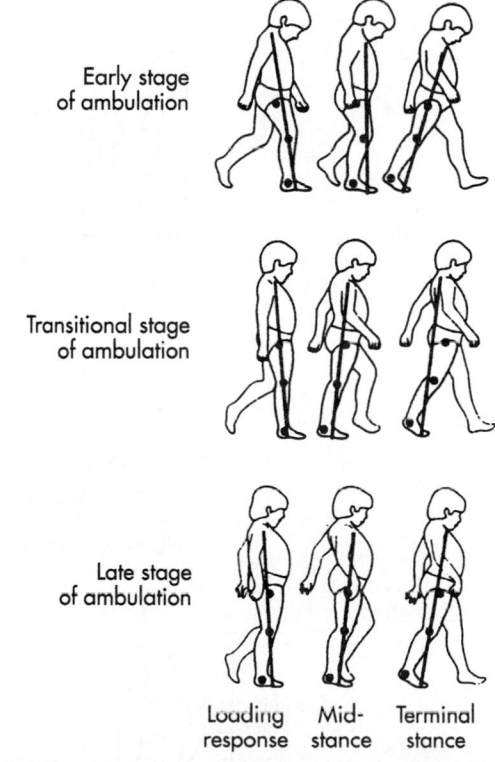

FIGURE 16-7 ■ Early through late stages of ambulation in DMD demonstrating changes in alignment at loading response, mid stance, and terminal stance phases of gait. (From Hsu JD, Furumasu J: Gait and posture changes in the Duchenne muscular dystrophy child, *Clin Orthop Rel Res* 288:122-125, 1993.)

affected before distal musculature. Functional changes related to weakness of upper-extremity musculature, however, usually lag behind those in the lower extremities by 2 to 3 years. The early weakness of the scapular stabilization muscles interferes with controlled movement of the arms and hands during reaching. The child gradually loses biceps and brachioradialis function, followed by continued deterioration of triceps and more distal musculature. The marked instability of scapular musculature is clearly evident when the child tries to elevate his trunk with his arms (e.g., when attempting to use crutches) or when he is lifted from under the shoulders.[234,237] A classic test of scapular stability is the test for the Meryon sign, in which the child slips from the examiner's grip as the child is being lifted from under the arms (Figure 16-8). Typical progression of upper-extremity weakness is shown by use of the reaching test (Figure 16-9).

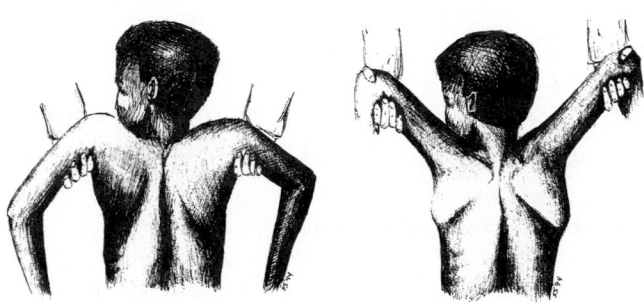

FIGURE 16-8 ■ Meryon sign shows lack of scapular stability as the child slips from the examiner's grip when lifted from under the arms.

By the time the child reaches stage 3 of the reaching test, he needs considerable help with eating, hair care, and oral hygiene. Because of major trunk involvement and marked lower-extremity weakness, the child will also be dependent for most ADLs, such as hygiene, dressing, and transferring. Typical functional stages in DMD are identified in Box 16-5. See Emery and Muntoni[224] for a comprehensive review of the clinical process of DMD.

Medical Intervention
Treatment of Primary Pathology

DMD has no cure. Some clinicians suggest that until an effective treatment can be found, the best way to decrease the number of children with DMD is through genetic counseling. Serum CK is elevated in the female carriers, and genetic molecular probes of possible carriers are now available to identify deletions within the Xp21 region (the short arm of the X chromosome) at a 95% accuracy level. Of course, some families may have belief systems that do not allow consideration of pregnancy termination to prevent having a boy with possible DMD. Those views must be respected. Prenatal diagnosis of DMD for women without a family history of the disease is not yet practical.[238] Despite much effort, an effective pharmaceutical agent has not been identified to treat DMD. Research was initiated in the 1980s to determine if the growth hormone inhibitor mazindol would slow weakness and contracture in DMD; however, no evidence was found to support that hypothesis.[239] In some cases, oral corticosteroids are effective to prolong ambulation,[240] although the results have been questioned because of

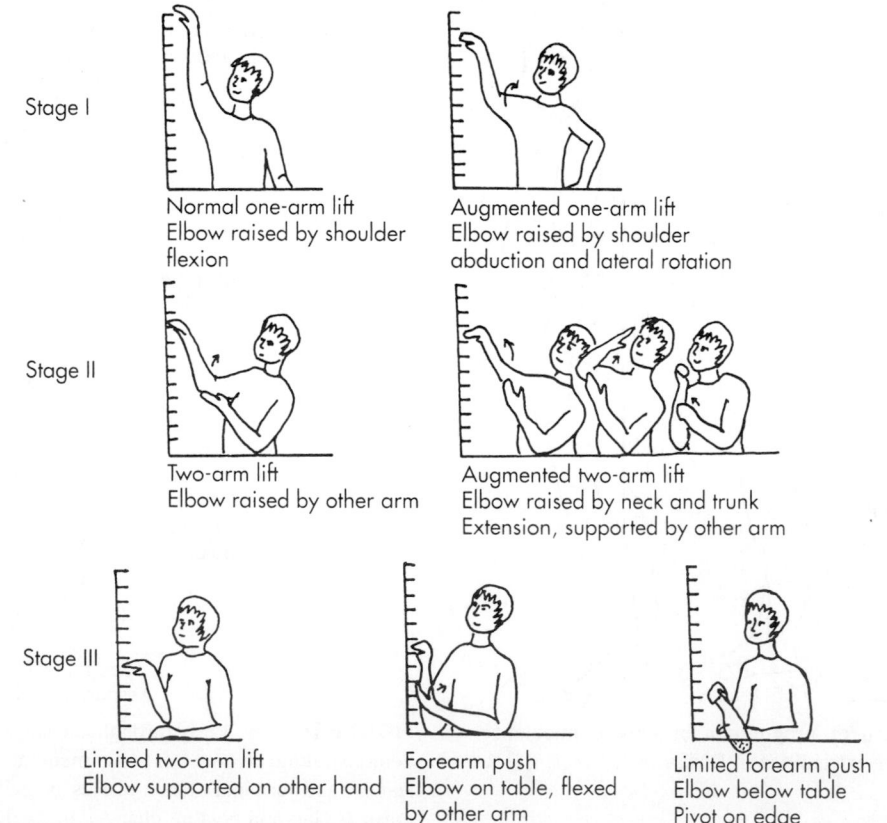

Stage I

Normal one-arm lift
Elbow raised by shoulder flexion

Augmented one-arm lift
Elbow raised by shoulder abduction and lateral rotation

Stage II

Two-arm lift
Elbow raised by other arm

Augmented two-arm lift
Elbow raised by neck and trunk
Extension, supported by other arm

Stage III

Limited two-arm lift
Elbow supported on other hand

Forearm push
Elbow on table, flexed by other arm

Limited forearm push
Elbow below table
Pivot on edge

FIGURE 16-9 ■ Method of evaluating the working hand as demonstrated by the reaching test.

BOX 16-5 ■ FUNCTIONAL TRANSITIONS IN PATIENT WITH MUSCULAR DYSTROPHY

1. Ambulates with mild waddling gait and lordosis. Can run with marked effort, gait problems magnified. Can ascend, descend steps, curbs.
2. Ambulates with moderate waddling gait and lordosis. Cannot run. Difficulty with stairs and curbs. Rises from floor using Gowers maneuver. Rises from chair independently.
3. Ambulates with moderately severe waddling gait and lordosis. Rises from chair independently but cannot ascend or descend curbs or stairs or rise from floor independently.
4. Ambulates with assistance or in some cases with bilateral KAFOs. May have had surgical release of contractures. May need assistance with balance. Needs wheelchair for community mobility. Propels manual chair slowly. Independent in bed and self-care, although may need help with some aspects of dressing and bathing because of time constraints.
5. Transfers independently from wheelchair. Unable to walk independently but can bear and shift weight to walk with orthoses if supported. Can propel self in manual chair but limited endurance. Motorized chair more functional. Independent in self-care with transfer assist for bath or shower.
6. Wheelchair independence in motorized chair. May need trunk support or orthosis. Needs assistance in bed and with major dressing. Can perform self-grooming but dependent for toileting and bathing. May need alternating pressure relief mattress.
7. Wheelchair independence in motorized chair but may need to recline intermittently while in chair. Dependent in hygiene and most self-care requiring proximal upper-extremity control.
8. As above; will also use two hands for single-hand activities: one hand supports working arm. May perform simple table-level hand activities, some self-feeding with arm support.
9. Sits in wheelchair only with trunk support and intermittent reclining or transfer to a supine position. Boys attending school may need to be on gurney for part of day. May benefit from nighttime ventilatory support or intermittent daytime PPV. (Some patients may have had an elective tracheostomy and need ventilatory support unit attached to wheelchair.) May have some hand control if arms supported. Will need help with turning at night.
10. Totally dependent. Unable to tolerate upright position, may elect home ventilatory support. Tracheostomy necessary for prolonged ventilation. Tracheostomy may be adapted for speech if oral musculature adequate. Needs 24-hour care. If around-the-clock home care cannot be arranged, patient must be hospitalized.

---

possible problems with research bias.[241] In a Cochrane Database Review, Manzur et al[242] concluded that glucocorticoid corticosteroid therapy improves muscle strength in the short term of 6 months to 2 years; however, adverse effects such as weight gain, excessive hair growth, osteoporosis, and behavioral problems were noted. Researchers have also attempted to implant the normal precursor muscle cells or myoblasts directly into dystrophic mice and, in several cases, into children with DMD to precipitate the proliferation of normal donor muscle cells into the host muscles of dystrophic subjects, but results have not led to significant improvement.[243] This finding was supported by Miller et al,[244] who implanted myoblasts into 10 boys with DMD. The myoblast implantation had no positive effect; however, muscle force generation from cyclosporine, the immunosuppressant drug used concomitantly with the myoblast implantation, did have a positive effect. Most recently, researchers have been working on recombinant adenovirus vector–mediated dystrophin gene transfer to patients with DMD.[245] Animal studies using helper-dependent adenoviral vectors for dystrophin gene transfer to muscles in dystrophic mice show promise for patients with DMD.[246] Although no cure for DMD is on the horizon despite the positive research on gene transfer, the functional status of the patient, quality of life, and life expectancy can be influenced with thoughtful, functionally based treatment and supportive care.

Treatment of Cardiopulmonary Factors

Respiratory failure is the cause of death in 70% to 80% of patients with DMD. Cardiac and other causes account for the remaining deaths.[241] Although cardiac involvement is evident early, because of limited physical activity the clinical impact of heart disease is not a significant problem until the adolescent years.[228] Once the child becomes wheelchair dependent, his cardiorespiratory fitness deteriorates markedly. With increasing weakness of the respiratory musculature and the development of scoliosis, physicians must be vigilant in their treatment of respiratory infections. The American Thoracic Society[225] consensus statement on the respiratory care of boys with DMD suggests the following:

- A child should be seen between the ages of 4 to 6 years for baseline pulmonary function testing.
- Patients should be seen by a pediatric respiratory physician twice a year after becoming wheelchair dependent if the FVC falls below 80% or the child is older than 12 years.
- Patients who need mechanically assisted airway clearance or mechanically assisted ventilation should be seen by a pulmonary specialist every 3 to 6 months.
- All patients should undergo cardiac and pulmonary assessments before any surgery.[225]

Sleep-disordered breathing and hypoventilation are common in the later stages of DMD, and the onset is often subtle. Early symptoms include repeated nighttime awakenings, early morning headache, and daytime sleepiness. Inexpensive oximetry can be used in the home to identify nighttime oxygen desaturation if polysomnography with continuous carbon dioxide monitoring is not available.[247]

Because sleep hypoxia is common in the later stages of DMD, intermittent positive-pressure ventilation (IPPV) by nasal mask is recommended to control oxygen desaturation at night. Oxygen alone should not be used to treat hypoventilation without IPPV.[225] Eventually most boys with DMD enter a stage of constant hypoventilation throughout the day and night and a decision needs to be made about the use of 24-hour ventilation support. Daytime ventilation should be considered when waking PCO_2 exceeds 50 mm Hg or hemoglobin saturation is lower than 92% while awake.[225] Several noninvasive options for sustaining life in the final stages of DMD other than ventilation by tracheostomy are available.[248] The most common system used today is mouthpiece-delivered IPPV assist-controlled ventilation.[249] Less commonly used options are the pneumobelt (see Appendix 16-B), which provides intermittent pressure on the abdominal area to create a forced expiration followed by a passive inspiration, and the cuirass negative pressure chest respirator, which was more commonly used with polio patients.

Once a patient with DMD requires day and nighttime ventilation and has severe bulbar muscle weakness, a decision must be made to elect ventilation by tracheostomy or palliative care. Ventilation by tracheostomy allows higher ventilation pressures and a better patient-ventilator interface.[250] However, use of a tracheostomy requires careful stoma hygiene to prevent infections and mucus plugs and requires 24-hour caregiver vigilance.[248] Although many patients and families adapt well to tracheostomy use, the ability to speak audibly may be affected. Consideration must be given to use of a speaking valve system.[225] Several cases of pneumothorax have been reported with long-term IPPV.[251] Also, as the number of patients use long-term tracheostomy-based ventilation, the potential for tracheal erosion or tracheobronchomalacia, which must be monitored to prevent hemorrhaging, is increasing.[252] As with patients with ALS, many significant treatment and ethical decisions must be made by the patient, family, and health care providers when submitting to prolonged HMV.[253] Patient autonomy and family input after adequate patient education about prolongation of life by tracheostomy ventilation must be respected.[225]

Cardiomyopathy seldom becomes symptomatic until end stages of DMD because the child's decreased activity level does not stress the weakened heart muscle. In later stages of the disease, however, cor pulmonale with right-sided heart failure may occur. Medical treatment of any cardiac symptoms generally follows the conventional interventions. Some boys with severe scoliosis that creates cardiac compression may require correction by spinal fixation.[254] Retrospective data suggest that children treated with deflazacort (a corticosteroid) have a lower incidence of cardiac involvement.[225]

Nutritional Concerns
Excessive weight gain that impairs functional ability is a frequent and difficult problem for children with DMD and their families. The typical active child needs approximately 2,400 calories daily to maintain weight and grow; however, the child with DMD who is more sedentary or who is wheelchair dependent may need 1,200 or fewer calories to maintain weight. Because of decreased esophageal and intestinal motility, exacerbated by weak or absent abdominal muscle strength, a healthy low-fat diet should be encouraged with adequate bulk foods, stool softeners, and fluids to facilitate bowel function and motility. Problems with obesity are often

related to the family's typical pattern of eating and nurturing. The child and family members may "feed" their anxiety or depression about the disease.[238] In many cases, family members and friends feel that the child's only pleasure may be eating. Although this may seem true, caring for a totally dependent obese teenager or young adult can become problematic for both the child and the caregivers. Before obesity becomes an issue, the child and his family should be referred for comprehensive nutritional advice from a specialist experienced in dealing with childhood obesity. Suggestions for adapting eating behavior and food choices will not be followed if they are too restrictive or unreasonable for the child's social situation.[255,256]

Although obesity is a common problem for children with DMD (greater than 54%), malnutrition is also common. Malnutrition usually occurs in the late stages of the disease as a result of dysphagia.[225] Special care must be taken to provide adequate nutrition after spinal surgery. In a retrospective study of 17 wheelchair-using boys who had spinal surgery and a control group that did not have spinal surgery, 9 of 17 boys lost more than 5% of their body weight after surgery. On review, weight loss was related to the inability to self-feed; therefore the investigators suggest that before surgery a feeding evaluation should be done and an appropriate plan should be put in place to prevent postsurgical malnutrition.[257]

As the disease progresses, some children develop problems swallowing. To decrease the possibility of aspiration, careful attention must be paid to food textures and chewing and swallowing functions (see page 484 for information on dealing with bulbar symptoms). Depending on the patient's and family's decisions about prolongation of life, some patients now elect to have a permanent percutaneous endoscopic gastrostomy (PEG) placed once self-feeding and swallowing become a problem rather than a pleasure. Even if the patient can still swallow and enjoys eating in the late stages of DMD, the patient may not be able to physically take in adequate calories; the PEG allows the delivery of needed calories and fluids beyond what the patient can take orally (see page 480 for information on dysphagia and eating issues). Consensus is that body weight and body mass index should be reviewed regularly and family education on nutrition should be an ongoing process. Evaluation of swallowing should be assessed by taking a history of choking episodes and observing the child eat different foods and fluids. Videofluoroscopy should be used to determine if aspiration is a problem, and appropriate adjustments in feeding should be instituted under the supervision of the appropriate therapist.[225]

Treatment of Orthopedic Factors
Scoliosis is a frequent complication of DMD, with a reported incidence of 49% to 93%. Consequences of severe scoliosis are increased respiratory problems in boys with respiratory compromise, chronic pain related to musculoskeletal problems, sitting tolerance difficulties, and caregiving issues. In a retrospective study of 88 patients with DMD, Lord et al[258] showed that scoliosis was identified in 30% of boys in the 8- to 14-year age group, 92% in the 15- to 20-year age group, and 64% in boys older than age 20 years. The decrease in the number of boys with scoliosis older than age 20 years suggested that boys without scoliosis have greater longevity,

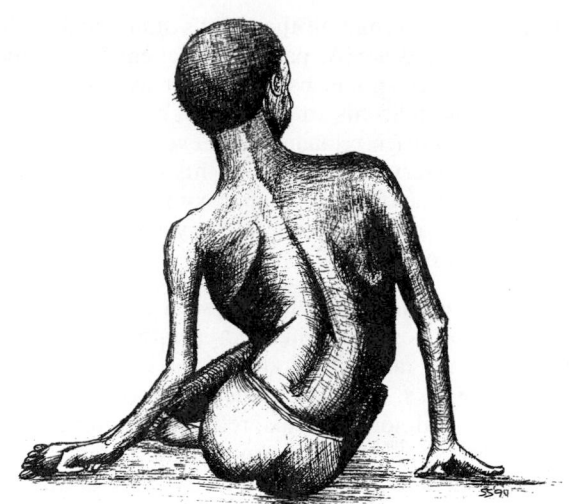

FIGURE 16-10 ■ Moderate scoliosis affecting sitting stability.

although the evidence was not conclusive. Figure 16-10 presents an example of a boy with moderate scoliosis that affects sitting posture. Note the pelvic asymmetry that would seriously affect sitting alignment.

Scoliosis tends to occur in two basic patterns: the early-onset form (seen in approximately 23%), which becomes evident before the child begins to use a wheelchair, and the late-onset form, which develops, on average, 4 years after wheelchair dependency. In the early-onset form the curve usually becomes severe and progressive, leading to pulmonary compromise and structural-based pain. In the late-onset form the course is usually mild. The traditional view of scoliosis development has been that the child's increasing weakness leads to abnormal sitting postures, which in turn lead to severe kyphoscoliosis. However, McDonald et al[259] and Lord et al[258] counter that scoliosis is an age-related condition closely associated with the adolescent growth spurt and is not necessarily causally linked to use of a wheelchair. Unfortunately, attempts to control sitting posture through the use of spinal orthosis and wheelchair seating inserts (inserts that place the child in lumbar lordosis to lock facets, thereby preventing rotation and lateral collapse or, more commonly, lumbar and thoracic lateral supports) have been disappointing.[258] Although DMD is generally thought to have a symmetrical pattern of weakness, recent evidence suggests an asymmetrical paraspinous involvement, which may be the cause of the severe scoliosis seen in some boys.[260] Bach[261] states that thoracolumbar bracing is never indicated to slow scoliosis development in DMD and it cannot substitute for surgical correction.

Efforts have been made to delay the time of onset of scoliosis with steroid treatment protocols. In a study of 88 ambulatory boys with DMD (66 in the therapy group and 22 in the control group), investigators found that a treatment regimen with oral prednisone (1.5 to 5 years' duration; mean, 2.5 years) significantly delayed the onset of scoliosis.[262] Another group of 54 ambulatory boys was assigned to prednisone treatment or nontreatment groups and followed up for 5 years. Evidence supported the hypothesis that onset of scoliosis would be delayed; however, a longer follow-up period would be required to determine if scoliosis could be prevented.[263]

Currently, surgical correction of scoliosis is the standard of care for boys in whom curves greater than 25 degrees have developed. Miller et al[254] reported on 68 patients with DMD who underwent posterior spinal fusion with instrumentation for severe scoliosis. (Over the course of the study, several different forms of fixation were used.) Although they found that the boys who underwent spinal fixation were more comfortable in their later years and were easier to care for, deterioration of pulmonary function was not slowed after surgery. The average age at death of the boys in the study was 18.3 years. This was the same as the average age at death reported for another similar group of boys who did not have spinal surgery.

In interviews with 42 end-stage patients with DMD who underwent scoliosis surgery or their caregivers, 35 caregivers believed that the instrumentation was beneficial, 6 believed that it was not, and 1 was uncertain. Of 15 patients interviewed, all thought that the surgery was helpful. Seventeen percent of the boys had pulmonary complications after surgery. On the basis of their experience, the authors suggest that an FVC of at least 35% of normal is necessary before surgery can be performed. They recommend that spinal stability is best achieved with segmental fixations rather than with Harrington rods because the segmental fixation systems allow immediate postoperative mobilization of the patient, which is essential to prevent marked disuse deterioration. Attention must also be given to how the spine is positioned with fixation. If the curve cannot be completely corrected, the curves should be balanced to create a horizontal pelvis. Maintenance of some lumbar lordosis (45 degrees) and thoracic kyphosis (25 degrees) is essential because it allows the boy to keep his head in a forward position to compensate for severely weakened anterior neck muscles.[254] Cervellati et al[264] reported on a study of 20 boys treated between 1985 and 1995 and concluded that early surgery significantly reduces the risk factors associated with severe spinal deformities. The period after spinal surgery requires careful coordination of medical, respiratory, and physical therapy services. Depending on the hospital culture, physical therapists may be responsible for the pulmonary drainage and breathing exercise programs as well as typical passive and active exercise programs while the child is in ICU and postsurgical care environments. Preferably, therapists should introduce postural drainage and breathing techniques as well as exercise expectations to the child before surgery to gain better cooperation after surgery.

Long bone fractures in children with DMD are a serious problem that can have a significant long-term impact on ambulation. In a study of 378 patients, 21% had incurred fractures, primarily from falling. Leg fractures predominated in independent ambulators and wheelchair users, whereas upper-extremity fractures more often occurred in boys using knee-ankle-foot orthoses. Twenty percent of those who had fractures lost the ability to ambulate.[265] Other orthopedic interventions to prolong ambulation are discussed in a later section.

Therapeutic Management
Therapeutic Evaluation
Ideally, a team of specialists should be involved in the long-term care of a child with DMD and his family. The

therapist's primary role is twofold: to perform serial evaluations of the child's movement capabilities and to adjust the child's intervention program accordingly to maximize function and quality of life as the disease progresses. A typical therapy evaluation should include assessment of muscle strength and ROM impairments with a comprehensive assessment of functional status and level of disability. In some facilities the therapist also collects data on the child's pulmonary status.[176]

Manual Muscle Testing. MMT is a reasonably reliable technique for measuring muscle strength of children with DMD if consecutive evaluations are made by the same rater. Reliability of scores in the gravity-eliminated position was shown to be highest.[266] DMD shows a linear pattern of decreased muscle strength without marked changes in the rate of deterioration in strength over time. The rate of actual muscle weakness is not influenced by bracing programs or wheelchair use,[237] although functional status may change. MMT after prolonged periods of immobility, however, may reflect increased weakness from disuse atrophy rather than the disease progress. Therefore marked, precipitous decreases in MMT scores may reflect a transitory situation that will respond to increased activity and exercise. A number of electronic muscle strength testing units are currently available and are appropriate for research protocols but are not necessary for clinicians skilled in MMT techniques.

Range of Motion. As with MMT, serial ROM evaluations should be completed by the same therapist because intrarater reliability is higher than interrater reliability.[267] Contractures in DMD are thought to be related to static positioning of the limbs. The lack of upright weight bearing and reliance on a wheelchair for mobility tends to accelerate contracture development; therefore therapists should be particularly vigilant about monitoring lower-extremity ROM as the child becomes more sedentary.[268] Some boys with significant shoulder girdle weakness begin to develop contractures even before they become wheelchair dependent. Therefore early attention should be paid to possible subluxation of the shoulder.[269]

Particular attention should be given to the accuracy of measuring hip ROM. Rideau et al[270] recommend the "dangling leg" test, in which the child is placed supine with his lower legs hanging over the end of the table. An inability to bring the thighs to midline indicates a contracture of the iliotibial band and hip abductors. One can quantify the contracture by measuring the distance of the thigh from the midline and from the surface of the table. Additionally, the therapist should note pelvic obliquity, preferably with serial photographs taken in the sitting and supine positions. Ideally, the patient can be photographed from the back in sitting position against a simple clear, framed plastic sheet with grid squares to allow easy, nonradiographic tracking of scoliosis.

Functional Status. The child's functional status continues to be relatively stable for some time even when MMT indicates that the child is losing strength. Because the weakness is gradual, many children develop remarkably adaptive adjustments in movement patterns to cope with the loss of strength. Brooke et al[271] and others[272] have described a func-

tional scale for determining the child's status and for predicting appropriate care. As part of the patient's assessment, adaptive behaviors should be noted. For example, a child may not be able to lift his arm overhead, but he may use his fingers (strength often remains intact even after respiratory support is necessary) to "crawl" up his chest to reach his head or he may lean forward to approximate his chest to his hand or use his other arm or a lever system to assist with activities (see Box 16-5).[261]

Respiratory Function. The physical therapist's role in evaluating respiratory status in children with DMD will vary depending on the facility and area of the country in which the therapist works. For more in-depth information regarding evaluating pulmonary status, refer to Chapter 35 or see Irwin and Tecklin.[176] At a minimum, the therapist should evaluate bulbar function, cough effectiveness, and FVC (a simple spirometer available in most clinics is adequate). For more sophisticated testing, the child should be seen by a pulmonary function specialist. In addition, the therapist may find testing the child's energy cost to be helpful during ambulation by using the Energy Expenditure Index described by Rose et al,[273] which divides walking heart rate minus resting heart rate by walking speed (EEI = WHR − RHR/D/T). By determining the child's work efficiency with this simple method, clinicians may be able to help the child, family, and treatment team determine when making the transition to a wheelchair is best. Additionally, in late stages the therapist may need to assess the child's bulbar function to prevent swallowing and aspiration problems caused by tongue and oral-facial muscle weakness.

Therapeutic Goals

The basic goals for a therapeutic program are straightforward: (1) to prevent contractures that can lead to further disability and pain, (2) to maintain maximal strength and prevent disuse atrophy, (3) to facilitate maximal functional abilities by using appropriate adaptive equipment, (4) to maintain maximal respiratory muscle strength and movement of secretions, and (5) to foster realistic child and family expectations within the context of the environment. These broad-based goals, however, may not be adequate for today's third-party payers, and the therapist may need to write more specific, time-oriented goals.

Therapeutic Interventions

In today's health care environment, younger children with disabilities are usually eligible for school-based therapy services. However, therapists increasingly act primarily in the role of consultant rather than direct service provider, especially for older children. Much of the child's exercise program must be carried out at home by parents or caregivers. When both parents work outside the home or when the child lives in a single-parent home with a working parent, compliance with home programs can be problematic. As many exercise activities as possible should be encouraged within the child's school day so that parents can focus on parenting, nurturing, general caregiving, and simple positioning and bedtime exercises. Under the supervision of a consulting therapist, the child's therapy often can be provided in some form at the child's school if on-site therapists, personal attendants, or adaptive physical education teachers are available.

Respiratory and Dysphagia Care. In the school therapy environment, where most children with DMD are monitored, the therapist should be prepared to provide the child and family with methods to improve breathing efficiency. In the early stages of the disease, the child and family can be taught simple breathing exercises stressing diaphragmatic breathing, full chest expansion, air shifts, and rib cage stretching. Most children enjoy playing with handheld incentive spirometer units and playing blowing games (e.g., bubbles, pinwheels). Preliminary evidence suggests that respiratory endurance can be improved in children with DMD.[274] More recently, in a study of 18 boys with DMD to determine the efficacy of respiratory endurance and strength training programs, the investigators found improvement in ventilatory muscle endurance but not in respiratory muscle strength.[275,276]

Respiratory exercise cannot reverse the process of respiratory failure; however, attention to pulmonary hygiene can help the child cope more effectively with respiratory infections and the discomfort accompanying respiratory compromise. Although inspiratory exercises tend to be the focus of interventions, expiratory inefficiency may play a major role in the inability to clear secretions.[277] Once the child begins to have difficulty clearing secretions, the family should be taught manual or mechanically assisted postural drainage techniques as long as the patient has an adequate cough. Patients who need support with coughing need to be taught "air stacking" techniques (taking a serious of breaths without exhaling between breaths) to increase intrathoracic pressure needed to cough effectively. Some patients respond well to manual coughing assistance. Increasingly, patients and caregivers are being taught to use a mechanical insufflator-exsufflator (positive pressure followed by negative pressure) to stimulate coughing.[278,279] These techniques should be reviewed and used aggressively whenever the child is bed bound for more than 1 or 2 days and before and after all surgical procedures.[225] Physical therapy interventions, such as postural drainage and breathing exercises, are invaluable in preventing early death from respiratory failure. The Muscular Dystrophy Association continually updates its information on breathing and respiratory care.[280,281]

In end stages of DMD when the child is dependent, dealing with oral-motor problems that may interfere with eating and swallowing is imperative. Techniques such as positioning, increased sensory input (texture, temperature), and volume changes in foods may improve the child's swallowing and allow the child to continue taking food orally.[282] The interventions are similar to those described for ALS and are clearly documented in most occupational and speech therapy manuals and texts.[64] The Muscular Dystrophy Association also publishes informational manuals dealing with dysphagia problems (see www.mdausa.org).

Prevention of Contractures. The two-joint muscles are most prone to developing significant contractures. Early in the course of the disease process, both parents and the child must be educated about the expected changes in muscle balance and how they can play an active role in preventing or limiting the impact of contractures caused by muscle imbalance. Because contractions at the hip, knee, and ankle interfere with the mechanical alignment necessary to stand erect and walk, each day the child should be encour-

aged to move his own limbs to end ranges through normal play activities to slow development of contractures related to sedentary positioning. Some research supports the view that the combination of positioning, stretching, and splinting should begin before contractures exist. For example, the child can be encouraged to watch television or play video games while lying prone with legs aligned out of the common "frog leg" pattern. Once a child has significant hip flexor or iliotibial band contractures, stretching techniques must be specific because simple prone positioning can force the lumbar spine into excessive lordosis. Although difficult to accomplish in some mainstreamed school environments, positioning the child in a standing frame during several class periods helps provide prolonged stretch to hip, knee, and ankle musculature.

In a prospective study of prevention of deformity in DMD, Scott et al[283] found that boys who had consistent treatment with AFOs and daily stretching were able to continue walking longer than boys who did not have a splinting and stretching program. These findings were supported by Brooke et al,[234] who found that night ankle splints, worn consistently in combination with stretching, minimized the rate of contracture development. Although some children will tolerate night splinting to control plantar flexion contractures, in reality few children will tolerate wearing long-leg orthotics at night to prevent knee flexion contractures or to align the hips (an additional bar between legs to control rotations).

At the first sign of loss of end ROM, the therapist should adjust the child's program to include specific stretches.[269,284] As active ROM becomes more difficult, parents will need to assist the child to move his limbs to the end ranges of all motions to stretch the muscles and periarticular structures. The stretching program should use static stretching techniques with prolonged, mild tension to affect both the viscoelastic and plastic properties of the muscle.[285] For example, in a recent randomized study of normal subjects, periodic stretching programs (stretches performed 5 days a week, once per day, held for 30 seconds for three repetitions over a 6-week time frame) produced significant changes in knee extension range of motion.[286] Unfortunately, no studies exist to identify the best stretching program for a DMD patient population. The best approach to contractures is to prevent them.[268] (See Grossman et al[287] for a review of the effect of immobilization on muscle and appropriate therapy interventions.)

Although development of contractures of the hip, knee, and ankle caused by muscle imbalance has been thought the cause of early loss of ambulation rather than muscle weakness,[288] others believe that weakness causes the loss of ambulation rather than contractures.[284]

Exercise and the Maintenance of Maximal Functional Level. In most progressive neuromuscular diseases peak oxygen uptake, pulmonary ventilation, work capacity, and endurance are reduced. In DMD, cardiomyopathy and restrictive lung disease, as well as the muscle fiber degeneration and deconditioning, may be primary underlying factors in poor functional exercise tolerance. The importance of improving muscular strength versus aerobic capacity to improve tolerance to activities of daily living in DMD, however, is unclear.[289] Hasson,[290] in a review of exercise studies of patients with muscular dystrophy, reports that oxygen consumption improved with endurance training, although whether repetitive endurance training at moderate or high intensity (70% of Vo2max) causes muscle damage is not clear.

Elder[291] reviewed animal studies suggesting that dystrophic mice trained on a treadmill showed increased damage to muscle tissue, whereas forced swimming in dystrophic mice had no adverse effect. In a case review of three generations of patients with facioscapulohumeral muscular dystrophy (seven cases and one suspected case), Johnson and Braddom[292] noted asymmetrical weakness of the upper extremities. They related the weakness to patterns of overuse (dominant side or side used most often in work activities). On the basis of their information and additional evidence that muscle-derived enzymes (CK and myoglobin concentrations in blood) were markedly elevated in patients with DMD after prolonged exercise,[293] they suggested that endurance exercise may be contraindicated.[294]

Other research has shown that judicious exercise may have a positive effect on function. For example, Vignos and Watkins[295] compared two groups of boys with DMD in 1966. One group participated in a 12-month home strengthening program that used graduated weights for maximal resistance. The control group continued normal activities and did not participate in the exercise program. The muscle strength of both groups had showed a decline during the year before the study. At the end of the study, the control group showed continued decline. The exercise group, however, showed a small increase in strength as measured by MMT. They noted that the initial strength of the muscles before the program was initiated was positively related to improvement in strength. Therefore the authors suggested that the exercise program should be started during the initial stages of the disease rather than waiting until the child has stopped ambulating. In another study, boys exercised one quadriceps isokinetically for 6 months. The contralateral leg was used as a control. At the end of the study, no evidence of overwork weakness was noted. A nonsignificant increase in muscle strength of the exercised quadriceps was noted compared with the nonexercised contralateral muscle, which was maintained for 3 months after cessation of exercise. The authors concluded that submaximal exercise did not negatively affect muscle tissue, but it may be of limited value in increasing strength.[296]

In a more recent study of endurance training of dystrophic hamsters, Elder[291] concluded that increased contractile activity associated with treadmill exercise had no detrimental effect on developing muscle and may have had a beneficial effect in young animals by improving fiber hypertrophy, increasing maximal tetanic force, and decreasing fiber degeneration. In children with DMD, Hasson[290] concluded that exercise consisting of brief periods of low- or high-intensity activity can improve strength for patients with minimal to moderate weakness. The increased recruitment of motor units from training effects also may improve muscle coordination and reduce disuse atrophy. However, exercise programs have no effect on strength of muscles already severely weakened.

In addition to active and resistive exercise programs, Scott et al[283] completed a small study of the effect of intermittent, long-term, low-frequency electrical stimulation on dystrophic anterior tibialis muscles. They demonstrated a significant increase in mean voluntary contraction force and suggested that electrical stimulation can have a beneficial effect if used with children whose muscles are not already markedly weakened. Zupan[297] supports this finding, but children under treatment were unable to maintain strength beyond 4 to 5 months.

Overall, the data from animal and human studies suggest that submaximal exercise is not harmful and it may be helpful in maintaining maximal movement function if the patient does not exercise into marked fatigue. Because muscle endurance and peak power are diminished in addition to muscle strength, a focus on program design related to functional exercises individualized to each child's functional requirements is recommended.[277]

Ideally, the child's exercise needs can be incorporated into pleasurable activities adapted for children with movement and weakness-related balance problems. Because endurance is a problem, aerobic-type programs are not appropriate in most cases, with the exception of respiratory endurance programs previously noted.[298] Many ambulatory children, however, enjoy ball activities, walking-based simple obstacle courses, parachute games, table tennis, cycling (preferably tandem), and especially swimming. Swimming is an excellent exercise for children with DMD because they often are quite buoyant because of their increased fat/muscle ratio. Many children can continue to float or swim independently on their backs well into the time they are able to move only distal musculature. The Muscular Dystrophy Association has an excellent guide to water-based exercises, *No Sweat Exercise: Aquatics.*[299]

A safe indicator of extent and intensity of exercise is that the patient should recover from exercise fatigue after a night's rest. An active exercise program did not benefit patients who were in later, dependent stages of DMD.[290] When designing an active play program, therapists should review the types of muscle contractions that the activity requires considering that most muscle damage occurs when muscles are active and functioning in an eccentric manner.[300] Those concerns about damage from eccentric muscle contractions were supported by Allen,[301] who found that dystrophic muscles are more susceptible to stretch-induced muscle damage. His work with mdx mice, testing whether blockades to stretch-activated ionic changes can protect against some of the features of DMD, may provide helpful information on appropriate exercises for damaged muscles. Figure 16-11 shows responses of normal and impaired muscle to exercise. (See Kilmer's[289] review and commentary on aerobic exercise training in human beings with neuromuscular diseases and Eagle's[302] report on exercise in neuromuscular diseases.) In a summary of findings on effects of physical exercise on conditioning in muscular dystrophy, Ansved[303] found that the scientific basis for clear recommendations on exercise prescription is poor, but evidence does show the importance of maintaining an active lifestyle with limitations on high resistance and eccentric training activities.[303]

Maintenance of Ambulation. As DMD progresses, the child's posture (a result of both weakness and contracture) and gait pattern abnormalities become extreme and he

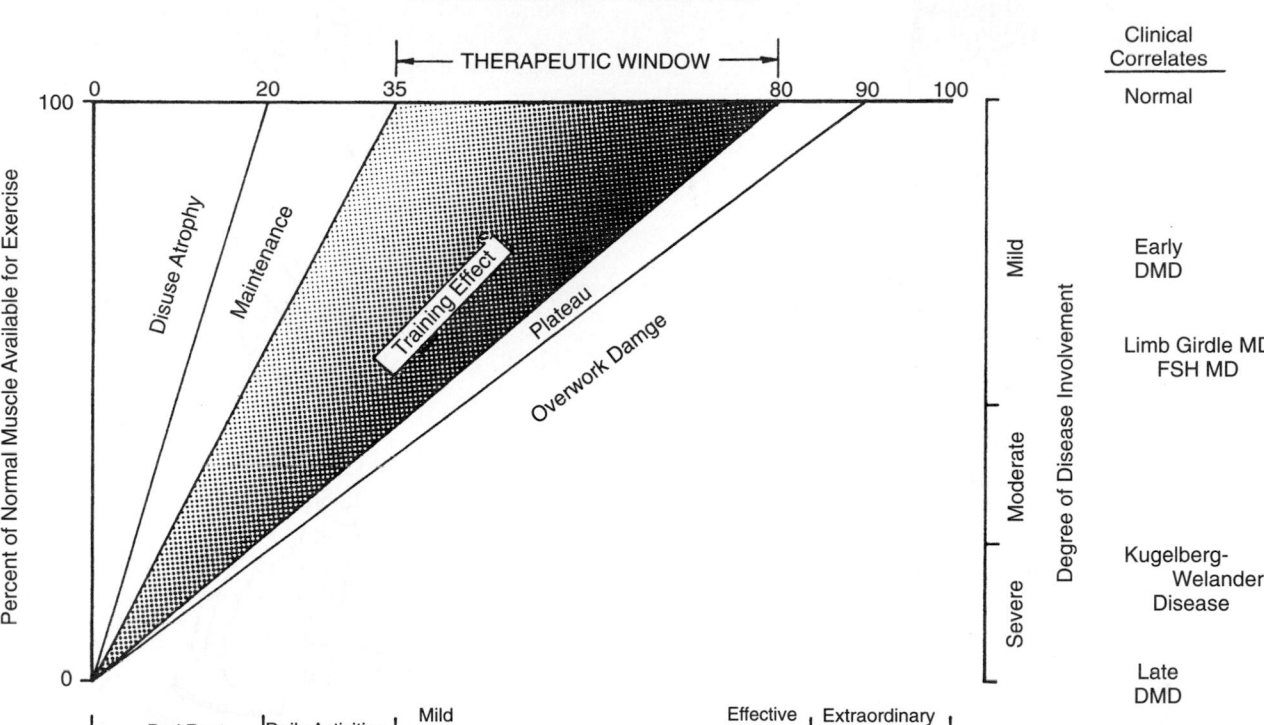

Percent of Maximum Potential Stress

FIGURE 16-11 ■ Idealized response of normal and impaired muscle to exercise. The therapeutic window of safe exercise narrows progressively. Activities (lower X axis) causing normal exercise effects in normal muscle (upper X axis) correlate with different effects in impaired muscle. (From Coble NO, Maloney FP: Effects of exercise on neuromuscular disease. In Maloney FP, Burks JS, Ringel SP, editors: *Interdisciplinary rehabilitation of multiple sclerosis and neuromuscular disorders*, New York, 1985, J.B. Lippincott.)

must work harder to maintain balance while walking. Most children gradually discontinue walking about a year after they lose their ability to deal with stairs or when daily ambulation time decreases to less than 30 minutes per day.[223] Toward the end of the child's independent walking stage, he has a marked anterior pelvic tilt with lordosis and a protuberant abdomen. His shoulders are retracted and he may hold his hands behind his hips or elevated in a mid-guard position to stabilize his hips. He has a severe waddling gait with a shortened stride, and he must carefully lock his knees at each step. He falls frequently, which may result in fractures of the lower or upper extremities.

If the child and his family have followed an aggressive ROM, positioning, and activity program, the child's walking time may be extended by months. In most cases, however, the contractures from muscle imbalance continue relentlessly and the child begins to need support when walking.[270] When contractures at the hip, knee, and ankle show evidence of interfering with the child's ability to stabilize each joint during stance, most children are referred for surgery to restore functional joint motion. Figure 16-12 shows the typical walking pattern of a boy with DMD who is being considered for release of contractures and bracing.

Bach and McKeon[304] studied 13 boys with DMD who had surgery to release lower-extremity contractures. Seven boys

were ambulating independently before surgery (early surgery group), and six boys were preparing to use or had begun to use a wheelchair before surgery (late surgery group). Depending on the contracture patterns, the boys underwent surgical procedures that typically included subcutaneous release of the Achilles tendons and hamstring muscles and fasciotomy of the iliotibial bands. Four patients had rerouting of the posterior tibialis to the dorsal surface of the second or third cuneiform to balance the foot and prevent the often severe varus position of the foot. Boys in the late surgical group required more extensive inpatient rehabilitation, whereas boys in the early surgical group were treated as outpatients after a short hospitalization. Physical therapy was started on the second postoperative day. The program consisted of general conditioning exercises of the trunk and extremities (e.g., rolling, trunk stabilization, neck and head control), stretching exercises, and intensive weight bearing in standing while wearing bilateral long-leg casts or below-knee casts, depending on the surgery. One child participated in a pool therapy program. Bach and McKeon[304] suggest that early surgery for contractures followed by intensive physical therapy can prolong brace-free ambulation. The number of falls experienced by the boys decreased markedly after the surgery and rehabilitation period. Boys in the early intervention groups benefited from the surgical

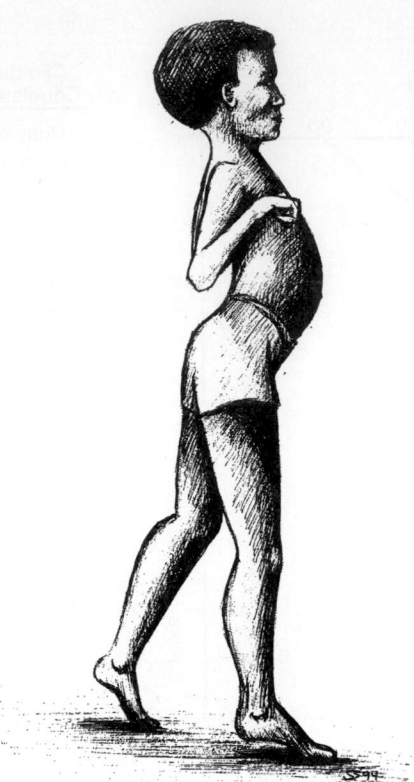

FIGURE 16-12 ■ Typical walking pattern of a boy with DMD who is being considered for release of contractures and bracing.

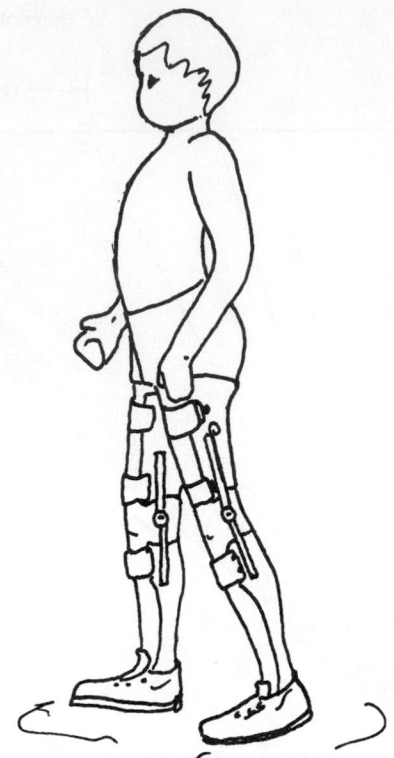

FIGURE 16-13 ■ Example of boy walking in KAFOs showing ischial weight–bearing quadrilateral socket, knee drop locks, and plastic ankle component.

interventions more than the boys in the later intervention groups. All patients and their families in the early surgery group thought that the procedures were helpful. Boys in the late surgery group, however, stated either that they would not have had the surgery if they had a chance to decide again or that they had no opinion. Roposch et al[305] reviewed the records of 91 boys with the typical equinovarus deformity in DMD and strongly recommended surgical intervention, including a posterior tibialis transfer over conservative, non-surgical treatment to maintain foot position and lengthen time of ambulation.

In current standard treatment protocols for children with DMD, bilateral knee-ankle-foot orthotics (KAFOs) are used in conjunction with surgical release of contractures.[306] Surgery is followed by an aggressive therapy program. The main criterion for the surgery-bracing program is the child's impending loss of ability to walk independently. When this occurs, the child has usually lost approximately 60% of his muscle mass and has a pattern of contractures that magnifies the effect of the weakness.[193] Ideally, the KAFO should be measured and fitted in final form before the surgery so the child can begin upright weight bearing in the KAFO the day after surgery. KAFOs are commonly fabricated of molded plastic thigh units (ischial weight-bearing quadrilateral socket) with metal joints at the knee (drop locks) and ankle (or a flexible plastic ankle component) (Figure 16-13).[307] If the orthoses are not immediately available, the child can begin the standing program in long-leg casts.

In the hospital, standing in bilateral KAFOs can be initiated on a tilt table. Most children are fearful after surgery

and report significant pain when their legs are moved or if they are placed upright. For therapy to be successful during this early standing stage and during passive ROM exercises, the child must have adequate pain medication. If the child is not properly medicated in the first few days after surgery, the therapist may have to deal with difficult, resistant behaviors of the child that persist long after the pain should have subsided. Pain protocols must be discussed before the child's surgical procedures. The child should be medicated at least 30 minutes before the therapist's visit.

Gait training is usually begun within 48 hours after surgery. Initial work focuses on helping the child regain his sense of standing balance because his old patterns of equinus, lordosis, and shoulder retraction may no longer be adaptive. The child should be allowed to find his own best center of balance, and he should be allowed to use compensatory gait deviations necessary to allow the best mobility and stability. Depending on the child's upper-extremity strength and control, he may progress from parallel bars for balance assist, to pushing a wheelchair or weighted walker, to balance assist from a therapist with a safety strap to prevent falls. Some children who seem to need a walker for balance transition do best if they use a walker with forearm rests and vertical hand grips, which seem to help them stabilize their arms more effectively than a standard walker. Fortunately, most children do learn to walk independently without support again after surgery, although they are unable to negotiate steps or inclines or rise from the floor independently.[308] Hyde et al[307] reported that 24 of 30 boys treated with KAFOs were able to achieve functional ambulation again. In another study, 15 of 17 boys with DMD who had ceased walking were able to ambulate again after release of contractures followed by use of KAFOs and physical therapy. Even though the children's walking speed was decreased after bracing and the children were not able to rise from the floor or negotiate stairs, the children's ability to move about independently at home or around the classroom was considered invaluable for their independence.[295] Vignos et al[309] report in a review of long-term treatment of DMD that a combination of operative procedures, orthotics, stretching, and a program of standing and walking extended walking until a mean age of 13.6 years and standing for 2 years after that. With the early use of surgery and bracing procedures to maintain ambulation, the expected deterioration in muscle strength and function as a result of becoming sedentary in a wheelchair is deferred.[310]

Because most children with DMD today are discharged home within a few days of surgery, physical therapists must provide options for continuing standing within the home. Standing frames are often available through the child's school district or therapy unit. If they are not, the therapist can help the family build a simple standing frame for home. This frame often can be made from a piece of plywood, or a gluteal strap system can be attached to a table at home. If possible the child should be positioned just forward of the line of gravity to encourage back extension with facet stability and to allow the child better head control in the presence of weak anterior neck muscles. Use of swivel walkers has been recommended by some therapists and physicians because the child does not need upper-extremity control for support. Although the concept of hands-free walking seems logical, boys with DMD had more difficulty using the walkers compared with children with paraplegia because of the more delicate postural adjustments needed by children with dystrophy and their greater sensitivity to the motion restriction of the swivel walker. In addition, older children with DMD are seldom willing to wear externally visible bracing outside the home or school system. Some therapists have reported success with the ORLAU variable center of gravity swivel walker (Mopac Ltd., Eau Claire, Wis.)[311]; however, support for its use is not widespread.

Although the standard of treatment for boys with DMD is to use a combination of surgery and bracing to extend the time of ambulation, Manzur et al[312] carried out a randomized, controlled trial of 20 boys with DMD (ages 4 to 6 years) to study the effect of early release of contractures. The boys were followed up for 12 months. Although the surgery corrected the contractions, no positive effect on muscle strength or functional status was noted, and some of the boys in the operated group showed more rapid deterioration. Therefore the authors did not recommend routine early surgery to relieve contractures. Bakker et al[313] carried out a review of the literature on the effectiveness of the treatment with surgery and KAFOs. They found that the scientific strength of the studies was poor. Although the treatment approach seemed to prolong the walking time, whether it extended functional walking was not clear. The children who benefited most were highly motivated and had slower rates of deterioration.

Transition to Wheelchair. Although surgical and orthotic interventions may prolong ambulation within the home and classroom past the predicted time for cessation of independent walking (8 to 12 years), most children begin to use a wheelchair for community mobility and long distances before this time. When children begin to spend more time in their chair, the rate of development of contractures, disuse weakness, and obesity increases.[193,307] Because of this more rapid deterioration in the child's functional skills, professionals and parents often discourage the child from using a chair for mobility. Children, however, tend to welcome use of the chair because they have more energy for their social interactions and learning tasks.[307]

Selection of the appropriate wheelchair is often difficult for the patient and family because of the multiple decisions that must be made. Few children with DMD can propel a manual wheelchair for more than a few years because of their increasing upper-extremity weakness. In addition, their propulsion speed in their manual chair is seldom adequate to keep up with their peers. Eventually, the child will need a motorized chair. Although this provides tremendous freedom for the child, a motorized chair presents problems to many families because transporting the chair requires a van and lift unit, which is seldom funded by insurance. Ideally, the child should have both a manual and a motorized chair; however, in today's health policy climate, parents often have to engage in protracted efforts to obtain adaptive equipment for their child.

An important consideration when purchasing a wheelchair is the trunk support system. Traditionally, boys with DMD are thought to develop a gravity collapse of the spine related to their functional sitting posture. To control the collapsing spine, spinal orthosis and seat inserts to lock the spine in extension (to prevent lateral bending and rotation) are frequently recommended. Unfortunately, the effectiveness of positioning devices to control the development of scoliosis has been disappointing.[258,261] Although Drennan[235] suggests that spinal fixation is necessary to control scoliosis, not all children are candidates for surgery. The therapist therefore should work with the child, family, and the orthopedist to determine the best system to maintain optimal spinal alignment and trunk stability as the child weakens. In addition, as the child becomes more physically dependent, the chair may need to be fitted with a pressure relief molded seat and trunk cushions, elevating leg rests, and a reclining back with a head rest.[314] The Tilt-in-Space chair (La Bac Systems, Inc, Denver) is a good example of a chair that can be motorized to allow mobility as well as maximal adjustment of seat position by using mouth control systems. It can also be adapted for respirator attachment. The decision about the type of power chair necessary in the later stages of disease progression takes considerable thought. Therapists, the patient, and the parents or caregivers must review environmental constraints, access issues, social goals, and work and recreational needs.

Because of the problems associated with increased wheelchair use, the therapist must work closely with the family and any school-based personnel to design a realistic plan to prevent rapid deterioration in strength and independent function. If possible, the child's standing program in KAFOs should be continued at school and at home as long as possible, with a goal of 3 to 5 hours of standing per day. With mainstreaming, however, continuing a standing program at school is sometimes difficult because attendants and equipment are not available, the child may need to move from room to room for different classes, and the child may not like being singled out for special treatment. It is helpful to caregivers if the child continues to wear his KAFOs when using the chair until he is totally dependent for transfers and can no longer be pivoted from chair to another surface.

If the child uses a motorized wheelchair, directional control systems must be adapted to each child's needs. Most young people with advanced DMD do well for years with a standard joystick hand control system; however, because of extended survival times relative to the long-term use of mechanical ventilation, many patients must have their control systems adjusted frequently to minimize the need for muscle control, such as pinch strength. The need for ventilation support while using the wheelchair was shown to not interfere with the ability to drive.[315] (See Cooper[316] for a comprehensive manual on wheelchair selection. This information is equally valuable for patients with ALS and GBS.)

When the child can no longer tolerate the sitting position, some children have continued to attend school on a gurney. Once the person with DMD is no longer able to attend school or work, the home environment will need to be adapted for maximal self-direction despite significant physical dependence. Both low- and high-tech environmental control systems are more readily available today than they were 10 years ago. Television control units, voice-activated telephones, switch-activated bed controls, and page turners are among the low-tech systems. Sip-n-puff, blink-operated, and voice-activated control units can be adapted to operate most electronic devices. Occupational and physical therapists can provide invaluable support to the person with DMD and the caregivers by making several home visits to suggest modifications and adaptive devices and systems. (See Cook and Hussey[121] for detailed information on assistive technology systems. Also see an excellent Web site for home automation, environmental control, and electronic aids for daily living [EADL]: http://www.makoa.org/ecu.htm.)

Psychosocial Issues

Psychosocial issues related to DMD are family issues. At the time of the child's diagnosis, the parents are often emotionally devastated and cycle back and forth through many phases of denial, anger, sadness, and active coping. This process tends to recur when the child does not meet expected normal physical and social milestones or when he reaches predicted stages of deterioration, such as the transition to a wheelchair. Early in the child's life, the family should be guided to encourage the child's independence and to discourage overprotection. Therapists can play an important role in helping the child and family identify realistic goals for independence. In addition, therapists can be instrumental in extending independence and the sense of self-direction by anticipating patient needs for adaptive equipment and identifying appropriate assistive devices and environmental control systems that empower the person with DMD and provide relief for caregivers from the constant attention required by a completely dependent person. Key to family support is access to a multidisciplinary clinic with specialists in neurology, pulmonology, orthopedics, rehabilitation services, psychology, social work, and dietetics. Only through comprehensive clinics do families of children and adults with DMD receive the level of education and support necessary to deal with the changing levels of function and demands on family systems.[225]

Psychosocial support should be made available to the child and family during predictable times of crisis. Major times of crisis occur around the age of 5 years when the child begins to realize his differences, between the ages of 8 to 12 years when the child loses the ability to walk independently, during the adolescent years when social interactions become restricted, and around the time of high school graduation when the child and family must face vocational limitations and almost certain death within the next decade.[317] Transition times are often accompanied by depression, withdrawal, and anxiety in the child and family members. Parents had a marked preoccupation with their sons and a diminished expression of enjoyment.[314] In a pilot study, 43 boys with DMD between the ages of 4 and 15 years completed human figure drawings (HFDs). HFDs have been used for 75 years as a projective tool to identify emotional factors that may not be verbalized clearly by the child. Using the process, the authors found that the children's drawings were characterized by emotional indicators suggesting physical inadequacy, body inadequacy, immaturity, and insecurity. Adolescents with DMD felt significantly isolated from mainstream life.[318]

Predictably, the integrity, strength, and intragenerational and intergenerational function and coping styles of the child's family contribute a great deal to the way the family responds to the child's progressive deterioration. Extended periods of anxiety and depression should be treated vigorously with cognitive interventions, support groups, respite care and, when appropriate, short-term anxiolytics and antidepressants. Repeated opportunities to discuss end-of-life care must be given to both the child and parents. Professionals, however, tend to underestimate the quality of life for patients with end-stage DMD; therefore patients and family members must be educated about long-term options for ventilatory support or palliative care well ahead of any respiratory emergency that might occur to ensure that the patients desires are respected.[225,319]

Because of the extended life opportunities for DMD patients who may now live into their 20s, home care requirements, the impact of in-home care on family members, and the financial impact must be fully reviewed and support systems put in place before caregiving stress becomes overwhelming. Increasingly, young men with DMD are attending college even though they may require 24-hour assistance with ADLs and monitoring of ventilation equipment. To date, parents are providing most of the care to their children with DMD by attending colleges or living in dorms or apartments with their child. With life extended with ventilation, parents and the young person with DMD should begin early to plan for a future with maximal decision making by the young adult with DMD. This mind set of a "future" requires considerable problem solving by all people involved in the care of the young adult. Parents of children with DMD should involve their child early in life to make appropriate decisions about their care, learn about medical needs and practices, and deal with finances necessary to run a home or hire an attendant. These issues related to independence (even though physically dependent) and caregivers are just being discussed by patients DMD and their caregivers.[320]

Parents and the child should be given the opportunity to discuss the impending death in an accepting environment with persons who are experienced in dealing with degenerative diseases. Because the child and family have long anticipated the child's death and have made transitions through many levels of grieving, the process of separation and mourning may have occurred before the child's death. Each child and family member should therefore be helped to deal with the process according to his or her own pace and in response to individual needs. The child's death is sometimes considered a welcome relief.[321] This feeling of relief, however, is often accompanied by survivor guilt and a tremendous sense of loss of life focus for the family members whose lives have been so intertwined with that of the child's. Ideally, arrangements should be made for the family to meet with the professionals with whom they feel most comfortable several weeks after the child's death and again several months later so that the family (and caregivers) can deal with their thoughts and feelings (Case Study 16-3).[322,323]

CASE STUDY 16-3 ■ JEREMY

Jeremy was 3 years old when he was diagnosed with DMD. He lived at home with his mother and a 5-year-old sister. There was no known family history of DMD, although family lore suggested that a cousin died quite young from pneumonia and a "wasting disease." Jeremy was referred for a medical evaluation when a playground supervisor at his preschool noted that he was clumsy when running and that he had difficulty on the playground climbing equipment and the slide. He also had difficulty rising from the ground and needed to hold on to a railing when stepping up a stair.

During a medical history, Jeremy's mother said that she had noticed that he was "slow to develop" but was not worried because she thought he was just a "late bloomer." A muscle biopsy was positive for a diagnosis of DMD. A physical therapy evaluation 3 months after diagnosis showed ROM to be within normal limits for all joints. Muscle weakness was evident on MMT with G– (4–) hip abduction and extension and quadriceps strength bilaterally. Hip flexion, knee flexion, dorsiflexion, and toe extension were in the G (4) range. Plantar flexion was G+ (4+) with evident hypertrophy. Shoulder abduction and flexion was in the G (4) range, although he had difficulty sustaining abduction for more than 5 seconds.

Jeremy had a moderate head lag when moving from supine to sitting due to G– (4–) anterior neck muscles. The therapist made an on-site school visit to help the teachers identify obstacles to Jeremy's full integration with his classmates. The school custodian built some ramps to help Jeremy use the playground equipment.

Jeremy ambulated independently until age 8 years. His gait pattern was typical of late-stage ambulation (marked equinus, knee hyperextension during stance, bilateral Trendelenburg on stance, marked lordosis with a protuberant abdomen with arms held posterior to hips). He had 40-degree hip flexion contractures with iliotibial band tightness, no knee contractures, and 25-degree plantar flexion contractures. MMTs showed the expected decrease in strength, with pelvic and shoulder girdle muscles being weaker than more distal musculature, except that the anterior tibialis and the peroneals were F+ (3+). He was unable to rise independently from the floor and needed assistance with stairs. Because his gait pattern was slow and he needed to rest frequently when walking more than 20 feet at school, Jeremy had been using a manual wheelchair for long-distance mobility since the age of 7 years.

On the recommendation of orthopedist consultants, Jeremy underwent bilateral percutaneous hip flexor lengthening, iliotibial band fasciotomy, and heel cord release. Bilateral KAFOs had been fitted before surgery, and Jeremy was placed in the braces after surgery. No casting was done. Despite his complaints, he was gradually brought to the full weight-bearing standing position by late afternoon on the day after surgery. Adjustments were made in his pain medication schedule to allow him to tolerate the process more comfortably. By the third hospital day, Jeremy participated in two therapy sessions per day and was standing on the parallel bars, where he was taught lateral and anteroposterior weight shifting in preparation for ambulation. Active assisted and passive ROM exercises were performed without the KAFOs twice a day. On the fourth hospital day, Jeremy began to take short steps using the parallel bars for balance. His mother was also taught his exercises so that Jeremy could have more than two therapy sessions a day. On the fourth day, he practiced walking for 10 minutes six times a day with full physical therapy treatment twice a day.

Because Jeremy was from a rural area and daily physical therapy would not be available on discharge, he was kept in the hospital for 3 additional days for intensive rehabilitation. An occupational therapist worked with Jeremy to provide adaptive equipment for reaching, self-care, and eating (he was unable to raise his arms above 45 degrees and needed his left arm to assist the right when reaching). He was discharged home on the eighth day. An Elks traveling therapist arranged to visit the family once a week for the next month to continue ambulation training and to guide the mother in a home positioning and ROM program. The therapist also helped the mother adapt the home environment and his school to adjust expectations of Jeremy so he was less prone to falling and excessive fatigue.

The family was lost to follow-up, but by report Jeremy continued to ambulate in his KAFOs for approximately 9 months after surgery when he chose to use his wheelchair full time. A motorized wheelchair

Continued

CASE STUDY 16-3 ■ JEREMY—cont'd

was recommended; however, his mother believed that Jeremy was easier to handle in his manual chair. The Muscular Dystrophy Association loaned Jeremy a motorized wheelchair for school use. He had developed moderate scoliosis but did not report pain. He refused to wear a molded spinal corset, but the padded thoracic pads fitted to his chair increased his comfort. By age 15 years, Jeremy was dependent for all care except feeding. He was able to sit with support in a large living room chair and he enjoyed watching television and playing card games with a few friends who visited his home. He was disinterested in continuing school and missed more days than he attended. He was not cooperative with his home-based teacher.

During his fifteenth year, Jeremy had repeated episodes of chest congestion and difficulty handling stringy foods. The visiting therapist taught his mother some postural drainage and breathing exercises for Jeremy; however, the mother did not follow through with the recommendations. Because his mother had to work full time, a public agency provided in-home care during the days when Jeremy was not at school or after he returned from school. The mother refused in-home nursing care, preferring to continue with the attendant, who was not comfortable carrying out Jeremy's exercises or pulmonary care. The family refused counseling or support from parents of other children with disabilities. Jeremy died at home after a brief bout with pneumonia.

SUMMARY

Three different diseases are described to depict the varied effects of neuromuscular pathology on a person's day-to-day function. ALS is an adult-onset degenerative disease of the upper and lower motor neurons; GBS is an inflammatory process affecting the peripheral nervous system of children and adults; and DMD is an inherited degenerative disease presenting in childhood that affects muscle tissue. In all three conditions the therapist is challenged to design a therapy program that will provide the patient with the impetus to become or remain as active as possible without causing possible muscle damage from excessive exercise demands or overwork.

Therapists must be aware of their own feelings and reactions to patients with severe neuromuscular diseases. Working with patients with GBS is usually a positive experience because most patients attain full recovery despite their often severe disability during the acute illness and long recovery period. Working with patients with degenerative terminal diseases, however, draws deeply on the therapist's emotional and spiritual strength. A typical response of health care professionals is to view these patients' conditions as hopeless and to assume that the patients must also perceive their existence as hopeless, depressing, and without value. Research does suggest an increased incidence of depression and demoralization in patients with degenerative, terminal diseases compared with nonaffected populations. Other research, however, has indicated that many patients perceive their own life satisfaction much more positively than professionals would believe.[319,324] Therefore therapists must tap into patients' positive energy to design treatment programs that respect patients' goals and life plans within the context of their environment.

Extensive literature documenting the most appropriate exercise and therapeutic intervention programs for patients with progressive neurological diseases does not exist. In addition, some concern exists that patients with a history of severe GBS may show age-related changes in muscle strength similar to those in patients with postpolio syndrome. Because few medical-clinical facilities see a large enough sample of patients, therapists must align with their professional organizations to institute nationwide, multisite research studies that will provide clear information about appropriate therapy programs.

REFERENCES

1. Caroscio JT: Amyotrophic lateral sclerosis: the disease. In Caroscio JT, editor: *Amyotrophic lateral sclerosis.* New York, 1986, Thieme Medical.
2. Felice KJ, North WA: Creatine kinase values in amyotrophic lateral sclerosis, *J Neurol Sci* 160(suppl 1):S30-S32, 1998.
3. Hirano A: In pursuit of the early pathological alterations in ALS. In Tsubaki T, Yase Y, editors: *Amyotrophic lateral sclerosis.* Amsterdam, 1988, Elsevier Science.
4. Bryant PR, Geis CC, Moroz A et al: Stroke and neurodegenerative disorders. 4. Neurodegenerative disorders, *Arch Phys Med Rehabil.* 85(3 suppl 1):S21-S33, 2004.
5. Berger M, Kopp N, Vital C et al: Detection and cellular localization of enterovirus RNA sequences in spinal cord of patients with ALS, *Neurology* 54:20-25, 2000.
6. Rosen DR: Mutations in Cu/Zn superoxide dismutase gene are associated with familial amyotrophic lateral sclerosis, *Nature* 362:59-62, 1993.
7. Norris FH, Smith RA, Denys EH: The treatment of amyotrophic lateral sclerosis. In Cosi V, Kato AC, Parletti I, editors: *Amyotrophic lateral sclerosis. Therapeutic, psychological and research aspects,* New York, 1987, Plenum Press.
8. Appel SH, Smith GR: Can neurotrophic factors prevent or reverse motor neuron injury in amyotrophic lateral sclerosis? *Exp Neurol* 124:100, 1993.
9. Milonas I: Amyotrophic lateral sclerosis: an introduction, *J Neurol* 245(suppl 2):S1-S3, 1998.
10. Dangond F: *Amyotrophic lateral sclerosis:* http://www.emedicine.com/neuro/topic14.htm. Accessed December 22, 2004. Last update, April 10, 2006.
11. Gue'gan C, Vila M, Rosoklija G et al: Recruitment of the mitochondrial-dependent apoptotic pathway in amyotrophic lateral sclerosis, *J Neurosci* 21:6569-6576, 2001.
12. Gue'gan C, Przedborski S: Programmed cell death in amyotrophic lateral sclerosis, *J Clinical Invest* 111:153-161, 2003.
13. Xu Z: Mechanism and treatment of motoneuron degeneration in ALS: what have SOD1 mutants told us? *Amyotroph Lateral Scler Other Motor Neuron Disord* 1:225-234, 2000.
14. Belsh JM: Diagnostic challenges in ALS, *Neurology* 53(suppl 5):S26-S30, 1999.

15. Wilbourn AJ: Clinical neurophysiology in the diagnosis of amyotrophic lateral sclerosis: the Lambert and the El Escorial criteria, *J Neurol Sci* 160(suppl 1):S25-S29, 1998.

16. Brooks BR: El Escorial World Federation of Neurology criteria for the diagnosis of amyotrophic lateral sclerosis, *J Neurol Sci* 124(suppl):96-107, 1994.

17. Rowland LP: Diagnosis of amyotrophic lateral sclerosis, *J Neurol Sci* 160(suppl 1):S6-S24, 1998.

18. Brooks BR: Introduction: defining optimal management of ALS: from first symptoms to announcement, *Neurology* 53(suppl 5):S1-S3, 1999.

19. *El Escorial revisited: revised criteria for the diagnosis of amyotrophic lateral sclerosis.* http://www.wfnals.org/guidelines/1998elescorial/elescorial1998.htm. Accessed June 29, 2006.

20. Mulder DW, Kurland LT: Amyotrophic lateral sclerosis (motor neuron disease): four clinical questions. In Tsubaki T, Yase Y, editors: *Amyotrophic lateral sclerosis,* Amsterdam, 1987, Elsevier Science.

21. Tashiro K, Moriwaka F, Matsuura T et al: Sensory findings in amyotrophic lateral sclerosis. In Tsubaki T, Yase Y, editors: *Amyotrophic lateral sclerosis,* Amsterdam, 1988, Elsevier Science.

22. Daube JR, Litchy WJ, Low PA et al: Classification of ALS by autonomic abnormalities. In Tsubaki T, Yase Y, editors: *Amyotrophic lateral sclerosis,* Amsterdam, 1988, Elsevier Science.

23. Lomen-Hoerth C: Characterization of amyotrophic lateral sclerosis and frontotemporal dementia, *Dement Geriatr Cogn Disord* 17:337-341, 2004.

24. Swash M: Early diagnosis of amyotrophic lateral sclerosis/motor neuron disease, *J Neurol Sci* 160(suppl 1):S33-S36, 1998.

25. Brooks BR, Sufit RL, DePaul R et al: Design of clinical therapeutic trials in amyotrophic lateral sclerosis. In Rowland L, editor: *Advances in neurology, vol 56,* New York, 1991, Raven Press, pp 521-546.

26. Sobue G, Sahashi K, Takahashi A et al: Degenerating compartment and functioning compartment of motor neurons in ALS: possible process of motor neuron loss, *Neurology* 33:654, 1983.

27. Brooks BR: What are the implications of early diagnosis? Maintaining optimal health as long as possible, *Neurology* 53(suppl 5):S43-S49, 1999.

28. Chou SM: Pathology of intraneuronal inclusions in ALS. In Tsubaki T, Toyokura Y, editors: *Amyotrophic lateral sclerosis,* Baltimore, 1979, University Park Press.

29. Ringel SP, Murphy JR, Alderson MK et al: The natural history of amyotrophic lateral sclerosis, *Neurology* 43:1316, 1993.

30. Armon C, Moses D: Linear estimates of rates of disease progression as predictors of survival in patients with ALS entering clinical trials, *J Neurol Sci* 160(suppl 1):S37-S41, 1998.

31. Hillel AD, Miller RM, Yorkston K, et al: Amyotrophic lateral sclerosis severity scale, *Neuroepidemiology* 8:142, 1989.

32. Hillel AD, Miller RM, Yorkston K et al: Amyotrophic lateral sclerosis severity scale. In Rose CF, editor: *Amyotrophic lateral sclerosis,* New York, 1990, Demos Publications.

33. Pradas J, Finison L, Andres PL et al: The natural history of amyotrophic lateral sclerosis and the use of natural history controls in therapeutic trials, *Neurology* 43:751, 1993.

34. Friedlander RM: Apoptosis and caspases in neurodegenerative diseases, *N Engl J Med* 348:1365-1375, 2003.

35. Cashman NR: Do the benefits of currently available treatments justify early diagnosis and announcement? Arguments for, *Neurology* 53(suppl 5):S50-S52, 1999.

36. Desai J, Sharief M, Swash M: Riluzole has no effect on motor unit parameters in ALS, *J Neurol Sci* 160(suppl 1):S69-S72, 1998.

37. Ludolph AC, Riepe MW: Do the benefits of currently available treatments justify early diagnosis and announcement? Arguments against, *Neurology* 53(suppl 5):S46-S49, 1999.

38. Bensimon G, Doble A: The tolerability of riluzole in the treatment of patients with amyotrophic lateral sclerosis, *Expert Opin Drug Saf* 3:525-534, 2004.

39. Gordon PH, Moore DH, Gelinas DF et al: Placebo-controlled phase I/II studies of minocycline in amyotrophic lateral sclerosis, *Neurology* 62:E22-E23, 2004.

40. Drachman M, Cudkowicz M: *Northeast ALS Consortium Celebrex study: Celebrex shows no benefit in ALS:* http://www.mdausa.org/research. Search for Celebrex. Accessed September 6, 2006.

41. Ascherio A, Weiskopf MG, O'Reilly EJ et al: Vitamin E intake and risk of amyotrophic lateral sclerosis, *Ann Neurol* 57:104-110, 2005.

42. Graf M, Ecker D, Horowski R, et al: High dose vitamin E therapy in amyotrophic lateral sclerosis as add-on therapy to riluzole: results of placebo-controlled double-blind study, *J Neural Transm* 112:649-660, 2005.

43. Orrell R, Lane J, Ross M: Antioxidant treatment for amyotrophic lateral sclerosis/motor neuron disease, *Cochrane Database Syst Rev* 2004 Oct 18;(4):CD002829. Update in: *Cochrane Database Syst Rev* 2005;(1):CD002829.

44. Amtmann D, Weydt P, Johnson KL et al: Survey of cannabis use in patient with amyotrophic lateral sclerosis, *Am J Hosp Palliat Care* 21:95-104, 2004.

45. Di Lazzaro V, Oliviero A, Pilato F et al: Motor cortex stimulation for amyotrophic lateral sclerosis. Time for a therapeutic trial? *Clin Neurophysiol* 115:1479-1485, 2004.

46. Ziemann U, Eisen A: TMS for ALS: why and why not, *Clin Neurophysiol* 115:1237-1238, 2004.

47. Houpt JL, Gould BS, Norris FH: Psychological characteristics of patients with amyotrophic lateral sclerosis, *Psychosom Med* 39:299, 1977.

48. Mackin GA: Optimizing care of patients with ALS: steps to early detection and improved quality of life, *Postgrad Med* 105:141-158, 1999.

49. Matheron L, Barrau K, Blin O: Disease management: the example of amyotrophic lateral sclerosis, *J Neurol* 245(suppl 2):S20-S28, 1998.

50. Beghi E, Mennini T: Basic and clinical research on amyotrophic lateral sclerosis and other motor neuron disorders in Italy: recent findings and achievements from a network of laboratories, *Neurol Sci Suppl* 2:41-60, 2004.

51. Traynor BH, Alexander M, Corr B et al: Effect of a multidisciplinary amyotrophic lateral sclerosis clinic (ALS) survival: a population based study, 1996-2000, *J Neurol Neurosurg Psychiatry* 74:1258-1261, 2003.

52. Ashworth NL, Satkunam LE, Deforge D: Treatment for spasticity in amyotrophic lateral sclerosis/motor neuron disease, *Cochrane Database Syst Rev* 1:CD004156, 2004.

53. Kesiktas N, Paker N, Erdogan N, et al: The use of hydrotherapy for the management of spasticity, *Neurorehabil Neural Repair* 18:268-273, 2004.

54. Ganzini L, Johnston WS, Hoffman WF: Correlates of suffering in amyotrophic lateral sclerosis, *Neurology* 52:1434-1440, 1999.

55. Norris FH, Denys EH: Nutritional supplements in amyotrophic lateral sclerosis. In Cosi V, Kato AC, Parletti I, editors: *Amyotrophic lateral sclerosis. Therapeutic, psychological and research aspects,* New York, 1987, Plenum Press.

56. Carpenter RJ, McDonald TJ, Howard FM: The otolaryngologic presentation of amyotrophic lateral sclerosis, *ORL* 86:479, 1978.

57. Mayberry JF, Atkinson M: Swallowing problems in patients with motor neuron disease, *J Clin Gastroenterol* 8:233-234, 1986.

58. Willig TN, Bach JR, Venance V et al: Nutritional rehabilitation in neuromuscular disorders, *Semin Neurol* 15:18-23, 1995.

59. Scott A, Heughan A: A review of dysphagia in four cases of motor neurone disease, *Palliat Med* 7(suppl 2):41-47, 1993.

60. Hillel AD, Miller RM: Management of bulbar symptoms in amyotrophic lateral sclerosis. In Cosi V, Kato AC, Parletti I, editors: *Amyotrophic lateral sclerosis. Therapeutic, psychological and research aspects,* New York, 1987, Plenum Press.

61. Hillel AD, Miller RM: Bulbar amyotrophic lateral sclerosis: patterns of progression and clinical management, *Head Neck* 11:51-59, 1989.

62. Hillel AD, Dray T, Miller R, et al: Presentation of ALS to the otolaryngologist/head and neck surgeon: getting to the neurologist, *Neurology* 53(suppl 5):S22-S25, 1999.

63. van den Berg MP, van den Berg JP, van Dessel EF et al: The symptomatic treatment of amyotrophic lateral sclerosis, *Ned Tijdschr Geneeskd* 148:513-518, 2004.

64. Appel V: *Meals for easy swallowing,* Tucson, AZ, 1986, Muscular Dystrophy Association.

65. ALS Association: Adjusting to swallowing and speech difficulties: diet. In *Living with ALS:* http://www.alsa.org/resources. Select desired manual. Accessed September 6, 2006.

66. Silani V, Kasarskis EJ, Yanagisawa N: Nutritional management in amyotrophic lateral sclerosis: a worldwide perspective, *J Neurol* 245(suppl 2):S13-S19, 1998.

67. Forbes RB, Colville S, Swingler RJ: Frequency, timing and outcome of gastrostomy tubes for amyotrophic lateral sclerosis/motor neurone disease—a record linkage study from the Scottish Motor Neurone Disease Register, *J Neurol* 251:813-817, 2004.

68. Kelly JH, Buccholz DW: Nutritional management of the patient with a neurologic disorder, *Ear Nose Throat J* 75:293-300, 1996.

69. Dworkin JP, Hartman DE: Progressive speech deterioration and dysphagia in amyotrophic lateral sclerosis: case report, *Arch Phys Med Rehabil* 60:423-424, 1979.

70. Koidis PT, Topouzelis N: Palatal lift prosthesis for palatopharyngeal closure in Wilson's disease, *Xc Res* 6:101, 2003.

71. Sufit R: Symptomatic treatment of ALS, *Neurology* 48(suppl 4):S28-S32, 1999.

72. Humberstone N: Respiratory assessment and treatment. In Irwin S, Tecklin JS, editors: *Cardiopulmonary physical therapy,* ed 3, Philadelphia, 1995, C.V. Mosby.

73. Oliver D: Ethical issues in palliative care—an overview, *Palliat Med* 7(suppl 2):15, 1993.

74. Sivak ED, Shefner JM, Mitsumoto H et al: The use of non-invasive positive pressure ventilation (NIPPV) in ALS patients. A need for improved determination of intervention timing, *Amyotroph Lateral Scler Other Motor Neuron Disord* 2:139-145, 2001.

75. Aboussouan LS, Khan SU, Arroliga AC et al: Effect of non-invasive pressure ventilation on pulmonary function in ALS, *Chest* 116:271S, 1999.

76. Pinto A, de Carvalho M, Evangelista T et al: Nocturnal pulse oximetry: a new approach to establish the appropriate time for non-invasive ventilation in ALS patients, *Amyotroph Lateral Scler Other Motor Neuron Disord* 4:31-35, 2003.

77. Bach JR, Bianchi C, Aufier E: Oximetry and indications for tracheostomy for amyotrophic lateral sclerosis, *Chest* 126:1502-1507, 2004.

78. Mitsumoto H: Patient choices in ALS: life-sustaining treatment versus palliative care, *Neurology* 53:248-249, 1988.

79. Miller RG, Rosenberg JA, Gelinas DF et al: Practice parameter: the care of the patient with amyotrophic lateral sclerosis (an evidenced-based review): report of the Quality Standards Subcommittee of the American Academy of Neurology: ALS Practice Parameters Task Force, *Neurology* 52:1311-1323, 1999.

80. Moss AH, Casey P, Stocking CB et al: Home ventilation for amyotrophic lateral sclerosis patients: outcomes, costs and patient, family and physician attitudes, *Neurology* 43:438, 1993.

81. Albert SM, Murphy PL, Del Bene ML, et al: A prospective study of preferences and actual treatment choices in ALS, *Neurology* 53:278-283, 1999.

82. Lechtzin N, Wiener CM, Clawson L et al: Use of noninvasive ventilation in patients with amyotrophic lateral sclerosis, *Amyotroph Lateral Scler Other Motor Neuron Disord* 5:9-15, 2004.

83. Russell J: Ethical considerations in disease management of amyotrophic lateral sclerosis: a cross-cultural, worldwide perspective, *J Neurol* 245(suppl 2):S4-S6, 1998.

84. Oppenheimer EA: Decision-making in the respiratory care of amyotrophic lateral sclerosis: should home mechanical ventilation be used? *Palliat Med* 7(suppl 2):49, 1993.

85. Kaub-Wittemer D, Steinbuchel N, Wasner M et al: Quality of life and psychosocial issues in ventilated patients with amyotrophic lateral sclerosis and their caregivers, *J Pain Symptom Management* 26:890-896, 2003.

86. Oliver D, Cardy P: *Motor neuron disease: death and dying,* North Hampton, UK, 1991, Motor Neuron Disease Association.

87. Mitsumoto H, Del Bene M: Improving the quality of life for people with ALS: the challenge ahead, *Amyotroph Lateral Scler Other Motor Neuron Disord* 1:329-336, 2000.

88. Onders RP, Schilz R, Katirji B et al: Early results of laparoscopic motor point diaphragm pacing in amyotrophic lateral sclerosis: can exogenous electrical stimulation impact respiratory failure? *Amyotrophic Lateral Sclerosis* 6(suppl 1):138-145, 2005.

89. Carver AC, Vickrey BG, Bernat JL et al: End-of-life care: a survey of US neurologists' attitudes, behavior, and knowledge, *Neurology* 53:284-293, 1999.

90. Vignos PJ: Physical models of rehabilitation in neuromuscular disease, *Muscle Nerve* 6:323, 1983.

91. Calzada-Sierra DJ, Gomez-Fernandez L: The importance of multi-factorial rehabilitation treatment in amyotrophic lateral sclerosis, *Revista de Neurologia* 32:423-426, 2001.

92. Sanjak M, Brinkmann J, Belden DS, et al: Quantitative assessment of motor fatigue in amyotrophic lateral sclerosis, *J Neurol Sci* 191:55-59, 2001.

93. World Federation of Neurology: *Amyotrophic lateral sclerosis,* http://www.wfnals.org. Accessed June 29, 2006.

94. Kilmer DD, Aitkens S: Neuromuscular disease. In Frontera WR, Dawson DM, Slovik DM, editors: *Exercise in rehabilitation medicine,* Champaign, IL, 1999, Human Kinetics, pp. 253-266.

95. Mazzini L, Mora G, Balzarini C, et al: The natural history and the effects of gabapentin in amyotrophic lateral sclerosis, *J Neurol Sci* 160(suppl 1):S57-S63, 1998.

96. Muller EA: Influence of training and of inactivity on muscle strength, *Arch Phys Med Rehabil* 51:449, 1970.

97. Appell HJ: Muscular atrophy following immobilization, *Sports Med* 10:42-58, 1993.

98. Spencer WA: *The treatment of acute poliomyelitis,* Springfield, IL, 1954, Charles C Thomas.

99. Bennett RL, Knowlton GC: Overwork weakness in partially denervated skeletal muscle, *Clin Orthop* 12:22, 1958.

100. Reitsma W: Skeletal muscle hypertrophy after heavy exercise in rats with surgically reduced muscle function, *Am J Phys Med* 48:237, 1969.

101. Francis K, Bach JR, DeLisa JA: Evaluation and rehabilitation of patients with adult motor neuron disease, *Arch Phys Med Rehabil* 80:951-963, 1999.

102. Sinaki M, Mulder DW: Rehabilitation techniques for patients with amyotrophic lateral sclerosis, *Mayo Clin Proc* 53:173-178, 1978.

103. Clarkson PM, Nokasa K, Braun B: Muscle function after exercise-induced muscle damage and rapid adaptation, *Med Sci Sports Exerc* 24:512-520, 1992.

104. Sanjak M, Reddan W, Brooks BR: Role of muscular exercise in amyotrophic lateral sclerosis, *Neurol Clin* 5:251, 1989.

105. Milner-Brown HS, Miller RG: Muscle strengthening through high-resistance weight training in patients with neuromuscular disorders, *Arch Phys Med Rehabil* 69:14-19, 1998.

106. Chan CW, Sinaki M: Rehabilitation management of the ALS patient. In Belsh JM, Schiffman PL editors: *Amyotrophic lateral sclerosis: diagnosis and management for the clinician,* New York, 1996, Futura.

107. Sanjak M, Paulson D, Sufit R, et al: Physiologic and metabolic response to progressive and prolonged exercise in amyotrophic lateral sclerosis, *Neurology* 37:1217-1220, 1987.

108. Jette DU, Slavin MD, Andres PL et al: The relationship of lower-limb muscle force to walking ability in patients with amyotrophic lateral sclerosis, *Phys Ther* 79:672-681, 1998.

109. Kilmer DD, McCrory MA, Wright NC et al: The effect of a high-resistance exercise program in slowly progressive neuromuscular disease, *Arch Phys Med Rehabil* 75:560-563, 1994.

110. Wright NC, Kilmer DD, McCrory MA et al: Aerobic walking in slowly progressive neuromuscular disease: effect of a 12-week program, *Arch Phys Med Rehabil* 77:64-69, 1996.

111. Dal Bello-Haas V: Physical therapy for a patient through six stages of amyotrophic lateral sclerosis, *Phys Ther* 78:1314-1324, 1998.

112. Drory, VE, Goltsman E, Reznik JG et al: The value of muscle exercise in patients with amyotropic lateral sclerosis, *Neurol Sci* 191:133-137, 2001.

113. Kirkinezos IG Hernandez D, Bradley WG et al: Regular exercise is beneficial to a mouse model of amyotrophic lateral sclerosis, *Ann Neurol* 53:804-807, 2003.

114. Aksu S, Citak-Karakaya I: Effect of exercise therapy on pain complaints in patients with amyotrophic lateral sclerosis, *Pain Clin* 14:353-359, 2002.

115. Mazzini L, Balzarini C, Colombo R, et al: Effects of creatine supplementation on exercise performance and muscular strength in amyotrophic lateral sclerosis, *J Neurol Sci* 19:139-144, 2001.

116. Sinaki M: Exercise and rehabilitation measures in amyotrophic lateral sclerosis. In Yase Y, Tsubaki T, editors: *Amyotrophic lateral sclerosis: recent advances in research and treatment,* Amsterdam, 1988, Elsevier Science.

117. Smith PS: Maintaining quality of life [letter], *Phys Ther* 79:423, 1999.

118. Simonds AK, Muntoni F, Heather S et al: The impact of nasal ventilation on survival in hypercapnic Duchenne muscular dystrophy, *Thorax* 53:949-952, 1998.

119. Murphy J: Communication strategies of people with ALS and their partners, *Amyotroph Lateral Scler Other Motor Neuron Disord* 5:121-126, 2004.

120. American Speech-Language-Hearing Association: *Dysarthria,* http://www.asha.org/public/speech/disorders/dysarthria.htm. Accessed June 29, 2006.

121. Cook AM, Hussey SM: *Augmentative and alternative communication systems,* New York, 1995, C.V. Mosby.

122. Kazandjian NS: Communication intervention. In Kazandjian NS, editor: *Communication and swallowing solutions for the ALS/MND community,* San Diego, 1997, Singular Publishing.

123. Neumann N, Hubler A: Training locked-in patients: a challenge for the use of brain-computer interfaces, *IEEE Trans Neural Syst Rehabil Eng* 11:169-172, 2003.

124. Cobble M: Language impairment in motor neurone disease, *J Neurol Sci* 160(suppl 1):S47-S52, 1998.

125. Borasio GD, Sloan R, Pongratz DE: Breaking the news in amyotrophic lateral sclerosis, *J Neurol Sci* 160(suppl 1):S127-S133, 1998.

126. McCluskey L, Casarett D, Siderowf A: Breaking the news: a survey of ALS patients and their caregivers, *Amyotroph Lateral Scler Other Motor Neuron Disord* 5:131-135, 2004.

127. Purtilo R, Haddad A: *Health professional and patient interaction,* ed 6, Philadelphia, 2002, Elsevier Science.

128. Goldstein LH, Adamson M, Jeffrey L et al: The psychological impact of MND on patients and careers, *J Neurol Sci* 160(suppl 1):S114–S121, 1998.

129. Ganzini L, Johnston WS, Silveira MJ: The final month of life in patients with ALS, *Neurology* 59:428-431, 2002.

130. Ganzini L, Silveira MJ, Johnston WS: Predictors and correlates of interest in assisted suicide in the final month of life among ALS patients in Oregon and Washington *J Pain Symptom Manage* 24:312-317, 2002.

131. Rabkin JG, Wagner GJ, Del Bene M: Resilience and distress among amyotrophic lateral sclerosis, *Psychosomat Med* 62:271-279, 2000.

132. Trail M, Nelson N, Van JN et al: Major stressors facing patients with amyotrophic lateral sclerosis: a survey to identify their concerns and to compare with those of their caregivers, *Amyotroph Lateral Scler Other Motor Neuron Disord* 5:40-45, 2004.

133. Damiano AM, Patrick DL, Guzman GI et al: Measurement of health-related quality of life in patients with amyotrophic lateral sclerosis in clinical trials of new therapies, *Med Care* 37:15-26, 1999.

134. Gelinas DF, O'Connor P, Miller RG: Quality of life for ventilator-dependent ALS patients and their caregivers, *J Neurol Sci* 160(suppl 1):S134-S136, 1998.

135. Smith EWL: A gestalt therapist's perspective on grief. In Stern EM, editor: *Psychotherapy and the grieving patient,* New York, 1985, Harrington Park Press.

136. Moore MJ, Moore PB, Shaw PJ: Mood disturbances in motor neurone disease, *J Neurol Sci* 160(suppl 1):S53-S56, 1998.

137. Carter JH, Nutt JG: Family caregiving: a neglected and hidden part of health care delivery, *Neurology* 51:1245-1246, 1998.

138. Vine P: *Families in pain,* New York, 1982, Pantheon Books.

139. Hallum A, Krumboltz JD: Parents caring for young adults with severe physical disabilities: psychological issues, *Dev Med Child Neurol* 35:24-32, 1993.

140. Guillain G, Barré JA, Strohl A: Sur un syndrome de radiculo-névrité avec hyperalbuminose du liquide cephalorachidien sans réaction cellulaire: Rémarques sur les caractères cliniques et graphiques des réflexes tendineux, *Bull Mem Soc Med Hop Paris* 40:1462, 1916.

141. Ouvrier R: Update on acute and chronic inflammatory polyneuropathy, *J Child Neurol* 14:53-57, 1999.

142. Hughes RAC, Swan A, van Doorn P: Cytotoxic drugs and interferons for chronic inflammatory demyelination polyradiculoneuropathy, *Cochrane Database Syst Rev* 2004 Oct 18;(4):CD003280.

143. Ng YS, Lo YL, Lim PAC: Characteristics and acute rehabilitation of Guillain Barré syndrome in Singapore, *Ann Acad Med* 33:314-319, 2004.

144. Pritchard J, Hughes, RAC: Guillain Barré syndrome, *Lancet* 363:2186-2188, 2004.

145. Domonville de la Cour C, Andersen H, Stalberg E et al: Electrophysiological signs of permanent axonal loss in a followup study of patients with Guillain Barré syndrome, *Muscle Nerve* 31:70-77, 2005.

146. Steck AJ, Schaeren-Wiemers N, Hartung HP: Demyelinating inflammatory neuropathies, including Guillain-Barré syndrome, *Curr Opin Neurol* 11:311-318, 1998.

147. Meythaler JM: Rehabilitation of Guillain-Barré syndrome, *Arch Phys Med Rehabil* 78:872-879, 1997.

148. Atanasova D, Ishpekova B, Muradyan N et al: Conduction block—the diagnostic value in the early stage of Guillain Barré syndrome, *Electromyogr Clin Neurophysiol* 44:361-364, 2004.

149. Kandel ER, Schwartz J, Jessell T: *Principles of neural science,* ed 4, New York, 2000, McGraw-Hill.

150. Hartung HP, van der Meche FGA, Pollard JD: Editorial review: Guillain-Barré syndrome, CIDP and other chronic immune-mediated neuropathies, *Curr Opin Neurol* 11:497-513, 1998.

151. Trojaborg W: Acute and chronic neuropathies: new aspects of Guillain-Barré syndrome and chronic inflammatory demyelinating polyneuropathy, an overview and an update, *Electroenceph Clin Neurophysiol* 107:303-316, 1998.

152. Visser LH, Schmitz PI, Muelstee JA et al: Prognostic factors of Guillain Barré syndrome after intravenous immunoglobulin or plasma exchange, *Neurology* 53:598-604, 1999.

153. Rees J: Guillain-Barré syndrome: the latest on treatment, *Br J Hosp Med* 50:226, 1993.

154. Pascuzzi RM, Fleck JD: Acute peripheral neuropathy in adults, *Neurol Clin* 15:529-547, 1997.

155. Zochodne DW: Autonomic involvement in Guillain-Barré syndrome: a review, *Muscle Nerve* 17:1145-1155, 1994.

156. Kandel ER, Schwartz JH, Jessell TM, editors: *Principles of neural science,* ed 4, New York, 2000, McGraw-Hill.

157. Ropper AH, Shahani BT: Pain in Guillain-Barré syndrome, *Arch Neurol* 41:511-514, 1984.

158. Ropper AH: Severe acute Guillain-Barré syndrome, *Neurology* 36:429-432, 1986.

159. French Cooperative Group on Plasma Exchange in Guillain-Barré Syndrome: Efficiency of plasma exchange in Guillain-Barré syndrome: role of replacement fluids, *Ann Neurol* 22:753, 1987.

160. Clague JE, MacMillan RR: Backache and the Guillain-Barré syndrome: a diagnostic problem, *BMJ* 293:325, 1986.

161. Pentland B, Daonald SM: Pain in the Guillain-Barré syndrome: a clinical review, *Pain* 59:159-164, 1994.

162. Meythaler JM, DeVivo MJ, Braswell WC: Rehabilitation outcomes of patients who have developed Guillain-Barré syndrome, *Am J Phys Med Rehabil* 76:411-419, 1997.

163. Smith M: Guillain Barré syndrome: a patient's experience [letter], *Dev Med Child Neurol* 43:69-70, 2001.

164. Ropper AH: The Guillain Barré syndrome, *N Engl J Med* 326:1130-1136, 1992.

165. de Jager AEJ, Minderhoud JM: Residual signs in severe Guillain-Barré: analysis of 57 patients, *J Neurol Sci* 104:151-156, 1991.

166. Vasjar J, Fehlings D, Stephens D: Long-term outcome of pediatric Guillain Barré syndrome, *J Pediatr* 143:305-309, 2003.

167. Bernson RA, Jager AE, Schmitz PI et al: Long-term sensory deficit after Guillain-Barré syndrome, *J Neurol* 248:483-486, 2001.

168. Bach JR, Ishikawa Y: GBS respiratory complications revisited [letter], *Arch Phys Med Rehabil* 79:115-116, 1998.

169. Guillain-Barré Syndrome Study Group: Plasmapheresis and acute Guillain-Barré syndrome, *Neurology* 35:1096, 1985.

170. Bouget J, Chevret S, Chastang C et al: Plasma exchange morbidity in Guillain-Barré syndrome: results from the French prospective, double-blind, randomized, multi-center study, *Crit Care Med* 21:651-658, 1993.

171. Bril V, Ilse WK, Pearce R et al: Pilot trial of immunoglobulin versus plasma exchange in patients with Guillain-Barré syndrome, *Neurology* 46:100-103, 1996.

172. Irani DN, Cornblath DR, Chaudhry V et al: Relapse in Guillain-Barré syndrome after treatment with human immunoglobin, *Neurology* 43:872-875, 1993.

173. Hughes RAC, Wijdicks EF, Barohn R et al: Practice parameter: immunotherapy for Guillain Barré syndrome: report of the quality standards subcommittee of the American Academy of Neurology, *Neurology* 61:736-740, 2003.

174. Karni Y, Archdeacon L, Mills KR et al: Clinical assessment and physiotherapy in Guillain-Barré syndrome, *Physiotherapy* 70:288-292, 1984.

175. Lewis CB, Bottomley JM, editors: *Geriatric physical therapy: a clinical approach,* East Norwalk, CT, 1994, Appleton & Lange.

176. Irwin S, Tecklin JS, editors: *Cardiopulmonary physical therapy: a guide to practice,* ed 4, St. Louis, 2004, Elsevier.

177. Logemann JA: *Evaluation and treatment of swallowing disorders,* Austin, TX, 1997, PRO-ED.

178. Sonies BC: Instrumental procedures for dysphagia diagnosis, *Semin Speech Lang* 12:185, 1991.

179. Ruttenberg N: Assessment and treatment of speech and swallowing problems in patients with multiple sclerosis. In Maloney FP, Burks JS, Ringel SP, editors: *Interdisciplinary rehabilitation of multiple sclerosis and neuromuscular disorders,* Philadelphia, 1985, JB Lippincott.

180. Long DM, Campbell J, Grucer G: Transcutaneous electrical stimulation for relief of chronic pain, *Adv Pain Res Ther* 3:593-598, 1979.

181. Thorsteinsson G, Stonnington HH, Stillwell GK et al: Transcutaneous electrical stimulation: a double blind trial of its efficacy for pain, *Arch Phys Med Rehabil* 58:8, 1977.

182. *Capsaicin,* http://en.wikipedia.org/wiki/Capsaicin#Medical. Accessed December 12, 2004.

183. Stillwell GK: Rehabilitative procedures. In Dyck PJ et al, editors: *Peripheral neuropathy,* ed 2, Philadelphia, 1984, W.B. Saunders.

184. Akeson WH, Amiel D, la Violette D et al: The connective tissue response to immobility: an accelerated aging response? *Exp Gerontol* 3:289, 1968.

185. Gitter AJ, Haselkorn JK: Landry Guillain Barré syndrome and heterotopic ossification: case report [abstract], *Arch Phys Med Rehabil* 71:823, 1990.

186. Meythaler JM, Korkor AB, Nanda T et al: Immobilization hypercalcemia associated with Landry Guillain-Barré syndrome: successful therapy with combined calcitonin and etidronate sodium, *Arch Intern Med* 146:1567-1571, 1986.

187. Soryal I, Sinclair E, Hornby J et al: Impaired joint mobility in Guillain-Barré syndrome: a primary or a secondary phenomenon? *J Neurol Neurosurg Psychiatry* 55:1014, 1992.

188. Lehmann JF, Masock AJ, Warren CG et al: Effect of therapeutic temperature on tendon extensibility, *Arch Phys Med Rehabil* 51:481, 1970.

189. Taylor DC, Dalton JD Jr, Seaber AV et al: Viscoelastic properties of muscle-tendon units: the biomechanical effects of stretching, *Am J Sports Med* 18:300, 1990.

190. Warren CG, Lehmann JF, Koblanski JN: Elongation of rat tail tendon: effect of load and temperature, *Arch Phys Med Rehabil* 52:465, 1971.

191. Warren CG, Lehmann JF, Koblanski JN: Heat and stretch procedures: an evaluation using rat tail tendon, *Arch Phys Med Rehabil* 57:122, 1976.

192. Warren CG: The use of heat and cold in the treatment of common musculoskeletal disorders. In Kessler RM, Hertling D, editors: *Management of common musculoskeletal disorders: physical therapy principles and methods,* Philadelphia, 1983, Harper & Row.

193. Spencer GE, Vignos PJ Jr: Bracing for ambulation in childhood progressive muscular dystrophy, *J Bone Joint Surg* 44-A:234, 1962.

194. Kessler RM: The shoulder. In Kessler RM, Hertling D, editors: *Management of common musculoskeletal disorders: physical therapy principles and methods,* Philadelphia, 1983, Harper & Row.

195. Salter R: Clinical application of basic research on continuous passive motion for disorders and injuries of synovial joints: a preliminary study, *J Orthop Res* 1:325, 1984.

196. Mays ML: Incorporating continuous passive motion in the rehabilitation of a patient with Guillain-Barré syndrome, *Am J Occup Ther* 44:750, 1990.

197. Hertling D, Jones D: Relaxation. In Kessler RM, Hertling D, editors: *Management of common musculoskeletal disorders: physical therapy principles and methods,* Philadelphia, 1983, Harper & Row.

198. Steinberg JS: *Guillain-Barré syndrome (acute idiopathic polyneuritis): an overview for the lay person,* Wynnewood, PA, 1987, The Guillain-Barré Syndrome Support Group International.

199. Herbison GJ, Jaweed MM, Ditunno JF Jr: Exercise therapies in peripheral neuropathies, *Arch Phys Med Rehabil* 64:201, 1983.

200. Bensman A: Strenuous exercise may impair muscle function in Guillain-Barré patients, *JAMA* 214:468, 1970.

201. Petajan JH, White AT: Recommendations for physical activity in patients with multiple sclerosis, *Sports Med* 27:179-191, 1999.

202. Blei ML, Fall AM, Kushmerick MJ: Energy balance for muscle function: principles of bioenergetics. In Frontera WR, Dawson DM, Slovik DM, editors: *Exercise in rehabilitation medicine,* Champaign, IL, 1999, Human Kinetics, pp. 3-22.

203. Bushbacher L: Rehabilitation of patients with peripheral neuropathies. In Braddom RL: *Physical medicine and rehabilitation,* Philadelphia, 1995, W.B. Saunders, pp. 972-989.

204. Fielding RA, Bean J: Physiological adaptations to dynamic exercise. In Frontera WR, Dawson DM, Slovik DM, editors: *Exercise in rehabilitation medicine,* Champaign, IL, 1999, Human Kinetics, pp. 41-54.

205. Guccione AA: Functional assessment. In *Physical rehabilitation: assessment and treatment,* Philadelphia, 1994, FA Davis, pp. 193-207.

206. van der Putten JJ, Hobart JC, Freeman JA et al: Measuring change in disability after inpatient rehabilitation: comparison of responsiveness of the Barthel Index and the Functional Independence Measure, *J Neurol Neurosurg Psychiatry* 66:480-484, 1999.

207. Schmitz TY: Environmental assessment. In *Physical rehabilitation: assessment and treatment,* Philadelphia, 1994, FA Davis, pp. 209-223.

208. Grand'Maison F, Feasby TE, Hahn AF et al: Recurrent Guillain-Barré syndrome, *Brain* 115:1093-1106, 1992.

209. Burrows DS, Cuetter AC: Residual subclinical impairment in patients who totally recovered from Guillain-Barré syndrome: impact on military performance, *Milit Med* 155:438, 1990.

210. Karper WB: Effects of low-intensity aerobic exercise on one subject with chronic-relapsing Guillain-Barré syndrome, *Rehabil Nurs* 16:96, 1991.

211. Pitetti KH, Barrett PJ, Abbas D et al: Endurance exercise training in Guillain-Barré syndrome, *Arch Phys Med Rehabil* 74:761, 1993.

212. Fehlings D, Vajsar J, Wilk B et al: Anaerobic muscle performance of children after long-term recovery from Guillain-Barré syndrome, *Dev Med Child Neurol* 46:689-693, 2004.

213. Tuckey J, Greenwood R: Rehabilitation after severe Guillain-Barré syndrome: the use of partial body weight support, *Physiother Res Int* 9:96-103, 2004.

214. Hesse S, Werner C, Seibel H et al: Treadmill training with partial body-weight support after total hip arthroplasty: a randomized controlled trial, *Arch Phys Med Rehabil* 84:1767-1773, 2003.

215. Lamontagne A, Fung J: Faster is better. Implications for speed-intensive gait training after stroke, *Stroke* 35:2543, 2004.

216. Joffe D, Watkins M,Steiner L et al: Treadmill ambulation with partial body weight support for the treatment of low back and leg pain, *J Orthop Sports Phys Ther* 32:202-213, 2002.

217. Bernsen RA, de Jaeger AE, Schmitz PI et al: Long-term impact on work and private life after Guillain-Barré syndrome, *J Neurol Sci* 201:13-17, 2002.

218. Skirrow P, Jones P, Griffiths D: Intensive care—easing the trauma, *The Psychologist* 14:640-642, 2001.

219. Baxter A: Posttraumatic stress disorder and the intensive care unit patient: implications for staff and advanced practice critical care nurses, *Dimens Crit Care Nurs* 23:145-150, 2004.

220. Hunt JM: The cardiac surgical patient's expectations and experiences of nursing care in the intensive care unit, *Aust Crit Care* 12:47-53, 1999.

221. Nagashima T, Nishimoto Y, Hirata K et al: Outcome after Guillain Barré syndrome: comparison of motor function status and changes in social life [in Japanese], *Rinsho Shinkeigaku* 44:50-53, 2004.

222. Carroll A, McDonnell G, Barnes M: A review of Guillain Barré syndrome in a regional neurological rehabilitation unit, *Int J Rehab Res* 26:297-302, 2003.

223. Dubowitz V: Forty years of neuromuscular disease: a historical perspective, *J Child Neurol* 14:26-28, 1999.

224. Emery A, Muntoni F: *Duchenne muscular dystrophy,* New York, 2003, Oxford University Press.

225. American Thoracic Society: Respiratory care of the patient with Duchenne muscular dystrophy: a consensus statement, *Am J Respir Crit Care Med* 170:456-465, 2004.

226. Jones KJ, North KN: Recent advances in the diagnosis of the childhood muscular dystrophies, *J Paediatr Child Health* 33:195-201, 1997.

227. Tidball JG, Wehling-Henrickds M: Evolving therapeutic strategies for Duchenne muscular dystrophy: targeting downstream events, *Pediatr Res* 56:831-841, 2004.

228. Backman E, Nylander E: The heart in Duchenne muscular dystrophy: a non-invasive longitudinal study, *Eur Heart J* 13:1239-1244, 1992.

229. Fukunaga H, Okubo R, Moritoyo T et al: Long-term follow up of patients with Duchenne muscular dystrophy receiving ventilatory support, *Muscle Nerve* 16:554-558, 1993.

230. Billard C, Gillet P, Signoret JL et al: Cognitive functions in Duchenne muscular dystrophy: a reappraisal and comparison with spinal muscular atrophy, *Neuromusc Disord* 2:371-378, 1992.

231. Billard C, Gillet P, Barthez M et al: Reading ability and processing in Duchenne muscular dystrophy and spinal muscular atrophy, *Dev Med Child Neurol* 40:12-20, 1998.

232. Wicksell RK, Kihlgren M, Melin L et al: Specific cognitive deficits are common in children with Duchenne muscular dystrophy, *Dev Med Child Neurol* 46:154-159, 2004.

233. Appel SH: The muscular dystrophies, *Neurol Clin* 1:7, 1979.

234. Brooke MH, Fenichel GM, Griggs RC et al: Duchenne muscular dystrophy: patterns of clinical progression and effects of supportive therapy, *Neurology* 39:475, 1989.

235. Drennan JC: Neuromuscular disorders. In Morrissy RT, editor: *Pediatric orthopaedics,* ed 3, Philadelphia, 1990, JB Lippincott.

236. Sutherland DH, Olshen R, Cooper L: The pathomechanics of gait in Duchenne muscular dystrophy, *Dev Med Child Neurol* 23:3, 1981.

237. Allsop KG, Ziter FA: Loss of strength and functional decline in Duchenne dystrophy, *Arch Neurol* 38:406, 1981.

238. Siegel IM: Update on Duchenne muscular dystrophy, *Comp Ther* 15:45, 1989.

239. Griggs RC, Moxley RT 3rd, Mendell JR et al: Randomized, double-blind trial of mazindol in Duchenne dystrophy, *Muscle Nerve* 13:1169-1173, 1990.

240. Brooke MH, Fenichel GM, Griggs RC et al: Clinical investigation of Duchenne muscular dystrophy: interesting results in a trial of prednisolone, *Arch Neurol* 44:812, 1987.

241. Heckmatt J, Rodillo E, Dubowitz V: Management of children: pharmacological and physicalPCDC (phosphatidylcholine deoxycholate) *Br Med Bull* 45:788, 1989.

242. Manzur AY, Kuntzer T, Pike M et al: Glucocorticoid corticosteroids for Duchenne muscular dystrophy, *The Cochrane Database of Systematic Reviews* 2004, Issue 2. Art. No.: CD003725. DOI: 10.1002/14651858.CD003725.pub2.

243. Partridge TA: Myoblast transfer: possible therapy for inherited myopathies, *Muscle Nerve* 14:197, 1991.

244. Miller RG, Sharma KR, Pavlath GK et al: Myoblast implantation in Duchenne muscular dystrophy: the San Francisco study, *Muscle Nerve* 20:469-478, 1997.

245. Petrof BJ: Respiratory muscles as a target for adenovirus-mediated gene therapy, *Eur Respir J* 11:492-497, 1998.

246. Dudley RW, Lu Y, Gilbert R et al: Sustained improvement of muscle function one year after full-length dystrophin gene transfer into mdx mice by a gutted helper-dependent adenoviral vector. *Hum Gen Ther* 15:145-156, 2004.

247. Kirk VG, Flemons WW, Adams C et al: Sleep-disordered breathing in Duchenne muscular dystrophy: a preliminary study of the role of portable monitoring, *Pediatr Pulmonol* 29:135-140, 2000.

248. American Thoracic Society: Care of the child with chronic tracheostomy, *Am J Respir Crit Care Med* 161:297-308, 2000.

249. Bach JR: Update and perspectives on noninvasive respiratory muscle aids. Part 1: the inspiratory aids, *Chest* 105:1230-1240, 1994.

250. Corrado A, Gorini M, DePaola E: Alternative techniques for managing acute neuromuscular respiratory failure, *Semin Neurol* 15:84-89, 1995.

251. Vianello A: Pneumothorax associated with long-term non-invasive positive pressure ventilation in Duchenne muscular dystrophy, *Neuromusc Dis* 14:355, 2004.

252. Baydur A, Kanel G: Tracheobronchomalacia and tracheal hemorrhage in patients with Duchenne muscular dystrophy receiving long-term ventilation with uncuffed tracheostomies, *Chest* 124:1307-1311, 2003.

253. Miller JR, Colbert AP, Schock NC: Ventilator use in progressive neuromuscular disease: impact on patients and their families, *Dev Med Child Neurol* 30:200-207, 1988.

254. Miller F, Moseley CF, Koreska J: Spinal fusion in Duchenne muscular dystrophy, *Dev Med Child Neurol* 34:775, 1992.

255. Edwards RHT: Weight reduction in boys with muscular dystrophy, *Dev Med Child Neurol* 26:384, 1984.

256. Griffith R, Edwards RHT: A new chart for weight control in Duchenne muscular dystrophy, *Arch Phys Med Rehabil* 63:1256, 1988.

257. Iannaccone ST, Owens H, Scott J et al: Postoperative malnutrition in Duchenne muscular dystrophy, *J Child Neurol* 18:17-20, 2003.

258. Lord J, Behrman B, Varzos N et al: Scoliosis associated with Duchenne muscular dystrophy, *Arch Phys Med Rehabil* 71:13, 1990.

259. McDonald CM, Abresch RT, Carter GT et al: Profiles of neuromuscular diseases: Duchenne muscular dystrophy, *Am J Phys Med Rehabil* 74:S70-S92, 1995.

260. Stern LM, Clark BE: Investigation of scoliosis in Duchenne dystrophy using computerized tomography, *Muscle Nerve* 11:775, 1988.

261. Bach JR: Therapeutic interventions and habilitation considerations: a historical perspective from Tamplin to robotics for pseudohypertrophic muscular dystrophy, *Semin Neurol* 15:38-45, 1995.

262. Yilmaz O, Karaduman A, Topaloglu H: Prednisone therapy in Duchenne muscular dystrophy prolongs ambulation and prevents scoliosis, *Eur J Neurol* 11:541-544, 2004.

263. Alman BA, Raza SN, Biggar WD: Steroid treatment and the development of scoliosis in males with Duchenne muscular dystrophy, *J Bone Joint Surg Am* 86-A:519-524, 2004.

264. Cervellati S, Bettini N, Moscato M et al: Surgical treatment of spinal deformities in Duchenne muscular dystrophy: a long term follow-up study, *Eur J Neurol* 13:441-448, 2004.

265. McDonald DG, Kinali M, Gallagher AC et al: Fracture prevalence in Duchenne muscular dystrophy, *Dev Med Child Neurol* 44:695-698, 2002.

266. Florence J, Pandya S, King WM et al: Intrarater reliability of manual muscle test grades in Duchenne muscular dystrophy, *Phys Ther* 72:115, 1992.

267. Pandya S, Florence JM, King WM et al: Reliability of goniometric measurements in patients with Duchenne muscular dystrophy, *Phys Ther* 65:1339, 1985.

268. McDonald CM: Limb contractures in progressive neuromuscular disease and the role of stretching, orthotics and surgery, *Phys Med Rehabil Clin North Am* 9:187-211, 1998.

269. Carter GT: Rehabilitation management in neuromuscular disease, *J Neurol Rehab* 11:69-80, 1997.

270. Rideau Y, Duport G, Delaubier A et al: Early treatment to preserve quality of locomotion for children with Duchenne muscular dystrophy, *Semin Neurol* 15:9-16, 1995.

271. Brooke MH, Fenichel GM, Griggs RC et al: Clinical investigations in Duchenne muscular dystrophy: II. Determination of the "power" of therapeutic trials based on the natural history, *Muscle Nerve* 6:91, 1983.

272. Vignos PJ, Spencer GE, Archibald KC: Management of progressive muscular dystrophy of childhood, *JAMA* 184:89, 1963.

273. Rose J, Gamble JG, Lee J et al: The energy expenditure index: a method to quantify and compare walking energy expenditure for children and adolescents, *J Pediatr Orthop* 11:571, 1991.

274. DiMarco AF, DiMarco MS, Jacobs J et al: The effects of inspiratory resistive training on respiratory muscle function in patients with muscular dystrophy, *Muscle Nerve* 8:284-290, 1985.

275. Martin AJ, Stern L, Yeates J et al: Respiratory muscle training in Duchenne muscular dystrophy, *Dev Med Child Neurol* 28:314, 1986.

276. Topin N, Matecki S, Le Bris S et al: Dose-dependent effect of individualized respiratory muscle training in children with Duchenne muscular dystrophy, *Neuromusc Disord* 12:576-583, 2002.

277. Gozal D: Pulmonary manifestations of neuromuscular disease with special reference to Duchenne muscular dystrophy and spinal muscular atrophy, *Ped Pulmonol* 29:141-150, 2000.

278. Bach JR: Mechanical insufflation-exsufflation: comparison of peak expiratory flows with manually assisted and unassisted coughing techniques, *Chest* 104:1553-1562, 1993.

279. Miske LJ, Hickey EM, Kolb SM et al: Use of mechanical in-exsufflator in pediatric patients with neuromuscular disease and impaired cough, *Chest* 125:1406-1412, 2004.

280. Horan S, Warren R, Stefans V: *Breath easy: respiratory care for children with muscular dystrophy:* http://www.mda.org/publications/breathe. Accessed September 6, 2006.

281. Robinson R: Breathe easy options offered for respiratory care, *Quest* 5(5):1998: http://www.mdausa.org/publications/Quest/q55breathe.html/1998. Accessed June 29, 2006.

282. Tilton AH, Miller MD, Khoshoo V: Nutrition and swallowing in pediatric neuromuscular patients, *Semin Pediatr Neurol* 5:106-115, 1998.

283. Scott OM, Vrbova G, Hyde SA et al: Responses of muscles of patients with Duchenne muscular dystrophy to chronic electrical stimulation, *J Neurol Neurosurg Psychiatry* 49:1427, 1986.

284. Vignos PJ: Management of musculoskeletal complications in neuromuscular disease: limb contractures and the role of stretching, braces and surgery, *Phys Med Rehab* 2:509-536, 1988.

285. Zachazewski JE: Improving flexibility. In Scully RM, Barnes MR, editors: *Physical therapy,* Philadelphia, 1989, JB Lippincott.

286. Reid DA, McNair PJ: Passive force, angle, and stiffness changes after stretching of hamstring muscles, *Med Sci Sports Exerc* 36:1944-1948, 2004.

287. Grossman MR, Sahrmann SA, Rose SJ: Review of length associated changes in muscle: experimental evidence and clinical implications, *Phys Ther* 62:1799, 1982.

288. Scott OM, Hyde SA, Goddard C et al: Prevention of deformity in Duchenne muscular dystrophy, *Physiotherapy* 67:177, 1981.

289. Kilmer DD: Response to aerobic exercise training in humans with neuromuscular disease, *Am J Phys Med Rehabil* 81(suppl):S148-S150, 2002.

290. Hasson SM: Progressive and degenerative neuromuscular disease and severe muscular dystrophy. In Hasson SM, editor: *Clinical exercise physiology,* St. Louis, 1994, Mosby.

291. Elder GCB: Beneficial effects of training on developing dystrophic muscle, *Muscle Nerve* 15:672, 1992.

292. Johnson EW, Braddom R: Over-work weakness in facioscapulohumeral muscular dystrophy, *Arch Phys Med Rehabil* 52:333, 1971.

293. Fowler WM Jr, Gardner GW, Kazerunian HH et al: The effect of exercise on serum enzymes, *Arch Phys Med* 49:554, 1968.

294. McCartney N, Moroz D, Garner SH et al: The effects of strength training in patients with selected neuromuscular disorders, *Med Sci Sports Exerc* 20:362-368, 1988.

295. Vignos PJ, Watkins MP: The effect of exercise in muscular dystrophy, *JAMA* 197:843-848, 1966.

296. de Lateur BJ, Giaconi RM: Effect on maximal strength of submaximal exercise in Duchenne muscular dystrophy, *Am J Phys Med* 58:26, 1979.

297. Zupan A: Long-term electrical stimulation of muscles in children with Duchenne and Becker muscular dystrophy, *Muscle Nerve* 15:362-367, 1992.

298. DiMarco A, Kelling J, DiMarco M et al: The effects of inspiratory resistive training on respiratory muscle function in patients with muscular dystrophy, *Muscle Nerve* 8:284-290, 1985.

299. Twardowshi B, Twardowshi J: No sweat exercise: aquatics, *Quest* 10(4):2003: http://www.mdausa.org/publications/Quest/html/1998. Accessed September 6, 2006.

300. Noonan TJ, Garrett J: Injuries at the myotendinous junction, *Clin Sports Med* 11:783-806, 1992.

301. Allen DG: Skeletal muscle function: role of ionic changes in fatigue, damage and disease, *Clin Exp Pharm Physiol* 31:485-493, 2004.

302. Eagle M: Report on the muscular dystrophy campaign workshop: exercise in neuromuscular diseases, *Neuromusc Disord* 12:975-983, 2002.

303. Ansved T: Muscular dystrophies: influence of physical conditioning on the disease evolution, *Curr Opin Clin Nutr Metab Care* 6:435-439, 2003.

304. Bach JR, McKeon J: Orthopedic surgery and rehabilitation for the prolongation of brace-free ambulation of patients with Duchenne muscular dystrophy, *Am J Phys Med Rehabil* 70:323, 1991.

305. Roposch A, Scher DM, Mubarak S et al: Treatment of foot deformities in patients with Duchenne muscular dystrophy [in German], *Z Orthop Ihre Grenzgeb* 141:54-58, 2003.

306. Bakker JPJ, De Groot IJ, De Jong BA et al: Prescription pattern for orthoses in The Netherlands: use and experience in the ambulatory phase of Duchenne muscular dystrophy, *Disabil Rehabil* 19:318-325, 1997.

307. Hyde SA, Scott OM, Goddard CM et al: Prolongation of ambulation in Duchenne muscular dystrophy by appropriate orthoses, PCDC (phosphatidylcholine deoxycholate) 68:105, 1982.

308. Harris SE, Cherry DB: Childhood progressive muscular dystrophy and the role of physical therapy, *Phys Ther* 54:4, 1974.

309. Vignos PJ, Wagner MB, Karlinchak B et al: Evaluation of a program for long-term treatment of Duchenne muscular dystrophy, *J Bone Joint Surg Am* 78:1844-1852, 1996.

310. Rideau Y, Gatin G, Bach J et al: Prolongation of life in Duchenne's muscular dystrophy, *Acta Neurol* 38:118, 1983.

311. Stallard J, Henshaw JH, Lomas B et al: The ORLAU VCG (variable centre of gravity) swivel walker for muscular dystrophy patients. *Prosthet Orthop Int* 16:46, 1992.

312. Manzur AY, Hyde SA, Rodillo E et al: A randomized controlled trial of early surgery in Duchenne muscular dystrophy, *Neuromusc Disord* 2:379-387, 1992.

313. Bakker JPJ, De Groot IJ, Beckerman H et al: The effects of knee-ankle-foot orthoses in the treatment of Duchenne muscular dystrophy: review of the literature, *Clin Rehabil* 14:343-359, 2000.

314. Eggers S, Zatz M: Social adjustments in adult males affected with progressive muscular dystrophy, *Am J Med Genet* 81:4-12, 1998.

315. Pellegrini N, Guillon B, Prigent H et al: Optimization of power wheelchair control for patients with severe Duchenne muscular dystrophy, *Neuromusc Disord* 14:297-300, 2004.

316. Cooper RA: *Wheelchair selection and configuration,* New York, 1998, Demos Medical Publishing.

317. Fowler WM Jr, Abresch RT, Koch TR et al: Employment profiles in neuromuscular diseases, *Am J Phys Med Rehabil* 76:26-37, 1997.

318. Witte RA: The psychosocial impact of a progressive physical handicap and terminal illness (Duchenne muscular dystrophy) on adolescents and their families, *Br J Med Psychol* 58:179, 1985.

319. Gibson B: Long-term ventilation for patients with Duchenne muscular dystrophy: physicians' beliefs and practices, *Chest* 119:940-946, 2001.

320. Medvescek C: Parent-caregivers learning to let go, *Quest* 11(6):2004: http://www.mdausa.org/publications/Quest/q116letgo.aspx. Accessed June 29, 2006.

321. Childress J: The dying child. In Kruger DW, editor: *Rehabilitation psychology,* Rockville, MD, 1984, Aspen Publishers.

322. Ahlstrom G, Gunnarsson L: Disability and quality of life in individuals with muscular dystrophy, *Scand J Rehabil Med* 28:147-157, 1996.

323. Ahlstrom G, Sjoden P: Coping with illness-related problems and quality of life in adult individuals with muscular dystrophy, *J Psychosomat Res* 41:365-376, 1996.

324. Bach JR, Campagnolo DI, Hoeman S: Life satisfaction of individuals with Duchenne muscular dystrophy using long-term mechanical ventilatory support, *Am J Phys Med Rehabil* 70:129-135, 1991.

APPENDIX 16-A ■ Scoot Guard Material

Product Type: Nonslip material
Function: Stabilizes household objects on tabletops.
Features: Trims easily with scissors. Roll measures to be $\frac{1}{16} \times 12 \times 12$ inches.
Considerations: Hand washable. Sold by the roll.
Suggested Price: $14.49.
Vendors: **Sammons Preston Rolyan** Patterson Company

270 Remington Blvd., Suite C
Bolingbrook, IL 60440-3593
Toll Free: 800-323-5547
Phone: 630-226-1300
Fax: 800-547-4333
Web site: http://www.sammonspreston.com

APPENDIX 16-B ■ Pneumobelt

Manufactured by RESPIRONICS, INC.

Request for Information Form	Contact Information
Company Name	RESPIRONICS, INC.
Address	1001 MURRY RIDGE LN.
City, State, Zip	MURRYSVILLE, PA 15668
Country	US
FDA Owner/Operator Phone	724-387-5200
FDA Medical Specialty Code	PM—Physical Medicine
FDA Product Code	KTD
FDA Classification Name	ORTHOSIS, ABDOMINAL
FDA Device Classification Code	General Controls
FDA Regulation Number	890.3490
FDA Common Generic Name	EXSUFFLATION BELT
FDA Proprietary Device Name	PNEUMOBELT
FDA Owner/Operator Number	2518422
FDA Owner/Operator Name	RESPIRONICS, INC.
FDA Establishment Registration Number	2518422
FDA Registered Establishment Name	RESPIRONICS, INC.
FDA Operation Code(s)	MM—Manufacturer MR—Remanufacturer RR—Repackager/Relabeller
FDA Listing Date	09-21-00
FDA Listing Status Code	Active
Differentiation	N/A
Keywords	N/A
Description	N/A
Brochure	N/A
Product Web site	N/A

CHAPTER 17

Traumatic Brain Injury

Patricia A. Winkler, PT, DSc, NCS

anticipatory responses
knowledge of results
learning theory
motor control
motor learning
motor skill
plasticity
systems theory
traumatic head injury

OBJECTIVES

After reading this chapter the student/therapist will be able to:
1. Understand the application of current concepts in motor control and motor learning theories.
2. Understand the meaning of impairment, activity limitation (functional limitation/disability), and participation limitation (handicap) and their interrelationships.
3. Describe methods of examining, evaluating, and developing interventions for clients with brain injuries on the basis of task, impairment, and functional problem/disability analysis.
4. Describe outcomes for clients with traumatic brain injury.
5. Differentiate between development of basic movement patterns and motor skills.
6. Understand the role of synergy formation, synergy selection and modification, and anticipatory and feedback information as used in motor skills.
7. Describe the learning concepts of knowledge of results, whole and part-task practice.

The Brain Injury Association of America (BIAUSA) provides the following definition of traumatic head injury[1,2]:

Traumatic brain injury is an insult to the brain, not of a degenerative or congenital nature but caused by an external physical force, that may produce a diminished or altered state of consciousness, which results in an impairment of cognitive abilities or physical functioning. It can also result in the disturbance of behavioral or emotional functioning. These impairments may be either temporary or permanent and cause partial or total functional disability or psychosocial maladjustment.

OVERVIEW OF BRAIN INJURY

Epidemiology of Traumatic Brain Injury

One and a half million people sustain a traumatic brain injury (TBI) every year.[1] One million people with brain injuries are treated in emergency departments every year, 230,000 with injuries severe enough to require hospitalization. Fifty thousand people die yearly of TBI, 80,000 injuries result in disabilities, and 5.3 million people are living with permanent disabilities from TBI. Brain injury is the leading killer and disabler of children and young adults.[3] Motor vehicle crashes cause 50% of all TBIs, falls cause 21%, violence causes 12% (the majority from firearms), and sports and recreation account for 10%. Child abuse accounts for 64% of infant brain injuries. Fifty thousand children sustain bicycle-related brain injuries, and 400 of these die.[4] Two thirds of firearm-related TBIs are suicidal. Falls are the leading cause of TBI in people aged 65 years and older, with

11% proving fatal. The incidence of TBI is 24.7 per 100,000 population, with 35% of those hospitalized having long-term disability.[3]

Population of Brain-Injured Clients

The incidence of brain injuries is higher for the male population than for the female population by more than 2 : 1. Most of those injured are between 15 and 24 years old.[3]

Cost

The estimated lifetime cost for each severely brain-injured individual exceeds $4 million. Annual costs for all TBIs in the United States exceed $35 billion dollars.[1]

Mechanisms of Injury

External forces hitting the head hard enough to cause brain movement cause TBI. Injuries include those with skull fracture and those without skull fracture (closed head injuries). Direct blows to the head can cause coup injuries (at the site of impact) and countercoup injuries (distant from the site of impact). Penetrating objects cause direct cellular and vascular damage. Injuries to the face and neck can cause brain injury by damaging the blood supply to the brain.[5]

Pathophysiology of Injury

Acceleration, deceleration, rotational forces, and penetrating objects act to cause tissue laceration, compression, tension, shearing, or a combination, resulting in primary injury.

Primary Damage

Contusion, which is a bruise or bleeding on the brain, and lacerations can occur with or without skull fractures. Either an object hits the head, neck, or face, or the head hits an object. Damage can be to any area of the brain. Occipital blows are more likely to produce contusions than are frontal or lateral blows. Areas in which the cranial vault is irregular, such as on the anterior poles, undersurface of the temporal lobes, and undersurface of the frontal lobes, are commonly injured. Lacerations of blood vessels within the brain itself or of blood vessels that feed the brain from the neck or face can be injured and reduce the flow of blood carrying oxygen to the brain.

Contusions and lacerations can also injure the cranial nerves. The most commonly injured are the optic, vestibulocochlear, oculomotor, abducens, and facial nerves. Lacerations of dura or arachnoid space may cause cerebrospinal fluid to discharge from the nose (cerebrospinal fluid rhinorrhea discharge increases with neck flexion, coughing, or straining).[6]

Diffuse axonal injury, or shearing injuries, may be one of the most common types of primary lesions in patients with brain trauma.[7,8] Unequal acceleration, deceleration, or rotation of tissues that differ in structure causes diffuse axonal injury and changes in the chemical process. Severing of the axons may be severe enough to result in coma. In milder forms, more spotty lesions are seen, including deficits such as memory loss, concentration difficulties, decreased attention span, headaches, sleep disturbances, and seizures. Damage often involves the corpus callosum, basal ganglia, brain stem, and cerebellum.[6,8]

Penetrating objects with high velocities, such as bullets, can cause additional damage remote from the areas of impact as a result of shock waves. Foreign objects such as sticks and sharp toys cause low-velocity injuries, directly damaging the tissues they contact.

Secondary Damage

Secondary injuries are mainly due to a lack of oxygen in the high-oxygen-demanding brain. Secondary problems may result from the following:

1. *Increased intracranial pressure* (resulting from swelling or intracranial hematoma). Swelling of the brain causes distortion because the brain is held in the skull, a rigid, unyielding structure. The resultant increased intracranial pressure can lead to herniation of parts of the brain. The most often seen herniations include cingulate herniation under the falx cerebri, uncus herniation, central (or transtentorial) herniation, and herniation of the brain stem through the foramen magnum.[9] Acute hydrocephalus occurs when blood accumulates in the ventricular system, expanding the size of the ventricles and causing increased pressure on brain tissue being compressed between the skull and the fluid-filled ventricles. The increased pressure can then result in changes in PCO_2, which is also harmful to nervous tissue. Increased intracranial pressure has been correlated with poorer outcomes and higher mortality rates.[10]

2. *Cerebral hypoxia or ischemia* (occurring when blood vessels are ruptured or compressed). Hypoxia can occur from a lack of blood to the brain or from lack of oxygen in the blood as a result of airway obstruction or chest injuries.

3. *Intracranial hemorrhage,* causing hypoxia to tissues fed by the hemorrhaging blood vessels and adding pressure and distortion to brain tissue. Metabolic products from damaged cells and blood bathe the brain. Cell death occurs within minutes after injury from ischemia, edema, necrosis, and the toxic effects of blood on neural tissues.

4. *Electrolyte imbalance and acid-base imbalance.* Secondary cell death occurs either by swelling and then bursting of the cellular membrane (necrosis) or by destruction from within the cell through changes in the DNA (apoptosis). Cell death can occur days, weeks, or months after injury.[11]

5. *Infection from open wounds.* Infection in brain tissue may cause swelling and cell death.

6. *Seizures from pressure or scarring.* Seizures are most common immediately after injury and between 6 months and 2 years after injury. The seizures can cause additional brain damage owing to high oxygen and glucose requirements.

Physiological, Cognitive, and Behavioral Changes after Brain Injury

Autonomic Nervous System[12]

Box 17-1 lists possible autonomic nervous system symptoms resulting from brain injury.

Motor, Functional, Sensory, and Perceptual Changes

Motor abnormalities after severe head trauma are common. More severe head injuries tend to manifest more persistent physical problems.[6] In at least two studies[6,13] a fourth of the cases had no neurophysical sequelae. Changes in muscle tone may reflect the physiological effects of changes in the amount of tissue compression or irritation.[14]

Box 17-2 lists motor changes and provides symptoms of sensory and perceptive involvement.

Cognitive, Personality, and Behavioral Changes

Cognitive and behavioral sequelae can result from generalized or focal brain injuries. Memory impairments are an aftermath of generalized lesions. Emotional changes may be seen with lesions in the orbitofrontal areas. Behavior may

---

BOX 17-1 ■ AUTONOMIC NERVOUS SYSTEM SYMPTOMS RESULTING FROM BRAIN INJURY

- Changes in pulse and respiratory rates or regularity
- Temperature elevations
- Blood pressure changes
- Excessive sweating, salivation, tearing, and sebum secretion
- Dilated pupils
- Vomiting

BOX 17-2 ■ MOTOR, FUNCTIONAL, SENSORY, AND PERCEPTUAL CHANGES RESULTING FROM BRAIN INJURY

Motor changes may include any or all of the following:
- Paralysis or paresis such as monoplegia or hemiplegia.
- Cranial nerve injury resulting in paralysis of eye muscles, facial paralysis, vestibular and vestibulo-ocular reflex abnormalities, slurred speech (dysarthria), swallowing abnormalities (dysphagia), and paralysis of the tongue muscles.
- Poor coordination of movement.
- Abnormal reflexes, including appearance of early reflexes such as tonic neck reflexes.
- Abnormal muscle tone: flaccidity, spasticity, or rigidity. (The terms "decorticate rigidity" and "decerebrate rigidity" are often used to denote abnormal posturing. Decerebrate rigidity denotes extension in all four limbs. Decorticate posturing includes flexion of the upper extremities and extension of the legs.)
- Combinations of asymmetrical cerebellar and pyramidal

signs and of bilateral pyramidal and extrapyramidal signs have all been reported.[13]
- Loss of selective motor control.
- Poor balance.
- Loss of bowel or bladder control.

Sensory and perceptive involvement may include any or all of the following:
- Hypersensitivity to light or noise
- Loss of hearing or sight
- Visual field changes
- Numbness and tingling (peripheral nerves are often injured)
- Loss somatosensory functions
- Dizziness or vertigo
- Visuospatial abnormalities
- Agnosia
- Agraphia

BOX 17-3 ■ COGNITIVE, PERSONALITY, AND BEHAVIORAL CHANGES RESULTING FROM BRAIN INJURY

Cognitive changes might include any or all of the following:
- Temporary or permanent disorders of intellectual function
- Memory loss
- Shortened attention span
- Concentration problem
- Confusion
- Changes in motivation
- Difficulty sustaining attention
- Executive function loss (executive functions are those that affect how behavior is regulated). Lezak[15] outlined four functions:
  1. Choosing a goal
  2. Developing a plan
  3. Executing a plan
  4. Evaluating the execution of the plan

- Reduced problem-solving skills
- Lack of initiative
- Loss of reasoning
- Poor abstract thinking
- Shortened attention span

Behavioral changes could include the following:
- Lability
- Uncontrolled anger
- Irritability
- Euphoria
- Intolerance
- Inappropriate sexual behavior
- Perseveration (repetition of movements or sounds)
- Impulsiveness
- Hyperactivity

---

be excessive and disinhibited. Septal area lesions result in rage and overall irritability. Pseudobulbar injuries can result in emotional lability of involuntary laughing or crying not associated with feelings of emotions. Behavioral changes can be present even without cognitive and physical deficits. Although actual psychoses can be sequelae, they appear to be neither common nor definitively related to the brain injury. The social consequences of inappropriate behavior can be disastrous and a stumbling block to achieving therapy goals. A correlation between preinjury personality and postinjury changes has not been established.[6] It does seem reasonable, however, that factors within an individual's psychological makeup may affect reaction to the injury. Head trauma frequently happens to adolescents—an age group

fraught with its own problems that may be aggravated by the injury. Box 17-3[15] lists both cognitive and behavioral changes resulting from brain injury.

Changes in Consciousness and Coma

Coma and changes in consciousness result from conditions in which there are diffusely extensive and bilateral cerebral hemispheric depression of function, direct depression or destruction of the brain stem–activating system that is responsible for consciousness or a combination of the two. In moderate or severe head injury, unconsciousness can be prolonged.

Plum and Posners' definitions[14] of various stages of acutely altered consciousness are briefly presented, intermingled with some insights from the descriptions offered by Gilroy and Meyer.[9] Plum and Posner[14] do not equate the presence or absence of motor responses with the depth of coma. These authors point out that the neural structures regulating consciousness differ from and are more anatomically distant from those regulating motor function.

Concussion. In mild concussion, the loss of consciousness may not occur or lasts a relatively short time (20 minutes or less) and there is little or no retrograde amnesia. A concussion can cause diffuse axonal injury and result in either temporary or permanent damage. The client may be irritable or distractible and have difficulty with reading and memory. There may be complaints of headache, fatigue, dizziness, and changes in personality and emotional disposition. This group of symptoms constitutes what is called posttraumatic syndrome. The effects of repeated concussions (second impact syndrome) are cumulative.[1,16]

Coma. Coma is defined as a complete paralysis of cerebral function; a state of unresponsiveness. The eyes are closed, and there is no response to painful stimuli. Within 2 to 4 weeks, nearly all clients in coma begin to awaken. Oculomotor and pupillary signs are valuable in assisting with the diagnosis, localizing brain stem damage, and determining the depth of coma.[14] In coma, brain stem responses may include grimacing to pain, which is frequently associated with a flexor or localizing motor response, loss of hearing or balance, abnormal palate and tongue movements, and loss or distortion of taste.

Stupor. Stupor is a condition of general unresponsiveness. However, the client, who is usually mute, can be temporarily aroused by vigorous and repeated stimuli.

Obtundity. Obtundity describes the condition of a client who sleeps a great deal and who, when aroused, exhibits reduced alertness, disinterest in the environment, and slow responses to stimulation.

Delirium. Delirium is often observed in recovery from unconsciousness after severe brain injury. Disorientation, fear, and misinterpretation of sensory stimuli characterize this state. The client is frequently loud, agitated, and offensive. *Clouding of consciousness* is a state of quiet confusion, distractibility, faulty memory, and slowed responses to stimuli.

Finally, no discussion of changes in consciousness would be complete without mention of those unfortunate enough to remain in a "persistent vegetative state." This state is characterized by a wakeful, reduced responsiveness with no evident cerebral cortical function. The vegetative state can result from diffuse cerebral hypoxia or from severe, diffuse white matter impact damage. The brain stem is usually relatively intact. Clients may track with their eyes and show minimal spontaneous motor activities that even appear purposeful, but they do not speak, nor do they respond to verbal stimulation.[17] Life expectancy can be weeks, months, or years.[18,19] Brain-injured clients who remain vegetative for 3 months rarely achieve an independent outcome. However, the term "persistent" should not be added to "vegetative state" until the injury has stabilized or the state has lasted for approximately 1 year.[20]

Recovery of consciousness, if it occurs, includes a gradual return of orientation and recent memory.[14] The duration of each of these stages is variable and can be prolonged. Improvement can stop at any point.

Two types of amnesia are frequently associated with brain injury: retrograde and posttraumatic.[21] Cartlidge and Shaw[12] define retrograde amnesia as a "partial or total loss of the ability to recall events that have occurred during the period immediately preceding brain injury." The duration of the retrograde amnesia may progressively decrease.

Posttraumatic amnesia is defined "as the time lapse between the accident and the point at which the functions concerned with memory are judged to have been restored."[12] The duration of posttraumatic amnesia is considered a clinical indicator of the severity of the injury.[12] An additional deficit can be the inability to form new memory, referred to as anterograde memory. The capacity for anterograde memory is frequently the last function to return after recovery from loss of consciousness.[22]

The client's inability to develop continuing short-term memory can be quite frustrating for the rehabilitation team as well as for the client because memory is an important component of learning.[23] There are two types of memory: declarative and procedural. Memory in which the client can recall facts and events of a previous experience is called declarative memory. Explicit learning, a conscious verbal learning, is based on declarative memory. However, many clients who cannot reproduce memories through conscious recollection do have the ability to learn new motor skills.

Implicit learning, a noncognitive type of learning in which clients can show changes in performance after prior experience, is based on procedural memory. Clients can show the ability to change motor, perceptual, or cognitive behaviors with practice or training but may lack declarative memory. That procedural memory may be present without declarative memory in clients with TBI has been demonstrated in several studies.[21]

Locked-In Syndrome. Locked-in syndrome occurs rarely and can be confused with coma. The client cannot move any part of the body except the eyes but is able to think and is conscious.[24]

Communication Disorders. Communication disorders include expressive and receptive language aphasia and dysarthria.

Other Complications. A list of the complications that may accompany brain injury would be limitless. In addition to any concomitant injuries, some of the diagnostic, monitoring, and therapeutic procedures themselves carry hazards. So does prolonged bed rest. Catheters, nasogastric tubes, and tracheotomies can cause iatrogenic injuries. Infections, contractures, skin breakdown, thrombophlebitis, pulmonary problems, heterotropic ossification, and surgical complications are but a few of the risks. Posttraumatic epilepsy is also a possible sequelae. See Box 17-4 for additional information.

Depression occurs frequently after brain injury, and it can alter functional outcome. It appears that a combination of neuroanatomical, neurochemical, and psychosocial

BOX 17-4 ■ **FACTORS THAT CAN INFLUENCE MANAGEMENT AND RECOVERY AFTER A TRAUMATIC BRAIN INJURY**

PREINJURY CHARACTERISTICS

A. Cognitive factors
  1. Intelligence*
  2. Memory
  3. Level of education
B. Behavioral factors
  1. Personality*
  2. Psychological status
C. Social factors
  1. Vocational skills
  2. Avocational skills
  3. Interpersonal skills
  4. Family/friends support systems
D. Physical factors
  1. Age*
  2. General health and physical fitness
  3. Existing physical deficits
  4. Morphology
  5. Level of **motor skill** development and capacity for motor learning

POSTINJURY CHARACTERISTICS

A. Static factors
  1. Trauma factors (neurological)
    a. Location(s) and extent of injury
    b. Cause and type of injury*
    c. Immediacy of injury*
  2. Cognitive factors
    a. Ultimate duration of retrograde amnesia*
    b. Ultimate duration of posttraumatic amnesia*
  3. Physical factors: extracranial injuries
B. Dynamic factors
  1. Trauma factors (neurological)
    a. Depth and duration of coma*
    b. Secondary brain damage
    c. Brain stem reflexes
    d. Special investigations (radiological and laboratory tests)
  2. Cognitive factors
    a. Rate of recovery of intellectual and memory functions*
    b. Quality of recovery of intellectual and memory functions*
    c. Communication disorders
  3. Behavioral factors
    a. Primary personality changes*
    b. Secondary personality changes*
    c. Psychological status
  4. Social factors
    a. Opportunity to reenter occupation/school
    b. Avocational reintegration abilities
    c. Reaction to family/friends
    d. Family adjustment and support capabilities*
  5. Physical factors
    a. Pattern and quality of sensorimotor recovery*
    b. Rate of recovery of sensorimotor function*
    c. Range of motion and muscle flexibility
    d. Cranial nerve deficits
    e. Concomitant disabilities
  6. Environmental factors
    a. Staff/facilities/equipment available
    b. Attitude of health care providers
    c. Expertise of health care providers
    d. Room/housing and treatment settings

*Discussed in the text.

factors are responsible for the onset and maintenance of the depression.[25]

Acute Care

The selection of tests depends on the availability of the special equipment required for testing, the reliability and validity of the tests, and on the perceived need for the tests. The results of some of these procedures may secondarily aid the therapist in the selection of intervention strategies. Conversely, other monitoring procedures may restrict the choice of therapeutic approaches.

Initially, a Glasgow Coma Scale[26] (GCS) (Box 17-5) is performed to test the function of the brain stem and the cerebrum through eye, motor, and verbal responses. It provides a measure of the level of consciousness. Scores range from 3 to 15, with lower scores associated with lower levels of function. Scores from 13 to 15 indicate a mild brain injury, 9 to 12 a moderate brain injury, and 8 or less a severe injury. According to the Brain Injury Association of America,[1] a mild injury is defined as a change in the mental status at the time of injury. The person is dazed, confused, or loses con-

sciousness. The change in mental status indicates that the person's brain functioning has been altered. With a moderate traumatic brain injury, the client experiences a loss of consciousness that lasts from a few minutes to a few hours, confusion lasts from days to weeks, and physical, cognitive, or behavioral impairments last for months or are permanent. A severe brain injury occurs when a prolonged unconscious state or coma lasts days, weeks, or months. The GCS is related to lesion size,[27] but lesion location is not a significant predictor of Glasgow Outcome Scale (GOS) scores (Box 17-6).

With the possible exception of the diagnosis and, hence, prognosis of diffuse white matter impact damage,[28] one third of clients hospitalized with brain injuries have extracranial injuries,[6] which are explored with a physical examination and appropriate special tests.

Additional testing depends on the client's particular dysfunctions. Computed tomography,[29] magnetic resonance imaging (MRI), positron emission tomography, radioisotope imaging, ventriculography, echoencephalography, electroencephalography, monitoring of intracranial pressure,

BOX 17-5 ■ GLASGOW COMA SCALE

EYE OPENING	E
Spontaneous	4
To speech	3
To pain	2
Nil	1

BEST MOTOR RESPONSE	M
Obeys	6
Localizes	5
Withdraws	4
Abnormal flexion	3
Extensor response	2
Nil	1

VERBAL RESPONSE	V
Oriented	5
Confused conversation	4
Inappropriate words	3
Incomprehensible sounds	2
Nil	1

COMA SCORE (E + M + V) = 3 TO 15

From Jennett B, Teasdale G: *Management of head injuries,* Philadelphia, 1981, FA Davis.

BOX 17-6 ■ GLASGOW OUTCOME SCALE

VEGETATIVE STATE
A persistent state characterized by reduced responsiveness associated with wakefulness. The client may exhibit eye opening, sucking, yawning, and localized motor responses.

SEVERE DISABILITY
An outcome characterized by consciousness, but the client has 24-hour dependence because of cognitive, behavioral, or physical disabilities, including dysarthria and dysphasia.

MODERATE DISABILITY
An outcome characterized by independence in activities of daily living and in home and community activities but with disability. Clients in this category may have memory or personality changes, hemiparesis, dysphagia, ataxia, acquired epilepsy, or major cranial nerve deficits.

GOOD RECOVERY
Client able to reintegrate into normal social life and able to return to work. There may be mild persisting sequelae.

Modified from Jennett B, Bond M: Assessment of outcome after severe brain damage: a practical scale, *Lancet* 1:480, 1975.

measurement of cerebral blood flow and metabolism, monitoring of cardiorespiratory and cardiovascular function, and cerebrospinal fluid and other biochemical studies all provide important information. Changes in electrocerebral potentials that occur in response to specific stimuli also are studied. Visual, auditory, and somatosensory evoked potential examinations are used with brain-injured clients but are more effective when combined with other examinations.[30] These examinations make it possible to observe the presence, evolution, and resolution of a lesion.[6]

Reflex motor responses in unconscious clients are tested by applying a noxious stimulus, such as pressure on a nail bed with a pencil or supraorbital pressure, and observing the response. Most responses generally fall into three categories: appropriate, inappropriate, or absent.[14]

Testing for cognitive and behavioral functions is usually done by neuropsychological tests. In some circumstances Intelligence Quotient tests, achievement tests, and Armed Forces tests may be available for comparison. Differentiating changes in cognitive and behavioral functions caused by brain injury from posttraumatic stress syndrome, conversion or hysterical reactions, malingering, depression, and anxiety is extremely important.

On the client's admission to the hospital, a neurosurgeon usually assumes initial and primary responsibility for the client. The first priority in medical care is resuscitation, after which baseline assessments are made and a history is obtained. Immediate surgery may or may not be indicated. Surgery is indicated in cases where blood and necrotic tissue are present in the cranial vault.

Early concerns may include the management of respiratory dysfunction, cardiovascular monitoring, treatment of raised intracranial pressure by means of pharmacological, mechanical, or surgical procedures,[12] and general medical care. Examples of general medical care are familiar: maintenance of fluid and electrolyte balance, nutrition, eye and skin care, prevention of contractures, postural drainage, and safety considerations.[6] The need for this type of care gradually lessens as the client responds, or it may continue if unconsciousness persists.

Pharmacological Interventions
Fulop et al[31] reviewed pharmacological interventions after brain injury. Their article separates the medications by symptoms to be treated as follows:

1. *Drugs that decrease intracranial pressure (ICP).* When ICP increases, changes in PCO_2 are seen. The maintenance of a PCO_2 between 30 and 40 mm Hg appears most appropriate. Osmotic agents such as mannitol are used to pull fluid from brain tissue back into the blood system, thus lowering ICP.

Intracranial pressure has, in the past, been lowered by intentional hyperventilation, which causes an increase in blood PCO_2 resulting in vasoconstriction of the central vessels and reduced cerebral blood flow. However, Muizelaar et al[32] as well as information from the traumatic coma data band[33] showed that dramatically reducing a client's PCO_2 in this manner resulted in a worse outcome than that in clients managed with medication. Therefore, hyperventilation is currently used only for nonresponsive cases and for short durations. Glucocorticoids have been used to treat cerebral edema (dexamethasone [Decadron], methylprednisolone [Solu-Medrol]), but most studies show no long-term changes in outcome.[34] Finally, barbiturates have been used to lower intracranial pressure, but they carry a high mortality rate.[11] See Chapter 36 for additional information.

2. *Drugs that control blood pressure.* Blood pressure control is important in brain-injured clients. In a study of

717 clients with TBI, systolic blood pressure below 90 mm Hg during resuscitation was a predictor of poor outcome.[11] Cerebral perfusion pressure[35] or adequate blood pressure to maintain cerebral blood flow against increased intracranial pressure is calculated by subtracting the ICP from the mean arterial pressure. If fluid management cannot keep the blood pressures elevated, then vasopressor drugs such as phenylephrine (Neo-Synephrine) are used to constrict peripheral vessels but not the vessels of the brain.

The brain produces neurotrophic agents[36] such as nerve growth factor in response to damage. These neurotrophins are thought to prevent neuronal death[36] and are being added to TBI regimens in a few cases. Substances that affect glial cell function are also being investigated. Endogenous glycolipid ganglioside has improved function in rats but has not been successful in humans.

3. *Drugs that affect the motor, behavioral, and cognitive functions* (see Chapter 36). Medications also may be prescribed for motor abnormalities involving increases in tone. Baclofen is now used more frequently with brain-injured clients; however, baclofen also can produce lethargy, confusion,[37] and reduction in attention span[38] in some clients. These effects are greatly reduced with implantation of a pump to deliver the drug. Dantrolene sodium is another medication used to decrease spasticity and rigidity. This drug works directly at the muscle level and therefore is less likely to cause cognitive disturbances but more likely to cause generalized weakness.[39] Botulinum toxin type A (Botox) is widely used to inject into specific muscles, such as the finger flexors, biceps, or gastrocnemius, to decrease that muscle's tone. Diazepam (Valium) initially was the drug most commonly administered for spasticity or high tone. However, diazepam also promotes drowsiness and decreased responsiveness and can increase muscle weakness and ataxia.[37] These side effects actually hinder rather than assist in rehabilitation. Glenn and Wrobewski[38] conclude that "rarely, if ever, are the benefits of diazepam's antispasticity effect great enough to justify its use in the brain-injured population."

Drugs to treat behavioral or cognitive dysfunction have not been particularly successful. Antidepressive drugs as well as carbamazepine (Tegretol) and propranolol (Inderal) have been used to treat aggression and agitation. Carbamazepine appears to reduce agitation or aggression in brain-injured clients.[40]

Sedative drugs prescribed in an attempt to control delirium may add to the client's confusion[6] and may also contribute to a decreased responsiveness. Later in the rehabilitative process, various antidepressants may be used to treat aggressive and disruptive behaviors. These, too, may have deleterious side effects. Antidepressants other than the tricyclics are apparently the most effective for treating depression.

Traumatically acquired neuroendocrine dysfunctions, such as hyperphagia and thermal regulation, also may be treated with pharmacological agents.[41]

Severe, intractable pain may be present in clients who have had injury to the thalamus. In these cases, some of the antiseizure drugs appear to be more effective, including phenytoin (Dilantin) and gabapentin (Neurontin). Late seizure control is usually through valproic acid (Depakote or Depakene).

For a variety of reasons, other pharmaceutical agents are prescribed as an adjunct to care. Antibiotics may be used with respiratory complications or with compound fractures.

Prognostic Indicators

Numerous problems are encountered in trying to predict outcome. Included among these problems are the validity and reliability of the tests used, the uniform implementation and interpretation of predictive factors, the percentage of error in prediction, the possible effects of intervention strategies and bias in treatment on the basis of predictions, and, finally, the definition of what constitutes a "successful" outcome. Understanding these problems is imperative because the therapist can provide persuasive suggestions as to the type and intensity of rehabilitative care after injury. The differences in operational definitions, types and sizes of populations, and length of time after injury when the outcome assessment was made contribute to the lack of consistency in studies of predictive factors for clients with brain injury. For example, several authors have found that clients younger than age 20 years usually recover better[42-44]; however, this has not been uniformly confirmed. A caution in using tests for prediction is the percentage of error in prediction. If prediction is 80% or even 90% accurate, there are still 10% to 20% of the clients with head trauma whose outcome may be predicted incorrectly.[45]

Lesion Size and Area

There is conflicting evidence regarding recovery outcomes on the basis of lesion size and area because the type of lesion and the rapidity with which lesions occur have an impact on both the deficits and the size. There is some evidence that lesion area rather than size is important. Van der Naalt et al[46,47] looked at 67 patients with brain injuries in the mild to moderate injury categories and found that frontal and frontotemporal lesions were predictive of poorer outcomes than other areas. However, Kurth et al[48] looked at number of acute hemorrhages, lesion volume, and location in traumatic brain injury using neuropsychological outcome measures and found no relationship between the numbers of hemorrhages and the volume of injury. Brain MRI in 80 adult patients (6 to 8 weeks after injury) was predictive of nonrecovery from persistent vegetative states at 12 months when the client had corpus callosum and dorsolateral brain stem lesions.[49]

Time since Lesion

Better functional outcomes were found in monkeys when rehabilitation occurred earlier after the lesion. Black et al[50] created lesions in motor cortex of 27 adolescent rhesus monkeys and then trained them on motor tasks involving the arm. Active postoperative training of the weak hand led to recovery of 82% of the preoperative function in 6 months if the therapy was initiated immediately. Recovery was only 67% of preoperative control if training was delayed 4 months.

Age

Age was an important factor in recovery. Beginning at age 40 years, older patients had significantly longer post-traumatic amnesia and worse functional outcome at any severity.[51]

Posttraumatic Amnesia

Posttraumatic amnesia (a neurophysiological process) duration was better related to outcome than either lesion area or size.[51] Postinjury amnesia had a predictable relationship to length of coma in patients with diffuse axonal injury. Duration of posttraumatic amnesia was strongly correlated with the GOS score at 6 and 12 months after injury in patients with diffuse axonal injury but poorly correlated in patients with primarily focal brain injury. Van der Naalt et al's[46] study of the GCS indicates that this scale, 12 months after injury, is a simple and consistent predictor of outcomes in clients with a score between 9 and 14 (mild to moderate brain injury).

Finally, several studies have reported that absence of substance abuse, absence of previous TBI,[35] a higher level of educational achievement, and stable work history also are positive preinjury variables for a better prognosis.[52] The Wechsler Adult Intelligence Scale (WAIS)-Revised intelligence quotient test may correlate with prognosis according to other studies.[52]

Motor disturbances resulting from brain injury generally have a good prognosis.[12] Of the physical deficits encountered, dysfunctions in the cerebral hemispheres and of the cranial nerves are the most common disorders, and these may partially resolve. Losses of these functions can be more permanent,[9,12] especially without skilled rehabilitation interventions. Complete recovery is rare except that with hearing, vestibular function, and smell.

In one Glasgow study, some degree of hemiparesis was present 6 months after injury in 49% of the 150 clients who regained consciousness after severe brain injury.[6]

Absence of brain stem reflexes usually indicates a poorer prognosis, but this is not necessarily a predictor of ultimate outcome.[12] Interpretation can be difficult, partially because of the variety of influences on these signs.[6]

Psychosocial outcomes vary after severe brain injury.[53] Psychosocial variables that significantly increased life satisfaction for persons with TBI were total family satisfaction, being employed, being married, having memory, bowel independence, and not blaming oneself for the injury. Those who do not blame themselves show a greater number of functional activities as indicators for their self-satisfaction.[54]

CONCEPTUAL FRAMEWORK FOR THERAPEUTIC INTERVENTION

Motor Control Theory

Motor control and learning theories try to explain how the central nervous system (CNS) accomplishes the miracle of coordinated, meaningful movement. Motor control theory and factors affecting effectiveness and speed of motor learning are reviewed in this section and are discussed in detail in Chapters 3 and 9. This chapter's examination, evaluation, and intervention techniques sections are based on that framework. A quick review of basic principles follows.

Synergistic Organization

Synergies, or motor patterns, were seen by Bernstein[55] as the basis of movement. The need for the brain to use synergistic organization comes from the infinite number of movement combinations that are available. By use of synergies, which decrease the number of degrees of freedom, speed and efficiency are added while flexibility of response is maintained. Force (amplitude) of contraction, velocity, and timing can still be changed to meet task demands.

Research suggests that synergies are shaped through experience and that they develop before birth (innate) and after birth (learned). Early experiments on motor learning demonstrate how synergies may develop. Payton and Kelley[56] showed that, with practice of a novel motor task, movements become more organized. In learning a new skill, movement begins with a "gross approximation" of the movement that includes agonist/antagonist cocontraction. As movement is refined, reciprocal movement replaces cocontraction.[57] In electrophysiological studies of skill acquisition, less electrical activity is seen on electromyography (EMG) and less time to peak activation of the muscle is noted in motor tasks after they are better learned. Additionally, fewer muscles are recruited for the same movement.[58] Positron emission tomographic scans have confirmed these EMG findings, demonstrating decreasing areas of brain activity after skill acquisition.

Neuronal changes brought about through long-term potentiation and long-term depression are a basis for learning new tasks and developing synergies and behavioral changes.[59] As neurons are repetitively fired at the same time, networks develop. These neuronetworks, or cell assemblies, are formed with increasing complexity and self-organization. The more they are used, the stronger and more permanent are the changes that occur. Finally, a specific stimulus now provokes a learned or skilled response as an organized synergy. The output of the networks is not a summation of individual functions but has "emergent properties" that are more than the sum of the output of individual neurons.

The best understood synergies are the balance and reaching patterns. Both appear to be basic innate synergies. Quiet standing in humans is maintained by somatosensory, visual, and vestibular inputs. It requires the coordination of many muscles, especially those of the hips, knees, and ankles, to maintain the body's center of gravity over its base of support. This complex coordination of muscle control is accomplished by sequences of stereotyped patterns mediated through the brain stem, cerebellum, and spinal cord. Somatosensory input during body sway stimulates the response in which posture is stabilized by small changes in the angle between the foot and the leg. For example, when length, force of contraction, or movement velocity of the calf muscles exceeds a preset threshold, somatosensory signals to the brain initiate rapid postural readjustments by triggering a synergistic response to decrease sway. For small center of gravity movements, these synergies are sequenced in a distal to proximal manner. The direction of sway determines the particular synergy elicited to correct for the shift in the center of gravity. In forward losses of balance, the posterior extensor muscles of the legs and trunk respond at about 100 milliseconds. In backward losses, the anterior muscles respond, including the anterior tibialis, hip flexors, and abdominals. The timing between muscle contractions and the proximal-to-distal sequence are preset. The amplitude of contraction varies with the environmental demands and the amount and velocity of sway. In greater losses of balance, a different synergy is used in which the person may bend at the hips and knees. If the balance loss is great enough, the person takes a step to maintain upright balance.[60] (For additional information, see Chapter 23 on balance and vestibular dysfunction.)

In gait, weight shifts from one leg to the other and stability after the weight shift are other aspects of dynamic balance performed through synergies. The movement pattern of the swing leg in gait is limited in the number of degrees of freedom at each joint and the sequence of movement by synergies. There is also a specific coordination and timing of swing leg movement in relation to the stance leg movement (interlimb timing and coordination).

In walking, the sequence of contraction of the leg muscle from ankle to hip, the time of onset of the contraction of each muscle, and a ratio of force for each muscle are all preset in the motor control program of the brain or spinal cord. If an increase in speed is needed, force can be increased within the synergy, but the basic synergies, or motor patterns, are what give identity to a gait pattern. Whether the person is walking quickly or slowly, there is an individually recognizable pattern.

In the reaching and grasping pattern, three components have been identified: the reaching portion (transport), the grasping or prehension portion, and the maintenance of balance. The reaching and maintenance of balance are accomplished through synergies.[61,62] The target determines the reaching pattern. Characteristics of the reaching synergy include a distal-to-proximal sequence of firing, and movement is in a straight line and has a bell-shaped velocity curve.[63] The prehension portion of reach and grasp is not a synergistic movement and the motor-sensory cortex helps with force production and selection of muscles[64] during hand movement to meet task demands. This may be why more severe deficits are seen in the hand after cortical injury.

Anticipatory and Adaptive Responses

To meet the motor task (external) requirements, synergies are used and modified through a feed-forward and feedback system of control. The brain adapts synergies to environmental constraints, such as obstacles, by modifying the basic synergies' velocity, intensity, or duration of contractions before the movement even begins.

Feed-forward, or anticipatory response (often from vision and past memory of successful movements) is the first muscle contraction that occurs during a movement. For example, before a forward reach, the gastrocnemius muscles will fire to reduce the amount of forward movement that would occur with the forward change in the center of gravity caused by the forward movement of the arm.[65]

For adaptive responses, sensory feedback (visual or proprioceptive are most commonly used) is used to check the effectiveness of the response and modify it, if needed. A final check is made to determine that the motor pattern matched the original "planned" pattern after movement occurred. These adaptive responses allow modification for environmental changes.

Sensory information helps fine tune the subsequent movements within a synergistic movement. For walking, the visual array moves in the peripheral visual field, the joints and muscles move, and the semicircular canals' hair cells fire. These sensory impulses drive motor system adaptations to the environment. In the reaching-prehension pattern, the target location is coded by the visual system. Both the spatial and temporal conditions for reach are present before the

movement begins. Once the hand is at the target, the hand has already been shaped for prehension. Initially, grip is determined by the visual system (anticipatory response) and past memory (learning) of the characteristics of the object to be picked up. Tactile input from the finger tips (feedback) is then used to make adjustments in grip force if the initial grip was not effective.[66] Once movement occurs, there is a final comparison of the original planned pattern with the executed pattern to see whether they match.

Dynamic Pattern Theory and New Patterns

Once called motor control theory, the dynamic pattern theory[67,68] addresses problems when motor behavior changes and also uses concepts of basic patterns of movement. This theory states that certain patterns are stable or unstable and that transition between patterns or to a new pattern depends on pattern stability. (See Giuliani[69] for a summary of this theory.)

The challenge for therapists is to identify what makes these "stuck" behaviors become unstable and perhaps amenable to change. Patterns that are "set" are much more difficult to change than those that are more variable. In fact, phase transitions between old and new patterns are noted by periods of increased variability. The client appears to vacillate between the old and the new behaviors during transition phases and before new behavior establishment points. Repetition is important to develop more consistent motor patterns and new establishment points.

Motor Learning

Byl[70] noted that motor cortex (M1) changes occurred (motor learning) when (1) new or novel tasks were used, (2) when movements were practiced together (spatial organization and temporally organized), (3) when movements were frequently repeated, and (4) when movements were important to the individual.

Three stages have been identified for motor learning: the cognitive stage during which the performer begins to understand the task, the associative stage where performances is refined, and the autonomous stage where the task performance is skilled. Many things affect motor learning (see Chapters 3 and 9), among which are knowledge of results and type of practice.

Interventions are designed to produce a task-oriented behavioral change that becomes permanent without continued therapist help or intervention. When this does not happen, the client performs well during therapy but does not seem to carry the improved performance outside the clinic. This difference between performance and learning is discussed by Schmidt[71,72] (see Chapters 3 and 9).

Knowledge of Results

Information on how successful the movement was in meeting the task goal is also basic to learning. Knowledge of results consists of extrinsic information over and above that provided by the task itself.[73] During the practice portion of most tasks, increasing any type of feedback appears to improve task performance.[74] But long-term learning may occur better when knowledge of results is provided less often. The relative frequency with which knowledge of results is provided in relation to the number of trials is important in learning. Bandwidth knowledge of results, in which information is given about trials falling outside a certain range, and a random schedule of feedback appear to be effective for many learning situations in therapy. Delaying knowledge of results also improves learning.[73]

Practice Type

The type of practice is important for clients who are learning new skills. A commonly used technique to simplify a task by practicing at a slower speed or practicing a part of a motor task is often not effective. For example, weight shifting is often practiced as a component of gait before walking is initiated. Winstein et al[75] demonstrated that this part-practice did not transfer to gait in a group of clients with stroke. In a study by Man et al,[76] a complex task was broken down into adaptive training methods (e.g., slower motions) and part-task training (on components of the task). Subjects who practiced the whole task had better performance than either of the other groups. A finding that practicing small components of a task does not make one better at the whole task is not too surprising. Many of us can jump, have good shoulder power, and can throw overhead but cannot, without practice, put this together to play basketball. A minimum basic amount of strength, range of motion (ROM), and inter-limb sequencing is necessary to play basketball but is not adequate to play without the actual practice of the sport.

Practicing other than the whole task may be possible. By use of the same task as that used by Man et al,[76] Newell et al[77] showed that part-task training was effective when it was conducted in natural subtasks of the whole. These subtasks are part of the whole task but are distinguished by changes in speed or direction. This area of skill acquisition has not been studied adequately to identify subtasks of most common movements.

Many therapy techniques that improve a client's performance inhibit learning because they are based on the external controls and support provided by the therapist's manipulations markedly changing the basic task. The type of feedback and the method in which it is provided are critical to learning new motor skills. For example, when the hip stabilization component of walking is externally provided by the therapist during gait training, the client has no need to develop his or her own hip stabilization patterns, and feedback lacks a basic component of gait.

To review, the conceptual framework for the evaluation and intervention of clients with TBI is based on distributed motor control theory, which states that movement is task- or goal-oriented and a result of combined systems working together to produce synergistic movement. Synergistic movement has an anticipatory component that is matched with sensory feedback and previous experience to contribute to task refinement through adaptation. Changes in motor behavior may be determined by how "set" patterns (dynamic pattern theory) are influenced by the type of practice, knowledge of the effectiveness of the results, and how the motor skills are broken down for practice.

EXAMINATION, EVALUATION, PROGNOSIS, DIAGNOSIS, AND INTERVENTION
Structure for Client Management

The American Physical Therapy Association has published levels of client management leading to optimal outcomes.[78]

The Association's *Guide to Physical Therapy Practice,* which uses examination, evaluation, diagnosis, prognosis, intervention, and outcomes as its basis, will be followed in this chapter. Although this is the terminology used by physical therapists, its application and integration into the profession of occupational therapy should be simultaneously acknowledged.

Examination should lead to an understanding of the underlying causes of the activity limitations or disabilities and should be the basis of the interventions program. Starting the examination at the functional level might be most useful. Once functional (activity) limitations are determined, a task analysis can be completed by having the client demonstrate the functional skill, such as walking. Tests and measures will be chosen on the basis of the therapist's knowledge of their importance in the task being performed. For example, a client might have elbow extension lacking 20 degrees, but this might not be critical in the task of feeding himself. The tests and measures should be reliable and valid and chosen on the basis of the hypothesis that the therapist generates from the task analysis. Tests and measures should cover all levels of dysfunction from impairment through participation limitation (handicap) because they establish a baseline by which to judge future improvement or lack thereof. This baseline should be quantified to permit measurement of the effectiveness of the intervention strategies. For the *components of examination,* see Box 17-7.

Evaluation identifies the problems that can be managed by the therapist and serves to "tease" out those factors that influence or restrict the choice of therapeutic approaches. Evaluation provides a qualitative means of determining reasons why a problem is present. It includes considerations of testing, motivation, and psychosocial areas. The evaluation thus determines intervention and goals. The purpose of the evaluation is to determine what prevents the client from performing in a functional, acceptable manner as identified by the client, the therapist, and society.

Diagnosis examines the various possible causes of the problem to determine which are most critical. The therapist has a multilevel task that includes (1) identification of the components that compose a complex task or activity; (2) evaluation of the degree to which a component's deficit contributes to impairment, activity limitation (functional limitation or disability), or participation limitation (handicap); and (3) evaluation of the ability of the client to recover the necessary improvement in a component or the need to provide substitutions.

Prognosis is used to determine the optimal level of improvement that may be attained. Prognosis includes short- and long-term goals.

The interventions are provided by skilled professionals to treat the impairments, functional problems, and participation limitations to achieve optimal outcomes.

An example of examination, evaluation, and diagnosis and prognosis would be as follows: A client comes to your clinic reporting that he falls several times a week and would like to improve his balance. The task analysis shows that he drags his toe in the initial swing phase of gait and that he has multiple deviations during straight and level walking. Examination reveals decreased strength in the anterior tibialis and gastrocnemius muscles (2+/5), decreased

BOX 17-7 ■ COMPONENTS OF EXAMINATION

I. History: injury, job, home environment, educational level, previous injuries, etc.
II. Client/family data: client and family goals, personal factors, socioeconomic factors relating to handicaps
III. Other health care team member assessments
IV. Tests and measurements
  A. Systems review
    1. Circulatory/respiratory
    2. Integumentary
    3. Musculoskeletal
    4. Nervous system
      a. Sensory
        (1) Primary
        (2) Integrated/perceptual
      b. Motor
        (1) Simple impairments
          ■ Tone
          ■ Muscle strength
          ■ Muscle flexibility
          ■ Response speed
          ■ Movement speed
          ■ Endurance and fatigue
        (2) Complex impairments
          ■ Basic synergies
          ■ Modification of synergies
          ■ Anticipatory reactions
          ■ Use of feedback
          ■ Variability of performance
        (3) Disabilities
      c. Vision
      d. Vestibular
    5. Autonomic nervous system-bowel, bladder
    6. Cognitive
    7. Language
    8. Emotional

dorsiflexion ROM (−10 degrees of dorsiflexion), increased tone (Ashworth 3) in the gastrocnemius/soleus, and use of the hip strategy for balance recovery regardless of conditions or amount of perturbation. He falls in tandem stance with his eyes closed. Evaluation conclusions might include (1) the hip flexion contracture and ankle strength together prevent the client from using normal ankle strategies and cause toe drag and (2) the client is not using proprioceptive or vestibular cues for balance recovery, resulting in balance losses and falling. Additional testing, specifically with force platform and sensory testing of the lower extremities, is recommended. This evaluation/diagnosis is based on being able to perform a (1) task analysis of balance and gait (i.e., knowing the components that make up balance), (2) knowing how to assess each of the components that would contribute to the task (i.e., what sensory systems contribute to balance and gait, what muscles contribute to balance reactions and gait), and (3) what tests and measures are reliable and valid to assess the components of balance and gait. Intervention of performing exercises to achieve ankle strengthening to the 4/5 manual muscle test level

might be in the intervention plan. Intervention would also include increasing the use of proprioceptive and vestibular information during balance and gait. The prognosis would be for a significant improvement in balance because strength and ROM, and proprioceptive and vestibular dysfunctions, are highly amenable to change and the client is motivated to improve. Outcomes might measure the number of falls, use force dynamometry for strength testing, goniometry for measuring ROM at the ankle, and a clinical test of sensory integration.[79]

The World Health Organization's International Classification of Impairments, Disabilities, and Handicaps, and the International Classification of Functioning, Disability, and Health

The World Health Organization provided a useful structure for client management in 1980 with the International Classification of Impairments, Disabilities, and Handicaps (ICIDH)[80] model of disablement. In the ICIDH model, impairment is the result of disease at the organ level, disability is the result of impairment at the functional or skill level, and handicap is the consequence of impairment at the societal level. In 2002 the World Health Organization established the International Classification of Functioning, Disability, and Health (ICF)[80a] model of health and disability. In the ICF model *functioning* refers to all body functions, activities, and participation, whereas *disability* is an umbrella term for impairments, activity limitations, and participation restrictions.[80a]

Currently, many health care entities place more emphasis on functional or activity limitations (disabilities) than on impairments. There is much debate by the insurance industry, case managers, and therapists about a client's right to have a therapist re-establish normal movement or functional skill. Until societies truly accept people whose physical movements vary from "normal," however, there will be deficits in the handicap area, even for those who have no functional deficits. Societies have been unable to accept people with physical disabilities such as paralysis, ataxia, and dysarthria as fully capable.

Impairments can be identified and evaluated for their contribution to a disability.[81,82] Some critical impairments will have more influences on a function than will others. For example, in children with cerebral palsy who have gait disabilities, Olney et al[83] demonstrated that poor force output by ankle plantarflexors during the late stance and (terminal swing) phases of gait was the most important factor in poor gait performance. Another example comes from Perry et al[84] who showed that to attain normal walking velocity, although cadence and stride length are important, a strength level of 3+/5 is a critical component in the ankle muscles. Deficiencies of timing, strength, or sequencing can contribute to poor hand function, but sensory deficits at the hand level, however, may be the critical impairment related to poor manipulation skills. Additionally, impairments in the circulatory, respiratory, integumentary, and musculoskeletal systems can account for disability in the brain-injured client (Figure 17-1).

Relative contributions of the impairments to the activity limitation or disability are addressed by the therapist's evaluation, task analysis, and diagnosis,[85] which then determine the focus of the intervention program.

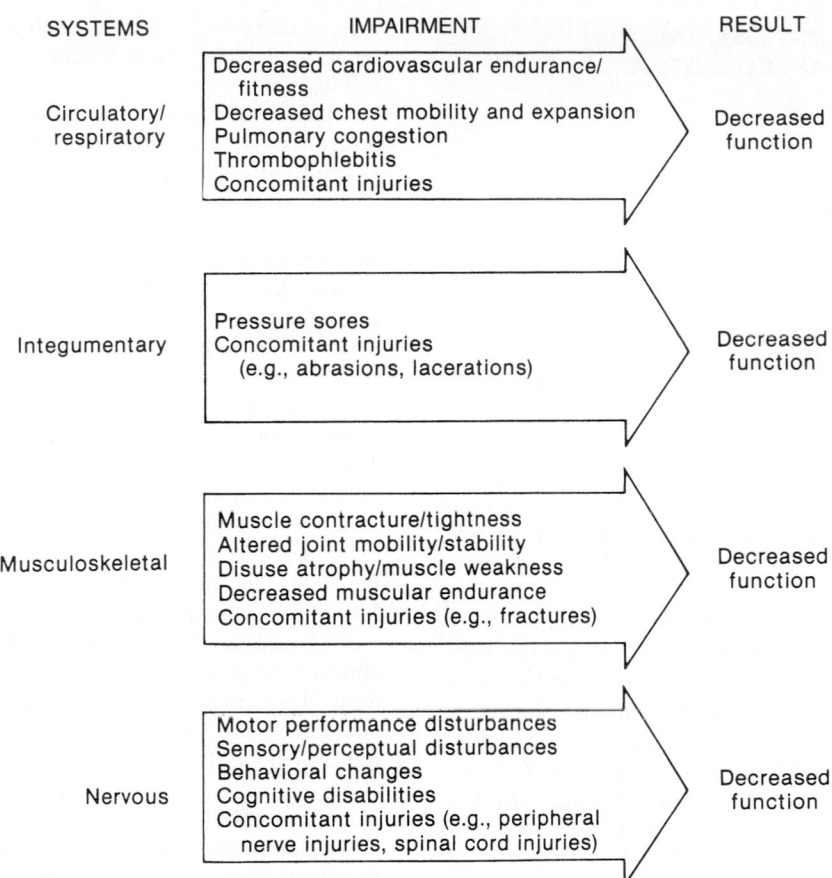

SYSTEMS   IMPAIRMENT   RESULT

Circulatory/
respiratory

- Decreased cardiovascular endurance/ fitness
- Decreased chest mobility and expansion
- Pulmonary congestion
- Thrombophlebitis
- Concomitant injuries

Decreased function

Integumentary

- Pressure sores
- Concomitant injuries (e.g., abrasions, lacerations)

Decreased function

Musculoskeletal

- Muscle contracture/tightness
- Altered joint mobility/stability
- Disuse atrophy/muscle weakness
- Decreased muscular endurance
- Concomitant injuries (e.g., fractures)

Decreased function

Nervous

- Motor performance disturbances
- Sensory/perceptual disturbances
- Behavioral changes
- Cognitive disabilities
- Concomitant injuries (e.g., peripheral nerve injuries, spinal cord injuries)

Decreased function

FIGURE 17-1 ■ Therapists develop intervention strategies to deal with functional deficits that may result from a variety of problems occurring primarily in one or more of the body systems depicted.

When problem resolution at the impairment level to improve the disabilities is not possible, the ICIDH system helps the therapist identify substitutions that can achieve the same functional goals (e.g., use of a wheelchair for the client who will not be able to walk or use of a feeding cuff for a client who will not develop adequate motor function in the hand for feeding).

Examination of Cognitive, Behavioral, and Communication Deficits

Figure 17-2 depicts the close association of cognitive, behavioral, and physical functioning soon after injury. The three domains gradually become more distinguishable in later stages of recovery and can be assessed more independently; however, their interrelationships remain exceedingly complex.

Cognition includes many aspects of function, including memory, learning, information processing, attention span, motivation, and initiation. Cognitive impairment was the primary contributor to disability in most brain-injured subjects who scored moderate to severe on the GOS.[86]

Neuropsychologists, speech pathologists, and occupational therapists usually perform testing of cognitive function. These tests may include word association, written word fluency, figural fluency, and card-sorting tests. Attention can be tested with tests such as the digit span and arithmetic tests on the WAIS[87] and by serial counting by 7. Information pro-

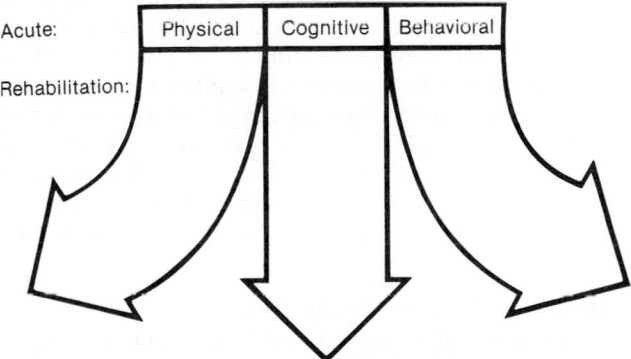

Acute: | Physical | Cognitive | Behavioral |

Rehabilitation:

FIGURE 17-2 ■ Schema representing the close association of cognitive, behavioral, and physical functioning soon after injury. The three domains gradually become more distinguishable in the later stages of recovery.

cessing is reflected in reaction time tests and digit symbol tests. Choice reaction time is an indicator of information processing and commonly remains below normal in brain-injured clients.[88]

Testing of intellectual functions is often done with the WAIS. However, formal testing of intellectual function can be hampered by inadequate perceptual, visual, and motor performance.

BOX 17-8 ■ RANCHO LOS AMIGOS HOSPITAL SCALE OF COGNITIVE FUNCTION

> I. No response
> II. Generalized response
> III. Localized response
> IV. Confused-agitated
> V. Confused-inappropriate
> VI. Confused-appropriate
> VII. Automatic-appropriate
> VIII. Purposeful-appropriate

Memory can also be tested with the WAIS and with the Galveston Orientation and Amnesia Test.[89] The Mini-Mental State Exam[90] is a memory screen often used by health care providers.

Language and cognitive problems are examined by speech pathologists and by use of neuropsychological tests that use naming tests, aphasia examinations, and tests of auditory comprehension and speed of comprehension.

A widely used system of cognitive function at the disabilities level is based on numerous observations of clients with brain injuries at Rancho Los Amigos Hospital. This has resulted in a descriptive categorization of various stages of "cognitive function," as shown in Box 17-8, with use of the Rancho Los Amigos Levels of Cognitive Functioning Test.

Examination of Motor Performance in the Brain-Injured Client

Although most of the following sections describe motor function, motor function is only a small part of the problem of the brain-injured client. Social and family problems will likely be the most devastating in the long term. Motivation, attention skills, emotional instability, memory, learning, and social deficits are all cognitive processes that prevent or retard clients' progress in the therapy program as well as in home and work environments. Working with professionals who specialize in these areas will improve the client's chances to escape deficits that are permanently handicapping.

Disabilities/Activity Limitations

Often the physical therapist begins the examination at the disability level. This usually involves observing those functions that the client identifies as problems. The physical or occupational therapist performs a task analysis of the impaired function by comparing the client's performance of the task with normal performance of the task. For example, the client who cannot stand from sitting independently may be having trouble in the pre-extension phase[91] with inadequate forward trunk momentum or in the extension phase perhaps because of poor hip extensor strength. Once the task analysis is performed, a hypothesis can be formed and tested, and interventions are then chosen to address the underlying problems.

Disabilities in brain-injured clients range over the entire spectrum of problems. They include loss of mobility in bed; loss of household and community ambulation; loss of activities of daily living (ADL) such as dressing, toileting, and feeding; and loss of instrumental ADL such as shopping and driving.

Wade[92] provides an in-depth presentation of examinations for the disability level. The Barthel Index[93] is an example of a simple tool for gross measurement of overall disability. It simply asks whether functional skills can be performed within a reasonable time limit. However, its usefulness sometimes is limited because it is not sensitive to change; the clients, therefore, must make large changes to show improvement in their scores. The Functional Independence Measure (FIM)[94] has six categories that evaluate independence. Twelve items relating to swallowing, community functions, and cognition (Functional Assessment Measure)[95] have been added to the FIM to make it useful for TBI clients. The Disability Rating Scale[11,96] is also widely used for clients with brain injuries.

Upper-extremity movement patterns and function can be examined with use of functional tests such as the Nine-Hole Peg Test,[97] the Frenchy Arm Test,[98] or the arm portion of the Motor Assessment Scale.[99]

These types of indexes should be chosen to address what abilities the client can accomplish. They are not intervention tools. Their purpose is to identify disabilities and monitor client progress. However, many are not effective in measuring changes in the client with higher-level functioning.

Impairments

Impairment at the Basic Component Level of Performance. Breaking motion down to its most basic components may be helpful, but two caveats are necessary. First, improvement in abnormal components may not lead to improvement in disabilities. Second, treating the individual impairments will not necessarily result in the client learning a skill. Skills result from an organization of many motor functions together. Conversely, not having a critical component, such as arm strength, may be the one factor preventing a person from learning to perform a skill (e.g., enough force cannot be generated to throw a ball 5 feet in the air to hit a basket).

Many examinations address the impairment level. These include muscle strength tests, flexibility (ROM) tests, and speed of motion, reaction time, sensation, vision, vestibular, tone, and proprioceptive examinations (see Chapter 8).

Strength or Force Production. Evidence consistently shows that traditional strengthening programs lead to functional improvements in clients with neurological injuries.[100]

In the case of upper motor neuron lesions, weakness can be a major problem. The number of motor neurons activated and the type of motor neurons and muscle fibers recruited affects force. Motor neurons in the motor cortex can be deficient, leading to disordered and reduced recruitment. Individuals with brain damage show early atrophy and loss of motor units, as well as motor units that fatigue easily.[101,102] Disuse, cast immobilization, joint dysfunction, improper nutrition, drugs, and aging can cause differential weakness with altered morphological, biochemical, and physiological characteristics within the muscle.[103] EMG studies by numerous investigators[104,105] suggest that reduced activity alters motor unit properties, discharge frequency, and recruitment patterns. Performance problems are reflected in the inability to generate force in different directions and against different loads as well as in problems sustaining force output.[9]

Changes in muscle length affect strength. In clients with a cerebrovascular accident, shortened muscles tend to be strong in short ranges and lengthened muscles are strongest in lengthened ranges but weak in shorter positions compared with the strength-length curves of normal muscles.[106]

Strength or force at the component level may be examined functionally (e.g., the client has enough strength to lift the arm overhead, out to the side, and up to the mouth or is able to go from sit to stand). In some cases, such as those in which the client is unable to perform balance reactions or has been on extended bed rest, testing individual muscles may be important. Traditional manual muscle testing with force transducers or strength testing with isokinetic testing[107] throughout the range provides good strength information. The level of testing chosen should be consistent with the deficit and the therapist's knowledge of its importance in contributing to the disability.

Flexibility. Flexibility at the muscle and joint level is important. Muscle atrophy occurs rapidly[101] and changes in muscle fiber type and function can be seen as early as 3 days. Viscoelastic properties change with paralysis so that the muscle feels stiffer.[108,109]

Examinations should determine the contribution of both tone and tissue factors in limiting flexibility. Active and passive motion should be compared because stiffness (not contracture) often prevents good function. For example, active dorsiflexion is often limited in clients who have full passive ROM because stiffness begins at neutral dorsiflexion. The functional result is foot drop or toe catch in the swing phase of gait because the anterior tibialis muscle cannot generate adequate force production to overcome the stiffness in the gastrocnemius/soleus. This restriction also may limit forward movement of the tibia over the foot during the stance phase of gait, resulting in hip retraction or an apparent balance loss. Knee hyperextension also can result from lack of forward motion of the tibia.

Flexibility measurements are done with goniometers, motion analysis systems, tape measures, inclinometers, photographs, or electronic devices. Taking both passive and active measurements is critical in identifying intervention approaches.

Tone. In the motor learning theories of today, many of the behaviors and resulting motor patterns after brain injury are seen as attempts by the CNS to compensate for loss. For example, spasticity (increased tone) may be the result of an attempt to compensate for the client's inability to increase force. When the amplitude of a contraction cannot be increased because of the injury, the CNS may increase the length of time the muscle fires or may recruit muscles not normally used in a particular pattern of movement; both are characteristics seen in spasticity.

Whatever the cause of increased tone, the therapist can evaluate tone at two levels: is it interfering with function, and, if so, can it be changed? Spasticity is not a single problem.[102-105,108,110-114] Spasticity includes the following:

Changes in response to stretch
Decreased ability to produce appropriate force for a specific task
Increased latency of activation
Inability to rapidly turn off muscles

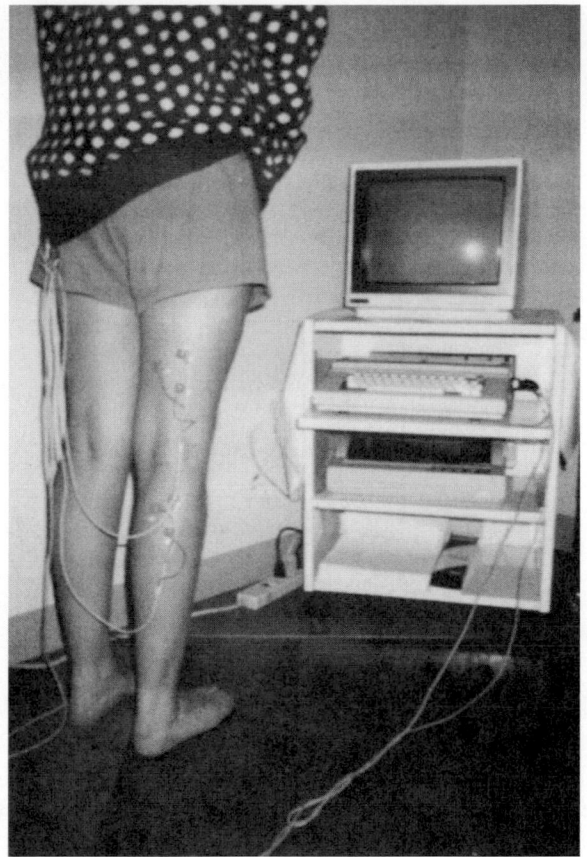

FIGURE 17-3 ■ Measurement of the sequence of contraction of gastrocnemius and hamstring in forward perturbation with dual-channel electromyographic surface electrodes.

Loss of reciprocal inhibition between spastic muscles and their antagonists
Changes in the intrinsic properties of the muscle fibers
Inability to generate enough antagonist power to overcome spastic muscles

Examination begins with identifying whether there is increased or decreased muscle tension at rest. If it is increased, is the tension at the muscle level (stiffness or sarcomere involvement) or the neurological level? Muscle stiffness resulting from tissue changes is common in the brain-injured client. If there is increased tone during movement, EMG may be beneficial to determine the nature of the tone. Is it a problem of cocontraction of agonist and antagonist at a joint? Is it a problem of prolonged contraction? Or is it poor sequencing, either temporally or spatially, of other muscles involved in the movement?

Spatial sequencing of movement involves the contraction of a preset group of muscles. Temporal sequencing involves muscles contracting in a fixed sequence. EMG and video analysis provide additional depth of information regarding the sequence and timing of movement patterns (Figure 17-3). For example, is the normal temporal sequencing in the distal-to-proximal manner present in the upper extremity during a reaching task? In a balance reaction, are the ankle, hip, and back extensors (spatial sequencing) all contracting in response to a forward perturbation? (See section on intervention for a discussion of modifying tone-related components.)

BOX 17-9 ■ MODIFIED ASHWORTH SCALE

Grade	Description
0+	No increase in muscle tone
1+	Slight increase in muscle tone, manifested by a catch and release or by minimal resistance at the end of the ROM when the affected part(s) is moved in flexion or extension
1+	Slight increase in muscle tone, manifested by a catch, followed by minimal resistance throughout the remainder (less than half) of the ROM
2	More marked increase in muscle tone through most of the ROM, but affected part(s) easily moved
3	Considerable increase in muscle tone, passive movement difficult
4	Affected part(s) rigid in flexion or extension

Reprinted from Bohannon R, Smith M: Interrater reliability of a modified Ashworth scale of muscle spasticity, *Phys Ther* 67:207; 1987, with permission of the American Physical Therapy Association.

The most commonly used tool in examination of tone is the Ashworth scale or Modified Ashworth scale[115] (Box 17-9). Testing of deep tendon reflexes identifies problems with stretch reflexes, and surface EMG can determine the presence of cocontraction, prolonged contraction, sequence and timing problems, and increases in latencies.

Speed of Motion. Research shows that seemingly different movements may actually be spatially the same (same muscles involved) but may appear different because of pauses within the movements, velocity, or speed.[116]

Measurements include how quickly a joint can be moved. Recording the number of repetitions of a movement in a specific time frame provides an easy clinical measurement. Isokinetic instruments can measure partial- and whole-extremity motion speed. Speed of movement at each joint in a synergistic movement (videotaped or movement analysis systems) can help to analyze function. Is poor performance to the result of speed of movement problems in just one part of the synergy or in all parts? Computerized motion analysis techniques can also help examine speed of motion relationships between and among limb segments, which is particularly useful in assessing upper limb movements such as reaching and grasping activities.

Reaction Time. How fast can the client begin motion? This parameter can be measured by EMG or with other computerized equipment.

Simple reaction time examination gives insight into the time for neurological processing because it is the measurement of time from a stimulus to a response. Rapid reaction times may be critical for many patterns to be effective, but especially for automatic patterns such as balance responses.

Endurance and Fatigue. Muscle endurance refers to the ability of a muscle to produce the same level of contraction over time. The subjective feeling of effort and weakness after fatiguing exercise may be related to the need to recruit more motor units and to increase the mean firing fre-

quency of the motor units to maintain constant force output.[117] EMG with medium-frequency analysis can test this type of fatigue. Fatigue can also be assessed by measurement of maximal voluntary force, maximal voluntary shortening velocity, or power.[117] Decreased force production, prolonged time to relaxation of muscle fibers, and recruitment of additional muscles during an activity are characteristic of fatigue.[118] Although repeated muscle testing can pick up decreased strength in specific muscles, in most instances, overwork fatigue is first noted by an altered pattern of movement of body segments during activity.

Cardiovascular endurance determines how effectively the body can use oxygen and how soon fatigue sets in. This type of endurance can be measured with several bicycle tests[119,120] and with treadmills with use of a Bruce[121] protocol or a branching protocol for clients with less endurance. A simple test is heart rate before and after activity; the less change and more rapid the return to resting rate, the better the client's fitness level. The 3- and 6-minute walk tests are also reliable and valid for endurance testing.

Fatigue, which is separate from impaired endurance, may result from increased energy requirements resulting from less efficient motor patterns or from more CNS activity.

Sensory Function. Various sensations can be impaired. Problems in the sensory system are often reflected in the motor system, creating distorted movement through faulty information in the feed-forward or feedback processes.

Two broad categories of sensations can be defined on the basis of the type of information: primary sensations and cortical (or integrative) sensations. This arbitrary division is useful functionally but it is not anatomically based. Primary sensations include exteroception and proprioception. The exteroceptors of smell, sight, and hearing are sometimes referred to as teloreceptors. Vision, hearing, olfaction, gustation, pain, touch, temperature, position sense, and kinesthesia are commonly checked primary sensations. Sensations cannot be clinically tested definitively without client participation. Further evaluations of sensation are provided in specific systems.

Proprioception, Light Touch, Two-Point Discrimination, and Stereognosis. Traditional evaluations of proprioception include the ability to distinguish motion and motion direction at each joint. Some clients who cannot distinguish direction or movement still function well. They may have proprioceptive function at the unconscious level (e.g., cerebellar) while not perceiving the input at the parietal level (conscious level).

Having the client close his or her eyes and then placing one of the limbs in a specific position and asking the client to copy the position with the other limb tests proprioception. Asking the client to close the eyes and identify when the therapist passively presents small movements of a joint while the client indicates specific direction of movement may also test proprioception.

Light touch is tested with a brush for localization and quality of sensation. For more definitive light touch discrimination, especially on the hands and feet to determine peripheral neuropathies, a monofilament test[122] can be used. Two-point discrimination can be tested with instruments specifically designed to measure how far apart two separate spots of contact need to be to identify them as distinct.

Stereognosis. Stereognosis, the ability to identify objects placed in the hand without visual assistance, may be critical to normal hand use.

Vision and Visual Perception. Vision is critical in recovery of many motor functions because it is responsible for much of the feed-forward or anticipatory control of movement. For example, balance can be maintained through the visual system by modifying synergy before surface change occurs. Feedback through the peripheral field by array movement can also trigger balance synergies. Some clients are able to use their hands for grasp and release, in spite of severe somatosensory deficits, when they able to use vision to guide the motion.

General visual functions can be screened by the physical or occupational therapist as follows:

1. Tracking is assessed by use of an "H" pattern of movement of the object being tracked. The examiner observes for any nystagmus or refixation saccades. Eye muscle paralysis can be observed during tracking if the client cannot move the eye(s) laterally, up, down, or medially.
2. Focus or accommodation can be checked by observing constriction and dilation of the pupil. Constriction occurs as an object is moved toward the nose and dilation as the object is moved away from the nose.
3. Binocular vision is controlled through feedback from blurred or doubled vision. This reflex signals whether the eyes and fovea are focused on a single point or target; do the images in both eyes fall on the same retinal points? A "cover test" can screen for binocular vision. The client stares at an object at about 18 inches from the nose. The therapist covers one eye. If there is movement to adjust the remaining uncovered eye back to the object, both retinas may not be focusing on the same point. Observing whether light reflections fall on exactly the same place on both pupils is also useful in evaluating binocular eye focus. Vergence testing can also be an indicator of binocular visual functions. A target is observed as it is moved toward the bridge of the nose. The client is asked to indicate when the object appears to double: a normal response is within 2 inches from the bridge of the nose. As the object is moved out, it should be seen as single again within 4 inches from the bridge of the nose.
4. Visual fields can be grossly tested by having the client look forward at a point (observer sits in front of the client to be sure client remains focused straight ahead, Figure 17-4). The client indicates when he or she first sees an object coming into the peripheral field from behind or the "spotter" notes when the client looks toward the object.
5. Visual interactions with the vestibular system are assessed through the vestibulo-ocular reflex. This reflex maintains a fixed gaze on a target as the head moves. The object should not appear to move or double during head motion at various speeds.
6. Perceptual tests that evaluate how visual information is used include visual memory tests, cancellation tests, and figure-ground tests.

Neuro-optometrists and neuro-ophthalmologists are appropriate referrals for clients needing in-depth visual workups, especially when visual perception is involved. See

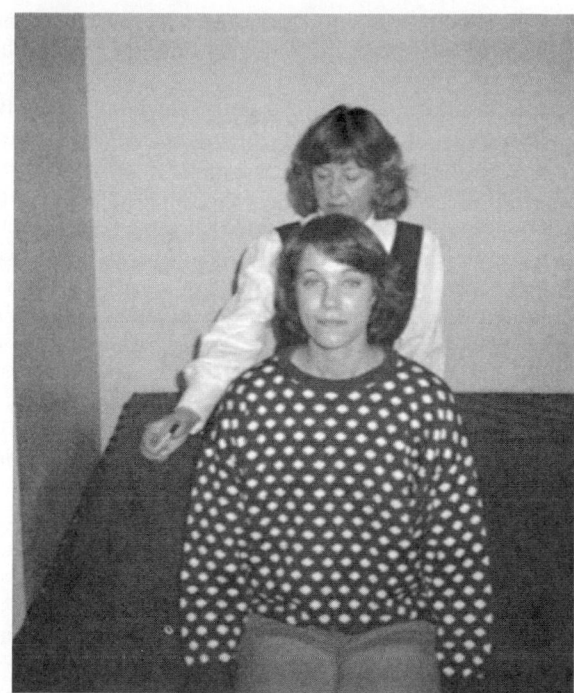

FIGURE 17-4 ■ Testing of peripheral visual fields from behind the client.

Chapter 30 for additional information on vision and visual testing.

Vestibular System. The vestibular system monitors the position of the head in space and helps distinguish when the body is moving from when the visual surround is moving. Vertigo, dizziness, eye/head incoordination, and postural and balance complications occur as a result of problems in the vestibular-cerebellar systems.

Vestibular tests can be performed at the screening level to note dizziness with body, head, or eye motions. A practical division includes testing head movement in lying, sitting, and standing positions. Vestibular System Evaluation and Training[123] is one such test. Symptoms occurring only with specific head movements can be an indicator of problems in the semicircular canals. Dizziness with head tilts might indicate problems in the otolithic system. In-depth evaluation tools may be used when clients are symptomatic. (See Chapter 23 for additional information on balance and vestibular dysfunctions.)

Impairment at Complex Task Level. Complex task evaluation, that of how movement works as a whole, asks different questions from those covered in component examination and requires extensive knowledge of abnormal and normal movement. Complex task evaluation, that of looking at larger movements involving many joints or even the entire body, may be considered from the point of view of motor control theory as follows:

1. **Are basic motor patterns available, accessible, and used appropriately?** Are basic reflexes such as swallowing, visual tracking, smiling, stretch and withdrawal reflexes intact? Injury at this level may often affect basic synergy production and sequencing. Are

automatic movement patterns present such as balance, walking and, running? Are volitional or voluntary movements present?

2. **Are the basic synergies being selected or modified to meet specific task requirements?** These functions are currently associated with cerebellar functions, which provide tone, timing, coordination, and amplitude of motions. The synergistic system smoothes out the motor program and provides adaptability. One of the contributions of synergy use is the ability to limit the degrees of freedom in a movement. Is the client able to use the basic synergies in a functional manner? Is the client able to modify and then accomplish activities such as rolling over, coming from sit to stand, standing, walking, reaching, picking up objects and ball catching? Is there good interlimb coordination as demonstrated by coordinated two-handed activities, good timing between limbs in walking, and jumping? Does the client appear to have the ability to coordinate motions (decrease the degrees of freedom) or are they limited by too few degrees of freedom? Does the client respond correctly to environmental changes or stimuli such as stepping over or around objects or being able to walk on different terrain? When synergies are used, are they appropriate for the stimulus? For example, is the hip strategy used for standing on moving or narrow surfaces during balance?

3. **Does the client show anticipatory reactions?** These reactions are dependent on learning. Anticipatory reactions require combining past information with present information to make motor responses appropriate to internal and external needs. Counterforces to our movements that must be anticipated are almost always necessary. For example, does the gastrocnemius muscle contract before forward-reaching activities? Does the client step over objects or shape the hand for picking up objects? Almost all motor functions have an anticipatory component. The sensory systems modify performance at this level of functioning. Component examination of visual, vestibular, and somatosensory systems may lead to understanding deficits at this level.

4. **Does the client use feedback correctly?** Feedback is used to modify and fine tune responses. Is activity corrected to meet changing environmental conditions? When not successful at task performance, does the client use the information to modify or adapt subsequent responses? Is the adaptation appropriate, or does it result in poorer performance?

5. **Does the client show variability of performance?** The plastic nervous system can adapt and change its motor output to meet different requirements. VanSant[124] showed that children and adults vary in the way they stand from supine, even under the same environmental conditions. She states that the most striking observation in nondisabled individuals is this variability of performance. The lack of variability has been suggested as a sign of system damage.[72] When the brain-injured client is assessed, the therapist should look for variability of performance in basic motor acts. Can the client accomplish the same task in several ways? Can the client adapt to different task demands? As the complex task is being performed, keep in mind that the extent of deficit is important. To what extent is the observed motor behavior involved? Is the behavior totally absent, is it deficient, or are there signs of substitution of function or adaptation?

Let's use an example of the examination process. Consider the client with difficulty in walking. Walking requires three complex elements; postural control, balance, and extensor strength.[125] First, a task analysis is performed. Postural control requires the client to be able to support the body in an upright position from the head down. This requires examination of force production. Is it adequate to maintain the body upright against gravity? Is force production in the lower extremities adequate to permit ambulation that requires a 3+/5 level of strength?[84] Are righting reflexes intact? Lean the client to the side with eyes closed or have the client lean to determine head-on-body righting. Is the head righted to the body or to gravity (as is normal in adults)? Examination for verticality would include lying, sitting or standing with the body vertical, both with eyes open where vision can control verticality and with eyes closed to examine somatosensory and vestibular control of posture and verticality. These patterns and synergies can be impaired after CNS injury.[65,111,112,126] Use of surface EMG on the leg muscles, will determine whether the client is using balance synergies with a temporal sequence of distal to proximal contraction (ankle strategy) during small perturbations. Does the client use only the appropriate muscles in balance responses (spatial sequence)? Or is the client cocontracting, indicating a temporal or spatial sequencing problem that disrupts the normal synergies? Is there efficient movement in the swing leg? Does it move in a straight line, and is foot placement on the floor appropriate (coordinated movement)? Does closing the eyes change the character of the movement? If it does, the client may be controlling movement by vision without regard to vestibular and somatosensory input. According to a gait analysis scale, is the movement and timing between the legs coordinated? Does the client step over objects placed or rolled in front of him (anticipatory and adaptation)? If not, was it because the client misjudged the height of the object (visual anticipatory responses) or misjudged the distance to move the leg (modification of the locomotion synergy at the amplitude level)? Is movement too disorganized (uncoordinated) to clear the object?

Tools for Examination of Gait and Balance. To monitor progress, many balance and gait examination tools exist. At the impairment level, the Romberg and Clinical Test of Sensory Interaction on Balance (CTSIB)[79] examines sensory components of balance; perturbation tests examine motor components. For gait, the Rancho Los Amigo Observational Gait Analysis analyzes kinematic aspects of the patterns of upper extremity, trunk, pelvis, and lower extremities in each phase of gait at the impairment level. The Barthel Index,[93] FIM,[94] Tinetti,[127] Gait Assessment Rating Scale,[128] and the Motor Assessment Scale[99] also examine different components of gait but more at the disability level. Speed of walking for functional activities such as crossing a street at a stoplight and endurance can be measured by distance and a stopwatch.[129] Endurance can be measured with a 6-minute walk test.[130]

INTERVENTION

Intervention Efficacy

The goal of intervention is the same: to help a client work in the environment to produce movements that are efficient, successful, and to some extent socially acceptable. Bach-y-Rita[131,132] states that long-term rehabilitation is key to improved motor control and that recovery can continue to occur as long as the brain is challenged.

The concept that the external environment influences structural neural changes is basic to physical and occupational therapy interventions; that is, activities in which a client participates change brain structure and organization. Evidence that mammalian brain anatomy and function are modifiable by environmental factors was first irrefutably demonstrated by Wiesel and Hubel,[133-135] who described the importance of environmental experience on functional development of brain cells in the visual cortex of kittens. These experiments showed that visual experiences determine the synaptic organization of neurons in the visual cortex. Devor et al[136] have demonstrated plasticity in other sensory systems.

That intervention makes a difference in recovery after brain injury has been shown in many studies. In studies by Mitchell et al,[137] kittens were deprived of sight by suturing one eye shut. Recovery of vision occurred in the sutured eye only if the animal was forced to use that eye. Similarly, Wolf et al[138] and Taub et al[139] showed that function in hemiplegic upper extremities is improved by forced use of the involved arm by constraining the uninvolved arm. Tower[140] demonstrated that when brain lesions caused limb dysfunction, monkeys did not use the involved limb, but if the remaining useful limb was restrained, the monkeys used the original "useless" limb for climbing and other activities.

Jones et al[141] looked at general versus complex exercise effects on plasticity by use of a general exercise of walking through a tunnel versus a complex exercise (acrobatics) in rats after cortical injury. She monitored recovery by looking at upper limb coordination tasks and also by the number of new synapses per neuron and the number of multisynapses formed. The rats doing complex exercise showed significantly more multisynaptic formations and better limb coordination. Avoiding excessive use of the intact limb may also prevent impaired recovery of involved limb, according to a study on rats by Jones and Schallert.[142] Forced use changes the motor cortex map for the hand[143] in patients with strokes. Whether this is from learned disuse, as suggested by Taub et al[139] or by deactivation of silent synapses is unknown.

Active participation is also important in motor learning, as Held's[144] experiments demonstrated. Activities that allow practice of the specific task have been proven effective. Walking on a treadmill with partial body weight support (Figure 17-5) provides practice of the walking pattern and has been widely effective in improving over ground gait parameters such as speed and improved pattern in a variety of neurological dysfunctions.[145,146]

Mental imaging and mental practice affects learning. Neuroimaging has shown that well-learned tasks stimulate similar areas of the brain even when done with different extremities (the hand versus the foot with writing, for example). Several authors have suggested that activation of the motor patterns by imaging movement[70] may be possible.

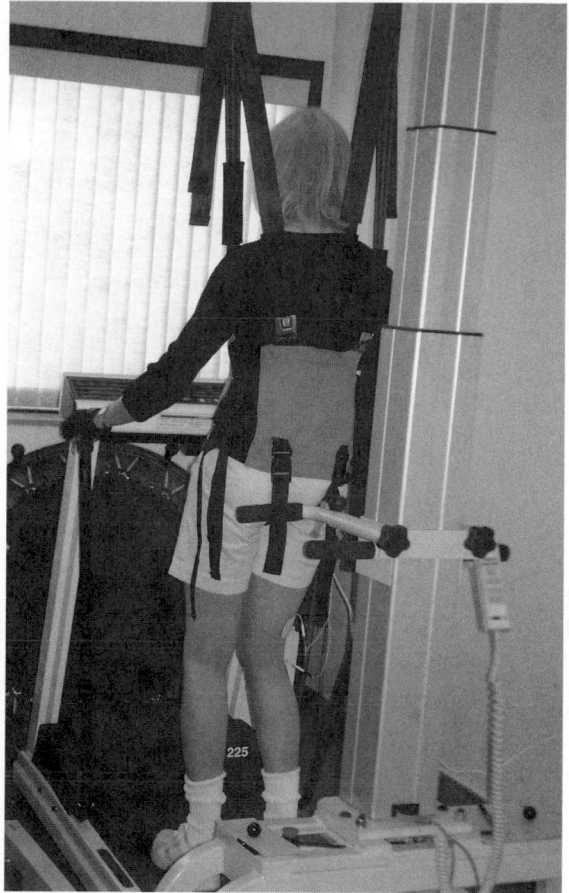

FIGURE 17-5 ■ Client using a partial body weight system on a treadmill intervention with FES on the right peroneal nerve to assist with dorsiflexion during swing phase of gait.

In a study by Porro et al[147] motor imaging activated the same regions of the brain as motor performance, but signal density was only 30% as great as real practice.

The neurophysiological mechanisms thought responsible for CNS recovery[81,141,143,148] after injury are discussed in earlier chapters.

Because the therapist can identify a deficit during the examination does not mean the deficit can be fixed. The ability to "fix" an impairment does not depend solely on the therapist's skills but includes inherent properties within the client such as the amount of physical damage, cognition, family support, and motivation. Just as critical are external constraints, for example, the availability of treatment devices such as electromyographs for biofeedback, stimulation devices, pools, and other equipment; travel to and from treatment; availability of qualified providers of care; and financial constraints on intervention.

Based on evaluation, two levels of intervention are likely to be continuing. At the impairment level, basic components of performance that are faulty and are contributing to lack of motor performance can be addressed. Loss of complex movements and synergies also will be part of the rehabilitation targets. At the disability level, substitutions for loss of function such as bracing, wheelchairs, functional electrical stimulation, ambulation devices and environmental changes such as ramps, chairs, bath benches, padding for skin care,

> **BOX 17-10 ■ DISABILITY: NOT ABLE TO WALK**
>
> **IMPAIRMENT: P+ + LOWER-EXTREMITY EXTENSOR STRENGTH**
> **Can improve:** Use weights, resistive exercises, antigravity work, etc.
> **Cannot improve (significantly):** Address at disability level; use wheelchair, cane, walker, bracing, etc.
>
> **IMPAIRMENT: DISRUPTED SEQUENCE OF MUSCLE CONTRACTION**
> **Can improve:** Use exercises to sequence muscles distally to proximally; use EMG feedback, etc.
> **Cannot improve:** Use bracing, electrical stimulation for bracing, wheelchair

> **BOX 17-11 ■ PROBLEMS AFTER TRAUMATIC BRAIN INJURY**
>
> - Impaired affect
> - Impaired arousal and attention
> - Impaired expressive or receptive communications
> - Impaired motor function, including oculomotor and oral motor
> - Altered muscle elastic properties
> - Impaired respiratory function
> - Impaired autonomic nervous system
> - Impaired cognition
> - Impaired learning
> - Impaired sensory integrity and perception
> - Impaired balance and anticipatory reactions

and reachers provide immediate change and improve the disability almost immediately. The reader must remember that colleagues often use this model to clarify areas needing improvement to reach the goals established by the patients that allow them to participate in the highest quality of life.

With use of the ICIDH model of impairment, disability, and handicap, the therapist determines whether improvement is possible at the level of impairment and then addresses these specific impairments. For example, for a client who is unable to roll over and is both weak and has contractures, strengthening, stretching, and casting may be done. If the problem is at the complex level, whole or part task practice of rolling may be used. In the client with a permanent contracture or paralysis, a cloth loop may be provided to allow rolling over by pulling with the arm for improving function at the disability level. This adaptation to rolling allows the patient independence and participation in daily living activities that lead to a quality of life that may not be attained without environmental adaptation.

An example of the ICIDH intervention model for walking is presented in Box 17-10.

To develop skill in an activity, many, many repetitions must be performed. Knowledge of results and feedback are also important in motor practice.[149] Attention span and motivation factors alone can impede skill acquisition.

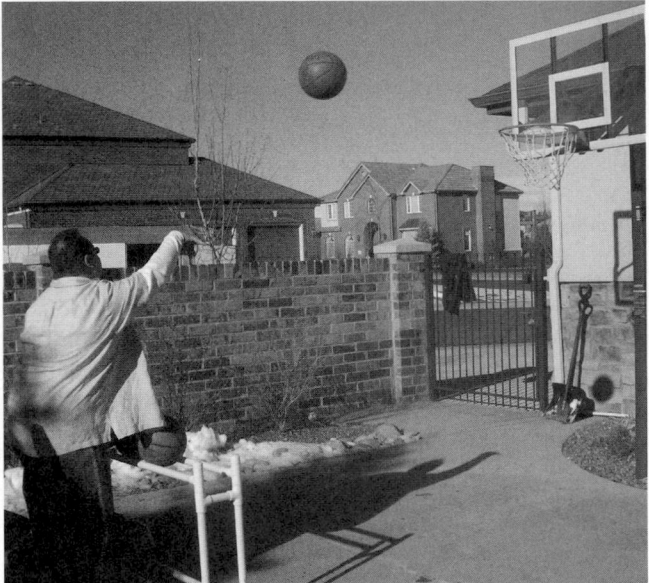

FIGURE 17-6 ■ Client with poor balance throwing a basketball to improve anticipatory and perturbation aspects of balance. Motivation for balance practice is high for this client, who loved to play basketball before his injury.

Areas of Intervention

Multiple problems may occur after brain injury, most of which are amenable to interventions. A partial list of the most common problems is in Box 17-11.

Motivation and Cognition and Memory

The motivational aspect of TBI may be one of the most difficult for the therapist to deal with. Clients' initiation and practice of movement are dependent on the internal control of the client and not easily dealt with from the external environment.

Working on client goals helps to establish motivation. Client goals that seem unrealistic should not be dismissed as inappropriate. The high school athlete who wants to play basketball next week and currently has no postural control can focus on how he will learn to sit, stand, walk, and run to play (Figure 17-6). Most clients who go through rehabilitation programs begin to assess their own potential more

appropriately once they have worked through part of the program. Many clients and their families believe that the brain heals like any other part of their body and expect full recovery provided a client tries hard enough.[150] Sometimes giving clients time out of therapy to experience everyday life at home and work helps them determine and readjust goals and skills and to set new priorities. The client who could not see doing "silly exercises" comes back asking to learn ADLs. In many cases it is the families who need help understanding their family member's social and behavioral changes.

Nearly as difficult to work with are alterations in attention span, confusion, and cognitive problems. The neuropsychological evaluation becomes crucial for treatment in the client with a short attention span and confusion. Early on, techniques to increase attention span will probably include removing distracting stimuli from the client's environment, including auditory, tactile, and visual distractions. But slowly, distracting stimuli need to be reintroduced and attention maintained. (See Chapter 9 for additional information.)

Exercises requiring active involvement in the problem-solving process (crossword puzzles, study, etc) may help with memory and perceived quality of life.[151] General fitness exercises may also affect cognitive functioning by influencing neurotransmitter functions that slow the decline in dopamine and muscarinic acetylcholinergic receptor density.[152] The total number of these receptors are associated with better mental function.

Component Level Intervention for Impairments

Although many interventions have a strong theoretical basis for their efficacy, there are several intervention techniques that are strongly supported in the literature that work for multiple impairments at the same time (such as functional electrical stimulation [FES] for improving force control, ROM, and coordination). At the component level are numerous and well-known approaches to intervention. A quick review of some of the current basis of component interventions and more nontraditional approaches may be useful.

Strength or Force Production. Muscle tension is increased and decreased by the number of motor units firing (spatial summation) and the rate at which they are fired (temporal summation).

FES for recruiting more nerve and motor fibers and changing type I back to type II[153,154] appears effective. FES applied to the peroneal nerve for improved dorsiflexion in gait should also improve force production. Surface EMG (sEMG) has also been shown effective in changing motor function after neurological injury.[155,156] Improving force control with sEMG has been shown to be more effective than feedback of angles of movement and traditional treatment in gait retraining.[157] Traditional strategies have also been effective. Movements that include resistance in eccentric and concentric contractions and movements through varying amplitudes effectively strengthen clients with neurological injury.[158] More functionally oriented tasks such as stepping up and down small and progressing to larger steps with proximal body weighting changes force production and requires both eccentric and concentric contractions. Changing lever arm length also changes the need for force production, for example, lifting the arm in overhead prehension with the elbow bent, straight, and with weighting during activity. Picking up and releasing (concentric and eccentric contractions) objects with differing sizes and weight such as weighted silverware, brushes, or cooking utensils are also effective. Holding large balls overhead and throwing to different targets can improve force control if done at different speeds. These tasks also may promote more interest and attention.

Improvements in strength are usually speed specific, so use of resistance at different speeds is critical. Body position in space may also be related to differences in force production. Current thought is that the brain uses different spatial maps for movement; therefore, use of the extremities and trunk in multiple positions is important to address all different types of patterns of muscle activation.

Consideration of weak muscles is important. Weak muscles sometimes fail to respond as rapidly if overworked.

Treatment in the pool or decreasing the number of repetitions and weight during strengthening may lead to more efficient strengthening and faster recovery. Production and practice of eccentric contractions are important in controlling speeds of movement and achieving accuracy of movement, especially in gait and upper-extremity reaching tasks. Using functional tasks for strengthening is often most effective. For example, practicing sit-to-stand will help strengthen the hips and knees.

Flexibility. Loss of sarcomeres and tissue shortening can occur rapidly in muscle and joints when clients are less active and in those with high levels of muscle tone. Flexibility can be addressed with traditional orthopedic techniques, including joint mobilization, stretching, and dynamic splinting as well as serial casting. Casting, splints, or ankle-foot orthoses may be used to prevent sarcomere loss and adaptive changes.[159] In length-tension curves shifting left or right, early attention to maintaining middle length of muscles is probably important. Additionally, electrical stimulation[154,155] is extremely effective in improving flexibility, especially in dorsiflexion. For example, a small spot electrode placed over the peroneal nerve at the fibular head and a 2-inch-square electrode medial to the lateral hamstring 2 to 3 inches above the knee works well. Use of this technique 10 to 20 minutes twice a day is usually adequate (Figure 17-7). Wrist flexor tightness has been treated with electrical stimulation with good results. However, electrical

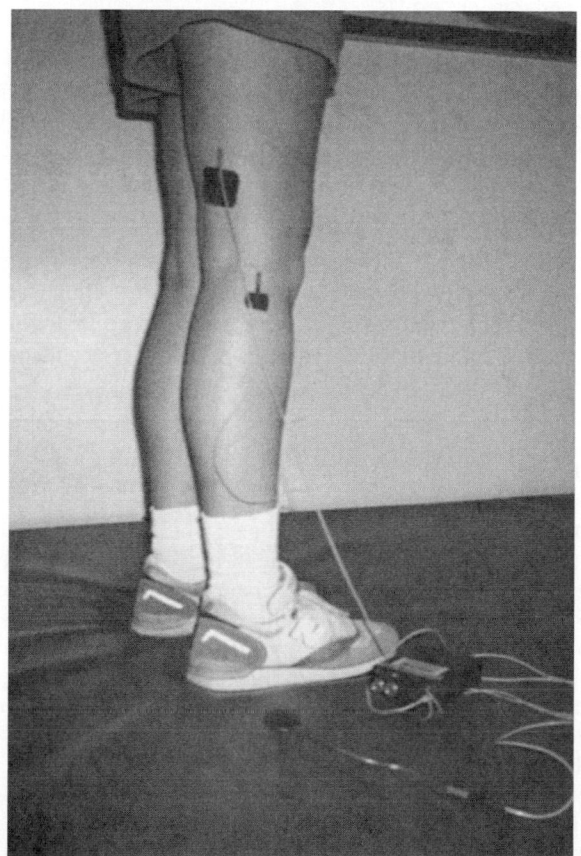

FIGURE 17-7 ■ Placement of electrical stimulation electrodes for peroneal nerve to attain dorsiflexion for stretching a tight gastrocnemius or for electrical bracing when used with a heel switch.

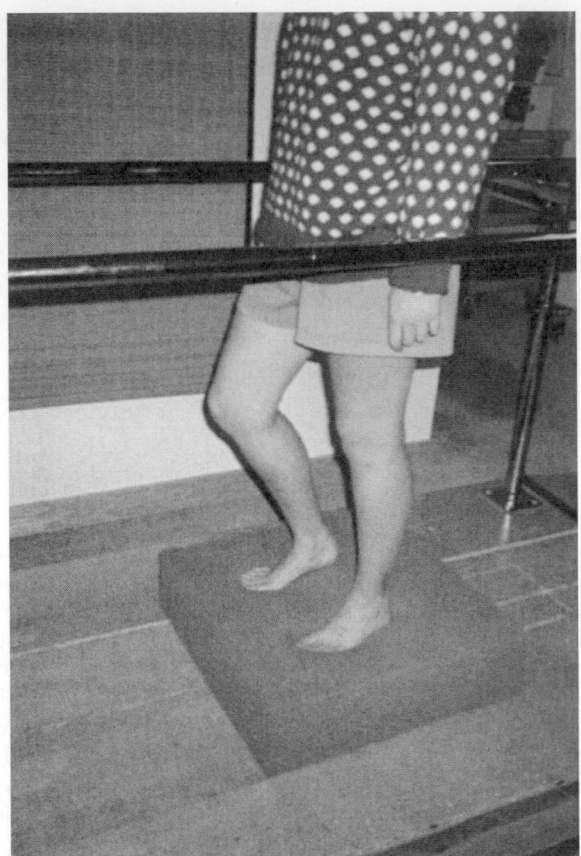

FIGURE 17-8 ■ Foam block to improve speed of motion and reaction time.

stimulation in the unconscious client with increased intracranial pressure or one who is agitated is usually contraindicated because noxious stimuli can increase these problems.

Speed of Movement. Speed of movement may be trained with isokinetic equipment, manually during resistive exercises or proprioceptive neuromuscular facilitation or with computerized equipment such as force platforms. Varying speed is important with activities. Many gait studies show that disability becomes most apparent when the speed of gait is increased. Walking at slow speeds, less than 50% of the normal gait velocity, results in disruption in the walking rhythm.[129]

Reaction Time. Reaction time training also can be done on force platforms with the client sitting or standing. In a pilot study by Winkler,[160] exercise performed while standing on foam pads (10 inches thick and of medium density, Figure 17-8) significantly improved reaction times during weight shifting to a visual stimulus in a group of eight clients with neurological deficits. Work on compliant surfaces may require that the client make faster corrections to avoid falling.

Endurance and Fatigue. Use of repetitions, increasing duration, and intensity can improve endurance. Upper-extremity ergometry can enhance cardiovascular conditioning in clients who are unable to walk or ride bicycles.

Somatosensory. Incorporating sensory function into movement is critical. Clients with poor tactile function can perform activities such as manipulation of objects, first in view and then out of view (nuts and bolts of different sizes are useful); using tactile discrimination to pick out objects from other objects (e.g., safety pins in a bowl of rice) is also challenging. The difficulty of the task can be increased by initiating treatment with visual and verbal cues and then removing all cues as the client progresses. To isolate the proprioceptive and muscle force feedback system, gloves can be used on the hands while grasp and release tasks are performed with and without visual guidance. Light, thin gloves can be changed for heavier, thicker gloves. Changing the surface of the objects that are manipulated from rough to increasingly smoother and slipperier also increases difficulty. Activities can progress from one-handed to two-handed tasks for interlimb coordination. Proprioception at the shoulder and elbow can be done by using a marking pen in the involved hand (a utility cuff may be required for securing) and then having the client practice writing and drawing on paper or a blackboard while sitting or standing. sEMG biofeedback can be used to help retrain the feeling of movement by having the client perform a movement based only on the EMG pattern and then reproduce the movement without vision. Lower-extremity sensory retraining can also use targets with and without vision and with shoes on and off.

Tone. As previously discussed, problems with tone are due to a variety of issues. Problems in spatial and temporal sequencing seem better addressed with multiple-channel sEMG (see Figure 17-3). The client can see both the level of muscle recruitment and the sequence in which the muscles function if dual channels are used (see Figure 17-3). Cocontraction can be decreased during functional activities such as gait or reaching by using EMG biofeedback. Activation of muscles omitted in the gait or reaching patterns can be enhanced and the ability to "turn off" muscles with prolonged contractions are also effectively treated by sEMG (see Chapter 31). In clients unable to use EMG biofeedback information to make changes, functional electrical stimulation may achieve some of the goals (see Figure 17-5). For example, gait training with use of an electrical stimulator on the dorsiflexor or plantarflexor nerves can achieve more normal activation patterns of the foot while providing some internal feedback information about sequencing. A heel switch and a unit with separate channel controls and ramp adjustment are necessary. Use of electrical stimulation on the gastrocnemius and hamstrings, with a slight delay of hamstring activation, has been effective in assistance with ankle strategy retraining. The goal is to slowly remove the "artificial" assistance over time. Strengthening exercises may also assist in improving central control of muscles and therefore improve tone control.

Vestibular System. Basic research has indicated a good response to treatment, especially for peripheral vestibular dysfunction.[161,162] Clients with sensory mismatches may require treatment that enhances input from the two normally functioning systems to adapt or retrain the faulty vestibular system. For example, the client who is dizzy when moving the head may need increased somatosensory input to provide information of the specific body motion that is occurring. The client can perform head motions while supine or sitting with feet and arms well supported (proprioceptive and tactile input) and eyes open. Progress in treatment occurs by decreasing the additional input as symptoms decrease so that the client is finally in standing positions and increasing the amount of movement without dizziness or imbalance occurring. Visual cues can be altered by adding movement in visual areas (movement in the visual surround). This causes the visual system to perceive body motion when there is none and forces the use of the somatosensory and vestibular systems to determine the real motion. Wearing bicycle glasses or taping the medial or lateral aspects of glasses can reduce peripheral visual input, enhancing vestibular and somatosensory input in clients with dizziness caused by visual movement or visual-vestibular conflicts. In clients whose vestibular systems no longer function, enhancing visual and proprioceptive information is critical. Working on the motor aspect of balance by using soft or inclined surfaces and narrow beams to facilitate hip strategies (see Figures 17-8 and 17-9) and using

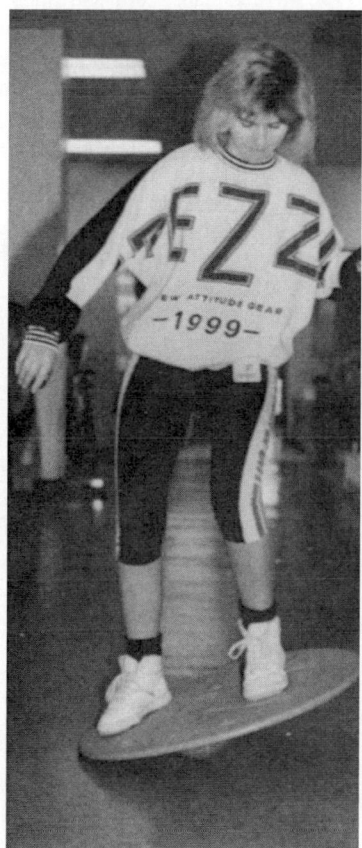

FIGURE 17-9 ■ Providing the appropriate sensory input is critical to stimulating the correct movement synergy or balance response. Although treatment of mechanoreceptive balance problems requires use of flat, firm surfaces, visual and vestibular balance problems are best treated on irregular, compliant, or moving surfaces, such as the multidimensional balance disk shown. The client should not be permitted to hold onto the therapist or to assistive devices because use of the arms changes the balance responses.

small perturbations and quick stops to facilitate ankle strategies are important.

Many brain-injured clients who have vertigo have benign positional vertigo and will need a canalith repositioning maneuver for effective treatment (see Chapter 23 for more in-depth discussion of treatment).

Visual System. The visual system can have impairments in the oculomotor areas of tracking, convergence/divergence, vestibulo-ocular reflex, saccadic motion, and so on. These can be treated with oculomotor exercises, such as looking from a near object to a far object or tracking while the client watches his or her own thumb for increased proprioceptive feedback, with eyes fixed on a target during head movement. Occipital lobe injuries generally result in more perceptual problems, those of making sense of the visual environment. Professionals specializing in this type of problem usually handle these best.

The visual system has separate pathways for movement, color, and form. Therapy can enhance visual input by increasing contrast between objects, such as light objects or print on dark backgrounds. Colors also can assist in easier object identification. Red is often a strongly recognized color in deficient systems. Moving visual targets are easier to perceive than stationary ones. Finally, objects with sharp edges and vertical or horizontal lines are easier to perceive than objects with less distinct or curved lines. (See Chapter 30 for more information on visual problems and treatments.)

Complex Level Treatment of Impairment

Synergies. In clients who have available the basic component functions, basic synergy or skill acquisition should be based on whole-task and natural subtask work. As stated earlier, using subtasks of a whole task improves performance. Identifying natural subtasks is difficult. Winstein[149] suggests that "natural breaks in the resultant velocity profile of a multisegment movement may signify the end of one subunit and may identify natural subtasks of a movement."

The variability shown in the task performance by nondisabled subjects also may help elucidate subtasks. Assessment of a task, as done by VanSant[124] in her supine to stand studies, may provide a model to identify subtasks. In VanSant's study, the upper-extremity patterns varied in six ways: push and reach to bilateral push, asymmetrical push, symmetrical push, symmetrical reach, asymmetrical push with thigh push, and push and reach to bilateral push with thigh push. The head and trunk movement patterns varied in five ways: full rotation abdomen down, full rotation abdomen up, partial rotation stomach down, partial rotation stomach up, and partial rotation; and the lower extremity patterns varied in five ways: kneel, jump to squat, half kneel, asymmetrical squat, and symmetrical squat.

A subtask exercise program to teach a client to get up from supine might work as follows: upper-extremity patterns of asymmetrical push with the trunk in partial rotation are practiced until successful; then lower-leg patterns are added; finally whole-task training is used. Natural subtask work probably will be more effective if it is performed in the environment in which the pattern is normally used.

In difficulty with sit-to-stand, sliding the hips forward and coming to partial standing appears to be a subtask unit and may be practiced. Dependent sit-to-stand is associated with institutionalization.[163] Sit-to-stand practice is outlined in other chapters in detail.

Ambulation training requires working in the upright position. One impairment for many clients is a slower swing phase in the involved leg. It is often accompanied by decreases in total knee flexion ROM leading to problems of toe clearance and increased time on the stance leg. The gait task may be broken down into more natural subtasks, for example, working on half a gait cycle by stepping from the fully extended position (initial swing) to initial contract position. Practicing pulling the thigh forward rapidly and changing speeds of thigh flexion can also be helpful to increase knee flexion.

Whole-task practice of gait in the brain-injured client leads to the question of safety. How does the therapist allow a client who cannot walk without falling to practice walking in light of research indicating that holding onto or using assistive devices changes the very skill the therapist is trying to teach? If the deficit is in balance, then walking without assistance may be critical to progress. The best the therapist may be able to do is to change the environment. Allowing a client to walk between parallel bars increases the likelihood that the client either catches himself or herself or that the therapist can catch the client during falls. Walking on mats may allow both for environmental stimulus for soft, uneven surface work and for safer falling. Falling may be critical in relearning ambulation. Little research is available in this area, but in a study by Cintas,[164] children who performed more daring gait activities fell more often (more problem-solving experiences?) but gained better gait skills. Use of a loose harness as used in unweighted treadmill walking may also be used for safety.

Goal-oriented tasks are mandatory in working with upper-extremity losses, just as with lower extremity problems (Figure 17-10). Many clients with minimal function can pick up and carry boxes. Often grip, but not release, is present. Again, EMG biofeedback is useful in helping develop release.[165] Functional release in clients with grip can be achieved by use of an electrical stimulator on the finger extensors with a hand switch. Some clients respond to a continuous low-level stimulation of the finger extensors and can learn to release by relaxing the grip. These activities are practiced while grasping and releasing objects. Feeding can be performed with this technique, as can other ADL tasks such as hair combing and opening doors.

The upper extremity also appears to use specific synergies for hand use in different positions. Clients can often open their hands in forward-reaching position but not with the wrist bent. Many clients with minimal functioning can be fitted with a utility cuff to hold writing instruments and write on boards or on tables while standing. This technique assists the shoulder in producing appropriate movement sequences for hand use but does not facilitate hand function. The intervention, however, does provide whole-task practice although some basic components are compensated through substitution. The therapist also may consider using a restraining device on the uninvolved side (with the client's permission) to force use of the involved extremity. Forced use by restraining the most commonly used extremity can also be effective in improving function. Games and other interesting activities, such as in Figure 17-11, may also be used.

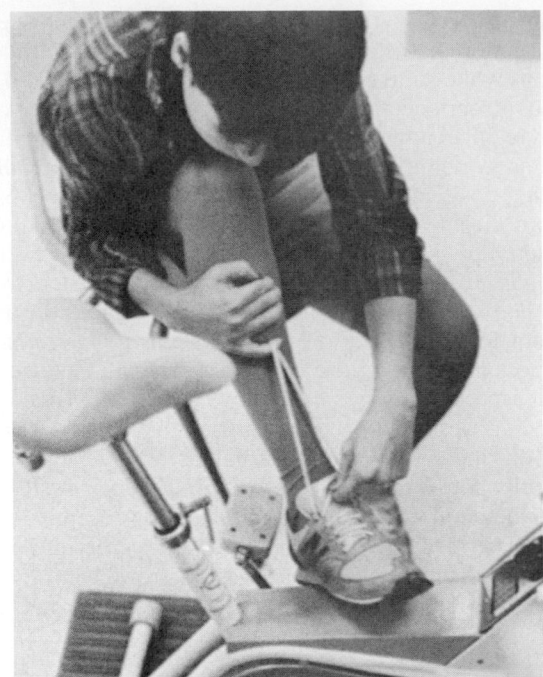

FIGURE 17-10 ■ Most clients seem to respond to functional activities such as dressing. Sitting and leaning forward (as to put on shoes) actively involves the client in the treatment. This is also an example of integrating components of movement into a meaningful activity and using the same activity to further develop motor components.

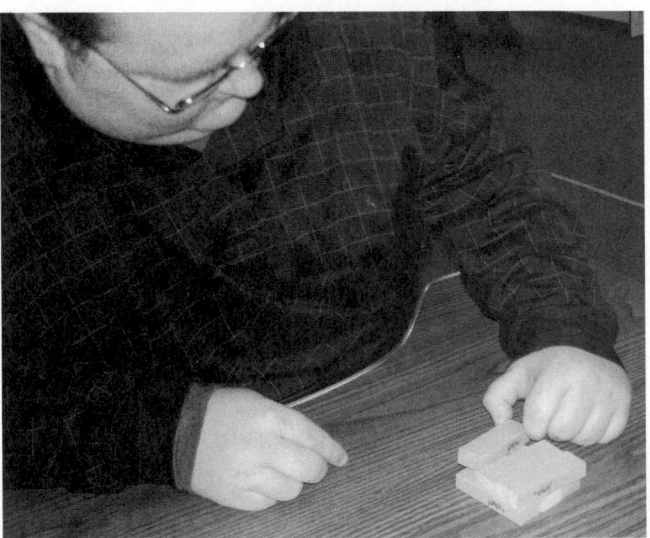

FIGURE 17-11 ■ Games that are challenging for both the mind and the hand provide interesting ways to work on upper extremity function. This client lacks refined prehension skills in the left hand.

The use of whole-task practice at each treatment session is critical for two reasons. First, it is the only legitimate feedback of performance. For example, when teaching a throwing motion for basketball, if practice of the arm motion and ball throwing is without a target, feedback may indicate that ball release is adequate. The skill of shooting the ball into the basket is placing the ball at a specific point in space. The feedback that the ball hit the target determines the accuracy of the motion. Throwing the ball into the air is not the same task and uses different motor and sensory information than that needed for basket shooting. Second, the forced use studies of Wolf et al[138] and Taub et al[139] demonstrate that motor skills improve better with functional use (whole-task practice). When they restrained the unaffected arm in clients with a cerebrovascular accident and monitored improvement in the involved arm, they found significant improvement in function in clients who had previous traditional arm rehabilitation.

Reversing tasks in some clients allows them to develop increased control but requires modifying a task or synergy and working muscles both eccentrically and concentrically. For example, slowly lowering a spoon from the mouth may improve lifting the spoon to the mouth by improving motor control of the biceps during eccentric contractions. Wrist weights can be added to improve somatosensory feedback. Changing control by having clients stop and start at different points in an activity or changing directions also develops improved responses as well as flexibility. The client is asked to stop without taking another step, to turn right, or to step backward during ambulation. These techniques provide external influences on motor activities, helping to establish flexibility into responses. Adding objects to the environment to avoid or manipulate and exposing the client to changing environments also develop adaptations and modifications to synergies. Finally, for clients who are unable to produce movement, handling techniques using righting reflexes may help with rolling and coming to sit or stand in clients who have lost basic synergies.[166]

Anticipatory Responses. More complex activities such as postural stability require work at the anticipatory response level and at the stability level. Moving the extremities (Figure 17-12), adding weights to extremities during forward movement, and increasing motion speeds are effective techniques. Pulling and pushing activities require an anticipatory set. More dynamic movement may be practiced with ball activities. Using punching, catching, throwing, and kicking activities with weighted balls and regular balls will change the force and speed involved, requiring the client to adapt responses to the changing environmental demands. Treadmills help clients to adapt their motion to environmental changes and to make anticipatory responses. But remember, treadmills cause sensory conflicts because the somatosensory system and vestibular systems report movement but the visual system reports no forward movement.

Variability. VanSant[124] also stated that variability of performance in her study had "something to do with body size, strength and ROM." Because force production (strength) and ROM may be critical components in variability, work in water or with weight to change force production and ROM may also enhance different responses. It is important to build environmental constraints so clients can perform functional movements in alternative ways.

Learning, Practice, and Feedback. According to Winstein,[149] knowledge-of-results research currently suggests a need to re-examine intervention approaches that

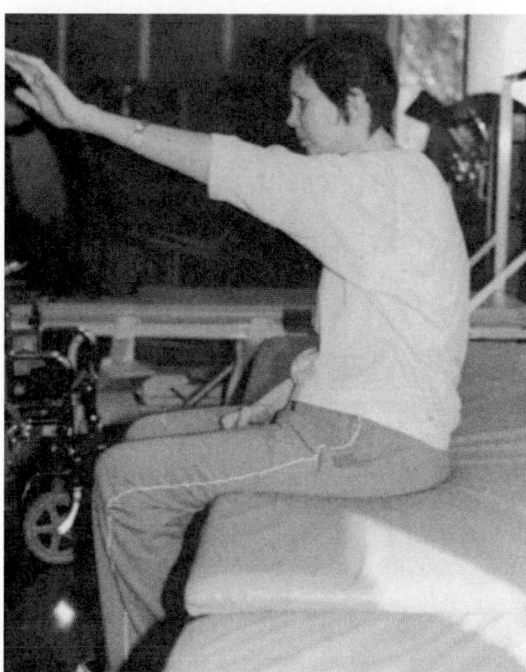

FIGURE 17-12 ■ Anticipatory trunk movements are essential to provide postural stability immediately before some extremity movements. For example, spinal extension and an anterior pelvic tilt usually accompany elevating an arm overhead. However, brain-injured clients frequently lack adequate preparatory movements and typically maintain trunk flexion while attempting this activity.

advocate performance accuracy, strong guidance (either manual, tactile, or verbal), frequent and continuous feedback, and avoidance of errors or "abnormal movements." The knowledge-of-results research findings are consistent with the motor control model that requires the client to be actively involved in problem solving through trial and error and adapting to new environmental situations. The higher-level client needs help to solve his or her own motor problems and thus needs less physical support but expanded environmental experiences.

Conversely, the client with minimal motor function or the client who is in an early recovery state may require a great deal of external help with basic components of movement before learning how to access or develop basic synergies and skill. Assisting movement is appropriate for the level of this client's functioning. For example, in training upper-extremity reaching patterns, this client may need trunk support intermittently, and then slowly decreasing the support will help develop the balance component necessary for successful reaching.

Because feedback is so critical to learning and improving motor performance, especially at the higher levels of functioning, the method of treating the highly functioning clients by assisting motion comes into question. Normal movement is unique in that it will change depending on the context in which it is performed and on the task constraints. The client being assisted in ambulation will not be making balance responses if the therapist is providing balance support.

The same problems may be inherent in the use of assistive devices such as canes and walkers. For example, Horak et al[65] showed that using a cane for balance disrupts the normal distal-to-proximal sequence in the lower extremities, and much of the balance responses are transferred to the arm, shoulders, and trunk. Canes also cause a shift in the center of gravity.[167] The same may be true of many externally guided motions. The therapist must provide the client with opportunities to practice all parts of the complex motor tasks, or the task requirements are not the same. Practice needs to be task specific, but changing environmental and task constraints can build in flexibility of response.

Disability (Functional) Level of Intervention

Mobility and prehension are the two most frequent disability losses after brain injury. In clients who will not be able to re-establish walking or prehension skills, functional devices are provided for substitution of the lost skills. This level also teaches functional tasks such as transfers, cooking, and self-care with assistive devices and modified techniques.

Retraining programs with emphasis on cognitive function, endurance, or social interactions are also available in larger communities.

Summary of Intervention Concepts

Evidence for the efficacy of interventions for clients with brain injury is strong for electrical stimulation, unweighted treadmill, mental imaging, and forced use.

In general, lower-level-functioning clients (those with losses of basic synergies, component impairments, or cognitive changes) need more hands-on help from the therapist while trying to develop basic motor programs. Intervention may need to focus at the component level, establishing strength, flexibility, timing, and sequencing of movements. In lower-level clients, assistive devices such as braces, neck supports, and postural seating systems are often used to substitute for missing components of function. Forced use may also play a role in higher-level clients who are able to accomplish complex-level work. For clients who cannot manage multiple tasks, such as balance, coordination of synergies, and anticipatory reactions, the therapist may choose to work in subtasks.

Many higher-level clients benefit from high-level functional activities. Square dancing, line dancing, karate, tai chi,[168] handball, and other sports often promote additional progress in balance, sequencing, and speed of movement. The clever therapist will tease out those components of the activities that best address the deficits in the client and structure enjoyable activities that provide specific training for the deficits in balance, gait, or upper extremity use.

No matter at what level the client is functioning, the teaching of functional skills is critical. The lowest-level client may learn to roll over and assist with eating or other ADL by using assistive devices. Modern equipment can enhance all types of function. Computers communicate for those with severe dysarthria, and power wheelchairs with switches to run lights, television, and so on are available. These devices assist clients in their societal interactions and reduce handicaps. Remember, the main purpose of motion is for exploration and getting the brain to a place it can be used!

OUTCOME

Leahy,[169] in a discussion of brain-injured adults, suggested a general categorization of clients for prognosis by a combination of levels of cognitive and physical functioning. Cognition is rated as low, moderate, or high level and physical dysfunction as severely impaired, moderately impaired, or minimally impaired. The therapist may use the GOS and the Rancho Los Amigos Hospital Scale of Cognitive Function to determine the categories. This system provides a means of predicting return of functional skills and long-term disability. As Leahy points out, clients with higher-level physical skills and moderate-level or low-level cognition skills are often the most difficult to reintegrate into the family and society. Therefore, they may have the higher levels of handicaps remaining after rehabilitation because family and coworker expectations are high on the basis of motor function, but it is the cognitive functions that make a person more successful in society.[88] These clients need aggressive help in the behavioral and cognitive areas early on. Neuropsychologists and counselors can suggest interventions that help with cognitive functions, especially techniques to deal with memory problems, attention span decreases, and inappropriate behavior. These programs can make a difference. Brotherton et al[170] documented long-term social behavior improvement in four severely brain-injured clients who had undergone traditional social skills training programs.

Clients with low-level motor skills and higher-level cognitive skills do better because there are available adaptive devices for these clients that help substitute for their loss of motor functions. These include head-, mouth-, or hand-controlled electric wheelchairs; computerized communications systems; electric lifts for vans and hand controls for driving; books on tape; and numerous upper- and lower-extremity devices to help with hand control and ADL. (See Chapter 19 on spinal cord injury for all types of substitution devices.)

SUMMARY

The following concepts summarize the theory, research, and intervention concepts presented in this chapter.

1. Intervention is based on the nervous system's ability to learn through environmental influences.
2. The client's goals must be addressed to provide motivation and persistence in exercise and practice.
3. As a starting point, examination and evaluation are done at the disability level.
4. A hypothesis is generated to explain the basic causes of the disabilities by identifying those impairments that are major contributors to the disability.
5. Tests and measures are performed in the examination to confirm the hypothesis.
6. Interventions for prevention of secondary complications such as contractures, skin breakdown, and muscle contractures begin early to prevent loss of function.
7. Strength or force production is critical in movement, and loss of this ability contributes significantly to disability; therefore, strengthening and controlled force exercises are important.

8. Changing speed of motion and varying the context and environment are necessary for thorough skill reacquisition.

9. Once components of movement are in place, the use of synergies or skill learning should be stressed through repetition of functional activities.

10. Interventions should be performed with the goal of the movement incorporated into the treatment.

11. Practice is necessary in multiple environments and conditions.

12. The client should be allowed to solve problems.

13. Physical assistance by the therapist to clients with moderate and minimal levels of disability should be kept to a minimum.

14. Variability in performance is normal.

15. sEMG biofeedback, functional electrical stimulation, isokinetic methods, and kinematic feedback should be used to modify responses that appear more resistant.

16. Environmental situations that cause changes in responses should be identified and used.

17. Feedback should be provided randomly and as a summary rather than on a continuous basis.

18. Substitution devices, assistive devices, and environmental changes should be provided for those clients who will not recover from their impairments.

19. Remember that the therapist's uniqueness lies in the ability to do evaluation and effective intervention.

QUALITY OF LIFE

A life has been saved. The job of the rehabilitation team is to help improve the quality of that life. But what is quality of life? Family members knew the client before injury. The "rehabilitated" client may be dramatically different from their expectation. The rehabilitation team members, who can contrast the client's progress only since the injury, may be quite pleased. Is quality measured by past performance, past potential, present performance, or future potential? Clients themselves may or may not have insight into past, present, or future performance and potential. What is the standard by which quality of life is measured? Is it income, reduction of dependence, contribution to society, or social interaction? Each of these indicators has been used as a standard. Ultimately, the determination of successful rehabilitation relies on the answer to these questions. Jennett and Teasdale[6] suggest six aspects of living: ADL, mobility and life organization, social relationships, work or leisure activities, present satisfaction, and future prospects. Most of these factors, although important, cannot be quantitatively measured, and they do not entirely answer the question of what is quality of life. However quality of life is estimated, those who have chosen to help rehabilitate clients with brain injury continue to pursue an ideal of quality for each life that has been saved and may, by doing so, enhance the quality of their own lives.

CASE STUDY 17-1 ■ MRS. E. K.

EXAMINATION
History
Mrs. E. K. is a 60-year-old woman who sustained a brain injury in a fall 1 year ago. Injury was to the cerebellum and brain stem resulting in left-sided body involvement and incoordination. She reports falling about two times monthly. She complains of feeling tired constantly and not having enough energy to even accomplish her housework. She lives with her husband and 29-year-old son in a two-story house 1.5 hours from a large western city. Her son is an alcoholic and unable to keep a job. Client goals included being able to sew again and to square dance with her club.

Task Analysis
Gait (With Use of the Observation Gait Analysis Based on the Rancho System)
Mrs. E. K. walks with a normal pattern on the right. She has minimal trunk rotation during right leg swing and a right pelvic drop in left leg stance. On the left during swing phase, hip flexion is limited, and the leg circumducts. The left knee has limited flexion and the foot has excessive plantar flexion. In stance phase on the left, there is limited hip extension during mid and late stance and flat foot contact at initial contact. The left arm is held tightly against her chest with the elbow in flexion and the forearm in full supination. When asked to put her arm to her side during ambulation, the arm swings uncontrolled in large arcs actually hitting her in the chest. Speed of walking is slow at 50 meters per minute. Cadence is 73 steps per minute with a 0.8-meter stride length.

Hypothesis 1
Gait
Gait is impaired in kinematics and speed as a result of poor force production in the left hip flexor and dorsiflexors complicated by quadriceps and gastrocnemius tone. Slowed gait is also present because of poor trunk rotation during arm-fixed gait and to instability when the arm is flailing. Flexibility of tissue in the quadriceps and gastrocnemius/soleus may also contribute to the poor movement patterns and there may be a disruption of the normal temporal sequencing of muscle firing in stance on the left. Question whether proprioceptive problems may be present because of poor foot placement in stepping. Mrs. E. K. may have anticipatory problems because gait is not compensated for by the arm movements.

Impairments-Component
Force production: Strength: 3+/5 left hip extensors and abductors, hamstrings, and ankle plantarflexors; otherwise within normal limits in lower extremities. Able to maintain upright posture in standing with only minimal deviations.

Flexibility: Left rectus femoris tight at 100 degrees knee flexion test in prone. The gastrocnemius/soleus is tight at neutral. Otherwise within normal limits.

Tone: Modified Ashworth level 3 in left quadriceps and gastrocnemius/soleus.

Continued

CASE STUDY 17-1 ■ MRS. E. K.—cont'd

Reaction time to weight shift delayed in the left leg when shifting left (tested on force platform).

Speed of motion slowed in left hip flexion and left foot dorsiflexion.

Proprioception is decreased when asking Mrs E. K. to note small changes in flexion and extension of the great toe and ankle. Within normal limits for knee and hip.

Impairments-Complex

Synergies are poor in trunk. There is no trunk rotation during walking, and a proximal to distal balance response during small perturbations (EMG). Visual-vestibular control of balance is poor; she cannot stand on 12-inch-thick foam pad without balance loss and cannot maintain narrow-base stance with eyes closed.

Anticipatory responses are poor as measured by rapid forward reaching resulting in forward balance loss in standing.

Mrs. E. K. falls on the CTSIB test on conditions 2, 3, 5, and 6.

Evaluation and Diagnosis

Poor walking ability and lack of automatic balance reactions as a result of decreased use of proprioceptive information, poor timing and force production in the hip extensors, abductors and gastrocnemius in gait, and increased tone and limited flexibility in the quadriceps/gastrocnemius and poor anticipatory responses disrupting balance when the upper extremities are moved rapidly or when the left arm flails.

Task Analysis

Sewing (large 4-inch needle with yarn through 1-inch square holes in plastic grid).

Ataxia and dysmetria are present as the needle approaches the hole during the task. Mrs. E. K. hits the hole with the needle about one in three attempts. The left hand does not work in a distal-to-proximal manner. The scapula and shoulder show excessive motion during the reaching phase of the movement, and dysmetria increases as the needle approaches the mat. The hand remains excessively supinated for the task.

Hypothesis 2

Poor timing and coordination of the scapula and shoulder muscles in addition to abnormal tone in the biceps are producing a discoordinated movement pattern.

Impairments-Component

Tone: Hypotonia throughout the left scapula and shoulder, normal tone in the forearm and hand (Ashworth 0).

Timing and coordination: Poor sequencing and timing of movement. Tremor of high frequency in the scapular stabilizers, especially the external rotators at rest and with movement. There are lower-frequency tremors of larger amplitude in the wrist flexors and extensors during voluntary motion. Cocontraction of the biceps occurs with all shoulder and hand motions. Examination was performed with sEMG.

Force production is good to normal throughout the limb.

Impairments-Complex

Modification of synergies is poor for upper-extremity reaching. Amplitudes of movement are far too large for tasks.

Evaluation and Diagnosis

Upper extremity is not being used functionally secondary to poor sequencing and timing of muscle firing during activities. Mrs. E. K. is unable to limit the degrees of freedom in the arm during upper extremity activities. The arm is held in cocontraction during walking and other activities to decrease the instability in balance caused by large movements of the entire arm.

Handicap

Decreased social interaction with friends.

Interventions

Mrs. E. K. was referred to a psychologist who diagnosed her with depression. Mrs. E. K.'s physician then prescribed an antidepressant medication.

Because Mrs. E. K. lived 70 miles from the treatment clinic, much of her treatment consisted of a home program. She was seen in the clinic once every 3 weeks for 3 months and then once a month for a year.

The initial home program focused on the basic impairments of reducing quadriceps and gastrocnemius/soleus tightness and increasing hip extensor, abductor, and gastrocnemius strength in the lower extremity with functional activities. These included sit-to-stand with the knees bent past 90 degrees, keeping the heels on the floor, and tall kneeling during upper extremity exercises. Mrs. E. K. worked on treadmill, walking starting at 1.2 miles per hour at home to increase her speed of walking and endurance. She practiced an imaging exercise for 10 minutes a day, using sewing as the task. sEMG was used in the clinic to improve scapular-humeral rhythm during functional activities such as drinking from a cup and her sewing task. sEMG was also used to decrease the cocontraction of the biceps during functional use of the arm. At first the sEMG provided continuous feedback with the client observing the screen. After she was able to achieve a particular goal for the day, the visual sEMG was only provided randomly to the client. Practice of activities was for short periods interspersed with different activities. To re-establish some control of amplitude of motion in the left arm, gross movement activities with the hand with the elbow stabilized and a wrist splint to limit the degrees of freedom were initiated. For example, drawing large circles with a pen and pulling long pieces of yarn through some large holes. She also used her left forearm to stabilize paper while writing, finally progressing to using the hand only for stabilization.

The remaining program focused on hand-guided movement activities such as sewing with yarn on a large (1-inch squares) mat, combing hair, molding clay,

CASE STUDY 17-1 ■ MRS. E. K.—cont'd

playing the organ, and other functional tasks. These activities were first performed with the elbow stabilized and a wrist splint, then with the elbow not stabilized, and finally without the wrist splint.

Lower-extremity work included improving the use of proprioceptive function. Standing exercises with the eyes closed or occluded progressed to stepping activities and finally walking. To increase proprioceptive use, Mrs. E. K. practiced identifying objects with her feet (e.g., pen, checker, modeling clay). Ankle strategies were promoted through rapid walking while the client's husband told her to stop abruptly and the client tried not to take a step after being told to stop.

Speed and range of dorsiflexion were facilitated through use of a rocker board (without holding on), jumping on foam, and walking with a longer step on the right. sEMG was used in standing to increase the force of contraction of the anterior tibialis.

As the amplitude of arm motion decreased with use, Mrs. E. K. was able to walk with her hands clasped behind her back and worked on trunk rotation coordinated with gait. When this was accomplished, she was able to allow her arm to hang freely at her side and had a natural trunk rotation in walking. Mrs. E. K. practiced line dancing with her husband, using an introduction videotape on line dancing. This activity promoted higher-level balance exercises and provided enjoyment.

Outcomes
At discharge, Mrs. E. K. had good synergies and improved pattern of motion in the left lower extremity. An articulated ankle-foot orthosis was used for long walks or when she was fatigued. She walked with 90 steps per minute with a 1.2-meter stride length. Tone was a level 2 Ashworth and reaction time was low normal. She performed within normal limits on the CTSIB. She was able to sew and use the left arm for most activities, although a much smaller tremor persisted with volitional movement. She only occasionally went to the square dancing club. Medication had controlled her depression and her fatigue was not as debilitating.

CASE STUDY 17-2 ■ P. H.

EXAMINATION
History
P. H., a 21-year-old woman, was in an automobile accident and sustained a severe brain injury and fractures of the left scapula, left radius, right ankle (fused), and jaw. She developed heterotopic ossification in the right elbow. P. H. was in a coma for 1 month and a stupor for 2 more months. Her GCS was 8/15 at 2 hours after the accident. Rancho Los Amigos Hospital Scale of Cognitive Function was a level V (confused, inappropriate).

Expressive language was minimal with severe expressive aphasia and dysarthria. P. H. appeared to understand well, following directions and nodding appropriately to questions.

Behavior was immature. For example, P. H. continuously hugged and kissed her boyfriend when he was in the room. She was easily frustrated by difficult tasks. At these times she became extremely agitated and scratched herself to the point of bleeding. Her memory was poor, as noted by her score of 19 on the Mini Mental State Exam.

Mobility was by wheelchair. P. H. was independent in transfers. She could roll and come to sit independently, but she needed moderate assistance to kneel and come to stand and maximal assistance to walk. She was unable to perform self-care such as personal grooming, hygiene, and dressing or to do household chores. Her chin rested on her chest except for 2 or 3 seconds after she lifted her head volitionally.

P. H.'s goals included use of the left arm to put on makeup and dance with her boyfriend.

Hypothesis 1
Weakness on the left side resulted from scapular fracture and disuse. Flexibility loss in the left elbow was the result of postoperative swelling from heterotopic ossification removal, problems with force production and gradation of force were the result of poor somatosensory function, and there was increased tone in the left arm. Poor perception of vertical and overstretch weakness of the neck with poor head righting responses were apparent.

Impairments-Components
1. Strength: Right arm—fairly normal in strength. Left arm—not able to actively abduct shoulder but able to actively hold if placed at 90 degrees. Shoulder external rotation and flexion and elbow flexion and extension—3/5, (but range was limited). Wrist extension—2+/5 (half range) and flexion 3+/5. Gross and fine finger control—present in the left hand. Neck extensors—3−/5.
2. Flexibility: Left shoulder—limited to 120 degrees of flexion and abduction, 45 degrees of external rotation. Left forearm supination—10 degrees. Right elbow—90 degrees of flexion, 20 degrees of extension.
3. Tone: Cervical hypotonia. Left biceps, triceps, wrist flexor, and finger flexors—3 (modified Ashworth scale). The tone in the left arm was of a cocontraction nature at the elbow. There was poor spatial sequencing throughout the limb.
4. Sensory: Light touch was intact in both upper extremities; proprioception was within normal limits in both arms except for the left hand, where

Continued

CASE STUDY 17-2 ■ P. H.—cont'd

movement was perceived correctly but direction was not consistent. P. H. identified 4 of 10 objects placed in the left hand. The left pupil was dilated. Visual tracking was poor; P. H. stopped tracking at midline when tracking to the left. She complained of diplopia.

5. Vestibular function appeared intact except for possible abnormality in perception of vertical (this did not appear to be a visual problem because eye-closed conditions did not change the impaired vertical position).

Impairments-Complex

1. Synergies appear intact except in the cervical area, where the head is not held upright to maintain the eye level.
2. Modification of synergies is poor in the left arm, where movement patterns were gross and poorly refined, and intralimb joint coordination was poor.
3. Anticipatory responses in reach and grasp: Did not show hand sizing to match object size.
4. Variability of performance: P. H. was able to reach and grasp and bend in many different ways with the right arm but had mainly an adducted, internal rotation pattern with elbow flexed on the left. She appeared limited in the degrees of freedom available at the forearm and hand.

EVALUATION AND DIAGNOSIS

Poor motor manipulation and prehension synergies in the left upper extremity resulted in nonuse of the left hand. Precision in grip was impaired by poor feedback from the fingers. Contributing to the lack of use of the hand was poor strength in the scapular stabilizers because of the scapular fracture and injury. Lack of adequate elbow ROM from heterotopic ossification in the right elbow prevented grooming, personal hygiene such as teeth brushing, and applying makeup with the right arm, which had fairly normal function. Prolonged bed rest had resulted in poor trunk postural muscle endurance and a forward lean when standing. Visual and synergy dysfunctions, as well as stretch weakness, resulted in flexed-forward head position. Perception of vertical was abnormal as a result of perceptual abnormalities in the visual and somatosensory systems.

Watching P. H. walk generated the following hypothesis of what might be wrong.

Hypothesis 2

Inability to ambulate independently is probably to the result of perceptual problems affecting verticality, somatosensory loss, excessive gastrocnemius/soleus tone, or flexibility causing toe touch at initial contact and poor head and trunk control. Additionally, P. H. had poor fitness and endurance as a result of prolonged inactivity and a low tolerance level for difficult activities.

Impairments-Components

1. Strength: 3 to 4/5 strength levels in right leg except 2/5 in the gastrocnemius; 3/5 strength in left leg except 2/5 in the right gastrocnemius; trunk

extensors were 3/5. Strength is 3/5 in the extensors of the mid and lower trunk muscles and 3–/5 in cervical extensors.
2. Flexibility: Gastrocnemius is tight at neutral on the left. Fusion of right ankle at +5 degrees of dorsiflexion. Forward trunk flexion is limited to 50% of normal by tightness in the lumbar extensors.
3. Tone: Modified Ashworth 3 in the left quadriceps and gastrocnemius. The left lumbar extensors have above-normal tone and often elicit an extensor spasm during forward bending.
4. Endurance was poor in trunk and lower extremity muscles; there was a reduction in amount of resistance tolerated after approximately 10 repetitions with isolated muscle testing on the quadriceps, hip extensors, back extensors, biceps and cervical extensor muscles.
5. Sensory/perceptual systems: Light touch and proprioception was intact in the right lower extremity; proprioception was decreased (needs larger movement for accuracy) in the left ankle, knee, and hip. P. H. has a left hemianopsia. No nystagmus was present. P. H. complained of double vision with head motion. Additional vestibular testing deferred until client can stand independently. (Vision and vestibular systems are also addressed under the disability.) Left tilt off vertical 15 degrees in standing with eyes open and with eyes closed.
6. Postural disability: Unable to hold head up consistently; no head righting reflexes to tilts. P. H. stood with weight on left leg leaning about 15 degrees to the left. Kyphosis of lumbar spine.

Impairments-Complex

1. Balance synergies to large and small perturbations: Appear intact, as measured with sEMG in the right lower extremity, but ankle strategy is absent in the left.

   Small perturbations in balance are responded to with synergies showing a proximal-to-distal firing beginning in the trunk flexors and extensors. Occluding vision during normal standing does not change balance, and balance degrades only slightly when on foam. Amplitude of balance correction was small even for large perturbations.
2. Modification of synergies: Left lower extremity shows a poor ability to modify walking patterns, resulting in large-amplitude movements at the hip and knee during walking. The right lower extremity shows modification of the hip strategy for different surfaces. Interlimb coordination in the lower extremities is poor. Modification of upright balance is poor and does not occur with changing visual feedback.
3. Anticipatory responses were generally absent in the left lower extremity and trunk during standing as the right leg lifted because P. H. fell to the right or forward.

4. Use of feedback was evident when feedback occurred through the tactile or auditory systems. Use of visual feedback was poor in modification of walking because P. H. tripped over objects placed in front of her. There appeared to be poor ability to vary the movement pattern in the left lower extremity during balance and walking (in the parallel bars). Variability of response was present depending on verbal cues but not spontaneously present in response to environmental cues. The gait pattern was fairly fixed and P. H. used a steppage-type gait with increased flexion at the left hip and knee in swing and increased extension at the hip, knee, and ankle throughout stance regardless of surface conditions of firm versus soft or on angled surfaces.

5. Attention span was about 2 minutes during therapy.

Disabilities/Activity Limitations

Barthel ADL Index 9/20. Unable to walk independently, dependent all self-care.

Handicap

Immature behavior and inappropriate anger and self-destructive responses resulting in loss of friends and inability to hold a job.

EVALUATION AND DIAGNOSIS

P. H. appears unable to walk without moderate to maximum assistance because of a lack of appropriate balance synergies in response to perturbations and lack of anticipatory responses to movements of her center of gravity. Poor left gastrocnemius strength probably contributes to lack of ankle strategy. Poor quality of movement in the left leg is a result of somatosensory loss and inability to gradate force.

P. H. has problems perceiving the vertical position in sitting and standing because of visual and proprioceptive losses. She has poor muscular endurance from prolonged bed rest, slowed movement, and decreased activity level over months. Walking is with hip strategy of knees and hips bent owing to poor production of torque on floor by the gastrocnemius muscles and poor use of walking synergies so the pattern is inconsistent. Ambulation is also impaired by poor anticipatory responses during right swing leg movement.

PROGNOSIS

Long-term goals were independent ambulation without an assistive device at home and with a cane in the community, as well as independence in all self-care and ADLs. P. H. will be able to participate in activities with appropriate emotional responses (no episodes of scratching herself). Her prognosis for meeting the goals was good because P. H. was young, had a supportive family (sister and mother), and showed more focal lesions on MRI. The literature shows that problems of force production, flexibility, and ambulation modification in clients with brain injury have shown good modification. Decreasing the overall frustration level by working on achievable short-term goals and doing behavior modification should result in more appropriate emotional responses.

INTERVENTIONS

Initial goals included addressing those impairments in the basic component level that did not allow higher levels of functioning. These were improvements in neck and trunk strength and endurance; gastrocnemius strength and flexibility; visual skills, particularly in tracking of objects into the left visual field; and awareness of vertical. Functional electrical stimulation to the posterior cervical muscles, intermittent use of a supportive collar to take the extensor muscles off stretch, and eye fixation exercises to focus on a single point were used to encourage visual control of head position. A high, firm collar was worn intermittently early in the program to help recover strength in the neck extensors and prevent additional stretch weakness. Complex neck activities to encourage basic synergy use and modification included seated activities in which P. H. wore a "hat" with a flat top from which she tried to prevent an object from falling off (first flat stable objects and later more rounded objects). This exercise was performed first on a firm, flat-seated surface and progressed to sitting on an exercise ball. The ball promoted automatic neck muscle synergies in which the body moves and the head is kept upright and still.

Traditional basic left upper-extremity strengthening exercises included the use of Theraband. Functional activities that required scapular use such as emptying the dishwasher with the left hand were assigned homework.

Electrical stimulation twice a day for 15 minutes to the right triceps gained 20 degrees of extension and 100 degrees of flexion. In the clinic, P. H. worked on picking up and manipulating objects of different sizes and shapes, throwing balls at targets, and two-handed carrying with a laundry basket. She sorted different-sized objects by retrieving them from a bucket also containing marble-sized balls with her vision occluded to force the use of stereognosis.

P. H. enjoyed cooking, so tasks were given that used elbow extension, such as rolling cookie dough. Exercises such as washing the dishes with hands in soapy water for proprioceptive feedback and practice of slip grip for enhancement of feedback through the finger tips were used. Setting the table with the left hand helped establish better functional use (plastic dishes).

Doing two-hand activities facilitated complex functions in manipulation with the left arm. P. H. used large mats to hook a small rug, and she had a list, as mentioned earlier, of chores to do that required lifting and manipulating with both hands. When able, she began trying two-handed typing. Two of the most motivating activities were applying makeup and inserting contact lenses.

Visual treatment used exercises that required visual fixation at different points in space and at different distances using letters and objects, while moving her head left and right with the goal of seeing only one image. These exercises advanced to include moving objects and head moving with a fixed object and

Continued

CASE STUDY 17-2 ■ P. H.—cont'd

progressed to both the object and head moving while maintaining a single image. Finally, full body movement with eyes fixed on moving object was accomplished.

Standing balance with ball throwing was used to develop anticipatory responses once standing balance was established. Balance exercises such as swaying around the ankles, getting from kneeling to standing, and working on a force platform with visual feedback for attaining and feeling vertical were successful. Trunk control neurological reeducation exercises were started by having P. H. take a full step on each foot. Goals were to keep the light worn at her waist from moving more than 2 inches side to side on a wall target in front of her. This was also facilitated by moving the parallel bars extremely close together and asking P. H. not to touch the bars with either hip as she practiced stepping.

Exercises to promote trunk and anticipatory responses early on used a Gymnastik ball, as well as wrist-weighted reaching exercises, ball kicking to a goal, ball catching, and ball throwing to a target. P. H. practiced walking over and around various objects, both stable and moving.

Spasticity was addressed with exercises to promote less cocontraction and distal-to-proximal sequencing in both the left leg and left arm. sEMG with a two-channel setup on the triceps/biceps and wrist flexors/wrist extensors was used with a faded schedule of feedback to teach decreased cocontraction during activities such as reaching and lifting. This was carried over to the home program.

P. H. used a NordicTrack machine for general cardiovascular fitness work. The gliding motion with toe loops allowed her to keep her feet near the ground when moving forward, and the arm work encouraged free movement of the trunk in rotation.

A partial weight-bearing system on the treadmill starting with 70% weight bearing was instituted in the clinic. In gait practice, a video camera recording from behind was used to teach P. H. to lift her foot so that "she could see her sole on the left foot" from behind; this approach resulted in increased left knee flexion in her gait pattern.

The goal she had when first starting therapy was "to dance with my boyfriend." To encourage functional use of postural and balance synergies, dancing was used. She started first with slow dancing with her boyfriend. Gradually, she was able to dance to faster music without being held, by using trunk and arm motion and a sidestepping motion. Finally, forward-backward movements and turning and bending were added. Additionally, P. H. agreed to model in the brain injury association fashion show, which provided motivation to walk independently.

Home exercises were not popular with P. H. A behavioral modification program was established so that she was given control to stop activities that were too stressful for her; and she participated in a volunteer program on a farm feeding and watering animals two to three times a week on a fixed schedule to establish personal responsibility and provide a positive learning environment. A program of rewards and withholding of reward was established to extinguish self-destructive behavior. Verbal feedback was provided with discussion when immature behavior was exhibited.

P. H. kept a diary of duties and accomplishments to help with memory and reinforce successes.

Motor learning was enhanced by using a program of blocked feedback to start, progressing to random feedback as P. H. was able to tolerate higher frustration levels.

OUTCOMES

P. H. reached the goals of independent household ambulation and community ambulation. She had normal posture and good assistive and gross independent use of the left hand and arm. Tone in the left arm and left quadriceps was at a level 2 at discharge. She was independent in all grooming and all but the most difficult of ADLs. Barthel Index was 19/20. P. H. had no episodes of scratching herself and much higher tolerance for more difficult tasks. She continued to have some immature behaviors, but the work at the farm helped her to assess her own deficits better. She made friends, had a strong social life, and participated in a fashion show as a fundraiser activity for the Brain Injury Foundation.

ACKNOWLEDGMENT

Thank you to Susan Smith, PhD, PT, and the author of this chapter in the first edition, for information included in this chapter.

REFERENCES

1. Brain injury of America (Website): www.biausa.org. Accessed January 2005.
2. National Head Injury Foundation. Annual report, Seattle, WA, 1985.
3. Centers for Disease Control and Prevention (Website): www.cdc.gov. Accessed January 2005.
4. Colorado Head Injury Foundation, Inc [brochure], *Head injury*, Denver, CO, 1993.
5. Gurdjian ES, Hardy WG et al: Closed cervical cranial trauma associated with involvement of carotid and vertebral arteries, *J Neurosurg* 20:418-427, 1963.
6. Jennett B, Teasdale G: *Management of head injuries*, Philadelphia, 1981, FA Davis.
7. Adams JH, Graham D, Murray LS et al; Diffuse axonal injury due to non-missile head injury in humans: an analysis of 45 cases, *Ann Neurol* 12:557-563, 1982.
8. Strich S: Lesions in the cerebral hemispheres after blunt head injury, *J Clin Pathol* 12(suppl 4):166-171, 1970.
9. Gilroy J, Meyer J: *Medical neurology*, ed 3, New York, 1979, Macmillan.
10. Signorini DF, Andrews PJ, Jones PA et al: Adding insult to injury: the prognostic value of early secondary insults for survival after traumatic brain injury, *J Neurol Neurosurg Psychiatry* 66:26-31, 1999.
11. Brain Trauma Foundation Report: The use of barbiturates in the control of intracranial hypertension, *J Neurotrama* 13:711-714, 1996.

12. Cartlidge N, Shaw D: *Head injury,* London, 1981, WB Saunders.

13. Roberts A: Long-term prognosis of severe accidental head injury, *Proc R Soc Med* 69:137-141, 1976.

14. Plum F, Posner J: *The diagnosis of stupor and coma,* ed 3, Philadelphia, 1980, FA Davis.

15. Lezak M: Neuropsychological assessment. In *Executive functions and motor performance,* New York, 1983, Oxford Press.

16. Salcido R, Costich J: Recurrent traumatic brain injury, *Brain Inj* 11:391-402, 1997.

17. Jennett B, Plum F: Persistent vegetative state after brain damage: a syndrome in search of a name, *Lancet* 1:734-737, 1972.

18. Jennett B, Teasdale G: Aspects of coma after severe head injury, *Lancet* 1:878-881, 1977.

19. Rosin A: Very prolonged unresponsive state following brain injury, *Scand J Rehabil Med* 10:33-38, 1978.

20. Berrol S: The Walter J. Zieter lecture: consideration for management of persist vegetative state, *Arch Phys Med Rehabil* 67:283-285, 1986.

21. Ewert J, Levin H, Watson M: Procedural memory during post-traumatic amnesia in survivors of severe closed head injury, *Arch Neurol* 46:911-916, 1989.

22. Russell W: Cerebral involvement in head injury a study based on the examination of two hundred cases, *Tr Med-Chir Soc* Edinburgh, 25-36, 1931.

23. Squire L: Neural organization and behavior. In Mountcastle VBPE, Gaiger S, editors. *Handbook of physiology, vol 5,* pp 295-370, Bethesda, 1987, American Physiological Society.

24. Malik K, Hess DC: Evaluating the comatose patient: rapid neurologic assessment is key to appropriate management, *Postgraduate Medicine* 111:38-40, 2002.

25. Rosenthal M, Christensen B, Ross TP: Depression following traumatic brain injury [review], *Arch Phys Med Rehabil* 79:90-103, 1988.

26. Jennett B, Snoak J, Brooks N: Disability after severe head injury: observation of the use of the Glasgow Outcome Scale, *J Neurol Neurosurg Psychiatry* 44:285-293, 1981.

27. Kido DK, Cox C, Hamill RW et al: Traumatic brain injuries: Predictive usefulness of CT, *Radiology* 182:777-781, 1992.

28. Zimmerman RA, Bilaniuk LT, Genneralli T: Computed tomography of shearing injuries of the cerebral white matter, *Radiology* 127:393-396, 1978.

29. Snoek J, Jennett B, Adams JH et al: Computerized tomography after recent severe head injury in patients without acute intracranial hematoma, *J Neurol Neurosurg Psychiatry* 42:215-225, 1979.

30. Wedkind C, Fischbach R, Pakos P et al: Comparative use of magnetic resonance imaging and electrophysiologic investigation for the prognosis of head injury, *J Trauma Injury Infect Crit Care* 47:44-49, 1999.

31. Fulop Z Wright D, Stein D: Pharmacology of traumatic brain injury: experimental models and clinical implications, *Neurol Rep* 22:100-109, 1998.

32. Muizelaar J Marmarou A, Ward JD: Adverse effects of prolonged hyperventilation in patients with severe head injury: a randomized clinical trial, *J Neurosurg* 75:731-739, 1991.

33. Gentry R: Imaging of closed head injury, *Radiology* 191:1-17, 1994.

34. Dearden N, Gibson J, McDowall D: Effects of high-dose dexamethasone on outcome from severe head injury, *J Neurosurg* 64:81-88, 1986.

35. Chestnut R, Marshall L, Klauber M: The role of secondary brain injury in determining outcome from severe head injury, *J Trauma* 34:216-222, 1993.

36. Hagg T, Vahlsing H, Manthorpe M: Nerve growth factor infusion into the denervated adult rat hippocampal formation promotes cholinergic reinnervation, *J Neurosci* 10:3087-3092, 1990.

37. Young RR, Delwaide P: Drug therapy: spasticity (second of two parts), *N Engl J Med* 304:96-99, 1981.

38. Glenn MB, Wroblewski B: Update on pharmacology: antispasticity medications in the patient with traumatic brain injury, *J Head Trauma Rehab* 1:71, 1986.

39. Young RR, Delwaide P: Drug therapy: Spasticity, Part I, *N Engl J Med* 304:28-33, 1981.

40. Mysiw WJ, Sandel M: The agitated brain injured patient, part 2: pathophysiology and treatment, *Arch Phys Med Rehabil* 78:213-220, 1997.

41. Glenn M: Update on pharmacology: antispasticity medications in the patient with traumatic brain injury, I, *J Head Trauma Rehab,* 3:87, 1988.

42. Berger MS, Pitts LH, Lovely M et al: Outcome from severe head injury in children and adolescents, *J Neurosurg* 62:194-199, 1985.

43. Leahy BJ, Lam C: Neuropsychological testing and functional outcome for individuals with traumatic brain injury, *Brain Inj* 12:1025-1035, 1998.

44. Stewart WA, Litton SP, Sheehe PR et al: A prognostic model for head injury, *Acta Neurochir* 45:199, 1979.

45. Gilchrist E, Wilkinson M: Some factors determining prognosis in young people with severe head injuries, *Arch Neurol* 36:355-359, 1979.

46. Van der Naalt J, van Zomeren A, Sluiter WJ et al: One year outcome in mild to moderate head injury: the predictive value of acute injury characteristics related to complaints and return to work, *Neurol Neurosurg Psychiatry* 66:207-213, 1999.

47. Van der Naalt J, Hew JM, van Zomeren AH et al: Computed tomography and magnetic resonance imaging in mild to moderate head injury: early and late imaging related to outcome, *Ann Neurol* 46:70-78, 1999.

48. Kurth SM, Bigler ED, Blatter DD: Neuropsychological outcome and quantitative image analysis of acute hemorrhage in traumatic brain injury: preliminary findings, *Brain Inj* 8:489-500, 1994.

49. Kampfi A, Schmutzhard E, Pfausler B et al: Prediction of recovery from post-traumatic vegetative state with cerebral magnetic-resonance imaging, *Lancet* 351:1763-1767, 1998.

50. Black P, Markowitz RS, Cianci SN: Recovery of motor function after lesions in motor cortex of monkey. In Black P, editor: *Outcome of severe damage to the central nervous system,* New York, 1975, Elsevier.

51. Katz DI, Alexander M: Predicating course of recovery and outcome for patients admitted to rehabilitation, *Arch Neurol* 51:661-670, 1994.

52. Evans R: Predicting outcome following traumatic brain injury, *Neurol Rep* 22:144-148, 1998.

53. Bond M: Assessment of psychosocial outcome of severe head injury, *Acta Neurochir* 34:57-70, 1976.

54. Warren L, Wrigley J, Yoles W et al: Factors associated with life satisfaction among a sample of persons with neurotrauma, *J Rehabil Res Dev* 33:404-406, 1996.

55. Bernstein N: *Coordination and regulation of movements,* New York, 1967, Pergamon Press.

56. Payton O, Kelley D: Electromyographic evidence of the acquisition of motor skill: a pilot study, *Phys Ther* 52:261-266, 1987.

57. Sale D: Influence of exercise and training on motor unit activation, *Exerc Sport Sci Res* 15:95-151, 1987.

58. Carey J, Allison J, Manudale M: Electromyographic study of muscular overflow during precision handgrip, *Phys Ther* 63:505-511, 1983.

59. Deadwyler S, Hampson R: The significance of neural ensemble codes during behavior and cognition, *Annu Rev Neurosci* 20:217-244, 1997.

60. Nashner L: Organization and programming of motor activity during posture control, *Prog Brain Res* 50:177-184, 1979.

61. Georgopolos A: On reaching. *Annu Rev Neurosci* 9:147-170, 1986.

62. Gordan J: Anticipatory guidance from a motor control perspective. Paper presented at: Annual Sensorimotor Integration Symposium, San Diego, 1992.

63. Marteniuk RG, MacKenzie CL, Jeannerod M et al: Constraints on human arm movement trajectories, *Can J Psychol* 41:365-378, 1987.

64. Evarts E: Role of motor cortex in voluntary movements in primates. In Brookhart JM, Mountcastle VB, editors. *Handbook of physiology,*

the nervous system—motor control, Bethesda, MD, 1981, American Physiological Society.

65. Horak FB, Esselman P, Anderson ME et al: The effects of movement velocity, mass displaced, and task certainty on associated postural adjustments made by normal and hemiplegic individuals, *J Neurol Neurosurg Psychiatry* 47:1020-1028, 1984.

66. Johansson RS, Westling G: Signals in tactile afferents form the fingers eliciting adaptive motor responses during precision grip, *Exp Brain Res* 66:141-154, 1987.

67. Kelso J, Schoner G: Self-organization of coordinative movement patterns, *Hum Move Sci* 7:27-46, 1988.

68. Schoner G, Kelso J: Dynamic pattern generation in behavioral and neural systems, *Science* 239:1513-1520, 1988.

69. Giuliani CA: Theories of motor control. In Lister M, editor: *New concepts for physical therapy in contemporary management of motor control problems,* Alexandria, 1991, American Physical Therapy Association.

70. Byl N: The neural consequences of repetition, *Neurol Rep* 24:60-70, 2000.

71. Schmidt R: *Motor control and learning: a behavioral emphasis,* Champaign, IL, 1988, Human Kinetics.

72. Schmidt R: A schema theory of discrete motor learning, *Psychol Rev* 82:225-260, 1975.

73. Schmidt R: Motor learning principles for physical therapy. In Lister M, editor: *Contemporary management of motor control problems,* Alexandria, 1991, American Physical Therapy Association.

74. Newell K: Knowledge of results and motor learning, *Exerc Sport Sci Rev* 4:195-228, 1974.

75. Winstein CJ, Gardner ER, McNeal DR, Barto PS, Nicholson DE: Standing balance training: Effect on balance and locomotion in hemiparetic adults, *Arch Phys Med Rehabil* 70:755-762, 1989.

76. Man AM, Adams JA, Donchin E: Adaptive and part-whole training in the acquisition of a complex perceptual-motor skill, *Acta Psychol (Amsterdam)* 71:179-196, 1989.

77. Newell KM, Carlton MJ, Fisher AT et al: Whole-part training strategies for learning the response dynamics of microprocessor driven simulator, *Acta Psychol (Amsterdam)* 71:197-216, 1989.

78. American Physical Therapy Association: *Guide to physical therapist practice, vol 81,* Alexandria, VA, 2001, The Association.

79. Shumway-Cook A, Horak, F: Assessing the influence of sensory interaction on balance, *Phys Ther* 66:1548-1550, 1986.

80. World Health Organization: *International Classification of Impairments, Disabilities and Handicaps,* Geneva, 1980, World Health Organization.

80a. World Health Organization: *International Classification of Functioning, Disability and Health.* Geneva, Switzerland: World Health Organization; 2002: http://www3.who.int/icf/beginners/bg.pdf. Accessed May 2003.

81. Johnson D, Almi C: Age, brain damage and performance. In Finger S, editor: *Recovery for brain damage,* New York, 1978, Plenum Press.

82. Kondraske GV, Jafari M, Carollo JJ: Human performance measurement: some perspectives, *IEEE Eng Med Biol Soc* 7:11-16, 1988.

83. Olney S, Costigan PA, Hedden DM: Mechanical energy patterns in gait of cerebral palsied children with hemiplegia, *Phys Ther* 67:1348-1354, 1987.

84. Perry J, Ireland M, Gronley J et al: Predictive value of manual muscle testing and gait analysis in normal ankles by dynamic electromyography, *Foot Ankle* 6:254-259, 1986.

85. Sahrmann S: Diagnosis by the physical therapist—a prerequisite for treatment: a special communication, *Phys Ther* 68:1703-1706, 1988.

86. Heinemann A: Functional states and therapeutic intervention during rehabilitation, *Am J Phys Med Rehabil* 74:315-326, 1995.

87. Wechsler D: *Wechsler memory scale—revised,* San Antonio, 1987, Psychological Corp.

88. Cecchini A: Functional assessment after traumatic brain injury, *Neurol Rep* 22:136-143, 1998.

89. Levin H, O'Donnell DV, Grossman R: The Galveston Orientation and Amnesia Test: a practical scale to assess cognition after head injured, *J Nerv Ment Dis* 167:675-684, 1979.

90. Folstein M, Folstein S, McHugh P: Mini-mental: a practical method for grading the cognitive state of patients for the clinician, *J Psychiatr Res* 12:189-198, 1975.

91. Carr J, Shepherd R: *Neurological rehabilitation, optimizing motor performance,* Woburn, 1999, Butterworh Heinemann.

92. Wade D: *Measurement in neurological rehabilitation,* New York, 1992, Oxford University Press.

93. Mahoney FI, Barthel D: Functional evaluation: the Barthel Index, *Md State Med J* 14:61-65, 1965.

94. Granger C, Hamilton B, Keith R: Advances in functional assessment for medical rehabilitation, *Top Geriatr Rehabil* 1:59-71, 1986.

95. Functional assessment measure, *J Rehabil Outcome Meas* 1:63-65, 1991.

96. Rappaport M, Hall KM, Hopkins K et al: Disability rating scale for severe head trauma: coma to community, *Arch Phys Med Rehabil* 63:118-123, 1982.

97. Weber K, Kashner L: Adult norms in nine hole peg test of finger dexterity, *Occup Ther J Res* 5:24-37, 1986.

98. DeSouza L, Langton T, Miller S: Assessment and recovery of arm control in hemiplegic stroke patients: Arm Function Test, *Int Rehab Med* 2:3-9, 1984.

99. Carr J, Sherperd R: Investigation of new motor assessment scale for stroke patients, *Phys Ther* 65:175-180, 1985.

100. Buchner D, deLatuer B: The importance of skeletal muscle strength in physical function in older adults, *Ann Behav Med* 13:12-21, 1991.

101. Dietz V, Ketelsen UP, Berger W et al: Motor unit involvement in spastic paresis: Relationship between leg muscle activation and histochemistry, *J Neurol Sci* 75:89-103, 1986.

102. Edstrom L, Grimby L, Hannerz J: Correlation between recruitment order of motor units and muscle atrophy pattern in upper motorneurone lesion: significance of spasticity, *Experientia* 29:560-561, 1973.

103. Rose SJ, Rothstein J: Muscle mutability, I: general concepts and adaptations to altered patterns of use, *Phys Ther* 62:1773-1787, 1982.

104. Rosenfalck A, Anderssen S: Impaired regulation and firing pattern of single motor units in patients with spasticity, *J Neurol Neurosurg Psychiatry* 43:907-916, 1980.

105. Tang A, Rymer W: Abnormal force-EMG relations in paretic limbs of hemiparetic human subjects, *J Neurol Neurosurg Psychiatry* 44:690-698, 1981.

106. Sahrmann S: Posture and muscle imbalance: faulty lumbar-pelvic alignment and associated musculoskeletal pain syndromes. In *Post-graduate advances in physical therapy: a comprehensive independent learning office study course,* Alexandria, VA, 1987, American Physical Therapy Association.

107. Watkins MP, Harris BA, Kozlowski BA: Isokinetic testing in patients with hemiparesis: a pilot study, *Phys Ther* 64:184-189, 1984.

108. Tardieu C, Lespargot A, Tabary C et al: For how long must the soleus muscle be stretched daily to prevent contracture? *Dev Med Child Neurol* 30:3-10, 1988.

109. Lindboe CF, Platou C: Effect of immobilization of short duration on the muscle fibre size, *Clin Physiol* 4:183-188, 1984.

110. Bourbonnais D, Vanden Noven S, Carey K et al: Abnormal spatial patterns of elbow activation in hemiparetic human subjects, *Brain* 112:85-102, 1989.

111. Craik R: Abnormalities of motor behavior. In Lister M, editor: *Contemporary management of motor control problems,* Alexandria, VA, 1991, American Physical Therapy Association.

112. Dietz V, Berger W: Interlimb coordination of posture in patients with spastic paresis: Imperial functions of spinal reflexes, *Brain* 107:965-978, 1984.

113. Knutsson E, Martensson A: Dynamic motor capacity in spastic paresis and its relationship to prime motor dysfunction, spastic reflexes and antagonistic coactivation, *Scand J Rehabil Med* 12:93-106, 1980.

114. Sahrmann SA, Norton B: The relationship of voluntary movement to spasticity in the upper motor neuron syndrome, *Ann Neurol* 2:460-465, 1977.

115. Bohannon R, Smith M: Interrater reliability of a modified Ashworth scale of muscle spasticity, *Phys Ther* 67:206-207, 1987.

116. Golani I, Fentress J: Early ontogeny of face grooming in mice, *Dev Psychobiol* 18:529-544, 1985.

117. Gandevia S: Spinal and supraspinal factors in human muscle fatigue, *Neurol Rev* 81:1725-1789, 2001.

118. Gandevia S: Neural control and muscle fatigue: changes in muscle afferents, moto neurons and moto cortical drive, *Scand Physiol Soc* 162:275-283, 1998.

119. World Health Organization: The 3-step ergometer test. In *The Future Fitness Measurement Guide,* Geneva, Switzerland, 1972, World Health Organization.

120. Astrand P: Quantification of exercise capacity and evaluation of physical capacity in man, *Prog Cardiovasc Dis* 19:51-67, 1976.

121. Bruce R: Exercise testing of patients with coronary artery disease, *Ann Clin Res* 3:323-332, 1971.

122. Matsushima M, Hironan S, Narumiya, M et al: Quantitative evaluation of Semmes-Weinstein Monofilament Pressure Perception Test in comparison with nerve conduction velocity, *Diabetes* 49:A196-197, 2000.

123. Smith-Weelock M, Shepard N, Telian SA: Physical therapy program for vestibular rehabilitation, *Am J Otol* 12:218-225, 1991.

124. VanSant AE: Rising from a supine position to erect stance: description of adult movement and a developmental hypothesis, *Phys Ther* 68:185-192, 1988.

125. Thelen E: Evolving and dissolving synergies in the development of leg coordination. In Wallace SA, editor: *Perspectives on the coordination of movement,* New York, 1991, Elsevier.

126. Badke MB, Duncan P: Patterns of rapid motor response during postural adjustment when standing in healthy subjects and hemiplegic patients, *Phys Ther* 63:13-20, 1983.

127. Tinniti M: Performance oriented assessment of mobility: problems in elderly patients, *J Am Geriatr Soc* 34:119-126, 1986.

128. Wolfson L, Whipple R, Amernan P et al: Gait assessment in the elderly: a gait abnormality rating scale and its relationship to falls, *J Gerontol* 45:m12-m19, 1990.

129. Perry J: *Gait analysis: Normal and pathological function,* Thorofare, NJ, 1992, Slack.

130. Butland J, Pang J, Gross E: Two-six and 12 minute walking tests in respiratory disease, *BMJ* 284:1607-1608, 1982.

131. Bach-y-Rita P: Brain plasticity as a basis for therapeutic procedures. In Bach-y-Rita P, editor: *Recovery of function: theoretical considerations for brain injury rehabilitation,* Baltimore, 1980, University Park Press.

132. Bach-y-Rita P: Brain injury, *Wall Street J* 1993.

133. Hubel DH, Wiesel T: The period of susceptibility to the physiological effects of unilateral eye closure in kittens, *J Physiol* 206:419-436, 1970.

134. Wiesel TN, Hubel D: Single-cell responses in striate cortex of kittens deprived of vision in one eye, *J Neurophysiol* 26:1003-1017, 1963.

135. Wiesel TN, Hubel D: Comparison of the effects of unilateral and bilateral eye closure on cortical unit responses in kittens, *J Neurophysiol* 28:1029-1040, 1965.

136. Devor M, Wall P: Dorsal horn cells with proximal cutaneous receptor fields, *Brain Res* 118:325-328, 1976.

137. Mitchell DE, Cynader M, Movshon JA: Recovery from the effects of monocular deprivation, *J Comp Neurol* 176:53-63, 1977.

138. Wolf SL, Lecraw DE, Barton LA et al: Forced use of hemiplegic upper extremities to reverse the effect of learned nonuse among stroke and head-injured patients, *Exp Neurol* 104:125-132, 1989.

139. Taub E, Miller NE, Novack TA et al: Technique to improve chronic motor deficit after stroke, *Arch Phys Med Rehabil* 74:347-354, 1993.

140. Tower S: Pyramidal lesions in the monkey, *Brain* 63:36-90, 1940.

141. Jones T, Chu C, Grande L et al: Motor skills training enhances lesion-inducted structural plasticity in the motor cortex of adult rats, *J Neurosci* 19:10153-10163, 1999.

142. Jones T, Schallert T: Use-dependent growth of pyramidal neurons after neocortical damage, *J Neurosci* 14:2140-2152, 1994.

143. Liepert J, Bauder H, Miltner W et al: Treatment-induced cortical reorganization after stroke in humans, *Stroke* 31:1210-1216, 2000.

144. Held R: Plasticity in sensory-motor systems, *Sci Am* 213:84-94, 1967.

145. Sullivan K, Knowlton B, Dobkin B: Step training with body weight support: Effect of treadmill speed and practice paradigms on post-stroke locomotor recovery, *Arch Phys Med Rehabil* 83:683-691, 2002.

146. Barbeau H, Norman K, Fung J et al: Does neurorehabilitation play a role in the recovery of walking in neurological populations? *Ann N Y Acad Sci* 860:377-392, 1998.

147. Porro C, Francescato MP, Cettolo V et al: Primary motor and sensory cortex activation during motor performance and motor imagery: a functional magnetic resonance imaging study, *J Neurosci* 16:7688-7698, 1996.

148. Nudo RJ, Plautz E, Frost SB: Role of adaptive plasticity in recovery of function after damage to motor cortex, *Muscle Nerve* 24:1000-1019, 2001.

149. Winstein C: Knowledge of results and motor learning: implications for physical therapy. In *Movement science, a monograph of the American Physical Therapy Association,* Alexandria, VA, 1991, American Physical Therapy Association.

150. Springer J, Farne J, Bower D: Common misconceptions about traumatic brain injury among family members of rehabilitation patients, *J Head Trauma Rehabil* 12:41-50, 1997.

151. Baatile J, Lanbein W, Weaver F et al: Effect of exercise on perceived quality of life of individuals with Parkinson's disease, *J Rehabil Res Dev* 37:529-534, 2000.

152. Fordyce D, Starnes J, Farrar R: Compensation of the age-related decline in hippocampal muscarinic receptor density through daily exercise or underfeeding, *J Geronotol* 46:B245-B248, 1991.

153. Clamann P: Motor unit recruitment and the gradation of muscle force, *Phys Ther* 73:830-843, 1993.

154. Benton L, Baker LL, Bowman BR et al: *Functional electrical stimulation: a practical clinical guide,* ed 2, Downey, CA, 1981, Rancho Los Amigos Rehabilitation Engineering Center.

155. Baker LL, Parker K: Neuromuscular electrical stimulation for the head injured patient, *Phys Ther* 63:1967-1974, 1983.

156. Wolf S, Baker M, Kerry JL: EMG biofeedback in stroke: effects of patient characteristics, *Arch Phys Med Rehabil* 60:69-102, 1979.

157. Colborne GR, Olney S, Griffin MP: Feedback of ankle joint angle and soleus electromyography in the rehabilitation of hemiplegic gait, *Arch Phys Med Rehabil* 74:1100-1106, 1993.

158. Bohannon R, Smith MB: Assessment of strength deficits in eight paretic upper extremity muscle groups of stroke patients with hemiplegia, *Phys Ther* 67:522-524, 1987.

159. Gossman R, Rose S, Sahrmann S et al: Length and circumference measures in one-joint and multijoint muscles in rabbits after immobilization, *Phys Ther* 66:516-520, 1986.

160. Winkler P: Use of the Sandune in exercise of multiple sclerosis patients [unpublished data], 1994.

161. Shepard N, Telian S: Vestibular and balance rehabilitation therapy, *Ann Otol Rhinol Laryngol* 102:198-205, 1993.

162. Konrad H, Tomlinson D, Stockwell CW et al: Rehabilitation therapy for patients with disequilibrium and balance disorders, *Otolaryngol Head Neck Surg* 107:105-108, 1992.

163. Branch L, Meyers A: Assessment of physical function in the elderly, *Clin Geriatr Med* 3:29-51, 1987.

164. Cintas H: The relationship of motor skill level and risk-taking during exploration in toddlers, *Pediatr Phys Ther* 165:59-63, 1992.

165. Cozean C, Pease WS, Hubbell SL: Biofeedback and functional electric stimulation in stroke rehabilitation, *Arch Phys Med Rehabil* 69:401-405, 1988.

166. Winstein CJ, Pohl P, Lewthwaite R: Effects of physical guidance and knowledge of results on motor learning: support for the guidance hypothesis, *Res Q Exerc Sport* 65:316-323, 1994.

167. Milczarek J, Kirby L, Harrison E et al: Standard and four-footed canes: their effect on the standing balance of patients with hemiparesis, *Arch Phys Med Rehabil* 74:281-285, 1993.

168. Hain TC, Fuller L, Weil L et al: Effects of T'ai Chi on balance, *Arch Otolaryngol Head Neck Surg* 125:1191-1195, 1999.

169. Leahy P: Head trauma in adults: Problems, assessment, and treatment. In Lister M, editor: *Contemporary management of motor control problems: Proceeding of II Step Conference,* pp 247- 252, Alexandria, VA, 1991, American Physical Therapy Association.

170. Brotherton FA, Thomas LL, Wisotzek IE et al: Social skills training in the rehabilitation of patients with traumatic closed head injury, *Arch Phys Med Rehabil* 69:827-832, 1988.

CHAPTER 18 Congenital Spinal Cord Injury

Kristin J. Krosschell, PT, MA, PCS
Mari Jo Pesavento, PT, PCS

KEY WORDS

Chiari malformation
crouch-control ankle-foot orthosis
diastematomyelia
hydrocephalus
lipomeningocele
myelodysplasia
myelomeningocele
reciprocating gait orthosis
sacral agenesis
spina bifida cystica
spina bifida occulta
standing A-frame
tethered spinal cord

OBJECTIVES

After reading this chapter the student/therapist will be able to:

1. Identify the various types of spina bifida.
2. Recognize the incidence and etiology of spina bifida.
3. Identify the clinical manifestations of myelomeningocele, including neurological, orthopedic, and urological sequelae.
4. Comprehend medical management in the newborn period and beyond.
5. Determine physical and occupational therapy evaluations, including manual muscle testing, range of motion, sensory testing, reflex testing, developmental and functional assessments, and perceptual and cognitive evaluations.
6. List the major physical and occupational therapy goals and appropriate therapeutic management for each of the following stages: (a) before surgical closure of sac, (b) after surgery during hospitalization, (c) preambulatory, (d) toddler through preschool age, and (e) primary school through adolescence.
7. Identify psychological adjustment to congenital spinal cord injury.

A spinal cord injury is a complex disability. When a spinal cord lesion exists from birth, an additional complexity is added. This congenital condition predisposes that many areas of the central nervous system (CNS) may not develop or function adequately. In addition, all areas of development (physical, cognitive, and psychosocial) that depend so heavily on central functioning will likely be impaired. The clinician therefore must be aware of the significant impact this neurological defect has on motor function as well as a variety of related human capacities.

A developmental framework and The Guide to Physical Therapy[1] have been used to aid in understanding the sequential problems of the child with spina bifida. The developmental model, however, must always stay in line with the functional model for adult trauma because the problems of the congenitally involved child grow quickly into limitations in functional activities and participation in life of the injured adult. With concentration on the present but with an eye to the future, appropriate management goals can be achieved.

OVERVIEW OF CONGENITAL SPINAL CORD INJURY

A congenital spinal cord lesion occurs in utero and is present at the time of birth. Understanding how this malformation develops requires an appreciation of normal nervous system maturation. The nervous system develops from a portion of embryonic ectoderm called the neural plate. During gestation, the neural plate develops folds that begin to close, forming the neural tube (Figure 18-1). The neural tube differentiates into the CNS, which is composed of brain and spinal cord tissue.[2] In the normal embryo, neural tube closure begins in the cervical region and proceeds cranially and caudally. Closure is generally complete by the twenty-sixth day.[2]

Types of Spina Bifida

Spina bifida involves a defect in the neural tube closure and the overlying posterior vertebral arches. The extent of the defect may result in one of two types of spina bifida: occulta or cystica. Spina bifida occulta is characterized by a failure of one or more of the vertebral arches to meet and fuse in the third month of development. The spinal cord and meninges are unharmed and remain within the vertebral canal (Figure 18-2). The bony defect is covered with skin that may be marked by a dimple, pigmentation, or patch of hair.[3] The common site for this defect is the lumbosacral area, and it is usually associated with no disturbance of neurological or musculoskeletal functioning.[4] Spina bifida cystica results when the neural and overlying vertebral arches fail to close appropriately. Cystic protrusion of the meninges or the spinal cord and meninges is present through the defective vertebral arches.

The milder form of spina bifida cystica, called meningocele, involves protrusion of the meninges and cerebrospinal fluid (CSF) only into the cystic sac (see Figure 18-2, *B*). The spinal cord remains within the vertebral canal, but it may exhibit abnormalities.[5] Clinical signs vary (according to spinal cord anomalies) or may not be apparent. This is a relatively uncommon form of spina bifida cystica.

A more severe form of spina bifida cystica, called myelocele or myelocystocele, is present when the central canal

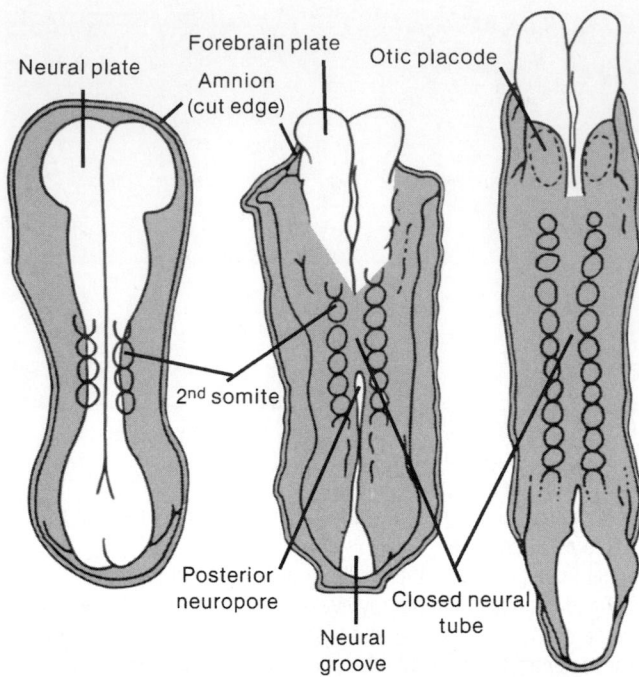

FIGURE 18-1 ■ Neural tube forming. (From Stark GD: *Spina bifida problems and management,* London, 1977, Blackwell Scientific.)

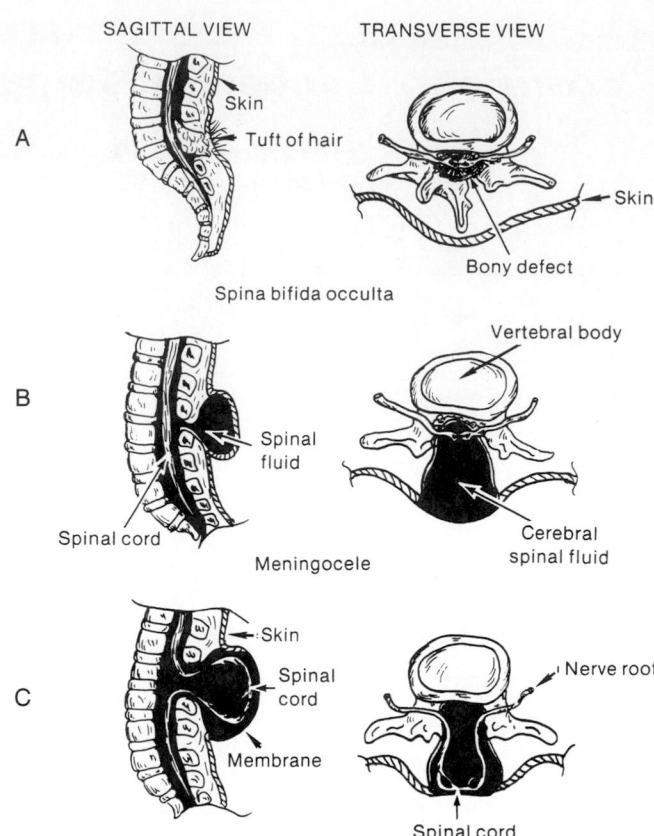

FIGURE 18-2 ■ Types of spina bifida. **A,** Spina bifida occulta. **B,** Meningocele. **C,** Myelomeningocele. (From McLone DG: *An introduction to spina bifida,* Chicago, 1980, Northwestern University.)

of the spinal cord is dilated, producing a large, skin-covered cyst. The neural tube appears to close normally but is distended from the cystic swelling. The CSF may ceaselessly expand the neural canal. Prompt medical attention is mandatory. This form of spina bifida is also rare.[6]

The more common and severe form of the defect is known as myelomeningocele, in which both spinal cord and meninges are contained in the cystic sac (see Figure 18-2, *C*). Within the sac, the spinal cord and associated neural tissue show extensive abnormalities. In incomplete closure of the neural tube (dysraphism), abnormal growth of the cord and a tortuous pathway of neural elements make normal transmission of nervous impulses abnormal. The result is a variable sensory and motor impairment at the level of the lesion and below.[3] In an open myelomeningocele, nerve roots and spinal cord may be exposed with dura and skin evident at the margin of the lesion.

Although spina bifida cystica can occur at any level of the spinal cord, myelomeningoceles are most common in the thoracic and lumbosacral regions. Myelomeningocele occurs in 94% of the cases of spina bifida cystica, and two thirds of open lesions involve the thoracolumbar junction.[3] The terms *spina bifida, myelodysplasia,* and *myelomeningocele* are frequently used interchangeably.[5]

Other forms of spinal dysraphism include diastematomyelia, lipomeningocele, and sacral agenesis. Diastematomyelia is present in 30% to 40% of patients with myelomeningocele and is secondary to partial or complete clefting of the spinal cord.[7] Lipomeningocele, another form of spina bifida cystica, is usually caused by a vertebral defect associated with a superficial fatty mass (lipoma or fatty tumor) that merges with the lower level of spinal cord. No associated hydrocephalus is present, and neurological deficit

is generally minimal; however, problems with urinary control and motor control of the lower extremities may be noted.[8] Neurological tissue invasion may be caused by a tethered spinal cord; therefore early lipoma resection is indicated for cosmesis and to minimize neurological sequelae. Lumbosacral or sacral agenesis may occur and is caused by an absence of the caudal part of the spine and sacrum. Children with this form of dysraphism may present with narrow, flattened buttocks, weak gluteal muscles, and a shortened intergluteal cleft. The normal lumbar lordosis is absent, although the lower lumbar spine may be prominent. Calf muscles may be atrophic or absent. The pelvic ring is completed with either direct opposition of the iliac bones or with interposition of the lumbar spine replacing the absent sacrum. These children may have scoliosis, motor and sensory loss and visceral abnormalities including anal atresia, fused kidneys, and congenital heart malformations. Management is started early and is symptomatic for each system.[9]

Failure of fusion of the cranial end of the neural tube results in a condition known as anencephaly. In this condition, some brain tissue may be evident, but forebrain development is usually absent.[4] Sustained life is not possible with this neural tube defect; therefore this condition is not discussed further.

Incidence and Etiology

Statistics about the incidence of spina bifida vary considerably in different parts of the world. In the United States the incidence is approximately 2 per 1000 births.[10] This is about midrange in world statistics, considering a spina bifida birth rate of 0.3 per 1000 in Japan and 4.5 per 1000 in certain parts of the British Commonwealth. Some evidence of seasonal variation exists, suggesting a positive relation between the occurrence of spina bifida and conceptions in March to May.[3,11,12]

Spina bifida is thought to be more common in females than in males, although some studies suggest no real sex difference.[5,13] The incidence of spina bifida is higher in those of Celtic origin and lower in Blacks and Asians.[11,14] A study of the association of race and sex with different neurological levels of myelomeningocele reported the proportions of whites and females to be significantly higher in thoracic level patients.[6] A significant relation also has been noted between social class and spina bifida: the lower the social class, the higher the incidence.[15,16]

Genetic factors seem to influence the occurrence of spina bifida. The chances of having a second affected child are between 1% and 2%, whereas in the general population the percentage drops to one fifth of 1%.[17,18] Although these factors are related to the incidence of spina bifida, the cause of this defect remains in question. Environmental conditions, such as hyperthermia in the first weeks of pregnancy, or dietary factors, such as canned meats, potatoes, or tea, have been implicated but not substantiated.[11,19,20] In addition, nutritional deficiencies, such as folic acid and vitamin A, have been implicated as a cause of primary neural tube defects.[21-24] Approximately 50% to 70% of neural tube defects can be prevented if a woman of childbearing age consumes sufficient folic acid daily before conception and throughout the first trimester of pregnancy. As a result of research findings in support of folic acid implementation, the United States Public Health Service has mandated folic acid fortification as a public health strategy. Genetic considerations, such as an Rh blood type, a specific gene type (HLA-B27), an X-linked gene, and variations in the many folate pathway genes have been implicated, but not conclusively.[25-27] Malformations are attributed to abnormal interaction of several regulating and modifying genes in early fetal development.[28] Environmental factors combined with genetic predisposition appear to trigger the development of spina bifida, although definitive evidence is not available to support this claim.[3,14,29]

The incidence of spina bifida has declined with the advent of amniocentesis. The presence of significant levels of alpha-fetoprotein in the amniotic fluid has led to the detection of large numbers of affected fetuses.[30] Currently, maternal serum alpha-fetoprotein levels have been effective in detecting approximately 80% of neural tube defects.[31] Prenatal screening can be most effective when a combination of serum levels, amniocentesis/amniography, and ultrasonography is used.[32-34] Although this screening is not yet performed routinely, it is suggested for those at risk for the defect. Knowledge of the defect allows for preparation for cesarean birth and immediate postnatal care. This includes mobilization of the interdisciplinary team who will continue to care for the child. For parents who decide to carry an involved fetus to term, adjustment to their child's disability can begin before birth, which includes mobilizing their own support system. Education from an integrated team regarding what will follow after delivery and neurosurgical closure is imperative to aid families in decision making and to allow families to assess and understand the child's disability and future care options.

Other advances in the field of prenatal medicine that affect spina bifida management and outcome include the in utero treatment of hydrocephalus and the in utero surgical repair to close the myelomeningocele. Treatment such as this, in conjunction with prenatal diagnosis, has been shown to have a positive impact on the incidence and severity of complications associated with spina bifida.[35-42] Limitations of current postnatal treatment strategies and considerations of prenatal treatment options continue to be explored. Ethics, timing of repair, and surgical procedures are all being investigated. In addition, continued assessment of outcomes from those who have undergone presurgical management requires continued exploration. The Management of Myelomeningocele Study (MOMS) was initiated in 2003 and is a large randomized, clinical trial that has been designed to compare both approaches to the treatment of infants with spina bifida (prenatal or fetal surgery and postnatal surgery) to determine if one approach is better than the other. An expected result of this study is the ability to better answer the question as to which treatment approach is most effective in management of the infant with myelomeningocele.[43]

Clinical Manifestations

The most obvious clinical manifestation of myelomeningocele is the loss of sensory and motor functions in the lower limbs. The extent of loss, while primarily dependent on the degree of the spinal cord abnormality, is secondarily dependent on a number of factors. These include the amount of traction or stretch resulting from the abnormally tethered spinal cord, the trauma to exposed neural tissue during delivery, and postnatal damage resulting from drying or infection of the neural plate.[3] Specific clinical impairments that commonly lead to functional limitations for the child with spina bifida are addressed in this section.

Sensory Impairment
Children with spina bifida have impaired sensation below the level of the lesion. The loss often does not match exactly the level of the lesion and needs to be carefully assessed. Sensory loss includes kinesthetic, proprioceptive, and somatosensory information. Because of this, children will often have to rely heavily on vision and other sensory systems to substitute for this loss.

Musculoskeletal Impairment
Weakness and Paralysis. Determining neurological involvement is not as straightforward as assumed. At birth, two main types of motor dysfunction in the lower extremities have been identified. The first type involves a complete loss of function below the level of the lesion, resulting in a flaccid paralysis, loss of sensation, and absent reflexes.[3,11] The extent of involvement can be determined by comparing the level of lesion with a chart delineating the segmental innervation of the lower limb muscles. Orthopedic defor-

mities may result from the unopposed action of muscles above the level of lesion. This unopposed pull commonly leads to hip flexion, knee extension, and ankle dorsiflexion contractures.

When the spinal cord remains intact below the level of lesion, the effect is an area of flaccid paralysis immediately below the lesion and possible hyperactive spinal reflexes distal to that area.[3,11] This condition is quite similar to the neurological state of the severed cord seen in traumatic injury. This second type of neurological involvement again results in orthopedic deformities, depending on the level of the lesion, the spasticity present, and the muscle groups involved.

Orthopedic Deformities. The orthopedic problems seen in myelomeningocele may be the result of (1) the imbalance between muscle groups; (2) the effects of stress, posture, and gravity; and (3) associated congenital malformations. Decreased sensation and neurological complications also may lead to orthopedic abnormalities.[44]

Besides the obvious malformation of vertebrae at the site of the lesion, hemivertebrae and deformities of other vertebral bodies and their corresponding ribs also may be present.[11,44,45] A lumbar kyphosis may be present as a result of the original deformity. In addition, as a result of the bifid vertebral bodies, the misaligned pull of the extensor muscles surrounding the deformity, as well as the unopposed flexor muscles, contribute further to the lumbar kyphosis. As the child grows, the weight of the trunk in the upright position also may be a contributing factor.[11,45] Scoliosis may be present at birth because of vertebral abnormalities or may become evident as the child grows older. The incidence of scoliosis is lower in low lumbar or sacral level deformities.[45,46] Scoliosis may also be neurogenic, secondary to weakness or asymmetrical spasticity of paraspinal muscles, tethered cord syndrome, or hydromyelia.[36] Lordosis or lordoscoliosis is often found in the adolescent and is usually associated with hip flexion deformities and a large spinal defect.[5,11,45] Many of these trunk and postural deformities exist at birth but are exacerbated by the effects of gravity as the child grows. They can compromise vital functions (cardiac and respiratory) and therefore should be closely monitored by the therapist and the family.

As has been alluded to previously, the type and extent of deformity in the lower extremities depend on the muscles that are active or inactive. In a total flaccid paralysis, in utero deformities may be present at birth, resulting from passive positioning within the womb. Equinovarus (clubfoot) and "rocker-bottom" deformity are two of the most common foot abnormalities. Knee flexion and extension contractures also may be present at birth. Other common deformities are hip flexion, adduction, and internal rotation, usually leading to a subluxed or dislocated hip.[11] Although many of these problems may be present at birth, preventing positional deformity (such as the frog-leg position), which may result from improper positioning of flaccid extremities, is of the utmost importance. Orthopedic care varies throughout the course of the child's life. Changes in clinical orthopedic management have evolved to establish evidence-based interventions.[47]

Osteoporosis. Because the paralyzed limbs of the child with spina bifida have increased amounts of unmineralized

osteoid tissue, they are prone to fractures, particularly after periods of immobilization.[48,49] Early mobilization and weight bearing can aid in decreasing osteoporosis.[45,50] Fortunately, these fractures heal quickly with appropriate medical management.

Neurological Impairment

Hydrocephalus. Hydrocephalus develops in 80% to 90% of children with myelomeningocele.[14,18,51] Hydrocephalus results from a blockage of the normal flow of CSF between the ventricles and spinal canal. The most obvious effect of the buildup of CSF is abnormal increase in head size, which may be present at birth because of the great compliance of the cranial sutures in the fetus, or it may develop postnatally.[52] Other signs of hydrocephalus include bulging fontanelles and irritability. Internally, a concomitant dilation of the lateral ventricles and thinning of the cerebral white matter are usually present. Without reduction of the buildup of CSF, increased brain damage and death may result.

Chiari Malformation. Patients with myelomeningocele have a 99% chance of having an associated Chiari II malformation.[7] This malformation is a congenital anomaly of the hindbrain that involves herniation of the medulla and at times the pons, fourth ventricle, and inferior aspect of the cerebellum into the upper cervical canal. The herniation usually occurs between C1 and C4 but may extend down to T1.[7,53,54] Not all Chiari II malformations are symptomatic. As a result of a symptomatic Chiari malformation, problems with respiratory and bulbar function may be evident in the child with spina bifida.[3,11,14] Paralysis of the vocal cords occurs in a small percentage of patients and is associated with respiratory stridor. Apneic episodes also may be evident, although their direct cause remains in question. Children with spina bifida also may exhibit difficulty in swallowing and have an abnormal gag reflex.[3] Problems with aspiration, weakness and cry, and upper-extremity weakness also may be present in children with a symptomatic Chiari II malformation.[55,56] Thus, depending on the orthopedic deformities present and the neurological involvement, severe respiratory involvement is possible in the affected child. These symptoms may be caused by significant compression of the hindbrain structures or dysplasia of posterior fossa contents, which can also occur in patients with Chiari II malformation.[7,57] This complex hindbrain malformation is a common cause of death in children with myelomeningocele despite surgical intervention and aggressive medical management.[58] Other common neurological problems for children with spina bifida include hydromyelia and tethered cord.

Hydromyelia. Between 20% and 80% of patients with myelomeningocele have hydromyelia.[59-61] Hydromyelia signifies dilation of the center canal of the spinal cord as hydrocephalus signifies dilation of the ventricles of the brain. The area of hydromyelia may be focal, multiple, or diffuse, extending throughout the spinal cord. The hydromyelia may be a consequence of untreated or inadequately treated hydrocephalus with resultant transmission of CSF through the obex into the central canal, with distention a result of increased hydrostatic pressure from above.[7] The increased collection of fluid may cause pressure necrosis of the spinal cord, leading to muscle weakness and scoliosis.[62] Common symptoms of hydromyelia include rapidly progressive scoliosis, upper-extremity weakness, spasticity, and ascending motor loss in the lower extremities.[7,63] Aggressive treatment of hydromyelia at the onset of clinical signs of increasing scoliosis is mandatory and may lead to improvement in or stabilization of the curve in 80% of cases. Surgical interventions may include revision of a CSF shunt, posterior cervical decompression, or a central canal to pleural cavity shunt with a flushing device.[7,57]

Tethered Cord. Tethered spinal cord is defined as a pathological fixation of the spinal cord in an abnormal caudal location (Figure 18-3). This fixation produces mechanical stretch, distortion, and ischemia with daily activities, growth, and development.[64] The presence of tethered cord syndrome should be suspected in any patient with abnormal neurulation (including patients with myelomeningocele, lipomeningocele, dermal sinus, diastematomyelia, myelocystocele, tight filum terminal, and lumbosacral agenesis). Presenting symptoms may include decreased strength (often asymmetrical), development of lower-extremity spasticity, back pain at the site of sac closure, early development of or increasing degree of scoliosis (especially in the low lumbar or sacral level child),[65,66] or change in urological function.[58,67-69] This clinical spectrum may be primarily associated with these dysraphic lesions or may be caused by spinal surgical procedures.[64] The cord may be tethered by scar tissue or by an inclusion epidermoid or lipoma at the repair site.[7] Surgery to untether the spinal cord (tethered cord release) is performed to prevent further loss of muscle function, decrease the spasticity, help control the scoliosis,[66,70] or relieve back pain.[71,72]

The effectiveness of a tethered cord release may be demonstrated by an increase in muscle function, relief of back pain, and stabilization or reversal of scoliosis.[66,70,72] Spasticity, however, is not always alleviated in all patients.[73] Selective posterior rhizotomy has been advocated for patients whose persistent or progressive spastic status after tethered cord repair continues to interfere with their mobility and functional independence.[58,59]

Bowel and Bladder Dysfunction. Because of the usual involvement of the sacral plexus, the child with spina bifida must commonly deal with some form of bowel and bladder dysfunction. Besides various forms of incontinence, incomplete emptying of the bladder remains a constant concern because infection of the urinary tract and possible kidney damage may result.[74] Regulation of bowel evacuation must be established so that neither constipation nor diarrhea occurs. Negative social aspects of incontinence can be minimized by instituting intervention that emphasizes patient and family education and a regular, consistently timed, reflex-triggered bowel evacuation.[75]

Cognitive Impairment and Learning Issues. The last major clinical manifestation resulting from the neurological involvement of myelomeningocele is that of impaired intellectual function. Although children with spina bifida without hydrocephalus may show normal intellectual potential, children with hydrocephalus, particularly those who have shunt infections, are likely to have below-average intelligence.[11,76-78] These children often demonstrate learning disabilities and poor academic achievement.[79] Even those with a normal IQ show moderate to severe visual-motor perceptual deficits.[14,80] This inability to coordinate eye and hand movements affects learning and may interfere with activities of daily living (ADLs), such as buttoning a shirt or opening a lunchbox.[81] Difficulties with spatial relations, body image, and development of hand dominance may also be evident.[3,81] Children with myelomeningocele demonstrate poorer hand function than age-matched peers. This decreased hand function appears to be caused by cerebellar and cervical cord abnormalities rather than hydrocephalus or a cortical pathological condition (see Chapter 15).[82]

Prenatal studies have shown that the CNS as a whole is abnormally developed in fetuses with myelomeningocele.[83-86] The impairment of intellectual and perceptual abilities has been linked to damage to the white matter caused by ventricular enlargement.[3,11] This damage to association tracts, particularly in the frontal, occipital, and parietal areas, could account for the often severe perceptual-cognitive deficits noted in the child with spina bifida.[87] Lesser involvement of the temporal areas may account for the preservation of speech, whereas the semantics of speech, which depend on association areas, are impaired. The "cocktail party speech" of children with spina bifida can be deceptive because they generally use well-constructed sentences and precocious vocabulary.[11] A closer look, however, reveals a repetitive, inappropriate, and often meaningless use of language not associated with higher intellectual functioning. Research on learning difficulties in children with spina bifida and hydrocephalus suggests that many of these children experience difficulties. Tasks and skills affected include memory, reasoning, math, handwriting, organization, problem solving, attention, sensory integration, auditory processing, visual perception, and sequencing.[84-86]

Integumentary Impairment

Latex allergy and sensitivity have been noted with increasing frequency among children with myelomeningocele, with frequent reports of intraoperative anaphylaxis.[88-92] These children have also been reported to have a higher than expected prevalence of atopic disease.[93] A 1991 Food and Drug Administration Medical Bulletin estimated that 18% to 40% of patients with spina bifida demonstrate latex

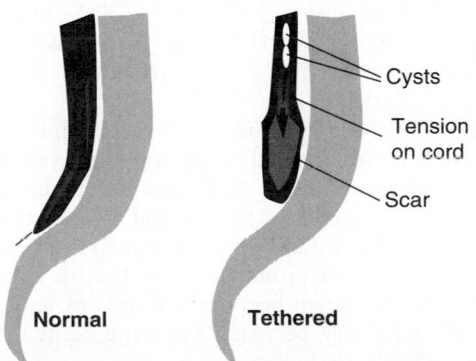

FIGURE 18-3 ■ Tethered cord in myelodysplasia. (From Staheli LT: *Practice of pediatric orthopedics,* Philadelphia, 2001, Lippincott Williams and Wilkins.)

sensitivity.[88,94] Within latex is 2% to 3% of a residual-free protein material that is thought to be the antigenic agent.[90] Frequent exposure to this material results in the development of the immunoglobulin E antibody. Children with spina bifida are more likely to develop the immunoglobulin E sensitivity because of repeated parental or mucosal exposure to the latex antigen.[95] Because of the risk of an anaphylactic reaction, exposure to any latex-containing products such as rubber gloves, therapy balls, or exercise bands should be avoided. Latex-free gloves, therapy balls, treatment mats, and exercise bands are now widely available and should be considered for standard use in all clinics treating children with spina bifida. Spina bifida, even in the absence of multiple surgical interventions, may be an independent risk factor for latex sensitivity. Latex-free precautions from birth are more effective in preventing latex sensitization than are similar precautions instituted later in life.[96,97] Latex sensitization decreased from 26.7% to 4.5% in children treated in a latex-free environment from birth.[97]

The presence of paralysis and lack of sensation on the skin places the child with spina bifida at major risk for pressure sores and decreased skin integrity. Various types of skin breakdown have occurred in 85% to 95% of all children with spina bifida by the time they reach young adulthood.[98] Common areas at risk for pressure sores include the lower back, kyphotic or scoliotic prominences, heels, feet, toes, and perineum. A pressure sore may result from excessive skin pressure that can cause reduced capillary flow, tissue anoxia, and eventual skin necrosis. Excessive pressure may manifest itself early as reactive hyperemia, a blister, and later as an open sore or overt necrosis. Chronic, untreated sores may lead to osteomyelitis and eventual sepsis.[93] Pressure sores often result in loss of time from school and work and can lead to financial hardship from medical treatment and hospitalizations. These negative consequences can largely be prevented with attention to education and instruction of the child and family. The goal of such education is to foster an understanding of the causes of skin breakdown and the necessary meticulous attention to skin care that must be carried out on a regular basis.

Growth and Nutrition

Nutritional intake and weight gain and loss have been found to be problematic in children with myelomeningocele. Early on, infants with spina bifida may have feeding issues as a result of an impaired gag reflex, swallowing difficulties, and a high incidence of aspiration.[3,56] Altered oral-motor function has been attributed to the Chiari II malformation.[99] These impairments may lead to nutritional issues and delayed growth and weight gain. Speech, physical, and occupational therapy are often needed to address these issues as a team.

Conversely, obesity can be a significant issue for children with spina bifida. This problem is complex and multifactorial.[100] Mobility limitations and decreased energy expenditure result in lower physical activity levels. In addition, decreased lower limb mass diminishes the ability to burn calories, which leads to weight gain. Decreased caloric intake as well as a lifelong engagement in rewarding and physically challenging physical activities are both necessary to enhance weight control and control obesity.

Children with myelomeningocele are short in stature. Growth in these children may be influenced by growth-retarding factors as a result of neurological deficit such as tethered cord.[101] Endocrine disorders and growth hormone deficiency have also been found to contribute to short stature in this population.[102] As a result of complex CNS anomalies (midline defects, hydrocephalus, Arnold-Chiari malformation), these children are at risk for hypothalamopituitary dysfunction leading to growth hormone deficiency.[103,104] Treatment with recombinant human growth hormone has proven successful in fostering growth acceleration in these children.[99,103,105,106]

Psychosocial Issues

Considering all the clinical manifestations resulting from this congenital neurological defect, social and emotional difficulties will arise for these children and their families. These will be considered as appropriate when discussing the stages of recovery and rehabilitation from birth through adolescence.

The preceding discussion concerning the clinical problems of the child with spina bifida is intended to inform, not overwhelm, the clinician. With a firm understanding of the difficulties to be faced, evaluation and intervention can be more efficient and effective.

Medical Management

At or before birth, the myelomeningocele sac presents a dynamic rather than static disability. The residual neurological damage will be contingent on the early medical management that the fetus or newborn receives.

Neurosurgical Management

Since the early 1960s the presence of a myelomeningocele has been treated as a life-threatening situation, and sac closure most often takes place within the first 24 to 48 hours of life.[3,107] Recent advances in treatment have led to investigational treatment in utero to repair the defect before birth.[35] The aim of either surgery is to replace the nervous tissue into the vertebral canal, cover the spinal defect, and achieve a watertight sac closure.[108] This early management has decreased the possibility of infection and further injury to the exposed neural cord.[14,21,108,109]

Progressive hydrocephalus may be evident at birth in a small percentage of children born with myelomeningocele. A greater majority, however, have hydrocephalus 5 to 10 days after the back lesion is closed.[108,110-112] With the advent of computed tomography (CT), early diagnosis of hydrocephalus can be made in the newborn without the need for clinical examination.

Although clinical signs are not always definitive, hydrocephalus may be suspected if (1) the fontanelles become full, bulging, or tense; (2) the head circumference increases rapidly; (3) a separation of the coronal and sagittal sutures is palpable; (4) the infant's eyes appear to look downward only, with the cornea prominent over the iris (sun-setting sign); and (5) the infant becomes irritable or lethargic and has a high-pitched cry, persistent vomiting, difficult feeding, or seizures (Table 18-1).[18,52,113]

If the results of CT confirm hydrocephalus, a ventricular shunt is indicated. This procedure involves diverting the

TABLE 18-1 ■ Signs and Symptoms of Shunt Malfunction

Infants	Bulging fontanelle
	Swelling along the shunt tract
	Prominent veins on scalp
	Downward eye deviation ("sunsetting")
	Vomiting/change in appetite
	Irritability or drowsiness
	Seizures
	High-pitched cry
Toddler	Headache
	Vomiting/change in appetite
	Lethargy or irritability
	Swelling along the shunt tract
	Seizures
	Onset of or increased strabismus
Older child	All the above, plus:
	Deterioration in school performance
	Neck pain/pain over MM site
	Personality change
	Decrease in sensory or motor functions
	Incontinence begins or worsens
	Onset of or increased spasticity

excess CSF from the ventricles to some site for absorption. In general, two types of procedures—the ventriculoatrial (VA) and ventriculoperitoneal (VP) shunt—are currently used, the latter being the most common (Figure 18-4). The shunt apparatus is constructed from Silastic tubing and consists of three parts: a proximal catheter, a distal catheter, and a one-way valve. As CSF is pumped from the ventricles toward its final destination, backflow is prevented by the valve system. In this manner intracranial pressure is controlled, CSF is regulated, and hydrocephalus is prevented from causing damage to brain structures.

Unfortunately for children with spina bifida, their problems do not end after the back is surgically closed and a shunt is in place. Management strategies in the care of shunted hydrocephalus varies.[114] Shunt complications occur frequently and require an average of two revisions before age 10 years.[14,51] The most common causes of complications are shunt obstruction and infection.[3,11] Obstructions can be cleared by revising the blocked end of the shunt. Infections may be handled by external ventricular drainage and courses of antibiotic therapy followed by insertion of a new shunting system.[3] The problem of separation of shunt components has been largely overcome by the use of a one-piece shunting system. The single-piece shunt decreases the complications of shunting procedures.

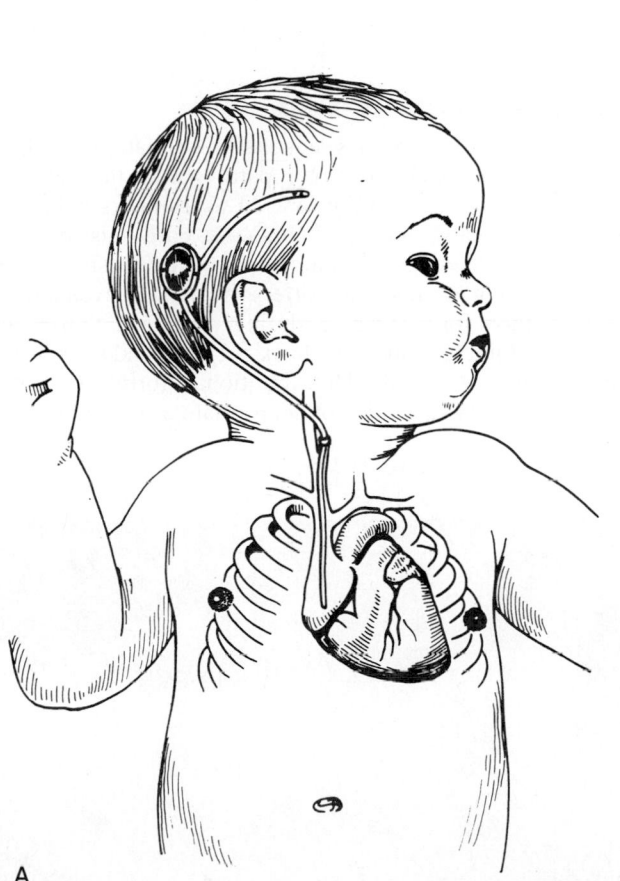

A

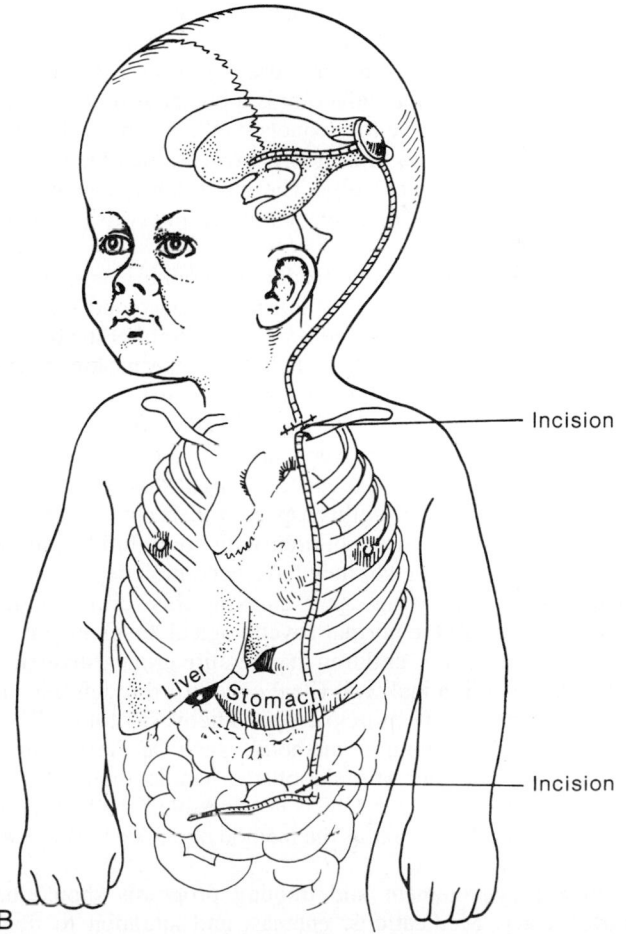

B

FIGURE 18-4 ■ A, Ventriculoatrial shunt. **B,** Ventriculoperitoneal shunt. (From Stark GD: *Spina bifida problems and management,* London, 1977, Blackwell Scientific.)

Prophylactic antibiotic therapy 6 to 12 hours before surgery and 1 to 2 days postoperatively is effective in controlling infection for both sac repair and shunt insertion.[14,61] This brief course of antibiotics has not led to resistant organisms. The main cause of death in children with myelomeningocele remains increased intracranial pressure and infections of the CNS.[14] With the use of antibiotics, shunting, and early sac closure, the survival rate has increased from 20% to 85%.[52,77]

Urological Management

Initial newborn workup should include a urological assessment. The urology team aims to preserve renal function and promote efficient bladder management. Initially, a renal and bladder ultrasound is performed to assess those structures.[83] Radiographic tests such as the voiding cystourethrogram or a cystometrogram can be performed to determine any blockage in the lower urinary tract. Functioning of the bladder outlet and sphincters, as well as ureteric reflux, also can be evaluated.[3,11,18] These tests, plus clinical observations of voiding patterns, help the urologist classify the infant's bladder function. If the bladder has neither sensory nor motor supply, a constant flow of urine is present. In this case infection is rare because the bladder does not store urine and the sphincters are always open.[62]

If no sensation but some involuntary muscle control of the sphincter exists, the bladder will fill, but emptying will not occur properly. Overflow or stress incontinence results in dribbling urine until the pressure is relieved. Because of constant residual urine, infection is a potential problem and kidney damage may be the sequela.[62] When some voluntary muscle control but no sensation is present, the bladder will fill and empty automatically. The child can eventually be taught to empty the bladder at regular intervals to avoid unnecessary accidents.

Regardless of the type of bladder functioning, urine specimens are taken to check for infection, and blood samples are taken to determine the kidney's ability to filter the body's fluids. On the basis of clinical findings, the urologist will suggest the appropriate intervention.

A program of clean intermittent catheterization (CIC) done every 3 to 4 hours prevents infection and maintains the urological system.[115-118] Parents are taught this method and can then begin to take on this aspect of their child's care. At the age of 4 or 5 years, children with spina bifida can be taught CIC. By doing so, they have become independent in bladder care at a young age. Achieving this form of independence adds to the normal psychological development of these children. Some children may require urinary diversion through the abdominal wall (ileal conduit), through the appendix (Mitrofanoff principle appendicovesicotomy),[119-121] or other less common methods, such as intravesical transurethral bladder stimulation, to handle their urinary condition.[115,122] Although CIC is not possible for all children with spina bifida, it remains the method of choice for bladder management.

Bowel management and training programs should be started early. Medications, enemas, and attention to fiber content in diet are all of value in establishing a bowel management program. The Malone ACE procedure is an important adjunct in the case of adults and children with problems of fecal elimination in whom standard medical therapies have failed.[123]

Orthopedic Management

Orthopedic management of the newborn with a myelomeningocele will generally concentrate on the feet and hips. Soft tissue releases of the feet may take place during surgery for sac closure. Casting the feet also has been effective in reducing clubfoot deformities (Figure 18-5). Early aggressive taping for clubfoot also is effective in the management of clubfoot deformities.[124,125] Short-leg posterior splints (ankle-foot orthoses [AFOs]) may be used to maintain range and prevent foot deformities.

The orthopedist also will evaluate the stability of the hips. In children with lower-level lesions, attempts to prevent dislocation are made by using a hip abductor brace (Figure 18-6, *A*) or a total-body splint (Figure 18-6, *B*) for a few months after birth. With higher-level lesions, dislocated hips are no longer treated because they do not appear to have an effect on later rehabilitation efforts.[113,126-128] Orthopedic management needs to be ongoing throughout the child's lifetime with continued assessment of orthopedic deformities and need for surgical intervention.

EVALUATIONS

In attempting to evaluate the child with spina bifida, a number of evaluations can be chosen, each designed to test specific, yet perhaps unrelated, components of function. The following section discusses those test procedures or specific standardized tests that would best define the complexity of the problem.

Manual Muscle Testing

The first and most obvious request for evaluation may be to determine the extent of motor paralysis. In the newborn, testing may be done in the first 24 to 48 hours before the back is surgically closed. In this case, care must be taken not to injure the exposed neural tissue during testing. Prone and side lying to either side offers the most convenient and safe position for evaluation during this time. Subsequent testing is done soon after the back is closed and as indicated throughout childhood. The traditional form of manual muscle testing (MMT) is not appropriate or possible for the

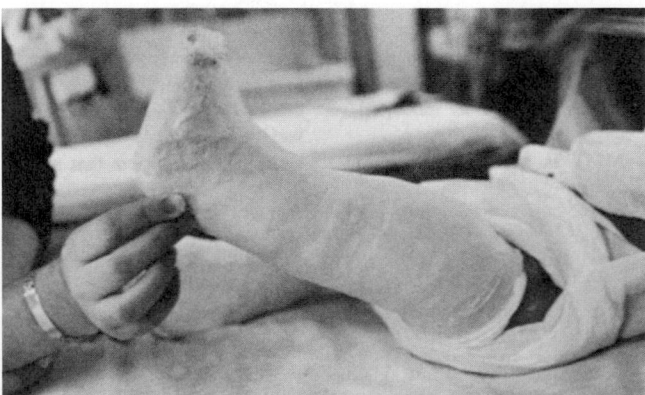

FIGURE 18-5 ■ Plaster cast of the foot and ankle to reduce clubfoot deformities.

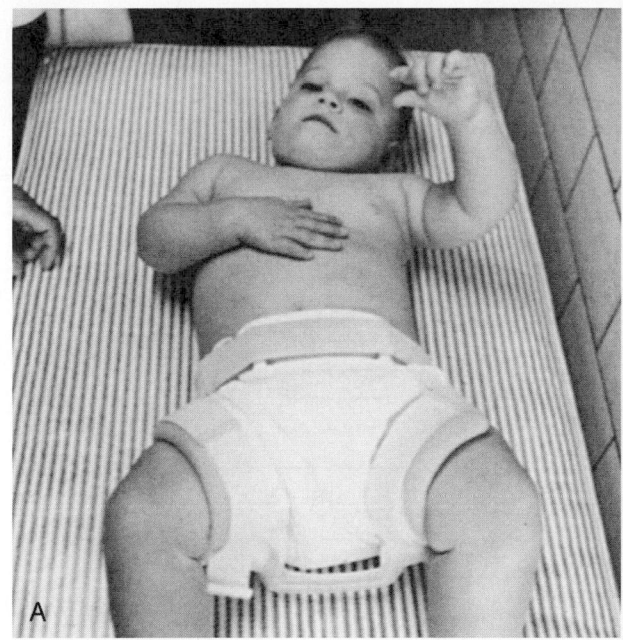

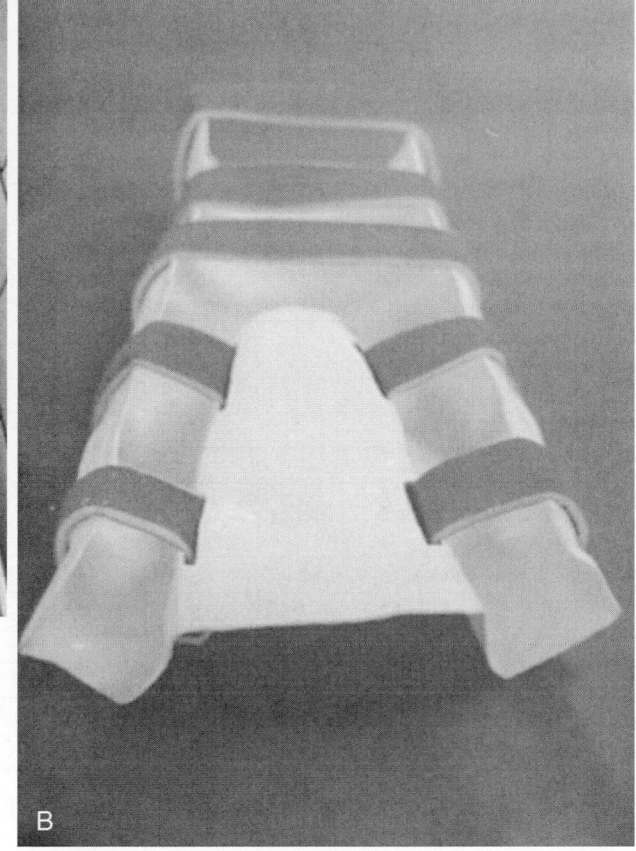

FIGURE 18-6 ■ **A,** Hip abductor brace. **B,** Total body splint.

infant or young child. Following is a discussion of how muscle testing can and must be adapted for this age group.

In evaluating the newborn, the importance of alertness is paramount. A sleeping or drowsy infant will not respond appropriately during the evaluation. The infant must be in the alert or crying state to elicit the appropriate movement responses. Testing hungry or crying infants provides an advantage because they are likely to demonstrate more spontaneous movements in these behavioral states.

The cumulative effect of a variety of sensory stimuli may be more effective in alerting the infant than using one made in isolation. For example, the infant may be picked up and rocked vertically to allow maximum stimulation to the vestibular system and to help bring the child to an alert state. In addition, the therapist may talk to the child to help him or her fixate visually on the therapist's face. Tactile stimuli above the level of the lesion further add to the child's level of arousal, thus contributing to more conclusive test results. In this way, the CNS receives an accumulation of information from a variety of sensory systems rather than relying on transmission from one system that may be weak or inefficient.

As the child is aroused, spontaneous movements can be observed and muscle groups palpated. Additional methods to stimulate movement may be necessary. For example, tickling the infant generally produces a variety of spontaneous movements in the upper and lower extremities. Passive positioning of children in adverse positions may stimulate them

to move. For example, if the legs are held in marked hip and knee flexion, the infant may attempt to use extensor musculature to move out of that position. If the legs are held in adduction, the child may abduct to get free. Holding a limb in an antigravity position may elicit an automatic "holding" response from a muscle group when spontaneous movements cannot be obtained in any other way.[129]

In grading muscle strength, differentiation between spontaneous, voluntary movement and reflexive movement is important. After severing of a spinal cord, distal segments of the cord may respond to stimuli in a reflexive manner. This results from the preservation of the spinal reflex arc and is known as distal sparing. If distal sparing of the spinal cord is present, the muscles may respond to stimulation or muscular stretch with reflexive, stereotypical movement patterns. The quality of this reflexive movement will be different from that of spontaneous movement and must be distinguished when testing for level of voluntary muscle functioning.

Muscle strength is generally graded for groups of muscles and can be graded by using either a numerical (1 to 5) or alphabetical designation (Figure 18-7) or simply by noting presence or absence of muscular contraction by a plus or a minus on the muscle test form. This latter method may be sufficient initially, but as the child matures a more definitive muscle grade should be determined.

By using an MMT form that lists the spinal segmental level for each muscle group, an approximate level of lesion

THE CHILDREN'S MEMORIAL HOSPITAL
PHYSICAL / OCCUPATIONAL THERAPY

MUSCLE EXAM - MM

PATIENT NAME _____ M.R. # _____

ATTENDING M.D. _____ PT. D.O.B. _____

DIAGNOSIS _____

_____

DATE: _____

P.T. NAME: _____

	*	LEFT	RIGHT	*	COMMENTS: (Include ROM limitations, spasticity, reflexive movements, etc.)
ILIOPSOAS (L$_1$ - 2)					
SARTORIUS (L$_1$ 3)					
HIP ADDUCTORS (L$_2$ - 4)					
TENSOR FASCIA LATA					
GLUTEUS MEDIUS (L$_4$ - S$_1$)					
GLUTEUS MAXIMUS (L$_5$ - S$_1$)					
QUADRICEPS (L$_2$ - 4)					
MEDIAL HAMSTRINGS (L$_4$ - S$_2$)					
LATERAL HAMSTRINGS (L$_4$ - S$_1$)					
ANTERIOR TIBIALIS (L$_4$ - L$_5$)					
POSTERIOR TIBIALIS (L$_4$ - L$_5$)					
PERONEUS LONGUS (L$_5$ - S$_1$)					
PERONEUS BREVIS (L$_5$ - S$_1$)					
GASTROC - SOLEUS (S$_1$ - S$_2$)					
EXT. HALLUCIS LONGUS (L$_5$ - S$_1$)					
FLEX. HALLUCIS LONGUS (S$_1$ - S$_2$)					
EXT. DIGITORUM LONGUS (L$_4$ - S$_1$)					
EXT. DIG. B. (L$_4$ - S$_1$)					
FLEX. DIGITORUM LONGUS (L$_4$ - S$_1$)					
FLEX. DIG. B. (L$_4$ - S$_1$)					
LUMBRICALES					

*INDICATE INCREASE (↑) OR DECREASE (↓) IN STRENGTH IN COMPARISON TO PREVIOUS TEST DATED _____

PLEASE NOTE ANY SIGNIFICANT INFORMATION ON OTHER MUSCLE GROUPS UNLISTED ABOVE (i.e., EHB; Flex. HB; Internal or External Rotators)

X	PRESENT	UNABLE TO BE GRADED
N	NORMAL	COMPLETE RANGE OF MOTION AGAINST GRAVITY WITH FULL RESISTANCE
G	GOOD	COMPLETE RANGE OF MOTION AGAINST GRAVITY WITH MODERATE RESISTANCE
G-	GOOD MINUS	COMPLETE RANGE OF MOTION AGAINST GRAVITY WITH SOME RESISTANCE
F+	FAIR PLUS	COMPLETE RANGE OF MOTION AGAINST GRAVITY WITH SLIGHT RESISTANCE
F	FAIR	COMPLETE RANGE OF MOTION AGAINST GRAVITY
F-	FAIR MINUS	INCOMPLETE (GREATER THAN 1/2 WAY) RANGE OF MOTION AGAINST GRAVITY
P+	POOR PLUS	LESS THAN 1/2 WAY AGAINST GRAVITY OR FULL ROM GRAVITY ELIMINATED PLUS SL RESISTANCE
P	POOR	COMPLETE RANGE OF MOTION WITH GRAVITY ELIMINATED
P-	POOR MINUS	INCOMPLETE RANGE OF MOTION WITH GRAVITY ELIMINATED
T	TRACE	CONTRACTION IS FELT BUT THERE IS NO VISIBLE JOINT MOVEMENT
O	ZERO	NO CONTRACTION FELT IN THE MUSCLE

FORM 354042790

FIGURE 18-7 ■ Muscle examination form using alphabetical designation. (Courtesy of Josefina Briceno, PT, Children's Memorial Hospital, Chicago.)

can be determined from the test results (see Figure 18-7). Because the spinal cord is often damaged asymmetrically, MMT does not always accurately reflect the level of lesion. If reflex activity is also noted on the form, the presence of distal sparing of the spinal cord can be determined. Muscle testing of the newborn gives the clinician an appreciation of muscle function and possible potential for later ambulation as well as an awareness of possible deforming forces. For example, if hip extensors or abductors are not functioning, then the action of hip flexors and adductors must be countered to prevent future deformities.

Muscle testing of the toddler or young child may require some of the techniques previously described. In addition, developmental positions can be used to assess muscle strength in an uncooperative youngster. For example, strength of hip extensors and abductors can be assessed as a child attempts to creep up steps or onto a low mat table. By adding resistance to movements, fairly accurate muscle grades can be determined. To elicit hip flexors in sitting, if an interesting toy or object is placed on the child's ankle or between the toes the child will often lift the leg spontaneously to reach for it. Ingenuity and creativity are prerequisites for muscle testing in the young child. Reliability of MMT in children with spina bifida younger than 5 years is difficult but has been demonstrated in a clinic setting where all therapists were trained in specific MMT technique to ascertain consistency in testing.[130] By the age of 4 or 5 years, muscle grades can generally be determined by traditional testing techniques, although the reliability of the test results will increase with the age of the child.[131]

Muscle testing is indicated before and after any surgical procedure and at periodic intervals of 6 months to 1 year to detect any change in muscle function. The level of innervation should not decrease throughout the life of the child with spina bifida. In the growing child or adolescent, an increasing weakness resulting from shunt malfunction, tethering of the spinal cord, or hydromyelia frequently can be substantiated by a muscle test of the lower extremities. The MMT is also valuable in determining the motor level so that potential future functional level can be determined (Figure 18-8).

Sensory Testing

Sensory testing of the infant and young child is simplified to determine the level of sensation as accurately as possible, with a minimal amount of testing. Full sensory tests are not possible until the child has acquired sufficient cognitive and language abilities to respond appropriately to testing.

In the newborn, sensory testing can best be done if the child is in a quiet state. Beginning at the lowest level of sacral innervation, the skin is stroked with a pin or other sharp object until a reaction to pain is noted. Although none of these methods is failsafe, they may be helpful in adapting a muscle test to a newborn or young infant. Repeated evaluation may be necessary to get an accurate picture of muscle function.

Because of dermatome innervation the pin is usually drawn from the anal area across the buttocks, down the posterior thigh and leg, then to the anterior surface of the leg and thigh, and finally across the abdominal muscles. Reactions to be noted are a facial grimace or cry, which indicates that the painful sensation has reached a cortical level. Care must be taken to see that each sensory dermatome has been

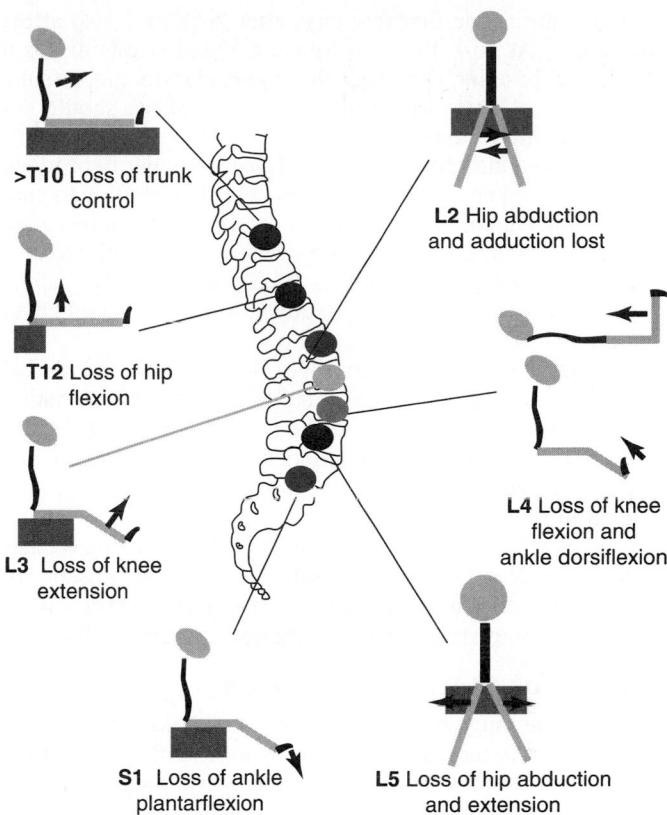

FIGURE 18-8 ■ Weakness related to level of spinal defect. (From Staheli LT: *Practice of pediatric orthopedics,* Philadelphia, 2001, Lippincott Williams and Wilkins.)

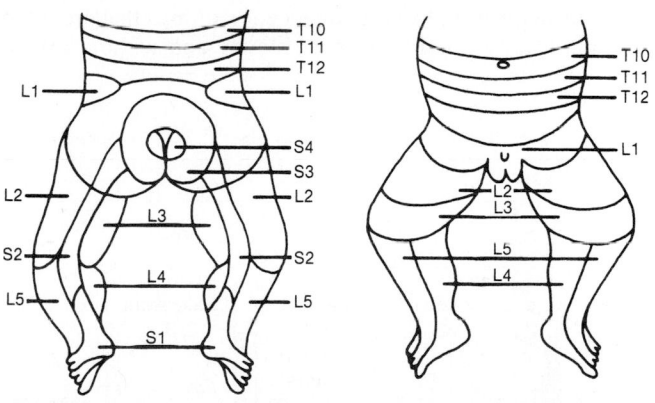

FIGURE 18-9 ■ Lower limb dermatomes. (From Brocklehurst G: Spina bifida for the clinician, *Clin Dev Med* 57:53, 1976.)

evaluated. Results can be recorded by shading in the dermatomes where sensation is present (Figure 18-9).

The therapist may be called on to evaluate the newborn before surgical closure of the spinal meningocele. Although sensory and motor levels can be determined as previously described, the infant's general condition should be considered when interpreting test findings. Any medication taken by the mother during labor and delivery may influence the neonate's performance and thus should be noted. In addition, the physiological disorganization normally seen in all infants during the first few days after birth may also affect testing.[132] At best, this presurgical evaluation establishes a tentative baseline, but significant changes in the infant's neurological status in the first few weeks of life should not be surprising to the clinician.

In the young child from 2 to 7 years of age, light touch sensation and position sense can be tested in addition to pain sensation. Again, the ingenuity of the therapist will be called forth to elicit an appropriate response and reliable test results. Using games such as "Tell me when the puppet touches you" may be more effective for the young child than traditional testing methods.

From age 7 years through adolescence, additional sensory tests of temperature and two-point discrimination may be added. Traditional methods are usually sufficient to ensure reliable testing, but a more behavioral approach may be indicated depending on the individual's cognitive functioning.

After testing, a survey of the sensory dermatome chart should indicate whether sensation is normal, absent, or impaired. MMT and sensory testing (dermatomes) can assist in determining spinal level of function (Figure 18-10).

Range of Motion Evaluation

A complete range of motion (ROM) evaluation of the lower extremities is indicated for the newborn with spina bifida. The therapist must be aware of normal physiological flexion that is greatest at the hip and knees. In the normal newborn these apparent "contractures" of up to 35 degrees are eliminated as the child gains more control of extensor musculature and kicks more frequently into extension.

In the child with spina bifida, contractures may be evident at multiple joints at birth because of unopposed musculature (Figure 18-11). Hip adduction should not be tested beyond the neutral position to avoid dislocation of hips that are often unstable. Range should be done slowly and without exces-

sive force to avoid fractures so often experienced in paralytic lower extremities. ROM should be checked with the same frequency as MMT. Active ROM of the upper extremities can be assessed by observation and handling the infant. A formal ROM evaluation for the upper extremities is not usually indicated. A baseline ROM and tone assessment of the upper extremities should be completed.

Reflex Testing

The purpose of reflex testing is twofold: to check for the presence of normal reflex activity and to check for the integration of primitive reflexes and the establishment of more mature reactions.[133] In the newborn, for example, strong rooting and sucking reflexes are expected. In the child with spina bifida, because of possible involvement of the CNS as previously described, these reflexes may be depressed or absent. Because these reflexes play an integral part in obtaining nutrients for the infant, their value is obvious. On the other hand, primitive reflexes, which persist past their expected span, also may indicate abnormality. For example, if the asymmetrical tonic neck reflex persists past 4 months, it will limit the infant's ability to bring the hands to midline for visual and tactile exploration.

As the primitive reflexes (initially needed for survival and to experience movement) become integrated, they are replaced by more mature and functional reactions. The righting and equilibrium reactions help the child attain the erect position and counteract changes in the center of gravity. Because these reactions depend on an intact CNS as well as a certain level of postural control, they may be delayed, incomplete, or absent in the child with spina bifida. For example, a child with a low thoracic spinal cord lesion may show an incomplete equilibrium reaction in sitting. This may be caused by the lack of a stable postural base or by lack of initiation of the reaction centrally. Both the neurological and muscular components of these reactions must be consid-

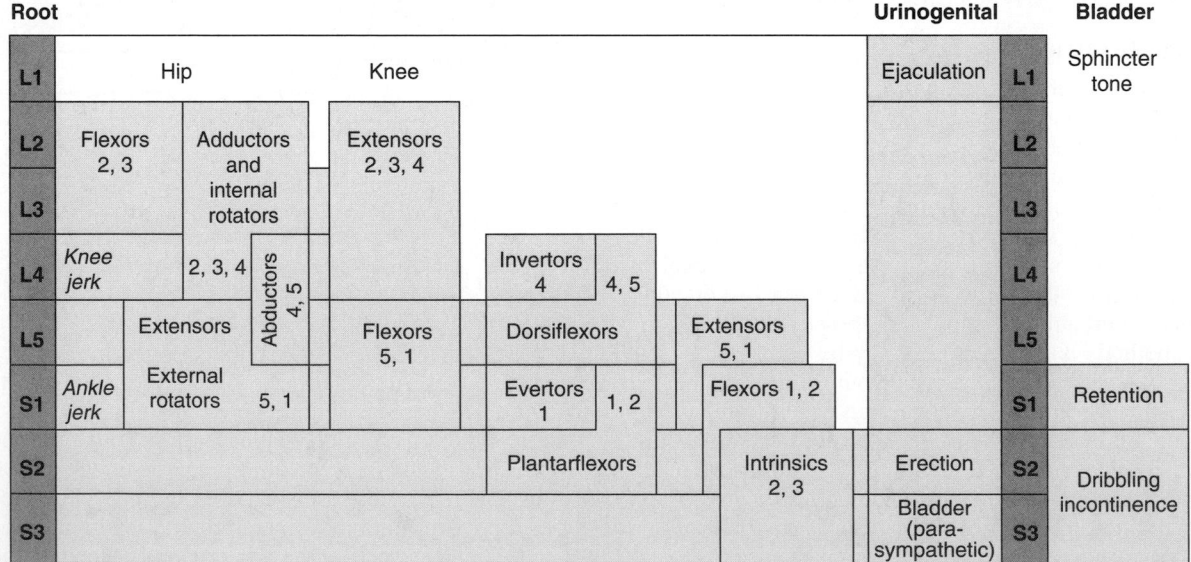

FIGURE 18-10 ■ Segmental nerve supply of the lower extremities. (From Stokes M: *Physical management in neurological rehabilitation,* London, 2004, Elsevier.)

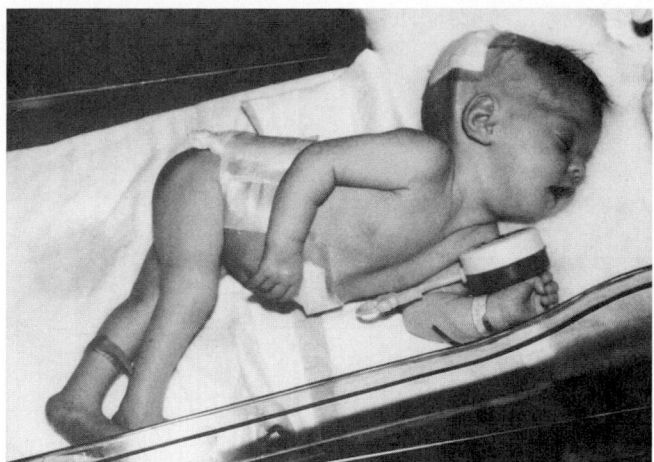

FIGURE 18-11 ■ Myelomeningocele infant with contractures. (From Molnar GE, Alexander MA: *Pediatric rehabilitation,* Philadelphia, 1999, Hanley and Belfus.)

ered.[133] Reflex testing for the child with spina bifida may not be as intensive as that for a child with cerebral palsy. It may, however, provide a check on the progress of normal development and as such reflect the integrity of the CNS (see Chapter 2).

Developmental and Functional Evaluations

Besides being aware of a child's sensory and motor levels, assessing the functional level is also important. Two important questions need to be asked: "Does the child show normal components of posture and movement synergies?" and "What is the child's level of function and mobility?" Several developmental and functional evaluations can be used with the child with spina bifida. The following are some suggestions for evaluation approaches or specifically designed tests to assist in assessment of this area.

Initially, a developmental sequence may be used to assess how a child is functioning. In each position used, both posture and movement are evaluated. The goals in using this type of assessment are to determine what a child can and cannot do, the quality of the action, and what is limiting the child. The progression begins in the supine position, rolling to prone, prone-on-elbows, prone-on-hands, up-to-sitting, hands-knees, kneeling, half-kneeling, standing, and walking. Both the ability to attain and the ability to maintain the positions should be assessed.

The way in which a task is accomplished is as important to evaluate as the accomplishment itself. For example, in rolling, is head righting sufficient to keep the head off the supporting surface? From the hands-knees position, can reciprocal crawling be initiated without the lower extremities being held in wide abduction? Can the child pull to stand easily by using trunk rotation? Assessing the quality of the child's abilities will assist the clinician in determining where therapeutic measures should begin and what the goals of such intervention will be.[134]

If a standardized assessment were desired, the Alberta Infant Motor Scale (AIMS) would be appropriate.[135] The

AIMS is designed to measure motor development from birth to 18 months of age. It is a 58-item observational test of infants in supine, prone, sitting, and standing positions. Each item includes detailed descriptions of the weight-bearing surface, the infant's posture, and antigravity movements expected of the infant in that position. The AIMS requires minimal handling of the infant and can be completed in 20 to 30 minutes. The test was normed on a cross-sectional sample of 2200 infants in Alberta, Canada. Interrater and test-retest reliability are high (0.95 to 0.99), as is concurrent validity with the Peabody Developmental Motor Scales (PDMS) (0.99) and the Bayley Scales of Infant Development (0.97). Predictive validity of the AIMS appears to be fair.[136] For the child with spina bifida the AIMS could be used to assess current motor development and track progress in motor development over time.

The Milani-Comparetti motor development screening test may also be useful in assessing the functional level of the child with spina bifida. This screening examination is designed to evaluate motor development from birth to 2 years of age (Figure 18-12).[137] It requires no special equipment and can be administered in 4 to 8 minutes. The test evaluates both spontaneous behavior and evoked responses. Spontaneous behavior includes postural control of the head and body in various positions as well as a sequence of active movement patterns. Primitive reflexes, righting, and equilibrium reactions comprise the evoked responses. The Milani-Comparetti test was normed on a sample of 312 children from Omaha, Nebraska. Interrater reliability percent of agreement was 89% to 95%. Test-retest reliability percent agreement was 82% to 100%. Predictive validity of the test has not been well established.[137] The Milani-Comparetti test should assist the clinician in evaluating each child's underlying postural mechanisms and his or her ability to attain the erect position. The test manual provides information on special examination procedures and scoring.

The Peabody Developmental Motor Scales-2 (PDMS-2) is another standardized assessment that may prove helpful in evaluating a child with congenital spinal cord injury.[138] The PDMS-2 consists of six gross and fine motor subtests from birth through 6 years of age. The two scales allow a comparison of the child's motor performance with a normative sample of children at various age levels. A stratified sample of 2003 children from 46 states in the United States was used to develop PDMS-2 test norms. Test-retest and interrater reliability are high. Content, construct, and concurrent validity have been well established. Although the child with activity limitations would not be expected to succeed on many of the gross motor items at the later age levels, the scale still serves as a reminder of expected gross motor performance at each age. The fine motor scale offers a chance to assess fine motor performance of children with congenital spinal cord injury. This area has been frequently overlooked in children with myelomeningocele. Fine motor development, however, may be affected because of congenital abnormalities in brain development associated with myelomeningocele or related to tethering of the spinal cord that can result in fine motor paresis. In addition, the PDMS-2 offers guidelines for administering the test to children with various activity limitations.[138]

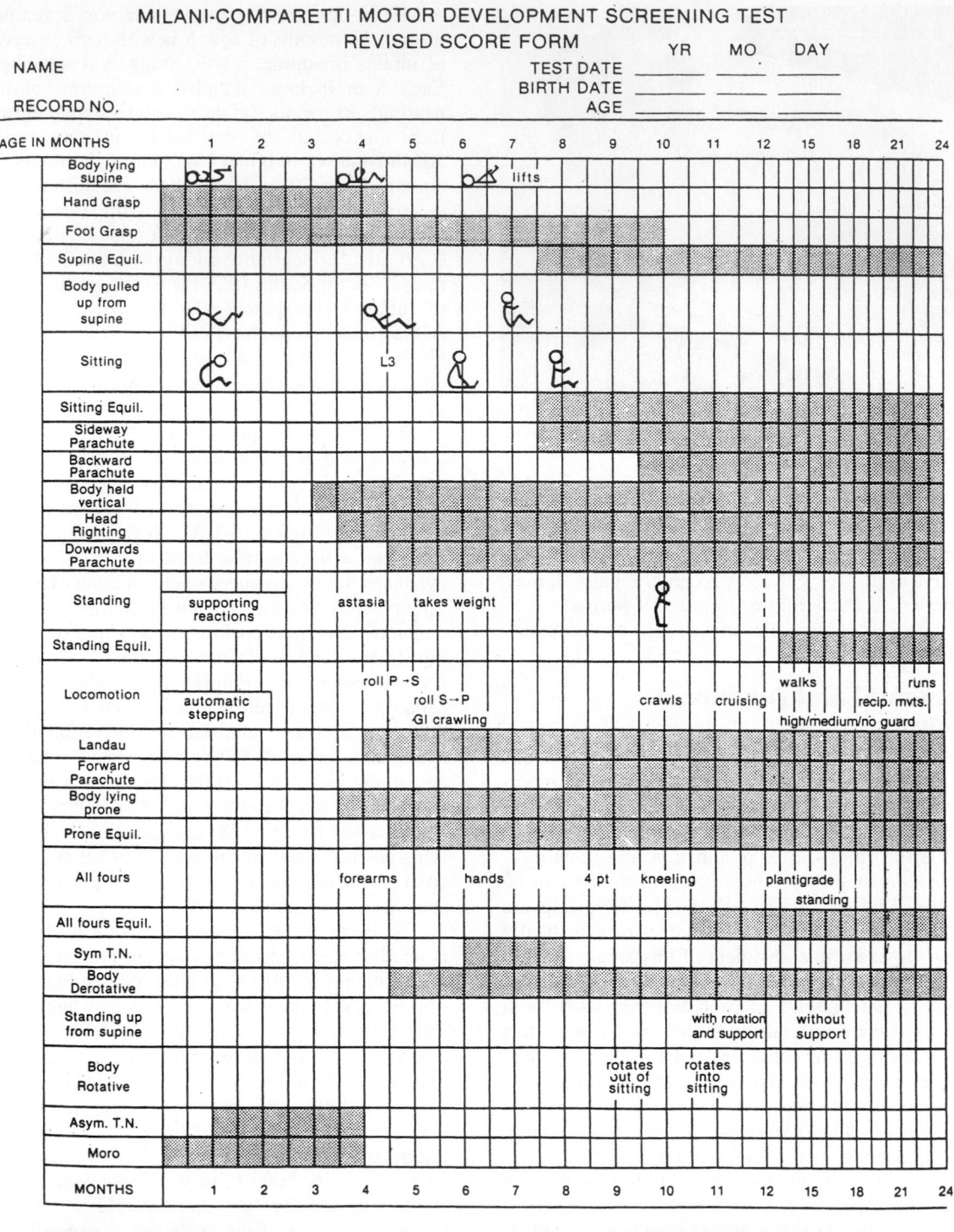

FIGURE 18-12 ■ Milani-Comparetti Motor Development Screening Test-Revised score form.

The Bruininks-Oseretsky Test of Motor Proficiency (BOTMP) can be used to evaluate the higher-level child with spina bifida.[139] Upper limb coordination tests and fine motor subtests of response speed, visual-motor control, and upper-limb speed and dexterity can be used to assist in evaluating areas of fine motor control and coordination difficulties. This test has been standardized on a large sample of children from age 4 through 14 years.[139]

Finally, the Pediatric Evaluation of Disability Inventory (PEDI) is a comprehensive assessment of function in children aged 6 months to 7 years.[140] The PEDI measures both capability and performance of functional activities in three areas: self-care, mobility, and social function. Capability is a measure of the functional skills for which the child has demonstrated mastery. Functional performance is measured by the level of caregiver assistance needed to accomplish a task. A modifications scale provides a measure of environmental modifications and equipment needed in daily functioning. The PEDI has been standardized on a normative sample of 412 children from New England. Some data from clinical samples (N = 102) are also available. Interrater reliability of the PEDI is high as demonstrated by high intraclass correlation coefficients (ICCs = 0.96 to 0.99). Concurrent validity of the PEDI with the Wee-FIM (child's version of the Functional Independence Measure) was also high (r = 0.80 to 0.97).[139] The PEDI can be administered in approximately 45 minutes by clinicians or educators familiar with the child or by structured interview of the parent. The PEDI should provide a descriptive measure of the functional level of the child with myelomeningocele as well as a method for tracking change over time.

Another assessment of motor performance that may be commonly used with the school-age child with spina bifida is the School Function Assessment (SFA). The SFA is standardized and was conceptually developed to reflect the functional abilities and needs of a student in elementary school. The three areas assessed include student's participation in school activities, task supports required by the student for participation, and the student's activity performance.[141,142]

Perceptual and Cognitive Evaluations

When evaluating a child with spina bifida, some assessment of perceptual and cognitive status is important to include. The appropriate assessment depends largely on the age of the child. The assessment may be performed by the physical, occupational, or speech therapist, depending on the setting.

For the newborn from 3 to 30 days old, the Brazelton Neonatal Behavioral Assessment scale may be adapted to assess the infant's organization in terms of physiological response to stress, state control, motoric control, and social interaction.[132] Ideally, the infant should be medically stable and free from CNS-depressant drugs before evaluation. Generally, this evaluation will occur after the back lesion is closed and a shunt is positioned to relieve the hydrocephalic condition.

Although test results may not have prognostic value because of the plasticity of the nervous system at this young age, they supply the clinician with information concerning the current status of the child. This information can be conveyed to the infant's caregivers—both medical personnel and parents—so that strengths can be appreciated and weaknesses anticipated and handled appropriately. Helping parents identify that their infant has his or her own unique characteristics and assisting them in dealing with these characteristics does a great deal to strengthen already precarious parent/infant bonding.

Repeated administration of the Brazelton Neonatal Behavioral Assessment scale in the first month of life may help monitor the infant's progress in organization and reflect the curve of recovery. Although the manual for this behavioral assessment is complete, proper administration scoring and interpretation require direct training with someone already proficient in using the scale.[132] Excellent training videos for the Brazelton Neonatal Behavioral Assessment scale are available through the Brazelton Institute for purchase or through the local university's learning resource centers.

A full developmental evaluation appropriate for the infant and toddler with spina bifida is the Bayley Scales of Infant Development, second edition (BSID-II).[143] The Bayley Scales, consisting of a mental and motor scale and a behavioral rating scale, can be used to test children from age 1 month to 42 months. The test provides information on gross motor, fine motor, language, personal-social, and cognitive development.

The BSID-II is well standardized and reliable and takes approximately 45 minutes to administer. It is not an easy test to learn and initially requires supervision of an experienced tester. This edition provides new normative data, extended age range, expanded content coverage, and improved psychometric qualities.

The BSID-II provides the clinician with a broader view of the child's total development. The gross motor information from this developmental assessment will not be specific enough for a therapist evaluating a child with spina bifida. The additional information on fine motor, language, personal-social, and cognitive development, however, is sufficient and will be important in planning a comprehensive intervention program. This test was recently revised to the Bayley Scales of Infant and Toddler Development-III (BSID-III) and became available commercially in 2006.[143a] The new version includes assessments in cognitive, motor, language, social-emotional, and adaptive behavior domains.

Various tests are available as screening tools to test visual-motor integration and perception. The Beery-Buktenica Developmental Test of Visual-Motor Integration (Beery-VMI) is an early screening tool to aid in diagnosis of learning problems in children. It assesses integration of visual perception and motor control of children from age 2 years through 18 years. The test takes 10 to 15 minutes to complete and requires the child to be able to copy designs. The Beery-VMI is norm referenced and was standardized on a large sample of children chosen from throughout the United States.[144]

Children with spina bifida often exhibit upper-extremity weakness in addition to probable sensory dysfunction. As a result, fine motor skills in children with spina bifida are often impeded by slowness and inadequate adjustment of manipulative forces, and a non–motor-perceptual test is often desired.[145-147] The Motor-Free Visual Perception Test-3 (MVPT-3)[148] and the Test of Visual Perceptual Skills, Non-Motor, Revised (TVPS-[n-m]-R)[149] can be used to determine the child's visual perceptual processing skills on the basis of a non–motor assessment of these skills. Both tests evaluate visual discrimination, visual memory, spatial relations, figure-ground, and visual closure. The TVPS-(n-m)-R also evaluates form constancy and sequential memory. The MVPT-3 can be used with individuals from 4 to 70 years of age, and the TVPS-(n-m)-R can be used with children from 4 to 17 years, 11 months of age. The TVPS-(n-m)-R has two levels; the lower level tests children from ages 4 to 12 years and the upper level tests children from ages 12 years to 17 years, 11 months. Both tests are easy and quick to administer (less than 15 minutes) and, based on the examiner's experience and training, interpretations can be made with prescription for remediation. The MVPT-3 was standardized on a nationally representative sample. The test-retest reliability of the MVPT-3 was 0.81.[148] Performance on the motor-free test has been shown to be independent of the degree of motor involvement when compared with other tests of visual perception.[148] The TVPS-(n-m)-R was standardized on a sample of 1000 children across the United States.[149]

With a firm database provided by a thorough physical and occupational therapy evaluation with referrals to other professionals as appropriate, a reasonable treatment plan can be developed and updated as necessary.

TREATMENT PLANNING AND REHABILITATION RELATED TO SIGNIFICANT STAGES OF DEVELOPMENT

Newborn to Toddler (Preambulatory Phase)

Stage 1: Before Closure of Myelomeningocele— Newborn

Physical therapy management of the infant in stage 1 is limited by his or her medical condition (Table 18-2). Attempts can be made, however, to prevent deformity and maintain ROM while giving stimulation to provide as normal an environment as possible. In addition to evaluation, the therapist may begin some early intervention (EI) measures that can be continued and expanded after surgery. ROM and positioning in prone or side lying may be initiated to prevent or decrease contractures in the lower extremities. If clubfeet are present, soft tissue stretching may be indicated. Stretching begins distally on the soft tissue of the forefoot and proceeds proximally toward the calcaneus. This is done to take advantage of the pliability of soft tissue structures and to minimize fixed deformity later. In addition, taping may be used to maintain optimal ROM and alignment between periods of stretching.[124] When treating the newborn before surgery, great care must be taken to avoid contaminating an open sac, which is usually covered with a sterile dressing and kept moist with a saline solution.[14]

Stage 2: After Surgery, During Hospitalization— Newborn to Infant

Therapeutic intervention during stage 2 is more aggressive than before surgery but is often limited by the infant's neurological and orthopedic status. A major goal during this stage is to prevent contractures and maintain ROM. Traditional ROM can be taught to nursing staff and family. It also can be carried out while the child is being held at the adult's shoulder or prone over the adult's lap. These positions allow closeness between the caregiver and infant, thus encouraging maximal relaxation and interaction between them.

Because of their medical conditions, hospitalized infants often experience early separation from their parents. Teaching the family to handle the child as described may enhance parent/infant bonding. Adequate bonding is essential for normal psychosocial development to occur.

When the child is not being handled, resting positions can be used to maintain ROM and enhance development. The prone position is the most advantageous because it prevents hip flexion contractures and encourages development of extensor musculature as the child lifts his or her head. Side lying, which allows the hands to come to midline and generally encourages symmetrical posture, can be used for alternate positioning. As much as possible, the supine position should be avoided because the child is most dominated by primitive reflexes and the effects of gravity in this position.

For example, for the child with spina bifida with CNS involvement the effects of the tonic labyrinthine reflex combined with paralytic lower extremities may make movement from the supine position extremely difficult.

A normal sensory experience should be presented to the child in spite of the hospital setting. Toys of various colors, textures, and shapes should be available. Musical mobiles held low enough for the child to reach provide a variety of sensory experiences. Stimuli such as squeaky toys or the human face and voice can be used to encourage visual and auditory tracking. Controlled stimulation relevant to the infant's neurological state, rather than overstimulation, should be the rule. Depending on the age of the child, appropriate learning situations must be presented to provide the child with as normal an environment as possible for perceptual and cognitive growth.

A major therapeutic goal is to guide the child through the developmental sequence, ultimately preparing him or her to assume the upright posture. In this immediate postsurgical stage, primary emphasis should be on attaining good head and trunk control and eliciting appropriate righting reactions. For example, the child can be seated on the therapist's lap, facing the therapist, and alternately lowered slowly backward and side to side. This action helps stimulate head righting and strengthen neck and abdominal muscles. Weight shifting in the prone-on-elbows position is another good activity for enhancing development of head and trunk control. Developmental handling may be limited by surgical interventions that limit mobility.

This second stage ends as the child is discharged from the hospital. The child should be monitored closely by the spina bifida team, which may include a neurosurgeon, an orthopedist, a urologist, a nurse clinician, a physical therapist (PT), an occupational therapist (OT), an orthotist, and a social worker. Before discharge, a definitive home program as well as referral to the local EI program should be given to the family because the child will most likely require ongoing therapy, including both PT and OT. Other professionals that may be involved in the child's EI program may include speech and language pathologists (SLP), developmental therapists (DT), social workers, and psychologists.

Stage 3: Condition Stabilized—Infant to Toddler (Preambulatory)

In this stage of rehabilitation, the major emphasis is on preparing the child mentally and physically for walking. Goals of preventing contractures and maintaining ROM will remain throughout the child's life. Unless this is done, ambulation becomes more difficult and often impossible. If possible, prone positioning during play and sleeping assists greatly in stretching tight musculature. Resting splints for the lower extremities or a total-body splint can be used as necessary to position and maintain ROM and alignment.

Assuming that the child has previously gained good head and trunk control, the next step is development of sitting equilibrium reactions. As sitting balance improves, fine motor and eye-hand coordination activities should be introduced. Upper-extremity functioning is often overlooked in the child with spina bifida, whose problems appear to be concentrated in the lower extremities. However, most children with spina bifida show decreased fine motor coordination,[14] and this problem should be addressed as

TABLE 18-2 ■ Summary of Treatment Planning and Rehabilitation Related to Significant Stages of Development

STAGE OF RECOVERY	MAJOR PHYSICAL THERAPY GOALS	PHYSICAL THERAPY MANAGEMENT
NEWBORN TO TODDLER (PREAMBULATORY PHASE)		
Stage 1: before surgical closure of myelomeningocele—newborn	Prevent contractures and deformity	ROM, positioning
	Encourage normal sensorimotor development	Graded auditory and visual stimuli
Stage 2: after surgery, during hospitalization—newborn to infant	Prevent contracture and deformity	ROM taught to hospital personnel and family
		Positioning in prone and side lying
	Encourage normal sensorimotor development	Provide toys of various colors, textures, and shapes
		Graded auditory and visual stimuli: music boxes, squeaky toys, brightly colored objects
		Therapeutic handling to encourage good head and trunk control
Stage 3: condition stabilized—infant to toddler	Encourage normal development sequence	Work in sitting on head righting and equilibrium reactions
		Eye-hand coordination activities
		Early weight bearing on lower extremities
		Encourage prone progression
		Weight shifting in standing frame
		Comprehensive home program
TODDLER THROUGH ADOLESCENT (AMBULATORY PHASE)		
Stage 4: toddler through preschool	Begin ambulation	Choose appropriate orthotic device
		Gait training
		Development and strengthening of righting and equilibrium reactions
	Continue development in cognitive and psychosocial areas	Consider referral to EI program
		Public preschool program
		Continue home program
	Collaborate on goals with other team members	Open communication with other team members
Stage 5: primary school through adolescence	Reevaluate ambulation potential	Replace orthotic device as necessary
		Wheelchair prescriptions as necessary
	Maintain present level of functioning	Teach locomotion activities
		Maintain strength in trunk and extremities
	Prevent skin breakdown as child becomes more sedentary	Teach skin care
	Promote independence in self-care skills	Work with team members to teach dressing, feeding, hygiene, and bowel and bladder care
	Remediate any perceptual-motor problems	Provide program and activities for sensorimotor integration
	Provide appropriate adaptive devices	Check for fit and proper use of adaptive devices
	Promote self-esteem and social-sexual adjustment	Collaborate with other team members in counseling efforts

developmentally appropriate. The normal infant begins to reach and grasp by 6 months of age[134]; therefore the child with spina bifida must be given ample opportunities to practice and perfect these same skills at an early age. Because many children with spina bifida may be receiving PT as their primary service through EI in these early months, referral to and consultation with an occupational therapist at this age is highly recommended.

Following a normal developmental sequence, the child with spina bifida will usually begin some form of prone progression as trunk and upper-extremity stability improve. This is a significant phase of development because it allows for the development of a sensorimotor base as the child expands

environmental horizons.[10] During this phase of high mobility, nonfeeling skin must be checked for injury frequently and often must be protected by heavier clothing. This may help prevent any major skin breakdown, which could significantly delay the rehabilitation process. For some children with high-level lesions in whom prone mobility is not safe or practical for long distances, a caster cart may be used (Figure 18-13).[10] This provides the child with a means of exploring the environment safely but independently.

Emphasis on head and trunk control and strengthening exercises in a variety of sitting postures is quite important in this early preambulatory phase. Development of adequate strength and motor control for trunk righting, equilibrium

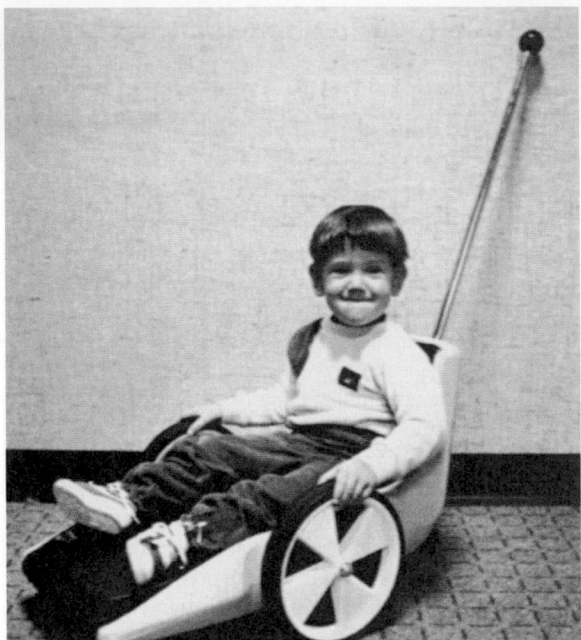

FIGURE 18-13 ■ Caster cart used for independent mobility.

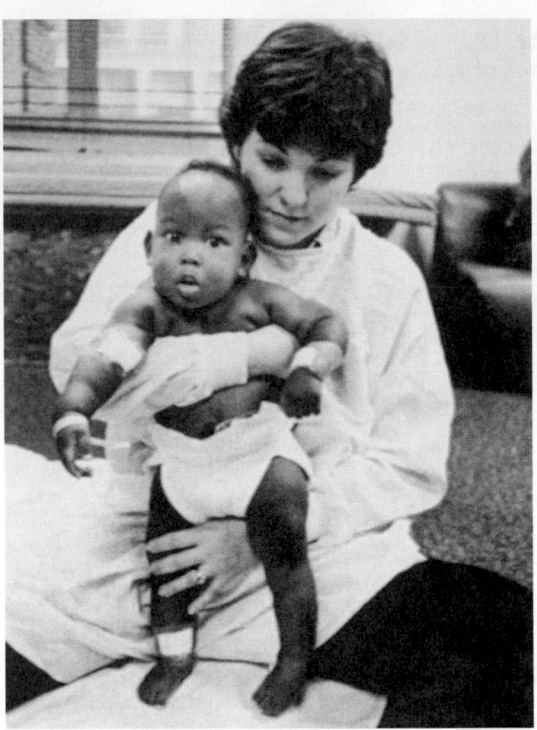

FIGURE 18-14 ■ Assisted standing with normal postural alignment.

reactions, and protective reactions will ultimately lead to improved sitting balance. Hands-free sitting with good balance is the optimal goal in this stage to allow for independence and freedom in play skills. In addition, hands-free sitting is a necessary precursor to ambulation with lower-extremity bracing and often is the determinant in deciding if a child will use a standing frame or will become a functional ambulator.

Early weight bearing is also of utmost importance, both physiologically and psychologically. The upright position has beneficial effects on circulation and renal and bladder functioning as well as on the promotion of bone growth and density.[50,150-152] Psychologically, weight bearing in an upright posture allows a normal view of the world and contributes to more normal perceptual, cognitive, and emotional growth. One way to achieve this weight bearing is in the kneeling position. This is developmentally appropriate because children 8 to 10 months old frequently use kneeling as a transition from all fours to standing.

Because young infants are frequently held in the standing position and bounced on their parents' laps, this form of weight bearing on the lower extremities is appropriate from birth onward. Failure to do so may deprive the child with spina bifida of the normal experience of standing at a very early age. When standing these children, however, care must be taken to see that the lower extremities are in good alignment and that undue pressure is not exerted on them (Figure 18-14). In this way the risk of fractures is minimized and a normal weight-bearing experience is provided.

Also in this phase of preambulation, transitions from one position to another should be assessed and facilitated. Teaching the child strategies for transitions will enhance his or her optimal functional independence. Compensations may be taught to substitute for weakened musculature. In addition, adaptive equipment and mobility devices may be recommended to enhance acquisition of age-appropriate milestones. Providing appropriate facilitation of mobility at a

level similar to that of their peers is important for psychosocial growth and development (Figure 18-15).

When the child attempts to pull to a standing position or would be expected to do so normally (at 10 to 12 months of age), the use of a standing device is indicated. Generally, a standing frame is the first orthosis chosen. This is a relatively inexpensive tubular frame to which adjustable parts are attached (Figure 18-16). Because it is not custom made, it can be fitted fairly quickly, although adjustments may be necessary to accommodate spinal deformities. This standing device offers support of the trunk, hips, and knees and leaves the hands free for other activities. Time spent in the standing frame should be increased gradually. This allows the child to adjust to the upright position in terms of muscle strength, endurance, blood pressure, and pressure on skin surfaces.

After children have built up a tolerance for standing, they may be taught to move in the device by shifting their weight from side to side. Initial shifting of weight onto one side of the body is necessary to allow the other side to move forward. This preliminary weight shift is also a prerequisite for developing equilibrium reactions in the standing position and thus will prepare the child for later ambulation. As the child shifts weight, the trunk musculature on the weight-bearing side should elongate and shorten on the non–weight-bearing side as muscle strength allows. This normal reaction to weight shifting also includes righting of the head and should be closely monitored by the therapist for completeness.

A therapy program must be designed to meet the individual's needs in each area. Age alone does not determine the appropriate therapeutic goals. Goals that are not suited for the child's cognitive and emotional needs, in addition to

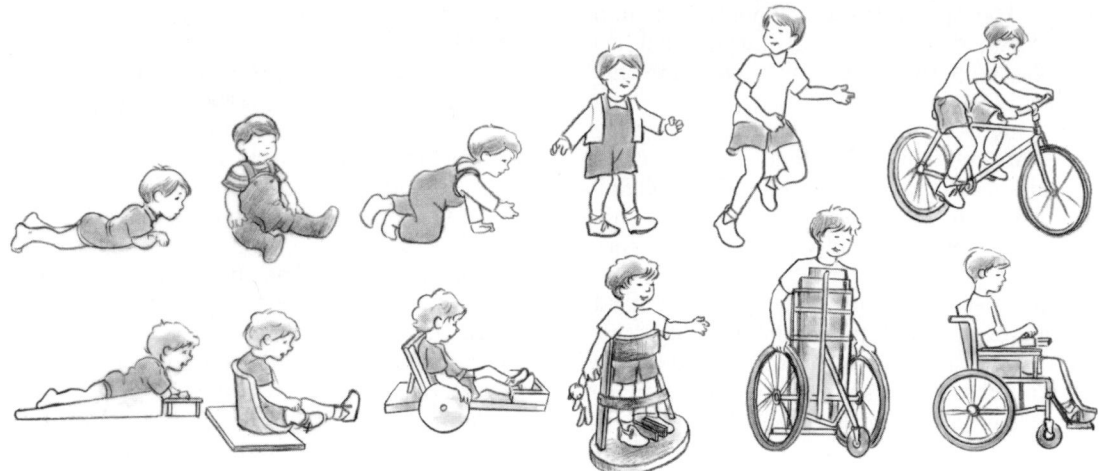

FIGURE 18-15 ■ Adaptive devices can help the young child with spina bifida reach major milestones at the same time as peers. (From Ratcliffe KT: *Clinical pediatric physical therapy,* St. Louis, 1998, Mosby.)

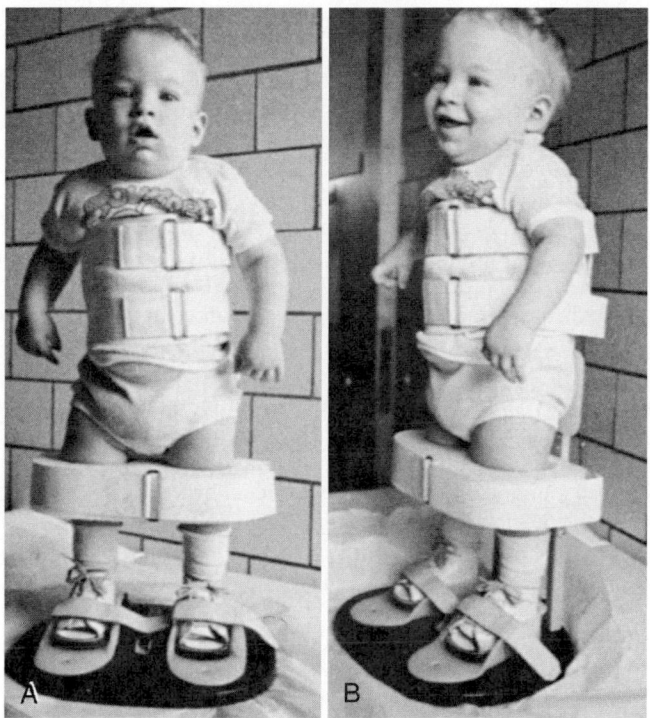

FIGURE 18-16 ■ Standing frame. **A,** Anterior view. **B,** Lateral view.

physical needs, will be doomed to failure before they are attempted. For example, an 18 month old may have the physical capabilities to ambulate independently with crutches and braces. The child may not, however, have the cognitive skills necessary to learn a four-point gait or be ready emotionally to separate from his or her mother for intensive therapy sessions. A more realistic goal may be to let the child walk holding onto furniture (cruising) while a wheeled walker for more independent ambulation is slowly introduced. Another alternative to using a conventional walker is to encourage the child to play with push toys such as grocery carts and baby buggies.

During this preambulatory stage therapy goals may be accomplished through a comprehensive home program, with frequent checks to note progress or problems and to change the program accordingly. For the more involved child, increased frequency of direct intervention may be indicated to achieve optimal developmental progress.

The program often must be reevaluated and goals changed if conditions such as shunt malfunctions or fractures occur. The warning signs for shunt dysfunctions are generally those previously described for suspected hydrocephalus. In addition, swelling along the shunt site may indicate a malfunction. Swelling and local heat or redness of a limb are the usual signs of a fracture. The limb may also look misaligned. Fever may accompany a fracture. As previously mentioned, these fractures generally heal quickly with proper medical intervention and minimally interrupt rehabilitation efforts.

Toddler through Adolescent (Ambulatory Phase)

Stage 4: Toddler through Preschool

This period in development marks the end of infancy and the beginning of childhood. For the typically developing child who has developed a strong sensorimotor foundation, physical development is marked by increased coordination and refinement of movement patterns. In addition, a great variety of motor skills will be achieved as the typically developing child learns to throw, catch, run, hop, and jump. This is also a period of great cognitive growth, as children's use of mental imagery and physical knowledge of their environments expand. Concepts of size, number, color, form, and space are all developing. Emotionally, most children are becoming more independent and begin to break away from the sheltered environment of the home. They are now more interested in interacting with others and become social beings to a greater extent.

All these changes in physical, cognitive, and emotional development will be evident in the child with spina bifida, although the degree depends on the extent of the functional limitations and their effect of the child's ability to participate in life. The characteristics of normal development must be understood so that cognitive, emotional, and motor behaviors can be nurtured and enhanced in the child with spina bifida.

Goals for this as for any other stage must address physical, cognitive, and emotional development. The most obvious goal at this stage is to help the child who is already standing to progress to an ambulatory status. Even the child with a low thoracic lesion can usually manage some form of ambulation.

Thus far, the child has learned to shift weight in the standing frame. By rotating the trunk toward the weighted side, the non–weight-bearing side can be shifted forward (Figure 18-17). By reversing the weight shift, the opposite side can be moved forward and a type of "pivoting forward" progression can be accomplished. To maintain balance while shifting, the child may initially use a two-wheeled walker. The therapist may help initiate weight shift and trunk rotation by alternately pulling the arms forward.[153] Once the child has gained this form of mobility, the type of permanent bracing chosen will depend on the level of the lesion and a variety of other factors.

The overall goal for ambulatory training is to promote efficient, independent mobility with the least amount of bracing while maintaining optimal joint integrity. Ambulatory potential as well as choice of bracing depends on many factors, including neurosegmental level of the lesion, motor power at the neurosegmental level, extent and degree of orthopedic deformity, balance, age, height, weight, sex, motivation, spasticity, design and effectiveness of the orthosis, effectiveness of PT intervention, environmental factors, upper extremity strength and control, and cognitive level.[154,155] The best prognosis for ambulation is most often seen in the child who is not shunted with good cognition, good quadriceps power, no deformity, stable neurological condition, and hands-free sitting balance. Factors that may limit potential for ambulation include hydrocephalus, high-level lesions, kyphosis or kyphoscoliosis, and unstable neurology.

For thoracic and high-level lumbar lesions, a parapodium is often chosen. The parapodium was developed by the Ontario Crippled Children's Center in 1970 and is similar to the standing frame except that hinges at the hips and knees allow for sitting and standing.[153] It, too, can be adjusted for growth and can accommodate orthopedic deformities. As with the standing frame, proper alignment of the parapodium is critical. The therapist, in conjunction with the orthotist, should check for correct standing alignment. The prevention of additional orthopedic deformities, development of good muscular control, and normal body image depend on a good-fitting orthosis.

After a pivoting gait is learned with the parapodium, a swing-to or swing-through gait can be attempted. By 4 to 5 years of age, a swing-through gait, with the child using Lofstrand crutches, can usually be accomplished. Variations of the parapodium allow for easier locking and unlocking of hip and knee joints. A swivel or pivot walker also may be attached to the footplate to allow for crutchless walking.

Another type of orthosis for the child with a thoracic or high lumbar lesion is the Orlau swivel walker. It consists of modular design similar to the standing frame, with a chest strap and knee blocks attached to swiveling foot plates.[156] Rather than the whole base moving forward, as when weight is shifted in the parapodium, in the swivel walker each footplate is spring loaded and is able to swivel forward independently. This allows for independent balance on one foot and therefore crutchless ambulation. The Orlau swivel walker is manufactured in the United Kingdom, and assembly kits may be ordered (see Appendix 18-A).[157]

Both the parapodium and swivel walker have had some problems with instability, ease of application, and cosmesis. New designs attempt to correct these problems.[158] Nevertheless, existing limitations in the parapodium and swivel walker, particularly energy cost of walking, slow rate of locomotion, and cosmesis, have limited their use, primarily to the younger child.[159] These devices, however, remain an effective means of preventing musculoskeletal deformities caused by long-term sitting, wheelchair positioning, and general immobility. They also enhance social-emotional development gained from the upright position.[156,159] Another option for the higher-level child with good sitting balance is the reciprocating gait orthosis (RGO).[160] This brace consists of bilateral long-leg braces with a pelvic band and thoracic extension, if necessary. The hip joints are connected by a cable system that can work in two ways: If the child has active hip flexors, he or she can activate the cable system by shifting weight and flexing the non–weight-bearing extremity. This brings the weight-bearing extremity into relative extension in preparation for the next step. Without hip flexors, the child extends his or her trunk over one extremity, thus positioning it in relative extension. By virtue of the cable system, the non–weight-bearing extremity moves into flexion, thus initiating a step. Several types of the RGO are in use, including the dual-cable LSU[160] or the horizontal-cable type.[161]

Most recently the Isocentric Reciprocal Gait Orthosis (I-RGO) (Center for Orthotics Design, Campbell, Calif.) has been used for children with high-level spina bifida. It has a more cosmetic and efficient design compared with the dual-

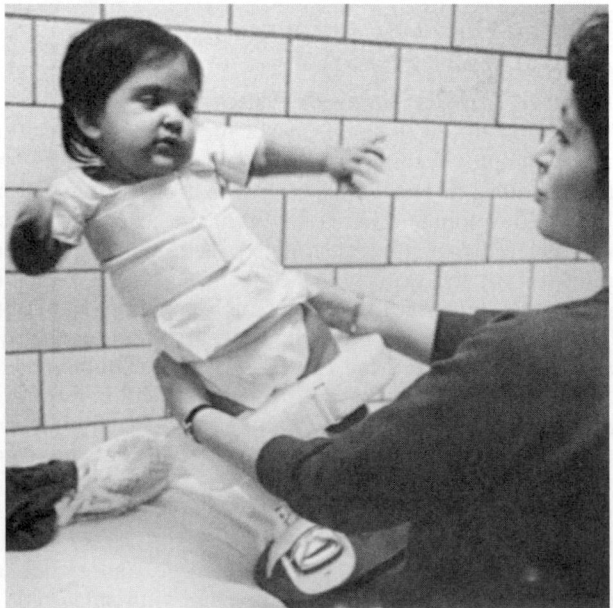

FIGURE 18-17 ■ Weight shift and forward rotation in standing frame.

cable LSU or horizontal-cable type RGO. This cableless brace has two to three times less friction and therefore is more energy efficient. The brace stabilizes the hip, knee, and ankle joints and balances the person, enabling him or her to stand hands free without the use of crutches or a walker (Figure 18-18).[161] Leg advancement for walking occurs through use of hip flexor or lower abdominal muscle contraction or through use of active or passive trunk extension.

A more common means of maintaining the upright position has been through the use of long- or short-leg braces. In the 1970s polypropylene braces largely replaced conventional metal bracing. These plastic orthoses are considerably lighter than metal bracing and therefore reduce the energy cost of walking for the child with spina bifida.[162] They allow close contact and can be slipped into the shoe rather than worn externally, thus affording the patient a better-fitting, more cosmetic orthosis.

The type of orthosis chosen (long-leg, with or without pelvic band, or short-leg) depends on the level of the myelomeningocele and the muscle power within that level (Table 18-3). Because lesions are frequently incomplete, muscle strength must be accurately assessed before bracing is prescribed. Independent sitting balance with hands free also is a prerequisite for use of long- or short-leg braces. Even children with L3 to L4 lesions who demonstrate incomplete knee extension may be able to use a short-leg brace with an anterior shell rather than requiring long-leg bracing.[163] This crouch-control AFO (CCAFO) will prevent a crouching gait pattern by improving knee extension during

gait (Figure 18-19).[164] The PT must work in conjunction with the orthopedist and orthotist to have each child fitted with the minimal amount of bracing that allows for joint stability and a good gait pattern (see Chapter 34).

Children with lower-level lesions (L5-S1) who use below-knee bracing often develop the ability to or choose to ambulate without assistive devices. However, recent studies have shown that crutch use may decrease excessive pelvic motion, which results in reducing abnormal joint forces.[165,166] Advocating for use of crutches may prevent abnormal joint forces, maintain joint integrity, and decrease the risk of additional orthopedic complications.

Children ambulating with AFOs often show excessive rotation at the knee because of the lack of functioning lateral hamstrings. Rather than going to a higher level of bracing, a twister cable can be added, which often decreases the rotary component during gait.[163] Twister cables can be heavy-duty torsion or more flexible elastic webbing, depending on function. Typically, the young child who is just beginning to pull to stand and remains reliant on floor mobility as the primary means of mobility should have elastic twisters prescribed to allow for ease of creeping and transitions. The older and more active child will require heavy-duty torsion cables. Rotational stresses may eventually lead to onset of late degenerative changes around the knee. A tibial derotation osteotomy may be indicated to prevent these changes from occurring.[167,168]

For children with low lumbar or sacral lesions who have at least fair strength in their dorsiflexors and plantar flexors, often a University of California Biomechanics Laboratory (UCBL) or polypropylene shoe insert to control foot position is the only bracing needed. These inserts fit snuggly inside the shoe and help control calcaneal and forefoot instabilities.[10] A supramalleolar orthosis (SMO) will also fit

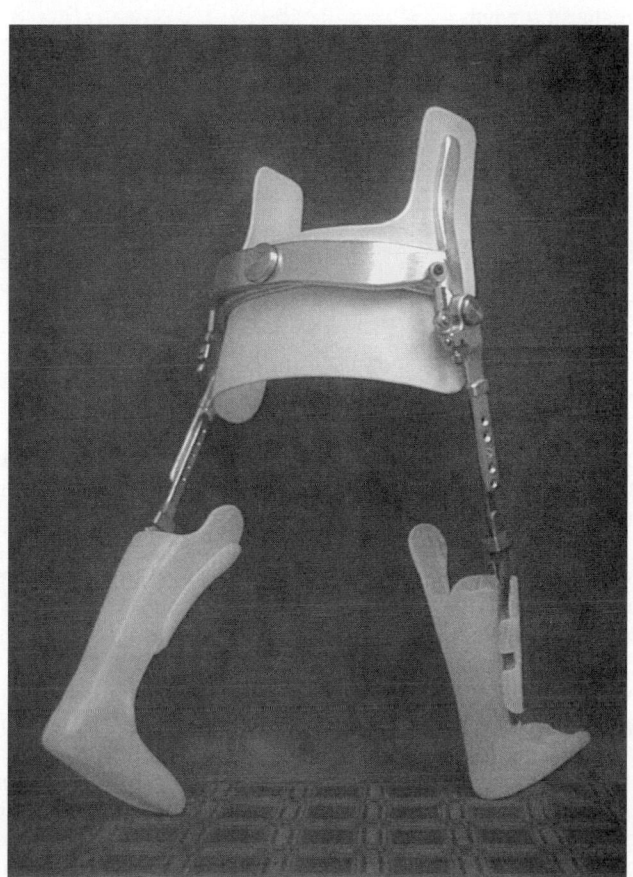

FIGURE 18-18 ■ RGO.

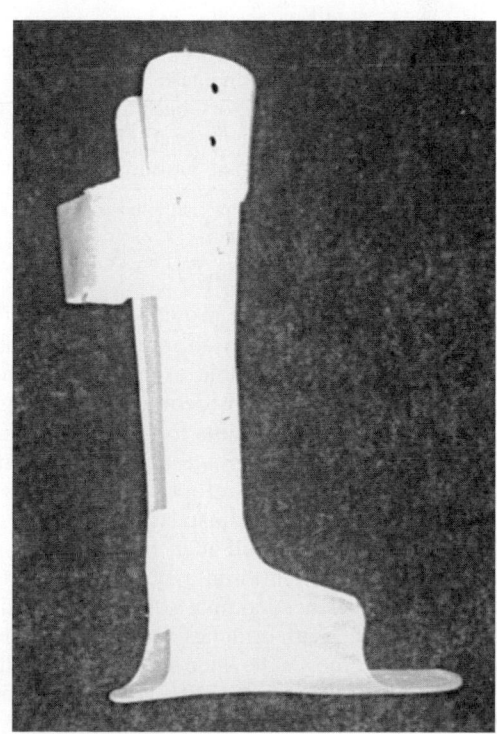

FIGURE 18-19 ■ Crouch control AFO.

TABLE 18-3 ■ **Common Gait Patterns and Levels of Assistance Required in Myelomeningocele**

LEVEL OF LESION	MUSCLE PERFORMANCE	RECOMMENDED LEVEL OF ASSISTANCE AND BRACING	AMBULATORY PROGRESSION
T8-L1 and above	Flaccid LEs with fair to poor trunk	Parapodium: Orlau, Toronto, Rochester Assistive devices often unnecessary with Orlau but may improve function with Toronto or Rochester braces	
L1-L2	Flaccid LEs with hip flexors present	Parapodium with progression to RGO RGO, ambulating with hips locked	Begin ambulating with a walker, progress to forearm crutches Four-point or swing-through gait
L3-L4	Fair quadriceps with weak or absent hamstrings	HKAFOs may be used with severe lordosis because of weak or absent gluteal musculature and decreased trunk control or to control rotation and abduction/adduction If quadriceps are less than fair strength, KAFOs may be needed As the patient progresses he or she may be cut down from KAFOs to AFOs; AFOs may be used with or without twister cables	Begin ambulating with a walker, progress to forearm crutches Four-point gait Begin ambulating with a walker and progress to forearm crutches In some rare cases the patient may progress to no assistive device at all depending on the gait pattern With increased use of trunk reversal the patient should be returned to forearm crutches to allow for a pattern that is more cosmetic and energy efficient Four-point gait pattern
L5	Good hip flexors and quadriceps; fair anterior tibialis; weak gluteus medius and maximus, toe extensors and gastrosoleus	AFOs with or without twisters depending on gluteal strength AFO is used to prevent a crouch gait pattern from weak gastrosoleus	Forearm crutches or no assistive devices Four-point gait
S1	Good hip flexors, quadriceps, gluteus medius, and toe extensors; weak gluteus maximus and gastrosoleus	AFO	Generally no assistive device is used unless decreased balance reactions or excessive lateral trunk flexion are present
S2-S3	Good hip flexors, quadriceps, gluteus medius and maximus, and gastrosoleus	Often no bracing needed	Often no assistive devices needed

LE, Lower extremity; *RGO,* reciprocating gait orthosis; *KAFO,* knee-ankle-foot orthosis; *HKAFO,* hip-knee-ankle-foot orthosis; *AFO,* ankle-foot-orthosis.

easily inside the shoe but will provide additional medial/lateral support and stability that an insert will not provide. Even though a child may be able to ambulate without an assistive device or bracing, consideration must be given to the stresses that occur at the joints that over time may lead to orthopedic deformity. The greatest risk of joint instability often occurs at the knee. Barefoot walking versus use of an AFO has shown increased instability, joint stress, and pain at the hip and knee as well as increased energy expenditure.[169-171] Even though children may be able to ambulate without the use of crutches, comparison of gait kinetics and kinematics of walking with crutches has shown a significant decrease of valgus forces at the knee and better overall alignment of the lower extremities.[165] Treatment aimed at strengthening gluteus medius and maximus strength to aid in increasing pelvic stability and reducing kinematic com-

pensations can also be important in the management of patients at this level to enhance their efficiency during ambulation.[172,173]

Gait training, begun as the child first starts to stand, can now continue in a more formalized manner. By using the appropriate orthosis and assistive devices (walker, crutches, or cane), each child must be helped to achieve the most efficient and effective gait pattern possible (see Table 18-3). As a part of gait training, the child should be taken out of the bracing and "challenged" so that righting and equilibrium reactions can be developed to their maximum. For example, having a child maintain balance while sitting on a ball or other movable surface (tilt board, trampoline) requires the participation of all available musculature, especially abdominal and trunk extensor muscles (Figure 18-20). Strengthening available musculature is a primary objective in this

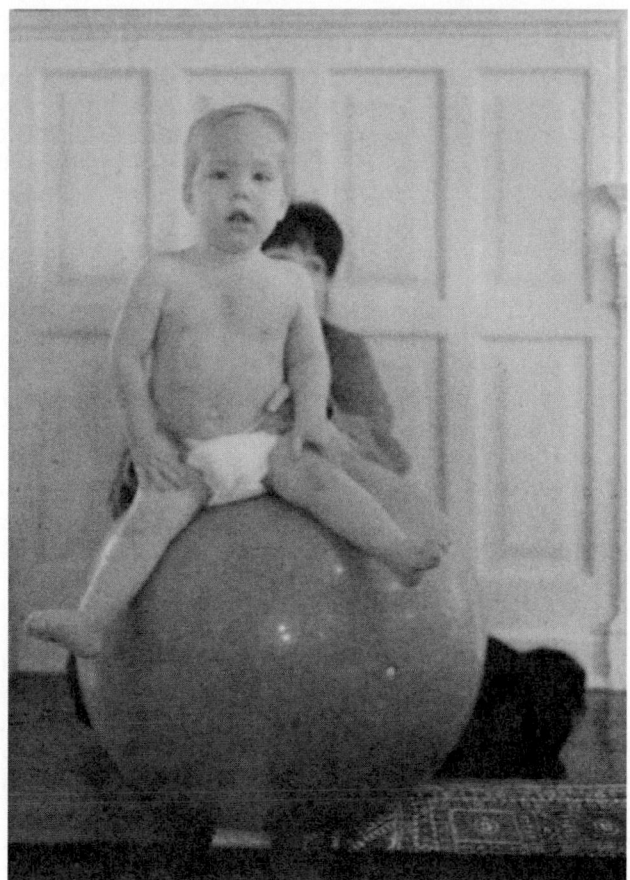

FIGURE 18-20 ■ Balance and strengthening exercises done on a movable surface.

phase of treatment. Often slow gains in muscle strength are the result of continued emphasis on strengthening during physical therapy. In addition to trunk muscles, the gluteus medius, gluteus maximus, and quadriceps are often targeted. Prone activities such as picking up toys while over a Swiss ball or moving around while prone on a scooter board requires use of these muscles while providing an enjoyable exercise for the child. Participation in equestrian therapy and aquatherapy programs at this age can also be beneficial. These unconventional gait-training techniques can be used to improve muscle strength in general and the gait pattern when bracing is reapplied. Regardless of the strengthening activities chosen, the pediatric therapist has the special task of using creativity to involve the child in therapeutic play activities. The ideas for creative activities are limitless but essential for combining therapy with age-appropriate cognitive abilities.

Sensory limitations may impede progress during early ambulation training. Because of limited kinesthesia and proprioception, available sensory systems must be augmented and the child taught to substitute with nonimpaired sensory systems. Impaired kinesthesia in children with myelomeningocele impedes their ability to anticipate changes in terrain and poses a safety problem. Vision may be the most relevant system to allow them to scan and preplan for changes in their walking environment.

Gait training and muscle strengthening are not the only consideration of the therapist. How cognitive and psy-

chosocial development can be enhanced during this stage of the child's development is also important. One appropriate solution is to place the child in a center-based EI program. Although these programs may vary in the services they provide, most usually include age-appropriate play activities and some type of parental counseling. In addition, many offer therapeutic intervention from physical, occupational, and speech therapists. This intervention may occur in groups or individually.

Besides the socialization that center-based EI programs provide for the child with myelomeningocele, they also teach the child age-appropriate ADLs, such as dressing and undressing. At this age ADL skills are more appropriately taught in a group setting than individually. For many children the EI program, along with individualized therapy, is sufficient to enhance development in the physical, cognitive, and psychosocial realms.

Presently, when children reach age 3 years, public school education becomes available to them. The preschool or early childhood (EC) program continues to offer the same fundamental benefits as the EI program. It is the role of the EI therapist to communicate the specific needs of each child entering the public school system. In this way continuity in the child's rehabilitation program is preserved.

The spina bifida team, usually headed by a pediatrician or clinical nurse specialist, continues to follow the child closely during this stage. The neurosurgeon checks shunt functioning and perform revisions as necessary. The orthopedist supervises bracing efforts to prevent and correct deformities in the spine and lower extremities. Well-child care and general medical treatment is the responsibility of the pediatrician on the team. The urologist continues to monitor renal functioning while keeping the child dry and free of infection. At this stage, the clinical nurse specialist will usually teach bowel and bladder training to the child and family. This clinician generally initiates this training according to age-appropriate developmental guidelines.

Bladder training usually consists of transferring the job of CIC from the parents to the child. Children as young as 3 years, but certainly by the age of 5 years, can learn CIC in a short period.[174] Children may first practice on dolls with male and female genitalia. Next, using mirrors to understand their own genital anatomy, they are able to accomplish the technique on themselves. CIC in conjunction with pharmacotherapy is useful in achieving continence in children with spina bifida.[115] Another method of bladder training recently being used in the United States is intravesical transurethral bladder stimulation. This technique has allowed children with neurogenic bladder to rehabilitate their bladder function so that they can detect bladder fullness and generate effective detrusor contractions, leading to improved continence.[83,175]

Bowel training can be achieved through proper diet, regular evacuation times, and appropriate use of stool softeners and suppositories.[83] Constipation (and resulting bypass diarrhea) can be prevented by proper habit training and use of fiber supplements. Stool softeners (not laxatives and enemas) and suppositories should be used to keep the stools soft and help stimulate evacuation. Finally, toilet training, which amounts to scheduled toileting in time with the stool stimulants, usually achieves bowel continence. Surgical procedures, such as the Malone ACE procedure,[74] may be necessary when other interventions have failed. The Malone ACE procedure, performed in conjunction with a Mitrofanoff procedure to gain urinary continence, can help these patients attain a better quality of life. Consistency at each step along the way is the key to successful bowel training. A therapist may be called on to assist the parents and child in obtaining independence in this ADL activity.

Other members of the team, such as the psychologist, social worker, and dietician, continue to function in their appropriate roles, interacting with the child and family as necessary. Physical and occupational therapists, as members of the team, must be sure that their treatment plans collaborate with the efforts of other team members.

Stage 5: Primary School Through Adolescence

This stage of development is marked by less rapid growth than earlier childhood but ends with a period of rapid physiological growth. Children in the 6- to 10-year age group are interested in a wider variety of physical activities as they challenge their bodies to perform. The adolescent, however, is going through a period of great sexual differentiation as primary and secondary sexual characteristics develop more fully.

Cognitively, children are able to solve problems in a more sophisticated manner, although they revert to illogical thinking with complex problems. As they reach adolescence, they become capable of hypothetical reasoning and their thought processes approach that of adults.

Emotionally, the 6 to 10 year old is in a period of relative calm. Children are interested in schoolwork and are eager to produce. During this period, they are building the skills of the future, preparing them for adult work. This is a prime time to introduce and teach new skills.

Adolescence is a stormy emotional period. Adolescents remain in turmoil as they seek their identities through sexual, social, and vocational activities. As their value systems develop, they feel less ambivalence between remaining as children and striving for independence. For the child with myelomeningocele, adolescence is not an optimal time to introduce new skills leading toward self-care and independence.[176]

As the energy cost of walking becomes too high, use of a wheelchair for locomotion often becomes appropriate. To a teenager whose emotional needs include a strong peer identity, being confined to a wheelchair may be devastating. Appropriate alternatives may be to delay the decision to use a wheelchair full time or limit ambulation to short distances or to those places most important to the child. Again, goals must be tailored to the child's needs and encompass his or her whole being.

In accordance with the child's growth spurts, frequent adjustment or reordering of bracing will be necessary. Continual reevaluation of orthotic needs may reveal that the level of bracing may decrease as the child grows and becomes stronger; the opposite development is also a possibility.

Usually during this stage, if it has not occurred previously, the evaluation of future ambulation potential occurs. The child whose larger size and limited abilities make ambulation more difficult each day frequently requests this evaluation. Strength does not increase in the same proportion as body weight.[107] Ambulation, although possible for the young child, may be impossible for that same person as a young adult.

Although no guidelines include every patient, generally children with thoracic-level lesions are rarely ambulators by the late teens.[10,126,177] Those with upper lumbar lesions may be household ambulators with long-leg bracing but will require wheelchairs for quick and efficient mobility as adults. With low lumbar lesions, most adults can become community ambulators. Patients with sacral-level lesions are usually able to ambulate freely within the community. Many require minimal bracing and ambulate without assistive devices.[10,126,177] It must be remembered that ambulatory status is not determined by level of the lesion alone. The muscle power available, degree of orthopedic deformity, age, height, weight of the patient and, of course, motivation are also determining factors.[10,68,128,163,178]

Because a large number of older children with spina bifida will become wheelchair dependent, potential problems connected with a sedentary existence must be explored. Skin care, always a concern for the child with spina bifida, becomes a priority for the constant sitter. Mirrors may be used for self-inspection of the skin twice daily. Well-constructed foam, gel, or air-cell seat cushions are essential for distributing pressure evenly. Children should be taught frequent weight shifting within the chair to relieve pressure areas. Clothing should not be constricting but heavy enough to protect sensitive skin from wheelchair parts. Children must also be taught to avoid extremes of temperature and environmental hazards, such as radiators, sharp objects, and abrasive surfaces. The therapist must reinforce the importance of skin care to prevent setbacks in the rehabilitation process that may result when skin breakdown develops.

Children with higher-level lesions may need spinal support to prevent deformities. A polyethylene body jacket or thoracolumbar sacral orthosis (TLSO) can be used to provide this support and, hopefully, prevent the progression of any paralytic deformities.[10] Whatever type of device or wheelchair padding is used, the therapist must check to see that weight is distributed equally through both buttocks and that the spine is supported as needed. Part of the therapeutic intervention is to provide strengthening exercises or activities to be done out of the supporting orthosis. This is necessary to maintain existing trunk strength and to preserve the child's present level of function.

Generally, in late childhood or early adolescence, orthopedic deformities that have been gradually developing require surgical intervention. Progressive scoliosis or kyphosis may require internal fixation when conservative methods fail.[179] Sectioning of tight or contracted muscles at the hip and knee is often required.[126] The iliopsoas, adductors, and hamstrings are frequently the offending muscles. These surgeries, followed by strengthening exercises and gait training, often add to the ambulatory life of the child with spina bifida. For example, in a child who displays an extreme lordotic posture, hip flexion contractures may be present and surgical lengthening of the tight muscles may be required to allow improved biomechanical alignment for standing and balance. Strengthening of the hip extensors and abdominals also helps prevent future muscle imbalances that may lead to contractures and tightness. A postoperative therapeutic program might include periods of prone lying to prevent future contractures and strengthening of hip extensors and abdominals that were previously overstretched by the lordotic position.

Of primary importance during this stage is preparing the child for independence in ADLs, which may be broken down into self-care, locomotion-related, and social interaction activities. In conjunction with the nurse, physical therapist, and occupational therapist, self-care skills of dressing, eating, and food preparation; general hygiene; and bowel and bladder care can be addressed. Because the adolescent is so concerned with achieving independence, he or she is more likely to comply with a regimen of strengthening exercises if shown how they relate to functional independence. A creative therapist may, for example, incorporate trunk stability and upper-extremity strengthening work in activities such as making popcorn or getting ready for a dance. In addition, fostering social and recreational independence through adaptive sports and fitness programs and leisure activities should not be overlooked. Participation in adaptive sports can aid immensely in improving strength, endurance, and self-esteem. Community adaptive recreational programs may include T-ball, martial arts, swimming, tennis, basketball, skiing, bowling, and many other common sports and leisure activities (Figures 18-21, 18-22, and 18-23).

Locomotion activities should include all gait-related skills, such as falling down, getting up, and ambulation on various terrains and stairs. Transfers of all types should also be included in locomotion activities. Again, a creative therapeutic program helps make achievement of skills more palatable. For example, school-aged children may enjoy a competitive relay race situation in which each child falls, gets up, walks across the room, and sits down in a chair safely. This type of activity combines gait-training activities with group socialization and may meet a variety of goals (motor and psychosocial) at the same time.

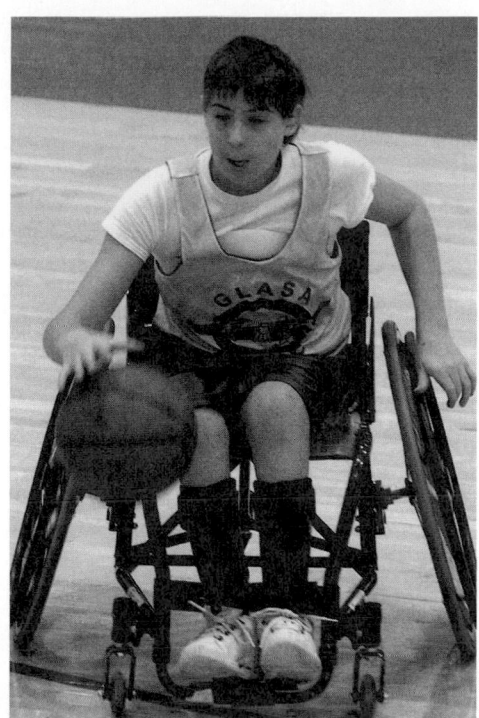

FIGURE 18-22 ■ Participation in wheelchair basketball. (Courtesy of Su Metzel.)

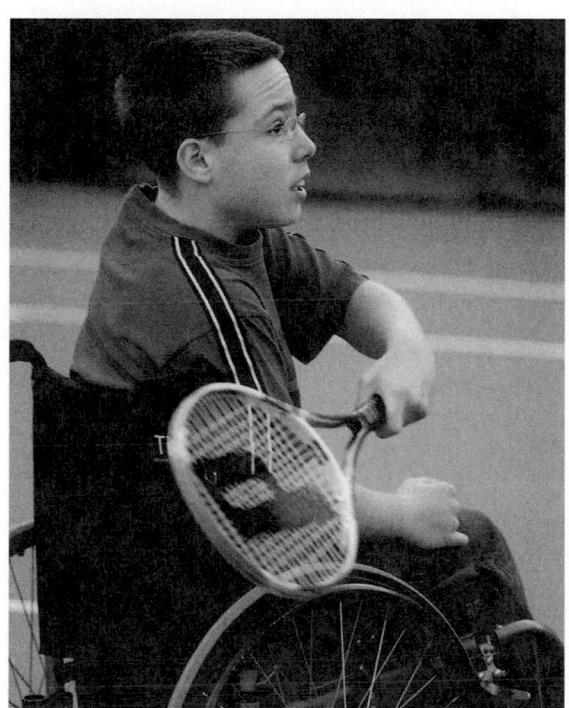

FIGURE 18-23 ■ Participation in adaptive tennis. (Courtesy of Su Metzel.)

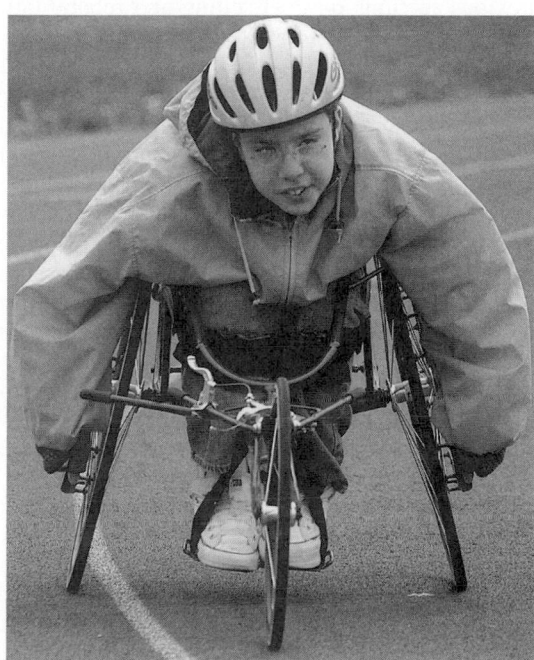

FIGURE 18-21 ■ Participation in wheelchair racing. (Courtesy of Su Metzel.)

Achievement of independence in ADLs for the child and adult with spina bifida does not depend solely on the level of paralysis. Also important are psychosocial and environmental factors. Mean ages for the achievement of various ADL activities have been developed and may assist the therapist in establishing realistic therapeutic goals in this area.[180]

Often during this stage of rehabilitation, the therapist may be asked to assist in assessing cognitive function. The perceptual and cognitive evaluations previously discussed may be administered and the results interpreted for parents and school personnel.

Also as previously discussed, children with spina bifida have a general perceptual deficit that can manifest itself in a variety of ways. First, the child may have difficulty recognizing objects and the relations that they have to each other. They may therefore perceive their world in a distorted manner, thus making their reactions unstable and unpredictable. These perceptual difficulties will most likely affect academic learning and may associate failure with the learning process. Difficulties in attaining independence in ADL activities are also linked to perceptual problems. Finally, emotional disturbances may be attributed in part to the perceptual difficulties of the child with spina bifida.[81]

Remedial programs, such as the Frostig Program for the Development of Visual Perception, have been effective in improving the visual perception of children with spina bifida.[81] Programs of this type are most effective when remediation begins early, preferably at or before the time the child enters school.

Children with spina bifida may also have difficulties with tasks requiring sensorimotor integration. Children requiring programs for sensorimotor integration should be referred to a therapist certified in this area. If one is not available, many appropriate activities for sensorimotor integration may be adapted from Ayres[181] or Montgomery and Richter.[182]

Regardless of the school setting chosen for the child, the therapist should be able to serve the classroom teacher as a consultant. Advice on adaptive seating and therapeutic goals appropriate for the classroom help ensure that the rehabilitation process will continue in the classroom as well as promote optimal conditions for learning.

When a child is moving from the preschool to elementary school setting, the support of the therapeutic team is essential and invaluable. The teacher's expectations, as created by the therapist regarding the child's special needs and abilities, often spell the difference between success and failure of complete academic and psychosocial integration within the school setting. Even though the child may no longer require direct therapeutic intervention, periodic consultation, including site classroom visits, are recommended to prevent minor problems from developing into major ones. For example, bowel and bladder accidents can be avoided by scheduling regular times for toileting. The teacher may be able to make minor adjustments in the teaching schedule to accommodate for this scheduling. Also, full-control braces (from hip to ankles) may seem overwhelming to the layperson. If the teacher is shown how the braces lock and unlock to allow the child to sit or stand to walk, he or she may feel more at ease if ever called on to assist the child.

The psychological perspective of the child colors therapeutic goals in this stage. As the child nears adolescence, these psychosocial aspects become of paramount importance. Although the therapist should not take on the role of the psychologist, collaborative efforts in the area of counseling will be necessary. Questions will arise many times during the physical/occupational therapy sessions, requiring factual answers that the therapist can and should provide.

Adolescents with spina bifida show great concern about self-esteem and social-sexual adjustment.[183,184] These concerns appear directly related to efficient bowel and bladder management.[185] Strategies to cope with bowel and bladder difficulties, as previously outlined, combined with appropriate emotional support from family and medical personnel help alleviate this concern.

Although great advances in medical management of children with myelomeningocele have occurred, a contrasting lack of improvement related to sexual function and reproductive issues exists. Five factors have contributed to delayed social and sexual growth in these adolescents: (1) severity of the mental handicap, (2) poor manual dexterity, (3) lack of education, (4) overprotective parents, and (5) limitations in health care personnel's ability to address sexuality with physically disabled patients and their families.[186] Questions about sexuality may be brought up by either the parents or the child. Parents of children with spina bifida realize the need to teach their children about sexuality, but they often feel inadequate about doing so and are reluctant to bring up questions to health care professionals.[187] The therapist must be open, informed, and able to provide resources to both parents and children.

Generally, the sexual capacity of the female with spina bifida is near normal; that is, she has potential for a normal orgasmic response, is fertile, and can bear children.[14,20,188] The pregnancy, however, may be considered high risk, depending on existing orthopedic abnormalities. Affected males are frequently sterile and have small testicles and penises. Their potential for erection and ejaculation depends on the level of the lesion. In many cases psychological problems may be a primary cause of sexual failure.[14] Sexuality is not merely a process involving the genitalia; it also depends on a positive body image and a feeling of self-esteem that is nurtured from birth.[113,189]

PSYCHOSOCIAL ADJUSTMENT TO CONGENITAL CORD LESIONS

The previous sections on goal setting and rehabilitation of the child with spina bifida have covered birth through adolescence. After adolescence, rehabilitation can be handled in much the same manner as an adult spinal cord injury. Keeping in mind the global effects of spina bifida on the growing child as he or she approaches adulthood is important, however.

Because of the congenital nature of spina bifida, psychological adjustment is somewhat different than adjustment to a traumatic spinal cord injury. The psychological adjustment to this congenital disability must be considered from the perspective of the parents, the family and, of course, the child.[190]

A longitudinal study concerning the psychological aspects of spina bifida showed that the parents go through a series of steps in the adjustment process. From birth to approximately 6 months of age, the parents experience shock and bewilderment. Information given during this time may be rejected or misinterpreted. Health care professionals therefore must be ready to repeat the same information to parents on several occasions during the first few years of the rehabilitation process. The period of 6 to 18 months of the child's life may be the most stressful on parents. Frequent hospitalizations during this time place increased pressure on the whole family. Parents are now able to comprehend fully the implications of their child's functional limitations and inability to participate in life. They begin to worry about the future and the impact of the disability on the rest of the family structure. The period from age 2 years through the preschool years is relatively peaceful. The parents are more concerned with toilet training, social acceptability, and general information on child rearing. They seem less aware of their child's cognitive limitations as he or she continues to develop into a relatively happy, well-adjusted child.

By the age of 6 years, children are becoming more aware of their limitations and parents are concerned about problems that may arise as their children enter elementary school. The child's psychological adjustment depends on the severity of the motor problems but primarily on the attitude of the parents and family and on the environmental conditions to which he or she is exposed.[185,191,192]

Because of their disabilities, children with spina bifida are often denied small tasks or chores that promote a sense of responsibility in the growing child.[107,183] To promote emotional growth and psychological well-being, caregivers must be persuaded to let go. Children with spina bifida must develop responsibility and independence by being given the chance to interact and even compete with their peers. As they approach adulthood, concerns regarding independent living situations and vocational placement must be addressed. With a foundation of strong support systems fostering emotional maturity, the future can be bright for the child with a congenital spinal cord injury (Case Study 18-1).

CASE STUDY 18-1 ■ MICHAEL

This case study focuses on the physical therapy management of Michael, a teenage boy with myelomeningocele (MM), a congenital spinal cord injury. Michael is now 16 years old and a sophomore in high school.

A spinal cord injury is a complex disability. When a spinal cord lesion exists from birth, an additional complexity is added. This congenital condition predisposes that many areas of the CNS may not develop or function adequately. In addition, all areas of development—physical, cognitive, and psychosocial—that depend so heavily on central functioning will likely be impaired. The clinician therefore must be aware of the significant impact this neurological defect has on motor function as well as a variety of related human capacities. Management can best be organized by using the *Guide to Physical Therapist Practice*. The following case study uses the concepts in the guide to discuss several episodes of care throughout Michael's life.

The *Guide to Physical Therapist Practice* is designed to provide a framework for the physical therapist to assist in client management.[1] During the infant to adolescent life span, Michael's specific PT needs will change. Michael's presentation of congenital spinal cord dysfunction may be best represented through the life span by preferred practice patterns, which may include the following[1]:

- 4F: Impaired joint mobility, motor function, muscle performance, ROM, and reflex integrity associated with spinal disorders
- 5C: Impaired motor function and sensory integrity associated with nonprogressive disorders of the CNS—congenital origin or acquired in infancy or childhood
- 6E: Impaired ventilation and respiration/gas exchange associated with ventilatory pump dysfunction or failure
- 7A: Primary prevention/risk reduction for integumentary disorders

Examination (evaluation) is a comprehensive screening and specific testing process that leads to a diagnostic classification required before intervention and is performed for all clients. It consists of three components: client history, systems review, and tests and measures. The physical therapist may identify impairments, functional limitations and disability, and changes in physical function or overall health status. The physical therapist synthesizes the findings to establish a working diagnosis (ICD-9 Code 741.0). Results from the evaluation are established and interventions with anticipated outcomes are made.[1] Refer to Tables 18-4 to 18-10 for a detailed synopsis of Michael's episodes of physical therapy during his 16 years. The occupational therapist should go through a similar process of screening and testing to develop a conceptual model for case management within the scope of occupational therapy. Many of the examination tools and intervention strategies may be the same, although the objective outcome may focus on different expectations.

NEWBORN EPISODE OF CARE

Michael was a term baby delivered by planned cesarean section with a prenatal diagnosis of myelomeningocele. The diagnosis was made during the second trimester after fetal ultrasound evaluation and amniocentesis. The family met with the neurosurgeon before delivery. Michael was delivered at 38 weeks of gestation and was transferred at 1 day of age to the local children's hospital for a planned surgical closure of his spina bifida. An orthopedic, urological, neurosurgical, and PT assessment occurred at 1 day of age before back closure. Michael was the second child for this family. His mother was diagnosed with breast cancer at his birth. His sister is 2 years older and lives at home. Both parents are professional working parents who have a nanny to assist with child care.

Presurgical MMT showed the presence of hip and knee musculature (L2-L4). Three days after the back closure, Michael required ventriculoperitoneal shunt insertion to control hydrocephalus. Postoperative MMT findings at 7 days of age were identical to preoperative results. Before discharge at 8 days of age parents were

Continued

CASE STUDY 18-1 ■ MICHAEL—cont'd

instructed in ROM exercises, positioning, and developmental handling. Michael would be monitored in an MM clinic twice a year for an MMT and functional assessment with a team of health care providers (Table 18-4).

EPISODE OF CARE: 6-MONTH FOLLOW-UP

At the age of 6 months Michael was readmitted to the hospital because of a shunt malfunction requiring ventriculoperitoneal shunt revision. After 2 weeks at home Michael returned to the clinic for postoperative follow-up. No medical concerns were present, but clinicians discovered that Michael had not yet begun to roll over. An evaluation with a standardized test was conducted. The AIMS was administered as well as additional tests of ROM, strength (by observation), reflexes, muscle tone, and endurance to establish a developmental baseline. At this visit a total-body night splint was fabricated to maintain hip alignment and prevent contractures of the lower extremities. Family education in latex precautions was provided. The need for assistive and adaptive devices was also assessed.

At this point, Michael had not received physical therapy because of the mother's health issues. Because of this situation, physical therapy that could be provided at home was recommended. The family was given a referral to their local EI system and a list of local pediatric physical therapy providers to obtain services (Table 18-5).

EPISODE OF CARE: EARLY INTERVENTION

The family contacted their local EI program after the previous clinic visit. An evaluation and assessment determined Michael was eligible for services. A variety of appropriate developmental assessments was used to determine eligibility (Table 18-6). At the individual family service plan meeting physical therapy intervention was determined to be the primary service at this time. Occupational, developmental, and speech therapies were not recommended. Michael received weekly physical therapy from 6 months through the age of 3 years. Therapy focused on developmental exercises to promote mobility, sitting and standing balance activities, strengthening available lower-extremity musculature, and orthotic assessment and gait training. The EI physical therapist instructed the family in activities to complement the weekly physical therapy program. Michael began crawling at 1 year. At 10 months he used a vertical stander to initiate an upright stand position and began gait training at 15 months. Michael began walking with AFOs and a forward walker at 30 months (see Table 18-6).

EPISODE OF CARE: EARLY CHILDHOOD

At age 3 years, Michael transitioned into an early childhood (EC) program at his local school. Physical therapy was a related service that was included as part of his individual educational plan (IEP). The transition meeting from EI to EC programming provided continuity of care unique to his needs. A global assessment tool to assess his mobility and self-care skills was administered. This test, the PEDI, was administered

by the physical therapist. Physical therapy management included ROM, strengthening, and gait training as it affected his ability to function in the preschool classroom and surrounding play areas. The school he attended was environmentally appropriate for his needs. It was one level, with wide doorways that allowed the use of his walker and then progressive use of forearm crutches with AFOs to advance his mobility skills. At the suggestion of his physical therapist in the outpatient MM clinic, Michael became involved in a toddler swimming program at the park district. A tricycle was adapted at the recommendation of the same therapist to assist with strengthening his lower extremities and to allow him to efficiently keep pace with his peers (Table 18-7).

Another framework that can organize the management of Michael's interventions is the International Classification of Function, Disability, and Health (ICF). The ICF identifies components of health and contextual factors that are important for achievement of desired outcomes.[193] Relationships between components of health and contextual factors change over time. An example is given for one episode of care, early childhood (Figure 18-24).

At age 5.5 years, an IEP meeting was conducted before he entered kindergarten. The family and school team decided that no resources or special adaptations were necessary to enhance his education. The school he was to attend was determined to be environmentally appropriate to meet his needs.

EPISODE OF CARE: TETHERED CORD EPISODE (AGE 6 YEARS)

At his semiannual visit to the MM clinic, the parents mentioned that Michael was falling frequently while using his forearm crutches and AFOs. Reddened areas at the left lateral calcaneus were noted. A routine MMT showed decreased strength in his left leg with an increase in muscle tone through his left leg. An MRI revealed a tethered spinal cord. A neurosurgical tethered cord release (TCR) was performed and his AFOs were revised. Two months after TCR Michael was again independent in ambulation and had progressed to stair climbing with one rail. His next routine 6-month MMT showed a return of strength to the level before his tethered cord episode (Table 18-8).

EPISODE OF CARE: PRE-ADOLESCENCE (7 TO 10 YEARS OF AGE)

Michael's physical conditioning continued to progress, and from ages 7 to 10 years he participated in adaptive sports and activities in his community. Swimming had become a favorite activity. He had been swimming to increase strength and endurance since he was a toddler at the suggestion of his physical therapist. Because of his activity level and independence in most functional activities, routine physical therapy had been discontinued with only biannual clinic visits. Michael and his family continued intensive stretching and a prone positioning program that they had been performing since Michael was a toddler. At his 10-year

CASE STUDY 18-1 ■ MICHAEL—cont'd

clinic visit, the therapist administered a formal MMT and ROM assessment and also carried out the PEDI. Scaled scores on the PEDI were used because he was above the age of normed standards for the test. An area of skin breakdown was noted on the left malleolus and decreased weight bearing was noted during gait. MMT and orthopedic examinations showed no changes. A brace check noted the AFO was too small and needed to be replaced. The brace was replaced and the physical therapist reviewed skin care and brace fit with Michael and his family (Table 18-9).

EPISODE OF CARE: ADOLESCENCE (AGE 13 YEARS)

At age 13 years Michael had gained a significant amount of weight that was limiting endurance for long-distance ambulation. Michael was referred to a nutritionist for counseling. The physical therapist in conjunction with the physician discussed with Michael and his parents the possibility of using a wheelchair for long-distance travel. After much discussion and initial resistance from Michael, Michael and his family decided to try a wheelchair. At age 16 years, Michael continues to be an independent ambulator and uses a wheelchair for long distances only. He continues to be monitored on an annual basis or as needed as problems arise. Michael's physical therapy has encouraged and continued to motivate him to maintain his participation in sports activities during his teenage years (Table 18-10).

TABLE 18-4 ■ Newborn Episode of Care for Child with Spina Bifida

PRACTICE PATTERNS	SYSTEMS TO REVIEW	TESTS AND RESULTS	INTERVENTIONS	ANTICIPATED GOALS AND EXPECTED OUTCOMES
4F	Musculoskeletal	**MMT:** No innervation below L4	Collaborate and coordinate systems review evaluation results with health care team.	Joint integrity and mobility improves.
7A	Integumentary	**Muscle length:** WFL	Document impairments, functional limitations, and strengths.	Postural control and muscle performance improves.
6E	Cardiopulmonary	**ROM:** WFL		Sensory awareness develops appropriately.
5C	Neuromuscular Cognition/ communication	**Skin integrity:** WFL **HR/RR/CE:** WFL **Reflexes:** Absent DTRs below knee (+) Suck/swallow (+) Galant **Muscle tone:** Flaccid below L4; low in trunk; upper extremities: WFL **Motor skills:** Informal testing turns head, kicks, clears head in prone **Observation:** Decreased pain in LEs	Prepare a plan of treatment. Therapeutic exercises to improve balance, muscle strength, and mobility. Family training: instruction in ROM; developmental positioning for function and enhancement of performance; instruction regarding sensory impairment and skin integrity and areas of pressure; and instruction in signs of VP shunt malfunction.	Risk prevention: parents understand signs and symptoms of VP shunt malfunction. Caregivers understand importance of checking skin for irritation and breakdown. Cognition and language develops appropriately. Improved infant/family sense of well-being. Stressors decrease.

WFL, Within functional limits; *HR,* heart rate; *RR,* respiratory rate; *CE,* cardiorespiratory endurance; *DTR,* deep tendon reflex; *LE,* lower extremity; *VP,* ventriculoperitoneal.

TABLE 18-5 ■ Six-Month Follow-up Episode of Care for Child with Spina Bifida

PRACTICE PATTERNS	SYSTEMS TO REVIEW	TESTS AND RESULTS	INTERVENTIONS	ANTICIPATED GOALS AND EXPECTED OUTCOMES
4F 7A 6E 5C	Musculoskeletal Integumentary Cardiopulmonary Neuromuscular Cognition/ communication	**MMT:** No innervation below L4 **Muscle length:** WFL **ROM:** WFL **Skin integrity:** WFL **HR/RR/CE:** WFL **Reflexes:** Absent DTRs below knee (+) Suck/swallow (+) Galant **Muscle tone:** Flaccid below L4; low in trunk; upper extremities: WFL **Motor skills:** AIMS completed; could not roll over, head righting emerging in prone and supported sitting **Observation:** Decreased pain in LEs VP shunt malfunction	Revised shunt: neurosurgery. Collaborate and coordinate systems review evaluation results with health care team. Document impairments, functional limitations, and strengths. Prepare a plan of treatment. Therapeutic exercises to improve balance and mobility. Family training: review instruction in ROM, positioning for function, signs of shunt malfunction, and latex precautions. Refer to EI program. Fabricate night splint for LE alignment. Transition to vertical stander at 10 months of age.	Joint integrity and mobility improves. Motor control and muscle performance improve. Established in physical therapy program. Risk prevention: parents understand signs and symptoms of VP shunt malfunction and importance of checking skin for irritation and breakdown. Latex precautions understood. Sensory awareness develops appropriately. Cognition and communication develop appropriately. Improved infant/family sense of well-being. Infant/family stressors decrease.

WFL, Within functional limits; *HR,* heart rate; *RR,* respiratory rate; *CE,* cardiorespiratory endurance; *DTR,* deep tendon reflex; *LE,* lower extremity; *VP,* ventriculoperitoneal, *EI,* early intervention; *AIMS,* Alberta Infant Motor Scales.

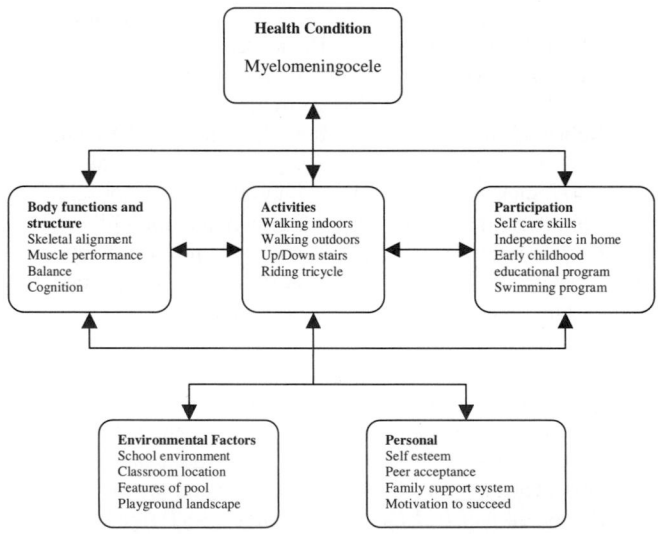

FIGURE 18-24 ■ Michael's early childhood episode of care as illustrated by the ICF model.

TABLE 18-6 ■ Early Intervention Episode of Care for Child with Spina Bifida

PRACTICE PATTERNS	SYSTEMS TO REVIEW	TESTS AND RESULTS	INTERVENTIONS	ANTICIPATED GOALS AND EXPECTED OUTCOMES
4F 7A	Musculoskeletal Integumentary	**MMT:** No innervation below L4 **Muscle length:** WFL	Collaborate and coordinate systems review evaluation results with health care team.	Joint integrity and mobility improves. Postural control and muscle performance improves.
6E 5C	Cardiopulmonary Neuromuscular Cognition/ Communication	**ROM:** WFL **Skin integrity:** WFL **HR/RR/CE:** WFL **Reflexes:** Absent DTRs below knee Emerging head and trunk righting **Muscle tone:** Flaccid below L4 low in trunk; upper extremities: WFL **Motor skills:** BSID-2 administered by PT with a 30% delay noted; fine motor domains of PDMS-2 administered by OT with no delays noted **Observation:** Decreased pain in LEs Hawaii Early Learning Profile (HELP) administered; WFL for age Oral-motor/language: WFL	Document impairments, functional limitations, and strengths. Prepare IFSP; case manager established PT as primary service by collaboration with developmental, occupational, and speech therapists. Therapeutic exercises to improve balance, mobility, and strength. Standing with vertical stander at 10 months, gait training with vertical stander and walker at 15 months, and progression to ambulation with AFOs and forward walker at 30 months. Family training: instruction in ROM and developmental activities to improve performance; sensory stimulation/body awareness activities; skin integrity; and assessment of adaptive equipment needs (vertical stander at 10 months, AFOs to position feet in standing, adjustment of stroller to provide leg support, and walker for progression of gait).	Risk prevention: parents understand developmental exercises, appropriate equipment use, and importance of checking for skin irritation and breakdown. Sensory awareness develops appropriately. Cognition and language develops appropriately. Improved infant/family sense of well-being. Infant/family stressors decrease. Developmental, occupational, and speech therapists will reassess at 6-month intervals and intervene if needed.

WFL, Within functional limits; *HR,* heart rate; *RR,* respiratory rate; *CE,* cardiorespiratory endurance; *DTR,* deep tendon reflex; *LE,* lower extremity; *IFSP,* Individual Family Service Plan, *BSID-2,* Bayley Scales of Infant Development, second edition; *PDMS-2,* Peabody Developmental Motor Scales, second edition; *ROM,* range of motion; *AFO,* ankle-foot-orthosis.

TABLE 18-7 ■ **Early Childhood Episode (3 to 5 Years) of Care for Child with Spina Bifida**

PRACTICE PATTERNS	SYSTEMS TO REVIEW	TESTS AND RESULTS	INTERVENTIONS	ANTICIPATED GOALS AND EXPECTED OUTCOMES
4F 7A 6E 5C	Musculoskeletal Integumentary Cardiopulmonary Neuromuscular Cognition/ communication	**MMT:** No innervation below L4 **Muscle length:** WFL **ROM:** WFL **Gait:** ambulates with AFOs and walker **Skin integrity:** WFL **HR/RR/CE:** WFL Established baseline walking distance/time with 6-minute walk test **Reflexes:** Absent DTRs below knee **Muscle tone:** Flaccid below L4; low in trunk; upper extremities: WFL **Motor skills:** PEDI carried out Independent walking with walker and AFOs ADLs are age appropriate with assist School function assessment (SFA) completed at 5 years of age **Cognition:** WFL PEDI social function section: WFL	Collaborate and coordinate systems review evaluation results with health care team. Document impairments, functional limitations, and strengths. Improve mobility in school environment through therapeutic exercise and progressive gait training with crutches. Family training: instruction in gait with crutches. Health and wellness: swimming and biking in community setting. Tricycle adapted. Educate family and Michael regarding latex precautions.	Joint and skin integrity maintained. Postural control and muscle performance improves. Mobility improves. Risk prevention: parents understand progression with crutches. Parents understand latex precautions in community environment and home. Sensory awareness develops appropriately. Improved child/family sense of well-being. Child/family stressors decrease.

WFL, Within functional limits; *HR,* heart rate; *RR,* respiratory rate; *CE,* cardiorespiratory endurance; *DTR,* deep tendon reflex; *LE,* lower extremity; *PEDI,* Pediatric Evaluation of Disability Inventory; *AFO,* ankle-foot-orthosis; *ADL,* activities of daily living.

TABLE 18-8 ■ Tethered Cord Episode of Care for Child with Spina Bifida (Age 6 Years)

PRACTICE PATTERNS	SYSTEMS TO REVIEW	TESTS AND RESULTS	INTERVENTIONS	ANTICIPATED GOALS AND EXPECTED OUTCOMES
4F 7A 6E 5C	Musculoskeletal Integumentary Cardiopulmonary Neuromuscular Cognition/ communication	**MMT:** decreased strength left leg **Muscle length:** WFL **ROM:** not WFL **Gait:** changed; weakness left side **Skin integrity:** redness lateral border of calcaneus **HR/RR/CE:** 6-minute walk test exhibits decreased pace **Reflexes:** Hyperreflexive DTRs below L3 on left Absent DTRs below knee on right **Muscle tone:** increased through left leg, flaccid below L4 on right, low in trunk Upper extremities: WFL **Motor skills:** falling more often Decreased ability to stand/walk; weight shifted toward right **Status:** unchanged	Collaborate and coordinate systems review evaluation results with physician. Physician ordered MRI, surgery for release of tethered spinal cord. Document impairments, functional limitations, and strengths. Prepare a plan of treatment. Increase therapeutic exercises, neuromuscular rehabilitation, and gait training to restore balance and gait with crutches. Family training: instruction in stretching for muscle length and developmental activity to progress/enhance performance. Refer to orthotist for brace adjustments.	Joint integrity, strength, and mobility are restored. Gait performance improves. Risk prevention: parents understand signs and symptoms of tethered cord. Skin integrity is maintained. Sensory awareness develops appropriately. Cognition and language skills develop appropriately. Improved child/family sense of well-being. Stressors decrease.

WFL, Within functional limits; *HR,* heart rate; *RR,* respiratory rate; *CE,* cardiorespiratory endurance; *DTR,* deep tendon reflex.

TABLE 18-9 ■ Preadolescent Episode of Care for Child with Spina Bifida (Age 10 Years)

PRACTICE PATTERNS	SYSTEMS TO REVIEW	TESTS AND RESULTS	INTERVENTIONS	ANTICIPATED GOALS AND EXPECTED OUTCOMES
4F 7A 6E 5C	Musculoskeletal Integumentary Cardiopulmonary Neuromuscular Cognition/ communication	**MMT:** Back to baseline; no innervation below L4 **Muscle length:** WFL **ROM:** WFL **Skin integrity:** WFL **HR/RR/CE:** WFL **Reflexes:** Absent DTRs below knee Balance/equilibrium appropriate for L4 spinal level **Muscle tone:** Flaccid below L4, low in trunk; upper extremities: WFL **Motor skills:** PEDI conducted; maximal score of 100 achieved Measured self-care, mobility, and social function **Observation:** WFL	Collaborate and coordinate systems review evaluation results with health care team. Document impairments, functional limitations, and strengths. Discharge from formal PT. Home program to continue and include intensive stretching and prone activities. Continue health and wellness programs, including swimming and community recreational programs. Continue to educate Michael on importance of skin integrity, latex sensitivity, and brace fit. Referred to orthotist for brace replacement.	Postural control and muscle performance are maintained. Joint integrity and mobility are maintained. Michael understands the importance of checking skin for irritation and breakdown and appropriate brace fit. Michael becomes active in the community adapted sports programs. Improved child/family sense of well-being. Client satisfaction.

WFL, Within functional limits; *HR,* heart rate; *RR,* respiratory rate; *CE,* cardiorespiratory endurance; *DTR,* deep tendon reflex; *PEDI,* Pediatric Evaluation of Disability Inventory.

TABLE 18-10 ■ Adolescent Episode of Care for Child with Spina Bifida (Age 13 Years)

PRACTICE PATTERNS	SYSTEMS TO REVIEW	TESTS AND RESULTS	INTERVENTIONS	ANTICIPATED GOALS AND EXPECTED OUTCOMES
4F 7A 6E 5C	Musculoskeletal Integumentary Cardiopulmonary Neuromuscular Cognition/ communication	**MMT:** No innervation below L4 **Muscle length:** WFL **ROM:** WFL **Skin integrity:** WFL Increase in height and weight **HR/RR/CE:** Increased HR and decreased distance traveled in 6-minute walk test; increased fatigue during long-distance ambulation **Reflexes:** Absent DTRs below knee **Muscle tone:** LEs, no change; UEs: WFL **Motor skills:** Decreased ability to keep pace with peers **Observation:** Increased social abilities	Collaborate and coordinate systems review evaluation results with health care team. Document impairments, functional limitations, and strengths. Prepare a plan of treatment. Assistive equipment/wheelchair evaluation; to be used for long distances. Short-distance ambulation with forearm crutches to continue at home/school. Client education: weight shifts every hour while using wheelchair for skin integrity. Refer to nutritionist. Design a plan to incorporate driver's education through high school as well as rehabilitation resources.	Joint integrity and walking mobility are maintained. Risk prevention: Michael understands signs and symptoms of decubitus pressure areas. Michael's long-distance mobility increases independence. Social and recreational opportunities increase. Improved client sense of well-being. Stressors decrease.

WFL, Within functional limits; *HR,* heart rate; *RR,* respiratory rate; *CE,* cardiorespiratory endurance; *DTR,* deep tendon reflex; *LE,* lower extremity; *UE,* upper extremity.

ACKNOWLEDGMENT
We acknowledge and dedicate this chapter to Jane W. Schneider, an author of previous editions of this chapter.

REFERENCES

1. APTA: Guide to physical therapist practice, *J Am Phys Ther Assoc* 81(1):738, 2001.
2. Pearson P, Williams C: *Physical therapy services in developmental disabilities,* Springfield, IL, 1976, Charles C Thomas.
3. Stark G: *Spina bifida: problems and management,* Boston, 1977, Blackwell Scientific.
4. Moore K: *Before we are born: basic embryological and birth defects,* Philadelphia, 1974, W.B. Saunders.
5. Menalaus M: *The orthopaedic management of spina bifida cystica,* ed 2, New York, 1980, Churchill Livingstone.
6. Greene WB, Terry RC, DeMasi RA et al: Effect of race and gender on neurological level in myelomeningocele, *Dev Med Child Neurol* 33(2):110-117, 1991.
7. Byrd S, Radkowski M: The radiological evaluation of the child with a myelomeningocele, *J Natl Med Assoc* 83:608-614, 1991.
8. Riegel D: Lipomeningocele, surgical indications and results. Presented at International Spina Bifida Symposium, May, 1990, Chicago.
9. Dounes E: Sacrococcygeal agenesis: a report of four new cases, *Acta Orthop Scand* 49:475-480, 1978.
10. Kupka J, Geddes N, Carroll NC: Comprehensive management in the child with spina bifida, *Orthop Clin North Am* 9(1):97-113, 1978.
11. Brocklehurst G: *Spina bifida for the clinician, vol 57,* Philadelphia, 1976, JB Lippincott.
12. Singer HA, Nelson MM, Beighton PH: Spina bifida and anencephaly in the Cape, *S Afr Med J* 53:626-627, 1978.
13. James W: The sex ratio in spina bifida, *J Med Genet* 16:384-388, 1979.
14. McLaughlin JF, Shurtleff DB: Management of the newborn with myelodysplasia, *Clin Pediatr (Phila)* 18(8):463-476, 1979.
15. Nesbit DE, Ziter FA: Epidemiology of myelomeningocele in Utah, *Dev Med Child Neurol* 21(6):754-757, 1979.
16. Nevin NC, Johnston WP, Merrett JD: Influence of social class on the risk of recurrence of anencephalus and spina bifida, *Dev Med Child Neurol* 23(2):155-159, 1981.
17. Lippman-Hand A, Fraser FC, Biddle CJ: Indications for prenatal diagnosis in relatives of patients with neural tube defects, *Obstet Gynecol* 51(1):72-76, 1978.
18. McLone D: *An introduction to spina bifida,* Chicago, 1980, Childrens' Memorial Hospital Myelomeningocele Service.
19. Hyperthermia and meningomyelocele and anencephaly [letter], *Lancet* 1:769-780, 1978.
20. Hyperthermia and the neural tube [editorial], *Lancet* 2:560-561, 1978.
21. McLone DG: Treatment of myelomeningocele: arguments against selection, *Clin Neurosurg* 33:359-370, 1986.
22. Smithells RW, Sheppard S, Schorah CJ et al: Apparent prevention of neural tube defects by periconceptional vitamin supplementation, *Arch Dis Child* 56(12):911-918, 1981.
23. Graf WD, Oleinik OE, Jack RM, et al: Plasma homocysteine and methionine concentrations in children with neural tube defects, *Eur J Pediatr Surg* 6(suppl 1):7-9, 1996.
24. Shurtleff DB: Epidemiology of neural tube defects and folic acid, *Cerebrospinal Fluid Res* 1(1):5, 2004.
25. Baker DA, Sherry CJ: Spina bifida and maternal Rh blood type, *Arch Dis Child* 54(7):567, 1979.
26. Burn J, Gibbens D: May spina bifida result from an X-linked defect in a selective abortion mechanism? *J Med Genet* 16(3):210-214, 1979.
27. Pietrzyk JJ, Turowski G: Immunogenetic bases of congenital malformations: association of HLA-B27 with spina bifida, *Pediatr Res* 13(8):879-883, 1979.
28. George TM, McLone DG: Mechanisms of mutant genes in spina bifida: a review of implications from animal models, *Pediatr Neurosurg* 23(5):236-245, 1995.
29. Finnell RH, Gould A, Spiegelstein O: Pathobiology and genetics of neural tube defects, *Epilepsia* 44(suppl 3):14-23, 2003.
30. Goldberg MF, Oakley GP Jr: Interpreting elevated amniotic fluid alpha-fetoprotein levels in clinical practice: use of the predictive value positive concept, *Am J Obstet Gynecol* 133(2):126-132, 1979.
31. Ferguson-Smith MA, Rawlinson HA, May HM et al: Avoidance of anencephalic and spina bifida births by maternal serum-alphafetoprotein screening, *Lancet* 1(8078):1330-1333, 1978.
32. Cochrane DD, Wilson RD, Steinbok P et al: Prenatal spinal evaluation and functional outcome of patients born with myelomeningocele: information for improved prenatal counseling and outcome prediction, *Fetal Diagn Ther* 11(3):159-168, 1996.
33. Griscom NT, Frigoletto FD, Harris GB: Amniography in second trimester diagnosis of myelomeningocele, *AJR Am J Roentgenol* 133(6):1151-1156, 1979.
34. Carstens C, Niethard FU: The current status of prenatal diagnosis of myelomeningocele—results of a questionnaire [in German], *Geburtshilfe Frauenheilkd* 53(3):182-185, 1993.
35. Meuli M, Meuli-Simmen C, Hutchins GM et al: The spinal cord lesion in human fetuses with myelomeningocele: implications for fetal surgery, *J Pediatr Surg* 32(3):448-452, 1997.
36. Tulipan N, Bruner JP: Myelomeningocele repair in utero: a report of three cases, *Pediatr Neurosurg* 28(4):177-180, 1998.
37. Bruner JP, Tulipan N, Reed G et al: Intrauterine repair of spina bifida: preoperative predictors of shunt-dependent hydrocephalus, *Am J Obstet Gynecol* 190(5):1305-1312, 2004.
38. Hamdan AH, Walsh W, Bruner JP et al: Intrauterine myelomeningocele repair: effect on short-term complications of prematurity, *Fetal Diagn Ther* 19(1):83-86, 2004.
39. Hamdan AH, Walsh W, Heddings A et al: Gestational age at intrauterine myelomeningocele repair does not influence the risk of prematurity, *Fetal Diagn Ther* 17(2):66-68, 2002.
40. Tulipan N: Intrauterine myclomeningocele repair, *Clin Perinatol* 30(3):521-530, 2003.
41. Tulipan N: Intrauterine closure of myelomeningocele: an update, *Neurosurg Focus* 16(2):E2, 2004.
42. Tubbs RS, Chambers MR, Smyth MD et al: Late gestational intrauterine myelomeningocele repair does not improve lower extremity function, *Pediatr Neurosurg* 38(3):128-132, 2003.
43. NICHD: Management of myelomeningocele study (website): *www.spinabifidamoms.com.* Accessed April 2, 2005.
44. Wescott M, Dynes MC, Remer EM et al: Congenital and acquired orthopedic abnormalities in patients with myelomeningocele, *Radiographics* 12:1155-1173, 1992.
45. Shaffer M, Dias L: *Myelomeningocele: orthopedic treatment,* Baltimore, 1983, Williams and Wilkins.
46. Muller EB, Nordwall A: Prevalence of scoliosis in children with myelomeningocele in western Sweden, *Spine* 17(9):1097-1102, 1992.
47. Dias L: Orthopaedic care in spina bifida: past, present, and future. *Dev Med Child Neurol* 46(9):579, 2004.
48. Drummond DS, Moreau M, Cruess RL: Post-operative neuropathic fractures in patients with myelomeningocele, *Dev Med Child Neurol* 23(2):147-150, 1981.
49. Ralis ZA, Ralis HM, Randall M et al: Changes in shape, ossification and quality of bones in children with spina bifida, *Dev Med Child Neurol Suppl* 37:29-41, 1976.
50. Quan A, Adams R, Ekmark E et al: Bone mineral density in children with myelomeningocele, *Pediatrics* 102(3):E34, 1998.
51. Dias MS, McLone DG: Hydrocephalus in the child with dysraphism, *Neurosurg Clin N Am* 4(4):715-726, 1993.
52. McLone DG: *An introduction to hydrocephalus,* Chicago, 1982, Childrens' Memorial Hospital.
53. McLone DG: The etiology of neural tube defects: the role of folic acid, *Childs Nerv Syst* 19(7-8):537-539, 2003.
54. McLone DG, Dias MS: The Chiari II malformation: cause and impact, *Childs Nerv Syst* 19(7-8):540-550, 2003.

55. Milerad J, Lagercrantz H, Johnson P: Obstructive sleep apnea in Arnold-Chiari malformation treated with acetazolamide, *Acta Paediatr* 81(8):609-612, 1992.

56. Vandertop P, Asai A, Hoffman HJ et al: Surgical decompression for symptomatic Chiari II malformation in neonates with myelomeningocele, *J Neurosurg* 77:541-544, 1992.

57. Oakes W: Developmental anomalies and neurosurgical diseases in children: Chiari malformations, hydromyelia, syringomyelia. In Wilkins R, Rengachary S, editors: *Neurosurgery,* New York, 1984, McGraw-Hill.

58. McLone DG, Knepper PA: The cause of Chiari II malformation: a unified theory, *Pediatr Neurosci* 15(1):1-12, 1989.

59. Alexander MA, Steg NL: Myelomeningocele: comprehensive treatment, *Arch Phys Med Rehabil* 70(8):637-641, 1989.

60. Byrd SE, Radkowski MA: The radiological evaluation of the child with a myelomeningocele, *J Natl Med Assoc* 83(7):608-614, 1991.

61. Charney EB, Melchionni JB, Antonucci DL: Ventriculitis in newborns with myelomeningocele, *Am J Dis Child* 145(3):287-290, 1991.

62. Cash J: *Neurology for physiotherapists,* ed 2, Philadelphia, 1977, JB Lippincott.

63. Hall P, Lindseth R, Campbell R et al: Scoliosis and hydrocephalus in myelocele patients. The effects of ventricular shunting, *J Neurosurg* 50(2):174-178, 1979.

64. Riegel D: Diagnoses and surgical treatment of tethered cord. Presented at International Spina Bifida Symposium, May 1990, Chicago.

65. McLone DG, Herman JM, Gabrieli AP, et al: Tethered cord as a cause of scoliosis in children with a myelomeningocele, *Pediatr Neurosurg* 16(1):8-13, 1990.

66. Reigel DH, Tchernoukha K, Bazmi B et al: Change in spinal curvature following release of tethered spinal cord associated with spina bifida, *Pediatr Neurosurg* 20(1):30-42, 1994.

67. Gabrieli AP, Dias L, Rosenthal A et al: Tethered cord syndrome in myelomeningocele: surgical treatment and results. Presented at International Spina Bifida Symposium, May 1990, Chicago.

68. Schopler SA, Menelaus MB: Significance of the strength of the quadriceps muscles in children with myelomeningocele, *J Pediatr Orthop* 7(5):507-512, 1987.

69. Cartwright C: Primary tethered cord syndrome: diagnosis and treatment of an insidious defect, *J Neurosci Nurs* 32(4):210-215, 2000.

70. Pierz K, Banta J, Thomson J et al: The effect of tethered cord release on scoliosis in myelomeningocele, *J Pediatr Orthop* 20(3):362-365, 2000.

71. McLone DG: Spina bifida today: problems adults face, *Semin Neurol* 9(3):169-175, 1989.

72. Sarwark JF, Weber DT, Gabrieli AP et al: Tethered cord syndrome in low motor level children with myelomeningocele, *Pediatr Neurosurg* 25(6):295-301, 1996.

73. Bergenheim AT, Wendelius M, Shahidi S et al: Spasticity in a child with myelomeningocele treated with continuous intrathecal baclofen, *Pediatr Neurosurg* 39:218-221, 2003.

74. Malone PS, Wheeler RA, Williams JE: Continence in patients with spina bifida: long term results. *Arch Dis Child* 70(2):107-110, 1994.

75. King JC, Currie DM, Wright E: Bowel training in spina bifida: importance of education, patient compliance, age, and anal reflexes, *Arch Phys Med Rehabil* 75(3):243-247, 1994.

76. Browne J, McLone DG: The effect of complications on intellectual function in 167 children with myelomeningocele, *Z Kinderchir* 34:117-120, 1981.

77. Junque C, Poca MA, Sahuquillo J: Neuropsychological findings in congenital and acquired hydrocephalus, *Neuropsychol Rev* 11:169-178, 2001.

78. Raimondi AJ, Soare P: Intellectual development in shunted hydrocephalic children, *Am J Dis Child* 127(5):664-671, 1974.

79. Friedrich WN, Lovejoy MC, Shaffer J et al: Cognitive abilities and achievement status of children with myelomeningocele: a contemporary sample, *J Pediatr Psychol* 16(4):423-428, 1991.

80. Friedrich WN, Shurtleff DB, Shaffer J: Cognitive abilities and lipomyelomeningocele, *Psychol Rep* 73(2):467-470, 1993.

81. Gluckman S, Barling J: Effects of a remedial program on visual-motor perception in spina bifida children, *J Genet Psychol* 136:195-202, 1980.

82. Muen WJ, Bannister CM: Hand function in subjects with spina bifida, *Eur J Pediatr Surg* 7 Suppl 1:18-22, 1997.

83. Kaplan W: Management of the urinary tract in myelomeningocele, *Prob Urol* 2:121-131, 1988.

84. Wills KE, Holmbeck GN, Dillon K et al: Intelligence and achievement in children with myelomeningocele, *J Pediatr Psychol* 15(2):161-176, 1990.

85. Lollar DJ: Learning patterns among spina bifida children, *Z Kinderchir* 45(suppl 1):39, 1990.

86. Culatta B, Young C: Linguistic performance as a function of abstract task demands in children with spina bifida, *Dev Med Child Neurol* 34(5):434-440, 1992.

87. Ito J, Saijo H, Araki A et al: Neuroradiological assessment of visuoperceptual disturbance in children with spina bifida and hydrocephalus, *Dev Med Child Neurol* 39(6):385-392, 1997.

88. Banta JV, Bonanni C, Prebluda J: Latex anaphylaxis during spinal surgery in children with myelomeningocele, *Dev Med Child Neurol* 35(6):543-548, 1993.

89. Gold M, Swartz JS, Braude BM, et al: Intraoperative anaphylaxis: an association with latex sensitivity, *J Allergy Clin Immunol* 87(3):662-666, 1991.

90. Slater JE: Rubber anaphylaxis, *N Engl J Med* 320(17):1126-1130, 1989.

91. Slater JE, Mostello LA, Shaer C et al: Type I hypersensitivity to rubber, *Ann Allergy* 65(5):411-414, 1990.

92. Kelly KJ, Pearson ML, Kurup VP et al: A cluster of anaphylactic reactions in children with spina bifida during general anesthesia: epidemiologic features, risk factors, and latex hypersensitivity, *J Allergy Clin Immunol* 94(1):53-61, 1994.

93. Banta JV, Lin R, Peterson M et al: The team approach in the care of the child with myelomeningocele, *J Prosthet Orthot* 2:263-273, 1990.

94. Gelb LN for United States Food and Drug Administration: Allergic reactions to latex containing medical devices, *Food and Drug Administration medical bulletin,* 1991.

95. Slater JE, Mostello LA, Shaer C: Rubber-specific IgE in children with spina bifida, *J Urol* 146(2 Pt 2):578-579, 1991.

96. Hochleitner BW, Menardi G, Haussler B et al: Spina bifida as an independent risk factor for sensitization to latex, *J Urol* 166(6):2370-2374, 2001.

97. Nieto A, Mazon A, Pamies R et al: Efficacy of latex avoidance for primary prevention of latex sensitization in children with spina bifida, *J Pediatr* 140(3):370-372, 2002.

98. Shurtleff D: Decubitus formation and skin breakdown. In Shurtleff D, editor: *Myelodysplasias and exstrophies: significance, prevention and treatment,* Orlando, FL, 1986, Grune and Stratton, pp. 285-298.

99. Mathisen BA, Shepherd K: Oral-motor dysfunction and feeding problems in infants with myelodysplasia, *Pediatr Rehabil* 1(2):117-122, 1997.

100. Mita K, Akataki K, Itoh K et al: Assessment of obesity of children with spina bifida, *Dev Med Child Neurol* 35(4):305-311, 1993.

101. Rotenstein D, Reigel DH, Lucke JF: Growth of growth hormone-treated and nontreated children before and after tethered spinal cord release, *Pediatr Neurosurg* 24(5):237-241, 1996.

102. Trollmann R, Strehl E, Dorr HG: Growth hormone deficiency in children with myelomeningocele (MMC)—effects of growth hormone treatment, *Eur J Pediatr Surg* 7(suppl 1):58-59, 1997.

103. Trollmann R, Strehl E, Wenzel D et al: Arm span, serum IGF-1 and IGFBP-3 levels as screening parameters for the diagnosis of growth hormone deficiency in patients with myelomeningocele—preliminary data, *Eur J Pediatr* 157(6):451-455, 1998.

104. Trollmann R, Strehl E, Dorr HG: Precocious puberty in children with myelomeningocele: treatment with gonadotropin-releasing hormone analogues, *Dev Med Child Neurol* 40(1):38-43, 1998.

105. Rotenstein D, Breen TJ: Growth hormone treatment of children with myelomeningocele, *J Pediatr* 128(5 Pt 2):S28-S31, 1996.

106. Rotenstein D, Reigel DH: Growth hormone treatment of children with neural tube defects: results from 6 months to 6 years, *J Pediatr* 128(2):184-189, 1996.

107. Perspectives in spina bifida, *Br Med J* 2(6142):909-910, 1978.

108. McLone DG, Dias MS: Complications of myelomeningocele closure, *Pediatr Neurosurg* 17(5):267-273, 1991.

109. McLone DG, Czyzewski D, Raimondi A et al: Central nervous system infections as a limiting factor in the intelligence of children with myelomeningocele, *Pediatrics* 70:338-342, 1982.

110. McLaurin R: *Myelomeningocele,* New York, 1977, Grune and Stratton.

111. Naidich TP, McLone DG, Mutluer S: A new understanding of dorsal dysraphism with lipoma (lipomyeloschisis): radiologic evaluation and surgical correction, *AJR Am J Roentgenol* 140(6):1065-1078, 1983.

112. Stein SC, Schut L: Hydrocephalus in myelomeningocele, *Childs Brain* 5(4):413-419, 1979.

113. Hendry J, Geddes N: Living with a congenital anomaly: how nurses can help the parents of children born with spina bifida to develop lasting patterns of creative caring, *Can Nurse* 74(6):29-33, 1978.

114. Li V, Dias MS: The results of a practice survey on the management of patients with shunted hydrocephalus, *Pediatr Neurosurg* 30(6):288-295, 1999.

115. American Academy of Pediatrics Action Committee on Myelodysplasia, Section on Urology: Current approaches to evaluation and management of children with myelomeningocele, *Pediatrics* 63(4):663-667, 1979.

116. Drago JR, Wellner L, Sanford EJ et al: The role of intermittent catheterization in the management of children with myelomeningocele, *J Urol* 118(1 Pt 1):92-94, 1977.

117. Lie HR, Lagergren J, Rasmussen F et al: Children with myelomeningocele: their urinary and bowel control, *Eur J Pediatr Surg* 1(suppl 1):40, 1991.

118. Lie HR, Lagergren J, Rasmussen F et al: Bowel and bladder control of children with myelomeningocele: a Nordic study, *Dev Med Child Neurol* 33(12):1053-1061, 1991.

119. Keating MA, Rink RC, Adams MC: Appendicovesicostomy: a useful adjunct to continent reconstruction of the bladder, *J Urol* 149(5):1091-1094, 1993.

120. Gonzalez R, Schimke CM: Strategies in urological reconstruction in myelomeningocele, *Curr Opin Urol* 12(6):485-490, 2002.

121. Sumfest JM, Burns MW, Mitchell ME: The Mitrofanoff principle in urinary reconstruction, *J Urol* 150(6):1875-1878, 1993.

122. Kaplan WE, Richards I: Intravesical bladder stimulation in myelodysplasia *J Urol* 140(5 Pt 2):1282-1284, 1988.

123. Koyle MA, Kaji DM, Duque M et al: The Malone antegrade continence enema for neurogenic and structural fecal incontinence and constipation, *J Urol* 154(2 Pt 2):759-761, 1995.

124. Hensinger R, Jones E: *Neonatal orthopedics,* New York, 1981, Grune and Stratton.

125. Noonan KJ, Richards BS: Nonsurgical management of idiopathic clubfoot, *J Am Acad Orthop Surg* 11(6):392-402, 2003.

126. Feiwell E: Surgery of the hip in myelomeningocele as related to adult goals, *Clin Orthop Relat Res* 148:87-93, 1980.

127. Feiwell E, Sakai D, Blatt T: The effect of hip reduction on function in patients with myelomeningocele. Potential gains and hazards of surgical treatment, *J Bone Joint Surg Am* 60(2):169-173, 1978.

128. Lee EH, Carroll NC: Hip stability and ambulatory status in myelomeningocele, *J Pediatr Orthop* 5(5):522-527, 1985.

129. Zausmer E: Evaluation of strength and motor development in infants. I, *Phys Ther Rev* 33(11):575-581, 1953.

130. Krosschell KJBA, Oren J, Schneider JW: Inter and intra-rater reliability of manual muscle testing children less than five years of age. Presented at American Academy of Developmental Medicine and Child Neurology, September 1990, Orlando, FL.

131. McDonald CM, Jaffe KM, Shurtleff DB: Assessment of muscle strength in children with meningomyelocele: accuracy and stability of measurements over time, *Arch Phys Med Rehabil* 67(12):855-861, 1986.

132. Brazelton T: *Neonatal behavioral assessment scale, vol 88,* ed 2, Philadelphia, 1984, J.B. Lippincott.

133. Fiorentino M: *Normal and abnormal development: the influence of primitive reflexes on motor development,* ed 2, Springfield, IL, 1980, Charles C. Thomas.

134. Colangelo C, Bergen A, Gottleib L: *A normal baby: the sensory motor processes of the first year,* ed 2, Valhalla, NY, 1986, Valhalla Rehabilitation Publications.

135. Piper M, Darrah J: *Motor assessment of the developing infant,* Philadelphia, 1994, W.B. Saunders.

136. Darrah J, Piper M, Watt MJ: Assessment of gross motor skills of at-risk infants: predictive validity of the Alberta Infant Motor Scale, *Dev Med Child Neurol* 40(7):485-491, 1998.

137. *The Milani-Comparetti motor development screening test: test manual,* ed 3, Omaha, NE, 1992, Meyer Children's Rehabilitation Institute.

138. Folio M, Fewell R: *PDMS-2: Peabody developmental motor scales,* Austin, 2000, PRO-ED.

139. Bruininks R: *Bruininks-Oseretsky test of motor proficiency examiner's manual,* Circle Pines, MN, 1987, American Guidance Services.

140. Haley S, Coster WJ, Ludlow LH et al: *Pediatric Evaluation of Disability Inventory (PEDI): development, standardization and administration manual,* Boston, 1992, Trustees of Boston University Health and Disability Research Institute, New England Medical Center Hospitals and PEDI Research Group.

141. Coster W: Occupation-centered assessment of children, *Am J Occup Ther* 52(5):337-344, 1998.

142. Mancini MC, Coster WJ, Trombly CA et al: Predicting elementary school participation in children with disabilities, *Arch Phys Med Rehabil* 81(3):339-347, 2000.

143. Bayley N: *Manual for the Bayley scales of infant development,* ed 2, San Antonio, TX, 1993, The Psychological Corporation.

143a. Bayley N: *Bayley scales of infant and toddler development,* ed 3, San Antonio, TX, 2006, Harcourt Assessment, Inc.

144. Beery K, Beery N: *The Beery-Buktenica developmental test of visual motor integration: administration, scoring and teaching manual,* Minneapolis, 2004, NCS Pearson.

145. Golge M, Schutz C, Dreesmann M et al: Grip force parameters in precision grip of individuals with myelomeningocele, *Dev Med Child Neurol* 45(4):249-256, 2003.

146. Norrlin S, Dahl M, Rosblad B: Control of reaching movements in children and young adults with myelomeningocele, *Dev Med Child Neurol* 46(1):28-33, 2004.

147. Norrlin S, Rosblad B: Adaptation of reaching movements in children and young adults with myelomeningocele, *Acta Paediatr* 93(7):922-928, 2004.

148. Colarusso R, Hammill D: *Motor-free visual perception test manual,* ed 3, Novato, CA, 2003, Academic Therapy Publications.

149. Gardner M: *Test of visual perceptual skills (non-motor)-revised,* Hydesville, CA, 1996, Psychological and Educational Publications.

150. Guttman L: *Spinal cord injuries: comprehensive management and research,* ed 2, Oxford, 1976, Blackwell.

151. Rosenstein BD, Greene WB, Herrington RT, et al: Bone density in myelomeningocele: the effects of ambulatory status and other factors, *Dev Med Child Neurol* 29(4):486-494, 1987.

152. Quan A, Adams R, Ekmark E et al: Bone mineral density in children with myelomeningocele: effect of hydrochlorothiazide, *Pediatr Nephrol* 18(9):929-933, 2003.

153. Gram M: *The parapodium: adjunct to habilitation of the child with spina bifida,* Woodridge, IL, 1991, MM Therapeutics, Inc.

154. Mazur JM, Kyle S: Efficacy of bracing the lower limbs and ambulation training in children with myelomeningocele, *Dev Med Child Neurol* 46(5):352-356, 2004.

155. Schoenmakers MA, Gulmans VA, Gooskens RH et al: Spinal fusion in children with spina bifida: influence on ambulation level and functional abilities, *Eur Spine J* 14(4):415-422, 2004.

156. Butler PB, Farmer IR, Poiner R et al: Use of the Orlau swivel walker for the severely handicapped patient, *Physiotherapy* 68(10):324-326, 1982.

157. Stallard J, Farmer IR, Poiner R et al: Engineering design considerations of the ORLAU Swivel Walker, *Eng Med* 15(1):3-8, 1986.

158. Stallard J, Lomas B, Woollam P et al: New technical advances in swivel walkers, *Prosthet Orthot Int* 27(2):132-138, 2003.

159. Rose G, Henshaw J: Swivel walkers for paraplegics- considerations and problems in their design and application, *Bull Prosthet Res* 10(20):62-74, 1973.

160. Durr-Fillauer Medical I-OD: *LSU reciprocating gait orthosis: a pictorial description and application model,* Chattanooga, TN, 1983, Durr-Fillauer Medical.

161. http://www.centerfororthoticsdesign.com/isocentric-rgo/index.html#rgo-introduction. Accessed on June 26, 2006.

162. Lindseth RE, Glancy J: Polypropylene lower-extremity braces for paraplegia due to myelomeningocele, *J Bone Joint Surg Am* 56(3):556-563, 1974.

163. De Souza LJ, Carroll N: Ambulation of the braced myelomeningocele patient, *J Bone Joint Surg Am* 58(8):1112-1118, 1976.

164. Berard C, Delmas MC, Locqueneux F et al: Anti-calcaneus carbon fiber orthosis in children with myelomeningocele [in French], *Rev Chir Orthop Reparatrice Appar Mot* 76(3):222-225, 1990.

165. Vankoski S, Moore C, Statler KD et al: The influence of forearm crutches on pelvic and hip kinematics in children with myelomeningocele: don't throw away the crutches, *Dev Med Child Neurol* 39:614-619, 1997.

166. Gupta RT, Vankoski S, Novak RA, et al: Trunk kinematics and the influence on valgus knee stress in persons with high sacral level myelomeningocele, *J Pediatr Orthop* 25(1):89-94, 2005.

167. Dunteman RC, Vankoski SJ, Dias LS: Internal derotation osteotomy of the tibia: pre- and postoperative gait analysis in persons with high sacral myelomeningocele, *J Pediatr Orthop* 20(5):623-628, 2000.

168. Vankoski SJ, Michaud S, Dias L: External tibial torsion and the effectiveness of the solid ankle-foot orthoses, *J Pediatr Orthop* 20(3):349-355, 2000.

169. Park BK, Song HR, Vankoski SJ et al: Gait electromyography in children with myelomeningocele at the sacral level, *Arch Phys Med Rehabil* 78(5):471-475, 1997.

170. Thomson JD, Ounpuu S, Davis RB et al: The effects of ankle-foot orthoses on the ankle and knee in persons with myelomeningocele: an evaluation using three-dimensional gait analysis, *J Pediatr Orthop* 19(1):27-33, 1999.

171. Vankoski SJ, Sarwark JF, Moore C et al: Characteristic pelvic, hip and knee patterns in children with lumbosacral myelomeningocele, *Gait Posture* 3:51-57, 1995.

172. Duffy CM, Hill AE et al: The influence of abductor weakness on gait in spina bifida, *Gait Posture* 4:34-38, 1996.

173. Bare A, Vankoski SJ, Dias L et al: Independent ambulators with high sacral myelomeningocele: the relation between walking kinematics and energy consumption, *Dev Med Child Neurol* 43(1):16-21, 2001.

174. Altshuler A, Meyer J, Butz MK: Even children can learn to do clean self-catheterization, *Am J Nurs* 77(1):97-101, 1977.

175. Katona F, Berenyi M: Intravesical transurethral electrotherapy in meningomyelocele patients, *Acta Paediatr Acad Sci Hung* 16(3-4):363-374, 1975.

176. Ito JA, Stevenson E, Nehring W et al: A qualitative examination of adolescents and adults with myelomeningocele: their perspective, *Eur J Pediatr Surg* (7 suppl 1):53-54, 1997.

177. Bannister CM, Russell SA, Rimmer S: Pre-natal brain development of fetuses with a myelomeningocele, *Eur J Pediatr Surg* (8 suppl 1):15-17, 1998.

178. Findley TW, Agre JC, Habeck RV et al: Ambulation in the adolescent with myelomeningocele. I: early childhood predictors, *Arch Phys Med Rehabil* 68(8):518-522, 1987.

179. Menelaus MB: Orthopaedic management of children with myelomeningocele: a plea for realistic goals, *Dev Med Child Neurol Suppl* (37):3-11, 1976.

180. Sousa JC, Telzrow RW, Holm RA et al: Developmental guidelines for children with myelodysplasia, *Phys Ther* 63(1):21-29, 1983.

181. Ayres A: *Sensory integration and the child,* Los Angeles, 1979, Western Psychological Services.

182. Montgomery M, Richter E: *Sensorimotor integration for developmentally delayed children: a handbook,* Los Angeles, 1977, Western Psychological Services.

183. Hayden PW, Davenport SL, Campbell MM: Adolescents with myelodysplasia: impact of physical disability on emotional maturation, *Pediatrics* 64(1):53-59, 1979.

184. Appleton PL, Minchom PE, Ellis NC et al: The self-concept of young people with spina bifida: a population-based study, *Dev Med Child Neurol* 36(3):198-215, 1994.

185. McAndrew I: Adolescents and young people with spina bifida, *Dev Med Child Neurol* 21(5):619-629, 1979.

186. Joyner BD, McLorie GA, Khoury AE: Sexuality and reproductive issues in children with myelomeningocele, *Eur J Pediatr Surg* 8(1):29-34, 1998.

187. Passo S: Parents' perceptions, attitudes, and needs regarding sex education for the child with myelomeningocele, *Res Nurs Health* 1(2):53-59, 1978.

188. Cass AS, Bloom BA, Luxenberg M: Sexual function in adults with myelomeningocele, *J Urol* 136(2):425-426, 1986.

189. Dorner S: Sexual interest and activity in adolescents with spina bifida, *J Child Psychol Psychiatry* 18(3):229-237, 1977.

190. Loomis JW, Javornisky JG, Monahan JJ et al: Relations between family environment and adjustment outcomes in young adults with spina bifida, *Dev Med Child Neurol* 39(9):620-627, 1997.

191. Nielsen HH: A longitudinal study of the psychological aspects of myelomeningocele, *Scand J Psychol* 21(1):45-54, 1980.

192. Rogers B: Comprehensive care for the child with a chronic disability, *Am J Nurs* 79:1106-1108, 1979.

193. Steiner WA, Ryser L, Huber E et al: Using the ICF model as a clinical problem-solving tool in physical therapy and rehabilitation medicine, *Phys Ther* 82:1098-1107, 2002.

APPENDIX 18-A ■ Orlau Swivel Rocker Distributors

United States
Mopac Ltd
206 Chestnut Street
Eau Claire, WI 54703
715-832-1685

United Kingdom
J. Stallard, Technical Director
Oswestry Orthopaedic Hospital
Shropshire, SY107AG
UK

CHAPTER 19

Traumatic Spinal Cord Injury

Myrtice B. Atrice, BS, PT
Sarah A. Morrison, PT
Shari L. McDowell, PT
Paula M. Ackerman, MS, OTR/L
Teresa A. Foy, BS, OTR/L

KEY WORDS

American Spinal Injury Association (ASIA)
autonomic dysfunction
autonomic dysreflexia
bulbocavernosus reflex
complete lesion
deep vein thrombosis (DVT)
Functional Independence Measure (FIM)
incomplete lesion
intermittent catheterization
lower motor neuron
mobile arm support
neuroprosthetics
offset feeder
orthostatic hypotension
paraplegia
pressure ulcer
pulmonary embolism (PE)
spinal cord injury (SCI)
tenodesis
tetraplegia
upper motor neuron

OBJECTIVES

After reading this chapter the student/therapist will be able to:
1. Describe the cause and demographics of spinal cord injury.
2. Discuss the acute medical management, surgical stabilization, and the current research efforts in spinal cord injury management.
3. Describe the secondary complications of spinal cord injury, the appropriate interventions, and the impact of complications on the rehabilitation process.
4. Identify the basic components of the examination process.
5. Identify problems based on the examination, set appropriate goals, and plan an individualized treatment program to reach the goals.
6. Describe adaptive equipment available to increase function.
7. Discuss client progression and the process of discharge planning throughout the rehabilitation process.
8. Describe functional expectations for individuals with complete spinal cord injuries.
9. Identify equipment needs for a given spinal cord injury lesion.

Spinal cord injury (SCI) is a catastrophic condition that, depending on its severity, may cause dramatic changes in the person's life. The effects of SCI have an impact not only on the lives of the client and family but also on society as a whole. SCI usually happens to active, independent people who at one moment are in control of their lives and in the next moment are paralyzed, with loss of sensation and loss of bodily functions and dependence on others for their most basic needs. Clients need a well-coordinated, specialized rehabilitation program consisting of a team of physicians and health care professionals to provide the tools necessary to develop a satisfying and productive post-injury lifestyle.[1,2]

The successful rehabilitation process is comprehensive. It includes prevention, early recognition, inpatient care, and outpatient care with the goal of community reintegration. The comprehensive rehabilitation team for SCI is composed of many health care professionals, including the physician, case manager, occupational therapist, physical therapist, therapeutic recreation specialist, prosthetist/orthotist, nurse, speech-language pathologist, dietitian, assistive technologist, respiratory care practitioner, psychologist, social worker, vocational counselor, engineer, and chaplain.[3-5]

Persons with SCI are best treated at tertiary care facilities that have a direct link to emergency medical services, including full trauma team availability, spine traumatologists, neurourologists, and on-site consultation by the staff of an accredited SCI rehabilitation program. A coordinated system of care shortens hospital stays and improves efficiency of functional gains made during rehabilitation.[6-9]

In this chapter a general overview is provided of the management of the client with SCI within the acute, rehabilitation, and postrehabilitation phases. The information is intended to aid health care professionals in the treatment of individuals with SCI by providing guidelines to maximize effective intervention. These guidelines must be modified with each client's input for the rehabilitation program to be truly successful in meeting individual needs.

SPINAL CORD LESIONS

SCI occurs when the spinal cord is damaged as a result of trauma, disease processes, or congenital defects. The clinical manifestations of the injury vary depending on the extent and location of the damage to the spinal cord.

Tetraplegia

Tetraplegia refers to impairment or loss of motor or sensory function as a result of damage to the cervical segments of the spinal cord. Function in the upper extremities, lower extremities, and trunk is affected.[10]

Paraplegia

Paraplegia refers to impairment or loss of motor or sensory function as a result of damage to the thoracic, lumbar, or sacral segments of the spinal cord. Depending on the level of the damage, function may be impaired in the trunk or lower extremities. This term does not refer to lumbosacral plexus lesions.[10]

Complete and Incomplete Lesions

In a complete lesion, there is total absence of sensory and motor function in the lowest sacral segment (S4-S5).[10] Complete injuries often damage the nerve root in the foramen.[11] Function of this root originating from the proximal intact cord can be expected to return within 6 months.[11]

With incomplete lesions, there is partial preservation of sensory or motor function below the neurological level and in the lowest sacral segment. Any sensation in the anal mucocutaneous junction, or deep anal sensation, indicates that the lesion is incomplete.[10]

Spinal shock occurs 30 to 60 minutes after spinal trauma; it is characterized by flaccid paralysis and absence of all spinal cord reflex activity below the level of the spinal cord lesion.[12] This condition can last anywhere from a few hours up to several weeks. The completeness of the lesion cannot be determined until spinal shock is resolved. The signs of spinal shock resolution are controversial; however, the return of reflexes may be a good indication.

MECHANISMS OF INJURY

Most spinal cord injuries occur as a result of trauma. The degree and type of force that are exerted on the spine at the time of the trauma determine the location and severity of damage that occurs.[12] Injuries to the vertebral column can be classified biomechanically as pure flexion or flexion-rotation injuries, hyperextension injuries, and compression injuries.[13] Penetrating injuries to the cord are usually the result of gunshot or knife wounds.[13]

Spinal cord damage can also be caused by nontraumatic mechanisms. Circulatory compromise to the spinal cord resulting in ischemia causes neurological damage at and below the involved cord level. Degenerative bone diseases can cause compression of the spinal cord, by prolapse of the intervertebral disk into the neural canal, and by various tumors and abscesses of the spinal cord or surrounding tissues. Congenital malformation of the vertebral canal, such as spina bifida, can also damage the spinal cord. Diseases that result in compromise of the spinal cord include Guillain-Barré syndrome, transverse myelitis, amyotrophic lateral sclerosis, and multiple sclerosis.

ASSOCIATED INJURIES

The incidence of multiple trauma in the client with a traumatic SCI is 55.2%.[14] The most common injuries are fractures (29.3%) and loss of consciousness (28.2%).[14] Traumatic pneumothorax/hemothorax are reported in 17.8%

of persons with SCI. Traumatic head injuries of sufficient severity to affect cognitive or emotional functioning are reported in 11.5% of all cases.[14] Skull and facial fractures, along with traumatic head injuries and vertebral artery and esophageal disruptions, are common in cervical injuries.[15] Limb fractures and intrathoracic injuries (rib fractures and hemopneumothorax) are frequent in thoracic injuries, whereas intraabdominal injuries to the liver, spleen, and kidneys are associated with lumbar and cauda equina injuries.[15]

DEMOGRAPHICS

The incidence of traumatic SCI in the United States is approximately 11,000 new cases per year.[16] Approximately 3000 new cases of spinal cord impairment resulting from disease and congenital anomalies occur each year.[17] The number of people living in the United States today with SCI is between 219,000 and 279,000.[16] Fifty-three percent of traumatic SCIs occur in persons between 16 and 30 years of age, with a mean age of 32.6 years.[16,18] Persons older than 60 years of age at injury have increased from 4.7% in the 1970s to 11.4% in 1990. This trend explains the increase in the median age during this same time period from 27.9 years to 35.3 years. Table 19-1 lists additional demographics.

In 2001, the average length of inpatient stay was 61 days (17 days in an acute care and 44 days in rehabilitation). The average yearly health care and living expenses vary according to severity of injury. In the first year, individuals with

TABLE 19-1 ■ SCI Demographics

Mean age at injury[16]	31.7 years
Most common age at injury[76]	19.0 years[14]
SEX	
Male	81.2%
Female	18.8%
CAUSES OF INJURY	
Motor vehicle accident	40.9%
Violent acts	21.6%
Falls	22.4%
Sports injuries	7.5%
Other	7.6%
NEUROLOGICAL CATEGORIES AT DISCHARGE (F&F)	
Incomplete tetraplegia	30.8%
Complete paraplegia	26.6%
Incomplete paraplegia	19.7%
Complete tetraplegia	18.6%
No deficits	0.7%
Unknown	1.7%
COMMON INJURY SITES[14]	
C5	15.7%
C4	12.7%
C6	12.6%
T12	7.6%
C7	6.3%
L1	4.8%

From *Spinal cord injury: facts and figures at a glance,* Birmingham, AL 1990, University of Alabama, National Spinal Cord Injury Statistical Center.

high tetraplegia spend $626,582, whereas individuals with paraplegia spend an average of $228,955.[16] Today 88.3% of persons with SCI are discharged to a noninstitutional residence. According to the National SCI Database, the leading causes of death after an SCI are pneumonia, pulmonary emboli, and septicemia.

CLINICAL SYNDROMES

Some incomplete lesions have a distinct clinical picture with specific signs and symptoms. An understanding of the various syndromes can be helpful to the client's team in planning the rehabilitation program. Figure 19-1 depicts the anatomy of the spinal cord.[11,13] This basic anatomy of the spinal cord can be referred to as the various syndromes are described.

Central Cord Syndrome. Hyperextension injuries usually result in a central cord syndrome.[13] This injury causes bleeding into the central gray matter of the spinal cord, resulting in more impairment of function in the upper extremities than in the lower extremities.[13] Most incomplete lesions result in this syndrome.[11] Approximately 77% of clients with central cord syndrome will attain ambulatory function, 53% bowel and bladder control, and 42% hand function.[19,20]

Anterior Spinal Artery Syndrome. This syndrome is usually caused by flexion injuries in which bone or cartilage spicules compromise the anterior spinal artery.[13] Motor function and pain and temperature sensation are lost bilaterally below the injured segment.[13] The prognosis is extremely poor for return of bowel and bladder function, hand function, and ambulation.[20]

Brown-Sequard Syndrome. Occasionally, as a result of penetrating injuries (gunshot or stab wounds), only one half of the spinal cord is damaged. The Brown-Sequard syndrome is characterized by ipsilateral loss of motor function and position sense and contralateral loss of pain sensation several levels below the lesion.[13] The prognosis for recovery is good. Nearly all clients attain some level of ambulatory function, 80% regain hand function, 100% have bladder control, and 80% have bowel control.[20]

Posterior Cord Syndrome. Posterior cord syndrome is rare, resulting from compression by tumor or infarction of the posterior spinal artery. Clinically, proprioception, stereognosis, two-point discrimination, and vibration sense are lost below the level of the lesion.[13]

Cauda Equina Syndrome. Damage to the cauda equina occurs with injuries at or below the L1 vertebral level. This syndrome results in a lower motor neuron lesion that is usually incomplete. This lesion results in flaccid paralysis with no spinal reflex activity present.[10,12]

Conus Medullaris Syndrome. Injury of the sacral cord and lumbar nerve roots within the neural canal results in a clinical picture of lower-extremity motor and sensory loss and an areflexic bladder and bowel.[13]

MEDICAL MANAGEMENT

Short-term medical treatment includes anatomical realignment and stabilization interventions and pharmacological management to prevent further neurological trauma and enhance neural recovery.

Surgical Stabilization

One of the first interventions after acute SCI is to stabilize the spine to prevent further cord or nerve root damage. In the emergency department, diagnostic studies reveal the severity of the spinal injury and the type and degree of the instability. On the basis of these findings, the physician, client, and family decide on treatment. Many options must be considered regarding the optimal operative strategy. Indications for surgical intervention include, but are not limited to, signs of progressive neurological involvement, type and extent of bony lesions, and degree of spinal cord damage.[21] The following discussion includes nonsurgical and surgical interventions.

Cervical Spine

At the scene of the accident, emergency medical technicians use extreme caution to immobilize the injured client and prevent excessive movement at the unstable spinal site. If there is compression of neurological tissue, vertebral fracture, or dislocation, reduction must occur to minimize ischemia and edema formation.[22] In the emergency department, reduction is accomplished by cervical traction with the goal of immediate and proper alignment of bone fragments and decompression of the spinal cord until further stabilization.[21,23,24] The most widely used traction is the Gardner-Wells tongs (Figure 19-2), which are inserted into the skull. Weights are added at approximately 5 pounds of traction per level of injury to achieve reduction of the dislocation and to maintain alignment.[23]

Certain precautions must be considered during therapy to prevent unnecessary movement at the injury site. The traction rope must be kept in alignment with the long axis of the cervical spine, and the weights must be allowed to hang freely. Cervical rotation must be prevented. In addition, care must be taken to ensure that continued traction is maintained at all times.

When surgical stabilization is indicated, common surgical protocols include posterior and anterior approaches. The posterior cervical fusion is the most commonly stabilization procedure. Unstable compression injuries are usually managed by a posterior procedure except when there is a deficient anterior column. Anterior approaches are indicated for patients with evidence of residual anterior spinal cord or nerve root compression and persistent neurological deficit.[21]

After cervical surgical stabilization, a hard collar such as a Philadelphia collar (Figure 19-3) or sternal-occipital-mandibular immobilizer brace (SOMI) is used until a solid

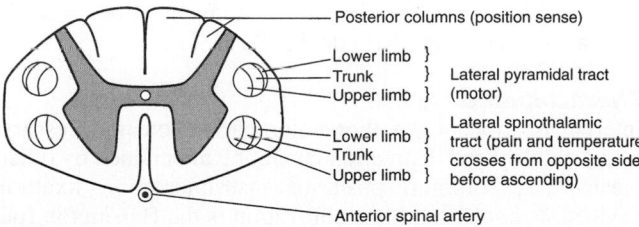

FIGURE 19-1 ■ Cross-sectional anatomy of the spinal cord.

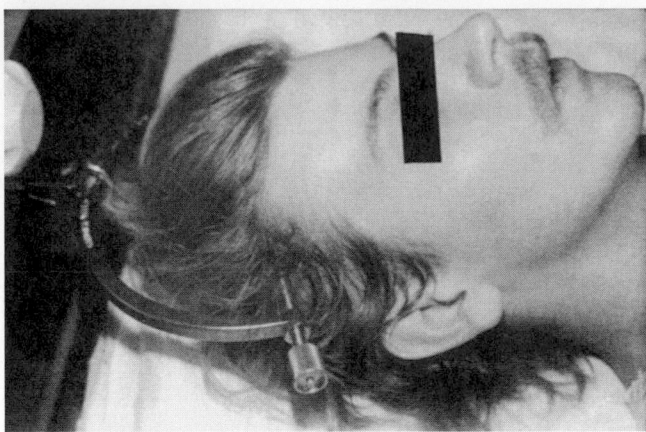

FIGURE 19-2 ■ Gardner-Wells tongs. Reduction is accomplished through weights attached to the traction rope. (Courtesy of Dr. H. Herndon Murray, Assistant Medical Director, Shepherd Spinal Center, Atlanta, Georgia.)

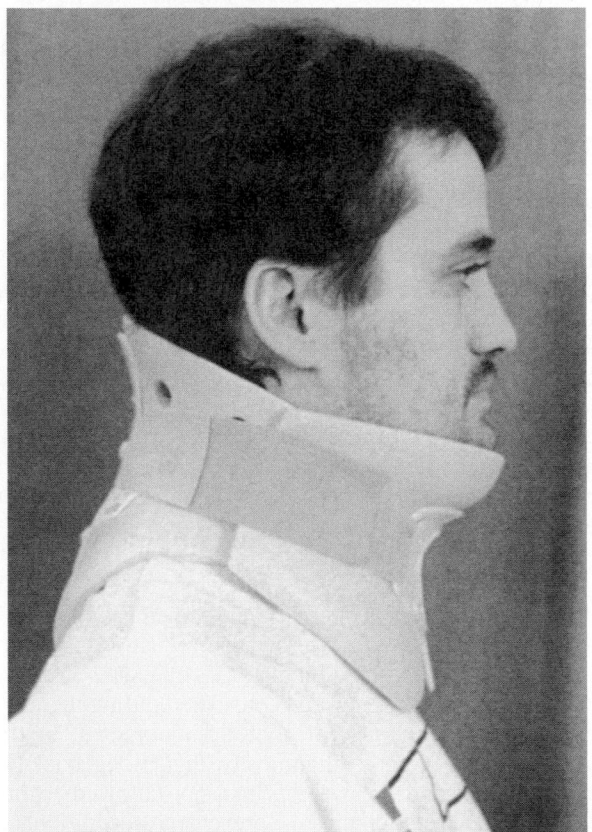

FIGURE 19-3 ■ Philadelphia collar. It is fabricated of polyethylene foam with rigid anterior and posterior plastic strips, it is easily applied via Velcro closures, and it limits flexion, extension, and rotary movements of the cervical spine.

bony fusion has developed. The solid bony fusion usually takes 6 to 8 weeks. Postoperatively, care must be taken to protect the bony fusion.

When surgery is not indicated, or when more postoperative stabilization is required, halo traction may be indicated. The halo restricts more movement in the upper cervical spine compared with the lower cervical spine.[25] The halo

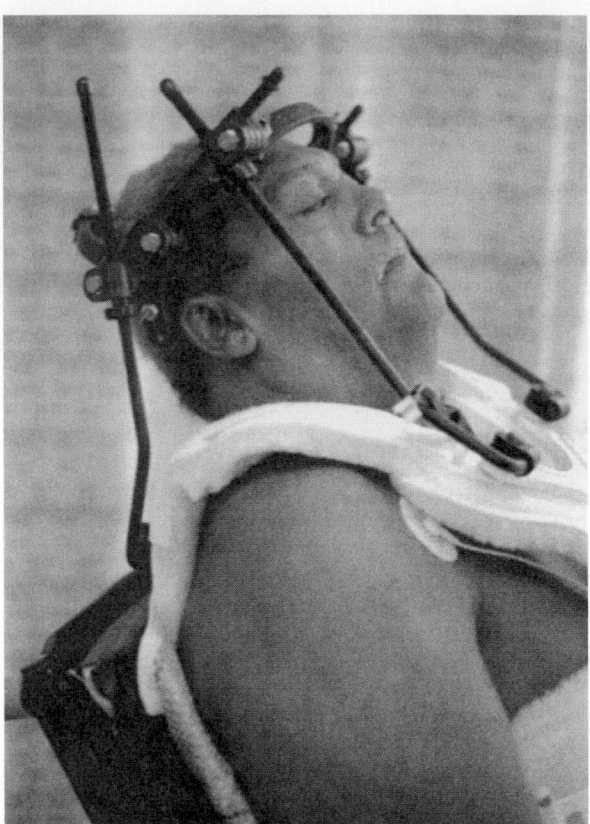

FIGURE 19-4 ■ Halo vest. Basic components are the halo ring, distraction rods, and jacket.

traction device consists of three parts: the ring, the uprights, and the jacket (Figure 19-4). The ring fits around the skull, just above the ears. It is held in place by four pins that are inserted into the skull. The uprights are attached to the ring and jacket by bolts. The jacket is usually made of polypropylene and lined with sheepskin. This equipment is left in place for 6 to 12 weeks until bony healing is satisfactory.[5] The advantage of using the halo device is the ability to mobilize the client as soon as the device has been applied without compromising spinal alignment. This allows the rehabilitation program to commence more rapidly. It also allows for delayed decision making regarding the need for surgery.

The disadvantage of the halo device is that pressure and friction from the vest or jacket may lead to altered skin integrity.[11] Special attention must be given to ensure the skin remains intact. During more active phases of the rehabilitation process, the halo device may slow functional progress because of its added weight and its interference with the middle to end range of upper-extremity movement. In a small percentage of clients, there are complications of dysphagia and temporomandibular joint dysfunctions associated with wearing the halo device.[11]

Thoracolumbar Spine
Internal fixation of the thoracolumbar region is necessary when stability and distraction cannot be maintained by other means.[26] A common posterior instrumentation fixation device for thoracolumbar stabilization is the Harrington rod (Figure 19-5). The Harrington rod is a rod-and-hook device

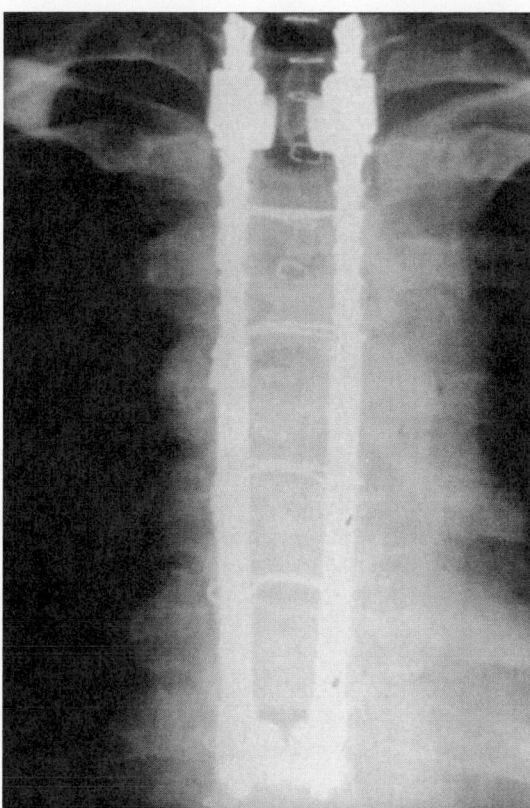

FIGURE 19-5 ■ Radiograph of Harrington rod instrumentation. (Courtesy of Dr. H. Herndon Murray, Assistant Medical Director, Shepherd Spinal Center, Atlanta, Georgia.)

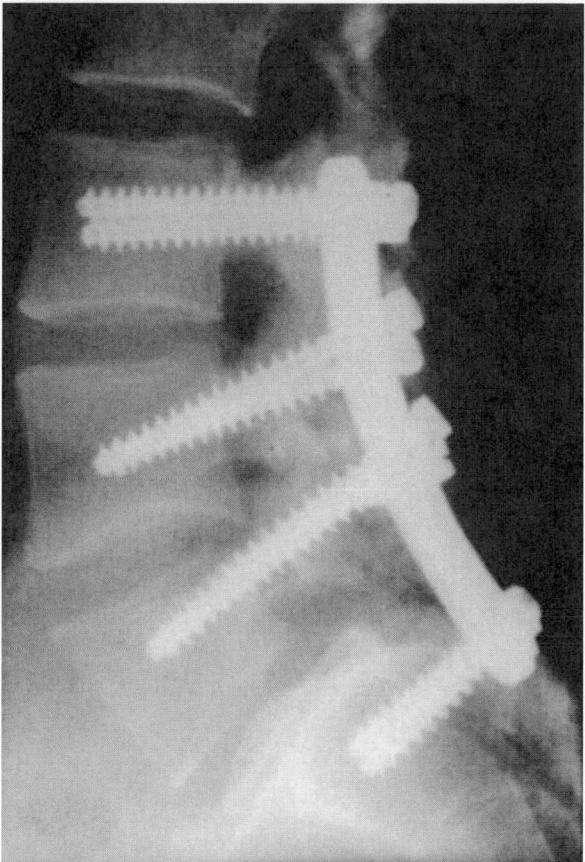

FIGURE 19-6 ■ Radiograph of transpedicular screws. (Courtesy of Dr. H. Herndon Murray, Assistant Medical Director, Shepherd Spinal Center, Atlanta, Georgia.)

that can offer compressive or distractive forces to the spine. Compressive forces are used to reduce fracture dislocations in the presence of an intact anterior column. Distractive forces are used to restore the height loss associated with burst fractures.[25] Other common thoracic stabilization procedures include transpedicular screws (Figure 19-6) or a hybrid type of instrumentation.

Postoperatively, an external trunk support is necessary to limit excessive vertebral motion and to maintain proper thoracic and lumbar alignment.[12,26] This may be achieved by a custom thoracolumbosacral orthosis (Figure 19-7) or a Jewett brace (Figure 19-8). Initially, the client's activity may be limited to allow for a complete fusion to take place and to minimize the possibility of rod displacement. All spinal limitations should be discussed with the surgeon postoperatively.

The goal of the operative procedures at any spinal level discussed is to reverse the deforming forces, to restore proper spinal alignment, and to stabilize the spine.[27] All these procedures have advantages and disadvantages. The surgeon, client, and family must be involved in the decision-making process to select the most appropriate method of treatment. This will allow the therapeutic rehabilitation process to begin.

Pharmacological Management

Neurological damage from SCI may be a result of (1) physical disruption of axons traversing the injury site, (2) local infarction as a result of ischemia or hypoxia, or (3) prevention of impulses by microhemorrhages or edema within the spinal cord at the injury site.[28,29] The initial trauma alone rarely causes anatomical transection of the spinal cord, even when there is a complete loss of sensory and motor function below the level of the injury.[29]

The injury often causes damage more centrally in the gray matter, with lesser damage occurring to the surrounding white matter.[29] This central contusion is believed to lead to secondary damage 24 to 72 hours after the injury. Investigators believe that secondary injuries to surrounding tissues can be lessened by pharmacological agents, specifically methylprednisolone and monosialotetrahexosyl-ganglioside (GM_1). To date, two major pharmacological clinical trials have been completed. The National Acute SCI Study[30] used high doses of methylprednisolone and showed significant improvements in sensory and motor function 6 months after injury.[31] Young and Flamm[32] showed that methylprednisolone enhanced the flow of blood to the injured spinal cords, preventing the typical decline in white matter, extracellular calcium levels, and evoked potentials. This acts to prevent progressive posttraumatic ischemia.[28,33-35]

GM_1 is a complex acidic glycolipid found at high levels in cell membranes in the mammalian central nervous system. Evidence suggests that GM_1 stimulates axonal growth.[29] The significant improvements in clients who

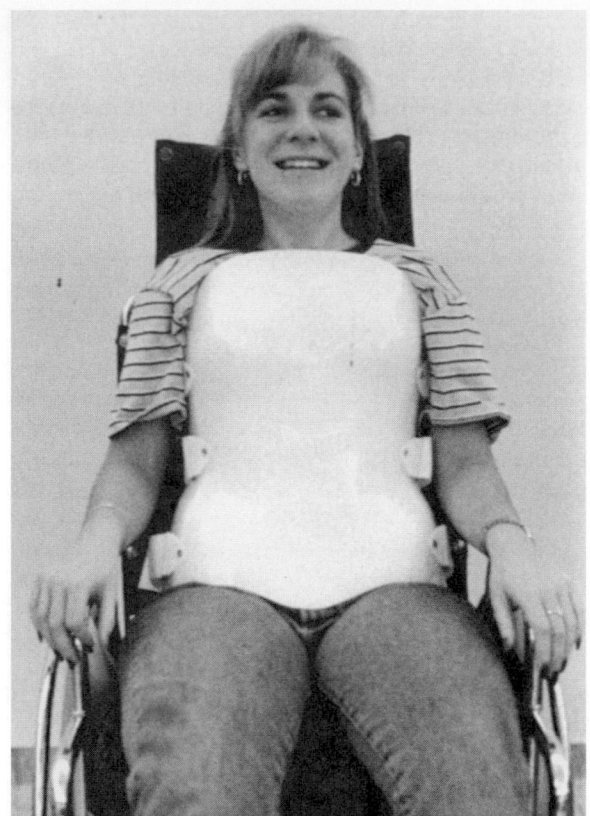

FIGURE 19-7 ■ Custom thoracolumbosacral orthosis. This molded plastic body orthosis has a soft lining on the interior. It controls flexion, extension, and rotary movements until healing of the bone occurs.

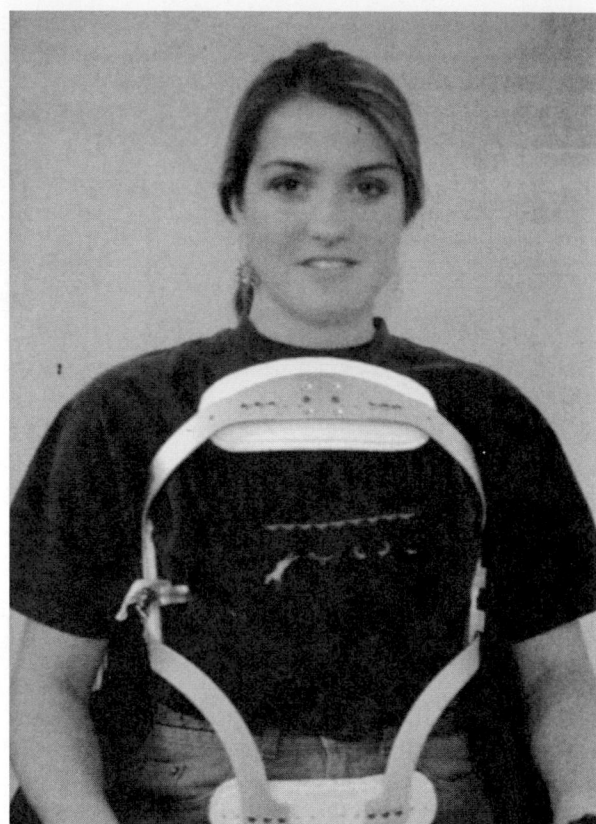

FIGURE 19-8 ■ Jewett hyperextension brace. A single three-point force system is provided by sternal pad, suprapubic pad, and thoracolumbar pad. Forward flexion is restricted in the thoracolumbar area.

received GM$_1$ were manifested in approximately 1 year, with some clinical changes seen as early as 1 day after receiving the drug. Motor function recovery was noted predominantly in the lower extremities. It is thought that neurological return was seen primarily in the lower extremities because GM$_1$ enhances the function of the surrounding white matter tracks to the lower extremities but not of the gray matter at the injury site.[28]

Theoretically, it may be more beneficial to combine the administration of these two drugs. Methylprednisolone would allow for initial survival of injured neurons, and GM$_1$ would enhance recovery in this larger number of surviving neurons.[29] In 2001, Geisler et al[35] completed a multicenter trial comparing methylprednisolone alone with methylprednisolone followed by GM$_1$ for 6 weeks. The treatment group that received both pharmacological agents showed faster recovery during the first 6 weeks, but both groups had similar recovery at 6 to 12 months.[35]

In addition to pharmacological management, there are promising clinical trials currently underway for both acute and chronic spinal cord injury. See Table 19-2[36-46] for summary of current spinal cord injury research.

THERAPEUTIC REHABILITATION CONTINUUM OF CARE

The therapeutic rehabilitation process is best described as a continuum of care. The continuum of care gives a frame-

work for how a client may progress through rehabilitation. Rehabilitation teams may use one of three models: multidisciplinary, interdisciplinary, and transdisciplinary.[3] As evidenced by standards set forth by the Commission on Accreditation for Rehabilitation Facilities (CARF) the interdisciplinary model of team structure is optimal in the rehabilitation setting.[47]

The continuum of care may be divided into several phases that include medical management (previously described), early rehabilitation, inpatient rehabilitation, and outpatient rehabilitation/community reintegration. The progression of a client through the rehabilitation process will vary greatly from one client to the next. The client may move back and forth throughout the continuum of care.

Early Rehabilitation

Early rehabilitation includes all therapeutic interventions during the critical and acute-care stages of rehabilitation. The primary emphasis of early rehabilitation is to lessen the adverse effects of neurotrauma and immobilization. This phase may last from a few days to several weeks, depending on the severity and level of injury and other associated injuries. Although therapeutic intensity may be limited, clients may begin out-of-bed activities. Goals during this phase should focus on prevention of secondary complications and preparing the client for full rehabilitation partici-

TABLE 19-2 ■ Summary of Spinal Cord Injury Research

AGENT/INTERVENTION	MECHANISM	PREVENT SECONDARY DEGENERATION	COMPENSATE FOR DE-MYELINIZATION	PROMOTE AXONAL REGENERATION	REPLACE DEAD CELLS
Methylprednisolone[36]	Antiinflammatory, blocks glutamate receptors, reduces accumulation of free radicals	X			
GM$_1$[37]	Neurotrophic factor limits cell death by buffering excitotoxicity and preventing apoptosis	X			
Activated macrophages[38]	Bolsters immune response, introduces nerve growth factors	X		X	
4-Aminopyridine[39]	Potassium channel blocker restores action potential conduction in demyelinated or poorly myelinated nerves; enhances synaptic transmission		X		
AIT-082 (Neotrofin)[40]	NGF promotes axonal sprouting			X	
Schwann cell transplants[41]	Myelin producers in peripheral nerves are known to cross into central nervous system at dorsal root; may be used to deliver trophic factors and as bridges to support axonal growth		X	X	X
Olfactory ensheathing glial cells[42,43]	Cells may function in three ways; bipolar form encourages cell migration; multipolar form guides direction of axon growth; ensheathing form provide a bridge or scaffold over cord damage			X	X
Fetal spinal cord transplants[44]	Experimental procedure for treatment of syringomyelia			X	X
Fetal pig neural stem cells[45]	Replace neural cells and promote differentiation				X
Umbilical cord blood stem cells[46]	Cells used in treatment of leukemia, autoimmune diseases (lupus erythematosus), and sickle cell anemia				X

Provided by Mike Jones, PhD, Vice President of Clinical Research of Crawford Clinical Research Center.

pation. The treatment team must begin discharge planning and family training in this phase.

Inpatient Rehabilitation

During inpatient rehabilitation, out-of-bed activities are tolerated for longer periods of time and the client begins to work toward specific long-term goals. In accordance with Medicare guidelines for rehabilitation, the client is able to participate in therapeutic programs a minimum of 3 hours a day.[48] The intensity of therapy may continue to be limited according to unresolved medical issues.

As medical issues resolve and endurance improves, the client will progress to a higher and more active level of participation. During inpatient rehabilitation, the client gains varying levels of independence in specific skills. The client may be taught advanced skills in performance of activities of daily living (ADL), transfers, and mobility skills. Community outings may be scheduled to refine advanced skills, identify further needs, and foster community reintegration. In addition, the following will be completed unless otherwise indicated by the rehabilitation team: (1) family training, (2) home and school or work evaluation, (3) vocational testing/planning, (4) delivery and fitting of discharge equipment, (5) instruction in home management, (6) instruction in home exercise programs, (7) referrals for continued services, and (8) driving evaluation. Discharge planning largely encompasses activities aimed at a smooth transition to home.

Outpatient Rehabilitation and Community Reentry

Discharge from an inpatient rehabilitation program marks only the beginning of the lifelong process of adjustment to disability and community reintegration. Inpatient rehabilitation provides an environment best suited for learning self-care skills, yet "the implications of living in the community with SCI can scarcely be anticipated accurately by the newly injured individual or the able-bodied staff."[49] Because of the shortened lengths of hospitalization, services provided after discharge are becoming increasingly important. A direct consequence of this shift results in outpatient treatment of clients who have more acuity, greater care needs, and fewer skills attained in the inpatient rehabilitation program before entry into the outpatient arena. Common outpatient therapy treatment programs have included advanced transfer training, advanced wheelchair mobility training, gait training, upgraded ADL training, and upgraded home exercise program instruction. This is a shift in the typical program structure because these skills were traditionally a part of the inpatient rehabilitation. This is a direct result of cost-containment efforts resulting in a shortened inpatient length of stay.

Services provided after inpatient discharge may include day programs, single-service outpatient visits, and routine follow-up visits and services. The primary purpose of these services is to provide a coordinated effort for the client to return to full reintegration into the community.

The "day program" concept has emerged to meet the demand for more comprehensive rehabilitation services. Clients who are medically stable, do not require skilled nursing services during the night, tolerate 3 hours or more of therapy per day, and need a coordinated approach for two or more services are good candidates for this type of program. A day program offers the same coordinated rehabilitation services as inpatient rehabilitation but is performed in an outpatient setting. The focus is not only on performance of functional skills but also on the transference of these skills into the community.

EXAMINATION AND EVALUATION

Regardless of where the client begins the rehabilitation process, an examination is completed on admission. The examination and evaluation will assist in establishing the diagnosis and the prognosis of each client as well as determine the appropriate therapeutic interventions. The client/caregivers participate by reporting activity performance and functional ability.[50] Any pertinent additions to the history stated by the client should be described. The client's statement of goals, problems, and concerns should be included.

The main areas of the examination are outlined here.

History

A review of the medical record is the first step toward the examination because it provides the background information and identifies medical precautions. The history should include general demographics, social history, occupation or employment, pertinent growth and development, living environment, history of current condition, functional status and activity level, completed tests and measures, medica-

tions, history of current condition if applicable, medical and surgical history, family history, reported client/family health status, and social habits.[51] If the history suggests a loss of consciousness or brain injury, the clinician should consider the possibility of compromised cognition and should include tests and measures during the examination and assessment appropriate to that impairment.

Systems Review

The physiological and anatomical status should be reviewed for the cardiopulmonary, integumentary, musculoskeletal, and neuromuscular systems. In addition, communication, affect, cognition, language, and learning style should be reviewed.[50]

Tests and Measures

Depending on the data generated during the history and systems review, the clinician performs tests and measures to help identify impairments, functional limitations, and disabilities and to establish the diagnosis and prognosis of each client. Tests and measures that are often used for persons with SCI are included in Box 19-1. For more detail related to specific tools, refer to the Guide of Physical Therapy Practice.[51]

Neurological Examination

American Spinal Cord Injury Association Examination

It is recommended that the international standards of the American Spinal Injury Association (ASIA) be used for the specific neurological examination after a spinal cord injury.[10] See Figure 19-9 for the ASIA Motor and Sensory Examination. Assessment of muscle performanc allows for specific diagnosis of the level and completeness of injury.

BOX 19-1 ■ TESTS AND MEASURES[51]

Aerobic Capacity and Endurance
Anthropometric Characteristics
Assistive and Adaptive Devices Assessment
Community and Work Integration or Reintegration
Environmental Home and Work Barriers Examination
Gait, Locomotion, and Balance
Integumentary Integrity
Joint Integrity and Mobility
Motor Function
Muscle Performance
Orthotic, Protective, and Supportive Devices
Pain
Posture
Range of Motion
Reflex Integrity
Self-Care and Home Management
Sensory Integrity
Ventilation, Respiration, and Circulation
Diagnosis of Impairment/Disabilities

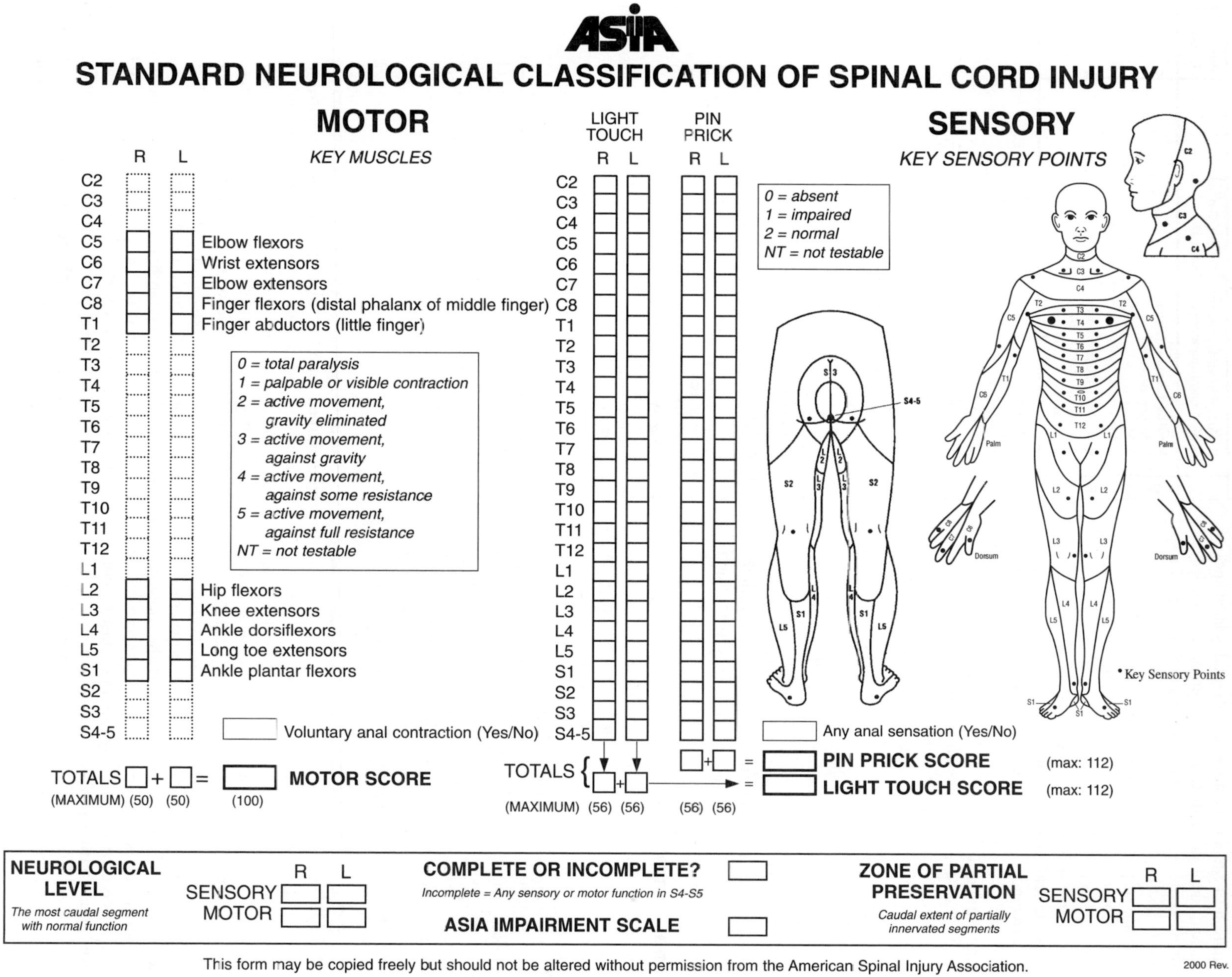

FIGURE 19-9 ■ ASIA Motor and Sensory Evaluation Form. (Courtesy of the American Spinal Injury Association, Atlanta, Georgia.)

The examination of muscle performance includes each specific muscle and identifies substitutions from other muscles.

A six-point scale is used to describe procedures for manual muscle testing[10]:

0 = no visible or palpable contraction is detected
1 = muscle contraction is palpable, but no limb movement is detected
2 = full movement of limb with gravity eliminated
3 = full movement of limb against gravity
4 = full movement with moderate resistance through range
5 = normal strength

Along with the strength of each muscle, the presence, absence, and location of muscle tone should be described. The Modified Ashworth scale is a common tool used to describe tone.[52]

The client's sensation is described by dermatome. The recommended tests include (1) sharp-dull discrimination or temperature sensitivity to test the lateral spinothalamic tract, (2) light touch to test the anterior spinothalamic tract, and (3) proprioception or vibration to test the posterior columns of the spinal cord. Sensation is indicated as intact, impaired, or absent per dermatome. A dermatomal map is helpful and recommended for ease of documentation.

Functional Examination

It is recommended that a complete functional assessment be performed on initial examination and thereafter as appropriate. A myriad of tools exist to assess functional skills. Many institutions develop functional assessments that address home, community, and institutional mobility and ADL functional skills. The Functional Independence Measure (Figure 19-10) is one of the more commonly used tools that is currently applied for many impairment diagnostic groups, including spinal cord injury.[53] Other tools, such as the Quadriplegia Index of Function (QUIF),[54] the Spinal Cord Independence Measure (SCIM),[55] and the Craig Handicap Assessment and Reporting Technique (CHART)[56] are options.

LEVELS		
	7 Complete Independence (Timely, Safely) 6 Modified Independence (Device)	No Helper
	Modified Dependence 5 Supervision 4 Minimal Assist (Subject = 75%+) 3 Moderate Assist (Subject = 50%+) **Complete Dependence** 2 Maximal Assist (Subject = 25%+) 1 Total Assist (Subject = 0%+)	Helper

	ADMIT	DISCH
Self Care		
A. Eating	☐	☐
B. Grooming	☐	☐
C. Bathing	☐	☐
D. Dressing-Upper Body	☐	☐
E. Dressing-Lower Body	☐	☐
F. Toileting	☐	☐
Sphincter Control		
G. Bladder Management	☐	☐
H. Bowel Management	☐	☐
Mobility		
Transfer:		
I. Bed, Chair, Wheelchair	☐	☐
J. Toilet	☐	☐
K. Tub, Shower	☐	☐
Locomotion		
L. Walk/Wheelchair	W ☐ C ☐ ☐	W ☐ C ☐ ☐
M. Stairs	☐	☐
Communication		
N. Comprehension	A ☐ V ☐ ☐	A ☐ V ☐ ☐
O. Expression	V ☐ N ☐ ☐	V ☐ N ☐ ☐
Social Cognition		
P. Social Interaction	☐	☐
Q. Problem Solving	☐	☐
R. Memory	☐	☐
Total FIM	☐	☐

NOTE: Leave no blanks; enter 1 if patient not testable due to risk.

FIGURE 19-10 ■ Functional Independence Measure. Guide for the Uniform Data Set for Medical Rehabilitation (Adult FIM) Version 4.0, Buffalo, New York: State University of New York at Buffalo, 1993.

GOAL SETTING

Goal setting is a dynamic process that directly follows the examination. Each problem identified should be addressed with specific short- and long-term goals. The clinician must interpret new information continuously, which leads to continuing reevaluation and revision of goals.[57] Goals are always individualized and should be established in collaboration with the treatment team, the client, and the caregiver, and with realistic consideration of anticipated needs on return to the home environment. Factors that must be considered in the goal-setting process include age, body type, associated injuries, premorbid medical conditions, additional orthopedic injury, cognitive ability, psychosocial issues, spasticity, endurance, strength, range of motion (ROM), funding sources, and motivation.

Long-term goals for the rehabilitation of clients with SCI reflect functional outcomes and are based on the strength of the remaining innervated or partially innervated musculature. Short-term goals identify components that interfere with functional ability and are designed to "address these limiting factors while building component skills"[11] of the desired long-term goals.[58]

Functional goals are established in the following areas: bathing, bed mobility, bladder and bowel control, communication, environmental control/access, feeding, dressing, gait, grooming, home management, ROM/positioning, skin care management, transfers, transportation/driving, wheelchair management, and wheelchair mobility. Refer to Table 19-3 for anticipated goals for each level of injury. Information presented in this table must be recognized as general guidelines because variability exists. These guidelines are most usefully applied to clients with complete SCI. Goal setting for individuals with incomplete SCI is often more challenging given the greater variability of client presentations and the uncertainty of neurological recovery. As with any client, continuing reevaluations provide additional insight into functional limitations or progression and potential and thereby direct the goal-setting process. In addition to specific functional goals and expectations, family training, home, work or school modifications, and community reentry must also be considered.

Rehabilitation teams may elect to hold a goal-setting or interim conference for each client during which team members, including the client, have the opportunity to

Text continued on p. 620

TABLE 19-3 ■ Functional Expectation for Complete SCI Lesions

FUNCTIONAL COMPONENT	OUTCOME POTENTIAL	ANTICIPATED EQUIPMENT TO ACHIEVE OUTCOMES
C1-4		
Sitting tolerance	80-90 degrees for 10-12 hours per day	Power wheelchair with power tilt/recline
Communication		Wheelchair cushion
Mouth stick writing	Minimal assist	Mouth sticks and docking station
ECU	Setup	ECU
Page turning	Minimal assist to setup	Book holder
Computer operation	Minimal assist to setup	Computer
Call-system use	Setup	Call system or speaker phone
Cuff-leak speech	Up to 2 hours	
Feeding	Dependent, but verbalizes care	
Grooming	Dependent, but verbalizes care	
Bathing	Dependent, but verbalizes care	Reclining shower chair
Dressing	Dependent, but verbalizes care	
Bowel management	Dependent, but verbalizes care	
Bladder management	Dependent, but verbalizes care	
Bed mobility		
Rolling side/side	Dependent, but verbalizes care	4-way adjustable hospital bed to assist
Rolling		caregiver with task
Supine/prone		
Supine to/from sit		
Scooting		
Leg management		
Transfers		
Bed	Dependent, but verbalizes care	Overhead lift system
Tub/Toilet		Hydraulic lift
Car		Slings
Floor		
Power wheelchair mobility		
Smooth surfaces	Modified independent	Power wheelchair with
Ramps	Modified independent	power recline/tilt system
Rough terrain	Modified independent	Lap tray
Curbs	Dependent, but verbalizes	Armrests, shoulder supports, and lateral trunk supports
Manual wheelchair mobility		
Smooth surfaces	Dependent, but verbalizes	Manual reclining/tilt wheelchair with same
Ramps		options as power wheelchair
Rough terrain		
Curbs		
Stairs		
Skin		
Weight shift	Modified independent with power wheelchair	Recline/tilt wheelchair
Padding/positioning	Dependent, but verbalizes	Wheelchair cushion
Skin checks	Dependent, but verbalizes	Pillow splints/resting splints
		Mirror
Community ADL		
Dependent passenger evaluation	Dependent, but verbalizes	Modified van
ROM to scapula, upper extremity, lower extremity, and trunk	Dependent, but verbalizes	
Exercise program	Independent for respiratory and neck exercises	Portable or bedside ventilator (C1-3 only)
C5		
Sitting tolerance	90 degrees for 10-12 hours per day	Power recline/tilt wheelchair
		Wheelchair cushion

Continued

TABLE 19-3 ■ Functional Expectation for Complete SCI Lesions—cont'd

FUNCTIONAL COMPONENT	OUTCOME POTENTIAL	ANTICIPATED EQUIPMENT TO ACHIEVE OUTCOMES
Communication		
Telephone use	Modified independent	Telephone adaptations
ECU	Setup	ECU
Page turning	Setup	Book holder, wrist support with cuff
Computer operation	Supervision	Computer
Writing/typing	Setup	Long Wanchik brace
Feeding	Minimal to setup assist	Mobile arm support or offset feeder
		Adaptive ADL equipment
Grooming		
Wash face	Minimal assist to setup	Mobile arm support or offset feeder
Comb/brush hair	Minimal assist	Wrist support with adapted cuff
Oral care	Minimal assist to setup	Adaptive ADL equipment
Bathing	Dependent, but verbalizes care	Upright or tilt shower chair
Dressing	Dependent, but verbalizes care	
Bowel management	Dependent, but verbalizes care	
Bladder management	Dependent, but verbalizes care	Automatic leg bag emptier
Bed mobility		
Rolling side/side	Maximal assistance to dependent and verbalizes care	4-way adjustable hospital bed to assist caregiver with care
Rolling		
Supine/prone		
Supine to/from sit		
Scooting		
Leg management		
Transfers		
Bed	Maximal assist to dependent for level transfers, verbalizes unlevel transfers	Overhead or hydraulic lift and slings
Tub/toilet		Possible transfer board
Car		
Floor		
Power wheelchair mobility	Recommended mode of locomotion	Power wheelchair with power recline/tilt system
Smooth surfaces	Modified independent	
Ramps	Modified independent	Recommend lap tray
Rough terrain	Modified independent	Armrests, shoulder supports, lateral trunk supports
Curbs	Dependent, but verbalizes	
Manual wheelchair mobility		
Smooth surfaces	Dependent, but verbalizes	Upright or reclining wheelchair with special back and trunk supports
Ramps		
Rough terrain		Consider manual wheelchair with power assist pushrims
Curbs		
Stairs		
Skin		
Weight shift	Modified independent with power wheelchair	Recline/tilt wheelchair and wheelchair cushion
Padding/positioning	Dependent, but verbalizes	Pillow splints/resting splints
Skin checks	Dependent, but verbalizes	Mirror
Home management		
Prepare snack	Moderate to maximal assistance	Wrist support with cuffs
		Adaptive ADL equipment
Community ADL		
Drive van	Independent	Highly adapted vehicle
Dependent passenger evaluation	Dependent	Modified van
ROM to scapula, upper extremity, lower extremity, and trunk	Dependent, but verbalizes	
Exercise program		Airsplints or light cuff weights
Upper extremity and neck	Minimal assistance	E-stim unit
C6		
Sitting tolerance	90 degrees for 10-12 hours per day	

TABLE 19-3 ■ Functional Expectation for Complete SCI Lesions—cont'd

FUNCTIONAL COMPONENT	OUTCOME POTENTIAL	ANTICIPATED EQUIPMENT TO ACHIEVE OUTCOMES
Communication		
Telephone use	Modified independent	Adaptive ADL equipment
Page turning		Tenodesis splint
Writing/typing/keyboard		Short opponens splint
Feeding	Modified independent	Adaptive ADL equipment
Grooming	Modified independent	Adaptive ADL equipment
		Tenodesis splint
Bathing		
Upper body	Minimal assist	Upright shower chair
Lower body	Moderate assist	Various bathing equipment
Dressing		
Upper body	Modified independent	Adaptive ADL equipment
Lower body (bed)	Moderate to minimal assist	
Bowel management	Moderate assist	Dil stick
		Adaptive ADL equipment
Bladder management	Male with minimal assist	Tenodesis
	Female with moderate assist	Adaptive ADL equipment
Bed mobility		
Rolling side/side	Minimal assist to modified independent	4-way adjustable hospital bed or regular bed with loops/straps
Rolling		
Supine/prone		
Supine to/from sit		
Scooting		
Leg management		
Transfers		
Bed	Minimal assist	Transfer board
Tub/toilet	Moderate assist	
Car	Moderate to maximal assist	
Floor	Dependent, but verbalizes procedure	
Power wheelchair mobility	Recommended mode of locomotion	Power upright wheelchair
Smooth surfaces	Modified independent	
Ramps	Modified independent	
Rough terrain	Modified independent	
Curbs	Dependent, but verbalizes	
Manual wheelchair mobility	Only if scapulae grades are 3 or better	Upright wheelchair
Smooth surfaces	Modified independent	May need adaptations to facilitate more efficient propulsion (i.e., push pegs, plastic-coated handrims)
Ramps	Modified independent	
Rough terrain	Moderate to minimal assist	
Curbs	Dependent but verbalizes procedure	Consider manual wheelchair with power assist pushrims
Stairs	Dependent but verbalizes procedure	
Skin		
Weight shift	Modified independent	Upright wheelchair with push handles
Pad/positioning	Moderate to minimal assist	Mirror
Skin checks	Moderate to minimal assist	
Home management		
Light home management	Minimal assist	Various adaptive ADL equipment
Heavy home management	Moderate assist	
Community ADL		
Driving vehicle	Modified independent	Modified vehicle
ROM to scapula, upper extremity, lower extremity, and trunk	Minimal assist	Leg lifter to assist with lower extremity ROM
Exercise program	Minimal assistance	Cuff weights
		Airsplints
		E-stim unit

Continued

TABLE 19-3 ■ **Functional Expectation for Complete SCI Lesions—cont'd**

FUNCTIONAL COMPONENT	OUTCOME POTENTIAL	ANTICIPATED EQUIPMENT TO ACHIEVE OUTCOMES
C7-8		
Sitting tolerance	90 degrees for 10-12 hours per day	
Communication		
Telephone use	Modified independent	Adaptive ADL equipment
Page turning		
Writing/typing/keyboard		
Feeding	Modified independent	Adaptive ADL equipment
Grooming	Modified independent	Adaptive ADL equipment
Bathing		
Upper body	Modified independent	Upright shower chair
Lower body	Modified independent	Various bathing equipment
Dressing (upper and lower body)	Modified independent for upper	Adaptive ADL equipment
In bed	Minimal assist to modified independent for	
In wheelchair	lower body dressing	
Bowel management	Modified independent	Dil stick
Bladder management		
Bed	Male with modified independent	Various bladder management/adaptive ADL
Wheelchair	Female with minimal assist to modified	equipment
	independent	
	Male with modified independence	
	Female with moderate assist	
Bed mobility		
Rolling side/side	Modified independent	Leg lifter
Rolling		
Supine/prone		
Supine to/from sit		
Scooting		
Leg management		
Transfers		
Bed	Modified independent	Transfer board
Tub/toilet	Modified independent	May not need transfer board for even surfaces
Car	Minimal assist for loading WC	
Floor	Maximal assist	
Power wheelchair mobility		
Smooth surfaces	Modified independent	Power upright wheelchair
Ramps	Modified independent	
Rough terrain	Modified independent	
Curbs	Dependent, but verbalizes	
Manual wheelchair mobility		
Smooth surfaces	Modified independent	Upright wheelchair
Ramps	Modified independent	
Rough terrain	Modified independent	
Curbs	Minimal to moderate assist	
Stairs	Maximal assist	
Skin		
Weight shift	Modified independent	Upright wheelchair with push handles
Pad/positioning	Minimal assist to modified independent	
Skin checks	Minimal assist to modified independent	Mirror
Home management		
Light home management	Modified independent	Various ADL equipment
Heavy home management	Moderate assist	
Community ADL		
Driving vehicle	Modified independent	Modified vehicle
ROM to scapula, upper extremity, lower extremity, and trunk	Modified independent	Leg lifter to assist with lower extremity ROM

TABLE 19-3 ■ Functional Expectation for Complete SCI Lesions—cont'd

FUNCTIONAL COMPONENT	OUTCOME POTENTIAL	ANTICIPATED EQUIPMENT TO ACHIEVE OUTCOMES
Exercise program	Modified independent	Cuff weights or e-stim unit
PARAPLEGIA		
Sitting tolerance	90 degrees for 10-12 hours per day	
Communication	Independent	
Feeding	Independent	
Grooming	Independent	
Bathing		
Upper body	Independent	Upright tub chair
Lower body	Modified independent	Long-handled sponge and handheld shower hose
Dressing (upper and lower body)		Adaptive ADL equipment
In bed	Modified independent	
In wheelchair	Modified independent	
Bowel management	Modified independent	Dil stick if positive bulbocavernous reflex
		Suppositories if negative bulbocavernous reflex
Bladder management	Modified independent	
Bed mobility		
Rolling side/side	Modified independent	
Rolling		
Supine/prone		
Supine to/from sit		
Scooting		
Leg management		
Transfers		
Bed	Modified independent	May need a transfer board
Tub/toilet		
Car		
Floor		
Upright wheelchair		
Manual wheelchair mobility		Upright wheelchair
Smooth surfaces	Modified independent	
Ramps		
Rough terrain		
Curbs	Moderate assist to modified independent	
Stairs (3-4)		
Ambulation	Depends on level of injury	
Smooth surfaces	Modified independent for T12 injuries and	Appropriate orthotics and assistive device(s)
Ramps	below. Will vary with higher thoracic	
Rough terrain	injuries.	
Curbs		
Stairs		
Skin		
Weight shift	Modified independent	
Pad/positioning		
Skin checks		Mirror
Home management		
Light home management	Modified independent	
Heavy home management	Modified independent	Various adaptive ADL equipment
Community ADL		
Driving vehicle	Modified independent	Hand controls for vehicle
ROM to left extremity and trunk	Modified independent	Leg lifter to assist with lower extremity ROM
Exercise program	Modified independent	Cuff weights, e-stim if any weakened lower extremity muscles

discuss the long-term goals that have been established. It may be useful to request that the client sign a statement acknowledging understanding of, and agreement to, all long-term goals.

EARLY REHABILITATION AND COMPLICATION PREVENTION

Early rehabilitation of the client with SCI begins with prevention. Preventing secondary complications speeds entry into the rehabilitation phase and improves the possibility that the client will become a productive member of society.

Table 19-4 describes an overview of the primary complications that can arise after a SCI. In this table any known etiology and common management is reviewed. Tests and measures used to determine or diagnose the complication and the recommended medical and ther-apeutic interventions are listed in the table. Although various reports of incidences are published, the largest database is the Model Spinal Cord Injury Care Systems report.[30] Because of their high incidence and potential effect on long-term outcomes, the following complications require further discussion: skin compromise, loss of ROM or joint contractures, and respiratory compromise after SCI.

TABLE 19-4 ■ Complications after SCI

COMPLICATION	CAUSE	DIAGNOSTIC TEST AND MEASURES	MEDICAL TREATMENT OR INTERVENTION	THERAPEUTIC INTERVENTION
CARDIOPULMONARY				
Pneumonia Atelectasis	Bacterial or viral infection, prolonged immobilization, prolonged artificial ventilation, general anesthesia	Radiographic studies, diagnostic bronchoscopy	Antibiotics, bronchodilator therapy, therapeutic bronchoscopy; suctioning	Chest physical therapy: percussion, vibration, postural drainage; mobilize the client; inspiratory breathing exercises
Ventilatory failure	Weakness or paralysis of the inspiratory muscles, unchecked bronchospasm	Pulmonary function tests (PFTs); arterial blood gases (ABGs), end-tidal CO_2 monitoring, pulse oximetry	Artificial ventilation and supportive therapy, management of underlying cause (i.e., pneumonia), oxygen therapy	Airway and secretion management treatment as above, early mobilization once stabilized, biofeedback to assist with ventilator weaning as appropriate
Deep vein thrombosis (DVT)*	Venous status, activation of blood coagulation, pressure on immobilized lower extremity, and endothelial damage[59,60,61]	Doppler studies, leg measurements, extremity visual observation and palpation, low-grade fever of unknown origin	Subcutaneous heparin[3,147] Prophylactic anticoagulation can decrease incidence to 1.3%[5] Vena cava filter for failed anticoagulant prophylaxis	Early mobilization and ROM for prevention, centripetal massage for prevention, compression garments, education about smoking cessation, weight loss, and exercise; avoid constricting garments and monitor overly tight leg bag straps and pressure garments (Paralyzed Veterans of America DVT guidelines)
Pulmonary embolus	Dislodging of DVT	Ventilation/perfusion lung scan, signs and symptoms including chest pain, breathlessness, apprehension, fever, and cough	Vena cava filter Anticoagulation therapy	None

*Consortium for Spinal Cord Medicine Clinical Practice Guidelines. Prevention of Thromboembolism in Spinal Cord Injury. Paralyzed Veterans of America, February 1997.

TABLE 19-4 ■ Complications after SCI—cont'd

COMPLICATION	CAUSE	DIAGNOSTIC TEST AND MEASURES	MEDICAL TREATMENT OR INTERVENTION	THERAPEUTIC INTERVENTION
Orthostatic hypotension	Vasodilation and decreased venous return, loss of muscle pump action in dependent lower extremities and trunk[144]	Monitor blood pressure with activity and changes in position, observation/signs and symptoms	Medications to increase blood pressure, fluids in the presence of hypovolemia	Gradient compression garments: Ace wraps, abdominal binders, appropriate wheelchair selection to prevent rapid changes in position early in rehabilitation
Apneic bradycardia	True origin unknown; believed to be caused by sympathetic disruption resulting in vagal dominance in response to a noxious stimuli or hypoxia[148]	Electrocardiogram Heart rate Respiratory rate	Hyperventilation	Remove noxious stimulus
INTEGUMENTARY SYSTEM				
Pressure ulcers	Prolonged external skin pressure exceeding the average arterial or capillary pressure[149]	Wound measurements staging classification, nutritional assessment[65]	Nutritional support as needed, surgical or enzymatic debridement, surgical closure, muscle flap, skin flap or graft, antibiotics as appropriate	Irrigation and hydrotherapy, dressing management, electrotherapy[65]
Shearing	Stretching and tearing of the blood vessels that pass between the layers of the skin[11]	See pressure ulcers	See pressure ulcers	Add protective padding during functional activities, skill perfection, correct handling techniques
Moisture	Excessive sweating below the level of injury, urinary and bowel incontinence, poor hygiene	See pressure ulcers	See pressure ulcers, treat possible urinary tract infection, medications for bladder incontinence	Protective barrier ointments and powders, establish effective bowel and bladder programs, educate for improved hygiene, and refine ADL skills
NEUROMUSCULAR				
Spasticity	Upper motor neuron lesion[66]	Ashworth or Modified Ashworth scale Deep tendon reflex spasticity scale evaluation	Antispastic pharmacological agents: baclofen, diazepam (Valium), dantrolene; surgical intervention: myelotomy, rhizotomy, peripheral neurotomy[66]; Botox injection Baclofen pump insertion[68]	Prolonged stretching; inhibitive positioning/ casting Cryotherapy, weight-bearing exercise and aquatic therapy
Flaccidity	Lower motor neuron lesion[11,13] Most often in injuries at L1 level and below	Deep tendon reflexes (would be absent)	None	None for treating flaccidity; however, secondary treatments that need to be considered include positioning to improve postural support,

Continued

TABLE 19-4 ■ Complications after SCI—cont'd

COMPLICATION	CAUSE	DIAGNOSTIC TEST AND MEASURES	MEDICAL TREATMENT OR INTERVENTION	THERAPEUTIC INTERVENTION
				education for skin protection and bracing and splinting to maintain joint integrity
Neurogenic bowel†	Refer to bowel management	Positive bulbocavernosus reflex: indicates reflexic bowel	Oral laxative, suppositories, and enemas	Establish comprehensive bowel program
Autonomic dysreflexia	Triggering of an uncontrolled hyperactive response from the sympathetic nervous system by a noxious stimulus[11]; noxious stimuli may include bowel or bladder distention, urinary tract infection, ingrown toenail, tight clothing, and pressure sore	Sudden rise in systolic blood pressure of 20-40 mm Hg above baseline[148] Observation of signs and symptoms: Sweating above level of injury Goose bumps Severe headache Flushing of skin from vasodilation above level of injury[148]	Catheterization of the bladder, irrigation of indwelling catheter, pharmacological management if systolic blood pressure is greater than 150 mm Hg Remove ingrown toenail if present	Immediately position the client in upright position, identify and remove noxious stimuli, check clothing and catheter tubing for constriction, and perform bowel program if fecal impaction is suspected
Ulcers/ gastrointestinal	Venous status, activation of blood	Radiographic studies, diagnostic	Medications to increase blood pressure	Gradient compression garments; Ace wrap
OTHER				
Thermoregulation problems	Interruption between communication with autonomic nervous system and hypothalamus Lack of vasoconstriction and inability to shiver or perspire[148]	Body temperature	Cooling or warming blanket if extreme	Education about risk and proper protection from elements; behavior modification, education for proper hydration and appropriate clothing
Pain	Radicular pain originating from the injury,[11,151,152] kinematic or mechanical pain, direct trauma, referred pain[152,153]	Pain scales functional assessment	Immobilization and rest, pain medications; injections for pain or antiinflammatory measures	Restore ideal alignment and posture; thermal and electromodalities; manual therapy, improve movement patterns
Urinary tract infections	Presence of excessive bacteria in urine	Urinalysis, urine culture and sensitivity, temperature	Antibiotics	Monitor fluid intake and educate for proper technique during bladder care

†Consortium for Spinal Cord Medicine Clinical Practice Guidelines. Neurogenic Bowel Management in Adults with Spinal Cord Injury. Paralyzed Veterans of America, March 1998.

TABLE 19-4 ■ Complications after SCI—cont'd

COMPLICATION	CAUSE	DIAGNOSTIC TEST AND MEASURES	MEDICAL TREATMENT OR INTERVENTION	THERAPEUTIC INTERVENTION
Contractures	Muscle imbalance around joint; prolonged immobilization, unchecked spasticity, pain	Goniometric measurements	Tendon release; Botox injection for isolated spasticity	ROM functional use of extremity, casting or splinting, achieving and maintaining optimal postural alignment
Heterotopic ossification (HO)	Unknown	Alkaline phosphatase levels (increase after 6 weeks)[154,155]; observation for sudden loss of ROM, local edema, heat, erythema, nonseptic fever	Etidronate disodium (Didronel): use prophylactically or during inflammatory stage Surgical resection	Maintain available ROM; avoid vigorous stretching during inflammatory stage; achieve and maintain optimal wheelchair positioning
Osteoporosis and degenerative joint changes	Bone demineralization[156]	Bone scan	None; calcium supplement for prevention	Weight-bearing techniques: amount and type unknown specific to SCI
Spinal deformities	Muscle imbalance or weakness around spinal column; poor postural support, asymmetrical functional activities	Posture evaluation, seating evaluation	If severe: surgical fixation, thoracic orthosis	Restore postural alignment, avoid repetitive asymmetrical activities, control spasticity
Gastroduodenal ulcers/ gastrointestinal bleeding	Acute: disruption of central nervous system, abdominal trauma or stress response to neuroendocrine system[157] Chronic: impairment of autonomic nervous system[11]	Hematocrit and hemoglobin; observation of gastrointestinal fluids	Surgical intervention; restore normal gastrointestinal function	Establish effective bowel program, establish high-fiber diet, provide education and stress management
Metabolic/ endocrine	Impairment of autonomic nervous system	Observe for fatigue, malaise; undesirable weight gain[57]	None known	Education, exercise, and weight control

Preventing and Managing Pressure Ulcers and Skin Compromise

After SCI and during the period of spinal shock, clients are at greater risk for development of pressure ulcers.[59,60] The use of backboards at the emergency scene and during radiographic procedures contributes to potential skin compromise.

Preventive skin care begins with careful inspection. Areas with a bony prominence are at greatest risk for acquiring a pressure sore.[61] Key areas to evaluate include the sacrum, ischia, greater trochanters, heels, malleoli, knees, occiput, scapulae, elbows, and prominent spinous processes. Turning at regular intervals is initiated immediately. The client's position in bed should be initially established for turns to occur every 2 to 3 hours.[60] This interval is gradually increased to 6 hours

with careful monitoring for evidence of skin compromise. Turning positions include prone, supine, right and left side lying, semiprone, or semisupine.[62,63] Secondary injuries such as fractures and the presence of vital equipment, such as ventilator tubing, chest tubes, and arterial lines, should be considered when choosing turning positions.

Pillows or rectangular foam pads are used to pad around the bony prominence and relieve potential pressure. Padding directly over a prominent area with a firm pillow or pad may only increase pressure and should be avoided. For clients who are not appropriate for rigorous turning schedules (e.g., clients with unstabilized fractures), specialty low-air-loss mattresses and flotation systems are available.[64] While the client is sitting, an appropriate pressure relief cushion is recommended and a pressure relief (weight shift) schedule is established and strictly enforced.

Although pressure is one of the most prevalent causes of skin compromise, other forces may lead to problems, including friction, shearing, excessive moisture or dryness, infection, and bruising or bumping during activities. This is especially true of clients with SCI because of altered thermoregulation, changes in mobility, decreased or absent sensation, and incontinence of bowel and bladder. In addition, as clients begin to learn functional skills, they may have poor motor control and impaired balance and must be carefully monitored to avoid injury.

Should skin compromise occur, the first intervention is to identify and remove the source of the problem. Modifications to the seating system or changing to a more pressure-relieving mattress system or cushion may be necessary. Examination and treatment will then need to focus on healing the wound and preventing other secondary complications that may occur as a result of potential immobility and delayed physical rehabilitation. The reader is encouraged to refer to *Pressure Ulcer Treatment: Clinical Practice Guideline* developed by the Agency for Health Care Policy and Research for examination tools, including the classification of pressure ulcers.[65]

Treatment interventions may include hydrotherapy, specialty wound dressings, electromodalities, and thermomodalities to increase circulation.[65] Mechanical, chemical, or surgical debridement may be necessary to obtain and maintain a viable wound bed. If the wound does not heal, surgical interventions with skin flaps or muscle flaps may be necessary for closure. Coordinated return-to-sit programs or protocols after such medical interventions are necessary to prevent opening of the surgical site. Such surgical procedures are costly and significantly delay functional rehabilitation.

After closure and healing of the wound, education becomes a priority to maintain skin integrity. The client must adhere to a more rigorous skin check program as rehabilitation continues, with special attention to the affected area. Prevention of skin compromise is critical and cannot be stressed enough to health care providers, clients, and caregivers.

Prevention and Management of Joint Contractures

The development of a contracture may result in postural malalignment or impede potential function. Daily ROM exercises and proper positioning may help prevent contractures.[60] Contracture prevention includes the use of splints for proper joint alignment, techniques such as weight bearing, ADLs, and functional exercises. Clients exhibiting spasticity may require more frequent range of motion intervention.[60,66]

Adaptive Shortening or Lengthening of Muscles

Although isolated joint ROM should be normal for all clients, allowing adaptive shortening or lengthening of particular muscles is recommended to enhance the achievement of certain functional skills.[63,67] Likewise, unwanted shorten-

ing or lengthening of muscles should be prevented. The following reviews a few examples of these concepts as they relate to SCI.

Tenodesis is described as the passive shortening of the two-joint finger flexors as the wrist is extended. This action creates a grasp, which assists performance of ADLs (Figure 19-11).[63,68] A client with mid to low tetraplegia may rely on adaptive shortening of these long finger flexors to replace active grip.[63] If the long finger flexors are stretched across all joints during ROM exercises, the achievement of some functional goals may be limited. ROM to the finger flexors should only be performed while the wrist is in a neutral position.

In the presence of weakened or paralyzed elbow extensors, adaptive shortening of the elbow flexors should be prevented because it will impair ADL function and transfer skills.[11,63] Contracted elbow flexors or pronator muscles in a client with SCI level of C6 can cost this client his or her independence.

The rotator cuff and the other scapular muscles should be assessed for their length-tension relationships and their ability to generate force. Normal length of these muscles should be maintained. For example, achieving external rotation of the shoulder (active and passive) is critical for clients with low-level tetraplegia. Shortening of the subscapularis and other structures can quickly result in a decrease in motion, limiting bed mobility, transfers, feeding, and grooming skills.

Clients with complete paraplegia who are candidates for ambulation require normal ROM in the lower extremities. If the hip flexors or knee flexors are allowed to adaptively shorten, achieving standing and ambulation goals will be difficult.

The combination of lengthened hamstrings and tight back extensor muscles provides stability for balance in the short- and long-sitting positions. This aids in the efficiency of transfers and bowel and bladder management. Balance in long sitting assists with lower-extremity dressing and other ADLs. Hamstrings should be lengthened to allow 110 to 120

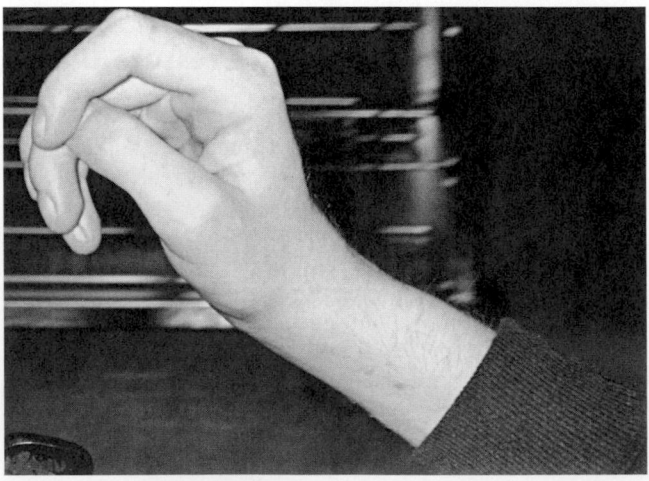

FIGURE 19-11 ■ Tenodesis grasp.

degrees of straight leg raising without overstretching back extensor muscles.

Splinting to Prevent Joint Deformity

Deformity prevention is the first goal for splinting.[69] In the absence or weakness of elbow extensors, a bivalve cast or pillow splint at night may be beneficial to prevent joint contractures. Another goal of splinting in the SCI population is to increase function.

Clients with cervical spinal cord injuries may have lost innervation to the musculature in their wrists or hands. Other clients may have partial innervation, which may lead to muscle imbalances. If the wrist and hand are not supported, function will be limited. Clients with C1 to C4 tetraplegia require resting hand splints to assist with proper positioning and maintain the support of the wrist and web space (Figure 19-12).[70] Clients with tetraplegia at the C5 level can only be independent with communication, feeding, and hygiene with an orthosis. They must have joint stability and support at the wrist and the hand to perform these skills. The splint is often adapted with a utensil slot or cuff so that the client can effectively perform the skills mentioned above.

Clients who are not strong enough to use their wrists for tenodesis may require splinting to support their wrists until they can use their wrists against gravity. Long opponens splints can be used to position the thumb for function but support the weak wrist (Figure 19-13). Once the wrist strengthens, the long opponens splint can be cut down to a hand-based short opponens to maintain proper web space and thumb positioning while maximizing tenodesis.

As mentioned previously, clients with injuries at the C6 level can use their wrists for a tenodesis grasp.[68,71,72] Critical components of the splint assessment for these clients are the positioning of the thumb, web space, and index finger observed during the grasp. Clients who are not splinted may not have the proper positioning to pick up objects because their tenodesis is "too tight" or "too loose." The client may want to have a more defined three-jaw chuck grasp in which the thumb is in alignment to oppose the first and second digit versus being limited to a lateral grasp.[72] There is controversy over shortening of the flexor tendons. Some clinicians argue that the client can develop a fixed flexion contracture of the proximal interphalangeal joints, interfering with future sur-

gical attempts to restore finger function.[25] However, if only used for tenodesis training, the splints may be discontinued and the client could resume daily stretching exercises if finger movement is in question.[70]

Clients with C8 to T1 injuries or clients who have incomplete injuries may have "clawing" or hyperextention of the metaphalangeal joints. This is caused by finger extensor musculature that is stronger than finger flexor musculature.[68,73] To prevent this, a splint can be made to block the metacarpophalangeal joints and promote weak intrinsic muscle function. Depending on the extent of the imbalance, these splints can be used during function or only worn at night. Cost, time, material, and clinician experience are important considerations when deciding between custom and prefabricated splints. A well-fitting, prefabricated splint can be as effective as a custom-fabricated splint in certain situations. Custom splints require additional resources and clinician expertise. One way to maximize time in fabrication of splints is to use a good pattern and premade straps. Finally, educating the client on the splint-wearing schedule, skin checks, and splint care is important in preventing skin breakdown.

Treatment for Joint Deformity

If a joint contracture occurs despite preventive measures, more aggressive treatments are necessary. This may include more aggressive use of splinting, plaster or fiberglass casting techniques, or botulinum toxin A (Botox) injections.[74-76] Surgical intervention may be recommended by an orthopedic physician in severe cases of joint contracture.[77] When splinting is not effective, fabrication of serial or bivalve casts may be indicated. The client with minimal ROM limitations may require only one cast. Most commonly, the client has a significant limitation and requires serial casts in which several casts would be applied and then removed over a period of

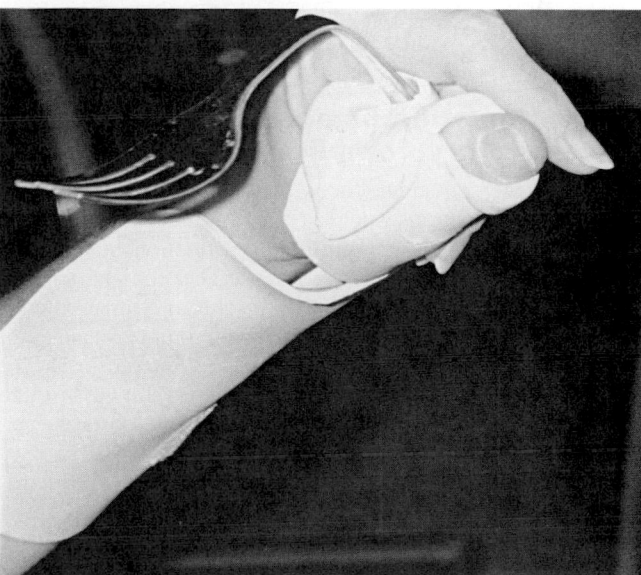

FIGURE 19-13 ■ Long opponens splint with fabricated utensil holder.

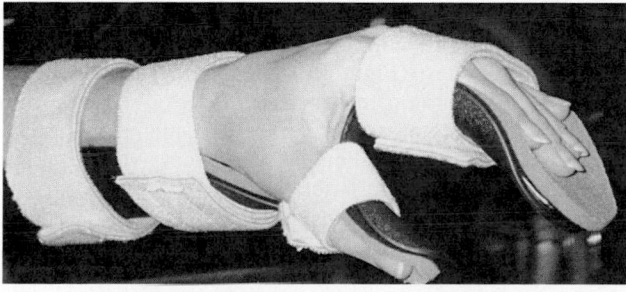

FIGURE 19-12 ■ Resting hand splint.

weeks to increase extensibility in the soft tissues surrounding the casted joint.[78] The involved joint would be placed at submaximal range of motion.[79] Once the cast is removed, the joint should have an increase of approximately 7 degrees of range of motion.[79] This process should continue until the deformity is minimized or resolved. The final cast is a bivalve so that the cast can act as a positioning device that can be easily removed. Casting contraindications are skin compromise over the area to be casted, heterotopic ossification, edema, decreased circulation, severe fluctuating tone, and inconsistent monitoring systems. The elbow, wrist/hand, and finger joints are the most common joints casted for clients with SCI. Casting for most of these clients may be the last resort to regain increased ROM before a client can begin feeding, grooming, or communication skills. Long-arm casts are used when elbow and wrist contractures must be managed simultaneously. If evaluation of the upper extremity reveals a pronation or supination contracture, a long-arm cast would also be the cast of choice. Dropout casts are used with severe elbow flexor or extensor contractures, but the patient should be in a position where gravity can assist. Wrist/hand and finger casts are indicated for contractures that prevent distal upper-extremity function. Most commonly, a client will have a wrist flexion/extension contracture or have finger flexor/extensor tone and will require a cast to use the tenodesis or individual fingers for fine motor skills. Sometimes wrist casts with finger shells or resting hand extensions on casts are needed to ensure that the hand, fingers, and web space are maintained in a position of optimal function. Casting is an expensive and labor-intensive treatment modality, but if indicated and used appropriately it can assist a client in regaining lost joint ROM needed for increased independence and function.

Botox may be used in conjunction with casting. In a study conducted by Corry et al[76] tone reduction was evident when botulinum toxin A was used; however, ROM and functional improvement varied among subjects. Pierson et al[75] found that, with careful selection, subjects who received botulinum toxin A had significant improvements with active and passive ROM. Research indicates that patients who have flexor spasticity without fixed contracture will benefit the most.

Prevention and Management of Respiratory Complications

Early management must focus heavily on preventing pulmonary complications such as pneumonia and atelectasis and enhancing available pulmonary function so that the client may perform functional tasks. The clinician should first determine which ventilatory muscles are impaired after the spinal cord injury. The primary ventilatory muscles of inspiration are the diaphragm and the intercostals. The diaphragm is innervated by the phrenic nerve at C3 through C5. The intercostals are innervated by the intercostal nerves positioned between the ribs. If the diaphragm is weak or paralyzed, its descent will be lessened, reducing the client's ability to ventilate.[80-83]

Accessory muscles of ventilation are primarily located in the cervical region.[84] The accessory muscles are used to augment ventilation when the demand for oxygen increases, as during exercise. Accessory muscles may also be recruited to generate an improved cough effort.[60] The most commonly cited accessory muscles are the sternocleidomastoids, the scalenes, the levators scapulae, and the trapezius muscles.[81,82] The erector spinae group may also assist by extending the spine, thus improving the potential depth of inspiration.[11,82]

The abdominals are the primary muscles used for forced expiration in such maneuvers as coughing or sneezing. The latissimus dorsi, the teres major, and the clavicular portion of the pectoralis major are also active during forced expiration and cough in the client with tetraplegia.[85] Alterations in the function of these muscles will have an impact on the client's ability to clear secretions and produce loud vocalization. Gravity plays a crucial role in the function of all ventilatory muscles.[82] Neural input to the diaphragm increases in the upright position in persons with intact nervous systems. As one moves into an upright position, the resting position of the diaphragm drops as the abdominal contents fall.[82] The diaphragm is effectively shortened, which makes generating a strong contraction more difficult. With intact abdominal musculature, however, a counterpressure is produced and adequate intraabdominal pressure is maintained, allowing the diaphragm to perform work. If weakness or paralysis of the abdominal wall is present, the client may need a binder or corset to maintain the normal pressure relationship.[63,80,86,87] Unless the SCI has affected only the lowest sacral and lumbar areas, some degree of ventilatory impairment is present and should be addressed in therapeutic sessions.

Many treatment techniques are available to address the myriad causes of ventilatory impairment. Decreased chest wall mobility and the inability to clear secretions should always be addressed. Interventions may include inspiratory muscle training, chest wall mobility exercises, and chest physical therapy.[63,67,83,88,89]

Inspiratory Muscle Training

Inspiratory muscle training is used to train the diaphragm and the accessory muscles that are weakened by partial paralysis, disuse from prolonged artificial ventilation, or prolonged bed rest. In general, the inspiratory muscles should be trained initially in the supine position[67,86,89] and progressed to the sitting position. When training a moderately weak diaphragm, gentle pressure during inspiration may be used to facilitate the muscle (Figure 19-14, *A* and *B*). Accessory muscle training may be facilitated with the client in the supine position while a slight stretch is placed on these muscles.[67] The stretch is accomplished by shoulder abduction and external rotation, elbow extension, forearm supination, and neutral alignment of the head and neck. A more challenging position incorporates upper thoracic extension. The clinician's hands are placed directly over the muscle to be facilitated. The client is instructed to breathe into the upper chest (Figure 19-15). As the treatment progresses, the diaphragm may be inhibited for short training periods by applying pressure over the abdomen in an upward direction. Care must be taken to avoid excessive pressure to prevent occlusion of vital arteries.

As the inspiratory muscles strengthen, resistive inspiratory devices may be used. The diaphragm also may be trained using weights on the abdominal wall. Derrickson et al[91] concluded that both inspiratory muscle training devices and abdominal weights were effective in improving

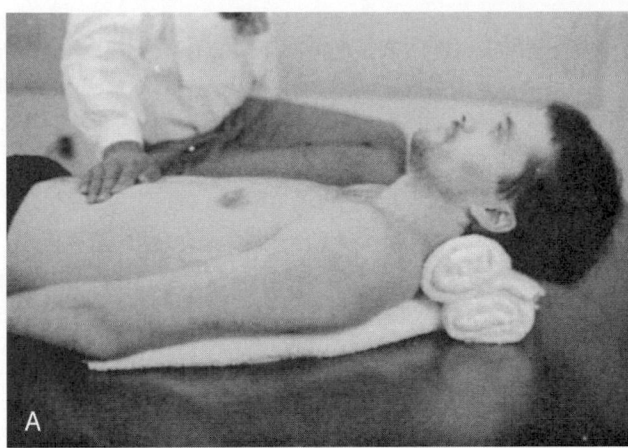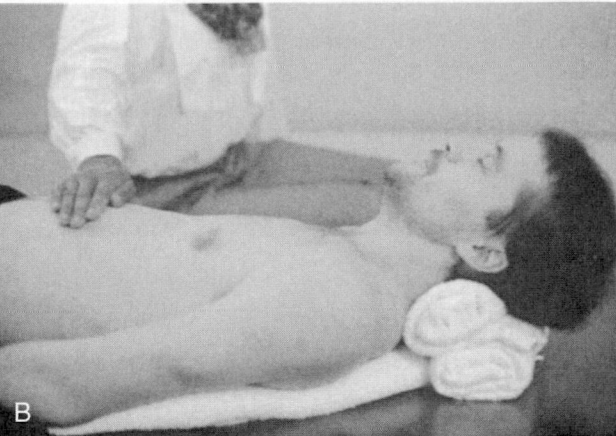

FIGURE 19-14 ■ Diaphragm facilitation. **A,** Hand placement and patient positioning to facilitate the diaphragm and inhibit accessory muscle activity. **B,** Firm contact is maintained throughout inspiration. The lower extremities are placed over a pillow in flexion to prevent stretching of the abdominal wall.

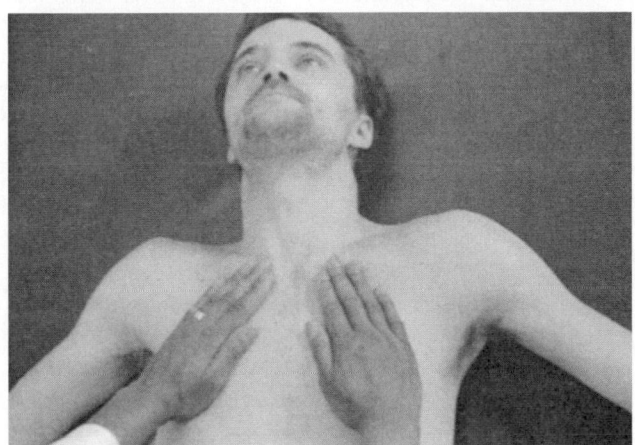

FIGURE 19-15 ■ Accessory muscle facilitation. Hand placement and patient positioning.

ventilatory mechanics. Muscle trainers, however, appear to promote more of an endurance effect than the use of abdominal weights.

Phrenic Nerve Pacing

When the primary inspiratory muscles are no longer volitionally active as a result of SCI, phrenic nerve pacing may be used to cause the diaphragm to contract. This may be indicated when the lesion is at or above the C3 level.[90-93] Electrical stimulation may be applied directly or indirectly through a vein wall or the skin or directly to the phrenic nerve. A more recent procedure allows for transdiaphragmatic pacing by laparoscopically inserting electrodes on the diaphragm.[94] This procedure is less invasive than an open thoracotomy procedure and may result in improved outcomes. However, this is still a new procedure and more evidence is needed to understand the long-term effects. Regardless of the procedure, caregivers and clients must receive extensive education to learn equipment management and emergency procedure plans in the event of pacer failure.

Most clients will still require some mechanical ventilation even after maximal tolerance is achieved so as not to overfatigue the phrenic nerve.

Glossopharyngeal Breathing

Glossopharyngeal breathing is another way of increasing vital capacity in the presence of weak inspiratory muscles.[83,86,89] By moving the jaw forward and upward in a circular opening and closing manner, air is trapped in the buccal cavity. A series of swallowing-like maneuvers forces air into the lungs, increasing the vital capacity. This technique has been reported to increase vital capacity by as much as 1 liter.[67] Although this technique is rarely used to sustain ventilation for long periods of time,[95] it may be used in emergency situations and to enhance cough function. The client with high tetraplegia should attempt to master this skill.

Secretion Clearance

Ventilatory impairment occurs when the client is unable to clear secretions.[80,96] Factors such as artificial ventilation and general anesthesia hamper secretion mobilization. With artificial ventilation, clients may require an artificial airway.[96,97] The presence of this airway in the trachea poses an irritant, and the client subsequently produces more secretions.[80] A description of various types and parameters of ventilation is beyond the scope of this chapter. Clinicians working with clients requiring artificial ventilation, however, are referred to other publications.[96,98]

Secretions are most commonly removed by tracheal suctioning, unassisted coughing, or assisted coughing. More recently, there has been a resurgence of previously used technologies that provide rapidly alternating pressures through a mouthpiece or an endotracheal tube to remove secretions. This is commonly referred to as inexsufflation. To date, conclusive research determining which single technique or combination of techniques achieves the best outcome is not available. Inexsufflation may result in fewer complications and is reported to be more comfortable to the client. Postural drainage, percussion or clapping, and shaking or vibration are used to assist with moving secretions toward larger airways for expectoration.[12,63,72]

Assisted coughing is typically used with people who are unable to generate sufficient effort.[89] The assistant places both hands firmly on the abdominal wall. After a maximal inspiratory effort, the client coughs and the assistant simply supports the weakened wall. A gentle upward and inward force may be used to increase the intraabdominal pressure, yielding a more forceful cough (Figure 19-16, *A* and *B*).[78,89] Excessive pressure over the xiphoid process should be avoided to prevent severe injury.

Clients may learn independent coughing techniques. In preparation for a cough, the client positions an arm around the push handle of the wheelchair, opening the chest wall to enhance inspiratory effort. The other arm is raised over the head and chest during inspiration. This procedure is followed by a breath hold, strong trunk flexion, and then a cough (Figure 19-17, *A* and *B*).[89] Another technique for independent coughing is accomplished by placing the forearms over the abdomen and delivering a manual thrust during cough. This technique is more difficult and may not provide an inspiratory advantage.

Early Mobilization

Getting the client upright as soon as possible promotes self-mobility and should be planned carefully. An appropriate seating system for pressure relief and support should be chosen. Most clients require a reclining wheelchair with elevating footrests when they are first acclimating to the upright position.[63,67,89]

The client is transferred initially to a reclining position and progressed to an upright position as signs and symptoms of medical stability allow. The client should be monitored for evidence of orthostatic hypotension. Dizziness or light-headedness is most common. Ringing in the ears and visual changes also may occur. Changes in mental function may indicate more serious hypotension, and the client should be reclined immediately. Assessing blood pressure before and during activities provides an objective measurement of the client's status.

Because the abdominal wall is not supporting the internal contents, abdominal binders or corsets should be applied to all clients with lesions above T12 to assist in venous return[67,87,89] and enhance ventilatory function. If the client has a history of vascular insufficiency or prolonged bed rest, wrapping the lower extremities with elastic bandages while applying the greatest pressure distally may be beneficial.

Abdominal binders and corsets are fitted so that the top of the corset lies just over the lower two ribs.[67] The bottom portion is placed over the anterior iliac spine and iliac crest (Figure 19-18). The corset or binder should be adjusted slightly tighter at the bottom to assist in elevating the abdominal contents.[63,67,89] Properly fitting the abdominal binder is essential. If placed too high or allowed to ride up, ventilation may be impaired by restricting chest wall excursion. If placed too low, it will not provide the necessary abdominal support.

The client can be transferred initially with a manual or mechanical lift. Lift systems may be advantageous because they allow total control of the client and give the assistant more time to ensure that monitoring devices, lines, or tubes attached to the client remain intact. Lift systems may be free-standing hydraulic lifts or electronic devices or may be mounted on the ceiling.

Once the client is out of bed, a weight shift or pressure relief schedule is immediately established. Initially, weight

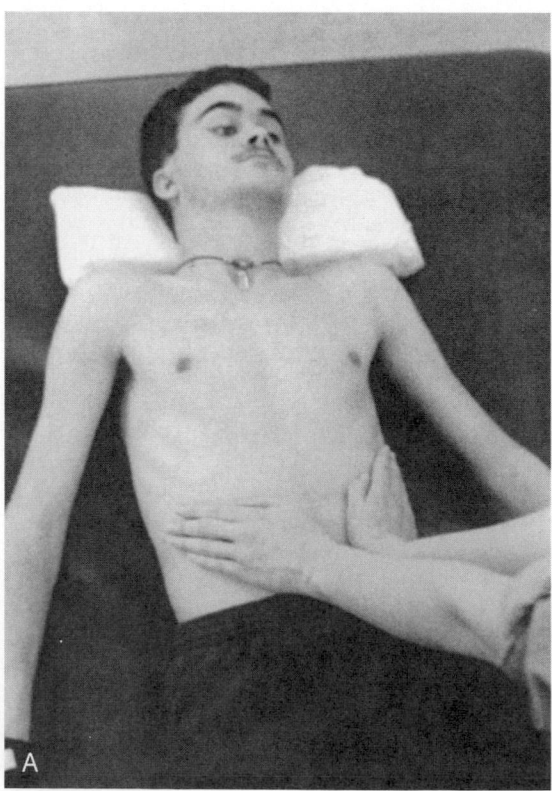

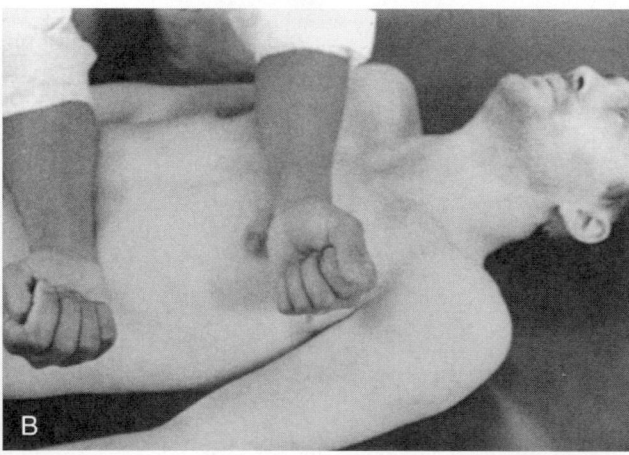

FIGURE 19-16 ■ Quad coughing. **A,** Hand placement for the Heimlich-like technique. **B,** Anterior chest wall quad coughing. The inferior forearm supination promotes an upward and inward force during the cough.

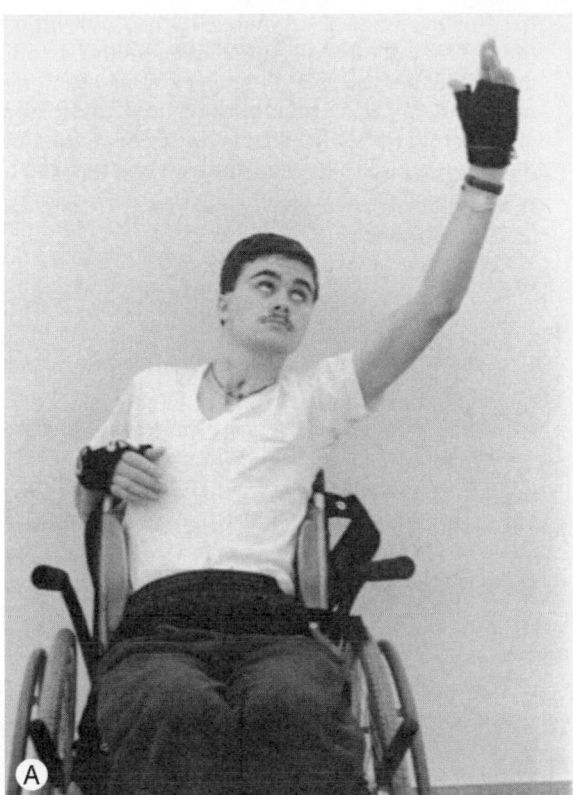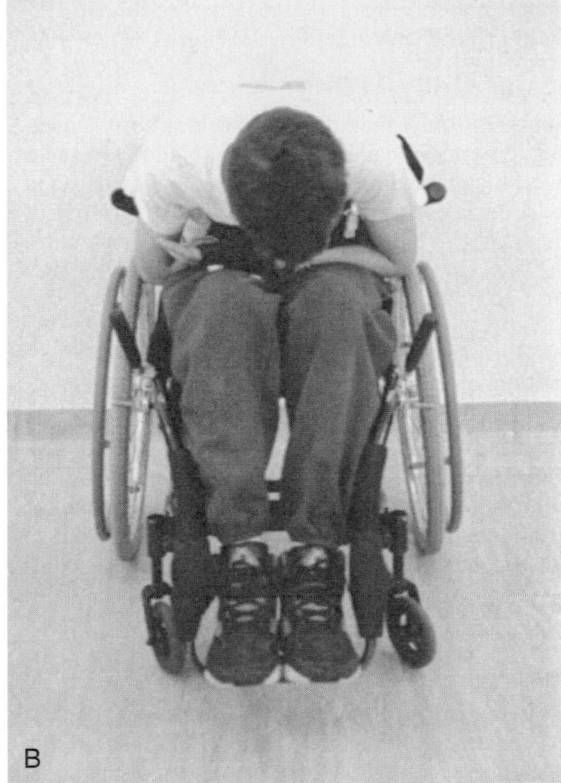

FIGURE 19-17 ■ Self quad coughing. **A,** Full inspiratory position. **B,** Expiratory/cough position.

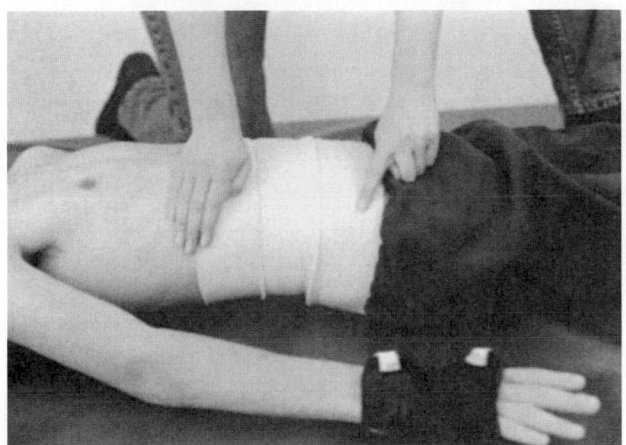

FIGURE 19-18 ■ Abdominal binder. Correct placement is over the anterior-superior iliac spine and at the level of lower rib cage. Custom corsets may be used if an elastic binder does not provide adequate support to enhance vital capacity.

shifts are performed at 30-minute intervals and modified according to skin tolerance.[61] A timer may be issued to ensure reminders for weight shifts. This is particularly important if the client has cognitive deficits. The skin is inspected thoroughly before and immediately after out-of-bed activities. Total sitting time is progressed according to tolerance.

REHABILITATION: ACHIEVING FUNCTIONAL OUTCOMES

Once secondary complications are managed and the client is able to tolerate out-of-bed activities, more aggressive rehabilitation begins. The following will address special considerations for functional progression related to SCI.

Optimal neck, shoulder, and upper-extremity strength and ROM are important factors when achieving functional outcomes. Neck musculature is typically painful and restricted in cervical injuries. Most clients will have a collar in place postoperatively to prevent rotation and flexion/extension. The client may be so tight that correcting forward head posture with stretching and proper positioning is the first goal. Soft tissue massage and manual therapy may be beneficial. Once cleared by the physician, the client can begin neck isometric exercises.

Key muscle groups in the shoulder to consider are the scapular stabilizers and movers, which allow for humeral flexion, adduction/abduction, shoulder internal and external rotation and scapular movements. Clients with high cervical injuries have the potential for development of tight upper trapezius muscles. Upper trapezius inhibitory or scapular taping to relax the tight muscles and facilitate the weak scapular musculature is beneficial. In the injury level above C7, the scapular musculature may not be fully innervated and thus positioning in the proper alignment and strengthening the innervated musculature is essential. Findings from the manual muscle test and goniometric examination will determine the appropriate stretching/strengthening program. Clients may need to begin with gravity-eliminated exercises with air splints, bilateral slings, skateboards, functional electric stimulation (FES), and side-lying exercises.

Activities of Daily Living

Activities of daily living include skills such as communication, feeding, grooming, bathing, dressing, bladder management, bowel management, and home management and community reentry. Depending on the level and severity of the SCI, clients will achieve varying levels of independence. Most of the ADL areas discussed below will address skill levels with a complete injury. Activities should be graded differently for an incomplete injury after completion of the ASIA and the manual muscle test.

Clients with high-level tetraplegia (C1-C4) will be dependent in most activities of daily living but will be able to verbalize how to safely perform all skills. Clients with low-level tetraplegia (C5-C8) may achieve some level of independence, but this will vary according to the amount of intact musculature. The ability of these clients to achieve maximum independence in all areas of ADL may be accomplished only through the use of appropriate orthoses or adaptive equipment. See Table 19-3 for functional expectations and Table 19-5 for orthotic indications.

Clients with injuries at the C5 or C6 level are especially challenging in this area of rehabilitation. These clients must have biceps function and adequate elbow ROM before any ADL goals can be achieved. To achieve these goals, clients also need to work toward supporting their body weight with simultaneous extension of the shoulder, elbow, and wrist, otherwise known as propping. Elbow positioning devices such as pillow splints, casts, or resting splints enhance alignment. Other orthotics to consider for maximizing function include definitive wrist supports and mobile arm supports (MAS). Appropriate wheelchair positioning with lap trays, armrests, wedges, or lateral trunk supports is important to maximize function for persons with C5 or C6 injuries.

Clients with C7 or C8 level of injury generally will not prove to be as challenging for the rehabilitation therapist. With the presence of triceps, the ADL skills are easier to achieve. Most clients, given the right body type, will be able to achieve these goals requiring only minimal assistance from a caregiver.

Clients with paraplegia usually obtain total independence with communication, feeding, and grooming. These clients may need adaptive equipment to perform some of these skills; however, they should be able to be performed without assistance from another person. Endurance is a major concern for the client's independence while performing ADLs. Some skills require a considerable amount of time and effort. If endurance becomes a factor, clients should choose to perform some activities while receiving assistance for other skills that are too challenging or time consuming.

Communication

Communication includes use of a call system, environmental control unit (ECU), telephone, and computer and the ability to perform writing, typing, and page turning. Clients at all levels of SCI can be independent with these skills after setup. Call systems, ECUs, and computers can be programmed to use pneumatic control (sip 'n' puff) or voice-activated controls for independence from bed and the wheelchair. There are switches that can be activated with head or eye control, allowing clients with little movement the ability to communicate. Clients with C1 to C4 injuries, depending on neck strength, can also use equipment such as mouth sticks for communication from the bed and wheelchair (Figure 19-19). Clients with C5 injuries begin to use their biceps, deltoids, and internal/external rotator strength in communication with use of an MAS. Adaptive splinting for support at the wrist can allow these clients to use their upper arms in writing, typing, page turning, and computer use (Figure 19-20). Clients with wrist function but no finger function can use cuffs on speakerphones or use their natural tenodesis in a wrist-driven hand brace to grasp objects (Figure 19-21). For injuries at the T1 level and below, communication in all areas should be independent.

Feeding

Clients with C1 to C4 tetraplegia are dependent in feeding but can verbalize this skill. Clients with C5 SCI with weak shoulders and biceps musculature require a dynamic orthosis to support the upper extremity during feeding. The most

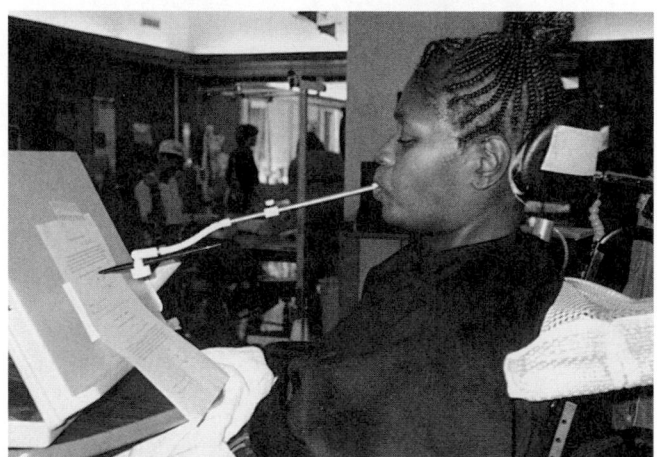

FIGURE 19-19 ■ Mouthstick writing can be accomplished with the client upright in the wheelchair and with the support of a bedside table and bookstand.

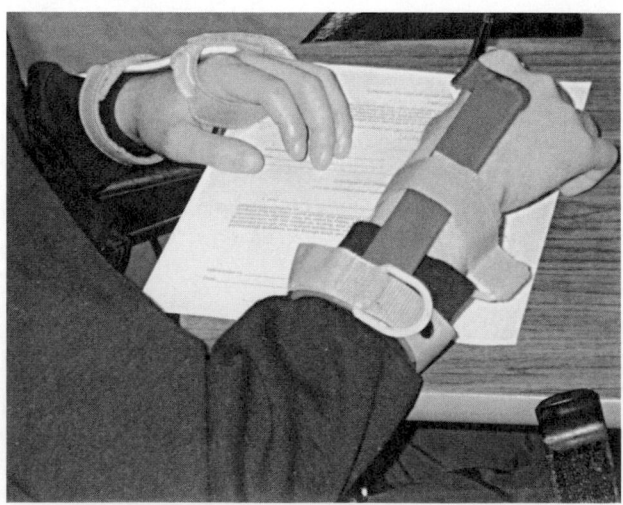

FIGURE 19-20 ■ Long Wanchick writing device.

TABLE 19-5 ■ Upper-Extremity Orthotics

LEVEL OF SPINAL CORD INJURY	SPLINT	RATIONALE
DYNAMIC ORTHOTICS		
Weak C5, incomplete injuries Also indicated with shoulder internal/external rotator muscle grades 2– to 3–/5 and bicep/supinator muscle grades of at least 2–/5	Mobile arm support (ball bearing and swivel arm use, allowing gravity to assist)	• Assists in reaching maximum range and use in horizontal and vertical planes • Increases functional ROM and strength • Independent feeding, hygiene after setup • Teaches correct movement patterns • Wheelchair trunk supports required for maximum benefit
C5, incomplete injuries Also indicated with shoulder external rotator muscle grades 3– to 3/5 in addition to biceps and supinator muscles grades of 3/5 or better		• Increases functional ROM and strength throughout • Independent feeding and hygiene after setup • Teaches correct movement patterns • Adjunct device for functional ADL training • Lateral wheelchair trunk supports may be required
C5, incomplete injuries Also indicated with shoulder external rotator grades 3 to 3+/5 but client fatigues and/or biceps grades of 3/5 or better	Overhead rod and sling (supports upper extremity with cuffs at elbow and wrist while attached to spring overhead)	• Increases ROM and strength • Can be used for driving wheelchair if shoulder strength is an issue • Independent for feeding and hygiene after setup • Lateral trunk supports may be required
16 STATIC UPPER-EXTREMITY SPLINTS/CASTS		
C1-C3	Resting hand	• Position • Prevents joint deformity • Cosmetic appearance
C4	Resting hand	• Position • Prevents joint deformity • Cosmetic appearance
C5	Resting hand	• Same as above • Preserves web space • Preserves balance between extrinsic and intrinsic musculature • Provides joint support at rest and prevents deformity
C5	Pillow (elbow)	• Position • Prevents elbow contractures from mild tone or muscle imbalance • Prevention of skin compromise
C5	Bivalve casts/elbow extension	• Position • Prevents skin compromise • Prevents elbow contractures from tone or muscle imbalance
C5	Rolyan tap (tone and positioning) splint (prefab)	• Position • Prevents supination/pronation contracture • Provides constant low-level stretch • Use with mild to moderate tone • Best with incomplete clients, gravity can assist to promote elbow extension
C5	Economy wrist support	• Function (slot for utensils, etc.) • Position • Prevents severe wristdrop • Prevents ulnar deviation initially • Not enough support long term (often ulnar deviation and some wristdrop develop) • If position is needed long term, consider permanent splint made by orthotist

Continued

TABLE 19-5 ■ Upper-Extremity Orthotics—cont'd

LEVEL OF SPINAL CORD INJURY	SPLINT	RATIONALE
C5	Long opponens	• Position • Can be dorsal or volar • Prevents wristdrop • Preserves web space and promotes proper thumb positioning • Function (with slot) • Prevents ulnar deviation and wristdrop • If position is needed long term, consider more permanent splint made by orthotist
C5	Wrist cockup	• Position • Supports or stabilizes wrist in extension • Allows for finger movement (incomplete injuries) • Preserves web space
C6	Short opponens	• Position • Thumb in opposition for functional activities • Improves prehension by providing stable post against which fingers can pinch during tenodesis • Preserves palmar creases and web space • Function (wear underneath wheelchair push gloves) • Consider permanent metal splint made by orthotist for long term
C6	Tenodesis	• Wrist-driven function • Enhances natural tenodesis action of wrist, allows for three jaw chuck or lateral pinch • Rehabilitation Institute of Chicago has pattern, or for more permanent metal splint consider orthotist to fabricate • Enhances writing, feeding, money, and catheter management
C6	Resting hand	• Same as for C5 • Usually worn only at night • Critical that wrist is supported and thumb and web space are well positioned for functional use
C6	Bivalve casts/elbow extension	• Position • Prevents skin compromise • Prevents elbow contractures from tone or muscle imbalance
C6	Thumb abduction strap	• Position • Thumb in opposition for functional activities • Easy to put on • Does not take up much space • Can be worn underneath wheelchair gloves
C7	Resting hand Short opponens	• Same as C5, C6 • Same as C6
C8, T1 (weak)	Metacarpophalangeal block	• Position • Can also be used for strengthening finger flexors • Prevents "claw hand" by blocking metacarpophalangeals • Protects weak intrinsic muscles • Joint stability

common orthoses used are the MAS (Figure 19-22) and the offset feeder (Figure 19-23). Clients with low-level tetraplegia may not have weakness in the shoulder that would affect feeding, but they may have weak wrist function. Some of the dorsal wrist supports have a cuff built in that can be functional. The client with no finger function can use a wrist-driven tenodesis brace for managing objects or to hold a feeding utensil (Figure 19-24). A universal cuff can be worn on the hand to hold feeding utensils (Figure 19-25). The client with weak finger function can use built up handles on the utensils.

Grooming
The basic components of grooming are washing the face, combing/brushing hair, oral care, shaving, and applying makeup. More advanced grooming activities may include

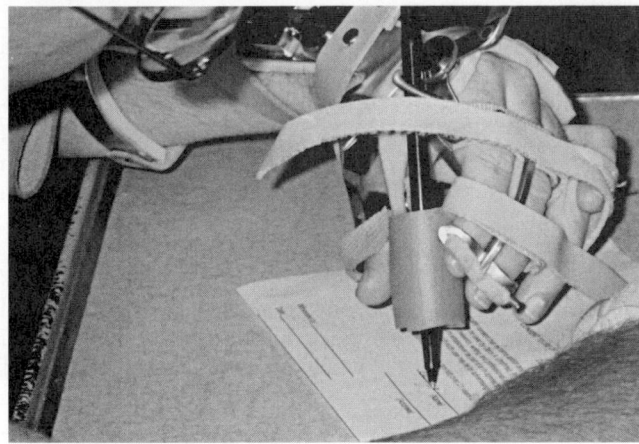

FIGURE 19-21 ■ Tenodesis brace writing by use of a pen with a built-up grip.

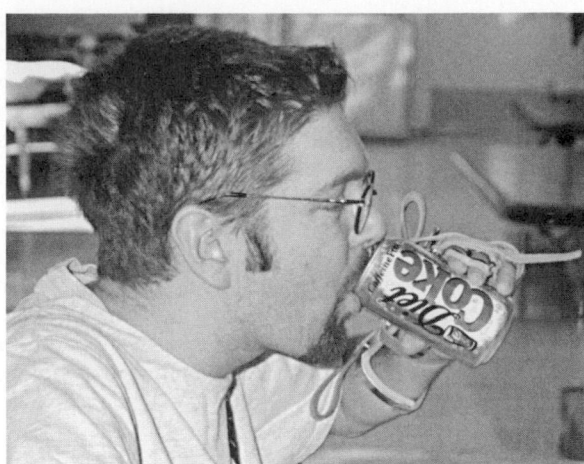

FIGURE 19-24 ■ Tenodesis braces have varying grasps. The largest grasp position allows the client to hold a soft drink can.

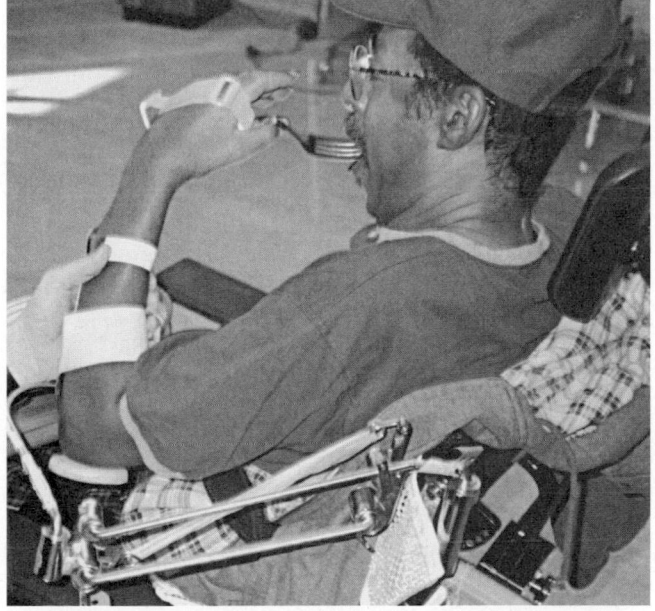

FIGURE 19-22 ■ Mobile arm support used during feeding.

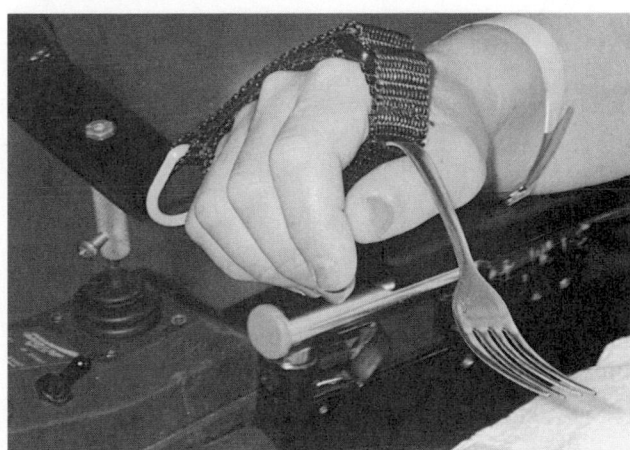

FIGURE 19-25 ■ Universal cuff used for feeding.

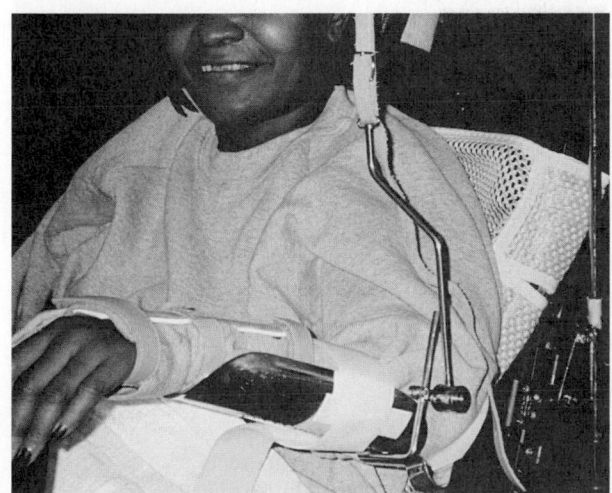

FIGURE 19-23 ■ Offset feeder orthosis.

nail care, donning/doffing contacts, or other hygiene tasks specific to the individual. Individuals with C1 to C4 tetraplegia are dependent but can verbalize these skills. Clients with C5 injuries perform these skills with some assistance but may require orthotic devices, such as an MAS or offset feeder for shoulder support and a splint for wrist support. Clients with low-level tetraplegia may need cuffs or builtup grips on razors, brushes, and toothpaste to be independent (Figure 19-26). A proper bathroom setup for optimal wheelchair positioning is important for all clients. Clients with tetraplegia often rely on the support of the elbows as an assist, so sink height should be considered. The proper positioning and adaptive equipment will be the difference between independence and dependence in these skills (Figures 19-27 and 19-28).

Bathing

Bathing includes washing and rinsing the upper and lower extremities and the trunk. Clients with C1 to C4 tetraplegia are dependent in bathing but are instructed to verbalize this skill. C5 clients can range from requiring maximal assistance to being dependent in bathing. Clients with low-level tetraplegia bathe with moderate assistance to total independence with use of adaptive devices. Clients with paraplegia are typically independent in bathing but may need adaptive devices. After examination of the client's upper-extremity strength, balance, spasticity, body type, endurance, and home accessibility, the therapy team can determine the appropriate bathing equipment and setup for the client (Figure 19-29). Clients with limited upper-extremity and trunk strength may need straps to assist with trunk support and adaptive cuffs to control the handheld shower. Basic bathing safety should be taught to all clients. Bathing safety includes checking the water temperature with a known area of intact sensation, skin checks before and after bathing, and skin protection during the transfers. These precautions are necessary to prevent burns and skin breakdown during the bathing process.

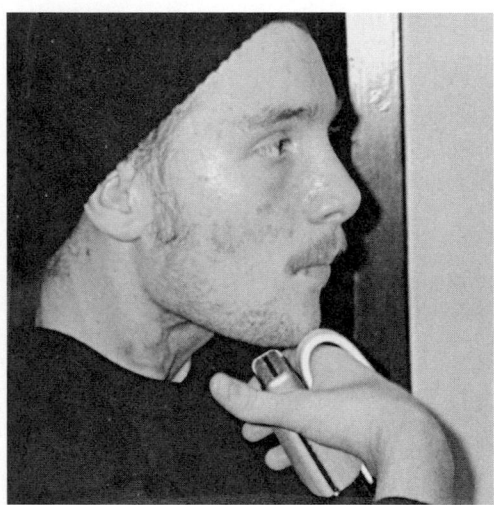

FIGURE 19-26 ▪ Client with a C5 spinal cord injury uses an electric razor with a wrist cuff.

Dressing

Dressing includes dressing and undressing the upper and lower extremities with clothing that fits the client's premorbid lifestyle. Clients with C1 to C5 tetraplegia are dependent, but they can verbalize safe techniques to perform all the dressing skills. Independence in this skill for clients with low tetraplegic and paraplegic injuries may depend on where the skill is performed (e.g., mat, bed, or wheelchair). Clients with low-level tetraplegia can perform upper body dressing/undressing independently with equipment such as a button hook, hook and loop fasteners (Velcro), or adapted loops. Lower body dressing is usually performed in bed (Figure 19-30) versus the wheelchair because of endurance, strength, and body type issues. Clients with paraplegia are expected to dress with total independence in the bed, but they may need equipment such as a leg lifter or a long-handled shoehorn for dressing in the wheelchair (Figure 19-31). This should be encouraged, if possible, for independence in the community.

Bladder Management

Bladder management includes determining and performing the program, clothing management, body positioning, setup/cleanup of equipment, and disposal of urine and cleanup of self. Water/video urodynamic studies are performed to determine the client's bladder status and the most optimal bladder training program. Clients often enter the rehabilitation program with an indwelling catheter as their bladder management program. The indwelling catheter should be removed as soon as possible because it is a risk for chronic urinary tract infections.[99]

On the basis of injury level, clients either have a reflex bladder (upper motor neuron lesions) or a nonreflex bladder (lower motor neuron lesions).[63] The reflex bladder reflexively empties when the bladder is full. The therapeutic goals for managing the reflex bladder include low-pressure voiding and low residual urine volumes. The nonreflex bladder will not empty reflexively and needs to be manually emptied at regular intervals. The goals for managing the

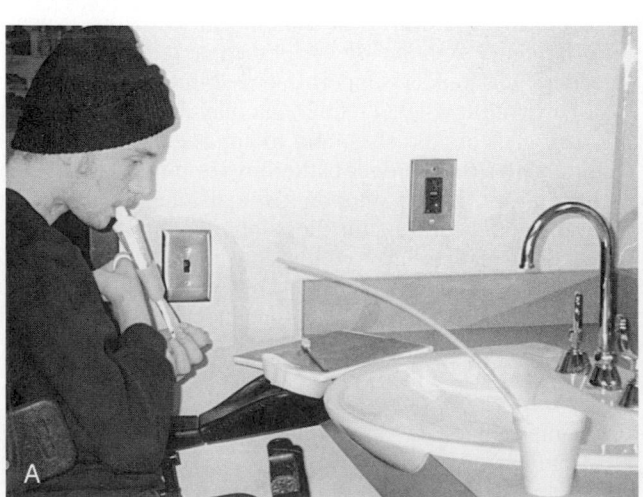
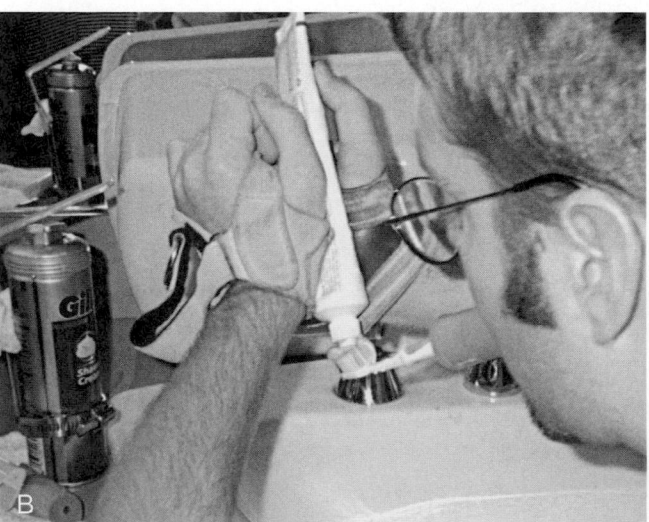

FIGURE 19-27 ▪ **A,** A client with a C5 spinal cord injury is able to brush his teeth with use of a cuff, adapted long straw, and proper wheelchair positioning at the sink. **B,** Client with C6 spinal cord injury uses bilateral tenodesis to support toothpaste while holding a toothbrush in his mouth.

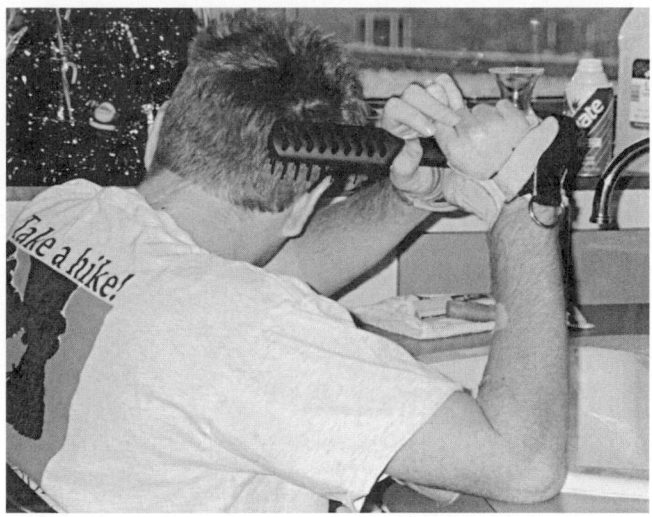

Figure 19-28 ■ Sink height can be important in assisting this client with C6 spinal cord injury to brush his hair.

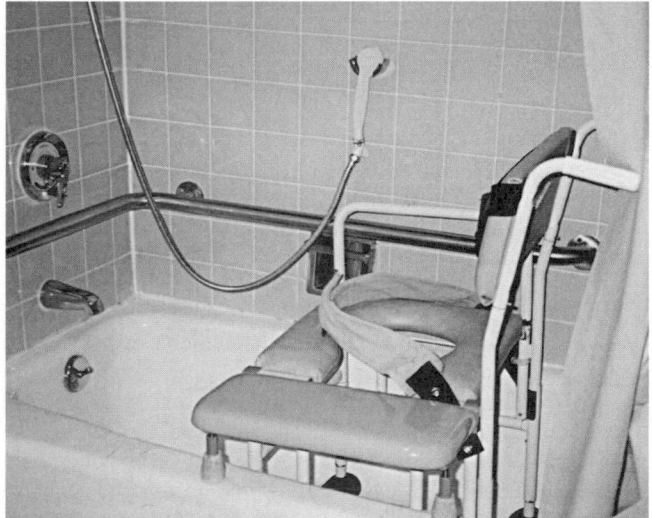

Figure 19-29 ■ Bathroom setup with shower/commode chair and handheld shower.

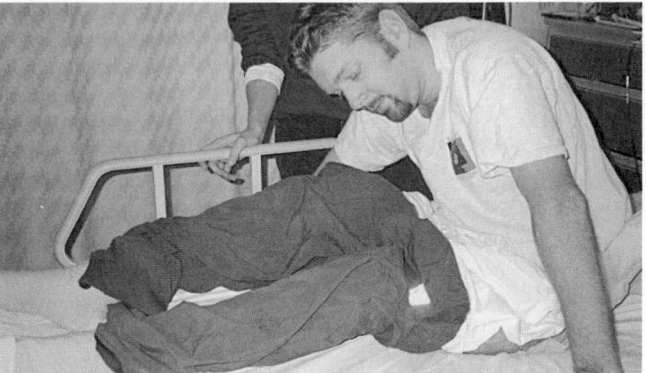

Figure 19-30 ■ Client with low-level tetraplegia maintains balance while performing lower-extremity dressing in bed.

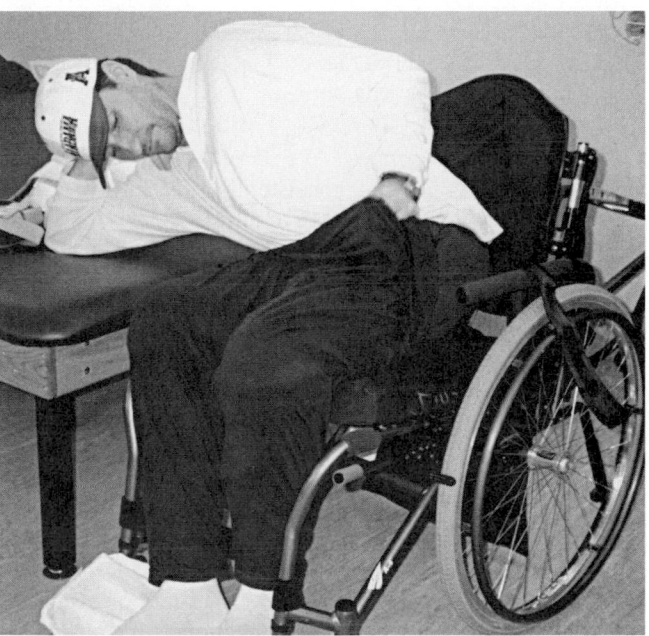

FIGURE 19-31 ■ Early practice when dressing in the wheelchair may involve leaning on a surface to assist with this skill.

nonreflex bladder include establishing a regular emptying schedule and continence between emptying. Management of a nonreflex bladder includes performance of intermittent catheterizations.

Clients with C1 to C5 tetraplegia are typically dependent in their bladder programs. An automatic leg-bag emptier can assist with just the elimination component of the bladder skill; however, the client will still be dependent in all of the other components of bladder management. Male clients with C6 level and below injuries may be able to complete portions of the bladder management. Clients with limited hand function may need adaptive devices such as orthoses to assist with catheter insertion, adaptive scissors to open bladder packages, leg bags with flip-top openers, and leg bag loops (Figure 19-32). Women with paraplegia will most likely need to begin their training in bed with a mirror to obtain the most ideal position. Touch technique can be taught so they will not be reliant on a mirror if they have

good finger sensation/use, and they may progress to using the touch technique in a wheelchair. Some people with SCI may decide to have a suprapubic catheter placed or a bladder augmentation procedure as a lifestyle choice.

Bowel Management

As described under bladder management, clients either have a reflex bowel or a flaccid bowel.[63] If the client has a positive bulbocavernosus reflex, this is indicative of a reflex bowel. With a reflex bowel, tone of the internal and external anal sphincter is present. Reflex bowel programs are most often managed by a 20-minute rectal digital stimulation program.

Flaccid bowel programs are much more difficult to regulate because there is no internal or external anal sphincter tone. Timing and diet are critical for the success of this program. A suppository may be required to assist with the process, and in this situation the rectum should be emptied before suppository insertion.[100] If the established bowel

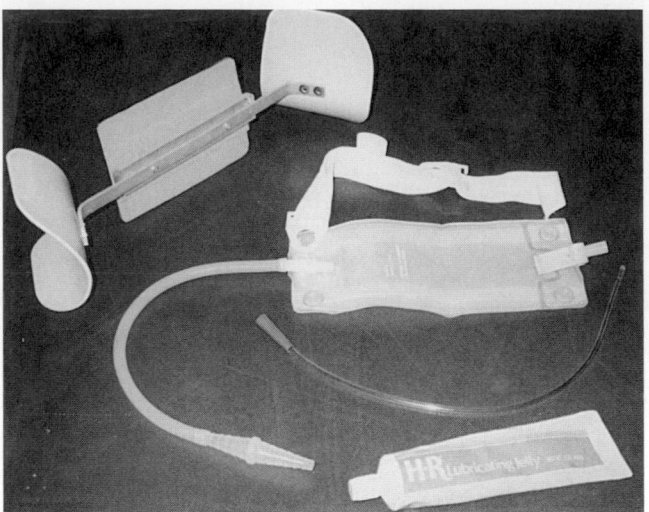

FIGURE 19-32 ■ Bladder management supplies may include knee spreader with mirror, leg bag with tubing and adapter, catheter, and lubricating jelly.

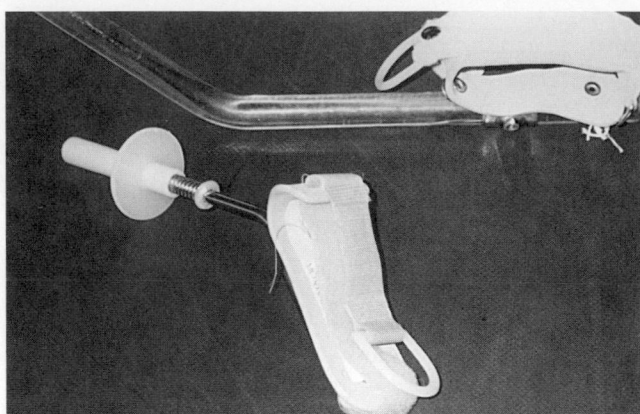

FIGURE 19-33 ■ Dil stick and suppository inserter with adaptive cuffs.

program is not followed consistently, involuntary bowel movements or impaction may occur.

Bowel management training must begin as soon as the patient is medically stable. The components of bowel management include clothing management, body positioning, setup/cleanup of equipment, performing the bowel program, disposing of feces, and cleanup of self. To establish the most effective bowel training program, the interdisciplinary team must work together. The team will need to discuss client medications that may affect the bowels, the time of day the client plans to perform the program, the physical appropriateness related to scapular strength and endurance, and all equipment that will be used.

Clients with injury levels above the C6 level will be dependent in performing the bowel program; however, they should be independent in the verbalization of the technique. Clients with limited hand (C6-C7) function may require a digital bowel stimulator and a suppository inserter with an adapted cuff or splint (Figure 19-33). In addition, a roll-in shower chair or upright shower/commode chair with a padded cutout in the seat will allow the client to reach the buttock area to perform the stimulation. For this level of injury, it may be advantageous to perform the bowel program in conjunction with the shower to conserve energy with transfers. For individuals with paraplegia, full independence is expected for completion of all bowel management skills. These programs are typically performed on appropriate bathroom equipment or the bed.

To increase the effectiveness of the bowel program the client should follow the guidelines identified in Box 19-2.

Home Management

Home management may be divided into two components: light home management and heavy home management. Light home management includes money management, preparing a snack in the kitchen, laundry, and making the bed. Heavy home management includes grocery shopping, preparing a complex meal in the kitchen, dusting, and vacuuming. The clinician should discuss the role the client

---

BOX 19-2 ■ **GUIDELINES FOR BOWEL PROGRAM**

1. Perform the bowel program at the same time each day.
2. Follow a diet high in fiber (25-35 g recommended).
3. Drink at least eight glasses of water per day.[105]
4. Drink a hot liquid 30 minutes before initiating the bowel program.
5. Perform the bowel program in an upright position.
6. Consider premorbid bowel schedule.

---

would like to assume at home. The client may want to resume previous home management roles or want to discuss changing roles with a family member or caregiver to have energy for other skills.

Clients with C1 to C5 tetraplegia will be dependent in home management. Clients with limited or no hand function will need adaptive kitchen devices, adapted utensils, and adapted cleaning equipment. Preplanning activities may be essential for independent function with clients at all levels of injury. Clients with hand function may require extended handles on equipment and must incorporate energy conservation techniques.

Mobility

Bed Mobility

The components of bed mobility include rolling side to side and supine to prone, coming to sit, and scooting in all directions while either long or short sitting. Initial training for bed mobility is usually conducted on the mat because the firmer surface is easier to learn on. Once the skills are mastered on the firmer surface, a softer surface, such as the bed, can be used. Bed mobility is a challenging skill for clients with tetraplegia to learn because of their limited upper extremity strength (Figure 19-34, A to C).[11,57] To accommodate for the loss of upper extremity musculature, compensatory strategies and assistive devices, such as bed loops, can be used. Clients with paraplegia often master bed mobility skills quickly and easily because of their intact upper extremity musculature.

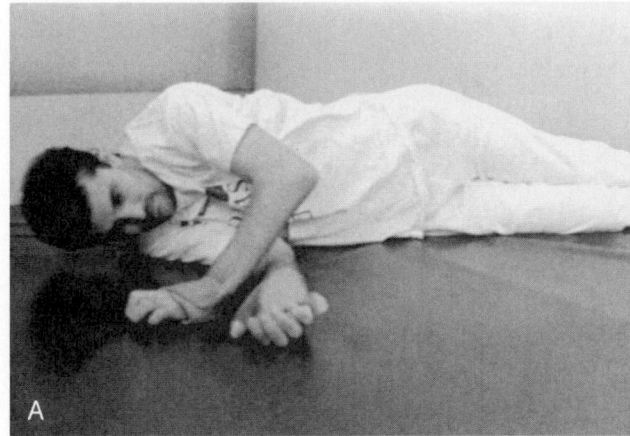
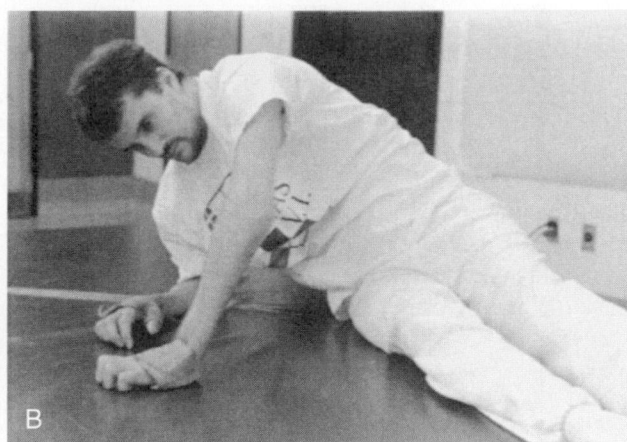
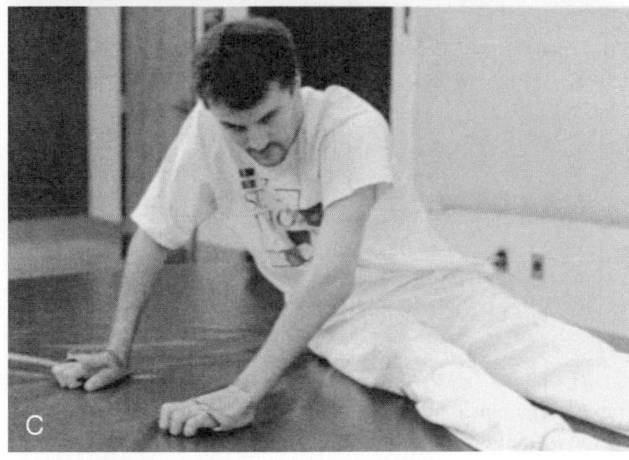

FIGURE 19-34 ■ Bed mobility. **A,** The patient gains enough strength to effectively roll from supine to side lying. **B,** He progresses to supporting his weight through the downside elbow and shoulder. **C,** The third step is shifting his upper body weight onto the upper extremity that is topside and using the head and shoulders to direct the position of the body as he performs a side pushup into the upright sitting position.

Pressure Relief in the Upright Position

The client with high tetraplegia achieves independent pressure relief in the wheelchair through appropriately prescribed specialty controls. For example, a pneumatic control switch may be used to activate the recline mode of a power wheelchair (Figure 19-35). When the client is unable to operate a specialty switch, an attendant control is used. When powered options are not feasible because of cognitive deficits, financial limitations, or other reasons, a manual recliner (Figure 19-36) or tilt wheelchair is used. When clients are dependent in performing pressure relief, they are taught to instruct others in this skill. Clients with mid- and low-level tetraplegia are taught to perform a side or forward lean technique for pressure relief if the shoulder musculature is within functional limits (Figures 19-37 and 19-38). The client with paraplegia is usually taught to perform a pushup (depression) for pressure relief (Figure 19-39).

The appropriate time to maintain the change in position is usually 60 seconds at intervals of 30 to 60 minutes. The treatment plan should include instructing the client in ways to ensure that the schedule for pressure relief is maintained in all settings. The use of watches, clocks, timers, and attendant care may be necessary.

Wheelchair Transfers

The physical act of moving oneself from one surface to another is described as a transfer. Wheelchair transfers may be accomplished in many different ways. The type of transfer used by a client is determined by the injury level, assistance needed, client preference, and safety of the transfer. When performing transfers, both the client and the person assisting must give attention to the use of appropriate body mechanics.

Dependent transfers may be accomplished with a power lift, hydraulic lift, manual pivot, transfer board, or manual lifts, which may require two or three people. A transfer with an overhead power lift is the least physically challenging on the part of the caregiver; however, these lifts are costly and are not easily transportable. The use of a hydraulic lift may be desirable if funding is not available for a power lift or the transfer needs to be done in an outdoor environment (i.e., car transfer). However, the hydraulic lift may not be the method of choice because the lift is bulky, difficult to store, and awkward to transport. Pivot transfers or manual lifts may be taught because of client or caregiver preference or when clients are smaller in stature.

Transfers can be performed with the use of a transfer board, depression-style or stand/squat pivot transfers. The mechanics of teaching an assisted transfer to a client with C7 tetraplegia is depicted in Figure 19-40. The client is taught to position the wheelchair, position the transfer board, use correct body mechanics to get the best leverage to effect movement in the desired direction, remove the board, and position his or her body appropriately.[11,57]

Wheelchair transfers are performed on many different surfaces. The training procedure begins with the easiest transfer and progresses to the more difficult transfer. Instructions for wheelchair transfers usually begin on level surfaces

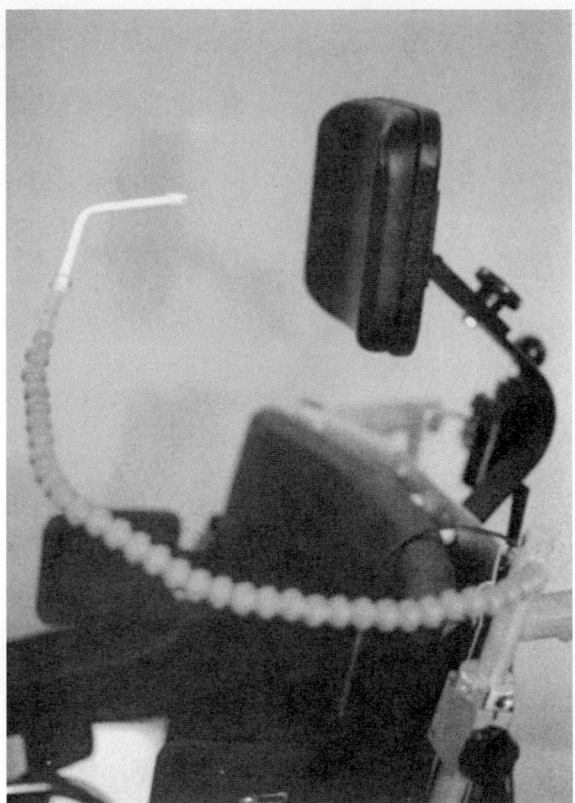

FIGURE 19-35 ■ The pneumatic control (sip 'n' puff straw) is usually ordered on a power reclining wheelchair. The straw is removable, and several are supplied with the wheelchair. The straw is attached to a flexible arm so that it is adjustable to different heights and angles to fit the needs of the patient.

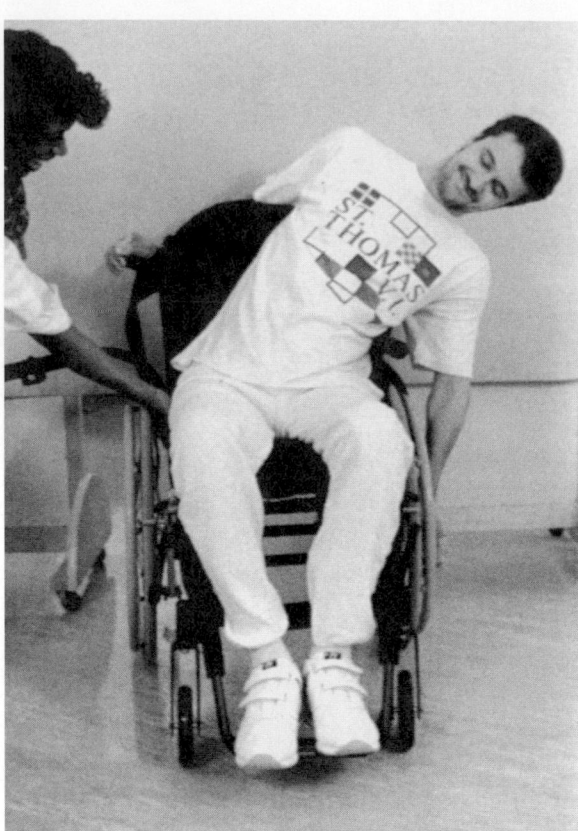

FIGURE 19-37 ■ Pressure relief: side lean. The C6/C7-level tetraplegic patient may use a side lean to achieve pressure relief over the ischial tuberosities. The patient hooks one upper extremity around the push handle of the wheelchair on one side and leans away from the hooked upper extremity until the ischium on the hooked side is clear of the wheelchair cushion. The position is maintained for 1 minute and repeated on the other side.

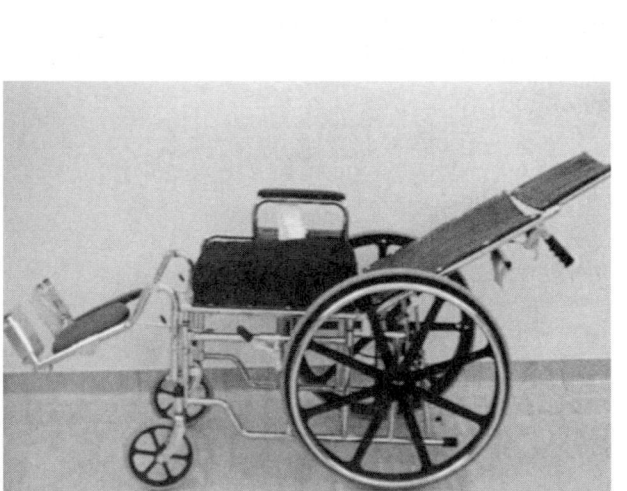

FIGURE 19-36 ■ The manual reclining wheelchair is a piece of durable medical equipment that is prescribed on a temporary or a permanent basis. The back of the wheelchair fully reclines and the legrests elevate to allow for effective pressure relief while the client is out of bed. Other features of the wheelchair are desk armrests, which may be adjustable in height; a removable headrest; and removable legrests. The wheelchair folds and may be transported in the trunk of a car.

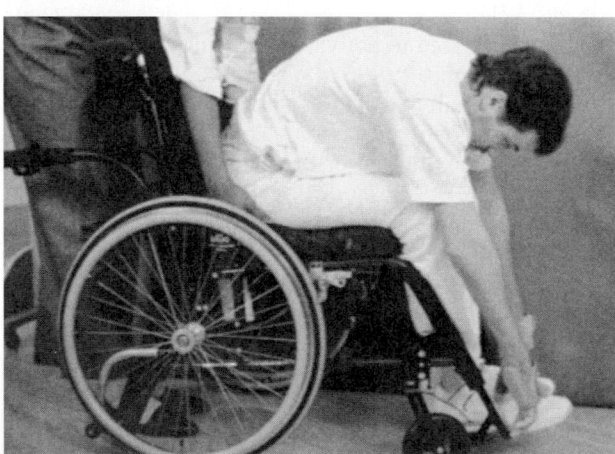

FIGURE 19-38 ■ Pressure relief: forward lean. The forward lean method of pressure relief is used for many different injury levels. The subject must have adequate ROM at the hips and in the lumbosacral spine to allow the ischia to clear the wheelchair cushion at the end range position.

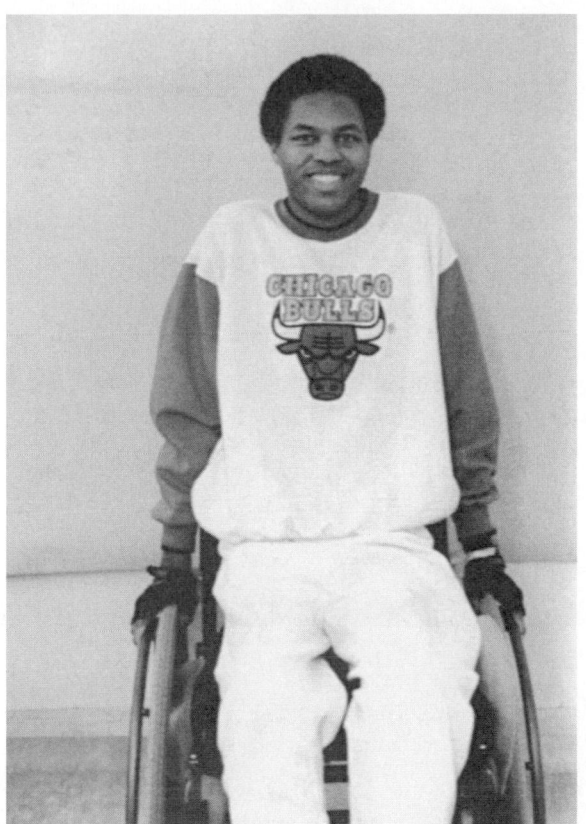

FIGURE 19-39 ■ Pressure relief: depression. This method of pressure relief is consistent with a full pushup in the wheelchair. Most paraplegic and some low tetraplegic patients are able to perform this method of pressure relief.

and progress to uneven surfaces as individual strength and skill allow.[11,57] Given these two principles, the list below is an example of how one might proceed with transfer training:

1. Mat transfer
2. Bed transfer
3. Toilet transfer
4. Bath transfer
5. Car transfer (Figure 19-41)
6. Floor transfer (Figure 19-42)
7. Other surfaces (e.g., armchair, sofa, theater seat, pool)

Wheelchair Mobility Skills

Instructions in the safe and appropriate use of the wheelchair begin before getting the client out of bed. The client is oriented to the wheelchair and its component parts.

Ideally, a power reclining or tilt wheelchair is supplied for clients with C1 to C5 tetraplegia to promote maximal independence. The most common drive-system options available for these clients includes, but is not limited to, chin drive, pneumatic systems, and head control. A client with mid- to low-level tetraplegia may be instructed in the use of both power and manual upright wheelchairs. The client with paraplegia is instructed in the use of a manual upright wheelchair unless there are extenuating circumstances. For example, a power wheelchair is appropriate for a client who is 50 years old and has severe rheumatoid arthritis.

A new breed of wheelchair that combines the benefits of a manual wheelchair with a power wheelchair is the pushrim-assisted power assist wheelchair[101] (Figure 19-43). This wheelchair may be best suited for clients who have some upper extremity weakness, joint degeneration, upper extremity pain from propelling a manual wheelchair, or reduced exercise capacity or endurance. This type of wheelchair could potentially delay secondary injuries of manual wheelchair users.[102] Both power and manual wheelchair mobility training begins on level surfaces. When a client is instructed on how to propel a manual wheelchair, it is suggested that a semicircular pattern is used to reduce the trauma to the upper extremities.[102] Training progresses toward more difficult skills as follows:

1. Mobility on level surfaces in open areas
2. Setup for transfers
3. Mobility in tight spaces
4. Mobility in crowded areas
5. On/off elevators
6. Up/down ramps
7. In/out doors
8. Wheelies (Figure 19-44)
9. Negotiation of rough terrain
10. Up/down curbs and steps (Figures 19-45 and 19-46)

Ambulation

"Will I ever walk again?" is a question often asked during SCI rehabilitation. The team must be empathetic toward and acknowledge the client's goals for ambulation, and the subject should be discussed openly. The professionals must be careful not to take hope away from the client. Hope is important to maintain positive survival skills in SCI rehabilitation. Clients who are not candidates for ambulation should receive an explanation of why these goals are not feasible. It is imperative that the rehabilitation team be made aware of all discussions regarding ambulation so that the team may support both the client and the involved team member.

When ambulation is an appropriate goal, the treatment program may be short and relatively uncomplicated for some and laborious for others. Treatment techniques may include therapeutic exercise, biofeedback, neuromuscular stimulation, balance training, standing, and pregait and gait activities. The clinician must consider the postdischarge environment and include those surfaces in training.

Equipment

In SCI rehabilitation, the use of equipment is necessary to achieve the expected outcomes. Clinicians work closely with the physician and other team members, including the rehabilitation technology supplier, to determine the most appropriate equipment to meet individual needs. It is important to have access to trial equipment so the client has the opportunity to practice with equipment similar to that which is prescribed. The rehabilitation technology supplier should be accessible to the rehabilitation team to allow for necessary adjustments to the equipment. Additionally, rehabilitation technology suppliers should be knowledgeable and responsible for educating rehabilitation professionals regarding new products. When possible, all equipment should be ordered from a single supplier to reduce

Text continued on p. 644

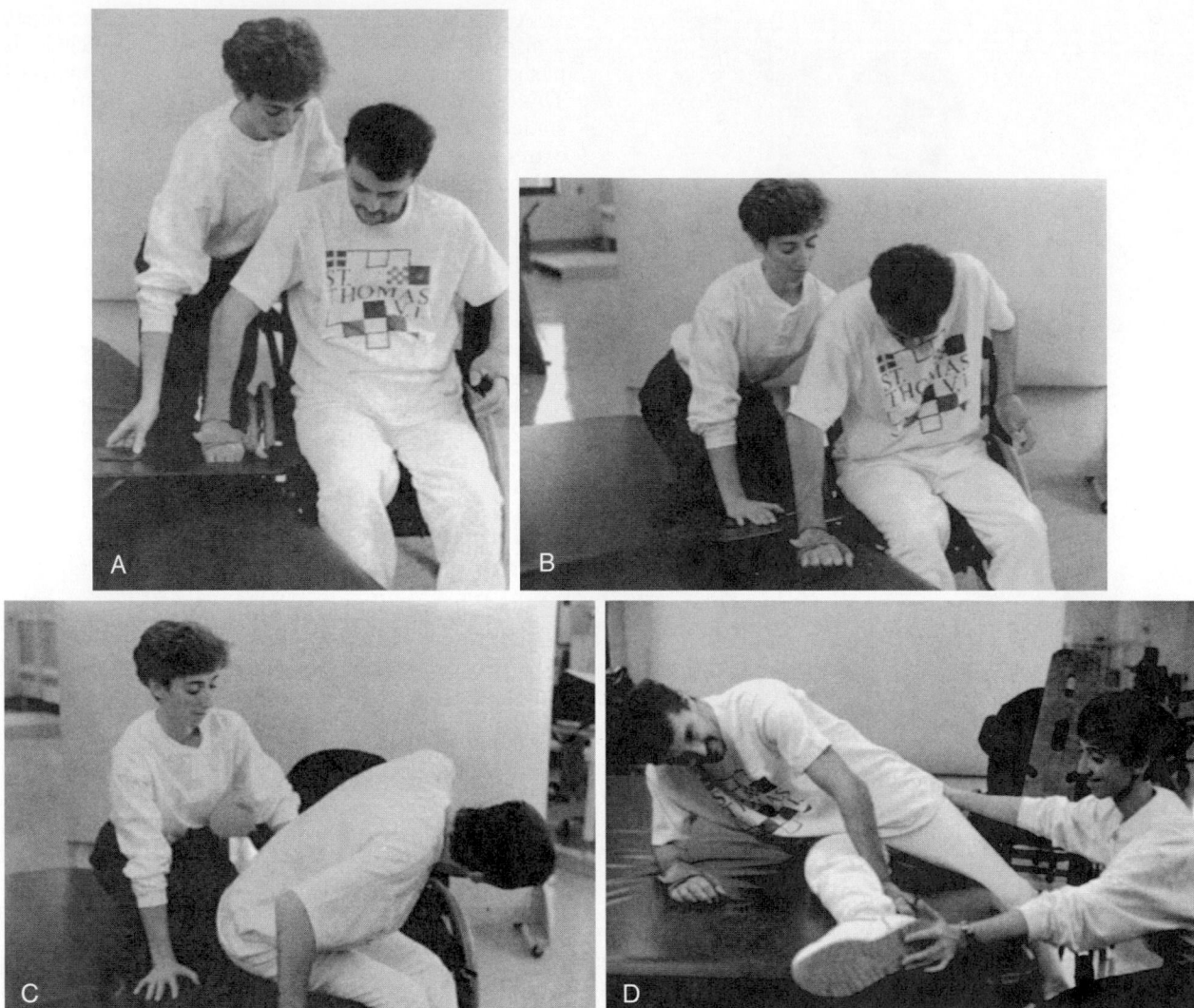

FIGURE 19-40 ■ Wheelchair transfer using a transfer board. **A,** The client positions the wheelchair at a 20- to 30-degree angle to the surface to which he is transferring and positions the board with assistance. **B,** The client positions the trailing hand close to the trailing hip and the lead hand on the transfer board or on the surface in a diagonal line. **C,** To achieve the appropriate mechanical leverage, the client is instructed to twist the upper body and look over the trailing shoulder as he pushes and lifts to effect movement across the board. **D,** When the client has achieved a safe position on the transferring surface, the transfer board is removed and the client is assisted to get his feet onto the surface.

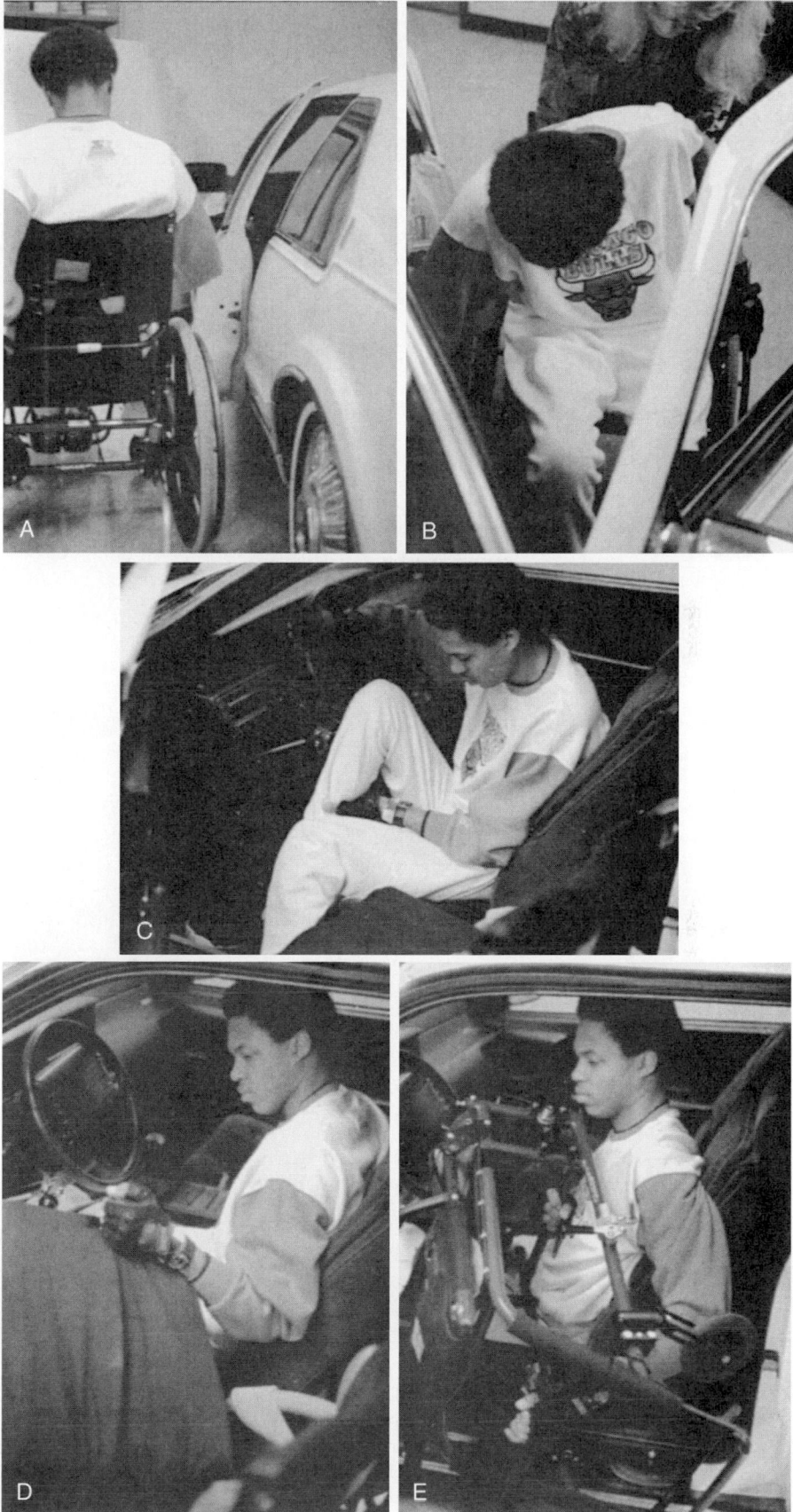

FIGURE 19-41 ■ Car transfer. Most paraplegic patients are independent (no equipment needed) in the performance of a car transfer. The client **(A)** approaches the car on the driver's side and opens the door, **(B)** positions the wheelchair and does a depression-style transfer onto the seat of the car, **(C)** positions his lower extremities, and **(D)** prepares to get the cushion and wheelchair into the car. Depending on the make/model of the automobile and the model of the wheelchair (folding vs. rigid) **(E)**, the wheelchair is placed on the back seat or transferred across the patient and onto the passenger seat. Transferring out of the car is the reverse process, beginning with the wheelchair.

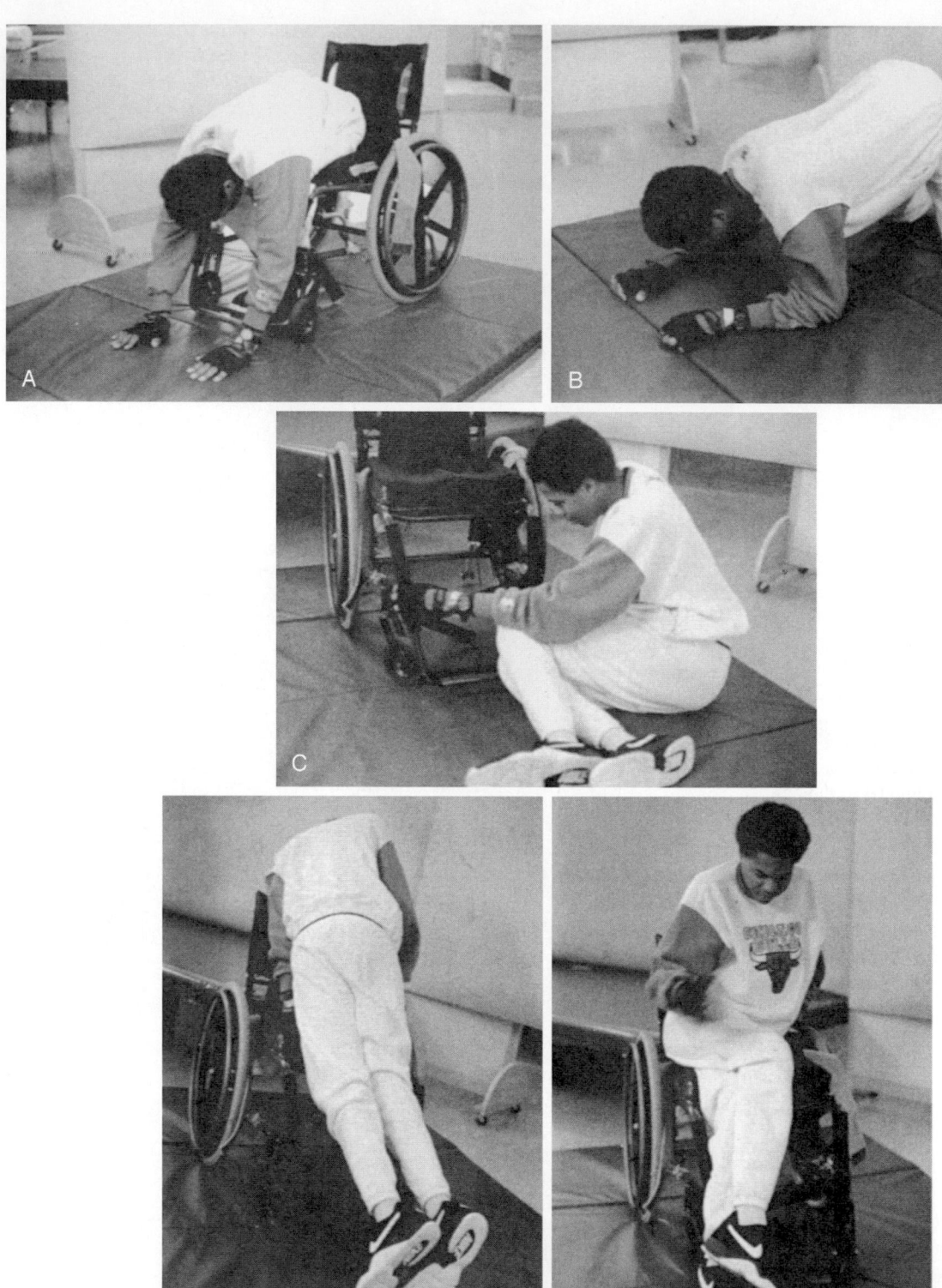

FIGURE 19-42 ■ Floor transfer. The independent performance of a floor transfer is a goal for most paraplegic patients. The patient may use different techniques to get onto the floor. **A,** Here the patient positions his feet off the footrest and moves forward onto the front edge of his cushion. **B,** He reaches for the floor with both hands, lowers his knees to the floor, and advances his hands forward until his body is clear of the wheelchair. **C,** To get back into the wheelchair he approaches the wheelchair in a forward position and (**D**) uses the front frame, seat, and/or back of the wheelchair to push himself up into the wheelchair (**E**), turning simultaneously to assume the balanced sitting position.

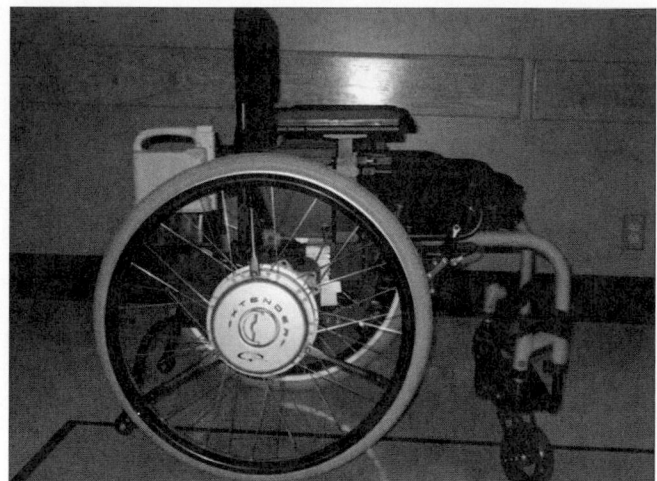

FIGURE 19-43 ■ Power assist system. The *Xtender* by Sunrise Medical is one of three power assist systems available. The motors are in the wheels. The battery extends off the back of the wheelchair. There is a connection between the motor of each wheel. The system is added to a manual wheelchair. There are two power assist levels.

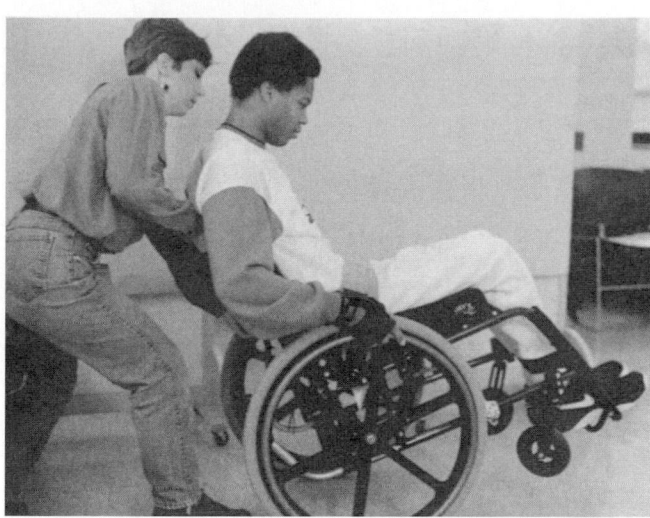

FIGURE 19-44 ■ A wheelie is a functional mobility skill that enhances functional independence. The performance of a wheelie is a precursor to negotiating steep ramps, curbs, steps, and rough terrain.

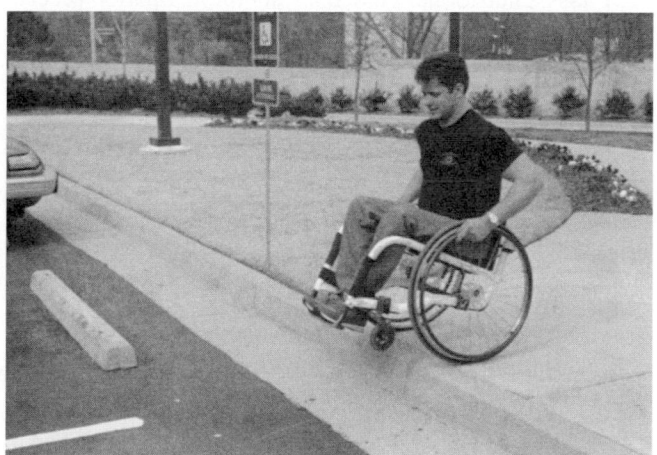

FIGURE 19-45 ■ Descending a curb is an advanced wheelchair mobility skill. This male T7 paraplegic assumes the balanced wheelie position and approaches the curb in a forward position. The wheelie position is maintained as he rolls off the curb.

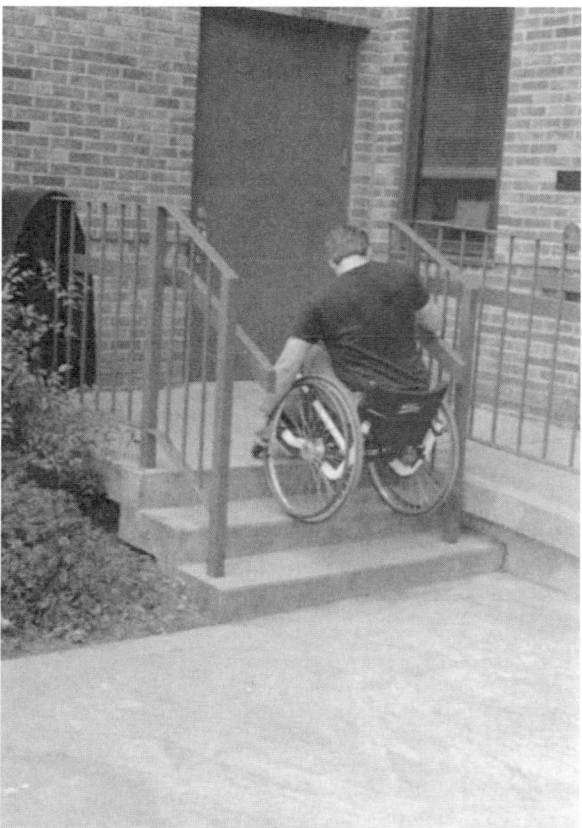

FIGURE 19-46 ■ Descending steps using one handrail. This T7 paraplegic person approaches the steps backward and, using the handrail on his right side and the hand rim of the wheelchair on his left side, lowers himself down three steps. This is one of several methods that may be used to negotiate steps.

TABLE 19-6 ■ Equipment Needs Correlated to Injury Level

INJURY LEVEL	EQUIPMENT	COST (IN DOLLARS)
C1 to C3	Ventilator (bedside)	14,700
	Ventilator (portable for wheelchair)	14,700
	Power tilt/recline wheelchair	17,000-26,000
	Manual recline wheelchair for transport	2100-4200
	Wheelchair cushion	450-600
	Reclining commode/shower chair	1800-3000
	ECU	1800-10,000
	Call system	700-800
	Bedside table	225
	Fully electric hospital bed	2000-3000
	Specialized mattress	800-10,000
	Adapted computer	2000-4000
	Communication devices	400-2000
	Overhead power lift	4000-15,000
	Hydraulic lift for transfers	1400-2000
C4 to C5	Power tilt/recline wheelchair	17,000-26,000
	Manual wheelchair for transport	2100-4200
	Lap tray	250-700
	Wheelchair cushion	450-600
	Bedside table	225
	ECU	1500-10,000
	Fully electric hospital bed	2000-3000
	Specialized mattress	800-10,000
	Commode/shower chair	1500-3000
	Communication devices	300-1500
	ADL equipment	400-1400
	Hydraulic lift for transfers	1400-2000
	Mobile arm support	500-800
	Upper extremity orthotics	700-1200
C6	Power upright wheelchair	7500-20,000
	Manual wheelchair	2000-4500
	Wheelchair cushion	450-600
	Bedside table	225
	ECU	250-7000
	Electric hospital bed	2000-3000
	Specialized mattress	800-10,000
	Commode/shower chair	1500
	ADL equipment	300-1500
	Tenodesis splint	1700
	Transfer board	100-200
	Hand control for car	500-800
	Bowel-bladder equipment	125-250
C7 to C8	Power upright wheelchair	7500-15,000
	Manual wheelchair	2000-6500
	Wheelchair cushion	450-600
	Bedside table	225
	ECU	250-1000
	Electric hospital bed	2000-3000
	Specialized mattress	600-10,000
	Commode/shower chair	1500
	Hand control for car	300-1500
	ADL equipment	300-1000
	Transfer board	100-200
	Bowel/bladder equipment	125-250
Paraplegia	Manual upright wheelchair	2000-5500
	Wheelchair cushion	450-600
	Raised/padded commode seat (cutout)	210
	Tub bench	220
	Hand controls for car	300-1500
	ADL equipment	100-300
	Bowel/bladder equipment	50-250
	Lower extremity orthotics (if ambulation is a goal)	4000-6000

Based on 2004 Atlanta, Ga., retail prices.

confusion when the need for repairs arises. To ensure that the most appropriate piece of equipment is prescribed, the following must be considered: durability, function, transportability, comfort, cost, safety, cosmesis, and acceptance by the user.[57] Generally, the higher the injury level, the more costly the equipment owing to the technology involved. Table 19-6 lists equipment according to injury level.

Ideally, equipment should be ordered as soon as possible so the client can be fitted before discharge. Shorter lengths of stay make early equipment ordering difficult. For example, a client may not have 3/5 wrist extension to be fitted with a tenodesis brace but with strengthening over time would be an excellent candidate. The clinicians need to negotiate with the funding source that equipment may be ordered in the outpatient setting. Equipment required for the SCI population is costly, requiring extensive review by third-party payers before funding is approved or denied. Many health care policies do not cover the funding of needed equipment. As a result of these factors, many clients are discharged without the equipment they need. Lack of appropriate equipment may result in (1) a feeling of loss of control, (2) contractures and postural deformities, (3) skin breakdown, (4) a loss of skills learned in rehabilitation, (5) a feeling of poor self-image, and (6) increased dependence on others.

Education

Education of the client and caregivers is an integral part of the rehabilitation process. Formal education includes group and individual instruction and family/caregiver training. Clients and caregivers are taught preventive skin care, bowel and bladder programs, safe ways to perform all ADL tasks, nutritional guidelines, thermoregulation precautions, pulmonary management, cardiopulmonary resuscitation, management of autonomic dysreflexia, equipment management and maintenance, transfer techniques, wheelchair mobility, ambulation, proper body positioning, ROM exercises, ADL basics, and leisure skills. Home programs are taught to maintain or increase strength, endurance, ROM, and function. Energy conservation techniques and proper body mechanics are incorporated into all aspects of training.

Clients are formally tested on their knowledge, and remedial instruction should be provided in deficient areas. During family training, caregivers are formally evaluated on their abilities to safely provide care to the client. Supervised therapeutic outings and passes allow the client, caregivers, and the team to identify problem areas and provide additional education in those areas.

Health Promotion and Wellness

The Surgeon General's Report on Physical Activity and Health identifies persons with disabilities as among the most inactive subgroup in the United States.[103] Physical activity after a spinal cord injury has been shown to improve muscle strength, endurance, mobility, the ability to fall asleep, self image, and blood lipid profiles and decrease the risk for premature death. In addition, exercise has been shown to decrease anxiety, loneliness, depression, stress, heart disease, blood pressure, respiratory illness, diabetes, obesity, and other medical complications.[104]

Clients with a spinal cord injury are at an increased risk for obesity.[105] This is due to clients being more sedentary and having a decreased working muscle mass and decreased metabolism by 10% to 30% below normal. Key components of a health and wellness program for persons with SCI are exercise, prevention of secondary complications, injury prevention, good nutrition, and good psychological support. Strict nutritional intake guidelines should be followed to prevent obesity. Nutritional intake guidelines for a person with a spinal cord injury are 40 ml/kg + 500 ml of fluid each day, 1.0 to 1.25 g/kg per day of protein if there is no skin compromise and 1.25-2.0 if there is skin compromise, 20 to 30 g of fiber per day, and 1,000 mg per day of calcium.[106]

An exercise program for persons with SCI must take into consideration the musculoskeletal, respiratory, cardiovascular, and autonomic nervous system changes that occur after a spinal cord injury. Components of an exercise program include flexibility, muscular strength, and cardiovascular endurance. Frequency of an exercise program ranges from two to five times per week with at least 1 day of rest between strengthening sessions. Duration of an exercise program has been shown to be beneficial with as little as 20 minutes[107] or as much as 90 to 120 minutes.[108] Intensity of exercise has ranged between 40% and 85% of maximal heart rate or within 13 to 15 on the Borg Rate of Perceived Exertion Scale.

Exercise programs, both in the clinic and home, may incorporate equipment. The literature on the types of equipment available for exercise testing or training in persons with SCI is well documented. Arm crank ergometers, wheelchair ergometers, wheelchair treadmills, lower extremity cycling with functional electrical stimulation, suspended ambulation protocols, and field test protocols are among the more widely used equipment in the clinic.[109,110] Exercise equipment varies in expense and technology and each clinic must choose the method that best fits its treatment setting and budget. Home exercise programs may be established with equipment such as weights/cuff weights, elastic bands and tubing, and hand cycles, and so forth.

Overuse syndromes are common among long-term wheelchair users. When any type of exercise program is established, factors that are specific to SCI should be considered. Long-term wheelchair use can lead to an increased incidence of carpal tunnel syndrome, elbow/shoulder tendonitis, early onset of osteoarthritis, and rotator cuff injuries. The motion and resistance of the upper extremity muscles during wheelchair propulsion can lead to an overdevelopment of anterior shoulder muscles, scapular protraction, and posterior shoulder weakness. This musculature imbalance may lead to elevation and internal rotation of the humeral head that may cause pain as a result of impingement. Injuries can be prevented or slowed if clients perform a proper warm up with stretching/flexibility exercises, wear protective equipment (i.e., helmet and padded gloves), alternate modes of exercise, and get proper rest between exercise sessions.

Through an established health and wellness program, a person with SCI has the potential to increase quality of life, improve ADLs, decrease secondary complications, decrease depression, and decrease the number of related hospitalizations. It is hoped that integration of individuals with SCI to wellness programs will become a standard in all facilities.

Psychosocial Issues

The immediate reaction to the onset of SCI is physical shock accompanied by anxiety, pain, and fear of dying. The response to such an injury varies greatly and depends on the extent of the injury, the premorbid activity level, the style of coping with stress, and family and financial resources. There may be great sensory deprivation from immobilization, neurological impairment, and the monotony of the hospital routine. Several psychological theories have been proposed to describe responses and coping mechanisms.[59] The process of coping with these changes is referred to as adjustment (see Chapter 5).

Rehabilitation personnel are becoming more aware of the need not only to teach functional skills but also to teach psychosocial and coping skills to the client and significant others. Education in the following areas facilitates the adjustment process: creative recreation, financial planning, negotiating community barriers, social skills, managing an attendant, creative problem solving, accessing community resources, fertility and child care options, assertiveness, sexual expression, vocational planning/training, and the use of community transportation. These skills may be introduced in the inpatient rehabilitation setting but will be developed further in the home and community environments. True adjustment and adaptation begin after discharge from rehabilitation.[111,112]

Sexual Issues

Altered sexual function is of concern to the SCI population.[113] The injury may result in impairment of erection, ejaculation, orgasm, male fertility, and vaginal lubrication.[114] Table 19-7 lists the relationship of the level of spinal injury to sexual function. Formal sexual counseling and education are indicated before discharge from a rehabilitation center. The educational program includes group sessions to address general issues and individual sexual function evaluations.[113] Sexual counseling, educational programs, and medical management provide opportunities to address the areas of sexual dysfunction, alternative behaviors, precautions, and other related areas.[114]

Treatment of sexual dysfunction is a coordinated effort between the client, significant other, psychologist, and urologist. Options may include surgical implantation of a penile prosthesis, vacuum erection devices, intracorporeal injection therapy, and the use of lubricants.[115] See Appendix 19-A at the end of this chapter for additional references regarding sexual function after SCI.

Discharge Planning

Discharge planning begins from the time the client is being considered for admission and continues through the rehabilitation program. It is a continuous process that includes the client, family, treatment team, and community resources, with the goal being successful community reintegration and a perceived good quality of life. The rehabilitation team must identify the specific needs of the client and structure

TABLE 19-7 ■ Relation of Level of Spinal Injury to Sexual Function

INJURY LEVEL	SEXUAL FUNCTION
Cauda equina/conus	Males
	Usually no reflex erections
	Rare psychogenic erection
	Ejaculation occasionally occurs
	Females
	Vaginal secretions often absent
	Patients generally fertile
Thoracic/cervical	Males
	Reflex erections predominate (usually short duration)
	Psychogenic erections generally absent
	Ejaculation occasional
	Females
	Vaginal secretions present as part of genital reflex
	Fertility preserved
	Sensation of labor pain absent

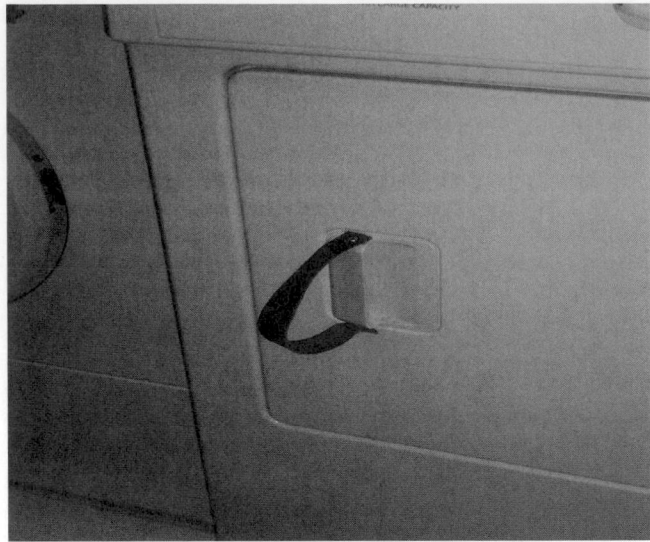

A

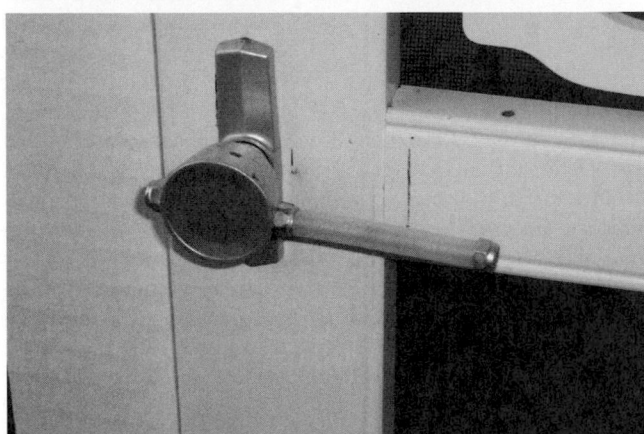

B

FIGURE 19-47 ■ Low tech home adaptations. **A,** Adding a strap, making clothes dryer door accessible. **B,** Drill hole and add handle on screen door knob.

the program to enhance the chance of success. Lengths of stay are getting shorter in response to pressure from third-party payers to contain costs. This requires the discharge planning process to be expedited so that procurement of needed equipment, completion of architectural modifications, and referrals to outpatient and community resources occur in a timely manner.

Architectural Modifications

Architectural barriers in the home, transportation system, workplace, or school may prevent access to opportunities. The architectural changes required by the person with SCI for independence in the home and community depend on the degree of impairment, financial resources, and client/family acceptance of modifications or equipment. The clinician should discuss equipment options with the client/family on the basis of the degree of modification they plan to make to their home. Thinking creatively about low-tech adaptations should be considered, part of the therapist's role. Problem solving with and by the client is vital to the process of identifying alternatives as problem solving ideas for the future (Figure 19-47, *A* and *B*).

Many available resources describe the dimensions of the basic wheelchair and specifications for making homes and facilities accessible to wheelchair users. See Appendix 19-A at the end of this chapter for resources on architectural modification.

Return to Work or School

Successful reintegration after SCI may include returning to work or school. Public school systems have a legal obligation to provide an appropriate school setting for a disabled child. At year 10 after injury, paraplegics (31.7%) have a slightly better employment outcome versus their tetraplegic counterparts, who are 26.4% employed.[30] Rehabilitation programs must emphasize returning to work throughout the process to improve a client's successful return to work and facilitate adjustment to the SCI.

Many individuals can return to their previous jobs after SCI.[116,117] The Americans with Disabilities Act of 1990 (PL 101-336) prohibits businesses with 15 or more employees from discriminating against "qualified individuals with disabilities" with respect to the terms, conditions, or privileges of employment.[118] Some situations may require modifications to the job site or a change in responsibilities. For those who are unable to perform previous jobs or who were unemployed before injury, many programs exist for training in vocational skills. The Department of Rehabilitation Services (DRS) evaluates clients for skills and functional abilities and provides funding for those qualifying for job training, job site modification, and the purchase of essential equipment that may include transportation. Services offered by the DRS vary from state to state. Each state agency has a list of resources available in the community, such as rehabilitation technology, independent living centers, and job training and placement programs. Individuals should refer to their state DRS for assistance with employment.

ADDITIONAL CLINICAL CONSIDERATIONS

Upper Extremity Restoration and Functional Electrical Stimulation

Improving hand and upper-extremity function plays a critical role in achieving independence with ADLs.[119,120] Surgical restoration of hand grasp, lateral pinch, or elbow extension in a patient with tetraplegia can be an option through tendon transfers.[121,122] Typically, before individuals are considered for surgery, their neurological function has plateaued, they are psychologically stable, and they have functional goals.[122] Individuals seeking restorative surgery to the upper extremity undergo a preoperative evaluation focusing on sensation, strength, and ROM. Before any surgical interventions, therapy may be recommended to ensure that the individual is a candidate for tendon transfer procedures.[122] Postoperative rehabilitation varies on the basis of specific procedures and may consist of 2 months or more.[123] Tendon transfer to improve the function of individuals with SCIs has been used for more than four decades and may be an option to improve upper-extremity function.[123]

The NeuroControl Freehand System is an implanted medical device that uses electrical stimulation to replace the brain's original nerve impulses when SCIs interrupt the neural pathway. This system allows clients with tetraplegia to regain the use of their paralyzed hands by using neural prosthetics with conventional reconstructive hand surgery. The system was approved by the Food and Drug Administration (FDA) in 1997. The system enables appropriately selected clients with SCI (C5-C6) to flex and extend the thumb, fingers, and elbow, allowing a useful pinch and grasp. Clients who otherwise required equipment to perform ADLs can now perform these same skills with no equipment, using their own hands. Electrodes are attached to muscles in the hands and forearms, and a pacemaker-type stimulator is surgically implanted in the chest. Signals come from the stimulator to the electrodes and cause muscles to contract and the hand to open and close. Externally, a transmitting coil is worn on the skin and the client uses simple shoulder movements to initiate hand function through a shoulder position sensor. An external controller is attached to the wheelchair as the power supply.

Ambulation Considerations

Orthotic disposition of clients with incomplete SCI is more challenging owing to the complexity of problems and varying degrees of impairment. These clients may have pain, ROM limitations, weakness, and spasticity. These problems sometimes preclude ambulation. Asymmetries, such as muscle shortening on the stronger side and lengthening on the weaker side, may lead to pelvic obliquity and scoliosis. An orthotic team approach is desirable for all orthotic dispositions to meet the needs of clients with incomplete SCI. Even if orthotic devices enable these clients to become independent, the energy costs, joint deterioration, and muscle stresses over the life expectancy of each individual need to be considered.

Advances in rehabilitation strategies include the use of body weight–supported treadmill training (BWSTT) to improve gait after incomplete spinal cord injuries. This technique of training is based on the activation of a neural network found at the spinal level of the cord. This network is collectively termed central pattern generators (CPG). The CPGs are thought to be responsible for the generation of the basic rhythmic muscle activity seen during ambulation. Research has shown evidence of CPGs in both humans and cats.[124-126] BWSTT allows the clinician to systematically train clients on a treadmill at increasing speeds. Research studies show several benefits of BWSTT. These benefits include improved speed, cadence, stride length, and weight acceptance both on the treadmill and during overground ambulation.[127-129]

The philosophy regarding the use of orthoses for ambulation for individuals with complete paraplegia varies greatly among rehabilitation centers. Some facilities encourage ambulation for these individuals, whereas others strongly discourage it, given that only a small percentage of these clients continue to use orthotics after training has been completed.[130,131]

When the philosophy of the rehabilitation center is to use braces for clients who are motor complete, criteria should be established so that both the client and the professional staff are consistent in the approach to ambulation. This gives the client specific information and clarifies goals to be attained, ensuring the most positive outcome (Box 19-3).

The ambulation trial gives the team and the client an opportunity to preview what the use of orthoses will be like. If the decision is made to order orthoses, specific goals are set. Goals range from standing and exercise ambulation to community ambulation. Most persons with complete injuries above the L2 level achieve only exercise ambulation because of the energy necessary for functional ambulation.

According to research performed at Rancho Los Amigos Hospital, the energy cost of ambulation for individuals with complete lesions at T12 or higher is above the anaerobic threshold and cannot be maintained over time. This study also concluded that ambulation for these individuals using a swing-through gait pattern are equivalent to "heavy work" or a variety of recreational and sporting activities.[131,132] Consequently, it is easy to understand why lower-extremity orthoses may end up in the closet unused.

The energy cost for ambulation is highest for persons with complete paraplegia who use a swing-through gait pattern and lowest for persons who use bilateral ankle-foot orthoses (AFO) or a combination of an AFO and a knee-ankle-foot orthosis (KAFO). Even individuals requiring only bilateral AFOs have a gait efficiency of less than 50% of normal,

---

BOX 19-3 ■ CRITERIA FOR AMBULATION TRIAL FOR COMPLETE INJURIES

- Expressed desire for ambulation with appropriate goals
- Body weight not to exceed 10% of ideal
- ROM: Hip extension 5 degrees, full knee extension, ankle dorsiflexion 5 to 15 degrees, passive straight-leg raise 110 degrees
- Intact skin
- Stable cardiovascular system
- Controlled spasticity
- Independent function at the wheelchair level

underscoring the importance of the hip extensor and abductor muscles required for normal ambulation. These muscles are severely or completely paralyzed in this population.

Given intact upper extremities, the energy cost of ambulation is progressively reduced when more residual motor function is present in the lower extremities. Conversely, the person with incomplete tetraplegia has higher energy costs for ambulation despite spared lower-extremity function because of upper- and lower-extremity weakness[131,132] (Boxes 19-4 and 19-5 and Figures 19-48 to 19-53).

BOX 19-4 ■ FOUR CATEGORIES OF AMBULATION[156]

1. Standing only
2. Exercise—Ambulates short distances
3. Household—Ambulates inside home or work, uses wheelchair much of the time
4. Community—independent on all surfaces; does not use wheelchair

---

BOX 19-5 ■ LOWER-EXTREMITY ORTHOSES[133]

HIP-KNEE-ANKLE-FOOT ORTHOSES
RGO (Figure 19-48)
Bilateral KAFOs with pelvic band

KNEE-ANKLE-FOOT ORTHOSES
Scott-Craig KAFOs (Figure 19-49)
Conventional KAFOs (metal uprights)
Polypropylene KAFOs (Figure 19-50)
Hybrid KAFOs (Figure 19-50)

ANKLE-FOOT ORTHOSES
Conventional AFOs (metal)
Custom polypropylene AFOs
Solid ankle (Figure 19-51)
Custom polypropylene AFOs, articulated ankle (Figure 19-52)
University of California Biomechanics Lab (UCBL) orthotic (Figure 19-53)

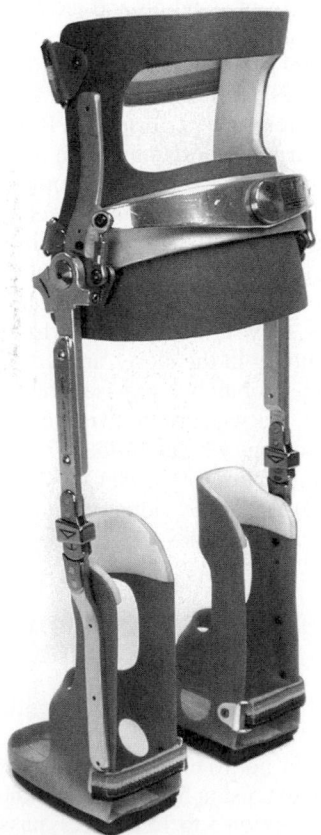

FIGURE 19-48 ■ The RGO, although generally used with children, is also used with the adult population. Its main components are a molded pelvic band, thoracic extensions, bilateral hip and knee joints, and lower limb segments that may be polypropylene construction with a solid ankle. The RGO uses a dual cable system to couple flexion of one hip with extension of the other.

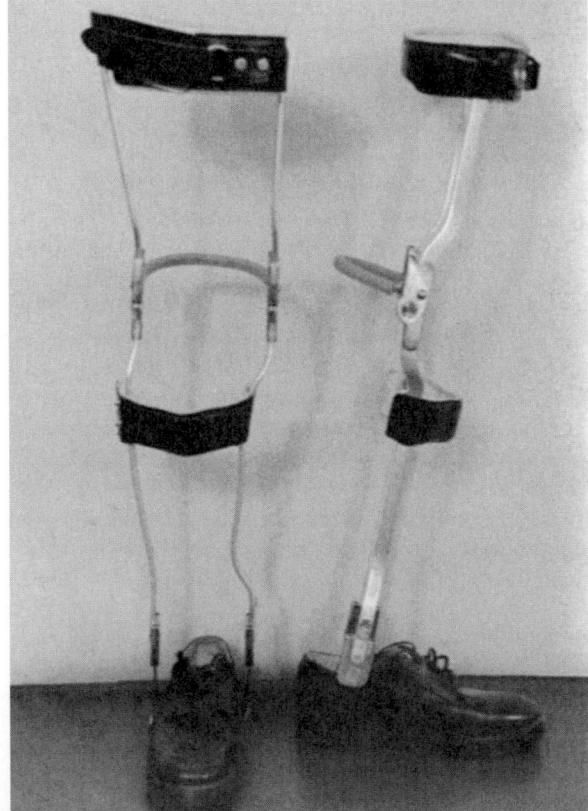

FIGURE 19-49 ■ Scott-Craig KAFO is a special design for spinal cord injury. The orthosis consists of double uprights, offset knee joints with pawl locks and bail control, one posterior thigh band, a hinged anterior tibial band, an ankle joint with anterior and posterior adjustable pin stops, a cushion heel, and specially designed longitudinal and transverse foot plates made of steel.

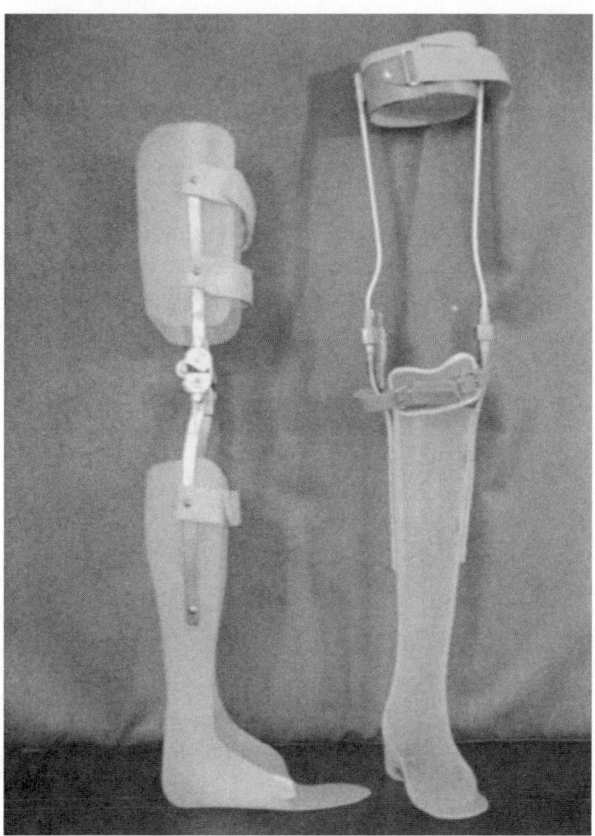

FIGURE 19-50 ■ Polypropylene KAFO and combination plastic and metal KAFO.

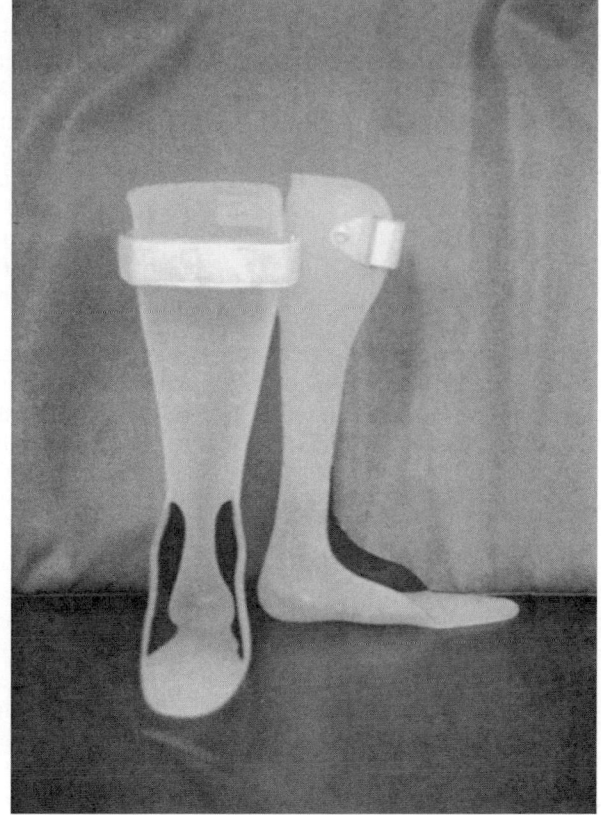

FIGURE 19-51 ■ Custom solid AFOs in 5 degrees of dorsiflexion with full footplates.

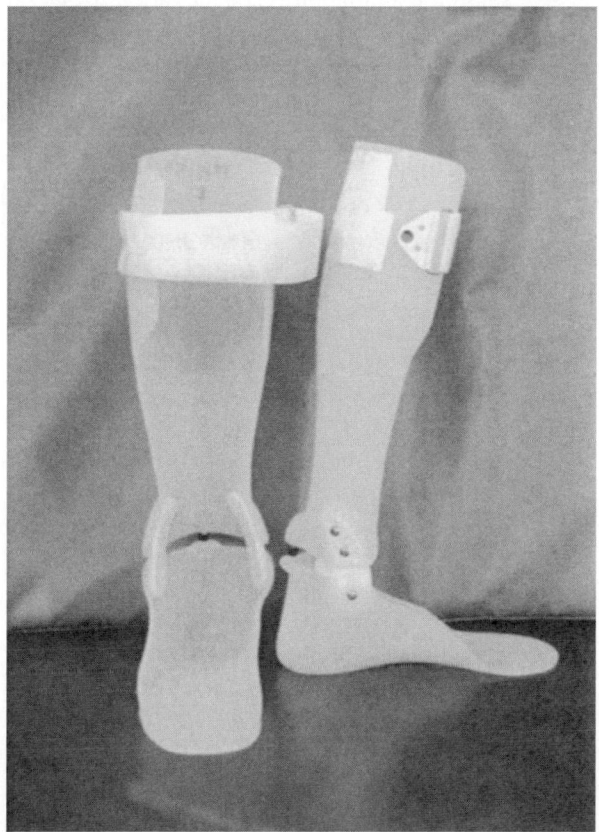

FIGURE 19-52 ■ Custom articulated AFOs with adjustable Oklahoma ankle joints.

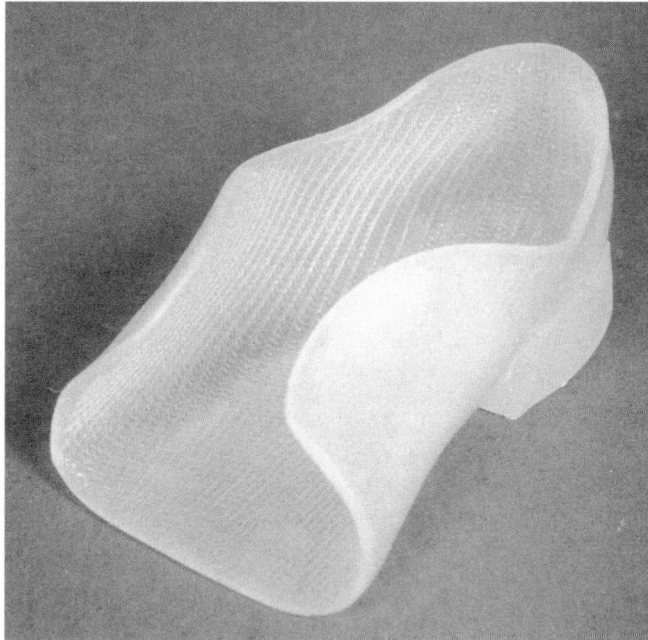

FIGURE 19-53 ■ University of California Biomechanics Laboratory orthosis. This orthosis is designed with a deep heel cup that holds the calcaneus securely. Additionally, the high medial and lateral trimlines support the joints of the midfoot and allows more optimal subtalar joint function. The orthosis also supports the longitudinal arch of the foot. (From Lusardi MM, Nielsen CC: *Orthotics and prosthetics in rehabilitation,* Woburn, MA, 2000, Butterworth Heinemann.)

Factors that affect orthotic selection are cost, injury level, residual motor function, experience, and bias of the clinician, and client acceptance. Generally, the hip, knee, ankle, and foot orthosis (HKAFO) is used when selected motions of the hip need control or the benefits of the reciprocating gait orthosis are desired, as is the case with the pediatric population. The use of a KAFO is indicated when the quadriceps muscle strength is less than 3/5. AFOs are indicated in the presence of ankle instability and weakness and to control hyperextension of the knee joint.[133] See Table 19-8 for correlation of complete injury levels and orthotic disposition.

The application of FES for standing and stepping is referred to as neuroprosthetics. Initial work with surface electrodes was performed in the 1970s and 1980s.[134] Principles developed by Slovenian investigators have formed the foundation for most of the continuing research in this field.[135] The first system to gain FDA approval was the Parastep II system developed by Sigmedic, Inc (Northfield, Ill.).[135]

These types of systems generally use two to twelve channels of stimulations. The system in its simplest form uses one set of electrodes placed over the quadriceps muscle and another set over the sural, saphenous, or peroneal nerve. The systems consist of a computer control box, lead wire, electrodes, and a cable connected to a walking device that houses the command switch(es) for step function. Other systems that use implanted electrodes are being investigated at this time, but none are FDA approved. The most promising work in progress is being done at the Veterans Administration Medical Center and Case Western Reserve University in Cleveland. Both FES systems, the surface electrode system and the implanted system, in their present state show promise for the future. However, these systems currently do not present a viable alternative to wheelchair use because of the high-energy requirement.[136,137] Additionally, there is limited research in the use of epidural spinal cord stimulation to facilitate ambulation.[138,139]

Hybrid FES orthosis systems are orthotic systems that incorporate FES. Usually the FES is a simple configuration of approximately four channels and uses surface stimulation. One such system, used with the reciprocating gait orthosis (RGO), was developed by Douglass and colleagues at Louisiana State University Medical School. Systems such as this offer the advantage of increased energy efficiency compared with the use of only orthoses or only FES. Conversely, the bulkiness of the systems impedes the completion of some ADLs, and donning and doffing is more difficult.[73,134,140] (See Chapter 31 for additional information on electrical stimulation intervention and Chapter 34 on orthotics.)

Seating Principles

Many individuals spend 8 hours or more per day in their wheelchairs after an SCI. Consequently, proper seating of these clients may be the most important intervention clinicians provide. The seating process should be addressed on admission, continually throughout the rehabilitation program, and regularly after discharge to help prevent and minimize complications.[11,141] The wheelchair is an integral part of the client's self-image and in many ways will help define personal lifestyle.[57] Goals for seating the client with an SCI are identified in Box 19-6.

Every seating session begins with a thorough examination, as described earlier. Trial simulations are essential to determine how the client will function and maintain posture over time in the seating system. Simulations help to avoid costly mistakes. The client must be involved in the decision-making process to ensure that the seating system will work.

The seating process may be complicated by impairment or loss of sensation and mobility. Great care must be taken to reduce pressure over bony prominences and to distribute pressure over as large an area as possible.[139] Pressure-distributing cushions should be evaluated clinically and with pressure-sensing devices to determine the optimal wheel-

TABLE 19-8 ■ Correlation of Complete Injury Levels and Orthotic Disposition

INJURY LEVEL	MUSCLES PRESENT	ORTHOSES	GOALS	BRACING RECOMMENDED
Above T2	Partial upper-extremity function	Standing frames RGOs	Standing Exercise ambulation	No
T2 to T6	Complete upper-extremity function	Standing frames RGOs KAFOs with spreader bar	Standing Exercise ambulation	No
T7 to T10	Partial function of trunk muscles	RGOs KAFOs with spreader bar	Standing Exercise ambulation	
T11 to T12	Almost complete function of trunk	RGOs KAFOs with spreader bar	Exercise ambulation	Sometimes
L1	Complete trunk function	RGOs KAFOs with spreader bar	Exercise or limited household ambulation	Usually
L2	Hip flexors	KAFOs	Exercise or limited household ambulation	Usually
L3	Quadriceps	Combination KAFO/AFO Bilaterally AFOs	Household or community ambulation	Yes
L4 and below	Quadriceps Partial hamstrings Partial ankle Partial hips	AFOs UCBL	Community ambulation	Yes

BOX 19-6 ■ GOALS FOR SEATING THE CLIENT WITH SCI

1. Maximize functional independence
2. Improve pressure distribution and relief of pressure
3. Optimize comfort
4. Enhance the quality of life
5. Optimize good postural alignment and sitting balance
6. Compensate for fixed deformities
7. Allow for transportation of the mobility system
   The following are basic seating concepts of proper postural alignment:
   - Neutral pelvic alignment
   - Symmetrical alignment of the trunk and neck
   - Neutral head positioning over the pelvis
   - Maintenance of a horizontal gaze
   - Maintain ankle in neutral alignment with full support of the foot
   - Maintenance of the thighs in neutral abduction/adduction with full contact with the cushion
   - Neutral shoulder positioning to avoid shoulder elevation, protraction, or retraction and to provide adequate upper-extremity support[141,142]
   - The elbow angle should approximate 100-120 degrees when the hand is resting at the top of the wheel or pushrim[101]

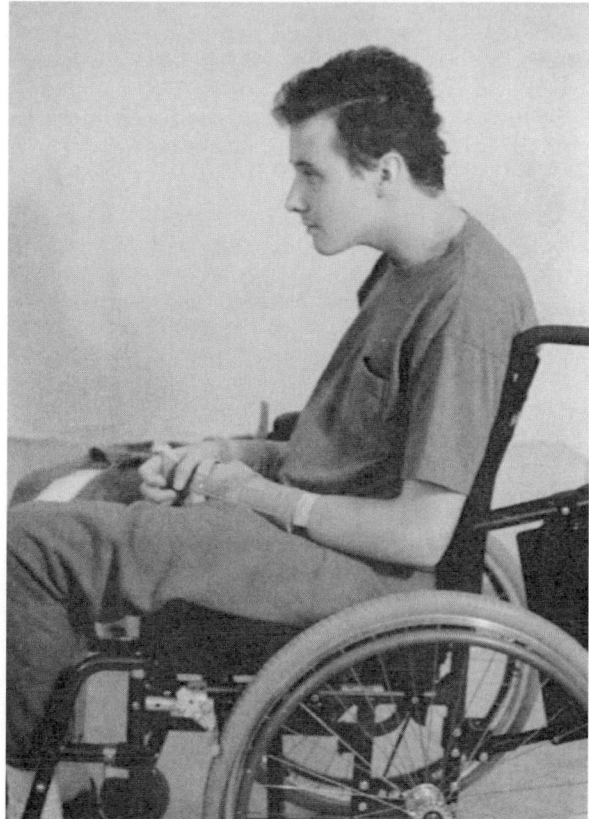

FIGURE 19-54 ■ Example of typical kyphotic C-curve posture in the patient with tetraplegia.

chair cushion for each individual.[141,142] Many clients with muscle paralysis of the trunk find that the effects of gravity in a sitting position pull the head and upper torso forward and over the pelvis, resulting in a long kyphosis or a C-curved posture (Figure 19-54).[142] Two resulting problems are increased weight bearing on the sacrum and development of a thoracic kyphosis, leading to neck hyperextension in an effort to maintain a horizontal gaze.[141] Unfortunately, this poor seating posture is quickly learned and difficult to correct.[141] This posture can often be prevented by tilting the wheelchair slightly backward while maintaining a fixed seat-to-back angle (Figure 19-55).[141] In this position, the effects of gravity augment sitting balance and facilitate good spinal alignment. The use of a sacral block, a firm wheelchair seat and back, and properly applied seat belts also aid in preventing the kyphotic posture.[141]

Asymmetrical muscle strength, asymmetrical spasticity, and power wheelchair propulsion using predominantly one upper extremity often result in poor trunk alignment. The use of lateral trunk supports, lateral pelvic supports, and properly applied seat belts may aid in maintaining symmetrical trunk posture.

Strong muscle spasms, combined with the effects of gravity, may cause the person with severely impaired mobility to slide down in the wheelchair, resulting in increased pressure on the sacrum and shearing of the skin. For these clients, a wheelchair with a fixed seat-to-back angle that tilts backward to allow for the performance of pressure relief may help to reduce this problem (Figure 19-56).

The size, weight, and portability of the seating system affect the individual's lifestyle. The client's home or work environment must be evaluated closely for accessibility so

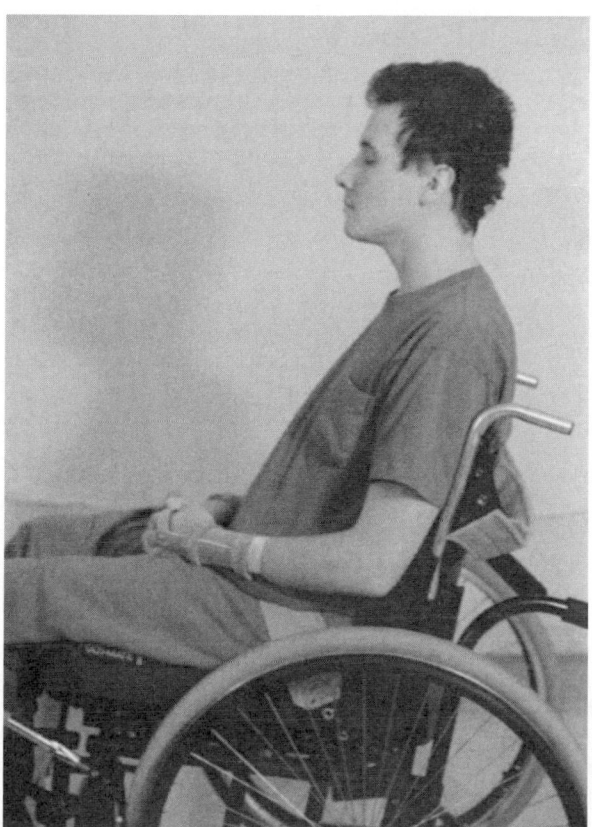

FIGURE 19-55 ■ Example of corrected C-curve posture.

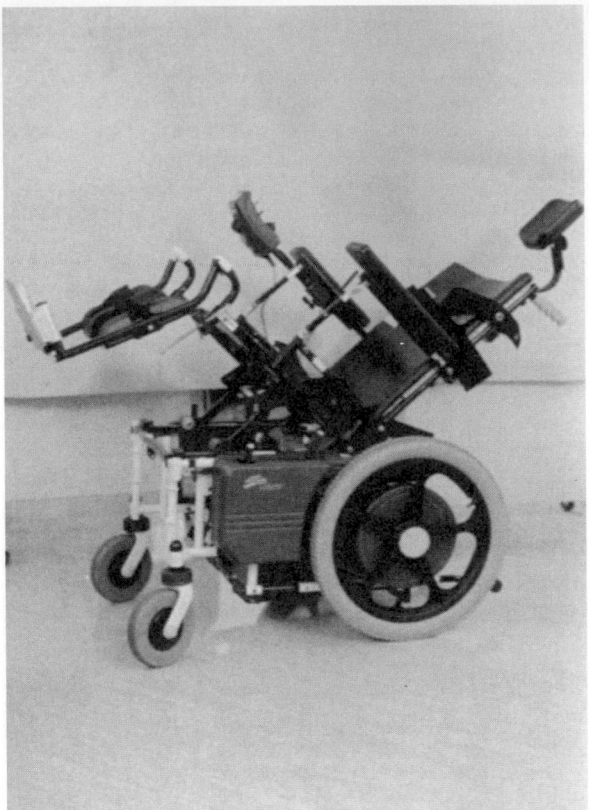

FIGURE 19-56 ■ Example of power-tilt-in-space wheelchair.

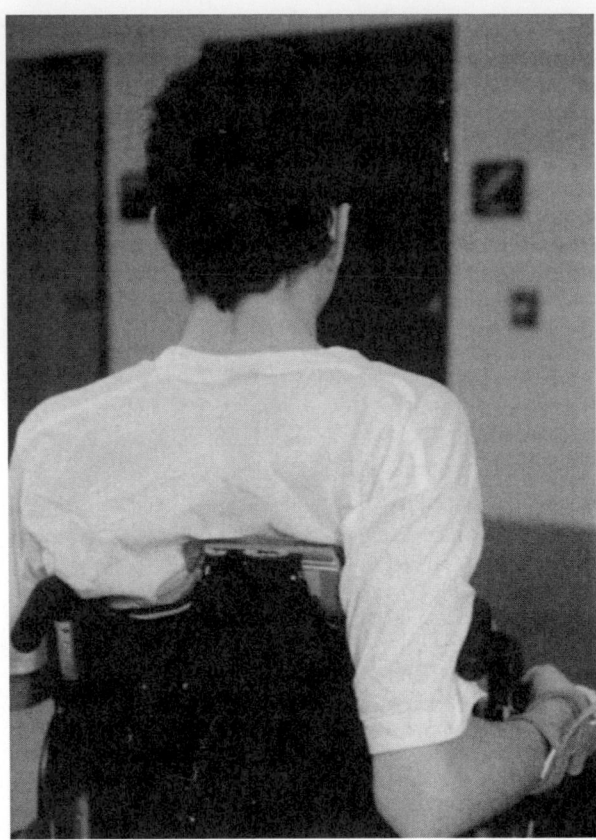

FIGURE 19-57 ■ Example of custom modification of a wheelchair back to allow a patient with tetraplegia to hook the push handle with one upper extremity.

that the seating system can be used effectively in those environments. The buildings must be structurally sound and spacious to accommodate heavy power wheelchair systems. The means of transportation of the wheelchair (car vs. van) determines whether a rigid or folding wheelchair frame is indicated and possibly whether a portable power wheelchair is the best choice.

The wheelchair must be as easy as possible to propel to reduce stress on upper-extremity joints. Many manual wheelchairs are lightweight (less than 35 pounds) and have multiple adjustments and choices of tires and casters that make manual wheelchair propulsion more efficient. The correct rear tire size reduces shoulder musculature fatigue. Rear tire size should be selected so that when the wheelchair user is seated with hands resting on the top of the push rims, there is 60 degrees of the elbow in the position of 30 degrees of flexion and no shoulder elevation.[143] In addition, shifting the distribution of the user's weight back over the rear axle (usually accomplished by moving the rear wheel axle forward) reduces the percentage of weight on the front casters, making propulsion more efficient.[143]

Distributing pressure over as large a surface area as possible without endangering function should be considered when taking wheelchair measurements. The width of the seat (wheelchairs are made with the same seat and back width) should be slightly more than that of the widest body part. The seat depth should come to within 1 inch of the popliteal fossae. The height of the back should reflect the client's motor function and be no lower than the presence of

functional musculature to provide appropriate trunk support. If the back is too high, it can restrict functional activities such as wheelchair propulsion and wheelies. Clients with tetraplegia who use the push handles of the wheelchair to hook while performing functional activities may require custom modification of the wheelchair back (Figure 19-57).

Finally, the impact of the wheelchair on the individual's self-image must be considered. The entire focus of their rehabilitation process is successful community reintegration. An attractive seating system is an integral tool for the client's success.

CONCLUSION

Comprehensive treatment of the individual with SCI continues to be a challenge to the rehabilitation team and to society as a whole. Health care reform issues force the rehabilitation team to explore new cost-efficient options to provide quality rehabilitation. New medical interventions improve the prognosis for return of function to a greater extent for the incomplete versus complete lesions. Additionally, the aging of this population presents new problems that require intervention and causes the team to examine past rehabilitation goals and treatment strategies. Passage of the Americans with Disabilities Act points out that community reintegration of individuals with disabilities is a responsibility of society. These and other issues will present many challenges for individuals with SCI in the future.

CASE STUDY 19-1 ■ C5-C6 FRACTURE

The client, a 24-year-old man, was drag racing while unrestrained on a country road. He had consumed several beers and lost control of his car. The car rolled several times and he was thrown approximately 20 feet from the vehicle. When the emergency medical services personnel arrived at the scene, the client was conscious and complaining of neck pain. He had a laceration across the left temporal area. A cervical collar was applied, and he was placed on a spine board for transportation to the closest emergency medical center.

On arrival, the client was reevaluated and the head laceration was cleaned and stitched. The physician ordered radiographs of the spine, skull, and chest, which revealed a C5-C6 fracture/subluxation and rib fractures laterally at ribs 4, 5, and 6 on the left; a skull fracture was ruled out. Physical examination revealed the following: client awake and alert, absent deep tendon reflexes below the C5 level (indicative of spinal shock), absent sensation below the nipple line, and no volitional movement in the upper or lower extremities except for shoulder shrugs and elbow flexion, and trace wrist extension.

Within 2 hours of the initial injury, methylprednisolone, 30 mg/kg, was administered intravenously. Additional emergency department treatment consisted of starting an intravenous catheter, inserting a Foley catheter, administering oxygen by means of a nasal cannula, and continuing immobilization in the cervical collar. Arrangements were made for transfer to a model SCI center.

On admission to the SCI center, the client was taken to the intensive care unit and evaluated by the attending physician. Confirmation of the previously established C5 motor level was made, and the sensory picture had improved, with impaired light touch present in the lower extremities and sacral dermatomes. The diagnosis of incomplete C5 tetraplegia was determined. The client was immediately placed in cervical traction with use of Gardner-Wells tongs and was transferred to the computed tomographic (CT) scanner for imaging of the abdomen, cervical spine, and skull. CT scans of the skull and the abdomen had negative results. CT scans of the cervical spine and the chest confirmed the initial diagnosis of fractures. A decision was made to manage the client with external fixation with halo traction. The client was placed on deep vein thrombosis prophylaxis, and the methylprednisolone protocol was continued.

Referrals were made to the rehabilitation team, including dietary services, occupational therapy, physical therapy, psychological services, respiratory therapy, social services, speech therapy, therapeutic recreation, and vocational counseling. The nursing staff initiated strict turning times with appropriate padding and positioning to prevent pressure ulcers and pulmonary complications.

All team members made initial contact with the client within 2 days of admission. The therapy evaluations were completed within 24 hours of admission and revealed the following neurological findings: the biceps and wrist extensors were 5/5; the triceps were a trace bilaterally; all other key muscles of the upper extremity were absent; a strong isometric contraction was noted in the trunk musculature (unable to fully test because of the halo vest; the hip flexor and extensor muscles were 2/5; knee extensors were 2/5; knee flexors were 1/5; and ankle dorsiflexors were 1/5 bilaterally. The motor neurological level was C6 bilaterally, and the ASIA impairment scale had improved to a classification of C (incomplete motor).

The client's vital capacity was 1200 ml, and he complained of left chest wall pain during inspiration. His cough was weak but productive. There was evidence of spasticity with sustained clonus in the right ankle. The Ashworth score was 2 on the left and 3 on the right. Initial treatment consisted of ROM exercises, deep breathing exercises, and a positioning program to prevent adaptive shortening. Out-of-bed orders were received on day 3 and inpatient rehabilitation began when the client tolerated 3 hours of therapy daily. All team members established rehabilitation goals with the client and family.

As the client's rehabilitation progressed, the functional strength of the triceps returned and weak hand intrinsics were noted. The lower extremities improved to functional strength on the left side; on the right there was continued weakness in the gluteal, hip flexor, and ankle musculature. He had normal bowel function. The client's bladder program was self-voiding; however, he performed intermittent catheterization for residual volume checks with use of a short opponens brace with a pincer grasp to assist.

The client was prescribed a rental hemiheight manual wheelchair in the seating clinic and was modified independent with propulsion on smooth surfaces and over rough terrain. He was evaluated in the brace clinic and began gait training on the parallel bars with the use of a right KAFO. The brace clinic team decided to delay ordering custom lower extremity orthotics until the muscle strength in the right quadriceps plateaued. He was independent in all transfers. The client required minimal assistance in meal preparation and was able to eat using utensils with built-up handles. He was able to dress his upper and lower extremities with use of a button hook and zipper pull. He was modified independent in all grooming and bathing skills. A tub bench was necessary during bathing to address balance and endurance deficits, and a long-handled sponge allowed access to hard-to-reach areas. The client was modified independent in written communication skills with adapted writing equipment (builtup pens/pencils or short Wanchik splint). A driving evaluation was completed, and the client was able to drive with minor modifications. The psychologist counseled the client and his wife on sexuality and sexual functioning.

Continued

CASE STUDY 19-1 ■ C5-C6 FRACTURE—cont'd

The home assessment was completed, and recommendations were made to accommodate the wheelchair yet leave flexibility for increased ambulation function. The client's work site, a car repair business, was also evaluated to ensure accessibility and safety. At the time of discharge from inpatient rehabilitation, the client was unable to perform his preinjury work duties as an auto mechanic because of hand weakness and the inability to lift heavy objects. The case manager contacted the vocational rehabilitation counselor to investigate other work opportunities at the client's current place of employment. Although the client's personal goal was to return to his previous duties, he would require a vocational evaluation after outpatient rehabilitation to determine the appropriateness of this goal.

At the time of discharge, the client and his family had completed family training and demonstrated appropriately the performance of all functional skills. The physical and occupational therapist provided the client with home exercise programs specific to his strengthening needs. The therapeutic recreation specialist enrolled him in a fitness program. Physical and occupational therapy outpatient referrals were made for gait and balance training, endurance training, upper extremity strengthening to become independent in all ADL skills, and hand rehabilitation.

After 6 weeks of outpatient therapy, the client's endurance and balance had improved, allowing full-time ambulation. The rental wheelchair was discontinued. The client was discharged from outpatient physical therapy with a revised home exercise program. The patient had achieved independence with all dressing and grooming skills. He could complete home management skills with modified independence and planned to continue only with hand rehabilitation. Follow-up assessments from all other team members occurred at 8 weeks after discharge from inpatient rehabilitation. He was scheduled for a 6-month evaluation to determine his return-to-work goals.

REFERENCES

1. Brown DJ: Spinal cord injuries: The last decade and the next, *Paraplegia* 30:77-82, 1992.
2. Whiteneck GG, Charlifue SW, Frankel HL et al: Mortality, morbidity, and psychosocial outcomes of persons spinal cord injured more than 20 years ago, *Paraplegia* 30:617-630, 1992.
3. DeLisa JA, Martin GM, Currie DM: Rehabilitation medicine: past, present, and future. In DeLisa JA, editor: *Rehabilitation medicine: principles and practice,* Philadelphia, 1988, JB Lippincott.
4. Dollfus P: Rehabilitation following injury to the spinal cord. *J Emerg Med* 11:57-61, 1993.
5. Nickel VL: The rationale and rewards of team care. In Nickel VL, Botte MJ, editors: *Orthopaedic rehabilitation,* ed 2, New York, 1992, Churchill Livingstone.
6. Apple DF, Hudson LM, editors: Spinal cord injury: the model. In Proceedings of the National Consensus Conference on Catastrophic Illness and Injury-the Spinal Cord Injury Model: Lessons Learned and New Applications, December 1989, Atlanta, 1990, Georgia Regional Spinal Cord Injury Care System, Shepherd Spinal Center.
7. Donovan WH, Carter RE, Bedbrook GM et al: Incidence of medical complications in spinal cord injury: patients in specialized compared with nonspecialized centers, *Paraplegia* 22:282-290, 1984.
8. Frost FS: Role of rehabilitation after spinal cord injury, *Urol Clin North Am* 20:549-559, 1993.
9. Heinemann AW, Yarkony GM, Roth EJ et al: Functional outcome following spinal cord injury: a comparison of specialized spinal cord injury centers vs general hospital acute care, *Arch Neurol* 46:1098-1102, 1989.
10. Marino RJ, Ditunno JF, chairmen: *International standards for neurological classification of spinal cord injury,* Chicago, 2003, American Spinal Injury Association.
11. Finkbeiner K, Russo SG, editors: *Physical therapy management of spinal cord injury: accent on independence,* Fisherville, VA, 1990, Woodrow Wilson Rehabilitation Center Project SCIENTIA.
12. Hanak M, Scott A: *Spinal cord injury: an illustrated guide for healthcare professionals,* New York, 1983, Springer.
13. Donovan WH, Bedbrook G: Comprehensive management of spinal cord injury, *Clin Symp* 34:2-36, 1982.
14. Stover SL, DeLisa IA, Whiteneck GG: *Spinal cord injury: clinical outcomes from the model systems,* Gaithersburg, MD, 1995, Aspen Publications.
15. Ryan M, Klein S, Bongard F: Missed injuries associated with spinal cord trauma, *Am Surg* 59:371-374, 1993.
16. *Spinal cord injury: facts and figures at a glance,* Birmingham, AL, 1990, University of Alabama, National Spinal Cord Injury Statistical Center.
17. Young JS, Northrup NE: *Statistical information pertaining to some of the most commonly asked questions about SCI* [monograph], Phoenix, 1979, National Spinal Cord Injury Data Research Center.
18. DeVivo MJ, Richards JS, Stover SL et al: Spinal cord injury rehabilitation adds life to years, *West J Med* 154(suppl):602-606, 1991.
19. DeVivo MJ, Rutt RD, Black KJ et al: Trends in spinal cord injury demographics and treatment outcomes between 1973 and 1986, *Arch Phys Med Rehabil* 73:424-430, 1992.
20. Bosch A, Stauffer ES, Nickel VL: Incomplete traumatic quadriplegia: a 10 year review, *JAMA* 216: 473-478, 1971.
21. Cervical Spine Research Society: *The cervical spine,* ed 2, Philadelphia, 1989, JB Lippincott.
22. Frymoyer JW: *The adult spine—principles and practice, vol 2,* New York, 1983, Raven Press.
23. Meyer RR: *Surgery of spine trauma,* New York, 1989, Churchill Livingstone.
24. Yashon D: *Spinal injury,* ed 2, Norwalk, 1986, Appleton-Century-Crofts.
25. McArdle CB, Crofford MJ, Mirfakhraee M et al: Surface coil NR of spinal trauma: preliminary experience, *AJNR Am J Neuroradiol* 7:885-893, 1986.
26. White AH, Rothman RH, Ray CD: *Lumbar spine surgery techniques and complications,* St. Louis, 1987, CV Mosby.
27. Errico TJ, Bauer RD: *Spinal trauma,* Philadelphia, 1991, JB Lippincott.
28. Geisler FH: GM-1 ganglioside and motor recovery following human spinal cord injury, *J Emerg Med* 2:49-55, 1993.
29. Geisler FH, Dorsey FC, Coleman PW: Recovery of motor function after spinal cord injury: a randomized, placebo-controlled trial with GM-1 ganglioside, *N Engl J Med* 324:1829-1838, 1993.

30. *Annual reports 9 and 10 for the Model Spinal Cord Injury Care Systems*, Birmingham, 1992, National Spinal Cord Injury Statistical Center.

31. Bracken MB: Pharmacological treatment of acute spinal cord injury: current status and future projects, *J Emerg Med* 2:43-48, 1993.

32. Young W, Flamm ES: Effect of high-dose corticosteroid therapy on blood flow, evoked potentials, and extracellular calcium in experimental spinal injury, *J Neurosurg* 57:667-673, 1982.

33. Hall ED: The neuroprotective pharmacology of methylprednisolone: a review article, *J Neurosurg* 56:106-113, 1982.

34. Hall ED, Wolf DL, Baughler JM: Effects of a single large dose of methylprednisolone sodium succinate on experimental post traumatic spinal cord ischemia—dose response and time-action analysis, *J Neurosurg* 61:124-130, 1984.

35. Geisler FH, Coleman WP, Grieco G et al; Sygen Study Group: Measurements and recovery patterns in a multicenter study of acute spinal cord injury, *Spine* 26(24 suppl):568-586, 2001.

36. Bracken MB: Methylprednisolone and acute spinal cord injury: an update of the randomized evidence, *Spine* 26(24 Suppl):547-554, 2001.

37. Geisler FH, Coleman WP, Grieco G et al: The Sygen multi center acute spinal cord injury study, *Spine* 26(24 suppl):587-598, 2001.

38. Schwartz M, Moalem G: Beneficial immune activity after CNS injury: prospects for vaccination, *J Neuroimmunol* 113:185-192, 2001.

39. Hansebout RR, Blight AR, Fawcett S et al: 4-Amino pyridine in chronic spinal cord injury: a controlled double-blind, crossover study in eight patients, *J Neurotrauma* 10:1-18, 1993.

40. Ramirez JJ, Parach T, George MN et al: The effects of Neotrofin on septodentate sprouting after unilateral entorhinal cortex lesions in rats, *Restor Neurol Neurosci* 20:51-59, 2002.

41. Bregman BS, Coumans JV, Dai HN et al: Transplants and neurotrophic factors increase regeneration and recovery of function after spinal cord injury, *Prog Brain Res* 137:257-273, 2002.

42. Li Y, Field PM, Raisman G: Repair of adult rat corticospinal tract by transplants of olfactory ensheathing cells, *Science* 227:2000-2002, 1997.

43. Ramon-Cueto A: Olfactory ensheathing glia transplantation into the injured spinal cord, *Prog Brain Res* 128:265-672, 2000.

44. Thompson FJ, Reier PJ, Utman B et al: Neurophysiological assessment of the feasibility and safety of neural tissue transplantation in patients with syringomyelia, *J Neurotrauma* 18:931-945, 2001.

45. Savitz SI, Rosenbaum DM, Dinsmore JH et al: Cell transplatation for stroke, *Ann Neurol* 52:266-275, 2002.

46. Saporta S, Kim JJ, Willing AE et al: Human umbilical cord blood stem cells infusion in spinal cord injury: engraftment and beneficial influence on behavior, *J Hematother Stem Cell Res* 12:271-278, 2003.

47. *Standards manual for organizations serving people with disabilities*, Tucson, AR, 1993, Commission on Accreditation of Rehabilitation Facilities.

48. CCH Business Law, editor: *Medicare and Medicaid guideline 1993*, Chicago, 1993, Commerce Clearing House.

49. Hammell KR: Psychological and sociological theories concerning adjustment to traumatic spinal cord injury: the implication for rehabilitation, *Paraplegia* 30:317-326, 1992.

50. Hammell KR: Psychosocial outcome following spinal cord injury, *Paraplegia* 32:771-779, 1994.

51. *Guide to physical therapy practice*, Alexandria, VA, 1997, American Physical Therapy Association.

52. Katz RT, Rovai P, Brait C et al: Objective quantification of spastic hypertonia: Correlation with clinical findings, *Arch Phys Med Rehabil* 73:339-347, 1992.

53. Hamilton BB, Laughlin JA, Granger CV et al: Interrater agreement of the seven level functional independence measure (FIM), *Arch Phys Med Rehabil* 72:115-119, 1991.

54. Gresham GE, Labi ML, Dittmar SS et al: The quadriplegia index of function (QIF): sensitivity and reliability demonstrated in a study of thirty quadriplegic patients, *Paraplegia* 24: 38-44, 1986.

55. Catz A, Itzkovich M, Agranov E et al: The spinal cord independent measure (SCIM): sensitivity to functional changes in subgroups of spinal cord lesion patients. *Spinal Cord* 39:97-100, 2001.

56. Whiteneck GG, Charlifue SW, Gerhart KA: Quantifying handicap: a new measure of long-term rehabilitation outcomes, *Arch Phys Med Rehabil* 73:519-526, 1996.

57. Nixon V: *Spinal cord injury: a guide to functional outcomes in physical therapy management*, Rockville, MD, 1985, Aspen Systems Corporation.

58. Stover SL: Review of forty years of rehabilitation issues in spinal cord injury, *J Spinal Cord Med.* 18:175-182, 1995.

59. Mawson AR, Biundo JJ Jr, Neville P et al: Risk factors for early occurring pressure ulcers following spinal cord injury, *Am J Phys Med Rehabil* 67:123-127, 1988.

60. Yarkony G: Spinal cord injury rehabilitation. In Lee BY, Ostrander LE, Cochran GVB et al, editors: *The spinal cord injured patient: comprehensive management*, Philadelphia, 1991, WB Saunders.

61. Madsen B, Barth P, Vistnes L: Pressure sores: overview. In Lee BY, Ostrander LE, Cochran GVB et al, editors: *The spinal cord injured patient: comprehensive management*, Philadelphia, 1991, WB Saunders.

62. Abruzzesse R: Pressure sores: nursing aspects and prevention. In Lee BY, Ostrander LE, Cochran GVB et al, editors: *The spinal cord injured patient: comprehensive management*, Philadelphia, 1991, WB Saunders.

63. Somers MF: *Spinal cord injury: functional rehabilitation*, ed 2, East Norwalk, 2001, Appleton & Lange.

64. Krouskop T: The role of mattresses and beds in preventing pressure sores. In Lee BY, Ostrander LE, Cochran GVB et al, editors: *The spinal cord injured patient: comprehensive management*, Philadelphia, 1991, WB Saunders.

65. Bergstrom N, Bennett MA, Carlson CE et al: *Pressure ulcer treatment: clinical practice guideline, quick reference guide for clinicians*, No. 15. Rockville, MD, 1994, U.S. Department of Health and Human Services, Public Health Service, Agency for Health Care Policy and Research. AHCPR publication No. 95-0653.

66. Young R, Shahani B: Spasticity in spinal cord injured patients. In Bloch RF, Basbaum M, editors: *Management of spinal cord injuries*, Baltimore, 1986, Williams & Wilkins.

67. Wetzel JL, Lidnsford BR, Peterson MJ et al: Respiratory rehabilitation of the patient with a spinal cord injury. In Irwin S, Tecklin JS, editors: *Cardiopulmonary physical therapy*, ed 2, St. Louis, 1990, CV Mosby.

68. Trombly CA: *Occupational therapy for physical dysfunction*, Boston, 1995, Boston University, Sargent College of Allied Professions.

69. Krajnick SR, Bridle MJ: Hand splinting in quadriplegia: current practice, *Am J Occup Ther* 46:149-156, 1992.

70. Curtin M: Development of a tetraplegic hand assessment and splinting protocol, *Paraplegia* 32:159-169, 1994.

71. Hill JP: *Spinal cord injury: a guide to functional outcomes in occupational therapy*, Rockville, MD, 1986, Aspen Publishers.

72. Tenney CG, Lisa JM: *Atlas of hand splinting*, Boston, 1986, Little, Brown.

73. Sykes L, Campbell IG, Powell ES et al: Energy expenditure of walking for adult patients with spinal cord lesions using the reciprocating gait orthosis and functional electrical stimulation, *Spinal Cord* 34:659-665, 1996.

74. Hill J: The effects of casting on the upper extremity motor disorders after brain injury, *Am J Occup Ther* 48:3, 219-224, 1994.

75. Pierson S, Katz DI, Tarsy D: Botulinum toxin A in the treatment of spasticity: functional implications and patient selection, *Arch Phys Med Rehabil* 77: 717-721, 1996.

76. Corry IS, Cosgrove AP, Walsh EG et al: Botulinum toxin A in the hemiplegic upper limb: a double blind trial, *Dev Med Child Neurol* 39:185-193, 1997.

77. Gschwind C, Tonkin M: Classification and operative procedure for pronation deformity, *J Hand Surg* [Br] 17B:391-395, 1992.

78. Cusick BD: *Serial casts,* Tuscon, 1988, Therapy Skill Builders.

79. Hill J: *Education series: RIC97,* Chicago, 2002, Rehabilitation Institute of Chicago.

80. Carter RE: Medical management of pulmonary complications of spinal cord injury, *Adv Neurol* 22:261-269, 1979.

81. Crane LD: Functional anatomy and physiology of ventilation. In Zadai CC, editor: *Clinics in physical therapy: pulmonary management in physical therapy,* New York, 1992, Churchill Livingstone.

82. Luce JM, Culver BH: Respiratory muscle function in health and disease, *Chest* 81:82-90, 1982.

83. Morgan M, Silver J: The respiratory system of the spinal cord patient. In Bloch RF, Basbaum M, editors: *Management of spinal cord injuries,* Baltimore, 1986, Williams & Wilkins.

84. DeVivo MJ, Black KJ, Stover SL: Causes of death during the first 12 years after spinal cord injury, *Arch Phys Med Rehabil* 74:248-254, 1993.

85. De Troyer A, Estenne M: Review article: the expiratory muscles in tetraplegia, *Paraplegia* 29:359-363, 1991.

86. Clough P, Lindenauer D, Hayes M et al: Guidelines for routine respiratory care of patients with spinal cord injury, *Phys Ther* 66:1395-1402, 1986.

87. McCool FD, Pichurko BM, Slutsky AS et al: Changes in lung volume and rib cage configuration and abdominal binding in quadriplegia, *J Appl Physiol* 60:1198-1202, 1986.

88. Griffin J, Grush K: Spinal cord injury treatment and the anesthesiologist. In Lee BY, Ostrander LE, Cochran GVB et al, editors: *The spinal cord injured patient: comprehensive management,* Philadelphia, 1991, WB Saunders.

89. Rinehart M, Nawoczenski D: Respiratory care. In Buchanan L, Nawoczenski D, editors: *Spinal cord injury: concepts and management approaches,* Baltimore, 1987, Williams & Wilkins.

90. Brownlede S, Williams S: Physiotherapy in the respiratory care of patients with high spinal injury, *Physiotherapy* 73(3):148-152, 1987.

91. Derrickson J, Ciesla N, Simpson N et al: A comparison of two breathing exercise programs for patients with quadriplegia, *Phys Ther* 72:763-769, 1992.

92. Lee B: Deep vein thrombosis. In Lee BY, Ostrander LE, Cochran GVB et al, editors: *The spinal cord injured patient: comprehensive management,* Philadelphia, 1991, WB Saunders.

93. Vincken W, Corne L: Improved arterial oxygenation by diaphragmatic pacing in quadriplegia, *Crit Care Med* 15:872-873, 1987.

94. Onders RP, DiMarco AF, Ignagni AR et al: Mapping the phrenic nerve motor point: the key to a successful laparoscopic diaphragm pacing system in the first human series, *Surgery* 136:819-826, 2004.

95. Bach JR: New approaches in the rehabilitation of the traumatic high level quadriplegic, *Am J Phys Med Rehabil* 70:13-19, 1991.

96. West JB: *Pulmonary pathophysiology: the essentials,* ed 4, Baltimore, 1992, Williams & Wilkins.

97. Biering-Sorensen M, Biering-Sorensen F: Tracheostomy in spinal cord injured: frequency and follow up, *Paraplegia* 30:656-660, 1992.

98. Grenvik A, Downs J, Rasanen J et al, editors: *Mechanical ventilation and assisted respiration: contemporary management in critical care,* New York, 1991, Churchill Livingstone.

99. Shepherd AM, Blannin JP: The role of the nurse. In Mandelstam D, editor: *Incontinence and its management,* ed 2, pp 160-163, Dover, NH, 1986, Croom Helm.

100. Kraft C: Bladder and bowel management. In Buchanan LE, Nawoczenski DA, editors: *Spinal cord injury: concepts and management approaches,* pp 81-98, Baltimore, 1987, Williams & Wilkins.

101. Boninger ML, Souza AL, Cooper RA et al: Propulsion patterns and pushrim biomechanics in manual wheelchair propulsion, *Arch Phys Med Rehabil* 83:718-723, 2002.

102. Department of Veteran Affairs: *Physical fitness: a guide for individuals with spinal cord injury,* Washington, DC, 1996, Department of Veteran Affairs.

103. Stotts KM: Health maintenance: paraplegic athletes and non-athletes, *Arch Phys Med Rehabil* 67:109-114, 1986.

104. Yamasaki M, Irizawa M, Komura T et al: Daily energy expenditure in active and inactive persons with spinal cord injury, *J Hum Ergol* 21:125-133, 1992.

105. Arva J, Fitzherals SG, Cooper RA et al: Mechanical efficiency and user power requirement with a pushrim activated power assisted wheelchair, *Med Eng Phys* 23: 699-705, 2001.

106. Consortium for Spinal Cord Medicine: *Pressure ulcer prevention and treatment following spinal cord injury: a clinical practice guideline for healthcare professionals,* Washington, DC, 2000, Paralyzed Veterans of America.

107. Hooker SP, Wells CL: Effect of low and moderate intensity training in spinal cord injured persons, *Med Sci Sports Exerc* 21:18-22, 1989.

108. Hicks AL, Martin KA, Ditor DS et al: Long term exercise training in persons with spinal cord injury: effects on strength, arm ergometry performance and psychological well being, *Spinal Cord* 41:34-43, 2003.

109. Franklin BA, Vender L, Wrisley D et al: Aerobic requirements of arm ergometry: implications for exercise training and testing, *Physician Sports Med* 11:81-90, 1983.

110. Vanderthommen M: Multistage field test of wheelchair users for evaluation of fitness and prediction of peak oxygen uptake, *J Rehab Res Dev* 39:655-692, 2002.

111. Trieschmann RB: Psychosocial research in spinal cord injury: the state of the art, *Paraplegia* 30:58-60, 1992.

112. Trieschmann RB: *Spinal cord injuries: Psychological, social and vocational rehabilitation,* ed 2, New York, 1988, Demos Publications.

113. Zigler JE: Rehabilitation of acute spinal cord injury. In Hochschuler SH, Cotler HB, Guyer RD, editors: *Rehabilitation of the spine: science and practice,* St. Louis, 1993, CV Mosby.

114. Ducharme S, Gill K, Bergman S et al: Sexual functioning: medical and psychological aspects. In DeLisa JA, editor: *Rehabilitation medicine: principles and practice,* Philadelphia, 1988, JB Lippincott.

115. Smith EM, Bodner DR: Sexual dysfunction after spinal cord injury, *Urol Clin North Am* 20:535-541, 1993.

116. Axelson P, Phillips L, Ozer M et al: *Spinal cord injury: a guide for patient and family,* New York, 1987, Raven Press.

117. Krause JS, Kjorsvig JM: Mortality after spinal cord injury: a four-year prospective study, *Arch Phys Med Rehabil* 73:558-563, 1992.

118. Gross GR: What your company could be doing now to implement Title I of the ADA, *Small Business News* May 1992.

119. Freehafer AA, Peckham PH, Keith MW: New concepts on treatment of the upper limb in the tetraplegic, *Hand Clin* 4:563-572, 1988.

120. Welch RD, Lobley SJ, O'Sullivan SB et al: Functional levels in quadriplegia: critical levels, *Arch Phys Med Rehabil* 67:235-239, 1986.

121. Mendelson LS, Peckham PH, Freehafer AA et al: Interoperative assessment of wrist extensor muscle force, *J Hand Surg* 13A:832-836, 1988.

122. Gansel J, Waters R, Gelman H: Transfer of pronator teres tendon to the tendons of the flexor digitorum profundus in tetraplegia, *J Bone Joint Surg* 72A:427-432, 1990.

123. Kelly CM, Freehafer AA, Peckham PH et al: Postoperative results of opponensplasty and flexor tendon transfer in patients with spinal cord injuries, *J Hand Surg* 10A:890-894, 1985.

124. Barbeau H, Rossignol S: Recovery of locomotion after chronic spinalization in the adult cat, *Brain Res* 412:84-95, 1987.

125. MacKay-Lyons: Central pattern generation of locomotion: a review of the evidence, *Phys Ther* 82:69-83, 2002.

126. Field-Fote EC: Spinal cord control of movement: implication for locomotor rehabilitation following spinal cord injury, *Phys Ther* 80: 477-484, 2000.

127. Finch L, Barbeau H, Arsenault B: Influence of body weight support on normal human gait: development of a gait retraining strategy, *Phys Ther* 71:842-856, 1991.

128. Behrman A, Harkema S: Locomotor training after human spinal cord injury: a series of case studies, *Phys Ther* 80:688-700, 2000.

129. Field-Fote EC, Tepavac D: Improved intralimb coordination in people with incomplete spinal cord injury following training with body weight support and electric stimulation, *Phys Ther* 82:707-715, 2002.

130. Bromley I: Rehabilitation: Some thoughts on progress, *Paraplegia* 30:70-72, 1992.

131. Perry J: *Gait analysis: normal and pathological function,* Thorofare, NJ, 1992, Slack.

132. Goldberg B, Hsu JD, editors: *Atlas of orthotics and assistive devices,* ed 3, St. Louis, 1997, CV Mosby.

133. Lusardi M, Nielsen C, editors: *Orthotics and prosthetics in rehabilitation,* Woburn, MA, 2000, Butterworth-Heinemann.

134. Kral A, Bajd T: *Functional electrical stimulation: standing and walking after spinal cord injury,* Boca Raton, 1989, CRC Press.

135. Triolo RJ, Bogie K: Lower extremity application of functional neuromuscular stimulation after spinal cord injury, *Topics Spinal Cord Injury Rehabil* 5:44-65, 1995.

136. Johnston TE, Betz RR, Smith BT et al: Implanted functional electrical stimulation: an alternative for standing and walking in pediatric spinal cord injury, *Spinal Cord* 41: 44-52, 2003.

137. Gallien P, Brissot R, Eyssette M et al: Restoration of gait by functional electrical stimulation for spinal cord injured patients, *Paraplegia* 33:660-664, 1995.

138. Marsolais EB, Edwards BG: Energy costs of walking and standing with functional neuromuscular stimulation and long leg braces, *Arch Phys Med Rehabil* 69:243-249, 1988.

139. Carhart MR, He J, Herman R et al: Epidural spinal-cord stimulation facilitates recovery of functional walking following incomplete spinal-cord injury, *IEEE Trans Neural Syst Rehabil Eng* 12:32-42, 2004.

140. Kobetoc R, Marsolais EB, Triolo FJ et al: Development of a hybrid gait orthosis: a case report. *J Spinal Cord Med* 26:254-258, 2003.

141. Kreutz DL: Seating and positioning for the newly injured, *Rehab Manag* 6:67-74, 1993.

142. Zarcharkow D: *Wheelchair posture and pressure sores,* Springfield, IL, 1984, Charles C Thomas.

143. Brubaker C: Ergonometric considerations, *J Rehabil Res Dev* 2(suppl):37-48, 1990.

144. Green D, Hull RD, Mammen EF et al: Deep vein thrombosis in spinal cord injury: summary and recommendations, *Chest* 102:633S-635S, 1992.

145. Mammen EF: Pathogenesis of venous thrombosis, *Chest* 102:640S-644S, 1992.

146. Merli GJ, Crabbe S, Doyle L et al: Mechanical plus pharmacological prophylaxis for deep vein thrombosis in acute spinal cord injury, *Paraplegia* 30:558-562, 1992.

147. Consortium for Spinal cord Medicine: *Prevention of thromboembolism in spinal cord injury,* Washington, DC, 2001, Paralyzed Veterans of America.

148. Bloch RF: Autonomic dysfunction. In Bloch RF, Basbaum M, editors: *Management of spinal cord injuries,* Baltimore, 1986, Williams & Wilkins.

149. Curry K, Casady L: The relationship between extended periods of immobility and decubitus ulcer formation in the acutely spinal cord injured individual, *J Neurosci Nurs* 24:185-189, 1992.

150. Lewis KS, Mueller WM: Intrathecal baclofen for severe spasticity secondary to spinal cord injury, *Ann Pharmacother* 27:767-774, 1993.

151. Coffey RJ, Cahill D, Steers W et al: Intrathecal baclofen for intractable spasticity of spinal origin: results of a long-term multicenter study, *J Neurosurg* 78:226-232, 1993.

152. Mariano AJ: Chronic pain and spinal cord injury, *Clin J Pain* 8:87-92, 1992.

153. Galer BS, Dworkin RH: *A clinical guide to neuropathic pain,* New York, 2000, McGraw Hill.

154. Stover SL: Heterotopic ossification after spinal cord injury. In Bloch RF, Bashaum M, editors: *Management of spinal cord injuries,* Baltimore, 1986, Williams & Wilkins.

155. Kuijk AA, Geurtz ACH, Kuppruelt HJM: Neurogenic heterotopic ossification, *Spinal Cord* 40:313-326, 2002.

156. Garland DE, Stewart CA, Adkins RH et al: Osteoporosis after spinal cord injury, *J Orthop Res* 10:371-378, 1992.

157. Seaton T, Hollingworth R: Gastrointestinal complications in spinal cord injury. In Bloch RF, Basbaum M, editors: *Management of spinal cord injuries,* Baltimore, 1986, Williams & Wilkins.

APPENDIX 19-A ■ Selected References

Sexual Issues

Althof SE, Levine SB: Clinical approach to the sexuality of patients with spinal cord injury, *Urol Clin North Am* 20:527-534, 1993.

Berard EJ: The sexuality of spinal cord injured women physiology and pathophysiology: a review, *Paraplegia* 27:99-112, 1989.

Charlifue SW, Gerhart KA, Menter RR et al: Sexual issues of women with spinal cord injuries, *Paraplegia* 30:192-199, 1992.

Drench ME: Impact of altered sexuality and sexual function in spinal cord injury: a review, *Sex Disabil* 10:3-14, 1992.

Farrow J: Sexuality counseling with clients who have spinal cord injuries, *Rehabil Couns Bull* 33:251-259, 1990.

Kettl P, Zarefoss S, Jacoby K et al: Female sexuality after spinal cord injury, *Sex Disabil* 9:287-295, 1991.

Lemon MA: Sexual counseling and spinal cord injury, *Sex Disabil* 11:73-97, 1993.

Lloyd LK, Richards JS: Medical and psychological considerations regarding the surgical or pharmacological treatment of impotence in males with spinal cord injury, *J Rehabil Res Dev* 28:419-420, 1991.

Nygaard I, Bartscht KD, Cole S: Sexuality and reproduction in spinal cord injured women, *Obstet Gynecol Surg* 45:727-732, 1990.

Robbins KH: Traumatic spinal cord injury and its impact upon sexuality, *J Appl Rehabil Couns* 16:24-27, 1985.

Sipski ML, Alexander CJ: Sexual activities, response and satisfaction in women pre- and post-spinal cord injury, *Arch Phys Med Rehabil* 74:1025-1029, 1993.

Tepper MS: Sexual education in spinal cord injury rehabilitation: current trends and recommendations, *Sex Disabil* 10:15-31, 1992.

Trieschmann RB: *Spinal cord injuries: psychological, social, and vocational rehabilitation,* ed 2, New York, 1988, Demos.

White MJ, Rintala DH, Hart KA et al: Sexual activities, concerns and interests of men with spinal-cord injury, *Am J Phys Med Rehabil* 71:225-231, 1992.

Architectural Modification

Accessibility in Georgia: a technical and policy guide to access in Georgia, Raleigh, NC, 1986, Georgia Council on Developmental Disabilities.

An accessible bathroom, Madison, WI, 1980, Design Coalition.

An accessible entrance: ramps, Madison, WI, 1979, Design Coalition.

Handbook for design: specially adapted housing, Veterans Administration pamphlet 26-13, Washington, DC, 1978, Department of Veterans Benefits, Veterans Administration.

Harber L, Mae R, Orleans P et al: *UFAS retrofit guide: accessibility modifications for existing buildings,* New York, 1993, Van Nostrand Reinhold.

Lebrock C, Behar S: *Beautiful barrier-free: a visual guide to accessibility,* New York, 1993, Van Nostrand Reinhold.

Mace RL: *The accessible housing design file,* New York, 1991, Van Nostrand Reinhold.

CHAPTER 20

Inflammatory and Infectious Disorders of the Brain

Judith A. Dewane, MHS, PT, NCS

Rebecca E. Porter, PhD, PT

KEY WORDS

brain abscess
encephalitis
functional activities
hypertonicity
hypotonicity
intervention goals
meningitis
postural control

OBJECTIVES

After reading this chapter the student/therapist will be able to:

1. Discuss the terminology for classifying different types of inflammatory and infectious disorders within the brain.
2. Discuss the range of neurological sequelae that occur.
3. Discuss the components of the comprehensive evaluation process and their interrelationships.
4. Structure the evaluation process to gather the information required to generate an intervention plan.
5. Discuss the general goals of the intervention process.
6. Plan the intervention process to meet the needs of the client.
7. Locate resources (both within this book and elsewhere) to assist with ideas for the intervention program.

The diversity of neurological sequelae that may occur after an inflammatory disorder in the brain (brain abscess, encephalitis, or meningitis) provides a range of challenges to the rehabilitation team. The therapist must identify the problems underlying the individual's movement dysfunctions without the template of the cluster of "typical" problems available with some other neurological diagnoses. Each client presents a combination of problems that is unique to that client and that requires the creative design of an intervention program. The following discussion of the therapeutic management of individuals recovering from an inflammatory disorder in the brain focuses on the process of designing an intervention plan to address the specific dysfunctions of the individual client. Because the management of the clinical problems is built on an understanding of the underlying pathological condition and because therapists may not be as familiar with these disease processes, an overview of the inflammatory disorders of the brain is presented.

OVERVIEW OF INFLAMMATORY DISORDERS IN THE BRAIN

Categorization of Inflammatory Disorders

Inflammatory disorders of the brain can be categorized based on the anatomical location of the inflammatory process and the cause of the infection, as shown below:

A. Brain abscess
B. Meningitis (leptomeningitis)
  1. Bacterial meningitis
  2. Aseptic meningitis (viral)
C. Encephalitis
  1. Acute viral
  2. Parainfectious encephalomyelitis
  3. Acute toxic encephalopathy
  4. Progressive viral encephalitis
  5. "Slow virus" encephalitis

In most individuals, the defense mechanisms of the central nervous system (CNS) provide protection from infecting organisms. Compromises of the protective barriers can result in CNS infections as complications of common infections. The response of the CNS to the infection depends on several factors, including the type of organism, its route of entry, the CNS location of the infection, and the immunological competence of the individual. CNS infections occur with greater frequency and severity in individuals who are very young or elderly, immunodeficient, or antibody deficient.

The inflammatory process may be a localized, circumscribed collection of pus; may involve primarily the leptomeninges; may involve the brain substance; or may involve both the meninges and the brain substance. The infecting agents may be bacterial, fungal, viral, protozoan, or parasitic. The most common agents producing meningitis are bacterial; the most common agents producing encephalitis are viral. However, bacterial encephalitis and viral meningitis also are disease entities. The following overview of the inflammatory processes within the brain is organized based on the anatomical location of the infection. More comprehensive discussions based on specific infecting organisms can be found in the references at the end of the chapter. The site of the infection will determine the signs and symptoms of the CNS infections, whereas the infecting organism determines the time course and severity of the problems.[1]

Brain Abscess

Brain abscesses occur when microorganisms reach brain tissue from a penetrating wound to the brain, by extension of local infection such as sinusitis or otitis, or by hematogenous spread from a distant site of infection. The route of infection influences the CNS region involved. The extension of a local infection tends to produce a solitary brain abscess in an adjacent lobe. Multiple abscesses may originate from the spread of microorganisms through the blood. The introduction of microorganisms by a penetrating trauma may result in an abscess soon after the trauma or several years later. As with the disorders presented in the subsequent discussions, circumstances that result in a compromised immune system (chronic corticosteroid or other immunosuppressive drug administration, administration of cytotoxic chemotherapeutic agents, or human immunodeficiency virus [HIV] infection) may predispose the individual to develop opportunistic infections.

Whereas the site and size of the abscess influence the initial symptoms, evidence of increased intracranial pressure, a focal neurological deficit, and fever is described as the classic presenting triad;[2] however, the classic triad occurs in less than 50% of patients.[3] Most individuals experience an alteration of consciousness. In 47% of the cases, the frontal, parietal, or temporal lobe is involved.[3] Medical management of the abscess typically consists of antibiotic therapy (depending on the infecting agent and size and site of the abscess) and, often, surgical aspiration or excision. Bharucha et al[2] describe neurological sequelae in 25% to 50% of the survivors, with 30% to 50% having persistent seizures, 15% to 30% with hemiparesis, and 10% to 20% with disorders of speech or language.

Meningitis

Meningitis (synonymous with leptomeningitis) denotes an infection spread through the cerebrospinal fluid (CSF) with the inflammatory process involving the pia and arachnoid maters, the subarachnoid space, and the adjacent superficial tissues of the brain and spinal cord. Pachymeningitis denotes an inflammatory process involving the dura mater. Meningitis can be caused by a wide variety of organisms, some of which cross the blood-brain barrier and the blood-CSF barrier. The CSF also can become contaminated by a wound that penetrates the meninges as a result of trauma or a medical procedure, such as implantation of a ventriculoperitoneal shunt. Once the organism compromises the blood-brain and blood-CSF barriers, the CSF provides an ideal medium for growth. All the body's typical major defense systems are essentially absent in the normal CSF. The blood-brain barrier may impede the clearance of infecting organisms by leukocytes and interfere with the entry of pharmacological agents from the blood. The infecting organism is disseminated throughout the subarachnoid space as the contaminated CSF bathes the brain. Entry into the ventricles occurs either from the choroid plexuses or by reflux through the exit foramen of the fourth ventricle. The spread of the organism through the CSF circulation accounts for the differences in the variety and extent of the neurological sequelae that can result from meningitis.

Bacterial Meningitis

Clinical Problems. The diagnostic categorization of meningitis depends on the infecting agent (e.g., *Haemophilus influenzae* meningitis, *Streptococcus pneumoniae* meningitis, and viral meningitis) and on the acute or chronic nature of the meningitis (acute, subacute, or chronic meningitis). The term *acute bacterial meningitis* denotes infections caused by aerobic bacteria (both gram-positive and gram-negative).[4] The most common infecting organism producing acute bacterial meningitis varies according to the age of the population. During the neonatal period and in the older adult, infections by gram-negative enterobacilli, especially *Escherichia coli,* and group B streptococci occur most frequently. Typical causative agents in children include *H. influenzae, Neisseria meningitidis,* and *S. pneumonia.*[5] *S. pneumoniae, N. meningitidis,* and *H. influenzae* are the most common causes of community-acquired meningitis.[5,6] Individuals with conditions such as sickle cell anemia, alcoholism, or diabetes mellitus, and individuals who are immunosuppressed are at increased risk.[7] Meningococcus bacterium has been implicated in meningitis that strikes young children most often but can also infect adolescents and young adults. Freshman who live in dormitories are almost four times more likely to get meningitis than other college students.

An example of an organism that uses a typical systemic route of bacterial infection is the *H. influenzae* organism that is a normal flora of the nose and throat. During an upper respiratory tract infection, the organism may gain entry to the blood. The route of transmission of the organism from the blood to the CSF is not well established.

The circulation of CSF spreads the infecting organism through the ventricular system and the subarachnoid spaces (Figure 20-1). The pia and arachnoid maters become acutely inflamed, and as part of the inflammatory response, a purulent exudate forms in the subarachnoid space. The exudate may undergo organization, resulting in an obstruction of the foramen of Monro, the aqueduct of Sylvius, or the exit foramen of the fourth ventricle. The supracortical subarachnoid spaces proximal to the arachnoid villi may be obliterated, resulting in a noncommunicating or obstructive hydrocephalus caused by the accumulation of CSF. As the CSF accumulates, the intracranial pressure rises. The increased intracranial pressure produces venous obstruction, precipitating a further increase in the intracranial pressure. The rise in the CSF pressure compromises the cerebral blood flow, which activates reflex mechanisms to counteract the decreased cerebral blood flow by raising the systemic blood pressure. An increased systemic blood pressure accompanies increased CSF pressure.

The mechanism producing the headaches that accompany increased intracranial pressure may be the stretching of the meninges and pain fibers associated with blood vessels. Vomiting may occur as a result of stimulation of the medullary emetic centers. Papilledema may occur as intracranial pressure increases.

Other routes of bacterial infection may involve a local spread as the result of an infection of the middle ear or mastoid air cells. Meningitis may occur as a complication of a skull fracture (open-head injury; Chapter 17), which exposes CNS tissue to the external environment or to the nasal cavity. Fractures of the cribriform plate of the ethmoid

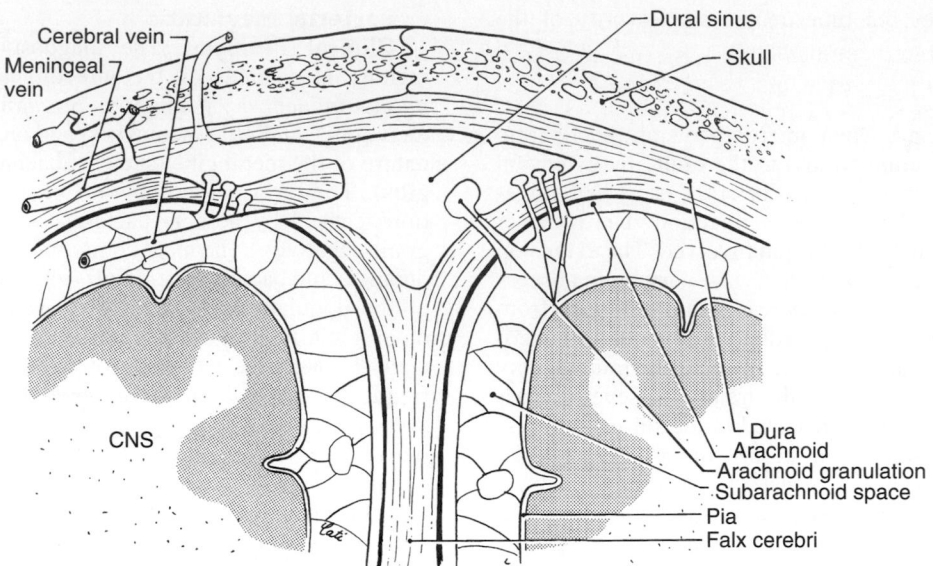

FIGURE 20-1 ■ The meninges, showing the layers of the dura, arachnoid, and pia mater and their relationship to the subarachnoid space and brain tissue. (From: Felten MD, Felten SY: A regional and systemic overview of functional neuroanatomy. In Farber SD, editor: *Neurorehabilitation: a multisensory approach,* Philadelphia, 1982, Saunders, p. 6.)

bone producing CSF rhinorrhea provide another route for infection. Meningitis may be a further complication to the clinical problems of a traumatic head injury.

Clinical features of acute bacterial meningitis include fever, severe headache, altered consciousness, convulsions (particularly in children), and nuchal rigidity. Nuchal rigidity is indicative of an irritative lesion of the subarachnoid space. Cervical flexion is painful because it stretches the inflamed meninges, nerve roots, and spinal cord. The pain triggers a reflex spasm of the neck extensors to splint the area against further cervical flexion; however, cervical rotation and extension movements remain relatively free.

Several clinical tests are used to demonstrate nuchal rigidity. The Kernig test consists of flexion of the cervical area with the client supine. Signs of pain indicate a positive test.[8] The Kernig sign refers to a test performed with the client supine in which the thigh is flexed on the abdomen and the knee extended (Figure 20-2). This pulls on the sciatic nerve, which pulls on the covering of the spinal cord, causing pain in the presence of meningeal irritation. The same results are achieved with passive hip flexion with the knee remaining in extension. This is the same procedure described by Hoppenfeld[8] as the straight-leg raising test for determining pathology of the sciatic nerve or tightness of the hamstrings. Passive hip flexion with knee extension can be painful because of meningeal irritation, spinal root impingement, sciatic nerve irritation, or hamstring tightness. Roos advocates performing the test for the Kernig sign with the individual sitting.[5] The Brudzinski sign refers to the flexion of the hips and knees elicited when cervical flexion (the Kernig test in supine) is performed[5] (Figure 20-2). These signs will not be present in the deeply comatose client who has decreased muscle tone and absence of muscle reflexes. The signs may also be absent in the infant or elderly patient.

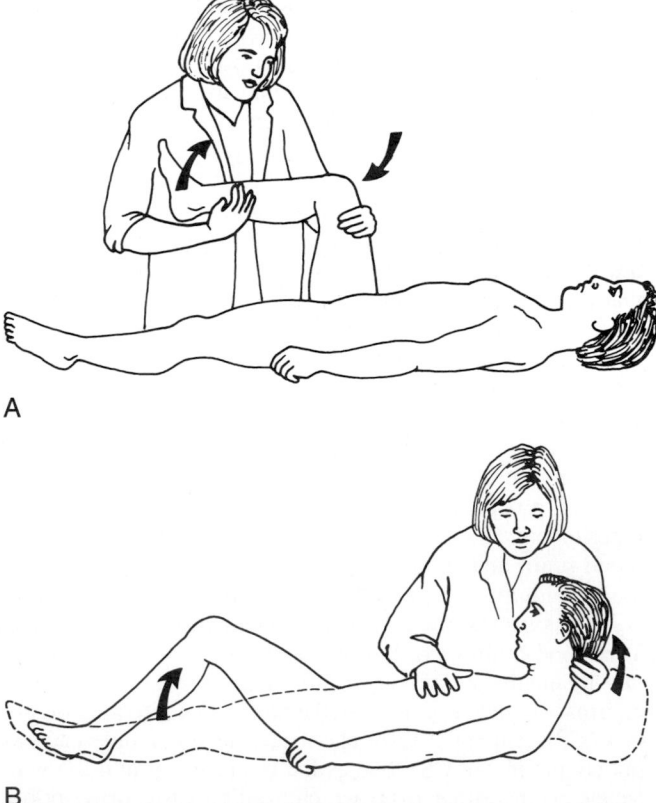

A

B

FIGURE 20-2 ■ Kernig's and Brudzinski's signs. (From: Felten MD, Felten SY: A regional and systemic overview of functional neuroanatomy. In Farber SD, editor: *Neurorehabilitation: a multisensory approach,* Philadelphia, 1982, Saunders, 1982, p. 6.)

The diagnosis of bacterial meningitis can be established based on blood cultures and a sample of CSF obtained by a lumbar puncture. CSF pressure is consistently elevated. The CSF sample in bacterial meningitis typically reveals an increased protein count and a decreased glucose level.

The type and severity of the sequelae of acute bacterial meningitis relate directly to the area affected, the extent of CNS infection, the age and general health of the individual, the level of consciousness at the initiation of pharmacological therapy, and the pathological agent involved. Some of the common CNS complications include subdural effusions, altered levels of consciousness, seizures, involvement of the cranial nerves, and increased intracranial pressure.

Medical Management. Medical management of bacterial meningitis consists of the initiation of the antimicrobial regimen appropriate to the infecting organism and procedures to manage the signs and symptoms of meningitis that have been described in the preceding paragraphs. Medical intervention strategies in both these areas change with the development of new pharmacological agents. Thus, medical management can change within short periods. The reader is encouraged to always review recent literature for additional information on current aspects of the medical management of the client with meningitis.

Prevention. Vaccination has significantly decreased the incidence of meningitis from *Haemophilus influenzae* type B in young children and infants. College freshmen who live in dormitories are four times more likely than other college students to develop meningococcus meningitis, and there is now a vaccine that has shown promise in reducing the outbreak rate.

Potential Neurological Sequelae. Even with optimal antimicrobial therapy, bacterial meningitis continues to have a finite mortality rate, which varies with the infecting organism, age of the individual, and time lapse to initiation of treatment, and has the potential for marked neurological morbidity. Neurological sequelae occur in 20% to 50% of the cases.[7] Bacterial meningitis is considered a medical emergency; delays in initiation of antibacterial therapy increase the risk of complications and permanent neurological dysfunction.[7]

Reports of the long-term outcome of individuals with bacterial meningitis indicate that up to 20% have long-term neurological sequelae.[2] The sequelae may be the result of the acute infectious pathological condition or subacute or chronic pathological changes. The acute infectious pathological condition could result in sequelae such as inflammatory or vascular involvement of the cranial nerves or thrombosis of the meningeal veins. Cranial nerve palsies, especially sensorineural hearing loss, are common complications. The risk of an acute ischemic stroke is greatest during the first 5 days.[7] Weeks to months after treatment, subacute or chronic pathological changes may develop, such as communicating hydrocephalus, which presents as difficulties with gait, mental status changes, and incontinence.[9] Approximately 5% of the survivors will have weakness and spasticity.[4] Focal cerebral signs that may occur either early or late in the course of bacterial meningitis include hemiparesis, ataxia, seizures, cranial nerve palsies, and gaze preference.[10] Cognitive slowness has been found in 27% of clients following pneumococcal meningitis, even with

good recovery as documented by a Glasgow Outcome Scale score of 5.[11]

Damage to the cerebral cortex can result in numerous expressions of dysfunction. Motor system dysfunction may be the observable expression of the damage within the CNS, but the location of the damage may include sensory and processing areas, as well as those areas typically categorized as belonging to the motor system. Perceptual deficits or regression in cognitive skills may present residual problems. Cranial nerve involvement is most frequently expressed as dysfunction of the eighth cranial nerve complex and produces auditory and vestibular deficits.

Aseptic Meningitis. Aseptic meningitis refers to a nonpurulent inflammatory process confined to the meninges and choroid plexus, usually caused by contamination of the CSF with a viral agent, although other agents can trigger the reactions. The symptoms are similar to acute bacterial meningitis but typically are less severe. The individual may be irritable, lethargic, and complain of a headache, but cerebral function remains normal unless unusual complications occur.[12] Aseptic meningitis of a viral origin usually has a benign and relatively short course of illness.[13,14]

A variety of neurotropic viruses can produce aseptic (viral) meningitis. The enteroviruses (echoviruses and the Coxsackie viruses), herpesviruses, and HIV are the most common causes.[5,15] The primary nonviral causes of aseptic meningitis are Lyme *Borrelia* and *Leptospira*.[16] The diagnosis of this type of aseptic meningitis may be established by isolation of the infecting agent within the CSF or by other techniques. The glucose level of the CSF in bacterial meningitis is usually depressed; however, the glucose level in viral meningitis is normal.[1]

Treatment of aseptic meningitis consists of management of symptoms. The condition does not typically produce residual neurological sequelae, and full recovery is anticipated within a few days to a few weeks.

Encephalitis

Clinical Problems. Encephalitis refers to a group of diseases characterized by inflammation of the parenchyma of the brain and its surrounding meninges. Although a variety of agents can produce an encephalitis, the term usually denotes a viral invasion of the cells of the brain and spinal cord.

Different cell populations within the CNS vary in their susceptibility to infection by a specific virus. (For example, the viruses responsible for poliomyelitis have a selective affinity for the motor neurons of the brain stem and spinal cord. Viruses such as Coxsackie viruses and echoviruses typically infect meningeal cells to cause the benign viral meningitis discussed in the previous section.) In acute encephalitis, neurons that are vulnerable to the specific virus are invaded and undergo lysis. Viral encephalitis presents a syndrome of elevated temperature, headache, nuchal rigidity, vomiting, and general malaise (symptoms of aseptic or viral meningitis), with the addition of evidence of more extensive cerebral damage such as coma, cranial nerve palsy, hemiplegia, involuntary movements, or ataxia. The difficulty in differentiating between acute viral meningitis and acute viral encephalitis is reflected in the use of the term *meningoencephalitis* in some cases.

The pathological condition includes destruction or damage to neurons and glial cells resulting from invasion of the cells by the virus, the presence of intranuclear inclusion bodies, edema, and inflammation of the brain and spinal cord. Perivascular cuffing by polymorphonuclear leukocytes and lymphocytes may occur as well as angiitis of small blood vessels. Widespread destruction of the white matter by the inflammatory process and by thrombosis of the perforating vessels can occur. Increased intracranial pressure, which can result from the cerebral edema and vascular damage, presents the potential for a transtentorial herniation. The likelihood of residual impairment of neurological functions depends on the infecting viral agent. Patients with mumps meningoencephalitis have an excellent prognosis, whereas 55% of the individuals with herpes simplex encephalitis treated with acyclovir have some neurological sequelae.[4] Because of the slow recovery of injured brain tissue, even in patients who recover completely, return to normal function may take months.[17]

Plum and Posner[18] discuss viral encephalitis in terms of five pathological syndromes. Acute viral encephalitis is a primary or exclusively CNS infection. An example would be herpes simplex encephalitis, in which the virus shows a predilection for the gray matter of the temporal lobe, insula, cingulate gyrus, and inferior frontal lobe. Also included are the mosquito-borne viruses. Parainfectious encephalomyelitis is associated with viral infections such as measles, mumps, or varicella. Acute toxic encephalopathy denotes an encephalitis that occurs during the course of a systemic infection with a common virus. The clinical symptoms are produced by the cerebral edema in acute toxic encephalopathy, which results in increased intracranial pressure and the risk of transtentorial herniation. Reye's syndrome is an example. Global neurological signs, such as hemiplegia or aphasia, are usually present rather than focal signs. The clinical symptoms of the previous three syndromes may be similar. Specific diagnosis may be established only by biopsy or autopsy.

Progressive viral infections occur from common viruses invading susceptible individuals, such as those who are immunosuppressed or during the perinatal to early childhood period. Slow, progressive destruction of the CNS occurs, as in subacute sclerosing panencephalitis. The final category of encephalitis syndromes consists of "slow virus" infections by unconventional agents (the prion diseases) that produce progressive dementing diseases such as Creutzfeldt-Jakob disease and kuru.[19]

Medical Management. The medical management of virally induced encephalitis has been, and with many infecting agents remains, primarily symptomatic. In some cases, intensive, aggressive care is necessary to sustain life. Pharmacological interventions are available to treat some viral infections, such as herpes encephalitis. The probability of neurological sequelae differs according to the infecting agent. Aggressive management of increased intracranial pressure is required because persistently elevated intracranial pressure is associated with poor outcome.[20] Further information concerning the clinical features, medical management, and potential for neurological sequelae of a specific type of encephalitis should be sought in the literature based on the infecting agent.

Clinical Picture of the Individual with Inflammatory Disorders of the Brain

An individual within the acute phase of meningitis or encephalitis or with residual neurologic dysfunction from these disorders may demonstrate signs and symptoms similar to generalized brain trauma, tumor disorder, or other identified abnormal neurological state. The variability in the clinical picture is reflected in the inclusion of the category of "infectious diseases that affect the central nervous system" in the *Guide to Physical Therapist Practice.*[21] Practice patterns for physical therapists that apply to this population include the following:

5C: Impaired Motor Function and Sensory Integrity Associated with Nonprogressive Disorders of the Central Nervous System—Congenital Origin or Acquired in Infancy or Childhood

5D: Impaired Motor Function and Sensory Integrity Associated with Nonprogressive Disorders of the Central Nervous System—Acquired in Adolescence or Adulthood

5I: Impaired Arousal, Range of Motion, and Motor Control Associated with Coma, Near Coma, or Vegetative State

5A: Primary Prevention/Risk Reduction for Loss of Balance and Falling

Although these patterns have been identified within the physical therapy practice patterns, the concepts and selection of evaluation and intervention procedures are just as applicable for occupational therapists and other individuals working on movement dysfunction. In the acute phase, the inflammatory process may result in impairments in arousal and attention, which range from an individual who is nonresponsive to an individual who is in an agitated state. The degree of agitation may range from mild to severe, depending on both the client's unique CNS characteristics and the degree of inflammation. The agitated state may be the result of alterations in the processing of sensory input, with the consequence of inappropriate or augmented responses to sensory input. The client may respond to a normal level of sound as though it were an unbearably loud noise. Low levels of artificial light may be perceived as extremely bright.

Perceptual and cognitive impairments may be present, resulting in a variety of functional limitations and disabilities. Clients may have distortions in their perception of events as well as memory problems. As their memory returns, accuracy of time and events may be distorted, leading to frustration and anxiety for both the client and those family and friends who are interacting within the environment.

In addition to alterations in mentation, the individual may demonstrate impaired affect, such as a hypersensitivity or exaggerated emotional responses to seemingly normal interactions. For example, when upset about dropping a spoon on the floor, a client may throw the tray across the table. When another individual was told his girlfriend would be a little late for her afternoon visit, the client became extremely upset and stated his intent to kill himself because his girlfriend did not love him anymore.

Because of the variety of pathological problems after acute inflammation, the client may have residual problems manifested as generalized or focal brain damage. The specifics of these impairments cannot be described as a typical clinical picture because they are extremely dependent on the individual client. These variations require the therapist to conduct a thorough examination and evaluation process to develop an appropriate individualized intervention program. Although content from the *Guide to Physical Therapist Practice* has been incorporated into the discussion of the examination, evaluation, and intervention processes, the model presented provides a structure that can accommodate the specific disciplinary expertise of both occupational and physical therapists.

EXAMINATION AND EVALUATION PROCESS

Just as the medical intervention with clients who have an inflammatory disorder of the CNS is, to a large extent, symptomatic, so is the intervention by therapists. Designing an individualized intervention program based on the client's problems necessitates a comprehensive initial and ongoing evaluation to define the impairments, functional limitations, and disabilities and to note changes in them. Although the discussion of examination procedures is separated from the discussion of intervention strategies, it must be recognized that the separation is artificial and does not reflect the image of practice. The evaluation process should be considered in relationship to both the long-term assessment of the individual's changes and the short-term within-session and between-session variations. For example, documentation of the level of consciousness of a client on day one of intervention will provide a starting point for calculation of the distance spanned at the time of discharge. Perhaps more critical to the final outcome is determination of the level of consciousness before, during, and after a particular intervention technique to determine its impact on the individual's level of arousal and ability to interact with the environment. The evaluation process is a constant activity intertwined with intervention. The observations and data from the process are periodically recorded to establish the course of the disease process and the success of the therapeutic management of the client.

Observation of Current Functional Status

The evaluation process should be conceptualized as a decision-making tree that requires the therapist to determine actively which components are to be included in a detailed examination and which can be eliminated or deferred. The first step in this process is the observation of the client's current functional status. If the client is comatose and nonmobile, the focus of the initial session might be an assessment of the stability of physiological functions, level of consciousness, responses to sensory input, and joint mobility. If the client is an outpatient with motor control deficits, the initial session might focus on defining motor abilities and components contributing to movement dysfunctions with a more superficial assessment of physiological functions and level of consciousness. The therapist must be alert to indications of the need for a more detailed evaluation of perceptual and cognitive function (e.g., the client cannot follow two-step commands, indicating the need to assess cognitive skills).

Some of the components discussed in the evaluation process may be assessment skills that are more typically possessed by other professions (e.g., assessment of emotional/psychological status). The inclusion of these items is not meant to suggest that the therapist must complete the formal testing. The items are included to indicate factors that will affect goal setting for the client and that will have an impact on the intervention strategy. Although the therapist may not be the health care team member who has primary responsibility for evaluation of these areas, he or she should recognize these areas as potential contributors to movement dysfunctions.

Observation of the current functional status of the client provides the therapist with an initial overview of his assets and deficits. This provides the framework into which the pieces of information from the evaluation of specific aspects of function can be fit. The therapist must not allow assumptions made during the initial observation to bias later observations. The therapist might note that the client is able to roll from the supine to the side-lying position to interact with visitors in the room. When the same activity is not repeated on the mat table in the treatment area, the therapist, knowing the client has the motor skill to roll, might conclude that he is uncooperative, or apraxic, or has perceptual deficits. The therapist may have failed to consider that the difference between the two situations is the type of support surface or the presence or absence of side rails, which may have enabled the client to roll in bed by pulling over to the side-lying position. It is characteristic of human observation skills that we tend to "see" what we expect to see. The therapist must attempt to observe behaviors and note potential explanations for deviations from normal without biasing the results of the subsequent observations.

The following discussion of the specific considerations within the evaluation process does not necessarily represent the temporal sequence to be used during the examination data collection process. As different items are discussed, suggestions for potential combinations of items will be made. The sequence of the process is best determined by the interaction of therapist and client. Figure 20-3 outlines the components that should be considered during the evaluation process and provides a synopsis of the following discussion.

The general philosophy in the evaluation of the client with neurological deficits as a result of brain inflammation is a whole-part-whole approach. General observations of the client's performance provide an overall description of the client's abilities while indicating deficits in his or her performance. The cause(s) of the deficits (impairments) is explored to provide the pieces of data defining her or his performance. These pieces of data then are arranged within the framework provided by the general observation to define the whole of the client's assets and deficits. As the whole picture is established (with the realization that it will be constantly adjusted), the process of goal setting is initiated. These goals need to incorporate the patient's and family's desires. The process presented for refining evaluation data into an intervention plan is applicable whether the client's neurological dysfunction is the result of a bacterial or viral infection, cerebrovascular accident, trauma, or other factors.

Evaluation of Physiological Responses to Therapeutic Activities

It is assumed that the therapist enters the initial interaction with a client after reviewing the available background infor-

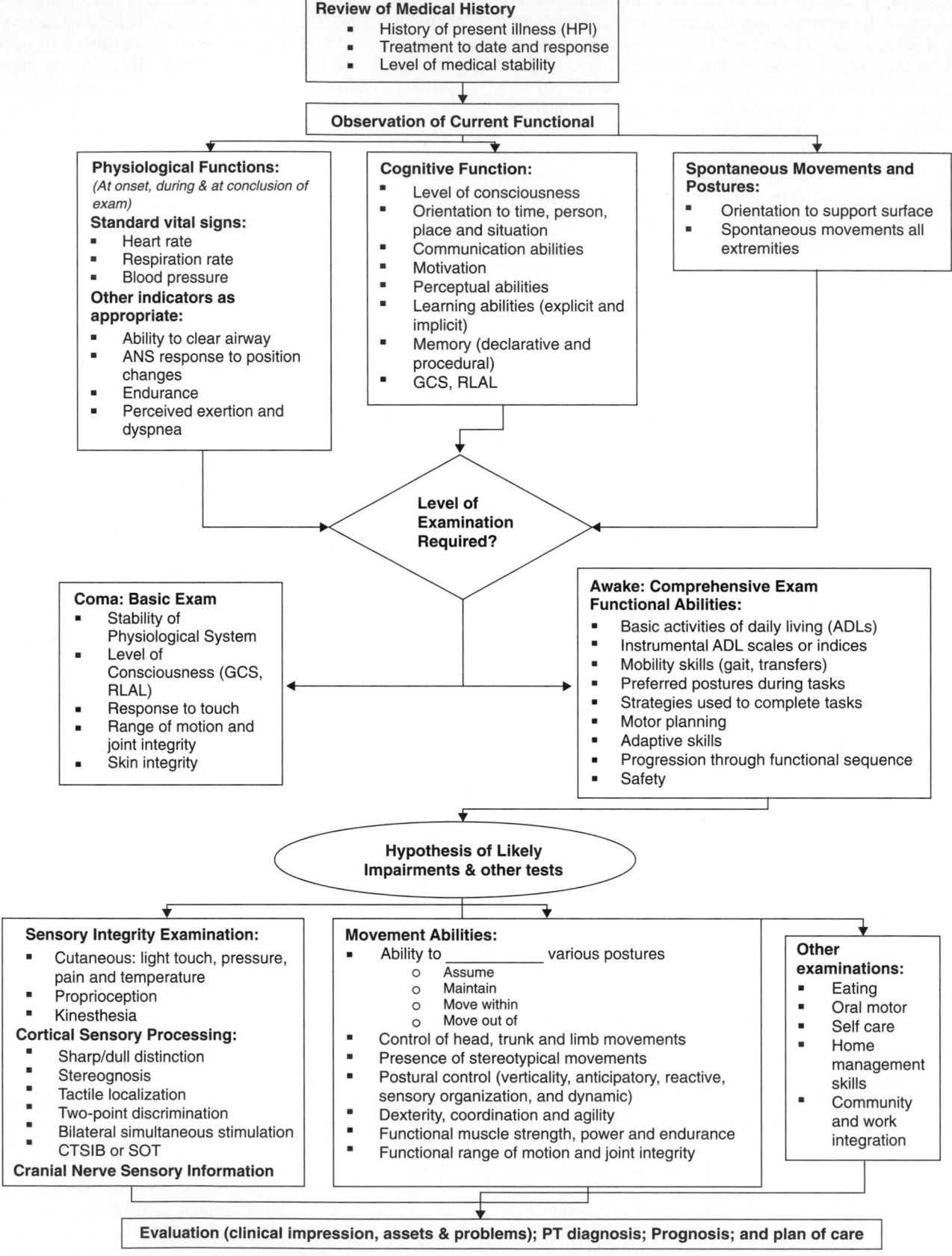

Review of Medical History
- History of present illness (HPI)
- Treatment to date and response
- Level of medical stability

Observation of Current Functional

Physiological Functions:
(At onset, during & at conclusion of exam)
Standard vital signs:
- Heart rate
- Respiration rate
- Blood pressure

Other indicators as appropriate:
- Ability to clear airway
- ANS response to position changes
- Endurance
- Perceived exertion and dyspnea

Cognitive Function:
- Level of consciousness
- Orientation to time, person, place and situation
- Communication abilities
- Motivation
- Perceptual abilities
- Learning abilities (explicit and implicit)
- Memory (declarative and procedural)
- GCS, RLAL

Spontaneous Movements and Postures:
- Orientation to support surface
- Spontaneous movements all extremities

Level of Examination Required?

Coma: Basic Exam
- Stability of Physiological System
- Level of Consciousness (GCS, RLAL)
- Response to touch
- Range of motion and joint integrity
- Skin integrity

Awake: Comprehensive Exam Functional Abilities:
- Basic activities of daily living (ADLs)
- Instrumental ADL scales or indices
- Mobility skills (gait, transfers)
- Preferred postures during tasks
- Strategies used to complete tasks
- Motor planning
- Adaptive skills
- Progression through functional sequence
- Safety

Hypothesis of Likely Impairments & other tests

Sensory Integrity Examination:
- Cutaneous: light touch, pressure, pain and temperature
- Proprioception
- Kinesthesia

Cortical Sensory Processing:
- Sharp/dull distinction
- Stereognosis
- Tactile localization
- Two-point discrimination
- Bilateral simultaneous stimulation
- CTSIB or SOT

Cranial Nerve Sensory Information

Movement Abilities:
- Ability to _____ various postures
  - Assume
  - Maintain
  - Move within
  - Move out of
- Control of head, trunk and limb movements
- Presence of stereotypical movements
- Postural control (verticality, anticipatory, reactive, sensory organization, and dynamic)
- Dexterity, coordination and agility
- Functional muscle strength, power and endurance
- Functional range of motion and joint integrity

Other examinations:
- Eating
- Oral motor
- Self care
- Home management skills
- Community and work integration

Evaluation (clinical impression, assets & problems); PT diagnosis; Prognosis; and plan of care

FIGURE 20-3 ■ Flow chart of the examination process.

mation. This may provide the therapist with information on the baseline status of the client's vital physiological functions. Any control problems in these areas should be particularly noted. Until the therapist determines that the vital functions, such as rate of respiration, heart rate, and blood pressure, vary appropriately with the demands of the intervention process, these factors should be monitored. The monitoring process should include consideration of the baseline rate, rate during exercise, and time to return to baseline. The pattern of respiration and changes in that pattern also should be noted.

Other tests and measures of the status of ventilation, respiration, and circulation may be indicated in specific individuals (refer to Chapter 35). Individuals with limited mobility or motor control of the trunk, or those with cranial nerve dysfunctions may demonstrate difficulty with functions such as moving secretions out of the airways. Inactivity during a prolonged recovery period may result in cardiovascular adaptations that compromise endurance and contribute to increases in the perceived exertion during activities.

Autonomic nervous system dysfunctions may be expressed as inappropriate accommodations to positional changes, such as orthostatic hypotension. Clients with depressed levels of consciousness may display temperature regulation dysfunctions. One mechanism for assessing the client's ability to maintain a homeostatic temperature is to review the nursing notes. The events surrounding any periods of diaphoresis should be examined. If no causative factors have been identified, then interventions, which involve thermal agents as discussed elsewhere in this text, should be used judiciously.

Evaluation of Cognitive Status

Because the evaluation process encompasses the stages of recovery from the critical acute phase through discharge from therapy, a range of aspects are included under the evaluation of cognitive status. As indicated previously, the observation of current functional status will direct the therapist toward the appropriate component tests and measures.

Acute bacterial meningitis and various forms of viral encephalitis may result in changes in the client's level of consciousness. *Consciousness* is a state of awareness of one's self and one's environment.[18] *Coma* can be defined as a state in which one does not open the eyes, obey commands, or utter recognizable words.[22] The individual does not respond to external stimuli or to internal needs. The term *vegetative state* is sometimes used to indicate the status of individuals who open their eyes and display a sleep-wake cycle but who do not obey commands or utter recognizable words. DeMeyer[23] presents a succinct description of the neuroanatomy of consciousness and the neurological examination of the unconscious patient. Plum and Posner[18] also provide extensive information in this area.

Several scales have been developed to provide objective guidelines to assess alterations in the state of consciousness. The Glasgow Coma Scale[22] assesses three independent items: eye opening, motor performance, and verbal performance. The scale yields a figure between 3 (lowest) and 15 (highest) that can be used to indicate changes in the individual's state of consciousness. The evaluation format is simple, and the scale demonstrates both interrater and intrarater reliability. The Rancho Los Amigos Scale assesses level of consciousness and behavior.[22] The therapist can use assessment tools such as the Glasgow Coma Scale and the companion Glasgow Outcome Scale to determine if the intervention program has resulted in any recordable changes in the client's level of consciousness. Ideally, the client with decreased levels of consciousness will be monitored at consistent intervals to determine changes in status. Any carryover or delayed effects of the intervention could then be noted. The record of the client's level of consciousness might also display a pattern of peak awareness at a particular point in the day. Scheduling an intervention session during the client's peak awareness time may maximize the benefit of the therapy.

In conjunction with the assessment of the client's state of consciousness is the determination of the individual's orientation to person, time, place, and situation. Because the individual's level of orientation (documented as oriented times 4) is frequently recorded by multiple members of the rehabilitation team, the information in the medical chart may provide insights into fluctuations over the course of a day or a week.

Gross assessment of the individual's ability to communicate—both the expressive and receptive aspects of the process—is an important component of the examination. If a dysfunction is present in the client's ability to communicate, the client should be evaluated by an individual with expertise in this area so that strategies for dealing with the communication deficit can be developed. Evaluation of the movement abilities of the client with communication deficits requires creative planning on the part of the therapist but usually can be accomplished if generalized movement tasks are used. With the client who cannot comprehend a verbal command to roll, the therapist should use an alternate form of communication, such as manual cueing or guidance. The therapist could structure the situation to elicit the desired behavior by activities such as placing the client in an uncomfortable position or positioning a desired object so that it can be reached only by rolling.

As the therapist progresses through the examination and intervention process, ongoing data collection should be occurring on factors that influence the motivation of the individual. Individuals with damage to certain areas within the frontal lobe will have difficulty with committing to long-term projects and may not be motivated to work during a therapy session by an explanation detailing the relationship of the current activity to the larger goal of returning home. In these situations, the therapist must create appropriate immediate rewards, such as a 2-minute rest break after completion of a specific movement task.

Deficits in cognition may be evident as problems in the area of explicit (declarative) or implicit (procedural) learning. Explicit learning is used in the acquisition of knowledge that is consciously recalled. This is information that can be verbalized in declarative sentences, such as the sequential listing of the steps in a movement sequence. Implicit or procedural learning is used in the process of acquiring movement sequences that are performed automatically without conscious attention to the performance. Procedural learning occurs through repetitions of the movement task. Because explicit and implicit learning use different neuroanatomical circuits, implicit learning can occur in the individuals with deficits in the components underlying explicit learning (awareness, attention, higher order cognitive processes).

The emotional and psychological aspects of the client and the higher order cognitive and retention skills of the client should be evaluated informally by the therapist, with referral to appropriate professionals if dysfunction in these areas is suspected. A coordinated team approach is necessary for clients with emotional and psychological, cognitive, perceptual, or communication problems or a combination of these problems. A consistent strategy used by all team members eliminates the necessity of the client to try to cope with different approaches by different people in an area in which she or he already has a deficit. The impact of cognitive deficits on the process of learning motor skills is further discussed in the next section on movement assessment. The assessment of the impact of perceptual dysfunctions is incorporated within the evaluation of sensory channels.

Evaluation of Functional Abilities

As indicated in the introduction to the evaluation of clients with inflammatory and infectious disorders of the brain, the examination process is not compartmentalized. As the therapist is examining the movement abilities of the individual through the format described in the previous section, he is also collecting information on the functional abilities of the individual. The components underlying the movement abilities of the client can be examined within the framework of the basic or instrumental activities of daily living (ADLs), depending on the functional level of the person. The treatment setting and documentation requirements within that setting will determine if the data on basic ADL and instrumental ADL skills are recorded with use of a formal scale or index, or are gathered through an individualized process.

The introduction of specific tasks provides the therapist with the opportunity to observe the preferred posture used to accomplish the different tasks. The therapist should construct situations that require the individual to respond to unexpected occurrences to provide some insight into the person's ability to adapt to the unexpected. Throughout the process of examining a patient's movement abilities and functional abilities, the therapist is assessing the individual's awareness of safety considerations and judgment in attempting tasks.

The presence of motor planning dysfunctions can be noted as the client attempts a movement sequence or a functional task. The therapist may have to cue the client physically to initiate the sequence, which then flows smoothly. The therapist may observe that the client has the correct components to a movement sequence, but that the sequence of the components is incorrect. Or the client may demonstrate the ability to produce a movement sequence under one set of conditions but not another. Indications of these types of motor planning problems can be observed during the initial interactions with the client. Similarly, the therapist also should be aware of indications of problems with dexterity, coordination, and agility, as well as with signs of cerebellar dysfunctions.

Another aspect of the evaluation process that can be integrated in the observations of movement abilities is identification of perceptual deficits. Aspects of the client's motor performance can provide indications for detailed perceptual testing to classify the deficits. This testing should be conducted by the health care team member qualified in the area of perceptual testing. During the general evaluation procedures, the therapist can screen the client for signs of perceptual deficits. Clients' abilities to cross their midlines with their upper extremities can be demonstrated in movement sequences, such as moving from the supine to the side-sitting to the sitting position (Figure 20-4). The quality of the integration of information from the two sides of the body can be indicated by the symmetry or asymmetry of posture in positions that should be symmetrical. The therapist may suspect that the client has a deficit in body awareness or body image by the poor quality of movement patterns that are within the motor capability of the individual. Spontaneous comments by the client as to how he or she feels when moving ("my leg feels so heavy") also add to the therapist's assessment of the client's body image. Problems with verticality can be seen with the client who lists to one side when in an upright posture. When the therapist corrects the list to a vertical posture, clients may express that they now feel that they are leaning to one side. Individuals who cannot appropriately relate their positions to the position of objects in their environments may have a figure-ground deficit or a problem with the concept of their position in space. When approaching stairs, these clients may fail to step up or may attempt to step up too soon. These examples should provide an indication of the observations that can indicate the need for detailed perceptual testing.

The preceding aspects of evaluation of movement abilities have focused on facets of motor performance. Within this process, the therapist should intertwine an appraisal of the individual's ability to learn motor tasks (or elements of the task). The therapist attempts to determine whether the client can maintain a change in the ability to perform a movement throughout a therapy session and into the next session. The client's ability to capture and integrate changes into the movement repertoire is fundamental to the success of the intervention program. The program can focus on the learning of movement sequences and the generalization of these sequences to movements within other contexts. Individuals with lowered levels of consciousness (typically Rancho Los Amigos Stages 1-3) will be unable to learn or have difficulty learning and generalizing new motor skills. Therapy sessions may be more successful if the focus remains on the performance of motor tasks that were previously "overlearned" and automatic. Although the therapist may be able to manually guide the individual in coming to sit on the edge of the bed, until the individual demonstrates a higher level of processing, it may be unrealistic to expect that she will consistently reposition the legs without cueing before attempting the movement sequence. From looking at the "whole" of function, the therapist needs to determine the impairments that require further examination.

Evaluation of Sensory Channel Integrity and Processing

The examination process must include an assessment of the channels for sensory input. Knowledge gained in the assessment of the sensory systems will be used in the program-planning process to select the intervention strategies that have the highest probability of success. Although movements can be performed (and in some cases even learned) in the absence of typical sensory feedback, the presence of

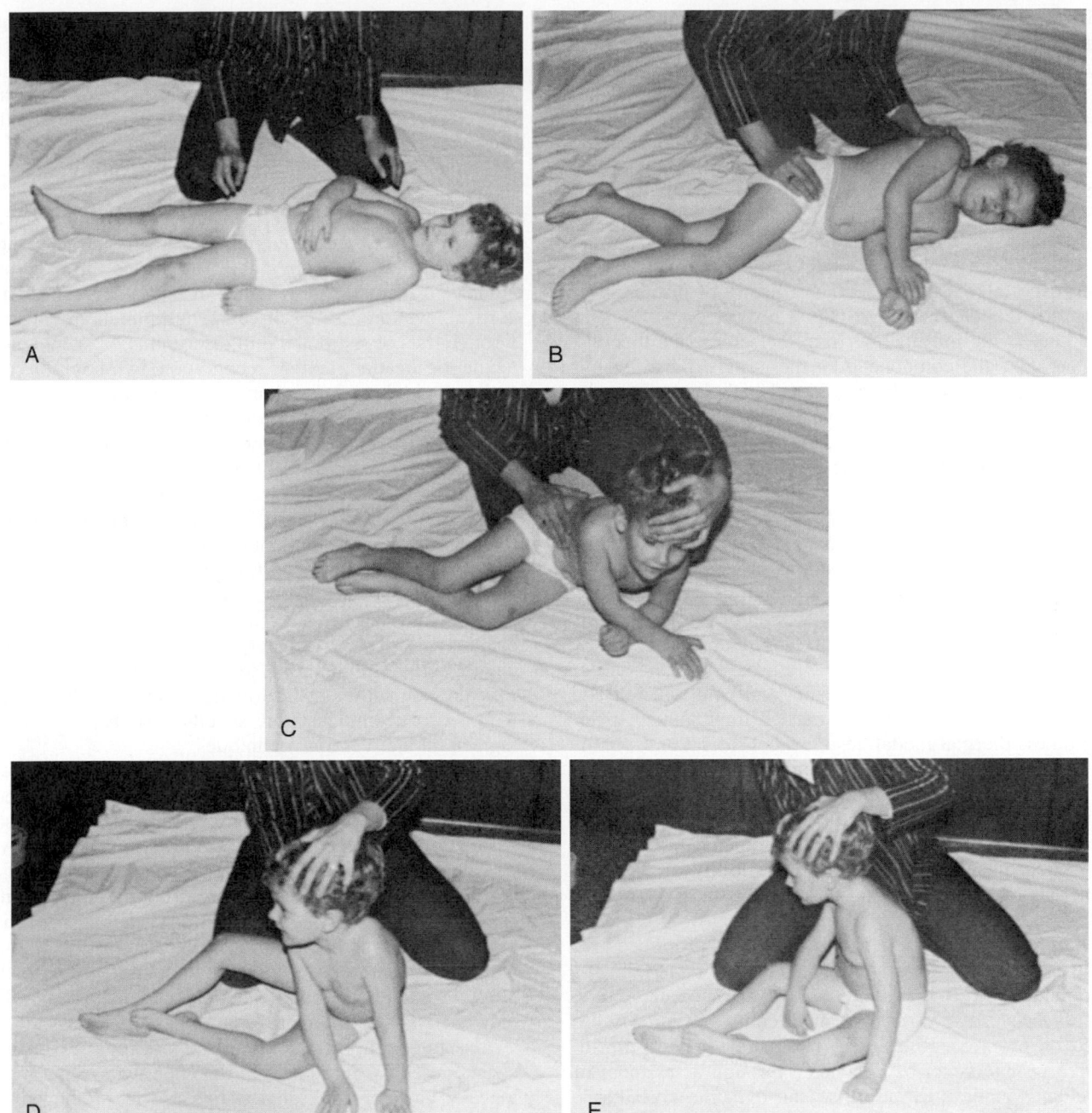

FIGURE 20-4 ■ Movement sequence from the supine to side-sitting to sitting positions. **A,** Supine position. **B,** Handling to side lying. **C,** Handling toward side sitting; arm positions are important. **D,** Side sitting; note propping patterns with arms. **E,** Handling to symmetrical sitting.

altered sensory function creates more challenges for both the client/learner and the therapist/teacher. The therapist assesses both the client's ability to perceive the sensory stimulus and the appropriateness of the response to the stimulus. Therefore, it is important to determine if the sensory modality is intact, impaired, or absent, and if it is impaired, is it hyperresponsive, hyporesponsive, or inconsistent. Tactile input could result in an appropriate activation of underlying muscles or a maladaptive increase of muscle activity in a stereotyped distribution.

Variations in the interpretation of sensory input may occur in some clients. Gentle tactile contact may be per-

ceived by the person as a noxious input. Some individuals will have difficulty processing and discriminating information with high levels of one type of sensory input (e.g., the noisy clinic area) or with multiple simultaneous inputs (e.g., talking to the therapist while walking down a hallway with people moving toward the individual). The therapist should be alert to indications of substitution of sensory feedback channels. The client with impaired proprioception tends to compensate through the use of visual information. Although this compensation may be functional within the constraints of isolated tasks, problems arise when vision is required to monitor other items, such as objects in the walking path.

During the evaluation process, the therapist must note the sensory inputs that elicit maladaptive behaviors so that these inputs can be either avoided within the intervention sequence or appropriately incorporated to progress toward an adaptive response.

The therapist should develop a systematic approach to the initial cursory screen of the sensory systems. Deficits identified in the initial examination will provide structure for scheduling more comprehensive evaluation of deficits in specific systems. The therapist must also monitor changes in the status of physiological vital functions during sensory input, especially if the client has a history of instability of heart rate, blood pressure, or rate of respiration.

Based on the information from the screen, the therapist will organize the components of the more detailed examination. Components to be considered include the integrity of the peripheral sensory circuits, the cortical level processing of the sensory information, the integrity of the cranial nerve sensory circuits, and the processing of multichannel input.

Cutaneous input has several aspects that must be assessed. Some of the inflammatory diseases of the brain may result in cutaneous distributions in which sensation is absent or diminished. These areas should be routinely evaluated for changes in distribution of level of sensation. Tests of light touch, pressure, and pain can be used if the client can communicate reliably. In most cases, inclusion of assessment of differentiation of hot and cold will not add appreciably to the information needed for treatment planning unless thermal modalities are a consideration.

A gross assessment of the intactness of the touch system can be made in the noncommunicative client by introducing a mildly adversive (not painful) stimulus, such as a light scratch, while monitoring the client for changes in facial expression, posture, or tonus. The possibility of a spinal-level reflex response should be kept in mind when interpreting the results of such a gross assessment.

Assessment of the client's response to proprioceptive input is incorporated within the assessment of the client's movement abilities and is intertwined with the intervention process because a variety of intervention techniques are based on proprioceptive input. Evaluation of the proprioceptive channels can be conducted through assessment of the client's static position sense and dynamic kinesthesia. These tests allow the therapist to make inferences concerning the client's cognitive abilities to interpret proprioceptive information. Inherent in the successful completion of these tests is the necessity for the client to be able to understand directions and to be able to communicate data to the therapist. Because information input, processing, and output are involved in these tests, failure to comply with the test instructions cannot be definitively attributed to dysfunction of the proprioceptive system. The therapist also should consider information obtained from watching the client move before drawing a conclusion concerning the intactness of the proprioceptive channels. Some of the factors to consider include disregard of an extremity and variations in quality of performance between visually directed and nonvisually directed movements. Although tests of position sense and kinesthetics provide one aspect of the evaluation of the proprioceptive system, the therapist also must be involved constantly in assessing the client's response to the intervention

techniques that are part of the treatment plan. This again illustrates the intermingling of assessment and intervention. Intervention places a demand for movement on the client. As the movement occurs, the therapist assesses the quality of the movement. If the quality is not appropriate, the therapist initiates intervention to improve the quality. If the technique does not produce the desired result, a second technique can be tried and the cyclic process continues.

In addition to determining the integrity of the peripheral sensory pathways and recognition of the input, it is important to assess the individual's ability to process more complex presentations of cutaneous input. Difficulties in the cortical level processing of cutaneous stimuli are identified through tests of sharp and dull discrimination, stereognosis, tactile localization, texture recognition, two-point discrimination, and bilateral simultaneous stimulation.

Central processing and integration of sensory information as it affects postural control can be examined using the Clinical Test of Sensory Integration of Balance (CTSIB)[24] or with computerized dynamic posturography using the Sensory Organization Test (SOT). With both tests, the effectiveness of using vision, somatosensory, or vestibular sensation at the appropriate time (sensory weighting), and changing from one sensory system to the other is examined.

Assessment of the integrity of the cranial nerve sensory channels is typically incorporated within the standard cranial nerve examination. Review of the physician's notes may provide sufficient information; however, the therapist may need to complete more specific tests before considering certain intervention techniques.

The olfactory channels are unique among the sensory input routes because the primary olfactory pathway directly synapses with the olfactory cortex within the limbic system before going to the thalamus. Olfactory inputs may provide a mechanism to elicit arousal in an otherwise unresponsive individual. The procedure for administering olfactory input as a component of evaluation and intervention regimens is discussed elsewhere in this text. Because of the potential hypersensitivity of any or all input systems, it is best to elicit arousal with pleasant odors rather than noxious odors, which may elicit a flight-or-fight response.

Gustatory sensory information is not typically an input channel used by therapists. In the client who is not receiving any gustatory stimulation because of prolonged tube feeding or in one who demonstrates dysfunction of the oral musculature, the gustatory avenue of sensory input should not be overlooked. Various tastes can be incorporated in the evaluation of the effects of sensory inputs on clients with depressed levels of consciousness. Gustatory input can be incorporated into an intervention plan with the goal of facilitating movement of the oral and facial musculature. The gustatory/tactile input of a small amount of peanut butter placed on the corner of the client's mouth may elicit tongue protraction with lateral deviation to remove the morsel. Introduction of a slightly sour taste may facilitate a pucker response of the orbicularis oris. The possibility of achieving desired goals through the inclusion of gustatory input should be considered during the evaluation process.

The complex functions of the vestibular system can be assessed through a variety of avenues. The integrity of the connections underlying a vestibularly induced nystagmus response is assessed by physicians through the caloric test (warm and cold water or air introduced into the ear channel to induce nystagmus). Therapists have used the Ayres Post-Rotatory Nystagmus Test[25,26] and variations of the test to gain information on the postrotatory nystagmus response. The postrotatory nystagmus tests provide information on the response of the extraocular muscles to vestibular input; however, they should not be overinterpreted as yielding insight about the integrity of the vestibular connections underlying postural responses.

Located in the utriculus and sacculus are the maculae, which record changes in the relationship of the head to the pull of gravity (position detectors) and changes in linear acceleration. This end organ is responsible for the tonic labyrinthine reflexes. By manipulating the position of the client's head in relation to the pull of gravity, the therapist can evaluate this aspect of the vestibular system by noting changes in the distribution of muscle activity. Verticality testing without vision can give the therapist information regarding the client's orientation to gravity. The effect of rapid linear accelerations and decelerations can be evaluated as potential activating mechanisms increasing the level of consciousness or level of muscle activity. An example is the Dynamic Gait Index, a functional test that incorporates changes in speed and head movements while walking.[27] Slow, rhythmical reversals of linear movements may have a calming effect on the client's behavior or level of muscle activation. Linear movements in all planes and diagonals should be explored. (Refer to Chapters 9 and 23 for additional information.)

Auditory and visual channels can be grossly assessed by the therapist. More detailed information on the intactness of the sensory channels can be obtained from other health care team members. The types of information available from other health care team members can vary from the assessment of brain stem-evoked potentials in response to auditory and visual inputs in the comatose individual to the identification of visual or auditory acuity deficits. Because the auditory and visual systems provide the therapist with a primary means of communicating with the client, and because they can be used to augment performance in the event of deficits in other sensory channels, these systems should be incorporated in the therapist's evaluation process. Simple visual system tests, such as identification of field deficits, assessment of tracking abilities, and a gross evaluation of visual acuity, can be performed quickly. Neurology textbooks can be consulted on the techniques for administering these tests. Simple tests for assessing auditory thresholds can include such techniques as rubbing fingers by the individual's ear, placing a ticking watch to the client's ear, or assessing the presence of a startle response to sounds in the client with altered states of consciousness. Although these quick tests of the visual and auditory systems will not yield quantifiable information, they should provide the therapist with the necessary data to design an intervention plan that accounts for the presence of the deficits or that can use the intact system to compensate for input missing from an impaired system.

During the evaluation of the client as well as during intervention with the client, the therapist must be aware of the potential to bombard him with sensory input and overload his or her ability to respond discriminatively to it. If the therapist detects that the client has difficulty in responding

appropriately to sensory input, as with a client in a lowered state of consciousness or an agitated state, or demonstrating tactile defensiveness, sensory input should be used selectively during the initial examination or intervention sessions. If multiple sensory inputs are used, the positive or negative effects cannot be attributed to a specific input or necessarily to the series of inputs. Evaluation as well as intervention with sensory inputs should proceed in a controlled fashion. Inclusion of additional sensory modalities in the intervention plan should occur systematically.

The individual's response to multichannel sensory conflict is typically assessed as a component of higher level balance assessment and locomotor abilities. A more thorough discussion of sensory assessment is discussed elsewhere in the text. The therapist should apply these concepts during the evaluation of all motor tasks. Consider the following example: a client who relies on visual input to supplement vestibular and somatosensory information is performing the task of sitting on the edge of the mat table. She remains relatively steady until someone walks directly toward her from across the clinic. This change in the environmental context of the performance requires her to assess whether she is moving toward the individual or the individual is moving toward her. Without reliable vestibular and somatosensory check points, the client may activate a postural response to the incorrect assessment. As this example demonstrates, the evaluation of the sensory channels is intertwined with the evaluation of the person's movement abilities.

Evaluation of Movement Abilities

The initial assessment of the individual's movement abilities is conducted by observing as she or he moves through a sequence of functional postures. The therapist determines the functional postures to be examined for a specific client, ranging from bed mobility activities (assessment of movement in prone and supine) through upright ambulation. The medical status of the individual, the extent of involvement, the intervention setting, and the age of the individual are considerations in determining the appropriate functional postures to be examined. The therapist gathers information on the movement abilities of the client as she moves into, within, and out of the position.

The assessment focuses on both the quantity and quality of motor performance. The quantitative aspect of the movement assessment refers to the number of different functional postures the individual can use. The quality of the movement abilities is assessed within the posture as well as in the process of moving between postures. For example, the therapist should assess the quality of the head, trunk, and extremity control demonstrated throughout the movement sequences. The use of stereotypical movement patterns should be noted because their presence may limit the adaptability of movements required to accomplish functional tasks. Other items relating to the client's movement abilities are assessed during this process.

Indications of abnormal ranges of movement of all joints can be obtained. The range may show a limitation of movement or an indication of joint instability. Once the gross deviations are identified, these joints can be examined to determine the source of the problem: joint capsular, ligamentous, bony, skin, or muscular and fascial dysfunction. Conducting the gross assessment of range while the client is moving eliminates the time spent in performing a joint-by-joint goniometric evaluation on articulations with normal excursions.

As the individual is moving (either independently or with the therapist assisting), an assessment of the distribution and fluctuations in muscle activity can be made and will provide information on functional muscle strength, power, and endurance. The timing, accuracy, and sequencing of muscle activation within the movement should be noted. The therapist can identify the postures that will be the most conducive to optimal motor performances and those that should be avoided. As the client is moving through various postures, the function of specific musculature can be examined. Muscle groups should be examined concerning their ability to function in both closed-chain (distal segment fixed) and open-chain (distal segment free) situations. Because numerous demands are being placed on each muscle group, therapists can assess their ability to perform isometric and isotonic (concentric and eccentric) contractions. Each different posture introduces a new set of variables; therefore, the performance of a muscle group must be reexamined as each new movement pattern is performed.

The therapist can identify postural control in a variety of functional positions. This includes the client's vertical orientation to the surface or to gravity as the situation dictates, anticipatory postural control, reactive postural control, sensory organization for postural control and dynamic balance for gait.

Within each posture, the therapist must examine the control the client displays over the posture. Because the assessment takes place as part of a dynamic sequence, the therapist can assess the client's ability to assume the posture. If the posture cannot be achieved independently, the therapist assesses the factors interfering with achieving the position, the type of assistance necessary to facilitate assumption of the posture, and the effect of the various intervention techniques used to assist the client in achieving the position. Once the client is in the posture, her or his ability to maintain the posture is examined. Factors that interfere with the performance are noted. The client's ability to move within the posture is identified. Movement demands placed on the client should include aspects of both static and dynamic equilibrium. Static balance in the sitting position (such as on the side of the bed) could be demonstrated by the individual matching the strength of a force attempting to displace him backward and maintaining the position when the force is suddenly released.

The presence of dynamic balance of the upper torso in the sitting position could be demonstrated by the individual reacting to a quick sideways displacement force administered to the shoulder by activating the trunk lateral flexors to compensate for the displacement. Equally important is the individual's ability to demonstrate appropriate equilibrium responses to self-imposed perturbations. The absence of anticipatory control in standing could be demonstrated by having the client do the rapid arm raise test with a 5-lb weight and noticing reactive stepping instead of doing a posterior weight shift in anticipation of the destabilizing force.

The final stage in examining the individual's movement abilities explores the individual's ability to move out of the posture. The client should have the ability to move out of the posture to a lower level posture and to a higher level posture before mastery of the posture is considered to have been achieved.

Many aspects of the client's performance are analyzed simultaneously. When the therapist assists the client in moving to a new posture, an analysis of the influence of facilitation and inhibition techniques is being conducted. The individual's response to these handling techniques cues the therapist in projecting the client's response to an intervention program. The therapist is constantly monitoring the client for changes in physiological functions or changes in the level of consciousness. Anything that results in expressions of pain by the client should be noted. Intervention programs should be a learning experience for clients. If they are attending to pain, they cannot attend to learning. The factor(s) producing the pain should be identified and measures instituted to eliminate the factor(s). If the factors producing the pain cannot be resolved, the intervention program should be designed to avoid triggering the pain or teaching the patient to self-monitor and identify when the severity of pain immobilizes the ability to move independently.

PROGNOSING AND GOAL SETTING

Ideally, the process of establishing the prognosis and setting the goals for a client is a coordinated effort that involves all members of the health care team, including the client (if feasible) and family. If the therapist is not functioning in a setting where involvement of many disciplines is viable, the therapist can progress through the goal-setting process in the context of his or her role in the client's care.

Having collected data from the examination process, the first steps are to establish two lists: one dealing with specific problems (impairments, functional limitations, and inability to participate in life) the client is encountering and one dealing with her or his assets. Formulating an asset list focuses on the positive data elicited from the evaluation process and is critical for prognosing outcomes. Items on the asset list could be observations, such as the client being able to assume the position of sitting on the side of the bed with set up assistance only, improved head control in this posture being facilitated by approximation, and controlled weight shifting being elicited by alternated tapping. The asset list provides a reference defining the postures and intervention techniques that are effective. This reference is used to develop the intervention goals and plan of care as well as an estimate of the time needed to reach these goals (prognosis). Formulating and recording a problem list and an asset list can be completed relatively quickly as one gains familiarity with the process. Whereas novice therapists will benefit from generating a written asset list, experienced clinicians may formulate a mental asset list while completing the written evaluation format required by the facility. Just as the evaluation process is ongoing, so are the steps involved in goal setting. The asset and problem lists are redefined as the client's status changes.

Having identified assets and problems, the next step is to establish the intervention steps to be taken to reach the expected outcomes from this episode of care. These outcome statements represent the general objectives toward which the intervention process is oriented. They identify the end point of the intervention process and the time needed to accomplish those goals. The exit criteria for terminating the episode of care are used when reassessing progress toward that end point.

TABLE 20-1 ■ Examples of Short-Term Objectives Relating to Mastery of Functional Activities in Sitting*

	CONDITION VARIABLES†	ACTIVITY	CRITERIA
1. When sitting on a mat	a. using the upper extremities for support	The client will maintain the posture	For _____ seconds.
2. When sitting on the edge of a mat table	b. using one upper extremity for support c. without using the upper extremities for support		
3. When sitting in a chair	d. with the therapist displacing the position of the: pelvis shoulders head lower extremities	The client will make postural adjustments of the head and trunk	Appropriate to the degree of displacement.
	e. leaning forward and returning to erect sitting	The client will bring the right foot to the left knee (as if to put on a shoe)	

*Outcome: The client will master functional activities in sitting. Short-term objective: Select one phrase from each column.
†Therapist needs to consider all aspects of each variable (i.e., 1—a, b, c, d, e; 2—a, b, c, d, e; 3—a, b, c, d, e).

The *Guide to Physical Therapist Practice* views outcomes in relationship to "minimization of functional limitations, optimization of health status, prevention of disability, and optimization of patient/client satisfaction," whereas goals "relate to the remediation (to the extent possible) of impairments."[21] The breadth of acceptance of these definitions with the neurorehabilitation professions remains to be determined. These definitions at least give professionals a place to start communicating with consistency. The ICF model of the World Health Organization (WHO) provides similar definitions with the focus being client centered. Although the *Guide to Physical Therapist Practice* still uses the Nagi model with the classification of impairment, functional limitations, and disability, quality of life and the ability to participate in life are current terminologies of the WHO and accepted by the world community of therapists. This current model focuses on empowerment of the patient and her or his ability to control the environment. (Refer to Chapter 1 for additional discussion of these models.)

Measurable, interim objectives should be established in relation to the outcome statements. To determine if the objective has been achieved, the objective should be measurable, either in terms of producing a numerical indicator of performance, such as time span, number of repetitions, distance covered, or accuracy of performance, or in terms of a precise description of the target motor behavior. The appropriate objective indicator must be carefully selected. Performing a movement more quickly may indicate that the individual is performing it with more normal control and, therefore, greater ease of movement, or it may indicate that the individual has become more skilled in using an abnormal pattern based on inappropriate muscle activation. If it is not appropriate to formulate the objective in terms of a numerical indicator, the objective can be formulated in terms of an observable behavior. The therapist can precisely describe body segment movements based on the component method of movement analysis presented by VanSant.[28,29] For example, the task of coming to standing from supine can be described in terms of the upper-extremity component, axial component, and lower-extremity component. Formulation

of an appropriate short-term objective could specify use of the upper extremities in a push-and-reach pattern during the task of coming to standing from supine. The interim objectives should be constructed so that observing the client's behavior will allow the therapist to state whether the criteria of the short-term objective were achieved. Table 20-1 gives an example of some components of short-term objectives leading to mastery of functional activities in sitting.

The outcome statements define the client's destination. The interim objectives define the mileposts. The therapist then uses the asset list to design the intervention program, which is the vehicle to get the client to his or her destination. From the asset list, the therapist knows the intervention techniques that have the highest probability of success. Adopting this process simplifies the task of outlining the strategy for intervention.

As the therapist considers the appropriate outcomes and goals for the client, a decision must be made as to whether the format of the intervention will focus on a "training" approach or a "motor learning" approach. During the assessment process, if the therapist concludes that the individual's level of cognitive function precludes the development of insight into movement errors (both the detection and correction of an incorrect performance) or the ability to retain the insight over time, then the therapist should delineate the outcomes and intervention plan to accommodate this limitation. The "training" approach requires more structure and repetition of activities within that structure. If it is more appropriate to design the intervention plan according to motor learning considerations, the therapist must consider the appropriate schedule and environmental context for the practice, the type and schedule for the feedback provided, and techniques to promote the generalization of the learning beyond the specific practice session.

General Goals for the Intervention Process

While the goal-setting process described earlier results in specification of the outcomes, goals, and objectives for a specific client, the general goals for the intervention process can be delineated to guide the process. As described in the overview of inflammatory disorders at the beginning of this chapter, the extent of the neurological sequelae may range from a single discrete problem to a devastating clinical picture composed of compromised functions in multiple areas. The goals for the intervention process address the problem areas that (1) jeopardize the efficiency and effectiveness of functional activities and (2) are the primary or secondary results of compromised neurological function. The listing of goals does not directly include consideration of secondary problems (such as decreases in joint range of motion [ROM], cardiovascular fitness, and endurance). The therapist should integrate these considerations in the overall assessment of the components of the movement problems.

The following goals are written as outcomes of the intervention process and not as goals for a specific client. Because of the broad nature of the goals, other professions also will contribute to the attainment of the goals. The goals of the therapeutic intervention program for clients with inflammatory CNS disorders are as follows:

Goal 1: Postural control is optimized as demonstrated by the ability to maintain a position against gravity and the ability to automatically adjust before and continuously during movement.

Goal 2: Selective, voluntary movement patterns within functional activities are optimized.

Goal 3: Performance of functional activities is enhanced.

Goal 4: Integration of sensory information is fostered.

Goal 5: Cognitive status and psychosocial responses are optimized.

Each of these goals is discussed in conjunction with the general therapeutic intervention procedures that can be used to achieve the goal.

GENERAL THERAPEUTIC INTERVENTION PROCEDURES IN RELATION TO INTERVENTION GOALS

■ *Postural control is optimized as demonstrated by the ability to maintain a position against gravity and the ability to adjust automatically before and continuously during movement.*

Because it is assumed that functional abilities are built on the base of the ability to control postures, the intervention goal of promoting optimal postural control underlies the ability to make selective, voluntary movement patterns (goal 2) and the performance of functional activities (goal 3). Optimization of a postural set includes the concepts of decreasing muscle activity that is too high to allow performance of movement sequences, augmenting activation that is too low to support the accomplishment of a movement sequence, and fostering proper timing of the postural responses. Intervention techniques to achieve this goal demand that the therapist constantly monitor the client's performance so that appropriate interventions are added when needed and continued only as long as they are needed.

Optimal postural control is defined by two elements. The client should have the ability to maintain a vertical orientation in regard to gravity and should be able to maintain his balance in the presence of both internal and external perturbations. Automatic adjustments in the postural set should occur in anticipation of and continuously during movements

(internal perturbations). Both elements should be performed with minimal physical or cognitive effort on the part of the client. Horak describes five components of normal postural control, including vertical orientation; anticipatory, reactive, sensory organization; and dynamic postural control for gait.[30] By looking at the subsets of postural control, interventions can be designed to specifically match the impairment (Table 20-2).

Verticality, or maintaining an upright posture, first requires the client to recognize the desired alignment. Augmenting internal feedback mechanisms with the use of mirrors, force plates or scales, or even using a flashlight attached to the client that shines on a target when he is vertical can be used effectively. Manual skills such as positioning the client and using approximation to reinforce the position can be added to the treatment. Progression of intervention strategies can be done by having the client maintain the posture and then begin to manipulate objects with his extremities. Research suggests that the CNS is organized around tasks and not movement patterns. So, as the client is learning to maintain vertical and move in and out of the position, designing a task will likely give a better outcome. For example, Paul developed encephalitis, which left him with residual deficits in verticality. The simple task of keeping a book balanced on his head while sitting or walking gave him the type of feedback he needed without constant cues to "stand up straight" being the focus. Further progression involves teaching the client to move to his limits of stability and find vertical again.

Anticipatory postural control involves the postural preset, which positions the trunk to allow skilled use of the extremities without loss of balance. It requires the client to recognize the situation and the likely destabilizing force that will result, and posturally preset so destabilizing will not occur. The process requires memory and the ability to recognize the critical environmental and task cues. Interventions focus on practicing both the postural adjustment and the focal action before the two components are combined. Table 20-2 also has suggested interventions for reactive, sensory integrative, and dynamic balance in gait problems. Postural control is affected as well by biomechanical constraints, such as tonal abnormalities.

The client's ability to demonstrate optimal postural control may be restricted by the presence of hypertonicity or hypotonicity in various muscle groups. These states may be relatively static or may fluctuate with the demands of a particular situation. Inappropriately high levels of muscle activity may be present in a stereotypical muscle distribution in the extremities, whereas the activity of the trunk musculature may be too low to support an antigravity posture. The therapist must design the interventions creatively to meet the shifting responses of the demands of a particular activity.

Being cognizant of the fact that spasticity is a reaction to initial peripheral instability, treatment needs to be selected that deals with the fact that as spasticity is modified, weakness or hypotonicity may be present. Inappropriately high levels of activity in a muscle group or groups may limit the client's ability to demonstrate optimal postural control (and optimal selective movements as addressed in the second goal). The therapist can select intervention techniques that are mediated through any of the sensory channels functional

TABLE 20-2 ■ Interventions for Postural Control Problems

POSTURAL CONTROL PROBLEM	POSSIBLE INTERVENTIONS
Malalignment and verticality problems	Augment sensory feedback: • Mirror • Static force plate • Flashlight on target • Videotape • Align without vision and check (knowledge of results) • Stepping with eyes closed
Limits of stability perception problems	• Computerized feedback of actual versus possible • Weight shifting exercise with feedback/targets (somatosensory, visual, both) • Surface orientation exercises (static, ankle sway, hip strategies)
Anticipatory control problems	• Hold on and slow down (lessen the need for anticipatory control—substitution) • Mental rehearsal (weight shift, then move) • Practice limb movements where balance must be controlled (start slow and get faster) 　—Interactions with the environment with a static BOS, such as reaching up in a cupboard, opening a door, opening a drawer, lifting a suitcase, lifting a bag of groceries, wearing a backpack 　—Interactions with the environment with a dynamic base of support (stepping up a step, kicking a ball, stepping over an object, stepping around an object, changing the pitch of the surface—inclines) • Practice rapid limb movements where balance must be controlled (opening a door, opening a drawer, lifting a briefcase, lifting a bag of groceries, lifting a suitcase, wearing a backpack). Practice order: 　—Practice the anticipatory postural adjustment 　—Practice the focal action while supported 　—Combine the anticipatory postural adjustment with the focal action unsupported (slow to fast) 　—Practice varying similar tasks (predictable to unpredictable) Example: after the patient is doing better on a lifting task of one object, work to be successful with several objects of different weights; first cognitively solve what must change to be successful in lifting one object versus another; then much repetition of alternating one object versus another, and eventually, work with a variety of objects in a varied pattern
Reactive postural control problems	• Work to regain balance strategies (ankle, hip, and stepping) • Remediate any biomechanical issues that affect use of balance strategies • Begin with self-perturbation and progress to reacting to external perturbations • Need to learn to match the magnitude and direction of perturbation • Physioballs, T-stools, tilt boards, reaching, weight shifting
Sensory integration problems	• If overreliant on vision, be sure you help patient with another strategy before you take vision away • Surface orientation exercises (tuning into somatosensory feedback) 　—Textured surface 　—Textured surface + visual tracking 　—Textured surface with vision occluded • Enhancing use of vestibular system: 　—Compliant surface with stationary visual target 　—Compliant surface + visual tracking 　—Compliant surface with moving visual background 　—Changing surface + head turns 　—Changing surface + head turns + moving visual background 　—Obstacle course with varying sensory demands
Dynamic balance problems in gait	• Alter the sensory contexts (e.g., resisted walking) • Walking and reading signs right and left • Carrying objects and looking at items carried • Walking with quick stops (predictable distances and reactive) • Practice falling without injury and getting up; practice slips and trips • Walking and negotiating obstacles (around and over) 　—Practice both around and over obstacles 　—Larger steps, standing on one foot, changing directions 　—Practice stopping quickly with feet in target 　—Practice shorter steps, on a slippery surface; braiding • Gesturing while walking

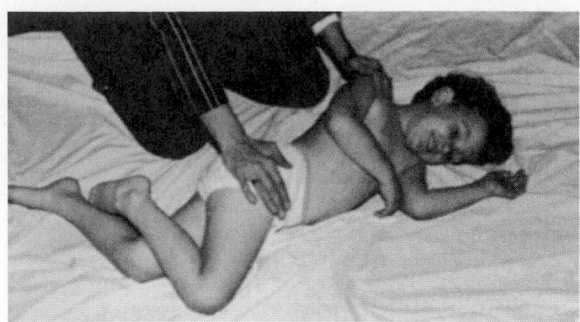

FIGURE 20-5 ■ Counterrotation of shoulder girdle backward (retraction) and the pelvis forward. Hand placement of therapist is important so that shoulder and hip movements can occur freely.

for that client. The choice of which channel or combination of channels to use for the input is based on the therapist's initial and continuing evaluation of the client's response to specific types of sensory input.

The therapist must address the hypertonicity influencing postural control as a generalized problem before demanding selective voluntary activation of specific muscle groups. Vestibular input that is slow and rhythmical may promote a generalized relaxation of skeletal muscle activity. In some clients, the trunk remains "stiff" in movement sequences in which a segmental response between the upper and lower trunk should occur. Repetitions of rhythmical movements in side lying where the therapist gently and progressively stretches the client's pelvis in one direction around the body axis while moving the shoulder girdle in the opposite direction, and then reverses the movement may effectively alter the biomechanical and neurological contributions to the stiffness (Figure 20-5).

For some clients, changing the dynamics of a spastic extremity may permit the emergence of more optimal levels of postural control. The appropriately designed ankle-foot orthosis (AFO) may alter the individual's need to rigidly control the position of the pelvis to remain upright (refer to Chapter 34). Use of a soft webbing thumb loop to alter the resting position of the first metacarpal may change the overactivity of musculature throughout the upper extremity and allow appropriate adjustment of the shoulder girdle as part of postural responses.

If the client is sufficiently alert so that attending to and understanding directions is a possibility, the therapist should direct the person to focus on the effects of the movement responses rather than focusing attention on the movement of the body.[31] As the person begins to appreciate the consequences of what is transpiring, he or she should be asked to assist in maintaining the changes that promote the more skillful movement response. Unless otherwise indicated by the client's status, interventions must actively involve the individual in the process of planning, initiating, completing, and evaluating the movement. Although the therapist may manipulate the environment (internal and external) in which the response is made, the client must be an active participant for learning to occur.

Although some clients will demonstrate a pattern of generalized overactivity of the postural muscles of the trunk, many will have difficulty generating sufficient activity in the appropriate groups to sustain a posture or to permit movement in the posture. With generalized hypotonia, temporary improvement in postural responses may occur by providing vestibular input that is characterized by rapid and irregular changes. The labyrinths should be stimulated by quick stops and starts with changes in direction. The program should include the introduction of movements in all planes. Approximation can be effective in developing appropriate postural activity from a state of either hypertonicity or hypotonicity. Empirically, it seems that more force is applied to increase than to decrease the postural response. Approximation appears to elicit a response in all the muscles surrounding a joint as preparation for responding to the demands to the erect posture or the demands of weight-bearing. Approximation lends itself to combination with other proprioceptive techniques, such as quick stretch or tapping. Although the changes evoked by these techniques may be of short duration, the alterations can evoke movement components that would not otherwise occur and thereby provide the opportunity for the individual to learn from the movement. (Refer to Chapter 9 for additional information and treatment ideas.)

As the therapist applies various techniques in an attempt to elicit a specific response, the therapist must evaluate the desired response in relationship to the environmental context. If the client is sitting on the edge of a mat table, the activity of the trunk musculature will vary, depending on whether the feet are flat on the floor, the client is engaged in an activity, the client is leaning on one arm for support, or the client is resting between activities. The client who slouches in sitting when fatigued, bored, or overwhelmed by the sensory input may present a different clinical picture when the appropriate factors are altered.

■ *Selective, voluntary movement patterns within functional activities are optimized.*

The concept of the influence of the environment on the quality of a movement response, discussed in relation to the first goal of the intervention process, is also incorporated in the second goal. Quality, selective, voluntary movement patterns are sought within the framework of functional activities, rather than as isolated and abstract movements. Optimization of the selective movement patterns may require a decrease in the stereotypical linkages of certain muscle groups, an increase in the ability to selectively activate certain muscle groups, the development of the ability to execute the movement in different postures, or a number of other variations.

Performance of functional activities requires that the individual have the capability of performing both mobility and stability patterns with the extremities. Mobility patterns are open kinetic chain movements in which the distal segment is free. These patterns are necessary for placing the extremities (e.g., swing phase of gait or reaching for a doorknob).

Clients who exhibit stereotypical posturing of the upper extremity with a restricted repertoire of available movement patterns require intervention to change the initial position of the extremity before movements are attempted. The influence of the spasticity that interferes with the repositioning of the extremity can be reduced by applying approximation through the long axis of the extremity. Preferably, the therapist's manual contacts for the application of the approximation force are on the weight-bearing surfaces of the hand. If the flexed position of the wrist prohibits application of the force to the heel of the palm, the approximation can be

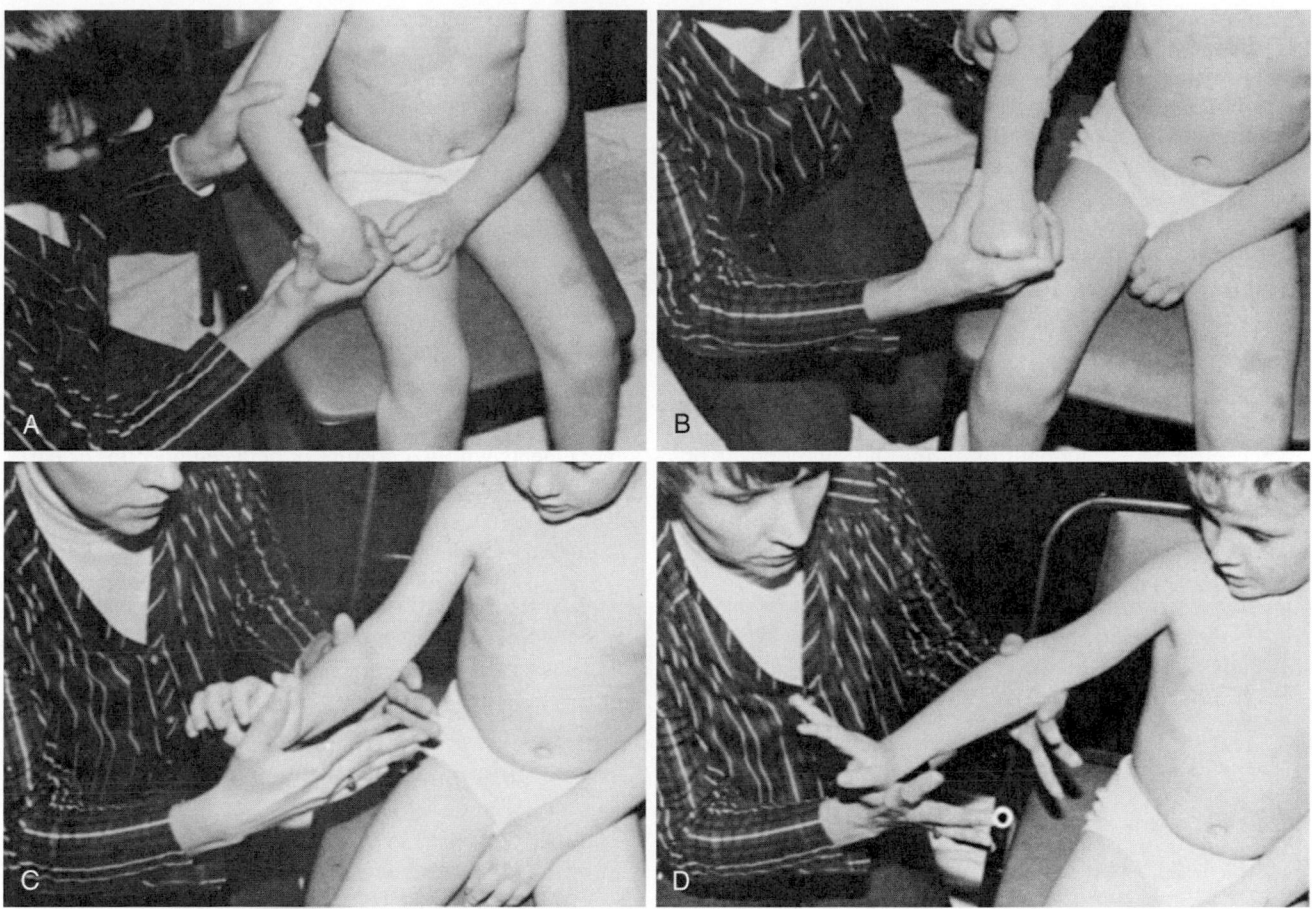

FIGURE 20-6 ■ Facilitating opening of the hand. **A,** Fisted hand; stretch to the extensors and approximation through hand, wrist, and elbow is applied. **B,** Approximation is continued; some resistance to the extensors may be applied. **C,** Approximation is applied to thenar eminence to further facilitate extensor tone. **D,** Full extension is achieved; approximation is maintained.

applied gradually through the fisted hand. As the resistance to passive movement diminishes, the wrist can be moved toward the neutral position so that the therapist can apply the approximation through the heel of the palm (Figure 20-6). The therapist is moving the extremity toward an alternative resting position so that a new movement sequence can be attempted. It is important to use an intervention technique, such as approximation, to reduce the level of spasticity before passive movement is attempted so that a more appropriate position can be assumed without inappropriately stretching the spastic muscles.

The client is asked to assist the therapist with the movement, with the person being cued to do so with a minimum of effort. Too often, clients attempt to make a selective movement through a massive effort and overactivation of the muscle groups, which compounds the underlying spasticity. Clients should be encouraged to make easy effortless movements—those they are instructed to perform with reduced effort so that they can relearn selective activation of motor units rather than mass firing patterns. Working "harder" often creates additional impairments versus increasing normal functional movement responses.

Electrical stimulation can be used as an adjunct to facilitate performance of a particular component of a mobility pattern. (Refer to Chapter 31.) The wrist extension compo-

nent of the proprioceptive neuromuscular facilitation (PNF) pattern of flexion, abduction, and external rotation can be reinforced by using a portable electrical stimulation unit with an adjustable surge duration. The electrical stimulation elicits the correct movement so that the client could learn from the feel of the correct pattern. Adjusting the practice schedule so that the pattern is performed with and without the electrical stimulation support of the movement avoids the potential problem of reliance on the device to produce the movement. Electromyographic (EMG) biofeedback can be a useful adjunct to achieve activation of specific muscle groups or to guide the client's attempts to reduce the level of activity of a muscle group. (Refer to Chapter 31.)

Mobility patterns in the upper extremity have as their foundation the freedom of the scapula to adjust appropriately to the position of the humerus. The mobility of the scapula can be addressed through techniques that result in a general decrease in muscle activity and diagonal movement patterns of the scapula. The scapular stabilizers, such as the rhomboids, trapezius, and serratus anterior, must be capable of allowing appropriate adjustment of the scapula, as well as providing the fixation base on which humeral elevation can occur.

In stability patterns, the distal segment of the extremity is fixed (closed kinetic chain). These patterns are used in the weight-bearing components of the functional activities, such as the stance phase of gait or creeping. The components of the stability patterns are enhanced by proprioceptive input, such as approximation. During the performance of both stability and mobility patterns, the therapist should control the situation so that the client learns the appropriate movement patterns and not those imposed on top of inappropriate muscle activation.

As the client performs mobility and stability patterns as components of functional activities, all categories of muscle contractions should be elicited from each muscle group. If a particular type of contraction poses a problem for a muscle group, the therapist can select an alternate posture in which to build on the ability of the muscle group to perform that type of contraction. For example, if the client has problems with eccentric hamstring control during the swing phase of gait, the pattern can be worked on as a component of the rolling sequence from the supine to the prone position

(Figure 20-7). Once the client gains control of the pattern within one movement context, the therapist must design activities to promote generalization of the pattern to other movement contexts to counter the specificity of strength training. The client who has difficulty with the cocontraction stability pattern of the upper extremity in the all-fours position may have more success with a forward propping position in sitting, which may allow more control of the amount of weight being supported by the upper extremity. After gaining control in the forward propped sitting, attempts can be made to generalize the response to positions such as side sitting and all fours.

Performance of movement patterns should progress toward an ability to easily reverse the direction of the movement. This can be promoted by incorporating rhythmical movements within a posture or between postures as early as possible in the intervention sequence. The end point at which the reversal is required should vary. In preparation for

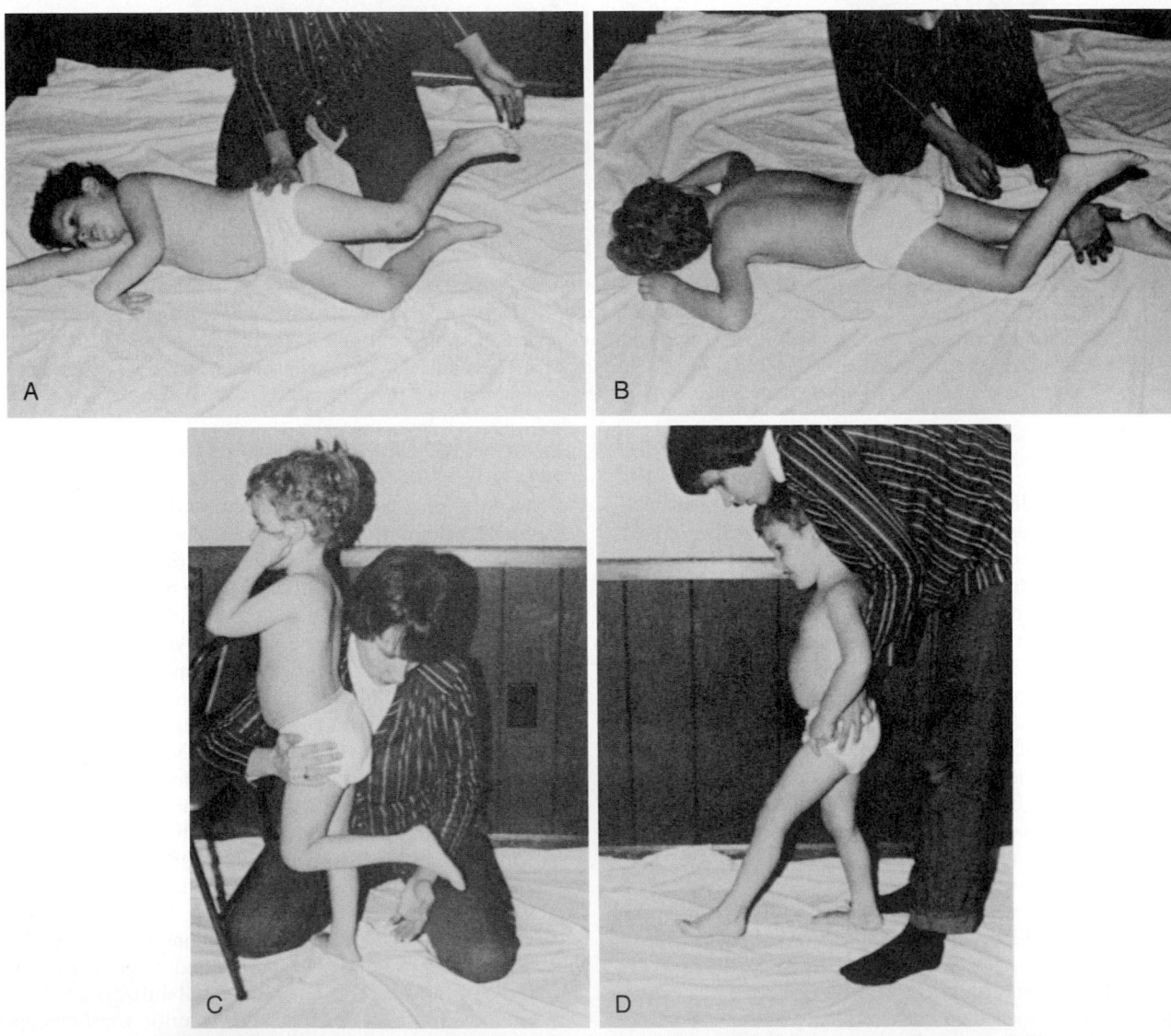

FIGURE 20-7 ■ Eliciting eccentric hamstring control within different movement contexts. **A,** Roll from the supine to side-lying position (beginning sequence). **B,** Roll from the side-lying to prone position with controlled lengthening of the hamstrings. **C,** Standing eccentric hamstring contraction. **D,** Controlled hamstring activity during swing phase of gait.

mastering the movements required to move from supine to sitting on the edge of the mat table, the client might be asked to move from the supine position to side sitting and back to supine; then the client could move from the supine position to side lying propped on one elbow (the halfway point in the overall movement), then reverse to supine. Incorporating reversal of movement patterns within the intervention program prepares the client to deal with situations that mandate unexpected adjustments in the movement sequence.

Clients who demonstrate problems with the sequencing of movements, such as those with motor dyspraxia, frequently perform better if the movement is performed at a speed that is close to normal. Clients who had normal movement sequences before the brain infection seem to be able to trigger better movement responses at normal speeds than at slower speeds. The slower movement speeds appear to disrupt the typical flow of the movement. In working with clients with sequencing problems, all team members should provide the same, consistent sensory cues to elicit a movement pattern. For example, the therapist may establish a coupling of the verbal cue "roll" with a quick stretch to the ankle dorsiflexors to elicit a rolling pattern. These same cues can be used by other team members to assist the client in changing positions in bed or in performing dressing activities. The consistency of cues may elicit a consistent response from the client. Once the pattern is well established, the intervention program can be designed to reduce the cues progressing toward the ability of the client to perform the activity in response to the demands of the situation rather than to externally imposed cues.

The flow of a movement pattern may be disrupted by problems categorized as incoordination. The origin of the coordination problems could be dysfunction of the visual-perceptual system, vestibular system, dyspraxia, or dysfunction caused by cerebellar damage. If possible, the factors involved in producing a lack of coordination should be identified.

■ Performance of functional activities is enhanced.

As the client develops more appropriate postural control and the ability to perform selective movement patterns within functional activities, she is developing the basis to perform increasingly challenging functional activities. The movement patterns (and the postural control that underlies them) provide the building blocks for mastering an expanding variety of activities.

As the therapist designs the expansion of activities within the intervention program, the demands of each new functional activity and posture must be scrutinized. The client's ability to meet these demands was examined in the evaluation process. The intervention strategy must focus on the quality of the client's ability to assume a posture, maintain the posture, move within the posture (static and dynamic equilibrium responses to both self-generated and external perturbations), and move out of the posture. The therapist will change the sequence of this progression of activities to meet the needs of the client. The client may achieve independence in maintaining a posture while still requiring assistance in assuming the posture.

This progression should be grounded within the context of functionally relevant activities. Unless the individual has difficulty tolerating change, activities should be practiced within different environments to enhance generalization of learning. The creative therapist can design a variety of functionally relevant activities that require similar movement components.

With infants, the therapist may choose to use the developmental sequence as a general model for the functional activities progression. Progression through the developmental sequence should be viewed as a dynamic process so that the intervention incorporates movement both within and between postures. For individuals through the remainder of the life span, the focus should be on the age-appropriate functional activities essential to the individual's daily life, such as bed mobility, sit to stand, stand to sit, ambulation, reaching, and manipulation.

Samples of handling techniques that can be adapted to enhance the individual's progression through the sequence of functional activities can be found in the works of Bobath,[32] Carr and Shepherd,[33,34] Duncan and Badke,[35] Levitt,[36] Ryerson and Levit,[37] Sullivan and Markos,[38] and Voss et al,[39] as well as throughout this book. These authors can provide the therapist with ideas for ways to enhance the client's performance within a specific activity.

■ *Integration of sensory information is fostered.*

At the same time that the therapist addresses the previous intervention goals, the goal of fostering integration of sensory input must be considered. Unless the therapist has advanced knowledge of sensory integration theories, this goal may be secondary rather than primary; nevertheless, it cannot be ignored.

The potential for an exaggerated and inappropriate response to sensory input was discussed as part of the clinical picture. Before the therapist expects the client to exhibit adaptive behavior to the potential bombardment of input from combinations of cutaneous, proprioceptive, auditory, and visual input, the therapist must assess the client's ability to respond to multisensory inputs. The ability to respond adaptively progresses from a response to a single sensory system input, to a response to the input in the presence of multiple system input, and then to an adaptive response based on inputs from two or more sources. The therapist must be sure that adding more sensory inputs augments an adaptive response rather than detracting from it. The client may respond to handling techniques that provide proprioceptive and cutaneous cues, but may demonstrate a deterioration of performance when auditory input is added. When verbal cues are added, the therapist should follow the philosophy that verbal commands should be concise, sparse, and appropriately timed.[39]

All sensory inputs should evoke the correct response on the part of the client, rather than cause her or him to sift through the jumble of inputs to recognize the appropriate inputs to which a response should be made. At the highest level, the client will demonstrate cross-modal learning in which input from one sensory system will evoke a response based on input previously obtained through a different system. Recognition of a comb by touch is based on the precept of "combness" usually obtained initially by visual input. If the therapist recognizes the hierarchy in the process of integrating sensory input, intervention situations that require too high a level of performance from the client can be avoided. The client who can respond adaptively to input from only one source will not be expected to perform in a crowded treatment area that presents extraneous visual and auditory input. The therapist will also recognize the need to include in the intervention plan situations that involve the controlled introduction of sensory inputs so that the client progresses toward the ability to deal with multiple inputs. Carr and Shepherd[34] discuss some general principles that can be used during the training of motor tasks in the presence of somatosensory and perceptual-cognitive impairments.

Dysfunctions in perceptual integration are addressed as the client moves through functional sequence activities. Although these movement activities would not provide the total program for an individual with a specific perceptual integration dysfunction, goals in this area can be addressed if the therapist is aware of indications of dysfunctions. The therapist must critically observe the performance of a movement sequence to identify substitute actions to compensate for problems such as inability to cross the midline. The therapist must then attempt to redesign the demands of the situation to elicit the desired behavior. The client who moves from the supine to the side sitting to the long sitting positions without the upper extremities crossing the midline could be required to side sit to the left and transfer objects with the right hand from the left side of the body to the right side (Figure 20-8). The therapist must determine whether the client is truly crossing the midline or rotating the midline of the body to continue to avoid crossing it.

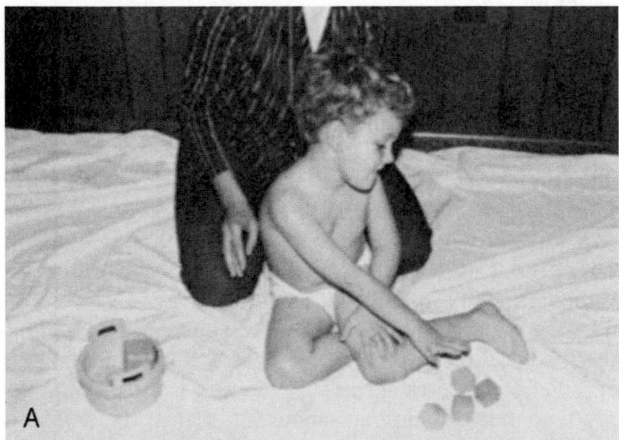

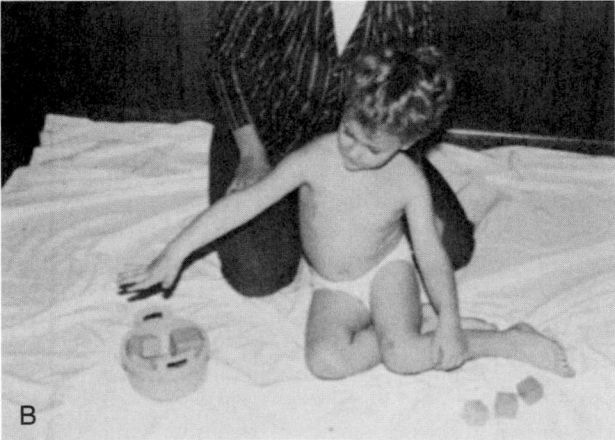

FIGURE 20-8 ■ Child crossing midline of body when transferring objects from left to right. **A,** Beginning act on contralateral side. **B,** Ending sequence by crossing midline and placing objects on ipsilateral side.

Therapists may be most aware of disturbances in the client's ability to integrate sensory information into an appropriate response when this dysfunction disrupts balance. The ability to maintain and move in upright postures requires successful processing of information from the sensory triad of postural control: the visual, vestibular, and somatosensory systems. When one component is missing, unreliable, or discrepant with the other two, the person is at risk for loss of balance. During the ongoing evaluation process, the therapist gathers information on the integrity of each system and any evidence of central processing difficulties. Incorporated within the practice of activities to develop postural control, to promote selective movements with functional activities, and to develop mastery of increasing difficult functional activities, is the simultaneous practice of integrating sensory information so that a successful response can be generated.

Clients who are performing at higher levels can be challenged to maintain balance when one element of the sensory triad is missing (e.g., vision occluded) or altered (e.g., sitting, standing, or walking on a soft, compliant surface). Successful maintenance of balance outside the protective environment of the therapy clinic requires the ability to switch the primary information source to any one of the three systems. Walking in the dark requires the person to rely on vestibular and somatosensory input. Standing on a moving bus looking out a window requires resolution of the conflict between visual input (the external world is moving), vestibular input (you are moving), and somatosensory input (you are stationary). Movement experiences within the therapy program should foster practice of this sensory integration process (see Table 20-2).

■ *Cognitive status and psychosocial responses are optimized.*

In addition to attending to the factors directly related to motor performance, the therapist also must attend to the client's psychosocial and cognitive responses. Although the therapist does not have primary responsibility in this area, a goal of the intervention process should be to enhance the individual's psychosocial and cognitive responses.

Particularly in the agitated state that may be a component of the response to the inflammatory process, the client may demonstrate exaggerated and inappropriate emotional responses to events. Dealing with these emotional fluctuations can become a major determinant in goal attainment in the other areas. Maintaining a positive, nonthreatening interaction allows the client to use the therapist as a reference for judging the appropriateness of emotional responses.

If the client's state of agitation is interfering with the intervention program, the therapist may alter the program to include techniques that have a calming effect. For example, the individual can be wrapped in a cotton sheet blanket and rocked in a slow, rhythmical, repetitive manner to decrease her agitation. Auditory and visual input should be controlled to avoid overloading sensory processing mechanisms.

Earlier in this text the psychosocial adjustment that occurs in the process of recovering from a neurological disability was discussed (see Chapter 5). The therapist must be aware of how the client's regression in affective and cognitive domains affects the intervention process. The therapist should seek assistance from the health care team members responsible for intervention in these areas to deal with the client constructively. The therapist must remember that both the family members and the client are in the process of adjusting to the client's changed and, it is hoped, changing status. Family members may be an asset or a liability to the client's recovery process. During the therapist's interactions with the family members in activities such as instructions in the client's home program, the therapist should be prepared to deal with expressions of the individual's difficulty in adjusting to the situation. The therapist also should be prepared to assist family members in identifying appropriate sources to help them deal with their problems. Ignoring family issues and assuming that the environment will self-correct reflect a model of empowering the therapist and medical team, not the patient and the family.

Changes in mentation, perception of events, and memory losses present challenges to both the client and the therapist. Repetition in the recounting of past events may help reorder past knowledge. Use of brief verbal or visual cues may assist the client in recalling safety instructions or the components of the exercise program. The therapist should try to generate a nonstressful environment when working on these deficits so that attention and recall are not overshadowed by emotional pressure. Chapter 28 discusses further intervention ideas that deal with individuals who have cognitive impairments.

As the therapist works with the client on an intervention program, situations arise that require problem solving to determine a way to accomplish a task. If the task is to accomplish an independent transfer from a wheelchair into a bathtub, decisions must be made concerning the sequence of movements. Therapists can approach this situation in two ways. They can instruct clients step by step in what to do, or they can involve clients to the extent possible in the process of deciding what to do. If the therapist instructs the client step by step, the client may seem to have mastered the task, but the client may not be able to perform it under different conditions or in a similar environment when instructions are not used as reinforcement. If the therapist involves the client in the decision-making process, the client may be learning not only how to accomplish the specific task, but also how to accomplish the task under varied conditions. The intervention process should lead to the ability to respond to the demands of a situation, and involvement of clients in the problem-solving process helps prepare them for independence. The therapist must structure the client's role in decision making to the level of the client's ability to participate so that the experience is not frustrating. Although the client's participation may initially increase the time required to complete a task, it promotes skills that may lead more quickly to independence of function.

INTERACTION WITH OTHER PROFESSIONALS

The therapist needs to design an intervention program that is coordinated with that of other members of the health care team. The recovery process of the client should be facilitated by a care plan in which each team member reinforces the goals of the other team members. The care of the person must be a collaborative effort. Each client deserves an intervention process that considers him or her as a whole person, not as a set of fragmented problems.

SUMMARY

This chapter has presented a brief discussion of the pathology and medical management of various inflammatory processes that affect the brain. The process of evaluation, the role of evaluation in designing an intervention program, the goals of the intervention process, and the means to meet those goals were presented to assist the reader in more effective management of clients with these diagnoses.

Although the problem-solving process presented in this chapter for evaluation, diagnosis, prognosis, goal identification, and treatment planning is not limited to clients with inflammatory supraspinal disorders, its application in the presence of typical neurological sequelae has been described. When dealing with inflammatory disorders of the brain, the variability of neurological sequelae is examined based on the anatomical location of the inflammatory process and the cause of the infection.

Although the neurological disorders discussed in this chapter are life threatening, many clients fully recover and return to their previous lifestyles. Clients will vary within the spectrum of minimal to severe involvement, from specific to generalized CNS dysfunction, and will demonstrate little to full recovery after the acute distress. Prognosis for recovery depends on the type of infecting organism and the extent of involvement. The therapist must remain flexible and willing to adjust every aspect of therapeutic intervention to meet the specific needs of each client while at the same time recognizing that learning requires active participation on the part of the client.

REFERENCES

1. Davis LE: Central nervous system infections, in Weiner WJ, Goetz CG, editors: *Neurology for the non-neurologist,* ed 4, Philadelphia, 1999, Lippincott Williams & Wilkins.
2. Bharucha NE, Bharucha EP, Bhabha SK: Bacterial infections, in Bradley WG, editor: *Neurology in clinical practice, vol 2,* Boston, 1996, Butterworth Heinemann.
3. Fritz DP, Nelson PB: Brain abscess. In Roos KL, editor: *Central nervous system infectious diseases and therapy,* New York, 1997, Marcel Dekker.
4. Weiner WJ, Goetz CG: *Neurology for the non-neurologist,* ed 4, Philadelphia, 1999, Lippincott Williams & Wilkins.
5. Roos KL: *Meningitis,* London, 1996, Arnold.
6. Roos KL: Bacterial meningitis. In Roos KL, editor: *Central nervous system infectious diseases and therapy,* New York, 1997, Marcel Dekker.
7. Davis LE: Infections of the central nervous system: acute bacterial meningitis. In Weiner WJ, Shulman LM, editors: *Emergent and urgent neurology,* Philadelphia, 1999, Lippincott Williams & Wilkins.
8. Hoppenfeld S: *Physical examination of the spine and extremities,* New York, 1976, Appleton-Century-Crofts.
9. Pruitt AA: Infections of the nervous system, *Neurol Clin* 16:419-447, 1998.
10. Roos KL, Bonnin JM: Acute bacterial meningitides. In Mandell GL, editor: *Atlas of infectious diseases, vol 3, central nervous system and eye infection,* Philadelphia, 1995, Churchill Livingstone.
11. Van de Beek D, Schmand B, deGans J et al. Cognitive impairment in adults with good recovery after bacterial meningitis. *J Infect Dis Soc Am* 186:1047-1052, 2002.
12. Gluckman SJ, DiNubile MJ: Infections of the central nervous system: acute viral infections. In Weiner WJ, Shulman LM, editors: *Emergent and urgent neurology,* Philadelphia, 1999, Lippincott Williams & Wilkins.

13. Bhabha SK, Bharucha NE, Bharucha EP: Viral infections. In Bradley WG, editor: *Neurology in clinical practice, vol 2,* Boston, 1996, Butterworth-Heinemann.

14. Johnson RT: *Viral infections of the nervous system,* ed 2, Philadelphia, 1998, Lippincott-Raven.

15. Roos KL: Viral meningitis and aseptic meningitis. In Roos KL, editor: *Central nervous system infectious diseases and therapy,* New York, 1997, Marcel Dekker.

16. Rotbart HA: Viral meningitis and the aseptic meningitis syndrome. In Scheld WM, Whitney RJ, Durach DT, editors: *Infections of the central nervous system,* ed 2, Philadelphia, 1997, Lippincott-Raven.

17. Cassady KA, Whitley RJ: Pathogenesis and pathophysiology of viral infections of the central nervous system. In Scheld WM, Whitney RJ, Durach DT, editors: *Infections of the central nervous system,* ed 2, Philadelphia, 1997, Lippincott-Raven.

18. Plum F, Posner JB: *The diagnosis of stupor and coma,* ed 3, Philadelphia, 1980, FA Davis.

19. McCarthy M, Weber T, Berger JR: Central nervous system diseases caused by unconventional transmissible agents and chronic viral infections. In Bradley WG, editor: *Neurology in clinical practice, vol 2,* Boston, 1996, Butterworth-Heinemann.

20. Schooley RT: Encephalitis. In Roper AH, editor: *Neurological and neurosurgical intensive care,* ed 3, New York, 1993, Raven Press.

21. *Guide to physical therapist practice,* ed 2, Alexandria, VA, 2001, American Physical Therapy Association.

22. Jennett B, Teasdale G: *Management of head injuries,* Philadelphia, 1981, FA Davis.

23. DeMeyer W: *Technique of the neurological examination,* ed 4, New York, 1994, McGraw-Hill.

24. Shumway-Cook A, Horak F: Assessing influence of sensory interaction on balance, *Phys Ther* 66:1548-1550, 1986.

25. Ayres JA: *Sensory integration and learning disorder.* Los Angeles, 1972, Western Psychological Services.

26. Ayres JA: *Southern California postrotatory nystagmus test,* Los Angeles, 1975, Western Psychological Services.

27. Shumway-Cook A, Woollacott MJ: *Motor control: theory and practical applications,* Philadelphia, 1995, Lippincott Williams and Wilkins.

28. VanSant AF: Analysis of movement dysfunction: usefulness of a component approach. In *Proceedings of the thirteenth annual Eugene Michels Researchers' Forum, Section on Research,* Alexandria, VA, 1993, American Physical Therapy Association.

29. VanSant AF: Rising from a supine position to erect stance—description of adult movement and a developmental hypothesis, *Phys Ther* 68:185-192, 1988.

30. Horak FB, Henry SB, Shumway-Cook A: Postural perturbations: new insights for treatment of postural control disorders, *Phys Ther* 77:517-533, 1997.

31. McNevin NH, Wulf G, Carlson C: Effects of attentional focus, self control, and dyad training on motor learning: implications for physical rehabilitation, *Phys Ther* 80:373-385, 2000.

32. Bobath B: *Adult hemiplegia: evaluation and treatment,* ed 3, London, 1990, William Heinemann Medical Books.

33. Carr JH, Shepherd RB: *Movement science-foundations for physical therapy in rehabilitation,* Rockville, MD, 1987, Aspen Publishers.

34. Carr JH, Shepherd RB: *Neurological rehabilitation—optimizing motor performance,* Boston, 1998, Butterworth Heinemann.

35. Duncan PW, Badke MB: *Stroke rehabilitation—the recovery of motor control,* St. Louis, 1987, CV Mosby.

36. Levitt S: *Treatment of cerebral palsy and motor delay,* ed 2, London, 1982, Blackwell Scientific.

37. Ryerson S, Levit K: *Functional movement reeducation: a contemporary model for stroke rehabilitation,* New York, Churchill Livingstone, 1997.

38. Sullivan PE, Markos PD: *Clinical decision making in therapeutic exercise,* Norwalk, CT, 1995, Appleton & Lange.

39. Voss DE, Ionta MK, Myers BJ: *Proprioceptive neuromuscular facilitation,* ed 3, Philadelphia, 1985, Harper & Row.

CHAPTER 21

Human Immunodeficiency Virus Infection: Living With a Chronic Illness

David M. Kietrys, PT, MS, OCS
Mary Lou Galantino, PT, PhD, MSCE

KEY WORDS

AIDS
human immunodeficiency virus (HIV)
psychoneuroimmunology

OBJECTIVES

After reading this chapter the student/therapist will be able to:
1. Appreciate the role of the immune system in chronic HIV disease.
2. Discuss the neuropathological features of HIV infection and understand potential neurocognitive and neuropsychological alterations that may occur.
3. Understand the various systems (integumentary, musculoskeletal, cardiopulmonary, and neurological) that affect function in HIV-infected adult and pediatric patients.
4. Appreciate the role of psychoneuroimmunology in HIV rehabilitation management.
5. Establish safe exercise parameters in the HIV-positive population.

IDENTIFICATION OF THE CLINICAL PROBLEM

Initially recognized in 1982, acquired immunodeficiency syndrome (AIDS) has been the leading cause of death among young adults in the United States since the 1990s. It has had a devastating impact on people in the developing world.[1,2] The epidemiology of human immunodeficiency virus (HIV) disease in industrialized nations, including the United States, has changed dramatically as a result of the development of medications used to treat the disease. Most epidemiologists and clinicians attribute improved life expectancy to the impact of new, highly active antiretroviral therapies (HAART). Implementation of these medications have resulted in a decline in AIDS deaths nationally.[3-5] However, the incidence of HIV disease, which demonstrated some decrease in the 1990s, demonstrated some increase from 1999 to 2006.[6] Because HAART regimens have fostered longevity for many, HIV infection has evolved into a chronic disease. Individuals previously disabled by the disease may have the potential to return to work through vocational rehabilitation. HIV disease has a great impact on rehabilitation medicine because multisystem involvement progresses slowly throughout the life span.

HAART has slowed the progression from HIV infection to AIDS and from AIDS to death.[3] In communities with access to antiretroviral medications, the incidence of perinatally acquired AIDS has declined significantly as a result of administration of HAART during pregnancy.[7] Unfortunately, perinatal transmission of the virus in developing nations continues to be a crisis.

The clinical and pathological information about this disease is constantly increasing. Certainly, our understanding of the disease process and advances in drug regimens will change between the writing and the publication of this book. Changes in terminology reflect this evolution of clinical knowledge. The definitions used throughout this chapter reflect current use.

The virus thought to be responsible for the transmission of AIDS was first identified in 1984, and it was named HIV (human immunodeficiency virus) in 1986 at the International Conference on AIDS in Paris. Because a second virus, HIV-2, was soon identified in western Africa, the strain originally identified was renamed HIV-1. Infection caused by HIV-2, less widely distributed, has since been established in Europe and in South, Central, and North America. Both HIV-1 and HIV-2 have resulted in AIDS, but evidence suggests that HIV-2 may be less virulent than HIV-1. In addition to these subtypes, several strains of HIV-1 have been identified. Different strains reflect variations in cellular affinities and resistance to medications. The context of discussion for the purpose of this chapter will be HIV-1, herein discussed as HIV.

In 1993 the Centers for Disease Control and Prevention revised its definition of AIDS and its classification system of HIV disease. To reflect current scientific knowledge, the new system elucidates the importance of T-helper (CD4) cell counts as indicators for pharmacological disease management. HIV disease had been staged, with the term AIDS being reserved for only the advanced stage of the disease. Advanced HIV disease, or AIDS, is now defined as HIV infection with CD4 cell counts below $200\,mm^3$/blood or as HIV infection with the presence of an opportunistic infection. In addition, three clinical conditions—pulmonary tuberculosis, recurrent pneumonia, and invasive cervical cancer—were added to the existing list of 20 AIDS-defining diseases.[8] The entire spectrum of illness from initial diagnosis to AIDS can be covered by the term *HIV disease*. The terms acute HIV infection, asymptomatic HIV disease, symptomatic HIV disease, and advanced HIV disease

(AIDS) are used throughout this chapter. Table 21-1 presents the various modifiers of quality of life throughout the various stages of HIV disease.

Epidemiology

AIDS (advanced HIV disease) has assumed the title of the leading cause of death in the world, according to the World Health Organization's World Health Report.[9] It is estimated that, in 2003, in the United States, there were approximately 1 million individuals living with HIV disease and approximately 18,000 deaths from AIDS-related illnesses.[6] It is estimated that, of the nearly 1 million HIV-positive individuals in the United States, approximately 25% of them do not know they are infected.[10] As of 2003, the global prevalence of HIV infections is estimated to be 40 million cases (37 million adults and 2.5 million children under the age of 15 years).[11] Adults and adolescents older than 13 years of age have accounted for almost 99% of the total AIDS cases. Fewer than 2% of cases (1.3%) have occurred in children younger than 13 years of age.[3] Globally, approximately 5 million new infections occurred in 2003 (4.2 million adults and 700,000 children under the age of 15 years). In the same year (2003), there were approximately 3 million deaths from AIDS (2.5 million adults and 500,000 children under the age of 15 years).[11]

HIV infection is the fourth leading cause of disability-adjusted life-years lost, a measure that assesses the impact of disease on both length and quality of life. Only perinatal diseases, acute respiratory infections, and diarrheal diseases cause more premature loss of life and function than that resulting from AIDS.[12]

Tuberculosis (TB), the former leading microbial killer, was estimated to have killed 1.8 million people in 1998, but 400,000 of these deaths were in HIV-infected individuals, and the World Health Organization credited these deaths to AIDS rather than to TB. HIV infection is now responsible for more than 20% of all deaths in people with TB.[12]

Normal Immunity

The immune system is complex and dynamic, comprising a multitude of components and subsystems, all of which interact continuously. The normal immune system has two main components, or lines of defense, against illness (Figure 21-1). The first is the innate, or inborn, component that includes the skin, the cilia and mucosal linings of the respiratory and digestive systems, the gastric fluids and

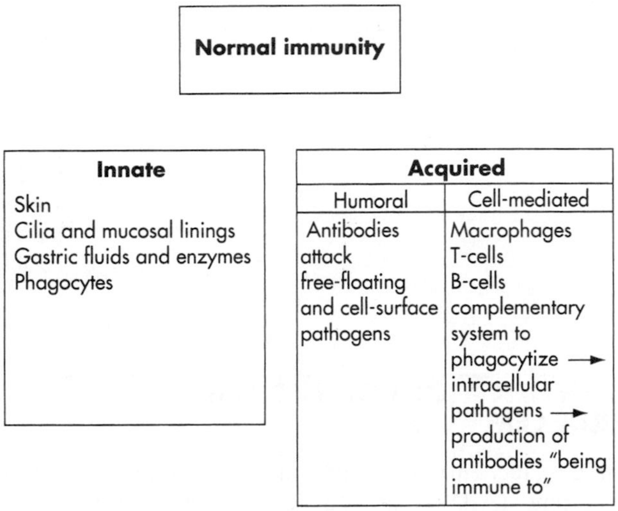

FIGURE 21-1 ■ Main components of immunity.

TABLE 21-1 ■ Quality of Life Issues for HIV Disease Stages

STAGE	CD4+ CATEGORY	PHYSICAL INDICATORS	MODERATORS OF QUALITY OF LIFE	GENERAL QUALITY OF LIFE ISSUES
Asymptomatic HIV infection	≤500 μl	May have persistent generalized lymphadenopathy	*Appraisals:* Anticipatory grieving, catastrophizing, and other cognitive distortions; changed expectations of future; identity and self-esteem issues *Coping:* Dealing with present and future uncertainties; at risk for denial, disengagement, substance abuse, risky sex, suicidality; issues of eliciting social support	*Emotional functioning:* Depression, anxiety, anger, often increasing at diagnosis and diminishing and recycling as individual confronts realities of living with HIV disease *Role functioning:* Often able to work; possible decrements in job mobility and career opportunities; job loss *Social functioning:* Fear, isolation, issues of trust in relationships; stigmatization; changes in social support networks because of deaths; relationship and sexual changes; isolation, withdrawal *Physical functioning:* Normal but may be altered because of depression or anxiety; may have hypervigilance regarding all physical symptoms *Spiritual functioning:* Opportunity to direct attention inward, thus yielding to contemplation of life's meaning, reassessment of spiritual and existential issues

TABLE 21-1 ■ Quality of Life Issues for HIV Disease Stages—cont'd

STAGE	CD4+ CATEGORY	PHYSICAL INDICATORS	MODERATORS OF QUALITY OF LIFE	GENERAL QUALITY OF LIFE ISSUES
Symptomatic HIV infection	201-499 μl	Emergence of symptoms such as thrush, night sweats, low-grade fevers, oral hairy leukoplakia, peripheral neuropathy; commonly taking antiretroviral drugs and/or *Pneumocystis carinii* prophylaxis	*Appraisals:* Anticipatory grieving, catastrophizing, and other cognitive distortions; changed expectations of future; identity and self-esteem issues related to threats to occupational and functional abilities *Coping:* Dealing with present and future uncertainties; at risk for denial, disengagement, substance abuse, and risky sex	*Emotional functioning:* Depression, anxiety, anger, often increasing on emergence of symptoms and then fluctuating with challenges and threats to present and future functioning *Role functioning:* Often able to work; may take on new roles as part of HIV support-related network *Social functioning:* Changes in social support networks due to deaths, isolation, withdrawal, relationship and sexual changes, and stigmatization *Physical functioning:* May have reduced energy levels; moderate symptomatology; possible cognitive deficits; pain; wasting *Spiritual functioning:* Anticipatory grieving, sense of relatedness to something greater than the self, unavoidable confrontation with one's own mortality
AIDS	<200 μl	Opportunistic infections such as extensive candidiasis, cryptococcal meningitis; Kaposi's sarcoma; tuberculosis; *Pneumocystis carinii* pneumonia; lymphomas; commonly taking antiretroviral drugs, chemotherapy, antibiotics, etc.	*Appraisals:* Facing chronic illness and death; grieving about current and anticipated losses; catastrophizing and other cognitive distortions; reassessment of spiritual and existential issues *Coping:* Coping strategies may be overwhelmed in dealing with current difficulties such as financial losses, medical costs, treatment and side effects, housing; may lose some traditional coping strategies such as recreational outlets	*Emotional functioning:* Depression, anxiety, anger may cycle according to fluctuations in disease status and appraisals; relief from uncertainty *Role functioning:* Diminished capacity for work; role changes—often need care instead of being a caretaker *Social functioning:* May have diminished social networks because of lack of mobility, illness, and deaths among friends *Physical functioning:* Self-care difficulties; fatigue; wasting; much time spent in medical care; debilitation from infection and treatments; possible cognitive deficits *Spiritual functioning:* Essential worth is to provide a framework from which to pose and seek responses to metaphysical questions generated by presence of life-threatening disease; integration and transcending of biological and psychosocial nature, which gives access to nonphysical realms as prophecy, love, artistic inspiration, completion, and healing actions

enzymes of the stomach, and the phagocyte cells. This innate component of the immune system keeps pathogens out of the body by creating barriers against them, by ejecting them, or by enveloping them and eliminating them. The second, the acquired component of the immune system, develops defenses against specific pathogens, starts in utero, and continues throughout life. It is acquired (or antibody) immunity that is most pertinent to understanding HIV infection and its progression.

Acquired Immunity

Acquired immunity is divided into humoral and cell-mediated responses. Humoral immunity depends on the production of antibodies. This response is effective for disposing of free-floating or cell-surface pathogens. The cell-mediated response is required to destroy infected cells, those with intracellular pathogens. Cell-mediated immunity is essential for destroying pathogens responsible for the opportunistic infections and neoplasms that are associated with AIDS.[13,14]

For the study of HIV pathology, it is important to consider three types of immune system cells: macrophages, T lymphocytes (T cells), and B lymphocytes (B cells). Macrophages originate in the bone marrow and then migrate to the organs in the lymphatic system. Macrophages recognize, and then phagocytize, antigens—substances deemed foreign to the body. All but a fragment of the antigen is digested by the macrophage. This remaining portion protrudes from the cellular surface, where it is recognized by T and B cells.[15]

Both of the lymphocytes originate in the bone marrow. Their differentiation into T and B cells depends on where they develop immunocompetence. T cells migrate to the thymus to perform this task. B cells complete it before leaving the bone marrow. T cells then travel to lymph nodes, the spleen, and connective tissue, where they wait to phagocytize the antigens in the manner previously described. B cells function in the same way against free-floating blood-borne pathogens.[15]

There are at least eight types of T cells with various functions. Two relevant types are helper T cells (CD4) and suppressor T cells (CD8). These cells are regulatory and complementary. On recognition of an antigen, CD4 cells chemically stimulate production and activation of other lymphocytes to destroy the foreign material. When the action of the T and B cells is sufficient, CD8 cells stop this action, thus preventing destruction of noninfected cells. The HIV virus destroys CD4 cells. Declining CD4 cell counts occur in untreated disease. However, because T-cell counts fluctuate somewhat under normal circumstances, the ratio of CD4 to CD8 cells is also considered a valuable laboratory value when the progression of the disease is tracked.

In the process of identifying and destroying these antigens, the acquired immune system also retains a memory of the antigen, which allows it to respond more rapidly and effectively to the pathogen if it is reintroduced into the body. Herein lies the pertinence of vaccination and the phenomenon of being immune to an illness.[15]

Psychoneuroimmunology: Prevention and Wellness in HIV Infection

Psychoneuroimmunology is that field that investigates the interrelationships among psychological constructs (e.g.,

stressors and mood states) of the neuroendocrine and immune systems. Although all the precise mechanistic links among these varied components of psychoneuroimmunology are not yet fully elucidated, psychoneuroimmunology does offer a useful framework for our understanding of how stressors play a role in immunomodulation. The progression of HIV disease can be modulated by psychosocial factors and by factors such as the viral strain, genetic characteristics of the host immune system, coinfections with other pathogenic organisms, and health maintenance habits (diet, exercise, medical treatments).[16] These effects may have a profound influence on the occurrence and progression of ill health in chronic diseases such as HIV infection or AIDS.

Psychoneuroimmunological findings show that it may be useful to evaluate the influence of behavioral factors on immune functioning and disease progression among HIV-infected individuals.[17-19] The stress response is physiologically mediated by certain immune parameters (catecholamines and glucocorticoid hormones). A study by Leserman et al[20] in 2002 concluded that "stressful life events, dysphoric mood, and limited social support" are correlated to the increased rate of progression from HIV to AIDS.[20] Behavioral interventions with immunomodulatory capabilities may help restore competence and thereby slow the progression of HIV disease, especially at the earliest stages of the infectious continuum.

A growing body of literature indicates that many different stressors have deleterious effects on the immune system.[21] It has been well documented in healthy individuals that changes in immune function and disease susceptibility are correlated with times of "psychic distress."[16] These stressors in the case of people living with HIV infection may be attenuated by an exercise training program. Research indicates that continued aerobic exercise training may result in increased CD4 cell counts, heightened immune surveillance, and a potential for a slowing of disease progression.[19] Other researchers have demonstrated similar benefits of exercise for individuals infected with HIV who are at more advanced stages of disease. However, these are studies conducted on traditional modes of exercise. Exercise within the context of psychoneuroimmunology appears to be a promising approach to the treatment of illness and promotion of health in chronic HIV disease.

PATHOGENESIS OF HIV INFECTION

HIV belongs to a class of viruses known as retroviruses, which carry their genetic material in the form of ribonucleic acid (RNA) rather than deoxyribonucleic acid. HIV primarily infects the mononuclear cells, especially CD4 and macrophages, but B cells are also infected.[22] HIV binds to the receptor sites on the surface of the lymphocytes, eventually fusing with and then entering the cells. Reverse transcriptase released from the HIV allows a deoxyribonucleic acid copy of the virus to be made within the host cell, which can then become integrated into the host cell genome. Other enzymes, such as integrase and protease, turn the lymphocyte into a "virus factory," and replicated virions bud out of the cell to infect others.

Within days of acute HIV infection, lymph nodes become sites of rampant viral replication, and viral loads in the blood are high. During the stage of acute HIV infection, the individual may remain asymptomatic or may experience non-specific and self-limited flu-like symptoms—fever, diarrhea, myalgias, and fatigue—for a period of 2 to 12 weeks. In the weeks following an acute infection, the body gradually produces an antibody response. The point at which antibodies can be detected with a blood test is known as seroconversion. Typically, seroconversion occurs within 3 months of the time of infection, but it can take as long as 12 months. Thus there is a period of time after HIV infection when an HIV antibody test (the most commonly used test to determine HIV status) will be negative.

The next stage is asymptomatic HIV disease. Individuals will have positive antibody tests during this stage. This stage may last between 1 and 20 years. Although generally asymptomatic, individuals in this stage may express periods of generalized lymphadenopathy.

Laboratory tests may reveal slowly declining immune dysfunction, as evidenced by abnormal CD4 cell counts and CD4/CD8 ratios. The viral load is typically at a "set point" during most of the asymptomatic stage of HIV disease. This set point is typically much lower than the viral load occurring during the period of acute infection. The viral load will inevitably escalate as the disease progresses.

As CD4 cell counts decline and viral load escalates, the individual will eventually enter the stage of symptomatic HIV disease. This stage of the disease may last from a few months to 5 years. CD4 cell counts are declining and viral loads are increasing. Concurrently with these laboratory value abnormalities, the individual begins to have one or more of an array of symptoms such as weight loss, fatigue, night sweats, fever, or neurological complications. When CD4 cell counts drop below 200/mm^3, the individual is diagnosed with an opportunistic infection or AIDS-defining illness, or the individual demonstrates wasting syndrome or HIV-related dementia, he/she is reclassified as having advanced HIV disease or AIDS. It is possible for patients in this stage to demonstrate remarkable recovery in terms of both laboratory values and function with HAART. Individuals who do not have access to HAART, or individuals who have failed HAART, will eventually die as a result of the effects of opportunistic infections that will inevitably occur. Quality-of-life issues throughout the stage of HIV disease are described in Table 21-1.

Medical Management

Cell Counts, Viral Load, and Prophylaxis

Pharmacological interventions to combat the opportunistic infections associated with HIV infection are beyond the scope of this chapter, but a simplified summary of clinical information is pertinent. Medical management of HIV infection is most often guided by the CD4 cell count and viral load.

For the healthy non–HIV-infected adult, the average CD4 cell count is approximately 1000 cells/mm^3. However, counts may vary widely and may range from 500 to 1500 cells/mm^3.[23] A CD4 cell count of 200 cells/mm^3 marks a critical point in the course of an HIV-infected individual. Multiple serious opportunistic infections occur once this level of immune depletion is attained.[24-26]

Exercise, stress, season, serum cortisol level, and the presence of acute or chronic illness have all been reported to affect CD4 cell counts. Thus, the initial CD4 lymphocyte

numbers should be confirmed by repeat testing. Caution should be exercised to avoid overinterpreting small changes in CD4 lymphocyte test results. The overall trend of CD4 counts is more important than any single value. Testing is typically done at a frequency of four times annually. In addition to CD4 cell counts, CD4/CD8 ratios are used to evaluate the status of the immune system. CD4 counts above 500/mm^3 usually indicate no need for antiretroviral therapy because individuals are generally asymptomatic. It is currently recommended that HAART should be initiated when CD4 levels are between 350 and 200/mm^3, with individual parameters influencing the decision.[27] CD4 cell counts below 200/mm^3 are an indication for prophylactic *Pneumocystis carinii* pneumonia (PCP) and toxoplasmosis measures. Persons with counts below 100/mm^3 may also receive prophylactic agents against cytomegalovirus (CMV) infection, infection with *Mycobacterium avium* complex (MAC), and fungal infections such as cryptococcosis and candidiasis.[13] Table 21-2 is a summary of common pharmacological agents prescribed to combat opportunistic infections and, most pertinent to rehabilitation, their potential side effects.

Viral Load Measurement

Testing for the amount of HIV in plasma by measuring viral RNA has become a standard component of the management of HIV-infected patients.[28] There are important prognostic implications for the amount of viral load in persons with HIV disease.[29] In patients with higher viral loads, disease progression is more rapid, both immunologically in terms of the rate of CD4 cell count decline and clinically in terms of development of AIDS-defining illness. Additionally, the plasma levels in HIV pregnant women directly correlate with the risk of perinatal transmission.[30] Viral load is an important useful marker for judging the effectiveness of various antiretroviral drug interventions.[31,32]

There are several assays available for testing HIV for resistance to antiretroviral agents. Genotype or phenotype testing is used to determine whether the virus has mutated. The results of genotype or phenotype testing provide important information about resistance to specific antiretroviral drugs. If a mutant form is resistant to a particular antiretroviral drug, the HAART regimen is changed so that the potential for viral suppression is maximized. Changes in drugs used for HAART in response to viral resistance is known as "salvage therapy." Like genotypic testing, phenotypic testing may not detect small subpopulations of resistant HIV.[33] Researchers continue to work on developing effective HAART components and vaccines. The primary goal of antiretroviral therapy is to achieve prolonged suppression of HIV replication.[28,34] In 1987, zidovudine (AZT), a nucleoside reverse transcriptase inhibitor (NRTI), was approved by the U.S. Food and Drug Administration. Since that time several more NRTI drugs have been approved.[35]

Additional drugs such as nevirapine and efavirenz also inhibit the reverse transcriptase enzyme, but they are not nucleoside analogs. These agents, known as nonnucleoside reverse transcriptase inhibitors (NNRTI) bind to the enzymatic binding pocket of the reverse transcriptase gene and block binding by nucleosides.[36]

Another drug target for anti-HIV agents is the protease enzyme. Protease inhibitors (PI) are structurally different

TABLE 21-2 ■ HIV Drug Classes

FI (FUSION INHIBITORS)		NRTI		NNRTI		PI (PROTEIN INHIBITORS)	
TRADE NAME	DRUG NAME	TRADE NAME	DRUG NAME	TRADE NAME	DRUG NAME	TRADE NAME	DRUG NAME
Fuzeon	Enfuvirtide	Combivir	Lamivudine or zidovudine	Rescriptor	Delavirdine	Agenerase	Amprenavir
		Emtriva	Emtricabine or FTC	Sustiva	Efavirenz	Crixivan	Indinavir
		Epivir	Lamivudine or 3TC	Viramune	Nevirapine	Fortovase	Saquinavir
		Hivid	Zalcitabine or ddC			Invirase	Saquinavir mesylate
		Retrovir	Zidovudine or AZT			Kaletra	Iopinavir or Ritonavir
		Trizivir	Abacavir sulfate or lamivudine or zidovudine			Lexiva	Fosamprenavir calcium
		Videx	Didanosine or ddl			Norvir	Ritonavir
		Videx EC	Didanosine or ddl			Reyataz	Atazanavir
		Viread	Tenofovir			Viracept	Nelfinavir
		Zerit	Stavudine or d4T				
		Ziogen	Abacavir sulfate				

from NRTI and NNRTI drugs and include agents such as ritonavir, indinavir, nelfinavir, and saquinavir.[37] HAART may be NNRTI or PI based (i.e., NNRTI and PI drugs are used in combination with a NRTI such as AZT). There has been a gradual evolution of pharmacology that has allowed for multiple drugs to be combined into one pill. Thus, the number of pills required per day as well as the dosing schedule has become increasingly more manageable over recent years. However, drugs from different classes (NRTI, NNRTI, and PI) are typically included in HAART.

Receptor site inhibitors such as T-20 may be used as part of salvage therapy. T-20 is a twice-daily injectable drug with a cost of more than $20,000 per year. Drugs in other classes, such as integrase inhibitors, are under study. Because of the rapidly evolving nature of HAART, the reader is advised to consult with the Centers for Disease Control and Prevention for the most current clinical practice guidelines.

Side effects and toxicities are common with drugs used to treat HIV disease. Purported side effects of NRTIs include peripheral neuropathy, myopathy, anemia, gastrointestinal (GI) disturbances, hepatomegaly, and pancreatitis. NNRTIs may cause rash, liver dysfunction, cognitive problems, and lactic acidosis. PIs may cause lipodystrophy, peripheral neuropathy, GI intolerance, hyperlipidemia, hyperglycemia, and liver toxicity. Injection site reactions are common with T-20. This list of side effects is cursory, and the full impact of these drugs on the various systems of the body is a continually emerging area. Occasionally an individual's HAART regimen is modified to mitigate the side effects that may occur with specific drugs.

Current medication regimens can significantly reduce the HIV level not only in the peripheral blood but also in the lymphoid tissue and the central nervous system (CNS).[38] The goal of HAART is to reduce HIV viral load to to undetectable levels. The greatest challenge with HAART is resistance to one drug in a class of agents, which may induce partial or complete resistance with other agents, depending on the specific mutations involved.[33,39] In a field that is rapidly changing, specific recommendations for antiretroviral therapy are difficult to make. The major therapeutic decisions include (1) when to initiate therapy and (2) when to change therapy and to which drugs. When PIs were introduced as a complement to already existing NRTI and NNRTI drugs, the mortality rate of HIV-infected patients and the incidence of opportunistic infections has dropped, both most likely as a result of the increased use of combination HAART.[40] The role of drugs with immunomodulating activity for use in combination with HAART is also undergoing extensive research.[41,42] Drug regimens for HIV disease are dynamic, and clinical practice guidelines are consistently updated; many changes in the approach to drug interventions can be expected as HIV infection continues to be a chronic disease.[43]

Vaccines. HIV-positive individuals respond less well than do uninfected persons to many vaccines. The degree of immunodeficiency present at the time of vaccination has an impact on the response to hepatitis A or B, pneumococcal, and influenza A and B vaccines.[44] Those who have a CD4 count of more than 200 cells/mm³ respond the best. Patients should be informed that the extent and duration of the protective efficacy of these vaccines are still uncertain.

Vaccination for HIV has the potential to prevent or control disease progression. The development of an effective preventative vaccine for HIV is an area of continuing research. The first human immunizations with potential a AIDS vaccine took place in 1986 in healthy seropositive volunteers in France and Zaire. Low levels of both humoral and cell-mediated immune responses resulted. One conclusion of this study is that booster vaccinations could be effective.[45] Several vaccine candidates have been developed and tested in human phase I or II trials. To date, at least 13 vaccine candidates have been created with use of different forms of recombinant proteins that target the HIV envelope. Research has found that the vaccine candidates introduced antibodies that rarely neutralized HIV progression, as evidenced by assessment of patient blood counts (i.e., CD4 counts). Furthermore, these recombinant proteins rarely produced a cellular response that would target and destroy cells already infected with HIV.[46] Currently there is no evidence of a vaccine that produces extended, high-titer neutralization across a variety of HIV strains.[46]

Genetic mutation of the virus further complicates attempts to disable it. Genetically similar but distinguishable strains of HIV can exist in one individual. Furthermore, drug-resistant strains of HIV have been identified.[47] Another difficulty with vaccination development is a lack of animal models. Chimpanzees replicate simian immune deficiency virus, a similar but not identical disease. In addition, an average of 12 years and $231 million is required for a new drug to gain Food and Drug Administration approval. Many major pharmaceutical companies seem wary of the immense research expenses and potential liability risks linked to vaccine development. The result is that smaller biotechnology companies with fewer resources are assailing the complicated problems of HIV infection.[13] It is estimated that a vaccine will not be readily available for another 5 to 10 years. This vaccine will ideally induce both humoral and cellular immune responses and have no toxic effects. It will protect against initial infection and retard disease onset in infected individuals.

Nutrition

Involuntary loss of more than 10% of baseline body weight and chronic diarrhea or unexplained weakness and fever constitute HIV wasting syndrome.[48] Retrospective demo-graphic research in the United States found that 17.8% of individuals with AIDS had wasting syndrome.[49,50] The ensuing malnutrition contributes to further immunosuppression.[51] It is important to have nutritional consultation not only for patients with wasting syndrome but also for prevention of disease and enhancement of the immune system.

Weight loss or reductions in lean body mass is also a problem for patients using HAART. Comprehensive nutritional intervention is advocated during the early stages of HIV infection to maintain nutritional status. HAART compromises nutrition in HIV patients because of complicated drug and nutrient interactions, excessive pill loads that must be consumed, and adverse side effects including diarrhea and nausea. Furthermore, HAART has been coupled with lipodystrophy, a syndrome marked by various combinations of insulin resistance, hyperlipidemia, visceral adiposity, loss of peripheral fat stores, or dorsocervical fat accrual. Lipodystrophy is a syndrome that makes the nutritional management of HIV more difficult and may require exercise, pharmacological intervention, and diet modifications.[52]

Systemic Manifestations
Integumentary System and Neoplasms

Cutaneous disorders develop in 64% to 90% of all individuals infected with HIV. Most HIV-induced skin findings develop only when the CD4 count falls below 500 cells/mm³. As the CD4 cell count decreases further, multiple cutaneous disorders may develop.[53] There are three AIDS-defining malignancies: Kaposi's sarcoma (KS), non-Hodgkin's lymphoma (NHL), and cervical cancer. KS was the first neoplastic condition to be related to HIV infection and it remains the most common. However, over the past decade the incidence of KS has diminished as a result of the use of more powerful antiretroviral therapy and maintenance of immune status.[53] KS can involve almost every part of the body, but the most common site of initial KS presentations is the skin or mucous membranes.[54] The disorder presents as cutaneous purple nodular lesions or as rife visceral lesions. AIDS-KS has been intimately associated with the lymphatic system, specifically, deficient lymphatic transport, nodal dysfunction, and tumors, which contribute to lymphedema that clinicians observe as swollen extremities.[55]

In KS there is a broad therapeutic spectrum from cryotherapy to systemic chemotherapy.[56] In NHL, early therapeutic intervention is necessary because of the fast progression of the tumor.[57] The cervical cancer in HIV-infected women seems to be more aggressive than in non-HIV-infected women and also needs early therapeutic intervention.[58] The cancer incidence in patients with HIV is reported to be higher among nonblack patients.[59]

There are several other tumors that occur with people with HIV infection: anorectal cancer, lung cancer, malignant testicular tumor, Hodgkin's lymphoma, basal cell carcinoma, and even malignant melanoma.[57,60] It is beyond the scope of this chapter to detail all aspects of cancer and dermatological concerns; however, the therapist needs to be aware of the importance of differential diagnosis because the skin is the first line of defense of the immune system and further workup may be warranted.

Musculoskeletal System

Musculoskeletal manifestations of HIV infection are not as common as manifestations seen in other parts of the body, including the CNS, pulmonary system, and GI tract. They tend to occur in advanced HIV disease. Knowledge of the different abnormalities that may occur in the musculoskeletal system is crucial to patient management and affects morbidity and mortality. Primary abnormalities are seen as osseous and soft tissue infections, polymyositis, myopathy, and arthritis. Secondary musculoskeletal complications are often due to the various compensatory patterns of gait as a result of HIV-related peripheral neuropathy syndrome or the change in biomechanics of the foot and ankle from KS and NHL.[61] This leads to potential spinal changes and back pain.

HIV-infected patients with acute myopathy typically have proximal muscle weakness and elevated creatine phosphokinase levels.[62] Patients may have initial symptoms of difficulty with basic activities of daily living (ADL), such as rising from a chair or climbing stairs.

Arthritis in HIV-infected persons has a wide spectrum of presentations ranging from mild arthralgias to severe joint disability.[63] Arthritides seen in patients with AIDS have been classified into five groups on the basis of clinical presentation: (1) painful articular syndrome, (2) acute symmetrical polyarthritis, (3) spondyloarthropathic arthritis (Reiter's syndrome, psoriatic arthritis), (4) HIV-associated arthritis, and (5) septic arthritis.[64]

Cardiopulmonary System

Pulmonary diseases continue to be important causes of illness and death in patients with HIV infection, but changes in therapy and demographics of HIV-infected populations are changing their manifestations. The risk for development of specific disorders is related to the degree of immunosuppression, HIV risk group, area of residence, and use of prophylactic therapies.[65] Sinusitis and bronchitis occur frequently in the HIV-infected population, more so than in the general public. The increasing population of HIV-infected drug users is reflected in the increasing incidence of TB and bacterial pneumonia.

Anti-*Pneumocystis* prophylaxis has reduced the incidence of and mortality from PCP. The PCP-causing organism is usually acquired in childhood, and between 65% and 85% of healthy adults possess PCP antibodies. Reactivation of latent infection is responsible for the recurrent fever, dyspnea, and hypoxia that characterize PCP.[66,67] Adjunctive corticosteroid therapy has improved the outlook for respiratory failure.[65]

Mycobacterial infections in HIV-infected individuals usually present as either MAC infection or TB.[5] Steadily increasing incidence of infection by *Mycobacterium tuberculosis* is likely the result of two factors: better medical management of HIV as a whole and the development of multidrug-resistant strains of mycobacteria.

MAC infection tends to appear late in the course of HIV infection. Initial infection involves the GI and pulmonary tracts and eventually disseminates throughout the body. This disorder probably is due not to latent reactivation of the organism but rather to primary infection by ingestion or inhalation.[68] Signs and symptoms of MAC infection include pneumonia, fever, weight loss, malaise, sweats, anorexia, abdominal pain, and diarrhea.

As in many other infections, initial signs and symptoms of TB include fever, weight loss, malaise, cough, lymph node tenderness, and night sweats. Pulmonary involvement accounts for between 75% and 100% of cases of TB infection in HIV-infected patients, but extrapulmonary infection, especially in lymph nodes and bone marrow, occurs in up to 60% of these individuals as well.[9,66-69] Other less common areas of infection include the CNS and cardiac and mucosal tissues.

TB is communicable, preventable, and treatable. Tuberculin skin testing should be available and routinely offered to individuals at HIV testing sites. Individuals at highest risk for concomitant HIV and TB infections include the homeless, intravenous drug users, and prisoners.[66,69] The risk of infection to health care personnel and to the general public is a concern. Isolation rooms that provide negative pressure, nonrecirculated ventilation, and specific air filters and air exchange rates offer the best protection to health care providers exposed to TB-infected individuals. Properly fitted face masks that filter droplet nuclei should be worn. Monitoring of personnel who work with these populations will identify the need for necessary preventive therapy.[66]

CMV can affect the GI and respiratory tracts but primarily targets optic structures and the CNS. Between 40% and 100% of healthy adults possess CMV antibodies.[70] However, an individual who is immunosuppressed becomes more vulnerable to symptoms of infection with CMV. Predominant consequences of HIV/CMV coinfection are unilateral or bilateral deficits in visual acuity, visual field cuts, and blindness.

Although most other organ system involvement has been extensively described in studies and reviews, cardiac complications related to HIV infection have remained less characterized. Most studies have described cardiac problems as postmortem findings, although some clinical series have been reported. It is now clear that cardiac involvement in people living with HIV infection is quite common. Pericardial effusion and myocarditis are among the most commonly reported cardiac abnormalities. Cardiomyopathy, endocarditis, and coronary vasculopathy have also been reported. It is now apparent that HIV infection itself, the medical management of HIV disease, and secondary opportunistic infections can all affect the myocardium, pericardium, endocardium, and blood vessels.[71,72]

Body fat changes and lipid abnormalities have been reported in individuals with HIV/AIDS.[73] Known as lipodystrophy, or fat redistribution syndrome, these body fat and metabolic changes have been connected to PI use.[74] These body fat changes may have strong implications for patients who receive rehabilitation intervention. Signs and symptoms of the syndrome vary, and not all need to be present in any particular patient. However, in both men and women, three main components of the syndrome have emerged. These include changes in body shape, hyperlipidemia, and insulin resistance. Clinically, distinct body shape changes are apparent. The most prevalent include increased abdominal growth, dorsocervical fat pad, benign symmetrical lipomatosis, lipodystrophy, and breast hypertrophy in women.[75,76] The increased abdominal growth is characterized by a redistribution and accumulation of fat in the central visceral areas of the body.[76,77] Corresponding symptoms include GI discomfort, bloating, distention, and fullness.[77]

In addition to visible signs and symptoms, adverse changes in lipid, glucose, and insulin levels have also been reported.[78] A number of studies revealed that hyperlipidemia was present in HIV-positive patients, many whom, but not all, were undergoing PI therapy.[79]

To date, the exact cause of lipodystrophy has not been determined, but two main theories have been hypothesized. Each is still in the process of being studied.[73,80] As individuals live longer with HIV disease, they are at greater risk for development of cardiac disease. Therapists need to be apprised of various changes in laboratory results and signs and symptoms of cardiac disease when designing an exercise program and facilitating return to function.

Neurological System

The neurological manifestations of HIV disease are numerous and they involve the autonomic nervous system (ANS), CNS, and peripheral nervous system (PNS).[81] Over the course of the disease, up to 70% of patients have some form of neurological symptom.[82] Significant progress in understanding and treating the neurologically involved HIV patient has been made over the past decade.[72] However, HIV continues to affect every division of the human nervous system (Box 21-1). Unfortunately, neurobehavioral dysfunction in early pediatric AIDS remains unchanged after therapy. Dementia develops in some adult patients in spite of the multidrug therapies, and other patients have subtle neurobehavioral changes that diminish the quality of their prolonged lives. Thus, HIV infection of the CNS remains an important clinical concern. Although much is known about the neuropathological features of HIV infection, major questions about neuropathogenesis remain. What is the neurotropism of HIV? What causes neuronal damage and loss? Is the CNS a reservoir of HIV?[72]

Autonomic Nervous System. Dysfunction of the ANS has been associated with HIV infection. This has implications for overall function and the design of a rehabilitation program for people living with HIV disease. In one study, individuals with the greatest ANS involvement also had dementia, myelopathy, and sensory peripheral neuropathy. Variations in heart rate, including resting tachycardia, were common. Abnormal blood pressure readings were identified in response to isometric exercise and positional changes (sit to stand and tilting).[83]

Central Nervous System. HIV enters the CNS during the early stages of the disease and is hypothesized to traverse the blood-brain barrier during the initial acute primary infection stage. Although the initial CNS invasion by HIV is asymptomatic in most individuals, affective and cognitive deficits may develop.[84] It is not possible in this context to discuss the neuropathological features of each of the many secondary infections and neoplasms of HIV illness. It is important to realize, however, that the clinical manifestations of these pathological processes overlap with one another and with the signs and symptoms of primary HIV infection of the CNS; lesions of the CNS can be the site of more than one opportunistic disease process simultaneously. In Table 21-3, a wide variety of organisms or conditions responsible for the neurological manifestations associated with HIV infection are listed. These include primary and

---

BOX 21-1 ■ NEUROPATHOLOGY OF HIV INFECTION

CENTRAL NERVOUS SYSTEM
Mechanism of CNS infection is unclear, but HIV seems unable to cross blood-brain barrier alone. It probably crosses in macrophages and T cells and most directly affects subcortical structures (basal ganglia, thalamus, brain stem).

AIDS dementia complex, a subcortical dementia, is different from cortical dementia such as Alzheimer's disease.

Estimated 70% of infected → cognitive, motor, and behavioral constellation that is AIDS dementia complex.

PERIPHERAL NERVOUS SYSTEM
Sensory—In early and middle stages, distal lower extremities are largely involved, with paresthesia and decreased temperature sensitivity. In advanced stages, the patient has decreased ankle and knee reflexes, diminished temperature and vibration sensitivity and proprioception, and hyperesthesia.

Motor—Most closely resembles Guillain-Barré syndrome (progressive muscle weakness → paralysis, decreased deep tendon reflexes). Splints and ankle-foot orthoses may prevent deformities.

AUTONOMIC NERVOUS SYSTEM
Arrhythmias, especially tachycardia

Abnormal blood pressure, orthostasis and with isometric exercises

ANS involvement has been associated with dementia, myelopathy, and peripheral sensory neuropathies.

---

secondary viral, protozoan, fungal, and *Mycobacterium* infections, as well as neoplasms and iatrogenic conditions. Infectious processes may cause large lesions in the brain, such as meningitis, encephalitis, or both. Such infections cause neurocognitive impairments that develop as dementia, amnesia, or delirium.[84] Thirty percent to 40% of healthy adults have contracted toxoplasmosis, caused by *Toxoplasma gondii*.[38,85] Unchecked by the immune system, toxoplasmosis results in CNS dysfunction, namely, altered cognition, headache, focal neurological deficits, encephalitis, and seizures. Cerebellar disorders associated with HIV infection are typically the result of discrete cerebellar lesions resulting from opportunistic infections such as toxoplasmosis and progressive multifocal leukoencephalopathy or primary CNS lymphoma.[86] CNS lymphoma results in cognitive dysfunction and presentation of fever, focal neurological impairments, headache, seizures, and motor deficits.[84]

A relationship between stroke and AIDS has been reported.[87,88] The most common cause of cerebral infarction in both clinical and autopsy series was nonbacterial thrombotic endocarditis. Intracerebral hemorrhages were usually associated with thrombocytopenia, primary CNS lymphoma, and metastatic KS.

HIV-related conditions in the spinal cord include not only HIV myelitis, opportunistic infections, and lymphomas but also vacuolar myelopathy, which affects predominantly the dorsolateral white matter tracts. The cause of vacuolar

TABLE 21-3 ■ Common Opportunistic Diseases in HIV Infection

DISEASE/PATHOGEN	SITES OF INFECTION	SYMPTOMS	MEDICATIONS AND SIDE EFFECTS	DISEASE-SPECIFIC PRECAUTIONS
PCP/*P. carinii,* a protozoan found in air, water, and soil, carried by domestic animals, and possibly latent in most people	Lungs, sometimes spreads to the spleen, lymph nodes, and blood	Fever, cough, shortness of breath, chills, chest pain, sputum production in late disease	Trimethoprim-sulfamethoxazole: rash, itching, Stevens-Johnson syndrome, extreme fatigue, dysphagia, fever, leukopenia, sore throat, thrombocytopenia, hepatitis, hematuria, diarrhea, dizziness, headache, anorexia, nausea, vomiting Intramuscular or intravenous pentamidine isethionate: azotemia, serum creatinine elevations, pain and induration at intramuscular sites, abscess or necrosis at injection sites, elevated liver function tests, leukopenia, nausea, vomiting, hypotension, syncope, blood sugar imbalances Aerosolized pentamidine isethionate: investigational Dapsone: nausea, vomiting, abdominal pain, vertigo, blurred vision, tinnitus, insomnia, fever, headache, phototoxicity, lupus, anemia Sulfadoxine-pyrimethamine: allergic skin reactions, nausea and vomiting, glossitis, stomatitis, headache, peripheral neuritis, mental depression, fatigue, weakness	None
Toxoplasmosis/*T. gondii,* a protozoan found in air, water, soil, and some cats and other animals. Most often acquired by ingestion of uncooked infected lamb or pork, unpasteurized dairy products, raw eggs, or vegetables. Mothers can give it to unborn children. Other human-human transmission does not occur.	Produces lesions in the CNS; may also involve heart and lungs	Fever, chills, headache, visual disturbances, lethargy, confusion, hemiparesis, seizures	Sulfadiazine: same as for trimethoprim-sulfamethoxazole Pyrimethamine: anorexia, vomiting, megaloblastic anemia, leukopenia, thrombocytopenia, glossitis	None

TABLE 21-3 ■ Common Opportunistic Diseases in HIV Infection—cont'd

DISEASE/PATHOGEN	SITES OF INFECTION	SYMPTOMS	MEDICATIONS AND SIDE EFFECTS	DISEASE-SPECIFIC PRECAUTIONS
Cryptosporidiosis/*Cryptosporidium,* a protozoan primarily acquired through oral contact with feces of an infected animal, or oral sexual contact with an infected person	GI tract	Copious diarrhea, abdominal pain, anorexia, nausea, vomiting, dehydration, weight loss, weakness, fever	Spiramycin: nausea, vomiting, diarrhea, abdominal pain Eflornithine: investigational	Gloves and gown/apron when handling feces. Private room when patient has poor hygiene.
Isosporiasis/*Isospora belli,* a protozoan primarily acquired through eating uncooked beef or pork or through oral sexual contact with an infected person	GI tract	Diarrhea, abdominal pain, nausea, vomiting, anorexia, weight loss, weakness, fever	Trimethoprim-sulfamethoxazole: see under *P. carinii*	Gloves and gown/apron when handling feces. Private room when patient has poor hygiene.
Mycobacterium avium-intracellulare infection/*M. avium-intracellulare,* a bacterium found in soil, water, animals, eggs, and unpasteurized dairy products and other foods. Infection is atypical and noncommunicable	Disseminated	Fever, malaise, night sweats, anorexia, diarrhea, weight loss	Isoniazid: paresthesia and peripheral neuropathy, elevated liver function test values, anorexia, nausea, vomiting, fatigue, malaise, weakness Rifabutin: hepatotoxicity, neutropenia, nausea, vomiting, diarrhea, rash, itching Clofazimine: reddish-brown discoloration of skin, conjunctiva, sweat, hair, urine, and feces; abdominal pain, diarrhea Ethambutol: reversible blurring of vision, anaphylaxis, skin irritation, nausea, vomiting, fever Cycloserine: convulsions, drowsiness, headache, tremor, other CNS disturbances Ethionamide: nausea, vomiting, peripheral and optic neuritis, mental depression, postural hypotension, rash Rifampin: urine discoloration, heartburn, nausea, vomiting, abdominal cramps, headache, drowsiness, fatigue	Gloves and gown/apron when handling wound drainage.

Continued

TABLE 21-3 ■ Common Opportunistic Diseases in HIV Infection—cont'd

DISEASE/PATHOGEN	SITES OF INFECTION	SYMPTOMS	MEDICATIONS AND SIDE EFFECTS	DISEASE-SPECIFIC PRECAUTIONS
			Streptomycin: nausea, vomiting, vertigo, numbness of the face, rash, fever, itching, elevated white blood cell count	
Candidiasis/*Candida albicans*, a fungus that inhabits the oropharynx, vagina, large intestine, and skin, causing no harm as long as immunity remains undamaged; may occur as a secondary infection in conjunction with herpes simplex virus lesions	Anywhere skin or mucous membrane is damaged, including intravenous therapy and pressure monitoring sites, etc.	Thrush, esophageal, perianal irritation, vaginitis, proctitis; inflammation around fingernails can be disseminated.	Clotrimazole: abdominal pain, diarrhea, nausea, vomiting Nystatin: diarrhea, nausea, vomiting, stomach pain Ketoconazole: hepatitis, gynecomastia, nausea, vomiting, decreased libido, diarrhea, dizziness, drowsiness, photophobia, rash, itching, sleepiness Amphotericin B	None
Cryptococcosis/*Cryptococcus neoformans,* a fungus found in air, water, soil, raw fruits and vegetables, and pigeon droppings and found on window ledges and nesting places; acquired by inhalation	CNS, lungs; can be disseminated	Altered cognition, low-grade fever, headache, nausea, vomiting, meningeal signs	Amphotericin B Ketoconazole: see under Candidiasis	None
CMV infection/cytomegalovirus, an organism found in saliva, semen, cervical secretions, urine, feces, blood, breast milk. It causes problems only when immunity is compromised.	Disseminated	Fever, profound fatigue, muscle and joint aches, night sweats, impaired vision, cough, dyspnea, abdominal pain, diarrhea	Ganciclovir: leukopenia, bone marrow, depression, elevated liver enzymes, edema, nausea, muscle aches, headaches, anorexia, disorientation, rash, phlebitis	Private room if the patient has enteritis and poor hygiene. Gloves and gown/apron for handling excretions and secretions if soiling is likely.
Herpes simplex virus (HSV) infection/HSV 1 is spread by contact with infected oral secretions. HSV 2 is spread by contact with infected genital secretions. Patient can spread either variety by touching lesions, then touching other body parts.	Mouth, perianal area; can be disseminated	Painful burning, itching vesicular lesions; sometimes colitis, pericarditis, esophageal infection	Acyclovir: rash, diarrhea, light-headedness, headache, nausea, vomiting, thirst, fatigue	Gloves and gown/apron for handling secretions from lesions. Private room if infection is disseminated or severe.
PML/JC virus; transmission routes unclear	Brain	Impaired speech, vision, and thought; ataxia and limb weakness; advanced disease can cause profound dementia	No known effective treatment	None

myelopathy is not understood, and it has not been unequivocally linked with HIV infection.[89] Unless it is treated with effective antiretroviral therapy, vacuolar myelopathy of the spinal cord associated with moderate clinical disability develops in many patients with AIDS.[90]

Treatment for CNS impairments includes an eclectic blend of rehabilitation strategies. Neuromuscular disturbances may first appear as movement disorders. Subtleties of altered movement can be detected early and during subsequent treatment phases. A neurological examination can be performed to provide a diagnosis and prognosis. This may include the level of the lesion, neuromuscular deficits, need for assistive devices, ADL, and functional abilities. Various quality-of-life assessments used with the HIV population can be found in Table 21-4.

Peripheral Nervous System. Possible neurological complications associated with HIV disease that may affect the PNS include meningitis, ataxia, myelopathy, and encephalitis. PNS diseases have been reported in up to 50% of HIV-infected individuals, resulting in distal polyneuropathy, Guillain-Barré syndrome, and mononueropathy.[91]

Distal symmetrical polyneuropathy (DSP) is the most common form of neuropathy in HIV infection. The most frequent complaints in DSP are numbness, burning, and paresthesias in the feet. These symptoms are typically symmetrical and often so severe that patients have contact hypersensitivity and gait disturbances. Involvement of the upper extremities and distal weakness may occur later in the course of DSP. Neurological examination shows sensory loss to pain and temperature in a stocking-glove distribution, increased vibratory thresholds, and diminished ankle reflexes compared with knee reflexes.[82,92] Patients with AIDS frequently have concurrent CNS disorders and neuropathy, characterized by hyperactive knee reflexes and depressed ankle reflexes.

The incidence of DSP increases with advancing immunosuppression, in parallel with decreased CD4 counts.[93] Thirty-five percent of patients with AIDS may have electrophysiological or clinical abnormalities.[94] Furthermore, pathological evidence of DSP is present in almost all patients who die of AIDS.[95] Various theories regarding the mechanism of DSP have been proposed. It was formerly thought that direct HIV invasion of the nervous system caused DSP[85]; however, most investigators now believe that this is not the case.[93] A "dying-back" neuropathy affecting all fiber types, with prominent macrophage infiltration of the peripheral nerve, has been described.[95] Cytokines, tumor necrosis factor, and interleukin-1 have been identified in the peripheral nerves of patients with AIDS.[96]

Balance and Postural Mechanisms. Balance disturbances may be seen with HIV involvement of either the CNS or the PNS. Polyneuropathy caused by AZT (AZT polyneuropathy) and CMV, which is a common pathogen in AIDS (inflammatory polyneuropathy), may manifest in the form of a generalized asymmetrical demyelination and chronic denervation of muscles.[97] Demyelination and denervation of nerves that supply postural muscles may weaken such muscles and result in balance problems (e.g., distal pain, paresthesia, or numbness). It is also possible that, apart from muscle demyelination and denervation, the pathologi-

cal process, which also includes macrophage infiltration of neural structures, could spread to affect the vestibular neural complex of the inner ear, which is important in the maintenance of both static and dynamic balance. Our clinical experience shows that sensory changes are common in the lower limbs of neuropathic HIV/AIDS patients. The balance problems of these patients are likely to be connected to a lack of adequate proprioception from the legs during stance, and it is well known that diminished sensory information makes gait control more difficult.

Peripheral neuropathy weakens the neuromuscular system and causes a limitation in functional activities. These effects on the neuromuscular system manifest in disturbances of postural control. An appropriate posture should be regarded as the starting position for a functional activity. However, compromise of the postural pattern is so characteristic of HIV peripheral neuropathy that it is diagnostic for HIV-1 infection.[98] The neurological abnormality resulting from peripheral neuropathy in HIV/AIDS produces postural disturbances[99] that may take various forms that exacerbate with the severity of the neuropathy[100] and compromise functional activity at various levels. This means that as the condition of HIV/AIDS patients deteriorates, balance deficits may increase.

According to Husstedt et al,[101] peripheral neuropathy in HIV disease progresses much more rapidly than that associated with diabetes or hereditary polyneuropathies. Again, because of demyelination as the HIV infection progresses, distal symmetrical peripheral neuropathy increases, resulting in a depression of certain motor functions such as gait and manual dexterity, and a worsening of the condition is due to demyelination.[101] There is therefore a need to treat HIV neuropathy as soon as it is diagnosed, to avoid complications.

Our group[61] has identified peripheral neuropathy and its complications as causes of functional derangement in HIV/AIDS. A patient who, for instance, has balance derangement resulting from peripheral neuropathy may not function effectively in ADL. It is well known that functional limitation is an important factor that takes people out of employment. The case is true for people with HIV/AIDS peripheral neuropathy. Pain may be the limiting factor in the ability to return to work. Any intervention that would reduce functional limitation should be applied.

Pain

Another factor closely related to the neuropathy of HIV/AIDS is pain. Pain is one of the most prominent and distressing symptoms in patients with HIV and it has a significant effect on quality of life and psychological state. Pain may affect patients at any stages of the disease process; however, it is more frequent during the advanced stages. The occurrence of pain during HIV infection varies between 30% and 80%. Pain is the result of a complex process that involves psychological and neurophysiological mechanisms and therefore it should be assessed with use of sensitive tools that examine its multidimensional nature. One model that evaluates the evaluative, affective, and sensory aspects of pain is the McGill Pain Questionnaire. This assessment tool is useful in evaluating HIV disease–related pain because different etiologies and nonsensorial factors related to the disease often make clinical assessment of pain difficult.[102]

TABLE 21-4 ■ Quality of Life Assessments in HIV Disease

INSTRUMENT	AUTHOR	DIMENSIONS	LENGTH	ADMINISTRATION
AIDS Health Assessment Questionnaire (AIDS-HAQ)	Lubeck and Fries (1991-1992)	Physical function, mental health, cognitive function, social health, energy/fatigue	30 items	Self-administered (5 minutes)
AIDS Specific Functional Assessment (ASFA)	Rapkin et al (1991-1993)	Evaluates usefulness of functional assessment	Varies	Self-administered, care provider
Individualized Functional Status Assessment (IFSA)	Rapkin et al (1991-1992)	Patient-generated activities associated with pursuit of following goal types: a. achievement b. problem-solving c. avoidance-prevention d. maintenance e. disengagement	75 items	Self-administered
Medical Outcomes Study HIV Instrument (MOS-HIV)	Wu et al (1991)	Health, pain, physical functioning, role functioning, social functioning, mental health, fatigue, energy, health distress, cognitive functioning, health transition, general quality of life	30 items	Self-administered (5 minutes)
HIV Patient- Reported Status and Experience (HIV-PARSE)	Berry et al (1991)	Physical health, mental health, general health	38 items	Self-administered (5 minutes)
Multidimensional Functional Evaluation of People with HIV	Marazzi et al (1992)	I ADL (4) Self-Care (8)	12 items	Self-administered
Neuropsychiatric AIDS Rating Scale (NARS)	Boccellari et al (1992)	Assesses patient's orientation, memory motor ability, behavioral changes, problem-solving ability, and ADL	Varies	Health care provider
HIV Overview of Problems Evaluation Systems (HOPES)	Schag et al (1992)	Global, physical, psychosocial, medical interaction, significant others, sexual	139 items	Self-administered (15 minutes)
HIV-Related Quality-of-Life Questions (HIV-QOL)	Cleary et al (1993)	Mental health, energy/fatigue, fever, limitations of basic ADL and intermediate ADL, disability days, all symptoms, sleep symptoms, neurological symptoms, memory symptoms, pain	30 items	Self-administered (5 minutes)
HIV-Quality Audit Marker (HIV-QAM)	Holzemer et al (1993)	Captures nurse data collector's judgment of status of patient based on observations, interviews, and recorded interviews	Varies based on duration of interview	Nurse
HIV Visual Analog Scale	Nokes et al (1994)	Rates HIV-related symptom severity and general well-being	Varies	Nurse Self-administered
HIV Assessment Tool (HAT)	Nokes et al (1994)	Physical symptoms related to HIV disease, social/role functioning psychological well-being, and personal attitudes related to well-being	34 items	Self-administered
Multidimensional Quality of Life Questionnaire for Persons with HIV (MQOL-HIV)	Avis and Smith (1994)	Mental health, physical health, physical functioning, social functioning, social support, cognitive functioning, financial status, partner intimacy, sexual functioning, medical care	40 items	Self-administered (10 minutes)

Most AIDS patients require various pain treatment interventions. Distal symmetrical peripheral neuropathy has been shown to be the most common peripheral neuropathy complaint in patients with HIV-1 infection.[103] Peripheral neuropathy is one of the most common types of pain suffered by HIV-infected men,[104] and peripheral neuropathies occur in as many as 40% to 60% of patients with HIV disease. Peripheral neuropathy is the most prevalent neurological complication associated with HIV. CNS or PNS involvement has been found in 30% to 63% of patients across the arena of HIV and it is often related to antiretroviral therapy.[105] When neuropathy results in distal painful paresthesia, imbalance in stance and gait may result from compensatory measures aimed at relieving pain in dynamic standing activities. Postural compensations may further exacerbate musculoskeletal, cervical, thoracic, or low back pain.

Pain management is a critical part of the overall care of individuals with HIV disease. Pain is the second most common reason for hospitalization of patients with AIDS.[106] A study of 72 AIDS patients found that 97% had pain related to the disease process.[107] Newshan and Wainapel,[107] who surveyed 100 patients who had pain associated with AIDS, showed that the two reported pain types were abdominal and neuropathic pain. In a longitudinal study of HIV-infected men, painful peripheral neuropathy was one of the most common types of pain suffered by these men.[104]

DSP exhibits painful paresthesias that are challenging to treat with pharmacological interventions. Oral gabapentin and cutaneous lidocaine patches are often prescribed to manage pain associated with peripheral neuropathy. Our clinical experience shows that conventional transcutaneous electrical nerve stimulation may exacerbate peripheral pain in HIV/AIDS. Another consideration for treatment is low-voltage electroacupuncture.[108] Manual therapy to improve ankle and foot range of motion along with other compensatory areas is recommended for pain management and return to function. (See Chapters 32 and 37 for additional information.)

Psychopathology

Medical and neuropsychiatric sequelae of HIV infection present a spectrum of diagnostic and treatment challenges to health care practitioners. Both HIV infection and the various opportunistic infections that manifest in patients as the result of an immunocompromised state also can affect the CNS. Therefore, therapists need to be familiar with the diagnosis and management of HIV infection–related medical and psychiatric disorders. This has great impact on the outcomes of rehabilitation.

Careful consideration of psychological function is warranted during clinical encounters with HIV-infected persons. AIDS-related psychopathologies mimic many previously described consequences of primary HIV infection, opportunistic infections, and drug side effects. These psychiatric complications can be affective or organic. Indicators include disturbances in sleep and appetite patterns, diminished memory and energy, psychomotor retardation, withdrawal, apathy, and emotional liability. Anxiety disorders (particularly posttraumatic stress disorder), adjustment reactions, reactive and endogenous depressions, and obsessive disorders frequently result.[109-111]

With use of the American Psychiatric Association's *Diagnostic and Statistical Manual of Mental Disorders,* third edition revised, one study found Axis I disorders (excluding substance abuse) in 61.9% of the subjects.[112] Indeed, the virus' affinity with subcortical structures of the CNS that regulate affect and mood support research indicate a prevalence of manic episodes that is ten times higher than that in the general population.[113] Manic syndrome has been identified at all stages of the disease process and may also occur in response to AZT therapy.[22,49,114] When associated with HIV infection, mania appears to be secondary to structural CNS changes.[115,116] Described manic episodes generally respond well to psychiatric medications and may not recur.[49,117-119]

Analyses of new-onset psychosis among HIV-infected individuals yielded the following information. Psychotic episodes are preceded by a period (days to months) of affective and behavioral changes.[120] Admitting diagnoses to psychiatric units included "undifferentiated schizophrenia, schizophreniform disorder, 'reactive psychosis,' atypical psychosis, depression with psychotic features and mania."[120] Some psychiatric diagnoses were revised during the course of hospitalization to "AIDS encephalitis, cryptococcal meningitis, or 'organic psychosis.'"[121] Eighty-seven percent of the subjects in one study displayed delusions that were usually persecutory, grandiose, or somatic. Affective disturbances were present in 81% of the subjects. Hallucinations and thought process disorders were each prominent in 61%. Several subjects received the diagnosis of AIDS during the psychiatric hospitalization.[121]

Remarkable progress has been made in recent years in the therapeutics of HIV-associated dementia. Viral replication in and outside the CNS has been reduced by HAART. This has resulted in partial repair of cellular immune function with improvement in, and the prevention of, neurological deficits associated with HIV disease.[122] Extensive use of PIs is associated with dramatic declines in overall mortality and morbidity, including HIV-associated dementia.[41,123]

Neuropathological abnormalities seen in the brain tissue of patients with HIV-associated dementia are usually diffuse and predominantly localized to the white and deep gray matter regions. Myelin pallor and inflammatory infiltrates composed of macrophages and multinucleated giant cells are the hallmarks of this disease process, although a spectrum of lesions has been identified from encephalitis to leukoencephalopathy.[124,125] The characteristic clinical feature of HIV-associated dementia is disabling cognitive impairment, often accompanied by behavioral changes, motor dysfunction, or both.[125] Degrees of impairment have been recorded, and a five-part staging system was subsequently developed.[126,126a,127] Motoric manifestations of AIDS dementia complex include gait disturbances, intention tremor, and abnormal release of reflexes.

Differentiation between psychiatric and physiological manifestations is complicated. Psychiatric and organic disorders are initially indistinguishable on the basis of behavior, and they may exist concurrently. Furthermore, other primary disease processes and drug reactions imitate psychopathological conditions. Differentiation is nonetheless essential because many disorders respond well to established therapies, both psychological and pharmacological, once differential diagnoses are established. Awareness of the intricate interplay of all factors is essential for competent rehabilitative efforts for those infected with HIV.

Pediatric HIV Infection

Pediatric HIV infection differs from that most commonly seen in adults. Symptoms develop much earlier in pediatric patients compared with adults. Children infected with HIV may be classified as "rapid progressors" or "slow progressors." "Rapid progressors" refers to children infected with HIV who present with symptoms within the first 12 to 24 months of life. These children progress quickly to AIDS-defining conditions and have a rapid decline in CD4 count. Children who are "slow progressors" have a more gradual progression of symptoms and are likely to show evidence of immune system compromise by 7 to 8 years of age. A small percentage of children remain healthy and have only nominal or no symptoms of the disease and a normal to slightly decreased CD4 count through 9 to 10 years of age.[128]

The prediction of 6 million pregnant women and 5 to 10 million children infected with HIV-1 by the year 2000[129] may have been an underestimate. An accurate understanding of the timing of HIV transmission from mother to fetus is important for the design of intervention strategies. The ACTG076 trial that included treatment from the fourteenth week of gestation in women with CD4 counts of more than 200/mm^3 prompts other considerations.[130] Onset of HIV-1 infection in children has a wide spectrum of clinical manifestations.[131] Thus prevention of transmission from mother to fetus via HAART is a critical component of managing this worldwide epidemic.

Pediatric HIV is neurotrophic in nature in that the virus most often initially affects the CNS rather than the PNS. As the virus spreads, pediatric HIV patients can have CNS disorders that include encephalopathy, pyramidal tract signs, language difficulties, cognitive deficits, and upper respiratory infections.[128]

In the first year of life, severe immunodeficiency develops in 15% to 20% of pediatric patients with serious recurrent infections or neurological dysfunction, whereas in school-age children the disease progresses more slowly and the risk for development of HIV-related encephalopathy becomes less.[132] Some infants have features of severe immunodeficiency, whereas others have nonspecific findings, such as hepatosplenomegaly, failure to thrive, unexplained fever, parotitis, and recurrent gastroenteritis. Adenopathy is common, and salivary gland enlargement occurs more frequently than in adults. Otitis media and measles, despite immunization, are also more frequent complications in children.[57,78] Cardiac involvement in children with HIV infection is a well-known entity and occurs clinically more often in patients with advanced disease.[133]

Children are susceptible to disorders seen in adults—herpesvirus infection, pneumonia, toxoplasmosis, meningitis, and encephalitis. HIV encephalopathy is noted to have the most serious side effects because of its progressive deteriorating pattern and associated CNS abnormalities,[23] although static encephalopathy can be characterized by severely delayed cognitive functioning and neuromotor skills without deterioration.[134] Manifestations in children include cerebral atrophy, ataxia, rigidity, hyperreflexia, and the inability to achieve or sustain developmental milestones.

Although the HIV-neurodevelopmental involvement causes a prognostic worsening, most studies about pediatric cases of neuro-AIDS demonstrate that an early diagnosis followed by adequate antiretroviral therapeutic regimens can lead to significant, even if temporary, improvement.[132]

Rehabilitation of the pediatric patient requires a multidisciplinary approach to meet the medical, emotional, and psychosocial needs of these children and their families. Children are encouraged to give form to their psychological experiences through play, writing or telling stories, and creating works of art.[135]

REHABILITATION INTERVENTIONS

The examination procedures for HIV illness are broadly outlined below. Of course, each case varies and the evaluation process is individualized according to the specific needs of the client (Box 21-2).

What is the relationship of the person with HIV infection to the environment, both at present and in the future? The rehabilitation therapist should keep this question in mind throughout the examination process. In this context, the term *environment* is meant to include not only the physical aspects of surroundings but also the psychological and emotional climate in which the individual functions (see Table 21-1).

The examination process has a different focus for different stages of the disease. If the client is in the early stages of the disease, the therapist should determine whether she or he is still managing in accustomed life roles. Important issues may include new or adapted vocational and leisure skills. During the advanced stage, the focus may change to more basic daily functional concerns. The therapist must remember, however, that the client may place more importance on participation in avocational interest than on independent self-care. This choice not only is valid but must be respected and supported by health care professionals. If the patient is evaluated in an inpatient setting, another crucial determination to be made is whether the person is to be discharged to home or some other supervised setting. In either case, it is critical to determine what kind of community-based support networks are available to the individual.

Astute evaluative questions about the psychosocial status of the client include the following:

Does the client's perception of his or her status and prognosis agree with that of the treatment team?

What is the client's predominant coping style?

Who are the client's caregivers?

What is the social support system?

The support system can be a critical issue for many people with HIV infection, especially those who are part of the high-risk groups, such as homosexual and bisexual men and intravenous drug users.[136] Many of these people have traditional networks of family, spouse, and friends; a significant number have equally strong nontraditional support systems. Some will be lacking in the kinds of support needed to cope with the devastating effects of the disease.

It is possible to use models developed for oncology and progressive neurological disorders for HIV involvement of the CNS and PNS. An orthopedic approach may be taken when pain is a presenting factor or biomechanical alterations are a result of other disease processes. Functional fluctuations that characterize HIV infection and secondary infec-

BOX 21-2 ■ EVALUATION PROCEDURES FOR HIV ILLNESS

A. Baseline data (premorbid functional level)
   1. Accustomed life roles
B. Stage in disease process
C. Psychosocial issues
   1. Coping mechanisms
   2. Social support system
D. Cognitive/perceptual status
   1. Reality orientation
   2. Memory
   3. Organizational skills
   4. Visual perception
   5. Motor planning
   6. Safety awareness
   7. Judgment
E. Communication
   1. Oral language
   2. Written language
F. Sensorimotor status
   1. Balance
   2. Gait
   3. Coordination
   4. Sensation/pain
   5. Muscle tone
   6. Strength
G. ADLs
   1. Grooming/hygiene
   2. Feeding
   3. Bathing
   4. Dressing
   5. Housework
   6. Community management
   7. Other self-care regimens (e.g., medications)
   8. Avocational interests
   9. Activity tolerance

BOX 21-3 ■ NEUROMUSCULAR REHABILITATION TREATMENT PROCEDURES FOR HIV INFECTION

A. Psychosocial intervention
   1. Facilitation of the expression of grief
   2. Validation and education of caregivers
B. Cognitive/perceptual intervention
   1. Rehabilitation
   2. Maintenance
   3. Compensation (including communication)
C. Sensory/motor intervention
   1. Sensory stimulation
   2. Maintenance of strength, range of motion, and endurance
   3. Tone normalization
   4. Functional mobilities (including ambulation equipment)
D. Pain control
   1. Psychological modalities
   2. Behavioral modalities
   3. Physical modalities
E. Training in ADLs
   1. Leisure or avocational skill development
   2. Community management skills
   3. Transfer training
   4. Recommendations for adaptive equipment
   5. Self-care retraining
   6. Energy conservation
   7. Work simplification
F. Continuity of care
   1. Discharge planning
   2. Community linkages

tions must be understood; therefore, the therapist must appreciate the effects that HIV infection has on various systemic complications.

The neurorehabilitation evaluation of an individual who has HIV disease should include standard cognitive, perceptual, and motor components of function. The idiosyncratic nature of the disease may necessitate more detailed evaluation of these specific areas. Recommended cognitive and perceptual evaluations are both formal and observational. Safety, judgment, and money management need to be assessed. In addition to the organicity of HIV-associated dementia, evaluation of the systemic complications of HIV infection is necessary for optimal rehabilitative planning and treatment team efficacy.

The ADL evaluation is best made within the context of the immediate and projected life roles of the individual. Maximal independent functioning is the goal of rehabilitation, whatever the stage of illness. If the person is at home or is being discharged to home, a crucial component of the ADL examination is the assessment of community management skills. Consider access to transportation, socialization opportuni-

ties, shopping, and banking; ability to negotiate health care and insurance systems; and community involvement. Many people with HIV infection and their caregivers have little experience with disability because of their age or social status. This, combined with the stressors of illness, can create unrealistic expectations and unnecessary frustrations.

Treatment Process

The neuromuscular rehabilitation treatment procedures for HIV infection and an overview of treatment techniques for opportunistic infections are presented in Boxes 21-3 and 21-4.

Cognitive deficits in attention, concentration, and memory require consistency, structure, and environmental cues to minimize confusion. Safety and judgment deficits can be countered by environmental adaptations. Lethargic clients benefit from sensory enhancement. Maintenance of endurance and strength and passive and active range of motion are important components of any motor function treatment plan. Neuromuscular facilitation and inhibition, positioning, and splinting are feasible modalities to normalize tone as needed. Gait training, the use of ambulatory aids, training in motor planning, and balance and endurance exercises may be appropriate.

In addition to techniques and modalities, active listening, empathy, and unconditional positive regard are important

BOX 21-4 ■ MOST COMMON OPPORTUNISTIC INFECTIONS AND REHABILITATION INTERVENTIONS IN HIV-INFECTED PATIENTS

PCP—Most common opportunistic infection. Infectious agent unclear but probable latent infection; 65% to 85% healthy adults possess PCP antibodies. Fever, dyspnea, and hypoxia → *diaphragmatic breathing, energy conservation.**

Candida albicans—Present in healthy people, immunocompromised status → yeast infections of oral, esophageal, and vaginal mucosal tissues → *teach good oral care with soft brush, bland diet, salt water rinses.*

Cryptococcus neoformans—Also a yeast but manifests in CNS as abscesses and meningitis. Headache, altered mental states, nausea, vertigo, somnolence, seizures, and coma → *pain management, safety and gait training, cognitive and sensory stimulation.*

Cryptosporidiosis—Infects gastrointestinal tract → chronic diarrhea and malabsorption, contributes to wasting syndrome → *nutritional and hydration strategies.*

Wasting syndrome—Involuntary loss of 10% of baseline body weight, weakness, chronic diarrhea, and unexplained fever. *Nutrition, hydration, energy conservation.*

Toxoplasmosis—Affects CNS in 30% to 40% of cases; headache, altered cognition, encephalitis, seizures, focal deficits → *imposed structure, concrete tasks, pain management.*

CMV—Present in 40% to 100% of healthy adults. Can affect GI and respiratory tracts, but most often affects ocular structures → unilateral or bilateral decreased visual acuity, field cuts and blindness → *compensatory skills, safety tasks and mobilities, home evaluation, supportive service referrals.*

Mycobacterial infections—Two are most pertinent: *M. avium*–MAC and *M. tuberculosis* (causes TB). MAC affects 18% to 56%, but autopsies reveal that this is a low estimate. MAC infection is not latent but is a primary infection. It appears late in HIV infection, begins in GI or respiratory tract, and then disseminates. Pneumonia, fever, weight loss, malaise, sweats, anorexia, abdominal pain, diarrhea may occur. TB appears early, with latent reactivation in 90% of HIV-infected patients. Pulmonary TB estimates 75% to 100% in HIV-infected persons infected with the TB bacillus. It also infects lymph nodes and bone marrow in 60% of these, and it also infects CNS, cardiac, and mucosal tissues. Fever, weight loss, malaise, cough, lymph node tenderness, and night sweats → *energy conservation, nutrition and hydration, and caregiver and patient education in safe management of infection. Is communicable; wear a mask, follow respiratory isolation protocol.*

AIDS-KS—Frequent neoplasm and most frequent in homosexual men; it is rare in women and intravenous drug users. There are purple skin or visceral lesions. Associated are deficient lymphatic transport, nodal tumors, and lymphedema → swollen, painful lower extremities. *Nutrition, pain management, task simplification, mobility and ADL training.*

---

*Italicized components identify potential treatment procedures recommended for the specific problem.

PCP, Pneumocystis carinii pneumonia; *CMV*, cytomegalovirus; *AIDS-KS*, AIDS–Kaposi's sarcoma.

---

aspects of therapeutic use of self. The clinician must set aside personal biases and beliefs to accurately hear the perspective of the individual client. The use of expressive modalities facilitates the development of coping skills while providing appropriate exploration and release of powerful emotions. Human touch can counter the powerful and isolating effect of fear of contagion. Rehabilitation therapists can demonstrate and educate caregivers about the safety and benefit of touch.

Motoric manifestations of AIDS dementia complex include gait disturbances, intention tremor, and abnormal release of reflexes.

Pain management is best approached with a behavioral and a physical approach. Pain reduction is achieved through training in breathing techniques, visualization, progressive muscle relaxation, autogenics, music, meditation, and engagement in meaningful activities. Electroacupuncture, thermal agents, and manual therapy are also therapeutic tools. (See Chapters 9, 32, and 37 for additional treatment ideas.)

The impact of HIV infection can be evident in cerebral, emotional, psychosocial, and other physical domains, affecting the patient infected with HIV and those around her or him. The prognosis and psychological and physical consequences of HIV infection are associated with significant emotional distress and clinical syndromes, such as adjustment disorders, depression, and anxiety in some patients.[137] Increasing focus is being placed on the potential impact of HIV infection–related stress on the course of infection because of the observed and postulated relationship between psychosocial stress, neuropsychological functioning, and immune status.[138] Minimizing stressful events throughout the management of chronic HIV infection can be approached in various ways, such as meditation, relaxation, and various forms of exercise.

Exercise

Exercise is an intervention commonly used by movement specialists to address a multitude of impairment and functional limitations. Thus, understanding of the implications of the HIV disease process on exercise prescription is important. A review of published studies[139] on the effects of exercise on individuals with HIV disease revealed the following: (1) although intense bouts of exercise may result in transient immunosuppression, there is no evidence that regular exercise in individuals with HIV disease results in a detrimental effect on the immune system over time, (2) some studies have shown actual improvement in immune system function in response to regular exercise, (3) improved cardiovascular function has been observed in response to aerobic exercise, and (4) resisted exercise may be effective in counteracting the effects of wasting syndrome and improving strength and lean body mass.

From a psychoneuroimmunological perspective, psychological stress has been implicated among the cofactors contributing to the immunological decline in HIV disease. Good evidence supports the stress management role of exercise training as a means to explain a buffering of these suppressive stressor effects, thereby facilitating a return of the CD4 cells. Early intervention with exercise, in compliance with guidelines, is most prudent to stave off opportunistic infections throughout the spectrum of HIV disease.

Precautions and Concerns during Exercise

It is important to address any orthopedic or neurological concerns before embarking on an exercise or movement therapy program. If musculoskeletal problems exist or other pain symptoms are present, a concerted effort to modulate pain is necessary for the successful completion of an exercise regimen.[140] If HIV-related peripheral neuropathy exists, it is important to implement proper foot care and supportive shoes when weight-bearing activities are performed.[61,141]

There is some concern about aerobic exercise increasing the body's metabolic rate and thus increasing additional muscle loss. However, with a balanced high-calorie diet and incorporation of a sound nutritional program, this should not pose a problem for the asymptomatic person with HIV disease. If wasting is present, the cause needs to be addressed and treatment rendered.[50] One study determined the contribution of total energy expenditure to weight changes in individuals with HIV infection-related wasting. The researchers observed a significant positive relation between total energy expenditure and the rate of weight change. During rapid weight loss, total energy expenditure fell from an average 2750 kcal per day to 2189 kcal per day. The key determinant of weight loss in HIV infection-related wasting they concluded was reduced energy intake, not increased energy expenditure.[142]

If fatigue is present as a symptom, a differential diagnosis including anemia, low testosterone levels, or specific vitamin deficiencies must be made before any exercise regimen is begun. Proper caloric intake must be adequate to meet the energy expenditure required for the activity. Seeking the advice of a nutritionist is recommended for proper guidance.

Evidence of autonomic neuropathy on provocative testing is common in HIV infection, with estimates of incidence ranging from 30% to 60%.[143,144] Underlying cardiac parasympathetic dysfunction may need to be assessed throughout the course of HIV disease. One method described by Mallet et al[145] is the use of the 4-second exercise test, which consists of pedaling an uploaded ergometer at maximal individual speed from the fourth to the eighth second of a 12-second maximal inspiratory apnea. From an electrocardiogram, vagal activity is estimated through a ratio. In that study, subjects were submitted to the respiratory sinus arrhythmia, which is a valid method to detect vagal dysfunction. The researchers found that there was a tendency for lower values of the vagal function test in HIV-infected subjects. Vital sign monitoring is prudent throughout any exercise regimen. Exercise can help control long-term side effects including altered body composition; elevated cholesterol, triglyceride, and blood glucose levels; and elevated blood pressure.[146] Some comorbidities associated with HIV disease, such as inflammatory myopathy, acute infectious arthritis, or cardiac status may result in restrictions on exercise prescription.[139]

A supervised training program should be consistent with recommendations by the American College of Sports Medicine. Guidelines have been established for the spectrum of the stages of HIV disease.[19] During the stage of asymptomatic HIV disease, there are no limitations on maximum graded exercise testing. Exercise should consist of resistance training, cardiovascular training, flexibility training, balance training, and mind-body training.[146] In this stage, all metabolic parameters are within normal limits for most individuals. Thus, unrestricted activity is generally encouraged. Most sports do not pose a significant risk of HIV transmission. However, sports such as boxing, where there is a risk of open wounds and contamination with infected blood should be viewed with great caution.[139]

Exercise is safe and beneficial for most individuals with HIV disease; however, caution is warranted with symptomatic HIV disease and advanced HIV disease. In symptomatic HIV disease, there may be reduced exercise capacity, Vo_2 max, and oxygen (O_2) pulse max. There may also be other cardiovascular problems, pulmonary problems, anemia, and peripheral muscle abnormalities. Pain, side effects of medications, psychosocial issues, and unplanned events may also create obstacles to exercise for individuals in the symptomatic stage of HIV disease. For individuals with cardiac myopathy or hyperlipidemia, submaximal aerobic capacity testing should be followed with a staged cardiac rehabilitation program[83] because of the risk of cardiac failure in patients with compromised cardiac status.[147]

Patients with advanced HIV disease, or AIDS, present with dramatically reduced exercise capacity, reduced vital capacity, Vo_2 max, and O_2 pulse max. Elevated heart rate and breathing reserve persists in this stage. Neurologic dysfunction, opportunistic infections, and progressive disability indicate a need for careful monitoring of the exercise program during this stage of the disease. In general, individuals with advanced HIV disease should remain physically active and exercise on a symptom-limited basis. Precautions related to comorbidities should be implemented. Individuals in this stage of the disease are at greater risk for exercise-induced injuries as a result of chronic tissue changes in both muscle and peripheral nerve. For individuals with severe morbidity and extensive disability, treatment should emphasize enhancement of basic functional tasks, ADLs, and energy conservation.[139]

Complementary Therapies in HIV Infection

There is substantial evidence to suggest that traditional exercise, particularly aerobic exercise, can provide notable physiological and psychological benefits for most individuals, especially those with chronic diseases. However, the mode, duration, and intensity of many traditional standardized exercise programs may not always be entirely appropriate during chronic illness. The stage of disease and the type of illness itself may preclude these more strenuous exercise activities at various times. During times like these, less traditional movement therapies may prove to be more appropriate and efficacious. In fact, movement therapy includes a number of similar constructs used in physical therapy and can be quite complementary to an individual's program of more traditional exercise.[148,149] Refer to Chapter 37 for additional information.

The HIV epidemic has witnessed an increasing use of alternative therapies, some more traditional than others.[147] The exploration outside the medical model has fostered investigations by the Office of Alternative Medicine at the National Institutes of Health.[150] Eisenberg et al[151] reported that prayer and exercise combined to account for more than 60% of all alternative therapies used. Other therapies include relaxation techniques (13%), massage (7%), imagery (4%), and spiritual healing (4%). Traditional exercise such as aerobic and weight training are incorporated in the medical model through exercise physiology and rehabilitation. However, various movement therapies (such as martial arts) are often viewed as less traditional and outside the established medical model. In a study by Bastyr University (1998), various movement therapies were used by people living with HIV disease. This study evaluated the use of alternative therapies within the past 6 months. Yoga was used by 15.5%, tai chi by 4.8%, and qigong by 3.6% of the participants. Recent research[148] demonstrated beneficial physiological and psychological effects of the use of tai chi and aerobic exercise (see Chapter 37). In 1993 researchers at the University of Maryland School of Nursing in Baltimore concluded that there was a positive correlation between patient health and participation in prayer and mediation. Relevant factors include: "perception of their physical, emotional, and spiritual health; and their participation in exercise and the use of special diets."[152] A study done at Rutgers University in 1999 looked at guided imagery and progressive muscle relaxation on HIV. Health status was significantly different after treatment. Guided imagery produced most positive effects more in the mid stage of the disease. The combination of imagery and muscle relaxation is suggested to improve health status and it should be initiated early in the disease process.[153]

Social Interactions and the Association with Disease Management

The process of grieving is often mistakenly associated solely with the death of another. It is a natural reaction to loss, including the loss of one's own health and diminished independence. Loss of abstract human qualities, such as perceived attractiveness and productivity, results in grief. Such emotions are often difficult for a client to articulate. It is the therapist's responsibility to be sensitive to the client's individualized grief pattern (see Chapter 5).

Placement issues accompany discharge planning from acute health care facilities. The rehabilitation professional is often called on to make recommendations regarding the level of assistance the client will need. All of the previously discussed areas of cognitive/perceptual, sensorimotor, and ADL management combined with available psychosocial and practical support influence these recommendations. Options include a return to independent living and work, assisted independent living by a loved one, home with supportive services (often supplied by community-based AIDS organizations), home with hospital-based home care, hospice, and extended care facility.

Literature on long-term survivors with AIDS is replete with anecdotal evidence linking survival to one or more of the following: (1) holding a positive attitude toward the illness, (2) participating in health-promoting behaviors, (3) engaging in spiritual activities, and (4) taking part in advocacy activities related to the HIV community.[154-156] Positive relationships have been demonstrated between hardiness and perception of physical, emotional, and spiritual health and participation in exercise and the use of special diets.[157-159]

Research provides support for the hypothesis that interpersonal relationships influence patterns of physiological functions. Data from experimental studies have shown that social contact can serve to reduce the physiological stress responses.[160,161] Community-based studies have also shown negative associations between reported levels of support and physiological parameters such as serum cholesterol, uric acid, and urinary epinephrine levels.[161] Studies of immune function have demonstrated that social relationships have both positive and negative impacts on immune function. Loss of a partner to cancer or HIV infection, family caregiving for patients with Alzheimer's disease, and divorce or poor marital quality all show negative associations with immune function, whereas more supportive relationships are associated with better immune function.[21]

Exercise and movement therapy in a group context may provide the socialization necessary to foster these physiological changes and adherence to an exercise regimen. Another area of potential socialization is the workplace. The quality-of-life issues for people with HIV/AIDS are becoming more complicated as more people with the disease achieve higher CD4 counts and lower viral load levels. Improvement in health status is directly related to the improved effectiveness of newer treatment regimens, and many individuals are improving enough to either continue working or re-enter the work force. Exercise and movement therapy may augment the stress and fatigue that may be associated with the adjustment to the workplace.

SUMMARY

Research and resultant treatments are extending lives so that more people require rehabilitative services that maximize function and quality of life. Medical management has focused on the treatment of reducing viral load, preventing the secondary illnesses, and improving the immunological status of chronic HIV disease. Examination of the neuromusculoskeletal system and interventions for individuals with HIV disease are similar to those for other progressive neuromusculoskeletal disorders. Advanced HIV disease, or AIDS, can be addressed like other diseases such as cancer, but with an emphasis on cognitive and perceptual function. Rehabilitation interventions focus on specific impairments, disabilities, and psychosocial ramifications of the disease. Compensation, mobility, ADL retraining, pain control, and community management skills constitute a well-developed treatment plan.

The epidemic is a major challenge on a personal as well as a professional level because of the continued natural fear of contagion. The illness originally appeared in subcultures that are often disenfranchised. Social, racial, and economic status and controversial behaviors contribute to prejudice, fear, and limited access to health care. Rehabilitation professionals have responded significantly to this challenge. Continued advocacy and compassion combined with professional enlightenment will, in a small way, alter the course of the disease.

Future Directions for Research

The issue of HIV disability warrants a careful investigation into our current health care system. Some long-term survivors of HIV disease who formerly received disability ranking are potentially ready to return to work. However, their grave concern about the long absence from work reflected on their resume and fears about potential opportunistic infections while on the job require specific strategies. Vocational rehabilitation and on-the-job counseling are necessary for optimal return to work. The systemic issues of acquisition of disability and the loss of all benefits when one relinquishes disability are quite complicated and overwhelming. The diagnosis of AIDS is the determining factor for disability, and many people living with HIV disease with CD4 counts less than 200/mm^3 have experienced considerable improvement in their immunological status with a concomitant drop in viral load. Prognosis for these individuals has great variability. Promoting quality of life may be greatly enhanced through the use of complementary therapies. An integral aspect of self-perception is often the role played in society. The workplace affords individuals a sense of identity and a self-sustaining purposefulness. Therefore, our health and governmental systems need to conduct further research on return-to-work outcomes, with ease of transition and on-the-job accommodations when necessary. Future directions in the AIDS epidemic as we see people living longer will be the full return to function in all domains of ADL and return to productive work.

CASE STUDIES

Three case studies are presented to help the reader understand and identify various stages of this clinical problem and how each stage may require a different therapeutic focus.

CASE STUDY 21-1 ■ ASYMPTOMATIC HIV DISEASE VERSUS SYMPTOMATIC HIV DISEASE: MARIO

EXAMINATION
History
Mario is a 48-year-old male chemistry teacher who tested positive for HIV 6 years ago. Currently, his absolute CD4+ cell count is 475/mm^3, and his viral load (HIV RNA) is 40,000 copies/ml. Mario runs 5 miles three times per week for exercise. Recently he began to experience some pain and tingling in the soles of his feet that is most noticeable after running. His weight has been stable. He has noticed a mild deficit in short-term memory over the past year, which he attributes to middle age. He has a history of rotator cuff tendonitis but is otherwise healthy and denies other symptoms. His wife and 28-year-old son serve as his primary emotional support system. The rest of his family live in Italy, his native country. He is a Roman Catholic and attends church regularly. Current medications: aspirin as needed after running.

Tests and Measurements
Left extremity sensation testing with Semmes Weinstein monofilaments (see reference) reveals diminished light touch sensation over the distribution of the medial plantar nerves bilaterally. A lower extremity neural tension test (straight leg raise with dorsiflexion) and a Tinel's test over the tarsal tunnel have positive results bilaterally and reproduce tingling along the medial arches of the feet. Screening of the lumbar spine, hips, and knees is negative. Foot and ankle range of motion and strength is normal. Pain is not provoked with passive stretching of the plantar fascia. Lower extremity reflexes are normal, and no abnormal reflexes are present. Excessive pronation is noted during the gait cycle; gait is otherwise normal. In standing, an excessive calcaneal valgus angle is noted; normal medial arches are observed in non–weight bearing. Foot pain on a visual analogue scale is 0/10 at rest, and 5/10 after running.

EVALUATION AND DIAGNOSIS
Bilateral distal sensory disturbances may be due to DSP in individuals with HIV disease. However, this is typically associated with side effects of HAART, and the patient has not yet been placed on these drugs. Furthermore, sensory loss with DSP typically involves multiple peripheral nerves and occurs first in the most distal distribution. The patient's toes have no sensory impairment. Myelopathy should be considered in patients with chronic HIV disease who appear to have peripheral neurologic symptoms; however, Mario does not demonstrate any signs that would suggest myelopathy as the cause of his foot symptoms. Examination is significant for signs and symptoms of flexible pes planus, which may be contributing to tarsal tunnel syndrome bilaterally. His gait pattern of excessive pronation is likely contributing to compression on the tibial nerve within the tarsal tunnel when he runs.

Prognosis, Goals, and Outcomes
Mario is expected to have full recovery with interventions directed at reducing biomechanical stress on the tarsal tunnel during running. Mario's goal is to run for 5 miles without any symptoms. Outcomes will be measured with patient's self-report of global improvement, the visual analogue scale for pain associated with running, and changes in clinical signs (lower extremity neural tension test, Tinel's test, and monofilament sensory testing).

Intervention Plan and Recommendations
Mario will receive Low Dye taping (see reference) to decrease his pronation and provide temporary relief of symptoms. Orthotics will be fabricated to reduce pronation and adverse stress on the tarsal tunnel. Mario will replace running with aerobic training on a stationary bike until his orthotics are adequately "broken-in" to resume running. Before discharge he will receive instruction in general lower extremity and plantar fascia flexibility exercises. If foot symptoms are recalcitrant to biomechanically based interventions, further consultation with Mario's HIV specialist will be warranted to rule out possible tibial nerve mononeuropathy related to his HIV disease. The therapist will encourage Mario to see a mental health professional because of the complaints of memory loss. A mental health professional may use the HIV Dementia Scale (see reference) or other instruments may be used to assess the patient's cognitive function and rule out the possibility of early signs of HIV dementia. If any of Mario's symptoms are determined to be related to his HIV disease, he will be restaged to symptomatic HIV disease.

CASE STUDY 21-2 ■ ADVANCED HIV DISEASE (AIDS) AND A PLAN FOR THE FUTURE: RUBY

EXAMINATION
History
Ruby is a 23-year-old woman of African American and Hispanic descent. Ruby has an 8-year history of intravenous drug abuse and bipolar disorder. She was tested for HIV disease 5 years ago, at which time she was hospitalized with a diagnosis of *P. carinii* pneumonia and oral thrush. At that time, her absolute CD4+ cell count was 15/mm^3 and her viral load was 750,000 copies/ml. Her opportunistic infections were successfully treated with antibiotics, and HAART was initiated. Within a few months, her viral load was undetectable, and her absolute CD4+ level had climbed to 400/mm^3. Since then, she has had intermittent periods of homelessness and is currently residing with a friend. She stopped adhering to her HAART regimen several months ago, during a period of depression. Recently, Ruby has worked as a prostitute to earn money for crack cocaine. Ruby was admitted to the hospital 12 days ago with complaints of abdominal bloating and severe left shoulder pain. Her behavior was clearly agitated. A large abscess was present over the left deltoid. Medical workup revealed that Ruby has a staphylococcal infection in the left anterior deltoid and infectious arthritis of the left glenohumeral joint. It was determined that she was 4 months pregnant. Her psychiatric status was significant for a manic episode. CD4 count was 175/mm^3 and viral load was 200,000 copies/ml. Ruby's shoulder infection has been treated with intravenous methicillin, and recent magnetic resonance imaging of the shoulder region was negative for osteomyelitis. Medical clearance for examination and interventions for the shoulder has been obtained from her infectious disease physician. She was placed on psychotropic medication for mood stabilization. Pending results of genotype testing, Ruby will be placed on a new regimen of HAART. Genotype testing is needed because she likely has mutant strains of the virus as a result of poor adherence to the previous course of HAART. HAART will be implemented quickly, with the goal of achieving undetectable viral loads by the time of birth. Consultation with nutrition services was ordered to ensure adequate nutrition during the remainder of her pregnancy. Ruby has disclosed that her arm infection was probably caused by injecting drugs. She has been referred to see an addiction counselor and the social worker. Current medications: none.

TESTS AND MEASUREMENTS
Ruby has a nonhealing wound over the left anterior deltoid region that was 1.5 cm × 1.1 cm with a depth of 0.5 cm. The wound appears to be clean with 100% granulation tissue, and the most recent laboratory report is negative for *Staphylococcus*. Ruby reports that the swelling and redness in her left shoulder have resolved, and no swelling or redness is observed during the examination. Left shoulder strength was 3/5 (fair) for abduction, internal rotation, and external rotation, and 4/5 (good) for other motions. Passive range of

motion (PROM) of the left is limited as follows: external rotation 70 degrees, abduction 160 degrees, and internal rotation 45 degrees. Her score on the Disabilities of the Arm, Shoulder, and Hand Questionnaire (DASH) (see reference) is 85/100 for the left upper extremity. Screening examination of the cervical spine is clear; however, hypertonicity is noted in the elbow and wrist, and finger flexors on the left side. PROM of the elbow, wrist, and hand is within normal limits; however, slight resistance is noted with quick passive stretching of flexor muscles. Ruby has weakness in grasp and demonstrates a mild flexor synergy pattern with attempts to elevate the left arm.

EVAULUATION AND DIAGNOSIS
As a result of the findings of the examination, neurology is immediately consulted and a brain MRI is performed. Magnetic resonance imaging reveals a mild right cerebrovascular accident involving the middle cerebral artery. Physical and occupational therapy will be initiated to address the following findings: impaired integumentary integrity associated with partial thickness skin involvement over the left anterior deltoid region; impaired glenohumeral joint mobility, muscle performance and range of motion associated with connective tissue dysfunction (adhesive capsulitis as sequela of infectious arthritis); impaired motor function (spasticity and weakness in the left upper extremity) associated with nonprogressive disorder (right cerebrovascular accident) of the CNS.

Prognosis, Goals, and Outcomes
Ruby's outcomes will be strongly influenced by her complex psychosocial status. She states that she is highly motivated to have a healthy baby and learn how to become a stable provider, which may help her adherence to HAART and drug rehabilitation. Continuing communication between all team members (infectious disease, obstetrics-gynecology, social work, addictions counseling, physical therapy, and occupational therapy) will be critical to optimize her care. Because of multisystem involvement and multiple impairments, it is expected that Ruby will require 6 to 8 weeks of therapy. Goals specific to physical therapy include the following: facilitate wound healing and prevent reoccurrence of infection, restore full PROM to the left shoulder, improve strength and function throughout the left upper extremity, and achieve independence with performance of ADLs with the left upper extremity, improve the DASH score (see reference), and minimal functional limitation as per the Barthel Index score (see reference). Outcomes will be measured with continuing assessment of wound characteristics, the DASH score (see reference), the Barthel Index score (see reference), shoulder PROM measurements, and strength assessment of upper extremity musculature.

Intervention Plan
Wound healing will be facilitated with dressing changes and use of topical agents as prescribed by her physician. Glenohumeral impairments will be addressed

CASE STUDY 21-2 ■ ADVANCED HIV DISEASE (AIDS) AND A PLAN FOR THE FUTURE: RUBY—cont'd

with joint mobilization, therapeutic exercises, and functional retraining. Upper extremity impairments involving tone and weakness will be addressed with motor learning techniques, functional activities, and strengthening exercises. Ruby will receive daily physical and occupational therapy until she is discharged from the hospital. Social work will facilitate discharge to a

structured group home for women because Ruby's current roommate is using drugs and working as a prostitute. On discharge from the hospital, Ruby will return for outpatient therapy at a frequency of three times per week. She will continue to follow up with the social worker regarding vocational counseling.

CASE STUDY 21-3 ■ ADVANCED HIV DISEASE (AIDS) AT THE END STAGE OF LIFE: WALTER

EXAMINATION
History
Walter is a 68-year-old man who was diagnosed with AIDS in 1987. He lost his life partner to the same disease in 1990. He has no living relatives. At the time of his diagnosis, Walter had toxoplasmosis, Kaposi's sarcoma, AIDS wasting syndrome, and anemia. He was one of the first patients to receive AZT, which, along with other medications used to treat the opportunistic infections, proved to be life saving. As new classes of drugs became available and were added to his regimen, Walter's viral loads and CD4 cell counts were usually stable. Over time, viral resistance developed to many of the drugs. Recently, he was placed on enfuvirtide (Fuzeon), an injectable receptor site inhibitor that is used when other forms or salvage therapy have been exhausted. His current CD4 count is 25/mm^3 with a viral load of 200,000 copies/ml. Walter has multiple side effects and complications of long-term HIV survival, including peripheral neuropathy in the hands and feet, chronic fibromyalgia, myelopathy, liver toxicity, and severe lipodystrophy. He has marked wasting of fat in the face and extremities, severe truncal obesity, and a dorsocervical fat mass. Walter has also been undergoing treatment for hypertension and hyperlipidemia. Over the past decade, Walter's Medical Outcome Survey HIV Health Survey (see reference) scores have indicated progressive disability and worsening quality of life. Walter has been hopeless and depressed about his physical appearance and level of function. Before admission to the hospital, Walter lived alone in a modest studio apartment. He employed a daily home health aide to assist with food preparation and personal hygiene. Walter had been ambulating short distances in his apartment, often using a walker because of fatigue and unsteadiness. Walter's gait became increasingly ataxic over the past month. Last week, he had a seizure that resulted in admission to the hospital. Testing revealed progressive multifocal leukoencephalopathy (PML). Walter's physician expects that this brain infection, combined with his immunosupression, will lead to death within a few months. Current medications: Fuzeon (enfuvirtide; HAART component), Kaletra (lopinavir and ritonavir; HAART component),

Truvada (emtricitabine and tenofovir disoproxil fumarate; HAART component), Oxycontin (oxycodone; for chronic pain), Norpramin (desipramine; a tricyclic antidepressant), Pravachol (pravastatin; a cholesterol-lowering agent), and Prinivil (lisinopril; an angiotensin-converting enzyme inhibitor/diuretic).

Tests and Measurements
Inspection of the integumentary system reveals redness over the sacrum; otherwise the skin is intact. Diminished light touch sensation is noted in a stocking/glove distribution over the hands and feet. A Hoffman's reflex, consistent with his myelopathy is present in the upper extremities. Walter rates his pain at rest as ranging from 4/10 to 6/10. His pain drawing indicates low back, bilateral hand, and bilateral foot pain. Pulse oximetry reveals 96% oxygen saturation. Vital signs sitting: heart rate 70 beats/min, blood pressure 130/70 mm Hg, and respiratory rate 16 breaths/min with no apparent distress. Rate of perceived exertion at rest (RPE, Borg Scale) is 1/10. Pitting edema (+1) is noted in the ankles and feet.

Walter is independent with all bed mobility. Sitting balance is good. Standing balance is fair. Contact guard is required for sit/stand transfer and for ambulation a distance of 10 feet with a rolling walker. Vital signs after ambulating 10 feet: heart rate 110 beats/min, blood pressure 150/70 mm Hg, respiratory rate 24 breaths/min, RPE 5/10, and oxygen saturation 96%. He demonstrates erratic foot placement and a wide base of support during gait. His Functional Independence Measure (FIM) (see reference) score is a 4. Because of fatigue and pain, strength and range of motion assessment is abbreviated. The following strength data are obtained (all measured bilaterally): shoulder abduction 3/5 (fair), elbow extension 4/5 (good), knee extension 3/5 (fair), and dorsiflexion and plantarflexion 4/5 (good). Passive range of motion data (bilateral): dorsiflexion = 5 degrees, knee flexion 125 degrees (full knee extension not available, 10-degree flexion contracture noted), hip flexion 120 degrees, hip extension 10 degrees, shoulder flexion and abduction 140 degrees, and elbow/wrist/hand within normal limits.

Continued

CASE STUDY 21-3 ■ ADVANCED HIV DISEASE (AIDS) AT THE END STAGE OF LIFE: WALTER—cont'd

EVALUATION AND DIAGNOSIS

Walter exhibits multiple impairments related to his advanced HIV disease (affecting multiple systems) and PML (a progressive disorder of the central nervous system). Summary: impaired integumentary integrity associated with superficial skin involvement, pain, impaired sensory integrity, impaired joint mobility and range of motion (knees, shoulders), impaired muscle performance, impaired gait, impaired balance, and impaired endurance.

Prognosis, Goals, and Outcomes

Walter's prognosis for survival is poor. It is likely that he will deteriorate slowly over the upcoming months. Goals and outcomes will thus focus on optimizing quality of life during Walter's remaining days. Specifically, goals are to reduce pain, prevent sequelae of immobility (such as pressure wounds, pneumonia, deep venous thrombosis, joint contracture, deconditioning, and atrophy), achieve independent sit/stand transfers and short distance (15 feet) ambulation with a wheeled walker, improved endurance (RPE of 2-3 after ambulation), maintain independence with bed mobility, and promotion of safety.

Intervention Plan

Physical therapy will first be provided at bedside. If the patient wishes, treatment may be provided in the physical therapy department. Interventions will include relaxation techniques, passive range of motion and grade I joint mobilization (knees and shoulders), gait training with a wheeled walker, and balance activities, and gentle strengthening and endurance exercises as tolerated. Occupational therapy will be consulted to address bed mobility and self-care tasks. Walter's vital signs will be closely monitored during therapy because it is possible that his ANS dysfunction may become evolved as a result of the CNS infection.

Walter's physician will be contacted regarding Walter's pain ratings. It is likely that increased dosage of pain medication is warranted as a result of reports of moderate pain at the current dosage. Walter will be seen by a dietician. The social worker will plan for transfer to a hospice setting.

In the hospice, physical therapy will focus basic functional activities, such as transfers, gait, and endurance. Palliative interventions (moist heat, gentle massage) will be provided as needed for pain control. Caregiver education will be provided re: prevention of the effects of immobility and safe functional mobility. In the hospice setting, Walter will have the opportunity to work with a spiritual counselor. Walter has expressed an interest in exploring Eastern medicine for pain control. Therefore a consultation with an acupuncturist will be arranged.

ACKNOWLEDGMENTS

We would like to acknowledge Laura LeCocq, Johnny Bonck, and Anne MacRae, the original authors of this chapter, for setting the foundation to this chapter and enlightening the readership through their case studies. We would like to thank the graduate students, Annemarie King, Melissa Nyzio, and Reena Varughese, from the Richard Stockton College of New Jersey for their editing work. We also thank our colleagues at the Early Intervention Program of Kennedy Health System/Garden State Infectious Disease Associates for their input. Mostly, we wish to acknowledge those living with HIV disease, who teach us so much through the many changing facets of the epidemic.

REFERENCES

1. Centers for Disease Control and Prevention: Update: Acquired immune deficiency syndrome—United States 1994, *MMWR Morb Mortal Wkly Rep* 44:64-67, 1995.
2. Quinn TC: Global burden of the HIV pandemic, *Lancet* 348:99-106, 1996.
3. Centers for Disease Control and Prevention: Update: Trends in AIDS incidence, deaths, and prevalence—United States, 1996, *MMWR Morb Mortal Wkly Rep* 46:165-173, 1997.
4. Centers for Disease Control and Prevention: Update: Trends in AIDS incidence—United States, 1996, *MMWR Morb Mortal Wkly Rep* 46:861-867, 1997.
5. Palella F, Moorman A, Delaney K et al: Dramatically declining morbidity and mortality in an ambulatory HIV-infected population. In Abstracts of the 5th Conference on Retroviruses and Opportunistic Infections, Chicago, February 1-5, 1998, abstract 198.
6. Centers for Disease Control and Prevention: 2003 Surveillance Report: http://www.cdc.gov/hiv/stats/2003surveillancereport.htm. Accessed May 30, 2004.
7. Centers for Disease Control and Prevention: Update: perinatally acquired HIV/AIDS—United States, 1997, *MMWR Morb Mortal Wkly Rep* 46:1086-1092, 1997.
8. Centers for Disease Control and Prevention: Projections of the number of persons diagnosed with AIDS and the number of immunosuppressed HIV-infected persons—United States, 1992-1994, *MMWR Morb Mortal Wkly Rep* 41(RR-18):1-29, 1992.
9. *World health report, 1999*, Geneva, 1999, World Health Organization.
10. Fleming P, Byers RH, Sweeney PA et al: HIV prevalence in the United States, 2000. Seattle, 2002, 9th Conference on Retroviruses and Opportunistic Infections.
11. AIDS epidemic update: December 2003. Geneva, 2003, World Health Organization.
12. Chaisson RE: HIV becomes world's leading infectious cause of death. In *The Hopkins HIV Report*, vol 11, No. 4, p 1, Baltimore, 1999, Johns Hopkins University AIDS Service.
13. Clerici M, Shearer GM: A $TH_1 \rightarrow TH_2$ switch is a critical step in the etiology of HIV infection, *Immunol Today* 14:107-111, 1993.
14. Cohen S, Iwane MK, Palensky JB et al: A National HIV community cohort: Design, baseline and follow-up of the AmFar Observational Database. American Foundation for AIDS Research Community-Based Clinical Trials Network, *J Clin Epidemiol* 51:779-793, 1998.
15. Marieb EN: *Human anatomy and physiology*, Redwood City, CA, 1989, Benjamin/Cummings.
16. McDaniel S, Gillenwater DR: Psychoneuroimmunology and HIV disease progression, *Psychiatr Times* (serial online): http://psychiatrictimes.com/p991063.html. Accessed June 7, 2006.

17. Antoni MH, Schneiderman N, Fletcher MA et al: Psychoneuroimmunology and HIV-1 [review], *J Consult Clin Psychol* 58:38-49, 1990.

18. LaPerriere A, Fletcher MA, Antoni MH et al: Aerobic exercise training in an AIDS risk group, *Int J Sports Med* 12(1 suppl):S53-S57, 1991.

19. LaPerriere A, Ironson G, Antoni MH et al: Exercise and immunology, *Med Sci Sports Exerc* 26:182-190, 1994.

20. Leserman J, Petitto JM, Gu H et al: Progression to AIDS, a clinical AIDS condition and mortality: psychosocial and physiological predictors, *Psycholl Med* 32:1059-1073, 2002.

21. Keicolt Glaser JK, Glaser R: Stress and immune function in humans. In Ader R, Felten DL, Cohen N, editors: *Psychoneuroimmunology,* ed 2, pp 849-867, New York, 1991, Academic Press.

22. Dauncey K: Mania in early stages of AIDS, *Br J Psychiatry* 152:716-717, 1988.

23. Reichert T, DeBruyere M, Deneys V et al: Lymphocyte subset reference ranges in adult Caucasians, *Clin Immunol Immunopathol* 60:190-208, 1991.

24. Crowe SM, Carlin JB, Stewart KI et al: Predictive value of CD4 lymphocyte numbers for the development of opportunistic infections and malignancies in HIV-infected persons, *J Acquir Immune Defic Syndr Hum Retrovirol* 4:770-776, 1991.

25. Masur H, Ognibene FB, Yarchoan R et al: CD4 counts as predictors of opportunistic pneumonias in HIV infection, *Ann Intern Med* 111:223-231, 1989.

26. Phair JP, Munoz A, Detels R et al: The risk of *Pneumocystis carinii* pneumonia among men infected with human immunodeficiency virus type 1, *N Engl J Med* 322:161-165, 1990.

27. Yeni PG, Hammer SM, Hirsch MS et al: Treatment for adult HIV infection: 2004 recommendations of the International AIDS Society-USA Panel, *JAMA* 292:251-265, 2004.

28. Centers for Disease Control and Prevention: Report of the NIH panel to define principles of therapy of HIV infection and guidelines for the use of antiretroviral agents in HIV-infected adults and adolescents, *MMWR Morb Mortal Wkly Rep* 47:1-83, 1998.

29. Mellors JW, Munoz A, Giorgi JV et al: Plasma viral load and CD4 lymphocytes as prognostic markers of HIV-1 infection, *Ann Intern Med* 126:946-954, 1997.

30. Dickover RE, Garratty EM, Herman SA et al: Identification of levels of maternal HIV-1 RNA associated with risk of perinatal transmission: effect of maternal zidovudine treatment on viral load, *JAMA* 275:599-605, 1996.

31. Hughes MD, Johnson VA, Hirsch MS et al: Monitoring plasma HIV-1 RNA levels in addition to CD4 lymphocyte count improves assessment of antiretroviral therapeutic response, *Ann Intern Med* 126:939-945, 1997.

32. Marschner IC, Collier AC, Coombs RW et al: Use of changes in plasma levels of human immunodeficiency virus type 1 RNA to assess the clinical benefits of antiretroviral, *J Infect Dis* 177:40-47, 1998.

33. Hirsch MS, Conway N, D'Aquila RT et al: Antiretroviral drug resistance testing in adults with HIV infection: Implications for clinical management, *JAMA* 279:1984-1989, 1998.

34. Havlir DV, Richman DD: Viral dynamics of HIV: implications for drug development and therapeutic strategies, *Ann Intern Med* 124:984-994, 1996.

35. Lipsky JJ: Antiretroviral drugs for AIDS, *Lancet* 348:800-803, 1996.

36. Spence RA, Katz WM, Anderson KS et al: Mechanism of inhibition of HIV-1 reverse transcriptase by non-nucleoside inhibitors, *Science* 267:988-993, 1995.

37. Flexner C: HIV protease inhibitors, *N Engl J Med* 38:1281-1292, 1998.

38. Schrager LK, D'Souza MP: Cellular and anatomical reservoirs of HIV-1 in patients receiving potent antiretroviral combination therapy, *JAMA* 280:67-71, 1998.

39. Arts EJ, Wainberg MA: Mechanism of nucleoside analog antiretroviral activity and resistance during human immunodeficiency virus reverse transcription, *Antimicrob Agents Chemother* 40:27-40, 1996.

40. Palella FJ, Delaney KM, Moorman AC et al: Declining morbidity and mortality among patients with advance human immunodeficiency virus infection, *N Engl J Med* 338:853-860, 1998.

41. Kovacs JA, Vogel S, Albert JM et al: Controlled trial of interleukin-2 infusions in patients infected with the human immunodeficiency virus, *N Engl J Med* 335:1350-1356, 1996.

42. Lederman NM: Host-directed and immune-based therapies for human immunodeficiency virus infections, *Ann Intern Med* 122:218-227, 1995.

43. Holtzer CD, Roland M: The use of combination antiretroviral therapy in HIV-infected patients, *Ann Pharmacother* 33:198-209, 1999.

44. Neilson GA, Bodsworth NJ, Watts N: Response to hepatitis A vaccination in human immunodeficiency virus infected and uninfected homosexual men, *J Infect Dis* 176:1064-1067, 1997.

45. Koff WC, Glass MJ: Future directions in HIV vaccine development, *AIDS Res Hum Retroviruses* 8:1313-1315, 1992.

46. Hoth DF, Bolognesi DP, Corey L et al: HIV vaccine development: a progress report, *Ann Intern Med* 121:603-611, 1994.

47. Stine GJ: *Acquired immune deficiency syndrome: Biological, medical, social and legal issues,* Englewood Cliffs, NJ, 1993, Prentice-Hall.

48. Centers for Disease Control and Prevention: Revision of the CDC surveillance case definition for acquired immunodeficiency syndrome, *MMWR Morb Mortal Wkly Rep* (suppl 2S), 1987.

49. Gabel RH, Barnard N, Norko M et al: AIDS presenting as mania, *Compr Psychiatry* 27:251-254, 1986.

50. Nahlen BL, Chu SY, Nwanyanwu OC et al: HIV wasting syndrome in the United States, *AIDS* 7:183-188, 1993.

51. Hellerstein MK, Kahn J, Mudie H et al: Current approach to the treatment of human immunodeficiency virus-associated weight loss: pathophysiologic considerations and emerging management strategies, *Semin Oncol* 17(9 suppl):17-33, 1990.

52. Brown D, Batterham M: Nutritional management of HIV in the era of highly active antiretroviral therapy: a review of treatment strategies, *Aust J Nutr Diet* 58:224-235, 2001.

53. Nunley JR: Cutaneous manifestations of HIV and HCV, *Dermatol Nurs* 12:163-169, 2000.

54. Krown SE: Acquired immunodeficiency syndrome-associated Kaposi's sarcoma, *Med Clin North Am* 81:471-494, 1997.

55. Witte MH, Witte CL, Way MF et al: AIDS, Kaposi sarcoma, and the lymphatic system: update and reflections, *Lymphology* 23:73-80, 1990.

56. Jie C, Tulpule A, Zheng T et al: Treatment of epidemic (AIDS-related) Kaposi's sarcoma, *Curr Opin Oncol* 9:433-439, 1997.

57. Brockmeyer NH, Pohl G, Mertins L: Combination of chemotherapy and antiviral therapy for Epstein-Barr virus-associated non-Hodgkin's lymphoma of high-grade malignancy in cases of HIV infection, *Eur J Med Res* 2:133-135, 1997.

58. Maiman M, Fruchter RG, Clark M et al: Cervical cancer as an AIDS-defining illness, *Obstet Gynecol* 89:76-80, 1997.

59. Johnson CC, Wilcosky T, Kvale P et al: Cancer incidence among an HIV cohort: pulmonary complications of HIV Infection Study Group, *Am J Epidemiol* 146:470-475, 1997.

60. Remick SC: The spectrum of non-AIDS defining neoplastic disease in HIV infection, *J Invest Med* 44:205-215, 1996.

61. Galantino ML, Jermyn RT, Tursi FJ et al: Physical therapy management for the patient with HIV: lower extremity changes, *Clin Podiatr Med Surg* 15:329-346, 1998.

62. Steinbach L, Tehranzadeh J, Fleckenstein J et al: Musculoskeletal manifestations of human immunodeficiency virus (HIV) infection, *Radiology* 186:833-838, 1993.

63. Rynes R: Painful rheumatic syndromes associated with human immunodeficiency virus infection, *Rheum Dis Clin North Am* 17:83, 1991.

64. Solomon G, Brancato L, Winchester R: An approach to the human immunodeficiency virus patient with a spondyloarthropic disease, *Rheum Dis Clin North Am* 17:44-52, 1991.

65. Rosen MJ: Overview of pulmonary complications, *Clin Chest Med* 17:621-631, 1996.

66. Bernard EM, Sepkowitz KA, Telzak EE et al: Pneumocystis, *Med Clin North Am* 76:107-119, 1992.
67. Kessler HA, Bick JA, Pottage JC Jr et al: AIDS, Part II, *Dis Mon* 38:691-764, 1992.
68. Kerlikowske KM, Katz MH: *Mycobacterium avium* complex and *Mycobacterium tuberculosis* in patients infected with the human immunodeficiency virus, *West J Med* 157:144-148, 1992.
69. Pitchenik AE, Fertel D: Tuberculosis and nontuberculous mycobacterial disease, *Med Clin North Am* 76:121-171, 1992.
70. Krech U: Complement-fixing antibodies against cytomegalovirus in different parts of the world, *Bull World Health Organ* 49:103-106, 1973.
71. Grody WW, Cheng L, Lewis W: Infection of the heart by the human immunodeficiency virus, *Am J Cardiol* 66:203-206, 1990.
72. Vitkovic L, Tardieu M: Neuropathogenesis of HIV-1 infection: outstanding questions, *C R Acad Sci Paris* 321:1015-1021, 1998.
73. Hanna L: Body fat changes: More than lipodystrophy, *Bull Exp Treat AIDS* 5:32-35, 1999.
74. Carr A, Cooper D: Lipodystrophy associated with an HIV protease inhibitor, *N Engl J Med* 339:1296, 1998.
75. Lo J, Mulligan K, Tai V et al: Body shape changes in HIV-infected patients, *J Acquir Immune Defic Syndr Hum Retrovirol* 19:307-308, 1998.
76. Miller K, Jones E, Yanovski J, Shankar R, Feuerstein I, Falloon J: Visceral abdominal-fat accumulation associated with the use of indinavir, *Lancet* 351:871-875, 1998.
77. Di Perri G, DelBravo P, Concia E: Protease inhibitors, *N Engl J Med* 339:773-774, 1998.
78. Henry K, Melroe H, Heubsch J et al: Severe premature coronary artery disease with protease inhibitors, *Lancet* 351:1328, 1998.
79. Sullivan A, Nelson M, Moyle G et al: Coronary artery disease occurring with protease inhibitor therapy, *Int J STD AIDS* 9:711-712, 1998.
80. Carr A, Samaras K, Chisholm DJ et al: Pathogenesis of HIV-1 protease inhibitor associated peripheral lipodystrophy, hyperlipidemia and insulin resistance, *Lancet* 351:1881-1883, 1998.
81. Berger J: Neurological complications of HIV disease, *PAAC Notes* 3:236-240, 1992.
82. Simpson DM, Tagliati M: Neurologic manifestations of HIV infection, *Ann Intern Med* 121:769-785, 1994.
83. Freeman R, Roberts MS, Friedman LS et al: Autonomic function and human immunodeficiency virus infection, *Neurology* 40:575-580, 1990.
84. Ungvarski PJ, Trzcianowska H: Neurocognitive disorders seen in HIV disease, *Issues Ment Health Nurs* 21:51-70, 2000.
85. Ho HH, Chung C, Liu T et al: A randomized controlled trial on the treatment for acute partial ischemic stroke with acupuncture, *Neuroepidemiology* 12:106-113, 1993.
86. Tagliati M, Simpson D, Morgello S et al: Cerebellar degeneration associated with human immunodeficiency virus infection, *Neurology* 50:244-251, 1998.
87. Pinto AN: AIDS and cerebrovascular disease, *Stroke* 27:538-543, 1996.
88. Roquer J, Palomeras E, Pou A: AIDS and cerebrovascular disease [letter], *Stroke* 27:1694, 1996.
89. Bell JE: The neuropathology of adult HIV infection, *Rev Neurol* 154:816-829, 1998.
90. Shepherd EJ, Brettle RP, Liberski PP et al: Spinal cord pathology and viral burden in homosexuals and drug users with AIDS, *Neuropathol Appl Neurobiol* 25:2-10, 1999.
91. McReynolds CJ, Garske GG: Current issues in HIV disease and AIDS: Implications for health and rehabilitation professionals, *Work* 17:117-124, 2001.
92. Simpson DM, Tagliati M, Grinell J et al: Electrophysiological findings in HIV infection: association with distal symmetrical polyneuropathy and CD4 level [abstract], *Muscle Nerve* 17:1113, 1994.
93. Simpson DM, Olney RK: Peripheral neuropathies associated with human immunodeficiency virus infection, In Dyck PJ, editor: *Peripheral neuropathy*, Philadelphia, 1994, WB Saunders.
94. So YT, Holtzman DM, Abrams DI et al: Peripheral neuropathy associated with acquired immunodeficiency syndrome: prevalence and clinical features based on a population-based survey, *Arch Neurol* 45:945-948, 1988.
95. Cornblath DR, McArthur JC: Predominantly sensory neuropathy in patients with AIDS and AIDS-related complex, *Neurology* 38:794-796, 1998.
96. Griffin JWI, Wesselingh S, Oaklander AL et al: MRNA fingerprinting of cytokines and growth factors: a new means of characterizing nerve biopsies [abstract], *Neurology* 43(2 Suppl):A232, 1993.
97. Morgello S, Simpson DM: Multifocal cytomegalovirus demyelinative polyneuropathy associated with AIDS, *Muscle Nerve* 17:176-182, 1994.
98. Petiot P, Vighetto A, Charles N et al: Isolated postural tremor revealing HIV-1 infection, *J Neurol* 240:507-508, 1993.
99. Arendt G, Maecker HP, Purrmann J et al: Control of posture in patients with neurologically asymptomatic HIV infection and patients with beginning HIV-1-related encephalopathy, *Arch Neurol* 51:1232-1235, 1994.
100. Boucher P, Teasdale N, Courtemanche R et al: Postural stability in diabetic polyneuropathy, *Diabetes Care* 18:638-645, 1995.
101. Husstedt I, Grotemeyer K, Heiner B et al: Progression of distal-symmetrical polyneuropathy in HIV infection: a prospective study, *AIDS* 7:1069-1073, 1993.
102. DelBorgo C, Izzi I, Chiarotti F et al: Multidimensional aspects of pain in HIV-infected individuals, *AIDS Patient Care STDS* 15:95-102, 2001.
103. Bradley WG, Venna A: Painful vasculitic neuropathy in HIV infection: relief of pain with prednisone therapy, *Neurology* 47:1446-1451, 1996.
104. Singer E, Zorilla C, Fahy-Chandon B et al: Painful symptoms reported by ambulatory HIV-infected men in a longitudinal study, *Pain* 54:15-19, 1993.
105. Nicholas PK, Demppainen JK, Holzemer WL et al: Self-care management for neuropathy in HIV disease, *AIDS Care* 14:763-771, 2002.
106. Lewis M, Warfield C: Management of pain in AIDS, *Hosp Pract* 30:51-54, 1990.
107. Newshan G, Wainapel S: Pain characteristics and their management in persons with AIDS, *J Assoc Nurses AIDS Care* 4:53-59, 1993.
108. Galantino ML, Eke-Okoro ST, Findley T et al: Use of noninvasive electroacupuncture for the treatment of HIV-related peripheral neuropathy: a pilot study, *J Altern Comp Ther* 5:135-142, 1999.
109. Fernandez F: Neuropsychiatric syndromes and their treatment in HIV infection. In *A psychiatrist's guide to AIDS and HIV disease*, Washington, DC, 1990, American Psychiatric Association.
110. Jacobsberg LB, Perry S: Psychiatric disturbances, *Med Clin North Am* 76:99-106, 1992.
111. Ostrow DG: *Psychiatric aspects of human immunodeficiency virus infection*, Kalamazoo, MI, 1990, Upjohn Pharmaceuticals, 1990.
112. Snyder S, Reyner A, Schmeidler J et al: Prevalence of mental disorders in newly admitted medical inpatients with AIDS, *Psychosomatics* 33:166-170, 1992.
113. Lyketsos CG, Hanson AL, Fishman M et al: Manic syndrome early and late in the course of HIV, *Am J Psychiatry* 150:326-327, 1993.
114. Schmidt U, Miller D: Two cases of hypomania in AIDS, *Br J Psychiatry* 152:839-842, 1988.
115. El-Mallakh RS: Mania in AIDS: Clinical significance and theoretical considerations, *Int J Psychiatry* 21:383-391, 1991.
116. Kieburtz K, Zettelmaier AE, Ketonen L et al: Manic syndrome in AIDS, *Am J Psychiatry* 148:1068-1070, 1991.
117. Buhrich N, Cooper DA, Freed E: HIV infection associated with symptoms indistinguishable from functional psychosis, *Br J Psychiatry* 152:649-653, 1988.
118. Maxwell S, Scheftner WA, Kessler HA et al: Manic syndrome associated with zidovudine treatment, *JAMA* 259:3406-3407, 1988.
119. O'Dowd MA, McKegney KP: Manic syndrome associated with zidovudine, *JAMA* 260:3587-3588, 1988.

120. Halstead S, Riccio M, Harlow P et al: Psychosis associated with HIV infection, *Br J Psychiatry* 153:618-623, 1988.

121. Harris MJ, Jeste DV, Gleghorn A et al: New-onset psychosis in HIV-infected patients, *J Clin Psychiatry* 52:369-376, 1991.

122. Carpenter CJ, Fishl MA, Hammer SM et al: Antiretroviral therapy for HIV infection in 1998: updated recommendations of the International AIDS Society-USA panel, *JAMA* 280:78-86, 1998.

123. Centers for Disease Control and Prevention: HIV/AIDS, *Surveill Rep* 9:1-44, 1997.

124. Budka H: HIV-associated neuropathology. In Gendelman HE, Lipton SA, Epstein L, Swindells S, editors: *The neurology of AIDS,* pp 241-260, New York, 1998, Chapman & Hall.

125. Lipton SA, Gendelman HE: Dementia associated with the acquired immunodeficiency syndrome, *N Engl J Med* 332:934-940, 1995.

126. Nunes JA, Raymond SJ, Nicholas PK et al: Social support, quality of life, immune function, and health in persons living with HIV, *Holistic Nurs* 12:174-198, 1995.

126a. Navia BA, Jordan BD, Price RW: The AIDS dementia complex, I: clinical features, *Ann Neurol* 19:517-524, 1986.

127. Price R, Brew B: The AIDS dementia complex, *J Infect Dis* 158:1079-1083, 1988.

128. Davis-McFarland E: Pediatric HIV/AIDS—Issues and strategies for intervention: http://www.asha.org/about/publications/leader-online/archives/2002/q1/020305e.htm. Accessed May 30, 2004.

129. Scarlatti G: Paediatric HIV infection, *Lancet* 348:863-868, 1996.

130. Centers for Disease Control and Prevention: Zidovudine for the prevention of HIV transmission from mother to infant, *MMWR Morb Mortal Wkly Rep* 43:285-287, 1994.

131. European Collaborative Study: Children born to women with HIV-1 infection: natural history and risk of transmission, *Lancet* 337:253-260, 1991.

132. Maccabruni A, Caselli S, Astori G et al: Evaluation of a protocol for the early diagnosis of HIV-related neurologic dysfunction [abstract 60697], *Int Conf AIDS* 12:1129, 1998.

133. Plein D, VanCamp G, Coysyns B et al: Cardiac and autonomic evaluation in a pediatric population with human immunodeficiency virus, *Clin Cardiol* 22:33-36, 1999.

134. Brouwers P, Belman AL, Epstein LG: Central nervous system involvement: manifestations and evaluation. In Pizzo PA, Wilfert CM, editors: *Pediatric AIDS: The challenge of HIV infection in infants, children and adolescents,* pp 318-335, Baltimore, 1991, Williams & Wilkins.

135. MacDougall DS: Pediatric HIV: Evaluation, management and rehabilitation, *J Int Assoc Physicians AIDS Care* 4:16-25, 1998.

136. Cohen S, Syme SL: *Social support and health,* Orlando, 1994, Academic Press.

137. Fitzgibbon ML, Cella DF, Humfleet G: Motor slowing in asymptomatic HIV infection, *Percept Motor Skills* 68:1331-1338, 1989.

138. Wolf TM, Dralle PW, Morse EV: A biopsychosocial examination of symptomatic and asymptomatic HIV-infected patients, *Int J Psychiatry Med* 21:263-279, 1991.

139. Kietrys D, Gillardon P, Galantino ML: Contemporary issues in rehabilitation of patients with HIV disease, III: The effects of exercise on individuals with HIV disease, *Rehabil Oncol* 20:10-14, 2002.

140. Galantino ML: *Clinical assessment and treatment in HIV disease: rehabilitation of a chronic illness,* Thorofare, NJ, 1992, Slack.

141. Galantino ML, Pizzi M, Lehmann M: Interdisciplinary management of disability in HIV infection. In O'Dell MW, editor: *HIV-related disability: assessment and management,* Philadelphia, 1993, Hanley and Belfus.

142. Macallan DC, Noble C, Baldwin C et al: Energy expenditure and wasting in human immunodeficiency virus infection, *N Engl J Med* 333:83-88, 1995.

143. Ruttimann S, Hilti P, Spinas GA et al: High frequency of human immunodeficiency virus-associated autonomic neuropathy and more severe involvement in advanced stages of human immunodeficiency virus disease, *Arch Intern Med* 152:485-501, 1991.

144. Villa A, Foresti V, Confalonieri F: Autonomic nervous system dysfunction associated with HIV infection in intravenous heroin users, *AIDS* 6:85-89, 1992.

145. Mallet AL, Soares PP, Nobrega AC et al: Cardiac parasympathetic function in HIV-infected humans [abstract 7333], *Int Conf AIDS* 8:104, 1992.

146. Preston GR: Warming up to HIV and exercise, *Body Positive:* http://www.phoenixbodypositive.org/index.shtml. Accessed October 21, 2004.

147. Acierno LJ: Cardiac complications in acquired immunodeficiency syndrome (AIDS): A review, *J Am Coll Cardiol* 13:1144-1154, 1989.

148. Galantino ML, Findley T, Krafft L et al: Blending traditional and alternative strategies for rehabilitation: measuring functional outcomes and quality of life issues in an AIDS population, Proceedings of the 8th World Congress of International Rehabilitation Medicine Association, Monduzzi Editore 1:713-716, 1997.

149. Sande MA, Volberding PA: Alternative therapies in HIV. In *Medical management of AIDS,* ed 4, Philadelphia, 1995, WB Saunders.

150. Office of Alternative Medicine: Functional description of the office, Bethesda, MD, 1993, National Institutes of Health.

151. Eisenberg DM, Kessler RC, Foster C: Unconventional medicine in the United States: Prevalence, costs and patterns of use, *N Engl J Med* 328:246-252, 1993.

152. Alternative and complementary therapies: Internet health library (website), 2001: http://www.internethealthlibrary.com/Health-problems/Aids-research-AltTherapies.htm. Accessed October 13, 2004.

153. HIV sufferers helped by guided imagery: Internet health library (website), 2001: http://www.internethealthlibrary.com/Health-problems/HIV_guided_imagery.htm. Accessed October 13, 2004.

154. Kendall J: Promoting wellness in HIV-support groups, *J Assoc Nurses AIDS Care* 3:28-38, 1992.

155. Lutgendorf S, Antoni MH, Schneiderman N et al: Psychosocial counseling to improve quality of life in HIV infection, *Patient Educ Couns* 24:217-235, 1994.

156. Nunes JA, Raymond SJ, Nicholas PK et al: Social support, quality of life, immune function, and health in persons living with HIV, *Holistic Nurs* 12:174-198, 1995.

157. Belcher AE, Dettmore D, Holzemer SP: Spirituality and sense of well-being in persons with AIDS, *Holistic Nurse Pract* 3:16-25, 1989.

158. Carson VB: Prayer, meditation, exercise and special diets: behaviors of the hardy person with HIV/AIDS, *J Assoc Nurses AIDS Care* 4:18-28, 1993.

159. Kendall J: Wellness spirituality in homosexual men with HIV infection, *J Assoc Nurses AIDS Care* 5:28-34, 1994.

160. Kamarck TW, Manuck SB, Jennings JR: Social support reduces cardiovascular reactivity to psychological challenge: a laboratory model, *Psychosom Med* 52:42-58, 1990.

161. Thomas PD, Goodwin JM, Goodwin JS: Effect of social support on stress-related changes in cholesterol level, uric acid level and immune function in an elderly sample, *Am J Psychiatry* 142:735-737, 1985.

REFERENCES FOR OUTCOME TOOLS*

Used throughout case studies, listed in the order in which they appear.
Semmes Weinstein Monofilaments
Bell-Krotoski J: Advances in sensibility evaluation, Hand Clin 7:527-546, 1991.

Low Dye Taping
Lange B, Chipchase L, Evans A: The effect of low-dye taping on plantar pressures, during gait, in subjects with navicular drop exceeding 10 mm, J Orthop Sports Phys Ther 34:201-209, 2004.

HIV Dementia Scale
Berghuis JP, Uldall KK, Lalonde B: Validity of two scales in identifying HIV-associated dementia, J Acquir Immune Defic Syndr 21:134-140, 1999.

DASH

Bot SD, Terwee CB, van der Windt DA, Bouter LM, Dekker J, de Vet HC: *Clinimetric evaluation of shoulder disability questionnaires: a systematic review of the literature, Ann Rheum Dis 63:335-341, 2004.*

Barthel Index Score

Granger CV, Hamilton BB, Gresham GE, Kramer AA: *The stroke rehabilitation outcome study, II: relative merits of the total Barthel index score and a four-item subscore in predicting patient outcomes, Arch Phys Med Rehabil 70:100-103, 1989.*

MOS HIV Health Survey

Grossman HA, Sullivan PS, Wu AW: *Quality of life and HIV: current assessment tools and future directions for clinical practice, AIDS Reader 13:583-590, 595-597, 2003.*

FIM

O'Sullivan SB, Schmitz TJ: *Physical rehabiliation—assessment and treatment, ed 4, p 321, Philadelphia, 1994, FA Davis Company.*

CHAPTER 22

Multiple Sclerosis

Debra I. Frankel, MS, OTR

KEY WORDS

autoimmune disease
Avonex (interferon beta-1a)
axonal damage
Betaseron (interferon beta-1b)
Copaxone (glatimer acetate)
cytokines
demyelination
encephalomyelitis
exacerbation
experimental allergic encephalomyelitis (EAE)
glial cells
immunosuppression
lesion
multiple sclerosis
myelin
plaques
remission
T cells
Tysabri (natalizumab)

OBJECTIVES

After the end of this chapter the student/therapist will be able to:

1. Describe the medical basis of multiple sclerosis, including epidemiology, etiology, signs and symptoms, diagnosis, and course.
2. Discuss the four categories currently used to describe the clinical course of multiple sclerosis.
3. Discuss current research strategies and findings regarding multiple sclerosis.
4. Identify options in the medical management of the patient with multiple sclerosis.
5. Appreciate the unique psychosocial and neuropsychological effects of multiple sclerosis.
6. Discuss appropriate rehabilitation goals, formulate a rehabilitation plan, and develop rehabilitation strategies to maximize function and quality of life.

OVERVIEW OF MULTIPLE SCLEROSIS

Pathophysiology

Multiple sclerosis (MS) is thought to be an autoimmune disease that affects the central nervous system (CNS): the brain, spinal cord, and optic nerves.[1] The disease was formally identified and established as a clinical pathological entity in 1868 by Jean Martin Charcot, a French neurologist. He called the disease *sclerose en plaques,* describing the hardened, patchlike areas found (on autopsy) disseminated throughout the CNS of individuals with the disease.[2]

Episodes of inflammation (also called attacks, relapses, or exacerbations) damage the myelin sheath (the fatty insulating substance surrounding nerve fibers in the white matter of the brain and spinal cord) causing scarring (also called plaques or lesions). The name *multiple sclerosis* comes from the *multiple* areas of scarring (*sclerotic* tissue) that characterize the disease process. Inflammatory lesions appear as distinct areas of myelin loss scattered throughout the CNS (Figure 22-1). Recent findings also indicate that axons become irreversibly damaged as a consequence of inflammation even early in the disease and may contribute to persistent neurological deficits and long-term disability.[3]

These inflammatory attacks—along with the scarring and axonal damage they produce—occur randomly, varying widely in severity, frequency, and duration from one person to another. The scars on the myelin sheath and damage to axons interfere with the transmission of nerve impulses, thereby producing the symptoms experienced by people with MS.

Etiology

Myelin damage is most likely mediated by the immune system.[1,4,5] Genetically susceptible individuals seem to have an abnormality in the immune response that results in an attack on the individual's own neural tissue—that is, an autoimmune response. A specific antigen—the target of the immune attack—has not yet been identified. Recently researchers have been able to identify which immune cells are involved in the attack, how these cells may be activated, and some of the sites on the attacking cells that seem to be attracted to the myelin to begin the destructive process. Researchers have proposed that a virus is the trigger of this abnormal immune response. However, the virus may infect a large number of people with only a few of the infected developing the secondary process (MS).[4,5]

Some investigators suggest that the immune system mistakes a portion of myelin protein for a virus that is structurally similar and targets it for destruction (molecular mimicry).[6] Others theorize that small amounts of myelin are released in the circulation after viral infection, resulting in autoimmunization.

Epidemiology

Although 90% of patients are diagnosed between the ages of 16 and 60 years, MS can develop in infancy or well after

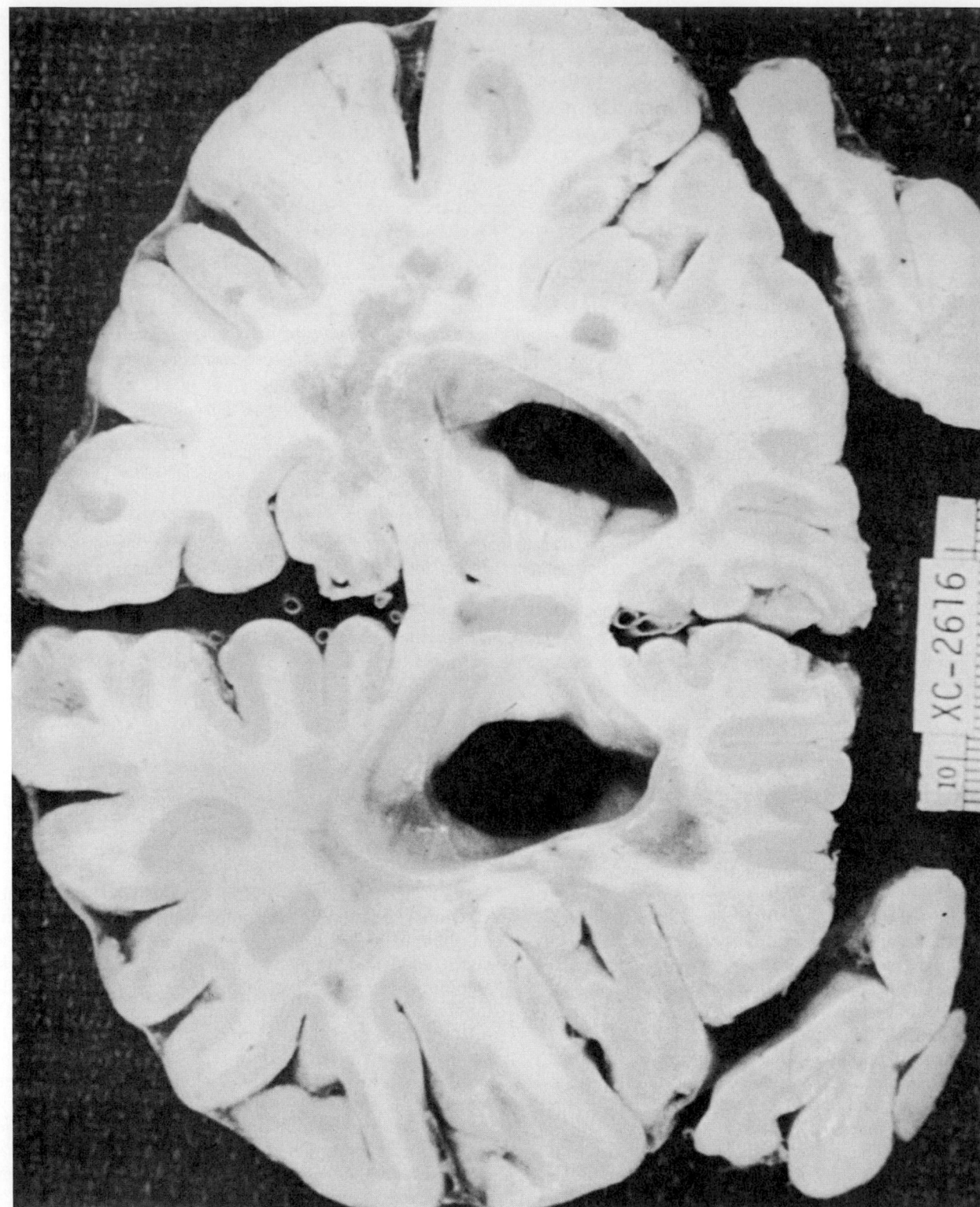

FIGURE 22-1 ■ Brain slice indicating MS plaques. (Reprinted from *Therapeutic claims in multiple sclerosis*, 1982, published under the auspices of the International Federation of Multiple Sclerosis Societies; courtesy of Cedric Raine, MD, Albert Einstein College of Medicine, Yeshiva University, New York.)

the age of 60 years. MS is more common in women than in men by a ratio of 2-3:1. MS is rare in some races (e.g., African blacks and Eskimos) and is most predominant in whites of northern European ancestry.

A number of studies have established geographical patterns of MS prevalence. MS appears more prominently in areas of the world farther from the equator (Figure 22-2). Migration patterns and epidemiological studies (that take into account variations in geography, socioeconomics, genetics, and other factors) have demonstrated that people who are born in an area of the world with a high risk of MS and move to an area with a lower risk before 15 years of age acquire the risk level of their new home. These data suggest that exposure before puberty to some environmental agent (e.g., a virus) may predispose a person to have MS.[7,8] Approximately 400,000 people in the United States have MS.[9] The worldwide estimate is approximately 2.5 million.[10]

Support for the conclusion that MS has a genetic component comes from the fact a first-degree relative of someone with MS (e.g., a parent or sibling) has a significantly greater risk of developing MS than a person with no MS in the family. Thus, although the risk of MS in the general population is about 1 in 750, that figure rises to 1 in 40 for a person who has a parent with MS, with the risk being higher for girls than boys and for children of a woman with MS than those of a man with MS.[11,12] Research has demonstrated a higher prevalence of certain genes in populations with high rates of MS. Common genetic factors have also been found in some families where more than one person has MS.

Disease Course

The course of the disease is unpredictable. The four categories currently used to describe the clinical course of MS are as follows (Figure 22-3):

1. Relapsing/remitting MS (characterized by clearly defined relapses, or episodes of acute worsening, followed by recovery and disease stability) (A)
2. Primary progressive MS (characterized by continuous worsening, or steady progression, not interrupted by distinct relapses) (B)
3. Secondary progressive (characterized by relapsing/remitting disease followed by progression with or without occasional relapse, minor remission, or plateau) (C)
4. Progressive relapsing (characterized by progressive disease from the onset with clear, acute relapses that may or may not resolve; periods between relapses are characterized by continued progression) (D)[13]

Efforts to identify factors that predict clinical course or long-term outcome have not been reliable, although the following factors may suggest a more-favorable outcome: female gender, onset before 35 years of age, monoregional versus polyregional attack, and complete recovery after attacks. The following factors are associated with a less-favorable outcome: male gender, brain stem symptoms (nystagmus, tremor, ataxia, and dysarthria), poor recovery after exacerbations, and high frequency of attacks.[14-16]

Various factors have been associated with exacerbations or temporary worsening (pseudoexacerbation). These include excessive fatigue, trauma, and rise in body temperature because of fever, hot bath, or hot weather conditions, the rise in body temperature likely having an impact on nerve conduction velocity and temporarily worsening symptoms. Recent evidence has been presented by researchers that MS is actually active and progressive from its earliest stages. Until recently, MS was thought to be active only during acute exacerbations or periods of acute worsening of symptoms. By using gadolinium to enhance magnetic resonance (MR) images, researchers have shown that even when the patient's symptoms are stable, their MS may be active. Gadolinium enhances MR images to indicate new and active lesions.[17]

Diagnosis

The diagnosis of MS is largely clinical. The basic diagnostic criteria are described in Table 22-1.[18] The use of MRI has hastened the diagnosis in many cases; however, MS cannot be diagnosed solely on the basis of this test. Some people confirmed to have MS on the basis of other criteria show no lesions on MRI. Conversely, many other diseases may cause lesions that appear on the MRI, and many healthy individuals also may exhibit unidentified bright spots on MRI.[19] Gadolinium, a chemical compound given during MRI that helps distinguish new (active) lesions from old, has been useful in monitoring disease activity. Studies using gadolinium enhancement indicate that the disease may be active even when functional status and neurological signs are stable.[17,20] See Figure 22-1 for an MRI image indicating MS lesions.

Evoked potentials may include visual evoked potentials (VEP), brain stem auditory evoked potentials (BAEP), and somatosensory evoked potentials (SSEP). These tests, which measure nerve conduction along visual, auditory, and sensory pathways, often provide evidence of altered nerve conduction that may not be apparent on neurological examination.[21]

Cerebrospinal fluid examination is not routine in diagnosing MS but may provide additional clues in complicated cases. Elevated gamma globulin levels are found in many cases of MS, and approximately one fourth of persons with active MS may show white blood cells in the cerebrospinal fluid.[15]

Because no specific test exists for MS, and the time between attacks can range from months to years, the diagnostic process can be a long and frustrating one. In addition, the symptoms are so variable and sometimes so subjective that people's symptoms may be ignored or misinterpreted as psychosomatic.

Symptoms

Because of the great variability of the anatomical location, volume, and time sequence of lesions in people with MS, the clinical manifestations of the disease vary among individuals. Symptoms may develop quickly, within hours, or slowly over several days or weeks. The most common symptoms are fatigue, motor weakness, paresthesia, unsteady gait, double vision, tremor, and bladder/bowel dysfunction (Boxes 22-1 and 22-2).[22] Other types of onset, such as hemiplegia, trigeminal neuralgia, and facial palsy, are less common. In many individuals, a history of vague functional impairment precedes definite symptoms.

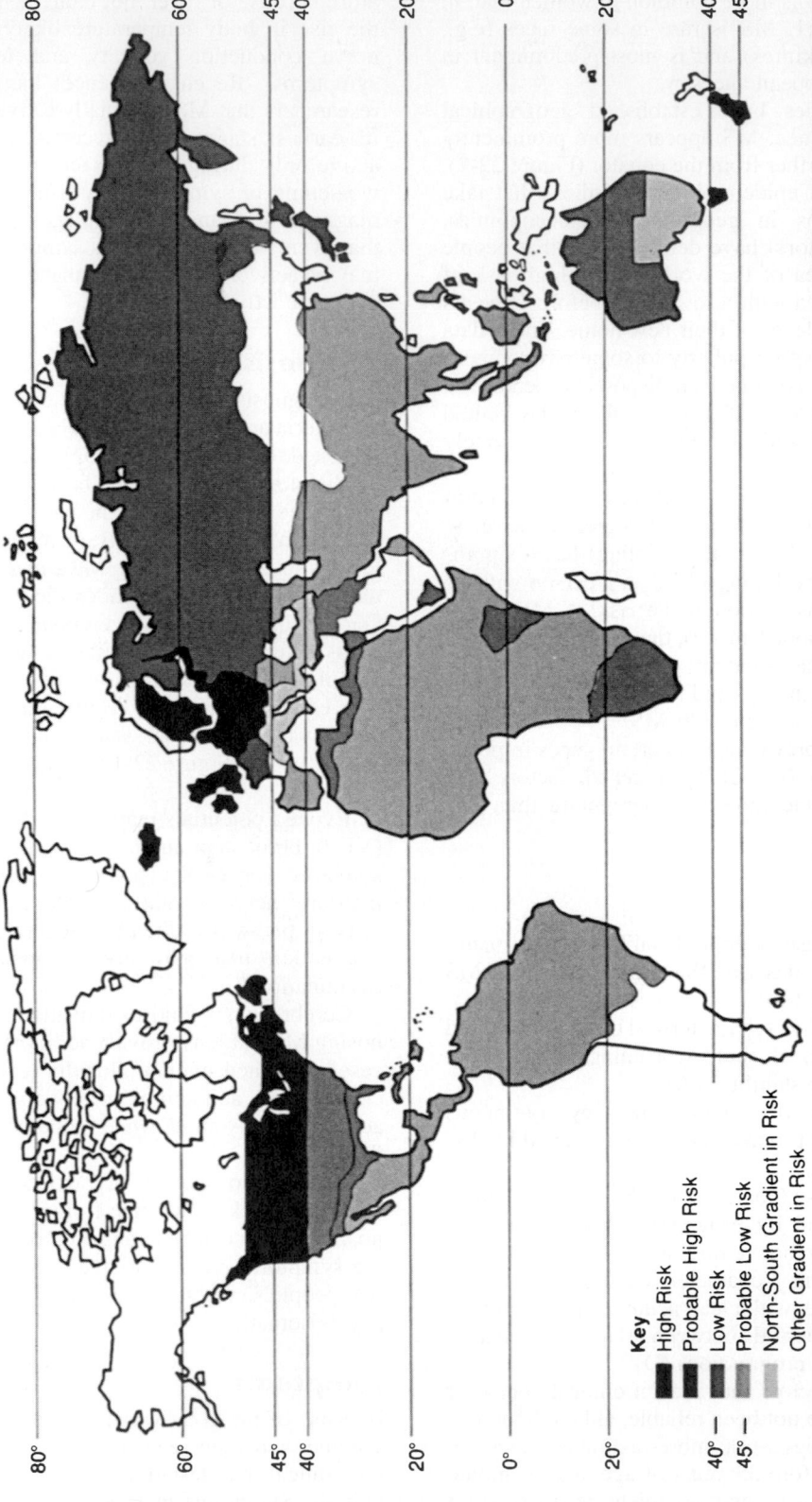

FIGURE 22-2 ■ World map indicating MS incidence. (Adapted from National Institute of Neurological and Communicative Disorders and Stroke: *Multiple sclerosis: hope through research,* publication No. 79-75, Washington, DC, 1981, National Institutes of Health.)

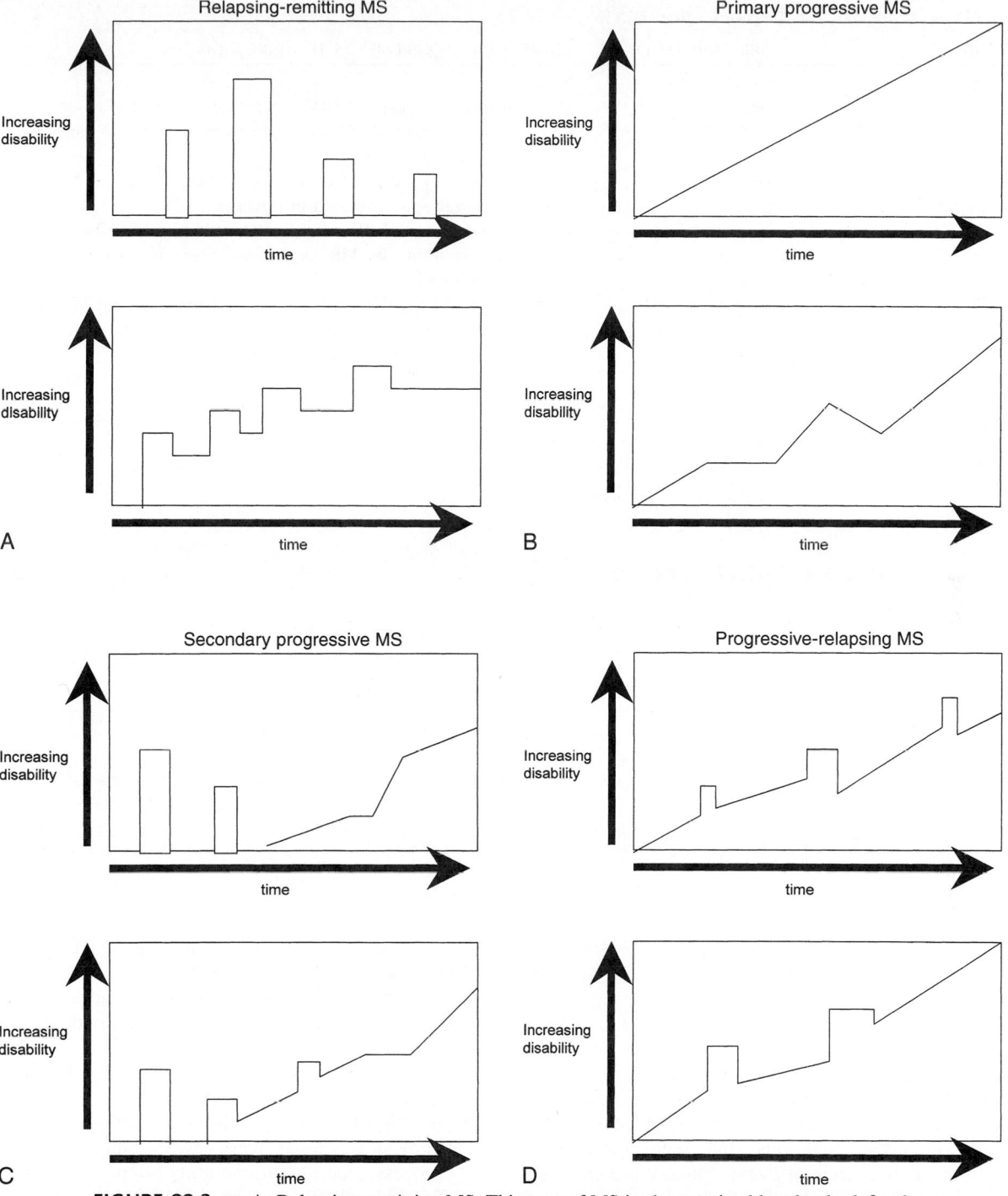

FIGURE 22-3 ■ **A,** Relapsing-remitting MS. This type of MS is characterized by clearly defined acute attacks with full recovery *(top)* or with residual deficits after recovery *(bottom)*. Periods between disease relapses are characterized by a lack of disease progression. **B,** Primary progressive MS. This type is characterized by progression of disability from the beginning without plateaus or remissions *(top)* or with occasional plateaus and temporary minor improvements *(bottom)*. **C,** Secondary progressive MS. This type begins with a relapsing-remitting disease course, followed by progression *(top)*, which may also include occasional relapses and minor remissions and plateaus *(bottom)*. **D,** Progressive-relapsing MS. Progression occurs from the beginning but with clear acute relapses, with *(top)* or without *(bottom)* full recovery. (Reprinted from Lublin F, Reingold S: Refining the course of multiple sclerosis, *Neurology* 46:907, 1996.)

TABLE 22-1 ■ Diagnostic Criteria for MS

CLINICAL (ATTACKS)	OBJECTIVE LESIONS	ADDITIONAL REQUIREMENTS TO MAKE A DIAGNOSIS
Two or more	Two or more	None
Two or more	One	Dissemination in space by MRI, or positive CSF and two or more MRI lesions consistent with MS or further clinical attack involving different site
One	Two or more	Dissemination in time by MRI or second clinical attack
One (monosymptomatic)	One	Dissemination in space by MRI or positive CSF and two or more MRI lesions consistent with MS *and* Dissemination in time by MRI or second clinical attack
None (progression from onset)	One	Positive CSF *and* Dissemination in space by MRI evidence of nine or more T2 brain lesions *or* Two or more cord lesions or four to eight brain and one cord lesion *or* Positive VEP with four to eight MRI lesions *or* Positive VEP with fewer than four brain lesions plus one cord lesion *and* Dissemination in time by MRI or continued progression for 1 year

MRI, Magnetic resonance imaging; *CSF,* cerebrospinal fluid; *VEP,* visual evoked response.
Reprinted from McDonald WI, Compston A, Edan G et al: Recommended diagnostic criteria for MS, *Ann Neurol* 50:121-127, 2001.

BOX 22-1 ■ MOST FREQUENT SYMPTOMS OF MS

Fatigue: 88%   Visual disturbances: 58%
Walking problems: 87%   Cognitive problems: 44%
Bowel and bladder problems: 65% Tremors: 41%
Pain and other sensations: 60%

From a study of 697 patients with MS.

Aronson K, Goldenberg E, Cleghorn G: Socio-demographic characteristics and health status of persons with multiple sclerosis and their care givers, *MS Management* 3(1):5-15, 1996.

The subject of cognitive and affective changes associated with MS has recently been formally addressed. About 50% of people with MS show evidence of some cognitive impairment.[23] Most of these individuals have mild impairment, with approximately 10% to 20% showing significant cognitive dysfunction. Research does not support the idea that the occurrence of cognitive symptoms is related to severity of physical symptoms or to duration of the disease.[24] Specifically, cognitive functions that seem most often affected are short-term memory, conceptual reasoning, and problem solving. Verbal fluency and speed of information processing are sometimes affected. Widespread deterioration of intellectual function in MS is rare.[23]

Depression appears more common in those with MS than in the general population or those with other medical conditions.[25-27] This probably results from an interaction of variables, including the pathophysiological features of the disease, the unique stressors that characterize MS, and the individual's particular circumstances.

Psychosocial Considerations

The personality, history, cultural background of the individual, and the family and community environment all influence the response to illness. The nature of the disability itself will also, of course, influence the emotional response.

MS is an emotionally challenging disease, and all members of the family feel its impact. Anxiety and grief accompany the diagnosis and may appear and reappear with the disease course and the individual's particular circumstances.

The following clinical aspects of MS influence the psychosocial impact of the disease:

1. **Ambiguity of diagnosis.** Although MRI and increased knowledge about MS have hastened the diagnostic process, a period of ambiguity often exists, during which the individual experiences symptoms without a clear explanation. During this time individuals may harbor fantasies of life-threatening or debilitating illness or may not be taken seriously by physicians or friends. Once a confirmed diagnosis of MS is made, some individuals report feeling relief of having an explanation, even though the implications of the diagnosis remain ambiguous.

2. **Unpredictability of the course.** The course of MS is uncertain. The disease may be benign for some but severely disabling for others. An individual may be free of symptoms for months or years and then unexpectedly experience an exacerbation. Symptoms may even vary from morning to evening of the same day. This unpredictability and the accompanying sense of loss of

BOX 22-2 ■ SUMMARY OF COMMON SIGNS AND SYMPTOMS

MOTOR SYMPTOMS
Spasticity and reflex spasms
Weakness
Contractures
Gait disturbance
Fatigue

Cerebellar and Bulbar Symptoms
■ Resultant swallowing/respiratory difficulties
■ Nystagmus
■ Intention tremor

SENSORY SYMPTOMS
Numbness
Pain (most often of musculoskeletal origin)
Paresthesia
Dysesthesia
Distortion of superficial sensation

VISUAL SYMPTOMS
Diminished acuity
Double vision
Scotoma
Ocular pain

BLADDER/BOWEL SYMPTOMS
Urgency
Frequency
Incontinence
Urinary retention
Constipation

SEXUAL SYMPTOMS
Impotence
Diminished genital sensation
Diminished genital lubrication

COGNITIVE AND EMOTIONAL SYMPTOMS
Depression
Lability
Disorders of judgment
Agnosia
Memory disturbance
Diminished conceptual thinking
Decreased attention and concentration
Dysphasia

---

control can frequently lead to depression, anxiety, and fear. Planning for the future becomes difficult and has an impact on family, work, and social interactions and activities.

3. **Covert symptoms.** Many symptoms of MS, including fatigue, double vision, bladder dysfunction, and paresthesias, are not visible to others yet can be disabling and disturbing to the individual. Many people find they are misunderstood, are seen as lazy or lacking initiative, and find explaining the effect of these hidden symptoms to others to be difficult. Some struggle with the decision to disclose their diagnosis to employers or friends. They fear job discrimination or alienating friends, but they may find that the diagnosis is a stressful and disturbing secret to keep.

The stress of MS is in many ways like the stress of any serious or chronic illness. A profound sense of vulnerability and exhausting self-concern underlies the coping process. The loss of a sense of control over one's body and lifestyle may precipitate an ongoing grieving process and an existential search to give meaning to such a distressing life event (see Chapters 4 and 5).

MEDICAL MANAGEMENT
Disease-Modifying Agents

In recent years, several disease-modifying agents (DMAs) have been approved by the U.S. Food and Drug Administration (FDA) for the treatment of MS. They are interferon beta 1a (Avonex), interferon beta 1b (Betaseron), glatiramer acetate (Copaxone), interferon beta 1a (Rebif), and mitoxantrone (Novantrone). Recently, natalizumab (Tysabri) has been approved to delay the accumulation of physical disability and reduce the frequency of relapses in those with relapsing multiple sclerosis, creating another new treatment option for individuals with relapsing forms of MS.

Four of the agents are administered by injection, and two are administered by intravenous infusion. (Avonex is administered weekly and intramuscularly; Betaseron is administered every other day and subcutaneously; Copaxone is administered daily and subcutaneously; Rebif is administered three times per week and subcutaneously; Novantrone is administered four times per year by intravenous infusion; and Tysabri is a monoclonal antibody given by intravenous infusion every 4 weeks.)

Table 22-2 shows the approved indications for each agent. All the agents are associated with side effects. Table 22-3 describes the side effects for each agent.

The development of these DMAs and the continued data collection on their effectiveness have made a significant impact on the treatment of MS. The agents have been shown in clinical trials to reduce the frequency and severity of attacks and may reduce future disability for many people with MS. All have been shown to limit development of lesions within the CNS. The drugs do not cure MS, but in some patients they may modify the expected course and prevent permanent damage to axons.

In September 1998 the National Multiple Sclerosis Society's medical advisors approved a statement regarding early intervention and access to these agents for patients with relapsing/remitting MS (Box 22-3). This disease management consensus statement was updated in 2004. As a result the drugs are becoming widely accepted as standard treatment for many patients with MS.

Treatment of Relapses and Symptoms

In addition to treatment with DMAs, medical management of MS focuses on the treatment of acute relapses,

BOX 22-3 ■ NATIONAL MULTIPLE SCLEROSIS SOCIETY DISEASE MANAGEMENT CONSENSUS STATEMENT

The Executive Committee of the Medical Advisory Board of the National Multiple Sclerosis Society has adopted the following recommendations regarding use of the current MS disease-modifying agents.

■ Initiation of therapy with an immunomodulator is advised as soon as possible after a definite diagnosis of MS with a relapsing course and may be considered for selected patients with a first attack who are at high risk for MS.

■ Patients' access to medication should not be limited by the frequency of relapses, age, or level of disability.

■ Treatment is not to be stopped while insurers evaluate for continuing coverage of treatment.

■ Therapy is to be continued indefinitely, except for the following circumstances: there is clear lack of benefit; there are intolerable side effects; new data reveal other reasons for cessation; or better therapy becomes available.

■ All FDA-approved agents should be included in formularies and covered by third-party payers so that physicians and patients can determine the most appropriate agent on an individual basis; failure to do so is unethical and discriminatory against a very small percentage of patients.

■ Movement from one immunomodulatory drug to another should be permitted.

■ Immunosuppressant therapy with mitoxantrone (Novantrone) may be considered for selected relapsing patients with worsening disease.

■ Most concurrent medical conditions do not contraindicate use of immunomodulatory drugs.

■ None of the four therapies has been approved for use by women who are trying to become pregnant, are pregnant, or are nursing mothers.

National MS Society Disease Management Consensus Statement, National Multiple Sclerosis Society. Updated 2004.

The Disease Management Consensus Statement is under review by the National Multiple Sclerosis Society's Medical Advisory Board to formulate changes in light of the FDA's recent approval of natalizumab (Tysabri) for relapsing forms of MS.

TABLE 22-2 ■ DMAs for MS and Indications

DRUG	PURPOSE
Avonex	For the treatment of all relapsing forms of MS and for a single clinical episode if MRI features consistent with MS are also present
Betaseron	For the treatment of all relapsing forms of MS
Copaxone	For the treatment of relapsing/remitting MS
Rebif	For treatment of all relapsing forms of MS
Novantrone	For treatment of worsening relapsing/remitting MS and for progressive relapsing or secondary progressive MS
Tysabri	A monotherapy treatment for relapsing forms of MS; generally recommended for patients who have had an inadequate response to, or are unable to tolerate alternative MS therapies

Reprinted from *Comparing the disease-modifying drugs*, Washington, DC, 2005, National Multiple Sclerosis Society; www.nationalmssociety.org/Brochures-Comparing.asp.

symptomatic management, improvement of function with rehabilitation therapies, and psychological support.

Treatment of Acute Relapses

Natural improvement of acute exacerbations frequently occurs within 4 to 12 weeks. The degree of improvement varies. For acute relapses, most physicians prescribe high-dose intravenous corticosteroids such as methylprednisolone (Depo-Medrol) over a 3- to 5-day period. This high-dose intravenous course may be followed by a gradually tapering dose of oral corticosteroid (e.g., prednisone). Oral corticosteroids also used to treat a mild or moderate relapse, although intravenous methylprednisolone is usually pre-

TABLE 22-3 ■ Side Effects of DMAs

DRUG	ADVERSE REACTIONS*
Avonex	Flulike symptoms after injection that lessen over time for many. Rarer: depression, mild anemia, elevated liver enzymes, allergic reactions, heart problems.
Betaseron	Flulike symptoms after injection that lessen over time for many. Injection site reactions, approximately 5% of which need medical attention. Rarer: allergic reactions, depression, elevated liver enzyme levels, low white blood cell counts.
Copaxone	Injection site reactions. Rarer: vasodilation (dilation of blood vessels); chest pain; a reaction immediately after injection that includes anxiety, chest pain, palpitations, shortness of breath, and flushing. This lasts 15 to 30 minutes and has no known long-term effects.
Rebif	Flulike symptoms after injection that lessen over time for many. Injection site reactions. Less common: liver abnormalities, depression, allergic reactions, and low red or white blood cell counts.
Tysabri	Potential increased risk of progressive multifocal leukoencephalopathy (PML), infusion reactions, headache, fatigue, joint and limb pain, abdominal discomfort, diarrhea, and rash.

Reprinted from *Comparing the disease-modifying drugs*, Washington, DC, 2005, National Multiple Sclerosis Society; www.nationalmssociety.org/Brochures-Comparing.asp.
*People with MS taking these drugs are generally able to successfully manage these side effects by working closely with their health providers and using specific strategies aimed at alleviating the particular reaction. Refer to the Web site for specific strategies. Also, many side effects decrease over time on the drug.

scribed for optic neuritis and retrobulbar neuritis. Although these antiinflammatory agents are used widely in acute attacks of MS, little evidence has shown that they alter the extent of residual disability or the overall course of the disease.[28] Long-term side effects of corticosteroids (osteoporosis, hypertension, cataracts, muscle wasting) are not generally associated with short-term use; nevertheless, side effects may include altered mood, frequent urination, and blurred vision. Mood changes are relatively common, with people reporting feeling "high," energetic, unable to sleep, or depressed, particularly as they come off the medication. A small percentage of people may experience quite severe disturbances in mood or behavior.[28,29]

Symptomatic Treatment

Spasticity. Baclofen (Lioresal) and tizanidine (Zanaflex) are the most commonly used medications to control *spasticity* in MS. Side effects such as increased weakness, lethargy, and fatigue may occur with baclofen. The surgical implantation of a pump to deliver a continuous dose of baclofen intrathecally has been significantly beneficial to many people with severe spasticity. The pump is implanted beneath the skin, usually on the lower abdomen, and the rate of drug delivery can be adjusted to meet individual need. Sodium dantrolene (Dantrium) may also be helpful, although it may induce weakness even at low doses. Diazepam (Valium) is also used, most frequently for spasms that occur at night. Cyclobenzaprine (Flexeril) is sometimes prescribed for back spasms and also may have an overall antispasticity effect. Botulinum toxin (Botox) injections have been shown to be effective in relieving spasticity in individual muscles for up to 3 months. Phenol blocks or tendon release surgical procedures may be required if severe spasticity interferes with personal hygiene and other activities of daily living (ADLs), although a combination of exercise, stretching, and medication can usually avoid these more extreme measures. Severe tremor may be treated with agents such as the antituberculosis agent isoniazid (INH), the antihistamine hydroxyzine (Atarax and Vistaril), the β-blocker propranolol (Inderal), the anticonvulsive primidone (Mysoline), the diuretic acetazolamide (Diamox), and anti-anxiety drugs buspirone (BuSpar) and clonazepam (Klonopin) with varying degrees of success.[28,29] Reducing spasticity generally results in improved mobility and function; however, a certain degree of spasticity may be beneficial to some individuals, especially when it aids in the support of weak legs. Physical and occupational therapy and a stretching regimen are also beneficial in reducing spasticity.

Fatigue. Fatigue is one of the most common symptoms of MS and may be significantly debilitating. Energy conservation, moderate exercise, rest, use of assistive devices, work simplification, and cooling may be effective in controlling fatigue in MS. Amantadine hydrochloride (Symmetrel) and modafinil (Provigil) are the most commonly prescribed medications. Although neither is approved specifically by the FDA for the treatment of MS-related fatigue, each has been shown in clinical trials to relieve the symptoms of fatigue for many people with MS. Some stimulants such as pemoline (Cylert) and methylphenidate (Ritalin) are also used. These stimulants may cause sleep-lessness or other side effects that must be monitored.[28] Depression may contribute to fatigue in some cases; when the underlying depression is alleviated, fatigue levels improve. The Multiple Sclerosis Council of the Paralyzed Veterans of America has developed clinical practice guidelines of managing fatigue in patients with MS. These present an evidence-based, systematic strategy for use by all health care providers and provide a framework for identifying appropriate care.[30]

Bladder Symptoms. Most bladder symptoms result from a neurogenic bladder; however, urinary tract infection must be considered because this may also cause changes in bladder function. Smooth muscle relaxants or nerve blockers such as propantheline bromide (Pro-Banthine), imipramine (Tofranil), and oxybutynin (Ditropan) may reduce spasms of the bladder. Urinary retention is frequently treated with bethanechol (Urecholine) or phenoxybenzamine (Dibenzyline). The Crede technique and intermittent catheterization are used with the bladder that does not sufficiently empty. If a bladder problem cannot be solved by medication or intermittent catheterization, continuous catheterization with a Foley catheter may be necessary.[31] Bladder infections caused by urinary retention are treated with an antibiotic specific to the bacteria present. Prevention of infection is the best approach by adding acidifying agents to the diet. The Multiple Sclerosis Council of the Paralyzed Veterans Administration has developed clinical practice guidelines in bladder management that are effective and widely used approaches to care (see Chapters 33 and 36).[31]

Absence of Good Bowel Control. Absence of good bowel control may lead to constipation or incontinence. Bulk formers such as hydrophilic colloid (Metamucil) or stool softeners such as docusate (Colace) may be recommended. Rectal stimulants such as glycerin or bisacodyl (Dulcolax) suppositories may also be effective. Frequent use of enemas should be avoided. A bowel program including dietary (adequate fluids and bulk) and drug regimens can usually control the constipation and incontinence of patients with MS.[28]

Pain. Although pain is not a hallmark of MS, many people with the disease have a variety of painful syndromes. Tic douloureux (trigeminal neuralgia), a sharp pain in the face stimulated by touch or facial movement, is most common. It is usually treated with carbamazepine (Tegretol), phenytoin (Dilantin), or baclofen (Lioresal). In extreme cases, surgical procedures may be used to sever the sensory root fibers of the trigeminal nerve. Many individuals with MS have dysesthetic pain, frequently described as a burning sensation. This pain may be treated with gabapentin (Neurontin). Dysesthesias may also be treated with an antidepressant such as amitriptyline (Elavil), which modifies how the CNS reacts to pain. Pain frequently associated with MS is caused by spasticity, poor posture, or abnormal use of muscles to compensate for loss of function. Physical and occupational therapy may play an important role in pain management of this type along with analgesics, nonsteroidal antiinflammatory drugs (NSAIDs) and, in the case of back spasms, drugs such as cyclobenzaprine (see Chapters 32 and 36).[28,32]

Sexual Function. MS can affect sexual function directly by causing neurological impairment that results in erectile difficulties, orgasmic dysfunction, or decreased libido. Indirectly, such symptoms as fatigue, spasticity, depression, and bladder and bowel dysfunction may interfere with sexual expression and intimacy. Sexual aids, prosthetic devices, counseling, and medications such as sildenafil (Viagra), vardenafil (Levitra), alprostadil (Muse), or prostaglandin injections for erectile dysfunction may improve function and satisfaction with sexual expression. For women, medications such as phenytoin (Dilantin) and carbamazepine (Tegretol) may reduce sensory discomfort that interferes with sexual enjoyment. Over-the-counter personal lubricants may also be useful (see Chapter 5).[28]

Dizziness and Vertigo. Dizziness and vertigo may accompany loss of balance. If vertigo is severe, medications such as meclizine (Antivert, Bonine) or Dramamine may be suggested. Skin patches that deliver scopolamine or the antinausea drug ondansetron (Zofran) may also be useful. In severe cases of dizziness or vertigo, a short course of corticosteroids may be needed (see Chapter 23).[28]

Cognitive Impairment. Neuropsychological testing can assist in determining the degree of cognitive impairment in patients with MS. Treatment of cognitive problems usually involves retraining and teaching of compensatory strategies. Cognitive dysfunction may be a major disabling feature of MS. Symptoms may be exaggerated by underlying depression or may be confused by communication deficits.

Depression. People with MS have a high incidence of depression along with a suicide rate that one study identified as 7.5 times higher than the general population.[25-27,32] Both organic and psychosocial factors contribute to depression and anxiety in MS. Counseling, support groups and, in some cases, antidepressant medications and psychotherapy may be helpful in addressing these issues in MS.

A large percentage of persons with MS show improvement in symptoms as a result of the natural history of the disease at various times, regardless of treatment. Additionally, complementary therapies (e.g., acupuncture, massage, movement therapies, diets, vitamin supplementation) are gaining popularity among people with MS as in the general population (see Chapter 37). Any complementary therapies patients use should be discussed to ensure no contraindications or negative interactions result.

RESEARCH CONSIDERATIONS

The search for the cause and cure of MS is the focus of efforts in the United States primarily by the National Multiple Sclerosis Society and the National Institutes of Health. Internationally, work is being conducted in academic and scientific institutions worldwide. The Multiple Sclerosis International Federation (MSIF) works to coordinate these efforts and facilitate communication among investigators. The primary areas of MS research include the following[33,34]:

■ Immunology: exploring the role of the body's complex immune system in the development, progression, and possible suppression of MS
■ Study of glial cells: investigating ways to repair myelin

■ Nerve physiology: exploring fundamental workings of nerve cells
■ Genetics: understanding genetic susceptibility in MS
■ Virology
■ Health-care delivery and policy: studying how health care for people with MS might be improved
■ Therapy: searching for treatments for MS with complimentary/alternative therapies
■ Rehabilitation of MS: exploring the role of rehabilitation therapies in treating and managing MS

Immunology

The most likely hypothesis about the cause of MS relates to immune dysfunction. New mechanisms are being tested for intervening with immune function, particularly with the function of T cells and B cells and antibodies, all of which play a role in MS. Work of this kind in the animal model of MS (i.e., experimental allergic encephalomyelitis [EAE]) has resulted in the development of highly specific immune system regulatory agents. These include monoclonal antibodies; synthetic peptides, which alter immune function and prevent EAE from occurring; and identification of cytokines, which are naturally occurring molecules that help regulate immune function.[34]

Glial Cell Biology

The study of oligodendrocytes, the glial cells that make and maintain myelin, offers the best hope for recovery of function. Efforts to transplant oligodendrocytes in mice and manipulate the immune system to accelerate remyelination are showing promise in improving function.[34]

Nerve Physiology, Pathology, and Repair

When myelin is inflamed or destroyed in MS, nerve fiber conduction is impaired or stopped. Moreover, the immune attack also damages or even severs the axons, ending their ability to function.

Nerves can remyelinate from cells within the CNS that are still capable of forming new myelin, and it can remyelinate from "immature" myelin-making cells, which, when myelin is lost, begin to divide, multiply, and produce new myelin. The problem in MS seems to be that myelin loss proceeds more aggressively and quickly than remyelination. Understanding the myelination process is thus a vital area of research.

Studies in animal systems show that growth or trophic factors, and some immune antibodies, may accelerate remyelination. Also, myelin-making cells can be transplanted from a healthy animal into one in which myelin-making cells are gone. These findings may drive future therapies.[34]

Genetics

Evidence suggests that many genes may contribute to susceptibility to MS. Some of these genes are important in determining immune system function and control, but others are not related to immune function. The fact that predisposition to MS likely involves different genes acting together makes understanding the genetic basis for this disease more complex than for other diseases.

Studies of families in which more than one member has MS, and of ethnically diverse populations with MS and groups with restricted geography and gene mixture, facilitate genetic research in MS.[34]

Virology

For decades scientists have been looking for the MS "trigger" to develop a vaccine or treatment that would eliminate the disease. Dozens of viruses and bacteria have been studied, but not one has shown a direct cause-and-effect relation with MS. Ultimately the problem may lie in the way that a person with a genetically predisposed immune system handles infections in general.[34]

Therapies

Although the ultimate objective is to find a cure for MS, the following are additional objectives[34]:

■ Inducing a remission of active disease
■ Prolonging remission so that the disease does not flare up again
■ Altering the course of the disease by slowing its progression or reducing the frequency of acute attacks
■ Providing relief from disease symptoms

Health Policy and Health Care Delivery Research

Understanding how MS care is delivered and what barriers exist to obtaining quality care is a major component required to change policy and service delivery. This includes acquiring data on the cost effectiveness of various treatments, understanding the impact of the disease on the family and the individual, and evaluating and improving access to care and health delivery systems.[34]

Rehabilitation Research

Members from all branches of the health care community are embracing evidence-based management strategies to improve patient outcomes and enhance quality assurance. Evidence-based medicine refers to systematic weighting of health care practices according to research or scientific evidence supporting those practices. Where scientific evidence is lacking, practice guidelines are developed and evaluated on the basis of expert opinion and consensus. This concept helps clinicians make treatment decisions informed by the best current evidence as opposed to relying solely on past experience, intuition, or anecdotal observation. Evidence-based practice closes the gap between research and clinical application.

The following summarizes some recent research in MS rehabilitation management. These findings will help inform the decisions made in determining rehabilitation goals, modalities, and techniques.

Researchers in Royal Oak, Mich., concluded that an interdisciplinary approach to MS rehabilitation (occupational and physical therapy) improved mobility of the patient, minimizing such symptoms as spasticity and fatigue as well as reducing complications of inactivity.[35] Researchers at the Institute of Neurology in London, in a study to determine if the benefits of inpatient rehabilitation of MS patients carried over to the community, found that benefits were partly maintained although declined over time, reinforcing the need for continuity of care between inpatient settings and the community.[36] Investigators at the Istituto Nazionale Neurologico in Milan, Italy, concluded, in a study of the effects of physical rehabilitation in patients with MS,

that despite unchanging impairment rehabilitation resulted in improvement of functional skills and had a positive impact on mental components of health-related quality of life measures and participation in life activities.[37] Another study at the Institute of Neurology in London attempted to identify the physical and cognitive variables affecting rehabilitation outcome in patients with MS.[38] The researchers concluded that verbal intelligence and cerebellar function are influential in determining rehabilitation outcomes.

Therapists at the Jimmie Heuga Center in Edwards, Colo., reported that physical fitness and emotional state improve in patients with MS with exercise training despite increases in functional limitations.[39] Neufeld[40] reported in preliminary findings that patients with MS in an exercise- and skills-based wellness course designed by an occupational therapist showed gains in self-efficacy for self-management, increasing use of self-management behaviors, and achievement of personal goals.

Patients with MS who received multidisciplinary rehabilitation in addition to intravenous steroids demonstrated increased improvement in functional status, mobility, quality of life, and disability over those who received steroids alone.[41] A study of the effect of inpatient rehabilitation on individuals with relapsing/remitting MS suggested that inpatient rehabilitation is useful for patients with incomplete recovery from relapses who have accumulated moderate to severe disability.[42] Another study showed a significant decrease in length of stay in a rehabilitation inpatient unit for patients who were given more intensive rehabilitation therapies.[43] Patients with progressive MS who received outpatient rehabilitation had reductions in fatigue and MS-related symptoms.[44] Furthermore, a physiotherapy program conducted at home or in a hospital outpatient clinic resulted in significant improvements in mobility, subjective well-being, and mood in patients with chronic MS.[45] This study suggests that ongoing physiotherapy might be necessary for sustaining benefit for improvement in mobility or prevention of deterioration. Other studies demonstrated positive impact of multidisciplinary rehabilitative care on the daily life of patients with MS.[36,37] Much research in rehabilitation and MS suggest positive benefit; however, all recommend additional research that uses rigorous study design and large sample sizes.

REHABILITATION MANAGEMENT

Although DMAs are now available to slow the progression of activity restrictions (functional limitations) in some persons with MS, many people with the disease have limitations in their ability to manage ADLs. Rehabilitation is directed toward maximizing function, preventing unnecessary complications, empowering individuals to realize their highest potential, and improving overall quality of life. Although rehabilitation interventions will not eliminate neurological damage in MS, they can reduce disability and enhance functioning. In 2004 the National MS Society published an expert opinion report recommending rehabilitation intervention for MS at all stages of the disease (Box 22-4).[46]

Rehabilitation Team and Setting

Involvement in a rehabilitation program may take several forms. From a practical point of view, fiscal considerations may dictate the frequency and duration of therapy visits as well as location, that is, whether the care is administered at

BOX 22-4 ■ NATIONAL MULTIPLE SCLEROSIS SOCIETY REHABILITATION: RECOMMENDATIONS FOR PERSONS WITH MULTIPLE SCLEROSIS

The National Multiple Sclerosis Society expert opinion and recommendations are:

Although the disease course cannot be altered by rehabilitation, a growing body of evidence indicates that improvement in mobility, ADLs, quality of life, prevention of complications, reduction in health care utilization, and gains in safety and independence may be realized by a carefully planned program of exercise, functional training, and activities that address the specific needs of the individual. Thus rehabilitation is considered a necessary component of comprehensive, quality health care for people with MS at all stages of the disease.

■ The physician* should consider referral of individuals with MS for assessment by rehabilitation professionals† when there is an *abrupt or gradual* worsening in functional limitations or increase in impairment that has a significant impact on the individual's mobility, safety, independence, or quality of life.

■ Patients who present with any functional limitation should have an initial evaluation and appropriate management.

■ Assessment for rehabilitation services should be considered early in the disease when behavioral and lifestyle changes may be easier to implement.

■ The complex interaction of motor, sensory, cognitive, functional, and affective impairments in an unpredictable, progressive, and fluctuating disease such as MS requires periodic reassessment, monitoring, and rehabilitative interventions.

■ The frequency, intensity, and setting of the rehabilitative intervention must be based on individual needs. Some complex needs are best met in an interdisciplinary, inpatient setting, whereas other needs are best met at home or in outpatient settings. The health care team should determine the most appropriate setting.

■ Research and professional experience support the use of rehabilitative interventions‡ in concert with other medical interventions for the following impairments in MS:

■ Mobility impairments (e.g., impaired strength, gait, balance, range of motion, coordination, tone, and endurance)

■ Fatigue
■ Pain
■ Dysphagia
■ Bladder/bowel dysfunction
■ Decreased independence in ADLs
■ Impaired communication
■ Diminished quality of life (often caused by inability to work, engage in leisure activities or to pursue usual life roles)
■ Depression and other affective disorders
■ Cognitive dysfunction

■ Appropriate assessments and outcome measures must be periodically applied to establish and revise goals, identify the need for treatment modification, and measure the results of the intervention.

■ Known complications of MS, such as contractures, disuse atrophy, decubitus ulcers, risk of falls, and increased dependence may be reduced or prevented by specific rehabilitative interventions.

■ In a fluctuating and progressive disease, maintenance of function, participation, and quality of life are essential outcomes.

■ Maintenance therapy includes rehabilitation interventions designed to preserve current status of ADLs, safety, mobility, and quality of life and to reduce the rate of deterioration and development of complications.

■ A thorough assessment for wheelchairs, positioning devices, other durable medical equipment, and environmental modification by rehabilitation professionals is recommended and will result in the use of the most appropriate equipment.

■ Regular and systematic communication between the referring health care provider and rehabilitation professionals will facilitate comprehensive, quality care.

■ Whenever possible, patients should be seen by rehabilitation therapists who are familiar with neurological degenerative disorders.

■ Third-party payers should cover appropriate and individualized restorative and maintenance rehabilitation services for people with MS

Reprinted from *Rehabilitation: recommendations for persons with multiple sclerosis,* New York, 2004, National Multiple Sclerosis Society.
*Or nurse practitioner or physician's assistant.
†Includes rehabilitation physician, occupational, physical, speech and language therapists, and others.
‡Includes exercise, functional training, equipment prescription, provision of assistive technology, orthotics prescription, teaching of compensatory strategies, caregiver/family support and education, counseling, and referral to community resources.

home or on an inpatient or outpatient basis. Unfortunately, the availability of third-party payment for therapy is often conditional, with many individuals ineligible for reimbursement, particularly for maintenance and preventive therapies. The above recommendations were developed by the National Multiple Sclerosis Society, in part to encourage third-party coverage of rehabilitation services for MS.

The place at which treatment is provided can often dictate the modalities used. An inpatient setting, for example, provides an opportunity for intensive therapies, a therapeutic community, multidisciplinary support, a comprehensive

treatment environment, and easy availability of equipment and modalities. Such a setting requires learning skills outside the home environment, transferring those skills after discharge, and adjusting psychologically to the home setting, where the client has the opportunity and responsibility to integrate his or her program into ADLs.

As an alternative, home-based treatment provides a familiar environment; however, availability of equipment or modalities may be limited. The treatment environment selected needs to be based on the client's needs, the availability of resources, and cost.

Treatment focuses on helping the patient achieve optimal functional independence and is best carried out by an interdisciplinary team. Members of the team include the physician, occupational therapist, physical therapist, speech therapist, nurse, dietitian, social worker, recreation therapist, vocational counselor and, of course, the patient and her or his family. Not all members will be involved at all times, and financial realities may prohibit involvement of all team members; however, the team approach is the most comprehensive approach to management. The team uses a variety of methods to reduce disability and improve the quality of life for a person with MS: physical treatment, education/training, advocacy, environmental changes, compensation with adaptive equipment, and counseling. Table 22-4 indicates how the interdisciplinary team might collaborate on many common MS problems.[47]

Evaluation

In 2001 The World Health Organization (WHO) approved an International Classification of Functioning, Disability and Health (ICF).[48] Functioning and disability are viewed as an interaction between health conditions of the individual and the contextual factors of the environment. The ICF provides a common framework and language that views impairment in relation to participation in life activities and in the context of the individual's physical and social environment. This language will likely find its way into evaluation tools in the near future.

The clinician must consider various factors when evaluating the individual with MS. Subjective perceptions of problems by the individual and family members may be of greater significance than objective measures. Functional assessment at times may not correlate with clinical measures; that is, MS lesions may be functionally silent in some cases yet in others significant functional impairment may result from apparently minimal clinical disease activity (as indicated by MRI). The individual with MS must be evaluated at intervals during the fluctuating course of the disease. Additionally, factors that influence performance such as heat and fatigue must be considered when the client is evaluated.

An assessment profile (Box 22-5) must be developed before establishing treatment goals. Ideally, a collaborative approach to assessment, pooling the various findings of the members of the rehabilitation team with the priorities of the individual, will provide direction for the rehabilitation process.

Each patient serves as her or his own baseline because the course of MS and severity of symptoms are so variable.

Measurement Tools

The rehabilitation assessment tools listed in Box 22-6 represent many of the tools commonly used in rehabilitation assessment of patients with MS.[49] Some are specific to the disease, (marked with an asterisk), whereas others will be familiar to therapists for use with other patients. The Kurtzke Scale (Box 22-7) is a common descriptor of level of disability and is frequently used in clinical trials and other clinical settings.

Some MS clinical centers have developed their own screening measures that draw from the various tools just

TABLE 22-4 ■ Examples of Team Interaction on Common MS Problems

PROBLEM	GOALS	TEAM*	PLAN
Weakness	Strengthen disuse component Maintain fitness	MD, nurse, OT, PT	Strengthening exercises, substitution, compensation, protective splints
Spasticity	Normalize tone without causing loss of support	MD, nurse, OT, PT	Medication, stretching, positioning, cold bath or spray, movement techniques, motor point block
Incoordination, tremor, impaired balance	Improve balance and control	MD, nurse, OT, PT	Medication, coordination and balance exercises, joint approximation, adaptive equipment, extremity weights, compensatory techniques, air splints, weighted canes or crutches, gait training
Impaired sensation	Enhance sensory awareness Teach precautions	MD, nurse, OT, PT	Education, visual compensation, developmental sequence exercises, joint approximation, tapping, brushing, weights
Pain	Decrease source of pain Decrease perception of pain	Biofeedback, counselor, MD, nurse, OT, PT	Medication, improve posture, transcutaneous nerve stimulation, increase activity, stress management, muscle relaxation, diminish pain behavior
Visual impairment	Improve vision Compensate for loss	Blind services, MD, nurse, OT, PT, ophthalmologist	Medication for acute optic neuritis, patch for double vision, compensatory techniques, talking books, home visits
Fatigue	Increase and conserve available energy	Biofeedback, counselor, MD, nurse, OT, PT	Teach energy conservation, treat depression, improve endurance, efficient compensatory techniques and equipment, stress management, patient record of activities and readjustment, rest periods at onset of fatigue

Continued

TABLE 22-4 ■ **Examples of Team Interaction on Common MS Problems—cont'd**

PROBLEM	GOALS	TEAM*	PLAN
Memory, cognitive impairment	Identify Compensate	Counselor, MD, nurse, OT, PT	Evaluation, education of patient and family, compensatory techniques, alteration of home environment
Ambulation, transfers	Safe and efficient mobility	Nurse, OT, PT	Decrease spasticity, strengthen and improve balance, improve trunk stability, gain training, gaiting aids, practice on ward, evaluate environment (hospital, home, work) for safety, accessibility, wheelchair evaluation, training
ADLs, community skills	Efficient and safe self-care Energy conservation Access to community	Driver education, nurse, OT, PT, recreation	Transfers; balance; bed mobility; home equipment; new skills; adaptive equipment; energy conservation; practice on ward, at home, and on supervised recreational outings
Bowel dysfunction	Regularity without constipation, diarrhea, incontinence	Dietician, MD, nurse, OT, PT	Diet, decrease constipating medications, manage bladder program, sitting balance, transfers, hand function, increase daily activity
Bladder dysfunction	Freedom from incontinence and infection	MD, nurse, OT, PT, urologist	Evaluation, medication, teach bladder program, sitting/standing balance, transfers, hand function, treat infections
Sexual dysfunction	Compensation Education	Counselor, MD, OT, PT, urologist	Evaluation, education, mobility, balance, decrease spasticity, contractures, hand function, bowel and bladder control, compensatory techniques, prosthesis, support, self-image
Dysarthria	Improve communication Maintain functional communication Compensation Energy conservation	Nurse, OT, PT, speech	Retraining, teach others to listen, abdominal breathing exercises, oral exercises, decrease spasticity, practice on ward, communication boards, hand function for boards
Dysphagia	Nutrition Safety Energy conservation	Dietician, MD, nurse, OT, speech	Diet, patient and family training and education, evaluation of alternative routes of nutrition if needed
Adjustment, motivation	Facilitate adjustment Appropriate independence/ dependence Prevent isolation Stress management	Biofeedback, counselor, MD, nurse, OT, PT, recreation, speech	Supportive counseling, alternative goals, success at valued tasks, improved ability to communicate, antidepressant medication, biofeedback, relaxation, positive social and recreational experiences
Medical complication: decubitus ulcer	Prevent, treat	Dietician, MD, OT, PT	Evaluate, educate patient and family, strengthen and position, decrease spasticity, improve nutrition, protective equipment, correct contractures
Medical complication: contractures	Prevent, decrease	MD, nurse, OT, PT, surgeon	Stretching, positioning, educate patient and family, equipment, strengthen, surgical release
Medical complication: nutrition	Maximize nutrition Avoid fads	Dietician, MD, nurse, OT, PT	Evaluate, educate, train in swallowing, body position, hand control, treat depression, proper diet
Medical complication: respiratory problems	Improve breath control Avoid respiratory illness	MD, nurse, PT	Breathing exercises, improve posture, increase activity, medical care if needed
Vocation Family adjustment Avocation Homemaking	Best and most interesting job and recreation available Strengthen family Mobilize community resources	Counselor, MD, nurse, OT, PT, recreation, speech, vocation counselor	Physical skills, motivation, help to overcome environmental barriers, build bridges to community resources, counseling

Reprinted from Maloney FP: *Interdisciplinary rehabilitation of multiple sclerosis and neuromuscular disorders,* Philadelphia, 1985, J.B. Lippincott
*Team members are listed in alphabetical order.
MD, Physician; *OT,* occupational therapist; *PT,* physical therapist; *speech,* speech/language pathologist; *biofeedback,* biofeedback technician; *recreation,* recreation therapist.

BOX 22-5 ■ ASSESSMENT PROFILE FOR MS

Mobility/gait
Transfers/bed mobility
Posture
Tone
Range of motion
Functional strength
Fatigue
Sensation
ADLs/independent ADLs
Work and leisure

Driving
Pain
Balance
Speech and swallowing
Cognition
Safety
Other: bladder/bowel, sexual function
Social and life phase activities
Emotional status

BOX 22-6 ■ REHABILITATION ASSESSMENT MEASURES IN MS

Ashworth and Modified Ashworth Spasticity Scale*: These are ordinal scales of tone intensity. The Ashworth rates tone on a scale of 0 to 4, whereas the Modified Ashworth was developed to further define the lower end of the scale, making it more discrete by adding the grade 1+. Reference: Lee KC, Carson L, Kinnin E, et al: The Ashworth scale: a reliable and reproducible method of measuring spasticity, *J Neurol Rehab* 3:205-209, 1989.

Barthel Index: An ordinal scale of function in 10 areas encompassing mobility, ADL function, and continence. Reference: Mahoney FI, Barthel DW: Functional evaluation: the Barthel index, *Maryland Med J* 14:61-65, 1965.

Berg Balance Scale: An ordinal scale of balance that is sensitive to change. Reference: Berg K, Wood-Dauphinee S, Williams JI, et al: Measuring balance in the elderly: validation of an instrument, *Can J Public Health* Jul-Aug(suppl 2):S7-S11, 1992.

Box and Block Test of Manual Dexterity (BBT): The Box and Block test was originally developed to evaluate the gross manual dexterity of adults with cerebral palsy. The test is made up of a box with a partition directly in the center, creating two equal sides. A number of small wooden blocks are placed in one side of the box. The subject being tested is required to use the dominant hand to grasp one block at a time and transport it over the partition and release it into the opposite side. The subject is given 60 seconds in which to complete the test, and the number of blocks transported to the other side is counted. The test is then repeated with the nondominant hand. It is suitable for persons with limited cognition and manual dexterity. Reference: Mathiowetz V, Volland G, Kashman N, et al: Adult norms for the box and block test of manual dexterity, *Am J Occup Ther* 39:386-391, 1985.

Canadian Occupational Performance Measure (COPM): An individualized, client-centered measure of three areas: self-care, productivity, and leisure. Information about this measure can be found at www.caot.ca/copm.

The Dallas Pain Questionnaire: This test was developed to assess the amount of chronic spinal pain that affects daily and work activities, leisure activities, anxiety and depression, and social interest. A 16-item self-report takes approximately 5 minutes to complete. Each item contains its own visual analog scale. The scales are divided into five to eight small segments in which the subject is asked to mark an "X" to indicate where her or his pain impact falls on the continuum. The visual scales are anchored at the beginning with words such as "no pain" (0%), "some" (50%), and "all the time" (100%) regarding where the experience of pain falls on the continuum. Reference: Lawlis G, Cuencas R, Selby D, et al: The development of the Dallas pain questionnaire, *Spine* 14(5):511-516, 1989.

Functional Independence Measure (FIM): This test is an ordinal scale of functioning in multiple areas, including feeding, grooming, bathing, dressing, toileting, transferring, locomotion, comprehension, expression, social interaction, and problem solving. Information about obtaining the FIM may be obtained from Uniform Data System for Medical Rehabilitation UB Foundation Activities at (716) 817-7800 or www.udsmr.org.

Health Status Questionnaire (SF-36): This is a 36-item patient self-report regarding the patient's perception of health and physical limitations. It is widely used in the United States. It is a component of the MS Quality of Life Inventory. It is a registered trademark of the Medical Outcomes Trust, Inc. (20 Park Plaza, Suite 1014, Boston, MA 02116). Additional references: About the SF-36 (website): www.mcw.edu/midas/health/SF-36.html and National Multiple Sclerosis Society: *Measures for use in clinical studies of MS: health status questionnaire (SF-36)* (website): www.nationalmssociety.org/MUCS_health.asp.

Kurtzke Functional System Scores (FSS) and Expanded Disability Status Scale (EDSS): The FSS and EDSS constitute one of the oldest and probably the most widely used assessment instruments in MS. On the basis of a standard neurological examination, the seven functional systems (plus "other") are rated. These ratings are then used in conjunction with observations and information concerning gait and use of assistive devices to rate the EDSS. Each of the FSS items is an ordinal clinical rating scale ranging from 0 to 5 or 6. The EDSS is an ordinal clinical rating scale ranging from 0 (normal neurological examination) to 10 (death from MS) in half-point increments. These tests may be found at www.nationalmssociety.org/MUCS_FSS.asp.

Continued

BOX 22-6 ■ REHABILITATION ASSESSMENT MEASURES IN MS—cont'd

Minimal Assessment of Cognitive Function in MS (MACFIMS): An expert panel convened by the Consortium of MS Centers in 2001 developed this neuropsychological assessment for patients with MS. This is a 90-minute battery of seven neuropsychological tests covering processing speed and working memory, learning and memory, executive function, visual-spatial processing, and word retrieval. Reference: Benedict RH, Fischer JS, Archibald CJ, et al: Minimal neuropsychological assessment of MS patients: a consensus approach, *Clin Neuropsychol* 16(3):381-397, 2002.

Modified Fatigue Impact Scale (MFIS): This test consists of 21 items to determine the effects of fatigue in terms of cognitive, physical, and psychosocial functioning. An abbreviated version consists of five items. The MFIS is part of the MS Quality of Life Inventory and can be downloaded in PDF format from www.nationalmssociety.org/MUCS_fatigue.asp.

Multiple Sclerosis Functional Composite (MSFC): This test includes the timed 25-foot walk (T25-FW), 9-hole peg test (9HPT), and the paced auditory serial addition test (PASAT): The MSFC administration and scoring manual can be downloaded in PDF format from the National Multiple Sclerosis Society Web site at www.nationalmssociety.org/MUCS_MSFC.asp.

Multiple Sclerosis Quality of Life-54 (MSQOL-54): This is a multidimensional health-related quality of life measure that combines the SF-36 and 18 items that are specific to MS, including fatigue and cognitive function. It can be downloaded in PDF format from www.nationalmssociety.org/MUCS_MSQOL-54.asp.

Multiple Sclerosis Quality of Life Inventory (MSQLI): This is a structured self report encompassing the following components: SF-36, Modified Fatigue Impact Scale, Pain Effects Scale (PES), Sexual Satisfaction Scale (SSS), Bladder Control Scale (BLCS), Bowel Control Scale (BWCS), Impact of Visual Impairment Scale (IVIS), Perceived Deficits Questionnaire (PDQ), Mental Health Inventory (MHI), and Modified Social Support Survey (MSSS). *MSQLI: A User's Manual* can be downloaded as a PDF file from www.nationalmssociety.org/MUCS_MSQLI.asp.

ROM and manual muscle test (MMT) and grasp dynamometry: ROM at selected joints is assessed by using a goniometer that measures the angle of the joint through its range. MMT uses a 6-point grading system (0 = no contractile ability; 5 = strength through full ROM with maximal resistance) to assess strength where the patient has selective joint control. Grasp dynamometer testing uses a dynamometer to measure grasp and pinch strength in pounds.

Tinetti Assessment Tool: This is an easily administered test that measures gait and balance. The test is scored on a 3-point scale to assess the patient's ability to perform specific tasks. Scores are combined to form three measures: an overall gait assessment score, an overall balance assessment score, and a gait and balance score. The scores can be interpreted with regard to risk for falls. Reference: Lewis C: Balance, gait test proves simple yet useful, *PT* Bulletin 2(10):9, 40, 1993; and Tinetti ME: Performance-oriented assessment of mobility problems in elderly patients, *JAGS* 34:119-126, 1986.

From: Multiple sclerosis: a course for occupational and physical therapists, *Rehabilitation assessment measures in MS*, New York, 2004, National Multiple Sclerosis Society.

BOX 22-7 ■ SPECIFIC SCORING OF THE DISABILITY SCALE: KURTZKE SCALE

0 = Normal neurological examination (all grade 0 in functional groups).

1 = No disability, minimal signs (Babinski, minimal finger-to-nose ataxia, diminished vibration sense) (grade 1 in functional groups).

2 = Minimal disability: slight weakness or stiffness, mild disturbance of gait, or mild visuomotor disturbance (one or two items functional grade 2).

3 = Moderate disability: monoparesis, mild hemiparesis, moderate ataxia, disturbing sensory loss, or prominent urinary or eye symptoms, or combinations of lesser dysfunctions (one or two items functional grade 3 or several grade 2).

4 = Relatively severe disability not preventing ability to work or carry on normal activities of living, excluding sexual function. This includes the ability to be up and about 12 hours a day (one item functional grade 4 or several grade 3 or less).

5 = Disability severe enough to preclude working, with maximal motor function walking unaided up to several blocks (one item functional grade 5 alone, or combination of lesser).

6 = Assistance (canes, crutches, braces) required for walking (one item functional grade 6 alone or combination of lesser).

7 = Restricted to wheelchair: able to wheel self and enter and leave chair alone (combinations with at least one item above functional grade 4).

8 = Restricted to bed but with effective use of arms (combinations usually functional grade 4 or above in several functional groups).

9 = Totally helpless bed patient (combinations usually functional grade 4 or above in most functional groups).

10 = Death from MS.

From Kurtzke JF: On the evaluation of disability in multiple sclerosis, *Neurology* 11:688, 1961.

BOX 22-8 ■ ASPECTS OF QUALITY OF LIFE

PSYCHOPHYSIOLOGICAL EQUILIBRIUM

Understanding of the disease, the symptoms, and how to manage them

Understanding of limitations and strengths; functioning up to but respecting limits

Maintenance of function with minimal effort and maximal safety (balancing rest and activity appropriately)

Functional improvement despite persistent neurological signs

Return to preexacerbation physical status

Altering environment to support independence, diminish disability

Wellness lifestyle

Mastery over potential uncertainty and loss of control

INTERRELATEDNESS

Having realistic expectations for patient and family

Preservation of family unit

Learning new ways to fulfill family and friendship roles

Knowing and practicing how to be realistically independent— not being a burden—but also being able to communicate when and how help is needed

Avoiding social isolation

Knowing and appropriately using community resources

PRODUCTIVITY

Developing alternative plans to already established vocational goals (job, education, other training)

Establishing a productive life (paid or volunteer)

CREATIVITY

Developing problem-solving skills

Developing avocational interests

Reaching important life goals; focusing on remaining possibilities

Developing an enjoyable, personally meaningful life (MS not being the focus of one's life)

Adapted from Maloney FP, Burks JS, Ringel SP, editors: *Interdisciplinary rehabilitation of multiple sclerosis and other neuromuscular disorders,* Philadelphia, 1985, J.B. Lippincott.

indicated. The Consortium of MS Centers, representing MS Clinical Centers in the United States and Canada, is an excellent resource to network with these MS centers (201-837-0727; www.mscare.org).

Setting Goals

A statement from *A Manual on Multiple Sclerosis* summarizes important guidelines in setting goals[50]:

In every rehabilitation program, the patient must be treated as a whole, the best physical and psychological condition under the circumstances must be achieved, complications eliminated as far as possible and realistic motivations exploited. This can only be accomplished by the well-coordinated teamwork of doctors, nurses, physiotherapists, occupational therapists, clinical psychologists, social workers, the patient and his family and friends, and organizations with a genuine interest and sense of responsibility for him.

The ideal rehabilitation model acknowledges the client's responsibility and resources. It recognizes both the client's and family members' priorities and values; it considers not only the home environment but also community resources, medical issues, history of the disease, and the cognitive and affective status of the individual.

Frequently in MS, the therapist's role is one of support in helping the patient solve problems to improve the quality of his or her interactions with the environment as opposed to offering therapeutic activities designed to restore function or ability per se. Problem solving and education are key aspects of the rehabilitation process in MS, particularly because restoration of abilities and reversal of clinical symptoms may not be realistic expectations.

Therefore the overriding principle in setting rehabilitation goals is to maximize independence, self-determination,

and quality of life within the context of the individual's lifestyle and abilities (Box 22-8).[47] Vital to achieving these goals, however, is concordance between the therapist's and patient's expectations. Unrealistic expectations and discrepancies between what "improvement" and "getting better" mean to the therapist and to the patient can lead to a disappointing rehabilitation experience.

Often, for more stable or clear-cut disabilities, goals are set according to a functional skill such as ambulatory or wheelchair level. This may not be appropriate for clients with MS. A large number may be ambulatory for short distances but require a wheelchair for more demanding tasks. Additionally, for periods of exacerbation, training in wheelchair mobility may be a temporary yet important necessity. The variations in MS confirm the need for ongoing reestablishment of goals in response to therapy and to changes in the client's condition, home environment, patient priorities, and the family situation (see Chapter 32).

Interventions for Specific Problems

Fatigue

Fatigue is one of the most common symptoms of MS: 75% to 95% report experiencing fatigue, and 50% to 60% report fatigue as their worst symptom. It can cause significant activity limitations, even in those with few other symptoms.[51,52] Fatigue is a major reason for unemployment in MS. Because of its impact on the workforce, fatigue is listed as a cause of MS disability in the Social Security Administration impairment guidelines. As an invisible symptom, friends, family, or employers frequently misunderstand fatigue. The pathophysiological basis for MS fatigue is not well understood and most likely has biological, emotional, environmental, pharmacological, and lifestyle origins.

The factors contributing to fatigue are sleep deprivation (sleep disturbance caused by urinary frequency or muscle spasms is common in MS), poor diet, deconditioning (loss of aerobic capacity, endurance, and muscle tone as a result of inactivity), movement limitations (more effortful and inefficient approaches to accomplishing daily activities because of ataxia, weakness, spasticity, etc.), depression, neuromuscular conditions (more energy consumption by demyelinated axons), and MS itself (some researchers and clinicians describe a lassitude that is unique to MS that worsens as the day progresses and prevents sustained physical activity).

Rise in body temperature during the course of the day may affect nerve conduction velocity, resulting in increased fatigue. Emotional stress has also been cited as associated with worsening of fatigue.

Because MS fatigue is multidimensional, so, too, is the approach to fatigue management, addressing the various contributing factors. In 1998, the Multiple Sclerosis Council for Clinical Practice developed an algorithm intended to guide clinicians in the evaluation and treatment of MS fatigue.[30] The guidelines include several self-report measures, a daily activity log, and sleep questionnaire to guide assessment. The Modified Fatigue Impact Scale (MFIS), a component of the MS Quality of Life Inventory (see Box 22-7),[53] is used to assess outcomes of intervention. Energy conservation techniques, adaptive equipment and assistive technology, and planned exercise and rest activities may compensate for fatigue. Adapting the work environment for energy conservation often allows the patient with MS to continue employment. In addition, exercise to increase general endurance, cardiovascular health, and overall conditioning may address this symptom. Pharmacological intervention includes amantadine, pemoline, and modafinil. Cooling may also be beneficial in reducing fatigue; aerobic exercise may help improve fatigue in some individuals.[54]

Weakness

Decreased strength results from several causes: upper motor neuron weakness, fatigue, disuse, compensatory movements, pain, and overriding spasticity in an antagonistic muscle. To enhance function in weak muscles, active assistive exercise, active exercise, and resistive exercise should be incorporated into a daily program. Progressive resistive exercise may also be effective in improving strength.[55] Although strengthening exercises will not alter neurological status, compensatory strengthening of unaffected muscle groups, preventing weakness from disuse, and strengthening agonist muscles to overcome spasticity in antagonistic muscle groups may improve function.

If compensatory strengthening proves to be limited in improving mobility, bracing may be effective in reducing gait abnormalities and improve the individual's ability to function with less effort. Ankle-foot orthoses (AFOs) are used to stabilize the ankle and compensate for footdrop and are commonly used for MS gait problems. Other orthotics also may compensate for weakness in both upper and lower extremities. See Boxes 22-9 and 22-10 for general principles of a strengthening program and bracing guidelines.[55]

BOX 22-9 ▪ GENERAL PRINCIPLES OF A STRENGTHENING PROGRAM

The following are common principles to remember while implementing a strengthening program:

1. Unaffected muscle groups should be maximally strengthened to allow maximal use of compensation techniques that involve unaffected limbs.
2. Use adaptive devices (e.g., canes and crutches) to allow the patient to remain ambulatory longer and maintain functional strength levels as long as possible.
3. Strengthening exercises must be safe and efficacious. Therapists must teach the patient a judicious balance between rest and exercise.
4. The patient should progress through the strengthening program slowly. For example, if she or he is starting at 8 to 10 repetition (reps) of each exercise, she or he can increase 1 to 2 reps every 2 to 3 weeks to 20 to 25 reps. One- to 2-pound weights may then be added and the reps decreased to 8 to 10, with the progression starting over. This slow increase in progression accompanied by good compliance will lead to successful strengthening. A cool atmosphere allows more efficient exercise because MS patients are often highly sensitive to heat.
5. Home programs for these exercises are essential; the effectiveness of any exercise program depends on its being carried out on an ongoing basis.
6. Before strengthening, stretching exercises should be performed to decrease spasticity, increase flexibility, and increase blood flow to the area.
7. To improve functional strength, exercises should be performed at submaximal resistance with frequent repetitions.
8. Emphasis should be placed on proximal strengthening to decrease energy consumption during functional activities.
9. Large fluid movements to enhance coordination should be used.
10. If a patient has difficulty initiating movement, try starting with large body/trunk movements, then moving from proximal to distal.
11. Light weights may help stabilization if a patient has significant tremors.
12. Combining strengthening exercises with aerobic, balance, or spasticity-reducing exercises whenever possible will maximize benefits within the patient's exercise tolerance.
13. Avoid excessive fatigue of a muscle: 1- to 5-minute rest periods throughout the exercise session will facilitate recovery of neurotransmission.
14. Set realistic goals and expectations with the patient. Be creative, realistic, and simplistic. The more enjoyable the exercises, the better the compliance.

From Schapiro R: *Multiple sclerosis: a rehabilitation approach to management,* New York, 1991, Demos Publications.

BOX 22-10 ■ BRACING

The most common braces used to brace the lower extremities in MS are standard polypropylene AFOs and those with an articulated joint. The following guidelines may be helpful. A standard AFO is indicated if the patient exhibits the following:

1. Consistent footdrop or toe drag
2. Poor knee control (especially hyperextension)
3. Weakness of grade 2 or 3 at the ankle with dorsiflexion testing
4. Minimal to moderate spasticity
5. Poor endurance in gait
6. Poor proprioception and sensory sense

The advantages of an AFO include the following:

1. Saves energy during gait because the patient does not work as hard to clear his or her toes during the swing-through phase of the gait
2. Improves footdrop or toe drag during the swing phase of gait
3. Improves general safety during walking by avoiding many falls because of the toe drag
4. Provides more knee control during mid-stance phase of gait by avoiding hyperextension of the knee
5. Provides greater ankle stability
6. Improves the overall gait pattern
7. Provides better cosmesis for the patient

The advantages of the AFO with an articulating joint include the following:

1. All the above listed for the standard AFO.
2. It allows some mobility at the ankle joint. This permits a more natural movement at the ankle during gait, which looks more normal. It allows the patient to drive while wearing the brace and allows more freedom for squatting down to reach objects on the floor.

3. It provides a plantar flexion stop to prevent the foot from further plantar flexion during the swing phase of gait.
4. It still allows for dorsiflexion assist and can be set up to 5 degrees of dorsiflexion to clear the foot during the swing-through phase.

Relative contraindications for these types of braces include the following:

1. Moderate or severe spasticity in the lower extremities
2. Severe foot edema
3. Severe weakness (muscle grades 2 or less) at the hips

A double-upright metal brace can provide some of the same advantages listed above and usually provides more adjustments for the ankle and the knee. However, this brace is usually not the preferred choice because of its weight and poorer cosmetic appearance.

The polypropylene AFOs may be set in a few degrees of dorsiflexion to provide better knee control. If hyperextension is severe, a Swedish hyperextension knee cage may be useful. In some people this device may be quite helpful, but it is decidedly more bulky and often moves down the leg, which decreases its effectiveness. Custom bracing of the knee can be the answer to this problem because effective orthotics may make up for instability of the joints, tendons, and ligaments. This usually requires the skills of a trained orthotist and is a topic beyond the scope of this text.

Some therapists have found rocker clog shoes to be of some help for those few people who need to have the plantarflexed position neutralized while the curved forefoot sole will initiate knee flexion. A skilled therapist should determine if this situation is present before purchase of this device is recommended.

For additional information on bracing, see Chapter 34.

From Schapiro R: *Multiple sclerosis: a rehabilitation approach to management*, New York, 1991, Demos Publications.

Spasticity

In managing spasticity, the therapist should consider reflex dominance, hypertonicity, and abnormal movement. Spasticity usually coexists with weakness and may present as phasic spasms or sustained increase in tone. Spasticity can interfere with mobility and may also cause pain, predispose the individual to contractures, interfere with breathing, interfere with hygiene, lead to poor posture, and be associated with sexual difficulties. Spasticity may have some advantages, however. A patient my have poor strength, but spasticity may assist in standing and ambulation. It may support circulation and help prevent deep vein thrombosis.

A stretching routine may be beneficial and should allow for slow elongation of the muscle through relaxation. The application of cold has been useful in some cases in reducing hypertonicity, as have other inhibitory relaxation techniques, including joint approximation, slow rolling from supine to side, slow rocking, slow stroking of the paravertebral muscles, and pressure on the tendinous insertion of the spastic muscle (see Chapter 9).

Reflex-inhibiting movement patterns and positioning (side lying) may inhibit abnormal postural reflex mechanisms (e.g., asymmetrical tonic neck reflex or tonic labyrinthine reflex and abnormal movements). Additionally, the use of functional exercise and weight bearing performed in various spatial positions may be helpful in normalizing movement. Daily active and passive range of motion (ROM) exercises will help maintain joint range. Training in self-ROM and encouragement of participation in functional tasks will aid in the prevention of contractures. Severe ROM limitations may require surgical intervention such as myotenotomy. Medications and implantable intrathecal baclofen therapy, as discussed earlier, may augment physical treatment (see Chapter 36).

Balance and Coordination

Cerebellar problems are common in MS and difficult to manage. Balance and coordination problems predispose the individual to falls. Ataxia, incoordination, dysmetria, and tremor that become exaggerated with movement may be present in all the extremities and trunk. Treatment sequences in functional activities may help improve balance in various positions. Progress is made from a wide to narrow base of support, from static to dynamic activities, and from a low to a high center of gravity. Additionally, strengthening the fixation musculature, visual cues, and biofeedback may improve balance and lessen tremor. For the most part, however, treatment is compensatory. The use of adaptive equipment in ADLs, weighted cuffs to reduce tremor, or weighted canes to reduce ataxia may prove useful. The use of weighted cuffs may increase imbalance, however, and, once removed, exaggerate the problem. Also, increased fatigue related to the extra weights may contraindicate their use. Tremors of the head and neck may be controlled with a collar or brace. Tremors in MS are frequently exaggerated by stress. Drug treatment, as discussed earlier, may augment compensatory training techniques but frequently has an unwanted sedating effect.[55]

Sensory Dysfunction

Impaired sensation is frequently a problem in MS. Treatment is aimed at compensating for the loss, maximizing safety, and increasing awareness of the sensory impairment. Inability to perceive temperature or pain must be attended to by training in visual compensation and safety techniques. Routine skin inspection and pressure relief techniques, particularly when significant immobility is present, should be taught, and appropriate wheelchair cushioning or mattresses should be provided. Unpleasant dysesthesias, such as burning or tight banding sensations, may respond to cold applications. Medications such as corticosteroids, phenytoin (Dilantin), amitriptyline (Elavil), or carbamazepine (Tegretol), may be useful if sensations are painful or interfere with function.[28,32]

Dysarthria and Dysphagia

Fatigue, weakness, tremors, incoordination, and abnormal tone may contribute to imprecise articulation, vocal harshness, slurring, changes in rate of speech, hypernasality, and other problems in oral communication. After evaluation, speech therapy generally focuses on compensating for dysfunction. Specific techniques of speech therapy include using pauses to improve speech that is slurred, rapid, and runs together; exaggerating articulation; reducing phrase length; increasing voice volume; using oral exercise to maximize ROM and strength of oral musculature; and using augmentative communication devices including writing, computer-driven systems, communication boards, and pointing. Those who have motor difficulties, however, may be limited in the use of some of these methods. Frequently a referral to a speech therapist is not made until severe dysarthria or dysphagia is present. Early intervention, as with all rehabilitation therapies, increases the potential for minimizing dysfunction and setting up the state for neuroplasticity.

Treatment for dysphagia focuses on body positioning (to prevent aspiration), the "think swallow" style of eating (a conscious swallow as opposed to dependence on reflexive swallowing), and food and liquid selection (semisoft, moist foods and thick liquids with progression to more challenging foods). Because fatigue can exacerbate swallowing problems, larger meals taken earlier in the day followed by smaller meals later may be easier to manage. Placement of feeding tubes may be required if a practical degree of swallowing cannot be achieved.

Ambulation and Mobility

Weakness, spasticity, impaired sensation, ataxia and proprioception, problems with balance, fatigue, visual problems, and incoordination influence gait in MS patients. In addressing ambulation, trunk control and balance should be addressed first, followed by normalization of tone and maximizing flexibility and ROM. Gait is often more functional when strength can be improved in the trunk and extremities. Some patients also may require a graduated sitting tolerance program, tilt-table routine, and graduated standing tolerance schedule before specific gait training. Visual and tactile cues may help compensate for sensory and proprioceptive loss. Specific ambulation aids can improve safety, decrease energy expenditure, and improve endurance. Upper-extremity strength and motor control, cognitive status, and emotional response to using the device must be considered in prescription.

In wheelchair prescription, the goal is proper positioning to be sure the pelvis, spinal column, and limbs are in correct alignment and the patient is secure in the chair. Seating may be modified by the use of foam inserts, clamp-on side supports, and customized contour seating systems. Footrests should be adjusted so that the thighs are parallel to the floor. A seat belt should be used for safety. Functional training should include propulsion, retropulsion, and maneuvering in narrow areas and on various terrains. Manipulation of armrests, leg rests, footrests, brakes, and other wheelchair accessories must be included in wheelchair mobility training, and tilt-in-space wheelchairs offer the benefit of relieving pressure and shifting weight when the individual cannot do so independently. A reclining chair may be most effective for those with head, neck, and trunk instability. Electric wheelchairs may be necessary when fatigue, weakness, or tremors make independent propulsion of a manual chair impossible. Three-wheel scooters are frequently used by people with MS with adequate trunk stability and upper-extremity function. The three-wheeler also offers greater ease of dismantling and loading into a car than a traditional electric wheelchair. Many people with MS find that the three-wheeled scooter carries less of a stigma and is more convenient than a traditional wheelchair. Cushion prescription to minimize skin breakdown and discomfort should be made with regard to the patient's risk for developing these problems.

Cognitive Dysfunction

Cognitive problems in MS result from demyelination in the cerebral tracts that connect with primary sensory, motor, speech, and integration areas of the cerebrum. This may result in poor recognition of deficits as well as an inability to store and retrieve new information, a combination that may present a major impediment to rehabilitation.

The most commonly affected functions are memory, attention, speed of processing, abstract reasoning, verbal fluency, and executive functions.[23,24,26] Interventions should be designed to improve a person's ability to function in all aspects of family and community life that are meaningful to the person with MS. Intervention should involve systematic, functionally oriented therapeutic activities that are based on understanding of specific deficits. Most commonly, compensatory strategies (i.e., using intact skills and/or external aids) are used to improve daily functioning. Examples include cognitive structuring (i.e., a learned, practiced approach used to turn the cognitive tasks in routine behaviors); substitution strategies (i.e., the learned use of intact cognitive abilities to circumvent or bolster impaired abilities, such as using intact visual memory in place of impaired verbal memory function); scheduling and timelines; use of recording devices; memory strategies (e.g., lists, mnemonics, clustering, visualization techniques); templates for repeated tasks; organizational strategies; assistive technology (e.g., handheld computers, electronic calendars, and memory logs), creating a structured environment; and conducting conversations and activities in quiet places to minimize distraction. Solution-focused, practical training in how to maximize function in spite of deficits that can be generalized to the individual's everyday environment is most desirable. In therapy, deficits in judgment, logical analysis, reasoning, and self-monitoring may require the use of clear, written, sequenced steps for exercises or adapted methods of performing ADLs, transfers, and ambulation. The therapist should be aware that what may appear to be low motivation or poor compliance in therapy may be the interference of cognitive deficits.

Research into the effectiveness of restorative approach to cognitive rehabilitation is largely inconclusive. Nonetheless, many individuals with MS would derive benefit from a neuropsychological evaluation. Such an evaluation could be helpful in several ways:

- The person with MS as well as family members can gain a better understanding of the nature and extent of the illness.
- The evaluation can identify impaired and intact functions.
- The evaluation may assist the person in developing realistic vocational and other life goals.
- The results can clarify misconceptions on the part of others who may incorrectly attribute cognitive problems to uncooperative or oppositional behavior.
- The results can suggest compensatory techniques.

General Conditioning and Fitness
A reduction in physical activity because of MS limitations may result in a general reduction in overall fitness. This reduction is characterized by the following[55]:

- Increased neuromuscular tension
- Increased pulse rate at rest
- Decreased muscular strength
- Decreased vital capacity at rest
- Decreased maximal vital capacity
- Increased fatigue
- Increased anxiety
- Increased depression

A physical conditioning program is not likely to have an impact on the course of MS. However, enhanced overall health and fitness can improve a sense of well-being, reduce fatigue, improve mood, and reduce the other secondary effects of inactivity.[39] With attention to body temperature, incoordination, cycles of fatigue, and safety, a conditioning program geared to the individual can offer a sense of control over some aspects of health and improve the quality of life. Aerobic exercises such as swimming, walking, stationary bikes, and rowers may be appropriate for some patients. Swimming and other water exercise can be ideal for those with MS, especially if the water temperature can be maintained to avoid overheating. All patients should have a car-diovascular examination by a physician before starting an aerobic program. This area should be addressed even when no obvious signs of disability are present and should be modified according to ability thereafter.

Activities of Daily Living
Functional improvement or maintenance of functional independence is a key goal of the rehabilitation program. Carryover of therapeutic exercise, mat exercises, and ambulation training to ADL tasks is vital. In addition, specific training in techniques of dressing, bathing, toileting, personal hygiene, feeding, and bed mobility can improve or maintain independence in ADLs. Adaptive equipment can be used to conserve energy and compensate for weakness and incoordination. For example, weighted silverware and plate guards can compensate for tremor and incoordination in self-feeding. Button hooks, reachers, stocking aids, and hook-and-loop fasteners may improve independence in dressing. Transfer training should be incorporated into functional activities. The use of a sliding board, hydraulic lift, or assistance from another individual must be geared to the client's ability and priorities regarding expenditure of energy.

Adapted tools for communication skills (e.g., writing or typing), such as built-up pencils, keyboard shield, adapted keyboard, or universal cuffs, may assist communication. Homemaking tasks and child care from a wheelchair level, ambulatory-assisted level, or ambulatory level can be practiced with the aid of assistive devices and energy-conservation techniques.

Driving often presents problems for the individual with MS. Diplopia or blurred vision, decreased coordination, weakness, spasticity, attention deficits, and reaction time may interfere with safe driving or require the use of hand controls or an adapted vehicle. Perceptual and cognitive considerations must be made in a predriving evaluation or in driver training along with physical assessment.

Employment
An estimated 90% of people with MS have worked at some point in their lives, and 65% were working at the time of diagnosis. However, only 25% to 35% remain in the workforce 5 to 10 years after diagnosis.[56] Many leave employment prematurely, perhaps under the advice of a health care provider or well-meaning family member during an acute exacerbation or for fear of disclosing their diagnosis at work, fear of asking for accommodation, or ignorance of their rights under the Americans with Disabilities Act. People who leave the workforce most commonly cite fatigue, cognitive dysfunction, visual problems, bowel and bladder dysfunction, and mobility problems as barriers to continuing employment.[56] Often the rehabilitation team can be of help in assessing how symptoms might be effectively managed at the workplace and accommodations made to help the individual retain employment. Common, reasonable accommodations for MS include a part-time or flex-time schedule, work-at-home options, accessible work environment (e.g., bathrooms, desk), special transportation, memory aids (e.g., day planners, tape recorders), vision aids (e.g., voice recognition software, large-print materials, voice mail), an office close to the elevator and/or restroom, hands-free telephone devices, air conditioning, wheeled carts for transporting

files, and mobility aids (e.g., scooters, walkers, wheelchairs). The therapist can play an important role in helping the individual stay employed as well as making decisions regarding retirement, career change, or temporary leave of absence.

Psychosocial Issues

The challenges of MS are formidable and ongoing. Despite new drug treatments, MS remains an incurable disease with an uncertain prognosis. Although many individuals and families cope quite effectively with the disease, the incidence of depression is high, and the impact on family and marital relationships, finances, work life, and social activities of the individual is pervasive.

The meaning of illness or disability in a family relates to culture, religion, and personal values and beliefs. For some, disability is associated with personal weakness, imperfection, and asexuality. For others, illness may be seen as a growth-inspiring experience, one that provides new insights and awareness of priorities. Individuals are influenced strongly by the viewpoints of friends, family, medical caregivers, and rehabilitation team members. The attitudes and beliefs of the therapist about disability are important to examine because therapists may communicate these beliefs in subtle ways to their patients.

Helping families cope with MS may involve an examination of their premorbid patterns of dealing with stress, conflict, and tragedy. MS often magnifies preexisting problems and tensions so that families who present "MS-generated" problems may have had these problems well before the diagnosis was made.

The relations among attitude, psyche, and physical wellness or disease are well documented.[57] Although stress itself cannot be implicated in causing exacerbations, the ability to manage stress can positively influence overall health and well being (see Chapters 4 and 5).

SUMMARY

MS is a chronic and often progressive disease of the CNS characterized by disseminated patches of demyelination and inflammation in the brain and spinal cord, resulting in multiple and varied neurological symptoms and signs. Destruction of myelin, accompanied by edema and inflammation and followed by tissue scarring and axonal damage, appears to be the underlying cause that impedes or prevents neurotransmission.

The clinical diagnosis of MS depends largely on evidence of two or more distinct CNS lesions, symptoms and signs that have appeared in distinct episodes or have progressed over time, and the exclusion of other neurological explanations. Laboratory and electrophysiological tests provide support of a clinical diagnosis; however, no test is currently pathognomonic for MS.

The course of the disease is characterized by an unpredictable series of exacerbations and remissions in some cases, progressive disability over time in other cases, or a combination of the two, often accompanied by periods of disease stability.

The cause of MS appears to be an autoimmune process in which myelin is destroyed. The trigger of this abnormal immune response is unknown, although a viral trigger is probable in genetically susceptible individuals.

Treatment of MS has improved with the availability of several DMAs (Avonex, Betaseron, Copaxone, Rebif, Novantrone, Tysabri) that appear to reduce the relapse rate and slow progression of disability in some patients. Symptomatic therapies and treatment of acute MS exacerbations are also effective. Many other therapeutic agents are under investigation.

Rehabilitative measures, including physical, occupational, and speech therapy, do not appear to alter the underlying pathological course of the disease. Therefore the overriding principle in setting rehabilitation goals for a person with MS is to maximize functional independence and safety, minimize complications and problems caused by decreased mobility, compensate for loss of function, and maximize quality of life. Psychosocial adjustment, vocational disposition, and family issues merit significant attention by the treatment team because MS may generate significant need in these domains.

REFERENCES

1. Compston DA: *McAlpine's multiple sclerosis*, ed 3, New York, 1998, Churchill Livingstone.
2. Rolak LA: *History of multiple sclerosis*, New York, 2003, National Multiple Sclerosis Society.
3. Trapp BD, Peterson J, Ransohoff RM, et al: Axonal transection in the lesions of multiple sclerosis, *N Engl J Med* 338(5):278-285, 1998.
4. Noseworthy JH: Progress in determining the causes and treatment of multiple sclerosis, *Nature* 399(6738 suppl):A40-A47, 1999.
5. Brankin AB: Pathogenesis of multiple sclerosis—the immune diathesis and the role of viruses, *J Neuropathol Exp Neurol* 52(2):95-105, 1993.
6. Gran B, Hemmer B, Vergelli M, et al: Molecular mimicry and multiple sclerosis: degenerate T-cell recognition and the induction of autoimmunity, *Ann Neurol* 45(5):559-567, 1999.
7. Alter M, Kahana E, Loewenson R: Migration and risk of multiple sclerosis, *Neurology* 28(11):1089-1093, 1978.
8. Kurtzke JF: Epidemiologic evidence for multiple sclerosis as an infection, *Clin Microbiol Rev* 6(4):382-427, 1993.
9. National Multiple Sclerosis Society (website): www.nationalmssociety.org. Accessed December 2004.
10. Multiple Sclerosis International Federation (website): *www.msif.org*. Accessed December 2004.
11. Baranzini SE, Oksenberg JR, Hauser SL: New insights into the genetics of multiple sclerosis, *J Rehabil Res Dev* 39(2):201-209, 2002.
12. Ebers GC, Dyment DA: Genetics of multiple sclerosis, *Semin Neurol* 18(3):295-299, 1998.
13. Lublin F, Reingold S: Defining the course of multiple sclerosis, *Neurology* 46(4):907-911, 1996.
14. Zaffaroni M, Ghezzi A: The prognostic value of age, gender, pregnancy and endocrine factors in multiple sclerosis, *Neurol Sci* 21(suppl 2):S857-S860, 2000.
15. Paty DW, Ebers GC: *Multiple sclerosis*, Philadelphia, 1998, FA Davis.
16. Kraft GH, Freal JE, Coryell JK, et al: Multiple sclerosis: early prognostic guidelines, *Arch Phys Med Rehabil* 62(2):54-58, 1981.
17. McFarland HF, Frank JA, Albert PS, et al: Using gadolinium-enhanced magnetic resonance imaging lesions to monitor disease activity in multiple sclerosis, *Ann Neurol* 32(6):758-766, 1992.
18. McDonald WI, Compston A, Edan G, et al: Recommended diagnostic criteria for MS, *Ann Neurol* 50:121-127, 2001.
19. Yetkin FZ, Haughton VM, Papke RA, et al: Multiple sclerosis: specificity of MR for diagnosis, *Radiology* 178:447, 1997.
20. Miller DH, Grossman RI, Reingold SC, et al: The role of magnetic resonance techniques in understanding and managing multiple sclerosis, *Brain* 121:3-24, 1998.
21. Gronseth GS, Ashman EJ: Practice parameter: the usefulness of evoked potentials in identifying clinically silent lesions in patients with sus-

pected multiple sclerosis (an evidence-based review): report of the Quality Standards Subcommittee of the American Academy of Neurology, *Neurology* 54:1720-1725, 2000.

22. Aronson K, Goldenberg E, Cleghorn G: Socio-demographic characteristics and health status of persons with multiple sclerosis and their care givers, *MS Management* 3(1):5-15, 1996.

23. Rao SM, Leo GL, Bernardin L, et al: Cognitive dysfunction in multiple sclerosis. I. Frequency, patterns, and prediction, *Neurology* 41(5):685-691, 1991.

24. Peyser JM, Edwards KR, Poser CM, et al: Cognitive function in patients with multiple sclerosis, *Arch Neurol* 37:577-579, 1980.

25. Minden SL, Orav J, Reich P: Depression in multiple sclerosis, *Gen Hosp Psychiatry* 9:426, 1987.

26. Minden SL, Schiffer R: Affective disorders in multiple sclerosis, *Arch Neurol* 47:98, 1990.

27. Mohr DC, Goodkin DE, Gatto N, et al: Depression, coping and neurological impairment in multiple sclerosis, *Multiple Sclerosis* 3:254, 1997.

28. Halper J, Holland N: *Comprehensive nursing care in multiple sclerosis*, ed 2, New York, Demos Publishers, 2002.

29. Kalb R, editor: *Multiple sclerosis: focus on rehabilitation*, New York, 2002, National Multiple Sclerosis Society.

30. Multiple Sclerosis Council for Clinical Practice Guidelines: *Fatigue and multiple sclerosis: evidence-based strategies for fatigue and multiple sclerosis*, Washington, DC, 1998, Paralyzed Veterans of America.

31. Multiple Sclerosis Council for Clinical Practice Guidelines: *Urinary dysfunction and multiple sclerosis: evidence-based strategies for urinary dysfunction in multiple sclerosis,* Washington, DC, 1999, Paralyzed Veterans of America.

32. Schapiro R: *Symptom management in multiple sclerosis*, ed 3, New York, 1998, Demos Publications.

33. National Multiple Sclerosis Society (website): www.nationalmssociety.org. Accessed December 2004.

34. Reingold SC: *Research directions in multiple sclerosis*, New York, 2004, National Multiple Sclerosis Society.

35. LaBan MM, Martin T, Pechur J, et al: Physical and occupational therapy in the treatment of patients with multiple sclerosis, *Phys Med Rehabil Clin North Am* 9(3):603-609, 1998.

36. Freeman JA, Langdon DW, Hobart JC, et al: Inpatient rehabilitation in multiple sclerosis: do the benefits carry over into the community? *Neurology* 52:50-56, 1999.

37. Solari A, Filippini G, Gasco P, et al: Physical rehabilitation has a positive effect on disability in multiple sclerosis patients, *Neurology* 52:57, 1999.

38. Langdon DW, Thompson AJ: Multiple sclerosis: a preliminary study of selected variables affecting rehabilitation outcome, *Multiple Sclerosis* 5:94, 1999.

39. Hutchinson B, Kushner S, Engstrom D, et al: *Increased physical fitness and emotional state with increased disability in multiple sclerosis,* Platform presentation, Kansas City, MO, Consortium of MS Centers, 1999.

40. Neufeld P: *Wellness course efficacy with MS*, Platform presentation, Kansas City, MO, Consortium of MS Centers, 1999.

41. Craig J, Young CA, Ennis M, et al: A randomised controlled trial comparing rehabilitation against standard therapy in multiple sclerosis patients receiving steroid treatment, *J Neurol Neuropsychol Psych* 74:1225-1230, 2003.

42. Liu C, Playford ED, Thompson AJ: Does neurorehabilitation have a role in relapsing remitting multiple sclerosis? *J Neurol* 250(10):1214-1218, 2003.

43. Slade A, Tennant A, Chamberlain MA: A randomised controlled trial to determine the effect of intensity of therapy upon length of stay in a neurological rehabilitation setting, *J Rehabil Med* 34(6):260-266, 2002.

44. Di Fabio RP, Choi T, Soderberg J, et al: Health-related quality of life for persons with progressive multiple sclerosis: influence of rehabilitation, *Phys Ther* 77(12):1704-1716, 1997.

45. Wiles CM, Newcombe RG, Fuller KJ, et al: Controlled randomized crossover trial of the effects of physiotherapy on mobility in chronic multiple sclerosis. *J Neurol Neurosurg Psychiatry* 70:174-179, 2001.

46. Medical Advisory Board of the National Multiple Sclerosis Society: *Rehabilitation: recommendations for persons with multiple sclerosis,* New York, 2004, National Multiple Sclerosis Society.

47. Maloney FP, Burks JS, Ringel SP, editors: *Interdisciplinary rehabilitation of multiple sclerosis and other neuromuscular disorders,* Philadelphia, 1985, J.B. Lippincott.

48. National Committee on Vital and Health Statistics (website): www.ncvhs.hhs.gov. Accessed December 2004.

49. Multiple sclerosis: a course for occupational and physical therapists. *Rehabilitation Assessment Measures in MS*, New York, 2004, National Multiple Sclerosis Society.

50. Bauer H: *A manual on multiple sclerosis*, Vienna, 1977, International Federation of Multiple Sclerosis Societies.

51. Freal JE, Kraft GH, Coryell JK: Symptomatic fatigue in multiple sclerosis, *Arch Phys Med Rehabil* 65:135, 1984.

52. Kraft GH, Freal JE, Coryell JK: Disability, disease duration, and rehabilitation service needs in multiple sclerosis: patient perspectives, *Arch Phys Med Rehabil* 67(3):164-168, 1986.

53. Fischer JS, LaRocca NG, Miller DM, et al: Recent developments in the assessment of quality of life in multiple sclerosis, *Multiple Sclerosis* 5:251, 1999.

54. DeLisa J, Gans B, Walsh NE, editors: *Physical medicine and rehabilitation: principles and practice*, ed 4, Philadelphia, 2003, JB Lippincott.

55. Schapiro R: *Multiple sclerosis: a rehabilitation approach to management*, New York, 1991, Demos Publications.

56. Rumrill P: *Employment issues and multiple sclerosis*, New York, 1996, Demos Publications.

57. Benson H: *The mind/body effect*, New York, 1979, Simon & Schuster.

CHAPTER 23

Balance and Vestibular Disorders

Leslie K. Allison, PhD, PT
Kenda Fuller, PT, NCS

KEY WORDS

anticipatory postural responses
automatic postural responses
balance
base of support
center of gravity
disability
impairment
limit of stability
motor learning stages
sensory conflict
sensory environment
strategies
systems model or systems approach
volitional postural movements

OBJECTIVES

After reading this chapter the student/therapist will be able to:

1. List common postural control impairments found in clients with neurological problems.
2. Describe both central and peripheral sensory and motor components of the postural control system.
3. Identify and analyze the function of the vestibular system in balance activities.
4. List commonly used balance tests.
5. Differentiate how test results are used to identify impairments and disabilities.
6. Analyze the interaction of individual, task, and environmental factors that affect balance.
7. Describe how to progress balance exercise programs to increase the use of, or compensation with, available sensory inputs.
8. Describe how to progress balance exercise programs to increase the control of center of gravity in upright postures and during gait.
9. Describe how to facilitate adaptation and central nervous system reorganization to regain control of balance and decrease dizziness.

No matter what the neurological diagnosis, a disease or injury that affects the nervous system is likely to compromise one or more of the postural control mechanisms. For example, clients with stroke, head trauma, spinal cord injury, peripheral neuropathy, multiple sclerosis, Parkinson's disease, cerebellar dysfunction, cerebral palsy, or Guillain-Barré syndrome frequently experience disequilibrium problems. The common thread among all these different medical diagnoses is the presence of balance impairments. Clients with different diagnoses may have the same balance impairments; and clients with the same diagnosis may have different balance impairments depending on which portions of the postural control system are involved.[1] To optimally understand and manage balance problems, an evaluation of each balance component and the interactive nature of the components is important. The traditional medical "diagnostic" model does not provide this information and is not the most beneficial model for balance rehabilitation interventions. The medical diagnosis is relevant: knowing whether deficits are permanent or temporary is critical, or whether recovery or progressive decline is expected. This medical prognostic information will assist in goal setting and intervention planning.

An alternative model, to the concept of "impairment" and "disability" described by the World Health Organization (WHO) (see Figure 1-1) is the Nagi model. It better describes the interactions of impairments and functional limitations seen in balance and postural movement dysfunction. This Nagi disablement model has been adopted by the American Physical Therapy Association and applied specifically to the rehabilitation of clients with neuromuscular disorders in *The Guide to Physical Therapist Practice.*[2] Balance impairments negatively affect function, leading to functional limitations and often reducing the individual's ability to participate in life.[3] These impairments often restrict activity levels, produce abnormal compensatory motor behavior, and may require support from devices or assistance from others. When imbalance is severe, falls can result, leading to secondary injuries. To avoid these consequences and advance the functional status of their clients, therapists should understand both the demands that various environments and functional tasks place on postural control systems and the impairments that may diminish the ability of those systems to respond adequately. The second WHO model incorporates the concepts of the first WHO model, as well as the Nagi model, but incorporates the role of the client and the importance of activities or movement function in relations to participation in life and those specific activities that the client wishes to participate in. This chapter embraces both the Nagi concept of functional limitations as well as the *international classification of functioning, disability and health (ICF)* WHO model, which stresses the importance of participation in and quality of life.[3a]

BALANCE

Definitions of Balance

Balance is a complex process involving the reception and integration of sensory inputs and the planning and execution of movement to achieve a goal requiring upright posture. It is the ability to control the center of gravity (COG) over the base of support in a given sensory environment.[4,5] The COG is an imaginary point in space, calculated biomechanically from measured forces and moments, where the sum total of all the forces equals zero. In a non–vertically challenged person standing quietly, the COG is located just forward of the spine at approximately the S2 level. With movement of the body and its segments, the location of the COG in space constantly changes. The base of support is the body surface that experiences pressure as the result of body weight and gravity; in standing it is the feet, in sitting it includes the thighs and buttocks. The size of the base of support will affect the difficulty level of the balancing task. A broad base of support makes the task easier; a narrow base makes it more challenging. The COG can travel farther while still remaining over the base if the base is large. The "shape" of the base of support will alter the distance that the COG can move in certain directions.

Any given base of support places a limit on the distance a body can move without either falling (as the COG exceeds the base of support) or establishing a new base of support by reaching or stepping (to relocate the base of support under the COG). This perimeter is frequently referred to as the limit of stability or stability limit.[4,6] It is the farthest distance in any direction a person can lean (away from midline) without altering the original base of support by stepping, reaching, or falling.

Environmental Context

This biomechanical task (keeping the COG over the base of support) is always accomplished within an environmental context, which is detected by the sensory systems. The sensory environment is the set of conditions that exist, or are perceived to exist, in the external world that may affect balance. Peripheral sensory receptors gather information about the environment, body position and motion in relation to the environment, and body segment positions and motions in relation to the self. Central sensory structures process this information to perceive body orientation, position, and motion and to determine the opportunities and limitations present in the environment. Gravity is one environmental condition that must be reckoned with to remain stable. For everyone except astronauts, it is a constant condition. Surface and visual conditions, however, may vary significantly and may be stable or unstable. Unstable surface conditions might include the subway, a sandy beach, a gravel driveway, or an icy parking lot. Common unstable visual conditions are experienced on mass transit, in crowds, or on a boat. Rapid head movements may render even a stable visual environment unusable for postural cues, and darkness may preclude the use of vision. The more stable the environment, the lower the demand on the individual for balance control. Unstable environments place greater demands on the postural control systems.

Balance is also affected by an individual's intentions to achieve certain goals and the purposeful tasks that are undertaken. Volitional balance disturbances are self-initiated almost constantly, such as shifting from foot to foot, reaching for the telephone, or catching an object that is falling from a high shelf. Even reactions to involuntary balance disturbances, such as a slip or trip, are modified on the basis of

the immediate task. A man carrying a bag of groceries who slips may drop the bag to reach with both hands and catch himself. If he is instead carrying his infant child, he may reach with only one hand or even suffer the fall if by doing so he can protect the infant from harm. Often in real life we perform several tasks at once, such as carrying a laundry basket while walking, or talking on a cellular phone while climbing a flight of stairs. When tasks are undertaken concurrently, attention must be divided between them, which may also affect balance abilities.

All these variables—the location of the COG, the base of support, the limit of stability, the surface conditions, the visual environment, the intentions and task choices—are inconstant, producing changing demands on the systems that control balance. The integrity and interaction of postural control mechanisms allow a wide range of movements and functions to be achieved without loss of balance.

HUMAN CONTROL OF BALANCE

Early studies of postural control mechanisms using selectively lesioned cats and primates focused on reflexive and reactive equilibrium responses that are relatively "hard wired."[7] These valuable studies brought to light certain stereotypical motor responses to specific sensory stimuli, such as the crossed extension reflex or tonic neck reflexes. Earlier balance treatment methods based on this neurophysiological science sought to inhibit abnormal reflexes and facilitate normal responses.[8,9] Controversy exists regarding the merit of these techniques, but recent research advances show that this view of the nervous system and resultant scope of treatment are too narrow.[10,11] Balance abilities are heavily influenced by higher-level neural circuitry and other systems (e.g., cognitive, musculoskeletal) as well.[6] In addition, the nervous system is widely understood to be influenced by and responsive to the demands placed on it by the tasks being accomplished and the environments in which those tasks are performed.[12-14] More recent theory includes all these facets in a systems model or systems approach to dynamic equilibrium.[15-17] Contemporary testing and treatment methods based on this systems model have consequently evolved.[16,18,18a] Prior techniques have been modified and expanded to allow for a more comprehensive approach.[19]

The Systems Approach

The dynamic systems model for dynamic equilibrium recognizes that balance is the result of interactions between the individual, the task the individual is performing, and the environment in which the task must be performed. These interactions are represented in Figure 23-1. Within the individual, both sensory inputs and processing systems (left side of figure) and motor planning and execution systems (right side of figure) are critical. Both peripheral components (lower part of figure) and central components (upper part of figure) of the systems are involved in the cycle. The cycle is driven both by purposeful choices of the individual (task) and demands placed on the individual by the environment. Successful function of the sensory systems allows recognition of body position and motion in relation to self and the world. The desired outcome from the motor systems is the generation of movement sufficient to maintain balance and perform the chosen task.

Dynamic equilibrium

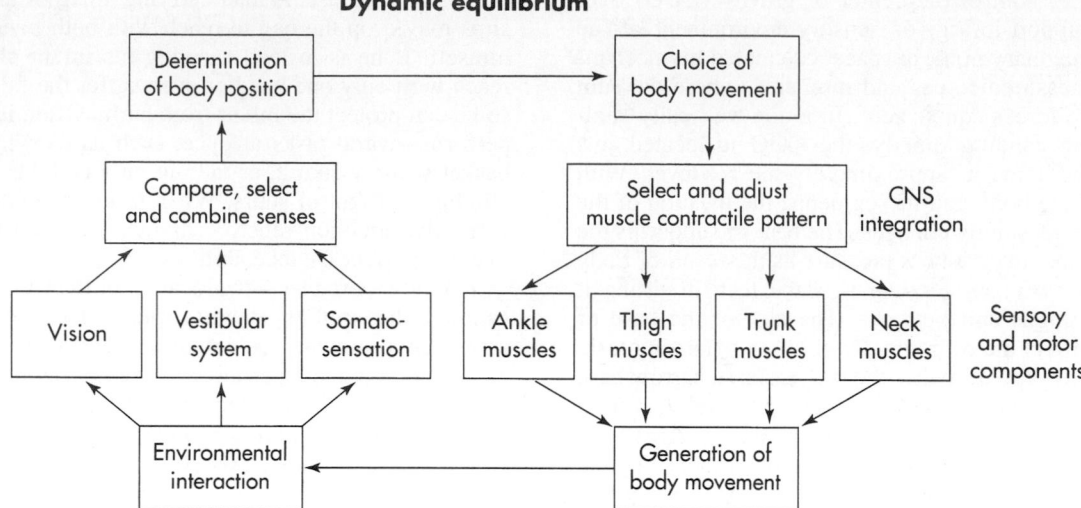

FIGURE 23-1 ■ The systems model of postural control illustrates the constant cycle that occurs simultaneously at many levels. (Reprinted with permission from NeuroCom International, Inc., Clackamas, OR.)

Peripheral Sensory Reception

The three primary peripheral sensory inputs contributing to postural control are the bilateral receptors of the somatosensory, visual, and vestibular systems.[5,15] Somatosensory receptors located in the joints, ligaments, muscles, and skin provide information about muscle length, stretch, tension, and contraction; pain, temperature, pressure; and joint position. The feet, ankles, knees, hips, back, neck, and eye muscles all furnish useful information for balance maintenance. Somatosensation is the dominant sense for upright postural control and is responsible for triggering automatic postural reactions. Somatosensory loss significantly impairs balance.

Visual receptors in the eyes perform dual tasks. Central (or focal) vision allows environmental orientation, contributing to the perception of verticality and object motion, as well as identification of the hazards and opportunities presented by the environment.[15] For example, a canoeist may see rocks in a stream as a hazard to be avoided, whereas a hiker who wants to cross the stream may see the same rocks as a welcome opportunity. Peripheral (or ambient) vision detects the motion of the self in relation to the environment, including head movements and postural sway, whereas central visual inputs tend to receive more conscious recognition.[15] Both are normally used for postural control. Vision is critical for feedforward, or anticipatory, postural control in changing environments.

The vestibular system provides the central nervous system (CNS) with information about the position and motion of the head. The position of the head in relation to gravity is detected through the otolith system. Horizontal and vertical accelerations, such as riding in a car or an elevator, are also detected by the otoliths (Figure 23-2).[20] Movements of the head are detected through the semicircular canals (Figure 23-3). Head movement stimulates both sets of semicircular canals, so that the vestibular nerve on one side becomes inhibited while the other becomes excited. The vestibular system provides sensory redundancy in the information obtained from each separate vestibular appara-

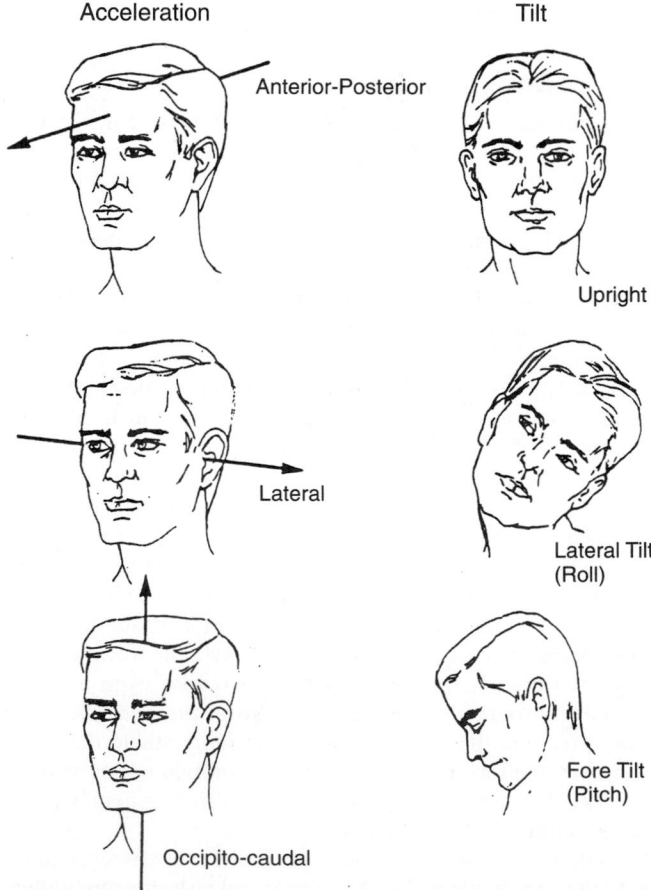

FIGURE 23-2 ■ The otoliths register linear acceleration and static tilt of the head. (From Hain TC, Ramaswany TS, Hillman MA: Anatomy and physiology of the normal vestibular system. In Herdman SJ, editor: *Vestibular rehabilitation,* Philadelphia, 2000, FA Davis.)

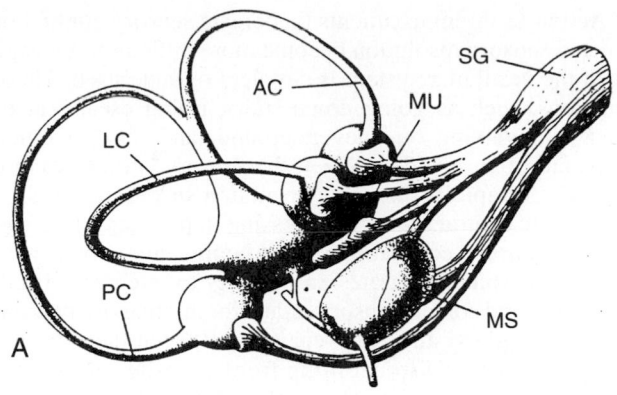

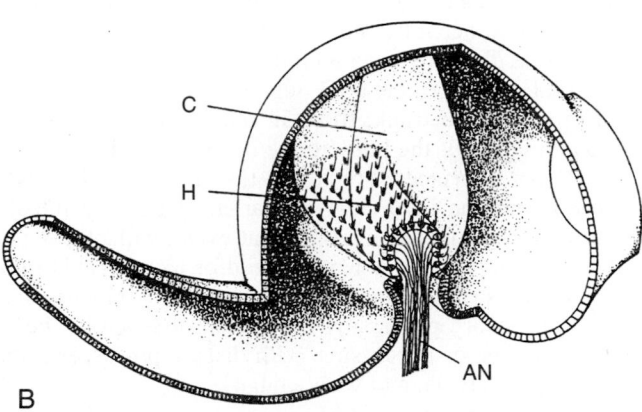

FIGURE 23-3 ■ **A,** The labyrinth system, including lateral or horizontal semicircular canal *(LC),* anterior semicircular canal *(AC),* posterior semicircular canal *(PC),* macula utriculi *(MU),* macula sacculi *(MS),* and Scarpa's ganglion *(SG).* **B,** Cross-sectional view of the semicircular canal. *C,* Cupula; *H,* hair cells; *AN,* afferent nerves. (Adapted from Barber HO, Stockwell CW: *Manual of electronystagmography,* St. Louis, 1976, C.V. Mosby.)

BOX 23-1 ■ SENSORY COMPONENTS OF THE VESTIBULAR SYSTEM

LABYRINTHS

- Semicircular canals are ring-shaped, fluid-filled structures containing hair cells that respond to fluid movement when the head moves.
- The canals are arranged so that when the head moves, the direction and velocity in each canal are compared with a mutually perpendicular canal on the opposite side of the head.
- The brain uses the relative change in firing from each side to identify the direction of rotation. This provides for sensory redundancy; the brain interprets motion by comparing information from each side to calculate the velocity and direction of head turns.
- The orientation of the three semicircular canals on each side corresponds to the directions of neck motion, flexion/extension, right/left rotation, and right/left side-bending. This relation supports the integration of vestibular inputs with somatosensory information from the cervical spine.

OTOLITHS

- Located in the vestibule or central component of the labyrinth. The otoliths respond to gravity and linear acceleration through hair cell deflection.
- These compartments contain multiple hair cells attached to the walls and connected to the vestibular nerve. These hair cells are embedded in a gel-like substance called the macula.
- Sitting on top of the macula are crystals of calcium carbonate, known as otoconia. The purpose of the otoconia is to establish mass so that the hair cells can measure the effects of gravity as well as movement.
- The otoliths respond to movement of the head by the shearing effect of the otoconia pressing on the macula and displacing the hair cell in the opposite direction of the movement. These signals from the otoliths are used to compare this motion with the resting tone established by gravity.

---

tus. If the vestibular system is damaged on one side, the information can be captured by the intact canals on the opposite side. The vestibular system is critical for balance because it uniquely identifies self-motion as different from motion in the environment. Box 23-1 describes the sensory components vestibular system.

Orientation to the wider environment, primarily from vision, allows feedforward, or anticipatory, adjustments. Detection of head movement by the vestibular and cervical somatosensory systems, and of body sway by somatosensory and peripheral visual systems, provides feedback for responsive actions.

Disease of, or damage to, any of the peripheral sensory receptors impairs or removes the detection capabilities of the system, rendering sensory information unavailable for use in postural control. Many patients with neurological diagnoses have peripheral sensory impairments. Peripheral somatosensory loss occurs after spinal cord injury, peripheral neuropathy, tabes dorsalis, amputation, and so forth. Peripheral vision loss may result from diabetic retinopathy, cataracts, macular degeneration, or glaucoma. Peripheral

vestibular loss is experienced with infectious neuronitis, temporal bone fracture, acoustic Schwannoma, Menière's disease, and other disorders.[20,21]

Central Sensory Perception

The brain processes all the environmentally available sensory information gathered by the peripheral receptors in varying degrees. This processing is usually referred to as multisensory integration or sensory organization.[5,15] Central sensory structures function first to compare available inputs between two sides and among three sensory systems. The somatosensory system alone is unable to distinguish surface tilts from body tilts. Also, the visual system by itself cannot discriminate movement of the environment from movement of the body.[20] The vestibular system by itself cannot tell if head movement through space is produced by neck motion or trunk/hip motion. Therefore the brain needs information from all three senses to distinguish correctly self-motion from motion in the environment. For example, as specific head movements increase the firing from one vestibular organ, they simultaneously decrease proportionately in the other. This is known as push-pull function, and the information is considered to "match." With the same example, if the eyes are open while the head moves, the rate of the visual flow will be equal and the direction of the visual flow will be opposite to the rate and direction information from the vestibular inputs. The inputs from the two systems are congruent. If both sides and all three systems provide compatible inputs, the process of sensory organization is simplified.

When changes in the environment occur, the relative availability, accuracy, and usefulness of information from the three sensory systems may also change. Sensory organization also includes an adaptive process, called multisensory reweighting, that permits the CNS to prioritize the sources of sensory information when environmental conditions change.[22,23] Available, accurate, and useful information is "upweighted," whereas unavailable, inaccurate, or less-useful information is "downweighted." For example, in dark environments vision would be downweighted and somatosensory and vestibular information would be upweighted. This adaptive process is imperfect, however, and balance is not as well controlled when any sense must be downweighted as it is when all three senses are available and accurate. Individuals with peripheral sensory loss or central sensory processing deficits may have difficulty reweighting quickly and fully, which impairs their ability to adapt to, and remain stable in, changing environments.[24]

Sensory conflict can arise when information between sides or between systems is not synchronous. Sensory organization processing then becomes more complex because the brain must then recognize any discrepancies and select the correct inputs on which to base motor responses. The vestibular system is used as an internal reference to determine accuracy of the other two senses when they conflict. For example, a driver stopped still at a red light suddenly hits the brake when an adjacent vehicle begins to roll. Movement of the other car detected by the peripheral visual system is momentarily misperceived as self-motion. In this situation, the vestibular and somatosensory systems do not detect motion, but the forward visual flow is interpreted as backward motion. Because the brain failed to suppress the (mismatched) visual inputs, the braking response was generated.

When the brain recognizes that the information coming from one sensory input is inaccurate, as is the case when the vestibular system is sending abnormal signals of head acceleration or rotation, it must depend on the remaining senses (in this case, somatosensation and vision) to determine position and motion in space. The brain then compares and uses information from senses it considers accurate for balance. An individual with the problem just described may compensate for the loss of vestibular function by becoming visually dependent for balance during movement. If vision or somatosensation subsequently also becomes disrupted, this individual may have loss of balance, dizziness, or both. Clients with this type of vestibular problem will limit head motion during walking and step with a flat foot to increase stability. When visual conditions do not provide stable cues, clients with vestibular loss will most often report vertigo, whereas those with somatosensory loss will report light-headedness and instability.

Activities or environments that create sensory conflict or demand sensory resolution become more difficult to manage when the vestibular system is deficient or underused. These situations, such as going down stairs, riding escalators or elevators, walking on uneven ground, and making quick turns, are often avoided. When the sensory conflict cannot be resolved rapidly, dizziness or motion sickness occurs.

Intrinsic central sensory processing impairments also can produce sensory conflict. An adult hemiplegic patient with pusher syndrome illustrates an inability to integrate visual, vestibular, and somatosensory inputs for midline orientation. Within a single system, discrepancies between the sides are also problematic. Unequal firing from opposite sides of the vestibular system, as in unilateral vestibular hypofunction, produces a mismatch that is subsequently interpreted as head rotation when head movement does not occur. This spinning sensation is known as vertigo.[20] Vertigo is resolved if the brain is able to adapt to the mismatch.

Finally, the central processing mechanisms combine any available and accurate inputs to answer the questions "Where am I?" and "How am I moving?" This includes both an internal relation of the body segments to each other (e.g., head in relation to trunk, trunk in relation to feet) and an external relation of the body to the outside world (e.g., feet in relation to surface, arm in relation to handrail). CNS disease or trauma involving the parietal lobe may impair these processing mechanisms so that even available, accurate sensory inputs are not recognized or incorporated into determinations of position and movement.[25,26] Impairments of central sensory processing may occur after stroke, head trauma, tumors, or aneurysms; with disease processes such as multiple sclerosis; and with aging.

Central Motor Planning and Control

Whereas sensory processing allows the interaction of the individual and the environment, motor planning underlies the interaction of the individual and the task. Aside from reflexive activity such as breathing and blinking, most motor actions are voluntary and occur because some goal is to be achieved. That is not to say that reflexes occur separately from volitional movements; for example, the vestibulo-ocular reflex is active concurrently with tracking activity, but most actions occur because of some purposeful intent.[20] These task intentions precede motor actions.[15,27] Wrist and hand movements vary depending on what is to be grasped (a cup vs. a doorknob); foot placement and trunk position vary depending on what is to be lifted (a heavy suitcase vs. a laundry basket). The initiation of volitional motor actions depends on intention, attention, and motivation.[15,28]

Once an objective ("Where do I want to be? What do I want to do?") has been chosen, the next step in motor planning is to determine how to best accomplish the goal given the many options that are potentially available. For example, when the task demands fine skills or accuracy, the dominant hand is preferred; when the task involves lifting a large or heavy object, both hands are preferred. In addition to which limbs, joints, and muscles will be used, motor planning also adjusts the timing, sequencing, and force modulation. This can be demonstrated in various reaching tasks. Reaching to remove a hot item from the oven will occur slowly, whereas reaching to put an arm through a sleeve will occur more quickly. Optimal motor plans are developed with knowledge of self (abilities and limitations), knowledge of task (characteristics of successful performance), and knowledge of the environment (risks and opportunities).[28]

The motor plan must be transmitted to the peripheral motor system to be enacted. A copy of the intended movement plan is sent to the cerebellum during the transmission. When the movement begins, incoming sensory inputs (feedback) about the actual movements and performance outcome are compared with the intended movements and performance outcome. Movement errors (the difference between the intended and the actual movement) and performance errors (desired goal not achieved) are detected, and plans for correction are then formed and transmitted. This process of error detection and error correction is the foundation of motor learning.

Clients with CNS disorders often have central motor planning and control impairments. After a stroke, clients may have hypertonus; clients with head trauma may have difficulty initiating or ceasing movements; clients with Parkinson's disease exhibit bradykinesia; and those with cerebellar ataxia display modulation problems.[29] The major outflow of the vestibular nuclei goes to the cerebellum. When the cerebellum is not functioning properly, the calibration of the vestibular reflexes is affected, and the ability to make corrective movements at the appropriate scale and speed is compromised.

Peripheral Motor Execution

Movement is accomplished through the bilateral joints and muscles. Normal range of motion (ROM), strength, and endurance of the feet, ankles, knees, hips, back, neck, and eyes must be present for the execution of the full range of normal balance movements. Decreased ankle dorsiflexion ROM, for example, restricts the forward limits of stability. Strength deficits are a primary cause of movement abnormalities in both central and peripheral nervous system disorders. In addition, weakness may be the result of force modulation deficits or disuse.[16] Balance is directly affected by loss of strength. For example, weakness of the hip extensors and abductors will impede successful use of a hip strategy for upright trunk control. Initially adequate toe clearance may diminish with fatigue. Many neurological clients also have stiffness and contractures as a result of persistent weakness or hypertonus. Restrictions in ROM also limit balance abilities.

The ability to achieve static postural alignment, although necessary for normal balance, is not sufficient to allow volitional functions. Adequate strength (to control body weight and any additional loads) through normal postural sway ranges is needed to permit dynamic balance activities such as reaching, leaning, and lifting. Postural control demands are increased during gait because the forces of momentum and the interaction between recruitment, timing, and velocity also must be regulated.[30] Traditionally considered orthopedic problems, deficits in strength, ROM, posture, and endurance have a great impact on balance abilities. Attention must be given to these musculoskeletal impairments in examination of and intervention for clients with neurological diagnosis.

Influence of Other Systems

Balance abilities are also influenced by other systems. Attention, cognition and judgment, and memory are critical for optimal balance function and are often impaired in hemi-plegic and head-injured clients as well as those who have progressive neurological disorders, including progressive vestibular loss. Attentional deficits reduce awareness of environmental hazards and opportunities, interfering with anticipatory postural control.[17] When balance is threatened, an inability to allocate attention to the necessary task of balance versus a secondary, less necessary task increases the risk for falls. Cognitive problems such as distractibility, poor judgment, and slowed processing also increase the risk of falls. Memory loss may preclude recall of safety measures. Depression, emotional lability, agitation, or denial of impairments also can increase the risks for loss of balance. In addition to having a direct impact on balance abilities themselves, these cognitive and behavioral problems impede motor learning processes, which are crucial for the relearning of balance skills.

Constant Cyclic Nature

The systems model of postural control previously presented illustrates the constant cycle that simultaneously occurs at many levels. Attention and intention allow feedforward processing for active sensory search of the environment and motor planning, both of which are needed for anticipatory postural control. Movements are initiated and executed with resultant sensory experiences and error detection, or feedback. Successful movements are repeated and refined; unsuccessful ones are modified. The nature of this cycle presents the clinician with opportunities for intervention after the appropriate examination of sensory, motor, and cognitive functions. Through feedback and practice, balance abilities can improve.[19]

Motor Components of Balance

Reflexes

Many levels of neuromuscular control must be functioning to produce normal postural movements. At the most basic level, reflexes and righting reactions support postural orientation. The vestibulo-ocular reflex (VOR) and the vestibulospinal reflex (VSR) contribute to orientation of the eyes, head, and body to self and environment.[15]

When motion of the head is identified by the semicircular canals it triggers a response within the oculomotor system called the VOR. This causes the eyes to move in the opposite direction of the head but at the same speed. Stimulation of the otoliths drives the eyes to respond to linear head movement. Quick movements of the head will trigger the VOR.[31]

The VOR allows the coordination of eye and head movements. When the eyes are fixed on an object while the head is moving, the VOR supports gaze stabilization. Visuoocular responses often work concurrently with the VOR. They permit "smooth pursuit" when the head is fixed while the eyes move and visual tracking when both the eyes and the head move simultaneously.[15]

The VSR helps control movement and stabilize the body. Both the semicircular canals and the otoliths activate and modulate muscles of the neck, trunk, and extremities after head movement to maintain balance. Abnormal muscular responses in the extremities are noted in the presence of an acute vestibular disorder. This can result in postural instability. Vestibular dysfunction can result in an unconscious lateral weight shift, most often to the side of the lesion. The VSR permits stability of the body when the head moves and is important for the coordination of the trunk over the extremities in upright postures. Righting reactions support the orientation of the head in relation to the trunk and the head position relative to gravity and include labyrinthine head righting, optical head righting, and body-on-head righting.[15]

Automatic Postural Responses

At the next level, automatic postural responses operate to keep the COG over the base of support. They are a set of functionally organized, long-loop responses that act to keep the body in a state of equilibrium.[4,5] Functionally organized means that the responses, although stereotypical, are matched to the stimulus in direction and amplitude. If the stimulus is a push to the right, the response is a shift to the left, toward midline. The larger the stimulus, the greater the response. Automatic postural responses always occur in response to an unexpected stimulus and are typically triggered by somatosensory inputs. Because they occur rapidly, in less than 250 msec, they are not under immediate volitional control.

Four automatic postural responses, or strategies, have been commonly identified. Ankle strategy describes postural sway control from the ankles and feet. The head and hips travel in the same direction at the same time, with the body moving as a unit over the feet (Figure 23-4). Muscle contractile patterns are from distal to proximal (i.e., gastrocnemius, hamstrings, paraspinals). This strategy is used when sway is small, slow, and near midline. It occurs when the surface is broad and stable enough to allow pressure against it to produce forces that can counteract sway to stabilize the body. Ankle strategy is typically used to control anterior/posterior sway because most of the degrees of freedom at the ankle are in this direction.

Hip strategy describes postural sway control from the pelvis and trunk. The head and hips travel in opposite directions, with body segment movements counteracting one another (Figure 23-4, B). Muscle contractile patterns are from proximal to distal (i.e., abdominals, quadriceps, tibialis anterior). This strategy is observed when sway is large, fast, and nearing the limit of stability or if the surface is too narrow or unstable to permit effective counterpressure. Hip strategy is used to control both anterior/posterior and medial/lateral sway.

Suspensory strategy describes a lowering of the COG toward the base of support by bilateral lower-extremity flexion or a slight squatting motion (Figure 23-4, C). By shortening the distance between the COG and the base of support, the task of controlling the COG is made easier. This strategy is often used when a combination of stability and mobility is required, as in windsurfing.

Stepping and reaching strategies describe steps with the feet or reaches with the arms in an attempt to reestablish a new base of support with the active limb(s) when the COG has exceeded the original base of support.

Misconceptions about these automatic postural reaction strategies are common. First, these strategies do not function in daily life as separately as they are described in the early research literature. In quiet standing, for example, frequency analysis of unperturbed postural sway in nonmotorically impaired adults reveals that both ankle and hip strategies occur in combination, simultaneously.[32] In perturbation studies, mixed use of strategies is often seen unless the perturbation is clearly below or above certain-sized thresholds. Second, these strategies occur in response to disturbances from all directions, not just in pure anterior/posterior or medial/lateral directions.[33] Third, although these strategies are stereotypical in humans, great individual variation in strategy selection and performance comes from other influential factors. For example, many people use stepping strategy for most perturbations unless specifically instructed not to step or unless the conditions do not permit a step. An anxious person may reach or step much sooner than a relaxed person with similar physical deficits. Lastly, all these strategies do *not* occur in sequence with every balance disturbance.[34,35] In other words, individuals normally do not try ankle strategy and wait until it fails before trying hip strategy and wait until it fails before trying stepping strategy (although early learning may involve such exploration). Because these responses must occur rapidly to prevent balance loss, such a sequential approach would be inefficient and ineffective. Instead, the normal response is the emergence of the single strategy best suited to the particular perturbation, the limitations of the individual, and the conditions in the environment.

Abnormal use of automatic postural responses is often observed in individuals with neurological disorders. Clients

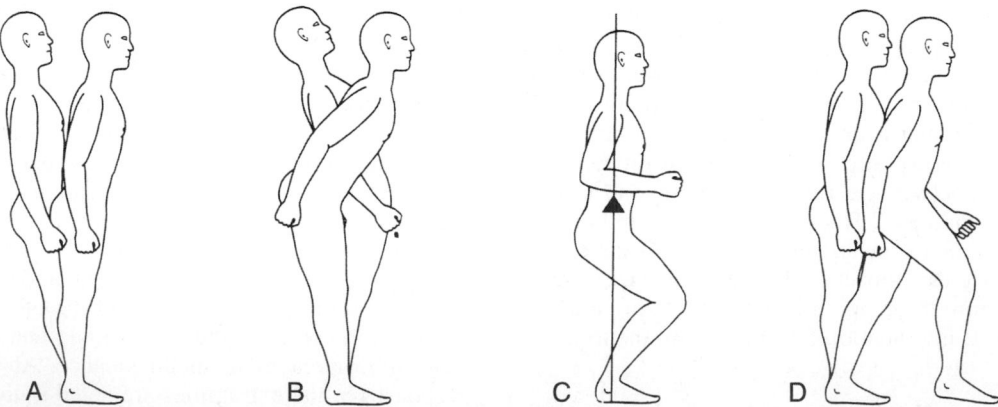

FIGURE 23-4 ■ Automatic postural strategies. **A,** Ankle strategy. **B,** Hip strategy. **C,** Suspensory strategy. **D,** Stepping strategy. (From Hasson S: *Clinical exercise physiology,* St. Louis, 1994, Mosby.)

with vestibular deficits typically rely on ankle strategy, which permits the head to remain aligned with the body and sustains congruence between vestibular and somatosensory inputs. Use of hip strategy may be modified or limited because when the head is moving in the opposite direction as the COG, vestibular and somatosensory inputs are not congruent. Activities that require use of hip strategy, such as standing in tandem or on one leg, can be a problem for clients with bilateral vestibular loss or an uncompensated vestibular lesion. However, some cases involve excessive use of hip strategy on a level surface when an ankle strategy would suffice.[36] This may reflect abnormal integration of the somatosensory and vestibular information. If somatosensation is impaired, or central sensory weighting of somatosensory inputs is inappropriate, it may not be able to assist the vestibular system in controlling the hip strategy.

Clients with somatosensory loss, distal lower extremity weakness or hypertonus, restricted ankle ROM, and/or reduced limits of stability typically rely on hip strategy. This occurs because the client cannot feel the surface or the feet well enough to modulate foot pressure against the surface, because the person cannot generate sufficient force against the surface with the ankle muscles, or because restricted ankle ROM prevents COG sway. The use of hip strategy is normal when the COG is at or near the limits of stability and a step is either not possible or desired.

When the hip or ankle strategy is not efficient enough to control the movement of the center of pressure, or if conditions and instructions permit a stepping response, stepping strategy may be preferred.

Anticipatory Postural Adjustments

Anticipatory postural adjustments are similar to automatic postural responses, but they occur before the actual disturbance.[27] If a balance disturbance is predicted, the body will respond in advance by developing a postural set to counteract the coming forces. For example, if an individual lifts an empty suitcase thinking it is full and heavy, the anticipatory forces generated before the lift (to counter the anticipated weight) will cause excessive movement and brief instability. Failure to produce these anticipatory adjustments increases the risk of sudden balance loss, creating the need to use rapid, reactive automatic postural responses to prevent a fall. For clients with deficits in reaction time or automatic postural responses, superior use of anticipatory postural control can help the client avoid the unexpected perturbations that make automatic postural responses necessary.

In balance laboratories, anticipatory postural adjustments are studied by using electromyography so that muscle activity before observable movement can be measured. In the clinic, problems with anticipatory adjustments may be observed when the client fails to counteract a predicted disturbance, such as "don't let me push you backward," or fails to integrate postural control tasks during other activities, such as the inability to step smoothly over an anticipated obstacle during gait or inability to maintain sitting balance when both arms are intentionally lifted overhead.

Volitional Postural Movements

Volitional postural movements are under conscious control. Weight shifts to reach the telephone or put the dishes in the dishwasher, for example, are self-initiated disturbances of the COG to accomplish a goal. Volitional postural movements can range from simple weight shifts to complex balance skills of skaters and gymnasts. They can occur after a stimulus or be self-initiated. Volitional postural movements can occur quickly or slowly depending on the goal at hand. The more complex or unfamiliar the task, the slower the response time. A variety of movements that might successfully achieve a goal is possible. Volitional postural movements are strongly modified by prior experience and instruction. Automatic and anticipatory postural responses allow the continuous unconscious control of balance, whereas volitional postural movements permit conscious activity. This level of postural motor control is the most frequently tested and treated in clinical practice, but it is by no means sufficient by itself to produce normal balance.

CLINICAL ASSESSMENT OF BALANCE
Objectives of Testing

When present, disabilities need to be identified and measured: functional scales are typically used to determine the presence and severity of disabilities. From these functional tests, decisions can be made about whether to treat and, if so, what tasks need to be practiced. If treatment is indicated, clinicians must make judgments about what to treat. Further testing to identify and measure impairments is then necessary to know what systems are involved. A comprehensive evaluation of balance includes both functional and impairment tests.[17] No single test of balance that adequately covers the many multidimensional aspects of balance is currently available.

No single, simple test for balance is possible because balance is such a complex sensorimotor process.[37] Many balance tests exist, but not all tests are appropriate for all clients. Different tests may be needed to answer specific questions. For example, several good tests have been developed to determine the risk for falls in elderly people. These would be insufficient to discern whether an injured dancer can resume practice or an injured roofer is ready to return to work. Clinicians should understand the advantages and limitations of different balance tests to be able to select appropriate evaluative tools.

In general, a balance test will not be useful unless it sufficiently challenges the postural control system being tested. Tests for stability (static balance) are appropriate for clients who are having difficulty simply finding midline or holding still in sitting or standing. They are of much less value for clients with higher-level abilities. Conversely, single-leg stance tests or sensory tests with a foam surface may be far too difficult for clients with lower-level abilities to perform.

A word of caution about interpreting test results is indicated. Most clinical tests rely on observations of motor behavior to arrive at some conclusion about impairments. Abnormal motor behavior has many causes, and clinicians should be careful before concluding that an observed behavior is caused by problems in a certain system. For example, the Romberg test is commonly assumed to test the use of vestibular inputs. Yet during the test both somatosensory and vestibular inputs are (normally) used for balance control. If balance control is impaired, is the vestibular system necessarily the culprit? Could somatosensory system deficits also result in a poor test result? Or, alternatively, because the Romberg test is performed with feet together, what effect would hip weakness have on the ability to stand with a narrowed base of support? When using a test whose results may be altered by problems in more than one system, any relevant system should be evaluated. If multiple system deficits exist, and they often do in neurological clients, then use caution in making commonly assumed conclusions on the basis of clinical test results.

Because so many balance tests are available, several questions must be asked to determine whether a test is appropriate for use.[37] For what purpose and population was the test designed? Can the test be used for a different purpose or with a different population? Is it valid? Is it repeatable by different examiners or by the same examiner multiple times? Are results reliable? In what populations are they reliable? What is the threshold for this test? That is, how large must changes be before this test can detect them? Are normative data available for comparison? Most of these questions have not been answered for clinical balance tests commonly used by therapists.

Types of Balance Tests

Balance tests can be grouped or classified by type. No single test can adequately measure all the components of balance. Different types of tests measure different facets of postural control (Table 23-1). Quiet standing (static) refers to tests in which the client is standing and the movement goal is to hold still. Disturbances to balance, called perturbations, may or may not be applied. Active standing (dynamic) tests also position the patient standing, but the movement goal involves voluntary weight shifting. Sensory manipulation tests use altered surface and visual conditions to determine how well the CNS is using and reweighting sensory inputs for postural control. Vestibular system tests use various body and head positions, eye movements, or stepping to stimulate or restrict visual, vestibular, and somatosensory inputs. Functional balance, mobility, and gait scales involve the performance of whole-body movement tasks, such as sit-to-stand, walking, and stepping over objects. A few test batteries offer a combination of the preceding tests. New dual-task tests have been developed to examine the effect of concurrent activities and divided attention on balance and mobility performance. A commonly accepted test for sitting balance in adults is not yet available, although clients with neurological problems may often need sitting balance retraining in early stages. Clinicians typically modify standing tests or pediatric sitting tests to assess sitting balance in adult neurological clients. For example, the functional reach test has been used to measure excursion in seated individuals with spinal cord injuries.[38]

Quiet Standing

The classic Romberg test was originally developed to "examine the effect of posterior column disease upon upright stance."[39] The client stands with feet parallel and together and then closes the eyes for 20 to 30 seconds. The examiner subjectively judges the amount of sway. Quantification of sway can be accomplished with a videotape or forceplate. Excessive sway, loss of balance, or stepping during this test is abnormal. The sharpened Romberg,[39] also known as the tandem Romberg, requires the client to stand with feet in a

TABLE 23-1 ■ Types of Balance Tests

TYPE	TESTS
Quiet standing (with or without perturbation)	Romberg
	Sharpened Romberg/tandem Romberg
	OLST
	Timed stance battery
	Postural sway
	Nudge/push
	Postural Stress Test
	Motor Control Test
Active standing	Functional reach
	Multidirectional Reach
	Limits of stability
Sensory manipulation	Sensory Organization Test (SOT)
	Clinical test of sensory interaction on balance (CTSIB)
Vestibular	Vertiginous positions
	Hallpike-Dix maneuver
	Nystagmus
	Semicircular canal function
	Visual-vestibular interaction
	Visual acuity
	Oculomotor tests
	Fukuda Stepping Test
	Dizziness Handicap Inventory
Functional scales	Berg Balance Scale
	Timed Up and Go test
	Tinetti performance oriented assessment of balance
	Tinetti performance oriented assessment of gait
	Gait Assessment Rating Scale (GARS)
	Dynamic Gait Index
	Functional Gait Assessment
Combination test batteries	Fregley-Graybiel ataxia test battery
	Fugl-Meyer sensorimotor assessment of balance performance
Dual task	Stops walking when talking
	Multiple tasks test

heel-to-toe position and arms folded across the chest, eyes closed for 60 seconds. Often four trials of this test are timed with a stopwatch for a maximum score of 240 seconds.

One-legged stance tests (OLSTs) are commonly used.[39,40] Both legs must be alternately tested, and differences between sides are noted. The client stands on both feet and crosses the arms over the chest, then picks up one leg and holds it with the hip in neutral and the knee flexed to 90 degrees. The lifted leg may *not* be pressed into the stance leg. This test is scored with a stopwatch. Five 30-second trials are performed for each leg (alternating legs), with a maximum possible score of 150 seconds per leg. Normal young subjects are able to stand for 30 seconds, but this may not be a reasonable expectation for older clients.[39]

In both the Romberg test and the OLST, problems in sensory organization processes can be observed. To determine how much of the stability is achieved through visual stabilization, each test can be repeated with eyes closed. The client with visual dependency for balance will often have an immediate loss of balance when the eyes are closed. (Remember, visual dependency may be a sign of somatosensory or vestibular loss.) As noted earlier, the client with vestibular loss may have difficulty producing the hip strategy necessary to perform these tasks.

A battery of timed stance tests has been developed by Bohannon and Leary.[41] This set of tests varies the foot position (apart, together, tandem, and single leg) and the availability of visual information (eyes open and closed) to produce eight different combinations. Maintenance of balance in each condition is timed for a maximum of 30 seconds; the assigned score is the total number of seconds that balance could be maintained. The best possible score on

this test is 240 seconds. This test is reliable, valid, and sensitive to change over time.[41]

Objective postural sway measures can be obtained by computerized forceplates.[42,43] The client is asked to adopt a standardized foot placement if possible (this varies by manufacturer) and to stand quietly with arms at the sides or hands on hips for 20 or 30 seconds. Sway with both eyes open and eyes closed is commonly measured. Graphic and numerical quantification is provided (Figure 23-5). Normative data may be provided. These measures are able to detect more subtle problems, and are more sensitive to change in performance after treatment, than are rating scales or timed measures.

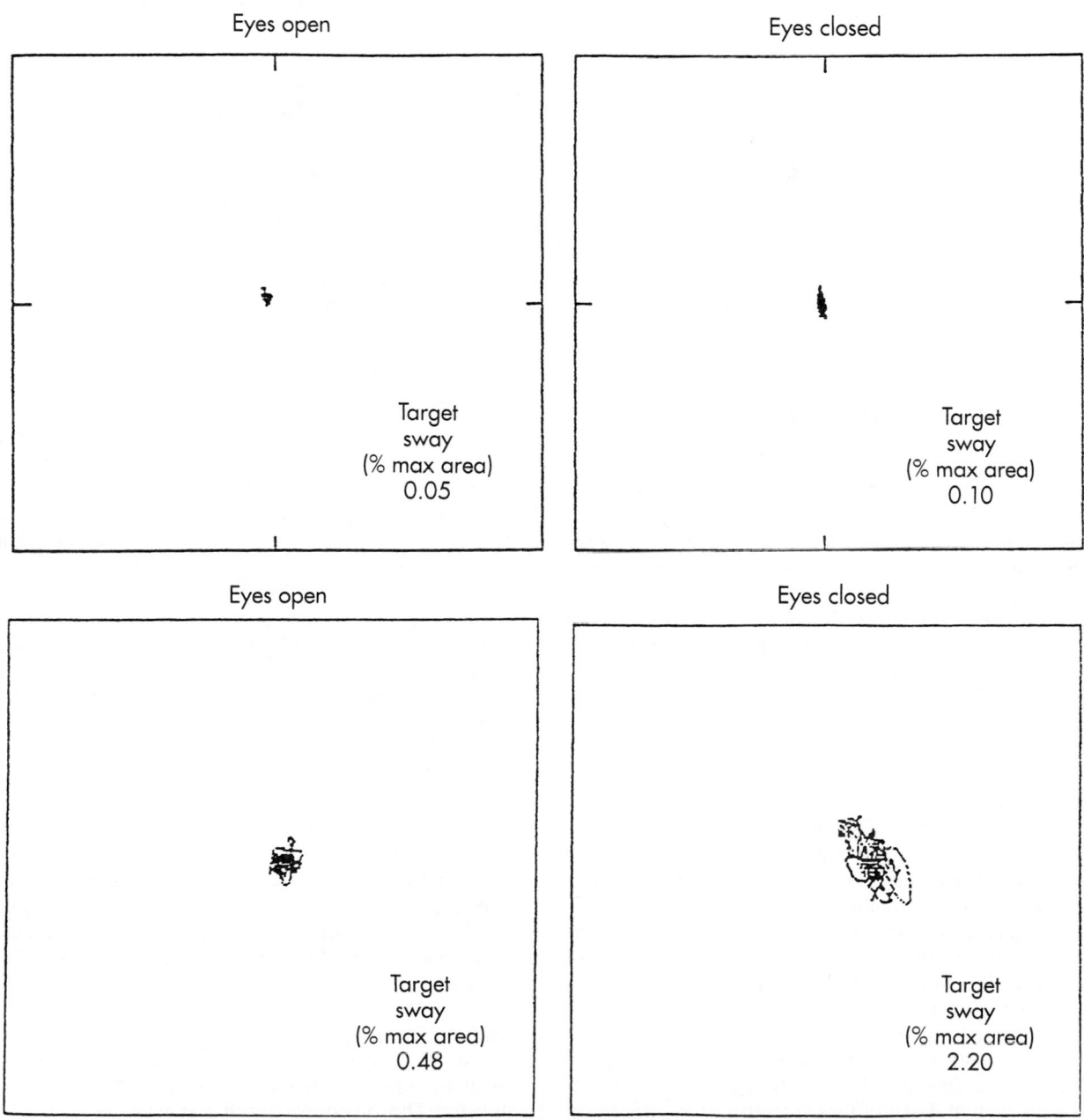

FIGURE 23-5 ■ Graphic and numeric postural sway measures using a computerized forceplate system. *Top left,* Normal subject, eyes open. *Top right,* Normal subject, eyes closed. *Bottom left,* Client with Parkinson's disease, eyes open. *Bottom right,* Client with Parkinson's disease, eyes closed. (Reprinted with permission from NeuroCom International, Inc., Clackamas, OR.)

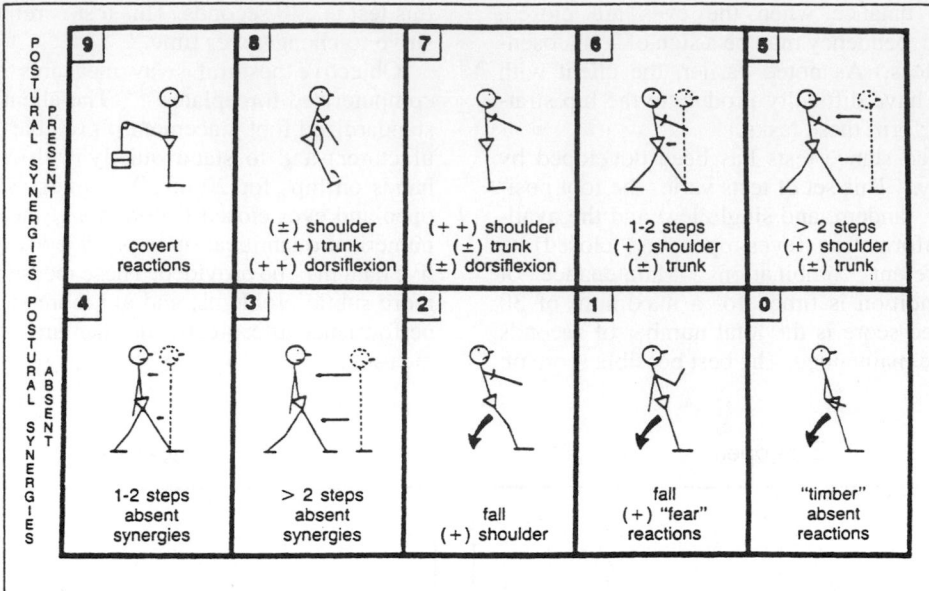

FIGURE 23-6 ■ Ratings of balance strategies used by elderly subjects during the postural stress test after a backward postural perturbation. (+) and (++), Very frequently visible and invariably visible synergistic responses, respectively. (±), Less frequently seen components. Frames 2 to 0 show essentially absent coordinated activity followed by a fall. (Reprinted from Whipple R, Wolfson LI: Abnormalities of balance, gait, and sensorimotor function in the elderly population. In Duncan P, editor: *Balance: Proceedings of the APTA forum,* Alexandria, VA, 1990, American Physical Therapy Association.)

Automatic postural responses are assessed by the client's response to perturbations. The client is asked to stand quietly, and the examiner disturbs the balance, either manually or with equipment. Nudge/push tests are most commonly used.[17] Although not without value, these tests are not quantifiable or repeatable and thus are not reliable measures. For this reason their use is discouraged. However, widely accessible and acceptably reliable alternatives to nudge/push tests have not been developed. Should the examiner decide to use such tests, the client is given slight to moderate pushes backward at the sternum or pelvis and then forward between the shoulder blades or at the pelvis. The clinician subjectively notes any losses of balance and the use of recovery strategies (e.g., ankle, hip, stepping). Scoring involves rating the responses as normal, good, fair, poor, or unable. If used, these nudge/push tests should be performed both predictably (i.e., "don't let me push you") to judge anticipatory postural control and unpredictably (no cues) to judge automatic postural responses. Perturbations of different sizes from multiple different directions should be given.

The postural stress test was developed to examine older adults and determine risk for falls.[18] It is essentially a quantifiable, repeatable nudge/push test that is known to be reliable with trained raters.[44] The client stands while wearing a waist belt attached posteriorly to a line that travels through a pulley and is attached on the other end to one of three weights. The weights are 1.5%, 3.0%, or 4.25% of the client's body weight. Each of these weights is dropped from a standard height, pulling the line that displaces the client backward. The expected response is a compensatory forward adjustment. Clients are videotaped, and the videotape is reviewed to assign scores to the balance responses from 0 (no response/fall) to 9 (appropriate response) (Figure 23-6). If a videotape cannot be made, a second examiner may be asked to observe the responses during the test. Although this test is more repeatable and reliable than nudge/push tests, it is not used often because it requires equipment, videotape or two trained testers, and additional time to perform.

The Motor Control Test (MCT) is a computerized test of automatic postural responses that perturbs the client through surface displacement (Figure 23-7).[4] The client stands on a dynamic (movable) forceplate with feet parallel and arms at sides. The support surface rapidly translates (slides) forward or backward. This surface displacement results in a rapid shift in the relation between the COG and the base of support. The expected responses are directionally specific (to the direction of the stimulus) forces generated against the surface to bring the COG back to the center. Response latencies, strength, and symmetry are measured. Normative data are available. This test can be used to look for abnormal stepping strategies when failure to select hip strategy occurs. The MCT is the most standardized and reliable test of automatic postural responses, but it is not widely used because it requires computerized equipment.

Active Standing

Volitional control of the COG is evaluated by asking the client to make voluntary movements that require weight shifting. The functional reach test was developed for use with older adults to determine risk for falls.[45] The client stands near a wall with feet parallel. Attached to the wall at shoulder height is a yardstick. The client is asked to make a fist and raise the arm nearest the wall to 90 degrees of shoul-

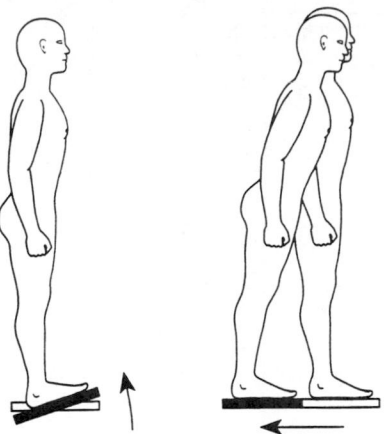

FIGURE 23-7 ■ Surface perturbations during the motor control test using computerized dynamic posturography. Forceplate measures include latency and amount of response and adaptation of the response to repeated perturbations. (From Hasson S: *Clinical exercise physiology,* St. Louis, 1994, Mosby.)

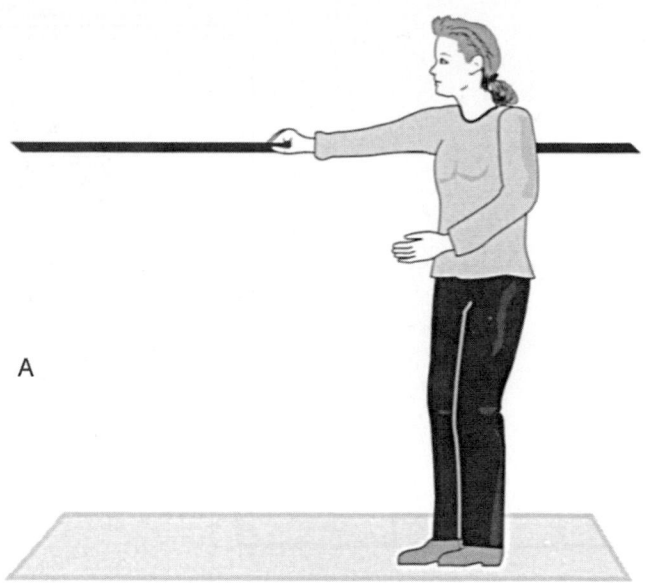

A

der flexion. The examiner notes the position of the fist on the yardstick. The client is then asked to lean forward as far as possible, and the examiner notes the end position of the fist on the yardstick (Figure 23-8). Beginning position is subtracted from end position to obtain a change unit in inches. Three trials are performed. Normative data are available, and the test is reliable. However, the standard error of measurement for this test may be as high as 2 inches, meaning that a change in score of less than 2 inches cannot be attributed to clinical improvement because it may reflect only measurement error. Subsequent studies have not shown that this test is useful for fall prediction.[46-48]

One serious limitation of the functional reach test is that it measures sway in only one direction (forward). An expansion of this test has been devised to measure sway in four directions.[49] The multidirectional reach test is conceptually equivalent but measures sway anteriorly, posteriorly, and laterally to both sides. This test should provide a more comprehensive picture of volitional COG control limitations. Validity and mean values have been established for community-dwelling older adults.[50]

The limits of stability test uses a computerized forceplate to measure postural sway away from midline in eight directions.[42,51] Clients assume a standardized foot position and control a cursor on the computer monitor by shifting their weight. They are asked to move the cursor from midline to eight targets on the screen (Figure 23-9). Measures include movement velocity, directional control (path sway), measures of excursion (length of the trajectory of the COG), and reaction time. This test should be performed once for familiarization, then a second time for scoring purposes. Second and subsequent tests are reliable. Normative data are available.

Sensory Manipulation

Sensory inputs play a critical role in postural control, but few tests to measure their use to produce a balance performance outcome have been developed. The sensory organization test (SOT) uses a computerized, movable forceplate

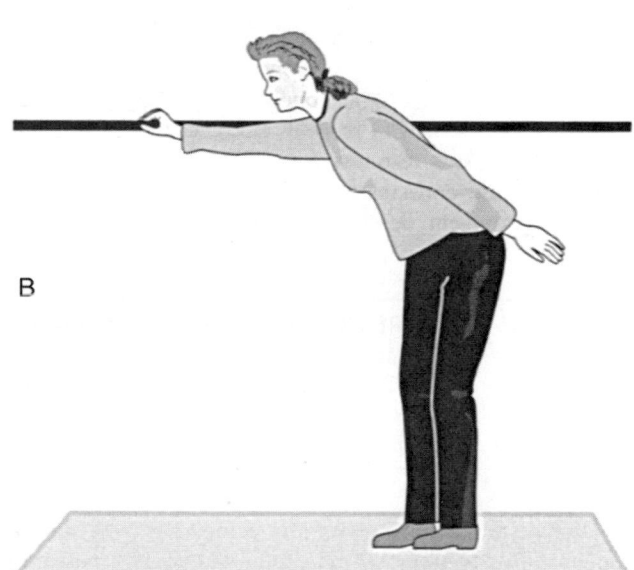

B

FIGURE 23-8 ■ During the functional reach test, the client is asked to reach forward as far as possible from a comfortable standing posture. The excursion of the arm from start to finish is measured by a yardstick affixed to the wall at shoulder height. **A,** Functional reach, starting position. **B,** Functional reach, ending position.

and movable visual surround to alter the surface and visual environments systematically.[4,5] The client stands on the forceplate with feet parallel and arms at the sides and is asked to stand quietly. Three 20-second trials under each of six sensory conditions are performed (Figure 23-10). In conditions one, two, and three the support surface (forceplate)

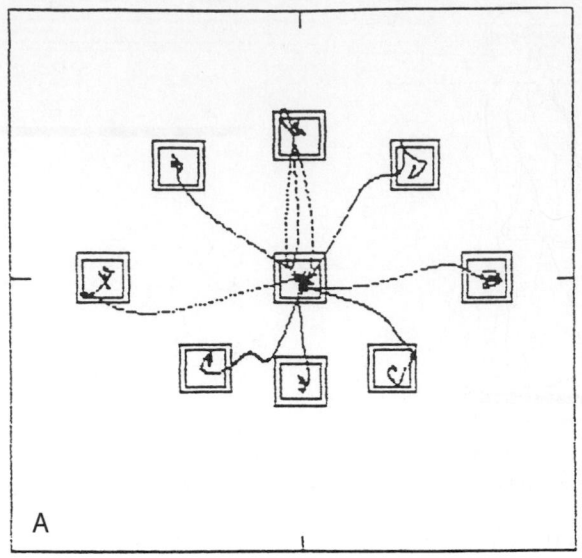

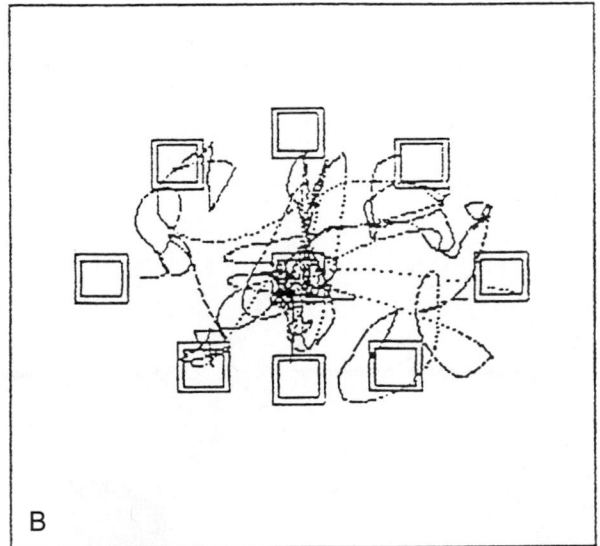

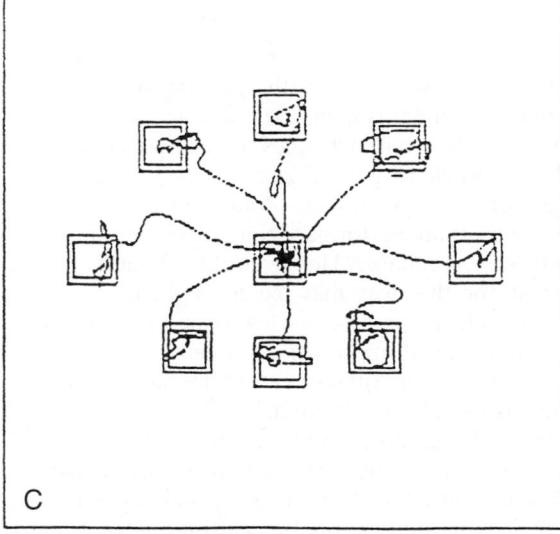

FIGURE 23-9 ■ Graphic postural sway measures from the limit of stability test using a computerized forceplate system (numerical measures not shown). Clients are asked to move away from and return to midline. **A,** Subject with normal postural sway. **B,** Hemiplegic client on initial evaluation. **C,** Hemiplegic client on discharge evaluation. (Reprinted with permission from NeuroCom International, Inc., Clackamas, OR.)

is fixed. During conditions four, five, and six the support surface is sway referenced to the sway of the client. In other words, the movement of the surface is matched to the movement of the client in a 1:1 ratio. This responsive surface movement maintains a near-constant ankle joint angle despite body sway, rendering the somatosensory information from the feet and ankles inaccurate for use in balance maintenance. Visual inputs are undisturbed in conditions one and four. Vision is absent (eyes are closed) in conditions two and five. The movable visual surround is sway referenced in conditions three and six. This responsive visual surround movement maintains a near-constant distance between the eyes and the visual environment despite body sway, rendering visual inputs from the eyes inaccurate for balance maintenance in those two conditions.

Under condition one, all three senses (vision, vestibular, and somatosensory) are available and accurate. Body sway is measured by the forceplate; this initial measurement forms the baseline against which subsequent measures are compared (Figure 23-11). Under condition two, the eyes are closed, so only somatosensory and vestibular cues remain. In an individual with normal movement function, the somatosensory inputs will dominate in this condition. By comparing sway during condition two to sway during condition one, detection of how well the client is using somatosensory inputs for balance control is possible. Clients with somatosensory loss from spinal cord injury, diabetes, or amputation have difficulty in condition two. Functional situations with inadequate lighting or unusable visual cues (e.g., busy carpeting) are similar to condition two.

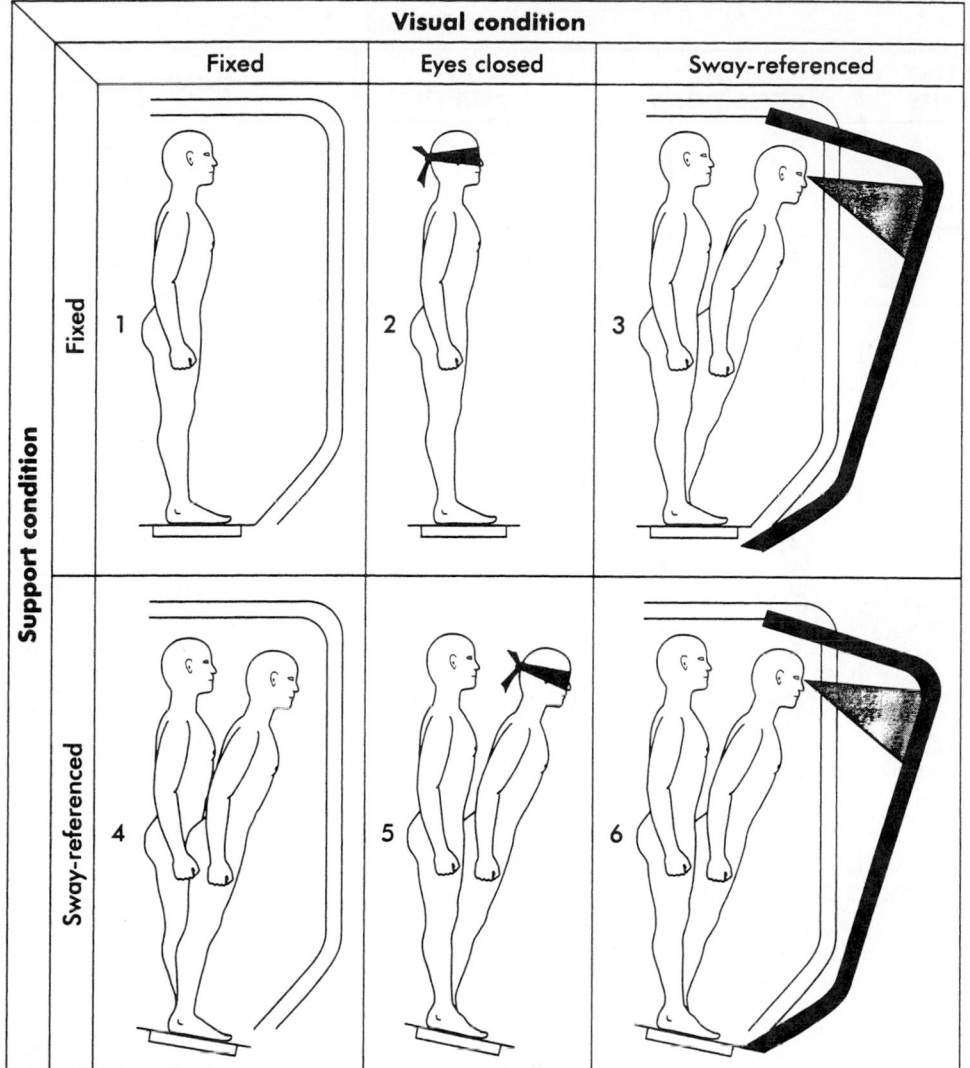

FIGURE 23-10 ■ The six sensory organization test conditions. The sensory organization test determines the relative reliance on visual, vestibular, and somatosensory inputs for postural control using computerized dynamic posturography. (From Hasson S: *Clinical exercise physiology,* St. Louis, 1994, Mosby.)

Under condition four, the support surface is sway referenced (somatosensory cues are available but are inaccurate), so only visual and vestibular cues remain useful. In a normal subject, the visual inputs will dominate in this condition. Comparing sway during condition four to sway during condition one indicates how well the client is using visual inputs for balance control. Clients with visual loss caused by diabetes, cataracts, or field loss have difficulty in condition four. Functional situations that correlate with condition four include compliant surfaces (beach, soft ground, gravel driveway) and unstable surfaces (boat deck, slipping throw rug).

Under condition five, the eyes are closed (visual cues are absent) and the support surface is sway referenced (somatosensory cues are inaccurate), leaving the vestibular inputs as the only remaining sense that is both available and accurate. Comparison of sway during condition five to sway during condition one indicates how well the client is using vestibular inputs for balance control. Clients with vestibular loss caused by head injury, multiple sclerosis, or acoustic

neuroma may have difficulty with condition five. Many elderly clients also may be unstable in this condition. Functional situations in which these clients may be at risk for falls would have both inadequate lighting and compliant or unsteady surfaces (e.g., walking on a gravel driveway or thick carpet in the dark).

Under both conditions three and six, the visual surround is sway referenced (visual cues are available but inaccurate). By comparing sway during these two conditions to sway in the absence of vision (conditions two and five, with eyes closed), determining how well the client can recognize and subsequently suppress inaccurate visual inputs when they conflict with somatosensory and vestibular cues is possible. Some clients with CNS lesions (e.g., head injury, stroke, tumor) may have difficulty with this condition. Clients who cannot recognize and ignore inaccurate visual cues cannot distinguish whether they are moving or the environment is moving. If they perceive that they are moving (away from midline) when they are not, they may often actively generate

SENSORY ANALYSIS			
RATIO NAME	**TEST CONDITIONS**	**RATIO PAIR**	**SIGNIFICANCE**
SOM Somatosensory	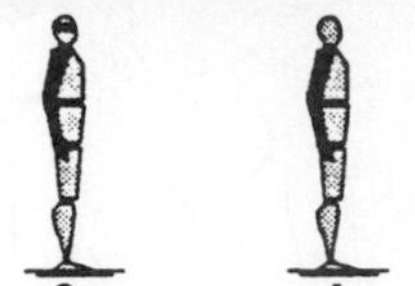 2 1	Condition 1 / Condition 2	Question: Does sway increase when visual cues are removed? Low scores: Patient makes poor use of somatosensory references.
VIS Visual	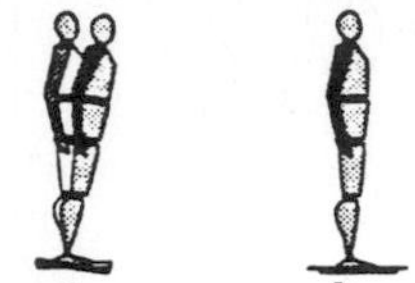 4 1	Condition 4 / Condition 1	Question: Does sway increase when somatosensory cues are inaccurate? Low scores: Patient makes poor use of visual references.
VEST Vestibular	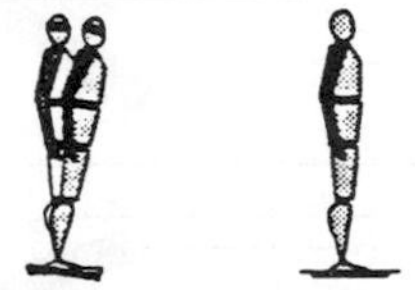 5 1	Condition 5 / Condition 1	Question: Does sway increase when visual cues are removed and somatosensory cues are inaccurate? Low scores: Patient makes poor use of vestibular cues, or vestibular cues unavailable.
PREF Visual Preference	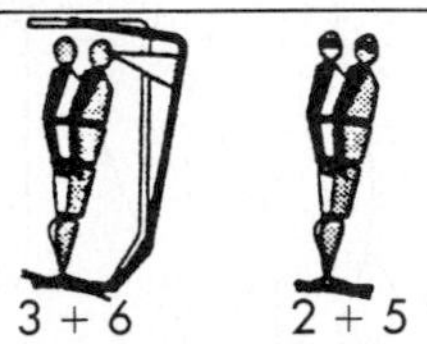 3 + 6 2 + 5	Condition 3 + 6 / Condition 2 + 5	Question: Do inaccurate visual cues result in increased sway compared to no visual cues? Low scores: Patient relies on visual cues even when they are inaccurate.

FIGURE 23-11 ■ Postural sway measures from each of the six sensory organization test conditions are compared and the ratios are used to identify impairments in the use of sensory inputs for postural control. (From Jacobson GP, Newman CW, Kartush JM: *Handbook of balance function testing,* St. Louis, 1993, Mosby.)

postural responses to "right" themselves. These responses, invoked to bring the COG to midline, then result in movement away from the midline. The inaccurate perception leads to a self-initiated loss of balance. Functional situations that correlate with this test condition include public transportation, grocery and library aisles, and moving walkways.

The SOT is valid and reliable in the absence of motoric problems, which increase sway for reasons unrelated to sensory reception and perception. Normative data are available.

The Clinical Test for Sensory Interaction on Balance (CTSIB) is a clinical version of the SOT that does not use computerized forceplate technology.[52] The concept of the six conditions remains intact (Figure 23-12). Instead of sway measures, the examiner uses a stopwatch and visual observation. A thick foam pad substitutes for the moving forceplate during conditions four, five, and six. In subjects and clients with peripheral vestibular lesions, measures with foam correlate to moving forceplate measures.[53] Originally, a modified Japanese lantern substituted for the moving visual surround in conditions three and six. Studies have not shown that measures using the Japanese lantern correlate with the moving visual surround measures. Most clinicians now perform the modified CTSIB with just four conditions, eyes open and closed on a firm surface and eyes open and

closed on the foam surface. The client is asked to stand with feet parallel and arms at sides or hands on hips. At least three and up to five 30-second trials of each condition are performed.[25] The watch is stopped if the client steps, reaches, or falls during the 30 seconds. A maximum score for five trials of each condition is 150 seconds. Subjects with normal movement function are able to stand without loss of balance for 30 seconds per trial per condition. The CTSIB may not be a reliable measure in clients with hemiplegia or other conditions that involve motor deficits in, or abnormal response time through, the lower extremities and trunk.[54] The clinician can use the information regarding client response in a variety of environmental conditions to determine intervention management strategies.[55]

Individuals with well-compensated vestibular system deficiencies may perform well on the standard SOT or CTSIB with eyes open and a static head position; however, having the individual perform head movements during these tests can indicate visual dependence (the need for gaze stabilization to maintain balance).

Vestibular System Tests

There are many types of common vestibular disorders. This chapter cannot provide a total discussion of all these disorders. They have been summarized in Appendix 23-A. Some

VISUAL CONDITIONS

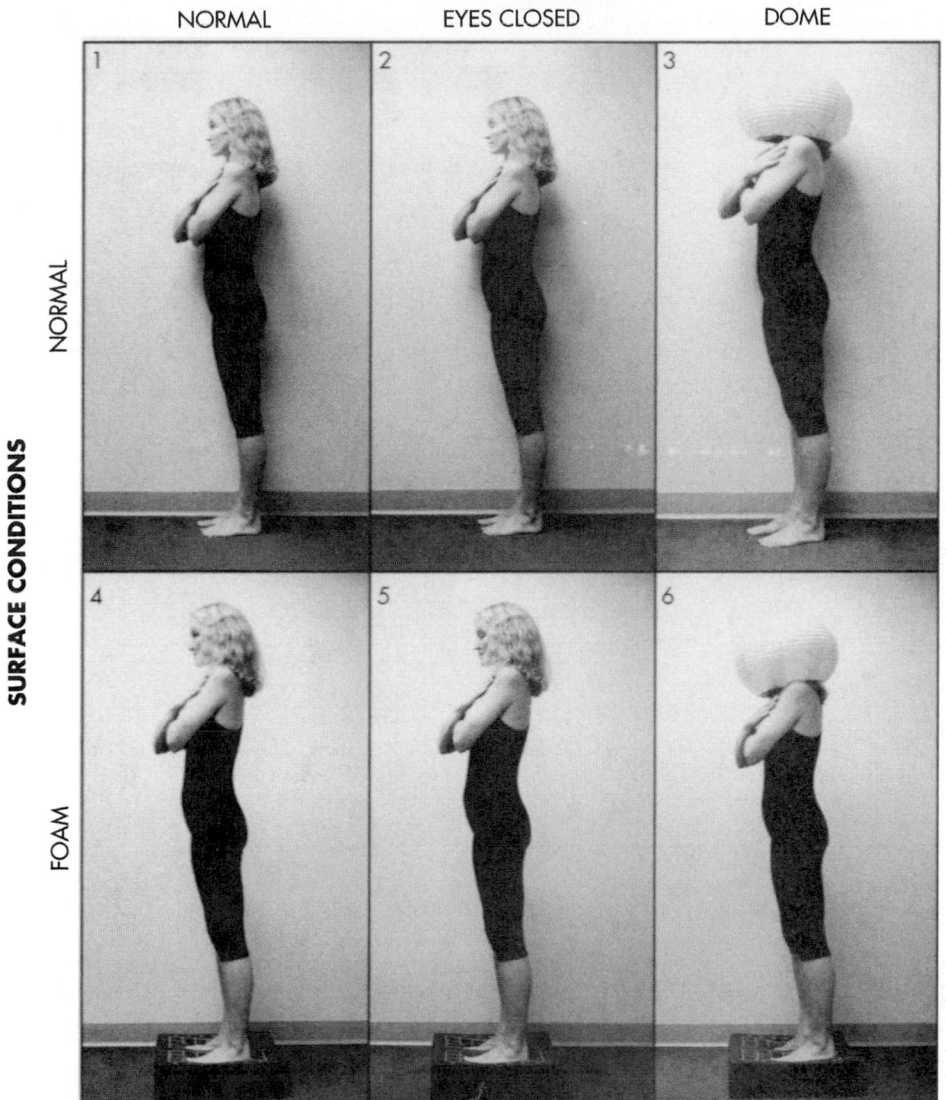

FIGURE 23-12 ■ The clinical test for sensory interaction in balance uses foam and a Japanese lantern to replicate the six sensory conditions. A stopwatch is used to time trials.

of the specific vestibular system tests are discussed within this section.

Nystagmus

Assessment of eye movement control can help diagnose dysfunction of the peripheral and central vestibular pathways through the medial longitudinal fasciculus. In particular, tests for a specific type of abnormal eye movement called nystagmus should be performed in clients with dizziness and those with known neuropathology involving these pathways. Nystagmus is nonvoluntary, rhythmic oscillation of the eyes, with movement in one direction clearly faster than movement in the other direction. The client with nystagmus will also usually report vertigo. There is more than one type of nystagmus; identification of the particular type can direct the clinician toward the area of dysfunction.[20]

Spontaneous nystagmus results from imbalance in the vestibular signals through their transmission to the oculo-motor neurons. This imbalance produces a constant drift of the eyes in one direction interrupted by brief, fast movement in the opposite direction. Spontaneous nystagmus occurs after acute vestibular lesions and usually lasts approximately 24 hours. Peripheral versus central lesions may be distinguished by asking the patient to fix his or her gaze on a stable target. Nystagmus from peripheral vestibular lesions is easily inhibited with visual fixation. Nystagmus caused by central lesions of the brain stem or cerebellum is not easily inhibited with visual fixation.

Positional nystagmus is induced by a change in head position. Nystagmus caused by stimulation of the peripheral semicircular canals lasts only seconds and then dissipates. Nystagmus caused by central vestibular system damage lasts minutes or longer before abating. Static nystagmus occurs with lesions to the peripheral otolith system through connections in the vestibular nuclei and cerebellum. It is provoked with change of head position in relation to gravity and continues as long as the position is maintained, although it

UNIVERSITY OF MICHIGAN VESTIBULAR TESTING CENTER HABITUATION TRAINING

NAME: _____ MRN: _____ AGE: _____ SEX: _____

DATE: _____	INTENSITY	DURATION	SCORE
BASELINE SYMPTOMS			
1. Sitting → Supine			
2. Supine → Left Side			
3. → → Right Side			
4. Supine → Sitting			
5. Left Hallpike			
6. → → Sitting			
7. Right Hallpike			
8. → → Sitting			
9. Sitting → Nose To Left Knee			
10. Sitting → Erect Left			
11. Sitting → Nose To Right Knee			
12. Sitting → Erect Right			
13. Sitting → Head Rotation			
14. Sitting → Head Flex. And Ext.			
15. Standing → Turn To Right			
16. Standing → Turn To Left			

INTENSITY: SCALE FROM 0 TO 5 (O=NO SX, 5=SEVERE SX)
DURATION: SCALE FROM 0 TO 3 (5-10 SEC=1 POINT, 11-30 SEC=2 POINTS, ≥30 SEC=3 POINTS)

MOTION SENSITIVITY QUOTIENT: $\dfrac{\text{POSITIONS} \times \text{SCORE}}{2048} \times 100 =$ _____ 28-12.

TOTAL

FIGURE 23-13 ■ An example of a standardized list of vertiginous positions tests. Intensity of dizziness is rated by the client, and duration of dizziness is measured with a stopwatch. (Courtesy of the University of Michigan Vestibular Testing Center, Ann Arbor, MI.)

can fluctuate in frequency and amplitude. Static nystagmus can be suppressed with visual fixation.

Gaze-evoked nystagmus occurs when clients shift the eyes from a primary central position to a second location. It is caused by the inability to maintain stable gaze position, and the eye drifts back toward the center or primary position. Usually indicative of a CNS problem, it is common in multiple sclerosis, brain injury, and congenital lesions.

The head-shaking nystagmus test is performed by the examiner passively moving the client's head. Starting with the head anteriorly flexed to 30 degrees (placing the lateral canal parallel to the ground), the head is moved side to side 45 degrees in each direction for 30 cycles with a velocity of 360 degrees per second. Normal individuals do not have nystagmus after this stimulus, but nystagmus occurs in clients with vestibular dysfunction. It can be immediate or with latency (delay of onset is usually about 10 seconds) and lasts for 5 to 20 seconds. This test can be easily performed in the clinic and is an indicator of vestibular dysfunction.[56]

Tests of Semicircular Canal Function

Tests that attempt to stimulate the vestibular semicircular canals are usually called vertiginous position tests because they move or place clients in various positions and monitor for vertigo, dizziness, nausea, and nystagmus.[20] No single list of positions is used consistently across sites, but in general most of these tests have 10 to 20 provoking movements performed from least to most disturbing (Figure 23-13). A standardized method of scoring is not used across sites, but the examiner usually monitors the number of positions that induce symptoms (e.g., 10 of 16), the number of repetitions of the maneuver that can be performed before symptoms begin to increase, the intensity of the symptoms as rated by the client (0 = no symptoms, up to 10 = severe symptoms with near vomiting), and the duration of the change in symptom level (e.g., client began at intensity level two and symptoms increased with the positioning maneuver to a level seven; it took 26 seconds for the symptoms to return to a level two). If a canal is hyperresponsive to head motion, the canal that is affected will be activated and cause dizziness when the head moves in the direction of that canal. For example, if the head is tipped forward and to the right, the right anterior canal and the right posterior canal will be activated. The response will most often be vertigo and will be brief (less than 1 minute). If the dizziness is persistent and does not decrease over time, the disorder may be central in nature. In

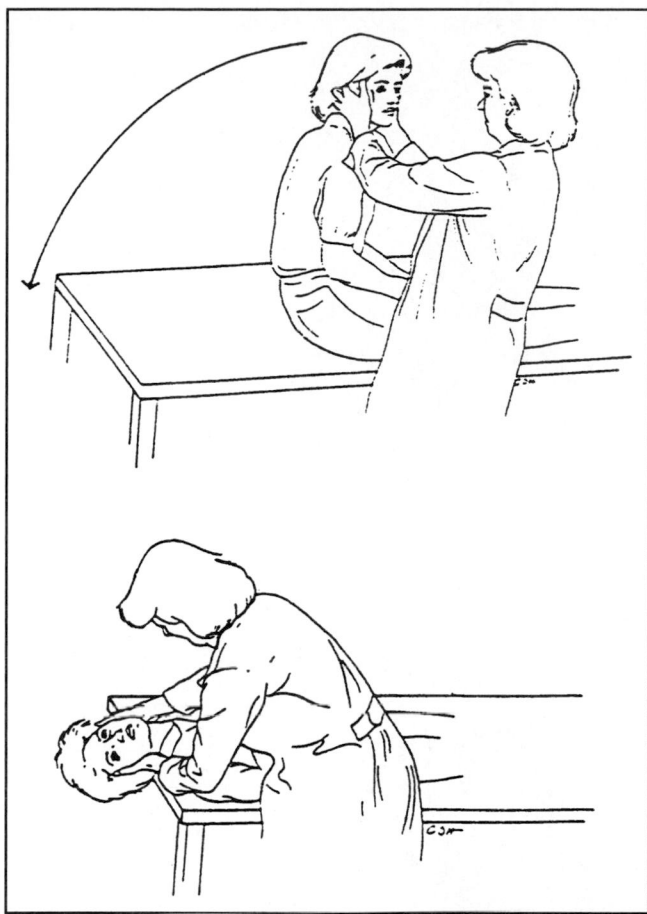

FIGURE 23-14 ■ The Hallpike-Dix maneuver. Moving the patient rapidly from a sitting to a supine position with the head turned so that the affected ear is 30 to 45 degrees below the horizontal stimulates the posterior canal and may produce vertigo and nystagmus. (From Herdman S: Treatment of benign paroxysmal positional vertigo, *Phys Ther* 70:381-388, 1990, with permission of the American Physical Therapy Association.)

this case the symptom may be vertigo or diffuse dizziness. With a central disorder the examiner may observe nystagmus during the change of positions, or the symptom may come as the client returns to the starting point. When symptoms are caused by canal hypersensitivity, improvement over time is noted by fewer provoking positions, a greater number of repetitions before symptom exacerbation, lower intensity of symptoms, and shorter duration of symptoms.[57]

The Hallpike-Dix maneuver is a vertiginous position test to stimulate the posterior semicircular canal (Figure 23-14).[20] This test is used to determine if otoconia are present in the semicircular canal. A positive response (vertigo and nystagmus) on this test leads to a diagnosis of benign positional vertigo (BPV). The client is positioned in long sitting on a mat or plinth such that, when supine, the head and neck extend over the upper edge of the surface. The examiner holds the head of the sitting client between both hands and then rapidly moves the client backward and down with the head turned to the side and the neck extended 30 to 45 degrees below the horizontal. The head is held in this position for 20 to 30 seconds. The examiner monitors for symptoms of vertigo and observes the eyes for nystagmus. If

nystagmus occurs, the direction of the nystagmus indicates whether the otoconia are free floating or adherent. When the quick phase of the nystagmus is toward the ground (geotropic), the otoconia are free floating. If the otoconia are adherent to the hair cells, the quick phase of the nystagmus is away from the ground (ageotropic).[58] In cases of BPV, the involved side is distinguished by which ear is toward the ground when the symptoms occur. The critical hallmark of BPV is that the vertigo usually starts after 5 to 10 seconds and resolves or fatigues within 20 to 40 seconds. Benign positional nystagmus or vertigo is a common sequela of head concussion, viral labyrinthitis, and vascular occlusion of the inner ear. It can also develop without a known external cause.[20]

BPV may involve any semicircular canal, although the posterior canal is most common because of its relation to the otoliths when the person is in the recumbent position. However, the horizontal canal can collect otoconia and the result is horizontal nystagmus generated with head movement. Horizontal canal BPV is tested in the supine position with the head held in 30 degrees flexion to keep the lateral canal perpendicular to the ground or in the neutral position for ease of positioning. The head is then turned in each direction and the eyes observed for horizontal nystagmus. This must be distinguished from static positional nystagmus by the fact that the nystagmus will fatigue if it is caused by movement of the otoconia but otherwise persists.[59]

Visual-Vestibular Interaction

The VOR test examines the interaction of the visual and vestibular systems for eye and head orientation. The ability to hold the eyes fixed on a target while the head is moving is known as gaze stabilization. The client is asked to perform these tasks in horizontal, vertical, and diagonal planes and at the speed of 2 Hz (Figure 23-15). If the image blurs, the gain of the system is abnormal, meaning that the vestibular system is unable to move the eyes at the exact speed in the opposite direction as the head movement. The ratio of eye velocity to head velocity is known as the gain of the VOR. The gain of an intact VOR is usually equal to one, which means movement of the eyes is equal to the movement of the head. The client with a vestibular disorder has usually self-limited the speed of head movement to accommodate for the abnormal gain. In some instances, the client will not describe blurring (a lack of gaze stabilization) with testing but will report dizziness while performing the test procedure. This is most likely related to the blurring of the visual field beyond the target, which is interpreted as motion. Blurring of the image during head movement may also be the result of an oculomotor dysfunction that limits convergent gaze.

The ability to synchronize simultaneous eye and head movements in the same direction is associated with the ability of the brain to suppress the VOR and is known as VOR cancellation. If the central integration capabilities are abnormal, the client will not be able to override the reflex activity and cannot keep the eye and head moving at the same rate in the same direction.

Visual Acuity Test

When the oculomotor system is unable to maintain clear visual targets as the eyes move, symptoms of dizziness, nausea, and headache may be present. Saccades, or the

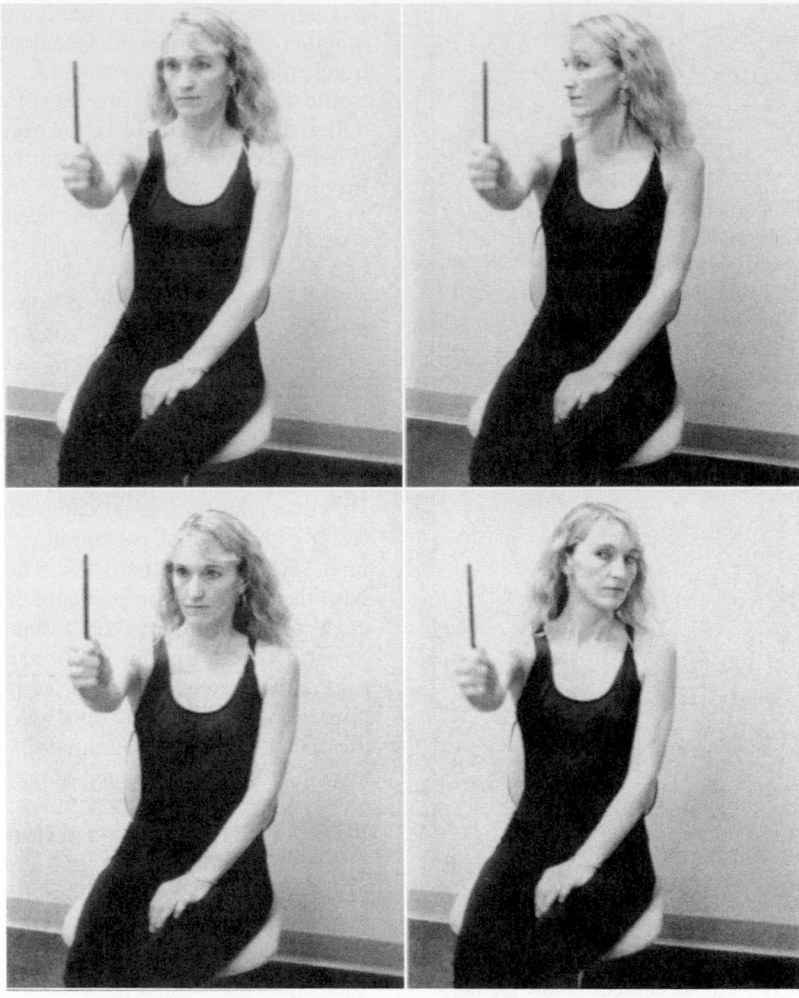

Head fixed, eyes tracking a moving object.

Eyes fixed on an object, head moving. (see corresponding sequence of photos)

Eyes and head and object moving while focusing on the moving object.

Vertical movements of the eyes with the head stable and moving.

Eyes diagonal with the head stable and moving.

Eye movements incorporated with trunk movements.

FIGURE 23-15 ■ Eye and head motions are assessed to determine whether symptoms associated with the vestibular-ocular reflex mechanism are present. (From Whitney S: Dizziness and balance disorders, *Clin Management* 11:42-48, 1991, with permission of the American Physical Therapy Association.)

ability for the eyes to move suddenly to locate a point in space, are tested by asking the client (head fixed) to look at one target. The examiner then presents a second target on the opposite side of the visual field. The client must look at this second target as quickly as possible without moving the head. In normal subjects, a single rapid jump of the eyes occurs. Abnormal responses include an undershooting or overshooting of the visual target, which must be adjusted with subsequent smaller jumps. The examiner observes for these multiple attempts to locate the visual target exactly. Smooth pursuit, or the ability for the eyes to move at various

speeds to follow a moving visual target, is tested by asking the client (head fixed) to follow a moving object held by the examiner. The examiner moves the object at different speeds and in different directions throughout the visual field and observes for any inability to follow the object. Normal subjects have no difficulty following the moving target (see Chapter 30).

Fukuda Stepping Test
The Fukuda stepping test was developed to assess labyrinth function.[39] A grid is drawn on the floor with two concentric

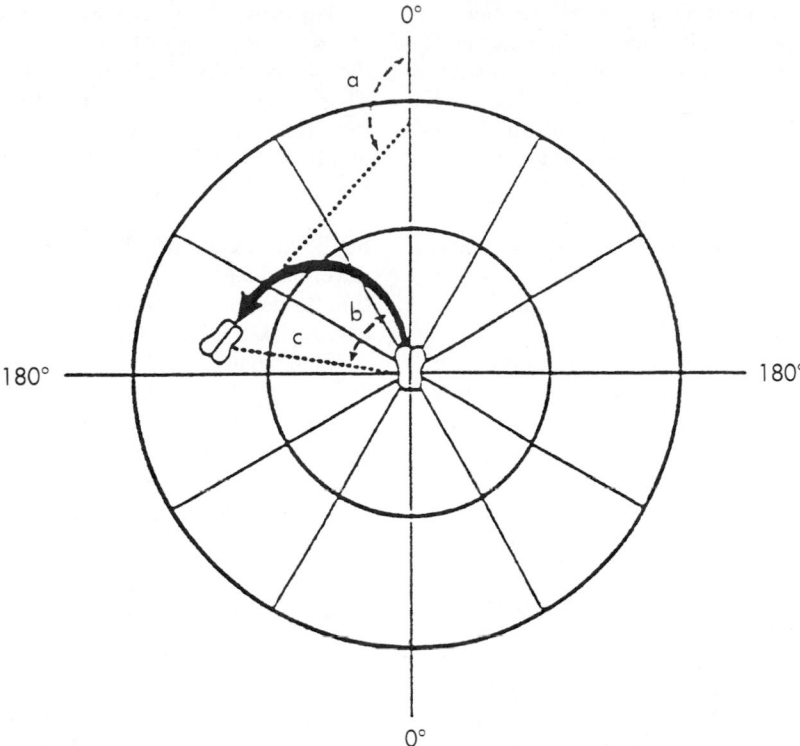

FIGURE 23-16 ■ The Fukuda stepping test for peripheral vestibular clients uses a floor grid to detect the extend of drift that occurs during an eyes-closed stepping task. (From Newton R: Review of tests of standing balance abilities, *Brain Inj* 3:335, 1989.)

circles (1 and 2 m in diameter, respectively) divided into 30-degree sections (Figure 23-16). The client is placed standing in the center of the circles, is blindfolded, and raises the arms outstretched to shoulder height. The examiner instructs the client to take 100 marching steps (knees high) in place, then observes for postural sway and deviations of position of the head, arms, and body. Once the client has stopped, the examiner quantitatively measures the angle of rotation, angle of displacement, and the distance of displacement. According to Fukuda, normal subjects are able to take 100 steps without traveling more than 1 m and without rotating more than 45 degrees, whereas clients with peripheral vestibular dysfunction deviate outside this range toward the side of the deficit. *Individuals with a normal vestibular system and no symptoms can also test positive on this test,* so it should be used for diagnostic purposes only in conjunction with other tests—never in isolation. Obviously, the client being tested must be at a high level motorically to perform this test, and the examiner must be sure that any observed deviations are not from motoric (versus vestibular) causes. The reliability of this test is poor, and its use is not recommended.[60] Performance of this test can be of some benefit to identify whether the client can identify movement without the use of visual information. If the otoliths cannot detect movement forward or to the side, the individual will most likely develop a visual dependency for balance during similar tasks such as walking.

Functional Scales

A comprehensive balance evaluation must include both impairment measures and disability measures. Functional scales help address the latter. By asking the client to perform functional tasks that demand balance skills, the clinician can determine the presence of disabilities and identify the tasks that the client needs to practice. Three mobility scales and three gait scales focus on postural control; five of these were developed for the elderly population to determine risk for falls. Many clinicians also are using them to assess neurological clients, although their usefulness with neurological populations has not been formally evaluated. Standardized tests for high-level balance skills have not been developed; some clinicians adapt tests used by athletes, but these are often at too high of a level for many neurologically involved clients.

The Berg Balance Scale is a list of 14 tasks that the client is asked to perform.[61] The examiner rates the client on each task by using a scale of 0 to 4, in which 0 is unable to perform and 4 is able to perform without difficulty. This test is highly reliable. Originally designed for assessing risk for falls in older adults, cutoff scores for fall risk vary depending on which of several studies is consulted.[62,63] Use of higher cutoff scores may erroneously identify nonfallers as fallers; use of lower cutoff scores may erroneously identify fallers as nonfallers. The Berg Balance Scale has also been used with clients after stroke.[64-67]

The original get-up-and-go test is made up of seven items and subjectively scored on a scale of 1 to 5, in which 1 is normal and 5 is severely abnormal.[68] This test has been modified by making it a timed measure to increase its objectivity and reliability, which is now high. The Timed Up-and-Go Test eliminates the "standing steady" segment and uses a stopwatch to time the performance.[69] Clients are asked to rise from a chair without arms, walk three meters as fast as they safely can, turn, walk back to the chair and sit down. This test may be performed with an assistive device; however, the use of a device will alter the speed at which the task can be accomplished, and any retesting must be done with the same device to produce comparable results. Originally designed to assess frailty in older adults, the test is now more commonly used to assess fall risk in this population. Young adults perform this task in 5 to 7 seconds, motorically normal older adults in 7 to 9 seconds (low risk), moderate-risk older adults in 10 to 12 seconds, and high-risk older adults in 13 seconds or more.[70,71]

The Tinetti Performance Oriented Assessment of Balance is a list of nine items scored on scales of either 0 to 1 or 0 to 2, with the higher numbers reflecting better (more normal) performance.[72] The score value is specific to the item. The best possible score is 16, with a score of 10 or lower indicating a high risk for falls.[72a]

Most balance and mobility scales have been developed to assess risk for falls in older adults. Many share similar items. See Table 23-2 for a summary of scale items.

The Tinetti Performance Oriented Assessment of Gait is a list of seven normal aspects of gait that are observed by the examiner as the client walks at a self-selected pace and then at a rapid but safe pace.[72] Scoring scales are again either 0 to 1 or 0 to 2, and higher numbers indicate better performance. Score values are specific to the item being observed (Table 23-3). The best possible score is a 12; scores of 8 or below indicate a high risk for falls. When combined, the Tinetti balance and gait scales offer a best possible score of 28, with scores of 19 or less indicating a high fall risk.

The original gait assessment rating scale (GARS) is a list of 16 abnormal aspects of gait observed by the examiner as the client walks at a self-selected pace (see Table 23-3).[18] These abnormalities are commonly seen in older adults who fall. The items are scored on a scale of 0 to 3, with lower numbers reflecting better (less abnormal) performance. The best possible score is 0. This gait scale provides some relative numerical indication of the quality of gait. A shorter, modified version of this test, the modified GARS, has been developed and provides equivalent sensitivity and takes less time to perform.[73] These two gait scales were developed to assess risk for falls in older adults.

The dynamic gait index is a more recently developed test specifically designed to look at postural control during gait.[17] It includes eight items requiring changes in gait speed, walking with horizontal and vertical head turning, whole-body turns during gait, stepping over and around obstacles, and stair ascent and descent. Items on this test are scored on a scale of 0 to 3, with 3 being normal performance and 0 indicating severe impairment. The best possible score on this test is a 24. The presence of head and whole-body turns in this test may help identify clients with potential vestibular dysfunction. The reliability of this test is high.[63,74,75] A modified and slightly more difficult version of this test, the functional gait assessment, has been developed specifically for use with patients with vestibular disorders.[76] The three tests listed previously are distinct from traditional gait tests because they focus on elements of postural control during gait.

Combination Test Batteries

Because no single test can give a complete picture of a client's balance abilities, three commonly used test batteries

TABLE 23-2 ■ Balance and Mobility Scale Items

ACTIVITY	BERG BALANCE	DYNAMIC GAIT INDEX	TIMED UP AND GO	TINETTI BALANCE
1. Sit unsupported	√			√
2. Sit-to-stand	√		√	√
3. Stand-to-sit	√		√	√
4. Transfers	√			
5. Stand unsupported	√		√	√
6. Stand with eyes closed	√			√
7. Stand with feet together	√			
8. Tandem stand	√			
9. Stand on one leg	√			
10. Trunk rotation while standing	√			
11. Retrieve object from floor	√			
12. Turn 360 degrees	√			√
13. Stool stepping	√			
14. Reach forward while standing	√			
15. Sternal nudge				√
16. Walk		√	√	
17. Abrupt stop		√		
18. Walk then turn		√	√	
19. Step over obstacle		√		
20. Stairs		√		
21. Walk at preferred and varied speeds		√		
22. Walk with horizontal and vertical head turns		√		
23. Step around obstacles		√		

combine several types of tests. The Fregley-Graybiel Ataxia Test Battery is a list of eight test items that the client must perform (Figure 23-17).[39] Standing trials in tandem stance both off and on a rail with eyes open and closed are timed. Timed single-leg stance trials also are performed for each leg. Walking 10 steps with eyes closed is included. Five trials of each task are given. Trials are stopped if the client uncrosses the arms, opens the eyes (during eyes-closed trials), steps (during standing trials), or falls. Trials are judged on a pass/fail basis. This test battery is valid for use with clients who have peripheral vestibular dysfunction. Normative data are available from a normative database composed primarily of young men. As noted earlier, clients

TABLE 23-3 ■ Gait Scale Items

GAIT ACTIVITIES	TINETTI GAIT SCALE	GAIT ASSESSMENT RATING SCALE
1. Initiation (hesitancy)	√	√
2. Step length	√	√
3. Step height	√	√
4. Step symmetry	√	√
5. Step continuity	√	√
6. Path deviation	√	√
7. Trunk	√	√
8. Walking-heel distance	√	
9. Staggering		√
10. Heel strike		√
11. Hip ROM*		√
12. Knee ROM*		√
13. Elbow extension*		√
14. Shoulder extension*		√
15. Shoulder abduction*		√
16. Arm-heelstrike synchrony		√
17. Forward head*		√
18. Shoulders held elevated*		√
19. Forward flexed trunk*		√

*During gait.

must be at a high level motorically to perform these tasks. This test is a good choice for clients with higher-level abilities because it does provide more demanding balance tasks. Interpretations regarding a client's use of sensory inputs when motor involvement is also present cannot be made with certainty.

The Fugl-Meyer Sensorimotor Assessment of Balance Performance is a subset of the Fugl-Meyer Physical Performance Battery, which was designed for use with hemiplegic clients (Figure 23-18).[25] Three sitting and four standing balance activities are listed. The items are scored on a 0 to 2 scale, with score values specific to each item. Higher scores indicate better performance; the maximum (best) score is 14. However, a client could achieve this score of 14 and still not have normal balance.

The Dizziness Handicap Inventory (DHI) was developed to identify specific functional, emotional, or physical problems associated with an individual's reaction to imbalance or dizziness.[77,78] The DHI assesses the client's perception of the effects of the balance problem and the client's level of emotional adjustment. It also looks at perceived physical limitations as a consequence of the disorder. Twenty-five items are divided into three subscales in this self-assessment inventory. Included are a nine-item functional scale, a nine-item emotional scale, and a seven-item physical scale. Each item is assigned a value of four points for a "yes," two points for a "sometimes," and zero points for a "no." This inventory is reliable, is easy to administer, and can be used to evaluate treatment outcomes.[79] Changes in scores on the functionally based DHI correlate highly with changes in scores on the impairment-based SOT.[77]

The DHI can be given before the initial evaluation to help determine which physical tests should be performed. An astute clinician can see patterns of dysfunction within the reported symptom level. For example, visual motion sensitivity and visual dependency can be indicated from the answers about grocery stores, crowds, riding in a car, or difficulty at night. Imbalance usually is indicated when the client has difficulty walking down a sidewalk and using stairs. When the client reports inability to perform vigorous activities and consistent dizziness, the problem may be

FREGLEY TEST

Condition	Trials				
	1	2	3	4	5
1. Sharpened Romberg, EC (60 sec; feet in tandem)					
2. Walk on Rail, EO (5 steps; best 3/5 trials)					
3. Stand on Rail, EO (3 trials; 60 sec/trial)				x	x
4. Stand on Rail, EC (3 trials; 60 sec/trial)				x	x
5. Stand on Right Leg, on Floor, EC (5 trials; 30 sec/trial)					
6. Stand on Left Leg, on Floor, EC (5 trials; 30 sec/trial)					
7. Walk on Floor, EC (3 trials; 10 steps each)				x	x
8. Stand sideways on rail (characterize sway)*					

*Added by the author to observe the movement strategy used by the individual
EO, eyes open; EC, eyes closed.

FIGURE 23-17 ■ A combination of tasks (Romberg, OLST, walking) and environments (eyes open, eyes closed, rail) are included in the Fregley-Graybiel ataxia test battery. (From Newton R: Review of tests of standing balance abilities, *Brain Inj* 3:335, 1989.)

FUGL-MEYER

Test	Scoring	Maximum Possible Score	Attained Score
1. Sit without support _____	0—Cannot maintain sitting without support 1—Can sit unsupported less than 5 minutes 2—Can sit longer than 5 minutes		
2. Parachute reaction, non-affected side _____	0—Does not abduct shoulder or extend elbow 1—Impaired reaction 2—Normal reaction		
3. Parachute reaction, affected side _____	Scoring is the same as for test 2		
4. Stand with support _____	0—Cannot stand 1—Stands with maximum support 2—Stands with minimum support for 1 minute		
5. Stand without support _____	0—Cannot stand without support 1—Stands less than 1 minute or sways 2—Stands with good balance more than 1 minute		
6. Stand on unaffected side _____	0—Cannot be maintained longer than 1–2 seconds 1—Stands balanced 4–9 seconds 2—Stands balanced more than 10 seconds		
7. Stand on affected side _____	0—Scoring is the same as for test 6		
	Maximum Balance Score		

FIGURE 23-18 ■ The Fugl-Meyer Sensorimotor Assessment of Balance Performance includes both low level and high level tasks. (From DiFabio RP, Badke MB: Relationship of sensory organization to balance function in patients with hemiplegia, *Phys Ther* 70:20, 1990.)

related to motion-provoked dizziness. Patients with chronic mild head injury often will report most activities as most provoking related to both the inability to integrate the sensory systems and poor motor control for balance.

If the individual has a new onset of BPV, she or he will report symptoms only with the questions related to head movement, such as rolling in bed, looking up, and bending forward. The DHI should be carefully examined in the individual who may be referred for BPV to assess for other indications of changes within the vestibular mechanism. If recurrent, motion-provoked dizziness is present along with visual dependency, the client may have developed compensation to manage symptoms in the past.

Dual-Task Tests

In everyday life tasks, normal balance is largely unconscious and does not compete for attentional resources. In clients with balance disorders, however, the challenge of maintaining postural control during gait is often sufficient to demand the use of attentional resources. The interaction of cognitive demands and postural control demands is examined in dual-task tests that add concurrent cognitive and motor tasks to a gait task. At the simplest level are the walking while talking (WWT) and stops walking when talking (SWWT) tests.[80-83] In these tests the client is asked to walk and, while walking, the clinician asks the client one or more questions and observes if the client must stop walking to answer the question(s). If so, the test result is positive; that is, the client must stop attending to the postural control demands of walking to reallocate attention to the cognitive task. A more formalized dual task test is the Multiple Tasks Test (MTT), which includes eight items involving gait plus other verbal cogni-

tive and motor tasks such as carrying a tray and avoiding obstacles.[84,85] Although these dual-task tests are a promising start to the examination of the interaction of cognition and balance, their reliability and validity are not well established, and disagreement in the literature exists regarding their usefulness. In clinical use, these tests appear to be able to detect clients with major balance problems but may not discriminate those with moderate or mild problems.

Considerations in the Selection of Balance Tests

To determine the type and level of challenge of the tests to be used during the examination, a thorough subjective history is critical. In describing the symptoms and the situations that cause dizziness or imbalance, the client offers clues to possible deficits and thereby the measures that will help identify them. Typical components of the history to be included in the evaluation of clients with dizziness are listed in Box 23-2.

Many of the functional scales previously reviewed were designed to determine whether balance is abnormal in elderly clients who have no diagnosis, in other words, as screening tools. Clinicians working with clearly diagnosed neurological clients often do not need such tools to establish that balance skills are abnormal because the deficits are patently obvious. These tools can be useful, however, to identify disabilities, establish a baseline, monitor progress, and document outcomes.

Many clinical facilities have their own therapy evaluation forms that include a section on balance. Items and scoring are usually defined by the facility. They are not standardized across sites, as are published scales, and are rarely tested for measurement quality such as validity and reliability. As rehabilitation professions evolve toward evidence-based practice, nonstandardized tests with unknown measurement quality are no longer acceptable. Clinicians should use standardized, objective, quantifiable, valid tests with high reliability, sensitivity, and specificity whenever possible. Facilities with their own tests should conduct research to ensure that they are valid, reliable, and sensitive to change over time. A functional balance rating scale is important in the evaluation of clients with neurological impairment. To be sensitive enough to measure changes in clients who clearly are not (and may never be) clinically normal, scales should have at least five, and perhaps seven, possible relative scores.

In addition, additional tests are necessary to assess the systems that may affect postural control to help identify and measure impairments (e.g., ROM, strength, sensation and sensory organization, motor planning, and control). These types of measures should be sensitive, objective, and quantifiable. Unfortunately, some systems do not have objective, quantifiable clinical measures (e.g., motor planning, coordination). In these cases, clinicians must continue to use subjective rating scales.

Other factors to include when deciding what tests to use are the time required to perform the test, the number of staff who must be present, and the space and equipment needed. Clinicians must weigh the potential benefits of technological tools (e.g., computerized forceplates, isokinetics, motion analysis, electromyography) against their cost and practicality (i.e., their cost effectiveness). The test must be suitable for the client's level of functioning (physical and cognitive). Many head-injured clients, for example, cannot initially participate in traditional forms of testing because of cognitive limitations.

PROBLEM IDENTIFICATION, GOAL SETTING, AND TREATMENT PLANNING

Clinical Decision Making

Treatment of clients with neurological diagnosis is based on the particular set of impairments and disabilities possessed by each individual. Remediation of balance deficits similarly must be specific to the involved systems and functional losses in each client. Clinicians should generate an overall problem list for each client; if imbalance is a listed problem, then a sublist of balance problems also can be developed (Figure 23-19).

To direct and establish priorities for treatment, clinicians must review the problem list and ask themselves the following questions (Figure 23-20): Which impairments are temporary and can be remedied? How much improvement can be expected? How soon will it occur? Which impairments are permanent and must be compensated for? What other systems can be counted on to substitute? What external compensations may be needed? For example, consider two clients, both with vestibular diagnosis. One client has unilateral peripheral vestibular hypofunction. This situation may be temporary; if permanent, the contralateral vestibular organ may be able to compensate. In either case the use of vestibular inputs for balance control could improve, so exercises to stimulate the vestibular system are indicated. The other client has total bilateral vestibular loss as a result of neurotoxic medication. This condition is permanent and no use of vestibular inputs is possible, so exercises must focus on improving the use of remaining inputs (somatosensory and visual).

With some clients with neurological impairments, knowing whether a problem is permanent or temporary is not possible, as in recovery from a stroke or head injury. In others with progressive diseases such as Parkinson's disease or multiple sclerosis, the rate of decline is unknown and abilities may fluctuate. In these cases the clinician should consider the following issues: Would a consult provide the required information? If so, referral is appropriate. Do any contraindications to treatment exist? What are the risks and benefits of providing versus withholding treatment? Is some amount of functional improvement possible? If no contraindications are present, the benefits outweigh the risks, and functional improvement is expected, then a trial of treatment may be given even if knowing for certain whether the problem(s) will respond to the treatment is not possible. In these cases especially, a baseline must be established against which to measure any change. Change for the worse or no change after a reasonable trial period indicates that treatment should be altered or discontinued.

EXAMPLE OF BALANCE PROBLEM LIST

General Problem List	Balance Problem List
1. Decreased strength (L) side	
2. Decreased ROM (L) shoulder	
3. Decreased endurance	
4. Impaired sensation (L) side	
5. Decreased balance	a. Decreased weight bearing on left (L) LE b. Unable to maintain midline orientation c. Extraneous sway with eyes closed d. Unable to stand on (L) LE e. Decreased limits of stability to 40/100% f. Unable to shift to (L) side g. Unable to establish stable base of support h. Unable to stand on unstable surface i. Unable to perform hip strategy
6. Increased tone (L) side	
7. Synergistic movement (L) side	
8. Min. assist transfers	
9. Mod. assist ambulation	

FIGURE 23-19 ■ An example of a balance-specific problem list (as a subset of a general problem list), which should be developed to guide balance rehabilitation treatments.

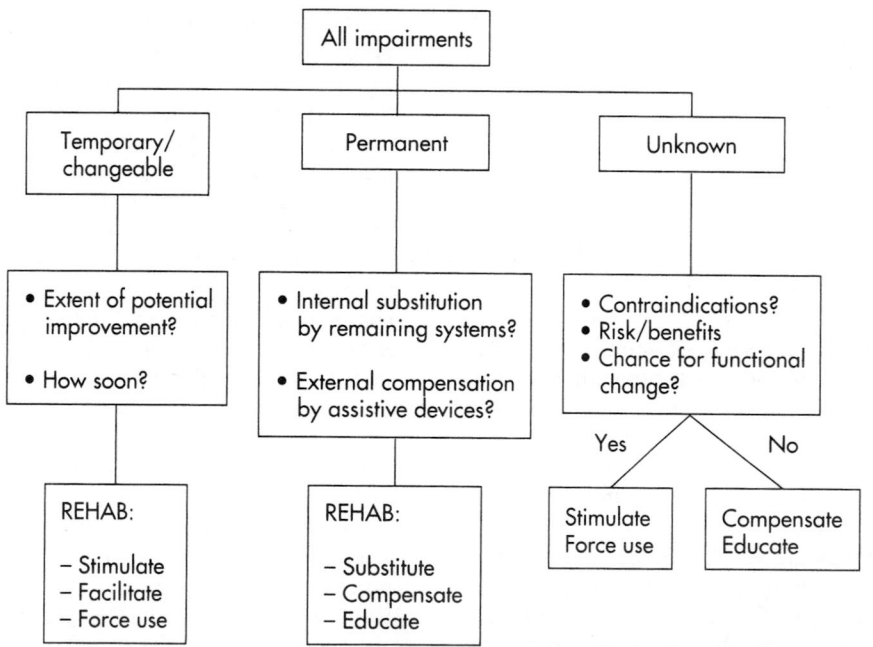

FIGURE 23-20 ■ A clinical decision-making tree to illustrate the treatment planning process in balance rehabilitation.

In some clients with vestibular impairments, the receptors or neurons that were damaged may recover. Spontaneous recovery after unilateral vestibular loss may occur as the resting tone of the system is reestablished and nystagmus is eliminated. Vestibular adaptation occurs when the vestibular system responds to facilitation and recovers function. This takes time and repeated exposure to the appropriate stimuli. Appropriate stimuli include activities that produce an error (mismatch) signal to provoke the brain to make the calibration changes necessary for adaptation.[86]

Using the Systems Model to Identify Postural Control Impairments

The systems approach is useful to develop a balance problem list because it can be applied to different diagnoses equally well and allows deficits in multiple systems to be recognized. Table 23-4 illustrates several examples of ways this framework is used to identify balance deficits in clients with different neurological diagnoses.

For each client, problems affecting postural control should be described in objective, measurable terms whenever possible. For example, the term "impaired vision" is too vague; "four-line drop on eye chart" is more specific. "Poor use of visual inputs for balance control" is an interpretation; the objective result could be stated "Loss of balance after less than 15 seconds on 5/5 trials of standing on foam, eyes open." Documenting problems in this manner makes goal writing (and consequent treatment planning) much easier.

Writing Goals on the Basis of Impairments and Disabilities

Goals also should be stated in objective and measurable terms so that their achievement can be judged. "improved balance" is open to any interpretation, whereas "able to stand on right leg for 30 seconds on 3/3 trials" and "walks tandem entire length of balance beam without misstep 7/10 times" are measurable goals. These types of goals may be helpful to the clinician who understands the link between impairments and function, but they may seem nonfunctional (and therefore unnecessary) to others who read them (e.g., case managers, third-party payers). From their standpoint, incorporating the functional task that will be positively affected by its achievement into the impairment goal is beneficial; for example, "able to stand on right leg for 10 seconds at a time so that stairs can be ascended/descended step-over-step without railing," or "walks tandem on balance beam to demonstrate ability to avoid falls using hip strategy." By describing the impairment/function relation in

the treatment objectives, clinicians force themselves to focus on functional outcomes and illustrate for others why these goals are meaningful. The need for and validity of the treatment are then more likely to be clearly perceived.

If a problem cannot be alleviated and requires compensation, the goal(s) should reflect this as well. For example, a client with diabetes has progressive peripheral neuropathy with somatosensory loss and ineffective ankle strategy. If the client's visual and vestibular sensory systems and proximal strength are relatively intact, however, then the goals might mention improved use of visual cues and successful substitution of hip and stepping strategies. Educational and environmental modification goals for safety also are appropriate in these situations.

Developing a Treatment Plan

Once the goals are listed and priorities are established, the treatment plan is developed. The most effective and efficient treatments focus first on those problems with the greatest impact on function and address more than one problem at a time. Training balance on an unstable surface contributes to the use of visual and vestibular inputs as well as to the use of hip strategy, increased lower-extremity strength, and increased motor control (skill) on that type of surface. Training gait on a treadmill with eyes closed or head movement increases the use of somatosensory and vestibular inputs, endurance, and lower-extremity strength. Creative clinicians develop comprehensive treatment plans with this type of multiple-problem approach to maximize the time available with clients.

The clinician must thoughtfully choose environments and tasks that together stimulate and challenge the appropriate postural control systems. To stimulate one sensory system,

TABLE 23-4 ■ Examples of Impairments and Diagnosis

IMPAIRMENTS FROM SYSTEMS MODEL	CLIENT WITH DIABETIC STROKE	CLIENT WITH PARKINSON'S DISEASE	CLIENT WITH INCOMPLETE PARAPLEGIA
PERIPHERAL SENSORY			
Vision	Retinopathy	Cataracts	
Vestibular		Hair cell loss	
Somatosensory	Peripheral neuropathy	Slowed transmission time	Complete loss
CENTRAL SENSORY			
Vision	Hemianopia	Vision dominant	Needs superior use to compensate
Vestibular	Failure to use inputs		Needs superior use to compensate
Somatosensory	Failure to use inputs	Failure to use inputs	
Strategy selection	Step dominant	Ankle dominant	Hip dominant
Perception of position in space	Midline shift with left neglect	Restricted limits of stability	
CENTRAL MOTOR			
Timing	Increased reaction time	Bradykinesia	
Sequencing	Disordered	Co-contraction	
Force modulation	Spasticity	Rigidity	
Error correction	Use right side only		
PERIPHERAL MOTOR			
Range of motion	Knee hyperextension	Bilateral ankle plantar flexor contractures	Hip flexion contractures
Strength	Decreased left side	Decreased bilateral extremities and trunk	Severe weakness bilateral lower extremities and trunk
Endurance	Severely impaired	Moderately impaired	Mildly impaired

the other systems must be placed at a disadvantage to force reliance on the targeted system. The environment is then structured to put the other systems at a disadvantage (i.e., training with eyes closed or in the dark puts vision at a disadvantage and forces the use of somatosensory and vestibular inputs). If one side or limb is significantly more affected, such as in hemiplegia, then the other side must be disadvantaged to force reliance on the targeted side. Tasks are then selected to disadvantage the less affected side. For example, placing the less affected leg on a step or small ball makes it more difficult to use for balance and forces the transference of weight to the more affected leg. To achieve optimal function, however, all systems and all sides must be capable of working together, so training to improve balance impairments must be incorporated and interspersed with training functional tasks. For carryover of improvements into real-life situations, training tasks should be varied enough to promote motor problem solving on the part of the client.[87] For example, sitting balance and transfers should be taught to stable and unstable surfaces, of different heights and firmnesses, with and without armrests and back supports, or to both right and left sides. This technique may improve the client's abilities to perform safe sitting and transfers in new situations not previously practiced in therapy.[19]

Tables 23-5 through 23-7 illustrate the process of test choice, problem identification based on test results, goal setting based on impairments and disabilities, and treatment planning based on goals in three different types of clients. Note that for each client only selected tests were performed. Goals were directly related to the problems that were identified by the tests, and treatment plans followed directly from the goals.

BALANCE RETRAINING TECHNIQUES

Motor Learning Concepts

Although covering the principles of motor learning is not within the scope of this chapter (refer to Chapters 3 and 9), the discussion of balance retraining methods is not possible without some consideration of several motor learning concepts that must be incorporated into treatment. The clinician must remember that successful treatments address the interaction of the individual, the task, and the environment (Figure 23-21).[17,19]

Individual

Therapists should know their clients' impairments: sensory and motor, peripheral, and central. Whenever possible, therapists should know which impairments can be rehabilitated and which require compensation or substitution. Because of the nature of neurological insult, this includes an awareness of cognitive and perceptual impairments that may affect the ability to relearn old skills or develop new ones. Optimal learning of skilled movement requires that the client have (1) knowledge of self (abilities and limitations), (2) knowledge of the environment (opportunities and risks), (3) knowledge of the task (critical components), (4) the ability to use those knowledge sets to solve motor problems, and (5) the ability to modify and adapt movements as the task and environment change. To the extent that a client is missing these characteristics, the clinician should attempt to support their

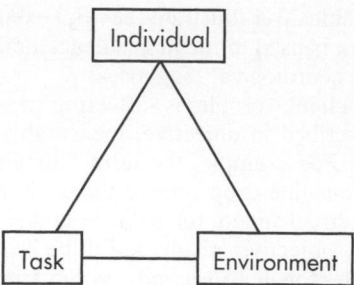

FIGURE 23-21 ■ Interactions of the individual, the environment, and the task are critical to postural control skills. Although they may be isolated in the mind of the clinician for assessment purposes, they are never isolated in the function of the client.

development or even supply them until they are present. Different types of clients vary regarding which characteristics are likely to be missing. For example, a cognitively impaired, head-injured client may lack awareness of self and environment, even though his or her physical abilities make modifying and adapting movements possible. Conversely, a quadriplegic client may be aware of his or her limitations, the environment, and the task demands but may initially have limited experience to know how to solve a motor problem and limited physical ability to modify movements.

The clinician must also ask what motor learning stage the client is in for different tasks. Skill acquisition is the first stage. The objective is for the client to "get the idea of the movement" to begin to acquire the skill.[88] In this stage, errors are frequent and performance is inefficient and inconsistent. Within the nervous system only temporary changes are occurring. Skill refinement is the second stage. The goal is for the client to improve the performance, reduce the number and size of the errors, and increase the consistency and efficiency of the movements. Skill retention is the final stage. The ability to perform the movements and achieve the functional goal has been accomplished, and the new objective is to retain the skill over time and transfer the skill to different settings. Retention and transfer are the hallmarks of true learning, where some relatively permanent changes have occurred within the nervous system. A client may have attained the skill retention phase for sitting balance tasks, be in the skill refinement stage for standing balance tasks, and be in the skill acquisition stage for locomotor balance tasks.

Therapists use practice and feedback to teach motor skills. Repetition is necessary to develop skill; feedback is necessary to detect and correct errors. During skill acquisition, frequent repetition of a movement or task and frequent feedback are beneficial to help the client begin to be able to perform the desired movements and tasks. As soon as the client progresses to the skill refinement stage (the clinician observes reduced errors and less variable performance), however, then practice should be varied and feedback briefly delayed. For example, the task of standing and reaching to one side to take an object from the therapist might initially be repeated to the same side and at the same height several times. Then the therapist should begin to vary the task demands gradually: reach farther or faster; take different objects of various weights, shapes, and sizes; and take the object from higher and lower heights and alternately reach

TABLE 23-5 ■ An Example of Test Selection, Problem Identification, Goal Setting, and Treatment Planning in a Client with Peripheral Vestibular Deficit

Patient profile: 50-year-old woman
Diagnosis: Uncompensated (R) unilateral peripheral vestibular deficit for 6-7 years
Course of examination and treatment: Otolaryngologist → psychologist → neuro-otologist → outpatient PT

TEST	PROBLEMS IDENTIFIED	GOALS SET	TREATMENT PLAN
Visual acuity	Four-line drop on Snellen eye chart	Able to read chart with only one-line drop	Gaze stabilization exercises
Ocular motor: Saccades Pursuit Nystagmus	Positive nystagmus with Frenzel lenses		
Gaze stabilization: Visual/vestibular interaction VOR cancellation	Unable to perform test ↓ Fixation with horizontal+ vertical head movements after 5-10 sec	Able to rotate head horizontally 2 min without problems Able to perform visual/vestibular interaction test	Gaze stabilization exercises
Hallpike SOT	Decreased use of somatosensory inputs 70/100 Decreased use of visual inputs 55/100 Absent use of vestibular inputs 0/100 Unable to resolve visual conflict 0/100	Somatosensory use 100/100 Vision use 90/100 Vestibular use 70/100 Visual conflict resolution 90/100	Sensory environment stimulation
Limits of stability	Restricted anteriorly and posteriorly to 35% limit of stability Slow movement time	Limits of stability expanded to 85% anterior and posterior at 5-sec pacing	COG control training
ROM/strength	None		
Gait: Eyes open Eyes closed Head turning Pivots Abrupt stops	Weaves side to side Deviates to (R) with eyes closed Dizzy with horizontal head turns Loss of balance and dizzy with (R) pivot Very unsteady with abrupt stop; feels "off"	Walks in a straight line with eyes closed Walks with only slight deviation with eyes closed and head turning Spins to (R), (L) with eyes closed Comes to abrupt stop steadily	Gait training

Reprinted with permission from NeuroCom International, Inc., Clackamas, OR.
(L), Left; *(R)*, right.

to right and left sides. This variation introduces a problem-solving demand for the client: modifications in timing, force, and sequencing are now necessary.[87]

Feedback, which is especially helpful for those with sensory reception or perception problems, initially may contain information to assist the client in detecting errors about the goal achievement (knowledge of results, such as "you did not lean far enough to reach this last time") or about a movement error (knowledge of performance, such as "you did not straighten your knee enough last time").[89] Early feedback also may contain cues about what to do better next time, such as "straighten your knee before you shift weight onto that leg." If feedback is always provided by an external source, such as the therapist, a mirror, or a computer monitor, then the client is not given the opportunity to develop internal error detection/error correction mechanisms and will not be as likely to retain or transfer the skill. By delaying the feedback and asking the client to estimate or describe her or his own errors, and afterward providing the feedback, the client is allowed to compare her or his own developing internal frame of reference with the correct external frame of reference. By asking clients to suggest what might be done to correct the errors, the error correction process shifts from the external source to the clients, supporting motor problem-solving processes. As clients progress to the skill retention level, variations should increase (including task and environmental demands) and feedback delays should be longer. The clinician must develop a sense of how to use practice variation and feedback delay therapeutically to progress clients through the stages of motor learning. Too much variation and too little feedback early on impede skill acquisition; insufficient variation and excessive feedback later on hamper skill retention and transfer.

Task

Functional rating scales performed as a part of the evaluation yield information about what tasks, or functional activities, are limited by the postural control impairments. Bed mobility, sitting, sit-to-stand, transfers, standing, walking, working, and sports participation may be affected. Repeat-

TABLE 23-6 ■ **Example of How Treatment Planning Flows from Test Results in an Elderly Client with Frequent Falls**

Patient profile: 72-year-old woman
Diagnosis: Disequilibrium of aging, frequent falls
Course of examination and treatment: Cardiologist → neurologist → outpatient PT

TEST	PROBLEMS IDENTIFIED	GOALS SET	TREATMENT PLAN
Peripheral sensory Somatosensory	Mildly decreased vibration sense bilateral lower extremity	Compensate for permanent sensory loss	Educate about safe surfaces and lighting Home safety evaluation
Vision	↓ Acuity, cataracts ↓ Depth perception		
SOT	Absent use of vestibular inputs 0/100	Increase use of vestibular inputs to 30/100	Somatosensory and vestibular stimulation*
	Decreased use of somatosensory inputs 60/100	Increase use of somatosensory inputs to 75/100	
	Dependent on vision		
Static postural sway	Excessive sway—2 standard deviations outside normal range for age	Standing sway within normal limits for age	COG control training
Nudge/push test	No use of ankle or hip strategy Steps immediately	Survives 5/10 pushes with hip strategy	Hip strategy exercises*
LOS	No ankle strategy—uses hip strategy Sway to 45% LOS anterior, 35% LOS posterior	Uses ankle strategy to reach 40% LOS anterior/posterior Reaches 8/8 targets at 75%	COG control training
	Slow movement time	LOS using hip or ankle strategy within 4 sec	
ROM	↓ Neck extension 0-10 degrees ↓ Lumbar extension 1-15 degrees ↓ Hip extension 0-5 degrees	↑ Spinal extension neck 0-20 degrees ↑ lumbar 0-20 degrees ↑ Hip extension 0-10 degrees	ROM exercises*
Strength	Flexion 4/5 (B) Hip abduction 3+/5, extension 3/5 (B) Knee extension 4+/5, flexion 4/5 (R) Ankle dorsiflexion 3−/5 (L) Ankle dorsiflexion 2/5 (B) Ankle plantar flexion 3+/5	↑(B) Hip abduction/extension to >4/5 ↑ (B) Ankle dorsiflexion and plantarflexion to 4−/5	Progressive resistive exercises, including bicycle*
Gait (GARS)	Score 25/51 Deviations Forward flexed trunk Double limb stance prolonged bilaterally Short step length	GARS scales 35/51 (I) Ambulation with walker in home/community	Gait training* 1—starts, stops, turns 2—treadmill 3—uneven surfaces, curbs, stairs, carpet, outdoors
Endurance	Fatigue after ambulating 60 ft	Ambulates >200 ft without stopping	Gait training as above
Tinetti balance scale	6/16 score	Tinetti balance score 10/16	Gait training as above
Tinetti gait scale	5/12 score Falls and catches self	Tinetti gait score 8/12	Gait training as above

Reprinted with permission from NeuroCom International, Inc., Clackamas, OR.
*Also included in home exercise program.
LOS, Limit of stability; *(B)*, bilateral; *(I)*, independent; *(L)*, left; *(R)*, right.

ing the problematic tasks over and over is one approach; however, analyzing the problematic tasks to determine what postural control demands are placed on the client when undertaking those tasks is far more productive for the clinician. Does a task demand predominantly stability? Mobility? Both? For example, standing to take a photograph demands the ability to hold still, standing to move laundry from the washer to the dryer requires weight shifting, and standing to don a pair of pantyhose calls for both steadiness and movement. All three are standing tasks, but each places different postural control demands on the client. By using task analysis, the therapist may consciously select or design tasks to place specific demands on the client such that the postural control systems that need improvement will be challenged to respond.

Analysis of mobility tasks includes attention to timing, force, and duration of movements. Consider the different timing demands for weight shifting and reaching to catch an item falling from a shelf, take a hot casserole out of the oven, or open a door. Compare the different amounts of force nec-

TABLE 23-7 ■ An Example of How Treatment Planning Flows from Test Results in a Client with Right Hemiparesis

Patient profile: 69-year-old woman
Diagnosis: Left cerebrovascular accident with right hemiparesis
Course of examination and treatment: Acute rehabilitation → home health → outpatient rehabilitation

TEST	PROBLEMS IDENTIFIED	GOALS SET	TREATMENT PLAN
Peripheral somatosensory	None		
SOT	Average overall stability 47/100 Absent use of vestibular inputs 0/100	Average stability 60/100 ↑ Use of vestibular inputs 15/100	Vestibular stimulation with forced use and head movements COG control training
Postural sway			
Functional reach	Forward lean restricted to 5 inches	Able to reach forward 8 inches	

Static balance	Weight shift asymmetry to left in static standing and medial/lateral sway, 25% LOS to left of midline	↑ Control of COG:
		  Stands midline
		    ↑ Forward LOS to 50%
		    ↑ Right LOS to 50%	

Limit of stability	Forward weight shift restricted to 25% LOS	↓ Extraneous sway scores by 50%	
Rhythmic weight shift	Extraneous sway off desired path		
OLST	Unable on right leg 30 seconds on left leg	Stands on right leg, 10 seconds	COG control training
Nudge/push (motor strategy selection)	Switch from ankle to hip strategy noted but unable to withstand perturbation	Able to stand upright after mild perturbations 5/10 times Able to "catch" self by stepping/reaching 5/10 times	Hip and stepping strategy training
Range of motion	None		
Strength: right leg	4/5 Knee extension 3/5 Knee flexion 2/5 Ankle dorsiflexion 3/5 Ankle plantar flexion	↑ RLE strength 5/5 Knee 4/5 Ankle	Progressive resistive exercises
Endurance	Standing tolerance less than 10 minutes	Able to stand unaided for 15 minutes	Standing tolerance tasks
Gait	↓ Step length—RLE ↓ Step height—RLE ↓ Heel strike—RLE ↓ Toe off—RLE	Symmetrical step height and length 5/10 times ↑ Heel strike RLE 5/10 times	Gait training on treadmill

Tinetti gait scale	4/12 score
	Unable to turn, reach, or bend without loss of balance
	Falls:
	  uneven surfaces
	  low lighting
	  head turning
	No community ambulation
	Requires cane
	Requires supervision for household ambulation
		8/12 score
		No falls
		Gait independent without cane in household; with cane in community
			Gait training on uneven surfaces, with head movements, with low lighting
			Safety education

Reprinted with permission from NeuroCom International, Inc., Clackamas, OR.
LOS, Limit of stability; *RLE,* right lower extremity.

essary to pick up a heavy suitcase, pick up a baby from a crib, or replace a ceiling light bulb. The duration of a balance demand may be brief, as in recovering from a trip, or extended, as in walking across an icy parking lot. Clinicians should choose tasks that vary these parameters to prepare clients for activities with various mobility demands. Activities that incorporate changing head positions will further challenge the individual with vestibular insufficiency.

Therapists also need to consider whether the elements of the task are predictable or unpredictable. In other words, will the postural control demand be a voluntary movement (e.g., sweeping the porch), an automatic postural response (e.g., missing the last step on a flight of stairs), or an anticipatory postural adjustment (e.g., preceding a lift)? Clients need to learn to respond in all three conditions, which are often combined. For instance, lifting is a voluntary movement. Predicting the load to be lifted leads to anticipatory postural preparation. Counteracting the destabilizing force of a greater-than-predicted load requires an automatic postural response. If, during therapy, the clinician says "don't let me push you" before nudging the client, the demand is for anticipatory postural adjustment. If the disturbance is provided without warning, the demand calls for automatic postural reactions. If the clinician requests a lean to the right, that is a voluntary postural adjustment. Activities that demand all three types of balance control, either one at a time or in combination, should be included in balance retraining programs.

Environment

Just as tasks can be purposefully selected to promote postural control responses, environmental conditions also must be included in the design of the therapy plan to stimulate the necessary systems. Gravity cannot be manipulated by the clinician, but the client needs to learn to counteract it at different speeds and from different positions, among other things. Familiarity with how gravity can aid movement, as in walking, is also important. The therapist can vary the surface conditions. They may be stable, even, and predictable (hospital hallway, sidewalk), unstable (boat, subway, gravel driveway), uneven (grass, curbs, stairs), or compliant (beach, padded carpeting). Visual conditions also may be manipulated. Visual cues may be available and accurate (daylight, fluorescent lighting), unavailable (darkness or poor lighting, or lack of environmental cues such as a busy carpet pattern on a stairway), unstable (moving crowd, public transportation), used for purposes other than balance (fixation on a ball in tennis), or dependent on head movements. Clinicians should help prepare their clients to function in the real world by training them to maintain balance under different combinations of surface and visual conditions. This includes situations where cues from the environment agree; that is, visual, somatosensory, and vestibular inputs are all sending the same message, so to speak, as well as in sensory conflict environments, where cues from one system may disagree (not match) with cues from the other sensory systems. Functional situations where sensory conflicts may exist include elevators, escalators, people movers, airplanes, and subways. An emphasis on being able to adapt to changes rapidly and effectively in environmental conditions is also important.

Intervention

Successful intervention for the individual with a balance disorder or dizziness depends on the ability of the clinician to identify the components of the problem. The therapist must create a program that addresses several components at a time, not just for efficiency, but because these systems should be able to function together to perform functional activities in real-world environments. Treatment is oriented toward multiple impairments, with tasks and environments selected to best stimulate involved or compensatory systems.

The intervention must be matched to the level and combination of impairments. For example, tasks related to the different functions of the vestibular system should be identified and not treated as a single impairment. The clinician should have a good idea of the level of stimulus during each exercise program so that the facilitation is as accurate as possible. Progression of the program follows the changes seen from one intervention to the next, and the exercise progression integrates activities that reflect those changes. This usually involves more complex movement skills in a greater range of gradually more challenging environments.

Sensory Systems

In general, the less sensory information available, the more difficult the task of balancing. A treatment progression might therefore start with full sensory inputs (vision, somatosensory, and vestibular: 3/3) available in the environment and perhaps augmented feedback if intrinsic sensory channels are deficient, as with somatosensory loss or a vestibular disorder. Challenge is added by manipulating either visual or somatosensory inputs, so that equilibrium must be maintained by using only two of three senses (vision and vestibular or somatosensory and vestibular). If both vision and somatosensory inputs are manipulated, then only the vestibular inputs are a reliable source of sensory information and balance is accomplished with only one of three senses.[57]

Most patients with vestibular or somatosensory losses naturally compensate and become visually dependent. In cases in which improving the use of somatosensory or vestibular inputs is necessary, the training of vision for stability can be counterproductive. On the other hand, visual retraining is entirely appropriate for the client with severely compromised somatosensation, as is common in persons with diabetes, and in the individual who has completely lost vestibular function, which rarely occurs. If an oculomotor dysfunction contributes to dizziness and imbalance, it should be corrected as quickly as possible. Clinicians should then progress to challenging the client with activities to reintegrate vision for balance.

To stimulate the use of visual inputs, environments are designed to disadvantage somatosensation while providing reliable visual cues (stable visual field with landmarks). Somatosensation cannot be removed as can vision, but it can be destabilized by sitting or standing on unstable surfaces (rocker board, biomechanical ankle platform system [BAPS] board, randomly moving platforms) or confused by sitting or standing on compliant surfaces that give way to pressure, such as foam, "space boots," or responsively moving platforms.

To stimulate the use of somatosensory inputs, environments are designed to disadvantage vision while providing reliable somatosensory inputs (stable surfaces). Having the client close the eyes or practice in low lighting or darkness removes or decreases visual inputs. For clients with an over-reliance on visual input for balance, the somatosensory system needs to be facilitated while the visual system is disrupted. This can be accomplished by having the client sit or stand on a stable surface while performing quick head turns. For the client with self-limited head movement, the intervention may begin with head movement during quiet standing and progress to head movements during weight shifts and then walking. Eyes-closed standing and weight shifting also increase the use of somatosensation for balance. Optokinetic stimuli in the visual surround stimulate use of somatosensory inputs and replicate the "grocery store dizziness" phenomenon.

In some clients the integration of vestibular and somatosensory inputs is so poor that they are not congruent even at rest. This results in the sensation of movement inside the head when the body is held at rest in supported sitting. In this instance, enhancing the somatosensory input by weighting through the spinal column or having the patient lie on a firm surface should be part of the initial intervention. This allows the vestibular system to calibrate appropriately to a zero level, which can then be facilitated from that point. On the other hand, if the use of weights increases the sensation of movement, the clinician should suspect abnormal central sensory weighting of somatosensory inputs.

To stimulate the use of vestibular inputs for adaptation of the CNS, environments are designed to disadvantage both vision and somatosensation while providing reliable vestibular cues (detectable head position). Practicing on unstable or compliant surfaces, with vision either absent (eyes closed), destabilized (eye movements or head movements), or confused (e.g., optokinetic stimulation) provides challenging combinations. Adding neck extension and rotation to place the vestibular organ at a disadvantaged angle can increase difficulty.

Adaptation of the VOR is accomplished by having the client move his or her head while trying to maintain gaze stabilization (keeping a stationary object in clear focus).[90,91] The speed of head movement is gradually increased, with the goal of achieving head movement at 2 Hz (cycles per second) without the object blurring. Initially, the client can focus on the thumb or a business card held at arm's length. The activity is progressed to a higher level of difficulty by adding background visual stimulus such as a television set or a visually complex environment. Gaze stabilization with head turns while standing on an uneven surface or while walking creates a higher-level challenge. Many clients have avoided head movement, so simply turning the head may initially trigger dizziness. Dizziness with head motion should not be confused with abnormal VOR; the criteria for VOR dysfunction is eyes that are not able to keep the object steady during testing.

The VSR is facilitated when the vestibular system is the primary input for balance, as is required during quick head displacements or motions, such as the increased head velocity after a person has tripped (VSR used to recover balance). For the vestibular inputs to become primary, both somatosensory and visual inputs must be placed at a disadvantage, as previously described. For example, the vestibular system becomes the primary input when the surface is compliant or the base of support is narrow (tandem or single-leg stance) and visual cues are unstable. Quick movements of the head, head tilts, or forward bending triggers vestibular signals to add input to the system. Combining these types of activities can create progressively more complex challenges. Standing on foam with eyes closed, weight shifts with eyes closed, and head and eye movement while walking all require vestibular input for successful performance.

Certain positions or movements of the head during upright activities can affect balance if abnormal function of just one part of the vestibular system is present. If the otoliths are damaged or hypersensitive, a voluntary lateral tilt of the head when standing with the eyes closed can cause destabilization. Deficient otolith function should also be suspected if ineffective head righting responses are seen during sharpened Romberg or standing on a narrow surface. When the position of the head cannot be accurately determined through vestibular inputs, the individual will attempt to use somatosensory inputs from the cervical spine, usually combined with visual inputs, to determine head position. Activities that require quick changes of position in a superior or inferior direction, such as a lunge or going up and down stairs, can also be difficult when the otoliths are damaged. Good program components for otolith stimulation are activities involving up-and-down body movements. Examples include sit-to-stand, seated bouncing on a Swiss ball, and standing bouncing on a mini-trampoline, all with eyes closed to eliminate use of vision for stability.

When the use of vestibular inputs has been minimized through self-limitation of head and eye movements to control dizziness and imbalance, the visual system often becomes dominant for balance. To train the client to use vestibular input versus vision, activities such as watching a ball being tossed from hand to hand while walking, walking backward, or walking with eye movements can be used. Clients with visual dependency often report excessive fatigue after activity because of the strain of using vision for postural stability. When these clients are in situations with excessive visual stimulation, reports of dizziness increase. The subtle eye movements associated with viewing a computer monitor cause more fatigue for the individual with vestibular disorder. These individuals also often avoid crowds as in a mall, grocery store, or airport. Attending church services, which are often characterized by low lighting, visual stimulation, and the need to stand with eyes closed or read a hymnal while singing challenges the vestibular system.

A vestibular adaptation program should challenge the patient at the limit of his or her ability. Clients often choose to do the easiest exercise and avoid the more difficult exercises if they are not educated about the need to trigger the symptoms. Conversely, if the challenge is too far above the ability of the patient, the CNS will fail to adapt.

Positional Dizziness

When the Hallpike-Dix test position indicates BPV, specific, highly effective procedures can be performed in the clinical setting to remediate the disorder.[59,92] Canalith repositioning is a series of passive movements designed to move loose debris (otoconia) through the canal and back into the otolith (Figure 23-22). The client is first brought down into the

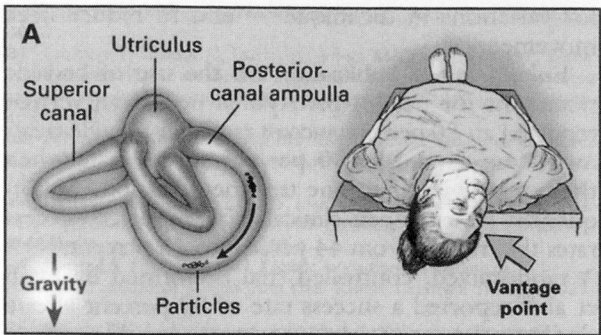

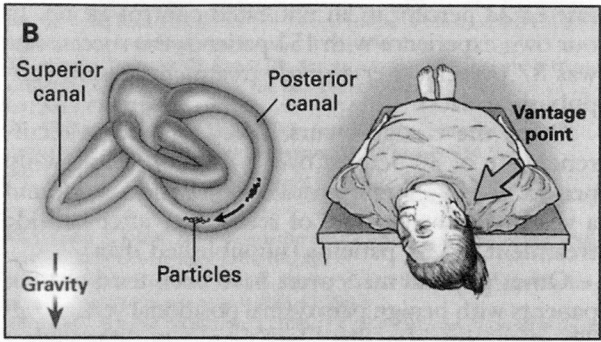

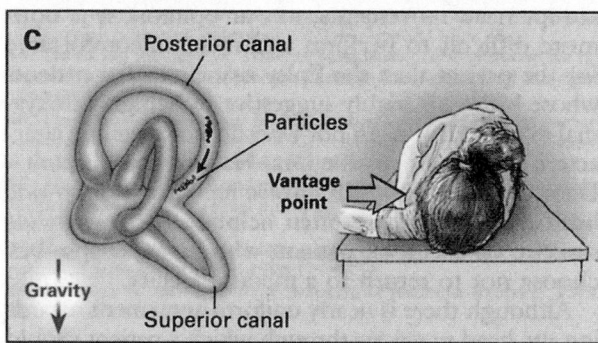

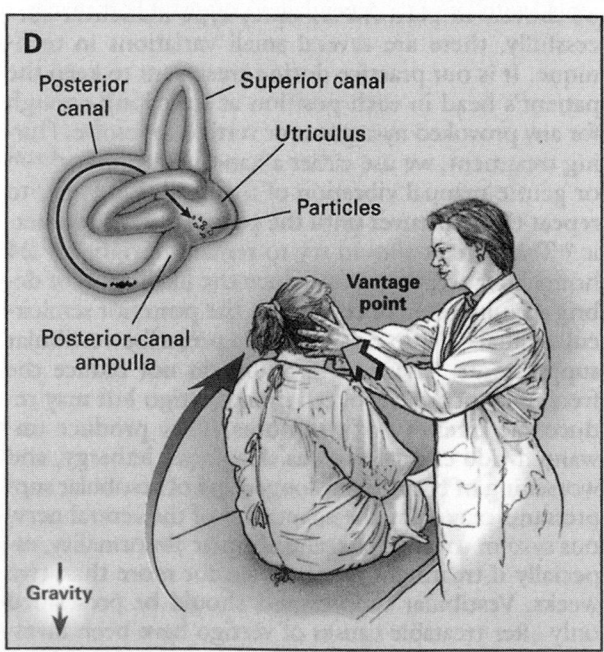

FIGURE 23-22 ■ Canalith repositioning maneuver for the patient with posterior canal BPV. Figure represents procedure for right-side BPV. Movement of particles through the canal is shown in each position. (From Furman JM, Cass SP: Benign paroxysmal positional vertigo, *N Engl J Med* 341:1590-1596, 1999. Copyright 1999 Massachusetts Medical Society. All rights reserved.)

extended and rotated position that causes the nystagmus and vertigo (the positive Hallpike-Dix position). The head is held in that position until the symptoms fade completely or for 60 to 90 seconds. The head is maintained in extension and then slowly rotated toward the unaffected side and kept in that position for an additional 1 to 2 minutes to allow movement of the otoconia through the canal. The client then rolls so that she or he is side-lying and the head is turned to a 45-degree position relative to the ground. This position often produces more vertigo and nystagmus as the otoconia continue to move through the canal. In the next movement, the head is tipped toward the chest and the client is assisted into the sitting position. The client must then follow specific instructions for 48 hours. These include avoiding forward, backward, or lateral head tilts or bending activities. Clients should also sleep with the head elevated to at least 30 degrees and avoid turning to the involved side.[55]

When the BPV is within the horizontal canal, dizziness or vertigo is reported when rolling, especially if the head is elevated on a pillow because that puts the canal in a position perpendicular to the ground. The symptoms are reported when the head is turned in either direction, but the side that triggers the worst symptoms is thought to be the side of the dysfunction.[93] The repositioning intervention then begins with the client supine with the head turned toward the most affected ear. The head is then turned away from the affected ear and the client is slowly rolled 360 degrees (essentially staying in the same place) until the head is returned to the original position. The client sits back up with the head tucked. Side tilts of the head, as well as forward and backward movements of the head and trunk, are avoided for 2 days.

Position-provoked dizziness that does not appear to be BPV may be related to canal sensitivity or abnormal firing through the brain stem. In this case, exercises should be done to increase the client's tolerance to the provoking position(s). This involves having the client perform the provoking positions to give the CNS the opportunity to adjust to the sensation that the position triggers. Spinning in a chair can help adapt when stimulation to the horizontal mechanism is disrupted or when maladaptation of the input of one labyrinth is present compared with the other. In addition to exercise sessions, incorporating the provoking positions into daily activities is also important.

Multisensory and Motor Control Dysfunction

Older clients often have dysfunction in all three sensory systems. Disease-related disruptions of the somatosensory or visual systems (e.g., a peripheral neuropathy or cataracts) are combined with age-related declines in the vestibular system. In some cases therapy aimed at increasing vestibular function can have a significant impact on postural stability. If the vestibular system cannot adapt, the client is classified as having a multisensory balance disorder. If sensory loss is permanent or progressive, safe function may require the use of an assistive device.[94] Choosing an assistive device for these clients can be a challenge. A single cane often does not allow for compensation for changes in direction of an impending fall, and a standard aluminum walker does not provide support when changing directions because it must be lifted. The ideal walker has four rotating wheels and thus the ability to change direction without being lifted. This device greatly increases stability, and the client usually describes a significant increase in confidence. Of course, the use of a walker also limits normal use of the upper extremities and trunk during gait and restricts the types of environments that can be negotiated.

Many neurological clients have temporary difficulty with head control early on in their recovery, and others have chronic head control problems. Their ability to orient the vestibular organs, eyes, and neck proprioceptors properly is impaired, which negatively affects the ability to perceive internal and environmental cues that could assist in balance maintenance. Clients with spasticity or contractures of the ankles and feet who cannot place their feet in full contact with the floor are at a biomechanical disadvantage and also have difficulty receiving somatosensory inputs that could support postural control processes. The more accurate and reliable sensory information available, the greater the chances that the sensoriperceptual processes that contribute to balance can fulfill their role. Treatment progressions should include attention to increasing the client's ability to receive and process sensory information pertinent to balance control through oculomotor, head, and peripheral limb positioning and movement.

Control of the Center of Gravity. Effective control of the COG depends on accurate awareness of body position and motion in space and the relation between body parts (perception) as well as biomechanical and musculoskeletal systems (execution). Trunk and head control abilities are primary. For clients with paralysis or degenerative disease that limits the ability of arms and legs to assist with postural stability, head and trunk control may be the dominant means of balance. Both the head and neck and trunk need to be able to achieve and hold a midline position, rotate around this midline axis, and move away from and return to the midline without loss of balance. The term "midline" here refers not to a line between right and left sides, but to a point where right/left and forward/backward components are centered in all planes—medial/lateral, anterior/posterior, rotary, and side bending (shortening/elongation on either side).

Sitting Balance. In sitting, the pelvis and posterior thighs form the primary base of support, with additional stability provided by the feet in contact with the floor. The axis of anteroposterior movement rotates around the greater trochanter, and forward/backward leans are achieved through pelvic and trunk movement. Anterior pelvic tilt with upper trunk extension allows forward reaching and begins the sit-to-stand transition. Lateral weight shifts with trunk elongation precede right/left reaching and scooting. Lateral weight shifts with trunk rotation permit cross-midline reaching and begin the sit-to-supine progression. The use of arms to prop in sitting is an extension of the base of support.

In standing, the feet form the base of support. The axis of anteroposterior movement rotates around the medial malleolus. Weight shifts move the COG through space for reaching and lifting tasks as well as in preparation for stepping. Ankle strategy is most effective for movement of the COG through the limits of stability on a stable surface. As the COG nears the sway boundary, hip strategy works to restrict its travel. If this fails, stepping or reaching strategies are used to reestablish a new base of support. During gait, the COG follows a sinusoidal path as forward progression of the body mass combines with alternating lateral weight shifts to the stance foot (Figure 23-23).[30] Each step creates

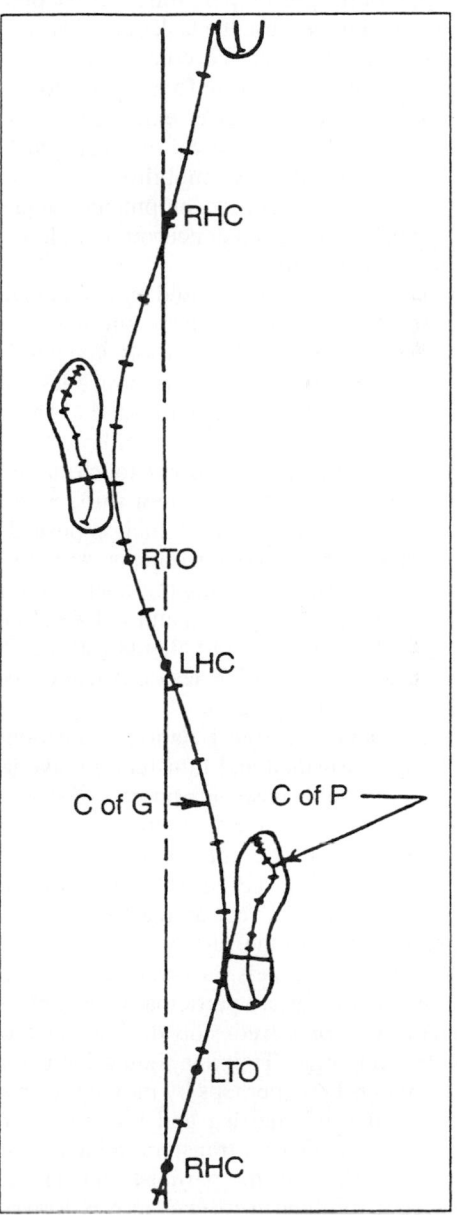

FIGURE 23-23 ■ The trajectory of the COG *(C of G)* and the center of pressure *(C of P)* during a gait cycle. *RHC,* Right heel contact; *RTO,* right toe-off; *LHC,* left heel contact; *LTO,* left toe-off. (From Palia AE et al: Identification of age-related changes in the balance control system. In Duncan P, editor: *Balance: Proceedings of the APTA forum,* Alexandria, VA, 1990, American Physical Therapy Association.)

a new base of support. Assistive devices such as canes, walkers, and crutches extend the base of support and thus reduce the demands on the intrinsic balance control system. In sitting, standing, and walking, control of the COG involves the ability to establish a stable base of support and transfer weight over it. Treatment progressions for COG control then involve training to establish, maintain, and reduce the base of support and to produce automatic, anticipatory, and voluntary postural responses to restrict or produce weight shifts.

Early treatment progression for COG control includes neurodevelopmental sequence activities (e.g., prone on elbows, all fours, kneeling, right/left side sitting, half-kneeling), not for the purpose of "reflex development" in the traditional sense but because the task demands are to balance with progressively less surface contact (i.e., shrinking the base of support). It also is useful for simultaneously addressing impairments such as lower-extremity extensor tone, trunk weakness and asymmetries, and head/neck extensor weakness. Functionally, bed mobility and floor-to-stand transfers are related to neurodevelopmental sequence exercises and should be practiced concurrently in low- and high-level clients, respectively.

Sitting balance can be progressed by (1) removing upper-extremity support (hands on firm surface to moveable surface [e.g., ball, bolster, rolling stool], one hand free, both hands free); (2) making the seating surface less stable (mat to bed to rocker board to Swiss ball); and (3) removing the use of one foot by crossing the leg or of both feet by raising the height of the seat so they do not touch the floor. Tasks might include multidirectional weight shifts with the hands in contact with a bolster or ball, which is pushed or pulled to and fro, reaching or passing objects, upper body tasks (grooming, dressing), and managing socks and shoes and wheelchair armrests and footrests, and so forth. Sitting activities can be the best place to start clients with vestibular dysfunction because they involve less challenge and a lower demand for sensory integration.

Sit-to-Stand and Transfer Balance. Transitional movements such as sit-to-stand and transfers involve large COG excursions over a stable base of support. For sit-to-stand, the base of support must change from the seat to the feet. The feet begin to accept the weight first by downward pressure through the heels as the pelvis rolls anterior. The weight moves to the front of the feet as the trunk comes forward and the pelvis lifts from the surface, then backward toward midline as the trunk extends into standing. The COG stays near midline if both legs are participating equally, but it will often deviate to a preferred side during the transition in clients with hemiplegia. Training should include disadvantaging the preferred leg (perhaps by moving it a bit forward) to allow the more affected leg and foot to experience the weight transference. During transfers, a lateral weight shift is required in addition to the partial stand. The COG does not remain near midline; it instead moves forward to load the feet and then laterally toward the side of the transfer. Progression of balance skills in sit-to-stand and transfer tasks may involve gradually lowering the height of the surface, removing armrests to preclude upper-extremity assist, and transferring to surfaces of different heights and firmnesses. Remember that velocity is a normal part of sit-to-stand movements because the momentum is used to assist the weight transfer from seat to feet, so the clinician must allow some speed during this task. If the client is unsteady on arising (cannot dampen or slow the speed in a controlled manner), working gradually from stand-to-sit initially may be beneficial before progression to sit-to-stand. Practice of sit-to-stand with the eyes closed can be an effective way to train clients who are overdependent on vision for balance. Without the use of vision for stability, integration of vestibular and somatosensory systems can be facilitated.

Standing Balance. Standing balance tasks also can begin with finding midline and becoming stable there. Controlled mobility (volitional) should be encouraged as soon as possible, first on a stable surface with slow, small weight shifts. Challenge is added by increasing the distance traveled away from midline, moving toward restricted regions of the limits of stability, altering speed of sway, adding combined upper-extremity activities (e.g., dribbling a basketball, reaching), and adding resistance (manual, flexible bands). Narrowing the base of support (Romberg, tandem, single leg) makes control of the COG more demanding. Placing the feet in a diagonal stride position is more desirable for pregait weight shifting than is symmetrical double stance. Attention should be given to the stance (loading) leg regarding pelvic protraction, hip and knee extension, and ankle dorsiflexion, with the tibia traveling forward over the foot. Focus on the swing (unloading) leg should include pelvic drop with knee flexion as the heel comes up and pressure through the ball of the foot and toes to load the opposite leg maximally. Standing balance exercises can be made more difficult by training on a less stable surface (carpet, foam, rocker board, BAPS board) and by adding combined head/eye movement tasks or closing the eyes. The goals for dynamic sitting and standing balance exercises are to increase the size and symmetry of the limits of stability and improve the ability to transfer weight to different body segments with control at different speeds and with varied amounts of force. To facilitate somatosensory and vestibular integration, these activities can be performed with decreased or distorted visual cues. Closing the eyes, turning the head quickly, turning the lights down low, or wearing sunglasses may decrease the use of vision for stabilization.

Strategy Training. Training ankle, hip, and stepping strategies may begin in a voluntary manner but must progress to an automatic level of use to develop more normal balance and prevent loss of balance. Before strategy training, the clinician should be sure that the client has the ability to develop the desired strategies. The observed dominance of other strategies is appropriately compensatory, not dysfunctional, if a missing strategy cannot be effectively executed. Clients use these strategies to prevent loss of balance, so the clinician must take care not to reduce reliance on an effective strategy but to add additional strategies to the repertoire.

Ankle strategy should be practiced on a firm, broad surface. Clients can be asked to sway slowly in anterior/posterior, right/left, and diagonal directions, first to and from midline, progressing to passing midline, and finally progressing to sway toward the periphery without return to midline. Head and pelvis should be traveling in the same direction at the same time. Clients can practice standing near a wall with a table in front of them, swaying forward to touch the table with the stomach (leading with the pelvis) and backward to touch the wall with the back of the head. Cues are given not to "bow" to the table and not to touch the wall with the buttocks. As soon as the client is able to perform this protocol, functional meaning should be added with maneuvers such as forward or lateral reaching tasks, hands over head to take things off shelves, and leaning backward to rinse hair in the shower. To improve anticipatory and automatic ankle strategy use, add slight perturbations to the body or the surface when midline, progress to gentle perturbation when away from midline, and finally progress from predictable to unpredictable perturbations.

Hip strategy is practiced on a narrow surface, such as standing sideways on a balance beam, 2 × 4, or a half-slice foam roller or on an unstable surface such as foam or a rocker board. The head and pelvis travel in opposite directions to counterbalance each other, in a forward bow/backward bending motion for anterior/posterior sway. Rapid sway is requested in forward/backward, right/left, and diagonal directions. By using the wall and table setting previously mentioned, clients can be cued to bow to touch the nose toward the table while simultaneously touching the wall with the buttocks. Lateral hip strategy can be trained similarly, with the client standing sideways to the wall, touching the table with one hip and the wall with the opposite shoulder. Sway close to the edge of the client's limit of stability should produce a shift from ankle to hip strategy, so to enhance the use of hip strategy the client should practice sway control as far away from midline as possible without stepping. As soon as the client demonstrates the ability to perform this strategy, it should be incorporated into functional tasks such as low reaching (e.g., trunk of car, laundry dryer). To promote anticipatory and automatic use of hip strategy, the client is in midline and given moderate, rapid perturbations to the body or the surface such that ankle strategy will be insufficient to counteract the force. Then the size of the disturbance is increased, and the client is positioned away from midline when the perturbation is given so that righting to midline is appropriate. The shift should be made from predictable ("don't let me make you step or fall") to unpredictable perturbations. Stepping strategy can be practiced first from atop a step, curb, or balance beam. Both legs should be included in training because real-life situations such as a slip or trip often preclude the use of one limb and demand the use of the other. Progress is made by stepping on a level surface and then to stepping up onto a step or curb or over progressively larger obstacles (appliance cord, shoe, phone book). All directions should be practiced. Large, rapid perturbations are given such that ankle and hip strategies will be inadequate and stepping/reaching is demanded. Again, progress should be made from predicted to unpredictable disturbances.

When the head righting reflex is inadequate, clients are reluctant to move into hip and stepping strategy because of the rapid head movement. The result is an overreliance on the upper extremities for balance responses that allows stability without movement of the head. Therapeutic activities should provide the maximal level of challenge that can be managed without the need for upper extremity support. If the client needs to hold on, then the activity is at too high a level and should be modified. Otherwise, what is being taught is a "hand strategy" that will not be useful if the client experiences loss of balance when nothing firmly fixed is available to grasp for stability. Extremely anxious clients may initially benefit from training with an overheard harness system that will permit hands-free motion but prevent a fall if balance loss occurs.

Gait Training. The initial focus for controlling the COG during gait is a stable base of support that can be continually reestablished quickly and reliably through stepping. Unlike standing balance, where the base is stable and the COG moves over it, during locomotion the base is moving and the COG moves to stay over the base. Achieving a symmetrical, smoothly oscillating COG movement is the objective, with the forces of gravity and momentum being exploited.

The training is begun first in the forward direction but also includes backward and sideways directions (sidestepping, braiding, or karaoke) to increase postural control demands. Challenge can be added by narrowing the base of support (tandem) or reducing the foot/surface contact (walk on toes or heels). Training to integrate postural control with locomotor skills is best accomplished not through continuous, steady pace walking, but by starting, stopping, turning, bending, varying the speed, and avoiding or stepping over obstacles. Difficulty is added by increasing the abruptness, frequency, and unpredictability of these types of tasks and by adding tasks such as carrying or reading while walking. Altered surface conditions (carpets, ramps, curbs, stairs, grass, gravel) or reduced lighting conditions also heighten the challenge. Head and eye movements while walking should be added as the client improves. Walking quickly while reading signs on the wall or room numbers, for example, or looking toward and away from the therapist while walking makes vision more difficult to use for stability. Walking in crowds or in busy, cluttered environments is also challenging. Locomotion training on the treadmill reduces some abnormal asymmetries and increases control of gait with increased extension of the trailing limb.[95]

Gait with head motion is important for the individual with vestibular dysfunction. Because head movement causes visual disturbances and dizziness, the client with a vestibular disorder will significantly limit head movement while walking. When visual cues are used predominantly for balance, the client will try to keep the body in line with vertical and horizontal visual targets. This will decrease the small, natural movements typically made during the gait cycle. Clients with potentially recoverable vestibular function should be trained to walk with eye and head movements, trunk rotation, and arm swing.

Permanent bilateral vestibular loss, however, requires superior use of somatosensation and vision to orient to the environment. Use of a cane or walking stick to increase use of somatosensation and allow more time to prepare for the next step can increase confidence in gait. Spatial memory and navigation deficits can develop over time in the client with bilateral vestibular loss because of changes in the hippocampus. This may contribute to difficulties with the patient's ability to move through environments that may have once been familiar.[96]

When the vestibular system does not accurately inform the client about the speed and direction of head movement, visual cues are used to determine movement speed and direction in relation to nonmoving objects. However, in environments with a lot of motion, or when someone approaches in the opposite direction, determining speed and direction of self-movement becomes more difficult. Clients often report dizziness and imbalance in a crowd. Changing visual environments can trigger imbalance in the client with visual dependency. Walking into a darkened room, especially if the surface is uneven (such as in a theater), can often trigger a fall or stumble. Clients with permanent vestibular loss should be educated about these potentially high-risk environments and taught compensatory strategies to ensure safe mobility. If improvement in vestibular function is anticipated, however, then progressive exposure to these busy environments is needed to prepare the client for real-world mobility.

To increase somatosensory input, clients with a vestibular disorder often put the whole foot down at once to get better input on the position of the body relative to the ground. The normal heel-toe weight progression over the ball of the foot is diminished. This is often seen in conjunction with increased step width while walking. This compensatory strategy is acceptable in clients with permanent loss but should be discouraged in those clients who do not need to be overreliant on somatosensation for balance control during walking. Walking on uneven surfaces can be a challenge if the client is primarily reliant on somatosensory input and has poor visual-vestibular interaction. This is one reason why walking indoors is less of a problem than walking outdoors. Again, clients who are not expected to recover vestibular function should be educated about these potentially hazardous environments and encouraged to develop compensatory mechanisms to permit safe mobility. Gait training on progressively less-stable surfaces is appropriate for clients who need to reduce overreliance on somatosensory cues and improve visual-vestibular interaction.

Other Considerations

Treatment Tools. Therapists use both high-technological and low-technological equipment in the remediation of balance deficits; each has advantages and disadvantages. High-technological options include forceplate systems with postural sway biofeedback, electromyographic biofeedback, optokinetic visual stimulation (from visual surround or moving lights), videotaping, and treadmills. Computerized systems allow advanced monitoring of progress and biofeedback, which supports motor learning.[97] Motorized systems provide the ability to manipulate the environment easily and efficiently and to graduate tasks and environmental challenges safely. Drawbacks to high-technological equipment include cost, space requirements, and operator training requirements. Low-technological options include mirrors, soft foam pads, hard foam rollers, rocker boards, BAPS boards, tilt boards, Swiss balls, mini-trampolines, balance beams, and wedges/incline boards. All these items are accessible (low cost, easy to obtain), portable, and easy to use. They do not provide novel feedback, objective scoring, or graphic recording; and clinicians must be skilled and creative in their use for appropriate gradation of task difficulty and environmental conditions.

Safety Education and Environmental Modifications. Remediation of balance deficits is not always possible, but the clinician is responsible for ensuring the safety of each client. When permanent deficits exist, the client and the family should be taught in what environments the client is at risk (e.g., a client with vestibular loss on a gravel driveway at night), what tasks are unsafe (e.g., ladder climbing, changing ceiling light bulbs), how the client can compensate (e.g., use a cane at night or in crowds), and what changes in the home or workplace are needed (e.g., night lights, stair stripes). Clinicians can ask the client (or family) to problem solve risky situations. What would the client do? Home evaluations should be followed by a list of recommended safety modifications. Falls are frightening and dangerous; clinicians should do their utmost to prevent them. If falls are likely, clients and families should be taught what to do if a fall occurs, including floor-to-stand or floor-to-furniture transfers. Home monitoring services such as LifeLine may be indicated if the client lives alone and is prone to falling. Hip protectors will not prevent falls but do significantly reduce the risk of hip fracture.

Home Programs. Strengthening, stretching, posture, and endurance exercises can all be performed safely at home so that time in the clinic can be spent on balance challenge exercises requiring supervision. Improvements in strength, ROM, posture, and endurance support improvements in balance. Many balance exercises can and should be performed at home if safety and compliance can be ensured; however, *unstable clients should always be supervised.* Standing balance tasks can be completed in a corner or near a countertop so that *in case of balance loss* the client can use the hands (reaching strategy) to prevent a fall if other automatic postural response strategies are inadequate. However, balance exercises should not be routinely done while holding onto countertops, furniture, or other surfaces. If the client needs to use her or his hands to perform the balance task, the task is too difficult and should be modified so that it can be safely performed without needing to hang on to a stable object. The community setting is ideal for postural control gait training. Grocery or library aisles, public transportation, elevators, escalators, grass, sandboxes or beaches, ramps, trails, hills, and varied environmental conditions in general provide both challenge and functional relevance.

Concurrent Tasks. Normal balance is largely subconscious. One objective in balance retraining is to force the nervous system to solve postural control problems at the automatic, subconscious level. A great deal of practice and dual-task training are necessary to accomplish this; the conscious brain is focused on accomplishing some other goal(s) and thus balance control must be achieved at a less-conscious level. Alternative tasks can be physical in nature, such as carrying a tray or dribbling a basketball, or cognitive, such as conversing or solving verbal or math problems, or a combination of physical and cognitive demands.

CASE STUDIES

Three case studies have been included to help the reader understand some of the issues, problems and solutions for individuals with various types of vestibular and balance problems.

CASE STUDY 23-1 ■ ANDY

Andy is a 27-year-old man who sustained a severe closed-head injury in a skiing accident. He was hospitalized for 2 months and resided at a long-term care facility for 6 months before cranial surgery for removal of bilateral subdural hygromas and revision of a ventriculoperitoneal shunt. After surgery he demonstrated marked improvement and was transferred to a rehabilitation unit. His initial physical therapy assessment revealed the following impairments, which had a negative effect on postural control:

1. Oculomotor deficits (difficulty tracking to the right and upward)
2. Disorientation
3. Delayed and slow responses
4. Bilateral ankle plantar flexion contractures (1 to 10 degrees left, 1 to 15 degrees right); limited right shoulder flexion (0 to 100 degrees) and external rotation (0 to 20 degrees)
5. Hypotonic trunk (right, moderate; left, mild), hypertonic (extensor) lower extremities (right, moderate; left, mild), hypertonic right upper extremity (mild)
6. Fair head control
7. Poor trunk control with right scapular atrophy, shortened right side, strength 3–/5
8. Left upper and lower extremity movement isolated and coordinated but slow, strength 4/5 at shoulder, 4+/5 elbow/wrist/hand, 4/5 hip and knee, 3+/5 ankle, able to place and hold for weight bearing
9. Right upper extremity rests and moves in synergistic pattern but can move out of synergy with request or demonstration; strength 3–/5 at shoulder and 4–/5 distally; coordination is poor; can place and hold for weight bearing if cued but not spontaneously
10. Left lower extremity moves in flexor/extensor pattern, grossly 3+/5 in hip and knee flexion, 2+ hip extension, 3+/5 knee extension, no isolated ankle movement, cannot place or hold for weight bearing

Functional tests found the following disabilities:
1. Minimum assist supine-to-sit
2. Sitting balance, poor
3. Moderate assist sit-to-stand
4. Standing balance, unable
5. Moderate assist transfers
6. Nonambulatory

Impairment goals were the following:
1. Increase ROM to within normal limits throughout
2. Increase trunk tone to normal and strength to 4+/5
3. Decrease right-sided tone to normal
4. Increase spontaneous use, isolated movement, and strength (4+/5) in right extremities
5. Able to place and bear weight on right lower extremity

Short-term functional goals were the following:
1. Independent in all bed mobility
2. Independent in wheelchair transfers
3. Good static and fair dynamic sitting balance
4. Contact guard sit-to-stand
5. Minimal assist static standing balance. Ambulation goals were temporarily deferred because of the ankle contractures and balance deficits.

Early treatments included the following:
1. Standing frame activities for head control, visual tracking, trunk control, reduced lower-extremity extensor tone, and heel cord stretching with ultrasound
2. Neurodevelopmental sequence activities for head and trunk control, trunk strengthening, decreased lower-extremity extensor tone, balance on all fours/heel-sitting/kneeling
3. Supine to and from sitting, especially over the right arm
4. Sitting balance with upper-extremity functional tasks (e.g., putting glasses on/off, taking shirt off/on, wiping nose with tissue), with focus on right visual tracking, right trunk elongation, and incorporation of right lower-extremity ground pressure for stability
5. Transfer training with incorporation of right upper extremity to push up, reach and grasp, and right lower-extremity placing and weight-bearing

As soon as Andy's ankle dorsiflexion ROM was near neutral on the right (was then 0 to 5 degrees on the left), neurodevelopmental activities were phased out and standing balance and pregait activities in the parallel bars were initiated with moderate assistance. He rapidly progressed to minimal assistance gait in the parallel bars but with significant scissoring of the lower extremities. Gait outside the bars was begun with a quad cane on the left, but Andy was not able to organize the sequence for cane use and did not use it when loss of balance occurred, so it was discontinued. Gait without an assistive device required moderate assistance from the therapist for balance. A line drawn on the floor provided a visual cue to remind him to keep his feet apart; when walking without this cue, approximately 25% of his steps were close or crossed.

At discharge, 2 months after admission, Andy had good visual tracking; normal ROM with the exception of right lower-extremity dorsiflexion, which was limited to 0 to 5 degrees; normal tone in the left extremities; mildly increased tone in the right extremities with slight extensor patterning in the leg; good head and trunk control; and strength grossly 4+/5 throughout. Functionally, he was independent in bed mobility, wheelchair mobility, and sitting balance. He required supervision for safety in transfers and standing activities and minimal to moderate assistance for indoor ambulation without an assistive device depending on his fatigue level.

CASE STUDY 23-2 ■ DORIS

Doris is a 73-year-old woman with a long history of Parkinson's disease who had fallen four times within the 6 months before referral to physical therapy. As a result of her most recent fall, during which she hit her head, Doris had ear pounding, lightheadedness, and headaches. After referral to an otolaryngologist, she was diagnosed with unspecified peripheral vestibular dysfunction and referred to outpatient therapy. Her therapist found that Doris reported increased lightheadedness and dizziness, with anterior/posterior head movements, rolling in bed, sit-to-stand, and the Hallpike-Dix maneuver (worse to the right). Multiple impairments that could be contributing to her instability and falls, as well as symptoms related to the vestibular disorder, were also noted. Doris had mildly decreased ROM in her left ankle, shoulders, and neck; mild left-sided weakness and lack of coordination; marked bilateral upper-extremity tremor; and moderate forward flexed posture.

She could not perform an ankle strategy at all and continually used hip strategy; she also used stepping strategy frequently with the least shift or sway. Static postural sway tests indicated that Doris had excessive sway when attempting to stand still and that she kept her COG slightly posterior and to the right of midline. Sway increased 10-fold with eyes closed, indicating poor use of somatosensory inputs for postural control. Doris could not perform repeated weight shifts in either anterior/posterior or medial/lateral directions. Her limits of stability were severely restricted to less than half of normal sway range anteriorly, and her movement time was slow.

Functional testing revealed that Doris had several disabilities. She had to use a walker or have manual assistance to ambulate and could negotiate level surfaces only. Without her walker or handhold assistance, Doris could stand for less than 30 seconds and take a maximum of 10 steps. For community ambulation, Doris needed minimum assistance with her walker and could go only short distances. She also required minimum assistance with bathing and household tasks.

Doris participated in therapy twice a week for 6 weeks and also performed a home exercise program daily. Her treatment plan included vestibular exercises for the dizziness and balance retraining exercises for instability and falls. The vestibular exercises she was given were designed to provoke her symptoms repeatedly and included head turning in supine and sitting (progressed to standing), rolling in bed, rocking in a rocking chair, and sit-to-stand practice. As her dizziness subsided, her home program was modified to increase the number and rate of head movements. To improve her use of somatosensory and vestibular inputs, Doris also practiced standing on a firm surface with eyes closed (with family supervision). In the clinic, Doris did stretching, strengthening, and postural extension exercises to address her musculoskeletal limitations. For increased use of somatosensory and vestibular inputs, she practiced standing and weight shifts with optokinetic stimulation. By using postural sway biofeedback, she practiced achieving the midline position, controlled anterior and left-sided weight shifts at progressively faster speeds, and ankle strategy. Gait training included starts, stops, turns, and obstacle avoidance and progressed to community ambulation tasks such as curbs and ramps. As her endurance improved, she also did gait training on the treadmill to increase the gait speed, stride length, hip strength, and use of vestibular inputs.

Despite her multiple problems, Doris was able to reduce the severity of her impairments and consequently improve her functional level. Her dizziness resolved completely. Although she still had excess sway during static standing, she was able to achieve and hold a midline position, and her sway with eyes closed reduced by more than half. Doris could shift her weight in both anterior/posterior and medial/lateral directions at moderate speeds by using ankle strategy without stepping. Her limits of stability were expanded from 35% to 80% of normal, and she was able to shift her weight much more quickly. Functionally, she could stand without the walker for 8 minutes and walk independently indoors on level surfaces without the walker for short distances. She was independent in community ambulation with the walker. At a 3-month follow-up visit, Doris reported that she had had no more falls.

CASE STUDY 23-3 ■ SARAH

Sarah is a 20 year old with a history of cystic fibrosis. During an acute episode she was treated with gentamicin, an antibiotic in the aminoglycoside family. Approximately 6 days later, she lost her balance when getting out of bed. As she tried to get up, the room began to feel like it was moving. She was unable to regain her balance. Although previously functionally independent, she became reliant on her family to assist her for all mobility. Evaluation by a neuro-otologist determined that she had lost 70% of her vestibular function in one ear and 65% in the other.

On her initial physical therapy evaluation she was unable to maintain focus on her outstretched thumb while turning her head side to side or up and down. She could move her eyes from target to target, but it made her dizzy. She reported dizziness with smooth pursuit of the eyes and had difficulty maintaining focus as the speed of the moving target increased.

She had an increased base of support in quiet standing and was unable to keep her balance with her feet touching. Even with a wide base of support, she lost her balance when she moved her head. She could not stand with her eyes closed, even on a firm surface. She fell immediately when trying to stand on foam; she was therefore not asked to try to close her eyes.

INITIAL TREATMENT

Because her ability to walk was so impaired, Sarah was given a cane to increase the somatosensory input and further increase her base of support. She was able to walk with the cane without assistance on smooth surfaces, but she needed help with stairs, curbs, and when walking on grass. Sarah was also given gaze-stabilization exercises, one of which was to look at a business card and move her head only as fast as she could while keeping the letters in focus. Each day she would try to move her head faster but not let the letters get fuzzy.

Sarah was instructed to stand in the corner, with her back approximately 4 inches from the wall. She was told to close her eyes and count. Each time that she fell against the wall she was to right herself and start her count over. Her goal was to stand for 30 seconds without touching the wall. When she could stand for 30 seconds, she would try to move her feet closer together.

She was also instructed to stand in the corner and begin to move her head as she was looking at a nonmoving object.

To avoid the oscillopsia associated with turning her head while walking, she was instructed to turn her body in the direction that she wanted to turn while she was focused on a stable object. Then she would close her eyes as she turned her head, using her somatosensation to maintain balance. She would refocus to move forward. She was instructed to return in 3 weeks.

PROGRESSION

At her next visit Sarah could move her head at approximately 1 Hz and maintain focus. Her ability to use somatosensation for balance improved with both eyes closed and turning her head while standing on a firm surface. She could stand with her feet close together with her eyes open on a firm surface. Her program was progressed to include standing on foam in the corner and beginning to turn her head while looking at a stationary target. She was instructed to begin a gentle sway while standing on a firm surface with eyes closed. For her gait training, she was instructed to use visual targets to maintain stability as she began to slowly move her head (called "hanging on with your eyes"). She continued to use her cane for community mobility. She could now move around her house without using the cane.

Three weeks later, she demonstrated gaze stabilization at 2 Hz. She was told then to start holding the card in front of the television while she turned her head to further challenge the ability to maintain gaze stabilization.

She could easily stand in the corner with eyes closed but felt uneasy with weight shifts. She could move her head at approximately 1 Hz while walking on a firm surface with gaze stabilization. Standing on foam was easy with head turns.

To progress her program further, she worked on a Profitter to shift from side to side as she maintained gaze stability. She began using the StairMaster with head turns. She started walking on the treadmill at 1.0 mph without upper-extremity support. She was encouraged to try to move outdoors as much as possible to be on uneven surface. She started to try reading while standing. She was given a ball to toss in the air and instructed to follow it with her eyes while maintaining her peripheral gaze on vertical and horizontal targets. Driving was addressed because she was hoping to return to school in the fall. Because she still demonstrated some oscillopsia and reported dizziness with head turns, she was instructed to look in the rear-view mirror and then close her eyes as she moved her head back to the front of the car. This eliminated the blurred vision during head turns, and she could do it quickly enough to be safe. She was warned not to drive during inclement weather, when the snow or rain would disrupt her vision.

Three months later, she returned for a follow-up evaluation before returning to school. She had spent the summer babysitting for two small children and played outside throwing and catching the ball. She stated they loved it when she fell down, but for her it was good training to incorporate head movements and gaze stabilization on uneven surfaces. She was able to walk in the community without an assistive device. She described difficulty when the wind was blowing (disrupting visual cues), when there was glare, and when she had to walk in a dark theater.

Although the physician reported no increase in her vestibular function, she had made significant improvement in her ability to move through her environment and return to her normal activities.

ACKNOWLEDGMENT

Thanks to Janet Helminski, PT, PhD; Linda Horn, PT, NCS; and Pat Huston, MS, PT, for their significant contributions to the development of this chapter. Gratitude is also extended to Darcy Umphred, PT, PhD, FAPTA, and our families for their patience and support.

REFERENCES

1. Allison L: Imbalance following traumatic brain injury: causes and characteristics, *Neurol Rep* 23:15, 1999.
2. American Physical Therapy Association: Guide to physical therapy practice. Second edition, *Phys Ther* 81:9-746, 2001.
3. Fields J: The disablement model: The relationships between and among impairment, functional limitation and disability in the elderly population, *Issues on Aging* 22:5, 1999.
3a. World Health Organization: *The international classification of functioning, disability and health (ICF),* Geneva, Switzerland, 2001, World Health Organization.
4. Nashner L: Evaluation of postural stability, movement, and control. In Hasson S, editor: *Clinical exercise physiology,* Philadelphia, 1994, Mosby.
5. Nashner L: Sensory, neuromuscular, and biomechanical contributions to human balance. In Duncan P, editor: *Balance: Proceedings of the APTA forum,* Alexandria, VA, 1990, American Physical Therapy Association.
6. Horak F, Shupert C, Mirka A: Components of postural dyscontrol in the elderly: a review, *Neurobiol Aging* 10:727-738, 1989.
7. Sherrington C: *The integrative action of the nervous system,* New Haven, CT, 1961, Yale University.
8. Bobath B: *Adult hemiplegia: Evaluation and treatment,* ed 2, London, 1978, William Heinemann.
9. Knott M, Voss D: *Proprioceptive neuromuscular facilitation: patterns and techniques,* ed 2, New York, 1968, Harper & Row.
10. Morris SL, Sharpe MH: PNF revisited, *Physiother Theory Pract* 9:43, 1993.
11. Van Sant AF: Should the normal motor developmental sequence be used as a theoretical model to progress adult patients? In Lister MJ, editor: *Contemporary management of motor control problems: Proceedings of the II-STEP conference,* Alexandria, VA, 1992, Bookcrafters.
12. Gibson JJ: *The senses considered as perceptual systems,* Boston, 1966, Houghton Mifflin.
13. Gordon J: Assumptions underlying physical therapy intervention: theoretical and historical perspectives. In Carr JH, Shepherd RB, Gordon J, editors: *Movement sciences: Foundations for physical therapy in rehabilitation,* Rockville, MD, 1987, Aspen Publishers.
14. Horak F: Assumptions underlying motor control for neurologic rehabilitation. In Lister MJ, editor: *Contemporary management of motor control problems: Proceedings of the II-STEP conference,* Alexandria, VA, 1992, Bookcrafters.
15. Barnes ML, Crutchfield ML: *Reflex and vestibular aspects of motor control, motor development, and motor learning,* Atlanta, 1990, Stokesville Publishing.
16. Schenkman M, Butler RB: A model for multisystem evaluation, interpretation, and treatment of individuals with neurologic dysfunction, *Phys Ther* 69:538-547, 1989.
17. Shumway-Cook A, Wollacott MH: *Motor control: theory and practical applications,* Baltimore, 2000, Lippincott Williams & Wilkins.
18. Horak F: Clinical measurement of postural control in adults, *Phys Ther* 67:1881-1885, 1987.
18a. Whipple R, Wolfson LI: Abnormalities of balance, gait, and sensorimotor function in the elderly population. In Duncan P, editor: *Balance: Proceedings of the APTA forum,* Alexandria, VA, 1990, American Physical Therapy Association.
19. Rose DJ, Clark S: Can the control of bodily orientation be significantly improved in a group of older adults with a history of falls? *J Am Geriatr Soc* 48:275, 2000.
20. Herdman S: *Vestibular rehabilitation,* ed 2, Philadelphia, 2000, FA Davis.
21. Arenberg IK: Menière's disease: diagnosis and management of vertigo and endolymphatic hydrops. In Arenberg IK, editor: *Dizziness and balance disorders,* New York, 1993, Kugler.
22. Jeka J, Oie K, Kiemel T: Multisensory information for human postural control: Integrating touch and vision, *Exp Brain Res* 134:107-125, 2000.
23. Oie KS, Kiemel T, Jeka JJ: Multisensory fusion: simultaneous reweighting of vision and touch for the control of human posture, *Brain Res Cogn Brain Res* 14:164-176, 2002.
24. Peterka RJ, Benolken MS: Role of somatosensory and vestibular cues in attenuating visually induced human postural sway, *Exp Brain Res* 105:101-110, 1995.
25. DiFabio RP, Badke MB: Relationship of sensory organization to balance function in patients with hemiplegia, *Phys Ther* 70:542-548, 1990.
26. Ingersoll C, Armstrong C: The effects of closed head injury on postural sway, *Med Sci Sports Exerc* 24:739-743, 1992.
27. Cordo P, Nashner L: Properties of postural adjustments associated with rapid arm movements, *J Neurophysiol* 47:287-302, 1982.
28. Schmidt RA, Lee TD: *Motor control and learning: a behavioral emphasis,* ed 3, Champaign, IL, 1999, Human Kinetics.
29. Charness A: *Stroke/head injury: A guide to functional outcomes in physical therapy management,* Rockville, MD, 1986, Aspen Publications.
30. Patla AE, Winter DA, Frank JS et al: Identification of age-related changes in the balance control system. In Duncan P, editor: *Balance: Proceedings of the APTA forum,* Alexandria, VA, 1990, American Physical Therapy Association.
31. Hain T, Ramaswamy T, Hillman M: Anatomy and physiology of the normal vestibular system. In Herdman S, editor: *Vestibular rehabilitation,* ed 2, Philadelphia, 2000, F.A. Davis.
32. Creath, R, Kiemel, T, Horak, F, et al: A unified view of quiet and perturbed stance: simultaneous coexisting excitable modes, *Neurosci Lett* 377:75-80, 2005.
33. Henry SM, Fung J, Horak FB: EMG responses to maintain stance during multidirectional surface translations, *J Neurophysiol* 80:1939-1950, 1998.
34. Maki BE, McIlroy WE: The control of foot placement during compensatory stepping reactions: Does speed of response take precedence over stability? *IEEE Trans Rehabil Eng* 7:80-90, 1999.
35. McIlroy WE, Maki BE: Age-related changes in compensatory stepping in response to unpredictable perturbations, *J Gerontol A Biol Sci Med Sci* 51:M289-M296, 1996.
36. Horak F, Shupert C: Role of the vestibular system in postural control. In Herdman S, editor: *Vestibular rehabilitation,* ed 2, Philadelphia, 2000, FA Davis.
37. Duncan P: Is there one simple measure for balance? *PT Magazine* 1:74-77, 1993.
38. Lynch SM, Leahy P, Barker SP: Reliability of measurements obtained with a modified functional reach test in subjects with spinal cord injury, *Phys Ther* 78:128-133, 1998.
39. Newton R: Review of tests of standing balance abilities, *Brain Inj* 3:335-343, 1989.
40. Bohannon RW: One-legged balance test times, *Percept Mot Skills* 78:801-802, 1994.
41. Bohannon RW, Leary KM: Standing balance and function over the course of acute rehabilitation, *Arch Phys Med Rehabil* 76:994-996, 1995.
42. Flores AM: Objective measurement of standing balance, *Neurol Rep* 16:17, 1992.
43. Moore S, Woollacott M: The use of biofeedback devices to improve postural stability, *Phys Ther Pract* 2:1, 1993.
44. Harburn KL, Hill KM, Kramer JF et al: Clinical applicability and test-retest reliability of an external perturbation test of balance in stroke subjects, *Arch Phys Med Rehabil* 76:317, 1995.

45. Chandler J, Duncan P: Balance and falls in the elderly: issues in evaluation and treatment. In Guccione A, editor: *Geriatric physical therapy*, St. Louis, 1993, Mosby.

46. Wallmann HW: Comparison of elderly nonfallers and fallers on performance measures of functional reach, sensory organization, and limits of stability, *J Gerontol A Biol Sci Med Sci* 56:M580-M583, 2001.

47. Behrman AL, Light KE, Flynn SM, et al: Is the functional reach test useful for identifying falls risk among individuals with Parkinson's disease? *Arch Phys Med Rehabil* 83:538-542, 2002.

48. Thomas JI, Lane JV: A pilot study to explore the predictive validity of four measures of falls risk in frail elderly patients, *Arch Phys Med Rehabil* 86:1636-1640, 2005.

49. Newton RA: Balance screening of an inner city older adult population, *Arch Phys Med Rehabil* 78:587-591, 1997.

50. Newton RA: Validity of the multidirectional reach test: a practical measure for limits of stability in older adults, *J Gerontol A Biol Sci Med Sci* 56:M248-M252, 2001.

51. Clark S, Rose DJ: Generalizability of the limits of stability test in the evaluation of dynamic balance among older adults, *Arch Phys Med Rehabil* 78:1078-1084, 1997.

52. Shumway-Cook A, Horak F: Assessing the influence of sensory interaction on balance, *Phys Ther* 66:1548-1550, 1986.

53. Weber PC, Cass SP: Clinical assessment of postural stability, *Am J Otol* 14:566-569, 1993.

54. Cromwell S, Held J: Test-retest reliability of three balance measures used with hemiplegic patients, *Neurol Rep* 17:24, 1994.

55. Furman JM, Cass SP: Benign paroxysmal positional vertigo, *N Engl J Med* 341:1590-1596, 1999.

56. Tseng H, Chao W: Head-shaking nystagmus: a sensitive indicator of vestibular dysfunction, *Clin Otolaryngol* 22:549-552, 1997.

57. Shumway-Cook A, Horak F: Vestibular rehabilitation: an exercise approach to managing symptoms of vestibular dysfunction, *Semin Hearing* 10:194, 1986.

58. Herdman S, Tusa R: Assessment and treatment of patients with benign paroxysmal positional vertigo. In Herdman S, editor: *Vestibular rehabilitation*, ed 2, Philadelphia, 2000, FA Davis.

59. Fife T: Recognition and management of horizontal canal benign positional vertigo, *Am J Otol* 19:345-351, 1998.

60. Bohannon M, Newton R: Test-retest reliability of the Fukuda stepping test, *Physiother Res Int* 3:58, 1998.

61. Berg K, Wood-Dauphinee S, Williams JI et al: Measuring balance in the elderly: Preliminary development of an instrument, *Physiother Can* 41:304, 1989.

62. Bolen JC, Friedman SM: Berg balance scale predicts fall risk in frail older adults, *J Am Geriatr Soc* 47:S66, 1999.

63. Shumway-Cook A, Baldwin M, Polissar NL, et al: Predicting the probability for falls in community-dwelling older adults, *Phys Ther* 77:812-819, 1997.

64. Niam S, Cheung W, Sullivan PE et al: Balance and physical impairments after stroke, *Arch Phys Med Rehabil* 80:1227-1233, 1999.

65. Berg K, Wooddauphinee S, Williams JI: The balance scale: Reliability assessment with elderly residents and patients with an acute stroke, *Scand J Rehabil Med* 27:27-36, 1995.

66. Qutubuddin AA, Pegg PO, Cifu DX, et al: Validating the Berg Balance Scale for patients with Parkinson's disease: a key to rehabilitation evaluation, *Arch Phys Med Rehabil* 86:2225-2226, 2005.

67. Whitney S, Wrisley D, Furman J: Concurrent validity of the Berg Balance Scale and the dynamic gait index in people with vestibular dysfunction, *Physiother Res Int* 8:178-186, 2003.

68. Mathias S, Nayak US, Isaacs B: Balance in the elderly patient: the "get up and go" test, *Arch Phys Med Rehabil* 67:387-389, 1986.

69. Podsiadlo D, Richardson S: The timed "up and go": a test of basic functional mobility for frail elderly persons, *J Am Geriatr Soc* 39:142-148, 1991.

70. Brooks D, Davis AM, Naglie G: Validity of 3 physical performance measures in inpatient geriatric rehabilitation, *Arch Phys Med Rehabil* 87:105-110, 2006.

71. Shumway-Cook A, Brauer S, Woollacott M: Predicting the probability for falls in community-dwelling older adults using the timed up & go test, *Phys Ther* 80:896-903, 2000.

72. Tinetti ME: Performance oriented assessment of mobility problems in elderly patients, *J Am Geriatr Soc* 34:119-126, 1986.

72a. Faber MJ, Bosscher RJ, van Wieringen PC: Clinimetric properties of the performance-oriented mobility assessment, *Phys Ther* 86:944-954, 2006.

73. VanSwearingen JM, Paschal KA, Bonino P et al: The modified gait abnormality rating scale for recognizing the risk of recurrent falls in community-dwelling older adults, *Phys Ther* 76:994, 1996.

74. Shumway-Cook A, Gruber W, Baldwin M, et al: The effect of multidimensional exercises on balance, mobility, and fall risk in community-dwelling older adults, *Phys Ther* 77:46-57, 1997.

75. Whitney SL, Hudak MK, Marchetti GF: The dynamic gait index relates to self-reported fall history in individuals with vestibular dysfunction, *J Vestib Res* 10:99-105, 2000.

76. Wrisley DM, Marchetti GF, Kuharsky DK, et al: Reliability, internal consistency, and validity of data obtained with the functional gait assessment, *Phys Ther* 84:906-918, 2004.

77. Jacobson GP, Newman CW, Hunter L et al: Balance function test correlates of the dizziness handicap inventory, *J Am Acad Audiol* 2:253-260, 1991.

78. Jacobson GP, Newman CW: The development of the dizziness handicap inventory, *Arch Otolaryngol Head Neck Surg* 116:424-427, 1990.

79. Newman C, Jacobson G: Balance handicap assessment. In Jacobson G, Newman C, Kartush J, editors: *Handbook of balance testing function*, St. Louis, 1993, Mosby–Year Book.

80. Bowen A, Wenman R, Mickelborough J, et al: Dual-task effects of talking while walking on velocity and balance following a stroke, *Age Ageing* 30:319-323, 2001.

81. Verghese J, Buschke H, Viola L, et al: Validity of divided attention tasks in predicting falls in older individuals: a preliminary study, *J Am Geriatr Soc* 50:1572-1576, 2002.

82. Lundin-Olsson L, Nyberg L, Gustafson Y: "Stops walking when talking" as a predictor of falls in elderly people, *Lancet* 349:617, 1991.

83. de Hoon EW, Allum JH, Carpenter MG, et al: Quantitative assessment of the stops walking while talking test in the elderly, *Arch Phys Med Rehabil* 84:838-842, 2003.

84. Bloem BR, Valkenburg VV, Slabbekoorn M, et al: The multiple tasks test: development and normal strategies, *Gait Posture* 14:191-202, 2001.

85. Southard V, Dave M, Davis MG, et al: The multiple tasks test as a predictor of falls in older adults, *Gait Posture* 22:351-355, 2005.

86. Shepard NT, Telian SA, Smith-Wheelock M et al: Vestibular and balance rehabilitation therapy, *Ann Otol Rhinol Laryngol* 102:198-205, 1993.

87. Rose DJ: *A multilevel approach to the study of motor control and learning*, Boston, 1997, Allyn & Bacon.

88. Gentile AM: A working model of skill acquisition with application to teaching, *Quest* 17:3, 1972.

89. Magill RA: *Motor learning: concepts and applications*, ed 5, Boston, 1998, McGraw-Hill.

90. Asai M, Wantanabe Y, Shimizu K: Effects of vestibular rehabilitation on postural control, *Acta Otolaryngol (Stockh)* 528:116-120, 1997.

91. Foster CA: Vestibular rehabilitation, *Ballieres Clin Neurol* 3:577-592, 1994.

92. Wolf M, Hertanu T, Novikov I et al: Epley's maneuver for benign paroxysmal positional vertigo: A prospective study, *Clin Otolaryngol* 24:43-46, 1999.

93. Baloh R, Honrubia V: *Clinical neurophysiology of the vestibular system*, ed 2, Philadelphia, 1990, FA Davis.

94. Lackner J, DiZio P, Jeka J et al: Precision contact of the fingertip reduces postural sway of individuals with bilateral vestibular loss, *Exp Brain Res* 126:459-466, 1999.

95. Rose DK, Guiliani CA: A comparison of overground walking and treadmill walking in patients with cerebral vascular lesion, *Neurol Rep* 17:23, 1993.

96. Brandt T, Schautzer F, Hamilton DA et al: Vestibular loss causes hippocampal atrophy and impaired spatial memory in humans, *Brain* 128:2732-2741, 2005.

97. Allison L: The role of biofeedback in balance retraining, *Biofeedback* 24:16, 1996.

APPENDIX 23-A ■ Common Vestibular Disorders

Infection: A common cause of dizziness associated with a vestibular disorder is infections that affect the vestibular nerve. Most often the infection is viral in nature and is known as neuronitis. It can be due to bacterial infection and should be treated by antibiotics.[93] The infection can be preceded by a systemic illness or an upper respiratory tract infection, or it can be an isolated infection affecting the nerve or labyrinths. This causes an acute, severe dizziness because the brain is suddenly provided with abnormal information coming from the involved vestibular end organ. The result is loss of normal postural reactions and the sensation of spinning known as vertigo. As the brain adapts to the change of status of the system, the vertigo begins to resolve. There can be residual problems with postural control and vertigo caused by rapid head turns.

Hydrops: Increased fluid pressure within the labyrinth, known broadly as hydrops, will cause vertigo. When the fluid pressure increases, the brain receives abnormal signals from the labyrinth on one side, and the result is the sensation of spinning. There is often concurrent loss of hearing related to the pressure in the cochlea. The episode can last from just a few minutes to a day but is usually between 2 and 4 hours in duration. The use of diuretics can sometimes control the fluid changes and decrease the number and intensity of symptoms. Ménière's disease is a type of hydrops that occurs intermittently, and the person has normal balance when not in episode.[3] Over time there appears to be a gradual degradation of the vestibular system, resulting in symptoms associated with chronic unilateral vestibular loss. These clients often have a diffuse dizziness and complain of imbalance. Intervention is targeted at adaptation of the abnormal vestibular responses, and this can improve symptoms, although it cannot remedy the disease itself. Traumatic hydrops can be the result of a blow to the head during a fall or whiplash injury. The mechanism is not fully understood, but it may be related to damage of the endolymphatic sac during the trauma, resulting in inflammation or scarring that limits the regulation of fluid in the sac.

Benign positional vertigo (BPV): When the otoconia in the vestibule is loosened, it can move into the semicircular canal and become a cause of vertigo. Benign positional nystagmus or vertigo is a common sequela of head concussion, viral labyrinthitis, hydrops, and vascular occlusion in the distribution that feeds the inner ear. It can also develop without a known external cause and is the most common cause of vertigo.[20] BPV may involve any semicircular canal, although the posterior canal is most common because of its relationship to the otoliths when the person is in the recumbent position. However, the horizontal canal can collect otoconia, and the result is horizontal nystagmus generated with head movement.

Despite the use of the term *benign,* the symptoms related to positional vertigo are intense and can cause significant disability. There is often a strong sense of falling or spinning out of control, even when the individual is lying on a bed. Before the individual is aware of the mechanism, it seems to be something that is uncontrollable because it is associated with head movement.

Vascular disorders: Ischemia in the areas of the vestibular system (brain stem, cerebellum, parietal-insular cortex) can cause dizziness and imbalance. Vertebral basilar artery insufficiency syndrome, for example, classically produces these problems. Ischemia is usually seen in individuals older than 50 years, but it can also be associated with bleeding disorders such as leukemia. Migraine headache can cause intermittent dizziness from compromise of blood flow in the areas of the vestibular system.

Neoplasia: This can compromise vestibular function when it occurs near any part of the vestibular system. Vestibular schwannoma (commonly, but mistakenly known as acoustic neuroma) can cause damage as it slowly grows on the sheath of the vestibular nerve. The schwannoma can grow into the pontocerebellar angle and cause symptoms typically associated with cerebellar lesions. Meningiomas (encapsulated tumors found most often deep in the brain) growing in the area of the temporal lobe can cause pressure on the vestibular mechanism. In some cases, damage to the vestibular nerve occurs as a result of surgical removal of the tumor.

Ototoxicity: Aminoglycosides, antibiotics used in cases of massive or systemic infection, can be ototoxic (causing damage to the vestibular hair cells). Although a small percentage of users experience this adverse effect, it can affect both sides of the bilateral vestibular apparatus and cause significant disability. Often the client does not begin to experience the symptoms until the medication has been used for more than a week.

Traumatic brain injury (TBI): This can affect the vestibular system in several ways. It can cause direct damage to the vestibular end organ (in the temporal bone); BPV; and, in many cases, disruption of the integration of the vestibular nuclei (in the brain stem) and cerebellum. Sensorimotor disturbances are common with TBI involving the cerebellum or parietal lobe. Visual dysfunction results from damage to brain stem areas such as the pontine gaze centers or central damage in the medial longitudinal fasciculus. Frequently, the third, fourth, or sixth cranial nerves are damaged, and this affects the ability to move the eyes for conjugate gaze. In some extensive TBI cases, the brain loses its ability to use any of the three sensory systems accurately. Dizziness and imbalance are prevalent complaints from client with TBI because there are often situations in which they cannot acquire accurate sensory information. Each system should be evaluated individually for its function. In patients with TBI, the adaptation of the vestibular system occurs more slowly and with more effort than for other clients with vestibular deficits. The client with vestibular problems associated with TBI requires significantly more intervention initially, and the outcomes are less favorable compared to other clients experiencing vestibular dysfunction.[86]

Allergies: Persons with allergies are often predisposed to episodes of dizziness. Foods, airborne allergens, and chemicals can trigger dizziness in these individuals.

Metabolic disorders: Vertigo and dizziness are often reported with metabolic disorders such as diabetes. Autoimmune diseases such as rheumatoid arthritis, lupus, and human immunodeficiency syndrome infection can also cause symptoms when the disease process damages components of the vestibular system.

CHAPTER 24

Metabolic, Hereditary, and Genetic Disorders in Adults with Basal Ganglia Movement Disorders

Marsha E. Melnick, PT, PhD

KEY WORDS

basal ganglia
Huntington's disease
Parkinson's disease

OBJECTIVES

After reading this chapter the student/therapist will be able to:
1. Describe the circuitry of the basal ganglia.
2. Relate the anatomy and physiology of the basal ganglia to its roles in sensorimotor and cognitive processes.
3. Use the information on anatomy, physiology, and pharmacology to explain the signs and symptoms seen in Parkinson's disease and Huntington's disease.
4. Develop an evaluation plan for patients with diseases of the basal ganglia.
5. Develop an intervention plan for these patients with the rationale for treatment methods.
6. Determine treatment effectiveness, especially in the case of degenerative diseases.
7. Integrate the information in this chapter with the information provided in Section I of this book to develop intervention plans for patients with metabolic or toxic disorders.

This chapter considers the degenerative, metabolic, hereditary, and genetic disorders that typically have their onset in adulthood, including Parkinson's disease, Parkinsonian syndromes, Huntington's disease, Wilson's disease, heavy metal poisoning, and drug intoxication. Because of the wide variety of diseases with a wide variety of causes, the concentration is on understanding the clinical problems and commonalities that exist within this grouping. In general, the practice parameter of the diseases discussed in this chapter fit the physical therapy diagnostic parameter 5E: Impaired Motor and Sensory Integrity associated with Progressive Disorders of the Central Nervous System of the *Guide to Physical Therapist Practice.*[1] Although the occupational therapy guide does not classify practice parameters in that manner, the concepts and clinical reasoning process can be used by both professionals. The predominant area of the brain affected by these disorders is the basal ganglia; this group of central nervous system (CNS) structures is therefore discussed in some detail.

THE BASAL GANGLIA

The most commonly seen disorders affecting the basal ganglia include Parkinson's disease, Huntington's disease, Wilson's disease, and dystonias, including drug-induced dyskinesias. All these medical diagnoses involve changes in muscle tone, a decrease in movement coordination and motor control, decreases in postural stability, and the presence of extraneous movement. Taken together, these disorders now affect approximately 1 million people.[2-5]

To understand how one interrelated area of the brain can account for such a wide variety of symptoms, the anatomy, physiology, and pharmacology of these structures must be considered.

Anatomy

The dorsal or sensorimotor basal ganglia are composed of three nuclei located at the base of the cerebral cortex—hence their name. These nuclei are the caudate nucleus, the putamen, and the globus pallidus. Two brain stem nuclei, the substantia nigra and the subthalamic nucleus, are included as part of the basal ganglia because they have a close functional relation to the forebrain nuclei. Other parts of the basal ganglia, the ventral basal ganglia, are intimately related to the limbic system and are discussed in Chapter 4. (The anatomical location of the various parts of the basal ganglia is shown in Figure 24-1.)

Embryologically, anatomically, and functionally the caudate nucleus and the putamen are similar structures and are often referred to together as the neostriatum—a term derived from striate and used to denote pathways from and to the caudate and putamen. The term corpus striatum refers to the caudate, putamen, and globus pallidus. The various connections and interconnections of this system are discussed according to these definitions.

Afferent Pathways

Functionally, the basal ganglia can be divided into an afferent portion and an efferent portion (Figure 24-2). The

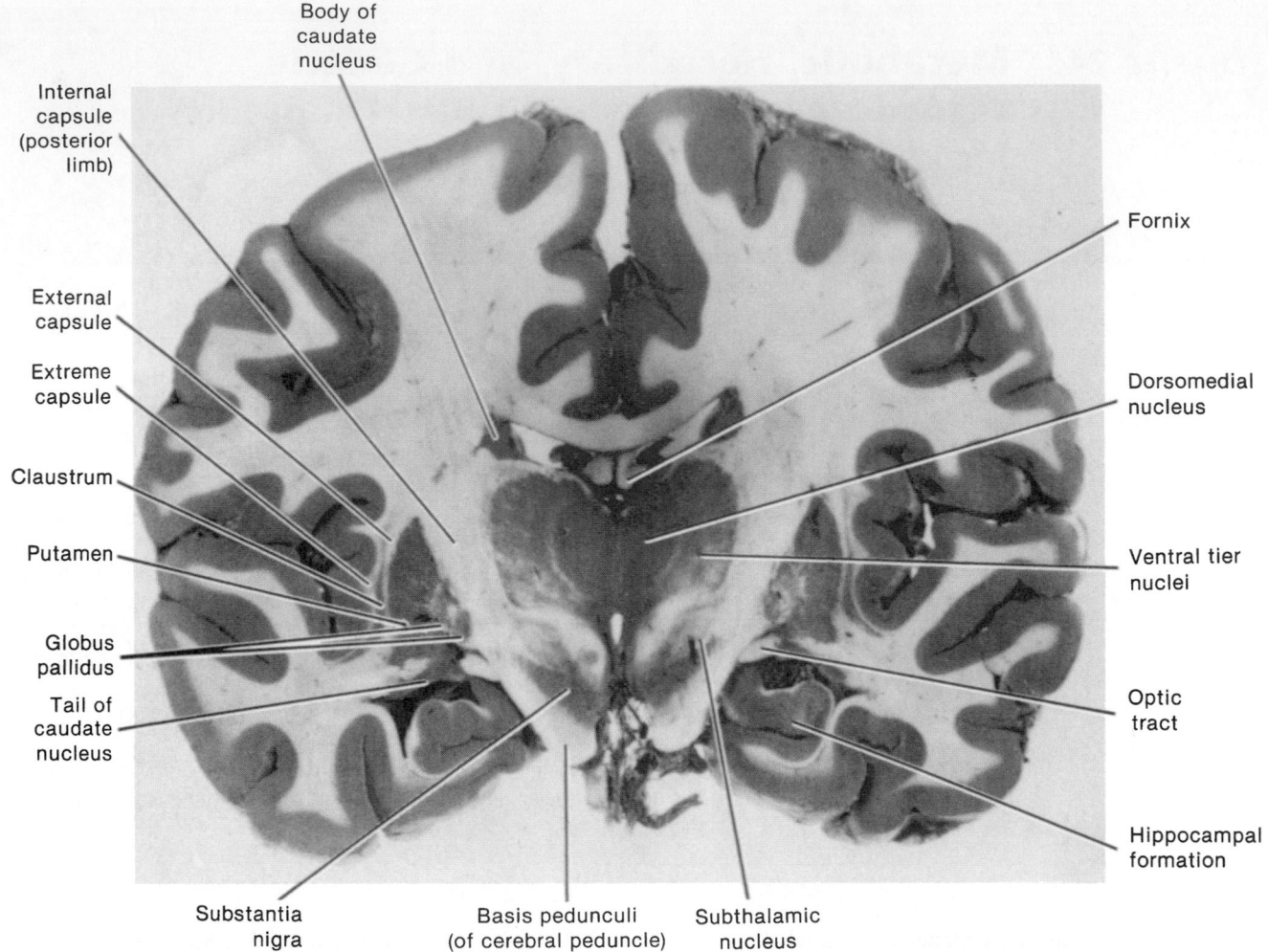

Body of
caudate
nucleus

Internal
capsule
(posterior
limb)

External
capsule

Extreme
capsule

Claustrum

Putamen

Globus
pallidus

Tail of
caudate
nucleus

Fornix

Dorsomedial
nucleus

Ventral tier
nuclei

Optic
tract

Hippocampal
formation

Substantia
nigra

Basis pedunculi
(of cerebral peduncle)

Subthalamic
nucleus

FIGURE 24-1 ■ A coronal section of the anatomical location of various parts of the basal ganglia. (Reprinted from Nolte J: *The human brain: an introduction to its anatomy,* St. Louis, 1981, C.V. Mosby.)

afferent structures are the caudate and putamen. They receive input from the entire cerebral cortex, the intralaminar thalamic nuclei, and the centromedian-parafascicular complex of the thalamus as well as from the substantia nigra and the dorsal raphe nucleus, both located within the brain stem. The projections from the cortex are systematically arranged so that the frontal cortex projects to the head of the caudate and putamen and the visual cortex projects to the tail. In addition, the prefrontal cortex projects mainly to the caudate, whereas the sensorimotor cortex projects mainly to the putamen.[6,7] Those projections from the cortical regions that represent the proximal musculature, and those from the premotor regions, may be bilateral.[2,8-10] These close and profuse connections between the cortex and the basal ganglia suggest a close interfunctional relation between the cortex and the neostriatum. The projections from the thalamus to the caudate-putamen are also somatotopically arranged. The heaviest projections are from the centromedian nucleus, which also receives massive input from the motor cortex.[6-9]

The somatotopic arrangement of the cortico-striatal-thalamic-cortical pathways is maintained throughout the loop. This finding has led to an important functional hypothesis that the basal ganglia form parallel pathways subserving specific sensorimotor and associative functions.[2,8] The putamen is linked to the sensorimotor functions and the caudate to the associative, including cognitive functions.

As knowledge of the circuitry of the basal ganglia has advanced, so has the knowledge regarding the microscopic structure. The caudate-putamen looks somewhat homogeneous because of the predominance of one cell type. Careful analysis by using precise staining methods has demonstrated the appearance of patches within these nuclei. Input can be segregated depending on whether the patches are innervated or the areas around the patches (matrix) are innervated.[11,12] The intrinsic structure of the caudate-putamen also suggests that at least nigral input occurs in a way that could immediately modulate the input coming from the cortex.[13,14]

Efferent Pathways

The input that has been processed in the caudate-putamen is then sent to the globus pallidus (pallidum) and substantia nigra (nigra), which comprise the efferent portion of the basal ganglia. The globus pallidus and substantia nigra are each divided into two regions. The globus pallidus has an external and an internal region; the substantia nigra consists of the dorsal pars compacta and the ventral pars reticulata. Embryologically and microscopically, the internal segment

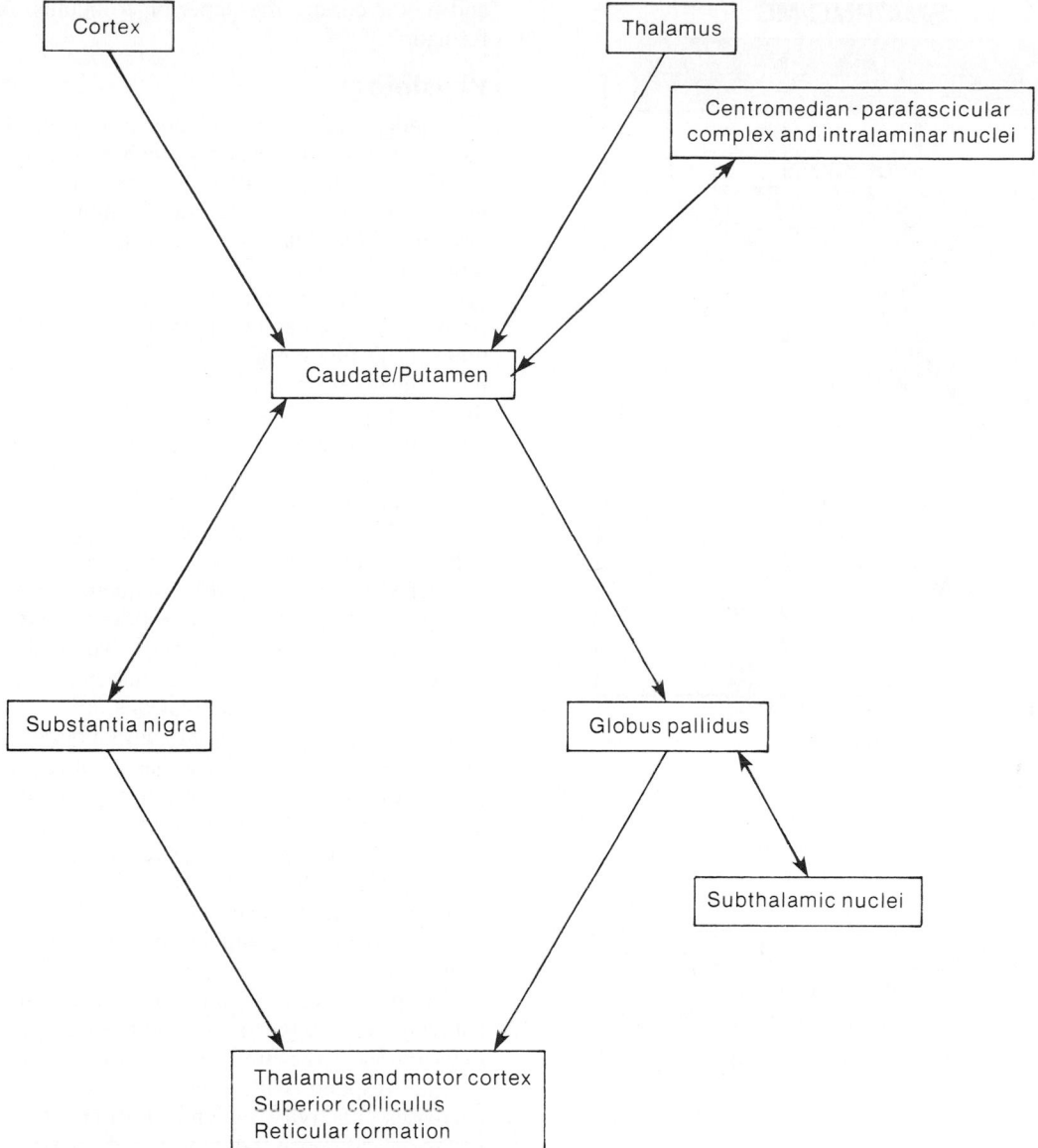

FIGURE 24-2 ■ Afferent and efferent portions of the basal ganglia.

of the globus pallidus and the pars reticulata of the substantia nigra are similar. These two regions are the primary efferent structures for the basal ganglia. The projections from the caudate and putamen to the pallidum and nigra maintain the somatotopic arrangement. The caudate projects primarily to the rostral and dorsal third of the pallidum and the anterior portion of the substantia nigra. The putamen projects to the caudal and ventral portions of the pallidum and the caudal nigra.[15,16] Evidence suggests that the projection from the caudate and putamen are separate in the pallidum and nigra.[9] From these structures the information is transmitted to the thalamus and then to the cortex. The pallidum projects to the lateral portions of the ventrolateral and ventroanterior nuclei of the thalamus. The nigra projects to the medial portions of these nuclei. The superior colliculus, the pedunculopontine nucleus (PPN), and other less defined brain stem structures (perhaps the reticular formation) also receive pallidal and nigral output. All output of the basal ganglia has then been processed through the globus pallidus and/or the substantia

nigra before proceeding to other areas of the brain (see Figure 24-2).

Pathways to the Motor System

Information processed in the basal ganglia can influence the motor system in several ways, but no direct pathway to the alpha or gamma motor neurons of the spinal cord exists. The first route is the projection to the ventroanterior and ventrolateral nuclei of the thalamus, which then projects predominantly to the premotor cortex. Another pathway is through the superior colliculus and then to the tectospinal tract. Pathways exist from the globus pallidus and substantia nigra that terminate in areas of the reticular formation (e.g., the PPN) and then through the reticulospinal pathways. Anatomically the basal ganglia are therefore in good position to affect the motor system at many levels.

The basic circuitry of the basal ganglia is composed of two loops.[6] The loops for the sensorimotor system are shown in Figure 24-3. The direct loop is the loop that begins in the

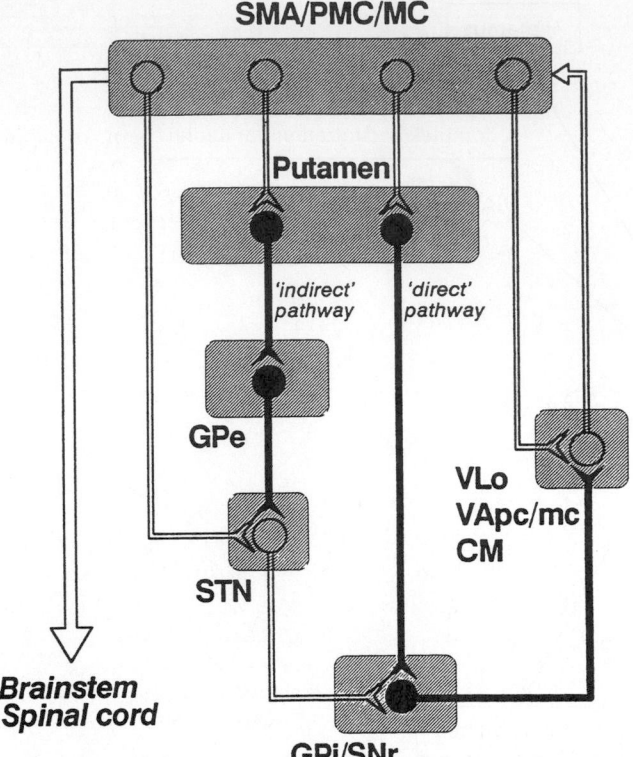

FIGURE 24-3 ■ Diagram of the sensorimotor portion of the basal ganglia depicting the direct and indirect pathways. *Black circles* represent inhibitory neurons; *open circles* represent excitatory neurons. *SMA,* Supplementary motor cortex; *PMC,* premotor cortex; *MC,* motor cortex; *GPe,* globus pallidus external segment; *GPi,* globus pallidus internal segment; *STN,* subthalamic nucleus; *VLo,* ventral lateralis pars oralis nucleus of the thalamus; *VApc/mc,* ventral anterior pars parvocellularis and pars magnocellularis of the thalamus; *CM,* centromedian nucleus of the thalamus; *SNr,* pars reticularis of the substantia nigra. (Reprinted from Alexander GE, Crutcher MD: Functional architecture of basal ganglia circuits: neural substrates of parallel processing, *Trends Neurosci* 13:266, 1990.)

motor regions of the cortex and projects to the putamen and then directly to the globus pallidus, internal segment, and on to the thalamus. The indirect pathway adds the subthalamic nucleus between the globus pallidus, external segment, and the thalamus. The subthalamic nucleus also receives direct input from the premotor and motor cortex as well as from the pallidum.[17,18] The darkened neurons represent inhibitory connections, and the open neurons represent excitatory connections. In general, the direct pathway, by disinhibition, activates the thalamocortical pathway; the indirect pathway inhibits the thalamocortical system. The role of these loops in normal and diseased states is clarified in the discussion of the physiology and pharmacology of the basal ganglia.

In summary, input from the motor cortex, all other areas of the cortex, parts of the thalamus, and the substantia nigra enter the basal ganglia through the caudate and putamen. Here they are processed and sent on to the globus pallidus and substantia nigra. The appropriate "gain" of the system is adjusted, for example, how large a movement is necessary and how much postural stability is needed. The information is sent to the muscles by way of the thalamus

and motor cortex, the superior colliculus, or the reticular formation.

Physiology

The understanding of the physiology of the interactions among areas of the basal ganglia has greatly increased in the last decade. The prevalent view initially was that the basal ganglia exerted an inhibitory influence on the motor system.[19] Most current studies show both excitatory and inhibitory influences.[20,21]

The caudate and putamen are composed of neurons that fire slowly, whereas the neurons in the globus pallidus fire tonically at fairly high rates. (The spontaneous activity of the caudate and putamen is therefore low, whereas that of the globus pallidus is high.) The low firing rates of neostriatal neurons are partially a result of the nature of thalamic synaptic inputs.[22]

Stimulation of the cortex, thalamus, and substantia nigra almost always produces excitatory postsynaptic potentials (EPSP) followed by longer inhibitory postsynaptic potentials (IPSP)—the EPSP-IPSP sequence. Furthermore, input from the cortex seems to have priority over input from the thalamus and substantia nigra.[23] These data provide evidence that the cortex is instrumental in regulating the responsiveness of caudate neurons.[24-26]

The influence of the basal ganglia on the cortex has been one of intense study.[27-29] The basal ganglia stimulation may prepare the cortex for subsequent inputs; this might be especially important when a response must be withheld until an appropriate stimulus occurs, such as keeping the foot on the brake until the light turns green.[30] Similarly, Mink[31] has hypothesized that the basal ganglia activate only the most necessary pathways and inhibit all unnecessary pathways (Figure 24-4).

The pattern of neuronal firing in the direct and indirect pathways also suggests that the basal ganglia modify input to the cortex. The neurons of the efferent portion of the basal ganglia respond with either phasic increases or phasic decreases in activity, which in turn affect the activity in the thalamus and hence the cortex. A decrease in activity of the internal segment of the globus pallidus removes inhibition to the thalamus and thus enables cortical activation. Whether the two pathways are activated concurrently or whether different activities activate the two pathways separately is not yet known. In the former possibility, the indirect pathway is seen as a "break" on ongoing activity; if the latter, the indirect pathway would act to decrease all other patterns in a form of lateral inhibition.[6] In both cases, the basal ganglia would have a role in cortical activation and modulation. In fact, one of the current views in relation to disease processes is that an underactive direct pathway and/or an overactive indirect pathway would lead to decreased activation of the cortex and hence bradykinesia and akinesia, whereas an overactive direct pathway and/or underactive indirect pathway would lead to the presence of extraneous movements (see Figure 24-3).[5,32]

How do these pathways relate to everyday function? Rigidity could be explained by too much muscle activity. The akinesia and bradykinesia of Parkinson's disease are due to insufficient excitation or too many conflicting patterns of movement. The increased extraneous movements are characteristic of basal ganglia diseases and can be attrib-

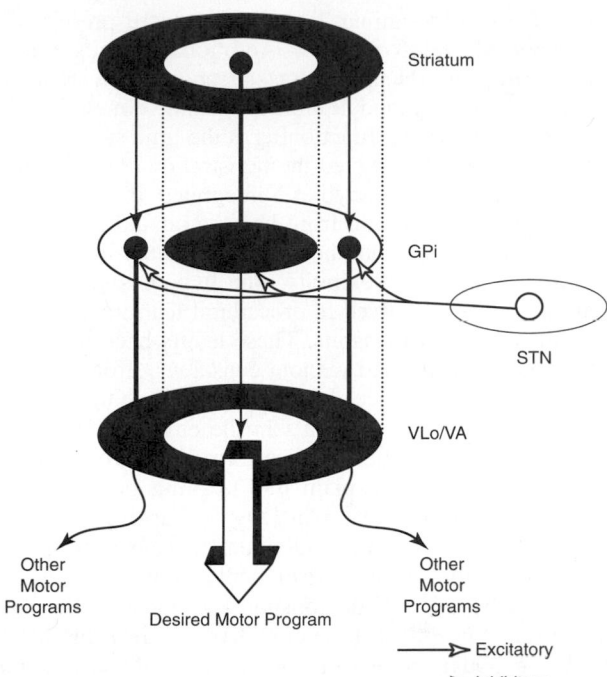

FIGURE 24-4 ■ The net effect of basal ganglia circuitry to produce an area of excitation (the desired program) surrounded by an area of inhibition (all other unnecessary programs). *GPi,* Globus pallidus internal segment; *STN,* subthalamic nucleus; *VLo/VA,* ventral lateralis oralis/ventral anterior. (Adapted from Mink JW: The basal ganglia: focused selection and inhibition of competing motor programs, *Prog Neurobiol* 50:381, 1996.)

uted to the dysfunctions within these pathways. Mink's[31] hypothesis also fits with the role of the basal ganglia in the selection of environmentally appropriate behaviors, specifically in selecting the correct amount of muscle activity in the correct sequence with the necessary timing.[33]

Relation of the Basal Ganglia to Movement and Posture

Lesion experiments; single-unit recording in awake, behaving animals; careful observations of the sequelae of human disease processes; and the results of functional magnetic resonance imaging and transcortical magnetic stimulation studies in human beings have provided some answers regarding the precise role of the basal ganglia in movement and posture.

Automatic Movement

The earliest view of the basal ganglia came from Willis in 1664. He hypothesized that the corpus striatum received "the notion of spontaneous localized movements in ascending tracts . . . Conversely, from here tendencies are dispatched to enact notions without reflection [automatic movements] over descending pathways."[34] Willis possessed great insights in the discussion of the signs and symptoms of basal ganglia disease. Magendie in 1841 demonstrated that removal of the striatum bilaterally produced compulsive movements, whereas removal of only one striatum produced no visible effect.[35] Studies by Nothnagel[36] demonstrated that destruction of the globus pallidus produced a twisting of the

spine with the convexity toward the side of the lesion, whereas lesions of the nigra tended to produce immobility. With the advent of the use of electrical stimulation in the late nineteenth century, further information on the function of the basal ganglia was gathered. Stimulation of the caudate nucleus did not (and does not) produce movement of muscles or limbs as occurs with stimulation of the motor cortex. However, at higher levels of current, total body patterns and postures were usually evoked. The earliest stimulation of the caudate nucleus produced an increase of flexion of the head, trunk, and limbs and tonic contraction of the facial muscles.[37] These early studies are still mentioned because of the insights they provide for the symptoms of these disorders even today. The study of basal ganglia stimulation continues to be investigated as a potential treatment for individuals with Parkinson's disease.[38]

Motor Problems in Animals

Contemporary experiments concerning lesions show a wide variety of motor problems in a variety of animals. Hypokinesia, a decrease or poverty of movement, and a tendency to remain or assume a fixed posture are the most common problems after a lesion in the basal ganglia. These motoric dysfunctions are seen whether the lesion is made by surgical resection, cooling, or pharmacological interventions.[39-45] In essence, movements are altered in scale (related to gain), take longer for completion, and may take place under altered conditions of antagonistic muscle interactions (e.g., cocontraction).[46]

Movement Initiation and Preparation

The hypothesis that the basal ganglia are involved in movement initiation and preparation is an area of some research disagreement. Kornhuber[47] described a "readiness potential" in recordings from the scalp of human beings that was not present in individuals with Parkinson's disease; he hypothesized that the generator was not in the motor cortex but in the subcortical basal ganglia. More recent studies of the readiness potential continue to implicate the basal ganglia and indicate that deficits in this potential are more apparent in complex than in simple movements.[48-50]

Neuronal recordings from awake, behaving animals have also been used to study movements and have indicated that the basal ganglia are active before electromyographic (EMG) activity of the prime movers of the task.[51-53] These findings indicate that basal ganglia are involved in aspects of the initiation and execution of movements. These early activity changes may be a form of movement readiness or "set"[28,54-56]; both "response set"[28] and "activating set" have been used to characterize the early activity of the basal ganglia. Response set was defined as "the ability to initiate and carry out smoothly and in proper sequence a set of movements that comprise a defined response."[22] Activating set has been defined as the "preparation of the mechanism preparatory to a motor performance *oriented to the environment*."[57] The difficulty in parkinsonism of initiating movements, in changing from one movement to another, or choosing the correct movement for the environmental conditions is an example of a disruption in these response set processes.

As previously mentioned, whether the basal ganglia are involved in movement initiation compared with movement execution is controversial. Some of the differences in results are related to tasks used in the experiments, especially whether an external cue is used. The basal ganglia appear more involved in internally generated movements as well as more complex movements.

Postural Adjustments and Postural Stability

The basal ganglia have been implicated in processes of posture and postural adjustments. People with diseases of the basal ganglia assume flexed or other fixed postures as the disease progresses. Additionally, these individuals have decreased postural stability and are therefore at risk for falls. Animal experiments indicate a deficit exists in determining response based on one's own body position, or "egocentric localization."[58,59] This deficit decreases the ability of a person with basal ganglia disease to modify a postural response to the precise environmental demands.

Martin,[60] in his extensive studies of individuals with Parkinson's disease, was the first to describe severe disturbances in posture, especially when vision was occluded. Melnick et al[61] showed that a decrease in static postural adjustments in persons with Parkinson's disease could be seen early in the disease process.[62] Bloem et al[63-65] and Visser et al[66,67] meticulously studied the reflexes involved in postural adjustments and described deficits in the longer loop reflexes but not in the short latency reflex associated with the stretch reflex.

Others have investigated the interactions of the sensory systems involved in balance in those with Parkinson's disease.[67-69] Bloem et al[65] and Visser et al[67] concluded that postural instability was caused by a decrease in proprioception. Other investigators have interpreted their data to show that decreased scaling of response explains loss of balance reactions.[70,71] Regardless of the physiological explanation, all researchers have demonstrated a loss of postural reflexes in all the various diseases affecting the basal ganglia.

Perceptual and Cognitive Functions

The basal ganglia are not solely motor structures. The basal ganglia have been shown to be involved in aspects of sensory integration, cognitive functions, and responses associated with reward.[42,43,72-75] Researchers found that learned movements were more affected by lesions than reflexes, that neurons in the basal ganglia were responsive to some sensory input, especially proprioceptive input, and that neurons in other parts of the basal ganglia were responsive to reward and anticipation of reward.[33,76,77] Klockgether and Dichgans[78] and Jobst et al[79] found that patients with Parkinson's disease had impairments in kinesthesia and that this impairment increased with distance from the center of the body. Schneider et al[80] found that animals that developed parkinsonian symptoms from a neurotoxin had deficits in operantly conditioned behavior. They suggested that the decrease in performance was caused by a "defect in the linkage" between a stimulus and the motor output centers. These sensory difficulties may be important factors in evaluation and treatment of basal ganglia diseases, especially those associated with dystonia.

The basal ganglia appear to be involved in the process of withholding a response until it is appropriate.[81] Animals, including human beings, have difficulty in performing alternation tasks after basal ganglia lesions.[82] One reason for these deficits is the animal's tendency toward preservation of a previously reinforced cue. Additional deficits exist in remembering or relearning tasks requiring a temporal sequence.[83] Livesey and Rankine-Wilson[83] concluded that interference in caudate functioning at the time such a task is learned selectively disrupted the registration of information generated internally. Graybiel[33] integrated the behavioral findings with information from her anatomical and chemical studies to suggest that the basal ganglia are important in providing behavioral flexibility. She hypothesizes that the basal ganglia are involved in procedural learning that leads to the development of habits. These habits become routine and are easily performed without conscious effort. Because these activities can proceed without thought, human beings are free to react to new events in the environment and to think. She and colleagues have performed electrophysiological experiments that explain this learning process; these studies demonstrate great plasticity in basal ganglia networks.[84] This enables the individual to select the proper movements in the proper environmental context. An elegant study by Brown et al[85] demonstrates a model of the basal ganglia that can reflect these cognitive and learning activities. Their model seems to integrate many of the functions of the basal ganglia with the physiology and pharmacology of the entire system. These cognitive dimensions are important to remember when developing a plan of care for patients with basal ganglia dysfunction.

Human beings with basal ganglia disease also show problems in perceptual abilities, including deficits in tasks that involve perception of interpersonal and intrapersonal space.[86] In pursuit-tracking tests individuals with Parkinson's disease had particular difficulties in correcting errors, which is consistent with Teuber's view that "the basal ganglia may play a role in the regulation of 'corollary' discharges, that is, in presetting of the motor system by sensory stimuli."[82] If the motor system is inflexibly set, corrections can be made only by a complete reprogramming.

The ability to perform cognitive activities involves integrating sensory information and, on the basis of this information, making an appropriate response. The basal ganglia seem to have a sensory integrative function, as evidenced by experiments that show a multisensory and heterotopic convergence of somatic, visual, auditory, and vestibular stimuli.[87-89] Segundo and Machne[90] observed unitary discharges of the basal ganglia to both somatic and vestibular stimuli. They hypothesized that the function of the basal ganglia was not subjective recognition of the stimuli but rather the regulation of posture and movements of the body in space and in the production of complex motor acts.[59] Although direct sensory pathways have not been found, the basal ganglia are generally believed to be involved in sensory perception.[68,91-93]

For movements to be controlled and sequenced properly, the two sides of the body need to be well integrated. Some anatomical evidence suggests some means of bilateral control for the basal ganglia. A lesion of one caudate nucleus or nigrostriatal pathway produces a change in the unit activity of the remaining caudate.[24,83] Studies of the dopaminergic pathway also indicate interactions between the two sides of the body.[24] For this reason deficits in function can be found even on the "uninvolved" side of an individual with disease of the basal ganglia. Diseases of the basal ganglia may also go unnoticed until damage is found bilaterally.

This summary of experimental results on the function of the basal ganglia illustrates several points. At least in some general way the basal ganglia are involved in the processes of movement related to preparing the organism for future motion. This may include preparing the cortex for approximate time activation, setting the postural reflexes or the gamma motor neuron system, organizing sensory input to produce a motor response in an appropriate environmental context, and inhibiting all unnecessary motor activity. The various parts of the basal ganglia may subserve different aspects of movement, which might account for the differences between an individual with Parkinson's disease and one with Huntington's disease. In a clinical assessment the loss of automatic postural adaptations appropriate for the task at hand must be carefully assessed. Perhaps one day it will no longer be necessary to say, "The exact nature and function of the large mass of basal gray matter known as the corpus striatum have hitherto constituted, it is no exaggeration to say, one of the unsolved problems of neurology."[94] The therapist's job will certainly be easier once the true functions and the specific integrative nature of the basal ganglia have been identified. Until then clinicians must carefully observe all aspects of movement (simple and complex) and postural tone during examination and treatment as well as the responses to treatment (see Chapter 9).

Neurotransmitters

Before a detailed analysis of the diseases of the basal ganglia can be considered, a brief description of the neurotransmitters of this region is necessary. The most prevalent diseases discussed in this chapter indicate a deficit in specific neurotransmitters. The pharmacological treatment of Parkinson's disease and, in the future, perhaps other "basal ganglia plus" diseases, is based on these neurochemical deficits. The basal ganglia possess high concentrations of many of the suspected neurotransmitters: dopamine (DA), acetylcholine (ACh), γ-aminobutyric acid (GABA), substance P, and the enkephalins and endorphins. This discussion, however, includes only the first three neurotransmitters. A diagram of the basal ganglia pathways, which includes the neurotransmitters, is shown in Figure 24-5.

DA is the major neurotransmitter of the nigrostriatal pathway. It is produced in the pars compacta of the substantia nigra. The axon terminals of these dopaminergic neurons are located in the caudate nucleus. Dopamine appears to be excitatory to the neurons in the direct pathway (GABA/substance P neurons) and inhibitory to the neurons in the indirect pathway (GABA/enkephalin neurons).[5] This dual effect means that a loss of DA will lead to a loss of excitation in the direct pathway and an excess of excitation of the indirect pathway, leading to a powerful decrease in activation of the thalamocortical pathway.

Several DA receptors exist; however, their chemical interactions permit the continued usage of D_1 and D_2 receptor classes.[11] The role of DA may modulate the effects of other neurotransmitters, such as glutamate. Many new drugs (called the DA agonists) influence only one of these receptors. Recent experiments have been trying to determine which behaviors are mediated by which DA receptor in the

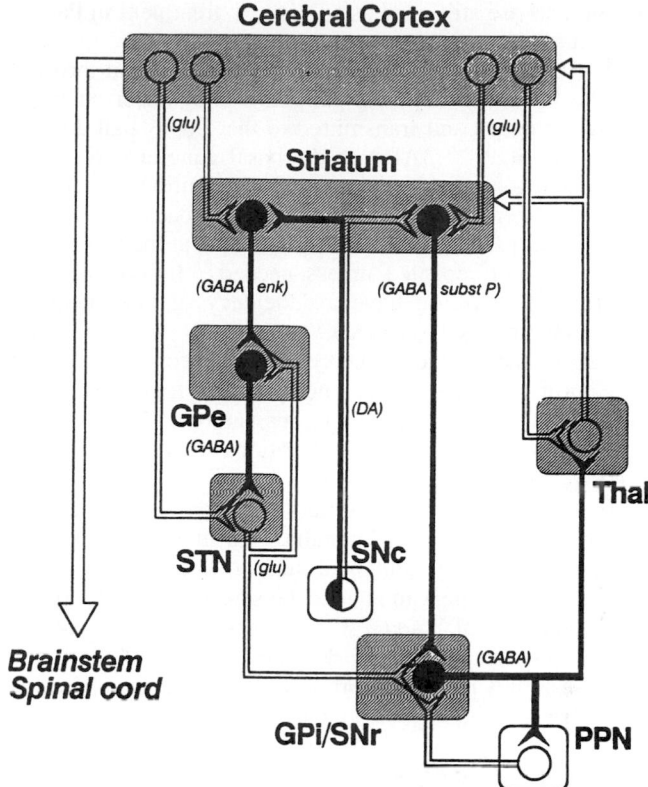

FIGURE 24-5 ■ The neurotransmitters of the direct and indirect pathways of the basal ganglia. *Black circles* represent inhibitory neurons; *shaded circles* represent excitatory neurons. *glu,* Glutamate; *enk,* enkephalin; *subst P,* substance P; *Thal,* thalamus; *GPe,* globus pallidus external segment; *GPi,* globus pallidus internal segment; *STN,* subthalamic nucleus; *SNr,* pars reticularis of the substantia nigra. (Reprinted from Alexander GE, Crutcher MD: Functional architecture of basal ganglia circuits: neural substrates of parallel processing, *Trends Neurosci* 13:266, 1990.)

hope that this research may lead to more effective drug treatment with fewer side effects.

Because various drugs and chemicals can act as agonists (similar to) and antagonists (block the action of) of DA, they are used in treating diseases involving the basal ganglia. Agonists include amantadine, apomorphine, and a class of drugs called the ergot alkaloids (e.g., bromocriptine). Amphetamine, which prevents the reuptake of DA, can enhance the effect of any DA present in the system. Antagonists include haloperidol, clozapine, and antipsychotic drugs of the phenothiazine class. With time these drugs may deplete the basal ganglia of DA and thus cause Parkinson's disease or tardive dyskinesia. Similar effects on the DA system are observed in a single dose of methamphetamine (see Chapter 36).[95]

ACh is believed to be the neurotransmitter of the small interneurons of the caudate and putamen. It is presumed to inhibit the action of DA in this region and classically must be "in balance" with DA (and GABA). Dopaminergic axon terminals are found on cholinergic neurons. Substances that increase dopaminergic activity decrease release of ACh and vice versa.[96] The antagonists of ACh, such as belladonna alkaloids and atropinelike drugs, were one of the first classes of drugs used in the treatment of Parkinson's disease. ACh antagonists are still used as adjuncts to treatment in Parkinson's disease.

GABA is an inhibitory neurotransmitter found throughout the brain. In the basal ganglia it is synthesized in the caudate nucleus and transmitted to the globus pallidus and substantia nigra.[97] GABA in the basal ganglia may permit movement to occur by allowing a distribution of neuronal firing. It also may provide a means of feedback inhibition in the efferent parts of the basal ganglia so that the program of activity is not repeated unless needed.[97] Individuals with Huntington's disease have a deficiency of this chemical. Although agonists of GABA exist (e.g., muscimol and imidazole-acetic acid), a successful drug for the treatment of Huntington's disease has not yet been found. This may be a result of either the ubiquitous nature of GABA or the complex circuitry and interrelations that exist among GABA, ACh, and DA.

In addition to the transmitters discussed, co-transmitters may be found in the basal ganglia. Two such co-transmitters are cholecystokinin and neurotensin. The interactions of these co-transmitters may alter the sensitivity of DA receptors. Fuxe et al[98] suggest that the interactions of co-transmitters may alter the "set point" of transmission in synapses. They may therefore be important in one of the side effects of DA therapy, supersensitivity.

SPECIFIC CLINICAL PROBLEMS ARISING FROM BASAL GANGLIA DYSFUNCTION

Parkinson's Disease

Parkinson's disease, first described by Parkinson in 1807, is a disease characterized by rigidity, bradykinesia (slow movement), micrography, masked face, postural abnormalities, and a resting tremor. As might be suspected from the review of functional physiology of the basal ganglia, the postural abnormalities include an assumption of a flexed posture, a lack of equilibrium reactions, especially of the labyrinthine equilibrium reactions, and a decrease in trunk rotation. Parkinson's disease is among the most prevalent of all CNS degenerative diseases. An estimated 800,000 people in the United States currently have this disease, an incidence of 4.5 to 20.5 and a prevalence of 31 to 347 per 100,000.[3] Incidence increases with advancing age, and men generally have an increased age-adjusted prevalence that persists across ethnicities compared with women.[99] An estimated one in three adults older than 85 years will have this disease.[2] The personal and societal burden of Parkinson's disease is great and includes the costs of actual treatment, the burden of caregiving, and the costs of lost earnings in those patients younger than 65 years.[100]

The pathology of Parkinson's disease consists of a decrease in the DA stores of the substantia nigra with a consequent depigmentation of this structure and the presence of Lewy bodies (intracellular inclusions). DA gives the substantia nigra its coloration (and hence its name); therefore the lighter the substantia nigra the greater the DA loss.

The etiology of Parkinson's disease remains unknown and the consensus is that it is multifactorial.[101,102] A slow viral process or long-term effects of early infection were implicated in postencephalitis parkinsonism. Some evidence shows that environmental factors are involved in the cause and that the interaction of environment and aging lead to a critical decrease in DA. Several investigators have found a link between growing up in a rural area and Parkinson's disease; the important factors include pesticide use, insecticide use, and well water.[103-109] The accumulation of free radicals, cell death from toxins to the excitatory neurons, and dysfunction of nigral mitochondria have been implicated in the pathological process. Genetics may also be a factor in Parkinson's disease.[3,110,111] Although twin studies indicate that a single gene may not be involved in Parkinson's disease, as in Huntington's disease, a family history is an important risk factor.[105] Other possible risk factors include a history of depression.[112]

In view of possible treatment effects for parkinsonism, a study by Sasco et al[113] found an inverse relation, albeit small, between participation in exercise or sports and later development of parkinsonism. Most researchers agree that the cause is an interaction of toxic exposure, genetics, and aging. The loss of DA from the substantia nigra (SN) leads to alterations in both the direct and indirect pathways of the basal ganglia, resulting in a decrease in excitatory thalamic input to the cortex and perhaps a decrease in inhibitory surround that leads to the symptoms of Parkinson's disease.

Symptoms

Bradykinesia and Akinesia. Bradykinesia (a decrease in motion) and akinesia (a lack of motion) are characterized by an inability to initiate and perform purposeful movements. They are also associated with a tendency to assume and maintain fixed postures. All aspects of movement are affected, including initiation, alteration in direction, and the ability to stop a movement once it is begun. Spontaneous or associated movements, such as swinging of the arms in gait or smiling at a funny story, are also affected. Bradykinesia is hypothesized to be the result of a decrease in activation of the supplementary motor cortex, premotor cortex, and motor cortex.[114] The resting level of activity in these areas of the cortex may be decreased so that a greater amount of excitatory input from other areas of the brain would be necessary before movement patterns could be activated. In the individual with Parkinson's disease, an increase in cortically initiated movement even for such "subcortical" activities as walking supports this hypothesis. Automatic activities are cortically controlled, and each individual aspect seems to be separately programmed. Associated movements in the trunk and other extremities are not automatic. This means that great energy must be expended whenever movement is begun.[115]

Bradykinesia and akinesia affect performance of all types of movements; however, complex movements are more involved than simple movements, such as multiple-joint motions compared with single-joint motions.[76,116-119] Additionally, patients with parkinsonism have increased difficulty performing simultaneous or sequential tasks, over and above that seen with simple tasks. Parkinsonian patients must complete one movement before they can begin to perform the next, whereas control subjects are able to integrate two movements more smoothly in sequence. This deficit has been shown in a variety of tasks, from performing an elbow movement and grip to tracing a moving line on a video screen. The patient with Parkinson's disease behaves as if one motor program must be completely played out before the next one begins, and no advance planning occurs for the next movement while the current movement is in progress.[116-118,120,121] Morris and Iansek[122] demonstrated a similar phenomenon in walking. Patients with parkinsonism were unable to walk while reciting a numerical sequence.

Sequential movements become more impaired as more movements are strung together; for example, a square is disproportionately slower to draw than a triangle, and a pentagon is more difficult to draw than a square.[4,116] These results indicate that patients with Parkinson's disease have difficulty with transitions between movements. Transitional difficulties are more impaired in tasks requiring a series of different movements than tasks requiring a series of repetitive movements. For example, an individual will have less difficulty continually brushing his teeth than a movement requiring transitions such as coming from a chair to stand and walking. (This fact is important when determining a client's disability as well as in planning a comprehensive treatment program. These deficits affect safety as well.) Clinically, remember that programming of movements in Parkinson's disease is task dependent and that familiarity with the task and the use of multisensory systems improve performance.

Bradykinesia is not caused by rigidity or an inability to relax. This was demonstrated in an EMG analysis of voluntary movements of persons with Parkinson's disease.[123] Although the pattern of EMG agonist-antagonist burst is correct, these bursts are not large enough, resulting in an inability to generate muscle force rapidly enough. Even in slow, smooth movements, however, these individuals demonstrated alternating bursts in the flexor and extensor muscle groups. This type of pattern, expected in rapid movements that require the immediate activation of the antagonist to halt the motion, interferes with slow, smooth, continuous motion. Other researchers have found an alteration in the recruitment order of single motor units.[124,125] These alterations included a delay in recruitment, pauses in the motor unit once it was recruited, and an inability to increase firing rates. These persons therefore would have a delay in activation of muscles and an inability to sustain muscle contraction properly for movement, and a decreased ability to dissipate force rapidly.[31,124,126] Such changes may account for decreases in strength that are seen in persons with Parkinson's disease. They are also important to remember in both treatment planning and the assessment of treatment efficacy.

Rigidity. The rigidity of Parkinson's disease may be characterized as either "lead pipe" or "cogwheel." The cogwheel type of rigidity is a combination of lead pipe rigidity (increased tone) with tremor. In rigidity an increased resistance to movement occurs throughout the entire range in both directions without the classic clasp-knife reflex that is characteristic of spasticity. Procaine injections can decrease the rigidity without affecting the decrease of spontaneous movements, confirming that rigidity is not the same phenomenon as bradykinesia.[127,128]

Rigidity is not caused by an increase in gamma motor neuron activity, a decrease in recurrent inhibition, or a generalized excitability in the motor system.[129] Long and middle latency reflexes are enhanced in parkinsonism, and the increase in long latency reflexes approximates the observable increase in muscle tone. Short latency reflexes (i.e.,

deep tendon reflexes), on the other hand, may be normal in persons with Parkinson's disease.

Tatton et al[130] found differences in certain cortical long-loop reflexes in normal and drug-induced monkeys with parkinsonian symptoms, which led them to speculate that the reflex gain of the CNS may lose its ability to adjust to changing environmental situations. For example, in persons with normal motor skills the background level of motor neuron excitability is different for the task of writing compared with the task of lifting a heavy object; in individuals with Parkinson's disease motor neuron excitability would be set at the same level. Similarly, the individual with normal movement function has a difference in excitability if the environmental demands were for excitation or inhibition of a muscle; for the individual with Parkinson's disease, similar motor neuron excitability would occur regardless of task demands. Furthermore, this lack of modulation may mean that the person with parkinsonism perceives to be moving farther than she or he is. It is also consistent with a decrease in system flexibility and an inability to adjust to equilibrium perturbations.[63,64,70]

An important aspect of rigidity is that it might increase energy expenditure.[131] This would increase the patient's perception of effort on movement and may be related to feelings of fatigue, especially postexercise fatigue.[132]

Tremor. The tremor observed in Parkinson's disease is present at rest, usually disappears or decreases with movement, and has a regular rhythm of approximately 4 to 7 beats/sec. Some people with Parkinson's disease may have a postural tremor. The EMG tracing of a person with such a tremor shows rhythmical, alternating bursting of antagonistic muscles. Tremor can be produced as an isolated finding in experimental animals that have lesions in various parts of the brain stem or that have been treated with drugs, especially DA antagonists. DA depletion, however, is not the sole cause of tremor. It appears that efferent pathways, especially from the basal ganglia to the thalamus, must be intact because lesions of these fibers decrease or abolish the tremor.[133] Poirier et al[133] proposed that tremor results from a combined lesion of the basal ganglia and cerebellar–red nucleus pathways. Because both the basal ganglia and the cerebellum project to the thalamus, a lesion of the thalamus can abolish the tremor regardless of the specific pathway(s). Although tremor may be cosmetically disabling, the tremor rarely interferes with activities of daily living (ADLs).

Postural Instability. Postural instability is a serious problem in parkinsonism that leads to increased episodes of falling and the sequelae of falls. More than two thirds of all patients with parkinsonism fall, and more than 10% fall more than once a week.[134] People with Parkinson's disease have a ninefold risk of recurrent falls compared with age-matched control subjects.[65,135-138] Patients have an increased likelihood of falling as the length or duration of the disease increases. Most falls are intrinsic, and 62% result in soft tissue damage, not fractures.[138] Drug treatment is not usually effective in reducing the incidence of falls. Unilateral pallidotomy is also ineffective in altering postural disturbance.[61] Deep brain stimulation (DBS) and exercise, on the other hand, have been shown to be effective on increasing functional skills or motor performance; these improvements may therefore decrease the number of falls.[139-139c] Future research needs to delineate these specific variables in relation to DBS and fall prevention.

Although the causes of balance difficulties are not known, several hypotheses exist. One explanation for postural instability is ineffective sensory processing. Several investigators have found deficits in proprioceptive and kinesthetic processing.[60,79,126] For example, Martin[60] found that labyrinthine equilibrium reactions were delayed in patients with Parkinson's disease. Studies of the vestibular system itself, however, have shown that this system functions normally. Pastor et al[140] studied central vestibular processing in patients with Parkinson's disease and found that the vestibular system responds normally and that patients can integrate vestibular input with the input from other sensory systems. This group hypothesized that the patients had an inability to adequately compensate for baseline instability. This theory is in partial agreement with studies by Beckley, Bloem, and others[63,64,70] demonstrating that patients with Parkinson's disease were unable to adjust the size of long and middle latency reflex responses to the degree of perturbation. These patients are therefore unable to activate muscle force proportional to displacement. Melnick et al[61] found that subjects with Parkinson's disease were unable to maintain balance on a sway-referenced forceplate. Glatt et al[141] found that patients with Parkinson's disease did not demonstrate anticipatory postural reactions and, in fact, behaved exactly as a rigid body with joints. Horak et al,[142,142a] in a variety of studies, reported similar findings and found defects in strategy selection as well; patients with Parkinson's disease chose neither a pure hip strategy nor a pure ankle strategy but mixed the two in an inappropriate and maladaptive response. Investigators have found that antiparkinsonian medications

could improve background postural tone but did not improve automatic postural responses to external displacements.[63,64,70,142,142b] Taken together, postural instability appears to result from inflexibility in response repertoire, an inability to inhibit unwanted programs as well as the interaction of akinesia, bradykinesia, and rigidity, with some disturbance in central sensory processing.

Gait. The typical parkinsonian gait is characterized by decreased velocity and stride length.[143,144] As a consequence, foot clearance is decreased, which again places the individual at greater fall risk.[145] In many patients, especially as the disease progresses, speed and shortening of stride progressively increase as if the individual is trying to catch up with his or her center of gravity; this is termed festination. Forward festination is called propulsion; backward festination is known as retropulsion. One hypothesis is that festinating gait is caused by the decreased equilibrium responses. If walking is a series of controlled falls and if normal responses to falling are delayed or not strong enough, then the individual will either completely fall or continue to take short, running-like steps. The abnormal motor unit firing seen with bradykinesia may also be the cause of ever-shortening steps. If the motor unit cannot build up a high enough frequency or if it pauses in the middle of the movement, then the full range of the movement would decrease; in walking this would lead to shorter steps. Festination may also be the result of other changes in the kinematics of gait.

The changes in gait kinematics include changes in excursion of the hip and ankle joints (Figure 24-6). Instead of a heel-toe progression, the patient may have a flat-footed or, with disease progression, a toe-heel sequence. The patient with Parkinson's disease appears to have lost the adult gait

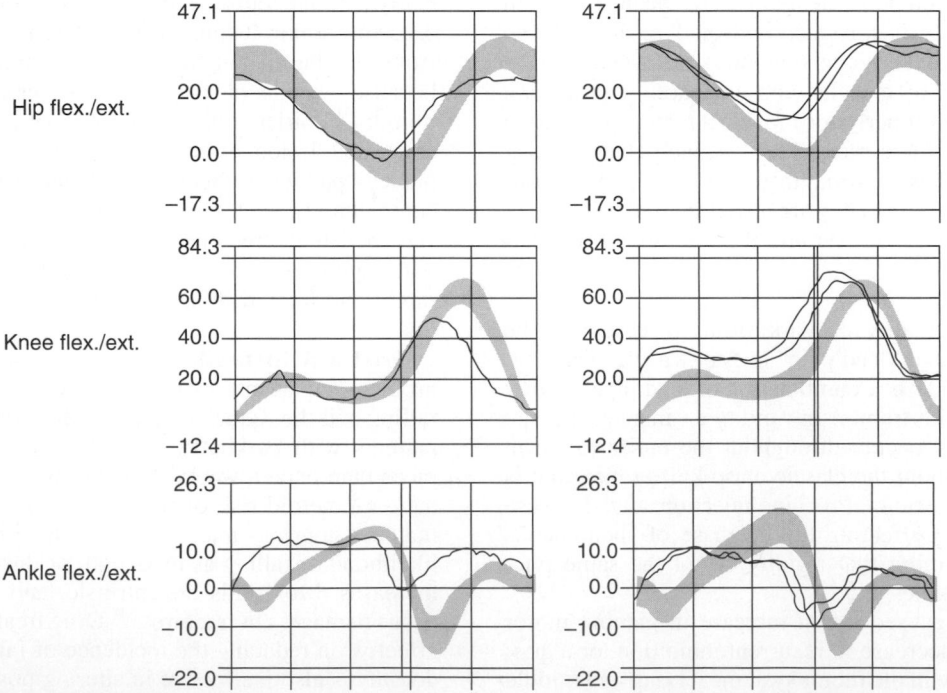

FIGURE 24-6 ▪ Angles of excursion during gait in a patient with Parkinson's disease. *Shaded areas* are mean ± standard deviations for adults with Parkinson's disease; *black line* represents a patient with Parkinson's disease. Movement shown for right and left lower extremities. Note decreases, especially in left lower extremity for extension and bilateral decreased plantar flexion.

pattern and is using a more primitive pattern. The flat-footed gait decreases the ability to step over obstacles or walk on carpeted surfaces. The use of three-dimensional gait analysis has shown a decrease in plantar flexion at terminal stance. Changes are also seen in hip flexion, which may alter ankle excursion. However, qualitative aspects of the timing of joint excursion appear intact.[143,146] Figure 24-6 illustrates the joint angles in a 55-year-old patient with Parkinson's disease compared with adults without basal ganglia dysfunction.

Gait and postural difficulties are the two impairments that cause the greatest handicap to persons with parkinsonism. They have been found to be the major elements of disability at home and work for these patients.[84]

Perception, Attention, and Cognitive Deficits. Especially in recent years, researchers have tried to address the cognitive and perceptual impairments of people with Parkinson's disease.[147-150] Whereas the movement deficits are hypothesized to be caused by a decrease in putamenal excitation of the cortex, the learning and perceptual deficits are hypothesized to be caused by a decrease in cortical excitation from the caudate nucleus.[121] The deficits are of frontal lobe function and include an inability to shift attention, an inability to quickly access "working memory," and difficulty with visuospatial perception and discrimination. Research attention has focused on the specific deficits of patients with Parkinson's disease compared with patients with Alzheimer's disease, patients with frontal lobe damage, and those with temporal lobe damage.[147,150,151] These perceptual deficits appear to increase with progression of the disease process. In general, patients have difficulty in shifting attention to a previously irrelevant stimulus,[152] learning under conditions requiring selective attention,[152] or selecting the correct motor response on the basis of sensory stimuli.[153-155] These impairments affect treatment strategies.

Learning deficits also have been found in patients with parkinsonism; procedural learning has been particularly implicated. Procedural learning is learning that occurs with practice or, as defined by Saint-Cyr et al,[155a] "the ability gradually to acquire a motor skill or even a cognitive routine through repeated exposure to a specific activity constrained by invariant rules." In their tests, patients with Parkinson's disease did poorly on tests of procedural learning, but their declarative learning was within normal limits. Pascual-Leone et al[121] studied procedural learning in more detail. They found that patients with Parkinson's disease could acquire procedural learning but needed more practice than control subjects did. They also found that the ability to translate procedural knowledge to declarative knowledge was more efficient if it occurred with visual input alone rather than the combination of visual input with motor task. This may be a rationale for more therapy, not less.

Other Symptoms. In addition to the motoric, sensory, and cognitive/perceptual problems, a number of other symptoms are also present in many people with Parkinson's disease. These include sleep disturbances and autonomic dysfunction. The patient commonly reports bowel and bladder problems, usually constipation and urinary frequency and urgency. The constipation may be caused by side effects of L-dopa. Consistent reports of bowel problems can be serious and cause obstruction; the therapist should there-

fore ask about these other side effects. Sexual dysfunction is also a side effect of Parkinson's disease and includes both impotency and loss of libido. Increased motor function sometimes decreases sexual dysfunction. Orthostatic hypotension is a frequent finding that is usually a side effect of L-dopa. When a patient reports being dizzy when she or he stands up after a meal, the therapist should record the blood pressure with the patient sitting and standing and then make any safety recommendations.

Sleep disorders are widespread in Parkinson's disease, especially daytime drowsiness and decreased sleep at night. The pathophysiology of sleep disorders is not known and may be medication related. However, even in those not on medication have decreased consolidation of sleep with decreased total sleep time as well as an increase in periodic leg movements (as in restless leg syndrome).[156] Daytime drowsiness may be a side effect of medication; however, it can also be exacerbated after therapeutic exercise, so a cooldown period is necessary before the patient sits down and relaxes.

Stages of the Disease

Parkinson's disease is a progressive disorder.[157] The initial symptom is usually a resting tremor or unilateral micrography (bradykinesia of the upper extremity). With time rigidity and bradykinesia are seen bilaterally; postural alterations then begin to occur. This commonly starts with an increase in neck, trunk, and hip flexion that, accompanied by a decrease in righting and balance responses, leads to a decreasing ability to maintain the center of gravity over the base of support.

While these postural changes are occurring, so does an increase in rigidity, which is most apparent in the trunk and proximal/axial musculature. Trunk rotation is severely decreased. No arm swing occurs during gait, no spontaneous facial expression occurs, and movement becomes more and more difficult to initiate. Movement is usually produced with great concentration and is perhaps cortically generated, therefore bypassing the damaged basal ganglia pathways. This great concentration then makes movement tiring, which heightens the debilitating effects of the disease.

Eventually the individual becomes wheelchair bound and dependent. In the late and severe stages of the disease, especially without therapeutic attention to movement, the client may become bedridden and may demonstrate a fixed trunk-flexion contracture no matter what position the person is placed in. This posture has been called the "phantom pillow" syndrome because, even when lying supine, the person's head is flexed as if on a pillow.

Throughout this progressive deterioration of movement, higher-level sensory processing also decreases. In addition, the patient can perform only one task at a time. Reports of dementia range from 30% to 93% of patients with Parkinson's disease.[158] The amount of dementia is frequently related to the age of the patient, and these patients may represent a subset of Parkinson's disease. The presence of dementia with Parkinson's disease may indicate involvement of Ach or the noradrenergic mesolimbic system. In this case, treatment with anticholinergic drugs may increase a tendency toward dementia, especially in older patients. Sometimes cognitive deficits are inferred because of slowed responses, spatial problems, sensory processing problems, and a masked face (see Chapter 36).

The most serious complication of Parkinson's disease is bronchopneumonia. Decreased activity in general, along with decreased chest expansion, may be contributing factors. The mortality rate is greater than in the general population, and death is usually from pneumonia.

Pharmacological Considerations and Medical Management

The knowledge that the symptoms of Parkinson's disease are caused by a decrease in DA led to the pharmacological management of this disease. Because DA itself does not cross the blood-brain barrier, levo-dihydroxyphenylalanine (L-dopa), a precursor of DA, has been used to treat Parkinson's disease since the late 1960s.[159-161] An inhibitor of aromatic amino acid decarboxylation (carbidopa) is usually given with L-dopa to prevent the conversion to DA before entering the brain. The decarboxylase inhibitor allows a reduction in dosage of L-dopa itself, which helps decrease the cardiac and gastrointestinal side effects of DA.

Amantadine is another drug that has been effective in treatment of Parkinson's disease. Although the mechanism of action of this antiviral medication is unknown, it may include a facilitation of release of catecholamines (of which DA is one) from stores in the neuron that are readily releasable. It is often administered in combination with L-dopa.

Treatment of Parkinson's disease with L-dopa in these various combinations is extremely helpful in reducing bradykinesia and rigidity. It is less effective in reducing tremor. Because Parkinson's disease involves the nigral neurons, the receptors and the neurons in the striatum (which are postsynaptic to DA neurons) remain intact and are initially somewhat responsive to DA.[162,163] With time, however, the receptors appear to lose their sensitivity, and the prolonged effectiveness (10 years or more) of L-dopa therapy is questionable.[164-166] A further complication of L-dopa therapy is the development of involuntary movements (dyskinesias) and the "on-off" phenomenon: a short-duration response resulting in sudden improvement of symptoms followed by a rapid decline in symptomatic relief and perhaps the appearance of dyskinesias or dystonias.[167] With time the "on" effect becomes shorter and shorter in duration.[164] The effectiveness of L-dopa does not appear to be closely correlated with the stage of the disease.

The use of L-dopa alone or in combination with carbidopa has not provided a cure or even prevented the degeneration of Parkinson's disease. Therefore many new drugs are being tested and tried. As scientists learn more about the DA receptors and their role in motor control, more effective medications may be found. Some of these newer drugs include bromocriptine and pergolide, both D_2 receptor agonists. Low doses of bromocriptine seem to decrease the wearing-off phenomenon of L-dopa and may also decrease the dyskinesia. The sensitivity of the brain to these pharmacological dosages may interact with neuroplasticity and will be a focus of future study.[168] However, the side effects include hallucinations, nausea, and vomiting. Pergolide also appears to be effective in treatment; however, double-blind studies seem to indicate recovery in placebo as well.[169] Newer D_2 or D_2/D_1 agonists will likely be developed. Other pharmacological interventions include drugs that prevent the breakdown (e.g., catechol-O-methyltransferase [COMT] inhibitors) or re-uptake of DA. Entacapone, a COMT inhibitor, has now been approved for use.

Another approach to pharmacological treatment of Parkinson's disease developed from research on a designer drug that contained the neurotoxin 1-methyl-4-phenyl-1,2,3,6-tetrahydropyridine (MPTP). Conversion of MPTP to the active neurotoxin MPP[+] was found to be prevented by monamine oxidase inhibitors such as deprenyl and pargyline.[170] Deprenyl (also known as selegiline) is now used before the initiation of, or in conjunction with, L-dopa/carbidopa. Although its mechanism of action is still not fully understood, it may act as a neuroprotective agent.[171-173] Neurotrophic factors such as brain-derived or glial-derived neurotrophic factors are also under investigation.

Stereotaxic surgery is an old technique that has made a comeback based on the new knowledge of basal ganglia connectivity and improvements in the instrumentation.* Three classes of surgery are presently under investigation and include lesions, DBS with implanted electrodes, and neural transplantation.[176] Lesions are made in specific areas of the globus pallidus and in the subthalamic nucleus.[174,175,177,178] After the appearance of these lesions, which are small and usually restricted to the posteroventral region of the globus pallidus, rigidity, bradykinesia, and akinesia improve. Patients spontaneously demonstrate associated reactions. In many cases dyskinesias also improve. Thalamic lesions are made in cases in which tremor is the most disabling symptom. DBS is another surgical alternative; it is now preferred because this electrical lesion is reversible and safer for bilateral surgeries. Sites include the thalamus for tremor and the globus pallidus and subthalamic nucleus (STN) for other symptoms of Parkinson's disease.[179,180] All sites have now been approved by the Food and Drug Administration. DBS of the globus pallidus or STN and pallidotomy have been shown to decrease all symptoms, especially dyskinesias.[180-182] The effects are greater for symptoms manifested in the "off" state. STN stimulation often leads to a decrease in amount on medication needed. DBS is usually performed bilaterally for STN stimulation; for globus pallidus stimulation the leads may be placed unilaterally or bilaterally. DBS has been demonstrated to decrease side effects of pharmacological treatment, improve gait,[62,181,183-186] and improve balance[61,187] and has been recently shown to improve movement velocity and speed of muscle recruitment for activity.[188,189] The proposed mechanism of action is interference with the abnormal neuronal firing.[190,191] Longer-term studies are underway and, depending on the symptom under investigation, effects remain for 5 years.[181,182] Therapists may find that intense treatment immediately after these surgeries may be able to take advantage of neural plasticity provided by DBS.

Fetal transplantation of the substantia nigra to the caudate nucleus is currently under investigation. A double-blind, placebo-controlled trial was completed with mixed results.[176,190,192,193] Studies continue, including those of dose, type of cell, and placement of cells. At this time, the American Academy of Neurology has made no recommendations for use of fetal transplantation.[77]

---

*References 5, 6, 81, 164, 174, 175.

Examination of the Client with Parkinson's Disease

The previous sections indicated the symptoms and hypothesized pathophysiological explanations for those symptoms. Examination of the client with Parkinson's disease should include the degree of rigidity, bradykinesia, balance and gait impairments, and how much these symptoms interfere with ADLs; that is, how do the symptoms influence the client's handicap? Examination of rigidity should extend to the muscles of respiration as well as the trunk and extremities. The tools used should be as objective as possible. The most commonly used descriptor for the patient's level of involvement is the Hoehn and Yahr scale (see Figure 24-6).[157] The most prevalent and one of the most comprehensive physician examination is the Unified Parkinson's Disease Rating Scale (UPDRS), which measures cognitive and emotional status, ADL ability, motor function, and side-effects of medication.[194-194b] This is an ordinal scale and, although it is used to measure efficacy of treatments, may not be ideal for physical therapy treatment planning. Another clinical scale is the Core Assessment Program for Intracerebral Transplantation (CAPIT), which includes timed tests.[195] This scale, as its name implies, is more time consuming and therefore tends to be used in research more than in the clinic.

Because of the effects of bradykinesia and difficulty with sequential movements associated with Parkinson's disease, the therapist must note whether the client can accomplish an activity as well as how long it takes to do so. Gait can be assessed by general pattern as well as speed and distance. Forward and backward walking as well as braiding should be evaluated. The effect of interfering stimuli and tasks is also a beneficial measure. Measurements of gait should include stride length, speed of walking, and cadence.[143,144] During periodic examinations, the therapist should measure the ability of the client to alter gait speed. Similarly, the time necessary to complete transitional movements such as moving from sitting to standing, standing to sitting, and supine lying to sitting and back again should be recorded. Handwriting should be periodically sampled. Active and passive range of movement, general strength, and chest expansion and/or functional capacity should also be measured.

A careful analysis of balance is imperative for the patient with Parkinson's disease. This must include assessment with and without vision and the differences in the two recorded (see Chapter 23). Assessing challenges to balance such as tandem walking or standing on a compliant surface is important, especially in the early stages of the disease. This may be the first sign of a balance impairment. Posturography is the most sensitive measure of postural instability, especially in the early (Hoehn and Yahr stages I and II) stages of the disease.[61] A clinically useful tool to assess dynamic balance is the functional reach test; recent studies have shown this to be an effective, predictive tool in people with Parkinson's disease as it is in the elderly.[196]

Another aspect of assessment includes the detailed observation of associated postural movements. For example, in rising from a chair, does the patient move forward in the chair, place the feet underneath the knees, and lean forward before rising? Ideally, the evaluation format should also include the performance of simultaneous and sequential tasks. An assessment of chest expansion and vital capacity should also be included. This is important because of the complication of pneumonia. A complete and easy-to-use form for evaluation does not currently exist for Parkinson's disease.

General Prognosis, Treatment Goals, and Rationale

As with all treatment, the prognosis (functional goals and established time parameters) is based on the general goals related to the findings on examination of each client and the client's expectations and functional requirements. Parkinson's disease must be understood as a degenerative disease when establishing the prognosis and treatment plan. Nonpharmacological and surgical interventions, especially physical therapy treatment, are especially important in the beginning of the disease.[197] In general, goals include increasing movement and range of motion in the entire trunk as well as the extremities, maintaining or improving chest expansion, improving balance reactions, and maintaining or restoring functional abilities. Increased movement may in fact modify the progression of the disease and prevent contractures.[198,199] It may further help to retard dementia. Although L-dopa decreases bradykinesia, it alone is not effective in increasing movement or improving balance; therefore aggressive intervention in the early stages is necessary. Increasing trunk rotation and increasing spinal extension go hand in hand with increasing range of movement and motion in general. The longer clients are kept mobile, the less likely they are to develop pneumonia and the longer they can maintain independence in ADLs. Ideally, physical therapy interventions should begin at the first sign of the disease, but this is not always possible. Treatment begun while the disease is still unilateral (Hoehn and Yahr stage I) is more advantageous to the patient.[200,201]

Treatment Procedures

In general, treatment interventions should be based on the pathophysiology and functions of the basal ganglia as previously discussed. Performing functional activities that incorporate complex motor activities, changing the sequence of activities, and participating in gait and balance activities are especially useful early in the disease progression. Practice is a critical variable for maintenance of functional skill.[202] Strengthening muscle groups in functional activities is more efficacious than nonfunctional strengthening exercises if the goal is carryover to ADLs.[135,203-208] As the disease progresses more specific interventions for the spine and breathing may be indicated. These activities may need to be modified for safety. Movement therapy may also be helpful in decreasing depression,[187,209-211] dementia,[211] and fatigue.[211]

Movement throughout a full range of motion is crucial, especially early in the disease process to prevent changes in the properties of muscle itself. In Parkinson's disease the contractile elements of flexors become shortened and those of the extensor surface become lengthened, enhancing the development of the flexed posture traditionally seen.[212] And for most patients, treatment proceeds better if rigidity is decreased early in the treatment session. In fact, movement therapy interventions appear to have more lasting effects when the treatment is during the "on" phase of medication.

To reduce rigidity, many relaxation techniques appear to be effective, including gentle, slow rocking, rotation of the extremities and trunk, and yoga (see Chapter 9). In the client with Parkinson's disease, success in relaxation may be better achieved in the sitting position because rigidity may increase in the supine position.[103] Furthermore, because the proximal muscles are often more involved than the distal muscles, relaxation may be easier to achieve by following a distal to proximal progression. The inverted position should be used with care. Initially this position facilitates some relaxation (increase in parasympathetic tone) and then increases trunk extension, which is important for the client with Parkinson's disease. Relaxation may also be effective in reducing the tremor of Parkinson's disease.

Once a decrease in rigidity is achieved through relaxation, movement must be initiated. For the client with Parkinson's disease this movement should be large and through the entire range. As with relaxation techniques, starting with distal motions first and gradually increasing the movement may be easier, bringing in proximal/axial and trunk muscles. Sitting is a good position from which to begin, starting perhaps with swinging of the arms in ever-increasing amplitude. Because bilateral symmetrical patterns are easier than reciprocal patterns, they should be used first and then followed with diagonal patterns. To add trunk rotation (which also helps decrease the proximal rigidity), proprioceptive neuromuscular facilitation (PNF) patterns and rhythmic initiation may be used.[213,214] Additionally, neurodevelopmental treatment (NDT) and mobilization techniques may be useful to increase scapular and pelvic mobility. Rhythm and auditory cues facilitate movement. Rhythm, especially as in a march, seems to enable the client to move continuously with alternating flexion and extension without becoming fixated. Clapping or music enhances this effect. At present no explanation can be given for this phenomenon, although one study found changes in the DA system with decreases in rigidity and bradykinesia with music.[215] Once the therapist has improved movement, functional activities should be practiced. The therapist must always remember that functional behavior is based on the patient's ability to perform the activity. Thus no matter what the therapeutic intervention, patient participation and practice are key to any long-term or interim effect with the motor system. No research has been done to identify the potential neuroplasticity within a brain during a slow, progressive degenerative process or disease. Thus a therapist must be familiar with the most current research and understanding of neuroplasticity to provide the best learning environment for the adult in care.[216]

Exercise is important for the person with Parkinson's disease. Longevity and physical activity are related.[217] Those who exercise have lower mortality rates.[217] Some evidence also indicates that exercise may alter the magnitude of free radicals and other compounds linked to aging and parkinsonism. Immunological function may also be improved with exercise. Sasco et al[113] demonstrated a link between a lack of exercise and development of parkinsonism. Finally, the role of aerobic fitness itself may be a factor in reducing dysfunction.[19] Recent animal data indicate that functional exercise decreased DA loss after a variety of lesion models.[138,200,201,218] Aerobic exercise may improve pulmonary function in patients with Parkinson's disease because these functions appear to suffer from deficiencies in

rapid force generation of the respiratory muscles, similar to limb musculature.[219] Exercise is most beneficial when it is begun early in the disease process, as is recommended in all books and pamphlets for the patient.[220] All research on the effects of exercise programs in parkinsonism indicates this point. When the use of forced functional activities was delayed too long, no beneficial effects of exercise on the DA system were shown in animal studies.[200,201] Hurwitz[221] found that patients who were still independently mobile at home and in the community benefited the most from a home program. Schenkman and Butler[212] also indicated that patients in the earlier stages of the disease had the best potential for improvement. If patients practice regular physical exercise in conjunction with disease-specific exercises, the ill effects of inactivity will not potentiate the effects of the disease process itself. Although most patients with parkinsonism can achieve an adequate exercise level, many clients have fitness levels that are poor or very poor before the medical diagnosis.[131] Exercise, even once a week, is effective in improving gait and balance in clients with Parkinson's disease.[222]

So far all but one study has found that exercise under the guidance of a therapist is effective. Few studies, however, have used random assignment with good controls.[223] A report by Palmer et al[207] used precise, quantitative measures to assess motor signs, grip strength, coordination, and speed as well as measurements of the long latency stretch reflex after two exercise programs in patients with Parkinson's disease: the United Parkinson Foundation program and karate training. Their results indicated improvement over a 12-week period in gait, grip strength, and coordination of fine motor control tasks but no change in a decline in movements requiring speed. The patients all felt an increase in general well being. The results of this careful study indicate that more research and careful documentation of exercise programs are needed. A study by Comella et al[224] as well as one by Patti et al[225] also found decreases in parkinsonian symptoms with physical and occupational therapy. However, these studies found no long-term carryover of therapy. The authors never explain the exercise program precisely or the instructions provided for a home program.

Another study used "sports activities" in a twice-weekly program.[155a] The program included exercises on land designed to improve gait and balance and exercises in the water to increase strength. These investigators reported significant improvements in the UPDRS, cognitive function, and mood in addition to ADLs and motor scores during the 14-week program. Interestingly, they also found decreases in dyskinesia. The greatest changes in exercise appeared early and were maintained up to 6 weeks after cessation of the exercise program. Hiking was effective in a study in Switzerland.[226] One effective program used dance and other weight bearing exercise. Marchese et al[227] used complex activities. All of the studies demonstrated similar improvements in balance and especially initiation of gait.[222,227]

Physical activity and movement appear to increase quality of life by decreasing depression and improving mood and initiative.[228,229] Group classes can serve as an extra support system for patients and their spouses.[84,229,230] Intensive exercise is beneficial in early stages of the disease.[208] Carefully structured low-impact aerobics program appears to be beneficial to patients even with longstanding disease.[222] One program begins with seated activities for upper extrem-

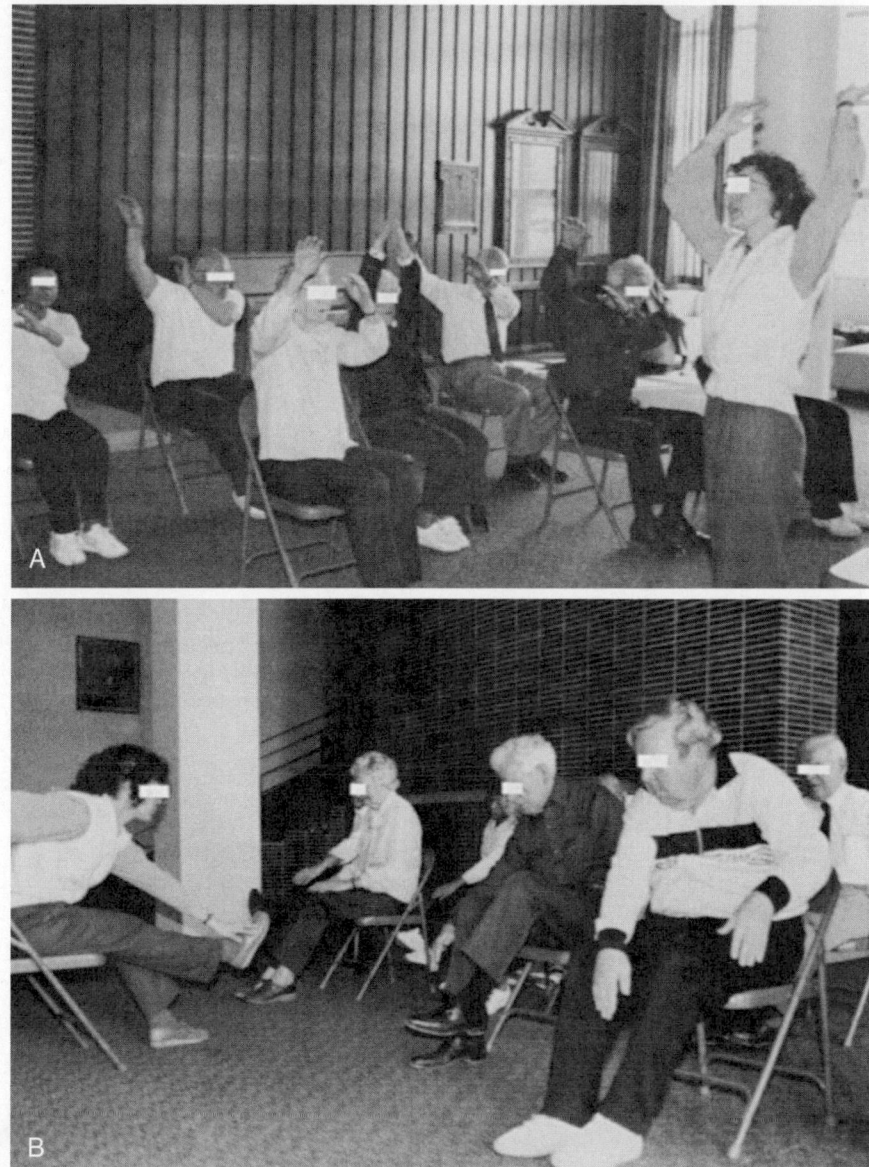

FIGURE 24-7 ■ Seated aerobics or warm-up exercises. **A,** Clients are using bilateral upper extremity patterns to facilitate trunk rotation. Instruction was to let the head follow the hands. **B,** This exercise encourages trunk rotation, large movements, and coordination of the upper and lower extremities. Clients are to reach with the arms and touch the opposite foot. This coordination is difficult for those with Parkinson's disease, and many clients initially could not move the arms and legs at the same time.

ities and then combination movements for warm-up (Figure 24-7). The participants then progress to standing and marching activities that incorporate coordinated movements of arms and legs as well as balance and trunk rotation (Figure 24-8). Throughout the program, the participants are encouraged to increase the size of their movements and to make them as "big as possible." External cueing and rhythm are critical to success of this program. Heart rate should be monitored periodically. Many Parkinson's disease associations also have audiotapes for exercises (e.g., United Parkinson Foundation).

Rhythmic exercise has been shown to decrease rigidity and bradykinesia and improve gait over time.* Ballroom

dancing is a form of rhythmic therapy for patients with Parkinson's disease that incorporates rhythmical movement, rotation, balance, and coordination. The waltz or fox trot is a good beginning dance because it is easy and somewhat slow (Figure 24-9). The mambo promotes separation of the pelvis from the trunk and increases coordination. A modified Charleston can be used to increase one-legged balance, as can modified tap dancing. The use of dance also facilitates changing direction. Some of the group activities and possible exercises are depicted in Figures 24-7 to 24-10. In patients who practice rhythmic exercise, the author has found a decrease in the time it takes the client to respond to a "go" signal and walk 3 feet and continue walking 20 feet. A concomitant increase in stride length also occurred. Balance improved for those patients who could not stand on

*References 84, 206, 209, 227, 228, 230-232.

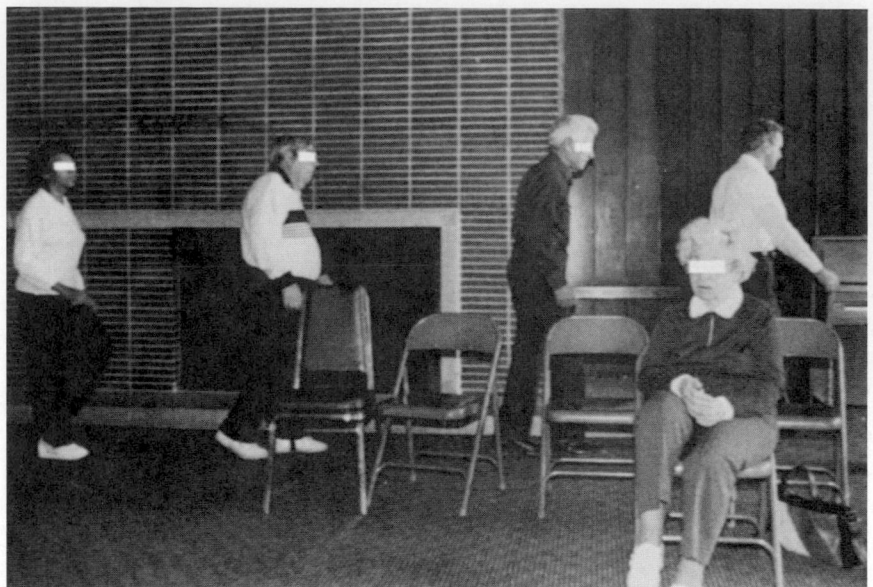

FIGURE 24-8 ■ Initial warm-up in standing. Clients are to walk with the head up, with the back as straight as possible, and to take large steps. When the group began, walking was the major aerobic activity and was used to increase endurance and encourage movement. Nonambulatory patients march in place while seated.

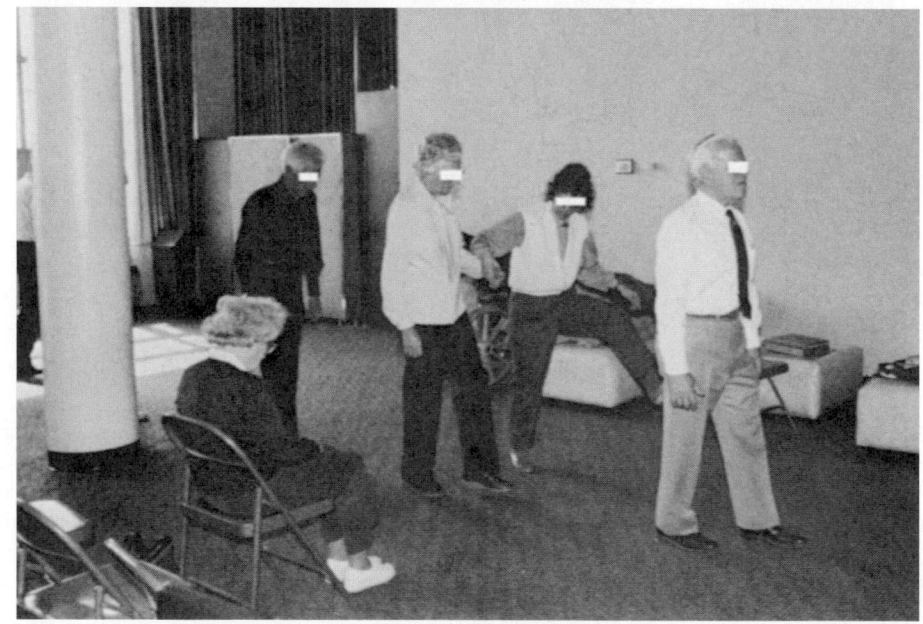

FIGURE 24-9 ■ Walking in a "waltz rhythm" (slow, quick, quick) emphasizes a big step for the slow step. Note lack of automatic arm swing. Also note flexed posture of seated patient during rest period.

foam at the start of the program. The authors also found that clients with more severe Parkinson's disease (Hoehn and Yahr stage III-IV) also demonstrated improvement in gait after a 6-week session of group exercise.

The most successful exercise programs to ameliorate many of the dysfunctions associated with parkinsonism appear to be those that incorporate context-dependent responses and a varied environment.* Examples of these

*References 135, 185, 203-205, 207-209, 222, 227, 229, 233-236.

activities are presented in Box 24-1. (Aerobic exercises that are not as effective in requiring context-dependent responses are presented in Box 24-2.) Research has shown the importance of adjusting the response to the specific task and has also demonstrated the importance of practice for the patient with Parkinson's disease.[155,237] The principles of motor learning are of paramount importance in the treatment program of these patients. Random practice may enable the patient to learn the correct schema by which to regulate the extent, speed, and direction of the movement. Random practice also

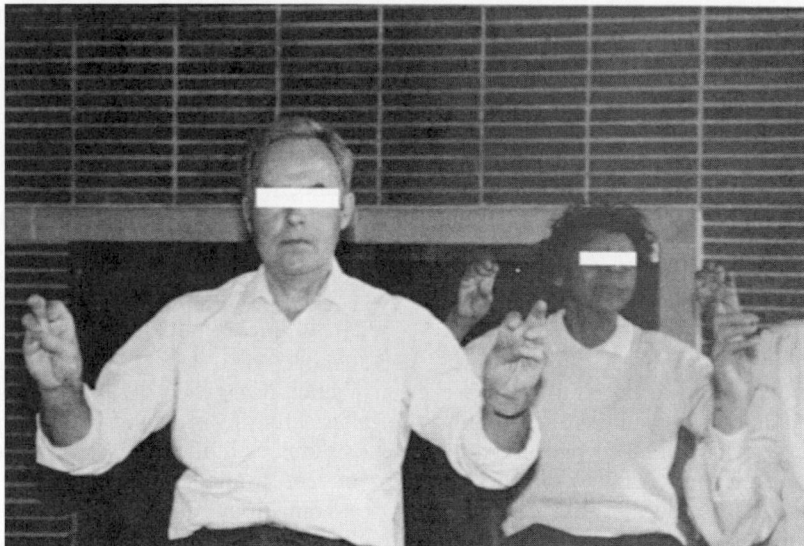

FIGURE 24-10 ■ Cool-down period allows time to work on fine finger movements. Thumb abduction with rounded fingers and various rhythms are used to increase coordination. Note "masked face" appearance.

BOX 24-1 ■ EXAMPLES OF EXERCISE REGIMENS THAT PROMOTE CONTEXT-DEPENDENT RESPONSES

Walking outdoors
Karate and other martial arts
Dancing (all forms)
All ball sports
Cross-country and downhill skiing
Well-structured, low-impact aerobics classes

This list is an example of activities; it should not be considered all inclusive.

BOX 24-2 ■ EXERCISE REGIMENS THAT PROMOTE FITNESS AND INCREASE IN RANGE OF MOTION BUT NOT CONTEXT-DEPENDENT RESPONSES

Walking on a treadmill
Riding a stationary bicycle
Using strengthening machines and free weights (with low weights or low resistance)
Using step exercises and stair climbers
Rowing on a machine
Swimming laps

This list is an example of activities; it should not be considered all inclusive.

---

may be important in facilitating the ability of the patient to shift attention and to learn to access "working memory." The patient with Parkinson's disease may benefit from visual instruction and mental rehearsal before performing the movement.[140,155] The research on sensory systems in Parkinson's disease indicates effectiveness in the use of multisensory cuing.

Strengthening exercises have been advocated for the patient with Parkinson's disease. With disuse comes decreased strength. Weakness occurs with initial contraction and also with prolonged contraction. Manual muscle testing may not reveal losses in strength; however, most successful exercise programs previously mentioned include strength training as part of the program. According to the literature, functional strength training seems to be more effective than weightlifting if the goal is improvement in ADLs.[155a] An important part of any strengthening program is the trunk musculature. Spinal extensors need to be exercised and spinal flexibility likewise encouraged.[238]

As the disease progresses, intensive exercise programs may need to be revised or altered. By stage 2.5, gait disorders are the most common diagnosis for which the person with Parkinson's disease will see a therapist. Many aspects of gait are amenable to treatment. The problems that cause the biggest handicap are freezing and small steps. Both auditory and visual stimuli have been used in treatment of parkinsonian gait disorders. Thaut et al[239] have demonstrated that a metronome or carefully synthesized music improve stride length and speed and that these improvements remain up to 5 weeks after the cessation of the auditory stimulus. Melnick et al[222] have also demonstrated both immediate and longer-lasting improvements in gait after a rhythmic exercise program once a week in patients needing assistance to walk.

People with Parkinson's disease find climbing stairs easier than walking on a flat surface because of the visual stimulation provided by the stairs. Visual stimuli have been effective in freezing episodes. These include the use of lines on the floor and stair climbing. Martin[60] found that parallel lines were more facilitating than other lines and that the space between lines was also important; the lines cannot be too close together. The use of visual stimuli, however, has scant evidence of carryover. One client has used visual stimuli in special glasses. These glasses provide constant lines for the client to step over. At present these glasses are not commercially available. Dunne et al[240] described a cane that could present a visual cue for the patient who has freezing episodes. Canes can be especially useful for patients who fall because of freezing. If a specialized cane is not available, the client can turn his or her own cane upside down. Other visual stimuli have been used to help initiate movement after freezing. One patient tosses pennies ahead of him and steps over them. (He does not bend to pick them up, which would again lead to freezing.) Another watches the movement of a person walking beside him; the movement of that person's feet encourages his feet to move. Morris et al[145] have tried to increase carryover of visual stimuli by incorporating them with a program of visualization. Their clients practiced walking with lines until the steps were near normal in size; the clients were then to visualize the lines on the floor as they walked. Their visualization program met with initial success. Increasing the magnitude of the step or the amplitude of the movement appears to be the most important component for improvement in gait and a decrease in freezing.[145] Both auditory and visual sensory cues have, as expected, met with excellent success. Additional improvements occurred in ADLs. Improvements were seen in postural stability as well as gait in a study that added tactile cues to visual and auditory cues.[236]

Gait rehabilitation must include walking in crowds, through doorways, and on different surfaces. Practice walking slowly and quickly is important, as is walking with differing stride lengths, because in the real world step length and speed must change with environmental demands. Although no controlled studies have yet been reported, the principles of motor learning presented in Chapter 3 appear to be helpful for facilitating carryover of the therapeutic effects in preliminary studies. One word of caution, however; the person with Parkinson's disease has increasing difficulty performing two tasks at once, such as walking and performing math problems or walking with a glass of water on a tray.[153] The patient may have to concentrate only on walking as the disease progresses to increase patient safety.

Balance disorder is another problem for which therapy is indicated, especially because drugs and surgical treatment are ineffective. This problem will eventually affect all persons with Parkinson's disease.[241] If at all possible, the client should be instructed in practicing balance exercises at the early stages of the disease. Equilibrium reactions in all planes of movement and under different controls should be encouraged. Rhythmical stabilization may be used to increase static balance if the use of resistance does not lead to an increase in truncal rigidity. The timing of the resistance must be gradual, allowing the client time to develop force in one set of muscles before increasing resistance and then switching directions. This alters the context of the environment and allows the client to practice a variety of variations of the original plan. If proper time is not allowed, the ther-apist may reinforce the already inefficient, ineffective patterns of motor activity. Techniques to increase dynamic balance should also be included, especially turning the body and turning the head. All three balance strategies need to be addressed and then practiced in a variety of environmental conditions. (See Chapter 23 for other procedures to improve balance.)

Rarely will the client with Parkinson's disease state that she or he has difficulty performing two tasks at once. Nonetheless, this is quite apparent in simple activities such as requiring the patient to count backwards and walk at the same time.[144,146] One solution is to instruct the client to attend to only one task at a time. Another is to have the client practice doing two things at the same time and constantly alter activities in a random practice mode during treatment. Differences in the efficacy of these two approaches had not yet been studied.

Transitional movements pose great problems for the client, especially by stage 3. This is most likely because normal postural adjustments are no longer automatic and they become a sequential task. Practice is helpful with frequent review. Some researchers report improvement in moving from a seated to a standing position after practicing techniques designed to increase forward weight shift (e.g., leaning on a chair while standing up).[242,243] Visualization of this task demonstrates carryover. Rolling in bed and rising from the supine position also become difficult and need practice and increased emphasis on trunk rotation.

Bed mobility is another important consideration for patients with Parkinson's disease. A firm bed may make getting in and out of bed easier. Most patients report that satin sheets with silk or satin pajamas make moving in bed far easier. This is true in both the early and later stages of the disease. Teaching the client to roll onto the side and lower the legs off the bed facilitates getting out of bed; the client may not be using this method, so relearning this movement is important. The patient may be able to roll in the clinic setting but then must practice with sheets and blankets as well. Beds with a head that can be raised electrically may be helpful as the disease progresses, but while sleeping the patient should lower the head as close to horizontal as possible. If getting up from a chair becomes too difficult, chairs with seats that lift up have been used effectively.

Breathing exercises are crucial for the patient with Parkinson's disease. As stated previously, the most common cause of death is pneumonia. Chest expansion may be included in upper-extremity activities such as swinging the arm. The clinician may also have the client shout—especially with a rhythmical chant, such as a simple "left, right" while walking. With disease progression, specific breathing exercises need to be incorporated. This is crucial for the patient who is no longer able to walk.

In addition to treatment in the therapy department, the client with Parkinson's disease also should be given a home program. The home program should encourage making moderate, consistent exercise a part of the normal day. Periodic checks may enhance compliance. Fatigue should be avoided and the exercise graded to the individual's capability. The therapist should keep in mind that learned skills such as various sports are sometimes less affected than automatic movements, perhaps because these skills may rely on cortical involvement.[16]

Fatigue is a frequent symptom among people with Parkinson's disease. Although it has been correlated with disease progression, depression, and sleep disturbances it also exists in a high percentage of those without depression or sleep difficulty (44% of patients in one study).[244] This fatigue is over and above that associated with the exertion of the exercise program and may be one reason those with Parkinson's disease no longer exercise. The client with Parkinson's disease frequently experiences postexercise fatigue. When a patient is more tired after exercise and cannot perform normal ADLs, exercise will not become a part of her or his daily routine. Documented postexercise fatigue is easily alleviated by extending a cool-down period and making certain that it is gradual.

Patients frequently ask about the timing of medication and exercise. For any form of exercise in parkinsonism to be effective, movement must be possible, especially movement through the full arc of the joint. Plausibly, exercise should therefore be performed during the "on" period. On the other hand, perhaps a more long-lasting effect would result if the patient with Parkinson's disease tried to exercise without medication. The question of the effects of exercise on DA agonist absorption were recently investigated by Carter et al.[245] They concluded that the effect was variable from patient to patient; however, the response of each patient was consistent. However, none of the patients exercised vigorously, which may have skewed the results. Reuter et al[246] interpreted the decrease in dyskinesia seen after their exercise program as indicative of more efficient DA absorption. Nevertheless, this study supports the concept that the patient needs to be "in tune" with his or her own response and adjust medications and exercise to a schedule accordingly. Patients appear to be able to integrate their exercise and medication schedule well.

The therapist is also involved in the prescription of assistive devices. The use of assistive devices in gait for patients with Parkinson's disease is an area with no clear-cut guidelines. Because coordination of upper and lower extremities is often difficult, the ability to use a cane or walker is often lacking. The patient may drag the cane or carry the walker. Walkers with wheels sometimes increase the festinating gait, and the patient may simply fall over the walker. Nonetheless, four-wheel walkers with push-down brakes appear to be work best for many clients. For those patients with a tendency to fall backwards, an assistive device may simply be something to carry backwards with them. Therefore the reason for using the assistive device must be carefully assessed. Walkers or canes can be helpful for the person with postural instability and the ability to walk with a heel-toe gait. The height of walker or cane should be adjusted carefully to promote extension and avoid an increase in trunk flexion. A walking stick, such as that used in hiking, is less likely to promote flexion than a cane. A survey by Mutch et al[231] in Ireland found that nearly half of the patients responding used some type of assistive device. These devices included devices for walking, reaching, and performing ADLs. Patients with Parkinson's disease may also benefit from assistive devices for eating and writing.

As Parkinson's disease progresses the patient may experience difficulty in swallowing and even chewing. Therapy for oral-motor control should be initiated, and a dietitian consult may be necessary to ensure adequate nutrition.

A dietitian may also be beneficial in guiding the patient's protein intake. A diet high in protein may reduce the responsiveness of the patient to DA replacement therapy.[144] Regulating the amount and timing of protein ingestion can improve the efficacy of drug treatment in some patients.

The resurgence of surgery as a treatment alternative in Parkinson's disease means that the therapist will face new and exciting challenges in treatment. After lesion creation, stimulation of deep brain sites, or fetal transplantation, the brain may have increased plasticity.[247] Many researchers have shown that fetal cells do survive and connect to target cells. However, initial results demonstrated negative side effects that outweighed the benefits. Intense therapy, especially incorporating complex motor skills, has been demonstrated to be effective in improving function after a lesion in animal studies.[248] This intensity of therapy after surgery may be necessary to maximize benefits from all surgeries in Parkinson's disease (and also Huntington's disease or dystonias).[33]

Finally, Parkinson's disease is a progressive, degenerative disease. Therapy and exercise may modify the progression but cannot halt or reverse it. Quality of life throughout the course of the disease may be enhanced, however, and the therapist can assist the client and family in coping with the constraints of this disease. As stated in one study of Parkinson's disease, the total cost of treatment must also include the cost to the spouse or other family members (Case Studies 24-1 and 24-2).

Differences between Parkinson's Disease and "Parkinson Plus" Syndromes: Theoretical and Practical Considerations

Several other disorders are lumped together as "Parkinson plus" syndromes. Clients with these syndromes usually do not respond to L-dopa. The most common of these is progressive supranuclear palsy (PSP). Symptoms of this disease include bradykinesia, gait instability with frequent falls, rigidity, and a vertical gaze palsy. These clients can be evaluated and treated in a manner similar to the client with Parkinson's disease. However, PSP usually involves more cognitive impairment and the progression is more rapid; within a decade the patient is typically immobile.

Multiple system atrophy (MSA), as the name suggests, is a degenerative disease that affects cortical and perhaps cerebellar pathways as well as the basal ganglia. This disease is characterized by bradykinesia and rigidity and a tendency to walk with a wide base of support. A person with MSA often has frontal lobe dysfunction and may have autonomic dysfunction as well. L-dopa is not effective in treating the symptoms.

Because these syndromes are rarer than Parkinson's disease and far more variable, no studies have been undertaken regarding treatment efficacy. Because accurate differential diagnosis is important in patient planning, a thorough evaluation by a neurologist is highly recommended.

Huntington's Disease

Huntington's disease (formerly known as Huntington's chorea) is another degenerative disease of the basal ganglia.[249] It is the classic disorder representing hyperactivity in the basal ganglia circuitry.[250] This disease gets its name from the family of physicians who described its patterns of

CASE STUDY 24-1 ■ MS. T

Ms. T. is a 55-year-old woman who was diagnosed with Parkinson's disease 1 year ago. The disease began in her left arm and leg when she noticed increasing stiffness and difficulty moving. She reports some instability in walking and recently has developed a slight resting tremor in the left hand. On initial evaluation she had full active and passive range of motion in all extremities, neck, and trunk. A mild resting tremor is present in the left hand. Mild cogwheel rigidity is present in the left upper and lower extremities; some intermittent resistance to passive movement in the right upper extremity is present as well. Strength is grossly within normal limits throughout. Sensation is intact throughout. Equilibrium reactions are delayed, but the patient demonstrates an ankle strategy on a flat surface and a hip strategy when standing on the balance beam; no mixing of the synergies is present, and her balance responses are appropriate to the degree of displacement.

The patient is able to stand in the sharpened Romberg position for 30 seconds with the eyes open and 20 seconds with the eyes closed. She can stand on the right leg for 30 seconds with the eyes open and 15 seconds with the eyes closed; she can stand on the left leg for 15 seconds with the eyes open and 10 seconds with the eyes closed. When walking, she has a heel-toe sequence, shortened stride length, and normal stride width. No arm swing occurs on the left and a diminished arm swing occurs on the right. The trunk is not rotated and slight trunk flexion is present throughout the gait cycle. Speed is within normal limits for a 25-foot walk. The patient is able to turn freely. She has recently begun to have foot dystonia, which is worse with fatigue. It has interfered with her daily walking program and her tennis, an activity she enjoys with her husband twice a week. Her only medication is deprenyl.

This patient is in Hoehn and Yahr stage I, with some beginning of bilateral symptoms and progression to stage II. She is young, employed full time, and has been involved in regular exercise for the past 10 years. Her symptoms are stiffness, slowed movements, and foot dystonia. Because her symptoms are mild at present and she has good balance in standing and walking, this patient should be encouraged to continue exercising regularly. She should try to keep playing tennis because it requires complex, sequential, context-dependent movements. Although tennis involves motor responses to external cues, it does necessitate rapid force generation and anticipatory movements. This should encourage continued motor learning. Additionally, she should be encouraged to continue walking outdoors and practice alternating speed of walking. The dystonia is more difficult to resolve. It may be tied to medication; differing medication schemes are now being tried. She is also on a program of stretching and strengthening of the ankle as well as a sensory stimulation program for the feet. Foam between the toes has helped decrease dystonia early in the day.

Ms. T. has also been informed about the importance of maintaining chest expansion and monitoring her breathing. This will be important as the disease progresses. She attends a support group for young patients with Parkinson's disease to increase her awareness of the disease, new treatments, and support. As the disease progresses, she will need a home program appropriate for her symptoms. The home program will be reassessed every 3 to 6 months.

---

inheritance. Huntington's disease is inherited as an autosomal dominant trait and affects approximately 6.5 in 100,000 people.[16] The defect is on the short arm of chromosome 4.[251] The altered genetic material has an increase in the cytosine-adenine-guanine (CAG) sequence; individuals without movement dysfunctions have 11 to 34 CAG triple repeats, but individuals with Huntington's disease have 37 to 86 repeats.[69] The longer the length of the CAG triple repeats, the earlier the onset of disease. The CAG repeat is related to glutamine. The target protein affected by the polyglutamine expansion has been named huntingtin. The length of the expansion is correlated with an earlier the age of disease onset. Huntingtin combines with ubiquitin and induces intranuclear inclusions and interference with mitochondrial function. The defect is characterized by severe loss of the medium spiny neurons and preservation of the ACh spiny neurons. Choline acetyltransferase (CAT) and Ach levels are decreased, as well as the number of muscarinic ACh receptors, glutamic acid decarboxylase, and substance P. No decrease in DA, norepinephrine, or serotonin (5HT) is usually found, although more recent studies with single-photon emission computed tomography (SPECT) indicate that DA does diminish significantly in the later stages of the disease.[252]

Huntington's disease is usually manifested after the age of 30 years, although childhood forms appear rarely. Those younger than 20 years with the disease account for approximately 10% of all people with Huntington's disease. Death from this disease occurs approximately 15 to 25 years after the onset of symptoms although, as in Parkinson's disease, the earliest symptom is not known.

A marker for the Huntington gene has been detected.[251] If the family pedigree is known and the chromosomes of the parents can be obtained, detection of which offspring have the faulty chromosome is possible presymptomatically. Of course, early detection of this disease involves ethical and practical issues. At present, although testing is available it is not widely used. Furthermore, testing for Huntington's disease is typically only available to those older than 18 years. Despite these problems, localization of the gene and the repeat is promising and offers hope for improved means of treatment.

Symptoms

Some of the signs and symptoms of Huntington's disease are similar to Parkinson's disease: abnormalities in postural reactions, trunk rotation, distribution of tone, and extrane-

CASE STUDY 24-2 ■ MR. R.

Mr. R. is a 68-year-old man with a 7-year history of Parkinson's disease. He now falls two to three times a day, has difficulty eating, and has noticed weakness in his right hand. He would like to return to full activity, including golf twice a week, swimming, and skiing. On evaluation he has moderate rigidity in all extremities; the right side is worse than the left. It is most marked in the right wrist, forearm, and hand. Shoulder flexion and abduction lack 15 degrees bilaterally. He has a 15-degree knee flexion contracture on the right; all other joints in the lower extremity have range within functional limits. Strength is a grossly 4 - 4+ throughout, including grip strength. Sensation is within normal limits throughout. Static and dynamic sitting balance is good.

The patient sits with a posterior pelvic tilt, rounded shoulders, and flexed neck. On rising to a standing position, he does move forward in the chair, which positions his feet under his knees. He does not lean forward as he stands. He momentarily loses his balance when rising from a chair. Static standing balance is fair; dynamic balance is fair. When pushed on the sternum, he takes one to two steps backward, even to a gentle push. When pushed from behind he takes several steps forward. He lost his balance and required assistance when trying to catch a large ball thrown to the side. His gait pattern is typical of a patient with Parkinson's disease. He has a shortened step and a flat-footed foot contact. He reports festination and freezing, but neither was observed during the evaluation. He turns en bloc.

No arm swing or trunk rotation is present. He walks slowly and was unable to increase his speed measurably in a 25-foot walk. He is taking L-dopa/carbidopa and deprenyl. He has tried another D_2 agonist but experienced hallucinations. He was able to ski until last winter. At that time, he found that he could not stand up once he fell down, and sometimes he fell without realizing that he was falling. He stated that he "did not think it was safe to ski." He also no longer swims because he has difficulty breathing in the pool and coordinating his breathing with the strokes. He does not play golf because it takes him so long.

This patient needs to be encouraged to continue to exercise and socialize while exercising. He has been encouraged to resume golf at times when his club is less crowded. Additionally, he has been given a home program consisting of activities performed in the seated and standing positions, which encourage trunk rotation and large movements and are coordinated with good breathing practices. He has been given some balance exercises that challenge his equilibrium in a safe environment. His home program will be monitored every 3 months because of the distance he must travel to come to the clinic. His wife was instructed to exercise with her husband and to exercise to music with him. He was referred to the speech pathologist for a swallowing evaluation and was given a joint program for his speech and breathing. He is able to play golf once a week; he is not yet ready to resume swimming or skiing.

---

ous movements. Individuals with Huntington's disease, however, are at the other end of the spectrum; rather than a paucity of movement, they exhibit too much movement, which is evident in the trunk and face in addition to the extremities. The gait takes on an ataxic, dancing appearance (in fact, "chorea" means to dance in Greek), and fine movements become clumsy and slowed.[253] As with the person with parkinsonism, associated movements are decreased (e.g., arm swing). The extraneous movements are of the choreoathetoid type, that is, involuntary, irregular isolated movements that may be from jerky and arrhythmic, as in chorea, to rhythmic and wormlike, as in athetosis. Usually, however, these extraneous movements occur sequentially so that the entire picture is one of complex movement patterns. The "movement generator" aspects of the basal ganglia seem to be continuously active, as would fit the hypothesis of a disruption in the indirect pathway. As the disease progresses, the choreiform movements may give way to akinesia and rigidity.

Gait patterns of the person with Huntington's disease are in some ways similar to that of Parkinson's disease. Gait velocity and stride length are decreased. The decrease in velocity is correlated with progression. Unlike the person with Parkinson's disease, however, the person with Huntington's disease has a decreased cadence as well.[254] The base of support is increased (again unlike the pattern seen in Parkinson's disease). In addition lateral sway is increased along with great variability in distal movements.

Disruptions in movement for the person with Huntington's disease reflect the role of the basal ganglia in movement. For example, the person with Huntington's disease, like the person with Parkinson's disease, has difficulty responding to internal cues; they also have difficulty with internal rhythms. Kinematic analysis of upper-extremity complex tasks demonstrates that the person with Huntington's disease must rely on visual guidance in the termination of a movement. This has been interpreted to indicate impairment in the development and fine tuning of an internal representation of the task.[255] These clients have increasing difficulty with more complex movements in the absence of advanced cues.[256,257] The lack of internal cuing in the person with Huntington's disease has been linked to the increased variability of response seen in these clients.[258]

The abnormal movements are seen in the muscles of speech, swallowing, and breathing. Speech lacks rhythm, as might be expected with decreased internal timing, and is often soft. Swallowing and therefore eating may also be difficult, which is a problem for individuals who are already thin. Weight loss is a common problem for individuals with Huntington's disease. A study by Pratley et al[259] found that sedentary energy expenditure was higher in the patient population than in age- and gender-matched control subjects;

however, sleeping metabolic rate was not different from the control subjects. They also found that the Huntington group was less active than the control group. The increase in energy expenditure was related to the severity of the disease. Some data suggest that a person with decreased body weight and a parental history of the disease is at greater risk.[260]

Eye movement is often the first sign of the disease. The person with Huntington's disease has difficult with initiation and control of saccadic eye movement.

In addition to the involvement of the motor systems, the individual with Huntington's disease also shows signs of dementia and emotional disorders that become worse as the disease progresses. Neuropsychological tests are therefore included in the United Huntington Disease Rating Scale. The client may show lack of judgment and loss of memory, deterioration in speech and writing (i.e., severe decrease in ability to communicate), depression, hostility, and feelings of incompetence. IQ decreases, with performance measures decreasing more rapidly than verbal levels. Evidence is present of ideomotor apraxia, especially as the disease progresses.[261] Suicide is fairly common.

The movement disorders of Huntington's disease are presumed to be related to degeneration of the striatal neurons, specifically the enkephalinergic neurons.[16] The dementia is associated with cortical destruction.

The exact mechanisms for the production of choreoathetoid movements are unknown. Because these extraneous movements are part of a person's normal repertoire of movement patterns, they may be "released" at inappropriate times and without any modulation. A postmortem examination showed a decrease in GABA that was greater in the globus pallidus external segment than in the internal segment. This agrees with the previously described current model.[5] Recent use of PET scans demonstrates loss of ACh and GABA neurons.[262] A pattern therefore may be released before it is necessary, and inappropriate portions of a movement pattern cannot be inhibited. Many years ago Petajan et al[263] found motor unit activity indicative of bradykinesia. Recordings of single motor units in the muscles indicate that persons with Huntington's disease have a loss of control evidenced by an inability to recruit single motor units.[263] As the efforts at control increased, these individuals demonstrated an overflow of motor unit activity that resulted in full choreiform movements. Those in the earlier stages of the disease demonstrated what the experimenters termed "microchorea," or small ballistic activations of motor units.[263] As in Parkinson's disease, difficulty occurs in modulating motor neuron excitability. Another finding in this experiment revealed motor unit activity indicative of bradykinesia. Yanagasawa[264] used surface EMG recordings to classify involuntary muscle contractions in patients with Huntington's disease with varying movement disorders from chorea to rigidity. He found brief, reciprocal, irregular contractions in those patients with classical chorea and tonic nonreciprocal contractions in those patients with rigidity. Presence of athetosis or dystonia was associated with slow, reciprocal contractions. During sustained contractions EMG activity demonstrated brief, irregular cessation of activity in the choreic patients. Thus patients with Huntington's disease have interruption of normal motor function at rest and during sustained activity (e.g., stabilizing contractions).

The abnormal postural reactions of the person with Huntington's disease may occur from a misinterpretation of sensory input, especially vestibular and proprioceptive (similar to the parkinsonian syndrome). However, the dementia of Huntington's disease precludes further testing.

Stages of the Disease

Huntington's disease is a progressive disorder. The initial symptoms are most often incoordination, clumsiness, or jerkiness. A classic test for eliciting choreiform movements in this early stage is a simple grip test. The client grips the examiner's hand and maintains that grip for a few seconds. The person with Huntington's disease displays what is descriptively called the "milkmaid's sign": alternate increases and decreases in the grip that are perhaps the equivalent of the EMG abnormalities seen during sustained contractions. Facial grimacing or the inability to perform complex facial movements also may be present early.

In many cases the dementia and psychological symptoms of Huntington's disease occur after the onset of the neurological signs. In those cases in which subtle personality changes occur first, the diagnosis may be more difficult. Such persons may appear forgetful or unable to manage appointments and financial affairs. They may be thought to have early senility, or they may show signs of severe depression or schizophrenia. Early diagnosis may be important, and SPECT is showing promise for early detection of the disease.[265]

With time, the combination of the psychological and neurological problems causes the individual to lose all ability to work and perform ADLs. This person eventually can be cared for only in an extended-care facility. By this time the choreiform movements have given way to rigidity and the patient is bedridden. Figure 24-11 shows the stages of Huntington's disease according to Shoulson and Fahn[266] and Shoulson et al.[267]

Pharmacological Considerations and Medical Management

The great advances in pharmacological management of Parkinson's disease have led to a great deal of research to find appropriate drugs for the management of Huntington's disease.[268-269d] At present, however, no fully effective medication is available for this disease. In fact, no evidence has shown that improvement of the chorea movements leads to functional improvement.

The symptoms of Huntington's disease indicate an increase in dopaminergic effect. At autopsy a decreased number of intrinsic neurons of the striatum that contain the neurotransmitter GABA or Ach are found. Biochemical studies reveal a definite decrease in GABA concentration in addition to a decrease in ACh concentration in the basal ganglia. Therefore drug therapy depends on drugs that are cholinergic or GABA-containing agonists and those that act as DA antagonists. To date the DA antagonists have been more effective in ameliorating neurological symptoms; however, these drugs have severe side effects, including Parkinson's disease—for example, bradykinesia and rigidity—and tardive dyskinesia.[268]

In general, pharmacological treatment is not started until the choreiform movements interfere with function because these drugs have side effects that may be worse than the

	Engagement in occupation	Score	Capacity to handle financial affairs	Score	Capacity to manage domestic responsibility	Score	Capacity to perform activities of daily living	Score	Care can be provided at	Score
Stage 1	Usual level	3	Full	3	Full	2	Full	3	Home	2
Stage 2	Lower level	2	Requires slight help	2	Full	2	Full	3	Home	2
Stage 3	Marginal	1	Requires major help	1	Impaired	1	Mildly impaired	2	Home	2
Stage 4	Unable	0	Unable	0	Unable	0	Moderately impaired	1	Home or extended care facility	1
Stage 5	Unable	0	Unable	0	Unable	0	Severely impaired	0	Total care facility only	0

FIGURE 24-11 ■ Functional stages of Huntington's disease. (Reprinted from Shoulson I, Fahn S: Huntington's disease: clinical care and evaluation, *Neurology* 29:2, 1979.)

chorea.[270] Perphenazine, haloperidol (Haldol), and reserpine are still the most commonly used medications (see Chapter 36). The first two block the DA receptors themselves; reserpine depletes DA stores in the brain. Side effects include depression, drowsiness, a parkinsonian type of syndrome, and sometimes dyskinesia. Drugs such as choline, which would increase ACh concentrations, have produced only transient improvement.[185] Many efforts have been undertaken to find a GABA agonist that would reduce the symptoms of Huntington's disease, but these have so far been unsuccessful.[270,271] The problem with finding a medication to increase GABA is that such a drug will probably cause inhibition throughout the brain, not just in the basal ganglia. Thus the individual's level of alertness and ability to function might be reduced—something the person with Huntington's disease can ill afford.[271]

Management of the dementia and personality problems interfere more with life tasks than the movement disorders do. Newer neuroleptic drugs are promising, and a combination of medications is frequently prescribed to treat the specific emotional and psychological symptoms. Cortical degeneration is most certainly involved, but disruption of the heavy corticostriate projections also may be a factor in the progression of this disease. Although alterations in DA have been implicated in psychotic problems such as schizophrenia, the role of the basal ganglia in thought processes is, at best, little understood. In the words of Woody Guthrie: "There's just not no hope. Nor not no treatment known to cure me of my dizzy called Chorea."[272]

At present the best hope for the person with Huntington's disease lies in a better understanding of the genetic mechanisms causing destruction of the GABA-containing cells in the striatum and cortical destruction. In the meantime correct and early diagnosis is important in providing the proper early intervention, which must include counseling.[273] The Committee for the Control of Huntington Disease has set up several research centers, including a brain and tissue bank, in an effort to facilitate research into the causes of the disease.

Transplantation is also a factor in clinical trials of Huntington's disease. As with Parkinson's disease, the tissue does survive, but the results are even more preliminary than for the person with parkinsonism.

Examination of the Client with Huntington's Disease

The standard medical evaluation is the United Huntington Disease Rating Scale (UHDRS).[274] This comprehensive evaluation examines cognitive function as well as motor function. The physical or occupational therapy evaluation of a person with Huntington's disease must include an assessment of the degree of functional ability and how the chorea interferes with function. Which extremities, including the face, are involved? Does the client have any cortical control of the chorea or any means of allaying these extraneous movements? What exacerbates the symptoms? What lessens them? A simple rating scale is the capacity to perform ADLs (see Figure 22-11). A standard ADL form with space to write in how the client performs these activities or why she or he cannot perform them is helpful.

Gait analysis can include a timed walk and cadence; stride length can then be calculated. A subjective assessment of variability and incoordination should also be made. Additionally, posture and equilibrium reactions should be tested. What associated reactions, if any, are present? In assessing posture, care should be taken to observe the posture of the extremities in addition to the trunk, head, and neck. Dystonic posturing should be carefully noted, especially if the client is taking medication. Any changes should be reported to the physician.

A gross assessment of strength should be made, with particular attention paid to the ability to stabilize the trunk and proximal joints. To reduce the effects of rigidity, ROM becomes important as the disease progresses.

In the assessment of the client with Huntington's disease, the stage of psychological involvement and mental state must be reliably assessed both during evaluation and treatment. SPECT and other computer tomography scans may give some clues to the amount of cortical and basal ganglia degeneration, which can assist in determining possible cortical functioning.

General Treatment Goals and Rationale

Maintaining an optimal quality of life is the most important goal for treatment of persons with Huntington's disease and their families, including maintenance of functional skills and advice to the family on adaptive equipment. Techniques that reduce tone may also reduce choreiform movements. Increasing stability about the shoulders, trunk, neck, and hips helps maintain function. Again, the evaluation results dictate treatment procedures.

Treatment Procedures

The Commission on the Control of Huntington Disease stated that affected individuals are underserved by physical and occupational therapy.[267] Peacock[275] surveyed physical therapists in one state. Of the 585 therapists who responded, 15.5% had worked with at least one patient with Huntington's disease and only 6.2% had worked with more than one patient, thus confirming the underuse of physical and occupational therapy. Hayden[272] and Peacock[275] suggest that therapy can improve the patient's quality of life. Yet few articles have been published on treatment procedures, and even fewer articles address treatment efficacy. Theories regarding which techniques may prove most beneficial are mentioned in this chapter with the warning that to date none has been documented (see Chapter 9 for specific treatment techniques).

The treatment of the person with Huntington's disease has some parallels with the treatment of cerebral palsy athetosis. These techniques, however, must be adapted to the adult. Of critical importance are the techniques for improving coactivation and trunk stability. Pivot-prone and withdrawal patterns of Rood are helpful, and their benefit may be increased with the use of Thera-Bands (the Hygenic Corporation, Akron, Ohio). Neck cocontraction and trunk stability may improve or at least maintain oral functions. Additionally, the techniques of rhythmical stabilization in all positions as well as heavy work patterns of Rood should be helpful.[214] Yet movements practiced out of context may not carry over into functional activities; thus practicing coactivation in functional patterns during treatment if at all possible is recommended. Whereas in Parkinson's disease the emphasis is on large-amplitude movements, movements for the person with Huntington's disease need to be of smaller amplitude with increased control.

Relaxation aids reduction of extraneous movements. In the early stages methods that require active participation of the client, such as biofeedback and traditional relaxation exercises, may be included. As dementia becomes more apparent, more passive techniques such as slow rocking and neutral warmth must be used. These techniques are also helpful in reducing the choreiform movements of the mouth and tongue, which may prove useful for the dentist and those responsible for proper nutrition of the client. In most cases of Huntington's disease, the individual is quite thin (almost emaciated) and begins to age rapidly as the disease progresses. The extraneous movements, especially as they become more severe, increase metabolic demands and nutrition therefore becomes increasingly important. Attention therefore must be paid to head, neck, and oral-motor control. Increased pressure on the lips may aid in lip closure and facilitate swallowing. Special straws with a mouthpiece similar to a pacifier may be useful. A dietitian should be consulted for assistance in teaching the family how to prepare balanced and appetizing meals and snacks that are still easy to swallow.

The degree of dementia influences the treatment. Conscious efforts to control extraneous movements are more difficult as cognitive function decreases. Furthermore, new memories and new patterns of movements are difficult to establish. The therapist therefore must use techniques that require subcortical control and keep in mind that the client can sometimes remember old, normal patterns of movement.

Peacock's[275] study suggests that group programs including strength, flexibility, balance, coordination, and breathing exercises may be quite successful, especially in the early stages of the disease. No amount of physical or occupational therapy, however, can prevent neuronal cell loss. Because Huntington's disease is a progressive, degenerative disease, the client will get worse. Eventually goals must be aimed at preventing total immobility and assisting caretakers in transfer techniques and advising them in the use of adaptive equipment. One aspect of treatment that cannot be measured but is important is the degree of hope offered simply by the fact that a health professional is providing ongoing care. This may lessen the client's degree of despair and depression and may help maintain quality of life.

The gait disorder of Huntington's disease has been shown to respond to rhythmic auditory stimuli.[276] The ability to respond decreases in those most severely involved, indicating that treatment in the later stages of the disease may not be amenable to rhythmic stimuli. Another finding of this study was that cadence was a larger problem than stride length, especially at normal and fast speeds (compare this to the findings in Parkinson's disease). Interestingly, people with Huntington's disease were able to modulate gait to a metronome but had more difficulty with musical cues even when the tempos were identical. Nevertheless, the subjects with Huntington's disease demonstrated short-term carryover of metronome auditory stimuli to gait without auditory stimuli. Although the long-term carryover was not studied, use of a metronome in gait training may be helpful in clients with Huntington's disease.

Animal research on the effects of forced use or increasing functional activity have only now begun. No data are yet available, in contrast to Parkinson's disease, regarding the effect of activity on neurotransmission or neuronal function in animal models of Huntington's disease.

Wilson's Disease

Wilson's disease, or hepatolenticular degeneration, is a disease caused by faulty copper metabolism. The toxic effects of copper lead to degeneration of the liver and the basal ganglia. Wilson's disease, inherited as an autosomal recessive trait, affects a small percentage of the population. If the disease is recognized and properly treated, the patient can function without restrictions.

Wilson's disease is characterized by an increase in the amount of copper absorbed from the intestinal tract, a subsequent elevation in the amount of copper in the blood serum, and an increase in the amount of copper deposited in tissue.[277] Ceruloplasmin is concomitantly reduced. The increase in tissue copper may interfere with various enzyme systems of particular cells. The connection of copper with DA metabolism may account for the basal ganglia involvement.

Neuronal degeneration is present in the globus pallidus and putamen and to a lesser extent in the caudate nucleus. Atrophy may also be present in the gray matter of the cortex and the dentate nucleus of the cerebellum.

Symptoms

The deposition of the excess copper in the cornea results in the classic diagnostic sign of Wilson's disease, the Kayser-Fleischer ring: a brownish-green or brownish-red colored ring found in the sclerocorneal junction.

Several forms of Wilson's disease have been classified on the basis of the constellations of signs and symptoms. One type entails only liver involvement and no neurological signs. A dystonic form is most common in those with an onset of the disease after age 20 years. The individual shows the same abnormal positioning of the limbs and trunk that characterizes the dystonia, rigidity, and bradykinesia seen in Parkinson's disease. Associated reactions and facial expressions are absent. Festinated gait and flexed posture are present. Tremor of the hand, head, and body may be present.[277]

If the onset of the disease occurs before age 20 years, the appearance of choreoathetoid movements of the face and upper extremities is usually present. The gait resembles that of the individual with Huntington's disease. This early-onset form is accompanied by rapid deterioration.[278]

Common to all forms of Wilson's disease that involve brain structures is difficulty in speaking and swallowing, incoordination, and personality changes. The personality changes are the first signs of the disease, especially emotional lability and impaired judgment. If the disease progresses, dementia and cirrhosis of the liver increase and motor function progressively decreases.[277,278]

The term dystonia is used for involuntary movements with a sustained contraction at the end of the movement.[16] Usually these movements involve a twisting of the extremity. If the contraction at the end of the movement is prolonged, the term dystonic posture is used. A peculiar aspect of dystonia is that it can be decreased with proprioceptive or tactile input.[16] Dystonia is usually seen with widespread involvement of the basal ganglia and intralaminar nuclei of the thalamus. The cerebellum also may be involved.[279]

Dystonia, like bradykinesia and choreoathetosis, belongs on a continuum of the extraneous movements present with basal ganglia involvement. The movement patterns are total and involve rotation of the limb. As in the other diseases of the basal ganglia previously discussed, normal associated movements are also decreased. As Wilson's disease progresses, the classic abnormal posture of increased flexion occurs, along with rigidity and, if severe enough, the total inability to move. As with other diseases of the basal ganglia, an imbalance or abnormal response in the neurotransmitters occurs; however, the precise imbalance is not yet known.

Stages of the Disease

The first symptom of Wilson's disease is usually a change in the individual's personality. When this becomes severe enough or when the movement disorder appears, a diagnosis can be made by the presence of the Kayser-Fleischer ring or by an analysis of copper metabolism. Because Wilson's disease is now treatable by chemical means, the full progression of this disease is usually not seen. If left untreated, the dystonia becomes worse and the person becomes more rigid. Additionally, muscle weakness can occur and progress, seizures may develop, and the dementia and personality disorder also become worse.

Medical Management

Wilson's disease is usually one of the first diseases to be ruled out when a patient presents with movement disorders and behavioral problems, especially in the younger patient. Because the signs and symptoms of Wilson's disease are caused by an increased absorption of copper, treatment consists of drugs that will inhibit this absorption. Concomitantly, copper intake in the diet should be restricted. Penicillamine is the drug of choice, usually in combination with vitamin B_6.[16] Penicillamine has some side effects, but these appear to be infrequent. If the copper imbalance is treated, the neurological signs do not progress.

Examination and Treatment Intervention

Because Wilson's disease is fully treatable and can be diagnosed early, it may not concern the therapist. If the client is referred for therapy, treatment techniques should be wholly based on symptoms. Examination is similar to that of the patient with Parkinson's disease or Huntington's disease. It consists of describing the type of extraneous movement present, when it is present, and factors that influence the degree of dystonia. Ease of movement also should be assessed, and it may be timed as for the client with Parkinson's disease. Additionally, range of movement and strength should be evaluated, especially if the disease is progressing.

Treatment is then designed to alleviate the problems. Extraneous movements may be reduced by any technique that reduces tone. Positioning is important. If bradykinesia is the major sign, then treatment is similar to that used in Parkinson's disease; if trunk stability is poor, the therapist proceeds as in Huntington's disease. The client with Wilson's disease has knowledge of what normal movement feels like and usually has good cognitive abilities at the time treatment is started. Because of the emotional lability, which is one of the first symptoms in this disease, the treatment session should be well planned and quite structured.

Tardive Dyskinesia

Tardive dyskinesia is a drug-induced disorder and thus is mentioned to indicate the problems that can arise from drug intoxication. In particular, this section concentrates on the problems associated with drugs that affect DA metabolism, including amphetamine, haloperidol, and classes of drugs used in treatment of psychotic disorders: the phenothiazines, butyrophenones, and thioxanthenes. As the use and misuse of drugs become more common, these types of disorders may become more frequent (see Chapter 36).

The use of phenothiazines (one of the neuroleptics) has become an effective and common treatment for schizophrenia. This treatment protocol has enabled many schizophrenics to leave the mental institution. These drugs are DA antagonists and thus decrease the amount of DA in the brain. The exact site of the brain involved in schizophrenia itself is not within the scope of this chapter, but the neurological signs that occur are discussed. As might be expected, they involve structures within the basal ganglia. Tardive dyskinesia is a gradual disease that occurs after long-term drug treatment. The most typical involvement is of the mouth, tongue, and muscles of mastication; therefore tardive dyskinesia may be called orofacial or buccolingual-masticatory (BLM) dyskinesia.

Symptoms

Dyskinesia is defined as an inability to perform voluntary movement.[273] In practical terms, however, dyskinesia is usually a series of rhythmical extraneous movements. In tardive dyskinesia this typically begins with, or may be confined to, the region of the face. These extraneous movements may include choreoathetoid or dystonic movements. Because of abnormality in basal ganglia function, abnormalities in postural tone and postural adjustments are also present. Instead of the typical flexed posture of Parkinson's disease, clients with tardive dyskinesia show extension of the trunk with increased lordosis and neck flexion.[280] This description of the disease is rather broad, but the problems of drug-induced movement disorders are varied. They may take the form of drug-induced Parkinson's disease or dystonia. In tardive dyskinesia, akinesia and rigidity similar to that seen in parkinsonism may exist simultaneously with the choreoathetoid-like movements. The key factor in tardive dyskinesia is its slow onset after the ingestion of neuroleptic medications.

Etiology

Although many people take neuroleptic medications, only a small percentage acquires tardive dyskinesia. Many factors may predispose an individual to movement disorders. One of these is age.[281] This might be expected because of the influence of aging processes on the concentration of DA. Sex may also be a factor; women are more at risk for tardive dyskinesia.[280] The fact that sex can affect DA levels is supported in studies of animals with brain lesions. In one study, female rats had a lower concentration of DA after early brain lesion than did their male litter mates.[282] The absolute amount of neuroleptic ingested may also be a factor, but to date definitive studies have not been completed. So far the length of time the individual takes medication does not appear to be a strong predisposing factor. As the biological abnormalities of schizophrenia become better understood, further understanding of the causes of tardive dyskinesia also may be elucidated. The development of tardive dyskinesia is hypothesized to be caused by supersensitivity.[3,273] With the use of drugs that deplete the brain of DA, the brain becomes more sensitive to it. And, in fact, in human beings the withdrawal of neuroleptics tends to heighten the disease; withdrawal of the DA antagonist essentially means that far more DA is able to act on these already sensitive terminals.[3,273,283]

Because of the effectiveness of long-term treatment for schizophrenia provided by neuroleptics, research into the underlying cause and therefore treatment of the major side effect, the motor disorders, has greatly increased.[283a] But as with Parkinson's disease and Huntington's disease, animal models are difficult to produce. For one thing, the normal function of the basal ganglia in movement is obscure. However, experimental evidence indicates that the basal ganglia are involved in movements about the face, especially the mouth, and buccolingual dyskinesia is the most frequently encountered symptom in tardive dyskinesia.[74,75] Lidsky et al[284] hypothesized that sensory input about the face was involved in the high number of globus pallidus units responsive to licking. Further experiments showed that basal ganglia stimulation could alter the threshold of mouth reflexes.[285] The response of basal ganglia neurons to sensory input shows increasing localization of response with age; the region about the mouth becomes increasingly sensitive.[75] Further research along these lines, both in normal animals and those with lesions, may answer the question of what is happening at a neuronal level. This would facilitate drug, physical, and occupational therapy intervention.

Pharmacological and Medical Management
Tardive dyskinesia is often irreversible. The withdrawal of medication, in fact, may increase the movement disorders. Or recovery may take even more time than that required for the onset of the disease. Strangely, sometimes the drug that caused the disease may be the drug that reduces the symptoms; that is, increasing the dose may lessen the movement disorder.[283a] This might be expected if supersensitivity to DA is involved. But again, with time the increased dose will also cause a reappearance of the symptoms.

The use of other drugs in conjunction with the neuroleptics has been tried in various animal models of the disease. As might be expected, anticholinergic drugs (which would worsen an imbalance between DA and ACh) worsen the dyskinesia. Lithium has been successful in one animal model of dyskinesia.[273] Some neuroleptic drugs seem to have less effect on movement than others; however, the side effects of one such drug, chlorpromazine, are life threatening. More research is needed into both the mechanisms of schizophrenia and the mechanisms for the production of the abnormal movements.

Evaluation and Treatment Intervention
The effectiveness of therapy intervention in drug-induced dyskinesia is, as yet, not completely known. However, because the neuroleptics do provide an effective long-term treatment of schizophrenia, therapists need to become aware of the problem and offer some assistance. Early drug holidays (time without taking drugs) may be of value in treat-

ment of tardive dyskinesia, and therefore early awareness of incipient changes in motor function may be of value. Assessment of patients receiving drug therapy could perhaps begin before treatment and then at prescribed intervals. The knowledge that postural adjustments are abnormal in most basal ganglia diseases means that analysis of posture statically and in motion might provide early clues of development of movement disorders. The same would be true for balance reactions and changes in tone with changes in position. Once movement disorders appear, an assessment of when and where the extraneous movements occur is important (see Chapters 8 for general examination tools and 23 specifically for tests of balance).

General treatment is similar to that used in Huntington's disease; oral treatment corresponds to that for the athetotic child with cerebral palsy. If a hyperreactivity to sensory stimulus exists, then oral desensitization may be of value.

Ameliorating the oral grimacing, of course, would be helpful for the schizophrenic person who is trying to return to society. The effectiveness of physical and occupational therapy treatment cannot be assessed until therapists become involved with these clients and record the effectiveness of their interventions. In cases in which the parkinsonian-like symptoms are stronger than the dyskinetic movements, treatment rationale should follow the plan for the individual with Parkinson's disease.

Other Considerations
Other drugs besides neuroleptics may also produce movement disorders. Amphetamine, for example, has been shown to cause long-term changes in brain function even from extremely small doses.[286-288] Adults who were hyperactive children sometimes show a decrease in the readiness potential.[289] Further longitudinal research and research utilizing PET scans and functional magnetic resonance imaging are underway to determine the role that medications such as methylphenidate (Ritalin), used in treating hyperactive children, might play in changing the architecture of the basal ganglia and causing movement disorders.[95] The problem of drug-induced movement disorders may become an ever-increasing one for the therapist.

In 1982 several young people were treated for rigidity and "catatonia" after the use of what they thought was heroin. Careful examination of these patients revealed that they had parkinsonian-like symptoms.[290,291] The chemical responsible for the symptomatology was L-methyl-4-phenyl-1,2,3,6-tetrahydropyridine (MPTP), a meperidine analog that was an impurity in the designer heroin. This discovery has enabled research in animals and clinical studies in human beings. Although some differences exist among idiopathic Parkinson's disease, MPTP-induced Parkinson's disease, and MPTP-induced parkinsonism, important similarities exist: MPTP selectively damages DA cells in the substantia nigra; L-dopa is effective in alleviating the symptoms; and the symptoms seen are irreversible and progressive. In animal studies, age does affect the degree of damage,[292,293] and in human beings, some of those who used the drug MPTP are now beginning to show symptoms of parkinsonism.[294] This delay in appearance of symptoms fits a model of Parkinson's disease that suggests that an initial insult to the DA system may not result in disease until a critical level is reached. The critical level of DA depletion may occur with age because of a gradual loss of DA in the aging process. The real importance of the discovery of MPTP-induced parkinsonism is that it may enable better understanding of the pathogenesis and, in turn, of the treatment of the disease. One hypothesized cause of Parkinson's disease implicated environmental toxins (because some herbicides such as paraquat resemble the chemical structure of MPTP) and the involvement of superoxide free radical.[104,171,173] Epidemiology studies are now underway to investigate Parkinson's disease in areas known for high herbicide usage, and α-tocopherol is under investigation as a protective agent.

Dystonia

Dystonia is a movement disorder characterized by sustained muscle contraction in the extreme end range of a movement, frequently with a rotational component. Inherited dystonias usually involve the entire body. These dystonias are most prevalent in those of European Jewish descent. Focal dystonias involve one joint, such as spasmodic torticollis or writer's cramp. Full-body dystonia is a disease of the basal ganglia, and the current view is that the focal dystonias also involve lesions of precise areas of the basal ganglia.[295-295c]

Symptoms

The person with generalized dystonia begins a movement (such as walking) and then experiences a torsional contraction of the trunk, upper extremity (especially at the shoulder), ankle, foot, and toes. These contractions may be so strong that further movement in impossible. Many patients experience pain because the muscles remain contracted for long periods of time.[296]

Spasmodic torticollis is the most common focal dystonia. The person with this disorder has involuntary contractions of neck muscles that result in head turning or head extension/flexion movements that are often sustained for long periods. Other common sites of focal involvement are the vocal cords, the tongue and swallowing muscles, the facial muscles (especially about the eye), the hand, and the toes. Writer's cramp is a task-specific dystonia, unlike other focal dystonias.[297]

An interesting phenomenon of dystonia is the fact that many patients develop a sensory or motor "trick" that decreases the severity of the muscle contractions and may even stop these movements. In all cases of dystonia excessive co-activation of agonists and antagonists occurs that interferes with the timing, execution, and loss of independent joint motions. Rarely are any abnormalities of muscle tone present, per se; that is, no increase in deep tendon reflexes or rigidity occur. Muscle strength and range of motion are usually within normal limits unless disuse leads to weakness.[186]

Etiology

The etiology of full-body dystonia is predominantly genetic, involving the *DYT* gene.[298] The etiology of the focal dystonias is unknown. Some people have suggested that focal dystonias may also be genetic; others speculate that they occur after injury. In addition to the motor component of the disease, strong evidence suggests that the sensory systems are involved. Byl et al[299] found that subjects with focal hand dystonia had difficulty in discriminative sensory processing

and frequently had an abnormal sensation of movement. Tinazzi et al[300] found a significantly higher sensory evoked potential in subjects with dystonia that they thought might be indicative of decreased activity in the putamen and that poor processing of sensory information in the basal ganglia-thalamus-cortical loop could lead to the motor dysfunction. Focal dystonia has also been linked to repetitive movements produced under high cognitive constraints and attention.[299] Rapid, high repetition might be interpreted as simultaneous contraction, and a learned sensorimotor dysfunction ensues.[301] Byl et al[302] have indeed developed an animal model of focal hand dystonia following repetitive movements and have demonstrated degradation in the sensory cortex after training.[303] Whether these results can be generalized to other focal dystonias is unknown.

Pharmacological and Medical Management

The most common medical treatment for the focal dystonias is injection of botulinum toxin. This toxin binds with the ACh receptors on the muscle and prevents muscle contraction. The injections are made under EMG guidance so that only those motor units involved in the production of the extraneous movements are paralyzed. However, the treatment does not cause permanent change, so the patient must have these injections every 3 to 4 months. At present only botulinum A is approved by the Food and Drug Administration and approved only for blepharospasm.[76] Some people have developed antibodies to the toxin, making it no longer effective. Therefore other botulinum strains are under investigation. Before understanding how other strains may affect focal dystonias, a clear comprehension of the differences between dystonias and their effects on specific functional movement need to be differentiated and understood from a pathophysiological perspective.[304,305]

Evaluation and Treatment Intervention

Evaluation of the person with full-body dystonia is similar to the evaluation of the person with tardive dyskinesia or Huntington's disease. Evaluation of the person with focal dystonia must involve some other aspects of the disease manifestation. The duration of the dystonia, the trigger, and the person's trick, if any, to decrease the dystonia must be noted. Tricks are sensory in nature and help relieve the pain often associated with the extreme movement. The Toronto Western Spasmodic Torticollis Rating Scale (TWSTRS) is one evaluation for the person with spasmodic torticollis.[306]

Several ADLs should be examined. For example, the person with writer's cramp has no difficulty holding a fork or a toothbrush, only a pen for writing. Additionally, a position dependence exists so that writing in the prone position may not evoke the dystonia despite severe inability to hold the pen at a desk.[301]

In addition to the full extent of the motoric abnormality, sensation, especially higher-level sensory processing such as precise localization of touch, graphesthesia, and kinesthesia, must be assessed. Recent evidence suggests that balance, particularly dynamic balance, should also be assessed in patients with torticollis.[307] These balance difficulties have not been relieved with botulinum toxin.

Movement therapy interventions are only now being developed. One successful program uses sensory integration and relearning techniques performed with attention.[299] Practice is a crucial element of treatment, and the client must be willing to practice the sensory tasks many, many times throughout the day for benefit. The client practices cognitively demanding sensory discrimination tasks throughout the day and uses only normal, tension-free movements.[301]

Treatment of those with torticollis must include a relearning of midline before the person can begin to practice normal movement away from midline. The client may find this relearning process easier after the botulinum injection.

Other Considerations

As with other extraneous movements associated with basal ganglia disorders, relaxation can reduce the muscle contraction. However, the time to incorporate the relaxation is before the full-blown development of the muscle contraction—a difficult task. This task requires a shift in paradigm to a health and wellness model and prevention (see Chapter 6). Therefore clients should practice relaxation on a regular basis. A psychological aspect to the focal dystonias frequently may need intervention from a psychiatrist or psychologist.

METABOLIC DISEASES AFFECTING OTHER REGIONS OF THE BRAIN

All alterations of metabolism, if allowed to continue, affect nervous system function. This includes alterations in sodium, water, sugar, and hormonal balance. Table 24-1 lists metabolic diseases that often have neurological sequelae. Proper treatment is usually medical management of the imbalance. Physical therapeutic intervention, if necessary, should address specific neurological symptoms.

Ingestion of or exposure to heavy metals may also lead to CNS disease. Methamphetamine also affects brain tissue,

even with one use, and the sequelae of movement disorders is now becoming more apparent (Table 24-2).

SUMMARY

This chapter focuses on the pathophysiology, evaluation, and treatment of genetic, hereditary, and metabolic diseases affecting adults. In all these diseases the therapist/movement specialist is an important (though sometimes underused) part of the rehabilitation team. Knowledge of the possible mechanisms involved in the production of the varying movement disorders may make the appropriate evaluation and subsequent intervention more meaningful. Even with degenerative, progressive disorders the therapist plays an important role in maintaining quality of life and assists the client and family in coping with the disease. The importance of documentation (see Chapter 10) and publication of cases and larger controlled studies cannot be overstressed. Both assist in the development of improved therapeutic techniques and may help researchers in planning and interpreting appropriate experimental studies. Establishment of effectiveness will be the first step toward evidence-based practice and a critical link in the evolution of professionals who have been identified as movement specialists.

With the advent of the Internet, many Web sites have been created to focus on the diseases mentioned in this chapter. In addition, the organization Worldwide Education and Awareness for Movement Disorders has a Web site for both patients and health care providers (www.wemove.org). These sites answer many questions for patients and provide information on making day-to-day life easier. Local support groups for these diseases also provide information and support for the patient and the caregiver.

TABLE 24-1 ■ Neurological Complications of Metabolic Disorders

METABOLIC PROBLEM	TREATMENT	NEUROLOGICAL COMPLICATION
Decreased sodium (too much water)	Restriction of water intake	Muscle twitching, seizures, coma
Increased sodium	Slow rehydration	Cerebral edema, muscle rigidity, decerebrate rigidity
Decreased potassium (hypokalemia), often caused by aldosteronism	Restoration of calcium levels after assessing primary cause	Changes in resting potential of neuron; hyperpolarization; muscle weakness and fatigue with eventual total paralysis
Magnesium imbalance	Improved diet, intravenous magnesium	Mental confusion, muscle twitching, myoclonus, tachycardia, hyperreflexia, extraneous movements, seizures
Diabetes mellitus	Proper control of diabetes	Peripheral neuropathy, pseudotabes, possible seizures and coma
Hypoglycemia	Treatment of primary cause; diet adjustment	Anoxia of the brain, seizures, mental confusion
Hyperthyroidism	Thyroid-blocking agents; intravenous fluids, hydrocortisone, and propranolol if patient is in thyroid crisis	Hyperkinesia, irritability, nervousness, emotional lability, symmetrical peripheral neuropathy
Hypothyroidism	Thyroid supplement	Sluggishness, mental and motor retardation, muscle weakness, sometimes muscle pain
Hypercalcemia	Treatment of primary cause, which is often hyperparathyroidism, vitamin D malignancy (therefore surgical removal)	Headache, weakness, fatigue, proximal neuropathy, rigidity, tremor, disorientation
Hypocalcemia	Intravenous administration of calcium (possible medical emergency)	Hyperexcitability of the peripheral and central nervous systems, which can lead to tetany and convulsions

TABLE 24-2 ■ Neurological Complications of Heavy Metal Poisoning

TYPE OF METAL	TREATMENT	NEUROLOGICAL COMPLICATION
LEAD Source: lead paint, industrial (fumes of molten lead)	Elimination of source, reduction of fluids, intravenous urea or mannitol, use of chelating agents	Interstitial edema and hemorrhage (especially in cerebellum) in acute poisoning; all levels of central nervous system affected in chronic long-term poisoning In children: seizures, mental retardation, behavior problems, hyperactivity In adults: spasticity, rigidity, dementia, personality changes Peripheral neuropathy may occur in adults and children
ARSENIC Source: paint and insecticides	Removal of source, gastric lavage, intravenous fluids, maintenance of electrolyte balance; penicillamine used in acute poisoning	Demyelinization of peripheral nerves in all extremities
MANGANESE Source: industrial if manganese dust is not removed; symptoms appear 2-25 yr after exposure	Levodopa	Neuronal loss in basal ganglia, substantia nigra, and cerebellum Initially psychiatric disturbances, including nervousness, irritability, and a tendency toward compulsive acts Later, muscular weakness and parkinsonian symptoms
MERCURY Rare, but may affect farmers and dental office workers	Penicillamine; function returns only with physical, occupational, and speech therapy	Loss of neurons, especially in cerebellum; also in cortex near calcarine fissure Alternating periods of confusion, drowsiness, and stupor with restlessness and excitability Ataxia, dysarthria, visual deterioration

REFERENCES

1. American Physical Therapy Association: *Guide to physical therapist practice,* ed 2, *Phys Ther* 81:9, 2001.
2. Aminoff MJ: Treatment of Parkinson disease, *West J Med* 161:303, 1994.
3. Tanner CM, Goldman SM: Epidemiology of Parkinson disease, *Neurol Clin* 14:317, 1996.
4. Agostino R, Berardelli A, Formica A et al: Sequential arm movements in patients with Parkinson disease, Huntington disease and dystonia, *Brain* 115:1481, 1992.
5. Albin RL, Young AB, Penney JB: The functional anatomy of basal ganglia disorders, *Trends Neurosci* 12:366, 1989.
6. Alexander GE, Crutcher MD: Functional architecture of basal ganglia circuits: neural substrates of parallel processing, *Trends Neurosci* 13:266, 1990.
7. Kunzle H: Projections from the primary somatosensory cortex to basal ganglia and thalamus in the monkey, *Exp Brain Res* 30:481, 1977.
8. Alexander GE, Crutcher MD, DeLong MR: Basal ganglia-thalamocortical circuits: parallel substrates for motor, oculomotor, "prefrontal" and "limbic" functions, *Prog Brain Res* 85:119, 1990.
9. Kemp JM, Powell TPS: The connexions of the striatum and globus pallidus: synthesis and speculation, *Philos Trans R Soc Lond B Biol Sci* 262:441, 1971.
10. Kunzle H: Bilateral projections from precentral motor cortex to the putamen and other parts of the basal ganglia: an autoradiographic study in Macaca fascicularis, *Brain Res* 88:195, 1976.
11. Ariano MA, Fisher RS, Smyk-Randall E et al: D2 dopamine receptor distribution in the rodent CNS using antipeptide antisera, *Brain Res* 609:71, 1993.
12. Graybiel AM: Functions of the nigrostriatal system, *Clin Neurosci* 1:12, 1993.
13. Baldessarini RJ, Tarsy D: Dopamine and the pathophysiology of dyskinesias induced by antipsychotic drugs, *Ann Rev Neurosci* 3:23, 1980.
14. Smith AD, Bolam JP: The neural network of the basal ganglia as revealed by the study of synaptic connections of identified neurones, *Trends Neurosci* 13:259, 1990.
15. Carlsson A: Some aspects of dopamine in the basal ganglia. In Yahr MD, editor: *The basal ganglia,* New York, 1976, Raven Press.
16. Fahn S: The extrapyramidal disorders. In Wyngaarden JB, Smith LH, editors: *Cecil's textbook of medicine,* ed 16, Philadelphia, 1982, WB Saunders.
17. Monakow KH, Akert K, Kunzle H: Projections of the precentral motor cortex and other cortical areas of the frontal lobe to the subthalamic nucleus in the monkey, *Exp Brain Res* 33:395, 1978.
18. Nauta HJW, Cole M: Efferent projections of the subthalamic nucleus: an autoradiographic study in monkey and cat, *J Comp Neurol* 180:1, 1978.
19. Mettler FA et al: The extrapyramidal system, *Arch Neurol Psychiatry* 41:984, 1939.
20. Glickstein SB, Schmauss C: Dopamine receptor functions: lessons from knockout mice, *Pharmacol Ther* 91:63, 2001.
21. Jackson DM, Westlind-Danielsson A: Dopamine receptors: molecular biology, biochemistry, and behavioral aspects, *Pharmacol Ther* 64:291, 1994.
22. Buchwald NA, Hull CD, Levine MS et al: The basal ganglia and the regulation of response and cognitive sets. In Brazier MAB, editor: *Growth and development of the brain,* New York, 1975, Raven Press.

23. Hull CD, Bernardi G, Price DD et al: Intracellular responses of caudate neurons to temporally and spatially combined stimuli, *Exp Neurol* 38:324, 1973.

24. Levine MS, Hull CD, Buchwald NA: Pallidal and entopeduncular intracellular responses to striatal, cortical, thalamic and sensory inputs, *Exp Neurol* 44:448, 1974.

25. Levine MS, Hull CD, Buchwald NA: The spontaneous firing patterns of forebrain neurons. II. Effects of unilateral caudate nuclear ablation, *Brain Res* 78:411, 1974.

26. Levine MS, Hull CD, Buchwald NA et al: The spontaneous firing pattern of forebrain neurons. III. Prevention of induced asymmetries in caudate neuronal firing rates by unilateral thalamic lesions, *Brain Res* 131:215, 1977.

27. Buchwald NA, Heuser G, Wyers EJ et al: The "caudate-spindle." III. Inhibition by high frequency stimulation of subcortical structures, *Electroencephalogr Clin Neurophysiol* 13:525, 1961.

28. Buchwald NA, Wyers EJ, Lauprecht CW et al: The "caudate-spindle." IV. A behavioral index of caudate-induced inhibition, *Electroencephalogr Clin Neurophysiol* 13:536, 1961.

29. Dieckmann G, Sasaki K: Recruiting responses in the cerebral cortex produced by putamen and pallidum stimulation, *Exp Brain Res* 10:236, 1970.

30. Hull CD, Bernardi G, Buchwald NA: Intracellular responses of caudate neurons to brainstem stimulation, *Brain Res* 22:163, 1970.

31. Mink J: Neurobiology of basal ganglia and Tourette syndrome: basal ganglia circuits and thalamocortical outputs. *Adv Neurol* 99:89, 2006.

32. Hallett M: Physiology of basal ganglia disorders: an overview, *Can J Neurol Sci* 20:177, 1993.

33. Graybiel AM: The basal ganglia and chunking of action repertoires, *Neurobiol Learn Mem* 70:119, 1998.

34. Willis T: Cerebri anatomic cui accessit nervorum descriptio et usus, 1664. Translated in *Assoc Res Nerv Ment Dis* 21:8, 1940.

35. Magendie M: Fonctions et maladies du systeme nerveux, Paris, 1841, Lecapalin. Translated in *Assoc Res Nerv Ment Dis* 21:8, 1940.

36. Nothnagel H: Experimentalle untersuchungen uber die funktion des geherns, *Virchows Arch* 57:184, 1873. Translated in *Assoc Res Nev Ment Dis* 21:8, 1940.

37. Ferrier D: *The functions of the brain*, London, 1876, Smith, Elder.

38. Montgomery EB, Jr: Effect of subthalamic nucleus stimulation patterns on motor performance in Parkinson's disease. *Parkinsonism Relat Disord* 11:167, 2005.

39. Bemelmans AP, Horellou P, Pradier L et al: Brain-derived neurotrophic factor-mediated protection of striatal neurons in an excitotoxic rat model of Huntington disease, as demonstrated by adenoviral gene transfer, *Hum Gene Ther* 10:2987, 1999.

40. Benita M, Conde H, Dormont JF et al: Effects of ventrolateral thalamic nucleus cooling on initiation of forelimb ballistic flexion movements by conditioned cats, *Exp Brain Res* 34:435, 1979.

41. Denny-Brown D: *The basal ganglia and their relation to disorders of movement*, Liverpool, England, 1962, Liverpool University Press.

42. Hore J, Vilis T: Arm movement performance during reversible basal ganglia lesions in the monkey, *Exp Brain Res* 39:217, 1980.

43. Hore J, Myer-Lohmann J, Brooks VB: Basal ganglia cooling disables learned arm movements of monkeys in the absence of visual guidance, *Science* 195:584, 1977.

44. Pan HS, Walters JR: Unilateral lesion of the nigrostriatal pathway decreases the firing rate and alters the firing pattern of the globus pallidus neurons in the rat, *Synapse* 2:650, 1988.

45. Stern G: The effect of lesions in the substantia nigra, *Brain* 89:449, 1966.

46. Woodlee MT, Schallert T: The interplay between behavior and neurodegeneration in rat models of Parkinson's disease and stroke, *Restore Neurol Neurosci* 22:153, 2004.

47. Kornhuber HH: Motor functions of cerebellum and basal ganglia: the cerebellocortical saccadic (ballistic) clock, the cerebellonuclear hold regulator, and the basal ganglia ramp (voluntary speed smooth movement) generator, *Kybernetik* 8:157, 1971.

48. Corcos DM, Chen CM, Quinn NP et al: Strength in Parkinson disease: relationship to rate of force generation and clinical status, *Ann Neurol* 39:79, 1996.

49. Low KA, Miller J, Vierck E: Response slowing in Parkinson's disease: a psychophysiological analysis of premotor and motor processes, *Brain* 125:1980, 2002.

50. Shibasaki H, Fukuyama H, Hanakawa T: Neural control mechanisms for normal versus parkinsonian gait, *Prog Brain Res* 143:199, 2004.

51. DeLong MR: Activity of basal ganglia neurons during movement, *Brain Res* 40:127, 1972.

52. DeLong MR, Strick P: Relation of basal ganglia, cerebellum and motor cortex units to ramp and ballistic limb movements, *Brain Res* 71:327, 1974.

53. Jog MS, Kubota Y, Connolly CI et al: Building neural representations of habits, *Science* 286:1745, 1999.

54. Melnick M, Hull CD, Buchwald NA: Activity of forebrain neurons during alternating movement in cats, *Electroencephalogr Clin Neurophysiol* 57:57, 1984.

55. Neafsey EJ, Hull CD, Buchwald NA: Preparation for movement in the cat. I. Unit activity in the cerebral cortex, *Electroenchephalogr Clin Neurophysiol* 44:706, 1978.

56. Neafsey EJ, Hull CD, Buchwald NA: Preparation for movement in the cat. II. Unit activity in the basal ganglia and thalamus, *Electroencephalogr Clin Neurophysiol* 44:714, 1978.

57. Denny-Brown D, Yanagesawa N: The role of the basal ganglia in the initiation of movement. In Yahr MD, editor: *The basal ganglia,* New York, 1976, Raven Press.

58. Olmstead CE, Villablanca JR: Effects of caudate nuclei or frontal cortical ablations in kittens: bar pressing performance, *Exp Neurol* 63:244, 1979.

59. Potegal M: The caudate nucleus egocentric localization system, *Acta Neurobiol Exp* 32:479, 1972.

60. Martin JP: *The basal ganglia and posture,* London, 1967, Pitman Books.

61. Melnick ME, Dowling GA, Aminoff MJ et al: Effects of pallidotomy on balance and motor function in patients with Parkinson's disease, *Arch Neurol* 56:1361, 1999.

62. Karlsen K, Larsen JP, Tandberg E et al: Fatigue in patients with Parkinson disease, *Mov Disord* 14:237, 1999.

63. Bloem BR, Van Dijk JG, Beckley DJ et al: Altered postural reflexes in Parkinson disease. A reverse hypothesis, *Medical Hypotheses* 39:243, 1992.

64. Bloem BR, Beckley DJ, Van Dijk JG et al: Influence of dopaminergic medication on automatic postural responses and balance impairment in Parkinson disease, *Mov Disord* 11:509, 1996.

65. Bloem BR, Grimbergen YA, Cramer M et al: Prospective assessment of falls in Parkinson's disease, *J Neurol* 248:950, 2001.

66. Visser JE, Bloem BR: Role of the basal ganglia in balance control. *Neural Plast* 12:161, 2005.

67. Visser M, Marinus J, Bloem BR et al: Clinical tests for the evaluation of postural instability in patients with Parkinson's disease, *Arch Phys Med Rehabil* 84:1669, 2003.

68. Almeida QJ, Frank JS, Roy EA et al: An evaluation of sensorimotor integration during locomotion toward a target in Parkinson's disease, *Neuroscience* 134:283, 2005.

69. Demirci M, Grill S, McShane L et al: A mismatch between kinesthetic and visual perception in Parkinson's disease, *Ann Neurol* 41:781, 1997.

70. Beckley DJ, Bloem BR, Remler MP: Impaired scaling of long latency postural reflexes in patients with Parkinson disease, *Electroencephalogr Clin Neurophysiol* 83:22, 1993.

71. Diener C, Scholz E, Guschlbauer B et al: Increased shortening reaction in Parkinson's disease reflects a difficulty in modulating long loop reflexes, *Mov Disord* 2:31, 1987.

72. Brooks VB: Roles of cerebellum and basal ganglia in initiation and control of movements, *Can J Neurol Sci* 2:265, 1975.

73. Crutcher MD, DeLong MR: Single cell studies of the primate putamen. II. Relations to direction of movement and pattern of muscular activity, *Exp Brain Res* 53:244, 1984.

74. Lidsky TI: Pallidal and entopeduncular single unit activity in cats during drinking, *Electroencephalogr Clin Neurophysiol* 39:79, 1975.

75. Schneider JS, Lidsky TI: Processing of somatosensory information in striatum of behaving cats, *J Neurophysiol* 45:841, 1981.

76. Berardelli A, Rothwell JC, Thompson PD, et al: Pathophysiology of bradykinesia in Parkinson's disease, *Brain* 124:2131, 2001.

77. Hallett M, Litvan I: Evaluation of surgery for Parkinson's disease: a report of the Therapeutics and Technology Assessment Subcommittee of the American Academy of Neurology. The Task Force on Surgery for Parkinson's Disease, *Neurology* 53:1910, 1999.

78. Klockgether T, Dichgans J: Visual control of arm movement in Parkinson disease, *Mov Disord* 9:48, 1994.

79. Jobst EE, Melnick ME, Byl NN et al: Sensory perception in Parkinson disease, *Arch Neurol* 54:450, 1997.

80. Schneider JS, Unguez G, Yuwiler A, et al: Deficits in operant behavior in monkeys treated with MPTP, *Brain* 111:1265, 1988.

81. Battig K, Rosvold HE, Mishkin M: Comparison of the effects of frontal and caudate lesions on discrimination learning in monkeys, *J Comp Physiol Psychol* 55:458, 1962.

82. Teuber HL: Complex functions of basal ganglia. In Yahr MD, editor: *The basal ganglia,* New York, 1976, Raven Press.

83. Livesey PJ, Rankine-Wilson J: Delayed alternation learning under electrical (blocking) stimulation of the caudate nucleus in the cat, *J Comp Physiol Psychol* 88:342, 1975.

84. Gauthier L, Dalziel S, Gauthier S: The benefits of group occupational therapy for patients with Parkinson disease, *Am J Occup Ther* 41:360, 1987.

85. Brown J, Bullock D, Grossberg S: How the basal ganglia use parallel excitatory and inhibitory learning pathways to selectively respond to unexpected rewarding cues, *J Neurosci* 19:10502, 1999.

86. Bowen FP: Behavioral alterations in patients with basal ganglia lesions. In Yahr MD, editor: *The basal ganglia,* New York, 1976, Raven Press.

87. Krauthamer GM, Albe-Fessard D: Electrophysiological studies of the basal ganglia and striopallidal inhibition of non-specific afferent activity, *Neuropsychologia* 2:73, 1964.

88. Matsunami K, Cohen B: Afferent modulation of unit activity in globus pallidus and caudate neurons and changes induced by vestibular nucleus and pyramidal tract stimulation, *Brain Res* 91:140, 1975.

89. Muskens L: The central connection of the vestibular nuclei with the corpus striatum and their significance for ocular movements and for locomotion, *Brain* 45:452, 1922.

90. Segundo JP, Machne X: Unitary responses to afferent volleys in lenticular nucleus and claustrum, *J Neurophysiol* 19:325, 1956.

91. Hallett M: Parkinson revisited: pathophysiology of motor signs, *Adv Neurol* 91:19, 2003

92. Nallegowda M , Singh U, Handa G et al: Role of sensory input and muscle strength in maintenance of balance, gait, and posture in Parkinson's disease: a pilot study, *Am J Phys Med Rehabil* 83:898, 2004.

93. Nowack DA, Rosenkranz K, Topka H et al: Disturbances of grip force behaviour in focal hand dystonia: evidence for a generalised impairment of sensory-motor integration? *J Neurol Neurosurg Psychiatry* 76:953, 2005.

94. Wilson SAK: An experimental research into the anatomy and physiology of the corpus striatum, *Brain* 36:427, 1914.

95. Wang GJ, Volkow ND, Chang L et al: Partial recovery of brain metabolism in methamphetamine abusers after protracted abstinence, *Am J Psychiatry* 161:242, 2004.

96. Nieoullon A, Cheramy A, Glowinski J et al: Interdependence of the nigrostriatal dopaminergic systems on the two sides of the brain in the cat, *Science* 198:416, 1977.

97. Roberts E: Some thoughts about GABA and the basal ganglia. In Yahr MD, editor: *The basal ganglia,* New York, 1976, Raven Press.

98. Fuxe K et al: Heterogeneities in the dopamine neuron systems and dopamine cotransmission in the basal ganglia and the relevance of receptor-receptor interactions. In Fahn S, Marsden CD, Jenner P et al, editors: *Recent developments in Parkinson disease,* New York, 1986, Raven Press.

99. Mayeux R, Denaro J, Hemenegildo N et al: A population based investigation of Parkinson's disease with and without dementia: relationship to age and gender, *Arch Neurol* 49:492, 1992.

100. Whetten-Goldstein K, Sloan F, Kulas E et al: The burden of Parkinson's disease on society, family, and the individual, *J Am Geriatr Soc* 45:844, 1997.

101. Calne DB, Teychenne PF, Claveria LE et al: Bromocriptine in parkinsonism, *Br Med J* 4:442, 1974.

102. Rajput AH, Uitti RJ, Stern W, et al: Geography, drinking well water chemistry, pesticides and herbicides and the etiology of Parkinson disease, *Can J Neurol Sci* 14:414, 1987.

103. Barbeau A, Roy M, Bernier G et al: Ecogenentics of Parkinson disease: prevalence and environmental aspects in rural areas, *Can J Neurol Sci* 14:36, 1987.

104. Barbeau A, Roy M, Cloutier T et al: Environmental and genetic factors in the etiology of Parkinson's disease, *Adv Neurol* 45:299, 1987.

105. Butterfield PG, Valanis BG, Spencer PS, et al: Environmental antecedents of young-onset Parkinson disease, *Neurology* 43:1150, 1993.

106. Koller W, Vetere-Overfield B, Gray C et al: Environmental risk factors in Parkinson disease, *Neurology* 40:1218, 1990.

107. Robertson C, Flowers KA: Motor set in Parkinson disease, *J Neurol Neurosurg Psychiatry* 53:583, 1990.

108. Sherer TB, Betarbet R, Testa CM et al: Mechanism of toxicity in rotenone models of Parkinson's disease, *J Neurosci* 23:10756, 2003.

109. Testa CM, Sherer TB, Greenamyre JT: Rotenone induces oxidative stress and dopaminergic neuron damage in organotypic substantia nigra cultures, *Brain Res Mol Brain Res* 24:109, 2005.

110. Bonifati V, Fabrizio E, Vanacore N et al: Familial Parkinson's disease: a clinical genetic analysis, *Can J Neurol* 22:272, 1995.

111. Tanner CM: Parkinson disease in twins: an etiologic study, *JAMA* 281:341, 1999.

112. Hubble JP, Cao T, Hassanein RE et al: Risk factors for Parkinson disease, *Neurology* 43:1693, 1993.

113. Sasco AJ, Paffenbarger RS Jr, Gendre I, et al: The role of physical exercise in the occurrence of Parkinson disease, *Arch Neurol* 49:360, 1992.

114. Pechadre JC, Larochelle L, Poirier LJ: Parkinsonian akinesia, rigidity and tremor in the monkey, *J Neurol Sci* 28:147, 1976.

115. Teasdale N, Phillips J, Stelmach GE: Temporal movement control in patients with Parkinson disease, *J Neurol Neurosurg Psychiatry* 53:862, 1990.

116. Benecke R, Rothwell JC, Dick JP et al: Disturbance of sequential movements in patients with Parkinson's disease, *Brain* 101:361, 1987.

117. Benecke R, Rothwell JC, Dick JP et al: Performance of simultaneous movements in patients with Parkinson disease, *Brain* 109:739, 1986.

118. Brown RG, Jahanshahi M, Marsden CE: Response choice in Parkinson disease: the effects of uncertainty and stimulus-response compatibility, *Brain* 116:869, 1993.

119. Vidailhet M, Stocchi F, Rothwell JC, et al: The Bereitschafts potential preceding simple foot movement and initiation of gait in Parkinson disease, *Neurology* 43:1784, 1993.

120. Montgomery EB Jr, Nuessen J, Gorman DS: Reaction time and movement velocity abnormalities in Parkinson's disease under different task conditions, *Neurology* 41:1476, 1991.

121. Pascual-Leone A, Grafman J, Clark K et al: Procedural learning in Parkinson's disease and cerebellar degeneration, *Ann Neurol* 34:594, 1993.

122. Morris ME, Iansek R. Characteristics of motor disturbance in Parkinson disease and strategies for movement rehabilitation, *J Hum Mov Sci* 15:416, 1996.

123. Hallett M, Shahani BT, Young RR: Analysis of stereotyped voluntary movements at the elbow in patients with Parkinson's disease, *J Neurol Neurosurg Psychiatry* 40:1129, 1977.

124. Grimby L, Hannerz J: Disturbances in the voluntary recruitment order of anterior tibial motor units in bradykinesia of parkinsonism, *J Neurol Neurosurg Psychiatry* 37:47, 1974.

125. Milner-Brown HS, Fisher MA, Weiner WJ: Electrical properties of motor units in parkinsonism and a possible relationship with bradykinesia, *J Neurol Neurosurg Psychiatry* 42:35, 1979.

126. Kunesch E, Schnitzler A, Tyercha C et al: Altered force release control in Parkinson's disease, *Behav Brain Res* 67:43, 1995.

127. Pollock LJ, Davis L: Muscle tone in parkinsonian states, *Arch Neurol Psychiatry* 23:303, 1930.

128. Walshe FMR: Nature of musculature rigidity of paralysis agitans and its relationship to tremor, *Brain* 47:159, 1924.

129. Lelli S, Panizza M, Hallett M: Spinal cord inhibitory mechanisms in Parkinson's disease, *Neurology* 41:553, 1991.

130. Tatton WG, Bawa P, Stein RB: Altered motor cortical activity in extrapyramidal rigidity. In Poirier LJ, Sourkes TL, Bedard PJ, editors: *Advances in neurology, vol 24*, New York, 1979, Raven Press.

131. Markus HS, Cox M, Tomkins AM: Raised resting energy expenditure in Parkinson's disease and its relationship to muscle rigidity, *Clin Sci (Lond)* 83:199, 1992.

132. Friedman J, Friedman H: Fatigue in Parkinson's disease, *Neurology* 43:2016, 1993.

133. Poirier LJ, Pechadre JC, Larochelle L et al: Stereotaxic lesions and movement disorders in monkeys, *Adv Neurol* 10:5, 1975.

134. Koller WC, Glatt S, Vetere-Overfield B, et al: Falls and Parkinson's disease, *Clin Neuropharmacol* 12:98, 1989.

135. Ashburn A, Stack E, Pickering RM et al: A community dwelling sample of people with Parkinson's disease: characteristics of fallers and non-fallers, *Age Ageing* 30:47, 2001.

136. Gray P, Hildebrand K: Falls risk factors in Parkinson's disease, *J Neurosci Nursing* 32:222, 2000.

137. Schrag A, Ben-Schlomo Y, Quinn N: How common are complications of Parkinson's disease? *J Neurol* 249:419, 2002.

138. Wood BH, Bilclough JA, Bowron A, et al: Incidence and prediction of falls in Parkinson's disease: a prospective multidisciplinary study, *J Neurol Neurosurg Psychiatry* 72:721, 2002.

139. Anderson VC, Burchiel KJ, Hogarth P et al: Pallidal vs subthalamic nucleus deep brain stimulation in Parkinson disease, *Arch Neurol* 62:554, 2005.

139a. Kleiner-Fisman G, Fisman DN, Sime E et al: Long-term follow up of bilateral deep brain stimulation of the subthalamic nucleus in patients with advanced Parkinson disease, *J Neurosurg* 99:489, 2003.

139b. Loher TJ, Burgunder JM, Pohle T et al: Long-term pallidal deep brain stimulation in patients with advanced Parkinson disease: 1-year follow-up study, *J Neurosurg* 96:844, 2002.

139c. Rodriguez-Oroz MC, Obeso JA, Lang AE et al: Bilateral deep brain stimulation in Parkinson's disease: a multicentre study with 4 years follow-up, *Brain* 128:2240, 2005.

140. Pastor MA, Day BL, Marsden CD: Vestibular induced postural responses in Parkinson's disease, *Brain* 116:1177, 1993.

141. Glatt S: *Anticipatory and feedback postural responses in perturbation in Parkinson disease*, Phoenix, 1989, Society for Neuroscience Abstract.

142. Horak FB, Frank J, Nutt J: Effects of dopamine on postural control in parkinsonian subjects: scaling, set, tone, *J Neurophysiol* 75:2380-2396, 1996.

142a. Horak FB, Dimitrova D, Nutt JG: Direction-specific postural instability in subjects with Parkinson's disease, *Exp Neurol* 193:504-521, 2005.

142b. Bigalke H, Wohlfarth K, Irmer A et al: Botulinum A toxin: dysport improvement of biological availability, *Exp Neurol* 168:162, 2001.

143. Morris ME, Iansek R, Matyas TA et al: The pathogenesis of gait hypokinesia in Parkinson's disease, *Brain* 117:1169, 1994.

144. Morris ME, Iansek R, Matyas TA et al: Stride length regulation in Parkinson's disease. Normalization strategies and underlying mechanisms, *Brain* 119:551, 1996.

145. Morris ME, Huxham FE, McGinley J et al: Gait disorders and gait rehabilitation in Parkinson's disease, *Adv Neurol* 87:347, 2001.

146. Morris ME, Huxham FE, McGinley J et al: The biomechanics and motor control of gait in Parkinson's disease, *Clin Biomech* 16:459, 2001.

147. Friedman JH: Behavioral function in Parkinson's disease, *Clin Neurosci* 5:87, 1998.

148. Kliegel M, Phillips LH, Lemke U, et al: Planning and realisation of complex intentions in patients with Parkinson's disease, *J Neurol Neurosurg Psychiatry* 76:1501, 2005.

149. Muslimovic D, Post B, Speelman JD et al: Cognitive profile of patients with newly diagnosed Parkinson disease, *Neurology* 65:1239, 2005.

150. Weintraub D, Moberg PJ, Culbertson WC et al: Evidence for impaired encoding and retrieval memory profiles in Parkinson disease, *Cogn Behav Neurol* 17:195, 2004.

151. Noe E, Marder K, Bell KL et al: Comparison of dementia with Lewy bodies to Alzheimer's disease and Parkinson's disease with dementia, *Mov Disord* 19:60, 2004.

152. Owen AM, Roberts AC Hodges JR et al: Contrasting mechanisms of impaired attentional set-shifting in patients with frontal lobe damage or Parkinson's disease, *Brain* 116:1159, 1993.

153. Bond J, Morris ME: Effects of goal-directed secondary task performance on gait in subjects with PD, *Arch Phys Med Rehabil* 81:110, 2000.

154. O'Shea S, Morris ME, Iansek R: Dual task interference during gait in people with PD: effects of motor versus cognitive secondary tasks, *Phys Ther* 82:888, 2002.

155. Stelmach GE, Worringham CJ, Strand EA: Movement preparation in Parkinson's disease: the use of advanced information, *Brain* 109:1179, 1986.

155a. Saint-Cyr JA, Taylor AE, Lang AE: Procedural learning and neostriatal dysfunction in man, *Brain* 111:941, 1988.

156. Comella CL: Sleep disturbances in Parkinson's disease, *Curr Neurol Neurosci Rep* 3:173, 2003.

157. Hoehn MM, Yahr MD: Parkinsonism: onset, progression and mortality, *Neurology* 17:427, 1967.

158. Jordan N, Sagar HJ, Cooper JA: Cognitive components of reaction time in Parkinson disease, *J Neurol Neurosurg Psychiatry* 55:658, 1992.

159. Cotzias GC, Papavasiliou PS, Gellene R: Modification of parkinsonism: chronic treatment with L-dopa, *N Engl J Med* 280:337, 1969.

160. Hornykiewicz O: The mechanisms of action of L-dopa in Parkinson's disease, *Life Sci* 15:1249, 1974.

161. Lloyd KG, Davidson L, Hornykiewicz O: The neurochemistry of Parkinson's disease: effect of L-dopa therapy, *J Pharmacol Exp Ther* 195:453, 1975.

162. Fahn S, Elton RL: Unified Parkinson disease rating scale. In Fahn S, Marsden CD, Jenner P et al, editors: *Recent developments in Parkinson disease, vol 2*, Florham Park, NJ, 1987, MacMillan Healthcare Information.

163. Jellinger K: Pathology of parkinsonism. In Fahr S, Marsden CD, Jenner P, editors: *Recent developments in Parkinson disease*, New York, 1986, Raven Press.

164. Kelly PJ, Gillingham FJ: The long-term results of stereotaxic surgery and L-dopa therapy in patients with Parkinson disease: a 10-year follow-up study, *J Neurosurg* 53:332, 1980.

165. Markham CH, Diamond SG: Evidence to support early levodopa therapy in Parkinson disease, *Neurology* 31:125, 1981.

166. Melmon KL, Morrelli HF: *Clinical pharmacology: basic principles in therapeutics*, ed 2, New York, 1978, Macmillan.

167. Nutt JG, Woodward WR, Hammerstad JP, et al: The "on-off" phenomenon in Parkinson's disease: relation to levadopa absorption and transport, *N Engl J Med* 310:483, 1984.

168. Morgante F, Espay AJ, Gunraj C et al: Motor cortex plasticity in Parkinson's disease and levodopa-induced dyskinesias, *Brain* 129:1059-1069, 2006.

169. Diamond SG, Markham CH: One year trial of pergolide as an adjunct to Sinemet in the treatment of Parkinson disease, *Adv Neurol* 40:537, 1984.

170. Heikkila RE, Manzino L, Cabbot FS et al: Protection against the dopaminergic neurotoxicity of 1-methyl-4-phenyl-1,2,5,6-tetrahydropyridine by monoamine oxidase inhibitors, *Nature* 311:467, 1984.

171. Cohen G, Heikkila RE: The generation of hydrogen peroxide, superoxide radical and the hydroxyl radical by 6-hydroxy dopamine, dialuric acid and related autotoxic agents, *J Biol Chem* 249:2447, 1974.

172. Gerlach M, Double K, Reichman H et al: Arguments for the use of dopamine receptor agonists in clinical and preclinical Parkinson's disease, *J Neural Transm* 65:167, 2003.

173. Kopin IJ, Markey SP, Burns RS et al: Mechanisms of neurotoxicity of MPTP. In Fahr S, Marsden CD, Jenner P et al editors: *Recent developments in Parkinson's disease,* New York, 1986, Raven Press.

174. Vitek JL, Bakay RA , DeLong MR: Microelectrode-guided pallidotomy for medically intractable Parkinson's disease, *Adv Neurol* 74:183, 1997.

175. Vitek JL, Bakay RA, Hashimoto T et al: Microelectrode-guided pallidotomy. Technical approach and its application in medically refractory Parkinson's disease, *J Neurosurg* 88:1027, 1998.

176. Olanow CW, Goetz CG, Kordower JH et al: A double-blind controlled trial of bilateral fetal nigral transplantation in Parkinson's disease, *Ann Neurol* 54:403, 2003.

177. Su PC, Tseng HM, Liu HM et al: Subthalamotomy for advanced Parkinson's disease, *J Neurosurg* 97:598, 2002.

178. Su PC, Tseng HM, Liu HM, et al: Treatment of advanced Parkinson's disease by subthalamotomy: one-year results, *Mov Disord* 18:531, 2003.

179. Benabid AL, Pollack P, Gao D et al: Chronic electrical stimulation of the ventralis intermedius of the thalamus as a treatment of movement disorders, *J Neurosurg* 84:203, 1996.

180. Deep Brain Stimulation for Parkinson's Disease Study Group: Deep brain stimulation of the subthalamic nucleus or pars interna of the globus pallidus in Parkinson's disease, *N Engl J Med* 345:956, 2001.

181. Goetz CG, Poewe W, Rascol O et al: Evidence-based medical review update: pharmacological and surgical treatments of Parkinson's disease: 2001 to 2004, *Mov Disord* 20:523, 2005.

182. Pahwa R, Factor SA, Lyons KE et al: Practice parameter: treatment of Parkinson disease with motor fluctuations and dyskinesia (an evidence-based review). Report of the Quality Standards Subcommittee of the American Academy of Neurology, *Neurology* 66:983, 2006.

183. Bastian AM, Kelly VE, Perlmutter JS et al: Effects of pallidotomy and levodopa on walking and reaching movements in Parkinson's disease, *Mov Disord* 18:1008, 2003.

184. Bastian AM, Kelly VE, Revilla FJ et al: Different effects of unilateral versus bilateral subthalamic nucleus stimulation on walking and reaching in Parkinson's disease, *Mov Disord* 18:1000, 2003.

185. Melnick ME, Radtke S, Alsbury N et al: Effects of unilateral deep brain stimulation on gait in patients with Parkinson's disease, *Mov Disord* 15:64, 2000.

186. Piper M, Abrams GM, Marks WJ Jr: Deep brain stimulation for the treatment of Parkinson's disease: overview and impact on gait and mobility, *Neuro Rehabil* 20:223, 2005.

187. Melnick ME, Dowling GA, Baum WC et al: Effects of rhythmic exercise on balance, gait, and depression in patients with Parkinson's disease, *Gerontol* 39:293, 2000.

188. Alberts JL, Elder CM, Okun MS et al: Comparison of pallidal and subthalamic stimulation on force control in patient's with Parkinson's disease, *Motor Control* 8:484, 2004.

189. Revilla FJ, Perlmutter JS, Mink JW: Different effects of unilateral versus bilateral subthalamic nucleus stimulation on walking and reaching in Parkinson's disease, *Mov Disord* 18:1000, 2003.

190. Nutt JG, Rufener SL, Carter JH et al: Interactions between deep brain stimulation and levodopa in Parkinson's disease, *Neurology* 57:1835, 2001.

191. Vitek JL: Mechanisms of deep brain stimulation: excitation or inhibition, *Mov Disord* 17:69, 2003.

192. Freed CR, Greene PF, Breeze RE et al: Transplantation of embryonic dopamine neurons for severe Parkinson's disease, *N Engl J Med* 344:710, 2001.

193. Freeman TB, Olanow CW, Hauser RA et al: Bilateral fetal nigral transplantation as a treatment for Parkinson's disease, *Ann Neurol* 38:379, 1995.

194. Goetz CG, Stebbins GT, Chmura TA et al: Teaching tape for the motor section of the unified Parkinson's disease rating scale, *Mov Disord* 10:263, 1995.

194a. Richards M, Marder K, Cote L et al: Interrater reliability of the Unified Parkinson's Disease Rating Scale motor examination, *Mov Disord* 9:89, 1994.

194b. Stebbins GT, Goetz CG: Factor structure of the Unified Parkinson's Disease Rating Scale: motor examination section, *Mov Disord* 13:633, 1998.

195. Langston JW, Widner H, Goetz CG et al: Core assessment program for intracerebral transplantations (CAPIT), *Mov Disord* 7:2, 1992.

196. Behrman AL, Light KE, Flynn SM, et al: Is the functional reach test useful for identifying falls risk among individuals with Parkinson's disease? *Arch Phys Med Rehabil* 83:538, 2002.

197. Olanow CW, Watts RL, Koller WC: An algorithm (decision tree) for the management of Parkinson's disease (2001): treatment guidelines, *Neurology* 56(11 suppl 5):S1, 2001.

198. Divac I: Neostriatum and functions of prefrontal cortex, *Acta Neurobiol Exp* 32:461, 1972.

199. Sunvisson H, Lokk J, Ericson K et al: Changes in motor performance in persons with Parkinson's disease after exercise in a mountain area, *J Neurosci Nurs* 29:255, 1997.

200. Tillerson JL, Cohen AD, Caudle WM et al: Forced nonuse in unilateral parkinsonian rats exacerbates injury, *J Neurosci* 22:6790, 2002.

201. Tillerson JL, Caudle WM, Reveron ME et al: Exercise induces behavioral recovery and attenuates neurochemical deficits in rodent models of Parkinson's disease, *Neuroscience* 119:899, 2003.

202. Behrman AL, Cauragh JH, Light KE: Practice as an intervention to improve speeded motor performance and motor learning in Parkinson's disease, *J Neurol Sci* 174:127, 2000.

203. Deanne KH, Jones D, Clark CE et al: A comparison of physiotherapy techniques for patients with Parkinson's disease, *The Cochrane Library* 3, 2001.

204. Deanne KH, Jones D, Clark CE et al: A comparison of physiotherapy techniques for patients with Parkinson's disease, *The Cochrane Library* 2, 2002.

205. de Goede CJ, Keus SJ, Kwakkel G et al: The effects of physiotherapy in Parkinson's disease: a research synthesis, *Arch Phys Med Rehabil* 82:509, 2001.

206. Melnick ME, Palmer G: Physical therapy. In Koller WC, Paulson G, editors: *Therapy of Parkinson disease*, New York, 1990, Marcel Dekker.

207. Palmer SS, Mortimer JA, Webster DD, et al: Exercise therapy for Parkinson's disease, *Arch Phys Med Rehabil* 67:741, 1986.

208. Suchowersky O, Gronseth G, Perlmutter J et al: Practice Parameter: neuroprotective strategies and alternative therapies for Parkinson disease (an evidence-based review): report of the Quality Standards Subcommittee of the American Academy of Neurology, *Neurology* 66:976-982, 2006.

209. Baum WC, Piper M, Rust L et al: *Effects of exercise on gait, balance, and depression in patients with Parkinson's disease,* 5th International Symposium on Parkinson's disease, London, 1999.

210. Melnick ME, Radtke S, Piper M et al: Effects of unilateral deep brain stimulation on balance in Parkinson's disease, *Neurol* 56:A275, 2001.

211. Melnick ME, Dowling GA, Dodd MJ: The Pro-Self program: exercise for Parkinson's disease, *Gerontology* 41:282, 2001.

212. Schenkman M, Butler RB: A model for multisystem evaluation treatment of individuals with Parkinson disease: rationale and case studies, *Phys Ther* 69:932, 1989.

213. Bobath B: *Adult hemiplegia: evaluation and treatment,* London, 1976, William Heinemann.

214. Knott M, Voss D: *Proprioceptive neuromuscular facilitation patterns and techniques,* ed 2, New York, 1968, Harper & Row.

215. Sutoo D, Akiyama K: Music improves dopaminergic neurotransmission: demonstration based on the effect of music on blood pressure regulation, *Brain Res* 1016:255, 2004.

216. Montgomery EB Jr: Rehabilitative approaches to Parkinson's disease, *Parkinsonism Relat Disord* 10(suppl 1):S43, 2004.

217. Kuroda K, Tatara K, Takatorige G, et al: Effect of physical exercise on mortality in patients with Parkinson's disease, *Acta Neurol Scand* 86:55, 1992.

218. Cohen AD, Tillerson JL, Smith AD et al: Neuroprotective effects of prior limb use in 6-hydroxydopamine-treated rats: possible role of GDNF, *J Neurochem* 85:299, 2003.

219. de Bruin PF, de Bruin VM, Lees AJ, et al: Effects of treatment on airway dynamics and respiratory muscle strength in Parkinson's disease, *Am Rev Respir Dis* 148:1576, 1993.

220. Duvoisin RC: *Parkinson disease: a guide for patient and family,* New York, 1978, Raven Press.

221. Hurwitz A: The benefit of a home program exercise regimen for ambulatory Parkinson disease patients, *J Neuro Nurs* 21:180, 1989.

222. Melnick ME, Dowling GA, Piper M et al: The effect of rhythmic exercise on gait, balance and depression in people with Parkinson disease, *J Am Geriatr Soc* 47: 1999.

223. Ball J: Personal communication, 1983.

224. Comella CL, Stebbins GT, Brown-Toms N et al: Physical therapy and Parkinson's disease: a controlled clinical trial, *Neurology* 44:376, 1994.

225. Patti F, Rocca WA, Meneghini F et al: Effects of rehabilitation therapy on Parkinsonian's disability and functional independence, *J Neurol Rehab* 10:223, 1996.

226. Kaakkola S, Teravainen H, Ahtila S et al: Effect of entacapone, a COMT inhibitor, on clinical disability and levodopa metabolism in parkinsonian patients, *Neurology* 44:77, 1994.

227. Marchese R, Diverio M, Zucchi F, et al: The role of sensory cues in the rehabilitation of parkinsonian patients: a comparison of two physical therapy protocols, *Mov Disord* 15:879, 2000.

228. Formisano R, Pratesi L, Modarelli FT, et al: Rehabilitation and Parkinson's disease, *Scand J Rehabil Med* 24:157, 1992.

229. Pacchetti A: Active music therapy in Parkinson's disease: an integrative method for motor and emotional rehabilitation, *Psychosom Med* 62:386, 2000.

230. McGeer PL, McGeer EG, Suzuki JS: Aging and extrapyramidal function, *Arch Neurol* 34:33, 1977.

231. Mutch WJ, Smith WC, Scott RF: A pilot study of patient rated disability and the need for aids in Parkinson disease, *Clin Rehabil* 3:151, 1989.

232. McIntosh GC, Brown SH, Rice RR et al: Rhythmic auditory-motor facilitation of gait patterns in patients with Parkinson's disease, *J Neurol Neurosurg Psychiatry* 62:22, 1997.

233. Baatile J, Langbein WE, Weaver F et al: Effect of exercise on perceived quality of life of individuals with Parkinson's disease, *J Rehabil Res Develop* 37:529, 2000.

234. Dam M, Tonin P, Casson S et al: Effects of conventional and sensory enhanced physiotherapy on disability in Parkinson's disease patients, *Adv Neurol* 69:551, 1996.

235. Ellis T, de Goede CJ, Feldman RG et al: Efficacy of a physical therapy program in patients with Parkinson's disease: a randomized controlled trial, *Arch Phys Med Rehabil* 86:626, 2005.

236. Muller V, Mohr B, Rosin R et al: Short-term effects of behavioral treatment on movement initiation and postural control in Parkinson's disease: a controlled clinical trial, *Mov Disord* 12:306, 1997.

237. Conner NP, Abbs JH: Task-dependent variations in Parkinsonian motor impairments, *Brain* 114:321, 1991.

238. Schenkman M, Cutson TM, Kuchibhatla M et al: Exercise to improve spinal flexibility and function for people with Parkinson's disease: a randomized, controlled trial, *J Am Geriatr Soc* 46:1207, 1998.

239. Thaut MH, McIntosh GC, Rice RR, et al: Rhythmic auditory stimulation in gait training for Parkinson's disease patients, *Mov Disord* 11:193, 1996.

240. Dunne JW, Hankey GJ, Edis RH et al: Parkinsonism: upturned walking stick as an aid to locomotion, *Arch Phys Med Rehabil* 68:380, 1987.

241. Smithson F, Morris ME, Iansek R: Performance on clinical tests of balance in Parkinson's disease, *Phys Ther* 78:577, 1998.

242. Dibble LE, Nicholson DE, Shultz B, et al: Sensory cueing effects on maximal speed gait initiation in persons with Parkinson's disease and healthy elders, *Gait Posture* 19:215, 2004.

243. Saint-Cyr JA, Taylor AE, Nicholson K: Behavior and the basal ganglia, *Adv Neurol* 65:1, 1995.

244. Alves G, Wentzel-Larson T, Larson JP: Is fatigue an independent and persistent symptom in patients with Parkinson disease? *Neurology* 63:1908, 2004.

245. Carter JH, Nutt JG, Woodward WR: The effect of exercise on levodopa absorption, *Neurology* 42:2042, 1992.

246. Reuter I, Engelhardt M, Stecker K et al: Therapeutic value of exercise training in Parkinson's disease, *Med Sci Sports Exerc* 31:1544, 1999.

247. Hashimoto T, Elder CM, Okun MS et al: Stimulation of the subthalamic nucleus changes the firing pattern of pallidal neurons, *J Neurosci* 23:1916, 2003.

248. Jones TA, Chu CJ, Grande LA et al: Motor skills training enhances lesion-induced structural plasticity in the motor cortex of adult rats, *J Neurosci* 19:10153, 1999.

249. Sotrel A, Williams RS, Kaufmann WE et al: Evidence for neuronal degeneration and dendritic plasticity in cortical pyramidal neurons of Huntington's disease: a quantitative Golgi study, *Neurology* 43:2088, 1993.

250. Storey E, Beal MF: Neurochemical substrates of rigidity and chorea in Huntington's disease, *Brain* 116:1201, 1993.

251. Harper PS: Localization of the gene for Huntington chorea, *Trends Neurosci* 7:1, 1984.

252. Leslie WD, Greenberg CR, Abrams DN et al: Clinical deficits in Huntington disease correlate with reduced striatal uptake on iodine-123 epidepride single-photon emission tomography, *Eur J Nucl Med* 26:1458, 1999.

253. Reynolds NC Jr, Myklebust JB, Prieto TE et al: Analysis of gait abnormalities in Huntington disease, *Arch Phys Med Rehabil* 80:59, 1999.

254. Koller WC, Trimble J: The gait abnormality of Huntington disease, *Neurology* 35:1450, 1985.

255. Georgiou N, Phillips JG, Bradshaw JL et al: Impairment of movement kinematics in patients with Huntington's disease: a comparison with and without a concurrent task, *Mov Disord* 12:386, 1997.

256. Georgiou N, Bradshaw JL, Iansek R et al: Reduction in external cues and movement sequencing in Parkinson's disease, *J Neurol Neurosurg Psychiatry* 57:368, 1994.

257. Georgiou N, Bradshaw JL, Phillips JG et al: Reliance on advance information and movement sequencing in Huntington's disease, *Mov Disord* 10:472, 1995.

258. Phillips JG, Bradshaw JL, Chiu E et al: Bradykinesia and movement precision in Huntington's disease, *Neuropsychologia* 34:1241, 1996.

259. Pratley RE, Salbe AD, Ravussin E et al: Higher sedentary energy expenditure in patients with Huntington's disease, *Ann Neurol* 47:64, 2000.

260. Djousse L, Knowlton B, Cupples LA et al: Weight loss in early stage of Huntington's disease, *Neurology* 59:1325, 2002.

261. Shelton PA, Knopman DS: Ideomotor apraxia in Huntington disease, *Arch Neurol* 48:35, 1991.

262. Feigin A, Leenders KL, Moeller JR et al: Metabolic network abnormalities in early Huntington's disease; an [(18)F]FDG PET study, *J Nucl Med* 42:1591, 2001.

263. Petajan JH: Motor unit control in Huntington's disease: a possible presymptomatic test. In Chase TN, Wexler NS, Barbeau A, editors: *Advances in neurology, vol 23,* New York, 1979, Raven Press.

264. Yanagasawa N: The spectrum of motor disorders in Huntington disease, *Clin Neurol Neurosurg* 94(suppl):S182, 1992.

265. Harris GJ, Codori AM, Lewis RF et al: Reduced basal ganglia blood flow and volume in pre-symptomatic, gene-tested persons at-risk for Huntington's disease, *Brain* 122:1667, 1999.

266. Shoulson I, Fahn S: Huntington disease: clinical care and evaluation, *Neurology* 29:1, 1979.

267. Shoulson I, Fahn S: Clinical care of the patient and family with Huntington disease. In *Commission for the control of Huntington disease and its consequences, vol 2,* Washington, DC, 1977, National Institutes of Health.

268. Feigin A, Zgaljardic D: Recent advances in Huntington's disease: Implications for experimental therapeutics, *Curr Opin Neurol* 15:483, 2002.

269. Alpay M, Koroshetz WJ: Quetiapine in the treatment of behavioral disturbances in patients with Huntington's disease, *Psychosomatics* 47:70, 2006.

269a. Berger Z, Ravikumar B, Menzies FM et al: Rapamycin alleviates toxicity of different aggregate-prone proteins, *Hum Mol Genet* 15:433, 2006.

269b. Hersch SM, Gevorkian S, Marder K et al: Creatine in Huntington disease is safe, tolerable, bioavailable in brain and reduces serum 8OH2'dG, *Neurology* 66:250, 2006.

269c. Stack EC, Smith KM, Ryu H: Combination therapy using minocycline and coenzyme Q10 in R6/2 transgenic Huntington's disease mice, *Biochim Biophys Acta* 1762:373, 2006.

269d. Tariq M, Khan HA, Elfaki I et al: Neuroprotective effect of nicotine against 3-nitropropionic acid (3-NP)-induced experimental Huntington's disease in rats, *Brain Res Bull* 67:161, 2005.

270. Shoulson I, Goldblatt D, Charlton M, et al: Huntington's disease: treatment with muscimol, a GABA-mimetic drug, *Trans Am Neurol Assoc* 102:124, 1977.

271. Bird ED: Biochemical studies on γ-aminobutyric acid metabolism in Huntington chorea. In Bradford HF and Marsden CD, editors: *Biochemistry and neurology,* London, 1976, Academic Press.

272. Hayden MR: *Huntington chorea,* Berlin, 1981, Springer-Verlag.

273. Klawans HL, Goetz CG, Perlik S: Presymptomatic and early detection in Huntington's disease, *Ann Neurol* 8:343, 1980.

274. Huntington's Study Group: Unified Huntington's Disease Rating Scale: reliability and consistency, *Mov Disord* 11:136, 1996.

275. Peacock IW: A physical therapy program for Huntington disease patients, *Clin Management* 7:22, 1987.

276. Thaut MH, Miltner R, Lange HW et al: Velocity modulation and rhythmic synchronization of gait in Huntington's disease, *Mov Disord* 14:808, 1999.

277. Walshe JM: Wilson's disease: the presenting symptoms, *Arch Dis Child* 37:253, 1962.

278. Strickland CT, Leu ML: Wilson's disease: clinical and laboratory manifestations in 40 patients, *Medicine* 54:113, 1975.

279. Cooper IS: *Involuntary movement disorders,* New York, 1969, Paul B. Hoeber.

280. MacKay AVP: Clinical controversies in tardive dyskinesia. In Marsden CD, Fahn S, editors: *Movement disorders,* Boston, 1981, Butterworth.

281. Smith JM, Baldessarini RJ: Changes in prevalence, severity and recovery in tardive dyskinesia with age, *Arch Gen Psychiatry* 37:1368, 1980.

282. Shellenberger MK: Persistent alteration of rat brain monoamine levels by carbon monoxide exposure: sex differences and behavioral correlation, *Neurotoxicology* 2:431, 1981.

283. Burt DR, Creese I, Snyder SH: Antischizophrenic drugs: chronic treatment elevates dopamine receptor binding in brain, *Science* 196:326, 1977.

283a. Margolese HC, Chouinard G, Kolivakas TT et al: Tardive dyskinesia in the era of typical and atypical antipsychotics. Part 2: Incidence and management strategies in patients with schizophrenia. *Can J Psychiatry* 50:703, 2005.

284. Lidsky TI, Labuszuski T, Avitable MJ et al: The effects of stimulation of trigeminal sensory afferents upon caudate units in cats, *Brain Res Bull* 4:9, 1979.

285. Labuszewski T, Lidsky TI: Basal ganglia influences on brain stem trigeminal neurons, *Exp Neurol* 65:471, 1979.

286. Levine MS, Hull CD, Garcia-Rill E et al: Long-term decreases in spontaneous firing of caudate neurons induced by amphetamine in cats, *Brain Res* 194:263, 1980.

287. Levine MS, Hull CD, Buchwald NA: Long-term behavioral and neurophysiological effects of neonatal δ-amphetamine administration in kittens, *Neurosci Abst* 8:965, 1982.

288. Mazloom M, Smith Y: Synaptic microcircuitry of tyrosine hydroxylase-containing neurons and terminals in the striatum of 1-methyl-4-phenyl-1,2,3,6-tetrahydropyridine-treated monkeys, *J Comp Neurol* 495:453-469, 2006.

289. Coons HW, Peloquin LJ, Kloman R et al: Effect of methylphenidate on young adult's vigilance and event-related potentials, *Electroencephalogr Clin Neurophysiol* 51:373, 1981.

290. Davis CG, Williams AC, Markey SP et al: Chronic parkinsonism secondary to intravenous injection of meperidine, *Psychiatry Res* 1:249, 1979.

291. Langston JW, Ballard P, Tetrud JW et al: Chronic parkinsonism in humans due to a product of meperidine analog synthesis, *Science* 219:979, 1983.

292. Melnick ME, Shellenberger MK, Hassanein R: Comparison of behavioral effects of MPTP in young adult and year-old rats. In Markey SP, Castognoli AJ, Trevorand IJ et al, editors: *MPTP: a neurotoxin producing a Parkinsonian syndrome,* Orlando, FL, 1986, Academic Press.

293. Wagner GC, Jarvis MF: Age-dependent effects of MPTP. In Markey SP et al, editors: *MPTP: a neurotoxin producing a Parkinsonian syndrome,* Orlando, FL, 1986, Academic Press.

294. Langston JW: MPTP neurotoxicity: an overview and characterization of phrases of toxicity, *Life Sci* 36:201, 1985.

295. Goto S, Lee LV, Munoz EL et al: Functional anatomy of the basal ganglia in X-linked recessive dystonia-parkinsonism, *Ann Neurol* 58:7, 2005.

295a. Hutchison WD, Lang AE, Dostrovsky JO et al: Pallidal neuronal activity: implications for models of dystonia, *Ann Neurol* 53:480, 2003.

295b. Pralong E, Debatisse D et al: Effect of deep brain stimulation of GPI on neuronal activity of the thalamic nucleus ventralis oralis in a dystonic patient, *Neurophysiol Clin* 33:169, 2003.

295c. Steigerwald F, Hinz L, Pinsker MO et al: Effect of propofol anesthesia on pallidal neuronal discharges in generalized dystonia, *Neurosci Lett* 386:156, 2005.

296. Chan J, Brin MF, Fahn S: Idiopathic cervical dystonia: clinical characteristics, *Mov Disord* 6:119, 1991.

297. Marsden CD, Sheehy MP: Writer's cramp: a focal dystonia, *Trends Neurosci* 13:148, 1990.

298. Bressman SB, Sabatti C, Raymond D et al: The DYT1 phenotype and guidelines for diagnostic testing, *Neurology* 54:1746, 2000.

299. Byl N, Wilson F, Merzenich M et al: Sensory dysfunction associated with repetitive strain injuries of tendonitis and focal hand dystonia: a comparative study, *J Orthoped Sports Phys Ther* 23:234, 1996.

300. Tinazzi M, Frasson E, Polo A et al: Evidence for an abnormal cortical sensory processing in dystonia: selective enhancement of lower limb P37-N50 somatosensory evoked potentials, *Mov Disord* 14:473, 1999.

301. Byl NN, Melnick ME: The neural consequences of repetition: clinical implications of a learning hypothesis, *J Hand Ther* 10:160, 1997.

302. Byl NN, Merzenich MM, Jenkins WM: A primate genesis model of focal dystonia and repetitive strain injury: I. Learning-induced dedifferentiation of the representation of the hand in the primary somatosensory cortex in adult monkeys, *Neurology* 47:508, 1996.

303. Wenger KK, Musch KL, Mink JW: Impaired reaching and grasping after focal inactivation of globus pallidus pars interna in the monkey, *J Neurophysiol* 82:2049, 1999.

304. Byl NN, McKenzie A, Nagarajan SS: Differences in somatosensory hand organization in a healthy flutist and a flutist with focal hand dystonia: a case report, *J Hand Ther* 13:302, 2000.

305. Rosenkranz K, Williamon A, Butler K et al: Pathophysiological differences between musician's dystonia and writer's cramp, *Brain* 128(part 4):918, 2005.

306. Tarsy D: Comparison of clinical rating scales in treatment of cervical dystonia with botulinum toxin, *Mov Disord* 12:100, 1997.

307. Moreau MS, Cauquil AS, Costes Salon MC: Static and dynamic balance function in spasmodic torticollis, *Mov Disord* 14:87, 1999.

CHAPTER 25 Brain Tumors

Corrie J. Stayner, MS, PT
Rachel M. Lopez, MPT, NCS
Karla M. Tuzzolino, PT, NCS

KEY WORDS

astrocytoma
biopsy
chemotherapy
Gamma knife
glioblastoma multiforme
hospice care
Karnofsky Performance Status Scale
meningioma
metastatic
radiation therapy
ventriculostomy

OBJECTIVES

Upon completion of this chapter the student/therapist will be able to:

1. Identify the categories of primary brain tumors.
2. Recognize and interpret signs and symptoms of primary brain tumors specific to tumor location.
3. Recognize current diagnostic tests used to detect brain tumors.
4. Identity the types of medical and surgical management for brain tumors and how that management will affect functional movement.
5. Describe the side effects associated with the treatment of brain tumors and recognize their impact on therapeutic intervention.
6. Discuss the multiple considerations necessary to plan and execute an intervention program for the client with a brain tumor.
7. Recognize the emotional and psychosocial impact of the disease process on the client, the client's support system, and the interdisciplinary team.

AN OVERVIEW OF BRAIN TUMORS

The rehabilitation clinician serves many different populations, including clients with brain tumors. Despite the prognosis for limited survival associated with primary brain tumors, these individuals have shown progress in the rehabilitation setting similar to that noted in clients with diagnoses of stroke or traumatic brain injury.[1-3] Advances in medical and surgical treatment for clients with cancer have resulted in improved survival rates and longer life expectancy. However, individuals are often faced with progressive functional impairments resulting from the disease process.[2] These impairments may be physical or cognitive, or both, and require an interdisciplinary team approach to best facilitate the individual's return to a meaningful lifestyle. In addition, clinicians must recognize the psychological and emotional needs of the individual given this diagnosis and be sensitive and flexible in accommodating these feelings. Improved quality of life, especially the opportunity to return home, remains the ultimate goal of the rehabilitation process.

The clinical presentation of clients with brain tumors mimics that of persons with other central nervous system (CNS) conditions. The location of the tumor or vascular accident determines the deficits the client will exhibit. However, in the brain tumor client, the burdensome effects of standard medical intervention and the aggressive nature of the disease course itself provide obstacles to therapeutic intervention. The client's probability of eventual physical and cognitive deterioration provides a challenge to the clinician attempting to formulate realistic goals and plan for future needs. Therefore, a thorough knowledge of the

tumor's natural history, the complications and side effects of treatment, and the neurological deficit the client exhibits will assist the clinician in best developing a comprehensive, individualized plan of care.

Incidence and Etiology

The incidence of adult brain tumors is on the rise in the United States, with an estimated 41,130 new cases of primary benign or malignant brain and CNS tumors for 2004. Of these, 18,400 are expected to be malignant, resulting in 12,690 deaths. The statistics for children include 3200 new cases of primary benign or malignant brain and CNS tumors for the same 12-month period.[4,5]

The exact cause of the increase in incidence of brain tumors is not known. Studies suggest that the increase is the result of more tumors being diagnosed with improved tumor imaging, rather than an actual increase in the occurrence of malignant brain tumors.[6,7]

In the United States, brain tumors typically afflict two distinct categories: (1) children aged 0 to 15 years and (2) adults in the fifth to seventh decades of life. In adults, white Americans have a higher incidence than black Americans, and in both pediatric and adult populations males are more frequently affected than females.[8,9] In children, a primary brain tumor is now the second most common cause of solid tumor cancer death in the 0- to 15-year-old age group.[5]

The frequently occurring meningioma, typically benign, accounts for nearly 29.2% of all primary brain tumors. Glioblastoma multiforme, a malignant tumor, accounts for 21% of adult primary tumors[10] (Figure 25-1). Pediatric

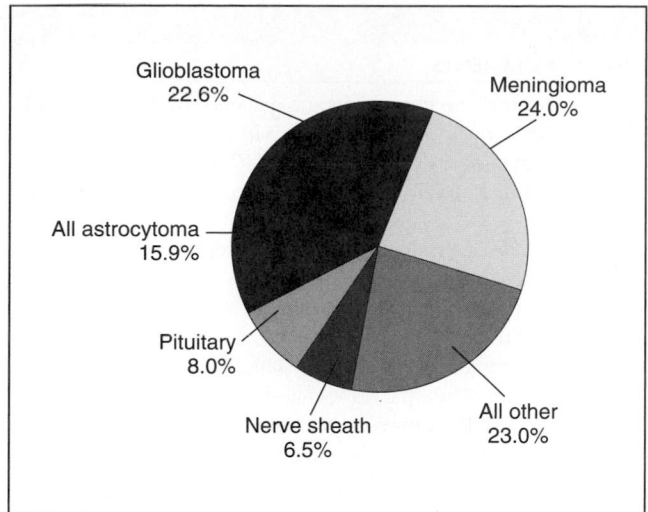

FIGURE 25-1 ■ Distribution of all primary brain and central nervous system tumors by histology. (From CBTRUS: *2004 statistical report: primary brain tumors in the United States, 1977-2001,* Chicago, Central Brain Tumor Registry of the United States.)

tumors, unlike adult tumors, are unique in their histology and behavior and are rarely metastatic. The predominant tumors in children are typically infratentorial in location; most specifically, cerebellar astrocytoma, medulloblastoma, and fourth ventricular ependymoma.[11]

The etiology of brain tumors remains unclear. Theories suggest that heredity is a contributing factor, but studies show familial incidence can be explained by a common toxic or infectious exposure.[12,13] Research indicates an association, but not a causal relationship, linking brain tumors to certain chemicals and materials (petrochemicals, organic solvents, rubber). These materials are frequently found in specific occupations, such as farming and manufacturing. Electromagnetic field exposure is associated with an increased incidence of brain tumor.[14] Ionizing radiation, used therapeutically in high doses to treat tumors, was found to have a causal relationship to the development of a second brain tumor.[15]

Continued investigation into possible causal relationships with potential risk factors is essential if the incidence and mortality rate associated with brain tumors is to decrease.

Classification of Tumors

The World Health Organization (WHO) first published a universal classification system for CNS tumors in 1979. This system classifies tumors according to their microscopic characteristics and has been accepted as the universal method for the classification of brain tumors.[16,17]

Primary tumors originate in the CNS, whereas metastatic or secondary tumors spread to the CNS from systemic cancer sites outside the brain. Characteristics of the most common brain tumors are discussed in the following paragraphs, with information provided regarding age at onset, location, medical treatment, and prognosis.

Gliomas are primary tumors that arise from supportive tissues of the brain and are frequently located in the cere-

bral hemispheres. These tumors may also occur in the brain stem, optic nerve, and spinal cord. In children, the cerebellum is a primary location for gliomas.[18] Gliomas have four primary categories and are classified by their predominant cellular components: astrocytomas and oligodendrogliomas originate from glial cells, ependymomas from ependymal cells, and medulloblastomas from primitive cells.[19]

Astrocytomas are derived from astrocytes, which are star-shaped glial cells, and are the most common primary brain tumor in adults and children.[20] Astrocytomas vary in morphology and biological behavior, from those that are diffuse and infiltrate surrounding brain structures to those that are circumscribed with a decreased likelihood of progression. Astrocytomas are typically found in the cerebrum, originating in the frontal lobe in adults, and in the cerebellum in children. In adults, the primary age at onset is typically in the third to fifth decades of life.[7,16]

Astrocytomas are further classified into four grades: well-differentiated, low-grade (grades 1 and 2) tumors; anaplastic, high-grade (grade 3) tumors; and glioblastoma multiforme, high-grade (grade 4) tumors. The higher the grade, the poorer the prognosis.[7]

Low-grade tumors (grade 2) grow slowly and are typically subtotally resected through surgery when accessible, whereas grade 1 tumors occur primarily in children and are typically cured with complete surgical resection. Recurrence is common as a result of incomplete resection.[7] If these tumors recur, their form and structure often change to that of an anaplastic astrocytoma or glioblastoma.[19]

Anaplastic, midgrade (grade 3) tumors grow rapidly, typically carry malignant cell traits, and routinely progress toward glioblastoma multiforme tumors.[16] Grade 4 tumors, glioblastoma multiforme, are discussed below.

Astrocytomas are typically treated with surgery, radiation therapy, and chemotherapy depending upon the grade, location of the tumor, age of the patient and Karnofsky performance scale score[7,18,21] (Table 25-1). On average, patients with astrocytomas have a 5-year survival rate of 30%.[22] Patients with grade 2 astrocytomas treated with radiation therapy and surgery have a 65% 5-year survival rate and a 40% 10-year survival rate.[23] Those with grade 3 astrocytomas have a 5-year survival rate of only 22% when treated similarly.[22]

Glioblastoma multiforme is the distinct name given to the highly malignant grade 4 astrocytoma. These tumors grow rapidly, invade nearby tissue, and contain highly malignant cells. Glioblastomas are predominantly located in the deep white matter of the cerebral hemispheres but may be found in the brain stem, cerebellum, or spinal cord. Fifty percent of these tumors are bilateral or occupy more than one lobe of a hemisphere. Like the astrocytoma, typical age at onset is during midlife, with males having a 2:1 incidence rate over females.[7,16,18] The medical prognosis is poor for persons with glioblastoma: less than 20% survive more than 1 year and only 2% survive 5 years after the tumor diagnosis was made.[22] The most important prognostic variables are age, tumor histology, and postoperative score on the Karnofsky performance status scale. These tumors are treated by surgical resection, radiation therapy, stereotactic radiosurgery, and chemotherapy.[7]

Oligodendrogliomas are slow growing but progressive tumors that typically develop over a period of several years,

TABLE 25-1 ■ Karnofsky Performance Status Scale

CONDITION	PERFORMANCE STATUS (%)	COMMENTS
A. Able to carry on normal activity and to work; no special care is needed	100	Normal; no complaints; no evidence of disease
	90	Able to carry on normal activity; minor signs or symptoms of disease
	80	Normal activity with effort; some signs or symptoms of disease
B. Unable to work; able to live at home, care for most personal needs; a varying degree of assistance is needed	70	Care of self; unable to carry on normal activity or to do active work
	60	Requires occasional assistance, but is able to care for most of personal needs
	50	Requires considerable assistance and frequent medical care
C. Unable to care for self; requires equivalent of institutional or hospital care; disease may be progressing rapidly	40	Disabled; requires special care and assistance
	30	Severely disabled; hospitalization is indicated, although death not imminent
	20	Very sick; hospitalization necessary; active supportive treatment necessary
	10	Moribund; fatal processes progressing rapidly
	0	Dead

From Karnofsky DA, Burchenal JH: The clinical evaluation of chemotherapeutic agents in cancer. In Macleod C, editor: *Evaluation of chemotherapeutic agents,* New York, 1949, Columbia University Press.

with 50% involving multiple lobes. Fifty percent of these tumors occur in the frontal lobe, 42% in the temporal lobe, and 32% in the parietal lobe. Many clients have seizures as the only clinical manifestation of the tumor.[16,24,25] Oligodendrogliomas typically appear in the fourth to sixth decades of life, and the ratio of affected males to females is 2:1.[26] The prognosis with oligodendrogliomas varies considerably and is dependent upon age at diagnosis and tumor grade. Positive prognostic indicators have been age at onset of less than 40 years and a tumor grade of 1 or 2. These patients have a median survival of 9 years with a 5-year survival rate of 60% to 75% and 10-year survival rate of 46%.[22,25,27] Negative prognostic indicators include age at onset over 40 years, hemiparesis, and cognitive changes.[27] The 5-year survival rate decreases to 36% with anaplastic oligodendroglioma.[22] Treatment is dependent upon symptoms and ranges from observation and seizure control with anticonvulsant drugs to surgical resection followed by radiation and chemotherapy.[7,18,19,24]

Ependymomas and *ependymoblastomas* are tumors arising from ependymal cells lining the ventricles that grow in the ventricles or in adjacent brain tissue.[18,19] Sixty percent to 66% of ependymomas are located in the posterior fossa.[7,26] Anaplastic ependymomas, also known as ependymoblastomas, are primarily located supratentorially, are more commonly seen in children, and have a tendency toward metastatic spread via the cerebrospinal fluid (CSF).[7,16,26] For 40% of infratentorial tumors, the age at onset is in the first decade of life, whereas for supratentorial tumors, the age at onset is evenly distributed across the life span.[26] Ependymomas are primarily treated with surgical resection followed by radiation therapy, but chemotherapy is also used.[7,18,19,26] These tumors frequently recur and prognosis is dependent upon the success of

resection, with a 5-year survival rate ranging from 58% to 68%.[15,28,29]

Medulloblastomas are malignant embryonal tumors thought to arise from primitive neuroectodermal cells in the granular layer of the cerebellum, but the exact cell of origin is unknown. These tumors are typically located in the posterior fossa, originating laterally in the cerebellar hemispheres in young adults and in the vermis in children.[16] Medulloblastomas typically grow into the fourth ventricle, blocking CSF flow, causing hydrocephalus and increased intracranial pressure (ICP).[7] These tumors primarily occur in children, accounting for 25% of childhood brain tumors.[16,18] Five-year survival rates range from 30% to almost 70%.[26] Systemic metastases occur in 5% of cases and bone metastases in 90%. Because of the increased incidence of metastases, the prognosis for children younger than age 4 is poor.[7] Prognosis is better for children younger than age 4, for tumors with complete resection, and with decreased metastases present. Treatment is surgery followed by radiation therapy and chemotherapy.[18]

Meningiomas are slow-growing tumors that primarily originate from cells located in the dura mater or arachnoid.[18,20,26] Frequently these tumors are found incidentally during imaging studies or at autopsy.[30] Approximately 25% are symptomatic when diagnosed.[20,30,31] The incidence increases with age and they occur in females in a 2:1 ratio over males.[3,10,32,33] Resectable tumors are primarily treated by surgery and recurring tumors are treated with surgery, radiation therapy, or stereotactic radiosurgery.[19] Patients with nonmalignant meningiomas have a 5-year survival rate of 70% versus a 5-year survival rate of 55% with malignant meningiomas.[22,34]

Pituitary adenomas are benign epithelial tumors originating from the adenohypophysis of the pituitary gland and frequently encroach on the optic chiasm.[16,19,26] These tumors are characterized by hypersecretion or hyposecretion of hormones.[7,18] Age at onset spans all ages, but pituitary adenomas are rare before puberty.[7] The female-to-male ratio of incidence is 2.25:1. These tumors are primarily treated by surgical resection and drug therapy.[7,18,19] Prognosis is related to size and cell type of the tumor.[28]

Schwannomas are encapsulated tumors composed of neoplastic Schwann cells that can arise on any cranial or spinal nerve.[18,19] The eighth cranial nerve is the cranial nerve usually involved, and a schwannoma here is called an *acoustic neuroma*.[16] Acoustic neuromas produce otological or focal or generalized neurological deficits, depending upon the location of the tumor. These tumors are typically located in the internal auditory canal but may extend into the cerebellopontine angle.[7,26] These tumors are frequently treated by surgical resection, but stereotactic radiosurgery is increasing in popularity as an alternative method of treatment.[18,35,36] The prognosis for patients with these tumors is good, yet complications can result from treatment, including facial paralysis, deafness, and equilibrium impairments. Resulting neurological deficits after surgery vary depending on the size and location of the tumor. Currently these tumors rarely result in death, and with the increasing use of noninvasive procedures, the eighth cranial nerve is being preserved more frequently.[36]

Primary central nervous system lymphoma is an aggressive non-Hodgkin's lymphoma that represents only a small percentage of tumors, although their incidence has tripled over the past two decades in the United States. These tumors have been found in immunocompetent and immunosuppressed individuals.[37,38] Congenital or acquired immunosuppression, particularly acquired, increases the risk of primary central nervous system lymphoma with the highest incidence occurring in patients with AIDs.[37] Currently no behavioral or environmental risk factors are known to increase the incidence of these tumors in immunocompetent individuals. These lymphomas peak in the sixth to seventh decades of life with the incidence slightly higher in men. Behavior and cognitive changes are the two most common symptoms and occur in approximately two thirds of patients, whereas hemiparesis, aphasia, and visual field deficits are found in 50% of patients at the time of diagnosis. Fifteen percent to 20% of patients present with seizures. Lymphomas are typically diagnosed by a stereotactic biopsy, with chemotherapy typically being the first treatment choice, as resection has not been shown to have a therapeutic role. Standard chemotherapy treatments used for systemic lymphomas are ineffective in the treatment of cerebral lymphomas. Although radiation was previously the primary method of treatment with a median survival of 12 to 18 months, cranial irradiation combined with methotrexate-based regimens has increased the median survival to 40 months with 25% of the patients surviving 5 years or longer. Caution must be used when combining radiation and chemotherapy with these patients, as delayed neurological toxicity has been shown to develop especially in patients older than age 60. Because of the delayed neurological toxicity, chemotherapy-only regimens are now being explored with some success.[38]

Metastatic brain tumors are secondary tumors that have spread to the brain, typically through the arterial circulation, from a primary systemic cancer site elsewhere in the body.[7]

The frontal lobe is the most common site for metastatic disease from primary systemic sources, including the lungs, breast, and kidneys, or from melanoma.[39] Approximately 20% to 30% of people with systemic cancer develop metastatic brain tumors.[40]

Treatment for these tumors is tailored to the individual and dependent upon the management of the systemic disease, the accessibility of the lesion, and the number of lesions present. The prognosis varies, with positive prognostic indicators including a Karnofsky performance scale score of 70 or greater, age 60 years or younger, remission or resolution of the primary cancer, and metastases located in the brain only. Typically, an individual will survive approximately 1 month after diagnosis without treatment.[23,40] With corticosteroids, survival increases to 2 months, and whole-brain radiation therapy extends survival to 3 to 5 months. Microsurgical resection of a single metastasis has been shown to increase survival to 9 to 14 months.[23,40,41] Survival increases to 16 months when surgical resection and whole-brain radiation are combined. In one study in which the systemic disease was controlled and solitary brain metastases occurred, a survival rate greater than 5 years was shown in 21% of cases.[42]

Signs and Symptoms

The clinical manifestation of a brain tumor can range from a decreased speed in comprehension or a minor personality change, to progressive hemiparesis or seizure, depending on the type and site of the tumor. Patients with brain tumors typically present with headaches, seizures, nonspecific cognitive or personality changes, or focal neurological signs.[26,43] Some may present with a general sign, a specific neurological symptom, or a combination of both.

General Signs and Symptoms

General signs and symptoms of the presence of a brain tumor include headache, seizures, altered mental status, and papilledema. *Headache* is the presenting symptom in 30% of cases and develops during the course of the disease in 70% of cases. These headaches are generally dull, intermittent, and nonspecific, and are usually on the same side as the tumor. They are often difficult to distinguish from migraine or cluster headaches. It is important to identify the specific nature of the headaches, because certain features often indicate the presence of a brain tumor. These features include the following:

1. The headache that interrupts sleep or is worse upon waking and improves throughout the day
2. The headache that is elicited by postural changes, coughing, or exercise
3. The headache of recent onset that is more severe or of a different type than usual
4. The new onset of headache in a previously asymptomatic person
5. The headache associated with nausea and vomiting, papilledema, or focal neurological signs[1,7]

The mechanism of the headache is not clearly understood but may be related to local swelling, distortion of blood vessels, direct invasion of the meninges, and increased ICP. When the tumor has grown to a volume large enough to cause compression and displacement of the brain, the onset and severity of the headache seems to correlate with changes in ICP.[44] With increased ICP, a bifrontal or bioccipital headache is present regardless of the tumor location.[26,45]

Seizure activity is the presenting symptom in one third of cases and is present in 50% to 70% of cases at some stage of the disease.[15,43] Approximately 10% to 20% of adults with new-onset seizure activity have brain tumors. Seizures are usually focal but may become generalized and cause loss of consciousness.[38] Frontal lobe gliomas produce seizures in 59% of all cases. The percentage of cases exhibiting seizures from gliomas in other lobes is as follows: parietal, 42%; temporal, 35%; and occipital, 33%.[43]

Altered mental status is the initial symptom in 15% to 20% of cases and is frequently present at the time of diagnosis. Mental status changes can range from subtle changes in concentration, memory, affect, personality, initiative, and abstract reasoning to severe cognitive problems and confusion.[43] Subtle changes may be incorrectly attributed to worry, anxiety, or depression.[26] Changes in mentation are common with frontal lobe tumors and in the presence of elevated ICP. Increased ICP causes drowsiness and decreased level of consciousness, which can progress to stupor or coma if treatment is not initiated.[43]

The incidence of *papilledema,* swelling of the optic nerve, is less frequent today because brain tumors are being diagnosed earlier with the use of sensitive imaging techniques. Papilledema is associated with symptoms of transient visual loss, especially with positional changes, and reflects evidence of increased intracranial hemorrhage transmitted through the optic nerve sheath. It is more common in children and with slow-growing tumors and posterior fossa tumors.[43] Other less common symptoms are vomiting and frank positional vertigo, usually accompanying tumors found in the posterior fossa.[26]

Specific Signs and Symptoms

Certain clinical features are related to functional areas of the brain and thus have a specific localizing value when diagnosing a brain tumor.[43] Therefore, it is essential that clinicians be familiar with the lobes of the brain and their distinct functions to manage effectively the deficits resulting from the tumor (Figure 25-2). These symptoms may vary among individuals and result in impairments that range from mild to severe.[44]

The *frontal lobe* is responsible for motor functioning, initiation of action, and interpretation of emotion, including motor speech, motor praxis, attention, cognition, emotions, intelligence, judgment, motivation, and memory.[46,47] Therefore, frontal lobe tumors may result in hemiparesis, seizures, aphasia, and gait difficulties. Initially, the tumor may be clinically silent. As the tumor grows, however, there may be

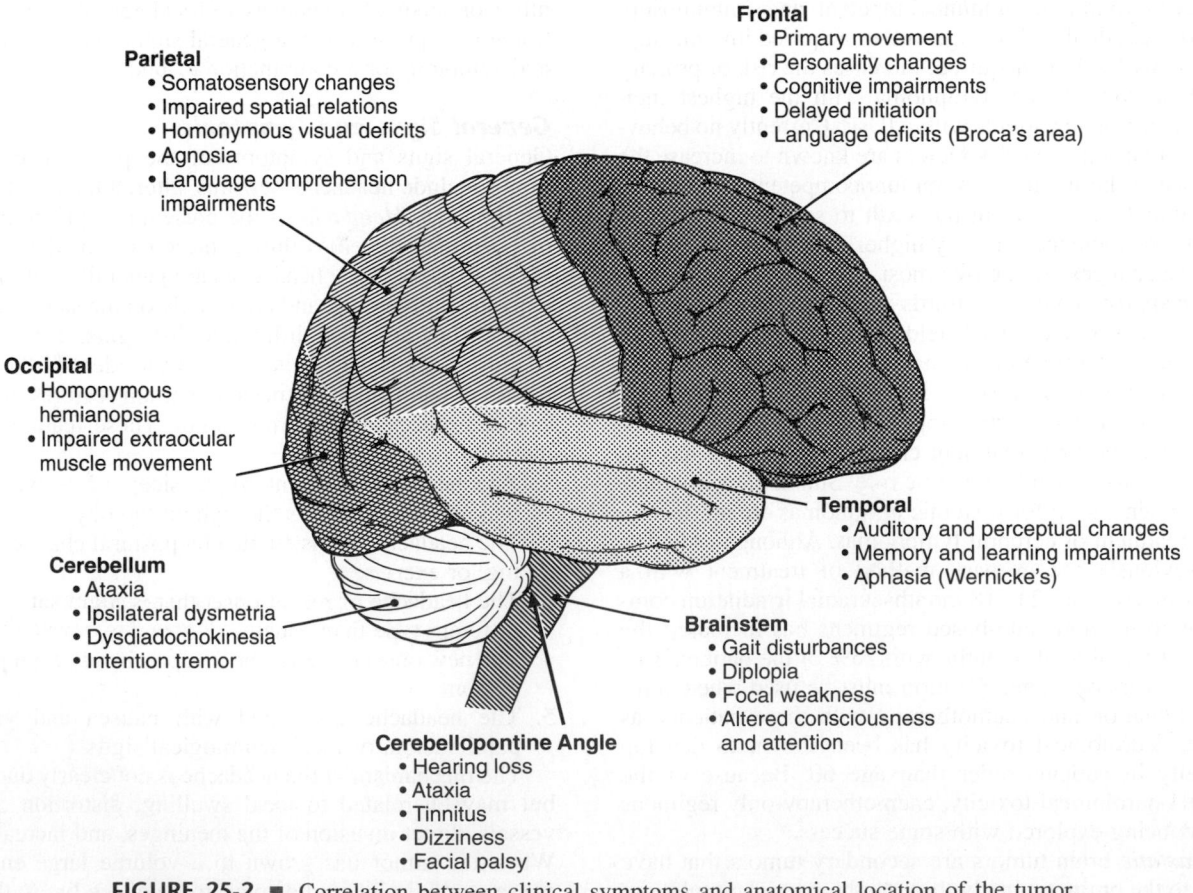

Parietal
- Somatosensory changes
- Impaired spatial relations
- Homonymous visual deficits
- Agnosia
- Language comprehension impairments

Frontal
- Primary movement
- Personality changes
- Cognitive impairments
- Delayed initiation
- Language deficits (Broca's area)

Occipital
- Homonymous hemianopsia
- Impaired extraocular muscle movement

Cerebellum
- Ataxia
- Ipsilateral dysmetria
- Dysdiadochokinesia
- Intention tremor

Temporal
- Auditory and perceptual changes
- Memory and learning impairments
- Aphasia (Wernicke's)

Brainstem
- Gait disturbances
- Diplopia
- Focal weakness
- Altered consciousness and attention

Cerebellopontine Angle
- Hearing loss
- Ataxia
- Tinnitus
- Dizziness
- Facial palsy

FIGURE 25-2 ■ Correlation between clinical symptoms and anatomical location of the tumor. (Used with permission from Barrow Neurological Institute.)

personality changes, including disinhibition, irritability, impaired judgment, and lack of initiative.[43,48] Bifrontal disease usually associated with infiltrative gliomas and primary CNS lymphomas may cause bilateral hemiplegia; spastic bulbar palsy; severe cognitive impairment; emotional lability; dementia; and prominent primitive grasp, suck, and snout reflexes.[44]

The *parietal lobe* processes complex sensory and perceptual information related to somesthetic sensation, spatial relations, body schema, and praxis. General symptoms of a parietal lobe tumor include contralateral sensory loss and hemiparesis, homonymous visual deficits or neglect, agnosias, apraxias, and visual-spatial disorders. If the dominant parietal lobe is involved, aphasia and seizures may be present. When the nondominant parietal lobe is involved, contralateral neglect and inability to recognize deficits may be apparent.[32,43,45]

The *occipital lobe* is the primary processing area of visual information. Therefore, lesions of the occipital lobe often result in disorders of eye movement and homonymous hemianopsia. If the parieto-occipital junction is involved, visual agnosia and agraphia are often present. Although less common, visual seizures may be present, characterized by lights, colors, and formed geometric patterns.[23,43,45] Bilateral occipital tumors may cause cortical blindness.[44]

The *temporal lobe* is responsible for auditory and limbic processing. Anterior temporal lobe lesions may be clinically silent until becoming quite large, resulting in seizures. If the lateral hemispheres are involved, auditory and perceptual changes may occur. When the medial aspects of the lobe are involved, changes in cognitive integration, long-term memory, learning, and emotions may be seen. When the dominant temporal lobe is involved, aphasia may be present. Anomia, agraphia, acalculia, and Wernicke's aphasia, characterized by fluent, nonsensical speech, are specific to left temporal lobe lesions.[23,43,45] In comparison to bifrontal tumors, bitemporal tumor involvement is rare and causes memory deficits and possible dementia.[44]

The *cerebellum* is responsible for coordination and equilibrium.[32] The most common symptoms of cerebellar tumors in adults include headache, nausea and vomiting in 40% of cases, and ataxia in 25% of cases. Lesions of the midline cause truncal and gait ataxia and lesions of the hemispheres cause unilateral appendicular ataxia, most commonly seen in the upper extremities. Lesions of either hemisphere may cause ipsilateral dysmetria, dysdiadochokinesia, and intention tremor. If the tumor involves the cerebellopontine angle, hearing loss, headache, ataxia, dizziness, tinnitus, and facial palsy may occur. If the tumor invades the meninges at the foramen magnum or increased ICP causes cerebellar tonsil herniation, nuchal rigidity and head tilt away from the lesion may be seen. Abnormal posturing of the head is observed in children but not adults.[44] Because the cerebellum is located in an extremely confined space, even minimal increases in pressure can cause death from cerebellar tonsil herniation.[7,43,44,49]

The *brain stem*, which communicates information to and from the cerebral cortex via fiber tracts, controls basic life functions. The reticular formation specifically controls consciousness and attention. Even small changes in tumors invading or compressing the brain stem can lead to death or devastating signs and symptoms. Symptoms of a brain stem tumor have an insidious onset and may include gait disturbances, diplopia, focal weakness, headache, vomiting, facial numbness and weakness, and personality changes.[7] If the dorsal midbrain is involved, Parinaud syndrome, characterized by loss of upward gaze, pupillary areflexia to light, and loss of convergence, may be seen. If the reticular system of the pons and medulla is involved, symptoms of apnea, hypoventilation or hyperventilation, orthostatic hypotension, or syncope may occur.[7,49]

The pituitary gland is an endocrine gland that secretes hormones that regulate many bodily processes. Pituitary tumors are typically large and affect pituitary function by compressing its structure or hypersecreting hormones. An enlarging tumor causes a loss of pituitary function and decreases hormone secretion, resulting in pituitary disorders specific to the type of hormone involved (Cushing disease, hypothyroidism, Addison disease, diabetes, etc.). As the tumor enlarges it may invade or compress nearby structures. Lateral extension involving the third and fourth cranial nerves causes diplopia; fifth cranial nerve involvement causes ipsilateral facial numbness; and internal carotid artery occlusion causes cerebral infarction. Upward extension is more common and may compress the optic chiasm, hypothalamus, or third ventricle. Downward extension may compress the sphenoid sinus, typically without clinical signs.[7]

Diagnosis of Disease/Pathology

Advances in research and the development of sophisticated diagnostic equipment have greatly improved brain tumor diagnosis. When a physician suspects a brain tumor, many specialized tests may be used to gather clinical, radiological, pathological, and laboratory information to confirm the diagnosis.[43]

Clinical Diagnosis

A clinical diagnosis consists of information the physician gathers during a comprehensive evaluation. First, a thorough medical history, including the specific nature of signs and symptoms, must be obtained. A neurological examination is then performed to assess visual, cognitive, sensory, and motor function, and test reflexes.[49] If the presence of a brain tumor is suspected after the neurological examination, the next diagnostic step, tumor imaging, is warranted.[26]

Radiological Diagnosis

The modern era of CNS imaging began with the introduction of computed tomography (CT) in 1973 and with magnetic resonance imaging (MRI) in 1979.[7] The availability of sensitive imaging allows for earlier tumor detection and has revolutionized the diagnosis and management of brain tumors.[43,50] Tumor imaging has continued to develop and can be classified into three categories: static imaging, dynamic imaging, and computer integration imaging.

Static Imaging. Static neurological imaging includes computed tomography (CT) and magnetic resonance imaging (MRI), which are noninvasive techniques that provide accurate anatomical and functional analysis of intracranial structures.[43] CT, which relies on the electron density and photon energy of tissues, was the first brain imaging technique to determine tumor size. Contrast enhancement helps to identify isodense tumor from surrounding parenchyma, hypodense lesions in edematous areas, and optimal sites for tumor biopsy.[7,43] Following surgical intervention, CT can be used to confirm the proper tissue biopsy site and determine the success of tumor resection. Although MRI has become the preferred method, CT scanning offers lower cost, shorter scanning time, and a more sensitive method to detect calcification bony involvement.

Magnetic Resonance Imaging (MRI). MRI is the initial diagnostic imaging procedure of choice. MRI scanning is superior to CT scanning in detecting and localizing brain tumors as well as evaluating edema, hydrocephalus, or hemorrhage.[44] CT scans can miss structural lesions, especially posterior fossa tumors and low-grade gliomas.[38] MRI is a more sensitive imaging modality than CT for identifying lesions and margin abnormalities by providing greater anatomical detail with thin slices and multiplanar images. With MRI, different signal intensities differentiate between normal brain and tumor. Contrast enhancement with gadolinium sharpens the definition of a lesion.[7,26,45] Under certain conditions, MRI enhanced with gadolinium can distinguish between tumor and edema. However, not all high-grade astrocytomas enhance with gadolinium, and MRI signals may imitate imaging abnormalities seen in low-grade astrocytomas or nonmalignant conditions. MRI also cannot accurately predict tumor type or grade of malignancy for which surgical biopsy is necessary.[7,43]

Dynamic Imaging. Dynamic functional imaging includes positron emission tomography (PET), single-photon emission computed tomography (SPECT), magnetic resonance spectroscopy (MRS), and echo planar MRI. *PET* is a noninvasive technique using a cyclotron and specific isotopes to obtain dynamic information about the metabolism and physiology of the brain tumor and the surrounding brain tissue. PET scans using fludeoxyglucose F18 (^{18}FDG) to measure glucose metabolism can be useful in determining the grade of primary brain tumors and in differentiating tumor regrowth from radiation necrosis.[9,45,51] However, recent studies suggest that ^{18}FDG-PET actually has a limited ability to differentiate recurrent tumor from radiation necrosis.[48,52] PET can also be helpful in studying the metabolic effects of chemotherapy, radiation therapy, and steroids on the tumor.[43] However, PET is less reliable in patients treated heavily with chemotherapy and radiation therapy.[7,26]

Single-Photon Emission Computed Tomography (SPECT). SPECT is a functional imaging technique evolved from PET that uses infused thallium (Tl), which localizes in tumor but not in necrotic or normal brain tissue.[7,26,43] SPECT is used to distinguish between high- and low-grade tumors and between tumor recurrence and radiation necrosis.[7,43] Along with ^{18}FDG-PET, SPECT is used preoperatively with static imaging to localize the highest metabolic area within tumor for biopsy. Although SPECT is a less sensitive method of obtaining physiological information on brain tumors, it is more readily available and less expensive.[7]

Magnetic Resonance Spectroscopy (MRS). MRS is a noninvasive technique used in conjunction with static MRI to measure the metabolism of brain tumors.[7] MRS has been proved to differentiate successfully normal brain from malignant tumor and recurrent tumor from radiation necrosis. It also has been used to document early treatment response and provide information regarding histological grade of astrocytomas.[53,54] In the future, MRS targeting may enhance the diagnostic yield of brain biopsy and possibly be a noninvasive alternative to surgical biopsy.[53,55]

Echo Planar MRI. Echo planar MRI, or functional MRI, uses a conventional MRI scanner fitted with echo planar technology. This technique maps cerebral blood flow at the capillary level. Its intended purpose is to provide information regarding the diffusion of contrast into tumor, resulting in better resolution of tumor and edema.[7]

Modern computer technology allows for the two- and three-dimensional reconstruction of identical planes in cranial space by combining tumor images from different modalities, including CT, MRI, PET, and SPECT. *Computed integration imaging* involves the simultaneous display of images from different techniques in a single imaging system that is transposed to a reference stereotactic frame. This development has resulted in significant advances in stereotactic biopsy, interstitial radiotherapy, and laser-guided stereotactic resection.[7] By improving targeting and visualization of tissues, stereotaxis provides a safer, more accurate method of tissue acquisition and biopsy. A correct tissue diagnosis can be made in 95% of cases with this technique.[56]

Biopsy

Surgical biopsy is performed to obtain tumor tissue as part of tumor resection or as a separate diagnostic procedure.[15] Stereotactic biopsy is a computer-directed needle biopsy. When guided by advanced imaging tools, stereotactic biopsy yields the lowest surgical morbidity and highest diagnostic information. This technique is frequently used with deep-seated tumors in functionally important or inaccessible areas of the brain in order to preserve function.[57]

Laboratory Diagnosis

Laboratory testing is often used to further assess focal deficits during the diagnosis and management of brain tumors. Perimetry is the measurement of visual fields used when evaluating tumors near the optic chiasm. Electroencephalography (EEG) is used to monitor brain activity and detect seizures but has limited value during screening because EEG is often normal in clients with brain tumors.[43] Lumbar puncture analyzes CSF, which is useful in the diagnosis and detection of dissemination of certain brain tumors. However, lumbar puncture is risky in patients with increased ICP and should be avoided in those cases.[26,43,45] Audiometry and vestibular testing are useful for diagnosing tumors in the cerebellopontine angle. Endocrine testing is used to examine endocrine abnormalities with tumors in the pituitary gland and hypothalamus.[43]

Medical and Surgical Management

After diagnosis of a brain tumor is confirmed, specific treatment must be selected. The ultimate goals of tumor management are to improve quality of life and extend survival, by preserving or improving neurological function.[58] These goals are accomplished by removing or decreasing the size of the tumor. Treatment techniques are determined by histological type, location, grade, and size of tumor; age at onset; and medical history of the patient.[7,15,19,58] Four types of treatment are discussed: (1) traditional surgery, (2) chemotherapy, (3) radiation therapy, and (4) stereotactic radiosurgery.

Traditional Surgery

The primary goal of traditional surgery is maximal tumor resection with the least amount of damage to neural or supporting structures.[7] Gross total resection is associated with longer survival rates and improved neurological function.[38] Benign tumors, if accessible, are resected completely, whereas malignant tumors are typically partially resected secondary to location or size of the tumor.[7,58] The *purposes* of surgery in the management of brain tumors include the following:

1. Biopsy to establish a diagnosis
2. Partial resection to decrease the tumor mass to be treated by other methods
3. Complete resection of the tumor
4. Providing access for other treatment techniques[18]

Biopsies are performed through open, needle, and stereotactic needle techniques. Open biopsies involve exposure of the tumor followed by removal of a sample through surgical excision. Needle biopsies involve insertion of a needle into the tumor through a hole in the skull and the excision of the tissue sample drawn through the needle. Stereotactic needle biopsies use computers and MRI or CT scanning equipment to assist in directing the needle into the tumor. This type of biopsy is useful for deep-seated or multiple brain lesions.[7,15]

Partial and *complete resections* are accomplished through craniotomy. Craniotomy involves removal of a portion of the skull and separation of the dura mater to expose the tumor. Stereotactic craniotomy uses recent technology to create computed three-dimensional pictures of the brain to guide the neurosurgeon during the procedure. CT scanning and, more recently, MRI scanners are used to provide an evaluation of the tumor resection during the procedure.[7,15,59]

Preoperative Management. Before surgery, clients are evaluated for general surgical risks and the possibility of tumors in additional locations. Unless medically contraindicated, steroids are administered before surgery if brain edema is present or if extensive manipulation will be occurring during surgery. Anticonvulsant medications are also administered preoperatively to prevent seizures during or after surgery.[7,58]

Intraoperative Management. During surgery, precautions are taken to prevent an increase in edema or intracranial pressure. Mannitol is used to shrink the surrounding brain tissue, thus providing easier access to the tumor. Steroid use is continued and antibiotics are administered to prevent infection. Hyperventilation, with a CO_2 level of 25 mEq/L, is also used to reduce intracranial pressure.[7,58]

Postoperative Management. Patients are observed in an intensive care unit for at least 24 hours for possible intracranial bleeding or seizures. Blood pressure is monitored continuously. Following surgery, patients are at risk for developing deep vein thrombosis or pulmonary embolism secondary to decreased muscle activity, but, because these patients are at risk for intracranial bleeding, anticoagulants cannot be given.[60] Therefore compression stockings are used prophylactically in an attempt to prevent deep vein thrombosis. Steroids are tapered after surgery over 5 to 10 days. Anticonvulsant medications are continued after surgery with the length of time dependent on the presence of seizure activity before and after surgery.[7,58] The primary limitations of traditional surgery include the following:

1. Medical complications such as hematoma, hydrocephalus, infection, and infarction from the surgical procedure
2. Complications resulting from general anesthesia
3. Increased cost of hospital stay and surgical procedure[23,36,58]

Chemotherapy

Chemotherapy is another treatment frequently used to manage brain tumors. It can be used independently or as an adjuvant to surgery or radiation. Chemotherapeutic drugs are not effective on all types of tumors. Certain tumors are known to be resistant to certain drugs, and other treatments are more effective for these tumors.

Chemotherapy drugs impede cellular replication of the tumor cells, interfering with their ability to copy DNA and reproduce. Once the replicating capability of the tumor cell is disrupted, it dies. In this way, the tumor is prevented from growing and is destroyed at the cellular level.[15]

One of the challenges in delivering cytotoxic drugs to the brain is the blood-brain barrier (BBB). The BBB is the brain's natural protective barrier against transmission of foreign substances from the blood into the brain.[15] One class of drugs that does permeate the BBB is the *nitrosoureas*. These include BCNU (carmustine) and CCNU (lomustine), which are lipid-soluble and cell cycle-specific. These drugs are given in high doses and typically are used for glioblastoma multiforme and anaplastic astrocytoma; however, often these high-grade tumors invade and destroy the blood brain barrier.

Methotrexate is a highly toxic drug and is usually paired with a drug called an antidote drug to reverse the side effects on normal cells. Leucovorin is used to counteract high-dose methotrexate.[61] Typically, this drug is used to treat cancer outside of the CNS. Methotrexate has been found to produce a high degree of neurotoxicity when used in combination with radiation therapy.[62]

Other drugs used to treat brain tumors include cisplatin, carboplatin, procarbazine, vincristine, etoposide (VP-16), and a newer drug called temozolomide.[51] Drugs can be given in combination to target all cell types present within the tumor. Because different drugs have different modes of action and side effects, combined drug therapy often proves to be one of the most effective treatments.[15]

Hormones. Tamoxifen hormone therapy appears to inhibit tumor growth. This estrogen antagonist is currently being tested for efficacy in tumor treatment.[15]

Administration. Chemotherapy can be administered in a number of different ways. Most agents are given intravenously through a peripheral IV or through a catheter such as a peripherally inserted central catheter (PICC) or Groshong catheter. Other drugs are placed directly into the tumor bed or are given intramuscularly, orally, or by means of an implanted device.

Chemotherapy agents such as BCNU can be placed in the tumor area in the form of wafers that release the drug over time. Neurotoxic to surrounding tissue, methotrexate and araC are drugs able to be introduced directly into the CSF through an intraventricular Ommaya reservoir.[44] The reservoir, implanted under the scalp, is filled by use of a syringe and the medication is then circulated through the ventricles to the brain.[15]

The drugs are typically given in a clinic setting by a registered nurse certified in chemotherapy administration. A patient's chemotherapy schedule varies depending on the drug given. An on/off cycle is used to allow the patient to recover from the toxic effects of the drug.

Biotherapy. When compared with conventional therapy for improving the survival of patients with astrocytoma, most available methods of biotherapy have not been successful. Methods investigated include the use of cytokines (interferons, interleukins, and tumor necrosis factor), interleukin-stimulated lymphokine-activated killer cells, antigens-stimulated lymphocytes, and monoclonal antibodies. Research grows in this area as newer agents are identified and biotherapy in combination with other treatment modalities is tested.[63] Other areas that hold promise include gene therapy, antiangiogenesis, inhibition of signal transduction, and growth factor inhibitors.[37]

Gene Therapy. One area of promising biological therapy for the treatment of malignant astrocytomas is gene therapy.[63] There are two major components to gene therapy: the delivery system and the therapeutic gene.[37,63] The delivery system, or vector, most commonly used is a virus. Predominant vectors include retroviruses, adenoviruses, and herpes viruses.[63] Gene therapy lends itself to treatment of brain tumors because the retroviruses insert themselves only into dividing cells and the tumors are localized, only rarely metastasizing outside the CNS.[37]

The most widely used therapeutic gene in brain tumor trials is the herpes simplex virus gene, thymidine kinase (TK). The TK gene is inserted into the tumor and replicated. The tumor cells now carrying the gene are destroyed when an antiviral agent such as ganciclovir is then introduced.[37]

Antiangiogenesis. Antiangiogenesis is a new area of research that looks at arresting the tumor's vascular supply. This inhibition of tumor-associated new blood vessel growth could retard tumor growth and become a potentially useful treatment modality.[37]

Radiation Therapy

Radiation therapy can be used alone or in conjunction with surgery or chemotherapy to treat malignant brain tumors. It is typically chosen as a treatment option for tumors that are too large or inaccessible for surgical resection and to eradicate residual neoplastic cells following a surgical debulking.

Radiotherapy consists of the delivery of high-powered photons, with energies in a much greater range than that of standard x-rays, as an external beam directly at the tumor site. The external beam is transmitted to the tumor through a linear accelerator or a cobalt machine that uses cobalt isotopes as the radiation source. External beam radiation is the most widely used form of radiation treatment.[7]

Conventional radiation therapy, as described above, is delivered in units called *fractions*.[15] This refers to the dose of radiation delivered at each treatment session. Often if a large fraction is to be delivered, the dose is divided and given more than once per day; this is called hyperfractionation. Hyperfractioned radiation therapy is believed to increase the efficacy and decrease the long-term side effects of radiation. More studies need to be completed to know its exact benefits. This form of delivery is being used to treat malignant gliomas.[30]

Conformal radiation is the utilization of high-dose external beam radiation, produced by a linear accelerator, to precisely match or "conform" to the tumor shape. One such method of conformal radiation delivery is the Peacock system. This method attempts to deliver a uniform amount of radiation to the tumor and minimize irradiation of healthy brain tissue.[15]

Another type of radiation therapy is focal radiation. Two types of focal radiation exist: interstitial brachytherapy and radiosurgery. *Brachytherapy* refers to the placement of radioactive iodine 125 in or near the lesion. Patients who have poor access to medical care or who will not tolerate other forms of radiation or chemotherapy are candidates for such radiation. The iodine can be delivered through transcranial catheters, or iodine seeds can be placed in the resected tumor bed. These implants can deliver low-dose radiotherapy for about 6 months.[7] Patients receiving this type of radiation are considered to be radioactive and precautions must be taken to protect others around them from radiation exposure. *Radiosurgery* involves relatively high-dose hypofractionated radiation beams directed at small tumor areas through the use of computer planning.[15] This type of treatment includes the Gamma knife, linear accelerators, and the cyberknife, which are discussed later.

Certain drugs have been found to increase (radiosensitizers) or decrease (radioprotectors) the effects of radiation on normal cells and are administered before radiation delivery. Currently these drugs are being tested in adults undergoing conventional radiation therapy.[15]

The radiation oncologist determines the dosage, frequency, and method of radiation delivery depending on tumor type, location, growth rate, and other medical issues for each client. A typical course of radiation therapy will last 6 weeks. Clients are irradiated for just 1 to 5 minutes, 5 days a week. The radiation is intended to kill the malignant cells and preserve healthy cells, but certain rapidly growing cells, those in skin tissue and mucosa, are killed as well. The side effects experienced by those undergoing treatment are a result of this destruction of healthy cells.

Radiation therapy has considerable limitations and disadvantages. There is an accepted maximum lifetime dosage of radiation that the brain and body can tolerate. As doses come close to this limit, the risk of radiation necrosis increases. Because the brains of young children are particularly vulnerable to radiation, other therapies, such as chemotherapy, are used until the developing brain is more tolerant of radiation. Metastatic lesions have invaded multiple organs or body systems, and a more systemic treatment such as chemotherapy is most effective for this type of brain cancer.[15]

Stereotactic Radiosurgery

Stereotactic radiosurgery is defined as delivery of a high dose of ionizing radiation, in a single fraction, to a small, precisely defined volume of tissue.[7,23,58,64] The high-energy accelerators involved with stereotactic radiosurgery improve the physical effect of radiation by allowing energy to travel more precisely in a straight line and penetrate deeper, before dissipating.[64] The goal of stereotactic radiosurgery is to arrest tumor growth.[65] This technique has been shown to be most beneficial for treating centrally located lesions less than 3 cm in size and for patients with increased surgical risk factors.[23,64] Advantages of stereotactic radiosurgery are as follows:

1. Noninvasive procedure utilizing local anesthesia and sedation to place the stereotactic frame
2. Avoids risks of general anesthesia and immediate postoperative risk such as bleeding, CSF leak, or infection
3. Lowers treatment cost and shortens hospital stays[7,36,64,66]

Stereotactic radiosurgery is used to treat benign and malignant tumors, vascular malformations, and functional disorders.[58,64] The primary modes of administration for stereotactic radiosurgery include the Gamma knife, linear accelerators, and cyberknife.[7,19,58]

The *Gamma knife* was first introduced in Sweden in 1968 and is now used worldwide at 65 sites (Figure 25-3). The Gamma knife uses 201 discrete sources of cobalt 60 that are focused precisely to one point in three-dimensional space within the cranium.[23,58,64,67] The Gamma knife is typically used for deeply embedded small tumors that require precise delivery of radiation.[23]

MRI, CT scanning, or angiography is used to identify the exact location of the lesion to be treated after the stereotactic frame is placed on the client's head. The stereotactic frame is then fixed to the machine and attached to a collimator helmet containing 201 holes for the radiation to pass through. The patient is then locked into position. The prescribed dose is given over 20 minutes to 2 hours. After treatment the frame is removed, the client is observed and is frequently discharged after 24 hours. Return to previous activity typically occurs within a few days.[23,36,58,67]

With the Gamma knife, the full dose of radiation is received only at the point where the 201 beams intersect, thereby giving only a minimal dose to uninvolved tissue when targeted accurately. Side effects are rare, but headache and nausea may occur.[7] The primary limitations of the Gamma knife are the limited brain volume that can be treated with one dose and the cost of the Gamma knife machine.[7,58]

Linear accelerators used for conventional radiation can be modified for stereotactic radiosurgery. The brain lesion to be targeted is stereotactically placed in the center of the arc of rotation of the machine. A single highly focused beam of radiation is delivered over multiple sweeps around the brain lesion. Linear accelerators can be used to treat larger tumors with precise shape while maintaining uniform dose. Because linear accelerators are used for conventional radiation, a quality check for beam accuracy is imperative before using the machine for stereotactic radiosurgery.[7,58]

The cyberknife uses a compact linear accelerator mounted on a robotic arm, with the robotic arm moving around the linear accelerator to multiple precalculated positions (Figure 25-4). At each position, the accelerator fires a beam of radiation at the tumor or lesion. A high cumulative dose of radiation is achieved at the tumor or lesion because of the convergence of the beams. This dose is typically strong enough to destroy the abnormal cells while minimizing the damaging effects of radiation to healthy surrounding tissue. The cyberknife differs from other stereotactic radiosurgery

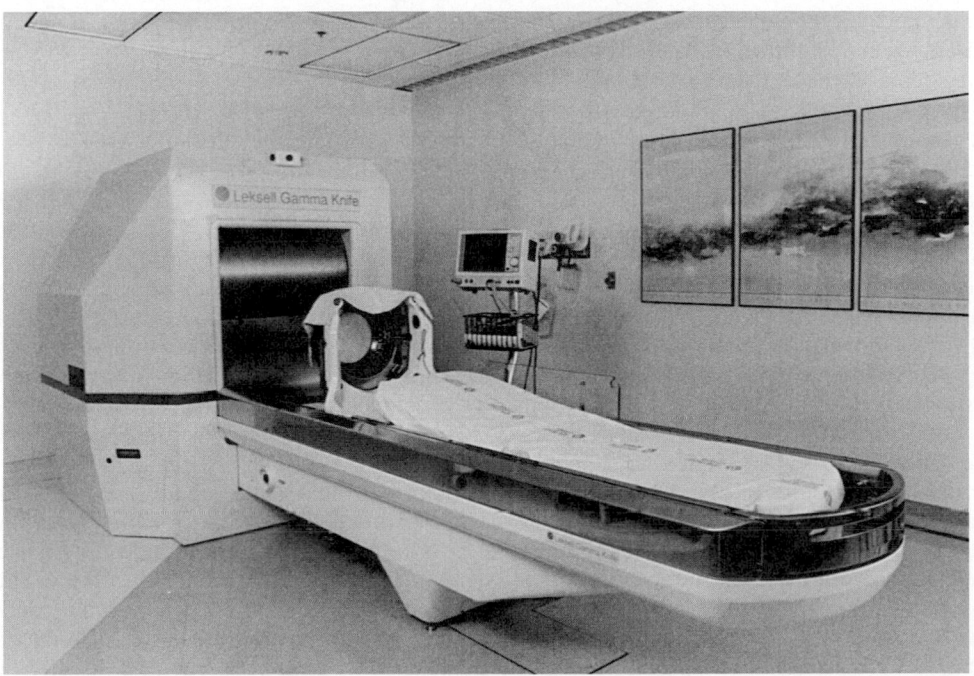

FIGURE 25-3 ■ The Leksell Gamma Knife.

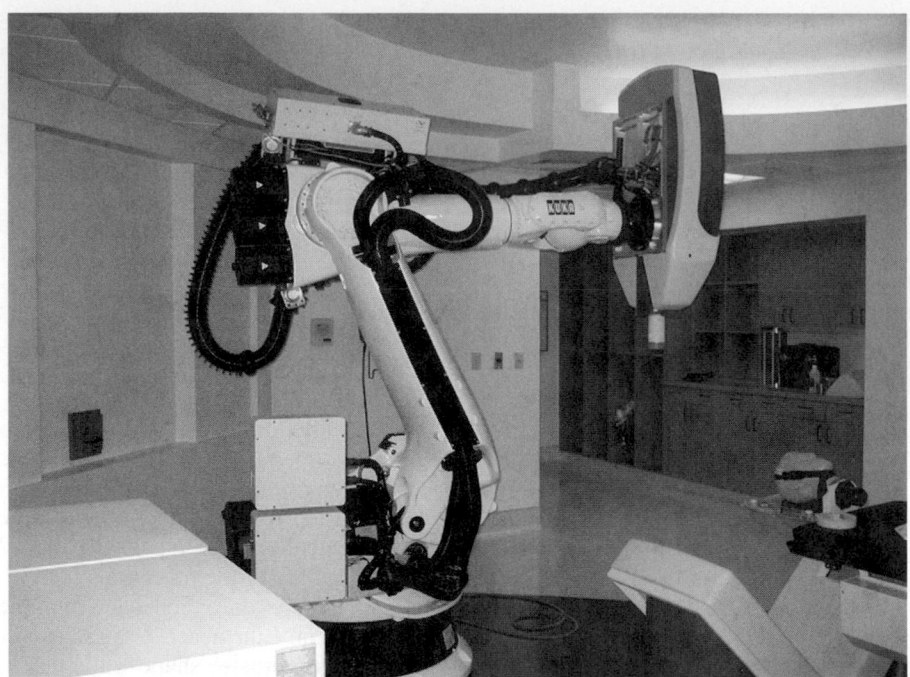

FIGURE 25-4 ■ The Cyberknife

because a linear accelerator is combined with an image guidance system. The robotic arm allows the cyberknife to target difficult-to-reach areas of the body, as well as adjust quickly for changes in target location during treatment. Another advantage of cyberknife is that it does not require the use of an invasive head frame like Gamma knife.

Several research studies have reported on the use of stereotactic radiosurgery, including the Gamma knife and linear accelerators, and compared this modality with microsurgery; however, studies involving cyberknife are limited. In patients with brain metastases, the Gamma knife is typically indicated for small lesions that are centrally located. Surgical resection is indicated for superficial lesions greater than 3 cm in diameter, when a significant mass effect of the tumor exists, or if edema is present in the cranium.[23] The Gamma knife has been shown to achieve tumor control rates as high as those for surgery and whole-body radiation therapy combined, and to halt or reverse neurological progression in 78% of patients treated.[68,69]

Microsurgical resection has shown a 90% cure rate for acoustic neuromas less than 3 cm in size. Stereotactic radiosurgery avoids the risk of an open procedure, but the tumor is controlled rather than removed. Thus far, a 92% tumor control rate has been noted, but the patients in this study have not had a 10-year follow-up.[35,36]

Research exists for both low- and high-grade gliomas, but large, controlled studies are few. With low-grade tumors, small studies have shown increased survival after stereotactic radiosurgery, but these studies are uncontrolled and limited by the small number of participants.[66] For high-grade tumors, recent studies found median survival rates ranging from 9.5 to 17 months with use of stereotactic radiosurgery.[47,70-72] For recurrent malignant gliomas, survival after fractionated and nonfractionated stereotactic radiosurgery was shown to be 8 to 11 months.[28,60,73,74] The addition of radiosurgery to surgery and radiation therapy produced only modest improvement when compared with surgery and radiation therapy alone.[66]

The preferred treatment for *meningiomas* is surgical resection, if complete resection is possible. When surgery is not an option and the tumor is less than 3 cm in size or 5 mm away from the optic nerve, stereotactic radiosurgery is indicated.[33,75,76] Four-year survival rates in 91% of benign meningiomas and 21.5% in malignant meningiomas have been demonstrated after use of the Gamma knife.[33,75] In a survey taken 5 to 10 years after radiosurgery, 96% of patients believed radiosurgery had provided a satisfactory outcome.[75]

REHABILITATION
Overview

Rehabilitation is a key component in the management of the client with a brain tumor. With advances in technology and treatment intervention, survival rates of people with cancer have improved. Consequently, people are living longer with physical impairments resulting from the disease or its treatment, necessitating interdisciplinary therapeutic intervention.[2] Rehabilitating the effects of brain tumors is challenging because the cognitive, communicative, behavioral, and physical deficits complicate the medical and psychological issues typically associated with cancer diagnosis.[21] By preventing complications, maximizing function, and providing support, rehabilitation specialists ultimately improve the client's quality of life.[21] The most effective rehabilitation plan is flexible, to allow for increasing disability, and sensitive, to accommodate the highly emotional impact that accompanies the diagnosis of a primary brain tumor. The tumor's invasion is marked by complaints of pain and growing functional deficits with daily activities. These functional consequences of the disease process are the target of the rehabilitation team. In addition to the side effects of therapeutic intervention, functional progress may be affected by cerebral edema, hydrocephalus, tumor regrowth, infection, and radiation necrosis.

The management of a client with a brain tumor is different from that of other CNS disorders, despite a similar clinical presentation. To establish an appropriate plan of care, the clinician must understand the nature of the specific tumor, consider the client's fluctuating neurological status, and prepare for the likelihood of progressive decline. The preferred approach is holistic, addressing quality of life issues such as physical, psychosocial, and emotional needs, incorporated into the systems model of motor control. Factors defining quality of life are unique to each individual and, therefore, clinicians should identify and use these factors to construct a meaningful treatment program.[77]

Evaluation, clinical analysis, intervention, discharge planning, and psychosocial issues specific to the management of the client with a brain tumor are discussed in the following sections.

Evaluation

The evaluation process must include a comprehensive examination and assessment of all systems in order to establish an appropriate impairment/disability diagnosis, problem list, prognosis, and plan of care. Before a neurological assessment is performed, a thorough review of the client's medical history and an understanding of the medical diagnosis are necessary. The client's occupation, support system, personal goals, and role in the family are important psychosocial factors that should be identified in the evaluation. These factors, along with a thorough functional and neurological examination, assist the clinician through the diagnostic process. This process includes identification of clinical problems, establishment of realistic and appropriate goals, selection of the most effective intervention, and discharge planning.

Although the neurological examination yields important information regarding strength, reflexes, sensation, vision, and cognition, it is important not to rely solely on its findings to determine an appropriate intervention. Because multiple systems interact to produce normal movement, it is difficult to examine isolated systems and apply the findings accurately to movement patterns. Therefore, clinicians are encouraged to examine all systems through functional tasks to understand how the impaired neurological, musculoskeletal, and cognitive systems are affecting the client's movement. During the evaluation process, the clinician notes systems that are functioning normally, identifies abnormal components of movement, and determines appropriate interventions to optimize motor recovery.[46] The progressive nature of the disease necessitates ongoing evaluation followed by accommodating intervention.

Goal Setting

The functional deficits and objective neurological findings provide the clinician with valuable information to assess prognosis, establish goals, and determine a treatment plan. Despite the progressive nature of the disease, treatment goals should maximize the potential for function, introduce effective, task-oriented movement strategies, and offer multiple movement options.[46]

To set realistic and client-oriented goals, it is important for the clinician to envision where the patient will be at discharge based on present level of function, prognosis, and disease course, while considering client/caregiver personal goals. Appropriate goals range from comprehensive caregiver training to independent mobility with transition back to a work environment. Goals need to challenge the client to attain an optimal level of function, but must also allow for fluctuations in potential resulting from the disease process. Clients who have the potential to return to work may require additional intervention from neuropsychology, vocational rehabilitation, or a multidisciplinary day program, depending on the nature of their job and their deficits.

Because the rehabilitation potential for clients with brain tumors varies greatly, it is imperative that the client, family members, rehabilitation team and third party payers understand and agree with the purpose of the client's rehabilitation program. Pathways can be extremely instrumental in clarifying rehabilitation goals and identifying the caregiver's role upon discharge (Table 25-2). If a client has a poor prognosis, the rehabilitation team can successfully train family and order equipment within 1 week if the family understands the goals and the need to be present during treatment sessions. The pathway serves as a guideline assisting the rehabilitation team in achieving the client's goals in an effective and efficient manner.

Functional Assessment

Historically persons with primary malignant brain tumors have not been considered rehabilitation candidates because of the progressive nature of their disease. Physicians, health care providers, and third-party payers have questioned the efficacy of rehabilitation in this population because of poor prognoses and limited survival rates. However, advances in medical diagnosis and intervention are resulting in longer survival of people with multiple functional deficits that require rehabilitation. Functional assessment scales provide objective evidence that rehabilitation is effective and worthwhile for these clients.[3,78]

The functional assessment is a critical component in the development of the treatment intervention. It provides a method of analyzing deficits, compiling a problem list, developing a treatment plan, and measuring functional outcomes. The Functional Independence Measure (FIM) is a functional assessment tool used to measure degree of disability, regardless of underlying pathology, and burden of care to demonstrate functional outcomes of rehabilitation and assist clinicians with discharge planning.[60]

Functional outcome scales like the FIM provide a means of documenting the client's response to therapy intervention for clinicians, physicians, and third-party payers in the rehabilitation setting. Research using FIM data demonstrates efficacy for inpatient rehabilitation of brain tumor clients similar to that noted in those with traumatic brain injury or stroke when matched by age, sex, and functional status on admission.[1,3,35,78]

Physicians use specific functional evaluation scales to measure the success of treatment. The Karnofsky performance scale, which rates patients' functional performance, is the tool most widely used in clinical research and treatment decisions (see Table 25-1).[21] The client receives a

TABLE 25-2 ■ Brain Tumor Clinical Pathway: One Week Stay

	DAY 1	DAY 2	DAY 3	DAY 4-5	DAY 6-7
Nursing	Medical and functional assessment Establish LOS with MD Initiate care plan with caregivers	Provide education re: sequelae of diagnosis and treatment Facilitate team meeting Collaborate with CM	Provide nutritional and dietary education prn Train caregiver with tube feedings prn	Skin care B&B training Home safety Address medical questions	Provide info re: medications (i.e., pain and antiepileptics) Review side effects of radiation/chemotherapy Refer to palliative care or hospice prn
Physicians	Provide education and handouts to patient and family re: diagnosis, prognosis, and treatment plan	Prescribe medications to minimize side effects (seizure, pain, etc.) and maximize rehabilitation potential	Maintain open communication between oncologist and rehabilitation physician		Recommend follow-up appointments and treatment
Physical Therapy	Functional evaluation Assess family support Schedule home evaluation prn	Provide education and handouts for caregiver body mechanics, physical therapy positioning and mobility techniques Determine and order equipment	Continue mobility training different types/surfaces Educate re: safety precautions and energy conservation	Caregivers return demonstrate competency with mobility techniques Home evaluation completed	Patient discharged if caregivers competent in all necessary mobility techniques and equipment obtained
Occupational Therapy	Functional evaluation Discuss home environment Schedule home evaluation prn	Provide education and handouts for caregiver body mechanics, extremity management & ADL techniques Determine adaptive equipment needs and order	Continue training Train caregivers in visual-perceptual needs	Caregiver return demonstrate competency with ADL techniques Home evaluation completed	Patient discharged if caregivers competent in all necessary ADL and mobility techniques and equipment obtained
Speech and Language Therapy	Bedside swallow evaluation performed Diet recommended MBS/FEES scheduled prn	MBS/FEES completed prn Provide education and handouts re: precautions and strategies for safe swallow, appropriate diet Signs of aspiration	Initiate cog/com evaluation Monitor diet Continue caregiver training for swallowing	Complete cog/com evaluation Provide family with ideas to modify environment to improve cog/com function Educate caregiver of signs of functional decline	Continue to monitor diet Continue caregiver education re: swallow, safety/judgment and cog/com function
Therapeutic Recreation Therapy	Evaluate patient's leisure interests		Leisure skill building with holistic approach	Review community resources	Discharge
Neuropsychology	If indicated				
Case Management/ Social Services	Initiate assessment	Complete assessment Inform physical therapy/caregiver of team recommendations and LOS	Order DME	Arrange for continued therapies prn	Review discharge plans and recommendations with patient & caregivers

Adapted with permission from Barrow Rehabilitation.

ADL, Activities of daily living; *B&B*, bowel & bladder; *cog/com*, cognitive/communication; *CM*, case manager; *DME*, durable medical equipment; *FEES*, fiberoptic endoscopic evaluation/swallowing, *LOS*, length of stay; *MBS*, modified barium swallow; *MD*, medical doctor; *prn*, when necessary.

score from 0 to 100 based on independence or level of assistance required for normal activity. The scale is used in research to evaluate an individual's physical response to treatment.[21,60,79,80]

Side Effects and Considerations

Through advances in chemotherapy and radiation therapy, the ability to reduce tumor mass has greatly improved. Unfortunately, despite the often favorable long-term results of these treatments, the immediate effects create physical and psychological challenges for the client and clinician. Clients who are being treated aggressively during the rehabilitation phase will probably experience a decline in neurological or hematological status. These declines often limit the individual's tolerance for treatment intervention and increase client and caregiver feelings of depression and hopelessness. Clinicians have the opportunity to provide more than physical restorative services and should offer psychosocial support to enhance successful rehabilitation.[81]

The side effects and special considerations that arise with this population range from physical, to cognitive, to psychosocial and emotional. The following paragraphs relate the spectrum of complications and side effects the client may experience when undergoing medical treatment, and the impact these may have on therapeutic intervention.

Not everyone undergoing chemotherapy or radiation treatment will experience physical side effects; the possibilities include hair loss, fatigue, nausea, skin burns or irritation, difficulty eating or digesting food, anorexia, and dry, sore mouth.[61,82] The side effects are caused by the toxic effects the drugs have on healthy, rapidly dividing cells, including bone marrow cells, cells lining the mucosa, and hair cells.[15,82]

The toxic effect chemotherapy has on bone marrow impairs the client's ability to produce red and white blood cells and platelets.[15] The client may develop anemia, infection, or a hemorrhage as a result of depressed hematological values.

The lining of the mouth, esophagus, and intestines may become inflamed and irritated and interfere with the ability to eat or digest food. The client may experience nausea, vomiting, diarrhea, or constipation, any of which will impair mobility and energy for daily activities.[19]

Hair loss is a common side effect of brain radiation and chemotherapy. This requires an especially difficult adjustment for most people because it causes a drastic change in appearance.[15]

Clinicians involved in the management of clients who are currently receiving radiation therapy or chemotherapy need to be mindful of these side effects when developing a plan of intervention. Fatigue, low blood count, and gastrointestinal complaints may limit a client's ability to fully participate in the planned therapy session or may call for a modification in activity or environment. Moreover, the clinician must use these factors to determine if the client's health or safety would be jeopardized by therapeutic intervention at any particular time. In addition, the clinician must be flexible to determine the optimal time when intervention is most effective and does not interfere with medications or meals.

Together with the physical side effects mentioned above, many clients with brain tumors have changes in cognition or personality as a result of the tumor's location. A patient with a frontal lobe tumor who was previously quiet and withdrawn may, over time, become loud and disinhibited as a result of tumor growth. Tumors that invade the speech language area cause communication and comprehension difficulties that create challenges for client and clinician. The client who has a left parietal tumor may be aphasic and not respond to verbal commands. In this case, the clinician must engage in alternative means of communication or provide therapeutic facilitation with tactile cues only. An observant, critical analysis of the client's physical deficits and impaired communication, comprehension, and feedback mechanisms is essential to select an effective, client-specific intervention plan.

Because of the emotionally charged nature of the disease process, psychosocial and emotional issues frequently arise. Clinicians should be sensitive to fluctuations in temperament and mood that the diagnosis itself and subsequent treatment strategies create. Clinicians can offer psychosocial support and direct the client and family to resources that may give direction and guidance during difficult periods.

Intervention

The ultimate goal of rehabilitation is to achieve maximum restoration of function, within the limits imposed by the disease, in the client's preferred environment. The clinician must recognize that the physical, cognitive, and emotional status of these individuals is inconsistent and changing as a result of the disease process or medical intervention. Treatment plans must be flexible to manage effectively fluctuations in the client's presentation. A comprehensive rehabilitation plan is individualized to accommodate progressive changes in functional mobility and provides problem-solving experiences to prepare the client and caregiver for these situations. The rehabilitation process typically begins in the intensive care unit and continues in the inpatient, outpatient, and home health settings.

In the intensive care unit, communication with nursing staff regarding the client's present medical status and an understanding of ICP, hemodynamic values, and monitoring devices is crucial to determining tolerance for therapy intervention (Figure 25-5). For a ventriculostomy, a catheter is placed in the third ventricle to drain CSF and to monitor ICP. Mobilizing a patient with a ventriculostomy is possible, but nursing staff must close the drain before any positional change and should inform the clinician of appropriate treatment measures. A client's dependence upon these monitoring devices does not prevent therapeutic intervention, but the critical status of these individuals must be considered. The monitoring equipment provides constant feedback that assists the clinician in assessing the client's tolerance to activity and his or her ability to proceed with treatment.

As the client becomes more medically stable, the clinician upgrades mobility and prepares the client for the next stage of rehabilitation. Despite clients' decreased medical acuity in the rehabilitation setting, clinicians must continually reassess functional and neurological status and alert physicians to any changes. Clinicians spend many hours with clients during their rehabilitation stay. This day-to-day interaction gives the clinician the opportunity to connect with the client on a personal level and observe her or him in many settings. Intuitive therapists are often the first to

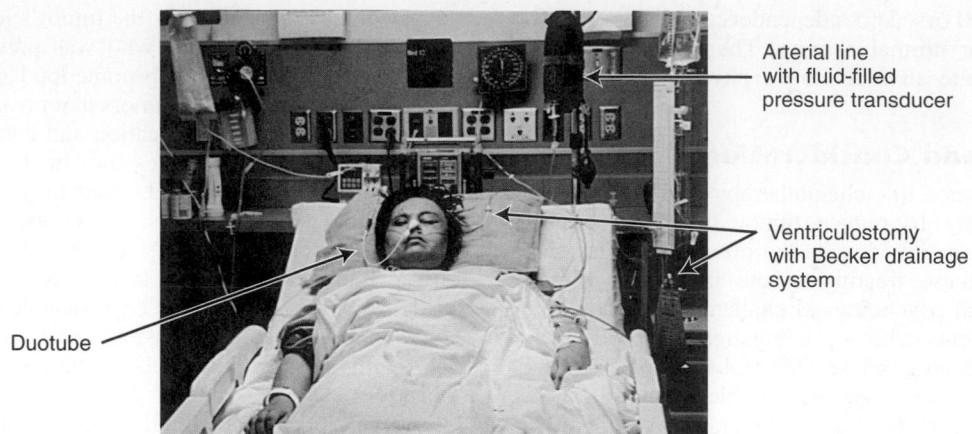

FIGURE 25-5 ■ A patient after a partial tumor resection. Labels indicate the equipment commonly seen in the neurological intensive care unit.

notice physical, cognitive, and emotional changes. Communication to the physician of significant changes is imperative for appropriate follow-up procedures and referrals to provide optimal care.

In the inpatient rehabilitation setting, treatment focuses on optimizing functional capabilities to prepare the client and family for discharge. Integrating the client's personal goals and interests into therapeutic intervention invests the client and family in the rehabilitation process. The incorporation of these quality-of-life issues encourages the pursuit of a meaningful lifestyle upon discharge. If clinicians believe the client's goals are unrealistic, gentle redirection is necessary to channel energy toward achievable goals. Goals for inpatient rehabilitation range from returning the client to an independent lifestyle to training family to be caregivers in the home environment.

The restoration of previous functional movement patterns is desired. The literature reports increasing evidence that the CNS has dynamic properties, including neural regeneration and collateral sprouting, which supports the concept of plasticity. Plasticity allows intact neural centers to recognize and assume functions of areas of the brain impaired or destroyed by the lesion or medical management.[83] The treatment focus may need to turn to compensatory strategies if the potential for motor recovery and learning is lacking. Once compensatory patterns are established, it is not clearly known whether recovery of normal movement will be achieved.[83] Compensatory techniques may be beneficial in increasing safety and efficiency with mobility and activities of daily living, or in providing more independence for the client.[60] Increasing independence can assist in improving quality of life for the client and may permit return to work or participation in previous recreational activity.[60] For example, an avid golfer with right-sided hemiparesis and impaired standing balance can modify his clubs and return to the game at the wheelchair level.

The rehabilitation program should prepare the client and caregivers for an efficient transition from the structured care setting to the home. Utilizing motor learning principles to teach functional mobility will best produce transfer of learning from a constant environment to an unpredictable home environment. Repetitive practice of specific parts of a skill

in fixed surroundings, with physical and verbal guidance throughout the movement, and frequent feedback during and following the completion of the task, are beneficial in teaching acquisition of a specific movement or activity.[84-86] Practicing the whole activity in a variable context, with irregular feedback and decreased physical and verbal guidance, expedites learning.[86-88]

Learning results in the ability to execute a task in any setting. Community outings and home passes naturally provide an environment that facilitates learning. The clinician can measure retention and transfer of learning by the client's performance in the community or at home. This information should be used to adjust the treatment plan and make recommendations for environmental modifications that minimize physical and cognitive demands on the client. A client whose individual treatment focus is transfers gains confidence when able to transfer from a wheelchair to a table chair in a crowded restaurant.

An interdisciplinary team approach is used for community reentry to provide a meaningful experience for the client. Recreational therapists play an integral part in identifying the individual's interests, reintegrating the client into the community, and modifying leisure activities to meet physical abilities. Activities addressed in daily therapy sessions are practiced in the community, and feedback is provided to the appropriate clinician as well as the client. Initial reentry into the community can be intimidating to the client and may cause changes in the client's behavior that will affect mobility performance. Therefore, it is necessary for the clinician to be sensitive and recognize the issues the client may be experiencing.

For caregiver training and education to be successful, a good rapport must be established between clinician, client, and the family members/caregivers. Caregiver training includes mobility training and education regarding the effect the tumor may have on the client's present and future mobility. Instruction should be given based on present level of function, but the probability of progressive decline should not be overlooked. An intuitive clinician should offer effective techniques and problem-solving situations to address potential obstacles created by the disease process. For example, when performing transfer training, the clinician may demonstrate a stand-pivot transfer, but may also suggest a squat-pivot transfer if physical or cognitive changes mandate increased assistance by the caregiver.

Discharge Planning

Discharge planning is initiated early, continues throughout the rehabilitation process, and must allow for changes in the client's functional status. Upon discharge from the rehabilitation setting, the client will make the transition to one of the following settings: home, skilled nursing facility, or hospice. The transition to home is typically preferred by the client, caregiver, and interdisciplinary rehabilitation team. If the client cannot be physically or medically managed at home, then placement in a skilled nursing facility may be necessary. The client may choose hospice care when medical treatment is no longer providing control of the tumor and the physical demands of the client are not manageable by the caregivers. The appropriate case management worker contacts insurance providers to determine coverage and, after conferring with the interdisciplinary team, gives the client and family information regarding discharge options.

Client and caregiver training and education constitute an integral part of discharge planning. Before discharge, the client and caregiver should be instructed in functional mobility and activities of daily living, informed of equipment needs and vendor resources, and provided with community resources for support and education. During individual training, the clinician is able to provide feedback to the caregiver and client to facilitate an easier transition to home. Documentation of caregiver education and training should be included in the progress and discharge notes. A sample form for interdisciplinary documentation of education is provided in Figure 25-6.

Equipment necessary to assist the client and family with mobility and activities of daily living is recommended by the appropriate clinician. When ordering equipment, fluctuations in the client's present status, as well as the probable progressive decline in function, are considered. If the client is functioning without equipment at discharge, resources such as equipment vendors or local charitable organizations for future equipment needs should be provided.

Local community and national resources specific to brain tumors also should be provided before discharge. These resources can be found on the Internet, in the local phone book, or through communication with previous patients or other health care professionals familiar with these organizations. Support groups provide the caregiver and the client with an opportunity to share experiences and information, prevent isolation, foster hope, discover coping skills, and offer emotional support.[89] A study conducted to describe experiences and needs of clients with brain tumors found that "attendance and participation in a support group empowers people to seek the most out of life following a brain tumor diagnosis."[89] National organizations can provide educational information and support to clients (Box 25-1). These organizations can help the client find local resources unfamiliar to the clinician.

Hospice Care

A time may come when traditional tumor treatment is ineffective and local control is no longer expected. Patient and family must make a decision regarding the living environ-

---

BOX 25-1 ■ NATIONAL ORGANIZATIONS

The Brain Tumor Society
124 Watertown St., Suite 3-H
Watertown, MA 02472
(617) 924-9997
http://www.tbts.org
e-mail: info@tbts.org

American Brain Tumor Association
2720 River Rd.
Des Plaines, IL 60018
(800) 886-2282
http://www.abta.org
e-mail: info@abta.org

National Brain Tumor Foundation
22 Battery St., Suite 612
San Francisco, CA 94111-5520
(800) 934-CURE
http://www.braintumor.org
e-mail: nbtf@braintumor.org

---

ment and type of care desired. One option available is hospice care. In the United States, the hospice movement in health care has evolved to include specific standards, licensure requirements, and certification. Providing physical, emotional, and psychosocial support to patients and their families in their final days is the intent of hospice care.[90] Hospice recognizes the impact terminal illness has on a patient's family system, and the demands, both physical and emotional, it places on the caregiver.[91] The use of hospice implies a holistic approach that allows families the opportunity to be directly involved in the patient's care, and encourages the expression of grief, love, support, and acceptance.

Inpatient hospice facilities provide continuous nursing care in a structured, supervised environment. Hospice services in these facilities offer ongoing pastoral counseling and emotional support to patient and family. However, if patient and family prefer, hospice care can be provided in the patient's home, with home health aides and nursing giving limited physical care or providing respite care.

Typically, mobility and caregiver training for the hospice patient are addressed by a therapist earlier in the patient's disease process. However, positioning, range of motion, and pain relief are important to the patient's continued comfort throughout the course of the disease and in any setting.

PSYCHOSOCIAL CARE

With many clients living extended lives with brain tumors, it is important to measure the efficacy of treatment not only in terms of functional outcome, but also in terms of its effect on quality of life. Quality of life is the individual's subjective sense of well-being as a whole and has been studied closely in the treatment of clients with brain tumor.[80] Quality of life is a multifaceted concept encompassing emotional and physical well-being, life satisfaction, material wealth, meaning of life, coping mechanisms, and social network. A single assessment to comprehensively evaluate a person's quality of life does not exist. Therefore, a multidimensional

**St. Joseph's Hospital
and Medical Center**
Mercy Healthcare Arizona

NEURO REHABILITATION UNIT

BRAIN TUMOR TEACHING GOALS

ADULT BRAIN TUMOR

* Please note: For the brain tumor patient who is able to completely or partially use his or her extremities and cognitive abilities, the emphasis on rehab is to maximize the patient's own ability to be independent. It is also to educate and teach the family or care giver appropriate care and safe assistance with the patient and his or her equipment. Efforts will be directed to facilitate the patient's return to home and to resume work (if able) in his or her community in the most efficient and practical manner possible for the patient and the family.

Initials = Full Name & Title

=	=	=
=	=	=
=	=	=

KEY

I	=	Instructed	RD	=	Return Demonstration	NI	=	Not available for instruction
D	=	Demonstrated	VD	=	Verbally directs care	NA	=	Not Applicable
C	=	Comprehended	DC	=	Discharge review			

PATIENT NAME: _____ DATE _____

NURSING

1. Anatomy and physiology of brain tumor
2. Application of braces-splints
3. Bowel elimination
4. Circulation
5. Depression / grieving
6. Family adjustment
7. Hydrocephalus
8. Medications
9. Nutrition
10. Safety
11. Seizures
12. Sensory stimulation
13. Skin integrity
14. Sexuality
15. Stress management
16. Tube feedings
17. Treatments
18. Urinary elimination
19. Other _____
20. Other _____

	PATIENT								CARE GIVER						
	I	D	C	RD	VD	DC	NI	NA	I	D	C	RD	DC	NI	NA
1.															
2.															
3.															
4.															
5.															
6.															
7.															
8.															
9.															
10.															
11.															
12.															
13.															
14.															
15.															
16.															
17.															
18.															
19.															
20.															

RESPIRATORY

1. CPR training
2. List emergency numbers
3. Suction (in hospital) - (in community)
4. Trach care
5. Other _____

	PATIENT								CARE GIVER						
	I	D	C	RD	VD	DC	NI	NA	I	D	C	RD	DC	NI	NA
1.															
2.															
3.															
4.															
5.															

FIGURE 25-6 ■ Interdisciplinary education inventory for brain tumor teaching. (From Barrow Neurological Institute, St. Joseph's Hospital and Medical Center, Phoenix, AZ.)

OCCUPATIONAL THERAPY (OT)

UPPER EXTREMITY

1. R.O.M. - exercise
2. Positioning
3. Splinting

	PATIENT							CARE GIVER						
	I	D	C	RD	VD	DC	NI	NA	I	D	C	RD	DC	NI	NA
1.														
2.														
3.														

SELF CARE

1. Swallowing
2. Self-feeding
3. Hygiene

	PATIENT							CARE GIVER						
	I	D	C	RD	VD	DC	NI	NA	I	D	C	RD	DC	NI	NA
1.														
2.														
3.														

PATIENT NAME: _____ DATE _____

OCCUPATIONAL THERAPY (OT)

4. Bathing
5. Dressing
6. Adaptive equipment - vendors
7. Home management
8. Cooking

	PATIENT							CARE GIVER						
	I	D	C	RD	VD	DC	NI	NA	I	D	C	RD	DC	NI	NA
4.														
5.														
6.														
7.														
8.														

TRANSFERS

1. Toilet - Commode
2. Tub - Shower

	PATIENT							CARE GIVER						
	I	D	C	RD	VD	DC	NI	NA	I	D	C	RD	DC	NI	NA
1.														
2.														

PHYSICAL THERAPY (PT)

1. Range of motion exercise
2. Bed mobility
3. Bed transfers
4. Car transfers
5. Wheelchair mobility and management
6. Ambulation
7. Safety precautions
8. Equipment vendor resources
9. Other _____

	PATIENT							CARE GIVER						
	I	D	C	RD	VD	DC	NI	NA	I	D	C	RD	DC	NI	NA
1.														
2.														
3.														
4.														
5.														
6.														
7.														
8.														
9.														

SPEECH LANGUAGE PATHOLOGY

1. Aphasia
2. Dysarthria
3. Dysphagia
4. Cognitive deficits due to tumor-surgical area
5. Cognitive deficits (generalized)
6. Other _____

	PATIENT							CARE GIVER						
	I	D	C	RD	VD	DC	NI	NA	I	D	C	RD	DC	NI	NA
1.														
2.														
3.														
4.														
5.														
6.														

THERAPEUTIC RECREATION

1. Community re-entry skills _____
2. Community leisure referrals _____
3. Adapted recreation resources and or referrals _____
4. Community mobility skills _____

	PATIENT							CARE GIVER						
	I	D	C	RD	VD	DC	NI	NA	I	D	C	RD	DC	NI	NA
1.														
2.														
3.														
4.														

PATIENT NAME: _____ DATE _____

SOCIAL SERVICES-CASE MANAGEMENT

Referrals to community resources:

1. _____
2. _____
3. _____
4. _____
5. _____

	PATIENT							CARE GIVER						
	I	D	C	RD	VD	DC	NI	NA	I	D	C	RD	DC	NI	NA
1.														
2.														
3.														
4.														
5.														

FIGURE 25-6, cont'd

approach incorporating multiple assessment tools is necessary.[80,92] Some of these tools include the Functional Living Index, the Karnofsky performance scale, the Index of Independence in Activity of Daily Living, the State-Trait Anxiety Inventory, and the Self-Rating Depression Scale.[92]

The development of a strong supportive relationship with client and caregivers is key to successful rehabilitation. This process begins with respecting the client's unique experience and involves continually evaluating and addressing his or her changing psychosocial needs.[83] The clinician must feel invested, demonstrate good communication skills, and exhibit self-confidence in discussing sensitive issues for a caring relationship to develop. By actively listening, the clinician can identify the client's true concerns and feelings and assist the client and family in coping with the cancer experience.[83] The clinician's consistent interaction with the client can foster a supportive and safe environment in which emotional and spiritual feelings can be shared. Once a trusting relationship is established, the clinician's empathy can help decrease common feelings of isolation and helplessness and support the client through the different stages of the disease.[83]

Hope is a key psychosocial need of the individual with cancer. It is an important coping strategy that can help clients with brain tumors face an uncertain and often fearsome future. Hope gives the client something to look forward to each day. Clinicians can create a hopeful environment by encouraging clients to share their expectations, identify realistic short-term goals, and acknowledge hopes, even if they are unrealistic. It is important to recognize that hope must be balanced with reality and honest disclosure regarding diagnosis and prognosis.[83,93]

Psychological and social problems are not identified in 80% of physically ill persons, possibly owing to clinicians'

personal behaviors or beliefs. Clinicians may find it easier to focus on the physical aspect of care to avoid becoming emotional or experiencing the client's distress. Persons with cancer often experience feelings of powerlessness and isolation, which may be increased by distancing behaviors demonstrated by clinicians. Before offering support to clients, clinicians need to examine their own thoughts, feelings, and past experiences with death and dying. This awareness may prevent the clinician from internalizing the client's grief, from protecting the client and family members from the pain of grieving, and from allowing personal values to adversely influence their psychosocial support.[93] By recognizing that psychosocial care involves holistic healing, clinicians will be able to develop the best environment for interventions to improve multiple aspects of the client's quality of life.[93]

SUMMARY

It is important for the clinician involved in the treatment of a client with a brain tumor to anticipate the functional limitations that will develop as a result of the medical intervention or the tumor itself. These limitations provide the foundation for treatment planning and goal setting. Improved quality of life is the goal of the rehabilitation process. This means restoring the client to maximal functional capacity with the least amount of assistance from others. Regardless of the client's life expectancy, the rehabilitation process should enable the client to pursue a productive and meaningful life. Case Study 25-1 is an example of the complexity of the problems faced by an individual with a CNS tumor. These problems include both the medical condition and the functional movement limitations caused by the tumor and/or the medical management.

CASE STUDY 25-1 ■ MEDICAL DIAGNOSIS: LOW-GRADE ASTROCYTOMA

Mrs. S. is a 46-year-old woman diagnosed 9 years ago with a low-grade astrocytoma in the right posterior frontal lobe. Before this diagnosis, she had a 4-year history of seizures. She underwent a partial resection of a microcystic pilocytic astrocytoma. Postoperative medical management focused on controlling seizure activity. Radiation therapy and chemotherapy were not provided. Physically, she presented with resultant left foot weakness and minor seizures characterized by tingling numbness and tremors in the left foot. She was able to continue to work, but a career change was necessary owing to cognitive changes, including the inability to perform fast calculations, impaired memory, and decreased recall.

Three years later, imaging studies revealed tumor enlargement and Mrs. S. underwent Peacock radiation therapy. She remained independent for an additional 2 years. Two weeks ago, she presented with left facial weakness, progressive left hemiparesis, and hyperreflexia on the left side. MRI scans revealed a lesion in the right midcerebral hemisphere below the original tumor site. A stereotactic biopsy confirmed a diagnosis of glioblastoma multiforme. She then

underwent a gross total tumor resection, received Gamma knife radiosurgery, and was subsequently treated with chemotherapy.

Mrs. S. was admitted to the neurological rehabilitation unit for comprehensive rehabilitation. During the examination, it was noted that her speech was fluent and she tended to be hyperverbal, distractible, and perseverative. Manual muscle testing revealed functional strength in the right hemibody and 0/5 strength in the left hemibody except for hip flexion of 2–/5. Decreased sensation to light touch and proprioception in the left hemibody was noted. Because of the location of the lesion, Mrs. S. experienced left seventh cranial nerve involvement, left homonymous hemianopsia, severe left-sided neglect, and right gaze preference. These visual-perceptual deficits greatly impaired her mobility. She was able to attend to the left side with maximal cues, but carryover was not observed.

Functionally, Mrs. S. required moderate assistance to assume sitting on the edge of the bed, where she demonstrated fair sitting balance. Owing to poor standing balance, she required maximal assistance to

CASE STUDY 25-1 ■ MEDICAL DIAGNOSIS: LOW-GRADE ASTROCYTOMA—cont'd

stand and pivot to her wheelchair. In standing, her head was rotated to the right and flexed, her pelvis was rotated to the right, her hips were flexed, her left knee was buckled, and her left foot was inverted. She was able to ambulate 15 feet in the parallel bars with maximal assistance to address these postural impairments and to advance the left leg. She was able to propel her wheelchair with her right arm and leg with much assistance and encouragement.

Mrs. S. refuses to use a wheelchair at home because her goal is to walk. She is married with three children and lives in a single-story house. Her husband works full-time, necessitating independent and safe mobility to return home. Mrs. S. and her family demonstrate poor understanding of her prognosis and express unrealistic goals. They frequently refer to her previous return to independence following her first resection and expect a similar outcome this time.

The clinician, in consideration of the client's goal to walk, incorporated standing, pregait, and gait training into treatment sessions. However, Mrs. S was encouraged to propel her wheelchair as a means of independent mobility on the rehab unit. A knee-ankle-foot orthosis (KAFO) was fabricated to provide stability in the left leg and assist in her goal of walking again.

Two weeks into her rehabilitation program, Mrs. S. began to demonstrate increased lethargy, decreased ability to participate in treatments, and increased weakness. She required more assistance with mobility. The clinician modified the treatment intervention to an appropriate, yet challenging level. Sitting balance and transfers became the focus rather than standing balance and gait. The therapy team notified the physician of these changes and the client was transferred to acute care. She underwent additional surgery to drain a cyst and remove necrotic tissue within the tumor.

Upon her return to rehabilitation Mrs. S. became more alert and able to participate in therapy sessions. She and her family expressed hope that this surgery would cure the tumor. The clinician expresses encouragement but gently reminds the client and family members that while the drainage of the cyst may allow for functional improvements, the tumor is still present. The client's strength continues to improve and functional gains are observed. In gait, her left leg is now able to stabilize during the stance phase; however, an Ace bandage is necessary to control foot drop. The client is able to ambulate household distances with minimal assistance.

The interdisciplinary team has provided the client and family with the appropriate resources to choose a facility where Mrs. S. can continue her therapy and the family can easily visit. They have also been provided with referrals regarding support groups and hospice care if needed in the future. At the time of discharge, Mrs. S. was delighted with her ability to walk but is disappointed that her left arm remains flaccid and that she is not returning home. The client and family continue to search for hope daily, but leave with a better understanding of the poor prognosis.

REFERENCES

1. Huang ME, Cifu DX, Keyser-Marcus L: Functional outcome after brain tumor and acute stroke: a comparative analysis, *Arch Phys Med Rehabil* 79:1386-1390, 1998.

2. Marciniak CM, Sliwa JA, Heinemann AW et al: Functional outcome following rehabilitation of the cancer patient, *Arch Phys Med Rehabil* 77:54-57, 1996.

3. O'Dell MW, Barr K, Spanier D et al: Functional outcome of inpatient rehabilitation in persons with brain tumors, *Arch Phys Med Rehabil* 79:1530-1534, 1998.

4. Ries LG, Kosary CL, Hankey BF et al, editors: *SEER Cancer Statistics Review 1973-1996*. Bethesda, MD, National Cancer Institute, 1999.

5. *United States Population Estimates by Age from Census Data 1997-2001*. Chicago, Central Brain Tumor Registry of the United States, 2004.

6. Desmeules M, Mikkelson T, Mao Y: Increasing incidence of primary malignant brain tumors: influence of diagnostic methods, *J Natl Cancer Inst* 84:442-445, 1992.

7. Greenberg HS, Chandler WF, Sandler HM: *Brain tumors*, New York, Oxford University Press, 1999.

8. Surawicz TS, McCarthy BJ, Kupelian V et al: Descriptive epidemiology of primary brain and CNS tumors: results from the Central Brain Tumor Registry of the US 1990-1994, *J Neurooncology* 41:14-25, 1999.

9. *United States Population Estimates by Age from Census Data 1992-1997*. Chicago, Central Brain Tumor Registry of the United States, 2000.

10. Landis SH, Murray T, Bolden S et al: Cancer statistics 1998, *CA Cancer J Clin* 48:10-27, 1998.

11. Salcman M: Epidemiology and factors affecting survival, in Apuzzo MLJ (ed): *Malignant Cerebral Glioma*. Park Ridge, IL, American Association of Neurological Surgeons, 1990.

12. Grossman SA, Osman M, Hruban RH et al: Familial gliomas: The potential role of environmental exposures, *Proc Am Soc Clin Oncol* 14:149, 1995.

13. Lossignol D, Grossman SA, Sheidler VR, et al: Familial clustering of malignant astrocytoma, *J Neurooncol* 9:139 145, 1990.

14. Thomas T, Inskip P: Brain and other nervous system. In *Cancer rates and risks*, ed 4, Publication No. 96-691, Bethesda, MD, National Cancer Institute, 1996.

15. Segal G: *A primer of brain tumors*, Des Plaines, IL, 1998, American Brain Tumor Association.

16. Kleihues P, Burger PC, Scheithauer BW: *Histological typing of the tumours of the central nervous system (international histological classification of tumours)*, Berlin, 1993, Springer-Verlag.

17. Mennel H: Grading of intracranial tumors following the WHO classification systems, *Neurosurg Rev* 14:249-260, 1991.

18. *Color me hope*, ed 3, Boston, 1997, Brain Tumor Society.

19. Rowland LP: *Merrit's textbook of neurology*, ed 9, Baltimore, 1995, Williams & Wilkins.

20. Hill JR, Kuriyama N, Kuriyama H et al: Molecular genetics of brain tumors, *Arch Neurol* 56:439-441, 1999.

21. Karnofsky DA, Burchenal JH: The clinical evaluation of chemotherapeutic agents in cancer. In Macleod C, editor: *Evaluation of chemotherapeutic agents*, New York, 1949, Columbia University Press.

22. Surawicz TS, Davis F, Freels S et al: Brain tumor survival: results from the National Cancer Data Base, *J Neurooncol* 40:151-160, 1998.

23. Smith KA: Metastatic brain tumors: gamma knife radiosurgery or microsurgical resection, *BNI Q* 13:22-29, 1997.

24. Grant R: Oligodendroglioma and oligoastrocytoma. In Gilman S, Goldstein G, Waxman S, editors: *Neurobase,* San Diego, 1996, Arbor Publishing Corporation.

25. Shaw EG, Scheithauer BW, O'Fallon JR et al: Oligodendrogliomas: the Mayo Clinic experience, *J Neurosurg* 76:428-434, 1992.

26. Adams RD, Victor M, Ropper AH: *Principles of neurology,* ed 6, New York, 1997, McGraw-Hill Information Services.

27. Mork SJ, Lindegaard KF, Halvorsen TB et al: Oligodendroglioma: incidence and biological behavior in a defined population, *J Neurosurg* 63:881-889, 1985.

28. Hall WA, Djalilian HR, Sperduto PW et al: Stereotactic radiosurgery for recurrent malignant gliomas, *J Clin Oncol* 13:1642-1648, 1995.

29. Sutton LN, Goldwein J, Perilongo G et al: Prognostic factors in childhood ependymomas, *Pediatr Neurosurg* 16:57-65, 1990-1991.

30. Radhakrishnan K, Mokri B, Parisi JE et al: The trends in incidence of primary brain tumors in the population of Rochester, Minnesota, *Ann Neurol* 37:67-73, 1995.

31. Chang Y, Horoupian DS: Pathology of benign brain tumors. In Morantz RA, Walsh JW, editors: *Brain tumors: a comprehensive text,* New York, 1994, Marcel Dekker.

32. Gillen G, Burkhardt A: *Stroke rehabilitation: a function-based approach,* St. Louis, 1998, Mosby.

33. Hakim R, Alexander E 3rd, Loeffler JS et al: Results of linear accelerator based radiosurgery for intra-cranial meningiomas, *Neurosurgery* 42:446-453, 1998.

34. McCarthy BT, Davis BJ, Freels S et al: Factors associated with survival in patients with meningioma, *J Neurosurg* 88:831-839, 1998.

35. Lunsford LD, Kondziolka D, Pollock BE et al: Gamma knife stereotactic radiosurgery for acoustic neuromas: what have we learned? *Neurosurgeons* 14:164-169, 1995.

36. Shetter AG: Gamma knife radiosurgery for the treatment of acoustic neuromas, *BNI Q* 13:30-36, 1997.

37. Belford K: Central nervous system cancers. In Yarbro CH, Frogge MH, Goodman M, editors: *Cancer nursing: principles and practice,* Sudbury, 2000, Jones and Bartlett.

38. DeAngelis L: Brain tumors, *N Engl J Med* 344:114-123, 2001.

39. Patchell RA: Brain metastases, *Neurol Clin* 9:817-824, 1991.

40. Williams J, Enger C, Wharam M et al: Stereotactic radiosurgery for brain metastases: comparison of lung carcinoma v. non-lung tumors, *J Neurooncol* 37:79-85, 1998.

41. Bindal RK, Sawaya R, Leavens ME et al: Surgical treatment of multiple brain metastases, *J Neurosurg* 79:210-216, 1993.

42. Smalley SR, Laws ER Jr, O'Fallon JR et al: Resection for solitary brain metastasis. Role of adjuvant radiation and prognostic variables in 229 patients, *J Neurosurg* 77:531-540, 1992.

43. Black P, Wen PY: Clinical, imaging and laboratory diagnosis of brain tumors. In Kaye AH, Laws ER, editors: *Brain tumors,* New York, 1997, Churchill Livingstone.

44. Louis DN, Cavenee WK: Neoplasms of the central nervous system. In DeVita VT, Hellman S, Rosenberg SA, editors: *Cancer principles and practice of oncology,* Philadelphia, 2001, Lippincott Williams & Wilkins.

45. Morantz RA, Walsh JW: *Brain tumors: a comprehensive text,* New York, 1994, Marcel Dekker.

46. Fisher B, Yakura J: Movement analysis: a different perspective, *Orthop Phys Ther Clin North Am* 2:1-4, 1993.

47. Masciopinto JE, Levin AB, Mehta MP et al: Stereotactic radiosurgery for glioblastoma: a final report of 31 patients, *J Neurosurg* 82:530-535, 1995.

48. Ricci PE, Karis JP, Heiserman JE et al: Differentiating recurrent tumor from radiation necrosis: time for re-evaluation of positron emission tomography? *AJNR Am J Neuroradiol* 19:407-413, 1998.

49. Kornblith PL, Walker MD, Cassady JR: *Neurologic oncology,* Philadelphia, 1987, JB Lippincott.

50. Byrne TN: Imaging of gliomas, *Semin Oncol* 21:162-171, 1994.

51. Brock CS, Newlands ES, Wedge SR et al: Phase I trial of temozolomide using an extended continuous oral schedule, *Cancer Res* 58:4363-4367, 1998.

52. Kahn D, Follet KA, Bushnell DL et al: Diagnosis of recurrent brain tumor: value of 210T1 SPECT vs F-fluorodeoxyglucose PET, *AJR Am J Roentgenol* 163:1459-1465, 1994.

53. Meyerand ME, Pipas JM, Mamourian A et al: Classification of biopsy-confirmed brain tumors using single-voxel MR spectroscopy, *AJNR Am J Neuroradiol* 20:117-123, 1999.

54. Norfray JF, Tomita T, Byrd SE et al: Clinical impact of MR spectroscopy when MR imaging is indeterminate for pediatric brain tumors, *AJR Am J Roentgenol* 173:119-125, 1999.

55. Hall WA, Martin AJ, Liu H et al: Brain biopsy using high-field strength interventional magnetic resonance imaging, *Neurosurgery* 44:807-813, 1999.

56. Rabb CH, Apuzzo MLJ: Stereotaxis in the diagnosis and management of brain tumors. In Kaye AH, Laws ER, editors: *Brain tumors,* New York, 1997, Churchill Livingstone.

57. Lunsford LD, Coffey RJ: Stereotactic surgery in the diagnosis and therapy of malignant intra-cranial gliomas. In Apuzzo MLJ, editor: *Malignant cerebral glioma,* Park Ridge, IL, 1990, American Association of Neurological Surgeons.

58. Ojemann RG: Surgical principles in the management of brain tumors. In Kaye AH, Law ER, editors: *Brain tumors,* New York, 1997, Churchill Livingstone.

59. Black PM, Moriarty T, Alexander E 3rd et al: Development and implementation of intra-operative magnetic resonance imaging and its surgical applications, *Neurosurgery* 41:831-845, 1997.

60. Freeman G: Brain tumors. In Umphred D, editor: *Neurological rehabilitation,* ed 3, St. Louis, 1994, Mosby.

61. Rottenburg DA: *Neurological complications of cancer treatment,* Boston, 1991, Butterworth-Heinemann.

62. Pizzo PA, Poplack DG, Bleyer WA: Neurotoxicities of current leukemia therapy, *Am J Pediatr Hematol Oncol* 1:127-140, 1979.

63. Belford K, Gargon-Klinger R: Astrocytoma. In Miaskowski C, Buchsel P, editors: *Oncology nursing assessment and clinical care,* St. Louis, 1998, Mosby.

64. Speiser B: Gamma knife stereotactic radiosurgery: an overview, *BNI Q* 13:4-10, 1997.

65. Subach BR, Kondziolka D, Lunsford LD: Stereotactic radiosurgery in the management of acoustic neuromas associated with neurofibromatosis Type 2, *J Neurosurg* 90:815-822, 1999.

66. Williams J, Zakhary R, Watts M et al: Stereotactic radiosurgery for human glioma: treatment parameter and outcome for low vs. high grade, *J Radiosurg* 1:3-8, 1998.

67. Fiedler JA: Physical aspects of stereotactic radiosurgery, *BNI Q* 13:11-21, 1997.

68. Alexander M, Friedrich WK, Gerhard AH: Surgery and radiotherapy compared with Gamma knife radiosurgery in the treatment of solitary brain metastases of small diameter, *J Neurosurg* 91:35-43, 1999.

69. Lavine SD, Petrovich Z, Cohen-Gadol AA: Gamma knife radiosurgery for metastatic melanoma: an analysis of survival, outcome, and complications, *Neurosurgery* 44:59-64, 1999.

70. Buatti JM, Friedman WA, Bova FJ et al: Linac radiosurgery for high grade gliomas: the University of Florida experience, *Int J Radiat Oncol Biol Phys* 32:205-210, 1995.

71. Gannett D, Stea B, Lulu B et al: Stereotactic radiosurgery as an adjunct to surgery and external beam radiotherapy in the treatment of patients with malignant gliomas, *Int J Radiat Oncol Biol Phys* 33:461-468, 1995.

72. Mehta MP, Masciopinto J, Rozental J et al: Stereotactic radiosurgery for glioblastoma multiforme: report of a prospective study evaluating prognostic factors and analyzing long term survival advantage, *Int J Radiat Oncol Biol Phys* 30:541-549, 1994.

73. Laing RW, Warrington AP, et al: Efficacy and toxicity of fractionated stereotactic radiosurgery in the treatment of recurrent gliomas (phase I/II study), *Radiother Oncol* 27:22-29, 1993.

74. Shrieve DC, Alexander E, Wen PY: Comparison of stereotactic radiosurgery and brachytherapy in the treatment of recurrent glioblastoma multiforme, *Neurosurgery* 36:275-282, 1995.

75. Kondziolka D, Levy EI, Niranjan A et al: Long-term outcomes after meningioma radiosurgery: physician and patient perspectives, *J Neurosurg* 91:44-50, 1999.

76. Lunsford LD: Contemporary management of meningiomas: radiation therapy as an adjuvant and radiosurgery as an alternative to surgical removal? *J Neurosurg* 80:187-190, 1994.

77. Kirshblum S, O'Dell MW, Ho C et al: Rehabilitation of persons with central nervous system tumors, *Cancer* 92(4 suppl):1029-1038, 2001.

78. Huang ME, Wartella J, Kreutzer J et al: Functional outcomes and quality of life in patients with brain tumours: a review of the literature, *Brain Inj* 15:843-856, 2001.

79. O'Toole DM, Golden AM: Evaluating cancer patients for rehabilitation potential, *West J Med* 155:384-387, 1991.

80. Stewart-Amidei C: Quality of life in the neuro-oncology patient: a symposium, *J Neurosci Nurs* 27:219-223, 1995.

81. Kuchler T, Wood-Dauphinee S: Working with people who have cancer: guidelines for physical therapists, *Physiother Cancer* 43:19-23, 1991.

82. *Radiation therapy and you: a guide to self-help during treatment,* revised ed. Bethesda, MD, 1993, National Cancer Institute, National Institutes of Health.

83. Loney M: Death, dying and grief in the face of cancer. In Sigler B, editors: *Psychosocial dimensions of oncology nursing care,* Pittsburgh, 1998, Oncology Nursing Press.

84. Carr JH, Shepherd RB: *Movement science: foundations for physical therapy in rehabilitation,* Rockville, MD, 1987, Aspen.

85. Schmidt RA: A schema theory of discrete motor skill learning, *Psychol Rev* 82:225-259, 1975.

86. Schumway-Cook A, Woolcott MH: *Motor control theory and practical applications,* Baltimore, 1995, Williams & Wilkins.

87. McCracken HD, Stelmach GE: A test of the schema theory of discrete motor learning, *J Motor Behav* 9:193-201, 1977.

88. Winstein CJ: Knowledge of results and motor learning implications for physical therapy, *Phys Ther* 71:140-149, 1991.

89. Leavitt MB, Lamb SA, Voss BS: Brain tumor support group: content themes and mechanisms of support, *Oncol Nurs Forum* 23:1247-1256, 1996.

90. Simpson DA, Pitorak E: Hospice or palliative care? *Am J Hospice Palliative Care* 15:122-123, 1998.

91. Enyert G, Burman M: A qualitative study of self-transcendence in caregivers of terminally ill patients, *Am J Hospice Palliative Care* 16:455-462, 1999.

92. Giovagnoli AR, Tamburini M, Boiardi A: Quality of life in brain tumor patients, *J Neurooncol* 30:71-80, 1996.

93. Sivesind DM, Rohaly-Davis JA: Coping with cancer: patient issues. In Sigler B, editor: *Psychosocial dimensions of oncology nursing care,* Pittsburgh, 1998, Oncology Nursing Press.

CHAPTER 26   Clients with Cerebellar Dysfunction

Marsha E. Melnick, PT, PhD

KEY WORDS

ataxia
cerebellar disease
cerebellum
therapeutic interventions for cerebellar disorder

OBJECTIVES

After reading this chapter the student/therapist will be able to:

1. Identify and discuss the anatomy, physiology, and function of the cerebellum.
2. Identify the signs and symptoms of cerebellar disorders.
3. Explain the physiology responsible for the clinical presentation of patients with cerebellar disorders.
4. Describe the relationship between the cerebellum and other parts of the brain and how the important feedback loops affect movement.
5. Select appropriate interventions for patients with a cerebellar disorder based upon potential for plasticity, principles of motor learning, as well as the patient's lifestyle and personal goals.

The signs of cerebellar disease are seen in specific diseases within the cerebellum, as well as in head trauma, cerebrovascular accidents, multiple sclerosis, and other neurological conditions. All conditions that lead to disruption of the cerebellum and its connections, whether degenerative or static, involve disorganization of movement, especially rapid movements, along with a decrease in balance and central postural control. Cerebellar symptoms are also common in the late stages of alcoholism and, for this reason, alcoholism is discussed in this chapter. Additionally—and this is, perhaps, the most devastating symptom—there is a loss of motor learning. In this chapter, the anatomy, physiology, and common diseases of the cerebellum will be presented as well as the examination and intervention suggestions for the specific symptoms of loss of cerebellar neurons and connections.

The word *cerebellum* means little brain, and yet this region of the brain contains more neurons than the rest of the brain put together.[1] This "little brain" also has a large role in motor control and motor learning. Loss of the cerebellum or its connections with the remainder of the brain results in many well-known motor problems that are difficult for the therapist and the physician to treat. These motor problems lead to loss in abilities to perform many functional activities and often decrease the individual's ability to participate in life.

OVERVIEW OF CEREBELLAR ANATOMY AND PHYSIOLOGY

Connections between the cerebellum and the rest of the brain occur in three large axonal bundles: the superior, middle, and inferior cerebellar peduncles. The cerebellum is a highly organized, three-layered structure, located in the posterior-inferior portion of the cranium. The cerebellar gray matter located on the outer rims of the cerebellum communicates with the rest of the brain through three pairs of deep cerebellar nuclei: the fastigial, interposed, and dentate. This general organization is similar to the basal ganglia, in that there is an afferent portion of the system and an efferent portion. Functionally, the cerebellum is divided into three parts based upon the afferent and efferent connections to and from other areas within the nervous system. Although most of the studies regarding function have been based upon animal data, evidence is now accumulating that there is a high correlation between these animal studies and the human cerebellum.[2-5] Anatomically the most medial and hindmost (inferior) portion of the cerebellum receives information from and projects directly to the lateral vestibular nuclei and the fastigial nucleus. These two nuclear masses project to areas of the brain including the vestibular nuclei concerned with balance (the vestibulocerebello-vestibular tract). This portion of the cerebellum is involved in the control of posture, balance, equilibrium, and locomotion.[6-8] Moving laterally, the intermediate or paramedian portion of the cerebellum, receives information from deep nuclei within the cerebellum and projects processed information back through the interposed nuclei. This system plays a predominantly motor regulatory aspect of the nervous system. It receives information from both peripheral receptors as well as the motor generator within the spinal (the spinocerebellum) and bulbar (bulbar-cerebellar) areas. This is the portion of the cerebellum that motorically controls discrete, ipsilateral limb movements and reflexes. The lateral portions of the cerebellar hemispheres connect primarily with the cerebral cortex through the dentate nucleus. The cerebellum receives information through the middle cerebellar peduncle as afferents from the pons (cerebropontocerebellum). Efferents leaving the cerebellum pass from the cerebellar cortex, synapsing within the dentate and then project via the superior peduncle to the contralateral thalamus and then to the frontal lobe. Some fibers also synapse at the red nucleus, thus impacting both the thalamic cortical connections and the ipsilateral rubro-spinal tract. The entire tract might be referred to as the cerebro-ponto-dento-cerebello-dento-rubro-thalamo-cerebral tract. The reader needs to remember that each synapse within a nuclear mass will be named within a tract name and represents a place where information may be modified. Complex, visually guided limb movements, as well as planning of those movements, are controlled by this portion of the cerebellum. Descending connections from the cerebellum to the spinal cord and brain stem are ipsilateral; those descending from within the cerebral cortex and other diencephalons and neocortical brain structures are contralateral. Therefore the cerebellum, through ipsilateral connections, has specific motor control over the same side of the body, but when communicating with the cerebral cortex those fibers need to cross over prior to ascending to the appropriate neurons within the cortical regions. This distinction is important when working with individuals with massive ipsilateral damage. The damage above any crossing or decussation from higher centers will affect the contralateral side of the body, while the damage at or below the descending fibers from the cerebellum will result in ipsilateral motor deficits. With damage throughout one side of the motor system, a patient might have specific motor loss on the contralateral side that is different but just as debilitating on the ipsilateral side. The gross anatomy of the cerebellum is presented in Figure 26-1. A view of the cerebellum within the cranium is shown in the magnetic resonance imaging (MRI) scan in Figure 26-2.

Input to the cerebellum is rapid; there are few synapses between the projection areas and the specific cerebellar location receiving the input. The cerebellum receives input regarding head, trunk, and extremity position and movement from peripheral receptors and the state of the motor pool itself, as well as extensive input from the cerebral cortex regarding the motor command. Its connections, therefore, allow it to compare ongoing movement of head, trunk, and limbs with the motor command and the intent of that command. Input to the cerebellum greatly exceeds output, which denotes that this is an integrative structure. Based upon the anatomical connections of the cerebellum, it is involved in balance and eye movements (vestibular and cerebropontocerebellum), integration of proprioceptive information (e.g., spinocerebello-fastigio-rubro-spinal) and control of voluntary movement (cerebropontocerebellum and spinocerebellum), and motor learning (all areas).

The cellular organization of the cerebellar cortex is precise. There are three layers with only five neuronal types. There is only one type of efferent neurons that leave or exit the cerebellar cortex, the large Purkinje cells, which are inhibitory to the three deep cerebellar nuclei and to the

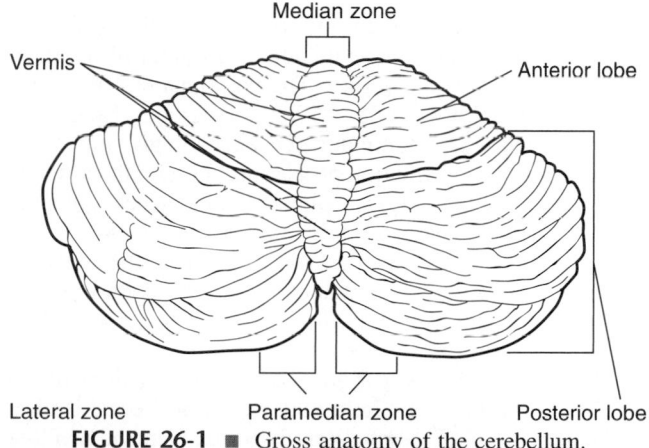

FIGURE 26-1 ■ Gross anatomy of the cerebellum.

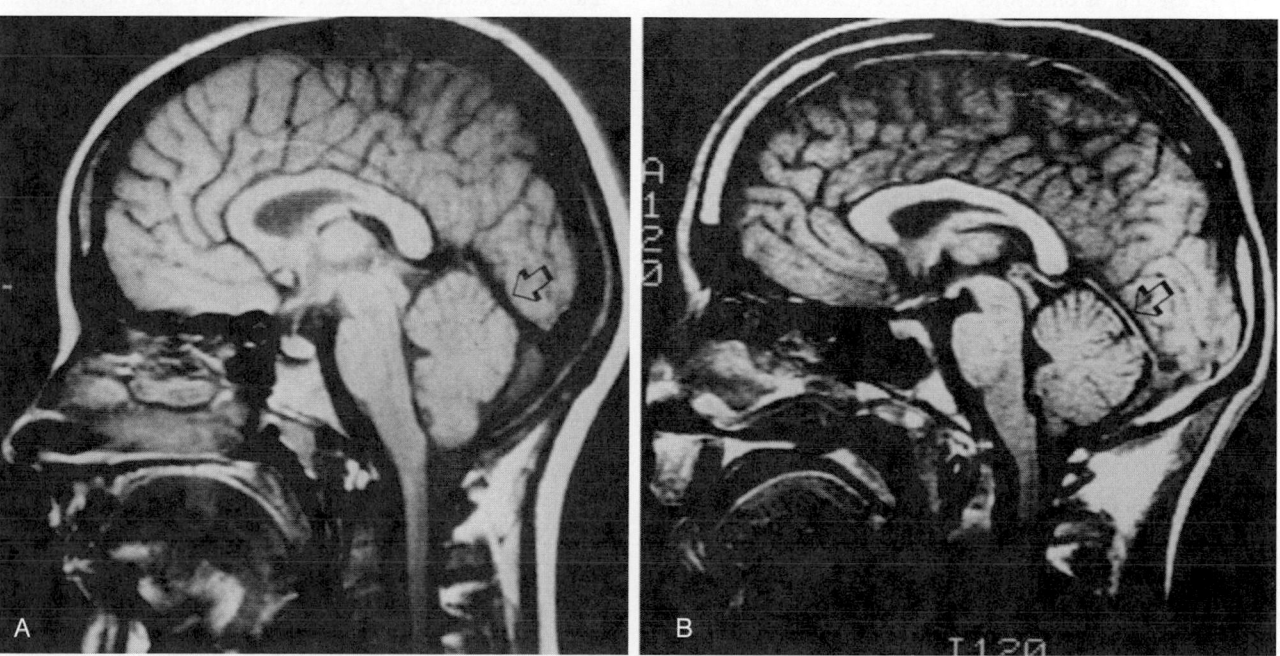

FIGURE 26-2 ■ **A,** Magnetic resonance imaging (MRI) of normal cerebellum. Note full solid white area as indicated by *arrow.* **B,** MRI of spinocerebellar atrophy. Note dark and branching areas of cerebellum as indicated by *arrow,* which denotes atrophy.

lateral vestibular nuclei. All input to the cerebellar cortex is excitatory and is through either climbing fibers from the inferior olivary complex in the medulla or via mossy fibers from everywhere else. All fibers send collaterals to the deep cerebellar nuclei in order to excite those gray matter clusters. The climbing fibers wrap around a Purkinje cell and form many synapses as they climb their way up the dendritic tree. A climbing fiber contacts only a few Purkinje cells (1-10 cells), and each Purkinje cell receives input from only one climbing fiber. This unique relationship will be important as we discuss the motor learning and cognitive functions of the cerebellum. Anatomical research indicates that the interactions between the climbing fibers and the Purkinje cells are somatotopically arranged, as is the output of the Purkinje cells. Mossy fibers, on the other hand, are distributed to many thousands of Purkinje cells via parallel fibers. The circuitry of the cerebellum is such that a strip of Purkinje cells is activated as those on either side of it are inhibited. This lateral inhibition is provided by the interneurons in the cerebellar cortex.

The Purkinje cells send inhibitory input to the deep cerebellar nuclei and vestibular nuclei. The output of the deep cerebellar nuclei is excitatory. The combinations of inhibition and excitation have led to the description of the cerebellum as a base two computer. It is exceedingly simple and yet allows rapid information processing. I prefer the description of the cerebellum as a player piano, which can play complex music just through the precise location and sequence of holes in the card, but can change the sound or action when new motor demands are placed upon it (cortical centers). Using this example, a piano player would be given a different music sheet to play.

Physiological investigations support the functions of the cerebellum in movement and motor control. Recent studies of the activity of the cerebellum during movement also link the cerebellum with the changes associated with plasticity of learning as well as emotions.[7,9] The cerebellum is vital in environmental adaptation and, if this structure is lost, it is likely that motor adaptation will be permanently lost or severely impaired. One hypothesis for the adaptive ability of the cerebellum comes from experiments by Llinas, who was able to demonstrate synchronous firing in Purkinje cells and in the olivary complex, which may enable cooperative behavior among Purkinje cells. These enclaves of cooperativity change as the motor behavior required changes.[10] Another important finding linking the cerebellum to learning is a process known as *long-term depression*. In long-term depression, there is a reduction in the response to subsequent excitatory input. Long-term depression appears to be selective in the cerebellum[11] and is time dependent, but it can last for hours. It is dependent upon a large influx of calcium that occurs with climbing fiber synapses.

The functional organization of the cerebellum will be discussed in more detail because of its relation to theories of treatment. The medial area (vestibulocerebellum) receives input from the inner ear, from both the semicircular canals and the utricle and saccule via the eighth cranial nerve, and relays information back to the vestibular nuclei and on to other nuclei within the brain stem. Outside of the deep cerebellar nuclei, the vestibular nuclei (not just the lateral vestibular nuclei) are the only nuclei within the brain to receive direct input from the Purkinje cells. Lesions of the

vestibulocerebellum, as might be expected, lead to difficulty with maintenance of balance, as well as inability to coordinate the eyes with head movements.[12] Movement in the distal parts of the extremities is difficult to execute without the ability to maintain one's balance. The person with dysfunction in the vestibulocerebellum is able to control the extremities in a supported (e.g., supine) position; however, the person is not able to do so in an upright position, such as walking, which requires both postural support as well as adequate balance reactions within axial trunk multisegmental patterns.

The spinocerebellum receives input from the spinal cord, including input from the proprioceptors within the muscles, namely the muscle spindle and Golgi tendon organs, and feedback input from the spinal motor generators. The spinocerebellum also receives information from the cortex regarding the motor command. Input from the lower extremities is greater than that from the upper extremities. The input is somatotopically arranged and there are two maps of the body. In these maps the trunk is represented in the medial cerebellum; this portion projects to the fastigial nucleus and on to the vestibular nuclei. These projections eventually make their way to the portion of the motor cortex that controls proximal musculature. Therefore the medial cerebellum is also involved in control of posture and balance.[13] There is also limb control from the more lateral portions of the spinocerebellum, which project to the interposed nuclei and then to the red nucleus decussating on its way to the motor cortex (via the thalamus). The input from the spinal cord travels to the cerebellum primarily in two pathways: the dorsal and ventral spinocerebellar tracts. The dorsal spinocerebellar tract relays precise information of individual muscle activity and provides sensory feedback during movements. The ventral spinocerebellar tract, on the other hand, appears to be more related to internally generated processes involved in rhythmic automatic movement, such as walking and other centrally generated patterns of movement. The spinocerebellum is in a position to compare the ongoing movements (inputs from the muscles and joints) with the intended movements (input from the cortex), both rhythmic patterns and precise voluntary movements. Posture and gait disturbances are therefore seen when the function of the spinocerebellum is impaired.[13]

Lesions of the spinocerebellum produce many of the symptoms seen in clients with cerebellar disease. One such problem is hypotonia. This is hypothesized to occur because of decreased excitation of the red nucleus and motor cortex and, in turn, a decreased activation of motor neurons excited by the rubrospinal and corticospinal pathways.

The interpositus nucleus is strongly related to properties of ongoing movement rather than those of intended movement.[14-16] A disruption of the interposed nuclei decreases the accuracy of reaching movements because of loss of control of the direction, extent, force, and timing of the movement. This is what is seen clinically as dysmetria.

Joint movements, especially multijoint movements, lose control in a way that movements tend to be curved instead of straight. This lack of precision and coordination is known as ataxia. Corrections of these imprecise or ataxic movements lead to further errors of timing and extent, which increases the ataxia, further increasing the error, and so on. The result is an oscillation at the end of a movement: an intention tremor. Unlike the tremor of Parkinson's disease, which occurs at rest, a cerebellar tremor occurs upon intentional movement and has its highest amplitude at the end of the movement. Oscillation at the end of movement is also seen in the deep tendon reflexes and, although the response to a tendon tap may be normal, the limb moves in a pendular manner after the initial response.

This exaggeration of movements has been studied recently in humans during both walking and stepping through three-dimensional motion analysis.[5,17,18] These studies showed that in comparison to those without cerebellar damage, those with cerebellar damage from several causes had exaggerated movements in both stepping and walking that were the result of excessive knee flexion. Further, this increased movement was greater during stepping (a nonautomatic movement) than during walking. Analysis of the kinetics of the excessive knee flexion led to overcompensation of deceleration torques, as if the individual needs to walk over a larger obstacle.

The cerebropontocerebellum is involved in complex motor tasks as well as performance of perceptual and cognitive tasks. It is this region of the cerebellum that has undergone the largest phylogenetic growth. It receives input from the cortex through pontine nuclei and projects back to the cortex, primarily the motor cortex, via the dentate nucleus and the ventrolateral nucleus of the thalamus. There also is a projection from the dentate to the red nucleus and inferior olive. Discharge of the dentate nucleus appears to be tightly related to properties of intended movements, as well as properties of ongoing movement.[14] Imaging of the brain indicates that these loops, especially the cerebellar-red nucleus-inferior olive-cerebellar loop, are especially active during the mental rehearsal of a movement.

Lesions of cerebropontocerebellum lead to a decomposition of movement. As in lesions of the spinocerebellum, there is a disruption in the timing of movements. Instead of several aspects of the movement being sequenced together, each part of the movement is sequenced separately. These disturbances are especially important in hand function. Loss of the dentate nucleus also leads to a slowing of reaction time and delayed initiation of movement. Single-unit recording studies have shown that the dentate nucleus is active prior to activation of electromyographic (EMG) activity.[15,19] There has been some thought that the cerebellum is especially important in initiation of rapid (i.e., ballistic) movements.

Timing of movements is but one of the deficits that occur as a result of cerebropontocerebellum lesions. The person's perception of timing is also impaired. For example, a person with a lesion in this region of the cerebellum is unable to determine which of two objects is moving faster. This finding led to investigations to determine the role of the cerebellum in cognitive functions. Results of studies by Dum and Strick[9] and by Gao et al[20] indicate that cerebellar processing is crucial to one's ability to solve spatial and temporal problems, as are needed, for example, in hitting a baseball with a bat. More recently Ito[7] has demonstrated some of the mechanisms used by the cerebellum for learning—both motor and "cognitive" learning. Involvement of the cerebellum in learning is an area of rapid investigation and may help to provide information that may increase both the effectiveness and the efficacy of treatment.

With that brief description of the anatomy, connectivity, and physiology of the cerebellum, the discussion will focus on the role of the cerebellum in motor control.

THE CEREBELLUM AND MOTOR CONTROL

Our understanding of the cerebellum's contribution to movement has come a long way from the original concept in 1839 that its only function was to maintain sexual potency.[21] Electrophysiological studies of the normal function and consequences of lesions of the cerebellum strongly suggest that the cerebellum controls the onset, level, and rate of force production by muscles. On the basis of these findings and the anatomical connections of the cerebellum, it has been suggested that the cerebellum acts as a comparator between sensory input and motor output.[22-24] Remember, there are far more axons projecting to the cerebellum (from the vestibular and proprioceptive systems as well as the motor cortex) than are exiting the cerebellum as output. The cerebellum, then, is in a good position to compare the voluntary command for movement with the sensory signals produced by the evolving movement. If the motor commands and evolving sensory signals are not appropriately matched, the cerebellum will provide corrective feedback to motor pathways capable of influencing the movement prior to the end of the movement.[22] Without such a function, movement will be inaccurate. To understand this concept, think about what a disaster it would be if the National Aeronautic and Space Administration (NASA) were unable to compare the location, speed, and trajectory of a rocket destined to land on the moon with the location and movements of the moon.

This idea of the cerebellum as a comparator has been refined in recent years. Rather than simply providing corrections to ongoing voluntary movement, the cerebellum is assumed to perform predictive compensatory modification of reflexes in preparation for movement.[25] The success of voluntary movement depends largely on the stability and adjustment of many different reflexes. For example, if the stretch reflexes of a limb are too sensitive, high-speed movements may be impeded by the constant response to stretch. Thus muscle spindle activity will have to be reduced before and during such movement. In other circumstances the sensitivity of muscle spindles may have to be increased before movement. The cerebellum may be the initiator of such compensatory modification of the stretch reflex, as well as many other reflexes.

A vital function of the cerebellum is its role in motor learning. Ito[26] proposed that the cerebellum acts as an adaptive feed-forward control system, which programs or models voluntary movement skills based on a memory of previous sensory input and motor output. According to this theory, an internal model stored in or triggered by the cerebellum controls learned movement. Imaging studies by Shadmehr and Holcomb[27] showed that the anterior cerebellum was active during consolidation of a learned internal model of a motor task. Other investigators have also demonstrated the role of the cerebellum in integrating multiple internal models for complex motor activities and transformations.[21,27a] If the cerebellum is damaged, the learned motor programs cannot be used. Movement will then be guided by slow sensory feedback loops through the cerebrum, just as in learning a new skill, and incoordination will result. Additionally, the ability to adapt to minor changes necessitated by environmental context or unusual circumstances cannot occur.[8,28-31]

If the cerebellum learns or memorizes movements, are programs retained for complex movements, such as a serve in tennis, or for simple qualities of movements? Brooks[14] suggested that the lateral and intermediate cerebellum act to sequence simple movements that make up complex actions. The cerebellum may thus learn small, simple programs, which are then triggered in the order needed to produce the complex motion. Hikosaka et al[32] hypothesize that the cerebellum, particularly the anterior cerebellum and the dentate nucleus, are important in the acquisition and execution of sequential procedures that comprise complex learned motor acts. Similarly Molinari et al[33] demonstrated impairments in procedural learning of a motor sequence and suggested that the cerebellum was important in the detection and recognition of event sequences. Ito[7] has shown that this process is dependent upon long-term depression.

Thach et al[34,35] first showed the role of the cerebellum in adaptation during trial-and-error learning in studies examining the changes that occur with prism glasses. Lang and Bastian[28] and others[29,31,36] studied the role of the cerebellum during catching. They examined the effects of learning to adapt to a change in ball weight in a catching task. In one study, the subject learned to catch a light ball and then had to catch an unexpectedly heavy ball. Following adaptation, the subject again had to catch the light ball. Lang and Bastian[28] found that those with cerebellar disease required almost 40 trials to learn to adapt to the change in ball weight, compared with less than two trials in the subjects with normal motor control. Further, when the ball weight was returned to the original weight, the subject with cerebellar disease demonstrated no negative after effect suggestive of adaptation. The EMG recordings indicated that the cerebellar subjects could not increase anticipatory activity to counteract the increased ball weight. Lang and Bastian[28] also reversed the presentation order and found no differences in adaptation ability if the heavy ball was used first. They concluded that the cerebellum was vital to controlling anticipatory muscle activity across several joints and vital to modification of response. It is important to remember that the client with cerebellar disease will require many more practice sessions than other clients and that alternative strategies for performance may have to be taught.

No one knows where and how learning in the cerebellum may take place; however, several ideas have been proposed that put heavy emphasis on the role of the inferior olivary nucleus.[3,37] Each olivary neuron is presumed to be activated by the cerebral cortex during a demand for an elemental or simple movement. Climbing fiber pathways are modulated during active movements in a way that prevents irrelevant sensory information from reaching the cerebellar cortex and facilitating the projection of relevant information.[38] The discharge of Purkinje cells is also affected by input from the mossy fibers, which reflects the sensory context in which the elemental movement is demanded. Possibly, the climbing fiber input potentiates the mossy fiber input so that mossy fiber input to the Purkinje cell may be able to evoke an elemental movement from the Purkinje cell in the absence of input from the cortex.[7]

Further research has demonstrated that sequence is the key to understanding the cerebellum.[33,39] The process whereby there is a row of excitation of Purkinje cells surrounded by rows of lateral inhibition has led to speculation that these "beams" respond to sequences of events in the sensory input and then produce sequences of output information. Braitenberg et al[39] noted that these beams were well tuned (much like FM radio stations) and were used to refine movement sequences for the adaptation necessary for the physics of multijoint movements. More recent studies on human subjects also showed that multijoint movements were more involved than single-joint motions and that combinations of movements, such as reach and grasp, were more disorganized than a single movement.[4,8,30]

The cerebellum has been shown to be active during mental imagery or mental practice. According to Ryding et al[40] mental imagery is a pure mental activity, requiring no muscle involvement and the same amount of time as the actual motor performance. The dentate nucleus and the cerebellar hemispheres are the cerebellar areas most involved during mental rehearsal. Patients who show damage in the lateral region of the cerebellar hemispheres have a reduced or absent capacity for anticipatory cues when performing a pretrained motor task and decreased ability to image a movement.[41] There is other evidence that the role of the cerebellum is not purely motor. Evidence is mounting that the cerebellum is involved in purely cognitive and emotional activities, including thinking and verbal encoding. For example, Akshoomoff and Courchesne[2] suggested that the cerebellum can affect voluntary control of a specific cognitive operation, such as rapid and accurate shifts of attention. Patients with damage to the cerebellum, such as those with astrocytoma, and idiopathic cerebellar atrophy, showed a deficit in shifting attention from one sensory domain to another when no motor action was involved. The implication is that cerebropontocerebellar action for cognitive processes does not necessarily depend on the motor control system. In essence, Akshoomoff believes that possibly the neocerebellum "helps us to effortlessly shift from one domain of thought to another (p. 737)."[2] Morton et al[5,18,30] have shown a similar process in movements. They showed that those with cerebellar damage/disease also have an inability to shift motor coordination in response to environmental demands or to make "context-dependent" movements.

No one is certain whether the cerebellum functions in all three of these capacities or predominantly in just one. If the cerebellum does perform all three of the described functions, different lesions may disturb one function more than another. Recognition of these theories and the consequences of their disruption may help a therapist more carefully examine a client and plan a therapeutic program. For example, if the cerebellum no longer functions as a comparator, movement will obviously be dysmetric. This individual will need time-consuming practice, but in selected activities that will be most useful for him or her, as opposed to practicing all movements. Even though the cerebellum may not automatically correct movement errors, the client may consciously be able to correct movement with practice, or the remaining central nervous system (CNS) may be able to assume a role of automatic correction. Compensatory strategies become more important in treating these patients, which may be crucial to independent functioning.

If the cerebellar function of a reflex compensator is lost, the client may display abnormal muscle tone, inappropriate postural adjustment, inappropriate magnitude of movement, and loss of associated limb movements, as well as being dysmetric. The therapist may need to evoke reflexes during an activity that would assist the postural stability and progression of movement. The presumption, again, is that the client can consciously learn to control the activity or that another part of the nervous system can begin to make the reflex adjustment automatically.

The concept of learning by the cerebellum is especially important for therapists to consider. If clients have lost "learned motor programs" controlled by the cerebellum, they will obviously be dysmetric. Therapy for any neurologically involved client is offered with the hope that a long-term modification of motor behavior will take place. However, if the cerebellum is the primary area where adaptive movement can be learned, the client may never receive much benefit from therapy. Currently, few studies[18,30,36] quantify the ability of clients with cerebellar lesions to learn new motor skills or relearn lost skills with training. Those that do exist use small numbers of patients and control subjects who have no motor involvement. Obviously, such research would be a valuable guide to therapists in providing activities that can achieve better motor performance. Therapists, however, need to recognize that even though the best therapeutic program possible is offered, the motor learning capabilities of some clients with cerebellar lesions may be limited and gains achieved slowly, at best.

The anatomy and physiology and theories of the role of the cerebellum in motor control have been reviewed. The focus of the next section is an understanding of the impairments that are seen in cerebellar disease.

BALANCE AND EQUILIBRIUM

As its anatomical connections may indicate, the cerebellum is a vital structure in the maintenance of the upright posture. Lesions of the cerebellum that include the vestibulocerebellum and/or the fastigial nucleus result in postural sway and delayed balance reactions. Use of vision is not effective in preventing loss of balance. Additionally, the person with cerebellar disease is unable to modulate long loop postural reflexes appropriately.[42] Nashner[42] studied the ability of patients with cerebellar disease to increase or decrease the size of the long loop reflex to environmental demands and demonstrated that postural adaptations were lost in the person with cerebellar damage. (See Chapter 24 for discussion in relationship to the basal ganglia and Chapter 23 to balance.) The person with cerebellar dysfunction does not modify the reflex even with repeated presentations of the appropriate stimulus(i). More recently, Morton, and Bastian[5] showed that gait difficulties, especially gait ataxia, were more related to difficulties with balance. Additionally, they concluded that cerebellar control of balance and gait are interrelated and could not be dissociated.

Oddly enough, patients with late cerebellar atrophy almost never fall, even though they have severe disturbances in stance and gait.[12] The absence of falling appears to be the result of intact intersegmental movements between the head, trunk, and legs. In fact, the person with cerebellar disease of the vestibular portion of the cerebellum (though rare) has good control of the limbs when supine, or fully supported.

CONTROL OF MUSCLE TONE

The spinocerebellum has been linked to the problem of decreased tone or hypotonicity. This is because of the decrease in excitation from the cerebellar deep nuclei to regions of the brain that excite alpha and gamma motor neurons.[43-46] The muscle itself feels less firm to palpation, and when the therapist examines passive range of motion, the limb will appear heavy. In fact, if the limb is suddenly dropped, the extremity will fall rapidly without correction. The limb will move through a greater arc of motion than does a normal limb when the limb is shaken. Hypotonicity is also demonstrated by asking the client to hold the arm out against gravity. One will observe either a slow falling of the arm or a postural tremor. The person with a cerebellar lesion can correct this movement impairment by attention. However, the effort needed to concentrate all the time on objects being held would be unrealistic and dysfunctional. In the lower extremities, the decrease in underlying muscle activity is seen in a wide, flat footprint.

Deep tendon reflexes are typically normal, but there is often a pendular movement of the limb after the initial muscle contraction response. This pendular reflex was first described by Holmes[47] in an EMG experiment of the knee jerk. The normal EMG response to quadriceps stretch is a recording of two peaks of tension (Figure 26-3, A). The initial peak is evoked by the tendon tap and is responsible for the brisk twitch of knee extension. Descent of the leg causes another stretch reflex of the quadriceps femoris muscle. The descent of the leg is actually slowed by this second contractile response. A client with a cerebellar lesion, on the other hand, displays only the early peak (Figure 26-3, B). The second response, which would brake or slow down the return of the limb, is not present, and the limb falls heavily. Thus, during a knee jerk, the leg behaves as a pendulum that falls by its own weight and oscillates momentarily because of momentum.

The problem with this is a resultant incoordination of limb movement. The client has decreased ability to contract

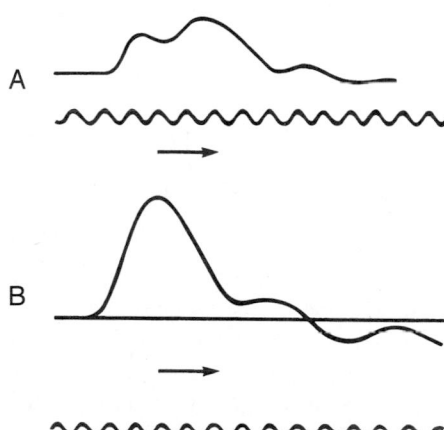

FIGURE 26-3 ■ Myogram of quadriceps muscle on normal knee-jerk response (**A**), and that evoked from a person with cerebellar lesion (**B**). Time indicated below each trace by vibrations of tuning fork at 25 Hz. Note absence of second peak of tension in response of person with cerebellar disease. (From Holmes G: The Croonian lectures on the clinical symptoms of cerebellar diseases and their interpretation, *Lancet* 1:1181, 1922.)

muscles and stabilize a limb. She or he may demonstrate good distal control if the limb has external support, as in sliding the arm along a table, but is unable to reach out in space in an open chain activity. This lack of muscle control is more apparent in multijoint movements when each segment of the limb must control the inertial forces of the other segments.[16] Indeed, the cerebellum is far more related to multijoint than to single-joint movements.

DYSMETRIA: LOSS OF DIRECTION, EXTENT, FORCE, AND TIMING OF MOVEMENTS

Dysmetria is defined as a deficit in reaching a target, usually a past pointing. It results from the deficit in defining accurately the direction, extent, force, and timing of the limb movement, one role of cerebellar function. A classic test for this is asking the patient to touch the examiner's finger and then her or his nose. Holmes[48] first described these deficits. He illustrated a slow onset in development of muscle tension, a reduced intensity, and a slow release compared to normal movement (Figure 26-4). Other aspects of the inability to regulate force of movements are seen in dyssynergia, also described by Holmes.[47] This is tested clinically by suddenly removing a restraining force from an isometrically contracting limb. In a person without motor deficits, the limb will not change position. In contrast, the limb of a person with a cerebellar lesion will move abruptly as if still opposing the resistance.

Other studies have extended the observations of Holmes and concentrated on the sequence of muscle activity.[16,49] A

ballistic motion uses a sequence of agonist-antagonist-agonist activity, a triphasic pattern (Figure 26-5).[50,51] The first burst from the agonist has a consistent duration of 50 to 110 msec. The antagonist muscle burst displays a consistent duration of 40 to 100 msec. The duration of the second agonist muscle burst varies. The amplitude of the first agonist burst is related to the distance moved and is thought to provide the impulsive force needed to start the movement.[52] The amplitude of the antagonistic muscle burst is not

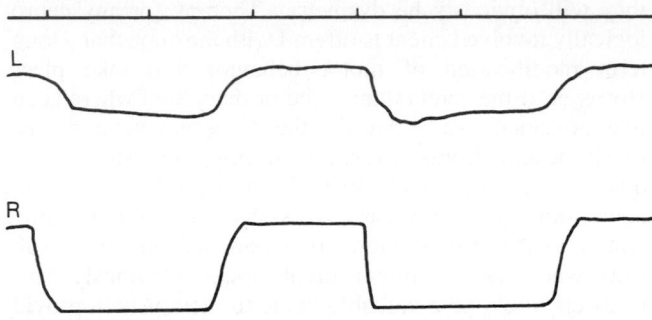

FIGURE 26-4 ■ Tracings on a slowly rotating drum of simultaneous depression of the right (*R*) and left (*L*) arms against springs of equal tension, from a man with a lesion of the left side of the cerebellum. The tracings show delay in starting and slowness in effecting the movements, reduced and irregular exertion of power, and slowness in relaxation on the affected side. Time in seconds. (From Holmes G: The cerebellum of man, *Brain* 62:10, 1939.)

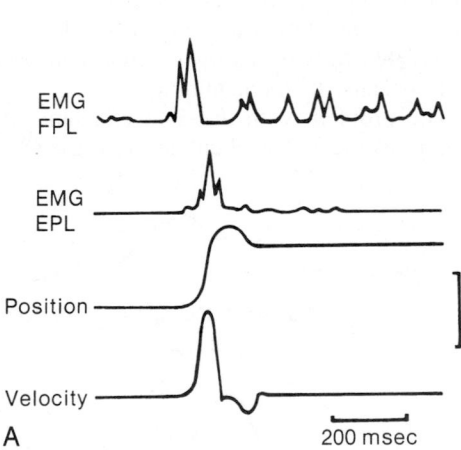

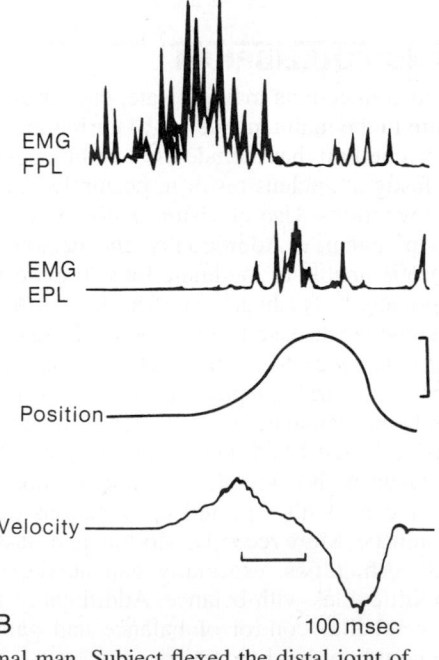

FIGURE 26-5 ■ **A,** Fast ballistic movements in a normal man. Subject flexed the distal joint of the thumb through 20 degrees. Records are, from top down, rectified EMG of flexor pollicis longus (*FPL*), rectified EMG of extensor pollicis longus (*EPL*), position, and velocity. Calibration is 200 ms and 20 μV, 27 degrees or 336 degrees/sec. **B,** Fast thumb flexion from a 62-year-old man with unilateral cerebellar ataxia resulting from stroke. Records from top down are ordered as in **A.** Calibration is 100 ms and 100 μV, 25 degrees or 313 degrees/sec. Note the slower movement, inability to hold final position, and prolonged bursts of activity in the agonist and antagonist muscle. (From Marsden CD et al: Disorders of movement in cerebellar disease in man. In Rose CF, editor: *Physiological aspects of clinical neurology,* Oxford, 1977, Blackwell Scientific.)

related to the amplitude of the movement or forces of deceleration, but probably does assist in checking the movement. The amplitude of the second agonist burst varies with accuracy of movements and might serve as a means of correction. The function of this second burst appears to be to dampen oscillations that might occur at the end of movement. This EMG pattern is a centrally programmed pattern; afferent inputs may modulate the activity but are not necessary for the activity. The study by Berardelli et al[52] showed that the cerebellum is important in the EMG bursts of voluntary movements and suggested that the cerebellum implemented the muscle force phasically. This may be related to the findings of Morton and Bastian,[5] which showed exaggerated movements to clear an obstacle when walking.

Agonist-antagonist-agonist EMG is lost with cooling (a transient lesion) of the interposed or dentate cerebellar nuclei.[53] Vilas and Hore[53] found that such lesions prevented anticipatory movements in response to perturbations. They concluded that the cerebellum operates in a feed-forward manner. Loss of feed-forward mechanisms would mean that the animal or person could only respond with slower, feedback responses. A lack of programmed deceleration was thought to be responsible for the overshoot of dysmetria and the oscillation around the end of a reaching movement. Multijoint movements were more affected than single-joint movements as control of the effects of movement of one segment on the other segments in a limb are lost. Movement of the shoulder, therefore, becomes separated from movement of the elbow.

Hallett et al[54,55] studied the sequence of muscle activation further. They found that when subjects with no motor impairments isometrically extend their elbows against a resistance and then are unexpectedly told to flex their elbows fast, activity in the triceps muscle ceases before the onset of the biceps activity. In subjects with cerebellar lesions, however, the triceps was continuously active, even during the biceps activity. This abnormal coactivation of the antagonists would lead to a delay in reversing resisted movement, and/or would produce an overshoot, or both. Abnormalities also are seen in the coordination of grip in the person with a cerebellar lesion.[27a] The client will use an abnormally high grip and appear to be unable to adjust the grip to the environmental or task-specific demands. When resistance abruptly ends the movement, the client demonstrates a longer latency before reacting. This is another example of improper regulation of the long-loop reflexes. Serrien and Wiesendager[27a] concluded that the cerebellum is involved in both proactive (as demonstrated above in the EMG recordings) and reactive mechanisms of movement.

In addition to the disruptions in force and extent of movement, the cerebellum has been implicated in the initiation and timing of movement. A person with a cerebellar lesion affecting the cerebropontocerebellum, the dentate nucleus, or both displays a delay in the initiation of movement and difficulty in movements that require bursts of speed. Therefore, rapidly alternating movements are severely impaired. This is referred to as *dysdiadokokinesia*.

Conrad and Brooks[56] temporarily cooled the dentate nucleus in monkeys who had been trained to perform fast-alternating flexion and extension of the ipsilateral elbow. Range of movement was limited by mechanical stops at the end of flexion and extension. During cooling, termination of the agonistic activity was delayed, but velocity or acceleration of motion was unaffected. For slower movements in which the spatial dimension of the movement was learned but not mechanically stopped, dentate cooling produced an overshoot or hypermetria, increased velocity, and acceleration of motion.[57] Cooling the interpositus nucleus in animals, on the other hand, leads to hypometria and decreased velocity of motion. Thus, circumscribed lesions of the cerebellum may cause different characteristics of dysmetria.[58] Specific research on human subjects is not available, but the assumption is that lesions similar to those studied in monkeys will cause similar symptoms in humans.

According to Brown et al,[59] the cerebellum has a coordinative role during oculomanual tracking tasks. When there is a lesion in the cerebellum, the patient takes longer to initiate purposeful limb movements on the affected side. When only the eyes are required to track a target, saccadic onset times are the same as those of individuals without cerebellar dysfunction. When initiation of eye and arm movements is coupled in the cerebellar patient, however, the initiation times are significantly prolonged. The cerebellum may be the center linking oculomotor and limb motor systems during a task requiring coordination of eye and limb movement.

MOVEMENT DECOMPOSITION

The person with a cerebellar lesion has difficulty performing a movement in one smooth pattern and may perform the movement in a sequence of steps. For example, if a client in supine position is asked to place a heel on the opposite knee, he or she may first raise the extended leg, then flex the knee, and finally lower the heel to knee. This breakdown in executing a movement as a whole is called *decomposition*.[60] Holmes[60] was the first to theorize that the cerebellum functions to sequence and time simple movements into one smooth, complex act. In the absence of this function, the movement becomes separated into individual components. Much investigation on the way in which the cerebellum acts to sequence movement has occurred since Holmes' time. Cooling the dentate nucleus will produce this decomposition in monkeys.[56]

Recent studies by Zackowski et al[31] investigated movement decomposition in humans with and without cerebellar disease. They measured reaching and grasp in isolation and combination. Their results indicated that those with cerebellar damage overestimated target size (similar to overestimating obstacle size). Patients with cerebellar dysfunction performed worse on isolated reach or grasp; however, on the combination movement they had deficits in the sequence of movements as well as the timing, especially of peak grip aperture. Interestingly, those in the patient group showed no decomposition in the fast-movement task compared to marked decomposition in the slow-movement task. On the other hand, the patient group did drop the target more often than controls and more often than in the slow-movement task. These researchers interpreted their findings to indicate that the cerebellum controls coupling of grasp and reach into a single motor program. The results of this study are not identical to those obtained in cooling parts of the cerebellum, but the human studies indicate that the cerebellum participates in multijoint movements and is involved in the organization of movement.

DYSDIADOCHOKINESIA

Many clients with cerebellar lesions are unable to perform rapidly alternating movements. This deficit can be demonstrated by having clients rapidly supinate and pronate their forearm or rapidly tap their hand on their knee. Compared with that of a person without a cerebellar lesion, the movement appears slow and quickly loses range and rhythm.

Holmes[48] attributed dysdiadochokinesia to an inability to stop ongoing movement rather than to a reduced velocity of motion. The use of EMG has revealed discrete, nonoverlapping bursts of antagonistic muscle activity during rapid, alternating movements in people with intact CNS.[61] In people with cerebellar lesions, however, antagonistic muscle activity typically overlaps, resulting in a braking action for movement, such that activities like brushing one's teeth or stirring food will become ineffective.

Dysdiadochokinesia is related to dysmetria, in that both result from the inappropriate timing of muscle activity. The inability to stop a goal-directed movement in one direction will be displayed as hypermetria, whereas the attempt to abruptly reverse the direction of movement will reveal dysdiadochokinesia.

In monkeys trained to perform rapid, rhythmic flexion and extension of the elbow, dentate cooling increased the duration of agonistic activity up to 0.1 to 0.2 seconds.[56] The onset of activity of the antagonist was delayed and often overlapped the activity of the agonist. No change in actual movement velocity was noted. Control of reciprocal motion by the cerebellum is also revealed by the observation that discharge of Purkinje cells in the intermediate zone of the cerebellum is related to reciprocal action of muscles. During cocontraction, these same Purkinje cells become inhibited.[62] If the cerebellum is damaged, such neural discharge patterns may not occur.

ATAXIA

Ataxia is one of the classic signs of cerebellar diseases. It appears in the trunk, extremities, head, mouth, and tongue (speech). As may be expected, multijoint and patterns of movement are more affected than single-joint movements. Most therapists have seen classic ataxia in the slurred speech and uncoordinated gait pattern of someone who is drunk.

In fact, ataxia is most often associated with disturbances of gait. Amici et al[63] found ataxic gait the most frequent symptom in their clients with cerebellar tumors. Gilman et al[64] likewise noted that 100 of 162 clients with cerebellar lesions displayed the phenomenon. The ataxic gait is one in which there is uneven step length, width is irregular, rhythm is absent, and the feet are often lifted too high. The individual cannot walk a straight line without lurching. The gait pattern becomes even more distorted by walking heel to toe, walking in a small circle, or walking backward. Arm swing is typically gone.

Gait may be altered without changes in limb movement, muscle tone, or equilibrium in some cases with late atrophy of the cerebellum or chronic severe alcoholism.[65,66] In these conditions the cortex of the anterior lobe of the cerebellum is selectively involved.

The cerebellum has anatomical connections that indicate that it can play a significant role in the generation of the pattern of locomotion. The cerebellum receives inputs from

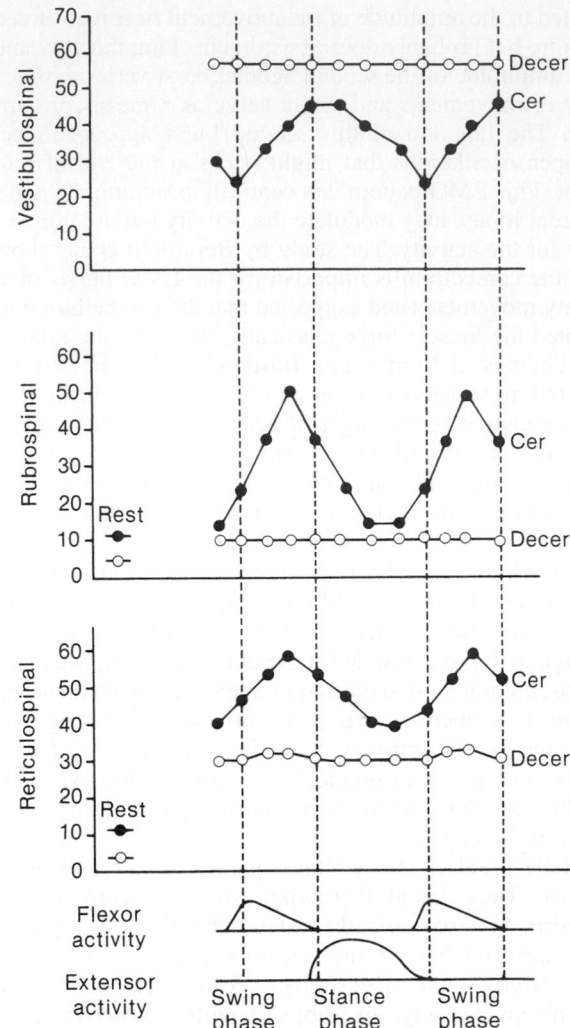

FIGURE 26-6 ■ Activity of descending tracts during locomotion. Mean values of the discharge rate of neurons of the vestibulospinal, rubrospinal, and reticulospinal tracts are plotted as a function of the hindlimb position (ipsilateral for vestibulospinal and reticulospinal tracts; contralateral for rubrospinal tract). Curves obtained in cats with the cerebellum intact (Cer) and those who have been decerebellated (Decer) are presented. A mean value of the resting discharge rate is also presented (Rest). Flexor and extensor activity is shown schematically. (From Orlovsky GN, Shik ML: Control of locomotion: a neurophysiological analysis of the cat locomotor system. In Porter R editors: *International review of physiology, neurophysiology II, vol 10,* Baltimore, 1976, University Park Press.)

the spinal cord relating to the locomotor pattern. The descending tracts, that is, rubrospinal, reticulospinal, and vestibulospinal, discharge in rhythm with swing and stance phases of gait.[67] After cerebellectomy, these rhythmic discharges disappear (Figure 26-6). In humans the clinical problem might be observed as a total disruption of the rhythm of gait: the stance and swing phase are totally irregular in duration, and the client cannot adjust for deviations in the surface on which he or she walks.

Gait disturbances can also occur as a result of incorrect programming of rate and force of muscle contraction, as in dysmetria. The inability to regulate posture will also decrease efficiency and smoothness of gait. Additionally, the lack of balance makes walking even more precarious.[4,5,8,17,68]

ASTHENIA

A lesion of the cerebellum can produce a condition of generalized weakness known as *asthenia*. Holmes[47] noted that, in people with traumatic unilateral injury to the cerebellum, muscle strength on the involved side of the body may be reduced by 50% when compared to the normal limb. Posture also may be poorly maintained in the client displaying asthenia. The clients complain of a sense of heaviness, excessive effort for simple tasks, and early onset of fatigue.[48] Asthenia is not as common as other symptoms accompanying cerebellar lesions. Amici et al[63] noted that the symptom occurred in only 10% of their clients with cerebellar tumors. Likewise, Gilman et al[64] noted it in only two of 162 clients with cerebellar lesions caused by a variety of problems.

The mechanism underlying asthenia is not clear. Hagbarth et al[69] performed an experiment that offered a possible model for cerebellar asthenia. They infiltrated lidocaine about the median nerve in subjects without CNS or motor dysfunction, producing weakness in the hand. Lidocaine blocks conduction in thin nerve fibers, including gamma motor neurons. During voluntary contraction, both alpha and gamma motor neurons to a muscle are normally coactivated. If the gamma motor neurons are blocked by lidocaine, an excitatory input to alpha motor neurons from muscle spindles will be reduced. Without the excitatory input from muscle spindles, the supraspinal drive to alpha motor neurons may have to increase to produce the voluntary movement. The normal perception of heaviness or force of effort is thought to be related to intensity of supraspinal signals required to produce the movement.[70] Thus any increase in the supraspinal drive to produce voluntary movement will be perceived as increased effort and fatigue, which is a common complaint in asthenic clients and one that can interfere with patient motivation (Case Study 26-1 at the end of the chapter).

A decrease in fusimotor activity is known to occur in cerebellar lesions and has been suggested as the mechanism for hypotonicity. Hypotonicity and asthenia, however, do not necessarily accompany one another. This suggests that although the conditions may share similar features, the mechanisms for them may not be identical.

Bremer[71] theorized that asthenia is caused by a loss of cerebellar facilitation to the motor cortex, which in turn could reduce the activity of spinal motor neurons during voluntary movement. A loss of facilitation of the cortex also has been suggested as a mechanism underlying hypotonicity. If loss of facilitation of the cerebral cortex is responsible for asthenia and hypotonicity, perhaps the areas of the cortex that are affected in asthenia and hypotonicity are not identical. Future research is required to untangle the similarities and differences of these two symptoms of cerebellar dysfunction.

TREMOR

People with cerebellar damage often display intention tremor, in which a hand oscillates back and forth as they try to touch their nose or the heel oscillates as they attempt to slide it down the opposite shin. The tremor has a frequency of 3 to 5 Hz and is typically enhanced during the termination of a goal-directed movement.[60]

Dentate dysfunction also influences oscillations that accompany voluntary movement. Normal movement is accompanied by very-low-amplitude oscillations, which are presumably the result of oscillating activity in long-loop feedback pathways. In monkeys performing a self-paced tracking task, dentate cooling causes a shift in the predominant peak of the power spectra of limb oscillation from 6 to 3 to 5 Hz.[72] As mentioned before, intention tremor in clients with cerebellar disease also has a frequency of 3 to 5 Hz. Thus, damage of the dentate nucleus could be involved in the generation of intention tremor. The slower oscillation of intention tremor might result from the time-consuming relay of sensory input to the motor cortex needed to modulate movement when the cerebellum no longer functions effectively.[53,73-75] A client with intention tremor may have trouble performing tasks requiring precision of limb placement and steadiness, such as drinking from a cup, placing a key in the door, or putting on makeup.

Another type of tremor may be seen when a person with cerebellar dysfunction is asked to maintain a posture, either to maintain position of the body as a whole or to hold an extremity against gravity. This type of tremor is referred to as postural tremor. For example a tremor may appear in an abducted arm but will disappear if support is provided at the axilla. The frequency of this oscillation is typically about 3 Hz, and both antagonistic muscles about a joint participate.[47,76,77] Postural tremor is an infrequent symptom, occurring in 9% (14 of 162 patients) studied by Gilman et al[64] and in 13.1% of patients studied by Amici et al.[63]

The mechanisms for postural tremor and intention tremor may not be identical. For example administration of L-dopa will relieve postural tremor but not intention tremor.[78] Also, the two tremors are not always coincident, postural tremor being much less common than intention tremor.[63,79] One possible mechanism for the postural tremor could be disruption of proprioceptive feedback loops. If the body shifts position, proprioceptors signal this change and, via a suprasegmental or long-loop pathway involving the cerebellum or another region in the brain, an automatic postural correction is made. When the limbs of a motorically normal person shift because of gravity, sensory input leads to a motor output that returns the limb automatically to the desired position. The motor output occurs in time to prevent a noticeable disruption of position. An oscillation can occur in this feedback system if there is a delay in the processing of sensory input or motor output because of a lesion, a disruption in the compensatory role of the cerebellum.

Mauritz et al[80] electrically stimulated the tibial nerve to excite muscle spindle afferent fibers and evoke segmental and suprasegmental stretch reflexes. They found that persons with postural tremor had delayed long-loop reflexes. Postural tremor was also produced by this stimulation technique in persons with incipient degenerative cerebellar disease. Marsden et al[81] also found disruption in the long-loop reflexes in those with cerebellar disease. In their experiments, clients with cerebellar disease displayed the early stretch reflex at the same latency as people without cerebellar disease; however, only one (instead of two) late response occurred with a long latency of 80 msec.

Postural tremor also may be explained by another hypothesis. Sensory feedback systems, which operate over supraspinal as well as spinal pathways, all oscillate, even in a normal person. For example, the spinal stretch reflex pathway oscillates at 8 to 12 Hz, the corticospinal pathway has an oscillation of 3 to 5 Hz, and the transcerebellar pathway has an oscillation of 4 to 6 Hz. In spite of these potentially oscillating circuits, a healthy person displays no visually obvious tremor, because none of the feedback pathways operate in isolation from the others. By acting together, these multiple pathways effectively dampen one another's oscillation so that little oscillation is actually expressed. If one of these multiple reflex pathways is absent or delayed, however, a noticeable oscillation of the body or limbs may occur. If the transcerebellar reflex path is absent, the spinal reflex path is ineffective in dampening the low frequency oscillation (3 to 5 Hz) induced by the corticospinal pathway.[82] Thus the body will tend to oscillate at the low frequency–that of postural tremor. This explanation is analogous to the ability of the cerebellum to adjust to the forces of movement in multiple joint segments so that smooth movement is produced.

Clients with postural tremor display the tremor only when attempting to hold a fixed position, not necessarily all the time. Any limb displays a mechanical oscillation, similar to that of a metal spring or tuning fork when perturbed. When a limb or joint changes in stiffness, as from relaxation to an attempt at stabilization against gravity, its properties of mechanical oscillation also change. The mechanical oscillations of a stabilized limb may actually reinforce the low-frequency oscillation of the limb in a client with cerebellar disease and lead to a noticeable postural tremor, but not necessarily a movement tremor.

SPEECH

Cerebellar lesions also disturb speech, which is a complex motor function. Grammar or word selection is not altered, but the melodic quality and the rhythm of speech are changed. The resultant disturbance is called *dysarthria*. Words or syllables are pronounced slowly, accents are misplaced, and pauses may be inappropriately short or long.[83] Lechtenberg and Gilman[84] noted that 19% of 162 clients with various cerebellar lesions developed dysarthria, and Amici et al[63] found dysarthria in 8.5% of a large population of clients with cerebellar tumors. Clients also may display explosive speech or staccato speech.[85] The voice can become invariant in pitch and loudness, tremulous, nasal, or soft.[47,86,87]

The mechanisms responsible for dysarthria are most likely similar to those producing dysmetria of the limbs. For example, inability of muscles of the larynx to initiate or stop contractions quickly or hypotonicity of the larynx could produce a slurring in the pronunciation of consonants and vowels, slow speech, prolonged pauses, or uneven stress on syllables.[86,88] Hypotonicity of the larynx may also be responsible for the inability to increase loudness or vary pitch of the voice.

Attempts to localize areas of speech function in the cerebellum have revealed a relatively high incidence of dysarthria in clients with damage in the left cerebellar hemisphere.[84] The left cerebellar hemisphere is influenced by the right (nondominant) cerebral hemisphere, which has among its functions perception of melodies, tone, and rhythm.[89,90]

If the left cerebellum plays a role in the melodic production of speech, input from the nondominant cerebral hemisphere seems appropriate in the context of this task.

CONTROL OF EYE MOVEMENTS AND GAZE

Although most physical and occupational therapists are not expected to treat deviations of eye movement, they will see a relatively high frequency of such problems in clients with cerebellar lesions stemming from tumors, head injuries, brain stem strokes, and specific cerebellar injury. An awareness of the variety of problems and the underlying mechanisms should be helpful in interacting with a client who displays such phenomena. Just like posture of the limbs, the resting position of the eyes is affected by cerebellar dysfunction. After an acute lesion of a cerebellar hemisphere, both eyes deviate toward the contralateral side.[23,91] After cerebellar lesions, the eyes display some of the same characteristics as seen in the extremities and the speech apparatus, in this case called *ocular dysmetria*. The client with a cerebellar lesion is unable to move the eyes accurately to a target in the periphery. When persons with normal control of the eyes direct their gaze toward an object in the periphery, their eyes move in a rapid step called a *saccade*. The amplitude of the saccade must be accurate to place the intended image on the fovea of the retina. After cerebellar damage, the saccadic movement of the eyes can become too large or too small, and corrective saccades will have to be made, resulting in ocular dysmetria.[68,92,93] Ocular dysmetria is related to the initial position of the eyes, such that hypermetria occurs when the eyes are eccentric to the target and hypometria occurs when the eyes move from neutral to a peripheral target.

Ocular dysmetria also can occur with pursuit movements of the eyes. When an individual with normal cerebellar control follows a slowly moving object, the eyes move in a smooth, continuous fashion but will stop abruptly if the object stops moving. However, if a client with cerebellar dysfunction visually pursues an object, the eyes may move only in saccades and will continue to move after the object stops.[94-96] Clients are also unable to initiate conjugate eye movement and must accomplish lateral gaze by vigorous head movements.[97] Normal subjects can shift their eyes 30 degrees without accompanying head motion, but clients with cerebellar dysfunction typically move their heads within the first 30 degrees of eye movement. This is clearly seen in a degenerative disease of the cerebellum called *ataxia telangiectasia*.[5]

The posterior vermis, that is, the flocculus and the paraflocculus and the fastigial nucleus, are involved in control of accuracy of saccades and to saccade adaptation. If either of these areas is lesioned, there is an initial hypometria in some directions, which does recover over time. However, individual saccades are less precise than before the lesion and rapid saccade adaptation is permanently lost. Without such adaptation, repetition of the same saccade results in a slow, continuous reduction in the size of the eye movement. This latter decrease in saccade size is important to consistent visual function without fatigue This adaptation allows an individual to pursue objects visually late in the day with the same precision as early in the day.[49]

Neurons that discharge before a saccade have been located in the thalamus, cerebellum, vestibular nuclei, superior colliculus, pontine reticular formation, and mesencephalic aqueductal gray matter. However, the area of the brain that appears primarily responsible for the generation of the saccades is the pontine paramedian reticular formation, because specific lesions at this region will produce permanent loss of saccadic eye movement.[98] Damage to this region disrupts the rapid phases of both vestibular and optokinetic nystagmus. Although the cerebellum does not initiate saccades, it does influence their accuracy. To initiate saccades, the neurons in the pontine reticular formation send a burst of activity to the motor neurons of the extraocular muscles. This burst is believed to code the difference in the visual target position and the actual eye position at the start of the saccade. Thus, for this burst to move the eye to the exact location needed, the pontine reticular formation must have accurate estimates of the starting position of the eye as well as any other short-term or long-term changes in the eye and its muscles because of fatigue, injury, or aging. The cerebellum appears to provide this feedback to the saccadic pulse generator in the brain stem.[99]

Another common disturbance in eye movement is gaze-evoked nystagmus.[97] As the eyes move voluntarily to gaze at an object in the periphery, they move quickly in the intended direction and then drift involuntarily to neutral. The sequence is repeated as long as the effort is sustained to keep the gaze deviated toward the periphery. Clients with cerebellar atrophy may display a permanent gaze-evoked nystagmus bilaterally, whereas those with an acute unilateral lesion may display nystagmus temporarily to the ipsilateral side.[100] A rebound nystagmus often appears if gaze deviation is maintained 20 seconds or longer. The nystagmus then occurs briefly in a direction opposite to the prior gaze when the eyes are voluntarily returned to neutral.[101]

Gaze-evoked nystagmus has been explained by the loss of a holding function provided by the cerebellum. When the eyes are held steady at the end of a normal saccade, the discharge of motor neurons innervating the extraocular muscles is proportional to the position of the eyes in the head. However, the sensory systems that influence eye position transmit signals of velocity. For example, the semicircular canals detect velocity of head movement and the retina detects the velocity of the image moving across it. These signals must undergo a "mathematical" integration to code position rather than velocity. This process of neurointegration does not appear to occur in the cerebellum and is believed to occur in the brain stem[102]; however, the cerebellum is essential for the normal integration of the velocity signals. If the cerebellum is damaged, the integration undergoes a rapid decay, which is reflected in poor maintenance of eye position. Thus the cerebellum is necessary to sustain or boost the output of the brain stem integrator of sensory signals influencing eye position.[103] The appearance of gaze-evoked nystagmus does not correlate with a specific cerebellar lesion in humans, although nystagmus occurring with downward gaze is particularly common in clients with the Arnold-Chiari malformation (refer to Chapter 18).[104] In addition, removal of the flocculus and paraflocculus in monkeys leads to a serious defect in the ability to sustain gaze in any direction.[103]

Cerebellar lesions also distort the vestibuloocular reflexes movements, as well as voluntary movements of the eyes. These reflexes are crucial to maintaining an accurate visual image during head movement. The sensitivity of the vestibuloocular reflex can be calculated by a ratio of eye velocity to head velocity. Although the sensitivity of the reflex is not universally altered in clients with cerebellar lesions, in such problems as the Arnold-Chiari syndrome and spinocerebellar degeneration, the ratio can exceed that of individuals without cerebellar lesions.[98,105]

The amplitude of the vestibulo-ocular reflex will adapt to changes in internal or external conditions. Unilateral damage to the vestibular apparatus results in spontaneous nystagmus toward the damaged side, which typically disappears in a few weeks.[106] For example if one moves the head and the object simultaneously, the vestibulo-ocular reflex nearly disappears in the person without a cerebellar lesion.[105] These adaptations are lost if the cerebellum is damaged.

When a person without movement dysfunction watches stripes on a revolving drum moving horizontally or vertically, nystagmus develops in which the eyes snap quickly (fast phase) in the direction opposite to that of the revolving drum. The eyes then drift back slowly (slow phase) and the sequence is repeated. This phenomenon is called optokinetic nystagmus. In acute lesions of the cerebellum, the amplitude of the optokinetic nystagmus is often decreased, whereas in chronic problems, the amplitude of both phases or just one of the phases of optokinetic nystagmus is often increased.[64]

Distortions of optokinetic nystagmus may be a result of disruption in the cerebellar systems, which control either smooth pursuit or saccadic movement of the eyes. For example, a client may display a loss of smooth pursuit movement and a disturbance of the slow phase of optokinetic nystagmus. Presumably, the cerebellar mechanisms responsible for these two features of eye movement are the same. Similarly, saccadic eye movement may be distorted as well as the fast phase of optokinetic nystagmus.

As might be expected, the client with a cerebellar lesion may complain of visual defects. These defects include blurred vision, diplopia, loss of perspective, and difficulty seeing when his or her body is in motion.[104,105] While these deficits are characteristic of cerebellar lesions, they also appear in lesions affecting the extraocular muscles or the vestibular system or connections between these areas.

RECOVERY FROM CEREBELLAR LESIONS

After a brain lesion, there is always some level of spontaneous recovery of compensation; the level depends on the severity and pathophysiological cause of the lesion and its location. For cerebrovascular accidents and head trauma, therapists do have some published guidelines for recovery patterns to which they can refer; however, such information has not been well documented for cerebellar lesions. For this reason, this chapter cannot provide a complete description of recovery patterns after cerebellar damage. Further, disruption of the cerebellum can occur in a variety of circumstances. The cerebellum can be lesioned as a result of a cardiovascular accident (CVA) or head trauma; it may be involved in degenerative diseases, such as multiple sclerosis or a variety of inherited disorders. The cerebellum is also a site for brain tumors. Lastly, the cerebellum may be damaged from many toxins, such as alcohol or environmental contaminants. Nonetheless, it is hoped that the information presented will provide therapists with some clarifying expectations for their clients.

Various investigators have attempted to study the recovery patterns that follow cerebellar damage with animal models.[106] Poirier et al[107] observed the motor behavior of monkeys for up to 1 year after various surgical lesions had been placed in the cerebellum. The most severe problems resulted from total cerebellectomy and included truncal ataxia, dysmetria of the limbs, hypotonicity, and postural tremor. These problems decreased in severity over the first 4 weeks after surgery, but improvement then reached a plateau. The animal was still severely compromised, dysmetria and postural tremor being the least obvious of the above symptoms. Goldberger and Growdon[108] bilaterally lesioned the dentate and interpositus nucleus in monkeys. The animals displayed gross oscillations of the limbs at a frequency of two per second, hypermetria of the limb, and primitive movement locomotion during the first 2 weeks. As the animals improved over the next 50 weeks, the limbs developed a smaller and faster amplitude tremor of 6 to 8 Hz and a marked improvement in gait and accuracy of movement of the extremities. In contrast, if only one cerebellar hemisphere is damaged with no nuclear involvement in a primate, the animal displays ipsilateral dysmetria, postural tremor, and awkward leaping gait for the first 1 to 2 weeks and becomes essentially normal over the next 2 months. If the midline structure of the cerebellum is involved, the animal's chief problem is truncal ataxia, which improves over the first 3 to 5 months, but the movement dysfunction never totally disappears. Therefore from animal work it appears that recovery is poor from a total cerebellectomy; a bilateral lesion is more devastating than a unilateral lesion; damage to the deep cerebellar nuclei is more serious than that to the cortex; and spontaneous compensation will be complete within 6 months to a year.

Although one cannot assume that humans will respond to acute cerebellar injury exactly as primates do, the information provided by animal work does indeed provide a general framework for humans. A feature of cerebellar lesions that cannot be readily studied in animals is the effect of a degenerative disease or an expanding tumor. If a client has a degenerative cerebellar disease or a tumor, the developing symptoms are generally milder than those produced by the same damage occurring acutely. Thus compensation appears to be concurrent with a steadily progressing lesion.

If compensation for a cerebellar lesion is possible, what other neurological structures are necessary for the compensation to take place? If the cerebellum is not totally destroyed, some available adaptation for the movement distortions may occur because of the remainder of the cerebellum. Evidence for this is the observation that compensation for a cerebellar lesion will be disrupted by a second lesion in which deficits are more serious than those that have occurred if the second lesion had been produced alone.[63] The motor cortex is also considered to be an essential structure upon which compensation for a cerebellar lesion depends.[52] On the other hand, there is recent evidence that there may be little compensation for the movement disorders after cerebellar dysfunction.[28,29]

EVALUATION AND GOALS

As for any neurologically involved client, the primary goal of therapy is to make the client as functional as possible under conditions of maximum safety, reasonable energy cost to the client, and cosmesis. In deciding how to achieve this goal, a therapist has to decide what basic functions the client cannot achieve and specific reasons why. Similarly, the therapist needs to work closely with the patient and family to determine the specific functional goals they see as important. Evaluation of a client with a cerebellar lesion therefore should include, but not be limited to an initial determination of basic functional capabilities such as the following:

■ Bed mobility and posture
■ Ability to sit up from a reclining position
■ Maintenance of sitting posture on surfaces normally used by the client
■ Ability to stand up from a sitting position and transfer to and from a commode as if the person was within the home environment.
■ Maintenance of standing posture
■ Ambulation and the environment within which the person will ambulate.
■ Ability to dress, groom, and eat as normal daily living activities

Description of performance can include assistance needed, level of effort involved, time to complete the activity, potential hazards to the client, and unusual accompanying movements or noticeable features unique to that client.

The International Cooperative Ataxia Rating Scale (ICARS) may be useful in the evaluation of the patient with cerebellar disease. This scale so far is used more in research studies than in the clinic, but does provide a consistent, organized way to demonstrate changes in patient function and motor control. The scale measures ataxia in four categories of movement: posture and gait, limb kinetics, speech, and eye movements.[109] There are 100 points on an ordinal scale and the higher the score the greater the impairment or limitation in functional.

The evaluation should include the patient's goals of treatment, the living situation as well as the likely progression. A thoughtful process of linking the movement disorders present with the tests are presented in Table 26-1. Both sides of the body need to be examined even if a unilateral cerebellar lesion has been diagnosed. Although therapists are not expected to provide detailed evaluations of eye movement or speech, brief notations of obvious distortions may help clarify the total problem facing the client and determine a need for referral. If the client has multiple sites of brain involvement, the symptoms caused by cerebellar damage may be masked by spasticity or sensory loss, and tests for these additional CNS problems will need to be added. The presence of an inherited disorder increases the likelihood of multisystem involvement.

The cerebellar movement disorders the client displays will help the therapist decide why any of the basic functions cannot be performed. The therapist can then select the therapeutic activities that would best correct the movement disorder, thereby improving the client's functional behavior. For example if an individual is hypotonic, her or his resting posture while reclining, sitting, and standing will be changed. The treatment for such a client would need to include activities that enhance tone of antigravity muscles. If asthenia exists, postural stability and ambulation will be affected; the patient's perceived perception of effort will affect compliance with a home program. Resistive exercises

TABLE 26-1 ■ Assessment of Movement Disorders

	SPECIFIC TESTS	POSITIVE
HYPOTONICITY	1. Muscle palpation	1. Reduced firmness
	2. Deep tendon reflexes	2. Pendular
	3. Passive shaking of limbs	3. Limbs move through greater arc of motion than does normal limb
	4. Wet footprint	4. Print broader on involved side
	5. Hold object while conversing	5. Drops object when distracted
	6. Voluntary flexion and extension of knee or elbow supported and unsupported	6. Ataxic when unsupported; controlled when supported
	7. Flex one finger only	7. All fingers flex
Observation	1. Resting posture	1. Slack, asymmetrical
ASTHENIA	1. Maintain arm(s) in 90-degree position of flexion or abduction	1. Arm(s) tire quickly
	2. Maximal resisted muscle contraction for major muscle groups	2. Weaker on involved side or unable to work against resistance, which is normal for size and age
	3. Repeat submaximal muscle contractions, such as rising on toes, pushups, squeezing tennis ball	3. Tires quickly
Observation	1. Everyday activities	1. Tires easily, complains of heaviness
BALANCE AND POSTURAL CONTROL	1. Hold limb against pull of gravity	1. Postural tremor
	2. Nudge client unexpectedly when sitting or standing	2. Loses balance easily
	3. Stand on one foot or walk backward	3. Loses balance easily
Observation	1. Standing posture	1. Feet apart, trunk flexed slightly, needs to hold for stability, postural tremor of legs
DYSMETRIA	1. Flex arms to 90-degree position, quickly elevate overhead, and then return to 90-degree position	1. Not able to resume 90-degree position without initial error
	2. Put peg in a hole, trace circle with pencil, trace circle on floor with big toe, slide heel down shin slowly, place feet on markers when walking	2. Intention tremor; undershoots, or overshoots target
	3. Therapist resists client's elbow flexion and releases unexpectedly	3. Arm rebounds
	4. Voluntarily flex and extend knee or elbow in supported and unsupported position	4. Limb ataxic whether supported or not
	5. Submaximal isometric effort against force transducer	5. Onset and release of force of involved limb delayed
	6. Electromyogram of antagonistic pair of muscles during ballistic contraction	6. Duration of triphasic pattern longer than 300 ms
GAIT DISTURBANCE	1. March to cadence	1. Unable to follow rhythm
	2. Walk on heels or toes	2. Loses balance and rhythm
	3. Walk clockwise and counterclockwise	3. Stumbles in one direction
	4. Walk on uneven ground	4. Cannot compensate and stumbles
Observation	1. Typical gait pattern	1. Slow, stumbles easily, not rhythmical, step length and height irregular
DYSDIADOCHOKINESIA	1. Tap hand on knee or toes on floor	1. Rapidly loses rhythm and range
	2. Walk as fast as possible	2. Gait becomes impaired only when fast
Observation	1. Activities of daily living	1. Unable to brush teeth, stir food, shake salt shaker
MOVEMENT DECOMPOSITION	1. Supine client touches heel to opposite knee	1. Movement broken up into separate phases, does not flow
Observation	1. Typical movement	1. Activity appears as if in slow motion, mechanical like a puppet

to antigravity muscles may improve such a client's posture and endurance in ambulation, but care must be taken to think about time of day for activities and duration of exercise, especially at the beginning. If a client does not display hypotonicity or asthenia but still has poor postural stability, dysmetria may be the major problem. In this situation the client needs many sessions of practice in the precise posturing of the trunk, upper extremities, or legs in an attempt to make posture an automatic function or, second best, a consciously controlled function. If a client displays gait disturbances but does not have dysmetria, hypotonicity, or asthenia, the cerebellar motor program for gait and balance may have been selectively disturbed and attention in therapy will need to be directed only toward gait. However, if dysmetria of isolated movements in the limbs is present along with gait abnormalities, selected coordination exercises for the extremities as well as gait training should be implemented. Inability to dress, feed, or groom oneself effectively may be caused by hypotonicity, dysmetria, or asthenia, but may also be specifically caused by movement discomposition or dysdiadochokinesia. The predominant distortion will need to become the focus of treatment.

Identification of both the intact and limited functional movement activities is critical in assisting the therapist to recognize specific impairments within the various systems. Given these functional movement diagnoses, prognosis of outcome can be estimated based on disease stability, area of anatomical lesions and potential for plasticity, motivation of the patient and family support, and the therapist's understanding and skill in creating the best environment to empower the patient to regain function.

INTERVENTION

The program described in this section is for the client with a relatively severe but stabilized lesion of the cerebellum, such as might be produced by trauma, cerebrovascular accident, or a tumor that has been surgically removed. Many parts of the program, however, could be used to help maintain function of the client with degenerative cerebellar disease or multiple sclerosis affecting the cerebellum of cerebellar pathways. The reader should be aware that the success of any of the following activities has not been well documented and that at present there is no "best treatment" based upon studies of effectiveness or efficacy. Thus the interventions presented are to be taken only as ideas for obtaining selective goals. The reader must always remember that for any chance of successful recovery, the client with cerebellar disorders, from whatever pathology, requires many, many repetitions of a task and task sequence.[110] This is true for execution of both slow movements and rapid movements. A recent study showed that the client with cerebellar degeneration demonstrated good retention of an acquired skill and improved at a faster rate in subsequent sessions than on the first day of training. Thus, Topka et al[110] concluded that clients with cerebellar degeneration can indeed learn to perform slow movements in a near-normal manner, although they may have more difficulty learning fast movements. They hypothesized that the difficulty was with refinement of the movement. On the other hand, recent investigations of Bastian and her colleagues[8,29,30,36] question this hypothesis, as they found that there was disordered movement in both fast and slow movements and that the

cause of the movement disruption might be different for fast and slow movements.

It is also important that complex motor skills involving movement of more than one joint be presented in treatment sessions. Isaacs et al[111] demonstrated that complex motor tasks increased the volume of parallel fiber input to the Purkinje cell. There was a concomitant increase in blood vessel supply and mitochondria to maintain this increase in volume. Klintsova et al[51] trained rats on complex motor tasks following neonatal alcohol exposure and compared them to rats who had the same alcohol exposure but were allowed to run or were sedentary. The rats given "rehabilitation" showed significant improvement in tests of motor skills and this was accompanied by an increase in parallel fiber synapses in the Purkinje cells in the paramedian area. The complex motor skills used included tasks demanding balance responses and coordination of the limbs. The use of complex motor tasks during treatment can be used in cerebellar rehabilitation. Several goals toward which a therapist can work with a client having a cerebellar lesion are (1) postural stability, (2) balance, (3) functional gait including clearance of obstacles, and (4) accuracy of limb movement incorporating placement of both upper and lower extremities when performing all functional activities.

Head and Trunk Control

A client with postural instability needs to be assisted in maintaining posture in all activities in which that person engages. In other words, if the patient needs to sit for many activities, then that individual needs to practice sitting. There is no evidence regarding the sequence of obtaining postural stability (i.e., prone to all fours to sitting to standing), but learning to sit on noncompliant surfaces versus compliant surfaces requires the cerebellum to process more proprioceptive input in the former and more vestibular input in the latter. Thus the therapist needs to determine both the processing skill of the client and the environment within which he or she will need to sit. Stretch reflex activation may be used to increase muscle contraction in the initial phases of treatment[112]; however, eventually the patient needs to be able to maintain muscle contraction in the core trunk muscles independently. Thera-band is a good adjunct to treatment that can be used to maintain resistance and joint approximation. Additional information on increasing head and trunk control are presented in Chapters 9, 12, and 17.

Biofeedback might be tried in an attempt to promote upright head position in the severely involved client. For example, the client could wear a helmet that provides a visual and auditory clue when the vertical position of the head is not maintained.[113]

Sitting Balance

When clients can hold their heads up and have had some trunk control in a static position, they need to be offered progressive challenges to sitting balance. Early on, this may include treatment on the edge of the mat table or in a chair without back or arm support. Joint approximation has been used traditionally to promote trunk stability, but more research is needed on the effectiveness of these methods in the patient with cerebellar dysfunction. Likewise, rhythmic stabilization for trunk rotation may be used to help a client sustain contraction of the trunk muscles. In this situation

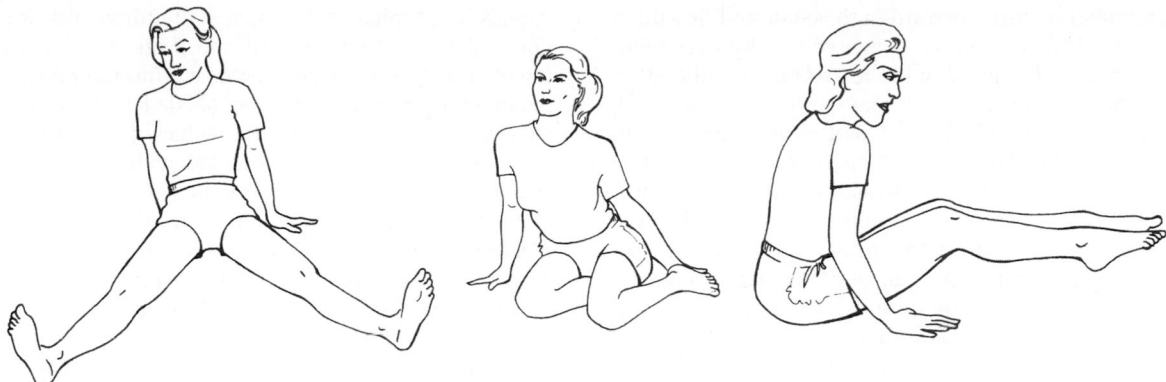

FIGURE 26-7 ■ Alternate positions in sitting to promote control of posture and balance.

rhythmic stabilization is provided not to increase strength but to give clients the sensation of stability, which they can then attempt alone. If clients cannot sustain a contraction requiring coactivation of the trunk muscles, a pattern of slow-reversal-hold over a steadily decreasing range of trunk rotation might be attempted instead.[114] Therapists can also help clients control balance by joining hands with them and having them meet a gentle resistance through their extended arms. Push-pull activities with hands joined or with a cane or pole are helpful as well in promoting coactivation needed for stability. A therapeutic ball also is a good activity as the client progresses. Gentle bouncing on the ball may promote activity in the small trunk extensors while helping the client regain an awareness of vertical.

Clients next need to practice weight shift in all directions while sitting. This can first be practiced with clients using both hands for support, progressing to no support from their hands. Clients also should try to sustain balance with their arms overhead and the trunk rotated, because this position will be used in activities of daily living. Although not essential, clients can be provided with practice in maintaining different sitting positions (Figure 26-7).[29] In all cases, the patient's lifestyle will provide information on what is functional for the patient. Given the evidence that there is little ability to generalize from one activity to another or to be able to shift focus,[29] functional activities are essential in the treatment setting. The more closely the treatment activities mirror the patient's life, the more likely the treatment will be successful.[115]

Rising from Supine or Prone Position to Sitting

At the same time the client has control of sitting balance, work on safe and efficient ways of moving from the lying to the sitting position will be necessary. The sequence(s) used will depend upon the way the patient sleeps as well as the client's weight, side of involvement, underlying muscle strength, age, and comorbid conditions. Ideally, the patient should be provided with a variety of ideas for rising from the bed; however, based upon the current literature indicating difficulty in adjusting to even a difference in ball weight, the patient should be provided with an optimum method for his lifestyle. Methods for rising from the floor should he fall can also be practiced with lying to sitting.

Independent Transfers between Various Sitting Structures

If clients have adequate sitting balance but are not considered candidates for safe ambulation, they should be taught as many independent transfers as possible. Transfers can be taught with the caregiver to increase follow-through and safety at home. A sliding transfer from a wheelchair to another chair or bed will be the safest. Swivel sliding boards may assist the caregiver for transfers in and out of a car. A trapeze over a bed or bars in the bath may increase the level of independence if the accuracy of limb movements allows such activity.

Preparing for Ambulation

If the goal is to progress clients toward ambulation, a series of preliminary activities would be beneficial before they attempt to stand. These activities may include exercises such as bridging. The patient may practice transferring from sit to stand many times through the day. A simple way to increase strength and practice in this activity is to have the patient stand after sitting one to five times every time she or he sits down or stands (except for when the patient is transferring to the toilet for hygiene. Moving from sit to stand and stand to sit can be increased by having patients use their hands on the table (before and after meals) or with the use of a walker or wheelchair if there is a need for using these assistive devices. Most adults are only on all fours when they fall; prone to stand using quadruped as an intermediate step may be practiced after the functional movements of sit-to-stand-to-sit. If the force generated when coming to stand from sit is exaggerated or disproportional, then a patient can be first placed in standing and asked to practice eccentrically lowering toward sit and then returning to stand. As control is reassumed, the client can lower farther toward sitting but needs to practice with control. Once stand to sit can be achieved smoothly, then the patient should be able to come to standing from sitting with the same integration.

If a client has been in a wheelchair or has been in bed for a long time, the therapist may need to prepare the person's cardiovascular system for being upright by placing him or her on a tilt table. Standing activities may be started in the parallel bars. Clients may not be able to assume a standing position without help. When standing up from sitting, clients need to remember to slide forward in the chair and flex their trunks considerably, placing the center of gravity over their feet. The trunk and legs should be extended only after gaining balance on the feet. This may be the most difficult step for an ataxic individual, who will either lean too far forward or extend the trunk too early and drop back into the chair. Another method of coming to stand early in a patient's recovery process is to place a medium or larger ball on a high/low table or mat. Have the patient place his or her arms over the ball. The therapist can assist both in placement of the arms as well as coming to stand while relaxing over the ball. The high/low mat can then be raised, which will bring the client to standing in a relaxed fashion. Once standing, a stand-to-sit pattern can be practiced with and without high/low mat assistance. Regardless of the starting point for coming to a standing position, the client will require a large amount of repetition as well as verbal feedback from the therapist. In addition to verbal feedback, viewing a videotape may help a client recognize and correct mistakes.

Once upright, the person should practice balancing, which can be reinforced by approximation through the hips and shoulders. Weights have been used to increase stability in standing and walking, although this has become controversial. A study by Widener indicated that small weights carefully placed for the individual was effective in improving standing balance[116]; others have stated that they are ineffective. The use of weights and the carryover when weights are removed will require more careful investigation and may, indeed, be patient or disease specific. The clinician must analyze whether the weights are increasing joint approximation in a closed chain or increasing joint distraction in an open chain. Closed chain enhancement may help the cerebellum, while open-chair distraction may increase the imbalance between agonist and antagonist during a movement pattern.

Rhythmic stabilization applied to rotation of the trunk also may be valuable in gaining stability. Further, biofeedback from a force platform may help the person control the center of gravity. It is hoped that the client can learn to come to and maintain standing without pulling on the bars; however, for some people this will be impossible. Those individuals who rely on the bars will not become independent in ambulation but may, with the assistance of another person or an assistive device, be able to get up and walk. Once standing and stable, the client needs to practice walking on a level surface, as well as walking over obstacles and uneven surfaces to be considered as functionally independent in ambulation.

Ambulation

When the person begins to walk within the parallel bars, he or she will need precise verbal feedback as to step length, body rotation, accessory movements, and trunk position. Sometimes, ambulation over the rungs of a ladder or lines on the floor can be used to increase visual cues and feedback regarding foot placement. As in the initial learning of a sport, the therapist will need to isolate one problem at a time and provide practice. When the person is ready to walk outside of the parallel bars, a decision will need to be made about an ambulatory aid. Aids, which may be necessary, may also be an obstacle because clients will now need to control position and movement of the device as well as themselves.

A walker is typically the most stable; however, it can be so only when all four legs of the walker are placed down together and at a correct distance from the body. For some patients, a visual cue will be needed to prevent the client from walking too far into the walker and falling backward. For many clients, a four-wheeled walker may be easier to manipulate than other walkers; this type of walker does not need to be lifted, just pushed forward like a grocery cart with which the patient is already familiar. Crutches or canes may be used but require reciprocal movement of the arms and legs with appropriate timing and placement; this too can be hard or impossible for some clients. The person may actually do better using a walking stick(s) for support rather than the typical cane or crutches. Therapists can measure a client's progress in ambulation by the number of times the client loses his or her balance in a treatment session, frequency of a specific error, the distance ambulated, or the level of assistance needed (see Chapters 17 and 23 for additional suggestions).

Activities for Temporary Reduction of Dysmetria

Clients with cerebellar lesions will be frustrated in many activities by the presence of dysmetria. A therapist attempting to modify this impairment needs to recognize that no therapeutic procedure will totally eliminate dysmetria; however, before clients practice specific functional activities, the therapist can have them perform activities that will temporarily decrease dysmetria. For example, use of proprioceptive neuromuscular facilitation (PNF) patterns of rhythmical stabilization or slow-reversal-hold for the lower extremities will allow clients to ambulate with better control.[117,118] Similarly, functional tasks involving the arms can be preceded by PNF patterns for the arms.[119] Frenkel's exercises, though old, are sometimes effective for some patients.[120] These exercises can be performed in the supine, sitting, or standing positions. Each activity is to be performed slowly, with the client watching the extremity carefully. When the client has gained reasonable control of one activity, she or he should proceed to the next. In a prescribed list of exercises such as Frenkel's (Box 26-1), the patient starts with moving a limb with support, to moving without support at one joint of a limb, to moving the limb as a whole.

The use of EMG or goniometrical biofeedback also may assist the client in receiving training in specific acts. For example, brushing the teeth may be impossible because the toothbrush misses the mouth or hits the teeth and once inside the mouth does not effectively clean the teeth. EMG feedback from the deltoids, biceps, wrist flexors and extensors, or goniometrical position of the shoulder and elbow may be relayed to clients as they try to learn a pattern that works for them or to duplicate the pattern of signals produced by individuals with normal motor control when brushing their teeth. Again, there is no research to indicate or refute the effectiveness or efficacy of this procedure. Weights have been used to decrease dysmetria; however, there is no evidence that they will increase skill of movement when they are removed.

ALCOHOLISM

One metabolic problem that specifically attacks the cerebellum warrants in-depth consideration: this is the

BOX 26-1 ■ FRENKEL EXERCISES

SUPINE

1. Flex and extend one leg, heel sliding down a straight line on table.
2. Abduct and adduct hip smoothly with knee bent, heel on table.
3. Abduct and adduct leg with knee and hip extended, leg sliding on table.
4. Flex and extend hip and knee with heel off table.
5. Place one heel on knee of opposite leg and slide heel smoothly down shin toward ankle and back to knee.
6. Flex and extend both legs together, heels sliding on table.
7. Flex one leg while extending other leg.
8. Flex and extend one leg while abducting and adducting other leg.

SITTING

1. Place foot in therapist's hand, which will change position on each trial.
2. Raise leg and put foot on traced footprint on floor.
3. Sit steady for a few minutes.
4. Rise and sit with knees together.

STANDING

1. Place foot forward and backward on a straight line.
2. Walk along a winding strip.
3. Walk between two parallel lines.
4. Walk, placing each foot in a tracing on floor.

drug-induced neurological disorder that arises from over-ingesting alcohol. Movement disorders involve the effects on the CNS of both alcohol and the nutritional deficiency that is part of the alcoholic syndrome. Alcohol, as a drug, has a direct effect on the nervous system. It has a profound effect on the developing brain and produces fetal alcohol syndrome. Additionally, the chronic effects of alcohol include vitamin and general nutritional deficiency. Alcohol has a high caloric value and, therefore, the chronic alcoholic tends to decrease food intake: the classic "drinking lunch or dinner." Thus acute intoxication, although not producing nutritional deficiency, contributes to it.

Signs and Symptoms of Acute Alcohol Intoxication

Most people are well aware of the symptoms of acute alcohol intoxication, perhaps through personal experience. Initially, alcohol produces relaxation and a loss of inhibitions. This is followed by a loss of judgment and coordination. If alcohol ingestion continues, a stuporous stage may be reached: the person "passes out" and awakens the next morning with a hangover. Drinking water and eating tend to alleviate the sick feeling, and the neurological signs are reversible at this stage. However, overly large volumes of alcohol can lead to coma and death. The symptoms of acute intoxication result from the direct effect of alcohol on the excitability of neurons, that is, inhibitory neurons become less excitable. Alcohol causes a decrease in membrane excitability. The cortex is usually affected first, and this effect descends the neuraxis. Coma is an indication of medullary involvement.

The individual with signs of acute intoxication will rarely, if ever, be seen in the clinic. The person with chronic alcohol intoxication, however, often will show neurological complications. The most prevalent problems involve cortical function, cerebellar function, and peripheral neuropathies. The cortical and cerebellar problems involve the combination of alcohol effects and nutritional deficiency; peripheral neuropathies are believed to be a result of nutritional deficiencies.[37] Because large neurons are more difficult to excite, it is possible that the large neurons of the cortex and cerebellum are more easily affected by decreases in excitability. The cerebellum and frontal lobes of the cerebral cortex are more sensitive to the deleterious effects of alcohol. The nutritional deficits further exacerbate these problems as the lack of food causes a decrease in glucose available for brain metabolism. Vitamin deficiency, especially of the B vitamins, is a further cause of the symptoms seen.

In addition to the effects of chronic alcohol use on the adult, alcohol can also be devastating to an unborn child. Because alcohol crosses the placenta, the developing brain with its high metabolic rate may be affected even in the absence of symptoms in the mother. Binge drinking by the mother can be as detrimental as abuse. This has become a great enough problem with enough similarities among affected infants that fetal alcohol syndrome is a recognizable disease at birth. In addition to a low birth weight and irritability, distinct facial anomalies also are associated with this disease. A long-term evaluation of these children will provide information on other neurological problems that may become more evident as they age. Animal research indicates that brain maldevelopment and delays in reflex and motor development are not reversible.[75] One of the areas showing a decrease in size is the frontal cortex.[75] (See Chapters 11, 12, and 13 for further information on pediatric problems.)

Signs and Symptoms of Chronic Alcoholism

The individual with chronic alcoholism can have neurological and psychological impairment. Neurological symptoms include ataxia (especially in the trunk and lower limbs), incoordination, and peripheral neuropathy. Seizures also may be a complication. The ataxia that occurs is the classic staggering, wide-base gait depicted on every television program showing an alcoholic. The person cannot perform a tandem gait (walking forward in heel-to-toe fashion on a straight line) and has difficulty maintaining an upright posture with the feet together. If weakness because of neuropathy is present, the ataxia, of course, is worsened. Vestibular deficits also are present and persist even after periods of abstinence. Abstinent alcoholics showed performance deficits on all sensory organization tests during dynamic posturography; these deficits reached statistical significance for those conditions that entailed proprioceptive conflict.[99]

The psychological problems also are fairly well known. These include delirium tremens (DTs), dementia, and the Wernicke-Korsakoff syndrome. DTs are most frequently seen in any withdrawal from alcohol. The individual is restless, irritable, disoriented, and often hallucinates when awake; speech may be unintelligible. Temperature is elevated, and the person is dehydrated. DTs are probably caused by a type of rebound phenomenon. The depressed neuronal firing initially observed as relaxed tone or inhibition over social behavior is freed from the alcohol and neurons are overly irritable. Deep tendon reflexes are also hyperactive.

Wernicke-Korsakoff syndrome (hyphenated because the two syndromes are usually seen together) is caused by frontal lobe involvement complicated by vitamin B_1 deficiency. In Korsakoff's syndrome there is a loss of memory, especially short-term and recent recall. The individual then tends to make up answers and may "remember" the physician or even the therapist as someone he or she met in a bar; a simple breakfast just completed may become a banquet feast. These confabulations are a classic sign of the chronic alcoholic. They are probably an attempt to function without recent memory. Wernicke's syndrome includes ataxia (already described), disorientation, dementia, and ophthalmoplegia. The eye problems include nystagmus followed by lateral rectus weakness and double vision.

The peripheral neuropathies exacerbate all these problems. The muscles are tender, and there may be a burning sensation in the hands and feet, which intensifies the irritability of patients with DTs. Muscle weakness will increase the apparent ataxia, and decreased sensation causes a further loss of proprioceptive cues the individual might otherwise use.

Pharmacological Considerations and Medical Management

The biggest factor in treatment for alcoholism and the residual functional loss is, of course, withdrawal from alcohol. Librium, which is synonymous with chlorpromazine and chlordiazepoxide, is used to keep the individual sedated and to reduce DTs. At the same time, the electrolyte and water balance of the body must be restored. Because alcohol usually causes dehydration, the body's fluids must be replaced, but refurnishing necessary electrolytes also requires attention. In addition, nutrition is important because the nutritional deficiencies are as harmful as the effects of alcohol itself. Large supplements of B complex vitamins should be added to the diet.

If the individual has been hospitalized fairly early, abstains from alcohol, and controls the diet, some of the cognitive and motor symptoms of the disease can be reversed. This is especially true of the eye involvement and of much of the ataxia. Permanent memory deficits, however, often occur; the longer the alcoholism, the worse the memory. The neuropathies, if they recover, recover slowly. Both the myelin sheath and the axon have been damaged. In long-standing alcoholism, the nerve roots also become involved, lessening the chances for regeneration and recovery. The best cure therefore is prevention.

Evaluation of Individuals with Alcoholism

Before proceeding with a neurological evaluation as one would for the person with cerebellar dysfunction, the therapist needs to assess the client's mental status. The following questions might be used as a guideline:

1. Is there any short-term retention? Can the individual's perception of sensation be trusted as accurate?
2. If the client cannot perform a task, is it because she or he did not understand the instructions, or has for-gotten them or does not have the motor control to perform the action?

All commands should be single commands and kept as short as possible. Because weakness and loss of sensation, especially proprioception, can produce signs similar to ataxia, it is a good idea to evaluate peripheral nerve function first. Nerve conduction tests are useful evaluation tools for the alcoholic patient. The faster myelinated nerves are the most sensitive to alcohol.[60] (Refer to Chapter 31.)

In assessing the degree of cerebellar involvement, static posture and movement need to be evaluated. This includes the ability to stand upright with the feet together, the width between the legs in standing or walking, and the presence or absence of balance reactions. Sometimes there is a delay in balance responses that needs to be recorded. Persistent involvement of the vestibular system means that tests of vestibular function, including vestibular-ocular reflex (VOR), optokinetic nystagmus (OKN), and balance should be performed. (Refer to Chapters 23 and 30.)

Treatment Considerations for Individuals with Alcoholic Syndrome

Treatment of the alcoholic adds a few problems that may not be encountered in these other cerebellar disease entities. The first problem encountered is one of setting goals cooperatively, because the client may not be sufficiently mentally alert to participate in that activity. Second, the degree of recovery is unpredictable; the therapist should strive for as much recovery as possible. Of course, the achievement of whatever goals are established depends on abstinence from alcohol.

In treatment of alcoholism, mental status is a crucial problem. If dementia is present, the client will not be able to use higher level thought processes or achieve cortical control over movement. Therefore techniques that require attention or learning may have limited success. In addition, carryover from one session to the next will be hampered because the client may have no recollection of the previous treatment or even of the therapist, nor can visualization or mental rehearsal between sessions be used. The lack of attention and memory also means that, just as during the evaluation, all commands must be brief and simple. The treatment session should be well structured so that the client's thoughts are not allowed to wander. Sometimes it may also be advisable to adjust the length of treatment to the individual's tolerance. The addition of both physical and occupational therapy may produce a more holistic treatment approach.

Another consideration in the treatment of the alcoholic is the effect of exercise on physical well-being in general, especially on any symptoms of asthenia. Even without neurological signs, alcoholic individuals may benefit from a carefully monitored program of physical activity—carefully monitored because these clients may be in a debilitated condition with generalized weakness and even respiratory problems. A study in Japan has shown that physical exercise can help the alcoholic's general rehabilitation progress.[121] All studies that involve inpatient or outpatient care of the alcoholic indicate that exercise is essential. The more specific the exercise for a patient's individual problems, the better the long-term results. Of course, unless the patient decreases or ceases alcohol intake, therapy that focuses upon movement function will not be as successful as it should be. As in all diseases discussed so far, the exact treatment procedures depend on the results of the evaluation. Documentation of the effects of therapy should be clear and, whenever possible, quantifiable (refer to Chapter 10).

This chapter has been concerned with the role of the cerebellum in movement and the effects of lesions of the cerebellum. One specific disease, alcoholism, also has been discussed. Because of the cerebellum's critical role in motor function, the prognosis of direct cerebellar damage versus indirect damage will generally be less optimistic. When tract loops going from and being sent to the cerebellum are neurologically involved, neuroplasticity may be more easily reinforced, but repetition of practice within the environment will always be extremely important.

CASE STUDY 26-1 ■ T. H.

T. H. is a 53-year-old man with a diagnosis of one of the spinocerebellar atrophies (SCA). He was referred for physical therapy to increase balance and to develop a home exercise program to improve strength and coordination and prevent deconditioning. The referral also requested that the therapist assist T. H. with information on assistive devices. When he came in for his appointment, his left forearm was in a cast as a result of a wrist fracture from a fall. He stated that he fell at least once a week.

HISTORY
About 2 years ago, T. H. began to notice that he was falling more and friends began to comment that he was weaving when he walked. He then began seeing the parade of doctors, which eventually led to diagnosis by a neurologist and confirmation of genetic changes by a geneticist. T. H. had to retire about a year ago because he did not think he could perform his job safely. He stated that he was able to walk without his cane on some days but not on others, and he did not know why he had "good days" and "bad days." He was not a person who liked to exercise and had not been active physically at any time in his life. T. H. was independent in his self care and was able to drive, but he was unable to participate in household chores and had decreased his leisure activities. He was able to continue activities with friends on most days.

COMPREHENSION
T. H. had no difficulty following complex commands and most conversations. He stated that if he was tired, he had difficulty following some complex conversations.

POSTURE AND GAIT
T. H. sat and stood symmetrically. He walked into the physical therapy clinic using a single point cane for balance. He walked with a wide-base gait with a shortened stride length and decreased cadence. He was able to decrease but not increase his speed, and he was unable to walk while turning his head. Additionally, he was unable to walk backward. He was able to walk without his cane; however, he slowed down even more and kept his hands in the air to catch himself. He scored 25/28 on the Tinetti Gait and Balance Test. He was able to walk on the treadmill at 1.6 mph with upper extremity support; he could not walk on the treadmill without the use of at least one arm.

BALANCE
In sitting, static and dynamic balance was within normal limits with the eyes open or closed. T. H. was able to stand without use of his arms although he took several seconds to become balanced. He was able to stand with his feet together with his eyes open for 30 seconds with moderate sway. He was able to stand with his feet together, eyes closed for 4 seconds maximum in three trials. He fell once to the left and twice to the back. He could not stand on one leg nor could he assume a tandem stance. He was able to turn his head slowly to either side in standing but could lean outside his base of support only for 8 cm. He did not complain of dizziness.

ROM AND STRENGTH
ROM was within normal limits. Strength was 4+/5 in all extremities except for the left upper extremity, which could not be tested because of the cast.

SENSATION
T. H. stated that light touch was even on the two sides. He was able to detect which fingers were touched with 100% accuracy. Kinesthesia and proprioception were mildly reduced. T. H. was able to identify the correct movement of the arms or legs, but required larger movements before he could accurately determine the direction of movement. This loss was equal proximally and distally. Vibration sensation also was decreased.

CRANIAL NERVES
There was no double vision or presence of loss in those cranial nerves that could be tested accurately.

DIAGNOSIS
PT

SYSTEMS/FUNCTION
T. H. demonstrated impairment in balance with decreased central sensory processing affecting gait consistent with involvement of the cerebellum as well as spinocerebellar tracts.

ACTIVITIES
T. H. was able to complete all self-care activities in a reasonable time. He was able to drive. He was not able to complete tasks requiring balance without upper extremity support, nor was he able to complete yard work or gardening.

PARTICIPATION
T. H. could participate in most leisure activities with friends unless he was fatigued. He was not a full partner in household tasks. It was difficult for him to play with his young grandchildren. His wife worked full time plus and, therefore, all therapeutic activities would have to be completed by T. H. without much assistance.

TREATMENT GOALS
1. T. H. would be able to participate in an exercise program that included walking in a safe environment independently.

Continued

CASE STUDY 26-1 ■ T. H.—cont'd

2. T. H. would be able to rise from the chair and walk from the main room to the kitchen independently.

3. T. H. would be able to participate in gardening activities with modification of the tasks. (Gardening was one of his favorite activities, and in the past, he had used this as a way to "unwind.")

T. H. was seen for outpatient treatment four times over a 2-month period. He was given a home program that included balance exercises in standing and on a ball, as well as strengthening with use of Thera-band and walking on his nonelectric home treadmill. Initially, he had asthenia and so was not able to exercise for long periods. He needed lots of motivation and small self-rewards to maintain his activity level.

Therapy sessions included walking on the treadmill with and without upper extremity support while reading, solving simple math problems, and turning his head. At the end of the four sessions, he was able to walk at 1.8 mph safely. All exercises were done with many repetitions and initially in a closed environment

with blocked practice. Even at the end of the four sessions, T. H. was unable to perform random practice of balance activities. T. H. did not respond well to any type of weights to increase proprioception or balance. Attempts at use of weights included ankle and wrist weights, a weighted belt, weighted vest, small weights in his pockets, and combinations. Efficacy of weights was evaluated with videotapes as well as by subjective findings of T. H. and the therapist.

At the time of discharge, T.H. was more comfortable in community activities and was able to tend to his plants independently. He was able to participate in leisure activities with friends and family with increased confidence. He did not want to know about available assistive devices but had resources when that time came. Psychology services were limited because of the rural setting in which T.H. lived. He also was reluctant to pursue such help because he was so well known in the community. His physician and therapist established a yearly re-evaluation schedule unless progression was more rapid.

REFERENCES

1. Dow RS, Moruzzi G: *The physiology and pathology of the cerebellum,* Minneapolis, 1958, University of Minnesota Press.

2. Akshoomoff NA, Courchesne E: A new role for the cerebellum cognitive operations. *Behav Neurosci* 106:731-738, 1992.

3. Albus JS: A theory of cerebellar function, *Math Biosci* 10:25, 1971.

4. Bastian AJ, Martin TA, Keating JG, et al: Cerebellar ataxia, *J Neurophysiol* 76:492-509, 1996

5. Morton SM, Bastian AJ: Contributions of limb incoordination and postural control deficits to cerebellar gait ataxia, *J Neurophysiol* 89:1844-1856, 2003.

6. Bastian AJ: Cerebellar limb ataxia: abnormal control of self-generated and external forces, *Ann N Y Acad Sci* 978:16-27, 2002.

7. Ito M: Mechanisms of motor learning in the cerebellum, *Brain Res* 886:237-245, 2000.

8. Thach WT, Bastian AJ: Role of the cerebellum in the control and adaptation of gait in health and disease, *Prog Brain Res* 143:353-366, 2004.

9. Dum RP, Li C, Strick PL: Motor and nonmotor domains in the monkey dentate, *Ann N Y Acad Sci* 978:289-301, 2002.

10. Llinas R: Functional significance of the basic cerebellar circuit in motor coordination. In Bloedel JR, Dichgans, J, Precht W, editors: *Cerebellar function,* Berlin, 1985, Springer.

11. Ito M: *The cerebellum and neural control,* New York, 1984, Raven.

12. Dichgans J, Mauritz K: Patterns and mechanisms of postural instability in patients with cerebellar lesions, *Adv Neurol* 39:633-643, 1983.

13. Chambers WW, Sprague JM: Functional localization in the cerebellum. I. Organization in longitudinal corticonuclear zones and their contribution to the control of posture, both extrapyramidal and pyramidal, *J Comp Neurol* 103:105-129, 1955.

14. Brooks VB: Control of intended limb movement by the lateral and intermediate cerebellum. In Asanuma H, Wilson VJ, editors: *Integration in the human nervous system,* New York, 1979, Igaku Shoin.

15. Strick PL: The influence of motor preparation on the response of cerebellar neurons to limb displacements, *J Neurosci* 3:2007-2020, 1983.

16. Thach WT: A role of the cerebellum in learning movement coordination, *Neurobiol Learn Mem* 70:177-188, 1998.

17. Earhart GM, Bastian AJ: Selection and coordination of human locomotor forms following cerebellar damage, *J Neurophysiol* 85:759-769, 2001.

18. Morton SM, Dordevic GS, Bastian AJ: Cerebellar damage produces context-dependent deficits in control of leg dynamics during obstacle avoidance, *Exp Brain Res* 156:149-169, 2004.

19. DeLong MR, Strick P. Relation of basal ganglia, cerebellum, and motor cortex units to ramp and ballistic movements, *Brain Res* 71:327-335, 1974.

20. Gao JH, Parsons LM, Bower JM, et al. Cerebellum implicated in sensory acquisition and discrimination rather than motor control, *Science* 272:545-547, 1996.

21. Flanagan JR, Nakano E, Imamizu H, et al: Composition and decomposition of internal models in motor learning under altered kinematic and dynamic environments, *J Neurosci* 19:RC34, 1999.

22. Eccles JC: The dynamic loop hypothesis of movement control. In Leibovic KN, editor: *Information processing in the nervous system,* New York, 1969, Springer.

23. Fisher CM, Picard EH, Polak A et al: Acute hypertensive cerebellar hemorrhage: diagnosis and surgical treatment, *J Nerv Ment Dis* 140:38-57, 1965.

24. Ruch TC: Motor systems. In Stevens SS, editor: *Handbook of experimental psychology,* New York, 1951, John Wiley & Sons.

25. MacKay WA, Murphy JT: Cerebellar modulation of reflex gain, *Prog Neurobiol* 13:361-417, 1979.

26. Ito M: Neurophysiological aspects of the cerebellar motor control system, *Int J Neurol* 1:162-176, 1970.

27. Shadmehr R, Holcomb HH: Inhibitory control of competing motor memories, *Exp Brain Res* 126:235-251, 1999.

27a. Serrien DJ, Wiesendanger M: Grip-load force coordination in cerebellar patients, *Exp Brain Res* 128:76-80, 1999.

28. Lang CE, Bastian AJ: Cerebellar subjects show impaired adaptation of anticipatory EMG during catching, *J Neurophysiol* 82:2108-2119, 1999.

29. Lang CE, Bastian AJ: Additional somatosensory information does not improve cerebellar adaptation during catching, *Clin Neurophysiol* 112:895-907, 2001.

30. Morton SM, Lang CE, Bastian AJ: Inter- and intra-limb generalization of adaptation during catching, *Exp Brain Res* 141:438-445, 2001.

31. Zackowski KM, Thach WT, Bastian AJ: Cerebellar subjects show impaired coupling of reach and grasp movements, *Exp Brain Res* 146:511-522, 2002.

32. Hikosaka O, Nakahara H, Rand MK et al: Parallel neural networks for learning sequential procedures, *Trends Neurosci* 22:464-471, 1999.

33. Molinari M, Leggio MG, Solida A et al: Cerebellum and procedural learning: evidence from focal cerebellar lesions, *Brain* 120:1753-1762, 1997.

34. Thach WT, Goodkin HP, Keating JG: Cerebellum and the adaptive coordination of movement, *Ann Rev Neurosci* 15:403-442, 1992.

35. Thach WT, Kane SA, Mink JW et al: Cerebellar output: multiple maps and modes of control in movement coordination. In Llinas R, Soto C, editors: *The cerebellum revisited*, New York, 1992, Springer Verlag.

36. Lang CE, Bastian AJ: Cerebellar damage impairs automaticity of a recently practiced movement, *J Neurophysiol* 87:1336-1347, 2002.

37. Marr D: A theory of the cerebellar cortex, *J Physiol* 202:437-470, 1969.

38. Apps R: Movement-related gating of climbing fibre input to cerebellar cortical zones, *Prog Neurobiol* 57:537-562, 1999.

39. Braitenberg V, Heck D, Sultan F: The detection and generation of sequences as a key to cerebellum function: experiments and theory, *Behav Brain Sci* 20:229-245, 1997.

40. Ryding E, Decety J, Sjoholm H et al: Motor imagery activates the cerebellum regionally. A SPECT rCBF study with 99mTc-HMPAO, *Cogn Brain Res* 1:94-99, 1993.

41. Lectenberg R: Ataxia and other cerebellar syndromes. In Jankovic J, Eduardo T, editors: *Parkinson's disease and movement disorders*. Baltimore, 1993, Williams & Wilkins.

42. Nashner LM: Adapting reflexes controlling human posture, *Exp Brain Res* 26:59, 1976.

43. Luciani L: *Il cervelletto: nuovi studi di fisiologia normale e patologica*, Florence, 1891, Le Monnier.

44. Luciani L: De l'influence qu'exercent les mutilations cerebelleuses sur l'excitabilite de l'ecorce cerebrale et sur les reflexes spinaux, *Arch Ital Biol* 21:190, 1894.

45. Rossi G: Sugli effetti consequenti alla stimolazione contemporanea della corteccia cerebrale e di quella cerebellare, *Arch Fisiol* 10:389, 1912.

46. Russell JSR: Experimental research into the functions of the cerebellum, *Philos Trans R Soc Lond* 185:819, 1894.

47. Holmes G: The Croonian lectures on the clinical symptoms of cerebellar diseases and their interpretation, *Lancet* 1:1177, 1922.

48. Holmes G: The cerebellum of man, *Brain* 62:1, 1939.

49. Barash S, Melikyan A, Sivakov A et al: Saccadic dysmetria and adaptation after lesion of the cerebellar cortex, *J Neurosci* 19:10931-10939, 1999.

50. Gilman S: The mechanism of cerebellar hypotonia: an experimental study in the monkey, *Brain* 92:621-638, 1969.

51. Klintsova AY, Goodlett CR, Greenough WT: Therapeutic motor training ameliorates cerebellar effects of postnatal binge alcohol, *Neurotoxicol Teratol* 22:125-132, 2000.

52. Berardelli A, Hallett M, Rothwell JC et al: Single-joint rapid arm movements in normal subjects and in patients with motor disorders, *Brain* 119:661-674, 1996.

53. Vilis T, Hore J: Effects of changes in mechanical state of limb on cerebellar intention tremor, *J Neurophysiol* 40:1214-1224, 1977.

54. Hallett M, Shahani BT, Young RR: EMG analysis of stereotyped movements in man, *J Neurol Neurosurg Psychiatry* 38:1154-1162, 1975.

55. Hallett M, Shahani BT, Young RR: EMG analysis of patients with cerebellar deficits, *J Neurol Neurosurg Psychiatry* 38:1163-1169, 1975.

56. Conrad B, Brooks VB: Effects of dentate cooling on rapid alternating arm movements. *J Neurophysiol* 37:792-804, 1974.

57. Brooks VB, Kozlovskaya IB, Atkin A et al: Effects of cooling dentate nucleus on tracking task performance in monkeys, *J Neurophysiol* 36:974-995, 1973.

58. Uno M, Kozlovskaya IB, Brooks VB: Effects of cooling the interposed nuclei on tracking-task performance in monkeys, *J Neurophysiol* 36:996-1003, 1973.

59. Brown SH, Kessler KR, Hefter H et al: Role of the cerebellum in visuomotor coordination, *Exp Brain Res* 94:478-488, 1993.

60. Holmes G: The Croonian lectures on the clinical symptoms of cerebellar diseases and their interpretation, *Lancet* 1:1231, 1922.

61. Terzuolo TA, Viviani P: Parameters of motion and EMG activities during some simple motor tasks in normal subjects and cerebellar patients. In Cooper IS, Riklan M, Snider RS, editors: *The cerebellum, epilepsy and behavior*, New York, 1973, Plenum Press.

62. Smith AM, Bourbonnais D: Neuronal activity in cerebellar cortex related to control of prehensile force, *J Neurophysiol* 45:286-303, 1981.

63. Amici R, Avanzani G, Pacini L: *Cerebellar tumors: clinical analysis and physiopathologic correlations*, New York, 1976, S Karger.

64. Gilman S, Bloedel JR, Lechtenberg R: *Disorders of the cerebellum*, Philadelphia, 1981, FA Davis.

65. Marie P et al: De l'atrophie cerebelleuse tardive lga predominance corticale, *Rev Neurol (Paris)* 38:849, 1082, 1922.

66. Victor M, Adams RD, Collins GH: A restricted form of cerebellar cortical degeneration occurring in alcoholic patients. *AMA Arch Neurol* 1:579, 1959.

67. Orlovsky GN, Shik ML: Control of locomotion: a neurophysiological analysis of the cat locomotor system. In Porter R, editor: *International review of physiology neurophysiology II, vol 10*, Baltimore, 1976, University Park Press.

68. Ritchie L: Effect of cerebellar lesions on saccadic eye movements, *J Neurophysiol* 39:1246-1256, 1976.

69. Hagbarth KE, Hongell A, Hallin RG et al: The effect of gamma fiber block on afferent muscle nerve activity during voluntary contractions, *Acta Physiol Scand* 79:27A, 1970.

70. McCloskey DI: Kinesthetic sensibility, *Physiol Rev* 58:763-820, 1978.

71. Bremer F: Le cervelet. In Roger GH, Binet L, editors: *Traite de physiologie normale et pathologique, vol 10*, Paris, 1935, Masson.

72. Cooke JD, Thomas JS: Forearm oscillation during cooling of the dentate nucleus in the monkey, *Can J Physiol Pharmacol* 54:430-436, 1976.

73. Allen GI, Tsukahara N: Cerebrocerebellar communications systems, *Physiol Rev* 54:957-1006, 1974.

74. Meyer-Lohmann J, Conrad B, Matsunami K et al: Effects of dentate cooling on precentral unit activity following torque pulse injections into elbow movements, *Brain Res* 94:237-251, 1975.

75. Vilis T, Hore J, Meyer-Lohmann J et al: Dual nature of the precentral responses to limb perturbations revealed by cerebellar cooling, *Brain Res* 117:336-340, 1976.

76. Dichgans J, Mauritz KH, Allum JH et al: Postural sway in normals and atactic patients, analysis of the stabilizing and destabilizing effects of vision, *Agressologie* 176:15-24, 1976.

77. Silfverskjold BP: A 3 sec leg tremor in a cerebellar syndrome, *Acta Neurol Scand* 55:385, 1977.

78. Goldberger ME, Growden JH: Tremor at rest following cerebellar lesions in monkeys: effect of l-dopa administration, *Brain Res* 27:183-187, 1971.

79. Nyberg-Hansen R, Horn J: Functional aspects of cerebellar signs in clinical neurology, *Acta Neurol Scand* 48(suppl 51):219, 1972.

80. Mauritz KH, Schmitt C, Dichgans J: Delayed and enhanced long latency reflexes as the possible cause of postural tremor in late cerebellar atrophy, *Brain* 104:97-116, 1981.

81. Marsden CD et al: Disorders of movement in cerebellar disease in man. In Rose CF, editor: *Physiological aspects of clinical neurology*, Oxford, 1977, Blackwell Scientific Publications.

82. Stein RB, Oguztoreli MN: Reflex involvement in the generation and control of tremor and clonus. In Desmedt JE, editor: *Physiological tremor, pathological tremor and clonus. Progress in clinical neurophysiology, vol 5*, Basel, Switzerland, 1978, Karger.

83. Cole M: Dysprody due to posterior fossa lesions, *Trans Am Neurol Assoc* 96:151-154, 1971.

84. Lechtenberg R, Gilman S: Speech disorders in cerebellar disease, *Ann Neurol* 3:285-290, 1978.

85. Zentay PJ: Motor disorders of the nervous system and their significance for speech. I. Cerebral and cerebellar dysarthrias, *Laryngoscope* 47:147, 1937.

86. Brown J, Darley FL, Aronson AE: Ataxic dysarthria, *Int J Neurol* 7:302, 1970.

87. Holmes G: The Croonian lectures on the clinical symptoms of cerebellar diseases and their interpretation, *Lancet* 2:59, 1922.

88. Kent R, Netsell R: A case study of an ataxic dysarthric: cineradiography and spectrographic observations, *J Speech Hear Disord* 40:115-134, 1975.

89. Oscar-Berman M, Goodglass H, Donnenfeld H: Dichotic ear-order effects with nonverbal stimuli, *Cortex* 10:270-277, 1974.

90. Shankweiler D: Effects of temporal lobe damage on perception of dichotically presented melodies, *J Comp Physiol Psychol* 62:115-119, 1966.

91. Nashold BS Jr, Slaughter DG, Gills JP: Ocular reactions in man from deep cerebellar stimulation and lesions, *Arch Ophthalmol* 81:538, 1969.

92. Kornhuber HH: Neurologie de kleinherns, *Zbl ges Neurol Psychiat* 191:13, 1968.

93. Selhorst JB, Stark L, Ochs AL, et al: Disorders in cerebellar ocular motor control. I. Saccadic overshoot dysmetria, *Brain* 99:497-508, 1976.

94. Chase RA, Cullen JK Jr, Sullivan SA et al: Modification of intention tremor in man, *Nature* 206:485-487, 1965.

95. Cogan DG: Ocular dysmetria: flutterlike oscillations of the eyes and opsoclonus, *Arch Ophthalmol* 51:318-335, 1954.

96. von Noorden GK, Preziosi TJ: Eye movement recordings in neurological disorders, *Arch Ophthalmol* 76:162-171, 1966.

97. Baloh RW, Konrad HR, Honrubia V: Vestibulo-ocular function in patients with cerebellar atrophy, *Neurology* 25:160-168, 1975.

98. Zee DS, Optican LM, Cook JD et al: Slow saccades in spinocerebellar degeneration, *Arch Neurol* 33:243-251, 1976.

99. Optican LM, Robinson DA: Cerebellar-dependent adaptive control of primate saccadic system, *J Neurophysiol* 44:1058-1076, 1980.

100. Jung R, Kornhuber HH: Results of electronystagmography in man: the value of optokinetic vestibular, and spontaneous nystagmus for neurologic diagnosis and research. In Bender MB: *The oculomotor system*, New York, 1964, Harper & Row.

101. Hood JD, Kayan A, Leech J: Rebound nystagmus, *Brain* 96:507-527, 1973.

102. Carpenter RHS: *Movement of the eyes*, London, 1977, Pion Ltd.

103. Zee DS, Yamazaki A, Butler PH et al: Effects of ablation of flocculus and paraflocculus on eye movements in primate, *J Neurophysiol* 46:878-899, 1981.

104. Zee DS, Friendlich AR, Robinson DA: The mechanism of downbeat nystagmus, *Arch Neurol* 30:227-237, 1974.

105. Zee DS, Yee RD, Cogan DG et al: Ocular motor abnormalities in hereditary ataxia, *Brain* 99:207-234, 1976.

106. Miles FA, Fuller JH: Adaptive plasticity in the vestibulo-ocular responses of the rhesus monkey, *Brain Res* 8:512-516, 1974.

107. Poirier LJ, Lafleur J, de Lean J et al: Physiopathology of the cerebellum in the monkey. II. Motor disturbances associated with partial and complete destruction of cerebellar structures, *J Neurol Sci* 22:491-509, 1974.

108. Goldberger ME, Growdon JH: Pattern of recovery following cerebellar deep nuclear lesions in monkeys, *Exp Neurol* 39:307-322, 1973.

109. Trouillas P, Takayanagi T, Hallett M et al: International cooperative ataxia rating scale for pharmacological assessment of the cerebellar syndrome, *J Neurol Sci* 145:205-211, 1997.

110. Topka H, Massaquoi SG, Benda N et al: Motor skill learning in patients with cerebellar degeneration, *J Neurol Sci* 158:164-172, 1998.

111. Isaacs KR, Anderson BJ, Alcantara AA et al: Exercise and the brain: angiogenesis in the adult rat cerebellum after vigorous physical activity and motor skill learning, *J Cereb Blood Flow Metab* 12:110-119, 1992.

112. Stockmeyer S: An interpretation of the approach of Rood to the treatment of neuromuscular dysfunction, *Am J Phys Med* 46:900-961, 1967.

113. Wooldridge CP, Russell G: Head position training with the cerebral palsied child: an application of biofeedback techniques. *Milbank Mem Fund Q* 57:407-414, 1976.

114. Knott M, Voss DE: *Proprioceptive neuro-muscular facilitation*, ed 2, New York, Harper & Row, 1968.

115. Winstein CJ, Wing AM, Whitall J: Motor control and learning principles for rehabilitation of upper limb movements after brain injury. In Grafman J, Robertson IH, editors: *Handbook of neurophysiology, vol 9*, ed 2, Amsterdam, 2003, Elsevier.

116. Widener G: Personal communication, 2005.

117. Kabat H: Studies on neuromuscular dysfunction. XII. Rhythmic stabilization: a new and more effective technique for treatment of paralysis through a cerebellar mechanism, *Permanente Found M Bull* 8:9, 1950.

118. Kabat H: Analysis and therapy of cerebellar ataxia and asynergia, *Arch Neurol Psychiatry* 74:375-382, 1955.

119. Nakamura R, Taniguchi R: Kinesiological analysis and physical therapy of cerebellar ataxia. In Sobue I: *Spinocerebellar degenerations,* Baltimore, 1978, University Park Press.

120. Krusen FH: *Handbook of physical medicine and rehabilitation*, ed 2, Philadelphia, 1971, WB Saunders.

121. Tsukue I, Shohoji T: Movement therapy for alcoholic patients, *J Stud Alcohol* 42: 144-149, 1981.

Hemiplegia

Susan D. Ryerson, DSc, PT

OBJECTIVES

After reading this chapter the student/therapist will be able to:

1. Identify the various types of neurovascular disease.
2. Identify the atypical patterns of movement in clients with residual hemiplegia.
3. Identify significant primary and secondary impairments that interfere with functional movement patterns.
4. Describe a reeducation intervention strategy for improving functional limitations in clients with stroke.
5. Identify various treatment procedures and analyze how they affect performance of functional movement.

OVERVIEW

The treatment of hemiplegia from vascular insult is controversial. Various treatment methods have been devised and advocated. Recent scientific theories have changed the focus of treatment from one of inhibition of abnormal tone and facilitation of normal movement to reeducation of control and weakness and functional retraining. In this chapter, pathological conditions, impairments, and intervention strategies for clients with hemiplegia from stroke are reviewed. Although hemiplegia from neurovascular pathological conditions is the focus of the chapter, therapists can use this information and apply it to hemiplegia in adults caused by other central nervous system (CNS) pathological conditions, such as tumor, trauma, multiple sclerosis, and demyelinating diseases. Movement components and their relationship to functional performance are used as the basis for selection of therapy techniques and training.

Definition

Hemiplegia, a paralysis of one side of the body, is the classic sign of neurovascular disease of the brain. It is one of many manifestations of neurovascular disease, and it occurs with strokes involving the cerebral hemisphere or brain stem. A stroke, or cerebrovascular accident (CVA), results in a sudden, specific neurological deficit. It is the suddenness of this neurological deficit—occurring over seconds, minutes, hours, or a few days—that characterizes the disorder as vascular. Although hemiplegia may be the most obvious sign of a CVA and a major concern of therapists, other symptoms are equally disabling, including sensory dysfunction, aphasia or dysarthria, visual field defects, and mental and intellectual impairment. The specific combination of these neurovascular deficits enables a physician to detect both the location and the size of the defect. CVAs can be classified according to pathological type—thrombosis, embolism, or hemorrhage—or by temporal factors, such as completed, in-evolution, or transient ischemic attacks (TIAs).

Epidemiology

In the United States, stroke is the third most common cause of death, with 160,000 dying each year.[1] The National Stroke Association estimates that 750,000 new or recurrent strokes occur each year. The incidence of stroke rises rapidly with increasing age: two thirds of all strokes occur in people older than the age of 65 years; and after the age of 55 years, the risk of stroke doubles every 10 years. With the over-50-years age group growing rapidly, more people than ever are at risk. In the United States, the incidence of stroke is greater in men than in women, and it is twice as high in blacks as in whites. Cerebral infarction (thrombosis or embolism) is the most common form of stroke, accounting for 70% of all strokes. Hemorrhages account for another 20%, and 10% remain unspecified. Stroke is the largest single cause of neurological disability. Approximately 4 million Americans are dealing with the impairments and disabilities from a stroke. Of these, 31% require assistance, 20% need help walking, 16% are in long-term care facilities, and 71% are vocationally impaired after 7 years.[1] One recent study reports that 12% of subjects have complete functional arm recovery and 38% have some dexterity 6 months after stroke. In addition, loss of leg movement in the first week after stroke and no arm movement at 4 weeks is associated with poor outcomes at 6 months.[2]

The three most commonly recognized risk factors for cerebrovascular disease are hypertension, diabetes mellitus, and heart disease. The most important of these factors is hypertension.[3] Because high blood pressure is the greatest risk factor for stroke, human characteristics and behaviors that increase blood pressure, including increased high serum cholesterol levels, obesity, diabetes mellitus, heavy alcohol consumption, cocaine use, and cigarette smoking, increase the risk of stroke.

Ostfeld[4] noted that mortality rates for stroke have declined, slowly at first (from 1900 to 1950) and then more quickly (from 1950 to 1970), with a sharp drop noted around 1974. Experts have speculated that the greater use of hypertensive drugs in the 1960s and 1970s started this decline, and the creation of screening and treatment referral centers for high blood pressure may account for the marked decline in the late 1970s.

Outcome

The long-term follow-up on the Framingham Heart Study revealed that long-term stroke survivors, especially those with only one episode, had a good chance for full functional recovery.[5] For those people left with severe neurological and functional deficits, studies have demonstrated that rehabilitation is effective and that it can improve functional ability.[6,7] It has been demonstrated that age is not a factor in determining the outcome of the rehabilitation process.[8] Currently, it is thought that clients should be given an opportunity to participate in the rehabilitation process, regardless of age, unless it is medically contraindicated.

The prediction of ultimate functional outcome has been hampered by the inaccuracy of commonly used predictors (medical items, income level, intelligence, functional level). Computed tomography (CT), functional magnetic resonance imaging, and regional cerebral blood flow studies are used in diagnosis and, increasingly, as predictors of functional recovery after stroke. Positron emission tomography and single-photon emission computed tomography are newer techniques that are used in research centers to define areas of dysfunctional but perhaps "salvageable" tissue.[2,9]

Pathoneurological and Pathophysiological Aspects

Classification

The pathological processes that result from a CVA can be divided into three groups—thrombotic changes, embolic changes, and hemorrhagic changes.

Thrombotic Infarction. Atherosclerotic plaques and hypertension interact to produce cerebrovascular infarcts. These plaques form at branchings and curves of the arteries. Plaques usually form in front of the first major branching of the cerebral arteries. These lesions can be present for 30 years or more and may never become symptomatic. Intermittent blockage may proceed to permanent damage. The process by which a thrombus occludes an artery requires several hours and explains the division between stroke-in-evolution and completed stroke.[10]

TIAs are an indication of the presence of thrombotic disease and are the result of transient ischemia. Although the cause of TIAs has not been definitively established, cerebral vasospasm and transient systemic arterial hypotension are thought to be responsible factors.

Embolic Infarction. The embolus that causes the stroke may come from the heart, from an internal carotid artery thrombosis, or from an atheromatous plaque of the carotid sinus. It is usually a sign of cardiac disease. The infarction may be of pale, hemorrhagic, or mixed type. The branches of the middle cerebral artery are infarcted most commonly as a result of its direct continuation from the internal carotid artery. Collateral blood supply is not established with embolic infarctions because of the speed of obstruction formation, so there is less survival of tissue distal to the area of embolic infarct than with thrombotic infarct.[2]

Hemorrhage. The most common intracranial hemorrhages causing stroke are those due to hypertension, ruptured saccular aneurysm, and arteriovenous (AV) malformation. Massive hemorrhage frequently results from hypertensive cardiac-renal disease; bleeding into the brain tissue produces an oval or round mass that displaces midline structures. The exact mechanism of hemorrhage is not known. This mass of extravasated blood decreases in size over 6 to 8 months.

Saccular, or berry, aneurysms are thought to be the result of defects in the media and elastica that develop over years. This muscular defect plus overstretching of the internal elastic membrane from blood pressure causes the aneurysm to develop. Saccular aneurysms are found at branchings of major cerebral arteries, especially the anterior portion of the circle of Willis. Averaging 8 to 10 mm in diameter and variable in form, these aneurysms rupture at their dome. Saccular aneurysms are rare in childhood.

AV malformations are developmental abnormalities that result in a spaghetti-like mass of dilated AV fistulas varying in size from a few millimeters in diameter to huge masses located within the brain tissue. Some of these blood vessels have extremely thin, abnormally structured walls. Although the abnormality is present from birth, symptoms usually develop between the ages of 10 and 35 years. The hemorrhage of an AV malformation presents a pathological picture similar to that for the saccular aneurysm. The larger AV malformations frequently occur in the posterior half of the cerebral hemisphere.[10]

Clinical Findings

The focal neurological deficit resulting from a stroke, whether embolic, thrombotic, or hemorrhagic, is a reflection of the size and location of the lesion and the amount of collateral blood flow. Unilateral neurological deficits result from interruption of the carotid vascular system, and bilateral neurological deficits result from interruption of the vascular supply to the basilar system. Clinical syndromes resulting from occlusion or hemorrhage in the cerebral circulation vary from partial to complete. Signs of hemorrhage may be more variable as a result of the effect of extension to surrounding brain tissue and the possible rise in intracranial pressure. Table 27-1 summarizes the clinical symptoms and the anatomical structures involved according to specific arterial involvement.

The frequencies of the three types of cerebrovascular disease—thrombosis, embolism, and hemorrhage—vary according to whether they were taken from a clinical study or from an autopsy study, but they rank in the order presented in this section. Ischemic strokes, thrombotic or embolic, account for 80% of strokes and hemorrhagic strokes account for 20%.[11] The clinical symptoms and laboratory findings for each type are condensed in Table 27-2.

Medical Management and Pharmacological Considersations

Acute Medical Care

Thrombosis and TIAs. Although infarcted tissue cannot at present be restored, medical management of the acute stroke from thrombosis or TIA is geared toward improving the cerebral circulation as quickly as possible to prevent ischemic tissue from becoming infarcted tissue. Cells that have 80% to 100% ischemia will die in a few minutes because they cannot produce energy, specifically adenosine triphosphate. This energy failure results in an activation of calcium, which causes a chain reaction resulting in cell death.[1] Around this area of infarction is a transitional area where the blood flow is decreased 50% to 80%. Cells in the transitional area are not irreversibly damaged.[12,13]

One of the newer drugs available for immediate stroke treatment is tissue plasminogen activator (t-PA) (see Chapter 36). It is most effective if used within 90 to 180 minutes of the onset of symptoms. Recent studies indicate that 42% of patients with stroke wait 24 hours before getting care, with the average being 13 hours.[13] The importance of community-wide programs to increase awareness of symptoms and effectiveness of emergency medical responses is immense for this drug's usage. The American Heart Association and the National Stroke Association are creating community campaigns to increase awareness of the medical emergency nature of stroke symptoms.

Anticoagulant drugs are used to prevent TIAs and may stop a stroke-in-evolution. Before anticoagulant drugs are used, an accurate differential diagnosis is necessary because of the danger of excessive bleeding if hemorrhage is present. Heparin is often used in the early stage of the stroke, and warfarin (Coumadin) is commonly used in the months after the stroke. Cerebral edema, if present, is managed pharmacologically during the first few days. Antiplatelet drugs such as aspirin, dipyridamole (Persantine), and sulfinpyrazone (Anturane) are used to prevent clotting by decreasing platelet "stickiness."[10]

Surgical treatment (thromboendarterectomy or grafting) is used when TIAs are the result of arterial plaques. Areas accessible to and suitable for surgery include the carotid sinus and the common carotid, innominate, and subclavian arteries. Although both surgery and anticoagulant therapy are used for TIAs, Adams and Victor[10] extensively reviewed the wide divergence of opinions. For clients who have had a stroke yet recovered quickly and well, medical care focuses on prevention. Prevention usually includes maintaining blood pressure and blood flow, monitoring hypotensive agents (if given), and avoiding oversedation, especially for sleep, to prevent cerebral ischemia.

Embolic Infarction. Management of embolic infarction is similar to that of thrombotic infarction. The primary emphasis is on prevention. Long-term anticoagulant therapy is effective in preventing embolic infarction in clients with cardiac problems such as atrial fibrillation, myocardial infarction, and valve prostheses. The diagnostic use of CT is important in anticoagulant therapy to rule out hemorrhage after the infarct.

Hypertensive Hemorrhage. Medical procedures for hypertensive hemorrhage parallel those for thrombosis and embolism. Surgical removal of the clot and lowering of the systemic blood pressure to decrease hemorrhage have generally not been helpful. Again, the preventive use of antihypertensive drugs in clients with essential hypertension is the soundest medical management available.[10]

Ruptured Aneurysm. Comatose clients are not good candidates for surgery. However, if the client survives the first few days and if the state of consciousness improves, surgical intervention, whether extracranial or intracranial, is the treatment of choice. Medical treatment consists of lowering arterial blood pressures. Bed rest for 4 to 6 weeks with all forms of exertion avoided is prescribed. Antiseizure medication may be used. Often a systemic antifibrinolysin is given to impede lysis of the clot at the site of rupture. Vasospasm, resulting in severe motor dysfunction, is present with the use of drugs such as reserpine (Serpasil) and kanamycin (Kantrex) (see Chapter 36).

Regardless of the cause of the stroke, comatose clients are managed by (1) treatment of shock; (2) maintenance of clear airway and oxygen flow; (3) measurement of arterial blood gases, blood analysis, CT, and spinal tap; (4) control of seizures; and (5) gastric tube feeding (if coma is prolonged). Hypertensive hemorrhage is one of the most common vascular causes of coma.[14]

Medical Management of Associated Problems

Spasticity. Spasticity and its treatment constitute a major medical problem after stroke because clients complain about it, it may fluctuate, and it does not respond to one fixed treatment. The relationship between spasticity and movement after stroke is an area of continued interest for researchers. Recent studies have refuted the earlier belief that spasticity was inversely related to voluntary movement.[15,16] Although therapists are more hesitant to treat spasticity now, physicians continue to treat it aggressively. Various pharmacological, surgical, and physical means are used to decrease spasticity. The pharmacological and surgical means are examined here, and therapy management is discussed later.

TABLE 27-1 ■ Clinical Symptoms of Vascular Lesions

AFFECTED VESSEL	CLINICAL SYMPTOMS	STRUCTURES INVOLVED
Middle cerebral artery	Contralateral paralysis and sensory deficit	Somatic motor area
	Motor speech impairment	Broca's area (dominant hemisphere)
	"Central" aphasia, anomia, jargon speech	Parieto-occipital cortex (dominant hemisphere)
	Unilateral neglect, apraxia, impaired ability to judge distance	Parietal lobe (nondominant hemisphere)
	Homonomous hemianopia	Optic radiation deep to second temporal convolution
	Loss of conjugate gaze to opposite side	Frontal controversive field
	Avoidance reaction of opposite limbs	Parietal lobe
	Pure motor hemiplegia	Upper portion of posterior limb of internal capsule
	Limb—kinetic apraxia	Premotor or parietal cortex
Anterior cerebral artery	Paralysis—lower extremity	Motor area—leg
	Paresis in opposite arm	Arm area of cortex
	Cortical sensory loss	Sensory area
	Urinary incontinence	Posteromedial aspect of superior frontal gyrus
		Medial surface of posterior frontal lobe
	Contralateral grasp reflex, sucking reflex	Uncertain
	Lack of spontaneity, motor inaction, echolalia	Uncertain
	Perseveration and amnesia	
Posterior cerebral artery		
Peripheral area	Homonymous hemianopia	Calcarine cortex or optic radiation
	Bilateral homonymous hemianopia, cortical blindness, inability to perceive objects not centrally located, ocular apraxia	Bilateral occipital lobe
	Memory defect	Inferomedial portions of temporal lobe
	Topographical disorientation	Nondominant calcarine and lingual gyri
Central area	Thalamic syndrome	Posteroventral nucleus ophthalmus
	Weber syndrome	Cranial nerve III and cerebral peduncle
	Contralateral hemiplegia	Cerebral peduncle
	Paresis of vertical eye movements, sluggish papillary response to light	Supranuclear fibers to cranial nerve III
	Contralateral ataxia or postural tremor	
Internal carotid artery	Variable signs according to degree and site of occlusion—middle cerebral, anterior cerebral, posterior cerebral territory	Uncertain
Basilar artery	Ataxia	Middle and superior cerebellar peduncle
Superior cerebellar artery	Dizziness, nausea, vomiting, horizontal nystagmus	Vestibular nucleus
	Horner syndrome on opposite side, decreased pain and thermal sensation	Descending sympathetic fibers
		Spinal thalamic tract
	Decreased touch, vibration, position sense of lower extremity greater than that of upper extremity	Medial lemniscus
Anterior inferior cerebellar artery	Nystagmus, vertigo, nausea, vomiting	Vestibular nerve
	Facial paralysis on same side	Cranial nerve VII
	Tinnitus	Auditory nerve, lower cochlear nucleus
	Ataxia	Middle cerebral peduncle
	Impaired facial sensation on same side	Fifth cranial nerve nucleus
	Decreased pain and thermal sensation on opposite side	Spinal thalamic tract
Complete basilar syndrome	Bilateral long tract signs with cerebellar and cranial nerve abnormalities	
	Coma	
	Quadriplegia	
	Pseudobulbar palsy	
	Cranial nerve abnormalities	

TABLE 27-1 ■ Clinical Symptoms of Vascular Lesions—cont'd

AFFECTED VESSEL	CLINICAL SYMPTOMS	STRUCTURES INVOLVED
Vertebral artery	Decreased pain and temperature on opposite side	Spinal thalamic tract
	Sensory loss from a tactile and proprioceptive	Medial lemniscus
	Hemiparesis of arm and leg	Pyramidal tract
	Facial pain and numbness on same side	Descending tract and fifth cranial nucleus
	Horner syndrome, ptosis, decreased sweating	Descending sympathetic tract
	Ataxia	Spinal cerebellar tract
	Paralysis of tongue	Cranial nerve XII
	Weakness of vocal cord, decreased gag	Cranial nerves IX and X
	Hiccups	Uncertain

Adapted from Adams RD, Victor M: *Principles of neurology,* New York, 1981, McGraw-Hill.

TABLE 27-2 ■ Clinical Symptoms and Laboratory Findings for Neurovascular Disease Ruptured Saccular Aneurysm

DISEASE TYPE	CLINICAL PICTURE	LABORATORY FINDINGS
THROMBOSIS	*Extremely variable*	Cerebrospinal fluid pressure is normal
	Preceded by a prodromal episode	Cerebrospinal fluid is clear
	Uneven progression	Electroencephalogram: limited differential
	Onset develops within minutes or hours or over	diagnostic value
	days ("thrombus in evolution")	Skull radiographs are not helpful
	60% occur during sleep—awaken unaware of problem,	Arteriography is the definitive procedure; it
	rise, and fall to floor	demonstrates site of collateral flow
	Usually no headache, but may occur in mild form	CT scan is helpful in chronic state when
	Hypertension, diabetes, or vascular disease elsewhere	cavitation has occurred
	in body	
TIAs	Linked to atherosclerotic thrombosis	Usually none
	Preceded or accompanied by stroke	
	Occur by themselves	
	Last 2-30 minutes	
	Experience a few attacks or hundreds	
	Normal neurological examination between attacks	
	If transient symptoms are present on awakening, may	
	indicate future stroke	
EMBOLISM	*Extremely variable*	
Cardiac	Occurs extremely rapidly—seconds or minutes	Generally same as for thrombosis except
Noncardiac	There are no warnings	for following:
Atherosclerosis	Branches of middle cerebral artery are involved most	If embolism causes a large hemorrhagic
Pulmonary thrombosis	frequently; large embolus will block internal carotid	infarct, cerebrospinal fluid will be bloody
Fat, tumor, air	artery or stem of middle cerebral artery	30% of embolic strokes produce small
	If embolus is in basilar system, deep coma and total	hemorrhagic infarct without bloody
	paralysis may result	cerebrospinal fluid
	Often a manifestation of heart disease, including atrial	
	fibrillation and myocardial infarction	
	Headache	
	As embolus passes through artery, client may have	
	neurological deficits that resolve as embolus	
	breaks and passes into small artery supplying small	
	or silent brain area	
HEMORRHAGE		
Hypertensive hemorrhage	Severe headache	CT scan can detect hemorrhages larger
	Vomiting at onset	than 1.5 cm in cerebral and cerebellar
	Blood pressure >170/90; usually "essential"	hemispheres; it is diagnostically superior
	hypertension but can be from other types	to arteriography; it is especially helpful
	Abrupt onset, usually during day, not in sleep	in diagnosing small hemorrhages that do
	Gradually evolves over hours or days according to	not spill blood into cerebrospinal fluid; with
	speed of bleeding	massive hemorrhage and increased pressure,

Continued

TABLE 27-2 ■ **Clinical Symptoms and Laboratory Findings for Neurovascular Disease Ruptured Saccular Aneurysm—cont'd**

DISEASE TYPE	CLINICAL PICTURE	LABORATORY FINDINGS
	No recurrence of bleeding	cerebrospinal fluid is grossly bloody; lumbar puncture is necessary when CT scan is not available
	Frequency in blacks with hypertensive hemorrhage is greater than frequency in whites	
	Hemorrhaged blood absorbs slowly—rapid improvement of symptoms is not usual	Radiographs occasionally show midline shift (this is not true with infarction)
	If massive hemorrhage occurs, client may survive a few hours or days as a result of brain stem compression	Electroencephalogram shows no typical pattern, but high voltage and slow waves are most common with hemorrhage
		Urinary changes may reflect renal disease
Ruptured saccular aneurysm	Asymptomatic before rupture	CT scan detects localized blood in hydrocephalus if present
	With rupture, blood spills under high pressure into subarachnoid space	Cerebrospinal fluid is extremely bloody
	Excruciating headache with loss of consciousness	Radiographs are usually negative
	Headache without loss of consciousness	Carotid and vertebral arteriography is performed only when diagnosis is certain
	Sudden loss of consciousness	
	Decerebrate rigidity with coma	
	If severe—persistent deep coma with respiratory arrest, circulatory collapse leading to death; death can occur within 5 minutes	
	If mild—consciousness regained within hours then confusion, amnesia, headache, stiff neck, drowsiness	
	Hemiplegia, paresis, homonymous hemianopia, or aphasia usually absent	

Adapted from Adams RD, Victor M: *Principles of neurology,* New York, 1981, McGraw-Hill.

Two types of drugs are used to counter the effects of spasticity: centrally acting and peripherally acting. Centrally acting drugs, such as diazepam, have been used to depress the lateral reticular formation and thus its facilitatory action on the gamma motor neurons. This form of drug is used widely to treat spasticity, although the greatest disadvantage of centrally acting drugs is that they depress the entire CNS. Drowsiness and anxiety are common side effects.

Peripherally acting drugs are used to block a specific link in the gamma group. Procaine blocks selectively inhibit the small gamma motor fibers, resulting in a relaxation of intrafusal fibers. The effect of procaine blocks is transient. Intramuscular neurolysis with the injection of 5% to 7% phenol has been used to destroy the small intramuscular mixed nerve branches.[17] Phenol blocks relieve hypertonicity and improve function, especially when followed by an intensive course of therapy.[18] It can provide relief from 2 to 12 months, and the effects have been documented to last as long as 3 years.[17,18] Disadvantages of phenol use include its toxicity to tissue and the complications of pain that occasionally result.

Botulinum toxin A (Botox) is also used to decrease the effects of hypertonicity on functional movement in hemiplegia.[19] Local injection of the toxin into spastic muscles produces selective weakness by interfering with the uptake of acetylcholine by the motor end plate. The effect of the toxin is temporary, depends on the amount injected, and is associated with minimal side effects. Repeat injections are recommended no sooner than 12 to 14 weeks to avoid antibody formation to the toxin. Researchers report positive functional results when botulinum toxin A injections are followed by intensive muscle reeducation and appropriate splinting.[19,20]

Dantrolene sodium is used to interrupt the excitation-contraction mechanism of skeletal muscles. Trials have shown that it has reduced spasticity in 60% to 80% of clients while improving function in 40% of these clients. The side effects—drowsiness, weakness, and fatigue—can be decreased through titration of dosage. Serious side effects, including hepatotoxicity, precipitation of seizures, and lymphocytic lymphoma, have been reported when the drug has been used in high dosages over a long time.[17]

Baclofen, in pill form, is used as a skeletal muscle relaxant to decrease spasticity. It can now be delivered intrathecally into the spinal cord with a pump that is surgically inserted into the body. It relieves spasticity with a small amount of medication (10 mg/20 mL, 10 mg/5 mL). Intrathecal baclofen has had dramatic results in cases of severe spasticity because it acts directly on the affected muscles instead of circulating in the blood. It is used for extremity spasticity that interferes with the ability to assume functional positions in patients with severe stroke, multiple sclerosis, head injury, and cerebral palsy.[21]

The surgical treatment of spasticity through tenotomy or neurectomy is considered when all other treatments fail, and it is used to correct deformity, especially of a hand or foot. A peripheral nerve block is often used as a diagnostic tool to evaluate the effect of surgical treatment. If anatomical or functional gains are made through a temporary nerve block, consideration is given to surgical release. The surgical treatment of spasticity does not necessarily result in increased movement control and, with the increased understanding of the causes of spasticity, does not seem appropriate in stroke.

Seizures. The highest risk for seizure after a stroke is immediately afterward; 57% of seizures occur in the first week and 88% occur within the first year.[22] Seizures after thrombotic and embolic stroke are usually of early onset, whereas seizures after hemorrhagic stroke are of late onset. The management of seizures after stroke is usually with antiseizure medication. Commonly used drugs include phenytoin (Dilantin), carbamazepine (Tegretol), gabapentin (Neurontin), and divalproex (Depakote).[23] Side effects that interfere with movement therapy include drowsiness, ataxia, distractibility, and poor memory.

Respiratory Involvement. Fatigue is a major problem for the person with hemiplegia. This fatigability, which interferes with everyday life processes and active rehabilitation, is attributed to respiratory insufficiency resulting from paralysis of one side of the thorax. Haas and colleagues[24] studied respiratory function in hemiplegia and found decreased lung volume and mechanical performance of the thorax to be significant factors, in addition to abnormal pulmonary diffusing capacity. Clients with hemiplegia consume 50% more oxygen while walking slowly (regardless of the presence or absence of orthotic devices) than that used by subjects without hemiplegia.[24] The decreased respiratory output and the increased oxygen demand that result from atypical movement patterns are responsible for early fatigue in persons with hemiplegia. Treatment objectives and techniques must reflect the understanding of this respiratory problem. The therapist should not overlook the use of standard respiratory functions as an objective measure of the efficacy of treatment techniques.

Trauma. If the hemiplegic client has severe trunk weakness with significant spinal asymmetries and relies exclusively on the nonparetic extremities for function, poor balance and falls are possible. Persons with stroke fall to the affected side when protective mechanisms are inadequate or absent. Common fracture sites are the humerus, wrist, and hip.[25]

Therapy intervention for a hip fracture with a hemiplegia is complicated by increased difficulty sustaining a symmetrical trunk posture over the fractured hip, decreased strength in the leg, pain, and spasticity. In addition to the loss of balance and protective mechanisms, the development of osteoporosis from disuse is a limiting factor for functional recovery after a fracture.[26]

Thrombophlebitis. Thrombophlebitis may occur in the early stages of rehabilitation. Vascular changes are often premorbid. Deep vein thrombosis is caused by altered blood flow, damage to the vessel wall, and changes in blood coagulation times. The vascular changes are aggravated by the inactivity and dependent postures of the weak extremities. Deep vein thrombosis is many times more common in the weak leg.[27]

Reflex Sympathetic Dystrophy. Medical treatment of reflex sympathetic dystrophy includes the use of chemical sympathetic blocks and oral or intramuscular corticosteroids. The use of blocks and corticosteroids often stops the burning pain. The length of time of the relief varies from client to client. Adverse reactions from block and corticosteroids occur about 20% of the time[28,29] (see Chapters 15 and 32).

Pain. The pharmacological management of pain (usually shoulder pain) includes the local injection of corticosteroids. (For additional information regarding pain and its management, see Chapter 32.)

Sequential Stages of Recovery from Acute to Adaptive Phase
Evolution of Recovery Process
The evolution of the recovery process from onset to the return to community life can be divided into three stages—acute, active (rehabilitation), and adaptation to personal environment.

The acute state involves the stroke-in-evolution, the completed stroke, or the TIA and the decision whether to hospitalize.

The stroke-in-evolution develops gradually with distinct demarcation of the damaged area over 6 to 24 hours. Thrombosis, the most common cause for stroke, results first in ischemia and finally in infarction. Its gradual onset has led researchers to believe that a "cure" may be found for this type of stroke. If ischemic tissue can be treated and saved before infarction occurs, the neurological damage may be reversible. Small hemorrhages also may become a stroke-in-evolution by effusing blood along nerve pathways and by attracting fluid.[30] A completed stroke has a sudden onset and produces distinct, nonprogressive symptoms and damage within minutes or hours. In contrast, the TIA has a brief duration of neurological deficit and spontaneous resolution with no residual signs. TIAs vary in number and duration.

The physician decides the extent of hospitalization. The trend to hospitalize is more common today than years ago.[31] However, a mild stroke or TIA may produce minimal physical-mental symptoms, and the person may not even seek medical help. Cost-containment measures in hospitals and managed care have led to decreased lengths of stay and the development of critical pathway plans to deliver services more efficiently. Critical pathways are plans that describe the duration and extent of services after a stroke. The inpatient length of stay for acute stroke is currently 2 to 4 days. After the inpatient stay, the client follows one of four pathways: he or she returns home with or without home care services, goes to a rehabilitation hospital for a 2- to 4-week stay, goes to a subacute facility to become strong enough for the rehabilitation regimen, or goes to a long-term care facility for rehabilitation or maintenance care.

Once the stroke is completed, the clinical symptoms begin to decrease in severity. A person with a stroke caused by an embolic episode may have symptoms that reverse completely in a few days; more frequently, however, improvement takes place very slowly with a marked deficit. The fatality rate is high within the first day but decreases substantially in the following months of recovery.[31] Evidence from efficacy studies of rehabilitation programs that aim at improving functional performance is limited. Studies by Bamford and colleagues[32] indicate that early rehabilitation intervention reduces disability and improves compensatory strategies.

The Framingham Heart Study has revealed that long-term stroke survivors have a good chance of returning to independent living. The greatest deficit in those persons with hemiplegia who have recovered basic motor skills and who have returned home is in the psychosocial and environmental areas.[5]

Recovery of Motor Function

Recovery of motor function after a stroke was thought historically to be complete 3 to 6 months after onset. Research has shown that functional recovery from a stroke can continue for months or years.[33]

The initial functional gains after the stroke are attributed to reduction of cerebral edema, absorption of damaged tissue, and improved local vascular flow. However, these factors do not play a role in long-term functional recovery. The brain damage that results from a stroke is thought to be circumvented rather than "repaired" during the process of functional recovery. The CNS reacts to injury with a variety of potentially reparative morphological processes. Two mechanisms underlying functional recovery after stroke are collateral sprouting and the unmasking of neuropathways: regeneration and reorganization.[33] Research continues to provide important insights into the fundamental capabilities of the brain to respond to damage. Methods of intervention that use the environment and help the client learn lead to long-term improved recovery.

The CNS has some predictable traits in response to injury. Twitchell, in his classic study, first documented the initial loss of voluntary function.[34] Although paralysis with flaccidity initially exists, there is seldom, if ever, total paralysis. He reported both an increase in deep tendon reflexes after 48 hours and the emergence of synergistic patterns of movement.[34] The synergistic movement patterns of the upper extremity and lower extremity have been described in detail by many.[35-37] Verbal description of a visual phenomenon often leads to differences in written and spoken communication, yet the visual array or behavioral patterns may be exactly the same.[38] Synergistic patterns may not be the same as movement combinations necessary for function. Although it is stated that the leg recovers more quickly or better than the arm, a leg that is bound by an extensor synergy and that is as "rigid as a pillar" during gait has not recovered more quickly and has no better function than an arm that is flexed and held across the chest and that can only grasp in a gross pattern with no ability to release.

Although studies are investigating the exact nature of the relationship between voluntary movement and spasticity, clinical evidence demonstrates that as voluntary function increases, the dependence on synergistic movement decreases.[16] With the knowledge that the CNS is capable of reacting to injury with a variety of morphological processes, we should no longer view the effect of a stroke as a fixed event. Because the brain immediately institutes neuromechanisms that reconstitute typical functions, therapy interventions should emphasize use of movement patterns on the affected side to maximize return and to help the client achieve the highest level of function.

Predictors of Recovery

Research in motor recovery shows that, although motor recovery may continue after 6 months, the functional status usually remains constant and that 86% of the variance in 6-month recovery is predictable at 1 month.[39]

Although 58% of patients regain independence in activities of daily living (ADL) and 82% learn to walk, 30% to 60% of patients have no arm function.[40] Initial return of movement in the first 2 weeks is one indicator of the possibility of full arm recovery. But failure to recover grip strength before 24 days is correlated with no recovery of arm function at 3 months.[40]

One problem inherent in prognostic research is the lack of a movement-based classification system. The clinical "predictors" in regression models are assumed to be static, whereas, in fact, they may change over time. Another problem is that there may be a lack in accuracy because of differences in researchers' objectives.[41]

As clinicians we can help minimize the problems in research methods by precisely formulating functional goals, stating movement components and significant impairments that interfere with functional performance, and following a model when making clinical decisions to postulate cause and effect during intervention.

Classification of Atypical Movement Patterns

Although the *Guide to Physical Therapist Practice* groups patients with neurological dysfunction according to pathological condition, therapy intervention rarely is directed by the diagnosis of stroke and resultant hemiplegia.[42] The World Health Organization (WHO) and Nagi models give us another option: classification by impairments.[43-45] These models have given therapists an organized structure for evaluation and treatment. They share the impairment category but use different terms to title "dysfunction in task performance" and "the societal implication" of this dysfunction (Table 27-3). The WHO has recently modified its designations from ones with negative connotations (ICIDH-1)—*disability* and *handicap*—to more positive language (ICIDH-2)—*activities* as the nature and extent of functioning and *participation* as the measure of involvement in life situations. In July 2005, the leaders of the III Step Neurologic Consensus Conference urged all participants to adopt the WHO model.

Impairment-related classification systems for stroke are just beginning to be researched.[46] Currently, atypical movement patterns in stroke are classified according to type of lesion (embolism, thrombosis, TIA) or side of weakness. The disease and disability classification models have made it easier for therapists to identify and define the focus of their intervention for the neurological patient. These models help us organize our interventions into two categories: (1) interventions that aim at improving relevant impairments that contribute to functional limitations/disability and (2) interventions that focus on the functional limitation/disability itself. The treatment interventions in this chapter are directed at the impairment category.

Although the main focus of this chapter is the evaluation and treatment of impairments that result in loss of movement control, a stroke may result in damage to other systems that affect the client's ability to perform functional skills.

TABLE 27-3 ■ **Comparison of WHO and Nagi Disability Models**

MODEL	DISEASE	LOSS OR ABNORMALITY	LIMITATION OF ACTIVITY	SOCIETAL CONSEQUENCE
Nagi	Pathology	Impairment Primary Secondary Composite	Functional limitation	Disability
WHO ICIDH-1	Pathology	Impairment Primary Secondary	Disability	Handicap
WHO ICIDH-2	Pathology	Impairment Primary Secondary	Activities	Participation

There may be deficiencies in sensory processing (vision, somesthetic sensation, and vestibular systems) and disorders of cognitive integration (arousal and attention, awareness of disability, memory, problem-solving, and learning), which all have a large impact on functional retraining. Depression and, most important, problems of language and communication also contribute to the client's ability to participate in a therapy program.

Impairments Contributing to Functional Limitation and Disability

Clients with hemiplegia from stroke have movement problems—impairments—that lead to functional limitations and disability. These movement problems manifest themselves as loss of movement in the trunk and extremities, atypical patterns of movement, compensatory strategies, and involuntary nonpurposeful movements of the affected side. These impairments interfere with normal functional movement and lead to loss of independence in daily life.

Impairments, as defined by both models, are the signs, symptoms, and physical findings that relate to a specific disease pathology. Schenkman and Butler were the first to apply a model of impairments to neurological physical therapy practice. Ryerson and Levit, using a similar format, specifically defined the impairment categories as primary, secondary, and composite[47,48] (Box 27-1).

Primary Impairments. Primary impairments are physical findings that are associated with the specific brain lesion. The primary impairments of stroke that relate to functional recovery of movement include changes in strength, changes in muscle tone, muscle activation or control changes (sequencing, firing, initiation), and changes in sensation. Cognitive/perceptual, emotional, and speech and language changes are also primary impairments that have an effect on function but are less of a focus of this chapter.

Secondary Impairments. Secondary impairments involve systems of the body other than the neurological system. They occur as a consequence of the stroke or because of other medical and environmental influences, such as a fall, pneumonia, or phlebitis. As they develop, they influence each other and the primary impairments. Secondary impairments influence the client's level of disability

BOX 27-1 ■ IMPAIRMENTS THAT INTERFERE WITH FUNCTIONAL MOVEMENT

PRIMARY IMPAIRMENTS
Changes in muscle strength
■ Paralysis or weakness
Changes in muscle tone
■ Hypotonicity
■ Hypertonicity-spasticity
Changes in muscle activation
■ Inappropriate initiation
■ Difficulty sequencing
■ Inappropriate timing of firing
■ Altered force production
Changes in sensation
■ Awareness
■ Interpretation
SECONDARY IMPAIRMENTS
Changes in alignment and mobility
Changes in muscle and soft tissue length
Pain
Edema
COMPOSITE IMPAIRMENTS
Movement deficits
Atypical movements
Undesirable compensations

Modified from Ryerson S, Levit K: *Functional movement reeducation: A contemporary model for stroke rehabilitation,* New York, 1997, Churchill Livingstone.

by contributing additional physical problems. There are four major categories of secondary impairments: orthopedic changes in alignment and mobility, changes in muscle and soft tissue length, pain, and edema.

Composite Impairments. Composite impairments are the combined effects of the primary and secondary impairments, motor recovery, effects of treatment, and behavioral factors. Movement deficits are the missing pieces of movement control that the client needs to move normally.

Atypical movements are movements that deviate from normal coordinated movement. Undesirable compensations are alternative severely one-sided strategies used to perform a functional activity because of loss of normal movement patterns.

Patterns of Recovery

In the 1970s, "neurophysiological" theories and approaches changed therapy treatment for adults with CNS lesions. The founders of these approaches described positions and patterns of trunk and extremity movement.[35-37] These patterns were described in terms of spastic synergies, reflexive patterns, and position. Extremity movements were described as patterns of flexor or extensor synergies, arm and leg patterns were changeable according to the influence of tonic reflexes, and trunk position was always short on the affected side with scapula and pelvic retraction. The intervention techniques followed the descriptions and understanding of the movement problems. As knowledge from orthopedics, manual therapy, and motor control grew, therapists looked more closely at movement patterns and body position in clients with hemiplegia and expanded the categories. As early as 1982, new descriptions emerged that combined synergistic patterns and biomechanical influences on the musculoskeletal systems.[49] Today, descriptions of position and patterns of movement follow the impairment categories. The composite impairment category used in this chapter has three generalized movement patterns that creates one model of classification: (1) *movement deficits,* (2) *atypical movements*, and (3) *undesirable compensatory patterns.*[47]

Movement deficits result from severe weakness or paralysis with either gradual, balanced return or no significant return. Functional movement patterns and levels of independence are based on the distribution and amount of return: trunk control greater than extremity control, extremity control greater than trunk control, distal extremity return greater than proximal extremity return or vice versa, and arm control greater than leg control or vice versa. These clients do not have problems with spasticity but, when weakness is severe, have long-term problems with the secondary impairments of muscle shortening and loss of joint range.

In the acute stage, the arm hangs by the side, the humerus is internally rotated, the elbow is extended, and the forearm is pronated. Inferior shoulder subluxation is common. The trunk is weak, the ribs flare, and posture is impaired with a convex lateral curve seen on the affected side. (Appearances of lateral trunk flexion with the concavity on the affected side exist with compensatory upper and lower trunk movements.) In standing, the client has problems recruiting strength on the affected leg. The pelvis lists downward, and the hip and knee flex. The hip and knee flexion combined with a tendency to place more weight on the stronger leg places the ankle in plantarflexion, and no weight is borne on the heel. As the client learns to walk, either the knee flexes because of weakness or the patient compensates and "locks" the knee in extension.

Over time, the heavy arm pulls the upper body into flexion, creating an appearance of a low shoulder. To stand and walk, a compensatory shift of the upper body onto a cane helps the client balance. This overshifting of the upper body also makes it easier for these clients to initiate stepping with the use of pelvic elevation (Figures 27-1 and 27-2).

Atypical movement patterns are found in clients with unbalanced muscle return and deficits in muscle activation. These clients have difficulty organizing and sequencing muscle return, quieting muscles after active firing, and grading strength of contractions. Clients with unbalanced return can be further divided into two subcategories: (1) those with greater weakness, that is, unbalanced return, with secondary problems of muscle shortening and poor alignment, and (2) those with greater return, with more problems of hypertonicity in the arm and leg.

These clients move and function with patterns that were formerly described as "spastic" or "synergistic." They have either anterior or superior shoulder subluxations, which determine the possibilities for fractionated movement in the arm. Common leg movement patterns used for walking include *swing*—proximal initiation patterns of pelvic hiking or rotation toward the affected side, hip flexion with internal rotation and knee extension, or pelvic posterior tilting with hip abduction and knee flexion—and *stance*—toe strike or foot flat, loss of hip extension, and loss of ability to use the leg to initiate forward progression.

Regardless of the proximal trunk and extremity patterns, the ankle/foot and wrist/hand patterns are predictable on the basis of the amount of distal return and the effects of proximal alignment. With weakness, the ankle plantarflexes and the wrist flexes. The foot/hand rotate on the ankle/wrist according to the pattern of and amount of return of proximal movements. Finger and toe patterns (curling/fisting or clawing) follow biomechanical rules of compensation or correlation (Figure 27-3, page 868).

Undesirable compensatory patterns are patterns of function that arise from either of the two previously described movement categories. Undesirable compensatory patterns are one sided; they rely on movements of the uninvolved arm and leg and do not use bilateral movements in the trunk. Because the patterns are one sided, balance is often precarious and external aids are required for support. These patterns create "learned nonuse" of the affected arm and leg, foster asymmetrical postural patterns, and lead to strong patterns of spasticity. Patients who come into therapy with strongly established undesirable compensatory patterns do not respond quickly to any type of intervention. Although therapists may be tempted to train a one-sided pattern in early rehabilitation to quickly meet a stated goal, the long-term effects of "learned nonuse of one side of the body" include increased severity of secondary impairments and poor balance with an increased chance of falls (Figure 27-4, page 869).

Although the main movement problems of stroke occur because of weakness, loss of movement control, and tonal problems of hypertonicity or flaccidity, other movement disturbances, such as ataxia, do occur. In clients with ataxia, the main movement problem is one of wide swings of tone and muscle activation disturbances. In these clients, there is trunk instability, excessive extremity movement, and overshooting of distal targets. Voluntary extremity movements are usually present but uncoordinated (see Chapter 26).

EVALUATION PROCEDURES

Evaluation is a process of collecting information to establish a baseline level of performance to plan interventions and to document progress. This section reviews medical evalu-

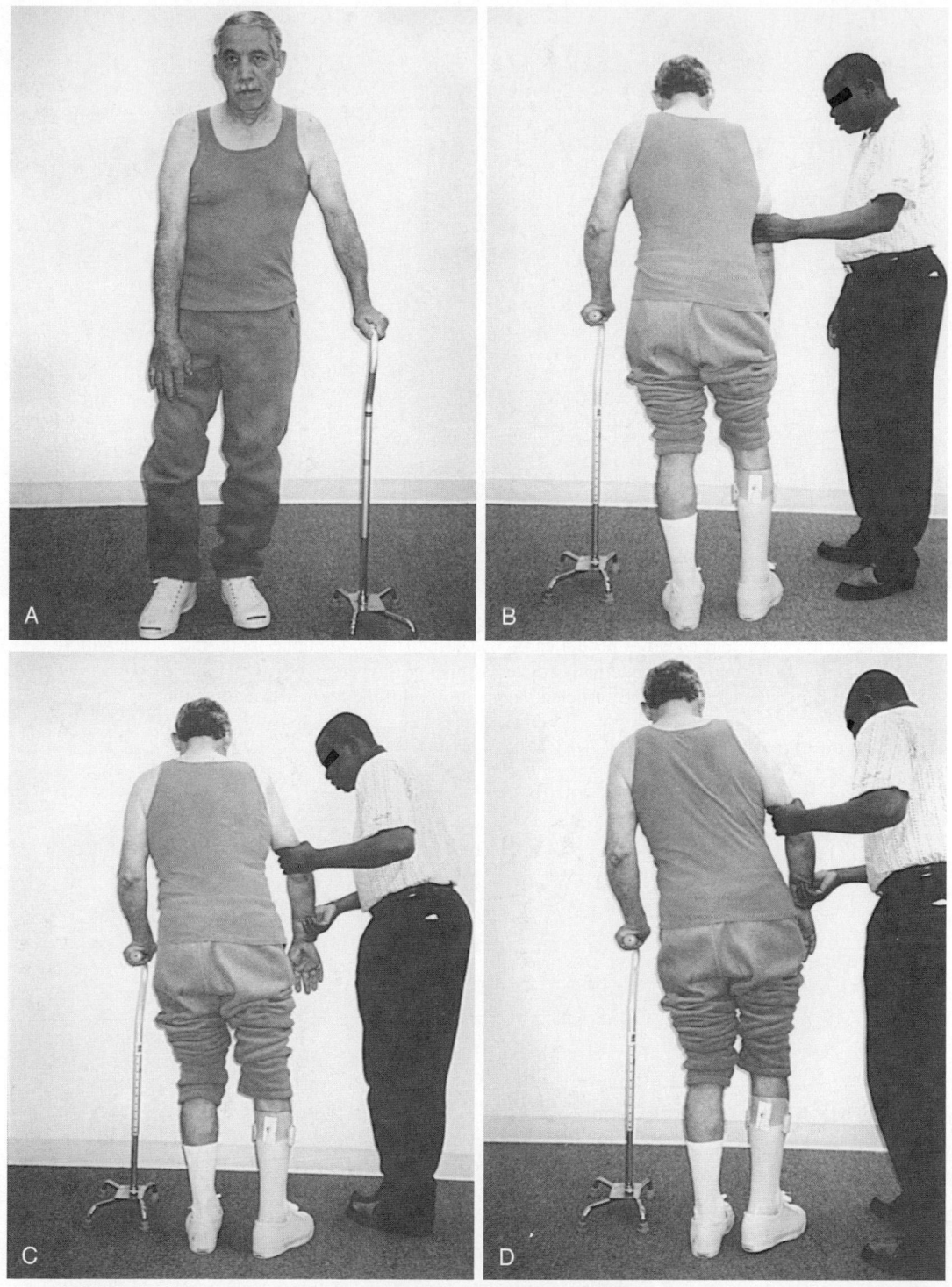

FIGURE 27-1 ■ **A,** Client with right hemiplegia. Movement deficit: paralysis; client was unable to move arm or leg in standing or sitting. **B,** Client uses cane and tries to shift to right as he gets ready to step forward with left leg. Note how the heavy weight of the right arm pulls the upper body into forward flexion and rotation left. **C,** Client prepares to step forward with right leg. Note that his attendant has corrected upper body position. **D,** Client leans heavily onto cane (upper body translates laterally to the left), to lessen weight on the right leg. He will accomplish the "step" by rotating his upper body to left, a compensation for the loss of leg control in standing.

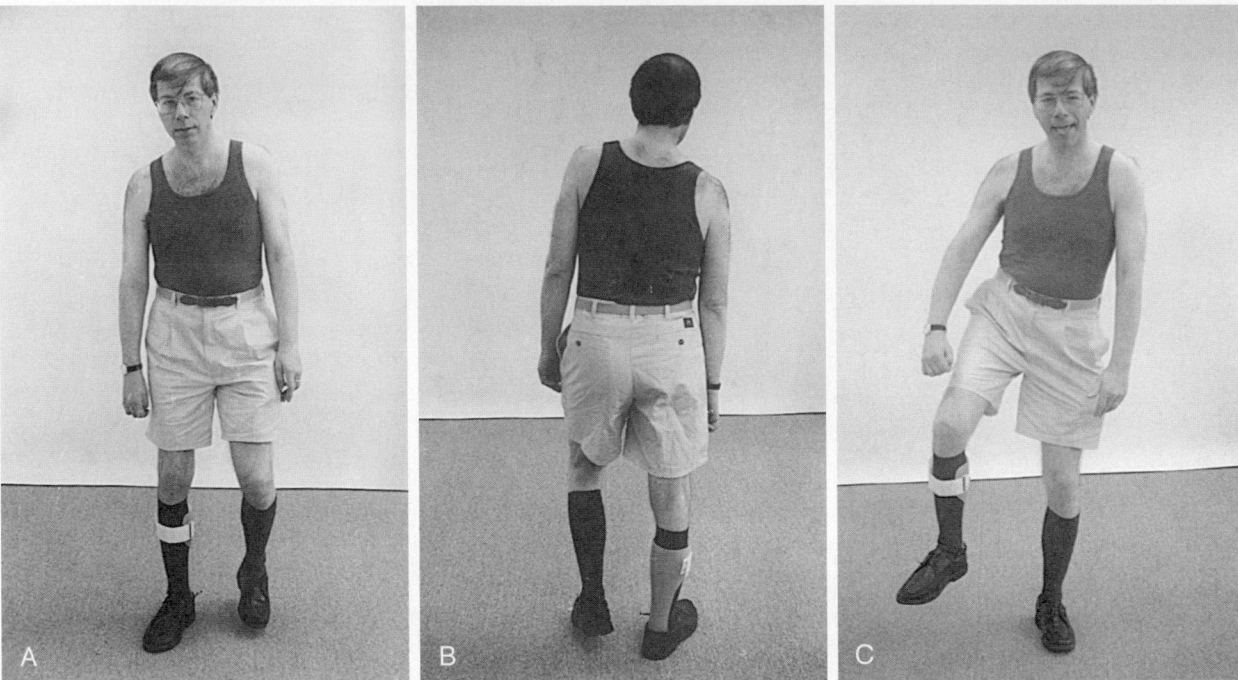

FIGURE 27-2 ■ **A,** Client with right hemiplegia. Movement deficit: weakness; client is able to walk with a brace and does not need a cane. **B,** During stance, his upper body moves laterally to the right and his right femur internally rotates as his knee hyperextends. **C,** He has enough trunk control to stand and balance and sufficient leg control to lift the leg with knee flexion.

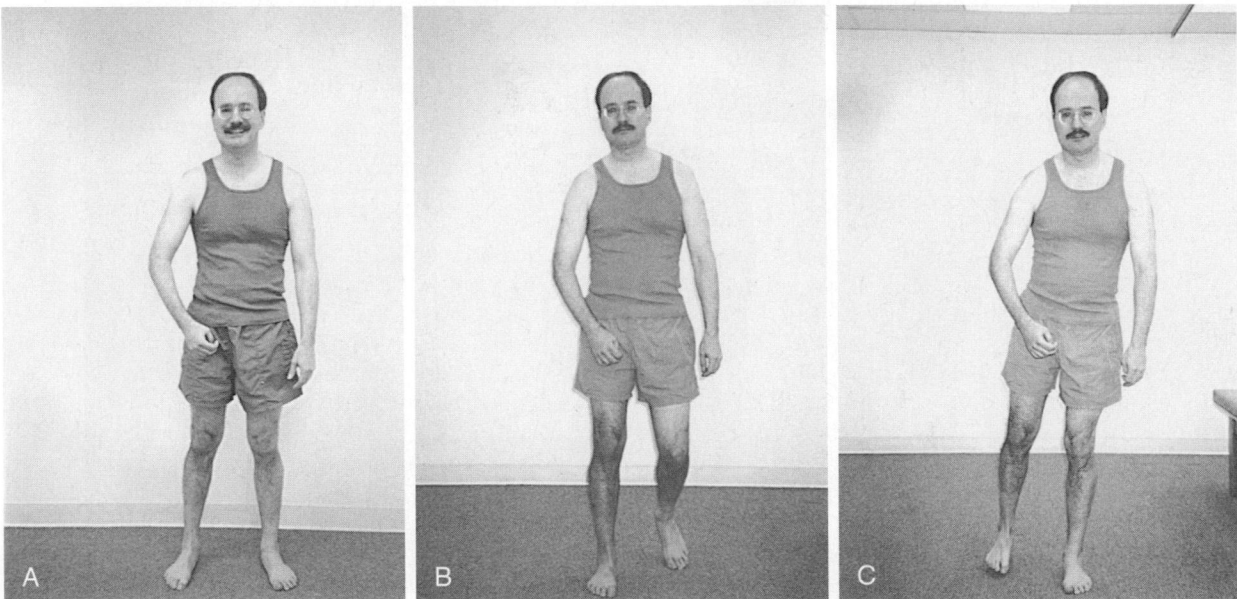

FIGURE 27-3 ■ **A,** Client with right hemiplegia. Movement deficit: loss of control of firing patterns, timing, and sequencing. **B** and **C,** Client walking.

ations, standardized evaluations of functional performance (disability scales), evaluation of motor function and balance, and evaluation of secondary impairments that interfere with motor performance.

Medical Evaluation

After or during the evolution of a stroke, a thorough medical examination is conducted. All systems are surveyed, with emphasis placed on the level of consciousness; mental, affective, and emotional states; communication; cranial nerves; perceptual ability; sensation; and motor function.

Levels of Consciousness

Scales of varying types are used to measure the client's level of consciousness, to assess the initial severity of brain damage, and to prognosticate recovery curves. The Glasgow

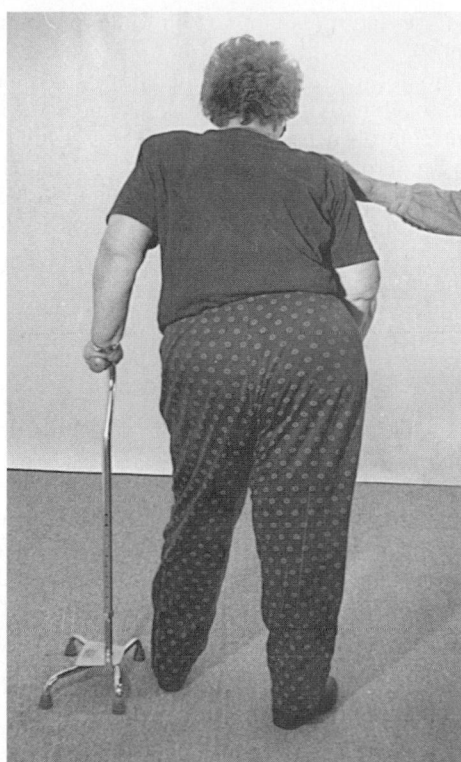

FIGURE 27-4 ■ Client with right hemiplegia. Severe compensatory patterns. She walks with a quad cane and standby assistance. Pelvis rotates to right, upper body rotates to left, hip flexes, and knee hyperextends. There is strong lateral translation of upper body to left (to the stable cane).

Coma Scale, devised by Teasdale and Jennett in collaboration with Plum,[50] has been used for nontraumatic comas caused by stroke, head injury, and cardiac disease. This scale records motor responses to pain, verbal responses to auditory and visual clues, and eye opening. It assigns numerical values according to graded scales. Plum and Caronna[51] and Levy et al[52] have also established criteria for correlating clinical signs of coma with prognosis.

The standard descriptions of level of consciousness—normal, semistupor, stupor, deep stupor, semicoma, coma, deep coma—are categorized by objective medical data but often leave a gap in the understanding of how the client functions in life.[50] This gap was closed by the creation of a scale, "Levels of Cognitive Functioning," devised at Rancho Los Amigos Hospital. This behavioral rating scale is not a test of cognitive skill but an observational rating of the client's ability to process information[53] (see Chapter 17).

Mental, Emotional, and Affective States

The history portion of the neurological evaluation leads to an assessment of the mental, emotional, and affective state. The client's ability to describe the illness gives information on memory, orientation to time and place, the ability to express ideas, and judgment. If the examiner suspects a particular problem, a more thorough review is undertaken of the higher cortical function: serial subtraction, repetition of digits, and recall of objects or names. Clients with right hemiplegia may be cautious and disorganized in solving a

given task, and clients with left hemiplegia tend to be fast and impulsive and seemingly unaware of the deficits present. These different response patterns stem from hemispheric involvement and prior hemispheric specialization.

Loss of emotional control often exists after a stroke. Crying is a common problem. Although excessive, inappropriate, or uncontrollable crying is usually a result of brain damage and a sign of emotional lability, crying can also be an expression of sadness as a result of depression. This difference is distinguishable by the ease with which the crying can be stopped. Other signs of emotional lability in persons with hemiplegia from stroke include inappropriate laughter or anger.

Communication

A general evaluation of communication disorders is noted while taking the history. Cerebral disorder resulting from infarct or hemorrhage can produce a loss of production or comprehension of the spoken word, the written word, or both. The therapist should be familiar with all types of communication disorders and with alternate modes of communication to establish a good client relationship.

Cranial Nerves and Reflexes

Thorough cranial nerve evaluation is necessary in hemiplegia because a deficit of a particular cranial nerve helps to determine the exact size and location of the infarct or hemorrhage. In hemiplegia, it is imperative to check for visual field deficits, pupil signs, ocular movements, facial sensation and weakness, labyrinthine and auditory function, and laryngeal and pharyngeal function.

Standard areas of reflex testing include the triceps, biceps, supinator, quadriceps, and gastrocnemius muscles. According to Adams,[10] there are four plantar reflex responses: (1) avoidance-quick, (2) spinal flexion-slow, (3) Babinski-toe grasp, and (4) positive support.

Perception

Perceptual deficits in clients with hemiplegia are complex and intimately linked to the sensorimotor deficit. Sensory integration theory has begun to establish normative values and objective data for testing and documenting perceptual deficits in children. Currently, norms and testing procedures for adults have not been standardized, but perceptual deficits have been identified in clients with hemiplegia. Common perceptual deficits found in left and right brain damage are listed in Box 27-2.

Perceptual retraining without standardized norms for the deficit is at best difficult. The soundest course currently available appears to be one that relates perceptual and motor learning rather than retraining perception in isolation (see Chapters 9 and 14).

Sensation

Traditional sensory testing is used to assess sensory deficits in the adult with hemiplegia: light touch, deep pressure, kinesthesia, proprioception, pain, temperature, graphesthesia, two-point discrimination, appreciation of texture and size, and vibration. A comparison of the differences in the two sides of the body and qualitative and quantitative measurements are important features of sensory testing. Sensory testing is difficult because it relies on the client's

---

BOX 27-2 ■ PERCEPTUAL DEFICITS IN CNS DYSFUNCTION

LEFT HEMIPARESIS: RIGHT HEMISPHERE— GENERAL SPATIAL-GLOBAL DEFICITS

Visual-perceptual deficits
- Hand-eye coordination
- Figure-ground discrimination
- Spatial relationships
- Position in space
- Form constancy

Behavioral and intellectual deficits
- Poor judgment, unrealistic behavior
- Denial of disability
- Inability to abstract
- Rigidity of thought
- Disturbances in body image and body scheme
- Impairment of ability to self-correct
- Difficulty retaining information
- Distortion of time concepts
- Tendency to see the whole and not individual steps
- Affect lability
- Feelings of persecution
- Irritability, confusion
- Distraction by verbalization
- Short attention span
- Appearance of lethargy
- Fluctuation in performance
- Disturbances in relative size and distance of objects

RIGHT HEMIPARESIS: LEFT HEMISPHERE— GENERAL LANGUAGE AND TEMPORAL ORDERING DEFICITS

Apraxia
- Motor
- Ideational

Behavioral and intellectual deficits
- Difficulty initiating tasks
- Sequencing deficits
- Processing delays
- Directionality deficits
- Low frustration levels
- Verbal and manual perseveration
- Rapid performance of movement or activity
- Compulsive behavior
- Extreme distractibility

---

interpretation of the sensation and on the client's general awareness and suggestibility and on the client's ability to communicate a response to each test item.

The presence and quality of sensory loss must be considered during the process of re-educating motor control. Although Sherrington established the principle of interdependence of sensation and movement, current researchers have refined the concept and hypothesize that sensation modifies continuing movement by providing feed-forward, feedback, and corollary discharge. They have provided evidence that sensation is not an absolute prerequisite for movement.[54]

Evaluation of motor function includes both standardized evaluation of functional performance and evaluation of movement control. Manual muscle testing, while used by physicians to provide a general level of strength, is not widely used by therapists to measure strength in individuals with CNS dysfunction because of the insensitivity of the test to loss of trunk/limb-linked control. New measures of manual muscle testing for stroke are now beginning to be investigated.

Standardized Evaluations

Functional Performance

During the initial interview, the therapist and the client together form a list of limitations and relate them to the client's goals and needs. The client can state his or her perceived functional limitations, or the therapist can ask the client to perform tasks. Commonly used standardized tests/scales for functional limitations/participation/disability are listed here, and additional information is found in Chapter 8.

Scales

The *Barthel Index* is one of the oldest measures of disability.[55] It has excellent validity and reliability and is profoundly simple, but it does not discriminate at higher levels of activity.

The *Motor Assessment Scale* (MAS) comes from the intervention theory of Carr and Shepherd.[56] Its reliability is high, it is simple to administer, and it only takes 15 minutes to perform. Although it mainly evaluates mobility skills, there is an arm and hand function section. The tests of arm function include movement patterns without tasks, and the hand function section uses object manipulation.

The *Function Independence Measure* (FIM) is commonly used in rehabilitation centers, takes 45 minutes to perform, and measures ADLs, mobility, cognition, and communication.[57,58] It has good to excellent reliability.

The *Rivermead Mobility Index* measures mobility only, takes 5 minutes to perform, and has been tested for reliability and validity.[59]

The *Assessment of Motor and Process Skills* (AMPS) is a standardized test that measures task performance abilities and efficiency during instrumental ADLs (IADL). This disability scale is used in occupational therapy evaluations.[60]

Tests of Motor Function and Balance

The *Fugl-Meyer Assessment* is weighted with items measuring arm movement more than leg movement, factors in reflexes and sensation, and has good validity and reliability, but it requires approximately 45 minutes to perform.[61] The movement patterns tested follow the Brunnstrom method of intervention.

The *Berg Balance Scale* is easy to administer, takes 5 minutes, and has norms specific to clients with stroke.[62,63]

The *Postural Assessment Scale for Stroke* is a clinical balance measure that has been found to have better psychometric characteristics than the Berg Balance Scale or the balance subtest of the Fugl-Meyer test for people with severe stroke during the acute recovery phase. It has excellent reliability and validity and is easy to perform.[64,65]

The *Functional Reach Test* provides a measure of balance in standing. It measures control only during anterior (forward reach) weight shifts. Reliability is high, and the test is fast and easy to perform.[66]

The *Wolf Motor Function Test* is used to measure upper extremity movements and functional tasks. It is a timed test, has been tested for reliability and validity, and is the assessment used in constraint-induced treatment studies.[67]

Gait

The evaluation of gait patterns includes the assessment of the temporal characteristics of each gait cycle, the description of gait deviations, and, ideally, the assignment of a numerical score representing the efficiency of ambulation. The *Functional Ambulation Profile* is a system that attempts to relate the temporal aspects of gait to neuromuscular and cardiovascular functioning and converts this relationship to a single numerical score.[68,69]

The Timed Up-and-Go test measures (in seconds) the ability to rise from a chair, walk 3 meters, turn, walk, and return to a seated position. It is frequently used in geriatric populations, but there is no validity testing for people post-stroke.[70]

The temporal characteristics of gait—step time, cycle time, step length, and stride length—can be measured with a piece of chalk and a stopwatch or with more sophisticated equipment such as a gait analyzer. These parameters provide an objective measurement of performance and a baseline from which the efficacy of treatment procedures and client progress can be assessed.

Gait deviations in persons with hemiplegia have been described according to their biomechanical and kinesiological abnormalities and in terms of the loss of centrally programmed motor control mechanisms.[71,72]

Perry[72] described common problems of the hemiplegic person's gait as loss of controlled movement into plantarflexion at heel strike, loss of ankle movement from heel strike to mid stance (resulting in loss of trunk balance and forward momentum for push off), and loss of the normal combination of movement patterns at the end of stance (hip extension, knee flexion, and ankle extension) and at the end of swing (hip flexion with knee extension and ankle flexion).

Knutsson and Richards[71] classified the motor control problems of the hemiplegic gait into three descriptive types. Type I is characterized by inappropriate activation of the calf muscles early in the gait cycle with corresponding low muscular activity in anterior compartment muscles. In the type I activation pattern, the calf musculature is activated before the center of gravity passes over the base of support. This thrusts the tibia backward instead of propelling the body forward in a pushoff as normally occurs. The client with hemiplegia compensates for the backward thrust of the tibia by anteriorly tilting the pelvis or flexing forward at the hip. Type II consists of an absence of or severe decrease in electromyographic activity in two or more muscle groups of the involved lower extremity. This pattern of markedly decreased muscular activity results in the adoption of compensatory mechanisms to gain stability. Type III activation patterns consist of abnormal coactivation of several limb muscles with normal or increased muscular activity levels in the muscle groups of the involved side. This type of pattern results in a disruption of the sequential flow of motor activity.

Evaluation of Movement Control

After the standardized testing is performed, the therapist continues on to a subjective evaluation of movement components, to gather information to answer the question "why" it is difficult for the client to perform specific movements or tasks.

Clients with stroke have difficulty moving the trunk and the arm and leg on the affected side because of the presence of primary and secondary impairments. Objective standardized measures for the primary impairments are few; standard muscle testing has been questioned for CNS deficits because of the numerous degrees of freedom available and the discrepancy in functional strength on the basis of the increasing degrees of difficulty of controlling linked trunk and extremity patterns as the body moves from function in supine, to function in sitting, to function in standing.

Active Movement/Strength

When active movement patterns in the trunk and extremities are assessed, the therapist measures both strength and control. Paralysis, weakness, and imbalanced return are determinates of strength. Initiation pattern, sequencing, and control of firing patterns are indicators of control. Weakness and paralysis after stroke have been largely ignored because of a lingering focus on spasticity. Some recent studies have shown that muscle weakness is, in fact, present and interferes with the ability to generate enough force to allow functional performance.[73-75] Motor weakness is present in 75% to 80% of clients after a stroke. There appears to be no difference in clients with left- or right-sided hemiplegia in terms of frequency or severity of weakness.[76] In contrast to these studies, Landau and Sahrmann[77] investigated the degree of functional impairment in strength that was a result of deficits in the contractile element of the affected muscles. Their findings from comparisons of maximal tetanic contraction of the anterior tibialis muscle suggest that maximal voluntary muscle strength was *not* impaired. Although recent research has moved weakness back into the impairment list, there is much more to learned about the nature of weakness in CNS dysfunction.

The assessment of active movement in hemiplegia is commonly documented by therapists through the use of the Fugl-Meyer Assessment Scale, which is derived from synergistic stages as outlined by Brunnstrom[36] by a modified version of Bobath's long evaluation form, which gradually builds series of selective/fractionated movement in the arm, trunk, and leg, in increasing levels of antigravity control.[78] The Wolf Motor Function Test, developed in conjunction with constraint-induced movement protocols, is a timed measure of upper extremity function, and is also incorporated into the Fugl-Meyer.[67] When assessing weakness and control of active movement patterns, the therapist should analyze and identify the client's patterns of posture and movement in the trunk and extremities by position (supine, side lying, sitting, and standing) and in linked combinations. Active movement control is evaluated in individual muscles, movement components, and movement sequences.[47] Verbal directions or demonstrations may be necessary to help the client understand what is desired. In this phase of the evaluation, the therapist should not physically assist the client's movement but should be prepared to prevent loss of balance.

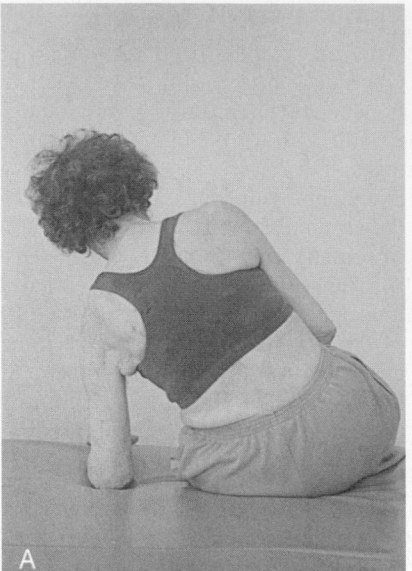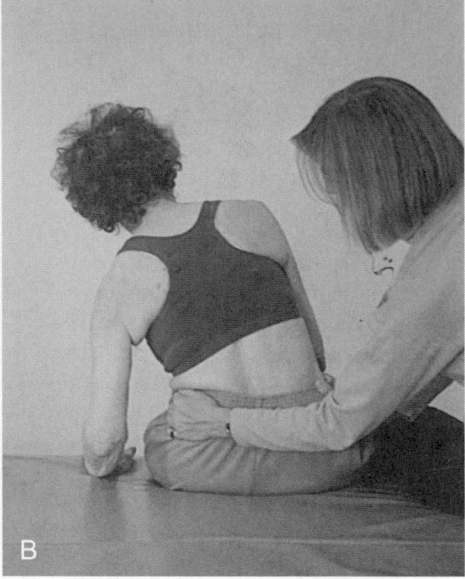

FIGURE 27-5 ■ **A,** Client with right hemiplegia trying to perform an upper body–initiated lateral weight shift to the left. Note the spine is straight and the right hip is off the surface. **B,** Therapist uses her hands to correct and stabilize the lower trunk as the client initiates the upper body lateral movement to the left. The therapist gains information about trunk and hip control and secondary impairments of trunk muscle tightness. Note the spine is beginning to curve as the client uses eccentric activity of the right lateral musculature to control the movement. Active stretching to the right quadratus lumborum/latissimus occurs if tight muscles are present.

While evaluating force production or weakness in all these categories, the therapist gathers information about sequencing movements in increasingly complex patterns, timing of muscle firing, and speed of movement. Muscle activation deficits in these categories may explain why some clients with good recovery of movement control and strength do not regain spontaneous functional use of the extremities.[47]

Assisted Movement

After the evaluation of active movement, therapists use their hands while retesting the movements to gain additional information about the relationships between impairments. Whereas the use of handling must be judicious, handling is used during an assessment for the following purposes:

1. To correct alignment to gather additional information about strength, control, and orthopedic impairments (Figure 27-5).
2. To limit degrees of freedom of one of the joints to assess relationships between intralimb segments.
3. To assist the movement of a weak muscle.
4. To block/stabilize a joint to assess the performance of a weaker muscle group or to limit the degrees of freedom of an intralimb segment[47] (Figure 27-6).

EXAMPLE

Step 1. *Assessment of forward reach in sitting by client with left hemiplegia.* Active movement patterns on left: client initiates movement proximally; shoulder flexes to 60 degrees, with internal humeral rotation; abducted, downwardly rotated scapula elevates during the movement; elbow flexes, forearm supinates to 10 degrees; wrist remains in flexion and radial deviation. Client leans trunk forward to assist with task but cannot reach arm forward to place it on table.

Step 2. *Clinical judgment/hypothesis 1:* weakness of scapula and humeral external rotators prevents antigravity use of elbow extensors during forward reach. Supination of forearm comes from strong proximal initiation and use of elbow flexors to lift arm. *Clinical judgment/hypothesis 2:* forearm/wrist/hand position prevents distal initiation and biases shoulder in internal rotation, thus blocking use of elbow extensors.

Step 3. *Test of hypothesis 1:* therapist uses her or his hands to externally rotate the humerus to neutral and asks client to reach again. *Result:* client activates elbow extension halfway through range with shoulder forward flexion and places wrist/hand on table. *Clinical intervention implication:* increased control of humeral external rotation and increased control of accompanying scapula pattern are important intervention goals to regain forward reach of arm. Retrain trunk/scapula/humeral movement patterns with emphasis on shoulder external rotation and scapular upward rotation. Assess secondary impairments of pectoral and rotator cuff tightness (rotator cuff is shortened if scapula is in an abducted position). *If result is unchanged, test hypothesis 2:* therapist supports wrist and hand with wrist splint or with his or her hand and asks client to reach again. *Result:* client activates elbow extension and places the wrist/hand on the table. *Clinical intervention implication:* prevention/blocking of wrist flexion limits the degrees of freedom, changes the internal rotation moment on the distal portion of the lever arm, and allows use of existing elbow extensors. Use light-weight

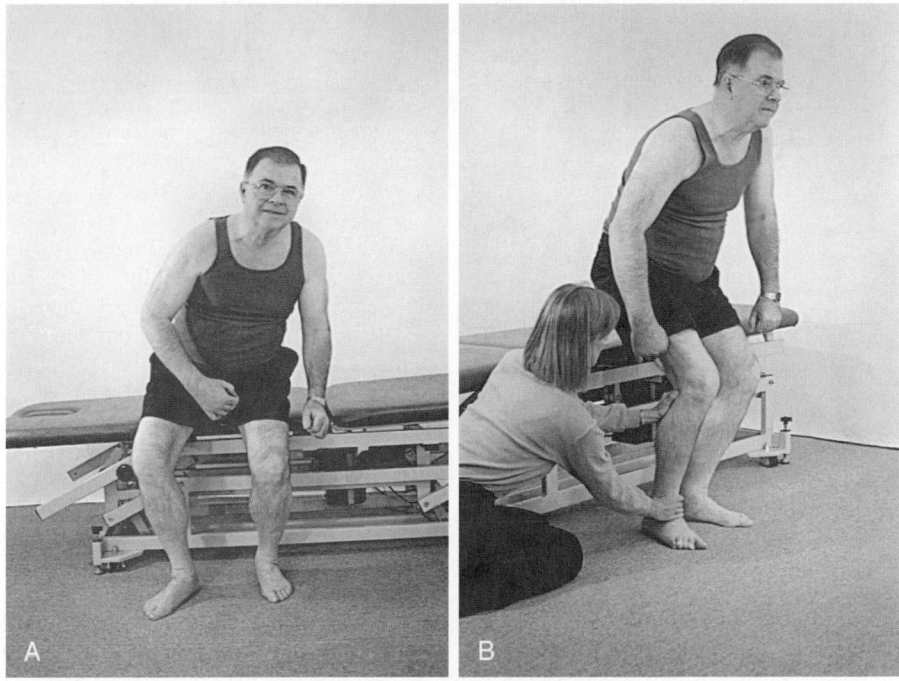

FIGURE 27-6 ■ **A,** Client with right hemiplegia moving from sitting to standing. Note the tendency to use the left leg more than the right, the left rotation of the upper body, and the position of the right arm. **B,** Therapist uses her hands to stabilize the lower leg and to assist lower leg movements as the client initiates sit to stand. Note the change in upper body position and the decrease in arm posturing.

wrist splint during independent practice or use object to assist/preset distal segment during practice.

Tone

The evaluation of postural mechanisms must always include an assessment of tone. Over the years, leading physiologists have split into two camps over the definition of tone. During the beginning of the century, tone was thought of as postural reflexes. In the 1950s the concept of tone was thought of as a state of light excitation or a state of preparedness.[79] Granit,[80] later, encouraged us to think of the relatedness of both these views. He believed that the same spinal organization is mobilized by the basal ganglia to produce both manifestations of tone, a state of preparedness and the postural reflexes.[80] In the 1980s, scientists challenged the concept that what led to a spastic movement pattern was hypertonicity resulting from an exaggerated stretch reflex.[81,82] A new construct emerged in the following years that acknowledged the contribution of both neural and nonneural elements to the phenomenon of "spasticity." This newer concept of spasticity explains why the stretch reflex/tendon tap response (performed in a passive condition—during rest) is an "epiphenomenon and is not the cause of the "spastic movement problem" that interferes with movement."[83] Although the Modified Ashworth Scale is an objective measure of spasticity caused by the stretch reflex,[84] it is not a measure of the functional problem that interferes with skilled movement. It is heartening to hear such discussions occurring among physiologists because therapists are also questioned about their notations of and changes in tone and they often have no objectively derived

standard clinical system for measurement. The debate over tone continues, but clients with CNS dysfunction clinically display changes of muscle tone that result in longer rehabilitation stays and problematic secondary impairments.[85]

The response of a spastic muscle to stretch differs during passive and active movements, leading some to question the usefulness of the classic numerical test of spasticity, the *Ashworth Scale*. The Ashworth Scale rates the severity of tone from 1 to 5.[86]

The first noticeable change in tone is the change from the premorbid state. Clients in the acute phase of hemiplegia exhibit, for varying periods of time, a lower than normal tonal state. Clients with paralysis of the extremities exhibit low tone or hypotonicity. The extremities feel like "dead weight" as the therapist moves them. As neuromuscular return slowly begins, the extremities feel heavy, but some "following" of passive movement patterns is detected.

As the client becomes more active, he or she uses all available movement patterns. Ryerson and Levit have described three specific situations, which in reality have overlap, wherein tone increases (see page 878 for a detailed discussion).[47] This increased tone, hypertonicity, or spasticity occurs in the arm and leg if the client's trunk control is less than the demand of the task, if altered joint alignment increases the tension of the muscle, or if the voluntary movement pattern of the extremity is unbalanced and disorganized.[47,87]

One clinical description of increased extremity tone put forth in the 1970s is still somewhat useful today: severe hypertonicity makes coordinated movements impossible; moderate hypertonicity allows movements that are characterized by great effort, slow velocity, and abnormal coordination; slight hypertonicity allows gross movement patterns to occur with smooth coordination, but combined, selective movement patterns are uncoordinated or impossible.[88]

Equilibrium and Protective Reactions

Equilibrium reactions help us to maintain or regain our balance by keeping the center of gravity within the base of support. Equilibrium reactions are often referred to as the body's first line of defense against falling. They occur when the body has a chance of winning the battle against gravity. If equilibrium reactions cannot preserve balance, the second line of defense emerges: protective reactions. One of the best known protective responses in the arm is the "parachute reaction." Protective responses in the leg in standing include hopping and stepping.

When assessing equilibrium or balance reactions in clients with hemiplegia, the therapist remembers the distinction between equilibrium reactions and protective reactions. Equilibrium reactions should be assessed while slowly moving either the limb or trunk away from the base of support. The amount of control in the trunk and supporting limb, the size of the base of support, and the available range of motion as well as the evaluator's handling skills affect the response (see Chapter 23).

Descriptive Analysis of Functional Activities

When evaluating functional activities, the therapist assesses three phases of the movement pattern. The first phase is the *initiation* of the act, which includes the body segment initiating the movement, the direction of movement, and the establishment of antigravity control. *Transition,* the second phase, represents the point in the functional activity at which there is a switch in the muscle groups that provide antigravity control. The third phase is the *completion* of the activity, involving a final weight shift and the ability to maintain postural control.[47]

If assistive devices are used, the following questions should be asked: Is the device always used? If not, when is it used? How is the device used? Could the device be used another way that would foster trunk symmetry and allow activity of the affected extremities?

Evaluation of Secondary Impairments

Loss of Joint Range and Muscle Shortening

In hemiplegia, loss of joint range is caused by muscle shortening from poor alignment that is the result of weakness or muscle activation problems. Loss of alignment occurs early in recovery, whereas muscle shortening and loss of range occur over time. When measuring joint range of motion and muscle shortening, the therapist must remember to consider the functional consequences of two-joint (multijoint) muscle tightness.

EXAMPLE. In sitting (knee bent), the client has ankle joint dorsiflexion range from 0 to 10 degrees; but in standing (knee and hip straight), ankle joint dorsiflexion range is −20 degrees. This functional loss of ankle range causes significant problems for standing and walking. Loss of ankle joint range in standing may be the result of gastrocsoleus, tensor fasciae latae, or hamstring muscle tightness (Figure 27-7).

Range of motion measurements should be documented in terms of functional position. Extremity muscles that cross multiple joints are the most common groups to shorten and limit joint range in hemiplegia. Muscle shifting (changes in the resting position of muscle bellies and tendons) occurs with prolonged changes in alignment and loss of joint range.

EXAMPLE. Long-standing wrist flexion may cause the ulnar wrist extensor to slip volarly and function as a wrist flexor. Similarly, a position of knee flexion with ankle plantarflexion and talar varus may lead to lateral shifting of the anterior tibial muscle belly. As the muscle shifts laterally, the tension increases distally and foot supination becomes more pronounced.

Pain

Two commonly used standardized pain measurement scales are the *Visual Analogue Pain Rating Scale* and the *McGill Pain Questionnaire.*[89,90] These scales focus primarily on the intensity of pain but provide an objective measure of intervention effectiveness. For an in-depth discussion of the topic of pain management, see Chapter 32.

The presence of pain in hemiplegia is devastating for the client and makes movement reeducation difficult. Shoulder pain is the most frequent pain complaint after stroke.[11,91] Pain must be evaluated specifically and should not be allowed to occur during intervention; the "no pain, no gain" message that is sometimes used in sports or orthopedic intervention should not be used in neurorehabilitation. Pain is an indicator that joint alignment or movements are incorrect. See Box 27-3 for general questions.

Motor Evaluation Forms

The foregoing information, once gathered, can be placed on an evaluation form in many ways. Every medical institution seems to have its own evaluation form and its own system of recording data. Active movement at the shoulder joint may be described in one institution in terms of percentages of synergistic stages, at another institution by a narrative of degrees and planes of movement, and at still another by functional outcomes of shoulder movement. At one hospital the documentation of pain may be descriptive, and at another

---

BOX 27-3 ■ **QUESTIONS FOR SUBJECTIVE EVALUATION OF PAIN**

Location: Where is the pain? Pinpoint the location.
Type: What does it feel like?
- Pins and needles
- Sharp and stabbing
- Aching
- Dull
- Pulling

Occurrence: When does the pain occur?
- At rest
- During movement
  - Range of motion exercises
  - Weight-bearing exercises
  - A specific part of the movement

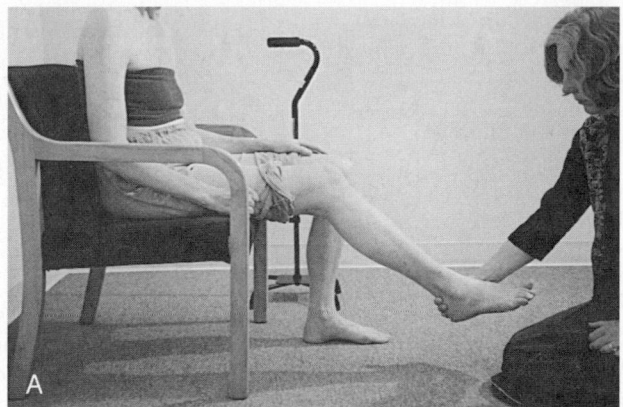

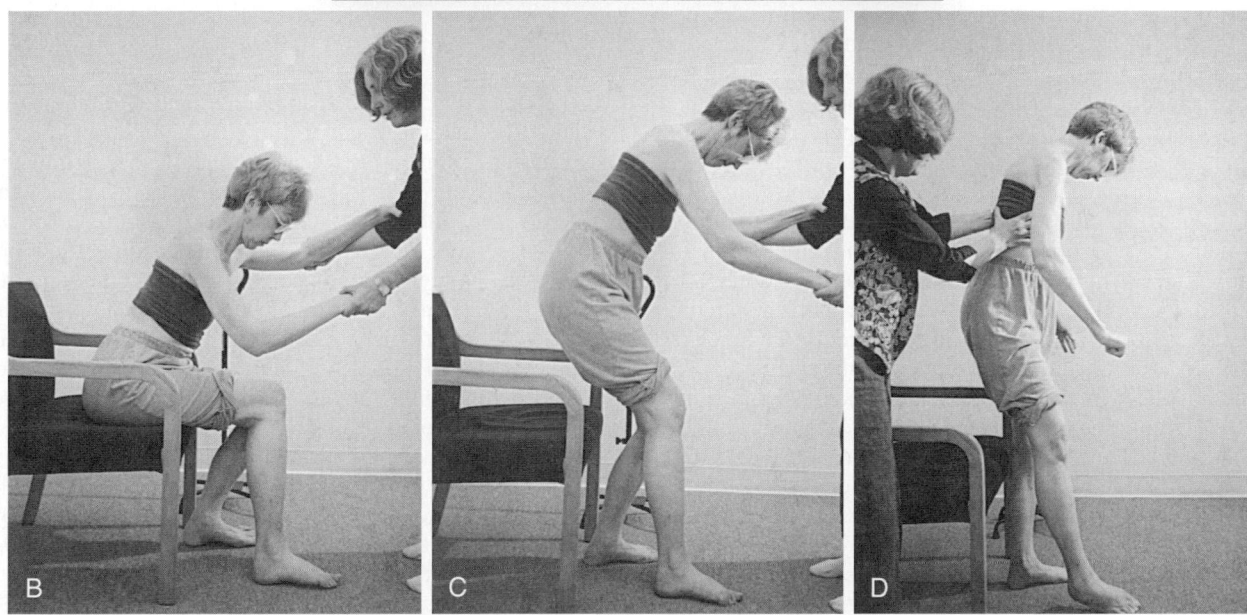

FIGURE 27-7 ■ **A,** Client with right hemiplegia with limited range in hamstring, tensor fasciae latae, and gastrocnemius/soleus muscles. **B,** Client has sufficient range at ankle to keep foot on the floor in sitting and as she initiates the rise to standing. **C,** As she stands and reaches the limit of range of these two muscle groups, her body compensates. The pelvis rotates right, and the tight medial hamstring adducts and internally rotates the femur and pulls the knee into extension as its medial insertion becomes more anterior to the joint. **D,** As the knee extends more, the calcaneus moves into equinus and varus. The foot supinates as a result of calcaneal varus and external tibial rotation from the tight tensor fasciae latae.

it may be numerical. It is important to keep in mind the substance of the evaluative material, not the form in which it is described. A detailed motor evaluation form is necessary for the establishment of realistic goals and for subsequent treatment planning, but the specific form depends both on the needs of the specific clinical setting and on the clinician's choice.

Recognizing Needs

The information obtained from the total evaluation provides the basis for answers to the following questions:

What movements and functions are possible?

What movements and functions are not possible?

How do the movement impairments and secondary impairments relate to functional performance?

By understanding the impairments and their relationship to functional limitations, the therapist can answer the following question: What significant movement components are missing? The answer to this question becomes the objective for treatment. How the possible is accomplished and why the impossible exists provide logical suggestions for selection of intervention techniques.

Therapy intervention occurs at either the level of activity (functional) limitation or at the level of movement-related primary and secondary impairments. The process of establishing goals and selecting activities for intervention begins with clinical decision making or problem solving.

CLINICAL DECISION MAKING/PROBLEM SOLVING

Problem solving is a process of gathering and analyzing evaluation information from task and movement analysis, organizing and reflecting on this information to develop hypotheses for causal relationships between significant impairments and functional performance, and establishing and prioritizing goals for therapeutic intervention. The problem solving process is also used to hypothesize how the movement problems of the trunk, arm, and leg are interrelated and how these problems relate to the ability to perform tasks. Movement control deficits, secondary impairments, and compensatory or atypical movement patterns should be identified for the trunk, arm, and leg in relation to each significant functional limitation.

Analyzing Evaluation Material

The relationship between functional performance and primary and secondary impairments in stroke has not been researched. Therefore, this relationship, which is the basis for therapy intervention, must be derived from clinical experience and judgment. Clinical intuition guides the evaluation process—what should be evaluated and how. As a result of the evaluation, the therapist has a list of functional skills that are difficult or impossible for the client to perform and a list of primary and secondary impairments that relate to the attempted performance of that task. The therapist analyzes this information with the goal of identifying common impairments in categories of tasks: Which primary impairments are major impediments in each task analyzed? Are there secondary impairments that interfere with the client's ability to perform specific critical movement components? What is the level of trunk-extremity control during task performance in each functional position evaluated? While analyzing the evaluation material, the therapist pays attention to all significant factors that limit performance of tasks, including cognitive, perceptual, and emotional problems.

EXAMPLE. A patient after an acute stroke with left hemiplegia cannot perform morning daily care activities at the sink while sitting in a wheelchair, cannot transfer from bed to chair, and cannot rise to stand. Common primary impairments include paralysis or weakness of the trunk and left arm and leg, inability to initiate arm movements, movements of the leg in supine against gravity but no ability to move the leg against gravity when sitting, and loss of proprioception, or the ability to distinguish touch. Secondary impairments that begin to appear by the end of the acute stay include excessive lateral trunk flexion with the convexity of the spinal curve on the left; inferior shoulder subluxation; loss of ankle joint dorsiflexion range; tightness in pectoralis, wrist flexors, and gastrocnemius; and edema in the hand and foot.

In the rehabilitation phase of care, the primary impairments of weakness and loss of control begin to improve. Clinical hypertonicity may be added to the primary impairment list at this time because of the increased activity level of the client. As the client performs tasks that exceed his level of trunk strength and control, tone in the arm and leg will increase as a strategy for maintaining balance or reinforcing trunk control. Secondary impairments of shoulder pain increase, along with increasing numbers and degrees of muscle tightness and continued loss of trunk-extremity alignment.

Developing Hypotheses for Significant Impairments

The process of motor performance evaluation results in a list of multiple impairments. However, not all these impair-

---

> ### BOX 27-4 ■ MOVEMENT COMPONENT CONTROL MODEL OF POSTURAL CONTROL
>
> Postural tone and stability
> Trunk control
>   Level I: Basic movement components
>   Upper body– and lower body–initiated movement
>   Anterior
>   Posterior
>   Lateral
>   Level II: Coordinated trunk and extremity patterns
>   Level III: Power production
> Equilibrium and protection

ments directly relate to each functional limitation of the client. The therapist, using clinical judgment, hypothesizes a causal relationship between frequently occurring limitations and functional performance. These impairments, called *significant impairments,* are the ones that must be changed for measurable changes in movement and function to occur.[47] The other impairments are not forgotten but are reevaluated later as improvement begins and new functional goals are chosen. The significant impairments are often used as the focus of short- and long-term impairment goals. Because functional movement depends on the linkage of trunk and extremity movements, the therapist develops hypotheses between impairments in the extremities and specific levels of trunk control to set goals that result in improved functional performance. If weakness and control deficits of the trunk, arm, and leg are treated separately, the client may see improvement in the impairments but not see a change in function (Box 27-4). (See Chapters 8 and 9 for further discussion.)

Goal Setting

Once the therapist reviews the impairment list and selects significant impairments that interfere with functional performance, the therapist and the client together choose a practical functional goal or a category of functional goals.

Functional Goals

Functional goals are based on the needs and desires of the client and on the functional impairments that have been identified by the therapist during the initial assessment. Functional goals should represent a significant change in the patient's level of independence, be practical, and reflect improvement in a specific functional limitation. They state the desired function and the expected level of performance.[47]

EXAMPLE. Client will stand independently and safely while performing self-care activities at the bathroom sink.

Long-Term Goals

A long-term goal should reflect a major improvement in a primary or secondary impairment or an increase in level of performance of an existing skill. The accomplishment of a long-term goal brings the client closer to the functional goal. The time it takes to accomplish a long-term goal varies tremendously depending on the frequency of treatment and

BOX 27-5 ■ COMPONENT GOALS IN FUNCTIONAL TRAINING

Component goal (power): Restore strength in trunk and extremity patterns (individual muscles, components, sequences)

Component goal (structure): Minimize/eliminate secondary impairments

Component goal (control): Reeducate patterns of control (sequencing/timing)

BOX 27-6 ■ REEDUCATION STRATEGY FOR INTERVENTION

Reeducating basic trunk movement components
Linking trunk/extremity patterns
■ Weight bearing
■ Movements in space
Preventing, minimizing, eliminating secondary impairments
Teaching appropriate compensations
Teaching independent practice routines

---

the length of time after stroke. The therapist may set many short-term goals to achieve one long-term goal. Long-term goals may be stated in functional terms, but they usually reflect a change in a primary impairment: an increase in strength, movement control, or balance.[47]

EXAMPLES. Functional goal: Client will be able to perform meal preparation activities in the kitchen safely (in standing)
Long-term goals:
1. Client will perform upper body-initiated movement (lateral and rotational) in standing while supporting hips against a kitchen counter.
2. Client will safely stand near the kitchen counter and maintain balance during far reach movements of the uninvolved arm.

Short-Term Goals

A realistic short-term goal should be achievable quickly and should be based on the result of the patient's response to handling during the evaluation of movement. Short-term goals should directly relate to the accomplishment of the long-term goal. There are multiple short-term goals that relate to one long-term goal. Short-term goals are compiled from the list of relevant secondary impairments or desired increases of strength or movement control. These goals are measurable but do not in and of themselves result in a functional change.[47]

EXAMPLE. Client will lengthen tight hamstring and gastrocnemius muscles in standing to allow the foot to remain flat on the floor during assisted upper body movements in standing.

When stated in terms of movement control rather than functional performance, these goals include the reestablishment of generalized movement patterns that link movement patterns of the trunk and extremities (Box 27-5).

Choosing Intervention Techniques

Once the problem-solving process of goal setting is finished, therapists can select specific intervention techniques and activities. Therapists have many techniques to choose from to meet their goals. Most clients with stroke will not fully regain normal movement patterns regardless of the type of intervention they receive.

Controversy exists as to the means of increasing functional mobility and performance in clients with stroke. One school of thought teaches compensatory patterns or hopes for some use of the affected side through task-specific practice

without direct intervention for the neurological impairments. The other prevalent practice pattern is to increase functional movement patterns on the affected side by increasing control and strength of movement sequences of the trunk and limb through specific levels of reeduction.[47,92-94]

A combination of these two practices may be useful: impairment-based intervention strategies to reeducate movement and training strategies to foster desirable compensations—a functional reeducation strategy. This type of intervention includes strengthening trunk/extremity-linked patterns of movement, minimizing or eliminating secondary impairments that interfere with regaining control, teaching appropriate compensations, and training the client to practice functional movement patterns in context of daily tasks[47,95] (Box 27-6). Research findings support a link between the trunk and upper extremity and the trunk and lower extremity during reaching activities.[96,97] One result of this research has been to design treatment interventions that restrain trunk movements during forward reach retraining to increase control of elbow extension movement in the paretic arm.[98,99]

For reeducation to be effective, therapists must allow the patient to initiate the active trunk/extremity pattern, must move from assisted practice to independent practice with the assistance of appropriately selected objects or verbal cues, and must teach the patient appropriately staged practice patterns. Studies, based on the "learned nonuse" phenomenon described by Taub, have shown that when patients are encouraged to use the affected arm, rather than receiving pessimistic messages about its potential, movement, and functional use, even if limited, are possible.[100-102]

Regardless of intervention type used, task-performance practice or a reeducation strategy, there comes a time in the recovery process when therapists help the client select practical compensatory strategies. Compensatory strategies are taught when the client needs to function independently and cannot yet use the affected arm because of insufficient recovery or the severity of damage. To be appropriate, the strategy should incorporate the use of the involved extremities and use appropriate trunk movement patterns to maximize the use of future return of movement. Undesirable compensations are patterns that are so asymmetrical that they fail to incorporate available movements of the affected trunk and extremities (Figure 27-8).

Although current literature generally applauds function-based techniques, therapists in clinical setting use hands-on approaches to increase muscle strength and control and to decrease impairments that block the emergence of new functional patterns.[47] As research in movement science and

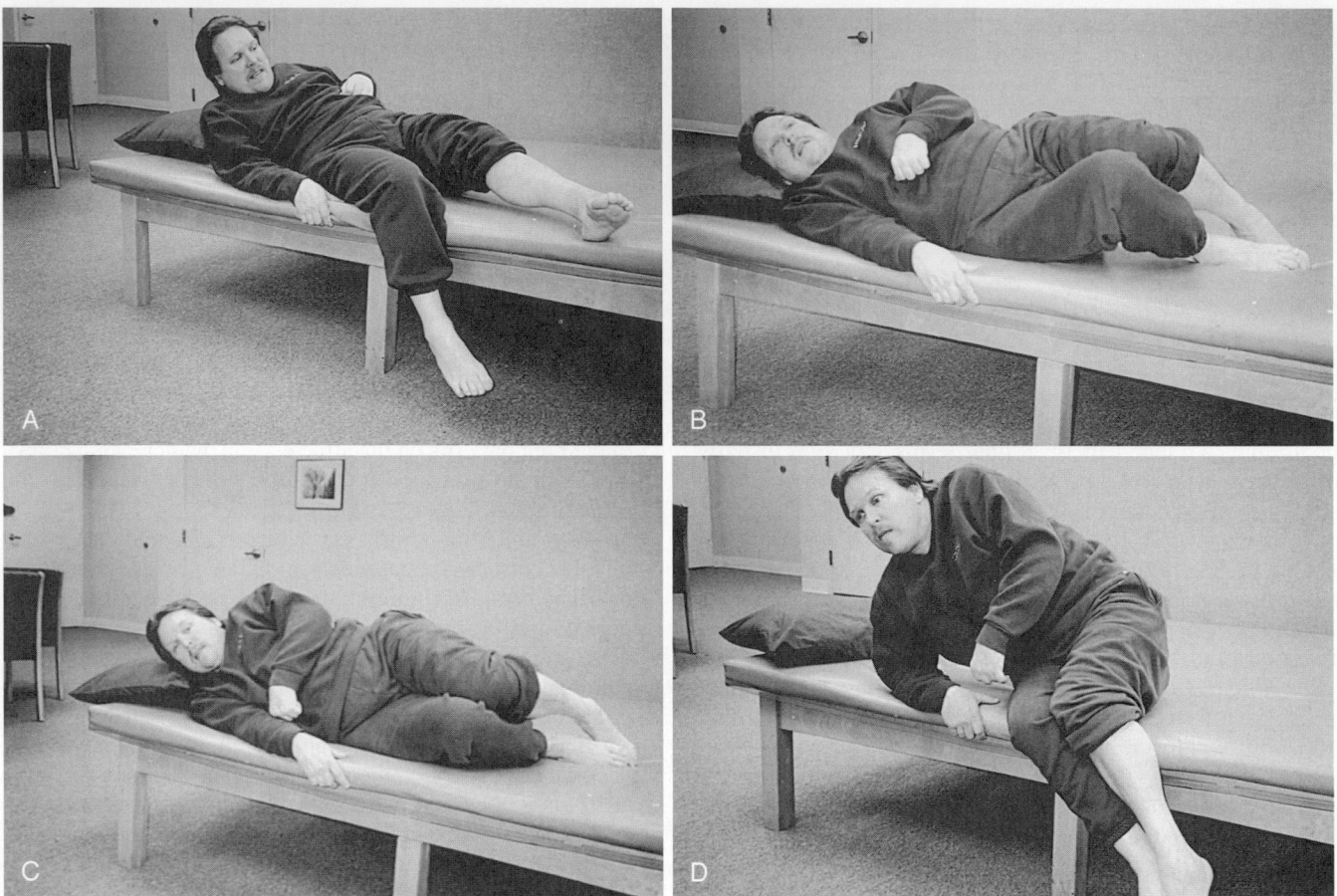

FIGURE 27-8 ■ **A,** Client with left hemiplegia using his right side to move to sitting and not incorporating movement of the left side—an undesirable compensation. **B** to **D,** Client moving to sitting while using as much control as possible on the left side to assist the movement to sitting.

recovery of movement increases, therapists must critically analyze research findings and compare them with their own clinical experience and intuition.

COMMON IMPAIRMENTS AND INTERVENTION SUGGESTIONS

Weakness and Loss of Control

Diminished muscle strength, either paralysis or weakness, is an important category of impairment in hemiplegia. A paralyzed muscle is unable to contract to produce enough force for movement. A weak muscle contracts insufficiently for joint or body segment movement or to allow functional performance.[73-75] In a client with a severe, acute stroke, the paralysis or weakness affects the majority of muscles and results in a loss of functional movement in the face, trunk, arm, and leg. In clients with less-severe strokes, some muscle groups are weak and produce movement, whereas other muscles are paralyzed and cannot be activated. Other stroke patients have no paralysis, only weakness.[43]

Weakness from stroke differs from generalized weakness and orthopedic weakness: it involves one entire side of the body and includes the trunk and extremities. Weakness in trunk muscles can exist with patterns of hypertonicity in the arm and leg. Muscle weakness in the trunk affects postural control and the ability to perform movement sequences.[102] Weakness in the extremities interferes with functional use in either weight bearing or movement in space.[47,103]

Model of Postural Control

Trunk control allows the body to remain upright, to adjust to weight shift, to control movements against the constant pull of gravity, and to change and control body position for balance and function. Therapy based on neurophysiological models stressed facilitation of trunk rotation to gain trunk control. Newer clinical models of postural and trunk control began appearing around 1990.[87,104,105] Information from motor control science has resulted in revision of therapists' thoughts on trunk control.[106-108]

In a movement component model of postural control, trunk control is part of postural control[109] (see Box 27-4). Trunk control has levels of increasing difficulty. Trunk control not only helps us remain upright but also allows weight transfer to free an arm or leg for function. For some functional movements, such as sitting, trunk control keeps the upper and lower trunk stable as we shift our weight and balance. For other tasks, such as reaching forward beyond the length of the arm, the upper trunk is stable and adjusts to the lower body-initiated anterior weight shift.[47]

Additional postural control models, based on a developmental or systems model, are well documented.[88,110-112]

TABLE 27-4 ■ Upper Body-Initiated Weight Shift Pattern: Sitting

WEIGHT SHIFT	SPINAL PATTERN	MUSCLE ACTIVITY
Anterior movement—reach down to floor	Flexes	Eccentric extensor activity
Posterior—to sit back up	Extends	Concentric extensor activity
Lateral—reach sideways and down to right	Laterally flexes with concavity on right	Eccentric lateral activity on left
Lateral—comes back up to middle	Spine moves back to neutral	Concentric lateral activity on left

Research in the field of postural control shows that the level of trunk control and trunk strength correlates with sitting balance, that extremity function correlates with trunk control, and that loss of trunk strength occurs in all planes.[102,113,114]

As a result of differences in testing methods, position, and design, there is no consensus on whether there is trunk muscle weakness after a stroke: some research findings indicate a loss of lateral paretic-side trunk strength,[115] others find no significant difference in lateral trunk strength,[116,117] and others find sight weakness in the trunk extensors.[118,119]

Postural Tone and Stability. Clients with hemiplegia frequently have alterations in both muscle tone and postural tone. Postural tone refers to the overall state of tension in the body musculature. Postural tone is tone that is "high" enough to keep the body from collapsing into gravity but "low" enough to allow the body to move against gravity. It is influenced by the input from the corticospinal tracts, the vestibular system, the alpha and gamma systems, and peripheral-tactile and proprioceptive receptors.[120] Normal postural tone allows a constant interplay between the various muscle groups in the body and imparts a constant readiness to move and to react to changes in the environment (internal and external). It provides us with an ability to adjust automatically and continuously to movements. These adjustments provide the proximal fixation necessary to hold a given posture against gravity while allowing voluntary and selective movements to be superimposed without conscious or excessive effort.

Trunk Control. Trunk control can be divided into levels of increasing complexity. The first level of trunk control is the ability to perform the basic movement components. Trunk strength and control at this level provides a base that allows extremity movement to be combined and used for function. Retraining strength and control of basic trunk movements in the three cardinal planes is a prerequisite for the coordination of trunk and extremity patterns for tasks.

Trunk movements in sitting are initiated from the upper trunk or the lower trunk according to the demand of the task. In standing, functional trunk movements are initiated from the upper trunk (if the head or arm is initiating a task) or the lower extremity. The two initiation patterns result in different spinal patterns, different types of muscular activity, and changes in the distribution of weight[47] (Tables 27-4 and 27-5). These basic movement patterns allow the body to be positioned for functional use.

EXAMPLES. While sitting, the client reaches down or sideways to the floor to pick up an object. As the arm reaches

TABLE 27-5 ■ Lower Body-Initiated Weight Shift Pattern: Sitting

WEIGHT SHIFT	SPINAL PATTERN	MUSCLE ACTIVITY
Posterior weight shift—	Flexion	Concentric flexor activity
Anterior weight shift—	Extension	Concentric extension activity
Lateral weight shift—to R	Lateral flexion—convexity to R	Eccentric lateral activity R Concentric lateral activity L

down, the upper body initiates the anterior weight shift. The lower body provides stability yet adjusts and adapts.

While sitting, the client lifts up a leg to tie a shoe. As the leg moves up, the lower body initiates a posterior weight shift. The upper body adjusts to the weight shift and to the demands of the arm and hand as they tie the shoe.

The second level of trunk control links trunk and extremity movements. This level of control allows the trunk to remain stable yet adapt to movement of the arms and legs. There are two different ways this happens: trunk movements occur as postural adjustments to extremity movement around midline, or trunk movements can precede voluntary movements to help extend the reach of the extremities. These coordinated movements can occur in supine, sitting, or standing.

EXAMPLES
1. In sitting, the lower trunk initiates a forward weight shift to extend the reach of the lifted arm. The upper body adjusts to the scapula/humeral demands and yet remains relatively stable and adjusts to the forward movement of the lower body.
2. In standing, upper trunk movements occur as postural adjustments to maintain balance and the trunk remains stable and adaptable to allow the legs to initiate the forward weight shift of walking.

The third level of trunk control allows strength and stability for power production from the arm or leg. The movement and control of the trunk are used to support power production in the extremities for propulsive activities such as stair climbing, jumping, running, throwing, hitting, and rowing.

The entire model is summarized in Box 27-4.

Extremity Weakness
Weakness in the arm and the leg results in ineffective and inefficient functional patterns in daily life. Intervention for

weakness in the extremities includes reeducation of movements in space, reeducation of weight-bearing movements, and training of and appropriate initiation and sequencing of movement. Most clients with hemiplegia regain enough control in the leg to stand and walk, but those same patients may not be able to use the arm for any purpose. Today, the concept of "learned nonuse" may help therapists understand why the discrepancy between arm and leg recovery exists. Wolf et al[101] conclude from studies of hemiplegic patients that learned nonuse does exist in some patients with stroke and suggest a program of "forced use" training. Although the research training model may not be directly transferable to the clinic, this study points out the benefits of incorporating the use of the affected side in intervention strategies.

Distal reeducation is an important component of early reeducation that has been neglected by therapists because of a previous belief that proximal return comes before distal. Distal reeducation trains the client to be able to initiate movements from the hand or foot, instead of the common proximal initiation patterns seen during attempted reach or stepping (Figure 27-9).

Weight bearing on either the forearm or the extended arm is used as a postural assist during transition activities such as side lying to sitting, or as a means of supporting the weight of the upper trunk in sitting or standing, and is used to stabilize objects during task performance. The activity of accepting weight through the arm is not passive but extremely active and dynamic. Forearm weight bearing in sitting or standing is used to activate trunk movements, to re-establish scapulohumeral rhythm, to maintain range of motion in the arm, or to strengthen movement sequences in the arm. It is not used to inhibit tone (Figure 27-10). The muscles of the arm are linked with trunk weight shifts during active weight bearing.[47] Table 27-6 presents the linked trunk/arm muscle activity during active weight bearing for one functional task.

The ability to support body weight on both legs for stability and movement control is important in sitting, standing, and walking retraining. Movements of the trunk in sitting and standing occur with constant changes of muscle activity in the legs as part of the base of support, to adjust to demands of weight shifts, and to increase activity levels of leg muscles to initiate standing weight shifts. Loss of control of weight bearing on both legs or on one leg has an immediate effect on balance. Problems of weight-bearing control of the leg may exist because of weakness; because of muscle shortening in the pelvis, hip, knee, or ankle; or because of posturing. When the leg cannot actively support

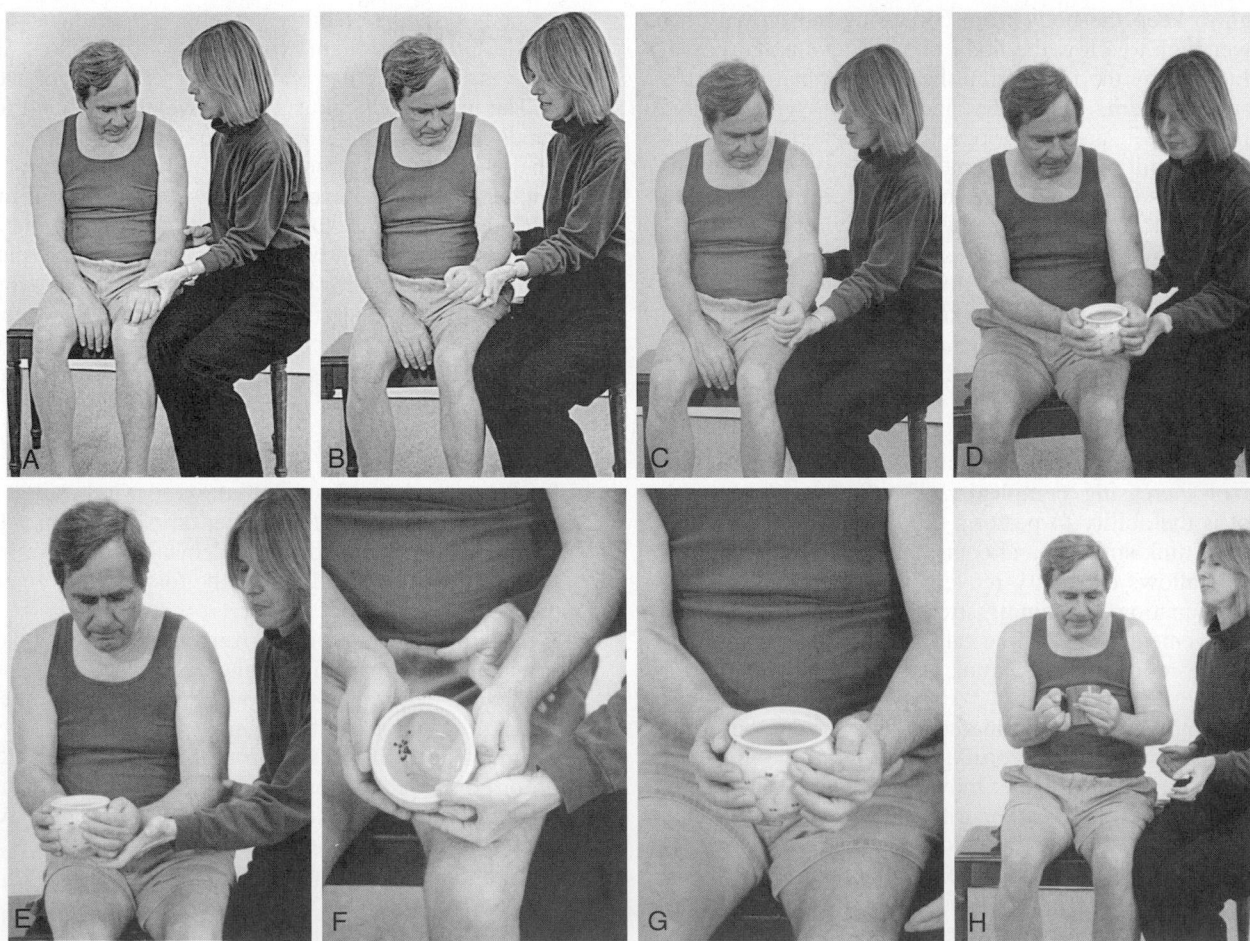

FIGURE 27-9 ■ **A** to **C,** Client with left hemiplegia. Therapist assists movements of forearm, wrist, and hand as client practices increasing distal arm control. **D** to **F,** Therapist introduces object and assists client as he learns to control the object and the movement. **G,** Independent practice. **H,** Client uses same movements with a similar object.

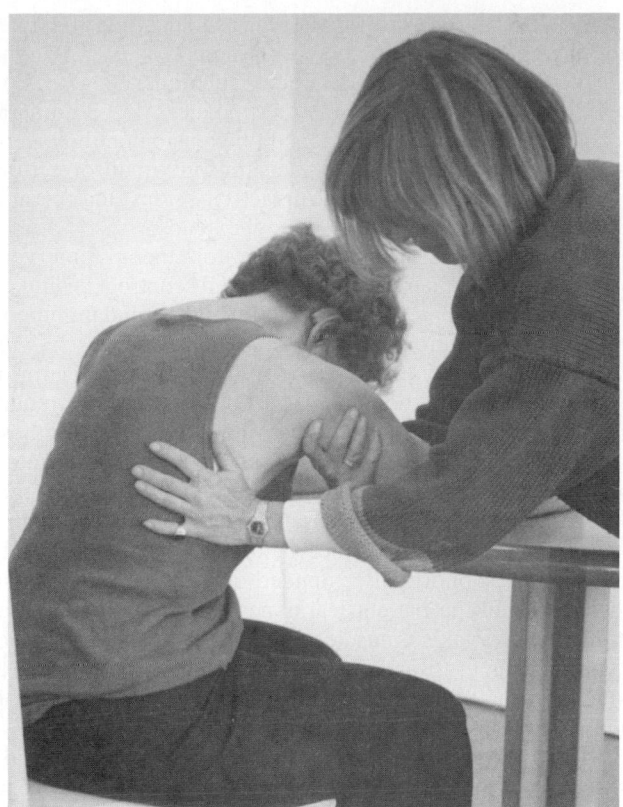

FIGURE 27-10 ■ Client performs lower body–initiated posterior movement during forearm weight bearing at a table. The therapist uses her hands to stabilize the humerus, and as the patient moves back, the therapist's left hand slowly stretches or releases tight tissue in the rotator cuff.

TABLE 27-6 ■ Trunk/Arm-Linked Movements in Forearm Weight Bearing

Functional task: Sit at a table with both forearms supported on the table. Keeping both arms on the table, move forward toward the table, and then move body back away from the table.

TRUNK/ARM LINK	BODY MOVES FORWARD	BODY MOVES BACK
Spine	Extends	Flexes
Scapula	Adducts and depresses	Abducts and elevates
Glenohumeral joint	Less flexion	More flexion
Elbow	Flexes	Extends

body weight, undesirable asymmetrical compensations result. A significant and often overlooked prerequisite for active control of the leg in weight bearing is a stable, aligned upper body. The use of forearm or extended-arm weight bearing in standing provides external stability to the upper body while allowing the therapist to reeducate control of bilateral or unilateral weight-bearing movements in the leg.

Muscle Activation Deficits

Common muscle activation deficits include improper initiation, the inability to grade timing and force production, and the inability to sequence muscles for task performance.

Improper initiation of movement occurs when the client attempts to move the arm or leg in space and substitutes the stronger proximal muscles for weaker distal muscles.[47]

EXAMPLE. If we ask a client to lift a hemiplegic arm and reach forward for an object, she or he often initiates the movement proximally instead of distally with the hand and forearm, using the stronger elevators/abductors instead of the weaker hand and forearm muscles.

This is also seen during walking.

EXAMPLE. The client initiates swing phase of gait proximally instead of distally with the foot, using the stronger pelvic elevators or rotators instead of the weaker ankle and foot muscles.

Inappropriate muscle selection for the task occurs when the client substitutes a strong muscle group for a paralyzed muscle although it is inappropriate for the function.

EXAMPLE. When the hamstrings are weak, the client may use the quadriceps to lift the leg up a step. This results in strong overshifting in the trunk and makes balance precarious.

Inappropriate sequencing includes improper initiation and excessive cocontraction. Excessive cocontraction occurs when the client activates too many muscles either at the same time or out of sequence for the task.

Excessive force production occurs when the patient activates muscles with inappropriate effort during voluntary movement. When force is excessive, the movement pattern is slow and the extremity feels stiff. Frequently, these muscles easily fatigue and the extremity slowly falls back to the starting position. Therapists often label this movement a "spastic" pattern and intervene with inhibition techniques. However, if this pattern is not from spasticity but from a muscle activation pattern, the intervention should focus on reeducation of control, not inhibition.[47]

Hypotonicity

Hypotonic muscles offer no resistance to passive movement and are clinically associated with paralysis and weakness. Clients who have had a severe stroke have paralysis in the trunk and extremities with low tone. As strength and control in the muscles of the trunk and extremities increase, the hypotonicity lessens. If weakness persists, they do not have problems with spasticity but have problems with the secondary impairments of poor joint alignment, muscle and soft tissue tightness, and, eventually, joint deformity or contracture.

Hypertonicity

There is considerable debate in the academic and clinical therapy community over the clinical relevance of spasticity, or hypertonicity, and the need to address it in treatment.[73,121] Characteristics of a spastic muscle include increased velocity-dependent resistance to stretch, a clasp-knife phenomenon, and hyperactive tendon responses. Schenkman[122] hypothesized an interesting distinction for clinical purposes: therapists can think of "hypertonicity" as tone that is higher than normal and that responds to intervention and can think of "spasticity," as researched in the laboratory, as a different type of high tone. The presence or a sudden increase of its intensity is easily recognized by the therapist and the client. If hypertonicity is left untreated, the task of muscle re-education becomes more difficult and additional secondary problems result, such as joint dysfunction, pain, and undesirable compensatory movements. In clients with hemiplegia from stroke, hypertonicity is found in the extremities, not the trunk. In severe head injury with decorticate or decerebrate posturing, trunk rigidity, a type of hypertonicity, may occur.

Clinical Hypertonicity

Although clinically the terms *spasticity* and *hypertonicity* are interchangeable, it is important to separate the types of hypertonicity that are changeable by physical and occupational therapy intervention. Therapists, although realizing that hypertonicity is not the *major* problem in hemiplegia, must understand the situations that cause it to occur. At least three different situations result in a client's increase in tone: (1) increased tone as a result of proximal instability, either insufficient trunk control for the task or instability of proximal limb musculature (e.g., hip weakness), (2) increased tension on a two-joint muscle owing to poor joint alignment and the resultant shortening or shifting of muscles, and (3) increased tone that is voluntarily produced during attempts at active movement, especially in the extremities.[47]

These situations are divided into three groups for ease of description, but, in reality, overlap occurs between groups. *Insufficient postural stability and control* in the trunk is the first explanation for arm and leg posturing. The extremity patterns of arm flexion or leg extension occur as an atypical balance strategy when the body is unstable.

EXAMPLE. If a client has sufficient trunk control in sitting, the arm and leg display normal resting positions. However, during the rise to stand, the arm postures in flexion. The arm postures most obviously during the transition phase of the stand when the hips are off the surface and the center of gravity of the body is behind the feet, the new base of support.

Treatment of the increased tone, in this case, would not be directed at the arm. Rather, intervention would focus on increasing stability of the upper body during lower trunk-initiated sit-to-stand patterns and on increasing strength and control of the leg in weight bearing. As the trunk and leg gain more control, the arm hypertonicity decreases (see Figure 27-6).

A second situation in which hypertonicity exists is when muscle tension increases in a two-joint muscle because of changes in alignment of one of the joints.

EXAMPLE. In sitting, tightness in the gastrocnemius muscle across the knee may not affect the ability to keep the heel on the floor. However, as the client extends the knee, the limit of tightness in the gastrocnemius is reached and the distal end of the tendon shortens and the ankle plantarflexes. When gastrocnemius tightness pulls the calcaneus into equinus, it also moves the calcaneus into varus because of the position of its insertion on the sustentaculi talus. The resultant position, ankle plantarflexion and foot supination, has been labeled a spastic foot position (see Figure 27-7).

However, after lengthening of the gastrocnemius across the ankle and knee in standing and correction of the calcaneal position, the patient can stand and keep the foot on the floor.

EXAMPLE. In an anterior shoulder subluxation, the anterior movement of the humeral head increases tension on the biceps proximally, resulting in elbow flexion. As the tension increases, the forearm begins to supinate. As the humeral head and scapula are repositioned, the tension on the biceps is diminished. If the therapist holds this proximal correction, the elbow and forearm posturing activity stops; the forearm slowly pronates and then the elbow extends.

For the posturing to permanently stop, therapy intervention must help increase strength and control in linked trunk/scapulohumeral patterns to prevent the malalignment.

The third situation, *inappropriate voluntary muscle activation,* occurs when the client is trying to move the arm or leg. The client uses the muscles that have returning strength in the only way he or she knows how. Historically, these patterns were labeled "spastic." This label resulted in intervention strategies of inhibition. If these patterns are thought of as unbalanced or inappropriately initiated, or inappropriately sequenced, therapy intervention is more appropriately directed. The abnormally extended or flexed leg movement changes when the patient learns new activation patterns or strengthens weaker muscle sequences. Often, these are "learned" patterns and are difficult to change. Early re-education should include training in these skills of controlling sequencing, intensity, and duration of firing.

The underlying cause of each of these situations is weakness or loss of control. Therefore, for changes in hypertonicity to last, treatment interventions must address the underlying causes. In each of these situations, the cause is weakness or loss of control of activation patterns.

In this model, generalized inhibition is inappropriate because it does not focus on the underlying cause. Intervention techniques that focus on global inhibition of extremity tone—maximal elongation, vibration, biofeedback, cold, or relaxation—rarely result in a permanent change in the tone. The temporary decrease of hypertonicity that occurs with any of these methods does not by itself directly lead to an increase in function. If used, they must be immediately followed by therapeutic exercise to create a learning environment that improves motor performance.[123,124]

Toe Posturing

There are two patterns of toe posturing: toe clawing and toe curling. Toe clawing, metatarsal hyperextension with phalangeal flexion, is a result of loss of alignment; and toe curling, metatarsal and phalangeal flexion, is a response to instability of the trunk and leg in during standing, that is, part of a balance response.[47]

Toe curling and toe clawing interfere with comfort during standing and walking. Problems of blistering on pads of the toes and on the top of the proximal interphalangeal joint and toe pain occur in the intermediate and long-term stage of hemiplegia as the result of the toes rubbing on the tops of the shoes and digging into shoe soles. Relief from pressure and pain on the toepads (tips) comes with use of commercially available "hammertoe crest pads" available from distributors (e.g., AliMed) or from medical pharmacies.

Loss of Alignment

Muscle weakness or abnormal tone in the trunk leads to atypical alignment patterns in the trunk and shoulder and pelvic girdles. This loss of alignment creates an atypical starting position for functional movement, interferes with muscle activation patterns, and limits weight transfer between extremities. Loss of alignment in the trunk in sitting and standing is analyzed and incorporated into intervention goals to re-educate functional trunk/limb-coordinated movements. The commonly described pattern of trunk shortening (lateral flexion with the concavity) on the affected side is only one of the possible alignment problems. More routinely, weakness of the trunk on one side results in a flaring of the rib cage and lateral flexion of the spine with the *convexity on the affected side*. The "appearance" of shortening on the side comes from a number of compensatory adjustments to balance or as a result of the heavy weight of a weak arm. Often therapists confuse the lower contour of the shoulder on the hemiplegic side with shortening of the trunk/concavity of the spine. The heavy weight of the weak arm pulls the upper quadrant into *excessive forward flexion*. In this position, the scapula elevates and tips forward on a flexed, rotated thoracic spine (Figure 27-11).

Another compensatory pattern is excessive spinal flexion throughout the spine, the convexity on the weak side, and *spinal rotation toward the affected side*. Clients with this asymmetry usually shift weight onto the stronger hip. This pattern viewed from the front or rear gives the appearance of a low shoulder. This pattern of rotation to the weak side does not occur acutely but develops over time in clients who sit more than they stand or walk.

Lateral translation of the thoracic spine from the hypermobile point of T10 occurs as a means of balancing when trunk weakness results in a lateral curve, with the convexity on the affected side. This asymmetry is common in sitting when the client is encouraged to stand by pushing up with the good arm without any weight on the affected leg. It occurs in standing when quad canes or hemiwalkers are used before standing control on both legs is re-educated. The stable external cane acts as a "third stable leg," and the "long, weak" side translates laterally as the unaffected arm pushes down into the cane for stability. This pattern creates a "skin fold" on the affected side that has been confused with shortening of the affected side (see Figures 27-1 and 27-4).

In standing, because the need for leg stability and movement control is much greater than in sitting, trunk alignment patterns change to accommodate the demands of the leg. Often the upper body and lower body patterns are opposite one another (i.e., *counterrotational*). If the leg is in a position of ankle plantarflexion and knee extension, the hip flexes with pelvic rotation toward the affected side. The upper body then counterrotates to provide an equal and opposite balance pattern to allow the client to stand. The opposite may also exist: if the pelvis and hip rotate toward the unaffected side because of learned compensatory swing and/or stance patterns, the upper body rotates toward the affected side to provide a counterrotation for balance (see Figure 27-4).

The atypical alignment pattern in one client may be different in sitting and standing as a result of the pattern of loss of control in the leg. In sitting, the hip is in flexion and provides support, a base, for the upper and lower trunk. Weakness in the knee and lower leg is not as critical to sitting balance and function as it is to standing functions. In standing, the hip demand is one of neutral extension to support the trunk; and complex combinations of knee, ankle, and foot movements are necessary for functional activities.

Shoulder girdle asymmetries are described in the sections on shoulder subluxation, and pelvic girdle and leg asymmetries are described in the sections on standing and walking.

Alignment problems in the distal extremity segments are related to loss of movement control and proximal alignment changes. Patterns in the distal arm and distal leg are strikingly similar. When the mid joint, elbow or knee, is extended, the proximal rotational alignment asymmetry translates down the lower segment into the hand or foot. Shoulder internal rotation translates across an extended elbow, causing the forearm to pronate and the hand to fall into carpal pronation (often confused with ulnar deviation) (Figure 27-12, *A*). Similarly, with knee extension, hip internal rotation asymmetries translate across the knee and cause tibial internal rotation and midfoot pronation. However, as the mid joints gain flexion activity, the proximal pattern no longer dictates distal asymmetries. The distal weight-bearing pattern or active initiation pattern causes a distal rotation that may be opposite to the proximal rotational pattern. When this occurs, the mid joint may posture with hypertonicity as a result of incompatible intralimb alignment.

EXAMPLE. As return occurs in the biceps muscle, it causes the elbow to flex and the forearm to supinate. The biceps internally rotates the shoulder joint, which may already be internally rotated from shoulder subluxation. Beginning forearm supination on an internally rotated shoulder produces elbow flexor hypertonicity and a pattern that has been labeled flexion/pronation spasticity (see Figure 27-12, *B*).

The weakness pattern of ankle plantarflexion and calcaneal equinovarus biases return in the anterior and posterior tibialis. During movements of the leg in space with hip and knee flexion, this distal supination pattern pulls the tibia into external rotation. To place the supinated foot on the ground, the client compensates proximally by rotating the pelvis and femur, as a unit, toward the unaffected side. This incompatible tibial external rotation and femoral internal rotation result in knee hyperextension.

Muscle and tissue tightness is a common result of alignment problems. Techniques of lengthening muscle and tissue tightness must be balanced with muscle reeducation. Isolated stretching does not result in a lasting improvement in range and may decrease functional ability if not combined with activities designed to increase control. In hemiplegia, slow stretching in functional positions through active weight shifting (i.e., functional stretching) is more effective than "orthopedic" stretching because it re-educates the weakness that underlies the loss of muscle length (Figure 27-13).

Because weakness is the underlying cause of loss of alignment and joint range, in the acute phase the *joints are hypermobile*. Over time, the tissues tighten around some joints and therapists often confuse that "feel" with joint hypomobility. Joint mobilization techniques are rarely needed because the weakness in hemiplegia renders the joints hypermobile. It is important to avoid excessive mobility in the intricate joints of the hand and foot. Tightness around a joint may indicate the need for lengthening exercises, but the joint almost never requires mobilization.

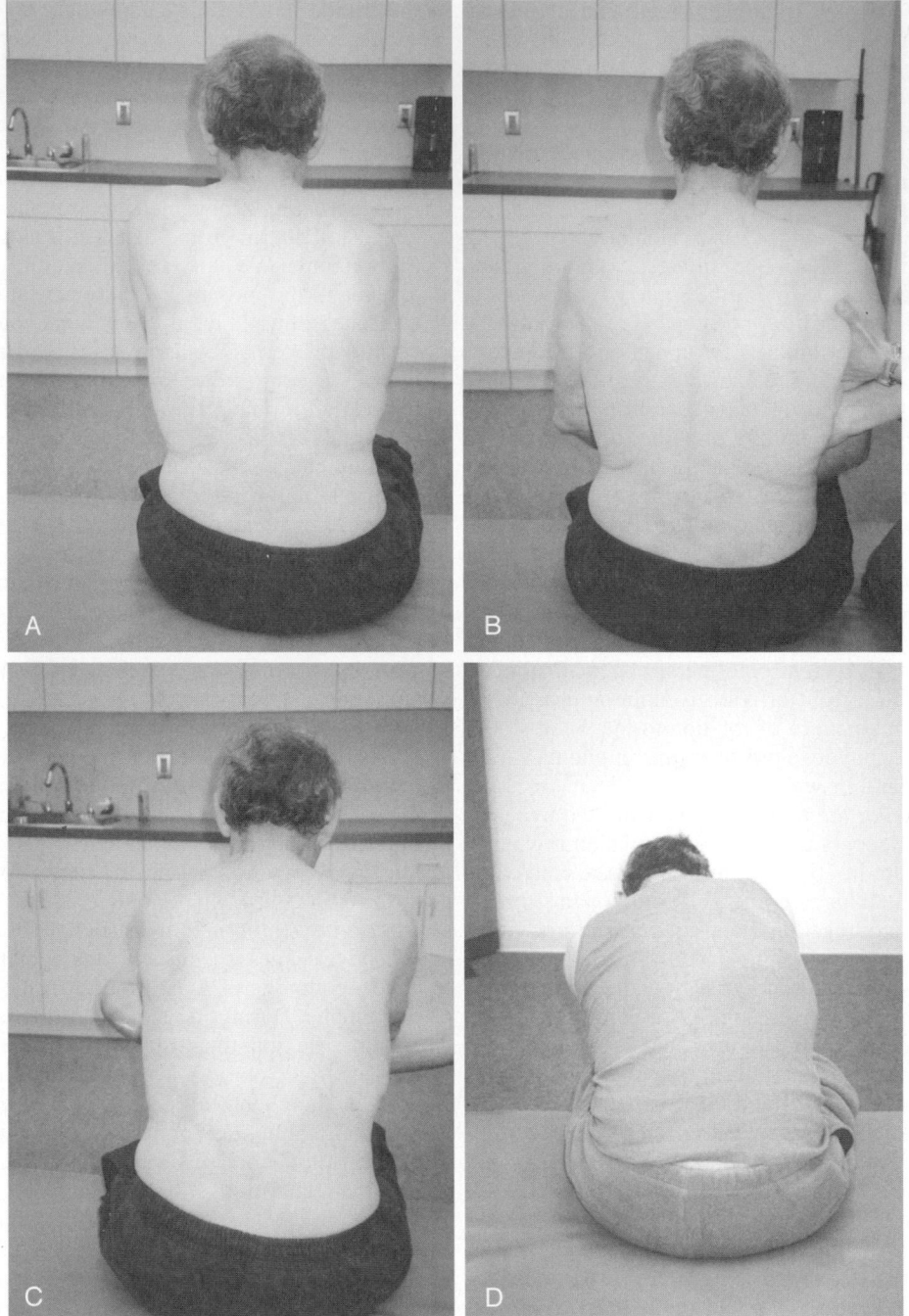

FIGURE 27-11 ■ **A,** Client with right hemiplegia. Contour of right shoulder appears lower and longer than the left. Pelvis lists downward on right. **B,** Therapist lifts client's upper body up out of forward flexion and corrects position of glenohumeral joint. Note that the contour of the right shoulder is now higher and shorter than left shoulder contour. Trunk is laterally flexed with the convexity on the right. These movement components, convexity of a lateral curve, high shoulder, and low pelvis, are compatible. **C,** Client's arms are supported symmetrically by a table. Note the convexity of the curve on the right and the low pelvis on the right. **D,** Same client moving forward and down with an upper body anterior weight shift. This position allows the therapist to evaluate the position of the trunk. Note the tendency to avoid weight on the right hip. The trunk is laterally flexed with the convexity on the right, and the right shoulder is higher than the left shoulder.

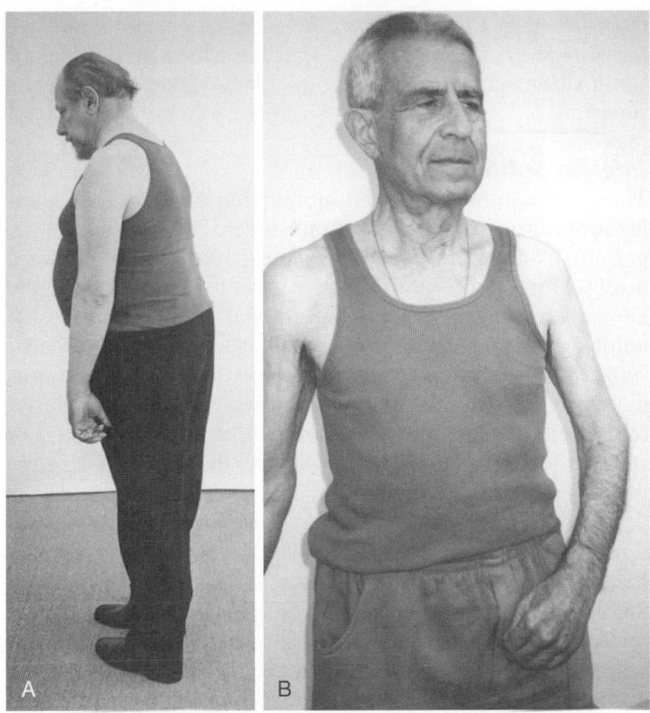

FIGURE 27-12 ■ A, Client with left hemiplegia and severe weakness. The left arm and hand is in shoulder internal rotation, elbow extension, and forearm pronation. The left wrist flexes, and the hand pronates and radially deviates on the wrist. **B,** Client with left hemiplegia with atypical movements. The left arm is positioned in shoulder internal rotation and elbow flexion. As the elbow flexes, the forearm begins to supinate on the internally rotated humerus. The wrist flexes and radially deviates with finger flexion.

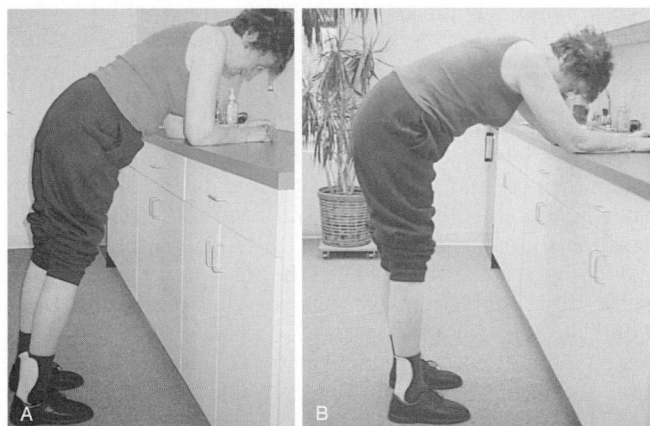

FIGURE 27-13 ■ A, Client with right hemiplegia practicing home program. During standing forearm weight bearing (providing upper body stability), she initiates a lower extremity forward/backward movement. As she moves her hips and lower leg forward, she thinks of keeping her knee straight and stretching her calf. **B,** As she moves her hips backward, she may feel a stretch in the back of her thigh, on the lateral aspect of her trunk, or under her axilla.

Pain

In the client with hemiplegia, arm pain can be caused by an imbalance of muscles, improper movement patterns, joint dysfunction, improper weight-bearing patterns, and muscle shortening or it may be related to diminished sensation and sensory interpretation. Although evidence-based approaches should be used to manage shoulder pain after stroke, systematic reviews show that there are few rigorous studies that can be used to guide treatment.[125]

Joint Pain

Joint pain is caused by poor shoulder joint mechanics during movement. Two common alignment problems are loss of scapula/humeral rhythm and insufficient humeral external rotation.[91,126] With a shoulder subluxation, the humeral head is not seated in the fossa and passive movements of the shoulder will not occur with scapulohumeral rhythm. At 60 to 90 degrees of forward flexion, impingement of the capsule will occur and the client will report sharp pain on the superior aspect of the shoulder joint. The pain ceases when the arm is lowered. The subluxation and loss of scapulohumeral rhythm result from loss of trunk/arm movements or muscle tightness from either persistent arm posturing or weakness.

If the client reports joint pain, the therapist should lower the humerus immediately, re-establish the mobility of the scapula, reseat the humerus if necessary, and maintain appropriate humeral rotation while moving the arm up again. Trunk movements in forearm weight bearing are used to teach a self-ranging practice routine that ensures scapulohumeral rhythm.

Muscle and Tendon Pain

When a hypertonic or shortened muscle is stretched too quickly or beyond available length, a strong "pulling" type pain is often reported in the region of the muscle belly being stretched. If the amount of stretch is decreased a few degrees, the reported pain subsides.

If the inappropriate stretching is not stopped, muscle pain progresses to tendon pain. Proximal biceps tendonitis, distal biceps tendonitis radiating into the forearm, and wrist flexor tendonitis are most common. The usual cause of tendonitis is improper weight bearing, with an inactive trunk and "hanging" on the arm with forced elbow extension and shoulder internal rotation. The treatment of tendonitis is rest and modalities (i.e., heat, ultrasound, or electrical stimulation) or injection of corticosteroids. When movement reeducation is restarted, it is important to avoid the "exercise" that caused the pain and to create a new intervention plan.

Shoulder-Hand Syndrome

The shoulder-hand syndrome begins with tenderness and swelling of the hand and diffuse aching pain from altered sensitivity in the shoulder and entire arm.[127] This pain interferes with the re-education of movement patterns and causes a general desire on the part of the client to "protect" the arm by not moving it. Limited shoulder and wrist and finger range of motion soon occurs.

The second stage of shoulder-hand syndrome includes further loss of shoulder and hand range of motion, severe edema, and loss of skin elasticity. This is followed by the third stage, which includes demineralization of bone, severe soft tissue deformity, and joint contracture.[127]

Not every edematous hemiplegic hand leads to shoulder-hand syndrome. Hand edema results from an upper extremity that remains dependent and that does not move for long periods of time. It is essential to teach the person with hemiplegia how to properly care for the hand and to give the responsibility for the care of the hand and arm to the client.

Ryerson and Levit[47] propose five steps for intervention of severe or chronic arm pain: (1) eliminate pain from intervention or the home program, (2) desensitize the arm and hand to touch, (3) eliminate hand edema, (4) introduce pain-free arm movements by re-establishing scapula mobility, and (5) beginning with guided arm movements below 60 degrees, gradually increase the variety and complexity of arm movements.

Edema

Edema in the hand and foot is another common secondary impairment that develops as a consequence of loss of movement control and hospitalization factors such as intravenous infiltrates and limb positioning. Edema limits joint range and tissue mobility. The edematous fluid places the skin on stretch and acts as an interstitial "glue" that bonds the skin, fascial tissue, muscle tissue, and tendons. Hand edema is associated with the development of shoulder-hand syndrome. Foot edema is as common as hand edema, limits ankle joint dorsiflexion range, and is often ignored during intervention programs. Edema begins on the volar surface of the hand and foot, progresses dorsally, and then continues proximally across the wrist or ankle.

Edema interferes with the retraining of functional movement patterns by preventing the smooth glide of tissues. It must be eliminated before active reeducation begins.

Edema has defined stages. When the involved tissue feels soft and fluid, the condition responds to retrograde massage and elevation. When the tissue is gelatinous and pitting, the edematous fluid cannot be physically expressed. At this stage, it begins to adhere to underlying tissues. The edema must be softened and liquefied through transtissue massage. The last stage of edema is characterized by hard, lumpy tissue that does not "pit" in response to manual pressure. This stage of edema requires gentle bilateral compression to break up the hard, solid areas into regions of softness. The soft regions then act as open spaces into which fluid released by massage of hard tissue is directed. The goal is to reverse the process of hardening—from hard, to pitting, to soft and fluid. In these last two stages, when the edematous tissue no longer feels fluid, elevation, elastic gloves or bandaging, and retrograde massage are not effective. When edematous tissue is soft and fluid, active and active assistive extremity movement patterns produce muscular contractions that assist venous and lymphatic return of the fluid.[47]

Shoulder Subluxation

Shoulder subluxation occurs when any of the biomechanical factors contributing to glenohumeral joint stability are interrupted. In persons with hemiplegia, subluxation is related to a change in the angle of the glenoid fossa occurring because of muscle weakness. In the frontal plane the scapula is normally held at an angle of 40 degrees. When the slope of the glenoid fossa becomes less oblique (and more vertical), the humerus will "slide" down and out of the fossa.[128] Ryerson and Levit[129] first described three types of subluxation in clients with hemiplegia: inferior, anterior, and superior.

Inferior Subluxation

The most common type of subluxation is an inferior subluxation. It occurs in clients with severe weakness and it is present in the acute stage. Weakness and the weight of a heavy arm result in downward rotation of the scapula. Downward rotation orients the glenoid fossa vertically, the unlocking mechanism of the capsule is lost, and the humerus subluxates inferiorly with internal rotation. As the humerus internally rotates, the bicipital tuberosity rolls anteriorly; this anterior prominence is often confused with an anterior subluxation.[47] As subluxation occurs, the shoulder capsule is vulnerable to stretch, especially when the humerus is dependent and resting by the side of the body. In this position, the capsule is taut superiorly, so any downward distraction of the humerus will place an immediate stretch on the upper part of the capsule. The coracohumeral ligament reinforces the superior portion of the capsule, which is crucial for shoulder stability. Jenson[130] has discussed the implications of rupture of this ligament as a result of forced abnormal passive motion as a cause of shoulder pain in subluxation.

Anterior Subluxation

Anterior subluxation occurs when the humeral head separates anteriorly from the glenoid fossa. Anterior shoulder subluxation occurs when the downwardly rotated scapula elevates and tilts forward on the rib cage and the humerus hyperextends with internal rotation. In an anterior subluxation, as tension increases on the proximal biceps tendon, the elbow flexes, and the forearm supinates. This subluxation is found in clients with atypical patterns of return and trunk rotational asymmetries.[47]

Superior Subluxation

A superior subluxation occurs when the humeral head lodges under the coracoid process in a position of internal rotation and slight abduction. The humeral head is "locked" in this position so that every movement of the humerus is accompanied by scapula movement. The scapula position in this subluxation is one of abduction, elevation, and neutral rotation. The forearm adducts across the body as the humeral abduction and elbow flexion increase. A superior subluxation occurs in clients with inappropriate muscle firing and cocontraction.

Subluxation is not painful but results in changes in muscle length-tension relationships, muscle shortening, and permanent stretch of the joint capsule. If a subluxation exists, the therapist reduces the subluxation by correcting trunk, scapula, and humeral alignment patterns before attempting to reeducate arm movement patterns. A discussion of these subluxations, accompanying trunk movement patterns, and intervention suggestions can be found in therapy literature.[47] As the client learns to move the arm in patterns of functional coordination, subluxation and associated arm posturing decrease.

Prevention of subluxation requires (1) proper assessment of secondary alignment problems (rib cage/scapula/humeral position), (2) early reeducation of trunk/arm-linked patterns in sitting and standing, and (3) prevention of shoulder capsule stretch, including support and positioning as the client sits, stands, and practices walking.

FUNCTIONAL ACTIVITIES

Functional mobility movement analysis, intervention techniques, unilateral compensatory strategies, and suggestions for task practice are documented in therapy literature.[131-133] In this section, representative mobility skills are selected in three functional positions: supine, sitting, and standing. For each task selected, the focus is on the basic trunk and extremity control patterns used, significant impairments in addition to weakness that make it difficult for the client to perform the task, and observations from the clinic that relate to intervention and practice. Detailed descriptions of each trunk and trunk/extremity-linked pattern can be found in the literature.[47]

Supine

Rolling

Basic trunk movements to be re-educated include (1) upper trunk flexion/rotation initiation, (2) lower trunk extension/rotation initiation, and (3) symmetrical lateral flexion initiation.

Trunk/Extremity-Linked Patterns. The upper-trunk flexion-rotation initiation pattern is linked with arm reach across the body. Active assistive patterns, using a bilateral arm reach, are encouraged when strength is insufficient to lift the arm against gravity or, through therapist handling, when arm muscle paralysis or weakness results in such a heavy feeling that the patient cannot control the extremity with the unaffected hand. If the therapist assists the arm, the goal of practice is for the client to initiate the active anti-gravity trunk pattern.

A lower trunk extension-rotation initiation pattern is coordinated with either a leg-reach pattern or a flexed-leg "push" pattern. Active assistive patterns can be implemented through therapist handling to help train the sequencing or to grade the firing patterns of the leg when it is pushing into the bed. Independent practice is performed when the control and strength in the affected leg return or both knees rotate with the pelvis and extending lower trunk. Independent practice also requires the upper body and arm to follow the movement of the lower body.

The symmetrical lateral flexion initiation pattern is known as "log rolling." In this pattern, the trunk does not rotate but is linked in a symmetrical pattern with arm and leg "reach or push" on the leading side.

Impairments That Interfere. Shoulder joint pain may occur when the client rolls onto the affected side. Pain occurs if the shoulder is trapped under the trunk as the client moves to side lying or when the humeral/scapula alignment causes the capsule to be impinged. The client should not continue to roll or lie on the painful shoulder.

In rehabilitative or outpatient care, muscle tightness in the latissimus, quadratus lumborum, biceps, or tensor fasciae latae may limit trunk rotation or trunk/extremity-linked movements.

Clinical Observations. Weakness in the extremities is a significant factor during rolling because the arm and the leg are used to assist the trunk initiation patterns. Rotational patterns are difficult in the acute stage because they require an integration and sequencing of flexor and extensor muscle patterns. Symmetrical rolling is an easier independent pattern to train. Active assistive strategies and strengthening need to be incorporated early in intervention. Clients have an easier time rolling to the affected side because they use the strength of the unaffected side to initiate the roll. But they may not want to stay on that side because of shoulder pain, instability of the hip, or decreased sensation and the fear that ensues. The client may prefer rolling to the unaffected side because it is easier to rest on, but initiating the movement is difficult because of loss of control.

The family is educated to understand the nature of the loss of movement and the loss of sensation and their effects on body awareness and early bed mobility. Family members are encouraged to sit with, visit, talk to, feed, and touch the person with the hemiplegia from the client's affected side. They are instructed in simple movements, such as rolling, to promote symmetry, midline control, and activation of trunk muscles. Because family members are often afraid to touch or move the client's affected side, they are educated quickly to be made a part of the intervention process.

Feeding and Swallowing

Although detailed facilitation and inhibition of oral and neck muscle movement for feeding and articulated language are a specialty of speech pathologists, the movement therapist activates trunk control to increase upper body stability to prepare for more automatic chew and swallow.

Basic trunk patterns to be re-educated include (1) lower body anterior/posterior movement control to move toward table and back into chair and (2) upper body anterior/posterior and lateral movement control to provide control for head and arm movement.

Impairments That Interfere

Oral problems include the following:
- Forward head, poor lip closure, loss of saliva and food
- Facial asymmetry during function greater than at rest
- Inability to swallow
- Inability to chew
- Inability to lateralize foods
- Inability to take liquids from cup or spoon
- Muscle weakness with hypotonia

Central problems are as follows:
- Asymmetry of trunk
- Poor postural control
- Upper body flexion with or without weight of weak arm
- Inability to feed self

Compensations include the following:
- Use of gravity—with head and neck extension the food flows down the throat
- Chewing on one side only
- Using the hand to place food in the mouth
- Using the hand to pull food from the cheek
- Using thicker food, which is much easier to handle than soft, liquid foods

Clinical Observations. Drooling occurs when upper trunk extensor weakness results in excessive upper trunk flexion. As the client tries to lift the head, it extends on the cervical spine in a forward position. As a result of the biomechanics of the forward head position, the jaw opens, automatic swallowing becomes difficult, and saliva runs out of the open mouth.

Drooling from one side of the mouth is annoying and embarrassing. The client may not be able to maintain lip closure and, in addition, may not feel the saliva running out or may not identify a need to swallow. Drooling lessens as upper body control increases.

In the majority of cases, swallowing problems are transient in persons with hemiplegia. After the initial insult and during the flaccid period, many clients exhibit a decreased gag reflex. In acute care settings, where liquid diets are often routinely given to persons with hemiplegia, education of hospital staff to the merits of using thicker foods should be considered. Thicker, chopped food is easier to swallow than soft food. Soft food is easier to swallow than liquids. Liquids with distinct taste or texture are easier to swallow than water. Specific feeding programs are noted in Chapters 9, 11, and 12.

Sitting

Function in sitting is based on the ability to maintain the trunk in an upright position, to automatically adjust the trunk when the arms or one leg moves around midline, and to control shifting of the trunk as the arm and leg extend their reach. Control in sitting is also used to help change position, such as sitting to standing, or lying down. The re-establishment of control in sitting for function is an important early goal in rehabilitation care.

Basic trunk movements to be reeducated include the following:

1. Anterior, posterior, and lateral upper body–initiated movements. Upper body movements are easier to retrain than lower body movements are because the base of support (contact of the buttocks and feet) remains on the surface.
2. Anterior and posterior lower body–initiated movements. With lower body–initiated movement, the upper body needs to be stable and yet adjust to and follow the movement of the lower body. The reeducation of upper body control allows the therapist to begin retraining lower body control.
3. Lateral lower body–initiated movements. These movements are the most difficult of the three movements required for sitting control because as the movement begins, the base of support narrows.
4. Rotational movements. In sitting, the easiest rotational patterns to reeducate are upper body rotation on a stable lower body.

Trunk/Arm-Linked Patterns (Representative Examples). Postural adjustments to arm movements around midline require the trunk to be upright, to be active, and to perform small adjustments. When the hand functions in front of the body, the trunk adjusts with small posterior weight shifts and increased flexor control, whereas as the hand(s) move to function behind the body, the trunk adjusts with a small anterior weight shift.

The trunk moves with an arm to extend reach. If the reach is forward and down to the floor, as if to reach a shoe, the upper body initiates an anterior weight shift and the spine moves into flexion with control from eccentric contraction of the spinal extensors. If the reach is forward as if to grab an object on the far side of a table, the lower body initiates an anterior weight shift as the upper body remains stable and adjusts to the demands of the arm movement.

Trunk/Leg-Linked Patterns (Representative Examples). Small trunk adjustments occur with leg movements around midline. If the feet move back under the hips, the trunk adjusts with a small amount of anterior weight shift. When one foot is lifted up to slide into a slipper, the lower body adjusts with a small lateral weight shift. Upper trunk stability allows lower trunk–initiated patterns when rising to stand. As the hips and knees extend to lift the buttocks off the chair, trunk adjustments accompany the changing leg pattern to provide balance.

Impairments That Interfere. Changes in alignment of the arm resulting from weakness and muscle shortening affect the position of the thoracic spine and rib cage. The weight of a flaccid or extremely weak arm pulls the upper trunk into forward flexion; an increase of flexor tone in the arm causes the scapula to elevate and the rib cage to rotate. Both of these alignment problems of the trunk interfere with the ability to increase strength in basic trunk movement patterns.

Shoulder subluxation results in muscle shortening (biceps, pectorals, latissimus, subscapularis), alters the line of muscle pull, and interferes with scapulohumeral rhythm. Muscle shortening contributes to loss of upper body alignment and interferes with strengthening trunk patterns.

Loss of trunk alignment as a result of trunk weakness creates an atypical starting position for movement and limits the number and type of movement patterns that can be safely produced.

Clinical Observations. Alignment changes in the arm influence strength and control of the upper body. Therefore, intervention techniques to restore alignment and control of the arm on the upper trunk must be included in the list of short-term goals to achieve the functional goal of safe, independent task performance in sitting.

Active control of the pelvis in a neutral position is necessary for the reeducation of lower body lateral and rotational weight shifts. Pelvic position influences leg position. If the pelvis is held in a posterior tilt, the leg initially tends to abduct; and if it is held in an anterior tilt, the leg initially adducts.

Clients with poor hip control do not regain functional trunk patterns in sitting until they can activate and strengthen hip muscles for stability during weight shifts. Weakness of the hip joint results in a desire to shift weight to the stronger side, thus creating a spinal or pelvic asymmetry. Clients who push to the affected side in sitting need strength from the weak leg for stability as a prerequisite for midline control of the trunk.

Lower body–initiated lateral weight shift patterns are difficult to train because they require a narrowing of the base of support. Forearm weight-bearing movement patterns are used to increase the base of support to allow practice of these patterns that are needed for functional activities such as scooting, toileting, and lifting one leg off the surface. This movement is difficult to practice without upper body stability (external or internal).

Transfers. Transfers in the half-stand, pivot pattern require upper body control over the lower body and combined trunk/leg control patterns. The squat, pivot position is trained when leg strength and control are weak and the goal is to train the client to use the affected leg. Transfers involve interim patterns that are trained before safe standing is possible.

The client practices transfers to different objects (chair, bed, toilet) to either side. This promotes symmetry, encourages the use of the affected leg, and allows practice with varying environmental constraints. Transfers to the unaffected side have the advantage of being familiar to hospital staff because they are the "traditional" textbook way of transferring the person with hemiplegia. Nevertheless, transfers to the affected side need to be trained by therapists to allow function in either direction.

Sit to Stand. Sit to stand is an important skill to retrain early after a stroke because it is used many times a day during functional activities. In a study investigating the relationship between sit to stand and walking, Chou et al[134] found that a critical component of sit to stand was vertical force displacement; the amount of weight transferred down into the floor. Those who had a maximal vertical force difference of less than 30% body weight between both legs displayed faster walking speeds and more typical gait parameters.

Two initiation patterns are commonly used, with or without the use of momentum, to train sit to stand. A lower body–initiated anterior weight transfer occurs with a straight spine as the shoulders move forward. Therapists should emphasize the forward weight shift component of this pattern rather than the anterior pelvic tilt component; the requirement of sit to stand is a forward shift of the upper body and shoulders. An anterior pelvic tilt usually results in a backward movement of the shoulders. The confusion over this movement occurs because clients often sit in a position of flexion with a posterior pelvic tilt. To come to upright, they must extend the spine and move the pelvis to neutral. Although individuals with a tendency for lumbar extension may have an anterior pelvic tilt as they shift forward, the anterior pelvic tilt is not as important a component as is a forward weight shift.

An upper body–initiated anterior weight transfer during sit to stand results in spinal flexion and eccentric activity in the spinal extensors. This pattern keeps body weight over the feet, the new base of support, but does not link the extension of the legs with the lower trunk. The demand on the trunk from lift off to stand is greater than in the previous pattern because muscle contraction type must change and there is a larger requirement for strength and control as the spine moves from flexion to standing. This pattern is used in rehabilitative and extended care centers because it allows caregivers to perform safe, maximal assist transfers. Use of both legs during sitting, transfers, and sit to stand increases strength in the legs ("forced use") and promotes

symmetry of the pelvis, thus enhancing control in the trunk.

During transfer and sit-to-stand training, techniques of directing manual pressure from the top of the knee through the tibia into the foot help the client remember to keep weight on both feet and increase the dorsiflexion movement at the ankle.

Full standing should not be attempted if loss of control in the leg results in nonuse. If the client cannot activate leg muscles in a weight-bearing position in attempts to stand, the stand will be precarious with undesirable trunk compensatory patterns.

Standing

Standing Control

Control in standing is a difficult early goal to achieve because the control demands of the trunk and leg are complex. Control of basic movement patterns in standing is divided into upper body–initiated control patterns and lower extremity–initiated control patterns.[112] Upper body control in standing includes the ability to move the upper trunk and arm in all planes with appropriate leg responses and the ability to respond and adjust to weight transfer to each leg and to provide postural stability for movements of each leg in space.

Lower extremity control in standing has a weight-bearing component and a movement in space component. As a prerequisite for reeducation of these movements, the upper body must have enough strength and control to provide stability and postural adjustments for movements of the leg.

Basic trunk movements to be re-educated include:
1. Upper body–initiated anterior, posterior, lateral, and rotational patterns with critical corresponding adjustments in the leg (either hip, knee, or ankle strategies).
2. Control of the upper body over the lower trunk during lower extremity–initiated weight-bearing movements.
3. Linked trunk/leg patterns during movements of the leg in space. This is easiest when the leg moves around midline, and it increases in difficulty as movement in space increases in amplitude or speed.
4. Increased upper body control to support power production of the arms for pushing, pulling, or lifting objects and increased lower body control to support power production of the legs for jumping, running, and stair climbing.

Trunk/Arm-Linked Patterns. These patterns include the following:
1. Upper body–initiated flexion movements that occur with forward and downward arm-reach patterns.
2. Upper body–initiated extension that occurs when the arm reaches up or up and back.
3. Upper body–initiated lateral flexion when the arm reaches down and to one side.
4. Upper body flexion/rotation when the arm reaches down and to one side.
5. Upper body extension/rotation when the arm reaches up and back to one side.

Trunk/Leg-Linked Patterns in Weight Bearing. Control of the upper and lower trunk during unilateral stance on either leg is one of the most difficult patterns to retrain. Control of the trunk in unilateral stance is linked with the need for abduction control on the stance leg. In clients with hemiplegia, the complicated control demands for leg and trunk control in standing combined with the presence of weakness and control problems result in loss of alignment in multiple joints and strong compensatory patterns.

Trunk/Leg-Linked Patterns as the Leg Moves in Space. When the leg moves in space in small ranges, the movement of the upper trunk is small and occurs as a postural adjustment. The movement pattern of the femur and pelvis is a linked rhythm similar to scapulohumeral rhythm. The first 30 to 45 degrees of hip flexion occur with no pelvic movements; from 45 to 90 degrees the pelvis moves with the flexing hip with a posterior tilt; with continued hip flexion the upper trunk flexes to maintain balance. This rhythm occurs in the other planes of movement as well. As the movement of the leg increases in range, such as when turning, the demand on the trunk increases.

1. Lower trunk flexion occurs when the leg reaches forward and up; stepping up.
2. Lower trunk extension occurs when the leg reaches back.
3. Lower trunk lateral flexion occurs when the leg lifts up and out to the same side.

Impairments That Interfere. In standing, loss of alignment in the upper body on the hemiplegic side creates compensatory patterns that interfere with functional standing movements and balance. Loss of upper body stability produces one of three common patterns: (1) forward flexion of the upper trunk, (2) upper body rotation toward the affected side, or (3) upper body rotation away from the affected side.

Loss of ankle joint dorsiflexion range blocks the ability of the body to use ankle strategies for leg responses to upper body–initiated movements or for leg movements and function. Loss of ankle joint dorsiflexion range is one cause of knee hyperextension in standing. Ankle range is lost within a few days after stroke and needs to be prevented to train early standing functions.

Loss of knee control during standing is the result of weakness of the trunk, pelvis, hip, ankle, or both. Loss of knee control from weakness is influenced by the position and movement control of the hip and ankle joints. Initially, the knee flexes as more weight is shifted to the unaffected side, and the pelvis lists downward. If the pelvic position is not corrected (leveled) and the client is encouraged to straighten the knee, the pelvis rotates toward the affected side to provide "length" for the knee movement. This pelvic rotation is accompanied by hip flexion as the client tries to straighten the "weak" knee. After standing and walking are practiced, the client may learn to "lock" the knee in hyperextension with unbalanced quadriceps firing as a means of gaining stability (Figure 27-14).

The cause of early arm flexor hypertonicity and leg extensor hypertonicity in standing is insufficient trunk control. Over time, leg extensor hypertonicity results from all three previously stated situations: insufficient trunk control, altered intralimb alignment, and unbalanced "learned" firing. If the therapist uses handling to change one of the three situations, the previously extended knee begins to "wobble," a sign of the underlying loss of control.

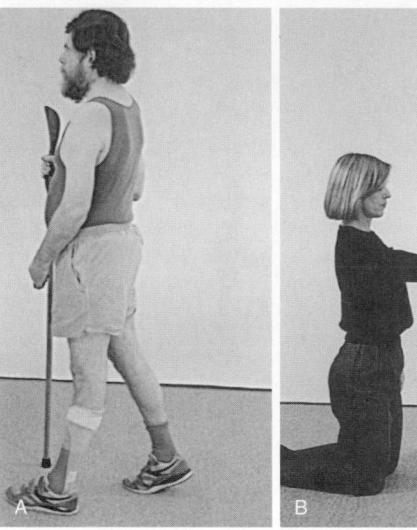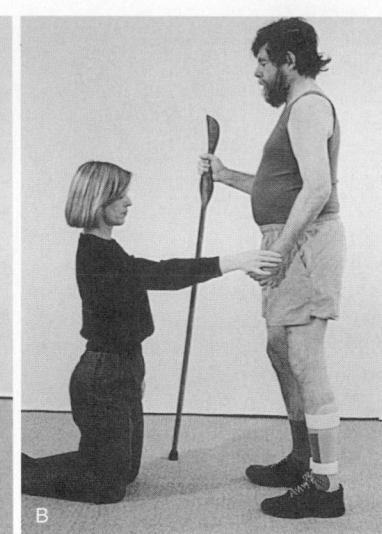

FIGURE 27-14 ■ **A,** Client with left hemiplegia with knee hyperextension wearing a lightweight prefabricated posterior leaf-spring brace that does not control his knee hyperextension. **B,** A solid ankle brace with foot control that decreases knee hyperextension by providing distal stability.

Clinical Observations. In the acute phase, therapists can help the client practice standing with the hips and shoulders back against a wall to provide support for the trunk and pelvis while allowing a safe situation to practice active self-initiated leg weight-bearing movements. The client can slide down the wall, activating eccentric control in the legs, and then slide back up, activating concentric control. By using the wall to assist the stand, the therapist frees his or her hands to help correct leg alignment problems and lets the client practice the initiation of movement early, independently, and safely.

The client can practice controlled lateral weight transfer with appropriate trunk activity in this position. Whereas one study concluded that there is no relationship between lateral weight shift and walking, therapists should not conclude that unilateral weight acceptance is inappropriate functional training.[135] During intervention and independent practice, many patients move laterally incorrectly by overshifting or without the prerequisite of upper body control. The main focus of weight-shift training for walking in hemiplegia should be an anterior weight shift.

Upper extremity forearm or extended-arm weight bearing provides upper trunk stability for lower extremity–initiated practice. This practice pattern also allows a means of self-ranging for the ankle, knee, hip, and pelvis. This position is used not to inhibit tone in the extremities but to activate and strengthen the trunk and legs in linked patterns.

Walking

Independent, functional, and safe walking is difficult to retrain in the early phases of intervention because it requires refined degrees of trunk and extremity control. It requires an advanced level of trunk control, linked trunk/leg movements, and enough strength and control in the leg to support body weight, to move the multiple joints of the leg in complex patterns, and to control speed, momentum, and balance. Walking patterns in clients with stroke are characterized by slow speed, uneven step and stride lengths, impaired balance with resulting arm and leg posturing, and reliance on adaptive equipment.

In the current health care environment with the emphasis on limited therapy visits, therapists are confronted with major intervention dilemmas: Should they force the client to walk without minimal prerequisites? Should they allow undesirable compensations although they predict future secondary problems? Should they use the benefits of the large health care systems to divide responsibility for continued gait training between therapy (inpatient, rehabilitation, home care, outpatient) divisions?

Prerequisites for functional, safe walking include the following:

- Upper body control to adjust to leg movements in unilateral stance and during movements of the leg in space
- Lower trunk control to prevent atypical pelvic alignment patterns during movements of the leg in space
- Strength and control of the leg to initiate weight shifts
- Strength and control in the leg to move in space

Because gait is the most extensively studied, analyzed, and discussed in terms of intervention, this section describes the prerequisites for walking training and common impairments that interfere with walking.[136-138] Common impairments that interfere with walking are separated into three divisions of the walking cycle: (1) forward progression, (2) single/double-limb support, and (3) swing.[139,140]

Impairments that interfere with functional walking are summarized in Box 27-7.

Research on and equipment for partial-body-weight supported treadmill walking training has increased over the past 4 years. In a 2004 review of randomized controlled studies, there was strong evidence for poststroke treadmill training with or without body weight support[141] (Figure 27-15, A and B). Task specificity, speed, intensity, and symmetry of practice in this type of equipment contribute to improved overground walking performance.[142]

Clinical Observations. If weakness in the foot and ankle creates difficulty clearing the foot during stepping, the body recruits a proximal initiation pattern: hip hiking, circumduction, or posterior pelvic tilting. If allowed to persist, this atypical initiation pattern results in a walking pattern that is difficult or impossible to change. This points to a need to consider minimal ankle/foot support during early walking as a means of creating appropriate distal initiation patterns and limiting the need for proximal compensation (Figure 27-16). (See Chapter 34 for additional suggestions.)

After the identification of significant impairments for swing phase and stance phase, specific intervention techniques are chosen.

EXAMPLE. After the description set forth by Knuttson and Richards,[71] in a type I motor control problem with premature activation of the calf muscles, intervention may stress lower extremity–initiated forward weight shift. Control of the ankle with appropriate knee activity allows the center of gravity to advance ahead of the foot before the activation of calf muscles pulls the lower leg backward. With a type II disturbance, training to improve control and power of the leg in standing or during sit to stand under varied conditions may be indicated. In a type III problem, intervention is

BOX 27-7 ■ SUMMARY OF SIGNIFICANT FUNCTIONAL IMPAIRMENTS

FORWARD PROGRESSION—HEEL STRIKE TO MIDSTANCE
Poor Trunk Control
- Loss of alignment of the upper trunk over lower trunk
- Loss of control of upper trunk as leg initiates weight shift forward

Lack of Proper Initiation Pattern and Direction
- Excessive forward trunk flexion
- Excessive lateral weight shift

Insufficient Ankle Joint Dorsiflexion Range
- Muscle tightness
- Loss of control
- Edema

Inappropriate Foot Contact
- Weakness of foot and ankle muscles
- Muscle tightness
- Foot posturing

SINGLE/DOUBLE LIMB SUPPORT
Insufficient Trunk Control to Maintain Position over One Leg
- Asymmetries during unilateral stance
- Loss of control of upper trunk over lower trunk

Poor Lower Extremity Control
- Hip instability
- Loss of knee control in unilateral stance
- Loss of ankle joint dorsiflexion range
- Toe clawing or curling

Loss of Ability to Transfer Weight Through Foot
- Inability to maintain leg on floor behind body
- Muscle tightness
- Weakness or inappropriate activation of leg muscles

SWING—EARLY AND LATE
Atypical Leg Muscle Firing Patterns
- Lack of proper initiation
- Loss of ankle and foot dorsiflexion
- Inability to control trunk and lower extremity initiation pattern
- Initiation pattern

Inability of the Body to Continue to Move Forward as Leg Swings
Foot Posturing

directed at achieving stability control of the upper trunk during lower extremity–initiated patterns.

EQUIPMENT

Equipment for persons with CNS dysfunction can be thought of as supports or as "extra" help to allow better alignment or stabilization so that the client can move and function more independently. Too much support or equipment prevents participation in an activity and hinders the development of new movement control. Equipment should never be a substitute for treatment and should not be given without practice during treatment. One-handed equipment

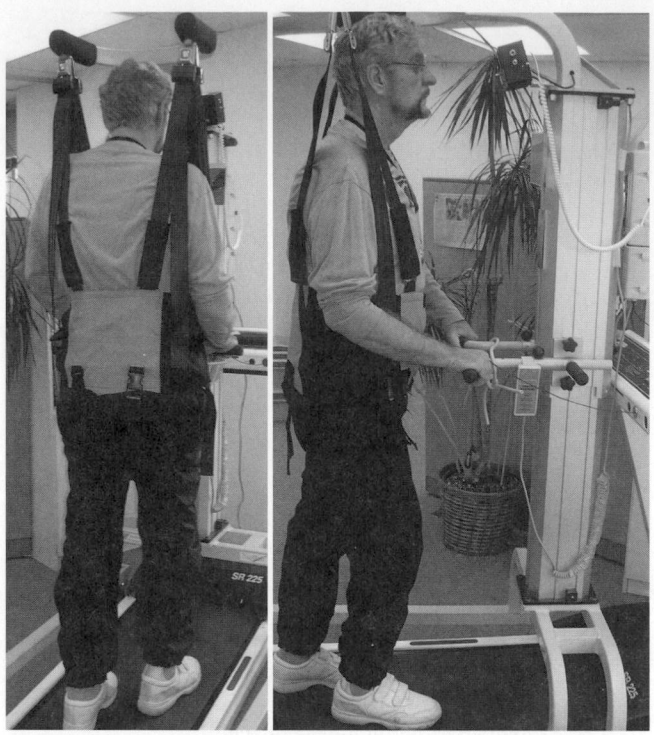

A   **B**

FIGURE 27-15 ■ **A** and **B,** Client with right hemiplegia walking on a treadmill with partial body weight support.

that is used as a substitute for trunk control is less successful than equipment that is used to compensate for loss of extremity function. Therapists should perform continuing assessments of the appropriateness of the equipment in relation to gains made in therapy.

EXAMPLE. A "reacher" compensates for loss of trunk/limb-linked control to allow the arm to extend its reach, whereas an electric can opener designed for one-handed use substitutes for the ability to use both hands.

Bedside Equipment

In acute and rehabilitation settings, pillows, blankets, or towels are used to position the client in bed. With the client in the supine position, the head pillow can be angled so that it slips under the shoulder and scapula to prevent loss of alignment. The therapist uses a pillow to support the humerus and makes sure the shoulder joint is not hyperextended. Hyperextension of the shoulder in supine results in elbow flexion by increasing biceps tension proximally. A soft towel roll or pillow under the greater trochanter or knee maintains alignment of the leg in the first few days after a stroke. Once the client begins to move to both sides in bed, the use of pillows for support is not necessary.

Wheelchairs

Wheelchairs must have a solid surface to sit on and, when possible, a supportive backrest. The soft, leather seats of transport chairs act as a sling and allow the pelvis to posteriorly tilt and the spine to flex. This reinforces the preferred position of the body with paralysis or severe weakness. Solid seats and backs allow the pelvis, trunk, and extremities to

be more normally aligned. Wheelchairs specifically for clients with hemiplegia who are not expected to walk have lower seat heights and one-armed drive (two hand rims on one wheel). These adaptations make it easier for clients to propel the chair with the unaffected hand and foot.

Support for the hemiplegic arm when sitting in a wheelchair reduces the effect of the downward pull of gravity on the weak or paralyzed arm. Lapboards support both arms and provide symmetry for the upper body. In some settings, they are considered a form of restraint and cannot be used. Half-lapboards or arm troughs are used to support the arm if the client has enough perceptual awareness to be able to limit trunk movements. The use of a pillow in the lap is another option for bilateral support of the arms. If an arm support is used, the client should be taught trunk movements in relation to the support and how to protect the arm and hand while on the support.

Slings

Slings are used to support the glenohumeral joint to prevent capsular stretch, to temporarily maintain alignment that is gained in treatment, and to take some of the weight of the paralyzed arm off the upper trunk as the client begins to learn to stand and walk. They cannot reverse an existing subluxation once the capsule is stretched. Because subluxation is not inherently painful, a sling should not be used to prevent pain. However, use of a sling can help break the cycle of pain from shoulder-hand syndrome.

Various reviews and comparisons of slings are available.[143,144] In the studies, shoulder joint position was examined without consideration of trunk or scapula position. There is no sling available that corrects a subluxation because no existing sling provides scapula upward rotation control. Slings only "hold" a correct scapulohumeral position that has been restored in treatment.

The ideal shoulder sling helps maintain the normal angular alignment of the glenoid fossa, decreases the tendency of the humerus to internally rotate, takes some of the weight of the arm off the upper trunk, and allows the upper extremity freedom of movement. Therapists should not prescribe slings that cradle the arm in front of the body, prevent any movement, and, in effect, teach learned nonuse. The orthopedic-type *envelope arm sling* was used in the 1950s and 1960s. In the 1970s, influenced by Bobath,[88] sling usage was thought to be undesirable. As more information about tone and movement became available, new slings were designed to allow the arm to be supported while movement was re-educated. Slings have different suspensions, provide different means of control for the arm, give differing "messages" to the arm and trunk, and have individual uses. Table 27-7, adapted from the work of Levit,[145] lists available slings and their characteristics.

Clients who come into therapy with a sling, but who do not require one, are weaned from a supportive sling into a less-controlling one. Clients state that the *clavicle support* provides support during household tasks that require upper body flexion, such as bed making or vacuuming. Clients who complain of "aching" in the arm at the end of the day may relieve this ache by using a support for a few hours around midday.

If the arm dangles or bangs against the body during active periods, the *shoulder saddle sling* can be adjusted to

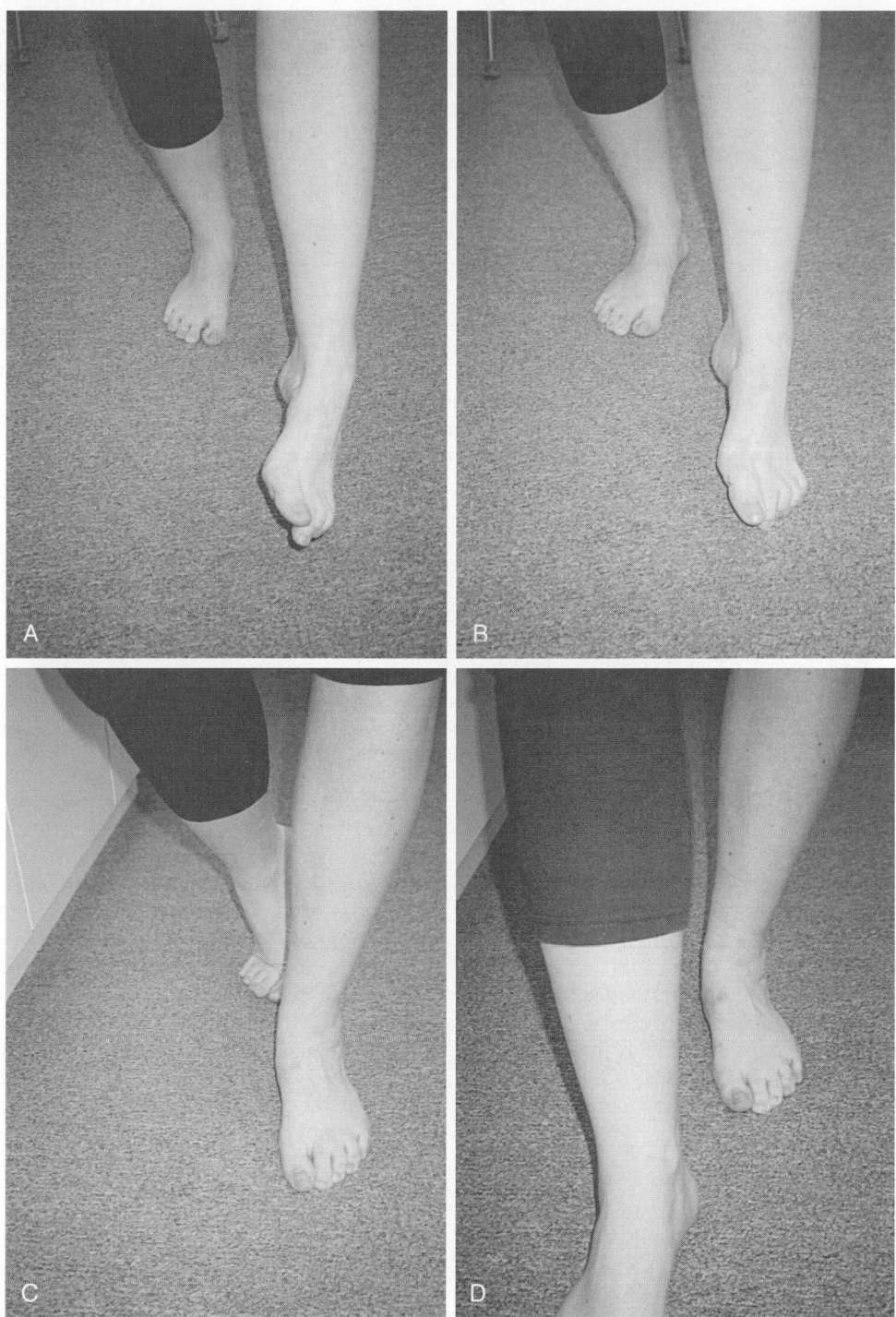

FIGURE 27-16 ■ **A** and **B,** Client with left hemiplegia. Supination of the foot during swing and during foot contact with ankle joint plantarflexion and calcaneal varus. **C** and **D,** Compensatory pronation of the midfoot to allow the foot to contact the ground during stance.

protect the arm from bruising. This sling is also helpful to clients with severe shoulder-hand pain because it allows full support of the arm and can be adjusted by the client to allow the elbow to extend as the pain subsides. The *humeral cuff slings* are the least practical from a functional standpoint because they do not affect the scapula or trunk but are frequently used in acute and rehabilitation care.

Canes

Canes are given to clients with hemiplegia to provide "extra" balance, not as a means to support body weight. Canes should be used after upper body control and lower extremity–initiated movements are practiced.

If quad canes or hemiwalkers are used before trunk and leg activity is minimally established, they encourage lateral translation of the spine or rotation of the spine and ribs.

TABLE 27-7 ■ Available Slings and Their Characteristics

BASIC TYPE	SUPPLIER	SUSPENSION	MESSAGE	COMMON USE
Clavicle support	DePuy (clavicle fracture sling with 1-inch soft foam axilla pad)	Figure-of-8 between scapulae	"Spine extend, scapula adduct"	Acute care
		Support under axilla		Minimal support
				To wean out of other supports
Humeral cuff	Rolyan Hemi Arm Sling	Figure-of-8 between scapulae	"Arm up"	Rehabilitative care
		Velcro cuff support to humeral shaft		
Unilateral shoulder orthosis	Bauerfeind Rolyan	Across body	"Lift humerus up"	Rehabilitative care
		Elastic or spandex cuff support to humeral shaft		
Shoulder-saddle sling	Sammons	Saddle sits on top of shoulder	Maximal support of arm	To prevent "banging" of flaccid arm in active patients or during sports activities
		Strap across body		To provide support for painful arm
		Forearm cuff— adjustable straps allow changes in elbow position		
Giv-Mohr sling	Giv-Mohr	Figure-of-8 between scapulae	Arm up	To relieve weight of "heavy" flaccid arm
		Plastic Cone in palm of hand		

When clients shift off the weak leg onto this stable cane, the cane acts functionally as a third leg. This one-sided compensation encourages learned nonuse of the affected leg.

Single canes provide a balance assist. Often clients use the cane while walking outdoors or in crowded situations but not inside their homes. Reliance on a cane for walking eliminates the possibility of carrying objects and makes it difficult to perform one-handed tasks such as opening a door. Wrist loops allow the client to use the unaffected hand without losing the cane.

Orthotics

Ankle-foot orthoses (AFOs) are used to allow foot clearance during walking, to ensure heel strike, to provide distal stability for early standing and walking in clients with severe weakness, to provide lateral lower leg stability in clients who need an assist to lateral hip weakness, and to control knee hyperextension caused by loss of ankle dorsiflexion control. Different design types provide different functions. Solid ankle bracing with plastic beyond the malleoli limits distal freedom but allows clients with severe weakness to practice gaining control of trunk and hip movements.

The use of polypropylene bracing to control foot posturing in adults began in the 1970s with information from pediatrics and podiatry. Foot control in a brace stops supination of the foot in swing and compensatory pronation of the foot in stance. This control is achieved through neutral rearfoot positioning and long medial and lateral foot counters. Techniques of Aquaplast fabrication have created new possibilities for inexpensive, immediate, remoldable bracing for the foot and ankle.[146]

Custom-made AFOs provide the best fit and control, but an excellent prefabricated polypropylene brace is available through DobiSymplex/Hanger, an orthotics company. Their orthoses have long medial and lateral foot edges for control of foot posturing, come in multiple models and sizes, and can be ordered with regular or long foot plates (DobiSymplex/Hanger, a division of Seattle Limb System).

Clients should be encouraged to spend time standing or walking short distances without the brace so that dependence is not established. Clients like to be able to walk to the bathroom at night without a brace. Orthopedic ankle and foot supports provide alternatives to plastic bracing. The Malleoloc ankle support controls rearfoot equinus and varus while allowing ankle and forefoot movement (Bauerfeind/AliMed). Clients with moderate supination posturing report a reassuring feeling of security with this support while walking short distances and during sports participation. This support, a substitute for the Aircast and Ace support, is a good choice for sports activities such as golfing, bicycling, jumping, and running.

Functions and limitations of commonly used braces are found in Table 27-8 and orthotic manufacturers in Appendix 27-A.

Movable Surfaces

Movable surfaces such as gymnastic balls of varying sizes, large rolls, and adjustable stools with casters are used as assistive devices to help clients increase trunk/extremity strength and control. To encourage trunk/leg activity, the client sits on the ball and moves it in small ranges to the limits of perceived balance. This is an activity that increases

TABLE 27-8 ■ AFOs Used in Clients With Hemiplegia From Stroke

ORTHOTIC DESIGN	FUNCTION	LIMITATIONS	PATIENT TYPES (CATEGORIES)
Solid ankle with foot control	Heel strike Distal stability Lateral hip stability Assists forward progression Assists knee control Stops foot posturing	No ankle mobility No toe break	Severe weakness in trunk and leg Need for distal stability
Modified solid ankle with foot control	Heel strike More distal mobility-less ankle control Stops foot posturing	Less knee control Less message of forward progression No control of knee	Increasing leg strength Increasing trunk/leg control
Posterior leaf spring	Toe clearance	No control of foot posturing	Good return of control in trunk and leg Need for minimal dorsiflexion assist
Articulated ankle	Free dorsiflexion Heel strike if plantar stop used	Limited control of foot posturing Bulky at ankle	Normal ankle range—if range is limited, the movement of brace is translated into foot Functional needs; climb hills, stairs, move to and from ground
Supramalleolar foot orthoses in Aquaplast	Foot control Assist heel strike Used for weaning from AFOs Sports	No knee control Short shelf life of material	Increasing leg control Desire to begin increasing activity level
Foot orthoses	Balance small asymmetries of foot	No control of foot posturing No ankle or knee control	Persistent but minimal rearfoot/forefoot asymmetries
Klenzak metal, double-upright	Toe clearance Reminder of forward progression	No foot control Control of ankle and foot through shoe	Used before creation of polypropylene to provide heel strike and stop foot supination

See Chapter 34 for additional suggestions.

trunk and leg control but does not lead directly to improvements in standing or walking. Gymnastic balls provide symmetrical support to the rib cage when used in the hands and knees position and are used to stretch specific tight tissues. Routines of lifting the ball with either the arms or legs strengthen extremity movements in space.

When spasticity was considered the major impairment in hemiplegia, therapists often placed clients prone over balls to "inhibit" tone. This is an inappropriate technique considering advances in understanding of movement control and recovery.

Hand Splints

The practice of splinting the hemiplegic hand is controversial. Historically, the hand in clients with hemiplegia was splinted in a "resting" position. After the introduction of neurophysiological approaches, splinting became "inhibitory" in design.[147-149] Now, with the understanding that spasticity is not the major problem, splinting the wrist and hand has undergone another change. A new splint designed in 1982 by Levit,[150] as a neutral functional splint, promotes functional retraining and hand use while minimizing secondary impairments. This splint, designed to hold the wrist and hand in a position of orthopedic neutral, decreases hypertonicity that occurs either from poor alignment or unbalanced muscle return. The splint promotes support of the wrist and hand to avoid the secondary impairments of muscle tightness, muscle shifting, and overstretching of weak wrist and finger muscles.

Therapists custom make the splints with the goals of supporting the wrist in neutral, preventing radial or ulnar deviation with long, high sides, and maintaining the palmar arches. The fingers are not incorporated into the splint but are left free to allow movement reeducation and practice.

The increased tone in finger flexors, previously labeled "spasticity," comes in part from incomplete return or weakness of finger muscle activity on a poorly aligned wrist. A position of wrist flexion results in a drop of the proximal row of carpals and a flattening of the palmar arches. If the wrist is supported in neutral and the arches are preserved, returning muscle activity is re-educated in functional patterns. Finger support in a splint should be used only when there is a serious deformity with a need to serially, systematically, and slowly lengthen tight tissues.

This functional type of splint is worn mainly during the day when arm posturing is greater and when support of critical joints allows beginning hand use. Hand posturing is less of a problem when the patient lies down because of decreased demands on the trunk and legs. Clients are instructed not to wear the splint at night.

Design Considerations. If joint range is limited, the therapist makes the splint to support available range. The splint can be revised as range increases. Alignment is corrected in three steps: (1) keeping the wrist in flexion, the lateral deviation is corrected by aligning the third metacarpal with the middle of the radius; (2) the carpal position is corrected (usually gently lifted up from a low position under the radius); and (3) the hand is moved to wrist neutral (see *Functional Movement Reeducation*[47] for a step-by-step analysis). The warmed, soft splinting plastic captures this corrected position as it cools. The length of palmar support is decided by the therapist after assessment of degree and distribution of muscle return and muscle tightness patterns. The thumb is supported at its base in a neutral position, not one of abduction. As beginning grip returns, the thumb hole is widened to allow function.

A variety of neutral functional splints have been designed. The neutral wrist/thumb hole splinting design is hard to keep on the hand of patients with severe weakness. They sometimes find ulnar or radial trough splints or wide opponens splints easier to keep on.

As wrist extension control against gravity emerges, the therapist can fabricate a wide opponens splint to maintain the palmar arches as the client begins practicing finger movements. The wide opponens splint supports the base of the hand and assists in maintaining carpal alignment. Patients can switch between the two splints as needed.

Clients with severe hand pain prefer a neutral wrist splint with a resting area for the thumb. This splint is fabricated with little or no correction initially but with gentle support for the wrist and palmar arches. As the pain decreases, this splint is modified to become the original neutral functional splint.

Although the move away from "inhibitory" splints and from night splinting to day-time functional splinting breaks many of the "rules" from the past, it is more compatible with concepts from research and clinical experts.

Recommended resources for practical solutions to one-handed functioning and devices that assist in independence are listed in Appendix 27-B at the end of this chapter.

PSYCHOSOCIAL ASPECTS AND ADJUSTMENTS

The suddenness of a stroke and the dramatic change in motor, sensory, visual, and perceptual performance and feedback may leave the person with hemiplegia confused, disoriented, angry, stressed, frustrated, and fearful. When a stroke occurs, time is not allowed for gradual adjustment to the resulting disability.

Psychosocial adjustments may be more detrimental than is any functional disability to long-term stroke survivors.[151] Decreased interest in social activity inside and outside the home and decreased interest in hobbies attributable to psychosocial disability hamper the hemiplegic person's return to a normal social life.[152] Feelings of rejection and embarrassment may interfere with the hemiplegic person's interaction with people outside the home environment. Individuals with long-standing hemiplegia often become clinically depressed with symptoms of loss of sleep and appetite, self-blame, and a hopeless outlook. Suicide can result. The usual psychosocial adjustments to disability are compounded in persons with hemiplegia resulting from stroke by the issues associated with aging.

Family members and spouses may have difficulty assessing the capabilities of the hemiplegic person and may be overprotective. Overprotection among spouses may be a sign of affection and support or a sign of guilt.[153] Long-standing marriages do not tend to dissolve when one member has a stroke. However, previous marriage problems and personality traits may become exaggerated as a result of

the presence of increased and changing demands and stresses that occur when the person returns home.

A comparison of occupational status of long-term stroke survivors in the United States and in Sweden reveals that 40% of the Swedes returned to a form of employment (including part-time work) but none of the U.S. group returned to work.[154] The scarcity of part-time work and a shorter treatment period dictated by third-party payers in the United States may account for this discrepancy.

Age is a general predictor for return to employment, and younger people are more attractive to employers. Barriers to return to work for the person with hemiplegia include speech, perceptual, and cognitive deficits along with a need for psychosocial support. Architectural barriers also can create severe problems for hemiplegic clients with regard to both work and recreational activities. Stroke clubs, usually organized through hospitals, the National Stroke Association or the American Heart Association, provide educational, social, and recreational support for the hemiplegic person and her or his spouse.

The impact of psychosocial disability and the need for its long-term treatment is great. Programs need to be established and continued for years to allow clients and their families to deal with the many problems that result from the stroke. Refer to Appendix 27-C for resources.

Sexuality

Most persons with hemiplegia experience a decline in sexuality through a decrease in frequency of sexual intercourse without a change in the level of prestroke sexual desire.[155] On return home, the person with hemiplegia faces uncertainty about sexual skills and the risk of failure. Sexual dysfunction that results from a stroke depends on the amount of cerebral damage and includes a decreased ability to achieve erection and ejaculation in men and decreased lubrication in women.[156] The sensory, motor, visual, and emotional disturbances of hemiplegia may cause awkwardness, but these disturbances can be overcome through the education of the spouse in alternate positioning and ways to provide appropriate sensory experiences. The normal factors of aging also interfere with the sexual performance of persons with hemiplegia. A person's prestroke sexual activity is a good indicator of poststroke sexual activity. The closeness between partners achieved through satisfactory sexual relationship can add to the quality of life after stroke (see Chapter 5).

SUMMARY

This chapter reviews the neuropathology of stroke, the evaluation of impairments that interfere with functional movement patterns, and intervention planning. Both evaluation of outcomes and evaluation of movement components are described. The chapter highlights significant impairments and provides clinical observations on critical areas of intervention. A detailed process of clinical problem solving helps the therapist organize and prioritize impairments to plan intervention programs that retrain movement components and train desirable compensatory patterns to help the client gain the highest level of functional performance and independence in daily life. An example of the synthesis of this chapter's concepts and ideas can be found in the following case study.

CASE STUDY 27-1

A client with left hemiplegia was seen 4 days after stroke on admission to a rehabilitation center. The classification of movement disorder was one of composite movement category/severe movement deficits.

FUNCTIONAL LIMITATION NO. 1: CLIENT IS UNABLE TO PERFORM MORNING SELF-CARE AT BEDSIDE OR SITTING IN WHEELCHAIR IN FRONT OF A SINK

Why? Client cannot perform anterior/posterior or lateral trunk movements in sitting without loss of balance and falling to left. Client cannot feel left arm, and it hangs by side.

Evaluation

Primary Impairments

Weakness in trunk

Weakness in left arm

Inability to initiate trunk movements

Weakness in left leg

Decreased sense of touch left arm, trunk, and leg

Secondary Impairments

Loss of trunk alignment in sitting (upper trunk flexion)

Left shoulder subluxation

Muscle tightness—pectorals, latissimus, wrist flexors

Loss of alignment of lower trunk and pelvis—left pelvis lists downward

Loss of 10 degrees of left ankle joint dorsiflexor range

FUNCTIONAL LIMITATION NO. 2: CLIENT IS UNABLE TO TRANSFER FROM BED TO CHAIR INDEPENDENTLY

Why? Client cannot perform lower body anterior weight shifts (stable upper body) to initiate transfer left. Upper body falls into flexion. Left arm hangs by side with an inferior shoulder subluxation. Left leg cannot move in sitting. Client sits up by pulling on edge of bed with right arm.

Primary Impairments

Weakness in upper trunk

Weakness in left leg and trunk/leg patterns

Inability to initiate lower trunk patterns

Secondary Impairments

Loss of left upper body alignment

Loss of left ankle joint dorsiflexion range

Tightness in left hamstrings and gastrocnemius

FUNCTIONAL LIMITATION NO. 3: CLIENT IS UNABLE TO STAND UP FROM CHAIR INDEPENDENTLY

Why? Client is unable to control upper body over lower trunk during lower body–initiated transfers and sit to stand. Client is unable to use left leg for support and movement during the transition of sit to stand. Client is unable to keep weight (depress leg into floor) on left foot in standing.

Primary Impairments

Weakness in upper trunk

Weakness in leg and trunk/leg patterns

Inability to initiate lower trunk patterns

Secondary Impairments

Loss of left upper body alignment

Loss of left ankle joint dorsiflexion range

Tightness in left hamstrings and gastrocnemius

SIGNIFICANT IMPAIRMENTS FOR FUNCTIONS EVALUATED

1. Loss of upper body alignment during lower body–initiated movements, especially anterior/posterior plane
2. Shoulder subluxation contributes to loss of upper body alignment
3. Loss of ankle joint dorsiflexion range
4. Loss of control and weakness of trunk and left arm and left leg

TREATMENT GOALS AND INTERVENTIONS

  I. Functional goals
   A. Transfer from chair to bed and back with contact guarding
   B. Perform morning self-care activities in wheelchair in bathroom independently
   C. Rise to standing with assistance of one person
 II. Long-term goals
   A. Sit safely while performing tasks with right arm and leg around midline; that is, perform upper body– and lower body–initiated trunk movements in sitting independently
   B. Use left arm as a weight-bearing assist during movements of the right arm and leg in sitting and standing; that is, increase upper body control to prepare for independent, safe, lower body–initiated movement patterns (extended-arm reach and sit to stand and standing balance)
   C. Transfer, rise to stand, and stand with minimal assistance to the upper body; that is, increase leg strength and control in trunk/leg patterns
   D. Establish a home program that the client performs independently
III. Short-term goals
   A. Perform basic trunk movement patterns in sitting with contact guarding
   B. Decrease trunk asymmetry; increase control in upper body to decrease shoulder subluxation
   C. Protect shoulder joint from excessive capsular stretch
   D. Be able to lift weak arm with unaffected arm, maintain sitting balance, and position arm for bathing
   E. Increase ankle joint dorsiflexion range in standing
   F. Increase strength in leg and in trunk/leg-linked patterns during lower body–initiated transfers, during sit to stand, and in supported standing to allow assisted practice with moderate support to upper body (to maintain symmetry)
IV. Treatment techniques
   A. Assisted trunk movements in sitting with assistance to correct alignment of upper body on lower body

Continued

CASE STUDY 27-1—cont'd

B. Independent practice of trunk movements (home program)
C. Independent practice of trunk movements during forearm weight bearing in sitting (home program)
   1. Practice basic trunk movements
   2. Maintain arm range of motion; stretch tight muscles
D. Independent practice of trunk/arm-linked movements
   1. In weight bearing—see earlier
   2. In space-modified cane exercises in patterns practiced in A

E. Standing, lower extremity—initiated movements with assistance to upper body
F. Assisted practice of leg movements in space in sitting
G. Standing lower extremity—initiated movements to increase length of tight gastrocnemius and hamstring muscles
   1. Forearm weight bearing in standing
   2. Standing against a wall
H. Support arm on pillow in wheelchair, use shoulder-saddle support during transfers, sit to stand, and standing

REFERENCES

1. National Stroke Association: www.stroke.org. Accessed July 2006.
2. Kwakkel G, Kollen B, van der Grond J, Prevo A: Probability of regaining dexterity in the flaccid upper limb, *Stroke* 34:2181-2186, 2003.
3. Bonita R: Epidemiology of stroke, *Lancet* 339:342-344, 1992.
4. Ostfeld A: A review of stroke epidemiology, *Epidemiol Rev* 2:136-152, 1980.
5. Gresham GE, Phillips TF, Wolf PA et al: Epidemiologic profile of long-term stroke disability: the Framingham study, *Arch Phys Med Rehabil* 60:487-491, 1979.
6. Jongbloed L: Prediction of function after stroke: a critical review, *Stroke* 17:765-776, 1986.
7. Kalra L, Dale P, Crome P: Improving stroke rehabilitation: a controlled study, *Stroke* 24:1462-1467, 1994.
8. Adler MK, Brown CC Jr, Acton P: Stroke rehabilitation: is age a determinant? *J Am Geriatr Soc* 28:499-503, 1980.
9. Cinnamon J, Viroslav AB, Dorey JH: CT and MRI diagnosis of cerebrovascular disease: going beyond the pixels, *Semin CT MRI* 16:212-236, 1995.
10. Adams RD, Victor M: *Principles of neurology,* New York, 1981, McGraw-Hill.
11. Roth EJ, Harvey RL: Rehabilitation of stroke syndromes. In Braddom RL, editor: *Physical medicine and rehabilitation,* Philadelphia, 1996, WB Saunders.
12. Simmoons ML et al: Individual risk assessment for intracranial hemorrhage during thrombolytic therapy, *Lancet* 342:1523, 1993.
13. Wardlaw JM, Warlow CP: Thrombolysis in acute ischemic stroke: does it work? *Stroke* 23:1826-1839, 1992.
14. Kistler JP, Ropper AH, Martin JB: Cerebrovascular disease. In Isselbacker KJ et al, editors: *Harrison's principles of internal medicine,* New York, 1994, McGraw-Hill.
15. Landau WM: Spasticity: The fable of a neurological demon and the emperor's new therapy [editorial], *Arch Neurol* 31:217-219, 1974.
16. Sahrmann S, Norton BJ: The relationship of voluntary movement to spasticity in the upper motor neuron syndrome, *Ann Neurol* 2:460-465, 1977.
17. Easton JKM, Ozel T, Halpern D: Intramuscular neurolysis for spasticity in children, *Arch Phys Med Rehabil* 50:155-158, 1979.
18. Petrillo CR et al: Phenol block of the tibial nerve in the hemiplegic patient, *Orthopedics* 3:871, 1980.
19. Snow BJ, Tsui JK, Bhatt MH et al: Treatment of spasticity with botulinum toxin: a double-blind study, *Ann Neurol* 28:512-515, 1990.
20. Das TK, Park D: Effect of treatment with botulinum toxin on spasticity, *Postgrad Med J* 65:208-210, 1989.

21. Penn RD, Savoy SM, Corcos D et al: Intrathecal baclofen for severe spasticity, *N Engl J Med* 320:1517-1521, 1989.
22. Norris JW, Hachinski VC: Misdiagnosis of stroke, *Lancet* 6:328-331, 1982.
23. Wiebe-Velasquez S, Blume WT: Seizures, *Phys Med Rehabil State Art Rev* 7:73-86, 1993.
24. Haas AL, Rusk HA, Pelosof H et al; Respiratory function in hemiplegic patients, *Arch Phys Med Rehabil* 48:174-179, 1967.
25. Mion LC, Gregor S, Buettner M et al: Falls in the rehabilitation setting: Incidence and characteristics, *Rehabil Nurs* 14:17-22, 1989.
26. Poplinger AR, Pillar T: Hip fracture in stroke patients: epidemiology and rehabilitation, *Acta Orthop Scand* 56:226, 1985.
27. Brandstater ME, Roth EJ, Siebens HC: Venous thromboembolism in stroke: literature review and implication for clinical practice, *Arch Phys Med Rehabil* 73(suppl):S379-S391, 1992.
28. Cailliet R: *The shoulder in hemiplegia,* Philadelphia, 1980, FA Davis.
29. Lankford LL: Reflex sympathetic dystrophy, In Hunter JM, MacKin EJ, Callahan AD, editors: *Rehabilitation of the hand,* ed 3, St. Louis, 1990, CV Mosby.
30. Marshall J: *The management of cerebrovascular disease,* ed 3, Oxford, 1976, Blackwell Scientific Publications.
31. Weinfeld D, editor: The national survey of stroke, *Stroke* 12(1 suppl):2, 1981.
32. Bamford J, Sandercock P, Dennis M et al: A prospective study of acute cerebrovascular disease in the community: the Oxfordshire Community Stroke Project 1981-1986, *J Neurol Neurosurg Psychiatry* 53:16-22, 1990.
33. Bach-y-Rita P: *Recovery of functions: Theoretical considerations for brain injury rehabilitation,* Baltimore, 1980, University Park Press.
34. Brooks VB: Motor programs revisited. In Talbott RE, Humphrey DR, editors: *Posture and movement,* New York, 1979, Raven Press.
35. Bobath B: *Adult hemiplegia: Evaluation and treatment,* ed 3, London, 1990, William Heinemann Medical Books.
36. Brunnstrom S: *Movement therapy in hemiplegia,* New York, 1970, Harper & Row.
37. Knott M, Voss DE: *Proprioceptive neuromuscular facilitation,* New York, 1976, Harper & Row.
38. Bizzi E, Polit A: Characteristics of motor programs underlying movement in monkeys, *J Neurophysiol* 42:183-194, 1979.
39. Skillbeck CE, Wade DT, Hewer RL et al: Recovery after stroke, *J Neurol Neurosurg Psychiatry* 46:5-8, 1983.
40. Heller A, Wade DT: Arm function after stroke: measurement and recovery over the first three months, *J Neurol Neurosurg Psychiatry* 50:714-719, 1987.
41. Kwakkel G, Kollen BJ, Wagenaar RC: Long term effects of intensity of upper and lower limb training after stroke: a randomised trial, *J Neurol Neurosurg Psychiatry* 72:473-479, 2002.

42. American Physical Therapy Association: Guide to Physical Therapist Practice. Second Edition. American Physical Therapy Association, *Phys Ther* 81:9-746, 2001.

43. Nagi SZ: Some conceptual issues in disability and rehabilitation. In Sussman MB, editor: *Sociology and rehabilitation,* Washington, DC, 1985, American Sociological Association.

44. World Health Organization: *International classification of impairments disabilities, and handicaps: a manual of classification relating the consequences of disease,* Geneva, 1980, World Health Organization.

45. Steiner WA, Ryser L, Huber E et al: Use of the ICF model as a clinical problem-solving tool in physical therapy and rehabilitation medicine, *Phys Ther* 82:1098-1107, 2002.

46. Sheets PK, Sahrmann SA, Norton BJ: Diagnosis for physical therapy for patients with neuromuscular conditions, *Neurol Rep* 23:158-161, 1999.

47. Ryerson S, Levit K: *Functional movement reeducation: a contemporary model for stroke rehabilitation,* New York, 1997, Churchill Livingstone.

48. Schenkman M, Butler RB: A model for multisystem evaluation, interpretation and treatment of individuals with neurologic dysfunction, *Phys Ther* 69:538-547, 1989.

49. Ryerson S: Development of abnormal patterns in adult hemiplegia, Lecture, Newark, NJ, 1984, Barbro Salek Memorial Symposium.

50. Teasdale G, Jennett B: Assessment of coma and impaired consciousness: a practical scale, *Lancet* 2:81-84, 1974.

51. Plum F, Caronna JJ: Can one predict outcome of medical coma? In *Outcome of severe damage to the central nervous system,* Ciba Foundation Symposium 34, Amsterdam, 1975, Ciba Foundation.

52. Levy DE, Bates D, Caronna JJ et al: Prognosis in nontraumatic coma, *Ann Intern Med* 94:293-301, 1981.

53. Malkmus D: *Levels of cognitive functioning,* Los Angeles, 1977, Ranchos Los Amigos Hospital.

54. Taub E: Movement in nonhuman primates deprived of somatosensory feedback, *Exerc Sport Sci Rev* 4:335-374, 1976.

55. Mahoney F, Barthel DW: Functional evaluation: the Barthel Index, *MD State Med J* 14:61-65, 1965.

56. Carr JH, Shepherd RB, Nordholm L et al: Investigation of a new motor assessment scale for stroke patients, *Phys Ther* 65:175-180, 1985.

57. Granger CV, Hamilton BB: The Uniform Data System for medical rehabilitation report of first admissions for 1990, *Am J Phys Med Rehabil* 71:108-113, 1992.

58. Keith RA, Granger CV: The functional independence measure: a new tool for rehabilitation. In Eisenberg MG, Grzesiak RC, editors: *Advances in clinical rehabilitation, vol 1,* New York, 1987, Springer-Verlag.

59. Collen FM, Wade DT, Robb GF et al: The Rivermead Mobility Index: a further development of the Rivermead Motor Assessment, *Int Disabil Stud* 13:50-54, 1991.

60. Fisher AG: *Assessment of motor and process skills,* Fort Collins, CO, 1995, Three Star Press.

61. Fugl-Meyer AR, Jaasko L, Leyman I et al: The post-stroke hemiplegic patient: a method for evaluation of physical performance, *Scand J Rehabil Med* 7:13-31, 1975.

62. Berg KD, Maki BE, Williams JI et al: Clinical and laboratory measures of postural balance in the elderly population, *Arch Phys Med Rehabil* 73:1073-1080, 1992.

63. Berg KD, Wook-Dauphinee S, Williams J: The balance scale: reliability assessment with elderly residents and patients with an acute stroke, *Scand J Rehabil Med* 27:27-36, 1995.

64. Benaim C, Perennou DA, Villy J et al: Validation of a standardized assessment of postural control in stroke patients: the Postural Assessment Scale for Stroke Patients (PASS), *Stroke* 30:1862-1868, 1999.

65. Mao H-F, Hsueh I-P, Tang P-T et al: Analysis and comparison of the psychometric properties of three balance measures for stroke patients, *Stroke* 33:1022-1026, 2002.

66. Duncan P, Weiner DK, Chandler J et al: Functional reach: a new clinical measure of balance, *J Gerontol* 45:192-197, 1990.

67. Wolf S, Catlin P, Ellis M et al: Assessing Wolf Motor Function Test as outcome measure for research in patients after stroke, *Stroke* 32:1635-1639, 2001.

68. Nelson AJ: Functional ambulation profile, *Phys Ther* 54:1059-1065, 1974.

69. Nelson AJ: Personal communication, November 1981.

70. Podsiadlo D, Richardson S: The timed "Up and Go" test: a test of basic functional mobility for frail elderly persons, *J Am Geriatr Soc* 39:142-148, 1991.

71. Knutsson E, Richards C: Different types of disturbed motor control in gait of hemiparetic patients, *Brain* 102:405-530, 1979.

72. Perry J: Clinical gait analyzer, *Bull Prosthet Res,* Fall:188-194, 1974.

73. Bohannon RW, Larkin PA, Smith MB et al: Relationship between static muscle strength deficits and spasticity in stroke patients with hemiparesis, *Phys Ther* 67:1068-1071, 1987.

74. Bohannon RW, Smith MB: Assessment of strength deficits in eight paretic upper extremity muscle groups of stroke patients with hemiplegia, *Phys Ther* 67:522-525, 1987.

75. Bourbonnais D, Vanden Noven S: Weakness in patients with hemiparesis, *Am J Occup Ther* 43:313-319, 1989.

76. Mohr JP et al: Hemiparesis profiles in acute stroke, *Ann Neurol* 12:156, 1984.

77. Landau WM, Sahrmann SA: Preservation of directly stimulated muscle strength in hemiplegia due to stroke, *Arch Neurol* 59:1453-1457, 2002.

78. Bobath B: *Evaluation and treatment,* London, 1970, William Heinemann Medical Books.

79. Granit R: Comments. In Granit R, editor: *Progress in brain research,* Amsterdam, 1979, North Holland Biomedical Press.

80. Granit R: Interpretation of supraspinal effects on the gamma system. In Granit R, editor: *Progress in brain research,* Amsterdam, 1979, North Holland Biomedical Press.

81. Dietz V, Muller R, Colombo D: Locomotor activity in spinal man: significant of afferent input from joint and load receptors, *Brain* 125:2626-2634, 2002.

82. Landau W: Spasticity: the fable of a neurological demon and the emperor's new therapy, *Arch Neurol* 31:217-219, 1974.

83. Dietz V: Spastic movement disorder: what is the impact of research on clinical practice? *J Neur Neurosurg Psychchiatry* 74:820-821, 2003.

84. Bohannon RW, Andrews W: Inter-rater reliability of a modified Ashworth scale of muscle spasticity, *Phys Ther* 67:206-207, 1987.

85. Feldman RD, Young RR, Koella WP, editors: *Spasticity: disordered motor control,* Chicago, 1980, Year Book.

86. Ashworth B: Carisoprodol in multiple sclerosis, *Practitioner* 192:540-542, 1964.

87. Levit K: Shoulder dysfunction. Presented at the third annual Magee Stroke Conference, Philadelphia, 1992.

88. Bobath B: *Adult hemiplegia: evaluation and treatment,* ed 2, London, 1978, William Heinemann Medical Books.

89. Huskisson EC, Jones J, Scott PJ: Application of visual analogue scales to the measurement of functional capacity, *Rheumatol Rehabil* 15:185-187, 1976.

90. Melzack R: The McGill Pain Questionnaire: major properties and scoring methods, *Pain* 1:277-299, 1975.

91. Bohannon RW, Larkin PA, Smith MB et al: Shoulder pain in hemiplegia: a statistical relationship with five variables, *Arch Phys Med Rehabil* 67:514-516, 1986.

92. Carr JH, Shepherd RB: *A motor relearning programme for stroke,* ed 2, Rockville, MD, 1982, Aspen Publishers.

93. Davies PM: *Steps to follow: a guide to the treatment of adult hemiplegia,* New York, 1985, Springer-Verlag.

94. Davies PM: *Right in the middle: selective trunk activity in the treatment of adult hemiplegia,* New York, 1990, Springer-Verlag.

95. Mathiowetz V, Bass Haugen J: Motor behavior research: implications for therapeutic approaches to central nervous system dysfunction, *Am J Occup Ther* 48:733-745, 1994.

96. Cirstea CM, Levin MF: Compensatory strategies for reaching in stroke, *Brain* 123:940-953, 2000.

97. Levin MF, Michaelsen SM, Cirstea CM et al: Use of the trunk for reaching targets placed within and beyond the reach in adult hemiparesis, *Exp Brain Res* 143:171-180, 2002.

98. Michaelsen SM, Luta A, Roby-Brami A et al: Effect of trunk restraint on the recovery of reaching movements in hemiparetic patients, *Stroke* 32:1875-1883, 2001.

99. Michaelsen SM, Levin MF: Short-term effects of practice with trunk restraint on reaching movements in patients with chronic stroke: a controlled trial, *Stroke* 35:1914-1919, 2004.

100. Taub E, Miller NE, Novack TA et al: Technique to improve chronic motor deficit after stroke, *Arch Phys Med Rehabil* 74:347-354, 1993.

101. Wolf SL, Lecraw DE, Barton LA et al: Forced use of hemiplegic upper extremities to reverse the effect of learned nonuse among chronic stroke and head injured patients, *Exp Neurol* 104:125-132, 1989.

102. Fisher B: Effect of trunk control and alignment on limb function, *J Head Trauma Rehabil* 2:72, 1987.

103. Gillian G: Upper extremity function and management. In Gillian G, Burkhardt AL, editors: *Stroke rehabilitation,* St. Louis, 1998, CV Mosby.

104. Mohr JD: *Management of the trunk in adult hemiplegia: topics in neurology,* Alexandria, VA, 1990, American Physical Therapy Association.

105. Ryerson S: Postural control: from movement to function. Presented at the NDTA annual conference, San Diego, 1989.

106. Cordo PJ, Nashner LM: Properties of postural adjustments associated with rapid arm movements, *J Neurophysiol* 47:287-302, 1982.

107. Shumway-Cook A, Woollacott M: *Motor control: theory and practical applications,* Baltimore, 1995, Williams & Wilkins.

108. Woollacott MH, Bonnet M, Yabe K: Preparatory process for anticipatory postural adjustments: modulation of leg muscles reflex pathways during preparation for arm movements in standing man, *Exp Brain Res* 55:263-271, 1984.

109. Levit K: Trunk control during functional performance. Presented at the American Occupational Therapy Association annual conference, Baltimore, 1997.

110. Horak FB: Clinical measurement of postural control in adults, *Phys Ther* 67:1881-1885, 1987.

111. Nashner LM: Adaptation of human movement to altered environments, *Trends Neurosci* 5:358, 1982.

112. Shumway-Cook A, Woollacott M: The growth of stability: postural control from a developmental perspective, *J Motor Behav* 17:131-147, 1985.

113. Bohannon RW: Recovery and correlates of trunk muscle strength after stroke, *Int J Rehabil Res* 8:162-167, 1995.

114. Bohannon RW, Cassidy D, Walsh S: Trunk muscle strength is impaired multidirectionally after stroke, *Clin Rehabil* 9:47-51, 1995.

115. Bohannon RW: Lateral trunk flexion strength: impairment, measurement reliability and implications following unilateral brain lesion, *Int J Rehabil Res* 15:249-251, 1992.

116. Dickstein R, Heffes Y, Laufer Y et al: Activation of selected trunk muscles during symmetrical functional activities in poststroke hemiparetic and hemiplegic patients, *J Neurol Neurosurg Psychiatry* 66:218-221, 1999.

117. Dickstein R, Sheffi S, Ben Haim Z et al: Activation of flexor and extensor trunk muscles in hemiplegia, *Am J Phys Med Rehabil* 79:228-234, 2000.

118. Tanaka M, Hachisuka K, Ogata H: Muscle strength of trunk flexion-extension in post-stroke hemiplegic patients, *Am J Phys Med Rehabil* 77:288-290, 1998.

119. Karatas M, Cetin N, Bayramoglu M et al: Trunk muscle strength in relation to balance and functional disability in unihemispheric stroke patients, *Am J Phys Med Rehabil* 83:81-87, 2004.

120. Scholtz J: *NDTA adult hemiplegia course manual,* Hartford, CT, 1982, NDTA.

121. Carr JH, Shepherd RB, Ada L: Spasticity: research findings and implications for intervention, *Physiotherapy* 81:421-426, 1995.

122. Schenkman M: Lecture notes: Recent developments in motor control and their relevance to intervention techniques in adults with CNS dysfunction, NDTA Certification Course in Adult Hemiplegia, Alexandria, VA, 1990.

123. Chan WY: Some techniques for the relief of spasticity and their physiological basis, *Physiother Can* 38:85, 1986.

124. Odeen I: Reduction of muscular hypertonus by long-term muscle stretch, *Scand J Rehabil Med* 13:93-99, 1981.

125. Price CI: Shoulder pain after stroke: a research challenge, *Age Aging* 31:36, 2002.

126. Roy CW, Sands MR, Hill LD: Shoulder pain in acutely admitted hemiplegics, *Clin Rehabil* 8:334, 1994.

127. Ryerson S, Levit K: The shoulder in hemiplegia. In Donatelli R, editor: *The shoulder in physical therapy,* ed 3, New York, 1997, Churchill Livingstone.

128. Basmajian JV: *Muscles alive: their functions revealed by electromyography,* Baltimore, 1978, Williams & Wilkins.

129. Ryerson S, Levit K: Glenohumeral joint subluxations in CNS dysfunction, *NDTA News* November 1988.

130. Jenson M: The hemiplegic shoulder, *Scand J Rehabil Med* 7(suppl):113, 1980.

131. Kane LA, Buckley KA: Functional mobility. In Gillen G, Burkhardt A, editors: *Stroke rehabilitation,* St. Louis, 1998, Mosby.

132. Schenkman M, Berger RA, Riley PO et al: Whole-body movements during rising to stand from sitting, *Phys Ther* 70:638-651, 1990.

133. VanSant A: Life span development in functional tasks, *Phys Ther* 70:788-798, 1990.

134. Chou S-W, Wong AM, Leong C-P et al: Postural control during sit-to-stand and gait in stroke patients, *Am J Phys Med Rehabil* 82:42-47, 2003.

135. Weinstein CJ et al: Balance training in hemiparetics, *Arch Phys Med Rehabil* 70:755-762, 1989.

136. Knutsson E: Gait control in hemiparesis, *Scand J Rehabil Med* 13:101-108, 1981.

137. Smidt G: Rudiments of gait. In Smidt GL, editor: *Gait in rehabilitation,* New York, 1990, Churchill Livingstone.

138. Winter D: *Biomechanical and motor control factors in gait,* Toronto, 1989, Waterloo Press.

139. Perry J: The mechanics of walking, *Phys Ther* 47:778-801, 1967.

140. Ryerson S: The foot in hemiplegia. In Hunt GC, McPoil TG, editors: *The foot and the ankle in physical therapy,* ed 2, New York, 1995, Churchill Livingstone.

141. Van Peppen RP, Kwakkel G, Wood-Dauphinee S et al: The impact of physical therapy on functional outcomes after stroke: what's the evidence, *Clin Rehabil* 18:833-862, 2004.

142. Sullivan K, Knowlton B, Dobkin B: Step training with body-weight support: effect of treadmill speed and practice paradigms on post-stroke locomotor recovery, *Arch Phys Med Rehabil* 83:683-691, 2002.

143. Moodie NB, Brisbin J, Morgan AM: Subluxation of the glenohumeral joint in hemiplegia: Evaluation of supportive devices, *Physiother Can* 38:151, 1986.

144. Smith RO, Okamoto G: Checklist for the prescription of slings for the hemiplegia patient, *Am J Occup Ther* 35:91-95, 1981.

145. Levit K: History of shoulder slings. Lecture notes, Advanced NDTA Upper Extremity Course, Alexandria, VA, 1992.

146. Ryerson S: Neurological and biomechanical considerations in lower extremity bracing in adults with CNS dysfunction. Presented at the APTA annual conference, Denver, 1992.

147. Farber S: Adaptive equipment. In Farber S, editor: *Neurorehabilitation: a multisensory approach,* Philadelphia, 1981, WB Saunders.

148. MacKinnon F et al: The MacKinnon splint: A functional hand splint, *Can J Occup Ther* 42:157, 1975.

149. Neuhaus B, Ascher ER, Coullon BA et al: A survey of rationales for and against hand splinting in hemiplegia, *Am J Occup Ther* 35:83-90, 1981.

150. Levit K: Treating the hemiplegic hand. Lecture notes, Arizona State OT conference, Phoenix, 1992.

151. Gresham GE, Phillips TF, Labi ML: ADL status in stroke: relative merits of three standard indexes, *Arch Phys Med Rehabil* 61:355-358, 1980.

152. Labi ML, Phillips TF, Gresham GE: Psychosocial disability in physically restored long-term stroke survivors, *Arch Phys Med Rehabil* 61:561-565, 1980.

153. Kinsella GJ, Duffy FD: Attitudes towards disability expressed by spouses of stroke patients, *Scand J Rehabil Med* 12:73-76, 1980.

154. Fugl-Meyer AR: Post-stroke hemiplegia-occupational status, *Scand J Rehabil Med* 7(suppl):53-67, 1980.

155. Fugl-Meyer AR, Jaasko L: Post-stroke hemiplegia and sexual intercourse, *Scand J Rehabil Med* 7(suppl):158-166, 1980.

156. Garden FH, Smith BS: Sexual function after cerebrovascular accident, *Curr Concepts Rehabil Med* 5:2-7, 1990.

APPENDIX 27-A ■ Product Manufacturers

DobiSymplex-Sea Fab
9561 Satellite Blvd.
Orlando, FL 32837

AliMed
P.O. Box 9135
Dedham, MA 32703

DePuy Orthotech
700 Orthopedic Dr.
Warsaw, IN 46581-0988

Smith and Nephew, Rolyan
One Quality Drive
Germantown, WI 53022-8205

Sammons Preston
P.O. Box 5071
Bolingbrook, IL 60440

APPENDIX 27-B ■ Resources for One-Handed Adaptations

One-Handed in a Two-Handed World
Tommye K. Mayer
Prince-Gallison Press

P.O. Box 23
Boston, MA 02113

Adaptive Resources: A Guide to Products and Services
National Stroke Association
8480 E. Orchard Rd.
Englewood, CO 80111

APPENDIX 27-C ■ Stroke Survivor Resources

Internet Links

National Stroke Association: www.stroke.org.
American Stroke Association: www.strokeassociation.org.
American Stroke Foundation: www.americanstroke.org.
Resource site: www.strokecenter.org.
Stroke journal: http://stroke.ahajournal.org.
Neurology stroke information: http://brainattacks.net.
Useful stroke information: www.strokehelp.com.

Audiovisual and Literary Resources

Films and Videotapes

Inner World of Aphasia, 35-minute film
American Journal of Nursing Film Library
267 W. 25th St.
New York, NY 10001
Candidate for Stroke, 35-minute film
American Heart Association
I Had a Stroke, 35-minute film
Filmmakers Library, Inc.
290 West End Ave.
New York, NY 10023
Living with Stroke
Rehabilitation Research and Training Center
The George Washington University
2300 I St., NW, Suite 714
Washington, DC 20037
Evaluation of the Hemiplegic Patient (sensory/motor)
Audio-Visual Department
School of Allied Health
University of Maryland
32 Greene St.
Baltimore, MD 21201

Books

CHILDREN
First One Foot, Then the Other, by Tomie de Paola. This book explores the feelings and fears of children about a relative who has had a stroke.
ADULT
How to Conquer the World with One Hand . . . and an Attitude, by Paul E. Berger. Merrifield, VA, 1999, Positive Power Publisher.

KEY WORDS

aging
Alzheimer's disease
caregiver training and support
dementia and delirium
function
physical/occupational therapy examination and
    intervention
problem solving
rehabilitation
therapeutic environment

OBJECTIVES

After reading this chapter the student/therapist will be able to:

1. Define the basic terminology and discuss the prevalence of cognitive disturbances seen in older persons.
2. Describe normative changes in brain function with normal aging and their relevance to the diagnoses of delirium and dementias.
3. Discuss how symptoms are altered with normal aging (specifically related to Arndt-Schultz principle, law of initial values, habitual biorhythms) for an individual.
4. Describe normal sensory changes with aging and how they alter a person's overall ability to adapt to stress.
5. Describe how, and for what type of patient, to use the Mini-Mental State Examination as a part of the physical/occupational therapy examination.
6. Describe common sensory changes with dementia and implications for adapting physical/occupational therapy evaluation and intervention.
7. Discuss common changes in learning styles with aging and implications for adapting physical/occupational therapy intervention to enhance patients' ability to perform at their highest functional level.
8. Describe how the environmental design and ergonomics can enhance patient performance in activities of daily living and instrumental activities of daily living.
9. Describe a strategy to evaluate patient's emotional capacity to participate in a learning task and its clinical relevance to both occupational and physical therapy outcomes.
10. Describe criteria for delirium and reversible dementia and sample strategies for modifying evaluation and treatment procedures.
11. Discuss symptoms and disease progression in irreversible dementia.
12. Discuss the therapist's role on the treatment team in educating key caregivers and support personnel and sample training strategies.
13. Discuss treatment skills that are helpful in working with persons who have irreversible dementia.
14. Describe research activities and new findings that affect physical evaluation and treatment of the patient with dementia or delirium.

STARTING POINT WITH OLDER PERSONS IN PHYSICAL/OCCUPATIONAL THERAPY

The older person can learn to adapt to new physical crises. The goal is to use the processes of habilation and rehabilitation to work so that caregivers (family, friends or staff) are trained to bring out the best functional performance in the older person. The people relating to the older person in a time of crisis facilitate and support them in adapting to the best of their capacity. The specifics in this process include the following:

1. Document the presence of lost functional skills
2. Evaluate and create specific measurable results (goals) for their functional capacity in their current physical, emotional, and social environment (if the caregiver changes, new goals or strategies may need to be developed because not all caregivers have the same capacity to relate to the older person)
3. Identify and train the older person in specific neuro-facilitation strategies to enhance self-image and kinesthetic awareness of self in space and use of skeletal support (self in body)
4. Screen for signs of reversible cognitive losses
5. Provide adaptations and training for performance of activities of daily living when chronic cognitive problems exist
6. Train caregivers and the older person in ways to adapt the activities of daily living (ADLs) and instrumental activities of daily living (IADLs) to maximize ability

7. Train caregivers in basic handling skills that take advantage of the habits of action, postures, and positioning to maximize ease of daily living

PARADIGM FOR AGING, THE BRAIN, AND LEARNING

Life is learning. The brain and human nervous system have at least 3×10^{10} parts. As Feldenkrais stated, "This is large enough for its balanced functions to obey the law of large systems. The health of such a system can be measured by the shock (stimuli) it can take without compromising the continuation of its processes."[1] Adaptability and health can be measured by the amount of stimuli or shock people can tolerate without their usual way of life being compromised. Aging is a process that requires ongoing adaptation to and compensation for the losses that are imposed on human beings from the world and the internal physiological changes that occur with the passage of time, physical activities, emotional state, fatigue, digestive and elimination processes, and habitual rest-activity cycle. If a person's health is altered by illness or trauma, then he or she goes through an adaptive process. If too many changes happen too quickly, the brain is not able to create a functional adaptive response and the individual must alter or simplify her or his life processes or face negative mental or physiological reactions. The literature demonstrates that regression periods and illness seem to be linked.[2-5] As human beings explore coping with unfamiliar experiences, they require more nurturing, rest, and physical contact that is perceived as empowering.

Human beings progress to adulthood through the millions of perceptions and choices that are recorded and responded to through the developmental years. Human beings are not born with the brain and nervous system having the skills of an adult. In infancy, the brain begins to learn during interactions with the environment. The kinesthetic and sensory connections provide the data about the internal and external environments.[6] Through this interactive learning process each human being (with a nondifferentiated nervous system) discovers new differentiations and thus new strategies for relating to the world. With advanced age comes a gradual decrease in the acuity of the kinesthetic and sensory information received. Some key concepts are common to interactive learning for both the child and the older adult: active participation has a positive impact on recall and learning,[7] predictable events support recall,[8] and ordered events are easier to recall. Differentiation for human beings does not happen uniformly.[9,10] As a person grows, the result of this lack of uniformity is that some adults prefer to relate to the world visually, others aurally, and still others by touch or kinesthetically. In other words, people specialize with their sensory processing and at the same time become vulnerable to issues of sensory adaptation and selection.[11]

The adult phase of brain and central nervous system development will, for most people, involve a gradual narrowing of the focus in the development of new skills as well as increased repetition of certain activities. The tendency is to have activity narrow more and more to the activities in which a person excels or feels comfortable. Intuitive or practical people continue to pursue self-knowledge and explore ways to maximize their talents. By accident or through mentoring, these people discover that lifelong learning is the gift

of life itself. Ongoing and ever-increasing self-awareness allows for enhanced adaptability at any age. What if rehabilitation after illness or trauma invited a guided examination of self-awareness and habitual strategies as the basis for inventing new functional adaptive strategies? The Feldenkrais Method is one model for neurological facilitation and enhancement of human learning and adaptability that is built on the concept of starting from the current habits of action of the person.[1,12,13] The Feldenkrais Method also uses several other basic learning strategies that make this approach helpful for the older patient: going slowly, simplifying the movement or stimuli, proceeding from the perception of the patient, learning to detect and respond to the smallest possible input, and increasing the awareness and use of the skeleton and the support it gives. Feldenkrais noted what a person automatically did during a crisis, such as a fall. He noted the automatic human response and then built in a self-defense response that took advantage of the innate reflex.[14] The result is that the exploratory learning is easy for the patient because it builds on the automatic response the person is already familiar with. The goal is to invent physical therapy interventions that encourage patient participation and that feel safe and useful to the patient.

In this chapter the paradigm for aging and lifelong learning presumes the following:

1. The brain and central nervous system are viewed as the master system and the controller of the other human systems (e.g., digestive, cardiovascular, muscular, hormonal).
2. Capacity exists for ongoing learning (self-awareness), self-regulation, and adaptability through the lifespan.
3. The whole (human being) is greater than the sum of its parts.
4. Language shapes reality and the experience and perceptions of life.
5. Enjoying a comfortable and easy pace for new learning is beneficial. Being able to learn new skills is important for adaptability and for lifelong well-being.
6. The mind and body are not separate.
7. Personal variations in learning style and preferences for relating can be used to maximize adaptation throughout life.
8. The activation of the limbic system for "fight or flight" is normal and when the crisis (real or imagined) is over, the ability to release the limbic activation and find the resting state becomes an important skill as people grow older.
9. Creation of environments that encourage safe exploration of new ideas and ways of self-expression can generate lifelong human growth and development.

FRAMEWORK FOR CLINICAL PROBLEM SOLVING

Therapists working with patients with cognitive impairments need to have received adequate advanced training in assessment of communication skills and neurological functioning as well as gerontology so they can work with maximal efficiency and enjoy the clinical interactions with each patient. In 37 BC the Roman poet Virgil wrote, "Age carries all things, even the mind, away."[15] Nearly 400 years ago, Shakespeare described the last stage of human life as "second childishness and mere oblivion, sans teeth, sans eyes, sans taste, sans everything."[16] This pessimistic view of the fate of the elderly persists among health care workers today despite the fact that significant cognitive deficits affect only between 6.1% and 12.3% of the elderly (older than age 65 years) in the United States.[17,18]

The clinician should not assume that an older person has impaired cognitive functioning. Perhaps the most crucial concept for clinical problem solving is that the clinician must not assume that the current abilities reflect the true capacity of the person. When a patient is observed to have altered brain function, description of the extent and type of the distortion of intellectual capacity and determination of the time of onset (sudden or gradual) are necessary to enable the provision of appropriate and effective treatment and care. The capacity to learn is a possibility, although the process of learning may be altered or different from unaffected older adults.[19-22] When age, illness, or medications create a temporary or permanent change in cognitive abilities, all functional training requires alteration to meet the unique cognitive abilities of the patient at the moment. For example, the son of a patient who needed physical and occupational therapy showed staff how to communicate with his mother so she did not get scared. The therapist walked slowly into the room and greeted the patient by touching her softly on the cheek with the back of her hand. The patient looked up and smiled. The therapist smiled back and stroked the patient softly on the top of her head. The patient smiled again. The therapist kneeled down so that she was eye to eye with the patient sitting in the wheelchair. She took the patient's hand in her own hand and with her other hand slowly stroked the back of the patient's hand. The patient smiled again. The therapy session had begun. For this patient words were actually confusing so they were avoided.[23] The need for tactile nurturing input stays and persists as people age.[24] Nurturing tactile input done at a pace that is pleasant for the patient can actually support a positive clinical outcome.[25]

Definition of Terms

Intellectual impairment falls into three categories: mental retardation, delirium, and dementia. A definition of terms is necessary to ensure that all personnel use the same framework for clinical problem solving.

A person with mental retardation (also called developmental disability) has had some degree of intellectual impairment all her or his life. A person with mental retardation also can develop delirium or dementia. Delirium or dementia differs from mental retardation in that a change from the baseline level of functioning has occurred in that person.

A person with delirium usually shows a change both in intellectual function and in level of consciousness.[26,27] The patient may be perplexed, disoriented, fearful, forgetful, or all of these. The patient is often less alert than normal and may be sleepy or obtunded; however, many patients with delirium are hypervigilant and may be extremely agitated and suspicious. Delirium frequently occurs in the presence of a concurrent dementia. Early identification of the symptoms and formal medical assessment and treatment are critical to ensure the return of a normal level of alertness and intellectual function and to prevent the development of secondary functional impairments and possible dementia.[28]

Dementia is the impairment of some or all aspects of intellectual functioning in a person who is fully alert. Some diseases that can cause dementia are treatable, and if treated early and aggressively, the patient's deterioration of intellectual function may be either reversed or halted. Dementia usually involves cognitive impairment affecting memory and orientation and at least one of the following[29]:
- Abstract thinking. This is a common loss and involves an altered ability to relate to anything other than tangible reality. In dementia or Alzheimer's disease, this skill is predictably missing in most cases. This is exacerbated by fear and anxiety.
- Judgment and problem solving. This capacity decreases in the first stage of Alzheimer's disease and is missing by the second stage.[30-32]
- Language. Use of language for communication becomes altered in the second stage of Alzheimer's disease, and by the third stage little verbal or no verbal communication is possible.[33]
- Personality. A complex of all the attributes—behavioral, temperamental, emotional, and mental—that characterize a unique individual. A person makes choices that, whether remembered or not, make up his or her personality. Human beings live through these choices, which become filters for all future life experiences, and they believe that they are the truth. Caregivers and therapists must be aware of how the world is perceived by the patient. The staff must respect patients and their beliefs and work to minimize confrontation and agitation despite a person's beliefs, prejudices, and biases.

Alzheimer's disease (AD) is not synonymous with dementia but rather is one of the many causes of dementia. The term should be used only as a diagnosis when a complete clinical evaluation has been performed, a diagnosis of dementia has been made, and all other possible causes of the dementia have been ruled out. Definitive diagnosis of this disease is not possible until an autopsy or brain biopsy has been performed. Although multiple putative causes of the disease have been proposed, the etiology and pathogenesis are unknown. No curative treatment for Alzheimer's disease is currently available. Some drugs appear to slow the process of cognitive deterioration in some patients, and patients and their families can be helped through rehabilitation to cope better with the vicissitudes of the disease (see Chapters 5 and 36).

Psychiatric problems may be present before old age or develop as a result of dementia and need to be assessed and treated along with the dementia. Depression, for example, can mimic dementia.

Epidemiology

Researchers estimate that by 2050 13.2 million Americans will have Alzheimer's disease (AD) if current trends continue and no cures are found.[34] Half the people aged 85 years and older will have some form of dementia (9.5 million in 2050).[35] Disorders causing cognitive deficits are expected to continue to be a growing public health problem for at least the next 50 years. The projected statistics, assuming no cures or effective means of preventing the common causes of dementia are discovered, are that by 2040 five times more individuals with dementia will be in society as today (7.4 million Americans). This increase is partially the result of the increased life expectancy of Americans.[36] The most rapid population growth in this country is in the oldest age group, thus the increase in the prevalence of severe dementia. The prevalence of dementia rises from approximately 3% at ages 65 to 74 years to 18.7% at ages 75 to 84 years and to 47% of those older than 85 years.[35] The increasing number of persons older than 85 years will be paralleled by an increase in the incidence of dementia.

More than 70 conditions are known to cause dementia.[37] Secondary behavioral problems in the patient with dementia can be interpreted as a response to somatic, psychological, or existential stress.[38] Because memory impairments, impairments of abstract thinking or judgment, or global cognitive impairments in an elderly person may be symptoms of acute physical illness, the patient's physical, emotional, social, and cognitive status and physical and social/caregiver environment need to be systematically evaluated.[39]

Gradual or sudden changes in intellectual capacity or memory function are not a normal part of the aging process. Any change, whether it develops slowly over time or happens suddenly, should be diagnosed and, when possible, the underlying cause(s) of the delirium or dementia should be treated. Even if the cause of the dementia is untreatable, teaching the patient and significant others strategies to make the patient's ADLs and IADLs easier to manage is always possible.

Physical and occupational therapists are an important part of the comprehensive evaluation, treatment, and caregiver training for patients with delirium or dementia. All treatment planning should occur as a part of a team effort in which the patient, the family or significant others, the physician, nurses, social worker, physical therapist, and occupational therapist collaborate so that a consistent treatment plan and orientation are followed. Inclusion of the day-to-day care giver(s) is crucial for all training because they most need to know and use the adaptations for the patient's personal style of communication and how to facilitate functional movement for ADLs and IADLs.

PHYSIOLOGY OF AGING: RELEVANCE FOR SYMPTOMATOLOGY AND DIAGNOSIS OF DELIRIUM AND DEMENTIAS

The Normal Brain

The brain of a normal person at age 80 years shows several significant anatomical, physiological, and neurochemical changes when compared with the brain of a younger person. Brain weight decreases with advancing age. For example, the mean brain weight for women aged 21 to 40 years is 1260 g, whereas for women older than 80 years it is 1061 g.[40] Brody and Vijayashankar[41] have noted that although the brain loses thousands of cells daily, the areas of the brain involved in language, memory, and cognition are relatively spared of significant loss of neurons. Normal age-related changes vary from person to person in degree and severity and can include the following:

- Disturbance in ability to register, retain, and recall certain recent experiences
- Slowed rate of learning new material[21]
- Slowed motor performance on tasks that require speed[21,42,43]

- Difficulties with fine motor coordination and balance[44-49]

A motivated elderly person who is not undergoing emotional stress will show few negative changes in intellectual capacity and may actually demonstrate an increase in intellectual functioning over time.[16,50-53]

Because many of the variables that need to be considered as part of the clinical evaluation of the rehabilitation potential of the person with dementia are affected by both aging and disease, therapists working with the aged patient should be aware of these variables. The therapist explores ways to compensate for these changes; as a result, the patient will have a greater possibility of achieving her or his potential for self-care and contentment.

A slowing of the natural pace of movement is commonly noted in people older than 80 years. This slowdown is manifested in the brain as a slowing of resting electroencephalogram (EEG) rhythms. At age 60 years, the mean frequency of the occipital rhythm is 10.3 Hz; at age 80 years, the mean frequency is 8.7 Hz. The average change in EEG frequency is approximately 1 cps per decade during these years.[54] The speed of nerve conduction in the elderly can be 10% to 15% slower than in younger persons.[55] Because of these physiological changes, if the process and structure of evaluation and care of the healthy older person emphasize speed of execution or timed activities, older adults will appear less capable than they really are. The therapist may need more time when working with persons older than 70 years than is generally required with the younger adult.

For a person's brain to function effectively, it requires a delicate synchronization of a large number of variables. To maximize intellectual function, the brain must have the following:

- No genetic defects
- A constant supply of nutrients, neurotransmitters, and other neurochemicals from a personally suitable diet
- Functional daily elimination
- An unfailing supply of oxygen (implying appropriate blood count, collateral circulation, normal respiratory exchange/rule out sleep apnea)
- Adequate cardiac output
- Fluid, rhythmic breathing that adapts to needed changes in posture and exertion of the activity
- Normal blood biochemistry, especially fluid and electrolytes, so that adequate fluid intake is critical; dehydration can contribute to altered brain function
- Normal hepatic and renal function
- Freedom from noxious stimuli such as trauma, infection (including periodontal/gum disease), or toxins (including medications)
- Optimal levels of sensory stimulation and emotional stimulation balance
- Optimal levels of intellectual stimulation
- Adequate rest and sleep

The brain is the most physiologically active organ in the body. The brain represents only 2% of the total body weight, yet it consumes up to 20% of the oxygen and 65% of the glucose available in the circulation in the entire body.[15] The minimal cardiovascular output required to deliver this is 0.75 L/min, which is equal to 20% of the total circulation (also dependent on body size). Because of the high level of nutrient use by the brain, it is one of the organs of the body most likely to be affected by any acute change in homeostasis. The homeostasis of the elderly brain is more vulnerable to disruption because of the normal age-related changes already discussed, as well as the increased permeability of the blood-brain barrier and increased sensitivity of neurons to the effects of outside agents such as drugs.[56]

Arndt-Schultz Principle

The Arndt-Schultz principle summarizes the differences between the ability of the younger brain and the aged brain to discriminate or respond to stimuli[57]:

1. The elderly require a higher level or a longer period of stimulation before the threshold for initial physiological safety response is reached. A related safety issue is that heat takes longer to be perceived, so the elderly are more likely to get a severe burn.
2. The physiological response in the aged is rarely as large, as visible, or as consistent as noted in younger age groups. In response to a heat pack, for example, the elderly may not turn bright red in response—they may turn white instead. When fever is present, they may not feel warm to the touch but instead may be very tired or clumsy.
3. The only similarity between the response of the young and the elderly to stimuli is that once the threshold is reached, then more stimuli predict an increase in responses.
4. On average, the range of safe therapeutic stimulation is narrower for the elderly than for the young.

The implication of the Arndt-Schultz principle for clinical problem solving is that the level of a stimulus (e.g., heat, cold, sound, light, or emotional input) needs to be adjusted to compensate for the altered physiology of the aging patient. A level of stimulus that is therapeutic for a young person may not be therapeutic for the older person. The stimuli may be too low so it does not reach the threshold for generating a physiological response, or it may go beyond the safe therapeutic range for the older adult and become harmful. Therefore, when an elderly patient does not respond to treatment or presents with an unusual physical response, the clinician needs to ascertain whether the strength of the stimulus is too strong or too weak and if modification of the stimulus is necessary because of factors associated with the aging process or the patient's cognitive deficits (he or she may be unable to accurately report the response because of a cognitive deficit). The older person with mild or moderate confusion needs small, slow clinical input and precise monitoring of the general response (heart rate, blood pressure, respiration) as well as local response. This is especially true for persons who are hearing impaired. Because the patient may not hear what is being spoken, the therapist may assume that the patient does not have the capability to comprehend what is being said. Never assume that a person does not comprehend when she or he may simply be unable to hear what is being spoken.

Law of Initial Values

The law of initial values is both a physiological and a psychological principle stating that, with a given intensity of stimulation, the degree of change produced tends to be greater when the initial value of that variable is low at the onset of stimulation. In other words, the higher the initial level of functioning, the smaller the change that can be produced.[58,59] The law of initial values, when defined and applied to younger persons, presumes that homeostasis is a stable and consistent process. When the law is used to describe physiological and psychological responses in older persons, it cannot be presumed that homeostasis for any variable is predictable or consistent from one person to the next, or even within a 24-hour period for the same individual. For example, an older person with mild dementia may eat only sweets if left without companionship at a meal. As a result, after the meal the individual may feel unsteady and afraid to walk back to the room. In the young, defining the average times of peak activity for most physiological processes as well as for intellectual capacity is possible. In the clinical assessment of the older persons, defining the peak times of day for awareness and intellectual capacity for each individual is necessary. For example, some patients are best able to participate in learning a new skill in the early morning and some only in the late afternoon.

Biorhythms

The body has a biological clock that controls all physiological functions in a precise temporal course, whether daily (e.g., secretion of some hormones), monthly (e.g., menstruation), or during a certain period of the life cycle (e.g., ability to become pregnant).[2,60] Before evaluating a geriatric patient who presents with dementia or disturbance of intellectual functioning, assessment of the patient's premorbid biorhythm is helpful. What was her or his daily schedule of activities before the crisis? The assessment involves a detailed description or time study that maps rest periods, activities and level of exertion, sleep/rest periods, mental stimulation, emotional stimulation, eating and elimination cycles, for example, across a 24-hour period. The patient assessment must allow for and assess the current and past variability of individual biorhythms. These biorhythms should be clearly documented and their stability evaluated and maintained as much as possible (critical if the patient will be going back to the family). For example, if a woman has worked for 40 years as a night nurse, being primarily active from 11 AM to 7 PM, she will most likely be alert and best able to participate in a rehabilitation program during those hours. In most cases the patient should be allowed to choose the best time for treatment. For those patients whose dementia is too severe to make this determination, the staff, by monitoring the patient's behavior, can choose a time for treatment when the person is most alert. For the elderly, and particularly for those who have dementia, the time of assessment and treatment must be documented to maximize the person's rehabilitation potential.[61,62]

Sensory Changes with Aging

Aging can also be defined in terms of adaptation. Aging is the progressive and usually irreversible diminution, with the passage of time, of the ability of a person or body part to perform efficiently or adapt to changes in the environment. The consequence of the process is manifested as decreased capacity for function and for withstanding stresses.[63] Because the rehabilitation evaluation identifies functional problems, therapists should examine the possibility that sensory losses or disturbances (e.g., vision, hearing, touch, taste, smell, proprioception, temperature, and kinesthesia) are contributing to the functional impairments.[57] A partial or total loss of one or more of the normal sensory inputs can result in disturbance of an individual's mental status.

The more sudden the loss of a sense, the more difficult is the adaptation to the sensory disability. This is especially true for elderly persons because several mild sensory changes are already taxing their capacity to adapt. Adaptation to a sensory loss in one modality is typically accomplished through an increased utilization of the other senses. For example, a young blind patient can adapt by using hearing and kinesthesia and usually learns to function well in spite of the loss of visual input. The older the patient is when blinded, however, the more difficulty she or he will have in making this adaptive crossover to other senses. At some time in any person's life, adaptive crossover from one sense to another becomes exceedingly difficult, if not impossible. Thus psychopathological or behavioral changes may occur if a sensory impairment develops.[64] This situation becomes more likely if the disruption is caused by a central nervous system deficit with multiple and abrupt simultaneous sensory input loss, such as might occur from a stroke.

The poliomyelitis epidemics of the early 1950s demonstrated the relationship between sensory input and abnormal behavior. Patients with poliomyelitis who were placed in tank-type respirators developed intermittent disruptions in mental state, including hallucinations, delusions, and dreamlike experiences while awake.[63] The patients were deprived of normative input to the senses (kinesthesia and proprioception) and had severely restricted vision and hearing because of the nature of the construction of and the noise that emanated from the respirator. Solomon and Shackson[65] and Solomon[66] called this problem sensory deprivation psychosis but this clinical situation may include cognitive changes in addition to psychotic symptoms. This type of problem often occurs today after a hip fracture when a patient is given a medication to control the pain that has the side effect of disrupting reality orientation to time and place. Until other medication can be tried to control the pain, the patient is described as "out of his or her mind," especially at night. The patient may try to remove all clothing or call out to people for help, often a mother or father. The psychosis stops when the medication is removed. Recovery is also enhanced when consistent nurturing is provided.

Sensory changes associated with normal aging can lead to the same degree of loss or distortion of significant sensory input as previously described.[67,68] A bilateral loss of vision may lead to agitation and disorientation. Elderly people with hearing impairments often have grave difficulty relating to the world. Elderly persons who become deaf commonly experience some episodes of paranoid behavior.[64] The problems for hearing-impaired elderly persons are often exacerbated by health care professionals who do not know how to place a hearing aid in a patient's ear, replace a battery, adjust the volume on the aid, remove excess ear wax from the aid, identify the need to trim ear hair, or consider the possibility of a malfunctioning aid. Finally, sensory impairments may become exacerbated by surgical or medical interventions.

Certain medications, as well as some diseases, also can distort kinesthesia or retard the activity and movement of the patient.[56] Movement is significant in the maintenance of an efficient nervous system. Anything that denies a person the ability to perform physical movement (e.g., drugs, restraints, traction, passive motion machine, positional props, or architectural designs not adapted to the elderly) hastens and increases the difficulty of adapting to functional limitations. The patient loses her or his freedom to move and may feel trapped and helpless. This can trigger memories of other trauma or violent experiences that involved feeling helpless or victimized. Movement is necessary for accurate sensation.[12,67] It has been demonstrated that if movement of the eyes does not occur properly, vision becomes ineffective. The same is true to a lesser degree for hearing. If movement does not occur in the course of the hearing process, hearing can become distorted and misrepresented at the central level.

New research on brain function in the elderly points to the following ideas for clinical consideration and possible modifications to enhance functional performance:

1. Evaluate the capacity to demonstrate the visual search response. This eye response is a tool to verify that the patient is relaxed and ready for new learning. A clinical example would be to have the person rest supine (with props for comfort as needed under the head, wrists, knees, ankles) and then begin a very slow passive roll of the head 1 to 4 degrees per second to one direction and observe the eye response. They eyes of a relaxed person will naturally follow objects in the visual field in a functional tracking response as the head is rolled. The skill of visual search is altered (i.e., eyes dart around in a rapid visual search process or rest passively and do not move passively in the direction of the rolling of the head) when limbic activation or actual brain damage is present (90% discrimination).[11,69,70] When the visual search is compromised, the Feldenkrais Method or other neurofacilitation can be used to normalize the resting pattern of the neck and chest and invite the enhanced functional response for eye-head righting. Therapeutic exercise and neurofacilitation to encourage eye participation and other eye/body coordination training strategies have shown good functional improvements for persons with AD.[71]

2. Evaluate the capacity to use symbols. Assess the capacity to use signage in the building; does the patient comprehend and demonstrate comprehension by performance? For example, when an arrow points left, does the patient turn left?

3. Evaluate the capacity to perform complex motor skills (e.g., consistent step-by-step sequence). Even if the skill is not mastered, does the patient show improvement in the speed of a repetition task or increased emotional ease and willingness to participate even if verbal or physical cuing is still needed? Even if the patient cannot perform some motor skill, she or he may still show normal capacity to learn another motor skill.

4. If anxiety is present, try to alleviate it because anxiety interferes with integration of sensory learning (e.g., try a hot pack to the belly area for 5 to 10 minutes to promote relaxation).

Cognitive Changes in Normal Aging

As previously noted, the idea that cognitive decline is a necessary part of aging is a myth. This belief has been debunked by research on crystallized and fluid intelligence.[72] Crystallized intelligence involves the ability to perceive relationships, engage in formal reasoning, and understand intellectual and cultural heritage. Crystallized intelligence can be affected by the environment and the attitude of the individual.[73,74] Crystallized intelligence can increase with self-directed learning and education as long as a person is alive. The measurement of crystallized intelligence is usually in the form of culture-specific items such as number facility, verbal comprehension, and general information.

Fluid intelligence, what has been called "native mental ability," is the product of the brain's information processing system. It includes attention and memory capacity and the speed of information processing used in thinking and acting.[75] It is not closely associated with acculturation. It is generally considered to be independent of instruction or environment and depends more on the genetic endowment of the individual.[7] The items used to test fluid intelligence include memory span, inductive reasoning, and figural relationships, all of which are presumed to be unresponsive to training. Because fluid intelligence involves those intellectual functions most affected by changes in neurophysiological status, it has been generally assumed to decline with age. Several studies have shown this to be untrue; one study noted that during middle age, scores on tests for fluid intelligence are similar to scores in mid-adolescence.[50,76] These changes, however, are primarily associated with processing speed and working memory and executive function.[10,77]

Recent studies that have looked at the effects of cognitive changes on action have shown that older people perform activities at a slower rate and use different areas of the brain in the process compared with younger people. Those additional areas of the brain used have mostly to do with monitoring and processing the ongoing activity.[11,78] Activities are therefore performed more in a feed-back rather than feed-forward manner, which also requires more time. So, if older adults are given time to complete tasks, they usually do well.

Botwinick[31] described the classic pattern of changes in intelligence with aging. In the adult portion of the life span, verbal abilities decline little, if at all, whereas psychomotor abilities decline earlier and to a greater extent (greater decline if not engaged in regular physical activity). The period between ages 55 and 70 years is a transition time, and some decreases in performance are noted on many cognitive tests. A substantial decline on laboratory tests of cognitive function is generally limited to those older than 75 years.[36] In these latter years, however, the decline in fluid intelligence is offset by the growth in crystallized intelligence for most people unless dementia is present. Thus although changes may be demonstrated in the laboratory, they may not be significant in the "real world," and the elderly may be as capable as the young of participating in rehabilitation training. For elderly people to benefit maximally, however, they must control the pace of training because the tasks that are the most difficult for older adults are those that are fast paced, unusual, and complex.[79] All physical and occupational therapy treatments with older patients need to be structured to encourage the patient to set his or her own pace. The goal is to have a pace that allows ease of breathing and a comfortable, functional upright posture so that the person can enjoy the experience. Interventions should be predictable and progress by adding one new concept at a time.

Terminal drop is another type of cognitive change that differs from those that occur in normal aging and in those with dementia. This involves a decline in IQ scores in persons within the year before their death. This change in intellectual function is thought to result from some predeath changes in brain physiology. Research studies that show drastic decreases in intellectual function with advanced age may have a large percentage of subjects who were near death as a part of the sample.[80] Subjects who did not experience this terminal drop would then appear similar to those in studies on normal elderly persons.

Stress and Intellectual Capacity

Selye[53] defined stress as the nonspecific response of the body to any demand made on it. All human beings require a certain amount of stress to live and function effectively. When a stressor (stimulus) is applied, the body predictably goes through the three stages of response called the "general adaptation syndrome" (GAS). The first response is a general alarm reaction, a "fight or flight" response that mobilizes all senses in an effort to make a judgment about the response needed. The older person is at a disadvantage because collecting and processing accurate sensory data due to short-term memory loss are decreased with normal aging. This will manifest in a patient asking the same question repeatedly during a crisis. The sensory memory in an older person lasts less than 1 second.[21] The next stage involves judgment and the selective adaptation to the stressor. A decision is made regarding which body action is needed, and all other body activities return to homeostasis. The older person is slower to search and retrieve the information from storage. If the stimulus continues and goes beyond the therapeutic/functional level, then the body system or part will gradually experience physiological exhaustion. A person in physiological exhaustion is likely to manifest abnormal responses to any new stimulus. Paradoxical reactions can result in unusual physiological or psychological responses to stimuli (e.g., an erythematous response when an ice pack is applied or a patient becoming more agitated after receiving a sedative).

When a person is under perceived stress (whether real or imagined), a predictable set of cognitive changes can occur. These cognitive functional changes can include preoccupation; forgetfulness; disorientation; confusion; low tolerance to ambiguity; errors in judgment in relation to work, distance, grammar, or mathematics; misidentification of people; inability to concentrate, solve problems, or plan; inattention to details or instructions; reduced creativity, fantasy, and perceptual field size; decreased initiative; decreased interest in usual activities, the future, or people; and irritability, impatience, anger, withdrawal, suspicion, depression, and crying. Differentiating whether the patient is having a stress reaction or truly experiencing dementia is critical. If the changes occur with a sudden onset, they are probably related to a medical or pharmaceutical problem and may be reversible.

With aging, the body undergoes physiological changes that make the older person less physiologically efficient in her or his response to stressors. The general alarm reaction is poorly mobilized and takes longer to become activated (Arndt-Schultz principle). The stage of resistance should yield a series of responses that allows the body to economize in its response to stress. In persons of all ages who receive too many different stimuli and in the elderly who experience normal levels of stimuli, the body becomes less efficient at turning off the general alarm response and replacing it with more appropriate and limited responses. When a person is overwhelmed by this type or level of stress, the individual may demonstrate mild global or specific cognitive impairments, especially mild short-term memory loss.

At this time, the historical clinical data become the only means of establishing a diagnosis because no tests are currently available to distinguish acute dementia from emotional exhaustion. In cases of domestic violence that have been kept secret for years, this can be a difficult problem. For example: A 90-year-old man had beaten his wife a few times early in their marriage. They later came to an agreement and their marriage had continued with only verbal abuse and no physical abuse. As he approached 85 years of age, however, he again began to get violent and would shove her during arguments. At one point she fell, broke her hip, and ended up in a nursing home for 8 weeks. Another time he was bringing her to therapy and on the way he became angry and let go of the wheelchair, and it ran into a wall. The wife chose to do nothing and say nothing. The only sign was that she always cried in physical therapy when she started to relax. The client eventually confided to the physical therapist and was referred to a crisis counselor to determine how to proceed. She saw the counselor weekly for more than 4 years. Another incident happened in which the wife was hurt and protective services were called. The patient refused to press charges and returned to the home, stopped all counseling, withdrew in embarrassment, and within several weeks became confused. The husband placed her in a nursing home and she was given the diagnosis of dementia and placed on haloperidol (Haldol). No other therapeutic services were offered. Access to one-on-one counseling and family therapy is critical. What if support had been offered? Could this situation have turned out differently? If the person had been 36 years old, a psychiatric evaluation would likely have been made and treatment could have reversed the confusion that masked the severe depression.

The assessment of an elderly person, with or without dementia, must include a determination of the type, number, and severity of the patient's current stressors. Positive life events (e.g., marriage or the birth of a grandchild) are also stressful life events. Scores that rate stressful life events can identify patients who are at greatest risk of physiological and emotional exhaustion.[81] Elderly patients, with their numerous psychosocial problems and chronic and acute illnesses, are likely candidates for physiological and emotional exhaustion and the development of psychopathology. Thus the environment and process of rehabilitation care need to be modified to counteract the effect of stress on the intellectual capacity of the older patient. Any action that modifies stress so that a deterioration of intellectual function is stopped or reversed is an efficient and cost-effective part of the total rehabilitation effort.

STRATEGIES FOR ASSESSING, PREVENTING, AND MINIMIZING DISTORTIONS IN INFORMATION PROCESSING

Each person acts on the available data perceived at a specific moment. This stimulus-response cycle has four major steps; each step contains a possibility for distortion or error.

When a person is presented with a stimulus, the brain processes all the data (physiological, psychological, sociological, and environmental) collected and then integrates it with data from past experience. Based on this process, a response is elicited, which is then followed by the behavior concomitant to this response.

At the outset of the process of patient assessment, examination is necessary regarding the amount of verbal and written stimuli processed by the patient in relation to the amount used as a part of the testing evaluation process. With an overview of the patient's cognitive capacity, the rehabilitation staff may be able to modify the process of evaluation to maximize the patient's performance (e.g., several 15-minute interactions spread over the 8-hour workday instead of an hour without rest; performing the assessment in the presence of a regular caregiver the patient trusts). A basic assessment of the patient's functional abilities (ADLs/ IADLs) at a given moment to allow a comparison of cognitive capacity at other times in the 24-hour cycle provides the clinician a specific description of what aspects of intellectual function appear to be impaired and pinpoints those aspects of intellectual functioning that are still intact. Based on this approach, the rehabilitation evaluation can proceed in a language (perhaps the native language of childhood) and at a pace that is comfortable for the patient.

Mini-Mental State Examination and Other Cognitive Scales

The Mini-Mental State Examination (MMSE) was developed as a result of a study noting that 80% of cognitive disorders among elderly people were not detected by the general practitioner.[17,82] It appears to be the most predictable test but is only helpful if all caregivers can monitor the cognitive state of the older patient. All caregivers must be part of the team effort to get a real 24-hour picture of the cognitive capacities of the patient. Most professionals on the rehabilitation team (physicians, nurses,[83,84] physical therapists[85] and social workers[86]) are likely to have had only minimal specialty training in gerontology and the unique symptoms and needs of the elderly.

The MMSE provides a screening test for identifying unrecognized cognitive disorders in the elderly (Figure 28-1).[18,87,88] The MMSE assesses only cognition and does not examine other aspects of the traditional mental status examination such as mood, delusions, or hallucinations. The test can identify if the patient is oriented; remembers (short term); and can read, write, calculate, and see and reproduce in drawing the relation of one object or figure to another. The examination is used to screen for cognitive dysfunctions, much as a measurement of blood pressure or blood sugar is used to screen for significant medical disorders. The MMSE also may be used in a serial fashion to quantify changes in a patient's cognitive status over time. This examination can be used as a springboard for planning how to carry out the traditional rehabilitation evaluation on a patient who has some intellectual dysfunction.[89,90]

The MMSE has been standardized for elderly persons living in the community. The scores on this test correlate significantly with the Weschsler Adult Intelligence Scale and the Weschsler Memory Test. The MMSE is reported to have a high test-retest reliability for both normal and psychiatric samples populations with $r = 0.89$ or greater. It has been

MINI-MENTAL STATE EXAMINATION

Maximum score	Score	
5	( )	**ORIENTATION** What is the (year) (season) (date) (day) (month)?
5	( )	Where are we: (state) (county) (town) (hospital) (floor)?
3	( )	**REGISTRATION** *Name* 3 objects: 1 second to say each. Then ask the client all 3 after you have said them. Give 1 point for each correct answer. Then repeat them until the client learns all 3. Count trials and record. TRIALS
5	( )	*Attention and calculation* Serial 7's. 1 point for each correct. Stop after 5 answers. Alternatively spell "world" backwards.
3	( )	*Recall* Ask for 3 objects repeated above. Give 1 point for each correct.
9	( )	*Language* Name a pencil and watch. (2 points) Repeat the following "No ifs, ands, or buts." (1 point) Follow a *3-stage command:* "Take a paper in your right hand, fold it in half, and put it on the floor." (3 points) *Read and obey* the following: "Close your eyes." (1 point) Write a sentence. (1 point) Copy design. (1 point)
30	( )	**TOTAL SCORE**

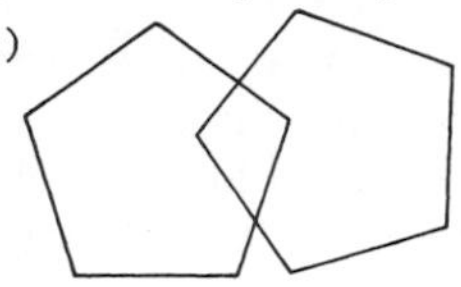

Assess level of consciousness along a continuum.

Alert   Drowsy   Stupor   Coma

FIGURE 28-1 ■ Form used for MMSE to assess cognition.

found that when a cut-off score of 24 is used for the detection of dementia, the MMSE had a sensitivity of 87.6% and a specificity of 81.6%.[87] Several studies have noted that interviews with informants are highly consistent with elderly persons' scores on the MMSE.[91]

The examination takes only a few minutes to administer, is scored immediately, and can be administered by any member of the rehabilitation team. The entire examination grades cognitive performance on a scale from 0 to 30. A score of 24 or less usually indicates some degree of cognitive dysfunction, but some patients with dementia may score above 24 and some with depression or delirium may score significantly below 24. A low score on this examination can mean that the patient probably has dementia, delirium, mental retardation, amnestic syndrome, or aphasia. A low score on the MMSE can indicate the areas of specific cognitive impairment and gives the rehabilitation team data

about how to best communicate with the patient. MMSE scores are also correlated with educational level, with scores dropping 10% to 20% for people with an eighth-grade education or less who are older than 70 years.[92] A shortened version of the MMSE has been developed that uses only 12 of the 20 original variables. Although the original study suggested that the shortened version of the MMSE is equally as effective as the full MMSE in identifying elderly patients with cognitive deficits, more recent studies have questioned these findings.

Older persons may show changes in mental abilities immediately after surgery, after hypoxia (low oxygenation), not being found after a fall, or after hitting the head during a fall or other trauma. The Glasgow Coma Scale and the Rancho Los Amigos Cognition Scales can be used in many ways to assess the cognitive status of an individual, especially if brain injury results from an impact to the head or severe whiplash, for example. First, the extra testing helps staff choose which patients can live safely and compatibly in the same unit. The Rancho Los Amigos Scale can help identify the need to segregate the patients who are prone to screaming incomprehensible words over and over. The coma state may be temporary as a result of medication, anxiety, or anesthesia. Test scores may be used to create a patient group that allows calm and functional use of the shared living space. Another purpose in using these additional tests is to create small groups where patients at level 4 (confused, agitated, alert, active, aggressive or bizarre behaviors, nonpurposeful motor movement, short attention span, inappropriate verbalization) are segregated from those at level 5 (agitated by too much stimuli, require continual redirection) to allow level 5 clients to live and function to their full capacity and allow level 4 patients to have room to move and express. A level 4 patient may become upset and cry on a unit that has mostly level 5 and a few level 3 (inconsistent response to commands, turns toward or away from sound) patients. The biggest factor is to use the test scores to target activities and recreation to a specific cognitive level so that satisfaction and social comfort are possible.

Sensory and Perceptual Changes with Dementia

Patients with dementia may have specific problems that inhibit the integration of sensory input. Aphasias and disruption of association pathways may inhibit the patient's ability to integrate accurately perceived sensory information in a meaningful way. Bassi et al[93] and Fozard[94] have demonstrated that patients with AD, multiinfarct dementia,[95] and alcoholic dementia may demonstrate disturbances in visual acuity, depth perception, color differentiation, and differentiation of figure from ground when compared with normal age-matched control subjects and normal younger subjects.

An assessment of specific sensory systems is necessary when a person demonstrates cognitive losses. The challenge in rehabilitation is to design a process and environment of care so that compensation and modification maximize the ability of the elderly patient with sensory deficits to adapt to most life situations. The example of visual deficits is a case in point. One of every two blind persons in the United States is older than 65 years.[96] Techniques of environmental adaptation and special measures to organize care to help elderly blind people have allowed many of them to live independently in the community.[97] However, many elderly people with visual impairments are not blind. Some of the structural changes that result in mild to moderate deficits of vision include yellowing; uneven growth, striation, and thickening of the lens; increasing weakness of the muscles controlling the eye; alteration in the perception of color (especially fine distinctions in tone and brightness); and slower adaptation to light.[94] Modifications of the environment can include adequate effective lighting (including adequate intensity and controlling of reflection), dark and clear large-print, low-vision aids (e.g., magnifying glass), verbal orientation and escort by persons accompanying patients in a new environment, consistent furniture placement, explanation when changes occur, clear hallways, a systematic storage system for clothes and toilet articles, and the use of consistent contrasting colors to identify doors, windows, baseboards, and corners.[70,72,83,94,98]

Older Adult Learning Styles and Communication

Learning occurs throughout life.[79] In physical and occupational therapy, habilitation occurs when the client learns new skills, and rehabilitation occurs when the person relearns old adaptive skills. As with intelligence, the learning process does not change abruptly when an individual reaches old age, but differences in performance have been reported. One challenge for rehabilitation therapy is to find ways to improve the efficiency of learning by the older person.

Botwinick[31] has noted that learning and performance are not the same. Poor performance on a learning task may mean that insufficient learning has occurred, that learning has not transferred to a new environment or task, or that the performance does not accurately reflect the extent of learning achieved.[7] The key variables that affect a person's ability to participate in a learning task can include intelligence, learning skills acquired over the years, and flexibility of learning style. Noncognitive factors also can have a strong bearing on an individual's performance. The noncognitive factors include visual and auditory acuity, health status, motivation to learn, level of anxiety, the speed at which stimuli and learning are paced, and the meaningfulness to the individual of the items or tasks to be learned. Research has shown that learning styles change over the life span and that people learn better when instructional approaches are matched to their learning style.[22] Therefore a rehabilitation assessment needs to include a review of the preferred learning style of the patient. This is particularly important before discharging a patient from a rehabilitation program. The rationale is that a lack of progress may not reflect the patient's lack of capacity for rehabilitation, but rather may reflect a dissonance between the patient's learning style and skills with the presentation of materials in the treatment program (e.g., verbal input has not been adapted to match the level or pace of comprehension of a person who may have a strong preference for visual learning and slower pace).

Interference

Interference can make the learning process less efficient in two major ways.[99] First, interference can result from a conflict between present knowledge and the new knowledge to be learned. Second, if the task to be learned has two or more components, secondary components may interfere with the learning of the primary components. This is particularly true if secondary components overlap in time or use the same sensory modality.[75] The elderly have special difficulties if they must concentrate on intake, attention, and retrieval processes at the same time. Therefore the process and therapeutic environment of rehabilitation for the elderly patient must not be disturbed by background noise, other stimuli in the environment, or anxiety. When learning a new task, the elderly patient may require a quiet room with no stimuli other than that offered by the therapist. The need to rid the environment of distractions is particularly important when working with an elderly patient with dementia because this patient will have greater difficulty filtering out irrelevant sensory inputs compared with elderly patients without dementia.

Pacing

The pacing of therapeutic intervention is a significant variable in helping an elderly person learn. Elderly persons (with or without dementia) perform best if they are given as much time as they need and when learning is self-paced.[31] The major drawback of a fast pace (**as perceived by the patient**) is that the elderly person generally chooses not to participate rather than risk making a mistake. A lack of response by the patient is often interpreted as apathy, poor motivation, or "confusion."[100] Patient participation is increased when extra time to complete a rehabilitation task is offered. After the individual assessment, group work (where concepts can be presented, reviewed, and examined at leisure) also can be used to reduce the psychological pressure of faster-paced 1-1 learning. The details of therapy must be planned carefully, including how questions are asked (this involves asking clear and precise questions in nonmedical language) and, most importantly, setting aside enough treatment time so the patient can respond at a manageable pace.

Organization

If data are organized in the brain as part of the learning process, the retrieval of these data becomes easier. Older persons are less likely than members of other age groups to organize data spontaneously to facilitate learning and later retrieval (memory) of that learning.[33] Elderly people who are highly verbal show fewer weaknesses in the ability to organize stimuli. Elderly persons with poor verbal skills show significant improvement in data retrieval when strategies for organization of data are provided by others (e.g., the therapist). Older learners have difficulty following content because they cannot anticipate what will be taught and do not see the "whole picture" of what is being presented.[101] This is an example of how an organization may influence the learning process.

Thus organizing therapy by beginning with an overview in outline form of the entire lesson is helpful. This presents the patient with a conceptual map of the upcoming experience. The use of purposeful organizing also can help bridge the gap between what the older person knows and the new information or task to be learned. The use of neurolinguistic programming (NLP) is especially effective with elderly patients and patients with cognitive deficits because it builds consciously—through language, kinesthesia, and visual input—a picture of a new concept from a known and familiar frame of reference.[101]

Inefficient learning, and at times an inability to learn, occurs in the older adult if material is presented in one way and the older person is expected to apply it in some other way. Instructions need to be provided in the format and context in which they are to be used. If possible, one piece of new data should be presented at a time. A conscious transition needs to be made by the therapist from the patient's current frame of reference to the understanding of the new data, and the pace needs to be set by the patient.

Several other strategies exist for maximizing the efficiency of older adult learners based on awareness of normal age-related changes. Some of the more frequently used techniques are summarized in Box 28-1.

Communication

Therapists can begin by inquiring into what the reality of the patient looks like. The first goal should be to communicate with words, gestures, positioning, and so on so that stimuli bring out functional responses in the patient. All people have

---

BOX 28-1 ■ **TECHNIQUES FOR MAXIMIZING THE EFFICIENCY OF OLDER ADULT LEARNERS**

1. Use mediators; the association of word, story, mnemonics, or visual inputs can help the person remember.
2. Choose learning activities that are meaningful for the client.
3. Use concrete examples to make learning easier.
4. Provide a supportive learning environment to prevent stress that can interfere with efficient learning.
5. Use supportive or neutral feedback and avoid feedback that is presented in a challenging tone.
6. Reward all responses but reward correct responses more than incorrect responses. This can encourage elderly persons to decrease the number of errors by omission, which are often interpreted as apathy or lack of cooperation.
7. Use combinations of auditory and visual input to facilitate the learning process. This is only effective if the data presented are similar because variation between the two kinds of messages can result in interference and a decrease in the efficiency of learning.
8. Active learning is more effective. A patient who moves the involved body part while receiving verbal and visual input is likely to better master the new skill.
9. Design the learning situation so that successful completion of the task is likely. Older people are more likely to focus on errors, which increases anxiety and lowers self-esteem. Worst of all, with all the energy focused on the error, there is a strong chance of repeating the error.

---

an ongoing internal dialogue. As a healthy adult, the therapist chooses to notice his or her own dialogue, hear the content, and then pursue the goals and commitments that enhance interaction with the patient.

The interaction with the patient needs to be grounded in the present moment. The power for action lies in the present moment. The patient will bring his or her authentic self to the conversation or the interaction. The therapist needs to be sensitive to the entire communication—what is said and what is withheld. The patient with cognitive problems may not understand the content but many still have the ability to sense and respond to the therapist's affective state at the moment. When beginning communication, be clear of all previous concerns and bring no extra or extraneous emotions into the interaction. Caregivers and therapists bring into the conversation the power of intention to create a therapeutic interaction and the choice to stay on task. Patients bring their own sets of concerns at any particular moment. Knowing something about the patients concerns helps the process.

Therapists and caregivers need to be self-aware. What is the therapist's favorite strategy for communication? What is the therapist's favorite sentence structure? Our habitual forms of presentation need to be assessed as to whether they are effective, because the patient needs to be the focus of attention. Honoring the communication habits of the patient is necessary if effective communication is to occur with a person with cognitive deficits. If the therapist chooses to speak to the patient as if there were no cognitive deficits, consistent results will not occur and the patient may be upset or agitated. The patient could be approached as if he or she were a person from another culture that has its unique customs, norms, and ways of communication. The patient-therapist interaction becomes an inquiry where success is measured by the achievement of functional outcomes that are needed and wanted (e.g., the patient transferring into bed and feeling safe).

Now the question becomes what is the specific process of interaction in which the patient appears to be most comfortable and feels safe? Every patient is different and it may depend on the time of day or whether the patient is tired or feeling threatened. Persons commonly respond best to one particular style of communication and are predictably upset or agitated by another style. If a patient wants to joke around and be playful, this should be a cue to staff that this is a workable style of communication. Another patient smiles whenever the tone of the conversation is soft, nurturing, and tender, and if staff is willing, this is where ease of relating can occur. Other patients relate best to rules and need predictable structures and boundaries. They love to know what is coming next. Still another category is people who can relate and communicate when definite admiration and respect are built into the conversation or when patient and therapist can agree to disagree. Each patient with cognitive problems needs to have caregivers develop a chart of what works to create a sense of relatedness and ease in communication. A challenge here for caregivers is that the patient's abilities can change; guidelines for communication when new caregivers are introduced to the patient can also be helpful. Someone who is familiar and enjoys interacting with the patient should introduce new staff to the patient.

For persons with cognitive disturbances, familiarity and rituals are keys to ease of adaptability. The basis for rituals is a well-organized documentation that all caregivers have access to and contribute to on an ongoing basis. This information needs to be filtered and organized so that each shift can see what is working for the patient today. Even a nonverbal patient can relate effectively to bathing if a ritual exists regarding dressing and undressing (e.g., the socks always come off first). Mace and Rabins[90] spelled out the details of the importance of caregivers being aware of the power of familiarity and rituals. Mintzer et al[102] reinforced the same idea in their research on the effectiveness of alternative care environments for agitated patients with dementia. Another detail that requires staff or caregiver attention, evaluation, and adaptation in daily care is *ideational apraxia*. LeClerc and Wells[103] described this as "a condition in which an individual is unable to plan movement related to an object because he or she has lost the perception of the object's purpose." This is especially important in relation to feeding, dressing, and bathing. The authors described a tool that can help caregivers assess the ideational apraxia and problem-solving compensations to prevent unnecessary agitation or disability and take actions to preserve existing abilities. Savelkoul et al[104] emphasized the importance of effective communication between staff and patients and the importance of routines for patient care to maximize functional behaviors for institutionalized elderly living in residential homes. Another key point noted was that staff corrected and tested residents too often, which can create

agitation and anxiety. This appeared to be related to lack of training and information on the part of the staff about the dementia and cognitive status of patients as well as a lack of support from other staff.

As a patient goes through gradual deterioration of cognitive status, as is common in AD, staff, family, and caregivers must be trained in nonverbal, positional, manual cues, and emotional communication techniques. Many patients come to a place in their lives with dementia when words are a source of confusion. Other strategies to communicate should then be used. Sign language is initially a possible tool until the associative functions begin to disappear. Accurate assessment needs to create adaptations in communication. Hand-guided communication may be necessary in which the patient is led through a task or parts of a task to get his or her cooperation. At this stage of communication, ease and trust are the most important goals. It may take 5 minutes of tenderly holding a patient's hand before the patient is ready to walk to the dining room or bathroom. This requires much patience on the part of staff. Positional communication can be used as well as simple touch. As patients begin to feel safe with their state of being, they will relax and choose to participate. At times patients have unique needs such as only wanting to be cared for by a female caregiver or a male caregiver. Honoring patient needs is critical because the cognitively impaired may not be able to learn or adapt to the demands of the staff member because of previous trauma (assault or incest, real or imagined).

As a way to summarize the considerations about communication with a person with cognitive impairment, therapists may find it useful to examine their own intentions from moment to moment. "What is my goal in this interaction?" "Who am I being at this moment?" The task may be important and the "doing" of it may be critical. For the patient with cognitive disturbance, therapists must provide life-enhancing stimuli on the basis of the patient's perceptions. If in the zeal to "do," the patient is accidentally scared, intimidated, or bullied, the damage may not be able to be undone. The cognitively impaired patient presents a unique challenge if a threat has been created because reestablishing their trust is often difficult. Often the patient may be afraid of the therapist and simply needs the therapist to leave the room for some time. The saving grace for many patients is that their short-term memory is poor so they may not remember the incident tomorrow. The problem with agitation occurs when other cognitively impaired clients in the area also get upset.

The solution to the crisis moment, when a breakdown in communication has occurred, is to redirect communication and the focus of the present moment effectively. For example, a staff member could purposely bump into a chair and knock it over, drop a cup of water or a book, start to sing, whistle loudly, or clap his or her hands. At that moment a distraction is created. If the distraction works, then the patient's attention is pulled away from his or her old thought and focused to a new topic. At that moment the staff needs to be intentional. The new focus needs to offer comfort or nurturing or a predictable sense of well-being (e.g., eating some food, looking at a picture of a favorite thing, holding a favorite item, touching a favorite comfort object, hugging).

The research findings and techniques previously discussed describe many of the aspects of the Feldenkrais approach to learning.[1,12] The *Feldenkrais Method* has been applied to the needs of elderly persons with good results. The principle that learning needs to be pleasurable is especially applicable to elderly clients (with or without dementia) because they are often under more stress and have fewer supportive resources to cope with a crisis. Despite changes in learning style, the older person (with or without dementia) can be helped to learn more efficiently through well-planned instruction. The use of techniques to increase learning efficiency in the elderly has been demonstrated to decrease the stress that at times may result in emotional or cognitive overload and abnormal cognitive reactions.

Ann[105] notes that because habits and procedural memory (behaviors learned by doing, including habits) are two of the last areas of the brain affected by AD and dementia, individuals with these diseases can often walk around after they are no longer able to be aware of their surroundings, consistently communicate, or reason. The Feldenkrais Method taps into an individual's habits, producing positive and lasting results through the capacity of the individual to still use procedural learning (even though she or he is not able to describe verbally or be consciously aware of the learning that is achieved). One example of how the Feldenkrais Method taps into procedural memory follows. Lee, an elderly man of 92 years with advanced dementia, was able to achieve changes in his behaviors, even though he was worked with while he was sleeping, which changed his behavior while he was awake. Because of Lee's constant walking and potentially combative behavior, working with him initially was difficult. When he was asked to sit or lie down, he complained loudly and told the therapist to get away. Instead, the therapist worked with him during his frequent naps. He walked bent over with his feet and legs turned out and a wide stance. He held both arms close to his sides, with his elbows bent and no arm swing. He was unable to move isolated areas of his torso; he therefore did not turn his head to look at something next to him. Instead, he turned his whole body. Lee would decide to sit down without looking to see if a chair was behind him, partially because he did not have safety awareness and partially because he did not have the capability to rotate his body. Immediately after waking up or finishing a meal, he would start to walk. As a result of these limitations and actions, Lee was constantly falling. Lee needed to learn how to differentiate the movement pattern of turning his head separate from his trunk. Lee had a pattern that was "un"differentiated in which he moved his head and trunk as a single unit of action; he had no choice to do anything else. Through gentle movements while Lee was lying on his back or side, the first several sessions involved exploring passive movement of his pelvis and spine. The focus was to explore with Lee his capacity to move in diagonal patterns and to create a kinesthetic relationship between his right shoulder and his left hip and vice versa, the sensation of elongating his spine and learning to twist his torso. He began to demonstrate the capacity to breathe by allowing his chest to expand in the lower rib area. The passive movement explorations involved exploring upper torso rotation, including head turning, shoulder blade differentiation, and the ability to move the shoulder blades independent of his ribs, and connecting movements of the ribs and chest to flow with the movements of the upper spine. After the third session, Lee stopped

falling while walking. Although he still exhibited rigid movements and difficulty moving his arms away from his body, he shifted weight a little more easily and demonstrated minimal trunk rotation for walking in both directions. Lee did not fall for several months until he stopped walking because of a sore on the ball of one foot. Lee gradually discovered how to allow the therapist to work with him and the protest stopped. This ability to learn to allow the therapist to sit next to him and touch him is an example of learning through use of his emotional memory, another type of memory which seems to work in conjunction with the procedural learning. Both procedural and emotional memory is preserved long after other memories are lost. Even without cognitive recognition, emotional memory capabilities in persons with AD allow them to communicate and establish trust with another human being and learn new functional ways to balance in gravity.

Another example follows. Dina was an 83 year old with advanced AD, Parkinson's disease, depression, and cataracts. The Feldenkrais sessions with her demonstrated the power of focusing the communication and interaction on keeping the activities pleasant and working within the comfort of the patient. The chief problem was that the patient had swollen knees and had not been able to straighten her knees past 90 degrees for the past 2 years. Dina had received traditional physical therapy in which the intervention included attempting to straighten the knees by placing a weight on top of them. Dina cried during this treatment and reported pain. She could not propel her own wheelchair, and it took two staff to transfer her to and from her wheelchair. Her reaction to their attempt to transfer her was to lift her legs off the floor and give them her entire weight. She did not rest her feet on the floor, even in sitting. Dina had difficulty lying in all positions. When on her back, her lower body twisted to the side. She stayed where she was placed and in the position she was placed in. Dina was unable to specifically point to a body part and say it hurt her. The focus of the first session was to explore how to help her rest more comfortably. The first efforts were to try to enhance mobility in her ribs and spine. After the first session, she was able to rest more fully on one side. After the second session she was able to rest more fully on both shoulder blades and on her pelvis evenly. After the fourth session, Dina began wheeling herself in the wheelchair with her feet and staff reported that later in the day they saw her stand up from the wheelchair for about 1 minute by herself. None of the sessions had involved direct work with her legs, and the progress in her ability to participate in her life points to the fact that movement deficits are not always the root of problems. The capacity to feel safe and allow touch and other physical and social communication can create improvements in the ability to live in gravity and assist caregivers with the chores of life. The *Feldenkrais Method* is an example of effective, functional communication/manual therapy/neurological rehabilitation that enhances daily living skills in people with AD and other dementias.[1,12,105]

ENVIRONMENTAL CONSIDERATIONS
Hypothermia

The temperature of the living environment must be carefully controlled because aged clients may not perceive that the environment is cold and may not experience shivering. Accidental hypothermia can develop in an older person even at temperatures of 60° F (15.5° C) to 65° F (18.3° C). Accidental hypothermia is a drop in the core body temperature to less than 95° F (35° C). Patients at risk for hypothermia are presented in Box 28-2.

The symptoms of hypothermia may include a bloated face, pale and waxy or pinkish skin color, trembling on one side of the body without shivering, irregular and slowed heartbeat, slurred speech, shallow and slow breathing, low blood pressure, drowsiness, and symptoms of delirium. The two principles of treatment of hypothermia are that the person will stay chilled unless the body temperature is slowly increased and that he or she should be evaluated by a physician, regardless of the apparent severity of the hypothermia.[7,106]

If a person continues to be at risk for hypothermia, specific measures can be taken to prevent subsequent distortions of cognitive status. First, the room temperature should be set to at least 70° F (21° C). Second, the person should wear adequate clothing; this may include long underwear and an undershirt. Adequate nutrition also may be a factor in preventing hypothermia.

Patients and their caregivers may attempt to save money by lowering room temperatures and thus inadvertently cause hypothermia. To prevent accidental hypothermia in institutions with central air conditioning, special accommodations for the elderly, such as a special wing of the building or individual temperature controls in the rooms, are required.[96]

Transplantation Shock

Some elderly persons seem to function well in a familiar environment but become severely disoriented and unable to perform ADLs if taken out of their own homes. As a general rule, these persons have mild symptoms of dementia that are not readily apparent when they remain in a structured, familiar, stable environment and maintain a consistent daily routine. When faced with the need to adapt to a new environment and bombarded with multiple unfamiliar sensory stimuli, however, their limited brain capacity is unable to make sense out of the large volume of new stimuli. If a patient was oriented before admission to an institution and then becomes disoriented, the patient's cognitive functioning will likely return to its baseline level of functioning on return

to the familiar environment. Therefore all moves by a patient from one hospital room to another or from one institution to another, and all changes in a treatment regimen, need to be carefully planned. If a change is anticipated, the patient should be involved in the decision making. If the change is a permanent move, the patient needs to have a chance for one or two trial visits before the actual move. The patient needs to be informed of all changes well in advance, and this information needs to be given repeatedly to the patient with dementia. The precautions mentioned can help the patient relocate without creating transplantation shock and the negative cognitive/emotional changes.

EMOTIONAL CAPACITY TO PARTICIPATE IN A LEARNING TASK

Many elderly persons who come for physical therapy are in a state of emotional overload, as evidenced by disorientation, depression, anger, or a withdrawn and apparently uncooperative attitude. A person who is at or near the point of emotional overload needs to be evaluated regarding his or her ability to be involved in learning tasks that require active participation. If the patient is in emotional overload, forms of therapeutic intervention that temporarily allow the patient to be a passive recipient of therapeutic intervention can be used. Various types of therapeutic interventions, including massage, connective tissue massage, heat, breathing exercises, relaxation exercises, and *Feldenkrais Functional Integration,* can promote a relaxation response, lower the anxiety level, reinforce self-pacing of activity, and thereby prepare the patient to participate in more physically active types of therapeutic exercise.[107] If asked directly, most patients will state whether they feel able to participate actively.[1,12,105]

If for any reason the patient is not able or willing to state his or her feelings, evaluating the patient's ability to participate is still possible. If the therapist can get a patient's cooperation, the following movements can be attempted and then evaluated. (These active movements should be used only if active diseases involving the eyes are not present and no pain occurs during the movements.) The therapist asks the patient to:

1. Close your eyes.
2. Close your eyes and keep them closed for 30 seconds, then for 1 minute.
3. Close your eyes; move only the eyes to the right and left slowly (slow movements with control is the goal).
4. Close your eyes; move your eyes diagonally: right and up, left and down, left and up, right and down.

If a patient is unable to perform these movements, feels they require too much effort, or experiences discomfort, a high level of tension is usually present. Another option is to create a screening of ease of movement and capacity for following increasingly complex directions using the mouth and tongue or movements involving the hands and face. When the patient is extremely tense, treatment should begin by using passive therapeutic procedures. If a person can comfortably execute the movements, she or he (i.e., the central nervous system and the body) is likely to be able to receive and integrate new data and act with ease. When the specific therapeutic intervention requires active participation by the patient, psychomotor readiness to participate can be explored using these kinds of screening activities.

Distortions in intellectual and emotional capacity to receive input, integrate input, and then act on the input affect a person's ability to participate in a learning task. This section has described the most common sources of distortion in information processing that are external to the patient and therefore under the direct control of the rehabilitation team. The rehabilitation team may choose to acknowledge the common age-related changes and common sources of stress response in the elderly and then design a learning process and environment of care that maximizes the elderly patient's potential.

DELIRIUM AND REVERSIBLE DEMENTIA: EVALUATION AND TREATMENT

The following discussion focuses on the patient's internal environment (physiological, psychological, spiritual, and pathological) and presumes that all unnecessary external environmental stressors have been removed. Delirium and dementia have been previously defined. Delirium can manifest suddenly or over a period of hours or days. Delirium may occasionally be chronic, but this is relatively infrequent. Dementia, whether reversible or irreversible, usually has a much longer time of onset, although an acute onset can occur.

The establishment of the diagnosis of the underlying cause of dementia or delirium is the key to effective care. Although the diagnostic process is primarily at the level of pathology, the therapist can obtain information, as part of a team evaluation, which will help establish the underlying diagnosis. Historical information needs to be obtained regarding the following:

- The amount of time that has elapsed since the onset of symptoms
- The progression or lack of progression of symptoms
- Associated functional impairments and associated medical signs and symptoms
- Use of prescription, over-the-counter, home remedies, and illegal drugs or alcohol, caffeine, and nicotine
- Exposure to toxins at work or during recreation
- Even in a patient with cognitive disturbances, this information can frequently be obtained and corroborated by obtaining a history from significant others.

The causes of delirium and reversible dementia are many. In the elderly person, however, certain causes are more common than others (Box 28-3). Alcohol and drugs (prescribed, over-the-counter, illegal, and home remedies) are prime offenders (see Chapter 36). The delirium may be the result of intoxication, side effects, or withdrawal syndromes.[65] Benzodiazepines are among the most commonly prescribed offenders; even a low dose (2 mg) may cause demonstrable cognitive changes.[52] Other common drugs that cause delirium or reversible dementia are alcohol, oral narcotics, psychotropic medications, steroids, antineoplastic drugs, digoxin, anesthetic agents, antiparkinsonian drugs, and antihistamines. However, all drugs have the potential to cause significant cognitive problems in the elderly.[108] These symptoms often resolve with discontinuation of the offending agent or treatment of the withdrawal syndrome. For some patients a medication holiday of longer than 24 hours may be needed before a positive change in cognition can be noted.[62]

BOX 28-3 ■ COMMON CAUSES OF DELIRIUM AND REVERSIBLE DEMENTIA

ALCOHOL/DRUG ABUSE OR DEPENDENCE
Intoxication
Toxicity
Side effects
Withdrawal

CARDIOVASCULAR/PULMONARY
Congestive heart failure
Cardiac arrhythmia
Hypertensive crisis
Hypoxia
Chronic obstructive pulmonary disease

METABOLIC/ENDOCRINE
Electrolyte disturbance (especially hyponatremia)
Hypercalcemia
Dehydration
Overhydration
Renal failure
Hypoglycemia
Diabetic ketoacidosis
Hypothyroidism
Hyperthyroidism
Malnutrition
Vitamin B_{12}/folate deficiency
Hepatic failure
Wernicke-Korsakoff syndrome
Cushing's syndrome

INFECTION
Urinary tract infection
Pneumonia/acute bronchitis
Tuberculosis
Other acute infections

NEUROLOGICAL
Stroke
Head trauma
Mass lesion (e.g., tumor, hematoma)
Seizure

PHARMACOLOGICAL
Benzodiazepines
Barbiturates and other sedative-hypnotics
Antidepressants
Neuroleptics
Antihistamines
Anticholinergics
Cardiac glycosides
Steroids
Antineoplastic drugs
Narcotics
Antiarrhythmics
Antihypertensives

MISCELLANEOUS
Sensory deprivation
Sensory overstimulation
Acute or chronic pain
Constipation/fecal impaction
Urinary retention

At times, the symptoms may be clearly correlated with the pharmacokinetic profiles of the medications taken by the client. The dose or frequency of administration of medications can be a contributing factor to a delirious state.[109] Every member of the rehabilitation team needs to document the patient's ability to participate in learning tasks and the time of the assessment because timing of medication administration can affect functional performance. The rehabilitation team needs the input of a clinical pharmacologist who can help the team focus on concepts such as biological half-life, clearance, bioavailability of drugs, and the time course of drug concentration in plasma as a function of dose and frequency.

Several medical diseases are likely to cause symptoms of delirium or reversible dementia, which will also reverse with treatment of the underlying disease. Urinary tract infections, more common in women, are the cause of delirium in 23% of elderly patients.[110] Fecal impaction is another common cause of acute cognitive change in elderly persons. Others are distended bladder caused by prostate enlargement or drug-induced urinary retention, dehydration, malnutrition, cardiovascular disorders,[106] metabolic disturbances (particularly undiagnosed diabetes mellitus),[15] endocrine diseases, renal diseases, hematological diseases, pneumonia or bronchitis,[106] and vitamin B_{12} deficiency.

Transient (and usually mild) cognitive deficits may be the result of a cerebrovascular accident (CVA). The cognitive deficits after a CVA are often reversible, although they may last for several months after the stroke. The rehabilitation team needs to evaluate and regularly reevaluate the patient's cognitive capacity and build a program of care around current abilities. A program of therapeutic intervention that allows the older person to work in a self-paced program for 1 to 3 months can yield good therapeutic results and also prevent unnecessary secondary deconditioning until part or all of the patient's cognitive capacity returns.[111]

Depression is commonly misdiagnosed as dementia in the elderly.[106,112] For many years depression was thought to be a form of "pseudodementia" or false dementia.[113] Depression can result in mild and subtle cognitive changes affecting immediate recall, attention, and the ability to perform basic ADLs. Some reports noted that as many as 31% of those thought to have dementia have depression instead.[114] However, recent research has clarified the close relationship between structural changes in the elderly brain and the onset of depression, thus bringing the concept of pseudodementia, or depression as a reversible dementia, into disrepute.[115,116] Depression is a treatable disorder, and many patients with cognitive impairments show some improvement in their cognitive functioning if the depression is treated; however, the underlying cognitive problem does not resolve with treatment of the depression.[117]

Because the presence of depression can interfere with the progress of rehabilitation through cognitive deficits or its effects on motivation, this disorder needs to be diagnosed early and accurately. The Geriatric Depression Scale, a 30-item yes/no questionnaire, screens for this disorder.[118] No arbitrary cutoff score signifies depression in this test, and most individuals with a score of 15 or higher have this disorder. The higher the score, the more likely that the patient has depression and the severity of the depression is greater.

Depression after a stroke can produce a reversible decline in cognitive performance.[72] Depression after a stroke is more likely to occur in patients with left hemisphere lesions and as the site of the lesion moves toward the frontal pole.[7] The relation between site of lesion and depression also has been noted on neuropsychological testing.[80]

The treatment of major depression generally involves pharmacotherapy, psychotherapy, and environmental manipulation, which can require support from the entire rehabilitation team.[117,119] In the treatment of a patient with depression, therapeutic techniques can promote a relaxation response, enhance upright posture, decrease anxiety level (massage, heat, or *Feldenkrais Functional Integration*) and help bring the patient to the point at which aerobic training is possible, which is known to have a beneficial effect. All aerobic training for the elderly needs to begin with a stress test, modified as necessary to determine the patient's exercise target heart rate. The modification most commonly required is use of the upper extremities to achieve the training effect because lower extremity function may be limited, or use of major ADLs involving the upper extremities as the stress test/training program.

The causes of delirium and reversible dementia are usually treatable, and if diagnosis and care are provided in a timely fashion, the patient can likely regain full command of his or her cognitive processes. When this does not happen, the patient probably had mild, irreversible dementia that remained hidden until the onset of an acute problem that uncovered the poor cognitive functioning. The length of time in an institution (hospital or nursing home) needs to be kept as short as possible to avoid learned dependency and learned helplessness,[119] which make a return to full cognitive functioning and independent living difficult.[112]

Therapy for elderly persons with delirium or reversible dementia consists of treating the underlying causes of the cognitive changes. A close working relationship among all members of the rehabilitation team, including a geriatric psychiatric consultant, is necessary. Even before the cause of the disorder is elucidated, the patient should receive the same emotional and physical support as any patient with an irreversible dementia. The therapist must adapt all activities to the extent and types of cognitive losses that are present. The patient needs to feel secure, live in an environment that has as few changes as possible, and have a consistent and stable schedule for activities.

IRREVERSIBLE DEMENTIA

The course of irreversible dementia is unique for each patient. The variation in clinical course occurs based on the cause of the underlying disease and superimposed biological and psychosocial factors, including medications, concurrent illness (including delirium), the nature of the social support system, and the patient's premorbid personality structure. The causes of irreversible dementia are summarized in Box 28-4.

Regardless of the cause of the dementia, the clinical course of these disorders has several commonalities.[76] Most of these diseases are progressive. Symptoms may be subtle early in the course of the illness, and the onset of disease is usually noted by the person with the disorder, family members, friends, or colleagues at work rather than by a physician. The signs of impairment of mental ability are typically memory loss, poor judgment, or incompetence at work. The patient can often succeed at hiding his or her symptoms for a while. The social consequences of the cognitive impairment usually bring the patient to the attention of health care professionals. In addition, the patient with dementia can manifest a variety of psychiatric symptoms, including mood disturbance, agitation, violent behavior, socially inappropriate behavior, delusions, hallucinations, catastrophic reactions, and perseveration.[90,120] The pattern of onset and the types of psychiatric symptoms are often directly related to the underlying pathological condition.

When a physician is finally consulted, the diagnostic process can begin. When a complete diagnostic evaluation—including history, physical examination, neurological examination, neuropsychological testing, and laboratory testing (Box 28-5)—is performed, an accurate diagnosis can be made in approximately 90% of patients, although experienced geriatric psychiatrists can make an accurate diagnosis in more than 95% of patients.[37]

Once the diagnostic process is completed, treatment can be started. Medications can assist in reversing underlying causes in only a small percentage of cases; patients in whom drug therapy is successful usually have potentially reversible dementia that has gone untreated and now have permanent sequelae of the disorder. Medications may only be able to slow down the process of an irreversible disorder (e.g., tacrine for Alzheimer's disease) or prevent further deterioration (e.g., aspirin for multiinfarct dementia). Psychotropic drugs may reverse depression or the behavioral symptoms associated with dementia.[114,119,121] Medical man-

agement also involves the prevention and treatment of other medical conditions and side effects of the new interventions as they are added.

Medical management of irreversible dementia focuses on maximizing the patient's remaining functions and roles, rehabilitating some lost functions, and providing family education and support.[90] Training caregivers to adapt to the patient (e.g., modifications for getting the patient out of bed, bathing), simplifying the individual's living space, and referring relatives to family support services are some of the issues to be addressed.[122] The treatment of irreversible dementia is a long-term process. Recent studies have found that the average duration of illness from first onset of symptoms to death was 8.1 years for AD, 6.7 years for multiinfarct dementia,[123] and 5.6 years for Pick's disease.[124] Medical and nursing care can extend the life expectancy of patients with dementia for up to 20 years or more.

In 1907, Alois Alzheimer[30] described the case and the neuropathology of a 54-year-old woman who developed morbid jealousy, which was followed by loss of memory, inability to read and understand, and death 4.5 years after onset of the illness. Since then it has been noted that 50% of patients with dementia have AD.[92] In making the diagnosis of AD, all other causes of cognitive dysfunction must be ruled out. The disease can occur at any age, but the onset of the disease is almost always after age 65 years. The prevalence of the disease gradually increases to a rate of 20% in persons older than 85 years.[125,126]

AD can be clinically staged. The use of staging enables the family and health care team to plan ahead for the individual's needs. Staging helps the family prepare longitudinally for the process of interacting with the patient. It allows the treatment team to plan for appropriate levels of services as the individual's abilities decline. Finally, it allows the health care team to quantify change in functional and cognitive abilities over time, which helps assess the effectiveness of the patient's treatment plan and establish evidence-based practice. The use of staging requires an accurate description of the patient's behavior (without the use of jargon) as well as an assessment of the patient's mental state.

Traditionally, the symptoms of AD have been thought to progress in three stages. Stage 1 lasts from 2 to 4 years and involves loss of functional skills or orientation, memory loss, and lack of spontaneity. The patient is often aware of the losses and is, in many cases, able to cover up the cognitive losses by talking around the issues. During this stage the patient and family may need to deal with the issue of giving up a job, hobbies, or other types of meaningful activity because of the patient's inability to carry them out safely and independently. The patient begins to lose the ability to handle money and a personal budget, drive a car safely, and tell time. The family or meaningful others may have to come to terms with the question of whether the patient can live alone. Depression is common during this stage of the disorder.[119]

Stage 2 is characterized by progressive memory loss and the presence of a variety of neurological symptoms. Aphasias, apraxias, wandering, repetitive movements and stereotypical behavior, increased or decreased appetite, constant movement, and a peculiar wide-based gait can manifest. Psychotic symptoms (especially paranoid delusions and hallucinations), agitation, violent behaviors, and uncontrollable screaming are common symptoms during this stage of the disorder.

In stage 3 the patient develops vegetative symptoms. The patient may become mute, stop eating, and become incontinent of bowel and bladder. Muscle twitches or jerks, spasms of the diaphragm, and an inability to walk generally occur. The patient may develop seizures, and emotional responsiveness, if present, is at a primitive level. Eventually, the patient dies from the disease.

The MMSE also may be used as a staging tool. Scores of 26 or more are generally associated with minimal, if any, dementia; scores of 21 to 25 are associated with mild dementia, scores of 15 to 20 with moderate dementia, scores of 10 to 14 with severe dementia, and scores of 9 or less with profound dementia. The severity of most other symptoms correlates well with the MMSE score.

Reisberg[127] and Reisberg et al[128] developed a scale that defines seven stages, many with substages, of AD. This scale is probably the most accurate staging system for AD. In addition, the staging used by this scale closely correlates with the progression of different sets of symptoms through the course of the disease.

The Barthel Index

The Barthel Index (Table 28-1) is a profile scale that rates 10 self-care, continence, and mobility criteria.[129] The specific rating guidelines used in scoring are presented in Appendix 28-A. The advantage of the Barthel Index is its simplicity and usefulness in evaluating patients before, during, and after treatment. It is functionally oriented and may be best used accompanied by a clinical evaluation.[80] The scale allows documentation of functional changes over time and is useful when discussing with families the need for help for the patient with daily self-care with families.

STRATEGIES FOR TREATMENT AND CARE

Most elderly people with decreased cognitive abilities live with family or friends and not in institutions. Because of this, the rehabilitation team needs to include the caregivers

TABLE 28-1 ■ Barthel Index

	WITH HELP	INDEPENDENT
1. Feeding (score as "with help" if food needs to be cut)	5	10
2. Moving from wheelchair to bed and return (including sitting up in bed)	5-10*	15
3. Personal toilet (wash face, comb hair, shave, clean teeth)	0*	5
4. Getting on and off toilet (handling clothes, wipe, flush)	5	10
5. Bathing self	0*	5
6. Walking on level surface (or if unable to walk, propel wheelchair)	10	15
7. Ascending and descending stairs	5	10
8. Dressing (includes tying shoes, fastening fasteners)	5	10
9. Controlling bowels	5	10
10. Controlling bladder	5	10

Adapted from Mahoney FI, Barthel DW: Functional evaluation: the Barthel index, *Md State Med J* 14:61, 1965.

A patient scoring 100 is continent, feeds, dresses, gets up and out of bed and chairs, bathes himself or herself, walks at least a block, and can ascend and descend stairs. This does not mean that he or she is able to live alone. The patient may not be able to cook, keep house, and meet the public but is able to get along without attendant care.

*A score of 0 is given in the activity when the patient cannot meet the criteria as defined (see Appendix 28-A).

and the patient as much as possible in treatment planning. The goal of rehabilitation is to ensure that the patient remains safe, independent, and able to perform ADLs and IADLs for as long as is reasonable. The planning to reach these goals is best done within the context of the patient's social support system.

The rehabilitation process begins while the diagnostic workup is still in progress. At this stage of treatment, the rehabilitation plan includes basic training for the patient in performing and adapting the ADL. It also includes caregiver training and support for significant others so they can make needed environmental modifications to ensure the safety of the patient with dementia.

Once the diagnosis is established, treatment planning for long-term care at home or in an institution must be carefully made. No matter where the patient will be living, involvement of the caregivers and significant others is essential to maximizing functional outcomes. The emotional, physical, and financial resources of the patient and family or significant others who will be the caretakers must be ascertained. A review of the caretakers' willingness to perform basic tasks or make visits, their willingness to learn and teach the necessary skills, and the realistic need for respites must be determined.[130] Family training and orientation manuals that deal with all the details of caring for a person with dementia are available.[90,131] The same detailed orientation is needed for institutional staff who care for elderly patients with dementia. The structure and process of care can help patients be maximally active in their self-care and prevent unnecessary anxiety and catastrophic reactions.

Supporting Families and Caregivers with Their Own Sense of Loss, Frustration, and Helplessness

Family, significant others, and caregivers go through their own coping and adaptive process as the patient experiences gradual or sudden cognitive disturbances.[132] These people have a history with the patient and have expectations about what the relationship and communication should be. As cognitive disturbance occurs, they experience a series of losses because the patient is no longer able to respond and interact as he or she has in the past. With progressive cognitive decline, family and friends experience ongoing losses because the patient is continually changing and less able to relate. For many patients with cognitive disturbances, at the final stage all communication disappears and the family is left with only nonverbal communication or no communication at all. Staff who work with a patient over a period of time also face their own personal reactions of loss, unfulfilled expectations, and a continual need to reassess how to relate effectively to the patient. **The entire burden of creating a positive relationship falls on the people who are interacting with the patient.** The family and caregivers themselves need training and ongoing support in learning how to nurture and maintain an ongoing relationship with the patient. This requires that caregivers and family members be aware that they are in a healing process as they relate to the loss of the relationship that previously existed.

Epstein: Stages of Healing for Caregivers

Epstein[133] provides a workable description of the stages of healing that occur when major trauma or loss occurs. Epstein defines *healing* as "putting right our wrong relation to our body, to other people and . . . to our own complicated minds, with their emotions and instincts at war with one another and not properly understood and accepted by what we call 'I' or 'me.' The process is one of reorganization, reintegration of things which have come apart."[133] When a patient experiences cognitive changes, the first stage of response by those who care for or love this person is suffering. Chaos exists during this traumatic time. For example, the patient suddenly cannot understand simple directions on how to operate the new electric cart and insists on getting the old one back. The family is upset and arguments ensue. The family and patient together eventually get a medical workup and they are told that "Mom has some type of degenerative cognitive problem." They all experience a profound sense that "something is wrong." The response to helplessness for most human beings is to resist. The lesson of this stage is acceptance. When acceptance is present, then detachment from the emotions is possible. With acceptance present, adaptation and compensation for losses are possible. In the example noted, this would mean that the family would return the new electric cart and have the old (familiar) model refurbished. The family would get training from the therapist in exactly what skills of interaction Mom does not have so that they can work to avoid creating situations in which she feels "stupid and helpless." When a cognitive loss is truly present, training in skills only creates frustration in the patient that may lead to anger and rage. The staff and family need to be trained to understand the exact nature of the losses and provide appropriate compensations in their oral communication and how they relate to the patient.

Stage 2 has been alluded to as a part of stage 1. Therapists, the family, and caregivers search for second opinions, see other types of physicians, and try alternative treatments to gain power over helplessness. The polarities and rhythms of this process define this stage. All persons involved, even the patient, eventually begin to note that the emotions of the interactions may actually be making things worse. Acceptance that no magic solution is available begins. Everyone involved looks with interest at the proposition, "What can I do to make *this* life—*this* person—cope more effectively and have a reasonable quality of life (regardless of my opinion about what cognitive loss means to me personally)?" The lesson at this stage is another level of acceptance.

The third stage invites an examination of the ways in which people are "stuck in a perspective." When overwhelming stimuli occur, people commonly resort to their favorite strategy from childhood. For some people the favorite strategy is to withdraw, for others it may be to eat to create a distraction, and for others it may be anger. The emotional and mental options created to adapt to a difficult situation are as varied as the human race itself. Human beings dwell in the desire to know why or how to fix something. The lesson of this stage is, again, another level of acceptance and insight about how involved individuals contribute to the problem by reactions at the moment.

Stage 4 begins the process of "reclaiming power." This is the stage at which people realize that the "script" (their internal dialogue) from the last three stages is not workable or even desirable. The anger is recognized and it brings an awareness that this reaction is not helping. Recognition begins that resisting is also not working because the condition of the patient is not affected in a positive way by the emotional reaction on the part of the caregiver(s). The truth of the matter is that the first four stages of healing often cause family and caregivers to be part of the problem and not part of the solution. The problem is how to support the patient to heal and adapt to the cognitive changes, whether temporary or permanent. Family and caregivers need to bring their healing process to their own support system separate from the patient. When caregivers attempt to share their frustration, suffering, sadness, or anger with the patient, the patient is usually upset because she or he cannot comprehend what the details of the issue really are. The patient only knows that people are upset. This will cause the patient to be further upset and agitated. The stages of healing in staff and family must be recognized and services created or referral to support groups made so the patient can interact with people who are able to adapt to his or her needs and not cause further upset.

Stage 5 is called "merging with the illusion" and represents the first step in being able to "relate to the facts in a powerful way" rather than resist or try to manipulate them. It is the step at which family and caregivers begin to integrate the facts into their view of the world. The adult son may say, "I hate the fact that my mom cannot live alone; it makes me feel so helpless or frustrated or angry or upset or inadequate." Many health care providers get upset when cognitive losses occur in their loved ones. The cognitive loss seems to be a failure that they take personally.

Stage 6 begins with active steps to prepare for the resolution of the emotions connected with the process. Many people describe this stage as the time when they really admit that their parents are never going to be able to give them advice again, baby-sit, or travel alone. The healing comes in allowing people to notice the emotions that come with accepting these big changes in reality.

Stage 7 brings the actual physical or emotional discharge. The process can be expressed as laughter, crying, fever, the urge to be physically active, sneezing, coughing, and so on. Resolution is marked by a deep sense of peace and inner strength. The person will have gone through the six stages, and the release of emotions or movement results in a deep shift away from resistance. **Family and caregivers need to create these healing experiences separate from or away from the patient with cognitive losses.** When therapists work with the patient with cognitive losses, they must create for the patient a world that works and is safe and respectful of his or her unique abilities. In most cases, the profound emotional and physical release that comes with resolution only tends to upset the patient.

At stage 8 affected individuals are emptied and the board has been wiped clean. In the space of nothingness is an opportunity for new possibilities for relating to the patient. **The relationship should not be based on the past but on moment-to-moment information that comes from the patient.** Therapists can now enjoy being with the patient and begin to feel gratitude. Family and caregivers begin to look for ways to make things work easier.

Stage 9 is a time when the caregivers and family relate to the energy of the universe and begin to see the connections to all life around them. At this stage, involved individuals begin to see that they are also a part of the great flow of time and energy and that an opportunity for joy exists. The process of illness and dying becomes the focus of awe and a reason to connect with other people and appreciate other people because they are a part of the whole process of life.

Stage 10 is the time to connect with the creative force of the universe. The spiritual process is brought to the issue at hand. A sense of great wisdom and oneness with all creation is felt. **When working from this state of being, the caregiver has the unique capacity to speak or act to bring out the best in others.** In health care, some caregivers have the special gift of allowing themselves to step into the mental world of the other person and thereby create communication that will be heard and that can be acted on even by those with limited mental capacities. The most interesting thing is that the patients can often tell if a caregiver is in this unique state because they will come and sit next to the caregiver or want to hold hands. This state of ease and connection can be learned. A possible resource for exploring these skills is an organization called Landmark Education ([415] 981-8850; www.landmarkeducation.com), which provides programs and courses that examine how people listen, what bias they bring to the communication process, and specific speech strategies to bring out the best in others.

Epstein's stage 11 is when people live day to day without being attached to the situation. Epstein notes that in this stage, "we communicate with ourselves and others through our wounds instead of from them." As healing progresses, caregivers become part of the solution in the care of the patient with cognitive losses. They know they can make a positive difference and take action to create what needs to be done. **They are able to sort out the facts of a situation from the first impression, which is often loaded with judgments and wishful thinking. As caregivers relate to the verifiable facts, they speak to the issues at hand with power and create positive outcomes in which "win-win" becomes the norm.**

In the last stage, caregivers bring their unique individuality to the service of the community. They become aware that the limits to what they can bring to the community are connected to the limits to their sense of wholeness. This insight sends them back to their earlier stages of healing to create further self-awareness and healing on other issues. Inservice training can offer a basic introduction to strategies for lifelong learning, healing, and self-awareness. "What works for me?" "What is the easiest way to learn new skills?" "What strategies enhance adaptability?" This type of learning is nonlinear and is the model a scientist uses to conduct an inquiry.

Nonlinear learning begins with the posing of a question. Then data and information are collected, and additional questions are generated that are related to the first question. At some point an "Aha!" moment or insight occurs. A new relationship is suddenly made possible that was not possible before. Nonlinear learning is not about small gradual steps of progress but occurs as learning balance occurs when riding a bicycle—one minute balance is impossible, and the next is the breakthrough moment. Nonlinear training offers precise strategies that can enhance communication with someone who has cognitive deficits. Nonlinear learning is built on scientific communication that operates on the basis of verifiable facts at the present moment. Nonlinear learning invites each person to examine all strategies for communication to be sure that problems are not occurring as a result of misinterpretation of the facts. Communication can occur without verbal language, and fear does not need to be present. When a patient has cognitive deficits, the art and science of human interaction need to be precise so that caregivers do not speak in words that are not understandable to the patient. What caregiver prejudgments are brought to the interaction with the patient needs to be understood: experiencing the stage of awe, sharing joy in the moment, or suffering because the person is "difficult"? The care and therapy provided to a person with cognitive disturbances need to be created based on the facts of the moment and carried out in a state of gratitude, vulnerability, and nurturing for the staff and the patient.

All persons with cognitive losses should have access to caregivers who are trained to manage emotional responses in order to provide precise strategies for communication with those with dementia. A gracious and secure existence is possible even when cognition is diminished if the caregivers are committed to adapting the environment and its demands to match the capacity of the patient. The challenge for health care is designing training programs that truly prepare families and caregivers to be effective, empowering communicators. All caregivers need training to create this experience for a person with cognitive deficits.

As a part of the rehabilitation program, caregiver training for this group of patients needs to emphasize reassurance, hands-on interventions, and communication to allow treatment to proceed at a pace perceived as reasonable by the patient.[62] In the early and middle stages of all dementias, physical therapy intervention usually can prolong the ability to move with ease in ADLs and IADLs and maintain the ability to participate in some social activities. This is extremely important for caregivers because deficits in the patient's ability to perform ADLs and IADLs often relate to the inability to physically perform these activities under supervision.[45] The ability to walk is lost late in most dementias, but gait and coordination disturbances are common and can benefit from physical therapy.[134-136] Therapy intervention to assist the patient and train the caregivers involves facilitation of ease of movement and motor planning and developing or refining environmental and cognitive cues to assist in carrying out complex tasks. Ultimately, caregivers require training in how to move, lift, and otherwise assist the patient.

Cognitive impairment is a key limiting factor in the performance of ADLs and IADLs as well as a limiting factor for participating in rehabilitation. Accurate assessment and training by the therapist helps the caregiver provide only the help that is absolutely needed, with patients continuing to perform for themselves as many ADLs as possible. For example, when brushing the teeth, the patient needs to be able to remember the command to brush, recognize the toothbrush, and perform a complex but repetitive motor action. The patient may only need the help of someone placing the toothbrush in his or her hand and slowly guiding it to the mouth to be able to safely brush the teeth.

The accurate assessment of IADLs and ADLs is more reliable than medical diagnosis for predicting the amount of assistance and interaction a person will need in a nursing home (see Table 28-1 and Appendix 28-A).[129] The first goal of rehabilitation for patients with dementia is to create a supportive emotional and physical environment. In other words, the environment must actively work to compensate for the patient's cognitive and functional losses as they occur. The ultimate goal is to help patients feel they are capable so that they will continue to try to do those things for themselves that they can do safely, whether they remain in their home or live in an institution. Orientation and training of significant others is also important so they feel comfortable allowing the patient to participate safely in activities and basic self-care tasks modified to their cognitive level.

The Alzheimer's Association (800-272-3900; www.alz.org) is a resource for professionals and caregivers of people with dementia. The goals of the association are the following:

- To support research related to the diagnosis, therapy, cause, and cure of Alzheimer's disease and related disorders
- To aid in organizing family support groups; to educate and assist affected families
- To sponsor educational programs for professional and laypersons on the topic of Alzheimer's disease
- To advise government agencies of the needs of the affected families and to promote federal, state, and private support of research
- To offer help in any manner to patients and their caregivers to promote the well-being of all involved

The Alzheimer's Association promotes the provision of humane care to the patient with dementia or related disorders throughout the course of the illness. Other support groups have been tried in communities where spouses have worked to develop ongoing respite care.[137]

As a member of the rehabilitation team, the physical or occupational therapist needs to conduct an inventory of services as a part of the annual review of the quality of care that is provided for patients with dementia. A survey of persons caring for patients with dementia listed the following services in their perceived order of importance[76,138]:

1. A paid companion who can come to the home a few hours each week to give caregivers a rest (respite)
2. Assistance in locating people or organizations to provide patient care
3. Assistance in applying for government programs, such as Medicaid, disability insurance, and income support programs
4. A paid companion who can come to the home for overnight care so caregivers can go away for one or more days (respite)
5. Personal home care for the person with dementia to help with activities such as bathing, dressing, or feeding in the home
6. Support groups composed of others who are caring for persons with dementia and other cognitive deficits
7. Special nursing home care programs only for persons with dementia and other cognitive deficits while the caregiver is away
8. Adult day care providing supervision and activities away from the home
9. Visiting nurse services for care at home

In the home care category, information about the availability of services and government programs and various forms of respite care were also ranked high in the survey. Overall, caregivers (family and friends) of the patient are often able and willing to provide care for the patient throughout the illness if appropriate professional consultation can help them cope with problematic situations and if adequate respite time is provided to the caregiver(s).

Not mentioned in this chapter was the need for psychological support for caregivers. The stress on caregivers is extreme, and symptoms of anxiety and depression are common. Because of the relative lack of counseling services for caregivers, however, the use of (and probable abuse of and dependence on) psychotropic medications by caregivers is high.[56,139] Because these medications may impair the cognitive functioning of caregivers, the risk of harm to the patient with dementia is also high.

DEMENTIA AND DELIRIUM: NEW FRONTIERS

Most current research in delirium and dementia is focused on AD. The Alzheimer's Association is the largest private foundation funding research on dementia, supporting almost 100 projects totaling almost $18 million in 2005 alone. Research is underway to explore possible causes of dementia, including work that examines the roles of neurotransmitters, structural brain changes, nutrition, viruses, drugs, immunological deficits, and heredity in the etiology of AD. Studies to increase the diagnostic accuracy of different forms of dementia, including a distinction between cortical and subcortical dementia, or the use of DSM-III-R criteria,[138,140] DSM-IV criteria,[141] or neuropsychological criteria, are also underway. Newer diagnostic models of dementia, including that caused by stage II or III human immunodeficiency virus infection, are also being studied.[142] New research that may shed light on the mechanisms of the early stages of AD relates to other neurodegenerative diseases. Persons with dementia who also have parkinsonian symptoms, delusions, and hallucinations have been reported to experience faster decline that those who do not.[143] This research team found a relation between the presence of Lewy bodies (abnormal structures in the brain that contain a protein called synuclein) and parkinsonian symptoms; affected individuals had lower survival rates than those with either symptom present by itself.

The most exciting area of research is pharmacology (see Chapter 36).[45] The advent of tacrine, a drug that slows down the progression of AD in some patients, has produced an explosion of research on drugs aimed at stabilizing or reversing the symptoms of this disease. Although no cures are available, some drugs, such as physostigmine, ondansetron, and nerve growth factor, have shown some promise. These studies have spawned a search for new drugs to treat both AD and the symptoms of other dementias.

Research is also being funded that is investigating the best ways to provide care and support in the home and at long-term residential settings.

SUMMARY

Why some people stay lively and creative in their older years is not known; Michelangelo designed St. Peter's when he was nearly 90; Picasso painted at 90; and Arthur Rubenstein, Pablo Casals, and Martha Graham all worked creatively in their older years. What is clear is that lonely, isolated older people are much more likely to be confused and disoriented than their peers who remain actively involved with family and friends. Perhaps what is needed is to invite the world to explore rules of conduct in which older persons are honored and included. As stated in Timothy 1:5 within the Christian Bible, "Rebuke not an elder, but entreat him as a father; . . . the elder women as mothers . . . honor widows. . . . But if any not provide for his own, and specifically for those of his own house, he hath denied the faith, and is worse than an infidel."

In working with an older person with dementia or delirium, the therapist can do much to make the quality of life better for the patient, family, and caregivers.[90] A thorough listing of the details needed to develop an environment and process of care for elderly persons with cognitive deficits can be found in other texts.[90,120,131]

Specific examples of modifications of physical and occupational therapy examination and treatment may include working in collaboration with the family, close friends, and other members of the rehabilitation team and developing a consultative relationship with key caregivers (professional and nonprofessional and all shifts of institutional staff) to encourage problem solving and patient participation in self-care. Another important modification includes the evaluation of each patient's communication abilities before the therapy assessment to adapt the assessment in such a way as to promote patient participation. Case Study examples are presented later in this chapter (refer to Case Studies 28-1 and 28-2) to provide clinical scenarios and corresponding physical and occupational therapy examination and treatment strategies.

Modifications of treatment include the use of gentle, nonverbal neurological rehabilitation techniques (e.g., the *Feldenkrais Method*). The key is to acknowledge the now well-established research finding that nondeclarative learning and memory (procedural) are available long after declarative learning and memory (ability to consciously learn and remember facts and events) are lost for a person with AD. Motor ability is one of the last areas to be affected by AD.[144] Assisting a person with AD to edit procedural memory and increase walking safety is therefore possible. The functional outcomes of this learning can include a decrease in abnormal muscle tone, enhanced sensory awareness and organization for the position of the eyes and head in space, an increase in the ease of movement, an increase in the ease of breathing, enhanced endurance, minimized anxiety, minimized resting muscle rigidity in the chest, and increased patient coordination. **The therapist needs to modify the process of neurological facilitation by decreasing patient effort and adding extra cuing and more frequent breaks for integration of learning.** Tasks may need to be simplified so that the patient can perform them, and the caregiver is trained to perform only those tasks that the patient cannot perform.

Each month the therapist, treatment team, patient, and caregiver(s) need to identify safe physical activities that the patient can be encouraged to perform for recreation, relaxation, and overall fitness. The goal is to enhance the performance of simple ADL and IADL tasks (e.g., washing socks, setting the table), which can enhance patient self-esteem. In addition, the physical therapist, along with other members of the rehabilitation team and caregivers, needs to monitor the patient for new signs and symptoms of concurrent delirium or reversible dementia so that treatment can be initiated early and further deterioration can be prevented.

Hospital and nursing home patient "Bill of Rights" define the minimal quality of care required for any patient. The concepts presented apply to the care of patients with cognitive deficits no matter what the setting. The provision of considerate and respectful care for the patient with dementia or other cognitive deficits is possible and necessary. Well-planned and gentle care prevents unnecessary distortions in cognitive function brought on by feelings of fear or being rushed and thereby maximizes all remaining cognitive function. To use his or her remaining emotional and cognitive resources, the patient with cognitive deficits needs to live in an environment and experience a process of care that is modified to meet the special needs created by delirium or dementia.

Major efforts are underway in research to discover a cure for AD. In 1997 a consensus conference on the diagnosis and treatment of AD and related disorders was organized by the American Association for Geriatric Psychiatry, the Alzheimer's Association, and the American Geriatrics Society. The conclusions of the conference included the statement,

"Alzheimer's disease is the most common disorder causing cognitive decline in old age and exacts a substantial toll on

society. Although the diagnosis of AD is often missed or delayed, it is primarily one of inclusion, not exclusion, and usually can be made using standardized clinical criteria. Most cases can be diagnosed and managed in primary care settings, yet some patients with atypical presentations, severe impairment, or complex co-morbidity benefit from specialist referral. Alzheimer's disease is progressive and irreversible, but pharmacologic therapies for cognitive impairment and non-pharmacologic and pharmacologic treatments for behavioral problems associated with dementia can enhance quality of life. Psychotherapeutic intervention with family members is often indicated, as nearly half of all caregivers become depressed. Health care delivery to these patients is fragmented and inadequate."[32]

Physical and occupational therapy are key resources for the creation of a therapeutic environment and for the effective and timely assessment and treatment of the patient with cognitive deficits (presuming that the therapy can take into account the need to affect procedural learning directly—i.e., the *Feldenkrais Method*). The goal of therapy is to create a process of care in which the patient feels safe and the caregivers are given training and support in problem solving to guide the patient to participate in self-care, ambulation, and recreation as long as it is safe and functionally possible.

Caregiver agreements can enhance capacity in older persons with dementia to participate in daily life—exploring the possibility of living a life with safety, dignity, and love. Following is a brief list of basic environmental supports for encouraging procedural memory to be activated:

1. I will ask my patient if they would like to pray or worship today and make arrangements to meet those needs.
2. I will speak or communicate in a way that is functional and workable for the patient.
3. I will repeat what I hear and perceive back to the patient to ensure that I capture her or his perspective.
4. I will encourage natural participation by creating a pace that is pleasant for the patient.
5. I will close doors quietly.
6. I will not raise my voice and shout except in a real emergency.
7. I will talk to someone on staff when I get upset or take something personally so I can have peace with co-workers, creating a positive atmosphere for the patients to live in.
8. I will offer a warm-up of their tea or coffee to all people I am serving when possible.
9. I will only create one choice at a time so the patient can understand and then choose yes or no.
10. I will know what "my" patient has eaten on my shift.
11. I will know my patients' timing for toileting so I can support their continence and dignity.
12. I will tell the patient I am going to touch them before I touch them to avoid surprises.
13. I will walk (rolling or ambulating) with every one of my patients outdoors as often as possible or at least every 3 days to encourage good sleep and mental and physical stimulation.
14. I will sit and visit with each of my patients for 10 minutes (every shift).
15. I promise to listen with an open heart to the patients' perception of life at the moment.
16. I promise to close the blinds in every room at night (unless the patient requests otherwise) and open blinds every morning to reinforce day/night orientation.
17. I will discover and use the "personal" get ready for bed routine for all patients so they sleep well.
18. I promise to talk and walk at a pace that encourages a sense of safety for my patients.
19. I promise to be self-nurturing and come to work well rested and ready to share myself.
20. I promise to avoid confrontational actions and body language except in an emergency.
21. I promise to respect the unique ergonomics of each patient and adapt as needed.
22. I promise to offer to add support to explore ways to increase comfort.
23. I promise to notice how my patients relate so no one agitates or bothers another.
24. I promise to be kind to myself, other staff, and my patients.
25. I promise to be of service and adapt to meet my patients needs.
26. I promise to report problems (equipment, environment, relationships) to the person who can do something about them.
27. I promise not to gossip (talk about others so that it leaves a negative impression and no resolution of the problem).
28. I promise to leave my workspace clean and restocked after I have taken care of the patient (or at least leave a note to alert the next shift what is not done yet).

CASE STUDY 28-1 ■ THE COMPLEXITY OF AGING

The patient was a 78-year-old woman who had the following deficits on the MMSE: was not aware of where she lived, date, or year; had poor short-term memory; could not spell the word "world" backwards; could not copy the two overlapping pentagons. The patient was generally happy and enjoyed having someone sit with her. The patient fractured her femur and because of the location of the fracture site, a surgical procedure was performed to allow total weight-bearing. The surgeon and the psychiatrist decided that partial weight-bearing would not be a concept that the patient could understand. The physical therapist and assistant worked together with the family and caregivers in the nursing home to develop a plan of care. At the initial care conference, the main question was whether the patient should receive physical therapy. The family

CASE STUDY 28-1 ■ THE COMPLEXITY OF AGING—cont'd

was fearful that the patient would fall again if she were taught how to walk. The focus of the conference was to educate the family and other staff regarding the importance of physical therapy so the patient could learn how to participate in and eventually perform transfers from wheelchair to toilet as well as to bed. The decision was made to begin physical therapy, with the initial goal being to achieve all functional ADL transfers with standby physical assistance.

The patient was not interested in walking and was fearful of falling. The key change in physical therapy intervention was in the style of communication used to teach basic bed mobility and the components of transfer skills. By using trial and error, the patient responded best to a smile, verbal encouragement, hand signals, and gentle manual pressure to indicate the desired task to be performed. If the task was broken down and components were identified, the patient became frustrated and refused to participate. If the patient was invited by manual cues and verbal reassurance to stand up and sit on the bed, the patient would hesitate for up to 1 minute and then she would attempt to perform the task. It became obvious that the patient needed at least 30 to 60 seconds of waiting time between verbal requests given by staff and when she was ready to act on the request. If additional time was given, the patient appeared to get frustrated and would refuse to cooperate. A sign was placed over her bed with instructions for communication: smile, reassure, use your hands to guide her to perform the desired action, and wait 60 seconds; let her feel there is plenty of time.

A sliding board was introduced in therapy, and the patient enjoyed the idea. The board allowed transfers for all ADLs to involve no lifting for the staff. The patient would lean her head on the shoulder of the staff member while sitting and then she would assist in sliding across on the board. All transfers for ADLs using the sliding board were possible within five visits of physical therapy. A bed was located that was 17 inches high to facilitate bed-to-wheelchair transfers. The bed could be raised to assist the nursing aide in cleaning activities. The decision was made to leave the bed at 17 inches unless the nursing staff needed to perform special in-bed procedures with the patient. The wheelchair foot rests were modified so that they formed a solid flat surface to allow the patient to rest in a natural position. The patient was only 5 feet 2 inches tall, and the standard wheelchair only allowed her to comfortably put both feet on one foot pedal and sit with her weight mostly on one buttock. A smaller wheelchair and the adapted footrest gave the patient an equal pressure on both sitting bones, and the patient began to sit at rest in a natural upright posture. The other goal of physical therapy was to teach the

patient wheelchair mobility by using her hands to push the chair. Once the patient was given gloves for her hands (she did not like germs), she was willing to try to push the wheelchair. The patient was instructed in the physical therapy department during two visits. The patient was next seen by the therapist on the unit to allow the nurse's aide to be a part of the physical therapy instruction. The rationale was that the nurse's aide would need to help reinforce the skills and encourage practice of wheelchair mobility skills as a part of daily activities. During the last visits the physical therapist watched daytime, afternoon, and evening staff practice with the patient and addressed new situations that arose. All caregivers on three shifts were trained to ensure consistency of verbal and manual cuing for the patient.

Before discharge to restorative nursing, the patient's current level of functional abilities was documented by using an ADL chart that specified time of day when tasks were easiest, task(s), equipment needs, special positioning, clothing and other assistive devices, verbal cuing, and other communication requirements for each critical task that had been mastered in physical therapy. The cataloging of functional skills reminded the nurse's aide of the ingredients involved for the patient to successfully perform ADLs. The other advantage of the detailed discharge summary to the nursing staff is that new staff could use the document and, as needed, contact physical therapy for clarifications if the patient suddenly were not able to perform the tasks (a signal of possible medical or psychosocial problems).

KEY POINTS

1. Common goals were identified and agreed on among all team members and the patient's significant others.
2. Education was provided as needed to allow for consistency of verbal and manual cuing to the patient.
3. Physical therapy treatment began in a quiet, undisturbed area where the patient could concentrate. As mastery of a skill was achieved, the skill was practiced with supervision and instruction of other staff was provided as needed.
4. Equipment and furniture were adjusted to help the patient perform tasks with minimal assistance.
5. Discharge from therapy involved providing nursing staff with a detailed description of functional abilities and the conditions required to help maximize patient participation, sense of safety, and control (as had already been reviewed with all aides working with patient).
6. The physical therapist was designated as a resource person for nursing staff for simplifying functional tasks in patient care, problem solving, communication, and movement-related issues.

CASE STUDY 28-2 ■ A CLIENT IN THE EARLY STAGE OF AD

The patient was a 64-year-old man who until 1 month ago was working. He was forced to retire because he kept forgetting the natural sequences of the work tasks. For example, his partner would see him direct someone to wait for him in the waiting room and then he would forget the person was in the waiting room. On the MMSE, he had difficulty with date and year and would try to redirect the question in an apparent attempt to cover up for loss of short-term memory. He could or would not spell the word "world" backward, and he poorly copied the overlapping hexagons (looked more like squares). He was a runner but now he apparently could not remember how to get home, and he would pretend to be hurt and get someone to drive him home. The man reported feeling restless.

The patient, his wife, and two sons were seen by the team at a psychiatric clinic. The wife was very upset and the family was asking for help. The role of therapy at this early stage of AD involved the following:

1. Functional assessment of basic ADLs/IADLs and home assessment.
2. Orientation of spouse and significant caregivers regarding the functional changes that may occur in the near future and how to compensate for current functional losses (e.g., patient had difficulty dressing in the morning and would get frustrated).
3. Orientation to the role of therapy in hands-on treatment related to techniques to help the patient relax. After initial evaluation, the team decided to teach caregivers massage techniques identified by the therapist as soothing and relaxing for the patient. (Note: The emphasis in hands-on intervention is to create slow, predictable, and nurturing contact that is perceived by the patient as soothing and relaxing.)
4. Orientation of caregivers to the use of manual contact and hand signals to communicate and reinforce the intention. Kinesthetic contact and the ability to follow kinesthetic cues can help the patient with ADL tasks at home. At this time the kinesthetic cuing may not be critical for the patient, but the caregivers need to get in the habit of cuing the patients as a compensatory tool for future cognitive losses.
5. Orientation of caregivers was given to the benefits of a ritualized schedule of daily events for the patient and assistance in developing the daily schedule. The predictability of the ritual will help the patient feel safe and in control. The ritualizing is especially helpful to address the frustrations with dressing in the morning.
6. Written information about local support groups, day treatment centers, and the availability of the rehabilitation team was given including therapy for problem solving.
7. Participation in evaluation of patient/family need for placement in a day treatment center or use of a home health aide was completed. Supervision was needed for cooking (would leave burners on), working in the woodshop (would leave power tools running), and in self-care to ensure his safety. Supervision in the home was decided, with family members sharing the load. The idea of going to a new place was not positively received by the patient. (Note: The patient may function better in the environment where he or she has lived for a long time because of the familiarity with the details of the surroundings.)
8. The therapist participated in development of the home care plan and provided for home visits to accomplish tasks described in items 1 through 7. The next contact that the family made with therapy was 1 month later to address the patient's inability to settle down and be able to go to sleep at night. A home visit was made to evaluate the bedtime ritual, the relaxation strategies being used, and communication with the physician about current medications taken. The patient disliked bathing and undressing for bed. After discussion with caregivers the patient was allowed to go to bed in his clothes without bathing and undressing (bathing and undressing would be carried out in the morning when he was less tired). Relaxation massage was modified to involve the face, neck, hands, and feet, and the caregivers were instructed and practiced during two visits under the supervision of the therapist. A satisfactory bedtime ritual was developed and home health care was workable for the patient and the caregivers.

The next request for therapy consultation came 4 months later when the wife and the daughter-in-law (who had been taking turns being the primary caregiver) both felt the need to hire and train an attendant/companion for the patient for 8 hours a day. At this time the patient preferred to be in the home, walk in the yard, or take long walks in the local park. The therapist, in cooperation with other team members, trained the patient and aide in how to sequence for ease in ADL tasks; use of kinesthetic cuing; how to facilitate ADLs, bathing, and dressing with a slow pace and ritualized format; and how to sequence the tasks and relaxation techniques to help the patient settle down and go to sleep. Foot massage was the only technique that the patient now allowed and appeared to enjoy. After three physical therapy visits over a 2-week period, the attendant was able to carry out home health care effectively for the patient.

The last request for help occurred when the family was concerned because the patient was trying to run away. The therapist made a home visit and found that the patient sat most of the day. The MMSE showed that he could not give his own first or last name and had no short-term memory. Based on the evaluation, the therapist proposed that the family/attendant go with the patient for a walk when the patient showed an interest in leaving the house. This strategy worked for a few months, but then the patient began to sit down on the sidewalk when he was tired. Another visit was made after a wheelchair was ordered to train the caregivers in

DEDICATION

A personal note: This chapter was written for my grandmother. She had depression and related cognitive disturbances after World War II. She gradually got worse and worse in her ability to remember new information, but she could hold my hand and show me how to feed the ducks. We were great friends. I helped her remember to turn off the stove, and I remembered where she put her glasses. She could make sandwiches, and I could always find her comb. We empowered each other. Over 15 years she gradually grew more and more helpless in the adult skills of life. Even then she could give great hugs and loved to sit and drink tea with me. I remember her as a very frail woman. I watched the nurse's aide tuck her in, kiss her on the cheek, and hold her hand while they said prayers. The aide hummed a familiar song as she left the room. It was like those familiar songs that come from our childhood, and they wrap us in a sense of warmth and love and safety—we declare that all is well with the world and we go to sleep and dream of peaceful things.

REFERENCES

1. Feldenkrais M: *On health,* Portland, OR, 1979, Feldenkrais Guild.
2. Ader R, Cohen N: Conditioning and immunity. In Ader R, Felten DL, Cohen N, editors: *Psychoneuroimmunology vol 2,* ed 3, New York, 2001, Academic Press, p. 3-34.
3. Heimann M: *Regression periods in human infancy,* London, 2003, Lawrence Erlbaum.
4. Helman CG: *Culture, health and illness. An introduction for health professionals,* ed 2, London, 1990, Wright.
5. Parkes CM: Psycho-social transitions: a field study, *Soc Sci Med* 5:101-115, 1971.
6. Schanberg SM, Field TM: Maternal deprivation and supplemental stimulation. In Field TM, McCabe PM, Schneiderman N, editors: *Stress and coping across development,* Hillsdale, NJ, 1988, Lawrence Erlbaum, p. 3-25.
7. Peterson D, Orgren RA: Older adult learning. In Jackson O, editor: *Physical therapy of the geriatric patient,* New York, 1983, Churchill Livingstone.
8. Polirstok SR, Dana L, Buono S et al: Improving functional communication skills in adolescent and young adults with severe autism using gentle teaching and positive approaches, *Top Lang Disorders* 23:146, 2003.
9. Schneiderman N, editor: *Stress and coping across development,* Hillsdale, NJ, 1988, Lawrence Erlbaum.
10. Schretlen D, Pearlson GD, Anthony JC, et al: Elucidating the contributions of processing speed, executive ability, and frontal lobe volume to normal aging-related differences in fluid intelligence, *J Int Neuropsychol Soc* 6:52-61, 2000.
11. Ward NS, Frackowiak RS: Age-related changes in the neural correlates of motor performance, *Brain* 126(part 4):873-888, 2003.
12. Feldenkrais M: *Awareness through movement,* New York, 1972, Harper & Row.
13. Feldenkrais M: *The elder citizen,* Berkeley, CA, 1989, Feldenkrais Resources.
14. Mattson A: Introduction. In Mattson A, editor: Neurobiological aspect of development, vulnerability, and adaptation to physical and behavioral disorders, *J Am Acad Child Psychiatry* 25:737, 1986.
15. Charatan FB: *Management of confusion in the elderly,* New York, 1979, Roerig.
16. Shakespeare: *As You Like It,* 2.7, New York, 1997, Washington Sugar Press.
17. Solomon K, Vickers R: Attitudes of health workers toward old people, *J Am Geriatr Soc* 27:186-191, 1979.
18. Folstein MF, Anthony JC, Parhad I, et al: The meaning of cognitive impairment in the elderly, *J Am Geriatr Soc* 33:228-235, 1985.
19. Ross E: Effect of challenging and supportive instructions in verbal learning in older persons, *J Educ Psychol* 58:261-266, 1968.
20. Schaie KW: Intellectual development in adulthood. In Birren JE, Schaie KW, editors: *Handbook of the psychology of aging,* ed 3, San Diego, 1990, Academic Press.
21. Williams ME: *American Geriatrics Society complete guide to aging and health,* New York, 1995, Harmony Books.
22. Van Wynen EA: A key to successful aging: learning-style patterns of older adults, *J Gerontol Nurs* 27:6-15, 2001.
23. Thomas SM, Jordan TR: Contributions of oral and extraoral facial movements to visual and audiovisual speech perception, *J Exp Psychol Hum Percep Perform* 30:873-888, 2004.
24. Calhoun RO, Gounard BR: Meaningfulness, presentation rate, list length and age in elderly adults paired association learning, *J Educ Gerontol* 4:49, 1979.
25. Moore MS: Disturbed attachment in children: a factor in sleep disturbance, altered dream production and immune dysfunction. 1. Not safe to sleep: chronic sleep disturbance in anxious attachment, *J Child Psychother* 15:99, 1989.
26. Light LA: Interactions between memory and language in old age. In Birren JE, Schaie KW, editors: *Handbook of the psychology of aging,* ed 3, San Diego, 1990, Academic Press.
27. Lipowski ZJ: Delirium in the elderly patient, *N Engl J Med* 320:578-582, 1989.
28. Lipowski ZJ: Delirium (acute confusional states), *JAMA* 258:1789-1792, 1987.
29. Rebok GW, Folstein MF: Dementia, *J Neuropsychiatry Clin Neurosci* 5:265-276, 1993.
30. Alzheimer A, Stelzmann RA, Schnitzlein HN et al: An English translation of Alzheimer's 1907 paper, "Uber eine eigenartige Erkankung der Hirnrinde," *Clin Anat* 8:429-431, 1995.

31. Botwinick J: *Aging and behavior—a comprehensive integration of research findings,* New York, 1978, Springer-Verlag.

32. Small GW, Rabins PP, Buckholtz NS et al: Diagnosis and treatment of Alzheimer's disease and related disorders. Consensus statement of the American Association of Geriatric Psychiatry, the Alzheimer's Association and the American Geriatrics Society, *JAMA* 278:1363-1371, 1997.

33. Arenberg D, Robertson-Tchabo EA: Learning and aging. In Birren JE, Schaie KW, editors: *Handbook of the psychology of aging,* New York, 1977, Van Nostrand Reinhold.

34. Hebert LE, Scherr PA, Bienias JL, et al: Alzheimer's disease in the U.S. Population: prevalence estimates using the 2000 census, *Arch Neurol* 60:1119-1122, 2003.

35. Evans DA, Funkenstein HH, Albert MS, et al: Prevalence of Alzheimer's disease in a community population of older persons: higher than previously reported, *JAMA* 262:2551-2556, 1989.

36. Hertzog C, Schaie KW: Stability and change in adult intelligence: simultaneous analysis of longitudinal means and covariance structures, *Psychol Aging* 3:122-130, 1988.

37. Katzman R: Alzheimer's disease, *N Engl J Med* 314:964-972, 1986.

38. Solomon K, Szwabo P: Psychotherapy for patients with dementia. In Morley JE, Coe RM, Strong R et al, editors: *Memory functioning and aging related disorders,* New York, 1992, Springer.

39. Agate J: *The practice of geriatrics,* ed 2, London, 1970, Heinemann.

40. Reichel W, editor: *Clinical aspects of aging,* Baltimore, 1978, Williams & Wilkins.

41. Brody H, Vijayashankar N: Anatomical changes in the nervous system. In Finch CE, Hayflick L, editors: *Handbook of the biology of aging,* New York, 1977, Van Nostrand Reinhold.

42. Bremner JG, Johnson SP, Slater A, et al: Conditions for young infants' perception of object trajectories, *Child Dev* 76:1029-1043, 2005.

43. Poe MK, Seifert LS: Implicit and explicit tests: evidence of dissociable motor skills in probable Alzheimer's dementia, *Percep Mot Skills* 85:631-634, 1997.

44. Cerella J: Aging and information-processing rate. In Birren JE, Schaie KW, editors: *Handbook of the psychology of aging,* ed 3, San Diego, 1990, Academic Press.

45. Spirduso WW, MacRae PG: Motor performance and aging. In Birren JE, Schaie KW, editors: *Handbook of the psychology of aging,* ed 3, San Diego, 1990, Academic Press.

46. Stern RG, Davis KL: Treatment approaches in Alzheimer's disease: past, present, and future. In Weiner MF, editor: *The dementias: diagnosis and management,* Washington, DC, 1991, American Psychiatric Press.

47. Wassenberg R, Feron FJ, Kessels AG, et al: Relationship between cognitive and motor performance in 5-6 year old children: results from a large-scale cross sectional study, *Child Dev* 76:1092-1103, 2005.

48. Willingham DB, Peterson EW, Manning C, et al: Patients with Alzheimer's disease who cannot perform some motor skills show normal learning of other motor skills, *Neuropsychology* 11:261-271, 1997.

49. Dick MB, Hsieh S, Bricker J, et al: Facilitating acquisition and transfer of a continuous motor task in healthy older adults and patients with Alzheimer's disease, *Neuropsychology* 17:202-212, 2003.

50. Heuninckx S, Wenderoth N, Debaere F, et al: Neural basis of aging: the penetration of cognition into action control, *J Neurosci* 25:6787-6796, 2005.

51. Licht S: *Therapeutic heat and cold,* New Haven, CT, 1960, Elizabeth Licht.

52. Salzman C, Fisher K, Nobel K et al: Cognitive improvement following benzodiazepine discontinuation in elderly nursing home residents, *Int J Geriatr Psychiatry* 7:89, 1992.

53. Selye H: *Stress without distress,* New York, 1974, JB Lippincott.

54. Wang HS: Special diagnostic procedures—the evaluation of brain impairment. In Busse EW, Pfeiffer E, editors: *Mental illness in later life,* Washington, DC, 1973, American Psychiatric Association.

55. Birren JE: *Handbook of aging and the individual,* Chicago, 1973, University of Chicago.

56. Meyers BS, Cahenzli CT: Psychotropics in the extended care facility. In Szwabo PA, Grossberg GT, editors: *Problem behaviors in long-term care: recognition, diagnosis, and treatment,* New York, 1993, Springer-Verlag.

57. Libow LS: Pseudo-senility: acute and reversible organic brain syndromes, *J Am Geriatr Soc* 21:112-120, 1973.

58. Wilder J: Basimetric approach to psychiatry. In Arieti S, editor: *American handbook of psychiatry,* New York, 1966, Basic Books.

59. Wilder J: *Stimulus and response: the law of initial value,* Bristol, UK, 1967, John Wright & Sons.

60. Schleifer SJ, Scott B, Stein M, et al: Behavioral and developmental aspects of immunity, *J Am Acad Child Psychiatry* 26:751-763, 1986.

61. Harper DG, Volicer L, Stopa EG, et al: Disturbance of endogenous circadian rhythm in aging and Alzheimer's disease, *Am J Geriatr Psychiatry* 13:359-368, 2005.

62. Jackson O: *Physical therapy and the geriatric patient,* New York, 1987, Churchill Livingstone.

63. Foley JM: Sensation and behavior. In Fields WS, editor: *Neurological and sensory disorders in the elderly,* New York, 1975, Stratton Intercontinental.

64. Kay DWK, Cooper AF, Garside RF, et al: The differentiation of paranoid from affective psychoses by patient's premorbid characteristics, *Br J Psychiatry* 129:207, 1976.

65. Solomon K, Shackson JB: Substance use disorders in nursing home patients. In Reichman WE, Katz PR, editors: *Psychiatric care in the nursing home,* New York, 1996, Oxford University.

66. Solomon P: *Sensory deprivation,* Cambridge, MA, 1961, Harvard University.

67. Fields WS, editor: *Neurological and sensory disorders in the elderly,* New York, 1975, Stratton Intercontinental.

68. Leighton DA: Special senses—aging of the eye. In Brocklehurst JC, editor: *Textbook of geriatric medicine and gerontology,* New York, 1985, Churchill Livingstone.

69. Gobetz GE: *Learning mobility in blind children and the geriatric blind,* Cleveland, 1967, Cleveland Society for the Blind.

70. Gobetz GE, Drane HW, Underwood EL: *Home teaching of the geriatric blind,* Cleveland, 1969, Cleveland Society for the Blind.

71. Drabben-Thiemann G, Hedwig D, Kenklies M et al: The effects of Brain Gym® on the cognitive performance of Alzheimer's patients, *Brain Gym J* vol 16, no 1, 2002. Discussed on www.BrainGym.org. Accessed August 7, 2006.

72. Grant I, Adams K, editors: *Neuropsychological assessment of neuropsychic disorders,* New York, 1986, Oxford University.

73. Cattell RB: Theory of fluid and crystallized intelligence—a clinical experiment, *J Educ Psychol* 54:1, 1963.

74. Elias MF, Elias PK: Motivation and activity. In Birren JE, Schaie KW, editors: *Handbook of the psychology of aging,* New York, 1977, Van Nostrand Reinhold.

75. Holtzer R, Stern Y, Rakitin BC: Age-related differences in executive control of working memory, *Mem Cognit* 32:1333-1345, 2004.

76. Office of Technology Assessment, U.S. Congress: *Congressional summary: losing a million minds: confronting the tragedy of Alzheimer's disease and other dementias,* Washington, DC, 1990, U.S. Government Printing Office.

77. Rabins PV, Fitting MD, Eastham J, et al: Emotional adaptation over time in care-givers for chronically ill elderly people, *Age Ageing* 19:185-190, 1990.

78. Holmes TH, Rahe RH: The Social Readjustment Rating Scale, *J Psychosom Res* 11:213-218, 1967.

79. Knox AB: *Adult development and learning,* San Francisco, 1977, Jossey-Bass.

80. Bolla-Wilson K, Robinson RG, Starkstein SE et al: Lateralization of dementia of depression in stroke patients, *Am J Psychol* 146:627-634, 1989.

81. Hultsch DF, Dixon RA: Learning and memory in aging. In Birren JE, Schaie KW, editors: *Handbook of the psychology of aging,* ed 3, San Diego, 1990, Academic Press.

82. Galasko D, Klauber MR, Hofstetter CR et al: The MMSE in the early diagnosis of disease, *Arch Neurol* 47:49-52, 1990.

83. Campbell ME: Study of the attitudes of nursing personnel toward the geriatric patient, *Nurs Res* 20:147-151, 1971.

84. Gunter LM: Student attitudes toward geriatric nursing, *Nursing Outlook* 19:466-469, 1971.

85. Jackson O: *Physical therapy and the geriatrics patient—a descriptive study of cross-cultural trends in Denmark and the United States* [thesis], Ann Arbor, 1979, University of Michigan.

86. Busse EW, Pfeiffer E, editors: *Mental illness in later life,* Washington, DC, 1973, American Psychiatric Association.

87. Folstein MF, Folstein SE, McHugh PR: "Mini-Mental State". A practical method for grading the cognitive state of patients for the clinician, *J Psychiatr Res* 12:189-198, 1975.

88. van der Cammen TJ, van Harskamp F, Stronks DL, et al: Value of the Mini-Mental State Examination and informants' data for the detection of dementia in geriatric outpatients, *Psychol Rep* 71:1003-1009, 1992.

89. Braekhus A, Laake K, Engedal K: The Mini-Mental State Examination: identifying the most efficient variables for detecting cognitive impairment in the elderly, *J Am Geriatr Soc* 40:1139-1145, 1992.

90. Mace NL, Rabins PV: *The 36 hour day—a family guide to caring for persons with Alzheimer's disease, related dementing diseases and memory loss in later life,* Baltimore, 1981, Johns Hopkins University.

91. Jackson JE, Ramsdell JW: Use of the MMSE to screen for dementia in elderly outpatients, *J Am Geriatr Soc* 36:662, 1988.

92. Allison RS: *The senile brain,* London, 1962, Edward Arnold.

93. Bassi CJ, Solomon K, Young D: Vision in patients with Alzheimer's disease, *Optom Vis Sci* 70:809-813, 1993.

94. Fozard JL: Vision and hearing in aging. In Birren JE, Schaie KW, editors: *Handbook of the psychology of aging,* ed 3, San Diego, 1990, Academic Press.

95. Robinson RG, Kubos KL, Starr LB, et al: Mood disorders in stroke patients, *Brain* 107:81-93, 1984.

96. Worden H: Aging and blindness, *New Outlook Blind* 70:433, 1976.

97. Gross AM: Preventing institutionalization of elderly blind, *Vis Impairment Blindness* 2:49, 1979.

98. Carroll K, editor: *Human development in aging—compensation for sensory loss,* Minneapolis, 1978, Ebenezer Center for Aging and Human Development.

99. Craik IM: Age differences in human memory. In Birren JE, Schaie KW, editors: *Handbook of the psychology of aging,* New York, 1977, Van Nostrand Reinhold.

100. Arenberg D: Concept problem solving in young and old adults, *J Gerontol* 23:279-282, 1968.

101. Bandler R, Grinder J: *Frogs into princes,* Cupertino, CA, 1979, Real People Press.

102. Mintzer JE, Colenda C, Waid LR, et al: Effectiveness of a continuum of care using brief and partial hospitalization for agitated dementia patients, *Psychiatr Serv* 48:1435-1439, 1997.

103. LeClerc CM, Wells DL: Use of a content methodology process to enhance feeding abilities threatened by ideational apraxia in people with Alzheimer's-type dementia, *Geriatr Nurs* 19:261-267, 1998.

104. Savelkoul M, Commissaris K, Kok G: Behavior and behavioral determinants in the management of demented people in residential homes, *Patient Educ Counseling* 34:33-42, 1998.

105. Ann J: Individuals with dementia learn new habits and become empowered through the Feldenkrais Method. Pending publication in *Alzheimer's Care Quarterly,* Fall 2006, vol 7, number 4.

106. Brocklehurst JC: *Textbook of geriatric medicine and gerontology,* ed 2, New York, 1985, Churchill Livingstone.

107. Crum RM, Anthony JC, Bassett SS, et al: Population-based norms for the Mini-Mental State Examination by age and educational level, *JAMA* 269:2386-2391, 1993.

108. Livingstone HA, Day AL: Comparing the construct and criterion-related validity of ability-based and mixed-model measures of emotional intelligence, *Ed Psych Measur* 65:757, 2005.

109. Simonton DK: Creativity and wisdom in aging. In Birren JE, Schaie KW, editors: *Handbook of the psychology of aging,* ed 3, San Diego, 1990, Academic Press.

110. Manepalli J, Grossberg GT: Recognition and treatment of depression. In Szwabo PA, Grossberg GT, editors: *Problem behaviors in long-term care: recognition, diagnosis, and treatment,* New York, 1993, Springer-Verlag.

111. Rodstein M: The characteristics of nonfatal myocardial infarction in the aged, *AMA Arch Intern Med* 98:84-90, 1956.

112. Solomon K: The elderly patient. In Spittel JA Jr, editor: *Clinical medicine, vol 12,* Hagerstown, MD, 1981, Harper & Row.

113. Levinson AJ, editor: *Neuropsychiatric side effects of drugs in the elderly,* New York, 1979, Raven Press.

114. May BJ: *An integrated problem solving curriculum for physical therapists,* Washington, DC, 1976, American Physical Therapy Association.

115. Grossberg GT, Manepalli J, Solomon K: Diagnosis of depression in demented patients. In Morely JE, Coe, RM, Strong R et al, editors: *Memory functioning and aging-related disorders,* New York, 1992, Springer-Verlag.

116. Krishnan KRR: Neuroanatomic substrates of depression in the elderly, *J Geriatr Psychiatry Neurol* 6:39-58, 1993.

117. Sunderland T, Alterman IS, Yount D, et al: A new scale for the assessment of depressed mood in demented patients, *Am J Psychiatry* 145:955-959, 1988.

118. Yesavage JA, Brink TL, Rose TL et al: The Geriatric Depression Rating Scale: comparison with other self-report and psychiatric rating scales. In Crook T et al, editors: *Assessment in geriatric psychopharmacology,* New Canaan, CT, 1983, Mark Powley Associates.

119. Solomon K: Psychosocial dysfunction in the aged: assessment and intervention. In Jackson OL, editor: *Physical therapy of the geriatric patient,* ed 2, New York, 1989, Churchill Livingstone.

120. Mace NL, editor: *Dementia care: patient, family, and community,* Baltimore, 1990, Johns Hopkins University.

121. Sky AJ, Grossberg GT: Aggressive behaviors and chemical restraints. In Szwabo PA, Grossberg GT, editors: *Problem behaviors in long-term care: recognition, diagnosis, and treatment,* New York, 1993, Springer-Verlag.

122. Winograd CH, Jarvik LF: Physician management of the demented patient, *J Am Geriatr Soc* 34:295-308, 1986.

123. Barclay LL, Zemcov A, Blass JP, et al: Survival in Alzheimer's disease and vascular dementias, *Neurology* 35:834-840, 1985.

124. Jung R, Solomon K: Psychiatric manifestations of Pick's disease, *Int Psychogeriatr* 5:187-202, 1993.

125. Kay DWK, Beamish P, Roth M: Old age mental disorders in Newcastle-Upon-Tyne: a study of prevalence, *Br J Psychol* 110:146, 1964.

126. McKahann G, Drachman D, Folstein M, et al: Clinical diagnosis of Alzheimer's disease, *Neurology* 34:939-944, 1984.

127. Reisberg B: Clinical presentation, diagnosis, and symptomatology of age-associated cognitive decline and Alzheimer's disease. In Reisberg B, editor: *Alzheimer's disease: the standard reference,* New York, 1983, Free Press.

128. Reisberg B, Ferris SH, de Leon MJ, et al: The Global Deterioration Scale (GDS): an instrument for the assessment of primary degenerative dementia (PDD), *Am J Psychiatry* 139:1136-1139, 1982.

129. Mahoney FI, Barthel DW: Functional evaluation: the Barthel index, *Md State Med J* 14:61-65, 1965.

130. Lang R, Jackson O: *Model demonstration of a comprehensive care system for older people,* Washington, DC, 1980, Administration on Aging.

131. McDowell FH, editor: *Managing the person with intellectual loss (dementia or Alzheimer's disease) at home,* White Plains, NY, 1980, Burke Rehabilitation Center.

132. Yankelovich S, White I: *Caregivers of patients with dementia,* Washington, DC, 1986, Office of Technology Assessment.

133. Epstein DM: *The twelve stages of healing,* San Rafael, CA, 1994, Amber-Allen.

134. Coons D, Robinson A, Spencer B et al: *Final report of project on Alzheimer's disease: subjective experience of families,* Ann Arbor, MI, 1983, Institute of Gerontology.

135. George LK: *The dynamics of caregiver burden,* Washington, DC, 1984, Association of Retired Persons, Andrus Foundation.

136. Katzman R: Clinical presentation of the course of Alzheimer's disease: the atypical patient. In Rose CF, editor: *Modern approaches to the dementias,* pt 2, Basel, Switzerland, 1985, Karger.

137. Brache CI: The aging client and their family network. In Jackson O, editor: *Physical therapy of the geriatric patient,* New York, 1983, Churchill Livingstone.

138. Rabbitt P, Diggle P, Holland F, et al: Practice and drop-out effects during a 17-year longitudinal study of cognitive aging, *J Gerontol B Psychol Sci Soc Sci* 59:84-97, 2004.

139. Clipp EC, George LK: Psychotropic drug use among caregivers of patients with dementia, *J Am Geriatr Soc* 38:227-235, 1990.

140. American Psychiatric Association: Organic mental syndromes and disorders. In *Diagnostic and statistical manual of mental disorders,* ed 3, revised, Washington, DC, 1987, American Psychiatric Association.

141. American Psychiatric Association: Delirium, dementia, amnestic and other cognitive disorders. In *DSM-IV draft criteria,* Washington, DC, 1993, American Psychiatric Association.

142. Morgan MK, Clarke ME, Hartman WL: AIDS-related dementia: a case report of rapid cognitive decline, *J Clin Psychol* 44:1024-1028, 1988.

143. 2003 progress report on Alzheimer's Disease, research advances at NIH, U.S. Department of Health and Human Services, National Institute of Health, National Institute on Aging, Washington, DC, 2004, U.S. Government Printing Office.

144. Sullivan KJ: Functionally distinct learning systems of the brain: implications for brain injury rehabilitation, *Neurol Rep* 22:126, 1998.

APPENDIX 28-A ■ Rating Guidelines for Barthel Index*

1. Feeding
   10 = Independent. The patient can feed himself or herself a meal when someone puts the food within reach. Patient must put on an assistive device if needed to cut up the food alone. The patient must accomplish this in a reasonable time.
   5 = Some help is necessary (with cutting up food, etc., as listed above).

2. Moving from wheelchair to bed and return
   15 = Independent in all phases of this activity. Patient can safely approach the bed in the wheelchair, lock brakes, lift footrests, move safely to bed, lie down, come to a sitting position in the wheelchair if necessary to transfer back into it safely, and return to the wheelchair.
   10 = Either some minimal help is needed in some step of this activity or the patient needs to be reminded or supervised for safety of one or more parts of this activity.
   5 = Patient can come to a sitting position without the help of a second person but needs to be lifted out of bed, or he or she transfers only with a great deal of help.

3. Doing personal toileting
   5 = Patient can wash hands and face, comb hair, clean teeth, and shave. He may use any kind of razor but must put in blade or plug in razor without help as well as get it from drawer or cabinet. Female patients must put on own makeup.

4. Getting on and off toilet
   10 = Patient is able to get on and off toilet, fasten and unfasten clothes, prevent soiling of clothes, and use toilet paper without help. If a bedpan is necessary instead of a toilet, patient must be able to place it on a chair, empty it, and clean it.
   5 = Patient needs help because of imbalance, handling clothes, or using toilet paper.

5. Bathing self
   5 = Patient may use a bathtub or a shower or take a complete sponge bath. Patient must be able to do all the steps involved in whichever method is used without another person being present.

6. Walking on a level surface
   15 = Patient can walk at least 50 yards without help or supervision. Patient may wear braces or prostheses and use crutches, canes, or a walker (but not a rolling walker). Patient must be able to lock and unlock braces, if used, assume the standing position and sit down, get the necessary mechanical aids into position for use, and dispose of them when sitting. (Putting on and taking off braces is scored under dressing.)
   10 = Patient needs help or supervision in any of the above but can walk at least 50 yards with a little help.

6a. Propelling a wheelchair
   5 = Patient cannot ambulate but can propel a wheelchair independently. Must be able to go around corners, turn around, maneuver the chair to a table, bed, toilet, etc. Must be able to push a chair at least 50 yards. (Do not score this item if the patient gets a score for walking.)

7. Ascending and descending stairs
   10 = Patient is able to go up and down a flight of stairs safely without help or supervision. Patient may and should use handrails, canes, or crutches when needed. Must be able to carry canes or crutches when ascending or descending stairs.
   5 = Patient needs help with or supervision of any one of the above items.

8. Dressing and undressing
   10 = Patient is able to put on and remove and fasten all clothing as well as tie shoelaces (unless adaptations are necessary). The activity includes putting on and removing and fastening corset or braces when these are prescribed.
   5 = Patient needs help putting on and removing or fastening any clothing. Patient must do at least half the work. Patient must accomplish this in a reasonable time. Women need not be scored on use of a brassiere or girdle unless these are prescribed garments.

9. Continence of bowels
   10 = Patient is able to control bowels and have no accidents. Can use a suppository or take an enema when necessary.
   5 = Patient needs help in using a suppository or taking an enema or has occasional accidents.

10. Controlling bladder
   10 = Patient is able to control his or her bladder day and night. Patients who wear an external device and leg bag must put them on independently, clean and empty bag, and stay dry day and night.
   5 = Patient has occasional accidents or cannot wait for the bedpan or get to the toilet in time or needs help with an external device.

Adapted from Mahoney FI, Barthel DW: Functional evaluation: the Barthel index, *Md State Med J* 14:63, 1965.

CHAPTER 29 Aging With Dignity and Chronic Impairment

Robert A. Eskew, PT, MS, PCS
Myla U. Quiben, DPT, PT, GCS, NCS
Ann Hallum, PT, PhD

KEY WORDS

acquired brain injury
adaptation
aging
cardiopulmonary complications
developmental disabilities
energy conservation
environmental modification
fatigue
orthotics
postpolio syndrome
traumatic brain injury

OBJECTIVES

After reading this chapter the student/ therapist will be able to:
1. Discuss the pathological considerations in people with lifelong functional limitations.
2. Analyze how the aging process may affect people with lifelong functional limitations and challenges in life participation.
3. Analyze the unique challenges faced by persons with chronic motor impairments such as cerebral palsy, neural tube defects, genetic malformations, postpolio syndrome, spinal cord injury, and traumatic/acquired head injury during the aging process.
4. Develop sensitivity and coping strategies when working with persons with intellectual disabilities.
5. Evaluate this population of clients with a sensitivity and skill that incorporates precautions and effectiveness of interventions.

INTRODUCTION

The conceptualization of this chapter has come from the increasing population of individuals who have survived an initial central nervous system (CNS) insult and the resulting chronic functional limitations and are now going through the aging process. Therapists over the last 30 years have been evaluating and establishing programs for a large group of individuals who had polio as children and have now developed a postpolio syndrome (PPS). Since the initial onset of the acute disease of polio, these individuals have aged and are now again being confronted with additional loss of components of functional activities. These losses have decreased their ability to participate in life activities, which they had done successfully in earlier adulthood.

Today, these problems of aging with chronic movement dysfunctions have grown to encompass not only individuals with postpolio syndrome but also individuals who came into life with neurological challenges, as well as those who have acquired CNS injury through either disease/pathological condition or trauma. Individuals who have been diagnosed with CNS damage at some time in their lives and who may have received extensive occupational, physical, and speech therapy at that time are now being challenged 20, 30, possibly 40 years after the insult with new functional limitations that are decreasing their ability to participate in life with the quality they expect. As with all human beings, the nervous systems of these individuals continue to age; however, their ability to adapt, accommodate, and modify to adjust to life's physical demands may be more limited as a result of the initial damage. The focus of therapy needs to be on energy conservation, environmental modifications, and mainte-

nance of function as opposed to an acceptance of the philosophy that working harder will lead to greater functional skill.

This chapter is divided into three sections. Section I discusses the challenges, problems, and solutions for individuals with developmental disabilities (DD) who are aging. Section II, as in the last edition, focuses on postpolio syndrome (PPS) or the late effects of polio. Section III encompasses individuals who have sustained a trauma somewhere within the CNS (spinal cord, brain stem, or higher centers) or those who have acquired CNS damage through disease or pathological condition.

Although individuals may fall under one of the three sections as the result of an initial medical diagnosis, there are commonalities to all these categories that need to be identified and analyzed from a long-term quality-of-life perspective. Individuals who are aging with these chronic functional limitations should be allowed to age with the dignity given to any other individual. The challenge to therapists will be to step out of the model of regaining functional skill through repetitive practice and into the model of maintaining function, energy conservation, and empowerment of that function to the individual needing service. The client is and should be the individual who determines what aspect of functional activities are critical to quality of life and what compensations are acceptable and unacceptable as part of an adult life expectation. From that information and the analytical understanding of what is happening to the CNS of these individuals, clients and therapists together can establish realistic goals and intervention strategies that will optimize and maintain the potential motor function of those individuals.

SECTION I

ADULTS WITH DEVELOPMENTAL DISABILITIES

Robert A. Eskew, PT, MS, PCS

OVERVIEW

Adults with DDs face unique challenges throughout their lives in various aspects of the aging process. One of the most vital in terms of experiencing a rich, full life is appropriate health care provided by trained professionals who understand these challenges. This is a broad topic due in part to the many conditions that are categorized as DDs. According to the Administration of Developmental Disabilities and the Administration of Children and Families, DDs are severe, chronic disabilities attributable to mental or physical impairments, that manifest before age 22 years, and that are likely to continue indefinitely. They result in substantial limitations in three or more areas: self-care, receptive and expressive language, learning, mobility, self-direction, capacity for independent living, and economic self-sufficiency, as well as the continuous need for individually planned and coordinated services.[1] Thus, this definition envelops a wide range of conditions leading to significant and lifelong disabilities. These conditions would include neuromuscular impairments such as seen in cerebral palsy (Chapter 12) and spina bifida (Chapter 18), as well as genetic malformations (Chapter 13) seen with individuals with Down syndrome. These individuals are frequently seen by therapists for various functional limitations that arise throughout their lives. However, the professional training that health care providers have received regarding the care of these individuals has focused on early childhood and school-aged children. As a result, many adolescents and adults with a DD have difficulty accessing appropriate health care information regarding secondary conditions resulting from their specific disabilities.

With improved neonatal medical services, science has dramatically improved the life expectancy of extremely premature infants with very low birth weights.[2] However, these infants are also at risk for development of a variety of conditions having lifelong sequelae (Chapter 11). Premature infants are at higher risk of intraventricular hemorrhage, putting them at a greater risk of neurological impairment with long-term consequences.[2] Retinopathy of prematurity is also a significant issue, although advances in laser correction have preserved sight that was once lost. Many of these children have continuing ophthalmic problems extending into their adult lives.[2-4] These visual disturbances lead to problems in processing information during early childhood that can interfere with cognitive development.

Pulmonary function is another area affected by premature birth (Chapters 11 and 35). Because of the natural development of lung tissue being interrupted, these infants also have a higher incidence of asthma and bronchopulmonary dysplasia. The administration of pharmaceutically engineered surfactants has lessened the effects of pulmonary issues. However, in studies of energy expenditure in individuals with cerebral palsy, it is clear that oxygen demand for the group is high. This variable is largely due to the inefficiency of movement and increased compensatory strategies, which lead to increased oxygen consumption. Any subsequent pathological process in this area could further limit functional status. As the individual ages and body size increases, pulmonary demand increases, which has the potential of decreasing functional ability. Clinicians working with adults with DDs should therefore obtain data on pulmonary status and endurance when planning treatment interventions or consulting with clients on how to maximize their functional potential and maintain this over time.

Rose et al[5] found that measuring heart rate was a reliable indicator of energy expenditure in children with cerebral palsy. Compared with nondisabled peer groups, the authors also found heart rate and oxygen uptake at various speeds had a linear relationship.[5] With additional studies this correlation was not substantiated.[5a,5b,5c] Data on heart rate can be used clinically for objective description of factors influencing the efficiency of functional gait. Therapists must also monitor oxygen uptake to make sure that the O_2 demands are not exceeded even when the heart rate is within normal parameter.

The model for providing services to persons with DDs has changed dramatically in the last 25 years. In the past, children with a profound DD were often separated from the community at large and were placed in residential facilities designed to provide for their every need. In these facilities, persons with a DD would remain throughout their lives with limited access to education and work. It was held that this was a population that needed to be cared for within a more traditional medical model and separation would lessen the perceived burden on individual families. This model of care created not only separation from educational opportunities or work training but also from a wide range of social experience. Indeed, many other problems were created by this model, including health issues such as poor nutrition, no separation between individuals who had severe emotional problems from those with severe motor limitations, and living in wards and close proximity to one another without separation when ill, thus increasing individuals' risks of physical trauma such as fractures, development of osteoporosis from disuse, and exposure to various pathogens.[6] The past has taught lessons to therapists, physicians, families, and clients. Today, the future of individuals with DDs comes with great hope for learning, neuroplasticity, and family environment to nurture a high quality of life. Because the life environment has changed, the number of children who have grown into adults and even into elderly citizens are increasing yearly and create challenges to therapists dealing with the integration of preexisting motor limitations and the aging body.

THE STRANGE ATTRACTORS OF DEVELOPMENTAL DISABILITY

The human body is a dynamic system with a high number of variables and many degrees of freedom. In the instance of DDs, one of the primary impairments is having one or more movement disorders. Along with having disturbances of postural tone, these individuals may have paralysis, hypotonia, ataxia, athetosis (or other dystonias), or spasticity. This disturbance in overall mobility sets in motion compensations within the body, which continue throughout life.

When looking at the management of activity limitations over the life span, one must consider the effect of abnormal forces, gravity, and ground-reaction forces over time. Normal movement development, which is characterized by effortless upright bipedal locomotion or normal upper body fine motor skills that are based on postural stability in the hips, trunk, and shoulder girdle muscles, is consistent with the development of a child not confronted with CNS damage. Once movement specialists begin to understand the interactions of the many subsystems involved in creating that picture of normal, a comprehension emerges of the challenges of aging with a DD. With many bodily functions designed around normal movement, a child with a DD is challenged from the start. For example, years of malaligned weight-bearing joints lead to bony changes and muscle imbalances causing pain and further disability. Similarly, disordered movement may disrupt other systems including circulatory, digestive, integumentary, skeletal, lymphatic, cardiopulmonary, urinary, and visual. By use of dynamic systems modeling, one can begin to predict disturbances within these systems before they are manifested clinically.

In the case of the circulatory system, it is fairly easy to conceptualize the effect of decreased mobility on fluid dynamics. Poor muscle contraction in the lower extremities coupled with mobility devices hold the lower extremities in an inactive dependent position. The venous return mechanism relies on contractive movement of muscular structures in the lower extremities for return blood flow. This process may be further disrupted after orthopedic surgery as a result of prolonged immobilization. This decrease in flow may continue for years without appropriate intervention. Without this activity, the body is forced to compensate or reorganize around a new set of control parameters (attractors). However, little is known about the long-term effects of these "attractors" on individuals with DDs. More studies are needed to investigate how these changes affect the individual's system over time. By better understanding the interaction of these changes, clinicians from all disciplines can more accurately identify current and potential problems, leading to improved preventive program planning. For example, if gravity and ground reaction forces lead to biomechanical changes in individuals with neuromuscular impairments, are there new methods of improving these changes earlier in life and avoiding future problems? Do these interventions alleviate or lessen further pathological conditions such as premature osteoarthritis? Specific parameters such as intensity, duration, and specificity of training need to be defined and clinical effectiveness established. This type of evidence-based practice would advance our understanding of neuromuscular disabilities and their impact on overall health throughout the life span.

MUSCULOSKELETAL MANAGEMENT

Box 29-1 lists the secondary conditions that may develop in an individual with cerebral palsy. The management of secondary musculoskeletal conditions in adolescents and adults with DDs is critical in preserving movement function. These impairment conditions not only cause pain but also limit mobility and interfere with performance of activities of daily living (ADLs) and leisure activities. Thus, a thorough evaluation of musculoskeletal status and periodic monitoring is imperative to maintaining quality of life and social participation for these individuals. Therapists are uniquely skilled to evaluate and design treatment interventions in conjunction with neurologists, orthopedists, physiatrists, and orthotists. Therapists' training in the areas of exercise, motor control, biomechanics, functional mobility, and pathokinesiology make their knowledge invaluable to individuals with developmental or other long-term chronic functional limitations.

BOX 29-1 ■ SECONDARY CONDITIONS DEVELOPED BY INDIVIDUALS WITH CEREBRAL PALSY

PATHOLOGICAL CONDITIONS
Fractures
Osteoporosis
Cardiovascular disorders
Degenerative joint disease
Spinal cord compression
Dental problems
Seizures
Pulmonary dysfunction

IMPAIRMENTS
Constipation
Contractures
Depression
Emaciation
Obesity
Incontinence (bowel and bladder)
Pain
Ulcers
Dysphagia
Gastrointestinal problems
Low self-esteem
Nerve entrapments
Overuse syndrome
Balance problems

FUNCTIONAL LIMITATIONS OR ACTIVITY RESTRICTIONS
Inability to indicate toileting needs
Dependency on others for ADLs
Limitations in mobility
Difficulties using public transportation

DISABILITIES OR LIMITATIONS IN LIFE PARTICIPATION
Difficulties living independently
Limited recreational opportunities
Problems with social relationships and intimacy
Social isolation
Difficulty with role as patient when medical professionals fail to make accommodations for treatment
Underemployment

Adapted from Gajdosik CG, Cicerello N: Secondary conditions of the musculoskeletal system in adolescents and adults with cerebral palsy, *Phys Occup Ther Pediatr* 21:49-68, 2001.

Several authors define secondary conditions as injuries, impairments, functional limitations, or disabilities that occur as a result of a primary condition or pathology.[7-12] Musculoskeletal problems account for many of these secondary conditions. Gajdosik and Cicerello[11] outlined numerous conditions that may affect the adult with cerebral palsy. Some are severe and can lead to significant loss in function and pain from complications such as fractures and osteoporosis. If this is further compounded by decreased sensation in the case of adults with neural tube defects, appropriate care may be delayed. The absence of any feedback/protective system such as pain may delay appropriate medical diagnosis, such as a urinary tract infection, and result in serious medical problems. Close monitoring by the adult individual, family members, and clinicians will help prevent these occurrences. Other musculoskeletal conditions, including scoliosis, subluxations, dislocations, patellae alta, foot deformities, pelvic obliquities, and contractures, further complicate the life progression of an adult with developmental disabilities.[11] Frequently, these chronic conditions may have their origins in childhood but, because of the lack of sensory awareness, may go undetected until later adolescence or adulthood when the body no longer has the ability to compensate for these abnormal biomechanical forces. Furthermore, as the aging process progresses, less regeneration of damaged tissue occurs leading to greater cumulative trauma in joints and other load sensitive structures.[12] Again, these conditions need to be closely monitored over time to ensure appropriate intervention optimizing an individual's function and minimizing damage to various tissues. Whenever possible, the client needs to participate in the decision making regarding goal setting and interventions to create the optimal environment for compliance.

Although these multiple concerns may be disconcerting to individuals and families, the environment can also be empowering from a prevention standpoint. Therapists and physicians should likewise be encouraged that, with early diagnosis of movement disorders and intervention, many of these functional limitations can be lessened or avoided altogether. By use of dynamic systems modeling, clinicians can be proactive by identifying parameters leading to pathokinesiological adaptations. With careful intervention and establishment of healthy lifestyles from an early age, individuals with DDs can lead healthy, rewarding lives with a life expectancy similar to that of the nondisabled population.

STRENGTH AND FITNESS

For much of the twentieth century, people with DDs were viewed through the lens of medicine as having active pathological conditions. Certainly, given the impairments, an individual may have medical intervention more frequently than in a nonmovement-impaired peer. However, to rely on this medical approach solely would prove inadequate to meet the complex needs of this unique population. As therapeutic procedures became based on motor control, motor learning, and neuroplasticity theories, strengthening spastic muscles may still be underused.[13,14] In the past, placing resistance on a spastic muscle was thought to increase the spasticity. This tenet was interpreted to preclude anyone from advocating strength training in these individuals.[13,15] Interestingly, the

literature identified that one of the major problems of cerebral palsy is weakness. Clinicians during the 1960s and 1970s believed that the answer to this weakness underlying spasticity was to increase proprioceptive and tactile stimulation.[13,15] Current research would say that true strengthening would not occur through feedback alone and resistance on muscle tissue was a necessary variable for strength training.[16-18] Damiano et al[19-22] have shown that resistance training does not affect spasticity negatively and, in fact, improves many functional measures of gait. On the basis of these findings, clinicians should evaluate individual patients to determine whether the level of weakness is affecting their functional performance or the attainment of personal goals. If indeed the individual's weakness is found to be clinically significant, then strength training is indicated. Strength training within functional patterns should lead to the greatest carryover.

For persons with abnormal biomechanical alignment resulting from spasticity, orthopedic deformation, or severe muscle imbalance, care must be taken to maintain proper alignment throughout the exercise. Additional positioning equipment may be required to assist the person in exercising independently. For example, persons with lower extremity spasticity frequently exhibit medial rotation of their femurs and bilateral pronation. Combined with asymmetrical patterns of weakness and tightness, a squatting motion produces an excessive valgus angle at the knee. By ensuring satisfactory alignment throughout the arc of motion, the efficacy of the exercise is improved. Conversely, without this attention to biomechanical alignment, these imbalances and deformities can be exacerbated. In some instances, persons with disabilities may need help from another person. Unfortunately, many fitness professionals lack knowledge of specific conditions and the unique challenges they present. In this area, physical and occupational therapists may be valuable as consultants to provide information and monitoring services for adolescents and adults with DDs and running exercise programs for the elderly.

Another factor that therapists need to consider is accessibility of exercise equipment for persons with limited mobility. Many manufacturers are beginning to consider this in the design of their products. As research supports fitness training for persons with DDs, more effort will be needed to maximize the availability of community-based facilities to meet the demand. Again, therapists can be instrumental in not only designing this equipment but advocating for their patients by educating governmental officials in the needs of those aging with DDs.

Today, adults with DDs have more of an opportunity to participate in sporting events and recreational activities. Therapists need to be involved in the process to ensure optimum benefit of these activities for clients to not only be successful but also be safe. Therapists not only possess the knowledge of the physiological affects of exercise but also understand biomechanical principles critical to ensuring safety in these activities. Therapists can work with these individuals on maximizing strength, flexibility, body mass indices, and cardiorespiratory reserves. This focus will not only increase functional capacity and social participation of the adult with functional limitations but will lower the risk of medical comorbidities associated with lower values in these four areas (Case Study 29-1).

CASE STUDY 29-1 ■ SPASTIC HEMIPLAGIC CEREBRAL PALSY: USE OF ADAPTIVE EQUIPMENT

B. S. is an 18-year-old man with left spastic hemiplegic cerebral palsy who is a high school senior preparing to begin university studies. While in high school, he was a member of the cross-country team (Figure 29-1). His orthopedic surgeon referred him at the request of his hand therapist to work on strengthening as it pertained to ADL performance. He was noted to have strong flexion synergy in his left upper extremity with limited hand function. He was "encouraged" to make a list of tasks he was unable to perform independently so preparations could be made for college. Although he was able to run with his cross-country teammates, B. S. had significant biomechanical challenges in his left lower extremity. Diffuse weakness was noted in the hip flexors and gluteals, including significant weakness of the left gluteus medius. This pattern of weakness caused excessive medial rotation of the left femur. He displayed left pronation with a secondary hallux valgus position and premature bunion formation. The left knee was in a valgus position with weakness of quadriceps, hamstrings, gastrocnemius/soleus complex, tibialis anterior intrinsics of the foot peroneals, and to a lesser degree, the adductors. His lower extremity spasticity, which measured 2/4 on the modified Ashworth Scale, was located in the hamstrings, adductors, and the gastrocnemius/soleus on the left.

Gait analysis revealed mild (<30 degree) spinal flexion with left shoulder flexion, internal rotation, and adduction. The elbow was flexed approximately 70 degrees with pronation of the forearm and flexion at the wrist. B. S. had decreased step length on the left with poor active hip flexion substituting lumbar flexion with a posterior pelvic tilt to advance the left lower extremity. As a consequence of the weak quadriceps and spastic (and weak) hamstrings, there was approximately 35-degree left knee flexion at midstance with little active push off on the left, again as a result of gastrocnemius/soleus weakness.

B. S.'s left hand function was severely limited, with a weak and inefficient prehensile grasp with the adducted thumb and forefinger. Figure 29-2 illustrates how an orthotic electroneuromuscular stimulator can be used to assist and teach B. S. to use his left hand as an assist to his right.

B. S. was highly motivated and looking forward to college. Discussions centered on ADL function allowing him to be independent, including shoe tying, tying a tie, fastening buttons and other fasteners, and typing.

Further, we spoke with B. S. regarding strengthening, flexibility, and cardiorespiratory function to both make his mobility faster and more efficient and identify areas that were vulnerable to degenerative changes such as the lumbar spine, left hip, left knee, and foot. Given the constant hinging of the lumbar spine during gait, over time stenotic and discal changes may create painful situations.[23]

It is of note that B. S. was very adept in identifying functional limitations but neither he, his family, nor other health care providers had discussed biomechanical issues in terms of secondary conditions associated with cerebral palsy.[8-10,23] Therapists can be invaluable to families by identifying potential problems before they happen and addressing these areas. Future research is necessary to guide therapists regarding how to best advise families.

B. S.'s treatment plan was designed around his high school schedule. He received instruction in stretching the tightened structure and techniques to self-mobilize his hip. His parents were also taught various techniques. Strengthening focused on the spine and posterior shoulder girdle on the left, triceps, hand and forearm, and abdominals including transversus abdominis, gluteals, quadriceps, hamstrings, and foot and ankle structures. Bilateral orthotics were obtained to improve the biomechanical position of both feet.

Partial body-weight supported treadmill training (PSBWSTT) with approximately 50 pound unloading allowed for aerobic training while mechanical forces were controlled on various joints. This type of gait training has been widely used by individuals with cerebral palsy. Frequently, they report decreased pain with improved fluidity of movement, which carries over after treatment.[24]

B. S. was also referred to an assistive technology center to inquire about voice-activated computer software. Although he had mild dysarthria with glossal spasticity, he was able to successfully use the software. He had been typing his high school assignments, which took excessive time and prevented him from having time in other areas of his life.

Providing assistive techniques to empower a person to greater independence is a critical point in working with persons with DDs and their families (Figure 29-3). Daily skills are arduous and time consuming, robbing people with disabilities of large portions of their life span while simultaneously placing unnecessary stress on their physical structures. As society struggles with how to best increase the participation of persons with DDs within their respective communities, scientific innovations designed to increase efficiency with these individuals will be needed. Attention needs to be given toward designing creative ways to incorporate people with DDs into the workforce and into the political process. Despite the passage of the Americans with Disabilities Act in 1990, concepts such as "reasonable accommodation" create anxiety for many employers.[25]

Therapists need to consider physical, attitudinal, and social obstacles when working with this population and look

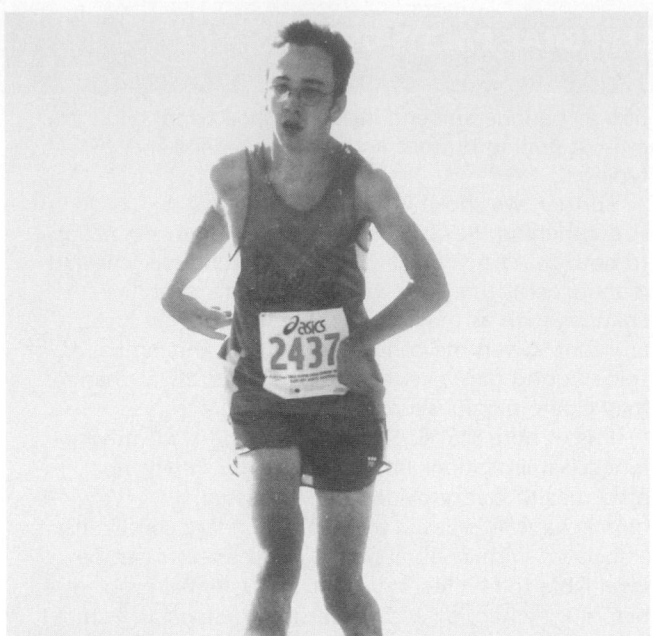

FIGURE 29-1 ■ Adolescent with cerebral palsy running cross-country with high school track team.

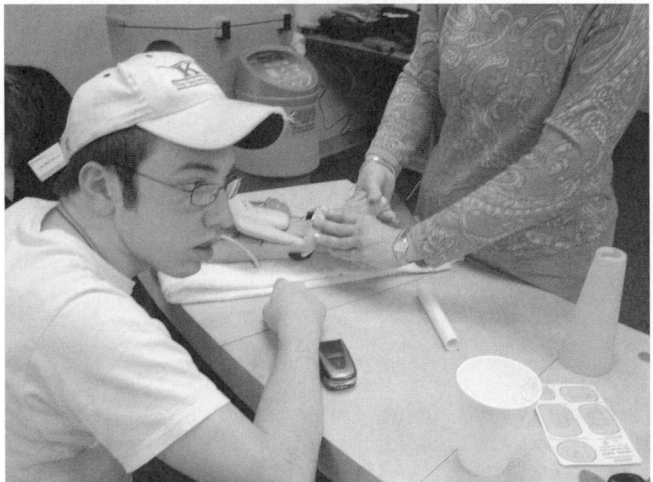

FIGURE 29-2 ■ Adult with spastic cerebral palsy wearing Bioness H200 neuromuscular hand splint using electrical stimulation to improve left hand functioning as a helper.

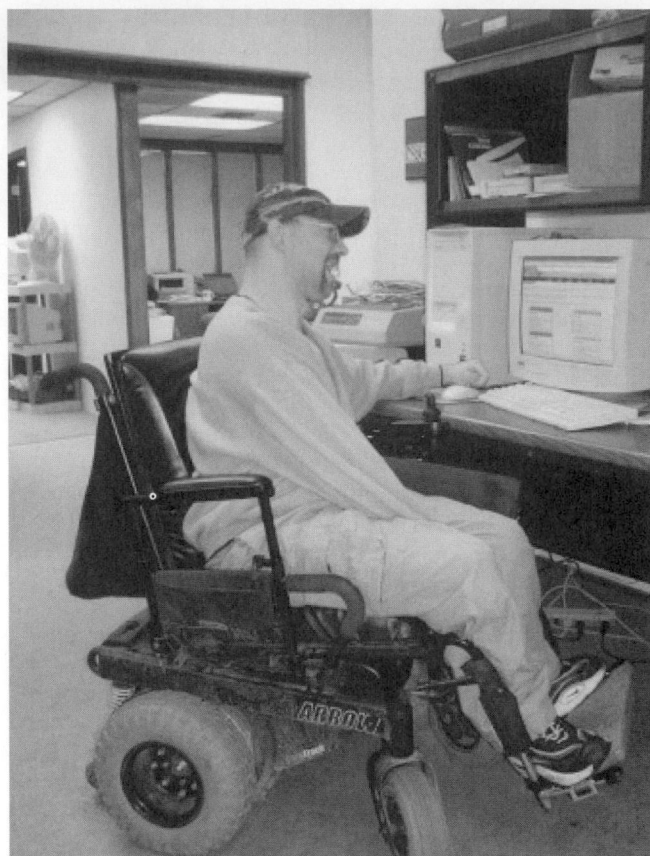

FIGURE 29-3 ■ Man with athetoid cerebral palsy working at his computer. His power chair has been modified with a back support and a seat cushion for proper positioning.

for ways to help them reclaim time and effort in the day. Therapists will need to use, and be instrumental in the development of, technology that can assist the individual with a DD. Only with the assistance of the scientific communities, the resolve of the political bodies, and the effort of dedicated professional clinicians and teachers, can the person with a DD lead a more productive and rewarding life, not only into young adulthood but also into middle age and beyond.

PAIN MANAGEMENT

Many types of DDs have a component of disordered movement from hypomobility in the case of spastic cerebral palsy to hypermobility in the case of Down syndrome. These abnormal joint stresses and strains cause long-term damage

to the musculoskeletal system.[4,11,26] Frequently, therapists will attempt to lessen these stresses through behavior programs designed to prevent such things as W sitting. One initial problem is that in a young, developing body these biomechanical misalignments are not painful and are more functionally stable given decreased muscle strength and control. The concept of future joint pain is abstract, which is difficult for both the family and the child to grasp, especially if the child is also cognitively impaired. Individuals with movement disorders resulting from DDs have fewer options when choosing movement patterns. In the case of W sitting, children need better options than long sitting, tailor sitting, or side sitting. Therapists need to work with the family and child on discovering effective choices to minimize long-term wear on joint structures.

Knowing that a natural degradation of joint structures with aging and weakness and abnormal ground reaction forces leads to higher incidence of musculoskeletal pain,[16,22,27] therapists should play a vital role in helping persons with DDs maintain their functional ability. These fundamental skills are critical in terms of fulfilling an individual's family and social responsibilities, which in turn leads to improved self-esteem. Community-dwelling participants have been shown to have a higher self-esteem than individuals never attaining that independence, although many do not described themselves as successful.[16] These dissonant findings suggest that this group of adults, although

CASE STUDY 29-2 ■ SPASTIC DIPLEGIC CEREBRAL PALSY: INTERVENTION USING BODY WEIGHT–SUPPORTED TREADMILL TRAINING

C. W. is a 54-year-old man with spastic diplegic cerebral palsy. He worked for many years in the automotive service industry until his mobility in his lower extremities and spine made it too difficult for him to continue. C. W. subsequently was legally classified as fully disabled. He was referred to physical therapy to regain as much mobility as possible. On initial evaluation, C. W. was found to be significantly obese with much of his excess weight distributed around the abdomen. He had severe limitations in overall hip mobility that dramatically affected his gait pattern. He was, however, ambulatory without an assistive device. Another of C. W.'s major complaints was consistent low back pain. Because of his weight gain, he had developed an increased lumbar lordosis and weakened abdominal muscles from overstretching. C. W. was also a moderately heavy smoker, which decreased his energy reserves and increased his back pain. The situation was further complicated by C. W.'s decreased mobility, preventing him from exercising effectively and aerobically to improve his fitness level. C. W. had good upper body strength and was motivated to work to the best of his ability. He was referred to a smoking cessation program as well.

Given his biomechanical concerns and his back pain, C. W. was started on a program of joint and soft tissue mobilization to maximize his available range of motion apart from any contractures. His spasticity was a 2 to 3 over 4 on the modified Ashworth scale and physical therapy worked with his medical team on oral control. Discussions also took place regarding intrathecal baclofen therapy; however, C. W. was reluctant to pursue this option.

He was started on PBWSTT with low back pain relief at 60 pounds of unloading. C. W. was then able to increase his treadmill ambulation by 15 to 20 minutes with lasting relief from his back pain and decreased perceived exertion. C. W. improved his community ambulation and overall endurance. He was also referred to a clinical dietician for nutrition counseling. Because he was on a fixed income, efforts were made to transition him from a traditional therapy model of care to a community fitness center to continue his progress. This met with resistance from a variety of government agencies that were restrictive in their allocations for services. However, progress in being made through NCPAD[28] as well as other advocacy programs around the country.

---

overall feeling positive about themselves, also feel many things have been left undone (Case Study 29-2).

SPASTICITY MANAGEMENT

One of the most emphasized areas in working with children and adults with upper motor neuron symptoms is spasticity management. Because the mechanism of spasticity lies in the CNS, it is inadvertently protected by the blood-brain barrier. Thus, oral medications remain marginally efficacious because of their difficulty crossing this protective barrier. In addition, because of their systemic nature, they can cause a variety of adverse effects. Of these, the most common is sedation.[29,30] For oral baclofen, diazepam, tizanadine, and dantrolene sodium, this is the dose-limiting factor. However, this does not mean that these medications are of no value. Indeed, for many persons with spasticity who are having pain with splints, positioning devices, spasms, or decreased mobility, the effects of these medications can be important (see Chapter 36).

Injection therapies such as botulinum toxin, are effective in treating focal spasticity and last 3 to 6 months before further injections are needed. Other preparations administered by injection include ethyl alcohol phenol. These chemicals reduce spasticity by neurolysis (denaturing proteins, causing tissue necrosis).[29] This frequently extends the efficacy of treatment by several months; however, it can have several unintended and significant adverse effects. These adverse effects include permanent peripheral nerve palsies, skin irritation; acute intoxication, painful necrosis of the muscle, chronic dysesthesia, vascular complications, sloughing of the skin, excessive motor weakness, permanent

sensory loss, and systemic side effects, including tremor, convulsions, CNS depression, and cardiovascular collapse.[30] Again, although many of the effects are rare, clinicians need to stay abreast of complicating factors that their patients may experience.

The most innovative method for dealing with the blood-brain barrier problem has been the development of continuous infusion techniques. For example, through the use of the Medtronic (Minneapolis, Minn.) intrathecal baclofen pump, baclofen is stored in a reservoir in a surgically implanted pump that then administers the medication directly into the cerebrospinal fluid. Because of this direct infusion, the dosages are reduced from milligrams to micrograms while efficacy is increased and side effects are decreased.[31]

As with all treatments for spasticity, a team approach with a clear delineation of the treatment(s), their effects and rehabilitation requirements is crucial for maximizing outcomes. Once again, this necessitates a team approach, including the individual with a disability. Determining the best treatment option, the expected outcome, and the need for further rehabilitation provides the best opportunities for functional use of the decrease in spasticity. For example, the use of intrathecal baclofen to reduce spasticity not only reveals the underlying weakness but also may cause increased weakness as well.[32] Thus, a strengthening program should be implemented as the effective dose is titrated to maximize the individual's function (Case Study 29-3).

MEDICAL/DENTAL CONCERNS

Therapists often see people with DDs more frequently than other health care professionals do. For this reason, a

CASE STUDY 29-3 ■ SPASTIC DIPLEGIC CEREBRAL PALSY: KEY FACTORS IN TREATMENT PLANNING

D. R. is a 22-year-old man with spastic diplegic cerebral palsy. He lives with his mother, father, and teenage brother in a supportive environment in which he is home schooled. The parents state that D. R. ambulated with a rolling walker until the age of 13 years. At that time, D. R. and his family judged the energy expense too high.

A physical therapist assisted the family in obtaining an ultralightweight sports-type wheelchair. He soon became independent with this in community settings and his overall mobility and participation in social outings improved as well.

By age 21 years, D. R. no longer had the ability to stand or ambulate for short distances, which concerned him. He was evaluated by a neurosurgeon who then placed him on intrathecal baclofen pump. He subsequently was followed up by a physiatrist for titration of the pump. The neurosurgeon also referred D. R. to physical therapy.

An initial examination revealed that D. R. had a 60-degree soft tissue contracture of both hamstrings (90 degrees against gravity) and 25 degrees at the hip flexors. The adductors were also shortened with severe weakness of the major muscle groups of the lower extremities. D. R. had no orthotics and both feet were severely pronated.

His intrathecal baclofen was titrated; however, minimal gains were made in passive ROM. By use of the modified Tardieu scale,[33,34] it was determined that D. R.'s problem was contracture versus spasticity. Weakness was also problematic; however, because of limited ROM, effective strengthening was difficult to perform.

D. R. and his family were referred to an orthopedic surgeon to improve his lower extremity biomechanics but declined. After realizing that significant functional improvement would be extremely difficult even with orthopedic intervention, D. R. chose to forego his standing goal in favor of wheelchair mobility.

This case illustrates the importance of several key factors in establishing an effective treatment plan for an adult with a DD.

First, it must begin in childhood. Health care providers need to be forward thinking prognosticators. For example, the wheelchair was a reasonable intervention. But at the time, D. R.'s spasticity was poorly managed and no standing and walking program was communicated to the family. Eight years in primarily a 90/90 hip and knee position allows for a significant amount of soft tissue shortening. Second, effective treatments applied at the incorrect time cease to be effective. Again, had the baclofen pump been implanted in early adolescence, D. R.'s outcome may have been different. As it was, he became a wheelchair user at 13 years when hamstrings are frequently at their tightest. Last, the team needs to communicate more effectively. In D. R.'s case, he went to providers who offered advice contained solely in their area of expertise. Without being part of a larger, coordinated plan, these individual strategies address only subsystems within a highly dynamic system and fall short of affecting system-wide behavioral change—in D. R.'s case, upright stance.

---

thorough examination including a detailed history including medications can be helpful to the person with the DD, the family, and other caregivers. As part of the evaluation, oral motor function is an important component in terms of sensation, speech, and swallowing. Particularly dysphagia and aspiration potential need to be carefully assessed because of its prevalence in people with DD. As a result of disturbances in muscle tone, these individuals often have difficulty with feeding, which may lead to serious medical complications and potential death. Recent advances in treatment including deep pharyngeal neuromuscular stimulation and neuromuscular electrical stimulation offer persons with poor motor control and weakness in pharyngeal musculature opportunities to improve safe oral feeding[2] (Figure 29-4). This is important because the ability to ingest food has been identified as a factor affecting the life expectancy of persons with cerebral palsy. The team of physicians and therapists need to work together to identify potential problems and establish a treatment plan. Dentition should also be noted with appropriate referral when indicated.

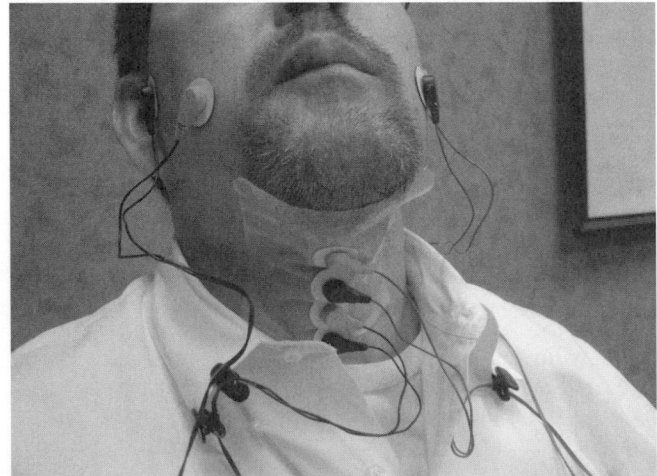

FIGURE 29-4 ■ Man with spastic cerebral palsy receiving neuromuscular electrical stimulation for facial and pharyngeal activation to improve swallowing and motor control in face.

Adults with DDs that have both motor and cognitive impairments often have increased difficulty maintaining good oral health through daily hygiene. Not only are there sensory concerns, but because of craniofacial abnormalities (Down syndrome, bruxism, malocclusion from tongue thrusting, increased mouth breathing, and finger sucking), additional secondary problems develop. Anticonvulsant medication may cause gingival hyperplasia that can lead to poor overall health of adults with DDs as a result of infection, poor nutritional status, and further social complications.

With the advent of deinstitutionalization, many more individuals with DDs have greater access to dental care in their communities. However, most predoctoral dental schools offer little education in the area of working with persons with DDs.[35,36] Special Olympics International began a program called "Special Smiles" to assist in training professionals in working with this population. They also have programs of a similar nature in orthopedics, nutrition, optometry, and physical/occupational therapy.

Therapists working with this population can be helpful in identifying problems not only with strategies for improving oral hygiene, such as desensitizing oral structures to make routine care more tolerable, but also through improving oral motor biomechanics as in the case of mandibular retraction in cerebral palsy. Another area in which therapists can be useful is as consultants to their community dental practices in terms of physical layout of the practice and positioning equipment to allow for increased comfort of the person with a DD and optimal positioning of the client for various dental procedures.

Spasticity management, familiar to both occupational and physical therapists, creates a unique expertise that can prove useful to dental professionals. For example, most dental professionals are used to asking the client to relax the tongue and move it toward the opposite side. Unfortunately, excessive effort often increases the stress and subsequently the muscle tone in the tongue. As the requests become louder and more insistent, one can see the vicious cycle emerge. By using some simple techniques learned from therapists, dental professionals will have better understanding and success when working with this population of individuals with DDs.

Behavioral management was once a limiting factor in providing comprehensive dental care.[35,37,38] Again, therapists can be an invaluable resource to dental professionals with environmental modifications and other calming strategies that will minimize the stress on the adult with a DD (Case Study 29-4).

CASE STUDY 29-4 ■ DOWN SYNDROME, TRISOMY 21: MAINTAINING FUNCTIONAL STATUS

R. D. is a 40-year-old man with Down syndrome, trisomy 21. He currently lives with his wife (of 8 months) in a two-bedroom house. They have 24-hour assistance on call because of his wife's seizure disorder. R. D. is ambulatory without an assistive device. He does require significant additional time to perform daily activities because of cognitive impairments and back pain.

R. D. is currently training at two jobs in the food industry (Figure 29-5). He performs inventory stocking and clean-up but would like to progress to food preparation. His family is involved in his care, keeping detailed records. From 1987 to 2004, R. D. had five dental appointments for various extractions with full extraction in June 2004. R. D. currently has full dentures. Medical history includes right Perthes disease with a Pemberton osteotomy performed in 1969, appendectomy, tonsillectomy, and cholecystectomy. R. D. has also had thermal injuries to his hands and ankles with no residual effects. He has struggled to maintain his weight throughout his life, with his highest recorded weight being 213 pounds. He is approximately 5'1" tall. R. D.'s I.Q. has been measured to be 56. He states that his learning difficulties and the slowness of processing are significant frustrations as well as his severe dysarthria. He augments his communication by signing. Current medications include those for hypothyroidism, reflux, insomnia, asthma, and seasonal allergies. R. D. states

that he and his wife have had to sacrifice privacy for safety by having a curtain on their bedroom entrance as opposed to a door. This fact, while affecting privacy, also provides some peace of mind for the couple. His primary hobby is bowling and he competes regularly in Special Olympics and in a community bowling league.[39] R. D. also enjoys fishing and occasionally golf. Another frustration is his inability to drive, making him more dependent on others as well as decreasing his overall leisure time. R. D. must factor in other schedules into his day because of limited public transportation in his community.

In terms of pain, R. D. reports cervical pain at C-7 (with no atlantoaxial instability) and lumbar pain when carrying heavy loads in front of him. He does report frequent exercise at home with a stationary bicycle with reciprocating handlebars.

Although R. D. is doing quite well overall, there are some areas in which consultation from a therapist would be helpful. Coordination with his job coach on biomechanics and ergonomics with a lumbar support at work may be beneficial. Also, orthotics therapy do not only control supination but also alleviate his pelvic obliquity stemming from his right hip osteotomy would ease some soft tissue strain and improve his stability as well. Most obvious, however, would be development of a realistic daily exercise program to target core strengthening and spinal stabilization to lessen his spinal pain.

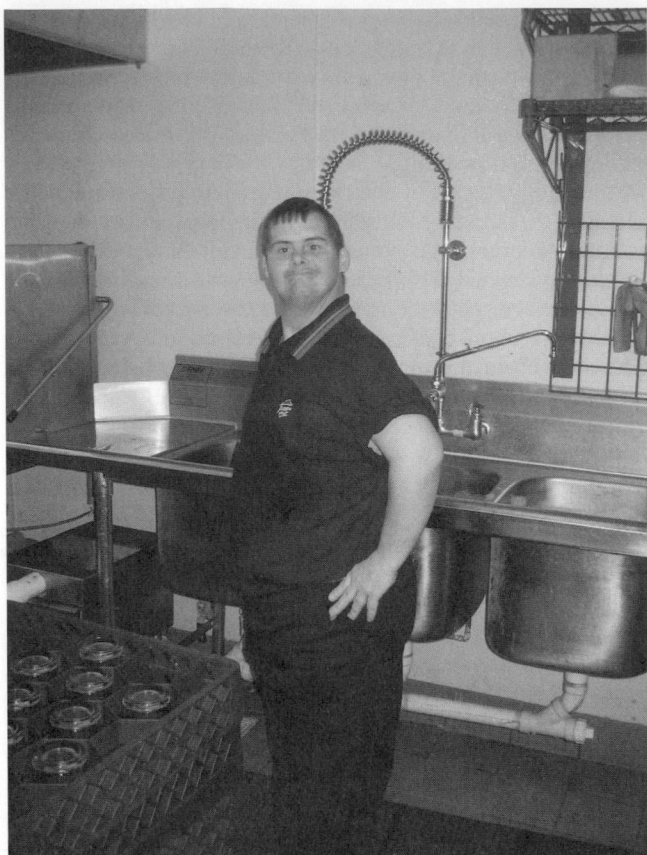

FIGURE 29-5 ■ Man with Down syndrome at one of his jobs. A lumbar support was recommended to help stabilize his spine during lifting and spinal stabilization exercises.

SECTION II
THE CHALLENGES OF THE LATE EFFECTS OF POLIO: POSTPOLIO SYNDROME
Myla U. Quiben, DPT, PT, GCS, NCS

OVERVIEW

Acute poliomyelitis, once a widely feared disease, has become a largely unknown medical entity, with current generations relating polio to vaccination. Although the war against polio has been largely successful, individuals who have seemingly conquered polio and are entering their mid to later years are now facing a new adversary in the form of new impairments hypothesized to be related to the initial infection. With these puzzling myriad of symptoms, individuals with the earlier medical diagnosis of polio face the possibility of losing their functional abilities and independence. The appearance of these late effects of polio, commonly known as postpolio syndrome (PPS), is a challenge for health care professionals who are responsible for understanding the complex processes and implications for an aging population of polio survivors.

In the realm of care for chronic disabilities, polio promises an enlightening example of the unique interaction among neurological and functional impairment, recovery, effects of aging, and health care. As a chronic condition, it can teach as much to reconsider our approach to individuals with activity limitations, impairments, ineffective postures and movements, and participation restrictions from chronic disease.

ACUTE POLIOMYELITIS

Poliomyelitis is a highly contagious disease caused by a small enterovirus that enters the body through the mouth. The primary symptoms of infection include headache, vomiting, fatigue, neck stiffness, sore throat, severe muscle pain, and flaccid paralysis or paresis. Spencer[40,41] outlined the specific symptoms of severe life-threatening poliomyelitis.

In most cases, the poliovirus is destroyed in the stomach or excreted through the intestinal tract without clinical manifestations. In some cases, the virus enters the bloodstream, produces flulike symptoms with recovery, minimal residual deficits, and development of immunity. In such cases, individuals are diagnosed with nonparalytic poliomyelitis. It is estimated that 10% to 15% of people who thought or were told they had polio did not, and many people with mild weaknesses were diagnosed as nonparalytic.[40,42,43]

The other clinical picture involves virus crossing the blood-brain barrier, where the functional consequence relates to primary destruction of specific cells in the brain, spinal cord, and brain stem. The distinctive characteristic of the poliovirus is its predilection for the motor nerve cells or motor neurons. Primarily affecting the nervous system with accuracy, the poliovirus attacks the anterior motor neurons while leaving intact adjacent cells that control sensation, sex, and bowel and bladder functions. During the 2 weeks of febrile illness, various motor neurons are infected and eventually destroyed while others fight off the virus and recover. Bodian[44] found that only 4% of the anterior horn cells were histologically normal at 2 to 6 days after onset, and by 14 days after onset the motor neurons were either destroyed or apparently normal in appearance. Clinically, there was no definitive distinction between normal muscle strength and slight muscle weakness. Historically, several individuals with mild paralytic poliomyelitis were reportedly diagnosed with nonparalytic polio.

Epidemics that swept across North America and Europe occurred from 1910 to 1959, with a major epidemic in New York in 1921 with a recorded 9,000 cases and 2,000 deaths.[44a] In 1937, then U.S. President Franklin D. Roosevelt, who contracted polio, formed the March of Dimes (National Foundation for Infantile Paralysis) to support the education, research, and campaign against polio. The introduction of inactivated vaccine by Salk in 1955 and live attenuated oral vaccine by Sabin in 1960 marked milestones in the fight against polio. The Global Polio Eradication Initiative spearheaded by the World Health Organization (WHO) targeted the eradication of poliovirus from the world by the end of 2000. Reported polio cases had dramatically dropped worldwide. WHO now identifies only six countries as polio endemic.[45] A poliomyelitis epidemic in 2002 with 407 new cases in India[45] emphasizes the need for continued vigilance in the face of difficulties in eradicating this disease. The goal of a poliofree world was initially moved to the end of 2005, highlighting the challenges in the fight against polio.[46] The considerable progress toward polio eradication made in 2005, along with new vaccines to combat the disease, have refocused antipolio efforts toward the final phase to meet the Global Polio Eradication Strategic Plan (2004-2008).[47]

Although polio cases still present in a smaller scale, it seems to have taken a back seat as a primary concern as medicine and health care faced newer diseases and disabilities.

Statistics from WHO indicate that approximately 20 million people worldwide have survived poliomyelitis with some degree of disability.[46]

An accurate number of individuals who had poliomyelitis is unavailable and most likely never will be available[42] because no national registry exists for individuals diagnosed with poliomyelitis. In a random survey of the U.S. population in 1987 from the National Center for Health Statistics, 1.63 million polio survivors were estimated.[42,48] Of this figure, Halstead[49] approximates the current number of survivors with paralytic polio at 600,000, with nonparalytic polio at 883,000, and the remaining of undetermined diagnosis. Of these estimates, an indeterminate percentage is at risk for the development of new, late symptoms of polio or may eventually demonstrate late effects of polio.

PHYSIOLOGICAL PROCESSES OF RECOVERY OF MUSCLE STRENGTH

The degree of initial paralysis or paresis is unpredictable and variable. During the 2 weeks of febrile illness a motor neuron, innervating 5 to 1,500 muscle fibers, could be unaffected, recovered, or destroyed with resulting denervation of the muscle fibers (Figure 29-6). The 100 to 1,000 motor neurons to a specific muscle may be unaffected or recovered; all the motor neurons to a muscle may be destroyed; or the muscle could be partially denervated with combinations of recovered and destroyed motor neurons. Fibrillation potentials from diagnostic electromyography (EMG) at this time would indicate recent denervation of muscle fibers.

Recovery is a continuing process of remodeling of motor units consisting of both denervation and reinnervation that eventually allows that the motor units reach a steady state of muscle strength. In convalescent poliomyelitis, muscle strength in partially denervated muscles increased to a maximum over a 2-year period, with 50% of the muscle strength recovery occurring in the first 3 months after onset and 75% in the first 6 months (Figure 29-7). The rate and magnitude of the recovery, however, could be compromised by misguided treatment, overactivity, and excessive exercise.[40,41,50,51] Muscle strength recovery and increase in functional ability occurred through the following four physiological processes:

1. Recovered neurons develop terminal axon sprouts to reinnervate orphaned muscle fibers[49,52-54] (see Figure 29-6). The growth of axon sprouts may be the body's response to maintain as many muscle cells functioning as possible. A single motor neuron is estimated to reinnervate up to five or more times its normal complement of muscle fibers, creating giant motor units. These extremely enlarged motor units enable fewer motor neurons to accomplish the work of many. Electromyographically, the action potentials of the single motor units are polyphasic with large amplitudes.

2. Innervated muscle fibers can be hypertrophied by intensive exercise and activity during the rehabilitation phase. This increase in muscle fiber size has been referred to as denervation hypertrophy.

3. Increased functional ability by neuromuscular learning whereby practice of an exercise or an activity leads to increased skill and performance without necessarily increasing muscle strength.[55]

4. Increased recruitment of the giant motor units for the task with use of the muscles at high levels of their already reduced capacity.

The profound neurological deficits caused by the disease are masked by such extensive compensatory physiological

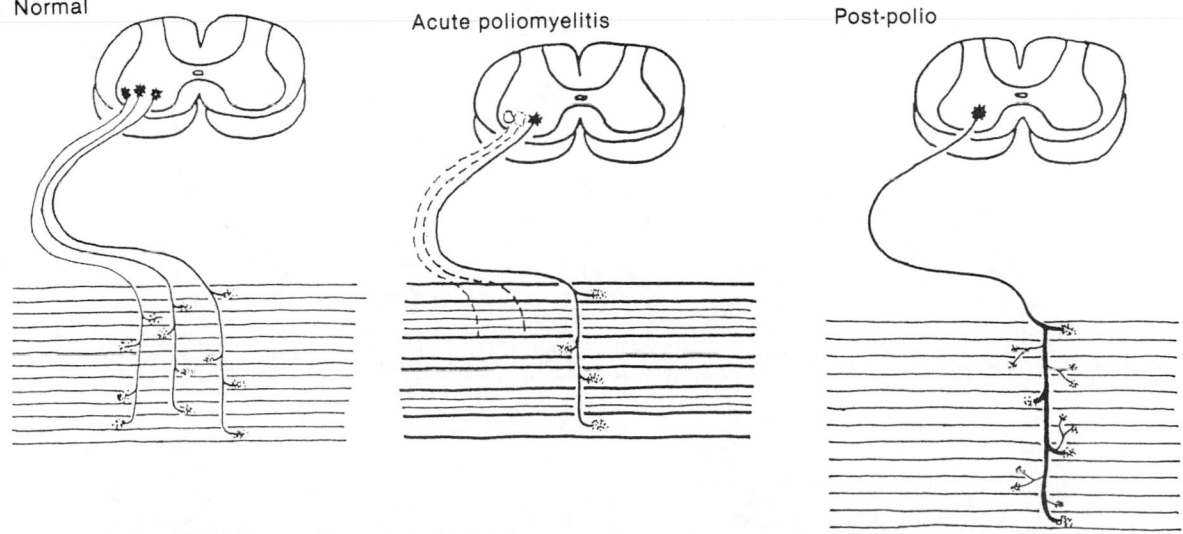

FIGURE 29-6 ■ Schematic representation of motor units to a muscle. *Normal* represents the 100 to 1,000 motor neurons of a muscle and the 5 to 1,500 muscle fibers each axon innervates. *Acute poliomyelitis* depicts viral destruction of some of the anterior horn cells with atrophy of denervated muscle fibers. *Postpolio* represents axon sprouting by recovered nerve cells with reinnervation of the orphaned muscle fibers and subsequent hypertrophy.

Percent chance of severely involved muscles recovering to "good" or "normal" eventual strength:

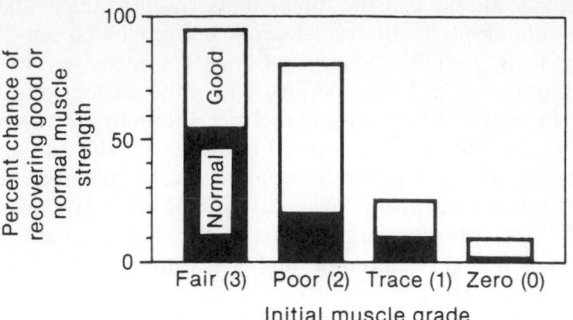

Rate of muscle recovery irrespective of the initial or final strength:

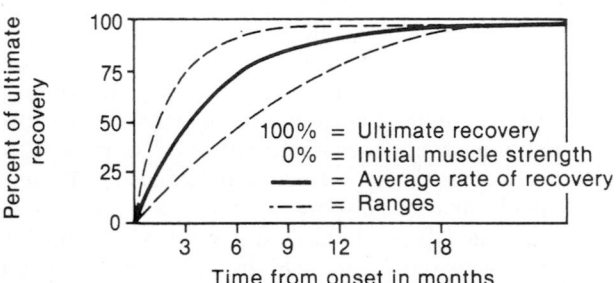

FIGURE 29-7 ■ The rate and extent of increase in manual muscle test scores in postacute poliomyelitis. Muscles showing some strength on initial examination will increase in strength unless they are overworked, in which case they may plateau or lose strength. The grade of Normal (5) is a clinical definition, not an indication of preillness strength. This grade can be recorded with loss of 60% of the anterior horn cells to a muscle. (Adapted from Spencer WA: *Treatment of acute poliomyelitis,* Springfield, IL, 1956, Charles C Thomas.)

processes. Sharrard[56] demonstrated this by counting the number of anterior horn cells for each muscle in the spinal cord of postpolio survivors who eventually died of other causes. He compared the percentage of cells present with previous manual muscle test grades in a scale of 0 to 5. Muscles graded 5 (normal) could have lost up to 60% of their anterior horn cells; muscles previously graded 4 (good) had lost 60% to 90% of their motor neurons; and muscles of grades 3 to 1 (fair, poor, or trace) lost 90% to 98%. It is truly remarkable how much polio survivors accomplished with so few motor units.

EARLY MANAGEMENT AND COMPENSATORY METHODS

Several individuals who recovered from polio during the early epidemics were encouraged to exercise for years and to use heroic compensatory methods for function. An exhaustive regimen of daily stretching and strengthening demanding compliance from individuals, and their support systems were strongly encouraged. Orthotics and assistive devices were promoted as a means toward independent mobility. The outcomes of rigorous training were individuals who adapted and compensated with their remaining capabilities. Compensations include use of muscles at high levels of their capacity, substitution of stronger muscles with increased energy expenditure for the task, use of ligaments for stability with resulting hypermobility, and malalignment of the trunk and limbs.

Figure 29-8 shows a boy diagnosed with acute poliomyelitis who appears to have a flail right lower extremity with nonfunctional muscle test grades of 3 (fair) to 0 and functional muscle strength of 5 (normal) or 4 (good) in the rest of his body. Walking shows excessive vertical and lateral movements of the center of gravity, and disproportionate movements of the upper extremities and lower extremities leading to abnormally high energy expenditure for the task.

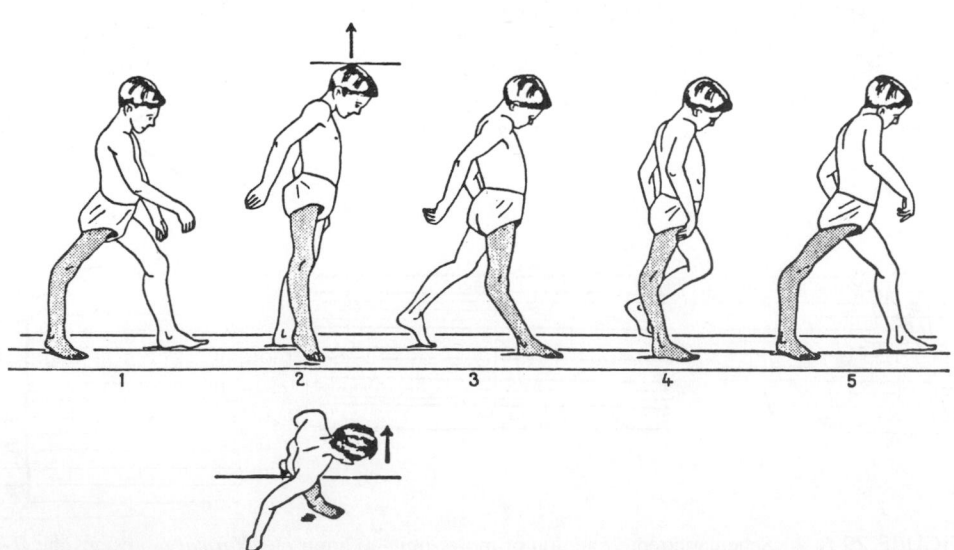

FIGURE 29-8 ■ The functional compensations of a boy with paralysis of the right lower extremity show increased energy expenditure and progressive ligamentous laxity. (Adapted from Ducroquet R, Darroquet J, Darroquet P: *Walking and limping—a study of normal and pathological salking,* Philadelphia, 1968, JB Lippincott.)

LATE EFFECTS OF POLIO, PPS

The historical epidemics of polio primarily infected children and adolescents, who are now entering their later years. With recovery from the symptoms and adaptation to deficits from the viral infection, individuals believed that their major challenges were behind them. For several years, most of these individuals lived active, healthy, and productive lives and careers.

However, in the 1970s and 1980s, some individuals with secondary disabilities stemming from the previous polio diagnosis started to experience new weakness, fatigue, and pain. Most of them turned to exercise programs only to find that they were not getting stronger but rather weaker and more fatigued. Literature has used the terms *late effects of polio, polio sequelae,* and more commonly *PPS* to describe the incidence of new symptoms. PPS is a clinical neurological syndrome that describes these new, late symptoms of weakness, fatigue, and pain in survivors of acute paralytic poliomyelitis.[42,49,52,57]

The estimates of individuals with new late manifestations of PPS vary in literature, with estimates in literature ranging from 28.5% to as high as 64% of polio survivors.[48,58,59] The final estimate of approximately 20% to 40% of individuals with PPS by Halstead and Naierman[59a] excluded individuals with a history of nonparalytic polio.[60] However, several individuals presenting with symptoms of PPS have no clear history of paralytic disease.[61] As such, Halstead recently stated that the diagnostic criteria for PPS should be modified to include a history of remote polio or findings in history, physical examination results, and laboratory studies compatible with polio damage of the CNS.[61]

It can be inferred from these recent changes that eventually an uncertain proportion of individuals with nonparalytic polio may in time present with PPS. Because there has been no attempt by organizations or institutions to gather accurate statistics on the number of polio survivors[60] on a worldwide basis or regional level, we are potentially facing a major health care challenge as more postpolio survivors continue to age.

An understanding of the issues involved with late effects of polio is necessary as individuals with new problems are seen for therapy. A paradigm shift from a purely medical approach to a functional rehabilitation approach that incorporates the individual's goals and quality of life is necessary in the attempt to help individuals with chronic conditions manage their problems.

SYMPTOMS

The most common late-onset symptoms catalogued by authors include such general complaints as fatigue, musculoskeletal manifestations such as muscle and joint pain, and neurological manifestations such as new weakness in previously affected or clinically unaffected muscle groups. Cold intolerance is a frequently reported symptom.[54,62] Other symptoms include breathing problems, sleep disorders, muscle cramps and fasciculations, muscle atrophy, swallowing difficulties, and hypoventilation. Most of the symptoms occur together, leading to new or increased difficulties in ADLs and physical mobility. These symptoms appear after a long period of neurological and functional stability after recovery from the acute polio infection.

TABLE 29-1 ■ Most Common New Health Problems in 132 Confirmed Postpolio Individuals with a Diagnosis of PPS

HEALTH PROBLEMS	NO.	%
Fatigue	117	89
Muscle pain	93	71
Joint pain	93	71
Weakness		
Previously affected muscles	91	69
Previously unaffected muscles	66	50
Cold intolerance	38	29
Atrophy	37	28
ADL PROBLEMS		
Walking	84	64
Climbing stairs	80	61
Dressing	23	17

Adapted from Halstead L, Wiechers D, editors: *Research and clinical aspects of the late effects of poliomyelitis,* White Plains, NY, 1987, March of Dimes, p 17.

The time from the acute infection to the onset of PPS is variable regardless of the age at the time of infection. The average time of onset of new symptoms is about 35 years from the initial acute poliomyelitis infection,[52] with a range from 8 to 71 years.[48] Individuals with greater disability after recovery from the initial polio are more likely to have PPS.

Symptoms typically develop insidiously over the course of several years. Halstead[49] notes that in several cases new problems seem to be precipitated by certain events, such as surgery, a fall, or a minor accident.

Generally, the apparent progression of new symptoms is comparatively slow, yet minor changes in the stability of motor neurons can result in disproportionate large losses of muscular function.[52] Some individuals may notice deterioration in performance two to three decades after the initial infection; others may not change for more than five decades.[62] When physiological reserves are low, it may take a relatively minor change in the stability of the systems to manifest evident symptoms and functional losses (Table 29-1).

PREDICTIVE FACTORS

The symptoms are typically nonspecific among individuals. As such, the exact course of PPS is unknown. Trojan et al[57a] examined predictive factors for the development of PPS. Their results show that significant risk factors included greater age, more weakness at acute polio, and a longer period since initial polio diagnosis.

The risk for PPS increased 1.8 for each decade of life and increased by 1.6 for each decade after polio. It appears that the length of time after the initial infection was more significant than age during the acute polio. Other predictive factors identified in the study included a longer time since the initial polio infection, more weakness during the acute polio, muscle pain specifically related to exercise, joint pain, and recent weight gain. Interestingly, age at acute polio, recovery after polio, physical activity, and sex did not appear to be contributing factors.[57a]

MEDICAL DIAGNOSIS

Differential medical diagnosis is critical in the diagnosis of PPS. Other diagnoses that may contribute to the symptoms need to be eliminated before a definitive diagnosis of PPS can be made.[42,54,63,64] The symptoms are so general and variable that all potential contributors to the new symptoms must be thoroughly explored. The common symptoms of fatigue, weakness, and pain are not specific to PPS alone and are typical in several conditions. A conclusive diagnosis of PPS becomes challenging as a result of the multifaceted condition, and diagnosis becomes primarily a diagnosis of exclusion.

Based on the recent literature, there appears to be some confusion regarding terminology pertaining to PPS. The complexity and nonspecificity of symptoms warrant consideration of all possible contributors to the symptoms of PPS. Medical practitioners must take into account the effects of existing comorbidities and aging. Compounding the general symptoms are the common problems in aging: decreasing muscle strength and endurance, joint problems, and a myriad of health deficits leading to functional losses. The aspects of physiological aging, overuse, and comorbidities play contributory factors in disrupting the state of stability after the initial infection.

McNaughton and McPhearson[64a] state that using simple descriptive labels "late problems after polio, of late deterioration after polio" are less-limiting terms and do not imply a direct link with the previous polio diagnosis. Post-Polio Health International[65] uses the terminology "late effects of polio and polio sequelae" to be the most inclusive category. Late effects of polio or polio sequelae pertains to health problems that are a result of chronic impairments from polio and may include degenerative arthritis from overuse, bursitis, or tendinitis. A subcategory under this heading is PPS leading to decreased endurance and decreased function.

Currently, no definitive test exists in literature to diagnose the late effects of polio or PPS. The diagnostic process for PPS is challenging and may be long. Halstead and Gawne[66] identified cardinal symptoms of PPS as new or increased muscle weakness, fatigue, and muscle and joint pain with neuropathic EMG changes in an individual with a definite diagnosis of polio. Diagnostic EMG may be required or used when the muscle pattern or history is atypical.

The criteria most commonly used for establishing a medical diagnosis of PPS were developed by Halstead[42] and are presented as follows:

1. A confirmed history of paralytic polio in childhood or adolescence,
2. Partial to complete muscle strength and functional recovery,
3. A period of at least 15 years of neurological and functional stability,
4. Onset of two or more new health problems listed in Table 29-2, and
5. No other medical conditions to explain these new health problems.

Dalakas[67] identified additional inclusion criteria in the diagnosis: residual asymmetrical muscle atrophy, with weakness, areflexia and normal sensation in at least one limb and normal sphincteric function and deterioration of func-

TABLE 29-2 ■ Major Postural Abnormalities in Sitting, Standing, and Walking in 111 Confirmed Postpolio Clinic Clients

POSTURE	ABNORMAL DEVIATION	NO.	%
Sitting (n = 111)	Absent lumbar curve	64	54
	Forward head (loss of cervical curves)	50	45
	Uneven pelvic base*	29	26
	Structural scoliosis	38	34
Standing (n = 76)	Absent lumbar curve	52	68
	Uneven pelvic base*	40	53
	Weight bearing on stronger leg	29	38
Walking (n = 76)	Abnormal gait deviations	76	100
	Major lateral trunk oscillations	33	43
	Obvious forward lean	40	53

Adapted from Smith L, McDermott K: Pain in post-poliomyelitis: addressing causes versus effects. In Halstead L, Wiechers D, editors: *Research and clinical aspects of the late effects of poliomyelitis,* White Plains, NY, 1987, March of Dimes.
*Pelvic asymmetry was $\frac{1}{2}$ inch or more.

tion after a period of functional stability unexplained by primary or secondary condition.

ETIOLOGY

The exact etiology of the PPS remains unknown on the basis of review of the literature. Although it is not clear what exactly causes the new symptoms, there appears to be a consensus that insufficient evidence implicates the reactivation of the previous poliovirus.[68] Underlying causes have been proposed in a variety of hypotheses from several authors.[49,69-72]

One hypothesis points to the loss of anterior horn cells during the initial polio as a factor.[68,69] Findings from Trojan et al[57a] support the hypothesis that the severity of the initial motor unit involvement, seen as weakness at acute polio, is critical in predicting PPS. Individuals at most risk for PPS had severe attacks of paralytic polio, although individuals with milder cases also had symptoms.[49]

The suggestion that aging contributes to PPS is supported in the literature.[57,69,73] By the fifth decade of life, loss of anterior horn cells begin, and by age 60 years, the loss of neurons may be as high as 50%.[74] Age-related changes superimposed with the already limited motor neuron pool after polio appear to be important factors in the development of PPS. With the effects of the normal aging process, the remaining anterior horn cells are further reduced to a point where the deficits caused by the initial insult cannot be overcome. The loss of even a few neurons from a greatly exhausted neuronal pool potentially results in a disproportionate loss of muscle function.[49,75] The loss of motor neurons from aging alone may not be a considerable factor in PPS because studies[49] have failed to link chronological age and the onset of new symptoms. Rather, it was the length of the interval between the onset of polio and the appearance of new symptoms that seems to be more critical.

Another plausible hypothesis alludes to overuse and fatigue of the already weakened muscles as a factor in the development of new muscle weakness.[52,57a,68] The study by

Trojan et al[57a] provides support to this hypothesis. Their results suggest that length of time since acute polio, joint and muscle pain, physical activity, and weight gain were factors associated with PPS. Years of overuse after recovery from polio causes a metabolic failure leading to an inability to regenerate new axon sprouts. The exact cause of degeneration of axon sprouts is not known. Evidence to support this hypothesis can be inferred from muscle biopsies, electrodiagnostic tests, and clinical response to exercise.[49]

McComas et al[76] suggested that neurons that demonstrated histological recovery from the initial virus were possibly not physiologically normal and potentially vulnerable to premature aging and failure.

Other proposed hypotheses include persistence of dormant poliovirus that was reactivated by unknown mechanisms, an immune-mediated response, hormone deficiencies, and environmental contaminants.[49] These hypotheses have not been completely examined and currently, the evidence is not strong enough to sustain any one possible cause. Clinically, it is difficult to assume that only one factor causes symptoms. The chronicity of the disease lends to the possibility that more than one factor contributes to the individual's symptoms.

The complexity of symptoms then warrants an interdisciplinary approach that integrates medical, social, and rehabilitative efforts to meet the unique problems of an aging population with chronic disability. A comprehensive physical therapist examination is a must. Should the patient's/client's symptoms fall outside either the physical or occupational therapist's scope of practice, appropriate referral or consultation is necessary. Only after this thorough movement analysis evaluation can a team of health-related professionals develop a comprehensive management plan that addresses the individual's specific needs based on the symptoms of chronic conditions and specific goals of the individual.

EXAMINATION: SYSTEMS MODEL

Overview

Aging with neuromuscular disorders is a challenge for both the individual and the health care professional. There is a small body of literature on the later life complications of early-onset acquired disabilities. Several problems result from complex interactions among physical, medical, environmental, behavioral, and psychosocial factors.

Aging may confound late-onset symptoms or magnify the deficits from the initial CNS insult. As the polio survivor population ages, there will be an increasing number of comorbidities, and sorting out the cause of each new symptom will be increasingly complicated. Bottomley[77] identifies essential components of a comprehensive geriatric assessment to include psychosocial, functional, mental, and social health. These components are applicable to postpolio patients, who with aging are experiencing new symptoms.

Examination Guidelines

Assessment of postpolio symptoms is challenging because of the nonspecific nature of symptoms and the complex interaction of several factors, including the heterogeneous effects of aging. Moreover, the absence of a specific medical diagnostic test lends to the dilemma, along with the continuing uncertainty of the underlying etiology and the lack of curative intervention. Health care professionals' limitations in knowledge of polio as an acute paralytic infection or as a chronic disabling condition with late manifestations also add to the complexity.

It is critical for the clinician to examine all possible contributors to symptoms reported by the individual with PPS. A thorough review of systems may identify symptoms that are related to the primary medical diagnoses, but equally important, it may identify symptoms that are associated to one or more existing comorbidities or factors.

Examination Pointers: PPS

- Comprehensive: A systems approach to address the number, complexity, and diversity of the deficits is a must. Essential components are physical, functional, mental, and social health.
- Interdisciplinary: Consideration for the functional, medical, vocational, and psychosocial issues warrants a coordinated evaluation of a team versed in addressing the unique needs of postpolio survivors.
- Patient/client centered: Factors that influence performance, such as fatigue, must be considered during the examination. Recognition of the individual's and family's values and goals is essential.
- Thorough: Assessment may take several hours and extend for two to four visits[47,78] to better integrate the evaluation process and allow the patient to fully participate and deal with the recommendations.

Physical therapists may develop diagnostic focuses regarding functional limitations different from those of occupational therapists. These variances depend on the functional activities limitations identified by the patient and the professional.[79,80] An example of the physical therapy diagnostic process can be found in Appendix 29-A.

Health History

Therapists typically collect health history information as part of a comprehensive examination. The history information along with the symptom investigation and review of systems and physical examination will provide guidance in the differential diagnosis process (see Chapters 8 and 9) and in the choice of examination and intervention techniques.

The information from the history will be useful in determining the possible cause of current symptoms (Box 29-2). Fatigue or pain may be present from unnecessary and inefficient movement strategies or from high levels of activity. Information on the habitual sleeping, sitting, standing, and walking postures along with ineffective use of devices may alert the clinician to possible factors contributing to the patient's symptoms.

Systems Review

A systems approach to the examination is essential because postpolio presentation is a complex interaction of all systems along with the effects of aging, previous interventions, and environmental, psychosocial, and medical aspects of care. The initial diagnosis of polio, which is critical in the diagnostic criteria, will need to be established. This may be problematic because approximately 10% to 15% of individuals who were believed to have or were diagnosed with polio

BOX 29-2 ■ COMPONENTS OF PATIENT/ CLIENT HISTORY

- Demographics
- Growth and developmental history (particularly in those diagnosed with polio as children)
- Current and past medical-surgical history (includes family history that may be critical in ruling out possible contributors to symptoms such as pain from rheumatoid arthritis)
- Social and vocational history
- Living environment
- History of current condition
- General health status
- Current functional status and activity level

did not, and several individuals with mild weakness were diagnosed as having nonparalytic polio.[42,43]

Boissonnault[81] discusses the review of systems as a vital component in the physical therapist's (PT) role in medical screening and differential diagnosis. Occupational therapists (OT) are responsible for this same vital component. Possible multisystem involvement warrants review of all systems to determine if current problems are associated with existing comorbid conditions, with occult disease, or are indeed late manifestations of polio.

The nonspecificity of symptoms lends credibility to the need for review of all body systems. Fatigue, for example, is a common symptom associated with several systems, such as endocrine, nervous, psychological, and cardiopulmonary involvement.

Tests and Measures

Through system assessment by the physical and/or occupational therapist, each individual with PPS should have an opportunity to participate in development of a unique clinical profile. This profile should reflect the strengths and limitations of that individual. Simultaneously these data should aid both the patient and the therapist in identifying realistic treatment goals and selection of the most appropriate intervention strategies. The choice of outcome measures will depend on the individual's current functional skills, the medical status and the desires and expectations of the individual. Because the severity of symptoms is variable and nonspecific, the clinician is strongly urged to perform a thorough examination and take into consideration factors that may influence performance specific to that individual's functional impairment problems, such as fatigue and pain.

Fatigue

Bruno et al[82] state that fatigue has been identified as the most commonly reported, most debilitating, and least studied symptom in the postpolio sequelae. Generalized fatigue is typically described as overwhelming exhaustion or flulike aching accompanied by marked changes in level of energy, endurance, and mental alertness.[49] The lack of energy with minimal activity is often described as "hitting a wall," thus the term "polio wall." Polio survivors differentiated between the fatigue associated with weakness and a "central

fatigue" that leads to attention and cognitive problems.[82] Severe fatigue affects not only physical function but mental function as well. Thus the controversial suggestion that the postpolio fatigue is caused by impaired brain function rather than the diffuse degeneration of motor units and motor junctions.[82]

Descriptors for fatigue associated with PPS are significantly different.[83] The fatigue of PPS may not appear at the time of the activity, and recovery does not occur with typical rest periods. It has also been described as a sudden and total wipeout. In a few instances, headaches and sweating appear suggestive of autonomic nervous system overload.[84] Fatigue commonly occurs in the late afternoon or early evening. Fatigue that tends to last all day is atypical in PPS[42] and should alert the therapist to consider other possible diagnoses.

Differential diagnoses for fatigue are extensive and may include disorders from several systems, including psychological, cardiopulmonary, neurological, endocrine disorders, and medication use. Specific conditions that may present with fatigue include depression, myasthenia gravis, hyperparathyroidism, congestive heart failure, sleep apnea, cancer, and infections. The challenge is to differentiate the fatigue from typical activities from the fatigue of PPS.

Pain

Pain that occurs with PPS may be muscular or it may be joint related, or both. The source of pain needs to be considered because pain may limit the individual's functional abilities and lead to further decline. Muscle pain is often described as a deep, aching pain similar to the pain experienced during the initial infection. The pain is frequently aggravated by physical activity, stress, and cold temperature. Pain is unusual in that it does not occur at the time of activity but rather 1 to 2 days after a precipitating event.

Joint pain in itself usually results primarily from long-term microtrauma from abnormal biomechanical forces. Joint pain is frequently associated with physical activity but is rarely associated with inflammation. Neck, shoulder, and back pain radiating to the hip and leg was reported by more than 65% of those with PPS.[84a] This pain is expected because the incidence of major postural abnormalities and gait deviations is also high, as shown in Table 29-2. Interventions are complicated by the presence of osteoporosis, lack of compensatory substitutions to rest the injured part, and, often, poor response to exercise. Failing joint fusions, uneven limb size, progressive scoliosis, poor posture, and abnormal mechanics may also contribute to pain.[48]

Differential diagnosis for muscle and joint pain includes consideration of chronic musculoskeletal conditions leading to wear and tear and disorders with significant muscle or joint manifestations. The list is extensive and may include osteoarthritis, tendinitis, bursitis, fibromyalgia, rheumatoid arthritis, and polymyalgia rheumatica.

Strength

Weakness may occur in both previously affected and clinically unaffected muscles; however, it is primarily prominent in muscles most severely affected in the initial infection.[42] It is typically asymmetrical and may be proximal, distal, or patchy.[48] Weakness is primarily observed in repetitive and stabilizing contractions rather than with single maximum efforts. The decreased ability of the muscles to recover rapidly after contracting may be a factor. Overuse of muscles in relation to their limited capacity has long been associated with these new problems.[50,85,86] New weakness and atrophy have been attributed to metabolic overload of the giant motor units, with more pruning of muscle fibers than axon sprouting.[54,87]

Recovery of quadriceps muscle strength after fatiguing exercise was significantly less in symptomatic PPS subjects compared with nonsymptomatic and control subjects.[88]

New muscle involvement may also present symptoms such as muscle fasciculations, cramps, atrophy, and elevation of muscle enzymes in the blood. Fasciculations occur at rest and during contraction and tend to persist even when muscle pain and fatigue have been resolved. Muscle cramps are common in fatigued muscles and are alleviated by decreased activity. The new weakness may or may not be accompanied by atrophy. New postpolio muscular atrophy of muscles is sometimes reported; it is most noticeable when it occurs in the gastrocnemius or the anterior tibialis. Elevation of muscle enzymes, indicative of muscle damage, has been found in individuals with PPS and has been related to the intensity of work.[85,89,90]

Manual muscle testing of the entire body is necessary to determine the muscular involvement. Gross muscle testing may mask the true involvement because several muscles that were initially believed to be uninvolved were truly subclinically affected by polio. The pattern of definitive manual test (spotty, flaccid, and asymmetrical paresis/paralysis) is also used to confirm the initial polio diagnosis. Muscle testing, however, may not always reveal the full extent of muscle involvement, and functional assessment may provide a better picture of individuals' potential and true difficulties.

Several polio survivors were able to function at high levels of activity on few strong muscle groups as a result of the random, diffuse nature of the motor deficits and the body's ability to compensate with uncommon muscle and joint function. This delicate balance has been maintained for years, and a disruption from late-onset weakness of a significant muscle group can lead to disproportionate functional losses.

Superimposed pathological problems have been proposed as a possible cause of late, new symptoms in postpolio survivors. Several conditions may contribute to weakness, including arthritis, fibromyalgia, deconditioning, from disuse, and coronary heart disease.[91]

Mobility and Posture
In individuals with chronic functional limitations, addressing inefficient alignments and postures is of critical importance, particularly if this area was not addressed early in their care. The dire effects of such malalignments and compensations described in the following text eventually affect functional abilities.

Asymmetrical or abnormal gait patterns, crutch walking, or propelling manual wheelchairs for several decades are frequently the major sources of the pain, weakness, and fatigue in people with PPS. The incidence of pain in a group of 114 patients with confirmed PPS increased from 84% in those who were ambulatory without orthotics to 100% for those who used crutches or wheelchairs for locomotion.[92] A high prevalence of osteoarthritis in patients with PPS was documented in the hand and wrist by radiography.[93] More than twice the number of subjects with PPS had osteoarthritis of the wrist or hand than would be expected in a healthy population of the same age. The risk factor was significantly increased with lower extremity muscle paralysis and use of assistive devices.[93]

In an EMG study of walking in clients with PPS, Perry et al[94] demonstrated overuse and substitution activity of the vastus lateralis, biceps femoris, and gluteus maximus muscles when the soleus is nonfunctional. Such substitution and overcompensation in the long term, however, leads to microtrauma of ligaments and joint structures and exhaustion of neuromuscular units.

In addition to sitting in poorly supporting chairs, sofas, auto seats, and wheelchairs, the individual with PPS may have trunk muscle paresis or asymmetries of the pelvic base and may spend up to 16 hours per day in the seated position. The typical posture is slumped, hanging on posterior vertebral ligaments with loss of lumbar and cervical curves. Neck, shoulder, and back pain are thus commonly reported.

Range of Motion and Muscle Length
Limitations of joint motion from muscle contractures and from shortening of ligamentous joint structures are common in individuals with PPS. Likewise, hypermobile joints may also result from compensatory techniques to allow more mobility. An evaluation of the individual's activity levels and goals is vital before intervening with muscle and joint deficits. In some instances during the convalescent stage of polio, selective tightness was allowed to give some stability to joints with paralyzed muscles. In addition, the body may develop useful contractures to maintain or regain function. Before attempts to stretch contractures, therapists should carefully evaluate the functions that may be lost if gains in range of motion (ROM) are achieved. Equally important is to evaluate what functions would be gained and what the cost would be. Consider that after 20 to 40 years these contractures resist any significant elongation, and aggressive intervention may cause more harm and loss of function.

Environmental Cold Intolerance
Sensory deficits per se are not hallmark features of polio; however, cold intolerance is a common reported late-onset symptom. Involved extremities in individuals with PPS are frequently abnormally cold as a result of sympathetic nerve cell involvement leading to decreased vasoconstriction and venoconstriction with heat loss to the environment. The impairment may become worse with PPS. Environmental adaptation can create an easy solution to this problem as long as the individual with PPS is aware first of the problem and second of the adaptations necessary to avoid thermoinstability within the extremities. Preventing versus responding to the inadequate vasoresponse to cold empowers the individual to environmental control.

Sleep Disturbances
More than 50% of individuals with PPS have been found to have sleep disturbances.[95] These disturbances may be caused by pain, stress, hypoventilation, or obstructive apnea.[96-98] A thorough history and review of systems may reveal the potential causes and guide the therapist in the clinical decision making process for referral and consultation.

The role of the therapist is primarily in the area of pain management.

Life-Threatening Conditions

Bulbar muscle dysfunction[48] may also result from the new weakness. Life-threatening conditions such as hypoventilation, dysphagia, sleep apnea,[99] and cardiopulmonary insufficiency require management by medical specialists.[40,96,100] These problems occur in people with previous bulbar poliomyelitis who may or may not be using ventilatory assistance and in those with severe kyphosis or scoliosis. Respiratory failure may occur primarily in individuals with residual respiratory insufficiency and minimal reserves.[101]

Functional Assessment

Performance in functional activities often provides a better picture of the losses stemming from new symptoms of PPS. Decreases in strength are not usually revealed in a single-effort maximum contraction such as required in the manual muscle test. Resistive force during testing is an necessary element for two grades, 5 (normal, "N") and 4 (good, "G"), whereas the other four grades are nonresistive and mostly nonfunctional, and few examiners are now tested for reliability.[102] In a 1-year follow-up using quantitative muscle force testing, no differences were found in muscle strength, work capacity, endurance capacity, or recovery from fatigue of the quadriceps in either nonsymptomatic or symptomatic groups with PPS.[103] Nevertheless, there is at best a slow decline in functional ability, which clients may describe as loss of muscle strength. Clinically, individuals seeking therapy report functional loss or limitation more easily rather than a specific loss of muscle strength.

Functional assessment of individuals with chronic movement limitations provides a more practical and clearer picture of the abilities and limitations related to the initial condition or stemming from new impairments. Functional activities are visible and reportable performances of relevant tasks in the context of the individual's culture.[104] Functional tasks imply a specific goal and can range from simple to complex activities. In functional motor performance, the specific task and environmental context is as important as the individual functional movement. Consideration for these factors is necessary during examination. Detailed functional assessment is outlined by Howle[105] and Zabel.[106]

Functional limitations describe difficulty in performing specific tasks. According to Agre and Rodriguez[107] postpolio survivors with significant weakness perform daily activities at a different level of effort than other individuals; muscles of polio survivors may have to work near maximal effort during activities that nonpolio individuals can execute at relatively lower levels of effort. Individuals with PPS commonly report difficulty in walking, stair climbing,[42] and dressing (see Table 29-2). Westbrook[107a] described a 5-year follow-up study examining physical and functional abilities and health status of 176 individuals with PPS. During the course of the study, most subjects reported increases in muscle weakness, muscle and joint pain, and changes in walking. Notably, the participants reported more difficulty in four of the eight daily living activities (stair climbing, walking on level surfaces, transfers in and out of bed, and meeting the demands of home or work). Most of the participants (87%) also reported problems in meeting the demands

of their job and completing household tasks. Clearly, the ability to perform motor tasks essential in completing ones' goals and desires is multifactorial. As such, functional limitations are usually related to a combination of systems impairments.

To determine whether the cause of the new weakness is overuse or possibly disuse, a detailed assessment is required of home, work, recreational, and community activities.[108] If the client is merely asked what his or her activity level is, the response may lead to assumptions that weakness is from disuse. With specific questioning, one usually finds that the client is doing an extraordinary amount of physical activity. It is vital to establish a total picture of the client's activities in sitting, standing, walking, lifting, carrying, climbing stairs, using a telephone or a computer, and activities such as cooking, mowing the lawn, playing tennis, or taking care of grandchildren.

PSYCHOSOCIAL CONSIDERATIONS

Several authors have addressed prevalence, etiology, and aging on the development of PPS over the past years. However, the psychological effects are not as widely addressed in the literature. Not much is known about the quality of life of older adults with congenital or childhood-acquired disabilities. Psychological adjustment is difficult with any disease with an unpredictable course, and differentiating organic psychological problems from adjustment issues may complicate the management of individuals after polio.

Although the physical manifestations and interventions for PPS are recognized, psychological symptoms become evident in polio survivors. Bruno and Frick[109] described psychological symptoms such as chronic stress, depression, anxiety, compulsiveness, and type A behavior in polio survivors, which not only cause distress but limit these individuals in making lifestyle changes to manage late-onset symptoms. Currie et al[91] made generalizations about adults with childhood-onset or congenital disabilities spanning a range of disability types. Understanding the background of individuals with PPS and a few of the myths that helped to shape their lives is beneficial in their care. Fear of the disease was rampant during the early epidemics. Despite safety measures, children and adolescents were afflicted with polio. Part of the coping strategy was encouraging the child to high levels of physical achievement; approval and rewards were gained by walking farther or faster and keeping up with or exceeding the performance of other children. The best treatment available provided to all polio victims at that time was the March of Dimes, which entailed hospitalization for months at a time away from their families and communities. The situation led to feelings of abandonment, anxiety, and total dependence on strangers. The "polio patient" was expected to be a "good patient" and to "work hard." Indeed, they did work hard to reeducate weakened muscles and compensate for lost function.[110-113] Courage, determination, and cheerfulness were attributes to be prized, self-pity was viewed unfavorably, and talking about the functional loss was not encouraged. Later in the recovery process, parents made the decisions to undergo multiple surgical procedures to allow removal of heavy braces for children so that they would look "normal and fit in." One can understand why clients react so negatively to the suggestion of orthotics.

Coping Strategies

The psychosocial issues confronting persons with PPS often are more disruptive than the physical problems.[43,70,71,114-116] An increasing population of polio survivors is experiencing, with aging, an unanticipated late onset of new symptoms. Associated with loss of physical function and independence are social and psychological problems stemming from the inability to perform personal and societal roles. Previous research suggests that well-established, often compulsive behavior patterns may impair the ability to deal effectively with the new threats to functional independence. Bruno and Frick[72] confirmed the presence of psychological stress in survivors, noting that type A behavior and stress could precipitate or exacerbate postpolio sequelae. In a later study in 1991,[109] the same researchers suggested that the acute experience conditioned survivors into lifelong patterns of compulsive type A behavior, a behavior pattern that impairs the ability to cope with new late postpolio symptoms. Kuehn and Winters[117] also noted that symptom distress and intensity were less in individuals with greater coping resources. In this study[117] in Sweden of 113 patients with postpolio sequelae, results revealed that the prevalence of distress was highest in the physical dimensions of physical mobility, pain, and energy and lowest in social isolation. The high scores for the triad of dimensions were similar to previous studies.[99]

Individuals with PPS developed several styles to cope with their disability. Maynard and Roller[118] described coping styles according to severity of muscular involvement. Survivors with little or no obvious physical involvement were able to hide atrophy with clothing and avoided activities that revealed the weakness. Many individuals invested much energy in projecting normality and were so adept at denial that they disconnected themselves from the polio experience; often spouses do not know of the history of polio. This group can develop the most severe cases of PPS. The denial renders them detached from other individuals with PPS and thus difficult to assist.

Polio survivors with obvious physical involvement such as a limp, an atrophied extremity, or who use an assistive device have usually pushed themselves to function at normal or supernormal levels. These individuals will suffer high levels of pain before acknowledging the late effects of polio. The third group, the most severely impaired of the individuals with PPS, may have respiratory involvement or more mobility deficits. Several use wheelchairs for mobility or have required great effort and persistence to gain independence in self-care activities. This group integrated their functional problems into their self-image and has led active, productive lives.

In a 5-year study of 176 individuals with PPS, it was unexpectedly found that participants' stress levels decreased over time.[107a] The author hypothesized that eventually, lifestyle modifications and treatment contributed to the coping process. Kuehn and Winters[117] in their study found that more than half of their subjects of working age had gainful employment. Moreover, no difference in employment rate as a result of distribution of polio involvement was found, implying that this was not a deciding factor. The authors hypothesize that persons with severe polio involvement were either forced to choose or encouraged to take up an appropriate profession early in life, whereas those with less involvement had not needed such planning. Nevertheless, vocational issues encompassing satisfactory accessibility and equipment are an important part of management.

Response to New Diagnosis

The response to the diagnosis of PPS can range from relief or despair. Relief comes to polio survivors who have been told their symptoms were psychosomatic. Despair occurs as a program of lifestyle changes and management suggestions that are opposed to the adage they followed during the initial infection. The proposed philosophy shift from "no pain, no gain" to that of energy conservation and rest may be viewed unfavorably or with disdain.

The stresses of the diagnostic process also add to the challenges. Most health care professionals have limited understanding of the initial polio experience and the late effects of polio, and as such, the diagnostic process of PPS may take time and involve a series of physician consultations.[110,111,119-121] Publicity from support groups has helped refer clients to PPS clinics or to specialists with knowledge of PPS.[121]

Fear of the threat to independence, inadequate knowledge about the physiological changes, and the expectation of functional loss may contribute to the anxiety of polio survivors. Individuals with PPS will feel anxious about the prospects of changing roles with their families, friends, and coworkers.[111,118,120] Defenses and coping strategies that have been successfully used for years have broken down, and the individual experiences overwhelming anxieties and conflicts.[120]

Compliance

The patient-clinician relationship is an important determinant of compliance. Several authors[72,109,122] have identified compliance as a significant problem in type A polio survivors. Although a few individuals with PPS readily accept suggestions for lifestyle changes, a few immediately make changes, and a few refuse to consider any changes at all, most will eventually make changes but will require support, patience, and time to process. Clinicians' sensitivity, support, and respect will play a major role in the patient/client's response to management suggestions. Acknowledging the individual's current activities, values, and goals is an important step in establishing a relationship with the patient/client. Allowing clients to express feelings about the new challenges, their prior high levels of physical achievement, and previous treatment is equally important.

A health care provider perceived to be knowledgeable, interested, and concerned significantly increases compliance with recommendations.[123] Compliance of the client with PPS may be improved by the therapist's ability to suggest management strategies that are accepted as conventional and the ability to alleviate pain in the initial examination. Conservative management should be attempted first before more aggressive or life-changing interventions such as orthosis, mobility changes, or motorized carts, which may have used in the past and eventually discarded. Therapists can also be a source of information about PPS support groups.[121] Support groups offer information about every facet of living with PPS, and these members may be positive role models to help the newly diagnosed individual in the transition process.

EVIDENCE-BASED APPROACH TO MANAGEMENT

Historical Perspective

Historically, polio survivors were placed on exhaustive regimens of intense strengthening and daily stretching that demanded compliance from both the patient and the family. The prevailing ideology stressed intense physical effort to achieve independence without mechanical assistance as much as possible. For independent mobility, bracing and assistive devices were initially encouraged and eventually discarded as the patient adapted or compensated with her or his remaining capabilities. The adage of "use it or lose it" allowed polio survivors to attain high levels of activity and productive lifestyles while ignoring pain in the process.

With the occurrence of late symptoms and the diagnosis of PPS presenting a possible "second disability," the adage and ideology used in initial polio management are not applicable. The principles used then are ineffective and will cause more harm if used to address late-onset symptoms. A review of current literature points to a paradigm shift in the management of PPS that promotes energy conservation, joint protection, nonfatiguing activities, and use of assistive mobility devices as necessary is in stark contrast to previously held principles and approaches. This necessary paradigm shift presents as a challenge to both health care professionals who may have limited understanding of polio or the experiences of the polio survivor and the patient who is facing a new intervention philosophy that is contrary to the previous approach in the earlier struggles and the lifelong attitude toward the physical limitations.

INTERVENTION STRATEGIES

The rehabilitation clinician is in a unique position to provide holistic care to the client with PPS. There is much to learn from the complex nature of the late effects of polio, and designing an intervention program may be as challenging as the evaluation because of the interactions of the systems and environmental, medical, and aging influences. Prior to beginning physical or occupational therapy it is necessary for the team to first identify and treat other medical and neurological conditions that may produce the reported symptoms.[64]

The heterogeneity of this population lends to the need for individualized management programs. The aging process is unique for each individual, as is the recovery process in PPS and the overall manifestation of late-onset symptoms. As such, intervention will be dependent on the individual's current symptoms, functional needs, level of activity limitations, and values or goals.

The individual's values and goals are the most significant variables to take into consideration in designing the interventions. Improvement will largely depend on the patient's commitment and thus compliance. Relatively simple interventions may result in distinctive positive changes. Conservative management should be attempted first before major life-changing interventions. Psychological considerations play a major role in designing an acceptable and appropriate management plan that will encourage compliance. Lifestyle modifications may not be favorably viewed by some individuals with PPS who have "conquered" the disease and pushed themselves to be independent. Prescription of interventions that are perceived to be "radical"

should be done with sensitivity and caution. The rationale for interventions should be carefully considered in light of the client's current functional status and goals. Introduction of orthoses, assistive devices, and mobility modifications is often difficult for the individual with PPS to accept, given the long, arduous effort expended over years to avoid such devices.

The long-term goals for individuals with PPS centers primarily on self-management of home exercise programs and appropriate lifestyle changes to reduce physical demands. No definite curative intervention currently exists; thus, symptom management is a key element in both short- and long-term *management*. Short-term goals focus on the symptoms present and may address the following areas:

- Lifestyle modifications
- Postural correction
- Energy conservation
- Modified strengthening and conditioning
- Mobility and locomotion
- Balance during functional activities
- Walking aids, mobility devices, orthoses
- Pain reduction
- Improved functional endurance
- Ability to transfer
- Respiratory care
- Weight control

The information is presented with an evidence-based approach. When possible those intervention approaches first offered should focus on several problems at one time (Table 29-3). The importance of individualized programs that address the variability of symptoms cannot be overemphasized. The reader is referred to specific references for further details on management prescriptions.

Pain Management

Pain management in the patient with PPS is dependent on the cause of the muscle or joint pain. Typical interventions for pain include activity reduction, therapeutic heating modalities, cryotherapy, stretching, or energy and joint conservation techniques.

If chronic overuse is the only or major underlying cause of the symptoms present, conservative measures can often slow or prevent further deterioration and may even lead to improved function. Conservative measures include reducing mechanical stress, pacing activities, supporting weak muscles, stabilizing abnormal joint movements, and improving biomechanics of the body. Interventions that address fatigue and weakness such as nonfatiguing functional activities, energy conservation,[108] more frequent rest periods, or change of activity[124] are also useful in pain management. Antiinflammatory agents have been used to supplement conservative measures.

Joint conservation techniques may include use of ergonomic devices, elevated chairs, bathtub bench or shower stool, and weight control. Recommendations for the neck and upper extremities include seating and workstation corrections, telephone headsets, rolling carts for carrying items, newspaper support for reading, ergonomic computer screens, wrist rests, and keyboards.

Successful intervention of joint pain, however, requires identification and elimination of the cause of the pain. This is frequently difficult because the person with PPS may not have the strength in other parts of the body to compensate

TABLE 29-3 ■ Evidence-Based Approach to the Management of PPS

GENERALIZED WEAKNESS

Lifestyle changes
Therapeutic nonfatiguing strengthening exercises
Aerobic exercise
Orthosis
Assistive devices
Avoidance of overuse
Weight loss

PAIN

Therapeutic heating modalities*
Cryotherapy*
Activity reduction and lifestyle changes
Pacing of activities
Stretching
Weight loss
Assistive devices
Orthosis
Motorized mobility devices
Nonsteroidal antiinflammatory drugs[†]

DYSPHAGIA

Dietary changes or restrictions
Breathing techniques
Swallowing techniques
Monitoring fatigue and timing eating when not fatigued

FATIGUE

Lifestyle changes
Energy conservation techniques
Nonfatiguing exercise programs
Lightweight orthosis and assistive devices
Pacing of activities
Frequent rest breaks
Naps during the day
Motorized mobility devices

CARDIOPULMONARY CONDITIONING

Aquatic exercise training
Endurance training
Cycle or arm exercises

PSYCHOSOCIAL CONCERNS

Postpolio support groups
Interdisciplinary approach
Counseling from psychologists, psychiatrists
Vocational counseling
Behavior modification

PULMONARY DYSFUNCTION

Preventive measures
Noninvasive ventilatory assistance
Pulmonary therapy
Breathing exercises: glossopharyngeal breathing

Adapted from Trojan D, Finch L: Management of post-polio syndrome, *Neurorehabilitation* 8:93-105, 1997 and Jubelt B, Agre J: Management of post-polio syndrome, *JAMA* 284:412-414, 2000.
*Effectiveness of heat and cold modalities are patient specific and must be used with caution.
[†]Antiinflammatory drugs have been shown to be effective in pain management in medical treatment of PPS. The specific drug and dosage must be prescribed by the physician.

and carry out an essential function, or the person may be unable or unwilling to make necessary lifestyle changes. Intervention techniques may include inhibiting muscle spasm, stretching fascia and muscles, decreasing edema and increasing nutrition in joint structures, and mobilizing or stabilizing joints.[125] At some point, relaxation, meditation, modified tai chi (see Chapters 28 and 37), underwater exercise, or body awareness techniques such as Feldenkrais[126] may be beneficial.

Local pain and dysfunction can be treated as athletic injuries from overuse, but they require major modifications and careful monitoring of performance, pain, and fatigue. Many joint pain problems can be relieved and controlled by home program interventions such as rest for the injured part, mechanical postural corrections, cold packs, nonsteroidal antiinflammatory drugs, orthotics, and pain-free ROM exercises.

Although no radiological evidence for McConnell taping show changes in actual alignment of bone, individuals (non-polio) have experienced a 50% to 78% reduction in patellofemoral pain during activities.[125,127] In The Institute for Rehabilitation and Research, Houston, Texas, Postpolio Clinic, these taping techniques relieved anterior knee pain for several months at a time in all individuals with PPS who were selected to receive the taping. Relief occurred although the ability to strengthen surrounding muscles was limited or impossible. The therapy program should also include assist-

ing the client in carrying out the home program and lifestyle changes, along with the development of a continuing program of appropriate exercises.

As with the management of fatigue, compliance of the individual with PPS with suggested recommendations plays a significant role in pain management. Peach and Olejnik[128] found that muscle pain was resolved in 28% and improved in 72% of people who complied with recommendations. In those who were noncompliant, muscle pain was improved in 14%, unchanged in 57%, and increased in 29%.

Alternative Pain Management

Pain sensitivity must be acknowledged by clinicians when providing therapy that may be perceived as painful, such as stretching, and in the treatment of acute pain.[128a] Several polio survivors underwent extensive orthopedic surgery in attempts to overcome their initial deficits, and some have pain or hypersensitivities at the surgical sites. Desensitization exercises may decrease the hypersensitivities if the client is willing to devote the necessary time. The most frequent old surgical sites of pain are in the trunk from surgery for scoliosis, the ankle near a subtalar arthrodesis, or the foot with hypermobility of the transverse tarsal joint. In most instances of foot pain, stabilization of the ankle and foot in a custom-made ankle-foot orthosis (AFO) and use of a rocker-bottom shoe has relieved the pain and permitted weight bearing and walking.[129] Custom-made corsets and trunk supports in chairs may help with the pain at previous surgical sites in the trunk. Transcutaneous electrical nerve stimulation may be helpful for pain control (see Chapters 31 and 32). Most individuals, however, stop using these devices because masking the pain permits them to physically overdo, leading to further injury to their bodies.

Static magnetic fields have become a familiar alternative approach in the treatment of athletic injuries as well as in persons with PPS who have localized pain. In a double-blind randomized clinical trial, Vallbona et al[130] applied active (300-500 Gauss) and placebo magnets in a group of 50 subjects with PPS and chronic pain. The magnets were applied to the palpable pain pressure point for 45 minutes. There was a significant ($P < .0001$) and prompt decrease of pain in the group receiving the active magnets compared with those who received the placebo.[130]

Fatigue Management

Use of muscles at high levels for extended periods will result in muscle overload. To perform the same activity with weak muscles, the muscles need to contract at a higher percentage of their capacity than is normally required. For example, in walking, clients with PPS contract their muscles at both higher intensities and for prolonged or even continuous periods in the gait cycle.[131] Energy expenditure for the task is increased, and the prolonged contractions keep the capillaries compressed to limit needed muscle nutrition. Clients with PPS are often observed using nearly maximum voluntary contractions to perform a daily activity. The muscles of individuals with PPS cannot maintain these high levels of activity indefinitely.

A general program addressing fatigue in PPS may include nonfatiguing daily activities and energy conservation techniques. Relaxation, breathing, and meditation exercises may also be useful. Lifestyle changes that incorporate methods that decrease physical demands and prevent further decline in function are the most efficacious way to target fatigue impairments. In a study by Agre and Rodriquez[132] symptomatic subjects with PPS demonstrated the ability to perceive muscular exertion. This is indicative of a mechanism to monitor local muscle fatigue that may be used to avoid exhaustion. Their study of pacing, defined as interspersed activity with rest, revealed less local fatigue and significantly greater strength recovery in subjects who paced their activities than when they worked at a constant rate to exhaustion. The Borg Rating of Perceived Exertion (RPE) is an outcome measure that may be used to judge effort (see Chapter 35). Finch et al[133] in a study of individuals with PPS found that after one training session subjects reliably used the RPE in an exercise test to monitor their effort and complete the test. Finch et al[133a] have gone on to establish reliability and construct validity on an effort-limited treadmill test for individuals with PPS.

Peach and Olejnik[128] on reevaluation found that compliance with recommendations affected fatigue; it was resolved or improved in a group who complied with recommendations or unchanged or increased in the group that did not.

Therapeutic Exercise

Strengthening and Conditioning

The literature clearly documents the benefits of physical activity, and in polio survivors with PPS, activity that falls

---

BOX 29-3 ■ FUNCTIONAL EXERCISE: KEY POINTS

1. Consult with a health care team prior to starting an exercise program. A physical and occupational therapist can provide valuable insight and recommendations on activity type and intensity.
2. AVOID overuse of muscle groups.
3. Judicious exercise programs of low to high intensity can result in positive results. Include warm-up and cool down periods.
4. Short periods of activity are encouraged.
5. Allow for adequate rest between bouts of activity.
6. Alternate days may be necessary for full recovery (depending on activity type).
7. Individualized therapy program to address unique needs is critical.
8. Use energy conservation and joint protection techniques in regular routines.
9. Incorporate breathing, relaxation, mental imagery, and meditation exercises into daily activities.
10. Be cognizant of the body's alignment during exercise and functional activities.
11. Incorporate postural exercises and correction to address malalignments and unnecessary use of muscles and joints.
12. Compliance with clinical recommendations can significantly reduce symptoms and prevent further decline.
13. Listen to your body—pain is typically your body's way of alerting you to slow down or to stop.

---

within a safe range is beneficial to the overall functional performance (Box 29-3). Generally, survivors with PPS who exercised and avoided overuse demonstrated positive results without detrimental effects. Several types of nonfatiguing strengthening exercises, aerobic exercise, and the evidence supporting them are provided. Specific exercise prescription is dependent on several factors such as the current level of function, other presenting symptoms, and the client's interests.

Jubelt and Agre[48] note that the most important advance in the treatment of weakness in PPS points to findings in several studies that mild to moderate weakness can be improved with nonfatiguing exercises. The benefits of nonfatiguing exercises using both submaximal and maximal contraction with limited number of repetitions are documented in literature.[48,134]

Isokinetic and isometric dynamometers have been used to record maximum muscle forces (or torques) in PPS subjects before and after resistive exercise programs designed to increase muscle strength. Two of the studies were of single cases,[135,136] and two had 12 and 17 subjects.[137,138] Both of the multisubject studies tested the quadriceps femoris. Einarsson[137] investigated the effects of a standardized 6-week, maximal effort and isometric strength training program on the quadriceps muscles of 12 individuals with postpolio muscles nine of whom met the criteria for PPS. They reported an average gain of 29% in isometric strength and 24% in isokinetic strength over a period of 6 weeks and muscle biopsy specimens revealed no muscle damage. In addition to the feeling of well-being during and after the training program from most of the subjects, 10 of 12 subjects stated a feeling of increased strength in the trained muscle. In subsequent follow-ups 6 to 12 months after intervention, gains in strength did not decrease and several subjects reported better performance in daily activities such as climbing stairs, walking, and standing from a chair.[137]

Fillyaw et al[138] reported a strength gain of 8% over a 2-year period. An isometric contraction was used for testing, and concentric-eccentric contractions were used for the exercise. These results do not compare with the strength gains of 100% and higher made by healthy subjects undergoing training but rather compare with serial testing when no exercise was done.[139,140] For example, Munin et al[139] measured the affected and nonaffected quadriceps muscle every 6 months over 3 years to document muscle weakness in persons with PPS. They reported increases in muscle strength up to 25%. In older persons without polio, test performance gains of the quadriceps increased an average of 174% in 90-year-old subjects[141] and 107% in 60- to 72-year-old men.[142] In these two studies, thigh muscle area (as documented by computed tomography) increased by 9% and 11%, respectively, indicating an increase in muscle bulk.

The effects of nonfatiguing resistance exercises are well documented in the literature. Fillyaw et al[138] in a study of 17 subjects with PPS concluded that muscle strength may be increased in individuals with PPS and suggested supervision of exercise programs by physical therapists and quantitative muscle testing every 3 months to guard against overuse weakness. Agre and Rodriguez[143] suggested that a supervised exercise program could safely increase strength in subjects with PPS with at least a grade 3+ strength. Their program of a supervised 12-week nonfatiguing quadriceps strengthening program with rest intervals revealed no detrimental effects. Most of the participants reported improvements in quadriceps strength, endurance, and work capacity and half noted increased strength recovery with rest periods after activity, walking, and stair climbing. A nonfatiguing weight lifting program for at least 24 weeks was examined in six subjects with PPS by Feldman and Soskolne.[144] The results showed increased strength in 14 of the 32 muscle groups with maintained strength in 17 muscles.

Alternate-day, low-intensity muscle strengthening quadriceps exercises showed no adverse effects with reported findings of increased endurance, strength, and work capacity. As a result of the low-intensity program, no increased muscle strength was found, although half of the participants sensed increased strength recovery after exercise.[145] The same protocol but with a more vigorous program of 4 days per week revealed improvements in muscular work performance and endurance without unfavorable effects noted.[145]

Because there are neural adaptations specific to the type of muscle contraction used for measurement and training, it is difficult to determine the differences in true increases in strength from the ability to increase a specific test performance. Another term for this phenomenon or increase in performance is motor learning (see Chapter 3). The theory states that the subject learns to perform the measurement or the exercise better without true gains in strength. This happens even with an apparently simple weekly maximum isometric contraction.[126] Evidence of this phenomenon can be seen when improvements are made in the opposite untrained muscle group (transfer of training), when the apparent strength gains are maintained for months after cessation of the training, and when there are no increases in the size of the muscle. The greatest increases in test performance occur when the muscle contraction is the same for both the test and the training. Smaller increases are seen when the measurement and training muscle contractions are different and when measures to decrease the effect of motor learning have been used.

The neural adaptation specific to the type of measurement or training is illustrated in the following study on older men.[142] Multiple tests to assess strength were performed. The training program required lifting and lowering 80% of the weight of one repetition maximum (1 RM), which was assessed weekly. After 12 weeks, there were average increases in quadriceps muscle strength of 104% for the 1 RM, 7% for maximum isometric, 8% for maximum isokinetic at 60 degrees per second, and 10% for isokinetic at 240 degrees per second. In addition, there was an increase in cross-sectional area of the quadriceps of 10%, and muscle biopsy showed approximately a 30% increase in muscle fiber size.[146] This study illustrates some of the complexities in designing or evaluating studies that attempt to measure changes in muscle strength.

Cardiopulmonary Conditioning

Aerobic testing using modified protocols to reduce fatigue has been used on the treadmill,[147] bicycle ergometer,[148] and arm ergometer.[149] There were no cardiorespiratory training effects in the first study, probably owing to the low intensity of the exercise, but the duration and distance of walking increased.[139] The two ergometry studies showed an increase in maximum oxygen consumption of 15% and 19%, which is a training effect comparable to normal values for age. There were, however, no changes in blood pressure or heart rate, particularly the expected decrease in resting heart rate that occurs with aerobic training. Although the intensity of the exercise protocols had to be reduced for some of the subjects, none had to terminate the exercise because of overuse symptoms, nor did these symptoms occur at the end of the studies. A problem in evaluating these studies is that it is not always clear whether the study subjects with PPS were asymptomatic, symptomatic (PPS), or mixed.

An endurance training program in subjects with PPS demonstrated beneficial cardiovascular and strength effects without adverse consequences.[150] Aerobic exercise such as bicycle ergometer, walking, or swimming may be useful but the client must be interested in the activity to increase compliance.[64] Willen et al[151] in a recent study of 28 individuals with late effects of polio found that a program of nonswimming dynamic exercise in warm water twice weekly resulted in decreased heart rate at submaximal work level, less pain, and positive functional impact. As with the previous studies on exercises, no adverse effects were noted. Their general fitness training, however, did not result in changes in muscle strength or endurance. Previous studies documenting improvements in muscle function and aerobic capacity were designed for three or more times per week; authors hypothesize that a twice-a-week program was not enough to show improvements in the subjects' aerobic capacities or muscle strength.

The literature indicates that exercise within constraints can lead to several beneficial physiological and psychological adaptations in individuals with PPS.[64,134] It appears that therapeutic exercise is beneficial when performed without causing undue pain and fatigue. As with any intervention, a comprehensive examination will assist in developing a well-rounded and individualized program tailored to the specific needs of the individual with PPS.

Decreasing the Workload of Muscles

Energy Conservation Techniques

Energy conservation techniques provide the easiest way to decrease the work of muscles without loss of function. Analysis of all activities by type, time, distance, and intensity is valuable in designing interventions. Such an inventory forms the basis for setting priorities and determining where and how individuals wish to use their limited neuromuscular capacity.[108]

Questions addressed include the following:

1. Can one trip do for two or three?
2. Can the activity be performed in a less strenuous way, such as by sitting or using a rolling basket?
3. Can the activity be broken up into parts with change of activity or rest?
4. Are there easier ways to perform the activity with modern comforts and technology, including motorization and electronics?
5. Can someone else perform some of the physical aspects of the activity?

Particular attention should focus on activities that produce fatigue and pain. Specific suggestions may address breaking tasks into subtasks, environmental adaptations such as work height and locations, using frequent rest breaks during activities, and use of adaptive or ergonomic equipment.

Orthotics and Assistive Devices

Reduction of muscular overuse and fatigue may be accomplished with lightweight splints and braces, adaptive equipment, walkers, or crutches.[48,91] However, unlike most rehabilitation clients, individuals with PPS may have strong and usually negative feelings about orthotics. The use of orthotics or assistive devices may be challenging for the individual newly diagnosed with PPS and facing a relatively "new disability." Polio survivors may have previously relied on devices or have refused such devices earlier in life and consenting to using them again may symbolize defeat and acceptance of losses.

As with every intervention, a thorough explanation of the specific rationale and goals for the intervention will not only be helpful in gaining the client's trust but will also improve compliance. Rationale for orthotic use includes preventing falls and potential fractures, limiting joint motion and preventing pain, restoring weight bearing on the weaker extremity to decrease the work of the less affected leg in locomotion, improving posture and decreasing back pain, and decreasing energy expenditure.

Thoughtful consideration for the appropriateness of orthosis or assistive devices is critical; such devices should not be haphazardly prescribed or given as the only intervention of choice. They should be prescribed cautiously.

Ineffective and inappropriate use of such devices will lead to malalignments, ineffective movement strategies, and postures that will cause more harm. Therapists should carefully evaluate the functions that may be lost or gained and the emotional and physical cost of their use.

Most individuals have long discarded braces and assistive devices and have relied on compensatory techniques for walking (see Figure 29-8). If an orthosis has been used and is essential for walking, it often becomes a part of the individual's body image; thus, the client may be resistant to changes in braces or devices. For other individuals prior attempts to use plastic orthosis may have been painful and of no functional use and thus they previously have rejected its potential. Thus, it may be difficult to persuade the person with PPS to consider orthoses or an orthotic change. When given the appropriate orthosis or prescription, however, polio survivors may benefit significantly enough to improve their current symptoms. A retrospective study of lower extremity orthotic management for ambulation in 104 postpolio clinic patients by Waring et al[151a] revealed that 78% of patients noted that the appropriate orthotic prescription improved the ability to ambulate, increased apparent walking safety, and decreased pain.

In instances where both the talocrural and subtalar ankle joints were fused surgically, the increased stresses on the posterior structures of the knee or the transverse tarsal joint for ambulation eventually leads to hypermobility and pain in these areas. Rocker bottom shoes may assist with restoring motion for walking. An AFO may address pain in the transverse tarsal joint, whereas a knee-ankle-foot orthosis (KAFO) may help with knee pain.

AFOs are recommended for dorsiflexor weakness resulting in dropfoot or slapfoot, for plantarflexor weakness with absent heel rise, and for mediolateral instability. Individuals with PPS have difficulty with solid AFOs because of the structural design; they are typically made with 5 to 10 degrees of dorsiflexion and are then placed in a shoe with a slight positive heel, thus increasing the angle of the posterior shell to the floor. In standing and walking, this causes a knee flexion torque, with potential buckling of the knee if the quadriceps muscle is weak. Clients may attempt to straighten the knee by pushing back against the posterior shell of the AFO, potentially causing pain. In such instances, AFOs should be made in slight plantarflexion so that the tibia is perpendicular to the floor in the usual shoes worn. This is the normal position of the ankle for toe and heel clearance.[152] In cases of plantarflexion contracture, more plantarflexion is required in the AFO. Most jointed AFOs are of limited value because of the bulk and weight. Moreover, they require a larger shoe and do not provide much control for the ankle. Jointed AFOs allow adjustment to find the best angle in function.

A floor reaction AFO prohibits all ankle motion and can place forces to control the knee.[153-155] The orthosis prevents dropfoot, promotes heel rise, provides an extension torque on the proximal tibia to supplement weak quadriceps muscles, and can limit hyperextension of the knee. It requires precision in fabrication for the knee extension torque to occur only when the tibia is perpendicular to the floor during gait. When used with rocker-bottom shoes, the client with a flail foot can walk with a more typical gait pattern. Subjects with ligamentous laxity of the knee, exces-

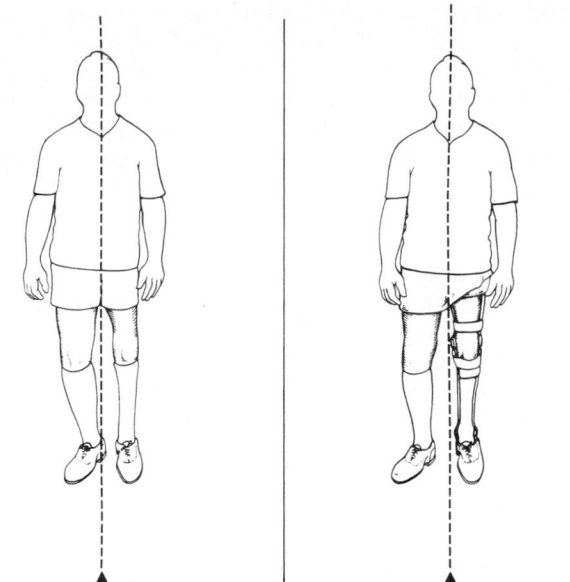

FIGURE 29-9 ■ This man has paralysis of the left lower extremity with severe fatigue, low back pain, pain and weakness in the right lower extremity, and decreased function. He can be seen to bear weight and stand on the right leg. Application of a left KAFO with a free knee joint (with a drop lock for use in prolonged standing and walking on rough terrain) and a limited-motion ankle joint unloaded his right leg and permitted him to walk in an erect posture. His pain disappeared and he has regained function at work and in social activities.

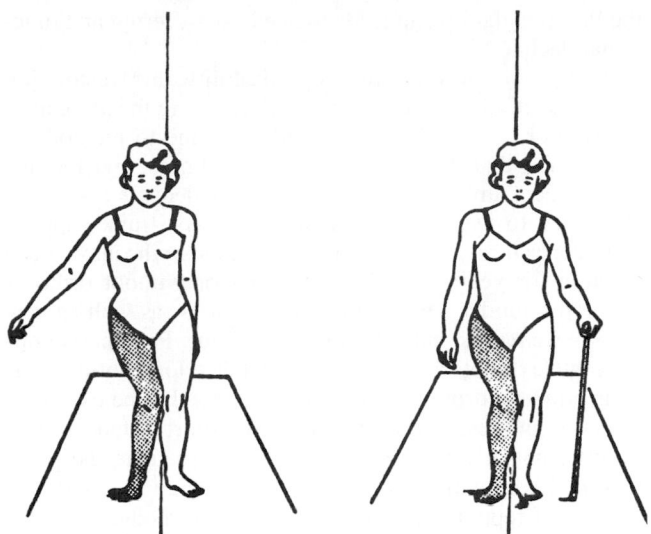

FIGURE 29-10 ■ Lateral trunk shift in a postpolio individual to illustrate abnormal forces occurring in the back, knee, and ankle with resulting joint dysfunction and pain. Prevention of these abnormal forces and some correction can be provided by use of a cane or forearm crutch. (Adapted from Ducroquet R, Darroquet J, Darroquet P: *Walking and limping—a study of normal and pathological walking,* Philadelphia, 1968, JB Lippincott.)

sive tibial torsion, or paralysis of the quadriceps muscles are poor candidates for this type of AFO.

Shoe inserts, heel lifts, and molded foot orthoses can provide a number of inconspicuous corrections. Positive heel shoes with a broad base, such as cowboy boots, stacked or Cuban heels, or the Swedish clog,[129] decrease the amount of dorsiflexion and plantarflexion motion and the work needed for ambulation. Rocker-bottom soles, which provide mechanical heel rise to assist the calf muscles, can be added to shoes and are commercially available. Work boots, dress boots, or basketball shoes may provide needed ankle stability.

Asymmetrical standing is typical in individuals with unilateral lower extremity paralysis or pain. Standing is accomplished with more weight on the stronger limb, which must perform continuous, high-level isometric contractions (Figure 29-9). Unloading the stronger leg requires restoration of weight bearing on the more involved leg using a KAFO or, in some instances, an AFO that prevents advancement of the tibia in the stance phase.[92,153-155]

Fifty percent of ambulatory individuals with PPS walk with an obvious forward-leaning posture. This posture requires continuous contraction of the erector spinae muscles and leads to back pain, often radiating to the hip and leg. The forward-leaning posture is found in people with quadriceps muscle paresis and in those with ankle weakness. Those with quadriceps weakness must move the center of gravity of the body anterior to the knee axis to lock the knee and prevent knee flexion in stance. This posterior force also produces ligamentous instability and genu recurvatum (see

Figure 29-8). In some instances, lightweight athletic knee braces allowing 10 to 15 degrees of hyperextension provide adequate control. More often, a KAFO with an offset knee joint allowing necessary hyperextension is required.[156,157,157a] People with dorsiflexor muscle paralysis or ankle instabilities walk in the forward-leaning posture to watch the floor and foot placement to avoid tripping and falling. Athletic ankle supports or boots may be sufficient to control some ankle instabilities. Molded and posted plastic AFOs with or without ankle joints are needed for more control. Flexible plastic AFOs and the dynamic spring dorsiflexion assists can correct simple dropfoot.[92] Once the forward-leaning posture is addressed, the individual can walk upright and back pain will lessen and may eventually disappear within days.

Walking with lateral trunk shift in the stance phase (gluteus medius gait) produces abnormal forces and joint dysfunction from the spine to the foot (Figure 29-10). Along with a strengthening program, these forces may be reduced with use of a forearm crutch or a cane.

Long-term crutch walkers with or without orthoses and those with slow, precarious, or labored gait should be evaluated for appropriateness for use of motorized vehicles as their primary form of locomotion, whereas orthotic corrections or applications may be indicated to assist with transfers and short-distance walking.

Changes in Locomotion

Despite severe difficulties with locomotion from overuse, asymmetrical gait patterns and movement, or ineffective use of assistive devices, changes or modifications are hard for many polio survivors to consider. As locomotion becomes more arduous or painful, many begin to limit outside activities rather than modify individual methods of locomotion. Resistance to lifestyle changes is common in the PPS population and leads to needless suffering and functional decline.[128]

Prevention of this spiraling disability and restoration of lost function requires a marked decrease in the amount of walking or propelling a chair and a change to methods of locomotion that do not cause pain, weakness, and fatigue. Independent ambulators or those with inadequate assistance may need to use a cane, forearm crutches, trunk support, shoe corrections, or new orthoses. Clients who have been walking for years with crutches with or without orthoses develop shoulder, elbow, and wrist injuries, as well as new muscle weakness, muscle pain, and fatigue. Personal mobility vehicles (motorized carts) for distance locomotion or as their primary form of locomotion may need to be explored, with walking reserved for transfers and short distances only. Lightweight manual wheelchairs only perpetuate the problems and eventually create new ones; use may lead to development of repetitive stress injuries of the shoulder, elbow, wrist, and hand. These people need to obtain electric wheelchairs or motorized carts if suitable. Manual wheelchairs at best only postpone problems. Motorized mobility devices will need to be explored to prevent fatigue, muscle overuse, and further damage to joints.

Use of motorized vehicles for locomotion should be considered and explored with sensitivity and caution. Specific rationales should be thoroughly understood by a seemingly resistant client and perceptions regarding its use should be addressed. Changes in methods of locomotion may be justified to increase safety and prevent costly falls, to reduce energy expenditure and decrease fatigue, to prevent further repetitive injury and pain, and, most important, to increase function and quality of life. Those who do make these difficult changes in their methods of locomotion seem to undergo a metamorphosis from pain and dysfunction to renewed activity and increased function.

Management of Postural Deviations

Common biomechanical deficits in polio survivors, which included genu recurvatum, genu valgum, inadequate dorsiflexion in swing, mediolateral ankle instability, and dorsiflexion collapse during stance, were described by Clark et al.[158] Strengthening exercises may be used to correct these impairments initially, with orthoses as an alternative management.

Postural exercises incorporated with breathing and stretching exercises is a way to address ineffective postures identified in all positions. Mental imagery, which may avoid impairments from fatigue, may be used early in addressing postural correction. Mechanical restoration of the lumbar curve in all seating at all settings and activities can address the problem if contractures do not limit motion. Properly fitted clerical chairs, ergonometric chairs, anterior tilt seats, gluteal pads, and several types of lumbar rolls, back supports, and seating systems may be beneficial.

Individuals with abdominal muscle paralysis may benefit from custom-made thoracolumbar corsets, with the posterior rigid stays bent to produce a normal standing lumbar curve. Paretic or paralyzed neck muscles can be rested and supported by soft foam collars or the supportive microcellular neck collars. People with severe trunk muscle paralysis or scoliosis with or without spinal fusion often support their trunk or relieve pain by pushing down with their hands or elbows on chairs, tables, and on their hips (see Figure 29-9). In time, such self-traction results in pain and weakness in their arms. Chair inserts and fixed supports as well as custom-made corsets, back braces, and molded body jackets should be considered. The rigid trunk supports, however, take away mobility used for function. Usually such supports can be worn for part of the day in activities where trunk mobility is not essential.

Weight Reduction

Weight reduction when appropriate is an effective way to decrease the muscle workload, but it is one of the most difficult. Weight loss is slow without exercise, but it can be accomplished. Weight control needs to be incorporated as a permanent modification of nutritional habits rather than achieved in a short-term diet. Dietetic counseling and support groups are important components of this challenging lifestyle modification.

Limitations in ROM

A thorough evaluation of muscle length and range of motion is critical in the overall management of life activities in individuals with PPS. The clinician should consider that not all tightness or limitations in motion are detrimental. Selective tightness may have provided some stability to otherwise unstable joints with paralyzed muscles, and useful contractures may have been developed by the body to achieve function. An excellent example can be seen in individuals who contracted polio as children. Muscle involvement was primarily in one lower extremity with a decrease in growth of that extremity as a result of diminished weight bearing forces. If the individual has at least a G- (4-) manual muscle test grade in the plantarflexors, the person will walk on the toes (in some plantarflexion) to decrease large drops in the center of gravity but resulting in increased energy expenditure for walking. Over the years, a plantarflexion contracture develops that can provide up to 3 to 4 inches for weight bearing on the shortened extremity. With a custom-made shoe, gait is similar to walking in a high-heeled shoe. This can be far more energy efficient than if motion were permitted to have dorsiflexion ROM.

Gentle myofascial release can also be beneficial for recent secondary impairments of muscles to decrease pain and muscle spasms, increase nutrition to the area, and slightly lengthen muscles.

Pulmonary Status

Older individuals with neuromuscular diseases may have increased vulnerability to respiratory complications.[91] Respiratory insufficiency and sleep apnea may mandate intermittent or constant use of ventilatory devices. Nighttime noninvasive positive pressure ventilation may be beneficial.[159] Pulmonary therapy and breathing exercises may help some individuals avoid tracheostomy.[91]

The role of the therapist is to modify activities and teach glossopharyngeal breathing, manually assisted coughing, or bronchial drainage as indicated.[160,161] If trunk supports are considered, vital capacity should be checked with and without an abdominal binder to determine the effect on breathing. The therapist's attention should also be directed toward prevention of problems that may occur from bed rest and maintaining as much function as can be permitted.

Sleep Disturbance

Several factors may contribute to reports of sleep disturbance, ranging from relatively apparent reasons to more medically complex reasons such as sleep apnea. Habitual sleeping patterns may provide important information. A history of pain or numbness that is worse at night or on rising points to sleeping surfaces that are too firm or sleeping with joints in close packed positions (usually the neck and shoulders). These problems are correctable with foam mattress covers or the new air pressure mattresses, cervical pillows, and modification of sleeping postures. More complex reasons for sleep disturbance such as sleep apnea may require referral to specialists (see section on pulmonary status).

Cold Intolerance

Most people have learned to control heat loss as best as they can with clothing, massage, and local heat. For interventions, however, cold intolerance can pose a potential problem with the use of cold modalities in the treatment of injuries and pain. Most people with PPS are hesitant to use local cold on any part of the body. They may typically use heating pads and hot water, which feels good at the time but may perpetuate or increase the edema, inflammation, and pain. Local cold is often more effective and is well tolerated by most people with PPS. Successful application of cold requires more client education about the use of cold and demonstration of the effects.

Other Interventions

A literature review of pharmacological approaches for PPS revealed that controlled trials of pyridostigmine and prednisone have not been beneficial.[57,162,163] Currently, there is no specific pharmacological agent widely recommended to address the multiple symptoms of PPS.

Specific management of dysphagia will warrant a thorough evaluation by a speech therapist. In general, intervention may consist of breathing exercises, swallowing techniques, monitoring fatigue levels, avoiding eating when fatigued, and dietary restrictions or changes (Case Study 29-5).

CASE STUDY 29-5 ■ PERSONAL REPORT: POSTPOLIO SYNDROME

Today my life is filled with optimism and hope. This was not the case long ago. I am 58 years old and have been diagnosed with postpolio syndrome. I contracted polio at the age of 2 years, but for the first time in my life with the medical diagnosis of PPS, I feel disabled.

It is difficult for me to determine when the symptoms began. My life over the last decades has been filled with caregiving. First my mother-in-law needed care and was ill for the last year of her life, and then my parents, who had special needs. I had a vague awareness that I was slowing down, not able to do some of the things that I had always done. But at that point in my life, the focus was not on me. It seems like when I was able to take a deep breath again; I was in a lot of pain.

I was able to see a doctor who specializes in postpolio syndrome. She recommended a new leg brace and she also recommended physical therapy. The new brace, while better for my body, is asking my motor system to change or learn new motor programs. I basically am trying to learn how to walk all over again. My pain stems from weakness and tight muscles in my unaffected limb. My unaffected leg has been stressed by many years of overuse. The pain I experience is mainly in my hip and occasionally in my knee within that leg. Because of the stress of this pain, my stamina is less than it once was; my balance is not good, and just the task of moving from point A to B is a challenge. I found that I needed to use crutches to help take weight off of my leg. The pain that I felt a little over a year ago became the focus of my life. It affected everything I did. My day was reduced to struggle to even shower and dress, let alone do anything else. I had to depend on my husband to do more and more.

During this period, I would allow myself, if I was having a really bad day, to just do nothing. Some days, I wouldn't even get out of bed until 11:00 AM. This didn't happen too often, but if it did, I allowed myself to not feel guilty. I think that this helped with my mental state. Yes, some days I would get frustrated, impatient and other days depressed, but it never lasted for too long. I have seen, on a personal level, what positive thinking can do. My parents were told that I would never walk again. I walked.

Having had polio, I learned at an early age how to "figure things out." If I couldn't do things one way, I perhaps could another. I think that this mind set has helped with my newest challenge. After meeting with my physical therapist, she helped to map out a plan to achieve my goals. My goals are simple: I want to walk without pain and without crutches. I want to cross my left leg over my right knee to tie my shoe. I want to build up my stamina so that I can go shopping. I want to be in the best health that I can be in. I want to remain independent.

I am learning that achieving my goals may be a long process. It has been a little over a year and I still have a long way to go. I have gained some strength, my stamina has increased, I am a bit more flexible, but more important, the pain level some days is just an afterthought. I am starting to regain my life.

I have learned in the past year how important it is to listen to your body. I have learned how to manage my work, rest, and exercise time. I understand that to achieve my goals it has and will take a lot of hard, sometimes painful, work. I also understand the importance of working toward my goal and achieving it. I consider myself to still be a relatively young woman who has a lot left to do in my life. Life is a gift, and that is what I want to do—live mine fully.*

---

*Orva Klopfer, as relayed to Holly Klopfer, PT, DPT.

ACKNOWLEDGMENTS
I thank Laura K. Smith, PhD, PT, and Carolyn Kelly, MS, PT, who contributed the chapter on *The Postpolio Syndrome* in the last edition of this text.

SECTION III

EFFECTS OF AGING ON THE FUNCTIONAL STATUS OF PATIENTS WITH SPINAL CORD INJURY, ACQUIRED BRAIN INJURIES, OR TRAUMATIC BRAIN INJURY

Ann Hallum, PhD

INTRODUCTION

In an excellent article on disability and wellness, Judy Kailes[164] asks, "Can disability, chronic conditions, health and wellness coexist?" She writes in her "white paper" that disability and health are typically seen as opposite ends of a health continuum. In this view, disability would exclude the experience of health or wellness. Because health professionals usually work within a medical environment, many come to believe the stereotypical view that people with a disability are sick. With continual reinforcement of the association between disability and illness, too few health professionals have paid attention to the issues of aging with a disability and the importance of maximizing a healthy lifestyle to prevent chronic diseases. As people with severe disabilities live longer, it is imperative that rehabilitation workers provide guidance and training on healthy living practices for people with disabilities who may be more vulnerable to aspects of the normal aging process. Kailes[164] recalls a friend's comment, "The lack of knowledge and understanding on the part of health care professionals concerning my disability and how it is affecting me as I age is extremely frightening to me. We are tired of reacting to pain and stiffness rather than preventing them."[164]

The typical process of aging leads to gradual decreases in joint mobility, muscle strength, and muscle flexibility and changes in endurance and balance. Although considerable research has shown that maintaining an active, healthy lifestyle can delay the decline and deterioration of physical and mental status as we age, there is an increased incidence of osteoarthritis, osteoporosis, and vascular change regardless of a healthy lifestyle. In nondisabled adults, more than one third of those over the age of 65 years fall each year, and 20% to 30% of those have injuries that impair mobility and independence. Healthy, but sedentary, older people reported more problems with ADL than did those who continued to be physically active and who had had a previously active lifestyle.[165-167] People living with disabilities undergo a similar aging process, but those natural changes are superimposed on the physical limitations caused by the previous and/or ongoing pathology or trauma.[168]

Until the last 10 to 15 years, little attention was paid to the long-term consequences of aging on the population of people with significant disabilities. Most health care providers believed that the life span of people with severe disabilities was decreased; therefore, many patients were led to believe that planning for the aging process or retirement was not necessary.[169] Because of that perception, many people with disabilities became passive in or disengaged from determining their own health outcomes, considering it beyond their control.[164] Yet, although people with disabilities such as spinal cord or brain injuries were expecting to die at a young age, many people who had contracted paralytic polio in the 1940s and 1950s were and are living well into old age. As stated within the previous PPS section, many of the people who had had polio as a child were finding that, as they aged, they struggled more with their usual ADLs as a result of increasing weakness and joint pain and marked fatigue. The experiences of those with polio stimulated the current interest on aging with a significant disability. For example, some clinicians have recently expressed concern that patients who had recovered from Guillain-Barré syndrome, particularly the axonal form, might have a problem with increased weakness and decreased functional abilities with aging similar to that experienced by some aging polio survivors.[170]

EFFECTS OF AGING

There is now an increasing awareness of the effects of aging on the functional status of patients with spinal cord (SCI) and acquired brain injuries (ABI) or traumatic brain injury (TBI). Because of medical advances, patients are now living 20 to 50 years past their time of injury. Numerous studies have been done describing quality of life issues for people with TBIs or ABIs; however, those studies seldom look specifically at changes in functional levels or what can be done to ameliorate the declines.[171-173]

McColl et al,[169] studying the impact of aging on people after a SCI, have identified major categories of problems related to aging, such as musculoskeletal problems and joint, sensory, and connective tissue changes; chronic urinary tract infections, heart, respiratory, and other chronic diseases; secondary complications of the initial lesions, such as syringomyelia; and problems related to social and cultural acceptance and access or barriers.

In a study of 150 people aging with an SCI, nearly 25% reported decreases in their ability to perform functional activities that they had been able to handle after the acute rehabilitation phase. The subjects reporting decreases in functional ability were generally older (45 years compared with 36 years) and had longer postinjury periods (18 years compared to 11 years). The most common symptoms reported by those who had a decrease in functional status were related to fatigue, pain, and muscle weakness. The ADLs reported to be more difficult were transfers, bathing, and dressing. People who had a decline in functional ability also reported needing additional equipment to maintain their functional levels.[174]

In another study of people 20 years after SCI, 22% of the subjects reported an increased need for support with ADLs. Compared with a general group of nondisabled men and women aged 75 to 84 years in which 78% of the men and 64% of women did not need help with ADLs, the population of people with SCI needed increasing support to remain independent, and the need for help occurred at a younger age. On average, those with quadriplegia required more help with ADLs around the age of 49 years, whereas those with paraplegia were able to maintain their functional level until age 54 years. The groups showing functional decreases reported greater fatigue, increased muscle weakness, pain, stiffness, and weight gain.[175] Other researchers support their findings that 5, 10, and 15 years after SCI there was an association with the need for additional help with increasing age.[176]

Liem et al,[177] referencing an international data set of people with SCI, studied a subset of 352 people who had had an SCI at least 20 years prior. Thirty-two percent of the subjects reported needing increased help with transfers and housework compared with their functional abilities at acute hospital discharge. Woman needed more help than men, possibly because more women with an SCI were single and relied on personal assistant support, whereas more men were married and had a spouse or parent who provided necessary caregiving. With increasing age, women also had a higher incidence of reported musculoskeletal impairments, which may have been related to biomechanical differences between men and women (e.g., 40% lower upper body strength). Women with preexisting functional limitations who are postmenopausal may show evidence of increased bone loss and an increase in heart disease that is compounded by mobility impairments and the resulting sedentary lifestyle patterns. Older women with mobility limitations and their health care providers need to be educated about preventive measures to decrease the incidence of fractures or heart disease.[178]

Neurogenic bowel and bladder symptoms also worsen with age in some people with SCIs. With changes in general health status, polypharmacy, decreased activity and poor nutritional patterns, bowel problems, particularly constipation, become more problematic. Although constipation seems like a minor issue relative to paralysis, people with SCIs reported significant abdominal distention and pain, an increased incidence of perineal and sacral skin breakdown, and, in some cases, autonomic dysreflexia. In addition to the discomfort of chronic bowel dysfunctions, the required bowel care programs may take more time, which can lead to increased psychosocial issues associated with anxiety about bowel accidents in social and work situations. The increased time required for bowel care also takes time away from social activities for both the person with an SCI and the caregiver. For some people with continuing bowel problems that interfere with life and work activities, a colostomy may be an option that increases independence from caregiver support during the bowel program.[179] Another complicating factor related to bowel dysfunction is the typical treatment of pain complaints. Because the origin of pain was often illusive, the most common treatment was related to use of oral medications rather than to referrals for therapeutic interventions. The recommendation of pain medications, especially opioids, increases gastrointestinal difficulties in nondisabled populations,[180] and the problem for patients with SCI is compounded. Therefore, for patients with SCI, prophylactic medications and nutritional recommendations to prevent or minimize constipation are essential.

In the study of Liem et al[177] constipation, pressure ulcers, female sex, and years since injury were most highly associated with decreased functional status, not increased weakness. Fortunately, bowel dysfunction, particularly constipation, and pressure ulcers can be prevented with a thoughtful rehabilitation and medical care plan. In addition, the ability to maintain transfer independence or to help with transfers can be improved by maintenance of ideal weight, management of spasticity, and appropriate hygiene. Because aging people with an SCI may have health problems similar to any aging population, primary impairments in muscle strength and endurance may be magnified. Therefore,

patients making repeat visits for medical problems (e.g., musculoskeletal, cardiac, respiratory, and renal diseases and diabetes) should have a referral to a comprehensive therapy program that focuses lifestyle changes rather than on reactions to secondary illnesses.

Drawing on the National Spinal Cord Injury Database of 7981 people with SCIs that occurred between 1973 and 1998, Charlifue et al[181] showed that there was a slight decrease in perceived health status the longer one lived after SCI. They also found evidence that those injured later in life had a higher number of rehospitalizations after injury than those injured at a younger age. Although there were problems with the statistical issues within the sample, the study clearly indicated that the best predictor of a complication is a previous history of that complication. On the basis of their results, Charlifue et al[181] suggest that prevention of complications is the best approach to improve quality of health and quality of life for people aging with SCI. That view coincides with the statement noted earlier that people with disabilities are "tired of reacting rather than preventing" secondary health problems.[164]

As an example of contributing to, but not preventing, secondary health problems, patients with SCI who complained of pain from musculoskeletal problems and overuse were seldom referred for therapeutic interventions but were treated primarily with prescription medications to treat painful conditions. This medical management often resulted in increased problems, such as constipation, fatigue, irritability, and frustration.[182] Preventive measures, especially interventions such as lifestyle changes and exercise, are major components of a program to counter negative aspects of aging. In the Wellness and SCI Project underway at the University of Michigan, Tate et al[183] are looking at barriers to continuing exercise in people with spinal cord injuries. One purpose of their randomized controlled trial is to help people who have survived an SCI prevent secondary conditions, such as pressure ulcers, carpal tunnel syndrome, and heart disease, which are partially associated with the primary diagnosis. The study is focused on identifying barriers, both physical and psychological, to exercise that prevent people with SCI from continuing exercise programs after leaving rehabilitation. Participants were assigned to a control group that had only physical examinations or to an intervention group that had regular physical examinations and workshops on exercise and wellness issues such as diet, stress management, and other lifestyle options. Data from a questionnaire on *Barriers to Physical Exercise and Disability* showed that 74% of people with SCI indicated that they wanted to participate in an exercise program, yet less than 46% do so. Those who were not exercising cited the same reasons as nondisabled people: lack of motivation and lack of energy. Most revealing was that fewer than 47% of their physicians had recommended that they engage in an exercise program. There was no mention that any of the study participants had been seen by or referred to a physical or occupational therapist. Nearly 50% of the study participants expressed concern that fitness center staff (not a rehabilitation site) would not know how to help develop an exercise program appropriate for their conditions and some expressed concern that exercising might worsen their conditions. Severity of SCI was not related to involvement or lack of involvement in an exercise program. The University of Michigan study, which is associated with one of the 16

Model Spinal Cord Injury Care Centers is ongoing. (See excellent, comprehensive Web site: http://www.med.umich.edu/pmr/modelsci/index.htm.)[184]

Intervention

Although no published studies were found on exercise plans and aging in SCI, the interest in promoting exercise and lifestyle changes to prevent secondary medical problems has been identified. The National Rehabilitation Hospital in Washington, DC, is currently involved in three major studies: a mail-based survey to determine the relationship between health and exercise/physical activity in people with SCI, a second study looking at cardiovascular disease risk screening and exercise testing, and a third study looking at secondary conditions and the relationship between health and exercise/physical activity in people with SCI. The Massachusetts Institute of Technology is currently engaged in an SCI decision-making study. The University of Miami's Center on Aging is engaging in a study to develop and evaluate new ways of assisting middle-aged and older persons living with the long-term effects of SCI. Information on these continuing studies can be found on the National Spinal Cord Injury Web site at http://www.spinalcord.org/.[184a]

The Rehabilitation Center at Penn State Milton S. Hershey Medical Center has posted suggestions for patients with SCI who want to begin an exercise program (Aging, Exercise, and Spinal Cord Injury; see http://www.hmc.psu.edu/rehab/services/spinalcord/).[184b] The suggestions recommend that patients establish a home exercise program on the basis of input from a rehabilitation specialist who can identify the appropriate equipment for home use and design a comprehensive program of exercise. As an alternative, they suggest working through a health club that has adapted equipment and personnel skilled in working with physical disabilities. Some of the recommended activities are swimming, arm-crank ergometers, wheelchair pushing on indoor rollers or outdoor paths, and functional electrical stimulation leg cycle ergometry (ESE). Neither the ESE nor the newer treadmill with body weight support systems now used for exercise with some disabilities is rarely available outside rehabilitation or research sites. They also recommend strength training to build muscle tone and endurance starting with low weight/high repetitions (15 repetitions/3 sets). The weights can be increased gradually, followed by increased repetitions. They caution that the same muscle group should not be exercised 2 days in a row and that a variety of activities be included in the program to prevent overuse/overwork injury of weakened muscles and structures (see section on exercise or overwork damage in amyotrophic lateral sclerosis section of Chapter 16). The unnamed authors of the document also offer suggestions to people with SCI about their body mass, aerobic capacity, temperature regulation, blood pressure, cardiovascular disease, contractures, joint pain, and pressure ulcers. Although the document is not research based, it does offer reasonable suggestions for maintaining a healthy lifestyle while aging.

The National Center on Physical Activity and Disability (NCPAD) (www.ncpad.org)[184c] has a series of excellent exercise videotapes on exercising with a disability. A tape specific to the needs of a person with an SCI, *"Exercise Program for Individuals with Spinal Cord Injuries: Paraplegia,"* includes segments on aerobics, strengthening, and flexibility, as well as precautions and information on how hard one should exercise.

Health promotion materials are available from many sources, but most refer only to the needs of nondisabled populations. Yet people with disabilities, who may be even more sedentary than nondisabled groups and who may underuse or overuse specific muscle groups, may have an even greater need for health promotion strategies because the aging process affects cell structure and functions. Although care must be taken not to overstress weakened muscles and structures related to the disability, research clearly indicates that we can improve efficiency of function by challenging our muscles, lungs, and heart to improve strength, flexibility, and endurance. Fortunately, SCI centers are now beginning to study the most appropriate types of exercise programs and lifestyle recommendations. (See Case Study 29-6 at the end of this section on p. 962 for a description of issues related to aging faced by Pete, who sustained a SCI at age 24 years.)

Another group of people often neglected by professional health care and insurance providers after the acute rehabilitation period are those who have recovered from TBIs. Levin[185] writes that, before 1980, people with brain injuries were considered "dead on arrival." People who would have died from the TBI several decades ago are now living into old age and are coping with the changes caused by the aging process superimposed on their physical limitations and cognitive problems. Of great concern is the possible relationship between a history of brain injury and increased cognitive changes along the dementia continuum.[186] Cognitive decline in the nondisabled population is problematic, but the additive effect for a person with a previous TBI may seriously impair the person's coping mechanisms when dealing with their own health and self-care needs.[187] Extensive work has been done on rehabilitation programs and quality-of-life issues related to head injury and to a lesser extent, cerebral vascular accidents.[188] (See also Chapter 17 for treatment interventions for head injury and Chapter 27 for treatment interventions related to hemiplegia.) Unfortunately, the focus of rehabilitation after a TBI has been on the acute and rehabilitation stages of treatment and not the chronic problems that follow this group of patients into their older years. Few patients see a therapist after they are discharged from rehabilitation unless they have acute events such as musculoskeletal problems, a seizure disorder, or internal medicine disorders. Across the United States, access to comprehensive rehabilitation services for TBI varies depending on geographic area and payment resources. The focus of treatment is primarily on having the person adapt to the environment, with less focus on modifications of the environment to enable people to participate more actively. Although TBI is a lifetime disability, little attention has been paid to the needs of aging people after a TBI who may have recurring needs for physical and cognitive rehabilitation and retraining over the life span. Also, patients who sustained a TBI after the age of 60 years may have different needs from those who were injured at a younger age. Those injured later in life had longer inpatient rehabilitation periods and lagged behind younger patients in functional status at the point of discharge; however, like the younger people who sustained a head injury, the over-60 patients showed measurable improvement during the 6-month study period. Therefore, aggressive management of older patients with TBI is recommended, and older patients may require continuing management because of the overlying issues of the aging process.[189] The National Institutes of Health (NIH) consensus document on the treatment of people with TBIs suggests that specialized interdisciplinary treatment programs need to be put in place to deal with the medical, rehabilitation, family, and social needs of people with TBIs who are over the age of 65 years. The document also concludes that access to and funding for long-term rehabilitation is necessary to meet long-term needs; however, it recognizes that changes in payment methods by private insurance and public programs may jeopardize the recommendations.[190]

Although the authors of the NIH document recognize the need to deal with the aging processes associated with TBI, there continues to be a lack of services and trained professionals available, especially at the community level.[191] As with the SCI population, work is now being done to investigate the relationships among TBI, aging, and health. Breed et al[192] found that older people with TBIs were more likely than their age-matched nondisabled peers to report metabolic, endocrine, sleep, pain, muscular, or neurological and psychiatric problems. Their findings support those of Hibbard et al[193] and Beetar et al[194] that suggest that medical personnel need to be prepared to treat a broad range of health issues in the aging TBI population. Fewer of the studies on long-term outcomes and issues in TBI extend to the 10- and 15-year postinjury periods that have been collected for patients with SCIs. In studies 5 years after TBI, improvement in physical and social functions were noted in most areas for at least the first 2 years after injury, with the exception that people with a history of alcohol or drug abuse did less well. One could assume that continued abuse of alcohol or drugs would bode ill for patients aging with a TBI.[195] In one study of 946 children and adolescents who sustained a TBI, Strauss et al[196] found that patients with severe and permanent mobility and feeding deficits had higher mortality rates with a 66% chance of surviving to age 50 years. In contrast, survivors with fair or good mobility had a life expectancy only 3 years shorter than that of the general population. However, because both severely and mildly injured individuals with a TBI can live well into and beyond their 50s, the impact of aging on the physical and cognitive deficits must be dealt with assertively to prevent superimposed disability.

Although few studies have been done on the impact of exercise or the best type of exercise for people aging with a TBI, Gordon et al[197] studied 240 people living in the community with a TBI. They compared exercisers and nonexercisers with a TBI and exercisers and nonexercisers without a TBI. Typical exercise activities were swimming, jogging, biking, or sports that increased heart rate for more than 30 minutes at least three times per week for a 6-month period. Their findings suggest that, although exercise did not decrease functional impairments related to the TBI, people who exercised complained of fewer physical, emotional (less depression), or cognitive complaints (sleep problems, irritability, memory problems, and disorganization). Of interest was that the exercisers in the group with a TBI had more severe brain injuries than those who did not exercise. In their online TBI consumer report, Gordon et al[198] recommend that aerobic and nonaerobic exercises are beneficial.

They also suggest that individuals with TBIs check out local exercise centers, independent living centers, or adult education classes and seek out videotapes that might provide encouragement or support for engaging in exercise. There is no mention of referrals to physical or occupational therapists for guidance in setting up exercise or lifestyle change programs or for resources within the community. See Case Study 29-7 at the end of this topic for clinical descriptions of typical situations faced by individuals aging with an ABI such as a stroke, an anoxic event, or a viral/bacterial infection (see Chapters 17, 20, and 27).

Although research and treatment centers have been established to deal with comprehensive care issues for individuals with disabilities,[199] Kailes'[164] statement that the lack of helpful information related to exercising while aging with a disability is disturbing. Considering the extensive evidence showing that many of the physical limitations that occur as part of aging in nondisabled people can be prevented or delayed by changing health habits, she suggests that people with disabilities need (1) appropriate fitness assessment measures that can be used with various types of disabilities, (2) exercise guidelines that are appropriate for age and types of limitations, (3) exercise facilities that are accessible, integrated, and not separate from those of nondisabled populations, and (4) exercise equipment the incorporates universal design features.

Unfortunately, in today's health care environment, many people with SCI, TBI, or ABI do not have access to specialists (therapists, neurologists, orthopedists, urologists, gastroenterologists, and wheelchair specialists) who understand the complex movement limitation–related needs and how that affects participation in life. Care is fragmented, and physicians and therapists, if involved in the care at all, seldom have a comprehensive picture of the person's needs. Although one might assume that the managed-care system would provide coordination of care within the provider system, more likely there are strong incentives to restrict access to care, particularly for disability-related care that may require a period of continuing rehabilitation treatment and retraining. Even providers within the group seldom communicate because the group is composed of practitioners who accept the insurance contract rather than a group composed of practitioners working together to improve health. Today few patients with SCI, ABI, or TBI (see Case Study 29-8) are followed up in comprehensive specialty centers or clinics as they age.[200,201]

The NCPAD is an example of an excellent center dealing with disability issues. The NCPAD provides leadership in the development of health promotion programs for people with disabilities. Recently, Rimmer et al[202] held focus groups across the United States with consumers with disabilities, architects, fitness and recreation professionals, and city planners and park district managers to identify various positive and negative factors associated with access and participation in fitness and recreation programs for people with disabilities. They identified a constellation of issues related to the natural environment, economic and resource issues, equipment barriers, emotional and psychological barriers, perceptions, and attitudes of both disabled and nondisabled people, including professional barriers related to the use and interpretation of guidelines, codes, regulations, and laws and policies and procedures both at the facility and community level. Clearly, the problem of access to exercise opportunities described by Pete (see Case Study 29-6) is a common problem across the country. The NCPAD Web site[184c] offers excellent resources for people with disabilities who want to begin an exercise or activity program. The site should be reviewed by all therapists who work with individuals who are aging with a disability to review summarized data on activity and exercise research and the extensive resources on exercise videos and pamphlets. Because of the lack of research related to lifestyle and exercise programs as modifiers of the aging process in individuals with disabilities, Kailes et al[164] at the NCPAD have made an extensive list of questions to stimulate research and service provisions, a few of which are identified here:

- Where do people with functional limitations go for fitness information that has a disability filter? How should they exercise? How much?
- What is the effect of exercise on preventing an increase in the functional limitations for specific types of groups with specific medical diagnoses and functional loss?
- How important is conditioning, flexibility, and endurance for people with preexisting functional loss? Is it more important that conditioning and flexibility

be maintained because many people work harder to physically function?
- Does active and consistent participation in various physical activities (e.g., sports, fitness) for people with movement limitations accelerate musculoskeletal injury or pain or does it slow or prevent pain or injury?
- How do people with functional limitations maintain cardiopulmonary conditioning, physical strength, bone density, coordination, and joint mobility?
- Should aerobic conditioning come before specific muscle strengthening or the reverse?
- What type of strengthening program is best for people with significant spasticity?
- Will osteoporosis become a major problem for people with mobility limitations? Should screening be conducted earlier for people with disabilities than for people without disabilities? What interventions are effective? When should they be started?[164]

The increasing interest in health in aging with a disability is reflected in the studies published in the February 2005 issue of *Archives of Physical Medicine and Rehabilitation Clinics of North America*. The documents were not available at the time of publication (Case Studies 29-6 to 29-8).[203-206]

CASE STUDY 29-6 ■ PATIENT WITH SPINAL CORD INJURY

Pete was an active 24-year-old competitive skier when he hit a tree while off-course skiing. Because he had been an excellent student before his injury, he adapted well by returning to college to study computer science. He also participated in an adapted skiing program but did not find it satisfying and decided that he could maintain his strength by using a manual rather than a motorized chair. He was successful using his manual chair because his work area and community were highly accessible. Pete had his car fitted with hand controls and was able to manipulate his chair into his vehicle. At age 31 years, he married and moved to a home designed for his needs. Pete and his wife tried repeatedly to have children and eventually adopted a girl and, 3 years later, a boy, both from China because they were unable to adopt successfully in the United States. Pete was an active father, easily lifting the children onto his lap during play. When he was 41 years old, he noticed that he had more difficulty roughhousing with the children and he also returned home from work every day tired, both significant changes. His wife, who was his primary caregiver, noted that his joints were stiffer and that he seemed to be developing more contractures, especially in the knees, which interfered with his care. Pete also complained of increasing hip, knee, and shoulder pain. Both he and his wife attempted to become more aggressive in the home exercise program that he had been given nearly 15 years earlier. Between the needs of the children and help with dressing and the extensive hygiene and bowel care required, Pete and his wife decided that they had to decrease their stress levels so they could focus more positively on their children. Seeking help from their primary care physician, they were told that

the changes were expected declines for someone with an SCI. After struggles with their insurance provider, they returned to their rehabilitation center more than 200 miles from their home. After an evaluation by a PT and OT, Pete decided to conserve energy by using a motorized chair, which required that he purchase a wheelchair-accessible van. His home exercise program of stretching and exercise with varied resistance elastic bands was reviewed, and the therapists recommended that he exercise at his local gym because he was not eligible for continuing therapy interventions in his health plan. With use of the manual chair only at home, Pete felt less shoulder pain and exhaustion at the end of the day. Because both Pete and his wife found the home exercise program "boring," he went to one of his local exercise centers; however, he was unable to use much of the equipment unless his wife helped with transfers and balance. No one at the facility was experienced in dealing with functional limitations and Pete felt that many of their suggestions were potentially harmful. The center's swimming pool was not accessible and the pool surfaces were abrasive, so Pete and his wife were concerned that their attempts to transfer him into the pool without a lift could cause skin damage. In addition, his wife felt that the 2 hours required to deal with changing clothes and catheters was more frustrating than helpful. Pete and his wife maintained a modest home exercise program and attempted to exercise as a family to a videotape of "chair exercise" designed for older people. However, his more sedentary lifestyle led to a significant increase in weight over the next 5 years. He, like most people, was not consistent in his exercise program. With his weight gain, he had his first significant pressure ulcer, which required a short

CASE STUDY 29-6 ■ PATIENT WITH SPINAL CORD INJURY—cont'd

hospital stay. Although he attempted to control his weight, he was not successful. His wife had more difficulty moving him for dressing and transfer assists and he began to have increasing problems with his bowel program. Bowel care that used to be completed in 30 minutes now required more than 70 minutes because of severe constipation and occasional diarrhea episodes. Pete and his wife contacted a dietitian who prescribed changes in his diet (increased fiber and water) with the addition of stool softeners and a bowel stimulant. The diet changes improved his sense of well-being and decreased his constant discomfort from abdominal distention. Over the next 5 years, Pete enjoyed his family and work life. Somewhere around the age of 51 years, he reported an overall sense of increasing fatigue and had more difficulty shifting his weight for pressure relief. He reentered the hospital for treatment of another pressure ulcer with a systemic infection. Because both he and his wife sensed increasing difficulties with his personal care and because his children were no longer home to help with lifting as they had as teenagers, his therapists and discharge nurse arranged for in-home support services to help with morning and evening care. Both Pete and his wife felt a great relief from the daily care requirements. Pete felt less stressed about the increased time it took for him and his wife to complete his bowel program. Although both found it frustrating to have "outsiders" in their home morning and evenings, they also found new energy to join a group exercise program recently offered by their local hospital therapy department. After 6 months of working with the hospital-based group (not covered by his insurance but priced at a reasonable rate for both of them), Pete and his wife continued their exercise program at home, feeling a renewed

spirit. At age 55 years, Pete fell from his chair when he missed a curb and fractured his femur. He considered this an enormous setback because he was discharged home needing total care and his insurance would not provide coverage for in-home nursing care. He continued to pay for 4 hours a day of in-home support services, and one of his children returned home to help with care during the day until his wife returned from work. Fortunately, once he was able to participate actively with physical and occupational therapy, his insurance company paid for home-based therapy services. The program included ROM, progressive resistive exercise for all active muscle groups, and aerobic exercises using an upper extremity ergometer. It took nearly 6 months for Pete to return to his prior functional level, although he feels that he gets more short of breath when he performs his daily routines. He again feels positive about his life, although concerned about falling again or causing injury to his wife because of lifting or moving him or his equipment. Both have been discussing long-term plans for dealing with the aging process. Fortunately, they are financially able to pay for some services not funded by their insurance. They are considering adding a room to their home so that they can have a full-time in-home caregiver when daily care routines and transfers become difficult for both of them. Both Pete and his wife are aware that most people with SCIs, especially those who are single, do not have their options to remain independent at home. They are clear that they do not want their children to be responsible for continuing attendant responsibilities. Both Pete and his wife have signed health care directives. Pete has indicated that he does not want life-sustaining care such as artificial ventilation should that become an issue.

CASE STUDY 29-7 ■ AN INDIVIDUAL WITH ACQUIRED BRAIN INJURY

I was 37 years old when I sustained an acquired brain injury. I was then the department head of Mt. Zion's occupational therapy department in San Francisco. I was independent, a single mother, extremely active, and never ill, except for minor asthma episodes. My injury was a result of an anoxic episode, status asthmaticus, resulting in diagnosis of a seizure disorder, myoclonus, and mild cognitive deficits.

I am currently 56 years old. And, yes, I am writing about the changes I am experiencing with aging. I do believe that being a wheelchair user, having a more sedentary lifestyle, being on multiple medications, having a compromised immune system, and being a woman, there are issues of aging and dependence I have to face.

PHYSICAL

■ Balance: I have poor to fair sitting and standing balance. In the past year I have had situations where

I was forced to sit in an armless meeting chair; I could not concentrate. Ten years ago this did not bother me. At times I cannot go to a public, even accessible, bathroom if the space is too large, because I teeter on the toilet. Recently at home, on occasion, I cannot maintain my balance, turn my trunk, lift my arm, and have the strength and ROM to flush the toilet.

■ Falls: I average at least one fall per month. I have osteopenia in my left hip. I am prescribed 1500 mg calcium/day as a result.

■ Somnolence: Usually this is an age-related problem. In my case, I believe it is due to medications. I have had the problem for years. Finding a balance between insomnia, tremors caused by respiratory drugs, and sedating drugs for seizure control that lull me, creating a vestibular component, has been difficult.

Continued

CASE STUDY 29-7 ■ AN INDIVIDUAL WITH ACQUIRED BRAIN INJURY—cont'd

■ Ambulation/endurance: Very limited. Weight bearing would help prevention of osteoporosis, but I am limited to the functional amount of time I can walk because of balance and endurance. I also have an odd psychophysical phenomenon that renders me with overload and I freeze in front of traffic or just fall. I have to have someone with me at all times.

ADLs

■ I am dependent in all household ADLs. I am independent in dressing except for back closures. I cannot tie any type of lace (decreased coordination and hand strength). There are increasing times I fall when transferring from my chair to bed, etc. At this point I would say I need minimal assistance with feeding, a change in the last 2 years. I have trouble with sandwiches, cups (cannot pick them up or keep proper grasp because I have a reflexive pinch/grasp when my hands touch an object hard or soft). I also

hit myself in the face with utensils as a result of the clonus.

PSYCHOSOCIAL

I have had a significant other for 16 years. It is a difficult situation having your caregiver be your significant other. You need him, and sometimes you wish you didn't. I can't imagine being 80 years old and being with him. I can't imagine being 80 years old. There is a sadness that I should be caring for my parents who are 80 years old, and they are still caring for me, even though we live separate active lives. I do not qualify for long-term care insurance because using a wheelchair disqualifies me. I believe it is a fact that right now is my early stage of being elderly, and even the doctors laugh when I say this, but I feel it within myself. It is nice to say, "think young, and you are," but it doesn't always work out that way; that is just a fact.

© 12/2004 Cheryl Damico

CASE STUDY 29-8 ■ INDIVIDUAL POST-TBI

Steve was 27 years old when he was hit on the left side of his head with a baseball bat in a robbery attempt. He was not expected to live because of severe brain swelling requiring the removal of part of his skull. Because of the intracranial pressure, he also suffered damage to the right side of his brain, resulting in a "double hemiplegia." After a 6-month coma period, he spent another 6 months in a rehabilitation center. At discharge, he was walking slowly with a walker, but he used a wheelchair for primary transportation by pushing with his more functional arm and leg. Although he had been engaged to be married, his fiancée left him 3 months after injury. He returned home to live with his parents, who were in their early 50s. His mother quit work to care for him, continuing his exercise programs and taking him to his many medical appointments. By the age of 35 years he had attempted and failed three job training programs with the Department of Rehabilitation. He returned to his local community college, which had a computer-based program to help with memory and problem solving. Although Steve had few friends outside his family, he was pleasant and cheerful while living at home. His family included him fully in all events and attempted to engage him in local activity programs for people with disabilities, such as bowling, kayaking, and swimming. Steve found the activities "boring" because he was unable to be truly active or participate.

Because of his major physical limitations, Steve gained more than 40 pounds by the time he was 39 years old. Despite repeated visits with a dietitian and participation in both medical and private diet programs, Steve continued to gain weight. Because of his weight gain, he had more difficulty walking and complained of

frequent back pain. Both parents noticed increased daytime sleepiness and, after testing, Steve was found to have sleep apnea and was started on a nasal continuous positive airway pressure system. The daytime sleepiness decreased and Steve was referred to physical therapy. Because of insurance limits, the programs designed were home based and Steve had difficulty getting on and off his exercise bike. He seldom attained an aerobic exercise level that would help with his weight problems and he had little personal motivation to maximize his exercise periods. He was then referred back to the community college, which had an adapted physical education program. He attended for several months, but this focus was on weight lifting rather than aerobic exercise. His parents offered to buy him a three-wheeled cycle, but after renting one, they realized that Steve was not willing to ride the cycle, even if accompanied by his parents.

Steve, now at age 50 years, has frequent bouts of disabling back pain because of his kyphotic sitting posture (repeated wheelchair inserts and adjustments have not helped). He walks infrequently and is now having more difficulty with knee flexion contractures that are making transfers more difficult. Steve's parents petitioned his insurance company for an in-patient rehabilitation program in which diet and exercise programs could be instituted and supervised over an extended time; however, they were denied. His parents, now in their 70s, are working with a local agency to identify the appropriate long-term living arrangements that will be necessary when they can no longer care for him. Steve does not have the capacity to plan for the future.

CHAPTER SUMMARY

There were three general medical categories discussed within this chapter: adults with developmental disabilities, individuals with PPS, and individuals with acquired CNS deficits (SCI, ABI, and TBI). Although the medical diagnosis made during each acute event has great variance as to the specific CNS lesions and their causes, the problems encountered by individuals as they age have great commonalities. All individuals initially have been encouraged to fully participate in life without consideration of the eventual effect that participation will have on the musculoskeletal, cardiopulmonary, or neuromuscular systems. When the effect of aging, individuals' chronic functional limitations after insult, and individuals' high level expectations on life participation is correlated, the result may change the models used by occupational and physical therapy when establishing long-term goals. There is no easy answer to early rehabilitations effect on future function or long-term extension of life participation. Yet, commonalities in (1) overuse requiring energy conservation, (2) pain stemming from malalignment in articulation surfaces and muscle imbalance, and (3) the psychosocial traumas from again losing motor function have become common themes in individuals aging with movement limitations. These future problems if understood during the initial rehabilitation of the acute problem might be avoided or delayed in onset as the person ages. Many of these areas discussed in this chapter will become the challenges of rehabilitation in the future. They need to be considered throughout the life of an individual who must face the challenges of living with functional limitations.

REFERENCES
Section I: Adults with Developmental Disabilities Across the Life Span

1. Developmental Disabilities Act, Public Law 98-527, U.S. Congress, Senate, 98th Congress; 1984.
2. Rapp CE, Torres MM: The adult with cerebral palsy, *Arch Fam Med* 9:466-472, 2000.
3. Connolly BH: Issues in aging in individuals with lifelong disabilities. In Connolly BH, Montgomery PC, editors: *Therapeutic exercise in developmental disabilities,* ed 3, Thorofare, NJ, 2004, SLACK, pp 505-530.
4. Connolly BH: Aging in individuals with lifelong disabilities, *Phys Occup Ther Pediatr* 21:23-47, 2001.
5. Rose J, Gamble J, Burgos A et al: Energy expenditure index of walking for normal children and for children with cerebral palsy, *Dev Med Child Neurol* 32:333-340, 1990.
5a. Hallum A: Disability and the transition to adulthood: issues for the disabled child, the family, and the pediatrician, *Curr Probl Pediatr* 25:12-50, 1995.
5b. Rose J, Gamble JG, Medeiros J et L: Energy cost of walking in normal children and in those with cerebral palsy: comparison of heart rate and oxygen uptake, *J Pediatr Orthop* 9:276-279, 1989.
5c. Rose J, Gamble JG, Lee J et al: The energy expenditure index: a method to quantitate and compare walking energy expenditure for children and adolescents, *J Pediatr Orthop* 11:571-578, 1991.
6. Jaffe JS, Timell AM: Prevalence of low bone density in institutionalized men with developmental disabilities, *J Clin Densitometry* 6:143-147, 2003.
7. Turk MA, Scandale J, Rosenbaum PF et al: The health of women with cerebral palsy, *Phys Med Rehabil Clin North Am* 12:153-268, 2001.
8. Overeynder JC, Turk MA: Cerebral palsy and aging: a framework for promoting the health of older persons with cerebral palsy, *Top Geriatr Rehabil* 13:19-24, 1998.
9. Turk MA, Geremski CA, Rosenbaum PF et al: The health status of women with cerebral palsy, *Arch Phys Med Rehabil* 78(5 suppl):S10-S17, 1997.
10. Murphy KP: Medical problems in adults with cerebral palsy; case examples, *Asst Technol* 11:97-104, 1999.
11. Gajdosik CG, Cicerello N: Secondary conditions of the musculoskeletal system in adolescents and adults with cerebral palsy, *Phys Occup Ther Pediatr* 21:49-68, 2001.
12. Strauss D, Ojdana K, Shavelli R et al: Decline in function and life expectancy of older persons with cerebral palsy, *Neurorehabilitation* 19:69-78, 2004.
13. Bobath B: The very early treatment of cerebral palsy, *Dev Med Child Neurol* 9:373-390, 1967.
14. Bobath K: The normal postural reflex mechanism and its deviation in children with cerebral palsy, *Physiotherapy* 57:515-525, 1971.
15. Thelen E, Fisher DM: Newborn stepping: an explanation for the "disappearing" reflex, *Dev Psychol* 18:760-775, 1982.
16. Damiano DL: Teaching effective ways to examine and treat spasticity and weakness and their effects in motor function, *Neurol Rep* 25:98-101, 2001.
17. Dodd KJ, Taylor NF, Damiano DL: A systematic review of the effectiveness of strength-training programs for people with cerebral palsy, *Arch Phys Med Rehabil* 83:157-164, 2002.
18. Fresher-Samways K, Roush SE, Choi K et al: Perceived quality of life of adults with developmental and other significant disabilities, *Disabil Rehabil* 25:1097-1105, 2003.
19. Damiano D: Reviewing muscle cocontraction: is it a developmental, pathological or motor control issue? *Phys Occup Ther Pediatr* 12:3-20, 1993.
20. Damiano DL, Kelly LE, Vaughn DL: Effects of quadriceps femoris muscle strengthening on crouch gait in children with spastic diplegia, *Phys Ther* 75:658-667, 1995.
21. Damiano DL, Martellotta TL, Sullivan. DJ et al: Muscle force production and functional performance in spastic cerebral palsy: Relationship of cocontraction, *Arch Phys Med Rehabil* 81:895-900, 2000.
22. Damiano DL, Martellotta T.L, Quinlivan JM et al: Deficits in eccentric versus concentric torque in children with spastic cerebral palsy, *Med Sci Sports Exerc* 33:117-122, 2000.
23. Carlson WE, Vaughan DL, Damiano DL, Abel MF: Orthotic management of gait in spastic diplegia, *Am J Phys Med Rehabil* 76:219-225, 1997.
24. Patel DR: Therapeutic interventions in cerebral palsy, *Indian J Pediatr* 72:979-983, 2005.
25. ADA Home Page (website): www.ada.gov. Accessed August 10, 2006.
26. Jensen MP, Engel JM, Hoffman AH et al: Natural history of chronic pain and pain treatment in adults with cerebral palsy, *Am J Phys Med Rehabil* 83:439-445, 2004.
27. Damiano DL, Abel MF: Relation of gait analysis to gross motor function in cerebral palsy, *Dev Med Child Neurol* 38:389-396, 1996.
28. National Center on Physical Activity and Disability (website): www.ncpad.org. Accessed August 10, 2006.
29. Boyd R, Delgado M, Heinen F et al: Options in the management of equinus in children with cerebral palsy, American Academy of Cerebral Palsy and Developmental Medicine Workshop, Washington, DC, 1999.
30. Katz RT, Rymer WL: Spastic hypertonia: mechanisms and measurements, *Arch Phys Med Rehabil* 70:144-155, 1989.
31. Guillaume D, Van Havenbergh A, Vloeberghs M et al: A clinical study of intrathecal baclofen using a programmable pump for intractable spasticity, *Arch Phys Med Rehabil* 86:2165-2171, 2005.
32. Latash ML: *Control of human movements,* Champaign, IL, 1993, Human Kinetics.
33. Morris S: Ashworth and Tardieu Scales: their clinical relevance for measuring spasticity in adult and paediatric neurological populations, *Phys Ther Rev* 7:753-62, 2002.
34. Mehrholz J, Wagner K, Meibner D et al: Reliability of the Modified Tardieu Scale and the Modified Ashworth Scale in adult patients with

severe brain injury: a comparison study, *Clin Rehabil* 19:751-759, 2005.

35. Waldman HB, Perlman SP, Swerdloff M: Orthodontics and the population with special needs, *Am J Orthod Dentofac Orthop* 118:14-17, 2000.

36. Waldman HB, Perlman SP: Providing general dentistry for people with disabilities: a demographic review, *Acad Gen Dent* 48:566-569, 2000.

37. Cooper SA: Meeting the mental health needs of older adults with intellectual disabilities, *Aging Ment Health* 7:411-412, 2003.

38. Lindemann R, Zaschel-Grob D, Opp S et al: Oral health status of adults from a California regional center for developmental disabilities, *Spec Care Dentist* 21:9-14, 2001.

39. Weiss J, Diamond T, Denmark J et al: Involvement in Special Olympics and its relation to self-concept and actual competency in participants with developmental disabilities, *Res Dev Disabil* 24:281-305, 2003.

Section II: The Challenges of the Late Effects of Polio: Postpolio Syndrome

40. Spencer WA: *Treatment of acute poliomyelitis,* Springfield, IL, 1956, Charles C Thomas.

41. Spencer WA, Jackson RB: Poliomyelitis, acute. In Conn HF, editor: *Current therapy,* Philadelphia, 1957, WB Saunders.

42. Halstead L: Assessment and differential diagnosis for post-polio syndrome, *Orthopedics* 14:1209-1217, 1991.

43. Halstead L, Wiechers D, editors: *Research and clinical aspects of the late effects of poliomyelitis,* White Plains, NY, 1987, March of Dimes Birth Defects Series 23.

44. Bodian D: The virus, the nerve cell, and paralysis, *Bull Johns Hopkins Hosp.* Available online at www.medicalarchives.jhmi.edu/jhbullindex/jhhb-40.htm. Accessed August 6, 2006.

44a. Cohn V: *Four billion dimes,* Minneapolis, MN, Minneapolis Star and Tribune, 1955.

45. Kumar S: Polio epidemic hits Uttar Pradesh, *BMJ* 325:617, 2002.

46. World Health Organization (website): http://www.who.int/topics/poliomyelitis/en/. Accessed November 18, 2005.

47. *Global polio eradication initiative* (website): http://www.polioeradication.org/content/publications/2004stratplan.pdf. Accessed August 3, 2006.

48. Jubelt B, Agre JC: Characteristics and management of postpolio syndrome, *JAMA* 284:412-414, 2000.

49. Halstead LS: Post-polio syndrome, *Sci Am* 278:42-47, 1998.

50. Bennett RL, Knowlton GC: Overwork weakness in partially denervated skeletal muscle, *Clin Orthop* 12:22-29, 1958.

51. Kendall H, Kendall F: Orthopedic and physical therapy objectives in poliomyelitis treatment, *Physiother Rev* 27:159-165, 1947.

52. Halstead LS, Wiechers DO, Rossi CD: Results of 201 polio survivors, *South Med J* 78:1281-1287, 1985.

53. Thompson W, Jansen JKS: The extent of sprouting of remaining motor units in partly denervated immature and adult rat soleus muscle, *Neuroscience* 2:523-535, 1977.

54. Wiechers D, Hubbel S: Late changes in the motor unit after acute poliomyelitis, *Muscle Nerve* 4:524-528, 1981.

55. Schenck J, Forward E: Quantitative strength changes with test repetitions, *Phys Ther* 45:562-569, 1965.

56. Sharrard WJW: The distribution of permanent paralysis in the lower limb in poliomyelitis: a clinical and pathological study, *J Bone Joint Surg Br* 37:540-548, 1955.

57. Trojan DA, Collet JP, Shapiro S et al: A multicenter randomized, double-blinded trial of pyridostigmine in post-polio syndrome, *Neurology* 53:1225-1233, 1999.

57a. Trojan DA, Cashman NR, Shapiro S et al: Predictive factors for post-poliomyelitis syndrome, *Arch Phys Med Rehabil* 75:770-777, 1994.

58. Ramlow J, Alexander M, La Prote R et al: Epidemiology of the post-polio syndrome, *Am J Epidemiol* 136:769-786, 1992.

59. Ivanyi B, Nollet F, Redekop WK et al: Late onset polio sequelae, *Arch Phys Med Rehabil* 80:687-690, 1999.

59a. Halstead L, Naierman N, editors: *Managing post-polio: a guide to living well with post-polio syndrome,* Washington, DC, 1998, NRH Press.

60. Salter C: Post-polio population statistics—a review, *Lincolnshire post-polio library production* (website): http://www.ott.zynet.co.uk/polio/lincolnshire/library/uk/pppopstats.html. Accessed November 17, 2005.

61. Halstead LS, Silver JK: Nonparalytic polio and postpolio syndrome, *Am J Phys Med Rehabil* 79:13-18, 2000.

62. Gandevia SC, Allen GM, Middleton J: Post-polio syndrome: assessments, pathophysiology and progression, *J Dis Rehabil* 22:38-42, 2000.

63. Maynard FM: Managing the late effects of polio from a life-course perspective, *Ann N Y Acad Sci* 753:354-360, 1995.

64. Trojan DA, Finch L: Management of post-polio syndrome, *NeuroRehabiliation* 8:93-105, 1997.

64a. McNaughton HK, McPherson KM: Problems occurring late after poliomyelitis: a rehabilitation approach, *Crit Rev Phys Rehabil Med* 15:295-308, 2003.

65. *Post-polio Health International* (website): http://www.post-polio.org/. Accessed November 20, 2005.

66. Halstead L, Gawne AC: NRH proposal for limb classification and exercise prescription, *Disabil Rehabil* 18;311-316, 1996.

67. Dalakas MC: The post-polio syndrome as an evolved clinical entity. Definition and clinical description, *Ann N Y Sci* 753:68-80, 1995.

68. Gordon PA, Feldman D: Post-polio syndrome: issues and strategies for rehabilitation counselors, *J Rehabil* 68:28-31, 2002.

69. Jubelt B, Cashman N: Neurologic manifestation of the post-polio syndrome, *Crit Rev Neurobiol* 3:199-200, 1987.

70. Trieschmann R: *Aging with a disability,* New York, 1987, Demos Publications.

71. Frick N: Post-polio sequelae and the psychology of second disability, *Orthopedics* 8:851-853, 1985.

72. Bruno RL, Frick NM: Stress and "type A" behavior as precipitants of post-polio sequelae. In Halstead LS, Weichers DO, editors: *Research and clinical aspects of the late effects of poliomyelitis,* White Plains, NY, 1987, March of Dimes.

73. McComas AJ, Quartly C, Griggs RC: Early and late losses of motor units after poliomyelitis, *Brain* 120:1415-1421, 1997.

74. Campbell MJ, McComas AJ, Petito F. Physiological changes in aging muscles, *J Neurol Neurosurg Psychiatry* 37:131-141, 1974. Cited in Guccione A: *Geriatric physical therapy,* ed 2, St. Louis, 2000, Mosby.

75. Tomlinson BE, Irving D: The numbers of limb motor neurons in the human lumbosacral cord throughout life, *J Neurol Sci* 34:213-219, 1977.

76. McComas AJ, Upton HRM, Sica REP: Motor neuron disease and aging, *Lancet* 2:1477-1480, 1973.

77. Bottomley JM: The geriatric population. In *Primary care for the physical therapist: examination and triage,* St. Louis, 2005, Elsevier, pp 288-306.

78. Weiss MT: *Physical therapy examination and treatment of the polio survivor* (website): http://www. post-polio.org/hlthpros.html. Accessed September 12, 2006.

79. American Physical Therapy Association: Guide to physical therapy practice, *Phys Ther* 81:9-746, 2001.

80. American Occupational Therapy Association: Standards of practice for occupational therapy in schools, *Am J Occup Ther* 34:900-903, 1980.

81. Boissonnault WG: *Primary care for the physical therapist: examination and triage,* St. Louis, 2005, Elsevier.

82. Bruno RL, Sapolsky R, Zimmerman JR et al: Pathophysiology of a central cause of post-polio fatigue, *Ann N Y Acad Sci* 753:257-275, 1995.

83. Berlly MH, Strauser WW, Hall KM: Fatigue in postpolio syndrome, *Arch Phys Med Rehabil* 72:115-118, 1991.

84. Smith E, Rosenblatt P, Limauro A: The role of the sympathetic nervous system in acute poliomyelitis, *J Pediatr* 34:1-11, 1949.

84a. Smith L, McDermott K: Pain in post-poliomyelitis: addressing causes versus effects. In Halstead L, Wiechers D, editors: *Research and clinical aspects of the late effects of poliomyelitis,* White Plains, NY, 1987, March of Dimes Birth Defect Series (23)4;121-134.

85. Peach PE: Overwork weakness with evidence of muscle damage in a patient with residual paralysis from polio, *Arch Phys Med Rehabil* 71:248-250, 1990.

86. Perry J, Fontaine J, Mulroy S: Findings in post-poliomyelitis syndrome, *J Bone Joint Surg Am* 77:1148-1153, 1995.

87. Trojan DA, Gendron D, Cashman N: Electrophysiology and electrodiagnosis of the post-polio motor unit, *Orthopedics* 14:1353-1361, 1991.

88. Rodriquez AA, Agre JC: Electrophysiological study of the quadriceps muscles during fatiguing exercise and recovery: a comparison of symptomatic and asymptomatic postpolio patients and controls, *Arch Phys Med Rehabil* 72:993-997, 1991.

89. Waring WP, McLaurin TM: Correlation of creatine kinase and gait measurement in the postpolio population: a corrected version, *Arch Phys Med Rehabil* 73:447-450, 1992.

90. Waring WP, Davidoff G, Werner R: Serum creatine kinase in the postpolio population, *Am J Phys Med Rehabil* 68:86-90, 1989.

91. Currie DM, Gershkoff AM, Cifu DX: Geriatric rehabilitation, 3: mid- and late-life effects of early-life disabilities, *Arch Phys Med Rehabil* 74: S413-S416, 1993.

92. Smith L, McDermott K: Pain in post-poliomyelitis: addressing causes versus effects. In Halstead L, Wiechers D, editors: *Research and clinical aspects of the late effects of poliomyelitis,* White Plains, NY, 1987, March of Dimes Birth Defect Series.

93. Werner RA, Waring W, Maynard F: Osteoarthritis of the hand and wrist in the post poliomyelitis population, *Arch Phys Med Rehabil* 73:1069-1072, 1992.

94. Perry J, Barnes G, Gronley JK: The postpolio syndrome: an overuse phenomena, *Clin Orthop* 233:145-162, 1988.

95. Fisher A: Sleep-disordered breathing as a late effect of poliomyelitis. In Halstead L, Wiechers D, editors: *Research and clinical aspects of the late effects of poliomyelitis,* White Plains, NY, 1987, March of Dimes Birth Defects Series.

96. Bach J, Alba AS, Bohatiuk G et al: Mouth intermittent positive-pressure ventilation in the management of postpolio respiratory insufficiency, *Chest* 91:859-864, 1987.

97. Hill R, Robbins AW, Messing R et al: Sleep apnea syndrome after poliomyelitis, *Am Rev Respir Dis* 127:129-131, 1983.

98. Sleeper G, Kignman P, Armeni M: Nasal continuous positive pressure for at-home treatment of sleep apnea, *Respir Care* 30:90, 1985.

99. Willen C, Grimby G: Pain, physical activity and disability in individuals with late effects of polio, *Phys Med Rehabil* 79:915-919, 1998.

100. Bach JR, Alba AS: Pulmonary dysfunction and sleep disordered breathing as post-polio sequelae: evaluation and management, *Orthopedics* 14:1329-1337, 1991.

101. Jubelt B, Drucker J: Poliomyelitis and the post-polio syndrome. In Younger DS, editor: *Motor disorders,* Philadelphia, 1999, Lippincott Williams & Wilkins, pp 381-395.

102. Iddings DM, Smith LK, Spencer WA: Muscle testing, II: reliability in clinical use, *Phys Ther Rev* 41:249-256, 1961.

103. Agre JC, Rodriquez AA: Neuromuscular function in polio survivors at one-year follow-up, *Arch Phys Med Rehabil* 72:7-10, 1991.

104. Gray DB, Hendershot GE: The ICIDH-2: Developments for a new era of outcomes research, *Arch Phys Med Rehabil* 81:S10-14, 2000.

105. Howle JM: *Neuro-developmental treatment approach: theoretical foundations and principles of clinical practice,* Laguna Beach, CA, 2002, Neuro-Developmental Treatment Association.

106. Zabel RJ: Techniques of functional muscle testing. In Reese NB, editor: *Muscle and sensory testing,* ed 2, St. Louis, 2005, Elsevier, pp 365-432.

107. Agre JC, Rodriquez AA: Neuromuscular function in polio survivors, *Orthopedics* 14:1343-1347, 1991.

107a. Westbrook MT: Changes in post-polio survivors over five years: symptoms and reactions to treatment. Proceedings of the twelfth World Congress, International Federation of Physical Medicine and Rehabilitation, Sydney, Australia. Cited in Gordon PA, Feldman D: Post-polio syndrome: issues and strategies for rehabilitation counselors, *J Rehabil* 68:28-31, 2002.

108. Young G: Energy conservation, occupational therapy, and the treatment of post-polio sequelae, *Orthopedics* 14:1233-1239, 1991.

109. Bruno RL, Frick NM: The psychology of polio as prelude to post-polio sequelae: behavior modification and psychotherapy, *Orthopedics* 14:1185-1193, 1991.

110. Bruno RL, Frick NM: The psychology of polio as prelude to post polio syndrome: behavior modification and psychotherapy, *Orthopedics* 14:1185-1193, 1991.

111. Conrady L, Wish JR, Agre JC et al: Psychological characteristics of polio survivors: a preliminary report, *Arch Phys Med Rehabil* 170:458-463, 1989.

112. Halstead L: The residual of polio in the aged, *Top Geriatr Rehabil* 3:9-26, 1988.

113. Scheer J, Luborsky ML: The cultural context of polio biographies, *Orthopedics* 14:1173, 1181, 1991.

114. Kaufert J, Kaufert PA: Aging and respiratory polio, *Rehabil Digest* 13:15-17, 1982.

115. Laurie G, Raymond J, editors: *Proceedings of Rehabilitation Gazette's Second International Post-Polio Conference and Symposium on Living Independently with a Severe Disability,* St. Louis, 1984, Gazette International Networking Institute.

116. Laurie G, Raymond J, editors: *Proceedings of Gazette International Networking Institute's Third Internation Polio and Independent Living Conference,* St. Louis, 1986, Gazette International Networking Institute.

117. Kuehn AF, Winters RKV: A study of symptom distress, health locus of control, and coping resources of aging post-polio survivors, *J Nurs Scholar* 26:325-330, 1994.

118. Maynard FM, Roller S: Recognizing typical coping styles of polio survivors can improve re-rehabilitation, *Am J Phys Med Rehabil* 70:70-72, 1991.

119. Hollingsworth L, Didelot MJ, Levington C: Post-polio syndrome: psychological adjustment to disability, *Issues in Mental Health Nursing* 23:135-156, 2002.

120. Backman ME: The post polio patient: psychological issues, *J Rehabil* 53:23-26, 1987.

121. *Post-polio directory—1993,* St. Louis, 1993, International Polio Network.

122. Creange S, Bruno RL: Compliance with treatment for post-polio sequelae: effect of Type A behavior, self-concept and loneliness, *Am J Phys Med Rehabil* 76:378-382, 1997.

123. McCord M: Compliance: self-care or compromise? *Top Clin Nurs* 7:1-8, 1986.

124. Agre JC, Rodriquez AA: Intermittent isometric activity: its effect on muscle fatigue in postpolio subjects, *Arch Phys Med Rehabil* 72:971-975, 1991.

125. Bockrath K, Wooden C, Ingersoll CD: Effects of patella taping on patella position and perceived pain, *Med Sci Sports Exerc* 25:989-992, 1993.

126. Ruth S, Kegerreis S: Facilitating cervical flexion using a Feldenkrais method: awareness through movement, *J Orthop Sports Phys Ther* 16:25-29, 1992.

127. Powers CM, Landel R, Sosnick T et al: The effects of patellar taping on stride characteristics and joint motion in subjects with patellofemoral pain, *J Orthop Sports Phys Ther* 26:286-291, 1997.

128. Peach P, Olejnik S: Effect of treatment and noncompliance on post-polio sequelae, *Orthopedics* 14:1199-1203, 1991.

128a. Bruno RL, Frick NM, Cohen J. Polioencephalitis, stress, and the etiology of post-polio sequelae, *Orthopedics* 14:1269-1276, 1991.

129. Perry J, Gronley JK, Lunsford T: Rocker shoe as a walking aid in multiple sclerosis, *Arch Phys Med Rehabil* 62: 59-65, 1981.

130. Vallbona C, Hazlewood C, Jurida G: Response of pain to static magnetic fields in postpolio patients: a double-blind pilot study, *Arch Phys Med Rehabil* 78:1200-1203, 1997.

131. Perry J, Fontaine J, Mulroy S: Findings in post-poliomyelitis syndrome, *J Bone Joint Surg Am* 77:1148-1153, 1995.

132. Agre JC, Rodriquez AA: Neuromuscular function in polio survivors at one-year follow up, *Arch Phys Med Rehabil* 72:7-10, 1991.

133. Finch L, Trojan D, Wilford C et al: A treadmill walking test in postpolio syndrome patients: preliminary results, *Physiother Can* 46:117, 1994 (abstract).

133a. Finch LE, Venturini A, Mayo NE et al: Effort-limited treadmill walk test: reliability and validity in subjects with postpolio syndrome, *Am J Phys Med Rehabil* 83:613-23, 2004.

134. Agre JC. The role of exercise in the patient with post-polio syndrome, *Ann N Y Acad Sci* 753:321-324, 1995.

135. Gross MT, Schuch CP: Exercise programs for patients with post-polio syndrome: a case report, *Phys Ther* 69:72-76, 1989.

136. Milner-Brown HS: Muscle strengthening in a post-polio subject through a high-resistance weight-training program, *Arch Phys Med Rehabil* 74:1165-1167, 1993.

137. Einarrson G: Muscle conditioning in late poliomyelitis, *Arch Phys Med Rehabil* 72:11-14, 1991.

138. Fillyaw MJ, Badger GJ, Gregory GD et al: The effects of long-term nonfatiguing resistance exercise in subjects with post-polio syndrome, *Orthopedics* 14:1253-1256, 1991.

139. Munin MC, Jaweed MM, Staas WE Jr et al: Postpoliomyelitis muscle weakness: a prospective study of quadriceps muscle strength, *Arch Phys Med Rehabil* 72:729-733, 1991.

140. Munsat TL, Andres P: Preliminary observations on long-term muscle force changes in the post-polio syndrome. In Halstead LS, Wiechers DO, editors: *Birth defects orig article series* 23:329-334, 1987.

141. Fiatarone MA, Marks EC, Ryan ND et al: High-intensity strength training in nonagenarians, *JAMA* 263:3029-3034, 1990.

142. Frontera WR, Meredith CN, O'Reilly KP et al: Strength conditioning in older men: skeletal muscle hypertrophy and improved function, *J Appl Physiol* 64:1038-1044, 1988.

143. Agre JC, Rodriguez AA, Franke TM et al: Effect of low-intensity, alternate day muscle strengthening exercise at home upon quadriceps muscle strength in post polio subjects, 1994. Cited in Agre JC: The role of exercise in the patient with post-polio syndrome, *Ann N Y Acad Sci* 753:321-324, 1995.

144. Feldman RM, Soskolne CL: The use of nonfatiguing strengthening exercises in post-polio syndrome. In Halstead LS, Weichers DO, editors: *Research and clinical aspects of the late effects of poliomyelitis,* White Plains, NY, 1987, March of Dimes Birth Defects Foundation,

145. Agre JC, Rodriguez AA, Franke TM, Knudtson ER et al Effect of low-intensity, alternate day muscle strengthening exercise at home upon quadriceps muscle strength in post polio subjects, 1994. Cited in Agre JC: The role of exercise in the patient with post-polio syndrome, *Ann NY Acad Sci* 753:321-324, 1996.

146. *Gazette international networking institute/international polio network* (website): www.post-polio.org. Accessed August 14, 2006.

147. Dean E, Ross J: Effect of modified aerobic training on movement energetics in polio survivors, *Orthopedics* 14:1243-1246, 1991.

148. Jones DR, Speier J, Canine K et al: Cardiorespiratory responses to aerobic training by patients with postpoliomyelitis sequelae, *JAMA* 261:3255-3259, 1989.

149. Kriz JL, Jones DR, Speier JL et al: Cardiorespiratory responses to upper extremity aerobic training by postpolio subjects, *Arch Phys Med Rehabil* 73:49-54, 1992.

150. Ernstoff B, Wetterqvist H, Kvist H et al: The effects of endurance training on individuals with post-poliomyelitis, *Arch Phys Med Rehabil* 77:843-848, 1996.

151. Willen C, Sunnerhagen KS, Grimby G: Dynamic water exercise in individuals with late poliomyelitis, *Arch Phys Med Rehabil* 82:66-72, 2001.

151a. Waring WP, Maynard F, Grady W et al: Influence of appropriate lower extremity orthotic management on ambulation, pain, and fatigue in a post-polio population, *Arch Phys Med Rehabil* 70:371-375, 1989.

152. Murray MP, Drought AB, Kory RC: Walking patterns of normal men, *J Bone Joint Surg Am* 46:335-360, 1964.

153. Lehmann J, Condon SM, de Lateur BJ et al: Ankle-foot orthoses: effect on abnormalities in tibial nerve paralysis, *Arch Phys Med Rehabil* 66:212-218, 1985.

154. Saltiel J: A one-piece laminated knee locking short-leg brace, *Orthot Prosthet* 23:68-75, 1969.

155. Yang GW, Chu DD, Ahn JH ct al: Floor reaction orthosis: clinical experience, *Orthot Prosthet* 40:33-37, 1986.

156. Clark D, Perry J, Lunsford T: Case studies—orthotic management of the adult post polio patient, *Orthot Prosthet* 40:43-50, 1986.

157. Perry J, Hislop H, editors: *Principles of lower extremity bracing,* Washington, DC, 1967, American Physical Therapy Association.

157a. Perry J, Fleming C: Polio: long-term problems, *Orthopedics* 8:877-881, 1985.

158. Clark DR, Perry J, Lunsford TR: Case studies—orthotic management of the adult post-polio patient, *Orthot Prosthet* 40:43-50, 1986.

159. Bach JR: Management of post-polio respiratory sequelae, *Ann N Y Acad Sci* 753:96-102, 1995.

160. Dail C: Clinical aspects of glossopharyngeal breathing: report of its use by 100 post-polio patients, *JAMA* 158:445-449, 1955.

161. Feigelson C, Dickinson DG, Talner NS et al: Glossopharyngeal breathing as an aid to the coughing mechanism in patients with chronic poliomyelitis in a respirator, *N Engl J Med* 254:611-613, 1956.

162. Dalakas MC: Why drugs fail in post-polio syndrome, *Neurology* 53:116-117, 1999.

163. Sonies BC, Dalakas MC, Dysphagia in patients with post polio syndrome. *N Engl J Med* 324:1162-1167, 1991.

Section III: Effects of Aging on the Functional Status of Patients with Spinal Cord Injury, Acquired Brain Injuries, or Traumatic Brain Injury

164. Kailes JI: Can disability, chronic conditions, health and wellness coexist? The National Center on Physical Activity and Disability, Rehabilitation Institute of Chicago, Department of Disability and Human Development, University of Illinois: http://www.ncpad.org. Accessed July 13, 2006.

165. Shupert CL: Balance in the elderly, *Vestibular disorders association, 1993* (website): http://www.vestibular.org/elderly.html/. Accessed January 2, 2005.

166. Svanborg A: Practical and functional consequences of aging, *Gerontology* 34(1 suppl):11-15, 1988.

167. National Center for Chronic Disease Prevention and Health Promotion: Healthy aging: preventing disease and improving quality of life among older Americans, 2004: http://www.cdc.gov/nccdphp/aag/aag_aging.htm. Accessed December 22, 2004.

168. McColl MA, Walker J, Stirling P et al: Expectations of life and health among spinal cord injured adults, *Spinal Cord* 35:818-828, 1997.

169. McColl MA, Arnold R, Charlifue S et al: Aging, spinal cord injury, and quality of life: structural relationships, *Arch Phys Med Rehabil* 84:1137-1144, 2003.

170. Meythaler JM, DeVivo MJ, Braswell WC: Rehabilitation outcomes of patients who have developed Guillain-Barré syndrome, *Arch Phys Med Rehabil* 76:411-419, 1997.

171. Dijkers MP: Quality of life after traumatic brain injury: a review of research approaches and findings, *Arch Phys Med Rehabil* 85(suppl 2):S21-S35, 2004.

172. Brown M, Vandergoot D: Quality of life for individuals with traumatic brain injury: comparison with others living in the community, *J Head Trauma Rehabil* 13:1-23, 1998.

173. Hicken BL, Putzke JD, Novack T et al: Life satisfaction following spinal cord and traumatic brain injury: a comparative study, *J Rehabil Res Dev* 39:359-365, 2002.

174. Thompson L: Functional changes in persons aging with spinal cord injury, *Assist Technol* 11:123-129, 1999.

175. Gerhart KA, Bergstrom E, Charlifue SW et al: Long-term spinal cord injury: functional changes over time, *Arch Phys Med Rehabil* 74:1030-1034, 1993.

176. Charlifue SW, Weitzenkamp DA, Whiteneck GG: Longitudinal outcomes in spinal cord injury: aging, secondary conditions, and well-being, *Arch Phys Med Rehabil* 80:1429-1434, 1999.

177. Liem N, McColl MA, King W et al: Aging with a spinal cord injury: factors associated with the need for more help with activities of daily living, *Arch Phys Med Rehabil* 85:1567-1577, 2004.

178. Vandenakker CB, Glass DD: 2001 Menopause and aging with disability, *Phys Med Rehabil Clin North Am* 12:133-151, 2001.

179. Randall N, Lynch AC, Anthony A, et al: Does a colostomy alter quality of life in patients with spinal cord injury? A controlled study, *Spinal Cord* 39:279-282, 2001.

180. Stewart DG, Phillips EM, Bodenheimer CF et al: Geriatric rehabilitation, 2. Physiatric approach to the older adult, *Arch Phys Med Rehabil* 85(3 suppl):S7-S11, 2004.

181. Charlifue SW, Weitzenkamp DA, Whiteneck GG: Aging with spinal cord injury: changes in selected health indices and life satisfaction, *Arch Phys Med Rehabil* 85:1848-1853, 2004.

182. Ehde DM, Jensen MP, Engel JM et al: Chronic pain secondary to disability: a review, *Clin J Pain* 19:3-7, 2003.

183. Tate D, Gater D, Scelza W: *People with spinal cord injuries need exercise too - but barriers to fitness persist, U-M study finds* (website): http://www.med.umich.edu/opm/newspage/2002/spineexercise.htm. Accessed July 13, 2006.

184. University of Michigan Health System. Department of Physical Medicine and Rehabilitation: *Model spinal cord injury care system* (website): http://www.med.umich.edu/pmr/modelsci/index.htm. Accessed July 13, 2006.

184a. The National Spinal Cord Injury Web site at http://www.spinalcord.org/. Accessed August 17, 1006.

184b. The Rehabilitation Center at Penn State Milton S. Hershey Medical Center: *Aging, exercise, and spinal cord injury* (website): http://www.hmc.psu.edu/rehab/services/spinalcord/. Accessed August 17, 2006.

184c. *The National Center on Physical Activity and Disability (NCPAD)* (website): www.ncpad.org. Accessed August 17, 2006.

185. Levin C: The effect of aging on people with brain injuries: TBI challenge, *Brain Inj Assoc Am* 4:1-5 2000.

186. Baker B: Head injury confers Alzheimer's risk regardless of apo E-4 status, *Clinical Psychiatry News*, vol. XXVIII, no. 1: 2. San Francisco: International Medical News Group, 2000.

187. Johnstone B, Childers MK, Hoerner J: The effects of normal aging on neuropsychological functioning following traumatic brain injury, *Brain Inj* 12:569-576, 1998.

188. Dijkers MP: Quality of life after traumatic brain injury: a review of research approaches and findings, *Arch Phys Med Rehabil* 2004; 85:4, S21-S35.

189. Mosenthal AC, Livingston DH, Lavery RF et al: The effect of age on functional outcome in mild traumatic brain injury: 6-month report of a prospective multicenter trial, *J Trauma* 56:1042-1048, 2004.

190. Rehabilitation of persons with traumatic brain injury, *NIH Consens Statement* 16:1-14, 1998.

191. Whiteneck G, Brooks CA, Mellick D et al: Population-based estimates of outcomes after hospitalization for traumatic brain injury in Colorado, *Arch Phys Med Rehabil* 85(suppl 2):S73-S81, 2004.

192. Breed ST, Flanagan SR, Watson KR: The relationship between age and the self-report of health symptoms in persons with traumatic brain injury, *Arch Phys Med Rehabil* 85(suppl 2):S61-S67, 2004.

193. Hibbard MR, Uysal S, Sliwinski M et al: Undiagnosed health issues in individuals with traumatic brain injury living in the community, *J Head Trauma Rehabil* 13:47-57, 1998.

194. Beetar JT, Guilmette TJ, Sparadeo FR: Sleep and pain complaints in symptomatic traumatic brain injury and neurologic populations, *Arch Phys Med Rehabil* 77:1298-1302, 1996.

195. Corrigan JD, Smith-Knapp K, Granger CV: Outcomes in the first 5 years after traumatic brain injury, *Arch Phys Med Rehabil* 79:298-305, 1998.

196. Strauss DJ, Shavelle RM, Anderson TW: Long-term survival of children and adolescents after traumatic brain injury, *Arch Phys Med Rehabil* 79:1095-1100, 1998.

197. Gordon WA, Sliwinski M, Echo J et al: The benefits of exercise in individuals with traumatic brain injury: a retrospective study, *J Head Trauma Rehabil* 13:58-67, 1998.

198. Research and Training Center, New York Traumatic Brain Injury Model System at Mount Sinai School of Medicine: TBI Consumer Reports. Issue 2, Aerobic Exercise Following TBI: http://www.mssm.edu/tbicentral/resources/publications/tbi_consumer_reports.shtml. Accessed July 13, 2006.

199. National Institute on Disability and Rehabilitation Research (website): www.ed.gov/about/offices/list/nidrr/index.html. Accessed September 13, 2006.

200. Batavia AI, Batavia M: Disability, chronic conditions, and iatrogenic illness, *Arch Phys Med Rehabil* 85:168-171, 2004.

201. Beatty PW, Hagglund KJ, Neri MT et al: Access to health care services among people with chronic or disabling conditions: patterns and predictors, *Arch Phys Med Rehabil* 84:1417-1425, 2003.

202. Rimmer J, Riley B, Wang E et al: Development and validation of AIMFREE: Accessibility Instruments Measuring Fitness and Recreation Environments, *Disabil Rehabil* 26:1087-1095, 2004.

203. Rimmer JH: Exercise and physical activity in persons aging with a physical disability, *Phys Med Rehabil Clin North Am* 16:41-56, 2005.

204. Cruise CM, Lee MH: Delivery of rehabilitation services to people aging with a disability, *Phys Med Rehabil Clin North Am* 16:267-284, 2005.

205. Cristian A: Aging with a disability, *Phys Med Rehabil Clin North Am* 16:xvii-xviii, 2005.

206. Kraft GH: Aging with a disability, *Phys Med Rehabil Clin North Am* 16:xiii-xv, 2005.

APPENDIX 29-A ■ Movement Diagnosis Process Used by Physical Therapists

The Guide to Physical Therapy Practice[79] outlines specific examination guidelines based on a diagnostic classification using preferred practice patterns. In the process of determining the appropriate physical therapy diagnosis, the pathophysiological features of poliomyelitis, current functional status, and impairments are invaluable. As an acquired viral disease that primarily affected the CNS, polio infected a broad age range, with the initial infection lasting a finite time. Individuals with PPS are then classified under the Neuromuscular Pattern and may fall under two categories:

Pattern C: Impaired Motor Function and Sensory Integrity Associated with Nonprogressive Disorders of the Central Nervous System–Congenital Origin or Acquired in Infancy or Childhood, Adolescence

Pattern D: Impaired Motor Function and Sensory Integrity Associated with Acquired Nonprogressive Disorders of the Central Nervous System Acquired in Adolescence or Adulthood

Individuals for whom the specific patterns are used *may not have all* of the symptoms listed as commonly reported. As Weiss[78] notes, although impaired sensory integrity is not a common deficit after polio, these patterns should still be more appropriate than any of the identified patterns that clearly apply to individuals without polio or patterns that specifically include polio in their exclusion criteria.

The examination element of the patient/client management model distinctly identifies three components: history, systems review, and test and measures (see Chapters 7 and 8). The application of these components in the management of individuals after polio follows can be found on page 945 within Chapter 29 beginning with Health History.

CHAPTER 30

Disorders of Vision and Visual-Perceptual Dysfunction

Laurie Ruth Chaikin, MS, OTR/L, OD

KEY WORDS

anatomy of the eye
eye diseases
functional visual skills
refractive error
strabismus
treatment
visual perceptual dysfunction
visual screening

OBJECTIVES

After reading this chapter the student/therapist will be able to:
1. Identify and analyze visual anatomy and physiology as they pertain to visual function.
2. Analyze the functional visual skills and how visual dysfunction may affect functional performance.
3. Identify the symptoms of visual dysfunction.
4. Develop the skill necessary to take a visual case history by use of behaviors and clinical observations.
5. Identify the difference between phoria and strabismus.
6. Identify and evaluate the difference between visual field loss and unilateral neglect.
7. Identify and differentiate various pediatric and age-related disease conditions that may affect vision.
8. Clearly differentiate nonoptical and optical assessment and intervention adaptations for patients with low vision.
9. Differentiate basic tools for vision screening.
10. Identify when and why to refer and the tools necessary to document that decision.

Vision is an integral part of development of perception. Some aspects of vision, such as pupillary function, are innate, but many other aspects are stimulated to develop by experience and interaction with the environment. Visual acuity itself has been demonstrated to rely on the presence of a clear image focused on the retina. If this does not occur, a "lazy eye," or amblyopia, will result. Depth perception develops as a result of precise eye alignment and will not occur unless eye alignment is corrected within the first 7 years of life. Research has demonstrated that, in fact, most visual skills such as acuity, binocular coordination, accommodation, ocular motilities, and depth perception are largely intact by age 6 months to 1 year.[1] Visual skill development parallels postural reflex integration and provides a foundation for perception.

Early in infancy visual input is associated with olfactory, tactile, vestibular, and proprioceptive sensations. The infant is driven to touch, taste, smell, and manipulate what he or she sees. Primitive postural reflexes such as the asymmetrical tonic neck reflex help to provide visual regard and attention.

At some point the young child is able to look at an object and determine both the texture and the shape without having to touch or taste it. In adults, vision has moved to the top of the sensory hierarchy, providing full multisensory associations from sight alone. Even the visualized image of eating an apple can recreate the smell, sound of crunching, taste, and feel of the experience.

Early visual impairment and later acquired impairment can affect the quality of the image presented to the brain and thus affect the learning process. In addition, damage to association centers involved with spatial perception, figure-ground, and directionality can interfere with learning and performance. Altered function may be the result of congenital and developmental disorders, birth trauma, physical trauma, or neurological or systemic diseases. It is important, therefore, to isolate the primary visual processes of seeing from the secondary or associational processes of perceiving in the evaluation of perceptual disorders. The identification of a vision problem becomes part of the differential diagnosis of a perceptual deficit. Visual screening must be done before perceptual evaluation so that visual problems do not bias or contaminate the perceptual testing. It is just as important to eliminate vision as a contributing factor to a perceptual problem as it is to find a possible vision problem.

ANATOMY OF THE EYE

An operational analogy of the eye as a camera may be useful up to a point in understanding the physical function of the structures. Once an image hits the retina and image enhancement begins, however, metaphors must change to match our ever-changing comprehension of brain function.

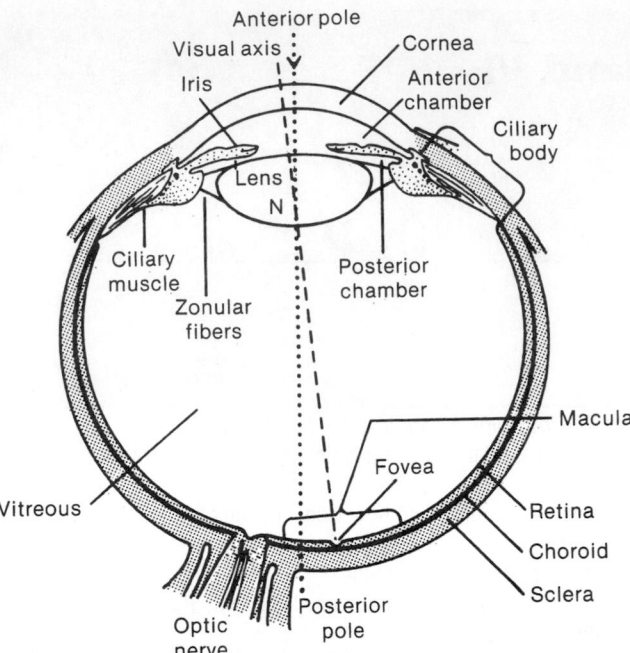

FIGURE 30-1 ■ Horizontal section of the eye. (Modified from Wolff E: *Anatomy of the eye and orbit,* ed 7, London, 1976, HK Lewis.)

Using computer analogies such as microprocessing of feature detectors comes closer. Many aspects of how we see remain a mystery inside the "black box" of our brain.

Eye Chamber and Lens

Structures and function are discussed from anterior to posterior (Figure 30-1). The first structure that light hits after it is reflected from an image is the cornea. (Technically, light first hits the tear layer, which has its own structure and rests on the corneal surface.) Corneal tissue is completely transparent. Light is refracted, or bent, to the greatest degree by the cornea because the light rays must pass through different media, which change in density, as in going from air to water.[2] The refraction of light can be observed by noting how a stick when placed into water appears bent where it enters the water (Figure 30-2).

Damage to the cornea from abrasions, burns, or congenital or disease-related processes can alter the spherical shape of the cornea and disturb the quality of the image that falls on the retina. Radial keratotomy, a surgical procedure done in the 1980s to reduce nearsightedness by placing spokelike cuts in the cornea, sometimes had the side effect of scarring the cornea and causing distorted vision. The newer surgeries such as LASIK are far superior in their reduction of refractive error (nearsightedness, farsightedness, or astigmatism) and induce no scarring or distortion. In keratoconus, the cornea slowly becomes steeper and more cone shaped, distorting the image and causing reduced vision.[3]

Iris

Behind the cornea is the iris, or colored portion, which consists of fibers that control the opening of the pupil, the dark circular opening in the center of the eye. The constriction and dilation of the pupil controls the amount of light enter-

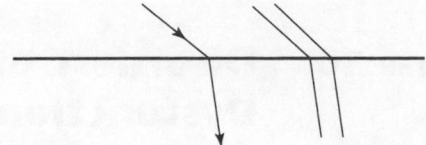

FIGURE **30-2** ■ Refraction: bending of light at air/water interface.

ing the eye in a similar fashion to the way the F stop on a camera changes the size of the aperture to control the amount of light and the depth of field.[4] Under bright light conditions the opening constricts, and under dim light conditions it dilates, allowing light in to stimulate the photoreceptor cells of the retina. This constriction and dilation are under autonomic nervous system (ANS) control with both sympathetic and parasympathetic components.[5] Under conditions of sympathetic stimulation (fight or flight) the pupils dilate, perhaps giving rise to the expression "eyes wide with fear." Under parasympathetic stimulation the pupils constrict. The effect of drugs that stimulate the ANS can be observed.[6] For example, someone who has taken heroin will have pinpoint pupils.

Exercise 30-1: Observation of Pupillary Constriction and Dilation

Observe pupillary dilation and constriction on a willing subject (or on yourself in a mirror) by flashing a penlight at her or his pupil. Observe the decreased size of the pupil. Remove the light and watch the pupil dilate.

Lens

Behind the iris is the lens. The lens is involved in focusing, or accommodation. It is a biconvex, circular, semirigid, crystalline structure that fine tunes the image on the retina. In a camera, the lens is represented by the external optical lens system. The ability to change the focus on the camera is achieved by turning the lens to change the distance of the lens from the film, which effectively increases or decreases the power of the lens, allowing near or distance objects to be seen more clearly. The same effect, a change in the power of the lens, is achieved in the eye by the action of tiny ciliary muscles, which act on suspensory ligaments, thereby changing the thickness and curvature of the lens. A thicker lens with a greater curvature produces higher power and the ability to see clearly at near. A thinner lens and flatter curvature produces less optical power, which is what is needed to allow distant objects to be clear (Figure 30-3). The process of lens thickening and thinning is accommodation.[4,5]

Ideally, the lens will bring an image into perfect focus so that it lands right on the fovea, the area of central vision. If the focused image falls in front of the retina, however, then a blurred circle will fall on the fovea (Figure 30-4). In this case the lens is too thick, having too high an optical power. This can be one cause of myopia (nearsightedness). The other causes of myopia are that the curvature of the cornea is too steep or that the length of the eyeball is too long. The result in each case is the same: the image comes to a focus point in front of the retina. One simple remedy is to place a negative (concave) lens externally in front of the eye in glasses (or contact lenses) to reduce the power of the internal lens and allow the image to fall directly on the fovea. A

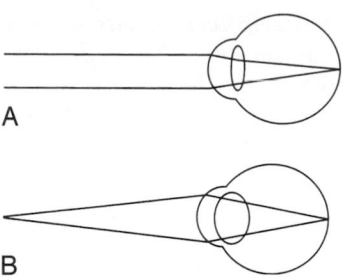

FIGURE 30-3 ■ Accommodation. *A,* Looking far away. *B,* Looking up close.

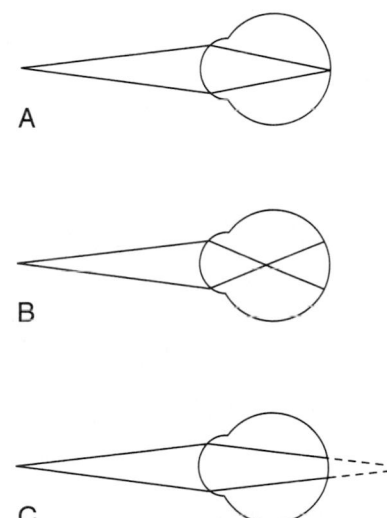

FIGURE 30-4 ■ Refractive error. *A,* Image focused on retina; no refractive error. *B,* A near-sighted or myopic eye. *C,* A far-sighted or hyperopic eye.

similar type of problem of blur can occur in hyperopia (far-sightedness), but now the image falls in back of the retina. In presbyopia (old eyes), the flexibility of the lens fibers decreases and the lens becomes more rigid.[7] Accommodation gets weaker until the image can no longer be focused on the retina. Normal-sighted individuals first begin to notice these changes in their early forties. When this occurs, a plus (positive) lens (or bifocals, progressive lenses, bifocal or monovision contact lenses) may be worn to aid in reading.[4]

Other solutions to the problems of aging can be implemented during the time of cataract surgery, where a bifocal implant may be inserted, or monovision implant correction in each eye.

The lens can be affected by the age-related process of cataract development, in which the general clarity of vision is impaired from a loss of transparency of the crystalline lens. Incoming light tends to scatter inside the eye, causing glare problems. When vision is impaired to such a degree that it affects function, it may be removed surgically and replaced with a silicone implant placed just posterior to the iris.

Vitreous Chamber

The space behind the lens, which is filled with a gel-like substance, is called the vitreous chamber.[5]

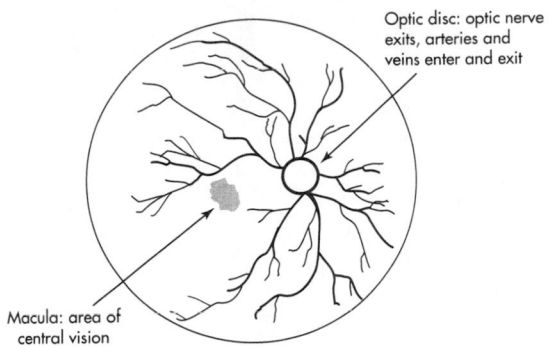

FIGURE 30-5 ■ Retinal topography.

Retina

The retina at the back of the eye is the photosensitive layer, like the film in a camera, receiving the pattern of light reflected from objects. The topography of the retina (Figure 30-5) includes the optic disc, which is where the optic nerve exits and arteries and veins emerge and exit. This is also the blind spot because there are no photoreceptor cells on the disc. The macula is temporal to the optic disc and contains the fovea, or central vision. The surrounding retina is considered peripheral vision and defines a 180-degree half-sphere.[5]

Exercise 30-2: Blind Spot

Your blind spot may be observed by doing the following: draw two dots 3 inches (7.5 cm) apart on a piece of paper. The dots can be $1/4$ inch (0.5 cm). Cover your left eye and look at the dot on the left. Starting at about 16 inches (40 cm), slowly bring the paper closer. Make sure you can see the two dots—one you are looking at directly and the other peripherally. At approximately 10 inches (25 cm) the dot on the right will disappear. This is your blind spot! Why can this exercise only be done monocularly (with one eye)?

Visual Pathway

The visual pathway begins with the photoreceptor cells, which begin a three-neuron chain exiting through the optic nerve. This chain consists of the rods and cones, which synapse with bipolar cells that synapse with ganglion cells (Figure 30-6).[5,8]

There are two types of photoreceptor cells: rods and cones. The cone or rod shape is the dendrite of the cell. Variation in shape and slight variation in pigment give each one different sensitivities. The rod cell has greater sensitivity to dim light but less sensitivity to color, whereas the cone cell has greater sensitivity to color and high-intensity light and less to reduced light conditions. The highest concentration of cone cells is in the fovea and macula, with decreasing concentration of cone cells and increasing concentration of rod cells moving concentrically away from the macula. The high degree of low light sensitivity can be most appreciated in conditions where you find yourself in survival mode such as lost in the woods on a moonless night. By swinging the eyes side to side one can maximize the image and keep the macula from interfering.

The phenomenon responsible for the high degree of neural representation of the foveal region and that accounts

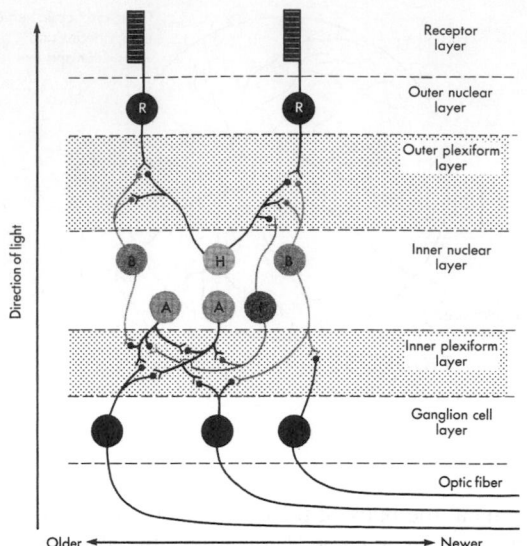

Direction of light

Receptor layer

Outer nuclear layer

Outer plexiform layer

Inner nuclear layer

Inner plexiform layer

Ganglion cell layer

Optic fiber

Older ◄——————► Newer

FIGURE 30-6 ■ The connections among retinal neurons and the significance of prominent layers. The neurons shown are photoreceptors *(R)*, horizontal cells *(H)*, bipolar cells *(B)*, interplexiform cells *(I)*, amacrine cells *(A)*, and ganglion cells *(G)*. It has been suggested that ganglion cells dominated by bipolar cell inputs represent newer circuitry. The arrow indicates the direction of light as it passes through the retina to reach the photoreceptors. (From Beme RM, Levy MN, editors: *Physiology*, p. 107, St. Louis, 1988, CV Mosby.)

for the tremendous conscious awareness of the central view is called convergence.[5] At the periphery of the retina the degree of convergence is great; many photoreceptor cells synapse on one ganglion cell, which accounts for poor acuity but high light sensitivity. The closer to the macula, the less the degree of convergence, until, finally, at the fovea there is no convergence. This means that one photoreceptor cell synapses with one bipolar cell and one ganglion cell.

The awareness of what is seen is directly related to the amount of convergence, which reflects the extent of neural representation. The 1:1 correspondence between photoreceptor and ganglion cell at the fovea means that there is a high degree of neural representation of the foveal image in the brain. It is even greater than the neural representation of the lips, tongue, or hands.[9] This accounts for the primary awareness of what is in the foveal field and secondary awareness of the peripheral field. Conscious awareness of the environment is whatever is in the foveal field at the moment. But continuous information about the environment is flowing over the peripheral retina, usually subconsciously. Attention quickly shifts from foveal to nonfoveal stimulation when changes in light intensity or rapid movement are registered. This type of stimulus arouses attention immediately because it could have specific survival value. For example, a person is driving down the street and senses rapid motion off to the right. The foveas swing around immediately to identify a small red ball bouncing into the street. This information goes to the association areas, in which "small ball" is associated with "small child soon to follow." Frontal cortical centers are aroused and a decision is made to initiate motor areas to take the foot off the accelerator and onto the brake.

Exercise 30-3: Peripheral Central Awareness

We have a unique ability to change our awareness by consciously shifting attention from our foveal or central awareness to our peripheral awareness. For example, as you read these words, become aware of the background surrounding the paper; notice colors, forms, and shapes; continue to expand your awareness to include your clothes, the floor, walls, and ceiling if possible. You are consciously stimulating your primitive, phylogenetically older visual system. The ability to do this has considerable therapeutic value because a typical pattern of visual stress is associated with a foveal concentration. The ability to expand the peripheral awareness at will is a skill that can help you to relax while you drive, can improve reading skills, and can be used in visual training techniques.

The moment light hits the retina, the photographic film model must be abandoned for the image processing or computerized image enhancement model. The primary visual pathway at the retinal level is a three-neuron chain. From back to front the first neuron is the photoreceptor cell, rods or cones. They synapse with a bipolar cell, which in turn synapses with a ganglion cell. The axon of the ganglion cell exits by means of the optic nerve. Image enhancement occurs at the two junctions between the three-nerve-cell pathway. Lateral cells at the neural junctions have an inhibitory action on the primary three-neuron pathway, and through the inhibition of an impulse the image is modulated. For example, at the first junction between photoreceptor cell and bipolar cell, there are horizontal cells. These cells enhance the contrast between light and dark by inhibiting the firing of bipolar cells at the edge of an image. This makes the edge of the image appear darker than the central area, which increases the contrast and thereby increases attention-getting value. After all, it is by perceiving edges that we are able to maneuver around objects. In a similar manner, amacrine cells act at the second neural junction between bipolar and ganglion cells to enhance movement detection.[10]

This image enhancement process continues throughout the visual pathway. The process has been likened to the way in which a computer enhances a distorted picture of outer space received from a satellite. The image goes through a series of processing stations in the inner workings of the computer. The computer-generated, enhanced image shown on the screen is like the end product in the brain: the perceived image.

The visual pathway continues through the brain (Figure 30-7). The ganglion cell axons exit the eyeball by means of the optic nerve, carrying the complete retinal picture in coded electrochemical patterns. From there the patterns project to different sites within the central nervous system (Figure 30-8). Projections to the pretectum are important in pupillary reflexes; projections to the pretectal nuclei, the accessory optic nuclei, and the superior colliculus are all involved in eye movement functions.[5] The largest bundle, called the optic tract, projects to the lateral geniculate body in the hypothalamus, where additional image enhancement and processing occurs. The next group of axons continues on to the primary visual cortex, and from there to visual association areas.

At what point does the retinal image become a perception, and with what part of the brain does one see? Current theory regarding visual perception is the result of Nobel

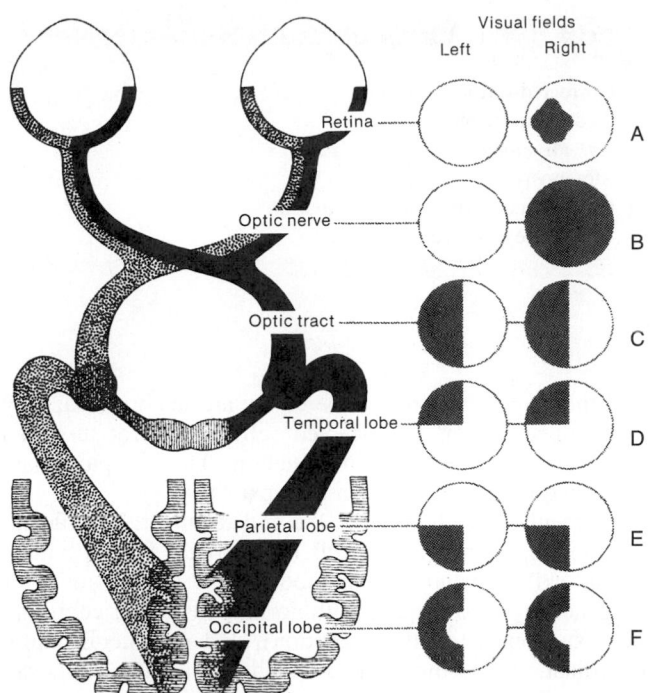

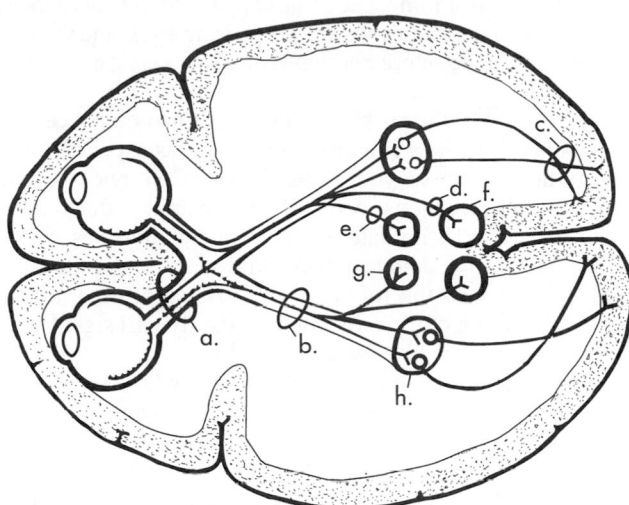

FIGURE 30-8 ■ Visual tract system: *a*, optic nerve; *b*, optic tract; *c*, geniculate-occipital radiators; *d*, retinocolliculo radiation; *e*, retinopretecto tracts; *f*, superior colliculus (midbrain); *g*, pretectal area (tegmentum); *h*, lateral geniculate.

FIGURE 30-7 ■ Visual field disturbances at various points along the optic pathway. *A*, Retinal lesion: blind spot in the affected eye. *B*, Optic nerve lesion: partial or complete blindness in that eye. *C*, Optic tract or lateral geniculate lesion: blindness in the opposite half of both visual fields. *D*, Temporal lobe lesion: blindness in the upper quadrants of both visual fields on the side opposite the lesion. *E*, Parietal lobe lesion: contralateral blindness in the corresponding lower quadrants of both eyes. *F*, Occipital lobe lesion: contralateral blindness in the corresponding half of each visual field but with macular sparing. (Courtesy of Smith, Kline & French Laboratories, Philadelphia, PA.)

prize–winning research by Hubel and Wiesel in the 1960s called the "receptive field theory."[11] This theory states that different neurons are feature detectors, defining objects in terms of movement, direction, orientation, color, depth, and acuity. Research in 1990 by Hubel and Livingstone[12] was able to locate a segregation of function at the level of the lateral geniculate body. They identified two types of cells, one type being larger and faster magno cells, which are apparently phylogenetically older and color blind but which have a high contrast sensitivity and are able to detect differences in contrast of 1% to 2%. They also have low spatial resolution (low acuity). They seem to operate globally and are responsible for perception of movement, depth perception from motion, perspective, parallax, stereopsis, shading, contour, and interocular rivalry. Through linking properties (objects having common movement or depth) emerges figure-ground perception. Much of this perception occurs in the middle temporal lobe.

The other type of cell, called the parvo cell, is smaller, slower, and color sensitive and has a smaller receptive field. These cells are less global and are primarily responsible for high-resolution form perception. Higher-level visual association occurs in the temporal-occipital region, where learning to identify objects by their appearance occurs. It appears that these two types of cells are functionally and structurally related to the two visual systems represented in retinal topography—the foveal (central) and peripheral visual systems.

Eye Movement System

The eye movement system consists of six pairs of eye muscles: the medial recti, lateral recti, superior and inferior recti, and superior and inferior obliques (see Figure 30-8). Together they are controlled by cranial nerves III (oculomotor), IV (trochlear), and VI (abducens). The eye movement system has both reflex and voluntary components. Reflexive movements are coordinated through vestibular interconnections at a midbrain level. The vestibular ocular reflex (VOR) functions primarily to keep the image stabilized on the retina. Through connections between pairs of eye muscles and the semicircular canals, movement is analyzed as being either external movement of an object or movement of the head or body. From this information the VOR is able to direct the appropriate head or eye movement.[5]

Two types of eye movements are the result. Smooth, coordinated eye movements are called pursuits, and rapid localizations are called saccades. Voluntary control of both these motions indicates cortical control. Pursuits are used for continuously following moving targets and they are stimulated by a foveal image. Saccades are stimulated by images from the peripheral system, where a detection of motion or change in light intensity results in a rapid saccadic eye movement to bring the object into the foveal field. Either difficulties in the eye movement system or underfunctioning of the vestibular system can affect the coordinated, efficient functioning of eye movement skills.

A third type of eye movement is specifically related to eye aiming ability. This is the coordinated movement of both eyes inward toward the nose, as in crossing the eyes, or outward toward midline, as when looking away in the distance. The inward movement is called convergence, and the outward movement is called divergence. The most important result of efficient vergence abilities is depth perception, or stereopsis.

Small errors in aiming can dramatically affect stereopsis. Problems such as double vision, wandering eyes, and strabismus are discussed in greater depth in a later section.

Exercise 30-4: Pursuits, Saccades, Convergence

Pursuits. Follow a moving target such as a pencil point as you move it across your field of gaze. Continue to move it in different directions, vertically, horizontally, diagonally, and circularly to stimulate all pairs of eye muscles. For a more challenging demonstration find a fly and follow its flight path around the room. If you lose sight of it, notice that the detection of the movement of the fly will signal your eye movement directly toward it.

Saccades. Hold two pencils about head width apart. Shift your eyes from pencil to pencil. Notice that your awareness is of the two pencils, not of the background between them. Generally, perception occurs the moment the eyes are still, rather than while moving during saccades. For a more challenging exercise, move the pencil you are not looking at, then shift quickly to it, move the other pencil while looking at the one you just moved. In other words, you will pick up the location of the other pencil peripherally and direct your eyes to the foveal region. The size and degree of blur of the peripheral image will tell the brain where the image is and how far to move the eyes. This ability again is due to the function of neural convergence, which is related to neural representation.

Convergence. Hold a pencil at arm's length along your midline. Slowly bring the pencil closer in toward you along your midline. Feel your eyes moving in (crossing). Try to bring the pencil to your nose, keeping the pencil visually single. (It is okay if you cannot.) Move the pencil away now, and your eyes are diverging.

FUNCTIONAL VISUAL SKILLS

Refractive Error

Before discussing binocular coordination and the individual visual skills, it is important to describe refractive errors and how they can affect binocular coordination. Three common types of refractive errors are myopia or nearsightedness, hyperopia or farsightedness, and astigmatism.[5,10]

The myopic eye is too long, so the focused image falls in front of the retina. It is easily corrected with a negative or minus lens, which optically moves the image back onto the retina.

The hyperopic eye is too short, and the focused image falls behind the retina. A positive or plus lens optically moves the image onto the retina.

An eye will have astigmatism if it is not perfectly spherical. An aspherical eye will cause the image to be distorted, where part of the focused image will be in front of the retina and part in back. A person with astigmatism may see vertical lines clearly and horizontal lines as blurry, depending on the specific aspherical shape. A cylindrical type of lens is used to correct astigmatism. This lens corrects the distortion of the image so that it is placed right on the retina.

The following are examples of different refractive errors:
−5.50 D.S. (diopter sphere): Myopia
+4.00 D.S.: Hyperopia
+1.50 c̄ − 1.50 × 180: Astigmatism.
Note: × stands for the axis of the cylinder correction.

When significant refractive errors are uncorrected, they can reduce vision. Uncorrected refractive error also can interfere with binocular coordination. The symptoms are described in greater detail in the next section.

Binocular coordination is the end result of the efficient functioning of the visual skills (Box 30-1). The individual visual skills include accommodation, eye alignment or vergence, eye movements with normal vestibular coordination, stereopsis (depth perception), and peripheral/central coordination. During normal activities, all the skills are inseparable.

Accommodation

Accommodation is the ability to bring near objects into clear focus automatically and without strain. Relaxation of accommodation allows distant objects to come into focus. The primary action is that of the ciliary muscles acting on the lens, and the primary system of control is the ANS with sympathetic and parasympathetic components.[5]

Accommodation is reflexly related to pupillary constriction and dilation.[4] As a person focuses on a near object, the lenses thicken, allowing the near object to come into focus. At the same time the pupils constrict to increase depth of field (just as in a camera). As a person looks into the distance, the lens gets flatter, relaxing accommodation, and the pupil dilates, decreasing the depth of field.

Accommodative ability is age related. A young child can focus on small objects just a few inches in front of the eyes. At about the age of 9 years, the accommodative ability slowly begins to decrease. By the mid 40s the reserve focusing power diminishes to the point that near objects begin to blur. At this stage, reading material is pushed farther away until the arms are not long enough, and then reading glasses are needed. This is called presbyopia (old eyes).

Problems in accommodation may contribute to myopia, hyperopia, and presbyopia. Symptoms include blurriness at either near or far, depending on the age and the problem.

Accommodation is important mainly for up-close activities: reading, hygiene, dressing (specifically, closing fasteners), use of tools, typing, tabletop activities, and games.

Exercise 30-5: Accommodation

Accommodation cannot be directly observed, but it can be implied indirectly through observation of pupillary constriction while doing an accommodative task. Cover one eye. Hold a finger in front at about 10 inches (25 cm). Focus on the finger, making sure that the fingerprint is clear. Shift focus to a distant object. Continue shifting far to near and near to far while a partner observes the pupil. The partner should be able to observe pupillary constriction/dilation as the focus is shifted.

Vergence

Vergence includes convergence and divergence. It is the ability to smoothly and automatically bring the eyes together along the midline to observe objects singly at near (convergence) or conversely to move the eyes outward for single vision of distant objects (divergence). Specific brain centers control convergence and divergence.

Vergence is reflexly associated with accommodation: convergence with accommodation, and divergence with relaxation of accommodation. The function of this reflex is to allow objects to be both single and clear, at either near or far. Vergence has both automatic and voluntary components. Most of the time it is not necessary to think about moving the eyes inward while looking at a close object; yet if asked to cross the eyes, most people can do this at will.

Problems can occur in vergence ability when the eye movement system is out of coordination with accommodation or from damage to cranial nerves III, IV, or VI. Problems can be slight, when there is merely a tendency for the eyes to converge in or out too far, or they can be gross. Tendencies to underconverge or overconverge are called phorias and are not visible to the affected person. An individual may be asymptomatic, but problems may be elicited under conditions of increased stress or fatigue such as excessive reading or working at computer terminal or from drug side effects (prescription and recreational).

Some phorias may worsen to the extent that binocularity breaks down, at which point the individual has a strabismus. There are two main types of strabismus: esotropia and exotropia. An esotropia is an inward turning of the eye, and an exotropia is a visible outward turning. A third, less common type of strabismus is hypertropia, in which one eye aims upward. Strabismus and dysfunctional phorias are discussed in greater detail in the next section.

Vergence ability is needed for singular binocular vision; thus, it is basic to all activities. At near, the patient may have difficulty finding objects; eye-hand coordination may be decreased, affecting self-care and hygiene tasks; and reading may be difficult. Distance tasks that may be affected include driving, sports, movies, communication, and, frequently, ambulation. Individuals with impaired vergence ability may also have difficulty focusing and may have decreased or no depth perception. Interpreting space can be quite difficult and confusing. If decreased vergence is a result of traumatic head injury or stroke, it may contribute to the patient's confusion, and he or she may not be able to identify or communicate the problem.

Exercise 30-6: Vergence

Hold a pencil in front of you at eye level at about 12 inches (30 cm). Look at the pencil. Look away into the distance. Looking at the pencil is convergence and looking into the distance is divergence. As you converge and diverge slowly back and forth notice any changes you may feel: changes in how relaxed you feel, how focused or spaced out you feel, feelings of dreaminess, or nothing at all. Observe a partner's eyes as they shift back and forth as well.

Pursuits and Saccades

Eye movement skills consist of pursuits and saccades. Pursuits are the smooth, coordinated movements of all eye muscles together, allowing accurate tracking of objects through space. Perception is continuous during pursuit movements. Saccades are rapid shifts of the eyes from object to object, allowing quick localization of movements observed in the periphery. The systems involved in eye movement skills are the oculomotor system with the VOR, in conjunction with coordination of the central and peripheral visual systems. The peripheral visual system is finely tuned for detecting changes in light levels and small movements.

Problems in pursuits and saccades can be the result of a dysfunctioning of any individual muscles or of the VOR. Because the VOR helps to stabilize the image on the retina and to differentiate image movement from eye movement, simple tracking can be more difficult. In addition, visual field loss, either central or peripheral, can dramatically affect localization ability. People with blind half or quarter fields can be observed to do searching eye movements rather than directly jumping to the object.

Activities affected include searching for objects, visually directed movement for fine motor tasks and gross movement and ambulation tasks, eye-hand coordination, self-care, driving, and reading.

Memory also may be affected by an eye movement dysfunction. Research by Adler-Grinberg and Stark[13] and Noton and Stark[14] examined patterns of eye movements as subjects looked at a picture. Distinct eye movement patterns, called scan paths, became apparent. When the subject was asked to recall the picture, the same eye movement pattern was elicited as the subject recalled the picture. Perhaps a type of oculomotor motor planning is involved in recall. Applying this idea to the clinical setting, if a patient has inaccurate eye movement, inability with undershooting and overshooting, or uses 32 saccades to scan a picture rather than 10, then perhaps the stored memory is less efficiently stored and consequently the image is more difficult to reconstruct from memory. Additionally, if a patient has a type of brain damage with generalized dyspraxia, the eye movement system could quite likely be affected and might be involved in the patient's perceptual dysfunction.

SYMPTOMS OF VISUAL DYSFUNCTION
History

The identification of a visual problem begins with case history. It is important to get some idea of the client's prior visual status or any history of eye injury, surgery, or diseases. Information can be elicited by direct questioning of the client or family members or by clinical observation. Sample questions include the following:

- Are you having difficulty with seeing, or with your eyes?
- Do you wear glasses? Contact lenses? For distance, near, bifocals, or monovision (one eye near, other distance)?
- Does your correction work as well now as before the (stroke, accident, etc.)?
- Have you noticed any blurriness? Near or far?

■ Do you ever see double? See two? See overlapping or shadow images?
■ Do you ever find that when you reach for an object that you knock it over or your hand misses?
■ Do letters jump around on the page after reading for a while?
■ Are you experiencing any eye strain or headaches? Where and when?
■ Do you ever lose your place when reading?
■ Are portions of a page or any objects missing?
■ Do people or things suddenly appear from one side that you didn't see approaching?
■ Do you have difficulty concentrating on tasks?

Clinical observations of the client while performing various activities are a valuable source of problem identification. Therapists in general are in an ideal position to observe clients in a variety of functional tasks that require near vision, far vision, spatial estimations, depth judgments, and oculomotor tasks. This situation varies considerably from the physician's observations in the more contrived environment of the examination room. Additionally, the therapist's initial observations can be used in documenting difficulties within the therapy realm that may be amenable to visual remediation in terms that can be applied to reimbursement of therapy.

Clinical observations include the following:
■ Head tilt during near tasks
■ Avoidance of near tasks
■ One eye appears to go in, out, up, or down
■ Vision shifts from eye to eye
■ Seems to look past observer
■ Closes or covers one eye
■ Squints
■ Eyes appear red, puffy, or irritated or have a discharge (Notify nurses or physician of these observations.)
■ Rubs eyes a lot
■ Has difficulty maintaining eye contact
■ Spaces out, drifts off, daydreams
■ During activity, neglects one side of body or space
■ During movement, bumps into walls or objects (either walking or in a wheelchair)
■ Appears to misjudge distance
■ Underreaches or overreaches for objects
■ Has difficulty finding things

Near Point Blur

The first area of symptoms is near accommodative problems. The primary symptom is near point blur. This symptom alone is not indicative of a problem in any one area, but it could indicate farsightedness (hyperopia), astigmatism, or reduced accommodative ability (insufficiency). The client may move objects or the head farther or closer, may complain of eye strain or headaches, may squint, or may even avoid near activities as much as possible. The therapist might observe excessive blinking, and the patient may complain of glasses not working well.

Distance Blur

The next problem could also indicate a number of different causes. Distance blur could indicate nearsightedness (myopia), a pathological problem (such as beginning cataracts or macular degeneration), or accommodative spasm. Most people have some experience with accommodative spasm. After spending long periods of time either studying or reading a novel and then glancing up at the wall across the room, it may be blurry and then clear up slowly. For some individuals, this spasm eventually becomes one component in their nearsightedness if the reading habits continue for a long time.

Clients with distance blur may make forward head movements and frequently squint in an attempt to see. They may not respond or orient quickly to auditory or visual stimuli beyond a certain radius. The therapist may also note excessive blinking and a withdrawn attitude because the patient cannot see well enough to interact with the environment.

Visual hygiene can be recommended to assist in the development of good visual habits. Good lighting and posture, taking frequent breaks, and monitoring the state of clarity of an environmental cue such as a clock across the room are all beneficial.

Phoria and Strabismus

The next area of eye alignment problems can be divided into two types of problems: phoria and strabismus. A phoria can be defined as a natural positioning of the eyes in which there is a tendency to aim in front of or behind the point of focus. It may or may not be associated with symptoms. Fusion is intact to some degree, and depth perception may also be intact.

Everyone has a phoria, just as everyone has a posture. It may be within normal range, or, just as someone may have scoliosis, a high phoria may cause problems. The following phorias may cause problems:
■ Esophoria: eyes are postured in front of the point of focus.
■ Exophoria: the eyes are postured in back of the point of focus.

Phoria is measured in units of prism diopters, which indicate the size of the prism needed to measure the eye position in or out from the straight-ahead position.[4]

Phorias tend to produce subtle symptoms. These include having difficulty concentrating, frontal or temporal headaches, sleepiness after reading, and stinging of the eyes after reading.

A strabismus, or tropia, is a visible turn of one eye, which may be constant, intermittent, or alternating between one eye and the other. The person may have double vision, or if the strabismus is long term, the person may suppress or "turn off" the vision in the wandering eye. Suppression is a neurological function that is an adaptation to the intolerable situation of double images. It is only exhibited in long-term strabismus because apparently the brain cannot learn to suppress past the time of peak plasticity (up to age 7 years). The developing brain must choose which eye has the visual direction, which is confirmed by motor and tactile inputs as being the "real" image. The other fovea's image is then neurologically suppressed. The peripheral vision in the suppressing eye is still normal, and the eye is not by any means blind.

Certain postures may facilitate fusion for some clients. The eye doctor will be able to determine which head position may be best. Frequently, many clients will automatically move around to the best position. At other times, however, head position will be used to avoid using one eye.

Head and body position, therefore, are important aspects to consider.

Many convergence problems are amenable to vision therapy,[15-17] but some are not.[18] Whether a particular problem can be helped by vision therapy can be determined by an eye doctor, who can prescribe specific exercises.

Oculomotor Dysfunction

If the client has a vestibular dysfunction, tracking activities should be combined as much as possible with vestibular stimulation. Vision therapy has been demonstrated to improve reading performance and comprehension.[19,20]

While doing any sort of tracking activity, the client is encouraged to maintain peripheral awareness. This technique will help the client keep her or his place. The oculomotor system is guided by the peripheral location of an object.

Hemianopsia

Hemianopsia is a loss of half of the visual field in each eye. Homonymous hemianopsia refers to the inner or nasal half and the outer or temporal half of each eye being affected. The retina itself is intact, but a neurological lesion has interrupted the ability of the visual cortex to receive recognition of the image. Vision processing may be occurring at lower centers, such as the lateral geniculate body, but if signals are not being received by the cortex, then they are not recognized as "seen." In 1979 Zihl and von Cramon[21] published their findings that damaged visual fields could be trained by use of a light stimulus presented repeatedly at the border of the visual field defect. Balliet et al[22] (when attempting to repeat the experiment, adding controls for oculomotor fixations) proposed that subjects were actually learning to make small compensatory eye movements rather than true improvements in the visual fields. Since then, in the 1980s and 1990s a group of German researchers developed a computer-based field training system for researching the question of visual field training. They found in their research that visual fields did expand on average by 5 degrees, with functional improvements noted by more than 80% of their patients (Figure 30-9).[23-26] These authors have also noted documentable and functional improvements in visual fields even when trained with less sophisticated methods.

Compensation training may also be required to allow the client to resume activities such as reading. Compensation techniques include use of margin markers and reading with a card with a slit in it (typoscope) to isolate one line or a couple of lines at a time. Holding reading material vertically also can help.

SUMMARY OF DISORDERS OF VISION

Table 30-1 summarizes primary visual deficits. Once a therapist or other specialist has eliminated the possibility of primary visual deficits, the clinician must assess whether the identified problem is due to central associative processing that is causing visual-perceptual dysfunction.

VISUAL-PERCEPTUAL DYSFUNCTION

This discussion of visual-perceptual disorders is divided into a number of categories: unilateral spatial inattention; cortical blindness, defective color perception, and visual agnosia; visual-spatial disorders; visual-constructive disorders; and

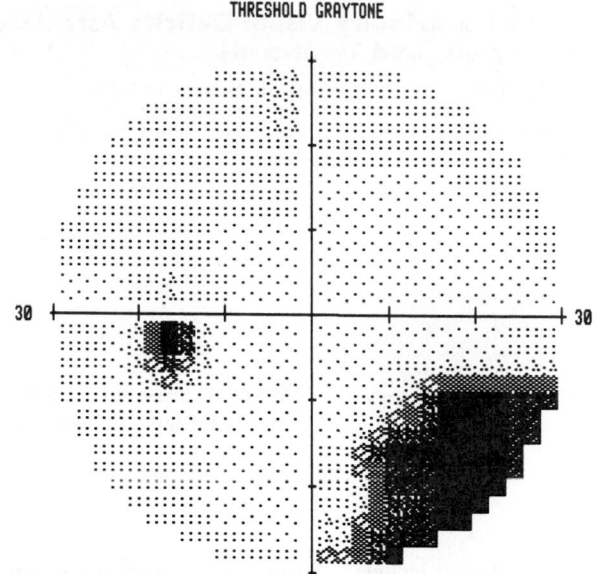

THRESHOLD GRAYTONE

FIGURE 30-9 ■ Visual field defect (inferior temporal) as measured on Humphrey visual field tester.

visual analysis and synthesis disorders. Cortical blindness is a disorder of primary visual input; however, because its variations may influence perceptual interpretation, it is discussed here. All other disorders listed involve direct problems with the interpretation of visual stimuli. Although each of these terms represents symptoms recognized by many authors, the reader is reminded that there are no clear boundaries between one deficit and another or one system and another. Apraxia and body image disorders are not discussed under separate categories because they are not considered "visual"-perceptual disorders per se although their presence may influence and complicate an already dysfunctional visual-perceptual system.

Problems of Unilateral Spatial Inattention
Identification of Clinical Problems

General Category. In its purest form, unilateral spatial inattention is defined as a condition in which an individual with normal sensory and motor systems fails to orient toward, respond to, or report stimuli on the side contralateral to the cerebral lesion. Although this condition is not often seen in its pure form, inattention has been documented in persons who demonstrate no accompanying visual field defect (homonymous hemianopsia) or limb sensory or motor loss.[27] In most cases, however, unilateral spatial inattention is not seen alone but is associated with (although not caused by) accompanying sensory and motor defects such as homonymous hemianopsia and decreased tactile, proprioceptive, and stereognostic perception along with paresis or paralysis of the upper limb.

It is easy to become confused by the numerous terms used in the literature, for example, unilateral spatial agnosia, unilateral visual neglect, "fixed" hemianopsia, hemi-inattention, or hemi-imperception. All terms describe the same deficit. *Unilateral spatial inattention* is used in this chapter because (1) in severe cases the syndrome most likely involves tactile and auditory as well as visual unawareness

TABLE 30-1 ■ Primary Visual Deficits Associated with Central Lesions, Functional Symptoms, Management, and Treatment

VISUAL DEFICIT	FUNCTIONAL DEFICIT	MANAGEMENT	TREATMENT
Decreased visual acuity (distance or near)	Decreased acuity for distance or near tasks (reading)	Provide best lens correction for distance and near	May not be correctable
Inconsistent accommodations	Inconsistent blurred near vision	Ensure appropriate lenses are worn for appropriate activities	Accommodation training may be appropriate
		Determine whether bifocal is usable; if not, provide separate lenses for distance and near	
		Enlarge target, control density, use contrast, task lighting	
Cortical blindness	Marked decrease in visual acuity	Evaluated by vision specialist to determine areas and quality of residual vision	Use headlamp to improve visual localization (i.e., functional use of residual vision)
	Severe blurring uncorrectable by lenses	Present targets of appropriate size/contrast in best area of visual field	
Visual field deficits include homonymous hemianopsias, quadrantanopsias, scotomas, visual field constrictions	Blindness or decreased sensitivity in affected area of visual field	Be aware of normal field position in all meridians of gaze	Scanning training to facilitate compensation
		Ask patient to outline working area before beginning task	Training in use of prism
		Partial press-on	
		Fresnel prism to facilitate compensation	
Pupillary reactions	Slow or absent pupillary responses	Sunglasses to control excess brightness	
Loss of vertical gaze (external ophthalmoplegia)	Inability to move eyes up or down	Raise target or working area to foveal level	Prism glasses to allow objects below to be seen as directly in front
		Teach patient head movement to compensate	
Conjugate gaze deviation	Inability/difficulty moving eyes from fixed gaze position		
Lack of convergence	Diplopia or blurred vision for near tasks		Convergence exercises prescribed by vision specialist
	Decreased depth perception for near tasks		
Oculomotor nerve lesion (strabismus)	Intermittent or consistent diplopia in some or all meridians of gaze	Fresnel prism to fuse image in select cases	Oculomotor and binocular exercises with prism use prescribed by vision specialist
	Loss of depth perception	Occlude deviant eye	
Pathological (motor) nystagmus	Movement/blur of image during reading/near activities/ decreased activities	Enlarge print/target to decrease blur	Rigid gas-permeable contact lens prescribed by vision specialist
		Contact lens provides feedback, reduces movement, and increases activity	
Poor fixations, saccades, or pursuits	Erratic scanning	Decrease density of material	Oculomotor exercises prescribed by vision specialist
	Unsteady fixation	Isolate targets during evaluation and treatment	Sensory integration activities
			Scanning training
			Use of kinesthetic and tactile systems to lead visual system (eye movements)

© Copyright by Mary Jane Bouska, OTR/L, 1988.
Modified by Laurie E. Chaikin, OD, OTR.

(i.e., a total spatial unawareness) and (2) the syndrome results in an involuntary lack of attention to stimuli contralateral to the lesion, whereas the term *neglect* implies a voluntary choice not to respond.

Unilateral spatial inattention occurs most frequently in individuals with a diagnosis of stroke (CVA), traumatic brain injury, or tumor. Most authors agree that unilateral spatial inattention occurs more often with right hemisphere than with left hemisphere lesions.[28-32] This frequency supports theories that the right hemisphere is dominant for visual-spatial organization. It is clear, however, that inattention may be present in individuals with left hemisphere lesions. The clinician should remember that, although the chances are statistically less, the client with right hemiplegia may exhibit inattention to right stimuli.

Unilateral spatial inattention has been associated with lesions in both cortical and subcortical structures. It is most commonly seen in inferior parietal lobe lesions[31] but has also been observed in lesions in the dorsolateral frontal lobe and in the cingulate gyrus,[33] and with thalamic[34] and putaminal hemorrhage.[35,36] Finally, lesions in the brain stem reticular formation have induced inattention in cats[36] and monkeys.[34]

Although a number of theories have been postulated regarding the mechanism underlying unilateral spatial inattention, no mechanism has been validly documented in human subjects. The one fact that is clear from all theoretical postulates is that inattention is a hemispheric deficit. LeDoux and Smylie[37] demonstrated this point effectively in an interesting case study of a right-sided lesion. During full visual exposure (bilateral hemispheric) of visual-perceptual slides, the affected individual made visual-spatial errors in left space. However, when the same slides were directed only to the right visual field (left hemisphere), performance improved substantially. It is as if the deficient hemisphere fails to receive or orient toward incoming information while the intact receiving hemisphere remains oblivious and goes about its own business. Treatment for inattention is problematic mainly because the mechanisms underlying unilateral spatial inattention are not clearly understood.

Theories on mechanisms underlying unilateral spatial inattention have attempted to explain it as an integrative associative defect as opposed to simply a problem of decreased sensory input. Theories include a unilateral attentional hypothesis, suggesting that inattention results from a disruption in the orienting response; that is, the corticolimbic hemisphere is underaroused during bilateral input and therefore stimuli presented to that hemisphere are neglected.[31,33] Another theory is the oculomotor imbalance hypothesis, which suggests that individuals with inattention have a visual-spatial disorder worsened by oculomotor imbalance. The hypothesis suggests that the lesion disconnects the frontal eye fields in the damaged hemisphere from their sensory afferent nerves, resulting in an oculomotor imbalance deviating the gaze toward the lesion. This imbalance can be compensated for only momentarily by a voluntary effort to gaze toward the opposite hemispace (i.e., neglected space).[38]

Unilateral Spatial Inattention with Homonymous Hemianopsia. Inattention occurs more commonly with visual field defects and is generally better when the macular projections are not involved. Individuals with pure hemi-

anopsia are aware of their visual loss and spontaneously learn to compensate by moving their eyes (foveae) toward the lost visual field to expand their visual space and thereby gather information right and left of midline. On visual examination other individuals may demonstrate no visual field defect on unilateral stimulation; however, during bilateral stimulation, they extinguish the target contralateral to the lesion. Other persons may perceive both targets simultaneously, yet when engaged in activity they may not respond to visual stimuli in one half of visual space contralateral to the lesion. These individuals are unaware of their inattention. Careful observation of their activity reveals few eye movements into the neglected space. The fovea does not appear to be directed to gather information in this space.

Unilateral Visual, Auditory, and Tactile Inattention. Inattention has been described as a multimodal sensory associative disorder involving not only visual but also tactile and auditory unawareness. Clinicians are well aware of the client with left inattention who continues to direct the head and eyes toward the right throughout an entire conversation although the therapist is standing on the client's left side. When one conceptualizes unilateral spatial inattention as a dynamic decrease or loss of sensory information within one half of the sensory-perceptual sphere (irrespective of hypothetical mechanism), the peculiar behaviors exhibited by these clients are more easily understood.

Unilateral Spatial Inattention and Body Image. Body image is often disturbed in individuals with inattention. The defect in these persons is unusual because it affects only that half of the body that is contralateral to the lesion, for example, the left side of the body in right-sided lesions. There appears to be a lack of spatial orientation and attention for one half of intrapersonal space. Those with severe inattention fail to recognize that their affected extremities are their own and function as though they are absent. They may fail to dress one half of the body or attempt to navigate through a door oblivious to the fact that the affected arm may be caught on the doorknob or door frame. In severe cases, individuals may deny their hemiparesis, or they may deny that the extremity belongs to them. This phenomenon is called anosognosia.

Behavioral Manifestations of Unilateral Spatial Inattention. Persons with inattention orient all their activities toward their "attended" space. The head, eyes, and trunk are rotated toward the side of the lesion during much of the time, including during gait. Careful observation of eye movements (scanning saccades) during activities indicates that all or almost all scanning occurs on only one side of the midline within the attended space; the individual never spontaneously brings the eyes or head past midline into contralateral "unattended" space. Oculomotor examination always shows full extraocular movements and no apraxia for eye movements.

Inattention, like all other perceptual disorders, may be viewed on a scale from mild to severe. Mild cases of inattention may go unrecognized unless behavior is carefully observed. Scanning is symmetrical except during tasks requiring increasingly complex perceptual and cognitive demands. Leicester et al[39] believe that inattention occurs mainly when the individual has a general perceptual problem with the material, that is, some other problem with processing the task. This performance difficulty or stress brings on the additional inattention behavior; for example, neglect for matching auditory letter samples is more common in those with aphasia than in those with right hemisphere involvement without aphasia.

Independence in activities of daily living is often impossible because of inattention to both the intrapersonal and extrapersonal environment. The individual may eat only half the food on the plate, dress only half the body, shave or apply makeup to only half the face, brush teeth in only half the mouth, read only half the page, fill out only one half a form, miss kitchen utensils, carpentry tools, or items in the store if they are located in the unattended space, collide with obstacles or miss doorways on the unattended side, and, when walking or driving a wheelchair, veer toward the attended space rather than navigating in a straight line.

Assessment

Because most tests used to measure cognitive, language, perceptual, and motor skills require symmetrical visual, auditory, and tactile awareness, it is most important to rule out inattention early in the evaluation process of any client with a central lesion. The two most common methods used to distinguish inattention from primary sensory deficits are double simultaneous stimulation testing and assessment of optokinetic nystagmus reflexes. Double simultaneous stimuli should be applied in three modalities: auditory, tactile, and visual. Initially, stimuli should be presented to the abnormal side. If primary sensation is impaired (e.g., a visual field loss), this evaluation cannot proceed because double simultaneous stimulation testing is invalid in that modality. If responsiveness is normal, however, bilateral simultaneous stimuli should be applied. Unilateral stimuli should be interspersed with bilateral stimuli to ensure valid responses. Lack of awareness (extinction) of stimuli contralateral to the lesion during bilateral stimulation should be noted. Clients with extinction in only one sensory system often do not demonstrate inattention behaviors; however, those with extinction in more than one modality (e.g., tactile and visual) often demonstrate these behaviors. If critical diagnosis of inattention is necessary, the client may be referred for optokinetic nystagmus testing.

One of the best evaluation tools is a keen sense of observation. The position of the client's head, eyes, and trunk should be observed at rest and during activity. Persistent deviation toward the lesion may indicate unilateral inattention. The individual should be asked to track a visual target from space ipsilateral to the lesion into contralateral space and maintain fixation there for 5 seconds. The therapist may ask the client to quickly fixate on visual targets both right and left of midline on command. Problems with searching for targets in contralateral space should be noted. Some erratic oculomotor searching is normal when making saccades into a hemianoptic field because saccades are centrally programmed by peripheral input. Slow searching or failure to search should be considered indicative of inattention.

Asymmetries in performance should be noted during spatial tasks. Specific spatial tasks have been designed to detect inattention, including the following:

- Cancellation tasks. The client may be given a sheet of paper with horizontal lines of numbers or letters and asked to cross out all the 8s or As.
- Crossing-out tasks. In this standardized test the client is asked to cross out diagonal lines drawn at random on an unlined sheet of paper.
- Line-bisection tasks. The client is asked to bisect a 4- to 8-inch line on a piece of paper placed at the midline.
- Drawing and copying tasks. The client may be asked to draw or copy a house, clock, or flower or to fill in the numbers of a clock drawn by the examiner. For copying tasks, it is important that the copy be placed in the client's attended space.

Clients with inattention demonstrate one or more of the following behaviors: failure to cancel figures or cross out lines in the unattended space; bisecting the line unequally, placing their mark toward the side of the midline ipsilateral to their lesion; placing their drawing toward the edge of the paper ipsilateral to their lesion rather than in the middle of the page; drawing only the right or left half of the house, flower, or clock; crowding all the numbers of the clock into the right or left half of the clock; or completing numbers on only one half of the clock (Figure 30-10). When interpreting performance, the examiner is looking specifically for asymmetries in performance. Clients with inattention often have other visual-perceptual deficits that result in faulty performance on these tasks; however, these deficits are always symmetrical, that is, evident in any space to which the individual attends.

Asymmetries in performance should be carefully observed during functional activities such as eating, filling out a form, reading, dressing, and maneuvering through the environment. The therapist may note unawareness of doorways and hallways in the unattended space; turns may be made only toward one direction. As a result, these clients lose their way in the hospital or even in the therapy clinic. This behavior should be distinguished from a topographical perceptual deficit in which the individual cannot integrate or remember spatial concepts well enough to find his or her way without getting lost. The Behavioral Inattention Test has recently been published as a standardized measure of functional inattention.[40]

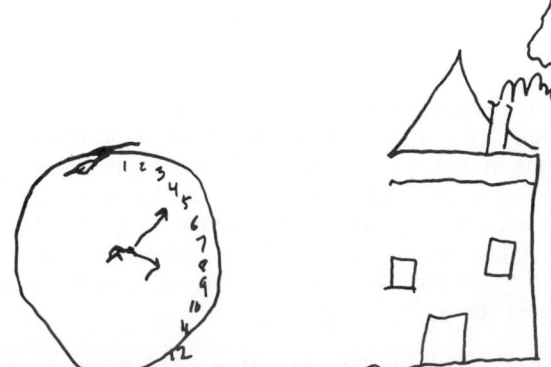

FIGURE 30-10 ■ Drawings of a clock and house by a client with a right hemisphere parietal lobe tumor. Note the left unilateral spatial inattention in the drawings.

Finally, various studies have shown that inattention may occur during testing that requires visual processing and therefore may invalidate test results.[28,41,42] Unresponsiveness to figures on one side of the page during visual, perceptual, cognitive, or language assessments may be subtle but must be documented to rule out the influence of inattention on raw score; *that is, if the patient did not see the entire test display in an item, that test item is invalid.* Responses to figures on the right half and left half of the test page should be counted. If the frequency of answers is noticeably less on one half of the page than would normally be expected, inattention may have occurred during testing. This may be used as additional evidence of inattention; but more important, this factor should be accounted for when computing the test score. Only those test items in which the correct answer was located in the attended space should be scored; that is, only those items in which the correct answer was right of midline in a client with left inattention should be scored.

Interventions

As previously stated, the mechanisms underlying unilateral spatial inattention have not been clearly elucidated. This has made development of treatment rationales difficult. A number of studies, however, have investigated the remediation of unilateral spatial inattention. They have attempted to (1) define effective remediation techniques and (2) measure changes in trained tasks and generalization to untrained tasks, that is, determine whether inattention training in one task carries over to other unrelated tasks such as activities of daily living. Treatment techniques used in all these studies resulted in less inattention in trained tasks.[29,43,44] An overview of these studies suggests that training may decrease inattention, although extent of change and generalization to other tasks may vary widely. Discrepancies in these results may be related to neurological variables in the various client samples, severity of inattention, sample size, or tasks measured. A discussion of general principles of remediation follows.

Efforts should be made to increase the client's cognitive awareness of the inattention. The individual should be made keenly aware of what a peripheral visual field loss is and how it is affecting her or his view of the world. The person with normal visual fields but with visual extinction should be treated the same as the individual with an actual visual field loss because the visual experience is similar. Pictures of the visual field deficit may be drawn for illustration. Actual performance examples in the environment should be pointed out to the client to demonstrate the biased field of view.

Visual scanning should be emphasized. Initially, the client should be made aware of how eye and eye-head movements may be used to compensate for the deficit. The individual should be trained to make progressively larger and quicker pursuits and saccades and longer fixations into the unattended space. Training may be accomplished with interesting targets held by the therapist, for example, targets secured to the tips of pencils, such as changeable letters, colored lights, or bright small objects. Pursuit or tracking movements of the target leading the eye from attended into unattended space should be stressed first, followed by saccades into the unattended space. Initially, the client may be allowed to move the head during scanning exercises;

however, eye movements without head movements should be the major goal. Individuals with inattention often move their head into the unattended space while their eye remains fixed on a target in the attended space (i.e., the visual field remains the same). The client should be taught to independently carry out a daily right-left scanning program with targets appropriately positioned by the therapist. Eventually, these targets can be moved farther into the unattended space.

Increased awareness and scanning abilities should be incorporated in increasingly complex visual-perceptual and visual-motor tasks. Because inattention often increases as task complexity increases, the therapist must select and structure tasks carefully. Examples of simple yet specific scanning tasks might include surveying a room repetitively, rolling toward and touching objects right and left of midline, assembling objects from pieces strewn on a table or the floor, completing an obstacle course, or selecting letters from a page of large print.

Scanning should be stressed during functional activities, for example, dressing, shaving, or moving through the environment. The client may be taught to constantly monitor the influence of inattention on functional performance, for example, "When something doesn't make sense, look into the unattended space and it usually will."

Diller[45] has designed a number of specific training techniques to decrease inattention during reading and paper and pencil tasks. With a little creativity, these techniques may be applied to other activities. For example, when the client is reading, a visual marker is placed on the extreme edge of the page in unattended space. The individual is instructed not to begin reading until he or she sees the visual marker. The marker is used to "anchor" the client's vision. As inattention decreases, the anchor is faded. Each line may also be numbered and the numbers used to anchor scanning horizontally and vertically. To control impulsiveness, which often accompanies inattention, clients are taught to slow down or pace their performance by incorporating techniques such as reciting the words aloud. Underlining and looping letters/words can also be used as a method to slow down impulsive scanning (Figure 30-11). Finally, the density of stimuli is reduced; decreased density appears to decrease inattention in these tasks.

To stimulate tactile awareness in clients with tactile extinction, Anderson and Choy[46] suggest stimulating the affected arm as the individual watches. A rough cloth, vibrator, or the therapist's or client's hand may be used. Eventually, this activity may be done before activities that require spontaneous symmetrical scanning, such as dressing or walking through an obstacle course.

During the early phases of treatment, when inattention is still moderate to severe, the client should be approached from the attended space during treatment for inattention or other deficits such as apraxia, balance, or speech. This ensures that the individual comprehends and views all demonstrations and treatment instructions. Subsequently, as orientation and scanning improve, activities should be moved progressively into the unattended space and the therapist should be positioned in the unattended space during treatment. In the final stages of treatment, the client should be able to symmetrically scan regardless of the therapist's position (i.e., the therapist should vary position).

```
               0  (1)   2    4    5    6    7    8    9    10

1.  (1)  2    3    5    4    9    7    8    0    6    3    2   10  (1)   2    3    5    4    9    7    1

2.   3    4    9    6    7   10    8   (1)   2    5    0    6    4    9    6    7   10    8    2    8    2

3.   8    0    6    2   (1)   3    5    4    7    9   10  (1)   8    0    6    2   (1)   3    5    7    3

4.   5    7    3    9    6   (1)   2    8    4   10    0    3    5    5    7    3    6   (1)   2    5    4

5.   6    5   (1)   4    2    3    8   10    9    7    9    0    6    5   (1)   4    2    3    8    9    5

6.   4    8   10    0    7    6    9    1    3    2    5    6    3    4    8   10    0    7    6    9    6

7.   9    6    5    3    8    4    2    0   10    1    7    2    4    9    6    5    3    8    2    4    7
```

FIGURE 30-11 ■ Underlining during visual discrimination tasks helps control eye movements (scanning).

To enhance the integration of scanning behavior during functional tasks such as gait and dressing, the client should be reminded of scanning principles and carried through a series of scanning exercises before initiation of the activity. If inattention reappears during the activity, the therapist should stop and assist the client in becoming reoriented before the activity is resumed. Inattention results in confusion, and confusion increases inattention. As will be pointed out repeatedly in the following pages, the therapist must control the perceptual environment continuously so that the client is able to sequence bits of information together meaningfully to learn or relearn.

Problems of Cortical Blindness, Color Imperception, and Visual Agnosia

Identification of Clinical Problems

Cortical Blindness. Cortical blindness is considered a primary sensory disorder as opposed to a secondary associative disorder. It is discussed here, however, because of the many variations of this lesion that may result in problems with interpretation of visual stimuli. Cortical blindness, also known as central blindness, is a total or almost total loss of vision resulting from bilateral cerebral destruction of the visual projection cortex (area 17). Similar destruction limited to one hemisphere results in hemianopsia.[27] The lesion may be ischemic, neoplastic, degenerative, or traumatic. The client may perceive the defect as a "blurring" of vision or as a marked decrease in visual acuity or may be unaware of the complete nature of the disability and even deny it, blaming the problem on eyeglasses that are too weak or a room that is too dark.

Color Imperception. Color perception may be impaired in the client with brain damage. This symptom is usually associated with right hemisphere or bilateral lesions.[47] This deficit is different from color agnosia, in which there is a problem with naming colors correctly. Clients with defective color perception may see colors as "muddy" or "impure" in hue, or the color of a small target may fade into the background, decreasing the ability to differentiate it from the background.[32,48] Total loss of color monochromatism is rare, but it can occur.

Visual Agnosia. A lesion circumscribed to the visual associative areas (areas 18 and 19) results in a number of unique visual disorders that are categorized as some form of visual agnosia. Lesions are usually bilateral with combined parietooccipital, occipitotemporal, and callosal lesions. Visual agnosia is defined as a failure to recognize visual stimuli (e.g., objects, faces, letters) although visual-sensory processing, language, and general intellectual functions are preserved at sufficiently high levels.[49] It also has been described as perception without meaning; perception apparently occurs, but the percept seems "disconnected" from previously associated meaning. In this pure form, visual agnosia is a relatively rare syndrome, and there is controversy as to whether it is simply an extension of primary visual sensory deficits (variations of cortical blindness) or whether it should be considered as a separate neuropsychological entity.

Three types of agnosia have been recognized: visual, tactile, and auditory. Agnosia is most often modality specific; that is, the individual who cannot recognize the object visually will usually give an immediate and accurate response when touching or hearing the object in use. In visual agnosia, then, poor recognition is limited to the visual sphere.

Visual agnosia is divided into a number of types: visual object agnosia, simultanagnosia, facial agnosia, and color agnosia. These deficits may be seen in isolation or in various combinations, depending on the size and location of lesion.

Visual Object Agnosia. During evaluation for the presence of visual object agnosia, the individual is presented with a number of common objects (e.g., key, comb, brush) and asked to name them. The evaluator may assume that the object is recognized if the client (1) names, describes, or demonstrates the use of the object or (2) selects it from among a group of objects as it is named by the examiner. If the person recognizes (describes or demonstrates) but is unable to name the object, failure is most likely a result of an anomia rather than an agnosic defect. Individuals with real visual agnosia have no concept of what the object is.[49]

Simultanagnosia. Along the same vein are visual disorders that constrict or "narrow" the visual field during active perceptual analysis (i.e., when perceptions are tested separately, the visual field is within normal limits). Simultanagnosia is a disorder in which the person actually perceives only one element of an object or picture at a time and is unable to absorb the whole. As the individual concentrates on the visual environment, there is an extreme reduction of visual span. The problem is functionally similar to tubular vision. The narrowing of the functional perceptual field decreases the ability to simultaneously deal with two or more stimuli. It appears as if the person has bilateral visual inattention with macular sparing although perimetric testing reveals full visual fields. A typical example is the individual whose visual attention is focused on the tip of a cigarette held between the lips and fails to perceive a match flame offered several inches away.[50]

Facial Agnosia. Another special type of agnosia that has been documented is failure to recognize familiar faces. The disorder is also known as prosopagnosia. The individual is able to recognize a face as a face but is unable to connect the face and differences in faces with people he or she knows. This person is unable to recognize family members, friends, and hospital staff by face. One must be careful not to confuse this with generalized dementia. There may be categorical recognition problems of items involving special visual experience, for example, recognition of cars, types of trees, or emblems. Facial agnosia is usually seen in combination with a number of other deficits, including spatial disorientation, defective color perception, loss of topographical memory, constructional apraxia, and a left upper quadrant visual field loss. These other symptoms are most likely not causative but rather a result of the similar neurological location of these functions.[51]

Color Agnosia. Finally, the individual may have difficulty recognizing names of colors, that is, an inability to name colors that are shown or to point to the color named by the examiner.[52] This defect is considered agnosic (as opposed to a defect in color perception) because the client is able to recognize all colors in the *Ishihara Color Plates*[53] and is also able to sort colors by hue. The determining factor here appears to be a problem with visual-verbal association. Color agnosia is most common in clients with left hemisphere lesions and is often accompanied by the syndrome of alexia without agraphia.[49]

Assessment

Cortical blindness and variations of it should be thoroughly assessed by the vision specialist. Assessment for agnosia must be preceded by a thorough assessment for visual acuity problems, visual field deficits, and unilateral visual inattention because these primary visual sensory and scanning deficits are often mistaken for agnosic performance. Next, basic color perception should be measured by use of the Ishihara Color Plates[53] and color-sorting or color-matching tasks. Individuals with defective color perception will have difficulty with some visual-perceptual tasks because contextual cues related to color and shading are unavailable to them. Agnosia is a valid diagnosis only if (1) the aforementioned primary visual skills are intact and (2) language skills are intact (i.e., there should be no word-finding difficulty in spontaneous speech).

Although there are no standardized tests for agnosia, commonly used assessment methods have been included. The presence of simultanagnosia is determined by keen observation of performance that indicates perception limited to single elements within objects, for example, describing only the wheel of a bicycle or, within the environment, describing only one part of a room or an activity.

Object agnosia is tested by placing common real objects (e.g., comb, key, penny, spoon) in front of the client and asking the client to name or point to the item chosen by the examiner. In pointing and naming tasks, the therapist must be sure that the client is fixating on the appropriate target. This response is considered normal if the object is named correctly or described or its functional use demonstrated. Abnormal responses will be confabulatory or perseverative, with the individual often giving the name of a previous or similar object. Responses may also be completely bizarre and unrelated. The examiner may also present objects at an unusual angle. Abnormal responses will show lack of recognition or rotation of the head or body to try to view the object in the "straight on" position. The diagnosis of visual object agnosia is further confirmed if the individual can identify the object by touch or by hearing it in use. Both should be done with vision occluded.

Color agnosia is evaluated by having the client name a color and point to colors named by the examiner. Facial agnosia is evaluated by presenting the individual with photographs of famous world figures, actors, politicians, and family members.[32]

Interventions

There are no reliable studies regarding treatment of cortical blindness, color imperception, or visual agnosia. Treatment principles presented here are based on the experience of Bouska and Biddle[41] and Bouska and Kwatny.[28] If cortical blindness or simultanagnosia is suspected, the therapist must first attempt to increase the client's knowledge of foveal versus peripheral vision, that is, where the client is fixating. A small headlamp attached to the client's forehead may be used under conditions of subdued lighting. This should not be used in a completely darkened room because the client needs to use normal spatial cues from the environment. The movement of the projected light in the environment and kinesthetic input from the neck receptors augment knowledge of where the eye is fixed. To carry out this task, the client must learn to position the eyes in midline of the head. The individual is asked to move the light (i.e., head and eyes) to locate and discriminate fairly large, bright stimuli placed on a plain background (e.g., yellow block on a brown table). As acuity and localization skills improve, stimuli and background should be made smaller and more complex (e.g., paper clip on a printed background or letters printed at different locations on a large page). The client should be encouraged to accurately point to or manipulate targets once located with the light or to keep the light on a target as he or she slowly moves the target with one hand. In this mode, the kinesthetic input from the limb can augment visual localization abilities.[43] In patients with color imperception, treatment should initially involve materials/tasks with sharp color contrasts with minimal detail and should progress to less contrast (more hues) with more detail.

If the assessment has revealed a narrowing of the perceptual field, treatment should be aimed at progressively increasing the perception of large, bright, peripheral targets. For example, the client may be asked to fixate on a centrally placed target while another bright target is brought in slowly from or uncovered in the periphery.[54,55] The individual is encouraged to maintain fixation on the central target while remaining alert for the presence of another target somewhere in the periphery. As the client improves, targets should be smaller, multiple, and exposed for briefer periods. Peripheral targets should always have bright surfaces that reflect light since the peripheral receptors in the retina are mainly rods (light as opposed to color receptors).

The treatment of clients with object agnosia should progress according to the abilities that return first in spontaneous recovery from agnosia. Common real objects should be used before line drawings in treatment. Presentations should be given "straight on" rather than at an angle or rotated. The client should be asked to point to objects named by the examiner before being asked to name them. Manipulation of the object with simultaneous visual input should be attempted. This may help recognition, or it may simply confuse the client; each case is unique. In general, tactile input with or without simultaneous visual input should be encouraged as a compensation method although it may not be helpful during treatment sessions.

Color and facial agnosia may be approached by simply drilling the individual with regard to two or three names of colors or names of faces of people important to her or him. The client may be helped to pick out or memorize cues for associating names with faces.[32]

Problems of Visual-Spatial Disorders

Identification of Clinical Problems

Individuals with brain lesions, particularly in the right posterior parietal and occipital areas, may have difficulties with tasks that require a normal concept of space.[27] Disorders of this nature have been termed visual-spatial disorders, spatial disorientation, visual-spatial agnosia, spatial relations syndrome, and numerous other names. Visual-spatial abilities are complexly interwoven within the performance of many perceptual and cognitive activities such as dressing, building a design, reading, calculating, walking through an aisle, and playing tennis. An attempt is made here, however, to discuss spatial disorders in their purest form—that is, basic disorders—before dealing with visual-constructive disorders and disorders of analysis and synthesis. Constructional tasks require spatial planning, a type of planning that involves the building up and breaking down of objects in two and three dimensions. Constructional apraxia is viewed as a particular type of spatial-perceptual disorder and therefore is discussed separately under visual-constructive disorders and disorders of analysis and synthesis. Similarly, although perceptual skills such as figure-ground, form constancy, complex visual discrimination, and figure closure involve spatial concepts, tasks involving these skills often require the intellectual operations of synthesis and deduction. They, too, are discussed in the section dealing with analysis and synthesis.

All visual-spatial disabilities involve some problem with the apprehension of the spatial relationships between or within objects. Benton[56] has categorized them as the following disabilities:

1. *Inability to localize objects in space, to estimate their size, and to judge their distance from the observer.* The client may be unable to accurately touch an object in space or indicate the position of the object (e.g., above, below, in front of, or behind). Relative localization may be impaired so that the individual may be unable to tell which object is closest. There may be difficulty determining which of two objects is larger or which line is longer. Holmes[57] reported cases of gross disorder in spatial orientation revealed through walking; affected individuals, even after seeing objects correctly, ran into them. In another example, a man, intending to go toward his bed, would invariably set out in the wrong direction. Difficulty in estimating distances may also extend to judgments of distances of perceived sounds and lead to overly slow and cautious gait or fear of venturing into public areas.

2. *Impaired memory for the location of objects or places.* An example is not being able to recall the position of a target previously viewed or the arrangement of furniture in a room. Individuals with this difficulty often lose things because they have no spatial memory to rely on for recall.

3. *Inability to trace a path or follow a route from one place to another.* Persons without this ability, known as topographical orientation, have difficulty understanding and remembering relationships of places to one another so that they may have difficulty finding their way in space, as in locating the therapy clinic in a hospital or locating the housewares department in a store previously familiar to them. Normally functioning individuals often have mild signs of topographical disorientation. Everyone is familiar with the disoriented feeling of not knowing how to get out of a large department store or losing a sense of direction in a familiar city. Many of the topographical errors made by clients result from unilateral spatial inattention. For example, someone with left inattention may make only right turns. Topographical disorientation, however, may be seen in a person with no signs of unilateral inattention. This individual will demonstrate route-finding difficulties at certain points and apparently randomly choose a direction.

4. *Problems with reading and counting.* These high-level tasks require directional control of eye movements and organized scanning abilities. Eye movements (saccades) during reading bring a new region of the text on the fovea, the part of the retina where visual acuity is the greatest and clear detail can be obtained from the stimulus. During reading, the line of print that falls on the retina may be divided into three regions: the foveal region, the parafoveal region, and the peripheral region. The foveal region subtends about 1 to 2 degrees of visual angle around the reader's fixation point, the parafoveal region subtends about 10 degrees of visual angle around the reader's fixation point, and the peripheral region includes everything on the page beyond the parafoveal region. Parafoveal and peripheral vision contribute spatial information that is used to guide the reader's eye.[58]

Visual-spatial disorders appear to interfere to varying degrees with the spatial schema of a page of type or numbers and the dynamic organizational scanning that must take place to gather information appropriately. Clients with unilateral spatial inattention will miss words or numbers located on one half of the page. Other spatial problems unrelated to unilateral inattention include skipping individual words within a line or part of a line, skipping lines, repeating lines, "blocking" or the inability to change direction of fixation, particularly at the end of a line, and generally losing the place on the total page. Performance usually deteriorates progressively as the individual continues to read. Eventually, such persons cannot make sense of what they read or, if counting, they complain of being lost or confused. This type of reading or counting disorder has nothing to do with recognition or interpretation of letters or numbers or their spatial configuration; rather, it represents a problem with dynamic sequential visual-spatial exploration during cognitive processing.

Other visual-spatial problems may include loss of depth perception, problems with body schema, and defective judgment of line orientation. There may also be difficulties with discrimination of right and left. Although unilateral spatial inattention is considered a visual-spatial disorder by many, it has been discussed separately in this chapter to increase clarity. Problems with judging line orientation (slant) or unilateral spatial inattention often interfere with a client's spatial ability to tell time with a standard watch or clock. Perception of the vertical may also be considered a visual-spatial skill. Verticality perception is the interpretation of internal and external cues to maintain body balance. This maintenance is a complex neuromuscular process involving visual, proprioceptive, and vestibular systems. Clients with right lesions, particularly in the parieto-occipital region, have more difficulty perceiving verticality than those with left lesions. This may affect posture and ambulation.[59]

Assessment

The client should be asked to accurately touch a number of targets in all parts of the visual field while fixating on a central point. Mislocalization should be noted as well as that part of the visual field in which it occurred. Mislocalization within the central field is infrequent; however, defective localization of stimuli on one or both extramacular fields is more frequently seen.[27] The client should be asked to determine which of a number of small cube blocks (placed perpendicularly in front of the client) is closest, which is farthest, and which is in the middle. Differences in binocular (stereoscopic) and monocular viewing should be measured in this and other tasks. Impairment in both of these types of depth perception and subsequent inaccuracy in judging distances have been described in individuals with brain injury.[56]

With regard to memory for the location of objects or places, clients should be asked to describe the position of objects in their room from memory. They may also be asked to duplicate from memory the position of two or more targets (on a table or piece of paper) that have been presented for a 5-second period. As the number of targets increases, individuals with short-term memory for spatial

> ### BOX 30-2 ■ TYPES OF STRABISMUS
>
> **Esotropia:** One eye turns in.
> **Exotropia:** One eye turns out.
> **Hypertropia:** One eye turns up relative to the other eye.
> **Intermittent:** The person is strabismic at times and phoric (fusing) at times. Fatigue or stress may bring out the strabismic state.
> **Alternating:** The person switches from using the right eye to using the left eye. The person also switches the suppressing eye. If using the right eye, the person suppresses the left, and while using the left eye, the person suppresses the right; otherwise the person would see double.
> **Constant strabismus:** One eye is always in or out (up or down), always the same eye.
> **Comitant/Noncomitant strabismus:** The amount of eye turn is the same regardless of whether the person is looking up, down, right, left, or straight ahead. People who have had the condition for a long time usually have comitant strabismus. New or acquired strabismics (i.e., from stroke or head injury) usually have noncomitant strabismus, in which the amount of eye turn changes depending on which direction the eyes are looking toward.

localization will begin to make errors in spatial placement. Visual memory per se should be ruled out as a conflicting variable.

The essential concept in understanding the difference between phoria and strabismus is that in strabismus fusion and depth perception are not present. Definitions of different types of strabismus are presented in Box 30-2. It is not a conclusive list; many other types and permutations are beyond the scope of this discussion. The intent here is to expose the therapist to different terms that may be used by the physician in diagnosing the type of strabismus.

In strabismus, one eye appears to go in, out, up, or down and there is frequently an obvious inability to judge distances, especially if the strabismus is of recent onset (acquired). The client may underreach or overreach for objects, cover or close one eye, complain of double vision, or exhibit a head tilt or turn during specific activities. He or she may appear to favor one eye, have difficulty reading, appear spaced out, or avoid near activities. Additionally, especially if the patient sees double but is unable or unwilling to talk about it, she or he may be confused or disoriented.

Oculomotor Dysfunction

A client with an oculomotor dysfunction will have difficulty with activities that require smooth pursuits, tracking, and convergence and divergence. During reading tasks these patients may lose their place, skip lines, or reread lines, or they may have poor ball skills, poor eye-hand coordination, decreased balance, and clumsiness.

Visual Field Loss

Visual field loss may indicate damage that is prechiasmic, at the optic chiasm, postchiasmic, in the visual radiations of the thalamus, or in the visual cortex. The resultant visual field loss is characteristic (even diagnostic) in each case. The visual field loss pattern will generally reflect the location of the lesion. It could be bitemporal (outer half of each field), half-field (hemianopsia) with or without macular involvement, or quarter-field loss (see Figure 30-7). Some symptoms of field loss are an inability to read or starting to read in the middle of the page, ignoring food on one half of the plate, and difficulty orienting to stimuli in a specific area of space.

Unilateral Spatial Inattention

Some clients also may have concomitant unilateral spatial inattention or neglect. Differentiating inattention from hemianopsia can be difficult. One test to differentiate between the two involves the extinction phenomenon. Presenting first stimuli on one side followed by simultaneous presentation of stimuli on both sides and comparing the results can differentiate hemianopsia from neglect if the client has neglect but not a hemianopsia. Please see the discussion on inattention later in the section on visual perception.

Generally, if the patient has a field loss, it will be possible to conduct a field test and obtain fairly reliable results. The client will be able to respond more easily and tell you where and when the test stimulus appears and disappears. Additionally, when doing compensation training, the client with a field loss can grasp the techniques, whereas a client with inattention cannot without frequent verbal reminders. The client with unilateral inattention frequently has proprioceptive and tactile loss on the neglected side, and that area of space including that half of the body does not provide feedback. Therefore if the client also has field loss, test results are unreliable and invariably inaccurate.

EYE DISEASES

Areas addressed in this section are common ocular and systemic diseases of the pediatric and geriatric populations, an introduction to low vision, and recommendations for adaptations of the treatment plan. If reduced vision (low vision) is a result of eye disease, the client may be assisted by magnification aids. Also, the therapy treatment program may need to be altered to accommodate any special visual needs of the client (lighting, working distance, inclusion of magnifiers, use of filters, contrast-enhancing devices).

Pediatric Conditions

Retinopathy of Prematurity
The incidence of retinopathy of prematurity is increasing because of the improved survival of premature infants as a result of improved ventilation.[60] Immature retinal vessels are sensitive to high oxygen tension. The effect on the vessels is vasoconstriction, eventually leading to obliteration of the vessels. This creates a state of ischemia, which stimulates the growth of new blood vessels. These small, fragile vessels bleed easily, leading to fibrosis and traction on the retina. As a result of the traction, the macula gets stretched, interfering with the function of central vision.

The temporal vessels are most affected because they develop last. The degree of damage may be mild or severe, depending on the amount of prematurity.[7]

Retinoblastoma
Retinoblastoma is the most common malignant tumor in children.[1] The current incidence is 1 in 20,000 live births, a rate that has been increasing over the past 30 years, apparently owing to inheritance of a mutated gene.

The young child may have a strabismus resulting from impaired vision in the eye with the tumor. As the tumor grows, the pupil may appear milky white. If not detected early, it will lead to loss of the eye; and if the tumor invades the brain, death will occur. Clearly, early detection is critical.

Mental Retardation
There are a higher number of visual problems in the mentally retarded populations.[1] These individuals have a higher incidence of refractive error (myopia, hyperopia, astigmatism), strabismus, nystagmus, and optic atrophy than that in children with normal intelligence.

Cerebral Palsy
Therapists who work with children with cerebral palsy may have noticed a high incidence of vision problems. Many studies confirm these observations. A study by Scheinman[60a] examining the incidence of visual problems in children with cerebral palsy and normal intelligence found the following incidences: strabismus in 69%, high phorias in 4%, accommodative dysfunction in 30%, and refractive errors in 63%.

Hydrocephalus
Various studies have found that the most common visual problem in children with hydrocephalus is strabismus, with an incidence of 30% to 55%. The strabismus may develop either from the hydrocephalus itself or from the shunting procedure.

Fetal Alcohol Syndrome
Children affected by fetal alcohol syndrome have several characteristic features and visual problems. They have a higher incidence of strabismus, myopia, astigmatism, and ptosis. These children frequently have some degree of mental retardation as well and are of small stature.

Age-Related Conditions
Cataracts. The most common malady affecting vision in elderly persons is cataracts. General clarity of vision is impaired from a loss of transparency of the crystalline lens of the eye.

In the senile cataract the lens slowly loses its ability to prevent oxidation from occurring, and liquefaction of the outer layers begins. The normally soluble proteins adhere together, causing light scatter.[3] Vision slowly declines as opacification and light scatter increase, until the lens must be removed.

Age-Related Macular Degeneration. Age-related macular degeneration is the leading cause of blindness in the Western world and is the most important retinal disease of the aged (affecting 28% of the 75- to 85-year-old age group).[7]

There is loss of central vision from fluid that leaks up from the deeper layers of the retina, pushing the retina up and detaching it from the nourishing layer. New vessel growth and hemorrhage and atrophy further destroy central vision.

This condition has significant implications for independent functioning. Mobility tends to be less impaired because the peripheral visual system is still intact. All activities involving fine detail such as reading, sewing, and cooking are affected. Safety also can be affected.

Arteriosclerosis. In arteriosclerosis, vision may or may not be affected. There is a hardening of the retinal arteries, which may eventually lead to ischemia, with the areas of retina deprived of sufficient oxygen eventually dying.

Hypertension. Hypertension is usually accompanied by arteriosclerosis. There may be retinal bleeding and edema, which can affect central vision if the macula is involved.

Diabetes. Diabetes can affect the lens. In the diabetic "sugar cataract," sorbitol collects within the lens, causing an osmotic gradient of fluid into the lens, which leads to disruption of the lens matrix and loss of transparency. As the fluid increases and decreases within the lens, the patient's vision also can fluctuate, depending directly on the sugar level. This makes prescribing glasses during this time quite difficult. The cataract will need to be removed if vision is worse than 20/40.

The retinal effects include microvascular damage and the development of microaneurysms. Central vision may be reduced as a result of retinal ischemia. The ischemia leads to new blood vessel growth (neovascularization). These new vessels are weak, frequently leaking and causing hemorrhage. The hemorrhage leads to fibrosis, which puts traction on the retina, pulling it off and leading to retinal detachment and blindness. Laser treatment of the bleeding retinal vessels will stop the bleeding but also burns photoreceptors, creating blind spots. This result is far preferable to total retinal detachment and blindness.

Glaucoma. Glaucoma occurs in 7.2% of the 75- to 85-year-old age group.[7] It is generally caused by an increase in the intraocular pressure. This pressure interferes with the inflow and outflow of blood and nutrients at the optic disc. As it progresses, glaucoma can cause tunnel vision and, in some, complete blindness. Because of the type of vision loss affecting the periphery, mobility and safety are significantly impaired. Try walking around holding a paper towel tube to your eye while closing the other eye, and see what happens to your ability to maneuver around obstacles or find your destination.

A less common type of glaucoma is low tension glaucoma, where the internal eye pressures are essentially normal. The mechanism is not understood, and it is treated with eye drops to lower internal pressure, just like the other types of glaucoma.

In one type of glaucoma, called open-angle glaucoma, the outflow of aqueous humor is reduced, leading to increased intraocular pressure. There are no overt symptoms. In another type, closed-angle glaucoma, the outflow is blocked by the iris. Symptoms are a painful, red eye, which may be confused with conjunctivitis.

Corticosteroids used to treat many conditions in the elderly for long periods of time may have side effects in some people, such as glaucoma and cataracts.

Eye Muscle Dysfunctions. Eye muscle dysfunctions causing double vision may result from several disease conditions including thyroid disease (Graves' disease and others), multiple sclerosis, myasthenia gravis, and tumors. The underlying condition must be diagnosed and treated.

Visual Field Loss. Visual field loss may be either central (macular degeneration glaucoma or retinal disease) or peripheral field loss from glaucoma, retinal damage, or stroke at any point in the visual pathway. This is potentially the most functionally disabling form of visual impairment (see Figure 30-7).

Implications for Functional Performance

Lighting

Lighting conditions are important and vary depending on the nature of the condition. The person with presbyopia requires more light because the aging pupil gets smaller. The smaller pupil has the advantage of increasing the depth of focus, allowing the presbyope to see clearly over a wider range, but it has the disadvantage of eliminating more light from the eye. Thus, providing a good source of direct lighting, especially on fine print, is helpful. Lighting for the low-vision client is critical. Direct sources of low-glare light such as halogen seem to work best. This is, however, quite individual, in that some clients actually see better in lower light conditions.

Glare

People who have problems with glare, such as those developing cataracts or other disease conditions, can be helped by several approaches. Incandescent or halogen lighting is preferred over fluorescent lighting. The use of a visor or wide-brimmed hat will reduce one source of glare, improving overall comfort. For some individuals who have trouble reading because of the glare coming off the white page, a black matte piece of cardboard with a horizontal slit in it (called a typoscope) can be used to reduce the surrounding glare and enhance reading. Various colored filters can be quite helpful; frequently a light amber color reduces glare while enhancing contrast. Other colors such as light green, plum, or yellow can be tried. The improvement noted is quite individual to the client. Special photochromic, tinted antiglare lenses developed by Corning are available by prescription through the ophthalmologist or optometrist. An antireflective coating may also help.

Low-Vision Aids

Many types of low-vision optical and nonoptical aids are available, usually by prescription by a low-vision specialist. Clients with damage to their central vision as in age-related macular degeneration or diabetic maculopathy and who still have some reduced central vision may be able to use various types of magnification aids.

Hand and Stand Magnifiers. One type is a stand magnifier, which is placed directly on the reading material and is useful for patients who have a tremor. Hand magnifiers are held in the hand and moved away from the page to the focal point of the lens, which may range from half an inch to 5 inches, depending on the amount of magnification.

Some are equipped with their own internal illumination, some with halogen lighting systems.

Telescopes. Telescopes can be used for a number of different functions. To increase independence in orientation and mobility, a "spotting" telescope is held in the hand and looked through to identify approaching bus numbers, public transportation signs, stop/walk signs, or aisle signs. There are also telescopes that are worn on the head for hands-free usage or for viewing the computer screen. A telescope system can be attached to the patient's glasses frames. Special driving telescopes called *bioptic* telescopes are ground into the patient's glasses, angled in such a way as to allow viewing straight ahead and, with a tip of the head, viewing through the scope to read a sign. The best corrected visual acuity needs to be at least 20/100, but regulations vary state to state. The greatest disadvantages of scopes are the small visual field and the additional training required to learn how to effectively use them.

Microscopes. Microscopes are high-powered reading glasses where the magnification is created in the glasses rather than in the hand. The disadvantage of these is the close viewing distance, depending on the power. The viewing distance could be as close as 1.5 inches, creating discomfort in reading for many.

Electronic Digital Magnifiers. The best systems for severely impaired clients are the electronic digital magnifiers such as closed-circuit television (CCTV). The CCTV system consists of a camera housed in a device that can be directed at the object to be viewed. The scope of magnification is significantly larger, ranging from low power to 50×. Additional benefits include no distortion like that caused by optical magnifiers and a field of view limited only by the size of the screen. The housing for the camera may be in a stand, with a screen above, or portable, held in the hand, or strapped to the head. Examples are the Merlin, Jordy, and Maxport by Enhanced Vision Systems.[61]

Nonoptical Aids. Nonoptical aids include large-print materials, available at many libraries, typoscopes, mentioned earlier, and reading stands. Talking books are available for those for whom reading is an important hobby. New developments include text-to-speech synthesizers, large-print computers, and image intensifiers.

Visual Field Expansion. For clients with field losses, specially designed prism or mirror systems may be used. These frequently require a training to get used to and are not useful for everyone. Compensation training also can be helpful, particularly in the use of eccentric viewing, or learning how to use a portion of the intact field by aiming the eye off center. Use of margin markers or reading slits and holding the book sideways so that the print is vertical are other helpful techniques.

Current Research. Areas of current research include mounting a video camera onto spectacles and then transducing the visual information to electrodes implanted in visual cortical centers. In one study this system allowed a low-vision patient to see the large E (20/400) and detect

large contours. This is an exciting area for further research and may hold significant potential for the blind.[62-64]

BOX 30-3 ■ KEY ELEMENTS IN VISION SCREENING

1. Distance and near visual acuities
2. Oculomotilities (pursuits, saccades, near point of convergence)
3. Some measure of eye alignment to detect a strabismus or high phoria
4. Some measure of depth perception (stereopsis)
5. Some measure of the visual fields

VISUAL SCREENING

Primary visual dysfunction must be differentiated from a visual-perceptual disorder so that appropriate treatment can be addressed for each problem. Gianutsos et al[65] found that more than half the individuals in their study admitted for general head injury rehabilitation who were eligible for cognitive services had visual sensory impairments sufficient to warrant further evaluation. Visual screening can identify the need for referral for a complete eye examination. The results of the examination become part of the differential diagnosis regarding a perceptual dysfunction. Box 30-3 presents key elements in vision screening.

This section describes vision screening tools and adaptations for various populations. The following principles should be kept in mind:
- *Acuities:* Acuities should always be tested first because decreased acuities will bias other tests except for ocular motilities and the peripheral field test.
- *Positioning:* The body and head should be in good alignment or straightened with positioning devices, with the head in midline.
- *Glasses:* If the client normally wears glasses, for either distance or near, the patient should be wearing glasses for tests for which spectacle correction is required. When in doubt, try it both ways, record the best response, and note whether glasses were worn.

Observations During Testing
The client's response during the test can provide important qualitative information about his or her visual system, including postural changes (head forward or back, body forward or back, head tilts or rotation [turning to either side]), squinting, closing one eye, excessive blinking, rubbing, signs of strain or fatigue, and holding the breath. Clients should be encouraged to relax, breathe normally, and not squint.

Distance Acuities
Equipment
Needed to measure distance acuity are a distance acuity chart, an occluder, a 20-foot measure, and the patient's corrective lenses if worn for distance.

Setup
A distance chart is taped on a well-lighted wall at the patient's eye level, and a distance of 20 feet is measured from the chart.

BOX 30-4 ■ INTERPRETATION/REFERRAL

20/20 is considered normal.

20/40 is required by the Department of Motor Vehicles (DMV) in most states for full-time day and night driver's license, although requirements vary in different states.

20/80 is required by the DMV for daytime driver's license.

20/40 or worse indicates referral to an eye doctor.

20/200 corrected (with spectacle prescription) is considered legally blind.

A difference of 2 lines or more between the two eyes indicates referral to an eye doctor (e.g., right eye is 20/20, left eye is 20/30).

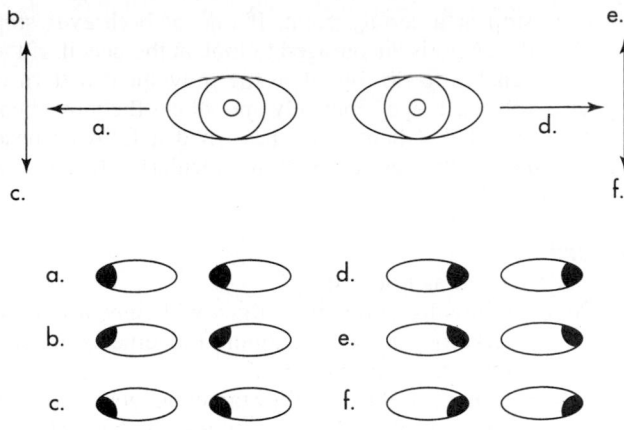

Then move from e→f, b→f, f→b, c→e to observe diagonal and midline pursuit patterns.

FIGURE 30-12 ■ Pursuit patterns.

Procedure

One of the patient's eyes is covered and the patient is asked to read the smallest letters that he or she can see. Exposing one letter or line at a time can help if tracking or attention is a problem. The examiner should encourage the patient to guess and instruct the patient not to squint. The number of letters that were missed on the smallest line that the patient is able to see is noted. The procedure is repeated by covering the patient's other eye, and then both eyes are tested unoccluded.

Record

The smallest line the patient was able to read is recorded. If the client missed any letters on that line then the number of letters missed is subtracted. For example, if the client read four letters correctly on the 20/30 line but missed the other two, then it is recorded as 20/30-2. The scores for the client's right eye, left eye, and both eyes together are recorded.

If the patient is unable to see the top line at 20 feet, the patient is asked to move forward until able to identify the top letters. Then the distance/letter size (top line) is recorded. For example, if the patient had to move up to 4 feet to see the top line, then 4/100 is recorded. To calculate 20-foot equivalence, an equation is used where x equals the size of the letter (e.g., $4/100 = 20/x$); thus, $4x = 2000$ and 2000, 4 = 500. The client's vision is 20/500 (Box 30-4).

For clients whose attention is poor, the testing distance may need to be as close as 2 feet. Other testing stimuli can be used for children, such as the Broken Wheel Test* or the Lighthouse cards.* Acuity in low functioning clients or infants can be evaluated by use of preferential looking methods. Targets are usually high-contrast grating patterns of decreasing size. One such type is the Teller cards.[†]

Implications

A patient who fails this test may require glasses or a change in the current prescription.

---

*Bernell/uso, 4016 N. Home Street, Mishiwaka, IN 46545; (800)-348-2225.

[†]Vistech Consultants, 4162 Little York Road, Dayton, OH 45414-2566.

Near Acuities

Equipment

A near-point test card, an occluder, and the client's corrective lenses if normally worn for near are needed.

Procedure

The procedure is the same as for distance acuity. The standard test distance is usually 16 inches (40 cm).

Record

The smallest line read is recorded.

Interpretation/Referral

A test result of 20/20 is considered normal, 20/40 is required for reading newspaper size print, and 20/100 is needed for large print. Referral to an optometrist or ophthalmologist should be made if vision is 20/40 or worse or if a difference of two lines exists between the two eyes. Neurological damage can affect the accommodative system. Sometimes it corrects itself spontaneously, but not always.

Visual retraining of the focusing system may be appropriate, depending on the patient's age. This can be determined by an optometrist familiar with vision therapy.

Pursuits

Equipment

Any target that holds the patient's attention can be used, such as a pencil or small toy.

Setup

The patient is seated facing the screener.

Procedure

One pencil is held 16 to 20 inches in front of the client, and the client is asked to look directly at one part, such as the eraser, and to keep the head still, holding it if necessary. The pencil is moved around in the pattern shown in Figure 30-12, which is designed to incorporate all directions of gaze. The examiner should observe for smooth following, noticing and recording jerks and jumps, where they occur, or if the eyes stop at a certain point. If one or both eyes stop tracking, the client is encouraged to look at the pencil. If the patient is unable to do this, then the movement pattern is repeated with each eye separately and where the movement stops is recorded. Clients who have had a CVA or head injury should be tested first monocularly (each eye separately).

Record

Results are rated as follows:
  Poor = Difficulty following target with any accuracy, jerky or jumpy, nystagmoid movements, incomplete range of motion
  Fair = Generally able to follow target but goes off target occasionally (one to two times), with slight jerkiness
  Good = Eye movements smooth with no jerkiness

If one eye stops tracking at a certain point or if the client reports double vision (diplopia) in certain directions, the examiner should record which eye or in which direction the problem is noticed (e.g., the right eye does not pass midline when moving from left to right, or diplopia is reported on upward right gaze). This specific information can be helpful to the ophthalmologist or optometrist.

Saccades

Equipment

Tracking pencils can be used, although a few saccadic tests are available. One is the King Devick Saccadic Test; the other is the Developmental Eye Movement Test.* These both require form perception (number reading) and may be difficult, depending on the client's cognitive level.

Setup

The patient is seated facing the screener.

Procedure

A pencil is held in each hand about 17 to 20 inches from the client, and the client is told that he or she is going to be asked to look at one pencil while the other pencil is moved but not to look at it until told to do so. The client is to move the eyes only, keeping the head still. While the client looks at the first pencil, the other pencil is moved as the screener says "shift" or "look at this pencil." The screener then moves the other pencil, says "shift," then moves the pencil, says "shift," then moves the pencil, and so on, until a pattern of movement can be discerned.

This call-shift is repeated about 10 times, moving into different fields of gaze. The screener continues until the client is seen to respond. The screener observes for overshooting or undershooting the target, for the ability to isolate the eyes from the head (hold head still), for controlled eye movement, and for ability to wait until the verbal command to look. It is important to observe for the client's ability to shift to all fields of gaze. A lower level of testing would be to ask the client to move the eyes from one target to the other as quickly as possible (Figure 30-13).

*Bernell/uso, 4016 N. Home Street, Mishiwaka, IN 46545; (800)-348-2225. Complete Vision Screening Kit: Laurie R. Chaikin, OD, OTR/L, 3717 Castro Valley Blvd, Castro Valley, CA 94546; (510)-538-3937.

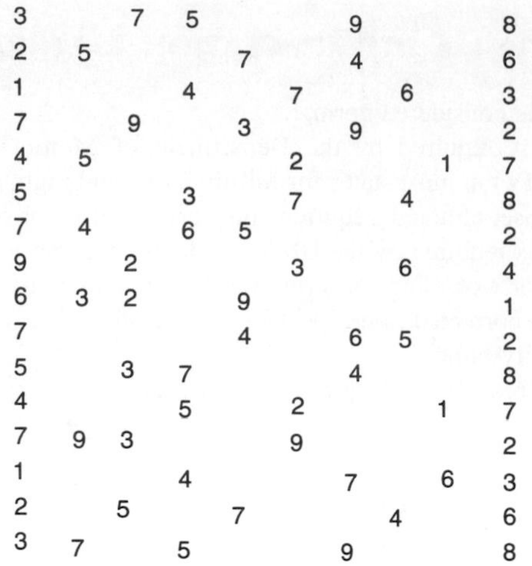

3		7	5			9			8
2	5			7		4			6
1			4		7		6		3
7		9		3		9			2
4	5			2				1	7
5			3		7		4		8
7	4		6	5					2
9		2			3		6		4
6	3	2		9					1
7				4		6	5		2
5		3	7			4			8
4			5		2			1	7
7	9	3			9				2
1			4			7		6	3
2		5		7			4		6
3	7		5			9			8

FIGURE 30-13 ■ Developmental Eye Movement Test.

Record

Results are rated as follows:
  Poor = Inability to control eyes with verbal command, consistent undershooting or overshooting, inability to isolate eyes from head
  Fair = Client able to maintain eyes on target with verbal command 50% of the time, with slight undershooting or overshooting, and able to isolate eyes from head with verbal reminders
  Good = Client able to follow verbal commands 90% of the time, with no undershooting or overshooting, and complete eye from head isolation

Near Point of Convergence

Procedure

A pencil is introduced about 20 inches away from the client's midline. The client is asked whether the pencil looks single. If it is not, it is moved farther away. The client is told that the pencil will be moved toward her or him and that it will be getting blurry but to keep watching it as far in as possible. When the pencil appears single, it is moved toward the nose at a moderately slow rate (but not too slow). The screener should watch the client's eyes. As long as the client's eyes are tracking the pencil, the pencil is kept moving toward the nose. At the point where one eye moves out, both eyes move out, or the eyes simply stop tracking, the distance of the pencil to the nose is measured. If the client is wearing bifocals, it is important to make sure the patient is looking through the reading segment.

Record

The break point is the distance at which the eyes were observed to stop tracking the pencil. If the client was able to track the pencil all the way to the nose, then record this fact.

Interpretation/Referral

A score of poor or fair on saccades or pursuits suggests the need for training. A near point of convergence with a break point of 5 inches or more is suggestive of convergence problems, and recommendations for referral should be made.

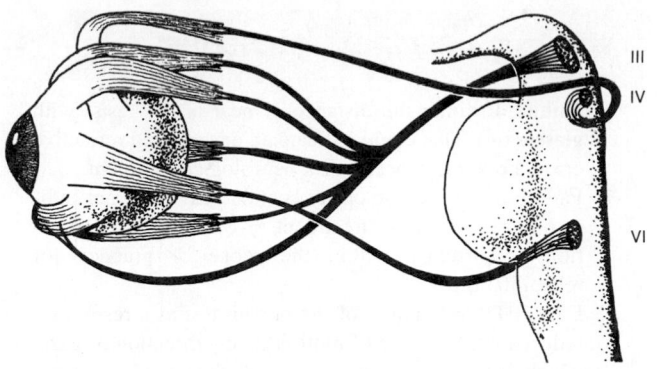

FIGURE 30-14 ■ Cranial nerves III, IV, and VI. Oculomotor, trochlear, and abducens nerves and their innervation of the extraocular muscles. (Courtesy of Smith, Kline & French Laboratories, Philadelphia, Pa.)

Implications

Difficulties with smooth pursuit, accurate saccades, or convergence can all present tracking difficulties for the patient. These difficulties can cause loss of place in reading, rereading of words or lines, skipping lines, and lower comprehension and concentration. Inaccurate eye movements also may affect visual memory.

An eye movement problem may be the result of direct damage to the eye muscles themselves (Figure 30-14) or to the nerves controlling them, as in the case of a head injury. Damage to the vestibular center also may involve visual components. Neurons from cranial nerves III, IV, and VI synapse in the vestibular nuclei. Reflex control of eye movements occurs through the VOR and the optokinetic system.

Cover Tests

Purpose

There are two cover tests. The cover/uncover test is used to determine whether a strabismus is present. The alternate cover test determines what type of phoria is present. The magnitude of the phoria generally determines the extent of the client's symptoms.

Equipment

An occluder and a tracking pencil or a small, distinct target is needed.

Setup

The client is seated facing the screener, who is also seated.

Procedure

A pencil is held approximately 16 inches in front of the client, and the client is asked to look directly at the target and to keep it in focus.

Near Cover Tests

Cover/Uncover. *The movement of the uncovered eye is observed.* The client's right eye is covered, and the left eye is observed for movement in, out, upward, or downward. This is repeated a few times, while allowing the eyes to be uncovered for about 2 seconds between trials. Then the left eye is covered to observe for movement in the right eye.

Alternate Cover Test. *Eye movement is observed as the eye is uncovered.* An occluder is held over the right eye for a few seconds while the client looks at a near target. The occluder is moved from the right eye to the left eye while the right eye is observed for movement in, out, up, or down. After a few seconds, the occluder is moved back to the right eye, observing the left eye for movement. This is repeated back and forth several times until the screener is sure of what is seen.

Far Cover Tests

The preceding procedure is repeated with the patient looking at a distant target.

Interpretation/Referral. Any visible eye movement seen during the cover/uncover test with good maintenance of fixation on the target indicates a strabismus. If there is no previous history of strabismus, referral is indicated. A large eye movement seen with the alternate cover test, along with the presence of symptoms such as eye strain, headaches, or apparent difficulty in making spatial judgments, also indicates referral. In the clinic the therapist may notice that the client has difficulty finding objects in a drawer, or that the client appears cross-eyed or seems to be looking past the target. He or she may have difficulty with spatial judgments in reaching for objects or in mobility, especially with stairs or curbs.

A visible eye movement may be part of a post-CVA client's premorbid pattern. This should be determined by asking the client or the family before making a referral. Or it may be the result of neurological damage to cranial nerve III, IV, or VI from CVA, head injury, or cerebral palsy. Eye muscles are striated muscles, under voluntary control. Like other striated muscles that can be affected by neurological damage, they may recover spontaneously, they may not recover at all, or they may benefit from visual retraining. Many learning-disabled children with vestibular dysfunction have poor binocular skills. An ophthalmologist or optometrist specially trained in visual remediation can determine a patient's potential for vision therapy. Some published research has demonstrated the success of vision therapy for post-CVA patients.[66]

Stereopsis (Depth Perception)

Equipment

Any test that uses either Polaroid or red/green filters can test for stereopsis ability. Examples are the Titmus Stereo Fly, Rheindeer, and Butterfly.*

Procedure

The client is asked to point to or say which test object appears closer. If the client is able to grasp for the object in space, some stereo ability is present.

Record

The client's response should be immediate. Long delays could indicate borderline ability.

---

*Bernell/uso, 4016 N. Home Street, Mishiwaka, IN 46545; (800)-348-2225. Complete Visual Screening Kit: Laurie R. Chaikin, OD, OTR/L 3717 Castro Valley Blvd, Castro Valley, CA 94546; (510)-538-3937.

Interpretation/Referral

If the client fails this test, a referral to an ophthalmologist or optometrist is recommended. The patient must have best-corrected acuities for this test; otherwise, the results are invalid.

Implications

A deficit in depth perception can interfere with all activities involving spatial judgments, in particular fine motor and eye-hand type activities in which judgments of relative depth are required (e.g., threading a needle, placing toothpaste on a toothbrush, hammering). Although ambulation itself may not be affected, ambulation involving curbs or stairs will be affected.

Vision therapy training can be helpful for clients with problems in binocular coordination. Proper diagnosis and therapy prescription are essential.

Visual Field Screening

Equipment

An occluder or eyepatch is required, and black dowels with white pins on the ends or just a wiggling finger can be used as a peripheral target.

Setup

The client is seated facing the examiner.

Procedure

The client holds the occluder over the left eye. The examiner explains that he or she is going to wiggle a finger out to the side and that the patient is to say "now" when he or she first detects the movement of the wiggling finger. The client should look at the screener's nose the entire time and ignore any arm movement. The test is begun with the examiner's hand slightly behind the client about 16 inches away from the client's head. The hand is brought forward slowly while a finger is wiggled. Different sections of the visual field are randomly tested in 45-degree intervals around the visual field. The left eye is then tested after the client's right eye is occluded. Alternatively, if a dowel is used, it is slowly brought in from the side until the client reports seeing the small pin at the end of the dowel.

These confrontation field tests are considered gross tests compared with a visual field perimeter test. Many clients cannot do the perimeter test because it requires a higher cognitive level. Confrontation fields will reveal a hemianopsia and a quadrantanopsia (quarter-field cut). For lower-functioning clients the examiner can observe eye movements in the direction of the target to get a general idea of peripheral function once clients have seen it.

Record

The portion of field missing for each eye is noted.

Interpretation/Referral

If any hemianopsia or quadrantanopsia is noted, the patient is referred to an optometrist or an ophthalmologist.

Implications

A visual deficit has significant implication for the safe performance of many functional activities, including driving and mobility. Visually guided movement through space

---

BOX 30-5 ■ REFERRAL GUIDELINES

1. Failure of either the distance or near acuity tests (with glasses on). This could indicate an uncorrected refractive error, a disease process, or a neurological problem.
2. Failure of the oculomotility section only does not indicate referral because treatment of oculomotor dysfunction is currently within the scope of practice for rehabilitation.
   EXCEPTION: Failure of the pursuit test as a result of a reduced ocular range of motion in any direction of gaze, which indicates cranial nerve involvement.
3. Failure on the cover/uncover test indicates a strabismus and is an indication for referral unless there is a history of an eye turn.
4. A large eye movement seen on the alternate cover test, along with apparent difficulties in stereopsis, such as spatial judgments, or symptoms, such as headaches, eyestrain, or difficulty with comprehension, constitutes an indication for referral.
5. Failure of the stereopsis test alone is an indication for referral if there is no history of an eye turn, and if there is movement on either cover test.
6. Quarter field loss and half field loss (hemianopsia) should be referred.

---

becomes impaired, as are efficient eye movements; if central field loss is present, reading and any other near activities are affected. The reader is referred to the discussion on assessment of unilateral inattention for differentiation between neglect and hemianopsia.

REFERRAL CONSIDERATIONS

The final outcome of the visual screening is referral to an ophthalmologist or optometrist. It is important not to make diagnostic statements but rather to indicate whether the client passed or failed the vision screening. By law, only optometrists or ophthalmologists can diagnose visual conditions.

It is not always clear when to refer a client or to whom. Many doctors do not test all areas of visual function. Generally, behavioral or developmental optometrists have a functionally oriented philosophy quite similar to occupational therapy models of functional performance.*

Recommended referral guidelines are shown in Box 30-5.

Rehabilitation Optometric Evaluation

Once the client has been referred for evaluation, the eye doctor will evaluate any changes in the refractive error and the need for new correction to achieve the best possible vision. The eye alignment will be quantified and it will be determined whether there is an eye muscle paresis, which cranial nerve is involved, whether strabismus or phoria is

---

*College of Optometrists for Vision Development has a list of behavioral doctors: 234 North Lindberg Blvd., Suite 310, St. Louis, MO 63141, or Optometric Extension Program, 1921 East Carnegie Ave, Suite 3L, Santa Ana, CA 92705-5510. Neuro-Optometer Rehabilitation Association, www.nora.cc/index.html.

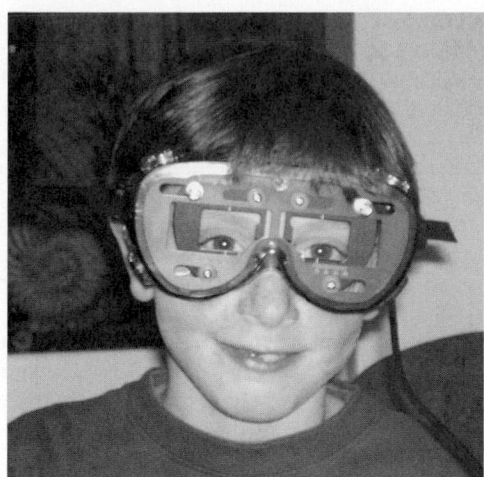

FIGURE 30-15 ■ The Visagraph (boy with goggles) measures eye movement while the subject is reading.

present, and whether the eye deviation is better or worse in particular directions of gaze.

Oculomotilities will be evaluated grossly, and more specific tests may be done. One test is the Developmental Eye Movement Test (see Figure 30-13). Another test is the Visagraph (Figure 30-15). This instrument records eye movements while the client is reading text. It will measure total reading rate, number of fixations and regressions per 100 words, span of recognition, and reading comprehension. The tool is excellent for in-depth evaluation and monitoring the progress of treatment over time.

Ocular health testing will include glaucoma testing, examination for cataracts, and retinal health evaluation. For visual field testing, either a screening field or a threshold visual field will be done on some type of automated perimeter such as the Humphrey Visual Field Analyzer or the Octopus. Threshold testing is done to determine the extent and depth of a defect, and it can help to determine whether there is potential for visual field retraining. In Figure 30-9 the black portions of the visual field are areas of absolute damage. The areas of white with small dots are intact visual fields. At the border of the damage area is a gray zone, which theoretically is amenable to training.[23-26]

The optometrist or ophthalmologist will deliver a report of the findings with recommendations for the treatment plan.

Visual Intervention

Early intervention is recommended when possible to identify ways in which a vision problem may be interfering with other therapies.[66-69] Some treatments may be applied early on as well. For example, if the client has an eye muscle paresis, range of motion exercises to the involved muscle can prevent the development of a contracture of the unopposed muscle.

In cases in which the client has double vision, a patching regimen can be instituted. One regimen is to alternate patching the eyes daily, allowing some time to experience diplopia, so that the eyes may attempt to make a fusion response. The stimulus to fusion is double vision. If one eye is always patched, spontaneous recovery may be slowed. Another patching regimen is binasal taping, and another is

to use partially opaque materials to allow peripheral vision in the occluded eye. The patching regimen should be prescribed by an optometrist or ophthalmologist.

In some cases of double vision, a temporary plastic (Fresnel) prism can be applied to the client's glasses to reduce or eliminate the diplopia. This may significantly enhance the client's functioning in other therapies, particularly when spatial judgments are being made (e.g., in fine motor tasks or ambulation).

Documentation

Vision problems should be documented in functional performance terms, that is, how the vision problem affects activities of daily living. Improvement can then be monitored according to function. This will also help in reimbursement. For example, a client with an eye muscle dysfunction will have difficulty with spatial judgments such as placing toothpaste on a toothbrush, spearing objects, reaching for a cup handle, doing pegboard tasks, and using vision for balance.

THERAPEUTIC CONSIDERATIONS

Once a referral has been made, the client has been seen, and the examination report has been received, what else can be done? How the dysfunction affects therapy can be considered and some visual training, prescribed by the optometrist, can be initiated.

Accommodative Dysfunction

If the client has an accommodative dysfunction, the treatment may be the prescription of glasses for reading or tabletop tasks or possibly near/far focusing exercises,[4] depending on the age of the client. "Flipper bars" are special lenses that exercise the focusing system.[70]

If the client needs glasses for near but cannot get them for some reason, the therapist can try moving the task farther away and increasing the lighting on the task.

Eye Alignment Dysfunction

If the client has a problem in the eye alignment system, several factors should be considered. If the client is able to fuse some of the time, but loses fusion, seeing double when stressed or tired, then the most difficult tasks should be attempted when the client is least fatigued. Otherwise, if the client has constant double vision, or the client is seeing double at the time the therapist is working with her or him, patching may be prescribed by the ophthalmologist or optometrist. This will reduce the client's confusion and increase attention to the task. For clients with an acquired double vision, however, it is important to provide time without a patch so that the eyes will attempt to regain fusion. Wearing the patch constantly will discourage any attempts by the brain to overcome the double vision.

Topographical sense is assessed by asking clients to describe a floor plan of the arrangement of rooms in their house or to describe familiar geographical constellations, such as routes, arrangement of streets, or public buildings. After therapy these persons may also be asked to find their way back to their rooms after being shown the route several times. Failure suggests a topographical orientation problem. Finally, such a client may be asked to locate states or cities on a large map of the United States. In all of these procedures, the examiner must be sure to separate unilateral spatial inattention errors from topographical errors.

The influence of spatial dysfunction on reading and counting written material may be measured simply by asking the client to read a page of regular newsprint. The examiner should observe performance carefully and document type and frequency of errors. If errors occur, eye movements should be observed to gather additional information. Pages of scanning material (letters or numbers) often give additional information on spatial planning during reading. These are pages of print in which the size and density of the print are controlled. Scanning behavior may be demonstrated by asking the client to circle specific letters. Switching direction in the middle of a line, skipping letters or lines, perseveration, or any other abnormal performance behavior should be noted. Benton's Judgment of Line Orientation Test[71] may be used to document problems with directional orientation of lines. If there is no indication of apraxia, the client may simply be given a ruler and asked to match it to the directional orientation of the examiner's ruler.

Interventions

Treatment for visual-spatial deficits should follow basic developmental considerations, progressing from simple to more complex tasks. As with children, if the evaluation suggests disorders in body scheme, tactile or vestibular input, or right-left discrimination, these should be dealt with first.

Clients who do not know where they are in space need to internalize a spatial understanding before they can make judgments regarding the space around them. In gross motor spatial training, clients can be asked to roll and reach toward various targets. In supine, prone, sitting, and standing, with vision occluded, clients should try to localize tactile stimuli (various body locations touched by the therapist) and auditory stimuli (e.g., snapping fingers or ringing a bell) presented above, below, behind, in front of, and right and left of their bodies. The individual should state where the stimulus is and then point, roll, crawl, or walk toward it; this verbal, kinesthetic, and vestibular input augments spatial learning. In the occupational therapy kitchen, the client, once oriented to the room, may be asked to retrieve one type of object (e.g., cup) from "the top cupboard above your head," from "the bottom cupboard below your waist," from "the table behind you," or from "the drawer on your right or left." These clients may also place objects in various positions within a room. They should then stand in the middle of the room, close their eyes, and from memory visualize, verbalize, and point to where the objects are in relation to themselves. Having localized them, the clients should then walk through the space and retrieve the objects in sequence. Functional carryover should always be emphasized, such as having individuals remember through visualization where they put their glasses in the living room before they begin searching. Visualization is defined as the internal "seeing" of something that is not present at that moment: a vision without a visual input or internal visual imagery.[72] Visualization (spatial and other) is part of all perceptual tasks and may be used effectively as a treatment strategy. As previously discussed, a small feedback light placed in the middle of the client's forehead can help teach spatial localization through eye-hand movements.

More complex spatial skills may be taught by asking clients to "partition" space and then localize within it. An excellent activity is one in which clients use a yardstick to divide a blackboard into four or more equal parts and then number each section.

Objects may be presented to clients, who must select the largest, the farthest away, or the one placed at an angle; they may be asked to place various objects in certain relationships to each other. As shape, size, and angle begin to "make sense" to these individuals, form boards, simple puzzles, and parquetry blocks may be added to training.

Topographical abilities should improve as clients begin to better conceptualize space; however, they may be trained directly. The therapist may help such clients organize a basic floor plan of the hospital room and the furniture within it while looking at the room. They may then be asked to do this from memory. Activities can progress to drawing plans or larger areas with a number of rooms. These clients should first "navigate" tactually through the area with a finger. Eventually, they should walk or wheel through the route themselves, visualizing and repeating the route until spatial concepts are learned. Imaginary routes also may be taken through maps of cities, states, or countries.

Organized visual-spatial exploration (eye movements) during reading or other scanning and cancellation tasks may be taught. Number and letter scanning sheets may be used for such training. Initially, the size of numbers and the spaces between numbers should be large; this places less stress on visual acuity while training scanning. Before beginning, clients should orient themselves to the page spatially by numbering the right and left edges of each line. These numbers are used as additional spatial localization cues if needed during the scanning task.[45] Clients should then be asked to circle a specific number (or numbers) whenever it occurs. To control erratic or impulsive eye movements, they should be instructed to use a pencil to underline each line and then loop the selected letter as it comes into view (see Figure 30-10). They may also be asked to read each letter. Underlining allows the kinesthetic and tactile receptors of the arm to control eye movements; verbalization allows the language and auditory systems to influence eye movements. Visual-spatial exploration exercises should progress to large-print magazines, books, or newspapers. The *New York Times* and *Reader's Digest* are both available in large print. In all training activities it is most important that, before the activity begins, clients fully comprehend the total space in which they will work. It is equally important that they reorient themselves at any point where errors occur. Those who lose their place during reading will eventually lose it again if the therapist simply points to where they should be. Chances are better that they will not lose their place again if they reorient themselves to the page spatially when an error occurs.

Problems of Visual-Constructive Disorders
Identification of Clinical Problems

Clients with lesions in either the right or left hemisphere may have problems when trying to "construct." Lesions in the parietal, temporal, occipital, and frontal lobes have been documented in individuals with visual-constructive disorders.[27,73] The normal ability to construct, also known as visual-constructive ability and constructional praxis, involves any type of performance in which parts are put together to form a single entity. Examples include assembling blocks to form a design, assembling a puzzle, making a dress, setting a table, and simply drawing four lines to form a square (graphic skills). The skill implies a high level of dynamic, organized, visual-perceptual processing in which the spatial relations are perceived and sequenced well enough among and within the component parts to direct higher-level processing to sequence the perceptual-motor actions so that eventually parts are synthesized into a desired whole. Visual-constructive ability may be compromised if any part of this process is disturbed.

Typical tasks used to measure this ability include building in a vertical direction, building in a horizontal direction, three-dimensional block construction from a model or a picture of a model, and copying line drawings such as house, flower, and geometric designs.[51]

Clients with visual-constructive deficits, especially those with right lesions, often also have visual-spatial deficits. These individuals may rotate the position of a part erroneously, place it in the wrong position, space it too far from another part, be oblivious to perspective or a third dimension, or simply be unable to complete more than two or three steps before becoming entirely confused. This is usually evidence of breakdown because of faulty or inadequate spatial information.

Other clients, usually those with left lesions, have an "executional" or apraxic problem; they seem to have difficulty initiating and conducting the planned sequence of movements necessary to construct the whole. The problem seems to be in planning, arranging, building, or drawing rather than in spatial concepts. This deficit in its purest form is known as constructional apraxia. Constructional apraxia lies clinically outside the category of most other varieties of apraxia and is considered a special kind of "perceptual" apraxia. It occurs frequently in aphasic individuals; therefore, the underlying mechanisms of aphasia and constructional apraxia may be related.[74]

Assessment

Constructional abilities are generally measured through tasks that require (1) copying line drawings such as a house, clock face, flower, or geometric designs (drawing may also be done without copy); (2) copying two-dimensional matchstick designs; (3) building block designs from copy or model; or (4) assembling puzzles. Table 30-2 lists common tests. The more complex the picture or design to be copied, the more complex is the constructional tasks. The following are examples of drawing and block construction deficits:

1. Clients may crowd the drawing or design on one side of the page or in one corner of the page or available space on the working surface, usually a result of the influence of unilateral spatial inattention.
2. Lines in drawings may be wavy or broken, too long or too short.
3. One line may not meet another accurately, or lines may transect each other; in block designs, parts may not be neatly placed but rather may have small gaps.
4. There may be "overdrawing" of angles or parts of the figure because of graphic perseveration (scribble), spatial indecision, or problems with executive planning.

TABLE 30-2 ■ Common Tests Used to Assess Visuoconstructive Skills

TEST	STANDARDIZATION
Drawing pictures or shapes with or withoutcopy	Not standardized
Reproducing matchstick designs	Not standardized
Assembling puzzles	Not standardized
Bender Visual Motor Gestalt Test	Standardized for children only
Kohs' Blocks Test	Standardized for adults
WAIS Block Design Test	Standardized for adults
Benton's Three-Dimensional Constructional Praxis Test	Standardized for adults

5. Clients may superimpose their copy on the model or superimpose one of their drawings on top of another. In block design construction, they may become confused between the model and their reproduction and use part of the model to complete their design. This has been termed the "closing-in" phenomenon, a failure to distinguish between model and reproduction.[27]
6. Parts of the drawing or design may be reversed. Horizontal reversals are more common than vertical reversals.

A note might be appropriate here regarding dressing apraxia. This problem occurs most frequently with right hemisphere damage. It is considered a "perceptual" apraxia rather than a motor apraxia because the inability to dress is believed to result from body scheme, spatial, and visual-constructive deficits rather than difficulty in motor execution. Persons with dressing apraxia cannot correctly orient their clothes to their body. They often put clothes on backward or inside out. Failure to dress one side of the body is also often noted and is directly related to unilateral spatial inattention.

Interventions

It must be remembered that both visual-constructive and visual analysis synthesis skills are often used almost simultaneously during task performance. Thus, treatment should not separate the two skills but rather should be a precise interrelationship of activities that require finer and finer levels of each facility. For example, arranging an office filing system is both an analytical/synthesis and a visual-constructive task. The individual must first analyze overall needs and translate them into an imagined visual-spatial plan (preliminary synthesis of the whole) that will help organization. Then the organizer begins to use the hands to categorize (segment visual space). This building is a visual-constructive task. Intermittently during building, new ideas of the whole surface, and visual-constructive tasks change in response to a "better idea" (final synthesis of the whole). Task performance, except for tasks that are rote, usually follows similar perceptual processes. Treatment therefore must be integral. Visual-constructive skills, however, may be emphasized more than visual analysis and synthesis skills or vice versa.

As previously mentioned, visual-constructive disorders are thought to result from different underlying problems in different individuals (e.g., visual-spatial disorders in persons with right hemisphere lesions and executive, planning, or synthetic disorders in those with left hemisphere lesions). There are few reliable studies on treatment strategies for visual-constructive disorders. One possible treatment strategy is known as *saturational cuing*.[75] This method involves presenting controlled verbal instruction on task analysis and sequence and presenting cues on spatial boundaries (cuing is also response related).

If there are problems with planning and sequencing of steps necessary to accomplish a visual-constructive task, the therapist should begin with simple tasks that require only three to four steps, such as positioning one place setting at a table. The client should discuss the plan and sequence of steps before initiating the activity, while looking at the parts to be used, such as silverware, plate, and glass. These steps may even be written down for additional input. The client should be helped to reorient the plan at any point during task breakdown. Eventually, tasks should increase in complexity (e.g., setting a table for five), and the client should be encouraged to function more independently. Another technique often used by clinicians is known as *backward chaining*. This involves presenting a partially completed task and asking the client to complete the final steps, for example, placing the knife and glass on a partially completed place setting. The perceptual cues of the task already begun appear to stimulate constructional abilities. As the client progresses, he or she should complete more steps.

Intervention for problems with spatial planning during visual-constructive tasks should begin with the simple spatial exercises discussed previously. If problems still exist, the individual may be asked to draw around shapes (blocks) one by one. These shapes should first have been placed in a simple two-dimensional design. The client is then asked to rebuild the design with the shapes alone. Therapy should progress from horizontal to vertical to oblique designs, from two-dimensional to three-dimensional designs, and from tasks with common objects to tasks involving abstract designs. For example, spatial problems with drawing, such as placing windows in a house or numbers on a clock face, are usually a result of underlying spatial disorder. The client should use a ruler or protractor to segment the space and plan placement before drawing. Dot-to-dot tasks may be designed that actually lead and sequence the drawing into a spatial whole. Simple puzzles also may be used to increase visual-spatial abilities during visual-constructive tasks. Finally, if task breakdown results from impulsive visual or motor behavior, these symptoms should be dealt with before further visual-constructive treatment continues.

Examples of visual-constructive tasks that may be designed for therapeutic use include the following:

- Setting a table for one to five people
- Wrapping a gift
- Assembling a piece of woodwork, a toy, a tool, a motor
- Changing a tire on a car
- Organizing a shelf in a library or a kitchen
- Organizing a filing system or cabinet
- Putting pieces of a sewing pattern together
- Addressing an envelope
- Rearranging furniture according to a preset plan
- Assembling a craft according to a preset plan
- Drawing from memory or copy
- Copying two-dimensional block designs
- Copying three-dimensional designs with oblique components

The key to effective visual-constructive learning, however, is not the task itself but rather how carefully the therapist organizes it and monitors performance. Clients with visual-constructive disorders are often visually or motorically impulsive; they often move or draw parts before analysis has taken place. Once a part is placed inappropriately, it begins to confuse the whole visual-perceptual process. This confusion increases anxiety and contributes to further breakdown in analysis and synthesis. Treatment should be directed at the underlying causes of task breakdown if these can be determined.

Problems of Visual Analysis and Synthesis Disorders

Identification of Clinical Problems

This separate discussion of visual analysis and synthesis is arbitrary. There is never any clear demarcation between the processes of visual-spatial orientation, visual-construction, and visual analysis and synthesis. Analysis of likes and differences, relationships of parts to one another, and reasoning and deduction occur simultaneously with more basic spatial and constructive percepts. The final visual concept of a task (e.g., what a place setting on a table should look like) is necessary before the task is begun. Similarly, synthesis of one part of a task may be necessary before synthesis of the entire task can occur. For example, the person who is setting a table for four people must be able to conceptualize one place setting before conceptualizing the table with four place settings. Those points during perceptual processing when there is a colligation or blending of discrete impressions into a single perception are known as synthesis. This final stage of coordination and interpretation of sensory data is thought to be deficient in many individuals with perceptual problems. Deficits may be present with either left or right hemisphere damage but are more common and more severe with right lesions.[32,76]

Visual-perceptual skills considered to be analytical and synthetic in nature include making fine visual discriminations, particularly in complex configurations; separating figure from background in complex configurations (figure-ground); achieving recognition on the basis of incomplete information (figure closure); and synthesizing disparate elements into a meaningful entity, as, for example, conceptualizing parts of a task into a whole.[5]

Assessment

Many tests have been designed to measure the capacity for analysis and synthesis. Test items include complex figures in which small parts of a figure differ from another figure. The client is asked to select the one that is different. Studies have shown that basic discrimination of single attributes of a stimulus such as length, contour, or brightness is intact in many clients.[77-79] The problem appears when these individuals are asked to discriminate between more complex configurations with subtle differences. Tests also measure

TABLE 30-3 ■ Common Tests Used to Assess Visual Analysis and Synthesis

TEST	USE
Hooper Visual Organization Test	Standardized for adults
Motor-Free Visual Perception Test	Standardized for adults
Raven's Progressive Matrices	Standardized for adults
Embedded Figure Test	Standardized for adults
Southern California Figure-Ground Test	Standardized for children only

figure-ground ability; the client must select the embedded figure from the background. Functional examples of this problem are the inability of a client to find her or his glasses if they are lying on a figured background, to find a white shirt on a white bedspread, and to find his wheelchair locks. Figure closure is measured by asking the client to complete an incomplete figure, such as part of the outline of a common shape. Finally, synthesis of parts into a whole, also known as visual organization, is measured by asking the client to conceptualize and organize the whole picture by, for example, looking at separate segments of the picture (e.g., cup or key) that have been divided and placed in unusual positions. This type of synthesis is necessary for high-level constructional tasks. Table 30-3 outlines examples of tests used to evaluate visual analysis and synthesis.

Interventions

Intervention for deficits in visual analysis and synthesis should follow developmental considerations described in the children's section. Visual discrimination tasks should begin with simple figures and obvious differences in complex figures. Color, size, texture, lighting, and verbal direction may help the client "cue in" on subtle differences among objects or figures. The therapist should determine the threshold at which the client is capable of discriminating differences and vary the dimension, contrast, and functional activity at this level. For example, if the individual cannot select a can of vegetables from a kitchen shelf stocked with cans of similar size, the therapist may simply change the task to fit that person's level of visual discrimination by removing some of the cans (decreasing the density of the display), replacing some of the cans with boxes of food (increasing the spatial contrast), moving the can to be selected forward or to one edge of the display (decreasing figure-ground difficulty), removing the label from the can (increasing the light and color contrast), or giving cues regarding what to search for (verbal direction). This example is described not as a method of compensation but rather as an approach to be used therapeutically in slowly building the client's visual discrimination abilities. Eventually, high-level visual discrimination skills should be incorporated within tasks requiring three or more steps, such as selecting a can of vegetables, opening the can (which involves selecting the can opener from the utensil drawer), and emptying the vegetables into a specific bowl (which involves selecting the bowl from among other bowls). Visual discrimination and figure-ground skills may appear normal until the client is required to do multiple-step activities, is given time constraints, or

becomes anxious or confused. Tabletop games that require high levels of visual discrimination along with cognitive strategies may be therapeutic and motivating. Examples include Monopoly and card games such as solitaire. Matching and sorting tasks also may be helpful in enhancing visual discrimination. Examples include matching picture cards and sorting laundry, tools, silverware, or files.

Drawings of figures with subtle differences also may be used for therapy. The client should be encouraged to point to, verbalize, or outline the subtle differences in two or more pictures; this enhances visual attention to detail. If the individual cannot select the discrepant detail(s) among three or more figures, the problem most likely results from an inability to select one feature and compare it with elements in the other figures. This is a fairly high-level skill that requires selective attention and analysis with internal visualization while the individual is still viewing the complete figures. This type of client should practice feature detection and then begin systematic comparisons of similarities and differences between two figures, eventually progressing to three or more figures. The therapist may number or outline similar areas of each figure to help the client (1) direct attention to similar areas of all figures and (2) sequence comparisons appropriately. The client should verbalize, draw, or write details concerning similarities and differences in individual aspects of the figures. This enhances visual analysis and also informs the therapist about how the individual is selecting and comparing features. Eventually, speed should be stressed, the highest level being presentation of tachistoscopic designs.

Visual organization may be emphasized by presenting the client with activities that have multiple parts that must be sequenced together into a whole. Activities involving this type of synthesis are discussed in the preceding section on treatment of visual-constructive disorders. Figure closure may be emphasized by presenting parts of figures or objects (e.g., half a plate covered by a towel) and asking the client for identification. Figure-closure task difficulty may be increased by placing many objects on a table, some of which partially occlude others. Identification of objects in such a task requires figure closure simultaneous with figure-ground abilities.

Visual analysis and synthesis deficits reflect a disruption in cognitive function with specific regard to visual-perceptual features. The affected client may function normally when analytical tasks require another system, for example, language. In others with generalized brain damage (e.g., traumatic head injury and senile dementia), general cognitive analysis and synthesis may be at fault rather than visual analysis. Because most cognitive performance requires visual processing, however, increased ability to analyze and synthesize visual-perceptual material often generalizes to an increase in cognitive function.

PERCEPTUAL RETRAINING WITH COMPUTERS

During the past 15 years, numerous computer programs have been developed for rehabilitation of brain damage symptoms, including cognition (e.g., attention, sequencing, or memory) and perception. Because the computer is so highly visual, it becomes an obvious tool for treatment of visual-perceptual dysfunction. Treatment with computers has been coined "computer-assisted therapy." No large treat-

BOX 30-6 ■ COMPUTER PROGRAMS FOR VISUAL-PERCEPTUAL TRAINING

HTS Home Therapy Systems: http://www.
  homevisiontherapy.com/
Visual Perceptual Diagnostic Testing and Training Programs
H. Greenberg and C. Chamoff
Educational Electronic Techniques, Ltd.
1886 Wantagh Avenue
Wantagh, NY 11793

Captain's Log Cognitive Training System
J. Sandford and R. Browne
Computability Corporation
101 Route 46 East
Pine Brook, NJ 07058

Psychological Software Services Programs
Odie Bracey
Psychological Software Services
P.O. Box 29205
Indianapolis, IN 46229

Life Science Associates Programs
R. Gianutsos
Life Science Associates
1 Fenemore Road
Bayport, NY 11705 (Diagnosis and Training)

Cognitive Rehabilitation Series
Hartley Courseware
2023 Aspen Glade
Kingwood, TX 77339

ment studies have yet defined the outcome significance of computer-assisted therapy versus conventional treatment programs. However, reports indicate that computer-assisted therapy is motivating for patients with poor attention and motivation. Advantages of computer-assisted therapy include control/flexibility of perceptual variables during treatment (e.g., number, size, speed), immediate feedback of performance, and automatic control for learning (i.e., items are repeated if incorrect to facilitate learning). Visual-perceptual training with computers, if used, should be viewed as one part of a patient's treatment program. One should always remember that the computer, monitor, and keyboard are just that: they do not require the many perceptual, vestibular, and motor responses typical of daily performance (e.g., scanning requirements may be bilateral, but they are not global and associated with head movement). A patient's total program may include computer-assisted therapy as an additional tool; however, it should never be substituted for more significant training within the multidimensional environment. Some computer programs for visual-perceptual training are listed in Box 30-6.

SUMMARY OF VISUAL-PERCEPTUAL DYSFUNCTION

Careful organized evaluation should delineate deficits well enough to result in a visual-perceptual function profile for each client, including both primary and associative visual skills. Clients rarely come with isolated visual-perceptual deficits; more often they exhibit a combination of visual-perceptual deficits usually interrelated with motor, language, and cognitive dysfunctions. For example, a visual-perceptual function profile may reveal strabismus, left unilateral visual inattention, visual-spatial deficits, visual-constructive deficits, and problems with visual analysis and synthesis, all affecting daily function. Treatment should be organized to progressively build skills, emphasizing one component more than another. The goal of treatment is eventual generalization of improvements in individual skills to spontaneous high-level function.

The presentation of information in this chapter is an attempt to use isolated and mechanistic terms to define a system that is extremely subtle, integrated, and complex. The reader is reminded that much of the normal and abnormal perceptual system has not been well defined. Preliminary studies cited throughout this chapter, however, suggest that disorders may be responsive to management and treatment. Research is needed to standardize evaluation procedures well enough to further define deficits and to investigate the effectiveness of various treatment approaches with various client populations.

REFERENCES

1. Rosenbloom DA, Morgan M: *Principles and practice of pediatric optometry,* San Francisco, 1990, JB Lippincott.
2. Keating M: *Geometric, physical and visual optics,* Boston, 1988, Butterworths.
3. Kanski JJ: *Clinical ophthalmology: a systematic approach,* ed 2, London, 1989, Butterworth-Heinemann.
4. Fannin T, Grosvenor T: *Clinical optics,* Boston, 1987, Butterworths.
5. Moses R, Hart W: *Adler's physiology of the eye, clinical application,* St. Louis, 1987, CV Mosby.
6. Bartlett J, Jaanus S: *Clinical ocular pharmacology,* ed 2, London, 1989, Butterworths.
7. Rosenbloom A, Morgan M, editors: *Vision and aging, general and clinical perspectives,* New York, 1986, Professional Press Books, Fairchild Publications.
8. Glaser J: *Neuro-ophthalmology,* Philadelphia, 1990, JB Lippincott.
9. Nilsson L: *Behold man,* Boston, 1973, Little, Brown.
10. Gregory RL: *Eye and brain,* ed 2, New York, 1972, World University Library, McGraw-Hill.
11. Hubel DH, Wiesel TN: Receptive fields and functional architecture of monkey striate cortex, *J Physiol* 195:215-243, 1968.
12. Hubel DH, Livingstone MS: Color and contrast sensitivity in the lateral geniculate body and primary visual cortex of the macaque monkey, *J Neurosci* 10:2223-2237, 1990.
13. Adler-Grinberg D, Stark L: Eye movements, scanpaths and dyslexia, *Am J Optom Phys Optics* 55:557-570, 1978.
14. Noton D, Stark L: Scanpaths in eye movements during pattern recognition, *Science* 22:171, 1979.
15. Gallaway M, Schieman M: The efficacy of vision therapy for convergence excess, *J Am Optom Assoc* 68:81-86, 1997.
16. Garriot RS, Heyman CL, Rouse MW: Role of optometric vision therapy for surgically treated strabismus patients, *Optom Vis Sci* 74:179-184, 1997.
17. Krohel GB, Kristen RW, Simon JW et al: Post-traumatic convergence insufficiency, *Am J Ophthalmol* 18:101-102, 104, 1986.
18. Carroll R, Seaber J: Acute loss of fusional convergence facility following head trauma, *Am Orthop J* 24:57-59, 1974.
19. Kulp MT, Schmidt PP: Effect of oculomotor and other skills on reading performance, a literature review, *Optom Vis Sci* 73:283-292, 1996.
20. Solan HA, Feldman J, Tujak L: Developing visual and reading efficiency in older adults, *Optom Vis Sci* 72:139-145, 1995.
21. Zihl J, von Cramon D: Restitution of visual function in cerebral blindness, *J Neurol Neurosurg Psychiatry* 42:312-322, 1979.

22. Balliet R, Blood K, Bach-Y-Rita P: Visual field rehabilitation in the cortically blind? *J Neurol Neurosurg Psychiatry* 48:1113-1124, 1985.

23. Kasten E, Poggel D, Sabel B: Computer-based training of stimulus detection improves color and simple pattern recognition in the defective field of hemianopic subjects, *J Cogn Neurosci* 12:1001-1012, 2000.

24. Kasten E, Wuest S, Behrens-Bamann W et al: Computer-based training for the treatment of partial blindness, *Nat Med* 4:1083-1087, 1998.

25. Kasten E, Mueller-Oering E, Sabel B: Stability of visual field enlargements following computer-based restitution training, *J Clin Expl Neuropsychol* 23:297-305, 2001.

26. Kerkhoff G: Restorative and compensatory therapy approaches in cerebral blindness—a review, *Restorative Neurol Neurosci* 15:225-271, 1999.

27. Critchley M: *The parietal lobes,* New York, 1966, Hafner.

28. Bouska MJ, Kwatny E: *Manual for application of the Motor-Free Visual Perception Test to the adult population,* Philadelphia, 1980, Temple University Rehabilitation Research and Training Center No. 8.

29. Diller L, Ben-Yishay Y, Gerstman LJ: *Studies in cognition and rehabilitation in hemiplegia,* Rehabilitation Monograph No. 50, New York, 1974, New York University Medical Center Institute of Rehabilitation Medicine.

30. Hacean T: Aphasic, apraxic and agnosic syndromes in right and left hemisphere lesions; Disorders of speech perception and symbolic behavior. In Vinken PJ, Bruyn GW, editors: *Handbook of clinical neurology, vol 4,* Amsterdam, 1969, North-Holland Publishing.

31. Heilman K, Valenstein E: Mechanisms underlying hemispatial neglect, *Ann Neurol* 5:166, 1979.

32. Seiv E, Freishat B: *Perceptual dysfunction in the adult stroke patient: a manual for evaluation and treatment,* Thorofare, NJ, 1976, Charles B Slack.

33. Heilman K: Neglect and related disorders. In Heilman K, Valenstein E, editors: *Clinical neuropsychology,* New York, 1979, Oxford University Press.

34. Watson RT, Heilman KM: Thalamic neglect, *Neurology* 29:690-694, 1979.

35. Hein DB et al: Hypertensive putomental hemorrhage, *Ann Neurol* 1:152, 1977.

36. Reeves AG, Hagaman WD: Behavioral and EEG asymmetry following unilateral lesions of the forebrain and midbrain of cats, *Electroencephalog Clin Neurophysiol* 30:83-86, 1971.

37. LeDoux JE, Smylie C: Left hemisphere visual processes in a case of right hemisphere symptomatology: implications for theories of cerebral lateralization, *Arch Neurol* 37:157-159, 1980.

38. Chedru F, Leblanc M, Lhermitte F: Visual searching in normal and brain-damaged subjects: contribution to the study of unilateral inattention, *Cortex* 9:94-111, 1973.

39. Leicester J, Sidman M, Stoddard LT, Mohr JP: Some determinants of visual neglect, *J Neurol Neurosurg Psychiatry* 32:580-587, 1969.

40. Wilson B, Cockburn J, Halligan P: *Behavioral inattention test,* Hants, England, 1988, Thames Valley Test.

41. Bouska MJ, Biddle E: The influence of unilateral visual neglect on diagnostic testing. Presented at the American Speech, Language and Hearing Association Annual Conference, Atlanta, November 1979.

42. Gianotti G, Tiacci C: The relationships between disorders of visual perception and unilateral spatial neglect, *Neuropsychologia* 9:451-458, 1971.

43. Kwatny E, Bouska MJ: *Visual system disorders and functional correlates: final report,* Philadelphia, 1980, Temple University Rehabilitation Research and Training Center No 8.

44. Stanton K: Teaching compensation for left neglect through a language-oriented program. Presented at the American Speech, Language and Hearing Association Annual Conference, Atlanta, November 1979.

45. Diller L: The development of a perceptual remediation program in hemiplegia. In Ince L, editor: *Behavioral psychology in rehabilitation medicine,* Baltimore, 1980, Williams & Wilkins.

46. Anderson E, Choy E: Parietal lobe syndromes in hemiplegia: a program for treatment, *Am J Occup Ther* 24:13-18, 1970.

47. Scotti G, Spinnler H: Colour imperception in unilateral hemisphere-damaged patients, *J Neurol Neurosurg Psychiatry* 33:22-28, 1970.

48. Meadows JC: Disturbed perception of colors associated with localized cerebral lesions, *Brain* 97:615-632, 1974.

49. Rubens A: Agnosia. In Heilman K, Valenstein E, editors: *Clinical neuropsychology,* New York, 1979, Oxford University Press.

50. Hacean T, de Ajuriaguera J: Balint's syndrome (psychic paralysis of visual fixation) and its minor forms, *Brain* 77:373, 1954.

51. Benton A: Visuospatial and visuoconstructive disorders. In Heilman K, Valenstein E, editor: *Clinical neuropsychology,* New York, 1979, Oxford University Press.

52. Nijboer TC, van Zandvoort MJ, de Haan EH: Covert colour processing in colour agnosia, *Neuropsychologia* 44:1437-1443, 2006.

53. Ishihara Color Plates, Tokyo, 1977, Kanehara. Available from Berneil Corp, P.O. Box 4637, South Bend, IN 46634-4637.

54. Balliet R: Rehabilitation of visual function in occipital lobe infarctions. Presented at the American Congress of Rehabilitation Medicine and the 43rd Annual Assembly of the American Academy of Physical Medicine and Rehabilitation, San Diego, November 1981.

55. Zihl J: Blindsight: Improvement of visually-guided eye movements by systematic practice in patients with cerebral blindness, *Neuropsychologia* 43:71-77, 1980.

56. Benton A: Disorders of visual perception, disorders of higher nervous activity. In Vinken PJ, Bruyn GW, editors: *Handbook of clinical neurology, vol 3,* Amsterdam, 1975, North-Holland Publishing.

57. Holmes G: Disturbances of visual orientation, *Br J Ophthalmol* 2:449, 1918.

58. Rayner K: Eye movements in reading and information processing, *Psychol Bull* 85:618-660, 1978.

59. DeCencio DV, Leshner M, Voron D: Verticality perception and ambulation in hemiplegia, *Arch Phys Med Rehabil* 51:105-110, 1970.

60. Gerontis C: Retinopathy of prematurity: www.emedicine.com/oph/topic413.htm. Accessed February 5, 2006.

60a. Scheinman A: Assessment and management of the exceptional child. In Rosenbloom A, Morgan M, editors: *Principles and practice of pediatric optometry,* San Francisco, 1990, JB Lippincott.

61. Merlin JM: Enhanced vision systems for closed circuit TVs: www.enhancedvision.com. Accessed February 5, 2006.

62. *Artificial vision:* http://jollyroger.com/retina. Accessed February 22, 2006, and July 26, 2006.

63. Brelen M, Duret F, Gerard B et al: Creating a meaningful visual perception in blind volunteers by optic nerve stimulation, *J Neural Engineering* 2:S22-S28, 2005.

64. OPTIV Optic Nerve Visual Prosthesis: electronic implant allows a blind patient to recover some vision: www.dice.ucl.ac.be/optivip. Accessed March 4, 2006.

65. Gianutsos R, Ramsey G, Perlin R: Rehabilitative optometric services for survivors of acquired brain injury, *Arch Phys Med Rehabil* 69:573-578, 1988.

66. Cohen A: Optometric management of binocular dysfunction secondary to head trauma: case reports, *J Am Optom Assoc* 63:569-575, 1992.

67. Aksionoff E, Falk N: Optometric therapy for the left brain injured patient, *J Am Optom Assoc* 63:564-588, 1992.

68. Cohen A, Rein L: The effect of head trauma on the visual system: the doctor of optometry as a member of the rehabilitation team, *J Am Optom Assoc* 63:530-536, 1992.

69. Gianutsos R, Ramsey G: Enabling survivors of brain injury to receive optometric services, *J Vis Rehabil* 2:37-58, 1988.

70. Andrezejewska W, Baranowska G: Accommodative disorders after head injury and cerebral contusion, *Klin Oczna (Poland)* 39:431, 1969.

71. Benton AL: Judgment of Line Orientation Test, Forms H and V, 1975, Department of Neurology, University Hospitals. Iowa City, University of Iowa Press.

72. Forrest EB: Visualization and visual imagery: an overview, *J Am Optom Assoc* 51:1005-1008, 1980.

73. Luria AR: *Higher cortical functions in man,* ed 2, New York, 1980, Basic Books.

74. Semenza C, Denes G, D'Urso V et al: Analytic and global strategies in copying designs by unilaterally brain-damaged patients, *Cortex* 14:404-410, 1978.

75. Ben-Yishay Y, Diller L, Mandleberg I: Ability to profit from cues as a function of initial competence in normal and brain-injured adults: a replication of previous findings, *J Abnorm Psychol* 76:378, 1970.

76. Warrington EK, James M: Visual apperceptive agnosia: a clinico-anatomical study of three cases, *Cortex* 24:13-32, 1988.

77. Nichelli EB, Spinnler H, Bisiach E: Hemispheric functional asymmetry in visual discrimination between invariate stimuli: an analysis of sensitivity and response criterion, *Neuropsychologia* 14:335-342, 1976.

78. Taylor AM, Warrington E: Visual discrimination in patients with localized brain lesions, *Cortex* 9:82-93, 1973.

79. Teuber HL, Weinstein S: Ability to discover hidden figures after cerebral lesions, *AMA Arch Neurol Psychiatry* 76:369-379, 1956.

ADDITIONAL READINGS

Arnadottir G: *Neurobehavioral assessment in adult CNS dysfunction,* St. Louis, 1989, CV Mosby.

Humphreys G, Riddoch MJ: *To see but not to see: A case study of visual agnosia,* Hillsdale, NJ, 1987, Laurence Erlbaum.

Scheiman M: *Understanding and managing vision deficits, a guide for the occupational therapist,* Thorofare, NJ, 1997, Slack.

Vision therapist: Hot topics, Santa Ana, CA, 1993, Optometric Extension Program.

Vision therapist: Working with the brain injured, Santa Ana, CA, 1993, Optometric Extension Program.

Zolton B, editor: Visual system dysfunction, *Head Trauma Rehabil* 4. 1989.

APPENDIX 30-A ■ **Resources**

Bernell/uso, 4016 N. Home Street, Mishiwaka, IN 46545; (800)-348-2225.

CCTVs: Enhanced Vision Systems, Optelec US, Inc, 321 Billerica Road, Chelmsford MA 01824, Humanware/Pulsedata: 175 Mason Circle, Concord, CA

Complete Visual Screening Kit: Laurie R. Chaikin, OD, OTR/L, 3717 Castro Valley Bld. Castro Valley, CA 94546; (510)-538-3937

Teller Cards: Vistech Consultants, 4162 Little York Road, Dayton, OH 45414-2566.

Helpful Web Sites

Annotated References List: www.vision-therapy.com/books.html.

College of Optometrists in Vision Development: www.covd.org.

Computerized home vision therapy system: www.homevisiontherapy.com.

Enhanced Vision Systems, for closed circuit TV's: www.enhanced-vision.com.

Neuro Optometric Rehabilitation Association: http://www.nora.cc/index.html.

Optometric Extension Program Foundation: www.oep.org.

Parents Active for Vision Education: www.pave-eye.com/~vision.

Position Statement on Optometric Vision Therapy (includes excellent reference list): www.aoanet.org/ia-op-vis-ther.html.

Vision Therapy Information and Referrals:
www.optometrists.org
www.vision3D.com
www.visionhelp.com

CHAPTER 31   Electromyography and Electrical Stimulation

George Wolfe, PT, PhD
Janet Marie Adams, PT, MS, DPT

KEY WORDS

electromyographic feedback
electroneuromyography
functional electrical stimulation
kinesiological electromyography
neuromuscular electrical stimulation
nerve conduction velocity

OBJECTIVES

After the end of this chapter the student/therapist will be able to:

1. Identify electroneural diagnostic tests performed on clients with neurological disorders.
2. Describe the instrumentation and general procedures for electroneural diagnostic testing.
3. Recognize normal and abnormal findings of various electroneural diagnostic tests.
4. Understand the differences in instrumentation, signal processing, and interpretation when performing electroneural diagnostic testing versus kinesiological electromyographic testing.
5. Understand the basic mechanism underlying functional neuromuscular stimulation, electrical stimulation, and electromyographic biofeedback.
6. Describe the appropriate instrumentation, signal processing, and interpretation for kinesiological electromyographic testing.
7. Describe the indications and contraindication for the use of neuromuscular stimulation, electrical stimulation, and electromyographic biofeedback.

The goal of this chapter is to enhance the clinician's ability to recognize indications for the most commonly used electrodiagnostic tests and to integrate knowledge of these test indications and findings into the management of clients with neuropathological dysfunction. The first section presents a basic description of the electrophysiological tests, including electroneuromyography (ENMG), kinesiological electromyography (KEMG), and the underlying neuroanatomical structures being tested. Normal and abnormal findings are discussed with emphasis on how knowledge of these tests can assist the therapist in client evaluation. The second section provides an introduction to the physiology, indications, contraindications, equipment, and applications of electrical muscle stimulation (EMS), neuromuscular electrical stimulation (NMES), and electromyographic biofeedback (EMGBF). The information integrates electrotherapeutic interventions into program planning for common neurological impairments and their subsequent functional limitations and disabilities. Published evidence examining efficacy is included to assist the therapist in making choices about the use of these tools in the clinic. The third section provides a series of five case studies that illustrate the usefulness of electromyographic (EMG) testing in patients with a variety of medical diagnoses.

ELECTRODIAGNOSIS

An informed perspective on the application of electrophysiological tests should benefit the therapist's interaction and communication with other members of the medical and health management community. These tests are part of differential diagnosis, and their results can guide decisions in planning and modification of programs for intervention from referrals or to create referrals back to other health care practitioners.

Electrodiagnostic tests are performed by medical practitioners (including physical therapists) who have education, training, and experience in these procedures. Most of the electrophysiological tests described involve the application of an external electrical stimulus to a nerve or muscle and observation and assessment of the muscle or nerve response. Other tests such as the electroneuromyogram (ENMG) and the single-fiber electromyogram (SFEMG) involve the monitoring and recording of the electrical activity produced by the muscle tissue at rest or during contraction.

Electrical tests commonly used at this time are motor and sensory nerve conduction tests, including F wave and H reflex measurements, repetitive stimulation, somatosensory evoked potential (SSEP) tests, and electromyography. The test for reaction of degeneration (RD) has been used in the past but is now rarely applied specifically. A review of the client's history, a relevant systems review, and a physical examination guide the examiner in the selection and sequencing of appropriate tests. Neurological signs, muscle strength and tone, sensation, range of motion (ROM), and cognition are important data in planning and administering electrical tests.

Reaction of Degeneration and Strength Duration Tests

A fundamental physiological feature of nerve and muscle is depolarization in response to an adequate electrical stimulus. To be adequate, an electrical stimulus must meet minimal criteria of amplitude (intensity) and duration.[1-5] The lowest amplitude of stimulus required to produce a response in nerve or muscle when using a pulse of long duration (>100 ms) is termed the *rheobase,* or threshold. When using a stimulus amplitude twice the rheobase value, the shortest pulse duration that can elicit a response is the *chronaxy.* The chronaxy of normal peripheral nerves is generally less than 0.5 ms. The chronaxy of muscle fibers is considerably longer. An innervated muscle will thus respond to stimuli less than 0.5 ms (the nerve fibers will respond and trigger the muscle contraction). A denervated muscle will not respond unless the duration of the pulse is much longer. This difference between the response of nerve and muscle formed the basis of the Reaction of Degeneration (RD) test. In the past, this qualitative test would be followed by a strength duration test in which the amplitude of stimulus needed to elicit a response at shorter and shorter pulse durations would be graphed, producing a strength duration curve for the gross muscle. The curve would then be evaluated to determine the degree of innervation or denervation (normal, partial degeneration/regeneration, or complete denervation). The RD and strength duration tests have generally been replaced by the more objective nerve conduction and EMG tests.

Most clinical electrical stimulators produce pulses less than 0.5 ms in duration. Muscles that are weak or paralyzed because of involvement of the central nervous system (CNS) should contract when NMES is applied. A failure of the muscle to respond may indicate involvement of the peripheral nervous system (PNS) and possible denervation. The therapist should then consider referral for electrodiagnostic examination.

Nerve Conduction Tests

A general overview of nerve conduction tests (NCTs) is presented to provide an understanding of their application and indications. Many excellent texts are available for details of the techniques.[6-10]

Motor and sensory NCTs can provide data that are helpful in establishing the presence and location of pathological conditions in the PNS. The tests may indicate the anatomical level, such as a plexopathy, versus a localized peripheral mononeuropathy. Individual and multiple nerves may be assessed and compared with responses of the same nerves contralaterally. The site of pathology may be localized, such as median nerve compression at the wrist versus lesion of the lateral cord of the brachial plexus.

Nerve conduction velocity is faster in myelinated fibers because of saltatory conduction. Disorders involving peripheral demyelination can thus be differentiated from impairments primarily involving axonal degeneration. A mild localized compressive disorder (neuropraxia) may be distinguished from a more severe lesion in which the nerve and surrounding connective tissue have been completely disrupted (neurotmesis).[8,11] In the event that the findings of NCT and EMG are normal the clinician may be able to rule out most conditions involving the PNS and look for CNS or other pathology. Knowledge of the rationale for NCT and EMG should help the therapist decide when the tests may be indicated and understand the reasoning behind reports of tests that have already been performed on their clients.

Motor Nerve Conduction

In motor NCTs (MNCTs), the peripheral nerve is stimulated at various sites and the evoked electrical response is recorded from a distal muscle supplied by the nerve (a measure of orthodromic conduction). Surface electrodes are usually used for both stimulating and recording. An example of electrode configuration for MNCT is shown in Figure 31-1. The response represents the electrical activity of muscle fibers under the recording electrodes and is called the compound muscle action potential (CMAP). It is also called the M wave or M response. Measurements are taken of latency (the time in milliseconds required for the impulse to travel from each stimulus site to the recording site), and the amplitude of the response in millivolts. The shape and duration of the response are assessed, and motor nerve conduction velocity (MNCV) is calculated for each segment of interest by dividing the distance between stimulus sites (in millimeters) by the difference in latency measured at each respective site.

Velocities, latencies, and the shape and amplitude of the responses are studied and compared with established normal values and often with values taken from tests of the uninvolved extremity (when possible). In infants and children, nerve conduction is slower than in adults and reaches adult values by age 4 years.[10] Nerve conduction velocities gradually slow after age 60 years but generally remain within the outer limits of normal.[8,10]

Sensory Nerve Conduction

Sensory nerve conduction can be measured from many superficial sensory nerves, such as the superficial radial and sural nerves. It can also be measured from mixed motor and sensory nerves. The stimulus is applied over the nerve in question and the recordings taken from electrodes placed over a distal sensory branch of the nerve. The recordings are called sensory nerve action potentials (SNAPs). An example of recording and stimulation sites is shown in Figure 31-2. Both orthodromic and antidromic conduction can be assessed. Response latencies and amplitudes are measured, and sensory nerve conduction velocities (SNCVs) are calculated for each segment by dividing the distance between two adjacent stimulus and recording sites, or two stimulus sites, by the latency (conduction time) between these same sites. Sensory nerve responses are considerably smaller than motor responses. Their amplitudes are generally measured in microvolts.

F Wave Latency

When a motor nerve is stimulated in the periphery both orthodromic (peripherally to the muscle) and antidromic (centrally toward the spinal cord) impulses are generated. A proportion of the antidromic impulses will return as a recurrent discharge along the same neurons to activate the muscle from which the recording is taken. This activity is termed the F wave and it is observed as a small wave occurring after the M wave.[5,8,10,12] No synapse is involved. Thus the F wave is not a reflex response, but rather only a measure of motor

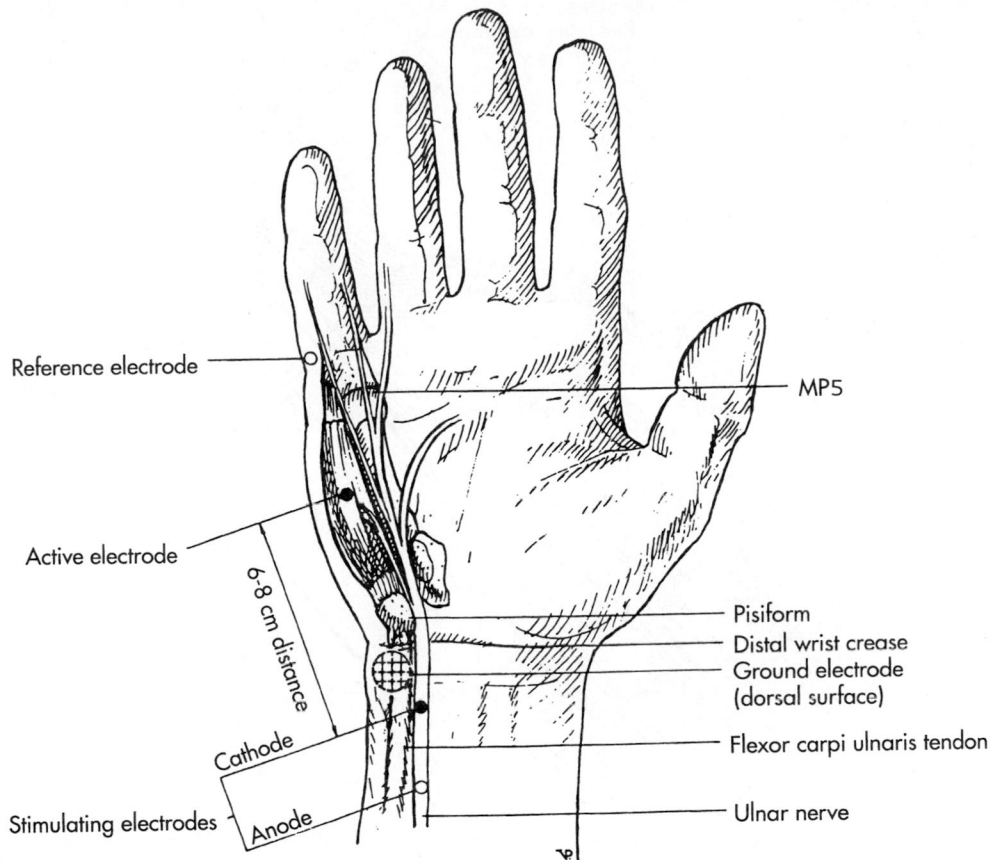

Reference electrode

MP5

Active electrode

6-8 cm distance

Pisiform
Distal wrist crease
Ground electrode
(dorsal surface)

Flexor carpi ulnaris tendon

Cathode

Ulnar nerve

Stimulating electrodes

Anode

FIGURE 31-1 ■ Electrode location for ulnar motor nerve conduction. *MP5,* Metacarpophalangeal joint 5. (Adapted from National Institute for Occupational Safety and Health: *Performing motor and sensory neuronal conduction studies in humans. Dept of Health and Human Services, publication no. 90-113.* Washington, DC, 1990, Centers for Disease Control and Prevention, p. 17.)

neuron conduction. Specific conditions of electropotential must exist at the somadendritic cell membrane to reactivate the efferent axon; therefore the occurrence of the F wave response is inconsistent and variable in latency and waveform.[12]

The F wave latency can be useful in evaluating conduction in conditions usually involving the proximal portions of the peripheral neurons (e.g., Guillain-Barré syndrome and thoracic outlet syndrome). Its value, however, has been questioned by some authors because of its variability. Normal values of F wave latency are 22 to 34 ms in the upper extremity (stimulating at the wrist), 40 to 58 ms in the lower extremity (stimulating at the ankle), and 12 ms central latency in the upper extremity with a bilateral difference in latency of no greater than 1 ms.[13]

H Reflex Response

The H reflex response latency is a measure of the time for action potentials elicited by stimulating a nerve in the periphery to be propagated centrally over the Ia afferent neurons to the spinal cord, to be transmitted across the synapse to alpha motor neurons, and then to travel distally over these neurons to activate the muscle. The response therefore measures conduction in both the afferent and efferent neurons.[8,10] It is also referred to as a "late" response.

The H wave is constant in latency and waveform, and it occurs with a stimulus usually below the threshold level required to elicit the M wave response (Ia afferent fibers are larger in diameter than alpha motor neurons and thus more sensitive to electrical stimulation). This monosynaptic reflex response is most easily found by stimulating the tibial nerve at the popliteal area and recording from the soleus muscle. Braddom and Johnson[14] reported a mean latency of 29.8 ms (± 2.74 ms) for the tibial nerve in normal adults, and a bilateral difference of no more than 1.2 ms. The H wave latency is a valuable measure of conduction over the S1 nerve root in differentiating suspected proximal plexopathy and radiculopathy from a herniated disk or foraminal impingement. Sabbahi and Khalil[15] have reported a technique for recording the H wave from the flexor carpi radialis muscle when stimulating the median nerve. In normal human beings older than 1 year, the H wave is usually seen only in the tibial and median nerves. It can be elicited from several nerves in infants and in conditions of CNS dysfunction in adults.

Repetitive Stimulation Tests

The repetitive stimulation (RS) test is used to evaluate transmission at the neuromuscular junction. RS tests are helpful in the differential diagnosis of disorders such as myasthenia gravis and bronchogenic carcinoma. One protocol uses a series of supramaximal electrical stimuli applied to a

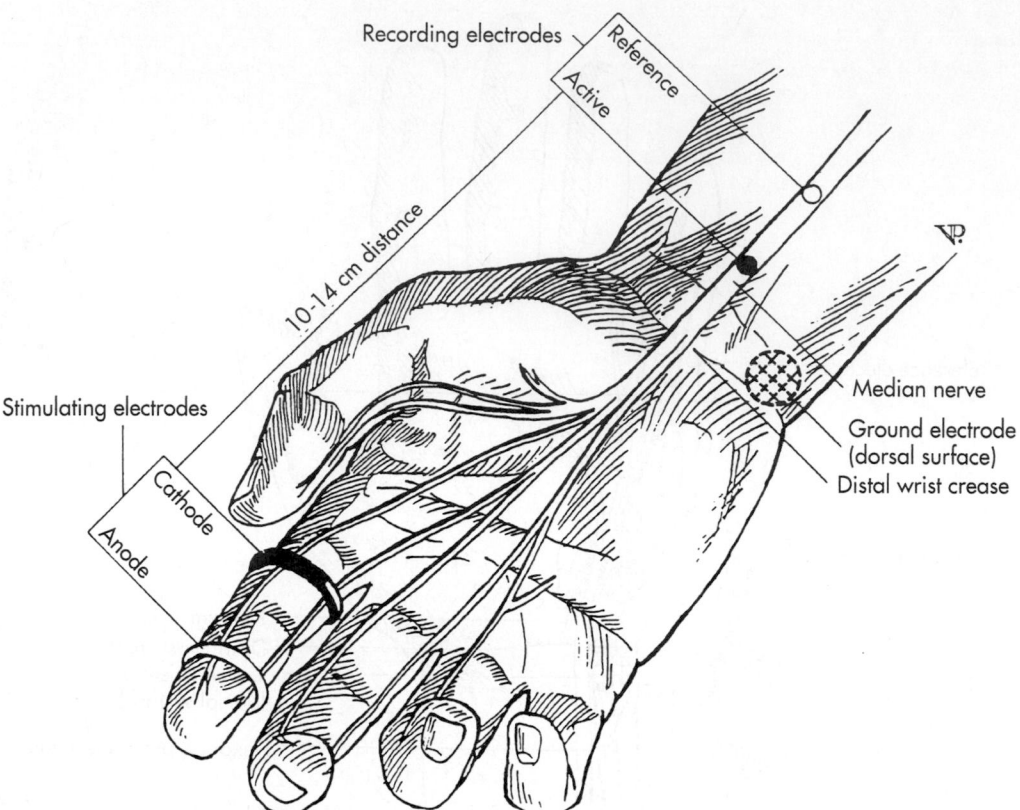

FIGURE 31-2 ■ Electrode location for median sensory nerve conduction. (Adapted from National Institute for Occupational Safety and Health: *Performing motor and sensory neuronal conduction studies in humans. Dept of Health and Human Services, publication no. 90-113.* Washington, DC, 1990, Centers for Disease Control and Prevention, p. 13.)

peripheral nerve at a distal site (e.g., median or ulnar nerve at the wrist) at a rate of three to five per second for five to seven responses. Changes in amplitude of the muscle response are assessed. Precise technical requirements are specified to prevent movement artifacts and other testing errors. Detailed descriptions of the RS test can be found in other texts.[8,16] Under normal conditions the amplitude does not change more than 10% from that of the initial response in a series of 10 stimuli recorded before and after resistive exercise. An amplitude decrease in the fifth or sixth response of more than 10% is considered abnormal and is compatible with a physiological defect at the postsynaptic receptor site of the neuromuscular junction, as in myasthenia gravis.

In another RS protocol, stimuli are applied to a nerve, first at a slow rate, then at a faster rate, usually 10 to 20 per second for up to 10 seconds. Normally, the amplitude can decrease up to 40% from the initial amplitude. In some defects at the presynaptic site, the response may be lower than normal during a slow stimulation rate but show a significant amplitude increase at the higher rate. Increases in amplitude greater than 100% over the initial response are consistent with presynaptic neuromuscular junction defects such as seen in small-cell bronchogenic carcinoma (Pancoast tumor) and in botulism. In 1957 Eaton and Lambert[17] reported this phenomenon as a myasthenic syndrome.

Gilchrist and Sanders[18] reported another protocol referred to as a double-step RS test. This test measures amplitude before and after a temporarily induced ischemia of the

extremity. They found the double-step RS test to be slightly more sensitive than the routine RS test, but only 60% as sensitive as the SFEMG technique. The RS test is a good alternative test for neuromuscular transmission when the SFEMG is not available, but the examiner must meticulously adhere to technical details when conducting the test.

Clinical Evoked Potentials

Electrical potentials elicited by stimulation of nerves or sense organs in the periphery can be recorded from various sites as the impulses are transmitted centrally along the neuronal pathway and from the representative area on the brain.[8,19-21] SSEP procedures are particularly useful in assessing the integrity of afferent pathways in the CNS. They are helpful in differentiating among lesions in areas such as the plexus, spinal cord, brain stem, thalamus, and cerebral cortex. Evoked potential tests have the advantage of providing data about the integrity of both peripheral and central neuronal pathways, including transmission across axodendritic synapses.

The SSEP is valuable in assessing damage and continuity of spinal cord tracts in early spinal cord injury (SCI). For example, if an electrical stimulus is applied at the popliteal area over the tibial nerve, responses can be recorded with surface electrodes placed over the spine at the L3 and C7 spinal segments and from the lumbar representation of the contralateral sensory cortical area. Conduction time and other parameters of the response waveforms can be measured from the recordings.

This simplified example of an SSEP illustrates how conduction over both motor and sensory peripheral nerves and afferent pathways to the cerebrum can be studied. The median nerve is usually tested to evaluate the integrity of peripheral and central pathways and their synaptic connections as the impulses travel from the upper extremity to the contralateral cortical area.

In visual evoked potential (VEP) procedures, visual stimuli such as variable light flashes of changing patterns are applied to one or both eyes under highly controlled conditions. The response is recorded from the scalp over the representative area of the cerebral cortex.[8,20,21] The term *pattern reversal evoked potentials* (PREPs), a more descriptive term for these procedures, is recommended by the American Electroencephalographic Society.[19] These tests and other VEP procedures are useful in assessing pathology of retinal photoreceptors, the optic nerve, and postchiasmal pathways. Abnormal conduction findings have been reported when using VEP studies in demyelinating disorders such as multiple sclerosis and optic neuritis. The examiner may conclude that the patient is cortically blind because no response is recorded on the visual cortex. Although many causes for a stimulus not reaching the visual cortex are possible, the end result is considered blindness. If the cause for cortical inactivity is swelling or a neurochemical imbalance within a nuclear relay structure, once corrected, the individual may experience normal vision. A change in the reaction of the patient to the visual environment may reflect increased awareness and a change in coma scale rating. Similarly, just because an individual turns toward a light or visual stimulus does not mean an evoked potential reaches the visual cortex. Instead, the eyes as receptors and the visual tract to the brain stem may be intact even though a problem in the synaptic connections between or within the thalamus and visual cortex may exist.

Auditory evoked potential tests are used to evaluate neurological function of the cochlear division of the auditory nerve (eighth cranial nerve), central auditory pathways and synapses in the brain stem, and the receptor areas on the cerebral cortex.[8,19-21] Brain stem auditory evoked potentials are frequently referred to as BAEPs. A series of high-intensity clicks is applied to auditory receptors in the ears through headphones, and several components of the response waveforms are recorded by using surface electrodes over the representative cortical areas. The BAEP is an effective test procedure for localizing and evaluating acoustic neuromas and other space-occupying lesions in the brain stem. This test is also used for assessment of brain damage in patients who are comatose as a result of traumatic brain injury. Robinson and Rudge[22] recommend caution when using BAEP tests for this purpose because other factors, such as defective receptor organs, can cause abnormalities in BAEPs.

The evoked potential tests described in this chapter all require application of appropriate external stimuli that are rapidly repeated many times. The response is electronically averaged to sort out the desired signal from interference signals. The conduction times (latencies), waveform shape and amplitude, and sometimes conduction velocities are measured and compared with normal values. Absence of a response, increased latencies, decreased amplitudes, and slowing of conduction velocities are all abnormal findings. Normal values and details describing techniques for the evoked potential tests are described elsewhere.[8,19-21]

Therapists with special interest and training more frequently administer the SSEP tests for neurological applications than other types of evoked potential tests. Because of the highly specialized techniques necessary to administer the VEP for ophthalmological applications and the BAEP for hearing dysfunction, they are usually performed by persons who specialize in these procedures.

Clinical Electroneuromyography

Unlike nerve conduction studies, which use the electrical stimulation of the motor nerves to elicit muscle contraction, clinical ENMG is used to record and analyze muscle activity at rest and during voluntary activation. It is particularly useful in identifying pathology of the lower motor neurons and of the muscle itself. EMG can also identify abnormalities of motor neuron recruitment that are associated with certain disorders of the CNS. The primary recording studied is the motor unit potential (MUP), which is produced by the depolarization of single motor units during voluntary or reflex activity. Spontaneous electrical activity of single muscle fibers is termed fibrillation and is diagnostic of denervation.

To record muscle activity, small-diameter needles are inserted within the muscles to be studied. Three electrodes are required: active (negative), reference (positive), and ground. The needles may be *monopolar,* requiring a second needle or surface electrode for reference, or *bipolar,* containing both the active and reference electrodes (usually concentric in cross section). The ground electrode is typically placed on the surface of the skin. Most commonly the needles used are disposable. The activity detected in the muscle is displayed on an oscilloscope (and can be stored and printed later). It may also be played through an audio amplifier. The electromyographer can often identify pathological conditions by the characteristic "sounds" of the electrical activity of the muscle. Many excellent resources are available for readers interested in details of the equipment and procedures for EMG.[6-8,23,24] Details of contraindications and special precautions are described by Currier et al.[24]

In an EMG examination, four conditions are evaluated at each location: (1) activity during needle insertion (normally a brief burst of high-frequency activity that abates when the needle ceases motion), (2) activity during rest (electrical silence is normal unless an electrode is placed directly over a motor endplate), (3) activity during minimal and gradually increasing voluntary contraction (biphasic or triphasic MUPs of small amplitude composed of slow-twitch fibers that increase in frequency and are joined by higher-amplitude potentials as larger predominately fast twitch motor units are recruited), and (4) activity during maximal activation (an *interference pattern* caused by the blending of potentials in which individual MUPs cannot be identified), characterized as full (complete), decreased, or absent. Several locations in an individual muscle may be studied. The specific muscles to be studied are determined by clinical findings, and results must always be interpreted in the context of the total complex of signs and symptoms. In determining the specific location of a lesion, muscles located both proximally and distally to the suspected lesion site must

TABLE 31-1 ■ **Characteristics of Normal and Abnormal EMG Potentials**

NEUROMUSCULAR STATUS	AT REST		MINIMUM CONTRACTION/ MOTOR UNIT POTENTIALS			STRONG CONTRACTION	
	INSERTION ACTIVITY	SPONTANEOUS ACTIVITY	AMPLITUDE	DURATION	WAVEFORM	RECRUITMENT PATTERN	AMPLITUDE
Normal	Brief discharges	None End Plate potentials	100 to 3000 μV	3-15 ms Avg 7 ms	Biphasic and triphasic 10% polyphasic	Full or complete interference (>75%)	*Concentric*: 2000-5000 μv or *monopolar*: 2000-8000 μV
Abnormal	Absent or decreased Increased or prolonged	Fibrillation Positive sharp waves Fasciculation Complex repetitive discharges Myotonic potentials on percussion	Absent or low or >5000 μV	<5 ms or >15 ms	Polyphasic >10%-15% or myotonic	Decreased (<75%) Discrete, single units Early recruitment	<2000 μV or *concentric*: >5000 μV or *monopolar*: >8000 μV

Adapted from Currier DP: Guidelines for clinical electromyography, *J Clin Electrophysiol* 5:2, 1993.

be assessed. Studies may be repeated at intervals to determine if changes consistent with recovery (such as reinnervation) or exacerbation are present. EMG is typically used to help determine the presence (and extent) of the following:

- Denervation
- Reinnervation
- Myopathic or neuropathic signs
- Distribution or specific location of peripheral nerve pathology

The primary findings in denervation and partial denervation include increased insertional activity, fibrillation potentials or positive sharp waves at rest, and a decreased or absent interference pattern. CNS dysfunction can result in no resting potentials, but if motor control was impaired a decreased or abnormal interference pattern might be apparent because of difficulty in recruitment (Table 31-1).

Although client cooperation during EMG testing is important, some aspects of muscle electrical activity can be studied in the client who is unable to move or who has only involuntary or reflex activity. Insertional and resting potentials can be evaluated. MUPs appear during the contraction of muscle fibers activated both voluntarily and involuntarily in both isotonic or isometric conditions. In normal conditions MUPs are seen with voluntary movement; however, reflex activation of muscle also produces MUPs with certain normal characteristics. In CNS disorders hypertonic or spastic muscles will produce recognizable MUPs when they are actively contracting. The myographer can elicit a contraction by tapping on the muscle or tendon. For example, consider a client who is recovering from a traumatic head injury with residual spastic hemiplegia. She is unable to cooperate with the EMG exam. The client has abnormal extensor responses in the lower extremity with the exception of the ankle and foot, which appear flaccid. An EMG of the leg and foot muscles detects abnormal resting potentials, including fibrillation and positive sharp waves in muscles innervated by the peroneal nerve. Tapping on the muscles fails to elicit MUPs. Muscles in the tibial nerve distribution have no resting potentials and respond with bursts of identifiable MUPs when the tendon is tapped. These findings would guide the physician and therapist in looking for a possible peripheral nerve lesion in addition to the CNS dysfunction. The treatment program in this situation would differ from that for a client without peripheral nerve pathology.

Justification and analysis of the basis principles and results after EMG studies should assist therapists managing clients with neurological dysfunction in planning and modifying therapeutic management programs. As electrical tests are being conducted, the findings are continuously studied and used by the physician and examiner as a guide in continuing with or modifying the plan for future tests based on whether they fit the characteristics usually identified with specific pathological conditions. As previously stated, the results of the electrodiagnostic tests must be correlated with other clinical findings and data.

Summary of Clinical Electroneuromyographic and Nerve Conduction Studies

Instruments with computer-assisted analysis are now commonplace for studying EMG signals in great detail.[8,25-27] Parameters of the waveform, including amplitude, duration, frequency spectrum, number of turns, or phase polarity reversals and area (the integral or total voltage of the waveform) can be automatically analyzed. The data are then compared electronically with predetermined patterns of electrical changes, which correlate with categories of neuromuscular disorders such as myelopathies and neuropathies.

The following is a summary of the more characteristic EMG and nerve conduction changes associated with selected groupings of neurological disorders. The intent is to assist in the understanding of reports of these studies and recognize changes that may be seen in sequential tests during the course of the disorders. The following is a simplified grouping of electrical changes; actual electrodiagnostic studies show considerably more detail and frequent variations of these findings.[6-8,23,24]

Electrical testing in CNS disorders typically shows normal motor and sensory nerve conduction. In the EMG, spontaneous activity is seen infrequently, and individual motor units seen on muscle contraction usually have normal parameters. The recruitment pattern may show a slower than normal MUP discharge frequency with an incomplete and irregular interference pattern. In the presence of tremor and other involuntary movements, bursts of MUPs occur consistent with the muscle contraction pattern. The tests are important in differential diagnosis between a CNS and a PNS problem, but often they are not used when clinical examinations demonstrate the problem to be definitively in the CNS.

In myelopathies, which include upper and lower motor neuron disorders (e.g., amyotrophic lateral sclerosis [ALS], poliomyelitis, cervical spondylitis, and syringomyelia), motor and sensory nerve conduction is usually normal, although mild slowing may be present.[8] The characteristic EMG changes, which usually appear in the more chronic stages of the disorders, are increased amplitude and duration of MUPs because of the variable impulse conduction time in sprouting axon terminals. An increased number of polyphasic potentials with increased duration are usually found. Spontaneous activity is often seen, and on strong contraction a reduced number of rapidly firing large MUPs are recruited, resulting in a single-unit or partial interference pattern.

Peripheral neuropathies show a variety of electrical changes depending on the type and location of the pathology. In a proximal pathology (e.g., radiculopathy), motor and sensory nerve conduction generally remain normal, except F waves and H reflex responses in specific spinal cord segments. If motor nerve roots are compromised, spontaneous activity and increased polyphasic potentials appear, and reduced recruitment of MUPs results in an incomplete interference pattern. In more chronic stages MUP amplitude and duration can be increased. As the lesion improves, spontaneous activity decreases and the recruitment patterns become more normal. If only sensory roots are injured, no EMG changes occur.

Lesions of peripheral nerves, which range from a focal mononeuropathy to plexopathy, frequently show abnormalities in motor and sensory nerve conduction depending on which components of the nerve are involved. In the EMG, spontaneous activity, particularly fibrillation and positive sharp waves, is common. If the lesion is complete, no MUPs are found. The presence of even a few MUPs suggests a more optimistic prognosis. Often the location of the lesion can be identified by the distribution of the electrical changes. With regenerating axons, low-amplitude polyphasic MUPs gradually appear. In the chronic stage, the amplitude and duration of MUPs are often increased. Spontaneous activity decreases with reinnervation, but it may persist for several years.

In generalized, systemic peripheral polyradiculoneuropathies of the primarily demyelinating type, such as Guillain-Barré syndrome, motor and sensory nerve conduc-

tion and F waves become markedly slow. EMG changes usually do not occur, except for a reduced recruitment pattern consistent with weak muscle contraction. With primarily axonal polyneuropathies, such as uremic neuropathy, isoniazid and cisplatin toxicity, and lead poisoning, motor and sensory nerve conduction is mildly slowed or may remain normal. The duration and amplitude of the response, however, decrease. During advanced stages, many polyneuropathies develop both demyelinating and axonal pathology (e.g., diabetic neuropathy). On EMG, spontaneous activity is commonly seen. These electrical changes generally become more severe with worsening of the pathology, but they also improve if the pathology is reversed.

With myopathic disorders, motor and sensory nerve conductions are generally normal unless neural tissue is also affected. In advanced stages, however, severely atrophied muscles can produce decreased amplitude and distorted nerve conduction responses. The characteristic findings on EMG are short-duration, low-amplitude potentials. Some spontaneous potentials, particularly fibrillations and positive sharp waves, may be found but are much more frequent in the inflammatory myopathies such as polymyositis. Spontaneous activity also is seen in some neuromuscular transmission disorders (e.g., botulism). Specific myotonic potentials appear in certain myopathic disorders (e.g., myotonia congenita). The recruitment pattern shows many low-amplitude MUPs, appearing in a full pattern, with little voluntary effort. This type of recruitment pattern is referred to as early recruitment.

Single-Fiber Electromyography

Electrical activity can be recorded from two or more muscle fibers innervated by the same motor unit by using a specially designed single-fiber needle electrode. SFEMG is, at this time, the most sensitive test for evaluation of neuromuscular transmission defects such as myasthenia gravis and myasthenic syndrome. It is also used to evaluate peripheral neuropathies, motor neuron diseases, and myopathies.

During a carefully controlled minimal voluntary contraction, a 25-µm-diameter needle is inserted into the muscle, and several potentials from muscle fibers within the recording area are stored. Equipment with a trigger and delay line is necessary to "time lock" the tracings of the potentials. The slightly different conduction time or interpulse interval (IPI) required for impulses to be transmitted from a single motor neuron to each of its terminal endplates, cross the neuromuscular junction, and activate the muscle fiber is called jitter. This time difference is collected from several tracings and is converted into a mean consecutive time difference (MCD), which normally ranges from 5 to 55 ms. Values shorter or longer than this range are considered abnormal. The impulses from some axons to their muscle fibers may fail to be transmitted. This is referred to as blocking. Another capability of SFEMG is the measure of fiber density, that is, the average number of muscle fibers within the needle recording area. Fiber density is increased in reinnervation and also with certain myopathies because of axonal collateralization or splitting.[25]

Macroelectromyography

A variation of SFEMG uses a macroelectrode to record the majority of muscle fibers of a single motor unit as they are triggered by an initial potential, which is then time locked with all the other muscle fiber potentials recorded from a different part of the same or a nearby needle.[8,26-29] Two recording channels are used. Maximal amplitude of the potentials from several muscles has been reported by Stalberg.[28] The findings are analyzed, along with findings of jitter, fiber density, and conventional EMG, to evaluate the status and prognosis of various neurological and neuromuscular disorders, such as motor neuron disease, peripheral nerve lesions, and myopathies.

Kinesiological Electromyography

Kinesiological electromyography (KEMG) measures muscle activation during movement whether it is purposeful, involuntary, dynamic, or relatively static. It is the method by which the therapist/examiner determines a muscle's (or muscle group) onset, cessation, relative intensity, and activation sequencing during functional activities such as walking. Because normal movement depends on the CNS's ability to execute motor programs through muscle action, KEMG provides the therapist with insight into motor function, motor control, and motor learning.

Persons with neuromuscular disorders typically exhibit control errors, including the inability to initiate, execute, or terminate movement. Selective control may be absent or abnormal with errors in muscle timing, intensity, and sequencing. Spasticity or synergistic muscle action may impede smooth execution of tasks and prevent purposeful movement. With increased emphasis on evidence-based practice, KEMG can provide objective documentation of abnormal control and intervention outcomes and provide insight into optimizing strategies for improved functional performance. Many orthopedic surgeons rely on KEMG testing to supplement clinical evaluation in planning surgical interventions (muscle transfers and releases) in children with cerebral palsy[30] and in patients with traumatic brain injury (TBI)[31] and stroke.[32]

KEMG interpretation depends on the examiner's understanding of the instrumentation chosen for testing, including electrode selection, recording techniques, signal processing, and time and intensity normalization.[33] Coupled with three-dimensional motion and force plate analysis, external moments are calculated that define internal force demands on muscles during functional activities such as walking. KEMG delineates the muscles that participate in meeting the internal force demand.

Recording Instrumentation

KEMG can be performed by using surface or fine wire electrodes (intramuscular). Controversy exists about the choice of electrodes with the selection dependent on the clinical or research question. If the examiner is interested in "muscle groups" (e.g., dorsiflexors, quadriceps) then surface electrodes are appropriate. Fine wire electrodes are optimal if activation of individual or deep muscles is desired (e.g., posterior tibialis, iliacus). Fine wire allows for specificity of muscle action required for surgical decisions related to muscle transfers, releases, or muscle lengthening.[30,31,34]

Needle/Fine Wire Electrodes (Indwelling or Intramuscular). A pair of 50-µg fine wire electrodes, also referred to as "indwelling or intramuscular" electrodes, are introduced through the skin and into the muscle with a 25-gauge hypodermic needle. The 50-µg, Teflon-coated wires are threaded through the needle's core. Two to 3 mm of the wire's distal end are stripped of insulation and, once inserted, record adjacent motor unit activity. Before insertion, the electrodes are sterilized. Inserted through the skin and into the muscle of interest, the barbed end "hooks" the muscle fibers when the needle is withdrawn. Accurate placement requires that the examiner have extensive knowledge of three-dimensional anatomy and excellent palpation skills. A maximal concentric voluntary contraction is elicited to anchor the wires into the muscle fibers, preventing displacement during subsequent contraction. This ensures sampling the same motor unit pool during subsequent tasks, trials, or conditions. Electrical stimulation is an essential testing element to verify electrode location. Wire electrodes allow a more precise definition of muscle timing (onset and cessation) by reducing the incidence of intramuscular crosstalk.[35] Disadvantages include decreased reliability and insertional pain caused by skin penetration.[36-38] In several states the examiner must possess specialized KEMG licensure to penetrate the skin with a needle.

Surface Electrodes. When the clinical question can be answered by using surface electrodes, electrical stimulation of motor points often defines optimal electrode placement over the muscle or group of muscles of interest. A maximal voluntary contraction is elicited to confirm that optimal placement is achieved. Standardizing electrode placement, size, interelectrode distance, and skin preparation enhance test-retest repeatability[39] with submaximal contractions more reliable than maximal contractions.[40] Skin displacement under the recoding site may introduce movement artifact, which can be minimized by securing the electrodes to the skin with tape. To improve interday reliability, electrode placement should be marked (with ink) and standardized electrodes used. When both recording electrodes are contained in the same housing, interelectrode distance is standardized and movement artifact attenuated. Advantages to using surface electrodes include improved reliability and the ease with which they can be applied without causing patient discomfort.[36-38] Specialized licensure is not required.

Instrumentation for KEMG Acquisition

KEMG signal acquisition requires either a telemetry unit (FM modulation) or a hard wire system that relies on a "cable" tethered to the subject to transmit signals from the electrode site to the receiver. The subject's performance and nature of movement strategies performed may be altered by the cabling. Telemetry allows the subject unrestricted movement; KEMG signals are transmitted through the air from a small unit worn around the subject's waist. The optimal characteristics of the receiver include a bandwidth frequency between 40 and 1,000 Hz and an overall gain of 1,000 Hz.[33]

Signal Processing. KEMG processing has become highly automated with the advent of high-speed computers and customized software programs. Once the signal is acquired, it is stored digitally and processed by various software programs. The "raw" signal is full wave rectified (all the negative values become positive) and a linear envelope generated within a designated time interval. The area under the curve is mathematically integrated and an average EMG profile is generated. Muscle-specific onset, cessation, and the relative intensity are defined with a variety of software programs. According to a recent study, KEMG timing (onset and cessation) is optimally identified by using the intensity filtered average (IFA) and packet analysis (PAC) when compared with ensemble average (EAV).[41] Despite a smaller recording volume with wires, Bogey et al[41] demonstrated no significant difference in signal amplitude when multiple insertion sites within the same muscle were compared.

Normalization. Any acquired "raw" EMG signal needs to be referenced to a standard value. This is accomplished by dividing the raw EMG during a functional task such as walking by a reference value. A maximal voluntary contraction (MVC) serves this purpose. Subjects exert a maximal voluntary effort for each muscle that determines the maximal EMG activity possible. All subsequent efforts are compared with this maximal effort and expressed as a percentage of maximum (%MVC). In patients with neurological dysfunction who lack selective motor control, a maximal effort can be elicited in either an extensor or flexor synergy by using the Upright Motor Control Test (UMC) developed at Rancho Los Amigos National Rehabilitation Center, grading the effort as "weak," "moderate," or "strong" in synergy.[42] Maximal efforts are elicited for 3 to 5 seconds and the software determines the maximal activity for a 1-second interval. The muscles activation during a functional activity is subsequently expressed as a percentage of MVC.

Interpretation of KEMG
Kinesiological EMG and Strength. KEMG testing does not directly measure muscle strength and the examiner should resist equating raw EMG signal amplitude directly with muscle force or torque output. Grading the strength (MMT or UMC) of each maximal effort must accompany the interpretation of the muscle participation during a functional task.[43] For example, patients with postpolio syndrome produce large-amplitude KEMG signals that often reflect the maximal exertion of a "weak" muscle (i.e., "MMT-Poor" or 2/5). Large-amplitude EMG signals represent activation of large motor units typical of reinnervation, not force output. Despite large-amplitude signals the muscle is functionally weak. In other words, a 100% MVC normalized KEMG record for a muscle may represent the maximal effort of a "poor or 2/5" muscle.

Muscle Tone versus Spasticity. Therapists should resist making inferences about *tone* from KEMG testing. As previously stated, KEMG reflects the contractile activity of motor units. Muscle tone refers to the amount of *resting* tension in a muscle because of its viscoelastic properties. Because tone is not a function of motor unit activity, it cannot be measured with KEMG.[33] In contrast, spasticity, defined as a hyperactive quick stretch response, can be recorded by KEMG because it reflects prolonged muscle activation (>0.1 seconds). Clonus has a distinct frequency characterized by a prolonged 5- to 8-Hz signal. Using signal duration in response to quick stretch, Cahan et al[44] identified significant decreases in spasticity in selected lower extremity muscles in children with cerebral palsy after selec-

tive dorsal rhizotomy. In these children spasticity interfered with agonist activation during walking.

In conclusion, KEMG is useful for delineating patterns of muscle activation in motor performance, reflecting the integrity of the neuromuscular control mechanism. The examiner's interpretation should also consider additional factors such as the type of contraction; speed of movement; joint acceleration; and a host of physiological, biomechanical, anatomical, and neurological elements beyond the scope of this chapter.

ELECTRICAL STIMULATION AND ELECTROMYOGRAPHIC BIOFEEDBACK

NEMS and, to a much lesser extent, EMS, are often used as tools in the management of neurological dysfunction. EMGBF is also used both alone and in conjunction with stimulation. The primary goal of use is improvement of function by improving voluntary motor control. To that end, strengthening and alteration of abnormal tone are also common goals of treatment. EMGBF is discussed later in this chapter. More detailed explication of treatment protocols is included in a variety of published work.[45-53]

Electrical stimulators may be either small, portable, battery-operated units or larger line-powered clinical instruments. The clinical units often will offer a variety of stimulus forms and options for modulation of currents. Portable units provide the ability for patients and caregivers to carry out prescribed stimulation at home. Clinical units allow the therapist to customize programs. The major difference between the two types of instruments is that battery-operated units may not provide the degree of power necessary to provide higher contractile forces when the goal is strengthening.[54] In many functional applications, however, strength is not the most important factor. Timing, endurance, and learning during the activity are more often paramount, and these situations do not require high levels of stimulation.

Parameters of Stimulation

Four parameters must be considered when applying therapeutic electrical stimulation: waveform, pulse (or phase) duration, pulse frequency, and pulse amplitude. Instruments are available that allow all of these to be independently adjusted. Other instruments may be less versatile. Modulation of the parameters are commonly used to enhance the effectiveness of the stimulation.

Waveform
The waveform of the stimulus produced by most NMES units is either a symmetrical or an asymmetrical biphasic pulse. The two phases of each pulse continually alternate in direction between positive and negative polarity. Some stimulators use a monophasic waveform. Although an ideal waveform has not been identified, most studies have shown the symmetrical biphasic waveform to be more comfortable than either the asymmetrical biphasic or the monophasic waveform.[45,55,56]

Duration
Stimulators with a phase duration of 1 to 300 μs (0.3 ms) can be used to activate muscles with intact innervation. A set duration of 300 μs has been reported as preferred

compared with shorter durations.[57,58] Shorter-duration waveforms require a greater current amplitude to produce a muscle contraction. They may be more comfortable but may not possess the charge needed for good contraction levels. Longer-phase durations may be used but are less comfortable. Denervated muscles require significantly longer phase durations (20 to 100 ms) because of the longer chronaxy of muscle cells compared with motor neurons.

Frequency

In applications seeking to provide muscle contraction, the stimulus rate should be at least 30 pps. This is a typical critical frequency at which a muscle will respond with a smooth contraction. In most applications a frequency of 50 pps is used. Higher frequencies than this can result in early onset of fatigue.

Amplitude

The amplitude (intensity) of the stimulus should be sufficient to achieve the desired strength of contraction. In line-operated units the intensity is typically measured in milliampules. Battery-operated units usually indicate the amplitude only in a relative way (nonquantitatively) because the output of the battery declines over time. Depending on the impedance of the electrodes, coupling agent, skin and soft tissue, the amount of current required at one location could be quite different than another to produce the same degree of muscle contraction. The client is usually asked to participate in the contraction during stimulation. The amplitude of stimulation should be graded based on the response of the patient, aiming at production of the clinically desired force output. In all situations, muscle fatigue should be avoided or minimized.

Electrical Muscle Stimulation

Electrical stimulation of denervated muscle is one of the oldest medical applications of electricity. A denervated muscle that is still viable will respond to stimulation if an adequate stimulus is used. As previously noted, muscle cells have a much longer chronaxy than do neurons. Innervated muscles contract when their motor neurons are depolarized with pulses of microseconds in duration. A pulse duration of at least 20 to 100 ms is required to produce responses in denervated muscle.[4,59] Many commonly used stimulators are not designed to administer pulses of that duration.

For clients with PNS dysfunction (e.g., peripheral nerve injuries or peripheral neuropathy), EMS may be helpful in preserving the contractility and extensibility of denervated muscle tissue and retarding muscle atrophy.[60-62] EMS will not prevent denervation atrophy and eventual death of the muscle cells if they are not reinnervated. Many animal studies[63-65] and a few in human beings[66-68] have demonstrated that electrical stimulation enhances nutrition, reduces (not prevents) muscle atrophy, and assists in maintaining the ROM and contractile properties of muscle. The goal of EMS, then, is to keep muscle tissue healthier and viable until reinnervation is established. Electrical stimulation does not hasten regeneration of injured nerve tissue.

In opposition are studies reporting that EMS may have the detrimental effect of retarding reinnervation at the terminal endplate and neuromuscular junction.[69,70] In addition, the time and cost of treatment are major factors because

regrowth of motor neurons at the rate of 1.5 to 2.0 mm/day dictates a recovery period of months or even 1 to 2 years. EMS has been used in cases of anterior horn cell pathology; however, a randomized placebo-controlled study in which 6 to 12 months of electrical stimulation was administered to muscles of children with spinal muscular atrophy resulted in no significant effect on quantitative myometry, manual muscle testing, excitable muscle mass (M-wave amplitudes), or function.[71]

If proceeding with EMS is chosen, pulse durations should be set at 20 to 100 ms and frequency at 10 to 30 pps. Bouts of five to 20 stimulations to each involved muscle should be followed by a rest time longer than the stimulation time (on-off time ratio of no less than 1:5). The bouts should be repeated two to three times a day. The intensity should be a strong muscle contraction (not maximal). If prognosis for regeneration is good and the blood supply is viable, EMS may be useful in maintaining optimal conditions of blood flow, nutrition, and muscle tissue contractility, so that if and when regeneration occurs, return of motor activation and function may be facilitated. The stimulation should be done at home with portable EMS units as a supplement to a carefully planned home exercise program.

Neuromuscular Electrical Stimulation

In NMES, muscle contraction is elicited by depolarization of the motor neurons. Electrodes may be placed over the muscle to be stimulated or over the motor nerve that controls the muscle. Firing order of neurons is a result of neuronal size, proximity of the electrical stimulus, and the intensity of stimulation.[72] Muscle recruitment patterns triggered by electrical stimulation differ from those observed in normal muscle activation. In a voluntary muscle contraction, motor units fire asynchronously, with a larger proportion of type I, fatigue-resistant muscle fibers of the smaller motor units being recruited first. The order of muscle fiber firing occurs as a result of motor neuron size and the anatomy of synaptic connections.[73] Conversely, an electrically stimulated muscle contraction elicits initial responses from larger motor units, which contain a greater number of fatigable, type II muscle fibers. The type II fibers are innervated by larger-diameter neurons that have a lower threshold for electrical stimulation than smaller neurons.[74] A study of healthy subjects demonstrated recruitment of these higher threshold motor units at relatively low NMES training levels. In voluntary exercise a much greater exercise intensity is required for activation of these larger motor units.[74]

Synchronous recruitment of muscle fibers is obtained with electrical stimulation. This does not occur with volitional activation. During a sustained volitional contraction motor units periodically "drop out" and then "drop in" to reduce fatigue. With NMES, once recruited the motor units will continue to fire until the stimulus is ended. This, coupled with the early recruitment of fatigable motor units, accounts for fatigue being a major problem in the use of NMES. It also is one reason functional activities performed under control by stimulation are much less smooth and balanced than when they are performed volitionally. At the same time, relatively low levels of NMES can recruit motor units that volitionally would be recruited only with maximal effort. This provides support for observed increases in strength with low NMES training intensities.[75] Numerous potential benefits are identified for NMES. Among them are improvement in ROM, edema reduction, treatment of disuse atrophy, and improvement of muscle recruitment for muscle reeducation.[48]

A pulse duration of 200 to 300 µs is typically preferred in NMES.[57,58] The stimulus frequency should be set at a rate sufficient to produce a smooth, sustained (tetanic) muscle contraction. Although this varies with different muscles, a frequency of 30 to 50 pps is usually effective, although lower frequencies may be used if a satisfactory contraction is obtained.[2] As previously noted, higher frequencies have the potential of causing early fatigue. During application, the amplitude of the stimulus is gradually increased until the desired strength of contraction is obtained. The client is typically asked to contract the muscle(s) in synchrony with the stimulation.

Modulations

In addition to the parameters of the basic individual stimulus pulses (e.g., waveform, phase and pulse duration, pulse frequency, and amplitude), several modulations are necessary to enhance the effectiveness of the NMES program. The stimulus is applied in a repetitive "train" of pulses, which can be periodically interrupted or turned on and off in rhythmical bursts or cycles, ramped, and delivered with preset duty cycles.

On Time and Off Time. NMES for facilitation of muscle contraction should be used to supplement exercise, and goals for stimulation should be consistent with the goals of the exercise program. To simulate isotonic or isometric muscle contractions, as in voluntary movement for exercise, the stimulator must have the capability of setting bursts (cycles of on and off times). Each period of muscle contraction is followed by a period of relaxation (Figure 31-3).[2,48] In most cases, a shorter on time than off time is desirable to avoid fatigue. For example, a 5-second on time may be followed by a 25-second off time in a cycle, resulting in an on-off ratio of 1:5. Packman-Braun[76] investigated ratios of stimulation to rest time with NMES for wrist extension in a group of hemiplegic patients. Results supported the on-off time of 1:5 as being the most beneficial in training programs of 20 to 30 minutes because of the deleterious

effects of fatigue with lower ratios (1:1, 1:2, 1:3, 1:4). If the goal is to reduce edema by providing a muscle pumping action, a ratio of 1:1 or 1:2 may be preferred.[76]

Ramping. Ramping is another modulation that can be set by the therapist. Ramp-up is the time it takes each train of pulses to increase amplitude or intensity sequentially from zero to maximum. Ramp-off is the period set at the end of the train of maximal intensity pulses to decrease sequentially from maximum to zero amplitude (see Figure 31-3). Ramp time can be adjusted so that the stimulation more nearly resembles a pattern of gradually contracting and relaxing muscles. For clients with hypertonicity or spasticity and a goal of facilitation and strengthening the antagonist muscle, a longer ramp-up time may avoid or minimize activation of the stretch reflex in the hyperactive agonist muscle. Shorter ramp times may be effective when the goal is to increase ROM or decrease edema.

Duty Cycle. The term *duty cycle* is sometimes confused with the on-off time ratio. Duty cycle is the percentage of time a series or train of pulses is on out of the total on and off time in a cycle.[2,45] For example, if the train of pulses is on 10 seconds and off 30 seconds, the total cycle time is 40 seconds. The duty cycle would be 25% (10 seconds of the total 40-second cycle). The actual on time and off time of the pulses in a cycle is a more informative description than either the duty cycle or the on-off ratio.

Muscle Reeducation

After an insult or injury affecting the CNS, problems with motor control are frequently manifested. One of the common goals of therapy is to facilitate movement in the areas where control is lacking. If active movement is not present, NMES allows movement to occur by stimulation, which may be followed by resumption of active movement, possibly triggered by the proprioceptive and sensory experience that accompanies the stimulation. When active movement is present but is weak or not well controlled, the therapist may choose to use NMES to supplement and strengthen the muscular contraction already present. Some evidence exists that NMES can increase activity in the somatosensory cortex and that the cortical activity is corre-

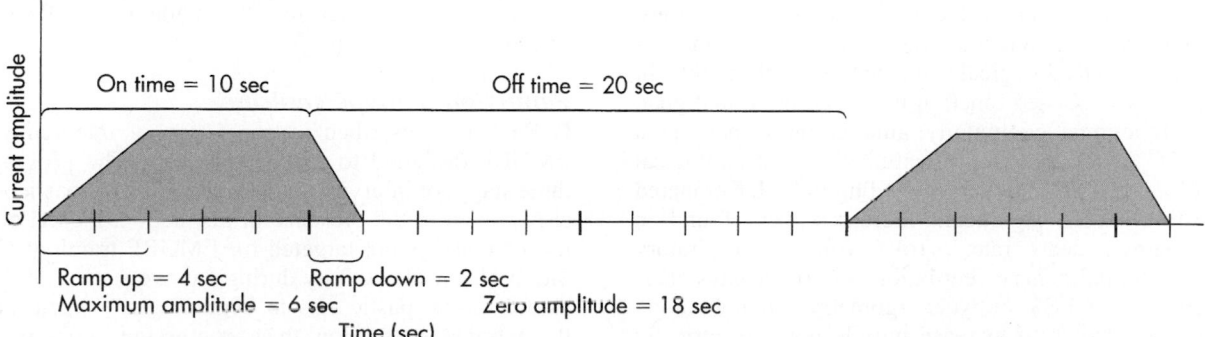

FIGURE 31-3 ■ Example of the relation between ramp times and on/off times. Each division on the horizontal axis equals 2 seconds. Note that the ramp-up time is considered part of the on time, whereas the ramp-down time is considered part of the off time. (Reprinted from DeVahl J: NMES in rehabilitation. In Gersh MR, editor: *Electrotherapy in Rehabilitation.* Philadelphia, 1992, FA Davis.)

lated with improvement in functional tasks.[77] In the presence of hypertonicity, the muscles serving as antagonists to the spastic muscle may be targeted for NMES, not only to strengthen the antagonist but to inhibit the spastic muscle by reciprocal inhibition.

Functional Electrical Stimulation

The term *functional electrical stimulation* (FES) has been used casually to describe various applications of NMES. However, FES is defined by the Electrotherapy Standards Committee of the Section on Clinical Electrophysiology as the use of NMES (on innervated muscles) for orthotic substitution.[2] Baker and Parker[78] use the term to describe external control of innervated, paretic, or paralytic muscles "to achieve functional and purposeful movements." Although NMES is generally considered to have therapeutic applications, such as increasing ROM, facilitation of muscle activation, and muscle strengthening, the key to application of FES is to enhance or facilitate functional control. It is used with clients with spinal cord injury (SCI), traumatic brain injury (TBI), cerebrovascular accident (CVA), and other CNS dysfunction who have intact peripheral innervation.

An example of FES application is the electrical stimulation of the peroneal nerve to enhance ankle dorsiflexion during gait in patients with hemiplegia.[79] Numerous other uses of FES have been described, ranging from isolated motor control activities, such as decreasing shoulder subluxation and reduction of scoliosis, to highly technical computerized gait and bicycling capabilities, sometimes referred to as computerized FES (CFES).[80-88] The trigger that activates muscle contraction in synchrony with the functional activity can be manually initiated by the client, set within the stimulator to automatically trigger on and off cycles, or programmed into a complex computer system for bicycling or gait.

Stimulation is generally applied in short-duration pulses with a frequency sufficient to provide smooth, tetanizing muscle contractions and adjusted to cycle on and off, with adequate ramp functions, as indicated by the speed and time needed to synchronize the stimulation with the functional activity. The length of the intervention depends on the purpose and may vary from a few contractions during the functional activity, building to multiple 30-minute sessions working up to several hours, repeated daily or three to five times per week. With the more complex computerized systems used with clients with complete spinal cord lesions, electrically activated functional movements are the mechanism to achieve physiological and psychological benefits. In some situations, assisted function is also an important goal, although functional community ambulation is not yet a reality.[84,86,89-96] Hooker et al[90] evaluated the physiological effects of use of FES-assisted leg cycling in SCI. Compared with resting levels, significant increases were found in cardiac output, heart rate, stroke volume, respiratory exchange rate, pulmonary ventilation, and other physiological phenomena. CFES for cycle ergometry and ambulation has also been shown to increase muscle mass, electrically induce muscle strength and endurance,[85,97,98] increase circulation and aerobic capacity, decrease edema, and have a beneficial impact on self-image.[86,98,99] Jacobs et al[96] compared the metabolic stress of FES-assisted standing versus frame supported standing. Cardiorespiratory stress was signifi-

cantly higher with FES, and the authors concluded that FES-assisted standing alone may provide a stress sufficient to meet minimal requirements for exercise conditioning.

The demonstrated benefits of FES clearly indicate that it is a valuable tool for supplementing functional activities. The practicality and cost of applications of the more complex computerized systems need further study, especially in terms of function in community activities.

Electromyographic Biofeedback

Biofeedback is a general term used to describe the use of visual or auditory representation of physiological processes to allow an individual to modify those processes. EMGBF makes available to the client information regarding the electrical activity of muscle. EMGBF has several well-documented applications, including alteration of physiological responses such as heart rate, temperature, and muscle tension.[46] These applications may prove beneficial for clients with neurological dysfunction. An example would be relaxation to modify pain perception. The focus of this review is the use of EMGBF for improvement of active movement, which may include hypertonicity reduction in addition to muscle reeducation. EMGBF units range from basic single-channel portable models to clinical units with multiple channels and multiple options for provision of feedback.

EMGBF may be used to assist a client in attaining greater levels of muscle activation in paretic muscle, decrease levels of muscle activation in spastic muscle, or attain a balance between agonist and antagonist muscle pairs.[100] For most practicing clinicians, EMG levels are monitored through the use of surface electrodes. Monitoring of activation of deep muscles is often not feasible. Attention to size and specific electrode placement is critical to ensure feedback that will be useful. Smaller electrodes allow specific placement, although higher impedance will be encountered. Skin must be carefully prepared to take this into account.[101] Because the EMG information recorded represents the sum of action potentials from motor units between the electrodes, large interelectrode distance will increase the area of muscle recorded. This may be desirable for large muscle groups or when minimal activity is present.

Smaller interelectrode distances are preferable if interference from "crosstalk" or "volume conduction" from muscles or motor units not part of the target group is a risk. Basmajian and Blumenstein[101] provide an excellent review of electrode placements.

Reduction of Hypertonicity

DeBacher[102] described a progression of intervention with EMGBF designed to reduce spasticity. The program uses three stages of intervention: (1) relaxation of spastic muscles at rest even in the presence of distraction, mental effort, or use of muscles not targeted for EMGBF training; (2) inhibition of muscle activity during passive static and dynamic stretch of the spastic muscle, beginning with static stretch at the extremes of motion, then progressing to passive movement speed at a speed of 15 degrees/sec; and (3) isometric contractions of the antagonist to the spastic muscle, with relaxation of the spastic muscle, progressing to prompt muscle contraction and relaxation of the spastic muscle, and grading of muscle contractions with movement for various force output requirements. Use of the technique in a small sample of young adults with cerebral palsy demonstrated improvement in resting levels of involuntary muscle activity.[103] Improvements in function, however, were not demonstrated.

Inhibition of a spastic muscle alone may not be enough to improve function. Weak antagonists to the affected muscle may contribute to the functional limitation. EMGBF to reinforce activity in the weak muscle may be done concurrently with its use to modify the tone in the agonist.[104] EMGBF can be useful in helping a client decrease abnormal muscle activation, but persistence of control problems may be related to lack of force production, deficits in speed of muscle activation, and lack of reciprocal interaction of muscle groups.[105]

Muscle Reeducation

Therapists may opt to use biofeedback to provide information about the quality of the muscle contraction directly to the client. The client can then attempt to alter the contraction in accordance with guidelines provided by the therapist, whether the focus is to facilitate stronger contraction, decrease apparent hyperactivity, or modulate a balance of muscle activity during a functional task.

Concurrent assessment of muscle activity (CAMA) is an application of EMGBF in which the therapist uses biofeedback as an adjunct in evaluation of client response to therapeutic exercise.[106] In this procedure the therapist decides which muscle group(s) are desired for activation and adjusts the position of the client or the therapist intervention accordingly to get the correct responses. CAMA allows for the judgment of the effectiveness of a particular activity based on actual EMG responses rather than presumptions of what the intervention should cause. In a placebo-controlled study of hemiplegic patients the addition of EMGBF to hand exercises based on the Brunnstrom approach resulted in significant improvement in active ROM in those using biofeedback compared with sham.[107]

Several authors suggest the use of biofeedback signals from homologous extremity muscles as a model for what the hemiplegic client needs to alter muscle activity in a particular function.[108,109] This has been described as a "motor copy" and was compared with a more targeted training procedure. Indications showed that the motor copy resulted in better carryover in function than the comparison therapy in follow-up evaluations. A similar training study showed indications of benefits of the procedure, but the results were not statistically significant because of the small group size.[108] At least two studies support patterning or copying EMG from other muscles as a potentially useful tool for individuals with C4-7 SCI.[110,111] A meta-analysis that compared EMGBF with conventional physical therapy for upper-extremity function in individuals after stroke reviewed only six studies and concluded that neither approach was superior to the other.[112]

Feedback Considerations

EMGBF has the benefit of being provided simultaneously with the client's movement, consisting of accurate and objective information about muscle activity (given careful electrode application), and not requiring the same level of therapist skill as verbal feedback provision. EMGBF there-fore may be beneficial for clients with deficient sensory feedback systems. The frequency of feedback provision, however, may require close scrutiny by the therapist.

Experiments examining feedback frequency in the learning of motor tasks support the use of less than 100% relative frequency for the subject to learn the task. Feedback provided on every trial may improve performance but degrades learning in normal subjects.[113] In a study of stroke patients attempting a pursuit tracking task biofeedback was used for the experimental group (electrodes over the spastic biceps) while the control group performed the task without feedback.[114] Posttests revealed that the use of continuous feedback had a negative transfer effect on learning of the movement task, suggesting that the experimental learners became dependent on the external feedback in performance of the task. The clinician must therefore carefully structure the use of external feedback so the client begins to develop a sense of muscle activation or relaxation that is present without the EMGBF apparatus. This may be accomplished by turning the screen away from the client and turning off the auditory signal as the patient progresses.

Integrating Neuromuscular Electrical Stimulation and Electromyographic Biofeedback

The use of EMG-triggered NMES, in which NMES is initiated once the client achieves a predetermined level of EMG activity in the targeted muscles, is an application that has shown to have merit.[115,116] Threshold levels of EMG activity could gradually be increased as the client gains the ability to activate muscles independently, with eventual discontinuance of the NMES as strength and active control allow. The success of this application has been shown in patients with hemiplegia in terms of increasing EMG activity and subsequent improvement in ROM and function in the involved arm and leg.[115] In another study, patients who had a stroke more than 1 year previously significantly improved wrist and finger extension strength and function after treatment with EMG-triggered stimulation compared with control.[116]

A variation of this application is NMES triggered by positional feedback, such that NMES is initiated once the patient actively moves through a portion of the available ROM at a joint.[117] The therapist my set the threshold angle in accordance with the patient's goals and abilities. This method was effective in improving wrist motion after stroke, although it was not as effective in altering control of the knee in a similar patient group.[118]

Although discussions of EMGBF, EMS, FES, and NMES are often presented separately, the use of these modalities can be intertwined to achieve desired muscle control. Processes of clinical decision making are represented in Figure 31-4, beginning with a determination of whether the movement control problem is a result of a CNS or a PNS lesion. NMES or FES may be initiated in the absence of active control (although lower levels of muscle activation may be discovered and facilitated with EMGBF). Once return of active control begins EMGBF may be used to refine the control. An increase in muscle EMG should not be assumed to translate automatically to an improvement in functional use of that muscle in daily activities. Consequently, NMES and EMGBF need to be integrated into daily

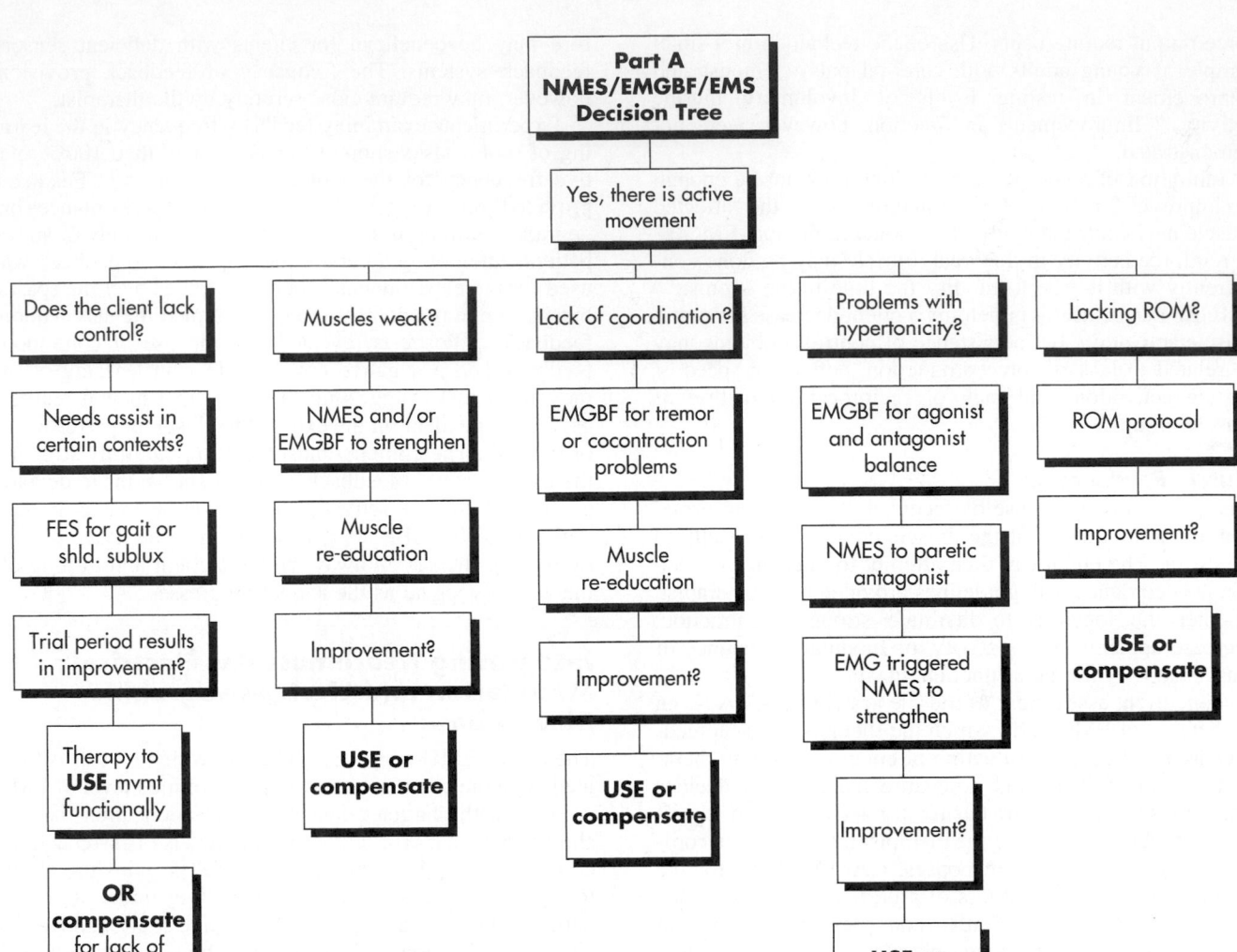

FIGURE 31-4 ■ **A,** Decision tree for clients that exhibit active movement in the targeted treatment area.

functional activities so that appropriate muscle activity is elicited and used in its appropriate functional context.

Applications

The application of the common principles of EMGBF and NMES to different patient populations emphasizes the role of the therapist in tailoring intervention to meet specific client needs. Many investigators have evaluated the use of NMES and EMGBF in clients with stroke.[104,119-121] FES has been used extensively with clients with SCI. Other populations that demonstrate neuromuscular impairment or dysfunction have not been as thoroughly studied. This may be because the heterogeneity of these groups may create difficulty in research design.

Wolf and Binder-Macleod[119] examined client characteristics that are critical to success with biofeedback training for upper- and lower-extremity control after stroke. In a group of 52 clients with stroke, no significant relations between outcome and age, sex, number of EMGBF treatments, or side of hemiparesis were found. Lower-extremity treatment

was associated with a greater probability of success, and this success did not seem related to chronicity of stroke sequelae. In contrast, success of upper-extremity treatment did appear to be related to length of time since onset of stroke, and poorer outcomes were noted if clients had received therapy to the involved arm for more than 1 year before EMGBF training. Improvements in elbow and shoulder function were obtained in this group of patients, but improvement in functional use of the hand was limited. Aphasia imposed a slight limitation to achieving improvement, but proprioceptive deficits were more significant in restricting functional gains. The role of client motivation in success with EMGBF training was emphasized. On follow-up over a 12-month period, the improvements made in the initial intervention were maintained in 33 of 34 clients evaluated.

A number of studies have been published discussing the muscle recruitment problems observed after CVA.[104,120,121] Knowledge of these problems is a prerequisite for determination of the appropriate application of EMGBF and NMES.

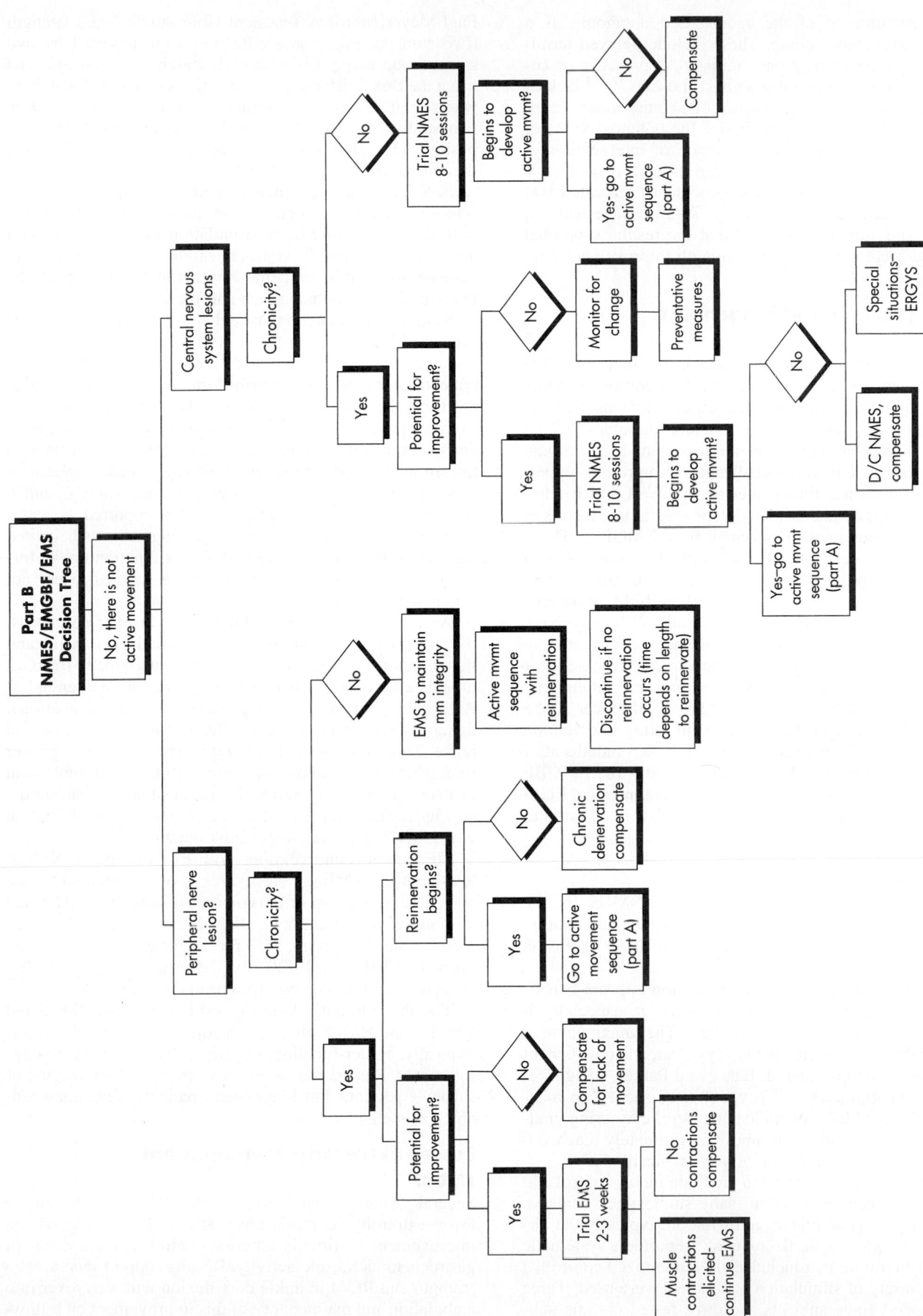

FIGURE 31-4, cont'd B, Decision tree for clients not yet demonstrating active movement as a result of peripheral nerve injury or CNS insult.

Delayed recruitment of the agonist and antagonist is a relatively consistent finding. These include delayed termination of muscle activity once initiated,[122] presence of co-contraction of agonist and antagonist muscles,[120,121] lack of co-contraction,[104] and maintenance of agonist muscle contractions.[120] These reports emphasize the potential value of EMGBF in determining the best mode of intervention. A meta-analysis of electrical stimulation and recovery of strength after stroke (four studies included) indicated that stimulation caused a statistically significant effect on strength. The authors concluded that the results supported use of electrical stimulation for strength improvement after stroke.

Upper Extremity Management

EMGBF

EMGBF has been extensively studied, but success of the treatment is mixed, with difficulty in interpretation. A reduction in co-contraction has been observed,[123] as well as improvement in several neuromuscular variables[119,124,125]; however, a lack of significant improvement in functional skill was noted. Given the challenge of improving upper-extremity functional ability after stroke, Wolf and Binder-Macleod[125] suggested consideration of several key factors in predicting which clients may benefit from EMGBF, "Those patients who achieve the most substantial improvement in manipulative abilities initially possess voluntary finger extension; comparatively greater active ROM about the shoulder, elbow, and wrist; and comparatively less hyperactivity in muscles usually considered as major contributors to the typical flexor synergy." Attention to the chronicity of motor dysfunction also appears critical in anticipating success with EMGBF, as clients 2 to 3 months after stroke demonstrated stronger functional gains after intervention with biofeedback compared with clients 4 to 5 months after stroke. A recent placebo-controlled study of EMGBF showed statistically significant improvement in active ROM of the hand in clients who received EMGBF in addition to exercise.[107]

NMES

Common upper-extremity applications of NMES for the stroke patient include reduction of shoulder subluxation (FES) and facilitation of elbow, wrist, and finger extension and motor control.

FES for shoulder subluxation reduction appears beneficial for prevention of pain and subluxation, especially if used during the early stages of recovery. The functional benefits over the long term are not always clear, and cost-benefit ratios need to be considered. Baker and Parker,[78] Faghri et al,[81] and Chantraine et al[126] have reported success in management of shoulder subluxation after stroke by using gradually increasing stimulation times that ultimately reached 6 to 7 hours per day. On-off ratios were typically 1:3.

Use of NMES after stroke to facilitate motor control and function has been studied, but many studies lack controls. The extensors of the fingers and wrist are typically the targeted muscle groups. de Kroon et al[53] reported a systematic review of literature that included six randomized controlled trials. A variety of stimulation parameters were used. Three studies tested acute subjects and three tested chronic subjects. Outcome measures for motor control included the Fugl-Meyer Motor Assessment (four studies) and strength (two studies). Functional outcomes were reported by two studies, one using the Action Research Arm test and one using the Box & Block test. The authors concluded that there was a positive effect of stimulation on motor control. Only two studies reported functional outcomes, but both were positive. Of significance is the fact that only six studies met the criteria for review in terms of rigor.[115-117,127-129]

FES has also been investigated as an upper-extremity orthosis after hemiplegia, using movement of the uninvolved shoulder to trigger stimulation of elbow extension and hand opening.[130] After an extensive training period, patients were able to demonstrate functional use of the involved hand for basic reach and grasp.

Systems with more than two channels of stimulation have proved difficult for patients to use.[131] Popovic et al[132] reported two studies in which they used NMES to treat patients after stroke. They termed the intervention functional electrical therapy (FET). The stimulation is used during an exercise program composed of voluntary arm movements and opening and closing, holding and releasing objects with the stimulation serving as an electric prosthesis. Treatment was 30 minutes daily for 3 weeks in one study[132] and 6 months in the other.[133] Outcomes were reported as better than controls. Initially higher functioning subjects benefited more than those who were rated as low functioning. Unfortunately, outcome measures in these studies were not standardized.

A study of use of daily NMES in the form of neuroprosthetic FES (NESS Handmaster) stimulation of hand and finger extensors in patients with subacute strokes (6 to 12 months after onset) was reported by Ring and Rosenthal.[134] All subjects were receiving physical and occupational therapy three times a week. The stimulator was used at home. Those receiving stimulation had significantly greater improvements in spasticity, active ROM, and functional hand test scores compared with control subjects. The authors concluded that supplementation of outpatient rehabilitation with NMES improves upper limb outcomes.[134]

Three-month interventions with EMG-triggered NMES, low-intensity NMES, PNF exercise, or no treatment were compared in a group of chronic stroke patients.[135] At 3 and 9 months after treatment, Fugl-Meyer scores improved 18% for the PNF group, 25% for the patients receiving low-intensity NMES, and 42% for the group receiving EMG-triggered NMES. The control group did not change.

The above findings lend support to the use of NMES and ENGBF and NMES alone as an adjunct to physical therapy. Typically, higher-functioning patients have shown the greatest impact. Results tended to show greater effect in acute or subacute patients, but longer-term patients sometimes benefited as well.

Lower-Extremity Management

EMGBF

Several studies evaluating EMGBF for retraining lower-extremity control after stroke have focused on improvement of tibialis anterior control and reduction of gastrocnemius muscle activity. Results support increases in strength and ROM in ankle dorsiflexion with carryover into ambulation and maintenance of this improvement on follow-up evaluation.[136-138]

Wolf and Binder-Macleod[119] examined a number of variables at the hip, knee, and ankle in a controlled group study of the effects of EMGBF. Subjects were assigned to one of four groups: lower-extremity FMGBF, upper-extremity EMGBF, general relaxation training, and no treatment. No significant changes were observed between experimental and control groups for EMG levels and ROM at the hip, but improvements were noted in knee and ankle active motion for the experimental group. Although subjects in the experimental group increased their gait speed, these changes were not significantly different from the comparison groups.

Use of EMGBF with the intent of improving ambulation may require use of feedback during the task of ambulation instead of during static activity, as demonstrated by this study. Positional biofeedback regarding ankle position and traditional EMGBF were compared in a group of hemiplegic subjects.[139] A computerized system provided audiovisual feedback during ambulation for both groups. Pretreatment and posttreatment measures of ankle motion, gait, and perceived exertion were conducted for the two treatment groups and a control group. The group receiving positional feedback increased walking speeds relative to the other groups, with improvements maintained at follow-up intervals of up to 3 months. The consideration of integrating feedback into functional ambulation bears further investigation.

Neuromuscular Electrical Stimulation

Peroneal nerve stimulation has been documented as an assistance for patients with hemiplegia to improve ambulation.[79,140-142] Long-term stimulation with implanted electrodes has proved effective in improving gait patterns, but difficulties in achieving balanced dorsiflexion, infection, and equipment maintenance were drawbacks.[142,143]

Shorter-term use of peroneal nerve stimulation as an adjunct to traditional physical therapy may be considered. In a controlled study examining the use of 20 minutes of peroneal nerve stimulation six times per week for 4 weeks, the stimulated group demonstrated dorsiflexion recovery three times greater than the control group, as measured by an average of 10 maximal dorsiflexion contractions. These improvements were regardless of site of lesion, age, or time since lesion.[140] Surface electrode stimulation is effective and gait parameters can be improved with its use.[144,145] If, however, a foot drop is the only major impediment to ambulation, lightweight plastic orthoses are a functional and much less expensive choice of intervention.

Multichannel electrical stimulation has been used in the management of ambulation in patients with stroke.[135,146-149] Although more effective than traditional gait training in some cases in terms of gait velocity and stride length, at follow-up evaluations 8 to 9 months after therapy the difference between groups had faded. However, the expense and availability of such systems make their use unlikely at this time.

NMES used for ankle dorsiflexion triggered by heel switch during gait and biofeedback to improve active recruitment of ankle dorsiflexors or relaxation of ankle plantar flexors was studied in hemiplegic clients.[150] Those patients who received a combination of these interventions demonstrated significantly improved knee and ankle range parameters more rapidly than those using a single modality. This improvement was maintained over a 1-month period.

Although all groups improved in gait cycle times, the combined group was better. This may be attributable to the synergy of biofeedback and stimulation.[43] Granat et al[151] also studied peroneal muscle stimulation effects on gait parameters after stroke. After intervention the subjects showed significant control of eversion on all surfaces. The Barthel Index score also improved after intervention. However, no improvement occurred when the patients were not using the stimulator.

Evidence-Based Practice

Much of the literature evaluating the use of EMGBF and NMES involves patients with CVA. Although these studies have shown many significant results, interpretation of these findings with relation to what is recommended for clinical intervention is not as clear cut. Improvements in generation of EMG activity and active movement are well documented, but the functional implications of these gains are not as well established. Clearly, in the current practice environment much of the focus is on function, so these techniques to improve muscle activation patterns must be put to functional use in the context of therapy. The therapist must consider the relevant factors that may predict success and critically evaluate outcomes during trial use of these modalities. Cost-benefit analyses must accompany any intervention using technology with the goal of regaining movement as quickly as possible and eliminating the use of equipment when practical.

Spinal Cord Injury

NMES has a variety of applications for clients who have sustained SCI. Muscle strengthening may occur for muscles innervated by segments just above a complete SCI, or a variety of strengthening applications may be appropriate in the case of incomplete SCI. EMGBF may be used to identify muscle activity in weak musculature, as a tool to judge improvement in muscle activation, and as a method of facilitating increased strength.[152] Applications of EMGBF for individuals with SCI also include facilitation of unassisted ventilation in high-level quadriplegia[153] and use of biofeedback for muscle reeducation with incomplete SCI in the acute stages when immobilization may be required.[154]

The use of NMES, EMGBF, and other physical therapy was examined in a group of clients with incomplete cervical SCIs over a total treatment period of 16 weeks. Clients were randomly assigned to one of four groups receiving either physical exercise, NMES, or EMGBF. Group 1 received EMGBF followed by physical exercise, group 2 received EMGBF followed by NMES, group 3 received NMES followed by physical exercise, and group 4 received 16 weeks of exercise only. Measurements of muscle strength, self-care ratings, mobility scores, and voluntary EMG were conducted at baseline, treatment midpoint, and conclusion of all interventions. All groups demonstrated improvement across the treatment period on all measures except voluntary EMG; however, no significant differences were seen among the four groups.[155] At least one other study compared conventional intervention, EMGBF, electrical stimulation, and combined stimulation with biofeedback over a 6-week period in individuals with quadriplegia. An examiner who was blinded to the intervention protocol evaluated 45 subjects in the four treatment groups. All groups improved in the parameters evaluated, and no significant difference between groups was noted.[156] These results again emphasize the need to consider carefully cost as well as time and effort for setup and equipment operation in intervention planning.

Upper-Extremity Management

The use of electrically stimulated hand orthotic systems for patients with C6 or higher-level SCI have been refined to allow greater functional independence for a select group of patients.[92,93,111,157-160] Because hand function does not occur in a cyclical pattern, the onset and termination of stimulation must be controlled by the patient in some manner, with a myoelectric or contact closing switch.[92] Multichannel stimulation is then applied with intramuscular electrodes for the flexors and extensors of the fingers and thumb, with computer-configured interplay between the different muscles to achieve a functional grasp. A chest-mounted position transducer (operated by shoulder elevation or depression and protraction or retraction) allows the user to initiate stimulation and lock the stimulation to maintain a grasp as well as unlock it for release. A toggle switch mounted on the chest allows a choice between electronically stimulated lateral or palmar grasp patterns.[93,157] Some investigators have used contralateral shoulder slings as well as elbow accelerometers to trigger the needed stimulation.[161,162] Multiple authors have described successful implantation and utilization, with a few drawbacks, of upper-extremity FES prostheses.[163-166] Use of this type of system may allow patients with SCI at the C5 level to operate at the same or even higher level of independence as those with C6 quadriplegia with tenodesis, gaining the ability to perform more activities of daily living (ADLs) without an attendant. Patients with SCI at the C6 level may be able to manipulate a greater variety of objects without special adaptations.

Lower-Extremity Management

Standing. In an excellent review of the use of FES for the purpose of standing patients with SCI, Gardner and Baker[167] described the easiest approach to stimulating the quadriceps femoris to allow paraplegic clients to stand. More complex systems may incorporate stimulation of the gluteus maximus, gluteus medius, hamstring, adductor magnus, gastrocnemius, and soleus muscles for longer-duration and better-quality standing performance. Multichannel surface and implantable systems have been and continue to be developed for assistance in sit-stand and transfer activities.[168-170] Surgical procedures, client selection, and technology are also factors cited in successful interventions. Despite these efforts, the duration of standing with electrically stimulated systems ranges from a few minutes to several hours. The client with SCI may be able to use this technology to perform functional activities that require standing. The use of these systems depends on the functions unavailable to a client without use of the technology, and the ease with which a system can be used and maintained. Peripheral to, but no less important, are the reactions of joints to these interventions. Two studies[170a,170b] have reported positive benefits to the structure and functions of lower-extremity joints of adolescents with SCI after participating in FES programs. A recent study has also identified that the physiological responses to standing in SCI may

provide a cardiorespiratory stress sufficient to meet minimal requirements for exercise conditioning.[96]

Cycling. The use of systems to stimulate reciprocal lower limb motions electrically has increased for stationary cycling. The benefits of these interventions for the client with SCI may relate to prevention of cardiovascular disease in the wheelchair-dependent client. Physiological changes noted with electrically stimulated cycling include improvement of peripheral muscular and cardiovascular fitness, as demonstrated by increased power output after training with leg cycle ergometry.[81,90,91,97,98] Combining FES and lower-extremity cycling with upper-extremity ergometry induced a higher level of cardiovascular fitness than lower-extremity ergometry alone.[171] Exercise session frequency as little as two times a week induced positive changes in cardiovascular fitness.[172] When testing of clients with paraplegia or quadriplegia is conducted with arm crank ergometry after a training program with electrically stimulated leg cycle ergometry, clients do not demonstrate differences in pretest and posttest measures of hemodynamic and pulmonary responses. These findings may relate to the specificity of the leg exercise training or the presence of a peripheral rather than a central circulatory response to the training procedure.[91] As previously noted, many cardiovascular factors can be improved and retained for at least 8 weeks after a program of FES ergometry.

Ambulation. As technology continues to progress, the use of electrically stimulated systems for ambulation may become more practical and useful for the patient with SCI.[94,173,174] Acceptance and use of the systems by clients outside the clinic have been mixed but shown to have positive effects on characteristics of ambulation.[143,175] Improvements in functional applications and use will also take place as the ability to select appropriate candidates improves.[176,177] Benefits of these systems may include increased muscle bulk, a reduced risk of pressure sores and osteoporosis, and psychological benefit. Generally, improvements in functional ability are expected to produce positive psychological factors. Addressing these factors directly, Bradley,[178] in a study measuring the effects of participation in an FES program on the affect of 37 individuals with SCI, demonstrated that positive affect was not significantly altered. Significant changes in negative affect occurred, however, with particular items of hostility and depression evident in those individuals in the treatment group who had unrealistic expectations. The author noted that these individuals need to be identified and monitored through the course of rehabilitation. Other drawbacks relate to the expense of the equipment and personnel and the lack of long-term efficacy studies. The speed with which a client with a complete SCI is able to walk with electrically stimulated systems remains relatively low (2 to 54 m/min) compared with normal rates of 78 to 90 m/min.[179,180] Many of the published reports do not provide information on the maximal distance patients are able to walk with these systems, but reported distances range from 100 to 400 m.

Some clients may perceive the technology of electrically stimulated standing and walking as moving them toward a cure for their paralysis. With a complete injury, however, the stimulation occurs passively, without expectation that voluntary control will return.[178] In cases of incomplete injury, electrically stimulated ambulation may assist the client in using and bolstering active control so that movement without the stimulation is more feasible. In considering use of electrically stimulated cycling and ambulation, discussion of the goals of treatment and the costs of the procedure must be done openly with the client to allow an educated choice to be made about the use of this expensive technology.

Traumatic Brain Injury

NMES may be a useful tool with clients having sustained brain injury, with potential benefits of managing contractures by increasing ROM, facilitating active control, and reducing spasticity by strengthening the antagonist of a spastic muscle.[181] In cases in which an understanding of the purpose and principles of NMES is not feasible for a client, the comfort of the stimulation may be critical in ensuring its continued use. Comfort may be enhanced by increasing the ramp-on time and selection of waveforms that allow stimulation at lower amplitudes yet still obtain the desired contraction.[29] Use of NMES with a client at Rancho Level IV and below is not appropriate because the client may not be able to understand the purpose and meaning of the stimulus and thereby perceive the stimulus as noxious.

EMGBF applications for clients with brain injury can be similar to those used with stroke, given similar motor presentations.[182] Therapists must consider residual cognitive deficits after brain injury in determining the appropriateness of EMGBF.

Guillain-Barré Syndrome

EMGBF in clients with Guillain-Barré syndrome demonstrated improvements in muscle strength in upper and lower extremities, although inconsistent improvement in functional use of the upper extremities was noted.[183,184] Treatment regimens consisted of EMGBF for 10 trials per muscle conducted in 45-minute treatment sessions twice a week, in one case for 78 weeks and in the other case for 46 weeks.[184]

Pediatric Applications

Special considerations for pediatric clients need to be understood when addressing the use of electricity. Although contraindications and precautions are the same as for adults, acceptance and tolerance of these devices are not. Fear and apprehension of electricity, for both child and parent, must be addressed. The clinician must take extra care in explanation and demonstration, perhaps on themselves and possibly the parent, before placing the device on the child. Allowing the child as much control as possible in device operation may assist with acceptance. Of course, the attention span of the child must also be addressed.

Cerebral Palsy

The use of NMES with children with cerebral palsy has been addressed to some degree, with several case study reports.[185-187] Carmick[185,186] described a variety of applications with children at 1.6, 6.7, and 10 years of age, integrating NMES into a treatment regimen that focused on a "task-oriented model of motor learning." Improvements were noted in upper- and lower-extremity movement and functional use across a variety of tasks appropriate to the age and movement dysfunction each child demonstrated.

Advancements in technology have allowed the use of EMGBF in increasing contexts, such as the computer-assisted feedback (CAF) system, which can be used to provide feedback about muscle activity during ambulation.[188] Data examining use of this system to provide feedback about the level of triceps surae activity during gait of children with cerebral palsy suggest potential improvements in gait symmetry, velocity, and appropriate muscle activation patterns as a result of this intervention. Use of this modality as an adjunct to physical therapy may prove beneficial.

Spina Bifida

Five subjects with spina bifida (aged 5 to 21 years) were treated with daily NMES over an 8-week period to strengthen the quadriceps femoris muscles. Increases in maximal quadriceps torque production were observed in two of the five subjects in the treated limb. Improvements in functional activity speeds were noted for all of the subjects. Lack of improvement in torque production by three subjects was speculated to be related to lack of adherence to the exercise regimen and the heterogeneity of the subject sample.[189]

Spinal Muscular Atrophy

One study has reported the use of low-intensity electrical stimulation in children with types II/III spinal muscular atrophy in an attempt to determine any effect on arm strength and function. After 6 to 12 months of stimulation no statistically significant differences were noted between experimental and placebo-control arms in strength, muscle mass, or function.[71]

Scoliosis

Axelgaard and Brown[190] demonstrated in the 1970s that surface NMES could reduce idiopathic scoliosis. Criteria for this treatment required curves measuring 20 to 45 degrees by the Cobb Method, at least 1 year of growth remaining, idiopathic and progressive nature of the curve, cooperative and psychologically stable and compliant patient, and tolerance of the stimulation. Electrodes were placed laterally over the midaxillary line on the convex side. A paraspinous location on the convex side was sometimes used. Settings included a pulse duration of 220 µs, frequency of 25 pps, and an on/off ratio of 6 seconds on and 6 seconds off. The treatment time was gradually increased to 8 hours of stimulation per day (the stimulation was typically done at night if tolerated). High success and low dropout rates were reported.[191] Others, however, reported much lower success rates.[192] Intolerance of the treatment resulting in low compliance may be the cause of these differences. This disorder is much more common in adolescent girls. At the time NMES first was introduced for scoliosis, the uncomfortable and cosmetically undesirable Milwaukee brace was still the norm for treatment. With more advanced materials and orthotic management that is much more acceptable cosmetically, the use of NMES in scoliosis management has significantly declined.

Contraindications and Precautions

Any electrical stimulation application is contraindicated for clients who have epilepsy or demand-type pacemakers. In addition, contraindications exist to applications over the transthoracic area or the uterus in pregnancy as well as in a cancerous area and the carotid sinus. Other factors require precaution but are not strict contraindications, such as sensory deficits, skin problems (sensitivity to stimulation, electrodes, or gel; edema; open wounds), tolerance of stimulation intensity sufficient to elicit muscle contraction, client's capability to participate in the training process, and financial considerations.[48-50,59]

Matthews et al[193] reported changes in blood pressure and heart rate suggestive of autonomic hyperreflexia when electrical stimulation was applied in seven subjects with SCI above the T6 level. FES to the quadriceps produced the noted changes as stimulation intensity was increased. The mechanism for this reaction is unclear. Clinicians should monitor vital signs in clients with SCI (and possibly all clients), at least during the initial application of electrical stimulation.

Use of stimulation modalities by clients outside clinical therapy sessions requires a degree of cooperation and motivation to take care of the stimulation unit, use it as instructed, and observe precautions. Long-term use of NMES (e.g., FES) may not be feasible for clients who do not have the financial resources (insurance or otherwise) to rent or purchase a unit or do not have reasonable access to support for equipment maintenance.

EMGBF does not require as many precautions because the procedure only monitors muscle activity. This form of feedback by the client requires a basic level of attention and cognitive skill to understand the meaning of, as well as act on, the feedback to change muscle performance. Client motivation and interest in use of this modality are also required because the client must be able to develop sensitivity to the degree of muscle activation independently so that feedback is no longer required. EMGBF may be used in some instances that do not require the cognitive skills of the client to use this information, such as an evaluative tool for the therapist to gather information about muscle activation to plan intervention strategies.

SUMMARY

The concepts, descriptions, and applications of electrodiagnosis presented in this chapter are intended to enrich the therapist's comprehension of these studies as applied to clients with neurological conditions. Integration of the results of these tests in differential diagnosis and in subsequent planning of intervention is invaluable.

Clearly the use of NMES and EMGBF has numerous possibilities with clients of all ages who have sustained neurological insult or injury. Improvement of motor control has been supported in some applications, although well-controlled group research in populations other than stroke and adult SCI is lacking. This underscores the need for further investigation to support the evidence for these modalities. As the therapy environment continues to change in response to time and funding constraints, therapists must carefully evaluate the benefits of a variety of available tools to assist their clients in regaining motor control and functional ability. A benefit of FES or EMGBF is the ability of the client to work autonomously (i.e., at home) after becoming familiar with the treatment regimen, with the therapist periodically updating a home program. This protocol allows physical and occupational therapy time to be used for direct intervention. NMES and EMGBF may efficiently assist in attaining improvement in control, and may also be used in the context of functional activities, but these tools alone will not create functional changes. Trial use of EMGBF or NMES for 2 to 4 weeks (daily to three times per week) with careful outcome assessment may assist the therapist in judging treatment effectiveness for each client. Case Studies 31-1, 31-2, 31-3, and 31-4 further integrate these concepts in actual patient scenarios.

CASE STUDY 31-1 ■ C8-T1 RADICULOPATHY

SUBJECTIVE EXAMINATION

A 48-year-old man was involved in a rear-end motor vehicle collision 6 months ago. He sustained a cervical strain/whiplash injury along with a contusion of the right medial elbow with no fracture. He had a brief bout (approximately 1 month) of headaches and cervical pain, both of which have resolved. For the past 3 months he has complained of weakness of his right hand, numbness, and pain and tingling in the medial three digits, resulting in difficulty with grasp and fine motor control and with typical ADLs.

OBJECTIVE EXAMINATION

Posture: Forward head; rounded shoulders, right greater than left.

ROM: Cervical flexion full, extension 50% with sharp central pain at end range, left rotation full, right rotation and left side-bending each decreased 25% with pain at upper trapezius, right side-bending full, but pain produced at C7-T1 and right scalenes on end range. Gross upper extremity ROM is without restrictions.

Strength (manual muscle test): Cervical and upper extremity isometric break tests are all 5/5 without pain.

Neurological: Reflexes C5-C6 biceps and C7 triceps present and equal bilaterally, C7-C8 wrist extension depressed on right; Sensory—light touch and sharp dull intact and equal bilaterally; diminished over medial forearm and medial three digits of right hand.

Special tests: Palpation. Tender to moderate palpation at right medial elbow, upper trapezius, scalenes, and C7-T1 facet areas. Thoracic outlet tests: Adson test, costoclavicular, and hyperabduction are negative. Tinel sign—ulnar nerve negative at wrist and elbow. Cervical axial compression in right side-bending, rotation, and extension is positive for pain locally at right C7-T1. Upper limb tension testing is positive to the right side.

CASE STUDY 31-1 ■ C8-T1 RADICULOPATHY—cont'd

IMPRESSION

Normal conduction in all nerves tested with exception of slow F wave latencies of right ulnar nerve. EMG abnormalities seen in muscles of right upper extremity innervated by C8-T1 spinal cord segment and right lower cervical paraspinals. No EMG abnormalities are seen in left upper extremity or left cervical paraspinals.

EVALUATION

Electrical test findings are consistent with a C8-T1 cervical radiculopathy on the right. Electrical changes do not indicate a peripheral plexopathy or a localized peripheral nerve lesion.

PROGNOSIS

Guarded; improvement expected during next 1 to 2 months with intervention depending on response to intervention and results of further imaging.

INTERVENTION

No electrical stimulation intervention is needed for functional or strengthening activities. Possible use of transcutaneous electrical nerve stimulation for pain control or high-voltage pulsed current in the cervical and medial elbow area for inflammation or healing could be considered. Other interventions could include postural exercise, stretching, and mobilization techniques. Their effects on the symptoms would determine these activities and their progression.

Electrophysiological Examination

NERVE CONDUCTION	DISTAL LATENCY (MS)			AMPLITUDE			VELOCITY (M/S)			F WAVE (MS)		
	R	L	NORM	R	L	NORM	R	L	NORM	R	L	NORM
Ulnar motor (above elbow to wrist)	2.8	2.6	<4.0	6	11	>5 mV	59	55	>45	34	29	<32
Ulnar sensory (digiti V to wrist)	2.8	3.1	<3.6	10	10	>6 µV	50	45	>38			
Median motor	3		<4.2	15		>5 mV	50		>45	30	30	>32
Median sensory	3.2		<3.6	18		>10 µV	43		>38			

R, Right; *L*, left.

ELECTROMYOGRAPHY	SPONTANEOUS ACTIVITY	MOTOR UNITS	RECRUITMENT
R abductor pollicis brevis	Fibrillations, positive sharp waves	Increased polyphasic potentials	Slightly reduced
Electromyography	Spontaneous activity	Motor units	Recruitment
R abductor digiti minimi	Fibrillations, positive sharp waves	Increased polyphasic potentials	Reduced
R first dorsal interosseus	Fibrillations, positive sharp waves	Increased polyphasic potentials	Reduced
R flexor carpi ulnaris	Fibrillations, positive sharp waves	Increased polyphasic potentials	Reduced
R abductor pollicis brevis	Fibrillations, positive sharp waves	Increased polyphasic potentials	Reduced
R extensor carpi ulnaris	Fibrillations, positive sharp waves	Increased polyphasic potentials	Reduced
R flexor pollicis longus	Fibrillations, positive sharp waves	Increased polyphasic potentials	Reduced
R flexor carpi radialis	None	Normal	Slightly reduced
R extensor carpi radialis	None	Normal	Normal
R biceps	None	Normal	Normal
R cervical paraspinals	Fibrillations, positive sharp waves in low cervical spine	Increased polyphasic potentials	Normal
L flexor carpi ulnaris	None	Normal	Normal
L abductor digiti minimi	None	Normal	Normal

R, Right; *L*, left.

CASE STUDY 31-2 ■ PERIPHERAL NEUROPATHY

J. R. is a 36-year-old woman with an 8-year history of renal disease. She has been receiving dialysis for 14 months. Over the past 4 to 5 months she has developed increasing weakness and decreased feeling in both lower extremities. She reports she has been falling recently.

EXAMINATION

Bilateral lower-extremity examination shows depressed deep tendon reflexes in quadriceps, hamstrings, dorsiflexors, and plantar flexors. Sensation of vibration and light touch is markedly decreased in a stocking pattern in legs beginning just below the knees. ROM is within functional limits. Muscle strength is 3+/5 in knee flexors and extensors and 1 to 2+/5 in muscles around the ankles. Toe muscle strength is 0/5 on the right and 1+/5 on the left. Sensation, range, and strength of upper extremities are within function limits and without symptoms. The client walks with a wide-based, shuffling gait with little or no push-off bilaterally.

IMPRESSION

NCT shows increased motor and sensory latencies and slow velocities of both lower extremities with normal conduction in the upper extremities. EMG shows abnormalities of fibrillations, positive sharp waves, and increased polyphasic potentials in distal leg muscles bilaterally.

EVALUATION

The pattern of clinical findings is suggestive of a peripheral polyneuropathy. Results of nerve conduction and EMG studies are consistent with incomplete axonal degeneration and confirm the clinical findings. EMG of upper extremities is normal. Review of medical management by the referring practitioner would be a key factor in treatment decisions for this client. Some of the pathological changes seen in peripheral neuropathies may be reversible or at least reduced with good compliance and clinical management.

PROGNOSIS

Depending on stabilization of renal function, functional improvement would be expected in gait status, strength, and sensation in the short term after beginning intervention. The long-term prognosis is unknown and depends on stabilization of disease process.

INTERVENTION

Ankle-foot orthoses (AFOs) for both lower extremities would enhance gait and also serve a protective function. The client's instructions should emphasize compliance with the medical plan and integumentary protective measures along with the exercise intervention.

NERVE CONDUCTION	DISTAL LATENCY (MS)			AMPLITUDE			VELOCITY (M/S)			F WAVE (MS)		
	R	L	NORM	R	L	NORM	R	L	NORM	R	L	NORM
Peroneal motor	No response	8.4	<5.5		1.2	>2 mV		27	>40	No response		>57
Tibial motor	7.8	7.2	<6	1.8	2	>2 mV	32	37	>40	68	66	<57
Sural	No response	5.9	<4.2	No response	3	>5 mV		24	>34			
Ulnar motor		3.1	<4.0		6.2	>5 mV		55	>45		26	<32
Median motor	3.5		<4.2	6.5		>5 mV	52		>45	27		<32
Ulnar sensory		2.7	<3.6		16	>6 μV		52	>38			
Median sensory	3		<3.6	19		>10 μV	47		>38			

ELECTROMYOGRAPHY R AND L	SPONTANEOUS ACTIVITY	MOTOR UNITS	RECRUITMENT
Tibialis anterior	3+ fibrillations and positive sharp waves	↑ Polyphasic potentials ↑ Duration	Markedly ↓
Peroneus longus	3+ fibrillations and positive sharp waves	↑ Duration	Markedly ↓
Gastrocnemius	3+ fibrillations and positive sharp waves	↑ Duration	Markedly ↓
Quadriceps	None	Normal	Normal
Hamstrings	None	Normal	Normal

R, Right; *L*, left; ↑, increased; ↓, decreased.

CASE STUDY 31-2 ■ PERIPHERAL NEUROPATHY—cont'd

EMGBF/NMES Options

CLIENT PROBLEM	GOALS	MODALITY PARAMETERS	MEASURES TO DETERMINE EFFICACY	CONSIDERATIONS
Lack of ankle dorsiflexion	Improve activation of intact motor units of the anterior tibialis to maximize dorsiflexion at heel-off and eccentric control at heel strike for distances approximating those at home.	FES two or three times daily for 10- to 15-minute sessions; sessions should be fatigue controlled. Because of extreme weakness begin 10:50-second on-off time with slow on-off ramping; advance to more aggressive 10:30 to 10:20 ratios if improvement is seen. Surface EMGBF could be a first choice for volitional enhancement of intact motor units with fatigability the signal for end of session; involve the peroneals depending on need to balance eversion with dorsiflexion.	Monitor each session for ability to dorsiflex foot against gravity; depending on disease progression or regression may or may not advance to use of a heel switch for gait control without AFO. Trial use 2 to 4 weeks, stopping if no improvement in status.	(1) Multiple daily sessions require rental of portable EMG or FES unit; cost of unit rental and supplies requires dual-channel units for bilateral activity. (2) A high level of client and family compliance is needed for success, requiring increased time to teach use of device; time may be recovered by use of units at home rather than during sessions. (3) Frequent use requires close monitoring of skin integrity as a result of reactions from stimulation or electrodes. (4) Electrode location for stimulation requires placement over area of compromised sensation; stimulation may require higher levels of intensity than usual; determine general levels of stimulation over nearest intact sensory area. (5) Partial denervation may produce areas of no reaction to FES; an increase in pulse duration, a decrease in frequency to 20 to 25 pps, and an increase in intensity to higher levels may be necessary. (6) Intense levels of contraction in a denervated muscle may be detrimental to reinnervation process if present.
Lack of ankle plantar flexion	Increase control of gastrosoleus for increased postural control as well as propulsion for short standing/gait time and distance.	EMGBF for enhanced activity during standing/stance especially for soleus; use increasing thresholds during activity as improvements in	Monitor standing balance for time and control, strength/endurance by level and number of contractions of plantar flexors.	Same as with dorsiflexion.

Continued

CASE STUDY 31-2 ■ PERIPHERAL NEUROPATHY—cont'd

EMGBF/NMES Options—cont'd

CLIENT PROBLEM	GOALS	MODALITY PARAMETERS	MEASURES TO DETERMINE EFFICACY	CONSIDERATIONS
		contractility are noted; 2- to 5-minute sessions involving body sway/ perturbations to activate postural control; FES parameters as with dorsiflexion.		
Weakness of quadriceps/ hamstrings	Maximize strength/ endurance of musculature for improved ambulation for distances approximating home.	Use of FES or EMG is potentially unnecessary because of strength level present; standard therapeutic exercise should be sufficient if situation stabilizes.	Standard muscle testing, monitor gait parameters.	Decrease of strength/ endurance may require further electrodiagnostic testing and consideration of electrotherapeutic programs.

CASE STUDY 31-3 ■ LEFT MIDDLE CEREBRAL ARTERY CVA

A 68-year-old woman is referred 3 weeks status post left middle cerebral artery CVA with residual right hemiparesis affecting the upper extremity to a greater degree than the lower extremity.

EXAMINATION

The client's left extremities appear well controlled with at least functional strength. She exhibits a two-finger breadth right shoulder subluxation, with pain at the extremes of shoulder flexion (150 degrees), abduction (135 degrees), and external rotation (30 degrees), and hypertonicity in a stereotypical flexor pattern affecting the shoulder horizontal adductors and internal rotators and elbow, wrist, and finger flexors. She is beginning to develop upper extremity movement with the ability to shrug her shoulder, abduct, and flex through partial range (with elbow flexed), full-range elbow flexion, partial-range elbow extension against gravity, and no wrist or finger extension. Right lower extremity ROM is within normal limits, although control is limited at the ankle (dorsiflexion only with hip and knee flexion, no eversion actively) and knee control is decreased (reduced eccentric quadriceps control, difficulty isolating knee flexion with hip extension). Ambulation is accomplished with the use of a quad cane and an articulating AFO on the right for limited distances with standby assistance. The complete absence of right wrist and finger extension raises the question of secondary radial nerve pathology. Nerve conduction and EMG studies are indicated to help differentiate this problem. This client lives at home with her husband, who is supportive of her rehabilitation. Both of them are retired, but they have an active calendar of participation

in volunteer and leisure activities. Insurance coverage is good.

IMPRESSION

Nerve conduction values are approaching the outer limits of normal but are within normal limits for the considered client's age. EMG shows no electrical evidence for peripheral denervation. A few single normal motor units were seen in wrist and finger extensors.

EVALUATION

The nerve conduction values are not unusual for clients older than 65 years. The normal nerve conduction is compatible with a CNS disorder. On EMG, spontaneous activity is rarely seen with upper motor neuron lesions, and if motor units are found, they generally have normal characteristics. Therefore the EMG findings are also consistent with a CNS rather than a PNS disorder.

The fact that radial nerve degeneration has been ruled out and the encouraging presence of some single motor unit potentials on EMG are important objective findings that should guide the therapist in management of this client.

PROGNOSIS

Independent or isolated motor function is promising for continued improvement in the condition of the client. The fact that peripheral nerve involvement does not seem to be present and motor units were found in the wrist and finger extensors would support return of function as expected with this type of CVA. Lower-extremity impairments are expected to be minimized as the return of motor control progresses. Quad cane use

CASE STUDY 31-3 ■ LEFT MIDDLE CEREBRAL ARTERY CVA—cont'd

should continue until isolated hip and knee action improves. A need for an AFO is expected for an indefinite period.

INTERVENTION

Interventions, including use of EMG or NMES, would assist in accelerating improvement in functional control.

Electrophysiological Examination

NERVE CONDUCTION	DISTAL LATENCY (MS)			AMPLITUDE			VELOCITY (M/S)		
	R	L	NORM	R	L	NORM	R	L	NORM
Radial motor	3.4	3.3	<3.5	3.5	3.2	>2.5 mV	47	47	>45
Radial sensory	3.2	3.3	<3.5	8.0	8.0	>10 μV	44	42	>40
Ulnar motor	3.7	3.8	<3.5	5.5	5.2	>5 mV	49	48	>45
Ulnar sensory	3.4	3.4	<3.5	7.0	7.5	>6 μV	40	41	>38

R, Right; *L*, left.

ELECTROMYOGRAPHY	SPONTANEOUS ACTIVITY	MOTOR UNITS	RECRUITMENT
R extensor digitorum	None	↓ Amplitude, normal duration and phase	Single units
R extensor carpi radialis	None	↓ Amplitude, normal duration and phase	Single units
R extensor pollicis brevis	None	↓ Amplitude, normal duration and phase	Single units
R extensor indicis	None	↓ Amplitude, normal duration and phase	Single units
R triceps	None	Normal	Moderately reduced, irregular pattern

R, Right; ↓, decreased.

EMGBF/NMES Options

CLIENT PROBLEM	GOALS	MODALITY PARAMETERS	MEASURES TO DETERMINE EFFICACY	CONSIDERATIONS
Shoulder subluxation	Decrease subluxation to 1 finger width, with pain manageable within patient's daily routine.	Portable FES for home use, begin with 10:30-second on/off ratio for 15-minute periods three times daily; amplitude to generate contraction without shoulder elevation. Increase on time and treatment time as tolerated so that reduction is maintained the majority of the day.	Trial use once per month. Measure amount of palpable subluxation, pain-free ROM; if improvement is not observed, discontinue FES, with instruction to maintain shoulder flexibility; consider lapboard or arm tray when sitting, support when standing.	(1) Requires rental of portable FES unit; patient/family compliance is needed for success in home program. (2) Cost of rental of FES and supplies. (3) Frequent use for reduction of subluxation requires close monitoring of skin for possible reactions to stimulation, gel, or electrodes. (4) Integrate scapular movement and stabilization exercises into program.
Lack of active ankle dorsiflexion	Increase active control of ankle dorsiflexion with knee extended, allowing heel strike without AFO for	FES twice daily for 15-minute duration; 10:20-second on-off ratio with slow ramping on-off; as active movement	Monitor each session for increased active dorsiflexion in sitting, standing, and ambulation. Integrate use of	(1) If client rents unit for shoulder subluxation, may also use stimulator at home instead of requiring time during therapy session.

Continued

CASE STUDY 31-3 ■ LEFT MIDDLE CEREBRAL ARTERY CVA—cont'd

EMGBF/NMES Options—cont'd

CLIENT PROBLEM	GOALS	MODALITY PARAMETERS	MEASURES TO DETERMINE EFFICACY	CONSIDERATIONS
	short-distance ambulation.	improves, consider EMGBF to focus attention on balanced dorsiflexion further (with eversion). Use of heel switch requires decreased ramp time to minimum patient can tolerate. Switch should activate at heel-off to control dorsiflexion through the swing phase.	heel switch during ambulation without AFO. Trial use over 2 to 3 weeks. Discontinue if not seeing increase in voluntary control; compensate with AFO.	(2) Similar cost and convenience issues as on previous page. (3) Additional education necessary if stimulator settings are to be switched for dorsiflexion and shoulder subluxation interventions.
Lack of full active wrist and finger extension	Control of active wrist and finger extension to allow release in gross grasp.	NMES and/or EMGBF twice daily. for 10-minute sessions initially, with gradual increase in duration up to 20 minutes if fatigue does not alter the quality of the contractions. Other parameters as described for ankle dorsiflexion.	Active movement in finger extensors with wrist in neutral position. Functional ability to release grasp of objects of varying shapes and sizes. Trial period of 2 to 3 weeks; discontinue if voluntary motion is not changing significantly.	May use portable stimulator as described for ankle or shoulder interventions, with similar considerations.
Muscle imbalance, lack of right upper extremity functional movement	Decrease hypertonicity in flexor muscle groups; increase extensor control for gross arm movements (i.e., positioning).	EMGBF to decrease flexor muscle activity (resting and with passive movement) and increase extensor activity. May utilize methodology described by DeBacher.[102]	Speed and control with reciprocal elbow motions, especially with extension. Use of this motion for functional activity (positioning the arm, reaching activity, etc.).	Focus on increased extensor control may prove more effective than simply decreasing flexor hyperactivity.

CASE STUDY 31-4 ■ CEREBRAL PALSY

EXAMINATION

A 9-year-old boy was referred with upper-extremity impairment secondary to a diagnosis of cerebral palsy. He has received physical therapy intervention for several years, which has currently brought him to a high level of activity with the exception of utilization of the forearm and hand. He has had no improvement in use of the wrist and hand for some time. Because no improvement occurred, his primary therapist discharged him to a home program. The client is involved in increasing levels of athletic activity, and he and his parents would like to explore the use of electrical stimulation as an avenue for improved use of the extremity. His goal is to use the hand in activities such as basketball.

OBJECTIVE

Independent function of the wrist, hand, and finger musculature; however, it is poorly coordinated. Grasp activities allow for closure of the fingers but without the needed wrist co-contraction and positioning. When the wrist was placed in the proper position he was able to maintain the needed wrist extension with a measured grip strength of 20 pounds, 50% of the opposite side. The wrist flexors are the primary movers, which leaves

CASE STUDY 31-4 ■ CEREBRAL PALSY—cont'd

the hand and wrist in a flexed position for most of the time. Increased intensity of requested action increases the pattern of wrist flexion.

IMPRESSION
Function at 3-month follow-up shows continuation of independent function of muscles. Challenge of grip and grasp of the wrist and hand automatically brought the limb into the proper position.

EVALUATION
At initial examination the client's ability to use the upper extremity in functional tasks was poor to nil as evidenced by the need for the therapist to position the part for proper use. The lower levels of individual muscle force and grip corroborated this. Follow-up visit showed improvements in strength and functional ability, but girth did not change.

PROGNOSIS
Initial: The client is an intelligent, active, and motivated individual. He is able to understand and comprehend the use of the device. He is also able to control his impulse to play with the device. The prognosis is unknown because no recent improvement with other therapy interventions has occurred. Whether he and his family are motivated enough to stay with the long-term requirements of the intervention is also unknown. A consistent intervention is expected to produce change within 2 to 3 months.

FOLLOW-UP
Continued improvement of functional ability and strength is expected. The client and family have shown themselves to be diligent in application of the

intervention, missing only a few of the requested daily sessions. Maximal level of improvement is unknown, as is carryover after cessation of the intervention. The program is expected to continue for at least 6 months total. If improvement continues, the recommendation is for purchase of the unit with continued use over the next 1 to 2 years.

INTERVENTION (DAILY)
Daytime exercise: Two-channel, neuromuscular stimulator with a symmetrical biphasic waveform. Channel 1 electrodes are placed on the motor points of the wrist extensors; channel 2 electrodes are placed to contract the finger flexors without activating wrist flexion. Electrode size was adjusted to achieve the desired results from the musculature. Timers were set so that channel 1 activated for wrist extension, followed approximately 2 to 3 seconds later by channel 2. Both channels shut off at the same time. The on-off ratio was at 10:30 seconds. The rate was 35 pps. The level of stimulation was at the maximal contraction tolerated. The client was asked to contract the muscles along with the stimulator and squeeze a small ball. Total time was 30 minutes for the exercise.

NIGHTTIME
As an adjunct, a nighttime program was added. The electrode setup was the same as the day program. Timers were adjusted to an on-off of 15:15 seconds and intensity was at the light sensory level only. The rate remained at 35 pps. The muscle did not contract. The client wore the unit throughout the night.

Measurements

MANUAL MUSCLE TEST	INITIAL	3-MONTH FOLLOW-UP
Elbow flexion/extension	4+/4+	5−/5−
Wrist flexion/extension	3+/3+	4/4
Thumb/finger	3+ all	3+ all
Girth (3 inches distal to lateral epicondyle)	6¾ inches	6¾ in.
Grip (dynamometer position 2)	20 pounds	26 pounds

ACKNOWLEDGMENTS
We would like to thank the chapter authors of the previous edition (Charlene Nelson, Jon D. Hacke, Karen L. McCulloch) and their families for their support.

REFERENCES
1. Cummings JP: Electrical stimulation of denervated muscle. In Gersh MR, editor: *Electrotherapy in rehabilitation,* Philadelphia, 1992, FA Davis.
2. American Physical Therapy Association Electrotherapy Standards Committee of the Section on Clinical Electrophysiology: *Electrotherapeutic terminology in physical therapy,* Alexandria, VA, 1990, American Physical Therapy Association.
3. Fischer E: Physiology of skeletal muscle. In Licht S, editor: *Electrodiagnosis and electromyography,* ed 3, New Haven, CT: 1971, Elizabeth Licht, p. 80.
4. Harris R: Chronaxy. In Licht S, editor: *Electrodiagnosis and electromyography,* ed 3, New Haven, CT, 1971, Elizabeth Licht.
5. Nelson C: Electrical evaluation of nerve and muscle. In Gersh MR, editor: *Electrotherapy in rehabilitation,* Philadelphia, 1992, FA Davis.
6. Dumitru D: *Electrodiagnostic medicine,* Philadelphia, 1995, Hanley & Belfus, p. 177.
7. Johnson EW, Pease WS: *Practical electromyography,* ed 3, Baltimore, 1997, Williams & Wilkins.
8. Kimura J: *Electrodiagnosis in diseases of nerve and muscle: principles and practice,* ed 2, Philadelphia, 1989, FA Davis.
9. National Institute for Occupational Safety and Health, Division of Safety Research: *Performing motor and sensory neuronal conduction studies in adult humans, 90-113,* Washington, DC, 1990, Centers for Disease Control and Prevention.
10. Oh SJ: *Clinical electromyography: nerve conduction studies,* ed 2. Baltimore, 1993, Williams & Wilkins.

11. Seddon HJ: Three types of nerve injury, *Brain* 66:237, 1943.

12. Shiller HH, Stalberg E: F responses studied with single fibre EMG in normal subjects and spastic patients, *J Neurol Neurosurg Psychiatry* 41:45, 1978.

13. Wu Y, Kunz JR, Putnam TD et al: Axillary central latency: simple electrodiagnostic technique for proximal neuropathy, *Arch Phys Med Rehabil* 64:117, 1983.

14. Braddom RL, Johnson EW: Standardization of H reflex and diagnostic use in S1 radiculopathy, *Arch Phys Med Rehabil* 55:161, 1974.

15. Sabbahi MA, Khalil M: Segmental H-reflex studies in upper and lower limbs of healthy subjects, *Arch Phys Med Rehabil* 71:216, 1990.

16. Ozdemir C, Young RR: The results to be expected from electrical testing in the diagnosis of myasthenia gravis, *Ann N Y Acad Sci* 274:203-235, 1976.

17. Eaton LM, Lambert EH: Electromyography and electrical stimulation of nerves in diseases of motor unit. Observations on myasthenic syndrome associated with malignant tumors, *JAMA* 163:1117, 1957.

18. Gilchrist JM, Sanders DB: Double-step repetitive stimulation in myasthenia gravis, *Muscle Nerve* 10:233, 1987.

19. Chatrian GE: American Electroencephalographic Society: guidelines for clinical evoked potential studies, *J Clin Neurophysiol* 1:3, 1984.

20. Chiappa KH: *Evoked potentials in clinical medicine,* ed 3, Philadelphia, 1997, Lippincott-Raven.

21. Halliday AM: *Evoked potentials in clinical testing,* ed 2, Edinburgh, 1992, Churchill Livingstone.

22. Robinson K, Rudge P: Centrally generated auditory potentials. In Halliday AM, editor: *Evoked potentials in clinical testing,* London, 1982, Churchill Livingstone.

23. Aminoff MJ: *Electrodiagnosis in clinical neurology,* ed 4, New York, 1999, Churchill Livingstone.

24. Currier DP et al: Guidelines for clinical electromyography, *J Clin Electrophysiol* 5:2, 1993.

25. Chu-Andrews J, Johnson RJ: *Electrodiagnosis: an anatomical and clinical approach,* Philadelphia, 1986, J.B. Lippincott.

26. Stalberg E, Chu J, Bril V et al: Automatic analysis of the EMG interference pattern, *Electroencephalogr Clin Neurophysiol* 56:672, 1983.

27. Stalberg E, Falck B, Sonoo M, et al: Multi-MUP EMG analysis—a two year experience in daily clinical work, *Electroencephalogr Clin Neurophysiol* 97:145, 1995.

28. Stalberg E: AAEE minimonograph #20, macro EMG, *Muscle Nerve* 6:619, 1983.

29. Zablotny C: Using neuromuscular electrical stimulation to facilitate limb control in the head-injured patient, *J Head Trauma Rehabil* 2:28, 1987.

30. Perry J: Preoperative and postoperative dynamic electromyography as an aid in planning tendon transfers in children with cerebral palsy, *J Bone Joint Surg Am* 59:531, 1977.

31. Perry J: The use of gait analysis for surgical recommendations in traumatic brain injury, *J Head Trauma Rehabil* 14:116, 1999.

32. Perry J: Determinants of muscle function in the spastic lower extremity, *Clin Orthop* 288:100-126, 1993.

33. Portney L, Roy S: Electromyography and nerve conduction velocity tests. In O'Sullivan S, Schmitz T, editors: *Physical rehabilitation: assessment and treatment,* ed 4, Philadelphia, 2001, FA Davis, pp. 213-256.

34. Waters RL, Frazier J, Garland DE et al: Electromyographic gait analysis before and after operative treatment for hemiplegic equinus and equinovarus deformity, *J Bone Joint Surg Am* 64:284, 1982.

35. Perry J, Schmidt Easterday C, Antonelli DJ: Surface versus intramuscular electrodes for electromyography of superficial and deep muscles. *Phys Ther* 61:7-15, 1981.

36. Young C, Rose S, Biden E et al: The effects of surface and internal electrodes on the gait of children with cerebral palsy, spastic diplegic type. *J Orthop Res* 7:732, 1989.

37. Giroux B, Lamontagne M: Comparisons between surface and intramuscular wire electrodes in isometric and dynamic conditions. *Electromyogr Clin Neurophysiol* 30:397-405, 1990.

38. Kadaba MP, Wootten ME, Gainey J et al: Repeatability of phasic muscle activity: performance of surface and intramuscular wire electrodes in gait analysis, *J Orthop Res* 3:350, 1985.

39. Komi PV, Buskirk E: Reproducibility of electromyographic measurements with inserted wire electrodes and surface electrodes, *Electromyography* 10:357-367, 1970.

40. Yang JF, Winter DA: Electromyography reliability in maximal and submaximal isometric contractions, *Arch Phys Med Rehabil* 64:417, 1983.

41. Bogey RA, Barnes LA, Perry J: Computer algorithms to characterize individual subject EMG profiles during gait, *Arch Phys Med Rehabil* 73:835, 1992.

42. Hislop HJ, Montgomery J: *Manual Muscle Testing,* Philadelphia, 2001, WB Saunders.

43. Adams J, Perry J: Gait analysis: clinical decision making. In Rose J, Gamble J, editors: *Human walking,* ed 3, Philadelphia, 2006, Lippincott Williams & Wilkins, pp. 165-184.

44. Cahan L, Adams J, Perry J et al: Instrumented gait analysis following selective posterior rhizotomy [abstract], *Phys Ther* 69:R144, 1989.

45. Baker LL, Wederich CL, McNeal DR et al: *Neuromuscular electrical stimulation: a practical guide,* ed 2, Downey, CA, 1993, Los Amigos Research and Education Institute.

46. Basmajian JV: *Biofeedback principles and practice for clinicians,* ed 3, Baltimore, 1989, Williams & Wilkins.

47. Delitto A, Robinson AJ: Electrical stimulation of muscle: techniques and applications. In Snyder-Mackler L, Robinson AJ: *Clinical electrophysiology: electrotherapy and electrophysiologic testing,* Baltimore, 1989, Williams & Wilkins.

48. DeVahl J: Neuromuscular electrical stimulation (NMES) in rehabilitation. In Gersh MR, editor: *Electrotherapy in rehabilitation,* Philadelphia, 1992, F.A. Davis.

49. Gersh MR: *Electrotherapy in rehabilitation,* Philadelphia, 1992, FA Davis.

50. Nelson RM, Hayes RW, Currier DP: *Clinical electrotherapy,* ed 3, Stamford, CT, 1999, Appleton & Lange.

51. Packman-Braun R: Electrotherapeutic applications for the neurologically impaired patient. In Gersh MR, editor: *Electrotherapy in rehabilitation,* Philadelphia, 1992, F.A. Davis.

52. Robinson AJ, Snyder-Mackler L: *Clinical electrophysiology, electrotherapy and electrophysiological testing,* ed 2, Baltimore, 1995, Williams & Wilkins.

53. de Kroon JR, van der Lee JH, Izerman MJ, et al: Therapeutic electrical stimulation to improve motor control and functional abilities of the upper extremity after stroke: a systematic review, *Clin Rehabil* 16:350-360, 2002.

54. Delitto A et al: Electrical stimulation of muscle. In Robinson AJ, Snyder-Mackler L, editors: *Clinical electrophysiology, electrotherapy and electrophysiological testing,* ed 2, Baltimore, 1995, Williams & Wilkins.

55. Baker LL, Bowman BR, McNeal DR: Effects of waveform on comfort during neuromuscular electrical stimulation, *Clin Orthop* 233:75-85, 1988.

56. McNeal DR, Baker LL: Effects of joint angle, electrodes and waveform on electrical stimulation of the quadriceps and hamstrings, *Ann Biomed Eng* 16:299-310, 1988.

57. Bowman BR, Baker LL: Effects of waveform parameters on comfort during transcutaneous neuromuscular electrical stimulation, *Ann Biomed Eng* 13:59-74, 1985.

58. Gracanin F, Trnkoczy A: Optimal stimulus parameters for minimum pain in the chronic stimulation of innervated muscle, *Phys Med Rehabil* 56:243-249, 1975.

59. Cummings J: Electrical stimulation of healthy muscle and tissue repair. In Nelson RM, Currier DP, editors: *Clinical electrotherapy,* ed 2, Norwalk, CT, 1991, Appleton & Lange.

60. Bergmans J, Senden R: Electrical stimulation of denervated muscle. In Gorio A et al, editors: *Posttraumatic peripheral nerve regeneration: experimental basis and clinical implications,* New York, 1981, Raven Press.

61. Eichhron KF, Schubert W, David E: Maintenance, training, and functional use of denervated muscle, *J Biomed Eng* 6:205-211, 1984.

62. Sunderland S: *Nerves and nerve injuries,* ed 2, Edinburgh, 1978, Churchill Livingstone.

63. Kosman AJ et al: The influence of duration and frequency in electrical stimulation of muscles, *Arch Phys Med* 29:559, 1948.

64. Pockett S, Gavin RM: Acceleration of peripheral nerve regeneration after crush injury in rat, *Neurosci Lett* 59:221-224, 1985.

65. Wakim KG, Krusen FH: The influence of electrical stimulation on the work output and endurance of denervated muscle, *Arch Phys Med Rehabil* 36:370-376, 1955.

66. Bowden REM, Gutmann E: Denervation and re-innervation of human voluntary muscle, *Brain* 67:273, 1944.

67. Rosselle N, De Meirsman J, De Keyser C et al: Electromyographic evaluation of therapeutic methods in complete peripheral paralysis, *Electromyogr Clin Neurophysiol* 17:179-186, 1977.

68. Valencic V, Vodovnik L, Stefancic M et al: Improved motor response due to chronic electrical stimulation of denervated tibialis anterior muscle in humans, *Muscle Nerve* 9:612-617, 1986.

69. Lobo R, Slater CR: Control of acetylcholine sensitivity and synapse formation by muscle activity, *J Physiol* 275:391, 1978.

70. Pinelli P et al: *In tibialis anterior reinnervation by collateral branching with or without electrotherapy.* Proceedings of the Fourth Congress of the International Society of Electrophysiology and Kinesiology, Boston, 1979.

71. Fehlings DL, Kirsch S, McComas A et al: Evaluation of therapeutic electrical stimulation to improve muscle strength and function in children with types II/III spinal muscular atrophy, *Dev Med Child Neurol* 44:741, 2002.

72. Gorman PH, Mortimer JT: The effect of stimulus parameters on the recruitment characteristics of direct nerve stimulation, *IEEE Trans Biomed Eng* 30:407-414, 1983.

73. Binder MD, Mendell LM: *The segmental motor system,* London, 1990, Oxford University Press.

74. Binder-Macleod SA, Snyder-Mackler L: Muscle fatigue: clinical implications for fatigue assessment and neuromuscular electrical stimulation, *Phys Ther* 73:902-910, 1993.

75. Trimble MH, Enoka RM: Mechanisms underlying the training effects associated with neuromuscular electrical stimulation, *Phys Ther* 71:273-280, 1991.

76. Packman-Braun R: Relationship between functional electrical stimulation duty cycle and fatigue in wrist extensor muscles of patients with hemiparesis, *Phys Ther* 68:51-56, 1988.

77. Kimberley TJ, Lewis SM, Auerbach EJ et al: Electrical stimulation driving functional improvements and cortical changes in subjects with stroke, *Exp Brain Res* 154:450-460, 2004.

78. Baker LL, Parker K: Neuromuscular electrical stimulation of the muscles surrounding the shoulder, *Phys Ther* 66:1930-1937, 1986.

79. Liberson WT, Holmquest HJ, Scot D, et al: Functional electrotherapy: stimulation of the peroneal nerve synchronized with the swing phase of the gait of hemiplegic patients, *Arch Phys Med Rehabil* 42:101-105, 1961.

80. Axelgaard J, Brown JC: Lateral electrical surface stimulation for the treatment of progressive ideopathic scoliosis, *Spine* 8:242-260, 1983.

81. Faghri PD, Glaser RM, Figoni SF: Functional electrical stimulation leg cycle ergometer exercise: training effects on cardiorespiratory responses of spinal cord injured subjects at rest and during submaximal exercise, *Arch Phys Med Rehabil* 73:1085-1093, 1992.

82. Grimby G, Nordwall A, Hulten B et al: Changes in histochemical profile of muscle after long-term electrical stimulation in patients with idiopathic scoliosis, *Scand J Rehabil Med* 17:191, 1985.

83. Keith MW, Peckham PH, Thrope GB et al: Functional neuromuscular stimulation neuroprostheses for the tetraplegic hand, *Clin Orthop* 223:25, 1988.

84. Ragnarsson KT: Physiologic effects of functional electrical stimulation-introduced exercises in spinal cord-injured individuals, *Clin Orthop* 233:53-63, 1988.

85. Ragnarsson KT, Pollack S, O'Daniel W Jr et al: Clinical evaluation of computerized electrical stimulation after spinal cord injury: a multicenter pilot study, *Arch Phys Med Rehabil* 69:672-677, 1988.

86. Sipski ML, Delisa JA, Schweer S et al: Functional electrical stimulation bicycle ergometry: patient perceptions, *Am J Phys Med Rehabil* 68:147-149, 1989.

87. Wang RY, Chan RC, Tsai MW: Functional electrical stimulation on chronic and acute hemiplegic shoulder subluxation, *Am J Phys Med Rehabil* 79:385-390, 2000.

88. Yan T, Hui-Chan CW, Li LS: Functional electrical stimulation improves motor recovery of the lower extremity and walking ability of subjects with first acute stroke: a randomized placebo-controlled trial, *Stroke* 36:80-85, 2004.

89. Faghri PD, Rodgers MM, Glaser RM et al: The effects of functional electrical stimulation on shoulder subluxation, arm function recovery, and shoulder pain in hemiplegic stroke patients, *Arch Phys Med Rehabil* 75:73-79, 1994.

90. Hooker SP, Figoni SF, Glaser RM et al: Physiologic responses to prolonged electrically stimulated leg-cycle exercise in the spinal cord injured, *Arch Phys Med Rehabil* 71:863-869, 1990.

91. Hooker SP, Figoni SF, Rodgers MM et al: Physiologic effects of electrical stimulation leg cycle exercise training in spinal cord injured persons, *Arch Phys Med Rehabil* 73:470-476, 1992.

92. Peckham PH, Marsolais EB, Mortimer JT: Restoration of key grip and release in the C6 tetraplegic patient through functional electrical stimulation, *J Hand Surg [Am]* 5:462-469, 1980.

93. Peckham PH, Keith MW, Freehafer AA: Restoration of functional control by electrical stimulation in the upper extremity of the quadriplegic patient, *J Bone Joint Surg [Am]* 70:144-148, 1988.

94. Petrofsky JS, Phillips CA, Larson P: Computer synchronized walking: an application of an orthosis and functional electrical stimulation, *J Neurol Orthop Med Surg* 6:219-230, 1985.

95. Twist DJ: Acrocyanosis in a spinal cord injured patient: effects of computer-controlled neuromuscular stimulation: a case report, *Phys Ther* 70:45-49, 1990.

96. Jacobs PL, Johnson B, Mahoney ET: Physiologic responses to electrically assisted and frame-supported standing in persons with paraplegia, *J Spinal Cord Med* 26:384-389, 2005.

97. Petrofsky JS, Phillips CA, Heaton HH: Bicycle ergometer for paralyzed muscles, *J Clin Eng* 9:13-19, 1984.

98. Phillips WT, Kiratli BJ, Sarkarati M et al: Effect of spinal cord injury on the heart and cardiovascular fitness, *Curr Probl Cardiol* 23:641-716, 1998.

99. Hirokawa S, Solomonow W, Baratta R et al: Energy expenditure and fatiguability in paraplegic ambulation using reciprocating gait orthosis and electrical stimulation, *Disabil Rehabil* 18:115-122, 1996.

100. Wolf SL, Binder-Macleod SA: Neurophysiologic factors in electromyographic feedback for neuromotor disturbances. In Basmajian JV, editor: *Biofeedback principles and practice for clinicians,* ed 3, Baltimore, 1989, Williams & Wilkins.

101. Basmajian JV, Blumenstein R: Electrode placement in electromyographic biofeedback. In Basmajian JV, editor: *Biofeedback principles and practice for clinicians,* ed 3, Baltimore, 1989, Williams & Wilkins.

102. DeBacher G: Biofeedback in spasticity control. In Basmajian JV, editor: *Biofeedback principles and practice for clinicians,* ed 3, Baltimore, 1989, Williams & Wilkins.

103. Neilson PD, McCaughy J: Self-regulation of spasm and spasticity in cerebral palsy, *J Neurol Neurosurg Psychiatry* 45:320-330, 1982.

104. Gowland C, deBruin H, Basmajian TV et al: Agonist and antagonist activity during voluntary upper-limb movement in patients with stroke, *Phys Ther* 72:624-633, 1992.

105. Landau WM, Hunt CC: Dorsal rhizotomy, a treatment of unproven efficacy, *J Child Neurol* 5:174-178, 1990.

106. Wolf SL, Edwards DI, Shutter LA: Concurrent assessment of muscle activity (CAMA): a procedural approach to assess treatment goals, *Phys Ther* 66:218-224, 1986.

107. Armagan O, Tascioglu F, Oner C: Electromyographic biofeedback in the treatment of the hemiplegic hand: a placebo-controlled study, *Am J Phys Med Rehabil* 82:856-861, 2003.

108. Wissel J, Ebersbach G, Gutjahr L et al: Treating chronic hemiparesis with modified biofeedback, *Arch Phys Med Rehabil* 70:612-617, 1989.

109. Wolf SL, Baker MP, Kelly JL: EMG biofeedback in stroke: a 1-year follow-up on the effect of patient characteristics, *Arch Phys Med Rehabil* 61:351-354, 1980.

110. Rakos M, Freudenschuss B, Girsch W et al: Electromyogram-controlled functional electrical stimulation for the treatment of the paralyzed upper extremity, *Artif Organs* 23:466-469, 1999.

111. Thorsen R, Ferrarin M, Spadone R et al: Functional control of the hand in tetraplegics based on residual EMG activity, *Artif Organs* 23:470-473, 1999.

112. Moreland J, Thompson MA: Efficacy of electromyographic biofeedback compared with conventional physical therapy for upper-extremity function in patients following stroke: a research overview and meta-analysis, *Phys Ther* 74:534-543, 1994.

113. Schmidt RA: Feedback and knowledge of results. In Schmidt RA, editor: *Motor control and learning,* ed 2, Champaign, IL, 1988, Human Kinetics.

114. Bate PJ, Matyas TA: Negative transfer of training following brief practice of elbow tracking movements with electromyographic feedback from spastic antagonists, *Arch Phys Med Rehabil* 73:1050-1058, 1992.

115. Francisco G, Chae J, Chawla H et al: Electromyogram-triggered neuromuscular stimulation for improving arm function of acute stroke survivors: a randomized pilot study, *Arch Phys Med Rehabil* 79:570-575, 1998.

116. Cauraugh J, Light K, Kim S et al: Chronic motor dysfunction after stroke: recovering wrist and finger extension by electromyography-triggered neuromuscular stimulation, *Stroke* 31:1360-1364, 2000.

117. Bowman BR, Baker LL, Waters RL: Positional feedback and electrical stimulation: an automated treatment for the hemiplegic wrist, *Arch Phys Med Rehabil* 60:497-502, 1979.

118. Winchester P, Montgomery J, Bowman BR et al: Effects of feedback stimulation training and cyclical electrical stimulation on knee extension in hemiparetic patients, *Phys Ther* 7:1096-1103, 1983.

119. Wolf SL, Binder-Macleod SA: Electromyographic biofeedback applications to the hemiplegic patient: changes in lower extremity neuromuscular and functional status, *Phys Ther* 63:1404-1413, 1983.

120. Hammond MC, Kraft GH, Fitts SS: Recruitment and termination of electromyographic activity in the hemiparetic forearm, *Arch Phys Med Rehabil* 69:106-110, 1988.

121. Hammond MC, Fitts SS, Kraft GH et al: Co-contraction in the hemiparetic forearm: quantitative EMG evaluation, *Arch Phys Med Rehabil* 69:348-351, 1988.

122. Sahrman SA, Norton BJ: Relationship of voluntary movement to spasticity in upper motor neuron syndrome, *Ann Neurol* 2:460-465, 1977.

123. Prevo AJH, Visser SL, Vogelaar TW: Effect of EMG feedback on paretic muscles and abnormal co-contraction in the hemiplegic arm, compared with conventional therapy, *Scand J Rehabil Med* 14:121-131, 1982.

124. Inglis J, Donald MW, Monga TN et al: Electromyographic biofeedback and physical therapy of the hemiplegic upper limb, *Arch Phys Med Rehabil* 65:755-759, 1984.

125. Wolf SL, Binder-Macleod SA: Electromyographic biofeedback applications to the hemiplegic patient: changes in upper extremity neuromuscular and functional status, *Phys Ther* 63:1393-1403, 1983.

126. Chantraine A, Baribeault A, Ubuelhart A et al: Shoulder pain and dysfunction in hemiplegia: effects of functional electrical stimulation, *Arch Phys Med Rehabil* 80:328-331, 1999.

127. Chae J, Bethoux F, Bohine T et al: Neuromuscular stimulation for upper extremity motor and functional recovery in acute hemiplegia, *Stroke* 29:975-979, 1998.

128. Sonde L, Gip C, Fernaeus SE et al: Stimulation with low frequency (1.7 hz) transcutaneus nerve stimulation (TNS) increases motor function of the post-stroke paretic arm, *Scand J Rehabil Med* 30:95-99, 1998.

129. Powell J, Pandyan AD, Granat M et al: Electrical stimulation of wrist extensors in post-stroke hemiplegia, *Stroke* 30:1384-1389, 1999.

130. Basmajian JV, Gowland C, Brandstater ME et al: EMG feedback treatment of upper limb in hemiplegic stroke patients: a pilot study, *Arch Phys Med Rehabil* 63:613-616, 1982.

131. Vodovnik L, Kralj A, Stanic U et al: Recent applications of functional electrical stimulation to stroke patients in Ljubljana, *Clin Orthop* 131:64-69, 1978.

132. Popovic MB, Popovic DB, Sinkjaer T et al: Restitution of reaching and grasping promoted by functional electrical therapy, *Artif Organs* 26:271-275, 2002.

133. Popovic MB, Popovic DB, Sinkjaer T et al: Clinical evaluation of functional electrical therapy in acute hemiplegic subjects, *J Rehabil Res Dev* 40:443-453, 2003.

134. Ring H, Rosenthal M: Controlled study of neuroprosthetic functional electrical stimulation in sub-acute post-stroke rehabilitation, *J Rehabil Med* 37:32-36, 2005.

135. Kraft G, Fitts SS, Hammond MC: Techniques to improve function of the arm and hand in chronic hemiplegia. *Arch Phys Med Rehabil* 73:220-227, 1992.

136. Basmajian JV, Kukulka CG, Narayan MG et al: Biofeedback treatment of foot-drop after stroke compared with standard rehabilitation technique: effects on voluntary control and strength, *Arch Phys Med Rehabil* 56:231-236, 1975.

137. Burnside I, Tobias HS, Bursill D et al: Electromyographic feedback in the remobilization of stroke patients: a controlled trial, *Arch Phys Med Rehabil* 63:217-222, 1982.

138. Santee J, Keister ME, Kleinman KM et al: Incentives to enhance the effects of electromyographic feedback training in stroke patients, *Biofeedback Self Regul* 5:51-56, 1980.

139. Mandel AR, Nymark JR, Balmer SJ et al: Electromyographic versus rhythmic positional biofeedback in computerized gait retraining with stroke patients, *Arch Phys Med Rehabil* 71:649-654, 1990.

140. Merletti R, Zelaschi F, Latella D et al: A control study of muscle force recovery in hemiparetic patients during treatment with functional electrical stimulation, *Scand J Rehab Med* 10:147-154, 1978.

141. Takebe K, Kukulka CG, Narayan MG et al: Peroneal nerve stimulator in rehabilitation of hemiplegic patients, *Arch Phys Med Rehabil* 56:237-240, 1975.

142. Waters RL, McNeal D, Perry J: Experimental correction of footdrop by electrical stimulation of the peroneal nerve, *J Bone Joint Surg* 57A:1047-1054, 1975.

143. Wieler M, Stein RB, Ladouceur M et al: Multicenter evaluation of electrical stimulation systems for walking, *Arch Phys Med Rehabil* 80:495-500, 1999.

144. Burridge J, Taylor P, Hagan S et al: Experience of clinical use of the Odstock dropped foot stimulator, *Artif Organs* 21:254-260, 1997.

145. Burridge J, Taylor P, Hagan S et al: The effects of common peroneal stimulation on the effort and speed of walking: a randomized controlled trial with chronic hemiplegic patients. Part 1: lower extremity, *Clin Rehabil* 11:201-210, 1997.

146. Bogataj U, Gros N, Malezic M et al: Restoration of gait during two to three weeks of therapy with multichannel stimulation, *Phys Ther* 69:319-327, 989.

147. Bogataj U, Gros N, Kljajic M et al: The rehabilitation of gait in patients with hemiplegia: a comparison between conventional therapy and multichannel electrical stimulation therapy, *Phys Ther* 75:490-502, 1995.

148. Malezic M, Kljajic M, Acimovic-Janezic R et al: Therapeutic effects of multisite electric stimulation of gait in motor-disabled patients, *Arch Phys Med Rehabil* 68:553-560, 1987.

149. Wolf LB: Use of biofeedback in the treatment of stroke patients, *Stroke* 21:22-23, 1990.

150. Cozean CD, Pease WS, Hubbell SL: Biofeedback and functional electrical stimulation in stroke rehabilitation, *Arch Phys Med Rehabil* 69:401-405, 1988.

151. Granat MH, Maxwell DJ, Ferguson AC et al: Peroneal stimulator, evaluation for the correction of spastic foot drop in hemiplegia, *Arch Phys Med Rehabil* 77:19-24, 1996.

152. Wolf SL: *Electromyographic feedback for spinal cord injured patients: a realistic perspective. Biofeedback principles and practice for clinicians,* ed 3, Baltimore, 1989, Williams and Wilkins.

153. Morrison S: Biofeedback to facilitate unassisted ventilation in individuals with high level quadriplegia: a case report, *Phys Ther* 68:1378-1389, 1988.

154. Nacht M, Wolf SL, Coogler CE: Use of electromyographic feedback during the acute phase of spinal cord injury: a case report, *Phys Ther* 62:290-294, 1982.

155. Klose K, Schmidt DL, Needham BM et al: Rehabilitation therapy for patients with long-term spinal cord injuries, *Arch Phys Med Rehabil* 71:659-662, 1990.

156. Kohlmeyer K, Hill JP, Yarkony GM et al: Electrical stimulation and biofeedback effect on recovery of tenodesis grasp: a controlled study, *Arch Phys Med Rehabil* 77:702-706, 1996.

157. Keith MW, Peckham PH, Thrope GB et al: Functional neuromuscular stimulation neuroprosthesis for the tetraplegic hand, *Clin Orthop* 223:25-33, 1988.

158. Prochazka A, Gauthier M, Wieler M et al: The bionic glove: an electrical stimulator garment that provides controlled grasp and hand opening in quadriplegia, *Arch Phys Med Rehabil* 78:608-614, 1997.

159. Saxena S, Nikolic S, Popovic D: An EMG-controlled grasping system for tetraplegics, *J Rehabil Res Dev* 32:17-24, 1995.

160. Scott T, Peckham PH, Kilgore KL: Tri-state myoelectric control of bilateral upper extremity neuroprostheses for tetraplegic individuals, *IEEE Trans Rehabil Eng* 4:251-263, 1996.

161. Smith B, Mulcahey MJ, Betz RR: Development of an upper extremity FES system for individuals with C4 tetraplegia, *IEEE Trans Rehabil Eng* 4:264-270, 1996.

162. Grill J, Peckham P: Functional neurouscular stimulation for combined control of elbow extension and hand grip in C5 and C6 quadriplegics, *IEEE Trans Rehabil Eng* 6:190-199, 1998.

163. Davis S, Mulcahey MJ, Smith BT et al: Self-reported use of an implanted FES hand system by adolescents with tetraplegia, *J Spinal Cord Med* 21:220-226, 1998.

164. Hart R, Kilgore KL, Peckham PH: A comparison between control methods for implanted FES hand grasp, *IEEE Trans Rehabil Eng* 6:208-218, 1998.

165. Kilgore K, Peckham PH, Keith MW et al: An implanted upper-extremity neuroprosthesis. Follow-up of five patients, *J Bone Joint Surg [Am]* 79:533-541, 1997.

166. Mulcahey M, Betz RR, Smith BT et al: Implanted functional electrical stimulation hand system in adolescents and spinal injuries: an evaluation, *Arch Phys Med Rehabil* 78:597-607, 1997.

167. Gardner E, Baker L: Functional electrical stimulation of paralytic muscle. In Currier DP, Nelson RM, editors: *Dynamics of human biological tissue,* Philadelphia, 1992, FA Davis.

168. Bijak M, Hofer C, Lammuller H et al: Personal computer supported eight channel surface stimulator for paraplegic walking: first results, *Artif Organs* 23:424-427, 1999.

169. Davis R, MacFarland WC, Emmons SE: Initial results of the nucleus FES-22-implanted system for limb movement in paraplegia, *Stereotact Funct Neurosurg* 6:192, 1994.

170. Triolo R, Bieri C, Uhlir J et al: Implanted functional neuromuscular stimulation systems for individuals with spinal cord injuries: clinical case reports, *Arch Phys Med Rehabil* 77:1119-1128, 1996.

170a. Johnston TE, Betz RR, Smith BT et al: Implanted functional electrical stimulation: an alternative for standing and walking in pediatric spinal cord injury, *Spinal Cord* 41:144-152, 2003.

170b. Johnston TE, Finson RL, Smith BT et al: Functional electrical stimulation for augmented walking in adolescents with incomplete spinal cord injury, *J Spinal Cord Med* 26:390-400, 2003.

171. Mutton D, Scremin AM, Barstow TJ et al: Physiologic responses during functional electrical stimulation leg cycling and hybrid exercise in spinal cord injured subjects, *Arch Phys Med Rehabil* 78:712-718, 1997.

172. Hooker SP, Scremin AM, Mutton DL et al: Peak and submaximal physiologic responses following electrical stimulation leg cycle ergometer training, *J Rehabil Res Dev* 32:361-366, 1995.

173. Cybulski GR, Penn RD, Jaeger RJ: Lower extremity functional neuromuscular stimulation in cases of spinal cord injury, *Neurosurgery* 15:132-146, 1984.

174. Kobetic R, Triolo RJ, Marsolais EB et al: Muscle selection and walking performance of multichannel FES systems for ambulation in paraplegia, *IEEE* 5:23-29, 1997.

175. Moynahan M, Mullin C, Cohn J et al: Home use of a functional electrical stimulation system for standing and mobility in adolescents with spinal cord injury, *Arch Phys Med Rehabil* 77:105-113, 1996.

176. Bajd T, Kralj A, Stefancic M et al: Use of functional electrical stimulation in the lower extremities of incomplete spinal cord injured patients, *Artif Organs* 23:403-409, 1999.

177. Konishi N, Shimada Y, Sato K et al: Electrophysiological evaluation of denervated muscles in incomplete paraplegia using macro-electromyography, *Arch Phys Med Rehabil* 79:1062-1068, 1998.

178. Bradley M: The effect of participating in a functional electrical stimulation program on affect in people with spinal cord injuries, *Arch Phys Med Rehabil* 75:676-679, 1994.

179. Murray M: Gait as a total pattern of movement, *Am J Phys Med Rehabil* 46:290-329, 1967.

180. Murray M, Kory RC, Sepic SB: Walking patterns of normal women, *Arch Phys Med Rehabil* 51:637-650, 1970.

181. Baker LL, Parker K, Sanderson D: Neuromuscular electrical stimulation for the head-injured patient, *Phys Ther* 63:1967-1974, 1983.

182. Lazarus J: Associated movement in hemiplegia: the effects of force exerted, limb usage and inhibitory training, *Arch Phys Med Rehabil* 73:1044-1049, 1992.

183. Cohen B, Crouch RH, Thompson SN: Electromyographic feedback as a physical therapeutic adjunct in Guillain-Barré syndrome, *Arch Phys Med Rehabil* 58:582, 1977.

184. Ince L, Leon M: Biofeedback treatment of upper extremity dysfunction in Guillain-Barré syndrome, *Arch Phys Med Rehabil* 67:30-33, 1986.

185. Carmick J: Clinical use of neuromuscular electrical stimulation for children with cerebral palsy. Part 1: lower extremity, *Phys Ther* 73:505-513, 1993.

186. Carmick J: Clinical use of neuromuscular electrical stimulation for children with cerebral palsy. Part 2: lower extremity, *Phys Ther* 73:514-527, 1993.

187. Dubowitz L, Finnie N, Hyde SA et al: Improvement in muscle performance by chronic electrical stimulation in children with cerebral palsy, *Lancet* 1:587-588, 1988.

188. Colborne G, Wright FV, Naumann S: Feedback of triceps surae EMG in gait of children with cerebral palsy: a controlled study, *Arch Phys Med Rehabil* 75:40, 1994.

189. Karmel-Ross K, Cooperman DR, Van Doren CL: The effects of electrical stimulation on quadriceps femoris muscle torque in children with spina bifida, *Phys Ther* 72:723-730, 1992.

190. Axelgaard J, Brown M: Lateral surface stimulation for the correction of progressive scoliosis, *Spine* 8:242-260, 1983.

191. Eckerson L, Axelgaard J: Lateral electrical surface stimulation for the treatment of idiopathic scoliosis, *Phys Ther* 64:483-490, 1984.

192. Durham J: Surface electrical stimulation versus brace in treatment of idiopathic scoliosis, *Spine* 15:888-891, 1990.

193. Matthews J, Wheeler JD, Burnham RS et al: The effects of surface anesthesia on the autonomic dysreflexia response during functional electrical stimulation, *Spinal Cord* 35:647-651, 1997.

194. Perry J, Young S, Barnes G: Strengthening exercise for post-polio sequelae, *Arch Phys Med Rehabil* 68:660, 1987.

195. Perry J: Poliomyelitis. In Nickel VL, Botte MJ, editors: *Orthopaedic rehabilitation,* New York, 1992, Churchill Livingstone, pp. 493-520.

CHAPTER 32 Pain Management

Annie Burke-Doe, PhD, MPT

KEY WORDS

ANS pain: complex regional pain syndrome
acute pain
behavioral manipulations: exercise; operant
  conditioning; hypnosis; biofeedback
chronic pain
CNS pain: thalamic pain
cognitive strategies: relaxation exercises; body
  scanning; humor
nociceptor
pain intensity measurements: visual analog scale
  (VAS); simple descriptive pain scale (SDPS); pain
  estimate; faces pain scale
pain localization tools: pain drawing
pain modulation: gate control theory;
  neurotransmitters; neuromodulators
pain pathway
pain quality measurements: McGill Pain
  Questionnaire (MPQ); pediatric verbal descriptor
  scale; caregiver checklists
point stimulation

OBJECTIVES

After reading this chapter the student/therapist will be able to:
1. Describe the pain pathways.
2. Describe how pain is modulated within the nervous system.
3. Identify the causes of acute and chronic pain.
4. List the signs and symptoms of CNS, ANS, and peripheral pain and give an example of each.
5. Perform a comprehensive pain evaluation, including taking a pain history, measuring pain intensity, measuring pain character, and examining the client.
6. Design a comprehensive pain management program that addresses the objective and subjective aspects of the pain experience.

Chronic pain has a profound impact on all aspects of an individual's life. It influences relationships with family members, friends, coworkers, and health care providers. It affects the ability to fulfill responsibilities, work, and participate in social activities. Perhaps more than any other factor, the presence of chronic pain and the response to it determine the overall quality of an individual's life.

Chronic pain is prevalent. The American Pain Society reports that 45% of all Americans seek medical care for chronic pain at some point in their lives,[1] and chronic back pain is the second most common reason people seek medical attention.[2] Yet, studies of physicians, nurses, and therapists who treat individuals with chronic pain show that most do not have even a basic understanding of the concepts of pain management.[3-5] The result is inadequate or inappropriate care[5-7] of individuals who complain of pain.

Many impairments within various body systems cause pain. The ability to identify different pathologies depends to a great extent on the clinicians' ability to identify different impairments that cause pain. This chapter deals with the complex issue of chronic pain management. In the first section, an overview of the anatomy and physiology of pain is presented. In the second section, examination and evaluation of pain is explained. In the third section, a number of treatment interventions are suggested. Finally, case studies are presented to guide clinicians through the problem-solving process when designing pain management programs.

DEFINING PAIN

Pain's primary purpose is protective to the body. It occurs whenever there is tissue damage and it causes the individual to react to remove the painful stimulus. Pain is also a sensation with more than one dimension. To the individual, pain is both an objective and a subjective experience. The objective dimension is the physiological tissue damage causing the pain. The subjective dimensions include[8] the following:

■ *A perceptual component:* the client's awareness of the location, quality, intensity, and duration of the pain stimulus.
■ *An affective component:* the psychological factors surrounding the client's pain experience, including the client's personality and emotional state.
■ *A cognitive component:* what the client knows and believes about the pain resulting from his or her cultural background and past pain experiences (both personal pain experiences and those of others).
■ *A behavioral component:* how the client expresses the pain to others through communication and behavior.

All of these components taken together constitute the client's pain experience. Thus, all must be addressed for a successful pain management program. When the subjective components of the pain experience are ignored, it is entirely possible that the client's underlying tissue damage is corrected without curing her or his pain perception.

In addition, recognizing that pain is more than simply a physical injury or disease process helps health professionals explain some of the inconsistencies observed in patients with chronic pain: Why is a client's pain report out of proportion to the magnitude and duration of the injury? Why is pain intolerable to one person and merely uncomfortable to another? And why is pain tolerable in one instance but overwhelming to the same individual when experienced at a different time?

The answers lie in the interconnectedness of the nervous system and the fact that pain transmission involves several higher centers. To select the most appropriate intervention, it is important for clinicians to have at least a general idea of the pain pathways. Therefore an overview of pain anatomy and physiology is in order.

PAIN ANATOMY

Pain arises from the stimulation of specialized peripheral free nerve endings called *nociceptors*. Injurious stimulation to the skin or tissue below can trigger these peripheral terminals whose cell bodies are located in the dorsal root ganglia and trigeminal ganglia. Nociceptors are extremely heterogeneous, differing in the neurotransmitters they contain, the receptors and ion channels they express, their speed of conduction, their response properties to noxious stimuli, and their capacity to be sensitized during inflammation, injury and disease.[9]

Nociceptors found in interstitial tissues become excited with extreme mechanical, thermal, and chemical stimulation,[10] whereas nociceptors found in vessel walls become excited with these stimuli plus marked constriction and dilation of the vessels.[11] These receptors respond directly to some noxious stimuli and indirectly to others by means of one or more chemicals (histamine, K+, bradykinin) released from cells in the traumatized tissues.[12]

Thermal nociceptors are triggered by intense temperatures hot or cold (>45° C or <5° C). They have fibers that are small diameter, thinly myelinated with moderately fast conduction signals between 5 and 30 m/sec. Mechanical nociceptors are triggered by intense pressures applied to the skin, such as a pinch. They also have thinly myelinated moderately conducting fibers between 5 and 30 m/sec.

Polymodal nociceptors are triggered by more than one sensory modality (mechanical, chemical, or thermal). These nociceptors have small-diameter, nonmyelinated fibers that conduct more slowly, generally velocities less than 1.0 m/sec. Stimulation of these receptors causes sensations of diffuse burning or aching pain. The difference in the fibers' size and lamination determines the speed that impulses will travel to the brain.

These three types of nociceptors are broadly distributed in the skin and tissues and may work together. One example would be, when you hit your shin against a table, a sharp "first pain" is felt immediately, followed later by a more prolonged aching, sometimes burning "second pain."[12] The fast, sharp pain is transmitted by A-delta fibers that carry information from thermal and mechanical nociceptors. The slow, dull pain is transmitted by C fibers that are activated by polymodal nociceptors.

Nociceptive input travels on A-delta and C fibers into the dorsal horn of the spinal cord, where the gray matter is laminated and organized by cytological features. The first-order A-delta and C fibers synapse with second-order neurons in lamina I (marginal layer), II (the substantia gelatinosa [SG]), and V. The second-order neurons do one of three things. A small number synapse with motor neurons causing reflex movements (e.g., withdrawing the hand from a hot object). Others synapse with autonomic fibers causing responses such as changes in heart rate and blood pressure and localized vasodilation, piloerection, and sweating. Most, however, travel a multisynaptic route to the higher centers by means of the ascending tracts.[10,13]

There are two major classes of neurons responding to pain in the dorsal horn: nociceptive-specific neurons and wide dynamic range neurons (WDR). Nociceptive-specific neurons are most abundant in superficial lamina and their receptor fields are discrete and vary from one to several square centimeters.[14] WDR neurons, in contrast, respond to a wide range of stimuli from A-delta, A-beta, and C fibers in a graded manner (i.e., the rate of firing escalates with increasing intensity of stimulation), can be found in all lamina, and are the most prevalent cells in the dorsal horn.[14] Because of their unique response to innocuous or nociceptive input, as well as their larger receptor field, WDR neurons play an important role in the central sensitization and the plasticity of the spinal cord.[14]

Nociceptive input crosses at the cord level to the anterolateral quadrant of the ascending contralateral spinothalamic tract (Figure 32-1). The axons of the anterolateral quadrant are arranged so that the sacral segments are most lateral, with the lumbar segments more medial and the cervical segments most central. This arrangement may be important clinically in that symptoms may be provoked according to dermatomal maps to some degree.[15] Pain dermatomes overlap to several adjacent dorsal roots so boundaries can be less distinct, requiring the clinician to distinguish the pain and dysfunction.

The anterolateral tract is divided into three ascending pathways: the spinothalamic, spinoreticular, and spinomesencephalic. The spinothalamic tract conveys information about painful and thermal stimulation directly to the ventral posterior lateral nucleus of the thalamus (location and intensity), as well as sends collaterals off at the brain stem to join the spinoreticular tract. Axons within the spinoreticular tract synapse on neurons of the reticular formation of the medulla and pons, which relay information to the intralaminar and posterior nuclei of the thalamus and to other structures in the diencephalon, such as the hypothalamus (emotional response to pain).

Axons in the spinomesencephalic tract relay information to the mesencephalic reticular formation and periaquaductal gray matter by way of the spinoparabrachial tract. It then projects to the limbic system, which is involved with the affective component of pain (central modulation of pain).

The thalamus relays and processes information to several higher centers.[11] Each projection serves a specific purpose. Axons of the spinothalamic tract project information to both the lateral and medial nuclear groups of the thalamus. The

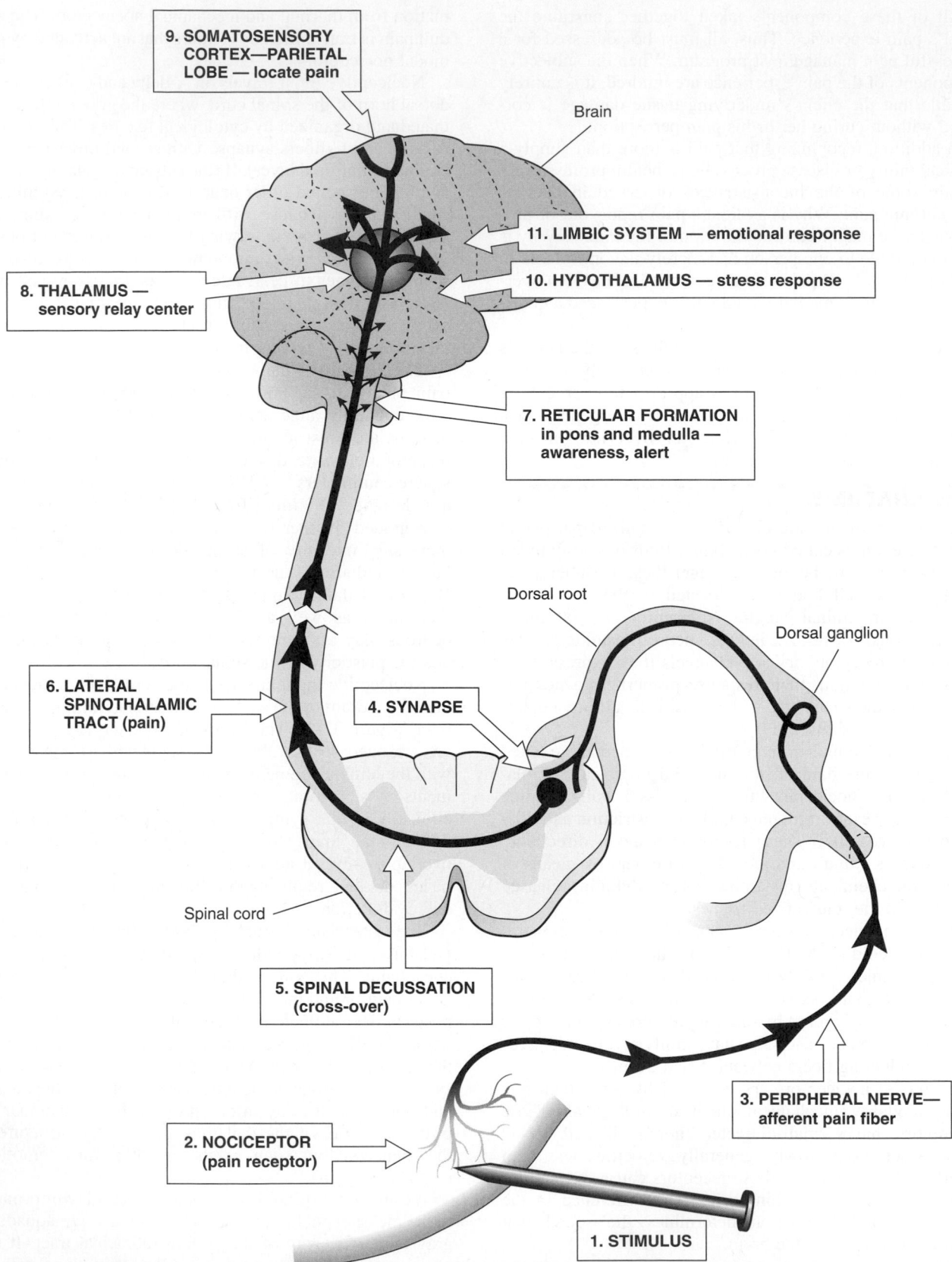

9. SOMATOSENSORY CORTEX—PARIETAL LOBE — locate pain

Brain

11. LIMBIC SYSTEM — emotional response

10. HYPOTHALAMUS — stress response

8. THALAMUS — sensory relay center

7. RETICULAR FORMATION in pons and medulla — awareness, alert

Dorsal root

Dorsal ganglion

6. LATERAL SPINOTHALAMIC TRACT (pain)

4. SYNAPSE

Spinal cord

5. SPINAL DECUSSATION (cross-over)

3. PERIPHERAL NERVE— afferent pain fiber

2. NOCICEPTOR (pain receptor)

1. STIMULUS

FIGURE 32-1 ■ Pain pathway. (From Gould BE: *Pathophysiology for the health professions,* ed 2, Philadelphia, 2002, WB Saunders.)

lateral nuclear group of the thalamus is where information about the location of an injury is thought to be mediated.[12] Injury to the spinothalamic tract and the lateral nuclear group of the thalamus causes central neuropathic pain, which is discussed in further detail below.

Projections from the spinoreticular tract to the medial nuclear group of the thalamus are concerned with processing information about nociception, and they also activate nonspecific arousal systems. These pathways project from the thalamus to the basal ganglia and many cortical areas.

Projections to the postcentral gyrus (sensory cortex) are responsible for pain perception. It is from this projection that pain can be localized and characterized. Projections from the thalamus to the frontal lobes and limbic system are concerned with pain interpretation. It is from all these projections that an individual perceives pain as hurting. Projections from the thalamus, as well as from the limbic system and sensory cortical areas, to the temporal lobes are responsible for pain memory; and projections from the thalamus to the hypothalamus are responsible for the autonomic response to pain.

PAIN TRANSMISSION

Ascending transmission of pain impulses is mediated by the action of chemical excitatory neurotransmitter glutamate (A-delta and C fibers) and tachykinins such as substance P (C fibers). Glutamate and neuropeptides have distinct actions on postsynaptic neurons, but they act together to regulate the firing properties postsynaptically.[12] Tachykinins' activity is thought to prolong the action of glutamate as levels are increased in persistent pain conditions.[14]

PAIN MODULATION

Nociceptive transmission is modulated at several points along the neural pathway by both ascending and descending systems.

The Gate Control Theory

The SG contains an ascending gating mechanism to block nociceptive impulses from leaving the dorsal horn of the spinal cord. The first-order neurons for both nociceptive and nonnociceptive information synapse with second-order neurons in the SG. The second-order neurons for both types of information project to specialized neurons named T (transmission) cells in lamina V. For pain transmission to occur, T cells must be stimulated while the SG is inhibited. The input from A-delta and C fibers stimulates the T cells and inhibits the SG (Figure 32-2). Therefore A-delta and C fiber input opens the gate, allowing pain transmission to the higher centers. On the other hand, when the SG and T cells are both stimulated, the T cells are inhibited and the gate is closed to pain transmission. The input from nonnociceptive A-beta fibers carrying information from pressoreceptors and mechanoreceptors stimulates both the T cells and the SG. Therefore A-beta fiber input closes the gate, blocking pain transmission.[15]

Thus one example would be the use of transcutaneous electrical nerve stimulation (TENS) in an area that overlaps the injury. It works to reduce chronic pain by activation of large-diameter A-beta fibers. This is also why shaking (vibration) your hand after hitting your thumb with a hammer temporarily relieves pain. The gate control theory

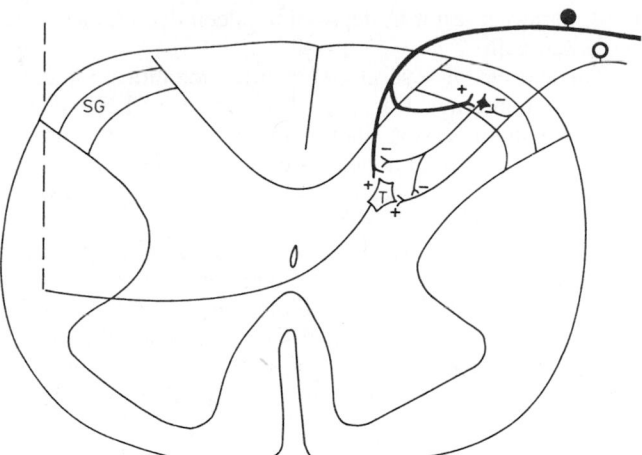

FIGURE 32-2 ■ Schematic representation of spinal structures involved in the gate control theory of pain transmission. Afferent input by means of both large- and small-diameter fibers is theorized to influence the transmission cell (T) directly and through small internuncial neurons located within the substantia gelatinosa (SG). (From Nolan MF: Anatomic and physiologic organization of neural structures involved in pain transmission, modulation, and perception. In Echternach JL, editor: *Pain,* New York, 1987, Churchill Livingstone.)

is thought to be the underlying mechanism for the effectiveness of the physical modalities in relieving pain.

Descending Pain Modulation System

There are at least two descending pain modulation systems. One involves the action of neurotransmitters, including serotonin, dopamine, norepinephrine, and substance P. High concentrations of brain serotonin108 and L-dopa (a precursor of dopamine)[16] have been found to inhibit nociception, whereas norepinephrine appears to enhance nociception.[17-20] The spinal mediators of descending nociceptive inhibitory influences include serotonin, norepinephrine, and acetylcholine. This may be relevant to the action of antidepressants in relieving pain in the absence of depression. Substance P is thought to be the neurotransmitter for neurons transmitting chronic pain.[21]

The second descending modulating system is mediated by neuromodulators—chemicals capable of directly affecting pain transmission. The neuromodulators include enkephalin and beta-endorphin, which are referred to as endogenous opiates because they have morphine-like actions and are found in areas of the central nervous system (CNS) that correspond to opiate-binding sites. Endogenous opiates are believed to modulate pain by inhibiting the release of substance P. They have been shown to have a profound effect on nociception and mood.[22-24] Their levels in the brain and spinal cord rise in response to emotional stress, causing an increase in the pain threshold and providing a possible reason that acute stress decreases acute pain.[25,26]

Although serotonin is not classified as an endogenous opiate, it exerts a profound effect on analgesia and enhances analgesic drug potency. High concentrations of serotonin lead to decreased pain by inhibiting transmission of nociceptive information within the dorsal horn,[27,28] whereas low concentrations result in depression, sleep disturbances, and increased pain.

The success of several therapeutic modalities, including noxious counterirritation (e.g., brief intense TENS or acupressure) and diversion (including hypnosis) is attributed to raising the level of endogenous opiates in the body.[26]

CATEGORIZING PAIN

Pain is grouped into several categories: acute, chronic, and referred and central neuropathic, autonomic, and peripheral.

Acute pain is the normal predicted physiological response and serves as a warning. It alerts the individual that tissues are exposed to damaging or potentially damaging noxious stimuli. Acute pain is localized, in proportion to the intensity of the stimuli, and lasts only as long as the stimuli or the tissue damage exists (1 to 6 months).[29] Although acute pain is associated with anxiety and increased autonomic activity (increased muscle tone, heart rate, and blood pressure),[30] it is usually relieved by interventions directed at correcting the injury. The pain experience is usually limited to the individual.[31]

Chronic pain is usually referred to as intractable pain if it persists for 6 or more months. It is defined as pain that continues after the stimulus is removed or the tissue damage heals. Physiologically, chronic pain is believed to result from hypersensitization of the pain receptors and enlargement of the receptor field in response to the localized inflammation that follows tissue damage.[32] Chronic pain is poorly localized, has an ill-defined time of onset, and is strongly associated with the subjective components outlined previously. It does not respond well to interventions directed solely at correcting the injury. Chronic pain patients frequently complain of other symptoms, such as depression, difficulty sleeping, poor mental and physical function, and fatigue. The effects of the pain experience extend beyond the individual and affect the family, the workplace, and the social sphere of the individual.[31]

Referred pain is felt at a point other than its origin. Pain can be referred from an internal organ, a joint, a trigger point, or a peripheral nerve to a remote musculoskeletal structure. Referred pain usually follows a specific pattern. For example, cardiac pain is frequently referred to the left arm or jaw and the referral pattern for trigger points is exact enough to be used as a diagnostic tool and often used by physicians to diagnosis pathology. Referred pain is the result of a convergence of the primary afferent neurons from deep structures and muscles to secondary neurons that also have a cutaneous receptive field.[33,33a]

Although it is now recognized that all neuropathic pain results in abnormal activity within the CNS,[34] pain initiated or caused by a primary lesion or dysfunction of the CNS[35] is referred to as *central neuropathic pain*. The involvement of the nervous system can be at many levels: nerves, nerve roots and central pain pathways in the spinal cord and brain. In this circumstance, there is permanent damage to the nervous system (usually a peripheral nerve) and likely anatomical reorganization of spinal terminations of surviving axons or ectopic activity from a neuroma that contributes paroxysmal, persistent input to the spinal cord.[36] In addition to anatomical reorganization in the spinal cord, there could be some reorganization in the rostroventral medulla (RVM) as well, but more likely there is prolonged input to the RVM

that sustains facilitatory influences that descend to the spinal cord. Less appreciated, descending facilitatory influences on spinal sensory processing could also be important to maintenance of chronic pain conditions, particularly those that persist in the absence of obvious tissue pathology.[36]

Central neuropathic pain is medically diagnosed by its defining neurological signs and symptoms; it is verified with neuroimaging tests that identify a CNS lesion and rule out other causes. It is important that the therapist be able to localize the level and differentiate between central and peripheral pain. Central neuropathic pain can be caused by vascular insult; traumatic, neoplastic, and demyelinating diseases; and surgery (including vascular compromise during surgery). Central neuropathic pain is distinct from nociceptive pain (nonneuronal tissue damage).

The onset of central neuropathic pain is usually delayed after the occurrence of the initial episode that results in damage to the CNS; onset of pain may occur during the phase of recovery from neurological deficits.[37] Pain originating from a cerebrovascular incident and spinal cord injury usually begins weeks or months after the insult, whereas pain originating from tumors may take years to begin.[34]

Individuals with central neuropathic pain may have difficulty describing their pain and report burning, aching, pricking, squeezing, or cutting pain after cutaneous stimulation, movement, heat, cold, or vibration. A normally nonnoxious stimulus, such as moving clothing across skin, becomes agonizing. In some cases the pain begins spontaneously.[38] Pain intensity varies, but it does seem to be associated to some degree with the location of the lesion.[34] Allodynia (pain from normally nonnoxious stimuli) and dysesthesia are common, and one of the characteristic features of central neuropathic pain is that the clinical symptoms persist long after the stimulus is removed.

Central neuropathic pain is topographical. The site of the lesion determines the location of the symptoms. The pain may involve half the body, an entire extremity, or a small portion of one extremity.[34] It is frequently migratory. Thalamic pain is the classic example of central neuropathic pain.

Central neuropathic pain is difficult to treat. Surgery is not helpful for most individuals with central neuropathic pain, and medications have not been effective in permanently relieving the symptoms.[10] Therefore the treatment of clients with central neuropathic pain stresses coping strategies and prevention of loss of functional activities and life participation. The ideal management of a chronic pain patient is by a multidisciplinary approach, including disciplines such as internal medicine, neurology, anesthesia, nursing, psychology, pharmacy, rehabilitation medicine, physical therapy, occupational therapy, and others. The limitation of this approach is that access to such a wide range of specialists is often available only at large medical centers and special pain clinics, which restricts access to a limited number of the patients.

Under normal conditions, there is a fine balance between the parasympathetic and sympathetic branches of the autonomic nervous system (ANS). Parasympathetic activity maintains homeostasis, whereas sympathetic activity functions to make "fight or flight" changes in response to stress. Stimulation of the autonomic efferent fibers is not normally painful. However, the balance between afferent input and the descending sympathetic nervous system is disrupted when there is injury, resulting in exaggerated and prolonged sympathetic activity, allodynia, and hyperalgesia (increased response to normally painful stimuli)—hence, *autonomic pain.*

Allodynia is a product of the phenomenon of central sensitization.[39] After injury, new axons sprout from the sympathetic efferent neurons. These fire spontaneously and, because they synapse on the cell bodies of the primary afferent neurons, cause them to fire as well. In addition, the dorsal horn neurons themselves become more excitable. They show an enlargement in their receptive field and become more sensitive to mechanical, thermal, and chemical stimulation. The result is an increase in the neuronal barrage into the CNS and the perception of pain with usually nonpainful stimuli.[12]

Complex regional pain syndrome (CRPS) is an example of pain that arises from abnormal activity within the ANS.[40] CRPS has been classified into two distinct types[41]: CRPS type I (formerly reflex sympathetic dystrophy) follows mild trauma without nerve injury, and CRPS type II (formerly causalgia) follows trauma with nerve injury. CRPS type I generally begins within the month after the injury, whereas CRPS type II can occur any time after the injury.[42]

The main features of CRPS type I are constant burning pain that fluctuates in intensity and increases with movement, constant stimulation, or stress. There are also allodynia and hyperalgia, edema, abnormal sweating, abnormal blood flow and trophic changes in the area of pain, and impaired motor function. CRPS type I is relieved by blocking the sympathetic nervous system, indicating that the pain is sympathetically maintained.[42]

CRPS type II occurs in the region of a limb innervated by an injured nerve. The nerves most commonly involved in CRPS type II are the median, sciatic, tibial, and ulnar; involvement of the radial nerve is rare. Pain is described as spontaneous, constant, and burning and is exacerbated by light touch, stress, temperature change, movement, visual and auditory stimuli, and emotional disturbances. Allodynia and hyperalgia are common and may involve the distribution of more than one peripheral nerve. As with CRPS type I, edema, abnormal sweating, abnormal blood flow, trophic changes, and impaired motor function occur. The symptoms spread proximally and can involve other areas of the body. Evidence also points to sympathetic involvement in CRPS type II.[42]

The treatment of CRPS is complex and must be carefully coordinated between an interdisciplinary team including the neurologist (medications), psychologist (behavioral), anesthesiologist (injections), and the therapist (functional recovery). The therapist provides the core treatment to improve function. Therapists need to pay close attention to the following aspects of the disorder: (1) the degree of motor abnormalities, including restricted active range of motion, abnormal posturing, spasm, tremor, and dystonia; (2) true passive range restriction; (3) hyperesthesia and allodynia; (4) swelling and vasomotor changes; and (5) evidence of osteoporosis by radiograph.[43] Please refer to Case Study 32-3 for interventions for clients with CRPS.

Peripheral pain results from noxious irritation of the nociceptors. The character of peripheral pain depends on the location and intensity of the noxious stimulation, as well as on which fibers carry the information into the dorsal gray matter. As noted previously, information carried on A-delta fibers is sharp and well localized, begins rapidly, and lasts only as long as the stimulus is present, whereas information carried on C fibers is dull and diffuse, has a delayed onset, and lasts longer than the duration of the stimulus. The treatment of peripheral pain is covered in detail in Chapter 15.

The management of central versus peripheral pain is determined by the type of pain: acute or chronic, and the clinical features present, including clinical localization; time of onset; laboratory study localization; response to analgesics, including narcotics; response to antidepressants; and response to nerve block or neurectomy.[37] Differentiation between features will drive the treatment plan, but because some peripheral and central forms can coexist, diagnosis may be difficult.

The multidimensional aspects of chronic pain make it important to evaluate the causative nature as well as the emotional and cognitive sequela.[44] Persistent pain is now considered to have a psychogenic component.[45] The longer an individual has pain, the more a psychological component may become dominant. Many emotional factors can strongly influence pain, such as pain thresholds, past experiences with pain, coping styles, and social roles. The emotional experience that we perceive with pain reflects the interaction of higher brain centers and subcortical regions, such as the amygdala and cingulate gyrus (limbic system).[46] Positron emission tomography of patients with chronic neuropathic pain demonstrates a shift of acute pain activity in the sensory cortex to regions such as the anterior cingulate gyrus.[47] Understanding the physical limitations of chronic pain is an area that therapists commonly assess; it is the mind-body connection that is often less articulated by the client and more difficult for the practitioner.

Treatment of chronic pain should include a patient-centered approach given the unique manifestations that occur in an individual's response to pain. Patient-centered models, such as the International Classification of Functioning, Disability and Health (ICF), provide a framework that embraces a multidisciplinary team approach practiced in pain clinics. In such models, chronic pain was noted to include psychological factors such as feelings of fear, anxiety, and depression,[48] which are known to have the ability to modulate and exacerbate the physical pain experience.[49] For example, a client with chronic pain who has the fear that movement will increase pain may alter his activity, causing muscular shortening, spasms, and a spiraling course of more pain and disability. The focus in treating clients with chronic pain should be on improving functional physical activity, decreasing peripheral nociception and central facilitation, and providing cognitive and behavioral strategies to help in resuming normal activities.

EXAMINATION OF THE CLIENT WITH PAIN

The examination of a client with pain can be challenging because the therapist must frequently weed through the individual's emotions, behaviors, and secondary gains in an attempt to identify the source of the symptoms. Many clients are not referred to therapy until they have participated in weeks, months, even years of failed interventions, and their expectations and patience are at low levels. They often approach therapy anticipating more instructions, more frustration, and more pain. Despite these obstacles, therapists must strive to complete pain evaluations that include measurable, reproducible information that identifies the source of pain and provides direction toward treatment that is both beneficial and cost effective, and that assists in establishing attainable goals.

Pain History

Every evaluation of a client with pain should begin with a comprehensive pain history. It is important to have a standardized format to decrease chances of missing important information and to minimize having the client "lead the interview." The following alphabetical mnemonic device may prove helpful:

- *Observation:* Observation of the client from the moment of entry until (and sometimes beyond) the moment of exit from the clinic. By observing the client outside of the evaluation, the therapist is able to assess the client's movement. The patient's nervous system will accurately express itself to the therapist, especially when the patient's attention is asked to focus on a topic other than pain and the patient is not aware that movement is being observed.
- *Origin/onset:* Date and circumstances of the onset of pain. How did the pain start? Gradually or suddenly? Was there a precipitating injury? If so, what was the mechanism of injury? If not, can the client correlate the onset to a particular activity or posture?
- *Position:* Location of the pain. Have the client demonstrate where the pain is located rather than relying on description alone. In addition to being more accurate, demonstration allows another observation of the client's ability and willingness to move. Clients can also be asked to draw their symptoms on a schematic, such as the pain drawing, which is described later.
- *Pattern:* Pattern of the pain. Is the pain constant or periodic? Does it travel or radiate? Which activities and postures increase or decrease the pain? Does medication or time of day have any effect on the pain? Have there been any recent changes in the pattern? Does the client believe that the pain is improving, worsening, or remaining the same?
- *Quality:* Characteristics of the pain. Does the client use adjectives indicating mechanical (pressing, bursting, stabbing), chemical (burning), neural (numb, "pins and needles"), or vascular (throbbing) origin? Two tools for describing pain character are described later.
- *Quantity:* Intensity of the pain. How has the pain intensity changed since the onset? Several methods that allow for monitoring change in pain intensity are presented later.
- *Radiation:* Characteristics of pain radiation. Does the pain radiate? What causes the pain to radiate? Can the radiation be reversed? How?
- *Signs/symptoms:* Functional and psychological components of the pain. Has the pain resulted in any functional limitations? Has it caused any changes in the client's ability to participate in life, including employment and recreational activities? Does the client's personality contribute to the pain, or has the pain caused changes in the client's emotional stability? Does the client benefit from the pain? How? It may be necessary to interview the

client's significant others or family members for an accurate picture.
- *Treatment:* Previous/current medical and therapeutic treatment and its effectiveness, including medications, home remedies, and recommendations for movement activities. It is also important to determine the client's attitude and expectations concerning therapy in addition to obtaining a treatment history.
- *Visceral symptoms:* Physical symptoms of visceral origin that can accompany and be responsible for the pain (Box 32-1). Visceral causes for pain require referral to the client's physician for further investigation before the initiation of treatment by a therapist.

Pain Measurement

Research has shown that pain memory does not provide an accurate measure of pain intensity.[51] Therefore pain measurement tools are designed to provide information about the intensity, location, and character of a client's symptoms *at the time of the evaluation.* This information can then be merged with the pain history, disease/pathology history, and the physical findings to identify the cause of pain. The disease/pathology management and its pain measurement will be the responsibility of the physician, whereas the movement limitations caused by the pain are the responsibility of the therapist. A number of pain measurement tools are available. These tools are used by professionals whose focus is pathology, as well as professionals whose responsibility is regaining functional activities and life participation. The applications and limitations of several are discussed.

Measuring Pain Intensity

Pain intensity rating tools are scales that have the client rate the current level of pain by marking a continuum or assigning a numerical value to the pain intensity (Figure 32-3).

Each of the first three tools described here has been found to be reliable over time when used to measure pain that is present at the time of the rating. In general, however, clients who are depressed or anxious tend to report higher levels of pain and clients who are not depressed or anxious tend to report lower levels of pain on all three of these scales.[52]

Visual Analog Scale (VAS). The client rates the pain on a continuum that begins with "no pain" and ends with "maximum pain tolerable." This tool provides an infinite number of points between the extremes, making it sensitive to small changes in pain intensity. However, it has not been found reliable for individuals who have impaired abstract thinking skills[53] and may be unable to translate their pain intensity into a corresponding point on a line.

Simple Descriptive Pain Scale (SDPS). The client rates the pain on a continuum that is subdivided using descriptors that gradually increase in intensity. Sample descriptors are "no pain," "mild pain," "moderate pain," "severe pain," and "maximum pain tolerable." This tool is more useful than the VAS for clients with impaired abstract thinking because it is easier for them to identify with the pain descriptors than with the line found in the VAS. However, clients have been found to favor the points

ment**1043**

BOX 32-1 ■ VISCEROGENIC BACK PAIN[50]

General signs and symptoms:
- Pain does not increase with spinal stresses/strains
- Pain is not relieved with rest
- Visceral symptoms accompany back pain
- Gastrointestinal tract signs and symptoms
- Pain is accompanied by altered bowel habits
- Pain is related to eating
- Peptic pain is relieved with vomiting

Kidney signs and symptoms:
- Increased pain with diuresis indicates hydronephrosis

Pelvic signs and symptoms:
- Low back pain associated with vaginal bleeding or discharge

Prostate signs and symptoms:
- Low back discomfort associated with micturition

Lung signs and symptoms:
- Posterior thoracic pain associated with respiration in chronic obstructive pulmonary disease

Vascular signs and symptoms:
- Deep, boring, pulsating low back pain associated with a palpable abdominal aortic aneurysm
- Back pain with/without calf pain after walking and relieved with standing still; possibly impaired lower extremity pulses and trophic skin changes associated with occlusive disease of the internal iliac artery or its branches

Adapted from Makofsky H, Willis GC: Non-mechanical and pathological causes of low back pain, *Phys Ther Forum,* May 15, p 12, 1989.

corresponding to each descriptor rather than the points between, resulting in a less sensitive tool than the VAS.[54]

Pain Estimate. The client assigns a numerical rating to the pain, staying within defined limits (most commonly between 0 and 100, where 0 represents no pain and 100 represents maximum pain tolerable). Because it provides a numerical range of scores, this tool is valuable for statistical analysis purposes. However, whereas some clients find assigning a numerical rating to their pain intensity easy, clients with impaired abstract thinking may have difficulty similar to that encountered with the VAS.

Faces Pain Scale. The client selects one of seven schematic faces representing gradually increasing pain intensities. The scale begins with a face representing no pain and ends with a face representing the most pain possible. This tool is designed for use with young children who do not have the ability to use any of the three previous tools. The Faces Pain Scale has been found to be valid across cultural lines[55] and to have a strong correlation with other pain measures.[53] It is simple to use, does not require verbal skills, and requires little instruction. It has been used successfully with children as young as age 3 and with individuals who are limited in verbal expression.

Localizing Pain Symptoms

Pain Drawings. The client is asked to draw his or her symptoms on a schematic of the human body using a provided list of symbols (Figure 32-4). The result is a diagram describing the nature and location of the client's pain that can be compared with the client's verbal report. In addition to providing a database, the pain drawing has been found to be useful in identifying individuals who have a heavy

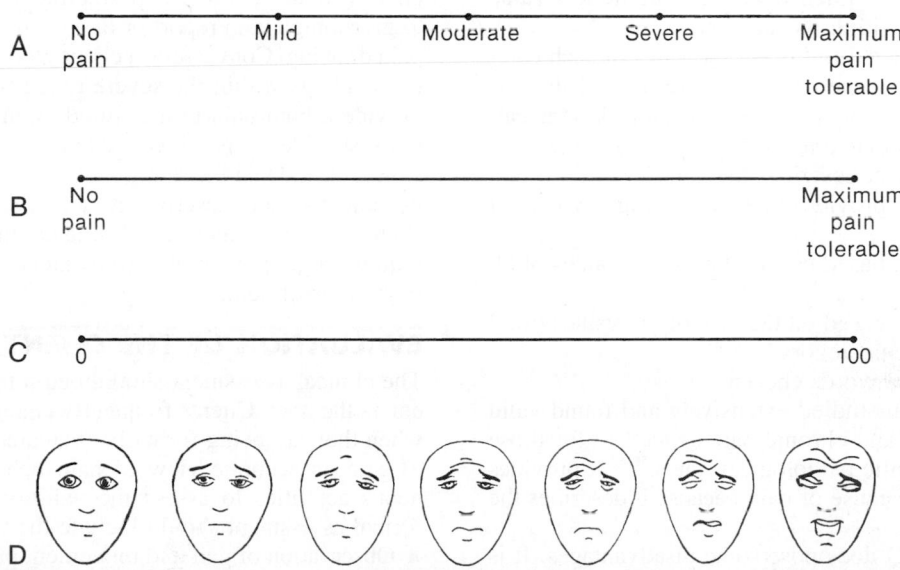

FIGURE 32-3 ■ Rating scales for measuring pain intensity. *A,* Simple descriptive pain scale (SDPS). *B,* Visual analog scale (VAS). *C,* Pain estimate. *D,* Faces pain scale. (*D,* Reprinted from Bieri D, Reeve DA, Champion GD et al: The faces pain scale for the self-assessment of the severity of pain experienced by children: development, initial validation, and preliminary investigation for the ratio scale properties, *Pain* 41:139-150, 1990, with permission from Elsevier Science.)

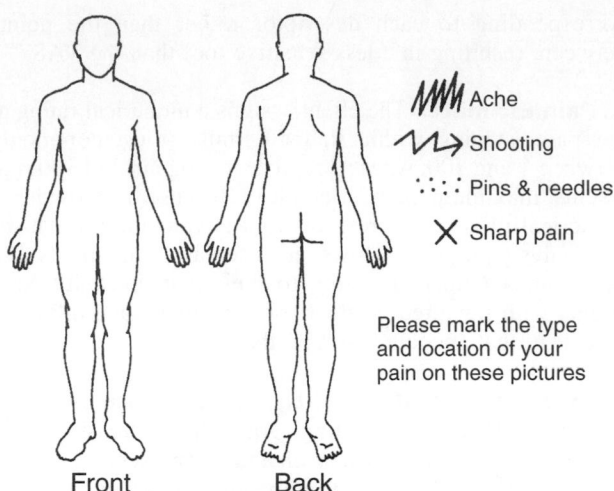

Ache

Shooting

Pins & needles

✗ Sharp pain

Please mark the type
and location of your
pain on these pictures

Front   Back

FIGURE 32-4 ■ Pain drawing for describing the nature and location of a client's pain symptoms. (From Cameron MH, editor: *Physical agents in rehabilitation,* Philadelphia, 1999, WB Saunders.)

psychological or emotional component to their pain, making it helpful also in identifying clients who would benefit from further psychological evaluation.[56]

Describing Pain Quality

McGill Pain Questionnaire (MPQ). One of the most popular scales to rate pain quality is the McGill Pain Questionnaire, which includes 20 categories of descriptive words covering the sensory (numbers 1 to 10), affective (numbers 11 to 15), and evaluative (number 16) properties of pain (Figure 32-5). Sensory properties are measured using temporal, thermal, spatial, and pressure descriptors. Affective properties are measured using fear, tension, and autonomic descriptors. Evaluative properties are measured using pain experience descriptors.[57] Each word has a numerical value based on its position within its category.

The client is instructed to "select the word in each category that best describes the pain you have now. If there is no word in the category that describes the pain, skip the category. If there is more than one word that describes the pain, select the word that best describes the pain."[57]

The MPQ can provide the following types of information[57]:

■ A pain-rating index based on the sum of the values of all the words selected
■ A pain-rating index based on the sum of the values of all the words in a given category
■ The total number of words chosen

The MPQ has been studied extensively and found valid for adults with acute and chronic pain as well as for those with a variety of specific pathological states.[58-60] It provides clues into the specific cause of pain because it describes the client's symptoms.

However, the MPQ does pose some disadvantages. It is time consuming, requiring more time to complete than any of the previously described rating scales. Thus, it is not appropriate for quick estimates of pain after treatment. Clients, especially children, are frequently unfamiliar with some of the descriptors and ask the evaluator to assist by

defining words. However, reliability and validity of this test are based on examiner objectivity and care must be taken to avoid the introduction of evaluator bias by helping the client to select appropriate descriptors.[57] This issue can be dealt with by telling the client, "If you do not recognize a word, it probably does not apply to you."

Pediatric Verbal Descriptor Scale. Because a child's description of pain is limited by a smaller vocabulary, Wilkie and associates[61] have developed a verbal descriptor scale specifically for use with children (Table 32-1). Their list includes 56 words commonly used by children aged 8 to 17 to describe their pain experience. The word list is divided into the four categories found in the MPQ. The evaluators' research has shown the list to be useful for children with a variety of diagnoses because it is relatively free of gender, ethnic, and developmental bias.

Caregiver Checklist. Clients who are unable to communicate verbally because of neurological disabilities may be unable to use any of the just-described pain measurement scales. However, because of pain associated with their medical conditions, extensive and repeated surgery, and behavioral oddities that might limit pain expression, these individuals are at high risk for having their pain go unrecognized. McGrath et al[62] have attempted to develop and categorize a checklist of demonstrated pain behaviors identified by caregivers of severely handicapped individuals. Although their list did not pass validity criteria, the researchers propose clinicians develop a client-specific checklist that could be used to gauge changes in the client's pain from the information gained during the caregiver interview portion of the evaluation of nonverbal handicapped clients.

In addition to qualifying and quantifying the client's pain, pain measurement tools have an additional value. They can be used to identify inconsistencies between a client's pain report and the clinician's objective findings. For example, a client with normal objective findings would not be expected to give a high pain report or draw symptoms over the entire pain drawing. Conversely, a client with a multitude of objective findings within the severe range would be expected to provide a high pain rating. In addition, as objective symptoms subside, it is expected that the client will report a similar decline on the rating scales. Inconsistencies between the client's pain descriptions and the therapist's findings should serve to alert the clinician that the client might require cognitive or affective intervention in addition to physical treatment.

EVALUATION OF THE CLIENT

The clinical assessment should begin the moment the client enters the door. Clients frequently change posture and affect when they are being formally evaluated, and it is important to gain an accurate view of pain behavior during spontaneous activities to assess the validity of complaints. The formal assessment should include the following:

■ Observation of gait and movement patterns, including the use of assistive devices
■ Notation of body type and anomalies
■ Assessment of sitting and standing posture, including both the normal posture and that assumed because of the pain (Observe the client during activities, if possible, to

What Does Your Pain Feel Like?

Some of the words below describe your present pain. Circle ONLY those words that best describe it. Leave out any category that is not suitable. Use only a single word in each appropriate category–the one that applies best.

1	2	3	4
Flickering	Jumping	Pricking	Sharp
Quivering	Flashing	Boring	Cutting
Pulsing	Shooting	Drilling	Lacerating
Throbbing		Stabbing	
Beating		Lancinating	
Pounding			

5	6	7	8
Pinching	Tugging	Hot	Tingling
Pressing	Pulling	Burning	Itchy
Gnawing	Wrenching	Scalding	Smarting
Cramping		Searing	Stinging
Crushing			

9	10	11	12
Dull	Tender	Tiring	Sickening
Sore	Taut	Exhausting	Suffocating
Hurting	Rasping		
Aching	Splitting		
Heavy			

13	14	15	16
Fearful	Punishing	Wretched	Annoying
Frightful	Grueling	Blinding	Troublesome
Terrifying	Cruel		Miserable
	Vicious		Intense
	Killing		Unbearable

17	18	19	20
Spreading	Tight	Cool	Nagging
Radiating	Numb	Cold	Nauseating
Penetrating	Drawing	Freezing	Agonizing
Piercing	Squeezing		Dreadful
	Tearing		Torturing

FIGURE 32-5 ■ The McGill Pain Questionnaire used to rate pain quality. (Reprinted from Melzak R: The McGill pain questionnaire: major properties and scoring methods, *Pain* 1:277, 1975, with permission from Elsevier Science.)

TABLE 32-1 ■ Pediatric Verbal Descriptor Scale

DIMENSION	WORD	DIMENSION	WORD	DIMENSION	WORD	DIMENSION	WORD
A	Annoying	S	Biting	S	Itching	A	Crying
	Bad		Cutting		Like a scratch		Frightening
	Horrible		Like a pin		Like a sting		Screaming
	Miserable		Like a sharp knife		Scratching		Terrifying
	Terrible		Pinlike		Stinging		
	Uncomfortable		Sharp			A	Dizzy
			Stabbing	S	Shocking		Sickening
E	Aching				Shooting		Suffocating
	Hurting	S	Blistering		Splitting		
	Like an ache		Burning			E	Never goes away
	Like a hurt		Hot	S	Numb		Uncontrollable
	Sore				Stiff		
		S	Cramping		Swollen		
S	Beating		Crushing		Tight		
	Hitting		Like a pinch				
	Pounding		Pinching	A	Awful		
	Punching		Pressure		Deadly		
	Throbbing				Dying		
					Killing		

Reprinted from Wilkie DJ, Holzemer WL, Tesler MD et al: Measuring pain quality: validity and reliability of children's and adolescents' pain language, *Pain* 41:151-159, 1990, with permission from Elsevier Science.
S, Sensory; *A*, affective; *E*, evaluative.

differentiate movement patterns altered by intent vs. automatic adjustments.)

■ Inspection of the skin for pliability, trophic changes, scar tissue, and other abnormalities

■ Palpation of the soft tissue structures to identify changes in temperature, swelling, tenderness, and areas of discomfort

■ Palpation of the anatomical structures to determine end feel–the sensation felt at the end of the available movement[63]

■ Bone-to-bone: hard normal, for example, at the end range of elbow extension

■ Spasm: muscular resistance abnormal

■ Capsular feel: rubbery normal at the extreme of full range of motion (ROM); abnormal when encountered before the end of ROM

■ Springy block: rebound abnormal

■ Tissue approximation: soft tissue normal at the extremes of full passive flexion

■ Empty feel: no physiological resistance, but client resists movement because of pain.

■ Measurement of ROM: active ROM is performed to assess the client's willingness to move and to identify any limitations or painful areas; passive ROM testing is used to further refine the observations.[63]

■ When active and passive movements are painful and restricted in the same direction and the pain appears at the limit of motion, the problem is arthrogenic.

■ When active and passive movements are painful or restricted in opposite directions, the problem is muscular.

■ When there is relative restriction of passive movement in the capsular pattern, the problem is arthritic.

■ When there is no restriction of passive movement but the client cannot perform the movement actively, the muscle is not functioning, either from intrinsic problems within the muscle or interruption in the neural pathway (central or peripheral).

■ Measurement of muscle strength:[63]

■ When the movement is strong and painful, there is a minor lesion in the muscle or tendon.

■ When the movement is weak and increases the pain, there is a major lesion that needs to be identified with further testing.

■ When the movement is weak but does not increase the pain, there is the possibility of either complete rupture of the muscle or tendon or a neurological disorder.

■ When all resisted movements are painful, the pain may be organic or the patient may be emotionally hypersensitive.

■ When movement is strong and painless, the test is normal.

■ Assessment of bilateral neurological function:

■ Reflexes: peripheral lesions tend to diminish deep tendon reflexes (DTRs). CNS lesions tend to intensify DTRs, and testing frequently elicits a clonic reaction.[64] Note any asymmetries in response.

■ Sensation: test light touch, sharp (noxious) touch, and vibration. Pressure on a nerve usually affects conduction on the large, myelinated fibers first. Therefore vibration is the first sensation to be diminished. Where there is decreased perception of touch and noxious stimuli, the lesion is more severe.[64] Note any asymmetries in response.

■ Allodynia and hyperalgesia: delineate areas of allodynia and hyperalgesia to touch, hot, and cold. Exact descriptions of these areas, along with areas of decreased perception of vibration, will provide information concerning A-beta versus C fiber involvement in the production of pain.[65]

■ Coordination.

■ Stretch and pressure tests to nerve trunks.

It is not always possible to complete a pain evaluation in one session. Clients may not be able to tolerate all the required activities at one time, or there may be enough inconsistencies for the therapist to want a second appointment to refocus on specific tests. However, with the limitations on number of visits common with managed care, the therapist may feel pressured to identify a cause for the client's pain in the initial visit. This is not necessary. It is far better to take more than one visit and be accurate than to take only one visit and develop a treatment plan that is not appropriate for the client's needs.

TREATMENT OF THE CLIENT WITH PAIN

There are three broad avenues of intervention for pain management: physical interventions, cognitive strategies, and behavioral manipulations.[66] Each avenue addresses a different aspect of the pain experience and each requires a different level of participation from the client.

Physical interventions are directed at the client's body with the goal of healing the tissue injury. Examples include medication, surgery, and the therapy modalities. Physical interventions are of use most frequently with acute pain or recurrent pain resulting from reinjury. Physical interventions are often passive and, for the most part, soothing. When used long term, they promote dependence on the clinician. Therefore it is best to use them as a short-term adjunct in the overall treatment program.

Cognitive strategies are directed at the client's thoughts with the goal of changing the client's pain paradigms. Cognitive strategies include body scanning and reinterpretation of self-statements. Cognitive strategies are self-initiated and performed independently; therefore they encourage personal responsibility and independence.

Behavioral manipulations involve a behavioral change on the part of the client to bring about the desired response. They include exercise, biofeedback, hypnosis, relaxation exercises, and operant conditioning. There is usually a brief learning period until the client becomes proficient with these techniques; however, once learned, behavioral manipulations can be initiated and performed independently. Behavioral manipulations also encourage personal responsibility and independence.

A brief review of the benefits, indications, contraindications, and precautions for many of the interventions provided by therapists should provide an overview of the complexity of pain management. The purpose of this section is to provide guidance in the selection of one treatment option over another so that intervention will be based on sound physiological principles. Readers who wish to explore an intervention in greater depth are directed to the references listed at the end of this chapter.

Physical Interventions

Thermotherapy

The physiological effects of heat depend on the method of application, the depth of penetration, and the rate and magnitude of temperature change. In terms of the use of thermotherapy to control pain, several mechanisms have been established. Muscle spasm decreases as a result of decreased activity in gamma motor efferents, decreased excitability of muscle spindles, and increased activity of Golgi tendon organs.[67,68] This modality will often decrease peripheral pain. Ischemic pain is relieved by the influx of oxygen-rich blood into the dilated vessels, and muscle tension pain is decreased by interruption of the pain/spasm cycle. In addition, the pain threshold itself rises through gating at the spinal cord level.[69,70]

Several textbooks[70a,71-74] on physical agents and rehabilitation discuss the physiological effects, precautions, contraindications, and method of application for these modalities. The reader is advised to refer to the textbooks for details.

Superficial heat can be applied by conduction, convection, or radiation. Conductive heating involves the exchange of heat down a temperature gradient by two objects that are in contact. The depth of penetration with conductive heating is usually 1 cm or less.[75] Moist heat packs and paraffin are examples of therapeutic conductive heating. Convective heating involves heat transfer through the flow of hot fluid. Therapeutic convective heating takes place during hydrotherapy and Fluidotherapy (Encore Medical Corp., Austin, Tex.). Molecules with a temperature greater than absolute zero are in an excited state and emit energy, thus creating radiant heat. Objects that are warmed by the energy are heated by radiation. Therapeutic radiant heat is applied with infrared or ultraviolet light. Because of the contraindications of ultraviolet light, this type of radiant heat is seldom used by therapists today in rehabilitation settings.

Clients can be taught how and when to apply superficial heat independently. Once they demonstrate independence, responsibility for the application of superficial heat should be transferred to the client or her or his caregiver.

The deeper tissues can be heated using conversion, the alteration of one form of energy into another. Examples of heating by conversion are applied with shortwave diathermy or ultrasound.

During **shortwave diathermy,** the client is placed into an oscillating magnetic field. The systemic ions create friction as they attempt to line up with the continuously reversing current, resulting in an increase in tissue temperature deep within the body. Shortwave diathermy is contraindicated for clients with metal implants because of the potential for the implant to become hot and burn the surrounding tissues. It is also contraindicated for clients with cardiac pacemakers because of the pacemaker's metal components and because the electromagnetic radiation may interfere with the pacemaker's operation. They should not be used for clients with cancer, multiple sclerosis or for those who are pregnant, and they should not be used over the eyes, the reproductive organs, or growing epiphyses. Female therapists should avoid prolonged exposure to shortwave diathermy because some research has demonstrated a possible negative effect on pregnancy outcome and fetal development.[76]

Ultrasound is another modality that heats deep tissues by conversion. As its name implies, ultrasound consists of sound waves delivered at a frequency too high to be perceived by human hearing. Sound waves are repeatedly refracted as they encounter tissues of differing acoustical resistance while traveling through the skin toward the bone (Figure 32-6). Tissues with high collagen content (tendon, ligament, fascia, and joint capsule) are heated more efficiently than tissues with low collagen content (fat, muscle). The extent of the temperature increase is related to the dosage of ultrasound delivered. As the dosage of ultrasound is increased by increasing the treatment duration or intensity, more energy is available to the tissues and the heating effect increases.[18] Moreover, the higher the frequency of ultrasound delivered, the more superficial the effect. Ultrasound delivered at 1 MHz heats tissues at depths to 5 cm, whereas ultrasound delivered at 3 MHz heats tissues in the upper 2 cm.[77]

The thermal effects of ultrasound can be used to increase tissue extensibility, cellular metabolic processes, and circulation; decrease pain and muscle spasm; and change nerve conduction velocity. The number of impulses traveling along the nerve decreases at low dosages but begins to rise slowly beginning at 1.9 W/cm^2. Sounding of C fibers yields pain relief distal to the point of application, whereas sounding of large-diameter A fibers brings relief of spasm by changing gamma fiber activity, making the muscle fibers less sensitive to stretch.[78] Because it is impossible to treat C or A fibers selectively, ultrasound provides both pain relief and relief from muscle spasm, making it effective in the treatment of peripheral neuropathies, neuroma, herpes zoster, and muscle spasm associated with musculoskeletal pathology, including sprains, strains, and contusions.[79]

In addition to thermal effects, ultrasound has nonthermal effects that come from the mechanical effects of the ultrasound wave on the tissues. Ultrasound causes cavitation, the development and growth of gas-filled bubbles, in the tissues. Ultrasound also causes tissue fluid to move or stream. The movement of fluid around the gas bubbles formed by cavitation is called *microstreaming,* and the movement of fluid

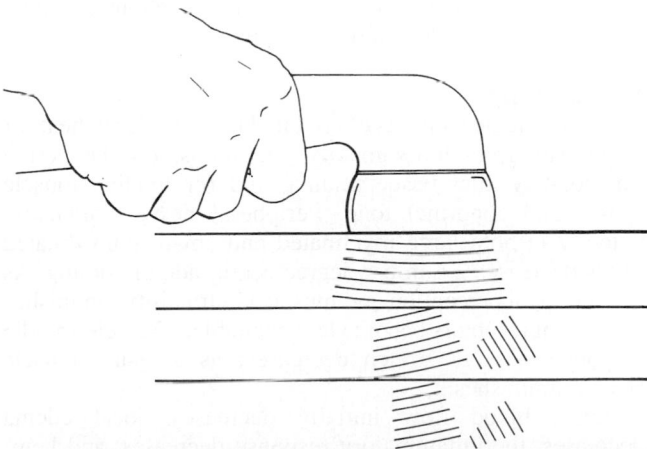

FIGURE 32-6 ■ The longitudinal wave of ultrasound is refracted at tissue interfaces where it encounters tissues of differing acoustical resistance. When the wave changes direction, energy is transferred to the tissues, resulting in the production of heat.

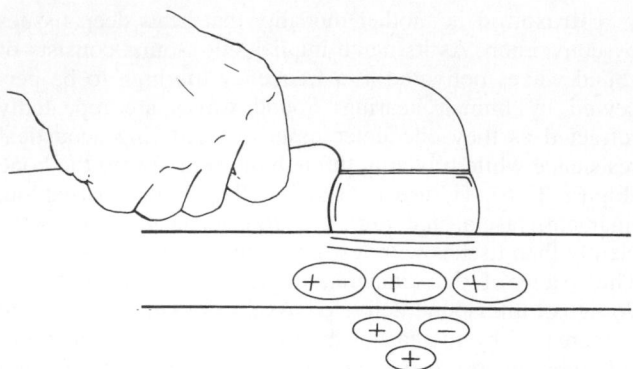

FIGURE 32-7 ■ Phonophoresis. Molecules of a substance are driven into the tissues by the ultrasound wavefront. They are not free for use by the body until they are broken down into chemical ions.

within the ultrasound delivery area is called *acoustic streaming.* The nonthermal effects of ultrasound include accelerating metabolic processes, enzyme activity, and the rate of ion exchange, as well as increasing cell membrane permeability and the rate and volume of diffusion across cell membranes. These effects are thought to explain the role of ultrasound in enhancing the healing of soft tissue and bone.[80-82] The nonthermal effects of ultrasound can be achieved without raising tissue temperature by applying ultrasound in the pulsed mode.

Phonophoresis is the use of ultrasound to deliver pain-relieving chemicals to the tissues. Chemicals are delivered to the cells by the ultrasound wave, where they are broken down into ions and taken up into the cells (Figure 32-7). Common pain-relieving chemicals that can be administered with phonophoresis include 5% Lidocaine ointment (Xylocaine) for acute conditions in which immediate pain relief is the primary goal; 10% or hydrocortisone cream or ointment, when pain is the result of inflammation.[83]

After phonophoresis, measurable quantities of these molecules have been found at tissue depths of up to 2 inches.[84] The contraindication to use of any chemical during phonophoresis is having an allergy to that chemical. Clients should be questioned about any adverse reactions to dental local anesthesia (lidocaine) or aspirin.

Cryotherapy

The physiological effects of cold make it superior to heat for acute pain from inflammatory conditions, for the period immediately after tissue trauma, and for treating muscle spasm and abnormal tone. Peripheral nerve conduction velocity in both large myelinated and small unmyelinated fibers decreases 2.4 m per degree centigrade of cooling. As a result, pain perception and muscle contractility diminish.[85] Peripheral receptors become less excitable.[85] Muscle spindle responsiveness to stretch decreases; as a result, muscle spasm diminishes.[78]

Local blood flow initially decreases, local edema decreases, the inflammatory response decreases, and hemorrhage is minimized. However, cold application for longer than 15 minutes results in increased local blood flow. Known as the "hunting response," this protective mechanism brings core temperature blood to the surface and prevents tissue

injury resulting from prolonged cooling.[75] Cellular metabolic activities slow. The oxygen requirements of the cell decrease.[85]

As with heat, several precautions must be taken when using cold as a therapeutic modality. Cryotherapy is contraindicated in individuals with Raynaud's phenomenon or cold allergy. Cryotherapy should not be used in individuals with rheumatic disease who, with the application of cold, have increased joint pain and stiffness. Cryotherapy should be used with caution in young, frail, or elderly individuals and those with peripheral vascular disease, circulatory pathological processes, or sensory loss.[86]

Cryotherapy is applied in three ways. Convective cooling involves movement of air over the skin (fanning) and is rarely used therapeutically. Evaporative cooling results when a substance applied to the skin uses thermal energy to evaporate, thereby lowering surface temperature. Most commonly, this substance is a vapocoolant spray. Conductive cooling uses local application of cold, either by ice packs, ice massage, or immersion. Cooling is accomplished as heat from the higher temperature object is transferred to the colder object down a temperature gradient. Conductive cooling is the most commonly used form of therapeutic cold application.

Because muscles, tendons, and joints respond differently, the best method of cold application depends on which tissues are causing the pain.[87] Acute injuries are best treated with cryotherapy along with rest, compression, and elevation (RICE). Muscle spasm is decreased with cold packs and stretching. Trigger points, irritable foci within muscles, are best treated with vapocoolant spray, deep friction massage, and stretching. Tendinitis responds well to ice massage and exercise. Cold packs are often the only source of pain relief in acute disk pathology. The inflamed joints of rheumatoid arthritis frequently respond to cold packs or ice massage with decreased inflammation, increased function, and long-lasting pain relief.[86,88]

Clients and caregivers can be taught how and when to perform cryotherapy independently. Once they demonstrate their proficiency, responsibility for the use of cryotherapy should be transferred to the client or the client's caregiver.

Transcutaneous Electrical Nerve Stimulation

TENS is the use of electricity to control the perception of pain. The exact mechanism by which TENS modulates pain still is not completely clear. It appears that, at a high rate, TENS selectively stimulates the low-threshold, large-diameter A-beta fibers, resulting in presynaptic inhibition within the dorsal horns,[89] either directly through the gating mechanism or indirectly through stimulation of the tonic descending pain-inhibiting pathways.[90] Research has shown that the neurons in the brain stem fire in synchrony with the TENS stimulation frequency,[91] and although the significance of this is not known at this time, it does indicate that the action of high-rate TENS is not limited to the dorsal columns. TENS delivered at a low rate is thought to facilitate elevation of the level of endogenous opiates in the CNS.[92]

Stimulation frequencies between 1 and 250 pulses per second (pps) decrease pain. Frequencies between 50 and 100 pps have proven most effective for sensory level (high rate) TENS, and frequencies between 2 and 3 pps are most effective for motor level (low rate) TENS.[28] Stimulation at exactly 2 pps causes an increase in the pain threshold.[51] As the frequency is decreased, more time is needed before the onset of relief, but the effects are more long-lasting.[93] Pulse width duration determines which nerves are stimulated. Sensory nerves are stimulated at widths between 20 and 100 msec and motor nerves between 100 and 600 msec.[94]

There are a variety of modes of TENS delivery. Each mode relieves pain through a specific physiological mechanism and is, therefore, most beneficial for a specific type of pain.

When TENS impulses are generated at a high rate (greater than or equal to 50 pps) with a relatively short duration, the stimulation is referred to as *sensory-level* or *conventional* or *high-rate TENS*. Sensory-level TENS produces mild to moderate paresthesia without muscle contraction throughout the treatment area. Sensory-level TENS is thought to control pain through the gating mechanism in the spinal cord. The onset of relief is fast (seconds to 15 minutes),[28] because the gate is closed at the onset of stimulation. The duration of relief after stimulation stops is short lived (at best up to a few hours). Sensory-level TENS has been found to be beneficial for acute pain syndromes and for some deep, aching chronic pain syndromes. Refer to Chapter 31.

When the impulses are generated at a low rate (less than or equal to 20 pps) and have a relatively long duration (100 to 600 pps), the stimulation is referred to as *motor-level* or *acupuncture-like* or *low-rate TENS*. Motor-level TENS produces strong muscle contractions in the treatment area with or without the perception of paresthesia. Motor-level TENS is associated with deployment of endogenous opiates within the CNS. The onset of relief is delayed 20 to 30 minutes, presumably the time it takes to deploy the opiates. Relief frequently lasts hours or days after treatment. Because motor nerves are not stimulated in isolation, sensory fibers are also excited, causing the gating mechanism to come into play.[94] Motor-level TENS has been found to be beneficial for chronic pain syndromes and where sensory level TENS has not been successful.

Stimulation using high-rate and long-duration impulses is called *brief-intense TENS*. Brief-intense TENS decreases the conduction velocity of A-delta and C fibers, producing a peripheral blockade to transmission.[28] Brief-intense TENS is useful in the clinical setting for short-term anesthesia during wound debridement, suture removal, friction massage, joint mobilization, or other painful procedures.

Modulating TENS parameters is one way to avoid the negative aspects of each of the treatment modes. Rate modulation is most commonly used to avoid neural accommodation during sensory-level TENS. By setting the initial pulse rate so that, even with the programmed decrement, it will remain within the treatment range, there will be continuous variation in the stimulus, and neural accommodation will be avoided.

Width modulation is most commonly used with motor-level TENS. By setting the initial pulse duration so that, even with the programmed decrement, the impulses are able to recruit the desired motor units, there will be a continuous variation in perceived strength of the muscle contraction, rendering motor level TENS more tolerable.

Stimulation in which the impulses are generated in pulse trains is called *burst TENS*. Burst TENS is another form of TENS modulation. The stimulator generates low-rate carrier impulses, each of which contains a series of high-rate pulses. Because burst TENS is a combination of high-rate and low-rate TENS, it provides the benefits of each. The low-rate carrier impulse stimulates endorphin release, and the high-rate pulse trains provide an overlay of paresthesia. The advantage to burst TENS is that muscle contractions occur at a lower, more comfortable amplitude, and accommodation does not occur. Burst TENS is beneficial whenever motor level TENS cannot be tolerated and sensory level TENS is ineffective because of neural accommodation.[95]

TENS, like all electrical stimulation, is contraindicated for clients with pacemakers, in the low back and pelvic regions of pregnant women, and over areas with thrombus. TENS should be used with caution for clients who have decreased sensation in the area being stimulated and for clients who have difficulty with understanding or expression. TENS electrodes should not be placed over areas of skin irritation, the eyes, or the carotid sinuses. It also should not be used in the immediate area of an operating diathermy unit.

TENS appears to be of greatest benefit for acute conditions with focal pain, chronic pain syndromes, postoperative incision pain, and during delivery. It has been found least effective with psychogenic pain[96] and pain of central origin.[96a] For additional information on TENS, see Chapter 31.

Clients and caregivers can be taught how and when to apply TENS independently. Once they demonstrate independence, responsibility for the use of TENS can be transferred to the client or to the caregiver.

Iontophoresis

Iontophoresis is a process in which chemical ions are driven through the skin by a small electrical current. Ionizable compounds are placed on the skin under an electrode which, when polarized by a direct (galvanic) current, repels the ion of like charge into the tissues. Once subcutaneous, the ions are free to combine with the physiological ions, resulting in a physiological effect dependent on the characteristics of the ion (Figure 32-8). Ions that are known to be effective analgesics are[97]:

■ 5% Lidocaine ointment (Xylocaine) administered under the positive electrode for an immediate, although short-lived, decrease in pain. Iontophoresis with lidocaine is

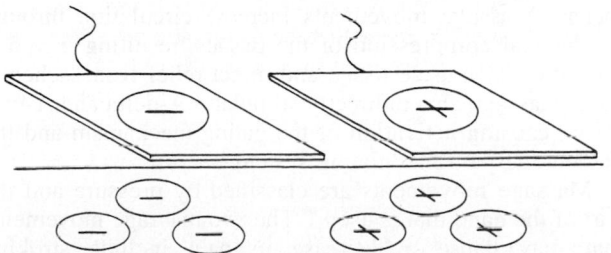

FIGURE 32-8 ■ Iontophoresis. Chemical ions are driven into the tissues by a small electrical current. Once subcutaneous, they are immediately free to take part in chemical reactions within the body.

recommended before ROM, stretching, and joint mobilization and when immediate relief of acute pain (as in bursitis) is the object of treatment.

■ 1% to 10% hydrocortisone administered under the positive electrode for relief of inflammatory pain in conditions such as arthritis, bursitis, or entrapment syndromes. Iontophoresis with hydrocortisone has a delayed onset but a prolonged effect, and it frequently eliminates the underlying cause of pain.

■ 2% magnesium (from Epsom salts) administered under the positive electrode for relief of pain from muscle spasm or localized ischemia. High levels of extracellular magnesium inhibit muscle contraction, including the smooth muscle found in the walls of the vessels, leading to localized vasodilation.

■ Iodine (from Iodex ointment [Lee Pharmaceutical Company, S. El Monte, CA 91733]) administered under the negative pole for relief of pain caused by adhesions or scar tissue. Iodine "softens" fibrotic, sclerotic tissue, thereby increasing tissue pliability.

■ Salicylate (from Iodex with methyl salicylate [Lee Pharmaceutical Company] or Gordogesic Creme [Gordon Labs, Upper Darby, PA 19082]) administered under the negative pole for relief of pain from inflammation. Salicylate is effective for arthritic joint inflammation, myalgia, and entrapment syndromes.

■ 2% acetic acid administered under the negative pole to dissolve calcium deposits.

■ 2% Lithium chloride or lithium carbonate administered under the positive pole to dissolve gouty tophi. In both acetic acid and lithium iontophoresis, the insoluble radicals in the deposits are replaced by soluble chemical radicals so the deposits can be broken down through natural processes.

The contraindication to the use of any ion is an allergy to that ion. Because most clients will not have had iontophoresis previously, it is important to inquire about experiences that might indicate an allergy. For example, intolerance to shellfish may be the result of an allergy to iodine, and a poor reaction to dental local anesthesia may indicate a problem with lidocaine.

Massage

Massage has been recognized as a remedy for pain for at least 3000 years. Evidence of its beneficial effects first appeared in ancient Chinese literature, and then in the writings of the Hindus, Persians, Egyptians, and Greeks. Hippocrates advocated massage for sprains and dislocations as well as for constipation.[98]

Massage decreases pain through both direct and indirect means. Massage movements increase circulation through mechanical compression of the tissues, resulting in reflex relaxation of muscle tissue and direct relief from ischemic pain. Massage also indirectly stimulates A-delta and A-beta fibers, causing activation of the gating mechanism and the descending pain modulating system.[31]

Massage movements are classified by pressure and the part of the hand that is used.[99] The two massage movements that may cause a decrease in pain include stroking (effleurage) and compression (kneading or pétrissage). Stroking involves running the entire hand over large portions of the body. Stroking causes muscle relaxation and

elimination of muscle spasm or improved circulation depending on the depth and force of the strokes. Compression is applied with intermittent pressure using lifting, rolling, or pressing movements meant to stretch shortened tissues, loosen adhesions, and assist with circulation.

Massage is useful in any condition in which pain relief will follow the reduction of swelling or the mobilization of the tissues. These include arthritis, bursitis, neuritis, fibrositis, low-back pain, hemiplegia, paraplegia, quadriplegia, and joint sprains, strains, and contusions. Massage is contraindicated over infected areas, diseased skin, and thrombophlebitic regions.

Clients or caregivers can be taught how and when to perform massage. Once they demonstrate independence in the appropriate technique, responsibility for the performance of massage should be given to the client or caregiver.

A specialized massage technique is lymphatic massage, which consists of light-pressure rhythmic strokes to encourage organizational flow of the lymphatic system. This type of massage can be beneficial with clients who have peripheral swelling with or without pain. A popular form of lymph massage, called manual lymphatic drainage (MLD) is used after surgical procedures to reduce swelling (for example, mastectomy for breast cancer). Evidence-based studies show conflicting results regarding the efficacy of this technique and more research needs to be done to validate it.[100-102]

Myofascial Release

Myofascial release (MFR) techniques are used to release the built-in imbalances and restrictions within the fascia and to reintegrate the fascial mechanism. The therapist palpates the various tissue layers, beginning with the most superficial and working systematically toward the deepest, looking for movement restrictions and asymmetry. Areas of altered structure and function are then "normalized" through the systematic application of pressure and stretching applied in specific directions to bring about decreased myofascial tension, myofascial lengthening, and myofascial softening,[103] thereby restoring pain-free motion in normal patterns of movement. MFR is useful in treating musculoskeletal injuries, chronic pain, headaches, and adhesions/adherent scars.[103a] MFR has been shown to be effective in the treatment of chronic prostatitis (CP) and chronic pelvic pain syndrome (CPPS) in conjunction with paradoxical relaxation therapy (PRT).[104]

MFR is contraindicated over areas with infection, diseased skin, thromboembolus, cellulitis, osteomyelitis, and open wounds. In addition, it should not be used with clients who have osteoporosis, advanced degenerative changes, acute circulatory conditions, acute joint pathology, advanced diabetes, obstructive edema, or hypersensitive skin.[103a] (See Chapter 37 for more in-depth information regarding MFR.)

Joint Mobilization

Joint mobilization consists of passive oscillations that allow the collagen fibers to rearrange and loosen, thereby restoring normal accessory movements.[105] In addition, the rhythmical repetition of the motions provides pain relief through the spinal gating mechanism.[106]

The oscillations involved in joint mobilization are presented in Chapter 9. Grades I and II oscillations are performed to maintain joint mobility and for pain relief, making them the choice for subacute conditions in which pain and potential loss of motion are the primary considerations. Grades III and IV oscillations are performed to increase joint mobility and are indicated for chronic conditions in which regaining lost motion is the goal. Grade V thrusts are performed to regain full joint mobility.[105]

Joint mobilization is contraindicated with rheumatoid arthritis, bone disease, advanced osteoporosis, and pregnancy (pelvic mobilization), as well as in the presence of malignancy, vascular disease, or infection in the area to be mobilized.[51]

Therapeutic Touch

A description of Therapeutic Touch can be found in Chapter 37. Therapeutic touch has been effective in treating painful conditions resulting from anxiety and tension. Ninety percent of individuals treated with therapeutic touch experienced tension headache relief, and 70% had continued relief for more than 4 hours; only 37% of the placebo group expressed sustained relief.[106a] A meta-analysis and systematic review on therapeutic touch revealed that the available studies have varying approaches and protocols on therapeutic touch, subject selection, and description. Although most of these studies confirm the efficacy of the technique, several studies also have demonstrated negative or mixed results.[107] Therapeutic touch, as well as other approaches, are being more widely accepted; however, the therapist must continue to be diligent in using outcome studies to substantiate the use of any complementary therapy. (See Chapter 37 for additional information.)

Point Stimulation

Refer to Chapter 37 for an in-depth discussion of point stimulation. It is interesting to note that acupuncture points frequently correspond in location to trigger points, which are tight, elevated bands of tissue that are extremely sensitive when palpated and have a characteristic pattern of radiation to remote regions of the body. Trigger points appear to be areas of "focal irritability" that are myofascial in origin and are usually the site of small aggregations of nerve fibers that produce continuous afferent input when stimulated.

Needling of acupuncture points stimulates the release of endorphins,[108] most probably through the central modulating pathway that originates in the periaqueductal gray matter.[11] Acupressure (i.e., finger pressure applied to acupuncture or trigger points) is thought to decrease their sensitivity through the same mechanism. The therapist applies deep pressure in a circular motion to each point for 1 to 5 minutes, until the sensitivity subsides. Pressure must be applied directly to each point for the treatment to be effective. Acupressure can be accompanied by the use of a vapocoolant spray to provide additional sensory stimulation.

Sensitive points also can be stimulated using electricity. A point locator is used to identify points along the appropriate meridians that are sensitive to stimulation or more conductive to electricity. Each is then stimulated at the client's level of pain tolerance for 30 to 45 seconds. The points farthest from the site of pain are treated first.

Points that are most sensitive to stimulation are beneficial sites for TENS electrode placement. When point stimulation alone does not provide sufficient pain relief, TENS can be used between sessions for continuous stimulation for more prolonged relief. (See Chapter 37 for additional information on electrical acupuncture.)

Cognitive Strategies

The extent to which an individual perceives and expresses pain is a result of his or her emotional state, expectations, personality, and cognitive view. Each individual feels and responds to pain differently. Melzak and Wall[106] identified the following three nonphysical components to pain that interact and determine how an individual will respond to pain:

1. The individual's sensory/discriminative interpretation of the pain
2. The individual's motivation and attitudes relating to the pain
3. The individual's cognitive/evaluative thoughts and beliefs concerning the pain experience.

Cognitive strategies are part of a holistic approach to health that looks at the total person and the interaction between the three components of body, mind, and spirit. Cognitive strategies recognize that the mind is not separate from the body, accept that there is a mental component to pain, and utilizes the inner resources of the mind to influence the pain experience.

Cognitive strategies work in two ways. First, they activate the descending cortical modulating systems and, second, they teach the individual to control, rather than be controlled by, the pain. Used in conjunction with other modalities necessary for physical relief, these approaches can play a significant role in long-term pain management and should not be overlooked when seeking a viable pain management alternative.

Relaxation Exercises

People who are in pain experience stress. Chronic stress can trigger increased pain. Both pain and stress cause an increase in sympathetic nervous system (SNS) activity, including increased muscle tension. Relaxation exercises can bring about muscle relaxation and a generalized parasympathetic response.[109] Benson[110] has named this effect *the relaxation response* and reports that it is accompanied by an increase in alpha brain waves.

Relaxation reduces ischemic pain by normalizing blood flow to the muscles by making way for more oxygen to be delivered to the tissues. In addition, relaxation reduces muscle tension, resulting in an interruption in the pain spasm cycle.[111]

Relaxation exercises all have two elements in common: a single focus and a passive attitude toward intruding thoughts and distractions. The end product of relaxation is a lowered arousal of the SNS and a lessening of the symptoms caused by or worsened by stress.[112]

Deep relaxation can be achieved through progressive relaxation and attention-diversion exercises. Progressive relaxation involves alternately tensing and relaxing the muscles until, eventually, the entire body is relaxed. This activity teaches the individual how to recognize and relieve muscle tension within the body.

Attention diversion is an active process in which the individual directs her or his attention to nonnoxious events or stimuli in the immediate environment to achieve distraction from the pain. Attention diversion is defined as passive or active. Passive attention diversion includes meditation and involves concentrating on a visual or auditory stimulus rather than the painful sensation, whereas active attention diversion involves active participation in a task (e.g., serial subtraction).

Meditation involves quieting the mind and focusing the attention on a thought, word, phrase, object, or movement. The individual becomes more alert to the constant stream of conversation taking place within the mind. Meditation calms the body through the relaxation response and keeps the attention focused in the present moment. Individuals in Eastern cultures have traditionally focused on a mantra, a word with spiritual meaning; however, there are no rules for where to focus the attention. The word or object should bring the individual a sense of peace and allow the attention to be pleasantly directed toward the immediate moment.

Imagery is another form of attention diversion. During imagery the individual uses his or her imagination to produce images with pain-weakening potential. This can take two forms. In one, the individual imagines experiences that are inconsistent with the pain (e.g., imagining rolling in snow to alleviate burning pain). In the other, the individual imagines experiences that modify specific features of the pain experience (e.g., imagining that the pain is the result of a sports injury or that the sensation is "numbness" rather than pain).

Attention diversion works by activating the relaxation response and by diverting the individual's attention from the pain. However, attention diversion also has been found to activate the higher brain centers and may have an inhibitory effect on pain through the spinal gating mechanisms.[41,66] Lautenbacher et al[113] found that individuals who used attention diversion for pain management reported decreased intensity and unpleasantness of their pain.

Clients can be taught to perform relaxation exercises independently and should be encouraged to perform them regularly because the benefits of these exercises are gained through regular practice.

Body Scanning

Clients with chronic pain frequently become one with their suffering; they do not view themselves as individuals with pain, but, rather, as painful individuals. Body scanning is a technique that endeavors to separate the individual from the pain.[114]

During body scanning, the client is taught to achieve a meditative state, then focus attention on each body area, one area at a time. The client is instructed to breathe into and out from each area, relaxing more deeply with each exhalation. When the area is completely relaxed, the client "lets go" of the region and dwells in the stillness for a few breaths before continuing. Painful areas are scanned in an identical manner as nonpainful areas. The client notes, but does not judge, changes in sensation, thoughts, and emotions during scanning of each area.

Individuals who practice this technique report new levels of insight and understanding concerning their pain experience. They separate the pain experience into the following three parts[114]:

1. An awareness of the pain sensation and their thoughts and feelings about it.

2. An awareness of a separation between the pain sensation and their thoughts and feelings about it.
3. An awareness of a separation between themselves and their pain, because they are able to examine objectively the sensation and their thoughts and feelings about it.

Once clients accept that they are not their pain or their reaction to the pain, they can determine how much influence and control pain will have in their lives.

Studies of chronic pain patients at the Stress Reduction Clinic at the University of Massachusetts Medical Center revealed that 72% of patients who used body scanning along with traditional medical interventions experienced at least a 33% reduction on their McGill-Melzak Pain Rating Index.[114] In addition, at the end of an 8-week training period, the individuals perceived their bodies in a more positive light, experienced an increase in positive mood states, and reported major improvements in anxiety, depression, hostility, and the tendency to be overly occupied with their bodily sensations.

Humor

Ever since Cousins[115] reported in his book, *Anatomy of an Illness,* that he used humor to manage pain and enhance sleep during his illness, the role of humor in healing has been well studied. Humor has been found beneficial for both acute and chronic pain management.[90,116]

Laughter increases blood oxygen content by increasing ventilation. It helps to exercise the heart muscle by speeding up the heart rate and enhancing arterial and venous circulation, resulting in more oxygen and nutrients being delivered to the tissues.[117] Laughter decreases serum cortisol levels (cortisol levels increase with stress and are thought to have a negative effect on the immune response),[118,119] and increases the concentration of circulating antibodies.[117] As little as 10 minutes of belly laughter a day has been found to decrease the erythrocyte sedimentation rate and provide 2 hours of pain-free sleep.[115] Finally, laughter releases energy and emotional tension and is followed by generalized muscle relaxation.[117,120]

Therapeutic humor can be used to provide distraction from pain and as a coping mechanism to decrease the anxiety and tension associated with chronic pain. The muscle-relaxing effect can be used to interrupt the pain-spasm cycle.

Therapeutic humor should not be used with individuals who do poorly with humor. This includes individuals who despise or misunderstand humor, individuals who find joy threatening or guilt inducing, and narcoleptic individuals who become cataleptic with laughter.[120a]

Very few clients will benefit from all these cognitive strategies, and it may take some trial and error to find the appropriate cognitive strategy for an individual client. Some clients will have no difficulty learning and practicing cognitive strategies, whereas others will not be able to perform any of these techniques independently. It may be beneficial to provide the client with an individualized relaxation tape or to have the client repeat coping affirmations over and over throughout the day. The success of cognitive strategies is dependent on applying the appropriate strategy to the appropriate client and fine-tuning the strategy so that it matches the client's needs.

In conclusion, it is important to reemphasize that all individuals with chronic pain have some degree of emotional or cognitive involvement, or both, in their pain experience. Many clients will live with pain regardless the treatment they receive. Therefore it is imperative for health care practitioners to address the emotional and cognitive components of each client's pain to allow her or him to function at the highest level and as comfortably as possible and to find joy in each day.

General Conditioning through Exercise

Deconditioning is a major source of disability with chronic pain. Pain causes an intolerance for activity, which in turn leads to physiological and pathological changes in the organ systems. Exercise improves overall functional performance by improving range of motion, muscle strength, neuromuscular control, coordination, and aerobic capacity, as well as offering higher self esteem.

All three types of exercise are beneficial for pain management. ROM and stretching exercises restore normal joint mobility and correct muscle tightness. The joints are held in normal alignment and are subjected to normal stresses during movement. ROM and stretching exercises are indicated where there is decreased mobility.

Strengthening exercises increase muscle strength and cardiovascular endurance. When performed with high intensity for a short duration, strengthening exercises result in increased muscle mass, improved neuromuscular control, and improved coordination. When performed at low intensity for a long duration, they increase the aerobic capacity of the muscles.

Aerobic exercises improve cardiovascular fitness. More oxygen is supplied to the tissues because there is an increase in the number and size of capillaries and a decrease in the diffusion distance between the capillaries and the muscles. The tissues use oxygen more efficiently, and the individual has a higher energy level.

All exercise has an analgesic effect through the gating mechanism by stimulation of the A-delta neurons and a pain-modulating effect through activation of the descending systems. Exercise of sufficient intensity has been known to increase circulating beta-endorphin levels, but exercise-induced beta-endorphin alterations are related to the type of exercise and special populations tested, and may differ in individuals with health problems.[121,121a]

It is important to include exercise in all pain management programs. Clients should be taught the appropriate exercises beginning with the first treatment session and encouraged to perform the exercises consistently when not at therapy. The ultimate end product of movement intervention is to empower the client to modulate and control all functional activities, enabling that individual to participate in life.

Operant Conditioning

Coping strategies are learned. Individuals with chronic pain express their pain with behaviors that provide them with consistent positive rewards. For example, wincing might result in attention from a family member or limping might allow the individual to avoid performing a particular task. Over time, the individual with pain becomes conditioned to perform certain behaviors for the behavior's rewards rather than as a reaction to the pain. Similarly, individuals with chronic pain also can condition their nervous systems through learning. If an individual expects to experience pain as the result of a particular level of activity, the individual will always experience pain at that level of activity.

Operant conditioning addresses the learned (or conditioned) aspects of pain.[122] Operant conditioning involves unlearning or separating the behavior and the response from the pain experience. If the goal of treatment is to lessen social reinforcement of the client's pain behaviors (and thus extinguish those behaviors), the client and the family or other involved individuals are shown how their behaviors and responses provide social reinforcement for the client's reaction to pain. The involved individuals are provided with specific new responses to the client's behavior. Family members might be instructed to ignore wincing, groaning, or the verbal report of pain. They might be told not to perform activities that are the client's responsibility just because the client reports pain. In time, the client will become conditioned to the new response, and pain in those situations will diminish.

If the goal of treatment is to increase the client's pain-free activity level, operant conditioning can be used to condition the nervous system to a higher level of activity before responding with pain. If the client's usual pattern is to remain active until the onset of pain (negative reinforcement for activity) and then rest (positive reinforcement for pain), the client is instructed to remain active to just below the pain threshold and then rest (positive reinforcement for activity). In this way the nervous system unlearns the connection between activity and pain, and the client's activity level increases.

Hypnosis

Hypnosis is a state in which the body and conscious mind are deeply relaxed while the subconscious mind remains alert, focused, and open to suggestion.[112] This has been demonstrated physiologically by electroencephalography, which shows an increase in the number of theta waves, which are associated with enhanced attention.[122a] When a hypnotized individual is given a suggestion that is in alignment with his or her existing belief system, it is accepted by the subconscious mind as reality. The suggestion is not filtered through the conscious mind, which is critical and judgmental. Hypnosis allows the individual to bypass her or his critical beliefs.[123] For example, if the individual believes that a certain activity will cause pain (critical belief), that activity is sure to cause pain. If, however, during hypnosis, the individual accepts the suggestion that the activity does not cause pain, the pain may decrease and even disappear.

When hypnosis is used for pain management, a client is first assisted to achieve complete relaxation, then given suggestions that reinterpret the pain experience. For example, a client might be guided to reframe the pain into a messenger and then be encouraged to listen to its message to gain understanding of the meaning behind the pain. Or a client might be guided to view the pain as an indication to stop a particular activity to avoid being injured. Or a client might be instructed to feel less pain. Finally, where harmless activities have become painful through learning, the client can be guided to disconnect the activity from his or her pain.

Biofeedback

Biofeedback is a training process in which the client becomes aware of and learns to selectively change physiological processes with the aid of an external monitor. A monitoring instrument is placed on the appropriate area of the body. The machine provides an initial readout. The client is instructed how to change the monitored process, and as change occurs, the machine "feeds back" that information. By mentally changing a biological function, the client learns to gain control over it. In time, the client learns to control the process without needing an assist from the instrument.

Muscle tension, pulse rate, blood pressure, skin temperature, and electromyography (EMG) and electroencephalography (EEG) readings are some of the physiological processes that can be consciously modified with biofeedback.[109]

Biofeedback is proving to be an effective pain management tool for headaches, muscle spasms, and other physical dysfunction that lead to or increase chronic pain (see Chapters 31 and 37).

GENERAL TREATMENT GUIDELINES

As noted earlier, chronic pain management using the medical model has not been found effective. Treatment limited to correcting pathology promotes dependence on the therapist, as well as making full resolution of symptoms the measure of success.

The disablement model addresses the functional losses associated with impairments. Therapeutic interventions are not focused on pathology, but they are directed at improving the individual's function and preventing or improving disability. This does not mean that the impairment is ignored, however. Most times, addressing the individual's functional losses involves treating the impairments that caused them.

For example, clients with chronic pain frequently become sedentary, leading to the impairments of limited ROM, muscle weakness, and deconditioning. These factors can then, of themselves, cause pain, creating a cycle that spirals upward until the individual becomes disabled. During therapy, interventions are directed at the impairments with the goal of restoring function. Therapeutic interventions are selected based on their ability to improve functional outcome. Impairments that do not affect function do not become the focus of therapy; therapeutic interventions that do not address functional deficits are not utilized.

The development of an appropriate treatment plan may seem overwhelming when the therapist is confronted with a client who has chronic pain that has not responded to previous interventions or who has a chronic condition that has pain as one of its characteristics. The key is to identify the client's functional deficits and then develop a treatment plan that addresses the causes of those deficits. In some cases this may mean not treating the pain itself but, rather, its causative factors.

For example, if the client has chronic pain because of joint hypomobility, the treatment plan includes interventions to increase joint mobility. Conversely, if the client's pain is due to joint hypermobility, the treatment plan includes interventions to increase support around the hypermobile joints. Merely addressing the joint pain by applying modalities will do little to resolve the pain because it does nothing to correct the precipitating cause.

When a client has pain because of a chronic disease and the treatment plan will include instruction in pain-relieving interventions, it is important for the therapist to understand the specific causes of the pain to select the appropriate intervention. For example, pain from rheumatoid arthritis most commonly is the result of either joint inflammation or biomechanical stress on unstable joints. A client would be instructed in pain-relieving modalities for the former and instructed to wear splints to support the joints for the latter. One intervention would not be appropriate for both causes.

CASE STUDIES

The following case studies (Case Studies 32-1, 32-2, and 32-3) demonstrate a problem-solving approach to the treatment of clients with chronic pain.

CASE STUDY 32-1 ■ FIBROMYALGIA

K. E. is a 35-year-old computer programmer with a diagnosis of fibromyalgia. She reports a 6-month history of generalized muscular pain and fatigue that increase when she performs repetitive motions or holds a position for a prolonged period. K. E. is currently unable to work because she is no longer able to perform data entry without increased neck and shoulder pain. She states she awakens from pain and leg cramps several times during the night. She awakens each morning with a headache and low back pain; she does not get much relief from pain medication. K. E. states she has not been out with friends in several months. She states she is "nervous, unable to concentrate, and depressed." She has been evaluated by several physicians. All medical tests are negative.

K. E.'s objective examination reveals pain with digital palpation to distinct points in the muscles of her neck and shoulder girdles, over both lateral epicondyles and greater trochanters, in her gluteal muscles, and just above the medial joint lines of the knees. Pain is referred from the tender points distally. K. E. sits and stands with a forward head and elevated protracted shoulders, and her cervical ROM is restricted slightly at end range because of her posture and muscle guarding. Muscle strength is 4/5 throughout. All other musculoskeletal and neurological tests are normal.

K. E. presents with the impairments of pain, poor posture, decreased cervical and shoulder ROM, and decreased endurance, resulting in the disabilities of interrupted sleep, decreased tolerance for activity, and the inability to work at her profession.

The long-term goals of treatment for K. E. are independence with self-management of pain, normalization of posture, restoration of normal sleep,

CASE STUDY 32-1 ■ FIBROMYALGIA—cont'd

independence with a home exercise program, and return to work and appropriate social activities. The short-term goals include decreasing K. E.'s pain, proper sleep positioning, correcting her postural abnormalities, improving her limited endurance, and assessing/correcting the ergonomics of her workstation. K. E. also needs intervention to address the emotional and cognitive aspects of her condition.

The lowered pain threshold and magnified pain perception seen with fibromyalgia results from a complex combination of muscle tissue microtrauma, neuroendocrine abnormalities, and changes in the levels of CNS neurotransmitters. The muscles of individuals with fibromyalgia show abnormal energy metabolism, poor tissue oxygenation, and localized hypoxia. Their blood shows decreased levels of the inhibitory neurotransmitter serotonin and increased levels of the facilitory neurotransmitter substance P. This combination, which is unique to fibromyalgia, is thought to cause changes in the dorsal horn neurons and, eventually, in the areas of the brain responsible for the sensory-discriminative and affective-motivational aspects of pain.[39]

Fibromyalgia pain has been shown to respond favorably to interventions that work through the gating mechanism. These include sensory-level TENS, light massage, muscle warming, and gentle stretching. K. E. can be taught to apply localized heat or to take a warm bath before gentle stretching of her tight muscles. She should be cautioned to stretch slowly to the point of resistance and to hold the stretch for 60 seconds to allow the Golgi tendon organs time to signal the muscle fibers to relax. Quick stretching to the point of pain will cause increased tightness and pain through the pain-spasm cycle. It is important for K. E. to understand that these measures address the pain of fibromyalgia but do not have any long-term effect on the course of her condition.

Individuals with fibromyalgia, and most individuals with chronic pain, experience a variety of emotions, including depression, anger, fear, withdrawal, and anxiety.[124] These individuals have been helped with hypnosis, biofeedback, and cognitive restructing.[39,124] In

addition to giving them a sense of control over their pain, these interventions are known to bring about an increase in the individual's level of endogenous opiates, thereby activating one of the descending pain modulation systems. K. E. can be taught to perform these techniques independently.

K. E. should be asked to demonstrate her sleeping posture. Because the muscles of individuals with fibromyalgia do not relax easily, K. E. should be shown how to use pillows to support her neck and back so that they are encouraged to relax while she sleeps. This will help to decrease the frequency of morning headaches and back pain and help her to sleep through the night. She might also benefit from a warm bath before going to bed.

K. E.'s therapist can use gentle MFR to help correct the biomechanical imbalances causing her poor posture. K. E. can then be taught to selectively stretch the shortened muscles of her neck and shoulder girdles using the technique already described and to selectively strengthen their weakened antagonists using light resistance. To counter deconditioning, K. E. should be placed on a nonimpact aerobic program (walking, pool exercises, or stationary bicycle) with a goal of 30 minutes three to four times a week at 70% maximum heart rate (220 minus her age). If she is unable to tolerate 30 minutes of exercise at one time, she can be started at 3 to 5 minutes twice or three times daily and gradually progressed to three sessions of 10 minutes, then two sessions of 15 minutes, and finally one session of 30 minutes. K. E. may require a significant amount of coaxing and education to motivate her to participate in exercise; many individuals with fibromyalgia do not wish to move because movement initially increases their pain.

Before she returns to work, K. E. should be assisted with the ergonomics of her workstation. Research[125] has shown that individuals who work at computers need to vary their positions throughout the day even if their sitting posture is appropriate. Further research[67,126,127] has shown that correct mouse placement is important to minimize stress to the arms and shoulders.

CASE STUDY 32-2 ■ PHANTOM LIMB PAIN

A. R. is a 60-year-old carpenter who underwent below-knee amputation of his right leg 4 weeks ago after a motor vehicle accident. He now reports a constant burning, piercing, throbbing sensation in the distal portion of his missing limb. He states that immediately after the amputation, he was aware of an itching or tickling in the missing portion of the leg, but the sensation gradually changed to pain. He notes that the leg feels as if it is shortening, as if the missing foot is moving closer and closer to his hip. A.R. has been fitted with a shrinker but does not wear it because of fear of increasing the pain. He does not believe he will be able to wear a prosthesis and is concerned because his employer will be unable to find work for him if he is wheelchair bound.

A. R.'s objective examination reveals a healing surgical incision and a poorly shaped stump. Right lower-extremity hip and knee strength are 3/5 and 2+/5, respectively. Sensation to light touch is diminished in the area of the incision. All other musculoskeletal and neurological tests are normal. A. R. ambulates short distances using a walker but relies on a wheelchair for locomotion outside his home.

A. R. presents with the impairments of a below-knee amputation, phantom limb pain, and decreased strength in the right lower extremity, resulting in the functional limitation and the inability to prepare his leg for a prosthesis, inability to ambulate, and inability to work in his profession.

The long-term goals of treatment for A. R. are independent use of a prosthesis and return to work with modified job tasks. The short-term goals include resolution of his phantom limb pain, preparation of his stump for a prosthesis, at least 4/5 right hip and knee strength, and, when appropriate, gait and balance training with the prosthesis.

There are two theories of the cause for phantom limb pain. At one time it was thought that it occurred as the result of the formation of a terminal neuroma at the site of the amputation[10]; however, this theory did not explain phantom phenomena in individuals with congenital amputations or individuals with complete spinal cord injuries who also experience painful and nonpainful sensations in their missing or anesthetic limbs. This led researchers to look at the role of the CNS in phantom phenomena, and the latest theories suggest the previously described changes in the dorsal horn neurons and changes in the spinal cord caused by the sudden loss of afferent impulses after amputation.[128]

These theories are supported by the effectiveness of interventions that stimulate the large nerve fibers and provide inhibitory input through the gating mechanism. Phantom limb pain is relieved by stroking, vibration, TENS, ultrasound, heat applications, and the use of a prosthesis. A. R. can be taught a progressive desensitization program. He should be encouraged to wear the shrinker both to prepare his stump for a prosthesis and to decrease pain. Because phantom limb pain is adversely affected by emotional stress, exposure to cold, and local irritants, he should be taught to avoid these factors as much as possible.

A. R.'s adjustment to a changed body image, a changed lifestyle, and the use of a prosthesis can be aided with any of the cognitive strategies described previously. He might also benefit from referral to an amputee support group.

It is important for A. R. to be aware of his abilities and limitations so that he remains safe when he returns to work. If appropriate, the therapist should accompany A. R. to his job and perform a job task analysis, making suggestions for necessary modifications. If this is not possible, the therapist could discuss needed modifications with A. R. based on his descriptions of his job tasks.

CASE STUDY 32-3 ■ COMPLEX REGIONAL PAIN SYNDROME

P. S. is a 45-year-old right-handed secretary who sustained a Colles fracture of the right wrist 6 months ago. The wrist was placed in a cast for 6 weeks, during which time P. S. avoided using the extremity. Two weeks after the cast was removed, P. S. developed pain, swelling, and stiffness in the wrist and hand. She returned to her physician who diagnosed CRPS type I. She has received four sympathetic nerve blockades. The first provided 4 weeks of pain relief. The second and third provided 2 weeks of relief each. She has just received her fourth injection along with a referral for therapy.

P. S. is wearing a sling. She presents with 30-degree flexion contractures of her right fingers, along with swelling and stiffness of the wrist and hand. Her right wrist, elbow, and shoulder show limited motion as well. P. S. describes constant burning pain that becomes worse with any stimulation, even air blowing over the skin. She rates her pain as 4/10 since the block, but she states the pain had slowly been escalating toward 10/10 before the injection. Her hand and wrist are cool, and the skin appears mottled and shiny. P. S. states she is not using her arm and needs assistance at home for activities of daily living and homemaking chores.

P. S. presents with the impairments of pain, swelling, stiffness, and decreased ROM of the right wrist and hand. These impairments cause activity limitations decreasing her ability to use the right upper extremity for any functional activities, including activities of daily living, job tasks, and homemaking activities. In addition,

CASE STUDY 32-3 ■ COMPLEX REGIONAL PAIN SYNDROME—cont'd

because she is not using the extremity and carries the arm in a sling, P. S. is at risk for developing shoulder-hand syndrome.

The long-term goal of treatment for P. S. is restoration of pain-free use of her right upper extremity. The short-term goals include quieting the SNS, decreasing P. S.'s pain and edema, and restoring normal ROM of the shoulder, elbow, wrist, and hand.

Successful treatment of CRPS involves a coordinated effort by the physician and the therapist. The treatment of choice is interruption of sympathetic activity with nerve blocks and movement therapy.[129]

Interventions included in a pain management program for CRPS should be chosen for their ability to quiet the SNS as well as accomplish the desired outcome. For example, thermotherapy is more beneficial than cryotherapy because of its ability to decrease pain without stimulating a sympathetic response.[129]

A successful rehabilitation program for CRPS cannot be limited to therapy visits. Clients need to be instructed in interventions that they then perform three, four, or even five times daily. Therefore the therapist needs to become a guide with the responsibility for performing the pain management program given over to the client or caregiver.

Pain reduction is the first priority. This can be accomplished through the gating mechanism or through the deployment of endogenous opiates. Thermotherapy and TENS have both been found effective for pain management with CRPS. If P.S. cannot tolerate electrode placement on the right arm, the electrodes can be placed on the opposite arm or along the spinal roots of the involved segments.[28,97] P.S. can be instructed in any of the superficial heating modalities. Stroking massage along the paravertebral muscles beginning in the cervical region and continuing to the coccyx has also been found effective in quieting the SNS.

Before P. S. can regain mobility of her wrist and fingers, the edema must be resolved. This can be accomplished with elevation, massage, lymphatic drainage and compression. P. S. can wear a compression glove or, if she is able to tolerate it, receive intermittent compression to the arm. She should be instructed to keep the arm above heart level as much as possible.

P. S. should be advised to discontinue use of the sling and begin frequent weight bearing through her arm. Immobility increases the symptoms of CRPS. Movement of the extremity is important to increase proprioception and circulation, both of which have an inhibitory effect on the SNS.[129] Therefore P. S. should be encouraged to begin using her hand as much as possible throughout the day. If she is reluctant to use the arm, the therapist can design a functional activity program that allows her to use the arm during simple activities, which can be progressed as her symptoms improve.

There are two forms of exercise that are beneficial in CRPS. The first is active ROM, which should be performed frequently throughout the day within the pain-free range to regain motion, increase circulation, and provide nonnociceptive input. Performance of the specific range of motion should be within functional activities. The activity itself will encouraging range of motion while the patient is concentrating on successfully completing the activity itself. The second form of exercise is stress loading,[130] which involves active compression and traction activities without joint motion. For example, P. S. can use a coarse-bristled brush to scrub a piece of plywood and apply as much pressure as possible without causing pain (compression activity). Or she can carry a briefcase or purse in her affected hand (traction activity). Compression and traction both provide increased proprioceptive input.

P. S. should also begin performing desensitization activities, which can be modified as she is able to tolerate more stimulation to her extremity. P. S. may benefit from biofeedback to gain control over the circulation in her arm and from relaxation activities to stimulate the relaxation response and enhance parasympathetic function.

Once P. S. becomes independent in the performance of her program, therapy can be decreased to once or twice weekly to monitor and modify her pain management regimen.

ACKNOWLEDGMENTS

We would like to acknowledge the contribution of Linda Mirabelli-Susens to the writing of this chapter in the previous edition.

REFERENCES

1. American Pain Society: *The facts on intractable pain,* Skokie, IL, 1994, American Pain Society.
2. Cypress BK: Characteristics of physicians' visits for back symptoms, a national perspective, *Am J Public Health* 73:389-395, 1983.
3. Bonica JJ: Importance of the problem. In Aronoff GM, editor: *Evaluation and treatment of chronic pain,* Baltimore, 1985, Urban & Schwarzenberg.
4. Bonica JJ: Cancer pain: a major national health problem, *Ca Nurs* 1:313-316, 1978.
5. Myers JS: Cancer pain: assessment of nurses' knowledge and attitudes, *Oncol Nurs Forum* 12:62-66, 1985.
6. Hauck SL: Pain: problem for the person with cancer, *Ca Nurs* 9:66-76, 1986.
7. Wolff MS, Michel TH, Krebs DE et al: Chronic pain: assessment of orthopedic physical therapist's knowledge and attitudes, *Phys Ther* 71:207-214, 1991.
8. Nolan MF: Pain: the experience and its expression, *Clin Management* 10:22, 1990.
9. Stucky C, Gold M, Zhang X: Mechanisms of pain. *Proc Natl Acad Sci U S A* 98:11845-11846, 2001.
10. Fine PG, Ashburn MA: Functional neuroanatomy and nociception. In Ashburn MA, editor: *The management of pain.* New York, Churchill Livingstone, 1998.

11. Swerdlow M: *The Therapy of Pain.* Philadelphia, JB Lippincott, 1981.

12. Kandel E, Schwartz J, Jessell T: *Principles of neuroscience,* New York, 2000, McGraw Hill/Appleton Lange.

13. Ignelzi RJ, Atkinson JH: Pain and its modulation: I. Afferent mechanisms, *Neurosurgery* 6:577-583, 1980.

14. Regan JM, Peng P: Neurophysiology of cancer pain, *Cancer Control* 7:111-119, 2000.

15. Nolan MF: Anatomic and physiologic organization of the neural structures involved in pain transmission, modulation and perception. In Echternach JL, editor: *Pain,* New York, 1987, Churchill Livingstone.

16. VanderWende C, Spoerlein MT: Role of dopaminergic receptors in morphine analgesia and tolerance, *Res Commun Chem Pathol Pharm* 5:35-43, 1973.

17. Nyborg WN, Ziskin MC: Biological effects of ultrasound, *Clin Diagn Ultrasound* 16:24, 1985.

18. Paalzow G, Paalzow L: Morphine-induced inhibition of different pain responses in relation to the regional turnover of rat brain noradrenaline and dopamine, *Psychopharmacologia* 45:9-20, 1975.

19. Torebjork E, Wahren L, Wallin G et al: Noradrenalin-evoked pain in neuralgia, *Pain* 63:11-20, 1995.

20. Wallin BG, Torebjörk E, Hallin R: Preliminary observations on the pathophysiology of hyperalgia in the causalgic pain syndrome. In Zotterman Y, editor: *Sensory functions of the skin in primates,* Oxford, 1976, Pergamon Press.

21. Nicolls ML: Transmission of chronic nociception by spinal neurons expressing the substance P receptors, *Science* 286:1558-1561, 1999.

22. Ignelzi RJ, Atkinson JH: Pain and its modulation: II. Efferent mechanisms, *Neurosurgery* 6:584-590, 1980.

23. Piercey MF, Folkers K: Sensory and motor functions of spinal cord substance P, *Science* 214:1361-1363, 1981.

24. Willer JC, Dehen H, Cambier J et al: Stress induced analgesia in humans: endogenous opioids and naloxone reversible depression of pain reflexes, *Science* 212:689-691, 1981.

25. Snyder SH: Opiate receptors and internal opiates, *Sci Am* 240:44-56, 1977.

26. Willer JC, Roby A, Le Bars D et al: Psychophysical and electrophysiological approaches to the pain-relieving effects of heterotrophic nociceptive stimuli, *Brain Res* 107:1095-1112, 1984.

27. Basbaum AI, Fields HL: Endogenous pain control systems: brainstem spinal pathways and endorphin circuitry, *Annu Rev Neurosci* 7:309-338, 1984.

28. Mannheimer JS, Lampe GN: *Clinical transcutaneous electrical nerve stimulation,* Philadelphia, 1984, FA Davis.

29. Woolf C: Generation of acute pain: central mechanisms, *Br Med Bull* 43:523-533, 1991.

30. Melzack R, Dennis SG: Neurophysiological foundations of pain. In Sternbach RA, editor: *The psychology of pain,* New York, 1978, Raven Press.

31. Wittink H, Michel TH: *Chronic pain management for physical therapists,* Boston, 1990, Butterworth-Heinemann.

32. Grubb BD: Peripheral and central mechanisms of pain, *Br J Anesth* 81:8-11, 1998.

33. Cervero F: *Persistent pain,* New York, 1983, Grune & Stratton.

33a. Slipman CW, Plastaras CT, Palmitier RA et al: Symptom provocation of fluoroscopically guided cervical nerve root stimulation. Are dynatomal maps identical to dermatomal maps? *Spine* 23:2235-2242, 1998.

34. Borsook D, LeBel A, Stojanovic M et al: Central pain syndromes. In Ashburn MA, editor: *The management of pain,* New York, 1998, Churchill Livingstone.

35. Merskey H, Bogduk N: *Classification of chronic pain,* ed 2, Seattle, 1994, IASP Press.

36. Gebhart GF: Descending modulation of pain, *Neurosci Biobehav Rev* 729-737, 2004.

37. Central neuropathic pain, *MedLink Neurology:* http://www.medlink.com. Accessed December 15, 2005.

38. Evans JH: Neurology and neurological aspects of pain. In Swerdlow M, editor: *Relief of intractable pain: monographs in anesthesiology, vol 1,* New York, 1974, Excerpta Medica.

39. Weigent DA, Bradley LA, Blalock JE, et al: Current concepts in the pathophysiology of abnormal pain perception. *Am J Med Sci* 315:405-412, 1998.

40. Bonica JJ: Causalgia and other reflex sympathetic dystrophies. In Bonica JJ, editor: *The management of pain,* ed 2, London, 1990, Lea & Febiger.

41. Mersky H, Bogduk N: *Classification of chronic pain syndromes and definitions of pain terms,* ed 2, Seattle, 1994, IASP Press.

42. Berger JN, Katz RL: Sympathetically maintained pain. In Ashburn MA, editor: *The management of pain,* New York, 1998, Churchill Livingstone.

43. Complex regional pain syndrome, *Medlink Neurology:* http://www.medlink.com. Accessed December 15, 2005.

44. Summers JD, Rapoff MA, Varghese G et al: Psychosocial factors in chronic spinal cord injury pain, *Pain* 47:183-189, 1991.

45. Weatherley CR, Prickett CF, O'Brien JP: Discogenic pain persisting despite solid posterior fusion, *J Bone Joint Surg Br* 68:142-143, 1986.

46. Vogt BA, Derbyshire S, Jones AK: Pain processing in four regions of human cingulate cortex localized with co-registered PET and MR imaging, *Eur J Neurosci* 8:1461-1473, 1996.

47. Hsieh JC, Belfrage M, Stone-Elander S et al: Central representation of chronic ongoing neuropathic pain studied by positron emission tomography, *Pain* 63:225-236, 1995.

48. Steiner WA, Ryser L, Huber E et al: Use of the ICF model as a clinical problem-solving tool in physical therapy and rehabilitation medicine, *Phys Ther* 82:1098-1107, 2002.

49. Ploghaus A, Narain C, Beckmann CF et al: Exacerbation of pain by anxiety is associated with activity in a hippocampal network, *J Neurosci* 21:98, 2001.

50. Makofsky H, Willis GC: Non-mechanical and pathological causes of low back pain, *Phys Ther Forum,* May 15, p 12, 1989.

51. Linton SJ, Melin L: The accuracy of remembering chronic pain, *Pain* 13:281-285, 1982.

52. Kremer E, Atkinson JH, Ignelzi RJ et al: Measurement of pain: patient preference does not confound pain measurement, *Pain* 10:241-248, 1981.

53. Bieri D, Reeve RA, Champion GD et al: The Faces Pain Scale for the self-assessment of the severity of pain experienced by children: development, initial validation, and preliminary investigation for ratio scale properties, *Pain* 41:139-150, 1990.

54. Huskisson EC: Measurement of pain, *Lancet* 2:1127-1131, 1974.

55. Stuppy DJ: The faces pain scale: reliability and validity with mature adults, *Appl Nurs Res* 11:84-89, 1998.

56. Ransford AO, Cairns D, Mooney V: The pain drawing as an aid to the psychologic evaluation of patients with low back pain, *Spine* 1:127-133, 1976.

57. Melzack R: The McGill Pain Questionnaire: major properties and scoring methods, *Pain* 1:277, 1975.

58. Byrne M, Troy A, Bradley LA et al: Cross-validation of the factor structure of the McGill pain questionnaire, *Pain* 13:193-201, 1982.

59. Kremer E, Atkinson JH Jr, Ignelzi RJ et al: Pain measurement: the affective dimensional measure of the McGill pain questionnaire with a cancer pain population, *Pain* 12:153-163, 1982.

60. Reading AE: A comparison of the McGill Pain Questionnaire in chronic and acute pain, *Pain* 13:185-192, 1982.

61. Wilkie DJ, Holzemer WL, Tesler MD et al: Measuring pain quality: validity and reliability of children's and adolescents' pain language, *Pain* 41:151-159, 1990.

62. McGrath PJ, Rosmus C, Canfield C et al: Behaviors caregivers use to determine pain in non-verbal, cognitively impaired individuals, *Dev Med Chil Neurol* 40:340-343,1998.

63. Cyriax J: *Textbook of orthopaedic medicine,* ed 8, London, 1984, Bailliere Tindall.

64. Kessler R, Hertling D: *Management of common musculoskeletal disorders,* Philadelphia, 1983, Harper & Row.

65. Weinstein SM: Physical examination. In Ashburn MA, editor: *The management of pain,* New York, 1998, Churchill Livingstone.
66. Fernandez E: A classification system of cognitive coping strategies for pain, *Pain* 26:141-151, 1986.
67. Albin T: To tell the truth, *Phys Ther Products* May-June:68-71, 1999.
68. Rennie GA, Michlovitz SL: Biophysical principles of heating and superficial heating agents. In Michlovitz SL, editor: *Thermal agents in rehabilitation,* Philadelphia, 1996, FA Davis.
69. Benson TB, Copp EP: The effects of therapeutic forms of heat and ice on the pain threshold of the normal shoulder, *Rheumatol Rehabil* 13:101-104, 1974.
70. Lehmann JF, Brunner GD, Stow RW et al: Pain threshold measurements after therapeutic application of ultrasound, microwave and infrared, *Arch Phys Med Rehabil* 39:560-565, 1958.
70a. Belanger AY: *Evidence-based guide to therapeutic physical agents,* Baltimore, 2002, Lippincott, Williams and Wilkins.
71. Bracciano A: *Physical agent modalities: theory and application for the occupational therapist,* Thorofare, NJ, 2000, Slack, Inc.
72. Hayes, K: *Manual for physical agents,* ed 5, Upper Saddle River, NJ, 1999, Prentice Hall Health.
73. Hecox B, Andemicael-Mehreteab T, Weisberg J et al: *Integrating physical agents in rehabilitation,* ed 2, Upper Saddle River, NJ, 2006, Pearson Education.
74. Prentice WE: *Therapeutic modalities in rehabilitation,* ed 3, New York, 2006, McGraw-Hill Medical.
75. Fischer E, Solomon S: Physiological responses to heat and cold. In Licht S, editor: *Therapeutic heat and cold,* Baltimore, 1972, Waverly Press.
76. Kallen B, Malmquist G, Moritz U et al: Delivery outcome among physiotherapists in Sweden: is non-ionizing radiation a fetal hazard? *Arch Environ Health* 37:81-84, 1982.
77. Draper DO, Castel JC, Castel D et al: Rate of temperature increase in human muscle during 1 MHz and 3 MHz continuous ultrasound, *J Orthop Sport* 22(A):142-150, 1995.
78. Eldred E, Lindsley DF, Buchwald JS et al: The effect of cooling on mammalian muscle spindles, *Exp Neurol* 2:144-157, 1960.
79. Shealy C: Transcutaneous electroanalgesia, *Surg Forum* 23:419-421, 1973.
80. Dyson M, Suckling J: Stimulation of tissue repair by ultrasound: survey of the mechanisms involved, *Physiotherapy* 63:105-108, 1978.
81. Heckman JD, Ryaby JP, McCabe J et al: Acceleration of tibial fracture healing by non-invasive, low intensity pulsed ultrasound, *J Bone Joint Surg Am* 76:26-34, 1994.
82. Pilla AA, Mont MA, Nasser PR et al: Non-invasive low-intensity ultrasound accelerates bone healing in the rabbit, *J Orthop Trauma* 4:246-253, 1990.
83. Kleinkort JA, Wood AF: Phonophoresis with 1% versus 10% hydrocortisone. *Phys Ther* 55:1320-1324, 1975.
84. Griffin JE: Physiological effects of ultrasonic energy as it is used clinically, *Phys Ther* 46:18-26, 1966.
85. Stillwell GK: Therapeutic heat and cold. In Krusen FH, Kottke FJ, Ellwood PM, editors: *Handbook of physical medicine and rehabilitation,* Philadelphia, 1971, WB Saunders.
86. Sherman M: Which treatment to recommend? Hot or cold? *Am Pharmacol* 20:46-49, 1980.
87. Cameron MH: Thermal agents: physical principles, cool and superficial heat. In Cameron MH, editor: *Physical agents in rehabilitation,* Philadelphia, 1999, WB Saunders.
88. Jacob J: Inflammation revisited: inflammatory pain and mode of action of analgesics, *Agents Actions* 2:634-636, 1981.
89. Bromage PR: Nerve physiology and control of pain, *Orthop Clin North Am* 4:897-906, 1976.
90. Bottorff J, Gogag M, Engelberg-Lotzkar M et al: Comforting: exploring the work of cancer nursing, *J Advanced Nurs* 22:1077-1084, 1995.
91. Wolf SL: Perspectives on central nervous system responsiveness to transcutaneous electrical nerve stimulation, *Phys Ther* 58:1443-1449, 1978.
92. Sjolund B, Eriksson M: Electro-acupuncture and endogenous morphines, *Lancet* 2:1085, 1976.
93. Richard RL: Causalgia: a centennial review, *Arch Neurol* 16:339, 1967.
94. Selkowitz DM: Electrical currents. In Cameron MH, editor: *Physical agents in rehabilitation,* Philadelphia, 1999, WB Saunders.
95. Mayer DJM, Price DD: Central nervous system mechanisms of analgesia, *Pain* 2:379-404, 1976.
96. Long D: *The comparative efficacy of drugs vs. electrical modulation in the management of chronic pain: current concepts in the management of chronic pain,* Miami, 1977, Symposia Specialists.
96a. Melzack R: Prolonged relief of pain by brief, intense transcutaneous somatic stimulation, *Pain* 1:357-373, 1975.
97. Kahn J: *Principles and practice of electrotherapy,* ed 3, New York, 1992, Churchill Livingstone.
98. Krusen F, Kottke FJ, Ellwood PM: *Handbook of physical medicine and rehabilitation,* Philadelphia, 1971, WB Saunders.
99. Wood E: *Beard's massage,* Philadelphia, 1974, WB Saunders.
100. Badger CMA, Peacock JL, Mortimer PS: A randomized, controlled, parallel-group clinical trial comparing multilayer bandaging followed by hosiery versus hosiery alone in the treatment of patients with lymphedema of the limb, *Cancer* 88:2832-2837, 2000.
101. Andersen L, Hojris I, Erlandsen M et al: Treatment of breast-cancer-related lymphedema with or without manual lymphatic drainage—a randomized study, *Acta Oncologica* 39:399-405, 2000.
102. Sitzia J, Sobrido L, Harlow W: Manual lymphatic drainage compared with simple lymphatic drainage in the treatment of post-mastectomy lymphoedema: a pilot randomised trial [with consumer summary], *Physiotherapy* 88:99-107, 2002.
103. Ward RC: *The myofascial release concepts .* Handout material from course entitled Myofascial Release Concepts, Palpatory and Treatment Skills, Lansing, MI, September, 1986.
103a. Barnes J: *MFR: a comprehensive evaluatory and treatment approach,* Paoli, PA, 1990, MFR Seminars.
104. Anderson RU, Wise D, Sawyer T et al: Integration of myofascial trigger point release and paradoxical relaxation training treatment of chronic pelvic pain in men, *J Urol* 174:155-160, 2005.
105. Saunders HD: *Evaluation, treatment, and prevention of musculoskeletal disorders,* Eden Prairie, MN, 1985, Author.
106. Melzack R, Wall P: Pain mechanisms: a new theory, *Science* 150:971-979, 1969.
106a. Keller E, Bzdek V: Therapeutic touch and headache, *Nurs Res* 35:101-105, 1986.
107. Winstead-Fry P, Kijek J: An integrative review and meta-analysis of therapeutic touch research, *Altern Ther Health Med* 5:58-67, 1999.
108. Tappan FM: *Healing massage techniques: holistic, classic and emergency methods,* Norwalk, CT, 1988, Appleton & Lange.
109. Isele FW: Biofeedback and hypnosis in the management of pain, *NY State J Med* 82:38-44, 1982.
110. Benson H: *The relaxation response,* New York, 1975, Avon Books.
111. Chapman SL, Shealy CN: Relaxation techniques to control pain. In Brena SF, editor: *Chronic pain: America's hidden epidemic,* New York, 1978, Atheneum Publishers.
112. Borysenko J: *Minding the body, mending the mind,* Reading, MA, 1987, Addison-Wesley Publishing Co.
113. Lautenbacher S, Pauli P, Zaudig M et al: Attentional control of pain perception: the role of hypochondriasis, *J Psychosom Res* 44:251-259, 1998.
114. Kabat-Zinn J: *Full catastrophic living,* New York, 1990, Delacorte Press.
115. Cousins N: *Anatomy of an Illness,* New York, 1979, Bantam Books.
116. Leise CM: The correlation between humor and the chronic pain of arthritis, *J Hol Nurs* 11:82-85, 1993.
117. Fry WF: The physiological effects of humor, mirth, and laughter, *JAMA* 267:1857-1858, 1992.
118. Berk LS: Modulation of human natural cells by catecholamines, *Clin Res* 2:115, 1984.

119. Berk L, Tau S: Neuroendocrine influences of mirthful laughter, *Am J Med Sci* 298:390-396, 1989.

120. Freud S: *Jokes & their relation to the unconscious,* Vienna, 1905, Deuticke.

120a. Cohen M: Caring for ourselves can be funny business, *Hol Nurs Prac* 4:1-11, 1990.

121. Goldfarb AH, Jamurtas AZ: Beta-endorphin response to exercise. An update, *Sports Med* 24:8-16, 1997.

121a. Schwarz L, Kindermann W: Changes in beta-endorphin levels in response to aerobic and anaerobic exercise, *Sports Med* 13:25-36, 1992.

122. Fordyce WE: *Behavioral methods for chronic pain & illness,* St. Louis, 1976, CV Mosby.

122a. Tambiev AE, Medvedev SD: The dynamics of the spatial synchronization of brain biopotentials in conditions of intense attention in the hypnotic state, *Neurosci Behav Physiol* 35:643-647, 2005.

123. Gannon C: *21st century medicine and hypnosis:* http://www. infinityinst.com/articles/med&hyp.html. Accessed Auguest 28, 2006.

124. Bennett R: *Principles of treating fibromyalgia:* http://www. myalgia.com/Treatment/treatment%20overview.htm. Accessed August 28, 2006.

125. Sauter SL, Schleifer LM, Knutson SJ et al: Work posture, work station design, and musculoskeletal discomfort in a VDT data entry desk, *Hum Factors* 33:151-167, 1991.

126. Harvey R, Peper E: Surface electromyography and mouse use position, *Ergonomics* 40:781-789, 1997.

127. Paul R, Nair C: Ergonomic evaluation of keyboard and mouse tray designs. Proceedings of the fortieth annual meeting of the Human Factors Society, Santa Monica, CA, 1996.

128. Hill A: Phantom limb pain: a review of the literature on attributes and potential mechanisms. *J Pain Symptom Management* 17:125-142, 1999.

129. Hooshmand H: *Chronic pain: reflex sympathetic dystrophy, prevention and management,* Boca Raton, FL, 1993, CRC Press.

130. Watson HK, Carlson L: Treatment of reflex sympathetic dystrophy of the hand with active stress loading program, *Am J Hand Surg* 12(5 pt 1):779-785, 1987.

CHAPTER 33

Pelvic Floor Treatment of Incontinence and Other Urinary Dysfunctions in Men and Women

Beate Carrière, PT, CIFK

KEY WORDS

clinical problem solving for pelvic floor dysfunction
evaluation of clients with incontinence
functional training exercises
recoordination of the functions of the abdominal
   compartment

OBJECTIVES

After reading this chapter the student/therapist will be able to:
1. Discuss the factors that lead to incontinence.
2. Understand the neurophysiology involved in pelvic floor dysfunctions.
3. Describe the different layers of the pelvic floor and their functional connections.
4. Correct faulty breathing patterns.
5. Understand why diaphragmatic breathing has to be coordinated with pelvic floor activity.
6. Apply motor learning/motor control principles when teaching exercises.
7. Select from various treatment approaches the most appropriate intervention to improve pelvic floor function.

OVERVIEW OF THE CLINICAL PROBLEM

History of Pelvic Floor Exercises

A different focus on how to view the pelvic floor and the problem of incontinence has evolved from new knowledge about neurophysiology, neuroplasticity, motor learning, and motor control. Kegel[1-3] is considered the great American pioneer who, in the late 1940s, recognized the importance of exercises to help women with urinary incontinence (UI). Dr. Kegel, a Los Angeles physician, found that many women did not have any awareness of the function of the pelvic floor and that they were not always successful with the exercise he prescribed: drawing in the perineum. He therefore developed a pneumatic apparatus, the perineometer, which measured each muscle contraction in a manner visible to the patient. He instructed his patients to perform the exercise for 20 minutes three times daily, or a total of 300 contractions, and suggested weekly visits for instruction.[1,2] Kegel also recognized that evidence of bladder weakness was present in some women before childbearing and emphasized the importance of training the pubococcygeus muscle to achieve continence.[2,3] Even though his approach to exercises demonstrates visual feedback combined with declarative learning, which must have been considered visionary at that time, the treatment has not changed much since.[4-7] Kegel exercises are stereotypical and highly repetitive (300 repetitions until improvement, then 80 per day for life) with little functional value. The pelvic floor works with many systems and subsystems of the body, such as the nervous system (central, peripheral, autonomic, sensory, and limbic), the musculoskeletal system, cardiopulmonary system, lymph system, and integumentary system as well as with different organs

in the abdominal cavity; it is also dependent on the environment.

Given the complexity of the role of the pelvic floor muscles, procedural learning, sensory awareness, and functional retraining are now part of the treatment, which may include breathing exercises, manual lymph treatment, visceral mobilization, and treatment of scars.

Prevalence of Incontinence

The prevalence of incontinence in men and women is high and costly. Although Fantl et al[8] reported in 1996 that 10% to 35%, or 13 million adult Americans, have UI, in 2000 Hu et al[9] estimated that 17 million community-dwelling persons had daily UI and 34 million overactive bladder (OAB) syndrome (but only 2.9 million of those had incontinence episodes).

In 1996 more than half of the 1.5 million nursing home residents in the United States were estimated to be incontinent; in addition, the most common reason for placing a family member in a home was incontinence[8-10]; The number of adults in institutional care has risen to 1.89 million in 2000 and 945,000 of those are estimated to have UI.[9] Women older than 60 years have twice the prevalence of incontinence than do men of that age.[8] The majority of patients with incontinence are parous women and older persons.[10] Britton et al[11] conducted a study of urinary symptoms in 578 men older than 60 years. Thirty percent of the men reported increased daytime frequencies, and 27% reported urgencies and a variety of other urinary symptoms, defined as OAB if nocturia (getting up at least once in the night to urinate) is included. Incontinence can also be found in the younger population. Nygaard et al[12] investigated UI in nulliparous elite athletes and found that gymnastics and sports that include jumping, high-impact landings, and running appear to score higher in the prevalence of UI than swimming or playing golf. Because exercises and activities during field training of soldiers can be strenuous, one third of 450 female soldiers experienced UI.[13] Baumann and Tauber[14] reported that 17% of boys between the ages 5 and 14 years are incontinent. Adedokun and Wilson[15] and Diokno et al[16] provided thorough epidemiological overviews, collecting data from various sources all over the world. Obesity can contribute to incontinence and make the treatment more difficult.[17] Cigarette smoking augments incontinence for three reasons: (1) it has been shown to interfere with collagen synthesis, (2) neuromuscular and anatomical changes likely occur from smoking, and (3) it causes coughing.[18] Smoking also cause erectile dysfunction, has an effect on sperm quality and, in women, is attributed to causing miscarriage, reduced chance of conception, and cervical cancer.[19] Smoking cessation, weight reduction, and regulation of bowel movements may reduce the risk of urinary incontinence.[20]

Individuals with neurological diseases often have urinary problems. The Agency for Health Care Policy and Research[21] reported that UI is most prevalent in persons with spinal cord injuries (SCIs) and people with multiple sclerosis (MS). Eighty percent of patients with SCI will have at least one urinary tract infection (UTI) by their sixteenth year post injury, and 70% to 90% of individuals diagnosed with MS develop bladder dysfunction, which places them at high risk for UTIs. Patients affected by spina bifida also can have various neurogenic urinary tract dysfunctions. Depending on the severity of the dysfunction, they may become socially dry with conservative therapy.[22] Hunter and Moore[23] state that an estimated 13% of seniors have diabetes, 32% to 45% of whom have associated bladder dysfunction, typically from decreased bladder sensation, increased bladder capacity, and impaired detrusor contractility.

In patients with Alzheimer's disease cognitive and central regulating mechanisms contribute to incontinence.[24] Brittain et al[25] state that urinary incontinence after a stroke is associated with poor outcome and depression in stroke survival and care. The prevalence of urinary incontinence is high in stroke patients admitted to the hospital. Individuals with Parkinson's disease, cerebrovascular disease, or traumatic brain injury can also have voiding dysfunction. Walters and Karram[26] provide a list of neurological diseases known to cause urinary problems, some of which are described in this chapter.

Cost of Incontinence

Hu et al[9] adjusted and reported the cost of UI and OAB in 2000: $19.5 billion and $12.6 billion, respectively. Thirty-four million individuals were affected by OAB syndrome and 17 million with UI. Because individuals with OAB have fewer incontinence episodes, the per-person cost is higher in patients with UI considering that 35% of patients with UI have stress urinary incontinence (SUI), which can involve expensive surgeries. However, the days spent in the hospital have declined since 1995.[9] The cost of UI escalated from 8.2 billion in 1984 to 16.4 billion in 1993 and to 26.3 billion, or $3565 per individual with UI, in 1995. According to Wagner and Hu,[27] this increase was attributed to the following three major changes in the last 10 years:

1. Introduction of more continence-related products to the market
2. Change in the age composition of the U.S. population
3. Change in prevalence of UI

The authors stated that the cost for people younger than 65 years was not included in the study and that the true cost may be much higher because UI is underreported.

Definition of Incontinence

Urinary incontinence is defined as involuntary loss of urine that is sufficient to be a problem.[8] Incontinence can have one or more causes, and in more than 90% of cases it can be improved or cured.[10] Treatment should only be instituted after a careful, thorough history and physical examination.[10] In nonneurological patients the most common forms of incontinence are stress urinary incontinence (SUI), OAB syndrome, urge urinary incontinence (UUI), and mixed incontinence. Weak pelvic floor muscles usually cause stress urinary incontinence. SUI occurs when the abdominal pressure is greater than the urethral pressure, resulting in a loss of urine with coughing, laughing, sneezing, lifting, and so forth. OAB syndrome, or detrusor overactivity, is associated with involuntary bladder muscle contraction during the filling phase, causing frequent urination; nocturia; and strong, sudden, and sometimes unpredictable urges to urinate but not always resulting in incontinence.[28]

Urge urinary incontinence can be caused by detrusor instability, an involuntary contraction of the muscle of the bladder before it is full. It is associated with a sudden urge to void. The urge can be so irresistible as to result in loss of urine before the individual reaches the bathroom. Mixed incontinence is the combination of SUI and UUI or urges.

ETIOLOGY

The causes of stress urinary and urge urinary incontinence in nonneurological clients are as follows (Figure 33-1):

1. Functional causes include the inability to undress in a timely fashion and being unable to reach a bathroom in a timely fashion because of obstacles (no light, cannot enter the bathroom with the walker without maneuvering, etc.).
2. Weakening of the pelvic floor structures can result from childbirth (overstretching of muscles, the pudendal nerve, or ligaments), hysterectomy, prolapse (rectocele, cystocele, vaginal prolapse), straining with constipation, and poor biomechanics when lifting, falls on the buttocks with shift of the pelvis affecting muscle length or stretching the nerves, poor coordination of the pulmonary diaphragm with the pelvic floor, scars in the perineal and pelvic area, aging (loss of muscle mass), obesity, smoking, poor posture, and pain in the pelvic area.
3. OAB syndrome and urge urinary incontinence can be caused by UTI and other conditions that irritate the bladder: neoplasia, status post bladder or bowel surgery, bladder outlet obstruction, anxiety, nervousness, and poor toileting habits. The condition can also be idiopathic. Some clients also have urges to eliminate the bowels.
4. Over-the-counter medications with anticholinergic agents can cause retention (an inability to empty the bladder completely), overflow (leakage of urine when the bladder is overextended), and frequency; antipsychotic

	Overview of bladder dysfunctions	
Non-neurological	**Stress:** *Weakness* of the pelvic floor muscles. Reasons: Injury from childbirth; decreased function because improper use when coughing, lifting, breathing; straining with constipation or fecal impaction, estrogen deficiency, genetic make-up (possible collagen deficiency)	
Bladder dysfunction	**Urge:** *Detrusor instability* Sudden urge to go to the bathroom, with or without loss of urine. Possible reasons: infection, prolapse of vagina, cystocele, weakness of the pelvic floor	
	Retention: *Inadequate emptying* of the bladder; can be associated with pressure/pain in the lower abdomen	**Overflow:** *Overdistention* of the bladder; it empties by constant dribbling of urine when the capacity is exceeded
Neurological	**1. Lesions in higher cortical areas and suprapontine:** *Possible causes:* MS, stroke, Parkinson's disease, traumatic brain injury (TBI), tumors, dementia, alcoholism, Alzheimer's disease, Huntington's disease	**Possible symptoms:** Retention, inability to control the micturation reflex resulting in detrusor hyperreflexia
	2. Lesions in the upper motor neuron (spinal cord): *Possible causes:* Spinal cord injury (SCI), MS, tumors, back injuries and prolapse of a disk, stenosis of the spinal canal, inflammatory and vascular diseases (e.g., transverse myelitis), infections (e.g., syphilis–tabes dorsalis), diabetes mellitus, cauda equina syndrome, herpes zoster	**Possible symptoms:** Detrusor sphincter dyssynergy with danger of urethrovesical reflux
	3. Lesions in the lower motor neuron, peripheral nervous system, and in the autonomic nervous system: *Possible causes:* Injuries to the spinal cord, radiculitis (e.g., herpes zoster), tabes dorsalis, radiation, radical abdominal/perineal surgeries, diabetes mellitus, autonomous neuropathy, Guillain-Barré syndrome	**Possible symptoms:** Areflexia of the detrusor muscle, decreased sensation, incontinence, void by straining. Autonomic nervous system symptoms can include diffuse pain
Other causes	**4. Psychogenic:** Non-neurogenic neurogenic bladder (Hinman syndrome), hysteria, schizophrenia, depression **5. Endocrine:** e.g., diabetes, hypothyroidism **6. Hormonal deficiencies:** e.g., lack of estrogen **7. Inflammatory:** e.g., cystitis, vulvovaginitis, and prostatitis **8. Obstructive:** e.g., tumor, prolapse **9. Pharmacological:** e.g., some over-the-counter medications, medication for treatment of hypertension, depression	**Possible symptoms:** Retention, frequency, urgency, and stress incontinence

FIGURE 33-1 ■ Overview of reasons for incontinence of nonneurological and neurological causes.

medications can cause sedation, rigidity, and immobility; and diuretics can worsen impaired continence. Medication for treatment of hypertension can also contribute to incontinence.[8,10,23,26,29]

5. Retention in nonneurological clients can occur in men with prostate problems; the enlarged prostate makes the passage of urine difficult.[11,30] Other causes in men and women are the hyperactive pelvic floor syndrome,[30a] an inability to relax the pelvic floor muscles. This can be caused by pelvic pain syndromes, by interstitial cystitis, or by bad habits: trying to void in a hurry, squeezing rather than relaxing the muscles, and the inability to void because of stressful situations.

6. An overdistended bladder can cause overflow incontinence. It can present as constant or intermittent dribbling, sometimes combined with urge or symptoms of stress incontinence. Patients often have high residuals and feel that their bladder does not empty properly.

7. Inadequate fluid intake (either too much or too little) and fluids that may be stimulants to the bladder can cause urge incontinence or frequent trips to the bathroom. Smoking, obesity, and postmenopausal estrogen deficiency contribute to the problem.[8,17,18,26,29]

Additional neurogenic causes of bladder dysfunctions are as follows:

1. Lesions in the higher cortical areas and suprapontine lesions can be found in patients with MS, stroke, Alzheimer's disease, Parkinson's disease, traumatic brain injury, tumors, and dementia. These diseases can cause retention and an inability to control the micturition reflex, resulting in detrusor hyperreflexia (overactive detrusor during filling phase) with coordinated urethral relaxation, because these diseases can interfere with normal tonic inhibition of the parasympathetic pathways and the balance between facilitatory an inhibitory mechanism in the pontine micturition center.[26,28,29,31]

2. Lesions in the upper motor neurons affect the spinal cord. Common problems resulting in urinary dysfunction are SCI, MS, cauda equina syndrome, tumors, inflammatory diseases such as transverse myelitis, infectious diseases such as syphilis (tabes dorsalis), injuries to the spinal column, prolapse of a disk, or stenosis of the spinal canal. A typical bladder problem is detrusor hyperreflexia without coordinated urethral relaxation (detrusor-sphincter dyssynergy.)[26,29,31,32]

3. Lesions to the peripheral or lower motor neurons such as injuries from childbirth, traumatic injuries, radiculitis (e.g., from herpes zoster), or tabes dorsalis can cause retention and detrusor areflexia. The inability to feel when the bladder is full can lead to an overflow bladder with symptoms of dribbling and incomplete or strained voiding. Patients may need to learn clean intermittent catheterization.[8,10,29,31,33]

4. Lesions stemming from injuries to the autonomic nervous system can be caused by surgery in the pelvic area, such as hysterectomy, rectum resection, and radical prostatectomy; injury; or inflammations such as chronic cystopathy in diabetic patients. Autonomic lesions can contribute to diffuse pain,[34] swelling, and altered sensory awareness. Urinary problems can cause the feeling of having cold feet.[35,36] Patients with diabetic cystopathy (DC)—in addition to their symptoms of weak stream, hesitancy in start-

ing urination, dribbling and overflow from high residual (caused by decreased bladder sensation and increased bladder capacity, and impaired contractility)—may also have other symptoms of autonomic dysfunction. These can include orthostatic hypotension, nocturnal fall of blood pressure, and changes in heart rate.[23]

5. Psychogenic causes of urinary dysfunction include schizophrenia and depression. Patients can have incontinence, hesitation, retention, and pain. A nonneurogenic neurogenic bladder is called Hinman syndrome.[26]

6. Endocrine causes are hypothyroidism and diabetes, which may lead to a flaccid or areflexic bladder and require clean intermittent self-catheterization.[26,33] Diabetes can also increase the frequency of urination.

ANATOMY AND PHYSIOLOGY OF THE PELVIC FLOOR

The pelvic floor consists of all the muscles that close the pelvic cavity. It is part of the abdominal compartment that can be defined by the pulmonary diaphragm cranially, the pelvic diaphragm and perineal membrane caudally, the muscles of the abdominal wall ventrally, and the muscles of the back dorsally. This compartment houses the internal organs and the viscera.[10,26,37,38] The pelvic floor is essentially composed of three layers: the endopelvic fascia, the pelvic diaphragm, and the perineal membrane.

Endopelvic Fascia

The endopelvic fascia suspends and supports the organs within the pelvis. It is a mesh of connective tissue composed of collagen, elastin, blood and lymph vessels, and nerves. A thick, fibrous part of the endopelvic fascia, the pubocervical fascia, attaches to the cervix in a slinglike fashion and assists in supporting the urethra and the bladder. Laterally it connects to the fascia white line, the tendinous arch of the levator ani muscle. Injuries to this important fascial support can contribute to weakness of the pelvic floor, prolapse, and leakage with increased abdominal pressure.[10,29,38]

Pelvic Diaphragm

The pelvic diaphragm consists mostly of the paired levator ani muscle (Figure 33-2). The levator ani is shaped like a hammock and has several parts. In the sagittal plane the muscle originates at the pubic bone and attaches to the coccyx, hence the name pubococcygeus muscle. The medial part of the pubococcygeus joins behind the rectum and therefore is named the puborectalis muscle. This part of the levator muscle provides continence of bowel by increasing the anorectal angle. Inability to relax the puborectalis therefore contributes to constipation in patients with hyperactive pelvic floor syndrome. Other fibers of the levator ani form a sling around the vagina or prostate (pubovaginalis and levator prostate muscles). Each side of the muscle meets in the midline with the other half and attaches to the perineal and anococcygeal bodies. The compressor urethrae muscle is part of the external urethral complex. It originates from the rami of the ischium and pubis and runs fanwise forward and medially to arch over the anterior part of the urethral surface. The sphincter urethrovaginalis is part of the puborectalis.[39]

The posterior part of the levator ani has two paired sections. The coccygeus (or ischiococcygeus) muscle covers

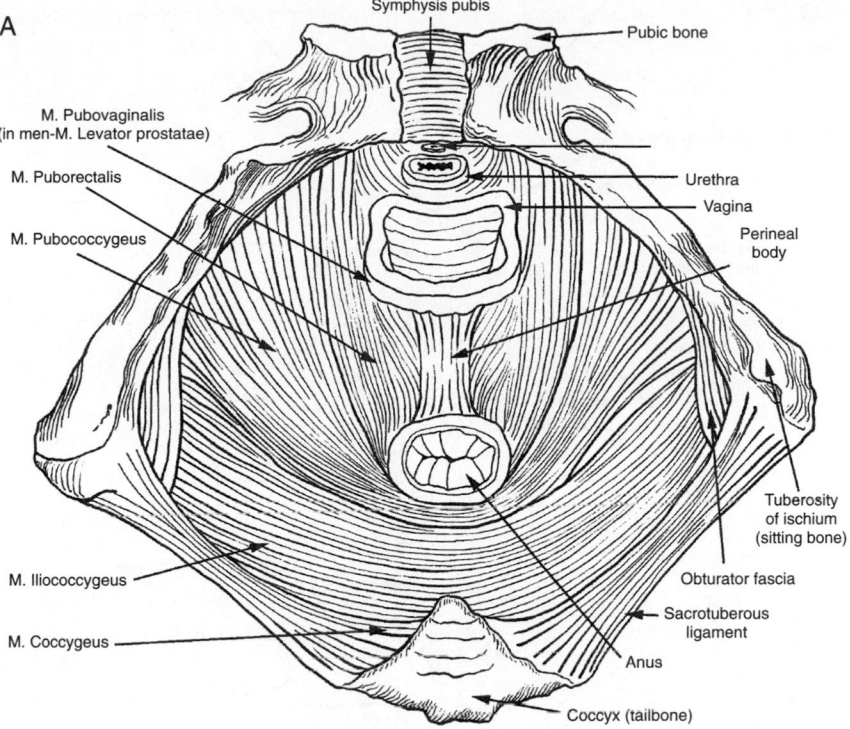

2nd layer of Pelvic Floor (Pelvic Diaphragm)
Levator Ani muscle
(viewed from above)

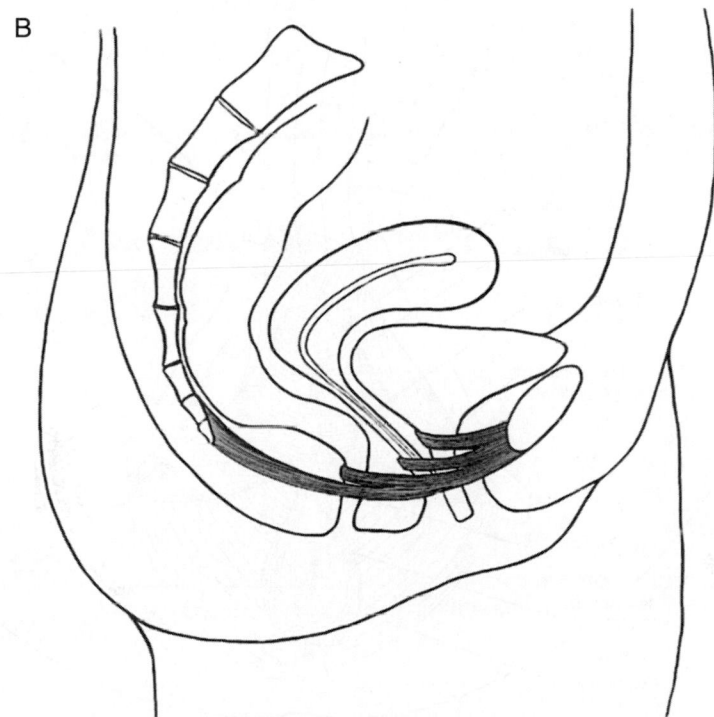

2nd layer of the Pelvic Floor
Pelvic Diaphragm
pubo-coccygeus, pubo-rectalis, pubo-vaginalis muscles
as part of the levator ani muscle
(viewed from the side)

FIGURE 33-2 ■ Anatomy of the pelvic floor. **A,** Second layer of the pelvic floor, pelvic diaphragm viewed from above. **B,** Second layer of the pelvic floor, pelvic diaphragm viewed from the side.

Continued

C

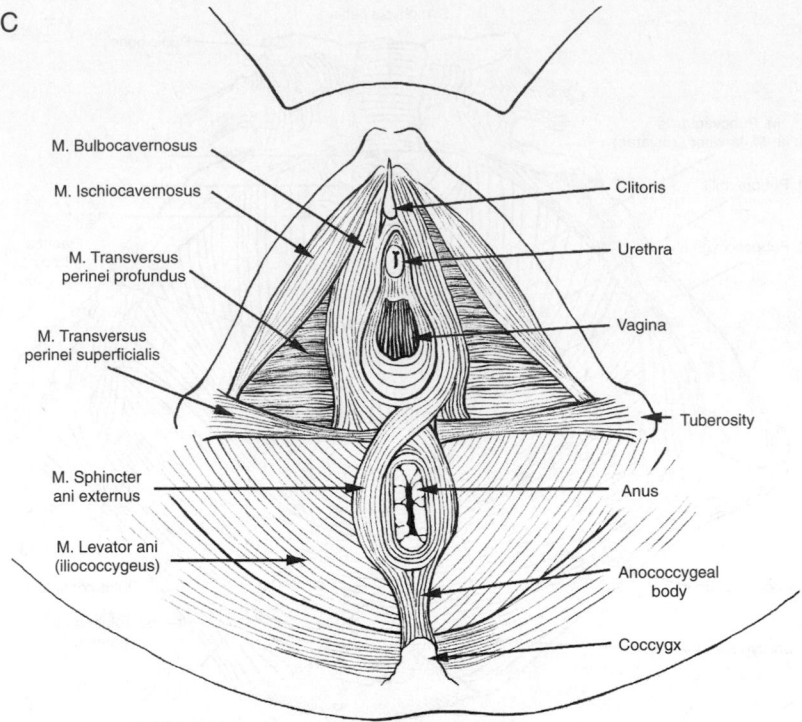

3rd layer of the Pelvic Floor
Perineal Membrane
(view from below)

D

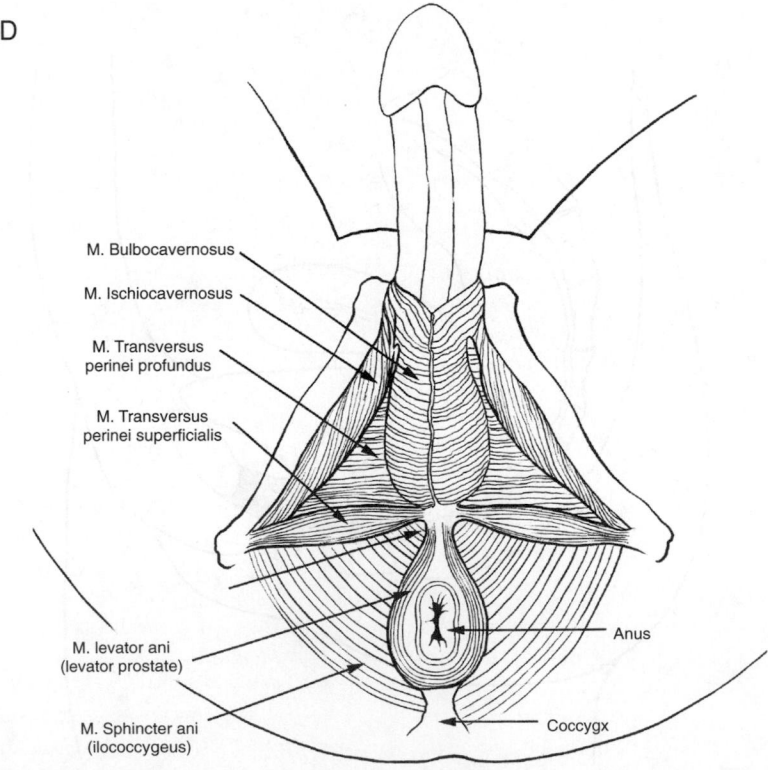

3rd layer of the Pelvic Floor
Perineal Membrane
(view from below)

FIGURE 33-2, cont'd C, Third layer of the pelvic floor perineal membrane viewed from below (female). **D,** Third layer of the pelvic floor, perineal membrane viewed from below (male).

the sacrospinous ligament. The muscle arises at the spine of the ischium and extends to the lowest part of the sacrum and the coccyx. The iliococcygeus lies between the coccygeus and the puborectalis and passes in a diagonal direction between the coccyx to the spine of the ischium and the tendinous arch of the levator ani. This fibrous band of the arcus tendineus is suspended between the pubic bone and ischial spine.[10,26,29,38-41] The levator ani is a skeletal muscle with a high resting tone; it consists of approximately 70% slow twitch fibers and 30% fast twitch fibers.[29,38,42-44] Wall et al[29] and Bump et al[42] consider the high resting tone critical for pelvic support and for keeping the hiatus of the levator closed. Because the levator ani muscle is under voluntary control, it can be actively contracted and provide closure during an increase in abdominal pressure, such as when coughing or sneezing.[29,43-45] According to Retzky and Rogers,[10] the innervation of the levator ani muscles is under dual control: on their pelvic surface by motor efferents of the sacral nerve from S2-S4 and on the perineal surface by the pudendal nerve.

Perineal Membrane

The perineal membrane (formerly urogenital diaphragm) is the outer layer of the pelvic floor. It is a thick, fibrous, and muscular layer of triangular shape immediately below the levator ani. In women the perineal membrane attaches the edges of the vagina to the ischiopubic ramus; in men it forms an uninterrupted sheet of tissue. The fibers of the deep and superficial transverse perineal muscles run primarily in a frontal plane and contain many fibrous tissues,[46] the ischiocavernosus muscle in a diagonal direction, and the bulbospongiosus muscle in a sagittal plane. The external sphincter muscle of the anus is part of the perineal membrane and is connected to the transverse perineal and bulbospongiosus muscle by the perineal body, which contains fibrous tissue. The dorsal attachment of the perineal membrane is achieved through the anococcygeal raphe, which connects the external anal sphincter to the coccyx.[29,40,43,46]

The muscles of the perineal membrane contain both smooth and striated muscles. The muscles become tight when the levator ani tone remains relaxed.[29] The anterior portion of the perineal membrane is closely connected to the urethral musculature. According to Wall et al,[29] the perineal membrane does not substantially contribute to pelvic support; it is mostly the levator ani that is much greater in strength and bulk and can exert upward traction when contracting to maintain outlet support. The ischiocavernosus, bulbospongiosus, and superficial transverse perineal muscles function mainly in sexual responsiveness, serving to enhance and maintain penile erection in males and maintaining erection of the clitoris in females.[29,38] Trigger points in these muscles can cause a degree of impotence and pain with intercourse. According to Claes et al,[47] Van Kampen et al,[48] and Dorey,[49] strengthening exercises of the muscles of the perineal membrane can significantly improve impotence. In women, the perineal membrane is often torn or injured during childbirth and, if not properly repaired, injuries can cause sexual dysfunction, pelvic floor pain, and low self-esteem.

The complicated autonomic innervation of the pelvic area and its clinical relevance, including the perineal area, has been well described by Wesselmann et al[34] as well as Fritsch

and Umphred.[46] The pudendal nerve diverges from the sacral plexus, intermingles with the autonomic nerves, and then branches into several directions, innervating the external anal sphincter and the anterior perineal muscles.

Mucosal Coaptation of the Urethra

In addition to the three pelvic floor layers, an important contributor to continence is the mucosal coaptation, which is the arteriovenous complex between the epithelial lining and the smooth muscle coat of the female urethra. It is sensitive to estrogen, and with deficiency of this hormone the resting pressure of the urethra can decrease and cause leakage.[10] Wall et al[29] compared it to an "inflatable cushion" helping to fill the urethral wall and sealing the 3- to 4-cm-long urethra in women. Because of possible serious side effects estrogen is only prescribed and applied to the vaginal area with great caution. It can help some menopausal women increase the resting tone of the urethra and improve closure. The male urethra is not estrogen dependent. Its mucosal coaptation is highly vascular and probably influenced by testosterone. In addition, the prostate gland and the length of the male urethra may contribute to a sealing effect.

Internal Sphincter of the Urethra

The internal sphincter muscle at the junction of bladder and urethra (urethrovesical junction) is an involuntary smooth muscle under autonomic control in both males and females. Its shape is circular and formed by the trigone, a smooth muscle in the bladder, and two U-shaped loops of muscles that derive from the bladder muscle. In females the urethra rests on a hammock of connective tissue (pubocervical fascia) and is held in a position that prevents descent into the vagina. The external sphincter muscle is able to close the middle portion of the female urethra.[10]

Incontinence usually happens when several factors come together. For example, men frequently leak after radical prostatectomy because the smooth internal sphincter urethra may have been damaged by the surgery and the pelvic floor muscles have to learn to substitute and provide closure of the urethra. A patient with dementia may not feel the need to go to the bathroom. Parkinson's disease may cause bladder outlet obstruction because of a noncontractile detrusor resulting in large volumes of residual urine.[50] In addition, the inability to undress fast complicates an already existing problem of incontinence in such a client.

In healthy individuals the external sphincter and levator ani muscles serve as a backup system for continence. However, weakness of these structures leads to decreased bladder neck and urethral support and can lead to incontinence, especially with activities that increase the abdominal pressure.

VOIDING MECHANISM OF THE BLADDER

Many of the neurophysiological connections involved in functioning of the bladder and the surrounding muscles are not fully understood. A complicated coordination of many systems is involved in a properly functioning bladder and other pelvic organs. Elaboration on all the neural interactions, which take place at all levels, is not possible in this chapter. Wesselmann et al[34] and Burnett and Wesselmann[51] provide comprehensive information about the neurobiology of the pelvis.

Sympathetic Innervation

The sympathetic innervation to the bladder, rectum, and sexual organs originates at the thoracolumbar segment of the spinal cord (T10 to L1-L2) as well as from the hypogastric plexus (the sympathetic hypogastric nerve), which descends from the aortic plexus (Figure 33-3). The hypogastric nerve feeds into the inferior hypogastric (pelvic) plexus, which is the major neuronal integrative center for multiple pelvic organs.[34,51] Both the sympathetic and parasympathetic divisions of the autonomic nervous system innervate the pelvic viscera, which are also innervated by the somatic and sensory nervous systems. The sympathetic innervation inhibits the bladder and increases bladder storage ability (it is sympathetic to be dry) and stimulates the muscles of the trigone and the internal sphincter muscles of the bladder as well as the muscles of the rectum. Attention should be paid to the T10 to L1-L2 segments in patients with tailbone pain and pain in the pelvic floor (e.g., testicular, buttock, scrotal pain) because the pain may be referred from that area. The author recalls a case in which tailbone pain disappeared instantly after treatment of the thoracolumbar area in a client who had fallen on the back in a flexed position. Doubleday et al[52] described a case report of a patient who for 5 years has complained of testicular and buttock pain along with posterior leg paresthesias. Treatment of the T10 to L1-L2 area (central disk protrusion T12-L1) with direct and guided physical therapy resulted in complete symptom resolution.

Parasympathetic Innervation

The parasympathetic innervation exits the spinal canal at the level of S2-S4. The nerves join the splanchnic nerve before entering the inferior hypogastric plexus (see Figure 33-3, A). The parasympathetic fibers stimulate the bladder and other pelvic organs, including the sexual organs.[34,51,53] The parasympathetic fibers ending in the bladder are especially sensitive to overstretching, infection, and fibrosis.[26] This explains the urge of wanting to urinate frequently under such conditions. The parasympathetic nerve helps bladder contraction by stimulating muscarinic receptors in the fundus of the bladder. Parasympathetic nerve activation also helps colonic mobility. Therefore, in a spinal cord injury (SCI) when the lower motor neuron (LMN) is injured (parasympathetic cell bodies in cauda equina and conus medullaris), slowed stool propulsion is the result with areflexic bowel. LMN injury causes constipation and increases the risk for incontinence from lax external anal sphincter (EAS) as described by Benevento and Sipski.[32]

In contrast an upper motor neuron (UMN) lesion causes hyperreflexia with no voluntary control over the EAS. The patient cannot relax the EAS to defecate even though reflex coordination and stool propulsion are present. Fecal retention and constipation are common in such UMN injuries.[32]

Detrusor sphincter dyssynergia (DSD), caused by impaired coordination between bladder contraction and external sphincter urethra, can be attributable to hyperreflexia or uncontrolled muscle spasm of the detrusor. This condition is common in patients with SCI[32] as well as MS but not in clients with cerebral vascular accident (CVA).

Somatic Innervation

The somatic innervation of the pelvic floor comes from the sacral plexus of S2-S4 (see Figure 33-3, A). The pudendal nerve leaves the spinal cord at S2-S4 and branches to innervate the striated muscles of the levator ani, the external sphincter muscles of both the urethra and rectum, and the muscles of the perineal membrane. The sacral plexus provides both efferent and afferent innervation; some of the fibers of the pudendal nerve intermingle with the autonomic pelvic nerves.[26,34,53] The somatic nerves can modulate the autonomic system. The complexity of the innervation of the pelvis and the influence of neurotransmitters in the bladder wall, as well as the control of higher central nervous system regulation (see Figure 33-3, B and C), can be appreciated when observing the filling and emptying phases of the bladder. Because of its topographical position the pudendal nerve is susceptible to nerve injury from stretching or compression from a fall on the buttocks, or slamming on the brake pedal during a motor vehicle accident (may alter pelvic alignment), or childbirth, especially during delivery of large babies,[10]

Sensory Innervation

The sensory innervation in the pelvic region is important to evaluate and restore in clients with motor control problems because sensation drives motor responses. The pudendal nerve carries both sensory and motor fibers. Absence of feeling in the perineal area can be due to stress and memory of pain (e.g., abuse). For example, a client with symptoms of incontinence and pain with sexual intercourse and a history of considerable continuous stresses stated after few treatments, "I thought my pelvic region was dead; I had no clue how little I could feel before sensory awareness training. Feeling the pelvic floor, I can now contract and relax the muscles much better." Sensory innervation of the bladder comes primarily from proprioceptive nerve endings in the bladder and urethra. The afferent neuronal visceral system probably enters the spinal cord by way of the sacral and lumber segments. These afferent nerve tracts may regulate pain, the absence of pain, and the feeling of having a full bladder.[26,53]

Filling/Storage Phase

The bladder is a smooth involuntary muscle with voluntary control. It stores the urine until it is emptied voluntarily. The normal bladder is a low-pressure system that accepts urine without a concomitant rise of internal pressure.[10,29] This is produced by sympathetic stimulation of the β-adrenergic receptors in the bladder wall. The sympathetic nervous system inhibits the parasympathetic activity at the same time sympathetic stimulation of the α-adrenergic receptors in the internal sphincter muscle cause constriction and a rise in urethral pressure.[10,29] During the filling phase the bladder is inactive until it holds approximately 350 to 500 ml of urine, even though a first sensation of filling may occur with 150 to 250 ml of urine in the bladder.[53] When the bladder is full the receptors send a signal to the cortical centers of the brain and, as a result, a voluntary micturition reflex is initiated to empty the bladder (see Figure 33-3, B).[10,29,53]

Involuntary contractions of the detrusor during the filling phase cause frequency and urgency (OAB syndrome). In neurological patients this is called hyperreflexia; if idiopathic, it is considered bladder instability.[26,29] Individuals with a hypersensitive bladder must empty their bladders frequently, which results in a functionally small bladder. When

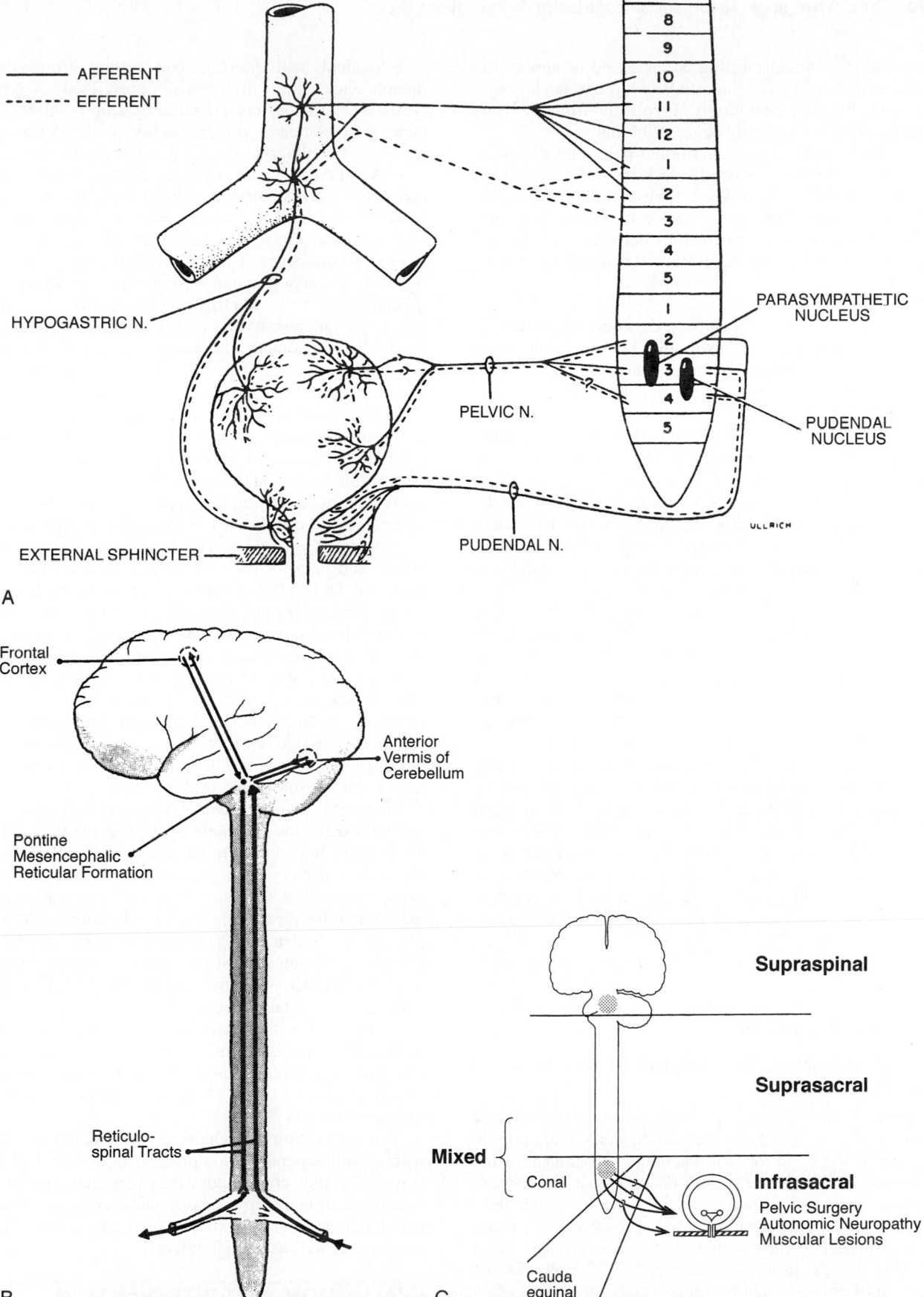

FIGURE 33-3 ■ Neurophysiology of the pelvic floor. (**A** from Blaivas JG: Management of bladder dysfunction in multiple sclerosis, *Neurology* 30:12, 1980; **B** from Bradley WE, Brantley SF: Physiology of the urinary bladder. In Harrison JH, Gittes RE, Perlmutter AD et al, editors: *Campbell's urology,* Philadelphia, 1978, WB Saunders, p. 106; **C** from Braddom RL: *Physical medicine rehabilitation,* ed 2, Philadelphia, 2000, WB Saunders.)

the sensation of bladder filling is decreased or absent, the bladder will overfill and urine can back up into the kidneys, causing dysfunction. Symptoms of overflow from the over-stretched bladder frequently cause dribbling.

Preconditions for a normal storage phase are described by Henscher[54] include good distensibility of the bladder, stable bladder without premature detrusor contractions (adequate bladder sensation, i.e., intact central and peripheral nervous systems), no obstruction between kidney and bladder, and positive urethral closure at rest and under load.

Emptying Phase

Micturition, or voiding, depends on the coordinated activity of the urethra and the detrusor muscle. The pelvic floor (levator ani and external sphincter muscles) has to relax when the detrusor muscle contracts. This occurs with activation of the parasympathetic cholinergic receptors in the bladder muscle. An afferent stimulus from the pelvic nerve (see Figure 33-3, A) reaches the pontine micturition center by way of the spinal cord. Efferent tracts inhibit the activity of the pudendal nerve, which results in relaxation of the external sphincter and levator ani. At the same time sympathetic activity at the bladder neck is inhibited and postganglionic parasympathetic neurotransmitters are stimulated. This results in detrusor contraction.[10,14,26,53]

From the pontine micturition center, signals are also sent to the cerebral cortex which allows voluntary control. An individual therefore can override the signal to empty the bladder and wait to empty it later, or can empty the bladder when there is no signal that it is full. Suprapontine control of bladder function is due to the modulating control of the brain stem, hypothalamus, and the cerebral cortex.[53]

Many reflexes are involved in urine storage and voiding at various levels. The sacral reflex, for example, can be elicited by light stroking at the lateral aspect of the anus and should result in a symmetrical contraction of the anal sphincter ("anal wink"). Absence of the anal wink can be an indication of a neurological problem at S2-S4, resulting in weakness or paralysis of the pudendal nerve.[10] The micturition reflex, on the other hand, depends on an intact pontine micturition center in the brain stem.[53]

Prerequisites for a normal emptying phase include intact neural control, adequate functioning of the detrusor, no increase in resistance to voiding by obstruction, and adequate pelvic floor relaxation.[54]

Pharmacological Treatment of Pelvic Floor Dysfunction

The great number of receptors in the bladder wall, as well as the ability to influence skeletal muscles with muscle relaxants, is the basis for pharmacological treatment of the symptoms found in patients with incontinence. Other treatments of urinary dysfunction address the hormonal deficiency. Estrogen, for example, was prescribed for many postmenopausal women with symptoms of leakage and a feeling of dryness in the vaginal area.[10,26,29,31] However, the treatment of oral estrogen is controversial and reports of its efficacy for treatment of urinary incontinence are mixed.[20] Topical vaginal application of Premarin and other drugs may be beneficial in the treatment of urinary incontinence because estrogen deficiency decreases the turgor of the submucosa around the urethra.

Individuals with enuresis (bed-wetting at night) or urge incontinence are frequently prescribed oxybutynin (Ditropan). Another prescribed drug is imipramine, an antidepressant. Patients with instability of the detrusor often receive anticholinergic agents or antispasmodic medications.

α-Adrenergic agents such as phenylpropanolamine or ephedrine increase striated muscle tone and are therefore used with stress urinary incontinence. α-Adrenergic antagonists, such as drugs for treatment of hypertension, can worsen incontinence. Caffeine, alcohol, and diuretics can increase urinary frequency, urgency, and stress urinary incontinence.[8,10,26,55] Antipsychotic agents are also α-adrenergic antagonists and reduce urethral pressure and can be used for treatment of urinary retention.[10] The problem with pharmaceutical treatment is the side effects, some which may affect the pelvic floor adversely (e.g., constipation). Other clients describe severe dryness in the mouth and to the need to drink or suck on a candy constantly. Many other side effects have been described by the people taking these drugs, including dizziness, blurred vision, somnolence, confusion, hypertension or hypotension, as well as dryness of the mucosal membranes of the mouth, vagina, and eyes.[23]

New drugs have entered the market promising fewer side effects and help for patients with OAB syndrome and frequencies. Duloxetine supposedly works at the level of the spinal cord, inhibiting serotonin and regulating noradrenaline and thereby increasing the time between voids.

Solifenacin succinate is an antimuscarinic agent blocking muscarine receptors on bladder smooth muscles, relaxing them. It is therefore indicated for relief of urinary frequency, urgency, and UI associated with OAB syndrome.

Anticholinergic compounds known as muscarinic receptor antagonists work on the overactive bladder by relaxing the smooth muscle tissue in the bladder.

For clients with MS anticholinergic medication is recommended for the treatment of neurogenic overactivity of the bladder. Intravesical treatments with vanilloids and botulinum toxin have been proposed as well and sublingual cannabinoids. Das Gupta and Fowler[56] also state that sildenafil citrate has been shown to be efficacious as a proerectile agent. Sildenafil (Viagra) has been shown to be efficacious in men with SCI; it also may improve arousal in women with SCI and is being evaluated for female patients with sexual arousal disorder.[57,58]

Intravesical resiniferatoxin (an analogue of capsaicin with more than 1000 times its potency in desensitizing C-fiber bladder afferent neurons) is a new therapy for detrusor hyperreflexia for SCI, MS, and other neurologically impaired patients.[59]

The motivation to achieve a functioning pelvic floor without full dependence on drugs is high. Physical therapy may be the main contributor to reaching that goal. The combination of drug therapy and physical therapy can be helpful, and the therapist should know which medications the client is taking as well as its side effects.

EVALUATION AND INTERVENTION
Medical Evaluation

Before a referral to physical therapy, a physician, preferably a urologist or gynecologist, should evaluate a patient with any urinary dysfunction. The patient's history will lead the physician to select appropriate diagnostic tests, including a urodynamic test, which helps explore the extent of the lesion, rule out causes that require other treatments, and determine if physical therapy may help.[10,26,29] Adams and Frahm[55] provide an excellent overview of the causes and the examination and intervention possibilities. Part of the evaluation process should be a bladder diary or voiding log completed over a several-day period so that a clear picture emerges about fluid input and output as well as when frequency and incontinence episodes occur and to what extent. If the physician has not done this it should be included in the physical therapy evaluation. Physicians should also include a muscle strength test of the levator ani when seeing a client with symptoms of UI to determine how much the muscle weakness contributes to the problem.[29,43,55] Therapists trained in women's health frequently assess the muscles of their clients by digital internal palpation. This may not necessarily take place on the first visit, and the patient must consent to such an evaluation. Because of the danger of retraumatization, internal examination and use of instruments in the vagina (such as biofeedback probes) should not be applied to clients who have been abused.[60,61] Therapists should be reminded that such patients may say yes when they mean no because of their past experiences. These therapists can perform external palpations with the consent of the client and use other tests for evaluation of the extent of leakage and weakness with stress incontinence such as the pad test, which can be performed by physicians or therapists.[26,29,55,62]

Conceptual Framework for Treatment

Therapy begins with an examination and evaluation, which are necessary to determine which structures and systems are involved and what kind of impairment or disability can be identified.[6,63,64] The information gathered leads to the prognosis and selection of the intervention and, hopefully, the most efficacious treatment.

Therapists working with female clients with incontinence have to ask about childbirth and related trauma or surgery, prolapses, and surgery such as hysterectomy or sling suspension. Different questions need to be asked when a male patient is evaluated because the reason for his pelvic floor dysfunction will likely be quite different.

Evaluation of Female Clients with Incontinence

An example of an evaluation process that might be used for female clients with incontinence is shown in Figure 33-4.

Question 1: This information gives the therapist a general idea of why the client was sent and how long the problem has existed.

Question 2: The therapist learns from this information whether damage to the muscles or nerves supplying the pelvic floor may be present as well as whether the surgery coincided with worsening, improvement, or the onset of symptoms. Because surgery produces scars, the possibility of scars being part of the problem should be considered.

Thought Process

If the heaviest child weighed 9 pounds at birth, pudendal nerve damage could be contributing to the pelvic floor problem. The question of diabetes is important in the medical history because diabetic mothers are known to sometimes have big babies. The scars must be evaluated, especially if the client reports pain or constipation. With a hysterectomy, the bladder is not "stabilized" by the vagina, which normally leans against the bladder.

Question 3: Scars, especially in the pelvic and abdominal region, can cause pain, which can radiate to the hips or pelvic region. They can also contribute to constipation.

Thought Process

Any surgery can cause scar tissue or muscle weakness in the area surrounding the pelvic floor. Observation and palpation of the abdominal cavity may be necessary. If the surgery was recent, vigorous exercises should be avoided, and a review of body mechanics and lifting may be indicated.

Question 4: Diabetes and heart conditions can lead to increased fluid input and output. Diabetes also often causes a decreased sensory awareness of the bladder. Cancer can cause bony involvement, swelling, pain, and so on. Back pain can be caused by injuries to the back or injuries to the pelvic area, including the viscera. Pulmonary conditions may cause frequent coughing.

Thought Process

Urine output can be increased in a patient with diabetes. A patient with frequent bladder infections may not drink enough water. The type of drink may stimulate the bladder, and the influence of medications on the medical condition may affect the muscle tone of the pelvic floor. Exercises need to be altered in clients with back pain or metastasis. Emphasis on tightening the pelvic floor before coughing needs to be addressed first in clients with pulmonary conditions.

Question 5: Remember that antihypertensive drugs, diuretics, antidepressants, and cough medicines can affect continence.

Thought Process

Is the client aware of what drugs may affect the incontinence problem?

Question 6: Information from this section gives information about the extent of the problem of the pelvic floor dysfunction and what other areas may need to be addressed.

Thought Process

Which impairment needs to be addressed first, and does the medical diagnosis match the symptoms? Are any physical or emotional reasons causing sexual dysfunction and pain?

Question 7: The pattern must be seen in light of the history and daily fluid intake. The information of the voiding diary should match the urinary pattern. Normal urination is six times per day at a volume of at least 250 ml (9 oz), with a maximum of 500 ml. Many adults normally get up once a night to urinate; elderly people may need to get up twice each night.[26]

Question 8: Women normally drink and void between 1500 and 2500 ml/day (50 to 80 oz). Except for water, all mentioned drinks are bladder irritants and can cause urgency or frequency.

Thought Process

A client who drinks below-average amounts of fluid may create frequency because the bladder is no longer used to

EVALUATION FORM

1. Medical Diagnosis:

Onset:

2. Childbirth information:
How many gestations?   births?
weight of heaviest child?
Cesarean, Y/N episiotomy
Vaginal/abdominal surgeries:
bladder suspension   hysterectomy
other?

3. General Surgical History:
Abdominal surgeries (please circle): hernia,
appendix, gallbladder, kidney, laparoscopy,
hemorrhoids, other?

4. Medical History:
Diabetes: Y/N heart problems Y/N
hypertension Y/N cancer Y/N
kidney/bladder infections Y/N
back pain Y/N neck pain Y/N asthma Y/N
bronchitis Y/N
other (e.g., neurological conditions)

5. Medications:

6. Current Symptoms:
Do you have (please circle if yes) any leakage:
with coughing, sneezing, straining?
While running and going up- or downstairs?
When resting? Are any other activities
causing leakage?
Do you have: hesitancy, urgencies, do you push
or strain?
(Please circle when applicable)
Does your problem cause you to have
sexual dysfunction?
Do you have any pain? If yes, please describe:

7. Urination pattern:
How often do you have to urinate?
day   night
How often do you leak?
daily   times a week   infrequent
Do you use one of the following during
the day (d) or night (n)?
(Please circle and indicate how many):
liners d n   pads d n
adult protection d n

8. Daily Fluid Intake (cups, glasses):
How much do you drink?
* water   coffee   tea   soda*
* alcohol   citrus*
* other:*

9. Bowel habits:
Regular Y/N incontinent of bowel Y/N
gas Y/N constipation Y/N Do you use
stool softenersY/N fiber rich-dietY/N

10. History of treatment:
Have you ever been treated for this condition
before? Y/N   Did you do Kegel exercises? Y/N
Other treatments? Y/N
Please describe:

11. Psychosocial history:
Current/previous employment: does it
involve lifting?
Hobbies, sports:

12. Treatment goal of client:

13. Objective:
(Evaluate posture, ability to do diaphragmatic breathing, pelvic tilt, ability to "feel" the activity of pelvic
floor muscles; evaluate muscle tone and strength of the pelvic floor muscles and of the surrounding
muscle if indicated; evaluate scar tissue when applicable; check for contraindications.)

14. Evaluation/Goal:

15. Intervention:

FIGURE 33-4 ■ Evaluation form.

store normal volumes. A person who drinks sodas or alcohol before going to bed needs to evaluate if a change of drinking habits affects the incontinence or urgency.

Question 9: Many reasons exist for constipation; it can be related to difficulty going to the bathroom at work, being always in a hurry, or not relaxing the pelvic floor because of improper leg support when sitting on the toilet.[65] Hyperactive pelvic floor syndrome (HPFS), eating hastily, and consuming constipating foods can contribute as well. Gastrointestinal problems, especially when combined with chronic pelvic pain or low back pain, can be the result of sexual abuse.[66]

Thought Process
Eating habits may have to be reviewed as well as behavior during defecation. Straining during defecation as a result of constipation weakens the pelvic floor muscles and does not help clients who have prolapse. The abdomen needs to be evaluated and possibly treated (e.g., teach client colon massage). Should sexual abuse be suspected for any reason?

Does the client appear to have low self-esteem? Are signs of fear or nervousness present during the evaluation, or a cluster of symptoms that could indicate sexual abuse?

Question 10: The therapist must find out if the patient has been treated for this condition before and whether the treatment was successful.

Thought Process

To motivate a patient, do not begin a treatment with exercises or modalities that have been used unsuccessfully in the past. The selection and explanation of the treatment intended are critical to success.

Question 11: Information about employment gives the therapist input about how work may contribute to the problem. How much does posture affect the pelvic floor dysfunction? How can exercises be integrated with activities at work? Hobbies and sports can be important motivational factors, but how the exercises or hobbies are done must be reviewed.

Thought Process

If poor postural alignment is part of the problem, stretching and strengthening exercises may have to be practiced to achieve a neutral posture. A client who can train the pelvic floor while doing his or her favorite exercises will be highly motivated. If the exercises can be incorporated while lifting at work, for example, the training effect will be greater.

Question 12: Client and therapist goals should ideally match.

Thought Process

If a great discrepancy is present, more explanations or other questions may be required in the objective evaluation. Try to set a goal with the client that is achievable within a reasonable time frame. Then set new goals. Initially, the goals can be having fewer episodes of wetness, sleeping through the night, having to wear a reduced number of pads, or urinating less frequently.

Question 13: Summarize the findings and consider the general cognitive status of the client and her or his mood. The therapist's goal should reflect the prognosis and the extent of the impairment or disability.

Thought Process

A client who is cognitively impaired may require a different treatment approach. Individuals with good body awareness usually learn exercises and correct breathing patterns much faster and may require fewer treatments before seeing changes.

Question 14: Many treatment possibilities are available to choose from. Often various concepts lead to the same goal. The selection also depends greatly on the therapist's experience and preference for a certain type of treatment.

CASE STUDIES

Case Studies 33-1 and 33-2 give insight into how Physical Therapy can help clients with incontinence. Before presenting another case study, the conventional treatment approach to incontinence is discussed briefly and then the Heller and Tanzberger concepts[67-73] are described in more detail.

Conventional Treatment Options for SUI, UUI, and Mixed Incontinence

Most therapists treating patients with incontinence are familiar with biofeedback, electrical stimulation, and vaginal cones, which are often used in combination with Kegel exercises. Kegel exercises have provided only limited success. Henalla et al[78] found that 65% to 69% of patients in two hospitals became dry or significantly improved with exercises only. Wall and Davidson[44] stated that exercise programs have a place in the treatment of genuine stress UI. Miller et al[45] demonstrated how tightening the pelvic floor muscles before a cough significantly diminished leakage from the bladder. Bø et al[79,80] found that intensive exercises taught by physical therapists over a long period provided better results, which was in agreement with a Danish study by Tilbæks.[81] Meaglia et al[82] stated that the motivation, close supervision, and encouragement are important for successful treatment. Holley et al[83] found that a great number of patients stopped exercising because of lack of motivation. Bump et al[42] found that brief verbal instructions in Kegel pelvic floor muscle exercises were not sufficient. Byl et al[84] investigated the effect of repetitive movements (three to 400 trials per day) in skeletal muscle in primates compared with variable repetitive movements and found that the repetitive movements caused interference with motor control. Repetitive movements are also a problem in patients with focal dystonia. Stereotypical and nearly simultaneous movement causes problems in the brain.[85,86] Variable trials preserved motor control. The question must be asked: Is performing Kegel exercises 300 times a day beneficial? The question is appropriate because these exercises train the muscle in isolation and not as part of a functional activity. Do individuals believe that Kegel exercises do not help and therefore discontinue them? Similarly, a therapist would not ask a client to perform isometric exercises of a skeletal muscle 300 times a day and continue 80 times a day for the rest of the client's life once improvement became noticeable. Thus this action does not seem any more appropriate if done with the pelvic floor muscles.

In a recent study by Salamey and Nof,[87] approximately 72% of the questioned therapists stated that they felt prepared to instruct patients in pelvic floor (Kegel) exercises. Only 18% of therapists were prepared to discuss UI with their patients, and the majority were not prepared to perform electrical stimulation, biofeedback, or other conservative treatments. Kegel exercises are what the majority of therapists learn in the United States as treatment for incontinence. Biofeedback and electrical stimulation, as well as vaginal cones, are recognized treatments for incontinence. They are used either in combination with exercises or alone.[80,88-90] The effect of electrical stimulation alone on stress and urge incontinence has been conflicting.[80,91] Bø[91] recommended its use only when a person is not able to contract the pelvic floor muscles and proposed continuing with the exercises when the individual is able to contract the pelvic floor muscles. Another study by Bø et al[80] found pelvic floor exercises superior to electrical stimulation, vaginal cones, and no treatment. The Tanzberger and Heller concepts, the most common form of exercises for continence taught in Germany,[67-73] have been introduced and taught in a modified version in the United States by Carrière[74,75]

CASE STUDY 33-1 ■ FEMALE CLIENT WITH INCONTINENCE

A 56-year-old woman was sent to therapy for biofeedback training and proper instruction in Kegel exercises. This alert librarian had a long history of mixed incontinence. Its onset was approximately 19 years ago but improved for 3 to 4 years after a hysterectomy and bladder suspension surgery in 1989. The client had two vaginal deliveries and one episiotomy, and her heaviest child was 8.5 pounds. The client had urges more than once an hour and used one or two pads a day; wetting occurred one to three times a week. The client drank one cup of coffee in the morning and approximately two sodas per day. Her diet was regular but she had constipation and took stool softeners.

The client liked to do brisk walking but had problems pursuing this activity because of the leakage. The client had received instructions for Kegel exercises elsewhere but they did not help her. She had a history of chronic back and sciatic pain. The objective evaluation revealed good sitting and standing posture. Because the client exhibited a sensory awareness of the pelvic floor muscles, a strength test at that time was deferred. Her general strength appeared to be good and the muscle tone of the abdomen was within functional limits.

IMPAIRMENT

The client had a poor awareness of a pelvic tilt motion and was a chest breather. There was incoordination of breathing with activity of the abdominal and back muscles and the pelvic floor muscles.

FUNCTIONAL LIMITATION

The client was unable to exercise without leakage and was required to wear one or two pads during the day. The assessment revealed a client who appeared motivated to achieve goals.

GOALS

Ability to cough and sneeze without leakage, not to have to wear pads during the day, and to resume walking. Ability to perform home exercises independently.

INTERVENTION

She received a total of 10 treatments within 3 months based on the Heller and Tanzberger concepts.[67-73] Breathing exercises, coordination of diaphragmatic breathing with pelvic floor contraction, instruction in Swiss ball exercises for strengthening the pelvic floor muscles in all planes and during bouncing.[72,74,75] Colon massage,[76] and treatment of scar tissue,[77] biofeedback or electrical stimulation were considered if no improvement with previous exercises would occur after three to five treatments.

The client returned 6 days after the initial visit and reported decreased leakage with laughing. She received a colon massage and gentle scar tissue massage as well as more challenging exercises with the Swiss ball and elastic bands. Instruction of proper lifting with contraction of the pelvic floor was part of the treatment. A return visit was scheduled 3 weeks later for an additional treatment for the abdomen and exercises. The client reported feeling better, with improvement of the back pain, which she had had for 2 years. The abdomen had felt much looser after the treatment and leakage with coughing and sneezing was further reduced. The plan was to review the exercises in 4 to 6 weeks. The client called 3 months later to report that she did not need further treatments. She was able to hold urine for 2 to 3 hours without wearing pads. She had no more wetting episodes and for safety she only wore pads when doing brisk walking for 45 minutes. Only occasionally did the client need to get up at night to urinate.

CASE STUDY 33-2 ■ MALE CLIENT WITH INCONTINENCE

Adjustments are required when taking the history when evaluating a man with pelvic floor problems (Figure 33-5). The client's answers are written in script typeface. Summary of treatment:

By the first return visit 4 weeks after the initial evaluation, the client was able to hold urine for longer periods and only needed to get up once during the night. The client also reported being able to attend water aerobics classes without loss of urine. He was exercising for approximately 20 to 30 minutes each day. The exercises, based on the Heller[69,70] and Tanzberger

concepts,[67,68,71-75] were reviewed with the client and new exercises were added. The client purchased a Swiss ball, and a return visit was scheduled approximately 3 weeks later. Before the next scheduled visit the client called, reported that he was doing fine, no longer had leakage, and did not need to wear pads at night. He resumed all other activities without problems. He was able to exercise at home independently and did not require further treatment. His next attempt was to maintain his condition without the bladder medication tolterodine (Detrol).

Evaluation of Male Clients with Incontinence including Treatment Example

Name: **DOB:** *1926, 72 years old*

Tel #

MD: **Therapist:**

Diagnosis: *Status post prostate surgery 10 years ago*

Onset: *1989*

Surgical history: Abdominal surgeries (please circle): hernia, appendix, gallbladder, kidneys, laparoscopy, prostate, hemorrhoids, other? *Hernia, appendix, radical prostatectomy 10 years ago; hip and knee surgery 3 years ago*

Medical history: DM: Y/Ⓝ heart problems Y/Ⓝ CA Y/Ⓝ pulmonary disease Y/Ⓝ bladder or kidney infections Y/Ⓝ history of bed-wetting? Y/Ⓝ other:

Medication: *Detrol for the urgency, Prilosec for heartburn, medication for depression; sleep medication causes urinary accident*

Current symptoms and examination process:

Do you have difficulty urinating because of strictures (scar tissues in urinary tract, enlargement of prostate)? Y/N If yes, does your doctor know? Was any procedure done? *Strictures from the surgery were treated several times*

Do you have (please circle if yes) any leakage; with coughing, sneezing, straining? while running and going up or downstairs? *With straining and lifting the legs* when resting? Are any other activities causing leakage? *No*

Do you have: hesitancy, dribbling, urgencies? do you push or strain? (Please circle if applicable) *urgencies*

Do you have erectile dysfunction? *No*

How often do you have to urinate during the day? *Within normal limits* **night?** *Two times*

Do you have any pain? (If yes, please describe):

Daily fluid intake: (cups, glasses) **How much do you drink?** *6-8 glasses*

Water *at night* coffee tea *herb* soda alcohol *1 martini* citrus other:

Do you urinate: sitting down? *At night* Or standing? (please circle)

Do you use one of the following during the day or night? (Please circle and indicate how many):

Liners: d n **pads:** d n **adult protection:** d Ⓝ *at night only*

Bowel habits: Regular: Ⓨ N incontinent of bowel Y/Ⓝ gas Y/Ⓝ constipation Y/Ⓝ Do you use stool softeners? Y/Ⓝ fiber-rich diet Ⓨ N

History of treatment:

Have you ever been treated for this condition before? Y/N **Did you do Kegel exercises?** *Yes, the exercises did not help.*

Other treatment? Y/Ⓝ describe:

Psychosocial history:

Current/previous employment: does it involve lifting? *Teaching night classes*

Hobbies, sports: *Water aerobics*

FIGURE 33-5 ■ Evaluation of male clients with incontinence, including treatment example.

Continued

Heller and Tanzberger Exercise Concepts

Heller and Tanzberger[67-73] developed exercises derived from Klein-Vogelbach[92-94] that use the Swiss ball for treatment of incontinence.[92] The goal of the exercises is to integrate the function of the entire abdominal compartment as a procedural program. Correct use of the pelvic floor muscles requires restoration of diaphragmatic breathing, as does coordination with all muscles of the abdominal compart-

ment.[74] The following elements are part of the Heller and Tanzberger concepts.

Client Education

A client needs to know where the pelvic floor muscles are, what their function is, and how they work with other systems of the body. The therapist should provide a clear picture of

EVALUATION PROCESS

What is your treatment goal? *To be able to lift legs and do water aerobics without leaking, not to have to wear "Healthdry" at night.*

Objective: (evaluate posture, ability to do diaphragmatic breathing, pelvic tilt, ability to "feel" the activity of pelvic floor muscles; evaluate muscle tone and strength of the pelvic floor or surrounding muscles when applicable; evaluate scar-tissue when applicable)

Patient with a good posture and good mobility of the pelvis. Because the patient became aware of his pelvic floor during the evaluation, muscle testing of the pelvic floor was deferred. The patient was also a chest-breather and was instructed in diaphragmatic breathing.

Impairment: *poor awareness of the pelvic floor muscles, dyscoordination of diaphragmatic breathing with the pelvic floor while lifting legs, coughing, etc.*

Functional Limitation: *unable to lift legs or do water aerobics without leakage of urine. Leakage at night, urgencies at night*

Assessment: *very motivated client who stated during the evaluation that he now understood the function of the pelvic floor.*

Intervention: *teaching of diaphragmatic breathing and coordination of breathing with the muscles of the entire abdominal compartment.*

Goal: *having to get up at night no more than once. No Healthdry at night; ability to lift legs, do water aerobics without leakage of urine.*

Plan: *teaching correct breathing and functional exercises based on the Tanzberger concept[71] to restore pelvic floor function in 6-8 treatments over 3 months or until patient feels independent with the home exercise program.*

SIGNATURE: _____ **Date:** _____

FIGURE 33-5, cont'd

these muscles so that the client can visualize them and understand their function.

Restoration of Proper Diaphragmatic Breathing

Every breath changes abdominal pressure. Forced exhalation increases the pressure; so does coughing and sneezing. Leaning forward or backward also changes abdominal pressure. Clients should learn to coordinate the contraction of the pelvic floor with changes of pressure. In addition, these activities cannot be done without the cooperation of the abdominal and back muscles. Exercises designed to restore pelvic floor function must therefore include coordination of all muscles involved. A great number of individuals with incontinence are chest breathers, possibly because of the poor habit of constantly pulling the stomach in to appear more slender. Restoration of diaphragmatic breathing is therefore the first priority for clients with incontinence.[74,75]

Better breathing patterns may also help provide more oxygen to the pelvic region. Knowing how to control breathing may help a client relax when nervous or anxious (Figure 33-6).

Sensory Awareness of the Pelvic Floor

The pelvic floor muscles are in the shape of a hammock. Their resting tone is high, and relaxing the pelvic floor is required during urination and defecation as well as during delivery and sexual activity.[43,46] Thus sensory awareness is an important aspect of retraining the pelvic floor muscles. For all individuals, activities such as coughing, sneezing, lifting, and sexual activity require contraction and relaxation of pelvic floor muscles. The ability to relax and contract these muscles is a problem for clients with incontinence. For individuals to regain this control and sensitivity within the pelvic floor, certain treatment protocols must be established.

First, a client can feel landmarks such as the coccyx, the pubic bones, and ischium. Sitting on a firm surface, the client can first contract the gluteal muscles, then relax them, then try to feel the contraction of the anal sphincter and the muscles around the vagina by imagining holding a small object with those muscles without activation of the gluteal muscles.

In the side-lying position, the client can place a hand over the gluteal muscles while touching the anal sphincter with a fingertip (Figure 33-7). The client can now try to pucker the anal sphincter, similar to puckering the mouth. The contraction can be faint but is correct if the gluteal muscles remain relaxed. Tightening of the levator ani can be palpated at the perineum, between anus and vagina, or at the side of the tip of the coccyx. It can also be palpated deep in the groin and often can be distinguished from a contraction of the

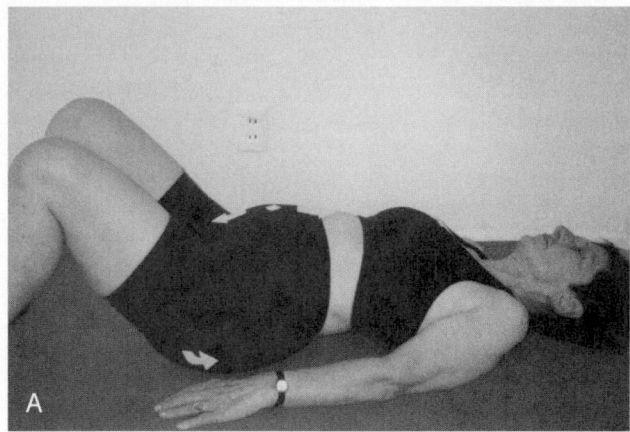

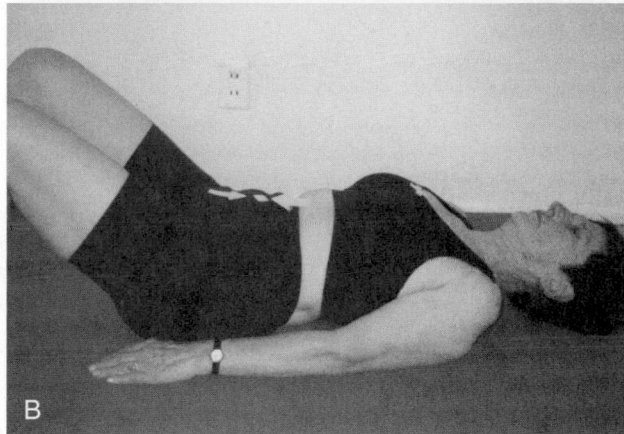

FIGURE 33-6 ■ Diaphragmatic breathing. **A,** Inhalation; **B,** exhalation.

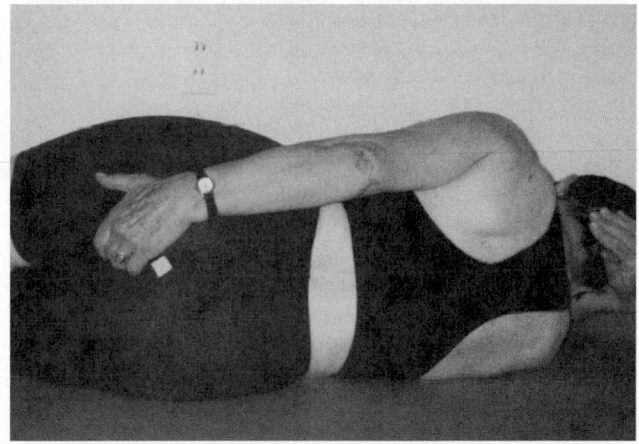

FIGURE 33-7 ■ Feeling the pelvic floor.

transverse abdominis. Clients learn that contraction of these muscles must precede any contraction of the surrounding pelvic floor muscles, such as the gluteal, adductor, and abdominal and back muscles. In the same position the client can also feel how a cough moves the pelvic floor muscles in a caudal direction. During proper breathing a gentle, rhythmical downward movement occurs during inhalation (eccentric for the pelvic floor and concentric for the pulmonary diaphragm). The client then tries to tighten the

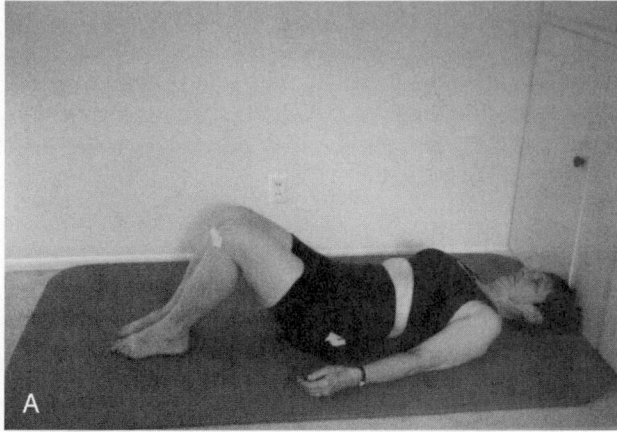

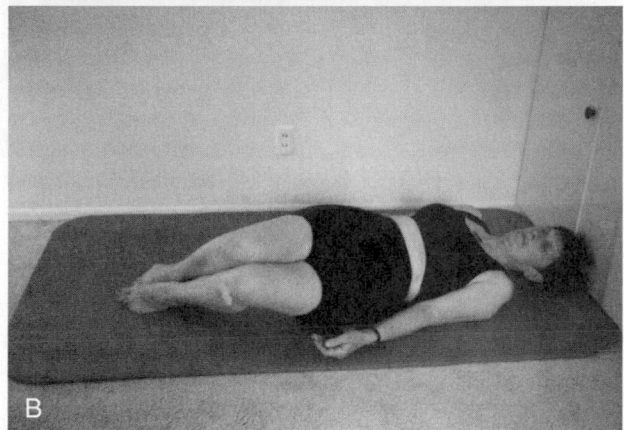

FIGURE 33-8 ■ Turning from lying on the back (**A**) to turning to the side while tightening the pelvic floor to the side (**B**).

pelvic floor muscles before coughing and feels less caudal movement of the pelvic floor muscles.[74,75] Sensory awareness of relaxation of the pelvic floor muscles may require education, visualization, and tactile feedback. It may be very difficult to learn to relax muscles that have been tight for a long time.

Coordination of Breathing with Pelvic Floor Muscle Activity

The client learns to contract the pelvic floor muscles while exhaling (eccentric for the pulmonary diaphragm, concentric activity for the pelvic floor muscles) and relax those muscles while inhaling. This can be done in different positions, such as supine, side lying, on all fours, sitting, or standing. When coughing, sneezing, lifting, and changing positions, such as from supine to side lying, the pelvic floor contraction must precede the activity (Figure 33-8). By contracting the pelvic floor before saying an explosive word such as a forceful "kick," then relaxing the pelvic floor by slowly saying "aaaaand," before tightening once more before saying "kick" again, the sequence of contraction and relaxation is learned.[74,75]

Strengthening Exercises

Strengthening exercises of the pelvic floor muscles must include fast twitch muscle fiber training with quick fast twitch muscle contraction, which can be done by bouncing on the ball as demonstrated in Figure 33-9.

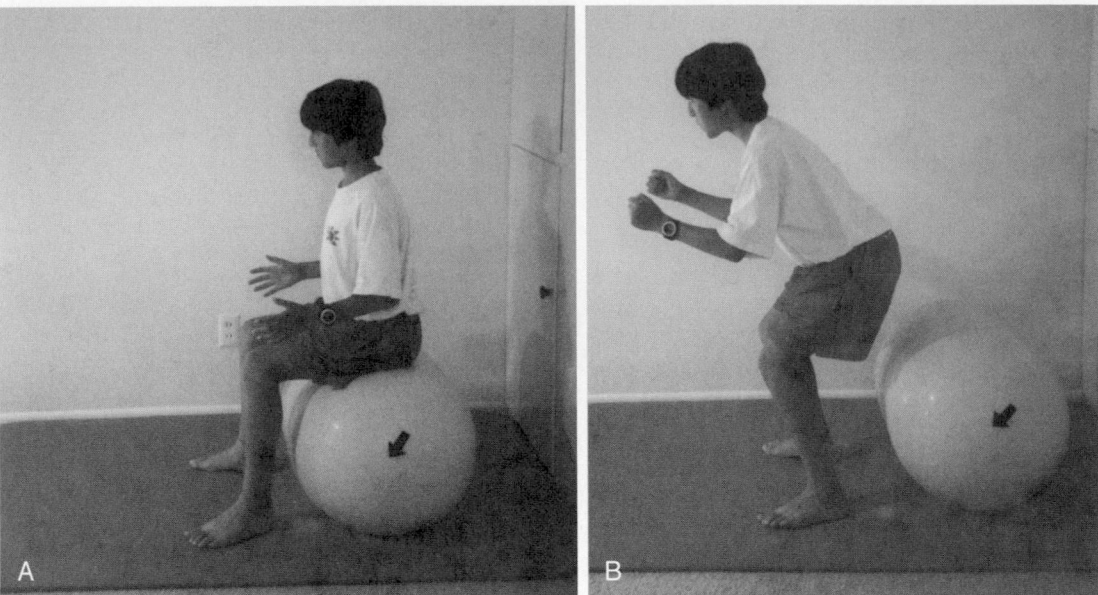

FIGURE 33-9 ■ **A,** Training fast fibers by bouncing on a double ball. **B,** Tightening the pelvic floor while lifting up.

Slow twitch muscle fiber training requires holding the contraction at the end for 5 to 10 seconds. This is demonstrated in Figure 33-10, where the client tightens the pelvic floor, gives herself resistance in a diagonal direction, and holds the contraction of the pelvic floor muscles for 5 to 10 seconds. The right ischial tuberosity initiates the movement toward the left knee, which should not move in space, as indicated by the *X*. The chest also is a "fixed" point marked by an *X*. All movement comes from the pelvis.

Because the pelvic floor muscle fibers run in a sagittal and frontal plane as well as in a diagonal direction, movements in different directions should be included to maximize the benefit of strengthening exercises. The Swiss ball allows movement in all directions as a functional activity. When two persons sit back to back on a ball (Figure 33-11), one person can pull the ischium in the direction of the knees, which do not move, while the other person tries to slow down the movement. This requires eccentric activity of the pelvic floor muscles. Isometric muscle activity occurs when both pull at the same time with the same force. In Figure 33-12, two 12-year-old children tighten their pelvic floor muscles during exhalation while pulling the ball with the feet. Many exercises with or without the ball can be adapted with the Heller and Tanzberger concepts.[67,70,72,74,75] Muscle strengthening is not done in isolation but is trained during functional movement activities such as lifting a grocery bag or hitting a tennis ball.

Teaching relaxation of the pelvic floor muscles is as important as strengthening exercises, especially in all clients with HPFS.

Programming of Functional Activities

Pelvic floor muscle activities must be tied to a function, such as getting up from a chair and tightening the pelvic floor muscles during exhalation (Figure 33-13). The exercises must be repeated many times in different combinations until they become automatic. The process of acquiring these skills

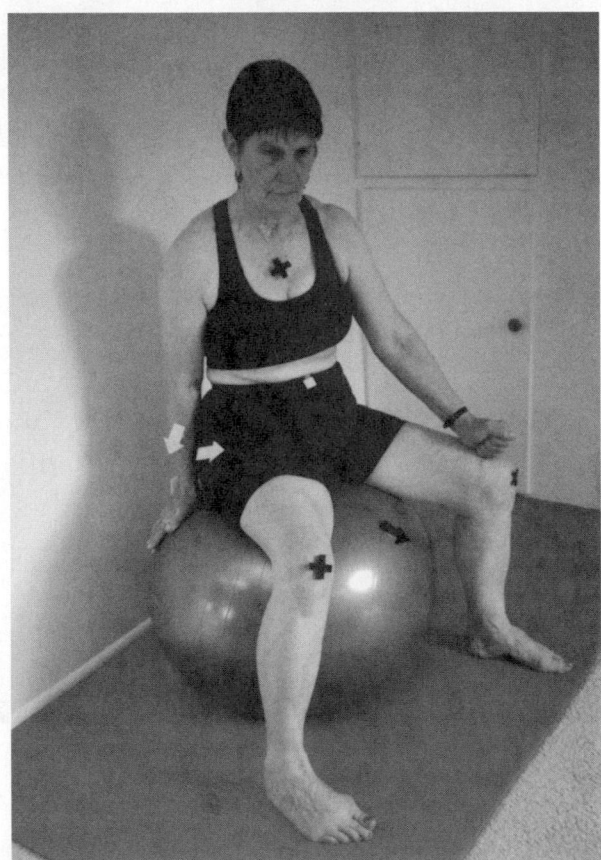

FIGURE 33-10 ■ Training of the slow muscle fibers by holding the contraction for 5 to 10 seconds at the end of the movement.

is part of procedural learning.[5,6,95-99] The client must be empowered to make changes in lifestyle activity and be motivated to achieve the changes. Only then will the client be willing to exercise for months until the task becomes automatic.[6,7,95-99] To improve motor control of a task, the exercises selected must be meaningful and varied as well as challenging. Mental practice, visualization, part-to-whole task practice, prepractice instructions, appropriate feedback, and guidance are all part of motor learning and are incorporated in the Heller and Tanzberger approaches.[95-99]

Precautions

For clients who do not feel safe on a ball, a double ball, a ball base, or a flat ball that fits onto a chair (Figures 33-14

and 33-15) can be used. All are commercially available. Exercises also can be performed between two chairs or in a corner so that the ball cannot roll away. When learning the exercise, a belt can be used at first to hold onto a client. The ball should not be used if a severe cognitive deficit in the client makes the activity unsafe. Any medical condition that endangers a client on a ball makes these exercises contraindicated and requires a change of exercise and equipment.[74,75,100] Many possibilities for functional exercises exist that are based on motor learning and motor control principles as described by Umphred.[86] The client can walk or perform favorite gym exercises by incorporating pelvic floor strengthening and breathing coordination. Functional training can also be achieved by incorporating the pelvic floor activity to certain movements that are done every day, such

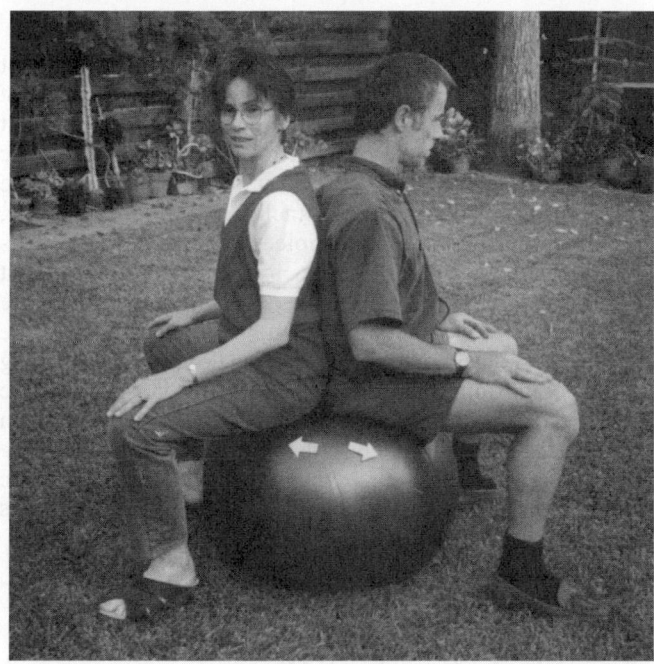

FIGURE 33-11 ■ Two adults sitting back to back on a ball doing eccentric and concentric pelvic floor contractions.

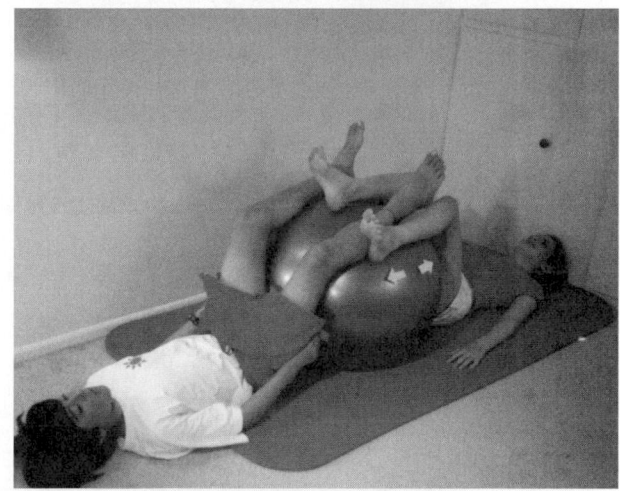

FIGURE 33-12 ■ Two children work on strengthening the pelvic floor during exhalation.

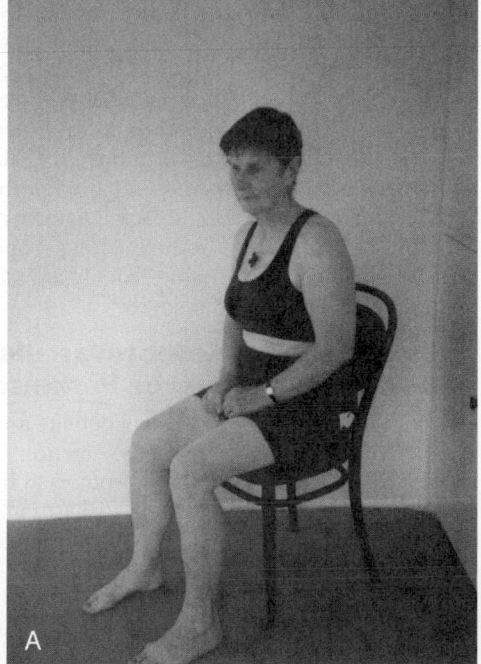
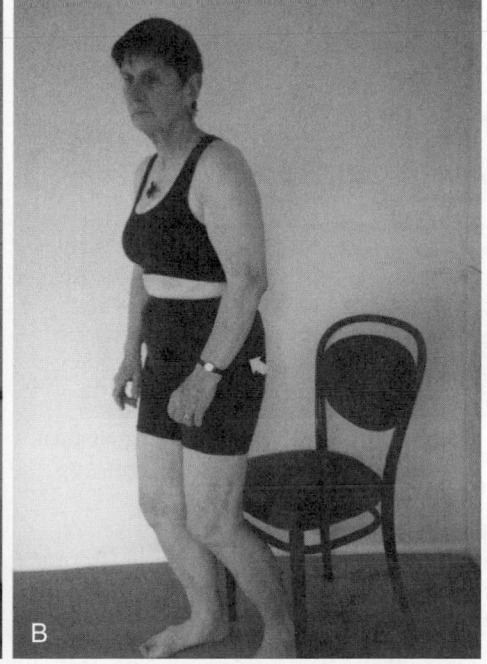

FIGURE 33-13 ■ **A** and **B,** Sit to stand can be done with integration of pelvic floor activity.

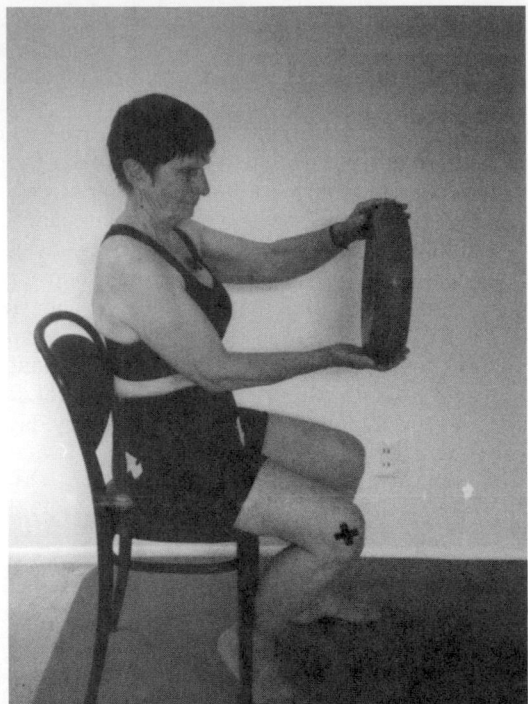

FIGURE 33-14 ■ Flat ball (sit fit).

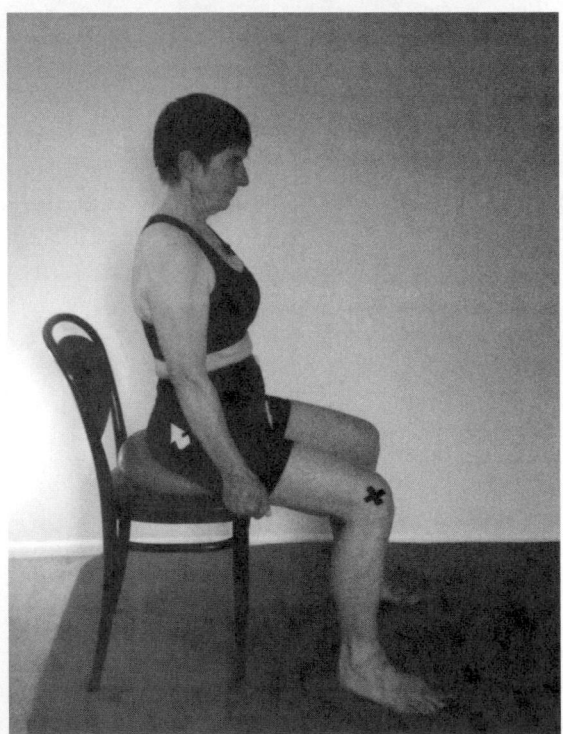

FIGURE 33-15 ■ Exercise for the pelvic floor; sitting on a flat ball.

as before lifting a child or grocery bag, getting up from a chair or out of a car, or turning in bed.

In addition, therapists must be aware of the involvement of other systems, such as the autonomic system or the limbic system. The patient may be nervous or fearful, depressed, and sleep deprived or have pain in addition to the incontinence problem.[86,101] Some clients may have been abused, which may be manifested in multisystem involvement.[66] An environment of trust, understanding, and sensitivity toward the client's problems must be created.

Clinical Application of the Heller and Tanzberger Concepts

After a therapist has defined the aspects of pelvic floor dysfunction that require retraining, a specific exercise program can be custom tailored to the patient.

Case Studies

None of the four clients discussed in this chapter underwent biofeedback or electrical stimulation for treatment, and most of the clients had performed Kegel exercises without success. In clients who are unable to learn to feel their pelvic floor muscles, electrical stimulation or biofeedback may be helpful. Functional activities, including proper breathing, should be performed during biofeedback. Isolated contractions of the pelvic floor muscles by using a device without incorporating functional activities does not seem to restore the many different functions of the pelvic floor. Therefore the use of cones without proper pelvic floor muscle training remains questionable. All the clients mentioned in the case studies were extremely motivated, which is not uncommon in patients who have pelvic dysfunctions. They are more than willing to follow their regimen. Problems arise when the client is cognitively impaired or when an illness affects motivation (Case Studies 33-3 and 33-4).

TREATMENT OPTIONS FOR PELVIC FLOOR DYSFUNCTION

Cognitively Impaired Clients

Adjustments must be made and functional barriers decreased to help cognitively impaired clients maintain or achieve continence (Table 33-1). Prompted voiding, timed voiding,[11,102-104] and medicine can be used when a client has cognitive problems and cannot go to the bathroom independently. In prompted voiding, clients (e.g., with Alzheimer's disease) are asked at regular intervals whether they have to go to the bathroom. In timed voiding, a client is placed on a commode or toilet at regular intervals. Many clients who are cognitively impaired probably would not be incontinent if they could reach a bathroom and if help were available to unbutton or unzip clothes, open a door, or assist in other aspects of toileting. Timely assistance could prevent falls and incontinent episodes.[105]

Clients with a Cerebrovascular Accident, Multiple Sclerosis, or Parkinson's Disease

Clients who have neurological deficits are usually not asked whether they have a urinary dysfunction. Not all clients with such diseases are incontinent; some had incontinence before the onset of the neurological disease. OAB syndrome and urge urinary incontinence are common in cerebrovascular accident,[25] MS, and other neurological diseases, whereas detrusor-sphincter dyssynergia is common in MS and SCI.[21,22] Patients with Parkinson's disease can also have retention. No matter what the cause, improvement can often be achieved by identifying the dysfunction, explaining the

CASE STUDY 33-3 ■ FEMALE CLIENT USING A WHEELCHAIR

A 25-year-old female client who used a wheelchair as a result of myelomeningocele, was referred to therapy for upper-extremity strengthening exercises. The diagnosis was left biceps tendonitis, left wrist strain, and lumbar discogenic pain. During treatment the young woman was questioned about her bladder and bowel condition.

The patient had a history of bladder surgery as a child; placement of a suprapubic catheter and bowel reconstruction surgery was done at age 15. She reported that 50% of the time she leaked loose stool and she frequently did not make it to the bathroom in time. She was wearing up to two pads per day.

The client was shown a model of the pelvic floor muscle to illustrate visually how to contract her pelvic floor muscles. Although her sensory awareness of the perineal area appeared to be reduced, she stated that she could feel a faint contraction when trying to pucker the anal sphincter. The client was a chest breather and was instructed in abdominal breathing techniques. She then was instructed to try to coordinate the puckering of her anus with exhalation and work on relaxation of the pelvic floor, especially during defecation. She was told to place a stool in front of the toilet so she could rest her short legs when sitting on the toilet.

The highly motivated client returned 3 weeks later and stated, "I am very happy, I do not leak anymore and did not have to use any pads the last few weeks. I also feel my sphincter muscle now." The client had a total of six treatments. Four treatments were devoted to her arm and trunk problems (which resolved) and the last two treatments to the pelvic problem. Treatment then was discontinued because all goals had been met.

CASE STUDY 33-4 ■ CLIENT WITH VAGINAL PROLAPSE, ANAL SPHINCTER WEAKNESS, AND MIXED INCONTINENCE

A 38-year-old woman was referred to therapy because of anal sphincter weakness and incontinence of flatus for 5 to 6 years. She stated that she also had a prolapse. The client reported having stress urinary incontinence when laughing and running and during sexual intercourse, which affected her self-esteem (as she explained during a later visit). She had urgency, which made her run to the bathroom every hour during the day and get up twice each night. The bladder was painful when full. She also had pain in the lower abdomen. The client had constipation and had to strain during defecation. The surgical history was remarkable for difficult labor and delivery, one with forceps and two others with episiotomies. The patient also had gallbladder surgery and hysterectomy over 10 years ago. The possibility of surgery for treatment of the prolapse and reconstruction of the vaginal area was discussed with the client and her physician. She had been instructed to perform Kegel exercises but they did not help. The client worked in an electrical assembly plant. The client's goals were to rid herself of the flatus and avoid surgery.

Objectively, she had decreased muscle tonus in the abdominal area and weakness of the abdominal and gluteal muscles. In addition, the client had incoordination between breathing and pelvic floor function. She developed some awareness of the pelvic muscles during the first evaluation. The impairment and the disabilities were considerable and the prognosis more guarded, but the goal was still to achieve anal continence, prevent surgery, and decrease urgency. The client was motivated.

The client was seen in therapy for 15 visits over a 7-month period, at first weekly, then every 2 weeks, and then for periodic reexaminations 3 to 4 weeks apart. Treatment began with teaching diaphragmatic breathing exercises and sensory awareness of the sphincter muscle. The client was able to distinguish between the activities of the anal sphincter and gluteal muscles and was also able to feel a faint contraction in the vaginal area. At first she had difficulty coordinating breathing with contraction and relaxation of the pelvic floor muscles, even when she practiced at home. At the second visit the client received a colon massage and gentle mobilization of the abdominal scars with connective tissue massage.[36,76,77] Home exercises for breathing and pelvic floor contraction and relaxation were reviewed with the client. At the third visit, the client reported that the flatus problem had improved and that the abdominal treatment lessened the constipation. New exercises were taught with the Swiss ball in supine and sitting positions. At the fourth visit, the client said, "I have less flatus, and I am able to control the sphincter. The pelvic floor is still a problem because of the prolapse; I have no more back pain after the visceral treatments." The client was also instructed regarding how to perform exercises with decreased load on the pelvic floor (supine, supine with the feet on the ball, side-lying, on all fours, etc.). The client was also instructed in how to self-massage the abdomen. At the fifth visit, the client said, "I am now taking medicine to help control the urgency and can hold urine now for 3 hours. My husband massages my abdomen, which decreases the constipation. The bowel movements are now every 1 to 2 days instead of once a week."

The client reported only occasional pain with a full bladder, a reduction in the number of times she had to get up at night, and her ability to hold urine for 3 hours without pressure from the prolapse. The grateful client stated that her self-image had improved because she was no longer leaking urine during intercourse. According to the client's wishes, surgery was deferred. As the strength of the pelvic floor improved, the client stopped taking medication for the urgency and was still able to hold urine for 3 hours and sleep through the night. The client continued occasional follow-up sessions to monitor her progress and provide her with more challenging exercises.

TABLE 33-1 ■ Possible Combinations of Treatment Options for Incontinence

	FUNCTIONAL EXERCISES AND BREATHING	BIOFEEDBACK	ELECTRICAL STIMULATION	CONES	PROMPTED VOIDING	TIMED VOIDING	ABDOMINAL TREATMENT, SCAR TREATMENT	SELF-CATHETERIZATION
Stress incontinence	X	(x)	(x)	(x)			(x)	
Urge incontinence	X	(x)					(x)	
Mixed incontinence	X	(x)	(x)				(x)	
Anal incontinence	X	(x)	(x)				(x)	
Constipation	X	(x)	(x)				X	
Retention of urine	X					X	(x)	(x)
Overdistention of bladder	X	(x)			(x)	X	(x)	(x)
Areflexia of bladder, anus	(x)	(x)	X		(x)	X	(x)	X

X means recommended therapeutic intervention; (x) means additional treatment option. These options may be a beneficial interventions, but evidence is mixed and outcomes may be patient specific.

anatomy and physiology to the client, and then offering treatment options. Coordination of diaphragmatic breathing with pelvic floor muscle activity can improve self-control to relax the pelvic floor and improve oxygen supply to the pelvic region. Improving the posture and sensory awareness training can also be integrated to varying degrees. The therapist can help the client improve afferent sensory input and use visualization to learn to contract and relax the muscles properly. A client with retention can learn to emphasize relaxation of the pelvic floor muscles during urination through breathing, proper seating on the toilet, and self-relaxation. Double voiding technique encourages the patient with an overextended bladder to time voiding to every 2 to 4 hours during the day. The patient then attempts to empty the bladder by staying on the toilet longer and trying to void more than once with each trip to the toilet, with supportive cues and timed voiding when the patients have cognitive impairment.[24,102,104] Often functional barriers can be eliminated or help can be provided. With clients who also need strengthening exercises for the pelvic floor and have difficulty sitting on a ball, a flat ball can be used in a chair, or exercises can be adapted to the client's ability without any devices.

Overdistended Bladder

Whether or not the overdistended bladder is neurogenic, the client must learn to time herself or himself to void at regular intervals. In other cases the client may learn to do clean intermittent catheterization and carefully monitor the output of urine. The residual urine in the bladder should be low, approximately 50 mL; measurements consistently higher require further evaluation by a urologist.[26] Proper relaxation of the pelvic floor is important; men often can relax the pelvic floor better when urinating in a seated position. Abdominal breathing and coordination with pelvic floor muscle activity are important for these clients and should be restored if a problem is present.

Areflexia

Education is always the most important part of intervention and is done at the beginning. Many clients may need to learn clean intermittent catheterization and timed intervals. In some clients electrical stimulation or biofeedback may help restore some function of the pelvic floor activity; exercise may improve the strength of the pelvic floor muscles once some function returns. Obviously, all therapeutic interventions depend on the extent of the lesion, but as described in Case Study 33-3, discussion with the client regarding the exploration of treatment options is important. This client probably could have been spared wearing diapers for the previous 10 years. She also could have been condemned to wearing diapers for the rest of her life without intervention. All that was needed in her case was to ask about the problem and instruct her in achieving continence.

Anal Incontinence

The inability to hold gas or leaking stool can occur in neurogenic and nonneurogenic disorders. Clients who have had resections of the colon may have anal urge incontinence. They must learn to evaluate what they ate, when the urge is appropriate, and when a signal is false. They often cannot distinguish gas, liquid stool, and solid stool. A client, after instruction and explanation of the defecation process, stated, "I got it; it is mind over matter." He was also instructed to use deep abdominal breathing and quick flicks (activation of the fast fibers) and distraction to control the urges. This helped him to stop and to control the need or motor program that could be identified as running to the bathroom every 30 minutes. He was asked to throw that program out consciously and replace it with breathing and reevaluation of each urge, which enabled him in a short time to regain control, sleep through the night, and increase the intervals during the day. As with all clients with pelvic floor dysfunction, careful evaluation and education must be completed before beginning the treatment. In the presence of constipation, a careful abdominal evaluation and possible treatment of the viscera,[106] such as colon massage,[76] may be indicated because constipation can also be present in clients who leak stool. The client needs to be educated about eating properly. Individuals who eat too much fiber need to drink large volumes of fluid to keep the stool soft. A client with a brain stem injury, for example, had bowel movements only every 5 days. When the family changed the breakfast to fruit and only minimal fiber the client had daily regular bowel movements.

Electrical stimulation or biofeedback can, in some cases, be an adjunct or precede treatment of functional exercises of the abdominal compartment. It can be used to re-train when to contract the pelvic floor muscles and also to improve sensory awareness.

SUMMARY

Every client with urinary incontinence, whether male or female, requires a thorough examination. To give the best possible chance for recovery, exercises must be custom tailored and modalities used with discretion. Electrical stimulation and biofeedback cannot replace functional exercises. Modalities may be helpful at the beginning of the treatment if the client has no sensory awareness of the pelvic floor but should be used in combination with exercises. Treatment of the viscera by a knowledgeable therapist should be considered in some clients to achieve full rehabilitation of the pelvic floor dysfunction.[106]

REFERENCES

1. Kegel AH: Progressive resistance exercises in the functional restoration of the perineal muscles, *Am J Obstet Gynecol* 8:238, 1948.
2. Kegel AH, Powell TO: The physiological treatment of urinary stress incontinence, *J Urol* 63:808, 1950.
3. Kegel AH: Physiologic therapy for urinary stress incontinence, *JAMA* 146:915, 1951.
4. Jewell MJ: Overview of the structures and function of the central nervous system. In Umphred DA, editor: *Neurological rehabilitation,* ed 3, St. Louis, 1995, Mosby.
5. Umphred DA: Classification of treatment techniques based on primary input systems. In Umphred DA, editor: *Neurological rehabilitation,* ed 4, St. Louis, 1995, Mosby.
6. Umphred DA: Introduction and overview. In Umphred DA, editor: *Neurological rehabilitation,* ed 4, St. Louis, 1995, Mosby.
7. Umphred DA: Limbic complex. In Umphred DA, editor: *Neurological rehabilitation,* ed 4, St. Louis, 1995, Mosby.
8. Fantl JA, Newman DK, Colling J et al: *Managing acute and chronic urinary incontinence, clinical practice guideline, no. 2, update,* Rockville, MD, 1996, U.S. Department of Health and Human Services.
9. Hu T-W, Wagner TH, Bentkover JD et al: Cost of urinary incontinence and overactive bladder in the United States: a comparative study, *Urology* 63:461, 2004.
10. Retzky SS, Rogers RM: Urinary incontinence in women, *Clin Symp* 47:3, 1995.
11. Britton JP, Dowell AC, Whelan P: Prevalence of urinary symptoms in men aged over 60, *Br J Urol* 66:175, 1990.
12. Nygaard IE, Thompson FL, Svengalis SL et al: Urinary incontinence in elite nulliparous athletes, *Obstet Gynecol* 84:184, 1994.
13. Sherman RA, Davis GD: Behavioral treatment of exercise-induced urinary incontinence among female soldiers, *Mil Med* 162:690, 1997.
14. Baumann M, Tauber R: Inkontinenz beim mann, *Krankengymnastik* 43:1372, 1991.
15. Adedokun AO, Wilson MM: Urinary incontinence: historical, global, and epidemiological perspectives, *Clin Geriatric Med* 20:399, 2004.
16. Diokno AC, Estranol MV, Mallett V: Epidemiology of lower urinary tract dysfunction, *Clin Obstet Gynecol* 47:36, 2004.
17. Dwyer PL, Lee ETC, Hay DM: Obesity and urinary incontinence in women, *Br J Obstet Gynaecol* 951:91, 1988.
18. Bump RC, McClish DK: Cigarette smoking and urinary incontinence in women, *Am J Obstet Gynecol* 167:1213, 1992.
19. Pincock S: BMA says smoking harms reproductive capability, *Lancet* 363:628, 2004.
20. Newman DK: Stress urinary incontinence in women, *AJN* 103:46, 2003.
21. Agency for Healthcare Quality and Research: *Prevention and management of urinary tract infections in paralyzed persons. Summary, evidence report/technology assessment,* Rockville, MD, 1999, Agency for Health Care Policy and Research.
22. Knoll M, Madersbacher H: The chances of a spina bifida patient becoming continent/socially dry by conservative therapy, *Paraplegia* 31:22, 1993.
23. Hunter KF, Moore KN: Diabetes-associated bladder dysfunction in the older adult, *Geriatr Nurs* 24:134, 2003.
24. Schultz-Lampel D: Bladder disorders in dementia and Alzheimer's disease. Rational diagnostic and therapeutic options, *Urologe A* 42:1579, 2003.
25. Brittain KR, Peet SM, Potter JK et al: Prevalence and management of urinary incontinence in stroke survivors. *Age Ageing* 8:509, 1999.
26. Walters MD, Karram MM: *Clinical Urogynecology,* St. Louis, 1993, Mosby.
27. Wagner TH, Hu TW: Economic costs of urinary incontinence in 1995, *Urology* 51:355, 1998.
28. Cannon TW, Damaser M: Pathophysiology of the lower urinary tract: continence and incontinence, *Clin Obstet Gynecol* 47:28, 2004.
29. Wall LL, Norton PA, DeLancey JOL: *Practical urogynecology,* Baltimore, 1993, Williams & Wilkins.
30. Barry MJ, Fowler FJ, O'Leary MP et al: The American Urological Association symptom index for benign prostatic hyperplasia, *J Urol* 148:1549, 1992.
30a. Ramakers MJ, van Lunsen RHW: Psychosocial influences. In Carrière B, Feldt CM, editors: *The pelvic floor,* Stuttgart, 2006 Thieme Verlag.
31. Cardenas DD, Mayo ME, King JC: Urinary tract and bowel management in the rehabilitation setting. In Braddon RL, editor: *Physical medicine rehabilitation,* Philadelphia, 1996, WB Saunders, pp. 555-572.
32. Benevento BT, Sipski ML: Neurogenic bladder neurogenic bowel, and sexual dysfunction in people with spinal cord injury, *Phys Ther* 82:601, 2002.
33. Mostwin JL: Urinary incontinence [editorial], *J Urol* 153:352, 1995.
34. Wesselmann U, Burnett AL, Heinberg LJ: The urogenital and rectal pain syndromes, *Pain* 73:269, 1997.
35. Enderlein K: Bindegewebsmassage—Behandlungshinweise und-voraussetzung, *Physikalische Ther* 3:71, 1985.
36. Schuh I: *Bindegewebsmassage,* Stuttgart, 1996, Gustav Fischer Verlag, pp. 62-253.
37. Tanzberger R: Der weibliche Beckenboden—Krankengymnastik bei Inkontinenzbeschwerden, *Krankengymnastik* 46:322, 1994.
38. Travell JG, Simons DG: *Myofascial pain and dysfunction, vol 2,* Baltimore, 1992, Williams & Wilkins, pp. 110-131.
39. Fritsch H, Lienemann A, Brenner E et al: *Clinical anatomy of the pelvic floor,* Heidelberg, 2004, Springer Verlag.
40. Clemente CD: *Gray's anatomy of the human body,* ed 33, Philadelphia, 1985, Lea & Febiger.
41. Acland RD, Riggs GH: The trunk. In *Human anatomy, videotape 3,* Baltimore, 1998, Williams & Wilkins.
42. Bump RC, Hurt WG, Fantl A et al: Assessment of Kegel pelvic muscle exercise performance after brief verbal instruction, *Am J Obstet Gynecol* 165:322, 1991.

43. McIntosh LJ, Frahm JD, Mallett VT et al: Pelvic floor rehabilitation in treatment of incontinence, *J Reprod Med* 38:662, 1993.

44. Wall LL, Davidson TG: The role of muscular re-education by physical therapy in the treatment of genuine stress urinary incontinence, *Obstet Gynecol Surg* 47:322, 1992.

45. Miller JM, Ashton-Miller JA, DeLancey JO: A pelvic muscle pre-contraction can reduce cough-related urine loss in selected women with mild SUI, *Am Geriatr Soc* 46:870, 1998.

46. Fritsch H, Umphred D: Anatomy. In Carrière B, Feldt CM, editors: *The pelvic floor*, Stuttgart, 2006, Thieme Verlag.

47. Claes H, Van Kampen M, Lysens R et al: Pelvic floor treatment of impotence, *Eur J Phys Med Rehabil* 2:42, 1995.

48. Van Kampen M, De Weerdt W, Claes H et al: Treatment of erectile dysfunction by perineal exercise, electromyographic biofeedback and electrical stimulation, *Phys Ther* 83:536, 2003.

49. Dorey G: *Pelvic floor exercises for erectile dysfunction*, London, 2003, G. Dorey Whurr.

50. Junemann KP, Melchior H: Disorder of bladder function in Parkinson syndrome, *Urologe A* 29:170, 1990.

51. Burnett AL, Wesselmann U: History of the neurobiology of the pelvis, *Urology* 53:1082, 1999.

52. Doubleday KL, Kulig K, Landel R: Treatment of testicular pain using conservative management of thoracolumbar spine: a case report, *Arch Phys Med Rehabil* 84:1903, 2003.

53. Jänig W: Vegetatives nervensystem. In Schmidt RF, Thews G, editors: *Physiologie des menschen*, ed 26, Berlin, 1995, Springer-Verlag, pp. 340-369.

54. Henscher U: Storage and emptying dysfunctions of the bladder. In Carrière B, Feldt CM, editors: *The pelvic floor*, Stuttgart, 2006, Thieme Verlag.

55. Adams C, Frahm J: Genitourinary system. In Myers RS, editors: *Manual of physical therapy practice*, Philadelphia, 1995, WB Saunders, pp. 459-504.

56. DasGupta R, Fowler CJ: Bladder bowel and sexual dysfunction in multiple sclerosis: management strategies, *Drugs* 63:153-166, 2003.

57. Berman JR, Berman LA, Toler SM, et al: Safety and efficacy of sildenafil citrate for the treatment of female sexual arousal disorder: a double-blind, placebo controlled study, *J Urol* 170:2333, 2003.

58. Marthol H, Hilz MJ: Female sexual dysfunction: a systematic overview of classification, pathophysiology, diagnosis and treatment, *Fortschr Neurol Psychiatr* 72:121, 2004.

59. Kim JH, Rivals DA, Shenot PJ et al: Intravesical resiniferatoxin for refractory detrusor hyperreflexia: a multicenter, blinded, randomized, placebo-controlled trial, *J Spinal Cord Med* 26:358, 2003.

60. Ramaker MJ, Lunsen R HW: Psychosocial influences. Treatment of sexual and pelvic floor dysfunctions, In Carrière B, Feldt CM, editors: *The pelvic floor*, Stuttgart, 2006, Thieme Verlag.

61. Raadgers M: Treatment of sexual and pelvic floor dysfunctions. Treatment of sexual and pelvic floor dysfunctions. In Carrière B, Feldt CM, editors: *The pelvic floor*, Stuttgart, 2006, Thieme Verlag.

62. Lose G, Rosenkilde P, Gammelgaard J et al: Pad-weighing test performed with standardized bladder volume, *Urology* 32:78, 1988.

63. American Physical Therapy Association: Guide to physical therapy practice, *Phys Ther* 77:1177, 1997.

64. Jette A: Physical disablement concept for physical therapy research and practice, *Phys Ther* 74:380, 1994.

65. Wennergren HM, Ölberg BE, Sandstedt P: The importance of leg support for relaxation of the pelvic floor muscles, *Scand J Urol Nephrol* 25:205, 1991.

66. Schachter CL, Stalker CA, Teram E: Toward sensitive practice: issues for physical therapists working with survivors of childhood sexual abuse, *Phys Ther* 79:248, 1999.

67. Tanzberger R: Incontinence. In Carrière B: *The Swiss ball*, Berlin, 1988, Springer-Verlag, pp. 327-358.

68. Tanzberger R: Beckenboden-/Sphinktertraining bei Dysfunktionen, *Krankengymnastik* 7:1174, 1998.

69. Heller A: *Geburtsvorbereitung Methode Menne-Heller*, Stuttgart, 1988, Thieme.

70. Heller A: *Nach der Geburt: Wochenbett und Rückbildung*, Stuttgart, 2002, Thieme.

71. Tanzberger R: Krankengymnastische Therapie bei Inkontinenz, *Krankengymnastik* 43:1364, 1991.

72. Tanzberger R, Kuhn A, Möbs G: *Der Beckenboden-Funktion, Anpassung und Therapie*, München, 2004, Urban und Fischer.

73. Tanzberger R: Krankengymnastik nach der Geburt, *Krankengymnastik* 43:967, 1991.

74. Carrière B: *Fitness for the pelvic floor*, Stuttgart, 2002, Thieme Verlag.

75. Carrière B: *Exercises for the pelvic floor [videotape]*, 1999, available from www.balldynamics.com.

76. Hüter-Becker A, Thom H: *Physiotherapie, vol 6, massage, Kolonbehandlung*, Stuttgart, 1996, Thieme Verlag, pp. 162-182.

77. Lörenz F: Ambulante krankengymnastische Behandlung nach Brustkrebsoperation, *Krankengymnastik* 50:1147, 1998.

78. Henalla SM, Kirwan P, Castleden CM et al: The effect of pelvic floor exercises in the treatment of genuine urinary stress incontinence in women at two hospitals, *Br J Obstet Gynaecol* 95:602, 1988.

79. Bø K, Hagen R, Kvarstein B et al: S: Pelvic floor muscle exercise for the treatment of female stress urinary incontinence, *Neurol Urodynamics* 9:489, 1990.

80. Bø K, Talseth T, Holme I: Single blind, randomised controlled trial of pelvic floor exercises, electrical stimulation, vaginal cones, and no treatment in management of genuine stress incontinence in women, *BMJ* 318:487, 1999.

81. Tilbæks S: Effekt af bækkenbundtræning hos stress og blandet stress/urge inkontinente kvinder, *Dan Fysioterapeuter* 2:10, 1994.

82. Meaglia JP, Joseph AC, Chang M et al: Post-prostatectomy urinary incontinence: response to behavioral training, *J Urol* 144:674, 1990.

83. Holley RL, Varner E, Kerns DJ et al: Long-term failure of pelvic floor musculature exercises in treatment of genuine stress incontinence, *South Med J* 88:547, 1995.

84. Byl NN, Merzenich MM, Cheung S et al: A primate model for studying focal dystonia and repetitive strain injury: effects on the primary somatosensory cortex, *Phys Ther* 77:269, 1997.

85. Byl NN, Nagajaran S, McKenzie AL: Effect of sensory discrimination training on structures and function in patients with focal hand dystonia: a case series, *Arch Phys Med Rehabil* 84: 1505, 2003.

86. Umphred D: The nervous system and motor control. In Carrière B, Feldt CM, editors: *The pelvic floor*, Stuttgart, 2006, Thieme Verlag.

87. Salamey J, Nof L: Physical practice pattern and perceptions related to urinary incontinence, *J Womens Health* 23:8, 1999.

88. Dumoulin C, Seaborne DE, Quirion-DeGiardi C et al: Pelvic floor rehabilitation. Pt 1: Comparison of two surface electrode placements during stimulation of the pelvic floor musculature in women who are continent using bipolar interferential currents, *Phys Ther* 75:1067, 1995.

89. Dumoulin C, Seaborne DE, Quirion-DeGiardi C et al: Pelvic floor rehabilitation. Pt 2: Pelvic floor reeducation with interferential currents and exercises in the treatment of genuine stress incontinence in postpartum women—a cohort study, *Phys Ther* 75:1075, 1995.

90. Knight S, Laycock J, Naylor D: Evaluation of neuromuscular electrical stimulation in the treatment of genuine stress incontinence, *Physiotherapy* 84:61, 1998.

91. Bø K: Effect of electrical stimulation on stress and urge urinary incontinence, *Acta Obstet Gynecol Scand Suppl* 168:3, 1998.

92. Klein-Vogelbach S: *Ballgymnastik zur funktionellen Bewegungslehre*, ed 3, Berlin, 1990, Springer-Verlag.

93. Klein-Vogelbach S: *Functional kinetics*, Berlin, 1990, Springer-Verlag.

94. Klein-Vogelbach S: *Therapeutic exercises in functional kinetics*, Berlin, 1991, Springer-Verlag.

95. Shumway-Cook A, Woollacott MH: *Motor control*, Baltimore, 1995, Williams & Wilkins, pp. 23-43.

96. Schmidt RA, Lange C: Optimizing summary knowledge of results for skill learning, *Hum Mov Sci* 9:325, 1990.

97. Schmidt RA, Young DE, Swinnen S, et al: Summary knowledge of results for skill acquisition, *J Exp Psychol* 15:352, 1989.

98. Winstein CJ: Knowledge of results and motor learning—implications for physical therapy, *Phys Ther* 71:140, 1991.

99. Winstein CJ, Pohl PS, Lewthwaite R: Effects of physical guidance and knowledge of results on motor learning: support for the guidance hypothesis, *Res Q Exerc Sport* 65:316, 1994.

100. Carrière B: *The Swiss ball,* Stuttgart, 1998, Springer-Verlag.

101. Rosenzweig BA, Hischke D, Thomas S et al: Stress incontinence in women: psychological status before and after treatment, *J Reprod Med* 36:835, 1991.

102. Colling J, Ouslander J, Hadley BJ, et al: The effect of patterned urge-response toileting (PURT) on urinary incontinence among nursing home residents, *J Am Geriatr Soc* 40:135, 1992.

103. Engbert S, McDowell BJ, Donovan N et al: Treatment of urinary incontinence in homebound older adults: interface between research and practice, *Ostomy Wound Manage* 43:18, 1997.

104. Schnelle JF: Treatment of urinary incontinence in nursing home patients by prompted voiding, *J Am Geriat Soc* 38:356, 1990.

105. Carrière B: Angst älterer Menschen vor einem Sturz, *Fisio active* 4:5, 2005.

106. Vleminckx M: Visceral mobilization. In Carrière B, Feldt CM, editors: *The pelvic floor,* Stuttgart, 2006, Thieme Verlag.

CHAPTER 34

Orthotics: Evaluation, Intervention, and Prescription

Walter Racette, CPO

KEY TERMS

ankle-foot orthosis (AFO)
anterior/toe lever arm
double-adjustable ankle joint
knee-ankle-foot orthosis (KAFO)
posterior/heel lever arm

OBJECTIVES

After reading this chapter the student/therapist will be able to:
1. Identify and analyze the force system produced by the use of an orthosis.
2. Comprehend the prescription rationale gained from an orthotic evaluation.
3. Identify and differentiate the variables considered by the orthotist to optimize outcome during orthotic intervention.

OVERVIEW

The advancements and access to medical technology has had a profound effect in the field of orthotics. The evolution of plastic, composite, and metals fabrication technology has dramatically improved the ability to control, support, and protect all areas of the human body. Today patients are fit for custom and prefabricated orthotic devices that provide a variety of functions in both a timely and cost effective manner. These factors have led physicians to routinely prescribe orthoses for a wide range of medical conditions; whereas in prior decades, lack of availability and shortage of experienced orthotist restricted patient access and narrowed the utilization of orthoses.[1] Today, orthoses are important options of treatment protocol for postoperative management, acute fracture management, and adjunct treatment, in addition to more traditional utilization interventions of the past decades. For many, the proliferation of the prefabricated orthosis signaled a dilution of quality orthotic care but the reality is, it has had just the opposite effect. These readily available, cost-effective orthoses have not taken orthoses out of the hands of the orthotist but have moved them into the minds of treating professionals. There has been continued growth of new and improved orthoses and expansion into other areas of treatment previously without orthotic use. Positional and corrective orthoses for premature and newborn infants, as well as a wide range of sizes of orthoses for all pediatric patients that before were only available in limited adult sizes are examples. As with any new technological advancement, there have been incorrect application and use. It is not that many of these prefabricated orthoses are difficult to apply; rather, a clear understanding has been lacking of the indications, contraindications, and limitations these devices present to the orthotist and other health professionals, such as occupational and physical therapists.

Advancements in technology have allowed the use of lighter, strong materials in the fabrication of lower extremity orthotics. Specifically, the substance termed *prepreg* is a graphite material with the exact amount of resin and catalyst already included and which, with the fibers properly directed over a model, can be formed with heat. Graphite has been used in both prosthetics and orthotics for years; however, it has limited acceptance in orthotics because it has not reduced the weight of the orthotic compared with other materials. It also lacks the ability to modify the orthosis after the lamination process. The prepreg graphite has dramatically reduced weight, still maintains strength, and gives the orthotist the possibility of using the dynamics of loading and response, similar to dynamic-response prosthetic feet. This allows for assistance in both the swing and stance phases (Figure 34-1). A clinical example at the end of this chapter will demonstrate this patient need. Another significant advancement in component technology has been the introduction of weight-activated orthotic knee joints. Although available in prosthetics for decades, the development of a lightweight, compact knee joint that would allow a patient to have knee stability during stance[2] and clearance during swing phase has been allusive, until recently. Prior to this, the mainstay of available knee joints for knee-ankle-foot orthoses (KAFO) was some type of locking mechanism that remained locked throughout the gait cycle. There are specific indications and contraindications, but early results are promising. This feature can significantly reduce energy output,[3] as it is not necessary to raise the center of gravity to clear the locked knee during swing phase, which offers patient safety when walking on uneven surfaces.

No discussion of the delivery of health care services within the United States would be complete or accurate without mentioning the effects of government and private regulations. The above discussion regarding a dramatic increase of utilization has raised the medical justification debate over the intervention of orthotics in all areas.

Government regulations have dramatically changed the course of the orthotic profession, beginning with the Medicare program, to diagnostic related groups (DRGs), managed care, and, soon, qualified providers. Medicare was the first national program to cover the cost of both orthotic and prosthetic devices. Prior to that point, only a special few had access to "braces and limbs." DRGs put the responsibility of paying for prescribed orthoses into the hands of the local hospital. Once the specific diagnosis was made, the

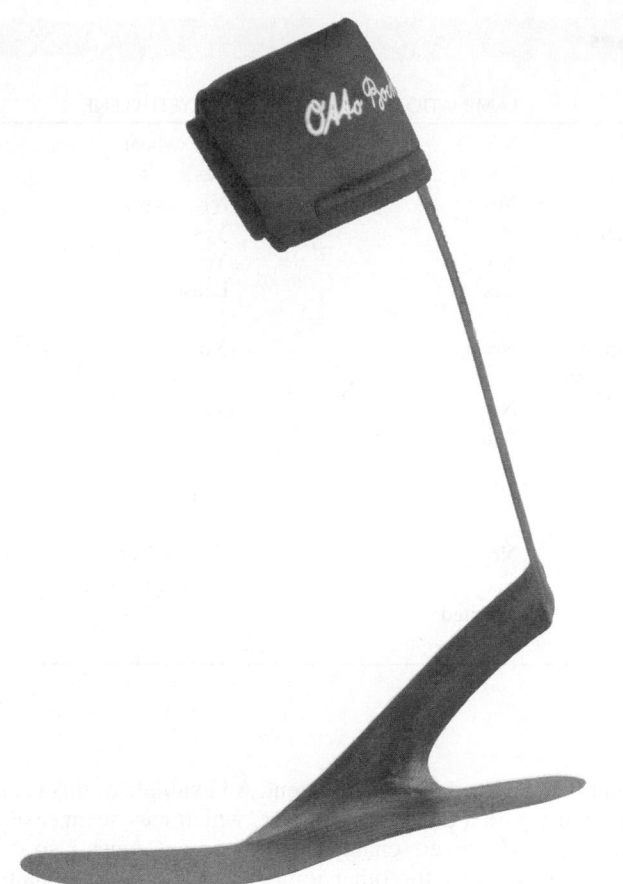

FIGURE 34-1 ■ New lightweight technology. (Courtesy of Otto Bock Healthcare.)

government would allow a specified amount for reimbursement, leaving the decision of how to do that with the physician/hospital. This policy change created many new innovations. Hospitals, interested in reducing the length of hospital stays, challenged the physicians to change the way they treated their patients. Patients no longer are immobilized for long periods in hospital beds and are sent home sooner, or to a less acute setting or skilled nursing facilities. The use of orthotic devices to expedite care and precautionary care while hospitalized has increased dramatically. The use of halo fixation systems, thoracic lumbar sacral orthoses (TLSOs), fracture orthoses, and contracture preventing orthoses are but a few examples that are helping to reduce length of stay. Another significant effect of the DRG decade on orthotics was the need to reduce delivery times and be as cost effective as possible. Orthoses needed to be delivered in hours, not days. Careful evaluation developed in regard to the use of prefabricated, custom-fit, or custom-made orthoses. Challenges to improve traditional methods of fabrication, better materials, and higher utilization spanned the rapid growth of a wide range of orthoses for patient care, and there is no reason to believe that this trend will slow down as our population ages.

Government-inspired changes in insurance coverage, health maintenance organizations, and insurance company consolidation have created wide-ranging effects—both positive and negative—on the entire medical delivery system. The full impact on the orthotic profession has yet to be seen, but several areas have changed patient care. Cost containment and "take it or leave it" contract options continue to stress both large and small facility providers. The pressure is to reduce customary fees to enable them to continue caring for long-term patients as the rush to join health maintenance organizations spreads throughout the country. For many professionals, the years of creating awareness, value, and benefit for providing orthoses is now challenged by an additional layer of administrative people with limited knowledge who questioned cost necessity but rarely medical necessity. The need to learn new rules required clinical staff to do less patient care and more administrative maneuvering at a reduced fee. Both the lack of ability to deal with these changes and the fear of failure had a profound effect on reshaping the orthotic and prosthetic profession. In a time when the orthotist saw many new technologies emerge and patient care outcomes were exceeding those of previous decades, managed care challenged our ability to make these advancements possible for most of our patients and restricted access through exclusive contracts with providers. Cost/value questions are essential in quality care. Unfortunately, our profession did not have the scientific data or justification ready for this health care revolution. Evidence-based care has been difficult for the profession to rationalize, identify, and develop and therefore is largely nonexistent. There is great importance in the professional relationship between physical/occupational therapy and orthotics as the evolution of managed care continues. Identifying patient functional goals and a variety of evidence-based care is critical for patient care and clinical outcomes. Orthotists must embrace the challenge of measured improvement and documentation in function from care they provide and use it to develop a standard of care, as has the rest of the medical profession. Orthotics and prosthetics have emerged from under the radar. Their use now must be based on proven evidence-based care specific to the profession. It is in that spirit that I challenge the wide-range understanding of the evaluation, prognosis, and intervention of orthotics in neurological rehabilitation.

An orthosis is an external device that when applied to the body produces a force that biomechanically affects the body in such a way as to correct, support, or stabilize the trunk, head, and/or extremity. The goals in patient care with orthotic utilization vary from permanent use, after other treatment to maintain improvement, to temporary use. Many factors enter into the decision on use and type of orthosis (to be discussed later), but it is essential that when the need for orthotic intervention is determined, the least complicated, cost-effective orthosis to fit patient needs be used. The rehabilitation team must build a priority list of desired outcomes and accept that at times, all of the items on the list may not be achieved by either the orthosis or the patient/team combination. At the very least care must be attempted in stages. As an example, an excessive amount of custom-made and custom-fit plastic ankle-foot orthoses have been used because they are "more cosmetic and lighter" than a metal and leather type ankle-foot orthosis. There are times when all higher priority goals can be achieved so that down the list, goal, cosmesis, and light weight can be considered (Table 34-1). However, in the case of neuropathy of the foot, one would take significant risk to provide a total-contact orthosis, such as a plastic ankle-foot orthosis, to keep it

TABLE 34-1 ■ Comparison of Metal and Plastic Orthoses

FACTOR	METAL AND LEATHER	POLYPROPYLENE	LAMINATION/GRAPHITE	POLYETHYLENE
Adjustability	Yes	Yes w/heat	No	Yes w/heat
Patient changes shoes	No	Yes	Yes	Yes
Strength weight bearing	Yes	Yes	Yes	No
Skin at risk	Yes	Yes, close observation	No	Yes
Best spinal use	No	Yes	No	Yes
Long-term wear	Yes	Less	Yes	Least
Weight (lightest = 1)	4	2	3	1
Adjustability to changing clinical picture	Yes	Limited, unless initial articulation fabricated	No	No
Short-term need	Yes	Yes	No	Yes
Requires corrective force with patient good sensation	Fair	Good	Fair	Good
Questionable patient compliance ability/direction	Best	Questionable	No	Fair
Clinician wants ability to change angulation, ankle or knee	Best	Limited*	No	Not indicated above for weight bearing
Upper extremity fabrication-direct mold highest frequency	Limited	Yes	Limited	Yes

*Used in combination with metal joints produces best results.

lightweight. A double upright metal ankle-foot orthosis with a well-fitted extradepth shoe with custom Plastazote insert would fit the patient's needs and take into consideration the sensory and motor changes within the lower extremity. Coordination between health-related professionals in development of patient treatment goals is essential during the evaluation process. Without communication, adequate care of the patient may be considered unsuccessful because of a design criteria omission as simple as placing a loop closure on the side the patient could not reach. A sound understanding of biomechanical and orthotic principles, as well as skilled patient management techniques must be used in this patient population to be successful. There are similarities in orthotic management of orthopedic and neurologically impaired patients; however, the neurological population presents additional factors that challenge prescription criteria and outcomes for the rehabilitation team. Lack of proprioception, sensation (hyper/hypo), and spasticity represent some of these special considerations. Other possible additional medical issues, problems with communication, and caregivers add to these patients' management complications.

BASIC ORTHOTIC FUNCTIONS

Alignment

Alignment of the extremities and spine is a common function in orthotic prescription. The orthosis can provide either temporary or permanent function. A TLSO may be prescribed for stabilizing alignment after spinal fusion in the case of an unstable spinal cord injury (refer to Chapter 19). A supramalleolar orthosis is commonly prescribed to hold the foot in proper alignment. When the goal of orthotic intervention is to correct alignment well tolerated by the overlying soft tissue and/or the malalignment being due to a muscle weakness, the new position should stabilize the joint. Remember that aligning one joint may result in the proximal or distal

joint being placed in malalignment. An example of this is an extremity with a genu valgum knee, which may seem easily corrected. However, changes in alignment must also be accommodated by the other joints up and down the chain. Thus questions such as "does the subtalar joint have the mobility to pronate?" must be asked and answered.

Stability

Stability is often required when caring for the patient with neurological deficits. These patients frequently lack the muscle control and strength necessary to maintain trunk balance or to ambulate. Patients with muscular dystrophy benefit from TLSOs to help maintain trunk stability, sitting balance, and safer transfers. However the decision regarding an orthosis must take into consideration maximum stability and flexibility while not restraining breathing capacity. An ankle-foot orthosis that limits both dorsi and plantarflexion can stabilize the ankle and the knee for the patient with cardiovascular accident (CVA). Although this patient may initially require medial lateral ankle stability, controlling the anterior posterior lever arms at the ankle can provide knee stability and prevent future knee impairments. The orthosis functions by producing a posterior force acting to extend the knee, as most patients requiring this type of stability function with a foot-flat gait instead of a normal initial heel-strike pattern.

Contracture Reduction

Contracture reduction is a goal of many orthotic uses in patients with neurological involvement. The increase in the use of these types of orthoses has been dramatic as even slight increases in contractures can make the difference between nonambulation function and community ambulation participation. Increased awareness and proactive orthotic use of prefabricated orthoses have become routine during periods of inactivity, associated surgical procedures, and "sound side" prevention. These type of orthoses are either dynamic or static and used in conjunction with different therapeutic modalities to reduce the contracture. Dynamic contracture-reducing orthoses use a spring-type mechanism that puts a low force over an extended period of time to gain range of motion. Static-type orthoses range from serial casts, where a manual stretch is placed over the joint, to custom-made cylinder devices designed to spread force over larger areas, to custom-fit devices with some type of quick adjustability. Dynamic-type orthoses are usually contraindicated for the patient with a neurological disorder. Low-tension stretch can trigger spasticity and create skin breakdown because of the high pressure on localized skin areas. The exception for this would be individuals with lower motor neuron-impairments and residual hypotonicity. Any tension orthoses needs to be monitored when there is sensory loss irrespective of the causation. To get results in contracture reduction, one must be cautiously aggressive as the amount of force required to get reduction often threatens the soft tissue's ability to tolerate the pressure of the orthosis. Experience, frequent sessions, and close communication with other members of the rehabilitation team and family/patient are critical factors in the success of the use of orthotic devices.

EVALUATION

The evaluation of the neurologically impaired patient must be comprehensive. One must not read a diagnosis and assume a total clinical picture. The diagnosis should alert the evaluator to movement patterns associated with the impairment, and these should be used to confirm potential findings. Complete patient evaluations do not end with range of motion, muscle testing, proprioception, and skin sensitivity or lack of same, or the integrity of the affected limb or spine. The individual ordering an orthotic device must assess the total picture to determine what limitations orthotic care may have on other important functions, activities, and patient participation in life. Last but not least, the evaluation must include a patient management assessment. What is the patient/family motivation? With how much componentry can the patient tolerate/function? What chance of success does the patient/family have once they leave the clinical setting? How significant are the risks associated with orthotic intervention? As stated, the total evaluation of the patient and patient environment is important in developing the treatment plan, as is the communication between the physical therapist, occupational therapist, and orthotist. Whether done together or, as is more realistic, at separate sites, the details of the treatment plan must be discussed. The patient with neurological impairment often presents a series of complex issues: biomechanical, communication, visualization, etc. Incomplete information or a lack of effort at communication among these professionals will not lead to a comprehensive treatment plan and ultimate outcome assessment.

During evaluation, review of the diagnosis and gathering of patient history are extremely valuable. A complete diagnosis will indicate important information to the team. For example, if a patient with poliomyelitis is to be seen, the orthotist is aware that it is a lower motor neuron lesion and that proprioception is intact (see Chapter 29). These patients initially have the benefit of skeletal balance and therefore require durable orthotic fabrication and components.

Compare this to a similar result in muscle testing and range of motion for an individual with an incomplete T12 level paraplegia. Assuming this is a complete lesion, patients with this upper motor neuron lesion lack proprioception. They require other stimulation to get a sense of standing balance and require a lightweight orthosis, as they rarely use orthoses as a major means of locomotion. Although gathering patient history is a vital part of the evaluation, it is, more importantly, an opportunity to establish a productive patient management environment. Patients and family members have important information regarding the initial injury, previous medical care, reasons they sought additional care, and desired outcomes of new treatment. Most of this information can be gathered efficiently as either the therapist or the orthotist begins other areas of professional evaluations. These are important patient/family management skills. One must hear from the patient/family why they came to see the health care professional and their expectations of care. The therapist should not assume the family's goals without asking, as often patient/family goals are higher than clinicians' expectations. Communicating at a level that is understandable is both vital and demonstrates to patient/family that the therapist is a concerned professional, thereby engendering trust and confidence (refer to Chapter 4). Complete and timely documentation of these findings is becoming increasingly vital to the evaluation and treatment plan. Whether communicating with others on the rehabilitation team, insurance carriers, or legal professionals, documentation and building medical justification are essential in treating all patients.

Evaluation of the Spine

Each area of the spinal column presents various combinations of motion and function. Beginning at the lumbar level as the base for upright position, the spinal column protects vital organs; serves as a supporting structure for the lungs to expand, for the upper extremities to reach, to carry objects; protects the nervous system pathway for the body; and controls the upright position and motions of the head. The individual segments of the spine have relatively few complicated orthotic challenges. However, it is rare that only one segment is involved in the patient with neuropathic impairments; it is more common that two or more segments of the spine will be involved in orthotic fitting. For example, supporting the head in a functional position is a major goal of orthotic intervention but to accomplish this, the orthosis must encompass the thoracic as well as the cervical spine in order to distribute the forces to tolerate skin pressure.

When evaluating the cervical spine and head one must, in addition to muscle testing, determine at what angulations upright position of the head cannot be recovered. Limiting the head from nonfunctional positions, that is, extreme extension, is an easier orthotic function than to have to fabricate an orthosis that will hold the head upright. Many patients with neurological problems may have the strength to move in a 15- to 20-degree range of flexion/extension, lateral bend, and rotation, but do not have the strength to recover the head from greater angles. Even the best soft tissue about the head does not tolerate long-term pressure from an orthosis; therefore intermittent control/relief is a critical design. Pressure directly on the ear is not tolerated at any time. Rare is the occasion that the thoracic and lumbar spine is treated separately with an orthosis in the patient with neurological deficient. The major reasons for orthotic intervention in this area are to stabilize the trunk for balance, to protect surgical correction/stabilization, and to maintain respiration. The pelvis is generally used as a base to prevent distal migration of the orthosis whether the patient is sitting our standing. For this reason, one must closely evaluate degree of deformity, prominence of bony structure, skin sensation, and condition of soft tissue coverage. Many neurologically impaired patients also have other medical conditions that need to be considered in orthotic design, such as colostomy, GI tubes, pressure sores, and others. Scoliosis and kyphosis are common biomechanical impairments within this patient group. Balance between correcting the spinal deformity to maintain respiratory function and doing so with a tightly fitting TLSO and the skin pressure it creates must be reached by the rehabilitation team. The evaluation of the spine and potential need for orthotic intervention would not be complete without recognizing the effect the desired orthosis may have on the extremities, whether the patient is ambulatory or non–weight bearing. What movements of the spine are present during ambulation and would immobilizing the spine significantly affect the patient? Will the orthosis restrict needed shoulder elevation and arm movements? Variation in materials used for fabrication of a spinal orthosis can often significantly improve the desired outcome, increase the wear time, ease the donning process, and improve skin care. From a patient/family management standpoint, one must consider many variables in potential design of the orthosis. Can the patient/family don the orthosis and remove when appropriate? Do they understand potential areas of pressure? What is the home situation like?

Evaluation of the Upper Extremities

Evaluation of the upper extremities requires multiple input from health care professionals, patients, family, and teachers because of the wide range of specific functions an individual performs daily. Unique to this area, multiple functions generally require multiple orthotic devices. Typical functions of orthoses of the upper extremity includes maintaining of functional wrist hand position, reducing contracture or tone, transfer of force available in one area to another, and supporting subluxations due to denervation in addition to various assistive orthoses necessary for activities of daily living. It is common that the neurologically impaired patient require several orthoses each with different functions for use throughout the day. Strength, range of motion, conditions of soft tissues, and sensation are all important evaluation factors. In addition, ambulatory status, bilateral or unilateral condition, status of vision, and condition of the spine and head must be factored into the indications and contraindications of formulation of the orthotic needs of the patient. Much more critical muscle tests must be made in the upper extremity as opposed to the lower extremity as minor increases or decreases in strength will dramatically alter orthotic need. For example, the C5 quadriplegic has the ability to function with a wrist hand orthosis with enough wrist extension to utilize the tenodesis effect that can produce a three-jaw-chuck grip. The difference between a functioning and nonfunctioning orthosis is minor not only because there is less muscle strength but also because minor inefficiencies in the tenodesis splint, either friction or

malalignment could reduce function to below acceptable levels. Patients with unilateral involvement have far different needs than the bilaterally involved. The patient with a CVA, being unilaterally involved, may have a typical intervention of a positional wrist hand orthosis to prevent contracture and prevent injury and a supporting shoulder orthosis to prevent shoulder subluxation. In these cases the other extremity becomes dominant and there is little need to fabricate complex orthoses for the use of the effected extremity. The patient with bilateral involvement presents a much different picture. Consideration for grooming, feeding, and mobility etc., must be factored into the desired expectation during evaluation. The patient with neurological impairments requiring orthotic intervention is complex as this patient typically has involvement in the trunk, head, and lower extremity. These patients require specialized wheelchairs and seating systems. Evaluation is most effective with all rehabilitation team members present to establish a treatment plan. Orthotic treatments maximize what little muscle strength and range of motion the patient may have. Orthoses that are used during the day to maximize function are often replaced with positional orthoses at night to preserve gains and prevent decline in range of motion. The occupational therapist provides most of functional and positional orthoses for the upper extremity. In today's rehabilitation environment, many occupational therapists work directly with orthopedic hand specialists and trauma physicians, using low-temperature materials to mold custom devices specifically designed for protecting surgical reconstruction, promoting or maintaining ROM, or for use as assistive devices.

Evaluation of the Lower Extremities

Evaluation of the lower extremity offers additional challenges due to the role of ambulation and its value to the independence for the patient and family members. Range of motion, strength, existing deformity, proprioception, muscle tone, and soft tissue condition and sensation must be evaluated and, where appropriate, weight-bearing/existing gait analysis done. Patient/family assessment as related to the ability to comprehend and follow instructions is extremely important, as the potential for injury may outweigh the benefit of orthotic intervention to transform a patient from non–weight bearing to limited ambulation. Lack of range of motion at the hip and knee will significantly decrease the duration of potential ambulation or may totally inhibit ambulation. Lack of range of motion at the hip and knee are more critical than lack of strength, and in the foot and ankle, the need for normal range of motion is more critical for efficient standing balance and ambulation. Orthoses of the lower extremity function by providing a combination of force lever arms acting about an axis: knee, hip, or ankle. These joints are significantly compromised by the lack of range of motion. These force lever arms within the lower extremities substitute for the lack of strength provided by the anterior lever arm. For example, by blocking dorsiflexion of the ankle the lever arm provides a posterior directed force that stabilizes the knee. If the patient lacks the ability to get the ankle even to neutral, this tightness provides its own lever arm, which will result in a variety of undesirable actions. Genu recurvatum, foot/ankle varus, shortened stride length on the nonaffected side, and the heel rising out of the shoe are common signs of this problem. These issues are further complicated when lack of proprioception, spasticity, and lack of sensation are present. This will be further discussed in the case study portion of the chapter. Lack of range of motion at the ankle creates many symptoms in the lower extremity but is often missed during evaluation as the cause of these problems. Genu varus and genu recurvatum are common deformities of the patient with neurological impairments. A number of factors create these problems. In addition to the ankle, leg length differences, lack of quadriceps strength, and lack of proprioception can create deformities about the knee. The patient with poliomyelitis may have both a short extremity and weak knee extensors, which lead to genu recurvatum and genu valgus. However, reducing the genu recurvatum without protecting against undesirable knee flexion would be a mistake. These patients with lower motor neuron disease have excellent proprioception, which is the reason they protect the unstable knee by hyperextending it using force within their upper extremity by pushing posterior on the femur. A similar patient with upper neuron impairments, for example a patient who has had a CVA, has a similar knee presentation; however, the usual cause of this patient's deformity is different. Reduced or lack of strength and range-of-motion limitations about the hip limit effective ambulation and leave the patient much more reliant on trunk stability and upper extremity ambulatory aids. Hip flexors are more critical than hip extensors, as they serve to advance the limb in reciprocal gait, whereas lack of hip extensors is substituted by the strong hip ligaments that tighten for stability in extension. A lack of range of motion to at least neutral extension about the hip creates major problems for the patient, even if the patient has excellent upper extremity strength. This lack of range will not allow stability in standing once force is removed from the upper extremity ambulatory aids. Creating hands-free standing balance is a highly desirable outcome resulting from orthotic intervention.

GOALS OF ORTHOTIC INTERVENTION

Evidence based care creates the framework for orthotic intervention. Unfortunately, the orthotic and prosthetic profession has been both reluctant and slow to respond in the generation of this body of work. With multiple types of clinical sites, mostly smaller private facilities, lack of any substantial literature base, and a perception that it does not apply to orthotics, the growth of evidence-based care has proceeded at glacial speed. Only with significant attention by the profession will this much-needed body of work be built, and then the goals of orthotic intervention can be much more predictable.

The patient evaluation and clinical experience must be used to create a plan of treatment expectation. The value of experience has not been tested as a predictor of the outcomes likely to occur after the treatment plan has been followed. Yet, through experience, professionals know that only a well-thought–out plan, thoroughly communicated to all participants, will be successful. All too frequently we, as health care providers, assume that the patient and family know the goals of orthotic intervention. We often do not listen to patient/family concerns before initiating the treatment plan. These are both major patient management mistakes. Several factors play key roles in the success of orthotic intervention.

Improved function without complication or patient risk: (1) the clinician must be sure to address the patient's major complaint; and (2) the reason the patient/family came to see either the therapist or orthotist must be clearly established to ensure compliance with orthotic intervention. It is important to establish a baseline of function, so that results of intervention are measurable. In some situations, the patient benefit is clear and immediate, whereas others require concentrated instruction, orthotic modification, and time before improved function can be observed or measured. The process of donning and doffing the orthosis as independently as possible enhances the overall goal for patient and family, and must be well thought out by the experienced clinician. Be conservative in setting these expectations. It is important to remember that what happens in the clinical setting may not be reproducible easily in the home situation. Protecting knee stability with use of the hamstrings during therapeutic instruction may be a risk in the home setting, whereas providing an ankle-foot orthosis with an anterior stop at the ankle would provide a mechanical knee stabilizing effect and prove much safer for the patient over the long term.

The orthotic interventions must be kept as simple as possible: what is the least amount of orthotic intervention that will provide the expected goal? Although an obvious statement, the balance between too much and not enough can challenge the clinician's skill and experience. The use of trial orthoses can provide valuable information during the evaluation and these are generally available commercially for short periods. The benefits of various types of thermomoldable plastics have been great for many individuals; however, at times, their use adds risk and complication without improvement, compared with traditional ankle-foot orthoses fabricated with metal and leather attached to the patient's shoe. For example, if the patient requires ankle and knee stability yet lacks sensation in the foot and ankle, the double upright metal orthosis attached to the patient's shoe creates much less risk for possible skin breakdown than a rigid total-contact plastic orthosis (see Table 34-1). With a plastic orthosis, the family must find a shoe big enough to easily fit the orthosis. Technological advancements have led to a number of additions to the arsenal of the orthotic profession. Prefabricated orthoses with better sizing and materials have given the clinician additional tools for both the evaluation and as permanent orthoses. Preimpregnated graphite ankle-foot orthoses are now available in sizes that provide toe pickup during swing phase and some knee stabilizing characteristics during stance phase. These orthoses play an important role, although very light weight, they provide a dynamic stance phase option. Introduction of biomechanical forces to the extremities may cause unwanted movements or restrictions, and careful selection of components is essential to keep the focus on the orthotic plan. For example, a patient with a CVA may need more anterior lever force for knee stability, so one would plantar flex the orthotic ankle joint. However, this knee stabilizing effect in stance phase would cause a toe drag during swing phase. A simple fix is to provide the opposite side with a $1/4$-inch heel-and-sole lift for additional clearance during swing phase of the affected extremity (Table 34-2).

Clinicians need to set realistic manageable patient-centered treatment goals. All too often, treatment plans are only in the minds of the clinicians and are either never or

TABLE 34-2 ■ Indications for Common Orthotic Modifications/Additions

MODIFICATION/ADDITION	DESCRIPTION
SACH modification	This modification is done by cutting out a triangular wedge in the heel of the shoe and securing a softer material. The solid ankle cushion heel (SACH) modification is used to dampen the effect of the heel/posterior lever arm at heel strike. This force produces an anterior force to destabilize the knee, which may be undesirable.
Heel and sole buildup	Adding a $1/4$-inch heel and sole buildup to the unaffected side can create additional swing clearance needed on the affected side. This modification is indicated if additional dorsiflexion of the orthotic joint creates knee instability or if the patient lacks dorsiflexion range of motion.
Rocker-bottom heel and sole modifications	There are several different styles of rocker-bottom buildup. Although the roll built into this modification may differ, the basic results are the same—to add motion and rotation of the center of gravity forward when the ankle and/or knee orthotic joint is locked.
Long tongue stirrup/extended steel shanks	A stirrup is the metal attachment to the shoe. The utilization of a long tongue (a steel extension that goes distal between the bottom of the shoe and the heel and sole) is necessary to transfer the force created by restriction of ankle motion. Without this type of fabrication, the force produced at midstance will not be controlled. The steel shank produces the same control but is not part of the stirrup and may be used alone in combination with a rocker bottom.
Medial/valgus control T-strap; lateral/varus control T-strap	These straps, leather on traditional double upright orthoses or plastic/padding modifications on plastic ankle-foot orthoses, produce a force to reduce valgus (a medial T-strap) or varus (a lateral T-strap). A medial T-strap attaches to the shoe medially, and the beltlike strap goes around the lateral upright and is tightened. The lateral T-strap is opposite.
Heel buildup	A heel buildup is used to accommodate heel cord tightness. The tibia must be at least 90 degrees to the floor for safe balance and ambulation. Common signs of the need to build up the heel are genu recurvatum and the heel slipping out of the shoe. The amount of heel buildup must be matched with the same heel and sole buildup on the opposite side.
Instep and figure-of-8 straps	This orthotic modification is used to keep the heel back in the shoe or plastic ankle-foot orthosis when a tight heel cord is present. These straps fit across the dorsum of the foot with a posterior attachment point.
Swedish knee orthosis	This prefabricated knee orthosis is an effective method to prevent genu recurvatum on a temporary basis. It is typically indicated after a cerebrovascular accident for the patient who lacks proprioception and whose knee pops back, creating pain and slack knee ligaments. It can be used temporarily as a training orthosis or permanently when persistent pain and instability are present.

too poorly communicated with the patient/family. One should expect that the patient, or the parents of the patient, will always expect that the benefits of the intervention will be far above what the therapist knows are possible. The time to address those gaps is certainly before treatment, not when the patient/family realizes expectations regarding functional gains may not become realistic. If failure is the reason why a patient recognizes the intervention was wrong, the therapists have lost the patient's trust and, thus, the potential for future intervention guidance. Discussing realistic achievable goals of treatment, assessing all factors, the home situation, and individual motivation with the patient/family in language they understand is critical if the success of orthotic intervention is to be achieved. The goal of orthotic care for a patient with CVA is to provide safe standing balance for transfer and minimal ambulation in the home. Patients and their families will realize the major benefit this will have on the home situation; however, without this identified as the goal prior to orthotic care; they may leave the therapeutic environment wondering why the patient cannot walk normally and participate in life activities that require longer

distance ambulation skills.[4] This clinical error is an all-too-frequent patient management mistake. Integrating orthotics with physical/occupational therapy motor relearning and neuroplasticity should help optimize functional recovery.

To provide a cost-effective orthosis in a timely manner, with today's vast number of orthotic devices, the orthotist must stay abreast of the wide array of choices at his or her disposal to meet the needs of the patient. The reality of cost containment is not a recent event in the orthotic profession, as funding for these devices has always been challenged. Rightfully so—and it has necessitated the development of more cost-effective alternatives, such as the prefabricated orthosis. The introduction of thermo-moldable plastics into orthotics in the late 1960s and early 1970s on a custom basis replaced, to a large extent, the need to mold leather and/or metal to fabricate an orthosis (see Table 34-1). This improved the total-contact fit and, at the same time, dramatically reduced the time and skill level for manufacturing. From this beginning, today's orthotist has a multitude of devices from which to choose to meet the needs of the patient. Options range from the custom-made fit using a patient mold, to the ready-made prefabricated custom fit. A thorough understanding of the indications and contraindications for each of these devices is essential in order to meet patient needs. A lack of understanding of biomechanical principles, of the limitations of prefabricated orthoses, and the knowledge of custom fitting can lead to failure and increase the impairment problems existing within the patient environment. All orthoses produce a force field, some desirable and some not. It requires an experienced clinician to make the most appropriate choices, as too often the failure of treatment is blamed on an orthosis. Usually, such failure is the result of an inappropriate initial selection of orthotic component, lack of custom made/custom fit, or misidentification of the patient as an orthotic candidate. Prefabricated custom-fit orthoses are only cost effective if they produce the desired goal over time. As a general rule, one should consider prefabricated custom-fit orthosis for patients who have an anatomically "normal" biomechanical structural environment and who will only use the orthosis for a short time. Custom-made orthosis for extremities/spine are usually prescribed for patients who have deformity, unusual size, or who must use it indefinitely.

CLINICAL EXAMPLES

Client with Paraplegia

Orthotic consideration for the paraplegic patient is generally considered at the T12 level in the complete lesion.[5] Complete lesions higher in the cord leave the patient without enough trunk stability to use bilateral orthoses effectively. Although a thoracic extension can be added to bilateral KAFOs, this addition greatly increases the difficulty of donning the orthosis independently, and most patients will have great difficulty getting from sitting to standing.

The orthoses for a T12 complete paraplegic are bilateral KAFOs. The patient generally uses a swing-to or swing-through gait, and successful use of orthoses requires excellent standing balance. There are three significant design requirements for these KAFOs: shallow thigh and calf bands, bail or French knee locks, and adjustable ankle joints with long tongue stirrups with strutter bars to the heads of the metatarsals (Scott-Craig design) (Figure 34-2). The shallow bands force the center of gravity forward, inducing lordosis so the patient can rest on the Y ligaments of Bigelow. The knee locks are automatic, because the patient requires the upper extremities for standing. The bail/French joint will lock as the patient stands and bends over the rigid ankle joint, forcing the knee joints into extension. The lock then will catch on the back of a wheelchair seat or other chair

and bend at the joint when the patient sits. The foot/ankle complex forms the basis for balance. A few degrees of adjustment at the double-adjustable ankle joint can make the difference between safe standing balance and limited standing balance. The long tongue stirrup extends at least to the heads of the metatarsals and farther if the patient is taller and heavier than normal (see Table 34-2). The use of a strutter bar from the upright of the stirrup extending to a transverse bar at the heads of the metatarsals ensures rigidity as complete as necessary. A point between effective standing balance and ambulation is reached after training and ankle adjustment. Patients must have full range of motion at the hips, knees, and ankles for use of these devices to be successful (Case Study 34-1).

Hemiplegia

Patients who have had a CVA can vary widely in their need for orthotic intervention, from a simple AFO to assist toe clearance, to an AFO to stabilize both ankle and knee, to an orthosis used temporarily for training purposes.[6,7] The use of

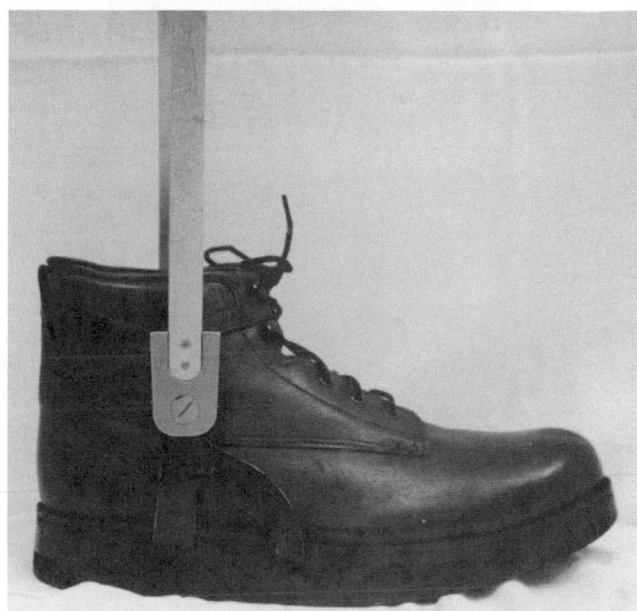

FIGURE 34-2 ■ Modifications necessary to control the ankle setting in a client with spinal cord injury (Scott-Craig shoe/stirrup modifications).

CASE STUDY 34-1 ■ A. M.

A. M. is a 21 year old with incomplete T12-level paraplegia secondary to a gunshot wound. A. M. has normal upper-extremity strength and ROM. He has had surgery for spinal fusion. Trunk strength is 4/5, left hip is 3/5, knee is 2/5, right hip is 1/5, and right knee is 0/5. ROM is full at hips, knees, and ankles. A. M. can transfer independently and has the goal of household ambulation, although he is aware that it "takes a lot of work." A. M. was fitted with a right KAFO with shallow bands, drop lock knee joints, and double-adjustable

ankle joints locked in 5 degrees of dorsiflexion (Figure 34-3). Drop locks were used instead of bail locks because of the use of a unilateral KAFO. A. M. had balance, strength, and a foot orthosis on the left side. The left lower extremity was fitted with an AFO, double upright, and double-adjustable ankle joints adjusted to match the right orthosis. The distal attachment to the shoes was with long tongue stirrups and strutter bars. The patient was able to ambulate with forearm crutches.

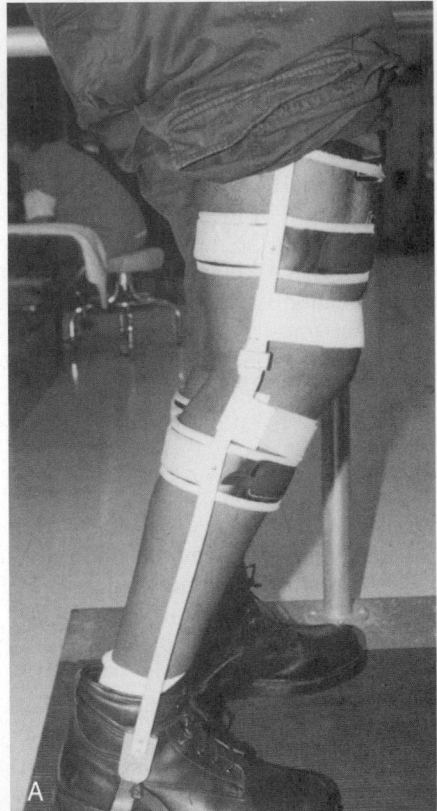

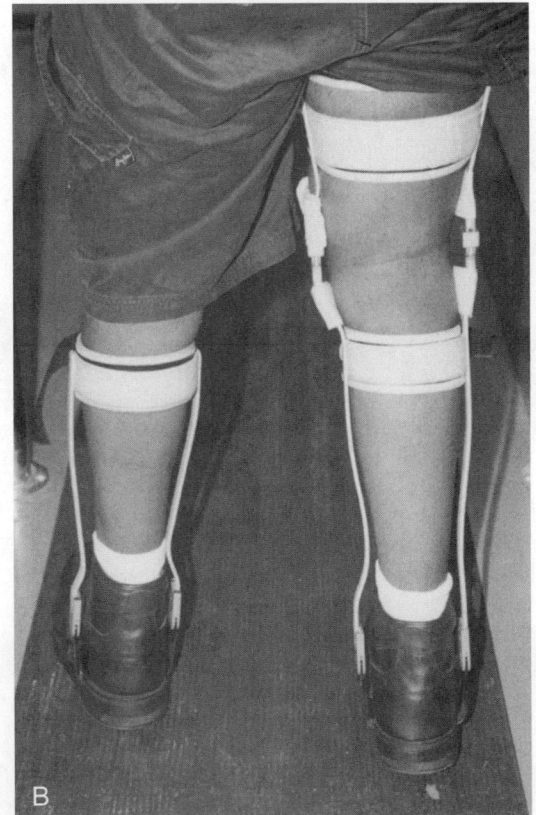

FIGURE 34-3 ■ Patient standing wearing a right knee-ankle-foot orthosis. **A,** Lateral view; **B,** posterior view.

a KAFO for the patient with hemiplegia is rarely indicated. Even though the more affected patient does not have knee stability, he or she rarely ambulates with a heel strike that would destabilize the knee and therefore can use an AFO with an anterior limited-range ankle joint. Additionally, patients cannot don the KAFO with the use of only one upper extremity. With the lack of hip flexors and knee instability on the affected side, the orthotic intervention may be to assist in transfers. As a general rule, orthotic intervention for the client with a CVA ranges from a static-toe pickup orthosis to a double-adjustable ankle joint with the ankle locked. The use of spring components is not effective, because they will initiate spasticity. The lack of ROM into dorsiflexion and even neutral causes the biggest problem for these patients. The ankle that lacks range prevents advancement of the center of gravity and produces a lever arm that induces genu recurvatum and pain, and either the heel comes out of the shoe or the ankle rolls into varus. Because these patients lack proprioception, this constant force directed posteriorly will, over the course of a few months, be significant, as the patient will hurt and not ambulate, the heel cord will shorten more, and the cycle will continue. Heel cords rarely gain length long term once the patient is discharged from the rehabilitation setting, and one must consider the family/home situation. Heel buildups on the affected side are used to bring the tibia into 90 degrees. Buildups of 1 to 1½ inches are not uncommon. Remember to balance the opposite shoe. If a patient is on the border between different orthotic components, it is best to choose the more stable orthosis. The use of trial orthoses during evaluation is invaluable and helpful initially as the patient improves, requiring less or no orthosis. A three-point pressure orthosis for the knee, such as a Swedish knee cage (Figure 34-4), is also a valuable training orthosis and, in the case of some post-CVA patients, is used daily when the degree of recurvatum exceeds the patient's ability to control the force. The stirrup, the metal attachment to the patient's shoe, must be firm and extend under the sole and heel to the heads of the metatarsals. Although this adds weight to the orthosis, it is necessary to transmit knee-stabilizing forces. Stirrups attached under the heel will only allow undesirable motion and will not provide the required stability (Case Study 34-2).

Paralytic Spine

Many neuropathic diagnoses affect the spinal column. Spinal muscle atrophy, teraplegia, myelomeningocele, and Duchenne's muscular dystrophy can all require orthotic intervention. Although materials, padding/no padding, trim lines, length of time used, and optional area openings can vary with different conditions, most spinal stabilizing orthoses are TLSOs. Orthoses used for postsurgical stabilization tend to be of more rigid material to support the healing spine. The paralytic spine that is not surgically stabilized can have either a flexible or rigid curvature. An orthosis for a patient with a rigid curvature is used to avoid further deformity and differs from that used by the patient with a flexible curvature. If the curve is flexible, the orthosis will be used to hold some of the correction that can be obtained. Patients with paralytic spine deformity are usually casted for custom orthoses, and although non–weight-bearing supine casts can greatly reduce the curve, many

CASE STUDY 34-2 ■ D. M.

D. M. is a 58 year old who had a left CVA, resulting in a right hemiplegia almost 2 years ago. She is being evaluated at the request of her physician because of increased knee pain and poor standing balance. D.M. was fitted with a plastic AFO fixed at 90 degrees 14 months ago. She is wearing the orthosis, but the heel will not stay in her shoe. Evaluation shows that the patient lacks 15 degrees from getting the foot to neutral (in plantarflexion), has no active dorsiflexion or plantarflexion, and has a fair minus knee extension and flexion. She also walks with the aid of a quad cane and has 10 degrees of genu recurvatum and slight genu varum at midstance. Her goal was to walk with less

pain and to be more stable. D. M. was fitted with bilateral upright, double-adjustable locked ankle joints with long tongue stirrups and a 1½-inch heel buildup (Figure 34-5). The left shoe was built up 1½ inches in the heel and sole to balance the right shoe (Figure 34-6). A Swedish knee orthosis also was used initially to help train the patient and be a positive hyperextension control. Although the double-adjustable ankle joint does give total flexibility to change the angle, a 90-degree posterior stop also can be used. Patients who lack this much range of motion provide an "anatomical" anterior stop.

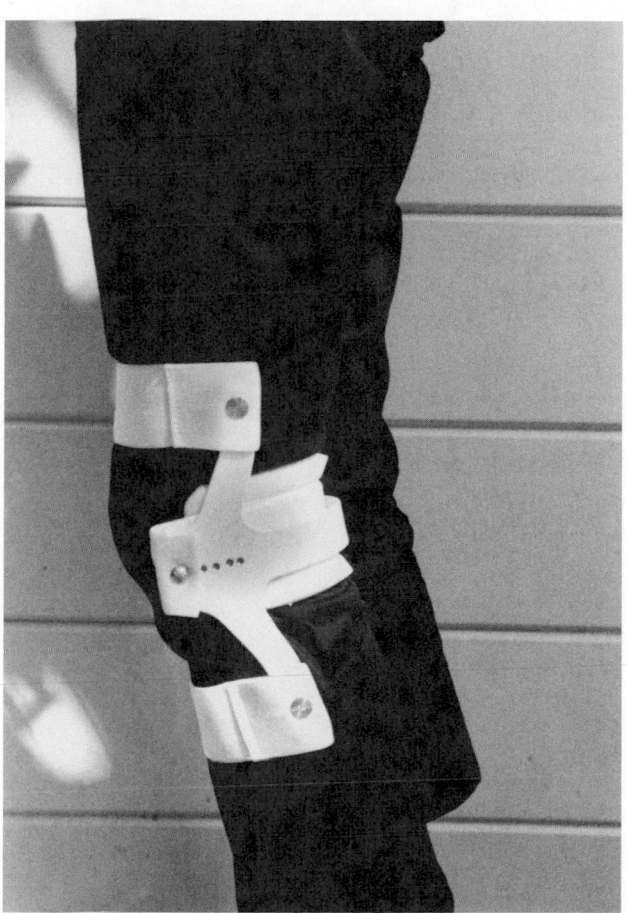

FIGURE 34-4 ■ Prefabricated three-point pressure knee orthosis (Swedish knee cage) to control genu recurvatum.

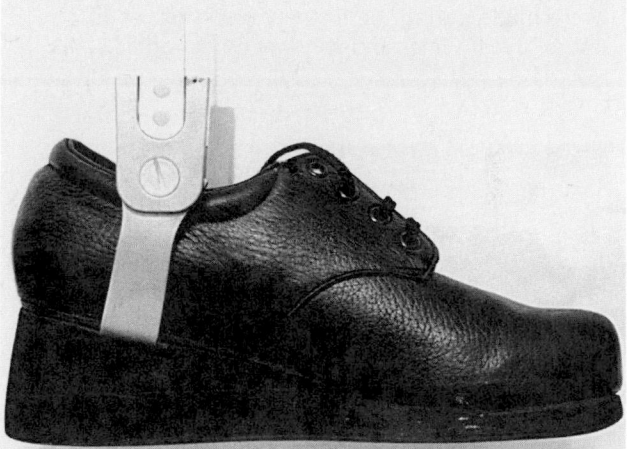

FIGURE 34-5 ■ Shoe modification with double-adjustable ankle.

Plastazote. Fabrication and fitting of these orthoses requires an experienced orthotist and adherence to detail. Establishing the distal and proximal trim lines of the orthosis will require a fine balancing act between providing enough length to support the spine without breaking down the skin in accomplishing that goal. Several clinic visits are necessary to obtain the desired outcome (Case Study 34-3).

Spastic Diplegic Cerebral Palsy

The goals of orthotic intervention in the cerebral palsy patient are to control tone, prevent contractures, and provide a secondary support after a surgical procedure.[8] Although it is not within the scope of this chapter to describe and discuss the current treatment protocol for cerebral palsy, orthotic intervention varies from region to region. What is clear is that careful evaluation, clinical experience, treating each patient individually, and a cohesive rehabilitation team are critical factors in successful orthotic intervention. As a general rule, the orthosis used to prevent contracture should be different from the orthosis used for ambulation. Some of the new designs incorporate modules that can key into each other or be used separately. This feature allows flexibility, assists in donning, especially in the spastic patient, and meets several treatment objectives. Modular articulating

patients will not tolerate the pressure once in the upright sitting position. Orthotic intervention usually has one or more of the following goals: improved sitting balance, support of surgical stabilization, prevention of further spinal deformity, and use as an assistive positional device for better utilization of head and upper extremities and improved respiratory function. Most TLSOs for these patients are total circumferential designs that use rigid materials (polypropylene) to less rigid materials (polyethylene) to combination padding with a rigid/semirigid frame to the heat-formable

CASE STUDY 34-3 ■ S. G.

S. G. is a 13 year old with spastic cerebral palsy with involvement of all four extremities. She is nonambulatory with significant scoliosis. Her hip range of motion is from minus 25 degrees to 135 degrees of flexion. S. G. is fully dependent and lacks upper-extremity use. The goal of orthotic intervention was to prevent further deformity, maintain the thoracic and lumbar column for internal organs, and provide trunk stability for seating balance in her wheelchair. She was fitted with a custom TLSO fabricated from a cast impression (Figure 34-7). It has ¼-inch padding with a polypropylene outer layer, which has been modified over bony prominences for skin tolerance. S. G. wears her TLSO not only while seated in her chair, but also in bed. Frequent checks of the skin were made during the first few weeks of use to establish trim lines and window type modifications.

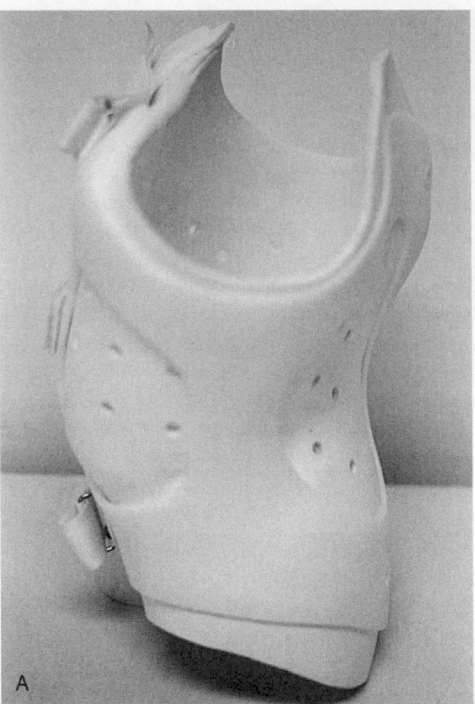

A

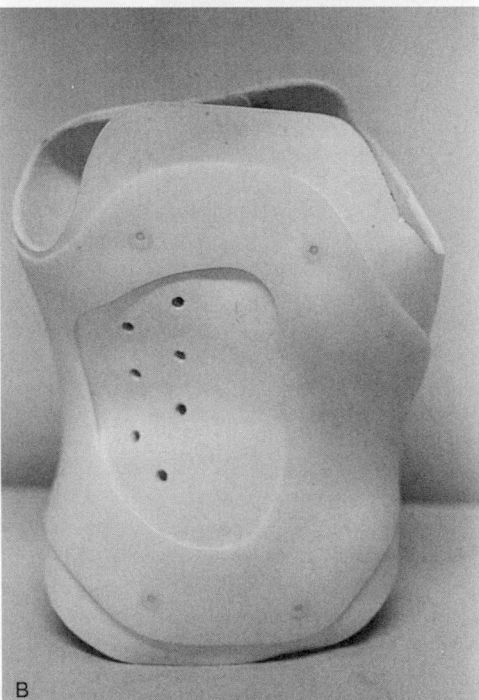

B

FIGURE 34-7 ■ Thoracolumbosacral orthosis with anterior opening. **A,** Lateral view. **B,** Posterior view. Cutouts in rigid plastic to inner soft foam are for expansion and comfort.

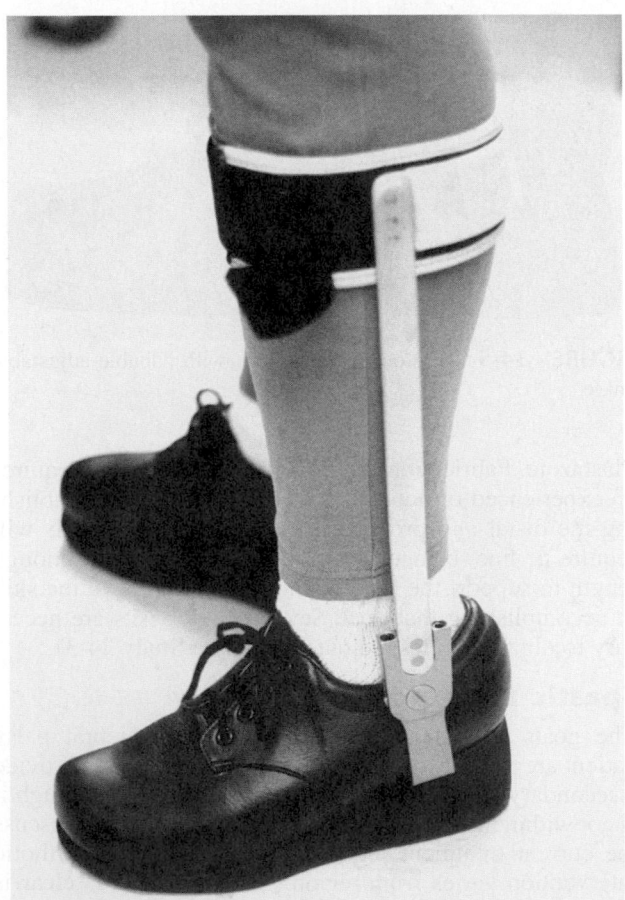

FIGURE 34-6 ■ Left double-upright, double-adjustable ankle-foot orthosis with balancing right buildup.

joints with various settings and functions to use with thermoplastic orthoses greatly increase the options that are available today. With the goals of orthotic intervention stated earlier, total-contact–type orthoses are generally the desired option. As with any total-contact orthosis and hypersensitive or hyposensitive skin, a cautious balance between correction/holding and skin tolerance must be reached. The fitting and follow-up of these types of orthoses requires experience, knowledge, and patience. Combinations of padding, wedging, straps, and heat relief are often necessary to enable the patient to wear the orthosis for a significant time on a daily basis. The spastic diplegic cerebral palsy patient relies heavily on her or his orthosis and wears it out faster than most other orthotic patients if, as in the case of a child, she or he does not outgrow it first. This should be considered in the design and fabrication (Case Study 34-4).

CASE STUDY 34-4 ■ R. B.

R. B. is a 41 year old with spastic diplegia cerebral palsy. She has tight heel cords bilaterally, minus 5 degrees. Plantarflexion strength is fair plus, and dorsiflexion is fair bilaterally. The patient has 5 to 7 degrees of varus in the calcaneus. The left lower extremity is asymptomatic. The right side has pain in the mid-femur and at the knee. She has a bilateral genu valgum deformity of 5 to 7 degrees (Figure 34-8, A). Range of motion at the knees is full, and strength of the quadriceps and hamstrings rate as good. Her hips are normal except for some internal rotation; leg lengths are equal and sensation is good. Because the right lower extremity was painful at the knee and ankle (see

Figure 34-8, B), the patient was fitted with an AFO that extended medially and proximally to the medial tibial condyle; ankle joints that had a posterior adjustment to limit plantarflexion; and a medial heel wedge and heel buildup of $^3/_8$ inch. The ankle was fitted with a submalleolar orthosis that fitted inside the AFO (see Figure 34-8, C and D). The submalleolar orthosis controlled enough pronation of the ankle along with the medial heel wedging and exerted a varus force at the knee (see Figure 34-8, E). The heel buildup reduced the posteriorly directed force from midstance to toe off. The patient's symptoms were reduced, allowing her to be more active (see Table 34-1).

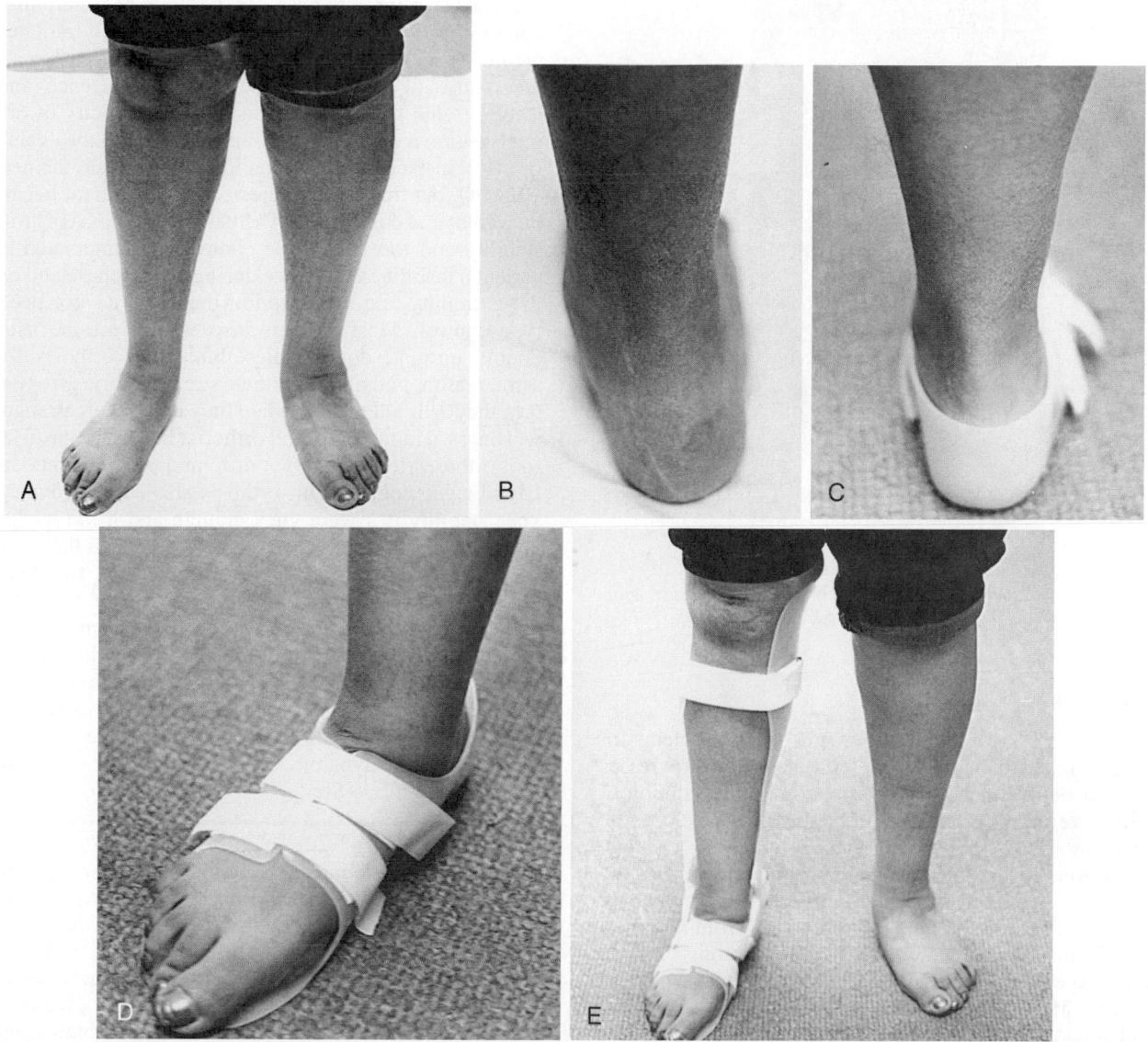

FIGURE 34-8 ■ **A,** Painful right genu valgus and pronation. **B,** Posterior view of right ankle. **C** and **D,** Client wearing submalleolar orthosis with pronation corrected. **E,** Patient in submalleolar ankle-foot orthosis extended to knee to control genu valgus.

CASE STUDY 34-5 ■ D. K.

D. K. is a 38-year-old female that is a mother of three young boys and works outside the home. She was diagnosed with multiple sclerosis at the age of 30. Until 4 years ago she was managing the symptoms with medication and having minimal ambulatory problems. With the birth of her son, she had to cease use of medication, and the symptoms have since reoccurred and weakness has increased. At age 36 her symptoms had increased and she was limiting her activity outside the home because of safety issues—she was falling and unstable. She was evaluated at that point and was fitted with a right ankle-foot orthosis as she had foot drop and knee instability, as well as the inability to recover if she caught her toe. A prefabricated graphite ankle-foot orthosis was fit to the patient (Figure 34-9). D. K. now has toe clearance during swing phase and dynamic knee extension during stance phase. Shortly after utilization of the orthosis she was able to walk safely on uneven ground and walk down stairs step over step for the first time in 3 years.

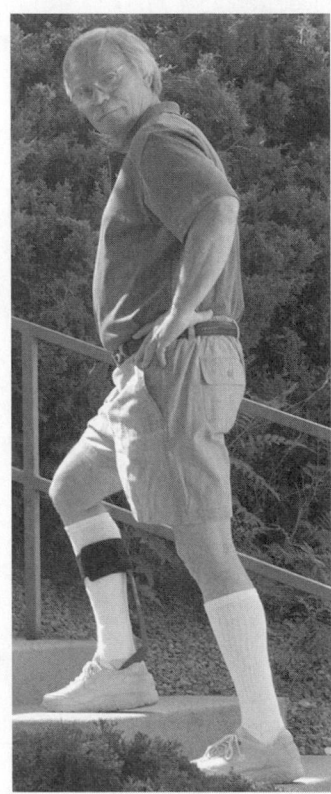

FIGURE 34-9 ■ AFO provides stance phase advantages in addition to swing phase. (Courtesy of Otto Bock Healthcare.)

Multiple Sclerosis

This upper motor neuron disease creates many problems for this neurological patient. As multiple sclerosis progresses and further demyelination occurs, increased interruption of normal nerve impulses creates problems of muscle control, vision, balance, sensation, and mental functions. Orthotic considerations for the multiple sclerosis patient vary as the patient's symptoms fade, reoccur and vary over the years of the disease. Therefore clinical pictures vary from month to month. Fatigue plays a major role in the symptoms, and the patient's expectation and willingness to use orthotic devices ebbs accordingly. The typical clinical picture is one of general weakness in the lower extremity, obtaining progressively lower muscle test scores as one goes from proximal to distal. One extremity is usually weaker than the other, albeit only slightly. Multiple sclerosis typically strikes patients in their late 20s to early 30s, when life activities are at their height. Typical patient reaction is reluctance to use any form of ambulatory aid or orthosis until safety is a major issue. Then, patients and family usually seek help when falls become more frequent. Toe clearance during swing phase and knee stability and push-off in stance phase are the most common problems, and although not entirely unilateral in nature, the contralateral side is slightly stronger. Because of the nature of symptom fade and reoccurrence and the increase with fatigue, the weight and simplicity of orthotic intervention must be a major consideration in the evaluation. In many instances, the evaluation will indicate the need for a KAFO, but this will be rejected by the patient because of its weight and complexity. The benefit of the KAFO for knee stability and foot and ankle control is counteracted by the patient's inability to advance during swing phase and control the extremity and a perception that they do not need that type control. Most patients also will reject the use of a double upright, double-adjustable metal orthosis for the same reason, and although their strength varies from day to day, they will judge need when they are at their strength, not weakness. Traditionally the orthotist has used plastic ankle-foot orthoses to control foot drop and provide some medial lateral ankle control. This orthosis also could provide some knee stability if it were thick enough and if the medial and lateral trim lines advanced anteriorly past the malleoli; however, because this anterior force stops the center of gravity's anterior motion at midstance, again, most patients reject this type of orthosis. Recent development of a prefabricated ankle-foot orthosis made of graphite with preimpregnated resin and catalyst has met the needs of these patients (see Figure 34-1). This ultralight orthosis fits inside the patient shoe. It will provide toe clearance during swing phase and some dynamic knee stability and push off during stance phase (Case Study 34-5).

SUMMARY

All orthoses create a force system. It is important to understand and integrate the appropriate force to achieve the desired outcome of intervention. A thorough initial evaluation and knowledge of the multiple orthotic options available are vital to reaching treatment goals. There has been a dramatic increase in material technology, far greater access to orthotics, and a much wider range of indications for orthotic intervention. This should challenge the rehabilitation team to establish measurable goals, and then to develop new goals leading from those treatment interventions with the most effective outcomes. This evidence-based practice will help provide better service for future patients.

REFERENCES

1 Otto J: Playing the numbers game: how demographics data impact orthotics and prosthetics, *O and P Business News*, January 2000, pp 1, 31-35.

2. Michael JW, Bowker JH: Prosthetics/orthotics research for the twenty-first century, *J Prosthet Orthot* 6:4, 1994.

3. Kaufman KR, Irby SE, Mathewson JW et al: Energy-efficient knee-ankle-foot-orthosis: a case study, *J Prosthet Orthot* 8:79-85, 1996.

4. Fish D: Characteristic gait patterns in neuromuscular pathologies, *J Prosthet Orthot* 9:163-167, 1997.

5. Freehafer A: Orthotics in spinal cord injuries. In *Atlas of orthotics*, St. Louis, 1985, CV Mosby, pp 287-297.

6. Waters R, Garland D, Montgomery J: Orthotic prescription for stroke and head injury. In *Atlas of orthotics*, St. Louis, 1985, CV Mosby, pp 270-286.

7. Yamamoto S, Ebina M, Miyazaki, Kubota T: Development of a new ankle-foot orthosis with dorsiflexion assist: I. Desirable characteristics of ankle-foot orthoses for hemiplegic patients, *J Prosthet Orthot* 9:174-179, 1997.

8. Bunch W, Dvonch V: Cerebral palsy. In *Atlas of orthotics*, St. Louis, 1985, CV Mosby, pp 259-269.

CHAPTER 35

Cardiovascular and Pulmonary Health and Fitness in Populations with Neurological Disorders

Marilyn MacKay-Lyons, PhD, PT

KEY WORDS

aerobic training
deconditioning
exercise tolerance
rating of perceived exertion

OBJECTIVES

At the end of the chapter, the student/therapist will be able to:
1. Explain the physiological principles related to cardiovascular responses to exercise testing.
2. Discuss the evidence behind cardiovascular fitness and describe the factors that contribute to the deconditioned state in adults with neurological disorders.
3. Explain the adaptive responses to aerobic training in populations with neurological disorders and the factors underlying these responses.
4. Discuss general guidelines when designing exercise programs to improve cardiovascular health and fitness.

INTRODUCTION

The cardiopulmonary health of individuals with residual movement dysfunction after a neurological insult has only recently become a topic of interest in neurorehabilitation. In traditional practice, the state of the neuromuscular system preoccupied the attention of clinicians in the quest to optimize neurological recovery. Most interventions were based on strategies to improve the capacity of that system—an approach that has met with limited success in terms of restoring functional independence. It is now becoming clear that recovery cannot be explained solely on the basis of improved neuromuscular function. For example, Roth et al[1] determined that less than one third of the variance in functional limitations after a stroke can be explained by the extent of neurological impairment.

The state of affairs in neurorehabilitation over the past decade has been somewhat paradoxical. Evidence has accumulated indicating that many people with neurological disabilities are woefully deconditioned. There has been widespread acknowledgment of the central role that aerobic exercise plays in improving cardiopulmonary health and fitness. Further, application of the principles of exercise physiology in cardiac rehabilitation has been widely endorsed. Yet neurorehabilitation clinicians have been observed to practice without full knowledge of their patients' cardiac status or without monitoring heart rate (HR) and blood pressure (BP).[2] Moreover, there is evidence to suggest that patients with neurological insults have not been challenged enough in therapy to induce the metabolic stress needed to enhance their cardiopulmonary fitness.[3] A troubling explanation offered for these observations is that clinicians lack either an understanding or an appreciation of the basic physiological principles of exercise.[4,5]

Fortunately, attention has now turned to the introduction of interventions that encompass the neuromuscular, cardiovascular, and pulmonary systems and promote a more holistic approach to neurorehabilitation. The challenge of improving cardiopulmonary health and fitness in these populations is not trivial. For individuals with chronic conditions, fitness is affected by a host of interacting influences such as the location and extent of the lesion, the presence of comorbidities (particularly cardiovascular disease), and the premorbid activity level. To complicate matters further, testing and training protocols for individuals with compromised motor and postural control need to be tailored to ensure safety and effectiveness.

This chapter begins with an overview of physiological principles related to cardiovascular responses to exercise testing. A summary of the evidence of cardiopulmonary fitness levels in adults with neurological disabilities is followed by a description of factors that contribute to the deconditioned state. Possible mechanisms responsible for reduced exercise capacity are then reviewed. Adaptive responses to aerobic training in patients with neurological conditions are examined and factors underlying these responses are examined. The chapter closes with a summary of guidelines for the design of exercise programs that can be used to improve cardiopulmonary health and fitness. Appendix 35-A at the end of this chapter clearly identifies the meanings of the abbreviations used throughout the chapter.

PHYSIOLOGICAL RESPONSES TO EXERCISE

At rest the human body consumes roughly 3.5 ml/kg/min of oxygen (O_2) or 1 metabolic equivalent (MET).[6] In the resting state, skeletal muscle activity accounts for less than 20% of the body's total energy expenditure; the brain, comprising only 2% of body weight, also consumes 20% of the available O_2.[7] Activities at rest such as breathing and contracting of the heart can be sustained indefinitely because the power demands of these activities are met by the rate of energy turnover. In other words, these activities occur well below

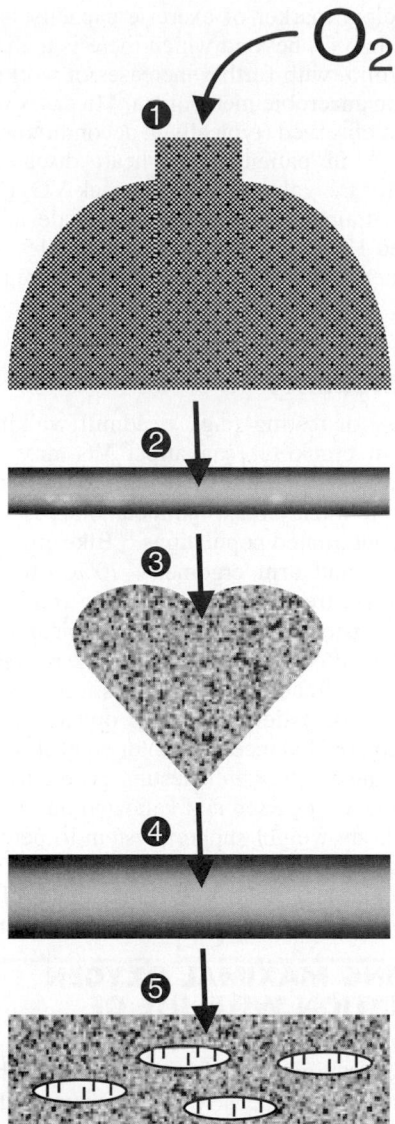

FIGURE 35-1 ■ Diagrammatic representations of the components of the O_2 transport system. (*1*) $\supseteq$ During inspiration O_2 from the air is delivered to the alveolar gas space by the process of respiration. (*2*) $\not\subset$ Transport of O_2 diffuses across the blood-gas barrier into the pulmonary capillary blood where almost all of the O_2 is bound to hemoglobin. (*3*) $\subset$ The heart acts as a pump and (*4*) $\subseteq$ the vascular system acts as the plumbing to transport O_2 to the various tissues, including the exercising muscle (*5*) ε where it diffuses from the red blood cells into the mitochondria within the myocytes. Reduced conductance of any component impairs O_2 transport whereas improved conductance of any component augments O_2 transport.

the *critical power* of the muscles, defined as the maximal rate of work that can be endured indefinitely.[8] Any physical activity beyond the resting state requires more O_2; the increase is dependent on the intensity of the effort involved. The rise in metabolism relies on O_2 transport by the pulmonary and circulatory systems and O_2 utilization by the active skeletal, cardiac, and respiratory muscles to convert chemical potential energy to mechanical energy.[9] The components of the O_2 transport system are outlined in Figure 35-1.

Selective distribution of the increased blood flow to regions with heightened metabolic demands—the working muscles—is due to local vasodilation mediated mainly by metabolites acting on the vascular smooth muscle (e.g., carbon dioxide [CO_2], hydrogen ions [H^+], nitric oxide, potassium ions, adenosine) and vasoconstriction in tissues with low metabolic demands.[10] Blood flow to other vascular beds either is unchanged or decreases (e.g., renal and splanchnic bed) through active vasoconstriction resulting primarily from increased sympathetic discharge. Cerebral autoregulation maintains regional and total cerebral blood flow and normal tissue oxygenation over a wide range of BPs[11]; thus, cerebral blood flow and O_2 delivery during exercise either remain stable[12,13] or increase slightly.[14,15] As exercise intensity increases, systolic BP (SBP) increases markedly while diastolic BP (DBP) either remains unchanged or lowers slightly, resulting in a moderate increase in mean arterial pressure.[16]

Extraction of O_2 from the muscle capillary blood to mitochondria is dependent on an adequate O_2 diffusion gradient. During a progressive increase in workload, the arterial hemoglobin saturation and arterial O_2 content remain relatively constant, whereas the venous O_2 content decreases substantially as a result of increased O_2 extraction in the active muscles.[17] As the metabolic rate rises, the minute ventilation (which equals respiratory rate by tidal volume) increases to remove CO_2 and to regulate pH balance of the active muscles. At low-intensity exercise, ventilation (mainly tidal volume) increases in a linear manner relative to the volume of O_2 use (VO_2) and CO_2 production (VCO_2). Above the critical power, the energy demand of the muscle exceeds the capacity of the aerobic process to supply energy for muscle contraction; the additional energy is supplied by the anaerobic glycolytic system.

During more intense exercise, ventilation is extremely variable among individuals; the respiratory rate increases without a substantial change in tidal volume.[16] The point at which the rate of glycolysis exceeds that of oxidative phosphorylation is called the *anaerobic threshold* (which approximates the ventilatory threshold or lactate threshold).[18] Pyruvic acid is converted to lactic acid, which completely dissociates to lactate and H^+, resulting in a rise in blood lactate levels and a fall in intramuscular pH. Exercise-induced muscular fatigue is due to the exponential accumulation of lactate and a drop in intramuscular pH, with negative effects on the actin-myosin turnover rate, enzyme activities, and excitation-contraction coupling.

Maximal oxygen consumption (VO_2max) is defined as the highest O_2 intake an individual can attain during physical work.[16] The Fick equation describes the relationship between cardiovascular function and VO_2max:

$$VO_2\text{max} = Q\text{max} \times \text{a-}vO_{2\text{diff}}\text{max},$$

where Qmax is the maximal cardiac output and a-$vO_{2\text{diff}}$max is the maximal arteriovenous O_2 difference.[19] Given that Qmax equals the product of maximal heart rate (HRmax) and maximal stroke volume (SVmax),

$$VO_2\text{max} = \text{HRmax} \times \text{SVmax} \times \text{a-}vO_{2\text{diff}}\text{max}.$$

Thus, VO_2max reflects both O_2 transport to the tissues and O_2 utilization by the tissues. Increases in VO_2 during exercise are due to increases in both cardiac output and a-vO$_{2diff}$, with HR and stroke volume (SV) increasing progressively over the lower third of the workload range. Thereafter, HR continues to increase while SV remains essentially constant,[20,21] resulting, at maximal effort, in a cardiac output three to six times greater than baseline levels. An increase in SV (50% over resting volume) is due to enhanced myocardial contractility and increased venous return resulting from compression of the veins by contracting muscles and reduced intrathoracic pressure.[22] At low-intensity exercise, the increase in HR is mainly due to decreased vagal tone, but, as exercise intensifies, sympathetic stimulation and circulating catecholamines play a greater role, yielding, at maximal workloads, a rise in HR 200% to 300% above the resting level.[23]

MEASUREMENT OF CARDIOPULMONARY FITNESS

Exercise (aerobic) capacity is the principal determinant of the ability to sustain the power requirements of repetitive physical activity. VO$_2$max is generally accepted as the definitive index of exercise capacity and cardiopulmonary fitness.[24] VO$_2$max is a relatively stable measurement; variability of repeated measures of VO$_2$max has been reported to be 2% to 4%[25] or 0.2 l/min.[26] Accurate determination of VO$_2$max requires (1) adequate duration and work intensity by at least 50% of total muscle mass, (2) independence from motivation or skill of the subject, and (3) controlled environmental conditions.[19] Also, because test performance is sensitive to time of day, the time of repeat testing should be consistent.

Before testing, a 2- to 3-minute warmup of slow treadmill walking on level grade or unloaded pedaling raises the metabolic rate twofold above resting,[27] preventing excessive local muscle fatigue from occurring before VO$_2$max is attained.[28] The intensity of exercise can be increased in a continuous, progressive manner (i.e., step or ramp protocol) or, less commonly, in a discontinuous, progressive manner (i.e., subject rests between stages). Throughout testing, continuous monitoring of the electrocardiogram and periodic monitoring of BP are essential. The optimal duration of a graded exercise test is 8 to 12 minutes, with testing terminated when the subject can no longer generate the required power, is limited by symptoms, or is unable to continue safely.[29]

Variables of interest during exercise testing include VO$_2$max expressed in absolute terms (liters of O$_2$ per minute) or relative to body mass (milliliters of O$_2$ per kilogram of body weight per minute), MET level, percent of predicted HRmax, respiratory exchange ratio (RER; ratio of VO$_2$ to CO$_2$), peak power, minute ventilation, tidal volume, respiratory rate, and rating of perceived exertion (RPE) according to the Borg scale.[30] Because there is considerable variability in HRmax among healthy individuals, the percent of predicted HRmax attained is not a robust indicator of exercise capacity.[31] Similarly, because both total exercise time and peak exercise intensity or power attained (i.e., peak treadmill speed and grade or peak power on bike) are dependent on the test protocol, neither is a reliable measure of exercise capacity.[32,33] In addition, noninvasive estimation of the anaerobic threshold by identifying the point of nonlinear increases in minute ventilation and VCO$_2$ can be highly subjective and, thus, unreliable.[34]

The principal marker of exercise capacity is attainment of a plateau in VO$_2$ beyond which there is a change of less than 100 ml/min, with further increases in workload dependent solely on anaerobic metabolism.[29] In cases where a VO$_2$ plateau is not observed (typically in deconditioned or elderly individuals or in patients with heart disease), the preferred term for the value obtained is peak VO$_2$ (VO$_2$peak).[35] Criteria for attainment of VO$_2$peak include achieving the age-predicted HRmax, RER in excess of 1.15, minute ventilation greater than the predicted maximal voluntary ventilation, tidal volume greater than 90% of the inspiratory capacity, and obvious patient exhaustion.[28]

Testing Modality

The modality of testing (e.g., treadmill walking, cycling, stepping, arm cranking) can affect VO$_2$max values. The treadmill has the greatest potential to recruit sufficient muscle mass to elicit a maximal metabolic response, particularly in deconditioned populations.[19] Bike ergometry yields 85% to 90%, and arm ergometry 70%, of the VO$_2$max achieved with a treadmill.[19] Ideally, the mode of exercise should be consistent with the patient's typical activity. Thus the treadmill is often preferred because the pattern of muscle activation during treadmill walking is similar to that of most mobility tasks. In patients with neuromuscular conditions, however, impaired balance and motor control often preclude the use of standard treadmill testing protocols. To resolve this limitation, we devised and validated an exercise protocol using a body weight support system to permit safe and valid testing of VO$_2$max early after stroke.[36] For subjects with paraplegia, tests with wheelchair treadmills are more functionally relevant than those using arm ergometry.

PREDICTING MAXIMAL OXYGEN CONSUMPTION WITH USE OF SUBMAXIMAL EXERCISE TESTS

Although submaximal tests do not measure the systemic response, they are inexpensive to administer and have a low risk of adverse events. The essentially linear relationship between VO$_2$ and HR permits the estimation of VO$_2$max from HR measurements taken during submaximal exercise. For example, for healthy people the HR increases approximately 50 beats per uptake of 1 liter of O$_2$, independent of sex and body size.[37] For unfit individuals and patients with cardiac impairment, the increases in HR are greater per liter, except for patients taking beta blockers, who demonstrate blunting of the HR response throughout exercise. The Åstrand-Ryhming nomogram is often used to predict VO$_2$max from submaximal HR.[38] The HR-VO$_2$ relationship is independent of the exercise protocol. However, HR, unlike VO$_2$max, is markedly affected by many stresses (e.g., dehydration, changes in body temperature, acute starvation), resulting in substantial error and inaccurate VO$_2$max estimations.[19] In fact, discrepancies between estimated and measured VO$_2$max in individuals with low exercise capacity can be as high as 25%.[39]

FITNESS LEVELS IN POPULATIONS WITH NEUROLOGICAL DISORDERS

Documentation of exercise capacity in populations with neurological disorders has been hindered by the lack of testing protocols that can safely and effectively accommo-

TABLE 35-1 ■ Exercise Capacity in Common Neurological Conditions

DIAGNOSIS	TIME SINCE DIAGNOSIS	NO.	SEX (% MEN)	AGE (Y)	TEST MODALITY	VO$_2$PEAK (ML/KG/MIN)	VO$_2$PEAK (% NORMAL)
Subacute stroke	15 ± 7 days[40]	12	100	59 ± 10	Cycle ergometer	8.3 ± 2	NR
	26 ± 9 days[41]	29	76	65 ± 14	Treadmill	14.4 ± 5	61
	29 ± 10 days[42]	17	76	61 ± 16	Semirecumbent ergometer	14.7 ± 4	51
	76 ± 3 days[43]	100	56	70 ± 10	Cycle ergometer	11.4 ± 3	NR
	120 ± 90 days[44]	8	100	52 ± 10	Cycle ergometer	16.1 ± 4	NR
Chronic stroke	>6 months[45]	42	55	56 ± 12	Cycle ergometer	15.8 ± 5	NR
	>6 months[46]	26	85	66 ± 9	Treadmill	15.6 ± 4	NR
	10 months[47]	30	100	54	Cycle ergometer	17.7 ± 4	NR
	>12 months[48]	63	59	6 ± 9	Cycle ergometer	22.0 ± 5	NR
Multiple sclerosis	3 ± 5 years[49]	10	40	39 ± 6	Arm-leg ergometer	39.0 ± 8	87
	7 ± 1 years[50]	46	33	40 ± 2	Arm-leg ergometer	25.2 ± 1	79
Paraplegia	102 ± 62 days[51]	80	75	41 ± 15	Wheelchair ergometer	14.7 ± 5	NR
	6 months[52]	39	100	30 ± 1	Arm ergometer	19.4 ± 1	69
	>3 years[53]	46	100	33 ± 9	Wheelchair ergometer	23.9 ± 5	NR
	7 ± 5 years[54]	6	100	36 ± 10	Arm ergometer	23.7 ± 3	NR
	21 ± 8 years[55]	9	100	30 ± 7	Arm ergometer	30.5 ± 8	71
Tetraplegia	108 ± 67 days[51]	22	74	39 ± 13	Wheelchair ergometer	12.1 ± 4	NR
	7 ± 6 years[56]	8	100	24 ± 4	Arm ergometer	12.1 ± 1	NR
Traumatic brain injury	17 ± 17 months[57]	36	78	32 ± 10	Cycle ergometer	22.3 ± 9	65
	2 ± 4 years[58]	40	73	33 ± 11	Treadmill	23.5 ± 7	NR
	NR[59]	14	93	29 ± 2	Treadmill	31.3 ± 2	67
Parkinson's disease	6 ± 3 years[60]	16	81	54 ± 5	Cycle ergometer	27.6 ±5	93
	9 ± 4 years[61]	20	65	64 ± 7	Cycle ergometer	22.0 ± 7	100
Postpoliomyelitis syndrome	11 ± 8 years[62]	68	34	53 ± 11	Cycle ergometer (n = 37), arm ergometer (n = 31)	23.1 ± 5 / 15.3 ± 5	63 / 65
	11-45 years[63]	20	50	43 ± 6	Cycle ergometer	17.7 ± 6	73
	46 ± 3 years[64]	32	50	50 ± 10	Cycle ergometer	20.5 ± 7	74
Guillain-Barré syndrome	3 years[65]	1	100	57	Leg-arm ergometer	27	NR

NR, Not reported; *VO$_2$peak % normal*, peak oxygen consumption expressed as a percentage of normative values.

date the motor and balance disturbances common to these populations. Not surprisingly, the limited evidence to date suggests that most individuals with neurological disabilities are significantly deconditioned. A summary of VO$_2$peak data from studies of common neurological conditions is presented in Table 35-1.[40-65] Variability in the results is due to a multitude of factors, including differences in testing protocols, as discussed in the previous section, and differences in subject characteristics; discussion of these points is found in the following section.

Impact of Low Fitness Levels on Health of Populations With Neurological Disorders

People with high fitness levels use only a small fraction of the *physiological fitness reserve*[66] of the cardiovascular, respiratory, and neuromuscular systems to respond to the metabolic challenge of activities of daily living (ADLs).[67,68] Thus, small declines in exercise capacity may not be noticeable in carrying out daily activities. In contrast, relatively minor reductions in capacity can substantially influence ADL performance of deconditioned individuals. Light instrumental ADLs require approximately 10.5 ml of O$_2$/kg/min (3 METs), whereas more strenuous activities have metabolic

costs of about 17.5 ml/kg/min (5 METs).[69] Cress and Meyer[70] reported that the VO$_2$peak of 20 ml/kg/min is needed for older adults to meet the physiological demands of independent living. From the data presented in Table 35-1, it is evident that many people living with neurological disabilities (particularly stroke, tetraplegia, and postpoliomyelitis syndrome) do not have the level of fitness required for the more strenuous ADLs and independent living. Moreover, relative exercise capacities (expressed as a percentage of normative values) associated with the disabilities in Table 35-1, with the exception of Parkinson's disease, are of concern, given that VO$_2$peak values less than 84% of normal are considered pathological.[16]

For individuals with neurological disabilities, the minimum VO$_2$ requirements for ADLs are actually greater than the previously mentioned levels because of the increased energy requirements resulting from gross motor inefficiencies and other related factors.[71-73] In other words, the percentage of VO$_2$peak required for activity at a fixed submaximal workload (termed *fractional utilization*) is increased. When the anaerobic threshold is exceeded prematurely and lactate accumulation is accelerated, accomplishment of low intensity ADLs is unsustainable for extended periods and achievement of mid- to upper-intensity ADLs is virtually impossible. Moreover, the combination of poor exercise capacity and elevated energy demands results in diminished reserves to support other activities. For example, in the case of people with postpoliomyelitis syndrome, the energy costs of walking are about 40% higher than for healthy peers and are highly correlated to lower extremity muscle strength.[74] Thus, in the calculation of fractional utilization for walking, the numerator (VO_2 during walking) is increased and the denominator (VO_2peak) is decreased; hence fractional utilization is substantially increased.

The population of individuals who have had a stroke creates the largest consumer group needing rehabilitation services.[75] This group has received the most attention in the literature in regard to functional capacity. Exercise capacities documented in this population are low—from 8.3 ml/kg/min in the subacute period[40] to 17.7 ml/kg/min in the chronic period.[44] As much as 75% to 88% of VO_2peak (almost twice that of the healthy control subjects) is required to perform household chores[76] and $1\frac{1}{2}$ to three times the VO_2 levels of healthy controls are needed to walk on level ground.[71,77,78] Not surprisingly, up to 70% of patients complain of fatigue after stroke[79] and rate poor energy levels ahead of mobility limitations, pain, emotional reactions, sleep disturbances, and social isolation as the area of greatest personal concern.[80]

In addition to contributing to reduced ADL performance and increased fatigability, low fitness levels are associated with higher mortality. Exercise capacity has been reported to be an independent predictor of mortality among persons with coronary artery disease (CAD), a comorbidity prevalent in some neurological populations.[81,82] Those with a VO_2peak <21 ml/kg/min are classified as the high mortality group and greater than 35 ml/kg/min as the excellent survival group.[83] Thus, the importance of determining an individual's VO_2peak cannot be understressed. Individuals who are being encouraged or are internally motivated to perform beyond their capacity and beyond the capabilities of the interaction of multiple systems are in a high-risk category. Conversely, individuals who are undermotivated or depressed and are performing below their capacity can be trained to self-monitor, which empowers them to reach goals that are safe and have the potential to improve the quality of their lives.

Factors Affecting Fitness Levels in Populations with Neurological Disorders

To identify appropriate measures to improve fitness levels in populations with neurological disorders, the myriad of factors at play that contribute to the deconditioned state must be considered. A useful conceptual framework to discuss the interaction of these factors is the International Classification of Functioning, Disability, and Health (ICF)[84] (see Chapter 1). The ICF uses a biopsychosocial approach to organize factors related to the health conditions into two components: (1) personal and environmental contextual factors and (2) functioning and disability, which are further subdivided into components of body functions and structures, activity, and participation (Figure 35-2). By applying the ICF framework, the complexity of interacting influences on cardio-

International Classification of Functioning, Disability and Health

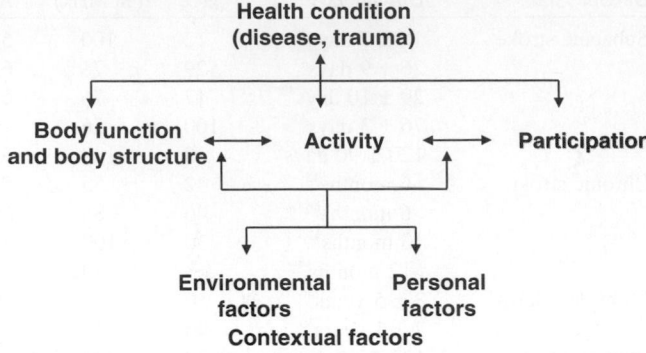

FIGURE 35-2 ■ Interaction of the various components of the ICF. The ICF is a conceptual framework that uses a biopsychosocial approach to organize factors related to the health conditions into two components: (1) personal and environmental contextual factors and (2) functioning and disability, which are further subdivided into components of body functions and structures, activity, and participation.

vascular and pulmonary health and fitness becomes more understandable.

Personal and Environmental Contextual Factors

For both able-bodied and disabled people, personal contextual factors contributing to individual differences in exercise capacity include age, sex, and lifestyle habits.

Age

A decline in VO_2max of approximately 1% per year (0.4-0.5 ml/kg/min/y) occurs between 25 and 75 years of age.[85] In accordance with the Fick equation, a reduction in VO_2max is due to both reduced O_2-transporting (i.e., Qmax) and utilization capacity (i.e., a-vO_{2diff}max) associated with cardiac, respiratory, and muscular changes. Decreased Qmax is the result of increasing myocardial stiffness and decreased left ventricular contractility, manifested by reductions in both ejection fraction and HRmax—hallmarks of cardiovascular aging.[86] In fact, HRmax is responsible for much of the age-associated decline in Qmax, decreasing 6 to 10 beats/min per decade.[87] Evidence also suggests that older adults have smaller SVmax[87] and that BP and systemic vascular resistance are higher during maximal exercise in older versus young adults.[88]

With advancing age, reduced elastic recoil of the lung and calcification and stiffening of the cartilaginous articulations of the ribs restrict compliance of the lungs, thus limiting increases in minute ventilation during exercise.[89] Age-related decline in oxidative capacity of the working muscles, and hence decreased a-vO_{2diff} during peak exercise,[90] have been attributed to alterations in mitochondrial structure and distribution, oxidative enzyme activity,[91] and skeletal muscle microcirculation, as well as sarcopenia resulting from a reduced number and size of fibers, particularly type II fibers.[92] Nevertheless, despite loss of aerobic capacity with aging, people without chronic health conditions retain adequate reserves for daily activities.

Sex

The absolute and relative VO_2max of women is about 77% of that of men, after adjustment for body weight and activity level.[93] Although older men and women generally exhibit similar responses to maximal exercise, older women tend to have lower SBP during maximal exercise.[88]

Lifestyle Factors

Smoking is one factor that has been shown to impair exercise capacity in the general population.[94] However, the lifestyle factor that has received the most attention in the literature is habitual activity. There is now irrefutable evidence of the link between physical activity and cardiopulmonary health and fitness.[95-97] Cardiovascular alterations resulting from physical inactivity (i.e., reduced VO_2max and Qmax) parallel, in many ways, the changes that occur with aging; in fact, sedentary lifestyles explain a significant proportion of these age-related declines. If physical activity levels and body composition remain constant over time, the expected rate of loss in aerobic power associated with senescence is reduced by almost 50%.[92] Nonetheless, people with chronic health conditions often rate poorly in terms of daily physical activity, in part because of underlying physical impairments (e.g., paralysis, pain). Some people with multiple sclerosis avoid physical activity to prevent elevated body temperature and minimize symptoms of fatigue.[98] Bernhardt et al[99] found that after a stroke, patients spend more than 50% of their time resting in bed. Short periods of bed rest cause rapid decreases in aerobic capacity—a 15% reduction in healthy, middle-aged men after 10 days of recumbency[100] and a 28% reduction in healthy young subjects after 3 weeks.[101] Inactivity-induced reductions in VO_2peak have been attributed to both central changes (decreased SV from impaired myocardial function and increased venous pooling) and peripheral changes characteristic of aerobically inefficient muscle fibers (decreases in oxidative enzyme concentrations, mitochondria, and capillary density).[23]

Environmental Factors

The influence of environmental factors such as social support and availability of community services on cardiovascular and pulmonary fitness of people with neurological disabilities has received little attention in the literature.

Health Condition

Exercise capacity reflects both systemic capacity and the health of the component systems. Thus, differences in VO_2peak across individuals with neurological disabilities are due not only to the contextual factors discussed above but also to pathological conditions involving the neuromuscular, cardiovascular, and pulmonary systems.

Neuromuscular System

For most individuals with neurological conditions, the existence of neuromuscular impairments confounds interpretation of VO_2peak testing. When people with an intact nervous system are tested, normal biomechanical efficiency is assumed; an impaired nervous system increases the complexity of physiological responses. Both primary effects of upper motor neuron damage (e.g., paralysis, incoordination, spasticity, sensory-perceptual disorders, balance disturbances) and secondary "peripheral" changes in skeletal muscle (e.g., gross muscular atrophy[102] and changes in muscle fiber composition[103]) affect the response to exercise. As a result, people with neurological disabilities manifest not only metabolic but also biomechanical efficiencies, both of which contribute to reduction in functional capacity. Consequently, the decline in exercise capacity is greater than expected (e.g., in people with postpoliomyelitis syndrome deterioration in VO_2peak over a 3- to 5-year period was 12% greater than the predicted decline[104]).

Paresis reduces the pool of motor units available for recruitment during physical work,[105] thereby reducing the metabolically active tissue and lowering the oxidative potential.[106] In the case of stroke, an estimated 50% of the normal number of motor units are functioning[107] and a strong relationship between bilateral thigh muscle mass and VO_2peak has been reported.[46]

Altered fiber composition and recruitment patterns of paretic muscle may also contribute to poor fitness.[103,108] Skeletal muscles are composed of fibers that express different myosin heavy chain (MHC) isoforms. Slow (type I) MHC isoform fibers have higher oxidative function, are more fatigue resistant, and are more sensitive to insulin-mediated glucose uptake; fast (type II) MHC fibers are recruited for more powerful movements, are more reliant on anaerobic or glycolytic means of energy production, fatigue rapidly, and are less sensitive to the action of insulin.[109] Although relatively equal proportions of slow and fast MHC isoforms are found in the vastus lateralis of healthy individuals,[106] elevated proportions of the fast, more fatigable fibers that are less glucose sensitive have been found in the paretic leg of people after a stroke.[103] Hence, it is likely that reduced insulin sensitivity and increased use of the anaerobic processes during dynamic exercise at the level of the muscle contribute to reductions in VO_2peak. Further, alterations in the structure of mitochondria[106] and reduced activity of oxidative enzymes (e.g., succinate dehydrogenase)[110] may contribute to the reduced oxidative capacity of paretic muscles.

Cardiovascular System

Cardiovascular comorbidities, prevalent in populations with neurological disorders, contribute to metabolic inefficiency. In fact, cardiovascular complications are the leading cause of death in persons with stroke,[111] multiple sclerosis,[112] and spinal cord injury.[113] About 75% of patients who have had a stroke are hypertensive[114] and the same proportion has underlying cardiovascular dysfunction.[115] The high prevalence of CAD in this population should not be surprising because these conditions share similar predisposing factors (e.g., age, hypertension, diabetes mellitus, cigarette smoking, sedentary lifestyle, and hyperlipidemia) and pathogenic mechanisms (e.g., atherosclerosis).[116] Indeed, most persons who have had a stroke have atherosclerotic lesions throughout their vascular system,[117] and a high correlation has been reported between the number and degree of stenotic lesions in the coronary and carotid arteries.[118,119]

Factors that elevate HR for a given VO_2, such as CAD, result in attainment of a peak HR (HRpeak) at a VO_2peak below that predicted for that individual. Cardiac dysfunction contributes to a lower aerobic capacity through two principal mechanisms: ischemia-induced reductions in ejection fraction and SV with exercise[120] and chronotropic incompetence—the inability to increase HR in proportion to the metabolic demands of exercise.[22] For persons who can attain HRmax within 15 beats/min of the predicted maximum, limitations in exercise capacity are probably not due to cardiovascular causes.

Impaired peripheral blood flow also contributes to reduced cardiovascular fitness. Inadequate blood flow to the periphery impairs O_2 transport and limits energy production in the working muscles, thereby compromising the ability to sustain physical activity. Both resting blood flow and postischemic reactive hyperemic blood flow have been found to be lower in the paretic leg of people post stroke.[121] Potential mechanisms responsible for reduced blood flow on the hemiparetic side include altered autonomic function,[122] enhanced sensitivity to endogenous vasoconstrictor agents,[123] and altered histochemical and morphological features of the vascular network itself.[124] However, the relative contribution of each of these factors is unknown. In addition, local metabolic mediators associated with changes in muscle fiber composition in the paretic limb (previously discussed) may contribute to impaired limb blood flow.[106]

Trauma to the spinal cord may disrupt the autonomic reflexes and sympathetic vasomotor outflow required for normal cardiovascular responses to exercise.[125] As a result, reduced venous return and cardiac output (referred to as *circulatory hypokinesis*) impair delivery of O_2 and nutrients to and removal of metabolites from working muscles, intensifying muscle fatigue.[126]

Pulmonary System

Typically, the lungs of people without chronic health conditions have a large reserve. Consequently, the pulmonary system rarely limits maximal aerobic power,[127] although at maximal workloads as much as 10% of VO_2max is needed to support the mechanical work of the diaphragm, accessory inspiratory muscles, and abdominal muscles.[128] In contrast, neurological populations may have limited O_2 availability for exercise as a result of pathological conditions involving the pulmonary system, either as a direct complication of neuromuscular condition (e.g., muscle weakness, impaired breathing mechanics) or as a result of cardiovascular dysfunction, comorbidity (e.g., chronic obstructive pulmonary disease), or lifestyle factors (e.g., physical inactivity, smoking habits).[129,130] These impairments can reduce the *ventilatory reserve,* defined as the difference between the maximal available ventilation and the ventilation measured at the end of exercise.[131]

As previously mentioned, minute ventilation is closely associated with VCO_2 during exercise. At peak exercise, a ratio of minute ventilation to VCO_2 above between 35[132] and 40[133] indicates an abnormal ventilatory response. Neu et al[134] reported an 87% incidence of obstructive pulmonary dysfunction in patients with Parkinson's disease, despite the finding that VO_2peak levels in this patient group tend to be in the normal range.[60,61] In the case of stroke, pulmonary function is usually affected to only a modest extent, notwithstanding acute respiratory complications (e.g., pulmonary embolism, aspiration pneumonia).[129] Impaired respiration may be attributed to cardiovascular dysfunction or lifestyle factors (e.g., physical inactivity, high incidence of smoking)[135] or a direct result of the stroke, particularly brain stem stroke. The overwhelming fatigue felt by some persons

after a stroke may be partly due to respiratory insufficiency as manifested by low pulmonary diffusing capacity, decreased lung volumes, and ventilation-perfusion mismatching.[136] Impaired breathing mechanics with restricted and paradoxical chest wall excursion and depressed diaphragmatic excursion have been also reported.[129,137] Expiratory dysfunction appears to be related to the extent of motor impairment (e.g., hemiabdominal muscle weakness), whereas inspiratory limitations appear to be related to the gradual development of rib cage contracture.[138]

To summarize, a host of interacting factors are associated with abnormally low cardiopulmonary fitness in populations with neurological disorders. Neuromuscular and respiratory dysfunctions are often superimposed on an already-compromised state as a result of comorbid cardiovascular disease and premorbid health- and lifestyle-related declines. Paresis and the subsequent reduction in lean muscle mass, changes in the muscle fiber phenotype, and increased reliance on anaerobic processes for energy production result in high metabolic costs of moving paretic limbs. As a consequence, cardiac reserves available for meaningful activity-level functions are limited and, in turn, have a negative impact on participation-level functions. Collectively, impairments in the neuromuscular, cardiovascular, and pulmonary systems converge to promote a sedentary lifestyle and reduced health-related quality of life, which, in turn, leads to further inactivity and further reductions in cardiopulmonary fitness. The contribution of skeletal system impairments to this downward spiral has received little attention. Recently, Pang et al[139] studied the relationship between bone health and physical fitness in the patients who had had a stroke and found a significant correlation between paretic femur bone mineral density and VO_2max. They concluded that further study is needed to determine the clinical implications of this finding.

ADAPTIVE RESPONSES TO AEROBIC TRAINING IN POPULATIONS WITH NEUROLOGICAL DISORDERS

It is now apparent that healthy young and old individuals who begin participating in regular activity even after years of inactivity can enjoy greater health and fitness than those who remain sedentary.[140] Training studies involving people with neurological disability, although limited in number and sample size and often lacking a control group, provide preliminary evidence of cardiopulmonary adaptations to physical work (Table 35-2). In populations with neurological disorders, cardiovascular adaptations in response to aerobic training enhance metabolic efficiency, and neuromuscular adaptations in response to strength and gait training improve mechanical efficiency. The result is improved functional capacity with lowered energy costs of ADLs, enhanced fatigue resistance, and increased exercise tolerance (Figure 35-3).

The magnitude of change in VO_2peak in training studies in Table 35-2 (mean gain of 20%) is comparable to the improvements of 10% to 30%[141,142] reported for healthy, sedentary adults and 13% to 15% for participants in cardiac rehabilitation.[143,144] The increases in VO_2peak for clinically stable individuals with CAD have been reported to be 12% to 46%.[145-147] Substantial intersubject variability in results is attributable to many factors, including differences in neuro-

TABLE 35-2 ■ Cardiopulmonary Adaptations to Aerobic Training Programs in Individuals with Common Neurological Disabilities

DIAGNOSIS	TRAINING MODE	NO.	PROGRAM WEEKS	FREQUENCY (×/WK)	DURATION (MIN)	INTENSITY	% VO$_2$PEAK CHANGE
Subacute stroke	Stationary bicycle[43]	E: 44 C: 48	12	3	20-30	40 rpm	E: +9 C: +0.5
	BWSTT[40]	E: 6 C: 6	3-Feb	5	20	NR	E: +35 C: +1
Chronic stroke	Stationary bicycle[45]	E: 19 C: 23	10	3	30	50-70 rpm	E: +13 C: +1
	Aerobic exercise[153]	E: 29	12	3	30	HR = (HR at RER = 1) − 15	E: +8
	Treadmill[66]	E: 23	26	3	20	<60% HRR	E: +10
	Aerobic exercise[48]	E: 32 C: 31	19	3	60	<80% HRR	E: +9 C: +1
	Water based[151]	E: 7 C: 5	8	3	30	<80% HRR	E: +23 C: +3
Multiple sclerosis	Arm-leg ergometry[50]	E: 21 C: 25	15	3	30	60% VO$_2$peak	E: +22 C: +1
C$_7$-T$_{12}$ SCI	FES-assisted rowing[154]	6 E	6	3	30	75%-80% VO$_2$peak	E: +11
Tetraplegia	FES-assisted ergometry[152]	E: 18	16-Dec	3	30	0-31 W	E: +23
	Arm ergometer[56]	E: 8	8	3	30	50%-60% of HRR or 60 rpm	E: +94
Traumatic brain injury	Low-intensity aerobic exercises[58]	E: 40	16	3	15-20	"Low"	E: +3
	Circuit training[59]	E: 14	16	3	45	70% of VO$_2$peak	E: +15
Postpoliomyelitis syndrome	Cycle ergometer[155]	E: 16 C: 21	16	3	15-30	70% HRmax	E: +15 C: +4
	Arm ergometer[63]	E: 10 C: 10	16	3	20	70%-75% HRR or 50-60 rpm or RPE$_{6-20}$ = 13	E: +19 C: −1
GBS	Arm-leg ergometer[65]	E: 1	16	3	20	75%-85% HRmax	E: +9

E, Experimental; *C,* control; *rpm,* revolutions per minute; *BWS,* body weight support; *FES,* functional electrical stimulation; *HRR,* heart rate reserve; *SCI,* spinal cord injury; *GBS,* Guillain-Barré syndrome.

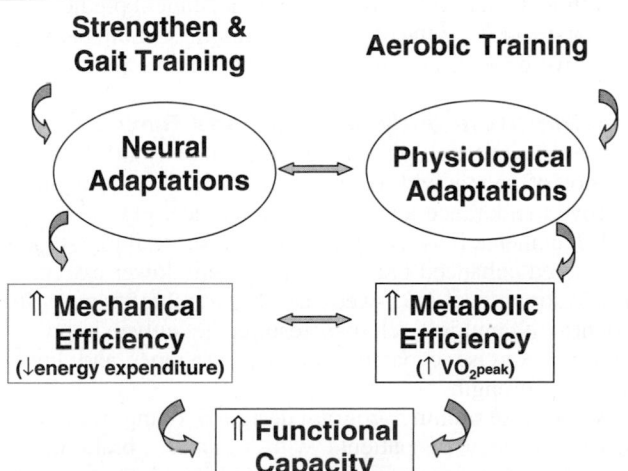

FIGURE 35-3 ■ Interaction of influences that enhance functional capacity. Neurorehabilitation interventions result in neural and physiological adaptations which, in turn, increase mechanical and metabolic efficiencies and ultimately improve functional capacity.

logical condition, severity, and time after insult, as well as variations in intensity of training, mode of exercise, and level of compliance with the exercise regimen. Within studies, considerable interindividual differences have been noted, of which only a small portion (about 11%) has been attributed to recognized covariates such as initial fitness status and an even smaller percentage (about 5%) to measurement error.[148] The most rapid improvements in exercise capacity are seen in previously sedentary people[16] and, similarly, the highest overall gains occur in individuals with the lowest initial values of VO2peak.[149] Age and sex have not been shown to have a substantial effect on exercise trainability.[150]

The dramatic increases in exercise capacity reported in some of the studies (e.g., improvements of 23%,[151,152] to 94%[40]) may not be possible for most people with neurological disabilities. Yet the subtle gains realized in other studies (e.g., 8%,[153] 11%,[154] 15%[155]) may yield meaningful dividends by extending the time in which muscle contraction can be sustained through oxidative processes, thus elevating the lactate threshold. Enhanced functional capacity could spell the difference between being dependent and independent. In other words, interventions that result in even small changes in aerobic capacity may be of practical significance for populations with neurological disorders.

Mechanism of Improved Exercise Capacity in Neurological Disorders

It remains unclear whether training-induced increases in VO_2peak in populations with neurological disorders result from central mechanisms or peripheral mechanisms. In healthy individuals, both peripheral and central adaptations occur and in those with CAD and an intact nervous system, central[156,157] and peripheral[146,156,158] adaptations have been variably reported. In accordance with the Fick equation, central adaptations rely on improved SV because HRmax remains unchanged with training. Enhanced myocardial contractility, together with decreased vasoconstriction in the nonworking muscles and improved venous return, account for the higher Qmax[159] without a concomitant increase in mean arterial pressure.[128] The effect of training on ejection fraction remains unclear[160] and lack of effect on blood hemoglobin content and coronary blood flow has been documented.[120]

Peripheral adaptations in the exercising muscle tissue include increases in capillary density,[161,162] size and number of mitochondria,[163] myoglobin levels, Krebs' cycle enzymes (e.g., succinate dehydrogenase), and respiratory chain enzymes (e.g., cytochrome oxidase).[23] As a consequence of these skeletal muscle adaptations, a-vO_{2diff}, and hence VO_2peak, increase.[85]

The possibility of "spontaneous" increases in exercise capacity during neurological recovery should not be overlooked. There have been several reports of non–exercise-induced adaptations after myocardial infarction.[164-166] Recently, we documented a significant increase (13%) in VO_2peak over the course of a stroke rehabilitation program that lacked an aerobic training component.[167] Recently, Haisma et al[51] reported that patients with tetraplegia and paraplegia demonstrated improvements in VO_2peak of 17% and 23%, respectively, over the course of inpatient spinal cord injury rehabilitation; however, the extent and mode of aerobic training was not indicated. The authors speculated that the improved capacity could be due, in part, to natural recovery and recuperation from trauma and complications. Dressendorfer et al[168] hypothesized that the metabolic demands of unregulated daily activities after myocardial infarction may have an insidious training effect. In support of this prospect, a recent review of the threshold exercise intensity to improve cardiorespiratory fitness indicated that, for deconditioned participants, an effective training intensity is lower than previously reported.[169]

Additional Benefits of Aerobic Training

In addition to increased exercise capacity, other benefits of endurance training realized by healthy populations appear to be attainable for individuals with neuromuscular disabilities. However, direct evidence of the impact on ICF-related domains remains limited.

Cardiopulmonary Function

Decreases in HR at a fixed submaximal workload after training have been attributed to increases in total blood volume[170] and vagal activity and to concomitant reductions in sympathetic-adrenergic drive and resting heart rate (HRrest).[171] However, according to Wilmore et al[170] the decrease in HRrest is of minimal physiological significance.

Potempa et al[45] reported reduction in SBP at submaximal workloads after a 10-week training program for people after stroke. Related to this finding, training can also reduce the rate-pressure product (product of HR and SBP) at submaximal loads,[87] which reflects improvement in cardiac efficiency.[172]

In patients with CAD, training has resulted in decreased ST segment depression (a marker of myocardial ischemia) during submaximal exercise performed at the same baseline rate pressure product,[157] thus raising the anginal threshold and extending the time that submaximal tasks can be performed without triggering myocardial ischemia. Cardiovascular and muscle adaptations also lower minute ventilation at a given submaximal workload, intimating improved ventilatory efficiency.[173] After training, VO_2 at a given submaximal workload is either unchanged[20] or modestly reduced[174] because the increased a-vO_{2diff} in trained muscles is offset by reduced blood flow to the working muscles and a less-pronounced decrease in blood flow to the nonexercising muscles resulting from depressed sympathetic reflex activity.[128]

Cardiovascular Risk Factor Reduction

Endurance exercise training lowers resting BP in both young and older hypertensive adults.[175] Training is also associated with lower fasting and glucose-stimulated plasma insulin levels and with improved glucose tolerance (if initially impaired) and insulin sensitivity.[176] Recent evidence suggests that populations with neurological disorders achieve similar training-induced improvements in lipid profile as previously documented for participants in cardiac rehabilitation.[177] Patients with multiple sclerosis showed reductions in triglyceride and very-low-density lipoprotein levels after a 15-week training program.[50] Similarly, an 8-week training program for individuals early after spinal cord injury led to improved lipid profiles, with more pronounced changes in response to high-intensity training.[178] However, these changes may be due to the result of training-induced reductions in body fat stores.[179] The potential for training to reduce intraabdominal fat is particularly significant because it is the body fat depot that increases the most with age and is associated with other cardiovascular disease risk factors.[180]

Although physical activity is an independent predictor of risk for stroke,[181-183] the capacity of exercise to confer similar protective benefits against stroke recurrence is unknown.

Impairments in Body Structure and Function

The benefits of training to impairments in body structure and function of people with neurological disabilities, other than improved endurance and exercise tolerance, have not been well documented. In patients with stroke, training studies have noted enhanced balance[43] and paretic lower extremity muscle strength.[152] A 15-week aerobic training program for patients with multiple sclerosis resulted not only in improvement in exercise capacity but also in upper and lower extremity strength.[50]

An exercise training program designed to improve ambulatory efficiency of patients with traumatic brain injury failed to reduce energy costs of walking despite a 15% improvement in VO_2peak.[59] In contrast, two studies reported mean reductions in energy costs of walking of 30%[77] and 23% after stroke rehabilitation,[78] and a pilot study reported a 32% reduction in the energy cost of walking in individuals with incomplete spinal cord lesions after a 12-week program of body weight–supported treadmill training.[184] Macko et al[66] interpreted gains observed in ambulatory workload capacity as a reflection of both improved exercise capacity and greater gross motor efficiency. The investigators postulated that central neural motor plasticity, mediated by the repetitive, stereotypic training, underlie these adaptations.

In recent years, the possible role that dynamic exercise may play in enhancing cognitive function has come under investigation. In 1995 Neeper et al[185] observed up-regulation of brain-derived neurotrophic factor (BDNF) in the cerebral cortex of rats housed in an environment with free access to a running wheel. Since then, several researchers have demonstrated increased BDNF production and synaptic plasticity in the brains[186,187] and spinal cords[188] of rodent models engaged in voluntary running. Tong et al[189] reported that these responses appear to be dose dependent. Van Praag et al[190] contributed to this line of inquiry by providing in vitro evidence of neurogenesis in the dentate gyrus of adult mice in response to an enriched environment that included voluntary wheel running. Gordon et al[191] drew on the findings from these animal studies by suggesting that the improved cognitive function observed in individuals with traumatic brain injury who exercised regularly may be attributed to exercise-induced increases in BDNF or other growth factors.

Activity, Participation, and Quality of Life

Few investigators have studied training-induced changes in activity, participation, and quality of life for people with neurological disabilities. In stroke survivors gains in walking capacity have been reported in terms of both gait speed[43,152] and walking tolerance.[43] Small improvements in VO_2peak can have a substantial impact on the ability to perform daily activities, particularly in individuals with limited cardiac or ventilatory reserves, but there is a lack of documentation of these benefits in populations with neurological disorders.

Aerobic Exercise Prescription to Optimize Fitness of People With Neurological Disabilities

Safety and Screening

In general terms, the risks imposed by lack of exercise are far greater than those imposed by exercise. Nevertheless, it is of paramount importance to recognize that symptomatic and asymptomatic cardiovascular disease, and related comorbidities such as diabetes, are much more prevalent in many neurological conditions than in the general population. Therefore thorough review of the health records of potential participants is critical to identify problems that may preclude safe participation in aerobic training programs. Cardiac screening, including a physician-monitored exercise stress test with continuous electrocardiographic (ECG) and periodic BP monitoring, is essential for those with known or suspected cardiac comorbidities. Table 35-3 provides a compilation of contraindications to testing and training.[27,192] Before an exercise program is implemented without preliminary exercise testing, the following should be considered: (1) careful screening for possible contraindications must be conducted, (2) training must be done under the close surveillance of trained personnel, (3) a period of continuous

ECG-telemetry at the initiation of training is recommended, (4) monitoring of BP, HR, and signs of exercise intolerance is essential. Furthermore, for subjects with pulmonary comorbidities such as chronic obstructive pulmonary disease, O_2 saturation levels should be monitored, with saturation levels less than 85% as the criterion to terminate exercise.[193]

In the past, clinicians were apprehensive about the possibility that the overload necessary to achieve an aerobic training effect could aggravate spasticity in patients with neurological disorders; however, such concerns have not been substantiated.[194-197] A recent study reported that the most patients (81%) in the subacute period after a stroke were nonspastic, leading the authors to suggest that focusing on spasticity may be out of step with its clinical importance.[197] Further, there is evidence from studies of cats[198] and humans after spinal cord injury[199] that treadmill training may, in fact, reduce spasticity by improving stretch reflex modulation.

Another concern raised regarding the implementation of aerobic training in neurological disorders is the potential for eliciting excessive fatigue. For people with multiple sclerosis, increased fatigue levels have been reported after high-intensity exercise[200]; however, exercising at an appropriate intensity has been shown to yield benefits without aggravating fatigue.[201] A preliminary study involving people with multiple sclerosis reported that, although fatigue was a significant problem for most subjects, a single bout of low- to moderate-intensity exercise had no deleterious effects on fatigue levels immediately after, and at 24 hours after, the exercise session.[202] Dawes et al[203] found that, for most of their subjects early after traumatic brain injury, increasing the workload during cycling exercises did not elicit a disproportionate increase in VO_2.

Initiation of Training

Most of the training studies on populations with neurological disorders have involved patients with chronic neurological impairments; however, the optimal time to introduce training is unknown. Macko et al[204] expressed caution about training in the early poststroke period, speculating that abnormal cardiovascular responses to exercise (e.g., hypotension, arrhythmia) may impede perfusion of ischemic brain tissue during the period when cerebral autoregulation is most often impaired. Nevertheless, in one study, training was initiated 8 to 21 days after stroke without complications.[40]

Training Environment

High-risk individuals, such as patients in the early stages of neurological recovery or with cardiac comorbidities, should be trained in a setting with quick access to emergency medical equipment and trained personnel. An adverse event protocol should be posted and rehearsed. Lower-risk individuals, after appropriate screening to ensure an appropriate response to exercise, can be trained in supervised community[205] or home-based[43] aerobic exercise programs. Regardless of the setting, certain safeguards are required. Because thermal dysregulation is common in patients with neurological disability, particularly multiple sclerosis[200] and spinal cord injuries,[55] the ambient temperature should be carefully controlled and fans, spray bottles, towels, and a water cooler

TABLE 35-3 ■ Contraindications to Exercise Testing and Aerobic Training

ABSOLUTE CONTRAINDICATIONS

Acute systemic illness or fever
Shortness of breath at rest
Suspected or known dissecting aneurysm
Suspected or known active myocarditis or pericarditis
Thrombophlebitis or intracardiac thrombi

RELATIVE CONTRAINDICATIONS

Myocardial infarction	Recent or complicated myocardial infarction
Heart surgery	Recent (within 3 months)
Angina	Unstable angina (within past 6 months), uncontrolled with medication, exertional angina at inexercise intensities <3 METs
Ventricular arrhythmia	Uncontrolled with medication
Atrial arrhythmia	Uncontrolled atrial arrhythmia that compromises cardiac function
Resting ST segment displacement	>2 mm displacement
Atrioventricular block	Third-degree block without a pacemaker
Sinus tachycardia	HRrest >120 beats/min
Pacemaker	Fixed rate pacemaker
Ventricular ectopy	Frequent or complex premature ventricular contractions at rest or during exercise
Congestive heart failure	Acute or uncompensated failure
Aortic stenosis	Moderate to severe aortic stenosis (peak systolic pressure gradient >50 mm Hg with aortic valve orifice <0.75 cm^2 in an average-size adult)
Carotid stenosis	Severe stenosis
Large vessel intracranial stenosis	Severe stenosis
Systemic or pulmonary embolus	Recent embolus
Emotional distress/psychosis	Significant emotional distress
Hypertension	Resting SBP >200 or resting DBP >110 mm Hg
Valvular disease	Moderate or severe valvular disease
Electrolyte abnormalities	Hypokalemia or hyperkalemia or hypomagnesemia
Metabolic diseases	Uncontrolled diabetes with resting blood sugar >400 mg/dl, thyroiditis, myxedema
Orthostatic hypotension	>20 mm Hg drop with symptoms
Sudden weight gain	>2 kg increase in previous 1-3 days
Cardiac	New York Heart Association functional class IV
Dizziness	Significant motion-induced dizziness/vertigo
Orthopedic conditions	Severe pain on weight bearing

are recommended. Hydration before and during exercise and rehydration after exercise should be monitored by use of a water bottle with volumetric indicators. The exercise area should be wheelchair accessible, free of obstacles and blunt objects, and sufficiently large to permit safe transfer to and from exercise equipment.

Preparation of Participants

Participants should be advised to avoid eating 2 hours before training and to empty bowel and bladder before training, when possible. Comfortable clothing and supportive footwear, appropriate for dynamic exercise, prepare the participant both physically and psychologically for training.

Scheduling of Sessions

Many patients with neurological involvement report a decline in energy levels in the afternoon. If fatigability is a concern, training should be scheduled for morning hours, when circadian body temperature is at its lowest. For certain patient groups, including people with Parkinson's disease, training should be coordinated with the timing of medication to optimize performance.

Duration of Program

A meaningful increase in aerobic capacity (i.e., greater than 10% improvement) of individuals without neurological impairment is unlikely to occur in less than 4 weeks.[206] The minimal exposure required for people with neurological disabilities has not been fully investigated. However, da Cunha et al[40] reported a mean improvement of 35% in VO$_2$peak after 2 to 3 weeks of treadmill ergometry in six people who were less than 1 month after stroke. Regardless of the minimum, participation in training must be sustained indefinitely to prevent returning to the deconditioned state measured at the beginning of the program. Therefore a maintenance program should be followed after termination of formal training sessions.

Frequency and Duration of Sessions

To optimize aerobic training, three to five sessions per week are required, although fitness can improve with twice weekly sessions.[207] A minimum of 20 minutes of exercise within the target zone for training per session is required to elicit a training effect.[207] For those with low fitness levels, training may be initiated with 5-minute exercise "bouts" with rest periods between bouts. Two additional 5-minute periods are required for warm up and cool down; hence, the minimal time required to complete a training session is 30 minutes. Incrementally increasing the duration to a target of 40 to 60 minutes of aerobic training is recommended. However, the greater the intensity of exercise, the shorter the duration needed to achieve improvement in cardiopulmonary fitness; conversely, low-intensity exercise can be compensated by longer duration.[208] As well, accumulation of 10- to 15-minute periods of activity throughout the day can yield similar physiological improvements, provided that the total volume of training is comparable.[209]

Mode of Training

To induce central adaptations, training must incorporate large muscle mass activities that require elevated levels of VO_2. Treadmill or overground walking is a preferred mode because of its direct functional nature; however, a variety of disabilities may preclude this approach. Suitable alternatives include the cycle ergometer with toe clips and heel straps, recumbent ergometer, arm-leg ergometer, wheelchair ergometer, stepping machine, and swimming. Although arm ergometry activates a smaller portion of total muscle mass, its effectiveness in the aerobic training of patients with quadriplegia has been demonstrated.[56] Recently, innovative approaches have been introduced to overcome limitations to exercise training imposed by upper motor neuron damage. For example, a combination of electric stimulation of lower extremity muscles and voluntary upper extremity rowing has been applied to augment the muscle activation of patients after spinal cord injury.[153] Our laboratory is currently investigating the use of body weight–supported treadmill training as an exercise mode for patients early after stroke when impairments in motor and postural control limit training options. Grealy et al[210] piloted use of a virtual reality recumbent ergometer with patients after traumatic brain injury, postulating that the interaction between the training apparatus and the participant might enhance attention to the task of exercising and increase the potential of structural changes in the brain.

A continuous, interval or circuit training regimen may be used. Typically, training studies involving patients with neurological disabilities have used short "bouts" of exercise with a gradual transition to continuous training. However, if continuous training results in either a lack of improvement or a plateau in response, interval training should be instituted.[142, 211]

Muscle Strengthening

Traditionally, aerobic training programs emphasized dynamic exercise. However, the addition of resistance training improves outcome.[195,212] Moreover, strength training decreases the cardiac demands of daily tasks such as lifting objects or carrying groceries while simultaneously increasing the endurance capacity to sustain these submaximal activities.[213] Muscle strengthening exercises should also be carried out 2 to 3 days per week. Key muscle groups (e.g., triceps, biceps, abdominals, hip and knee flexors and extensors, hip abductors, ankle dorsiflexors, and plantarflexors) should be strengthened with one set of 10 to 15 repetitions starting at a low weight and avoiding a Valsalva maneuver.[27]

Intensity of Training

Determining an appropriate intensity is the most challenging aspect of exercise prescription. The cardiovascular system responds to overload; hence, the metabolic load must be sufficient to provoke central and peripheral adaptations. However, excessive stress imposed on the heart and contracting skeletal muscles can evoke abnormal clinical signs or symptoms. The initial exercise intensity and progression must be individualized, using the participant's HR or VO_2peak data (Table 35-4). The RPE can serve as a valid proxy to more physiological measures,[30] with ratings of 11 ("fairly light") to 13 ("somewhat hard") on the RPE 6-20 scale is recommended to initiate training.[27] Despite considerable interindividual variation in RPE,[214] the ratings have been shown to correlate well with exercise intensity, even in patients taking beta-blockers.[215] When exercise intensity is being established, other variables (e.g., anginal symptoms, arrhythmias) should also be considered. Continuous monitoring of HR and periodic monitoring of BP and RPE will ensure that an appropriate intensity is sustained during training.

American College of Sports Medicine guidelines recommend light- to moderate-intensity physical activities to optimize *cardiopulmonary health*.[209] In fact, a recent meta-analysis revealed that for very unfit patients (which would include many people with chronic neurological conditions), the initial intensity can be much lower than previously recommended.[216] However, the only consistent beneficial cardiovascular response to low levels of training is reduction in BP in older hypertensive adults. To reduce cardiovascular risk factors and increase *cardiopulmonary fitness,* moderate- or high-intensity exercise appears to be

TABLE 35-4 ■ Formulae Used to Determine Threshold Intensity for Exercise Training

FORMULA	COMMENTS
Karvonen method: HRrest + $x\%$ of heart rate reserve (HRR), where HHR = Predicted HRmax* − HRrest	Training intensities of 40%-85% HHR are recommended[207] but for unfit patients intensities of 30% HHR can be effective.[216]
$x\%$ of predicted HRmax = 220 − Age, where Predicted HRmax = 220 − Age; if on beta-blockers, Predicted HRmax = 164 − 0.7 × age[217]	Deconditioned individuals can benefit from intensities as low as 55%-64% of predicted HRmax.[207]
HRrest + x beats	The recommended intensity postmyocardial infarction is HRrest + 20 beats and for postcardiac surgery is HRrest + 30 beats.[27]
$x\%$ of VO_2peak	Deconditioned individuals can benefit from intensities as low as 40%-50% of VO_2peak.[27]

TABLE 35-5 ■ Guidelines for Determining the Initial Intensity of Training of People Post Stroke

	LOW INTENSITY	MODERATE INTENSITY	HIGH INTENSITY
Intensity	Minimum target HR = HRrest + 40% HRR	Minimum target HR = HRrest + 50% HRR	Minimum target HR = HRrest + 60% HRR
Cardiac signs	Mild-moderate abnormalities on ECG ± BP ± HR responses	Borderline abnormalities on ECG ± BP ± HR responses	Normal ECG ± BP ± HR responses
Fitness level	VO₂peak <40% predicted	VO₂peak 40%-60% predicted	VO₂peak >60% predicted
Motor control	Chedoke-McMaster Stage of Leg: 1-2	Chedoke-McMaster Stage of Leg: 3-4	Chedoke-McMaster Stage of Leg: >4

necessary.[180] Nevertheless, light- to moderate-intensity physical activity programs may prove to adequate to reduce the rate of age-associated deterioration in a variety of physiological functions and, in the long run, improve both quantity and quality of life.[180]

For many people with neurological involvement, determination of an appropriate intensity of exercise is confounded not only by cardiac status but also by the extent of neurological impairment. We have derived guidelines for determining the initial intensity of treadmill training for people after stroke, based on baseline cardiac signs, prescription of beta-adrenergic blockage therapy,[217] fitness level, and motor control of the involved lower extremity (i.e., Chedoke-McMaster Stage of Recovery of the Leg)[218] (Table 35-5).

Music to Pace Exercise

Music, if properly selected, can be helpful in pacing the repetitive, alternating movements characteristic of aerobic exercise such as walking or cycling. Rossignol and Jones[219] found that with close matching of the cadence of music and alternating movements, music can potentiate muscle activation. Similarly, McIntosh et al[220] reported that music facilitated the gait pattern of people with Parkinson's disease. (Refer to Chapters 4, 24, and 37 for additional information.)

Progression of Training Program

Exercise progression must be individualized because people with neurological disabilities have a wide range of functional capacities. Progression usually occurs over a 3- to 6-month period from an initial conditioning phase, to a training phase, and then to a maintenance phase. Generally, the first goal of training is to reach a target frequency (i.e., a minimum of 3 days/week), then duration (minimum of 20 minutes), and finally an appropriate intensity (40%-60% of heart rate reserve, or 11-13 on the Borg scale). Subsequently, exercise duration should be increased as tolerated, every 1 to 3 weeks, with a goal of achieving 20 to 30 minutes of continuous exercise before increasing the intensity.[27] Patients with higher baseline fitness levels can be progressed more rapidly than those with lower initial capacities.

Laboratory Outcome Measures

Laboratory tests are useful not only to identify limitations in exercise capacity and establish exercise training protocols but also to evaluate the effectiveness of a training program. The principal indicator of a training effect is attainment of

a higher VO₂peak than was achieved in the pretrained state. The greatest increments occurring in individuals with the lowest initial VO₂peak.[149] Ideally, VO₂peak should be measured directly because indirect methods of predicting exercise capacity are more variable and prone to error. However, because VO₂peak testing requires special equipment and trained personnel, clinicians often resort to clinical measures of functional capacity.

Clinical Outcome Measures

6-Minute Walk Test. The distance walked in 6 minutes is sometimes used as a clinical surrogate for VO₂peak testing. However, the systemic response to the 6-Minute Walk Test (6MWT) is less than that of an incremental test using a treadmill cycle[221] or cycle ergometer.[222,223] Subjects tend to walk at a constant speed, achieve a VO₂ steady-state condition after the first few minutes of exercise, and, with practice, walk at a pace approaching critical power.[223,224] Pang et al[225] found a low correlation ($r = 0.402$) between 6MWT distance and VO₂ in patients after stroke, concluding that the 6MWT alone should not be used as an indication of cardiopulmonary fitness after stroke. The same laboratory recommended that, to enhance the usefulness of the 6MWT, BP and HR should be recorded at initiation and termination of the test.[226] Reference equations for the 6MWT can be used to compute the percent of predicted total distance walked in the 6MWT: for men, Distance (m) = (7.57 × Height [cm]) − (5.02 × age [yr]) − (1.76 × weight [kg]) − 309; for women, distance (m) = (2.11 × height [cm]) − (5.78 × age [yr]) − (2.29 × weight [kg]) + 667.[227]

Shuttle Walk Test. The shuttle walk test is a standardized incremental test during which walking is initiated at an audio-guided set pace for a prescribed length of time.[228] Walking speed is increased at each stage until the subject can no longer maintain the required pace. Peak systemic responses have been reported to be consistent with those achieved during a progressive cycle test.[223] A variation of this test, the endurance shuttle walk test, involves walking as far as possible at a constant speed determined in a previously performed progressive walk test.[229]

Adherence to Program

The benefits of training are lost unless some form of training stimulus is maintained. A decrease in mobility or inactivity can lead to rapid loss of cardiovascular and pulmonary fitness; for example, a 25% reduction in maximum oxygen uptake is observed in healthy young adults after 3 weeks of bed rest.[230] Strategies to enhance long-term exercise adherence include gradually progressing the exercise intensity, establishing regularity of training sessions, minimizing the risk of muscular soreness, exercising in groups, emphasizing enjoyment in the program, providing continuing positive reinforcement, and using activity logs and charts to record participation and progress. Training sessions should be scheduled at a convenient time and in an accessible location, and if feasible, assistance with transportation and child care should be offered. As therapeutic management is quickly incorporating the concept of patient-centered care, having a client identify why she or he wants to regain skill, endurance, and the participatory interactions in life will help to motivate cardiovascular and pulmonary fitness as a life activity and not an exercise program only done within a medical environment or rehabilitation setting.

Lifestyle Modifications
Aerobic training alone is not sufficient to optimize the health and fitness of people with neurological disabilities. Education and counseling regarding daily physical activity, nutrition, energy conservation techniques, smoking cessation, and coping strategies are essential.

CONCLUSION

Several conclusions can be made based on available evidence. Neuromuscular, cardiovascular, and pulmonary impairments associated with most neurological conditions interact with contextual factors and the health condition itself to adversely affect exercise capacity and cardiovascular fitness. Aerobic training is now unequivocally regarded as an effective intervention to reduce the functional decline associated with the deconditioned state. Research, albeit limited, suggests that, although patients with neurological impairments generally manifest poor cardiopulmonary fitness, they have the capacity to respond to exercise training in essentially the same manner as individuals without impairments. Trainability is evidenced by their ability to increase exercise capacity or VO$_2$peak in response to the metabolic stress imposed by aerobic exercise. While not abundant, research findings also suggest that involvement in aerobic exercise can also improve walking capacity and reduce risk factors for secondary complications. On the basis of the positive results of training studies, more aggressive training programs are now being introduced into neurorehabilitation, with the goal of interrupting the cycle of debilitation and enhancing neurological recovery. There is an obvious need for further, properly controlled research to examine the impact of aerobic training on all domains of function and quality of life, especially within a population where chronic impairments might be diminished and quality of future life improved. Patients with neurological insults clearly have compounding system variables that interact when they are trying to perform any movement. A clinician who is assisting individuals to regain functional control over movement to improve their quality of life cannot afford to ignore the cardiovascular and pulmonary system regardless of the medical diagnosis.

REFERENCES

1. Roth EJ, Heinemann AW, Lovell LL et al: Impairment and disability: their relation during stroke rehabilitation, *Arch Phys Med Rehabil* 79:329-335, 1998.
2. Roth EJ, Mueller K, Green D: Cardiovascular response to physical therapy in stroke rehabilitation, *Neurorehabil* 2:7-15, 1992.
3. MacKay-Lyons M, Makrides L: Cardiovascular stress during stroke rehabilitation: is the intensity adequate to induce a training effect? *Arch Phys Med Rehabil* 83:1378-1383, 2002.
4. Lamb S, Frost H: Exercise—the other root of our profession, *Physiotherapy* 79:772, 1993.
5. Paley CA: A way forward for determining optimal aerobic exercise intensity? *Physiotherapy* 84:620-624, 1998.
6. Jette M, Sidney K, Blumchen G: Metabolic equivalents (mets) in exercise testing, exercise prescription, and evaluation of functional capacity, *Clin Cardiol* 13:555-565, 1990.
7. Zauner A, Daugherty WP, Bullock MR et al: Brain oxygenation and energy metabolism: 1—biological function and pathophysiology, *Neurosurgery* 51:289-302, 2002.
8. Clingeleffer A, McNaughton LR, Davoren B: The use of critical power as a determinant for establishing the onset of blood lactate accumulation, *Eur J Appl Physiol* 68:182-187, 1994.
9. Conley KE, Kemper WF, Crowther GJ: Limits to sustainable muscle performance: interaction between glycolysis and oxidative phosphorylation, *J Exp Biol* 204:3189-3194, 2001.
10. Saltin B: Hemodynamic adaptations to exercise, *Am J Cardiol* 55:42D-47D, 1985.
11. Busija DW, Heistad DD: Factors involved in the physiological regulation of the cerebral circulation, *Rev Physiol Biochem Pharmacol* 101:161-211, 1984.
12. Madsen PL, Sperling BK, Warming T et al: Middle cerebral artery blood velocity and cerebral blood flow and O2 uptake during dynamic exercise, *J Appl Physiol* 74:245-250, 1993.
13. Hellstrom G, Fischer-Coltrie W, Wahlgrin NG et al: Carotid artery blood flow and middle cerebral artery blood flow velocity during physical exercise, *J Appl Physiol* 81:413-418, 1996.
14. Linkis P, Jorgensen LG, Olesen HL et al: Dynamic exercise enhances regional cerebral artery mean flow velocity, *J Appl Physiol* 78:12-16, 1995.
15. Pott F, Ray CA, Olesen HL, Secher NH: Middle cerebral artery blood velocity, arterial diameter and muscle sympathetic nerve activity during post-exercise muscle ischemia, *Acta Physiol Scand* 160:43-47, 1997.
16. Wasserman K, Hansen JE, Sue DY et al: *Principles of exercise testing and interpretation,* Philadelphia, 1999, Lippincott Williams & Wilkins.
17. Wasserman K, van Kessel A, Burton GG: Interaction of physiological mechanisms during exercise, *J Appl Physiol* 22:71-85, 1967.
18. Wasserman K, Hansen JE, Sue DY et al: *Principles of exercise testing and interpretation: including pathophysiology and clinical applications,* Philadelphia, 2005, Lippincott Williams & Wilkins.
19. Rowell LB: Human cardiovascular adjustments to exercise and thermal stress, *Physiol Rev* 54:75-103, 1974.
20. Hartley LH, Grimby G, Kilbom Å et al: Physical training in sedentary middle-aged and older men, 3: cardiac output and gas exchange at submaximal and maximal exercise, *Scand J Clin Lab Invest* 24:335-344, 1969.
21. Higginbotham MB, Morris KC, Williams RS: Regulation of stroke volume during submaximal and maximal upright exercise in normal man, *Circ Res* 58:281-291, 1986.
22. Camm AJ: Chronotropic incompetence, 1: normal regulation of the heart rate, *Clin Cardiol* 19:424-428, 1996.
23. Whipp BJ: The bioenergetic and gas exchange basis of exercise testing, *Clin Chest Med* 15:173-192, 1994.
24. Foster C, Crowe AJ, Daines E et al: Predicting functional capacity during treadmill testing independent of exercise protocol, *Med Sci Sports Exerc* 28:752-756, 1996.
25. Taylor HL, Buskirk E, Henschel A: Maximal oxygen uptake as an objective measure of cardiorespiratory performance, *J Appl Physiol* 8:73-80, 1955.
26. Marciniuk DD, Watts RE, Gallagher CGT: Reproducibility of incremental maximal cycle ergometer testing in patients with restrictive lung disease, *Thorax* 48:894-898, 1993.

27. American College of Sports Medicine: *Guidelines for exercise testing and prescription,* Baltimore, 2005, Lippincott Williams & Wilkins.

28. American Thoracic Society/American College of Chest Physicians: ATS/ACCP statement on cardiopulmonary exercise testing, *Am J Respir Crit Care Med* 167:211-277, 2003.

29. Jones NL: *Clinical exercise testing,* Philadelphia, 1997, WB Saunders.

30. Borg GA: Psychophysical bases of perceived exertion, *Med Sci Sports Exerc* 14:377-381, 1982.

31. Robergs RA, Landwehr R: The surprising history of the "hrmax = 220-age" equation, *J Exerc Physiol Online* 5:1-10, 2005.

32. Revill SM, Beck KE, Morgan MDL: Comparison of the peak exercise response measured by the ramp and 1-min step cycle exercise protocols in patients with exertional dyspnea, *Chest* 121:1099-1105, 2002.

33. Dolmage TE, Goldstein RS: Principles of aerobic testing and training, *Physiother Can* 58:8-20, 2006.

34. Davis JA, Vodak P, Wilmore JH et al: Anaerobic threshold and maximal aerobic power for three modes of exercise, *J Appl Physiol* 41:544-550, 1976.

35. Howley ET, Bassett DR, Welch HG: Criteria for maximal oxygen uptake: review and commentary, *Med Sci Sports Exerc* 27:1292-1301, 1995.

36. MacKay-Lyons M, Makrides L, Speth S: Effect of 15% body weight support on exercise capacity of adults without impairments, *Phys Ther* 81:1790-1800, 2001.

37. Eschenbacher WL, Mannina A: An algorithm for the interpretation of cardiopulmonary exercise tests, *Chest* 97:263-267, 1990.

38. Åstrand PO, Ryhming I: A nomogram for calculation of aerobic capacity (physical fitness) from pulse rate during sub-maximal work, *J Appl Physiol* 7:218-221, 1954.

39. Davies CT: Limitations to the prediction of maximum oxygen intake from cardiac frequency measurements, *J Appl Physiol* 24:700-706, 1968.

40. da Cunha Filho IT, Lim PA, Quershy H et al: A comparison of regular rehabilitation with supported treadmill ambulation training for acute stroke patients, *J Rehabil Res Dev* 38:245-255, 2001.

41. MacKay-Lyons M, Makrides L: Exercise capacity early after stroke, *Arch Phys Med Rehabil* 83:1697-1702, 2002.

42. Kelly JO, Kilbreadth SL, Davis GM et al: Cardiorespiratory fitness and walking ability in subacute stroke patients, *Arch Phys Med Rehabil* 84:1780-1785, 2003.

43. Duncan P, Studenski S, Richards L et al: Randomized clinical trial of therapeutic exercise in subacute stroke, *Stroke* 34:2173-2180, 2003.

44. Bachynski-Cole M, Cumming GR: The cardiovascular fitness of disabled patients attending occupational therapy, *Occup Ther J Res* 5:233-242, 1985.

45. Potempa K, Lopez M, Braun LT et al: Physiological outcomes of aerobic exercise training in hemiparetic stroke patients, *Stroke* 26:101-105, 1995.

46. Ryan AS, Dobrovolny CL, Silver KH et al: Cardiovascular fitness after stroke: role of muscle mass and gait deficit severity, *J Stroke Cerebrovasc Dis* 9:185-191, 2000.

47. Fujitani J, Ishikawa T, Akai M et al: Influence of daily activity on changes in physical fitness for people with post-stroke hemiplegia, *Am J Phys Med Rehabil* 78:540-544, 1999.

48. Pang MYC, Eng JJ, Dawson AS et al: A community-based fitness and mobility exercise program for older adults with chronic stroke: a randomized, controlled trial, *J Am Geriat Soc* 53:1667-1674, 2005.

49. Ponichtera-Mulcare JA, Mathews T, Glaser RM et al: Maximal aerobic exercise of individuals with multiple sclerosis using three modes of ergometry, *Clin Kinesiol* 48:4-13, 1995.

50. Petajan JH, Gappmaier E, White AT et al: Impact of aerobic training on fitness and quality of life in multiple sclerosis, *Ann Neurol* 39:432-441, 1996.

51. Haisma JA, Bussmann JB, Stam HJ et al: Changes in physical capacity during and after inpatient rehabilitation in subjects with a spinal cord injury, *Arch Phys Med Rehabil* 87:741-748, 2006.

52. Lin KH, Lai JS, Kao MJ et al: Anaerobic threshold and maximal oxygen consumption during arm cranking exercise in paraplegia, *Arch Phys Med Rehabil* 74:515-520, 1993.

53. Paré G, Noreau L, Simard C: Prediction of maximal aerobic power from a submaximal exercise test performed by paraplegics on a wheelchair ergometer, *Paraplegia* 31:584-592, 1993.

54. Jacobs PL, Mahoney ET, Nash MS et al: Circuit resistance training in persons with complete paraplegia, *J Rehabil Res Dev* 39:21-28, 2002.

55. Price MJ, Campbell IG: Thermoregulatory responses of spinal cord injured and well-bodied athletes to prolonged upper body exercise and recovery, *Spinal Cord* 37:772-779, 1999.

56. DiCarlo SE: Effect of arm ergometry training on wheelchair propulsion endurance of individuals with quadriplegia, *Phys Ther* 68:40-44, 1988.

57. Bhambhani Y, Rowland G, Farag M: Reliability of peak cardiorespiratory responses in patients with moderate to severe traumatic brain injury, *Arch Phys Med Rehabil* 84:1629-1636, 2003.

58. Mossberg KA, Kuna S, Masel B: Ambulatory efficiency in persons with acquired brain injury after a rehabilitation intervention, *Brain Inj* 16:789-797, 2002.

59. Jankowski LW, Sullivan SJ: Aerobic and neuromuscular training: effect on the capacity, efficiency, and fatigability of patients with traumatic brain injury, *Arch Phys Med Rehabil* 71:500-504, 1990.

60. Canning CG, Alison JA, Allen NE et al: Parkinson's disease: An investigation of exercise capacity, respiratory function, and gait, *Arch Phys Med Rehabil* 78:199-207, 1997.

61. Stanley RK, Protas EJ, Jankovic J: Exercise performance in those having Parkinson's disease and healthy normals, *Med Sci Sports Exerc* 31:761-766, 1999.

62. Stanghelle JK, Festvag L, Aksnes AK: Pulmonary function and symptom-limited exercise stress testing in subjects with late sequelae of poliomyelitis, *Scand J Rehabil* 25:125-129, 1993.

63. Kriz JL, Jones DR, Speirer JL et al: Cardiorespiratory responses to upper extremity aerobic training by postpolio subjects, *Arch Phys Med Rehabil* 73:49-54, 1992.

64. Willén C, Cider A, Stibrant Sunnerhagen K: Physical performance in individuals with late effects of polio, *Scand J Rehabil Med* 31:244-249, 1999.

65. Pitetti KH, Barrett PJ, Abbas D: Endurance exercise training in Guillain-Barre syndrome, *Arch Phys Med Rehabil* 74:761-765, 1993.

66. Macko RF, Smith GV, Dobrovolny CL et al: Treadmill training improves fitness reserve in chronic stroke patients, *Arch Phys Med Rehabil* 82:879-884, 2001.

67. Westerterp KR, Plasqui G: Physical activity and human energy expenditure, *Curr Opin Clin Nutr Metab Care* 7:607-613, 2004.

68. Passmore R, Durnin JV: Human energy expenditure, *Physiol Rev* 35:801-840, 1955.

69. Ainsworth BE, Haskell WL, Whitt MC et al: Compendium of physical activities: an update of activity codes and met intensities, *Med Sci Sports Exerc* 32:S498-S516, 2000.

70. Cress ME, Meyer M: Maximal voluntary and functional performance levels needed for independence in adults aged 65 to 97 years, *Phys Ther* 83:37-48, 2003.

71. Corcoran PJ, Jebsen RH, Brengelmann GL et al: Effects of plastic and metal leg braces on speed and energy cost of hemiplegic ambulation, *Arch Phys Med Rehabil* 51:69-77, 1970.

72. Gersten JW, Orr W: External work of walking in hemiparetic patients, *Scand J Rehabil Med* 3:85-88, 1971.

73. Mol VJ, Baker CA: Activity intolerance in the geriatric stroke patient, *Rehabil Nurs* 16:337-343, 1991.

74. Brehm M-A, Nollet F, Harlaar J: Energy demands of walking in persons with postpoliomyelitis syndrome: relationship with muscle strength and reproducibility, *Arch Phys Med Rehabil* 87:136-140, 2006.

75. American Heart Association: *Heart and stroke facts,* Dallas, 2002, American Heart Association.

76. Bjuro T, Fugl-Meyer AR, Grimby G et al: Ergonomic studies of standardized domestic work in patients with neuromuscular handicap, *Scand J Rehabil Med* 7:106-113, 1975.

77. Dasco MM, Luczak AK, Haas A et al: Bracing and rehabilitation training: Effect on the energy expenditure of elderly hemiplegics; a preliminary report, *Postgrad Med* 34:42-47, 1963.

78. Hash D: Energetics of wheelchair propulsion and walking in stroke patients, *Orthop Clin North Am* 9:372-374, 1978.

79. Schepers VP, Visser-Meily AM, Ketelaar M et al; Poststroke fatigue: Course and its relation to personal and stroke-related factors, *Arch Phys Med Rehabil* 87:184-188, 2006.

80. Johansson BB, Jadback G, Norrving B et al: Evaluation of long-term functional status in first-ever stroke patients in a defined population, *Scand J Rehabil Med* 26(Suppl.):105-114, 1992.

81. Rokey R, Rolak LA, Harati Y et al: Coronary artery disease in patients with cerebrovascular disease: A prospective study, *Ann Neurol* 16:50-53, 1984.

82. Iseri LT, Smith RV, Evans MJ: Cardiovascular problems and functional evaluation in rehabilitation of hemiplegic patients, *J Chron Dis* 21:423-434, 1968.

83. Morris CK, Ueshima K, Kawaguchi T et al: The prognostic value of exercise capacity: a review of the literature, *Am Heart J* 122:1423-1430, 1991.

84. World Health Organization: ICD-10: International statistical classification of diseases and related health problems, Geneva, 1992, World Health Organization.

85. Åstrand PO, Rodahl K: *Textbook of work physiology: physiological bases of exercise,* New York, 1986, McGraw-Hill.

86. Stratton JR, Levy WC, Cerqueira MD et al: Cardiovascular responses to exercise: effects of aging and exercise training in healthy men, *Circulation* 89:1648-1655, 1994.

87. Ogawa T, Spina RJ, Martin WH et al: Effects of aging, sex, and physical training on cardiovascular responses to exercise, *Circulation* 86:494-503, 1992.

88. Fleg J, O'Connor F, Gerstenblith G et al: Impact of age on the cardiovascular response to dynamic upright exercise in healthy men and women, *J Appl Physiol* 78:890-900, 1995.

89. Frontera WR, Evans WJ: Exercise performance and endurance training in the elderly, *Top Geriatr Rehabil* 2:17-32, 1986.

90. Beere PA, Russell SD, Morey MC et al: Aerobic exercise training can reverse age-related peripheral circulatory changes in healthy older men, *Circulation* 100:1085-1094, 1999.

91. Coggan AR, Spina RJ, King DS et al: Histochemical and enzymatic comparison of the gastrocnemius muscle of young and elderly men and women, *J Gerontol* 47:71-76, 1992.

92. Jackson AS, Beard EF, Wier LT et al: Changes in aerobic power of men ages 25-70 yr, *Med Sci Sports Exerc* 27:113-120, 1995.

93. Bruce RA, Kusumi F, Hosmer D: Maximal oxygen intake and nomographic assessment of functional aerobic impairment in cardiovascular disease, *Am Heart J* 85:546-562, 1973.

94. Huie MJ: The effects of smoking on exercise performance, *Sports Med* 22:355-359, 1996.

95. Laughlin MH: Physical activity in prevention and treatment of coronary disease: the battle line is in exercise vascular cell biology, *Med Sci Sports Exerc* 36:352-363, 2004.

96. Hu G, Barengo NC, Tuomilehto J et al: Relationship of physical activity and body mass index to the risk of hypertension: a prospective study in Finland, *Hypertension* 43:25-30, 2004.

97. Ketelhut RG, Franz IW, Scholze J: Regular exercise as an effective approach in antihypertensive therapy, *Med Sci Sports Exerc* 36:4-8, 2004.

98. Ng AV, Kent-Braun JA: Quantification of lower physical activity in persons with multiple sclerosis, *Med Sci Sports Exerc* 29:517-523, 1997.

99. Bernhardt J, Dewey H, Thrift A et al: Inactive and alone: physical activity within the first 14 days of acute stroke unit care, *Stroke* 35:1005-1009, 2004.

100. Convertino V: Cardiovascular response to exercise in middle-aged men after 10 days of bedrest, *Circulation* 65:134-140, 1982.

101. Saltin B, Blomquist G, Mitchell JH et al: Response to exercise after bed rest and after training: a longitudinal study of adaptive changes in oxygen transport and body composition, *Circulation* 38(7 suppl):1-78, 1968.

102. Ryan AS, Dobrovolny CL, Smith GV et al: Hemiparetic muscle atrophy and increased intramuscular fat in stroke patients, *Arch Phys Med Rehabil* 83:1703-1707, 2002.

103. De Deyne PG, Hafer-Macko CE, Ivey FM et al: Muscle molecular phenotype after stroke is associated with gait speed, *Muscle Nerve* 30:209-215, 2004.

104. Stanghelle JK, Festvåg L: Postpolio syndrome: a 5 year follow-up, *Spinal Cord* 35:503-508, 1997.

105. Dietz V, Ketelsen U, Berge W et al: Motor unit involvement in spastic paresis: Relationship between leg muscle activation and histochemistry, *J Neurol Sci* 75:89-103, 1986.

106. Landin S, Hagenfeldt L, Saltin B et al: Muscle metabolism during exercise in hemiparetic patients, *Clin Sci Mol Med* 53:257-269, 1977.

107. McComas AJ, Sica RE, Upton AR et al: Functional changes in motoneurones of hemiparetic patients, *J Neurol Neurosurg Psychiatry* 36:183-193, 1973.

108. Jakobsson F, Edstrom L, Grimby L: Disuse of anterior tibial muscle during locomotion and increased proportion of type ii fibers in hemiplegia, *J Neurol Sci* 105:49-56, 1991.

109. Daugaard JR, Richter EA: Relationship between muscle fibre composition, glucose transporter protein 4 and exercise training: possible consequences in non-insulin-dependent diabetes mellitus, *Acta Physiol Scand* 171:267-276, 2001.

110. Saltin B, Landin S: Work capacity, muscle strength, and sdh activity in both legs of hemiparetic patients and patients with Parkinson's disease, *Scand J Clin Lab Invest* 35:531-538, 1975.

111. Matsumoto N, Whisnant JP, Kurland LT et al: Natural history of stroke in Rochester, Minnesota, 1955 through 1969: an extension of a previous study, 1945 through 1954, *Stroke* 4:20-29, 1973.

112. Sadovnick AD, Eisen K, Ebers GC et al: Cause of death in patients attending multiple sclerosis clinics, *Neurology* 41:1193-1196, 1991.

113. Kennedy EJ: *Spinal cord injury: Facts and figures,* Birmingham, AL, 1986, University of Alabama at Birmingham.

114. Leonardi-Bee J, Bath PM, Philips SJ et al: Blood pressure and clinical outcomes in the International Stroke Trial, *Stroke* 33:1315-1320, 2002.

115. Roth E: Heart disease in patients with stroke, 1: classification and prevalence, *Arch Phys Med Rehabil* 74:752-760, 1993.

116. Roth E: Heart disease in patients with stroke, 2: impact and implications for rehabilitation, *Arch Phys Med Rehabil* 75:94-101, 1994.

117. Wolf PA, Clagett GP, Easton JD et al: Preventing ischemic stroke in patients with prior stroke and transient ischemic attack: A statement for healthcare professionals from the stroke council of the American Heart Association, *Stroke* 30:1991-1994, 1999.

118. Young W, Gofman JW, Tandy S: Quantification of atherosclerosis within and between the coronary and cerebral vascular bed, *Am J Cardiol* 6:300-308, 1960.

119. Mitchell JRA, Schwartz CJ: Relationship between arterial disease in different sites, *BMJ* 1:1293-1301, 1962.

120. Clausen JP, Klausen K, Rasmussen B et al: Central and peripheral circulatory changes after training of the arms and legs, *Am J Physiol* 225:675-682, 1973.

121. Ivey FM, Gardner AW, Dobrovolny CL et al: Unilateral impairment of leg blood flow in chronic stroke patients, *Cerebrovasc Dis* 512:283-289, 2005.

122. Herbaut AG, Cole JD, Sedgwick EM: A cerebral hemisphere influence on cutaneous vasomotor reflexes in humans, *J Neurol Neurosurg* 53:118-120, 1990.

123. Bevan R, Clemenson A, Joyce E et al: Sympathetic denervation of resistance arteries increases contraction and decreases relaxation to flow, *Am J Physiol* 264:H490-H494, 1993.

124. Kozak P: Circulatory changes of the paretic extremities after acute anterior poliomyelitis, *Arch Phys Med Rehabil* 49:77-81, 1968.

125. Glaser RM: Physiologic aspects of spinal cord injury and functional neuromuscular stimulation, *Cent Nerv Syst Trauma* 3:49-62, 1986.

126. Davis GM, Shephard RJ: Cardiorespiratory fitness in highly active versus inactive paraplegics, *Med Sci Sports Exerc* 20:463-468, 1988.

127. Wagner PD: Why doesn't exercise grow the lungs when other factors do? *Exerc Sport Sci Rev* 33:3-8, 2005.

128. Clausen JP: Effect of physical training on cardiovascular adjustments to exercise in man, *Physiol Rev* 57:779-815, 1977.

129. Vingerhoets F, Bogousslavsky J: Respiratory dysfunction in stroke, *Clin Chest Med* 15:729-737, 1994.

130. Wiercisiewski DR, McDeavitt JT: Pulmonary complications in traumatic brain injury, *J Head Trauma Rehabil* 13:28-35, 1998.

131. Clark TJ, Freedman S, Campbell EJ et al: The ventilatory capacity of patients with chronic airways obstruction, *Clin Sci* 36:307-316, 1969.

132. Sun XG, Hansen JE, Garatachea N et al: Ventilatory efficiency during exercise in healthy subjects, *Am J Respir Crit Care Med* 166:1443-1448, 2002.

133. Blackie SP, Fairbarn MS, McElvaney NG et al: Normal values and ranges for ventilation and breathing pattern at maximal exercise, *Chest* 100:136-142, 1991.

134. Neu HC, Connolly J, Schwertley F et al: Obstructive respiratory dysfunction in Parkinson's patients, *Am Rev Respir Dis* 95:33-47, 1967.

135. Harvey RL, Roth EJ, Heinemann AW et al: Stroke rehabilitation: clinical predictors of resource utilization, *Arch Phys Med Rehabil* 79:1349-1355, 1998.

136. Haas A, Rusk HA, Pelosof H et al: Respiratory function in hemiplegic patients, *Arch Phys Med Rehabil* 48:174-179, 1967.

137. Fugl-Meyer AR, Grimby G: Respiration in tetraplegia and hemiplegia: a review, *Int Rehabil Med* 6:186-190, 1984.

138. Fugl-Meyer A, Linderholm H, Wilson AF: Restrictive ventilatory dysfunction in stroke: its relation to locomotor function, *Scand J Rehabil Med Suppl* 9:118-124, 1983.

139. Pang MYC, Eng JJ, McKay HA et al: Reduced hip bone mineral density is related to physical fitness and leg lean mass in ambulatory individuals with chronic stroke, *Osteoporosis Int* 16:1796-1779, 2005.

140. Hu FB, Stampfer MJ, Colditz GA et al: Physical activity and risk of stroke in women, *JAMA* 283:2961-2967, 2000.

141. Samitz G, Bachl N: Physical training programs and their effects on aerobic capacity and coronary risk profile in sedentary individuals, *J Sports Med Phys Fitness* 31:283-293, 1991.

142. American College of Sports Medicine: American College of Sports Medicine position stand: the recommended quantity and quality of exercise for developing and maintaining cardiorespiratory and muscular fitness, and flexibility in healthy adults, *Med Sci Sports Exerc* 30:975-991, 1998.

143. Franklin BA, Besseghini I, Goldn LH: Low intensity physical conditioning: effects on patients with coronary heart disease, *Arch Phys Med Rehabil* 59:276-280, 1978.

144. Mertens DJ, Kavanagh T: Exercise training for patients with chronic atrial fibrillation, *J Cardiopulm Rehabil* 16:193-196, 1996.

145. Hung C, Daub B, Black B et al: Exercise training improves overall physical fitness and quality of life in older women with coronary artery disease, *Chest* 126:1026-1031, 2004.

146. Ades PA, Waldmann ML, Meyer WL et al: Skeletal muscle and cardiovascular adaptations to exercise conditioning in older coronary patients, *Circulation* 94:323-330, 1996.

147. Ehsani AA, Martin WH, Heath GW et al: Cardiac effects of prolonged and intense exercise training in patients with coronary artery disease, *Am J Cardiol* 50:246-254, 1982.

148. Shephard RJ, Rankinen T, Bouchard C: Test-retest errors and the apparent heterogeneity of training response, *Eur J Appl Physiol* 91:199-203, 2004.

149. Saltin B: Physiological effects of physical conditioning, *Med Sci Sport* 1:50-56, 1969.

150. Lewis DA, Kamon E, Hodgson JL: Physiological differences between genders: implications for sports conditioning, *Sports Med* 3:357-369, 1986.

151. Chu KS, Eng JJ, Dawson AS et al: Water-based exercise for cardiovascular fitness in people with chronic stroke: a randomized controlled trial, *Am J Phys Med Rehabil* 85:870-874, 2004.

152. Hooker SP, Figoni SF, Rodgers MM: Physiologic effects of electrical stimulation leg cycle exercise training in human tetraplegia, *Arch Phys Med Rehabil* 73:470-476, 1992.

153. Rimmer JH, Riley B, Creviston T et al: Exercise training in a predominantly African-American group of stroke survivors, *Med Sci Sport Exerc* 32:1990-1996, 2000.

154. Wheeler GD, Andrews B, Lederer R et al: Functional electric stimulation-assisted rowing: increasing cardiovascular fitness through functional electric stimulation rowing training in persons with spinal cord injury, *Arch Phys Med Rehabil* 83:1093-1099, 2002.

155. Jones DR, Spier J, Canine K et al: Cardiorespiratory responses to aerobic training by patients with postpoliomyelitis sequelae, *JAMA* 261:3255-3258, 1989.

156. Williams RS, McKinnis RA, Cobb FR et al: Effects of physical conditioning on left ventricular ejection fraction in patients with coronary artery disease, *Circulation* 70:69-75, 1984.

157. Ehsani AA, Biello DR, Schultz J et al: Improvement of left ventricular contractile function by exercise training in patients with coronary artery disease, *Circulation* 74:350-358, 1986.

158. Detry JM, Rousseau M, Vandenbroucke G et al: Increased arteriovenous oxygen difference after physical training in coronary heart disease, *Circulation* 44:109-118, 1971.

159. Willenheimer R, Erhardt L, Cline C et al: Exercise training in heart failure improves quality of life and exercise capacity, *Eur Heart J* 19:774-781, 1998.

160. Franklin BA, Gordon S, Timmis GC: Amount of exercise necessary for the patient with coronary artery disease, *Am J Cardiol* 69:1426-1431, 1992.

161. Cotter M, Hudlicka O, Vrbova G: Growth of capillaries during long-term activity in skeletal muscle, *Bibl Anat* 11:395-398, 1973.

162. Hudlicka O, Dodd L, Renkin EM et al: Early changes in fiber profile and capillary density in long-term stimulated muscles, *Am J Physiol* 243:H528-H535, 1982.

163. Essen B, Jansson E, Henriksson J et al: Metabolic characteristics of fiber types in human skeletal-muscle, *Acta Physiol Scand* 95:153-165, 1975.

164. Savin WM, Haskell WL, Houston-Miller N et al: Improvements in aerobic capacity soon after myocardial infarction, *J Cardiac Rehabil* 1:337-342, 1981.

165. DeBusk RF, Houston N, Haskell W et al: Exercise training soon after myocardial infarction, *Am J Cardiol* 44:1223-1229, 1979.

166. Sheldahl LM, Wilke NA, Tritani FE et al: Heart rate responses during home activities soon after myocardial infarction, *J Card Rehabil* 4:327-333, 1984.

167. MacKay-Lyons M, Makrides L: Longitudinal changes in exercise capacity after stroke, *Arch Phys Med Rehabil* 85:1608-1612, 2004.

168. Dressendorfer RH, Franklin BA, Cameron JL et al: Exercise training frequency in early post-infarction cardiac rehabilitation: influence on aerobic conditioning, *J Cardiopulm Rehabil* 15:269-276, 1995.

169. Swain DP, Franklin BA: VO$_2$ reserve and the minimal intensity for improving cardiorespiratory fitness, *Med Sci Sports Exerc* 34:152-157, 2002.

170. Wilmore JH, Stanford PR, Gagnon J et al: Endurance exercise training has a minimal effect on resting heart rate: the heritage study, *Med Sci Sports Exerc* 28:829-835, 1996.

171. Casaburi R: Physiologic responses to training, *Clin Chest Med* 15:215-227, 1994.

172. Nelson RR, Gobel FL, Jorgenson CR et al: Hemodynamic predictors of myocardial oxygen consumption during static and dynamic exercise, *Circulation* 50:1179-1189, 1974.

173. Jones NL: Dyspnea in exercise, *Med Sci Sports Exerc* 16:14-19, 1984.

174. Gardner AW, Poehlman ET, Corrigan DL: Effect of endurance training on gross energy expenditure during exercise, *Hum Biol* 61:559-569, 1989.

175. Hagberg J, Blair S, Ehsani A et al: Position stand: Physical activity, physical fitness, and hypertension, *Med Sci Sports Exerc* 25:i-x, 1993.

176. Seals D, Hagberg J, Allen W et al: Glucose tolerance in young and older athletes and sedentary men, *J Appl Physiol* 56:1521-1525, 1984.

177. Taylor RS, Brown A, Ebrahim S et al: Exercise-based rehabilitation for patients with coronary heart disease: systematic review and meta-analysis of randomized controlled trials, *Am J Med* 116:682-692, 2004.

178. De Groot PCE, Hjeltnes N, Heijboer AC et al: Effect of training intensity on physical capacity, lipid profile, and insulin sensitivity in early rehabilitation of spinal cord injured individuals, *Spinal Cord* 41:673-679, 2003.

179. Katzel L, Bleecker E, Colman E et al: Effects of weight loss vs. aerobic exercise training on risk factors for coronary disease in healthy, obese, middle-aged and older men, *JAMA* 274:1915-1920, 1995.

180. Mazzeo RS, Cavanagh P, Evans WJ et al: ACSM position stand on exercise and physical activity for older adults, *Med Sci Sports Exerc* 30:992-1008, 1998.

181. Gordon NF, Gulanic M, Costa F et al: Physical activity and exercise recommendations for stroke survivors: An American Heart Association scientific statement, *Circulation* 109:2031-2041, 2004.

182. Lee CD, Folsom AR, Blair SN: Physical activity and stroke risk: a meta analyses, *Stroke* 34:2475-2481, 2003.

183. Kurl S, Laukkanen JA, Rauramaa R et al: Cardiorespiratory fitness and the risk of stroke in men, *Arch Intern Med* 163:1682-1688, 2003.

184. Protas EJ, Holmes SA, Quereshy H et al: Supported treadmill ambulation training after spinal cord injury: a pilot study, *Arch Phys Med Rehabil* 82:825-831, 2001.

185. Neeper SA, Gomez-Pinilla F, Choi J et al: Physical activity increases mRNA for brain-derived neurotrophic factor and nerve growth factor in rat brain, *Brain Res* 726:49-56, 1996.

186. Molteni R, Ying Z, Gomez-Pinilla F: Differential effects of acute and chronic exercise on plasticity-related genes in the rat hippocampus revealed by microarray, *Eur J Neurosci* 16:1107-1116, 2002.

187. Farmer J, Zhao X, Van Praag H et al: Effects of voluntary exercise on synaptic plasticity and gene expression in the dentate gyrus of adult male Sprague-Dawley rats in vivo, *Neuroscience* 124:71-79, 2004.

188. Gomez-Pinilla F, Ying Z, Roy RR et al: Voluntary exercise induces a BDNF-mediated mechanism that promotes neuroplasticity, *J Neurophysiol* 88:2187-2195, 2002.

189. Tong L, Shen H, Perreau VM et al: Effects of exercise on gene-expression profile in the rat hippocampus, *Neurobiol Dis* 8:1046-1056, 2001.

190. Van Praag H, Kemperman G, Gage FH: Running increases cell proliferation and neurogenesis in the adult mouse dentate gyrus, *Nat Neurosci* 2:266-270, 1999.

191. Gordon WA, Sliwinski M, Echo J: The benefits of exercise in individuals with traumatic brain injury: a retrospective study, *J Head Trauma Rehabil* 134:58-67, 1998.

192. American College of Sports Medicine: *ACSM's exercise management for persons with chronic diseases and disability.* In Durstine JL, Moore GE, editors. Champaign, IL, 2003, Human Kinetics.

193. Mengelkoch LJ, Martin D, Lawler J: A review of the principles of pulse oximetry and accuracy of pulse oximeter estimates during exercise, *Phys Ther* 74:40-47, 1994.

194. Smith GV, Silver KHC, Goldberg AP et al: "Task-oriented" exercise improves hamstring strength and spastic reflexes in chronic stroke patients, *Stroke* 30:2112-2118, 1999.

195. Teixeira-Salmela LF, Olney SJ, Nadeau S et al: Muscle strengthening and physical conditioning to reduce impairment and disability in chronic stroke survivors, *Arch Phys Med Rehabil* 80:1211-1218, 1999.

196. Saunders DH, Greig CA, Young A et al: Physical fitness training for stroke patients, *Cochrane Database Syst Rev* CD003316, 2004.

197. Sommerfeld DK, Eek E, Svensson A-K et al: Spasticity after stroke: its occurrence and association with motor impairments and activity limitations, *Stroke* 35:134-140, 2004.

198. Coté MP, Ménard A, Gossard JP: Spinal cats on the treadmill: changes in load pathways, *J Neurosci* 23:2789-2796, 2003.

199. Trimble MH, Kukulka C, Behrman AL: The effect of treadmill gait training on low-frequency depression of the soleus h-reflex: comparison of a spinal cord injured man to normal subjects, *Neurosci Lett* 246:186-188, 1998.

200. Ponichtera-Mulcare JA: Exercise and multiple sclerosis, *Med Sci Sports Exerc* 25:451-465, 1993.

201. Kent-Braun JA, Sharma KR, Weiner RG: Effects of exercise on muscle activation and metabolism in multiple sclerosis, *Muscle Nerve* 7:1162-1169, 1994.

202. Smith RM, Adeney-Steel M, Fulcher G et al: Symptom change with exercise is a temporary phenomenon for people with multiple sclerosis, *Arch Phys Med Rehabil* 87:723-727, 2006.

203. Dawes H, Bateman A, Culpan J et al: The effect of increasing effort on movement economy during incremental cycling exercise in individuals early after acquired brain injury, *Clin Rehabil* 17:528-534, 2003.

204. Macko RF, Katzel LI, Yataco A et al: Low-velocity graded treadmill stress testing in hemiparetic stroke patients, *Stroke* 28:988-992, 1997.

205. Eng JJ, Chu KS, Kim CM et al: A community-based group exercise program for persons with chronic stroke, *Med Sci Sports Exerc* 35:1271-1278, 2003.

206. Saltin B, Henriksson J, Nygaard E et al: Fiber types and metabolic potentials of skeletal muscles in sedentary man and endurance runners, *Ann N Y Acad Sci* 301:3-29, 1977.

207. American College of Sports Medicine: *Guidelines for exercise testing and prescription,* Baltimore, 2000, Williams & Wilkins.

208. Pollock ML, Gaesser GA, Butcher JD et al: The recommended quantity and quality of exercise for developing and maintaining cardiorespiratory and muscular fitness, and flexibility in healthy adults, *Med Sci Sports Exerc* 30:975-991, 1998.

209. Pate RR, Pratt M, Blair SN et al: Physical activity and public health: a recommendation from the centers of disease control and prevention and the American College of Sports Medicine, *JAMA* 273:402-407, 1995.

210. Grealy MA, Johnson DA, Rushton SK: Improving cognitive function after brain injury: the use of exercise and virtual reality, *Arch Phys Med Rehabil* 80:661-667, 1999.

211. Eddy DO, Sparks KL, Adelizi DA: The effects of continuous and interval training in women and men, *J Appl Physiol Occup Physiol* 37:83-92, 1977.

212. Pierson LM, Herbert WG, Norton HJ et al: Effects of combined aerobic and resistance training versus aerobic training alone in cardiac rehabilitation, *J Cardiopulm Rehabil* 21:101-110, 2001.

213. Hickson RC, Rosenkoetter MA, Brown MM: Strength training effects aerobic power and short-term endurance, *Med Sci Sports Exerc* 12:336-339, 1980.

214. Whaley MH, Brubaker PH, Kaminsky LA et al: Validity of rating of perceived exertion during graded exercise testing in apparently healthy adults and cardiac patients, *J Cardiopulm Rehabil* 17:261-267, 1997.

215. Pollock ML, Lowenthal DT, Foster C et al: Acute and chronic responses to exercise in patients treated with beta blockers, *J Cardiopulm Rehabil* 11:132-144, 1991.

216. Swain DP, Franklin BA: VO_2 reserve and the minimal intensity for improving cardiorespiratory fitness, *Med Sci Sports Exerc* 34:152-157, 2002.

217. Brawner CA, Ehrman JK, Schairer JR et al: Predicting maximum heart rate among patients with coronary heart disease receiving beta-adrenergic blockade therapy, *Am Heart J* 148:910-914, 2004.

218. Gowland C, Van Hullenaar S, Torresin W et al: *Chedoke-McMaster stroke assessment: development, validation, and administration*

manual, Hamilton, 1995, Chedoke-McMaster Hospitals and McMaster University.

219. Rossignol S, Jones GM: Audio-spinal influence in man studied by the h-reflex and its possible role on rhythmic movements synchronized to sound, *Electroenceph Clin Neurophysiol* 41:83-92, 1976.

220. McIntosh GC, Brown SH, Rice RR: Rhythmic auditory-motor facilitation of gait patterns in patients with Parkinson's disease, *J Neurol Neurosurg Psychiatry* 62:22-26, 1997.

221. Kervio G, Carre F, Ville NS: Reliability and intensity of the six-minute walk test in healthy elderly subjects, *Med Sci Sports Exerc* 35:169-174, 2003.

222. Gayda M, Temfemo A, Choquet D et al: Cardiorespiratory requirements and reproducibility of the six-minute walk test in elderly patients with coronary artery disease, *Arch Phys Med Rehabil* 85:1538-1543, 2004.

223. Onorati P, Antonucci R, Valli G et al: Non-invasive evaluation of gas exchange during a shuttle walking test vs. a 6-min walking test to assess exercise tolerance in COPD patients, *Eur J Appl Physiol* 89:331-336, 2003.

224. Troosters T, Vilaro J, Rabinovich R et al: Physiological responses to the 6-min walk test in patients with chronic obstructive pulmonary disease, *Eur Respir J* 20:564-569, 2002.

225. Pang MYC, Eng JJ, Dawson AS: Relationship between ambulatory capacity and cardiorespiratory fitness in chronic stroke: influence of stroke-specific impairments, *Chest* 127:495-501, 2005.

226. Eng JJ, Chu KS, Dawson AS et al: Functional walk tests in individuals with stroke: relation to perceived exertion and myocardial exertion, *Stroke* 33:756-761, 2002.

227. Enright PL, Sherrill DL: Reference equations for the six-minute walk in healthy adults, *Am J Resp Crit Care Med* 158:1384-1387, 1998.

228. Singh SJ, Morgan MD, Scott S et al: Development of a shuttle walking test of disability in patients with chronic airways obstruction, *Thorax* 47:1019-1024, 1992.

229. Revill SM, Morgan MD, Singh SJ et al: The endurance shuttle walk: a new field test for the assessment of endurance capacity in chronic obstructive pulmonary disease, *Thorax* 54:213-222, 1999.

230. Saltin B, Blomqvist G, Mitchell JH et al: Response to submaximal and maximal exercise after bed rest and training, *Circulation* 38 (suppl 7):1-78, 1968.

APPENDIX 35-A ■ Abbreviations Commonly Used when Discussing Cardiovascular and Pulmonary Problems and Their Effect on Function

6MWT: 6-Minute walk test
ADL: Activities of daily living
a-vO$_{2diff}$: Arteriovenous oxygen difference
a-vO$_{2diff}$max: Maximal arteriovenous oxygen difference
BP: Blood pressure
CAD: Coronary artery disease
CO$_2$: Carbon dioxide
DBP: Diastolic blood pressure
ECG: Electrocardiogram
H$^+$: Hydrogen ions
HR: Heart rate
HRmax: Maximal heart rate
HRpeak: Peak heart rate
HRrest: Resting heart rate
HRR: Heart rate reserve
ICF: International Classification of Functioning, Disability, and Health
MET: Metabolic equivalent
O$_2$: Oxygen
Q: Cardiac output
Qmax: Maximal cardiac output
RER: Respiratory exchange ratio
RERpeak: Peak respiratory exchange ratio
RPE: Rate of perceived exertion
SPB: Systolic blood pressure
SV: Stroke volume
SVmax: Maximal stroke volume
VCO$_2$: Carbon dioxide production per minute
VO$_2$: Oxygen consumption per minute
VO$_2$max: Maximal oxygen consumption per minute
VO$_2$peak: Peak oxygen consumption per minute

CHAPTER 36

Impact of Drug Therapy on Patients Receiving Neurological Rehabilitation

Annie Burke-Doe, PhD, MPT
Howell I. Runion, PA, MS, PhD
Timothy J. Smith, RPh, PhD

KEY WORDS

adverse drug reactions
disease
drug interactions
drug therapy
impairment
pharmacist

OBJECTIVES

After reading this chapter the student/therapist will be able to:

1. Identify how drugs may positively or negatively affect behavior of individuals within a neurological rehabilitation setting.
2. Given a disease state, comprehend how drugs may affect that disease state and the implications on an individual's potential for neurological rehabilitation.
3. When considering one or more impairments, recognize the influence of drug therapy on these impairments and on an individual's potential for neurological rehabilitation.
4. Recognize the importance of a collaborative approach in resolving drug-related issues and how those issues affect an individual's potential for neurological rehabilitation.

INTRODUCTION

Pharmaceutical interventions are expanding into all arenas of health care. Only rarely will an occupational or physical therapist manage a client who is not receiving drug therapy for conditions either related or unrelated to the therapist's scope of practice. Drugs used for the management of a wide variety of disease states may have unintended or undesirable effects on a therapeutic plan for a client receiving neurological rehabilitation. Although the occupational or physical therapist may not be responsible for monitoring all aspects of a client's therapeutic plan, the scope of drug-related complications must be recognized. A client's pharmacist, who is acutely aware of the prescribing practices of the client's physician(s), may be instrumental in resolving the drug-related impact of any medication on a therapeutic plan. The client will benefit greatly from an effective collaboration that includes the therapist and a pharmacist. Focusing on drug effects, diseases, and impairments, the discussion in this chapter addresses these interactions from two perspectives. First, a disease or pathology-driven model focuses on the pharmacological approaches used in drug therapy of major diseases that are often concurrent with rehabilitation. Second, an impairment/functional limitation–driven model focuses on the effects of drugs on the impairment and resulting functional deficit and the impact on the therapeutic plan. Although defining every problem associated with a class of drugs or among patients with a particular impairment is not possible within the scope of this chapter, highlighting common difficulties is important.

DISEASE PERSPECTIVE

A number of diseases and their treatment regimens may be concurrently managed while a client is in a neurological rehabilitation environment. The pharmacological interventions for these conditions and their implications from both a physiological and disease/pathology model are addressed. Although not a comprehensive list, these include Parkinson's disease, cancer, seizure disorders (epilepsy), cardiovascular disorders, disorders of mood, autoimmune disorders, diabetes, infectious diseases, pulmonary diseases, and gastrointestinal disorders.

Parkinson's Disease

Parkinson's disease is a degenerative disorder involving a progressive loss of dopaminergic neurons in the substantia nigra. This deficit in dopaminergic function results in resting tremor and difficulty in the control of voluntary movement. Cardiovascular function, bowel motility, and cognitive function are often compromised. Although not directly associated with the motor system pathology, the functional deficits are emotionally devastating to the patient, resulting in depression and other mood disorders. The predominant pharmacological approach in the management of Parkinson's disease is the enhancement of dopaminergic function in the affected brain regions. Among the earliest successful approaches was the use of L-dopa, a precursor of dopamine in the central nervous system (CNS). The use of this agent (as with all agents to date) only enhances the dopaminergic function in remaining neurons. This approach has no effect on the progressive loss of neurons. In addition to central conversion of L-dopa to dopamine in the substantia nigra, a similar conversion occurs in the limbic system, a brain center associated with the regulation of behavior. Excessive dopaminergic influence in the limbic system has been associated with aberrant behaviors, including paranoia, delusions, hallucinations, and related psychiatric disturbances that may influence sleep and mood. These behavioral changes are obviously antagonistic to any therapeutic plan. In addition to L-dopa, a dopamine precursor, agents that inhibit the breakdown of dopamine, enhance the release of dopamine, or have dopaminergic agonist activity will have similar behavioral effects (Box 36-1). Dopaminergic agents may produce postural hypotension and syncope by virtue of their ability to produce vasodilation on the basis of CNS and peripheral actions.[1,2] If clients are unable to take their medication, an increasing danger exists (with extended therapy) that movement may be impossible and the normal chest wall expansion and contraction may be compromised (see Chapter 24).

Because Parkinson's disease is progressive in nature, clients may present differently depending on the stage of the disease and the presence of pharmacological interventions. In the early months of the disease, the motor signs may be particularly subtle and patients may only report slowness, stiffness, and trouble with handwriting. Particular attention to the history of tremor, slowness of fine motor control, a hunched and slightly flexed posture, and micrographia may lead the physician to diagnose Parkinson's disease in its early phases.[3] As Parkinson's disease advances, patients have increasing difficulty in activities of daily living and gait as well as bradykinesia and distal tremor.

Once a definitive diagnosis has been made, controlling symptoms of the disease and the side effects of medications is balanced with the level of functional involvement. The physician and client may discuss the option of a number of medications (see Box 36-1) but must determine the best approach on the basis of the clinical presentation. One limitation is the side effect of involuntary movements (dyskinesias). These dyskinesias can be difficult to control and are different from the involuntary movements caused by the

disease itself. As mentioned earlier, dopamine agonists can also be prescribed without causing dyskinesias, but their effect on symptoms is not as potent.[4] Often physicians may begin treatment of a dopamine agonist and continue with the agonist as long as symptoms are satisfactorily controlled. Later the physician can initiate treatment with L-dopa when the disease is in the advanced stages. With the elderly client who has cognitive deficits, combination therapy may be the initial choice. Once a medication regimen has been initiated the client and therapist may notice improvement in Parkinson disease symptoms and therefore functional abilities. After taking medications over time clients may find that the effect of the medication begins to wear off before the next dose is scheduled. At this point consultation with the rehabilitation team is recommended to potentially change the medication timing or release ability or combine the treatment with other antiparkinsonian medications.

Great emphasis is placed on treating the motor features of Parkinson's disease, but clients may have nonmotor manifestations, including depression, anxiety, cognitive impairment, and dementia. Often the client does not mention these difficulties because they do not link them to Parkinson's. Clients may demonstrate some of these difficulties, and the therapist should recognize the symptoms and refer the client for further follow-up.

The major problems that patients have after 5 years of treatment for Parkinson's disease are fluctuations (both motor and nonmotor), dyskinesias, and behavioral or cognitive changes.[5] The mechanisms behind these complications relate both to the underlying Parkinson's disease and to the effects of medications.[6] Motor fluctuations take several forms. Most commonly, a predictable decline in motor performance occurs near the end of each medication dose ("wearing off"). Patients change gradually from "on" with a good medication response into an "off" period 30 minutes to 1 hour before the next medication dose is due. Often patients have involuntary movements (dyskinesias) as a peak-dose complication, and sometimes similar movements occur at the end of the dose. sudden and severe cataclysms of motor fluctuation occur rarely, with ambulatory patients becoming immobilized over a period of seconds ("sudden on-off").[7] Because these fluctuations occur throughout the day, accurate detection requires cooperation by the patient, who must be trained to complete diaries of function.[8] These journals generally divide the 24-hour day into 30-minute segments to detect good medication response ("on"), poor medication response ("off"), disabling dyskinesias, and sleep.

In general, therapists working with clients taking antiparkinsonian medication must be aware of both the positive and negative side effects of medications to meet functional goals and outcomes effectively. Learning the difference between tremor and dyskinesia is crucial. The therapist must coordinate therapy sessions during good medication response times to assist optimal outcomes. Additionally, clients should be monitored for postural hypotension, dizziness, and cognitive changes. Therapists have the unique opportunity to determine best timing, frequency, and duration of their treatment and understand the impact of the clients' drug regimen will only enhance the outcome. Therapists must also be aware that exercise increases metabolism. Increased metabolism may use up the medication faster; thus an individual who generally remains symptom free (no off times between dosages) will again exhibit signs of the disease (distal tremors and axial/proximal rigidity). These increases in symptoms may be a drug dosage problem, not signs of further degeneration of the basal ganglia. All changes in symptoms should be discussed with both the pharmacist and the physician.

Cancer

Cancer may interfere with neurological rehabilitation in various ways. Tumors within the brain may interfere with cognitive and motor function as well as autonomic and metabolic control (see Chapter 25). Peripherally, tumors may interfere with peripheral nerve function and associated motor control or produce pain. In addition, drugs that reduce cancer pain may interfere with cognitive and motor function.[9] Among these, morphine and related opiate derivatives are notable (Box 36-2). A significant degree of tolerance to the CNS depressant effects of these agents will develop with long-term administration. In cancer chemotherapeutic regimens, many antiemetic agents are used. These include dopaminergic antagonists (which may produce motor deficits similar to Parkinson's disease), dronabinol (a chemical component of marijuana, which can affect cognitive function), as well as high-dose corticosteroids (affecting mood). Some antitumor agents may be neurotoxic. These include a reduction in deep tendon reflex, paresthesias, and demyelination associated with vincristine (Oncovin).[10] Naturally, any change in drugs that involves a cancer treatment regimen (directly or indirectly) requires the approval of the client's oncologist.

The main role of rehabilitation specialists is to help cancer patients recover from the physical changes that accompany their illness, promote function in activities of daily living, and help provide adaptations to activities within the limits of each patient's function and the illness. Clinicians should be aware of chemotherapy side effects and the

side effects for medications given to treat the toxic effects of chemotherapy.

A number of chemotherapeutic and nonchemotherapeutic medications are used to fight cancer. Most therapies against cancer operate on the simple principle that because cells in tumors are actively dividing, agents that kill dividing cells will kill tumor cells.[11] Tissues that rapidly divide in the body are therefore at risk, including hair, mucosal lining, bone marrow, immune cells, and skin epithelial cells. Nonchemotherapy medications called biologic response modifiers (BRMs) are naturally made by the body but delivered in large quantities and at higher doses than what the body is capable of producing.[12] Interferon and interleukin are two of the most commonly used medications. Monoclonal antibodies are also used as chemotherapy to suppress the immune system.

Chemotherapy often has side effects that affect the integumentary, gastrointestinal, hematological, and neurological systems. Each type of therapy has potential side effects as well as more general side effects of the treatment regimen. As a result of chemotherapeutic treatment of cancer, the patients often have muscular weakness, fatigue, pain, immobility, and reduced flexibility. Often the therapist will have to be supportive and flexible with treatment plans to accommodate for changing physiological, psychological, and social factors during treatment.

Gastrointestinal symptoms such as nausea and vomiting may occur, and medications such as Compazine and Reglan may be given to help these control episodes. Symptoms of diarrhea may be addressed through prescriptions or the use of over-the-counter medications including milk of magnesia and magnesium citrate. The development of mucositis or esophagitis is also possible. A prescription solution of three medications (Benadryl/Nystatin/viscous lidocaine) can help relieve the pain, inflammation, and potential associated fungal infections. Bone marrow suppression from chemotherapeutic regimens may lead to increased risk of infections, increased risk of bleeding, and increased fatigue and lack of exercise capacity resulting in musculoskeletal weakness. Patients undergoing chemotherapy may receive one or more medications to signal the bone marrow to increase output of white blood cells (Neupogen), stimulate the production of red blood cells (Epogen), and stimulate increased production of platelets (Neumega). These therapies may be instituted to help the patient more quickly reverse suppression of bone marrow and allow the chemotherapy to continue without interruption.[13] Generalized symptoms include fever, body aches and pains, and feelings of ill health and fatigue. No specific medications are used to improve these symptoms. In general, taking medications for fever and pain such as acetaminophen, ibuprofen, or narcotics may help. Currently, the use of exercise as an adjunct therapy for cancer treatment–related symptoms has gained favor in oncology rehabilitation as a promising intervention.[14,15] Exercise is thought to help improve endurance and functional abilities.[14] The major side effects associated with BRMs and monoclonal antibodies are generalized as well and include fever and flulike symptoms with associated arthralgia and myalgia. Other side effects include lymphedema characterized by fluid retention caused by disruption of lymphatic drainage or removal of lymph nodes. As mentioned earlier, neurological changes may occur with

---

BOX 36-2 ■ EXAMPLES OF NARCOTIC ANALGESICS, MORPHINE, AND RELATED AGENTS*

alfentanil (Alfenta)
buprenorphine (Buprenex)
butorphanol (Stadol)
codeine
fentanyl (Duragesic)
hydrocodone (Vicodin)
hydromorphone (Dilaudid)
levorphanol (Levo-Dromoran)
meperidine (Demerol)
methadone (Dolophine)
morphine (Contin-MS)
nalbuphine (Nubain)
oxycodone (Roxicodone)
oxymorphone (Numorphan)
pentazocine (Talwin)
propoxyphene (Darvon)
tramadol (Ultram)

*Effects on motor systems are systemic or indirect.

BOX 36-3 ■ ANTICONVULSANTS*

acetazolamide (various brand names)
carbamazepine (Tegretol)
clonazepam (Klonopin)
ethosuximide (Zarontin)
felbamate (Felbatol)
gabapentin (Neurontin)
lamotrigine (Lamictal)
levetiracetam (Keppra)
oxcarbazepine (Trileptal)
phenobarbital (various brand names)
phenytoin (Dilantin)
primidone (Mysoline)
tiagabine (Gabitril)
topiramate (Topamax)
valproic acid (Depakene)
vigabatrin (Sabril)
zonisamide (Zonagen)

*Effects on motor systems are direct and may decrease tone at higher doses. Direct effects on muscle are minimal. This list does not include benzodiazepines that have antiseizure applications.

the development of neurological signs as well as forgetfulness, suicidal ideation, and depression.[16] The rehabilitation professional is an important team member in oncology by potentially affecting quality of life.

Seizure Disorders (Epilepsy)

Epilepsy is associated with a diverse group of neurological disorders resulting in motor, psychic, and autonomic manifestations. Many antiseizure medications may produce drowsiness, ataxia, and vertigo (Box 36-3). Some may produce cognitive disorders in children and adults.[17,18] Although these adverse effects may be exhibited throughout therapy, they are most troublesome during initiation of drug therapy, addition of a drug, and dosage escalation. Sudden discontinuation of antiseizure medications may result in status epilepticus, which may be fatal. Many antiseizure medications are finding successful applications outside epilepsy, especially in the area of pain management.

The practicing clinician working with clients who have a history of seizure disorders must be prepared for the onset of a seizure and be aware of any adverse side effects of medications. Adverse side effects are typically determined on a clinical basis, signifying the importance of recognition by the health care provider. Many of the common side effects, such as those listed in Box 36-4, can also have negative

BOX 36-4 ■ COMMONLY USED ANTIHYPERTENSIVE AND CARDIOVASCULAR DRUGS*

BETA-ADRENERGIC BLOCKING DRUGS
acebutolol (Sectral)
atenolol (Tenormin)
betaxolol (Kerlone)
bisoprolol (Zebeta)
carvedilol (Coreg)
labetalol (Trandate)
metoprolol (Lopressor)
nadolol (Corgard)
penbutolol (Levatol)
pindolol (Visken)
propranolol (Inderal)
sotalol (Betapace)
timolol (Blocadren)

AGENTS AFFECTING ALPHA AND/OR BETA-ADRENERGIC SYSTEMS
clonidine (Catapres)
guanfacine (Tenex)
guanabenz (Wytensin)
guanadrel (Hylorel)
methyldopa (Aldomet)
doxazosin (Cardura)
prazosin (Minipress)
terazosin (Hytrin)

CALCIUM-CHANNEL BLOCKING DRUGS
amlodipine (Norvasc)
bepridil (Vascor)
diltiazem (Cardizem)

felodipine (Plendil)
isradipine (DynaCirc)
nicardipine (Cardene)
nifedipine (Procardia)
nisoldipine (Sular)
verapamil (Calan)

AGENTS AFFECTING THE RENIN-ANGIOTENSIN SYSTEM
Angiotensin Converting Enzyme Inhibitors
benazepril (Lotensin)
captopril (Capoten)
enalapril (Vasotec)
fosinopril (Monopril)
lisinopril (Zestril)
moexipril (Univasc)
perindopril erbumine (Aceon)
quinapril (Accupril)
ramipril (Altace)
trandolapril (Mavik)

Angiotensin Antagonists
candesartan (Atacand)
eprosartan (Teveten)
irbesartan (Avapro)
losartan (Cozaar)
olmesartan (Benicar)
telmisartan (Micardis)
valsartan (Diovan)

*Effects on motor systems are predominantly systemic or indirect.

implications for motor learning, especially while the client is getting used to the medication or the dosage is elevated or tapered.[19]

The treatment of seizure disorders with pharmacotherapy is typically intended to control the seizure activity completely without producing unwanted side effects.[20] Pharmacological intervention usually begins with one medication (monotherapy); if this drug is unsuccessful a second is added while the first is tapered. Or, a combination may be needed. The effects of the medications vary and may include enhancing the inhibitory affects of γ-aminobutyric acid (benzodiazepines), reducing posttetanic potentiation thereby reducing seizure spread (iminostilbenes), or modulating neuronal voltage-dependent sodium and calcium channels (hydantoin).[21] The overall result is a reduction in abnormal electrical impulses in the brain. The choice of antiseizure drugs primarily depends on the seizure type and, if possible, the diagnosis of a specific syndrome.[22] If seizures are recurrent and occur during critical periods of childhood, adolescence, and early adulthood, they may result in significant impairments in function and increase disability.

Some side effects may be slow to develop and difficult to diagnose because seizures can often be confused for sedation or cognitive dysfunction, especially in children who may not report drug side effects. Practitioners can also mistakenly accept reversible drug toxicity as a necessary consequence of seizure disorder. The number of seizures occurring during physical or occupational therapy should be tracked to assist in determining appropriate pharmacotherapy.

One common antiseizure medication, valproic acid (Depakene), may cause nausea, vomiting, hair loss, tremor, tiredness, dizziness, and headache. Valproic acid has also been reported to aggravate absence seizure in clients with absence epilepsy.[23] Metabolic side effects may include an increase in glucose-stimulated pancreatic insulin secretion, which may be followed by an increase in body weight.[24] Long-term valproic acid use is known to increase bone resorption in adult epileptic patients and lead to a decreased bone mineral density.[25]

Another seizure medication, carbamazepine (Tegretol), is considered a safe drug but has a long list of adverse events, most commonly ataxia and nystagmus.[26] Other systems frequently involved are the skin, the hematopoietic system, and the cardiovascular system. Gabapentin (Neurontin) is another well-tolerated antiseizure medication with proven clinical efficacy and a low incidence of adverse events in clinical trials.[27] Common side effects may include dizziness, fatigue, and headache. Phenytoin (Dilantin) has adverse reactions including ataxia, nystagmus, slurred speech, confusion, dizziness and, in high doses, peripheral neuropathy.

Benzodiazepines (e.g., Diazepam) are useful in managing status epilepticus, but their effects are not long lasting so they are often used along with a primary anticonvulsant. The most frequent side effects are dose-related sedation, difficulty with concentration, dizziness, and difficulty walking.

Pharmacological adverse events that occur under the influence of seizures medications must be recognized by the rehabilitation specialist to participate in a team approach to patient care. Therapists can assist in determination of effectiveness of a specific treatment regimen, appropriate timing of rehabilitation interventions, and the overall progress of the client during rehabilitation.

Stroke, Hypertension, and Related Disorders

Stroke, by virtue of the interference of blood flow and oxygenation, produces both reversible and irreversible neurological deficits (see Chapter 27). To reduce the damage associated with thromboembolism in such cases, tissue plasminogen activator has been recommended. However, this agent is most effective when given within an hour after the vascular insult. Drugs with other mechanisms used to improve the prognosis of stroke are under development. However, drugs used for concurrent conditions (atherosclerosis and hypertension) before and after a stroke are complicating factors for optimal outcomes from rehabilitation. These drugs include beta-adrenergic antagonists, which reduce heart rate and correspondingly reduce exercise tolerance. Occasionally, calcium channel blockers, alpha-adrenergic blockers, and related agents may cause similar effects, including weakness, dizziness, syncope, and cognitive disorders. Changes in serum electrolytes induced by diuretics and the angiotensin converting enzyme inhibitors may affect the heart, the vasculature, and skeletal muscle and ultimately affect impairments such as strength of contraction.[28,29] Box 36-4 lists many of these drugs. Many of the cholesterol synthesis inhibitors (agents used to reduce serum cholesterol) may induce muscle weakness (Box 36-5).[30,31] Abrupt discontinuation of antihypertensive medications may result in a hypertensive crisis, dramatically increasing the risk of stroke and related disorders.

Clinicians caring for patients with stroke, hypertension, and cardiac disorders will benefit from understanding the impact of any medication on the therapeutic plan. These clients may be taking any number of medications to manage the acute and subacute complications of cardiovascular impairments and their resulting sequelae. Other complications after stroke that may require pharmacological intervention include urinary tract infections, musculoskeletal pain, deep vein thrombosis, pressure sores, shoulder subluxation, and depression.[32] All these medications have their own concerns, and health care providers must be aware of adverse events and any alteration in function of the heart that may occur in relation to exercise.

Anticoagulants such as heparin, warfarin, and aspirin (so-called blood thinners) are used to prevent another stroke after the first one has occurred.[33] Side effects may include

---

BOX 36-5 ■ HYPOLIPIDEMIC DRUGS (HMG-COA REDUCTASE INHIBITORS)*

atorvastatin (Lipitor)
fluvastatin (Lescol)
lovastatin (Mevacor)
pravastatin (Pravachol)
rosuvastatin (Crestor)
simvastatin (Zocor)

*May rarely produce muscle damage through a direct effect on the muscle.

bleeding, allergic reactions, thrombocytopenia and, in the case of aspirin, stomach irritation.[34] Blood thinners make the client more susceptible to bruising; therefore care must be taken in client handling and choice of activity. Antiarrhythmics are used to restore normal conduction patterns of the heart.[35] Antiarrhythmic drugs may make some clients experience lightheadedness, dizziness, or faintness when they get up after sitting or lying down (orthostatic hypotension).[36] *Antiarrhythmic drugs may also cause low blood sugar or changes in thermoregulation.*[37,38] The most common side effects are dry mouth and throat, diarrhea, and loss of appetite.[39] These problems usually go away as the body adjusts to the drug and do not require medical treatment. Therapists must be prepared for hypotensive events and the need to educate clients on positions that will reduce the effects of orthostatic hypotension.

Hypertension is a common disorder that will be frequently encountered when treating patients in the rehabilitation environment. Antihypertensive medications are used to lower blood pressure (see Box 36-4) by limiting plasma volume expansion, decreasing peripheral resistance, and decreasing plasma volume. Often clients under medical management will undergo changes in dose and additions or deletions of medication, which may lead to problems during rehabilitation. Side effects of these medications may include increased frequency of urination, increased urinary excretion of potassium, orthostatic hypotension, hypotension, dehydration, tiredness, fatigue, cold hands and feet, and dizziness.[40] When working with clients taking antihypertensive medications, health care providers should monitor for side effects, clinical signs, and the clients perceived exertion. Generally, people on antihypertensive medications require careful cardiovascular monitoring during any physical activity.

Many clients may become depressed after a neurological disorder such as stroke or a cardiac event.[41] It may be attributable to a natural loss of physical function or a neurochemical response to changes in brain chemistry. Clients with signs and symptoms of depression (sadness, anxiousness, hopelessness, suicidal ideation) should be referred for further follow-up by the physician. Many antidepressant medications take at least 2 weeks to achieve a therapeutic level. Antidepressants may cause temporary side effects (sometimes referred to as adverse effects) in some people. These side effects are generally mild. Any unusual reactions, side effects, or behaviors that interfere with functioning should be reported to the doctor immediately. The most common side effects of tricyclic antidepressants are dry mouth, constipation, bladder problems, sexual problems, blurred vision, dizziness, and drowsiness.[42] The newer antidepressants have different types of side effects, including headache, nausea, nervousness, insomnia, agitation, and sexual problems.[43] Therapists working with clients who are depressed may need to delay rehabilitation until the depression is well managed.

Hyperlipidemia is considered a modifiable risk factor for heart disease and stroke. Many clients may be receiving this pharmacological treatment to reduce their cardiovascular risk. Several types of drugs are available for cholesterol lowering, including statins, bile acid sequestrants, nicotinic acid, and fibric acids.[44] The statins are considered first-line drugs and are generally well tolerated but can produce myopathy under some circumstances.[44] An elevation of creatine kinase level is the best indicator of statin-induced myopathy and should be checked when clients report leg pain. Bile acid sequestrants also produce moderate reductions in cholesterol. Sequestrant therapy can produce a variety of gastrointestinal symptoms, including constipation, abdominal pain, bloating, fullness, nausea, and flatulence.[45] Nicotinic acid (niacin) therapy can be accompanied by a number of side effects. Flushing of the skin is common with the crystalline form and is intolerable for some persons. However, most persons have tolerance to the flushing after more prolonged use of the drug. The fibrates have the ability to lower serum triglycerides and are generally well tolerated in most persons. Gastrointestinal symptoms are the most common reports, and fibrates appear to increase the likelihood of cholesterol gallstones.[44]

Overall, clients taking cardiovascular medications need careful monitoring for any drug impact on cardiorespiratory or metabolic responses in relation to rehabilitation activities. Thus the effects of drugs must be considered when developing the rehabilitation plan (see Chapter 35).

Anxiety and Depression

Agents used in the management of anxiety, whether from acute or chronic disease, must be carefully titrated. Among these agents are the benzodiazepines, whose anxiolytic (anxiety-reducing) dosage range immediately precedes a dose that may affect motor skills and cognitive function (Box 36-6). In subjects of all ages, but especially the geriatric population, administration of benzodiazepines may produce paradoxical excitement, confusion, and behavioral changes.[46] Geriatric subjects also have an increased incidence of injury from falls concurrent with benzodiazepines and other sedative-hypnotic drugs. Although benzodiazepines may have variable effects on learning and declarative memory, these effects may differ among the benzodiazepines, displaying considerable variation among individuals. If producing sleep alone is desired, zolpidem (Ambien) and zaleplon (Sonata) are attractive alternatives because these agents do not have anxiolytic effects.[47] Although the anxiolytic agent buspirone (BuSpar) is relatively free of benzodiazepine-like effects, the onset time for the desired anxiolytic effect is characteristically delayed.[48] Lack of compliance with anxiolytic agents may increase panic attacks and reduce effective interactions with a therapist.

BOX 36-6 ■ ANXIOLYTIC BENZODIAZEPINES*

alprazolam (Xanax)
chlordiazepoxide (Librium)
clorazepate (Tranxene)
diazepam (Valium)
halazepam (Paxipam)
lorazepam (Ativan)
oxazepam (Serax)

---

*Note that benzodiazepines indicated for sleep induction are not included in this list. The above agents reduce muscle tone through a direct effect on motor systems at higher doses.

The emergence of the serotonin-selective reuptake inhibitors (SSRIs) has revolutionized the treatment of depression. The older agents, such as the tricyclic antidepressants (TCAs) are just as effective in the management of several forms of depression; however, their adverse effect profile is somewhat different. TCAs often produce drowsiness and orthostatic hypotension, effects that complicate any rehabilitation regimen.[49] Although these effects may be produced by SSRIs, their incidence is much reduced. Certain TCAs, by virtue of their ability to inhibit the reuptake of norepinephrine in adrenergic nerve terminals, may be used at lower doses for neuralgia.[50] Although these low-dose regimens are usually not associated with the side effects previously mentioned, some patients may be more sensitive to these effects than others. This requires increased vigilance for the care team in determining iatrogenic versus pathological sources of somnolence and syncope. A partial list of antidepressants is presented in Box 36-7. Noncompliance with antidepressant therapy may result in lack of interest in any therapeutic regimen.

Patients with stroke and other neurological diagnoses often have depression, which reduces motivation and decreases compliance with a therapeutic regimen. Although obviously linked, the degree of functional restoration after a stroke does not always correlate with resolution of depression.

Many patients with neurological disorders are diagnosed with or experience anxiety and depression. The cause of affective symptomatology can be the result of cognitive and emotional deficits or a result of the impairment of brain function from the existing pathology.[41] In the rehabilitation environment many patients may show signs and symptoms of anxiety or depression that can make the process of recovery more difficult. The rehabilitation professional must recognize the manifestations of both anxiety and depression such as fear of dying or "going mad," heart palpitations, shortness of breath, difficulty concentrating, depressed mood, diminished interest or pleasure in activities, sleep disturbance, changes in appetite, psychomotor retardation and agitation, and suicidal ideation.[51] Anxiety and depression may limit the client's full participation in recovery of function and is associated with poorer outcomes.[43,52]

Anxiety and depression can be managed well when treated with the medications discussed above, but some drugs—including centrally acting hypotensives (methyldopa), lipid soluble beta blockers (propranolol), benzodiazepines, and other CNS depressants—may cause a depressed mood.[53] Therefore review of the medication regimen in someone with depression is useful in case one of the medications may be implicated.

Pharmacological treatments for anxiety and depression should be dosed and timed to ensure the best patient response during rehabilitation treatments. Antianxiety medications (see Box 36-6) act within a short time after ingestion, producing their effects of sedation and relaxation and thereby reducing anxiety. Higher levels may cause drowsiness, sleep, and anesthesia and are associated with falls, which may not be ideal when trying to promote recovery of function. Antidepressant medications (see Box 36-7) typically take weeks for therapeutic levels to be achieved in the brain and an improvement in mood to be demonstrated. Rehabilitation may be appropriate for this client when medications have improved mood and outlook. Side effects of antidepressants can also cause some difficulties, including lightheadedness, drowsiness, short-term memory loss, disturbed sleep, clumsiness, sedation, and low blood pressure.

Some evidence has shown that recovery from brain injury may be positively influenced by antidepressants[54,55] and that antidepressants can play a role in brain plasticity.[9] These studies suggest that recovery of function after brain injury can be influenced through experience and pharmacological intervention. Rehabilitation specialists need to be prepared to assess responses to pharmacotherapy, recognize adverse effects, manage minor side effects, and seek appropriate assistance for adverse events.

Arthritis and Autoimmune Disorders

In the management of rheumatoid arthritis, the therapeutic approach may influence the progress of rehabilitation. Aggressive treatment with glucocorticoids may reduce joint pain and facilitate movement, but it may produce changes in mood and muscle wasting.[56] Although this is reversible and limited to systemic administration of high-dose corticosteroids, its impact cannot be overlooked and certainly affects physical or occupational therapy prognosis. Prednisone and related glucocorticoids may often produce a false sense of well-being that may exceed the ability of the patients to engage safely in certain exercise regimens. From the patient's perspective, this pharmacological effect is perceived as a "cure" and does not provide the motivation to continue with exercise therapy. The same problems may exist with the use of corticosteroids in other autoimmune disorders.[57]

Nonsteroidal antiinflammatory agents (NSAIDs) (Box 36-8) have long been used for the relief of pain with arthritis; however, depletion of prostaglandins in the gastric mucosa produces bleeding that has limited their usefulness.[58] The development of newer agents that are more

BOX 36-8 ■ COMMONLY USED NSAIDs AND SALICYLATES*

GENERAL NONSTEROIDAL AGENTS AND SALICYLATES

aspirin or acetylsalicylic acid
diclofenac (Voltaren)
diflunisal (Dolobid)
etodolac (Lodine)
fenoprofen (Nalfon)
flurbiprofen (Ansaid)
ibuprofen (Advil, Motrin, Nuprin)
indomethacin (Indocin)
ketoprofen (Orudis KT, Oruvail)
ketorolac (Toradol)
meclofenamate (various trade names)
mefenamic acid (Ponstel)
meloxicam (Mobic)
nambutone (Relafen)
naproxen (Aleve, Naprosyn)
oxaprozin (Daypro)
piroxicam (Feldene)
sulindac (Clinoril)
tolmetin (Tolectin)

*Only at higher doses will these agents affect motor systems directly. Most problems are through systemic or indirect effects.

selective for isoforms of cyclooxygenase (COX-2 inhibitors) that are involved in joint inflammation are a major advance. An example is celecoxib. Although bleeding disorders are dramatically reduced, the incidence of ataxia with these agents may be increased.[59] Unfortunately, cardiovascular toxicity risk has led to the withdrawal of most of the COX-2 inhibitors from the market. Clients with neurological diseases or pathological processes with problems requiring antiinflammatory medications may develop side effects that interact and confound existing motor deficits. Failure to comply with arthritis medications will likewise reduce effective movement.

Clinically, clients with the onset of rheumatoid arthritis (RA) may have a number of systemic manifestations, including fatigue, anorexia, generalized weakness, and musculoskeletal symptoms followed by synovitis. These forewarning symptoms may continue over weeks or months before more specific symptoms occur. The initial evaluation of the patient with RA should document symptoms of active disease (e.g., presence of joint pain, duration of morning stiffness, degree of fatigue), functional status, objective evidence of disease activity (e.g., synovitis, as assessed by tender and swollen joint counts, and the erythrocyte sedimentation rate), mechanical joint problems (e.g., loss of motion, crepitus, instability, malalignment, or deformity), the presence of extraarticular disease, and damaged detected radiographically.[60] Neurological complications of rheumatoid arthritis may occur in the CNS (cerebral vasculitis), the peripheral nervous system (nerve compression), neuromuscular junction (myasthenic syndrome), and muscle (myopathy).[61] Depending on the stage of involvement the client may be undergoing nonpharmacological modalities (education,

weight loss, range of motion) and pharmacological therapy, including analgesics, NSAIDs, steroids, disease modifying antirheumatic drugs (DMARDs), and BRMs.

The goals of pharmacological treatment of RA are to prevent or control joint damage, prevent loss of function, decrease pain, and improve joint function.[60] NSAIDs assist in analgesia and decrease inflammation, thus allowing the therapist to work on range of motion and strengthening, but they do not alter the disease process. Because NSAIDs regulate the production of chemicals (prostaglandins) in the body that help trigger inflammation by inhibition of an enzyme (cyclooxygenase), they sometimes lead to unwanted side effects previously discussed. Data suggest that although selective COX-2 inhibitors have a significantly lower risk of serious adverse gastrointestinal effects than do nonselective NSAIDs, they are no more effective than nonselective NSAIDs, are related to cardiovascular events, and may cost as much as 15 to 20 times more per month of treatment than generic NSAIDs.[62,63]

Steroids are synthetic forms of naturally occurring hormones produced by the adrenal glands that are typically administered orally or by injection. They provide rapid and powerful reduction of pain and inflammation, thus resulting in improved function. Recent evidence suggests that low-dose glucocorticoids slow the rate of joint damage and therefore appear to have disease-modifying potential.[64] Side effects include blood sugar elevations, cataracts, hypertension, increased susceptibility to infection and bruising, osteoporosis, and weight gain, depending on the dosage and length of treatment. They are often used at disease onset or with disease flares as a temporary aid in obtaining control.[65] Disabling synovitis frequently recurs when glucocorticoids are discontinued, even in patients who are receiving combination therapy with one or more DMARDs. Therefore many patients with RA are functionally dependent while taking glucocorticoids and continue them long term.[60]

An important foundation in the treatment of RA are DMARDs, a term that refers to a number of medications that reduce signs and symptoms, reduce or prevent joint damage, and preserve the structure and function of the joints. Their use alone or in combination is also attributed to allowing patients to remain active and productive.[66] The most common DMARDs in current use include methotrexate, sulfasalazine, hydroxychloroquine, leflunomide, and cyclosporine. Others include gold salts, azathioprine, and D-penicillamine. Side effects may include diarrhea, eye damage, liver damage, nausea, and vomiting and depend on the DMARD taken.

Finally, BRMs are a newly developed class of medicines that restore or stimulate the immune system to fight disease. BRMs target specific parts of the immune system that destroy joints. Some do so by blocking the effects of tumor necrosis factor (TNF), a protein involved in RA through the inflammatory cascade, and are credited with improving signs, symptoms, and function in patients with RA.[67]

Rehabilitation therapy is important in maintaining physical function in clients with RA. With combinations of medications, health care providers can reach goals of increasing or maintaining joint mobility; decreasing pain; improving functional abilities; improving cardiovascular fitness; and educating clients on the use of assistive devices, joint protection, and energy conservation.

Infectious Diseases

Both bacterial and viral diseases may produce neurological disorders (see Chapter 20). The neurological impact of treatments and prophylactic measures must be understood. Although this may be readily apparent for drugs, vaccines have also been implicated in causing similar problems. The association of a hypotonic-hyporesponsive episode with the pertussis vaccine is such an example.[68]

In the course of treating bacterial diseases, many antibiotics and antiinfective agents may compromise sensory, motor, and cognitive function. These functions may be compromised temporarily or permanently and may be patient specific. First, in the critically ill patient, aminoglycosides (gentamicin, tobramycin, and amikacin) and vancomycin may produce ototoxicity, such as hearing loss (reversible and irreversible) and vestibular damage (dizziness, vertigo, and ataxia). Minocycline is also associated with vestibular toxicity.[69] Extra precautions may be necessary to prevent falls during and after therapeutic exercise sessions. Fall prevention programs must be developed in these cases as well as with the use of sedative-hypnotics, as previously noted.

A wide variety of viral diseases interfere with neurological function. Polio is historically the most widely recognized (see Chapter 29). Acquired immunodeficiency syndrome (AIDS) may be manifest as a wide variety of neurological disorders (see Chapter 21). A recent finding is that protease inhibitors, which reduce the assembly of viral particles, may dramatically reduce and possibly reverse the neurological manifestations of AIDS.[70] Although adverse effects associated with antiviral and antibiotic agents may be intolerable, noncompliance may result in increased resistance of the virus or microorganism to retreatment.

The guiding principle of chemotherapy for infection is selective toxicity, in which the agent must cause more harm to the pathogen than to the host. Problems facing antimicrobial therapy include resistance to drugs, side effects, allergies, and suppression of normal flora. Clinicians therefore ask clients to exercise under conditions in which they may potentially have a compromised immune response because of trauma, pathological condition, or surgery. These conditions may make clients more susceptible to infection, slow healing, and slow recovery.[71]

An increasing number of strains of antibiotic-resistant bacteria are now emerging, in large part because of the overuse and misuse of antimicrobial drugs by health care providers.[72] Overuse of antimicrobial drugs exerts a selective pressure among bacteria, encouraging the emergence of antibiotic-resistant strains by eliminating antibiotic-sensitive strains and promoting the establishment of bacterial with rare mutations of resistance and permitting the spread of resistant strains from infected individuals.[73,74] One example is the use of antibiotics for upper respiratory tract infections caused by viruses. This has been shown to have no beneficial impact on the course of the disease.[75] Infection control in the rehabilitation environment is essential to stop the spread of disease. Therapists must be vigilant with infection control procedures such as handwashing, updating vaccinations, only treating patients who may spread infections, and cleaning all equipment. Educating clients to use antibiotics only when needed and complete the entire course of medication can potentially slow the proliferation.

Common adverse effects from the use of antimicrobials and antiviral drugs may include nephrotoxicity and ototoxicity (aminoglycosides), gastrointestinal complications (cephalosporins, clindamycin), thrombophlebitis and vertigo (tetracyclines), jaundice (erythromycin), photophobia (vidarabine), neurotoxicity (metronidazole), and allergic reactions (beta-lactam antibiotics). The therapist must be aware of adverse side effects to assist with early recognition and referral to the physician.

Antibiotics kill various normal commensal bacteria in the gut, altering the balance and allowing overgrowth of pathogens.[76] This change of bacterial flora is believed to result in increased toxins from pathogens and can cause infection with resistant microbes.[76] When clients are taking drugs to fight infection or undergoing procedures or surgeries that place them at risk for infection (indwelling catheters), they can be more susceptible to infectious agents. Abscesses or contamination as a result of the normal flora into a normally sterile body side is often the reason for perioperative antimicrobial prophylaxis.[77] Rehabilitation specialists will most likely see many clients who are undergoing chemotherapy with antiinfective medications and play a crucial role in preventing and controlling infectious disease in the health care setting. Therapists need to update their knowledge foundation with evidence-based protocols for specific diagnosis and treatments as well as understand when infections may or may not need antimicrobial medications. Additionally, education of patients about why antimicrobial agents are not indicated in specific situation, how to alleviate symptoms, and what signs indicate further follow-up may help them understand the growing problem of antibiotic resistance.

Diabetes

The development of peripheral neuropathy (see Chapter 15) is a progressive problem in patients with diabetes. This neuropathy compromises sensory and motor control. In addition to long-term management of diabetes from a glucohomeostatic perspective, other agents show promise. Treatment of diabetic neuropathy with trazodone and mexiletine are examples.[78,79]

A more acute problem is swings in blood glucose level from inappropriate diet, exercise, insulin, and oral hypoglycemic drug administration. The balance of these factors is important, and monitoring of blood glucose level is essential. Swings in blood glucose level are often associated with changes in behavior and sensorium. This may pose a safety concern because cognitive and motor function may be impaired as a result. An increase in exercise will decrease the blood glucose concentration, thereby reducing insulin requirements. These factors should be carefully considered in any exercise regimen for the client with diabetes.[80] A list of oral hypoglycemic agents is presented in Box 36-9. Lack of glucose control because of noncompliance with medications that are useful in controlling diabetes will only return the client to an accelerated course to peripheral neuropathies and related sequelae.

In the clinical setting the health care practitioner must remember that the main goal of diabetes management is to prevent both the small-vessel (e.g., retinopathy and neuropathy) and large-vessel (e.g., heart disease and amputation) complications of the disease linked with elevated blood

BOX 36-9 ■ ORAL HYPOGLYCEMIC AGENTS*

SULFONYLUREAS
acetohexamide (Dymelor)
chlorpropamide (Diabinese)
tolazamide (Tolinase)
tolbutamide (Orinase)
glimepiride (Amaryl)
glipizide (Glucotrol)
glyburide (Micronase)

RELATED AGENTS
repaglinide (Prandin)
nateglinide (Starlix)

*May produce direct and indirect effects on motor systems through hypoglycemia.

glucose levels. Diabetes is therefore often controlled through intensive, tailored treatment regimens of diet and physical activity, oral agents, and insulin.[81] Each of these regimens is designed to potentially reduce hyperglycemia and can result in hypoglycemia if not monitored.

Initially, the physician and client with diabetes can work together on a treatment plan to manage the disease. An important first step is diet, physical activity, and a program to reduce body weight by 5% to 10%.[82] The effects of exercise as a cause of hypoglycemia deserve particular consideration because physical activity represents the most variable factor in the routine of many clients, especially those in rehabilitation.[83] With vigorous exercise, glucose use can increase severalfold, and this increase can persist long after the completion of the exercise, resulting in a fall in blood glucose long after its completion. Although diet and activity are important cornerstones for diabetes care, oral agents and/or insulin may eventually be required to achieve glycemic control.

Five classes of oral agents are available to help or make the body use its own insulin, including sulfonylureas (chlorpropamide), meglitinides (Repaglinide), biguanides (metformin), glitazones (rosiglitazone), and alpha glucosidase inhibitors (acarbose). These classes of medications have specific regimens and may be prescribed as monotherapy or taken in combination that may include insulin. Side effects vary from weight gain to gastrointestinal symptoms to hypoglycemia. Hypoglycemia as a side effect of pharmacotherapy is of concern in the rehabilitation setting because abnormally low glucose levels can cause alterations in cognition, cardiovascular hemodynamic changes, and a increased risk of physical injury.[84] The signs and symptoms of hypoglycemia can vary from person to person and may depend on how fast the blood sugar drops. Early signs include shaking, sweating, fatigue, and weakness. Later signs may manifest as confusion, combativeness, and exhaustion that inhibits eating, which may lead to loss of consciousness.

Insulin is a primary therapy in type 1 diabetes, in which the body has no ability to produce its own insulin. When oral antidiabetic agents no longer assist in maintaining glycemic

targets, insulin is usually instated in the diabetic with low production or resistance to insulin (type 2 diabetes).[85] Many forms of insulin are available, and administration is typically through subcutaneous injection or insulin pumps. Insulin can be long acting or short acting and is often used in combinations to maintain the optimal level of glycemic control. Hypoglycemia is the primary problem associated with inulin use because of its ability to lower blood sugar.[85]

Health professionals working with clients who have diabetes should consider a number of strategies for prevention of hypoglycemia and be able to analyze the risk and benefits of exercise. Because glycemic control is individualized each client must be addressed uniquely, and as a member of the health care team the rehabilitation specialist can potentially assist in education of all those involved in the care of the client. The following are guidelines published by the American Diabetes Association (ADA) and should be implemented in clients with known type 2 diabetes.[86] Medical evaluation of the client before exercise begins in important to determine the extent of involvement and complications present. Prepare the client for exercise by monitoring glycemic control before, during, and after exercise. Exercise is contraindicated if fasting glucose levels are more than 250 mg/dl and ketosis is present; use caution if glucose levels are greater than 300 mg/dl and no ketosis is present. The patient should ingest added carbohydrate if glucose levels are less than 100 mg/dl. Document when changes in insulin or food intake are necessary and learn the glycemic response to different exercise conditions (e.g., light, moderate, heavy). Food intake should include consumption of carbohydrates as needed to avoid hypoglycemia. Carbohydrate-based foods should be readily available during and after exercise.

Clinicians need to have an understanding of what causes diabetes, the effects of medications and exercise on the regulation of blood sugar levels, signs of symptoms of hypoglycemia, and what should be done in a diabetic emergency.

Pulmonary Diseases

Many clients with neurological problems have pulmonary disease as well (see Chapter 35). The treatment of pulmonary diseases presents an unusual challenge. Many drugs used for treatment of asthma, emphysema, and chronic obstructive pulmonary disease (COPD) are intended to have direct effects on the lung, yet systemic effects are often unavoidable. Adrenergic bronchodilators, such as albuterol, epinephrine, and metaproterenol, may increase heart rate and tremor.[87] If tremor is first manifested because of a neurological insult, then these drugs may exaggerate the motor impairment. Although ipratropium is an anticholinergic with bronchodilator properties, the associated systemic anticholinergic effects (such as urinary retention with prostatic hypertrophy) are not well tolerated in geriatric men.[88] Prednisone and related corticosteroids may dramatically reduce the degree of pulmonary hyperresponsiveness but often produce systemic effects as previously noted. These are often reduced (but not necessarily eliminated) with the use of inhaled corticosteroids such as beclomethasone, budesonide, flunisolide, and triamcinolone. Although the use of xanthines in asthma is declining, theophylline in asthma and obstructive pulmonary diseases can produce changes in cognitive function, including delusions and hallucinations with higher doses. General CNS stimulation, including nervousness, insomnia, and seizures, is well recognized.[89] Tremor and nausea are often produced with theophylline, even with clinical dosage regimens commonly accepted. Finally, the increase in diuresis by theophylline in patients with prostatic hypertrophy is certainly troublesome.[90] The metabolism of this drug is often changed by other medications, which complicates therapy. These changes in drug metabolism may increase toxicity or decrease efficacy.[91,92] A newer class of disease-modifying agents known as the leukotriene modifiers (montelukast and zafirlukast) are being favored in many regimens for the management of asthma. Although cardiovascular and neurological side effects of these drugs appear to be dramatically reduced when compared with other agents, they have been implicated in several important drug interactions.[93,94] Lack of compliance with these medications decreases pulmonary gas exchange, ultimately decreasing motor performance.

Clients may have signs and symptoms of lung dysfunction during exercise, including nonproductive cough, dyspnea, alterations in breathing rate and chest expansion, changes in skin color, auscultation and percussion. Symptomatic pharmacotherapy may be required to reduce disease-related symptoms such as shortness of breath and improve exercise tolerance.[95] The clinician should begin exercise after medications to improve exercise tolerance.[96] Often with chronic lung disease exacerbations may be caused by an infection; therefore antibiotics may be prescribed.[97] Additionally, thinning and mobilization of secretions in airways with mucolytics and chest therapy may be necessary.[98] Oxygen therapy is a secondary therapy that may be necessary for hypoxemic patients.[97] This therapy reduces the hematocrit level to more normal levels, moderately improves neuropsychological factors, and ameliorates pulmonary hemodynamic abnormalities.[99] Oxygen therapy may be indicated for patients during exercise in those whose levels become desaturated during low-level activity.[100] Understanding the use of pharmacological treatments for pulmonary dysfunction can assist the rehabilitation professional in promoting improved strength, exercise tolerance, and functional abilities in clients with pulmonary dysfunction.

Gastrointestinal Disorders

Among the wide variety of agents used in the treatment of gastrointestinal (GI) disorders, problems with agents affecting GI motility are among the most frequently encountered. Antiemetics that are dopaminergic antagonists, such as prochlorperazine (Compazine), chlorpromazine (Thorazine), and promethazine (Phenergan), may produce extrapyramidal side effects resembling Parkinson's disease through the drug's actions in the basal ganglia.[101] Dronabinol (Marinol), a cannabinoid derivative from marijuana, is an effective antiemetic but may produce cognitive and sensory disturbances, including drowsiness, dizziness, ataxia, disorientation, orthostatic hypotension, and euphoria.[102] The serotonin-selective antagonists dolasetron (Anzemet), granisetron (Kytril), and ondansetron (Zofran) are effective and valuable antiemetics, especially in cancer chemotherapy. The most common adverse effect is severe headache.[103] The benzodiazepine lorazepam is an effective adjunct for control of emesis. Problems associated with benzodiazepines have been previously discussed. Corticosteroids such as dexamethasone should be included among the antiemetic agents; their adverse effects have also been previously discussed.

In producing normal motility, metoclopramide (Reglan), domperidone (Motilium), and cisapride (Propulsid) are often used. The adverse effects of metoclopramide are primarily through dopaminergic antagonism. Domperidone was developed to reduce these CNS effects and has been used to treat diabetic gastroparesis with some success.[104] Cisapride, a restricted use prokinetic agent, may have a wide variety of CNS effects, including dizziness, mood disorders, vision changes, hallucinations, and amnesia, although with low incidence compared with concerns of arrhythmias induced by this drug.[105] Compliance with medications that reduce problems with the GI system may have little direct effect on motor performance but may prove troublesome to the client's quality of life.

In the rehabilitation setting, GI signs and symptoms are common problems for many clients. The side effects of drugs reported in formularies show that almost all oral preparations are the potential cause of some form of GI disturbance.[106] Symptoms include upper GI effects such as nausea, vomiting, indigestion, gastric reflux, and stomach pain or lower GI effects such as diarrhea, constipation, colonic pain, and blood in stools. These symptoms may be caused by an underlying GI condition (gallstones and acid reflux) or side effects from medications (nausea and vomiting). Because GI problems can be prevalent and challenging, cause poor compliance, and be a signal for a more serious condition, the causes and potential approaches used to ameliorate the symptoms must be understood.

Medications can modify GI absorption, cause dysmotility, damage the mucosal lining, or change the bioavailability and resulting effectiveness of drugs. Some drugs modify the absorption or activity of nutrients, ions, and drugs. Drugs such as metformin (used in the treatment of diabetes) may reduce the absorption of vitamin B_{12}, with the potential development of megaloblastic anemia, resulting in exercise precautions.[107] Other drugs that damage the mucosal lining (methotrexate, allopurinol, neomycin, colchicine, methyldopa) may reduce nutrient absorption, leading to deficiencies.[76] One class of agents, NSAIDs, is estimated to be regularly used by 5% to 10% of the U.S. population, with more than 70 million prescriptions filled annually[94] and more than 30 billion over the counter (OTC) tablets sold.[108,109] These drugs are implicated in patients reporting gastric dyspepsia (pain or discomfort in the upper abdomen), and concomitant administration of proton pump inhibitors (which block production of stomach acid) and prostaglandin analogues (which protect stomach lining) may often reduce mucosal erosion.[76]

Drugs that cause dysmotility of the small intestine such as TCAs (for depression), anticholinergics (for asthma), calcium channel blockers (for heart failure), and opiates (for pain) may be commonly administered to patients within the rehabilitation population.[76] The large intestine is more likely to have reduced motility, with abdominal pain, constipation, nausea, vomiting, and abdominal distention present. Many patients require increased activity, change of dietary habits, or laxatives to improve motility.[110] Precautions must be taken because of the potential for chronic use of laxatives, fluid and electrolyte imbalance, steatorrhea, protein-losing gastroenteropathy, osteomalacia, and vitamin and mineral deficiencies.[76]

It is important to note that some supplements and fluids (e.g., grapefruit juice) taken with medications can potentially cause changes in the bioavailability of drugs. Concurrent ingestion of iron causes a marked decrease in the bioavailability of a number of drugs such as tetracycline (an antibiotic), methyldopa (an antihypertensive agent), levodopa (for Parkinson's disease), and ciprofloxacin (an antimicrobial).[111] Grapefruit juice is also known to change the bioavailability of some medications, leading to an elevation of their serum concentrations; these include cyclosporine (an immunosuppressive agent), calcium antagonists (for hypertension), and coenzyme A reductase inhibitors (statins).[112]

Most medications have the potential to cause some form of GI difficulties, whether taken systemically, topically applied, or given by the parenteral route.[76] Most adverse effects can be reduced with identification of the causal relation, proper administration of the drug, and administration according to all the guidelines on the label. Therapists may suggest specific timing of medications to relieve symptoms and increase participation in therapy. The role of physical and occupational therapists should be recognized in observing adverse drug events to warn patients of early signs of potential problems, provide education, and refer for further follow-up by the pharmacist or physician.

AN IMPAIRMENT PERSPECTIVE

In this section of the chapter, different forms of neurological impairments are discussed and appropriate drugs are identified that either reduce or increase the degree of impairment. Although not a comprehensive list, these impairments include sensory, motor, cognitive, balance and coordination, cardiovascular, muscle tone, and a brief overview of neuroplasticity. Remember that pharmacists have been educated and work closely with physicians who have been educated in a disease/pathology model. A large portion of physicians' practice is related to drug therapy as it is related to disease and pathology. Looking at drugs from an impairment, functional activity, life participation model is not the role of either the physician or the pharmacist. Thus movement specialists, whose model for care is based on function and quality of life, need to bridge the gap between these concepts because the outcome of the interactions dramatically affect the potential of the individual after any CNS dysfunction.

Sensory Impairment

Drugs that affect hearing, vision, and touch may influence any type of sensory, cognitive, and motor impairment. In any impairment, the processing of accurate sensory information is crucial to modify and adjust procedural programming during movement. A subject must be able to visually, manually, or through auditory cues (even through olfactory means) relate to or recognize the relevance of the external environment, engage the specific motor programming centers that reach consensus regarding the specific motor response, and produce the series of signals that may progress uninterrupted through spinal mechanisms and the motor endplate to a regional muscle group for an appropriate response. Any impairment or drug that affects any compo-

nent within these systems, whether early or late in this sequence, will affect the motor performance. As previously discussed, certain drugs may influence hearing (as previously indicated regarding infectious diseases) or produce tinnitus (e.g., aspirin), which may be distracting and thus ultimately affect motor performance.[69] Changes in the visual field (e.g., ethambutol and anticonvulsants) are likewise important. Analgesics and topical anesthetics may dangerously affect surface heat/cold discomfort and undermine avoidance cues. However, elimination of excessive pain (peripheral and central) may enhance cognitive focus and learning as well as allow an individual to move as part of daily living, which will help maintain power, range, balance, and thus quality of life. The CNS functions with the consensus of multiple interactions. Because the branched as well as sequential nature of systems link sensory and motor functions, the peripheral effects of drugs commonly modify the function of central systems. This is a relatively unappreciated reason why drug therapy can modify rehabilitation techniques both positively and negatively (see Chapter 9, Neuroplasticity and Somatosensory Retraining).

Cognitive and Central Motor Control Impairment

Disorders of mood (anxiety and depression) reduce initiative in the rehabilitation process. In this context, anxiolytics and antidepressants may have a positive impact. However, if the dose is not carefully titrated, drowsiness and anterograde amnesia will cloud effective response and learning. Both antidepressants and many of the benzodiazepines may exhibit these effects, as previously discussed. Behavioral disorders, especially those associated with untreated psychoses or dementia, impede cognitive function. Although antipsychotics may correct these disorders, the dopaminergic antagonism associated with these may interfere with the function of the basal ganglia and facilitation of movement. Many newer antipsychotic agents (also known as the atypical antipsychotics) have, in addition to dopaminergic antagonism, serotonin antagonist activity, which may reduce the extrapyramidal side effects of the earlier agents when analyzed as movement dysfunction (Box 36-10) (see Chapter 24).

Vertigo, Dizziness, Balance, and Coordination

Many agents with histamine antagonist and anticholinergic activity have been used for treatment of vertigo and dizziness. Meclizine and related antihistamines are primary examples.[113] Occasionally, sinus congestion can result in impaired vestibular function and dizziness. In the absence of hypertension or related autonomic dysfunction, an indirect-acting adrenergic agonist such as ephedrine or pseudoephedrine can reduce this congestion and improve this condition (see Chapter 23).[114]

Cardiovascular Impairment

In the management of hypercholesterolemia, the 3-hydroxy-3-methylglutaryl coenzyme A (HMG-CoA) reductase inhibitors (see Box 36-5) may produce myopathies to various degrees. Changes in hemodynamics caused by antihypertensive regimens must be monitored because these agents can produce syncope and lower exercise tolerance.

BOX 36-10 ■ EXAMPLES OF ANTIPSYCHOTIC AGENTS

STANDARD ANTIPSYCHOTICS*
   chlorpromazine (Thorazine)
   fluphenazine (Prolixin)
   haloperidol (Haldol)
   loxapine (Loxitane)
   molindone (Moban)
   perphenazine (Trilafon)
   thioridazine (Mellaril)

ATYPICAL ANTIPSYCHOTICS
   aripiprazole (Abilify)
   clozapine (Clozaril)
   olanzapine (Zyprexa)
   quetiapine (Seroquel)
   risperidone (Risperdal)
   ziprasidone (Geodon)

*May produce a parkinsonian-like effect through dopaminergic antagonism.

BOX 36-11 ■ MUSCLE RELAXANTS AND ANTISPASMODICS*

baclofen (Lioresal)
carisoprodol (Soma)
chlorzoxazone (Paraflex)
cyclobenzaprine (Flexeril)
dantrolene (Dantrium)†
metaxalone (Skelaxin)
methocarbamol (Robaxin)
orphenadrine (Norflex)
tizanidine (Zanaflex)

*Direct effects on motor systems to reduce tone.
†Direct effects on muscle to reduce tone.

Weakness from intermittent claudication is a challenge that can be managed in part with cilostazol.[92] Any drug that is used to decrease spasticity as a consequence of stroke and related cerebrovascular disorders may impair motor control and thus affect motor learning. A discussion of these drugs is outlined in the next section (see also Chapters 27 and 35).

Spasticity and Muscle Tone

Muscle spasms may be controlled with centrally acting and peripherally acting agents, all of which produce drowsiness, dizziness, and muscle weakness to various degrees.[115] Commonly used agents are listed in Box 36-11. Pharmacological management of muscle tone, spasticity, and coordination of movement is of primary importance in neurological rehabilitation.

With regard to spasticity, several additional options are available. Tizanidine (Zanaflex) is the newest of the alpha-adrenergic agonists available to reduce spasticity, primarily through activation of descending noradrenergic inhibitory pathways.[116] Clonidine (Catapres) has similar actions. Intrathecal administration of baclofen (Lioresal) produces an antispasmodic effect through enhancement of gamma-aminobutyric acid (GABAergic) function, both central and spinal.[117] Likewise, enhancement of GABAergic function and reduced spasticity can be realized through the anti-seizure drug gabapentin.[118] Selective motor neurons can be inactivated through local injection of botulinum toxins.[119] These agents inhibit the release of acetylcholine at the neuromuscular junction. The investigational agent 4-aminopyridine has been shown to reduce spasticity in spinal cord injury.[120]

The involvement of serotonin in maintenance of muscle tone and spasticity is complex and controversial. Cyproheptadine, a relatively nonselective serotonergic antagonist, can reduce spasticity and maintain muscle tone.[121] However, SSRIs used as antidepressants may occasionally increase spasticity,[122] and clozapine (Clozaril), a serotonin-selective antagonist, may produce muscle weakness.[123]

In addition to spinal cord injuries, multiple sclerosis may exhibit spasticity as a complication. Although several interferons have been used in the management of multiple sclerosis, interferon beta$_{1b}$ has been shown to increase spasticity (see Chapters 19 and 22).[124]

Neuroplasticity

The effects of drugs on plasticity is highly controversial. In Alzheimer's disease a loss of plasticity may be realized through deficits in hippocampal and cortical function leading to memory loss (see Chapters 3, 4, and 9). Many anticholinesterase agents improve memory and may provide evidence of a class of agents that may enhance neuroplasticity.[125] This rapidly evolving area of research may provide interesting avenues for treatment of other neurological disorders in addition to Alzheimer's disease.

RESEARCH AND DEVELOPMENT PROSPECTS

The prediction of which areas of pharmacological research will have the most valuable impact on the management of neurological disorders and the resulting residual impairments is difficult. Drug development is a continuous process, although this text must have a definitive end point. Many drugs with outstanding promise for treating neurological diseases will have adverse effects that may be less acceptable than the neurological problem (or in fact may be lethal in rare cases) and may require removal from the market. In spite of these disappointments, many reasons for optimism exist.

Among the burgeoning areas of biotechnology that will have an influence on neurology will be the discovery, characterization, and application of neuronal growth factors, related growth modifiers, and cellular implants, which may have the long-term promise of either partially or completely restoring nerve function. Although these developments are unlikely to have extensive application within the next few years, over a period of decades these and related developments will take root and revolutionize our understanding and treatment of a wide variety of neurological disorders.

The pharmacist stands as a valuable resource for physical and occupational therapists today as well as in the future. Pharmacists must participate in the management of drug therapies that may be related to each area discussed in this chapter. Therapists should consult the pharmacist about new drug developments and discuss potential problems that these new drugs may have on neurological rehabilitation. This is especially true when new drugs not mentioned in this text are being administered to clients. These discussions can illuminate intended and adverse effects that may affect interventions and change patient outcomes. They may show improvements as well as exacerbations in movement function. Some of those changes are disease or pathology related. Other changes are attributable to spontaneous return, new learning, and neuroplasticity within the CNS. Changes can also occur because of drug therapy. Those changes as stated can be both positive and negative. The scope of practice for occupational and physical therapists does not involve differentiating which change is caused by which process, but these professionals certainly can recognize functional changes. When changes are positive the team needs to be aware and most likely everyone will take credit for the changes. When the changes take away function, families and therapists are often the first to identify those changes. The pharmacist and physician will need to determine why the system is deteriorating. The therapist is responsible for sharing those negative behavior changes with the team and following through with monitoring decisions of future change when drug regimens have been altered.

SUMMARY

In the therapeutic jungle of drug therapies, the clinician must be wary of trouble that lurks ahead. This degree of vigilance can yield greater rewards for the client in terms of affective management of multiple diseases and reduced interference with rehabilitation. Resolving problems with therapies requires a team approach. When drugs are involved with management of these problems, the client's physician, pharmacist, therapist, nurse, and caregiver must be aware that drugs pose a certain degree of risk with every positive step. The team must work closely to address adequately inquiries into possible drug problems and opportunities for therapeutic success.

CASE STUDIES

In a previous edition of this text, two patients in case studies were pharmacologically managed for cognitive decline with donepezil HCl (Aricept) 10 mg (1 tablet) daily. This information was shared with their physical therapists, and their therapy was successfully maintained until their deaths. Important lessons can be learned since the last edition from the management of these two cases that have also changed the way one author (H. R.) now writes referrals for physical or occupational therapy for any patient identified with a cognitive problem. This recommendation should be applied to any patient who is treated for memory loss or is suspected of having a cognition loss. The plan for physical or occupational therapy intervention must also consider the mental-cognitive abilities of those who will care for the patient at home, the spouse, other family members or an outside care provider. Sometimes home programs are not always completed because the patient does not understand or the family member in charge forgets the instructions or does not remember to have the patient do activities that help regain functional movement and thus activities of daily living. The primary care provider may also be in the early stages of

dementia. The plan should include illustrations and clear and easy-to-follow pictorial instructions of the exercises or functional activities. These must be given and discussed with the care provider for more effective reference and follow-up. If, in the course of a scheduled medical and occupational or physical therapy visit, the care provider does not come with the patient, request that the care provider accompany the patient on subsequent visits.

Other drugs related to donepezil are available for dementia. These need closer attention to titration to acceptable dosage levels (e.g., rivastigmine [Exelon] 1.5 mg, 3 mg, 4.5 mg, and 6 mg, administered twice daily); galantamine [Rementyl] 4 mg, 8 mg, and 12 mg, administered twice daily); and memantine HCl [Namenda] 5 and 10 mg, administered twice daily). The combination of Aricept and Namenda is well accepted for extending cognitive function. Regardless of the drug used, the impact of progressive dementia will exceed drug efficacy and adversely affect occupational and physical therapy. This reinforces the necessity for family and care provider involvement in all phases of therapy.

The two case studies presented in this section illustrate the importance of obtaining complete medical history before initiating therapy. Unfortunately, and all too often, physical and occupational therapists are asked by the referring physician to look only at a specific problem, for example, "improve upper limb mobility," and are not given background medical history other than perhaps a one-word descriptor such as "stroke," or a short note, "weakness in upper and lower extremities." Unless the therapist has access to a full medical history, including prescription and OTC drugs, the therapy requested may be less than fully successful because many drugs have adverse side effects that may alter cognitive function or the patient's ability to learn and redevelop impaired motor functions.

Therapists must know and understand the underlying pathophysiology of the referred patient's diagnosis to evaluate the impairment that is causing motor dysfunction. In addition, therapists need to understand how drugs affect the specific physical impairment that is altering the quality of life of day-to-day activity—in some cases hour by hour—functioning. For example, drugs given to patients can either alter or promote their depression and can interfere with intellectual, cognitive, and pain levels, all of which can alter their ability to fully participate in physical and occupational therapy. Often patients' cognitive abilities are modified by either their organic problem or the medical drug therapy. If a cognitive impairment is present, the therapist needs to assess how severe it is to adjust instructions and plan of therapy to a level at which the patient can succeed. The cognitive level, along with the primary medical diagnosis, shapes the physical and occupational therapy prognosis.

Knowledge of the drugs currently being used by the patient provides guidance in structuring therapy and may determine whether the plan of care will be effective. For example, will a patient taking pain medicine have a cognitive level that permits a full understanding of what is being asked during therapy? Will drug therapy provide adequate pain management to enable physical manipulation by either the therapist or the patient in response to the commands? When is the pain medication administered, and is the time in relation to the appointment appropriate? How long does the drug work, and does it have negative effects on cognition?

These are only a few examples of the kind of questions that therapists need to ask to design and implement therapy programs that enhance the patients' abilities to recover motor functions, prevent physical regression, and perhaps even retard or stop some aspects of mental regression caused by either drug therapy or endogenous depression. Clinicians must keep in mind the potential for both positive and negative drug-induced changes and ways that these can alter or improve the overall physical and mental status of the patient. The following case studies further illustrate the interactions of the disease, pharmacological management, and physical/occupational therapy interventions.

CASE STUDY 36-1 ■ MULTIPLE SCLEROSIS

C. G. is a 42-year-old white man with relapsing remitting multiple sclerosis (MS) who had an Extended Disability Status Score (EDSS) of 1 when first seen. He now has an EDSS score of 3.1. C. G. is no longer able to work. He had been a building contractor, and for a short period after his MS diagnosis he continued working until he lost the use of his legs. He is currently confined to a wheelchair, is incontinent for both bowel and bladder, has lost the ability to stand, and is unable to dress or transfer from any seated position, such as to toilet himself or shower independently. In addition, he is no longer able to prepare his own meals during the 8 to 10 hours per day he spends alone from his family.

HISTORY

C. G. had been treated unsuccessfully with two of the interferon drugs (interferon beta$_{1a}$ and beta$_{1b}$ [Avonex and Betaseron]) used to retard MS progression. He is now taking glatiramer acetate (Copaxone), a third MS suppressive drug, and is currently stabilized. Unfortunately, he has sustained considerable damage to both his brain and spinal cord.

Although MS is a crippling disease of motor and cognitive functions, C. G. remains cognitively intact but has slowed thinking. He also has lapses in immediate recall and occasional indiscretions of judgment that result in inappropriate conversation with outside family members. He expressed suicidal ideation and was treated effectively with paroxetine hydrochloride (Paxil) for his depression. Paxil, an SSRI, was specifically chosen because of its minimal cognitive blunting effects.

All of C. G.'s identified disabilities occurred gradually, but with a sudden progression of his disease his motor impairments progressed from poor lower extremity ambulation and postural control to involvement of his upper extremities and dependence on a wheelchair. He needed therapy initially for ambulation and more recently for wheelchair use and transfer techniques. As his MS status deteriorated, control of his upper extremities began to decline. Again therapy was ordered to teach him alternate ways to accommodate to these new losses in upper motor control and strength. He was retaught how to get dressed, use the toilet, shower, and feed himself.

Drugs used in the management of MS patients must be considered in any therapy plan, but most clinicians do not share this information or only list it as a part of the patient's chart. At the initial referral of C. G. for gait training, he was taking baclofen (Lioresal) for management of muscular spasms and associated pain. This drug, however, has the potential to increase weakness and fatigue as well as introduce some CNS depression. This is important information because C. G.'s MS was already responsible for motor weakness, but the need to reduce painful muscle spasticity outweighed the loss of muscle strength. If the therapist had not known that C. G. was taking baclofen, the physical therapy plans would have been significantly jeopardized because the therapist would have assessed C. G. as being weak simply because he had MS. The therapy plan needs to include exercises and maneuvers that compensate for the drug-induced motor weakness. C. G. was also taking oxybutynin chloride (Ditropan) for bladder control, a drug that has a potential side effect of drowsiness; in C. G.'s case the Ditropan dose was minimal and was not a cognitive concern. As noted, he had been placed on paroxetine, which also can contribute to muscle weakness, but in his case this did not increase his upper extremity weakness.

C. G. was referred to therapy for functional training, such as transferring from his wheelchair to a bed, shower stool, or toilet; dressing; and eating. Understanding the patient's environmental status, which includes his family situation, is also important in creating a therapy plan. C. G.'s therapy was through home health and incorporated a plan appropriate to C. G.'s environment. C. G. is married and has two children. His wife must work to support the family. The children are not yet in high school and are gone much of the day. Thus C. G. must manage self-care while the family is away during the day. Understanding how drug therapy enhances or interferes with physical or occupational therapy interventions is the only way to optimize the interaction of both and enhance the quality of life for C. G.

POSTSCRIPT

Unfortunately with MS, the demyelinating of neurons is relentless and progressive. At this writing, C. G. has begun to lose additional upper extremity mobility after an MS exacerbation 6 months after his last occupational therapy treatments. He has recently been taught to use assistive tools to grasp and pull items to him, such as books, utensils, and doorknobs. The assistive tools were introduced by the therapist treating C. G., thus extending C. G.'s self-reliance and security during time alone.

CASE STUDY 36-2 ■ PARKINSON'S PLUS SYNDROME

Mrs. N.'s background is that she is a 72-year-old married woman with Parkinson's plus syndrome whose disease status has progressed over the past 5 years, resulting in impaired gait, periods of severe rigidity, dystonia, occasional oculomotor dysfunction, significant behavioral and cognitive changes, and some speech impairment. She is a highly educated woman who had been a speech and special education therapist and administrator. In addition to the aforementioned problems, she now has attention span difficulty, is emotionally labile, and tends to ramble on tangentially to questions posed or simply on her own. Mrs. N. is still oriented to time and place, but to a large extent she is now housebound.

Mrs. N. is currently wheelchair dependent and has had extensive therapy over the past 5 years to keep her mobile and reduce muscle atrophy. She has been given hydrotherapy to facilitate both limb motion and flexibility. Her right hand and both arms are frequently immobilized for short periods of time by rigidity as a result of levodopa blood level peaks. These have been recently modulated by the addition of ropinirole (Requip, a dopamine agonist), and this drug, along with therapy to decrease upper extremity impairments, has improved her ability to carry out voluntary hand and arm movements. Mrs. N's limb movements are characteristically slow and deliberate as a result of the pathological features of Parkinson's disorders. She does not have any cogwheeling of the biceps, hands, or head frequently seen in Parkinson's patients. Her muscle mass is reduced as a result of disuse atrophy and noncompliance with home-instructed daily exercise. She continues, with poverty of motion, to feed herself but depends on her husband for assistance in dressing and transferring from her wheelchair to the toilet, bed, and shower despite the fact she could do these maneuvers on her own if she chose to do so.

She remains in a long-term stable relationship with a highly supportive husband, who is slowly being driven to exhaustion by her constant demands for attention. She scores well on mental status examinations and does not yet demonstrate marked signs of dementia but frequently has appeared slightly groggy. Mrs. N.'s chief complaint has been one of poor motor control and strength in both her upper and lower extremities. She is still able to stand but now requires assistance during walking. She is unable to sleep normally, finds rolling over or changing position in bed to be difficult, and wakes her husband to rotate her frequently throughout the night.

Her Parkinson's is less than successfully treated with standard antiparkinsonian therapy, that is, levodopa/carbidopa. With the addition of Requip, she has improved somewhat. One of the telltale characteristics of a Parkinson's plus syndrome is that patients do not respond as well to levodopa therapy as do persons with pure Parkinson's disease. Thus the

importance of adjunctive physical and occupational therapy to assist Mrs. N. in maintaining mobility cannot be overstated.

Mrs. N. has several other problems that affect her quality of life and her therapy. She, like many other patients with a parkinsonian syndrome, has significant joint pain for which she uses OTC drugs (NSAIDs) in addition to gabapentin (Neurontin, an anticonvulsant drug with neuropathic pain-relieving properties). Mrs. N. has painful muscle spasms that have been moderately well managed with baclofen. She has a nocturnal sleep problem that is lessened by using zolpidem tartrate (Ambien), which helps her get 3 to 4 hours of quality sleep. However, her daytime inactivity has resulted in significant night-time sleep disturbance that even zolpidem does not always cover.

Unfortunately, Mrs. N., like so many patients with chronic problems, has sought secondary sources of pain and fractured sleep relief without informing her medical and physical/occupational therapy team until she began to experience a new set of problems caused by polypharmacy, prescriptive, or OTC agents. She has been reluctant in the past to disclose her use of these additional agents, several of which have clouded assessment of her therapy. This is not an uncommon occurrence with patients who have progressively degenerative conditions.

Clinicians must routinely ask about patients' drugs and specifically about the use of OTC drugs at each visit. For example, Mrs. N. reported at one recent visit that she was having a hard time following her therapist's instructions and participating in the sessions. She was sure the therapist was "not paying proper attention to my needs." This not being the case, the therapist asked, "So, Mrs. N., refresh my mind and save me some time from looking it up. What medicines are you now taking?" She responded, "Sinemet, as you told me to; Requip; Ambien at bedtime; Synthroid; Klonopin; and a new pill I got at the health food store for sleep." She was taking two drugs—Klonopin and the OTC drug melatonin—both of which would account for the therapist's response that Mrs. N. appeared groggy and was not able to follow directions. The Klonopin she got from a psychiatrist friend of the family. She had put herself on these three sleep drugs, one long-acting and the other two short-acting, but in combination additive. In addition to this, the drug gabapentin, which was managing her neuropathic pain, and in a dose of 1200 mg/day, contributed to her level of drowsiness—a known side effect of gabapentin. Mrs. N. was already on the short-acting non–sensorium-clouding zolpidem that had been given to her for her sleep disorder. Zolpidem does not cause daytime hangover drowsiness. The key to her new daytime lethargy was found in the Klonopin and melatonin.

The offending drugs were discontinued with an explanation of why she should not add drugs. Mrs. N. subsequently returned to therapy, and her therapist

CASE STUDY 36-2 ■ PARKINSON'S PLUS SYNDROME—cont'd

found her once more able to participate in the therapy plans that had been worked out for her. Asking patients to review the drugs they are on is vital to the entire health care team and to their ultimate success.

With the recently confirmed diagnosis of Mrs. N.'s Parkinson's plus syndrome, all that can now be offered to her is supportive therapy, both medical and physical. She is in a class of Parkinson's patients who do not

respond well to the antiparkinsonian drugs. Her medical management now depends on her participation in physical and occupational therapy and her resisting the temptation to add other drugs that will only cloud her senses and not improve the underlying pathology. Mrs. N. and her husband have now accepted this, and she is doing better.

REFERENCES

1. Kostic VS, Marinkovic J, Svetel M, et al: The effect of stage of Parkinson's disease at the onset of levodopa therapy on development of motor complications, *Eur J Neurol* 9:9-14, 2002.
2. Mendis T, Suchowersky O, Lang A, et al: Management of Parkinson's disease: a review of current and new therapies, *Can J Neurol Sci* 26:89-103, 1999.
3. Becker G, Muller A, Braune S, et al: Early diagnosis of Parkinson's disease, *J Neurol* 249(suppl 3):III-40-48, 2002.
4. KK Jain: Carbamazepine. MedLink Neurology: MedLink Corporation: www.medlink.com. Accessed November 15, 2004.
5. Witjas T, Kaphan E, Azulay JP et al: Non motor fluctuations in Parkinson's disease: frequent and disabling, *Neurology* 59:408-413, 2002.
6. Kunin C: The responsibility of the infectious disease community for the optimal use of antimicrobial agents, *J Infect Dis* 151:388-398, 1985.
7. De Jong GJ, Meerwaldt JD, Schmitz PI: Factors that influence the occurrence of response variations in Parkinson's disease, *Ann Neurol* 22:4-7, 1987.
8. Hauser RA, Friedlander J, Zesiewicz TA et al: A home diary to assess functional status in patients with Parkinson's disease with motor fluctuations and dyskinesia, *Clin Neuropharmacol* 23:75-84, 2000.
9. Foley KM: Misconceptions and controversies regarding the use of opioids in cancer pain, *Anticancer Drugs* 6(suppl 3):4-13, 1995.
10. Postma TJ, Benard BA, Huijgens PC, et al: Long-term effects of vincristine on the peripheral nervous system, *J Neurooncol* 15:23-27, 1993.
11. Moore AR, O'Keeffe ST: Drug-induced cognitive impairment in the elderly, *Drugs Aging* 15:15-28, 1999.
12. *Medical immunology,* ed 9, New York, 1997, Lange Medical Books/McGraw-Hill.
13. Nirenberg A: Managing hematologic toxicities: novel therapies, *Cancer Nurs* 26(6 suppl):32S-37S, 2003.
14. Dimeo F: Exercise for cancer patients: a new challenge in sports medicine, *West J Med* 173:272-273, 2000.
15. Watson T, Mock V: Exercise as an intervention for cancer-related fatigue, *Phys Ther* 84:736-743, 2004.
16. Verstappen CC, Postma TJ, Hoekman K, et al: Peripheral neuropathy due to therapy with paclitaxel, gemcitabine, and cisplatin in patients with advanced ovarian cancer, *J Neurooncol* 63:201-205, 2003.
17. Bourgeois BF: Antiepileptic drugs, learning, and behavior in childhood epilepsy, *Epilepsia* 39:913-921, 1998.
18. Read CL, Stephen LJ, Stolarek IH et al: Cognitive effects of anticonvulsant monotherapy in elderly patients: a placebo-controlled study, *Seizure* 7:159-162, 1998.
19. Luef GJ, Lechleitner M, Bauer G et al: Valproic acid modulates islet cell insulin secretion: a possible mechanism of weight gain in epilepsy patients, *Epilepsy Res* 55:53-58, 2003.
20. Maxwell CJ, Hogan DB, Ebly EM: Calcium-channel blockers and cognitive function in elderly people: results from the Canadian Study of Health and Aging, *Can Med Assoc J* 161:501-506, 1999.
21. McNamara J: Drugs effective in the therapy of the epilepsies. In Hardman JG, Limbird LE, Goodman M et al, editors: *Goodman and*

Gilman's the pharmacological basis of therapeutics, ed 10, New York, 2001, McGraw-Hill, pp. 521-547.
22. Lichtenstein DR, Wolfe MM: Nonsteroidal anti-inflammatory drugs and the gastrointestinal tract: the double edged sword, *Arthritis Rheum* 38:5-18, 1995.
23. Levy RH, Meldrum BS, Perucca E, editors: *Antiepileptic drugs,* ed 5, Philadelphia, 2002, Lippincott Williams & Wilkins.
24. Maksimowicz-McKinnon K: Rheumatoid arthritis. In T.C.C. Foundation, editor: *Disease management project,* Cleveland, 2004, The Cleveland Clinic.
25. Sato Y, Kondo I, Ishida S et al: Decreased bone mass and increased bone turnover with valproate therapy in adults with epilepsy, *Neurology* 57:445-459, 2001.
26. Jarvis B, Coukell AJ: Mexiletine: a review of its therapeutic use in painful diabetic neuropathy, *Drugs* 56:691-707, 1998.
27. Bialer M: Comparative pharmacokinetics of the newer antiepileptic drugs, *Clin Pharmacokinet* 24:441-452, 1993.
28. Daniels V, Casey A: Antihypertensives, *Phys Med Rehabil Clin North Am* 10:319-335, 1999.
29. McKay D: Can CAM therapies help reduce antibiotic resistance? *Alt Med Rev* 8:28-42, 2003.
30. Kalra L, Yu G, Wilson K et al: Medical complications during stroke rehabilitation, *Stroke* 26:990-994, 1995.
31. Thompson PD, Zmuda JM, Domalik LJ et al: Lovastatin increases exercise-induced skeletal muscle injury, *Metabolism* 46:1206-1210, 1997.
32. Kane GC, Lipsky JJ: Drug-grapefruit juice interactions, *Mayo Clin Proc* 75:933-942, 2000.
33. Effect of lazabemide on the progression of disability in early Parkinson's disease. The Parkinson Study Group, *Ann Neurol* 40:99-107, 1996.
34. Lerman-Sagie T, Watemberg N, Kramer U et al: Absence seizures aggravated by valproic acid, *Epilepsia* 42:941-943, 2001.
35. Koller WC, Rueda MG: Mechanism of action of dopaminergic agents in Parkinson's disease, *Neurology* 50(6 suppl 6):S11-S14, 1998.
36. Blackshear JL, Kopecky SL, Litin SC, et al: Management of atrial fibrillation in adults: prevention of thromboembolism and symptomatic treatment, *Mayo Clin Proc* 71:150-160, 1996.
37. Kingery WS: A critical review of controlled clinical trials for peripheral neuropathic pain and complex regional pain syndromes, *Pain* 73:123-139, 1997.
38. Tabor PA: Drug-induced fever, *Drug Intell Clin Pharm* 20:413-420, 1986.
39. Roden D: Antiarrhythmic drugs. In Hardman LL, Gilman JG, Goodman A, editors: *The pharmacological basis of therapeutics,* New York, 2001, McGraw Hill, pp. 953-970.
40. Oates JA: Antihypertensive agents and the drug therapy of hypertension. In Hardman LL, Gilman JG, Goodman A, editors: *The pharmacological basis of therapeutics,* New York, 2001, McGraw Hill, pp. 871-900.
41. Silver JM, Hales RE, Yudofsky SC: Psychopharmacology of depression in neurologic disorders, *J Clin Psychiatry* 51(suppl):33-39, 1990.
42. Baldessarini R: Drugs and the treatment of the psychiatric disorders: depression and anxiety disorders. In Hardman LL, Gilman JG,

Goodman A, editors: *The pharmacological basis of therapeutics,* New York, 2001, McGraw Hill, pp. 447-483.

43. Glassman A, Shapiro P: Depression and the course of coronary artery disease, *Am J Psychiatry* 155:4-11, 1998.

44. Panel on Detection, Evaluation and Treatment of High Blood Cholesterol in Adults: *Third report of the National Cholesterol Education Program (NCEP) expert,* Bethesda, MD, 2001, National Heart Lung and Blood Institute. pp. 163-186.

45. Liesker J, Wijkstra PJ, Ten Hacken NH: A systematic review of the effects of bronchodilators on exercise capacity in patients with COPD, *Chest* 121:597-608, 2002.

46. Mintzer MZ, Griffiths RR: Triazolam and zolpidem: effects on human memory and attentional processes, *Psychopharmacology* 144:8-19, 1999.

47. Minagaurd A: Neurologic manifestations of rheumatoid arthritis. In Gilman S, editor: *MedLink Neurology,* San Diego, 2005, MedLink Corporation.

48. Pecknold JC: A risk-benefit assessment of buspirone in the treatment of anxiety disorders, *Drug Safety* 16:118-132, 1997.

49. Pollock BG: Adverse reactions of antidepressants in elderly patients. *J Clin Psychiatry* 60(suppl 20):4-8, 1999.

50. Kirwan JR: The effect of glucocorticoids on joint destruction in rheumatoid arthritis. The Arthritis and Rheumatism Council Low-Dose Glucocorticoid Study Group, *N Engl J Med* 333:142, 1995.

51. American Psychiatric Association, editor: *Diagnostic and statistical manual of mental disorders (DSM),* ed 4, Washington, DC, 1994, American Psychiatric Association.

52. Wing RR, Phelan S, Tate D: The role of adherence in mediating the relationship between depression and health outcomes, *J Psychosom Res* 53:877-881, 2002.

53. Hardman JG, Gilman AG, Limbird LE, editors: *The pharmacological basis of therapeutics,* ed 9, New York, 1995, McGraw-Hill.

54. Dam M, Tonin P, De Boni A et al: Effects of fluoxetine and maprotiline on functional recovery in poststroke hemiplegic patients undergoing rehabilitation therapy, *Stroke* 27:1211-1214, 1996.

55. Goldstein LB: Pharmacology of recovery after stroke, *Stroke* 21(11 suppl):III 139-142, 1990.

56. Shanahan EM, Smith MD, Ahern MJ: Pulse methylprednisolone therapy for arthritis causing muscle weakness, *Ann Rheum Dis* 58:521-522, 1999.

57. Brown ES, Suppes T: Mood symptoms during corticosteroid therapy: a review, *Harv Rev Psychiatry* 57:239-246, 1998.

58. Lauter JL, Lynch O, Wood SB, et al: Physiological and behavioral effects of an antivertigo antihistamine in adults, *Percept Mot Skills* 88(3 pt 1):707-732, 1999.

59. Goldenberg MM: Celecoxib, a selective cyclooxygenase-2 inhibitor for the treatment of rheumatoid arthritis and osteoarthritis, *Clin Ther* 21:1497-1513, 1999.

60. American College of Rheumatology Subcommittee on Rheumatoid Arthritis Guidelines: Guidelines for the management of rheumatoid arthritis: 2002 update, *Arthritis Rheum* 46:328-346, 2002.

61. Murray AW, Hunt T: *The cell cycle: an introduction,* New York, 1993, Oxford University.

62. Bombardier C, Laine L, Reicin A et al: Comparison of upper gastrointestinal toxicity of rofecoxib and naproxen in patients with rheumatoid arthritis. VIGOR Study Group, *N Engl J Med* 343:1520, 2000.

63. Silverstein FE, Faich G, Goldstein JL, et al: Gastrointestinal toxicity with celecoxib vs nonsteroidal anti-inflammatory drugs for osteoarthritis and rheumatoid arthritis: the CLASS study: a randomized controlled trial. Celecoxib Long-term Arthritis Safety Study, *JAMA* 284:1247, 2000.

64. Kochiadakis GE, Igoumenidis NE, Hamilos MI et al: Long-term maintenance of normal sinus rhythm in patients with current symptomatic atrial fibrillation: amiodarone vs propafenone, both in low doses, *Chest* 125:377-383, 2004.

65. Marks WJ Jr, Garcia PA: Management of seizures and epilepsy, *Am Fam Physician* 57:1589-1600, 1998.

66. Cannella AC, O'Dell JR: Is there still a role for traditional disease-modifying antirheumatic drugs (DMARDs) in rheumatoid arthritis? *Curr Opin Rheumatol* 15:185-192, 2003.

67. Fleischmann RM, Baumgartner SW, Tindall EA et al: Response to etanercept (Enbrel) in elderly patients with rheumatoid arthritis: a retrospective analysis of clinical trial results, *J Rheumatol* 30:691-696, 2003.

68. Braun MM, Terracciano G, Salive ME et al: Report of a US Public Health Service workshop on hypotonic-hyporesponsive episode (HHE) after pertussis immunization, *Pediatrics* 102:E52, 1998.

69. Tange RA: Ototoxicity, *Adverse Drug React Toxicol Rev* 17:75-89, 1998.

70. Tepper VJ, Farley JJ, Rothman MI et al: Neurodevelopmental/neuroradiologic recovery of a child infected with HIV after treatment with combination antiretroviral therapy using the HIV-specific protease inhibitor ritonavir, *Pediatrics* 101:E7, 1998.

71. Shephard RJ, Shek P: Immune response to inflammation and trauma: a physical training model. *Can J Physiol Pharmacol* 76:469-472, 1998.

72. Duman RS, Malberg J, Nakagawa S et al: *Neuronal plasticity and survival in mood disorders, Biol Psychiatry* 48:732-739, 2000.

73. Laszlo A, Kelly JP, Kaufman DE et al: Clinical aspects of upper gastrointestinal bleeding associated with the use of nonsteroidal antiinflammatory drugs, *Am J Gastroenterol* 93:721-725, 1998.

74. Swartz M: Use of antimicrobial agents and drug resistance, *N Engl J Med* 337:491-492, 1997.

75. Soyka LF, Robinson DS, Monaco J: The misuse of antibiotics for treatment of upper respiratory tract infections in children, *Pediatrics* 55:552-556, 1975.

76. Balon D: Managing GI effects, *Chemist Druggist* Jan 18:17, 2003.

77. Hanssen AD, Osmon DR: The use of prophylactic antimicrobial agents during and after hip arthroplasty, *Clin Orthop Relat Res* 36:124-138, 1999.

78. Jeppesen U, Gaist D, Smith T et al: Statins and peripheral neuropathy, *Eur J Clin Pharmacol* 54:835-838, 1999.

79. Wilson RC: The use of low-dose trazodone in the treatment of painful diabetic neuropathy, *J Am Podiatr Med Assoc* 89:468-471, 1999.

80. Gonder-Frederick LA, Clarke WL, Cox DJ: The emotional, social, and behavioral implications of insulin-induced hypoglycemia, *Semin Clin Neuropsychiatry* 2:57-65, 1997.

81. Ross S: Controlling diabetes: the need for intensive therapy and barriers in clinical management, *Diabetes Res Clin Pract* 65S:S29-S34, 2004.

82. American Diabetes Association: Evidence based nutrition principles and recommendations for treatment and prevention of diabetes and related complications, *J Am Diet Assoc* 102:109-118, 2002.

83. Hopkins D: Exercise-induced and other daytime hypoglycemic events in patients with diabetes: prevention and treatment, *Diabetes Res Clin Pract* 65S:S35-S39, 2004.

84. Frier BM: Morbidity of hypoglycemia in type 1 diabetes, *Diabetes Res Clin Pract* 65S:S47-S52, 2004.

85. Warren R: The stepwise approach to the management of type 2 diabetes, *Diabetes Res Clin Pract* 65S:S3-S8, 2004.

86. American Diabetes Association: Diabetes mellitus and exercise, *Diabetes Care* 25(suppl 1):S64, 2002.

87. Pringle TH, Riddell JG, Shanks RG: Characterization of the beta-adrenoreceptors that mediate the isoprenaline-induced changes in finger tremor and cardiovascular function in man, *Eur J Clin Pharmacol* 35:507-514, 1988.

88. Pras E, Stienlauf S, Pinkhas J, et al: Urinary retention associated with ipratropium bromide, *DICP* 25:939-940, 1991.

89. Baker MD: Theophylline toxicity in children, *J Pediatr* 109:538-542, 1986.

90. ACC/AHA/ESC guidelines for the management of patients with atrial fibrillation: executive summary, *Circulation* 104:2118-2150, 2001.

91. Cupp MJ, Tracy TS: Cytochrome P450: new nomenclature and clinical implications, *Am Fam Physician* 5:107-116, 1998.

92. Beebe HG, Dawson DL, Cutler BS et al: A new pharmacological treatment for intermittent claudication: results of a randomized, multicenter trial, *Arch Intern Med* 159:2041-2050, 1999.

93. Walsky RL, Gaman EA, Obach RS: Examination of 209 drugs for inhibition of cytochrome P450 2C8, *J Clin Pharmacol* 45:68-78, 2005.

94. Chambers CV: A cohort study of NSAID use and the management of related gastrointestinal symptoms by primary care patients, *P&T* 7:28, 2003.

95. Weiner P, Magadle R, Berar-Yanay N et al: The cumulative effect of long-acting bronchodilators, exercise, and inspiratory muscle training on the perception of dyspnea in patients with advanced COPD, *Chest* 3:672-678, 2000.

96. Lippe S, Lassonde M: Neuropsychological profile of intractable partial epilepsies, *Rev Neurol (Paris)* 160:S144-S153, 2004.

97. Tiep B: Disease management COPD with pulmonary rehabilitation, *Chest* 112:1630-1656, 1997.

98. Poole PJ, Black PN: Mucolytic agents for chronic bronchitis or chronic obstructive pulmonary disease, *Cochrane Database System Review* 2:CD001287, 2006.

99. Zielinski J: Indications for long term oxygen therapy: a reappraisal, *Monaldi Arch Chest Dis* 54:178-182, 1999.

100. Hoo GW: Nonpharmacologic adjuncts to training during pulmonary rehabilitation: the role of supplemental oxygen and noninvasive ventilation, *J Rehabil Res Dev* 40:81-97, 2003.

101. Caligiuri MP, Lacro JP, Jeste DV: Incidence and predictors of drug-induced parkinsonism in older psychiatric patients treated with very low doses of neuroleptics, *J Clin Psychopharmacol* 19:322-328, 1999.

102. Beal JE, Olson R, Laubenstein L et al: Dronabinol as a treatment for anorexia associated with weight loss in patients with AIDS, *J Pain Symptom Manage* 10:89-97, 1995.

103. Shuster J: Ondansetron and headache, *Nursing* 29:66, 1999.

104. Barone JA: Domperidone: a peripherally acting dopamine$_2$-receptor antagonist, *Ann Pharmacother* 33:429-440, 1999.

105. Gibson D: A review of the adverse effects of cisapride, *J Ark Med Soc* 95:384-386, 1999.

106. Balon D: Is it the drugs? *Chemist Druggist* 1:19, 2003.

107. Wulffele MG, Kooy A, Lehert P et al: Effects of short term treatment with metformin on serum concentrations of homocysteine, folate and vitamin B12 in type 2 diabetes mellitus a randomized, placebo controlled trial, *J Intern Med* 254:455-463, 2003.

108. Wolfe MM, Lichtenstein DR, Singh G: Gastrointestinal toxicity of non steroidal anti-inflammatory drugs, *N Engl J Med* 340:1888-1899, 1999.

109. Lipid research clinics program, *JAMA* 252:2545-2548, 1984.

110. Schaefer DC, Cheskin LJ: Constipation in the elderly, *Am Fam Physician* 58:907-914, 1998.

111. Campbell NR, Hasinoff BB: Iron supplements a common cause of drug interactions, *Br J Clin Pharmacol* 31:251-255, 1991.

112. Katial RK, Stelzle RC, Bonner MW et al: A drug interaction between zafirlukast and theophylline, *Arch Intern Med* 158:1713-1715, 1998.

113. Lepor NE: Changing the guard in long-term anticoagulation: clinical and economic implications, *Rev Cardiovasc Med* 5(suppl 5):S22-S29, 2004.

114. Baser B, Kacker SK: A simple, effective method of treating vertigo patients, *Auris Nasus Larynx* 17:165-171, 1990.

115. Borenstein DG, Lacks S, Wiesel SW: Cyclobenzaprine and naproxen versus naproxen alone in the treatment of acute low back pain and muscle spasm, *Clin Ther* 12:125-131, 1990.

116. Wagstaff AJ, Bryson HM: Tizanidine: a review of its pharmacology, clinical efficacy and tolerability in the management of spasticity associated with cerebral and spinal disorders, *Drugs* 53:435-552, 1997.

117. Gianino JM, York MM, Paice JA et al: Quality of life: effect of reduced spasticity from intrathecal baclofen, *J Neurosci Nurs* 30:47-54, 1998.

118. Gruenthal M, Mueller M, Olson WL et al: Gabapentin for the treatment of spasticity in patients with spinal cord injury, *Spinal Cord* 35:686-689, 1997.

119. Palmer DT, Horn LJ, Harmon RL: Botulinum toxin treatment of lumbrical spasticity: a brief report, *Am J Phys Med Rehabil* 77:348-350, 1998.

120. Segal JL, Pathak MS, Hernandez JP et al: Safety and efficacy of 4-aminopyridine in humans with spinal cord injury: a long-term, controlled trial, *Pharmacotherapy* 19:713-723, 1999.

121. Norman KE, Pepin A, Barbeau H: Effects of drugs on walking after spinal cord injury, *Spinal Cord* 36:699-715, 1998.

122. Stolp-Smith KA, Wainberg MC: Antidepressant exacerbation of spasticity, *Arch Phys Med Rehabil* 80:339-342, 1999.

123. Galletly C: Subjective muscle weakness and hypotonia during clozapine treatment, *Ann Clin Psychiatry* 8:189-192, 1996.

124. Bramanti P, Sessa E, Rifici C et al: Enhanced spasticity in primary progressive MS patients treated with interferon beta-1b, *Neurology* 51:1720-1723, 1998.

125. Allain H, Bentue-Ferrer D, Gandon JM et al: Drugs used in Alzheimer's disease and neuroplasticity, *Clin Ther* 19:4-15, 1997.

Alternative and Complementary Therapies: Beyond Traditional Approaches to Intervention in Neurological Diseases, Syndromes, and Disorders

Darcy A. Umphred, PT, PhD, FAPTA
Jennifer M. Bottomley, PT, MS, PhD
Carol M. Davis, PT, EdD, MS, FAPTA
Mary Lou Galantino, PT, PhD, MSCE
Therese Marie West, PhD, MT-BC, FAMI

KEY WORDS

alternative/complementary/transdisciplinary models
energetic-based theories
evidence-based practice
integrating theories
movement therapies

OBJECTIVES

After reading this chapter the student/therapist will be able to:
1. Differentiate the four worldviews of health care delivery.
2. Analyze how complementary/alternative-based health care practices overlap with an allopathic medical delivery model.
3. Analyze how mind, body, and spiritual interactions have the potential to lead to health and healing.
4. Compare and contrast the various models discussed and identify similarities and differences between them and the traditions of Western medical practice.
5. Appreciate the role of complementary and alternative approaches in the examination and intervention of individuals with neurological disorders.

The use of complementary and alternative methods (CAM) in the treatment of neurological disorders is evolving into common practice as clinicians and patients/clients seek nontraditional approaches for relieving signs and symptoms of neurological diseases, syndromes, and disorders and attempt to alter the progression of diseases of the central nervous system (CNS) through unconventional movement and manual therapies. It is important that professionals working within a traditional rehabilitation environment understand the principles and practices of transdisciplinary, complementary, and alternative approaches to treatment beyond traditional Western medical interventions because many of these therapeutic approaches are being proposed as options in the management of functional limitations resulting from neurological problems. The clinician needs to be cautious in the application of these treatment modalities. We do not want to get drawn through belief into alternative therapies as intervention solutions without significant evidenced-based research substantiating the use of these approaches. The reader must also be reminded that evidence comes from effectiveness, and many complementary approaches have established effectiveness.[1]

This chapter presents a sampling of alternative therapeutic models and philosophies that are available for potentially assisting patients/clients who have CNS movement dysfunction. Although most of the techniques discussed in this chapter have been firmly established by sound research, some less-evidenced-based models are also included, such as therapeutic touch and medical intuitive diagnostics. Clinicians are continually being exposed to the therapeutic

potentials of these less scientifically established theories and therefore need to be aware of their existence and potential. Creating evidence-based practice is not an all-or-none principle, nor do we suggest that models that do not have a strong research base are ineffective. We do suggest that to adopt a model because of belief or the charisma of the founder will be and should be challenged by colleagues today and in the future. Models whose theoretical constructs are based on sound rationale or that link effective-based practice across multiple areas, yet have not established efficacy, need to be scrutinized and approached cautiously but should not be nullified as potential alternatives. In time, if those models maintain their sound base, more research will be developed and their efficacy established. New models will also be created in the future that link and integrate theories with practice, and our professions will continue to evolve and offer better-quality care to the consumer.

HISTORICAL PERSPECTIVE

Jennifer M. Bottomley, PT, MS, PhD
Darcy A. Umphred, PT, PhD, FAPTA

A historical perspective of how complementary and alternative therapeutic approaches have evolved to become increasingly part of the medical and rehabilitation landscape can be helpful to obtaining a broader comprehension. The language and rationale encountered in alternative methods can seem confusing and foreign to clinicians unfamiliar with modalities outside the realm in which they were taught. With many of our patients/clients seeking alternative methods of intervention beyond the traditional Western medical model, the time has arrived for us to explore and understand the scientific basis for the apparent effectiveness of these interventions. The positive results experienced by many of our patients/clients who have received alternative interventions cannot be ignored. This is the impetus for the growing acceptance by the general public and many health care practitioners of alternative forms of therapy. Can we explain scientifically the effects of complementary and alternative interventions? And if so, how can we best integrate CAM approaches into our accepted, current, and changing approaches to neurological rehabilitation?

In their book, *The Second Medical Revolution,* Laurence Foos and Kenneth Rothenberg described levels of academic learning as being three tiered.[2,3] Starting at the top, the third tier is the applied studies and subjects for therapists, such as therapeutic exercise and electrotherapy. The second tier is the pure sciences on which these subjects are founded, such as anatomy, chemistry, physiology, and biology. The first tier is the "assumption of reality" (day-to-day observations) on which the pure sciences are based. This first tier is the basic assumptions found in "worldviews" today. Different worldviews yield different scientific bases, whether pure or applied. Alternative methods in medicine and rehabilitation are well established in "premodern" and "postmodern" worldviews. This is in contrast to the "modern worldview" customarily taught in current Western medical training. To present these methods in overview, it would be helpful to discuss these worldviews and how physical and occupational therapy may fit into the scheme.

Essentially, there are four worldviews[4]: the premodern, modern, "fracturing or splintering," and postmodern views.

The first worldview developed during prehistoric times and lasted until the sixteenth century. This is called the premodern view. In this perspective, time is cyclical rather than linear. In other words, the sun, the moon, and the stars circle around the earth, the tides ebb and rise cyclically, and the seasons circle back again and again, using the same patterns each time, connecting with "deep time." Deep time is compared with profane time. Profane time is tangible, as in the time it takes rice to boil; or visible, as in the sundial; or sensible, as in the heartbeat. In deep time such perceptions are suspended, profane time stands still, and one becomes a part of time. It is in deep time that premodern man finds reality. Infused in this thinking is that life and death, the earth and the sky, are mysterious or mystical. In other words, they contain truth beyond human comprehension.

This is a hard perspective for many to grasp, yet the role of the scientist is to be a passive observer. Numbers were used to describe observed events, such as the days between the circling of the sun and the moon, the number of hours between the ebb and high tide, but "there was no widespread assumption in the western world that natural processes in general had any intrinsic relation to numbers, to mathematics."[5] In other words, in Western science, these perspectives were not tangible, visible, or sensible . . . and so, historically, science moved on.

The second worldview, which began with Copernicus, is known as the modern worldview. It is the one with which the majority of the Western population would be most familiar and feel at home. In this view time is linear, progressing from start to finish. "The world is a rational, predictable, clockwork universe. Every bit of it can be predicted if you know one part of it. Purpose in life is to describe, generalize, predict, and control. Human beings are fairly mechanistic, separate, discrete entities from the rest of the universe."[4]

René Descartes (1596-1650) French philosopher and mathematician, and Isaac Newton (1642-1727), were two of the most important figures ushering in the "modern era." To Descartes, the world was logical, predictable, and intrinsically expressible through mathematics. The whole was obviously equal to the sum of the parts—categorical and hierarchical. The role of the scientist became that of an active, experimental, objective observer. If the numbers did not fit, it could not be real.

The modern era of the second worldview spanned the 1500s through the twentieth century. However, the near perfection of the view began to falter in the early 1900s with important discoveries in the field of physics. Although the hold of the second worldview on Western culture is still immense, it is splintering, as can be seen within our own professions.

Worldview 3 is about this fracturing, about the realization that the categorical, orderly clockwork is not a complete or necessarily accurate picture. It is a prelude to worldview 4. A small but growing number of people see the world in worldview 3, and fewer yet in worldview 4, but the effects are starting to be felt.

Worldview 4, postmodern, is complex, integrated, and nonlinear. It is about self-organizing and self-regulating systems, looking for patterns, and knowing that a small variation in the pattern can produce large changes. Time is a dimension, interwoven with the dimensions of space. Time and space can change, expand or shrink, speed up and slow down. Rituals are an important means for creating order. The whole is greater than the sum of the parts, and "we know and yet don't know." Worldview 4 has a lot of similarities with worldview 1. The pure sciences that arise from this worldview include systems theory, quantum physics, cybernetics, string theory, and fractal mathematics, which in turn affect many other fields of study, such as meteorology, ecology, business and economics, medicine, theology, movement science, and computer science, to name but a few. Research parameters, technology, and interpretation differ significantly from the assumptions of worldview 2 because scientific description is no longer considered purely objective, but rather *epistemology* (the view from which knowledge is gathered) is becoming "an integral part of every scientific theory."[6]

Today we practice within the paradigms of our professions, which have in the past aligned with Western medicine. Thus, for our ease, we can first start where we are, look at the medical profession, and discuss models or strategies that parallel the worldviews.

The roots of Western medicine extend back to Hippocrates, 400 BCE, who provided a holistic picture of the state of health, writing that "Health depends upon a state of equilibrium among the various internal factors which govern the operations of the body and the mind, the equilibrium in turn is reached only when man lives in harmony with his external environment (p. 23)."[2] The basic assumption in this perspective is that health depended on a balance with mind-body and nature or the environment, and disease was a disturbance of this balance. Preserving the balance was the priority for the practitioner. Three means were used to ascertain the characteristics of an illness: a dialogue with the patient, observational assessment of the patient's appearance, and palpation of the soft tissues and pulses. The most important component of this approach was considered the dialogue with the patient/client. It was believed that the patient's/client's meaning of the illness, attitude, and expectation was a valuable diagnostic and prognostic factor.

The shift from a preservative approach for mind-body-environment integrity to the conventional curative thinking found in medicine today was largely initiated by Descartes. He conceptualized reality as having two separate domains, one the body or matter, the other the mind. "The body is a machine," said Descartes, "so built up and composed of nerves, muscles, veins, blood and skin, that though there were no mind in it at all, it would not cease to have the same [functions]" (p. 32).[2] His ideas were closely tied to Newtonian physics, which conceives the universe as a harmonious and well-ordered machine. These concepts gave rise to the view that matter and nature were separate from humans, and thus one could observe without affecting what was being observed. The physician, then, could have complete objectivity when assessing the patient. The patient could be viewed as a biological organism whose function was reducible to interrelating physical parts.

The resulting medical model, known as biomedicine, was fully in place by the middle of the nineteenth century. Its characteristics may be considered as follows:

1. Disease or dysfunction is a "deviation from the norm of measurable biological parameters" (p. 23).[2] A patient/client is a biological organism whose dysfunction is reduced to the identified deviations. Treatments or procedures are then used to cure or at least improve the deviations, which in turn improves the biological condition.
2. Objectivity provides the basis for diagnosis or assessment and the subsequent rationale for treatment. Patients'/clients' descriptions of what they are experiencing and the clinician's observation are considered "subjective" and not given as great a value as the "objective" findings, such as laboratory or other measured tests.
3. Eventually biomedicine can address virtually all medical problems at least adequately, if not fully, through more knowledge and research.

It goes without saying that the biomedical model has produced stunning and tremendous accomplishments. Yet its restriction to physical causes of disease, in light of diseases and dysfunctions that are more widely recognized as having multiple causes, is creating a search for other answers. More of the public and some physicians and other health professionals are turning to alternative forms of intervention and healing. As stated in *Life* magazine in September 1996, "Why have alternative therapies in this country started to migrate from the margins to the center? One reason is that as allopathic medicine, a term commonly used to describe western techniques, becomes better at what it *can* do well, its limitations become more conspicuous. Allopathy is clearly superb at dealing with trauma and bacterial infections. It is far less successful with asthma, chronic pain and autoimmune diseases."[7]

Many of the alternative practices used in a medical setting today clearly come from premodern worldview sources, such as acupuncture, yoga, meditation, herbal remedies, and prayer. Just how some of these therapies work to restore health is difficult to perceive from a linear worldview 2 perspective. Frequently what happens is that alternative approaches are used to address areas of limitations in the biomedical model, in a complementary fashion. Alternative practices used this way do not supplant traditional medicine; rather, they support and enhance the options available in health care. A new worldview and medical model would not necessarily arise from this relationship, yet the conceptual framework is no longer cohesive. Ideas from ancient sources, as well as postmodern sources, are changing the previously complete-and-adequate image of the second worldview and consequent medical model. Grappling with these issues places one in worldview 3.

Evidence of these dynamics is apparent in the professions of physical and occupational therapy. In neurorehabilitation, for example, proprioceptive neuromuscular facilitation and neurodevelopmental techniques were developed in the middle of the twentieth century at a time when "rehabilitation" was being established as an integral part of unquestioned biomedical order. Both approaches, in their early form, worked primarily with the nervous system, and both used hierarchy and order. Patients/clients were to progress through a sequence of skills, such as the *developmental sequence,* that was invariable. The hierarchy was also found regarding the role of the therapist as the professional who could identify the pathokinesiology and "fix" it with the appropriate technique. The patient was the recipient of the treatment. With the advent of *motor control, motor learning, and neuroplasticity theories* over the last couple of decades, these fixed approaches have changed because the new concepts have influenced them. The developmental sequence, now termed *learning sequence,* no longer uses a strict hierarchy based on movement development of a child. Its treatment approach is moving away from emphasizing the therapist's role in identification and resolution of pathological movement and moving toward a science of functional movement that is based to a large extent on the role of the patient in his or her own capacity to problem solve, self-monitor the motor control system, and help establish outcome expectations on the basis of function, not pathological conditions. Last, an entirely new entity of neurorehabilitation has been formed recently as a result of concepts from motor control, motor learning, dynamical systems theory, and the understanding of neuroplasticity, which is known as the "task-oriented or functional approach."

One of the tenets of dynamical systems theory, as noted in the journal of the American Physical Therapy Association in 1990, is that "biological organisms are complex, multidimensional, cooperative systems. No one subsystem has logical priority for organizing the behavior of the system" (p. 770).[8] The nervous system, then, is no longer a dominant subsystem with neurological patients. Rather, it is part of a self-organizing system that has multiple subsystems such as arousal, gravity, learning style, weight, center of gravity, cardiovascular function, and so on. "No one subsystem contains the instructions for [an action]. . . . The behavior of the system is instead an emergent property of the interaction of multiple subsystems" (p. 771).[8] (See Chapters 3 through 5.)

Added to these developments was the emergence in the 1980s of a new field of therapy intervention: vestibular habilitation posture and balance, which is multisystem and multifunctional and inherently demands the use of motor control and learning principles and understanding of the mechanism of neuroplasticity and interactive systems theories. Systems concepts are used for both balance and the task-oriented approach, the concept being that "movement emerges from an interaction between the individual, the task, and the environment."[9] (See Chapters 17 and 23.)

Orthopedic, or manual, physical therapy appears to be firmly committed to the biomedical model, yet there is interest found in "being holistic" and treatment and exercise approaches are continually being developed that endeavor, to various degrees, to work with movement and function in a broader and more integrated manner. (See Chapter 15.)

Thus we find that today therapists are incorporating into practice systems concepts, motor control, and motor learning theories and experimenting with ancient sources of healing, such as yoga, tai chi, acupressure, and meditation, as well as refining skills in the traditional biomedical aspects of therapy. For our professions, holistic approaches have and will continue to create change and change can be confusing, threatening, and exciting all at the same time.

Worldview 2 still remains the dominant model within the Western allopathic health care delivery system. Two distinct observations may be made that show the prevalence of a worldview 2 approach. The first is that many colleagues continue to consider ourselves to be objective observers separate from our patients. The second is that we endeavor to understand ancient, modern, and postmodern therapeutic concepts and research, frequently from a linear, mechanistic, categorical worldview 2 epistemology. Yet such a view at times does not suffice to explain what is happening. That is the dilemma of worldview 3.

Further changes will be experienced when a critical mass of the population turns fully, in all aspects of personhood, to "worldview 4," which, again, has great similarities to worldview 1. A big difference, though, is that at this time in history, we have scientific methods for understanding our nonlinear, complex, evolving, multidimensional, multilevel, continually interacting, irreducible world. Through systems theory we can handle, with sophistication, this multitude of complex detail, by working with its "sweeping simplicity and order in overall design."[3] Throughout the twenty-first century, as the growth of worldview 4 continues to evolve on many levels and in many fields of endeavor, it is entirely possible that it and its sciences will indeed replace, and not simply complement, worldview 2. And from there, the future has yet to be conceptualized and belongs to future students willing to venture beyond what is comfortable to best meet the health care needs of a world society.

ALTERNATIVE MODELS AND PHILOSOPHICAL APPROACHES

Darcy A. Umphred, PT, PhD, FAPTA
Approaches to patient management that do not fall within a traditional allopathic medical model are often considered alternative or complementary. Although many of these therapeutic approaches have not been able to show effectiveness or efficacy in totality as an approach to medical management, neither has Western medicine. Although the evidence-based method of medicine is the accepted term for equating outcome measures by reliable and valid instrumentations

and interventions, there is controversy within the literature as to the reality base of evidence-based medicine.[10-15] Future research will help validate many aspects of Western medicine and areas will be discarded. Similarly, research will show the effectiveness of many components of complementary approaches, although some components will need to be eliminated and new creative ideas and therapeutic techniques developed. One research problem encountered with complementary approaches is that these approaches consistently focus on the patient as a total human being with all the interactions of all bodily systems. This philosophy of the whole does not coincide with the linear, reductionistic physical research accepted by Western medicine. Until research models are developed and instrumentation becomes available that measures multiple systems at multiple levels of consciousness simultaneously, it will be difficult to prove the strengths of many aspects of alternative approaches to patient management. That does not mean the evidence is not there. It means our research skill may not have developed to the level of measuring all the influences that are interacting simultaneously during a complementary approach intervention. Finding those research models with supporting instrumentation is and will continue to be a challenge to therapists who choose to incorporate these interventions as part of their professional management of patients with neurological disabilities.

All the models presented in this chapter for patient management have a common thread. All approaches focus on helping the patient/client maintain or regain a quality of life that is within that person's potential. The specific philosophy or conceptual framework embraced by any one approach varies. As various approaches are introduced in the following sections, subheadings will help the reader categorize similarities of philosophies.

Movement Therapy Approaches
Feldenkrais Method of Somatic Education
James Stephens, PhD, PT, CFP
The Feldenkrais method is about learning:

I do not treat patients. I give lessons to help people learn about themselves. Learning comes from the experience. I tell them stories (and give them experiences of movement) because I believe learning is the most important thing for a human being" (p. 117)[16] (parentheses added by the author).

Development of the Feldenkrais Method. As a boy in Palestine, Moshe Feldenkrais developed a method of hand-to-hand combat that was used by settlers for self-defense. Later, as a student in Paris where he trained in physics at the Sorbonne, he studied judo and became the first person in Europe to receive a black belt. When he injured his knee playing soccer, he relearned pain-free walking on his own. Later he studied with F. M. Alexander, Elsa Gindler, and Gurdieff. He also studied psychology, progressive relaxation, bioenergetics, and the hypnosis methods of Milton Erickson. And he was familiar with the physiology of his day: Sherrington, Magnus, Fulton, and Schilder. With this background, Feldenkrais developed two approaches to facilitating learning that are now known as Awareness Through Movement (ATM) and Functional Integration (FI).[17]

Feldenkrais was ultimately interested in the development of human potential. He saw that, although all people encounter trauma and difficulty in their lives, those who are most successful develop new, adaptive behaviors to overcome those difficulties. He proposed that a type of learning that reconnected the brain to the control of the musculoskeletal system would be the most effective way to approach this problem of adaptation. His initial thinking in this area is set out in his first book, *Body and Mature Behavior: a Study of Anxiety, Sex, Gravitation, and Learning.*[18]

Background Theory—Dynamic Systems Theory.

For Feldenkrais, learning was an organic process in which cognitive and somatic aspects were completely integrated and interactive. Presented first in 1949, this idea prefigured our current sense of dynamic systems functioning of the brain and body.[19] The learning should proceed at its own pace in an individualized way following the learner's intention and guided by the learner's perception that the performance of the task, movements of the body, and interaction with the environment become easier.[18] This interactive cycle of action and perception has been described well by the motor learning model proposed by Newell.[20]

Learning is a complex process with overlays from the intention of the learner, interference from environmental distraction, misperception of the task and the body, desire related to self-image, fear of injury, or incorrect performance. Thus it is possible to learn poorly, incorrectly, or in such a way as to interfere with performance and not improve it. This kind of process has been suggested by Byl et al[21] as the underlying cause of focal dystonia. One of the definitions Feldenkrais gave for learning took this process into account: "Learning is the acquisition of the skill to inhibit parasitic action (components of the action unrelated to the intention behind an action but resulting from a secondary intention) and the ability to direct clear motivations as a result of self-knowledge."[18] An adult engaged in learning to walk again after a stroke with a fear-related reluctance to weight bear on the involved limb would be an example of such a secondary intention.

The process of learning proposed by Feldenkrais is one of discovery. The outcome desired is one of increased awareness. Vereijken and Whiting[22] have proposed that discovery learning, in which learners are free to explore any range of solutions to learning a task that they want in any way that they want, is as or more effective than any formal approach to motor learning involving controlled schedules of practice or feedback. This process of discovery has the added dimension of allowing learners to focus on the perceptual understanding of the body/task/environment as a component of the learning process. In the Feldenkrais method this discovery and perceptual learning process is explicit.

Our understanding of how experience and learning restructure almost all areas of the CNS is expanding rapidly.[23] A large focus of current thinking in rehabilitation is how to translate neuroplasticity concepts into more effective techniques for rehabilitation.[24,25] The method developed by Feldenkrais and practiced by people around the world who are trained in this method is clearly explained by these new principles, creating new approaches to rehabilitation.

Approaches to Feldenkrais Method.

The two approaches to facilitating learning created by Feldenkrais, ATM and FI, are similar in principle and process although differ in practice. They are essentially two methods for communicating a sensory experience that the client can consider and act on. The first requirement of the process is to create an environment that is comfortable, safe, and conducive to learning, whether the learner is being moved passively or creating the movement experience voluntarily. The second requirement is that the amount of effort associated with making the movements be reduced greatly so that it is possible to make fine discriminations about the effects of force acting on the system from outside, from inside or both. The goal is to develop a rich understanding of changes throughout the system produced by small perturbations. This understanding becomes the basis for creating new solutions to movement problems as the client progressively approaches functional movements that she or he desires to perform.[26]

In FI, the practitioner will manually introduce small perturbations into the learner's system after placing the learner into a safe position closely approximating some desired activity to be learned. Here the practitioner is providing the force inputs and the client is asked to attend to the changes created in response to the perturbation. For example, the practitioner might press gently into the bottom of the client's foot and ask the client to notice where in the body movement and pressure is felt as a result. This will be repeated a number of times and then some other forces/ movements will be introduced. The guiding idea for the practitioner might be to build sensory experiences in the body that are associated with a particular movement, such as rolling. This goal is rarely explicitly expressed to the client and left to emerge in the client's understanding of the experience: "Oh, now I am rolling," or "This feels like rolling to me." Also there is no strict expectation by the practitioner about what specific movement might emerge. Thus, it is possible to create novel and unexpected outcomes of how a particular task might be best performed by this particular person. This allows for a process of assessment that is continually evolving as the intervention is unfolding.[26]

In ATM, the practitioner verbally provides suggestions for movements for a client to explore and asks the client to focus on the sensory outcomes throughout the body. Thus, the client introduces the experimental forces into his or her own system with the intention of understanding how the body as a whole responds. The underlying idea, however, is the same. In my practice, I use FI as a form of communication when clients do not understand how a force might act on the body or when they are unable to produce a range of movements that we might desire to explore. An example might be in a case where spasticity prevents fine discrimination in both sensory and motor realms.

In practice with an individual client, it is common to move back and forth between ATM and FI during the same session. The session is usually focused on the development of understanding and performing a specific function: turning, rolling, standing, stepping, etc. ATM is a verbal process in which clients direct their own movement; thus, a practitioner can work with many individuals simultaneously. At the same time individuals within the learning group are free to respond differently from each other in ways that may be appropriate only for them as individuals.[27] Because ATM is under the active control of the client, in the end this method is a closer approximation to voluntary movement and thus may be a more powerful tool in reestablishing voluntary control (Case Study 37-1).

Evidence of Effectiveness. The theory underlying the Feldenkrais method predicts that there should be changes in perception of the body or body image. Although there have not been a lot of studies in this area, there are several that support this prediction. Elgelid[28] reported positive changes in body perception, as evaluated by the semantic differentiation scale in a group of four subjects after a series of ATM lessons. Dunn et al[29] reported that subjects who had had a unilateral sensory imagery ATM lesson perceived their

experimental sides to be longer and lighter and demonstrated increased forward flexion on that side, linking the changes in perception to changes in motor control.

There is not a lot of literature evaluating the efficacy of the Feldenkrais method in general and even less specifically for people with neurological diagnoses, as a result of the complexity of the problems and the multiple system involvement of the individuals. Evidence-based studies on effectiveness are more easily identified. In a recent review, Stephens and Miller[26] divided the literature into four different areas: pain management, postural and motor control, functional mobility, and psychological and quality-of-life impact. Much of the literature is in case report format. A small amount of the literature is controlled study format, with some of that using randomized control groups. The

---

CASE STUDY 37-1 ■ SUE: HEREDITARY SPASTIC PARAPLEGIA

Sue was a toe walker as a young child. She remembered her father sitting in a chair all the time, his legs too stiff and weak to walk. In her mid 20s, she too began to develop weakness and stiffness in her legs. At the age of 36 years she was diagnosed as having "uncomplicated" hereditary spastic paraparesis (HSP).

Uncomplicated HSP involves extreme spastic weakness, some loss of sensation in the lower extremities, and hypertonic bladder reflexes. It progresses slowly over many years without exacerbations or remissions. Individuals experience progressive difficulty walking and often require canes, walkers, or wheelchairs. They typically retain normal strength and dexterity of the upper extremities, have no involvement of speech, chewing, or swallowing, and have a normal life expectancy.[393]

Sue was first seen in our outpatient clinic when she was 38 years old. She worked as an office manager at a local college. Her office was up a set of stairs that was becoming more difficult to negotiate. She also owned a horse that she had not been able to ride because she was no longer able to mount because of her increased spasticity. Sue was a large, muscular woman at 5 feet 10 inches and 175 pounds.

On initial examination she reported pain in her right knee with weight bearing (8/10) and pain in her low back (5/10). Her proprioception appeared to be intact. She had decreased passive range of motion (ROM) in dorsiflexion bilaterally and hyperextension of her knees bilaterally, greater on the right. There was tightness in the iliotibial band and hip adductors, flexors, and rotators bilaterally and the extensors of the back from the lumbar through the cervical spine. Her muscle strength was 3+ to 4–/5 at all joints of the both lower extremities, with the right being generally weaker than the left. She also had mild weakness in her trunk flexors (3+/5). There was sustained clonus in plantar flexors bilaterally and one beat clonus in her quads on the right. She had normal active range of motion throughout her upper extremities with normal (5/5) strength throughout. Sue stood statically with her hips externally rotated, knees hyperextended, hips forward

with her back extended in a stiff swayback posture. Her shoulders were retracted and tight. She was unstable to a moderate challenge and reported falling frequently. Her gait was stiff with knees hyperextended and toe drag bilaterally. She achieved swing by doing a lateral trunk tilt with contralateral circumduction with each leg, no arm swing and a foot flat landing. She used a straight cane for balance. Her self-paced gait speed was ≈75 feet/minute. (1 mph = 88 feet/min). She reported "it feels like I have a stick up my back and if I try to go faster, my knees lock and I'm really in trouble." Sue was assessed to be a good candidate for a Feldenkrais intervention and a series of Functional Integration and Awareness Through Movement lessons was planned.

The first Functional Integration lesson was an exploration of the organization of turning and rolling from supine. I began this exploration with Sue supine and observed her postural organization in that position. She lay with her arms flat at her sides, palms up. Her legs were adducted and externally rotated and her back arched away from the mat table. I put a small towel roll under her neck and back and a 4-inch roller under her knees to allow her extensors to relax somewhat. I began the exploration by rolling her head gently and found a lot of resistance to that movement. Attempts to do small amounts of turning of a leg or bending of the knee also met with similar resistance. I then began working through a process of manually shortening muscles that were tight and overworking. I began with neck extensors by gently holding the cervical spine in a slightly more extended position progressing to the extensors of the trunk by compressing the ribs from the side to cause a slight lateral flexion first on the right then on the left. The relaxation focused last on the legs by holding the knee and hip in a slightly more externally rotated and flexed position first on the right, then on the left. Going back to the neck, pressure was exerted down through the first rib on the right to cause a slight lateral flexion to the left through the spine. This movement was now easier than before with force being translated further down the spine into the lumbar area. Next the pressure was combined with rolling of the

Continued

CASE STUDY 37-1 ■ SUE: HEREDITARY SPASTIC PARAPLEGIA—cont'd

head to the right, first passively, then with small active movements. The instruction was to turn the head only as much as could be done with almost no effort. The same process of compression of the spine and turning of the head was repeated from the left side of the neck. The interaction then progressed to the right leg by pushing through the right foot so that the force translating up the leg caused lateral flexion of the spine to the left, then again from the left leg. The right foot was then turned to initiate external rotation and flexion of the right leg first passively and then actively. Sue began to be able to control that small movement on the right leg with minimal effort and then repeated on the left. We then began to link the movement of the legs, trunk, and head together in a sequence in which she began to be able to roll her head to the right, flex her right leg and left leg together toward the right, and allow her trunk to flex and turn toward the right. During this process, Sue's attention was directed to sensing the movement and timing of different body segments; to feel the forces created in her body by the movement of one segment and how they impeded or facilitated movement of other segments. This lesson ended with Sue being able to roll more easily onto her side from supine than she had been able to do in a long time. This session took about 45 minutes during which I was doing some work with another patient at the same time. When Sue came up to standing after this lesson, she reported feeling like she was stuck into the ground solidly. She felt shorter, softer, and better balanced. Her feet were flatter on the floor and when she walked she did not drag her toes on the floor.

At the beginning of the second session on the following day, Sue was tested again on the treadmill and was now able to walk about 120 feet/minute. The second lesson began again in supine and reinforced and developed the movements of the first lesson. Sue learned to slowly roll to her right side, moving her arms at the same time so that she could take weight on them, flex her legs until they came over the side of the mat table and then push herself up to sitting all in one motion and then reverse this process slowly until she was lying supine again. She learned to roll herself into a fetal position back and forth from the left to the right without her legs stiffening in between, and when she sat up she was able to actively flex her legs up to put her shoes on, which she had not been able to do for at least a year. After this lesson she reported that she had been able to move her foot easily from the gas to the brake in the car without slipping and that she was able to get onto and ride her horse for the first time in several years.

In the third lesson, we worked more purely with Awareness Through Movement because Sue was now able to control more movement more easily herself. During this lesson Sue learned to roll with minimal

effort to the left and right while holding her knees and then to reach to her ankles and roll while holding her ankles without stiffening her neck in the process. Flexing her hips had become easy.

The fourth lesson involved standing, weight shifting, and turning. The instructions related to keeping movements small and slow and maintaining a feeling of softness that she now had developed. She explored movements of allowing her knees to flex while she shifted weight to one foot and moving her body over the weight-bearing foot to get a sense of how she could distribute weight differently across her foot on the basis of changing the configuration of her upper body and movements of her hips. These movements included exploring the effects of intentionally stiffening and softening her back and neck to feel any changes that happened in control of her weight bearing, knee flexion, and ankle. Weight on one side was increased while the other was unweighted, and the unweighted leg was lifted in a controlled manner, easy and effortless, feeling the support of the skeleton for the process of lifting. At the end of this lesson, Sue was able to lift her foot easily up onto the 19-inch high surface of the mat table and bring it back to the floor without disturbing her balance. At home she was now able to step up onto her horse from a low step without other assistance.

In the fifth and final session, more time was spent doing an Awareness Through Movement lesson related to standing balance, turns in walking and bending to the floor. In this session and at the end of the previous one, we also spent time in transfer training with toilet, tub, car, and floor transfers and gait training on smooth and uneven surfaces and for speed on the treadmill. She still used a cane for balance (or a single hand support on the treadmill) but now was able to walk on the treadmill at 175 feet/minute, well more than double her initial speed without dragging her toes or hyperextending her knees. She did complain of some back pain and calf pain, but this was determined to be from exercising muscles that had not been used in years and resolved after several days. I recorded the Awareness Through Movement lessons with a lapel microphone and recorder as we did them and gave her the tapes to use at home as part of her home exercise program.

Three months after discharge, as a passenger in her sister's car, Sue was in an auto accident and sustained a herniated disk at C5-6. After this she had decreased mobility for several months. During this time she lost her understanding of how to control her movement and returned to us 6 months after her initial visit to review what she had done earlier. After several series of lessons over a period of several months, she achieved a level of function higher than previously so that she was able to walk and go up and down stairs with any support.

work on pain management suggests that the Feldenkrais method may be especially effective in treating pain that is biomechanical in origin. This concept may be applied to work with pain in patients with neurological diagnoses, especially pain caused by biomechanical malalignment. No research has been done in this area with neurological patients. Hall et al[30] found improvements in balance (Berg), mobility (Timed Up-and-Go [TUG]), functional activity (Frenchay, Short-Form-36 [SF-36]), and vitality (SF-36) in a large group of elderly women compared with control subjects as a result of a 16-week ATM intervention. There were similar findings (TUG) by Bennett and colleagues,[31] also using ATM with a group of elderly women. In the areas of psychological and quality-of-life impact, Kerr et al[32] have shown decrease in state anxiety in subjects who participated in ATM lessons, and Laumer et al,[33] working with young women with eating disorders, have demonstrated positive changes in self-concept, self-confidence, and behavior resulting from participation in ATM lessons. Many of these findings are beginning to be reproduced in clinical populations with neurological diagnoses. Most of the studies to date have been done with people with multiple sclerosis. Colleagues are beginning to look at ATM effectiveness in patients after a stroke (CVA).

Multiple Sclerosis. The initial study, done in Germany, looked qualitatively at the effects of a 30-day ATM experience on a group of people with multiple sclerosis. The investigators concluded that ATM improved overall well-being, resulted in greater self-reliance of the participants, and led to better self-acceptance and a more positive self image.[34] Johnson et al[35] studied the effects of FI in people with multiple sclerosis. Although they did not find any significant mobility changes, they did report a decrease in perceived stress in the FI compared with the massage controls. Stephens et al[36] reported the cases of four individuals who participated in the same ATM classes over a period of 10 weeks. Three of four reported large improvements in their Index of Well Being score. All subjectively reported improvements in gait. However, there were no measures of gait that consistently improved across the group. Instead, it was found that changes were appropriate to the participant's individual needs and resulted in a greater sense of control. In a follow-up to this study, using a randomized control group design, Stephens et al[36] found improvements in postural control and balance confidence measures, along with a strong tendency toward an increase in self-efficacy and decreased falling. The same authors[37] also found that the ATM group had significant improvements in memory of recent events and perception of positive social support. Interestingly, they also had an increase in pain effects. Perhaps there was a trade off of increased mobility and confidence for increased awareness of pain.

Cerebrovascular Accident. The original publication in this area is the classic work, *The Case of Nora*, in which Feldenkrais explained his work in great detail and described improvements in sensation, perception, and mobility of a woman several years after a right-sided CVA.[38] More recently, results from pilot studies are just beginning to be reported in patients with diagnoses of CVA. Connors and Grenough[39] reported a decrease in spatial neglect as measured by line and star cancellation tests in a patient after a series of ATM lessons. Nair et al[40] reported the recovery of

upper extremity function and the return to playing golf in a 68-year-old man after an 8-week program of ATM/FI. This Feldenkrais program was begun only after the end of a 9-month program of traditional rehabilitation had left him with a nonfunctional hand. The Feldenkrais program included mental imagery and bimanual activities. This subject was also studied before, during, and after the Feldenkrais program with functional magnetic resonance imaging. The magnetic resonance imaging analysis showed that there was a return to higher activity in the involved contralateral primary motor cortex with activity of the right hand compared with higher activity in the ipsilateral M1 and SMA that has been shown in other reports of CVA recovery[41] before the Feldenkrais sessions began. This finding suggests a return to more normal brain function even after a period of 1 year after the stroke. A small pilot study (three subjects)[42] found an average 33% decrease in movement times on the Wolf Motor Function Test. In another pilot with four subjects, Batson[42a] found significant improvements in Dynamic Gait Index ($P = .033$, 55% average) and the Berg Balance Scale ($P = .034$, 11% average) and a 35% improvement on the Stroke Impact Scale. A larger study is in progress to further assess these findings.

Other Medical Diagnoses. There are some preliminary findings with other neurological diagnoses. Shelhav-Silberbush[43] reported improvements in motor, sensory, kinesthetic, perceptual, and learning functions in two case studies of children with cerebral palsy. Shenkman et al[44] reported improvements in balance, gait, and functional movement in two people with Parkinson's disease as a result of interventions that were based partly on a Feldenkrais approach. Gilman and Yaruss[45] have reported significant improvements in several young children who had problems with stuttering. Ofir[46] reported improvements in flexibility, mobility, and level of dependence in two young women who had sustained traumatic brain injuries.

Conclusion. The Feldenkrais method, in its two forms, embodies a process of somatic learning that aims to develop the perceptual capabilities of clients as it underlies the control on movement. Recent literature suggests that predicted results of improved body perception and motor control are supported in work with people with neurological diagnoses. These findings are encouraging and suggest that Feldenkrais method might make positive contributions to our understanding and methods of rehabilitation. However, we must approach these findings with caution because many are case studies or pilot studies done with a small number of people. Research is underway to substantiate these claims at a higher evidence-based level. Refer to Box 37-1.

The Pilates Method

Brent D. Anderson, PhD, PT, OCS
Matthew N. Butler, DPT, CSCS

German-born Joseph H. Pilates developed his unique form of movement therapy in the early 1900s. As a young man, Pilates suffered from a multitude of illnesses that left him physically weak. In an effort to strengthen his frail body, Pilates studied yoga, martial arts, Zen meditation, and ancient Greek and Roman exercise. His experiences led him to develop his own unique method of physical and mental

cally designed apparatus: the Reformer (Figure 37-1), the Cadillac table (Figure 37-2), the Wunda chair (Figure 37-3), and the ladder barrel (Figure 37-4). The apparatus regimen evolved from Joseph Pilates' original mat work which was shown to be too difficult for many injured individuals. On the apparatus, springs and orientation to gravity are modified to assist an injured individual to successfully complete movements that would otherwise be difficult or limited. Ultimately, by altering the spring tension or increasing the challenge of gravity, an individual may progress

conditioning. In 1926, Pilates brought his movement exercise program with him to New York City. Joseph Pilates' studio was soon embraced by many artists and choreographers from the dance companies of Martha Graham, George Balanchine, and Jerome Robbins. At the time, traditional physical therapy lacked the knowledge of how to restore dancers to their prior level of activity. Pilates encouraged nondestructive movement early in the rehabilitation process and worked to correct underlying biomechanical problems. This early movement intervention without pain was believed to hasten the healing process and allowed dancers to quickly return to the stage.

Almost a century later, the Pilates method has gained popularity within the rehabilitation setting because of its assistive nature in restoring functional movement. Rehabilitation practitioners are currently using the method in a variety of fields including orthopedics, pain management, neurological rehabilitation, and geriatrics. Most Pilates exercises in the rehabilitation setting are performed on specifi-

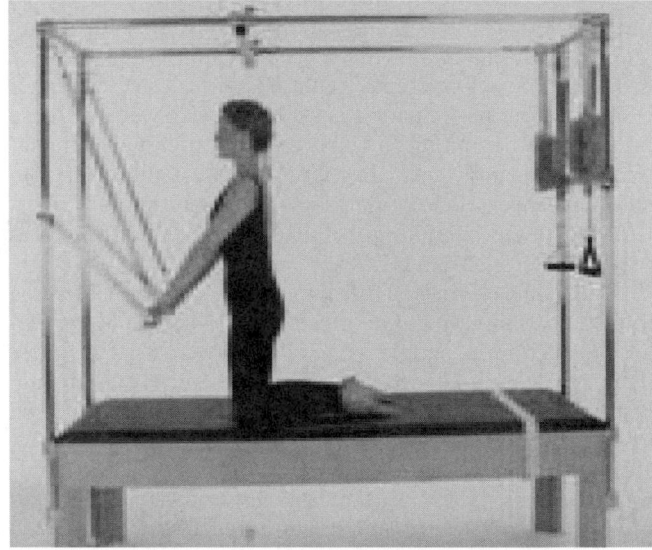

FIGURE 37-2 ■ Apparatus labeled "Cadillac" table.

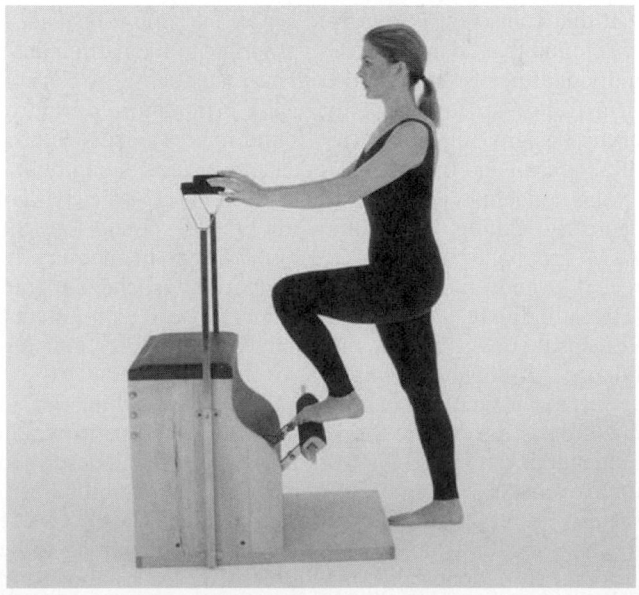

FIGURE 37-3 ■ Apparatus labeled the "Wunda" chair used in Pilates.

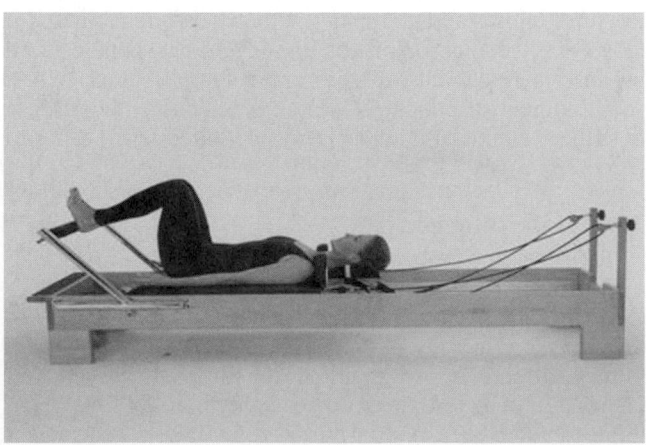

FIGURE 37-1 ■ The Reformer Apparatus used in Pilates.

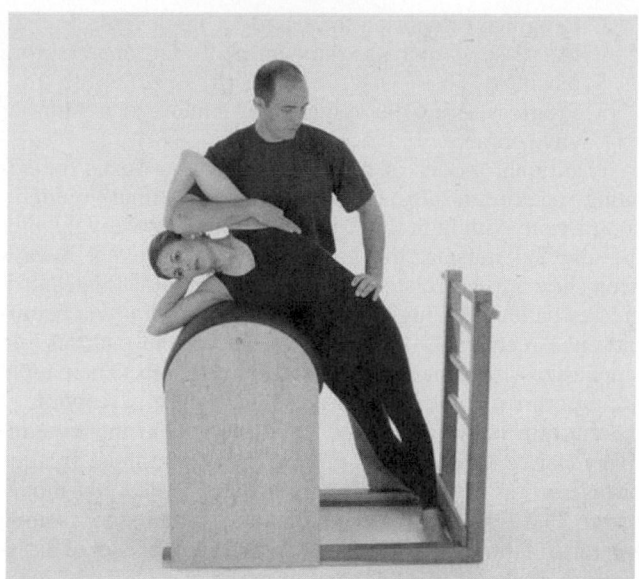

FIGURE 37-4 ■ Apparatus labeled the "ladder barrel" used in Pilates.

toward functional movement safely, efficiently, and without pain.

Pilates Principles. Although Joseph Pilates did not espouse any specific principles for his exercise regimen, the Pilates method has been classically taught using eight movement principles. These Pilates principles have been used as guidelines to examine and critique movement quality. They consist of concentration, control, precision/coordination, isolation/integration, centering, flowing movement, breathing, and routine. Polestar Pilates has modified the initial eight principles into six principles that have a greater practicality in the rehabilitation environment and stronger scientific support than the classic principles. The six Polestar Pilates principles include breathing, core control and axial elongation, efficiency of movement, spine articulation, alignment, and movement integration.

Breathing. Faulty breath patterns can be associated with complaints of pain and movement dysfunction.[47] Pilates movements create an environment where breath facilitates improved air exchange, breath capacity, and posture. During Pilates exercise, breathing is used to facilitate stability and mobility of the spine and extremities. Because of the movement of the rib cage on the thoracic spine, breath can facilitate either spinal extension or flexion depending on the movement. Breath assists with stability of the spine through the coordinated contraction of the diaphragm and the lower abdominal muscles, which both attach to the lumbar spine.[48,49]

Core Control and Axial Elongation. Core control is the optimal recruitment of the trunk musculature required to perform a given task in relation to the anticipated load. The transversus abdominus, internal abdominal obliques, external abdominal obliques, multifidi, erector spinae, diaphragm, and pelvic floor muscles are key organizational muscles that work together during movement in healthy individuals.[50-52] Motor control studies indicate that the coordinated, subthreshold contraction of these local and global stabilization muscles modulate the level of spinal stability required to safely perform activities of daily living.[53]

Axial elongation is the proper alignment of the head, spine, and pelvis that provides optimal joint spacing during movement. Correct joint spacing avoids working or resting at the end of range, which can place undue stress on the inert and contractile structures of the trunk and extremities.[54,55] By emphasizing axial elongation of the spine and maintaining appropriate joint spacing, soft tissue surrounding the joint can move more freely and the risk of injury can be minimized.

Efficiency of Movement. Efficiency of movement is the minimization of unnecessary muscle contractions that tend to interfere with healthy movement. The excessive recruitment of antagonist muscles is obstructive and significantly increases the amount of energy required to perform a task.[56,57] This principle can be applied to functional movement skills as well as performance skills. Inefficient motor recruitment can often be recognized by the amount of tension or faulty posture in the head, face, neck, and shoulder girdle, in relation to the thoracic spine and trunk.

Spine Articulation. Spine articulation is the equal distribution of movement throughout the cervical, thoracic, and lumbar spine. It has been suggested that repetitive movement at a hypermobile spinal segment may result in microtrauma or macrotrauma.[58-60] Hypermobility is often to the result of a lack of movement in a neighboring segment or joint.[61] Pilates exercise attempts to facilitate a change in movement strategy during functional tasks. Patients are trained to distribute movement in the spine over a greater number of spinal segments, thereby decreasing potentially harmful forces at the hypermobile segment. The ability to segmentally move the spine decreases unwanted stress and sheer of the spinal segments and increases the efficiency and fluidity of movement.

Alignment and Weight Bearing of Extremities. Alignment and posture are concepts often incorporated in the field of rehabilitation. The Pilates principle of alignment refers to the most energy-efficient posture of the body for a given task. Proper postural organization can significantly decrease energy expenditure during daily activities by improving mechanical advantage.[62,63] Faulty alignment in the extremities and the spine can be a source of decreased range of motion, early fatigue of muscle groups, or abnormal stresses on inert structures and may potentially cause injury.[64,65]

Pilates provides a closed-chain environment that facilitates compression and decompression forces on the axial skeleton and extremities through a full range of motion. The amount of load can be altered by adjusting the spring resistance or patient's orientation to gravity. The ability to regulate load on the basis of an individual's physiological limits, set by age or pathological condition, allows practitioners to more safely and effectively stress the skeletal and soft tissue systems. Theoretically, these forces can help stimulate osteoblastic activity and provide nutrition to a larger surface area of the joint and its surrounding connective tissue.[66-68]

Movement Integration. Many forms of rehabilitation focus on treating limitations of anatomical structures and neglect the neuromuscular reeducation required to learn to regain the motor control necessary to perform a complex task. Pilates provides a holistic approach by emphasizing the synthesis of mind and body to achieve fluid movement. Mobility, control, and coordination of the extremities on the trunk and the trunk on the extremities, are trained through motor learning and repetition of practice. In addition to the physical and mental capacity to complete a task, the environment in which a task is performed can greatly affect the success of movement organization.[69,70] Pilates provides an environment that can be modified on the basis of a patient's impairments and limitations, providing a safe, successful, and pain-free movement experience.

Clinical Application. Within the Pilates environment, faulty movement strategies are broken down into components and addressed through task-oriented interventions. By adaptation of the environmental constraints, such as gravity, assistance, and base of support, the degrees of freedom that must be controlled by the nervous system are reduced.[71] The successful manipulation of the environment can hasten the functional reeducation process and allow exercises to be safely and comfortably progressed until the desired outcome is achieved. It has been suggested that successful, pain-free movement, in addition to enhancing physical attributes, helps to alleviate anxiety.[72,73] By decreasing anxiety levels and improving self-efficacy, the development of chronic pain and dysfunction related to the injury may be prevented.[74-76]

The potential causes of faulty movement patterns include congenital defects and abnormalities, habitual adaptations, and compensation because of injury. Motor control problems associated with the pathological condition need to be addressed before the application of therapeutic interventions that are temporary cover-ups to problems that have deeper roots. For example, a pathological condition at the L4/L5 segment could be a result of faulty movement patterns in the hips and other lumbar vertebrae. The lack of movement in surrounding joints might be the mechanism of the lesion; however, treatments are often focused on the sight of the lesion, rather than the mechanism of the lesion.

One problem often encountered in the rehabilitation setting is flawed movement progression. On a spectrum of movement progression, practitioners often jump from passive movement to resistive movement too quickly. By facilitating assistive movement, a pattern can be practiced without irritating the lesion. Assisted movement with the use of springs can allow for a decrease in unwanted muscle activity or guarding that is often associated with pain, weakness, or abnormal tone. As the pattern progresses and symptoms decrease, assistance decreases and dynamic stabilization can be emphasized to challenge the newly acquired mobility or stability in a more functional and gravity-dependent position. Resistive movements are introduced only after adequate dynamic stability of the trunk is demonstrated through controlled movements that prevent excessive loading of the injured tissue. The five environmental conditions in Pilates that are altered to allow a therapist to facilitate motor changes are the following[69,77]:

1. Narrow or widen the base of support.
2. Raise or lower the center of gravity.
3. Lengthen or shorten the length of the levers.
4. Decrease or increase the degree of assistance (spring tension).
5. Progress from a foreign environment to a familiar environment.

Traditional modes of muscle conditioning focus on isolating specific muscles and producing a maximal voluntary contraction. Although this has been found to positively alter the targeted muscle, the gains achieved have not always been shown to correlate with functional return. Pilates progresses patients through stages of motor learning via neuromuscular reeducation of functional movement patterns and emphasizes efficient recruitment of motor units. The patient is first trained to become aware of or gain a perception of current movement strategies. Then the patient must cognitively learn a new strategy. Finally, the patient must practice or take action until efficient with the new strategy of movement. Task-specific interventions are progressed from a foreign to familiar environment by altering the level of assistance and the patient's orientation to gravity.

Summary. Pilates is an effective exercise system that works well in conjunction with traditional physical and occupational therapy practice. The Pilates-evolved apparatuses allow patients to safely perform exercises that improve strength, flexibility, balance, coordination, and motor control in an environment that can be easily progressed as they advance in their rehabilitation process. In addition, Pilates is thought to address the psychosocial components of an injury that lead to chronic pain or disability by decreasing anxiety and improving self-efficacy.[74,75] Early return of functional movement after an injury helps to physically and mentally empower individuals over the demands of life and is crucial in the long-term success of patient outcomes. The Pilates environment is a clinical tool that can be used by practitioners to provide patients with a safe, successful, and pain-free way of restoring function and quality of life.

Tai Chi

Jennifer M. Bottomley, PT, MS, PhD

Tai chi is an alternative therapeutic approach that can greatly enhance the practice of physical therapy. It is a form of exercise that recognizes the mind-body connection.[78] The movements are graceful, the tempo is slow, and the benefits are great. It can positively augment physical therapy programs aimed at improving balance and posture, coordination, and integration of movement, endurance, strength, flexibility, and relaxation. It has been demonstrated that tai chi can increase handgrip strength, flexibility, and peak expiratory flow rate, in addition to lowering resting heart rate.[79] Tai chi exercise has cardiovascular,[80-83] neuromuscular,[84-89] and psychological[90,91] benefits that are clinically observed. It is a form of exercise that allows the individual to assume an active role in obtaining maximal health and focus on the prevention of disease, rather than the passive acceptance of illness as a consequence of life, aging, fate, or genetics. It is an exercise form that is particularly helpful in an elderly population because of its slow, controlled, nonimpact-type movement that displaces, thereby "exercising," the center of gravity. This exercise form incorporates all of the motions that often become restricted with inactivity and aging. It improves respiratory status, stresses trunk control, expands the base of support, improves rotation of the trunk and coordination of isolated extremity motions, and helps to facilitate awareness of movement and position.[79,84-90] An additional benefit is the social interaction because most tai chi is done in group settings.

What is tai chi? Tai chi is an ancient physical art form, originally a martial art, where the defendant actually uses the attacker's own energy against the attacker by drawing the attack, sidestepping the attacker, and throwing the opponent off balance. There are numerous forms of tai chi[92] involving as many as 108 postures and transitions of controlled movement, each based on slightly different philosophical foundations. Family surnames came to be associated with the different styles of tai chi that have been passed on from generation to generation (e.g., Wu style, Yang style, Ch'en style, Chuan style). Each style is distinctive, but all follow classic tai chi principles.

Tai chi is a way of life that has been practiced by the Chinese for thousands of years. It is a Taoist philosophical perspective that forms the foundation of an exercise regimen developed to balance mind and body. Unlike Western civilization, which separates body from mind and allows spiritual development only in terms of religions and mystical beliefs, tai chi integrates the connections between mind, body, and spirit in a quest for the highest form of harmony in life through the combination of exercise and meditation.[93-95] The Chinese conceived the human mind to be of an unlimited dimension and focused on simplification of beliefs. They also viewed the human body as limitless in its physical capabilities. These beliefs were the keystone for the evolution of what we know today as tai chi chuan.[94]

Since ancient times, Taoist philosophy has been concerned with the question of how to reproduce and maintain the essential kind of energy required to prolong life and enhance the creativity of the individual. The answer can be found in the tai chi methods of Taoist meditation, in which a combination of movement, breathing, and mental concentration is used to purify the essential life energies, distill out its pure yang aspect, the vital energy (chi), and transmit it through the eight body-mind channels to every cell in the body. The regular practice of these methods has been shown to result in longevity, good health, vigor, mental alertness, and creativity far beyond what is experienced by most people.[96]

To obtain the full benefit from the practice of tai chi, it is essential to understand the principles underlying the methods. Hence, the aim of this section is not only to describe the methods of meditation and exercise but also to explain how they are based on the philosophy of Taoism.

The "spiritual" component of tai chi is what makes many Westerners uncomfortable with this and other Eastern practices.[93-95] However, the concentration required to accomplish the rhythmical and coordinated movement patterns and to integrate these motions with respiration in tai chi induces a level of concentration that edges on meditation.[78,91] Movement is vital to preventing disability and maintaining health and well-being. The capability of cognitively understanding the movements is an essential element in the successful practice of the tai chi exercise form. Tai chi requires practice (preferably throughout the life cycle) and commitment.[90,91] There would be a total lack of consistency and benefit from this exercise form if the mind-body connection were not made.

Philosophical Background. Behind every tai chi movement is the philosophy of yin and yang. The yin-yang principle has been the basis of the Chinese understanding of health and sickness since ancient times. Good health requires a balance between opposing forces within the body. If one or the other is too predominant, sickness results. It is the aim of Eastern medical practices, including acupuncture, qi gong, and herbal medicine, to discover the source of the imbalance and restore the forces to their proper proportions. In the Western world, exercise concentrates on outer movements and the development of the physical body. Tai chi develops both the mind and body.[78] It embodies a philosophy that not only promotes health but can be applied to every aspect of life. Tai chi emphasizes the development of the whole person, promoting personal growth in all areas.[97]

Tai chi means "the ultimate" energy. This ultimate power is *chi*. According to the legendary theory of yin and yang, chi exercises its power by creating a balance between the positive and negative energies of nature.[92] Tai chi's philosophical basis is directed toward improving and progressing toward the unlimited and immense interrelationship between the self and all other things in existence. Tai chi is guided by the theory of opposites: the yin and the yang, the negative and the positive. This is the *original principle* of Taoist thought. According to the tai chi theory, the abilities of the human body are capable of being developed beyond their commonly conceived potential. Creativity has no boundaries, and the human mind should have no restrictions or barriers placed on its capabilities.

The fundamental principle of Taoist philosophy, the joining together of opposites, is the basis for the practice of tai chi. The Taoist philosophy that underlies tai chi exercise and meditation is somewhat more complex in its application of the relationship between yin and yang within the body. It is not denied that a general balance is necessary to avoid illness; however, it is the aim of meditation to greatly increase the yang and to reduce and diminish the yin. One of the fundamental beliefs of Taoist philosophy is that the reason people become old and weak and eventually die is that they lack essential energy (chi) that sustains life.[95-97] Thus, the goal of exercises is to greatly reduce yang and to increase and enhance life's energy.[96,97] The combined practice of meditation and exercise balances these opposing energies.

One reaches the ultimate level of health and physical and mental well-being through exercise and meditative means of balancing the opposing powers and their natural motions: yin, the negative (yielding) power, and yang, the positive (action) power. The theory is that the interplay and balance between opposite, yet complementary, forces of equal strength promote health. These two opposing manifestations have universal significance and apply to the phenomena of the cosmos as well as to the operations of the human body. On the largest scale, heaven is yang, while earth is yin. Day is yang, while night is yin. Bright and clear weather is yang; dark and stormy weather is yin. On the scale of living things, the male is yang, the female yin. Spirit is yang, body yin. This opposition applies to the parts of the body and their functions as well. In the circulatory system, the arteries are yang, the veins are yin. Muscle contraction is yang, relaxation is yin. In breathing, exhalation is yang, inhalation is yin. In human activities, movement is yang, rest is yin.[98]

Hundreds of years ago, those who searched for a way to elevate the human body and spirit to their ultimate level developed the ingenious system known as tai chi exercise. It has since proved to be the most advanced system of body exercise and mind conditioning ever to be created.[92,98-100] It makes intuitive sense from a clinical perspective to apply the idea of a natural harmony and a balancing of life forces to the integration of body and mind.

Principles. An important insight to be attained through an understanding of Taoist philosophy concerns the way in which the practice of exercise, such as tai chi chuan, and meditation should complement one another. The relationship between them manifests as a subtle interweaving of opposite tendencies. This relationship can be seen in the famous diagram known as the tai chi t'u, the Diagram of the Supreme Ultimate (Figure 37-5). This diagram represents rest; the black portion is called the "greater yin," and the white portion, representing movement, is called the "greater yang." Within each figure there is a smaller circle of the opposite color. The black circle within the white figure is called the "lesser yin" and the white circle within the black portion is called the "lesser yang." This inner component represents the way in which each of the opposing forces, yin and yang, contains its opposite and continuously originates from its opposite. Tai chi, essentially a form of movement, is yang—the white portion. Meditation, which involves quiet and rest, is yin—the black segment. This distinction takes into account only the external aspects of these activities. To perform tai chi exercise effectively requires inner peacefulness and quiet while executing outwardly visible movements. Conversely, the meditator uses breath and mental concentration to move the vital energy through the psychic channels while remaining externally at rest. Thus, the inner aspect of each of these practices is opposite to its outer aspect. In other words, just as the greater yang contains the lesser yin within it, the greater yin embraces the lesser yang. The diagram is a pictorial representation of how exercise and meditation grow out of one another as alternating practices. The movements of tai chi tend to increase the yang side of the yin-yang balance. When the yang reaches a high point of energy and vitality, it generates the need to sit quietly—meditation, which produces a more peaceful condition and increases the yin side of balance. This is cyclical. When yin reaches its peak, it generates a need to increase the yang once again. Thus, it is through the alternate practice of these two opposite methods that one obtains the beneficial effects of this form of exercise/meditation: tai chi.[96-100]

The traditional Chinese concept of the human body differs somewhat from the Western one. Physiological foundations are based on descriptions of chi, or vital energy. The body is hypothetically composed of eight energy (psychic) channels and has 12 meridians that run along the surface of the body. These channels and meridians form the basis of the highly sophisticated theories of acupuncture and acupressure.[93,95,96]

The eight channels systematically include all parts of the trunk and extremities. These energy channels are represented in Figure 37-6. The *tu mo*, or channel of control, runs along the spinal column from the coccyx through the base of the skull and over the crown of the head to the roof of the mouth. The *jen mo*, or channel of functions, goes through the center and front of the body from the genital organs to the base of the mouth. The *tai mo*, or belt channel, circles the waist from the navel to the small of the back. The *ch'ueng mo*, or thrusting channel, passes through the center of the body between tu mo and jen mo, extending from the genitals to the base of the heart. The *yang yu wei mo* is the positive arm channel beginning at the navel, passing through the chest, and going down the posterior aspect of the arms to the middle fingers, while the *yin yu wei mo*, or negative arm channel, extends along the inner aspect of the arms from the palms, ending in the chest. Likewise, there are positive and negative channels for both lower extremities. The *yang chiao mo* is the positive channel that goes down the sides of the body and down the outer aspect of the lower extremity, ending at the soles. The negative channel, called the *yin chiao mo*, starts in the soles and extends upward on the inside of the legs through the center of the body to a point just below the eyebrows.[99]

Twelve "psychic centers" of the human body are identified in Taoist thought.[92,98,101] They are represented in the *I Ching*[97] by 12 hexagrams that signify not only the 12 pathways in the body but also the 12 months of the year and the 12 times of the day. According to Taoist thought, the circulation of energy through these 12 psychic centers reflects the cyclical pattern of the universe that brings about the alternation of light and darkness and the changing of the seasons.[98] Figure 37-7 relates the 12 psychic centers to the 12 hexagrams that symbolize them and indicates how the cycle reflects the times of the day and year and the center of the body that they represent.

According to Chinese astrologers, the yang movement begins with the eleventh month, which is identified with fu. This yang movement increases through the twelfth month up to the fourth month as represented by the increase in solid lines in the hexagrams. At the fifth month, the yang

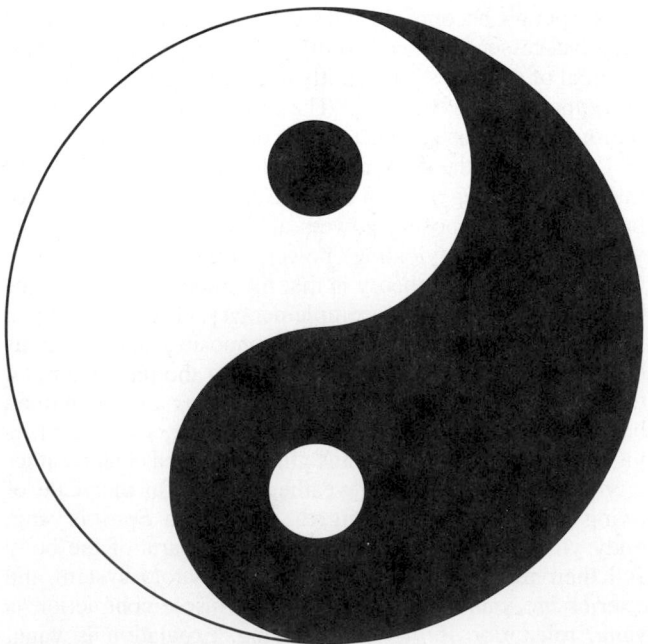

FIGURE 37-5 ■ Yin and yang: diagram of the Supreme Ultimate: tai chi t'u.

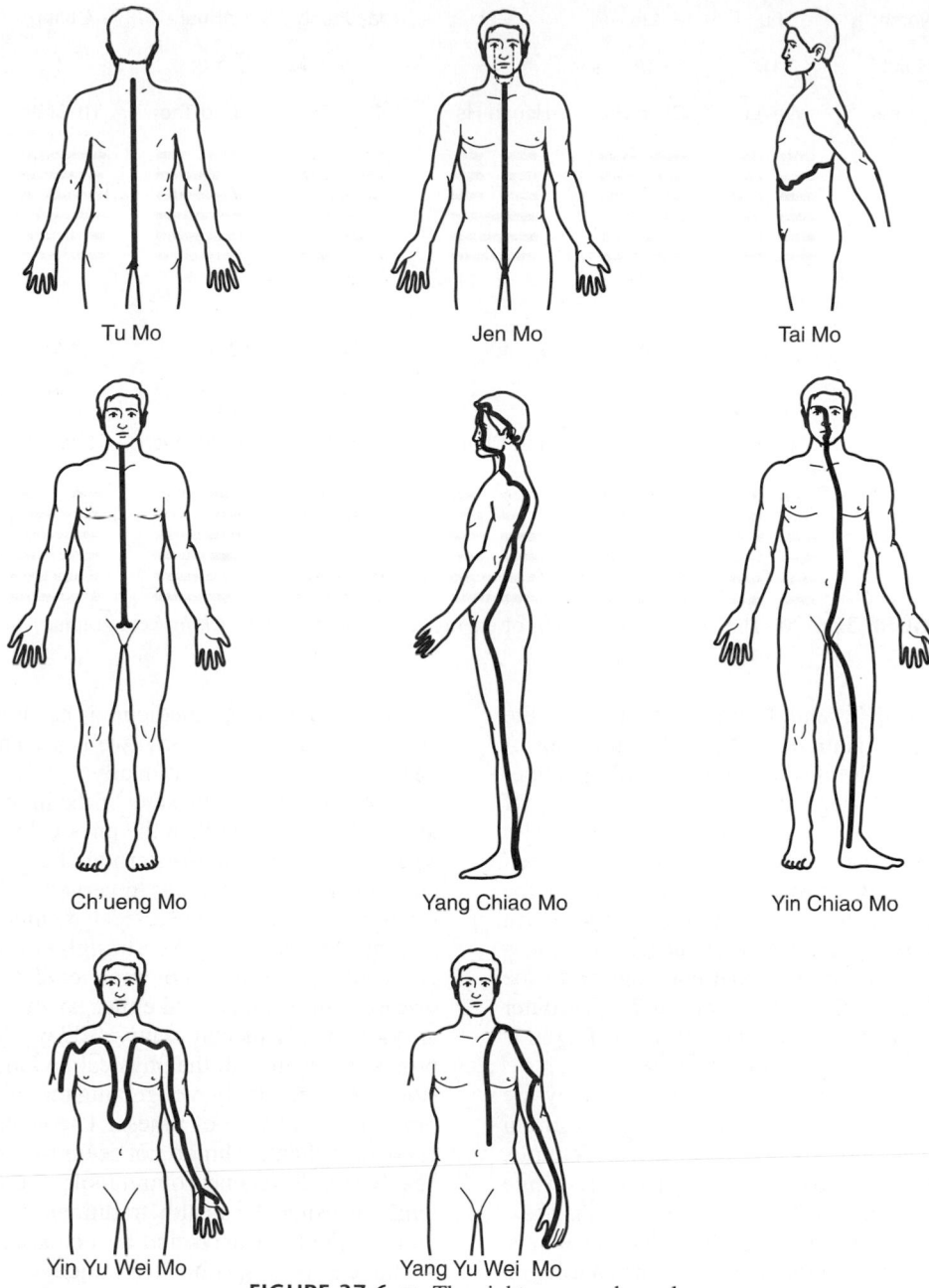

Tu Mo

Jen Mo

Tai Mo

Ch'ueng Mo

Yang Chiao Mo

Yin Chiao Mo

Yin Yu Wei Mo

Yang Yu Wei Mo

FIGURE 37-6 ■ The eight energy channels.

movement begins to decrease until it reaches the tenth month, when yin reaches complete dominance. The yin movement is the opposite of the yang.[96,98,101]

In addition to the psychic centers, there are 12 pathways of energy at the surface of the body, called meridians. The 12 pathways take their names from the specific inner organs to which they correspond. The development of the tai chi postures and movements is related to these meridians in the human body.[92,96,98] The transition from one posture to the next, combined with breathing, reflects the flow of energy through these meridians.

The importance of breathing techniques has long been stressed in Chinese medicine as a means of preventing illness, prolonging youth, and achieving longevity.[102] The

rationale behind this is that, besides oxygen, the air we breathe contains many other essential elements, such as iron, copper, zinc, and magnesium[92,96-98,102,103] and that the combination of exercise and breathing provides an efficient and effective method of taking these precious elements in and getting rid of wastes and poisons. It is believed that the breathing technique of abdominal or "inner" breathing facilitates the flow of energy throughout the body. Inhalation "stores" energy, whereas exhalation "releases" energy.[103]

The classic methods of tai chi combine movement with breathing. The movements are performed to assist and guide the circulation of vital energy, chi, through the eight channels and 12 meridians. The mind consciously "lifts" the energy during inward breathing from the solar plexus region,

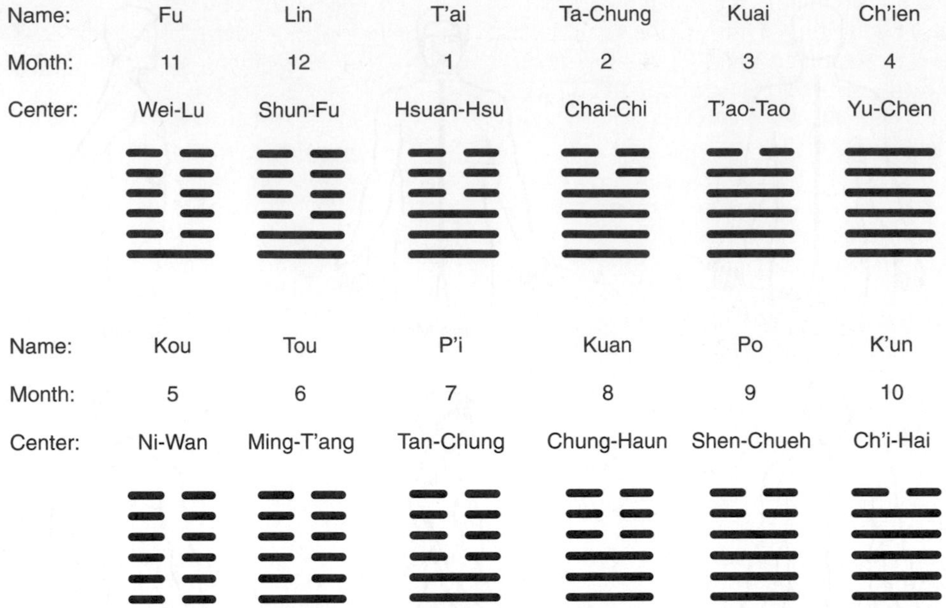

Name:	Fu	Lin	T'ai	Ta-Chung	Kuai	Ch'ien
Month:	11	12	1	2	3	4
Center:	Wei-Lu	Shun-Fu	Hsuan-Hsu	Chai-Chi	T'ao-Tao	Yu-Chen

Name:	Kou	Tou	P'i	Kuan	Po	K'un
Month:	5	6	7	8	9	10
Center:	Ni-Wan	Ming-T'ang	Tan-Chung	Chung-Haun	Shen-Chueh	Ch'i-Hai

FIGURE 37-7 ■ The waxing and waning of energy represented by the *I Ching* hexagrams.

which is considered the central energy source of the body.[92,97,98,103] During exhalation, concentrated directing of the energy is from the solar plexus region toward the lower abdomen.[92,96-98,103] It is through this conscious directing of the energy that each of the eight channels is supplied with energy during the movement of tai chi. It is hypothesized that in tai chi exercise the circulation of chi through the channels does not occur automatically as a result of the arm and leg movements combined with breathing. Rather, it is the mind's power of concentration that combines with the breathing to move the chi through the channels. The outer movements aid and guide the inner concentration. Tai chi is regarded as a method of "moving meditation."[97,98]

Both the movements of the limbs and the way they are coordinated with the breathing cycle constitute the tai chi form of exercise. The movements are relatively simple, involving only the bending and unbending of the knees while the hands are lowered or raised. The movements are an effective way of directing the flow of energy through the channels. Several kinds of movement of the body and limbs during tai chi exercise involve movements such as shifting the weight from one leg to another, rotating the body to the right or left, taking a step, moving forward or backward, and fine hand and foot movements, all put together and coordinated in more or less complicated combinations and sequences.

Preventive Qualities. More than 80% of all illness has been shown to have stress-related causes.[104] Medical and rehabilitation practices that seek only to "fix" the physical symptoms (body) without addressing the impact of emotional well-being on disease are missing the target. Although the origins of tai chi exercise are based on ancient Eastern philosophy, it is a suitable form of exercise for tense Westerners. It has the advantage of regular exercise combined with an emphasis on the gracefulness and slowness of pace that Western society so conspicuously lacks. Tai chi can provide those who live in a fast-paced environment a compensating factor in their lives.

In ancient Chinese medicine it has long been recognized that there are mental as well as physical aspects of disease.[99,100,102-104] Traditionally, according to Eastern philosophies, the mental state of the individual is considered to be *more* important than the physical symptoms. Recently, a new basic science of Western medical research, called psychoneuroimmunology, has emerged.[78,90,91,104] This area of science is the study of the effects of emotions on the immune system. The new studies strongly indicate that virtually every illness, from a common cold to cancer and heart disease, can be influenced either positively or negatively by an individual's mental status. Today, Western health care professionals in both the physical and mental health professions are increasingly recognizing the role of the mind in the prevention and cure of illness. The health practitioner may encounter clients who do not seem to respond to traditional health care. Psychoneuroimmunology confronts these problems by using the health traditions of other cultures and viewing the body and mind as a balanced whole.[78]

Tai chi is a specific technique for attaining peaceful mental states and therefore, by extrapolation, it may help prevent or reverse disease processes. Tai chi integrates the body and mind through breathing and movement. The open and closed movements of tai chi are coordinated with breathing. The benefits seem to be based on the fundamental combination of movements and breathing techniques in the basic tai chi exercise routines. The entry level of exercise has many similarities with medical treatments for respiratory illness (e.g., deep breathing exercises, segmental expansion exercises) and with walking exercise, the most recommended aerobic exercise for patients with coronary artery disease.[105-110]

In a study by Lai et al,[107] it was determined that the elderly tai chi exercisers showed a significant improvement in the volume of oxygen utilization (VO_2) uptake compared with an age-matched control group of sedentary elders. The authors concluded that the data substantiated the practice of tai chi as a means of delaying the decline in cardiorespiratory function commonly considered "normal" for aging individuals. In addition, tai chi was shown to be a suitable aerobic exercise for older adults.[107] A subsequent study by Lai et al[108] further substantiated that tai chi exercise is aerobic exercise of moderate intensity. In the past, it was believed, although never studied, that tai chi exercise forms did not have a significant cardiorespiratory component and therefore were deemed nonaerobic. A short style of tai chi chaun was found to be an effective way to improve many fitness measures. In fact, tai chi was found to be significantly better than brisk walking in enhancing certain measures of fitness including lower extremity strength, balance, and flexibility.[108a] It has been clearly demonstrated in these studies that, despite the slow, steady, smooth pace of tai chi exercise routines, there is a significant positive effect on the cardiorespiratory system.[105-110]

The potential value of tai chi exercise in promoting postural control, improving balance, and preventing falls has also been substantiated by several researchers.[95,111-114] Tse and Bailey[115] found that tai chi practitioners had significantly better postural control than did sedentary nonpractitioners. Province et al[86] found that treatments directed toward flexibility, balance, dynamic balance, and resistance, all components of tai chi exercise, reduced the risk of falls for elderly adults.[116-118] Tai chi has been found to enhance neuromuscular responses controlling the ankle joint of the perturbed leg when balance is lost.[119] Fast, accurate, neuromuscular activation is crucial for efficacious response to slips or trips. Wolfson et al[120] demonstrated that short-term exposure to "altered sensory input or destabilizing platform movement" during treatment sessions, in addition to home-based tai chi exercises, elicited significant improvements in sway control and inhibited inappropriate motor responses. The outcome measure of functional balance improved more substantially in the exercise group that combined the treatment sessions with the home program of tai chi. Wolf et al[121] compared a balance training group, in which balance was stressed on a static-to-moving platform using biofeedback, with a group of tai chi exercisers. A third group served as a control for exercise intervention. This article did not provide information on the results of the effects of the two different exercise approaches on balance and frailty measures, although it provided a superb set of assessment tools for measuring balance. In a subsequent interview with Wolf, he spoke positively about the therapeutic value of exercise forms such as tai chi in delaying or possibly preventing the onset of frailty.[122] The benefits of tai chi in prevention of falls has also been supported by a study by Judge et al,[112] who demonstrated improvements in single-stance postural sway in older women after tai chi exercises. A recent study demonstrates the positive influence that tai chi has on decreasing the fear of falling.[122a] Improving older adults' physical function, as well as their fear of falling, may reduce negative outcomes. Tsang and Hui-Chan[123] demonstrated that long-term tai chi practitioners had better knee muscle strength, less body sway in perturbed single-leg stance, and greater confidence. Significant correlations among these measures uncover the importance of knee muscle strength and balance control during perturbed single-leg stance in older adults' balance confidence in their daily activities.

Data exist to support the contention that tai chi specifically targets the impairments, functional limitations, dis-

ability, and quality of life associated with peripheral vestibulopathy.[124] In addition, tai chi appears to be useful for a variety of nonvestibulopathy etiological balance disorders, and it is safe.[117-124]

The stress reduction effects of tai chi exercise, as measured by heart rate, blood pressure, and urinary catecholamine and salivary cortisol levels, were compared with the levels in a group of brisk walkers, meditators, and quiet readers[91] In general, it was found that the stress-reducing effect of tai chi characterized those physiological changes produced by moderate exercise. Heart rate, blood pressure, and urinary catecholamine changes for the tai chi exercise group were similar to these changes occurring in the walking group. Additionally, it was reported that the tai chi group expressed the enhancement of "vigor" and a reduction in anxiety states. In a study by Brown et al,[90] unequivocal support is provided for the hypothesis that tai chi exercise, which incorporates a cognitive strategy as part of the training program, is more effective than exercise lacking a structured cognitive component in promoting psychological benefits.

A 3-week tai chi class resulted in improvement on all flexibility, strength, and balance measures in a patient with Parkinson's disease and may be a viable option for improving balance in patients with parkinsonism.[125]

Osteoporosis may also be influenced by tai chi. Studies have demonstrated that tai chi has a positive influence on bone mass density. Qin et al[126] showed, in the first case-controlled study, that regular tai chi chuan exercise may help retard bone loss in the weight-bearing bones of postmenopausal women. In another study, the tai chi group showed higher bone mass density in the lumbar spine and proximal femur and better neuromuscular function in postmenopausal women, including lower extremity strength and flexibility measures, compared with a control group.[127]

The elderly people who regularly practiced tai chi not only showed better proprioception at the ankle and knee joints than sedentary controls did, but also better ankle kinesthetic sense compared with swimmers and runners.[128] The large benefits of tai chi exercise on proprioception may result in the maintenance of balance control preventing many of the orthopedic conditions we encounter clinically.

Rheumatoid arthritis (RA) is another frequently seen problem in all clinical settings. The results of a study by Han et al[129] suggest that tai chi does not exacerbate symptoms of RA. In addition, tai chi had statistically significant benefits on improving joint range and decreasing pain in people with RA (Case Study 37-2).

An exciting area of research has evolved. This is the evaluation of complementary and alternative approaches to dementia. Many therapies in popular use have yet to be supported by best-evidence trials or meta-analysis and are clearly suboptimal. Among alternative practices that have been found effective in Alzheimer's disease, tai chi holds an important place in decreasing falls and promoting function, even as the disease progresses.[129a]

Conclusions. The increasing body of research related to the use of tai chi as a valuable therapeutic intervention substantiates our need as professionals, in a cost-containment arena, to evaluate the merits of this exercise

CASE STUDY 37-2 ■ MR. K.

Mr. K. is an 84-year-old white man admitted to the nursing home from home in a markedly deconditioned state, with a diagnosis of coronary heart disease, tuberculosis, confusion, a recent history of falls, depression, and malnutrition. He was referred to physical and occupational therapy for screening and recommendations. Screening by physical therapy resulted in an initial evaluation that revealed a significantly compromised cardiopulmonary response to any activity, flexed posturing in standing with occasional loss of balance during directional changes, ambulation with moderate assistance of one requiring verbal cuing, and a fluctuating cognitive status. He was quite congested and occasionally expectorated blood, especially with exertion. He had remarkable shortness of breath at rest and significant rubor of all extremities with 1+ pulses distally. He was withdrawn, minimally verbal, and obviously quite depressed. On the basis of our assessment, his prognosis was deemed poor for functional recovery to his premorbid state and discharge unlikely.

Mr. K. was placed on a fall prevention program that included trunk extensor strengthening, extremity strengthening, and flexibility exercises. Deep breathing exercises were initiated and a reconditioning walking program using a 12-minute test protocol was started. Buerger-Allen exercises were initiated for his circulation and to promote postural changes and mobility. He was also referred to a nutritionist, and the nursing staff was consulted regarding his skin and circulatory status. Patient's gains were marginal in both physical and occupational therapy over a 3-week period. He continued to require minimal to moderate assistance during ambulation, had a poor physiological response to activity of any sort, remained short of breath at rest, and was still withdrawn, now being virtually nonverbal and severely depressed.

As a result of the restrictions placed on duration of intervention in a managed care delivery system driven by critical pathways, aggressive "skilled" intervention could no longer be justified. The insurer agreed to a 4-week trial of tai chi exercises to be done 5 days per week in a group setting. The patient was initially instructed in breathing techniques and standing postures using a set of tai chi movements that did not significantly displace his center of gravity. Remarkable improvements were noted in respiratory status (i.e., he was no longer short of breath at rest) and standing

posture was distinctly improved by the end of the first week. It was noted that this elderly man was much more alert and responsive to his surroundings and appeared to be less depressed. The tai chi routine was expanded to encompass his increasing capabilities, and weight-shifting postures were started, although one-legged stance tai chi activities were still omitted from his routine. By the end of the second week, the patient was walking to and from all activities with standby assistance and no verbal cuing. His extremity pulses had improved to 2+ with no extremity rubor. He still had shortness of breath on exertion, although he was no longer short of breath at rest and was not expectorating blood. He was noted to be spontaneously telling stories and joking with the staff and other residents. He reported amiably "where" his energy was going from time to time and stated that he was "eating everything on my plate."

Mr. K. continued to progress in all areas of functional status. By the end of the third week he was walking to all activities independently and safely. He was alert and obviously happy. We were able to start one-legged stance postures in his tai chi routine. He was independently taking a shower (which pleased him no end). He was fondly appreciated by his fellow residents for his sense of humor, optimism, and compassion for their concerns.

By the end of the fourth week, Mr. K., a happy man, was discharged on a home program that included tai chi exercises. Since his discharge, he has enrolled in a tai chi program at a local martial arts facility, in which he participates for 2 hours, three times a week. He comes back to the nursing home twice a week to assist as an instructor in the tai chi classes.

Perhaps Mr. K.'s progress sounds too good to be true, but the reality of his improvement has been observed in many of our patients who participate in the tai chi classes. Beyond the physical aspects of this exercise form, the most notable improvement appears to be in the area of "outlook." Elderly individuals participating in the tai chi classes express pure enjoyment in the slow, rhythmic movements and the group interaction. They report that they "feel stronger," "more balanced," and that they feel as if they were "dancing, not exercising." And, the insurers are overwhelmed with the functional successes that seem to be inherent in this mode of exercise. Tai chi is a low-cost, low-tech group activity.

form.[80-82,86-89,96,107,108] Tai chi is viewed as an "alternative" therapy, has been observed clinically, and has been shown to enhance function in our elderly patients. Recently, the use of tai chi has been identified by the National Institutes of Health as one of a list of "alternative therapies" that will be targeted for research funding as a legitimate area for investigation. We should seize the opportunity to provide leadership in this emerging area in rehabilitative medicine. Tai chi, although it is a "nontraditional" approach to therapeutic

intervention, merits further scientific analysis to quantify its apparent therapeutic validity.

Tae Kwon Do

Clinton Robinson, Jr., 8th Degree
Darcy A. Umphred, 4th Degree, PT, PhD, FAPTA

Philosophy. The overall philosophy of Tae Kwon Do (TKD) can be summed up in the student oath recited by all practitioners at the beginning of each class: "I shall observe the tenets of taekwondo: courtesy, integrity, perseverance, self-control, and indomitable spirit." The tenets are to be practiced outside as well as inside the training hall in all aspects of life. All aspects of these tenets reflect CNS control and neuroplasticity and incorporate the cognitive, emotional, and motor aspects into an integrated whole. The oath continues with, "I shall respect the instructors and seniors," which refers to having respect for all people, our teachers, our parents, our peers, our students, our patients, which reflects all individuals with whom the student may interact through a lifetime. "I shall never misuse Tae Kwon Do." No matter what motor skill a student develops, it is not to be used to build one's ego or to injure another unnecessarily. "I will be a champion of freedom and justice." Individuals are expected to develop a sense of responsibility for those less fortunate than themselves and be an active participant in the development of mankind as a whole. These are basic philosophies of both occupational and physical therapy. Empowerment of others to overcome their movement limitations and once again participate in life should be the goals of all therapeutic treatment outcomes. "I will build a more peaceful world." Understanding that change begins with self, thus by developing and integrating the mind, body, and spirit while helping others do the same, will set an example not only in the classroom but in our society, so that others may improve themselves. The profession of occupational therapy has identified similar educational criteria outcomes after a professional educational program accredited by the respective body. Physical therapy has begun to integrate the mind, body, and spirit into outcomes but as of today has not embraced those interactions as part of the Commission on Accreditation of Physical Therapy Education (CAPTE) accreditation criteria. The overall goal of TKD training is the development of self-sufficiency through rigorous physical and mental practice. With this training, an inner balance or peace can be attained thus balancing all aspects of a person's life. Students are expected to strive for their own personal excellence versus comparing that skill with another's. Thus, individuals with physical challenges are always encouraged to participate. Their challenges and expectations are different, but achieving personal excellence gives them the same respect and confidence that any other student would receive. Thus, TKD as a movement science empowers participants to gain or regain a feeling of empowerment over the mind, the spirit, and the physical body.

Philosophy of Training. Training in TKD consists of three primary components: forms, breaking of solid objects, and sparring. The practice of tai chi focuses on the first component, but with practice a TKD student would have the skill to perform both breaking and sparring.

Poomsee. Poomsee is a prearranged dance of defensive and offensive techniques against an imaginary opponent. The practice of poomsee increases the practitioner's memory, coordination, balance, and body awareness. All poomsee components have predetermined patterns of movement that include various stances and hand and kicking techniques, along with a proper beginning and ending point. The complexity and difficulty of these forms increases as the student progresses. As beginners are challenged by simple movement and combinations of patterns, the highest ranking black belt will also be challenged by movements and com-

binations of complex patterns appropriate for that level of study. Thus, all individuals studying TKD are challenged to be in a state of growth and learning.[130]

Kyukpa. Kyukpa is breaking of solid objects such as boards, concrete, and bricks using a body part as a weapon. Kyukpa represents overcoming limitations and obstacles and facing fear. It requires tremendous concentration and belief in one's abilities. Additionally, it allow its practitioners to demonstrate the power they have attained, thereby increasing self-confidence. Self-confidence is the primary attribute in conflict resolution skills and leads to the understanding that there are few situations in life in which physical confrontation is necessary. Board breaking helps teach the learning that an obstacle is only an obstacle if you empower it to that role. Once the board is broken and the limb has passed through its obstacle it no longer is an obstacle. This philosophy reflects life and plays a role in establishment of values and motivation by learning to going beyond the known and through the obstacles that life poses.

Kyorugi. Kyorugi is actual sparring between two people using both defensive and offensive techniques learned through fundamental TKD practice. Kyorugi can be further broken down into two types: (1) In one-step sparring, the practitioners take turns initiating a prearranged attack while the other defends. This allows the practitioners to engage each other without risk of injury to either party. It also allows them to practice proper distancing and execution of the techniques. This develops confidence in the ability to use the techniques properly if the need arises. (2) In free sparring, neither opponent knows what the other is going to do. Although free sparring may appear dangerous to one untrained in TKD, it is a relatively safe activity. Free sparring requires respect for your partner and absolute controlled motions at all times. It is an exercise in which the aim is for all involved to increase their skill level.[131] It develops the practitioner's reflexes, confidence in his or her abilities, and overall awareness as well as a cooperative learning environment.

Although both offensive and defensive techniques are viewed as equally important, all training is begun with blocking techniques to indicate that TKD never allows any initial offensive attack in its technique. Blocking techniques are practiced diligently so that they may function equally as offensive techniques. This way one can defeat an opponent, whether in the classroom or in real life, without either suffering or inflicting serious injuries. This builds self-confidence and replaces a perception of the "role of a victim."[132] Defensive techniques are not only power against power but truly reflect power of the attacker and deflection by the opposition. This deflection can either stop the attacker, redirect the power back onto the attacker, or incapacitate the attacker in order for the opposition to get away. The skill in redirecting the force and intent of an attacker is not too different from redirecting a patient's motor pattern into a direction that would be functional as a motor program. The TKD practitioner and the therapist is working with the pattern of movement presented to them. The intent of the TKD student would be to disempower the attacker while the intent of the therapist would be to empower the patient.[133-135]

In TKD training, all students begin in the same place. There is no concern for one's status in life. The white belt is used to denote the beginning student. With all students beginning at that level, it allows another aspect of training that is critical to all students and individualized. Training encompasses setting and achieving goals or empowering oneself to one's own quality of life. In TKD, there is a belt ranking system and the object is to progress through the various levels of proficiency, culminating in the black belt. Everyone, regardless of social status or physical skill, has the same opportunity to advance in TKD. Students who persevere and obtain a first-degree black belt learn that they have only begun their circle of growth and learning. With additional years of training, students may advance in black belt ranks that should reflect a greater understanding and acceptance of those initial tenets. The circle of growth will always lead to further integration of mind, body, and spirit and an inner peace and balance.[136] The balance of mind, body, and spirit is the core of other complementary therapy paradigms and ultimately seems to be an element linked to health and healing.[137]

Tae Kwon Do and Complementary Therapy.[136,138-143] Although TKD is a martial arts style whose original intent was not to heal a disease pathological condition or to regain a functional movement activity lost after some acute health care crisis, the concepts and procedures learned, repetitively practiced, and transformed into life behavior have established the foundation for health and healing in individuals. Most students in TKD fall within a health and wellness model of life, but most have impairments within some aspect of their musculoskeletal systems. Many adults starting out this training have impairments within the CNS as a result of life activities that have forced the CNS to adapt and accommodate to prior physical limitations such as ligamentus tear or trauma from bullying in school. These experiences create change whether the deficits are motor, cognitive, or affective.[144,145] Similarly, with identified chronic motor limitations such as functional limitations after a birth trauma, an external head trauma, or an internal insult, TKD can help maintain motor function, cognitive integrity, emotional balance, and a feeling of self-worth in the face of a long-term and possibly progressive neurological problem.

As in all martial arts, TKD requires active participation by the student. When any TKD movement pattern is examined, certain motor control components are seen to be interacting. There are a variety of activities that generally occur during a class. First, there are warmup exercises, after which the student will work on (1) her or his respective form or poomsee or hyung (dancelike patterns that may have 18 to 100 different movement sequences), depending on the level of advancement; (2) sparring, which is either done with one partner moving with an identified pattern while the other stays in one position or with both moving and learning to respond to the movements or feints of the other; or (3) learning to focus and perform specific strikes or blows that will lead to skills in board or brick breaking or defending oneself against a life-threatening attack.

During warmup, a student stretches and builds up power, using specific movement, balance, timing, concentration, and cardiopulmonary functions that set the stage for the remainder of the class. When doing the forms, the student will need to work on balance, postural tone, the state of the motor generator, synergistic patterns of movement, trajectory, speed, force, directionality, sequencing, reciprocal patterns, and the context within which the movement is being done. Similarly, memory of the specific pattern, movement sequences, and direction of the movements requires concentration. As the student progresses in rank, the specific patterns become more and more complex, increase in number of specific movements, and frequently change from quick movements to slow, controlled patterns. This repetition of practice and increase in difficulty leads to higher skill and cortical representaion.[146,147] If other students are also practicing in class, then each individual needs to be aware of the total environment to respect the space of all other students. This unique individual experience during a group activity allows for variance during each class and thus should lead to greater motor learning and cortical represenation.[147,148]

When students are learning and practicing either one-step sparring or free sparring, they are not only working on learning combinations of movement patterns and how they interact or conflict with those of their partners, but they are also learning how to control their emotional responses to threatening situations. Little in life is worth hurting another—a basic principle of TKD. During sparring, the potential of injury is directly correlated with the control over the force and direction of movement of each team. That control can be dramatically affected by emotion (see Chapter 4). Once students learn to control the emotional aspect, their skill and techniques become procedural, which allows their cognitive analytical ability to drive responses (see Chapter 9). The student is then ready to begin study of the mind, body, emotional, and spiritual connections that need to intertwine and become harmonious if the student is to learn the true meaning of TKD. Sparring is a controlled environment in which injury or damage to another person is never acceptable. The instructor is never to spar above the skill level of the student, nor is the student to enter into a sparring match with the intent to show the teacher just how good he or she is. In reality, when a student does take that emotional stance, the motor skills only reflect just how much more that student needs to learn. Feedback from others is a powerful learning tool for students at all levels. Board and brick breaking is the time a student can demonstrate force production as it interlocks with trajectory, speed, and position in space. If any of these perceptual or motor variables are incorrect, the student will not succeed at going through the obstacle. These skills are taught and practiced not to damage or destroy the wood or brick, but rather to learn to go beyond or through the obstacle. Once the specific body part used as a trajectory goes beyond the obstacle, it no long remains an obstacle and the student feels great satisfaction. In reality, to be successful at these tasks, the hand, elbow, or foot that is used to go through the brick or wood is only an extension of the body. Success is based on the learner's ability to tie the entire body's motor response, its rotation, its balance, its trajectory, its force, and its speed into a motor program that will project through one or more obstacles as a knife cuts butter. If the student, emotionally, believes that the obstacle will not break, it will not! The student will stop the movement before completing the task and often empower the wood or brick as a successful obstacle versus empowering herself or himself to overcome that obstacle as if it were never there. This concept is a critical element of TKD. It is also a critical component of any client's learning of any motor program and turning the program into a functional activity and improving one's quality of life and ability to participate in that life's adventure. If a patient's CNS is convinced that the movement is not possible, then that individual will fail. Without internal motivation by an individual to accept the possibility of success, acceptance of failure is embraced. This internal environment plays a key role in any individual's overcoming what he or she perceives as an obstacle in life.[149] It is the role of the TKD teacher and the therapist teacher to empower the student to the possibility of success while creating an external environment that will enhance the probability of that success.[130,146] To ask TKD students to perform motor skills above their level of competence can lead to injury and embrace failure. Failure often stops the motivation to continue to learn. Patients in a therapeutic environment are no different. They need an environment that creates safety, promotes success, and empowers the individual to overcome life obstacles.

Those who respond best to TKD training to maintain motor function are individuals who are motivated to move, enjoy interactions with others, have cognitive integrity, and have some control over their motor system. When instructing a TKD club of individuals who had all had traumatic head injuries, the teacher (TKD instructor) and a therapist who had worked for more than 25 years in the area of neurological rehabilitation found that using therapeutic skills through TKD movement patterns augmented the students' learning and helped them to regain motor function through guided activities without the students ever realizing there was therapeutic intervention. To those students, they were learning and advancing in a martial arts style, tested and judged according to their development of skills, and feeling accomplishment as adults participating in adult activities. Carryover and improvement in balance, postural integrity, reciprocal patterns of movement, and control of trajectory, force, and speed, as well as development of emotional stability and confidence, could be easily identified and evaluated by use of standard objective measurement tools if so desired. Expected outcomes would be improvement in those areas of motor control just mentioned. As long as the student continued training, improvement would be expected and carryover into other life activities anticipated. These are the principles of neuroplasticity and have meaning both within the pre–disease/pathology model as seen in TKD[150,151] and after acute injury, disease, or insult to the CNS,[152-156] which may lead to movement dysfunction seen by physical and occupational therapists.

Energetic Therapy Approaches

Therapeutic Touch

Pat Winstead-Fry, RN, PhD
Rebecca M. Good, MA, RNC, ACRN, LPC, QTTT

Definition and Uses. Therapeutic touch (TT), a contemporary interpretation of several ancient healing practices, is practiced by nurses, physical therapists, occupational therapists, and other professionals in hospitals and health care settings. TT is an intentionally directed process of energy exchange during which the practitioner uses the hands as a focus to facilitate the rebalancing of another's energy field in support of healing. It is a complementary integrative therapy that works effectively with a wide variety of patient conditions. TT is effective in eliciting a relaxation response,

reducing anxiety, decreasing pain, increasing a sense of well-being, and accelerating the body's ability to heal from wounds and surgery.

TT is valuable for people of all ages, from neonates to the elderly. Indications for TT include, but are not limited to, preoperative and postoperative care, maternal and child care, cancer and all related therapies, many types of emotional and physical illnesses, human immunodeficiency virus (HIV) infection/acquired immunodeficiency syndrome, chronic illnesses, multiple sclerosis, Parkinson's disease, cancer, fibromyalgia, and death and dying. TT is as much a wellness therapy as it is a complementary therapy. It helps restore balance and order in all aspects of the individual: body, mind, emotion, and spirit.

Background. Dr. Dolores Krieger and Mrs. Dora Kunz developed the contemporary form of TT from the ancient practice of "laying on of hands." In the late 1960s, Mrs. Kunz, a noted natural healer, invited Dr. Krieger to watch Mr. Oscar Estabany treating patients with laying on of hands. Dr. Krieger was amazed that Mr. Estabany could help more than 95% of the patients he treated. Krieger and Kunz planned to study the use of hands in healing over time.

Most of the healers of the time thought healing was a God-given gift that could not be learned. Indeed, healers such as Mr. Estabany had little or no knowledge of anatomy, physiology, or medical diagnoses. In spite of this, Mrs. Kunz began to think that healing might be taught and learned. She began to teach Dr. Krieger how to heal.

By 1974, Dr. Krieger was proficient enough that she could develop a course entitled "Frontiers of Nursing" that was approved by the New York University School of Education curriculum committee. "Frontiers of Nursing" was taught for the first time in 1975. It has been taught every semester since then. It is a graduate level course, so the nurses who enroll in it are practicing nurses. These nurses could implement what they learned into their clinical care of patients.

There are several assumptions on which TT is based. One that draws on the work of nursing theorist Martha Rogers states that each person is a localized concentration of energy within a larger field that connects all living organisms.[157] The interconnection and openness of each individual system allows life energy to be directed from one person to another. Another assumption is that there is a universal healing field on which each TT therapist draws to make this energy available to patients. An assumption shared by many cultures is that symptoms of illness are actually indications of energy imbalance. Another assumption is that all healing is ultimately self-healing.

Krieger and Kunz hypothesized that the ability to facilitate healing in another person is an innate human potential, which could be actualized through training and practice.

TT is an important addition to nursing interventions. It is one answer to the National Institute of Nursing's mandate to reduce the burden of illness by developing and applying interventions. Nurses and other health care providers want to develop a group of noninvasive interventions that can easily and inexpensively be learned and implemented.

The North American Nursing Diagnosis Association (NANDA) recognizes TT as a nursing intervention under the NANDA diagnosis "Disturbed Energy Field."[158] Other professional organizations such as the American Nurses

Association and the National League for Nursing support TT as a nursing intervention on the basis of its extensive research. The National Institutes of Health's National Center Office for Complementary and Alternative Medicine recognizes TT worthy of receiving funding for further research, as does the U.S. Department of Defense.[159,160]

Therapeutic Touch—The Dynamic Process. The four phases of TT are learned as a sequence of distinct steps or phases, which typically evolve into a simultaneous, synchronized process as the therapist continues to practice.

The TT process is always individualized and can be done with the person sitting in a chair or lying down, whichever is more comfortable. It is not necessary for the client to disrobe. The practitioner will generally pass her or his hands over the person's body from head to toe, over the front and back of the body, holding the hands 2 to 6 inches from the skin. The practitioner will assess and then use rhythmical sweeping motions with the hands as explained below. The practitioner may or may not physically touch the person.

Throughout the session, the therapist holds the intention of the client/patient's wholeness. Compassion and intentionality are two guiding principles in the TT process.

The Four Phases of Therapeutic Touch. The TT process is dynamic, not linear. In the beginning, though, it is easier to understand when it is explained in phases or steps.[161]

Centering. The therapist begins by **centering** himself or herself; that is, the therapist brings body, mind, and emotions to a quiet, focused state of consciousness. Characteristics of this state may include finding an inner sense of equilibrium, a personal reference of physical, emotional, and intellectual stability; quieting the body, mind, and emotions; connecting with one's inner core of wholeness and stillness; feeling integrated; and, being nonjudgmental. The therapist continues through the entire TT interaction in a state of "sustained" centeredness. This state is unique to TT.

Assessment. In the second phase or step, **assessment,** also referred to as "scanning," the hands are used to determine the nature of the dynamic energy field of the patient. The therapist holds the hands 2 to 6 inches away from the patient's body while moving from the head to the feet in a rhythmic, symmetrical manner. The intent is to observe the nature of the flow of energy throughout the patient's field on the basis of the assumption that in health the flow is generally open and balanced. The therapist senses carefully for any differences in this flow. The sensory cues, which are received intuitively, cognitively, and energetically, vary for each practitioner but may include sensations of tingling, pulsation, or temperature changes.

Intervention/Rebalancing. The third phase or step, **intervention,** is also referred to as **balancing** or **rebalancing.** The intention of the therapist is to facilitate the symmetrical and rhythmic flow of energy through the patient's field by using the techniques of unruffling, directing, and modulating energy on the basis of the cues perceived in the assessment, thereby helping reestablish the symmetrical balance, rhythm, and flow in the field. In using "unruffling" or clearing, the therapist again moves the hands through the patient's field with the intention of facilitating the flow, allowing the field to clear itself of congestion or disruption

and return to a more balanced flow. This helps to free non-flowing energy and allows access to underlying imbalances.

In choosing to "direct" and "modulate," the therapist consciously makes the intention to bring energy through herself or himself into the field of the patient to bring balance to areas of imbalance. Energy may be directed through specific areas of the body on the basis of assessment and reassessment.

While directing energy, the therapist uses modulation to adjust the flow of energy during the TT intervention. As the therapist maintains the state of sustained centering, he or she does not push, force, or constrict the flow, but with gentle awareness allows the recipient's field to draw the needed energy. The therapist also recognizes the need to modulate the flow of energy on the basis of the recipient's sensitivity to the interaction.

Sensitive populations such as the very ill, elderly, very young, or those with psychological disturbances require an especially light, gentle flow of energy during modulation. Throughout the session the therapist holds the intention of the client/patient's wholeness.

Evaluation or Closure. In the final phase or step, **evaluation** or **closure,** the therapist uses professional, informed, and intuitive judgment to determine when the session has come to a close. Reassessment is a continuing process. When evaluation reveals balanced, symmetrical, and rhythmical order within the system or when the bioenergy field has absorbed all it can during the session, the practitioner ends the session. It is helpful if the patient can rest for a short period before resuming usual activities.

Frequency and Duration. The frequency and duration of a TT session varies according to the practitioner's assessment, but it is usually no longer than 20 to 25 minutes. It is shorter depending on the age and condition of the recipient. For example, neonates, children, pregnant women, and the elderly and debilitated are more sensitive and require shorter sessions.

Adverse Effects/Precautions. There have been no recorded adverse effects, but it is important for the practitioner to be knowledgeable and skilled in the TT process.

Qualifications for a Therapeutic Touch Practitioner. In this section we will talk briefly about what to look for in a TT practitioner or teacher. We cannot emphasize enough the importance of standards and scope of practice, credentialing, and a specific professional organization representing the complementary therapy.

TT has standards and a scope of practice, policy, and procedure for the practice of TT and ethics and a credentialing program for practitioners and teachers. Dr. Dolores Krieger and a group of TT practitioners and teachers formed Nurse Healers-Professional Associates International (NH-PAI), the official organization of TT in the late 1970s. NH-PAI sets the standards, policies, and procedures and the credentialing standards for the teaching and practice of TT.

According to NH-PAI, the credentialing program for practitioners begins when one takes a minimum 12-hour basic class from a teacher recognized by NH-PAI as a qualified TT teacher (QTTT). The student then enters into a mentoring program with a QTTT for a minimum of 1 year.

CASE STUDY 37-3 ■ MRS. P. G.

Mrs. P. G., a 59-year-old woman, presented herself at our Therapeutic Touch Clinic at the Cancer Wellness House last April 18, 2005. On September 23, 2004, she had a hemangioblastoma surgically removed from her cerebellum. The neurologist told her this slow-growing tumor had wrapped itself around her cerebellum. Her postsurgical course required the usual pain medicine and some physical therapy for motor imbalance and to increase ROM in her neck after surgery with little success. Mrs. P. G. reported that her physicians told her that, because of the size, location, and pressure of the tumor, she would be left with residual neurological damage.

She presented for Therapeutic Touch therapy with the following complaints: continuous motor imbalance, minimal ROM of her neck with severe pain, continuing dizziness especially on movement, and feeling "spacy" much of the time. She did not like taking pain medicine because it made her drowsy and she felt "doped up."

Mrs. P. G. is divorced and lives alone. She has little family support. Her two adult children are busy with families and careers. She has a brother in the area who is some support emotionally. She is her only source of income. She returned to work at a support desk job at an airline after being out of work for 9 months. She is involved with the Cancer Wellness House and participates in the activities there for emotional and wellness support.

She could only attend TT sessions once a month. She received TT monthly for 7 months. During TT sessions, she was given gentle relaxation and breathing prompts to do between sessions. It was also recommended that in addition she do gentle yoga, using a chair as needed, which was also offered at the Cancer Wellness House.

When Mrs. P. G. first started TT she was 7 months postoperative. She presented at the initial session holding her neck in a stiff and protective manner. She did not turn her neck because of the pain but protected it by turning her whole body instead. Her left neck in the area of the incision was tender and she was also protective of this area. The area of the incision was still raised and swollen. When ambulating, she would hold onto furniture, walls, and other structures to help maintain her balance as she made her way through the room and building. Initially, her reported pain levels before a TT session on the Likert scale averaged 8 to 10. At the end of the session she reported it as a 4 to 5.

As the sessions progressed, it was noted that she was able to ambulate without holding onto furniture or other objects to maintain stability and balance. She became progressively less protective of her neck. Her pain level before the TT session on the Likert scale averaged a 2 to 4. At the end of the session she reported it as between 0 and 2. With each TT session the ROM improved to where, at the seventh session, she proudly demonstrated full ROM with little pain.

After the first three sessions of TT, the incision area was no longer swollen or tender to touch. She no longer protected it when the practitioner's hands were near that area. She reported that TT helps her think more clearly and her "spacy" feeling is improved after TT, but this benefit does not last more than a few days. She still has problems with imbalance, which worsen when she is tired. However, as noted, her symptoms are significantly better than before she started TT therapy.

It was recommended that Mrs. P. G. continue to receive TT monthly for continuing neurological rehabilitation and wellness therapy.

After completing the mentoring program and a minimum 14-hour intermediate-level TT class from a QTTT, one may apply to NH-PAI to become recognized as a qualified TT practitioner (QTTP). One maintains the credential as a QTTP by satisfying specific requirements as set forth by the NH-PAI.

To become a QTTT, it is necessary to satisfy the requirements for a QTTP and take a minimum of three advanced level classes in TT from QTTTs. In addition, one enters into a minimum of a 1-year teacher-mentoring program, which may begin after the first advanced TT class. Under the guidance of the QTTT mentor, the individual will develop a teaching program. Among many other experiences in the teacher-mentoring program, one may assist in teaching under the supervision of a mentor. After satisfying the teacher preparation requirements and having practiced TT regularly for a minimum of 5 to 7 years, one may make application to NH-PAI to become recognized as a QTTT. There are specific requirements to maintain the QTTT credential as set forth by the NH-PAI.

As with any other professional one sees for therapy or as a teacher, it is important that there is a sense of comfort and

trust. If for some reason there is not this feeling, it is wise to seek out another practitioner or teacher (Case Study 37-3).

Research Findings. This section is divided into two sections. First we present a general review of the research on TT and its efficacy in treating various conditions. The focus is on quantitative research because this research tests hypotheses, is generalizable, and supports assumptions about the efficacy of TT for various problems. The second section presents an expanded report of a selected research study, which allows the reader to evaluate the quality of TT research in more depth. There are also qualitative studies of TT, most of which deal with the practitioner's characteristics and experiences, the patient's experience of receiving TT, and other subjective aspects of TT. These are not included here but help by increasing our understanding of the processes involved in an energetic treatment such as TT.

General Review of TT Research. Research on TT falls into several categories. For purposes of this presentation the following categories will be used: stress, pain or discomfort in medical and rehabilitation populations, and addictions. In

1979, a few years after TT was introduced at New York University, Dr. Patricia Heidt completed the first doctoral dissertation on TT.[162]

Stress. Although the mechanism by which TT achieves its effects is not known, it is probably in some way related to the relaxation response. Most practitioners and patients note a state of relaxation within a few minutes of beginning a TT treatment. One of the first studies by Krieger et al[163] demonstrated a patient relaxation response to TT by means of electroencephalogram, electrocardiogram, and palmar galvanic skin response as well as patient self-reports confirming a state of relaxation. Patient self-reports agreed that they were relaxed. Eight other studies supported similar findings with different patient groups, including hurricane survivors, hospitalized children, and HIV-positive persons.[164-171]

Pain or Discomfort in Medical and Rehabilitation Populations. Most of the studies in this category involved reducing anxiety or pain. Eleven studies demonstrate that TT decreases anxiety at a statistically significant level.[159,172-181] The population samples studied have included HIV-positive children, hospitalized adults, elders, and burn patients. Eight studies demonstrate the effectiveness of TT in reducing pain from differing sources.[159,172-188] Two studies demonstrated that TT increases functional ability in patients with osteoarthritis.[188,189] Smith et al[189] used TT with patients undergoing bone marrow transplant. These patients reported that TT provided comfort.

Addictions. Hagemaster[190] reported that TT increased periods of abstinence for persons who abuse alcohol and other drugs. Larden et al[191] reported that TT decreases anxiety in pregnant inpatients undergoing drug withdrawal.

Alzheimer's Disease. Several studies demonstrate that TT can reduce problematic behaviors in patients with Alzheimer's disease (AD).[192-195] Use of TT also can allow the staff to experience positive emotional connectedness with patients who are in varying stages of dementia and who are verbally uncommunicative.

A Study in Depth: Therapeutic Touch and Alzheimer's Disease. To give the reader a better sense of the state of TT research, a study by Woods and Dimond will be presented in more detail.[194] These researchers explored the efficacy of TT in decreasing salivary and urinary cortisol levels and the frequency of agitated behaviors in elders with AD. The agitated behaviors exhibited by patients with AD present a major challenge to nursing home staff. These behaviors include rhythmic, but purposeless, movement of the hands, trying to escape from restraints, searching and wandering through rooms and drawers, banging and tapping hands and feet, and continuous, mumbled vocalizations. These behaviors are difficult for other residents to tolerate and can create a barrier to effective staff-patient interactions. Because most patients with AD have other conditions that require medication, effective options for treating agitation with environmental or behavioral interventions are highly desirable.

Salivary and urinary cortisol measures are indicators of stress, relating to circulating levels of this stress hormone. Recent studies demonstrate that chronic stress and aging increase cortisol levels, which may lead to damage to neurons. Although this research is in its infancy, it seems possible that there may be a relationship between high cortisol levels and agitated behaviors.

Ten residents with AD on a special care unit were the participants in the study. All were 71 to 84 years of age; they had resided on the unit for at least 2 months, they were stabilized on antipsychotic medication; they were going to live on the unit for the length of the study, and they had been diagnosed with AD according to the *Diagnostic and Statistical Manual of Mental Disorders* (fourth edition). Persons newly diagnosed with AD, persons with acute physical or psychiatric illness, persons newly diagnosed with AD, or at the end stage of AD were excluded from the study.

Nursing staff used the Brief Agitation Rating Scale to document agitation during a 2-week period. The families of patients who demonstrated such behaviors were sent a letter describing the study. The families who responded to the letter were called by the principal investigator, who solicited informed consent.

The study design was a within-subject, interrupted time series study. Samples of salivary and urinary cortisol were taken every 24 hours. Participants were monitored 24 hours a day for physical activity and every 20 minutes from 8 AM to 6 PM for agitated behaviors. There were 630 total observations for each participant. TT was administered twice a day from 5 to 7 minutes each.

The data were organized into six equal time periods of 3 days. Day 1 was dropped because it was the adaptation time for the study. Days 2 to 4 were baseline data. Days 5 to 7 were the TT treatment days. Days 8 to 10, 11 to 13, and 14 to 16 were three posttreatments periods. After day 16, no data were collected for 18 days; this was considered the washout period. Data were again collected on days 36 to 38, the postwashout phase.

Repeated-measures analysis of variance was used to test three hypotheses: (1) TT would decrease agitated behavior, (2) TT would reduce the levels of salivary and urinary cortisol, and (3) there would be a positive relationship between cortisol levels and agitated behavior.

Hypothesis one was partially supported in that during the TT treatments vocalization and pacing were decreased at a statistically significant level. Both behaviors gradually increased after the treatments ended. Hypothesis two was not statistically supported. TT was not shown to decrease urinary or salivary cortisol levels. Hypothesis three was partially supported in that there was a positive, but not statistically significant, correlation between urinary ($r = 0.152$) and salivary ($r = .0.102$) cortisol levels and agitated behaviors. Although there was a trend for a decrease in cortisol levels, it failed to reach statistical significance. The authors present a discussion of their findings and the possible factors that may have confounded the experiment, for example, several participants came down with the flu, which may have affected agitated behaviors. They also discuss the lack of statistically significant findings with salivary and urinary cortisol levels, which may be related to methodological issues having to do with the collection of the samples in the study.

Although the study has limitations and needs to be replicated, the findings suggest that the use of TT, a noninvasive modality, is a potentially valuable alternative tool for dealing with agitation and pacing in patients with AD. Nurses and other staff in nursing homes find vocalizations particularly vexing and often request medication to treat it.

Pharmacological remedies are of limited efficacy and have side effects.

Evaluation of the Research: Meta-Analyses and Future Indications.

Four meta-analyses of alternative healing modalities have been conducted. Two of them refer to "healing" and to "distant healing."[195,196] These analyses include TT and other modalities. Peters[197] and Winstead-Fry and Kijek[198] conducted meta-analyses of the TT research and came to similar conclusions.

Winstead-Fry and Kijek[198] report a meta-analysis of TT research conducted up to 1997. They used 13 of the 18 experimental studies in the literature. The 13 studies were used because they reported means and standard deviations for treatment and control groups. They found that the average effect size *(d)*, weighted for sample size, was 0.39, which Cohen considers a moderate effect size.[199] The confidence limits for *d* ranged from 0.18 to 0.50, which can be interpreted as low to moderate positive values.

There was tremendous diversity in approaches to TT research.[197,198] Of the 29 studies that tested hypotheses of the efficacy of TT reviewed by Peters and Winstead-Fry and Kijek, 10 rejected hypotheses and 19 hypotheses were supported either fully or in part. Some studies did not follow (or did not report) the steps of TT as defined by Krieger and Kunz. Some studies did not report assessing the field or the TT was administered through a plastic shield or only one appendage was treated. These studies seriously deviated from TT practice. Studies that used healthy research participants did not support the hypotheses. Some TT treatments were given for only 5 minutes when most advanced TT practitioners report they usually treat for about 20 minutes.[198]

As a result of the meta-analysis, Winstead-Fry and Kijek recommend that the researcher not be the TT practitioner, that TT be administered on the basis of the assessment of the patients (not a 5-minute treatment), that ill persons be the research participants, and that more outcomes be more broadly explored. In her meta-analysis, Peters came to essentially the same conclusions.[197] Astin et al[196] examined 11 studies of "distant healing" (including TT) that had true randomization and placebo control. They concluded that a major weakness in TT research is the use of single-blind, rather than double-blind, control. However, Astin et al[196] point out that this cannot be overcome in TT research because practitioners have to know they are delivering TT. To offset this inevitable weakness in TT research, they recommend using larger sample sizes so that more sophisticated statistical designs can be used. They also recommend doing TT more frequently during the study, thus increasing the likelihood of TT having a more pronounced effect.

Other Developments in Therapeutic Touch

Continuous Quality Improvement Study. In 1999, a Department of Holistic Care Services was created at St. John's Riverdale Hospital in New York.[200] The department used the Krieger-Kunz method of therapeutic touch as part of its usual nursing care and patients are treated at no cost. Patients may be referred by health care providers, family or friends, or by themselves.

Evaluation of TT was part of the continuous quality improvement initiative within the hospital. To do the evaluation, a standardized tool had to be created. The tool has two parts, a patient satisfaction Survey (PSS) and a TT performance improvement tool (TTPIT). The PSS consists of six questions and has a space for patients to write comments. All patients who have received two TT treatments were asked to answer the PPS anonymously and send it by preaddressed envelope. The TTPIT is completed by the TT practitioner at the end of TT treatment. It notes among other things changes in patient discomfort, calmness, nausea, pain, falling asleep, and comments by the patient about the treatment.

By August 2000, 605 patients had received TT. Most had one treatment (373 patients). Others had as many as five or more treatments. A decrease in pain was reported by 48% of the 259 patients who had pain. Ninety percent rated TT as very helpful or helpful. Comments were generally favorable.

Subjective Experience of Therapeutic Touch Scale. The initial development of the Subjective Experience of Therapeutic Touch Scale (SETTS) was conducted as part of a project in the Nursing Research Emphasis Grant for Doctoral Programs in Nursing.[201] One reviewer questioned how we knew the TT practitioner was really doing TT. The SETTS was developed to assess whether practitioners were performing TT. The original scale consisted of 68 items that has a practitioner answer questions such as how the energy field is perceived, what they feel as they assess the energy field, and how they direct energy. Initial testing showed the SETTS had an alpha reliability of .98. There was some support for predictive validity because the scales could distinguish experienced practitioners (more than 3 years) from novice practitioners.

Ferguson undertook further assessment of the psychometric properties of the SETTS.[202] She studied four groups of TT practitioners: (1) experienced TT practitioners, 2) novice TT practitioners, (3) non-TT practitioners who mentally simulated doing TT, and (4) nurses who practiced routine nursing touch. She found a reliability of .97, meaning the test consistently measured the experience of TT. She found that the experienced TT practitioners were statistically significantly different from groups 2, 3, and 4. The inexperienced TT practitioners were different from groups 3 and 4.

Ferguson[202] also established construct validity, content validity, and predictive validity for the SETTS. The SETTS has been used by teachers of TT to assess improvement in students over time. It has been used in research to validate the practice of TT.

Winstead-Fry and Kijek[198] are conducting a study to decrease the number of items in the SETTS, to create a more manageable short form of the measure. This revised scale should be available in 2006.

Conclusion. This presentation has focused on the practice and the research relevant to TT. Guidelines for the qualifications to be a TT practitioner are important to ensure the quality of the treatment and to uniformity in practice, which provides a foundation for research evaluating the efficacy of TT. The research demonstrates that TT is useful for many age groups and diagnoses. Future research will contribute to our developing understanding of the processes and efficacy of TT. Refer to Box 37-2.

BOX 37-2 ■ ABOUT THERAPEUTIC TOUCH

American Holistic Nurses' Association
P.O. Box 2130
Flagstaff, AZ 86003
800-278-AHNA
e-mail: AHNA-flag@flaglink.com
http://www.ahana.org
Nurse Healers-Professional Associates International
The Official Organization of Therapeutic Touch
P O Box 158
Warnerville, New York 12187-0158
website: WWW.therapeutic-touch.org
email: nh-pai@therapeutic-touch.org
phone: 518-325-1185
fax: 509-693-3537

Medical Intuitive

Carol Ritberger, PhD, Medical Intuitive

The practice of medicine as traditionally defined is undergoing an exciting transformation. Through modern technology and research, many ancient concepts are being validated. No longer are those involved in the health and healing modalities able to ignore the effectiveness of ancient therapeutic and diagnostic tools, nor are they able to deny the presence of the subtle energy body. The use of intuitive diagnosis is re-emerging as a complementary method of identifying illness. Intuitive diagnosis works with the human energy system for the purpose of identifying imbalances and malfunctions in the physical body.[203]

The human energy system (the aura) is in actuality an extended sensory system that is an integral part of the communication network connecting the mind and the body.[204] It is electromagnetic in nature and acts as an antenna that is sensitive to both internal and external stimuli. The primary function of this energy system is to receive, interpret, transmit, and store information. It is rich in both biographical and biological information. Biographically, its electromagnetic interpretation instructs the cellular structure of the body, through an electrochemical dialogue, to store all emotional reactions of our thoughts and experiences. Biologically, it directly reflects the DNA structure and the state of all of body's major systems. The energy body, like the physical body, has predetermined communication pathways that instruct it in how to make known the state of health or lack of it in the physical body.[205]

The pathways of the energy body include the endocrine and chakra systems. In the physical body, the master glands of the endocrine system manufacture the major hormones that control the chemical production of the body and, as a result, the biochemical dialogue in our cellular structure.[206] The locations of the seven major endocrine glands are also the locations for the seven major spiritual centers of the body. These spiritual centers are called chakras. The chakras function at the etheric and subtle levels. Consequently, the chakra and endocrine systems pair up to act as energetic pathways (transducers) from the subtle level to the physical level.[207,208]

Persons who have developed their intuitive skills to the point that they can access the information found in the human energy system are called medical intuitives. The role of the medical intuitive is to read the body both energetically and physically and to link all the information together to provide a comprehensive analysis of a person's state of health and overall well-being. As a diagnostician, a medical intuitive looks at the physiological, psychological, and psychospiritual characteristics of the energy system. Through the use of intuition, a medical intuitive is able to analyze a person's energy for the following purposes:

- Identifying where energetic imbalances are occurring
- Determining the origin sites of the imbalances
- Clarifying what is triggering the imbalances, for example, emotional, psychological, or spiritual issues
- Identifying how these imbalances are affecting the physical body
- Analyzing all the parts of the body that are being affected
- Determining what needs to be done to restore energetic and physical balance
- The primary goal of this type of diagnostic process is to lead a person to self-knowledge and then to describe ways for that person to facilitate the healing process.

Medical intuitives can do the following:

- They can provide a comprehensive picture of what is creating the potential for illness because they work with all aspects of a person's well-being: physical, mental, emotional, and spiritual.
- They can offer insight into the deeper struggles in a person's life that are creating blockages.
- They can reveal what needs to be done to restore balance to a person's life.
- They can help the person connect with issues that are preventing her or him from having the life and health desired (Case Study 37-4).

Complementary Medical Teams of the Future. As we move forward in the twenty-first century, there appears to be an open-mindedness toward the integration of complementary healing modalities. Many major teaching institutions and hospitals are currently offering a complementary medical clinic with teams including physicians and alternative practitioners (medical intuitives being one). In essence, the combination of allopathic medicine and alternative medicine can be of great value to the patient for the following reasons:

1. Each practitioner brings particular expertise, skills, and training to the diagnostic and healing process. The physician and the healing practitioner work with the patient to restore balance and health to the physical body, and the medical intuitive assists in providing a more comprehensive assessment of the root cause of the illness.
2. Each practitioner has a way of gathering the necessary information to determine the cause of illness. The physician works with the standard medical history of the person, and the medical intuitive works with the person's beliefs and biographical history.
3. The physician works to heal the body, the medical intuitive assists to determine the origin of the

CASE STUDY 37-4 ■ MICHAEL

Michael, aged 56 years, is an example of how a medical intuitive assesses the energy body for the purpose of diagnosis.

ENERGY ANALYSIS

Michael shows overall depletion of the energy system. He has physical exhaustion and shows signs of chronic fatigue. There are electrical storms in the head area. Other signs are mental disarray, chemical imbalance in the brain, and damage to and malfunction of areas in the right side of the brain. There is very little energy activity on the right side of the brain. Energy flow in both arms is erratic, more so on the left side. He has tremors in both hands, but more so in the left hand. There is red energy protrusion in the area of the brain where the brain stem originates. This energy buildup is affecting motor skills, causing energy blockages in the upper spine, primarily the second, third, fourth, and fifth cervical vertebrae. There are signs of nerve degeneration. He has severe muscle tension in the shoulder area and midback. Auric colors indicate buildup of toxins and waste in muscle structure. He has signs of depression. Reddish-brown color as seen by the medical intuitive indicates the CNS is affected. Most of his energy is focused in the upper torso area. Lower extremities show little energy flow. He has poor circulation in the legs and feet. His weak sites are the chest, neck, upper shoulders (fourth and fifth chakras),[207] and specifically the cerebrospinal nervous system.

MEDICAL DIAGNOSIS

Michael was examined by an allopathic physician 4 months after the medical intuitive evaluation. The diagnosis was Parkinson's disease.

PSYCHOLOGICAL AND PSYCHOSPIRITUAL CAUSES

Michael showed extreme unwillingness to deal with change and an overwhelming need to control. He believed that if he did not have complete control of everything, his life would fall apart. He lacked belief in himself and had emotional issues pertaining to low self-esteem, a lack of drive, and lack of courage to go after what he wanted. He always felt he was not worthy of having what he had. Childhood experiences and the negative emotions he attached to them affected his self-worth. He believed that his life had no meaning or purpose. He lived with the belief that it was a mistake that he was ever born. His mother told him at a young age that she never wanted to have him. Michael had lived his life on the basis of the erroneous perception that he would never be loved or be worthy of getting what he desired.

There was a strong energy loss around his spiritual belief system. This was contradictory because Michael was raised in a structured and strict religious belief system that should have strengthened rather than disconnected him from his beliefs. Michael said that he felt that his God had abandoned him because he was an unwanted child.

The session revealed that Michael was afraid of change and that he never took the time to re-evaluate the beliefs that were limiting him. As a result, he was not able to get in touch with his insecurities. The struggle between his emotional and spiritual issues caused him to disconnect from himself. His life focus was more on existing than on discovering his true talents. It also represents a feeling of being alone and feeling unsafe in an uncaring world.

In clinical terms, the use of medical intuition as a diagnostic tool is effective when a multitude of illnesses are analyzed. Because medical intuitive diagnosis is not a treatment modality, it does not require repeated visits. Some clients do choose, however, to continue to work with a medical intuitive as a means of evaluating the progress of treatment processes.

---

malfunction, and the alternative practitioner works to heal both body and spirit.

4. When each practitioner's assessment is part of the evaluation and diagnostic process, then the treatment process can be potentially accelerated because the recommended approaches will treat both cause and effect.

Thomas Edison stated, "The doctor of the future will give no medicine, but will interest his patients in the care of the human frame, in diet, and in the cause and prevention of disease."[209]

Medical Intuitive Diagnostics as a Profession. Medical intuition as a profession is in its infancy in terms of its acceptability by allopathic medicine. There is not, at the time of this writing, a national organization with a referral listing base of medical intuitives. It was not until the late 1990s that the use of medical intuition came into awareness and the medical profession began to use these services.

There are currently educational programs being developed that will teach medical intuitive diagnostics.

Physical Body Systems Approaches

Craniosacral Therapy

John Upledger, DO
Mary Lou Galantino, PT, PhD, MSCE

Introduction. Craniosacral therapy (CST) is a gentle, noninvasive, yet powerful and effective treatment approach that relies primarily on hands-on evaluation and treatment. It focuses in the normalization of bodily functions that are either part of or related to a semiclosed hydraulic physiological system, which has been named the craniosacral system.

Structure of the Craniosacral System. The anatomy of the craniosacral system includes a water-tight compartment formed by the dura mater, the cerebrospinal fluid

(CSF) within this compartment, the inflow and outflow systems that regulate the quantity and pressure of the bones to which the dura mater attaches, the joints or sutures that interconnect these bones, and other bones not anatomically connected to the dura mater. The bones of the cranium and the second and third cervical vertebrae, the sacrum, and the coccyx are also included in the structures of the craniosacral system.[210,211] In combination with the message sent to the patient through the intentional touch of the therapist is the corrective work that is done on a basic physiological level by gentle hands-on manipulations applied both directly and indirectly to the craniosacral system. The semiclosed hydraulic system includes the dural sleeves, which invest the spinal nerve roots outside the vertebral canal as far as the intervertebral foramina, and the caudal end of the dural tube, which ultimately becomes the cauda equina and blends with the coccygeal periosteum. The fluid within the semiclosed hydraulic system is CSF. The inflow and outflow of CSF are regulated by the choroids plexuses within the brain's ventricular system and arachnoid granulation bodies, respectively. CSF outflow is not rhythmically interrupted, but its rate may be adjusted by intracranial membrane tension patterns, which are broadcast primarily by the falx cerebri and tentorium cerebelli to the anterior end of the straight venous sinus, where an aggregation of arachnoid granulation bodies is located. This concentration of arachnoid granulation bodies is known to affect venous backpressure, which has an effect on the rate of reabsorption of CSF into the blood-vascular system.[212-214]

Technique. The therapist, after mobilization bony restrictions, focuses on the correction of abnormal dural membrane restrictions, perceived CSF activities, and energy patterns and fluctuations as they relate to the craniosacral system. It is during this time that the patient often moves from a phase of being corrected and having obstacles removed to a phase of self-healing, with the therapist serving as a facilitator of the process. The tenets of CST include the concept that the dura mater within the vertebral canal (dural tube) has the freedom to glide up and down within that canal for a range of 0.5 to 2.0 cm. This movement is allowed by the slackness and directionality of the dural sleeves as they depart the dural tube and attach to the intertransverse foramina of the spinal column.[210]

A basic assumption in CST, as it has evolved, is that the patient's body contains the necessary information for the discovery of the cause of any health problem. The treatment relies primarily on hands-on evaluation and treatment. The hands-on contact is tender and supportive. It is accompanied by a sincere intention to assist the patient in any way that is possible. In short, the therapist serves primarily as a facilitator of the patient's own healing processes. The rapport that develops during the patient-therapist interaction lends itself powerfully to the positive therapeutic effect that many patients experience.

Western medicine imparts a therapeutic modality for curative measures, whereas CST fosters facilitation, wherein the client directs the treatment session. The inherent participation of the patient through CST promotes a holistic approach to healing. Conventional medical diagnosis will usually be more closely related to what the therapist views as the result rather than the cause. For example, the therapist would search for a cause of strabismus within the intracranial membrane system and the motor control system of the eyes, rather than considering the strabismus as a diagnosed condition to be corrected by surgery. The cause of strabismus can be found as an abnormal tension pattern in the tentorium cerebelli. The therapist then searches for the cause of the abnormal tentorial tension pattern. Quite often, these tension patterns are referred from the occiput or from the low back or the pelvis. If this is the case, the CST "diagnosis" would be intracranial membranous strain of the tentorium cerebelli as a result of occiput or low back or pelvic dysfunction, individually or severally, resulting in secondary motor dysfunction of the eyes (strabismus). The therapist would focus on the sacrum, the pelvis, the occiput, and then the tentorium cerebelli. Correct evaluation and treatment would be signified by a "spontaneous correction" of the strabismus.

Somatoemotional release is a technique that involves the bodily, and usually conscious, reexperiencing of episodes, the energies for which have been stored in the totality of body tissues. A powerful emotional content is typically connected with this technique and it has proved to be extremely effective in cases of severe posttraumatic stress disorder. It was tested through qualitative research with a group of six Vietnam veterans in 1993. It proved to be successful in all six of these patients.[210,211,215,216]

Outcomes. Objective responses to CST are based on the removal of obstructions to smooth and easy physiological motions of the patient's body, the absence of energy cysts, the free movement of the dural tube in the spinal/vertebral canal and the rate and quality of the craniosacral rhythm, the absence of pressing responses during the somatoemotional release process, and statements from the deeper levels of consciousness through dialogue with various images encountered in the session that "all is well."[210,211,215]

Subjectively, clients report an increased sense of well-being, improved sleep patterns, reduced manifestation of stress, reduction or disappearance of pain, increased energy levels, and fewer episodes of transitory illness. How long it takes to achieve these results is extremely variable and dependent on the complexity of the layers of adaptation, the defense mechanism, and the level of spiritual evolution of the patient.

Use in Treatment Intervention. CST is useful as a primary treatment modality and as an adjunct to a wide variety of visceral dysfunctions. It works well to balance autonomic function, specifically reducing sympathetic nervous tonus. It has proved beneficial in chronic headache problems, temporomandibular joint problems, whiplash sequelae, and chronic pain syndromes. We have used it as an intensive treatment for persons rehabilitating from head injuries, craniotomies, spinal cord injuries, poststroke syndromes, transient ischemic attacks, seizure disorders, and a wide variety of rare brain and spinal cord dysfunctions.[217-219a] Little positive effect has been reported in amyotrophic lateral sclerosis. However, there has been some remarkable success seen in multiple sclerosis.[219]

In children, CST has been used extensively and effectively in a high percentage of persons with spastic cerebral palsy, seizure disorders, Down syndrome, and a wide variety of motor system disorders, including problems with the oculomotor system, learning disabilities, attention deficit disorder, speech problems, childhood allergies, and autonomic dysfunction.[220-222]

We have used CST for people living with HIV disease who have HIV-related peripheral neuropathy and other chronic musculoskeletal and neurological problems. Pain management techniques can be used by the therapist and also taught to the family members to implement for a home program.[223] Future studies addressing the interaction of the immune system with the craniosacral system would be helpful in elucidating the neuroendocrine response to this technique.

The latest research includes using CST along with other osteopathic techniques to treat chronic lateral epicondylitis as opposed to treating it with traditional orthopedic techniques. The results revealed increased strength and decreased pain for both osteopathic and orthopedic groups. The assumption is that osteopathic techniques such as CST can be successful in treating chronic lateral epicondylitis[224]; however, future studies will need to isolate CST to ultimately reveal its efficacy in treatment for this problem.

To date, there are several studies refuting the value of CST. One example is the Review of Alternative Medicine. According to this group of researchers, interexaminer reliability among CST practitioners is zero.[225] Other studies suggest that the sutures in which CST practitioners are attempting to mobilize are fused in the adult population and are therefore ineffective.[226-230] For CST to achieve recognition as a valid and reliable treatment option, future studies are necessary.

Training. The prerequisites for training in CST by the Upledger Institute, Inc, are quite simple. It is believed that any kind of therapist who has a license to see and treat patients/clients might find CST, in its more basic form, a useful adjunct to practice. Therefore a license as a health care practitioner is all that is required to enroll in the Upledger Institute's CST seminar series.

There are six levels of training within the series that are required before one can enroll in the advanced-level workshops. The workshops are all 4 or 5 days in length and are about evenly divided between academic work and hands-on supervised practice. The training program is designed to develop the sense of touch, motion, and energy perception slightly before the academic material is presented. A certification process started in 1995 is now in place.

There is a newly formed International Association of Healthcare Practitioners of which the American Cranio-Sacral Therapy Association is a subdivision. The American CranioSacral Therapy Association, a nonprofit organization, was founded by a group of therapists and concerned laypersons in 1994. Its stated objectives are to bring CST into public awareness, to enhance networking between practitioners who use CST to develop a certification program that will result in the recognition of CST as a specialty for persons who are licensed as health care practitioners in other fields, and to ultimately develop CST as an independently licensed and free-standing profession.

Reimbursement by third-party carriers is done largely on a case-by-case basis. A few insurance companies have recognized CST, but there is much work to be done on this front. The Upledger Institute published a book listing all the practitioners who have completed training. It is available to all health care professionals.

Myofascial Release (Barnes Method)

Carol M. Davis, PT, EdD, MS, FAPTA

Myofascial release is a manual energetic therapy designed to treat the fascia that surrounds every cell and tissue in the body. John Barnes, the physical therapist credited for developing this holistic treatment technique, has pointed out that it is a mistake to think of muscle as being a tissue in and of itself. Just as we now recognize that the mind and body cannot be separated, we also realize that there is no such entity as muscle; rather, the fascial-muscle unit is the more accurate anatomical and physiological entity. As Janet Travell[231] first described it, the fascia that surrounds each muscle fiber and fibril is inextricably interconnected with the muscle, and it is impossible to treat the muscle alone. Until the fascial barriers are released, the muscle, no matter how often stretched or contracted, will tend to resume its original shape. If that shape is distorted by a central or peripheral nervous system pathological condition, as is so often the case with our clients, or distorted from hypertonicity, if the muscle group has taken a postural position of ease from prolonged positioning or emotional protection, or if the fascia surrounding the cells of skin nearby is contorted from a surgical scar, then the muscle is not free to contract in the way it was created to function.

It is also important to point out that fascia has been referred to as the structural base of the "living matrix" of all cells in the body.[232] Fascia surrounds not only skin and muscle cells, but surrounds each and every cell in our bodies and even penetrates each cell as a cytoskeleton. In sum, the cellular matrix is connected with the extracellular matrix by way of fascia. Thus, as therapists when we touch the skin, "we contact a continuous interconnected webwork that extends throughout the body" (p. 47).[233]

The Physiology of the Fascial System. To understand how myofascial release is administered and why it seems to result in such positive outcomes to patients, it is necessary to understand the physiology of the fascial system. Fascia, as described previously, exists as a three-dimensional web surrounding all our cells, from the top of our head to the bottom of our feet. Functional biomechanical movements depend on intact, properly distributed fasciae.[233] There are three different types of fascia, but each is composed of a web of connective tissue of similar structure. The fascia just below the dermis is known as *superficial* fascia. The fascia that surrounds and fuses with bone, muscle, nerves, blood vessels, and organs is termed *deep* fascia. The third type of fascia is the *dura,* which surrounds the brain and spinal cord. All fascia is composed of collagen, elastin, and a ground substance of polysaccharide composition. It is the connective tissue that plays a largely unrecognized but vital role in holding the body together. Without fascia, the body could not remain intact and erect, supported by bones, joints, tendons, and ligaments alone. The fascia functions much like the stays of a tent, supporting the structure of the body and also facilitating metabolism and blood and lymph flow and separating organs and other structures from each other, down to the cellular level.[233]

Intervention. In contrast to traditional stretching of tissue, during myofascial release practitioners and their clients experience a sensation of softening, or melting similar to melting butter, or stretching, like pulling taffy under the palms of the therapist. Once tight tissue is located by palpation or observation, the slack is taken out of the tissue under the hands, and the therapist gently leans into his or her hands and waits for the tissue to respond. Within 90 to 120 seconds, the therapist's hands will sink deeper, and a feeling of flow results. The therapist then simply follows that twisting and deepening flow of tissue until it stops (indicating a fascial barrier), when she or he again waits, maintaining slight tension until the tissue begins to flow again, and the therapist can follow the fascia, as it flows or releases, to the next collagenous barrier. The collagen fibers seem to be rearranging themselves back to a position of alignment, or self-correction. Often an area of heat and redness under the release occurs, but curiously, at times an area of erythema occurs distant from the release itself.[234] It is hypothesized that the feeling of flow occurs when the polysaccharide ground substance of the fascia becomes more in solution, less gel-like, by way of a piezoelectric effect. Mechanical pressure from the therapist's hands is converted to chemical energy. Recent research has shown that "actin filaments and microtubules, . . . could function as conduits for the spread of biochemical agents" once they are mechanically stimulated. In other words, human cells were filmed instantly messaging each other by way of mechanical energy being transmitted to biochemical messages.[235]

The effect of myofascial release can be enhanced by prolonged, corrective positioning with use of postural wedges or therapeutic balls, or both, to sustain the appropriate pressure to release the fascia over time. For example, for a rotated pelvis, wedges will sustain a correcting derotation while the patient is lying supine or prone.[235] In addition, once fascia has been released, it is important to exercise muscles to strengthen resistance to the fascia tightening up once again in gravity.

The purpose of myofascial release is to lengthen the fascia that has been abnormally constricted, thus allowing a more efficient and effective contraction of muscles, a more barrier-free blood and lymph supply to nerves and organs, an upright posture that responds in a neutral way to the forces of gravity, and a body/mind that is in more in balance from a less-restricted flow of body energy, or chi. Myofascial release, along with soft tissue mobilization, therapeutic exercise, and movement reeducation is an excellent holistic therapeutic approach for musculoskeletal, neuromuscular, and integumentary disorders in function.

Myofascial Release Intervention. Myofascial release treatment consists of a thorough examination of the client, including an in-depth history of symptoms and a thorough musculoskeletal and neuromuscular examination, noting pain, impairments in strength, range of motion endurance, and any disorders in function. The client's posture and, specifically, the position of the pelvis are noted. In many people, the hips will appear uneven, palpation of the anterior superior iliac spines will reveal an iliac rotation, and many times there will be a leg length discrepancy associated with pelvic rotation. In the case of stroke, traumatic brain injury, or cerebral palsy, abnormal tone will have resulted in

fascia frozen along with their spastic muscles as a result of disorganized nerve conduction. No matter what the cause of the fascial tightening, the treatment remains to release the connective tissue, the fascia. This is done with manual releases, soft tissue mobilization techniques, positioning on wedges, facilitating whole-body release (unwinding or somatoemotional release), craniosacral techniques, and a technique called "rebounding." The technique of rebounding, which is especially useful with CNS pathological conditions, involves a passive rocking of tissue, exploiting the hydrophilic aspect of tissue to the maximum. As the therapist rhythmically rocks chest, legs, thorax, or arms, the tissue reverberates with the rhythm of the motion, often resulting in a spontaneous release of tense and hypertonic tissue. Patients respond positively to this technique.

The actual techniques of myofascial release, a holistic complementary therapy, may at first appear to be exactly like mechanical manual therapies, but soon the novice recognizes the need to quiet the mind and body, learns to wait and feel gently with an enhanced proprioceptive sense for the tissue to "move up into the hands," and then gently to follow it as it twists and turns. It is an art that is greatly enhanced by a calm and centered proprioceptive listening that is not linear or mechanical in nature but energetic and holistic.[236] Palpating for the cranial rhythm takes the same centered, quiet "listening with one's hands." Eventually, we learn to feel with the whole self.[237]

Models of Health Care Belief Systems
Traditional Acupuncture
Jeffery Kauffman, MD, Certified Acupuncturist

Introduction. It has been gratifying to see Western medicine, as it is practiced by allopathic physicians, come around to include many of the holistic practices that were once considered quackery. This is happening with chiropractic, massage, and other forms of body work; nutrition and diet; and exercise practices such as hatha yoga and tai chi, and so on. A research study designed by David Eisenberg of Harvard Medical School, published in the *New England Journal of Medicine* in 1993 and again in 1998,[238,239] showed just how extensive alternative or holistic practices are and how a large percentage of patients are using these practices, with or without knowledge of their personal physicians. Alternative health therapeutic modes are on the rise, are being used by more and more of the general population of the United States, and are being more and more accepted by Western medical practitioners. Many medical schools now have courses teaching alternative healing practices to medical students.

The question arises as to why people are drawn to therapeutic approaches outside the medical sphere. The answer is relatively straightforward. They are not getting everything they need in health care from traditional allopathic, Western-trained medical doctors. People are looking for something that works better. More and more people are disenchanted by the lack of compassion of a large percentage of the medical profession. This involves the patient being approached by the physician as a disease rather than a person, as a gallbladder case or a case of appendicitis or chronic fatigue instead of Sherri Jackson or Marvin Jones. This involves the hurried 5- to 10-minute visits created and encouraged by health maintenance organizations. It involves the use of pharmaceuticals over the use of any other therapeutic modality. The side effects of such medications add to the problem. Along with the decrease in or lack of compassion comes the inability of many physicians to develop rapport with their patients.

There is one other important principle that separates allopathic medicine as it is practiced in the United States from holistic healing, and that is the attention paid to the symptoms. Allopathic medicine traditionally treats the symptoms. In fact, the diagnosis is usually the symptom with the name changed to something that has "-itis" on it at the end as a suffix. For example, *arthritis* means inflammation of the joints, *appendicitis* means inflammation of the appendix, and *iritis* means inflammation of the iris. Tension headache or migraine headache is simply a headache. It means an ache or pain in the head. Western medicine is essentially treating the symptoms, most commonly with drugs. Even the medications are named after the symptoms for example, antiinflammatories, antihypertensives, antimetabolites, antacids, antiarrhythmic agents, and diuretics (to increase output of fluid through the urine).

On the other hand, holistic healing is aimed at determining the cause of the disease (even the Western medical term *disease* means dis-ease or lack of ease). In determining the cause of disease, one looks for the underlying imbalances that all human beings have. None of us is born with a perfect body-mind that never breaks down. We all have an underlying imbalance or constitutional imbalance that is the weak or vulnerable area of our body-mind that will always be the first to show symptoms and illness when under pressure or stress.

The pressure or stress coming from the outside world, outside of our body, can be in the form of physical agents like physical trauma (accidents), which cause bruised tissues, strained or torn ligaments, or broken bones, toxic agents from the environment, such as poison or chemicals in the water or foods or air, carcinogens from contaminants, or poor nutrition and poor diet, not taking in enough nutrients or taking in too much of a particular kind. There are also external causes that are related to weather, such as excessive exposure to heat or cold or humidity or dryness or wind or dampness, being struck by lightning, or near drowning. Then there are the much more common causes of illness that come from the inside. These would be in the mental or emotional spheres. Generally, it is an emotion that is in excess or deficient in the person's life, such as too much fear or not enough, too much grief or not enough expression of grief, too much anger or not enough, too much joy (that's right, too much joy or inappropriate joy) or not enough, too much sympathy or not enough. Feelings and emotions that are in excess or in deficient states affect particular organs that, in turn, can cause imbalance, symptoms, and disease in a particular organ, which then manifests as a heart attack or arthritis or constipation or cancer, and so on. This occurs with our thoughts as well, where we can focus to excess on particular negative thoughts that then create imbalance, illness, and disease.

There is also the most important sphere for all human beings, which is the spirit, and there can be, and often are, imbalances in this realm that have everything to do with not recognizing one's true value, which means not acknowledging the spirit that lives inside each and every human being. When one is aware of the spiritual energy inside and focuses on it daily, then that person knows and experiences the infinite energy of spirit whose nature is bliss. Unfortunately, most human beings have lost sight of this and consequently are suffering deep inside because of a lack of recognition of self-worth or self-esteem. This, in turn, causes physical or mental disease.

There are also genetic causes of disease that are not adequately addressed. Generally, this is rather a cross that the person must bear and balancing of the body, mind, and spirit integration still helps that person lead an enjoyable and valuable life. Imbalances can also come from excess or deficiencies of other things such as too much work or not enough, too much exercise or not enough, too much sex (or not enough?), too much food or not enough. These are usually related to underlying emotional imbalances as well. Holistic modes of therapy address either these external causes or the internal causes, or preferably both.

Once alternative health practices are well entrenched in medical training in medical colleges, their efficacy could be proved easily over a 5-year period by simply measuring monies spent on pharmaceuticals and the quantities of pharmaceuticals used before, during, and after holistic programs are introduced. This would also include measuring and comparing outpatient visits to physicians, visits to emergency departments, hospital admissions, need for surgery, and some kind of standard for measuring quality of life. Some of these categories have already been proved in research studies done by Herbert Benson, MD,[240] noting the effect on patients using his relaxation response (a form of meditation) on a daily basis for 3 years.

History. Acupuncture as it is practiced in the United States is a huge conglomerate of different styles of acupuncture coming from China, Japan, Korea, Thailand, Vietnam, and Western Europe. The styles differ radically depending on who is doing the acupuncture, where he or she learned it, and how much of individuality has been instilled into the practice. Within this discussion, the similarities between practices are described, followed by an in-depth analysis of the style that I use.

Acupuncture is one of the five categories that make up Chinese medicine. The other four are herbal medicine, diet and nutrition, exercise, and massage. Acupuncture is a healing method that tunes a human being. Just as a piano tuner tunes a piano or one tunes a guitar or an auto mechanic does a tuneup on your car, it is possible to tune a human being. After this process, or intervention, is done, the body-mind functions more efficiently in a balanced, harmonious fashion. As a result, the aches and pains often are eliminated and illnesses and diseases reversed. Acupuncture can be used by itself and, even better, in combination with other holistic and traditional Western medical methods.

Methods. Acupuncture involves the use of tiny needles made of stainless steel, their diameter two or three times the width of a human hair, sharpened by a diamond. These needles are put into particular points on the surface of the body. There are at least a thousand of these points all over the human body. They have a lower electrical potential compared with the surrounding skin, as is evidenced by a galvanometer. These points are also known as acupuncture points, acupressure points, trigger points, and perhaps by other names as well. These points are about 1 mm in diameter and are located pretty much in the same place for everyone, according to bony landmarks, skin landmarks, anatomical structures such as nipples, umbilicus, fingernails and toenails, eyes, ears, nose and mouth, and so on. The points can be found easily by the trained finger. There are electrical instruments that can help locate these points but their reliability has not been established. Needles are put into these acupuncture points, and after being inserted, the needles are turned either clockwise or counterclockwise one revolution. They are either taken out immediately or left in for a period of time, depending on the individual patient's imbalance and illness.

Examination and Evaluation. Deciding where to insert the needles is really the key and the most difficult and important part of acupuncture diagnosis. This is where styles of acupuncture come into play. There is a spectrum of acupuncture styles or methods that ranges from completely symptomatic to perfectly holistic, just as there is in traditional Western medicine. The symptomatic methods are simply putting needles into acupuncture points at anatomical sites that are specifically related to symptoms. For example, for shoulder pain, or arthritis or bursitis, an acupuncturist using a symptomatic method would select acupuncture points that are in or around the shoulder area. Headache would be treated with needles in the head area. Constipation would be treated with needles in the belly area. Hemorrhoids would be treated with needles around the anus and coccygeal area. This method pays little attention to where the constitutional imbalance exists within each person. An opposite philosophy, which is called holistic acupuncture, treats the underlying constitutional imbalance within the person. Described earlier, these are considered the vulnerable, or weak, links in the chain in each human being, that part that always gives out first because it is not as strong or disease resistant as the rest of the body-mind. The type of acupuncture I use is a holistic form. Specifically, it is called five-element acupuncture. It is based on the Law of Five Elements, which is a law of nature that comes from Chinese philosophy and is one of the basic foundations of Chinese medicine. It is sometimes known as the Five Phases and is considered the most holistic form of acupuncture available.

The Law of Five Elements. The Law of Five Elements states that there are five elements in nature (fire, earth, metal, water, and wood) and that these elements all relate to one another in a particular fashion (Figure 37-8). The diagram in Figure 37-8 shows an outer creative cycle (known as Shen) that goes in a clockwise fashion and demonstrates that fire creates earth, earth creates metal, metal creates water, water creates wood, and wood creates fire again. Also, a star-shaped control, or destructive cycle (known as K'o) shows that fire destroys or controls metal, metal does the same to wood, wood to earth, earth to water, and water to fire. These two cycles, the creative and destructive cycles, are necessary to keep balance in nature. These five elements are also found in human beings because the body is composed of elements that come from nature and return to nature when the body dies. The emotions and feelings in our per-

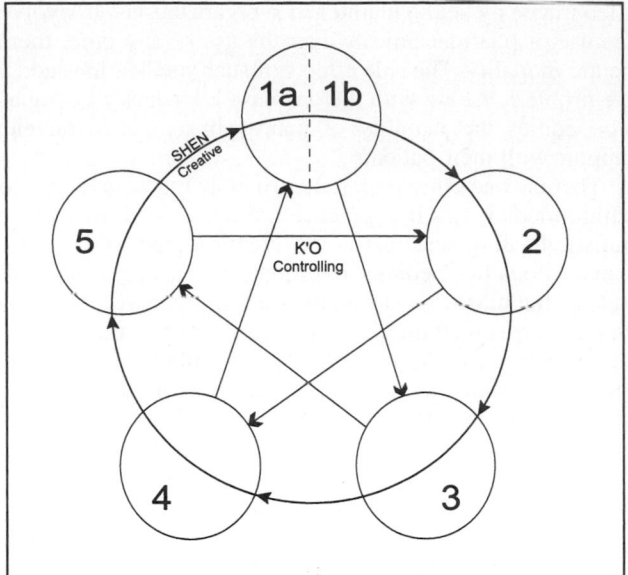

FIGURE 37-8 ■ Law of five elements: demonstrating the Shen (creative) and K'o (controlling) cycles.

	1a	1b	2	3	4	5
Element	Fire		Earth	Metal	Water	Wood
Meridian / Organ	Small Intestine	Three Heater	Stomach	Colon	Bladder	Gall Bladder
	Heart	Heart Protector	Spleen	Lung	Kidney	Liver
Color	Red		Yellow	White	Blue	Green
Emotion	Joy		Sympathy	Grief	Fear	Anger
Odor	Scorched		Fragrant	Rotten	Putrid	Rancid
Sound	Laughing		Singing	Weeping	Groaning	Shouting

FIGURE 37-9 ■ Law of five elements linking fire, earth, metal, water, and wood with interlocking variables.

sonality align themselves with these same elements (Figure 37-9).

People in Western society have not been taught to think of their bodies in elemental forms, but nevertheless these elements are there. The concept of fire is present in each and every cell. The cells burn glucose to survive and this is referred to as "burning calories." It is this burning that causes our body temperature to remain at 98.6° F throughout most of our lives. It is not difficult to picture each cell of the body having a little bonfire in the center with mitochondria sitting around roasting pieces of glucose on a stick. Obviously, water is present in our bodies. Students in grammar school are taught that our bodies are 98% water with all the tears and urine and lymph and blood. Similarly, metal can be found in the body in the form of calcium in the bones and iron in the blood, in our teeth, and so on. The concept of wood is most easily seen in the fingernails and toenails, which are similar to the bark of a tree. Also, the ligaments and tendons are much like a strong fiber. The concept of earth is best seen in the gastrointestinal tract. Picture taking a microscopic journey down the gastrointestinal tract starting from the mouth, going down the esophagus into the stomach and the intestines; the further down you get, the more the material seems earthlike, until it is excreted into the outside world.

Each of the elements has a particular color that emanates from the facies, a particular emotion that comes from the personality, a particular odor that comes from the body, and a particular sound that comes from the voice, as well as a particular taste, season, climate, secretion, and body part or system that it fortifies.

Every human being has a constitutional imbalance in one of these elements. The explanation for how this happens lies in spiritual law. Suffice it to say that this imbalance is well engrained some time during the first 5 years of life. Diagnosing this constitutional imbalance is both an art and a science and is done primarily by determining the color, emotion, odor, and sound belonging to each human being. The reader probably has noticed these colors, emotions, odors, and sounds previously with friends or even with strangers. Yet the realization that these are diagnostic clues that reveal a person's constitutional imbalance may not be as self-evident. The person who is always angry, no matter what, is displaying the emotion that goes with the wood element. The person who is always happy, joyful, bubbling over goes with the element of fire. The person who is always sympathetic and loves to take care of you or is always caring for children is displaying the emotion of sympathy and that goes with earth. The person who is always grieving, has tremendous loss and cannot seem to get over it, goes with the element of metal. And the person who is always fearful, paranoid, and afraid of life fits into the water element. People have different sounds to their voice. People who laugh excessively and are always humorous go with the fire element. People who shout a lot, their voices very powerful and strong, knocking you over, go with the wood element. People who have a singsong quality to their voice go with the earth element; groaning goes with the water element; and a weeping sound of the voice, although the person is not crying, goes with the metal element. You have probably smelled people who have a strong body odor and wondered why they didn't bathe or use deodorant. There are five different odors and each one belongs to one of these elements. And perhaps you have seen a person who is green with envy or ash white, white as a sheet, or has pallor in the face. Each one of these colors goes with an element as described in the diagram (see Figure 37-9).

Each element also has organs germane to it, with energetic pathways, called meridians, that are housed by that element. These pathways, or meridians, are just under the surface of the skin, throughout the body, and serve as channels for an electrical form of energy that flows in all human beings. This energy is the life force. In Chinese it is called chi. In the East Indian culture it is known as prana. This life force is always circulating round and round the body-mind along these pathways. And the acupuncturist can get in touch with this energy at certain points on these meridians, which are the acupuncture points.

Intervention. Once the examination is complete and the diagnosis is made, with the elemental constitutional imbalance determined, it is simply a matter of treating the points along the meridians that are housed by that element on a week-to-week basis. Generally, this tunes the human

being and everything starts to function more efficiently and more harmoniously, enhancing the person's quality of life.

There are 12 major meridians, two in each element, except for fire, which has four. Each of these meridians is named after the organ that it is connected to, which is also described in the diagram. Each meridian has from 9 to 67 points on it. Each point has a name described by the Chinese that has been translated into English. It is the names and the functions of the different points that allow the acupuncturist to decide which points are to be used on which day and time and treatment. Taking the history at each visit, and determining blockage of the chi energy flowing in the meridians, is used as well to select the points used in treatment.

As patients get better, not only do their symptoms decrease in intensity and dissolve and often totally disappear with time, their emotional and feeling states also change for the better. People tend to become more happy and peaceful and calm, more able to handle stress. They often will say, "I feel better in myself." The reason for this is that the patient is not just having her or his symptoms treated. This form of acupuncture, the five-element style, treats the body, the mind, and the spirit and integrates these three spheres of the human being. The point names are particularly revealing. There are names connected to nature and physical objects such as "small sea," "greater mountain stream," "blazing valley," "sea of chi," and "skull breathing." There are also point names that have to do with emotions and feelings, such as "palace of weariness," "gate of hope," "rushing the frontier gate," "intermediary," "little merchant," and "abdominal sorrow." And then there are the points that relate to the spiritual qualities of life, such as "spirit burial ground," "heavenly ancestor," "heavenly pond," "heavenly window," "gate of destiny," "inner frontier gate," "soul door," and "spirit deficiency." When these spirit points are used, the person's spirit is buoyed up, turns back on.

Each treatment lasts 15 to 60 minutes, depending on the individual practitioner. The practitioner can also include any of the following in the treatment sessions: conversation, history taking, massage, joint adjustments, instructions on diet and nutrition, psychosocial counseling, exercise recommendations, and so on. The initial visit takes longer because a history and physical examination are done and sometimes the initial treatment as well. This depends on the technique and abilities of the practitioner. Generally, the treatments are done twice a week for the first two to four visits and then once a week as the patient starts to get better. The interval continues to lengthen to every 2 to 4 weeks and, as the patient improves, the optimal interval is once every 3 months or once every season, the patient coming in for a tuneup for maintenance and prevention. Generally, a series of 10 treatments is a good way to start this type of therapy. Improvement in the patient's condition may be noticed as soon as the first treatment is done. It may take 5 or 10 treatments before it is noticed by the patient. Depending on the ability of the practitioner, improvement in the patient's condition generally occurs in 80% to 90% of patients. This, of course, also depends on the severity of the patient's imbalance and illness.

When acupuncture treatment is combined with psychosocial counseling, nutritional advice, exercise instruction, massage, or other forms of body work, in which the person is touched with warmth, peace, and love by another human being, great healing can take place.

Benefits of Intervention. Five-element acupuncture can be used for all sorts of clinical problems: physical, mental, emotional, and spiritual. Any and every type of person can and does respond. There are always exceptions to this, but the general rule is one of success. This includes acute problems and chronic problems, outpatients and hospitalized patients. In China, all patients with stroke are automatically treated with acupuncture as well as the more traditional Western methods. It works on babies, toddlers, adolescents, and the elderly. It can be used as a primary form of therapy to which other therapies are added or it can be an adjunct to surgery, radiation, and medication, or to other holistic therapies.

Future Treatments. The amount of time it takes for a person to heal depends on how long the person has been been ill. A rule of thumb is that for every year a person has had a particular physical or mental problem, it is going to take about a month's worth of treatment, with each session done weekly. So, if a person has had arthritis for 20 years, 20 months of treatment should be expected.

On the other hand, if symptoms have been present for only a month or two, it is possible that they could go away with one or two treatments unless it is some kind of serious illness, such as the sudden onset of cancer or heart disease or something that has been present for 1 or 2 years but has been subclinical. The general average is 10 treatments over a 4- to 8-week period, with a good possibility of illness being relieved partially or almost completely during that period, depending on the severity.

Summary. In summary, acupuncture is a healing therapy that is both an art and a science, that comes from the Orient, specifically starting in China approximately 4500 years ago. There are many styles of acupuncture, and the most holistic style is known as five-element acupuncture. It truly helps to integrate the body, mind, and spirit. When acupuncture is combined with teaching the patient how to live a more healthy lifestyle, including diet, reducing stress, making healthy choices, thinking healthy thoughts, and including fun and relaxation, true healing can occur. Because of the chronic and degenerative nature of many illnesses in the United States, it is possible that total healing would not occur. Nevertheless, this type of therapy, along with the adjuncts mentioned earlier, should definitely help to create a more healthy human being.

American Indian Healing Traditions of North and South America

Richard Voss, DPC, MSW

American Indians are understandably wary of the written word. Some may criticize the inclusion of this section in this chapter. This criticism is understandable because the written word objectifies understandings out of the cultural context and can be manipulated outside the relationship in which the understanding was shared. However, not to include a discussion of American Indian views about medicine and health care is also a concern because it perpetuates the invisibility of American Indian peoples. The purpose here is to honor the continuing journey of understanding between medical science practitioners and traditional American Indian medicine practitioners to see how these two medicine paths can help restore health to the people and to bring about increased understanding—*wo 'wableza*—among peoples.

Contemporary American Indian Health Care and Traditional Healing: North and South American Indian/Indigenous Perspectives. In a report to the National Institutes of Health, *Alternative Medicine: Expanding Medical Horizons,*[241] the Lakota (a Sioux people) were cited for the use of healing ceremonies by specialists who are essentially shamanic in their approach to treatment. To understand American Indian medicine ways, one cannot rely solely on written accounts. Although written ethnographical studies may provide a wealth of descriptive data, it is best to talk to authoritative sources personally. Professionals interested in learning more about traditional approaches to help and healing should contact any one of the federally recognized tribal headquarters and the tribally sponsored American Indian colleges and universities for more specific information. Many colleges conduct summer courses on Lakota culture and philosophy that are open to non–American Indians, as well as American Indians, interested in learning the culture. This information may be found on the Internet under tribal colleges and federally recognized tribes.

Today, many of the old American Indian healing traditions are experiencing a renaissance and are beginning to be viewed with a renewed sense of respect and credibility as an alternative and complement to more invasive or secular Western medical models of treatment.[241-247] For example, on the Cheyenne River Sioux Indian Reservation at Eagle Butte, South Dakota, the tribe has incorporated traditional methods and approaches in its alcohol treatment programs and delinquency prevention programs, and other youth programs where such problems are viewed in the context of historical trauma with important social, emotional, physical, and spiritual dimensions.[243,244,246,247] These traditional methods include the *inipi*, or purification ceremony (popularly called the "sweat lodge"), the *hanblecaya*, or pipe fast (often called the "vision quest"), and the *wiwang wacipi*, or the Sundance. The inclusion of these ceremonies within the treatment process has collectively been called the "Red Road approach."[243,244,247]

A number of medical facilities on various reservations include medicine men as consultants on a formal and informal basis,[247-250] and the use of traditional ceremonies in health care settings is encouraged and respected.[251] Where the ceremonial burning of sage (a common medicinal herb burned for purification) had been discouraged in the past, hospital staff report increased acceptance of this practice and now arrange appropriate space for traditional ceremonial practices both within the health care facility and outside on hospital grounds.[250-252] One Lakota friend commented on his recent hospitalization at an allopathic hospital. He was visited by a medicine man who placed a bundle of sage under his pillow. This made him feel better and showed how simple cooperation among allopathic medicine, health care practices, and alternative, complementary health care practices can be.

A Lakotacentric Perspective on Health. A traditional American Indian perspective on health care and medicine begins with the spiritual reality of the human being who is part of all creation and dependent on creation. Traditional understanding views human beings as intimately related to plants and all other creations in the natural world that sustain life. Reality is not linear, it is circular. Everything is connected to everything else. Good and bad, sickness and health, physician and patient are not separate processes, they are all related aspects and part of the whole. For the Lakotas and other traditional American Indian peoples there is no split or dualism in reality or creation. This traditional view challenges the intervention model and offers a prevention model as the starting place for social health and assistance. The emphasis from a Lakotacentric view is on building up the immune system and seeing the important role of the community in promoting good health care and well-being, a cultural emphasis often overlooked in conventional health care practices.

Traditional Lakota values of health and well-being emphasize the participation of the family in the healing process, including the extended family and the larger kinship community, to bring about good health to the individual. The health of the individual is connected to the health of the community, so there is an important tribal dimension to this understanding. For traditional Lakota people the help and healing process in not impersonal but highly personalized and individualized around specific needs. The roles of medicine practitioners are multidimensional and include those of healer, counselor, politician, and priest.

Another important contribution of the Native American perspective on health is that it provides a rich topology of spirit. The human creation, like all creations, is a spirit being composed of multilayered aspects of spirit. "Spirit" here is not some supernatural reality outside the human being but an intrinsic dimension of everything that is, including the human creation (person). To speak of human beings is to speak of spiritual reality. For traditional American Indians, medical treatment or any kind of social, human, or mental health service is first and foremost a spiritual endeavor.

Traditional Indian peoples of South America have similar and yet distinctive traditions of help and healing where the rain forest provides the pharmacopoeia of medicinal plants, bark, herbs, and vines. Of course, the forest itself is viewed as a powerful source of spiritual healing. During a recent field study to the Tambopata River area of the southeastern Peruvian Amazon (through the Amazon Center for Environmental Education and Research), I had an opportunity to meet with various shamans, their patients, and public health care representatives at a local community center where the regional public school and health care station are located. Interestingly, the entire health care staff all rotate, making visits to the area community members, including both indigenous traditional people, who mainly live dispersed through the forest (Amazon) and mestizo or mixed-blood settlers, many of whose families have lived in the river settlements since the mid-1970s.[253] Both indigenous natives and mestizo settlers seek assistance from the shaman, the curanderos, and the health station outpost, staffed by nurses and a visiting physician. The South American indigenous community I visited in the Tambopata River region of the southeast Peruvian Amazon used both herbal remedies and spirit-calling ceremonies, often incorporating the use of forest tobacco and other vegetation gathered from the forest as a means of purification. The use of *ayahuasca,* a concoction or tea made from various plants, tree bark, and vines gathered from the forest, is administered to both patient and shaman and is a common shamanic practice throughout Amazonia, according to the shamans I interviewed.[253] A detailed description of an *ayahuasca* ceremony is reported by Salak,[254] providing a fascinating participant observer's experience of an *ayahuasca* ceremony. A brief audio-video capture of the beginning of an *ayahuasca* ceremony may be viewed at www.nationalgeographic.com/adventure. Clinical applications of *ayahuasca* are being studied by Jacques Mabit, Director del Centro de Rehabilitacion de Toxicomanos (Rehabilitation and Detoxification Center) at the Takiwasi Center, Peru. Riba et al[255] (2004) have published their neuropsychobiology study on the effects of ayahuasca, so traditional medicine has captured both the imagination and the attention of medical science.

It is time for the diverse medical and health care disciplines to learn more about American Indian ways of healing and health from both North and South American Indian/indigenous peoples. The benefits of this cross-cultural collaboration affect not only American Indian people but everyone in the larger culture as well who will benefit from greater access to a more holistic health care model that recognizes the physiological and the spiritual causes of disease and sickness, as well as the efficacy of biological and spiritual remedies.

Allopathic Links to Models of Health Care Belief Systems

Electroacupuncture

Mary Lou Galantino, PT, PhD, MSCE

Acupuncture, a part of traditional Chinese medicine, has been used for more than 4500 years. Mapping of 12 meridian points, which are named primarily after the visceral organs they transverse, incorporates 361 regular points. There are also "Ashi points," which are typically tender points that are used for treatment of pain syndromes.[256] The acupuncturist must make a decision as to which acupuncture points to stimulate on the basis of a specific diagnosis. The goal is to balance chi, which is considered vital energy. If there is an imbalance caused by disease, the altered flow of chi can be detected and subsequently treated through needles or electric stimulation over specific acupuncture points.

The use of acupuncture is growing in popularity in most Western countries,[257] and the effectiveness of electroacupuncture as a modality for the treatment of pain has been shown by significant decreases in visual analog scale scores.[258] The therapeutic effects of acupuncture have generally been for the treatment of pain; with the increasing acceptance of acupuncture as an effective modality for pain relief, the scope of research on this modality has widened considerably to include other health care conditions. The intensive research efforts on other therapeutic effects of acupuncture have produced encouraging results.[259-261] These results point to a reduction in pain, improvement in motor function, better balance, improved gait; the results therefore have a neurophysiological interpretation. The effect of spasticity has been explored by researchers for multiple diagnoses such as spinal cord injury and stroke. Electroacupuncture has been found to have more of an effect on spasticity the earlier treatment is implemented, ideally within 3 weeks of injury. Findings reveal positive short- and long-term effects[262-264]; however, future research needs to include frequency of treatment and specific points of stimulation for a more comprehensive understanding. Some of the possible mechanisms by which acupuncture may affect motor function include the following:

1. A stimulation of the release of endogenous opoids.[265]
2. Changing the amplitude of end plate potential and thus facilitating the events at the neuromuscular junctions. It has been suggested that peripheral factors contributing to the potentiation of a reflex (e.g., the H reflex) may affect the afferents and the neuromuscular junction.[266]
3. Stimulation of the sensory system will result in integrative actions at the spinal cord level where acupuncture may facilitate the stretch reflex arc through both the gamma and alpha motor neurons. Facilitation may depend on the intensity and timing of the stimuli used to activate muscle afferents.[267]
4. Neuroimaging of acupuncture in patients with chronic pain reveals changes in cerebral blood flow associated with pain and acupuncture analgesia that correspond to areas of the brain involved in such phenomena.[267]

Training for acupuncture is varied throughout the United States. Because needling is considered an invasive technique, physical therapists are prohibited from using it. Therefore an alternative to needle acupuncture is noninvasive electroacupuncture. Concerning the effects of electrical neurostimulation, there are various interpretations of the methods and underlying physiological mechanisms. One mechanism is neural.[268] Another study indicated that electrical stimulation applied to acupuncture points may activate neurological and endocrine functions that control pain.[268] Anderson and Lundeberg's study supported the release of beta-endorphin and oxycotin, which are important for the control of pain and the regulation of blood pressure and body temperature.[268]

Research on the effects of electroacupuncture on HIV-related neuropathy found significant reduction in pain, which suggests an excitatory effect on the neuromuscular system. Such an effect may be on membrane potential (possibly through influencing ionic transport) and improvement in body fluid circulation.[269] The effect on the sympathetic system is often reported and more or less explained. The same explanation is proposed for the action of electrical stimulation on pain, with some effects on pain-mediating neurotransmitters at the level of the spinal cord and an endogenous modulation from the brain stem.[270]

Although there may be several mechanisms underlying the physiological mechanisms of electroacupuncture, it would be prudent for physical therapists to consider maximizing the benefits of electrical modalities in various musculoskeletal and neurological disorders.[271] One prospective study[272] investigated the physiological effects of stimulation of ST36 and ST39 with Dynatron 200 microcurrent. Hemodynamic functions and skin temperature were monitored, with no significant differences found. However, further research is necessary to elucidate the nature of physiological effects of specific surface electrodes and various types of stimulation to determine the efficacy of electroacupuncture treatment.

Biofeedback
Jennifer M. Bottomley, PT, MS, PhD

The suggestion that hemiplegia, migraine and tension headaches, asthma, hypertension, cardiac arrhythmias, torticollis spasms, pain, hyperkinesis, and functional disorders of any of the body's systems may be relieved by a single form of treatment sounds more like a nineteenth century pitch for snake oil than a true reflection of research. Yet biofeedback has been investigated extensively and has promising clinical applications in an astounding number of conditions.

The last two decades have seen an increasing convergence of body and mind therapies. These new therapies are often labeled psychosomatic or psychophysical medicine.[273] As both names imply, these approaches to healing deal with the effect of the mind on the body. With them, tremendous strides have been made in understanding mental influences on body systems ranging from the muscular to the immune system. This has led to treatment procedures that exploit this connection between mind and body. Biofeedback techniques for stress-related disorders and dysfunction and mental imaging using autogenic (a method of mind-over-body control based on a specific discipline for relaxing parts of the body by means of autosuggestion) feedback to enhance the responsiveness of the autonomic nervous system or the immune system response[274,275] are two good examples of this process. Biofeedback is one of the earliest and most accepted ways that rehabilitation professions have used that integrates rather than separates the mind and body.[276]

Biofeedback is a process of electronically using information from the body to teach an individual to recognize what is going on inside the own brain, nervous system, and muscles. Biofeedback refers to any technique, be it visual, auditory, or kinesthetic, that uses instrumentation to give a person immediate and continuing signals on changes in a bodily function that he or she is not usually conscious of, such as fluctuations in blood pressure, brain wave activity, or muscle tension. Theoretically, and often in practice, information input enables the individual to learn to control the "involuntary" function.

Biofeedback acts as an output-input system whereby output is based in the motor unit and the input is through sensory pathways comprising proprioceptors, exteroceptors, and interoceptors.[276] Biofeedback provides a means of measurement of a physiological response with an electronic device. It aids the sensory side of a feedback mechanism assisting a compensated sensation, as with a CVA or other brain injury, in responding appropriately (i.e., motor unit training) by increasing conscious awareness of intact, but usually unfelt, sensation. Basically, biofeedback acts as a sixth sense by providing an artificial proprioception feedback. By operant conditioning a new association between a stimulus and a response is developed. The action the learner takes is voluntary and under her or his own control. The response is instrumental in producing a reward or removing a negative stimulus, and this reinforcement shapes behavior and function with successive stages.

Biofeedback transfers the responsibility for final success to the patient. Often, individuals seek medical help, hoping to place the responsibility of "curing" their problems on the clinician, while the patient takes an almost passive role in the treatment process. This is commonly known as an external locus of control. Patients should understand that they have the ability, with assistance from the appropriate medical professionals, to help themselves. Biofeedback provides a modality to accomplish this.

Principles of Biofeedback. The prefix *myo-* is derived from the Greek word for muscle. In combination with the Greek word *graphos,* to write, and the additional prefix, *electro-,* the word becomes electromyograph (EMG), an instrument for recording the electrical activity of the muscles. EMG biofeedback is a modality for measuring and displaying muscle activity, and it is used primarily where any modification of muscular behavior is indicated. With its use, an individual can learn to become more aware of his or her own muscle activity and thus gain more complete control of functional activity. It also provides an ideal method for rehabilitation practitioners to record a patient's day-to-day progress.

The biofeedback device imparts objective information about the degree of activity occurring in a muscle through surface electrodes, in audio, visual, or audiovisual form, in much the same way that an electrocardiogram provides information about cardiac activity or an electroencephalogram displays brain wave activity. In an EMG biofeedback system, the electrical signal originating in the muscle under study is amplified and then translated into sound and visual readings, which correspond to increased and decreased muscle activity. EMG is the process of recording and interpreting the electrical activity of muscle. When a muscle contracts, it produces a characteristic spike (pulse) waveform that can be detected easily by placing an electrode on the skin over the muscle belly. For example, if you grasp an object tightly in your hand, the muscles in your arm will generate a specific electrical voltage, usually measured in millivolts or microvolts. As you squeeze the object tighter, the electrical voltage will increase as more motor units are recruited. As you relax your hand, the electrical voltage will decrease dramatically. EMG is therefore a direct physiological index of muscular activity and the state of relaxation.

The motor unit is a basic configuration of neuromuscular activity. It consists of a collection of muscle fibers controlled by a singe nerve fiber. When the nerve provides the "triggering" electrical impulse, the muscle fibers contract practically simultaneously. A motor unit may have only a few muscle fibers or thousands, and many motor units are needed to provide the mechanical force required to impart movement to the body[276,277] (see Chapter 31).

Both surface and needle electrodes have been used in EMG. Although the voltage from a single muscle fiber can be monitored by the use of a fine-tipped needle electrode, surface electrodes are commonly used for biofeedback in the rehabilitation setting. The voltage picked up by the surface electrodes is actually an average of the many muscle fibers below and near the electrodes. Although muscle action potentials as picked up by the electrodes could possibly be as high as 1000 µV, values between 100 and 500 µV are more representative.[277]

The principal advantage of needle electrodes is their high sensitivity to individual motor unit potentials, usually without interference from nearby muscles.[276] Therefore they are usually used for diagnostic purposes. However, because therapists normally use EMG biofeedback for muscle reeducation and relaxation purposes, surface electrodes have a number of advantages. For example, they eliminate the necessity of keeping all materials sterile and can be used easily at home by the patient.

Surface EMG (SEMG) protocols have been described within a neurological framework. A neuroanatomical pathway is used, including muscular disease, neuromuscular junction conditions, peripheral neuropathy, radiculopathy, myelopathy, brain stem disorders, cerebellar disorders, and subcortical and cortical disease.[278] SEMG findings within the clinical presentation of those pathological conditions are aimed at improving the diagnostic process and serve to focus the SEMG neuromuscular reeducation (biofeedback) component of the overall treatment plan.

EMG biofeedback has been reported as being a successful procedure for assisting with the rehabilitation of patients with a wide variety of neuromuscular problems, providing muscle reeducation or muscle relaxation in conditions that may include the following:

- Relaxation in spasmodic torticollis[276]
- Migraine headache pain[279-287]
- Tension headache pain[279-287a]
- Improvement of functional deficits in paraplegia and quadriplegia[288,289]
- Improvement of postural instability, proprioception, and reduction in falls[290-292]
- Treatment of children with cerebral palsy for muscle reeducation and relaxation[293,294]
- CVA rehabilitation[295-303]
- Muscular training after nerve, muscle, ligament, or tendon injury, repair, or transfers[304-308]
- Temporomandibular disorder[308a]
- Carpal tunnel syndrome, rotator cuff and other shoulder conditions, lateral epicondylitis, thoracic outlet syndrome, patellofemoral pain, and Achilles tendon repairs[304-308]
- Early joint mobilization after surgery[304-307]
- Total joint replacements and other orthopedic surgeries[309,310]
- Fibromyalgia[311]
- Ergonomic interventions[311a]
- Measurement of endurance with sustained activity[312-316]
- Functional training and reduction of myoclonus after brain injury[315,317,318]
- Control of urinary incontinence and other pelvic floor disorders[319-322a]
- Control of fecal incontinence[322b]
- Relaxation for intractable constipation symptoms[323-326]
- Respiratory control in asthma, emphysema, and chronic obstructive lung disease[327-332]
- Modification of hypertension[333-337]
- Autogenic training of temperature control in diabetes, vascular disease, and symptoms of intermittent claudication[338-340]
- Parasympathetic control of cardiac arrhythmia[341]
- Stress management[342-348]

- Intervention for dysphagia and other swallowing disorders and speech and swallowing problems[349-351]
- Muscle reeducation after Bell's palsy[352,353]
- Pain management and reduction in chemotherapy-related symptoms in patients with cancer[354-360]

It is well recognized that biofeedback treatment offers short-term, cost-effective approaches for many problems, such as chronic pain, irritable bowel syndrome, insomnia, incontinence, and asthma.[360a] It is an efficacious service in primary care practices to a wide variety of patients.

Conclusion. As a literate civilization, we are now more than 5000 years old. Physical needs have always kept the mind well occupied. Technologies have given us a modicum of control over our environment. Yet these technologies are costly. It is clear that medical problems can be caused or aggravated by the mental status of the individual. Western medicine has concentrated its efforts on developing extensive drugs and elaborate surgical techniques to deal with physical and mental compensations. With the evolution of managed care, the trend is now to seek less costly alternative care. This involves reaching inward and developing technologies that will allow us some insight into our inner world. It is time to balance the scales and attempt to solve some of the physical manifestations of pathological conditions from within.

Biofeedback has shown a remarkably positive benefit on the functional and treatment outcomes of numerous conditions.[361] Biofeedback instrumentation has been a growing part of physical therapy practice for more than 20 years, and physical therapists have contributed to researching its efficacy in treating various conditions. Sophisticated contemporary equipment does much more to quantify the worth of biofeedback techniques than was originally envisioned. The importance of relating quantified movement-based data to functional measures has influenced the level of appropriate reimbursement for physical therapy services that use biofeedback. Physical and occupational therapies, as integral members of the medical community, need to continue to investigate self-awareness and self-control as a probable rehabilitative tool in the treatment of a multitude of conditions.

Music Therapy
Therese Marie West, PhD, MT-BC, FAMI
Music therapy is the clinical and evidence-based use of music interventions to accomplish individualized goals within a therapeutic relationship by a credentialed professional who has completed an approved music therapy program.[362]

Although music is not a "universal language" in the sense that a particular piece of music would have the same meaning and effect for any person anywhere, music *is* a universal human phenomenon. Most people today could describe ways in which music might be used to enhance health or well-being, and we find evidence of the use of music as part of healing practices throughout history.[363,364] Within a first worldview perspective, magical or mystical powers were attributed to music, and healing occurred within a context of social structures and shared beliefs. Music was often a part of rituals conducted by a shaman or healer who served as a spiritual intercessor or guide in a process designed to reestablish balance and harmony for the

individual. Music, sometimes with dance, served as a gateway to altered states of consciousness and entry to deep altered states of consciousness, where creative experiences manifested multiple sources of information not available through observation alone. This process supported insights about the causes and remedies for physical, emotional, social, and spiritual imbalance. Where patient, healer, family, and community members participated together in healing rituals involving the use of music, treatment occurred within the natural environment and social fabric of everyday life. Examples of music healing within a first worldview perspective can still be found within indigenous cultural groups to this day.

The rise of the second worldview brought new values that emphasized logical and rational approaches to the use of music to address health issues. During this phase in history, we see the first examples of published work asserting the theory that music could influence emotions and mood states and thereby improve physical or mental health (see reference 363). Anecdotal evidence and case reports were used to support emerging theories and practices into the early twentieth century. In the latter part of the twentieth century, we begin to see the scientific method applied systematically to the study of music in relation to single variable changes in (1) disease/pathological states or (2) functional activities and willingness to participate in rehabilitation treatment settings. Researchers continue to explore possible mechanisms through which music may contribute to improved physical or mental health via its influence on various factors such as emotional responses, mood states, relaxation, activation, or motivation.

In the United States, music therapy began to develop as a profession after World War II, when it was found that music could facilitate both physical rehabilitation and recovery from emotional trauma in veterans returned from the war. Although early music therapists were often musician volunteers, music educators, or musician-physicians, it had become clear that specific education and training was needed, and music therapy curricula and academic programs were developed beginning in the mid 1940s. The first professional music therapy organization (the National Association for Music Therapy [NAMT]) was formed in 1950. A second professional organization, the American Association for Music Therapy (AAMT) formed in 1971. The NAMT and AAMT merged in 1998 to form the American Music Therapy Association (AMTA). The AMTA sets standards for education and clinical training in music therapy programs accredited at more than 70 colleges and universities in the United States and Canada. The Certification Board for Music Therapy was accredited in 1986 by the National Commission for Certifying Agencies and certifies music therapists to practice throughout the United States. This is a competency-based certification process, which includes specialized coursework, 1200 hours of supervised clinical training, and a certification board examination. There are currently more than 4000 music therapists maintaining the MT-BC (Music Therapist, Board Certified) credential and participating in at least 100 hours of continuing education and for recertification every 5 years to maintain and increase competencies for practice in this rapidly developing field. The development of music therapy in the United States parallels the stages of health care development as discussed earlier (see "Historical Perspective" in this chapter). Stage 2 worldviews were dominant during the formative years of music therapy as a profession in the United States. The concurrent emergence of behavioral psychology, along with a need to provide validation of specific music therapy treatments, led to an emphasis on outcomes understood via behavioral measurements. Meanwhile, the complex and multifaceted interactions between humans and their music remained mysterious as clear evidence for mechanisms eluded early researchers. Although basic science study is now part of the continuing research, applied or clinical research has continued to dominate the literature in music therapy, and there is a great deal of work ahead to better understand many of the powerful effects of music observed in clinical settings. Therapists observe that patients who are unable to speak as a result of stroke or Alzheimer's disease are often able to sing coherently when presented with familiar music. How is it that the gait of a patient with Parkinson's disease improves markedly in the presence of a rhythmic auditory stimulus?[365] How does music-evoked imagery (such as experienced with the Bonny Method of Guided Imagery and Music) alter physiological and psychological indicators of stress?[366,367] Modern research developments in brain neuroscience, gait assessment technology, and psychoneuroimmunology are improving researchers' ability to study mechanisms as well as treatment outcomes. Meanwhile, an important focus in the field of music therapy is the development of clinically validated treatments for specific problems and populations.

In the United States, music therapy is now recognized as "an established healthcare profession that uses music to address physical, emotional, cognitive, and social needs of individuals of all ages."[368] Standley[369] conducted a meta-analysis of music research in medical and dental treatment, examining effects for 233 dependent variables, including physiological, self-report, and behavioral measures reported across 92 studies. She reports a large overall mean effect size of 1.17 for music treatments within the pooled results. Although this finding must be interpreted carefully in light of possible methodological issues not revealed by the meta-analysis, there is promising evidence that music therapy may positively affect a number of important clinical parameters in various medical treatment settings. Further research investigations, including replication studies, are needed.

Music therapists develop specialized areas of practice, treating across the life span from perinatal to palliative care, in schools, hospitals, skilled nursing, rehabilitation, outpatient, or community settings. The goals they address support progress in developmental tasks, rehabilitation of physical and cognitive functioning, adaptation and coping, pain management, recovery from trauma, and quality of life. Music therapists work in private practice, as members of interdisciplinary teams, and as consultants and collaborators. West is one of many music therapists who has worked in rehabilitation settings in cotreatment, consultation, or collaboration with speech-language pathologists, physical therapists, and occupational therapists, as well as with a wide range of practitioners from other professions in medicine and mental health arenas. During early clinical collaborations in rehabilitation settings from the mid 1980s to the early 1990s, West found little research to support an understanding of observed phenomena in the rehabilitation clinic setting and

had to depend largely on basic skills of music therapy assessment, careful documentation, and evaluation of treatment outcomes and effectiveness. In recent years, the music therapy profession has focused on increasing the quality and scope of research to support empirically validated "best practices" with reliable outcomes for a number of specific populations of interest to professionals in rehabilitation settings. Rehabilitation music therapists now have the benefit of empirically supported treatment protocols and continuing research regarding effectiveness and safety of music therapy methods.

Music Therapy in the Neonatal Intensive Care Unit. Low-birth-weight and premature infants are at high risk for developmental disabilities, and given the vulnerabilities of their neurological systems, early sensory experiences in the neonatal intensive care unit (NICU) environment are of particular interest to music therapy researchers. A number of studies have explored the uses of music in the NICU, and results suggest that various clinically significant outcomes may result from carefully controlled application of music treatments for the premature infant. Physiological (autonomic nervous system) responses related to infant stress states (blood pressure, heart rate, respiration rate) have been shown to respond to various music stimuli, with favorable responses to sedative music.[370,371] Improvements in behavior state, weight gain, and decrease in length of hospital stay have been reported after treatment with recorded vocal music[372] and parent training in music and multimodal stimulation.[373] A collection of writings on basic theories, research, and clinical practice of music therapy in the NICU from 16 different countries offers an overview of the development of this practice area around the world.[374] Jayne Standley, a senior researcher and collaborator in the development of empirically supported treatments for premature and low-birth-weight infants in the United States, proposed specific music therapy protocols for pacification, stimulation, and parent-infant interaction.[375] Music therapy treatment protocols have been further reviewed and refined with particular attention to audiological issues and safety concerns[376] and with attention to nursing care models designed to meet individual developmental needs of newborn infants.[377] Research is continuing, and as longitudinal studies are conducted, we will know more about longer-term developmental outcomes that may correlate with the immediate benefits associated with music therapy in the NICU.

Music Therapy in Neurological Rehabilitation. Music therapists have been working in neurological rehabilitation settings in the United States for more than 25 years. Tomaino[378] describes her long professional collaboration with the neurologist Dr. Oliver Sacks and shares insights developed through extensive clinical application of music in the individualized assessment and treatment of various neurological diseases and injuries. Music can access intact neurological functions and is used to facilitate relaxation, to increase attention and motivation, to improve the readiness for (priming) and timing of motor activities, and to enhance communication and emotional expression while providing supports for coping and adaptation. Tomaino[378] describes the music therapy process from assessment and treatment planning through treatment and evaluation of outcomes, focusing not only on physical/behavioral changes but also on the engagement of the whole person through a trust-based therapeutic relationship. Familiar music can provide the patient a sense of safety, with predictable elements of rhythm, melody (prosody), words/lyrics, and structure across time within socially and culturally relevant contexts. Musical elements are systematically applied to support functioning in cognition/memory, speech/communication, gait, and upper extremity activities. One particularly interesting discovery is that the rhythmic elements of music can influence the timing and execution of motor sequences in both gross motor and fine motor activities.

A neuroscience approach to understanding potential effects of rhythmic auditory stimulation (RAS) in neurological rehabilitation is supported by a well-developed body of basic research and clinical studies with a number of rehabilitation populations,[379,380] which provide detailed discussions of the body of supporting research, theories, and development of mathematical models to describe motor-rhythm synchronization phenomena. In normal subjects, rhythmic auditory cuing has been shown to improve left/right leg stride rhythmicity and to change a number of parameters in gastrocnemius muscle activity as measured by EMG, suggesting that RAS may induce more focused motor unit recruitment patterns.[381] Studies using rhythmic cuing with hemiparetic stroke patients have resulted in similar findings as well as additional improvements in a number of other gait parameters related to differences between affected and nonaffected sides.[382,383] Another study demonstrated the ability of RAS to enhance treatment when it is added to a conventional physical therapy gait program for acute hemiparetic stroke patients.[384] These patients showed significant increases in velocity, stride length, and reductions in EMG amplitude variability of gastrocnemius muscle in the RAS-enhanced treatment group compared with the standard physical therapy (control) group.[384] Studies have also demonstrated benefits of RAS treatments in gait rehabilitation for patients with traumatic brain injury[385] and Parkinson's disease.[386] Research continues to investigate possible applications or RAS in other areas of rehabilitation, such as speech motor control in patients with Parkinson's disease, where the largest improvements were found in patients with the most severe impairments and only minimal benefits were found for mildly affected patients.[387] These findings highlight the importance of careful diagnostic assessment and an understanding of specific evidence-based best practices for music therapy or any other complementary or alternative treatment. Research continues to support the development of music therapy treatment protocols that demonstrate reliable physical outcomes for specific problems encountered in neurological rehabilitation settings.

Other kinds of music therapy investigations commonly conducted at earlier points along the pathway to empirical validation include qualitative research, case studies, and pilot studies. Although empirical research investigates specific outcomes, music therapists often look to qualitative research to help them identify and analyze processes and refine treatments on the basis of their effectiveness. A group of Australian music therapists investigated themes in songs written by patients with traumatic brain injury.[388] Such investigations give clinicians insight into the inner experience of the patient and may enable the practitioner to be more effective and supportive of patients' coping and recovery processes.

Case studies illustrate the potential of music therapy to enhance coping and adaptation to enormous losses experienced by CVA patients. Erdonmez[389] describes the piano performance–based treatment of a 54-year-old man whose quality of life as a successful general medical practitioner, linguist, and talented keyboard player was abruptly changed by a CVA with massive damage in left temporal and parietal lobes. New motoric skills were developed, as he learned to master with his functional left hand the complex musical tasks originally composed for the right hand. He learned new music and new adaptive skills, and treatment resulted in improvements in speed and manual dexterity. The results of this case study reinforce today's concepts of neuroplasticity and encourage further research into the possibility that music therapy may facilitate development of new neurological pathways and motor strategies. Simultaneously, music therapy gently supports the patient in coping with losses, adapting to limitations, and reconstructing a life with meaning and enjoyment. McMaster[390] describes a course of individual music therapy treatment for a woman in her early 40s who, after the rupture of a tumor in her heart resulting in a CVA, was blind, without speech, and severely disabled in many areas of functioning. Through a music therapy program, this woman was able to protest and grieve her many losses, discovered and received validation of her inner resources and creativity, and experienced new accomplishments. These experiences supported her sense of self and enabled her to mobilize her physical, emotional, and spiritual strengths to face life in a body that would never return to what she had always known.

Although loss of short-term memory and other cognitive limitations resulting from neurological insult may be considered contraindications for traditional psychotherapy approaches, Goldberg et al[391] explored the use of music-evoked imagery with a brain-damaged woman whose behavioral problems had resulted in psychiatric hospitalization. This adaptation of the Bonny Method of Guided Imagery and Music (GIM) supported a creative interaction between the patient and therapist. These interactions allowed the patient to explore in novel ways losses, role changes, and challenges in accepting help from others. Although these researchers were not able to gather follow-up data, immediate positive behavioral changes observed in the milieu suggested that the imagery may have facilitated psychological processing and change not accessible by verbal therapy alone. Short[392] suggests that the Bonny Method, through the spontaneous imagery process, can allow patients to convey information about how they are feeling physically and emotionally in regard to the rehabilitation process. She also proposes that the content of the images evoked by the music can be analyzed by the GIM therapist, to discover emergent themes relevant to the clinical treatment. More research is needed to help music therapy researchers, educators, and clinicians understand how music imagery treatments affect neurological functioning.

Meanwhile, music therapy continues to play an important role in holistic care, even while some phenomena yet elude our scientific methods. West was asked to assess two different teenage boys, hospitalized and in comatose states after head injuries. The treating neurologist was preparing to recommend longer-term follow up disposition for these young patients, and while considering all the medical evidence at his disposal, this physician also wanted to see what music therapy might discover in terms of responsiveness to stimuli. Although one patient showed no response of any kind to any auditory or tactile stimuli, the second patient proved to be a most interesting example of the mysterious recovery. His neurological tests indicated that his prognosis would be very poor; "persistent vegetative state" was the expectation. In the absence of any evidence that he could benefit from more intensive rehabilitation services, he would be sent to a facility where he would receive long-term custodial care but no therapies. During the music therapy assessment, this young man began to show signs of responsiveness to musical stimuli. A professional skeptic, West was reluctant to consider his eye gaze changes, head movement, and smiling to be meaningful responses to the music without additional testing. These could be random events coincident with the stimuli. West presented music in a popular style familiar to the patient (according to family sources) and gently applied tactile rhythmic stimulation to his hands, arms, legs, and feet in time with the music. The patient began to move his own extremities in rhythmic time to the music and continued to do so when the therapist removed her hands. The therapist carefully documented the procedures and patient responses and returned a report to the referring physician. Over the next few days, the patient's responsiveness increased dramatically. The neurologist had this young man placed in a rehabilitation treatment setting. A month later, he had begun to walk and showed promise of significant recovery of functions in a number of areas, including speech. This patient was initially medically evaluated as having little potential for recovery, yet after music therapy he was interactive and a participant in life. This case is a good example of how music can access and bring forward what is yet intact (whole) within a person whose body is damaged by illness or injury.

Although basic and clinical research activities are increasing an understanding of "how" and "for what, when, and for whom" music therapy can be of specific benefit in neurological rehabilitation and medicine, music therapists are also facing the new challenges and opportunities of new worldviews. Music therapy is among the complementary modalities provided as part of a response to increasing demand for holistic and patient and family-centered health care. Because music interacts with every domain of human experience (physical, cognitive, emotional, social, and spiritual), it has the potential to influence multiple needs simultaneously, in a unified way that respects both the uniqueness of the individual and the deep common ground of the person within the whole.

CASE EXAMPLE OF INTEGRATION OF VARIOUS APPROACHES

Carol M. Davis, PT, EdD, MS, FAPTA
Darcy A. Umphred, PT, PhD, FAPTA
Therese Marie West, PhD, MT-BC, FAMI

The intervention with the following patient reflected awareness by the therapist of using myofascial release, CST, and the Feldenkrais method, as well as more traditional therapeutic interventions (Case Study 37-5). The reader must remember that any one of the other approaches presented within this chapter might also have been implemented as part of this client's treatment given another therapist's experience, education, and therapeutic sensitivity, as well as the cultural biases of the client and family. No judgment is being placed on the method or methods selected for this client or any other. What is critically important are the objective outcome measures after the intervention.

CONCLUSION

Darcy A. Umphred, PT, PhD, FAPTA

Before anyone embraces any complementary approach, each clinician needs to identify which philosophy or paradigm matches her or his own belief system and emotional safety issues. Tethering an understanding of any approach to an established scientific base will allow clinicians to stretch beyond their respective comfort paradigm. When treating patients, clinicians are not recommended to jump from one theory to another or from one intervention strategy to another without clinically reasoning why those choices have been made. Therapists, during their professional education, are taught to focus on the Western medical model of disease

---

CASE STUDY 37-5 ■ MRS. P. K.

Mrs. P. K., a 66-year-old woman, presented herself 2 years ago, once she let her diagnosis of Parkinson's disease penetrate her consciousness. It was inconceivable to her that she might have the same illness that affected her grandmother and the same illness that the attorney general could not seem to mask in front of the public. As a seasoned lobbyist, she worked with politicians and traveled in powerful circles. Using her intellect and her considerable skill in negotiation, she successfully persuaded powerful people to see things her way for the benefit of her clients. A woman of small stature, (5 feet tall and 105 pounds), Mrs. P. K. feared that her illness would be seen as a weakness and was adamant that under no

circumstances was anyone to know that she had Parkinson's disease. Fortunately for her, her only symptom was a slight right upper extremity tremor on waking each morning and some "stiffness," especially in flexion and extension of her right shoulder and extension of her right knee. This aspect of the case is critical. Her endless motivation to exercise was based on this fear of exposure, which she regarded, in spite of her therapist's attempts to work through this with her, as a death knell for her professional life.

Mrs. P. K. had exercised much of her life and walked a mile on her treadmill each morning at 3.8 miles per hour. Her husband was familiar with massage and Rolfing, and, at her request, he stretched her hips and

Continued

CASE STUDY 37-5 ■ MRS. P. K.—cont'd

lower extremities each day as prophylaxis against the return of a low back pain problem years earlier. Initial examination revealed the following deficits:

Active right shoulder flexion 130/170

Active right wrist flexion 45/85

Cervical rotation, right 60/80

Cervical rotation, left 45/80

Gait. Mrs. P. K. tended to walk with a narrow stance, heels close together, but with good heel strike. She was unable to ascend or descend stairs, looking straight ahead without severe slowing. She had little head movement or thoracic rotation; her gait looked rather robotic.

Skin. There was slight edema on the right side of the face, with slight swelling of the upper right lip.

Posture. Mrs. P. K.'s pelvis was rotated down to the right, she had a slightly forward head, and although she did not have rounded shoulders per se, the fascia was drawn tight over her pectorals toward her sternum. The fascia of her legs was taut, and revealed a lack of tissue hydration.

Mrs. P. K. had no limitations in function. Her primary clinical goal was to prevent physical manifestations of the onset of the rigidity caused by Parkinson's disease. If and when the disease itself progressed, we reasoned that the more fluid her tissue was, and the more physically fit she was, the less the impact of a dopamine deficiency, and the more efficient her medication (selegiline) would be in reducing the impact of a dopamine deficiency and controlling the progression of her symptoms. An intervention plan was developed that included a combination of traditional exercises for Parkinson's disease, complemented by myofascial release and CST, and Feldenkrais exercises to increase her awareness of her movement.

After we received the referral from her neurologist, her treatments were scheduled for twice monthly, with home exercises. We explained how myofascial release "works" to keep the fascia loose but how it seems to facilitate a sense of calm and peacefulness when done in conjunction with craniosacral rhythm was not known. Given the lack of basic science evidence, she still willingly signed her informed consent. The plan of intervention integrated myofascial release techniques (along with Feldenkrais exercises) with her traditional therapeutic interventions focusing on the impairments caused by Parkinson's disease. These exercises stressed active rotation, spinal segmental exercises, and controlled, active relaxation of the antagonists. Her prognosis was good, for she was beginning intervention in the early stages of the disease, which would preclude secondary complications; she was fully functional and she was physically fit, if not well hydrated, and was motivated. She was encouraged to drink more water.

Treatment began with several minutes of bouncing on the Swiss ball, working on spinal segment articulation and spinal proprioception, and on lateral and backward balancing to relearn where her center of gravity was in her cone of stability. Next, with the assistance of the

therapist, she moved to the bolster where she lay supine with knees flexed and worked on lower extremity extension and balance. On the mat she worked with Feldenkrais exercises and rotation of her shoulders and hips in opposite directions, with head rotation, and reviewed the pelvic exercises in her home program to help her differentiate her pelvis from her hips and to keep her lumbosacral junction and sacroiliac joints mobile.

From there she moved to the plinth, where wedges were positioned to derotate her pelvis in the supine position. Myofascial treatment then began by gently palpation of her cranial rhythm, asking her to relax, take three large breaths, and in her mind's eye, "go on vacation." (Music therapy could be easily introduced at this time to assist her nervous system with relaxation.) This was difficult for her, for her mind is active, constantly thinking about work. As she relaxed, her breathing slowed, and her cranial rhythm became more pronounced. At this point, the thoughts of the clinician became centered and progressed through various activities. First, there was focused intention and reflective thought that asked that energy from the clinician be used to bring about the highest good for the client. Conscious centering included taking deep breaths and visualizing a grounding of the clinician and by seeing that energy flow deep into the earth. Next, the clinician focused attention within the heart (heart chakra according to medical intuitives) and felt deep appreciation for the client, and for the opportunity to help her by use of holistic techniques.

This exchange of healing energy was an important moment for both client and clinician. It might be conjectured that the therapist consciously tapped into the universal healing energy that surrounds all of us at all times and became a kind of transformer for that energy to be used to facilitate the flow of the client's own chi or healing energy that has been disrupted. No matter the verbal explanation used for this interaction, it created a strong bond of trust and respect that would continue to influence the outcome of the interventions.

The clinician continued treatment by moving into an occipital lobe release, followed by cranial releases and a sphenoid release, reasoning that this would assist the myofascia in the cranium to help ensure proper alignment of the cranial bones and to facilitate blood supply to and from the CNS. At this point in the treatment, the clinician would usually allow clinical perception or clinical intuition to guide decision making regarding the next movement. In reality, the therapist might just follow the guidance of the client's innate healing or centering aptitude. Occasionally, more time was spent on neck and upper thorax, with supine or side-lying scapular releases and cervical spine work. Sometimes, after the wedges were removed and the symphysis pubis was in place, a leg pull or diaphragm release was done. If the clinician noticed tightness or imbalance, or if the client indicated that the "fascial voice" was speaking to her, for example, along her right rib cage as the leg pull was carried out, the

CASE STUDY 37-5 ■ MRS. P. K.—cont'd

clinician would follow the lead of what was happening in the body of the client, disregarding any obvious symptoms that needed attention.

This concept is an important facet of myofascial release and many other complementary medical practices. Myofascial release would prescribe that, clinically, it is often shortsighted to go directly to the area of symptoms for treatment, for the problem is often caused by fascial restrictions distant from that area. Specifically, myofascial release as a type of complementary therapy seems to involve subtle or low-intensity nonmaterial stimuli known as "energy medicine." Although various explanations are offered for energy medicine in terms of a vital force or life energy, there is no agreed on scientific understanding or precise meaning of these ideas in Western scientific concepts. Two proposed mechanisms for healer interventions are (1) that consciousness is causal, that is, the conscious intention of the healer through prayer or other means may physically improve the health and well-being of the patient and (2) subtle energies may be exchanged or otherwise be involved, for instance, a condition of physical resonance between the energy fields of healer and patient, which may mediate the beneficial effects.

During the 2 years of Mrs. P. K.'s, treatment, she had a partial left rotator cuff tear and pain in the right fibular head area of her knee, both of which responded positively to myofascial release: cross-hands release work and soft tissue mobilization. Routinely, her right wrist was mobilized after an arm pull, and both scapulae were released in side lying after cross-hands release to the pectoral area.

On days when the pelvic area stiffness could not be relieved, 5 to 10 minutes of the myofascial release technique of rebounding was used, where her body and extremities were passively rocked back and forth. This helped the stiffness to release, after which Mrs. P. K. always remarked how much more "alive" her body felt. The treatment usually ended on the plinth with a side-lying dural tube release, helping her balance her energy gently.

Once the myofascial release and craniosacral work was completed, Mrs. P. K. might be asked to lie prone for further scapular extension exercise or go onto all fours for "cat and camel" spinal mobility work, with wrist extension, along with partial push-ups to work on active elbow extension. From there she would go to the stairs where she practiced step-over-step maneuvers, forward and back and with "grapevine twists," working on fluidity of motion and on masking her tendency to keep her right fingers extended in a parkinsonian posture. A critical component of her intervention was working on her ability to trust herself without needing to watch her feet.

Her home program consisted of pelvic mobility exercises and opposite rotation of arms and legs with cervical rotation. Extra shoulder exercises were added

for her rotator cuff injury, and passive lower extremity stretch over the side of the bed for iliotibial band release for her knee problem, along with fibular head mobilizations. She also lay supine on a 6-inch rubber ball, which she would roll segmentally up her spine to music to help with segmental mobilization. She then walked the treadmill for 1 mile.

The 3-month follow-up on impairment outcomes revealed the following:

Active right shoulder flexion 45/180

Active right wrist flexion 5/85

Cervical rotation, right 70/80

Cervical rotation, left 60/80

Gait: There was improved distance between heels. Stair agility was much improved, with ability to ascend and descend on most days looking straight ahead. Her braiding motion was smooth and continuous without needing to look at her feet. In Mrs. P. K.'s own words: "I feel stronger and more limber inside and outside. I feel I look better and function better."

Skin: The edema in the face was reduced and on most days was not noticeable at all.

The degenerative progression of Parkinson's disease varies with the individual, but Mrs. P. K. has been fortunate. With careful regulation of her medication, her home program, and her twice-monthly therapy sessions, there has been extraordinary success in preventing any obvious signs of rigidity from becoming manifest, which was her goal and thus a primary target outcome for the clinician. No one knows how much of the relief of symptoms was due to her medication, although she was taking the medication for 3 months before she began therapy without showing the results achieved with therapeutic intervention. With this therapeutic intervention demonstrating effective outcomes, it could be argued by both clinician and client that myofascial release and CST helped keep the fascial system elongated and functioning in a self-corrective way. Similarly, integrating traditional personalized exercises with complementary interventions has enhanced the accomplishment of the client's goals for therapy and helped her to regain and maintain a higher quality of life.

The case of Mrs. P. K. offers an opportunity to consider how other complementary and alternative therapies might also be added to her overall plan of care. For instance, music therapy could potentially support three areas of her treatment: (1) music-assisted relaxation during the myofascial treatment, (2) music added as a reinforcing and motivating element for her home exercise program, and (3) individual music therapy to support emotional coping and adaptation during the course of the Parkinson's disease.

The music therapist would first assess Mrs. P. K.'s responses to music and her music preferences, as well as her comfort in using musical experiences for relaxation or for emotional expression. For treatment

Continued

CASE STUDY 37-5 ■ MRS. P. K.—cont'd

areas 1 or 2, the music therapist would work in consultation and collaboration with the treating physical/myofascial therapist. A cotreatment approach is ideal, but the music therapist can also serve as a consultant, providing musical materials to be used by the physical or occupational therapist. It is important to consider musical elements such as rhythm, harmony, and tone qualities, as well as highly individualized responses such as nonmusical memories and associations that are elicited by the music. A music therapist is able to perform live music and compose or improvise original music, which creates infinitely more flexibility than is available with commercially available recordings. Once the music is developed and refined with input from the patient, this music may be recorded for the patient to use during clinic treatments or at home. The music therapist carefully selects appropriate musical styles and instrumentation and matches the music to the breathing rate, tension level, and other individual parameters to enhance relaxation responses. For goal 2, the flow, tense-release, and tempos in the music are carefully selected to support movements during exercising and to provide a pleasant, energizing, and motivating stimulus. Finally, as mentioned in goal area 3, music therapy may augment rehabilitation team treatments by supporting the patient in tasks related to the psychological and emotional aspects of coping with disease and assist the individual to continue experiencing well-being and quality of life. Music may enhance the sensory richness of mental imagery and can support sensory-kinesthetic imagery and body awareness. An advanced technique such as the Bonny Method of Guided Imagery and Music can be used to develop an increased awareness of bodily states through the language of imagery. This work can help the patient develop more sensitive awareness of the body's unique and individual form of nonverbal communication. This approach can facilitate the psychological work of bringing resources from mental, emotional, and spiritual aspects of self into a more integrated approach for adaptation to challenge, where one can move beyond merely coping, to thriving and living to full potential. Finally, music therapy can continue to provide familiar, comforting, and soothing support when the patient eventually enters the palliative care phase. Certainly, other complementary approaches discussed within this chapter could also be integrated into the previous case. It is not within the scope of this chapter to integrate and synthesize all complementary approaches as if a large holistic approach was available to everyone. However, it is within the hopes of the authors that colleagues will recognize that integration has the potential of existing in future health care environments, but will only evolve where therapists who are willing to accept that there is always more to

learn. There are always more options for the patient than any one therapist has available and new approaches will continue to evolve and become options in the future.

The final case study of Mrs. P. K. was presented not to negate but rather to integrate traditional therapeutic interventions with complementary approaches. With limitations in health care benefits, consumers experience frustration regarding access to providers such as physical, occupational, speech, or music therapists. Many chronic problems remain unanswered by allopathic medicine. Many clients are looking elsewhere for answers and for hope. When individuals no longer can look toward the Western medical system to regain or maintain health or healing, the only available options exist outside traditional Western medicine. As individual practitioners we can be part of that transition or be left behind with traditional Western medicine. It is interesting that branches of Western medicine are turning toward complementary philosophies and some medical schools are incorporating this training into student physicians' education. If physical and occupational therapy remain tethered to the portion of Western medicine that is linear, reductionistic, and focuses on research that is univariable, not system interaction–based, then these two professions have the same potential future as traditional medicine. That future is not clear, but certainly traditional medicine is going to play a significantly reduced role in health care delivery. Our future in neurorehabilitation is up to the breadth and limitations of our leaders and to the willingness of our younger colleagues to follow or become leaders themselves. The future possibilities for both professions are enormous, not only in integrating complementary and alternative medicine into intervention of clients with chronic and degenerative illnesses, but also in acute care and in health and wellness maintenance. The answers to what is the best evidence-based practice lie in functional outcome measurements. Innovative research will play a role in the future direction of competency-based interventions. Until the measurement tools are available to analyze the interactions of multivariables, clinicians are going to have to use objective outcomes measures as to effectiveness to determine whether the intervention should be stopped, continued, or altered. Selecting intervention strategies on the basis of belief only without simultaneously measuring objective outcomes will always lead to questions regarding whether the intervention was worth the financial investment. The challenge will be to remain open and willing to discover new alternatives while keeping grounded in the ethical responsibility to establish an evidence base for the practice of physical and occupational therapy.

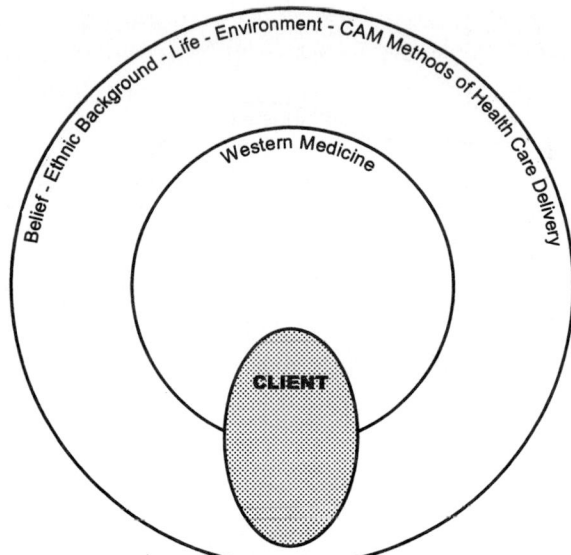

FIGURE 37-10 ■ Client enters Western medicine owing to disease/pathological condition or disability/impairment.

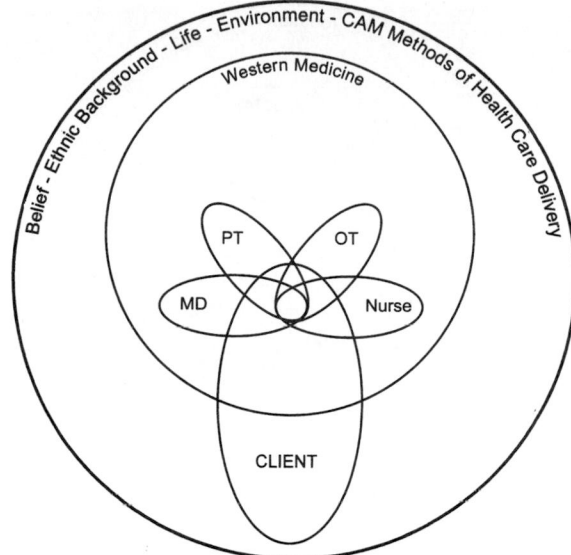

FIGURE 37-11 ■ Transdisciplinary interactions within Western medical model.

and pathology, and the client and the therapeutic variables that might influence the quality of movement of that client are considered external to medical management (Figure 37-10). At the same time, students are taught to accept that there is a transdisciplinary interaction between professional disciplines and that each profession not only uniquely affects the client but also has an interactive effect that is dependent on other professions and their respective impact on the patient's health, wellness, and potential to attain a maximal quality of life (Figure 37-11). When complementary and alternative approaches to health care are introduced into this model, then our colleagues need to determine which approaches interact with Western medicine and which do not (Figure 37-12). Why one approach interacts with the patient and another does not is based on the client's beliefs, needs, and responses to intervention. Because the professions of occupational and physical therapy have always been tethered to Western medicine, therapists need to critically analyze the interactions of those approaches that clearly overlap with our existing paradigm before we let go of the tether and venture totally into the unknown (Figure 37-13). Those components of alternative approaches that obviously overlap with acceptable practice need to be identified and their effectiveness established (Figure 37-14). With the establishment of those clear clinical correlations, the remaining components of identified alternative paradigms seem naturally to become part of the established delivery system. As a result, a new model for Western health care practice as identified by physical and occupational therapy is formed, which continues to allow the therapist to be tethered while enlarging or stretching a professional comfort zone to encapsulate alternative models without feeling as if the grounded neuroscience background is jeopardized (Figure 37-15). A clinician must always be cognizant of the fact that no matter what methods, philosophies, or interventions he or she selected to help a client reach a desired functional outcome, there is no way to eliminate the fact that other aspects of human system processing may also be active and affecting the outcome. For a century,

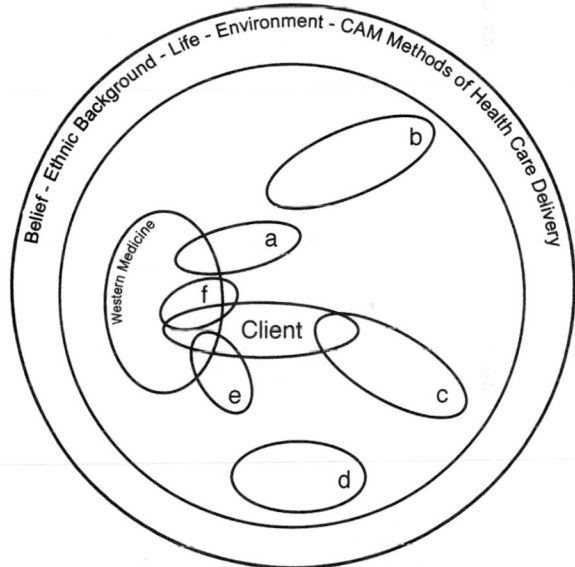

FIGURE 37-12 ■ CAMs of health care delivery. a, Some CAMs interact with Western medicine: a, f, e; b, Some alternative models do not interact with Western medicine: b, c, d; c, Some alternative models meet needs of the client: c, e, f; d, Some alternative models do not meet the needs of the client: a, b, d.

master clinicians have been observed treating clients. Often colleagues comment that, although those masters seem to use the same methods, they get different outcomes. The question is, are those masters using other alternative interventions without those techniques ever being brought to consciousness? That is, if as a therapist I use myofascial techniques along with traditional intervention, am I also affecting craniosacral rhythm, or affecting chakras and energy fields and setting the stage for the nervous system to learn by narrowing the window and allowing it to select better options for motor responses? If so, what truly is

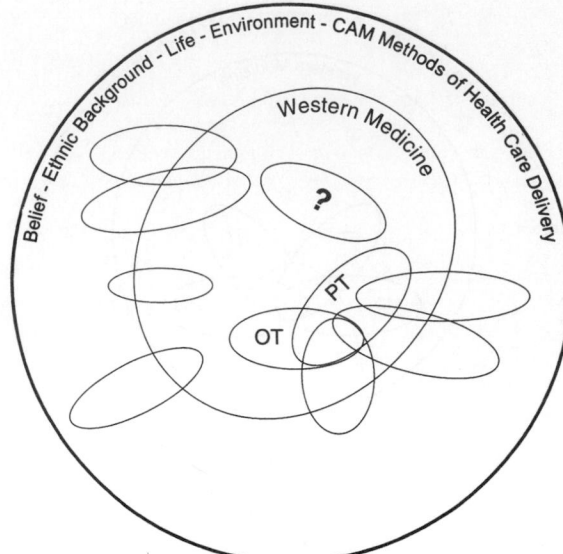

FIGURE 37-13 ■ CAMs interacting with Western medicine. Some models interact to a large extent with Western medicine and some to a small extent. Some models interact with both Western medicine and other complementary models. The extent of complementary interactions with either physical or occupational therapy or both reflect which models fall within respective scopes of practice and thus become part of the professional's treatment tools.

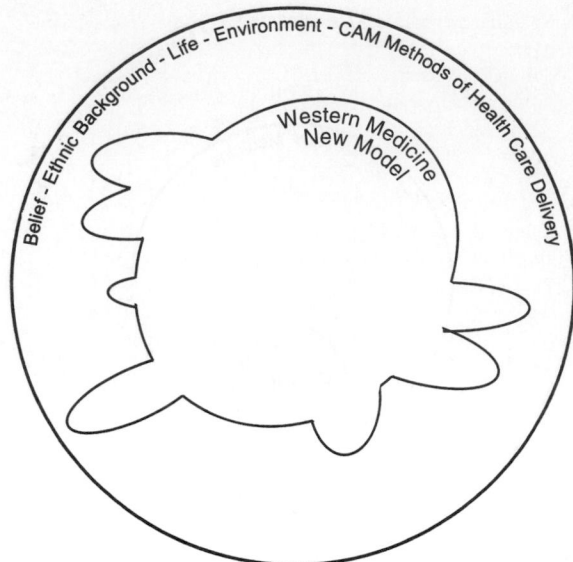

FIGURE 37-15 ■ New model of Western health care delivery beyond complementary therapies. As the overlapping components of each alternative model are accepted as part of existing Western health care delivery practice, the barriers to the remaining aspects of these models become transparent. With barriers disappearing a new model with a different shape and different alternative becomes what will be known as traditional medicine in the future.

leading to somatosensory retraining, motor learning, and neuroplasticity? It may be that master clinicians use *all* approaches but only verbalize the paradigm she or he is most comfortable with and capable of verbally explaining. The adventure is a process of learning, enlarging one's skill to provide the best service to clients and differentiating what is effective within the clinical setting from what is believed to be effective. Differentiating true behavior on a client-by-client basis from what one is taught should happen is the reason for effectiveness of master clinicians. Best practice is constantly evolving and changing. As movement specialists we have the responsibility to evolve as well. That change needs to come flexibly tethered to knowledge, motor skill, emotional openness, and freedom to venture beyond a comfort zone while objectively measuring positive change in the functional abilities of our clients and, thus, improve their quality of life.

REFERENCES

1. Portney LG, Watkins MP: *Foundations to clinical research: applications to practice,* ed 2, Upper Saddle River, NJ, 2000, Prentice Hall Health.

Historical Perspective

2. Foos F, Rothenberg K: *The second medical revolution,* Boston, 1987, Shambala.
3. Laszlo E: *The systems view of the world,* Cresskill, NJ, 1996, Hampton Press.
4. Jones J: Presented to the Feldenkrais Professional Training Program, Eugene, OR, June 16, 1995. Razummy D, Razummy E, editors: Berkeley, CA, Movement Studies Institute.
5. Dossey L: *Time, space, and medicine,* Boston, 1982, Shambala, 1982.
6. Capra F, Steindl-Rast D: *Belonging to the universe,* New York, 1991, HarperCollins.

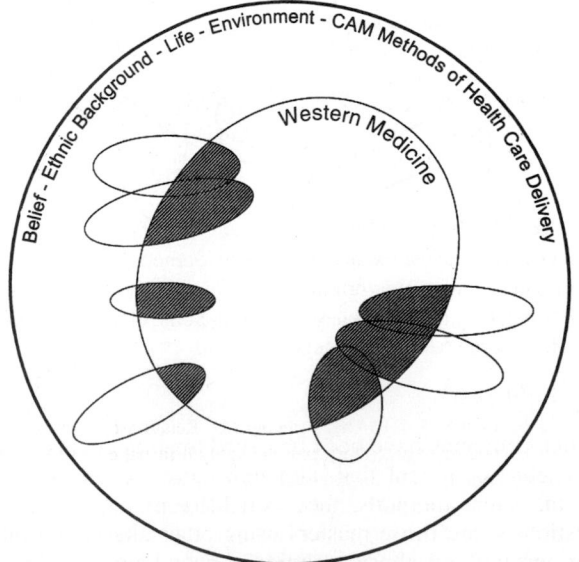

FIGURE 37-14 ■ The portion of each alternative or complementary model that overlaps with allopathic medicine and traditional occupational and physical therapy has been the focus of this chapter. As efficacy is established for those components that interlock, therapists will more readily accept these approaches as part of their practice.

7. Colt GH: See me, feel me, touch me, heal me, *Life* September 1996, p. 36.
8. Kamm K, Thelen E, Jensen JL: A dynamical systems approach to motor development, *Phys Ther* 7:763-775, 1990.
9. Reynolds JP: Balance strategies: 2000 and beyond, *PT Magazine* 5:24-31, 1997.

Alternative Models and Philosophical Approaches

10. Cohen AM, Stavri PZ, Hersh WR: A categorization and analysis of the criticisms of evidence-based medicine, *Int J Med Inform* 73:35-43, 2004.
11. Haynes RB: What kind of evidence is it that evidence-based medicine advocates want health care providers and consumers to pay attention to? *BMC Health Serv Res* 2:3, 2002.
12. Mykhalovskiy E, Weir L: The problem of evidence-based medicine: directions for social science, *Soc Sci Med* 59:1059-1069, 2004.
13. Parker M: False dichotomies: EBM, clinical freedom, and the art of medicine, *Med Humanit* 31:23-30, 2005.
14. Parker M: Whither our art? Clinical wisdom and evidence-based medicine, *Med Health Care Philos* 5:273-280, 2002.
15. Saarni SI, Gylling HA: Evidence based medicine guidelines: a solution to rationing or politics disguised as science? *J Med Ethics* 30:171-175, 2004.

Movement Therapy Approaches
Feldenkrais References

16. Feldenkrais M: *The elusive obvious,* Cupertino, CA, 1981, Meta Publications.
17. Newell G: Moshe Feldenkrais: a biographical sketch of his early years, *Somatics* 7:33-38, 1992.
18. Feldenkrais M: *Body and mature behavior: a study of anxiety, sex, gravitation, and learning,* London, 1949, Routledge and Kegan Paul.
19. Buchanan PA, Ulrich BD: The Feldenkrais Method: a dynamic approach to changing motor behavior [review, tutorial], *Res Q Exerc Sport* 72:315-323, 2001.
20. Newell KM: Motor skill acquisition, *Annu Rev Psychol* 42:213-237, 1991.
21. Byl NN, Merzenich MM, Cheung S et al: A primate model for studying focal dystonia and repetitive strain injury: effects on the primary somatosensory cortex, *Phys Ther* 77:269-284, 1997.
22. Vereijken B, Whiting HT: In defence of discovery learning, *Can J Sport Sci* 15:99-106, 1990.
23. Ioffe ME: Brain mechanisms for the formation of new movements during learning: the evolution of classical concepts [review], *Neurosci Behav Physiol* 34:5-18, 2004.
24. Kleim JA, Jones TA, Schallert T: Motor enrichment and the induction of plasticity before or after brain injury [review], *Neurochem Res* 28:1757-1769, 2003.
25. Ward NS: Functional reorganization of the cerebral motor system after stroke [review], *Curr Opin Neurol* 17:725-730, 2004.
26. Stephens J, Miller TH: Feldenkrais method: learning to move through your life with grace and ease (Or optimizing your potential for living). In Davis C, editor: *Complementary therapies in rehabilitation: evidence for efficacy, prevention and wellness,* Thorofare, NJ, 2004, Slack Inc.
27. Stephens J, Call S, Evans K et al: Responses to ten Feldenkrais awareness through movement lessons by four women with multiple sclerosis: improved quality of life, *Phys Ther Case Rep* 2:58-69, 1999.
28. Elgelid HS: Feldenkrais and body image unpublished master's thesis, Conway, AR, 1999, University of Central Arkansas.
29. Dunn PA, Rogers DK: Feldenkrais sensory imagery and forward reach, *Percept Mot Skills* 91:755-757, 2000.
30. Hall SE, Criddle A, Ring A et al: *Study of the effects of various forms of exercise on balance in older women,* unpublished manuscript Healthway Starter Grant, File #7672, Nedlands, Western Australia, 1999, Department of Rehabilitation, Sir Charles Gardner Hospital.
31. Bennett JL, Brown BJ, Finney SA et al: Effects of a Feldenkrais based mobility program on function of a healthy elderly sample, *Issues on Aging* 21:27, 1998 (abstract). Poster presented at Combined Sections Meeting, Boston, February 1998.
32. Kerr GA, Kotynia F, Kolt GS: Feldenkrais awareness through movement and state anxiety, *J Bodywork Movement Ther* 6:102-107, 2002.
33. Laumer U, Bauer M, Fichter M et al: Therapeutic effects of Feldenkrais method "Awareness Through Movement" in patients with eating disorders, *Psychother Psychosom Med Psychol* 47:170-180, 1997.
34. Bost H, Burges S, Russell R et al: *Feldstudie zur wiiksamkeit der Feldenkrais-Methode bei MS—betroffenen,* Saarbrucken, Germany, 1994, Deutsche Multiple Sklerose Gesellschaft.
35. Johnson SK, Frederick J, Kaufman M et al: A controlled investigation of bodywork in multiple sclerosis, *J Altern Complementary Med* 5: 237-243, 1999.
36. Stephens J, DuShuttle D, Hatcher C et al: Use of awareness through movement improves balance and balance confidence in people with multiple sclerosis: a randomized controlled study, *Neurol Rep* 25:39-49, 2001.
37. Stephens J, Cates P, Jentes E, Perich A, Silverstein J, Staab E, duShuttle D, Hatcher C, Shmunes J, Slaninka C: Awareness through movement improves quality of life in people with multiple sclerosis [abstract], *J Neurol Phys Ther* 27:170, 2003.
38. Feldenkrais M: *The case of Nora,* New York, 1977, Harper & Row.
39. Connors K, Grenough P: Redevelopment of the sense of self following stroke, using the Feldenkrais method. Poster presented at the Feldenkrais Annual Research Forum, August, 2004, Seattle, WA.
40. Nair DG, Fuchs A, Burkart S et al: Assessing recovery in middle cerebral artery stroke using functional MRI, *Brain Inj* 19:1165-1176, 2005.
41. Cramer SC, Bastings EP: Mapping clinically relevant plasticity after stroke, *Neuropharmacology* 39:842-851, 2000.
42. Batson G: Effect of Feldenkrais "Awareness Through Movement" on balance and upper extremity function in patients with chronic stroke: a pilot study. American Physical Therapy Association poster presented at CSM, Nashville, TN, February 2004 and personal communication.
42a. Batson G, Deutsch JE: Effects of Feldenkrais awareness through movement on balance in adults with chronic neurological deficits following stroke: a preliminary study, *Complementary Health Practice Review* 10:203-210, 2005.
43. Shelhav-Silberbush C: The Feldenkrais method for children with cerebral palsy, Master's thesis, Berkeley, CA, 1988, Boston University School of Education, Feldenkrais Resources.
44. Shenkman M, Donovan J, Tsubota J et al: Management of individuals with Parkinson's disease: rationale and case studies, *Phys Ther* 69:944-955, 1989.
45. Gilman M, Yaruss JS: Stuttering and relaxation: applications for somatic education in stuttering treatment, *J Fluency Disord.* 25:59-76, 2000.
46. Ofir R: A heuristic investigation of the process of motor learning using Feldenkrais method in physical rehabilitation of two young women with traumatic brain injury, unpublished doctoral dissertation, New York, 1993, Union Institute.

Pilates References

47. Ozgocmen S, Cimen OB, Ardicoglu O: Relationship between chest expansion and respiratory muscle strength in patients with primary fibromyalgia, *Clin Rheumatol* 21:19-22, 2002.
48. Hodges P, Kaigle HA, Holm S et al: Intervertebral stiffness of the spine is increased by evoked contraction of transversus abdominis and the diaphragm: In vivo porcine studies, *Spine* 28:2594-2601, 2003.
49. Hodges P, Gandevia S, Richardson C: Contractions of specific abdominal muscles in postural tasks are affected by respiratory maneuvers, *J Appl Physiol* 83:753-760, 1997.
50. Comerford M, Mottram S: Masterclass: Functional stability re-training: principles and strategies for managing mechanical dysfunction, *Manual Ther* 6:3-14, 2001.

51. Richardson C, Jull G, Hodges P: Local muscle dysfunction in low back pain. In *Therapeutic exercise for spinal segmental stabilisation in low back pain,* London, 1999, Churchill Livingstone.

52. Richardson C, Jull G, Hodges P: Overview of the principles of clinical management of the deep muscle system for segmental stabilization. In *Therapeutic exercise for spinal segmental stabilisation in low back pain,* London, 1999, Churchill Livingstone.

53. Porterfield J: Dynamic stabilization of the trunk, *J Orthop Sports Phys Ther* 6:271-279, 1985.

54. Gibbons S, Comerford M: Strength versus stability, 1: Concept and terms, *Orthop Div Rev* 1:21-27, 2001.

55. Gibbons S, Comerford M: Strength versus stability, 2: Limitations and benefits, *Orthop Div Rev* 1:28-33, 2001.

56. Detrembleur C, Vanmarsenille JM, De Cuyper F et al: Relationship between energy cost, gait speed, vertical displacement of centre of body mass and efficiency of pendulum-like mechanism in unilateral amputee gait, *Gait Posture* 21:333-340, 2005.

57. Unnithan VB, Dowling JJ, Frost G et al: Role of cocontraction in the O2 cost of walking in children with cerebral palsy, *Med Sci Sports Exerc* 28:1498-1504, 1996.

58. Panjabi M: The stabilizing system of the spine, I: Function, dysfunction, adaptation, and enhancement, *J Spinal Disord Tech* 5:383-389, 1992.

59. Panjabi M: The stabilizing system of the spine, II: Neutral zone and instability hypothesis, *J Spinal Disord Tech* 5:390-396, 1992.

60. Panjabi M, Abumi K, Duranceau J et al: Spinal stability and intersegmental muscle forces: A biomechanical model, *Spine* 14:194-200, 1989.

61. Cats-Baril W, Frymoyer J: Identifying patients at risk of becoming disabled because of low-back pain: the Vermont rehabilitation engineering center predictive model, *Spine* 16:605-607, 1991.

62. Brondel L, Mourey F, Mischis-Troussand C et al: Energy cost and cardiorespiratory adaptation in the "Get-Up-and-Go" test in frail elderly women with postural abnormalities and in controls, *J Gerontol A Biol Sci Med Sci* 60:98-103, 2005.

63. McDaniel J, Subudhi A, Martin JC: Torso stabilization reduces the metabolic cost of producing cycling power, *Can J Appl Physiol* 30:433-441, 2005.

64. Austin G, Benesky W: Thoracic pain in a collegiate runner, *Manual Ther* 7:168-172, 2000.

65. Hennessey L, Watson A: Flexibility and posture assessment in relation to hamstring injury, 27:243-246, 1993.

66. Englund U, Littbrand H, Sondell A et al: A 1-year combined weight-bearing training program is beneficial for bone mineral density and neuromuscular function in older women, *Osteoporos Int* 16:1117-1123, 2005.

67. Roos EM, Dahlberg L: Positive effects of moderate exercise on glycosaminoglycan content in knee cartilage: a four-month, randomized, controlled trial in patients at risk of osteoarthritis, *Arthritis Rheum* 52:3507-3514, 2005.

68. Yung PS, Lai YM, Tung PY et al: Effects of weight bearing and non-weight bearing exercises on bone properties using calcaneal quantitative ultrasound, *Br J Sports Med* 39:547-551, 2005.

69. Anderson B: Pilates rehabilitation. In Davis C, editor: *Complementary therapies in rehabilitation,* Thorofare, NJ, 2004, Slack Incorporated, pp 219-232.

70. Shumway-Cook A, Woolacott M: Motor control: Issues and theories. In *Motor control theory and practical applications,* pp. 1-25, Baltimore, 2001, Lippincott Williams & Wilkins.

71. Horak FB. Assumptions underlying motor control for neurological rehabilitation: Contemporary management of motor control problems. Presented at II STEP Conference American Physical Therapy Association, 1991, Norman, OK.

72. Cowan T, Lackner J, Anderson B et al: *A pilot study of Pilates exercise for rehabilitation of sub acute low back pain patients,* Miami, 2003, Polestar.

73. Mannion AF, Junge A, Taimela S et al: Active therapy for chronic low back pain, 3: Factors influencing self-rated disability and its change following therapy, *Spine* 26:920-929, 2001.

74. Guzman J, Esmail R, Karjalainen K et al: Multidisciplinary bio-psycho-social rehabilitation for chronic low back pain, *Cochrane Database Syst Rev* 1:CD000963, 2002.

75. Jensen M, Turner J, Romano J: Self-efficacy and outcome expectancies: relationship to chronic pain coping strategies and adjustment, *Pain* 44:263-269, 1991.

76. Lackner JM, Carosella AM, Feuerstein M: Pain expectancies, pain, and functional self-efficacy expectancies as determinants of disability in patients with chronic low back disorders, *J Consult Clin Psychol* 64:212-220, 1996.

77. Anderson B: *Polestar education instruction manual: Polestar approach to movement principles,* Miami, 2001, Polestar.

Tai Chai References

78. Wanning T: Healing and the mind/body arts: massage, acupuncture, yoga, t'ai chi, and Feldenkrais, *AAOHN J* 41:349-351, 1993.

79. Jones AY, Dean E, Scudds RJ: Effectiveness of a community-based tai chi program and implications for public health initiatives, *Arch Phys Med Rehabil* 86:619-625, 2005.

80. Lai JS, Wong MK, Lan CL et al: Cardio-respiratory responses of t'ai chi chuan practitioners and sedentary subjects during cycle ergometer, *J Formos Med Assoc* 92:894-899. 1993.

81. Lai JS, Lan C, Wong MK, Teng SH: Two-year trends in cardio-respiratory function among older t'ai chi chuan practitioners and sedentary subjects, *J Am Geriatr Soc* 43:1222-1227, 1995.

82. Ng RK: Cardiopulmonary exercise: a recently discovered secret of t'al chi, *Hawaii Med J* 51:216-217, 1992.

83. Chan KM, Chen WT, Wang JJ et al: Frail elders' view of tai chi, *J Nurs Res* 13:11-20, 2005.

84. Xu DQ, Li JX, Hong Y: Effect of regular tai chi and jogging exercise on neuromuscular reaction in older people, *Age Ageing* 34:439-444, 2005.

85. Judge JO, Lindsey C, Underwood M et al: Balance improvements in older women: effects of exercise training, *Phys Ther* 73:254-265, 1993.

86. Province MA, Hadley EC, Hornbrook MC et al: The effects of exercise on falls in elderly patients. A preplanned meta-analysis of the FICSIT Trials. Frailty and injuries: cooperative studies of intervention techniques, *JAMA* 273:1341-1347, 1995.

87. Tse SK, Bailey DM: T'ai chi and postural control in the well elderly, *Am J Occup Ther* 46:295-300, 1992.

88. Wolf SL, Kutner NG, Green RC et al: The Atlanta FICSIT study: two exercise interventions to reduce frailty in elders, *J Am Geriatr Soc* 41:329-332, 1993.

89. Wolfson L, Whipple R, Judge J et al: Training balance and strength in the elderly to improve function, *J Am Geriatr Soc* 41:341-343, 1993.

90. Brown DR, Wang Y, Ward A et al: Chronic effects of exercise and exercise plus cognitive strategies, *Med Sci Sports Exerc* 27:765-775, 1995.

91. Jin P: Efficacy of t'ai chi, brisk walking, meditation, and reading in reducing mental and emotional stress, *J Psychosom Res* 36:361-370, 1992.

92. Liao W: *T'ai chi classics: New translations of three essential texts of t'ai chi chuan,* Boston, 1990, Shambhala.

93. Kronenberg F, Mallory B, Downey JA: Rehabilitation medicine and alternative therapies: new words, old practices, *Arch Phys Med Rehabil* 75:928-929. 1994.

94. Lynoe N: Ethical and professional aspects of the practice of alternative medicine, *Scand J Soc Med* 20:217-225, 1992.

95. Wardwell WI: Alternative medicine in the United States, *Soc Sci Med* 38:1061-1068, 1994.

96. Jou TH: *The tao oftT'ai chi chuan way to rejuvenation,* Shapiro S, translator and editor, Warwick, NY, 1988, Tai Chi Foundation.

97. Da L: *T'ai chi ch'uan and I Ching,* New York, 1987, Harper & Row.

98. Da L: *T'ai chi ch'uan and meditation,* New York, 1991, Schocken Books.

99. Huai-chin N: *Tao and longevity,* New York, 1984, Weiser.

100. Legge J: *The texts of taoism,* vol 1, New York, 1962, Dover.

101. Blofeld J (translator and editor): *I Ching: the book of change,* New York, 1965, EP Dutton.

102. Fung Y: *A history of Chinese philosophy, vol 2,* Princeton, NJ, 1953, Princeton University Press.

103. Sohn RC: *Tao and t'ai chi,* Rochester, VT, 1989, Destiny Books.

104. Kirsta A: *The book of stress survival: identifying and reducing stress in your life,* New York, 1986, Simon & Schuster.

105. Tsai JC, Wang WH, Chan P et al: The beneficial effects of tai chi chaun on blood pressure and lipid profile and anxiety status in a randomized controlled trial, *J Altern Complement Med* 9:747-754, 2003.

106. Wolf SL, O'Grady M, Easley KA et al: The influence of intense tai chi training on physical performance and hemodynamic outcomes in transitionally frail, older adults, *J Gerontol A Biol Sci Med Sci* 61:184-189, 2006.

107. Lai JS, Wong MK, Lan CL et al: Cardiorespiratory responses of t'ai chi chuan practitioners and sedentary subjects during cycle ergometer, *J Formos Med Assoc* 92:894-899, 1993.

108. Lai JS, Lan C, Wong MK, Teng SH: Two-year trends in cardiorespiratory function among older t'ai chi chuan practitioners and sedentary subjects, *J Am Geriatr Soc* 43:1222-1227, 1995.

108a. Audette JF, Jin YS, Newcomer R et al: Tai Chi versus brisk walking in elderly women, *Age Ageing* 35:388-393, 2006.

109. Yeh GY, Wood MJ, Lorell BH et al: Effects of tai chi mind-body movement therapy on functional status and exercise capacity in patients with chronic heart failure: a randomized controlled trial, *Am J Med* 117:541-548, 2004.

110. Ng RK: Cardiopulmonary exercise: a recently discovered secret of t'al chi, *Hawaii Med J* 51:216-217, 1992.

111. Tsang WW, Wong VS, Fu SN et al: Tai chi improves standing balance control under reduced or conflicting sensory conditions, *Arch Phys Med Rehabil* 85:129-137, 2004.

112. Judge JO, Lindsey C, Underwood M et al: Balance improvements in older women: effects of exercise training, *Phys Ther* 73:254-265, 1993.

113. Fong SM, Ng GY: The effects on sensorimotor performance and balance with tai chi training, *Arch Phys Med Rehabil* 87:82-87, 2006.

114. Tsang WW, Hui-Chan CW: Effects of exercise on joint sense and balance in elderly men: Tai chi versus golf, *Med Sci Sports Exerc* 36:658-667, 2004.

115. Tse SK, Bailey DM: T'ai chi and postural control in the well elderly, *Am J Occup Ther* 46:295-300, 1992.

116. Li F, Harmer P, Fisher KJ, McAuley E et al: Tai chi and fall reductions in older adults: a randomized controlled trial, *J Gerontol A Biol Sci Med Sci* 60:187-194, 2005.

117. Tsang WW, Hui-Chan CW: Effect of 4- and 8-wk intensive tai chi training on balance control in the elderly, *Med Sci Sports Exerc* 36:648-657, 2004.

118. Choi JH, Moon JS, Song R: Effects of Sun-style tai chi exercise on physical fitness and fall prevention in fall-prone older adults, *J Adv Nurs* 51:150-157, 2005.

119. Gatts SK, Woollacott MH: Neural mechanisms underlying balance improvement with short term Tai Chi training, *Aging Clin Exp Res* 18:7-19, 2006.

120. Wolfson L, Whipple R, Judge J et al: Training balance and strength in the elderly to improve function, *J Am Geriatr Soc* 41:341-343, 1993.

121. Wolf SL, Kutner NG, Green RC et al: The Atlanta FICSIT study: Two exercise interventions to reduce frailty in elders, *J Am Geriatr Soc* 41:329-332, 1993.

122. Reynolds JP: Profiles in alternatives: East and West on the information superhighway: t'ai chi, *PT Magazine* 2:52-53, 1994.

122a. Zhang JG, Ishikawa-Takata K, Yamazaki H et al: The effects of Tai Chi Chaun on physiological function and fear of falling in the less robust elderly: an intervention study for preventing falls, *Arch Gerontol Geriatr* 42:107-116, 2006.

123. Tsang WW, Hui-Chan CW: Comparison of muscle torque, balance, and confidence in older tai chi and healthy adults, *Med Sci Sports Exerc* 37:280-289, 2005.

124. Wayne PM, Krebs DE, Wolf SL et al: Can tai chi improve vestibulopathic postural control? *Arch Phys Med Rehabil* 85:142-152, 2004.

125. Venglar M: Case report: Tai chi and parkinsonism, *Physiother Res Int* 10:116-121, 2005.

126. Qin L, Au S, Choy W et al: Regular tai chi chuan exercise may retard bone loss in postmenopausal women: a case-control study, *Arch Phys Med Rehabil* 83:1355-1359, 2002.

127. Qin L, Choy W, Leung K et al: Beneficial effects of regular tai chi exercise on musculoskeletal system, *J Bone Miner Metab* 23:186-190, 2005.

128. Xu D, Hong Y, Li J, Chan K: Effect of tai chi exercise on proprioception of ankle and knee joints in old people, *Br J Sports Med* 38:50-54, 2004.

129. Han A, Robinson V, Judd M et al: Tai chi for treating rheumatoid arthritis, *Cochrane Database Systematic Reviews:* http://www.cochrane.org/reviews/en/ab004849.html. Accessed August 12, 2005.

129a. Sierpina VS, Sierpina M, Loera JA et al: Complementary and integrative approaches to dementia, *South Med J* 98:636-645, 2005.

Tae Kwon Do References

130. Hasselmo ME: A model of prefrontal cortical mechanisms for goal-directed behavior, *J Cogn Neurosci* 17:1115-1129, 2005.

131. Stanne MB, Johnson DW, Johnson RT: Does competition enhance or inhibit motor performance: a meta-analysis, 125:133-154, 1999.

132. Mueller BM: Tae kwon do: a therapy adjunct, *Clin Manage* 11:64-66, 1991.

133. Katula JA, Sipe M, Rejeski WJ et al: Strength training in older adults: an empowering intervention, *Med Sci Sports Exerc* 38:106-111, 2006.

134. Rejeski WJ, Brawley LR: Functional health: innovations in research on physical activity with older adults, *Med Sci Sports Exerc* 38:93-99, 2006.

135. Slootmaker SM, Chin A, Paw MJ et al: Promoting physical activity using an activity monitor and a tailored web-based advice: design of a randomized controlled trial, *BMC Public Health* 5:134, 2005.

136. Postollec ML: Complementary movement therapies, *Adv Phys Ther* 8:8-10, 1998.

137. Lipton B: *The biology of belief: unleashing the power of consciousness matter and miracles,* Santa Rosa, CA, 2005, Elite Books.

138. Berger D: A mind/body approach, *PT Magazine* 1:66-75, 1994.

139. Fosnaught M: The quest for wellness, *PT Magazine* 1:38-44, 1994.

140. Jackson WO: Not a hamster on a wheel: the Feldenkrais method, *PT Magazine* 1:58-65, 1994.

141. Moyers B: *Healing and the mind,* Garden City, NY, 1993, Doubleday.

142. Reichley ML: What's a crane doing in PT? *Adv Phys Ther* 2:10-11, 1993.

143. Reynolds JP: Profiles in alternatives: East and West on the information superhighway, *Tai Chi. PT Magazine* 1:52-59, 1994.

144. Kandel ER, Schwartz JH, Jessel TM: *Principles of neural science,* ed 4, New York, 2000, McGraw Hill.

145. Schmidt RA: Motor learning principles for physical therapy. In Lister MJ, editor: *Contemporary management of motor control problems,* Norman, OK, 1990, Foundation for Physical Therapy.

146. Kleim JA, Hogg TM, VandenBerg PM et al: Cortical synaptogenesis and motor map reorganization occur during late, but not early, phase of motor skill learning, *J Neurosci* 24:628-633, 2004.

147. Remple MS, Bruneau RM, VandenBerg PM et al: Sensitivity of cortical movement representations to motor experience: evidence that skill learning but not strength training induces cortical reorganization, *Behav Brain Res* 123:133-141, 2001.

148. Luft AR, Manto MU, Ben Taib NO: Modulation of motor cortex excitability by sustained peripheral stimulation: the interaction between the motor cortex and the cerebellum, *Cerebellum* 4:90-96, 2005.

149. Mills N, Allen J: Mindfulness of movement as a coping strategy in multiple sclerosis: a pilot study, *Gen Hosp Psychiatry* 22:425-431, 2000.

150. Kleim JA: Neuroplasticity. III STEP Conference, Salt Lake City, Utah. July 17, 2005.

151. Monfils MH, Plautz EJ, Kleim JA: In search of the motor engram: motor map plasticity as a mechanism for encoding motor experience, *Neuroscientist* 11:471-483, 2005.

152. Bayona NA, Bitensky J, Salter K et al: The role of task-specific training in rehabilitation therapies, *Top Stroke Rehabil* 12:58-65, 2005.

153. Chu CJ, Jones TA: Experience-dependent structural plasticity in cortex heterotopic to focal sensorimotor cortical damage, *Exp Neurol* 166:403-414, 2000.

154. Nudo RJ: Adaptive plasticity in motor cortex: Implications for rehabilitation after brain injury, *J Rehabil Med* 41(suppl):7-10, 2003.

155. Teasell R, Bayona NA, Bitensky J: Plasticity and reorganization of the brain post stroke, *Top Stroke Rehabil* 12:11-26, 2005.

156. Teasell R, Bitensky J, Salter K et al: The role of timing and intensity of rehabilitation therapies, *Top Stroke Rehabil* 12:46-57, 2005.

Energetic Therapy Approaches
Therapeutic Touch References

157. Rogers ME: Nursing science of unitary, irreducible, human beings: update 1990. In Barrett EAM, editor: *Visions of RogerssScience-based nursing,* New York, 1990, National League for Nursing.

158. North American Nursing Diagnosis Association: *Nursing diagnoses: definitions and classifications 2005-2006,* Philadelphia, 2006, North American Nursing Diagnosis Association.

159. Turner JG, Clark AJ, Gauthier DK, Williams M: The effect of therapeutic touch on pain and anxiety in burn patients, *J Adv Nurs* 28:10-20, 1998.

160. White House Commission on Complementary and Alternative Medicine Policy: *Final report:* http://www.whccamp.hhs.gov/tl.html. Accessed March 26, 2002.

161. Nurse Healers-Professional Associates International, Inc: nhpai@earthlink.net.

162. Heidt P: Effect of therapeutic touch on anxiety level of hospitalized patients, *Nurs Res* 30:32-37, 1981.

163. Krieger D, Peper E, Ancoli S: Therapeutic touch: search for evidence of physiological change, *AJN* 79:660-665, 1979.

164. Sneed NV, Olson M, Bubolz B et al: Influences of a relation intervention on perceived stress and power spectral analysis of heart rate variability, *Prog Card Nurs* 16:34-40, 2001.

165. Cox C, Hayes J: Physiologic and psychodynamic responses to the administration of therapeutic touch in critical care, *Comp Ther Nurs Midw* 5:87-92, 1999.

166. Garrad CT:. The effect of therapeutic touch on stress reduction and immune function in persons with AIDS, *Diss Abs Int* 3692B: Univ Microfilms No. 8909162, 1995.

167. Olson M, Sneed N, Bonadonna R et al: Therapeutic touch and post-85 hurricane Hugo stress, *J Hol Nurs* 10:120-136, 1992.

168. Olson M, Sneed N. LaVia M et al: Stress-induced immunosuppression and therapeutic touch, *Alt Ther Health Med* 3:68-74, 1997.

169. Kramer NA: Comparison of therapeutic touch and casual touch in stress reduction of hospitalized children, *Pediatr Nurs* 16:483-485, 1990.

170. Aucott S, Donohue PK, Atkins E et al: Neurodevelopmental care in the NICU, *Ment Retard Dev Disabil Res Rev* 8:29803-29808, 2002.

171. Fedoruk RB: Transfer of the relaxation response: therapeutic touch B as a method for reduction of stress in premature neonates, *Diss Abs Int* 978B: Univ Microfilms No. 8509162, 1984.

172. Cox CL, Hayes JL: Reducing anxiety: the employment of therapeutic touch as a nursing intervention, *Comp Ther Nurs Midw* 3:163-167, 1997.

173. Gagne D, Toye R: The effets of therapeutic touch and relaxation therapy in reducing anxiety, *Arch Psych Nurs* 8:184-189, 1994.

174. Hale EH: A study of the relationship between therapeutic touch and the anxiety levels of hospitalized adults, *Diss Abs Int* 28995B: Univ Microfilms No. 8900128, 1986.

175. Heidt P: Effect of therapeutic touch on the anxiety level of hospitalized patients, *Nurs Res* 30:32-37, 1981.

176. Ireland M: Therapeutic touch with HIV-infected children: a pilot study, *J Assn Nurs AIDS Care* 9:68-77, 1998.

177. Parkes BS: Therapeutic touch as an intervention to reduce anxiety in elderly hospitalized patients, *Diss Abs Int* 573B: Univ Microfilms No. 8609563, 1986.

178. Quinn JF: The effects of therapeutic touch done without physical contact on state anxiety of hospitalized cardiovascular patients, *Diss Abs Int* 1797B: Univ Microfilms No. 8226788, 1982.

179. Shuzman E: The effect of trait anxiety and patient expectations of therapeutic touch on the reduction of state anxiety in preoperative patients who receive therapeutic touch, *Diss Abs Int* 1808B: Univ Microfilms No. 9423009, 1993.

180. Simington JA, Laing OP: Effects of therapeutic touch on anxiety in the institutionalized elderly, *Clin Nurs Res* 2:438-450, 1993.

181. Lin YS, Gill TA: Effects of therapeutic touch in reducing pain and anxiety in an elderly population, *Integr Med* 1:155-162, 1999.

182. Philcox P, Rawlins L, Rodgers L: Therapeutic touch and its effect on phantom limb and stump pain, *J Aust Rehabil Nurs Assoc* 5:17-21, 2002.

183. Blankfield RP, Sulzmann C, Fradley LG et al: Therapeutic touch in the treatment of carpal tunnel syndrome, *J Am Board Fam Pract* 14:335-342, 2001.

184. Peck SD: The effectiveness of therapeutic touch for decreasing pain in elders with degenerative arthritis, *J Holist Nurs* 15:176-198, 1997.

185. Denison B: Touch the pain away: new research on therapeutic touch and persons with fibromyalgia syndrome, *Holist Nurs Pract* 18:142-151, 2004.

186. Smith DW, Arnstein P, Roas KC, Wells-Federman C: Effects of integrating therapeutic touch into a cognitive behavioral pain treatment program, *J Holist Nurs* 20:367-387, 2002.

187. Gordon A, Merenstein JH, D'Amico F et al: The effects of therapeutic touch on patients with osteoarthritis of the knee, *J Fam Pract* 47:271-277, 1998.

188. Peck SD: The efficacy of therapeutic touch for improving functional ability in elders with degenerative arthritis, *Nurs Sci Q* 11:123-132, 1998.

189. Smith MC, Reeder F, Daniel L et al: Outcomes of touch therapies during bone marrow transplant, *Alt Ther Health Med* 9:40-49, 2003.

190. Hagemaster J: Use of therapeutic touch in treatment of drug addictions, *Holist Nurs Pract* 14:14-20, 2000.

191. Larden CN, Palmer ML, Janssen P: Efficacy of therapeutic touch in treating pregnant inpatients who have a chemical dependency, *J Holist Nurs* 22:320-332, 2004.

192. Snyder M, Egan EC, Burns KR: Interventions for decreasing agitation behaviors in persons with dementia, *J Geront Nurs* 21:34-40, 1995.

193. Woods DL, Craven R, Whitney J: The effect of therapeutic touch on disruptive behaviors of individuals with dementia of the Alzheimer's type, *Alt Ther* 2:95-96, 1996.

194. Woods DL, Dimond M: The effect of therapeutic touch on agitated behavior and cortisol levels in persons with Alzheimer's disease, *Biol Res Nurs* 4:104-114, 2002.

195. Abbot NC: Healing as a therapy for human disease: a systematic review, *J Alt Comp Med* 2:159-169, 2000.

196. Astin JA, Harkness E, Ernst E: The efficacy of "distant healing": a systematic review of randomized trials, *Arch Intern Med* 11:903-910, 2000.

197. Peters RM: The effectiveness of therapeutic touch: a meta-analytic review, *Nurs Sci Q* 12:52-61, 1999.

198. Winstead-Fry P, Kijek J: An integrative review and meta-analysis of therapeutic touch research, *Alt Ther Health Med* 5:58-67, 1999.

199. Cohen J: *Statistical power analysis for the behavioral sciences,* ed 2, Englewood Cliffs, NJ, 1979, Lawrence Erlbaum.

200. Newshan G, Schuller-Civitella D: Large clinical study sows value of therapeutic touch program, *Holist Nurs Pract* 17:100-103, 2003.
201. Krieger D, Winstead-Fry P: *Manual for subjective experience of therapeutic touch scale (SETTS),* ed 2, 1998. Available from Winstead-Fry, 2708 Herrick Brook Road, Pawlet, VT 05761.
202. Ferguson CK: Subjective experience of therapeutic touch survey (SETTS): psychometric examination of an instrument, *Diss Abs Int* Univ Microfilms No.8618464, 1986.

Medical Intuitive References

203. Ritberger C: *Your personality, your health,* Carlsbad, CA, 1998, Hay House.
204. Tiller W: *Science and human transformation,* Walnut Creek, CA, 1997, Pavior.
205. Tiller W: *Energy fields in medicine,* Kalamazoo, MI, 1989, John A. Fetzer Foundation.
206. Bailey AA: *Esoteric healing: a treatise on the seven rays, vol 4,* New York, 1977, Lucis.
207. Leadbetter CW: *The chakras,* Wheaton, IL, 1969, Theosophical Publishing House.
208. Powell AE: *The etheric double,* London, 1960, Theosophical Publishing House.
209. Ackerman JM: *The biophysics of the VAS in energy fields of medicine,* Kalamazoo, MI, 1989, John A. Fetzer Foundation.

ADDITIONAL RECOMMENDED REFERENCES FOR MEDICAL INTUITIVE DIAGNOSTICS

Davis-Floyd R, Davis E: Intuition as authoritative knowledge in midwifery and homebirth, *Med Anthropol Q* 10:237-269, 1996.
Higgins JP: Nonlinear systems in medicine, *Yale J Biol Med* 75:247-260, 2002.
Kerfoot K: Learning intuition—less college and more kindergarten: the leader's challenge, *Pediatr Nurs* 29:470-472, 2003.
McCraty R, Atkinson M, Bradley RT: Electrophysiological evidence of intuition, 2: a system-wide process? *J Altern Complement Med* 10:325-336, 2004.
McCutcheon HH, Pincombe J: Intuition: an important tool in the practice of nursing, *J Adv Nurs* 35:342-348, 2001.
Mykhalovskiy E, Weir L: The problem of evidence-based medicine: directions for social science, *Soc Sci Med* 59:1059-1069, 2004.
McKinnon J: Feeling and knowing: neural scientific perspectives on intuitive practice, *Nurs Stand* 20:41-46, 2005.
Parker M: False dichotomies: EBM, clinical freedom, and the art of medicine, *Med Humanit* 31:23-30, 2005.
Petros P: Non-linearity in clinical practice, *J Eval Clin Pract* 9:171-178, 2003.
Stitzman L: At-one-ment, intuition and "suchness," *Int J Psychoanal* 85:1137-1155, 2004.

Physical Body Systems Approaches
Craniosacral Therapy References

210. Upledger JE: *Craniosacral therapy II,* Seattle, 1987, Eastland Press.
211. Upledger JE, Vredevoogd J: *Craniosacral therapy,* Chicago, 1983, Eastland Press.
212. Retzlaff EW, Roppel RM, Becker-Mitchell FL et al: Craniosacral mechanisms, *J Am Osteopath Assoc* 76:288-289, 1976.
213. Retzlaff EW, Mitchell FL, Upledger JE et al: Nerve fibers and endings in cranial sutures: research report, *J Am Osteopath Assoc* 77:474-475, 1978.
214. Upledger JE, Karni Z: Mechano-electric patterns during craniosacral osteopathic diagnosis and treatment, *J Am Osteopath Assoc* 78:782-791, 1979.
215. Upledger JE: *Somatoemotional release and beyond,* Palm Beach Gardens, FL, 1990, UI Publishing.
216. The Vietnam veteran's interview videotapes. Palm Beach Gardens, FL, 1993, Upledger Institute.

217. Retzlaff EW, Upledger JE: Cranial suture pain, *J Am Osteopath Assoc.*
218. Retzlaff EW, Vredevoogd J, Upledger JE: A proposed mechanism for drugless pain control, *J Am Osteopath Assoc,* 1997.
219. Upledger JE: The therapeutic value of cranial sacral system, *Massage Therapy J,* 21:32-33, 1988.
219a. Upledger JE: Craniosacral therapy, *Phys Ther* 75:328-330, 1995.
220. Gilmore NJ: Right brain, left brain asymmetry, *ACLD Newsbriefs* July/August, 1982.
221. Upledger JE: Cranial therapy proves successful with some ADD children, *Assoc for Retarded Citizens Advocates Newsletter* 1980.
222. Upledger JE: Craniosacral function in brain dysfunction, *Osteopath Ann* 11:318-324, 1983.
223. Upledger JE: Thermographic view of autism, *Osteopath Ann* 118:356-359, 1983.
224. Geldschlager S: Osteopathic versus orthopedic treatments for chronic epicondylopathia humeri radialis: a randomized controlled trial, *Forsh Komplementarmed Klass Naturheilkd* 2:93-97, 2004.
225. Hartman SE, Norton JM: Interexaminer reliability and cranial osteopathy, *Sci Rev Altern Med* 6:23-40, 2002.
226. Cohen MM Jr: Sutural biology and the correlates of craniosynostosis, *Am J Med Genet* 47:581-616, 1993.
227. Melson B: Time and mode of closure of the spheno-occipital synchondrosis determined on human autopsy material, *Acta Anat* 83:112-118, 1972.
228. Madeline LA, Elster AD: Suture closure in the human chondrocranium: CT assessment, *Radiology* 196:747-756, 1995.
229. Okamato K, Ito J, Tokiguchi S et al: High resolution CT findings in the development of spheno-occipital synchondrosis, *Am J Neuroradiol* 17:117-120, 1996.

Myofascial Release (Barnes Method) References

230. Perizonius WRK: Closing and non-closing sutures in 256 crania of known age and sex from Amsterdam (A.D. 1883-1908), *J Hum Evol* 13:201-216, 1984.
231. Travell J: *Myofascial pain and dysfunction,* Baltimore, 1983, Williams & Wilkins.
232. Oschman J: *Energy medicine—the scientific basis.* Edinburgh, 2000, Churchill Livingstone.
233. Barnes JF: Myofascial release—The missing link in traditional treatment. In Davis C, editor: *Complementary therapies in rehabilitation—holistic approaches for preventions and wellness,* Thorofare, NJ, 1997, Slack.
234. Hall D: The aging of connective tissue, *Gerontology* 13:77-89, 1968.
235. Wang Y, Botvinick E, Zhao Y et al: Visualizing the mechanical activation of Src, *Nature* 434:1040-1045, 2005.
236. Rubik B: Energy medicine and the unifying concept of information, *Altern Ther Health Med* 1:34-39, 1995.
237. Rubik B, Pavek R, Greene E et al: Manual healing. In Swyers J, et al [11 member editorial board], editors: *Expanding medical horizons: Report to the NIH on alternative medicine,* publication No. 94-066, pp. 113-157, Washington, DC, 1996, US Government Printing Office.

Models of Health Care Belief Systems
Traditional Acupuncture References

238. Eisenberg DM, Kessler RC, Foster C et al: Unconventional medicine in the United States, *N Engl J Med* 328:246-252, 1993.
239. Eisenberg DM, Davis RB, Ettner SL et al: Trends in alternative medicine use in the United States: 1990-1997, *JAMA* 28:1569-1575, 1998.
240. Benson H, Stark M: *Timeless healing: the power and biology of belief,* New York, 997, Fireside.

ADDITIONAL RECOMMENDED READING FOR TRADITIONAL ACUPUNCTURE

Audette JF, Ryan AH: The role of acupuncture in pain management, *Phys Med Rehabil Clin North Am* 15:749-772, 2004.

Audette JF, Wang F, Smith H: Bilateral activation of motor unit potentials with unilateral needle stimulation of active myofascial trigger points, *Am J Phys Med Rehabil* 83:368-377, 389, 2004.

Baldry P: Superficial versus deep dry needling, *Acupunct Med* 20:78-81, 2002.

Chang QY, Lin JG, Hsieh CL: Effect of manual acupuncture and transcutaneous electrical nerve stimulation on the H-reflex, *Acupunct Electrother Res* 26:239-251, 2001.

Chiu JH, Chung MS, Cheng HC et al: Different central manifestations in response to electroacupuncture at analgesic and nonanalgesic acupoints in rats: a manganese-enhanced functional magnetic resonance imaging study, *Can J Vet Res* 67:94-101, 2003.

Farber PL, Tachibana A, Campiglia HM: Increased pain threshold following electroacupuncture: analgesia is induced mainly in meridian acupuncture points, *Acupunct Electrother Res* 22:109-117, 1997.

Itoh K, Katsumi Y, Kitakoji H: Trigger point acupuncture treatment of chronic low back pain in elderly patients—a blinded RCT, *Acupunct Med* 22:170-177, 2004.

Irnich D, Behrens N, Gleditsch JM et al: Immediate effects of dry needling and acupuncture at distant points in chronic neck pain: results of a randomized, double-blind, sham-controlled crossover trial, *Pain* 99:83-89, 2002.

Kuo TC, Lin CW, Ho FM: The soreness and numbness effect of acupuncture on skin blood flow, *Am J Chin Med* 32:117-129, 2004.

Langevin HM, Yandow JA: Relationship of acupuncture points and meridians to connective tissue planes, *Anat Rec* 269:257-265, 2002.

Lee MS, Jeong SY, Lee YH et al: Differences in electrical conduction properties between meridians and non-meridians, *Am J Chin Med* 33:723-728, 2005.

Lee MS, Kim YC, Moon SR et al: Hydrodynamic analysis of waveforms induced by vibrational stimuli at meridian and non-meridian points, *Am J Chin Med* 32:977-984, 2004.

Lee MS, Lee YH, Shin BC et al: Is there any energy transfer during acupuncture? *Am J Chin Med* 33:507-512, 2005.

Lee TN: Thalamic neuron theory: Meridians = DNA. The genetic and embryological basis of traditional Chinese medicine including acupuncture, *Med Hypotheses* 59:504-521, 2002.

Lee YH, Lee MS, Shin BC et al: Effects of acupuncture on potential along meridians of healthy subjects and patients with gastric disease, *Am J Chin Med* 33:879-885, 2005.

Li Z, Wang C, Mak AF et al: Effects of acupuncture on heart rate variability in normal subjects under fatigue and non-fatigue state, *Eur J Appl Physiol* 94:633-640, 2005.

Mayer-Gindner A, Lek-Uthai A et al: Newly explored electrical properties of normal skin and special skin sites, *Biomed Tech (Berl)* 49:117-124, 2004.

Molsberger AF, Mau J, Pawelec DB et al: Does acupuncture improve the orthopedic management of chronic low back pain—a randomized, blinded, controlled trial with 3 months follow up, *Pain* 99:579-587, 2002.

Omura Y: Connections found between each meridian (heart, stomach, triple burner, etc.) and organ representation area of corresponding internal organs in each side of the cerebral cortex: release of common neurotransmitters and hormones unique to each meridian and corresponding acupuncture point and internal organ after acupuncture, electrical stimulation, mechanical stimulation (including shiatsu), soft laser stimulation or QI Gong, *Acupunct Electrother Res* 14:155-186, 1989.

Sutherland JA: Meridian therapy: current research and implications for critical care, *AACN Clin Issues* 11:97-104, 2000.

Wu MT, Hsieh JC, Xiong J et al: Central nervous pathway for acupuncture stimulation: localization of processing with functional MR imaging of the brain—preliminary experience, *Radiology* 212:133-141, 1999.

Yan B, Li K, Xu J et al: Acupoint-specific fMRI patterns in human brain, *Neurosci Lett* 383:236-240, 2005.

Zhou W, Fu LW, Tjen-A-Looi SC et al: Afferent mechanisms underlying stimulation modality-related modulation of acupuncture-related cardiovascular responses, *J Appl Physiol* 98:872-880, 2005.

Native American Healing References

241. *Alternative medicine: Expanding medical horizons. A report to the National Institutes of Health on alternative medical systems and practices in the United States,* Washington, DC, 1992, US Government Printing Office.

242. Babor TF: Alcohol treatment in American Indian populations: an indigenous treatment modality compared with traditional approaches, *Ann N Y Acad Sci* 472:168-178, 1986.

243. Chante P: *The red road to sobriety* [videotape], San Francisco, 1995, Kiraru Productions.

244. Chante P: *The red road to sobriety video talking circle* [videotape], San Francisco, 1995, Kiraru Productions.

245. Hall R: Distribution of the sweat lodge in alcohol treatment programs, *Anthropology* 26:134-135, 1985.

246. Red Dog L: Personal communication, June 24, 1997. Member of Cheyenne River Sioux Tribe, On the Tree, SD.

247. Thin Elk G: Appendix: Wounded warriors: a time for healing. In *The red road approach,* St. Paul, MN, 1995, Little Turtle Publications, pp 319-320.

248. Clifford M: Personal communication, June 10, 1997. Member of Pine Ridge Sioux Tribe, Rapid City, SD.

249. Douville V: Personal communication, June 12, 1997. Member of Rosebud Sioux Tribe, Sinte Gleska University, Mission, SD.

250. Erikson J: Personal communication, 1997. Intake Social Worker, Indian Health Services Hospital, Rosebud, SD.

251. Richards M: Personal communication, June 16, 1997. Social Worker and Discharge Planner, Rapid City Regional Hospital, Rapid City, SD.

252. DuBray W, Sanders A: Interactions between American Indian ethnicity and health care, *J Health Soc Policy* 10:67-84, 1999.

253. Ese'eja community members, Infierno, Peru, March 9-11, 2005.

254. Salak K: Hell and back. In *National Geographic adventure,* pp. 55-58, 88-91, New York, 2006, National Geographic Society.

255. Riba J, Anderer P, Jane F et al: Effects of the South American psychoactive beverage *ayahuasca* on regional brain electrical activity in humans: a functional neuroimaging study using low-resolution electromagnetic tomography, *Neuropsychobiology* 50: 89-101, 2004.

ADDITIONAL RECOMMENDED READINGS FOR AMERICAN INDIAN HEALING

Braswell M, Wong E, Wong HD: Perceptions of rehabilitation counselors regarding Native American healing practices, *J Rehabil* 60:33-43, 1994.

Means R, Wolf MJ: *Where white men fear to tread: the autobiography of Russell Means,* New York, 1995, St Martin's Press.

Allopathic Links to Models of Health Care Belief Systems
Electroacupuncture

256. Xinnong C, editor: *Chinese acupuncture and moxibustion,* Beijing, 1987, Foreign Languages Press.

257. Senior K: Acupuncture: can it take pain away? *Mol Med Today* 2:150-153, 1996.

258. Kumar A, Tandon OP, Bhattacharya A et al: Somatosensory evoked potential changes following electroacupuncture therapy in chronic pain patients, *Anaesthesia* 50:411-414, 1995.

259. Chen A: Effective acupuncture therapy for stroke and cerebrovascular diseases, part 1, *Am J Acupunct* 21:105-122, 1993.

260. Naeser MA, Alexander MP, Stiassy-Elder D et al: Laser acupuncture in the treatment of paralysis in stroke patients: A CT scan lesion site study, *Am J Acupunct* 23:13-28, 1995.

261. Shoukang L: Acupuncture therapy for apoplectic hemiplegia, *Int J Acupunct* 2:333-335, 1992.

262. Cheng PT, Wong MK, Chang PL: A therapeutic trial of acupuncture in neurogenic bladder of spinal cord injured patients—a preliminary report, *Spinal Cord Inj* 36:476-480, 1998.

263. Moon SK, Whang YK, Park SU et al: Antispastic effect of electroacupuncture and moxibustion in stroke patients, *Am J Chin Med* 31:467-474, 2003.

264. Wong AMK, Leong C, Su T et al: Clinical trial of acupuncture for patients with spinal cord injuries, *Am J Phys Med Rehabil* 82:21-27, 2003.

265. Hans JS, Terenius L: Neurochemical basis of acupuncture analgesia, *Annu Rev Pharmacol Toxicol* 22:193-220, 1982.

266. Eke-Okoro ST: The H-reflex studied in the presence of alcohol, aspirin, caffeine, force and fatigue, *Electromyogr Clin Neurophysiol* 22:579-589, 1982.

267. Alavi A, LaRiccia PJ, Sadek AH et al: Neuroimaging of acupuncture in patients with chronic pain, *J Altern Complement Med* 3:S47-S53, 1997.

268. Anderson S, Lundeberg T: Acupuncture-from empiricism to science: functional background to acupuncture effects in pain and disease, *Med Hypoth* 45:271-281, 1995.

269. Galantino ML, Eke-Okoro ST, Findley TW et al: Use of noninvasive electroacupuncture for the treatment of HIV-related peripheral neuropathy: a pilot study, *J Altern Complement Med* 5:135-142, 1999.

270. Camels P: A scientific perspective on developing acupuncture as a complementary medicine, *Disabil Rehabil* 21:129-130, 1999.

271. Balogun JA, Biasci S, Han L: The effects of acupuncture, electroneedling and transcutaneous electrical stimulation therapies on peripheral haemodynamic functioning, *Disabil Rehabil* 20:41-48, 1998.

272. Shrode LH: Treatment of facial muscles affected by Bell's palsy with high voltage electrical muscle stimulation, *J Manipulative Physiol Ther* 16:347-352, 1993.

Biofeedback References

273. Ford CW: *Where healing waters meet,* Tarrytown, NY, 1989, Station Hill Press.

274. Gruber BL, Hersh SP, Hall NR et al: Immunological responses of breast cancer patients to behavioral interventions, *Biofeedback Self Regul* 18:1-22, 1993.

275. McIntosh LJ, Frahm JD, Mallett VT et al: Pelvic floor rehabilitation in the treatment of incontinence, *J Reprod Med* 38:662-666, 1993.

276. Peper E, editor: *Mind/body integration: essential readings in biofeedback,* New York, 1979, Plenum.

277. Wirth DP, Barrett MJ: Complementary healing therapies, *Int J Psychosom* 41:61-67, 1994.

278. Sella GE: Neuropathology considerations: clinical and SEMG/biofeedback applications, *Appl Psychophysiol Biofeedback* 28:93-105, 2003.

279. Arena JG, Bruno GM, Hannah SL et al: A comparison of frontal electromyographic biofeedback training, trapezius electromyographic biofeedback, and progressive muscle relaxation therapy in the treatment of tension headache, *Headache* 35:411-419, 1995.

280. Blanchard EB: Psychological treatment of benign headache disorders, *J Consult Clin Psychol* 60:537-551, 1992.

281. Grazzi L, Bussone G: Effect of biofeedback treatment on sympathetic function in common migraine and tension-type headache, *Cephalalgia* 13:197-200, 1993.

282. Grazzi L, Bussone G: Italian experience of electromyographic-biofeedback treatment of episodic common migraine: preliminary results, *Headache* 33:439-441, 1993.

283. King TI: The use of electromyographic biofeedback in treating patients with tension headaches, *Am J Occup Ther* 46:839-842, 1992.

284. Penzien DB, Holroyd KA: Psychosocial interventions in the management of recurrent headache disorders: description of treatment techniques, *Behav Med* 20:64-73, 1994.

285. Sheffied MM: Psychosocial interventions in the management of recurrent headache disorders: policy considerations for implementation, *Behav Med* 20:73-77, 1994.

286. Rokicki LA, Houle TT, Dhingra LK et al: A preliminary analysis of EMG variance as an index of change in EMG biofeedback treatment of tension-type headache, *Appl Psychophysiol Biofeedback.* 28:205-215, 2003.

287. Kaushik R, Kaushik RM, Mahajan SK et al: Biofeedback assisted diaphragmatic breathing and systematic relaxation versus propranolol in long term prophylaxis of migraine, *Complement Ther Med* 13:165-174, 2005.

287a. Kanji N, White AR, Ernst E: Autogenic training for tension type headaches: a systematic review of controlled trials, *Complement Ther Med* 14:144-150, 2006.

288. Klose KJ, Needham BM, Schmidt D et al: An assessment of the contribution of electromyographic biofeedback as an adjunct in the physical training of spinal cord injured persons, *Arch Phys Med Rehabil* 74:453-456, 1993.

289. Moore S, Woollacott MH: The use of biofeedback devices to improve postural stability, *Phys Ther Pract* 2:1-19, 1993.

290. Hawken MB, Jantti P, Waterston JA: The effect of sway feedback and loss of sensory cues in older women with a history of falls. In Woollacott MH, Horak F, editors: *Posture and gait-control mechanisms, vol 2,* Eugene, OR, 1992, University of Oregon Books, pp 263-266.

291. Leonhardt C: Posture biofeedback for improved sitting [in German], *Fortschr Med* 110:33-34, 1992.

292. Hegeman J, Honegger F, Kupper M et al: The balance control of bilateral peripheral vestibular loss subjects and its improvement with auditory prosthetic feedback, *J Vestib Res* 15:109-117, 2005.

293. Nashner LM, Shumway-Cook A, Marin O: Stance posture control in select groups of children with cerebral palsy—deficits in sensory organization and muscular coordination, *Exp Brain Res* 49:393-409, 1983.

294. Woolridge CP, Russell G: Head position training with the cerebral palsied child: an application of biofeedback techniques, *Arch Phys Med Rehabil* 57:407-414, 1976.

295. Howard S, Varley R: Using electropalatography to treat severe apraxia of speech, *Eur Disord Commun* 30:246-255, 1995.

296. Leplow B, Schluter V, Ferstl R: A new procedure for assessment of proprioception, *Percept Mot Skills* 74:91-98, 1992.

297. Moreland J, Thomson MA: Efficacy of electromyographic biofeedback compared with conventional physical therapy for upper-extremity function in patients following stroke: a research overview and meta-analysis, *Phys Ther* 74:534-547, 1994.

298. Schleenbaker RE, Mainous AG III: Electromyographic biofeedback for neuromuscular re-education in the hemiplegic stroke patient: a meta-analysis, *Arch Phys Med Rehabil* 74:1301-1304, 1993.

299. Shumway-Cook A, Anson D, Haller S: Postural sway biofeedback—its effect on reestablishing stance stability in hemiplegic patients, *Arch Phys Med Rehabil* 69:395-400, 1988.

300. Sunderland A, Tinson DJ, Bradley EL et al: Enhanced physical therapy improved recovery of arm function after stroke. A randomized controlled trial, *J Neurol Neurosurg Psychiatry* 55:530-535, 1992.

301. Wolf SL, Binder-MacLeod SA: Electromyographic biofeedback applications to the hemiplegic patient, *Phys Ther* 63:1404-1413, 1983.

302. Geiger RA, Allen JB, O'Keefe J et al: Balance and mobility following stroke: effects of physical therapy interventions with and without biofeedback/forceplate training, *Phys Ther* 81:995-1005, 2001.

303. Armagan O, Tascioglu F, Oner C: Electromyographic biofeedback in the treatment of the hemiplegic hand: a placebo-controlled study, *Am J Phys Med Rehabil* 82:856-861, 2003.

304. Palmerund G, Kadefors R, Sporrong H et al: Voluntary redistribution of muscle activity in human shoulder muscles, *Ergonomics* 38:806-815, 1995.

305. Reynolds C: Electromyographic biofeedback evaluation of a computer keyboard operator with cumulative trauma disorder, *J Hand Ther* 7:25-27, 1994.

306. Thomas RE, Vaidya SC, Herrick RT et al: The effects of biofeedback on carpal tunnel syndrome, *Ergonomics* 36:353-361, 1993.

307. Young MS: Electromyographic biofeedback use in the treatment of voluntary posterior dislocation of the shoulder: a case study, *J Orthop Sports Phys Ther* 20:171-175, 1994.

308. Neblett R, Mayer TG, Gatchel RJ: Theory and rational for surface EMG-assisted stretching as an adjunct to chronic musculoskeletal pain rehabilitation, *Appl Psychophysiol Biofeedback* 28:139-146, 2003.

308a. Medlicott MS, Harris SR: A systematic review of effectiveness of exercise, manual therapy, relaxation training, and biofeedback in the management of temporomandibular disorder, *Phys Ther* 86:955-973, 2006.

309. Kuiken TA, Amir H, Scheidt RA: Computerized biofeedback knee goniometer: acceptance and effect on exercise behavior in post-total knee arthroplasty rehabilitation, *Arch Phys Med Rehabil* 85:1026-1030, 2004.

310. White SC, Lifeso RM: Altering asymmetric limb loading after hip arthroplasty using real-time dynamic feedback when walking, *Arch Phys Med Rehabil* 86:1958-1963, 2005.

311. Van Santen M, Bolwijn P, Verstappen F et al: A randomized clinical trial comparing fitness and biofeedback training versus basic treatment in patients with fibromyalgia, *J Rheumatol* 29:575-581, 2002.

311a. Verhagen A, Karels C, Bierma-Zeinstra S et al: Ergonomic and physiotherapeutic interventions for treating work-related complaints of the arm, neck or shoulder in adults, *Cochrane Database Syst Rev* 3:CD003471, 2006.

312. Hatfield BD, Spalding TW, Mahon AD et al: The effect of psychological strategies upon cardiorespiratory and muscular activity during treadmill running, *Med Sci Sports Exerc* 24:218-225, 1992.

313. Hawken MB, Jantti P, Waterston JA: The effect of sway feedback and loss of sensory cues in older women with a history of falls. In Woollacott MH, Horak F, editors: *Posture and gait-control mechanisms, vol 2,* Eugene, OR, 1992, University of Oregon Books, pp 263-266.

314. Howard S, Varley R: Using electropalatography to treat severe apraxia of speech, *Eur Disord Commun* 30:246-255, 1995.

315. Klose KJ, Needham BM, Schmidt D et al: An assessment of the contribution of electromyographic biofeedback as an adjunct in the physical training of spinal cord injured persons, *Arch Phys Med Rehabil* 74:453-456, 1993.

316. Leisman G, Zenhausern R, Ferentz A et al: Electromyographic effects of fatigue and task repetition on the validity of estimates of strong and weak muscles in applied kinesiological muscle-testing procedures, *Percept Mot Skills* 80:963-977, 1995.

317. Kwolek A, Pop T: Use of biological vicarious biofeedback in the rehabilitation of patients with brain damage [in Polish], *Neurol Neurochir Pol* 1(suppl):321-327, 1992.

318. Duckett S, Kramer T: Managing myoclonus secondary to anoxic encephalopathy through EMG biofeedback, *Brain Inj* 8:185-188, 1994.

319. Jones KR: Ambulatory bio-feedback for stress incontinence exercise regimes: a novel development of the perineometer, *J Adv Nurs* 19:509-512, 1994.

320. Burgio KL, Goode PS, Locher JL et al: Behavior training with and without biofeedback in the treatment of urge incontinence in older women: a randomized controlled trial, *JAMA* 288:2293-2299, 2002.

321. Aukee P, Immonen P, Laaksonen DE et al: The effect of home biofeedback training on stress incontinence, *Acta Obstet Gynecol Scand.* 83:973-977, 2004.

322. Pages IH, Jahr S, Schaufele MK et al: Comparative analysis of biofeedback and physical therapy for treatment of urinary stress incontinence in women, *Am J Phys Med Rehabil* 80:494-502, 2001.

322a. Lopes AA, Andrade J, Macedo A et al: Nonpharmacological treatment of lower urinary tract dysfunction using biofeedback and transcutaneous electrical stimulation: a pilot study, *BJU Int* 98:166-171, 2006.

322b. Hosker G: Biofeedback and/or sphincter exercises for the treatment of fecal incontinence in adults, *Cochrane Database Syst Rev* 3:CD002111, 2006.

323. Mahoney RT, Malone PA, Nalty J et al: Randomized clinical trial of intra-anal electromyographic biofeedback physiotherapy with intra-anal electromyographic biofeedback augmented with electrical stimulation of the anal sphincter in the early treatment of postpartum fecal incontinence, *Am J Obstet Gynecol* 191:885-890, 2004.

324. Heymen S, Jones KR, Ringel Y et al: Biofeedback treatment of fecal incontinence: a critical review, *Dis Colon Rectum* 44:728-736, 2001.

325. Anismus and biofeedback [editorial], *Lancet* 339:217-218, 1992.

326. Turnbull GK, Ritvo PG: Anal sphincter biofeedback relaxation treatment for women with intractable constipation symptoms, *Dis Colon Rectum* 35:530-536, 1993.

327. Blanc-Gras N, Esteve F, Benchetrit G et al: Performance and learning during voluntary control of breath patterns, *Biol Psychol* 37:147-159, 1994.

328. Mass R, Dahme B, Richter R: Clinical evaluation of respiratory resistance biofeedback training, *Biofeedback Self Regul* 18:211-223, 1993.

329. Nahmias J, Tansey M, Karetzky MS: Asthmatic extrathoracic upper airway obstruction: laryngeal dyskinesis, *N J Med* 91:616-620, 1994.

330. Lehrer P, Vaschillo E, Lu SE et al: Heart rate variability biofeedback: effects of age on heart rate variability, baroreflex gain, and asthma, *Chest* 129:278-284, 2006.

331. Lehrer PM, Vaschillo E, Vaschillo B et al: Biofeedback treatment for asthma, *Chest* 126:352-361, 2004.

332. Giardino ND, Chan L, Borson S: Combined heart rate variability and pulse oximetry biofeedback for chronic obstructive pulmonary disease: Preliminary findings, *Appl Psychophysiol Biofeedback* 29:121-133, 2004.

333. McGrady A: Effects of group relaxation training and thermal biofeedback on blood pressure and related physiological and psychological variables in essential hypertension, *Biofeedback Self Regul* 19:51-66, 1994.

334. Vasilevskii NN, Sidorov YA, Kiselev IM: Biofeedback control of systemic arterial pressure, *Neurosci Behav Physiol* 22:219-223, 1992.

335. Del Paso GA, González MI: Modification of baroreceptor cardiac reflex function by biofeedback, *Appl Psychophysiol Biofeedback* 29:197-211, 2004.

336. Vaschillo E, Lehrer P, Rishe N et al: Heart rate variability biofeedback as a method for assessing baroreflex function: a preliminary study of resonance in the cardiovascular system, *Appl Psychophysiol Biofeedback* 27:1-27, 2002.

337. Nakao M, Yano E, Nomura S et al: Blood pressure-lowering effects of biofeedback treatment in hypertension: a meta-analysis of randomized controlled trials, *Hypertens Res* 26:37-46, 2003.

338. Fiero PL, Galper DI, Cox DJ et al: Thermal biofeedback and lower extremity blood flow in adults with diabetes: is neuropathy is limiting factor? *Appl Psychophysiol Biofeedback* 28:193-203, 2003.

339. Rice BI, Schindler JV: Effect of thermal biofeedback-assisted relaxation training on blood circulation in the lower extremities of a population with diabetes, *Diabetes Care* 15:853-858, 1992.

340. Sheffied MM: Psychosocial interventions in the management of recurrent headache disorders: policy considerations for implementation, *Behav Med* 20:73-77, 1994.

341. Reyes del Paso GA, Godoy J, Vila J: Self-regulation of respiratory sinus arrhythmia, *Biofeedback Self Regul* 17:261-275, 1992.

342. Lehrer PM, Carr P, Sargunaraj D et al: Stress management techniques: are they all equivalent, or do they have specific effects? *Biofeedback Self Regul* 19:353-401, 1994.

343. Van Zak DB: Biofeedback treatments for premenstrual affective syndromes, *Int J Psychosom* 41:53-60, 1994.

344. Blumenstein B, Breslav I, Bar-Eli M et al: Regulation of mental states and biofeedback techniques: effects on breathing pattern, *Biofeedback Self Regul* 20:169-183, 1995.

345. Freedman RR, Keegan D, Rodriguez J et al: Plasma catecholamine levels during temperature biofeedback training in normal subjects, *Biofeedback Self Regul* 18:107-114, 1993.

346. Lehrer PM, Carr P, Sargunaraj D et al: Stress management techniques: are they all equivalent, or do they have specific effects? *Biofeedback Self Regul* 19:353-401, 1994.

347. Montgomery GT: Slowed respiration training, *Biofeedback Self Regul* 19:211-225, 1994.

348. Shahidi S, Salmon P: Contingent and non-contingent biofeedback training for type A and B healthy adults: can type A's relax by competing? *J Psychosom Res* 36:477-483, 1992.

349. Crary MA, Carnaby Mann GD, Groher ME et al: Functional benefits of dysphagia therapy using adjunctive sEMG biofeedback, *Dysphagia* 19:160-164, 2004.

350. Sukthankar SM, Reddy NP, Canilang EP et al: Design and development of probable biofeedback systems for use in oral dysphagia rehabilitation, *Med Eng Phys* 16:430-435, 1994.

351. Bryant M: Biofeedback in the treatment of a selected dysphagic patient, *Dysphagia* 6:140-144, 1991.

352. Segal B, Zompa I, Danys I et al: Symmetry and synkinesis during rehabilitation of unilateral facial paralysis, *J Otolaryngol* 24:143-148, 1995.

353. Segal B, Hunter T, Danys I et al: Minimizing synkinesis during rehabilitation of the paralyzed face: Preliminary assessment of a new small-movement therapy, *J Otolaryngol* 24:149-153, 1995.

354. Middaugh SJ, Pawlick K: Biofeedback and behavioral treatment of persistent pain in the older adult: a review and a study, *Appl Psychophysiol Biofeedback* 27:185-202, 2002.

355. Harden RN, Houle TT, Green S et al: Biofeedback in the treatment of phantom limb pain: a time-series analysis, *Appl Psychophysiol Biofeedback* 30:83-93, 2005.

356. Ahles TA: Psychological approaches to the management of cancer-related pain, *Semin Oncol Nurs* 1:141-146, 1985.

357. Blum RH: Hypothesis: a new basis for sentry-behavioral pretreatments to ameliorate radiation therapy-induced nausea and vomiting [review], *Cancer Treat Rev* 15:211-227, 1988.

358. Contanch PH: Relaxation techniques as an independent nursing intervention for oncology patients [review], *Cancer Nurs* 10(suppl 1):58-64, 1987.

359. Ferrell BR, Ferrell BA: Easing the pain. *Geriatr Nurs* 11:175-178, 1990.

360. Stoudemire A, Cotanch P, Laszlo J: Recent advances in the pharmacologic and behavioral management of chemotherapy-induced emesis [review], *Arch Intern Med* 144:1029-1033, 1984.

361. Cassetta RA: Biofeedback can improve patient outcomes, *Am Nurse* 25:25-27, 1993.

361a. Patrick GJ: Neurotherapy: using biofeedback for difficult health problems, *Topics in Adv Prac Nurs* 2:1-8, 2002.

Music Therapy References

362. American Music Therapy Association: What is music therapy? *Frequently asked questions about music therapy:* http://www.musictherapy.org/faqs.html. Accessed October 2, 2005.

363. Hodges DA, Haak PA: The influence of music on human behavior. In Hodges DA, editor,: *Handbook of music psychology,* San Antonio, 1999, MMB Music, pp 469-555.

364. Davis WB, Gfeller KE: Music therapy: A historical perspective. In Davis D, Gfeller K, Thaut M, editors: *An introduction to music therapy theory and practice,* Boston, 1999, McGraw-Hill, pp 15-34.

365. Thaut MH, McIntosh GC, Rice RR, Miller RA, Rathbun J, Brault JM: Rhythmic auditory stimulation in gait training for Parkinson's disease patients, *Movement Disord* 11:193-200, 1996.

366. Körlin D: A neuropsychological theory of traumatic imagery in the Bonny Method of Guided Imagery and Music (BMGIM). In Bruscia KE, Grocke DE, editors: *Guided imagery and music: the Bonny Method and beyond,* Gilsum, NH, 2002, Barcelona, pp 379-415.

367. McKinney C: Quantitative research in guided imagery and music (GIM): a review. In Bruscia KE, Grocke DE, editors: *Guided imagery and music: the Bonny Method and beyond,* Gilsum, NH, 2002, Barcelona, pp 449-466.

368. American Music Therapy Association: *What is music therapy?* http://www.musictherapy.org/. Accessed October 2, 2005.

369. Standley JM: Music research in medical/dental treatment: an update of a prior meta-analysis. In Furman CE, editor: *Effectiveness of music therapy procedures: documentation of research and clinical practice,* ed 2, Silver Spring, MD, 1996, NAMT.

370. Cassidy JW, Standley JM: The effect of music listening on physiological responses of premature infants in the NICU, *J Music Ther* 28:208-227, 1995.

371. Lorch CA, Lorch V, Diefendorf AO et al: Effect of stimulative and sedative music on systolic blood pressure, heart rate, and respiratory rate in premature infants, *J Music Ther* 31:105-118, 1994.

372. Caine J: Effects of music on the selected stress behaviors, weight, caloric and formula intake, and length of hospital stay of premature and low birth weight neonates in a newborn intensive care unit, *J Music Ther* 28:180-192, 1991.

373. Whipple DH: The newborn individualized developmental care and assessment program (NIDCAP) as a model for clinical music therapy interventions with premature infants, *J Music Ther* 37:250-268, 2000.

374. Nöcker-Ribaupierre M, editor: *Music therapy for premature and newborn infants* (S. Weber, translator), Philadelphia, 2004, Barcelona.

375. Standley JM: The role of music in pacification/stimulation of premature infants with low birth weights, *Music Ther Perspect* 9:19-25, 1991.

376. Cassidy JW, Ditty KM: Presentation of aural stimuli to newborns and premature infants: an audiological perspective, *J Music Ther* 35:70-87, 1998.

377. Abromeit DH: The newborn individualized developmental care and assessment program (NIDCAP) as a model for clinical music therapy interventions with premature infants, *Music Ther Perspect* 21:60-68, 2003.

378. Tomaino CM: Active music therapy approaches for neurologically impaired patients. In Dileo C, editor: *Music therapy and medicine: theoretical and clinical applications,* pp 115-122, Silver Spring, 1999, American Music Therapy Association.

379. Thaut MH: *Rhythm, music and the brain: scientific foundations and clinical applications,* New York, 2005, Routledge.

380. Thaut MH, Miller RA, Schauer LM: Multiple synchronization strategies in rhythmic sensorimotor tasks: phase vs. period correction, *Biol Cybernetics* 79:241-250, 1998.

381. Thaut MH, McIntosh GC, Prassas SG et al: Effect of rhythmic auditory cuing on temporal stride parameters and EMG patterns in normal gait, *J Neurol Rehabil* 6:185-190, 1992.

382. Thaut MH, McIntosh GC, Prassas SG et al: Effect of rhythmic auditory cuing on temporal stride parameters and EMG patterns in hemiparetic gait of stroke patients, *J Neurol Rehabil* 7:9-16, 1993.

383. Prassas S, Thaut M, McIntosh G et al: Effect of auditory rhythmic cuing on gait kinematic parameters of stroke patients, *Gait Posture* 6:218-223, 1997.

384. Thaut MH, McIntosh GC, Rice RR: Rhythmic facilitation of gait training in hemiparetic stroke rehabilitation, *J Neurol Sci* 151:207-212, 1997.

385. Hurt CP, Rice RR, McIntosh GC et al: Rhythmic auditory stimulation in gait training for patients with traumatic brain injury, *J Music Ther* 35:228-241, 1998.

386. Thaut MH, McIntosh GC, Rice RR et al: Rhythmic auditory stimulation in gait training for Parkinson's disease patients, *Movement Disord* 11:193-200, 1996.

387. Thaut MH, McIntosh KW, McIntosh GC et al: Auditory rhythmicity enhances movement and speech motor control in patients with Parkinson's disease, *Funct Neurol* 16:163-172, 2001.

388. Baker F, Kennelly J, Tamplin J: Themes in songs written by patients with traumatic brain injury: Differences across the lifespan, *Aust J Music Ther* 16:25-42, 2005.

389. Erdonmez D: Rehabilitation of piano performance skills following a left cerebral vascular accident. In Bruscia K, editor: *Case studies in music therapy,* Philadelphia, 1991, Barcelona, pp 561-670.

390. McMaster N: Reclaiming a positive identity: music therapy in the aftermath of a stroke. In Bruscia K, editor: *Case studies in music therapy,* Philadelphia, 1991, Barcelona, pp 547-559.

391. Goldberg FS, Hoss TM, Chesna T: Music and imagery as psychotherapy with a brain damaged patient: a case study, *Music Ther Perspect* 5:41-45, 1988.

392. Short A: Enhancing the health care team: GIM and physical illness or injury. In Proceedings of the inaugural conference of the Music and Imagery Association of Australia, Lower Plenty, Victoria, 2002, MIAA, pp 9-22.

ADDITIONAL RECOMMENDED READING AND WEBSITES FOR MUSIC THERAPY

Association for Music and Imagery/AMI: *The Bonny method of guided imagery and music:* http://www.bonnymethod.com/ami. Accessed October 2, 2005.

American Music Therapy Association/AMTA: *Standards of clinical practice committee news:* http://www.musictherapy.org/membersonly/official/com_standards.html. Accessed October 2, 2005.

Standley JM: Music research in medical/dental treatment: an update of a prior meta-analysis. In Furman CE, editor: *Effectiveness of music therapy procedures: documentation of research and clinical practice,* ed 2, Silver Spring, MD, 1996, NAMT.

Standley JM: *Music therapy with premature infants: research and developmental interventions,* Silver Spring, MD, 2003 American Music Therapy Association.

Glossary

abnormal movement strategies Movement patterns that are inefficient, exaggerated or stereotypic when an individual uses that movement either in an activity or an isolated volitional movement.

abulia A loss or deficiency of will power.

acquired brain injury Brain injury that occurred after birth. The individual was considered to have a normal CNS prior to that injury.

ACTH (adrenocorticotropic hormone) A hormone released by the adenohypophysis, which stimulates the adrenal cortex to secrete its entire spectrum of hormones. Thought to be immunosuppressive and antiinflammatory in treating multiple sclerosis.

acute That period of time immediately following spinal cord injury when the management of all primary injuries and the prevention of further complications are the emphasis of care.

acute pain Pain that arises from stimulation of the nociceptors and functions as a warning system of impending or actual tissue injury.

adaptation The process or state of changing to fit new circumstances or condition.

adaptive response An appropriate response to an environmental demand. Adaptive responses require good sensory integration; they also allow the sensory integrative process to progress.

adjustment The ongoing process of responding to the world with a positive adaptive response that allows the person and significant others to grow and mature in regard to all aspects of life.

adverse drug reactions An unexpected reaction following administration of a specific drug which has potentially negative affects on some system within the patient.

agraphia Loss of ability to write.

aging A normal process of changing with time, especially during the later part of life.

AIDS A disease of the immune system caused by infection with the retrovirus HIV, which destroys certain white blood cells and is transmitted through blood or bodily secretions such as semen.

alcoholism A disease characterized by chronic, heavy consumption of alcohol, which may lead to peripheral nerve disease, cerebellar degeneration, and other systemic and psychiatric symptoms that impair health and function.

alexia Word blindness: inability to recognize or comprehend written or printed words.

Alzheimer's disease A term used as a diagnosis when, based on the symptoms of confusion and impaired intellectual functioning, all other possible causes have been eliminated. It is not possible to ascertain whether a client has this disease until an autopsy or brain biopsy has been done. At present, there is no known cause or treatment for Alzheimer's disease, but clients and families can be helped to cope better with the presenting losses of intellectual functioning.

amblyopia Dimness of vision not caused by refractive error or organic disease of the eye.

Amigo A scooterlike, battery-operated vehicle.

amniocentesis A procedure in which a needle is passed through the mother's abdomen into the amniotic sac of the fetus. Amniotic fluid is withdrawn and analyzed to detect a variety of abnormalities.

amygdala A nuclear mass within the anterior portion of the temporal lobe involved with limbic function, especially arousal, motivation, and declarative learning.

amyotrophic lateral sclerosis A fatal degenerative disease of the central nervous system marked by axonal death in the lateral columns of the spinal cord which residual muscle weakness and atrophy. It is also called Lou Gehrig's disease.

angiography The visualization of blood vessels by injection of a nontoxic radiopaque material.

ankle-foot orthosis (AFO) An external device which controls the foot and ankle complex, and can be utilized to generate forces about the knee.

ANS (autonomic nervous system) pain Pain arising from injuries within the sympathetic or parasympathetic nervous systems.

anterior/toe lever arm An orthotic device that creates a substitute for the lack of strength the anterior lever arm provides.

anterograde amnesia The inability to establish new memories.

anticholinergic Blocking the passage of impulses at cholinergic postsynaptic receptor sites; also an agent that so acts.

anticipatory responses The use of information about the environment and from past experience to plan and program intended actions for the immediate future.

anxiolytic An agent that reduces anxiety.

aphasia An impairment caused by brain damage, which interferes with the ability to process language symbols. It is disproportionate to impairment of other intellectual functions and is not caused by dementia, sensory loss, or motor dysfunction.

apraxia of speech An articulatory disorder resulting from the inability to program the position of speech muscles and the sequence of muscle movements in order to volitionally produce speech. The disorder results from an impairment arising from brain damage.

Arnold-Chiari malformation A deformity in which the medulla and pons are reduced in size, and the cerebellum herniates into the spinal canal.

ASIA American Spinal Injury Association

aspiration The act of inhaling fluids or substances into the lungs or the removal of fluids and gases from a cavity by suction.

asthenia Chronic lack of strength and energy.

astrocytoma A nerve-tissue tumor composed of astrocytes which are comparatively large much-branded.

ataxia Loss of muscular coordination.

ataxia-telangiectasia An inherited disorder characterized by progressive ataxia, oculocutaneous dilation of terminal arteries and capillaries, sinopulmonary disease, and abnormal eye movements.

athetosis From the Greek origin of the word: "without posture"; a dyskinetic condition that includes inadequate timing, force, accuracy, and coordination of movement in the limbs and trunk.

atypical movements Not conforming to the usual type or expected pattern of movement

augmented intervention The use of therapeutic intervention strategies, such as the therapist's hands, to augment or enhance the patient's ability to perform or participate in a functional activity or therapeutic procedure.

autism A disorder that in childhood is characterized by withdrawal behavior, reduced socialization, perseveration, bizarre behavior, lack of purposeful verbal communication, and echolalia.

autogenic movement patterns (AMPs) Movements of body segments (e.g., head, limbs, trunk) that are the result of spontaneous activity of motor neurons; in contrast to reflexive or volitional (voluntary) movements.

Autoimmune Disease in which the body produces a disordered immunological response against its own tissue. Antibodies against normal parts of the body are produced to an extent that causes tissue injury.

automatic postural responses Functionally organized, long-loop responses that produce muscle activation to bring the body's center of gravity into a state of equilibrium. Examples: ankle strategy, hip strategy.

automatic speech Words or phrases spoken without voluntary control, such as curse words, expletives, and greetings.

autonomic dysfunction An uncompensated reaction from either the parasympathetic or sympathetic division of the autonomic system following disease, injury, or chemical imbalances; more often observed within the sympathetic system as a reaction to a noxious stimulus that exhibits itself as a visceral response, such as sweating or increased heart rate.

autonomic dysreflexia An uninhibited and exaggerated reflex response of the autonomic nervous system to stimulation. It is often referred to as autonomic hyperreflexia.

autonomic hyperreflexia A reaction of the autonomic (involuntary) nervous system to over-stimulation. This reaction may include high blood pressure, change in heart rate, skin color changes (pallor, redness, blue-gray coloration), and profuse sweating.

Avonex (interferon beta-1a) Is used to treat the relapsing forms of multiple sclerosis (MS). This medicine will not cure MS, but it may slow some disabling effects and decrease the number of relapses of the disease.

axonal damage Damage to a section of the nerve between the cell body and the presynaptic cleft or presynaptic junction.

axonotmesis Interruption of the axon with subsequent wallerian degeneration; connective tissue of the nerve, including the Schwann cell basement membrane, remains intact.

babbling A stage in speech development characterized by the production of strings of speech sounds in vocal play.

balance The ability to control the center of gravity over the base of support in a given sensory environment.

ballistic movement High-velocity movement, such as a tennis serve or boxer's punch, requiring reciprocal organization of agonistic and antagonistic synergies.

basal ganglia A collection of nuclei at the base of the cerebral cortex. It includes the caudate nucleus, putamen, globus pallidus, and functionally includes the substantia nigra and subthalamic nucleus.

base of support The surfaces of the body that experience pressure as a result of body weight and gravity, and the projected area between them.

behavioral manipulations The use of modifications within the external environment such as exercise or the modification of the internal environment using tools such as hypnosis, operant conditioning and biofeedback which will change the pain behavior of the patient.

Betaseron (interferon beta-1b) A drug distributed by Berlex Labs (Richmond, CA) licensed by the U.S. Food and Drug Administration in 1993 for the treatment of relapsing/remitting multiple sclerosis (MS). The drug is based on interferon beta, which is a protein formed by the body when cells are exposed to viruses. The drug has an immunomodulatory effect and in clinical trials reduced disease activity in relapsing/remitting MS.

biasing motor generators Modulatory influence through synaptic excitation and inhibition over the resting state of the motor generators.

biofeedback A cognitive treatment technique in which the client becomes aware of and learns to selectively change physiological processes with the aid of an external monitor

biopsy The removal of a sample of tissue from a living person for laboratory examination

bite reflex This pathological reflex is a swift biting action produced by stimulation of the oral cavity. The bite may be difficult to release in some cases when an object such as a spoon or tongue depressor has been introduced into the mouth.

body scanning A cognitive treatment technique in which clients are taught to view their pain objectively in order to separate themselves from their pain.

bonding The process of creating a connection that results in trust and respect between two or more individuals.

brain abscess A localized collection of pus in a cavity formed by the disintegration of brain tissue.

bulbocavernosus reflex A reflexive response of the bowel triggered by fecal material. In patients with SCI a positive bulbocavernosus reflex is reflex bowel which means tone of the internal and external anal sphincter is present.

capitation a fixed amount of a payment or fee that can be charged or will be paid for a medical or therapeutic service.

caregiver checklists A list of activities to be practiced as a home program given to the caregiver

cardiopulmonary complications Systems or medical complications that arise within the cardiac and/or pulmonary system. Complications can arise from internal disease or pathology or from the environmental demands placed upon the individual during life activities.

caregiver training and support (1) Organizing educational experiences to assist caregivers to be better able to assist or perform needed tasks for patients; (2) organizing experiences (group or individual) to assist caregivers to cope with the challenges of performing as a caregiver. The support can be in the form of physical assistance or psychosocial activities.

causalgia ANS pain characterized by intense burning and hyperesthesia throughout the distribution of an incompletely damaged peripheral nerve.

center of gravity An imaginary point in space about which the sum of the forces and moments equals zero (equilibrium).

cerebellar atrophy (spinocerebellar degeneration) A general term for several familial disorders in which the cerebellum deteriorates.

cerebellum The part of the brain located directly below the occipital lobe and posterior to the other cerebral hemispheric lobes. Its main function is to control and coordinate muscular activities during motor programs such as balance.

cerebellar disease Disease within the cerebellum that results in medically significant movement problems in a human.

cerebral evoked potentials (EPs) Study of potentials evoked from the cortex, including visually evoked potentials (VEPs) stimulated by light, auditory evoked potentials (AEPs) stimulated by sound, and somatosensory evoked potentials (SSEPs) stimulated by electrical stimulation of the peripheral sensory nerves.

cerebral palsy A diagnostic term applied principally to a history of anoxia for a variety of reasons shortly before, during, or after the birth process, up to 2 years of age. The same conditions or experiences are often labeled with alternate diagnostic terms that vary with the geographical area and the clinic policy.

chemotherapy The use of chemical agents to treat disease, infections, and other disorders, especially cancer.

chewing reflex Pathological signs elicited in brain-damaged adults when the mouth is stimulated and repetitive chewing motions ensue.

childhood aphasia A disturbance of the capacity to process language resulting from brain dysfunction in childhood.

chorea Involuntary movements of the face and extremities that are of short duration, spasmodic, irregular; frequently involve a component of rotation.

chronic pain Pain that occurs without a clear stimulus to the nociceptors, in response to innocuous stimulation or in a prolonged exaggerated fashion to noxious stimulation.

climbing fibers One of two fiber types carrying input to cerebellar cortex; terminates in 1:1 relationship on a Purkinje cell.

clinical electromyography An electrophysiological evaluation encompassing the observation, recording, analysis, and interpretation of bioelectric muscle and nerve potentials detected by means of needle electrodes inserted into the muscles for the purpose of evaluating the integrity of the neuromuscular system.

clinical problem solving A method of analyzing specific questions that are difficult or perplexing, whose solution will be founded on actual observation and treatment of a patient as distinguished from data or facts obtained by experimentation or pathology.

closure Visualization of the whole figure when only a portion is visible.

CMS An abbreviation for Centers for Medicare and Medicaid Services.

CNS pain Pain arising from central nervous system lesions.

cognition The mind processes that allow the individual to perceive and be aware of the self, objects, and others in a person's internal or external environment.

cognitive-behavioral methods Treatment methods that deal with the sensory/discriminative, motivational/affective, and cognitive/evaluative aspects of pain.

cognitive strategies Relaxation exercises; body scanning; humor: strategies taught to a patient using the patient's cognition and understanding of how to relax the motor system.

cold application The use of cooling modalities to accomplish a therapeutic goal.

coma A complete paralysis of cerebral function, a state of unresponsiveness. Clients do not obey commands, speak, or open their eyes.

communication A reciprocal act of social interaction and sending/receiving information through conventional symbol systems (e.g., language) and affective messages (e.g., smiling). Customary rules of communication are established within individual social cultures.

complete lesion A lesion in which there is absence of sensory and motor function in the lowest spinal segment.

complex regional pain syndrome (CRPS) An example of pain that arises from abnormal activity within the ANS. CRPS has been classified into two distinct types: CRPS type I (formerly reflex sympathetic dystrophy) follows mild trauma without nerve injury, and CRPS type II (formerly causalgia) follows trauma with nerve injury. CRPS type I generally begins within the month after the injury, whereas CRPS type II can occur any time after the injury

complex spatial relations Relationship of one figure or part of a figure to another.

composite impairments The combined effects of the primary and secondary impairments, motor recovery, effects of treatment, and behavioral factors.

computed axial tomography (CT or CAT scan) An x-ray technique designed to show detailed images of structures on separate planes of tissue. When combined, these images can often detail multiple sclerosis lesions and other neurological deficits.

concentric contraction Controlled shortening of the muscle.

conceptual disorders A disturbance in thought processes, in cognitive activities, or in the ability to formulate concepts.

configuration Overall shape or enclosure of a figure.

constancy The invariant quality of distinctive features in spite of valuation in location, rotation, size, or color.

contrecoup injury Injury to the brain produced distant to the part sustaining the blow.

Copaxone (glatiramer acetate) An artificial protein that resembles a natural myelin protein. It is not known exactly how the medication works, but it may help people who have multiple sclerosis by preventing the body's immune system from attacking the myelin coating that protects nerve fibers. It is used with relapsing-remitting MS which is a form of MS in which symptoms randomly flare up (relapse) and then improve or fade (remission).

coping Behaviors used to respond to positive or negative stressors in a person's environment in an effort to overcome or deal with them.

copolymer 1 (Copaxone, glatiramer) A drug under study by TEVA Pharmaceuticals (Kulpsville, PA), which in clinical trials is reported to reduce the frequency of exacerbations in early exacerbating/remitting MS.

cor pulmonale Heart disease due to pulmonary hypertension secondary to lung disease with right ventricular hypertrophy.

cortisone, prednisone Synthetic adrenal glucocorticoids, used in multiple sclerosis to reduce edema and other aspects of inflammation. They are immunosuppressive and have also been shown to be useful in improving nerve conduction in demyelinated fibers.

coup injury Injury to the brain at the site of the impact.

CPT An abbreviation for "current procedural terminology" and is published by the American Medical Association. It is a code set designed to identify the interventions and other services performed by health care providers.

crouch-control ankle-foot orthosis A ankle-foot orthotic device that is controlled at the pelvis.

cryosurgery   Technique of exposing tissues to extreme cold to produce well-demarcated areas of cell destruction. The cold is usually produced by use of a probe containing liquid nitrogen; in rare cases, used to destroy thalamic tissue in persons with MS to control severe tremor and other involuntary movements.

Cytokines   Any of a class of immunoregulatory proteins (as interleukin, tumor necrosis factor, and interferon) that are secreted by cells especially of the immune system

declarative memory   The mental registration, retention, and recall of past experiences, sensations, ideas, knowledge, and thoughts. This memory has a high cognitive basis to it. The original data must relay through the amygdala or hippocampal nuclear structures before long-term storage is possible.

Deconditioning   A process that negatively impacts the ability to perform activities of daily living and participate in life that occurs to the human body following disuse.

decorticate rigidity   A term derived from animal transections, sometimes used to describe abnormal posturing in humans, that is characterized by exaggerated flexor responses in the upper extremities and exaggerated extensor responses in the lower extremities. In reporting, it is preferable to describe the posture observed.

decubitus ulcer   An ulcer resulting from pressure to an area of the body, usually from a bed or chair; the heels, sacrum, ischia, and trochanters are most prone to the development of these ulcers.

deep vein thrombosis   The existence of a blood clot within a deep vein.

Deiter nucleus   One of the vestibular nuclei, also known as the lateral vestibular nuclei; located in the brain stem.

delayed language   Failure of language to develop at the expected age because of any number of causes such as hearing loss, emotional disturbance, or brain injury.

delegation   The giving of some power or responsibility to an assistant, an aide or a family member

delirium   A delirious person shows both a change in intellectual function and in the level of consciousness. The client is less alert than normal and may be confused, disoriented, forgetful, and/or sleepy. Other commonly used terms to describe this condition are acute brain syndrome and reversible brain syndrome. If the underlying medical or emotional problem(s) is treated in a timely fashion, the level of alertness and intellectual function will return to normal.

dementia   An impairment in some or all aspects of intellectual functioning in a person who is clearly awake. Other terms used to describe this condition are organic brain syndrome, senility, senile dementia, hardening of the arteries, and shrinking of the brain. Some diseases that can cause dementia are treatable. In these diseases the distortion of intellectual capacity is reversed when treatment is given and/or the intellectual functioning is prevented from becoming worse.

demyelination   The process of breakdown or destruction of the myelin sheath surrounding the axons of nerve tissue.

dentate nucleus   One of the deep cerebellar nuclei; found lateral to the emboliform nucleus, within the cerebellar hemisphere; receives fibers from the lateral zone of the cerebellar cortex; fibers leave nucleus via brachium conjunctivum; is considered part of the neocerebellum.

developmental coordination disorder   Problems with movement coordination that manifest themselves when an individual is a child.

developmental disabilities   Problems that limit one's functional ability that have been caused from lack of development or damage to the nervous system that affect the child and later the adults ability to participate various activities of life.

developmental dyspraxia   A disorder of sensory integration characterized by an impairment in the ability to plan skilled nonhabitual movement.

developmental handling   Moving a child through part or all of the developmental sequence to enhance the expression of normal movement patterns (i.e., righting and equilibrium reactions).

developmental theory   Characterized as a systematic statement of principles and generalizations that provides a coherent framework for studying development.

diagnosis by a physical or occupational therapist   The conclusions drawn following a thorough examination that clearly identify the functional limitations of the individual and the system and subsystem impairments that are causing those limitations. These profession-specific conclusions are measurable and lay the foundation for prognosis and selection of treatment interventions and are based on disablement/enablement or human performance-based models.

diagnostic model: examination, evaluation, diagnosis, prognosis, intervention   A diagnostic model used by movement specialists to describe the process used when analyzing clients with movement dysfunction in order to identify impairments, functional limitation (where a patient has and does not have activity limitations) and how intervention would increase the clients ability to participate in life and increase that quality.

diastematomyelia   Congenital division of all or part of the spinal cord

Differential Diagnosis Phase 1   The first aspect of differential diagnosis when a therapist does medical screening to identify whether the movement problems fall within their respective scope of practice or should be referred to another practitioner.

Differential Diagnosis Phase 2   The second aspect of differential diagnosis when a therapist has identified that the movement dysfunction falls within his/her scope of practice, and the therapist must examine, evaluation, identify the movement problems, prognose the potential durations and outcome of treatment and clearly identify with the assistance of the patient and/or family the treatment protocol that will best match the desired outcomes.

dioptric power   Unit of measurement of the refractive power of an optic lens.

diplopia   Double vision.

direct intervention   Hands-on therapy to enhance the possibility of new motor learning when movement and postural control is inadequate.

disability   Any restriction or lack of ability to perform an activity in a normal manner or within the normal range. Examples: requires a cane to walk, requires assistance to transfer, etc.

disablement model   An evaluation and treatment model based on the specific impairment, functional loss, and quality of life attainable, not on the medical diagnosis of the injury or disease process.

distal sparing   The spinal cord below the congenital lesion remains intact. The reflex arc through the spinal cord therefore remains but is unmodified by supraspinal influences. This results in spastic movements distal to the level of the lesion.

disuse atrophy Reduction in muscle size and number in response to lack of use of that muscle in normal activities of daily living

disease A condition that results in medically significant symptoms. Disease can be acute or chronic and usually has recognizable signs and symptoms often having a known cause.

double-adjustable ankle joint An orthosis that is both adjustable and supports the ankle joint on both the lateral and medial sides

drug interactions The effect a drug has upon various bodily systems or the summation of the effects of various drugs upon bodily system. These drug interactions can be positive and negative depending on the body systems reaction to its influence.

drug disposition Refers to the absorption, distribution, metabolism, and excretion of a drug.

drug therapy The use of a natural or artificial substance to treat, prevent, or diagnose a disease; to lessen pain; or to modify an abnormal movement response during activities.

Duchenne muscular dystrophy A form of muscular dystrophy that attacks the muscles of the upper respiratory and pelvic areas first, with a higher incidence in boys than girls.

ductions Movements of one eye from the primary position into the secondary or tertiary positions of gaze.

dynamic equilibrium Ability of clients to adjust to displacements of their center of gravity by appropriately changing their base of support.

dysarthria A disorder of articulation resulting from impairment of the central or peripheral nervous system in the control of the muscles of speech—errors in articulation of speech sounds.

dysdiadochokinesia Inability to perform rapidly alternating motion.

dysesthesias Sensation is impaired, but not absent. Often used when referring to "pins and needles" sensation.

dyskinesia A defect in voluntary movements.

dysmetria An inability to position the limbs accurately with respect to another object.

dysphagia A disorder of swallowing.

dystonia An abnormal involuntary sustained movement or posture involving the contraction of a group of muscles.

dystrophin Protein that is missing or defective in Duchenne muscular dystrophy which is localized to the sarcolemma of the muscle cell membrane. Its absence results in abnormal cell permeability, which may lead to cell destruction.

eccentric contraction Controlled lengthening of a muscle.

echolalia Automatic reiteration of words or phrases that have been heard.

ecology Study of the environmental relations of organisms.

edema An abnormal buildup of serous fluid between tissue cells.

effectiveness in practice Results of an intervention that demonstrates through objective measurement that the intervention selected was effective.

ego-dystonic Destructive to self-enhancement.

ego-syntonic Supportive of self-enhancement.

electrical stimulation Study of muscle response to electrical currents including reaction of degeneration (RD), rheobase and chronaxy, strength-duration (SD), and galvanic-tetanus ratio tests.

electroencephalography (EEG) Study of the electrical activity of the brain.

electroglottography Process of measuring changes in electrical potential across membrane of the glottal tissue.

electromyographic biofeedback (EMGBF) Use of electronic instrumentation to elevate normally subconscious electromyographic potentials to a conscious level through auditory or visual signals, so that muscle contractions may be facilitated, inhibited, or coordinated for neuromuscular activity.

electroneuromyography (ENMG) The electrical activity of the muscles and their associated motor and sensory nerves.

electronystagmography Study of eye movements to evaluate vestibular function.

electrophoresis The movement of charged particles through the medium in which they are dispersed as a result of changes in electric potential; useful in analysis of protein mixtures because protein particles move with different velocities.

electroretinography Study of the potentials produced by the light-sensitive tissues of the retina.

emboliform nucleus One of the deep cerebellar nuclei in humans; receives input from intermediate zone of the cerebellum; involved in control of posture and voluntary movement.

emotional behavior Motor behavior activated by chemical reactions induced by emotional responses. The motor patterns activated by specific emotions elicit specific pattern generators.

empowerment The process by which power or authority over all aspects of self is reassumed by the client.

enablement model A model whose major focus is on the functional abilities and potential of a patient with movement dysfunction to engage empower that individual in success with activities of daily living and participation in life.

encephalitis Inflammation of the brain tissue.

encephalomeningitis Inflammation of the meninges and the brain substance.

end-feel Sensation experienced by therapist at the end of a patient's passive range of motion. May be springy or an abrupt halt, bone-to-bone, capsular, or tissue approximation.

endogenous opiates Naturally occurring substances that produce opiate-like effects, including analgesia.

endoscopy Examination of organs accessible to observation through an endoscope (small tube with light camera), which is inserted through the mouth.

energetic-based theories Theories based on the assumption that there is an energy field around and through the human body which can be used as a therapeutic modality to help the patient and/or practitioner correct the energy imbalances that are causing health issues. Once these balances are corrected healing will begin and continue as long as the imbalance is not reassumed.

energy conservation Movement activities that reduce the amount of energy needed by the individual when participating in life.

environmental modification External changes within the environment of the patient that will empower that individual or the family to function with less stress, physical demands, and/or frustration.

epicritic Pertaining to the somatic sensations of fine discriminative touch, vibration, two-point discrimination, stereognosis, and conscious and unconscious proprioception.

ergotropic Combinations of cortical alpha rhythm, sympathetic nervous system activity, and somatic muscle activation; activity or work state.

evaluation A process used by therapists to analyze the results of examination and determine the best course of intervention given all the internal and external environmental variables.

evidence-based practice Interventions that are selected because of the objective and identifiable evidence available to justify those decisions. Evidence can be based either on effectiveness as measured through objective, reliable, and valid instrumentation or through controlled efficacy studies.

evoked potentials The electrical manifestation of the brain's reception of and response to an external stimulus; a way of measuring efficiency in the CNS.

exacerbating-remitting An unpredictable disease course characterized by episodes of symptom appearance or worsening followed by partial or complete recovery.

exacerbation An increase in the symptoms of a disease or pathology.

examination A set of identifiable measures used to collect objective data regarding the individual's functional limitations or system/subsystem deficits (impairments)

exercise Physical or mental activity or movement, especially when intended to keep a person alert, fit, and healthy. A series of actions, movements or tasks performed repeatedly or regularly as a way of practicing and improving a skill or procedure.

exercise tolerance The ability of the individual to perform exercise without harm or danger to any system such as the heart, lungs, circulatory system.

experimental allergic encephalomyelitis (EAE) An inflammatory autoimmune disease that has been induced in laboratory animals and especially mice by injecting them with diseased tissue from affected animals or with myelin basic protein and that because of the similarity of its pathology to multiple sclerosis in humans is used as an animal model in studying the condition.

experimental autoimmune encephalomyelitis (EAE) An induced, laboratory model of multiple sclerosis characterized by inflammation and demyelination.

exteroceptive Receptors activated primarily by stimuli from the external environment.

extrafusal muscle Striated muscle tissue found outside the muscle spindle.

extrinsic ophthalmoplegia Paralysis of the extrinsic ocular muscles.

eye disease Any systemic or local disease that affects visual function; may cause a reduction in visual acuity (being able to see clearly with central vision), or some type of visual field defect.

faces pain scale An established and reliable pictorial example of facial expressions to help the patient identify his/her level of discomfort.

F2ARV continuum This continuum begins with fear or frustration and proceeds to anger, range, and violence in that order. This is a highly volatile emotional reaction and escalates as the emotions mount.

family A group of people living together such as parents and children or a group of people who are closely related by birth, marriage, or adoption.

family involvement The interactions of significant others in a person's life that relate to an individual's development and coping.

family network A large and distributed group of people that support the family and work together as a unit or system

family priorities Importance of services and intervention goals based on family values and preferences.

fast pain The sensation first perceived after injury; it is localized, easily qualified, and lasts as long as the duration of the stimulus.

fastigial nucleus One of the deep cerebellar nuclei; receives input from the medial zone of the cerebellum; involved in the control of equilibrium and posture.

fatigue Extreme tiredness resulting from physical or mental activity with a temporary inability of an organ or part such as a muscle or nerve cell to respond to a stimulus and function normally, following continuous activity or stimulation.

fine motor coordination Motor behaviors involving manipulative, discrete finger movements, and eye-hand coordination; require corticospinal tract innervation for intentional fine motor control.

flaccidity The absence of voluntary, postural, and reflex movements resulting in muscle laxity and lack of resistance to passive stretch; this condition results from destruction of all or practically all peripheral motor fibers supplying a muscle.

forced use The term used for an intervention strategy that requires the patient to use an extremity while participating in a functional activity. It may require either restraining the opposite extremity or require bilateral use of two extremities.

function An action or use for which something is suited or designed. For example, the heart's function is to pump blood through the lungs for oxygenation and again through the body to get that oxygen to the cells for metabolism and retrieval of waste produces from those same cells.

functional activities Activities normally performed by an individual as part of daily life such as dressing, eating, bathing, grooming, socially interacting, and working.

functional electrical stimulation (FES) Use of electrical stimulation of the peripheral nervous system to activate muscle contractions to assist in functional activities, such as walking or upper extremity function.

Functional Independence Measure (FIM) A reliable, valid measurement of an adult's ability to perform various daily living skills.

functional limitations Those normal daily living activities that an individual has difficulty performing.

functional skills Ability to accomplish necessary daily activities.

functional training The intervention strategy that uses a functional activity as the treatment itself and assumes that the functional movement strategy necessary for that activity is available to the patient to practice.

functional visual skills These include eye aiming, eye alignment or eye posture, oculomotilities, and depth perception.

gag reflex Also known as the pharyngeal reflex, this involuntary contraction of the pharynx and elevation of the soft palate is elicited in most normal individuals by touching the pharyngeal wall or back of the tongue.

Gamma knife Trademark used for a medical device that emits a highly focused beam of gamma radiation used in noninvasive surgery.

gate control theory The pain modulation theory developed by Melzak and Wall, who proposed that presynaptic inhibition in the dorsal gray matter of the spinal cord results in blocking of pain impulses from the periphery.

gaze-evoked nystagmus Abnormal oscillation of the eyes when attempting to fixate gaze on an object.

gestalt form, space, concept   The configuration of separate units into a pattern that itself seems to function as a unit or a whole.

general adaptation syndrome (GAS)   A protective response of the autonomic nervous system which causes relaxation with stress versus anxiety and high blood pressure.

genetic disorders   errors with the human gene that are found in specific disease states and can cause functional limitations in an individuals development.

glial cell   A supportive cell in the brain and spinal cord. Glial cells do not conduct electrical impulses as opposed to neurons. They surround neurons and provide support for them and insulation between them. Glial cells are the most abundant cell types in the CNS. There are three types of glial cells: astrocytes, oligodendrocytes and microglia.

glioblastoma multiforme   A highly malignant, rapidly infiltrating, primary brain tumor with tentacles that may invade surrounding tissue. This provides a butterfly-like distribution pattern through the white matter of the cerebral hemispheres. The tumor may invade a membrane covering the brain (the dura) or spread via the spinal fluid through the ventricles of the brain.

gliosis   An excess of astroglia in damaged areas of the central nervous system.

globose nucleus   One of the four deep cerebellar nuclei in humans; receives input from intermediate zone of the cerebellar cortex; involved in control of posture and voluntary movement.

goal setting   The establishment of realistic outcomes from a specific interventions strategy which can be goals within a specific time frame or steps toward a desired long term functional outcome following an extended plan of care.

goal-oriented movements   These used to be called voluntary movements in contrast to reflexive movements. These are movements that are organized around behavioral goals, environmental context, and task specificity.

gross motor coordination   Motor behaviors concerned with posture and movement, ranging from early developing behavioral patterns to finely tuned, highly complex functional activities. Based on axial/trunk movement patterns versus distal control and requires the regulation over the ventral/medial and lateral descending motor tract systems.

Guillain-Barré syndrome   A rare nervous system disorder that results from nerve damage caused by the body's own defenses (immune system), usually in response to an infection or other illness. GBS causes muscle weakness, loss of reflexes, and numbness or tingling in the arms, legs, face, and other parts of the body. It may progress to complete paralysis and is the most common medical cause of acute paralysis.

habilitate   To supply with the means to develop maximum independence that has never been obtained.

handling   In this context refers to physical contact with the client's body to guide directly the movement and postural adaptation to a more normal pattern; usually refers to functional movement patterns used in daily care.

heat application   The use of heating modalities to accomplish a therapeutic goal.

hemiplegia   Paralysis on one side of the body that causes movement dysfunction in the arm and leg. This movement problem can also involve the face, swallowing, eye function, and language. It is often caused by a cerebral vascular event within the central nervous system.

higher cortical processing   Refers to the functions of the many association areas of the cerebral cortex. This includes memory, learning, and associating multiple information from a variety of sensory and motor sources. Outcomes of this processing include something as relatively simple as stereognosis or complex as mathematical processing, abstract thinking, or art. Simply stated, higher cortical processing results in gnosis (knowing).

high-risk clinical signs   Clinical signs that are present and highly predictive of the child having cerebral palsy. At 1 to 2 months after term (40 weeks of gestation) stiff, jerky movements or a paucity of movement are considered high-risk; while at 4 months of age, hypertonicity of the trunk or extremities are recognized as high-risk clinical signs.

hip-knee-ankle-foot orthosis (HKAFO)   Essentially a device to control all lower extremity segments.

HIPAA   An abbreviation for Health Insurance Portability and Accountability Act

hippocampus   A nuclear complex forming the medial margin of the cortical mantle of the cerebral hemisphere. It forms part of the limbic system and projects by way of the fornix to the septum, anterior nucleus of the thalamus, and the mamillary body.

holistic   The spiritual dimension of a health care model.

holistic model for health care delivery   A delivery of health services that embraces all forms of potential clinical management, has the patient as the central focus, and empowers the patient and family to the responsibilities that entails.

homeostasis   The maintenance of a steady state, in particular, the maintenance of the internal (physiological milieu) and the maintenance of safety or viability in the external environment.

homonymous hemianopsia   Loss of the same side of the field of vision in both eyes.

hospice care   Assistance given to the family and patient during the final stages of life. Hospice care focuses on quality of life not on recovery.

human immunodeficiency virus (HIV)   Either of two strains of retrovirus that destroys the immune system's help T cells, the loss of which causes AIDS.

humoral   Pertaining to any fluid or semifluid of the body.

Huntington disease   An inherited disease with degeneration of the basal ganglia and cerebral cortex; characterized by choreiform movements and loss of cognitive functions.

hydrocephalus   An abnormal increase of cerebrospinal fluid around the brain, resulting in infants in an enlargement of the head because the bones of the skull are still unfused. In adults hydrocephalus is usually caused by a trauma or inflammation within the brain that causes an excessive production of cerebrospinal fluid. Without a release for that fluid secondary trauma can cause damage to peripheral gray matter affecting all aspects of cortical function.

hyperbaric oxygen   Oxygen under greater pressure than at normal atmospheric pressure (usually at $1\frac{1}{2}$ to 3 times absolute atmospheric pressure). Thought to be immunosuppressive in treating multiple sclerosis.

hypermetria   Distortion of target-directed voluntary movement, in which the limb moves beyond the target.

hypertonicity   The quality or state of being hypertonic.

hypesthesias   Abnormally decreased sensitivity to stimulation.

hypnosis   A cognitive treatment technique that involves changing pain perception while the client is deeply relaxed.

hypometria Distortion of target-directed voluntary movement, in which the limb falls short of reaching the target.

hypotonicity Reduced resistance to passive stretch; displayed as inability to hold resting posture against gravity; limp, "floppy" extremities during passive movement.

ICD-9-CM An abbreviation for *International Classification of Diseases, Ninth Revision, Clinical Modification*. It is a tabular list of medical diagnoses approved for use by the CMS and is based on the World Health Organization's ICD-9 originally published in 1977.

immunoglobulin Any one of several proteins that are capable of acting as antibodies. May be found in plasma, urine, and cerebrospinal fluid. IgG is an immunoglobulin.

immunosuppression The inhibition of the immune response, usually deliberately by administrating drugs to prevent rejection of transplanted organs but sometimes resulting from disease as in the case of AIDS

impairment Any loss or abnormality of psychological, physiological, or anatomical structure or function. Examples: loss of joint mobility, weakness, sensory loss.

impairment training An intervention strategy that assumes that with specific system or subsystem training, the individual will regain control over a specific or multiple functional activities.

imprinting casting The application of casting material to subject the body part to consistent input for a specified period of time. This allows the central nervous system to "learn" the warranted response.

incomplete lesion A lesion in which partial preservation of sensory and/or motor function is found below the neurological level and includes the lowest sacral segment.

incontinence An inability to control urination or defecation, so that either may take place involuntarily.

indirect intervention Instruction of parents and other caregivers to modify their daily care of the child or individual to open new possibilities for motor learning and preventing expression of abnormal movement patterns.

inferior olivary nucleus A large nucleus in the anterolateral medulla; origin of climbing fibers to the cerebellum.

inpatient services Services delivered to the patient during hospitalization.

input systems or modalities The ways specific information enters into the nervous system to inform the brain about the external world.

integrating theories A process of analyzing and coordinating separate elements within different theories and creating a balanced whole that includes those components that are compatible or work together while also identifying those aspects that contradict or seem to be in conflict.

intention tremor An abnormal tremor of 4 to 6 Hz that occurs during voluntary, goal-directed movement.

interferon A protein formed when cells are exposed to viruses and other stimuli. Noninfected cells exposed to interferon are protected against viral infection. Thought to be of use in treating multiple sclerosis.

intermediate region of the cerebellum cortex A longitudinal zone of the cerebellar cortex; located on either side of the median zone; involved in the control of posture and voluntary movement; projects to globose and emboliform nucleus in humans and the interpositus nucleus in lower animals.

intermittent catheterization Intermittent placement of an external device or sterile tube between the urethra and the bladder to eliminate urine from the body.

internal ophthalmoplegia Paralysis of the intrinsic muscles of the eye—those of the iris and ciliary body.

interoceptive receptors Receptors activated by stimuli from within visceral tissues and blood vessels.

interpositus nucleus One of the deep cerebellar nuclei in lower animals (globose and emboliform in humans); receives input from intermediate region of the cerebellar cortex; involved in the control of posture and voluntary movement.

intrafusal muscle Striated muscle tissue found within the muscle spindle.

Intuition The state of being aware of or knowing something without using known sensory input systems or without actual evidence for that knowledge.

iontophoresis The use of electricity to drive chemical ions into the body for therapeutic purposes.

isometric contraction Muscle tension without shortening.

isotonic contraction Contraction associated with shortening or lengthening of the muscle tissue; can be either concentric or eccentric.

jaw jerk Closure of the mouth caused by striking the lower jaw while it hangs passively open. This reflex is rare in normal individuals.

joint mobilization Graded passive oscillations at a joint for the purpose of increasing range of motion.

Karnofsky Performance Status Scale A functional performance scale designed as a functional measurement prognostic tool specifically for individuals who have undergone surgery for a brain tumor. The specific scale can be found in Table 25-1.

knee-ankle-foot orthosis (KAFO) An orthoses or brace that controls the movement function and interaction between the knee, ankle, and foot.

kinesiological electromyography Study of the muscle activity produced on motion.

knowledge of results Augmented information provided about success or errors in achieving environmental goals.

kyphosis The exaggeration or angulation of the normal posterior curve of the spine.

language A code for representing feelings and ideas about the world through a conventional system of signals (such as sign language) or symbols (such as spoken or written words). Language includes understanding and producing the conventional symbols and the rules for combining and using symbols.

language disorder A complete or partial disruption in the ability to understand and produce the conventional symbols or words that constitute one's native language, not directly attributable to sensory loss (e.g., blindness, hearing loss) or motor impairments.

laser A device that produces a coherent, monochromatic beam of light that can be used therapeutically for pain management, as well as for surgical procedures.

lateralization The tendency for certain processes to be more highly developed on one side of the brain than on the other. In most people, the right hemisphere develops the processes of spatial and musical thoughts, and the left hemisphere develops the areas for verbal and logical processes.

lateral region of the cerebellar cortex A longitudinal zone of the cerebellar cortex; located lateral to intermediate zone; comprises bulk of cerebral hemispheres; involved in the control of skilled voluntary movement; receives projection from motor cortex and has output to dentate nucleus.

learning disability A disorder in one or more of the basic physiological processes involved in understanding or using spoken or written language. This may be manifested in disorders of listening, thinking, talking, reading, writing, spelling, or doing arithmetic. They include conditions that have been referred to as, for example, perceptual handicaps, brain injury, minimal brain dysfunction, dyslexia, and developmental aphasia. They do not include learning problems that are primarily caused by visual, hearing, or motor handicaps, mental retardation or emotional disturbance, or environmental disadvantage.

learning environment All the conditions (internal and external), circumstances, and influences surrounding and affecting the learning of the client.

learning theory The theoretical basis used to describe changes in behavior or performance, whether declarative, procedural, or some combination of both.

lesion A physical change in a body part that is the result of illness or injury such as a head trauma that damages brain cells and creates lesions that can be measured objectively as change to the CNS.

leptomeningitis Inflammation of the arachnoid and pia mater layers of the meninges. The same condition may be referred to as meningitis.

life span disability A mental or physical limitations that will prevent the individual from participating in activities either considered normal for daily living or social interaction throughout the life span of that person.

ligation Application of a ligature (a ligature being any material used for tying a vessel or to constrict a part).

limbic system A group of brain structures that include amygdala, hippocampus, dentate gyrus, cingulate gyrus, and their interconnections with hypothalamus, septal areas and brain stem.

limits of stability (LOS) The boundary or range that is the farthest distance in any direction a person can lean away from vertical (midline) without changing the original base of support (stepping, reaching, etc.) or falling.

lipomeningocele A mild form of spina bifida. There is a fatty tumor over the spine. There may not be much nerve damage, but there may be urinary and bowel problems.

lipofuscin Any of a class of fatty pigments formed by the solution of a pigment in fat.

long-loop stretch reflex Stretch reflex mediated through centers above the spinal system.

loss and grief The process of dealing with the removal of function or roles in a person's life.

lower motor neuron A motor neuron whose cell body is located with the nervous system and whose axons leaves the CNS toward a preestablished destination such as a myoneural junction of striated muscle, to smooth muscle or to an organ.

magnetic resonance imaging (MRI) A scanning technique using magnetic fields and radio frequencies to produce a precise image of the body tissue; used for diagnosis and monitoring of disease.

massage Manipulation of the soft tissues of the body for the purpose of affecting the nervous, muscular, respiratory, and circulatory systems.

McGill pain questionnaire A pain character measurement tool in which clients are asked to select words that describe their pain from a series of word categories.

medial zone of cerebellar cortex The longitudinal zone of the cerebellar cortex, which includes the vermis and the flocculonodular lobe; involved in control of equilibrium and posture; projects to fastigial and vestibular nuclei.

medical screening A process used by physical and occupational therapists as part of their health screening for each patient in order to differentiate problems that are within a OT/PT's scope of practice and those clinical signs that should guide the therapist to refer the patient to another medical practitioner.

Medicaid A program funded by the U.S. and state governments that pays for medical expenses of people who are unable to pay some or all of their expenses.

Medicare A health insurance program in the U.S. under which medical care and hospital treatment for people over 65 or individuals who are considered disabled.

Meningioma A slow-growing benign tumor that affects the meninges of the brain or spinal cord and may cause serious damage by compression of the nervous system within its skeletal frame.

meningitis Acute inflammation of the meninges covering the brain and spinal cord.

metencephalon The cephalic part of the rhombencephalon, giving rise to the cerebellum and pons.

minimal brain dysfunction A mild or minimal neurological abnormality that causes learning difficulties in the child with average intelligence.

mobile arm support An orthotic device that supports the upper extremity and allows the individual to move the extremity with limited motor function.

model of human occupation A model that addresses the motivation for occupation, the patterning of occupational behavior into routines and lifestyles, the nature of skilled performance, and the influence of environment on occupational behavior.

modulation A variation in levels of excitation and inhibition over sensory and motor neural pools.

morphogenesis The morphological transformation including growth, alterations of germinal layers, and differentiation of cells and tissues during development.

mossy fibers One of two fiber types carrying information to the cerebellar cortex.

motor control The ability of the central nervous system to regulate and/or direct the musculoskeletal system in purposeful acts.

motor control theory Theoretical basis for understanding how the motor system is controlled within the human body.

motor coordination Functions that are traditionally defined as motoric. Includes gross motor, fine motor, and motor planning functions.

motor dysfunction, motor deficit, motor disorder, motor disturbance Generic terms for any type of disorder found in learning-disabled children that has a motor component.

motor lag A prolonged latent period between the reception of a stimulus and the initiation of the motor response.

motor learning The acquisition of skilled movement based on previous experience and functional outcomes.

motor learning stages The process through which a learner acquires, refines, and retains a new motor skill, in which performance of the skill occurs with diminishing errors and greater efficiency and flexibility.

motor learning theory Theoretical basis for understanding how the central nervous system learns to control, modify, and regulate the motor system in order to respond and react to the internal and external environment within which that body functions.

motor planning (praxis) The ability to plan and execute skilled nonhabitual tasks.

motor skill The ability to execute coordinated motor actions with proficiency.

MOVE (*m*otivation/*m*emory, *o*lfaction, *v*isceral [ANS], *e*motional) An acronym representing the functions of the limbic system in cognitive learning and motor control.

movement decomposition Distortion of voluntary movement in which the movement occurs in a distinct sequence of isolated steps, rather than in a normal, smooth, flowing pattern.

movement deficits Functional movement problems that prevents the individual from performing movement in an effortless fashion

movement speed The time elapsed between the initiation of a movement and its completion.

movement therapies Therapeutic practices and protocols that focus on the individual patient participating in functional movement activities with the help of a assistant when necessary to maintain what would be considered efficient and effective motor control.

multiple sclerosis A chronic disease of the white matter of the central nervous system characterized by inflammation, demyelination, and the development of hardened plaques. The symptoms and signs are numerous; the course is erratic; its etiology appears to be autoimmune.

muscle activation deficits Problems between the motor neuron cell body and contraction of the striated muscle fiber, which prevent the muscle fiber from contracting.

myelencephalon The lower part of the embryonic hindbrain from which the medulla oblongata develops.

myelin A fatlike substance forming the principal component of the sheath of nerve fibers in the CNS.

myelin basic protein (MBP) A protein component of myelin which has been the subject of considerable study in MS research. An injection of MBP can induce a demyelinating condition reminiscent of MS in animals called experimental allergic encephalomyelitis (EAE).

myelination The process of forming the "white" lipid covering of nerve cell axons; myelin increases the conduction velocity (speed) of the neuronal impulse; forms the white matter of the brain and spinal cord (as opposed to the gray matter).

myelodysplasia A developmentally anomaly of the spinal cord

Myelomeningocele Spina bifida in which neural tissue of the spinal cord and the investing meninges protrude from the spinal column forming a sac under the skin

myelography Radiographic inspection of the spinal cord by use of a radiopaque medium injected into the intrathecal space.

myasthenia gravis A disorder of neuromuscular function, thought to be due to the presence of antibodies to acetylcholine receptors at the neuromuscular junction. Clinically, there is fatigue and exhaustion of the muscular system with a tendency to fluctuate in severity and without sensory disturbance or atrophy.

myofascial release Manipulation of the soft tissues of the body for the purpose of interrupting built-in imbalances and restrictions within the fascia and reintegrating the fascial mechanism.

natural environments All integrated community settings.

neocerebellum Those parts of the cerebellum that receive input via the corticopontocerebellar pathway.

neologism A new, meaningless word, often spoken by fluent aphasic clients.

neonatal neuropathology A disease or pathology of the nervous system identified while the child was in utero or once a child is born prematurely.

neonatal intensive care unit environment (NICU) A critical care hospital unit where specialized health care practitioners treat and care for premature or very young babies that are in health crisis.

nerve conduction tests Measurement of the electrical conductivity of motor and sensory nerves by application of an external electrical stimulus to the nerve and evaluation of parameters such as nerve conduction time, velocity, amplitude, and shape of the resulting response, as recorded from another site on the nerve or from a muscle supplied by the nerve.

nerve conduction velocity The speed at which an impulse will travel down a neuron.

neural irritability Hypersensitivity of the receptor sites or outer wall of a neuron which causes that neuron to respond at a high rate that expected.

neural mobility The ability of the neuron or nerves to lengthen and shorten as the limb moves and the muscles contract and relax.

neural sensitization Axons that become inflamed, hypoxic, or demyelinated can enter a hyperexcitable state. A nerve in a hyperexcitable state can begin to discharge spontaneously, become mechanosensitive, or develop a sustained rhythmic discharge after stimulation, all of which can result in the production of pathological pain. If the change in sensitivity or threshold allows what were once subthreshold stimuli to evoke pain then suprathreshold stimuli may evoke exaggerated pain.

neurapraxia Interruption of nerve conduction without loss of continuity of the axon.

neurodevelopmental treatment A type of movement therapy that bases its theories on the function of the nervous system, how it learns, and how it normally changes over time.

neurography Study of the action potentials of nerves.

neurological assessment A specific examination tool that focuses on the various functions of the sensory and motor systems controlled and modified by the central nervous system.

neuromechanism A neurological system whose component parts work together to produce central nervous system function.

neuromodulators Chemicals capable of directly affecting pain transmission. The neuromodulators include enkephalin and beta-endorphin, which are referred to as endogenous opiates because they have morphine-like actions.

neuromotor assessment Examination of motor control system through the use of movement responses.

neuromotor intervention Treatment desired and delivered by occupational and physical therapists to create an environment that allow the client to learn and control normal functional movement.

neuromuscular electrical stimulation The use of an electrical impulse for the purpose of examination of the neuromuscular system and intervention when appropriate as biofeedback.

neuronal sprouting The process of regrowing a neuronal process (e.g., axon) in an injured neuron attempting to reestablish innervation with a target structure.

neuropathy Any disease or dysfunction of the nerves.

neuroplasticity Anatomical and electrophysiological changes in the central nervous system in response to demands from the internal and external environment.

neuroprosthetics The use of the existing neural pathways to control and run a specific prosthetic device.

neurotmesis Damage to the axon and the endoneurial tube with the nerve remaining macroscopically intact, or complete transection of the nerve. Regeneration is less successful than in axonotmesis.

neurotransmitter A specific chemical agent that is released from presynaptic cells and travels across the synapse to stimulate or inhibit postsynaptic cells, thereby facilitating or inhibiting neural transmission.

neurotrophic Nutrition and maintenance of tissues as regulated by nervous influence.

neurovascular entrapment Scarring, swelling, or abnormal tissue growth of connective tissue that traps or compresses both the vascular and nervous system creating dysfunction and pain.

nociceptor A peripheral nerve ending that appreciates and transmits painful or injurious stimuli.

nonverbal learning disabilities Learning disabilities in children that affect nonverbal learning strategies such as visual-spatial and perceptual reasoning.

normal movement strategies Motor programs can be available to the CNS at birth or learned throughout life. The variability of these programs and the amount of practice an individual has had to perform the movements determines the movement strategies available given any environmental context. The range of strategies that are used to perform the motor activity in an effortless, fluid, energy efficient manner is a range of behaviors that are defined as "normal." Thus normal movement strategies are a range of behaviors that are considered normal for a person of that age, activity level, and experience.

nosocomial Hospital-acquired.

nuchal rigidity Reflex spasm of the neck extensor muscles resulting in resistance to cervical flexion.

nystagmus A series of automatic, back-and-forth eye movements. Different conditions produce this reflex. A common way of producing them is by an abrupt stop following a series of rotations of the body. The duration and regularity of postrotary nystagmus are some of the indicators of vestibular system efficiency.

occupational-based performance Involves performance that requires the individual to have competence.

occupational therapy The therapeutic use of purposeful and meaningful goal-directed activities (occupations), which engage the individual's body and mind in meaningful, organized, and self-directed actions that maximize independence, prevent or minimize disability, and maintain health.

ocular dysmetria Inability to fix gaze on an object or follow a moving object with accuracy.

offset feeder One of the two most common orthosis used to assist in feeding to allow an individual with a C5 cervical spinal cord injury to independently feed. Refer to Figure 19-23 for a visual image.

oligoclonal banding A process by which cerebrospinal fluid IgG is distributed, following electrophoresis, in discrete bands. Approximately 90% of clients with multiple sclerosis show oligoclonal banding.

oligodendroglia Myelin-producing cells in the CNS.

operant conditioning A cognitive treatment technique in which a voluntary, nonautomatic behavior is paired with a new stimulus through reinforcement or punishment.

ophthalmoplegia Paralysis of ocular muscles.

opisthotonus Position of extreme hyperextension of the vertebral column caused by a tetanic spasm of the extensor musculature.

optokinetic nystagmus Nystagmus induced by watching stripes on a drum revolving around one's face.

oral myelin (Myloral) An oral bovine myelin therapy for MS currently under study by Autoimmune, Inc. (Lexington, MA), which is based on the theory of "oral tolerance" to reduce immune activity against myelin. Oral tolerance refers to the ability of the immune system associated with the digestive tract to protect against immunoreactions to foreign proteins that are ingested.

orthostatic hypotension A dramatic fall in blood pressure when a patient assumes an upright position, usually caused by a disturbance of vasomotor control decreasing the blood supply returning to the heart.

orthosis An external device utilized to apply forces to a body part to limit movement, increase the velocity or power of a movement, stop movement, or hold the body part in a particular position. Previously called brace or splint.

orthotics An external device that assists in the stability and/or mobility of a specific limb or joint.

outpatient Services provided to the patient following discharge from inpatient hospitalization, or services provided to a patient referred to the therapist directly from the physician.

overwork damage Damage to human tissue (neural or muscular) that is caused because the body forced the system to function beyond its normal capabilities.

pachymeningitis Acute inflammation of the dura mater.

pain character measurement Any of the tools used to define the character of a client's pain.

pain drawing A way to allow the patient to identify and express the level of pain that he or she perceives.

pain estimate A pain intensity measurement in which clients rate pain on a scale of 0 to 100.

pain intensity measurement Any of the scales used to quantify pain intensity.

pain intensity rating tools Scales that have the client rate the current level of pain by marking a continuum or assigning a numerical value to the pain intensity

pain localization tools Also referred to as pain measurement tools and are designed to provide information about the intensity, location, and character of a client's symptoms *at the time of the evaluation*. This information can then be merged with the pain history, disease/pathology history, and the physical findings to identify the cause of pain. Body diagram screening symptom location can be used to have the patient identify and the therapist mark where is pain is located. Figure 7-6 is an example of such a diagram chart.

pain mechanisms Pain mechanisms include CNS anatomy where the pain is recognized, process and interpreted, the sensory, motor and interneural pain pathways, pain modulation

pain modulation Variation in the intensity and appreciation of pain secondary to CNS and ANS effects on the nociceptors and along the pain pathways, as well as secondary to external factors such as distraction and suggestion.

pain pathway The route along which nerve impulses arising from painful stimuli are transmitted from the nociceptor to the brain, including transmission within the brain itself.

pain quality measurements McGill Pain Questionnaire (MPQ).

papilledema Edema of the optic disk.

paradigm An example that serves as a pattern or model for something, especially one that forms the basis of a methodology or theory.

parallel talk A form of speech used during play therapy with children in which the clinician verbalizes actions such as what is happening or what the child is doing without requiring answers from the child. For instance, "I'm making a cake. Mine is good. You're making a cake, too." The clinician often repeats utterances of the child correctly and parallels the child's activities.

paranodal myelin intussusception The ultrastructural change that occurs at Ranvier node because of acute focal compression of a nerve, resulting in a neuropraxic lesion.

paraplegia The impairment or loss of motor and/or sensory function in the thoracic, lumbar, or sacral (but not cervical) segments of the spinal cord, secondary to damage of neural elements within the spinal canal.

paraxial Lying near the axis of the body.

parent instruction An identified process used to guide and direct the parents in a functional activity or handling skill they will be doing or using with their child.

paresthesia An abnormal spontaneous sensation such as burning, pricking, tickling, or tingling.

Parkinson disease; parkinsonism A degenerative disease of the substantia nigra; cause is unknown for idiopathic parkinsonism; disease is characterized by slow movements, rigidity, a resting tremor, and postural instability.

patient referral The act or process of sending a patient to a medical specialist or a medical specialist sending that patient to a physical or occupational therapist for an evaluation and possible intervention.

patterned responses The programs either preprogrammed or created by the motor system to succeed at the presented task in the most efficient and integrated response possible at that moment in time.

pediatric verbal descriptor scale for pain A process where specific words are introduced to a child and the child responds in relation to his/her perceived pain

pelvic floor dysfunction Sensory and/or motor functional problems within the smooth and striated muscles of the pelvic floor leading to problems in volitional control of urination and defecation especially during activities such as exercise, sneezing, coughing, and any other activity that places pressure on the pelvic floor musculature.

pendular knee jerk Upon elicitation of the deep tendon reflex of the knee, the lower leg oscillates briefly like a pendulum after the jerk, instead of returning immediately to resting position.

perceptions The process of using the senses to acquire information about the surrounding environment or situation; any of the neurological processes of acquiring and mentally interpreting information from the senses.

perceptual-motor The interaction of the various channels of perception with motor activity, including visual, auditory, tactual, and kinesthetic channels.

perceptual-motor match The process of comparing and collating the input data received through the motor system and through perception.

peripheral pain Pain arising from injury to a peripheral structure.

phantom limb pain The sensation that an amputated part is still present, often associated with painful paresthesia.

pharmacist A professional trained and licensed to dispense medicinal drugs and to advise the patient and the doctor on their use.

phenol block An injection of phenol (hydroxybenzene) into individual nerves; used as a topical anesthetic and produces a selective block of these nerves; sometimes used to control severe spasticity in specific muscle groups.

phonophoresis The use of ultrasound waves to drive chemical molecules into the tissues for therapeutic purposes.

physical therapy A profession with an established theoretical base and widespread clinical application in the preservation, development, and restoration of optimal physical function. Interventions focus on movement function and dysfunction, which encompass treating musculoskeletal, cardiopulmonary, integumentary, and neuromuscular problems that affect the individual during life activities such as work, leisure time, or daily living skills.

physiological and musculoskeletal risks Dangers that injury, damage, or loss will occur to any physiological or musculoskeletal system because of the external environment or stressors placed on the patient's body from medical/therapeutic interventions.

physiological flexion The excessive amount of flexor tone that is normally present at birth because of the existing level of CNS maturation and fetal positioning in utero.

plaque A multiple sclerosis lesion characterized by loss of myelin and hardening of tissue.

plasmapheresis A process by which whole blood is removed from the client, plasma is discarded and replaced by normal plasma or human albumin, and reconstituted blood is then returned to the client. In treating multiple sclerosis this process is believed to rid the blood of antibodies or substances that are damaging to myelin or that impair nerve conduction.

plasticity The ability to change (refer to neuroplasticity when discussing nervous system plasticity).

pneumoencephalogram Radiographic examination of ventricles and subarachnoid spaces of the brain following withdrawal of cerebrospinal fluid and injection of air or gas via lumbar puncture.

point stimulation The stimulation of sensitive areas of skin using electricity, pressure, laser, or ice for the purpose of relieving pain.

polyradiculoneuropathy An inflammatory disorder (as Guillain-Barré syndrome) affecting peripheral nerves and the nerve roots of the spinal nerves and marked by demyelination or axon degeneration.

polyradiculopathy Inflammation of multiple nerve roots.

polysomnography Monitoring of physiological activity during sleep.

position in space Direction in which figures point, relationship of one body part to another, or the entire body's relationship to objects or others in space.

posterior/heel lever arm An orthotic device at the ankle the produces a posterior force acting to extend the knee and provides knee stability and prevents future knee impairment.

postpolio syndrome A condition that affects former poliomyelitis patients long after recovery from the initial acute disease and that is characterized by muscle weakness, joint and muscle pain, and fatigue.

posttraumatic amnesia The time elapsed between a brain injury and the point at which the functions concerned with memory are determined to have been restored.

postural and movement compensation Compensatory movement programs used by or taught to the patient to try to control both the postural and movement motor programs within any functional activity.

postural background movements   The subtle, spontaneous body adjustments that make overt movements of the hands easier, for example, reaching for a distant object. These postural adjustments depend on good vestibular and proprioceptive integration.

postural control   Those motor programs designed to stabilize joints during postural activities and to control coactivation of agonist and antagonists during movement at the joint(s).

postural tremor   A pathological tremor of 3 to 5 Hz that appears in a limb or the trunk when either is working against the pull of gravity.

posture   In the strictest sense, the position of the body or body part in relation to space and/or to other body parts. Functionally, the anticipation of and response to displacement of the body's center of mass.

pragmatics   The study of language as it is used in context.

praxis   The ability to plan and execute a motor program as a functional activity

predictors of recovery   Signs/ symptoms, cognitive processing, or motor control that would be indications that function is returning

prefrontal lobe   The area of the frontal lobe that is anterior and inferior to the premotor and supplementary motor cortex.

pressure ulcer   A slow-healing sore on the surface of the skin that may result in destruction of tissue that was the result of maintained pressure to the skin and lack of circulation/oxygenation to those tissues.

primary impairments   The main system or subsystem that is diseased or damaged that is preventing an individual from performing normal functional activities of daily living.

problem solving   The process of logically or intuitively overcoming barriers in an individual's environment.

procedural memory   The specific motor programs learned and retained to run motor programs or combinations of programs in order to perform functional activities

prognosis   In the area of movement analysis, it is an opinion as to the likely course and outcome following intervention.

prospective payment system (PPS)   A payment structure with in which the acute hospitals were initially paid a set amount per patient. The amount depended on the medical diagnosis and related morbidities. Today the PPS, extends beyond acute hospital services to inpatient rehabilitation and skilled nursing facilities, home health agencies, and long-term care hospitals.

proprioceptive   Receptors that respond to stimuli originating primarily from muscle spindles, Golgi tendon organs, and joints.

protopathic   Pertaining to the somatic sensations of fast, localized pain; slow, poorly localized pain; and temperature.

Pro-Ven   A processed mixture of cobra, krait, and water moccasin venoms developed by Florida physicians to treat multiple sclerosis. The FDA has banned the sale of Pro-Ven until it is tested for safety and effectiveness.

psychoneuroimmunology   A field of medicine that deals with the influence of emotional states (as stress) and nervous system activity on immune function especially in relation to their effect on the onset and progression of disease.

pulmonary embolism   An obstruction of the pulmonary artery or one of its branches usually caused by an embolus from a lower extremity thrombosis.

Purkinje cells   Large neurons found in the cerebellar cortex that provide the only output from the cerebellar cortex after the

cortex processes sensory and motor signals from the rest of the nervous system.

quadriplegia   Term used to describe paralysis in all four extremities; often used when describing the movement dysfunction in individuals following cervical neck spinal cord injury.

radiation therapy   The treatment of disease using radiation x-rays or beta rays directed at the body from an external source or emitted by radioactive materials placed within the body

reaction of degeneration   The condition in which a short-duration electrical stimulus (usually less than 1 ms) applied to a motor nerve results in a sluggish or absent muscle response, rather than the normally brisk contraction. The reaction may be partial or complete, depending on the extent of neuropathology. This electrophysiological reaction can be used as a screening assessment of peripheral nerve integrity.

reasonable and necessary   Words used to define a billing standard based on averages determined from local coverage standards. These standards along with ICD-9-CM codes are used to establish fees for services within various geographic areas and service environments.

rebound phenomenon   Inability to stop a resisted muscle contraction, such that movement of the limb occurs when the resistance is unexpectedly withdrawn from the limb.

reciprocating gait orthosis   an orthotic device that reciprocally moves one leg forward while stabilizes the weight bearing limb to propel the legs forward in an upright gait pattern.

recoordination of the functions of the abdominal compartment   The abdominal compartment plays and integral role in the normal functioning of the pelvic girdle. Recoodination of the function between the abdominal compartment and the pelvic girdle is an important element of pelvic girdle sensory and motor training. For example, when a person sneezes, the abdominal contraction is strong and must work in coordination with the pelvic girdle to simultaneously cause pelvic girdle contraction. Given this example, without this coordination the force from the abdominal system may cause a strong force on the bladder and release of urine, a situation termed incontinence.

red nucleus   Large, vascular nucleus found in mescncephalon, involved in transmission of cerebellar communications to the motor cortex and thalamus.

reflux   Backflow of urine from bladder to ureters.

refractive error   Nearsightedness (myopia), farsightedness (hyperopia), astigmatism, or presbyopia. All conditions are improved with corrective lenses.

rehabilitation   The restoration of a disabled individual to maximum independence commensurate with his or her limitations.

relaxation techniques   A cognitive treatment technique that addresses muscle tension accompanying pain.

remission   A lessening of the symptoms of a disease or their temporary reduction or disappearance of the functional limitations.

research   Methodical investigation into a subject to discover facts, to establish or revise a theory, or to develop a plan of action based on the facts discovered. Depending on the research design, the results can lead to effectiveness of treatment or efficacy of a specific variable in relation to change following a course of intervention. Both effectiveness and efficacy lead to evidence-based practice through research.

response speed   The time elapsed between presentation of a stimulus and the client's initiation of movement.

retardation A retarded person has had some degree of mental impairment all his or her life. A retarded person can also develop a delirium or dementia. A delirium or dementia differs from retardation in that there has been a change from what was normal for that person.

retrograde amnesia The inability to recall events that have occurred during the period immediately preceding a brain injury.

reverberating loops or circuits A process by which closed chains of neurons when excited by a single impulse will continue to discharge impulses from collateral neurons back onto the original neuronal pool. The end result may produce a higher level of excitation than the original input itself.

review of systems screening A screening process that systematically goes through screening of each bodily system to eliminate or identify potential signs and symptoms that would alert the examiner to potential system problems.

rhizotomy A neurosurgical intervention at the level of the cauda equina, or lower level of the spine, to interrupt abnormal sensory feedback that appears to maintain hypertonus. The procedure was developed in 1908 and has been modified by a series of neurosurgeons, with the objective of reducing hypertonus associated with CNS dysfunction to allow the expression of functional postural control.

rigidity Resistance to passive range of motion that is not velocity-dependent and affects the muscles on both sides of the joint.

rooting reflex This normal reflex in infants up to 4 months of age consists of head turning in the direction of the stimulus when the cheek is stroked gently.

saccadic eye movement An extremely fast movement of the eyes, allowing the eyes to accurately fix on a still object in the visual field.

saccadic fixations A rapid change of fixation from one point in a visual field to another

sacral agenesis An incomplete development or total absence of the sacral aspect of the pelvis.

scanning speech An abnormal pattern of speech characterized by regularly recurring pauses.

scoliosis Lateral curvature of the spine; this usually consists of two curves, the original abnormal curve and a compensatory curve in the opposite direction.

secondary impairments System problems that either have developed from the primary impairments or have developed along with the primary problems and may create further dysfunction if ignored.

sensorimotor therapy Therapy planned to enhance the integration of motor learning and the emergence of voluntary motor behaviors concerned with posture and movement.

sensory conflict Situations in which sensory signals that are expected to match ("agree") do NOT match, either between systems (vision, somatosensory or vestibular) or within a system (two proprioceptive inputs such as the joint and the muscle).

sensory deprivation An enforced absence of the usual repertoire of sensory stimuli. The continued decrease or absence of adequate, normal stimuli can produce severe cognitive, motor, and emotional changes, including hallucinations, anxiety, depression, neglect of an extremity or body part, and inadequate motor response to the environment.

sensory environment The sensory conditions that exist in the real world around us that affect balance (e.g., darkness, visual movement, compliant surfaces).

sensory integration The organization of sensory input for use, a perception of the body or environment, an adaptive response, a learning process, or the development of some neural function.

sensory integrative dysfunction A disorder or irregularity in brain function that makes sensory integration difficult. Many, but not all, learning disorders stem from sensory integrative dysfunctions.

sensory integrative therapy Therapy involving sensory stimulation and adaptive responses to it according to a child's neurological needs. Treatment usually involves full body movements that provide vestibular, proprioceptive, and tactile stimulation. It usually does not include desk activities, speech training, reading lessons, or training in specific perceptual or motor skills. The goal is to improve the brain's ability to process and organize sensations.

sensuality Responding to sensory input in a positive manner, resulting in the person deriving bodily or sensory pleasure.

septicemia Systemic disease associated with the presence and persistence of pathogenic microorganisms or toxins in the blood.

serial speech Overlearned speech involving a series of words such as counting and reciting the days of the week.

sexuality The behaviors that relate psychological, cultural, emotional, and physical responses to the need to reproduce.

shoulder pain Pain that is located with the axial aspect of the upper thorax or proximal upper limb

shoulder subluxation A partial dislocation of the humerus from the shoulder joint that leaves them misaligned but still in some contact with each other

significant impairments Impairments that have a major or important effect on functional activities.

simple descriptive pain scale (SDPS) A client rating scale for pain that is on a continuum that is subdivided using descriptors that gradually increase in intensity. Sample descriptors are "no pain," "mild pain," "moderate pain," "severe pain," and "maximum pain tolerable."

slow pain The second sensation perceived after injury; it is poorly localized and outlasts the duration of the stimulus.

skilled services Services that require special abilities developed and practiced over time

smooth pursuit movement of the eyes When the eyes are following a slowly moving object, they move together at a steady velocity, not in saccades.

soft neurological signs Mild or slight neurological abnormalities that are difficult to detect.

somatosensory retraining An intervention strategy used to retrain the somatosensory association areas in order to remap the sensory component of functional activities; used most often following repetitive strain injuries which result in distal focal dystonia.

spastic diplegia An increase in postural tonus that is distributed primarily in the lower extremities and the pelvic area.

spastic quadriplegia An increase in postural tonus that is distributed throughout all four extremities. These findings are often coexistent with relatively lower tone in the trunk and severe difficulty in controlling posture.

spasticity A motor disorder characterized by a velocity-dependent increase in tonic stretch reflexes with exaggerated tendon jerks, resulting from hyperexcitability of the stretch reflex. Spasticity is one component of the upper motor neuron syndrome.

speech The meaningful production and sequencing of sounds by the speech sensorimotor system (e.g., lips, tongue) for the transmission of spoken language.

speech pathology Speech/language pathology, speech therapy, or communicative disorders: terms used to specifically identify the professional scope of practice that focuses upon communication as a receptive, interactive, and expressive function of humans. This profession deals with the cognitive, emotional, and motor impairments that deal with human language and communication.

spina bifida cystica A fault in the spine where the bones of the back fail to form properly, leaving a gap. That gap can allow spinal fluid to fill in a sac that forms a cyst.

spina bifida occulta A mild often asymptomatic form of spinal bifida in which there is no hernial protrusion in the meninges or spinal cord. There is a bone defect but no nerve damage.

spinal cord injury (SCI) An insult to the spinal cord that results in neurological deficits.

spirituality That aspect of human thought and communication that focuses on the belief that man has more than a physical body and that aspect does or may join a universal energy that has a higher power source than any one individual. This may or may not have a direct connection with formal religion.

spirometry (pneumatometry) The measurement of air inspired and expired.

stages of motor development A series of progressive stages of motor learning that provides the foundation for movement development. It is often based on behavioral responses of children who are consider to be progressing, maturing and demonstrating motor skill appropriate for children of that chronological age.

standardized evaluations of function A test of movement function administered according to standardized procedures and compared with a acceptable standard of functional responses.

standing A-frame One of the first orthotic devices used with children with spina bifida. It is a relatively inexpensive tubular frame to which adjustable parts are attached. This standing device offers support of the trunk, hips, and knees and leaves the hands free for other activities. Refer to Figure 18-16 for a visual image.

static equilibrium Ability of an individual to adjust to displacements of his or her center of gravity while maintaining a constant base of support.

stereognosis The ability to recognize the sizes, shapes, and weights of familiar objects without the use of vision.

stereopsis Quality of visual fusion.

strabismus Oculomotor misalignment of one eye.

subspecialty training A very narrow or specialized field of study within an existing specialty.

strategies Carefully devised plan of action to achieve a goal or the art of developing or carrying out such a plan.

sudomotor Denoting the nerves that stimulate the sweat glands.

support systems Specific groups, family members, or friends that provide emotional, spiritual, and physical help to the patient.

synaptogenesis The process of forming synaptic connections between nerve cells, or between nerve cells and muscle fibers; the basis of neuronal communication.

synergy Fixed set of muscles contracting with a present sequence and time of contraction.

systems interactions The ways the various CNS systems affect or interact with one another to provide a more integrative and functional nervous system.

systems model A conceptual representation which incorporates a set of major functional divisions or systems within the CNS which interlock and interrelate to create the functional whole. Although each division may be considered a whole in and of itself with multiple subsystems interlocking to form its entire division, each major component or division influences and is influenced by all others and thus the totality of the CNS is based on the summation of the interactions, not individual function.

systems model/approach An interactive framework for understanding movement and postural control which includes (1) environmental stimuli; (2) sensory reception, perception, and organization; and (3) motor planning, execution, and modification.

systems theory A theory describing movements emerging as a result of an interaction among many peripheral and central nervous system components with influence changing depending on the task.

tactile defensiveness A sensory integrative dysfunction characterized by tactile sensations that cause excessive emotional reactions, hyperactivity, or other behavior problems.

T cells A subgroup of lymphocytes with two subpopulations CD8 and CD4+. CD4+ T cells are the middlemen of the immune response and the target of the virus leading to HIV infection.

telereceptive The exteroceptors of hearing, sight, and smell that are sensitive to distant stimuli.

tenodesis The operation of suturing the end of a tendon to a bone, or the pattern of wrist extension with tight wrist flexors which causes the hand to close.

tenotomy Surgical section of a tendon used in some cases to treat severe spasticity and contractures.

TENS (transcutaneous electrical nerve stimulation) The use of electricity for pain management.

tethered spinal cord syndrome A disorder characterized by progressive neurological deterioration that results from compression of the lowermost bundle of nerves of the spinal cord (cauda equina). It is most commonly associated with a defective closing the neural tube during embryonic development.

tetraplegia Impairment or loss of motor and/or sensory function in the cervical segments of the spinal cord due to damage of neural elements within the spinal canal.

thalamic pain CNS pain caused by injury to the thalamus and characterized by contralateral and sometimes migratory pain brought on by peripheral stimulation.

therapeutic environment Organizing all aspects of the environment in a systematic way so that they enhance a patient's ability to perform desired tasks and activities (mental, emotional, functional).

therapeutic interventions Specific interventions that are designed by occupational and physical therapists whose outcome should have a therapeutic value and assist the patient in regaining functional control or compensating for loss of function in activities of daily living.

therapeutic touch The exchange of energy from one person to another for the purpose of healing.

thermotherapy The use of heat or cold for therapeutic purposes.

third-party payer The organization or health care service payer that provides payment for services provided by physical and occupational therapy. This payer is an entity that was not present and did not receive the therapeutic intervention.

thrombophlebitis Inflammation of a vein associated with thrombus formation.

thyrotropin-releasing hormone A hormone from the hypothalamus which stimulates the anterior lobe of the pituitary gland to release thyrotropin.

tongue-thrust swallow An immature form of swallowing in which the tongue is projected forward instead of retracted during swallowing.

topognosis The ability to localize tactile stimuli.

total lymphoid irradiation (TLI) Radiation therapy targeted to the body's lymph nodes; in the treatment of multiple sclerosis, the goal is to suppress immune system functioning (reduce the number of lymphocytes in the blood).

transcutaneous nerve stimulation (TNS) A procedure in which electrodes are placed on the surface of the skin over specific nerves and electrical stimulation is carried out. Stimulation of the CNS in this manner is thought to improve CNS function, reduce spasticity, and control pain.

traumatic head injury An insult to the brain caused by an external physical force that may produce a diminished or altered state of consciousness resulting in impairment of cognitive abilities, emotional control, or functioning.

treatment Application of or involvement in activities/stimulation to affect improvement in abilities for self-directed activities, self-care, or maintenance of the home.

treatment strategies Therapeutic approaches used during neurological rehabilitation that incorporate impairment training, functional training, hands-on interventions, somatosensory retraining, and compensatory training, which are based on the internal potential, external environment, and specific goals of the client.

trophotropic Combination of parasympathetic nervous system activity, somatic muscle relaxation, and cortical beta rhythm synchronization; resting or sleep state.

truncal ataxia Uncoordinated movement of the trunk.

trunk/arm-linked movements Movement that are synergistically tied as motor programs that link arm and trunk movements during a functional activity

trunk control Control of proximal muscles of the spine and trunk that stabilize the trunk when the body is responding to gravity either in quiet balance patterns or during a movement or position change in space.

trunk/leg-linked movements Movement that are synergistically tied as motor programs that link leg and trunk movements during a functional activity

Tysabri (natalizumab) Used to prevent episodes of symptoms in patients with relapsing forms of multiple sclerosis, a disease in which the nerves do not function properly and patients may experience weakness, numbness, loss of muscle coordination and problems with vision, speech and bladder control. Natalizumab has not been shown to help patients with chronic progressive MS. Natalizumab is in a class of medications call immunomodulators and works by preventing the damage to the brain and nerves that causes the symptoms of MS.

ultrasound A therapeutic modality using sound waves.

undesirable compensations Movement or behavior responses that exaggerate or increase the deficit or functional limitation.

universal cuff An adaptive device worn on the hand to hold items such as utensils, shaver, or pencil, allowing an individual with weak grasp to participate in self-care activities.

upper motor neuron A neuron that is located within the central nervous system and whose function is to relay information from one part to the other or to modulate control within nuclear bodies.

ventriculostomy A surgical establishment of an opening in a ventricle of the brain to drain cerebrospinal fluid, especially in hydrocephalus

verbal rating scale A pain intensity measurement in which clients rate pain on a continuum that is subdivided from left to right into gradually increasing pain intensities.

vergence Movement of the eyes in the opposite direction.

vermis Forms the unpaired medial region of the cerebellum.

version Movement of the eyes in the same direction.

vestibular-bilateral disorder A sensory integrative dysfunction characterized by short-duration nystagmus, poor integration of the two sides of the body and brain, and difficulty in learning to read or compute. The disorder is caused by underreactive vestibular responses.

vestibulo-ocular reflex A normal reflex in which eye position compensates for movement of the head, induced by excitation of vestibular apparatus.

visual analog scale (VAS) A pain scale that the patient marks on a continuum that begins with "no pain" and ends with "maximum pain tolerable." This tool provides an infinite number of points between the extremes, making it sensitive to small changes in pain intensity.

visual analytical problem solving The ability to look at a complex array of visual stimuli, identify the critical attributes, and then use appropriate strategies to solve simple to complex problems.

visual-motor coordination The ability to coordinate vision with the movements of the body or parts of the body.

visual-motor function The ability to draw or copy forms or to perform constructive tasks.

visual-perceptual dysfunction May include deficits in any of the areas of visual perception: figure-ground, form constancy, or size discrimination; distinct from deficits in functional visual skills and tested separately.

vision screening Can include distance and near visual acuities, oculomotilities, eye alignment or posture, depth perception, and visual fields.

volitional postural movements or control Movement patterns under volitional control that relate specifically to controlling the center of gravity, as in skating, ballet, gymnastics, etc.

wallerian degeneration The physical and biochemical changes that occur in a nerve because of the loss of axonal continuity following trauma.

wholistic A model or approach to health care that takes into account all internal and external influences during the process. It incorporates the mind, the body, and the spirit as a total or whole.

zero-to-three infant stimulation groups Groups that provide therapeutic services for children from birth to 3 years of age, since this age group is not yet eligible for public school placement.

Index

Page numbers followed by f indicate figures;
t, tables; b, boxes.

1209